Chinese Herbal Formulas and Applications

Pharmacological Effects & Clinical Research

John K. Chen • Tina T. Chen

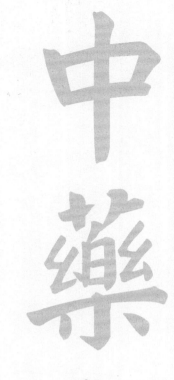

Chinese Herbal Formulas and Applications

Pharmacological Effects & Clinical Research

John K. Chen • Tina T. Chen

中藥方劑學

Authors
John K. Chen, Ph.D., Pharm.D., O.M.D., L.Ac.
Tina T. Chen, M.S., L.Ac.

Co-authors
Eric K. Chen, Ph.D., O.M.D., L.Ac., J.D.
Victor Meng-Chau Jang, L.Ac.
Delicia Liu, L.Ac.
Minh T. Nguyen, L.Ac.
Shenying Tang, L.Ac.

Editors
Minh T. Nguyen, L.Ac.
Lily Huang, L.Ac.

Associate Editors
Laraine Crampton, L.Ac.
Thad Ekdahl, L.Ac.
Catherine Lu, L.Ac.

Copy Editors
Abba Anderson, L.Ac.
Colleen Burke, L.Ac.
Lily Huang, L.Ac.
Dave Karaba, L.Ac.
Cathy McNease, Dipl.CH.
Marguerite Valance, L.Ac.

Draft Editors
Linda Joy Stone, L.Ac.
Kevin Inglis, L.Ac.

Consultants
Jize Li, L.Ac.
Huabing Wen, L.Ac.

Research Associates
Wei Chien
Lily Kathleen Ko, L.Ac.
Janice Lee, L.Ac.
Delicia Liu, L.Ac.

Chinese Language Consultant
Estella Huei-Mei Liu

Cover Design
Charles O. Funk

Book Design
Rick Friesen
Chien-Hui Liao

Portraits
Jimmy Wei-Yen Chang, L.Ac.

Copyright © 2009 by Art of Medicine Press, Inc.
Copyright © 1995, 1990 by John K. Chen and Eric K. Chen
All Rights Reserved. No part of this publication may be
reproduced, stored in a retrieval system, or transmitted,
in any form or by any means, electronic, mechanical,
photocopying, recording, or otherwise, except for brief review,
without the prior written permission of Art of Medicine Press, Inc.

Protected under the Berne Convention.

International Standard Book Number (ISBN)-10: 0-9740635-7-6
International Standard Book Number (ISBN)-13: 978-0-9740635-7-7
Standard Address Number (SAN): 255-3376
Library of Congress Control Number (LCCN): 2007905563

Art of Medicine Press, Inc.
P.O. Box 90878
City of Industry, CA 91715-0878

Website: www.aompress.com
Email: editor@aompress.com

Chinese Herbal Formulas and Applications

Abbreviated Table of Contents

Preface ·· XXIII
Acknowledgement ··· XXVII
Contributors ·· XXVIII
Using This Book ·· XXXII

Part I Overview ··· 1

Chapter 1 The History of Chinese Herbal Formulas ····························· 5
Chapter 2 Treatment Methods and Formulas ···································· 9
Chapter 3 Classification of Formulas ··· 11
Chapter 4 Composition of Formulas ·· 14
Chapter 5 Dosage Forms ··· 16
Chapter 6 Preparation and Administration of Decoctions ·················· 19
Chapter 7 Weights and Measures ·· 22
Chapter 8 Concurrent Use of Herbal Medicines and Pharmaceuticals ····· 24

Part II Formula Monographs ·· 25

Chapter 1 Exterior-Releasing Formulas ·· 29
Chapter 2 Downward Draining Formulas ·· 145
Chapter 3 Harmonizing Formulas ··· 197
Chapter 4 Exterior- and Interior-Releasing Formulas ·························· 277
Chapter 5 Heat-Clearing Formulas ··· 309
Chapter 6 Summer-Heat-Dispelling Formulas ··································· 429
Chapter 7 Interior-Warming Formulas ·· 451
Chapter 8 Tonic Formulas ·· 507
Chapter 9 *Shen*-Calming Formulas ·· 703
Chapter 10 Orifice-Opening Formulas ·· 739
Chapter 11 Astringent Formulas ··· 765
Chapter 12 Qi-Regulating Formulas ··· 815
Chapter 13 Blood-Regulating Formulas ·· 863
Chapter 14 Wind-Expelling Formulas ··· 959
Chapter 15 Dryness-Relieving Formulas ··· 1017
Chapter 16 Damp-Dispelling Formulas ··· 1059
Chapter 17 Wind-Damp Dispelling Formulas ····································· 1149
Chapter 18 Phlegm-Dispelling Formulas ··· 1201
Chapter 19 Reducing, Guiding, and Dissolving Formulas ····················· 1259
Chapter 20 Antiparasitic Formulas ·· 1285
Chapter 21 Emetic Formulas ··· 1305
Chapter 22 Formulas that Treat Abscesses and Sores ························· 1317

Part III Additional Resources ··· 1389

Appendix 1 Cross-reference Based on Traditional Chinese Medicine Diagnosis ····· 1393
Appendix 2 Cross-reference Based on Western Medicine Diagnosis ········· 1397
Appendix 3 Formulas Offering Beneficial Effects to Support Pregnancy ····· 1433
Appendix 4 Formulas Offering Beneficial Effects for Postpartum Care ······ 1434
Appendix 5 Cautions / Contraindications for the Use of Formulas During Pregnancy ···· 1435
Appendix 6 Dosing Guidelines ·· 1437
Appendix 7 Weights and Measures: Chinese, British and Metric Systems ····· 1439
Appendix 8 Convention on International Trade in Endangered Species (CITES) ···· 1441
Appendix 9 Cross-reference of Single Herb Names ····························· 1442
Appendix 10 Cross-reference of Herbal Formula Names ······················· 1464
Appendix 11 Tables of Famous Doctors ·· 1481
Bibliography of Historical Texts ··· 1485
Bibliography of Contemporary References ·· 1493
Glossary ·· 1505
Index ·· 1529
About the Authors ·· 1619

V

Table of Contents

Preface ·· XXIII
Acknowledgement ··· XXVII
Contributors ··· XXVIII
Using This Book ··· XXXII

Part I Overview ··· 1
Biography of Huang Di ··· 2

Chapter 1 The History of Chinese Herbal Formulas ···················· 5
Chapter 2 Treatment Methods and Formulas ······························ 9
Chapter 3 Classification of Formulas ····································· 11
Chapter 4 Composition of Formulas ······································· 14
Chapter 5 Dosage Forms ·· 16
Chapter 6 Preparation and Administration of Decoctions ············ 19
Chapter 7 Weights and Measures ··· 22
Chapter 8 Concurrent Use of Herbal Medicines and Pharmaceuticals ··· 24

Part II Formula Monographs ··· 25
Biography of Shen Nong ·· 26

Chapter 1. Exterior-Releasing Formulas ···································· 29
Biography of Zhang Zhong-Jing ··· 30

Section 1. Acrid and Warm Exterior-Releasing Formulas ············· 39
Ma Huang Tang (Ephedra Decoction) ·· 39
  Ma Huang Jia Zhu Tang (Ephedra Decoction plus Atractylodes) ········ 42
  Ma Xing Yi Gan Tang (Ephedra, Apricot Kernel, Coicis, and Licorice Decoction) ··· 43
  San Ao Tang (Three-Unbinding Decoction) ································· 43
Da Qing Long Tang (Major Bluegreen Dragon Decoction) ···················· 45
Hua Gai San (Canopy Powder) ·· 48
Jin Fei Cao San (Inula Powder) ·· 49
Gui Zhi Tang (Cinnamon Twig Decoction) ······································ 51
  Gui Zhi Jia Ge Gen Tang (Cinnamon Twig Decoction plus Kudzu) ······· 55
  Gui Zhi Jia Hou Po Xing Zi Tang (Cinnamon Twig Decoction plus Magnolia Bark and Apricot Kernel) ··· 55
  Gui Zhi Jia Shao Yao Tang (Cinnamon Twig Decoction plus Peony) ······· 55
  Gui Zhi Ma Huang Ge Ban Tang (Combined Cinnamon Twig and Ephedra Decoction) ··· 56
Ge Gen Tang (Kudzu Decoction) ·· 59
  Jing Fang Yi Hao (Neck Formula One) ···································· 62
  Jing Fang Er Hao (Neck Formula Two) ···································· 62
Jiu Wei Qiang Huo Tang (Nine-Herb Decoction with Notopterygium) ········ 64
  Da Qiang Huo Tang (Major Notopterygium Decoction) ··················· 66
Xiang Su San (Cyperus and Perilla Leaf Powder) ······························ 67
  Jia Wei Xiang Su San (Augmented Cyperus and Perilla Leaf Powder) ····· 69
  Xiang Su Cong Chi Tang (Cyperus, Perilla Leaf, Scallion, and Prepared Soybean Decoction) ··· 69
Xing Su Yin (Apricot Kernel and Perilla Leaf Decoction) ····················· 70
Shi Shen Tang (Ten-Immortal Decoction) ·· 72
Xiao Qing Long Tang (Minor Bluegreen Dragon Decoction) ·················· 74
  Xiao Qing Long Jia Shi Gao Tang (Minor Bluegreen Dragon Decoction plus Gypsum) ··· 78
  Jia Jian Xiao Qing Long Tang (Modified Minor Bluegreen Dragon Decoction) ··· 78
She Gan Ma Huang Tang (Belamcanda and Ephedra Decoction) ·············· 80
Cang Er Zi San (Xanthium Powder) ·· 82
Xin Yi San (Magnolia Flower Powder) ··· 84
  Xin Yi San (Magnolia Flower Powder) ···································· 85
  Jia Wei Xin Yi San (Augmented Magnolia Flower Powder) ············· 85
Qing Bi Tang (Clear the Nose Decoction) ······································· 86
  You Bi Tang (Benefit the Nose Decoction) ······························· 87

Chinese Herbal Formulas and Applications

Table of Contents

Section 2. Acrid and Cold Exterior-Releasing Formulas · **89**
Sang Ju Yin (Mulberry Leaf and Chrysanthemum Decoction) · 89
Yin Qiao San (Honeysuckle and Forsythia Powder) · 92
  Yin Qiao Tang (Honeysuckle and Forsythia Decoction) · 94
  Yin Qiao Jie Du San (Honeysuckle and Forsythia Powder to Relieve Toxicity) · 95
Ma Huang Xing Ren Gan Cao Shi Gao Tang (Ephedra, Apricot Kernel, Licorice, and Gypsum Decoction) · · · · · · · · · 96
  Jia Wei Ma Xing Gan Shi Tang (Augmented Ephedra, Apricot Kernel, Licorice, and Gypsum Decoction) · · · · · 99
Yue Bi Tang (Maidservant from Yue Decoction) · 101
  Yue Bi Jia Zhu Tang (Maidservant from Yue Decoction plus Atractylodes) · 102
Sheng Ma Ge Gen Tang (Cimicifuga and Kudzu Decoction) · 103
  Sheng Ma Ge Gen Tang (Cimicifuga and Kudzu Decoction) · 104
  Xuan Du Fa Biao Tang (Dissipate Toxins and Release the Exterior Decoction) · 104
Zhu Ye Liu Bang Tang (Lophatherum, Tamarisk and Arctium Decoction) · 106
Chai Ge Jie Ji Tang (Bupleurum and Kudzu Decoction to Release the Muscle Layer) · 107
  Chai Ge Jie Ji Tang (Bupleurum and Kudzu Decoction to Release the Muscle Layer) · · · · · · · · · · · · · · · · · 110
Cong Chi Jie Geng Tang (Scallion, Prepared Soybean, and Platycodon Decoction) · 111
  Cong Chi Tang (Scallion and Prepared Soybean Decoction) · 112
  Huo Ren Cong Chi Tang (Scallion and Prepared Soybean Decoction from the Book to Safeguard Life) · · · · · 112
Ning Sou Wan (Quiet the Cough Pill) · 113
Dun Sou San (Long-Bout Cough Powder) · 115
Zhi Sou San (Stop Coughing Powder) · 116
  Zhi Ke Tang (Stop Coughing Decoction) · 118
Jing Jie Lian Qiao Tang (Schizonepeta and Forsythia Decoction) · 120
Xin Yi Qing Fei Yin (Magnolia Decoction to Clear the Lung) · 122

Section 3. Supporting [the Upright] and Releasing [the Exterior] Formulas · · · · · · · · · · · · · · · · **124**
Bai Du San (Overcome Pathogenic Influences Powder) · 124
  Ren Shen Bai Du San (Ginseng Powder to Overcome Pathogenic Influences) · 126
  Cang Lin San (Old Rice Granary Powder) · 127
Shen Su Yin (Ginseng and Perilla Leaf Decoction) · 128
Zai Zao San (Renewal Powder) · 130
Ma Huang Fu Zi Xi Xin Tang (Ephedra, Asarum, and Prepared Aconite Decoction) · 132
  Ma Huang Fu Zi Gan Cao Tang (Ephedra, Prepared Aconite, and Licorice Decoction) · · · · · · · · · · · · · · · · 134
Cong Bai Qi Wei Yin (Scallion Decoction with Seven Ingredients) · 135
Jia Jian Wei Rui Tang (Modified Polygonatum Odoratum Decoction) · 137
  Wei Rui Tang (Polygonatum Odoratum Decoction) · 138

Exterior-Releasing Formulas (Summary) · **139**

Chapter 2. Downward Draining Formulas · **145**
Biography of Zhang Jing-Yue · 146

Section 1. Cold Purgatives · **152**
Da Cheng Qi Tang (Major Order the Qi Decoction) · 152
  Fu Fang Da Cheng Qi Tang (Revised Major Order the Qi Decoction) · 155
  Jia Jian Cheng Qi Tang (Modified Order the Qi Decoction) · 156
Xiao Cheng Qi Tang (Minor Order the Qi Decoction) · 158
Tiao Wei Cheng Qi Tang (Regulate the Stomach and Order the Qi Decoction) · 160
Da Xian Xiong Tang (Major Sinking into the Chest Decoction) · 161
  Da Xian Xiong Wan (Major Sinking into the Chest Pill) · 163
Yi Zi Tang (Yi Word Decoction) · 164
  Qing Chang Tang (Clear the Intestines Decoction) · 165

Section 2. Warm Purgatives · **166**
Da Huang Fu Zi Tang (Rhubarb and Prepared Aconite Decoction) · 166
Wen Pi Tang (Warm the Spleen Decoction) · 169

VII

Table of Contents

San Wu Bei Ji Wan (Three-Substance Pill for Emergencies) ·· 171

    San Wu Bai San (Three-Substance White Powder) ·· 172

Section 3. Moist Laxatives ·· **174**

Ma Zi Ren Wan (Hemp Seed Pill) ··· 174

    Wu Ren Wan (Five-Seed Pill) ·· 176

Run Chang Wan (Moisten the Intestines Pill) ··· 177

    Run Chang Wan (Moisten the Intestines Pill) ··· 178

    Ma Zi Run Chang Wan (Hemp Seed Pill to Moisten the Intestines) ····························· 178

Ji Chuan Jian (Benefit the River [Flow] Decoction) ··· 179

Section 4. Harsh Expellants (Cathartics) ··· **181**

Shi Zao Tang (Ten-Jujube Decoction) ·· 181

    Kong Xian Dan (Control Mucus Special Pill) ·· 182

Zhou Che Wan (Vessel and Vehicle Pill) ·· 184

Shu Zao Yin Zi (Spread and Unblock Decoction) ··· 185

Section 5: Purgative and Tonic Formulas ··· **187**

Huang Long Tang (Yellow Dragon Decoction) ·· 187

    Xin Jia Huang Long Tang (Newly-Augmented Yellow Dragon Decoction) ······················· 189

Zeng Ye Cheng Qi Tang (Increase the Fluids and Order the Qi Decoction) ···························· 190

    Cheng Qi Yang Ying Tang (Order the Qi and Nourish the Nutritive Qi Decoction) ················ 192

Downward Draining Formulas (Summary) ··· **193**

Chapter 3. Harmonizing Formulas ·· 197

Biography of Wu You-Xing ··· 198

Section 1. *Shaoyang* Harmonizing Formulas ··· **206**

Xiao Chai Hu Tang (Minor Bupleurum Decoction) ··· 206

    Chai Hu Zhi Jie Tang (Bupleurum, Bitter Orange, and Platycodon Decoction) ··················· 215

    Chai Hu Jie Du Tang (Bupleurum Decoction to Relieve Toxicity) ································· 215

Chai Hu Gui Zhi Tang (Bupleurum and Cinnamon Twig Decoction) ·································· 219

Chai Ling Tang (Bupleurum and Poria Decoction) ·· 222

Chai Xian Tang (Bupleurum Decoction to Raise the Sunken) ··· 226

Hao Qin Qing Dan Tang (Artemisia Annua and Scutellaria Decoction to Clear the Gallbladder) ····· 227

Chai Hu Da Yuan Yin (Bupleurum Decoction to Reach the Membrane Source) ······················ 230

    Da Yuan Yin (Reach the Membrane Source Decoction) ·· 231

    Qing Pi Yin (Clear the Spleen Decoction) ··· 231

Section 2. Liver and Spleen Harmonizing Formulas ·· **233**

Si Ni San (Frigid Extremities Powder) ··· 233

    Zhi Shi Shao Yao San (Immature Bitter Orange and Peony Powder) ······························ 236

Chai Hu Shu Gan San (Bupleurum Powder to Spread the Liver) ······································ 238

Shu Gan Tang (Spread the Liver Decoction) ··· 241

Chai Hu Qing Gan Tang (Bupleurum Decoction to Clear the Liver) ··································· 243

    Chai Hu Qing Gan Tang (Bupleurum Decoction to Clear the Liver) ······························ 244

    Zhi Zi Qing Gan Tang (Gardenia Decoction to Clear the Liver) ·································· 245

Yi Gan San (Restrain the Liver Powder) ·· 245

Xiao Yao San (Rambling Powder) ··· 247

    Hei Xiao Yao San (Black Rambling Powder) ·· 252

Jia Wei Xiao Yao San (Augmented Rambling Powder) ·· 254

    Shi Wei Xiao Yao San (Ten-Ingredient Rambling Powder) ·· 256

Tong Xie Yao Fang (Important Formula for Painful Diarrhea) ··· 257

Section 3. Intestines and Stomach Harmonizing Formulas ··· **261**

Ban Xia Xie Xin Tang (Pinellia Decoction to Drain the Epigastrium) ·································· 261

VIII

Chinese Herbal Formulas and Applications

Table of Contents

Sheng Jiang Xie Xin Tang (Fresh Ginger Decoction to Drain the Epigastrium) ·········· 268
Gan Cao Xie Xin Tang (Licorice Decoction to Drain the Epigastrium) ················· 269
Huang Lian Tang (Coptis Decoction) ···································· 271

Harmonizing Formulas (Summary) ··································· **274**

Chapter 4. Exterior- and Interior-Releasing Formulas ············ 277
Biography of Liu Yuan-Su ·· 278

Section 1. Exterior-Releasing and Interior-Attacking Formulas ········· 283
Da Chai Hu Tang (Major Bupleurum Decoction) ························· 283
   Chai Hu Tang (Bupleurum Decoction) ····························· 287
Hou Po Qi Wu Tang (Seven-Substance Decoction with Magnolia Bark) ······· 289
Fang Feng Tong Sheng San (Saposhnikovia Powder that Sagely Unblocks) ····· 291
   Shuang Jie Tong Sheng San (Double Relieve Powder that Sagely Unblocks) ··· 294

Section 2. Exterior-Releasing and Interior-Clearing Formulas ········· 295
Ge Gen Huang Qin Huang Lian Tang (Kudzu, Coptis, and Scutellaria Decoction) ··· 295
   Ge Gen Huo Xiang Shao Yao Tang (Kudzu, Pogostemon, and Peony Decoction) ·· 298
Shi Gao Tang (Gypsum Decoction) ······························· 299

Section 3. Exterior-Releasing and Interior-Warming Formulas ········· 301
Wu Ji San (Five-Accumulation Powder) ····························· 301
   Wu Ji San (Five-Accumulation Powder) ························· 303
Chai Hu Gui Zhi Gan Jiang Tang (Bupleurum, Cinnamon Twig, and Ginger Decoction) ·· 304

Exterior- and Interior-Releasing Formulas (Summary) ·············· 306

Chapter 5. Heat-Clearing Formulas ·························· 309
Biography of Ye Gui ··· 310

Section 1. *Qi* (Energy) Level-Clearing Formulas ················· 321
Bai Hu Tang (White Tiger Decoction) ······························ 321
   Bai Hu Jia Gui Zhi Tang (White Tiger plus Cinnamon Twig Decoction) ···· 323
   Bai Hu Jia Cang Zhu Tang (White Tiger plus Atractylodes Decoction) ····· 323
Bai Hu Jia Ren Shen Tang (White Tiger plus Ginseng Decoction) ········· 325
Zhu Ye Shi Gao Tang (Bamboo Leaves and Gypsum Decoction) ·········· 326

Section 2. *Ying* (Nutritive) Level-Clearing and Blood-Cooling Formulas ·· 330
Qing Ying Tang (Clear the Nutritive Level Decoction) ················· 330
Xi Jiao Di Huang Tang (Rhinoceros Horn and Rehmannia Decoction) ······· 333
   Shen Xi Dan (Magical Rhinoceros Special Pill) ··················· 335
   Qing Re Liang Xue Tang (Clear Heat and Cool the Blood Decoction) ······ 335
   Fu Zheng Yi Yan Tang (Support the Upright and Suppress Cancer Decoction) ·· 336

Section 3. *Qi* (Energy) and *Xue* (Blood) Levels-Clearing Formulas ···· 337
Qing Wen Bai Du Yin (Clear Epidemics and Overcome Pathogenic Influences Decoction) ·· 337
   Hua Ban Tang (Transform Blotches Decoction) ··················· 339

Section 4. Heat-Clearing and Toxin-Eliminating Formulas ·········· 341
Huang Lian Jie Du Tang (Coptis Decoction to Relieve Toxicity) ·········· 341
   Lian Qiao Jie Du Tang (Forsythia Decoction to Relieve Toxicity) ········ 345
Huang Lian Shang Qing Wan (Coptis Pill to Clear the Upper) ··········· 347
Qing Shang Fang Feng Tang (Clear the Upper and Guard the Wind Decoction) ··· 349
   Qing Re Jie Du Tang (Clear Heat and Relieve Toxicity Decoction) ······· 350
Liang Ge San (Cool the Diaphragm Powder) ······················· 351
Qing Liang Yin (Clearing and Cooling Decoction) ··················· 354

IX

Table of Contents

Pu Ji Xiao Du Yin (Universal Benefit Decoction to Eliminate Toxin) ⋯⋯⋯⋯⋯⋯ 355
Da Qing Tang (Isatis Decoction) ⋯⋯⋯⋯⋯⋯⋯⋯⋯⋯⋯⋯⋯⋯⋯⋯⋯⋯ 358
San Huang Xie Xin Tang (Three-Yellow Decoction to Sedate the Epigastrium) ⋯⋯⋯ 359
San Huang Shi Gao Tang (Three-Yellow and Gypsum Decoction) ⋯⋯⋯⋯⋯⋯⋯ 361
San Huang Shi Gao Tang (Three-Yellow and Gypsum Decoction) ⋯⋯⋯⋯⋯⋯⋯ 362
Liu Shen Wan (Six-Miracle Pill) ⋯⋯⋯⋯⋯⋯⋯⋯⋯⋯⋯⋯⋯⋯⋯⋯⋯⋯ 363

Section 5. *Zang Fu*-Clearing Formulas ⋯⋯⋯⋯⋯⋯⋯⋯⋯⋯⋯⋯ **365**

Dao Chi San (Guide Out the Red Powder) ⋯⋯⋯⋯⋯⋯⋯⋯⋯⋯⋯⋯⋯⋯ 365
Qing Xin Lian Zi Yin (Lotus Seed Decoction to Clear the Heart) ⋯⋯⋯⋯⋯⋯⋯ 368
Zhi Zi Chi Tang (Gardenia and Soja Decoction) ⋯⋯⋯⋯⋯⋯⋯⋯⋯⋯⋯⋯ 370
Long Dan Xie Gan Tang (Gentiana Decoction to Drain the Liver) ⋯⋯⋯⋯⋯⋯⋯ 371
  Xie Qing Wan (Drain the Green Pill) ⋯⋯⋯⋯⋯⋯⋯⋯⋯⋯⋯⋯⋯⋯⋯ 376
  Long Dan Jiang Ya Pian (Gentiana Pill to Lower [Blood] Pressure) ⋯⋯⋯⋯⋯ 376
  Long Dan Jie Du Tang (Gentiana Decoction to Relieve Toxicity) ⋯⋯⋯⋯⋯⋯ 376
  Zhi Zi Jiang Huo Tang (Gardenia Decoction to Descend Fire) ⋯⋯⋯⋯⋯⋯⋯ 377
Dang Gui Long Hui Wan (Tangkuei, Gentiana, and Aloe Pill) ⋯⋯⋯⋯⋯⋯⋯⋯ 379
Xi Gan Ming Mu San (Wash the Liver and Brighten the Eyes Powder) ⋯⋯⋯⋯⋯ 381
Xie Bai San (Drain the White Powder) ⋯⋯⋯⋯⋯⋯⋯⋯⋯⋯⋯⋯⋯⋯⋯ 383
  Ting Li Da Zao Xie Fei Tang (Descurainia and Jujube Decoction to Drain the Lung) ⋯⋯ 384
Qing Xin Li Ge Tang (Clear the Epigastrium and Benefit the Diaphragm Decoction) ⋯⋯ 386
  Qing Xin Li Ge Tang (Clear the Epigastrium and Benefit the Diaphragm Decoction) ⋯⋯ 387
Xiang Sheng Po Di San (Loud Sound Powder for a Broken Flute) ⋯⋯⋯⋯⋯⋯⋯ 388
Zuo Jin Wan (Left Metal Pill) ⋯⋯⋯⋯⋯⋯⋯⋯⋯⋯⋯⋯⋯⋯⋯⋯⋯⋯ 389
  Wu Ji Wan (Wu Ji Pill) ⋯⋯⋯⋯⋯⋯⋯⋯⋯⋯⋯⋯⋯⋯⋯⋯⋯⋯⋯⋯ 391
  Xiang Lian Wan (Aucklandia and Coptis Pill) ⋯⋯⋯⋯⋯⋯⋯⋯⋯⋯⋯⋯ 391
  Qing Wei Tang (Clear the Stomach Decoction) ⋯⋯⋯⋯⋯⋯⋯⋯⋯⋯⋯⋯ 392
Qing Wei San (Clear the Stomach Powder) ⋯⋯⋯⋯⋯⋯⋯⋯⋯⋯⋯⋯⋯⋯ 393
Xie Huang San (Drain the Yellow Powder) ⋯⋯⋯⋯⋯⋯⋯⋯⋯⋯⋯⋯⋯⋯ 396
Yu Nu Jian (Jade Woman Decoction) ⋯⋯⋯⋯⋯⋯⋯⋯⋯⋯⋯⋯⋯⋯⋯⋯ 398
Gan Lu Yin (Sweet Dew Decoction) ⋯⋯⋯⋯⋯⋯⋯⋯⋯⋯⋯⋯⋯⋯⋯⋯ 401
Shao Yao Tang (Peony Decoction) ⋯⋯⋯⋯⋯⋯⋯⋯⋯⋯⋯⋯⋯⋯⋯⋯⋯ 402
  Shao Yao Yi Yi Ren Tang (Peony and Coicis Decoction) ⋯⋯⋯⋯⋯⋯⋯⋯⋯ 405
  Shao Yao Hou Po Tang (Peony and Magnolia Bark Decoction) ⋯⋯⋯⋯⋯⋯⋯ 405
Huang Qin Tang (Scutellaria Decoction) ⋯⋯⋯⋯⋯⋯⋯⋯⋯⋯⋯⋯⋯⋯⋯ 406
Bai Tou Weng Tang (Pulsatilla Decoction) ⋯⋯⋯⋯⋯⋯⋯⋯⋯⋯⋯⋯⋯⋯ 408
  Bai Tou Weng Jia Gan Cao E Jiao Tang (Pulsatilla Decoction plus Licorice and Ass-Hide Gelatin) ⋯ 410

Section 6. Deficiency-Heat Clearing Formulas ⋯⋯⋯⋯⋯⋯⋯⋯⋯ **412**

Qing Hao Bie Jia Tang (Artemisia Annua and Soft-Shelled Turtle Shell Decoction) ⋯⋯ 412
  Zi Yin Qing Re Tang (Nourish Yin and Clear Heat Decoction) ⋯⋯⋯⋯⋯⋯⋯ 414
Qin Jiao Bie Jia San (Gentiana Macrophylla and Soft-Shelled Turtle Shell Powder) ⋯⋯ 416
Qing Gu San (Cool the Bones Powder) ⋯⋯⋯⋯⋯⋯⋯⋯⋯⋯⋯⋯⋯⋯⋯ 418
Dang Gui Liu Huang Tang (Tangkuei and Six-Yellow Decoction) ⋯⋯⋯⋯⋯⋯⋯ 420
Zi Yin Jiang Huo Tang (Nourish Yin and Descend the Fire Decoction) ⋯⋯⋯⋯⋯ 422

Heat-Clearing Formulas (Summary) ⋯⋯⋯⋯⋯⋯⋯⋯⋯⋯⋯⋯⋯⋯ **424**

Chapter 6. Summer-Heat-Dispelling Formulas ⋯⋯⋯⋯⋯⋯⋯⋯ **429**

Biography of Wu Tang ⋯⋯⋯⋯⋯⋯⋯⋯⋯⋯⋯⋯⋯⋯⋯⋯⋯⋯⋯⋯⋯ 430

Qing Luo Yin (Clear the Collaterals Decoction) ⋯⋯⋯⋯⋯⋯⋯⋯⋯⋯⋯⋯⋯ 435
Xiang Ru San (Mosla Powder) ⋯⋯⋯⋯⋯⋯⋯⋯⋯⋯⋯⋯⋯⋯⋯⋯⋯⋯ 436
  San Wu Xiang Ru Yin (Mosla Three Decoction) ⋯⋯⋯⋯⋯⋯⋯⋯⋯⋯⋯⋯ 438
  Shi Wei Xiang Ru Yin (Ten-Ingredient Decoction with Mosla) ⋯⋯⋯⋯⋯⋯⋯ 438
Xin Jia Xiang Ru Yin (Newly-Augmented Mosla Decoction) ⋯⋯⋯⋯⋯⋯⋯⋯⋯ 439
Liu Yi San (Six-to-One Powder) ⋯⋯⋯⋯⋯⋯⋯⋯⋯⋯⋯⋯⋯⋯⋯⋯⋯⋯ 441

X

Chinese Herbal Formulas and Applications

Table of Contents

Liu Yi San (Six-to-One Powder) ·· 442
Yi Yuan San (Benefit the Basal Powder) ·· 443
Bi Yu San (Jasper Powder) ·· 443
Ji Su San (Peppermint Powder) ··· 443
Gui Ling Gan Lu Yin (Cinnamon and Poria Sweet Dew Decoction) ························· 444
Qing Shu Yi Qi Tang (Clear Summer-Heat and Augment the Qi Decoction) ············· 446
  Qing Shu Yi Qi Tang (Clear Summer-Heat and Augment the Qi Decoction) ··········· 448

Summer-Heat-Dispelling Formulas (Summary) ··· **449**

Chapter 7. Interior-Warming Formulas ··································· 451
Biography of Wang Shu-He ·· 452

Section 1. Middle-Warming and Cold-Dispelling Formulas ························ 459
Li Zhong Wan (Regulate the Middle Pill) ·· 459
  Ren Shen Tang (Ginseng Decoction) ·· 462
  Li Zhong Hua Tan Wan (Regulate the Middle and Transform Phlegm Pill) ············ 462
Fu Zi Li Zhong Wan (Prepared Aconite Pill to Regulate the Middle) ······················ 463
Gui Zhi Ren Shen Tang (Cinnamon Twig and Ginseng Decoction) ························· 466
Wu Zhu Yu Tang (Evodia Decoction) ·· 467
Xiao Jian Zhong Tang (Minor Construct the Middle Decoction) ···························· 471
  Dang Gui Jian Zhong Tang (Tangkuei Decoction to Construct the Middle) ············ 473
Huang Qi Jian Zhong Tang (Astragalus Decoction to Construct the Middle) ············· 475
Gui Qi Jian Zhong Tang (Tangkuei and Astragalus Decoction to Construct the Middle) ·· 479
Da Jian Zhong Tang (Major Construct the Middle Decoction) ······························ 480
An Zhong San (Calm the Middle Powder) ··· 484

Section 2. Yang-Resuscitating Formulas ··· 486
Si Ni Tang (Frigid Extremities Decoction) ··· 486
  Si Ni Jia Ren Shen Tang (Frigid Extremities Decoction plus Ginseng) ·················· 488
  Tong Mai Si Ni Tang (Unblock the Pulse Decoction for Frigid Extremities) ··········· 488
  Bai Tong Tang (White Penetrating Decoction) ··· 489
  Shen Fu Tang (Ginseng and Prepared Aconite Decoction) ····································· 489
Hui Yang Jiu Ji Tang (Restore and Revive the Yang Decoction) ···························· 490
Hei Xi Dan (Lead Special Pill) ·· 492

Section 3. Channel-Warming and Cold-Dispersing Formulas ··················· 494
Dang Gui Si Ni Tang (Tangkuei Decoction for Frigid Extremities) ························· 494
  Dang Gui Si Ni Jia Wu Zhu Yu Sheng Jiang Tang (Tangkuei Decoction for Frigid Extremities plus Evodia and Fresh Ginger) ····· 498
Huang Qi Gui Zhi Wu Wu Tang (Astragalus and Cinnamon Twig Five-Substance Decoction) ··· 500

Interior-Warming Formulas (Summary) ·· **504**

Chapter 8. Tonic Formulas ··· 507
Biography of Qian Yi ·· 508

Section 1. Qi-Tonifying Formulas ·· 522
Si Jun Zi Tang (Four-Gentlemen Decoction) ·· 522
  Yi Gong San (Extraordinary Merit Powder) ··· 525
  Bao Yuan Tang (Preserve the Basal Decoction) ·· 525
Liu Jun Zi Tang (Six-Gentlemen Decoction) ·· 527
Xiang Sha Liu Jun Zi Tang (Six-Gentlemen Decoction with Aucklandia and Amomum) ··· 531
  Xiang Sha Liu Jun Zi Tang (Six-Gentlemen Decoction with Cyperus and Amomum) ··· 533
Xiang Sha Yang Wei Tang (Nourish the Stomach Decoction with Aucklandia and Amomum) ·· 534
Shen Ling Bai Zhu San (Ginseng, Poria, and Atractylodes Macrocephala Powder) ······· 535
  Qi Wei Bai Zhu San (Seven-Ingredient Powder with Atractylodes Macrocephala) ····· 539
  Shen Ling San (Ginseng and Poria Powder) ·· 539

XI

Table of Contents

Qi Pi Wan (Guide the Spleen Pill) ·· 540
Bu Zhong Yi Qi Tang (Tonify the Middle and Augment the Qi Decoction) ················· 542
  Ju Yuan Jian (Lift the Source Decoction) ··· 548
  Sheng Xian Tang (Raise the Sinking Decoction) ·· 549
Yi Qi Cong Ming Tang (Augment the Qi and Increase Acuity Decoction) ················· 551
Sheng Mai San (Generate the Pulse Powder) ·· 554
Ren Shen Ge Jie San (Ginseng and Gecko Powder) ·· 557
  Ren Shen Hu Tao Tang (Ginseng and Walnut Decoction) ·································· 559
  Ren Shen Chong Cao Tang (Ginseng and Cordyceps Decoction) ························· 559
Bu Fei Tang (Tonify the Lung Decoction) ·· 560

Section 2. Blood-Tonifying Formulas ··· 562

Si Wu Tang (Four-Substance Decoction) ·· 562
  Sheng Yu Tang (Sage-Like Healing Decoction) ··· 567
  Sheng Yu Tang (Sage-Like Healing Decoction) ··· 567
  Jia Wei Si Wu Tang (Augmented Four-Substance Decoction) ···························· 568
  Zhuang Jin Tang (Strengthen the Tendon Decoction) ····································· 568
  Tiao Jing Yi Hao (Regulate Menses Formula One) ··· 568
  Tiao Jing Er Hao (Regulate Menses Formula Two) ·· 568
  Tiao Jing San Hao (Regulate Menses Formula Three) ····································· 569
  Tiao Jing Si Hao (Regulate Menses Formula Four) ·· 569
Tao Hong Si Wu Tang (Four-Substance Decoction with Safflower and Peach Pit) ········· 571
Wen Qing Yin (Warming and Clearing Decoction) ··· 575
  Wen Qing Yin (Warming and Clearing Decoction) ··· 577
  Wen Qing Yin (Warming and Clearing Decoction) ··· 577
Guo Qi Yin (Delayed Menstruation Decoction) ··· 578
Dang Gui Bu Xue Tang (Tangkuei Decoction to Tonify the Blood) ·························· 580
Gui Pi Tang (Restore the Spleen Decoction) ··· 583
  Gui Pi An Shen Tang (Restore the Spleen and Tranquilize the Spirit Decoction) ······ 587
Zhi Gan Cao Tang (Honey-Fried Licorice Decoction) ·· 589
  Jia Jian Fu Mai Tang (Modified Restore the Pulse Decoction) ·························· 591
Nu Ke Bai Zi Ren Wan (Platycladus Seed Pill for Females) ····································· 592
Dang Gui Shao Yao San (Tangkuei and Peony Powder) ··· 594
  Ren Shen Dang Shao San (Ginseng, Tangkuei, and Peony Powder) ···················· 598
Shao Yao Gan Cao Tang (Peony and Licorice Decoction) ·· 599
  Jia Wei Shao Yao Gan Cao Tang (Augmented Peony and Licorice Decoction) ········· 603

Section 3. Qi- and Blood-Tonifying Formulas ······························· 604

Ba Zhen Tang (Eight-Treasure Decoction) ·· 604
Shi Quan Da Bu Tang (All-Inclusive Great Tonifying Decoction) ····························· 609
  Da Bu Tang (Great Tonifying Decoction) ·· 613
  Ren Shen Da Bu Tang (Ginseng Great Tonifying Decoction) ···························· 613
Ren Shen Yang Ying Tang (Ginseng Decoction to Nourish the Nutritive Qi) ·············· 615
Tai Shan Pan Shi San (Powder that Gives the Stability of Mount Tai) ······················ 618
Bao Chan Wu You Fang (Preserve Pregnancy and Care-Free Decoction) ·················· 621
Dang Gui San (Tangkuei Powder) ·· 623
Xiong Gui Tiao Xue Yin (Cnidium and Tangkuei Decoction to Regulate Blood) ········· 624

Section 4. Yin-Tonifying Formulas ·· 627

Liu Wei Di Huang Wan (Six-Ingredient Pill with Rehmannia) ································· 627
  Er Long Zuo Ci Wan (Pill for Deafness that Is Kind to the Left [Kidney]) ·············· 633
  Ming Mu Di Huang Wan (Improve Vision Pill with Rehmannia) ······················· 633
  Ming Mu Di Huang Wan (Improve Vision Pill with Rehmannia) ······················· 633
Zhi Bai Di Huang Wan (Anemarrhena, Phellodendron, and Rehmannia Pill) ············· 636
  Shi Wei Di Huang Wan (Ten-Ingredient Pill with Rehmannia) ························· 639
Qi Ju Di Huang Wan (Lycium Fruit, Chrysanthemum, and Rehmannia Pill) ············· 640
Mai Wei Di Huang Wan (Ophiopogonis, Schisandra, and Rehmannia Pill) ··············· 642

Table of Contents

Chinese Herbal Formulas and Applications

Du Qi Wan (Capital Qi Pill) ·· 644
Zuo Gui Wan (Restore the Left [Kidney] Pill) ························· 645
   Zuo Gui Yin (Restore the Left [Kidney] Decoction) ·············· 647
   Jia Wei Zuo Gui Wan (Augmented Restore the Left [Kidney] Pill) ··· 647
Da Bu Yin Wan (Great Tonify the Yin Pill) ···························· 649
Hu Qian Wan (Hidden Tiger Pill) ·· 651
   Hu Qian Wan (Hidden Tiger Pill) ···································· 653
Er Zhi Wan (Two-Ultimate Pill) ·· 654
   Sang Ma Wan (Mulberry Leaf and Sesame Seed Pill) ··········· 656
Yi Guan Jian (Linking Decoction) ·· 657
Shi Hu Ye Guang Wan (Dendrobium Pill for Night Vision) ········· 661
Zi Yin Di Huang Wan (Rehmannia Pill to Nourish Yin) ············· 663
Zi Shen Ming Mu Tang (Nourish the Kidney to Brighten the Eyes Decoction) ··· 664
Zi Shen Tong Er Tang (Nourish the Kidney to Unblock the Ears Decoction) ··· 666

Section 5. Yang-Tonifying Formulas ······························· **668**
Jin Gui Shen Qi Wan (Kidney Qi Pill from the Golden Cabinet) ··· 668
   Shi Bu Wan (Ten-Tonic Pill) ··· 671
Ba Wei Di Huang Wan (Eight-Ingredient Pill with Rehmannia) ··· 672
Ji Sheng Shen Qi Wan (Kidney Qi Pill from Formulas that Aid the Living) ··· 675
You Gui Wan (Restore the Right [Kidney] Pill) ······················ 678
   You Gui Yin (Restore the Right [Kidney] Decoction) ············ 680
   Jia Wei You Gui Wan (Augmented Restore the Right [Kidney] Pill) ··· 680
Huan Shao Dan (Return to Youth Pill) ··································· 681
   Huan Shao Di Huang Wan (Rehmannia Pill to Return to Youth) ··· 683
   Bu Shen Tang (Tonify the Kidney Decoction) ···················· 683
Er Xian Tang (Two-Immortal Decoction) ······························· 684
   Er Xian Bu Shen Tang (Two-Immortal Decoction to Tonify the Kidney) ··· 686

Section 6. Yin- and Yang-Tonifying Formulas ················ **687**
Gui Lu Er Xian Jiao (Tortoise Shell and Deer Antler Syrup) ······· 687
   Bu Shen Wan (Tonify the Kidney Pill) ······························ 689
   Bu Gu Wan (Tonify the Bone Pill) ·································· 689
Qi Bao Mei Ran Dan (Seven-Treasure Special Pill for Beautiful Whiskers) ··· 690
   Shou Wu Pian (Polygonum Pill) ···································· 692
Di Huang Yin Zi (Rehmannia Decoction) ······························· 693

Tonic Formulas (Summary) ··· **696**

Chapter 9. *Shen*-Calming Formulas ·························· **703**
Biography of Bian Que ·· 704

Section 1. Sedative Formulas that Calm the *Shen* (Spirit) ··· **710**
Zhu Sha An Shen Wan (Cinnabar Pill to Tranquilize the Spirit) ··· 710
   Sheng Tie Luo Yin (Iron Filings Decoction) ····················· 711
Zhen Zhu Mu Wan (Mother of Pearl Pill) ···························· 712
Ci Zhu Wan (Magnetite and Cinnabar Pill) ··························· 714
Chai Hu Jia Long Gu Mu Li Tang (Bupleurum plus Dragon Bone and Oyster Shell Decoction) ··· 715
   Chai Hu An Shen Tang (Bupleurum Decoction to Tranquilize the Spirit) ··· 720

Section 2. Nourishing Formulas that Calm the *Shen* (Spirit) ··· **722**
Suan Zao Ren Tang (Sour Jujube Decoction) ·························· 722
   Ding Zhi Wan (Settle the Emotions Pill) ························· 723
Tian Wang Bu Xin Dan (Emperor of Heaven's Special Pill to Tonify the Heart) ··· 725
   Tian Wang Bu Xin Dan (Emperor of Heaven's Special Pill to Tonify the Heart) ··· 728
   Tian Wang Bu Xin Dan (Emperor of Heaven's Special Pill to Tonify the Heart) ··· 728
   Bai Zi Yang Xin Wan (Biota Seed Pill to Nourish the Heart) ··· 729

Table of Contents

Yang Xin Dan (Nourish the Heart Pill) ·· 729
Zhen Zhong Dan (Pillow Special Pill) ··· 729
Gan Mai Da Zao Tang (Licorice, Wheat, and Jujube Decoction) ································· 731
An Shen Tang (Tranquilize the Spirit Decoction) ·· 733
Yang Xin Tang (Nourish the Heart Decoction) ··· 735

***Shen*-Calming Formulas (Summary)** ·· **737**

Chapter 10. Orifice-Opening Formulas ·· **739**
Biography of Hua Tuo ··· 740

Section 1. Cold Orifice-Opening Formulas ·· **746**
An Gong Niu Huang Wan (Calm the Palace Pill with Cattle Gallstone) ······················ 746
Niu Huang Qing Xin Wan (Cattle Gallstone Pill to Clear the Heart) ·························· 748
Zhi Bao Dan (Greatest Treasure Special Pill) ·· 749
Ju Fang Zhi Bao San (Greatest Treasure Powder from the Imperial Grace Formulary) ···· 751
Zi Xue (Purple Snow) ·· 752
Xiao Er Hui Chun Dan (Return of Spring Special Pill [Pediatric]) ···························· 754
Xing Jun San (Troop-Marching Powder) ·· 756

Section 2. Warm Orifice-Opening Formulas ·· **758**
Su He Xiang Wan (Liquid Styrax Pill) ··· 758
Guan Xin Su He Wan (Coronary Styrax Pill) ··· 760
Zi Jin Ding (Purple Gold Special Pill) ·· 760

Orifice-Opening Formulas (Summary) ··· **762**

Chapter 11. Astringent Formulas ··· **765**
Biography of Fu Shan ··· 766

Section 1. Exterior-Stabilizing Formulas to Stop Perspiration ··································· **773**
Yu Ping Feng San (Jade Windscreen Powder) ·· 773
Huang Qi Fang Feng Tang (Astragalus Decoction to Guard the Wind) ······················· 775
Mu Li San (Oyster Shell Powder) ·· 776

Section 2. Lung-Restraining Formula to Relieve Cough ··· **779**
Jiu Xian San (Nine-Immortal Powder) ··· 779

Section 3. Intestine-Binding Formulas to Stop Leakage ··· **781**
Zhen Ren Yang Zang Tang (True Man's Decoction for Nourishing the Organs) ············· 781
Si Shen Wan (Four-Miracle Pill) ··· 784
Tao Hua Tang (Peach Blossom Decoction) ··· 787
Chi Shi Zhi Yu Yu Liang Tang (Halloysitum and Limonite Decoction) ······················ 788

Section 4. *Jing* (Essence)-Stabilizing Formulas to Stop Leakage ······························ **789**
Jin Suo Gu Jing Wan (Metal Lock Pill to Stabilize the Essence) ································· 789
Shui Lu Er Xian Dan (Water and Earth Two Immortals Special Pill) ·························· 790
Liu Wei Gu Jing Wan (Rehmannia Six and Lotus Stamen Pill) ································· 791
Sang Piao Xiao San (Mantis Egg-Case Powder) ·· 792
Suo Quan Wan (Shut the Sluice Pill) ·· 795
Fu Tu Dan (Poria and Cuscuta Special Pill) ·· 797
Gui Zhi Jia Long Gu Mu Li Tang (Cinnamon Twig Decoction plus Dragon Bone and Oyster Shell) ···· 798
Zhi Zhuo Gu Ben Wan (Treat the Turbidity and Guard the Root Pill) ······················· 800

Section 5. Womb-Stabilizing Formulas to Stop Leakage ··· **802**
Gu Jing Wan (Stabilize the Menses Pill) ·· 802
Gu Chong Tang (Stabilize *Chong* [Thoroughfare Channel] Decoction) ······················ 803

XIV

Table of Contents

Zhen Ling Dan (Rouse the Spirits Special Pill) ·· 805
Wan Dai Tang (End Discharge Decoction) ·· 806
   Yi Huang Tang (Change the Yellow [Discharge] Decoction) ···························· 809
   Qing Dai Tang (Clear the Discharge Decoction) ·· 809
Ba Wei Dai Xia Fang (Eight-Ingredient Formula for Leukorrhea) ··························· 810

Astringent Formulas (Summary) ·· **812**

Chapter 12. Qi-Regulating Formulas ·· 815
Biography of Li Shi-Zhen ·· 816

Section 1. Qi-Moving Formulas ·· 822
Yue Ju Wan (Escape Restraint Pill) ·· 822
   Xiang Fu Wan (Cyperus Pill) ·· 824
Jin Ling Zi San (Melia Toosendan Powder) ·· 825
   Yan Hu Suo San (Corydalis Powder) ·· 826
   Yan Hu Yi Hao (Corydalis Formula One) ·· 826
   Yan Hu Er Hao (Corydalis Formula Two) ·· 826
Ban Xia Hou Po Tang (Pinellia and Magnolia Bark Decoction) ···························· 827
Zhi Shi Xie Bai Gui Zhi Tang (Immature Bitter Orange, Chinese Chive, and Cinnamon Twig Decoction) ··· 831
   Gua Lou Xie Bai Bai Jiu Tang (Trichosanthes Fruit, Chinese Chive, and Wine Decoction) ··· 832
   Gua Lou Xie Bai Ban Xia Tang (Trichosanthes Fruit, Chinese Chive, and Pinellia Decoction) ··· 832
   Jia Wei Gua Lou Xie Bai Tang (Augmented Trichosanthes Fruit and Chinese Chive Decoction) ··· 832
Ju He Wan (Tangerine Seed Pill) ·· 833
Tian Tai Wu Yao San (Top-Quality Lindera Powder) ·· 835
   San Ceng Hui Xiang Wan (Fennel Seed Pill with Three Levels) ······················· 836
   Dao Qi Tang (Conduct the Qi Decoction) ·· 837
Nuan Gan Jian (Warm the Liver Decoction) ·· 838
Hou Po Wen Zhong Tang (Magnolia Bark Decoction for Warming the Middle) ··········· 840
   Liang Fu Wan (Galangal and Cyperus Pill) ·· 841

Section 2. Qi-Descending Formulas ·· 842
Su Zi Jiang Qi Tang (Perilla Fruit Decoction for Directing Qi Downward) ··········· 842
   San Zi Jiang Qi Tang (Three-Seed Decoction for Directing Qi Downward) ········· 844
Ding Chuan Tang (Arrest Wheezing Decoction) ·· 845
Shen Mi Tang (Mysterious Decoction) ·· 847
Si Mo Tang (Four Milled-Herbs Decoction) ·· 849
   Wu Mo Yin Zi (Five Milled-Herbs Decoction) ·· 850
Xuan Fu Dai Zhe Shi Tang (Inula and Hematite Decoction) ································· 851
   Gan Jiang Ren Shen Ban Xia Wan (Ginger, Ginseng, and Pinellia Pill) ··········· 853
Ju Pi Zhu Ru Tang (Tangerine Peel and Bamboo Shaving Decoction) ················· 854
   Ju Pi Zhu Ru Tang (Tangerine Peel and Bamboo Shaving Decoction) ··········· 855
   Xin Zhi Ju Pi Zhu Ru Tang (Newly-Formulated Tangerine Peel and Bamboo Shaving Decoction) ··· 856
Ding Xiang Shi Di Tang (Clove and Persimmon Calyx Decoction) ····················· 856
   Shi Di Tang (Persimmon Calyx Decoction) ·· 858
Sheng Yang San Huo Tang (Raise the Yang and Disperse the Fire Decoction) ········· 858

Qi-Regulating Formulas (Summary) ·· **860**

Chapter 13. Blood-Regulating Formulas ·· 863
Biography of Wang Qing-Ren ·· 864

Section 1. Blood-Invigorating and Stasis-Removing Formulas ························· 873
Tao He Cheng Qi Tang (Peach Pit Decoction to Order the Qi) ···························· 873
   Xia Yu Xue Tang (Drain Blood Stasis Decoction) ·· 876
Tong Qiao Huo Xue Tang (Unblock the Orifices and Invigorate the Blood Decoction) ··· 877
Xue Fu Zhu Yu Tang (Drive Out Stasis in the Mansion of Blood Decoction) ········· 879

Table of Contents

San Jiao Zhu Yu Tang (Drive Out Blood Stasis in Three *Jiaos* Decoction) ············· 883
Ge Xia Zhu Yu Tang (Drive Out Blood Stasis Below the Diaphragm Decoction) ············· 885
Shao Fu Zhu Yu Tang (Drive Out Blood Stasis in the Lower Abdomen Decoction) ············· 889
Shen Tong Zhu Yu Tang (Drive Out Blood Stasis from a Painful Body Decoction) ············· 893
Zhu Yu Tang (Drive Out Blood Stasis Decoction) ············· 895
Fu Yuan Huo Xue Tang (Revive Health by Invigorating the Blood Decoction) ············· 897
Po Bu Zi Ye Tang (Cordia Decoction) ············· 900
Huo Xue Shun Qi Tang (Invigorate the Blood and Smooth the Qi Decoction) ············· 900
Zheng Gu Zi Jin Dan (Purple and Gold Pill for Righteous Bones) ············· 901
Huo Xue Zhi Tong Tang (Invigorate the Blood and Stop Pain Decoction) ············· 902
Qi Li San (Seven-Thousandths of a Tael Powder) ············· 903
Bu Yang Huan Wu Tang (Tonify the Yang to Restore Five Decoction) ············· 905
Nao Wei Kang Wan (Benefit Brain Atrophy Pill) ············· 909
Shi Xiao San (Sudden Smile Powder) ············· 911
Shou Nian San (Pinch Powder) ············· 913
Wen Jing Zhi Tong Tang (Warm the Channel and Stop Pain Decoction) ············· 913
Huo Luo Xiao Ling Dan (Fantastically Effective Pill to Invigorate the Collaterals) ············· 914
Gong Wai Yun Fang (Ectopic Pregnancy Formula) ············· 917
Dan Shen Yin (Salvia Decoction) ············· 917
Wen Jing Tang (Warm the Channels Decoction) ············· 919
Ai Fu Nuan Gong Wan (Mugwort and Cyperus Pill for Warming the Womb) ············· 923
Sheng Hua Tang (Generation and Transformation Decoction) ············· 925
Tong Ru Wan (Unblock the Breast Pill) ············· 927
Gui Zhi Fu Ling Wan (Cinnamon Twig and Poria Pill) ············· 928
Duo Ming Wan (Life-Taking Pill) ············· 931
Cui Sheng Tang (Birth-Hastening Decoction) ············· 931
Zhe Chong Yin (Break the Conflict Decoction) ············· 933
Bie Jia Jian Wan (Soft-Shelled Turtle Shell Pill) ············· 935
Da Huang Zhe Chong Wan (Rhubarb and Eupolyphaga Pill) ············· 937

Section 2. Stop-Bleeding Formulas ············· 939

Shi Hui San (Ten Partially-Charred Substances Powder) ············· 939
Zhi Xue Tang (Stop Bleeding Decoction) ············· 941
Si Sheng Wan (Four-Fresh Pill) ············· 942
Ke Xue Fang (Coughing of Blood Formula) ············· 943
Huai Hua San (Sophora Japonica Flower Powder) ············· 944
Huai Jiao Wan (Sophora Japonica Fruit Pill) ············· 946
Xiao Ji Yin Zi (Cirsium Decoction) ············· 946
Huang Tu Tang (Yellow Earth Decoction) ············· 948
Jiao Ai Tang (Ass-Hide Gelatin and Mugwort Decoction) ············· 950

Blood-Regulating Formulas (Summary) ············· 953

Chapter 14. Wind-Expelling Formulas ············· 959

Biography of Wang Tao ············· 960

Section 1. External-Wind Releasing Formulas ············· 967

Xiao Feng San (Eliminate Wind Powder) ············· 967
Qu Feng San (Dispel Wind Powder) ············· 969
Dang Gui Yin Zi (Tangkuei Decoction) ············· 970
Chuan Xiong Cha Tiao San (Ligusticum Chuanxiong Powder to be Taken with Green Tea) ············· 973
Ju Hua Cha Tiao San (Chrysanthemum Powder to be Taken with Green Tea) ············· 976
Qian Zheng San (Lead to Symmetry Powder) ············· 977
Zhi Jing San (Stop Spasms Powder) ············· 979
Jia Wei Qian Zheng San (Augmented Lead to Symmetry Powder) ············· 980
Yu Zhen San (True Jade Powder) ············· 981
Wu Hu Zhui Feng San (Five-Tiger Powder to Pursue Wind) ············· 982

XVI

Table of Contents

Chinese Herbal Formulas and Applications

Xiao Xu Ming Tang (Minor Prolong Life Decoction) ·················· 983
   Xiao Xu Ming Tang (Minor Prolong Life Decoction) ·················· 985
Xu Ming Tang (Prolong Life Decoction) ·················· 986
Da Qin Jiao Tang (Major Gentiana Macrophylla Decoction) ·················· 988
Wu Yao Shun Qi San (Lindera Powder to Smooth the Flow of Qi) ·················· 990

Section 2. Internal-Wind Extinguishing Formulas ·················· **993**
Ling Jiao Gou Teng Tang (Antelope Horn and Uncaria Decoction) ·················· 993
   Gou Teng Yin (Uncaria Decoction) ·················· 995
Gou Teng San (Uncaria Powder) ·················· 996
Zhen Gan Xi Feng Tang (Sedate the Liver and Extinguish Wind Decoction) ·················· 999
Jian Ling Tang (Construct Roof Tiles Decoction) ·················· 1002
Tian Ma Gou Teng Yin (Gastrodia and Uncaria Decoction) ·················· 1004
   Tian Ma Jiang Ya Pian (Gastrodia Pill to Lower [Blood] Pressure) ·················· 1006
E Jiao Ji Zi Huang Tang (Ass-Hide Gelatin and Egg Yolk Decoction) ·················· 1007
Da Ding Feng Zhu (Major Arrest Wind Pearl) ·················· 1009
   Xiao Ding Feng Zhu (Minor Arrest Wind Pearl) ·················· 1011
   San Jia Fu Mai Tang (Three-Shell Decoction to Restore the Pulse) ·················· 1011
   San Jia An Shen Wan (Three-Shell Pill to Tranquilize the Spirit) ·················· 1011

Wind-Expelling Formulas (Summary) ·················· **1013**

Chapter 15. Dryness-Relieving Formulas ·················· 1017
Biography of Tao Hong-Jing ·················· 1018

Section 1. Dispersing and Moistening Formulas ·················· **1025**
Xing Su San (Apricot Kernel and Perilla Leaf Powder) ·················· 1025
Sang Xing Tang (Mulberry Leaf and Apricot Kernel Decoction) ·················· 1027
   Qiao He Tang (Forsythia and Mint Decoction) ·················· 1028
Qing Zao Jiu Fei Tang (Eliminate Dryness and Rescue the Lung Decoction) ·················· 1029

Section 2. Nourishing and Moistening Formulas ·················· **1033**
Yang Yin Qing Fei Tang (Nourish the Yin and Clear the Lung Decoction) ·················· 1033
Bai He Gu Jin Tang (Lily Bulb Decoction to Preserve the Metal) ·················· 1036
Bu Fei E Jiao Tang (Tonify the Lung Decoction with Ass-Hide Gelatin) ·················· 1039
   Yue Hua Wan (Moonlight Pill) ·················· 1040
Qiong Yu Gao (Beautiful Jade Paste) ·················· 1041
Mai Men Dong Tang (Ophiopogonis Decoction) ·················· 1043
   Mai Men Yang Yin Tang (Ophiopogonis Decoction to Nourish the Yin) ·················· 1045
Sha Shen Mai Dong Tang (Glehnia and Ophiopogonis Decoction) ·················· 1047
Yu Ye Tang (Jade Fluid Decoction) ·················· 1049
   Xiao Ke Fang (Wasting and Thirsting Formula) ·················· 1051
Yu Quan Wan (Jade Spring Pill) ·················· 1052
Zeng Ye Tang (Increase the Fluids Decoction) ·················· 1054

Dryness-Relieving Formulas (Summary) ·················· **1057**

Chapter 16. Damp-Dispelling Formulas ·················· 1059
Biography of Wang Ken-Tang ·················· 1060

Section 1. Damp-Drying and Stomach-Harmonizing Formulas ·················· **1068**
Ping Wei San (Calm the Stomach Powder) ·················· 1068
   Chai Ping Tang (Bupleurum and Calm the Stomach Decoction) ·················· 1071
Jia Wei Ping Wei San (Modified Calm the Stomach Powder) ·················· 1072
Xiang Sha Ping Wei San (Cyperus and Amomum Powder to Calm the Stomach) ·················· 1073
   Xiang Sha Ping Wei San (Cyperus and Amomum Powder to Calm the Stomach) ·················· 1075
Bu Huan Jin Zheng Qi San (Rectify the Qi Powder Worth More than Gold) ·················· 1075

XVII

Table of Contents

Fu Ling Yin (Poria Decoction) ··· 1077

Huo Xiang Zheng Qi San (Agastache Powder to Rectify the Qi) ································· 1079

Liu He Tang (Harmonize the Six Decoction) ·· 1082

 Liu He Tang (Harmonize the Six Decoction) ·· 1083

Ge Hua Jie Cheng San (Pueraria Flower Powder for Detoxification and Awakening) ················ 1084

Section 2. Heat-Clearing and Damp-Dispelling Formulas ····················· **1086**

Yin Chen Hao Tang (Artemisia Scoparia Decoction) ·· 1086

 Zhi Zi Bai Pi Tang (Gardenia and Phellodendron Decoction) ·· 1089

 Yin Chen Si Ni Tang (Artemisia Scoparia Decoction for Frigid Extremities) ··············· 1089

 Yin Chen Pai Shi Tang (Artemisia Scoparia Decoction to Expel Stone) ························· 1089

Yin Chen Wu Ling San (Artemisia Scoparia and Five-Ingredient Powder with Poria) ··············· 1090

San Ren Tang (Three-Nut Decoction) ··· 1092

 Huo Po Xia Ling Tang (Agastache, Magnolia Bark, Pinellia, and Poria Decoction) ········· 1095

 Huang Qin Hua Shi Tang (Scutellaria and Talcum Decoction) ·· 1095

Gan Lu Xiao Du Dan (Sweet Dew Special Pill to Eliminate Toxins) ································· 1096

Lian Po Yin (Coptis and Magnolia Bark Decoction) ·· 1099

Can Shi Tang (Silkworm Droppings Decoction) ··· 1101

Ba Zheng San (Eight-Herb Powder for Rectification) ·· 1103

 Jia Wei Ba Zheng San (Augmented Eight Herb Powder for Rectification) ···················· 1105

 Fu Fang Ba Zheng San (Revised Eight-Herb Powder) ··· 1105

 San Jin Pai Shi Tang (Three Gold Decoction to Expel Stone) ·· 1106

Wu Lin San (Five-Ingredient Powder for Painful Urinary Dysfunction) ····················· 1107

 Huo Xue Tong Lin Tang (Invigorate the Blood to Unblock Dysuria Decoction) ·········· 1107

 Qing Re Tong Lin Tang (Clear Heat to Unblock Dysuria Decoction) ·························· 1108

Section 3. Water-Regulating and Damp-Resolving Formulas ················· **1109**

Wu Ling San (Five-Ingredient Powder with Poria) ·· 1109

 Si Ling San (Four-Ingredient Powder with Poria) ·· 1112

 Bai Mao Gen Tang (Imperata Decoction) ·· 1112

 Fu Ling Tang (Poria Decoction) ·· 1112

Wei Ling Tang (Calm the Stomach and Poria Decoction) ·· 1113

Zhu Ling Tang (Polyporus Decoction) ··· 1115

Fang Ji Huang Qi Tang (Stephania and Astragalus Decoction) ·· 1118

 Fang Ji Fu Ling Tang (Stephania and Poria Decoction) ··· 1120

Wu Pi San (Five-Peel Powder) ··· 1121

 Wu Pi San (Five-Peel Powder) ·· 1123

Jiu Wei Bing Lang Jia Wu Fu Tang (Areca Nine Decoction plus Evodia and Poria) ··············· 1123

Mu Fang Ji Tang (Cocculus Decoction) ··· 1125

Fen Xiao Tang (Separate and Reduce Decoction) ··· 1127

Dao Shui Fu Ling Tang (Poria Decoction to Drain Water) ··· 1129

Section 4. Warm Formulas that Dissolve Dampness ····························· **1131**

Ling Gui Zhu Gan Tang (Poria, Cinnamon Twig, Atractylodes Macrocephala, and Licorice Decoction) ······ 1131

Gan Cao Gan Jiang Fu Ling Bai Zhu Tang (Licorice, Ginger, Poria and Atractylodes Macrocephala Decoction) ··· 1133

Zhen Wu Tang (True Warrior Decoction) ··· 1135

 Fu Zi Tang (Prepared Aconite Decoction) ·· 1137

Shi Pi San (Bolster the Spleen Powder) ··· 1138

Bi Xie Fen Qing Yin (Dioscorea Hypoglauca Decoction to Separate the Clear) ··············· 1140

 Bi Xie Fen Qing Yin (Dioscorea Hypoglauca Decoction to Separate the Clear) ············ 1141

 Bi Xie Fen Qing Yin (Dioscorea Hypoglauca Decoction to Separate the Clear) ············ 1142

Damp-Dispelling Formulas (Summary) ··· **1143**

Chapter 17. Wind-Damp Dispelling Formulas ································ **1149**

Biography of Sun Si-Miao ··· 1150

XVIII

Chinese Herbal Formulas and Applications

Table of Contents

Section 1. Wind-Damp Dispelling Formulas **1156**
Qiang Huo Sheng Shi Tang (Notopterygium Decoction to Overcome Dampness) 1156
Juan Bi Tang (Remove Painful Obstruction Decoction) 1158
   Jian Bi Tang (Remove Painful Obstruction in the Shoulders Decoction) 1160
Du Huo Ji Sheng Tang (Angelica Pubescens and Taxillus Decoction) 1161
   Yao Tong Fang Yi Hao (Low Back Pain Formula One) 1164
   Yao Tong Fang Er Hao (Low Back Pain Formula Two) 1164
   Xi Tong Fang Yi Hao (Knee Pain Formula One) 1165
   Xi Tong Fang Er Hao (Knee Pain Formula Two) 1165
   Ji Tong Tang (Spine Pain Decoction) 1165
San Bi Tang (Three-Painful Obstruction Decoction) 1167
Shu Jing Huo Xue Tang (Relax the Channels and Invigorate the Blood Decoction) 1169
Shu Jin Li An San (Relax the Tendons and Instill Peace Powder) 1171
Yi Yi Ren Tang (Coicis Decoction) 1173
Shang Zhong Xia Tong Yong Tong Feng Wan (Upper, Middle, and Lower General Use Pill for Wind-Pain) 1175
   Tong Feng Wan (Wind-Pain Pill) 1176

Section 2. Damp-Cold Dispelling Formulas **1177**
Xiao Huo Luo Dan (Minor Invigorate the Collaterals Special Pill) 1177
   Da Huo Luo Dan (Major Invigorate the Collaterals Special Pill) 1179
   Jia Wei Huo Luo Dan (Augmented Invigorate the Collaterals Special Pill) 1180
Da Fang Feng Tang (Major Saposhnikovia Decoction) 1181
Ji Ming San (Powder to Take at Cock's Crow) 1183

Section 3. Damp-Heat Dispelling Formulas **1186**
Gui Zhi Shao Yao Zhi Mu Tang (Cinnamon Twig, Peony, and Anemarrhena Decoction) 1186
   Sang Zhi Shi Gao Zhi Mu Tang (Mulberry Twig, Gypsum, and Anemarrhena Decoction) 1187
Er Miao San (Two-Marvel Powder) 1188
   San Miao Wan (Three-Marvel Pill) 1190
   Si Miao Wan (Four-Marvel Pill) 1190
Dang Gui Nian Tong Tang (Tangkuei Decoction to Lift the Pain) 1191
   Nian Tong Tang (Lift the Pain Decoction) 1193

Section 4. Damp-Phlegm Dispelling Formula **1195**
Er Zhu Tang (Two-Atractylodes Decoction) 1195

Wind-Damp Dispelling Formulas (Summary) **1197**

Chapter 18. Phlegm-Dispelling Formulas **1201**
Biography of Zhu Zhen-Heng 1202

Section 1. Damp-Drying and Phlegm-Dissolving Formulas **1209**
Er Chen Tang (Two-Cured Decoction) 1209
   Dao Tan Tang (Guide Out Phlegm Decoction) 1211
   Di Tan Tang (Scour Phlegm Decoction) 1212
   Zhi Suo Er Chen Tang (Two-Cured Decoction with Aurantium and Cardamon) 1212
Wen Dan Tang (Warm the Gallbladder Decoction) 1213
   Shi Wei Wen Dan Tang (Ten-Ingredient Decoction to Warm the Gallbladder) 1216
Zhu Ru Wen Dan Tang (Bamboo Decoction to Warm the Gallbladder) 1217
Fu Ling Wan (Poria Pill) 1219
Xiao Ban Xia Jia Fu Ling Tang (Minor Pinellia and Poria Decoction) 1220

Section 2. Heat-Clearing and Phlegm-Dissolving Formulas **1222**
Qing Qi Hua Tan Wan (Clear the Qi and Transform Phlegm Pill) 1222
   Hua Tan Wan (Transform Phlegm Pill) 1223
Qing Fei Yin (Clear the Lung Drink) 1224
Qing Fei Tang (Clear the Lung Decoction) 1225

XIX

Table of Contents

Qing Fei Tang (Clear the Lung Decoction) ⋯⋯⋯⋯⋯⋯⋯⋯⋯⋯⋯⋯⋯⋯⋯⋯⋯ 1227

Zi Wan Tang (Aster Decoction) ⋯⋯⋯⋯⋯⋯⋯⋯⋯⋯⋯⋯⋯⋯⋯⋯⋯⋯⋯⋯ 1229

Jie Geng Tang (Platycodon Decoction) ⋯⋯⋯⋯⋯⋯⋯⋯⋯⋯⋯⋯⋯⋯⋯⋯ 1230

Ren Shen Xie Fei Tang (Ginseng Decoction to Sedate the Lung) ⋯⋯⋯⋯⋯⋯ 1231

Gua Lou Zhi Shi Tang (Trichosanthes Fruit and Immature Bitter Orange Decoction) ⋯⋯⋯⋯⋯ 1233

Xiao Xian Xiong Tang (Minor Sinking into the Chest Decoction) ⋯⋯⋯⋯⋯ 1235

   Chai Hu Xian Xiong Tang (Bupleurum Decoction for Sinking into the Chest) ⋯⋯⋯⋯ 1237

Gun Tan Wan (Vaporize Phlegm Pill) ⋯⋯⋯⋯⋯⋯⋯⋯⋯⋯⋯⋯⋯⋯⋯⋯ 1238

Section 3. Dryness-Moistening and Phlegm-Dissolving Formula ⋯⋯⋯⋯⋯ 1240

Bei Mu Gua Lou San (Fritillaria and Trichosanthes Fruit Powder) ⋯⋯⋯⋯⋯ 1240

Section 4. Warm Formulas that Dissolve Cold Phlegm ⋯⋯⋯⋯⋯⋯⋯⋯ 1242

Ling Gan Wu Wei Jiang Xin Tang (Poria, Licorice, Schisandra, Ginger, and Asarum Decoction) ⋯⋯⋯ 1242

   Leng Xiao Wan (Cold Wheezing Pill) ⋯⋯⋯⋯⋯⋯⋯⋯⋯⋯⋯⋯⋯⋯⋯ 1243

   San Jian Gao (Three Constructive Paste) ⋯⋯⋯⋯⋯⋯⋯⋯⋯⋯⋯⋯⋯ 1244

San Zi Yang Qin Tang (Three-Seed Decoction to Nourish One's Parents) ⋯⋯⋯⋯ 1245

Section 5. Wind-Expelling and Phlegm-Dissolving Formulas ⋯⋯⋯⋯⋯⋯ 1247

Ban Xia Bai Zhu Tian Ma Tang (Pinellia, Atractylodes Macrocephala, and Gastrodia Decoction) ⋯⋯⋯ 1247

   Ban Xia Bai Zhu Tian Ma Tang (Pinellia, Atractylodes Macrocephala, and Gastrodia Decoction) ⋯⋯⋯ 1250

Ding Xian Wan (Arrest Seizures Pill) ⋯⋯⋯⋯⋯⋯⋯⋯⋯⋯⋯⋯⋯⋯⋯⋯ 1251

   He Che Wan Fang (Placenta Pill Formula) ⋯⋯⋯⋯⋯⋯⋯⋯⋯⋯⋯⋯⋯ 1253

Phlegm-Dispelling Formulas (Summary) ⋯⋯⋯⋯⋯⋯⋯⋯⋯⋯⋯⋯⋯⋯ 1254

Chapter 19. Reducing, Guiding, and Dissolving Formulas ⋯⋯⋯⋯⋯⋯⋯ 1259

Biography of Li Gao ⋯⋯⋯⋯⋯⋯⋯⋯⋯⋯⋯⋯⋯⋯⋯⋯⋯⋯⋯⋯⋯⋯⋯ 1260

Section 1. Reducing, Guiding, and Dissolving Formulas that Treat Food Stagnation ⋯⋯⋯ 1266

Bao He Wan (Preserve Harmony Pill) ⋯⋯⋯⋯⋯⋯⋯⋯⋯⋯⋯⋯⋯⋯⋯⋯ 1266

   Da An Wan (Great Tranquility Pill) ⋯⋯⋯⋯⋯⋯⋯⋯⋯⋯⋯⋯⋯⋯⋯ 1268

   Shan Zha Tang (Crataegus Decoction) ⋯⋯⋯⋯⋯⋯⋯⋯⋯⋯⋯⋯⋯⋯ 1268

   Shan Zha Hua Tan Tang (Crataegus Decoction to Transform Phlegm) ⋯⋯⋯⋯⋯ 1269

Zhi Shi Dao Zhi Wan (Immature Bitter Orange Pill to Guide Out Stagnation) ⋯⋯⋯ 1270

Mu Xiang Bing Lang Wan (Aucklandia and Betel Nut Pill) ⋯⋯⋯⋯⋯⋯⋯⋯ 1272

Zhi Zhu Wan (Immature Bitter Orange and Atractylodes Macrocephala Pill) ⋯⋯⋯⋯ 1274

   Zhi Zhu Tang (Immature Bitter Orange and Atractylodes Macrocephala Decoction) ⋯⋯⋯ 1275

   Qu Mai Zhi Zhu Wan (Medicated Leaven, Barley Sprout, Immature Bitter Orange, and Atractylodes Macrocephala Pill) ⋯⋯⋯ 1275

   Ju Ban Zhi Zhu Wan (Tangerine Peel, Pinellia, Immature Bitter Orange, and Atractylodes Macrocephala Pill) ⋯⋯⋯ 1276

   Xiang Sha Zhi Zhu Wan (Aucklandia, Amomum, Immature Bitter Orange, and Atractylodes Macrocephala Pill) ⋯⋯⋯ 1276

Jian Pi Wan (Strengthen the Spleen Pill) ⋯⋯⋯⋯⋯⋯⋯⋯⋯⋯⋯⋯⋯⋯ 1277

   Zi Sheng Wan (Nourish Life Pill) ⋯⋯⋯⋯⋯⋯⋯⋯⋯⋯⋯⋯⋯⋯⋯⋯ 1278

Section 2. Reducing, Guiding, and Dissolving Formula that Relieves Distention ⋯⋯⋯ 1280

Zhi Shi Xiao Pi Wan (Immature Bitter Orange Pill to Reduce Focal Distention) ⋯⋯⋯ 1280

Reducing, Guiding, and Dissolving Formulas (Summary) ⋯⋯⋯⋯⋯⋯⋯ 1283

Chapter 20. Antiparasitic Formulas ⋯⋯⋯⋯⋯⋯⋯⋯⋯⋯⋯⋯⋯⋯⋯ 1285

Biography of Ge Hong ⋯⋯⋯⋯⋯⋯⋯⋯⋯⋯⋯⋯⋯⋯⋯⋯⋯⋯⋯⋯⋯ 1286

Wu Mei Wan (Mume Pill) ⋯⋯⋯⋯⋯⋯⋯⋯⋯⋯⋯⋯⋯⋯⋯⋯⋯⋯⋯⋯ 1292

   Li Zhong An Hui Tang (Regulate the Middle and Calm Roundworms Decoction) ⋯⋯⋯ 1295

   Lian Mei An Hui Tang (Picrorhiza and Mume Decoction to Calm Roundworms) ⋯⋯⋯ 1295

Fei Er Wan (Fat Child Pill) ⋯⋯⋯⋯⋯⋯⋯⋯⋯⋯⋯⋯⋯⋯⋯⋯⋯⋯⋯⋯ 1296

   Jin Jian Fei Er Wan (Golden Pill to Construct a Fat Child) ⋯⋯⋯⋯⋯⋯⋯⋯ 1298

Table of Contents

Chinese Herbal Formulas and Applications

Bu Dai Wan (Cloth Sack Pill) ··· 1299
Hua Chong Wan (Dissolve Parasites Pill) ·· 1300
Fa Mu Wan (Quell Wood Pill) ··· 1302

Antiparasitic Formulas (Summary) ··· 1303

Chapter 21. Emetic Formulas ··· 1305
Biography of Zhang Cong-Zheng ·· 1306

Gua Di San (Melon Pedicle Powder) ·· 1311
   San Sheng San (Three-Sage Powder) ··· 1312
Jiu Ji Xi Xian San (Urgent Powder to Dilute Saliva) ···································· 1313
Yan Tang Tan Tu Fang (Salt Decoction to Induce Vomiting) ···························· 1314

Emetic Formulas (Summary) ·· 1315

Chapter 22. Formulas that Treat Abscesses and Sores ···················· 1317
Biography of Gong Ting-Xian ·· 1318

Section 1. External Abscesses and Sores ······································ 1325
Xian Fang Huo Ming Yin (Sublime Formula for Sustaining Life) ························ 1325
   Zhen Ren Huo Ming Yin (True Man's Decoction to Revitalize Life) ················· 1330
   Huo Ming Yin (Revitalize Life Decoction) ··· 1330
   Lian Qiao Bai Du San (Forsythia Powder to Overcome Pathogenic Influences) ········ 1331
Niu Bang Jie Ji Tang (Arctium Decoction to Release the Muscle Layer) ················· 1332
Jing Fang Bai Du San (Schizonepeta and Saposhnikovia Powder to Overcome Pathogenic Influences) ··· 1334
   Jing Fang Bai Du San (Schizonepeta and Saposhnikovia Powder to Overcome Pathogenic Influences) ··· 1335
   Jing Fang Bai Du San (Schizonepeta and Saposhnikovia Powder to Overcome Pathogenic Influences) ··· 1336
Wu Wei Xiao Du Yin (Five-Ingredient Decoction to Eliminate Toxins) ·················· 1337
   Yin Hua Jie Du Tang (Honeysuckle Decoction to Relieve Toxicity) ·················· 1340
Shi Wei Bai Du Tang (Ten-Ingredient Decoction to Overcome Pathogenic Influences) ······ 1341
   Bai Du Tang (Overcome Pathogenic Influences Decoction) ·························· 1343
Si Miao Yong An Tang (Four-Valiant Decoction for Well-Being) ························ 1344
   Wu Shen Tang (Five-Miracle Decoction) ··· 1347
   Shen Xiao Tuo Li San (Miraculous Powder for Supporting the Interior) ·············· 1347
Zi Cao Gen Mu Li Tang (Arnebia and Oyster Shell Decoction) ························· 1348
Xi Huang Wan (Cattle Gallstone Pill) ·· 1350
   Xing Xiao Wan (Awake and Disperse Pill) ·· 1351
   Chan Su Wan (Toad Venum Pill) ·· 1351
Hai Zao Yu Hu Tang (Sargassum Decoction for the Jade Flask) ························ 1352
Xiao Luo Wan (Reduce Scrofula Pill) ·· 1355
San Zhong Kui Jian Tang (Disperse the Swelling and Break the Hardness Decoction) ······ 1357
   San Zhong Kui Jian Tang (Disperse the Swelling and Break the Hardness Decoction) ···· 1358
   Xiao San Tang Yi Hao (Dissolve and Disperse Decoction Formula One) ·············· 1359
   Xiao San Tang Er Hao (Dissolve and Disperse Decoction Formula Two) ············· 1359
Shi Liu Wei Liu Qi Yin (Sixteen-Ingredient Decoction to Flow Qi) ····················· 1360
   Shi Liu Wei Liu Qi Yin (Sixteen-Ingredient Decoction to Flow Qi) ·················· 1361
Tou Nong San (Discharge Pus Powder) ··· 1362
   Tuo Li Tou Nong Tang (Drain the Interior and Discharge Pus Decoction) ············ 1363
Pai Nong San (Drain the Pus Powder) ·· 1364
Qian Jin Nei Tuo San (Drain the Interior Powder Worthy of a Thousand Gold) ············ 1365
Tuo Li Xiao Du Yin (Drain the Interior and Detoxify Decoction) ······················· 1367
   Tuo Li Xiao Du Yin (Drain the Interior and Detoxify Decoction) ·················· 1368
Nei Bu Huang Qi Tang (Tonify the Interior Decoction with Astragalus) ················· 1369
Yang He Tang (Yang-Heartening Decoction) ·· 1370
   Zhong He Tang (Middle-Heartening Decoction) ···································· 1373
Xiao Jin Dan (Minor Gold Special Pill) ··· 1374

XXI

Table of Contents

Section 2. Internal Abscesses and Sores ··· **1377**

Wei Jing Tang (Reed Decoction) ··· 1377

Da Huang Mu Dan Tang (Rhubarb and Moutan Decoction) ··· 1378

   Qing Chang Yin (Clear the Intestines Drink) ··· 1381

Yi Yi Fu Zi Bai Jiang San (Coicis, Prepared Aconite, and Patrinia Powder) ··················· 1382

   Yi Yi Ren Tang (Coicis Decoction) ··· 1383

Formulas that Treat Abscesses and Sores (Summary) ···························· **1385**

Part III Additional Resources ··· 1389

Biography of Wu Shang-Xian ··· 1390

Appendix 1 Cross-reference Based on Traditional Chinese Medicine Diagnosis ··············· 1393

Appendix 2 Cross-reference Based on Western Medicine Diagnosis ····························· 1397

Appendix 3 Formulas Offering Beneficial Effects to Support Pregnancy ························ 1433

Appendix 4 Formulas Offering Beneficial Effects for Postpartum Care ······················· 1434

Appendix 5 Cautions / Contraindications for the Use of Formulas During Pregnancy ······· 1435

Appendix 6 Dosing Guidelines ··· 1437

Appendix 7 Weights and Measures: Chinese, British and Metric Systems ····················· 1439

Appendix 8 Convention on International Trade in Endangered Species (CITES) ··············· 1441

Appendix 9 Cross-reference of Single Herb Names ··· 1442

Appendix 10 Cross-reference of Herbal Formula Names ·· 1464

Appendix 11 Tables of Famous Doctors ··· 1481

Bibliography of Historical Texts ··· 1485

Bibliography of Contemporary References ··· 1493

Glossary ·· 1505

Index ··· 1529

About the Authors ··· 1619

XXII

Chinese Herbal Formulas and Applications

Preface

The nomenclature for some herbs has been changed since the publication of *Chinese Medical Herbology and Pharmacology* in 2004. Most changes correspond to the 2005 edition of 中华人民共和国药典 *Zhong Hua Ren Min Gong He Guo Yao Dian* (Pharmacopoeia of the People's Republic of China), which is the official pharmacopoeia in China, as well as our primary reference for nomenclature. Changes have been made to:

- accurately reflect the part of the plant used, from *Ba Dou* (<u>Fructus</u> Crotonis) to *Ba Dou* (<u>Semen</u> Crotonis)
- correctly pronounce the *pinyin* name, from *Huang <u>Bai</u>* (Cortex Phellodendri) to *Huang <u>Bo</u>* (Cortex Phellodendri Chinensis)
- precisely describe the processing method, from *Zhi Gan Cao* (Radix Glycyrrhizae <u>Praeparata</u>) to *Zhi Gan Cao* (Radix et Rhizoma Glycyrrhizae <u>Praeparata cum Melle</u>)
- be more specific: *Kun Bu* (Thallus <u>Laminariae seu Eckloniae</u>) is separated into *Hai Dai* (Thallus <u>Laminariae</u>) and *Kun Bu* (Thallus <u>Eckloniae</u>)
- be more inclusive: from *Shan Ci Gu* (Pseudobulbus <u>Cremastrae</u>) to *Shan Ci Gu* (Pseudobulbus <u>Cremastrae seu Pleiones</u>)
- adapt to the current rules and regulations, from *Xi Xin* (<u>Herba</u> Asari) to *Xi Xin* (<u>Radix et Rhizoma</u> Asari). Note: The aerial parts of asarum contain aristolochic acid, and have been banned by many countries around the world. As a result, the root and rhizome of asarum are now used, as they are believed to have little or no aristolochic acid.[1]
- and lastly, to humbly correct our previous errors, such as replacing the incorrect *Mu Fang Ji* (Radix <u>Couulus</u> Trilobus) with *Mu Fang Ji* (Radix <u>Cocculi</u> Trilobi).

Chinese Medical Herbology and Pharmacology	Chinese Herbal Formulas and Applications
Ba Dou (Fructus Crotonis)	*Ba Dou* (Semen Crotonis)
Ba Yue Zha (Fructus Akebiae)	*Yu Zhi Zi* (Fructus Akebiae)
Bai Dou Kou (Fructus Amomi Rotundus)	*Dou Kou* (Fructus Amomi Rotundus)
Bai Dou Kou Ke (Pericarpium Amomi Rotundus)	*Dou Kou Ke* (Pericarpium Amomi Rotundus)
Bai Hua She (Bungarus Parvus)	*Jin Qian Bai Hua She* (Bungarus Parvus)
Bai Hua She She Cao (Herba Oldenlandia)	*Bai Hua She She Cao* (Herba Hedyotis)
Bai Ji Li (Fructus Tribuli)	*Ji Li* (Fructus Tribuli)
Bai Qian (Rhizoma Cynanchi Stauntonii)	*Bai Qian* (Rhizoma et Radix Cynanchi Stauntonii)
Bai Wei (Radix Cynanchi Atrati)	*Bai Wei* (Radix et Rhizoma Cynanchi Atrati)
Bei Mu (Bulbus Fritillaria)	*Bei Mu* (Bulbus Fritillariae)
Bei Wu Jia Pi (Cortex Periploca Sepium Radicis)	*Xiang Jia Pi* (Cortex Periplocae)
Bi Ba (Fructus Piperis Longi)	*Bi Bo* (Fructus Piperis Longi)
Bi Xie (Rhizoma Dioscoreae Hypoglaucae)	*Fen Bi Xie* (Rhizoma Dioscoreae Hypoglaucae)
Bian Dou (Semen Lablab Album)	*Bai Bian Dou* (Semen Lablab Album)
Can Sha (Excrementum Bombycis Mori)	*Can Sha* (Faeces Bombycis)
Chi Fu Ling (Poria Rubrae)	*Chi Fu Ling* (Poria Rubra)
Chi Shao (Radix Paeoniae Rubrae)	*Chi Shao* (Radix Paeoniae Rubra)
Chong Wei Zi (Semen Leonuri)	*Chong Wei Zi* (Fructus Leonuri)
Chuan Xiong (Rhizoma Ligustici Chuanxiong)	*Chuan Xiong* (Rhizoma Chuanxiong)
Chun Gen Pi (Cortex Ailanthi)	*Chun Pi* (Cortex Ailanthi)
Ci Wu Jia (Radix et Caulis Acanthopanacis Senticosi)	*Ci Wu Jia* (Radix et Rhizoma seu Caulis Acanthopanacis Senticosi)
Da Hui Xiang (Fructus Anisi Stellati)	*Ba Jiao Hui Xiang* (Fructus Anisi Stellati)
Da Ji (Herba seu Radix Cirsii Japonici)	*Da Ji* (Herba Cirsii Japonici)

XXIII

Preface

Chinese Medical Herbology and Pharmacology	Chinese Herbal Formulas and Applications
Dai Zhe Shi (Haematitum)	*Zhe Shi* (Haematitum)
Dan Shen (Radix Salviae Miltiorrhizae)	*Dan Shen* (Radix et Rhizoma Salviae Miltiorrhizae)
Dang Gui (Radicis Angelicae Sinensis)	*Dang Gui* (Radix Angelicae Sinensis)
Dang Gui Shen (Corpus Radicis Angelicae Sinensis)	*Dang Gui Shen* (Corpus Radix Angelicae Sinensis)
Dang Gui Tou (Caput Radicis Angelicae Sinensis)	*Dang Gui Tou* (Caput Radix Angelicae Sinensis)
Dang Gui Wei (Extremitas Radicis Angelicae Sinensis)	*Dang Gui Wei* (Extremitas Radix Angelicae Sinensis)
Di Bie Chong (Eupolyphaga)	*Tu Bie Chong* (Eupolyphaga seu Steleophaga)
Duan Shi Gao (Gypsum Fibrosum Preparata)	*Duan Shi Gao* (Gypsum Fibrosum Praeparatum)
Fen Fang Ji (Radix Stephaniae Tetandrae)	*Fang Ji* (Radix Stephaniae Tetrandrae)
Fu Xiao Mai (Semen Tritici Aestivi Levis)	*Fu Xiao Mai* (Fructus Tritici Levis)
Gan Cao (Radix Glycyrrhizae)	*Gan Cao* (Radix et Rhizoma Glycyrrhizae)
Gan Song (Radix seu Rhizoma Nardostachys)	*Gan Song* (Radix et Rhizoma Nardostachydis)
Gan Sui (Radix Euphorbiae Kansui)	*Gan Sui* (Radix Kansui)
Gao Ben (Rhizoma Ligustici)	*Gao Ben* (Rhizoma et Radix Ligustici)
Ge Gen (Radix Puerariae)	*Ge Gen* (Radix Puerariae Lobatae)
Gu Zhi Hua (Semen Oroxyli)	*Mu Hu Die* (Semen Oroxyli)
Gua Lou Ren (Semen Trichosanthis)	*Gua Lou Zi* (Semen Trichosanthis)
Gua Lou Shi (Fructus Trichosanthis)	*Gua Lou* (Fructus Trichosanthis)
Guan Bai Fu (Rhizoma Aconitum Coreanum)	*Guan Bai Fu* (Radix Aconiti Coreani)
Guan Ye Lian Qiao (Herba Hypericum)	*Guan Ye Jin Si Tao* (Herba Hyperici Perforati)
Guan Zhong (Rhizoma Dryopteridis)	*Mian Ma Guan Zhong* (Rhizoma Dryopteridis Crassirhizomatis)
Hai Ge Fen (Concha Meretricis seu Cyclinae)	*Ge Qiao* (Concha Meretricis seu Cyclinae)
Hai Jin Sha (Herba Lygodii)	*Hai Jin Sha* (Spora Lygodii)
Han Fang Ji (Radix Stephaniae Tetandrae)	*Fang Ji* (Radix Stephaniae Tetrandrae)
Han Lian Cao (Herba Ecliptae)	*Mo Han Lian* (Herba Ecliptae)
Hei Cha (Folium Camelliae Nigrum)	*Hei Cha* (Folium Camelliae Nigrum)
Hei Dou (Semen Glycine Max)	*Hei Dou* (Semen Sojae)
Hong Dou Kou (Fructus Alphiniae Galangae)	*Hong Dou Kou* (Fructus Galangae)
Hong Teng (Caulis Sargentodoxae)	*Da Xue Teng* (Caulis Sargentodoxae)
Hu Jiao (Fructus Piper)	*Hu Jiao* (Fructus Piperis)
Hu Zhang (Rhizoma Polygoni Cuspidati)	*Hu Zhang* (Rhizoma et Radix Polygoni Cuspidati)
Huai Niu Xi (Radix Achyranthis Bidentatae)	*Niu Xi* (Radix Achyranthis Bidentatae)
Huang Bai (Cortex Phellodendri)	*Huang Bo* (Cortex Phellodendri Chinensis)
Huang Teng (Caulis Fibraurea)	*Huang Teng* (Caulis Fibraureae)
Huo Xiang (Herba Agastache)	*Huo Xiang* (Herba Agastaches)
Huo Xiang Ye (Folium Agastache)	*Huo Xiang Ye* (Folium Agastaches)
Jin Bo (Native Gold)	*Jin Bo* (gold foil)
Jin Yin Hua (Flos Lonicerae)	*Jin Yin Hua* (Flos Lonicerae Japonicae)
Jing Jie Sui (Flos Schizonepetae)	*Jing Jie Sui* (Spica Schizonepetae)
Jing Sui (Flos Schizonepetae)	*Jing Jie Sui* (Spica Schizonepetae)
Ju He (Semen Citri Rubrum)	*Ju He* (Semen Citri Reticulatae)
Ju Luo (Fibra Citri Rubrum)	*Ju Luo* (Vascular Citri Reticulatae)

Preface

Chinese Medical Herbology and Pharmacology	Chinese Herbal Formulas and Applications
Ju Ye (Folium Citri Rubrum)	Ju Ye (Folium Citri Reticulatae)
Ku Shen Gen (Radix Sophorae Flavescentis)	Ku Shen (Radix Sophorae Flavescentis)
Kun Bu (Thallus Laminariae seu Eckloniae)	Kun Bu (Thallus Eckloniae)
Long Dan Cao (Radix Gentianae)	Long Dan (Radix et Rhizoma Gentianae)
Lu Cha (Folium Camellia Sinensis)	Cha Ye (Folium Camelliae)
Lu Feng Fang (Nidus Vespae)	Feng Fang (Nidus Vespae)
Lu Han Cao (Herba Pyrolae)	Lu Xian Cao (Herba Pyrolae)
Lu Jiao Jiao (Gelatinum Cornu Cervi)	Lu Jiao Jiao (Colla Cornus Cervi)
Lu Jiao Shuang (Cornu Cervi Degelatinatium)	Lu Jiao Shuang (Cornu Cervi Degelatinatum)
Ma Huang Gen (Radix Ephedrae)	Ma Huang Gen (Radix et Rhizoma Ephedrae)
Mai Men Dong (Radix Ophiopogonis)	Mai Dong (Radix Ophiopogonis)
Mi Jiao (Cornu Elapnurus)	Mi Lu Jiao (Cornu Elaphuri)
Mi Rong (Cornu Elapnurus Parvum)	Mi Lu Rong (Cornu Elaphuri Pantotrichum)
Ming Fan (Alumen)	Bai Fan (Alumen)
Mu Fang Ji (Radix Couulus Trilobus)	Mu Fang Ji (Radix Cocculi Trilobi)
Niu Xi (Radix Cyathulae seu Achyranthis)	Niu Xi (Radix Achyranthis Bidentatae)
Pao Jiang (Rhizoma Zingiberis Preparatum)	Pao Jiang (Rhizoma Zingiberis Praeparatum)
Qian Cao (Radix Rubiae)	Qian Cao (Radix et Rhizoma Rubiae)
Qian Jin Zi (Semen Euphorbiae Lathyridis)	Qian Jin Zi (Semen Euphorbiae)
Ren Dong Cao (Herba Lonicerae)	Ren Dong Cao (Herba Lonicerae Japonicae)
Ren Dong Teng (Caulis Lonicerae)	Ren Dong Teng (Caulis Lonicerae Japonicae)
Ren Gong Niu Huang (Calculus Bovis Syntheticum)	Ren Gong Niu Huang (Calculus Bovis Artifactus)
Ren Shen (Radix Ginseng)	Ren Shen (Radix et Rhizoma Ginseng)
Rui Ren (Semen Prinsepiae)	Rui Ren (Nux Prinsepiae)
San Qi (Radix Notoginseng)	San Qi (Radix et Rhizoma Notoginseng)
Sang Shen Zi (Fructus Mori)	Sang Shen (Fructus Mori)
Shan Ci Gu (Pseudobulbus Cremastrae)	Shan Ci Gu (Pseudobulbus Cremastrae seu Pleiones)
Shan Dou Gen (Radix Sophorae Tonkinensis)	Shan Dou Gen (Radix et Rhizoma Sophorae Tonkinensis)
Sheng Di Huang (Radix Rehmanniae)	Di Huang (Radix Rehmanniae)
Shi Chang Pu (Rhizoma Acori)	Shi Chang Pu (Rhizoma Acori Tatarinowii)
Shi Hu (Herba Dendrobii)	Shi Hu (Caulis Dendrobii)
Shu Di Huang (Radix Rehmanniae Preparata)	Shu Di Huang (Radix Rehmanniae Praeparata)
Shui Chang Pu (Rhizoma Acori Calami)	Zang Chang Pu (Rhizoma Acori Calami)
Su Geng (Caulis Perillae)	Zi Su Geng (Caulis Perillae)
Su Ye (Folium Perillae)	Zi Su Ye (Folium Perillae)
Su Zi (Fructus Perillae)	Zi Su Zi (Fructus Perillae)
Suan Zao Ren (Semen Zizyphi Spinosae)	Suan Zao Ren (Semen Ziziphi Spinosae)
Tian Men Dong (Radix Asparagi)	Tian Dong (Radix Asparagi)
Tu Bei Mu (Bulbus Bolbostemma Paniculatum)	Tu Bei Mu (Rhizoma Bolbostematis)
Tu Niu Xi (Radix Achyranthes Longifolia)	Tu Niu Xi (Radix Achyranthis Longifoliae)
Wan Nian Song (Herba Selaginellae)	Juan Bai (Herba Selaginellae)
Wei Ling Xian (Radix Clematidis)	Wei Ling Xian (Radix et Rhizoma Clematidis)

Preface

Chinese Medical Herbology and Pharmacology	Chinese Herbal Formulas and Applications
Wu Ling Zhi (Excrementum Trogopteri seu Pteromi)	*Wu Ling Zhi* (Faeces Trogopteri)
Wu Long Cha (Folium Camellia Sinensis Fermentata)	*Wu Long Cha* (Folium Camelliae Fermentata)
Xi Xin (Herba Asari)	*Xi Xin* (Radix et Rhizoma Asari)
Xiang Ru (Herba Elsholtziae seu Moslae)	*Xiang Ru* (Herba Moslae)
Xiao Ji (Herba Cirisii)	*Xiao Ji* (Herba Cirsii)
Xing Ren (Semen Armeniacae Amarum)	*Ku Xing Ren* (Semen Armeniacae Amarum)
Xu Chang Qing (Radix Cynanchi Paniculati)	*Xu Chang Qing* (Radix et Rhizoma Cynanchi Paniculati)
Xuan Ming Fen (Matrii Sulfas Exsiccatus)	*Xuan Ming Fen* (Natrii Sulfas Exsiccatus)
Ye Jiao Teng (Caulis Polygoni Multiflori)	*Shou Wu Teng* (Caulis Polygoni Multiflori)
Ye Ming Sha (Excrementum Vespertilionis Murini)	*Ye Ming Sha* (Faeces Vespertilionis Murini)
Yi Tang (Saccharum Granorum)	*Yi Tang* (Maltosum)
Yi Zhi Ren (Fructus Alpiniae Oxyphyllae)	*Yi Zhi* (Fructus Alpiniae Oxyphyllae)
Yin Chen Hao (Herba Artemisiae Scopariae)	*Yin Chen* (Herba Artemisiae Scopariae)
Yin Guo Ye (Folium Ginkgo)	*Yin Xing Ye* (Folium Ginkgo)
Yuan Ming Fen (Matrii Sulfas Exsiccatus)	*Xuan Ming Fen* (Natrii Sulfas Exsiccatus)
Zang Hong Hua (Flos Crocus Sativus)	*Xi Hong Hua* (Stigma Croci)
Zhen Zhu Mu (Concha Margaritaferae)	*Zhen Zhu Mu* (Concha Margaritiferae)
Zhi Gan Cao (Radix Glycyrrhizae Preparata)	*Zhi Gan Cao* (Radix et Rhizoma Glycyrrhizae Praeparata cum Melle)
Zhi Ke (Fructus Aurantii)	*Zhi Qiao* (Fructus Aurantii)
Zhi Mu (Radix Anemarrhenae)	*Zhi Mu* (Rhizoma Anemarrhenae)
Zi Cao Gen (Radix Lithospermi)	*Zi Cao* (Radix Arnebiae)
Zi Wan (Radix Asteris)	*Zi Wan* (Radix et Rhizoma Asteris)
Zong Lu Pi (Fibra Stipulae Trachycarpi)	*Zong Lu* (Petiolus Trachycarpi)

[1] Wu KM, Farrelly JG, Upton R, Chen J. Complexities of the herbal nomenclature system in traditional Chinese medicine (TCM): Lessons learned from the misuse of Aristolochia-related species and the importance of the pharmaceutical name during botanical drug product development. Phytomedicine 2007;14:273-279.

Acknowledgement

We would like to thank all of our teachers, who have taught us everything we know, especially Drs. Chang Wei-Yen (Jimmy), Tan Teh-Fu (Richard), Zhang Xiao-Ping, Zhang Hua-Long, Jiao Shu-De, Sam Liang, Liu Zhi-Tong, Charlis Tsai and Tsai Wen-Qi.

Our thanks to Dan Bensky, Randall Barolet, Andrew Gamble, Giovanni Maciocia, Subhuti Dharmanada, Him-che Yeung, Nigel Wiseman and Feng Ye for their contributions to traditional Chinese medicine in the western worlds.

Our thanks to the team of co-authors, Eric Chen, Victor Jang, Delicia Liu, Minh Nguyen and Shenying Tang. Without their contributions, this book would still be a work in progress.

Our utmost appreciation to a team of many fine editors, Minh Nguyen, Thad Ekdahl, Catherine Lu, Laraine Crampton, Abba Anderson, Colleen Burke, Lily Huang, Cathy McNease, Marguerite Valance, Linda Joy Stone, and Kevin Inglis. You help to make this book a pleasure to read.

We warmly appreciate all of the other contributors and peer-reviewers, for your invaluable comments and suggestions.

Most importantly, we would like to thank our family: our father, for his vision and inspiration; our mom, for her endless love and support; and our family for reminding us to stop and smell the herbs throughout the twenty-year journey of writing this book.

The publication of *Chinese Herbal Formulas and Applications* would not have been possible without the help of everyone who has contributed. This book belongs to all of us.

John K. Chen
Tina T. Chen

First and foremost, I want to thank John and Tina for inviting me to participate and contribute to this exciting project. I feel honored to have had the opportunity to work and share my ideas with such an outstanding team of scholars, researchers, editors and visual artists.

Needless to say, editing a book of this size is impossible without the tremendous help, input and patience of many hardworking and talented people. My sincere thanks to all those who were involved; your hard work made my job a joy to fulfill. Very special thanks to my associate editors, Thad Ekdahl and Catherine Lu, for putting up with my demanding schedule. I also want to express admiration and deep gratitude to Laraine Crampton for her high editing standards and intelligent suggestions; this book is much more polished because of her input.

Heartfelt thanks and appreciation to all of my teachers, past and present, who shared their knowledge and joy of learning with me. In particular, I want to thank Wang Chiao-Nien for sharing his clinical experience and knowledge; he taught me the importance of touch and feeling, and, in doing so, taught me the wonders of healing. Much love and deepest appreciation to the wonderful, extraordinary people at Pangea Farm meditation center: Brother Norman Rosenberg, Tisha Roth and Laura Rosenberg. In opening up your door and hearts to me ten years ago, you guided me to Chinese medicine and healing. In teaching me the simple, but profound lessons of ground and breath, you showed me the incandescent beauty and infinite mysteries of life.

Minh Nguyen

Contributors

Authors
John K. Chen, Ph.D., Pharm.D., O.M.D., L.Ac.
Tina T. Chen, M.S., L.Ac.

Co-Authors
Eric K. Chen, Ph.D., O.M.D., L.Ac., J.D.
Victor Meng-Chau Jang, L.Ac.
Delicia Liu, L.Ac.
Minh T. Nguyen, L.Ac.
Shenying Tang, L.Ac.

Editors
Minh T. Nguyen, L.Ac.
Lily Huang, L.Ac.

Associate Editors
Laraine Crampton, L.Ac.
Thad Ekdahl, L.Ac.
Catherine Lu, L.Ac.

Copy Editors
Abba Anderson, L.Ac.
Colleen Burke, L.Ac.
Dave Karaba, L.Ac.
Cathy McNease, Dipl.CH.
Marguerite Valance, L.Ac.

Draft Editors
Linda Joy Stone, L.Ac.
Kevin Inglis, L.Ac.

Consultants
Jize Li, L.Ac.
Huabing Wen, L.Ac.

Research Associates
Wei Chien
Lily Kathleen Ko, L.Ac.
Janice Lee, L.Ac.
Delicia Liu, L.Ac.

Chinese Language Consultant
Estella Huei-Mei Liu

Legal Advisor
Eric K. Chen, Ph.D., O.M.D., L.Ac., J.D.

Cover Design
Charles O. Funk

Book Design
Rick Friesen - birdbrainArts
Chien-Hui Liao

Portraits
Jimmy Wei-Yen Chang, L.Ac.

Assistants
Nina Luu
Nam Hoang

Peer Review Committee
Mazin Al-Khafaji, D.C.M. (China)
Clinical Centre of Chinese Medicine
East Sussex, England

Kabba Anand, D.Ac.
Makawao, Hawaii USA

Abba Anderson, L.Ac.
Berkeley, California USA

Scott Anderson, L.Ac.
Phoenix Institute of Herbal Medicine and Acupuncture
Phoenix, Arizona USA

Simon Becker, L.Ac., Dipl. C.H.
Horgen, Switzerland

Dennis Boyles, L.Ac.
Portland, Oregon USA

James Brooks, M.D., L.Ac.
Fairfield, Iowa USA

Jilann Brunett, L.Ac., Dipl. Ac.
Manassas, Virginia USA

Jane Burch-Pesses, L.Ac.
Forest Grove, Oregon USA

Melonie H Burgess, L.Ac.
New Braunfels, Texas USA

Bruce Canning, O.M.D., L.Ac.
Pico Rivera, California USA

Meriam Chaheen, L.Ac.
Calabasas, California USA

Judith Chaleff, R.N., L.Ac.
Newburgh, New York USA

Julie Chambers, L.Ac.
Yo San University
Santa Monica, California USA

Contributors

Peishan Chen, L.Ac.
Bellevue, Washington USA

Pei Chun Chin, L.Ac.
Minnesota College of Acupuncture and Oriental Medicine
Bloomington, Minnesota USA

Nalini Chilkov, O.M.D., L.Ac.
Santa Monica, California USA

Elizabeth Chen Christenson, M.D., FAAMA, FCAP, ABHM, L.Ac., Dipl. Ac.
John A. Burns School of Medicine, University of Hawaii
Kailua, Hawaii USA

Yvonne Corcoran, D.O.M.
Southwest Acupuncture College
Albuquerque, New Mexico USA

Deirdre K. Courtney, M.T.C.M., C.Ac., Dipl.Ac.
Co. Dublin, Ireland

Beverly Cowan, M.A.O.M., L.Ac.
Scottsdale, Arizona USA

Ken Faber, M.A.O.M., L.Ac.
Portland, Oregon USA

Gena Lee Fleming, M.S.O.M., L.Ac.
Lytle, Texas USA

Cary Friedman, L.Ac.
Santa Cruz, California USA

Mark Frost, L.Ac.
American College of Traditional Chinese Medicine
Alameda, California USA

Francesca Gentile, L.Ac.
Aesch, Switzerland

Steve Given, D.A.O.M., L.Ac.
Bastyr University
Seattle, Washington USA

Thomas Grauer, M.D.
Zurich, Switzerland

Glenn Grossman, L.Ac.
Lansing, Michigan USA

Cally Haber, M.A., L.Ac., Dipl. Ac.
Santa Cruz, California USA

Ron Hershey, L.Ac., Dipl. Ac., Dipl. C.H.
Croton On Hudson, New York USA

Ingrid Hnerlimann, M.D.
Winterthn, Switzerland

Alexa Bradley Hulsey, M.S., L.Ac.
Yo San University
Los Angeles, California USA

Danny Johnson, L.Ac.
Santa Cruz, California USA

Robert Kaneko, L.Ac.
Oregon College of Oriental Medicine
Portland, Oregon USA

David Karaba, L.Ac.
Whittier, California USA

Elizabeth Ko, L.Ac.
Five Branches Institute
San Jose, California USA

Armin Koch, M.D.
Sarnen, Switzerland

Michelle Kuroda, L.Ac.
San Francisco, California USA

Doris Lei, M.D.
Zurich, Switzerland

Gidon Levenbach
Portland, Oregon USA

Yueling Li, M.D. (China), L.Ac.
Pacific College of Oriental Medicine
New York, New York USA

Zhenbo Li, Ph.D. (China), L.Ac.
Oregon College of Oriental Medicine
Portland, Oregon USA

Gwen Lovetere, M.A.O.M., L.Ac.
Oregon College of Oriental Medicine
Portland, Oregon USA

Contributors

Zaoxue Lu, Ph.D. (China), L.Ac.
Oregon College of Oriental Medicine
Portland, Oregon USA

Yunpeng Luo, M.Med. (China)
Oregon College of Oriental Medicine
Portland, Oregon USA

Giovanni Maciocia, C.Ac. (Nanjing)
Buckinghamshire, England

Michelle Maddrell
Portland, Oregon USA

George Mandler, M.A.O.M., Dipl.O.M., L.Ac.
Boston, Massachusetts USA

Anita Chen Marshall, Ph.D., Pharm.D., L.Ac.
Alameda, California USA

Keith E. Maust, D.O.M., A.P., D.Ac.
Key West, Florida USA

Kathryn McCarthy, L.Ac.
Portland, Oregon USA

Cathy McNease, Dipl.CH.
Ojai, California USA

Jack Miller
Pacific College of Oriental Medicine
San Diego, California USA

Sadie Minkoff, M.S.O.M., L.Ac.
Austin, Texas USA

Ueli Moos, M.D.
Uster, Switzerland

Will Morris, D.A.O.M., MSEd, L.Ac.
Academy of Oriental Medicine at Austin
Austin, Texas USA

Lyle Najita, L.Ac., CMT
Davis, California USA

David Nevins, M.S., A.P.
Aventura, Florida USA

Catherine Niemiec, L.Ac., J.D.
Phoenix Institute of Herbal Medicine and Acupuncture
Phoenix, Arizona USA

Szu Lin Pai, M.S.O.M., BSN, RN, L.Ac.
Austin, Texas USA

Wen-Chiang Pai, O.M.D., L.Ac., M.D.
Taiwan, R.O.C.

Michael Pope, L.Ac.
Medford, Oregon USA

Heather Price, L.Ac.
Roseburg, Oregon USA

Michael Dinesh Quatrochi, L.Ac.
San Diego, California USA

Elizabeth Ralph, L.Ac.
Miami, Florida USA

Guido Rampa, M.D.
Facharzt Fur Allgemeine Medizin
Zurich, Switzerland

Linda Robinson-Hidas, L.Ac.
Amherst, Massachusetts USA

Carola Rossi, M.D.
Solothurn, Switzerland

Douglas & Vanessa Rutkowski, L.Ac., M.S.O.M.
Austin, Texas USA

Silvio Schaller, M.D.
Zurich, Switzerland

William Schecher, Ph.D., M.Ac, L.Ac.
Hallowell, Maine USA

Bill Schoenbart, D.A.O.M., M.T.C.M., L.Ac.
Five Branches Institute
Santa Cruz, California USA

Michelle Schreiber, M.S.O.M., L.Ac.
Austin, Texas USA

Gerhard Schwestka, M.D.
Austrian Society for Acupuncture at Vienna
Vienna, Austria

Tim Sharpe, L.Ac.
Columbus, Ohio USA

Contributors

Miki Shima, O.M.D., L.Ac.
Corte Madera, California USA

Jane Sipe, L.Ac.
Graton, California USA

Lucio Sotte, M.D.
Matteo Ricci Foundation for TCM
Civitanova Marche, Italy

Al Stone, D.A.O.M., L.Ac.
Emperor's College
Santa Monica, California USA

Fransiscus Sulistyo
Witten-Herdeck University
Witten-Herdeck, Germany

Yorgen Synnergren
Port Townsend, Washington USA

Lia Tang, M.T.O.M., L.Ac.
Emperor's College
Santa Monica, California USA

Carol Taub
Oregon College of Oriental Medicine
Portland, Oregon USA

Tracy Thorne, L.Ac.
Portland, Oregon USA

Mark Tryling, L.Ac., Dipl. Ac., Dipl. C.H.
Bedford, Texas USA

Roy Upton, R.H.
American Herbal Pharmacopoeia
Soquel, California USA

Karene Villaronte, R.N., Dipl.Ac.
Philadelphia, Pennsylvania USA

Anthony Von Der Muhll, M.T.C.M., L.Ac.
Five Branches Institute
Santa Cruz, California USA

Amber Weiss, DNBAO, L.Ac.
Soquel, California USA

Yufang Xue, Ph.D. (China), L.Ac.
Oregon College of Oriental Medicine
Portland, Oregon USA

Mercy Yule, L.Ac.
Ithaca, New York USA

Pamela Zilavy, M.A., M.S., L.Ac.
Acupuncture & Integrative Medicine College
San Francisco, California USA

Using This Book

Chinese Herbal Formulas and Applications is a compendium designed to be used with Chinese Medical Herbology and Pharmacology. Both texts have been created for use in the clinic, in the classroom, in research, and to preserve and convey valuable historical information that may yet prove crucial in our future. Written to empower practitioners to become better clinicians, it offers detailed discussion of traditional applications, Chinese therapeutic actions, clinical manifestations, clinical applications, modifications, cautions and/or contraindications, suggested concurrent acupuncture treatments, and a contemporary expansion of clinician training: potential herb-drug interactions. All of these features also serve students and faculty in academic settings. Research professionals and clinicians will find invaluable *in vitro* information on pharmacological effects and toxicology, and practical *in vivo* information from clinical and research studies.

Proper translation and use of Traditional Chinese Medicine (TCM) terminology is a challenging issue. Because Traditional Chinese Medicine and Western medicine have distinct cultural and philosophical influences, it is sometimes difficult to accurately convey some TCM terms and concepts by using English or allopathic clinical language. We have made sincere efforts to provide consistent standards for terms and concepts to bridge the gap, as follows:

> *The glossary at the end of this text provides definitions, as well as a cross-reference to Chinese characters, pinyin names, and the terminology used by Wiseman and Ye.*

- Terms that have become an accepted part of English language discourse and are well understood by the general public, such as qi, yin, and yang, are not italicized or capitalized.
- Terms unique to the profession, understood primarily by TCM practitioners, are given in *pinyin*, italicized and translated but not capitalized; such as *bi zheng* (painful obstruction syndrome), *xiao ke* (wasting and thirsting syndrome), and *lin zheng* (dysuria syndrome).
- It is important to note that anatomical organ names in TCM imply functions distinct from their common understanding in Western medicine. Therefore, organ names are capitalized when discussed within the context of TCM, but <u>not</u> when referring exclusively to anatomical function. For example, *Qing Fei Tang* (Clear the Lung Decoction) is commonly used to clear **Lung** heat, a disorder of the **lungs** with such biomedical diagnoses as bronchitis, pneumonia, or bronchiectasis.
- Nouns distinct to herbal medicine are italicized, capitalized and translated, such as *Ren Shen* (Radix et Rhizoma Ginseng) and *Bu Zhong Yi Qi Tang* (Tonify the Middle and Augment the Qi Decoction).
- Translations are omitted after the first full use of the term in one monograph or segment of a monograph, unless repetition is necessary to insure clarity and safety in discriminating between substances or concepts.
- To avoid confusion, formulas other than the principal formula under consideration in a given monograph will be listed with their full *pinyin* and common names at each use, unless mentioned multiple times within a given paragraph.
- In some instances, we felt that rendering a highly precise translation of a Chinese word misses the common professional meaning/usage of the term. In these cases, the common usage has been chosen for the body of the text, while precise translation is offered in the glossary.
- The glossary provides additional information on individual terms and definitions. A cross-reference with the terminology chosen by **Wiseman** and **Feng** is also offered.

Although pertinent to the history, practice, and research of Chinese herbal medicine, not all herbs and formulas discussed herein are commercially available. Some rare or potentially-lethal medicinal substances that are *not* in contemporary use are included and discussed only to illustrate important concepts or historical value in traditional Chinese medicine. The discussion of these herbs and formulas <u>in no way</u> advocates resumption of use, or, in the case of endangered or at-risk species, further destruction of species or resources. These substances are included only to offer the accurate history of their critically important usage in traditional herbal medicine, and to serve as models for appropriate usage of effective herbal <u>*substitutes*</u>.

Readers are strongly encouraged to know and respect the rules and regulations for use of these substances in their own states and/or countries. Among these are:

Using This Book

- Endangered species, such as *Hu Gu* (Os Tigris) in *Hu Qian Wan* (Hidden Tiger Pill), and *Xi Jiao* (Cornu Rhinoceri) in *Xi Jiao Di Huang Tang* (Rhinoceros Horn and Rehmannia Decoction).
- Heavy metals, such as *Zhu Sha* (Cinnabaris) in *Zhu Sha An Shen Wan* (Cinnabar Pill to Tranquilize the Spirit), and *Hei Xi* (Lead) in *Hei Xi Dan* (Lead Special Pill).
- Illegal substances, such as *Ying Su Ke* (Pericarpium Papaveris) in *Jiu Xian San* (Nine-Immortal Powder).

One of the goals of this text is to bridge understanding between Traditional Chinese Medicine and Western medicine. To accomplish this goal, tremendous efforts have been made to research and discuss the Western scientific information available on herbal medicines, such as pharmacological effects, clinical studies and research, toxicology, and herb-drug interactions. Information is presented using the following parameters and general understandings:

- **References:** It has been our intention to cite from original and credible sources whenever possible. Selection of references was based on relevance, strong study design, English language, and use of human subjects whenever and wherever possible, with preference given to randomized, blinded, controlled studies over observational reports. However, not all references met our selection criteria, mostly because studies on Chinese herbs have been done predominately in China, and in Chinese. Therefore, instead of restricting ourselves and the readers to the limited amount of information that fit these strict criteria, we decided to use our best judgment in including relevant information from credible sources. Another limitation we encountered during the compilation of this text is the inaccessibility of some original articles, texts, and references—some are out of press and others simply cannot be located. Although some literature was not always as complete, detailed or current as we would prefer, we have made our best effort in all cases to convey as much information on the original source as possible, and occasionally have judged even limited information to be of some value.
- **Scientific and Medical Terminology**: For the occasional allopathic term that readers might find puzzling, we recommend accessing any standard allopathic medical dictionary. Since there is no need for translation or interpretation of these terms, we concluded that it was unnecessary and cumbersome to include such terms in the glossary of this text.
- **Medical Abbreviations and Symbols** are used in accordance with *Dorland's Illustrated Medical Dictionary*, 28th edition, published by Saunders.
- **Drug Names** are designated in this text by generic (proprietary) names only, or a combination of generic names. The generic names are referenced according to *Drug Facts and Comparisons*, which is updated monthly by Facts and Comparisons, a Wolters Kluwer company.

In addition to the general concepts described above, a brief explanation of headings found in each formula monograph is provided below.

IDENTIFICATION

Each formula is identified by four traits at the beginning of each formula monograph. **Chinese Characters** in both traditional and simplified forms are listed first. In cases where the traditional and simplified characters are identical, only one will be listed. *Pinyin Name* with Mandarin tone markings is provided to identify and pronounce the names as accurately as possible. The **Literal Name** is the name translated directly from its *pinyin* name. **Original Source** refers to the traditional text or reference in which the formula was first documented. This is an important aspect of identification because the original source then allows one to learn when, where, and by whom this formula was first developed. Lastly, when applicable, alternate names are given for formulas that have different pinyin, literal, or commercial names.

Accurate identification of herbal formulas is reasonably straightforward in most cases. Most formulas discussed in this text have distinct Chinese characters, *pinyin* names, and common names, and can be accurately identified. However, it is important to remember that Chinese herbal medicine has developed over two thousand years, across many dynasties,

> Chinese herbal medicine has developed over two thousand years, across many dynasties, and by physicians separated by both time and geography. Therefore, it is not uncommon for one or more herbal formulas to have identical names, with similar or completely different compositions and functions.

Using This Book

and by physicians separated by both time and geography. Therefore, it is not uncommon for one or more herbal formulas to have identical names, with similar or completely different compositions and functions. Under such circumstances, the original source text must be stated to accurately differentiate the identities of the herbal formulas. We have listed two examples to illustrate this potential confusion:

- Example One: There are two formulas called *Chai Ge Jie Ji Tang* (Bupleurum and Kudzu Decoction to Release the Muscle Layer). Both have similar actions and compositions.
  - *Chai Ge Jie Ji Tang* (Bupleurum and Kudzu Decoction to Release the Muscle Layer) from *Shang Han Liu Shu* (Six Texts on Cold-Induced Disorders) focuses more on relieving the muscles, and consists mainly of exterior-releasing and muscle-relieving herbs.
  - *Chai Ge Jie Ji Tang* (Bupleurum and Kudzu Decoction to Release the Muscle Layer) from *Yi Xue Xin Wu* (Medical Revelations) is better at clearing heat, and consequently contains more heat-clearing herbs.

- Example Two: Two formulas sharing the name of *Yi Yi Ren Tang* (Coicis Decoction) have distinctly different compositions and functions.
  - *Yi Yi Ren Tang* (Coicis Decoction), from *Ming Yi Zhi Zhang* (Displays of Enlightened Physicians) by Huang Fu-Zhong in the 16th century, is a formula that dispels wind-dampness from the exterior to treat *bi zheng* (painful obstruction syndrome).
  - *Yi Yi Ren Tang* (Coicis Decoction), from *Zheng Zhi Zhun Sheng* (Standards of Patterns and Treatments) by Wang Ken-Tang in 1602, is a formula that dispels dampness from the Intestines, to treat intestinal abscess.

COMPOSITION

This section details the composition of the herbal formula, listing the ingredients and doses. The names of the herbs are given in *pinyin* and pharmaceutical names, following the same standards as the terminology listed in *Chinese Medical Herbology and Pharmacology*. Herbs that require special preparation are stated accordingly, with preparation methods defined in detail in the glossary. The doses of the herbs are given using standard metric weights and measurements. In cases in which the doses are unavailable from the source text, or if the contemporary doses are different, the suggested doses are provided in brackets.

While the authors hope that reading this section is easy and straightforward, writing it at times was quite difficult and challenging because of the wide variety of substance names. To streamline the writing and learning processes, we chose to use standardized names. The standardized *pinyin* names of herbs refer to the ones established by *Zhong Hua Ren Min Gong He Guo Yao Dian* (Chinese Herbal Pharmacopoeia by the People's Republic of China), published by the People's Republic of China, 2005. We used this reference as the standard for nomenclature of *pinyin* and pharmaceutical names because this text offers the most precise, accurate, and current information on the identification of Chinese herbs and other medicinal substances.

This decision obviously has its advantages and disadvantages. The main advantage in standardizing the nomenclature is to facilitate learning and minimize confusion and avoid errors. However, a true disadvantage is that the reader loses an historical sense of how an herb was originally used in the formula. We tried to compensate for this disadvantage with a brief explanation in **Authors' Comments** when appropriate. We believe this approach has more advantages than disadvantages, and hope the reader will understand and forgive us for taking such liberty. Listed below are two examples of how the herb names were standardized, along with short illustrations of their advantages and disadvantages.

- Example One: *Bing Pian* (Borneolum Syntheticum) is used as the standard nomenclature whereas in the past it may have been named as *Long Nao* or *Mei Pian*, and cited in such formulas as *Zhi Bao Dan* (Greatest Treasure Special Pill) and *An Gong Niu Huang Wan* (Calm the Palace Pill with Cattle Gallstone). *Long Nao* and *Mei Pian* are alternate *pinyin* names of *Bing Pian* (Borneolum Syntheticum),

XXXIV

Using This Book

Chinese Herbal Formulas and Applications

neither of which are used frequently today. This gradual historical drift in names may require some additional time to cross-reference in order to correctly identify these alternate names elsewhere.

• Example Two: *Shao Yao* (Radix Paeoniae) is a general name that may refer to either *Bai Shao* (Radix Paeoniae Alba) or *Chi Shao* (Radix Paeoniae Rubra). While keeping the general name will retain its historical context, providing the specific name will be more clinically relevant and helpful. Since the main emphasis of this text is on herbal formulas and their clinical applications, we kindly ask your pardon when we recommend *Bai Shao* (Radix Paeoniae Alba) in *Shao Yao Gan Cao Tang* (Peony and Licorice Decoction), and *Chi Shao* (Radix Paeoniae Rubra) in *Gui Zhi Fu Ling Wan* (Cinnamon Twig and Poria Pill). Please see these two formulas for additional explanation.

Historically, the doses of herbs are stated using units from the Chinese system (such as *liang, qian,* and *fen*) or general descriptive terms, such as a certain number of pieces of *Ku Xing Ren* (Semen Armeniacae Amarum) or pills the size of egg yolks. While the general market place may still use such units and terms, academic and healthcare institutions have converted doses of herbal medicine to the metric system. Therefore, when necessary, we have also chosen to convert and present doses in metric weights and measurements. For additional background information on this conversion, *see* **Part 1, Chapter 7: Weights and Measures.**

DOSAGE / PREPARATION / ADMINISTRATION

This section describes the traditional methods for preparation and administration of the formula. Contemporary methods of preparation and administration are also discussed when applicable. The dosage here refers to that of the formula as a whole, not the dose of each ingredient.

Some formulas given as decoction do not have additional instructions on preparation or administration. In these cases, simply follow the generic method to prepare and administer the decoction, as described in **Part 1, Chapter 6: Preparation and Administration of Decoction.**

Some formulas commonly given as pills have lengthy, detailed descriptions of how to manufacture these products in large quantities. While this information may be interesting to some, it is not useful or practical to most. In these cases, readers may use their professional judgment and switch the dosage forms (e.g., from pills to decoction) and convert the doses of the ingredients accordingly.

CHINESE THERAPEUTIC ACTIONS

These are the treatment strategies that link the disease diagnosis with the therapeutic effects of the formulas.

CLINICAL MANIFESTATIONS

This section focuses on diagnosis of the disorder, and associated signs and symptoms. Tongue and pulse diagnoses are essential parts of TCM diagnosis and are listed here when applicable. The information presented in this section is drawn primarily from the original source texts and sometimes from the standard herbal formula textbooks used in mainland China. The diagnosis of the disorder and associated signs and symptoms are further elaborated upon and explained in the **Explanation** section.

CLINICAL APPLICATIONS

This section summarizes the primary clinical applications of the formula in terms of allopathic (biomedical) disease. Additional information justifying the formula's use for such conditions is found under **Pharmacological Effects** and **Clinical Studies and Research**.

Please note that this is not a comprehensive inclusive/exclusive list, but only a partial account of the most commonly used clinical applications. Inclusion of a biomedical disease in this list of applications does not imply that a given formula can be used indiscriminately for that particular disease. Similarly, the lack of mention of a biomedical disease here does not mean a given formula is ineffective for this condition. Listing of allopathic disease is designed to serve as a guide to assist practitioners in selecting the best possible formula. It is extremely important that the practitioner has

XXXV

Using This Book

a complete and thorough understanding of the formula, and that he or she uses it to treat appropriate Chinese medical presentations, whether of specific allopathic conditions or not.

EXPLANATION

This section is divided into two main sections: explanation of the etiology of the disease, and the strategy underlying the herbal treatment. A chart is also provided to summarize the relationship of the formula to its diagnosis, signs and symptoms, treatment strategies, and functions of the herbs within the formula.

MODIFICATIONS

This section details how to modify the principal formula to treat complications and variations of the target condition.

CAUTIONS / CONTRAINDICATIONS

While it may be self-evident to experienced practitioners, new students and researchers or healthcare professionals from other fields will want to note in particular the cautions and/or contraindications mentioned for use of each formula. However, if there are none reported in the literature or known within the tradition, none will be mentioned. Careful observation of these cautions and/or contra-indications ensures the safe and effective practice of Chinese herbal medicine with a minimum of unwanted side effects.

Information cited in this section is derived primarily from classic source texts, current textbooks, and research journals and articles. Cautions and contraindications are associated directly with the formulas as a whole, and not based on "cut and paste" information from individual ingredients. It is important to note that the cautions and contraindications of the formula as a whole are not the same as the sum of all cautions and contraindications of its individual ingredients. These formulas are carefully crafted with appropriate herbal checks and balances to ensure safety and efficacy. Thus, a particular herb that might individually be cautioned for use in a disease presentation may appear safely within a well-crafted formula to treat that disease pattern.

PHARMACOLOGICAL EFFECTS

Most pharmacological studies focus on the anatomical and physiological influences of the herbs on the body or against pathogens. For example, many formulas are described as having antihypertensive effects, as their administration leads directly to a decrease in blood pressure. Others are said to have antibacterial effects, for introduction of the formula leads to the inhibition or death of bacteria. However, it is extremely difficult to understand the exact mechanisms of action of the herbal formulas; each formula contains many herbs and each herb has many chemical constituents. As a result, most research information on individual herbs focuses on pharmacological effects, while research information on herbal formulas focuses on clinical studies.

CLINICAL STUDIES AND RESEARCH

This section briefly outlines the use of Chinese herbal formulas to treat allopathic (biomedical) diseases. The research methodologies vary from formula to formula and from disease to disease. While the use of the formula without modification may be appropriate in certain disorders, more complicated diseases will often require modifications in order for the formula to be effective. Although the traditional goal of research is to limit the number of variables and identify the causal relationships, this is often not possible with Chinese herbal medicine. Chinese herbs are used in <u>multiple herb formulas</u> to treat patients. Thus, most clinical studies and research cited include the use of many herbs, not simply a single substance under consideration. Although this increases the number of variables influencing the outcome, it nonetheless reflects the actual practice of Chinese herbal medicine and the basis on which centuries of refinement have been effectively carried forward.

Using This Book

Chinese Herbal Formulas and Applications

HERB-DRUG INTERACTION

Herb-drug interaction is a critically important subject, yet there is, at this point in time, little definitive information available. A basic understanding of this topic can be found in Part I of *Chinese Medical Herbology and Pharmacology*, Chapter 8: "Concurrent Use of Herbal Medicines and Pharmaceuticals." Documented interactions between formulas and drugs are discussed in each formula monograph when relevant. Theoretical or hypothetical interactions are not included because they involve too much assumption and speculation. Where formula monographs do not contain any herb-drug interaction information, there was no known or documented interaction available to include in timely fashion at the time of publication. However, readers are strongly encouraged to stay updated, as new information on herb-drug complementarities and conflicts is published regularly.

Note: *Chinese Medical Herbology and Pharmacology* documents interactions between individual herbs and drugs, while *Chinese Herbal Formulas and Applications* records interactions between herbal formulas and drugs. Readers are urged to check both sources as needed to assure the safety and compatibility of herb and drug therapies.

TOXICOLOGY

In most cases, the toxicology of herbal formulas is reported based on *in vitro* studies. Readers are advised to examine and understand these reports with the same attention to context, proportion, and clinical application as they would in reviewing toxicology and/or *in vitro* studies for any medicine or supplement.

RELATED FORMULA(S)

These formulas have similar compositions and/or functions to the principal formula, or have grown out of the broader application of the principal formula. This section highlights the contrasting differences between the principal and related formula(s) without restating overlapping similarities.

AUTHORS' COMMENTS

This closing segment provides additional insights, clinical experience, and relevant information that do not clearly fall under the other categories. This section also offers detailed comparison and contrast of formulas when appropriate.

This section occasionally offers clinical insights on the formulas from contemporary practitioners. It should be noted that these insights were originally presented in the context of educational seminars, and not in published works; hence, there is often or usually no cited reference in these instances.

REFERENCES

Reference material is embedded in the text for ease of access via endnotes in each monograph. The key information from all of these notes has been carefully consolidated into two thorough bibliographic resources.
• The complete names of historical books (given in Chinese characters, *pinyin* names, and English names) are listed in the Bibliography of Historical Texts.
• The complete names of recent journals, articles and books are listed in the Bibliography of Contemporary References.

ADDITIONAL RESOURCES

In a text involving so many hundreds of pieces of information as *Chinese Herbal Formulas and Applications*, it is inevitable that on any given page a reader might find information that inspires curiosity about specific details that are not included in that particular monograph. The authors want to provide as much information as possible and to avoid overwhelming students and practitioners with excessive repetition and complexity that obscure key concepts and bog down progress through the general text.

XXXVII

Using This Book

For this reason, the reader will find in Part III, ten specialty appendices that provide intensive bodies of information at the close of the text, followed by a thorough glossary and the two bibliographies mentioned above. Each of these is self-contained and self-explanatory.

The authors are proud and grateful to have had an excellent gathering of committed and experienced professionals contributing to, and evaluating, the content of this textbook. We invite the reader to appreciate the wealth of training and experience these contributors, who are listed in the beginning of the text, have brought to bear on behalf of *Chinese Herbal Formulas and Applications*.

Last but not least, there is an extensive index at the close of Part III, linking terminology and topics throughout the text for the convenience of students, practitioners and researchers.

It is our hope that these features will contribute to the greatest accessibility and convenience in your use of this volume.

DISCLAIMER

Great care has been taken by the authors, editors, and other contributors to maintain the accuracy of the information contained in *Chinese Herbal Formulas and Applications*. All information has been evaluated, double-checked and cross-verified. However, in view of the potential for human, electronic, or mechanical error, neither the authors, the publisher, nor any contributors involved in the preparation or publication of this text warrant that the information contained herein is in every aspect accurate, and they are not responsible for any errors or omissions, nor for the results obtained from the use of said information.

Chinese Herbal Formulas and Applications is intended as an educational guide for healthcare practitioners, as professional training and expertise are essential to the safe practice of herbal medicine, in both recommendation of, and effective guidance of, the use of herbs. We cannot anticipate all conditions under which this information may be used. In view of ongoing research, changes in governmental regulation, and the constant flow of information relating to Chinese and Western medicine, the reader is urged to check with other sources for all up-to-date information. In recognition of that fact that practitioners accessing information in this text will have varying levels of training and expertise, we accept no responsibility for the results obtained by the application of the information within this text. Neither the publisher, authors, editors, nor contributors can be held responsible for errors of fact or omission, or for any consequences arising from the use or misuse of the information herein.

It is our intention to continually update and improve this text to maintain and enhance its usefulness. We welcome and encourage your comments and suggestions.

Part 1

— Overview

黄帝 Huǎng Dì

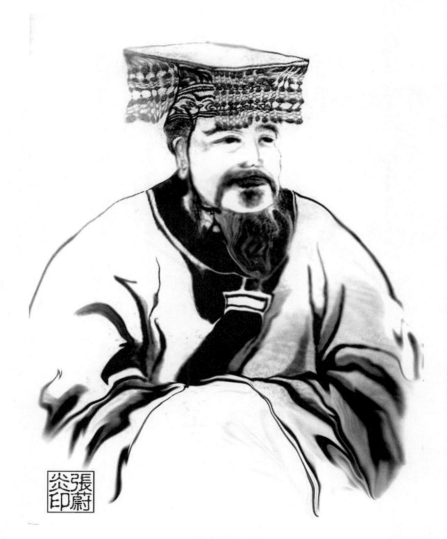

黄帝 Huǎng Dì, dates unknown.

Chinese Herbal Formulas and Applications

黄帝 Huǎng Di

Huang Di, also known as the "Yellow Emperor," was the first leader to unite all of the tribes in ancient China at the dawn of recorded civilization. Huang Di treated all citizens in his kingdoms like his own sons and daughters, and he suffered great distress when they were ill. To improve healthcare, Huang Di personally learned medicine from many of his deputies. According to legend, Huang Di inquired about all aspects of medicine: this conversation was later recorded and published as *Huang Di Nei Jing* (Yellow Emperor's Inner Classic).[1] The deputies that Huang Di consulted included 岐伯 *Qi Bo*, an authority in medicine; 桐君 *Tong Jun*, an expert in herbal medicine; 雷公 *Lei Gong*, the founder in the processing of herbs; 少俞 *Shao Yu*, an expert in acupuncture; and 伯高 *Bo Gao*, who knew pulse diagnosis in great detail. Of all the deputies, *Qi Bo* was considered the most knowledgeable, and was regarded by many as 天师 the Heavenly Physician.

Huang Di Nei Jing (Yellow Emperor's Inner Classic), also abbreviated as *Nei Jing* (Inner Classic), is organized into two volumes: 素问 *Su Wen* (Basic Questions) and 灵枢 *Ling Shu* (Magic Pivot). It assembled and presented the fundamental theories of traditional Chinese medicine, including 阴阳 yin and yang, 五行 the five elements, 脏腑 the *zang fu*, and 经络 the channels and collaterals. In addition to solidifying the fundamental theories of traditional Chinese medicine, the text was crucial in shaping the study of Chinese herbal formulas. Beyond the basic concepts, the text strongly emphasized the importance of holistic medicine, that the human body is a small universe within a bigger universe represented by the environment, each having close and inseparable connections within itself and to each other. Lastly, it stressed the importance of the prevention and treatment of disease, and discouraged belief in superstition and witchcraft.

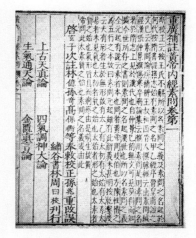

黄帝内经 *Huang Di Nei Jing* (Yellow Emperor's Inner Classic) compiled in the first or second century CE.

[1] This legend, however, is only folklore. In actuality, *Huang Di Nei Jing* (Yellow Emperor's Inner Classic) is believed to be a compilation of work by many physicians during the first and second century CE. They named it after *Huang Di* (Yellow Emperor) to honor his contribution to civilization in China.

Dynasties & Kingdoms	Year
Xia Dynasty 夏	**2100-1600 BCE**
Shang Dynasty 商	1600-1100 BCE
Zhou Dynasty 周	1100-221 BCE
Qin Dynasty 秦	221-207 BCE
Han Dynasty 汉	206 BCE-220
Three Kingdoms 三国	220-280
Western Jin Dynasty 西晋	265-316
Eastern Jin Dynasty 东晋	317-420
Northern and Southern Dynasties 北南朝	420-581
Sui Dynasty 隋	581-618
Tang Dynasty 唐	618-907
Five Dynasties 五代	907-960
Song Dynasty 宋	960-1279
Liao Dynasty 辽	916-1125
Jin Dynasty 金	1115-1234
Yuan Dynasty 元	1271-1368
Ming Dynasty 明	1368-1644
Qing Dynasty 清	1644-1911
Republic of China 中華民國	1912-Present Day
People's Republic of China 中華人民共和國	1949-Present Day

Table of Contents

Part I Overview ··· **1**

Biography of Huang Di ··· 2

Chapter 1 The History of Chinese Herbal Formulas ··· 5

Chapter 2 Treatment Methods and Formulas ·· 9

Chapter 3 Classification of Formulas ··· 11

Chapter 4 Composition of Formulas ·· 14

Chapter 5 Dosage Forms ·· 16

Chapter 6 Preparation and Administration of Decoctions ····································· 19

Chapter 7 Weights and Measures ··· 22

Chapter 8 Concurrent Use of Herbal Medicines and Pharmaceuticals ··················· 24

Chapter 1

— The History of Chinese Herbal Formulas

In the course of gathering food, humans discovered that certain plants, animals, and mineral substances have medicinal properties. Through trial and error in using these medical substances to treat various diseases, the Chinese discovered that combining substances was often more effective than using them individually. Such observations and experiences have been inventoried for thousands of years, and have led empirically to Chinese herbal medicine as it is practiced today.

五十二病方 *Wu Shi Er Bing Fang* (Prescriptions for Fifty-Two Kinds of Diseases) is the oldest record documenting the use of herbal formulas. It was unearthed in 1973 from the Number 3 Han Tomb at Ma Wang Dui, Changsha, in Hunan Province, and is estimated by archeologists to have been written in approximately the third century B.C. These medical writings, inscribed on silk fabric, include 280 herbal prescriptions to treat 52 kinds of diseases. While authorship remains unknown, this is the first known documentation to clearly outline the relationship between diseases and their corresponding treatments. The discussion of this relationship, however, lacks detail and explanation, and, without assigning names to formulas, contains only simple descriptions of herbs, doses, and dosage forms. While only briefly explaining the yin-yang relationship, it makes no reference to Five-Element theory or *zang fu* (solid and hollow organs) relationships. Although *Wu Shi Er Bing Fang* (Prescriptions for Fifty-Two Kinds of Diseases) is not a complete text by any means, it does represent a significant beginning in Chinese herbal medicine.

神农本草经 *Shen Nong Ben Cao Jing* (Divine Husbandman's Classic of the Materia Medica), compiled by numerous authors in the second century, A.D., is one of the first and most authoritative texts on Chinese herbal medicine. It contains information on 365 herbs, including details such as the taste, thermal property, doses, and toxicity. One of the earliest records of Chinese herbal medicine, it focuses primarily on individual herbs, not on herbal formulas.

黄帝内经 *Huang Di Nei Jing* (Yellow Emperor's Inner Classic), compiled in the first or second century A.D., is divided into two volumes: 素问 *Su Wen* (Basic Questions) and 灵枢 *Ling Shu* (Magic Pivot). Usually abbreviated as *Nei Jing* (Inner Classic), this text establishes the fundamental theories of Traditional Chinese Medicine. It documents thirteen herbal formulas, most of which are no longer used today; seven types of formulas (large, small, mild, urgent, odd-numbered, even-numbered, and composite); and dosage forms (decoction, pill, powder, paste, pellet, and medicinal wine). Additionally, it contains information on diagnosis, treatment methods, and principles, as well as the herbal formulas with accompanying explanations. In short, *Nei Jing* (Inner Classic) solidified the fundamental theories of Traditional Chinese Medicine, and was crucial in shaping the study of Chinese herbal formulas.

伤寒杂病论 *Shang Han Za Bing Lun* (Discussion of Cold-Induced Disorders and Miscellaneous Diseases), written by Zhang Zhong-Jing in the Eastern Han dynasty, is deemed to be one of the most important texts in all of traditional Chinese medicine. This text is considered the "ancestor" of contemporary herbal formulas, and the author is regarded as the "father" of traditional Chinese medicine. Zhang Zhong-Jing was the first doctor to discuss, in a systematic manner, the importance of and relationship among theory, strategy, formulas, and substances; and, moreover, to assert that all four components must be accurately developed and implemented to achieve successful treatment. This text contains a thorough, detailed discussion of 314 herbal formulas that were crafted with the utmost care and precision. Many of these formulas have stood the test of time and are still widely used today.

Part I – Overview

Chapter 1 — The History of Chinese Herbal Formulas

Shang Han Za Bing Lun (Discussion of Cold-Induced Disorders and Miscellaneous Diseases) was later rearranged and edited during the Jin dynasty by Wang Shu-He, who divided it into two parts: 伤寒论 *Shang Han Lun* (Discussion of Cold-Induced Disorders), which focused on externally-contracted diseases, and 金匮要略 *Jin Gui Yao Lue* (Essentials from the Golden Cabinet) which emphasized internally-generated disorders.

During the Jin and Tang dynasties, 肘后备急方 *Zhou Hou Bei Ji Fang* (Emergency Formulas to Keep Up One's Sleeve) was written by Ge Hong in 341 A.D. This reference elucidated valuable descriptions of diseases and their corresponding treatments using herbs that were inexpensive, readily available, and effective. Herbal treatments included both single-herb remedies and composite herbal formulas.

During the seventh century Tang dynasty, Sun Si-Miao wrote 备急千金要方 *Bei Ji Qian Jin Yao Fang* (Thousands of Golden Prescriptions for Emergencies). This reference text discussed many different subjects, including general medical theories, diet, materia medica, herbal formulas, and acupuncture. It also included specific information on pediatrics, gynecology and obstetrics. 千金翼方 *Qian Jin Yi Fang* (Supplement to the Thousand Ducat Formulas), written by Sun Si-Miao in 682 A.D., is a complement to *Bei Ji Qian Jin Yao Fang* (Thousands of Golden Prescriptions for Emergencies). Together, these two texts contain 7,300 herbal formulas (5,300 in the original text, and 2,000 in the supplemented text), and are considered the representative medical works of the Tang dynasty.

Also during the Tang dynasty, 外台秘要 *Wai Tai Mi Yao* (Arcane Essentials from the Imperial Library) was compiled by Wang Tao in 752 A.D. This text contains approximately 6,000 herbal formulas derived from various sources, and is one of the most extensive texts compiled during that era. It serves as an important reference in the study of Chinese herbal medicine. Many of the formulas listed in this text are still in use today.

During the Song dynasty, two of the most comprehensive texts on Chinese herbal formulas were written. 太平圣惠方 *Tai Ping Sheng Hui Fang* (Holy Grace Formulary of the Tai Ping Era) was compiled by Wang Huai-Yin and other medical officials of the Imperial Medical Department. This text is 100 volumes long, and contains 16,834 herbal formulas. It includes detailed explanations on pulses, diagnosis (based on yin and yang, excess and deficiency), and treatment principles. The second extensive text published during this era is 圣剂总录 *Sheng Ji Zong Lu* (General Collection for Holy Relief), written by a staff of court physicians of the Northern Song dynasty around 1111-1117. This 200-volume text contains over 20,000 formulas. Sources of the formulas include secret recipes from within the imperial palace, as well as recipes submitted by physicians throughout the entire country. This text covers topics such as internal and external medicine, gynecology, pediatrics, acupuncture, osteopathy, and disorders of the five sensory organs (nose, eyes, lips, tongue, and ears). While the massive number of herbal formulas recorded is the strength of these two texts, it is also their main weakness. The girth of the texts compromises their practical value, and the sheer number of formulas dilutes their clinical significance.

> **The 200-volume *Sheng Ji Zong Lu*, from the Northern Song dynasty, covered internal and external medicine, gynecology, pediatrics, acupuncture, osteopathy, and disorders of the five sensory organs.**

Finally, the Imperial Medical Department complied and published 太平惠民和济局方 *Tai Ping Hui Min He Ji Ju Fang* (Imperial Grace Formulary of the Tai Ping Era) in 1078-85. The original text contained only 297 herbal formulas, but the number increased to 788 in subsequent edits. Though this is not necessarily the most extensive record of herbal formulas, it is one of the most valuable ones. All the formulas listed were submitted by the best physicians in the country, with the clinical efficacy of each formula tested, reviewed, and confirmed by physicians in the Imperial Medical Department. Because this text was used as the official reference from which all herbal products were made, it became the first official pharmacopoeia in Chinese history published by the government. Many herbal formulas from this text are still in use today.

Chapter 1 — The History of Chinese Herbal Formulas

The Song dynasty also marks the continued development of pediatrics and gynecology. 小儿药症直决 *Xiao Er Yao Zheng Zhi Jue* (Craft of Medicinal Treatment for Childhood Disease Patterns), written by Qian Yi in 1119, contains two parts. Part one focuses on discussion of theories and etiologies of childhood diseases; part two emphasizes the herbal formulas for treating these diseases. 妇人大全良方 *Fu Ren Da Quan Liang Fang* (Complete Fine Formulas for Women), written by Chen Zi-Ming in 1237, was the most comprehensive work of its time on gynecology and obstetrics. Both of these works also contain practical clinical experiences on treatment.

伤寒论明理论 *Shang Han Lun Ming Li Lun* (Clarification of the Theory of Cold-Induced Disorders), written by Cheng Wu-Ji in 1156, is a relatively small, yet significant text. Although it lists only 20 formulas for treating *shang han* (cold damage) disorders, it dissects and analyzes every aspect of each formula. The first text to establish the theories and understanding of herbal formulas, it has made a significant impact on Chinese herbal medicine.

The Jin and Yuan Dynasties are characterized by the birth and development of four contrasting schools of thought. Liu Yuan-Su proposed the use of cold and cool substances, and complied 宣明论方 *Xuan Ming Lun Fang* (Discussion of Dispersing and Brightening Formulas). Zhang Cong-Zheng promoted the use of downward-draining substances, and wrote 儒门事亲 *Ru Men Shi Qin* (Confucians' Duties to their Parents). Li Gao emphasized the use of Spleen and Stomach tonifying substances, and published 脾胃论 *Pi Wei Lun* (Discussion of the Spleen and Stomach). Lastly, Zhu Zhen-Heng focused on using yin-nourishing substances, and wrote 丹溪心法 *Dan Xi Xin Fa* (Teachings of [Zhu] Dan-Xi). The main significance of these four contrasting schools of thought is that they represent the emergence of specialties within Traditional Chinese Medicine. Each school provided great insight into the etiology of each disease and offered corresponding treatments. Many formulas from these four schools are still in use today.

> The main significance of [the] four contrasting schools of thought is that they represent the emergence of specialties within TCM.

The Ming dynasty marks another step forward in the history and understanding of Chinese herbal formulas. 普济方 *Pu Ji Fang* (Formulas of Universal Benefit), a voluminous medical book compiled by Teng Hong, et al. under the auspices of Prince Zhu Su of the Ming dynasty, inventoried 61,739 herbal formulas in use at various medical branches. This text contains documentations of nearly all the formulas developed prior to this era, and has the most entries of any herbal formula reference.

The Qing dynasty marks the birth of the theory of *wen bing* (warm disease), another new school of thought proposing its own ideas of the origin of disorders and their complementary treatments. Many valuable theories and herbal formulas were developed during this time. Notable published works include 疫疹一得 *Yi Zhen Yi De* (Achievements Regarding Epidemic Rashes), by Yu Shi-Yu in 1794; 温病条辨 *Wen Bing Tiao Bian* (Systematic Differentiation of Warm Disease), by Wu Ju-Tong in 1798; and 温热经纬 *Wen Re Jing Wei* (Warp and Woof of Warm-Febrile Diseases), by Wang Meng-Ying in 1852.

Part I – Overview

Chapter 1 — The History of Chinese Herbal Formulas

Table 1. Summary of Important Historical Texts on Chinese Herbal Formulas

Name	Author	Time	Description
Wu Shi Er Bing Fang (Prescriptions for Fifty-Two Kinds of Diseases)	Unknown	Third century B.C.	Earliest documentation of herbal formulas with 280 herbal prescriptions to treat 52 kinds of diseases
Shen Nong Ben Cao Jing (Divine Husbandman's Classic of the Materia Medica)	Numerous authors	Second century, A.D.	Contains information on 365 herbs, but no herbal formulas
Huang Di Nei Jing (Yellow Emperor's Inner Classic)	Unknown	First or second century A.D.	Documents 13 herbal formulas, seven types of formulas, and various dosage forms
Shang Han Za Bing Lun (Discussion of Cold-Induced Disorders and Miscellaneous Diseases)	Zhang Zhong-Jing	Eastern Han dynasty	One of the most important texts of Traditional Chinese Medicine; it contains thorough, detailed discussions on 314 herbal formulas
Zhou Hou Bei Ji Fang (Emergency Formulas to Keep Up One's Sleeve)	Ge Hong	341 A.D.	Valuable description of diseases and their corresponding treatment using herbs that are inexpensive, readily-available, and effective
Bei Ji Qian Jin Yao Fang (Thousands of Golden Prescriptions for Emergencies)	Sun Si-Miao	Seventh century A.D.	Documents 5,300 herbal formulas and many different subjects in TCM, including general medical theories, diet, materia medica, herbal formulas, and acupuncture
Qian Jin Yi Fang (Supplement to the Thousand Ducat Formulas)	Sun Si-Miao	682 A.D.	Documents 2,000 herbal formulas, as a supplement to *Bei Ji Qian Jin Yao Fang* (Thousands of Golden Prescriptions for Emergencies)
Wai Tai Mi Yao (Arcane Essentials from the Imperial Library)	Wang Tao	752 A.D.	Contains approximately 6,000 herbal formulas derived from various sources
Tai Ping Sheng Hui Fang (Holy Grace Formulary of the Tai Ping Era)	Wang Huai-Yin	Song dynasty	Contains 16,834 herbal formulas with detailed explanation of pulses, diagnosis (based on yin and yang, excess and deficiency), and treatment principles
Sheng Ji Zong Lu (General Collection for Holy Relief)	Staff of court physicians	Northern Song dynasty	Documents 20,000 formulas on topics such as internal and external medicine, gynecology, pediatrics, acupuncture, osteopathy, and disorders of the five sensory organs
Tai Ping Hui Min He Ji Ju Fang (Imperial Grace Formulary of the Tai Ping Era)	Imperial Medical Department	1078-85	A pharmacopoeia published by the Imperial Medical Department containing 788 herbal formulas that were officially tested, reviewed, and approved
Xiao Er Yao Zheng Zhi Jue (Craft of Medicinal Treatment for Childhood Disease Patterns)	Qian Yi	1119	First specialized text on pediatrics
Fu Ren Da Quan Liang Fang (Complete Fine Formulas for Women)	Chen Zi-Ming	1237	First specialized text on gynecology and obstetrics
Shang Han Lun Ming Li Lun (Clarification of the Theory of Cold-Induced Disorders)	Cheng Wu-Ji	1156	Contains detailed explanations and analyses of 20 formulas for treating *shang han* (cold damage)
Xuan Ming Lun Fang (Discussion of Dispersing and Brightening Formulas)	Liu Yuan-Su	Jin and Yuan dynasties	Part of the four contrasting schools of thought that focused on the use of cold and cool substances
Ru Men Shi Qin (Confucians' Duties to their Parents)	Zhang Cong-Zheng	Jin and Yuan dynasties	Part of the four contrasting schools of thought that focused on the use of downward-draining substances
Pi Wei Lun (Discussion of the Spleen and Stomach).	Li Gao	Jin and Yuan dynasties	Part of the four contrasting schools of thought that focused on using Spleen and Stomach tonifying substances
Dan Xi Xin Fa (Teachings of [Zhu] Dan-Xi)	Zhu Zhen-Heng	Jin and Yuan dynasties	Part of the four contrasting schools of thought that focused on the use of yin-nourishing substances
Pu Ji Fang (Formulas of Universal Benefit)	Teng Hong et al.	Ming dynasty	The most comprehensive text inventorying 61,739 herbal formulas of various medical branches
Yi Zhen Yi De (Achievements Regarding Epidemic Rashes)	Yu Shi-Yu	1794	An important text on *wen bing* (warm disease) theory
Wen Bing Tiao Bian (Systematic Differentiation of Warm Disease)	Wu Ju-Tong	1798	An important text on *wen bing* (warm disease) theory
Wen Re Jing Wei (Warp and Woof of Warm-Febrile Diseases)	Wang Meng-Ying	1852	An important text on *wen bing* (warm disease) theory

Chapter 2

— Treatment Methods and Formulas

The treatment method is the bridge between any disease and its effective herbal remedy. As such, a successful treatment requires accurate diagnosis of the disease, strategic planning of treatment methods, and careful consideration of which herbal formula to prescribe.

Treatment methods have been well-documented throughout the history of Chinese herbal medicine. The *Huang Di Nei Jing* (Yellow Emperor's Inner Classic) was the first text to discuss treatment methods of herbal formulas. Zhang Zhong-Jing further elaborated on this concept in *Shang Han Za Bing Lun* (Discussion of Cold-Induced Disorders and Miscellaneous Diseases). Most recently, in the Qing dynasty, Cheng Zhong-Ling sorted the most commonly-used treatment methods into eight methods in his text *Yi Xue Xin Wu* (Medical Revelations). Cheng stated that "the sources of illness are either externally contracted or internally generated," "the characteristics of the disease are differentiated into cold or hot, excess or deficiency, exterior or interior, and yin or yang," and the "treatment methods include sweating, vomiting, draining downward, harmonizing, warming, clearing, reducing, and tonifying."

八法 *Ba Fa* (The Eight Treatment Methods)

1. 汗法 *Han fa* (sweating) induces a mild sweat by ventilating and dispersing Lung qi, and regulating and harmonizing the *ying* (nutritive) and *wei* (defensive) levels. Herbs that ventilate and disperse Lung qi release the exterior and dispel pathogenic factors from the superficial areas of the body. Herbs that regulate and harmonize the nutritive and defensive levels ensure proper opening and closing of skin pores, thereby allowing the release of exterior pathogenic factors via sweat. It is important to remember that the objective of sweating is not to induce heavy perspiration, but only to obtain mild diaphoresis. To promote sweating itself is not the objective, but rather, the escape of sweat is a process that indicates that Lung qi has been ventilated and dispersed, that the nutritive and defensive levels have been regulated and harmonized, and that exterior pathogenic factors have been dispelled.

    Sweating is primarily used to expel pathogenic factors at the exterior (skin) level. Clinical applications include the common cold, influenza, the early stages of measles, acute edema (especially above the waist), abscesses and sores with fever and chills, dysentery with exterior signs and symptoms, and many others.

    Since complications frequently extend or worsen disease, and patients have differing constitutional strengths, sweating may often need to be modified to address these concerns. Exterior conditions characterized by cold are treated with acrid and warm herbs to release the exterior, while those characterized by heat are treated with acrid and cold herbs. Individuals who have an exterior condition accompanied by underlying deficiencies need to be treated with both sweating and tonifying methods concurrently. Those affected by both exterior and interior conditions may require both sweating and downward-draining methods.

2. 吐法 *Tu fa* (vomiting) induces emesis to eliminate phlegm, stagnant food, or toxic materials from the throat, chest and diaphragm, or epigastrium. Vomiting induces qi to move upwards and outwards. Therefore, use of this method commonly results in concurrent vomiting and sweating.

    Clinical applications of vomiting include treatment for ingestion of poisonous substances, severe cases of food stagnation, sudden turmoil disorder with vomiting and diarrhea, mania and withdrawal caused by phlegm accumulation, and *zhong feng* (wind stroke) with phlegm accumulation.

    Vomiting is a potent and drastic treatment method that can easily damage Stomach qi. Accordingly, it is generally reserved for acute and excess conditions, and in patients who are otherwise strong and healthy. Vomiting must be used with extreme caution in individuals who have underlying weakness and deficiency, such as pediatric, geriatric, or pregnant patients.

Chapter 2 — Treatment Methods and Formulas

3. 下法 *Xia fa* (**draining downward**) cleanses the Stomach and Intestines, induces defecation, and eliminates pathogenic accumulation from the body, such as stagnant food, dry stools, cold accumulation, hot accumulation, blood stasis, phlegm stagnation, water stagnation, parasitic infestation, and many others.

    Draining downward is usually achieved with the use of four types of herbs: cold herbs that drain downward, hot herbs that drain downward, herbs that moisten the Intestines and drain downward, and harsh expellants (cathartics). Proper selection of herbs requires careful consideration of both the disease characteristics and the patient's constitution. Moreover, the method of draining downward should be modified if there are complications of the disease or changes in the constitution of the patient. For example, individuals with underlying deficiency may require concurrent treatment with both draining downward and tonifying.

4. 和法 *He fa* (**harmonizing**) regulates and accords complicated patterns of disease that affect multiple parts of the body. "Complicated patterns of disease" refers to concurrent presentation of hot and cold, or of deficiency and excess. "Multiple parts of the body" refers to a presentation of disease at both the exterior and interior, or affecting both *zang* (solid organs) and *fu* (hollow organs). Because of this complexity, it is insufficient to use only one of these eight methods of treatment.

    Harmonizing is generally used to treat such disorders as *shaoyang* syndrome, *mo yuan* (membrane source) disorders, disharmony of the Liver and Spleen, concurrent presentation of heat in the Stomach and cold in the Intestines, irregularities of qi and blood, and disharmony of the nutritive and defensive levels.

5. 温法 *Wen fa* (**warming**) method warms the interior, dispels cold, restores yang, and unblocks the channels and collaterals. Warming is usually used to treat the presence of cold affecting the normal functions of *zang fu* organs, or stagnation of cold blocking the channels and collaterals.

    Warming often needs to be modified since a disease may have different characteristics and patients have different body constitutions. Cold disorders may occur as a result of external invasion or internal injury and may reside in various parts of the body (such as in the upper, middle, or lower *jiaos*; *zang fu* organs; and channels or collaterals). It is also well known that cold typically affects individuals who have an underlying yang deficiency. In short, optimal treatment requires careful consideration of disease characteristics as well as patient conditions, and selection of appropriate treatment method or methods is of the utmost importance.

> **Selection of appropriate treatment methods is of the utmost importance.**

6. 清法 *Qing fa* (**clearing**) method clears heat, purges fire and cools the blood to treat diseases characterized by warmth, heat, fire, and toxins. It is also used in cases of heat with complications, such as damp-heat and yin-deficient fire.

    Clearing generally needs to be modified to achieve optimal clinical results, since heat disorders may affect different parts of the body and cause various complications. "Different parts of the body" here refers to *qi* (energy) level, *ying* (nutritive) level, and *xue* (blood) level, as well as the *zang fu* organs. "Complications" refers to the presence of heat drying or damaging yin and body fluids. Therefore, optimal treatment requires proper selection of herbs to clear heat at the diseased area, and concurrent utilization of clearing and tonifying in individuals who have heat with underlying deficiencies.

7. 消法 *Xiao fa* (**reducing**) dissolves and disperses hardnesses and nodules to treat accumulation and stagnation of various substances, such as food, qi, blood, phlegm, water, and parasites. Reducing may be used to treat a wide variety of illness due to various causes.

    In contrast to draining downward, which is generally used to treat acute and excess conditions via defecation, reducing is usually employed to address chronic conditions characterized by both deficiency and excess. These diseases are often located in the *zang fu* organs, channels and collaterals, or in the muscle tissues, and they are often present in some form of hardness or nodule that cannot be quickly eliminated. Thus, it becomes necessary to use reducing method to slowly dissolve and disperse the hardness and nodules. When necessary, reducing can be combined with tonifying or draining-downward method.

Chinese Herbal Formulas and Applications

Chapter 2 — Treatment Methods and Formulas

8. 补法 *Bu fa* (**tonifying**) nourishes, enriches, supplements, and benefits qi, blood, yin, and yang in the *zang fu* organs. Deficiency of qi, blood, yin, and yang seldom occur singularly; therefore, concurrent use of various tonics may be necessary to address such deficiencies. For example, chronic deficiency of qi often leads to decreased production (i.e., deficiency) of blood; and deficiency of yin is often accompanied by deficiency of yang. Furthermore, imbalance of the *zang fu* organs often occur together; likewise, concomitant use of various tonics may be required to address such imbalances. For example, Liver and Kidney yin deficiencies often occur together, and Heart and Spleen blood deficiencies generally accompany each other.

Tonifying must be used with caution in individuals with concurrent exterior excess and interior deficiency. With such conditions, sweating and tonifying must be used together to simultaneously release the exterior and supplement the interior. Use of sweating only may induce profuse perspiration and lead to more deficiency, while solely tonifying may complicate the illness by drawing the pathogenic factors from the exterior into the interior.

These eight treatment methods are all well-documented within the history of Chinese herbal medicine. Vomiting, however, has not been widely used, if at all, outside of mainland China. While vomiting may still be applicable, it is not as popular as the other seven methods. As stated earlier, it is often necessary to utilize more than one method when treating patients, as any one disease may have quite a few complications and may affect different parts of the body, while patients may have different underlying conditions.

Chapter 3
— Classification of Formulas

Many different systems have been proposed over the past two thousands years to organize and classify Chinese herbal formulas. Among the many different systems proposed are classifications based on characteristics of the formulas, treatment methods, primary function of the formulas, diseases, and special branches of medicine. The examples listed below are just some of the many systems documented in the history of Chinese herbal medicine.

七方 *Qi Fang* (**Seven Types of Formulas**), documented in *Huang Di Nei Jing* (Yellow Emperor's Inner Classic), is the first and the earliest attempt to describe and classify herbal formulas. It refers specifically to the following seven types of formulas: 大 *da* (large), 小 *xiao* (small), 缓 *huan* (mild), 急 *ji* (urgent), 奇 *qi* (odd-numbered), 偶 *ou* (even-numbered), and 复 *fu* (composite). *Da* (large) and *xiao* (small) refer to the number of ingredients and their doses within the formula.

Da (large) formulas contain a large number of ingredients and/or high dosages, and are designed to treat severe illnesses; and *xiao* (small) formulas contain a small number of ingredients and/or low dosages, and are designed to treat mild illnesses. *Huan* (mild) and *ji* (urgent) refer to the characteristic of the formula. *Huan* (mild) formulas are used to treat chronic diseases and must be taken for a long period of time, and *ji* (urgent) formulas are used to treat acute diseases and must be discontinued when the desired effects are achieved. *Qi* (odd-numbered) and *ou* (even-numbered) describe the number of ingredients in the formula. Examples of *qi* (odd-numbered) formulas include *Wu Ling San* (Five-Ingredient Powder with Poria) and *Qi Bao Mei Ran Dan* (Seven-Treasure

11

Part I – Overview

Chapter 3 — Classification of Formulas

Special Pill for Beautiful Whiskers), and examples of *ou* (even-numbered) formulas include *Si Jun Zi Tang* (Four-Gentlemen Decoction) and *Liu Wei Di Huang Wan* (Six-Ingredient Pill with Rehmannia). Lastly, *fu* (composite) formulas describe use of multiple herbs or formulas to treat more complicated illnesses, such as *Ba Zhen Tang* (Eight-Treasure Decoction) which is a *fu* (composite) formula composed of *Si Jun Zi Tang* (Four-Gentlemen Decoction) and *Si Wu Tang* (Four-Substance Decoction).

Qi Fang (Seven Types of Formulas) is a valuable tool that describes the general characteristic of the formulas and their clinical applications (such as severe or mild, acute or chronic, and simple or complicated illnesses). However, this method of classification is not very informative nor accurate, since it does not offer useful insights regarding the specific details of the formula nor the disease. Furthermore, certain statements from the original text do not seem to have any rational basis. For example, it stated that "diaphoretic formulas should not have even number of ingredients, and downward-draining formulas should not have odd number of ingredients." Today, texts use *Qi Fang* (Seven Types of Formulas) to **describe**, not to **classify** the herbal formulas.

十刹 *Shi Ji* (**Ten Types of Formulas**), first mentioned by Xu Zhi-Cai in the sixth century, describes the ten primary functions of the formula: 宣 *xuan* (disseminate), 通 *tong* (unblock), 补 *bu* (tonify), 泄 *xie* (drain), 轻 *qing* (light), 重 *zhong* (heavy), 涩 *se* (stabilize and bind), 滑 *hua* (lubricate), 燥 *zao* (dry) and 湿 *shi* (moisten). Descriptions of these primary functions were further explained by Li Shi-Zhen in *Ben Cao Gang Mu* (Materia Medica), in which he stated "*xuan* (dissemination) treats clogging, *tong* (unblocking) treats stagnation, *bu* (tonifying) treats weakness, *xie* (draining) treats obstruction, *qing* (light) lifts and eliminates excess, *zhong* (heavy) anchors and controls anxiety, *se* (stabilizing and binding) treats *tuo zheng* (abandoned syndrome), *hua* (lubricating) eliminates retention, *zao* (drying) treats dampness, and *shi* (moistening) treats dryness."

Finally in the Jin dynasty, Zhao Ji used the rationale in *Shi Ji* (Ten Types of Formulas) to formally classify formulas based on these primary functions in his work *Sheng Ji Jing* (Holy Relief Reference). This strategy of classifying herbal formulas based on their primary function was reiterated again in the Jin dynasty by Cheng Wu-Ji in his work *Shang Han Ming Li Yao Fang Lun* (Clarification of the Formulas and Herbs of Cold Induced Disorders). This marks the beginning and the consensus of classifying herbal formulas based on their primary functions.

Although this method provides an insightful description, the vastly different characteristics of the formulas cannot be categorized into these limited categories. As a result, the number of categories expanded over the years. 十二刹 *Shi Er Ji* (**Twelve Types of Formulas**) was proposed by Kou Zong-Shi in 1116 in his text *Ben Cao Yan Yi* (Extension of the Materia Medica). In addition to the pre-existing ten types, 寒 *han* (cold) and 热 *re* (hot) formulas were added to treat hot and cold diseases, respectively. Furthermore, Liao Zhong-Chun in the Ming dynasty added 升 *sheng* (ascending) and 降 *jiang* (descending) formulas to treat disorders in the upper and lower body, respectively.

Finally, Xu Si-He proposed 二十四刹 *Er Shi Si Ji* (**Twenty-Four Types of Formulas**) in his work *Yi Xue Quan Shu* (Complete Book of Medicine). In addition to the pre-existing ten types, fourteen more were added: 调 *tiao* (regulating), 和 *he* (harmonizing), 解 *jie* (releasing), 利 *li* (promoting), 温 *wen* (warming), 寒 *han* (cooling), 暑 *shu* (summer-heat), 火 *huo* (fire), 平 *ping* (pacifying), 夺 *duo* (guiding or despoliating), 安 *an* (calming), 缓 *huan* (mild), 淡 *dan* (bland), and 清 *qing* (clearing) formulas. *Er Shi Si Ji* (Twenty-Four Types of Formulas) represents the most complex system using this same rationale.

When Zhang Jing-Yue attempted to classify ancient and contemporary formulas, he recognized that eight arrays are insufficient to classify such a wide variety of formulas.

八阵 *Ba Zhen* (**Eight Arrays of Formulas**) was originally proposed by Zhang Jing-Yue in the Ming dynasty, and it classifies the formulas based on their characteristics. According to *Jing Yue Quan Shu* (Collected Treatises of [Zhang] Jing Yue), the eight arrays of formulas and their primary functions include 补 *bu* (tonic) formulas to treat deficiency, 和 *he* (harmonizing) formulas to treat disharmony, 攻 *gong* (attack) formulas to treat excess,

12

Chapter 3 — Classification of Formulas

散 *san* (disperse) formulas to disperse exterior conditions, 寒 *han* (cold) formulas to clear heat, 热 *re* (hot) formulas to dispel cold, 固 *gu* (stabilize) formulas to stop loss (of body fluids), and 因 *yin* (pattern-specific) formulas are used to treat specific disorders. However, when Zhang Jing-Yue attempted to classify 1,516 ancient and 186 contemporary formulas, he recognized that eight arrays were insufficient to classify such a wide variety of formulas. As a result, he added four additional categories: women's disorders (186 formulas), pediatric disorders (171 formulas), rashes (174 formulas), and external medicine (391 formulas).

The value of this method is that prior to this time, although many texts had been published on the classification of herbal formulas, many of them were not clinically useful because they were either too complex or overly simplified. *Ba Zhen* (Eight Arrays of Formulas) was an effective way to classify herbal formulas as it established a quick and meaningful way to find a useful formula to treat a given disease and/or patient.

二十二剂 *Er Shi Er Ji* (**Twenty-Two Types of Formulas**) was devised in 1682 during the Qing dynasty by Wang Ang in his work *Yi Fang Ji Jie* (Analytical Collection of Medical Formulas). Wang emphasized classifying herbal formulas based on the primary function of the formula, etiology of the disease, and specific branches of medicine. The 22 categories include 补养 *bu yang* (tonify and nourish), 发表 *fa biao* (disperse the exterior), 涌吐 *yong tu* (induce vomiting), 攻里 *gong li* (attack the interior), 表里 *biao li* (simultaneous treatment of the exterior and interior), 和解 *he jie* (harmonize and relieve), 理气 *li qi* (regulate the qi), 理血 *li xue* (regulate the blood), 祛风 *qu feng* (dispel wind), 祛寒 *qu han* (dispel cold), 清暑 *qing shu* (clear summer-heat), 利湿 *li shi* (resolve dampness), 润燥 *run zao* (moisten dryness), 泻火 *xie huo* (drain fire), 除痰 *chu tan* (eliminate phlegm), 消导 *xiao dao* (eliminate and guide out stagnation), 收涩 *shou se* (stabilize and bind), 杀虫 *sha chong* (kill parasites), 明目 *ming mu* (improve the vision), 痈疡 *yong yang* (abscesses and sores), 经产 *jing chan* (menstruation and childbirth), and 救急 *jiu ji* (emergencies).

The classification proposed by Wang Ang is regarded by many as one of the more comprehensive and clinically viable categorizations of herbal formulas. Many subsequent texts (including most textbooks today) follow these established guidelines with minor modifications. Today, textbooks on herbal formulas follow various rationales and systems as described above. Most textbooks contain approximately 18 to 21 categories. Many categories also have sub-categories to further delineate the similarities and differences among these formulas.

Part I – Overview

Chapter 4

— Composition of Formulas

Principles of Formulation

Successful treatment requires an accurate differential diagnosis, a strategic treatment plan, and effective herbal formulas. To ensure efficacy of the herbal treatment, *Huang Di Nei Jing* (Yellow Emperor's Inner Classic) used the system of *Jun Chen Zuo Shi* (Chief, Deputy, Assistant, Envoy) as the guiding principle in herbal formulation. Although the general concept has been expanded since then, the basic principles remain the same. The system consists of four components, each playing an important and essential function within the formula.

- 君药 *Jun yao* (**chief herb**) is used to treat the key disease or symptom. It is the essential ingredient that must be present in every formula. *Jun yao* (chief herb) is used at a large dose to maximize the effect.
- 臣药 *Chen yao* (**deputy herb**) has two main functions: 1) it reinforces the effect of *jun yao* (chief herb) to treat the key disease or symptom; and 2) it treats the associated or coexisting diseases or symptoms.
- 佐药 *Zuo yao* (**assistant herb**) has three main functions: 1) it reinforces the effect of *jun yao* (chief herb) or *chen yao* (deputy herb) to treat the disease, or directly treats the secondary symptoms; 2) it counteracts the toxicity or minimizes the drastic effects of the *jun yao* (chief herb) or *chen yao* (deputy herb); and 3) has an opposite effect as, but works in synergy with, the *jun yao* (chief herb) to treat the most serious and complex disorders.
- 使药 *Shi yao* (**envoy herb**) has two main functions: 1) it acts as a channel-guiding herb to direct the formula to the affected channels/areas of the body; and 2) it harmonizes all of the herbs within the formula. *Shi yao* (envoy herb) is usually used only in small doses.

> The *Jun Chen Zuo Shi* (Chief, Deputy, Assistant, Envoy) system is to be used flexibly, and in accordance with the condition of the patient.

The chief herb is the most essential component in every formula. Generally speaking, every formula has only one or two chief herbs used at a large dose to treat the key disease or symptom. The use of multiple chief herbs or at a lower dose is not desirable, since such practice will compromise the overall effectiveness of the formula. The other three components all have two or more functions, and are generally used at lower doses when compared to the chief herb.

It is important to note that *Jun Chen Zuo Shi* (Chief, Deputy, Assistant, Envoy) is a system to be used flexibly, and that the formulas must be prescribed in accordance with the condition of the patient. Thus, it is not necessary for all formulas to contain all four components. For example, for illnesses of simple etiology, use of one chief herb and two deputy herbs will often suffice to treat the condition. Or, in cases in which the chief herb is not toxic and does not have drastic effects, it is unnecessary to use an assistant herb to counteract the toxicity or minimize the drastic effects of the chief herb. Lastly, in cases in which the chief herb also enters the diseased channel or affected area of the body, the use of an envoy herb as a channel-guiding herb is not needed.

Please refer to *Ma Huang Tang* (Ephedra Decoction) for an explanation of *Jun Chen Zuo Shi* (Chief, Deputy, Assistant, Envoy) and how these terms apply within an herbal formula.

Chinese Herbal Formulas and Applications

Chapter 4 — Composition of Formulas

Modifications of Formulation

While it is extremely important to follow the essential guidelines in composing an herbal formula, it is just as important to remain flexible and customize the treatment to the individual conditions and needs of the patient. Factors that require additional consideration include age, body weight, clinical presentations of the disease, and the underlying constitution of the patient. Ingredients, doses, and the dosage forms may be adjusted to optimize the treatment results.

• **Ingredients:** The formulas listed in this text are designed to treat certain conditions. However, many patients will not clinically show such textbook presentations. Use of a fixed formula without modification to address the varied condition will produce suboptimal results. Therefore, it is necessary to modify the formula to properly and adequately address the variations of each condition. For example, *Ma Huang Tang* (Ephedra Decoction) is designed to treat exterior-excess, wind-cold syndrome, and is composed of four ingredients: *Ma Huang* (Herba Ephedrae), *Gui Zhi* (Ramulus Cinnamomi), *Ku Xing Ren* (Semen Armeniacae Amarum) and *Zhi Gan Cao* (Radix et Rhizoma Glycyrrhizae Praeparata cum Melle). When needed, herbs may be added or removed to address the variation of this condition. *Ma Huang Jia Zhu Tang* (Ephedra Decoction plus Atractylodes) is designed to treat exterior-excess, wind-cold syndrome with damp accumulation, and is composed of the same four ingredients plus *Bai Zhu* (Rhizoma Atractylodis Macrocephalae) to dry dampness. *San Ao Tang* (Three-Unbinding Decoction) is designed to treat exterior wind-cold affecting the Lung, and is composed of *Ma Huang* (Herba Ephedrae), *Ku Xing Ren* (Semen Armeniacae Amarum) and *Gan Cao* (Radix et Rhizoma Glycyrrhizae). The removal of *Gui Zhi* (Ramulus Cinnamomi) decreases the diaphoretic and exterior-releasing effects of the formula, and shifts its emphasis more toward ventilating the Lung.

• **Dosages:** Dosages of ingredients play an important role in the overall function of the formula. Generally speaking, large doses are used for acute or severe conditions, and smaller doses are used for chronic or mild conditions. Furthermore, dosage adjustments are needed for pediatric or geriatric patients, or individuals with larger or smaller body weights. In some cases, without changing the ingredients, changes in dosages will alter the overall function of the formula. For example, *Si Ni Tang* (Frigid Extremities Decoction) and *Tong Mai Si Ni Tang* (Unblock the Pulse Decoction for Frigid Extremities) contain the same three ingredients, but have different clinical functions and applications. *Si Ni Tang* (Frigid Extremities Decoction) contains a small amount of *Fu Zi* (Radix Aconiti Lateralis Praeparata) and *Gan Jiang* (Rhizoma Zingiberis), and is used to restore the depleted yang and rescue the patient from collapse. On the other hand, *Tong Mai Si Ni Tang* (Unblock the Pulse Decoction for Frigid Extremities) contains larger doses of *Fu Zi* (Radix Aconiti Lateralis Praeparata) and *Gan Jiang* (Rhizoma Zingiberis), and is used to treat true-cold, false-heat syndrome (true presence of cold in the interior and false symptoms of heat at the exterior). Please see *Si Ni Tang* (Frigid Extremities Decoction) for detailed explanation of the differences between these two formulas and syndromes.

• **Dosage forms:** Herbs may be given in various dosage forms, including but not limited to decoction, powder, pills, etc. Each form has its own advantages and disadvantages, and selection will depend on condition, constitution and compliance. Condition of the disorder often plays an important role in deciding what dosage form to use. For example, *Li Zhong Wan* (Regulate the Middle Pill) and *Ren Shen Tang* (Ginseng Decoction) have the exact same ingredients and doses, and differ only in dosage form, which is dictated by change in clinical indication. *Li Zhong Wan* is given as pills to treat the chronic condition of deficiency and cold of the middle *jiao*. *Ren Shen Tang* is administered as decoction to treat the acute condition of *xiong bi* (painful obstruction of the chest). Please refer to the next chapter, which provides a detailed discussion of various dosage forms.

Part I – Overview

Chapter 5

— Dosage Forms

Discussion of dosage forms was first documented in *Huang Di Nei Jing* (Yellow Emperor's Inner Classic) during the first or the second century A.D. This historical text provides a description of many dosage forms such as decoction, pills, powder, soft extracts, medicinal wine, and pellets. Although this description comprised a noble beginning, over the next two thousand years, many additional dosage forms have been developed and used. Listed below are many of the most commonly-used contemporary dosage forms, along with a brief discussion. While this text focuses on the traditional preparations of herbal formulas listed in *Huang Di Nei Jing* (Yellow Emperor's Inner Classic), readers are encouraged to use their own creativity to devise the best possible dosage form according to their patients' needs.

Please note that the information below represents the general description for each dosage form. Specific, detailed information is found in each formula monograph, under the section **DOSAGE / PREPARATION / ADMINISTRATION.**

> Decoctions may be applied topically as an herbal wash or soak, as well as gargled or swallowed.

汤剂 *Tang ji* (**decoction**) is one of the most commonly-used dosage forms for administering Chinese herbs. The general protocol for preparation is to first soak the herbs in water, cook them at a certain temperature for a certain amount of time (depending on the herbs), filter and save the decoction liquid while discarding the herb residue, and administer the decoction while warm. The exact instructions for preparing each decoction vary, depending on the formula purpose and the herbs used. The advantages of decoction include quick absorption, fast onset of action, and flexibility to customize herbal formulas for each patient. In addition to oral ingestion, decoction may also be applied topically as an herbal wash, an herbal soak, and a solution for mouth gargle. Examples of formulas historically given in decoction include *Ma Huang Tang* (Ephedra Decoction) and *Da Cheng Qi Tang* (Major Order the Qi Decoction). Note: Additional information on preparation and administration of decoctions is listed in **Part I Overview, Chapter 6: Preparation and Administration of Decoctions.**

散剂 *San ji* (**powder**) is also a frequently-used dosage form, and is prepared by grinding and blending all of the ingredients into small particles. Powdered herbs may then be used either internally or externally. For internal use, if only a small dose is needed, such as *Qi Li San* (Seven-Thousandths of a Tael Powder), mix the powder with warm water and ingest without modification. If a large dose is needed, such as *Xiang Su San* (Cyperus and Perilla Leaf Powder), cook the coarse powder in water and take the decoction. For external use, the powder is applied directly to the affected area (skin, throat, and other areas). The advantages of powder include simplified preparation, quick absorption, fast onset of action, and, in comparison to decoction, a longer shelf life. Examples of formulas historically given in powder include *Xiao Yao San* (Rambling Powder) and *Yu Ping Feng San* (Jade Windscreen Powder).

丸剂 *Wan ji* (**pill**) is a solid dosage form prepared by first grinding the herbs into powder, mixing the powder with an aqueous medium such as water, honey, alcohol, vinegar or others, and then shaping the resultant mixture into pills. Because pills require disintegration and dissolution prior to absorption, they have a slower onset but prolonged duration of action. Thus, pills, such as *Zuo Gui Wan* (Restore the Left [Kidney] Pill) or *You Gui Wan* (Restore the Right [Kidney] Pill), are generally used to treat chronic conditions that require long-term treatment.

However, some pill-based formulas are specifically made to treat an emergency situation rather than a chronic condition, such as *Su He Xiang Wan* (Liquid Styrax Pill) and *An Gong Niu Huang Wan* (Calm the Palace Pill with Cattle Gallstone). These formulas are given in pills for two main

Chapter 5 — Dosage Forms

reasons: 1) They are immediately available when needed during the emergency; and 2) many ingredients in these formulas are easily destroyed by heat and cannot be cooked in decoction.

Lastly, certain formulas have potent, drastic functions that are inappropriate for decoction, such as *Zhou Che Wan* (Vessel and Vehicle Pill). Administration of such formulas in decoction results in quick absorption and fast onset of action, which often causes unwanted side effects and adverse reactions. Therefore, these formulas are given as pills, which are better tolerated because they slowly exert their therapeutic effect over a longer period of time.

Other advantages of pills include increased patient compliance, convenient storage, and long shelf life. Depending on how they are made, there are four subcategories of pills:

- Honey pills are made by mixing fine herbal powder with honey and forming the resultant paste into small pills. In addition to serving as a binding agent, honey has tonifying and moistening effects within the formula. Honey pills are most suitable for treating chronic illnesses. Examples include *Shi Quan Da Bu Tang* (All-Inclusive Great Tonifying Decoction) and *Shi Hu Ye Guang Wan* (Dendrobium Pill for Night Vision).
- Water pills are made by mixing fine herbal powder with water, grain-based liquor, vinegar, or juice from fresh herbs and formed the mixture into small pills. Water pills disintegrate easily, which is both an advantage and a disadvantage. Clinically, fast disintegration means quicker absorption and faster onset of action. Commercially, however, easy disintegration means the pills break easily during transportation. *Bao He Wan* (Preserve Harmony Pill) is one example.
- Glue pills are made by mixing fine herbal powder with rice or cooked and mashed noodles, and then forming the mixture into small pills. Glue pills disintegrate more slowly than honey or water pills, thus allowing gradual absorption and prolonged duration of action. Moreover, rice or noodle pills are well-tolerated, and generally do not cause gastrointestinal side effects. An example includes *Xi Huang Wan* (Cattle Gallstone Pill).
- Extract pills are made by grinding a portion of the herbs into a fine powder, cooking the rest in water to obtain a dense liquid extract, and finally blending the two portions together using a medium. The advantages include high potency, smaller dosage (as it is already concentrated), and easy ingestion.

膏剂 *Gao ji* (**soft extract**) is prepared by cooking herbs with water or vegetable oil to concentrate the herbs into a soft extract, which may be used internally or topically. For internal use, the soft extract may be taken alone, or mixed with water immediately prior to ingestion. For topical use, the soft extract can be applied directly to the affected area. *Qiong Yu Gao* (Beautiful Jade Paste) is one formula historically given in this topical dosage form.

丹剂 *Dan ji* (**pellet**) is a solid dosage form, generally considered to be a type of *wan ji* (pill). Pellets are made the same way as pills, i.e., by mixing the fine herbal powder with a binding agent and shaping into pellets. The distinction between pellets and pills is that pellets are generally smaller in size but stronger in potency. Pellet is the preferred dosage form for herbs that are very valuable and expensive, and for ingredients that have been greatly condensed and concentrated. Examples of this dosage form include *Zhi Bao Dan* (Greatest Treasure Special Pill) and *Tian Wang Bu Xin Dan* (Emperor of Heaven's Special Pill to Tonify the Heart).

酒剂 *Jiu ji* (**medicinal wine**) uses grain-based alcohol as the solvent to extract the active constituents from the herbs. The medicinal wine may be prepared simply by soaking the herbs in grain-based liquor at room temperature, or by cooking the herbs in a mixture of water and liquor. After filtering out the herb residue, the medicinal wine may be administered internally or topically. In addition to working as a solvent to extract herbs, liquor also functions to promote blood circulation and open channels and collaterals. Therefore, medicinal wine is most appropriate for treatment of generalized weakness and deficiency, *bi zheng* (painful obstruction syndrome) due to wind-cold-damp, and external or traumatic injuries. However, medicinal wine should not be used for individuals who have yin-deficient fire, or damp accumulation.

Part I – Overview

Chapter 5 — Dosage Forms

茶剂 *Cha ji* (**tea**), as the name implies, is the administration of herbs in tea form, making tea by soaking herbs in hot water. In this case, the herbs are generally ground into a coarse powder and placed in a tea bag. While this method is convenient and commonly used for beverages, it is not very effective therapeutically, as the active constituents in many herbs cannot be effectively extracted simply by soaking the herbs in hot water.

药露 *Yao lu* (**distillation**) is a method used to capture the essential oils that are present in many fragrant and aromatic herbs. This method is generally used only when fresh herbs are available.

锭剂 *Ding ji* (**lozenge**) is made by first grinding the herbs into a fine powder, followed by mixing the powder with a binding agent (such as honey) to make into a solid dosage form. Lozenges may be taken orally, or applied topically to the affected area. One example is *Zi Jin Ding* (Purple Gold Special Pill).

灸剂 *Jiu ji* (**moxa**) is prepared by crushing and rolling *Ai Ye* (Folium Artemisiae Argyi) in a piece of paper to form a stick that resembles the shape of a cigar. Upon burning the moxa stick, heat and the effects of the herb are delivered locally to the affected area or the targeted channel.

糖浆剂 *Tang jiang ji* (**syrup**) refers to the addition of cane sugar to liquid dosage forms to mask the taste and improve patient compliance. Because of the sweet taste, this dosage form is used for individuals who are not accustomed to the taste of herbs.

片剂 *Pian ji* (**tablet**) is a contemporary dosage form. Tablets are made by combining the herbs (raw form or concentrated powder) and excipient(s) and pressing them into tablets. The advantages of tablets include improved patient compliance, precise dosage, and long shelf life. If necessary, a clear coating may be applied to the outside of the tablets to protect against moisture, or a sugar coating may be applied to mask any unpleasant taste. Furthermore, an enteric coating may be applied to ensure that the tablets disintegrate and dissolve in the intestines and not the stomach in order to minimize stomach irritation or prevent degradation of the herbs by gastric acid. Many classic formulas are now made and sold as tablets.

胶囊剂 *Jiao nang ji* (**capsule**) is also a contemporary dosage form. Capsules are made by filling empty gelatin capsules with the herbs, whether in raw form or concentrated powder. Since capsules dissolve relatively quickly in the stomach, this approach offers rapid absorption and a fast onset of action. The advantages of capsules include improved patient compliance, precise dosage, and long shelf life. Many classic formulas are now made and sold as capsules.

冲服剂 *Chong fu ji* (**granule or powder**) is another contemporary dosage form. Powder or granules are made by cooking the herbs in water, extracting the active constituents, and mixing the extraction with certain excipients (such as corn, rice or potato starch). This granular or powdered extract may be administered by mixing it with warm water, or it can be transformed easily into tablets or capsules. The advantages of granular or powdered extract include quick absorption, fast onset of action, improved patient compliance, flexibility in customizing the treatment for each patient, and long shelf life.

> **Injection delivers fast action, precise dosing, and the absence of interference from gastrointestinal absorption, but there is no room for error.**

针剂 *Zhen ji* (**injection**) is a method that delivers herbs via intravenous, intramuscular or subcutaneous injection. The preparation method of herbal injection varies according to the herbs. The advantages include extremely fast onset of action, precise dosing, and the absence of interference from gastrointestinal absorption. Although injection is a powerful way to deliver herbs, preparation must be done with extreme caution, and administration must be performed with exact precision, as there is no room for error.

In clinical practice, it is important to keep an open mind when selecting the dosage form. In most cases, dosage forms can be interchanged with comparable results. For example, if preparation and ingestion of decoction is inconvenient or undesirable, the

18

Chapter 5 — Dosage Forms

same formula can easily be prepared and given as powder or pills. On the other hand, if a product is only available in capsules or tablets but the patient cannot swallow this dosage form, the patient can simply open the capsules or crush the tablets and ingest the powder with water. In addition to all the dosage forms listed above, herbs may also be administered via other routes (such as topical, vaginal, or rectal). Proper selection of dosage forms and route of administration not only improves patient compliance but also clinical results.

Chapter 6

— Preparation and Administration of Decoctions

Preparation of Decoctions

Decoction is the most common way to administer Chinese herbs. Proper preparation is essential to ensure both safety and efficacy of the herbal decoction.

- **Equipment**: Ceramic or clay pots are generally used to prepare the decoction, as these types of material are inexpensive, readily available, and will not interact with the herbs or their constituents. In the past, the use of metal containers, especially iron, copper and aluminum, was contraindicated because such metals can cause unknown chemical reactions with the herbs and their constituents. Today, high quality stainless steel pots are used by many practitioners and herbal manufacturers without any unwanted effects.

- **Water**: It is important to use clean, unpolluted water to cook the herbs. In the past, Chinese people often used water from a running river or a clean well. Today, tap water, filtered water, or distilled water suffice. The amount of water used varies, depending on the total quantity of herbs. The general rule of thumb on the amount of water needed is to first place all the herbs in the pot, then add enough water to cover all the herbs by one *cun* (approximately 3-5 cm). In most cases, the herbs may be cooked twice, using more water in the first cooking process than in the second. The desired amount of decoction obtained should generally be between 100-150 mL.

- **Temperature**: Two types of heat are generally used to cook the herbs: 武火 *wu huo* (military fire) describes a high flame or high intensity fire, and 文火 *wen huo* (civilian fire) describes a low flame or low intensity fire. *Wu huo* (military fire) is usually used first to bring the decoction to a boiling temperature, and then *wen huo* (civilian fire) is used to cook and extract active constituents from the herbs.

Method of Decoctions

Chinese herbal medicine encompasses thousands of plant parts, animal substances, and minerals—all with unique characteristics. Therefore, in addition to the generic method of decoction, specific methods of decoction vary depending on the herbs used. The generic method is to first place all of the herbs in the pot, fill the pot with enough water to cover the herbs, allow the herbs to soak in the water for 20 to 30 minutes, and then cook the mixture to obtain the decoction. As described above, a high temperature is generally used first to bring the decoction to a boiling temperature, followed by a low temperature to extract the active constituents. The decoction should not be cooked at

Part I – Overview

Chapter 6 — Preparation and Administration of Decoctions

boiling temperature for an extended period of time, so as to avoid evaporating too much water and "drying up" the decoction. Moreover, the lid of the cooking pot should not be opened repeatedly during cooking, because this allows evaporation of water and essential oils. When the cooking process is finished, the herb residue is filtered and discarded, while the liquid is kept, and the resultant decoction is served while warm. In addition to this generic method, certain types of herbs must be processed with specific care as follows:

- 先煎*Xian jian* (**pre-decoction**) is a process by which some herbs are cooked for an extended period of time prior to the addition of others. Mineral substances and animal shells are hard to extract because they are generally sold in large pieces and have low water solubility. To ensure maximum effect, they must be crushed into smaller particles first to increase the surface area, and then boiled for 10 to 20 minutes before the addition of the other herbs. Examples of mineral substances and animal shells that require pre-decoction include *Ci Shi* (Magnetitum), *Shi Gao* (Gypsum Fibrosum), *Zhe Shi* (Haematitum), *Gui Ban* (Plastrum Testudinis), *Bie Jia* (Carapax Trionycis), *Shi Jue Ming* (Concha Haliotidis), *Long Gu* (Os Draconis), and *Mu Li* (Concha Ostreae).

  In addition to these mineral substances and animal shells, certain tonifying herbs and toxic herbs are also pre-decocted, although for opposite reasons. Tonic herbs are pre-decocted at *wen huo* (civilian fire) for a prolonged period of time to ensure the complete extraction of active constituents. In contrast, herbs that are toxic are pre-decocted at *wen huo* (civilian fire) for a prolonged period of time in order to deactivate and destroy toxic constituents.

  Lastly, herbs that contain a large amount of soil, such as *Fu Long Gan* (Terra Flava Usta), or herbs that are lightweight and very bulky, such as *Lu Gen* (Rhizoma Phragmitis), *Bai Mao Gen* (Rhizoma Imperatae), or *Xia Ku Cao* (Spica Prunellae), are decocted first, and the resultant liquid is retained, filtered, and used as the solvent to cook the rest of the herbs. Pre-decoction in these two cases helps to eliminate unnecessary components such as soil, and make room for other herbs in the pot (lightweight, bulky herbs sometimes completely fill the pot).

- 后下*Hou xia* (**post-decoction**) is a specific instruction to add particular herbs at the end of the decoction process and cook them for only a short period of time (approximately 5 to 10 minutes). Generally speaking, exterior-releasing herbs, heat-clearing herbs, aromatic herbs, and certain downward-draining herbs should be cooked at *wu huo* (military fire) for a short period of time to preserve their potency and prevent excessive evaporation of the active constituents. Specifically, acrid or aromatic herbs, such as *Bo He* (Herba Menthae) and *Huo Xiang* (Herba Agastaches), contain essential oils that evaporate easily if cooked at high temperature for a prolonged period of time. Furthermore, herbs that contain constituents that are easily deactivated by heat, such as *Da Huang* (Radix et Rhizoma Rhei) and *Fan Xie Ye* (Folium Sennae), are also added at the end of the cooking process to preserve the integrity of the active components. It is important to note that to facilitate extraction of active ingredients, these herbs should also be soaked in water for 20 to 30 minutes first, prior to adding them to the pot for post-decoction.

- 包煎*Bao jian* (**decocted in gauze**) describes the process by which the herbs are wrapped in gauze or cheesecloth during the cooking process. This is done for herbs that may irritate the throat and cause gagging or coughing, or may irritate the gastrointestinal tract, causing nausea and vomiting. Examples of these herbs include *Xin Yi Hua* (Flos Magnoliae), *Xuan Fu Hua* (Flos Inulae), *Che Qian Zi* (Semen Plantaginis), *Chi Shi Zhi* (Halloysitum Rubrum), and *Hua Shi* (Talcum).

- 另煎*Ling jian* (**separately decocted**) or 另炖*ling dun* (**separately simmered**) is generally reserved for herbs that are overly expensive or difficult to extract. These herbs are usually cut into very small pieces or thin slices and separately decocted or simmered for 2 to 3 hours to ensure maximum extraction and minimum waste. Examples include wild-crafted *Ren Shen* (Radix et Rhizoma Ginseng), *Ling Yang Jiao* (Cornu Saigae Tataricae), and *Xi Jiao* (Cornu Rhinoceri).

- 熔化*Rong hua* (**dissolution**) is a process used for substances which cannot or should not be cooked. Substances that are sticky tend to bind to other herbs in the pot and decrease the extraction process, and they also create a mess by binding to the pot and becoming burned. Instead of being cooked, these substances are placed in the already strained, hot decoction. The decoction is administered when these substances are completely dissolved. Examples of such sticky substances

20

Chinese Herbal Formulas and Applications

Chapter 6 — Preparation and Administration of Decoctions

include *Yi Tang* (Maltosum), *E Jiao* (Colla Corii Asini), *Feng Mi* (Mel), and *Lu Jiao Jiao* (Colla Cornus Cervi).

- 冲服*Chong fu* (**take drenched**) describes the process by which the herbs are mixed with the strained decoction immediately before ingestion, such as *Mang Xiao* (Natrii Sulfas), and juices from fresh herbs such as *Zhu Li* (Succus Bambusae) and *Sheng Jiang* (Rhizoma Zingiberis Recens). Substances that are aromatic and very expensive are also taken via infusion, such as *Niu Huang* (Calculus Bovis), *She Xiang* (Moschus), and *San Qi* (Radix et Rhizoma Notoginseng).

Administration of Decoctions

Frequency and timing of administering the herbs affect the efficacy of the formula. Factors to consider when deciding frequency and timing include the constitution of the patient, the stage or severity of the illness, and the dosage forms.

- **Timing**: Generally speaking, herbs are given on an empty stomach one hour before meals for optimal absorption. However, this is not always appropriate. If herbs tend to irritate the stomach, either due to their properties or due to patient sensitivity, they should be taken after meals. Tonic herbs that are cloying in nature should be taken on an empty stomach. Herbs that treat malaria should be taken approximately two hours before the outbreak. Herbs that calm the *shen* (spirit) should in general be taken before bedtime. Herbs for treating acute conditions are given as needed, and preferably in liquid dosage form for faster absorption. Herbs for treating chronic conditions are given at a fixed schedule, and preferably in solid dosage form for better patient compliance. Lastly, some formulas require a specific time of administration, such as *Ji Ming San* (Powder to Take at Cock's Crow), which should be given at room temperature on an empty stomach before dawn for optimal effect.

- **Frequency**: Frequency of dosing varies depending on the condition of the patient and the severity of the illness. Generally speaking, each pack of herbs may be cooked in water twice, and the two resultant decoctions are mixed together and given in two or three equally-divided doses. However, in acute or severe cases, the two resultant decoctions from one pack of herbs may be given in one dose for faster and stronger effects. And when necessary, two packs of herbs may be given in the same day. It is important to note that increase in dose and dosing frequency should be done carefully, and only when necessary, in order to avoid overdosage of herbs, especially if the herbs are toxic or have drastic, potent effects.

> ∼
> **Increases in dosage and dose frequency should be made carefully, and <u>only</u> when necessary, in order to avoid over-dosing.**
> ∼

- **Administration**: As a general rule, herbal decoctions are given while warm. Exterior-releasing formulas are usually given as warm decoction to induce mild perspiration. Disorders characterized by cold should be treated by hot herbs given as warm decoction, while disorders characterized by heat or fire should be treated with cold herbs given as room-temperature decoction. However, patients with conditions complicated by the presence of both heat and cold may reject warm decoctions if they experience nausea and vomiting. In such cases, the decoction should be given at room temperature. In other situations in which the patients experience nausea and vomiting with a warm decoction, these reactions may be alleviated by any of the following methods: add a small amount of *Sheng Jiang* (Rhizoma Zingiberis Recens) juice to the decoction; rub a thin slice of *Sheng Jiang* (Rhizoma Zingiberis Recens) on the tongue; chew a small piece of *Chen Pi* (Pericarpium Citri Reticulatae); or simply administer the decoction at room temperature.

- **Additional instructions**: In addition to timing and frequency, other instructions are required for some formulas to achieve maximum results. For example, in addition to serving *Ma Huang Tang* (Ephedra Decoction) as a warm decoction, the patients are also instructed to avoid exposure to wind, and to cover the body with a blanket to induce mild sweating. In cases of *Gui Zhi Tang* (Cinnamon Twig Decoction), administration of the formula should be followed by ingestion of a bowl of hot rice porridge to tonify the underlying deficiency and induce mild perspiration. Lastly, certain conditions require herbal treatment as well as diet and lifestyle changes, such as avoiding some foods or refraining from certain activities. When applicable, such additional instructions are stated in the monograph of each individual formula.

21

Part I – Overview

Chapter 7

— Weights and Measures

istorically, the Chinese have used their own system for weights and measurements. Though this system is still used by some in the general market place, academic and healthcare institutions have all adopted the metric system as the standard for weights and measurements. Accordingly, this text also uses the metric system as the standard to describe weight and volume. As a reference, the charts below summarize the Chinese system and its conversion to the metric system.

1. **Measure of Weight (Chinese System)**

   1 *jin* (斤) = 16 *liang* (两)
   1 *liang* (两) = 10 *qian* (钱)
   1 *qian* (钱) = 10 *fen* (分)
   1 *fen* (分) = 10 *li* (厘)

2. **Measure of Volume (Chinese System)**

   1 *shi* (石) = 10 *dou* (斗)
   1 *dou* (斗) = 10 *sheng* (升)
   1 *sheng* (升) = 10 *he* (合)
   1 *he* (合) = 10 *shao* (勺)

3. **Conversion (Chinese to Metric System)**

   Weight Conversion (Chinese Units : Metric)

Chinese Units	Grams
1 *jin*	500
1 *liang*	31.25
1 *qian*	3.125
1 *fen*	0.3125
1 *li*	0.03125

   Volume Conversion (Chinese Unit : Metric)

Chinese Unit	Liter
1 *sheng*	1

~

Chinese units vary from dynasty to dynasty: one *liang* in the Qin dynasty is 16.14 grams, while one *liang* in the Qing dynasty is 37.21 grams; one *sheng* in the Qin dynasty is equivalent to 340 mL, but one *sheng* in the Qing dynasty is equivalent to 1035.5 mL.

~

Additional Comments

Unfortunately, interpreting doses from historical texts is not as simple or as straight-forward as it may seem. It is important to remember that Chinese herbal medicine developed over a few thousand years, covering many different dynasties, and across various regions of China. All these variables contribute to variations in weights and measures, as exact values vary according to time and geographic location of the original source texts. Although the terms remain the same, their actual value can be significantly different. For example, one *liang* in the Qin dynasty is equivalent to 0.5165 *liang* today, while one *liang* in the Qing dynasty is equivalent to 1.194 *liang* today. Furthermore, one *sheng* in the Qin dynasty is equivalent to 0.34 *sheng* today, while one *sheng* in the Qing dynasty is equivalent to 1.0355 *sheng* today.

Chapter 7 — Weights and Measures

Additionally, the doses of herbs described in many historical texts were not necessarily in standard weights and measures, but rather, in descriptive terms. For example, *Da Zao* (Fructus Jujubae) is prescribed in pieces, *Ku Xing Ren* (Semen Armeniacae Amarum) in kernels, and *Sheng Jiang* (Rhizoma Zingiberis Recens) in slices. Lastly, the dose of the formulas may be described as "one pinch," such as in *Shou Nian San* (Pinch Powder), or the size of the pills may be described as the size of an "egg yolk."

Descriptions of doses are sometimes imprecise: fruits are described in pieces, seeds in kernels, fresh ginger in slices, powder in "pinch" and pills as being the size of "egg yolk" or "chicken head."

Despite the best efforts by scholars to interpret doses from historical source texts and convert them to contemporary measurements, information is sometimes simply unavailable to confirm or convert original doses. Even though the metric system is used as the standard for weights and measurements in this text, readers are encouraged to use their own judgments in deciding the best doses based on age, body weight, disease condition, and constitution of the patients.

The traditional system of measurement in China is significantly different from the British and metric systems. Listed below are conversions between the traditional Chinese system and the metric system:

Period (Dynasty)	Historical Weight	Contemporary Weight	Metric Weight	Historical Volume	Contemporary Volume	Metric Volume
Qin (221-207 BCE)	1 *liang*	0.5165 *liang*	16.1406 g	1 *sheng*	0.34 *sheng*	340.0 mL
Western Han (206 BCE- 24 CE)	1 *liang*	0.5165 *liang*	16.1406 g	1 *sheng*	0.34 *sheng*	340.0 mL
Eastern Han (25-220)	1 *liang*	0.4455 *liang*	13.9219 g	1 *sheng*	0.20 *sheng*	200.0 mL
Jin (265-420)	1 *liang*	0.4455 *liang*	13.9219 g	1 *sheng*	0.21 *sheng*	210.0 mL
Sui and Tang (581-907)	1 *liang*	0.5011 *liang*	15.6594 g	1 *sheng*	0.58 *sheng*	580.0 mL
Song (960-1279)	1 *liang*	1.0075 *liang*	31.4844 g	1 *sheng*	0.55 *sheng*	550.0 mL
Ming (1368-1644)	1 *liang*	1.1936 *liang*	37.3000 g	1 *sheng*	1.07 *sheng*	1070.0 mL
Qing (1644-1911)	1 *liang*	1.194 *liang*	37.3125 g	1 *sheng*	1.0355 *sheng*	1035.5 mL

Note: Because descriptions of doses in the classic formulas vary significantly, it is not always possible to determine the exact original dose or convert them to the precise metric units. Therefore, when applicable, we state the original doses in accordance to the source text, and insert recommended doses in metric units in brackets. We feel this is the best solution, as stating the original doses keeps the formulas true to their origins, and suggesting the metric doses helps to make this book more informative and clinically useful for practitioners.

Part I – Overview

Chapter 8

— Concurrent Use of Herbal Medicines and Pharmaceuticals

Herb-drug interaction is a critically important subject, yet there is little extensively definitive information available. Basic understandings of this topic are detailed in Chapter 8 in the first part of *Chinese Medical Herbology and Pharmacology* under "Concurrent Use of Herbal Medicines and Pharmaceuticals." Documented interactions between formulas and drugs are discussed in each formula monograph when relevant. Potential interactions are not included because they require too much assumption and speculation. Formula monographs that do not contain herb-drug interaction information imply that there was no known or documented interaction at the time of publication. Nevertheless, readers are strongly encouraged to stay updated however they can, as new information on herb-drug complementarities and conflicts is being published regularly.

Note: *Chinese Medical Herbology and Pharmacology* documents interactions between <u>individual herbs</u> and drugs, while *Chinese Herbal Formulas and Applications* records interactions between <u>herbal formulas</u> and drugs. Readers are urged to check both sources as needed to assure the safety and compatibility of herb and drug therapies.

Part II

— Formula Monographs

Part II – Formula Monographs

神农 Shén Nóng

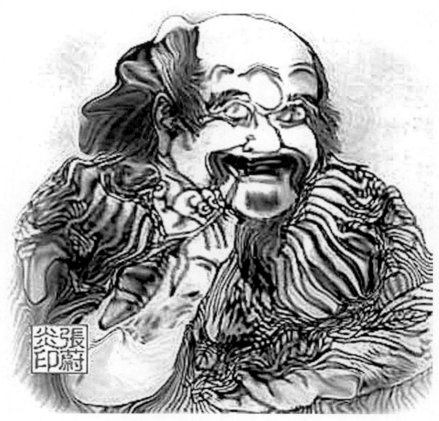

神农 Shén Nóng, dates unknown.

神农 Shén Nóng

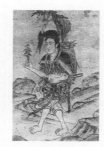

Shen Nong personally picking herbs.

According to folklore and legend, Shen Nong, also known as the "Divine Husbandman," was the person credited for converting the nomads in ancient China from seasonal wanderers into a settled, agricultural society. He taught people what plants to consume as food, when to plant seeds and harvest crops, and how to make tools. In addition, he dedicated his life to searching for herbal medicines to treat disease. He traveled all throughout ancient China, and personally collected and tasted each and every medicinal substance. After years of personal trial and error, he gained an uncommon understanding of the therapeutic effects and side effects of many medicinal substances. He reportedly ingested as many as 70 poisonous substances per day, but used *Cha Ye* (Folium Camelliae) to successfully neutralize these poisons. Unfortunately, Shen Nong died when he experimented with an extremely toxic herb called 断肠草 *Duan Chang Cao*.[1] To commemorate Shen Nong and his contributions to medicine, numerous authors and physicians compiled and published *Shen Nong Ben Cao Jing* (Divine Husbandman's Classic of the Materia Medica) in his name.

Shen Nong Ben Cao Jing (Divine Husbandman's Classic of the Materia Medica) is the first, and one of the most authoritative, texts on Chinese herbal medicine. It contains information on 365 medicinal substances (252 plants, 67 animals, and 46 minerals) including details such as taste, thermal properties, dosages, and toxicity. It also includes descriptions of how to cultivate the herbs, process the herbs, and distinguish true from false herbs. This is one of the earliest records of Chinese herbal medicine, and much of its documentations still holds true today, such as the use of *Ma Huang* (Herba Ephedrae) to treat wheezing and dyspnea, *Hai Zao* (Sargassum) to treat goiter, *Huang Lian* (Rhizoma Coptidis) to stop diarrhea, *Gua Di* (Pedicellus Cucumeris) to induce vomiting, *Lei Wan* (Omphalia) to kill parasites, *Huang Qin* (Radix Scutellariae) to reduce fever, and so on.

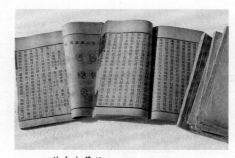

神农本草经 *Shen Nong Ben Cao Jing* (Divine Husbandman's Classic of the Materia Medica) compiled during the second century CE.

[1] 断肠草 *Duan Chang Cao*, literally "break the intestines herb," is a name given to many herbs that are toxic. Historians believe that the actual herb that poisoned and killed Shen Nong was *Gou Wen* (Herba Gelsemii Elegantis). The toxicity of this herb was later documented in great detail in *Ben Cao Gang Mu* (Materia Medica) by Li Shi-Zhen in 1596.

Dynasties & Kingdoms	Year
Xia Dynasty 夏	**2100-1600 BCE**
Shang Dynasty 商	1600-1100 BCE
Zhou Dynasty 周	1100-221 BCE
Qin Dynasty 秦	221-207 BCE
Han Dynasty 汉	206 BCE-220
Three Kingdoms 三国	220-280
Western Jin Dynasty 西晋	265-316
Eastern Jin Dynasty 东晋	317-420
Northern and Southern Dynasties 北南朝	420-581
Sui Dynasty 隋	581-618
Tang Dynasty 唐	618-907
Five Dynasties 五代	907-960
Song Dynasty 宋	960-1279
Liao Dynasty 辽	916-1125
Jin Dynasty 金	1115-1234
Yuan Dynasty 元	1271-1368
Ming Dynasty 明	1368-1644
Qing Dynasty 清	1644-1911
Republic of China 中華民國	1912-Present Day
People's Republic of China 中華人民共和國	1949-Present Day

Table of Contents

Part II Formula Monographs **25**

Biography of Shen Nong 26

Chapter 1 Exterior-Releasing Formulas 29
Chapter 2 Downward Draining Formulas 145
Chapter 3 Harmonizing Formulas 197
Chapter 4 Exterior- and Interior-Releasing Formulas 277
Chapter 5 Heat-Clearing Formulas 309
Chapter 6 Summer-Heat-Dispelling Formulas 429
Chapter 7 Interior-Warming Formulas 451
Chapter 8 Tonic Formulas 507
Chapter 9 *Shen*-Calming Formulas 703
Chapter 10 Orifice-Opening Formulas 739
Chapter 11 Astringent Formulas 765
Chapter 12 Qi-Regulating Formulas 815
Chapter 13 Blood-Regulating Formulas 863
Chapter 14 Wind-Expelling Formulas 959
Chapter 15 Dryness-Relieving Formulas 1017
Chapter 16 Damp-Dispelling Formulas 1059
Chapter 17 Wind-Damp Dispelling Formulas 1149
Chapter 18 Phlegm-Dispelling Formulas 1201
Chapter 19 Reducing, Guiding, and Dissolving Formulas 1259
Chapter 20 Antiparasitic Formulas 1285
Chapter 21 Emetic Formulas 1305
Chapter 22 Formulas that Treat Abscesses and Sores 1317

Chapter 1

— Exterior-Releasing Formulas

解表剂

张仲景 Zhāng Zhòng-Jǐng

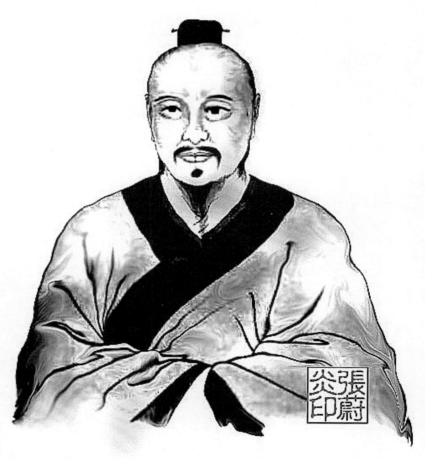

张仲景 Zhāng Zhòng-Jǐng, also known as 张机 Zhāng Jī, 150 – 219 CE.

张仲景 Zhāng Zhòng-Jǐng

Zhang Zhong-Jing, also known as Zhang Ji, was born near the end of the Eastern Han dynasty. During the transition from the collapse of the Eastern Han to the beginning of the Three Kingdoms era, China was ravaged by constant civil war, and people suffered from crime, poverty, infection and death. During a ten-year period near the end of the Eastern Han, two-thirds of the population fell ill and died. Seventy percent of the fatalities were due to *shang han* (cold damage). Although Zhang was from a wealthy family of over 200 members, even his family members could not escape the common fate and many succumbed to the epidemic. Greatly affected by the loss of his family members and the devastating impact of widespread losses in the community and nation, Zhang dedicated his entire life to studying and practicing medicine.

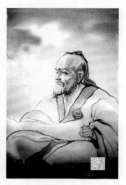

Zhang Zhong-Jing with his manuscripts.

伤寒杂病论*Shang Han Za Bing Lun* (Discussion of Cold-Induced Disorders and Miscellaneous Diseases) is the most famous work by Zhang. This original work later was divided by Wang Shu-He into two volumes: 伤寒论*Shang Han Lun* (Discussion of Cold-Induced Disorders) and 金匮要略 *Jin Gui Yao Lue* (Essentials from the Golden Cabinet).

- *Shang Han Lun* (Discussion of Cold-Induced Disorders) emphasized external disorders, and classified them according to *Liu Jing Bian Zheng* (Six Stages Differentiation).
- *Jin Gui Yao Lue* (Essentials from the Golden Cabinet) focused on internal and miscellaneous diseases, and classified them according to *Ba Gang Bian Zheng* (Eight Principle Differentiation).

Zhang's work clearly established the relationships among disease, progression, complications, treatment strategies, dosage forms, and herbal formulas. Zhang Zhong-Jing forever changed the practice of traditional Chinese medicine. Over 1,700 years after their original publication, his works are still studied as required textbooks in schools of Traditional Chinese Medicine around the world. Many of the formulas he used are still considered to be the standard herbal treatment, such as *Bai Hu Tang* (White Tiger Decoction) for fever, *Bai Tou Weng Tang* (Pulsatilla Decoction) for dysentery, *Yin Chen Hao Tang* (Artemisia Scoparia Decoction) for jaundice, and *Gua Lou Xie Bai Ban Xia Tang* (Trichosanthes Fruit, Chinese Chive, and Pinellia Decoction) for chest pain.

Because of his lasting influence, Zhang Zhong-Jing has always been remembered as 医圣 the Sage of Medicine.

伤寒论*Shang Han Lun* (Discussion of Cold-Induced Disorders)

Dynasties & Kingdoms	Year
Xia Dynasty 夏	2100-1600 BCE
Shang Dynasty 商	1600-1100 BCE
Zhou Dynasty 周	1100-221 BCE
Qin Dynasty 秦	221-207 BCE
Han Dynasty 漢	**206 BCE-220**
Three Kingdoms 三國	220-280
Western Jin Dynasty 西晉	265-316
Eastern Jin Dynasty 東晉	317-420
Northern and Southern Dynasties 北南朝	420-581
Sui Dynasty 隋	581-618
Tang Dynasty 唐	618-907
Five Dynasties 五代	907-960
Song Dynasty 宋	960-1279
Liao Dynasty 遼	916-1125
Jin Dynasty 金	1115-1234
Yuan Dynasty 元	1271-1368
Ming Dynasty 明	1368-1644
Qing Dynasty 清	1644-1911
Republic of China 中華民國	1912-Present Day
People's Republic of China 中華人民共和國	1949-Present Day

Examples of formulas of Zhang Zhong-Jing that are in common use today include:
- *Gui Zhi Tang* (Cinnamon Twig Decoction)
- *Da Cheng Qi Tang* (Major Order the Qi Decoction)
- *Xiao Chai Hu Tang* (Minor Bupleurum Decoction)
- *Bai Hu Tang* (White Tiger Decoction)
- *Li Zhong Wan* (Regulate the Middle Pill)
- *Jin Gui Shen Qi Wan* (Kidney Qi Pill from the Golden Cabinet)
- *Mai Men Dong Tang* (Ophiopogonis Decoction)
- *Wu Mei Wan* (Mume Pill)

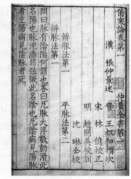

金匮要略 *Jin Gui Yao Lue* (Essentials from the Golden Cabinet)

Chinese Herbal Formulas and Applications

31

Chapter 1 – Exterior-Releasing Formulas

Table of Contents

Chapter 1. Exterior-Releasing Formulas ·· **29**
Biography of Zhang Zhong-Jing ··· 30

Section 1. Acrid and Warm Exterior-Releasing Formulas ······························· **39**
Ma Huang Tang (Ephedra Decoction) ·· 39
  Ma Huang Jia Zhu Tang (Ephedra Decoction plus Atractylodes) ································· 42
  Ma Xing Yi Gan Tang (Ephedra, Apricot Kernel, Coicis, and Licorice Decoction) ······· 43
  San Ao Tang (Three-Unbinding Decoction) ·· 43
Da Qing Long Tang (Major Bluegreen Dragon Decoction) ·· 45
Hua Gai San (Canopy Powder) ·· 48
Jin Fei Cao San (Inula Powder) ·· 49
Gui Zhi Tang (Cinnamon Twig Decoction) ··· 51
  Gui Zhi Jia Ge Gen Tang (Cinnamon Twig Decoction plus Kudzu) ··························· 55
  Gui Zhi Jia Hou Po Xing Zi Tang (Cinnamon Twig Decoction plus Magnolia Bark and Apricot Kernel) ····· 55
  Gui Zhi Jia Shao Yao Tang (Cinnamon Twig Decoction plus Peony) ························· 55
  Gui Zhi Ma Huang Ge Ban Tang (Combined Cinnamon Twig and Ephedra Decoction) ····· 56
Ge Gen Tang (Kudzu Decoction) ·· 59
  Jing Fang Yi Hao (Neck Formula One) ··· 62
  Jing Fang Er Hao (Neck Formula Two) ··· 62
Jiu Wei Qiang Huo Tang (Nine-Herb Decoction with Notopterygium) ···························· 64
  Da Qiang Huo Tang (Major Notopterygium Decoction) ·· 66
Xiang Su San (Cyperus and Perilla Leaf Powder) ·· 67
  Jia Wei Xiang Su San (Augmented Cyperus and Perilla Leaf Powder) ························ 69
  Xiang Su Cong Chi Tang (Cyperus, Perilla Leaf, Scallion, and Prepared Soybean Decoction) ···· 69
Xing Su Yin (Apricot Kernel and Perilla Leaf Decoction) ··· 70
Shi Shen Tang (Ten-Immortal Decoction) ·· 72
Xiao Qing Long Tang (Minor Bluegreen Dragon Decoction) ·· 74
  Xiao Qing Long Jia Shi Gao Tang (Minor Bluegreen Dragon Decoction plus Gypsum) ····· 78
  Jia Jian Xiao Qing Long Tang (Modified Minor Bluegreen Dragon Decoction) ············ 78
She Gan Ma Huang Tang (Belamcanda and Ephedra Decoction) ·· 80
Cang Er Zi San (Xanthium Powder) ·· 82
Xin Yi San (Magnolia Flower Powder) ··· 84
  Xin Yi San (Magnolia Flower Powder) ·· 85
  Jia Wei Xin Yi San (Augmented Magnolia Flower Powder) ·· 85
Qing Bi Tang (Clear the Nose Decoction) ·· 86
  You Bi Tang (Benefit the Nose Decoction) ··· 87

Table of Contents

Chinese Herbal Formulas and Applications

EXTERIOR-RELEASING FORMULAS

1

Section 2. Acrid and Cold Exterior-Releasing Formulas · **89**

Sang Ju Yin (Mulberry Leaf and Chrysanthemum Decoction) · 89

Yin Qiao San (Honeysuckle and Forsythia Powder) · 92

   Yin Qiao Tang (Honeysuckle and Forsythia Decoction) · 94

   Yin Qiao Jie Du San (Honeysuckle and Forsythia Powder to Relieve Toxicity) · · · · · · · · · · · · 95

Ma Huang Xing Ren Gan Cao Shi Gao Tang (Ephedra, Apricot Kernel, Licorice, and Gypsum Decoction) · · · · 96

   Jia Wei Ma Xing Gan Shi Tang (Augmented Ephedra, Apricot Kernel, Licorice, and Gypsum Decoction) · · · · 99

Yue Bi Tang (Maidservant from Yue Decoction) · 101

   Yue Bi Jia Zhu Tang (Maidservant from Yue Decoction plus Atractylodes) · · · · · · · · · · · · · · 102

Sheng Ma Ge Gen Tang (Cimicifuga and Kudzu Decoction) · 103

   Sheng Ma Ge Gen Tang (Cimicifuga and Kudzu Decoction) · 104

   Xuan Du Fa Biao Tang (Dissipate Toxins and Release the Exterior Decoction) · · · · · · · · · · · · 104

Zhu Ye Liu Bang Tang (Lophatherum, Tamarisk and Arctium Decoction) · · · · · · · · · · · · · · · · · 106

Chai Ge Jie Ji Tang (Bupleurum and Kudzu Decoction to Release the Muscle Layer) · · · · · · · · · · · 107

   Chai Ge Jie Ji Tang (Bupleurum and Kudzu Decoction to Release the Muscle Layer) · · · · · · · · · 110

Cong Chi Jie Geng Tang (Scallion, Prepared Soybean, and Platycodon Decoction) · · · · · · · · · · · · 111

   Cong Chi Tang (Scallion and Prepared Soybean Decoction) · 112

   Huo Ren Cong Chi Tang (Scallion and Prepared Soybean Decoction from the Book to Safeguard Life) · · · 112

Ning Sou Wan (Quiet the Cough Pill) · 113

Dun Sou San (Long-Bout Cough Powder) · 115

Zhi Sou San (Stop Coughing Powder) · 116

   Zhi Ke Tang (Stop Coughing Decoction) · 118

Jing Jie Lian Qiao Tang (Schizonepeta and Forsythia Decoction) · 120

Xin Yi Qing Fei Yin (Magnolia Decoction to Clear the Lung) · 122

Section 3. Supporting [the Upright] and Releasing [the Exterior] Formulas · · · · · · · · · · · · · **124**

Bai Du San (Overcome Pathogenic Influences Powder) · 124

   Ren Shen Bai Du San (Ginseng Powder to Overcome Pathogenic Influences) · · · · · · · · · · · · · 126

   Cang Lin San (Old Rice Granary Powder) · 127

Shen Su Yin (Ginseng and Perilla Leaf Decoction) · 128

Zai Zao San (Renewal Powder) · 130

Ma Huang Fu Zi Xi Xin Tang (Ephedra, Asarum, and Prepared Aconite Decoction) · · · · · · · · · · · 132

   Ma Huang Fu Zi Gan Cao Tang (Ephedra, Prepared Aconite, and Licorice Decoction) · · · · · · · · 134

Cong Bai Qi Wei Yin (Scallion Decoction with Seven Ingredients) · 135

Jia Jian Wei Rui Tang (Modified Polygonatum Odoratum Decoction) · · · · · · · · · · · · · · · · · · · 137

   Wei Rui Tang (Polygonatum Odoratum Decoction) · 138

Exterior-Releasing Formulas (Summary) · **139**

33

Chapter 1 — Overview

— Exterior-Releasing Formulas

Definition: Exterior-releasing formulas induce perspiration, release exterior factors from the skin and muscles, and/or promote the eruption of measles. This method of treatment is known as *han fa* (sweating), one of the *ba fa* (eight treatment methods) described in the *Huang Di Nei Jing* (Yellow Emperor's Inner Classic) in the first or second century A.D. The eight treatment methods are outlined in Part I, Chapter 2, of this text.

The term "exterior syndrome" refers to the invasion at superficial parts of the body by one or more of the *liu yin* (six exogenous factors), namely wind, cold, summer-heat, dampness, dryness, and fire. These six exogenous factors attack superficial areas of the body via the skin, mouth or nose. This causes a number of exterior signs and symptoms, such as aversion to cold, fever, headache, muscle aches, a thin, white or yellow tongue coating, and a superficial pulse. While most exterior-releasing formulas are indicated for either wind-cold or wind-heat syndromes, they also treat other disorders, such as abscesses and sores, edema, dysentery or malaria, measles, and the early stages of *wen bing* (warm disease).

> The exterior-releasing method is the most appropriate way to expel disease factors from the skin and muscle layers.

At this early stage of illness, which the disease factor is located at the exterior, the treatment plan should focus on expelling the disease factor from the skin and muscle levels. The exterior-releasing method is the most appropriate method for achieving this goal. If the *liu yin* (six exogenous factors) are not released from the exterior, they may proceed inward to attack the *zang* (solid) and *fu* (hollow) organs, which leads to more serious illness. Thus, treat exterior conditions immediately with exterior-releasing formulas, to prevent complications and deterioration.

SUBCATEGORIES OF ACTION

Since the range of exterior factors interacts with individual constitutional differences, the course and severity of exterior invasion illnesses vary widely. Exterior-releasing formulas are divided into three subcategories, to reflect the characteristics of the herbal formulas appropriate for treatment according to the nature of the disorder and patient constitution.

1. Acrid and Warm Exterior-Releasing Formulas

These formulas treat exterior wind-cold syndromes. Common symptoms when wind and cold invade include aversion to cold, fever, headache, neck and/or shoulder stiffness, soreness and pain of the muscles and extremities, the absence of thirst, no perspiration (or, fever and aversion to cold that persist after perspiration), a thin, white tongue coating, and a superficial, tight or superficial, moderate pulse.

Herbs commonly used to release exterior wind-cold include *Ma Huang* (Herba Ephedrae), *Gui Zhi* (Ramulus Cinnamomi), *Fang Feng* (Radix Saposhnikoviae), *Jing Jie* (Herba Schizonepetae), and *Zi Su Ye* (Folium Perillae). Formulas commonly used to release exterior wind-cold include *Ma Huang Tang* (Ephedra Decoction), *Gui Zhi Tang* (Cinnamon Twig Decoction), *Xiao Qing Long Tang* (Minor Bluegreen Dragon Decoction), and *Jiu Wei Qiang Huo Tang* (Nine-Herb Decoction with Notopterygium).

Chinese Herbal Formulas and Applications

Chapter 1 — Overview

2. Acrid and Cold Exterior-Releasing Formulas

These formulas treat exterior wind-heat syndromes marked by the following commonly seen clinical manifestations: fever, perspiration, slight aversion to wind and cold, headache, thirst, a sore throat, cough, a thin, white or thin, yellow tongue coating, and a superficial, rapid pulse.

Herbs commonly used to release exterior wind-heat include *Bo He* (Herba Menthae), *Niu Bang Zi* (Fructus Arctii), *Sang Ye* (Folium Mori), *Ju Hua* (Flos Chrysanthemi), and *Ge Gen* (Radix Puerariae Lobatae). Formulas commonly used to release exterior wind-heat include *Sang Ju Yin* (Mulberry Leaf and Chrysanthemum Decoction), *Yin Qiao San* (Honeysuckle and Forsythia Powder), and *Ma Huang Xing Ren Gan Cao Shi Gao Tang* (Ephedra, Apricot Kernel, Licorice, and Gypsum Decoction).

3. Supporting [the Upright] and Releasing [the Exterior] Formulas

These formulas are used for constitutionally-deficient patients who are attacked by *liu yin* (six exogenous factors). This situation presents two dilemmas. First, exterior-releasing formulas induce diaphoresis to dispel exterior exogenous factors, but may, in the process, damage yin and body fluids, especially in individuals who already have underlying deficiencies. Second, individuals who have underlying deficiencies often do not have enough *zheng* (upright) *qi* and body fluids (sweat), and are often unable to push out the exterior pathogens, even when they take exterior-releasing herbs.

Therefore, in order to safely dispel exterior pathogenic factors in deficiency patients, the underlying constitution must be supported simultaneously. Supporting and releasing formulas usually consist of both exterior-releasing herbs and qi- or yang-tonifying herbs, to accomplish both goals.

Herbs commonly used to support *zheng* (upright) *qi* include *Ren Shen* (Radix et Rhizoma Ginseng) and *Gan Cao* (Radix et Rhizoma Glycyrrhizae). Formulas that simultaneously support the upright and release the exterior include *Bai Du San* (Overcome Pathogenic Influences Powder), *Zai Zao San* (Renewal Powder), and *Cong Bai Qi Wei Yin* (Scallion Decoction with Seven Ingredients).

CAUTIONS / CONTRAINDICATIONS

- Exterior-releasing formulas are generally taken as warm decoctions to induce perspiration. Mild perspiration over the whole body is ideal. The body may be covered with a blanket to ensure and facilitate perspiration. However, profuse sweating should be avoided, since it may deplete qi and yin, and, in severe cases, cause qi or yang collapse.

~ **Profuse sweating may deplete qi and yin, and, in severe cases, cause qi or yang collapse.** ~

- After taking the decoction, avoid exposure to wind to prevent recurrent attacks.

- Avoid foods that are raw, cold, oily or greasy, as they may decrease absorption and compromise the therapeutic effects of these formulas.

- If interior symptoms are observed along with exterior symptoms, the normal treatment plan is to treat the exterior first, then the interior condition second, or treat both interior and exterior conditions at the same time.

- Exterior-releasing formulas are contraindicated if the disease factor has fully progressed into the interior. These formulas are also contraindicated in the presence of ulcerated sores, erupted measles, deficiency-type edema, and dehydration from vomiting or diarrhea.

PROCESSING

Many exterior-releasing formulas contain acrid herbs to induce sweating. These formulas should not be overcooked, since the essential oils that give these herbs their acrid, aromatic, and diaphoretic effects evaporate very easily. Therefore, many exterior-releasing herbs are post-decocted, added for the last five to ten minutes of cooking.

35

Chapter 1 — Overview

PHARMACOLOGICAL EFFECTS & CLINICAL APPLICATIONS

While exterior-releasing formulas have a wide range of clinical applications, they are primarily used to treat various respiratory and infectious disorders.

Essential oils, which give these herbs their acrid, aromatic, and diaphoretic effects, evaporate very easily.

1. **Cough**: Many exterior-releasing formulas have antitussive effects to suppress cough. *Ma Huang Tang* (Ephedra Decoction) arrests stubborn coughing that manifests after recovery from an exterior condition.[1] *Ma Huang Xing Ren Gan Cao Shi Gao Tang* (Ephedra, Apricot Kernel, Licorice, and Gypsum Decoction) alleviates coughing and dyspnea in cases of asthma or respiratory tract infection.[2] As an active ingredient in both formulas, *Ku Xing Ren* (Semen Armeniacae Amarum) has an inhibitory effect on the respiratory center of the brain, thereby producing antitussive and antiasthmatic effects.[3]

2. **Wheezing and dyspnea**: *Xiao Qing Long Tang* (Minor Bluegreen Dragon Decoction) and *Da Qing Long Tang* (Major Bluegreen Dragon Decoction) are exterior-releasing formulas used to treat wheezing and dyspnea. Several clinical studies have shown *Xiao Qing Long Tang* (Minor Bluegreen Dragon Decoction) to be effective in treating wheezing and dyspnea in patients with acute and chronic bronchial asthma.[4] Other studies indicate that *Da Qing Long Tang* (Major Bluegreen Dragon Decoction) effectively treats wheezing and dyspnea arising from chronic tracheitis.[5]

3. **Asthma**: Many exterior-releasing formulas have marked antiasthmatic effects, and may be used to treat asthma.[6,7] The proposed mechanisms of action include: 1) stimulating beta-adrenoceptors to achieve bronchorelaxation; and 2) inhibiting infiltration of eosinophils into the airway.[8,9] Two formulas that can treat asthma are: *Xiao Qing Long Tang* (Minor Bluegreen Dragon Decoction) and *She Gan Ma Huang Tang* (Belamcanda and Ephedra Decoction).

4. **Bronchitis**: Many exterior-releasing formulas are effective in treatment of bronchitis and related symptoms. *Xiao Qing Long Tang* (Minor Bluegreen Dragon Decoction) has both antibiotic and antiasthmatic effects, and is an excellent formula for treating bronchitis in both children and adults.[10,11,12,13,14] *Ma Huang Xing Ren Gan Cao Shi Gao Tang* (Ephedra, Apricot Kernel, Licorice, and Gypsum Decoction) treats both acute and chronic bronchitis,[15,16] with antitussive qualities to suppress cough,[17] bronchodilating effects to relieve wheezing and dyspnea,[18] and antiallergic influence to reduce swelling and inflammation.[19]

5. **Pneumonia**: Exterior-releasing formulas can treat both the cause and symptoms of pneumonia. For example, *Xiao Qing Long Tang* (Minor Bluegreen Dragon Decoction) and *Yin Qiao San* (Honeysuckle and Forsythia Powder) have antibiotic effects to treat lung infections.[20,21] In addition, *Xiao Qing Long Tang* (Minor Bluegreen Dragon Decoction), *Yin Qiao San* (Honeysuckle and Forsythia Powder), and *Ma Huang Xing Ren Gan Cao Shi Gao Tang* (Ephedra, Apricot Kernel, Licorice, and Gypsum Decoction) address associated symptoms of pneumonia, such as aversion to cold, fever, cough, dyspnea, chest congestion, and the presence of sputum.[22,23]

6. **Respiratory tract disorders**: Exterior-releasing formulas treat various types of respiratory tract disorders. In addition to the examples listed above, indications include rhinitis,[24] allergic rhinitis,[25,26] nasosinusitis,[27] tonsillitis,[28,29] pharyngitis,[30,31] and others.

7. **Nasal disorders**: Exterior wind-releasing formulas effectively treat various nasal disorders, such as sinusitis,[32] rhinitis,[33] and nasal polyps.[34] The mechanisms of action are attributed to antiallergic effects,[35] mast cell stabilizing effects,[36] and anti-inflammatory action, that suppress inflammation of the nasal mucosa.[37] Two representative formulas for treatment of nasal disorders are *Cang Er Zi San* (Xanthium Powder) and *Xin Yi San* (Magnolia Flower Powder).

8. **Fever**: Many formulas in this category have antipyretic effects to treat fever. The mechanisms of the antipyretic effects vary. *Ma Huang Tang* (Ephedra Decoction) and *Gui Zhi Tang* (Cinnamon Twig Decoction) have regulatory effects on body temperature to reduce fever.[38,39] *Ge Gen Tang* (Kudzu Decoction) lowers body temperature by suppressing interferon-induced interleukin-1alpha production.[40] *Yin Qiao San* (Honeysuckle and Forsythia Powder) has a broad spectrum of antibiotic effects to treat infection and fever.[41,42]

Chapter 1 — Overview

Chinese Herbal Formulas and Applications

9. **Common cold and influenza:** Exterior-releasing formulas are frequently used to treat viral infections such as common cold and influenza, with answers to both cause and symptoms. *Ge Gen Tang* (Kudzu Decoction) has antiviral effects to treat infection, and antipyretic and anti-inflammatory effects to alleviate fever and muscle aches and pains.[43,44,45] *Xiao Qing Long Tang* (Minor Bluegreen Dragon Decoction) is useful as both prophylaxis and treatment for influenza viral infection, since its antiviral effects stimulate and increase production of anti-influenza virus antibodies.[46] Lastly, *Yin Qiao San* (Honeysuckle and Forsythia Powder) is one of the most frequently-used formulas for common cold and influenza, since it treats both the cause and symptoms of viral infection with its antibiotic, analgesic, anti-inflammatory and antipyretic activities.[47,48,49]

10. **Infectious disorders:** In addition to the infections listed above, exterior-releasing formulas effectively treat herpes zoster,[50] measles,[51] viral myocarditis,[52] infectious meningitis, and many other disorders.

References

1. *Si Chuan Zhong Yi* (Sichuan Chinese Medicine) 1998;2:29.
2. *Jiang Su Zhong Yi Za Zhi* (Jiangsu Journal of Chinese Medicine) 1965;11:15.
3. Life Sci 1980;27(8):659.
4. *Shan Dong Zhong Yi Xue Yuan Xue Bao* (Journal of Shandong University School of Chinese Medicine) 1992;1:43.
5. *Shi Yong Zhong Xi Yi Jie He Za Zhi* (Practical Journal of Integrated Chinese and Western Medicines) 1998;2:146.
6. *Si Chuan Zhong Yi* (Sichuan Chinese Medicine) 1998;9:42.
7. *Shi Yong Zhong Yi Yao Za Zhi* (Journal of Practical Chinese Medicine and Medicinals) 1997;5:14.
8. Kao ST, Lin CS, Hsieh CC, Hsieh WT, Lin JG. Effects of xiao-qing-long-tang (XQLT) on bronchoconstriction and airway eosinophil infiltration in ovalbumin-sensitized guinea pigs: in vivo and in vitro studies. Allergy 2001 Dec;56(12):1164-71.
9. *Zhong Yi Fang Ji Xian Dai Yan Jiu* (Modern Study of Medical Formulae in Traditional Chinese Medicine) 1997;(1):62.
10. Nagai T, Yamada H. In vivo anti-influenza virus activity of kampo (Japanese herbal) medicine "sho-seiryu-to" and its mode of action Int. J. Immunopharmacol 1994;16:605-13.
11. Kao ST, Lin CS, Hsieh CC, Hsieh WT, Lin JG. Effects of xiao-qing-long-tang (XQLT) on bronchoconstriction and airway eosinophil infiltration in ovalbumin-sensitized guinea pigs: in vivo and in vitro studies. Allergy 2001 Dec;56(12):1164-71.
12. *Zhong Yi Fang Ji Xian Dai Yan Jiu* (Modern Study of Medical Formulae in Traditional Chinese Medicine) 1997;(1):62.
13. *Si Chuan Zhong Yi* (Sichuan Chinese Medicine) 1986;12:15.
14. *Shan Xi Zhong Yi* (Shanxi Chinese Medicine) 1997;4:174.
15. *Shang Hai Zhong Yi Yao Za Zhi* (Shanghai Journal of Chinese Medicine and Herbology) 1986;1:26.
16. *Shang Hai Zhong Yi Yao Za Zhi* (Shanghai Journal of Chinese Medicine and Herbology) 1986;1:26.
17. *Zhong Cheng Yao Yan Jiu* (Research of Chinese Patent Medicine) 1987;(4):47.
18. Kao ST, Yeh TJ, Hsieh CC, Shiau HB, Yeh FT, Lin JG. The effects of Ma-Xing-Gan-Shi-Tang on respiratory resistance and airway leukocyte infiltration in asthmatic guinea pigs. Immunopharmacol Immunotoxicol 2001 Aug;23(3):445-58.
19. Shichijo K, Saito H. Effect of Chinese herbal medicines and disodium cromoglycate on IgE-dependent histamine release from mouse cultured mast cells. Int J Immunopharmacol 1997 Nov-Dec;19(11-12):677-82.
20. Nagai T, Yamada H. In vivo anti-influenza virus activity of kampo (Japanese herbal) medicine "sho-seiryu-to" and its mode of action. Int. J. Immunopharmacol 1994;16:605-13.
21. *Zhong Cheng Yao* (Study of Chinese Patent Medicine) 1990;12(1):22.
22. *Hu Bei Zhong Yi Za Zhi* (Hubei Journal of Chinese Medicine) 1982;1:55.
23. *Zhong Yi Fang Ji Xian Dai Yan Jiu* (Modern Study of Medical Formulae in Traditional Chinese Medicine) 1997;(1):113.
24. *Nan Jing Zhong Yi Yao Da Xue Xue Bao* (Journal of Nanjing University of Traditional Chinese Medicine and Medicinals) 1995;(4):14.
25. *Xin Jiang Zhong Yi Yao* (Xinjiang Chinese Medicine and Herbology) 1996;4:20.
26. *Si Chuan Zhong Yi* (Sichuan Chinese Medicine) 1991;10:46.
27. *Zhong Yi Ming Fang Lin Chuang Xin Yong* (Contemporary Clinical Applications of Classic Chinese Formulas) 2001;646.
28. *Hu Bei Zhong Yi Za Zhi* (Hubei Journal of Chinese Medicine) 1998;2:41.
29. *Fu Jian Zhong Yi Yao* (Fujian Chinese Medicine and Herbology) 1999;4(3).
30. *Jiang Xi Zhong Yi Yao* (Jiangxi Chinese Medicine and Herbology) 1989;4:36.
31. *Fu Jian Zhong Yi Yao* (Fujian Chinese Medicine and Herbology) 1956;(2):13.
32. *Zhe Jiang Zhong Yi Za Zhi* (Zhejiang Journal of Chinese Medicine) 1989;10:454.
33. Yang SH, Hong CY, Yu CL. The stimulatory effects of nasal discharge from patients with perennial allergic rhinitis on normal human neutrophils are normalized after treatment with a new mixed formula of Chinese herbs. International Immunopharmacology 2002 Nov;2(12):1627-39.
34. *Fu Jian Zhong Yi Yao* (Fujian Chinese Medicine and Herbology) 1991;6:17.
35. *Zhong Guo Yao Li Xue Bao* (Chinese Herbal Pharmacology Journal) 1990;5:34.
36. Shichijo K, Saito H. Effect of Chinese herbal medicines and disodium cromoglycate on IgE-dependent histamine release from mouse cultured mast cells. Int J Immunopharmacol 1997 Nov-Dec;19(11-12):677-82.

Chapter 1 — Overview

37. Yang SH, Hong CY, Yu CL. The stimulatory effects of nasal discharge from patients with perennial allergic rhinitis on normal human neutrophils are normalized after treatment with a new mixed formula of Chinese herbs. International Immunopharmacology 2002 Nov;2(12):1627-39.

38. *Zhong Yi Za Zhi* (Journal of Chinese Medicine) 1984;(8):623.

39. *Zhong Yao Yao Li Yu Ying Yong* (Pharmacology and Applications of Chinese Herbs) 1987;3(2):1.

40. Kurokawa M, Kumeda CA, Yamamura J, Kamiyama T, Shiraki K. Antipyretic activity of cinnamyl derivatives and related compounds in influenza virus-infected mice. Eur J Pharmacol 1998 May 1;348(1):45-51.

41. *Zhong Cheng Yao* (Study of Chinese Patent Medicine) 1990;12(1):22.

42. *Liao Ning Zhong Yi Za Zhi* (Liaoning Journal of Chinese Medicine) 1994;12:548.

43. Kurokawa M, Tsurita M, Brown J, Fukuda Y, Shiraki K. Effect of interleukin-12 level augmented by Kakkon-to, a herbal medicine, on the early stage of influenza infection in mice. Antiviral Res 2002 Nov;56(2):183-8.

44. Kurokawa M, Kumeda CA, Yamamura J, Kamiyama T, Shiraki K. Antipyretic activity of cinnamyl derivatives and related compounds in influenza virus-infected mice. Eur J Pharmacol 1998 May 1;348(1):45-51.

45. Ozaki Y. Studies on antiinflammatory effect of Japanese Oriental medicines (kampo medicines) used to treat inflammatory diseases. Biol Pharm Bull 1995 Apr;1(4):559-62.

46. Nagai T, Yamada H. In vivo anti-influenza virus activity of kampo (Japanese herbal) medicine "sho-seiryu-to" and its mode of action. Int. J. Immunopharmacol 1994;16:605-613

47. *Zhong Cheng Yao* (Study of Chinese Patent Medicine) 1990;12(1):22.

48. *Zhong Yi Za Zhi* (Journal of Chinese Medicine) 1986;27(3):59.

49. *Zhong Yao Tong Bao* (Journal of Chinese Herbology) 1986;11(1):51.

50. *Xin Zhong Yi* (New Chinese Medicine) 1977;51.

51. Huang SP, Shieh GJ, Lee L, Teng HJ, Kao ST, Lin JG. Inhibition effect of shengma-gegen-tang on measles virus in Vero cells and human peripheral blood mononuclear cells. American Journal of Chinese Medicine 1997;25(1):89-96.

52. *Hu Nan Zhong Yi Za Zhi* (Hunan Journal of Chinese Medicine) 1997;4:29.

Chinese Herbal Formulas and Applications

Section 1

幸温解表剂
— Acrid and Warm Exterior-Releasing Formulas

EXTERIOR-RELEASING FORMULAS

1

Má Huáng Tāng (Ephedra Decoction)
麻黄湯
麻黄汤

Pinyin Name: *Ma Huang Tang*
Literal Name: Ephedra Decoction
Alternate Names: Ma-huang Decoction, Mahuang Combination
Original Source: *Shang Han Lun* (Discussion of Cold-Induced Disorders) by Zhang Zhong-Jing in the Eastern Han Dynasty

COMPOSITION

Ma Huang (Herba Ephedrae)	9g [6g]
Gui Zhi (Ramulus Cinnamomi)	6g [4g]
Ku Xing Ren (Semen Armeniacae Amarum)	70 kernels [9g]
Zhi Gan Cao (Radix et Rhizoma Glycyrrhizae Praeparata cum Melle)	3g

DOSAGE / PREPARATION / ADMINISTRATION

The source text instructs to cook *Ma Huang* (Herba Ephedrae) first with 9 cups [1,800 mL] of water until 7 cups [1,400 mL] of the liquid remain. Remove the foam from the top, add in the other ingredients, and cook until the liquid is reduced to 2.5 cups [500 mL]. Take 0.8 cup [160 mL] of the warm, strained decoction and cover the body with blankets to promote slight perspiration. Today, the decoction may be prepared using the doses suggested in brackets.

CHINESE THERAPEUTIC ACTIONS

1. Induces diaphoresis and releases the exterior
2. Ventilates the Lung and relieves dyspnea

CLINICAL MANIFESTATIONS

Exterior-excess, wind-cold syndrome: aversion to cold, fever, headache, neck stiffness, body aches and pains, absence of perspiration, dyspnea, a thin, white tongue coating, and a superficial, tight pulse.

CLINICAL APPLICATIONS

Fever, upper respiratory tract infection, common cold, influenza, bronchitis, pneumonia, asthma, wheezing and dyspnea, cough, peripheral neuropathy, enuresis, mastitis, anhidrosis, allergic rhinitis, and acute nephritis.

EXPLANATION

Ma Huang Tang (Ephedra Decoction) was first cited in the *Shang Han Lun* (Discussion of Cold-Induced Disorders) for the treatment of *taiyang* cold syndrome. This syndrome refers to attack by wind-cold at the exterior, with cold being the dominant factor. Because the location of the wind-cold attack is at the exterior or superficial level of the body, *wei* (defensive) *qi* is the main force of defense.

When cold attacks the exterior of the body, it causes the whole body to constrict. The constriction impedes the circulation of *wei* (defensive) *qi* at the exterior and *ying* (nutritive) *qi* in the interior. The impeded circulation leads to blockage of qi and blood in the channels, which then causes headaches, body aches, pain, and other symptoms. Fever and aversion to cold occur as a result of the battle between *wei qi* and the wind-cold factor.

Since the Lung is usually the first target organ of the exterior pathogenic factors, dyspnea may occur as a result of cold constricting the Lung and causing the Lung qi to flow in a reversed direction. Since the body is constricted by cold and the skin pores are closed, there will be no perspiration. A superficial, tight pulse is a sign of exterior excess cold. The tongue coating, which is not affected

39

Chapter 1 – Exterior-Releasing Formulas   *Section 1 – Acrid and Warm Exterior-Releasing Formulas*

Má Huáng Tāng (Ephedra Decoction)

Ma Huang Tang (Ephedra Decoction)

Diagnosis	Signs and Symptoms	Treatment	Herbs
Exterior-excess, wind-cold syndrome	• Fever and aversion to cold: exterior wind-cold condition • Absence of perspiration and a tight pulse: exterior excess condition • Dyspnea: reversed flow of Lung qi • Body aches and pains: blocked circulation of qi and blood • Superficial, tight pulse: exterior wind-cold condition	• Induces diaphoresis and releases the exterior • Ventilates the Lung and relieves dyspnea	• *Ma Huang* (Herba Ephedrae) induces diaphoresis, releases exterior wind-cold, and relieves dyspnea. • *Gui Zhi* (Ramulus Cinnamomi) disperses wind-cold and unblocks the channels and collaterals. • *Ku Xing Ren* (Semen Armeniacae Amarum) guides Lung qi downward and relieves dyspnea. • *Zhi Gan Cao* (Radix et Rhizoma Glycyrrhizae Praeparata cum Melle) harmonizes the herbs.

because the disease is still located at the exterior, remains thin and white.

Ma Huang (Herba Ephedrae), the chief herb, is acrid, bitter and warm. It effectively dispels cold and releases the exterior through diaphoresis. In addition, it relieves dyspnea and cough by expanding the Lung and soothing Lung qi. *Gui Zhi* (Ramulus Cinnamomi), the deputy herb, helps the chief herb disperse the wind-cold factor. It unblocks stagnation in the *ying* (nutritive) level and pushes the pathogenic factors outward to the *wei* (defensive) level. Because *Gui Zhi* (Ramulus Cinnamomi) is acrid and warm in nature, it alleviates pain by promoting the circulation of qi and blood in the channels and collaterals.

Ku Xing Ren (Semen Armeniacae Amarum), the assistant herb, helps *Ma Huang* (Herba Ephedrae) relieve dyspnea by guiding Lung qi downward. Together, the ventilating property of *Ma Huang* (Herba Ephedrae) and the descending property of *Ku Xing Ren* (Semen Armeniacae Amarum) regulate the functioning of the Lung to restore normal respiration.

Zhi Gan Cao (Radix et Rhizoma Glycyrrhizae Praeparata cum Melle) serves three functions in this formula. As the envoy herb, it tonifies the middle *jiao*. It also moderates the potent exterior-releasing effects of *Ma Huang* (Herba Ephedrae) and *Gui Zhi* (Ramulus Cinnamomi), so that these two herbs can induce perspiration without damaging *zheng* (upright) *qi*. Lastly, it harmonizes the contrasting directional tendencies of *Ma Huang* (Herba Ephedrae) to ventilate outward and *Ku Xing Ren* (Semen Armeniacae Amarum) to guide qi downward.

MODIFICATIONS

• For muscle aches and pains caused by exterior attack of wind, cold, and dampness, add *Cang Zhu* (Rhizoma Atractylodis) and *Yi Yi Ren* (Semen Coicis).
• If a sore throat is present, reduce the dose of *Gui Zhi* (Ramulus Cinnamomi) by half; and add *Tian Hua Fen* (Radix Trichosanthis) and *She Gan* (Rhizoma Belamcandae).
• For coughing, profuse sputum, dyspnea, and chest fullness caused by wind-cold affecting the Lung, remove *Gui Zhi* (Ramulus Cinnamomi); and add *Zi Su Zi* (Fructus Perillae), *Sang Bai Pi* (Cortex Mori), *Chi Fu Ling* (Poria Rubra), and *Chen Pi* (Pericarpium Citri Reticulatae).

CAUTIONS / CONTRAINDICATIONS

• *Ma Huang Tang* is extremely acrid and warm, and, if used incorrectly, may induce profuse perspiration and damage the qi and yin of the body. Therefore, it should only be used in conditions having all of the following characteristics: wind, cold, exterior, and excess.
• This formula should be used with caution in the following patients: elderly patients and individuals with generalized weakness.
• This formula is not recommended for the following syndromes: exterior wind-heat syndrome; exterior febrile conditions; transformation of wind-cold to wind-heat; interior heat; damp-heat accumulation; and qi or blood deficiency.
• This formula is not suitable for individuals with the following conditions: thirst caused by deficiency of body fluids; spontaneous sweating due to *wei* (defensive) *qi* deficiency, weak pulse from deficient conditions, rapid pulse from excess conditions; and palpitations and a sensation of heaviness in the body as a result of misuse of herbs.

40

Má Huáng Tāng (Ephedra Decoction)

- This formula is contraindicated in the following conditions: individuals with ulceration, abscesses and sores; *lin zheng* (dysuria syndrome); and patients with bleeding or excessive bleeding on the verge of collapse.
- This formula should be taken as a warm decoction to induce diaphoresis. Once the desired effect is achieved, it should be discontinued immediately. However, if exterior symptoms and signs still persist after sweating, *Gui Zhi Tang* (Cinnamon Twig Decoction) should be administered instead to harmonize the *wei* (defensive) and *ying* (nutritive) levels, and to mildly induce diaphoresis. On the other hand, if the use of *Ma Huang Tang* causes excessive and prolonged perspiration, sweating must be stopped to avoid collapse. For this purpose, use astringent herbs such as *Ma Huang Gen* (Radix et Rhizoma Ephedrae), calcined *Long Gu* (Os Draconis), and calcined *Mu Li* (Concha Ostreae).
- After taking this formula, some patients may notice nosebleeds or signs of irritability, which indicate transformation of wind-cold into heat. Should this happen, reduce the dose of the formula, and the heat will dissipate spontaneously. If the symptoms become worse, however, *Ma Huang Tang* should be discontinued, and an appropriate heat-clearing formula should be given.
- Rare cases of allergic rash have been reported following the use of *Ma Huang Tang*.[1]

PHARMACOLOGICAL EFFECTS

1. **Effect on temperature regulation**: In rabbits with artificially-induced fever, intravenous injection of a *Ma Huang Tang* preparation at the dose of 1 g/kg was effective in reducing the body temperature within 30 minutes. In mice with normal body temperature, intraperitoneal injection of a *Ma Huang Tang* preparation at the dose of 5 g/kg reduced the body temperature by 5°C after 30 minutes.[2]
2. **Antitussive**: In a laboratory study evaluating the effect of *Ma Huang Tang* in relieving cough, a number of mice were divided into herb-group or placebo-group. The mice in the herb-group received intraperitoneal injection of the herbs at the dose of 5 g/kg, while the placebo group received saline injection. The mice were exposed to ammonia to induce cough. After 5 minutes, the mice in the herb-group coughed an average of 17.70 times, while the mice in the placebo-group cough 44.96 times.[3]
3. **Antibiotic**: According to *in vitro* studies, *Ma Huang Tang* demonstrated inhibitory effects against *E. coli* and *Staphylococcus aureus*, and antiviral effects against respiratory syncytial virus.[4,5]
4. **Cardiovascular**: In one *in vitro* study, intravenous administration of *Ma Huang Tang* at 2-3 g/kg in rabbits was associated with an initial drop in blood pressure, followed by a rise of 10-20 mmHg. It was noted that repeated administration was associated with tolerance, and that use of a larger dose was associated with increased depth and rate of respiration as well as increased heart rate.[6] In one *in vivo* study involving 7 healthy human males (age, 22.3 +/- 1.8 years old), administration of *Ma Huang Tang* induced an increase in blood pressure, heart rate, stroke volume, cardiac output and cardiac index, but a decrease in total peripheral resistance. The study speculated that comprehensive mechanisms of *Ma Huang Tang* were not only dependent of ephedrine, the main active constituent of *Ma Huang* (Herba Ephedrae), but also dependent on the vasodilatory action of *Gui Zhi* (Ramulus Cinnamomi).[7]
5. **Radioprotective**: Intraperitoneal injection of *Ma Huang Tang* was associated with marked protective effects in mice against skin injury induced by irradiation.[8]

CLINICAL STUDIES AND RESEARCH

1. **Fever**: Thirteen children with high fever ranging between 38-40.1°C (100.4-104.2°F) were treated with 6 doses of *Ma Huang Tang* with reduction of body temperature in all patients.[9]
2. **Upper respiratory tract infection**: Two hundred and ninety-two children with upper respiratory tract infection and fever over 38°C / 100.4°F were treated with *Ma Huang Tang* with satisfactory results. The study reported complete recovery in 196 cases within 24 hours, 86 cases within 48 hours, and 10 cases with no improvement. The overall rate of effectiveness was 96.5%.[10]
3. **Cough**: Use of modified *Ma Huang Tang* to treat stubborn cough after recovery from an exterior condition demonstrated a rate of effectiveness of 92%. The herbal treatment contained this formula plus *Pi Pa Ye* (Folium Eriobotryae) and others as the base formula, with addition of *Dan Nan Xing* (Arisaema cum Bile) and *Ban Xia* (Rhizoma Pinelliae) for profuse sputum; *Huang Qin* (Radix Scutellariae) and *Shi Gao* (Gypsum Fibrosum) for yellow, sticky sputum; *He Zi* (Fructus Chebulae) and *Tian Hua Fen* (Radix Trichosanthis) for a sore throat and a hoarse voice; *Xuan Shen* (Radix Scrophulariae), *Mai Dong* (Radix Ophiopogonis), and *Sha Shen* (Radix Glehniae seu Adenophorae) for the presence of thick, sticky sputum that is difficult to expectorate and a red tongue body with a thin coating; and *Huang Qi* (Radix Astragali) and *Fang Feng* (Radix Saposhnikoviae) for fatigue and profuse perspiration. Of 26 patients, the study reported complete recovery in 18 cases, improvement in 6 cases, and no improvement in 2 cases.[11]
4. **Peripheral neuropathy**: Use of modified *Ma Huang Tang* to treat 38 patients with peripheral neuropathy resulted in an effectiveness rate of 68.75%. The herbal formula contained *Ma Huang* (Herba Ephedrae), *Gui Zhi* (Ramulus

Chapter 1 – Exterior-Releasing Formulas   *Section 1 – Acrid and Warm Exterior-Releasing Formulas*

Má Huáng Tāng (Ephedra Decoction)

Cinnamomi), *Zhi Gan Cao* (Radix et Rhizoma Glycyrrhizae Praeparata cum Melle), and *Ju Luo* (Vascular Citri Reticulatae). The treatment protocol was to administer the herbs in powder form three times daily for 3 weeks. Clinical improvements included increased physical sensation and reduced pain and numbness. Of 38 patients, the study reported significant improvement in 4 patients, moderate improvement in 22 patients, and no benefit in 12 patients.[12]

5. **Enuresis**: Administration of modified *Ma Huang Tang* was effective in treating enuresis in 10 children between 6-12 years of age with 3-9 years history of illness. The herbal formula contained *Ma Huang* (Herba Ephedrae) 5g, *Gui Zhi* (Ramulus Cinnamomi) 3g, *Sang Piao Xiao* (Ootheca Mantidis) 3g, *Jin Ying Zi* (Fructus Rosae Laevigatae) 3g, and *Gan Cao* (Radix et Rhizoma Glycyrrhizae) 2g. The dose of *Ma Huang* (Herba Ephedrae) was decreased to 4g in the summer, and increased to 6g in the winter. In addition to this base formula, *Dang Shen* (Radix Codonopsis) 6g was added for qi deficiency; and *Ba Ji Tian* (Radix Morindae Officinalis) 3g and *Yi Zhi* (Fructus Alpiniae Oxyphyllae) 3g were added for yang deficiency. The treatment protocol was to cook all the herbs together, and administer the decoction in two equally-divided doses daily. The study reported complete recovery in 9 of 10 patients within 3 to 6 packs of herbs.[13]

6. **Mastitis**: Modified *Ma Huang Tang* effectively treated 71 patients with acute mastitis with elevated white blood cells count and fever (58 patients with temperature over 38°C / 100.4°F). The base formula included *Ma Huang Tang* plus *Pu Gong Ying* (Herba Taraxaci) and *Jin Yin Hua* (Flos Lonicerae Japonicae), with the addition of *Lou Lu* (Radix Rhapontici) for obstructed flow of breast milk. The herbs were given in decoction, with most patients having significant improvement to complete recovery within 2 days. The overall rate of effectiveness was 98%.[14]

HERB-DRUG INTERACTION

Interferon-induced adverse reactions: Concurrent use of two separate herbal formulas reduced the adverse effects of interferon in hepatitis C patients. Of 28 patients with chronic hepatitis C, 8 patients in Group A received both interferon-beta and *Ma Huang Tang*, and 4 patients in Group B received both interferon-beta and *Da Qing Long Tang* (Major Bluegreen Dragon Decoction), and 16 patients in Group C received only interferon-beta. Adverse effects were evaluated and monitored by clinical and laboratory examinations. At the end of the treatment, patients in Group A and B had significantly lower incidences than Group C of discomfort, fever, general malaise, paresthesia and arthralgia. HCV-RNA was negative in all patients. Based on this information, the study concluded that the use of these two formulas may reduce the adverse effects accompanying interferon-beta treatment in patients with chronic hepatitis C without reducing the antiviral effects.[15]

Another study also reported positive results using *Ma Huang Tang* and interferon-beta in 18 patients with chronic hepatitis C. The treatment protocol was to administer *Ma Huang Tang* immediately before, immediately after, and 1 hour after interferon-beta administration. The study reported that patients who received both herbs and drug had significantly less adverse reactions such as general malaise, arthralgia and discomfort, compared to patients in the control group who did not receive the herbs. *Ma Huang Tang* did not affect plasma concentrations of interleukin-1beta and TNF-alpha. The study concluded that *Ma Huang Tang* was effective in reducing the flu-like symptoms accompanying interferon-beta and in improving the biochemical response rate.[16]

TOXICOLOGY

The LD_{50} of *Ma Huang Tang* in mice administered via intraperitoneal injection is 28.51 g/kg within 24 hours.[17]

RELATED FORMULAS

Má Huáng Jiā Zhú Tāng

(Ephedra Decoction plus Atractylodes)

麻黃加術湯
麻黄加术汤

Pinyin Name: Ma Huang Jia Zhu Tang
Literal Name: Ephedra Decoction plus Atractylodes
Original Source: *Jin Gui Yao Lue* (Essentials from the Golden Cabinet) by Zhang Zhong-Jing in the Eastern Han Dynasty

Ma Huang (Herba Ephedrae)	9g [6g]
Gui Zhi (Ramulus Cinnamomi)	6g [4g]
Ku Xing Ren (Semen Armeniacae Amarum)	70 kernels [9g]
Zhi Gan Cao (Radix et Rhizoma Glycyrrhizae Praeparata cum Melle)	3g
Bai Zhu (Rhizoma Atractylodis Macrocephalae)	12g [9g]

The source text states to cook *Ma Huang* (Herba Ephedrae) with 9 cups [1,800 mL] of water until 7 cups [1,400 mL] of liquid remain. Remove the foam on the top, add in the other ingredients, and cook until the liquid is reduced to 2.5 cups [500 mL]. Take 0.8 cup [160 mL] of the warm, strained decoction and cover the body with blankets to promote slight perspiration. Today, the decoction may be prepared using the doses suggested in brackets.

Ma Huang Jia Zhu Tang (Ephedra Decoction plus Atractylodes) induces diaphoresis, releases the exterior, disperses

42

Má Huáng Tāng (Ephedra Decoction)

cold, and dispel dampness. It treats exterior-excess, wind-cold syndrome with damp accumulation. Dampness may form inside the body following a wind-cold attack and block the qi flow, causing aches and pains and a feeling of heaviness all over the body. *Bai Zhu* (Rhizoma Atractylodis Macrocephalae) is added to dry dampness, relieve the aches and pains, and dispel the sensation of heaviness caused by cold and dampness.

Ma Huang Jia Zhu Tang treats wind-cold invasion with damp accumulation. It is best for patients with pre-existing dampness, who experience a wind-cold invasion. These patients tend to be heavier in weight or have Spleen qi deficiency. *Bai Zhu* (Rhizoma Atractylodis Macrocephalae) dries dampness, enhances the water-dispelling action of *Ma Huang* (Herba Ephedrae), and prevents profuse perspiration. This formula should never be prescribed to someone who has wind-heat invasion or deficiency manifesting in perspiration. Ideally, after taking the formula, the patient should feel a sensation of warmth and experience a slight perspiration. The dose of *Ma Huang* (Herba Ephedrae) should never be increased to induce profuse perspiration, since this may cause yin deficiency.

Má Xìng Yì Gān Tāng

(Ephedra, Apricot Kernel, Coicis, and Licorice Decoction)
麻杏薏甘湯
麻杏苡甘汤
Pinyin Name: Ma Xing Yi Gan Tang
Literal Name: Ephedra, Apricot Kernel, Coicis, and Licorice Decoction
Alternate Names: *Ma Huang Xing Ren Yi Yi Gan Cao Tang, Ma Hsing I Kan Tang, Ma Xing Yi Gan Tang,* Ephedra, Apricot, Coix and Licorice Decoction; Ma-huang and Coix Decoction, Mahuang and Coix Combination
Original Source: *Jin Gui Yao Lue* (Essentials from the Golden Cabinet) by Zhang Zhong-Jing in the Eastern Han Dynasty

Ma Huang (Herba Ephedrae)	1.5g [6g]
Ku Xing Ren (Semen Armeniacae Amarum), *chao* (dry-fried)	10 kernels [6g]
Zhi Gan Cao (Radix et Rhizoma Glycyrrhizae Praeparata cum Melle)	3g
Yi Yi Ren (Semen Coicis)	1.5g [12g]

The source text states to grind the ingredients coarsely, then cook 12g with 1.5 large bowls of water until the liquid is reduced to 80%. Take the strained decoction while warm. If sweating occurs after taking the formula, avoid exposure to wind. Today, this formula may be prepared as a decoction with the doses suggested in brackets.

Ma Xing Yi Gan Tang (Ephedra, Apricot Kernel, Coicis, and Licorice Decoction) releases the exterior and dispels dampness. Clinically, patients will have pain all over the whole body, and fever that is most prominent in the afternoon. The exterior-releasing effect of this formula is not as strong as *Ma Huang Tang*, since *Gui Zhi* (Ramulus Cinnamomi) is omitted from the formula, and the doses of all the herbs are drastically reduced.

Wind-cold generally turns into wind-heat if not treated properly. This formula does not contain warm herbs, such as *Gui Zhi* (Ramulus Cinnamomi) or *Bai Zhu* (Rhizoma Atractylodis Macrocephalae). Instead, a cool herb, *Yi Yi Ren* (Semen Coicis), is used instead to dispel dampness. Clinical applications of this formula include rheumatic arthritis, rheumatism, neuralgia, general aches and pains of the muscles and joints, keratosis, palmaris, keratosis plantaris, warts, and eczema.

Sān Ăo Tāng (Three-Unbinding Decoction)
三拗湯
三拗汤
Pinyin Name: San Ao Tang
Literal Name: Three-Unbinding Decoction
Original Source: *Tai Ping Hui Min He Ji Ju Fang* (Imperial Grace Formulary of the Tai Ping Era) by the Imperial Medical Department in 1078-85

Ma Huang (Herba Ephedrae)
Ku Xing Ren (Semen Armeniacae Amarum)
Gan Cao (Radix et Rhizoma Glycyrrhizae)

The source text instructs to grind equal portions of all three herbs into a coarse powder. Cook 15g of the powder with 5 slices of *Sheng Jiang* (Rhizoma Zingiberis Recens) in 1.5 large bowls of water until it is reduced to 1 bowl. After taking the strained decoction, the patient is advised to go to bed and stay covered until a mild perspiration has been induced.

San Ao Tang (Three-Unbinding Decoction) treats exterior wind-cold invasion by ventilating the Lung and expelling exterior factors. Clinically, it treats common colds caused by wind, and characterized by symptoms such as stuffy nose, a sensation of heaviness in the body, hoarseness of voice, headache, vertigo, lethargy, coughing with sputum, chest fullness, and shortness of breath.

Chapter 1 – Exterior-Releasing Formulas   *Section 1 – Acrid and Warm Exterior-Releasing Formulas*

Má Huáng Tāng (Ephedra Decoction)

AUTHORS' COMMENTS

Although *Ma Huang Tang* can treat common cold, influenza, acute bronchitis, and asthma caused by excess wind-cold invasion, it is rarely prescribed today. Rather, it serves as a foundation formula, to which other herbs are added.

"*Ma Huang Tang* must have *Gui Zhi* (Ramulus Cinnamomi) and *Gui Zhi Tang* (Cinnamon Twig Decoction) must **not** have *Ma Huang* (Herba Ephedrae)" is the classic guiding principle of these two formulas for the following reasons.

- *Ma Huang Tang* treats an exterior-excess, wind-cold condition with pathogenic factors affecting the *wei* (defensive) level and reaching the *ying* (nutritive) level. *Ma Huang Tang* needs *Gui Zhi* (Ramulus Cinnamomi) to harmonize the *wei* (defensive) and *ying* (nutritive) levels, so that *Ma Huang* (Herba Ephedrae) can safely and effectively dispel wind-cold from the exterior.
- *Gui Zhi Tang* (Cinnamon Twig Decoction) treats an exterior-deficient, wind-cold condition with perspiration. *Ma Huang* (Herba Ephedrae) must **not** be used to avoid profuse perspiration and excessive loss of body fluids. The use of *Ma Huang* (Herba Ephedrae) in someone who is already deficient will only worsen their condition and contribute to greater deficiency.[18]

Ma Huang Tang and *Gui Zhi Tang* (Cinnamon Twig Decoction) are two representative formulas for treating exterior wind-cold. Both formulas contain *Gui Zhi* (Ramulus Cinnamomi) and *Zhi Gan Cao* (Radix et Rhizoma Glycyrrhizae Praeparata cum Melle). The differences are as follow:

- *Ma Huang Tang* contains *Ma Huang* (Herba Ephedrae) and *Ku Xing Ren* (Semen Armeniacae Amarum) to treat exterior-***excess*** wind-cold condition affecting the Lung functions, causing dyspnea, cough and wheezing. After taking the herbal decoction, patients should cover up to induce more sweating.
- *Gui Zhi Tang* contains *Bai Shao* (Radix Paeoniae Alba) and *Da Zao* (Fructus Jujubae) to treat exterior-***deficient***, wind-cold invasion with disharmony of the *ying* (nutritive) and *wei* (defensive) levels. Because of deficiency, patients should eat porridge after taking the decoction to strengthen the body and to promote sweating.[19]

Ma Huang Jia Zhu Tang (Ephedra Decoction plus Atractylodes) and *Ma Xing Yi Gan Tang* (Ephedra, Apricot Kernel, Coicis, and Licorice Decoction), both derived from *Ma Huang Tang*, are indicated for pain with dampness associated with wind-cold invasion.

- *Ma Huang Jia Zhu Tang* contains *Bai Zhu* (Rhizoma Atractylodis Macrocephalae) to dry dampness and relieve pain that is associated with damp accumulation. In addition, *Bai Zhu* (Rhizoma Atractylodis Macrocephalae) prevents over-sweating from the use of *Ma Huang* (Herba Ephedrae). This formula is suitable for those patients with aversion to cold, fever, and absence of perspiration.
- *Ma Xing Yi Gan Tang* treats pain of lesser severity than *Ma Huang Jia Zhu Tang*. Besides pain, patients often experience fever that is more severe in the afternoon, which indicates that the wind-cold condition is turning into heat. For this reason, *Bai Zhu* (Rhizoma Atractylodis Macrocephalae) and *Gui Zhi* (Ramulus Cinnamomi), both warm in property, are not used, but instead, *Yi Yi Ren* (Semen Coicis) is selected.[20]

References

1. *Jiang Xi Yi Yao Za Zhi* (Jiangxi Journal of Medicine and Herbology) 1985;(10):32.
2. *Zhong Yi Za Zhi* (Journal of Chinese Medicine) 1984;(8):623.
3. *Zhong Yi Za Zhi* (Journal of Chinese Medicine) 1984;(8):623.
4. *Zhong Yuan Yi Kan* (Resource Journal of Chinese Medicine) 1955;(10):36.
5. *He Han Yi Yao Xue Hui Zhi* (Hehan Journal of Medicine and Herbology) 1986;3(3):364.
6. *Zhong Yi Za Zhi* (Journal of Chinese Medicine) 1982;(8):623.
7. Xu FH, Uebaba K. Effect of Kampo formulations (traditional Chinese medicine) on circulatory parameters. Acupuncture & Electro-Therapeutics Research 1999;24(1):11-28.
8. Wang CM, Ohta S, Shinoda M. Studies on chemical protectors against radiation. XXIX. Protective effects of methanol extracts of various Chinese traditional medicines on skin injury induced by X-irradiation. Yakugaku Zasshi 1990 Mar;110(3):218-24.
9. *Nei Meng Gu Zhong Yi Yao* (Traditional Chinese Medicine and Medicinals of Inner Mongolia) 1990;(1):28.
10. *Quan Guo Zhong Yi Er Ke Xue* (National Chinese Pediatrics) 1987;12(8):49.
11. *Si Chuan Zhong Yi* (Sichuan Chinese Medicine) 1998;2:29.
12. *Zhe Jiang Zhong Yi Xue Yuan Xue Bao* (Journal of Zhejiang University of Chinese Medicine) 1996;1:24.
13. *Si Chuan Zhong Yi* (Sichuan Chinese Medicine) 1996;3:38.
14. *Zhong Yuan Yi Kan* (Resource Journal of Chinese Medicine) 1990;4:9.
15. Kainuma M, Hayashi J, Sakai S, Imai K, Mantani N, Kohta K, Mitsuma T, Shimada Y, Kashiwagi S, Terasawa K. The efficacy of herbal medicine (kampo) in reducing the adverse effects of IFN-beta in chronic hepatitis C. American Journal of Chinese Medicine 2002;30(2-3):355-67.
16. Kainuma M, Sakai S, Sekiya N, Mantani N, Ogata N, Shimada Y, and Terasawa K. The effects of a herbal medicine (Mao-to) in patients with chronic hepatitis C after injection of IFN-beta. Phytomedicine 2004 Jan;11(1):5-10.
17. *Zhong Yi Za Zhi* (Journal of Chinese Medicine) 1984;(8):623.
18. Wang MZ, et al. *Zhong Yi Xue Wen Da Ti Ku* (Questions and Answers on Traditional Chinese Medicine: Herbal Formulas).
19. Wang MZ, et al. *Zhong Yi Xue Wen Da Ti Ku* (Questions and Answers on Traditional Chinese Medicine: Herbal Formulas).
20. Wang MZ, et al. *Zhong Yi Xue Wen Da Ti Ku* (Questions and Answers on Traditional Chinese Medicine: Herbal Formulas).

Chinese Herbal Formulas and Applications

Dà Qīng Lóng Tāng (Major Bluegreen Dragon Decoction)

大青龍湯
大青龙汤

Pinyin Name: *Da Qing Long Tang*
Literal Name: Major Bluegreen Dragon Decoction
Alternate Name: Major Blue Dragon Combination
Original Source: *Shang Han Lun* (Discussion of Cold-Induced Disorders) by Zhang Zhong-Jing in the Eastern Han Dynasty

COMPOSITION

Ma Huang (Herba Ephedrae)	18g [12g]
Gui Zhi (Ramulus Cinnamomi)	6g [4g]
Ku Xing Ren (Semen Armeniacae Amarum)	40 kernels [6g]
Shi Gao (Gypsum Fibrosum), *fen sui* (pulverized)	egg yolk in size [12g]
Zhi Gan Cao (Radix et Rhizoma Glycyrrhizae Praeparata cum Melle)	6g [5g]
Sheng Jiang (Rhizoma Zingiberis Recens)	9g [9g]
Da Zao (Fructus Jujubae), *bo* (opened)	12 pieces [3 pieces]

DOSAGE / PREPARATION / ADMINISTRATION

The source text instructs to cook *Ma Huang* (Herba Ephedrae) first with 9 cups [1,800 mL] of water until 7 cups [1,400 mL] of the liquid remain. Remove the foam from the top, add the other ingredients, and cook until the liquid is reduced to 3 cups [600 mL]. Take 1 cup [200 mL] of the strained decoction while warm to promote mild sweating. Discontinue the formula once perspiration occurs. Today, the decoction may be prepared using the doses suggested in brackets.

CHINESE THERAPEUTIC ACTIONS

1. Induces diaphoresis and releases the exterior
2. Clears heat and relieves irritability

CLINICAL MANIFESTATIONS

Exterior wind-cold syndrome with interior heat: fever and aversion to cold of equal severity, a superficial and tight pulse, body aches, absence of perspiration, irritability, and restlessness.

CLINICAL APPLICATIONS

Common cold, influenza, asthma, wheezing and dyspnea, fever, bronchitis, pneumonia, meningitis, measles, urticaria, erysipelas, arthritis, anhidrosis, allergic rhinitis, acute nephritis, and edema caused by nephritis.

EXPLANATION

Da Qing Long Tang (Major Bluegreen Dragon Decoction) is a variation of *Ma Huang Tang* (Ephedra Decoction), and treats severe *taiyang* cold syndrome with interior heat formation. Aversion to cold, fever, absence of perspiration, and a superficial, tight pulse all indicate *taiyang*

cold syndrome of exterior-excess and wind-cold. Because of the severe cold constriction at the exterior, the yang qi is unable to disperse and circulate; the blockage of yang qi circulation eventually produces interior heat. As a result, patients experience irritability and restlessness. Therefore, optimal treatment requires the use of herbs to release wind-cold from the exterior and clear heat from the interior.

In this formula, the dose of *Ma Huang* (Herba Ephedrae) is double the dose found in *Ma Huang Tang* (Ephedra Decoction) because this syndrome involves a more severe form of wind-cold. The increase in dose greatly enhances the exterior-releasing effect through diaphoresis. *Gui Zhi* (Ramulus Cinnamomi) helps *Ma Huang* (Herba Ephedrae) dispel exterior wind-cold and relieve body aches. *Ku Xing Ren* (Semen Armeniacae Amarum) smoothes the qi flow of the Lung to relieve dyspnea. *Shi Gao* (Gypsum Fibrosum) clears interior heat and relieves irritability and restlessness. It also prevents the warm property of *Ma Huang* (Herba Ephedrae) from creating more heat in the body. The dose of *Zhi Gan Cao* (Radix et Rhizoma Glycyrrhizae Praeparata cum Melle) is also increased to counter any body fluid loss caused by interior heat.

Sheng Jiang (Rhizoma Zingiberis Recens) and *Da Zao* (Fructus Jujubae) harmonize the *ying* (nutritive) and *wei* (defensive) levels and moderate the contrasting properties of *Ma Huang* (Herba Ephedrae) and *Shi Gao* (Gypsum Fibrosum). Moreover, they tonify qi and harmonize the middle *jiao*. Since this formula has a very strong exterior-releasing action, it should be discontinued as soon as mild perspiration is obtained.

EXTERIOR-RELEASING FORMULAS

1

45

Chapter 1 – Exterior-Releasing Formulas　　　　　*Section 1 – Acrid and Warm Exterior-Releasing Formulas*

Dà Qīng Lóng Tāng (Major Bluegreen Dragon Decoction)

Da Qing Long Tang (Major Bluegreen Dragon Decoction)

Diagnosis	Signs and Symptoms	Treatment	Herbs
Wind-cold syndrome with interior heat	• Fever and aversion to cold: exterior condition • Absence of perspiration and a tight pulse: exterior excess condition • Body aches and pains: blocked qi and blood circulations • Irritability and restlessness: interior heat • Superficial, tight pulse: exterior condition	• Induces diaphoresis and releases the exterior • Clears heat and relieves irritability	• *Ma Huang* (Herba Ephedrae) strongly dispels wind-cold and induces diaphoresis. • *Gui Zhi* (Ramulus Cinnamomi) dispels exterior wind-cold and relieves body aches. • *Ku Xing Ren* (Semen Armeniacae Amarum) smoothes the qi flow of the Lung to relieve dyspnea. • *Shi Gao* (Gypsum Fibrosum) clears interior heat and relieves irritability. • *Zhi Gan Cao* (Radix et Rhizoma Glycyrrhizae Praeparata cum Melle) prevents loss of body fluids caused by interior heat. • *Sheng Jiang* (Rhizoma Zingiberis Recens) and *Da Zao* (Fructus Jujubae) tonify qi, strengthen the middle *jiao*, and harmonize the *ying* (nutritive) and *wei* (defensive) levels.

MODIFICATIONS

• For headache and pain in the extremities, add *Chuan Xiong* (Rhizoma Chuanxiong) and *Bai Zhi* (Radix Angelicae Dahuricae).

• For signs of fever and fatigue, add *Mai Dong* (Radix Ophiopogonis) and *Wu Wei Zi* (Fructus Schisandrae Chinensis).

• If there is dryness and thirst caused by Lung heat, add *Xie Bai San* (Drain the White Powder).

CAUTIONS / CONTRAINDICATIONS

• *Da Qing Long Tang* is a strong exterior-releasing formula that may induce too much perspiration and damage yang qi. Therefore, this formula is contraindicated in patients who have spontaneous perspiration, aversion to wind, a weak pulse, or generalized deficiency. It should be used only as needed and discontinued when the desired effects are achieved. Do not use for a prolonged period of time or at exceedingly large dosages.[1]

• Profuse sweating may consume yang and cause weakness, irritability, aversion to cold, and inability to sleep. To stop perspiration, the source text instructs to apply powder to the body. Note: Traditionally, the powder of *Long Gu* (Os Draconis), *Mu Li* (Concha Ostreae), or *Nuo Mi* (Oryza Glutinosa) was used. Today, baby powder may be used as a substitute.

PHARMACOLOGICAL EFFECTS

1. **Effect on temperature regulation**: Oral ingestion of *Da Qing Long Tang* at 14 mL/kg (equivalent to 45.9g of dried herbs) reduced body temperature in rabbits with artificially-induced fever. The average onset of action was 90 minutes after oral ingestion. The average reduction of temperature was 0.96°C, measured 120 minutes after oral ingestion of the herbs.[2]

2. **Antibacterial**: *Da Qing Long Tang* demonstrated inhibitory effects against *E. coli* and *Staphylococcus aureus*.[3]

CLINICAL STUDIES AND RESEARCH

1. **Asthma**: Forty-six patients between 26-72 years of ages with asthma were treated with a slightly modified *Da Qing Long Tang* with marked improvement in 18 cases, moderate improvement in 23 cases, and no improvement in 5 cases. The rate of effectiveness was 89.1%.[4]

2. **Wheezing and dyspnea**: One study reported 93.3% effectiveness using modified *Da Qing Long Tang* to treat wheezing and dyspnea caused by chronic tracheitis. The herbal treatment consisted of *Da Qing Long Tang* plus *Hou Po* (Cortex Magnoliae Officinalis), *Di Long* (Pheretima), *Bai Guo* (Semen Ginkgo) and others as the base formula. *Huang Qin* (Radix Scutellariae) and *Gua Lou* (Fructus Trichosanthis) were added for cough with sticky, yellow phlegm; and *Xi Xin* (Radix et Rhizoma Asari), *Ban Xia* (Rhizoma Pinelliae), and *Sheng Jiang* (Rhizoma Zingiberis Recens) were added for cough with clear, watery phlegm. Out of 74 patients, the study reported relief of wheezing and dyspnea in 33 cases, marked improvement in 25 cases, slight improvement in 11 cases, and no improvement in 5 cases.[5]

3. **Fever**: *Da Qing Long Tang* was used successfully to treat patients with fever without perspiration. The treatment protocol was to cook one pack of herbs in water, and drink the decoction in three equally-divided doses daily.

Dà Qīng Lóng Tāng (Major Bluegreen Dragon Decoction)

Most patients responded within 2-3 packs, while those with severe fever may require up to 4-5 packs. Out of 300 patients, the study reported complete recovery in 273 cases, improvement in 21 cases, and no benefit in 6 cases. The overall effectiveness was 98%.[6]

4. **Anhidrosis**: Use of modified *Da Qing Long Tang* was effective in treating 12 patients with abnormal deficiency or absence of sweating caused by improper use of air conditioning or heating systems. The herbal treatment used *Da Qing Long Tang* plus *Ge Gen* (Radix Puerariae Lobatae) and *He Huan Pi* (Cortex Albiziae) as the base formula, with the addition of *Qiang Huo* (Rhizoma et Radix Notopterygii) and *Jie Geng* (Radix Platycodonis) for anhidrosis in the upper body; *Chuan Niu Xi* (Radix Cyathulae) for anhidrosis in the lower body; *Chuan Lian Zi* (Fructus Toosendan) for anhidrosis in the right side of the body; and *Zhi Mu* (Rhizoma Anemarrhenae) for fidgeting and irritability. The study reported complete recovery in all 12 cases within 3-9 packs of herbal treatment.[7]

5. **Allergic rhinitis**: Modified *Da Qing Long Tang* was effective in treating allergic rhinitis. In addition to the formula, *Huang Qi* (Radix Astragali) and *Bai He* (Bulbus Lilii) were added for generalized deficiency; *Xi Xin* (Radix et Rhizoma Asari) and *Lu Lu Tong* (Fructus Liquidambaris) were added for nasal obstruction; and *Bai Zhi* (Radix Angelicae Dahuricae) and *Chuan Xiong* (Rhizoma Chuanxiong) were added for headaches. The treatment protocol was to administer the herbs in decoction daily, and the average duration of treatment was 12 doses (days). Out of 32 patients, the study reported complete recovery in 19 cases, marked improvement in 7 cases, improvement in 5 cases, and no benefit in 1 case.[8]

6. **Acute nephritis**: One study reported good results using modified *Da Qing Long Tang* to treat acute nephritis. The herbal treatment included *Da Qing Long Tang* plus *Chan Tui* (Periostracum Cicadae), *Di Long* (Pheretima), *Bai Mao Gen* (Rhizoma Imperatae), *Yi Mu Cao* (Herba Leonuri), *Che Qian Zi* (Semen Plantaginis) and others as deemed necessary. The treatment protocol was to cook the herbs in water to obtain a decoction, and administer the decoction in five equally-divided doses daily, for 2 weeks per course of treatment. Out of 43 patients, the study reported recovery in 37 cases, improvement in 4 cases, and no benefit in 2 cases.[9]

HERB-DRUG INTERACTION

Interferon-induced adverse reactions: Concurrent use of herbs reduced the adverse effects of interferon in hepatitis C patients. Of 28 patients with chronic hepatitis C, 8 patients in Group A received both interferon-beta and *Ma Huang Tang* (Ephedra Decoction), and 4 patients in Group B received both interferon-beta and *Da Qing Long Tang*, and 16 patients in Group C received only interferon-beta. Adverse effects were evaluated and monitored by clinical and laboratory examinations. At the end of the treatment, patients in Group A and B had significantly lower incidences than Group C of discomfort, fever, general malaise, paresthesia and arthralgia. HCV-RNA was negative in all patients. Based on this information, the study concluded that the use of these two formulas may reduce the adverse effects accompanying interferon-beta treatment in patients with chronic hepatitis C, without reducing the antiviral effects.[10]

AUTHORS' COMMENTS

The key symptoms in *Da Qing Long Tang* are absence of sweating and presence of irritability and restlessness. Absence of sweating indicates an exterior-excess condition in a constitutionally strong patient. Irritability and restlessness imply heat formation in the interior. Exterior cold coupled with interior heat is the primary diagnosis for selecting *Da Qing Long Tang*.

According to Dr. Chang Wei-Yen, *Da Qing Long Tang* can be combined with *Shi Shen Tang* (Ten-Immortal Decoction) to treat common cold characterized by wind-cold and manifesting in symptoms of aversion to cold, and nasal obstruction or clear, watery nasal discharge.

References

1. *Si Chuan Zhong Yi* (Sichuan Chinese Medicine) 1986;(5):10.
2. *Si Chuan Zhong Yi* (Sichuan Chinese Medicine) 1985;(3):17.
3. *Zhong Yuan Yi Kan* (Resource Journal of Chinese Medicine) 1955;(10):36.
4. *Guo Wai Yi Xue* (Foreign Medicine) 1987;(2):39.
5. *Shi Yong Zhong Xi Yi Jie He Za Zhi* (Practical Journal of Integrated Chinese and Western Medicines) 1998;2:146.
6. *Tian Jin Zhong Yi* (Tianjin Chinese Medicine) 1988;6:45.
7. *Shan Dong Zhong Yi Za Zhi* (Shandong Journal of Chinese Medicine) 1999;5:210.
8. *Si Chuan Zhong Yi* (Sichuan Chinese Medicine) 1991;10:46.
9. *Zhong Yi Ming Fang Lin Chuang Xin Yong* (Contemporary Clinical Applications of Classic Chinese Formulas) 2001;48.
10. Kainuma M, Hayashi J, Sakai S, Imai K, Mantani N, Kohta K, Mitsuma T, Shimada Y, Kashiwagi S, Terasawa K. The efficacy of herbal medicine (kampo) in reducing the adverse effects of IFN-beta in chronic hepatitis C. American Journal of Chinese Medicine 2002;30(2-3):355-67.

Huá Gài Sǎn (Canopy Powder)

華蓋散
华盖散

Pinyin Name: *Hua Gai San*
Literal Name: Canopy Powder
Alternate Names: *Hua Kai San*, Ma-huang and Morus Formula, Mahuang and Morus Formula
Original Source: *Tai Ping Hui Min He Ji Ju Fang* (Imperial Grace Formulary of the Tai Ping Era) by the Imperial Medical Department in 1078-85

COMPOSITION

Ma Huang (Herba Ephedrae)	30g [9g]
Sang Bai Pi (Cortex Mori), *mi zhi* (fried with honey)	30g [9g]
Zi Su Zi (Fructus Perillae), *chao* (dry-fried)	30g [9g]
Ku Xing Ren (Semen Armeniacae Amarum), *chao* (dry-fried)	30g [9g]
Chi Fu Ling (Poria Rubra)	30g [9g]
Chen Pi (Pericarpium Citri Reticulatae)	30g [9g]
Zhi Gan Cao (Radix et Rhizoma Glycyrrhizae Praeparata cum Melle)	15g [6g]

DOSAGE / PREPARATION / ADMINISTRATION

The source text states to grind the ingredients into powder and cook 9g with one large bowl of water until 70% of the liquid remains. Take the warm, strained decoction after meals. Today, this formula may be prepared as a decoction with the doses suggested in brackets.

CHINESE THERAPEUTIC ACTIONS

1. Ventilates the Lung and releases the exterior
2. Dispels phlegm and stops coughing

CLINICAL MANIFESTATIONS

Wind-cold attacking the Lung: cough, dyspnea, profuse sputum, fullness and discomfort in the chest and diaphragm, nasal obstruction, stiff neck and upper back, and a superficial, rapid pulse.

CLINICAL APPLICATIONS

Common cold, influenza, coughing, nasal obstruction, stiff neck and upper back, asthma, wheezing, dyspnea, bronchitis, and other respiratory symptoms.

EXPLANATION

Hua Gai San (Canopy Powder) is a variation of *Ma Huang Tang* (Ephedra Decoction); it treats wind-cold attacking the Lung. Clinical manifestations include coughing and dyspnea with profuse sputum, and fullness and discomfort in the chest and diaphragm.

Hua Gai San (Canopy Powder)

Diagnosis	Signs and Symptoms	Treatment	Herbs
Wind-cold attacking the Lung	• Coughing and dyspnea with profuse sputum, and fullness and discomfort in the chest and diaphragm: wind-cold factor attacking the Lung • Superficial pulse: exterior condition	• Ventilates the Lung and releases the exterior • Dispels phlegm and stops coughing	• *Ma Huang* (Herba Ephedrae) releases exterior wind-cold and smoothes the flow of the Lung qi. • *Sang Bai Pi* (Cortex Mori) and *Zi Su Zi* (Fructus Perillae) relieve coughing and eliminate phlegm. • *Ku Xing Ren* (Semen Armeniacae Amarum) redirects Lung qi downwards to relieve coughing and dyspnea. • *Chi Fu Ling* (Poria Rubra) dispels dampness, eliminates phlegm, and strengthens the Spleen to stop phlegm production. • *Chen Pi* (Pericarpium Citri Reticulatae) regulates qi flow, relieves coughing, and eliminates phlegm. • *Zhi Gan Cao* (Radix et Rhizoma Glycyrrhizae Praeparata cum Melle) harmonizes the herbs.

Huá Gài Sǎn (Canopy Powder)

Ma Huang (Herba Ephedrae) releases exterior wind-cold and smoothes the flow of Lung qi. *Sang Bai Pi* (Cortex Mori) and *Zi Su Zi* (Fructus Perillae) relieve coughing and eliminate phlegm. *Ku Xing Ren* (Semen Armeniacae Amarum) redirects Lung qi downward to relieve coughing and dyspnea. *Chi Fu Ling* (Poria Rubra) dispels dampness, eliminates phlegm, and strengthens the Spleen to prevent further production of phlegm. *Chen Pi* (Pericarpium Citri Reticulatae) regulates qi flow, relieves coughing, and eliminates phlegm. *Zhi Gan Cao* (Radix et Rhizoma Glycyrrhizae Praeparata cum Melle) harmonizes the herbs.

MODIFICATIONS

- If there is more phlegm and accompanied by shortness of breath, add *Di Gu Pi* (Cortex Lycii) and *Jie Geng* (Radix Platycodonis).
- For severe cough and wheezing, add *Zhi Mu* (Rhizoma Anemarrhenae) and *Zhe Bei Mu* (Bulbus Fritillariae Thunbergii).
- With nasal congestion and a low-pitched voice, add *Fang Feng* (Radix Saposhnikoviae) and *Bo He* (Herba Menthae).

AUTHORS' COMMENTS

The literal name of this formula is "Canopy Powder," because anatomically, the lungs resemble a canopy that covers all of the internal organs. Since this formula focuses specifically on treating lung disorders, it is named *Hua Gai San*.

Jin Fèi Cǎo Sǎn (Inula Powder)

金沸草散
金沸草散

Pinyin Name: Jin Fei Cao San
Literal Name: Inula Powder
Alternate Names: *Chin Fei Tsao San*, Schizonepeta and Pinellia Formula
Original Source: *Tai Ping Hui Min He Ji Ju Fang* (Imperial Grace Formulary of the Tai Ping Era) by the Imperial Medical Department in 1078-85

COMPOSITION

Xuan Fu Hua (Flos Inulae)	90g [9g]
Jing Jie Sui (Spica Schizonepetae)	120g [12g]
Ma Huang (Herba Ephedrae)	90g [9g]
Qian Hu (Radix Peucedani)	90g [9g]
Ban Xia (Rhizoma Pinelliae), *xi* (washed) with liquid 7 times and *jin* (soaked) in ginger juice	30g [3g]
Chi Shao (Radix Paeoniae Rubra)	30g [3g]
Gan Cao (Radix et Rhizoma Glycyrrhizae), *chao* (dry-fried)	30g [3g]

DOSAGE / PREPARATION / ADMINISTRATION

The source text states to grind all of the ingredients into powder. Cook 9g of the powder with 3 slices of *Sheng Jiang* (Rhizoma Zingiberis Recens) and 1 piece of *Da Zao* (Fructus Jujubae) in 1.5 large bowls of water until the liquid is reduced by 20%. Take the strained decoction while warm. Today, this formula may be prepared as a decoction with doses the suggested in brackets.

CHINESE THERAPEUTIC ACTIONS

1. Releases exterior wind-cold
2. Ventilates the Lung and directs rising qi downward
3. Stops cough and dyspnea

CLINICAL MANIFESTATIONS

Wind-cold syndrome with severe Lung dysfunction: cough and dyspnea, profuse sputum, thick and sticky nasal discharge and sputum, a low-pitched voice, dizziness, headache, neck pain, body aches, aversion to cold and fever, fullness and a stifling sensation in the chest and diaphragm, and other Lung-related symptoms.

CLINICAL APPLICATIONS

Common cold, influenza, asthma, wheezing, dyspnea, bronchitis, and cough.

Chapter 1 – Exterior-Releasing Formulas　　　　*Section 1 – Acrid and Warm Exterior-Releasing Formulas*

Jīn Fèi Cǎo Sǎn (Inula Powder)

EXPLANATION

Jin Fei Cao San (Inula Powder) treats exterior wind-cold syndrome with severe Lung dysfunction. Exterior wind-cold is characterized by symptoms such as headache, neck pain, body aches, and aversion to cold and fever. Exterior wind-cold may affect the normal functioning of the Lung, causing symptoms such as cough, dyspnea, feelings of fullness and stifling sensation in the chest and diaphragm, and profuse sputum.

Xuan Fu Hua (Flos Inulae), the chief herb, ventilates the Lung, directs Lung qi downward, and dissolves phlegm. *Jing Jie Sui* (Spica Schizonepetae) and *Ma Huang* (Herba Ephedrae) dispel wind-cold and induce diaphoresis to eliminate the exterior pathogenic factors. *Qian Hu* (Radix Peucedani) dissolves phlegm and directs Lung qi downward. *Ban Xia* (Rhizoma Pinelliae) dries dampness and eliminates phlegm. Bitter and slightly cold, *Chi Shao* (Radix Paeoniae Rubra) controls the warming and drying herbs in this formula from consuming yin and body fluids. *Sheng Jiang* (Rhizoma Zingiberis Recens), *Da Zao* (Fructus Jujubae), and *Gan Cao* (Radix et Rhizoma Glycyrrhizae) strengthen the middle *jiao* and harmonize the formula.

MODIFICATIONS

- If there is more phlegm, add *Fu Ling* (Poria) and *Chen Pi* (Pericarpium Citri Reticulatae).
- For more severe cough, dyspnea, and chest congestion, add *Ku Xing Ren* (Semen Armeniacae Amarum) and *Hou Po* (Cortex Magnoliae Officinalis).

- If there is a feeling of fullness, distention and oppression underneath the heart, add *Zhi Qiao* (Fructus Aurantii) and *Jie Geng* (Radix Platycodonis).
- With signs of perspiration and cough, add *Ku Xing Ren* (Semen Armeniacae Amarum) and *Wu Wei Zi* (Fructus Schisandrae Chinensis).
- If the headache is more severe, add *Chuan Xiong* (Rhizoma Chuanxiong) and *Bai Zhi* (Radix Angelicae Dahuricae).

AUTHORS' COMMENTS

Hua Gai San (Canopy Powder) and *Jin Fei Cao San* treat wind-cold syndrome with severe Lung dysfunction. Both formulas relieve cough, eliminate phlegm, and treat various Lung-related signs and symptoms.

- *Hua Gai San* effectively dispels phlegm and directs Lung qi downward.
- *Jin Fei Cao San* strongly releases the exterior, and thus is reserved for severe cases of wind-cold syndrome affecting the Lung.

This formula is called *Jin Fei Cao San* because the chief herb in this formula was traditionally *Jin Fei Cao* (Herba Inulae). However, *Jin Fei Cao* (Herba Inulae) has only a mild potent action to direct qi downward and dissolve phlegm. Consequently, *Jin Fei Cao* (Herba Inulae) is now commonly replaced by *Xuan Fu Hua* (Flos Inulae), another herb from the same plant with more potent functions.

Jin Fei Cao San (Inula Powder)

Diagnosis	Signs and Symptoms	Treatment	Herbs
Wind-cold syndrome with severe Lung dysfunction	- Headache, neck pain, body aches, aversion to cold, fever, and nasal obstruction: exterior wind-cold - Cough and dyspnea with profuse sputum, feelings of fullness and a stifling sensation in the chest and diaphragm: exterior wind-cold affecting the Lung	- Releases exterior wind-cold - Ventilates the Lung and directs rising qi downward - Stops cough and dyspnea	- *Xuan Fu Hua* (Flos Inulae) ventilates the Lung, directs Lung qi downward, and dissolves phlegm. - *Jing Jie Sui* (Spica Schizonepetae) and *Ma Huang* (Herba Ephedrae) dispel wind-cold and induce diaphoresis. - *Qian Hu* (Radix Peucedani) dissolves phlegm and directs Lung qi downward. - *Ban Xia* (Rhizoma Pinelliae) dries dampness and eliminates phlegm. - *Chi Shao* (Radix Paeoniae Rubra) controls the warming and drying herbs from consuming yin and body fluids. - *Sheng Jiang* (Rhizoma Zingiberis Recens), *Da Zao* (Fructus Jujubae) and *Gan Cao* (Radix et Rhizoma Glycyrrhizae) strengthen the middle *jiao* and harmonize the herbs.

50

Chinese Herbal Formulas and Applications

Gui Zhī Tang (Cinnamon Twig Decoction)

桂枝湯
桂枝汤

Pinyin Name: *Gui Zhi Tang*
Literal Name: Cinnamon Twig Decoction
Alternate Names: *Kuei Chih Tang*, Cinnamon Decoction, Cassia Twig Decoction, Cinnamon Combination
Original Source: *Shang Han Lun* (Discussion of Cold-Induced Disorders) by Zhang Zhong-Jing in the Eastern Han Dynasty

COMPOSITION

Gui Zhi (Ramulus Cinnamomi)	9g
Bai Shao (Radix Paeoniae Alba)	9g
Zhi Gan Cao (Radix et Rhizoma Glycyrrhizae Praeparata cum Melle)	6g
Sheng Jiang (Rhizoma Zingiberis Recens), *qie* (sliced)	9g
Da Zao (Fructus Jujubae), *bo* (opened)	12 pieces [3 pieces]

DOSAGE / PREPARATION / ADMINISTRATION

The source text states to coarsely crush the ingredients and cook with 7 cups [1,400 mL] of water over low intensity fire until 3 cups [600 mL] of the liquid remain. Take 1 cup [200 mL] of the warm, strained decoction, followed by 1 cup [200 mL] of hot porridge, to promote and enhance the therapeutic effect of the herbs. For best results, have the patient sweat slightly all over the body but do not induce profuse sweating. Once slight sweating has been achieved, stop taking the formula. If perspiration does not occur, repeat the dose one or two more times, progressively reducing the time interval between doses within half of a day.

If the patient's condition is severe, administer the dose twice daily (morning and night), and progressively add another two to three doses if no sweating has been induced after taking the formula for two hours. Today, this formula may be prepared as a decoction with the doses suggested in brackets.

CHINESE THERAPEUTIC ACTIONS

1. Releases the exterior and muscle layer
2. Regulates and harmonizes *ying* (nutritive) *qi* and *wei* (defensive) *qi*

CLINICAL MANIFESTATIONS

Exterior-deficient, wind-cold syndrome: headache, fever, perspiration, aversion to wind, nasal congestion, dry heaves, absence of thirst, a thin, white tongue coating, and a superficial and moderate, or superficial and weak pulse.

Disharmony of the *ying* (nutritive) and *wei* (defensive) levels: feverish sensations with spontaneous sweating and aversion to wind in constitutionally-weak, chronic and debilitating, or postpartum patients.

CLINICAL APPLICATIONS

Fever, common cold, influenza, respiratory tract infections, allergic rhinitis, bronchial asthma, atrioventricular block, testicular pain, hernia, appendicitis, sciatica, allergic purpura, itching, frostbite, eczema, urticaria, enuresis, and hyperactivity disorder.

EXPLANATION

Gui Zhi Tang (Cinnamon Twig Decoction), first presented in the *Shang Han Lun* (Discussion of Cold-Induced Disorder), is designed to treat *taiyang* wind syndrome. *Taiyang* wind syndrome refers to attack by wind-cold pathogenic factors at the body's exterior, with wind being the dominant pathogen. Unlike cold, which constricts the body, wind is dispersing and highly mobile in character. Wind usually attacks the exterior of the body and leaves after the attack, taking with it some of the body's *wei* (defensive) *qi*.

Wei (defensive) *qi* controls the opening and closing of the skin pores; the subsequent depletion of *wei qi* impairs the body's regulation of the skin pores. The pores are left open after the wind invasion, which allows yang qi to leak out of the body, carrying body fluids with it. Hence, patients will experience perspiration and aversion to wind. Note that perspiration, one of the key characteristics of this syndrome, is absent in *taiyang* cold syndrome, as discussed in *Ma Huang Tang* (Ephedra Decoction).

Since cold is also involved in *taiyang* wind syndrome, stagnation of qi and blood and obstruction of the channels may also occur, causing headache and neck stiffness. However, the severity of the headache and neck stiffness seen in *taiyang* wind syndrome is much less than that found in *taiyang* cold syndrome. Since the disease is at the exterior, the tongue coating is still normal. The pulse,

EXTERIOR-RELEASING FORMULAS

1

51

Gui Zhī Tāng (Cinnamon Twig Decoction)

Gui Zhi Tang (Cinnamon Twig Decoction)

Diagnosis	Signs and Symptoms	Treatment	Herbs
Exterior-deficient, wind-cold syndrome	• Fever and aversion to wind: exterior wind-cold with deficiency of *wei* (defensive) *qi* • Perspiration: disharmony of the *ying* (nutritive) and *wei* (defensive) levels • Thin, white tongue coating: exterior wind-cold • Superficial and weak pulse: exterior condition with underlying deficiency	• Releases the exterior and the muscle layer • Regulates and harmonizes *ying* (nutritive) *qi* and *wei* (defensive) *qi*	• *Gui Zhi* (Ramulus Cinnamomi) releases wind-cold from the exterior and muscle layer. • *Bai Shao* (Radix Paeoniae Alba) consolidates the interior (yin and body fluids). • *Zhi Gan Cao* (Radix et Rhizoma Glycyrrhizae Praeparata cum Melle) relieves aches and pains, benefits yin, and harmonizes the herbs. • *Sheng Jiang* (Rhizoma Zingiberis Recens) and *Da Zao* (Fructus Jujubae) benefit the middle *jiao* and tonify qi.

superficial and moderate, or superficial and weak, indicates an exterior-deficiency syndrome.

Gui Zhi Tang contains only five ingredients, but it has multiple functions: disperse, tonify, release, and constrict. *Gui Zhi* (Ramulus Cinnamomi), the chief herb, releases wind-cold from the exterior and muscle layer to relieve body aches and pains. *Bai Shao* (Radix Paeoniae Alba), the deputy herb, consolidates the body's interior (e.g., yin and body fluids). Used together, *Gui Zhi* (Ramulus Cinnamomi) and *Bai Shao* (Radix Paeoniae Alba) harmonize *wei* (defensive) *qi* and *ying* (nutritive) *qi*. *Gui Zhi* (Ramulus Cinnamomi) is acrid and warm; *Bai Shao* (Radix Paeoniae Alba) is sour and cool. The former is dispersing in nature, while the latter is nourishing.

Zhi Gan Cao (Radix et Rhizoma Glycyrrhizae Praeparata cum Melle), double in dose compared to *Ma Huang Tang* (Ephedra Decoction), serves as both assistant and envoy herb. As an assistant, it helps *Gui Zhi* (Ramulus Cinnamomi) relieve aches and pains and helps *Bai Shao* (Radix Paeoniae Alba) benefit yin; as an envoy, it harmonizes the formula. *Sheng Jiang* (Rhizoma Zingiberis Recens), besides helping *Gui Zhi* (Ramulus Cinnamomi) to dispel exterior wind and cold, stops nausea and relieves dry heaves. *Da Zao* (Fructus Jujubae) tonifies qi and body fluids. *Sheng Jiang* (Rhizoma Zingiberis Recens) and *Da Zao* (Fructus Jujubae) work synergistically to benefit the middle *jiao* and assist in qi production.

Lastly, this formula also treats disharmony of *ying* (nutritive) *qi* and *wei* (defensive) *qi* brought on by major illnesses, child delivery, and qi or blood deficiency. Clinical manifestations in such cases include slight feverish sensations with perspiration and aversion to wind.

MODIFICATIONS

• For aversion to cold and absence of perspiration, add *Ma Huang* (Herba Ephedrae) and *Ge Gen* (Radix Puerariae Lobatae).

• With more fever than aversion to cold, add *Shi Gao* (Gypsum Fibrosum) and *Zhi Mu* (Rhizoma Anemarrhenae).

• For neck and shoulder pain, add *Ge Gen* (Radix Puerariae Lobatae).

• If there is headache, add *Gao Ben* (Rhizoma et Radix Ligustici), *Chuan Xiong* (Rhizoma Chuanxiong) and *Bai Zhi* (Radix Angelicae Dahuricae).

• For sneezing, runny nose, and nasal obstruction, add *Jing Jie* (Herba Schizonepetae), *Fang Feng* (Radix Saposhnikoviae) and *Xin Yi Hua* (Flos Magnoliae).

• If accompanied by coughing and wheezing, add *Hou Po* (Cortex Magnoliae Officinalis) and *Ku Xing Ren* (Semen Armeniacae Amarum).

• If there is profuse, white phlegm, remove *Bai Shao* (Radix Paeoniae Alba) and *Da Zao* (Fructus Jujubae), and add *Ban Xia* (Rhizoma Pinelliae) and *Chen Pi* (Pericarpium Citri Reticulatae).

• For convalescing patients with wind-cold invasion, add *Xiao Chai Hu Tang* (Minor Bupleurum Decoction).

CAUTIONS / CONTRAINDICATIONS

• Since *Gui Zhi Tang* is indicated for patients with exterior-**deficiency**, wind-cold syndrome, porridge should be consumed after taking this formula to strengthen the body and prevent the sweating from damaging body fluids. In the case of *Ma Huang Tang* (Ephedra Decoction), which is indicated for exterior-**excess**, wind-cold syndrome, the intake of porridge is not necessary, since there is no deficiency.

• This formula is contraindicated in *taiyang* cold syndrome, because *Gui Zhi* (Ramulus Cinnamomi) is not strong enough to dispel excess cold; moreover, the consolidating

52

Gui Zhī Tāng (Cinnamon Twig Decoction)

Chinese Herbal Formulas and Applications

characteristic of *Bai Shao* (Radix Paeoniae Alba) may actually lead cold into the interior.

- This formula is contraindicated in patients with wind-heat syndrome, exterior cold and interior heat, absence of perspiration with irritability, exterior excess conditions without perspiration, or beginning stages of febrile disorders with fever, sore throat, and thirst.
- During the course of the disease, avoid foods that are raw, cold, greasy, sticky, fatty, spicy, spoiled, or rotten. Foods such as alcohol, meat, cheese, garlic, leeks, scallions, onions, and products that are fermented or preserved should also be avoided.
- This formula is contraindicated in patients who drink alcohol frequently, since alcohol tends to cause damp-heat accumulation. Ingestion of the decoction may cause vomiting, since *Zhi Gan Cao* (Radix et Rhizoma Glycyrrhizae Praeparata cum Melle) and *Gui Zhi* (Ramulus Cinnamomi) are both sweet and warm herbs that can aggravate the damp-heat condition.

PHARMACOLOGICAL EFFECTS

1. **Effect on sweating regulation**: Use of *Gui Zhi Tang* in rats was associated with a bidirectional modulating effect on perspiration. *Gui Zhi Tang* reduced sweating in polyhidrosis induced by aminopyrine, and promoted sweating in hypohidrosis induced by atropine.[1]

2. **Effect on temperature regulation**: *Gui Zhi Tang* has marked effects to reduce body temperature in cases of fever and normal body temperature. According to laboratory studies, oral ingestion of this formula reduced body temperature for up to five hours in rats with fever, and up to four hours in rats with normal body temperature.[2] Another study in rabbits and mice on the pharmacokinetics of this formula stated that the initial onset of action was observed 60 minutes after administration, and reached the peak effect after 120 minutes. The average reduction of temperature was 3.8°C.[3,4]

3. **Anti-inflammatory**: Intraperitoneal injection of *Gui Zhi Tang* at 7.5 g/kg demonstrated marked anti-inflammatory effect in mice with swollen feet. The onset of effect began one hour after the injection, and lasted for approximately 24 hours.[5] According to another study in mice, the anti-inflammatory effect of *Gui Zhi Tang* (25.32 g/kg) was stronger than aspirin (100 mg/kg).[6]

4. **Analgesic and sedative**: Intraperitoneal injection of *Gui Zhi Tang* in mice at doses of 7.5 g/kg and 15 g/kg showed marked analgesic and sedative effects. Though effective, delayed onset of effect up to 120 minutes was observed.[7]

5. **Antibiotic**: According to *in vitro* studies, administration of *Gui Zhi Tang* was associated with inhibitory effects against *Helicobacter pylori*, *Staphylococcus aureus*, *Salmonella typhi* and *Mycobacterium tuberculosis*.[8]

6. **Cardiovascular**: Administration of *Gui Zhi Tang* induced an increase of systolic blood pressure and stroke volume in 7 healthy adult males (age, 22.3 +/- 1.8 years old).[9]

CLINICAL STUDIES AND RESEARCH

1. **Fever**: In one clinical study, *Gui Zhi Tang* was evaluated for its effect to reduce body temperature in subjects with fever due to infectious diseases. Out of 24 cases with high fever, the temperature was reduced to normal in 16 cases, reduced to mild fever in 4 cases, and no effect in 2 cases. Two cases were excluded from the study as the causes of fever were determined later to be other than infectious disorders.[10]

2. **Common cold**: In one study involving 42 patients with common cold in the summertime, administration of *Gui Zhi Tang* was associated with complete recovery within 2-3 packs of herbs.[11]

3. **Bronchial asthma**: One study reported 97.5% effectiveness using modified *Gui Zhi Tang* plus *Hou Po* (Cortex Magnoliae Officinalis) to treat bronchial asthma in 40 infants (29 males and 11 females, between 2-10 years of age, with 7 days to 6 months history of illness). The duration of treatment ranged from 1-5 days. Of 40 patients, the study reported recovery in 36 cases, improvement in 3 cases, and no effect in 1 case.[12]

4. **Atrioventricular block**: One study reported success using modified *Gui Zhi Tang* to treat atrioventricular block. The herbal treatment contained *Gui Zhi Tang* plus *San Qi* (Radix et Rhizoma Notoginseng) and *Huang Qi* (Radix Astragali) as the base formula, with addition of *Suan Zao Ren* (Semen Ziziphi Spinosae) for palpitations, and *Yu Jin* (Radix Curcumae) and *Gua Lou Pi* (Pericarpium Trichosanthis) for feeling of chest oppression. Of 30 patients, the study reported recovery in 28 cases and improvement in 2 cases after 14-21 days of treatment.[13]

5. **Testicular pain**: Use of modified *Gui Zhi Tang* was associated with marked relief in treating 20 patients with testicular pain. The herbal treatment contained *Gui Zhi Tang* plus *Chuan Lian Zi* (Fructus Toosendan) and *Mian Ma Guan Zhong* (Rhizoma Dryopteridis Crassirhizomatis) as the base formula. Additional modifications were made as follows: for severe pain, add *Ju He* (Semen Citri Reticulatae) and *Yan Hu Suo* (Rhizoma Corydalis); for redness and swelling of the testicles with burning sensations and pain, add *Long Dan* (Radix et Rhizoma Gentianae), *Mu Tong* (Caulis Akebiae), *Cang Zhu* (Rhizoma Atractylodis), and a large dose of *Mian Ma Guan Zhong* (Rhizoma Dryopteridis Crassirhizomatis); for testicular pain caused by trauma with blood stagnation, add *Tao Ren* (Semen Persicae), *Hong Hua* (Flos Carthami) and *Mu Xiang* (Radix Aucklandiae); and for fatigue, add *Dang Shen* (Radix Codonopsis). The duration of treatment ranged from 6-32 days.[14]

Guì Zhī Tāng (Cinnamon Twig Decoction)

6. **Sciatica**: Use of modified *Gui Zhi Tang* was associated with a 94.1% rate of effectiveness in treating 34 patients with sciatica characterized by deficiency and cold. The herbal treatment contained *Gui Zhi Tang* plus *Chuan Xiong* (Rhizoma Chuanxiong), *Mu Gua* (Fructus Chaenomelis) and others as the base formula. Modifications to the original formula included addition of *Huang Qi* (Radix Astragali) for qi deficiency; *Fu Zi* (Radix Aconiti Lateralis Praeparata) and *Xi Xin* (Radix et Rhizoma Asari) for cold lower extremities; *Du Zhong* (Cortex Eucommiae) and *Wei Ling Xian* (Radix et Rhizoma Clematidis) for severe low back pain; and *Ji Xue Teng* (Caulis Spatholobi) and *Di Long* (Pheretima) for chronic pain or blood stagnation. Of 34 patients, the study reported complete recovery in 24 cases, improvement in 8 cases, and no benefit in 2 cases.[15]

7. **Allergic purpura**: One study reported complete recovery in 33 of 35 patients with allergic purpura using *Gui Zhi Tang* plus *Dan Shen* (Radix et Rhizoma Salviae Miltiorrhizae) for 3-5 packs of herbs.[16]

8. **Itching**: Modified *Gui Zhi Tang* showed effectiveness in treating itching of the skin in geriatric patients. The herbal treatment contained *Gui Zhi Tang* plus *Fang Feng* (Radix Saposhnikoviae), *Ji Xue Teng* (Caulis Spatholobi) and *Dang Gui* (Radix Angelicae Sinensis). The treatment protocol was to cook the herbs in water, and administer the decoction orally in two equally-divided doses in the morning and at night. The same herbs were cooked one more time, and the resultant solution was applied topically to the affected area as an herbal wash. Of 31 patients, the study reported complete recovery in 19 cases, improvement in 9 cases, and no effect in 3 cases. The overall rate of effectiveness was 90.3%.[17]

9. **Frostbite**: One study reported good results using modified *Gui Zhi Tang* to treat 43 patients with frostbite. The herbal treatment contained *Gui Zhi Tang* plus *Chi Shao* (Radix Paeoniae Rubra) and grain-based alcohol as the base formula. *Ma Huang* (Herba Ephedrae) and *Xi Xin* (Radix et Rhizoma Asari) were added for presence of cold; *Huang Qi* (Radix Astragali) for qi deficiency; *Fu Zi* (Radix Aconiti Lateralis Praeparata), *Xi Xin* (Radix et Rhizoma Asari) and a higher dose (20g) of *Gui Zhi* (Ramulus Cinnamomi) for yang deficiency and aversion to cold; *Dan Shen* (Radix et Rhizoma Salviae Miltiorrhizae) and *Hong Hua* (Flos Carthami) for blood stagnation; and topical application to the affected area using *Ma Bo* (Lasiosphaera seu Calvatia) powder mixed with sesame oil for ulcers and sores.[18]

10. **Enuresis**: One study reported great success in treating enuresis in young children using modified *Gui Zhi Tang*. The herbal treatment contained *Gui Zhi* (Ramulus Cinnamomi) 10g, *Bai Shao* (Radix Paeoniae Alba) 10g, *Sheng Jiang* (Rhizoma Zingiberis Recens) 3 slices, *Da Zao* (Fructus Jujubae) 5 pieces, *Zhi Gan Cao* (Radix et Rhizoma Glycyrrhizae Praeparata cum Melle) 6g, *Yi Zhi* (Fructus Alpiniae Oxyphyllae) 15g, *Tu Si Zi* (Semen Cuscutae) 15g, *Wu Yao* (Radix Linderae) 10g, and *Mu Gua* (Fructus Chaenomelis) 2 pieces. Of 30 infants, the study reported complete recovery in 4 cases, significant improvement in 15 cases, and moderate improvement in 11 cases. The overall effectiveness was 100%.[19] Another study reported marked effectiveness in treating enuresis in 10 of 15 children using *Gui Zhi Tang* plus *Suo Quan Wan* (Shut the Sluice Pill). The average duration of treatment was 10 packs of herbs.[20]

11. **Hyperactivity disorder**: One study reported a 93.3% rate of effectiveness using *Gui Zhi Tang* to treat hyperactivity in 30 children (between 2-13 years of age, with up to 4 years history of illness). In addition to hyperactivity, other signs and symptoms included muscle spasms and cramps, grinding of the teeth, restless legs, poor sleeping patterns, and enuresis. The duration of treatment was 7 days per course, for a total of 2-3 courses. Of 30 children, the study reported complete recovery in 8 cases, significant improvement in 17 cases, slight improvement in 3 cases, and no benefit in 2 cases. The study reported that the success of treatment was directly proportional to the duration of illness. The two cases that did not respond to treatment both had over 3 years history of hyperactivity disorder.[21]

HERB-DRUG INTERACTION

Gonadotropin-releasing hormone agonist-induced menopause: One study evaluated the therapeutic effects of certain herbal medicines on menopausal symptoms induced by gonadotropin-releasing hormone agonist therapy in Japanese women with endometriosis, adenomyosis, or leiomyoma. Menopausal symptoms induced by gonadotropin-releasing hormone agonist therapy in 13 patients were successfully treated with *Dang Gui Shao Yao San* (Tangkuei and Peony Powder), *Shao Yao Gan Cao Tang* (Peony and Licorice Decoction), *Gui Zhi Fu Ling Wan* (Cinnamon Twig and Poria Pill), *Jia Wei Xiao Yao San* (Augmented Rambling Powder), *Tao He Cheng Qi Tang* (Peach Pit Decoction to Order the Qi) or *Gui Zhi Tang*. Of 11 patients with hot flashes, *Dang Gui Shao Yao San* (Tangkuei and Peony Powder) provided some relief in all 11 cases, and total relief in 4 cases. Most importantly, there was no significant change in serum estradiol levels after treatment with these herbal medicines. The researchers concluded that these herbal medicines could be recommended for menopausal symptoms induced by gonadotropin-releasing hormone agonists without a negative effect on serum estradiol levels.[22]

TOXICOLOGY

The LD_{50} of *Gui Zhi Tang* in mice is 28.125 g/kg within 72 hours via intraperitoneal injection.[23]

Guì Zhī Tāng (Cinnamon Twig Decoction)

RELATED FORMULAS

Guì Zhī Jiā Gě Gēn Tāng

(Cinnamon Twig Decoction plus Kudzu)

桂枝加葛根湯
桂枝加葛根汤

Pinyin Name: *Gui Zhi Jia Ge Gen Tang*
Literal Name: Cinnamon Twig Decoction plus Kudzu
Original Source: *Shang Han Lun* (Discussion of Cold-Induced Disorders) by Zhang Zhong-Jing in the Eastern Han Dynasty

Gui Zhi (Ramulus Cinnamomi)	6g
Bai Shao (Radix Paeoniae Alba)	6g
Zhi Gan Cao (Radix et Rhizoma Glycyrrhizae Praeparata cum Melle)	6g
Sheng Jiang (Rhizoma Zingiberis Recens), *qie* (sliced)	9g
Da Zao (Fructus Jujubae), *bo* (opened)	12 pieces [3 pieces]
Ge Gen (Radix Puerariae Lobatae)	12g

The source text states to cook the ingredients with 8 cups [1,600 mL] of water until 3 cups [600 mL] of the liquid remain. Take 1 cup [200 mL] of the warm, strained decoction and cover the body with blankets to promote mild sweating. Patients do not need to consume hot porridge after taking this formula. Please refer to *Gui Zhi Tang* (Cinnamon Twig Decoction) for additional information on administration and contraindications. Today, this formula may be prepared as a decoction with the doses suggested in brackets.

Gui Zhi Jia Ge Gen Tang (Cinnamon Twig Decoction plus Kudzu) treats *taiyang* wind syndrome with severe neck stiffness. The addition of *Ge Gen* (Radix Puerariae Lobatae) relieves muscle tension and neck stiffness. Other symptoms include perspiration with aversion to wind.

Guì Zhī Jiā Hòu Pò Xìng Zǐ Tāng

(Cinnamon Twig Decoction plus Magnolia Bark and Apricot Kernel)

桂枝加厚樸杏子湯
桂枝加厚朴杏子汤

Pinyin Name: *Gui Zhi Jia Hou Po Xing Zi Tang*
Literal Name: Cinnamon Twig Decoction plus Magnolia Bark and Apricot Kernel
Original Source: *Shang Han Lun* (Discussion of Cold-Induced Disorders) by Zhang Zhong-Jing in the Eastern Han Dynasty

Gui Zhi (Ramulus Cinnamomi)	9g
Bai Shao (Radix Paeoniae Alba)	9g
Zhi Gan Cao (Radix et Rhizoma Glycyrrhizae Praeparata cum Melle)	6g
Sheng Jiang (Rhizoma Zingiberis Recens), *qie* (sliced)	9g
Da Zao (Fructus Jujubae), *bo* (opened)	12 pieces [3 pieces]
Hou Po (Cortex Magnoliae Officinalis), *zhi* (fried with liquid)	6g
Ku Xing Ren (Semen Armeniacae Amarum)	50 kernels [6g]

The source text states to cook the ingredients with 7 cups [1,400 mL] of water until 3 cups [600 mL] of the liquid remain. Take 1 cup [200 mL] of the warm, strained decoction and cover the body with blankets to promote mild sweating. Today, this formula may be prepared as a decoction with the doses suggested in brackets.

Gui Zhi Jia Hou Po Xing Zi Tang (Cinnamon Twig Decoction plus Magnolia Bark and Apricot Kernel) is usually used in the following two situations: 1) dyspnea associated with reversed flow of Lung qi as a result of inappropriate treatment of an exterior wind-cold syndrome with downward draining herbs; and 2) wind-cold invasion in patients with pre-existing asthma. In these two situations, *Gui Zhi Tang* treats the exterior-deficiency wind-cold syndrome, and *Hou Po* (Cortex Magnoliae Officinalis) and *Ku Xing Ren* (Semen Armeniacae Amarum) are added to direct Lung qi downward and relieve dyspnea.

Guì Zhī Jiā Sháo Yào Tāng

(Cinnamon Twig Decoction plus Peony)

桂枝加芍藥湯
桂枝加芍药汤

Pinyin Name: *Gui Zhi Jia Shao Yao Tang*
Literal Name: Cinnamon Twig Decoction plus Peony
Original Source: *Shang Han Lun* (Discussion of Cold-Induced Disorders) by Zhang Zhong-Jing in the Eastern Han Dynasty

Gui Zhi (Ramulus Cinnamomi)	9g
Bai Shao (Radix Paeoniae Alba)	18g
Zhi Gan Cao (Radix et Rhizoma Glycyrrhizae Praeparata cum Melle)	6g
Da Zao (Fructus Jujubae), *bo* (opened)	12 pieces [3 pieces]
Sheng Jiang (Rhizoma Zingiberis Recens), *qie* (sliced)	9g

Gui Zhi Jia Shao Yao Tang (Cinnamon Twig Decoction plus Peony) treats patients with *taiyang* syndrome who have been improperly treated with downward draining methods. In these situations, the downward draining methods damage Spleen qi, allowing the Liver to attack the deficient Spleen. As the exterior wind-cold condition moves into the interior, the *taiyang* syndrome is now complicated by *taiyin* syndrome. Clinically, this condition is characterized by both exterior and interior signs and

Guì Zhī Tāng (Cinnamon Twig Decoction)

symptoms: aversion to cold, fever, perspiration, abdominal fullness, distention and pain, and diarrhea.

Gui Zhi Jia Shao Yao Tang (Cinnamon Twig Decoction plus Peony) is a modification of *Gui Zhi Tang*. The ingredients and the doses of the two formulas are exactly the same, with the exception of *Bai Shao* (Radix Paeoniae Alba). The dose of *Bai Shao* is doubled in *Gui Zhi Jia Shao Yao Tang*, making it a formula for treating interior disharmony instead of exterior conditions. Today, *Gui Zhi Jia Shao Yao Tang* is used to treat abdominal pain and cramps, enteritis, and food poisoning.

Guì Zhī Má Huáng Gè Bàn Tāng
(Combined Cinnamon Twig and Ephedra Decoction)

桂枝麻黄各半湯
桂枝麻黄各半汤

Pinyin Name: *Gui Zhi Ma Huang Ge Ban Tang*
Literal Name: Combined Cinnamon Twig and Ephedra Decoction
Alternate Name: Cinnamon and Mahuang Combination
Original Source: *Shang Han Lun* (Discussion of Cold-Induced Disorders) by Zhang Zhong-Jing in the Eastern Han Dynasty

Gui Zhi (Ramulus Cinnamomi)	4.5g
Bai Shao (Radix Paeoniae Alba)	3g
Sheng Jiang (Rhizoma Zingiberis Recens), *qie* (sliced)	3g
Zhi Gan Cao (Radix et Rhizoma Glycyrrhizae Praeparata cum Melle)	3g
Ma Huang (Herba Ephedrae)	3g
Da Zao (Fructus Jujubae), *bo* (opened)	4 pieces
Ku Xing Ren (Semen Armeniacae Amarum)	24 pieces [3g]

The source text instructs to cook *Ma Huang* (Herba Ephedrae) first, remove the foam from the top, and then add in the rest of the ingredients. Take the warm, strained decoction in three equally-divided doses.

Gui Zhi Ma Huang Ge Ban Tang (Combined Cinnamon Twig and Ephedra Decoction) is indicated for patients who still have *taiyang* syndrome eight to nine days after the initial onset. Clinical presentation at this time may include symptoms such as flushed face, generalized itching, alternate spells of fever and aversion to cold two to three times daily, more fever than aversion to cold, headache, absence of nausea, and normal bowel movement. Generally speaking, exterior pathogenic factors do not stay at the *taiyang* stage for as long as eight to nine days. The disease commonly progresses to either the *yangming* or *shaoyang* syndrome.

Differential diagnosis is absolutely critical to obtain effective treatment. *Yangming* syndrome is characterized by excess interior heat with constipation as a key symptom; *shaoyang* syndrome is characterized by nausea; and malaria is characterized by alternating spells of aversion to cold and fever every two to three days. In this case, normal bowel movement rules out *yangming* syndrome; absence of nausea rules out *shaoyang* syndrome; and alternating spells of fever and aversion to cold two to three times daily (instead of every two to three days) rule out malaria. Additionally, patients will still show somewhat typical *taiyang* syndrome with such symptoms and signs as fever and aversion to cold, more fever than aversion to cold, and headache. With more fever than aversion to cold, patients are likely to have flushed face; and with wind-cold residing at the exterior blocking the skin pores, patients are likely to experience generalized itching.

The treatment strategies for patients with *taiyang* syndrome lasting eight to nine days after the initial onset are to dispel exterior wind-cold and harmonize the *wei* (defensive) and *ying* (nutritive) levels. In selecting an appropriate herbal formula, neither *Ma Huang Tang* (Ephedra Decoction) nor *Gui Zhi Tang* is appropriate. *Ma Huang Tang* (Ephedra Decoction) dispels wind-cold, yet its effects are too strong for someone who has had *taiyang* syndrome for eight to nine days. Furthermore, *Ma Huang Tang* (Ephedra Decoction) does not harmonize the *wei* (defensive) and *ying* (nutritive) levels. *Gui Zhi Tang*, on the other hand, can harmonize the *wei* (defensive) and *ying* (nutritive) levels. However, it is not strong enough to dispel wind-cold. Therefore, the ideal herbal formula is a combination of both *Ma Huang Tang* (Ephedra Decoction) and *Gui Zhi Tang*.

Appropriately, the literal name of this formula is "Combined [half each of] Cinnamon Twig and Ephedra Decoction." For additional and detailed explanation, please refer to *Ma Huang Tang* (Ephedra Decoction) and *Gui Zhi Tang* (Cinnamon Twig Decoction).

The clinical applications of this formula include common cold, influenza, bronchitis, pneumonia, eczema, and urticaria.

AUTHORS' COMMENTS

For *Gui Zhi Tang*, extreme care must be taken in the use of *Gui Zhi* (Ramulus Cinnamomi) and *Sheng Jiang* (Rhizoma Zingiberis Recens) to induce perspiration in a deficient individual who is already sweating. The chief manifestations for *Gui Zhi Tang* include fever, headache, sweating,

Guì Zhī Tāng (Cinnamon Twig Decoction)

aversion to wind, dry heaves, nasal obstruction, absence of thirst, a superficial, moderate pulse, and a white tongue coating. The sweating that occurs in this wind-cold invasion with deficiency is the result of a weak *wei* (defensive) *qi* not being able to retain fluids inside the body. Consequently, body fluids leak out in the form of sweats.

This sweating as a result of constitutional deficiency, however, does not expel the pathogenic wind-cold that lingers at the skin level. For this reason, *Gui Zhi* (Ramulus Cinnamomi) and *Sheng Jiang* (Rhizoma Zingiberis Recens), mild exterior-releasing herbs, are used to induce a small additional amount of sweating, enough to expel the pathogenic factors. *Da Zao* (Fructus Jujubae) helps harmonize the *ying* (nutritive) and *wei* (defensive) levels, to prevent *Gui Zhi* (Ramulus Cinnamomi) and *Sheng Jiang* (Rhizoma Zingiberis Recens) from inducing too much sweating. If only harmonizing herbs are used to address the disharmony of the *ying* (nutritive) and *wei* (defensive) levels, the wind-cold factor would linger and further damage *wei* (defensive) *qi*.[24]

Gui Zhi Tang is a formula with dual moderating effects: it induces perspiration to release the exterior; and it harmonizes the *wei* (defensive) and *ying* (nutritive) levels to stop perspiration caused by *wei* (defensive) *qi* deficiency. Ideally, mild sweating is the objective in order to dispel pathogenic wind-cold without damaging *wei* (defensive) and *ying* (nutritive) *qi*. *Gui Zhi* (Ramulus Cinnamomi) and *Sheng Jiang* (Rhizoma Zingiberis Recens) induce perspiration and release the exterior. *Bai Shao* (Radix Paeoniae Alba) and *Da Zao* (Fructus Jujubae) harmonize the *wei* and *ying* levels to stop perspiration and prevent over-sweating. After the pathogenic factor is dispelled and the *wei* and *ying* levels are harmonized, the patient no longer will have sweating due to deficient *wei qi*. This is why *Gui Zhi Tang* is referred by some as a formula that stops sweating.[25]

Within the context of *Gui Zhi Tang*, perspiration is both a "disease condition" and a "therapeutic outcome," and must be differentiated and monitored carefully. Perspiration as a "disease condition" has the following characteristics: it is caused by deficiency of *wei* (defensive) *qi*; it occurs at specific regions of the body (such as around the neck or in the back only); sweating occurs with a feeling of cool or cold sensation; it is accompanied by signs and symptoms of wind-cold (e.g., fever, headache, or nasal discharge); and finally, perspiration does not alleviate the condition. On the other hand, perspiration as a "therapeutic outcome" has different characteristics: sweating occurs evenly throughout the entire body and is accompanied by a feeling of warmth in the body; sweating occurs after the ingestion of herbs; and the patient's overall condition improves greatly after the perspiration.[26]

Gui Zhi Tang can be used in deficient patients who show both wind-cold and wind-heat symptoms. These mixed symptoms may include aversion to cold, fever, aversion to wind, perspiration, a sore throat, headache, and other conflicting symptoms. When it is difficult to diagnose whether the patient has wind-cold or wind-heat, many times the condition is transitioning from wind-cold to wind-heat, and then to Lung heat. Right in the stage between wind-cold and wind-heat, mixed symptoms such as the ones described will be present and the *ying* (nutritive) and *wei* (defensive) levels will be disrupted. *Gui Zhi Tang* is often combined with *Yin Qiao San* (Honeysuckle and Forsythia Powder) in a 1:1 ratio to help expel the exterior pathogenic factors of both wind-cold and wind-heat.

In the clinic, patients may not show all the signs, or it may be difficult to match the exact symptoms. The key to selecting *Gui Zhi Tang* is to identify the main symptoms: aversion to wind, perspiration, and a superficial, moderate pulse. Deficient patients often catch colds frequently as their *wei* (defensive) *qi* is low. They often will wear more clothing to cover up their body, since they dislike being exposed to the wind. In addition to the traditional applications, *Gui Zhi Tang* can also be used in convalescing, pregnant, and postpartum patients with spontaneous sweating, a slight feverish sensation, or aversion to wind and cold.

Gui Zhi Tang and *Yu Ping Feng San* (Jade Windscreen Powder) both treat spontaneous perspiration and aversion to wind, but have completely different clinical applications.

- *Gui Zhi Tang* is an exterior-releasing formula that treats wind-cold invasion with disharmony between the *ying* (nutritive) and *wei* (defensive) levels, causing symptoms such as fever, headache, stuffy nose, and a superficial pulse. This formula is used for patients who currently suffer from exterior condition.
- *Yu Ping Feng San* is an astringent formula that also treats perspiration and aversion to wind. However, these symptoms are caused by *wei* (defensive) *qi* deficiency and its inability to consolidate the exterior. Besides leakage of body fluids, other symptoms include frequent catching of common colds, pale complexion, generalized weakness, and a deficient pulse. This formula is appropriate for patients who frequently suffer from exterior condition but do not currently have one.[27]

Gui Zhī Tāng (Cinnamon Twig Decoction)

Gui Zhi Tang and *Xiao Jian Zhong Tang* (Minor Construct the Middle Decoction) contain very similar ingredients, but have drastically different applications. *Xiao Jian Zhong Tang* is comprised of *Gui Zhi Tang* plus *Yi Tang* (Maltosum). However, because of dose differences, the main functions of the two formulas differ significantly.

- *Gui Zhi Tang* is an exterior-releasing formula. It contains *Gui Zhi* (Ramulus Cinnamomi) and *Bai Shao* (Radix Paeoniae Alba) as chief and deputy herbs to release the exterior and harmonize the *ying* (nutritive) and *wei* (defensive) levels.

- *Xiao Jian Zhong Tang* is an interior warming formula. It contains *Yi Tang* (Maltosum) as the chief herb to warm and tonify the Spleen to relieve pain. As deputy herbs, *Gui Zhi* (Ramulus Cinnamomi) warms yang qi and *Bai Shao* (Radix Paeoniae Alba) relieves pain.

- Although both formulas contain similar ingredients, *Gui Zhi Tang* primarily expels exterior wind-cold invasion, while *Xiao Jian Zhong Tang* (Minor Construct the Middle Decoction) warms and tonifies the middle *jiao* to relieve pain.

References

1. Fu HY, He YZ. Studies on the hidropoiesis of the decoction of gui-zhi tang in mice and rats. *Zhong Xi Yi Jie He Za Zhi* 1991 Jan;11(1):34-6.
2. *Zhong Yao Yao Li Yu Ying Yong* (Pharmacology and Applications of Chinese Herbs) 1987;3(2):1.
3. *Zhong Cheng Yao Yan Jiu* (Research of Chinese Patent Medicine) 1983;(3):25.
4. *Zhong Yi Za Zhi* (Journal of Chinese Medicine) 1984;8:63.
5. *Zhong Cheng Yao Yan Jiu* (Research of Chinese Patent Medicine) 1983;(3):25.
6. *Zhong Yao Yao Li Yu Ying Yong* (Pharmacology and Applications of Chinese Herbs) 1987;3(2):1.
7. *Zhong Cheng Yao Yan Jiu* (Research of Chinese Patent Medicine) 1983;(3):25.
8. *Zhong Yao Yao Li Yu Ying Yong* (Pharmacology and Applications of Chinese Herbs) 1987;3(3):1.
9. Xu FH, Uebaba K. Effect of Kampo formulations (traditional Chinese medicine) on circulatory parameters. Acupuncture & Electro-Therapeutics Research 1999;24(1):11-28.
10. *Jiang Su Yi Yao* (Jiangsu Journal of Medicine and Herbology) 1979;(1):43.
11. *Zhong Yi Ming Fang Lin Chuang Xin Yong* (Contemporary Clinical Applications of Classic Chinese Formulas) 2001;547.
12. *Si Chuan Zhong Yi* (Sichuan Chinese Medicine) 1998;9:42.
13. *Jiang Xi Zhong Yi Yao* (Jiangxi Chinese Medicine and Herbology) 1999;6:56.
14. *Zhe Jiang Zhong Yi Za Zhi* (Zhejiang Journal of Chinese Medicine) 1985;3:109.
15. *Shan Xi Zhong Yi* (Shanxi Chinese Medicine) 1993;2:78.
16. *Zhe Jiang Zhong Yi Za Zhi* (Zhejiang Journal of Chinese Medicine) 1994;3:33.
17. *Shan Dong Zhong Yi Za Zhi* (Shandong Journal of Chinese Medicine) 1988;6:23.
18. *Zhong Hua Yi Xue Za Zhi* (Chinese Journal of Medicine) 1956;19:978.
19. *Ji Lin Zhong Yi Yao* (Jilin Chinese Medicine and Herbology) 1998;4:36.
20. *Shi Yong Zhong Xi Yi Jie He Za Zhi* (Practical Journal of Integrated Chinese and Western Medicines) 1992;1:44.
21. *Hu Bei Zhong Yi Za Zhi* (Hubei Journal of Chinese Medicine) 1994;3:33.
22. Tanaka T. Effects of herbal medicines on menopausal symptoms induced by gonadotropin-releasing hormone agonist therapy. Clin Exp Obstet Gynecol 2001;28(1):20-3.
23. *Zhong Cheng Yao Yan Jiu* (Research of Chinese Patent Medicine) 1983;(3):25
24. Wang MZ, et al. *Zhong Yi Xue Wen Da Ti Ku* (Questions and Answers on Traditional Chinese Medicine: Herbal Formulas).
25. Wang MZ, et al. *Zhong Yi Xue Wen Da Ti Ku* (Questions and Answers on Traditional Chinese Medicine: Herbal Formulas).
26. Wang MZ, et al. *Zhong Yi Xue Wen Da Ti Ku* (Questions and Answers on Traditional Chinese Medicine: Herbal Formulas).
27. Wang MZ, et al. *Zhong Yi Xue Wen Da Ti Ku* (Questions and Answers on Traditional Chinese Medicine: Herbal Formulas).

Chinese Herbal Formulas and Applications

Gě Gēn Tāng (Kudzu Decoction)

葛根湯
葛根汤

Pinyin Name: *Ge Gen Tang*
Literal Name: Kudzu Decoction
Alternate Names: *Ko Ken Tang*, Pueraria Decoction, Pueraria Combination
Original Source: *Shang Han Lun* (Discussion of Cold-Induced Disorders) by Zhang Zhong-Jing in the Eastern Han Dynasty

COMPOSITION

Ge Gen (Radix Puerariae Lobatae)	12g
Ma Huang (Herba Ephedrae)	9g
Gui Zhi (Ramulus Cinnamomi)	6g
Bai Shao (Radix Paeoniae Alba)	6g
Zhi Gan Cao (Radix et Rhizoma Glycyrrhizae Praeparata cum Melle)	6g
Sheng Jiang (Rhizoma Zingiberis Recens), *qie* (sliced)	9g
Da Zao (Fructus Jujubae), *bo* (opened)	12 pieces [3 pieces]

DOSAGE / PREPARATION / ADMINISTRATION

The source text states to cook *Ma Huang* (Herba Ephedrae) and *Ge Gen* (Radix Puerariae Lobatae) first with 10 cups [2,000 mL] of water until 8 cups [1,400 mL] of the liquid remain. Remove the foam from the top, add in the other ingredients, and cook until the liquid is reduced to 3 cups [600 mL]. Take 1 cup [200 mL] of the strained decoction while warm to promote mild sweating.

CHINESE THERAPEUTIC ACTIONS

1. Releases the exterior and muscle layer
2. Promotes generation of body fluids

CLINICAL MANIFESTATIONS

Taiyang syndrome with wind-cold invasion: severe muscle stiffness of the neck and back, aversion to cold, with or without fever, aversion to wind, absence of perspiration, and diarrhea.

CLINICAL APPLICATIONS

Fever, common cold, influenza, infectious parotitis, upper respiratory tract infection, allergic rhinitis, chronic rhinitis, neck and shoulder stiffness and pain, periarthritis of shoulder, tendonitis or bursitis of the shoulders, soft tissues injuries, facial paralysis, Bell's palsy, meningitis, encephalitis, tension headache, scleroderma, urticaria, painful gynecomastia in liver cirrhosis, aqueous flare elevation after complicated cataract surgery, and diarrhea.

EXPLANATION

Ge Gen Tang (Kudzu Decoction) treats *taiyang* syndrome with wind-cold invasion. In comparison to the symptoms and conditions applicable to *Ma Huang Tang* (Ephedra Decoction) and *Gui Zhi Tang* (Cinnamon Twig Decoction), the distinguishing symptom for the use of this formula is the severe stiffness and pain in the neck and back. The severe neck stiffness and pain are caused by cold constriction, and lack of body fluids which fail to nourish the muscle layer. Other signs and symptoms of *taiyang* syndrome with wind-cold invasion include fever, aversion to cold, aversion to wind, and absence of perspiration.

Ge Gen Tang is formulated by adding *Ge Gen* (Radix Puerariae Lobatae) and *Ma Huang* (Herba Ephedrae) to *Gui Zhi Tang* (Cinnamon Twig Decoction). *Ge Gen* (Radix Puerariae Lobatae), however, acts as the chief herb. It promotes generation of body fluids and relieves muscle stiffness. *Ma Huang* (Herba Ephedrae) and *Gui Zhi* (Ramulus Cinnamomi) release wind and cold from the exterior. Also, the sweet and acrid properties of *Gui Zhi* (Ramulus Cinnamomi) help to relieve body aches and pains. *Bai Shao* (Radix Paeoniae Alba), the deputy herb, consolidates the interior (yin and body fluids) of the body. Used together, *Gui Zhi* (Ramulus Cinnamomi) and *Bai Shao* (Radix Paeoniae Alba) harmonize qi at the *wei* (defensive) and *ying* (nutritive) levels. *Zhi Gan Cao* (Radix et Rhizoma Glycyrrhizae Praeparata cum Melle) serves as both an auxiliary and envoy herb. As an auxiliary herb, it relieves aches and pains and promotes the production of body fluids; as an envoy herb, it harmonizes the formula. *Sheng Jiang* (Rhizoma Zingiberis Recens) helps *Gui Zhi* (Ramulus Cinnamomi) to dispel exterior wind-cold. *Da Zao* (Fructus Jujubae) tonifies deficient qi and body fluids.

EXTERIOR-RELEASING FORMULAS

1

59

Gě Gēn Tāng (Kudzu Decoction)

Ge Gen Tang (Kudzu Decoction)

Diagnosis	Signs and Symptoms	Treatment	Herbs
Taiyang syndrome with wind-cold invasion	• Neck stiffness and pain: cold constriction and lack of body fluids • Fever, aversion to cold, aversion to wind, and absence of perspiration: taiyang syndrome with exterior wind-cold	• Releases the exterior and muscle layer • Promotes generation of body fluids	• *Ge Gen* (Radix Puerariae Lobatae) promotes generation of body fluids and relieves muscle stiffness. • *Ma Huang* (Herba Ephedrae) and *Gui Zhi* (Ramulus Cinnamomi) release wind and cold from the exterior. • *Gui Zhi* (Ramulus Cinnamomi) and *Bai Shao* (Radix Paeoniae Alba) harmonize *wei* (defensive) and *ying* (nutritive) levels. • *Zhi Gan Cao* (Radix et Rhizoma Glycyrrhizae Praeparata cum Melle) relieves aches and pains and promotes the production of body fluids. • *Sheng Jiang* (Rhizoma Zingiberis Recens) dispels exterior wind and cold. • *Da Zao* (Fructus Jujubae) tonifies deficient qi and body fluids.

MODIFICATIONS

• For nausea and vomiting caused by reversed flow of Stomach qi, add *Ban Xia* (Rhizoma Pinelliae) and *Fu Ling* (Poria).
• If there are signs of fever and thirst, add *Zhi Mu* (Rhizoma Anemarrhenae) and *Shi Gao* (Gypsum Fibrosum).
• If accompanied by severe pain of the shoulders, add *Fu Ling* (Poria), *Bai Zhu* (Rhizoma Atractylodis Macrocephalae) and *Fu Zi* (Radix Aconiti Lateralis Praeparata).
• For abdominal pain and diarrhea with burning sensations, add *Huang Qin* (Radix Scutellariae) and *Huang Lian* (Rhizoma Coptidis).
• When there is itching of the skin, add *Jiang Can* (Bombyx Batryticatus).

CAUTIONS / CONTRAINDICATIONS

Please refer to *Ma Huang Tang* (Ephedra Decoction).

PHARMACOLOGICAL EFFECTS

1. **Antibacterial**: According to *in vitro* studies, *Ge Gen Tang* demonstrated an inhibitory effect against *E. coli* and *Staphylococcus aureus*, but only at high concentration.[1]
2. **Antiviral**: One study reported marked effectiveness using *Ge Gen Tang* to treat mice with early stage of influenza infection. The dose of the formula was 5.0 mg per mouse three times daily. The mechanism of this action was attributed to significant enhancement of interleukin-12 correlated with the reduction of virus yields in bronchoalveolar lavage fluid in the early phase of infection.[2]
3. **Antipyretic**: Administration of *Ge Gen Tang* effectively reduced fever in mice infected with influenza virus. The mechanism of the antipyretic effects was attributed to the suppression of interferon-induced interleukin-1-alpha production.[3]
4. **Anti-inflammatory**: Oral administration of *Ge Gen Tang* was associated with inhibition of the inflammatory processes in both the early exudative stage and the late proliferative stage. This study stated *Ge Gen Tang* was useful in treating stomatitis, tonsillitis, cold and chronic inflammatory diseases.[4]
5. **Cardiovascular**: In anesthetized dogs and cats, intravenous injection of *Ge Gen Tang* at 0.25-0.5 g/kg was associated with dilation of the blood vessels and increased blood perfusion to the brain. The duration of action was approximately one hour.[5]
6. **Chronotropic and inotropic**: *Ge Gen Tang* has positive chronotropic and inotropic effects via direct stimulation of the beta-adrenoceptor and/or the norepinephrine released from postganglionic nerve terminals in the heart.[6]
7. **Immunostimulant**: Continuous administration of extract of *Ge Gen Tang* in mice was associated with a significant influence to the immune system. Increase in phagocytic activity of the immune cells was observed in mice with suppressed immune system. However, a suppression of the immune response was observed in mice with hyperactive immune system.[7,8] In another study involving 10 subjects, use of *Ge Gen Tang* daily was associated with an increase of natural killer (NK) cells.[9]
8. **Hepatoprotective**: *Ge Gen* (Radix Puerariae Lobatae), the main ingredient in *Ge Gen Tang*, inhibited the elevation of alanine aminotransferase (ALT) activity at the dose of 90 mcg/mL in rats with immunological liver injury.

Gě Gēn Tāng (Kudzu Decoction)

The antihepatotoxic activity was attributed primarily to soyasaponin I and kudzusaponin, the representative saponins.[10]

CLINICAL STUDIES AND RESEARCH

1. **Fever**: One hundred and ten children with fever were effectively treated with modified *Ge Gen Tang*. The study reported reduction of body temperature in 66 cases (60%) after 1 dose, 43 cases (39%) after 2 doses, and 1 case (0.9%) after 3 doses. Minor modifications to the original formula were made based on the clinical manifestations of the patients.[11]

2. **Upper respiratory tract infection**: In one study, *Ge Gen Tang* demonstrated a rate of effectiveness of approximately 80% in releasing the pathogenic factor from the exterior. The main improvements were seen in runny nose, sneezing, and aversion to cold.[12]

3. **Meningitis**: Thirteen patients with infectious meningitis were treated with *Ge Gen Tang* with complete recovery in all cases. Resolution of symptoms and signs range from 40 hours to 15 days. No complications were reported.[13] It has also been reported that this formula is also effective in treating encephalitis, though treatment must begin within the first two days.[14]

4. **Neck and shoulder pain**: Seventy patients with neck and shoulder disorders were treated with a modified *Ge Gen Tang* with complete recovery in 9 cases, significant improvement in 30 cases, moderate improvement in 29 cases, and no improvement in 2 cases. *Ge Gen Tang* was modified by increasing the doses of *Ge Gen* (Radix Puerariae Lobatae) and *Gui Zhi* (Ramulus Cinnamomi).[15] Another study reported a 94% rate of effectiveness using modified *Ge Gen Tang* to treat 50 patients between 40-60 years of age, with neck and shoulder pain with history of illness ranging from 5 days to 10 years. The duration of treatment ranged from 30-50 days. Of 50 patients, the study reported complete recovery in 16 cases, significant improvement in 25 cases, moderate improvement in 6 cases, and no benefit in 3 cases.[16]

5. **Periarthritis of shoulder**: Forty-eight patients with periarthritis of the shoulder was treated for 10-20 days with complete recovery in 34 cases, significant improvement in 8 cases, and no benefit in 6 cases. The herbal treatment contained *Ge Gen Tang* plus *Xi Xin* (Radix et Rhizoma Asari), *Qiang Huo* (Rhizoma et Radix Notopterygii), *Fang Feng* (Radix Saposhnikoviae) and others.[17]

6. **Soft tissues injuries**: One study reported a 96.88% rate of effectiveness using modified *Ge Gen Tang* to treat soft tissues injuries in 32 patients (25 males and 7 females), between 10-55 years of age, and 1 hour to 1½ year history of illness. The herbal treatment consisted of *Ge Gen Tang*, with the dose of *Ge Gen* (Radix Puerariae Lobatae) increased to 50g. Of 32 patients, the study reported complete recovery in 19 cases, significant improvement in 12 cases, and no benefit in 1 case.[18]

7. **Facial paralysis**: Use of modified *Ge Gen Tang* was associated with varying degrees of improvement to complete recovery in all 216 patients with facial paralysis. The herbal treatment contained *Ge Gen Tang* plus *Bai Fu Zi* (Rhizoma Typhonii), *Jiang Can* (Bombyx Batryticatus), *Quan Xie* (Scorpio), and others as needed. The herbs were given in decoction daily, for 5 packs of herbs per course of treatment. The duration of treatment ranged from 5-35 packs of herbs.[19] Another study reported 97.67% effectiveness in treating 86 patients with facial paralysis. The herbal treatment contained *Ge Gen Tang* plus *Qian Zheng San* (Lead to Symmetry Powder), with addition of *Fu Ling* (Poria) and *Cang Zhu* (Rhizoma Atractylodis) for presence of dampness; and addition of *Chai Hu* (Radix Bupleuri) and *Huang Qin* (Radix Scutellariae) for fever. After 3-5 packs of herbs and induction of perspiration, the herbal treatment was modified by adding *Hong Hua* (Flos Carthami), *Dang Gui* (Radix Angelicae Sinensis) and *Huang Qi* (Radix Astragali); and eliminating *Ma Huang* (Herba Ephedrae), *Gui Zhi* (Ramulus Cinnamomi), *Qiang Huo* (Rhizoma et Radix Notopterygii) and *Ge Gen* (Radix Puerariae Lobatae). Upon stabilization and during the recovery phase, the herbal treatment was switched to *Shi Quan Da Bu Tang* (All-Inclusive Great Tonifying Decoction) for consolidation and maintenance. Of 86 patients, the study reported complete recovery in 79 cases, improvement in 5 cases, and no benefit in 2 cases.[20]

8. **Bell's palsy**: Seventy-eight patients with Bell's palsy were treated with *Ge Gen Tang* with marked effectiveness. The study reported a 53.8% rate of effectiveness (42 of 78 patients) within 5 doses.[21]

9. **Tension headache**: Powdered extract of *Ge Gen Tang* at 7.5 g/day, given in three equally-divided doses, was 80% effective in treating tension headache.[22]

10. **Scleroderma**: Use of modified *Ge Gen Tang* in 7 patients with scleroderma was associated with near-recovery in 5 cases and improvement in 2 cases. The herbal treatment contained *Ge Gen* (Radix Puerariae Lobatae) 30-60g, *Gui Zhi* (Ramulus Cinnamomi) 10-20g, *Ma Huang* (Herba Ephedrae) 6-10g, *Sheng Jiang* (Rhizoma Zingiberis Recens) 6-10g, *Bai Shao* (Radix Paeoniae Alba) 15-30g, *Gan Cao* (Radix et Rhizoma Glycyrrhizae) 15-30g, and *Da Zao* (Fructus Jujubae) 15-30g. The doses of herbs were adjusted to achieve mild perspiration after administration of the decoction. The duration of treatment was 15 days per course, for 4 courses total.[23]

11. **Painful gynecomastia in liver cirrhosis**: One study reported marked success using *Ge Gen Tang* to treat 4 patients with liver cirrhosis who complained of painful

Gě Gēn Tāng (Kudzu Decoction)

gynecomastia. After oral ingestion of *Ge Gen Tang*, relief of pain was reported in 3 patients in one week, and 1 patient in 4 weeks. The palpable induration diminished or disappeared, but the size of gynecomastia did not change significantly on mammography. Serum levels of estrogen, progesterone, testosterone, and other sex hormones were not affected by the herbs. The study suggested that *Ge Gen Tang* could be used for painful gynecomastia that is occasionally seen in cirrhotic patients.[24]

12. **Cataract surgery**: Use of *Ge Gen Tang* and *Huang Lian Jie Du Tang* (Coptis Decoction to Relieve Toxicity) was found to help reduce aqueous flare elevation after complicated cataract surgery. The treatment protocol was to administer powdered extract of *Ge Gen Tang* (7.5 g/day) and *Huang Lian Jie Du Tang* (Coptis Decoction to Relieve Toxicity) (7.5 g/day) for 3 days before surgery, the day of surgery, and for 7 days after surgery. In comparison to the control group that did not receive any herbs, oral administration of these two formulas was effective in decreasing aqueous flare elevation after small-incision cataract surgery.[25] Another study also reported that *Ge Gen Tang* reduced aqueous flare elevation after surgery for complicated cataract. The treatment protocol was to administer the herbs in granules, 7.5g daily for 3 days before surgery, the day of surgery, and for 7 days after surgery. Diclofenac eyedrops were also used in all patients.[26]

HERB-DRUG INTERACTION

Acetaminophen: One study evaluated the pharmacokinetics of acetaminophen under co-administration of *Ge Gen Tang* in human volunteers. The pharmacokinetic parameters were calculated from the blood acetaminophen concentration-time curves. No significant differences were noted between the group that received only acetaminophen and the group that received both acetaminophen and *Ge Gen Tang*.[27]

TOXICOLOGY

Ge Gen Tang is relatively safe, even at a high dosage. No side effects or toxicities were observed following oral administration of this formula at 2.5 g/kg in mice. Furthermore, adverse reactions were not observed following oral administration of this formula to mice at a dosage equivalent to seventeen times the normal adult human dose.[28] In humans, administration of this formula in extract at 7.5 g/day was associated with mild nausea, vomiting, fatigue and constipation.[29]

RELATED FORMULAS

Jǐng Fāng Yī Haò (Neck Formula One)
頸方一號
颈方一号
Pinyin Name: *Jing Fang Yi Hao*
Literal Name: Neck Formula One
Original Source: *Tian Jin Zhong Yi Xue Yuan* (Tianjin University of Chinese Medicine) in 1989

Ge Gen (Radix Puerariae Lobatae)
Bai Shao (Radix Paeoniae Alba)
Gan Cao (Radix et Rhizoma Glycyrrhizae)
Chuan Xiong (Rhizoma Chuanxiong)
Dang Gui (Radix Angelicae Sinensis)
Hong Hua (Flos Carthami)
Wei Ling Xian (Radix et Rhizoma Clematidis)
Qiang Huo (Rhizoma et Radix Notopterygii)
Yan Hu Suo (Rhizoma Corydalis)

This formula treats acute and severe neck and shoulder pain. It contains herbs to activate qi and blood circulation, dispel qi and blood stagnation, open the channels and collaterals, and relieve pain.

Jǐng Fāng Èr Haò (Neck Formula Two)
頸方二號
颈方二号
Pinyin Name: *Jing Fang Er Hao*
Literal Name: Neck Formula Two
Original Source: *Tian Jin Zhong Yi Xue Yuan* (Tianjin University of Chinese Medicine) in 1989

Ge Gen (Radix Puerariae Lobatae)
Bai Shao (Radix Paeoniae Alba)
Gan Cao (Radix et Rhizoma Glycyrrhizae)
Chuan Xiong (Rhizoma Chuanxiong)
Dang Gui (Radix Angelicae Sinensis)
Hong Hua (Flos Carthami)
Lu Lu Tong (Fructus Liquidambaris)
Dan Shen (Radix et Rhizoma Salviae Miltiorrhizae)
Di Gu Pi (Cortex Lycii)
Mu Gua (Fructus Chaenomelis)
Chuan Niu Xi (Radix Cyathulae)
Qiang Huo (Rhizoma et Radix Notopterygii)
Qin Jiao (Radix Gentianae Macrophyllae)
Sang Ji Sheng (Herba Taxilli)
Wu Jia Pi (Cortex Acanthopanacis)
Xu Duan (Radix Dipsaci)
Di Huang (Radix Rehmanniae)
Tao Ren (Semen Persicae)
Yan Hu Suo (Rhizoma Corydalis)

Gĕ Gēn Tāng (Kudzu Decoction)

This formula treats chronic neck and shoulder pain. It contains herbs to activate qi and blood circulation, dispel qi and blood stagnation, and open the channels and collaterals. In addition, this formula contains many herbs to nourish Liver and Kidney yin to strengthen the soft tissues and facilitate recovery.

AUTHORS' COMMENTS

Historically, *Ge Gen Tang* has been used for *taiyang* syndrome with wind-cold, and accompanied by stiffness of the neck and shoulders. Today, it is commonly used to treat neck and shoulder stiffness and pain associated with musculoskeletal injuries, with or without *taiyang* syndrome or wind-cold condition. For best results, combine *Ge Gen Tang* with *Shao Yao Gan Cao Tang* (Peony and Licorice Decoction) to treat neck and shoulder stiffness and pain.

Ge Gen Tang can be used at a low dose to complement the effects of *Qi Bao Mei Ran Dan* (Seven-Treasure Special Pill for Beautiful Whiskers) for hair growth. It helps guide the effects of *Qi Bao Mei Ran Dan* upward by relaxing the muscles around the neck, so that the tonic herbs can reach and nourish the scalp area directly.

References

1. *Zhong Yi Za Zhi* (Journal of Chinese Medicine) 1955;(10):36.
2. Kurokawa M, Tsurita M, Brown J, Fukuda Y, Shiraki K. Effect of interleukin-12 level augmented by Kakkon-to, a herbal medicine, on the early stage of influenza infection in mice. Antiviral Res 2002 Nov;56(2):183-8.
3. Kurokawa M, Kumeda CA, Yamamura J, Kamiyama T, Shiraki K. Antipyretic activity of cinnamyl derivatives and related compounds in influenza virus-infected mice. Eur J Pharmacol 1998 May 1;348(1):45-51.
4. Ozaki Y. Studies on antiinflammatory effect of Japanese Oriental medicines (kampo medicines) used to treat inflammatory diseases. Biol Pharm Bull 1995 Apr;18(4):559-62.
5. *Zhong Yao Yao Li Yu Ying Yong* (Pharmacology and Applications of Chinese Herbs) 1987;4(4):33.
6. Sugiyama A, Takahara A, Satoh Y, Yoneyama M, Saegusa Y, Hashimoto K. Cardiac effects of clinically available Kampo medicine assessed with canine isolated, blood-perfused heart preparations. Jpn J Pharmacol 2002 Mar;88(3):307-13.

7. *Guo Wai Yi Xue* (Foreign Medicine) 1993;15(3):23.
8. *Guo Wai Yi Xue* (Foreign Medicine) 1995;17(3):64.
9. *Han Fang Yi Xue* (Kampo Medicine) 1985;9(5):12.
10. Arao T, Udayama M, Kinjo J, Nohara T, Funakoshi T, Kojima S. Preventive effects of saponins from puerariae radix (the root of Pueraria lobata Ohwi) on in vitro immunological injury of rat primary hepatocyte cultures. Biol Pharm Bull 1997 Sep;20(9):988-91.
11. *Yun Nan Zhong Yi Za Zhi* (Yunan Journal of Chinese Medicine) 1987;8(2):35.
12. *Zhong Yi Fang Ji Xian Dai Yan Jiu* (Modern Study of Medical Formulae in Traditional Chinese Medicine) 1997;63(6):2007.
13. *Jiang Su Zhong Yi Za Zhi* (Jiangsu Journal of Chinese Medicine) 1963;(11):17.
14. *Fu Jian Zhong Yi Yao* (Fujian Chinese Medicine and Herbology) 1956;(2):13.
15. *Liao Ning Zhong Yi Za Zhi* (Liaoning Journal of Chinese Medicine) 1983;(6):34.
16. *Zhong Yi Han Shou Tong Xun* (Reports of Chinese Medicine) 1993;3:42.
17. *Hu Bei Zhong Yi Za Zhi* (Hubei Journal of Chinese Medicine) 1995;2:31.
18. *Zhong Yi Ming Fang Lin Chuang Xin Yong* (Contemporary Clinical Applications of Classic Chinese Formulas) 2001;677.
19. *Hu Nan Zhong Yi Za Zhi* (Hunan Journal of Chinese Medicine) 1992;1:43.
20. *Ji Lin Zhong Yi Yao* (Jilin Chinese Medicine and Herbology) 1995;1:18.
21. *Hu Nan Zhong Yi Za Zhi* (Hunan Journal of Chinese Medicine) 1989;5(3):26.
22. *Guo Wai Yi Xue* (Foreign Medicine) 1995;17(3):28.
23. *Zhe Jiang Zhong Yi Za Zhi* (Zhejiang Journal of Chinese Medicine) 1997;4:176.
24. Motoo Y, Taga H, Su SB, Sawabu N. Effect of gegen-tang on painful gynecomastia in patients with liver cirrhosis: a brief report. American Journal of Chinese Medicine 1997;25(3-4):317-24. erratum appears in Am J Chin Med 1998;26(1):114.
25. Ikeda N, Hayasaka S, Nagaki Y, Hayasaka Y, Kadoi C, Matsumoto M. Effects of traditional Sino-Japanese herbal medicines on aqueous flare elevation after small-incision cataract surgery. J Ocul Pharmacol Ther 2001 Feb;17(1):59-65.
26. Ikeda N, Hayasaka S, Nagaki Y, Hayasaka Y, Kadoi C, Matsumoto M. Effects of kakkon-to and sairei-to on aqueous flare elevation after complicated cataract surgery. American Journal of Chinese Medicine 2002;30(2-3):347-53.
27. Qi J, Toyoshima A, Honda Y, Mineshita S. Pharmacokinetic study on acetaminophen: interaction with a Chinese medicine. Journal of Medical & Dental Sciences 1997 Mar;44(1):31-5.
28. *Guo Wai Yi Xue* (Foreign Medicine) 1993;15(3):23.
29. *Guo Wai Yi Xue* (Foreign Medicine) 1989;11(1):52.

Chapter 1 – Exterior-Releasing Formulas   Section 1 – Acrid and Warm Exterior-Releasing Formulas

Jiŭ Wèi Qiāng Huó Tāng (Nine-Herb Decoction with Notopterygium)

九味羌活湯
九味羌活汤

Pinyin Name: *Jiu Wei Qiang Huo Tang*
Literal Name: Nine-Herb Decoction with Notopterygium
Alternate Names: *Chiu Wei Qiang Huo Tang, Jiu Wei Chiang Huo Tang,* Nine-Flavour Chiang-hou Decoction, Notopterygium Decoction with Nine Herbs, Notopterigium Nine Herb Combination
Original Source: *Ci Shi Nan Zhi* (Hard-Won Knowledge) by Wang Hao-Gu in 1308

COMPOSITION

Qiang Huo (Rhizoma et Radix Notopterygii)	4.5g [6g]
Fang Feng (Radix Saposhnikoviae)	4.5g [6g]
Cang Zhu (Rhizoma Atractylodis)	4.5g [6g]
Xi Xin (Radix et Rhizoma Asari)	1.5g [2g]
Chuan Xiong (Rhizoma Chuanxiong)	3g
Bai Zhi (Radix Angelicae Dahuricae)	3g
Di Huang (Radix Rehmanniae)	3g
Huang Qin (Radix Scutellariae)	3g
Gan Cao (Radix et Rhizoma Glycyrrhizae)	3g

DOSAGE / PREPARATION / ADMINISTRATION

The source text states to grind the ingredients coarsely and cook the coarse powder in water to make a decoction. Today, this formula may be prepared as a decoction with the doses suggested in brackets. In addition, 3 slices of *Sheng Jiang* (Rhizoma Zingiberis Recens) and 3 stalks of *Cong Bai* (Bulbus Allii Fistulosi) can be added to enhance the effects of unblocking yang qi and releasing the exterior.

CHINESE THERAPEUTIC ACTIONS

1. Induces diaphoresis and dispels dampness
2. Clears interior heat

CLINICAL MANIFESTATIONS

Wind, cold and dampness at the exterior and heat in the interior: aversion to cold, fever, absence of perspiration, headache, neck stiffness, soreness and pain of the body and limbs, a bitter taste in the mouth, thirst, a white tongue coating, and a superficial pulse.

CLINICAL APPLICATIONS

Common cold, influenza, arthritis, rheumatoid arthritis, sciatica, urticaria, muscle aches and pains, migraines, and headache.

EXPLANATION

Jiu Wei Qiang Huo Tang (Nine-Herb Decoction with Notopterygium) treats wind, cold and dampness

constricting the exterior and heat forming in the interior. Aversion to cold, fever, and absence of perspiration are caused by wind-cold constricting the pores and blocking the yang qi from reaching the *wei* (defensive) level. The wind, cold and dampness at the exterior block qi and blood circulation in the channels and collaterals, which results in headache, neck stiffness, body aches, and pain. Constriction at the exterior can lead to heat formation in the interior, causing a bitter taste in the mouth and thirst. However, the disease location is mainly at the exterior, as indicated by the white tongue coating and the superficial pulse. Treatment should thus focus primarily on releasing the exterior, and secondarily on clearing interior heat.

Acrid, aromatic and warm, *Qiang Huo* (Rhizoma et Radix Notopterygii) enters the *taiyang* channel and disperses wind, cold and dampness at the exterior. It releases wind-cold, dispels wind-dampness, benefits the joints, and relieves pain. *Fang Feng* (Radix Saposhnikoviae) helps dispel wind, and *Cang Zhu* (Rhizoma Atractylodis) dries dampness. *Xi Xin* (Radix et Rhizoma Asari), *Chuan Xiong* (Rhizoma Chuanxiong), and *Bai Zhi* (Radix Angelicae Dahuricae) dispel wind-cold factor, disperse dampness, activate qi and blood flow, and relieve headache and body aches. *Di Huang* (Radix Rehmanniae) prevents the acrid and warm herbs from damaging body fluids. *Huang Qin* (Radix Scutellariae) clears interior heat. *Gan Cao* (Radix et Rhizoma Glycyrrhizae) harmonizes the herbs.

64

Chinese Herbal Formulas and Applications

Jiǔ Wèi Qiāng Huó Tāng (Nine-Herb Decoction with Notopterygium)

Jiu Wei Qiang Huo Tang (Nine-Herb Decoction with Notopterygium)

Diagnosis	Signs and Symptoms	Treatment	Herbs
Exterior wind, cold and dampness, with interior heat	• Fever and aversion to cold: exterior wind-cold • Soreness and pain in the body and extremities: exterior wind-dampness causing qi and blood stagnation • White tongue coating and a superficial pulse: exterior condition • Thirst and a bitter taste in the mouth: interior heat	• Dispels exterior wind, cold and dampness • Clears interior heat	• *Qiang Huo* (Rhizoma et Radix Notopterygii) disperses wind, cold and dampness at the exterior. • *Fang Feng* (Radix Saposhnikoviae) dispels wind and cold. • *Cang Zhu* (Rhizoma Atractylodis) dries dampness. • *Xi Xin* (Radix et Rhizoma Asari), *Chuan Xiong* (Rhizoma Chuanxiong), and *Bai Zhi* (Radix Angelicae Dahuricae) dispel wind-cold factor, disperse dampness, and activate qi and blood flow. • *Di Huang* (Radix Rehmanniae) prevents the acrid and warm herbs from damaging body fluids. • *Huang Qin* (Radix Scutellariae) clears interior heat. • *Gan Cao* (Radix et Rhizoma Glycyrrhizae) harmonizes the herbs.

MODIFICATIONS

• If there is severe pain caused by more damp accumulation, increase the dose of *Qiang Huo* (Rhizoma et Radix Notopterygii) and *Cang Zhu* (Rhizoma Atractylodis).

• If the pain is moderate or mild because there is less damp accumulation, remove *Cang Zhu* (Rhizoma Atractylodis) and *Xi Xin* (Radix et Rhizoma Asari).

• When there is a feeling of fullness and oppression in the chest caused by damp accumulation, remove *Di Huang* (Radix Rehmanniae); and add *Zhi Qiao* (Fructus Aurantii) and *Hou Po* (Cortex Magnoliae Officinalis).

• If there is severe headache, add *Gao Ben* (Rhizoma et Radix Ligustici).

• If there is no bitter taste in the mouth or thirst, lower the dose or remove *Di Huang* (Radix Rehmanniae) and *Huang Qin* (Radix Scutellariae).

• With clear or watery nasal discharge, add *Xin Yi San* (Magnolia Flower Powder).

• If accompanied by cough, add *Ku Xing Ren* (Semen Armeniacae Amarum) and *Zhi Sou San* (Stop Coughing Powder).

• For vomiting or thirst, add *Zhi Shi* (Fructus Aurantii Immaturus) and *Jie Geng* (Radix Platycodonis).

• To enhance the exterior-releasing functions, add *Cong Bai* (Bulbus Allii Fistulosi) and *Sheng Jiang* (Rhizoma Zingiberis Recens).

CAUTIONS / CONTRAINDICATIONS

• *Jiu Wei Qiang Huo Tang* contains many warm, acrid, and drying herbs. It should be used with caution in patients with yin, qi or body fluid deficiencies.

• This formula is contraindicated in patients with wind-heat, yin-deficient heat, or generalized weakness and deficiency with heat.

PHARMACOLOGICAL EFFECTS

1. **Antipyretic**: Administration of *Jiu Wei Qiang Huo Tang* was effective in reducing body temperature in rabbits with artificially-induced fever. The antipyretic effects of the herbs started 2 hours after ingestion, and lasted for 6 hours. The reduction of body temperature was 0.7°C after 4 hours. The study also noted that the potency of the formula was similar to 0.2 mg/kg of aspirin.[1]

2. **Analgesic and anti-inflammatory**: One study reported that both water and alcohol extracts of *Jiu Wei Qiang Huo Tang* had marked analgesic and anti-inflammatory effects in mice.[2]

CLINICAL STUDIES AND RESEARCH

1. **Sciatica**: Modified *Jiu Wei Qiang Huo Tang* was used to treat 38 patients with sciatica with an overall effectiveness rate of 94.7%.[3]

2. **Headache**: Administration of modified *Jiu Wei Qiang Huo Tang* was associated with up to 92.86% effectiveness in treating headache characterized by wind-dampness. Out of 28 patients, the study reported complete recovery in 12 cases, improvement in 14 cases, and no effect in 2 cases. The herbal formula included *Jiu Wei Qiang Huo Tang* plus

65

EXTERIOR-RELEASING FORMULAS

Chapter 1 – Exterior-Releasing Formulas　　　　　　*Section 1 – Acrid and Warm Exterior-Releasing Formulas*

Jiǔ Wèi Qiāng Huó Tāng (Nine-Herb Decoction with Notopterygium)

Ge Gen (Radix Puerariae Lobatae) and *Dang Gui* (Radix Angelicae Sinensis) as the base formula. Modifications included the addition of *Tian Ma* (Rhizoma Gastrodiae), *Gou Teng* (Ramulus Uncariae cum Uncis) and *Ju Hua* (Flos Chrysanthemi) for severe dizziness; *Huang Qi* (Radix Astragali), *Dang Shen* (Radix Codonopsis) and *Bai Zhu* (Rhizoma Atractylodis Macrocephalae) for generalized weakness and deficiency; *Tao Ren* (Semen Persicae), *Hong Hua* (Flos Carthami) and *Quan Xie* (Scorpio) for chronic headache; *Chai Hu* (Radix Bupleuri) and *Long Dan* (Radix et Rhizoma Gentianae) for migraine headache; *Man Jing Zi* (Fructus Viticis) and *Gui Zhi* (Ramulus Cinnamomi) for occipital headache with neck stiffness and pain; and *Gao Ben* (Rhizoma et Radix Ligustici) for vertex headache.[4]

3. **Acute urticaria**: In one study, 144 of 152 patients with acute urticaria were treated successfully using modified *Jiu Wei Qiang Huo Tang*. The treatment protocol was to administer 3-10 packs of the herbs in decoction. The formula was modified by adding *Lu Dou* (Semen Phaseoli Radiati) and a large dose of *Gan Cao* (Radix et Rhizoma Glycyrrhizae) for urticaria caused by drug allergy; *Bing Lang* (Semen Arecae) and *Wu Mei* (Fructus Mume) for parasites; *Chan Tui* (Periostracum Cicadae), *Fu Ping* (Herba Spirodelae) and *Di Fu Zi* (Fructus Kochiae) for recurrent outbreaks; and elimination of *Xi Xin* (Radix et Rhizoma Asari) for the presence of wind-heat.[5]

RELATED FORMULA

Dà Qiāng Huó Tāng (Major Notopterygium Decoction)

大羌活湯
大羌活汤

Pinyin Name: *Da Qiang Huo Tang*
Literal Name: Major Notopterygium Decoction
Original Source: *Ci Shi Nan Zhi* (Hard-Won Knowledge) by Wang Hao-Gu in 1308

Qiang Huo (Rhizoma et Radix Notopterygii)	9g
Du Huo (Radix Angelicae Pubescentis)	9g
Fang Feng (Radix Saposhnikoviae)	9g
Xi Xin (Radix et Rhizoma Asari)	9g
Fang Ji (Radix Stephaniae Tetrandrae)	9g
Huang Qin (Radix Scutellariae)	9g
Huang Lian (Rhizoma Coptidis)	9g
Cang Zhu (Rhizoma Atractylodis)	9g
Zhi Gan Cao (Radix et Rhizoma Glycyrrhizae Praeparata cum Melle)	9g
Bai Zhu (Rhizoma Atractylodis Macrocephalae)	9g
Zhi Mu (Rhizoma Anemarrhenae)	30g
Chuan Xiong (Rhizoma Chuanxiong)	30g
Di Huang (Radix Rehmanniae)	30g

The source text specifies to coarsely grind the ingredients and cook 15g of the powder with 2 large bowls of water until 1.5 bowls of liquid remain. Remove and discard the herb residue. Take one large bowl of the warm, strained decoction. Patients may take an additional three to four doses until the condition is resolved. If there are any other remaining symptoms, use corresponding treatment as described in the *Shang Han Lun* (Discussion of Cold-Induced Disorders).

Da Qiang Huo Tang (Major Notopterygium Decoction) treats exterior wind, cold and dampness accompanied by interior heat. This formula releases wind-cold from the exterior, dispels dampness, and clears heat. Clinically, patients may show such symptoms as headache, fever, aversion to cold, a dry mouth, a bitter taste in the mouth, thirst, and irritability.

Qiang Huo (Rhizoma et Radix Notopterygii) releases wind-cold from the *taiyang* channel, while *Du Huo* (Radix Angelicae Pubescentis) releases wind-cold from the *shaoyin* channel. *Fang Feng* (Radix Saposhnikoviae), *Chuan Xiong* (Rhizoma Chuanxiong), and *Xi Xin* (Radix et Rhizoma Asari) release the exterior and relieve headache. *Huang Qin* (Radix Scutellariae) and *Huang Lian* (Rhizoma Coptidis) clear interior heat. *Zhi Mu* (Rhizoma Anemarrhenae) and *Di Huang* (Radix Rehmanniae) promote the generation of yin and body fluids and relieve thirst. *Fang Ji* (Radix Stephaniae Tetrandrae) regulates water circulation and dispels dampness. *Cang Zhu* (Rhizoma Atractylodis) and *Bai Zhu* (Rhizoma Atractylodis Macrocephalae) dry up dampness. *Zhi Gan Cao* (Radix et Rhizoma Glycyrrhizae Praeparata cum Melle) tonifies qi and harmonizes the formula.

Jiu Wei Qiang Huo Tang and *Da Qiang Huo Tang* (Major Notopterygium Decoction) have similar functions to release exterior wind, cold and dampness, and clear interior heat.
- *Jiu Wei Qiang Huo Tang* focuses on releasing wind, cold and dampness from the exterior.
- *Da Qiang Huo Tang* emphasizes clearing heat from the interior.

AUTHORS' COMMENTS

Jiu Wei Qiang Huo Tang is a formula that can be used in all four seasons to treat conditions characterized by wind, cold, and damp factors at the exterior, with heat in the interior. The main diagnostic symptoms include fever, aversion to cold, headache, absence of sweating, muscle aches and pains, a bitter taste in the mouth, and slight thirst.

Jiŭ Wèi Qiāng Huó Tāng (Nine-Herb Decoction with Notopterygium)

Jiu Wei Qiang Huo Tang and *Qiang Huo Sheng Shi Tang* (Notopterygium Decoction to Overcome Dampness) both contain *Qiang Huo* (Rhizoma et Radix Notopterygii) as the main ingredient, and both treat wind-dampness at the exterior. Their differences are as follows:

- *Jiu Wei Qiang Huo Tang* dispels wind, cold, and damp factors from the exterior, and clears heat from the interior. It mainly treats individuals who have both exterior and interior conditions, with such symptoms as fever, aversion to cold, mild aches and pains, a bitter taste in the mouth, and slight thirst.

- *Qiang Huo Sheng Shi Tang* strongly dispels wind-dampness. It primarily treats heaviness, immobility, and pain in the head and upper body.

References

1. *Zhong Yao Tong Bao* (Journal of Chinese Herbology) 1986;11(1):51.
2. *Zhong Cheng Yao* (Study of Chinese Patent Medicine) 1992;14(2):25.
3. *Shang Hai Zhong Yi Yao Za Zhi* (Shanghai Journal of Chinese Medicine and Herbology) 1988;7:23.
4. *Si Chuan Zhong Yi* (Sichuan Chinese Medicine) 1999;8:35.
5. *Shang Hai Zhong Yi Za Zhi* (Shanghai Journal of Chinese Medicine) 1982;4:21.

Xiāng Sū Săn (Cyperus and Perilla Leaf Powder)

香蘇散
香苏散

Pinyin Name: *Xiang Su San*
Literal Name: Cyperus and Perilla Leaf Powder
Alternate Names: *Hsiang Su San*, Cyperus and Perilla Powder, Cyperus and Perilla Formula
Original Source: *Tai Ping Hui Min He Ji Ju Fang* (Imperial Grace Formulary of the Tai Ping Era) by the Imperial Medical Department in 1078-85

COMPOSITION

Zi Su Ye (Folium Perillae)	120g [6-9g]
Xiang Fu (Rhizoma Cyperi), *chao* (dry-fried)	120g [6-9g]
Chen Pi (Pericarpium Citri Reticulatae)	60g [3-6g]
Zhi Gan Cao (Radix et Rhizoma Glycyrrhizae Praeparata cum Melle)	30g [3-6g]

DOSAGE / PREPARATION / ADMINISTRATION

The source text states to grind the ingredients coarsely and cook 9g with one large bowl of water until 70% of the liquid remains. Take the warm, strained decoction in three equally-divided doses any time during the day. This formula may also be prepared as a fine powder form and taken 6g per dose with a pinch of salt. Today, this formula may be prepared as a decoction with the doses suggested in brackets. A small amount of *Sheng Jiang* (Rhizoma Zingiberis Recens) and *Cong Bai* (Bulbus Allii Fistulosi) may be added to enhance the exterior-releasing effect.[1]

CHINESE THERAPEUTIC ACTIONS

1. Regulates qi
2. Releases the exterior

CLINICAL MANIFESTATIONS

Wind-cold factor at the exterior with qi stagnation in the interior: aversion to cold, fever, headache, absence of perspiration, fullness and distention of the chest and epigastrium, lack of appetite, a thin, white tongue coating, and a superficial pulse.

CLINICAL APPLICATIONS

Common cold, stomach influenza, acute gastroenteritis, chronic gastritis, and globus pharyngeus.

EXPLANATION

Xiang Su San (Cyperus and Perilla Leaf Powder) treats wind-cold condition with qi stagnation in the interior. Wind-cold causes symptoms such as aversion to cold, fever, headache, and absence of perspiration. Qi stagnation in this syndrome refers to qi stagnation in the middle *jiao*, which may produce fullness and rigidity of the chest and epigastrium, and lack of appetite. The thin, white tongue coating and the superficial pulse suggest that the disease is primarily at the exterior.

Xiāng Sū Săn (Cyperus and Perilla Leaf Powder)

Xiang Su San (Cyperus and Perilla Leaf Powder)

Diagnosis	Signs and Symptoms	Treatment	Herbs
Exterior wind-cold with interior qi stagnation	• Fever and aversion to cold: exterior wind-cold • Superficial pulse: exterior condition • Fullness and distention of the chest and epigastrium: qi stagnation	• Releases exterior wind-cold • Regulates interior qi circulation	• *Zi Su Ye* (Folium Perillae) dispels exterior wind-cold and relieves chest congestion. • *Xiang Fu* (Rhizoma Cyperi) activates qi circulation and relieves qi stagnation. • *Chen Pi* (Pericarpium Citri Reticulatae) regulates qi circulation and harmonizes the middle *jiao*. • *Zhi Gan Cao* (Radix et Rhizoma Glycyrrhizae Praeparata cum Melle) strengthens the middle *jiao* and harmonizes the herbs.

The chief herbs of this formula are *Xiang Fu* (Rhizoma Cyperi) and *Zi Su Ye* (Folium Perillae). *Xiang Fu* (Rhizoma Cyperi) activates qi circulation and relieves qi stagnation. *Zi Su Ye* (Folium Perillae), acrid, warm, and aromatic, dispels exterior wind-cold and relieves chest congestion. It is often used to treat digestive dysfunctions such as stomach flu, by harmonizing the middle *jiao*. *Chen Pi* (Pericarpium Citri Reticulatae) helps *Xiang Fu* (Rhizoma Cyperi) regulate the qi flow and harmonize the middle *jiao*. *Zhi Gan Cao* (Radix et Rhizoma Glycyrrhizae Praeparata cum Melle) harmonizes the herbs in the formula and strengthens the middle *jiao*.

MODIFICATIONS

- For cough that is continuous, add *Ban Xia* (Rhizoma Pinelliae), *Ku Xing Ren* (Semen Armeniacae Amarum), and *Sang Bai Pi* (Cortex Mori).
- With coughing and dyspnea, add *Jie Geng* (Radix Platycodonis) and *Qian Hu* (Radix Peucedani).
- If there is severe headache, add *Qiang Huo* (Rhizoma et Radix Notopterygii) and *Cong Bai* (Bulbus Allii Fistulosi).
- If there is severe headache, body aches, and neck stiffness, add *Jing Jie* (Herba Schizonepetae), *Qin Jiao* (Radix Gentianae Macrophyllae), *Fang Feng* (Radix Saposhnikoviae), *Man Jing Zi* (Fructus Viticis), *Chuan Xiong* (Rhizoma Chuanxiong), and *Sheng Jiang* (Rhizoma Zingiberis Recens).
- With stuffy nose and clear nasal discharge, add *Sheng Jiang* (Rhizoma Zingiberis Recens), *Dan Dou Chi* (Semen Sojae Praeparatum), and *Cong Bai* (Bulbus Allii Fistulosi).
- With stuffy nose and dizziness, add *Qiang Huo* (Rhizoma et Radix Notopterygii) and *Jing Jie* (Herba Schizonepetae).

- For poor appetite, add *Shan Zha* (Fructus Crataegi) and *Mai Ya* (Fructus Hordei Germinatus).
- For indigestion, add *Sha Ren* (Fructus Amomi) and *Qing Pi* (Pericarpium Citri Reticulatae Viride).
- If there is food stagnation, add *Shen Qu* (Massa Fermentata), *Ji Nei Jin* (Endothelium Corneum Gigeriae Galli), *Gu Ya* (Fructus Setariae Germinatus) and *Mai Ya* (Fructus Hordei Germinatus).
- When there is abdominal pain, add *Mu Xiang* (Radix Aucklandiae).
- If there is more fullness and distention of the chest and epigastrium as a result of severe qi stagnation, add *Hou Po* (Cortex Magnoliae Officinalis) and *Zhi Shi* (Fructus Aurantii Immaturus).
- If there is diarrhea and dysentery, add *Bai Zhu* (Rhizoma Atractylodis Macrocephalae) and *Fu Ling* (Poria).

CLINICAL STUDIES AND RESEARCH

1. **Chronic gastritis**: One hundred and twenty-two patients with chronic gastritis were treated with modified *Xiang Su San,* with complete recovery in 98 cases, improvement in 19 cases, and no benefit in 5 cases. The modifications included addition of *Bai Shao* (Radix Paeoniae Alba), *Ji Nei Jin* (Endothelium Corneum Gigeriae Galli), and others when deemed necessary.[2]

2. **Globus pharyngeus**: Administration of *Xiang Su San* was effective in treating globus pharyngeus, an abnormal throat sensation without any pathological cause. Of 23 patients treated at a dose of 7.5 g/day for at least 14 days, symptoms disappeared in 18 cases and improved in 3 cases (a 91.3% rate of effectiveness).[3]

Xiāng Sū Sǎn (Cyperus and Perilla Leaf Powder)

RELATED FORMULAS

Jiā Wèi Xiāng Sū Sǎn

(Augmented Cyperus and Perilla Leaf Powder)

加味香蘇散
加味香苏散

Pinyin Name: *Jia Wei Xiang Su San*
Literal Name: Augmented Cyperus and Perilla Leaf Powder
Original Source: *Yi Xue Xin Wu* (Medical Revelations) by Cheng Guo-Peng in 1732

Zi Su Ye (Folium Perillae)	4.5g
Chen Pi (Pericarpium Citri Reticulatae)	3.6g
Xiang Fu (Rhizoma Cyperi)	3.6g
Zhi Gan Cao (Radix et Rhizoma Glycyrrhizae Praeparata cum Melle)	2.1g
Jing Jie (Herba Schizonepetae)	3g
Qin Jiao (Radix Gentianae Macrophyllae)	3g
Fang Feng (Radix Saposhnikoviae)	3g
Man Jing Zi (Fructus Viticis)	3g
Chuan Xiong (Rhizoma Chuanxiong)	1.5g
Sheng Jiang (Rhizoma Zingiberis Recens)	3 slices

The source text instructs to coarsely grind the ingredients and prepare as a decoction. Take the warm, strained decoction and cover the body with blankets to promote mild sweating.

Jia Wei Xiang Su San (Augmented Cyperus and Perilla Leaf Powder) releases the exterior and induces diaphoresis. Clinical manifestations include headache, neck stiffness, stuffy or runny nose, body aches, fever, aversion to cold, aversion to wind, absence of perspiration, a thin, white tongue coating, and a superficial pulse.

Clinically, this formula can treat the common cold in all seasons in the elderly and children, or in individuals with weakened immunity. The cold in this case is not very severe, and strong exterior-releasing herbs such as *Ma Huang* (Herba Ephedrae) and *Gui Zhi* (Ramulus Cinnamomi) are not appropriate. Instead, *Zi Su Ye* (Folium Perillae) and *Jing Jie* (Herba Schizonepetae) serve as the chief herbs to release the exterior and induce mild diaphoresis. Their potency is only moderate, however, so they do not carry the risk of damaging qi and body fluids.

Xiāng Sū Cōng Chǐ Tāng (Cyperus, Perilla Leaf, Scallion, and Prepared Soybean Decoction)

香蘇蔥豉湯
香苏葱豉汤

Pinyin Name: *Xiang Su Cong Chi Tang*
Literal Name: Cyperus, Perilla Leaf, Scallion, and Prepared Soybean Decoction

Original Source: *Tong Su Shang Han Lun* (Plain Version of Discussion of Cold-Induced Disorders) by Yu Gen-Chu in the Qing Dynasty

Xiang Fu (Rhizoma Cyperi), *zhi* (prepared)	4.5-6g
Chen Pi (Pericarpium Citri Reticulatae)	4.5-6g
Cong Bai (Bulbus Allii Fistulosi), fresh	2-3 pieces
Zi Su Ye (Folium Perillae)	4.5-9g
Zhi Gan Cao (Radix et Rhizoma Glycyrrhizae Praeparata cum Melle)	1.8-2.4g
Dan Dou Chi (Semen Sojae Praeparatum)	9-12g

Xiang Su Cong Chi Tang (Cyperus, Perilla Leaf, Scallion, and Prepared Soybean Decoction) mainly treats wind-cold. This formula induces diaphoresis, releases the exterior, and regulates the middle *jiao*. *Xiang Fu* (Rhizoma Cyperi), *Zi Su Ye* (Folium Perillae), and *Chen Pi* (Pericarpium Citri Reticulatae) regulate the middle *jiao* to enhance the functioning of the Spleen and Stomach, and thereby relieve nausea, bloating, and distention. *Cong Bai* (Bulbus Allii Fistulosi) and *Dan Dou Chi* (Semen Sojae Praeparatum) are very mild exterior-releasing herbs. *Zhi Gan Cao* (Radix et Rhizoma Glycyrrhizae Praeparata cum Melle) harmonizes the formula and also assists the first three herbs in treating nausea and vomiting.

Xiang Su Cong Chi Tang (Cyperus, Perilla Leaf, Scallion, and Prepared Soybean Decoction) treats wind-cold condition in all four seasons. It has a mild to moderate potency, and may be used by women during menstruation or pregnancy. However, because of its mild to moderate potency, it is insufficient for treating severe cases of wind-cold, since such conditions require modifications of herbs and doses, or the selection of another formula altogether.

AUTHORS' COMMENTS

The original text prescribes *Xiang Su San* for the treatment of both febrile disorders and cold-induced disorders in all four seasons. Today, it is generally used in mild cases of common cold, influenza, stomach flu, and other gastrointestinal disorders.

References

1. *Tai Ping Hui Min He Ji Ju Fang* (Imperial Grace Formulary of the Tai Ping Era) by the Imperial Medical Department in 1078-85.
2. *Zhong Hua Ren Min Gong He Guo Yao Dian* (Chinese Herbal Pharmacopoeia by People's Republic of China) 1990;369.
3. Motoo Y, Taga H, Su SB, and Sawabu N. Effect of Koso-san on globus pharyngeus. American Journal of Chinese Medicine 1999;27(2):283-8.

Chapter 1 – Exterior-Releasing Formulas　　　　　*Section 1 – Acrid and Warm Exterior-Releasing Formulas*

Xíng Sū Yǐn (Apricot Kernel and Perilla Leaf Decoction)

杏蘇飲
杏苏饮

Pinyin Name: *Xing Su Yin*

Literal Name: Apricot Kernel and Perilla Leaf Decoction

Alternate Names: *Er Ke Xing Su Yin* (Pediatric Apricot Kernel and Perilla Leaf Decoction), Apricot Seed and Perilla Pediatric Formula

Original Source: *Yi Zong Jin Jian* (Golden Mirror of the Medical Tradition) by Wu Qian in 1742

COMPOSITION

Zi Su Ye (Folium Perillae)	[3-6g]
Ku Xing Ren (Semen Armeniacae Amarum), *chao* (dry-fried)	[3-6g]
Mai Dong (Radix Ophiopogonis)	[3-6g]
Jie Geng (Radix Platycodonis)	[3-6g]
Ju Hong (Exocarpium Citri Reticulatae)	[1-3g]
Qian Hu (Radix Peucedani)	[3-6g]
Zhi Qiao (Fructus Citri Aurantii), *chao* (dry-fried) with bran	[3-6g]
Zhe Bei Mu (Bulbus Fritillariae Thunbergii)	[3-6g]
Huang Qin (Radix Scutellariae)	[3-6g]
Sang Bai Pi (Cortex Mori), *chao* (dry-fried)	[3-6g]
Gan Cao (Radix et Rhizoma Glycyrrhizae)	[1-3g]

DOSAGE / PREPARATION / ADMINISTRATION

The source text states to decoct the ingredients with *Sheng Jiang* (Rhizoma Zingiberis Recens). Note: The doses of herbs are unavailable from the source text. Suggested doses are listed above in brackets. Actual doses vary, depending on the condition and age of the pediatric patients.

CHINESE THERAPEUTIC ACTIONS

1. Dispels wind-cold
2. Ventilates the Lung and dissolves phlegm

CLINICAL MANIFESTATIONS

Wind-cold at the exterior in children: headache, fever, aversion to cold, nausea, vomiting, drooling, sticky nasal discharge, sneezing, and cough.

CLINICAL APPLICATIONS

Common cold, influenza, and upper respiratory tract infection.

EXPLANATION

Xing Su Yin (Apricot Kernel and Perilla Leaf Decoction) is specifically designed to treat children who have wind-cold attacking the exterior. If wind travels to the upper parts of the body, patients may have headache. If cold blocks the normal flow of qi, patients may experience aversion to cold, cough, nasal obstruction, and sneezing.

Zi Su Ye (Folium Perillae) warms the exterior and dispels wind-cold. *Ku Xing Ren* (Semen Armeniacae Amarum) redirects the reversed flow of Lung qi and relieves cough. *Mai Dong* (Radix Ophiopogonis) nourishes yin and fluids of the Lung and Stomach. *Jie Geng* (Radix Platycodonis), *Ju Hong* (Exocarpium Citri Reticulatae), and *Qian Hu* (Radix Peucedani) ventilate Lung qi and relieve cough. *Zhi Qiao* (Fructus Aurantii), *Zhe Bei Mu* (Bulbus Fritillariae Thunbergii), and *Qian Hu* (Radix Peucedani) dissolve phlegm and eliminate stagnation. *Huang Qin* (Radix Scutellariae) and *Sang Bai Pi* (Cortex Mori) clear heat from the Lung, and prevent the wind-cold condition from turning into Lung heat. *Gan Cao* (Radix et Rhizoma Glycyrrhizae) and *Sheng Jiang* (Rhizoma Zingiberis Recens) harmonize the formula and relieve nausea and vomiting.

Xīng Sū Yǐn (Apricot Kernel and Perilla Leaf Decoction)

Xing Su Yin (Apricot Kernel and Perilla Leaf Decoction)

Diagnosis	Signs and Symptoms	Treatment	Herbs
Wind-cold at the exterior in children	• Headache, fever, aversion to cold, sticky nasal discharge, and sneezing: exterior wind-cold • Nausea and vomiting: wind-cold affecting Stomach qi flow • Coughing: wind-cold affecting Lung qi flow	• Dispels wind-cold • Ventilates the Lung and dissolves phlegm	• *Zi Su Ye* (Folium Perillae) warms the exterior and dispels wind-cold. • *Ku Xing Ren* (Semen Armeniacae Amarum) corrects the reversed flow of Lung qi and relieves cough. • *Mai Dong* (Radix Ophiopogonis) nourishes yin and fluids of the Lung and Stomach. • *Jie Geng* (Radix Platycodonis), *Ju Hong* (Exocarpium Citri Reticulatae), and *Qian Hu* (Radix Peucedani) ventilate Lung qi and relieve cough. • *Zhi Qiao* (Fructus Aurantii), *Zhe Bei Mu* (Bulbus Fritillariae Thunbergii), and *Qian Hu* (Radix Peucedani) dissolve phlegm and eliminate stagnation. • *Huang Qin* (Radix Scutellariae) and *Sang Bai Pi* (Cortex Mori) clear heat from the Lung, and prevents the wind-cold condition from turning into Lung heat. • *Gan Cao* (Radix et Rhizoma Glycyrrhizae) and *Sheng Jiang* (Rhizoma Zingiberis Recens) harmonize the formula and relieve nausea and vomiting.

MODIFICATIONS

- For exterior conditions caused by more wind-cold, add *Fang Feng* (Radix Saposhnikoviae) and *Jing Jie* (Herba Schizonepetae).
- When there is cough and dyspnea, add *Zi Su Zi* (Fructus Perillae) and *Ting Li Zi* (Semen Descurainiae seu Lepidii).
- For cough caused by wind-cold, add *Ding Chuan Tang* (Arrest Wheezing Decoction).
- For cough caused by phlegm, add *Er Chen Tang* (Two-Cured Decoction).

AUTHORS' COMMENTS

Xing Su Yin is also known as *Er Ke Xing Su Yin* (Pediatric Apricot Kernel and Perilla Leaf Decoction). It is a gentle formula that safely and effectively treats exterior wind-cold condition in children.

Chapter 1 – Exterior-Releasing Formulas   *Section 1 – Acrid and Warm Exterior-Releasing Formulas*

Shi Shén Tāng (Ten-Immortal Decoction)

十神湯
十神汤

Pinyin Name: *Shi Shen Tang*
Literal Name: Ten-Immortal Decoction
Alternate Names: *Shih Shen Tang*, Ten Spirits Decoction, Mahuang and Cimicifuga Combination
Original Source: *Tai Ping Hui Min He Ji Ju Fang* (Imperial Grace Formulary of the Tai Ping Era) by the Imperial Medical Department in 1078-85

COMPOSITION

Ma Huang (Herba Ephedrae)	120g
Ge Gen (Radix Puerariae Lobatae)	420g
Bai Zhi (Radix Angelicae Dahuricae)	120g
Zi Su Ye (Folium Perillae), remove any thick twigs	120g
Sheng Ma (Rhizoma Cimicifugae)	120g
Chuan Xiong (Rhizoma Chuanxiong)	120g
Chen Pi (Pericarpium Citri Reticulatae)	120g
Xiang Fu (Rhizoma Cyperi)	120g
Chi Shao (Radix Paeoniae Rubra)	120g
Zhi Gan Cao (Radix et Rhizoma Glycyrrhizae Praeparata cum Melle)	120g

DOSAGE / PREPARATION / ADMINISTRATION

The source text advises to grind the ingredients into a fine powder. Cook 9g of the powder with 5 slices of *Sheng Jiang* (Rhizoma Zingiberis Recens) in 1.5 bowls of water until the liquid is reduced to 70%. Take the warm, strained decoction any time during the day.

CHINESE THERAPEUTIC ACTIONS

Releases wind-cold from the exterior

CLINICAL MANIFESTATIONS

Exterior wind-cold: headache, aversion to cold, fever, chest congestion, hypochondriac distention, absence of perspiration, cough, dyspnea, and nasal obstruction.

CLINICAL APPLICATIONS

Common cold and influenza.

EXPLANATION

Shi Shen Tang (Ten-Immortal Decoction) treats exterior wind-cold. While most symptoms and signs are classic indications of exterior wind-cold, some patients may also complain of chest congestion and hypochondriac distention.

Many herbs in this formula specifically release exterior wind-cold, such as *Ma Huang* (Herba Ephedrae), *Ge Gen* (Radix Puerariae Lobatae), *Bai Zhi* (Radix Angelicae Dahuricae), *Zi Su Ye* (Folium Perillae), *Sheng Ma* (Rhizoma Cimicifugae), and *Sheng Jiang* (Rhizoma Zingiberis Recens). *Chuan Xiong* (Rhizoma Chuanxiong) helps *Bai Zhi* (Radix Angelicae Dahuricae) relieve headache. *Chen Pi* (Pericarpium Citri Reticulatae) and *Xiang Fu* (Rhizoma Cyperi) activate qi circulation to relieve chest congestion and hypochondriac fullness. *Chi Shao* (Radix Paeoniae Rubra) preserves yin and prevents the excessive loss of body fluids that can result from the actions of the exterior-releasing herbs. Lastly, *Zhi Gan Cao* (Radix et Rhizoma Glycyrrhizae Praeparata cum Melle) harmonizes the herbs.

Shi Shén Tāng (Ten-Immortal Decoction)

Shi Shen Tang (Ten-Immortal Decoction)

Diagnosis	Signs and Symptoms	Treatment	Herbs
Exterior wind-cold	• Headache, aversion to cold, and fever: exterior wind-cold • Chest congestion and hypochondriac distention: wind-cold causing constriction • Absence of perspiration: exterior excess • Cough, dyspnea, and nasal obstruction: wind-cold obstructing qi flow	• Releases wind-cold from the exterior	• *Ma Huang* (Herba Ephedrae), *Ge Gen* (Radix Puerariae Lobatae), *Bai Zhi* (Radix Angelicae Dahuricae), *Zi Su Ye* (Folium Perillae), *Sheng Ma* (Rhizoma Cimicifugae), and *Sheng Jiang* (Rhizoma Zingiberis Recens) release exterior wind-cold. • *Chuan Xiong* (Rhizoma Chuanxiong) activates qi and blood circulation to relieve headache. • *Chen Pi* (Pericarpium Citri Reticulatae) and *Xiang Fu* (Rhizoma Cyperi) activate qi circulation to relieve chest congestion and hypochondriac fullness. • *Chi Shao* (Radix Paeoniae Rubra) preserves yin and prevents the excessive loss of body fluids. • *Zhi Gan Cao* (Radix et Rhizoma Glycyrrhizae Praeparata cum Melle) harmonizes the herbs.

MODIFICATIONS

• With fever and headache, add *Cong Bai* (Bulbus Allii Fistulosi).

• With chest fullness, add *Zhi Qiao* (Fructus Aurantii).

• With epigastric fullness and distention, add *Zhi Shi* (Fructus Aurantii Immaturus) and *Ban Xia* (Rhizoma Pinelliae).

• With poor appetite, add *Bai Zhu* (Rhizoma Atractylodis Macrocephalae), *Sha Ren* (Fructus Amomi) and *Mu Xiang* (Radix Aucklandiae).

• With cough and increased respiration, add *Sang Bai Pi* (Cortex Mori), *Jie Geng* (Radix Platycodonis) and *Ban Xia* (Rhizoma Pinelliae).

• With constipation, add *Da Huang* (Radix et Rhizoma Rhei) and *Mang Xiao* (Natrii Sulfas).

• With nausea and vomiting, add *Huo Xiang* (Herba Agastaches) and *Ban Xia* (Rhizoma Pinelliae).

• With diarrhea, add *Bai Zhu* (Rhizoma Atractylodis Macrocephalae) and *Fu Ling* (Poria).

• With dysentery, add *Zhi Qiao* (Fructus Aurantii) and *Huang Lian* (Rhizoma Coptidis).

• With abdominal pain, add *Bai Shao* (Radix Paeoniae Alba).

AUTHORS' COMMENTS

The source text uses *Chi Shao* (Radix Paeoniae Rubra) as one of the ingredients in this formula. Today, however, *Chi Shao* (Radix Paeoniae Rubra) is generally replaced with *Bai Shao* (Radix Paeoniae Alba), because the latter more effectively preserves yin and prevents the excessive loss of body fluids that can occur from the actions of the exterior-releasing herbs.

Chapter 1 – Exterior-Releasing Formulas   *Section 1 – Acrid and Warm Exterior-Releasing Formulas*

Xiǎo Qīng Lóng Tāng (Minor Bluegreen Dragon Decoction)

小青龍湯
小青龙汤

Pinyin Name: *Xiao Qing Long Tang*
Literal Name: Minor Bluegreen Dragon Decoction
Alternate Names: *Hsiao Ching Lung Tang, Xiao Ching Long Tang*, Minor Blue Dragon Decoction, Minor Blue Dragon Combination
Original Source: *Shang Han Lun* (Discussion of Cold-Induced Disorders) by Zhang Zhong-Jing in the Eastern Han Dynasty

COMPOSITION

Ma Huang (Herba Ephedrae)	9g
Gui Zhi (Ramulus Cinnamomi)	9g [6-9g]
Xi Xin (Radix et Rhizoma Asari)	9g [3-6g]
Gan Jiang (Rhizoma Zingiberis)	9g [3-6g]
Ban Xia (Rhizoma Pinelliae), *xi* (washed)	0.5 cup [9g]
Bai Shao (Radix Paeoniae Alba)	9g
Wu Wei Zi (Fructus Schisandrae Chinensis)	0.5 cup [3-6g]
Zhi Gan Cao (Radix et Rhizoma Glycyrrhizae Praeparata cum Melle)	9g [6g]

DOSAGE / PREPARATION / ADMINISTRATION

The source text instructions are to cook *Ma Huang* (Herba Ephedrae) with 10 cups [2,000 mL] of water until the liquid is reduced to 8 cups [1,600 mL]. Remove the foam from the top, add the other ingredients, and cook until the liquid is reduced to 3 cups [600 mL]. Take 1 cup [200 mL] of the warm, strained decoction. Today, the decoction may be prepared using the doses suggested in brackets.

CHINESE THERAPEUTIC ACTIONS

1. Releases the exterior and dispels *yin* (invisible phlegm)
2. Relieves wheezing and coughing

CLINICAL MANIFESTATIONS

Wind-cold at the exterior with water accumulation in the interior: aversion to cold and fever, absence of perspiration, coughing and wheezing with profuse, clear, watery sputum, a stifling sensation in the chest, heaviness and pain of the body, edema of the face and limbs, a white, slippery tongue coating, and a superficial pulse.

CLINICAL APPLICATIONS

Pulmonary disorders, common cold, influenza, bronchitis, bronchitis in children, pneumonia, pulmonary emphysema, bronchiectasis, pulmonary tuberculosis, wheezing and dyspnea, asthma, cough, whooping cough, congestive heart failure, rhinitis or sinusitis, and acute nephritis.

EXPLANATION

Xiao Qing Long Tang (Minor Bluegreen Dragon Decoction) treats conditions characterized by wind-cold invasion at the exterior and water accumulation in the interior. Individuals who have pre-existing water accumulation in the interior generally have Spleen and Lung qi deficiencies. After being attacked by wind-cold at the exterior, patients may experience dysfunctioning of the Lung and Spleen, causing more water retention, especially in the epigastrium and the chest. Water retention in the chest causes a stifling sensation in the chest and the inability to breath properly when lying in a horizontal position.

Aversion to cold, fever, and absence of perspiration are caused by the wind-cold factor at the exterior. Cough, dyspnea and wheezing are the result of reversed flow of Lung qi, which is secondary to wind-cold attack and phlegm accumulation. Profuse, watery sputum, heaviness and pain of the body, swollen face and extremities, and a white, slippery tongue coating all suggest water accumulation and the failure of the Lung to metabolize water. The superficial pulse indicates that the disease is located at the exterior.

In this syndrome, the exterior and the interior must be treated at the same time. If only exterior herbs are used, the interior water accumulation remains. If only water-regulating herbs are used to address the water accumulation, the exterior condition remains untreated, and there may be further complications as the pathogenic factors move inward.

74

Xiǎo Qīng Lóng Tāng (Minor Bluegreen Dragon Decoction)

Xiao Qing Long Tang (Minor Bluegreen Dragon Decoction)

Diagnosis	Signs and Symptoms	Treatment	Herbs
Exterior wind-cold, interior water accumulation	• Fever, aversion to cold and absence of perspiration: exterior-excess wind-cold condition • Profuse, clear, watery sputum and edema of the face and limbs: water accumulation • Coughing, dyspnea and wheezing: reversed flow of Lung qi • Heaviness and pain of the body: damp and phlegm accumulation	• Relieves exterior wind-cold • Dispels water accumulation and phlegm • Relieves wheezing and coughing	• *Ma Huang* (Herba Ephedrae) and *Gui Zhi* (Ramulus Cinnamomi) dispel the exterior wind-cold. • *Xi Xin* (Radix et Rhizoma Asari) releases wind-cold from the exterior and warms the Lung in the interior. • *Gan Jiang* (Rhizoma Zingiberis) warms the middle *jiao* to dispel cold. • *Ban Xia* (Rhizoma Pinelliae) eliminates phlegm, directs Stomach qi downward, and harmonizes the middle *jiao*. • *Bai Shao* (Radix Paeoniae Alba) and *Wu Wei Zi* (Fructus Schisandrae Chinensis) prevent the acrid and warm herbs from damaging qi, yin, and body fluids. • *Zhi Gan Cao* (Radix et Rhizoma Glycyrrhizae Praeparata cum Melle) tonifies qi and harmonizes the herbs.

Ma Huang (Herba Ephedrae) and *Gui Zhi* (Ramulus Cinnamomi), the chief herbs, dispel exterior wind-cold factor through diaphoresis. *Ma Huang* (Herba Ephedrae) also smoothes Lung qi flow to relieve cough, dyspnea, and wheezing. *Gui Zhi* (Ramulus Cinnamomi) warms the yang and eliminates cold. *Xi Xin* (Radix et Rhizoma Asari), acrid and hot, enters the *shaoyin* channel and warms the Lung to resolve phlegm accumulation. It also assists *Ma Huang* (Herba Ephedrae) and *Gui Zhi* (Ramulus Cinnamomi) in releasing the exterior. *Gan Jiang* (Rhizoma Zingiberis) enters the *yangming* channel to warm the yang of the middle *jiao* to dispel cold. *Ban Xia* (Rhizoma Pinelliae) eliminates phlegm, directs Stomach qi downward, and harmonizes the middle *jiao*.

If only arid and warm herbs are used in this syndrome, however, the Lung qi may become dispersed or lost, and yin may be injured. For this reason, *Wu Wei Zi* (Fructus Schisandrae Chinensis) is added to contain and prevent the leakage of Lung qi. *Bai Shao* (Radix Paeoniae Alba) nourishes yin, tonifies the blood, and prevents the acrid herbs from drying up body fluids. Both *Wu Wei Zi* (Fructus Schisandrae Chinensis) and *Bai Shao* (Radix Paeoniae Alba) are used only in small doses, as large doses might interfere with the exterior-releasing effect. *Zhi Gan Cao* (Radix et Rhizoma Glycyrrhizae Praeparata cum Melle) supplements qi and harmonizes the exterior-releasing and astringent herbs in this formula.

MODIFICATIONS

• With cough and dyspnea, add *Ku Xing Ren* (Semen Armeniacae Amarum) and *Hou Po* (Cortex Magnoliae Officinalis).

• With fever and sore throat, add *Jie Geng* (Radix Platycodonis) and *Shi Gao* (Gypsum Fibrosum).

• With irritability arising from heat, add *Shi Gao* (Gypsum Fibrosum).

• With thirst as a result of Lung heat, add *Shi Gao* (Gypsum Fibrosum) and *Huang Qin* (Radix Scutellariae).

• With absence of sweating and severe aversion to cold, increase the dose of *Ma Huang* (Herba Ephedrae) and *Gui Zhi* (Ramulus Cinnamomi).

• With sweating and severe aversion to cold, increase the dose of *Gui Zhi* (Ramulus Cinnamomi) and *Bai Shao* (Radix Paeoniae Alba), and add *Sheng Jiang* (Rhizoma Zingiberis Recens) and *Da Zao* (Fructus Jujubae).

• If the exterior symptoms are not severe, remove *Gui Zhi* (Ramulus Cinnamomi) and use honey-fried *Ma Huang* (Herba Ephedrae) instead.

CAUTIONS / CONTRAINDICATIONS

• *Xiao Qing Long Tang* should not be taken for a prolonged period of time. It should be discontinued when the desired effects have been achieved.

• This formula is contraindicated in the following situations: heat condition with a sore throat or a rapid pulse; wind-heat or beginning stages of *wen bing* (warm disease); yin deficiency with dry cough or thirst; phlegm-heat

Chapter 1 – Exterior-Releasing Formulas   *Section 1 – Acrid and Warm Exterior-Releasing Formulas*

Xiăo Qīng Lóng Tāng (Minor Bluegreen Dragon Decoction)

conditions with thick, yellow sputum; cough with streaks of blood in the sputum; and cough with thick, yellow sputum, thirst, a red tongue with yellow tongue coating, and a rapid pulse.

- Because this is a relatively strong formula, caution must be used when prescribing this formula. *Xi Xin* (Radix et Rhizoma Asari) must be prescribed carefully because it is potentially toxic at a high dose. *Wu Wei Zi* (Fructus Schisandrae Chinensis) must not be used at a large dose to avoid retaining the pathogenic factors inside the body with its astringent effect.

- Use of *Xiao Qing Long Tang* has been associated with only a few side effects, such as dry mouth, sedation and drowsiness, due mainly to the blockage of histamine H1 and muscarinic receptors in the salivary glands and the brain.[1,2]

- Use of *Xiao Qing Long Tang* has been associated with rare cases of gastrointestinal discomfort (nausea, vomiting, and diarrhea) and skin itching. These reactions were self-limiting and resolved upon the discontinuation of the formula.[3]

PHARMACOLOGICAL EFFECTS

1. **Antiasthmatic**: *Xiao Qing Long Tang* has marked antiasthmatic effects, and has been used for centuries to treat bronchial asthma. There are two proposed mechanisms of the antiasthmatic effects. One, it stimulates the beta2-adrenoceptors to produce bronchorelaxation. Two, it inhibits the infiltration of eosinophils into the airway. Thus, *Xiao Qing Long Tang* is useful for both prevention and treatment of asthma.[4,5]

2. **Antiallergic**: One study reported that *Xiao Qing Long Tang* has antiallergic effects and may be useful and reasonable for controlling allergic diseases including bronchial asthma, allergic asthma and allergic rhinitis.[6] One demonstrated mechanism of the antiallergic effects was the inhibitory activity on histamine release and suppression of Th2 differentiation at the stage of antigen-presenting cells (APCs)-CD4(+)T cell interaction.[7] Another demonstrated mechanism is the inhibition of mast cell activities.[8] Lastly, it has been shown to control the allergen-induced inflammatory process by substantially inhibiting the allergen-induced synthesis of TNF-alpha.[9]

3. **Antiviral**: One study found *Xiao Qing Long Tang* to be useful for both prophylaxis and treatment of influenza virus infection in patients with allergic pulmonary inflammation, such as bronchial asthma. The mechanism of this action was attributed to the effects of the formula to augment the antiviral IgA antibody titer in the nasal and broncho-alveolar cavities, activate T-cell in Peyer's patch lymphocyte, and stimulate the production of anti-influenza virus IgA antibody in nasal lymphocyte.[10]

Xiao Qing Long Tang, however, has not shown direct action against the virus.[11] Clinically, *Xiao Qing Long Tang* can be used to prevent influenza virus infection by cross-protection of subtypes of influenza A virus and B virus. It is also useful for the treatment of influenza virus infection in elderly patients, and individuals with a history of influenza virus infection, influenza vaccination, and allergic pulmonary inflammation.[12,13]

4. **Immunomodulatory**: Administration of *Xiao Qing Long Tang* has immunomodulatory effects in reducing bronchial inflammation in allergen-sensitized mice. *Xiao Qing Long Tang* suppressed airway inflammation by decreasing the number of total cells and eosinophil infiltration in the bronchoalveolar lavage fluid, and down-regulated the allergen- or mitogen-induced intrapulmonary lymphocyte response of sensitized mice as compared to those of controls.[14]

5. **Effect on the adrenal cortex**: Administration of *Xiao Qing Long Tang* has marked effect on the plasma concentration of cortisol and ACTH. Following oral ingestion of the formula at 0.05 g/kg, plasma levels of cortisol and ACTH were measured at 30, 60, and 120 minutes. The study reported increases of 36%, 30% and 25% for cortisol, and 18%, 18% and 23% for ACTH, respectively. In control group that received placebo, no significant changes were noted with plasma concentrations of cortisol or ACTH.[15]

6. **Sympathomimetic**: Administration of *Xiao Qing Long Tang* was associated with increased respiratory rate, heart rate, blood pressure, systolic pressure, diastolic pressure, and decreased blood flow in dogs at all doses of 0.5, 1 and 2 g/kg via duodenal administration.[16]

CLINICAL STUDIES AND RESEARCH

1. **Pulmonary disorders**: In a clinical study, 258 patients between 6 to 67 years of age with various pulmonary disorders for over one month characterized by cough and dyspnea were examined and treated. According to western diagnosis, 120 patients had acute pneumonia, 68 had chronic pneumonia, 60 had acute asthma, 4 had pulmonary emphysema, 4 had pleurisy, 1 had pulmonary tuberculosis and 1 had pulmonary carcinoma. Patients with the first four diagnoses were treated with herbs only, while those with the last three diagnoses were treated with both herbs and drugs. The herbal treatment was based on *Xiao Qing Long Tang*, with minor modifications when necessary. The study reported significant improvement to complete recovery within 4-6 doses in all patients except ones with tuberculosis and carcinoma.[17]

2. **Bronchitis**: Use of modified *Xiao Qing Long Tang* was effective in treating bronchitis. Of 51 patients, the study reported significant improvement in 27 cases, moderate improvement in 15 cases, and no benefit in 1 case.[18]

Xiǎo Qīng Lóng Tāng (Minor Bluegreen Dragon Decoction)

3. **Bronchitis in children**: Modified *Xiao Qing Long Tang* demonstrated a 96% rate of effectiveness in treating bronchitis in children. The herbal treatment contained *Xiao Qing Long Tang* plus *Chuan Bei Mu* (Bulbus Fritillariae Cirrhosae), *Jie Geng* (Radix Platycodonis), *Zi Wan* (Radix et Rhizoma Asteris) and others as the base formula. Modifications were made as follows: *Jin Yin Hua* (Flos Lonicerae Japonicae), *Zhi Zi* (Fructus Gardeniae) and *Shi Gao* (Gypsum Fibrosum) were added for heat; *Jing Jie* (Herba Schizonepetae) and *Bai Qian* (Rhizoma et Radix Cynanchi Stauntonii) were added for wind-cold; *Ku Xing Ren* (Semen Armeniacae Amarum), *Niu Bang Zi* (Fructus Arctii) and *Xuan Shen* (Radix Scrophulariae) were added for repetitive cough with a hoarse voice; and *Cang Zhu* (Rhizoma Atractylodis) and *Huo Xiang* (Herba Agastaches) were added for profuse dampness and phlegm. Of 65 patients, the study reported complete recovery in 57 cases, improvement in 6 cases, and no benefit in 2 cases.[19]

4. **Pneumonia**: Use of modified *Xiao Qing Long Tang* effectively treated 72 of 89 patients with pneumonia within 2 weeks. Seventeen patients who did not respond were then treated with concurrent herb and drug therapy. The herbal treatment contained *Xiao Qing Long Tang* plus *Yu Xing Cao* (Herba Houttuyniae), *Huang Qin* (Radix Scutellariae) and *Ku Xing Ren* (Semen Armeniacae Amarum) as the base formula. For presence of sticky cold phlegm, *Bai Jie Zi* (Semen Sinapis), *Zi Su Zi* (Fructus Perillae) and *Xuan Fu Hua* (Flos Inulae) were added, and *Huang Qin* (Radix Scutellariae) and *Bai Shao* (Radix Paeoniae Alba) were removed. For accumulation of hot phlegm in the Lung, *Shi Gao* (Gypsum Fibrosum) and *Chuan Bei Mu* (Bulbus Fritillariae Cirrhosae) were added, and *Gan Jiang* (Rhizoma Zingiberis), *Gui Zhi* (Ramulus Cinnamomi) and *Xi Xin* (Radix et Rhizoma Asari) were removed. For generalized deficiency and weakness, *Ren Shen* (Radix et Rhizoma Ginseng), *Bai Zhu* (Rhizoma Atractylodis Macrocephalae), *Dang Gui* (Radix Angelicae Sinensis) and *Shu Di Huang* (Radix Rehmanniae Praeparata) were added, and *Huang Qin* (Radix Scutellariae) and *Ma Huang* (Herba Ephedrae) were removed.[20]

5. **Wheezing and dyspnea**: *Xiao Qing Long Tang* has been shown in many studies to effectively treat wheezing and dyspnea. One study reported 86.7% effectiveness using this formula in liquid form three times daily for 1-3 weeks to treat 30 patients with bronchial asthma.[21] Another study with 39 patients noted that *Xiao Qing Long Tang* was effective for both acute and chronic bronchial asthma.[22] Lastly, in one study of pediatric patients with bronchial asthma, the use of modified *Xiao Qing Long Tang* was associated with 64.5% rate of effectiveness.[23]

6. **Cough**: Sixty patients with cough characterized by wind-cold were treated with modified *Xiao Qing Long Tang* with marked success within 3-6 packs of herbs. The herbal treatment included *Xiao Qing Long Tang* plus *Sha Shen* (Radix Glehniae seu Adenophorae), *Zi Wan* (Radix et Rhizoma Asteris) and others as deemed necessary. *Zhi Mu* (Rhizoma Anemarrhenae) was added for fever. *Huang Qi* (Radix Astragali) was added for qi deficiency with profuse sweating. Lower doses of *Xi Xin* (Radix et Rhizoma Asari) and *Gan Jiang* (Rhizoma Zingiberis), and addition of *Shi Gao* (Gypsum Fibrosum) and *Huang Qin* (Radix Scutellariae), were used for presence of scanty thick yellow sputum.[24]

7. **Rhinitis**: Fifty-three patients with a past history of rhinitis between 2 weeks to 12 years were treated with *Xiao Qing Long Tang*. Clinical presentation included sneezing, itching and irritation of the nose, and profuse, clear and watery nasal discharge. The study reported an overall rate of effectiveness of 94.3%, with complete recovery in 26 cases, moderate improvement in 24 cases, and no benefit in 3 cases.[25]

8. **Allergic rhinitis**: *Xiao Qing Long Tang* plus *Chai Hu* (Radix Bupleuri) was used to treat 386 patients with allergic rhinitis with marked effectiveness in 164 cases, moderate effect in 177 cases, and no effect in 45 cases. The overall rate of effectiveness was 88.3%.[26]

HERB-DRUG INTERACTION

- **Fluticasone**: Forty-two asthma patients were divided into three groups: one group treated with *Xiao Qing Long Tang*, one group treated with fluticasone inhalation, and one group treated with both. The study reported that concurrent administration of fluticasone and *Xiao Qing Long Tang* was associated with superior results based on pulmonary function and serum interleukin (IL)-16 levels, in comparison with the other two groups. The study concluded that the combination (of inhaled fluticasone and oral *Xiao Qing Long Tang*) could become an important therapeutical method in treating mild and severe asthma patients.[27]

- **Carbamazepine**: One study evaluated the potential herb-drug interaction between *Xiao Qing Long Tang* and carbamazepine in rats. With simultaneous oral administration, *Xiao Qing Long Tang* delayed the oral absorption of carbamazepine, but did not influence the peak plasma concentration, area under the plasma concentration-time curve, or terminal elimination half-life ($T\frac{1}{2}$). With 1-week pre-treatment with *Xiao Qing Long Tang*, the Tmax and the elimination rate constant for carbamazepine were significantly increased, but the protein binding was not affected.[28]

Chapter 1 – Exterior-Releasing Formulas　　　　*Section 1 – Acrid and Warm Exterior-Releasing Formulas*

Xiǎo Qīng Lóng Tāng (Minor Bluegreen Dragon Decoction)

RELATED FORMULAS

Xiǎo Qīng Lóng Jiā Shí Gāo Tāng
(Minor Bluegreen Dragon Decoction plus Gypsum)

小青龍加石膏湯
小青龙加石膏汤

Pinyin Name: Xiao Qing Long Jia Shi Gao Tang

Literal Name: Minor Bluegreen Dragon Decoction plus Gypsum

Original Source: *Jin Gui Yao Lue* (Essentials from the Golden Cabinet) by Zhang Zhong-Jing in the Eastern Han Dynasty

Ma Huang (Herba Ephedrae)	9g
Bai Shao (Radix Paeoniae Alba)	9g
Xi Xin (Radix et Rhizoma Asari)	9g [3-6g]
Gan Jiang (Rhizoma Zingiberis)	9g [3-6g]
Zhi Gan Cao (Radix et Rhizoma Glycyrrhizae Praeparata cum Melle)	9g [6g]
Gui Zhi (Ramulus Cinnamomi)	9g [6-9g]
Ban Xia (Rhizoma Pinelliae), *xi* (washed)	0.5 cup [9g]
Wu Wei Zi (Fructus Schisandrae Chinensis)	0.5 cup [3-6g]
Shi Gao (Gypsum Fibrosum)	6g [9g]

This formula treats wind-cold at the exterior, with accumulation of water and heat in the interior. Clinically, patients may show irritability in addition to all the symptoms and signs listed under *Xiao Qing Long Tang*. *Shi Gao* (Gypsum Fibrosum), with its acrid, sweet, and cold qualities, is added to clear Lung heat and relieve irritability.

Xiao Qing Long Jia Shi Gao Tang is a strong herbal formula, comprised of *Xiao Qing Long Tang* and *Shi Gao* (Gypsum Fibrosum). The doses listed above are intended for a normal and generally healthy person. Children and individuals who are weak should have the doses adjusted accordingly.

Jiā Jiǎn Xiǎo Qīng Lóng Tāng
(Modified Minor Bluegreen Dragon Decoction)

加減小青龍湯
加减小青龙汤

Pinyin Name: Jia Jian Xiao Qing Long Tang

Literal Name: Modified Minor Bluegreen Dragon Decoction

Original Source: *Tian Jin Zhong Yi Xue Yuan* (Tianjin University of Chinese Medicine) in 1989

Ma Huang (Herba Ephedrae)

Ku Xing Ren (Semen Armeniacae Amarum)

Zhi Gan Cao (Radix et Rhizoma Glycyrrhizae Praeparata cum Melle)

Bai Jie Zi (Semen Sinapis)

Ban Xia (Rhizoma Pinelliae)

Cang Er Zi (Fructus Xanthii)

Zi Wan (Radix et Rhizoma Asteris)

Hou Po (Cortex Magnoliae Officinalis)

Bai Shao (Radix Paeoniae Alba)

Gan Jiang (Rhizoma Zingiberis)

Gui Zhi (Ramulus Cinnamomi)

Wu Wei Zi (Fructus Schisandrae Chinensis)

Jia Jian Xiao Qing Long Tang (Modified Minor Bluegreen Dragon Decoction) treats wheezing, dyspnea and coughing caused by wind-cold attacking the exterior and invading the Lung. This formula contains herbs that release wind-cold, eliminate the phlegm, dilate the Lung, and relieve wheezing and dyspnea. Clinically, it can treat a wide variety of respiratory tract disorders, such as common colds, influenza, asthma, bronchitis, and emphysema.

AUTHORS' COMMENTS

Xiao Qing Long Tang is frequently used today to treat wind-cold invasion with interior water retention, a condition that usually occurs in individuals who live in colder climates or who are constitutionally more cold or damp in nature. It has extremely strong dispersing and warming effects. Thus, accurate diagnosis is necessary before prescribing this formula. Chief diagnostic signs for selecting this formula include profuse, clear or white nasal discharge or sputum with aversion to cold, absence of sweating, dyspnea or cough with a white tongue coating. There should be no signs and symptoms of heat. Moreover, it should not be used for a prolonged period of time, since the warm herbs may change the condition from cold to heat. Patients should also be monitored closely as exterior wind-cold condition can turn into wind-heat condition rather quickly. As soon as signs of heat are evident, immediately stop the use of the formula and select a more appropriate formula.

Other uses of this formula today include respiratory symptoms of sneezing, clear or white nasal discharge in those who are exposed to cold environments, such as with water sports (swimming) or outdoor activities in winter (skiing). The sudden or prolonged exposure to cold weather may give rise to aversion to cold and fever (wind-cold) with sneezing and profuse nasal discharge (water retention). The use of *Xiao Qing Long Tang* in this situation is extremely effective and offers immediate relief so that the condition does not progress inward. *Xiao Qing Long Tang*, however, is not designed for long-term use. Building the immune system by using a formula such as *Yu Ping Feng San* (Jade Windscreen Powder) to strengthen the *wei* (defensive) *qi* is crucial to preventing exterior pathogenic attacks.

Xiǎo Qīng Lóng Tāng (Minor Bluegreen Dragon Decoction)

Ma Huang Tang (Ephedra Decoction) and *Xiao Qing Long Tang* both treat cough, but have the following differences:

- *Ma Huang Tang* treats exterior-excess, wind-cold condition; its chief function is to induce perspiration to expel pathogenic factors. It is not designed to treat asthma or to relieve cough. The dyspnea, cough, or wheezing are secondary symptoms of wind-cold attacking the Lung, giving rise to respiratory difficulties.

- *Xiao Qing Long Tang* treats exterior wind-cold attack with interior water accumulation. It has dual functions to release exterior wind-cold and resolve interior water accumulation. Its main function is to warm the Lung to resolve water accumulation. Therefore, along with cough, dyspnea, and wheezing, there are additional key symptoms such as profuse, clear sputum that may be frothy, as well as clear or white nasal discharge.[29]

Da Qing Long Tang (Major Bluegreen Dragon Decoction) and *Xiao Qing Long Tang* both release the exterior and arrest wheezing to treat exterior-excess conditions characterized by dyspnea and the absence of perspiration. Both formulas treat exterior and interior excess, and contain *Ma Huang* (Herba Ephedrae) and *Gui Zhi* (Ramulus Cinnamomi). Their differences are as follows:

- *Da Qing Long Tang* is based on *Ma Huang Tang* (Ephedra Decoction), but the dose of *Ma Huang* (Herba Ephedrae) is double that of the dose in *Ma Huang Tang* (Ephedra Decoction). Moreover, it contains *Shi Gao* (Gypsum Fibrosum) to clear Lung heat. It is most suitable for exterior excess, wind-cold condition with interior Lung heat. Other key signs include heat sensations, irritability, and the absence of perspiration.

- *Xiao Qing Long Tang* is also based on *Ma Huang Tang* (Ephedra Decoction), but it omits *Ku Xing Ren* (Semen Armeniacae Amarum) and adds *Xi Xin* (Radix et Rhizoma Asari), *Gan Jiang* (Rhizoma Zingiberis), *Wu Wei Zi* (Fructus Schisandrae Chinensis), *Ban Xia* (Rhizoma Pinelliae), and *Bai Shao* (Radix Paeoniae Alba). The dose of *Ma Huang* (Herba Ephedrae) is low, because wheezing and dyspnea are not the primary symptoms of this formula. Rather, the key symptoms are coughing with profuse, clear, white sputum and nasal discharge. *Xiao Qing Long Tang* is most suitable for exterior-excess, wind-cold with interior cold-phlegm accumulation.[30]

References

1. Sakaguchi M, Mase A, Iizuka A, Yuzurihara M, Ishige A, Amagaya S, Komatsu Y, Takeda H, Matsumiya T. Further pharmacological study on Sho-seiryu-to as an antiallergic. Methods Find Exp Clin Pharmacol 1997 Dec;19(10):707-13.

2. Sakaguchi M, Iizuka A, Yuzurihara M, Ishige A, Komatsu Y, Matsumiya T, Takeda H. Pharmacological characteristics of Sho-seiryu-to, an

antiallergic Kampo medicine without effects on histamine H1 receptors and muscarinic cholinergic system in the brain. Methods Find Exp Clin Pharmacol 1996 Jan-Feb;18(1):41-7.

3. *Zhong Yao Ming Fang Yao Li Yu Ying Yong* (Pharmacology and Applications of Famous Herbal Formulas) 1989;44-45.

4. Kao ST, Lin CS, Hsieh CC, Hsieh WT, Lin JG. Effects of xiao-qing-long-tang (XQLT) on bronchoconstriction and airway eosinophil infiltration in ovalbumin-sensitized guinea pigs: in vivo and in vitro studies. Allergy 2001 Dec;56(12):1164-71.

5. *Zhong Yi Fang Ji Xian Dai Yan Jiu* (Modern Study of Medical Formulae in Traditional Chinese Medicine) 1997;(1):62.

6. Tanno Y, Shindoh Y, Takishima T. Modulation of human basophil growth in vitro by xiao-qing-long-tang (syo-seiryu-to), chai-pu-tang (saiboku-to), qing-fei-tang (seihai-to), baicalein and ketotifen. American Journal of Chinese Medicine 1989;17(1-2):45-50.

7. Ikeda Y, Kaneko A, Yamamoto M, Ishige A, Sasaki H. Possible involvement of suppression of Th2 differentiation in the antiallergic effect of Sho-seiryu-to in mice. Jpn J Pharmacol 2002 Dec;90(4):328-36.

8. Sakaguchi M, Mase A, Iizuka A, Yuzurihara M, Ishige A, Amagaya S, Komatsu Y, Takeda H, Matsumiya T. Further pharmacological study on Sho-seiryu-to as an antiallergic. Methods Find Exp Clin Pharmacol 1997 Dec;19(10):707-13.

9. Tanaka A, Ohashi Y, Kakinoki Y, Washio Y, Yamada K, Nakai Y, Nakano T, Nakai Y, Ohmoto Y. The herbal medicine shoseiryu-to inhibits allergen-induced synthesis of tumour necrosis factor alpha by peripheral blood mononuclear cells in patients with perennial allergic rhinitis. Acta Otolaryngol Suppl 1998;538:118-25.

10. Nagai T, Yamada H. In vivo anti-influenza virus activity of kampo (Japanese herbal) medicine "sho-seiryu-to" and its mode of action. Int. J. Immunopharmacol 1994;16:605-613.

11. Nagai T, Yamada H. In vivo anti-influenza virus activity of Kampo (Japanese herbal) medicine "sho-seiryu-to"--stimulation of mucosal immune system and effect on allergic pulmonary inflammation model mice. Immunopharmacol Immunotoxicol 1998 May;20(2):267-81.

12. Yamada H, Nagai T. In vivo anti-influenza virus activity of Kampo medicine Sho-seiryu-to through mucosal immune system. Methods Find Exp Clin Pharmacol 1998 Apr;20(3):185-92.

13. Nagai T, Urata M, Yamada H. In vivo anti-influenza virus activity of Kampo (Japanese herbal) medicine "Sho-seiryu-to"--effects on aged mice, against subtypes of a viruses and B virus, and therapeutic effect. Immunopharmacol Immunotoxicol 1996 May;18(2):193-208.

14. Kao ST, Wang SD, Wang JY, Yu CK, Lei HY. The effect of Chinese herbal medicine, xiao-qing-long tang (XQLT), on allergen-induced bronchial inflammation in mite-sensitized mice. Allergy 2000 Dec;55(12):1127-33.

15. *Han Fang Yi Xue* (Kampo Medicine) 1982;6(82):12.

16. Amagaya S, Iizuka A, Makino B, Kubo M, Komatsu Y, Cheng FC, Ruo TI, Itoh T, Terasawa K. General pharmacological properties of Sho-seiryu-to (TJ-19) extracts. Phytomedicine 2001 Sep;8(5):338-47.

17. *Shan Dong Zhong Yi Za Zhi* (Shandong Journal of Chinese Medicine) 1994;13(8):342.

18. *Si Chuan Zhong Yi* (Sichuan Chinese Medicine) 1986;12:15.

19. *Shan Xi Zhong Yi* (Shanxi Chinese Medicine) 1997;4:174.

20. *He Bei Zhong Yi* (Hebei Chinese Medicine) 1998;2:114.

21. *Shang Hai Zhong Yi Yao Za Zhi* (Shanghai Journal of Chinese Medicine and Herbology) 1993;9:25.

22. *Shan Dong Zhong Yi Xue Yuan Xue Bao* (Journal of Shandong University School of Chinese Medicine) 1992;1:43.

23. *Guo Wai Yi Xue Zhong Yi Zhong Yao Fen Ce* (Monograph of Chinese Herbology from Foreign Medicine) 1979;1:33.

24. *He Bei Zhong Yi* (Hebei Chinese Medicine) 1999;2:16.

Chapter 1 – Exterior-Releasing Formulas   *Section 1 – Acrid and Warm Exterior-Releasing Formulas*

Xiǎo Qīng Lóng Tāng (Minor Bluegreen Dragon Decoction)

25. *Nan Jing Zhong Yi Yao Da Xue Xue Bao* (Journal of Nanjing University of Traditional Chinese Medicine and Medicinals) 1995;(4):14.

26. *Xin Jiang Zhong Yi Yao* (Xinjiang Chinese Medicine and Herbology) 1996;4:20.

27. Zhang X, Wang L, Shi Q. Effect of fluticasone inhalation combined with xiaoqinglong decoction on pulmonary function and serum interleukin-16 level in asthma patients. Zhongguo Zhong Xi Yi Jie He Za Zhi 2003 Jun;23(6):426-9.

28. Ohnishi N, Yonekawa Y, Nakasako S, Nagasawa K, Yokoyama T, Yoshioka M, Kuroda K. Studies on interactions between traditional herbal and Western medicines. I. Effects of Sho-seiryu-to on the pharmacokinetics of carbamazepine in rats. Biol Pharm Bull 1999 May;22(5):527-31.

29. Wang MZ, et al. *Zhong Yi Xue Wen Da Ti Ku* (Questions and Answers on Traditional Chinese Medicine: Herbal Formulas).

30. Wang MZ, et al. *Zhong Yi Xue Wen Da Ti Ku* (Questions and Answers on Traditional Chinese Medicine: Herbal Formulas).

Shè Gān Má Huáng Tāng (Belamcanda and Ephedra Decoction)

射幹麻黃湯
射干麻黄汤

Pinyin Name: *She Gan Ma Huang Tang*
Literal Name: Belamcanda and Ephedra Decoction
Alternate Name: Belamcanda and Mahuang Combination
Original Source: *Jin Gui Yao Lue* (Essentials from the Golden Cabinet) by Zhang Zhong-Jing in the Eastern Han Dynasty

COMPOSITION

Ma Huang (Herba Ephedrae)	12g [9g]
She Gan (Rhizoma Belamcandae)	9g [6-g]
Sheng Jiang (Rhizoma Zingiberis Recens)	12g [9g]
Xi Xin (Radix et Rhizoma Asari)	9g [3g]
Zi Wan (Radix et Rhizoma Asteris)	9g [6g]
Kuan Dong Hua (Flos Farfarae)	9g [6g]
Ban Xia (Rhizoma Pinelliae)	0.5 cup [9g]
Wu Wei Zi (Fructus Schisandrae Chinensis)	0.5 cup [3g]
Da Zao (Fructus Jujubae)	7 pieces [3 pieces]

DOSAGE / PREPARATION / ADMINISTRATION

The source text states to cook *Ma Huang* (Herba Ephedrae) with 12 cups [2,400 mL] of water and bring to a boil twice. Remove the foam from the top, add the other ingredients, and cook until the liquid is reduced to 3 cups [600 mL]. Take the warm, strained decoction in three equally-divided doses daily. Today, the decoction may be prepared using the doses suggested in brackets.

CHINESE THERAPEUTIC ACTIONS

1. Ventilates the Lung and dispels phlegm
2. Directs Lung qi downward and stops coughing

CLINICAL MANIFESTATIONS

Tan yin (phlegm retention) with reversed flow of Lung qi: excessive coughing, dyspnea, profuse, clear, watery sputum, rattling sounds in the throat, a feeling of fullness and stifling sensation in the chest and diaphragm, heaviness and pain of the body, swollen face and extremities, and a white, slippery tongue coating.

CLINICAL APPLICATIONS

Cough, asthma, asthmatic bronchitis, pulmonary emphysema, and whooping cough.

EXPLANATION

She Gan Ma Huang Tang (Belamcanda and Ephedra Decoction) is a modification of *Xiao Qing Long Tang* (Minor Bluegreen Dragon Decoction); it treats *tan yin* (phlegm retention) with reversed flow of Lung qi, and is suitable for conditions characterized by severe phlegm and water retention. Clinically, the cough and sputum are more severe in this case than that found in *Xiao Qing Long Tang*.

Ma Huang (Herba Ephedrae) ventilates the Lung and relieves dyspnea. *She Gan* (Rhizoma Belamcandae)

Chinese Herbal Formulas and Applications

Shè Gān Má Huáng Tāng (Belamcanda and Ephedra Decoction)

She Gan Ma Huang Tang (Belamcanda and Ephedra Decoction)

Diagnosis	Signs and Symptoms	Treatment	Herbs
Tan yin (phlegm retention) with reversed flow of Lung qi	• Profuse, clear, watery sputum and rattling sounds in the throat: *tan yin* (phlegm retention) • Severe coughing and dyspnea: phlegm accumulation blocking Lung qi circulation • White, slippery tongue coating: water accumulation	• Ventilates the Lung and dispels phlegm • Redirects Lung qi downward and stops coughing	• *Ma Huang* (Herba Ephedrae) ventilates the Lung and relieves dyspnea. • *She Gan* (Rhizoma Belamcandae) dispels *tan yin* (phlegm retention). • *Sheng Jiang* (Rhizoma Zingiberis Recens), *Xi Xin* (Radix et Rhizoma Asari), *Zi Wan* (Radix et Rhizoma Asteris), *Kuan Dong Hua* (Flos Farfarae), and *Ban Xia* (Rhizoma Pinelliae) dissolve phlegm, clear the throat, and direct the rising qi downward. • *Wu Wei Zi* (Fructus Schisandrae Chinensis) contains the leakage of Lung qi and stops coughing. • *Da Zao* (Fructus Jujubae) harmonizes the middle *jiao*.

dispels *tan yin* (phlegm retention). *Sheng Jiang* (Rhizoma Zingiberis Recens), *Xi Xin* (Radix et Rhizoma Asari), *Zi Wan* (Radix et Rhizoma Asteris), *Kuan Dong Hua* (Flos Farfarae), and *Ban Xia* (Rhizoma Pinelliae) dissolve phlegm, clear the throat, and redirect the rising qi. *Wu Wei Zi* (Fructus Schisandrae Chinensis) contains the leakage of Lung qi and stops coughing. *Da Zao* (Fructus Jujubae) harmonizes the middle *jiao*.

She Gan Ma Huang Tang is modified from *Xiao Qing Long Tang*, with the removal of *Gui Zhi* (Ramulus Cinnamomi), *Bai Shao* (Radix Paeoniae Alba), and *Gan Cao* (Radix et Rhizoma Glycyrrhizae), and the addition of *She Gan* (Rhizoma Belamcandae), *Zi Wan* (Radix et Rhizoma Asteris), *Kuan Dong Hua* (Flos Farfarae), and *Da Zao* (Fructus Jujubae). These additional herbs enable *She Gan Ma Huang Tang* to strongly dispel phlegm and direct Lung qi downward to treat cough and dyspnea.

MODIFICATIONS

- For Lung heat from respiratory tract infection, add *Yu Xing Cao* (Herba Houttuyniae), *Jin Yin Hua* (Flos Lonicerae Japonicae), *Lian Qiao* (Fructus Forsythiae), and *Huang Qin* (Radix Scutellariae).
- If there is high fever, add *Shi Gao* (Gypsum Fibrosum) and *Geng Mi* (Semen Oryzae).
- With chest and abdominal fullness and distention, add *Hou Po* (Cortex Magnoliae Officinalis) and *Lai Fu Zi* (Semen Raphani).
- For dysuria, add *Fu Ling* (Poria) and *Ze Xie* (Rhizoma Alismatis).
- When there is profuse sputum, add *Gua Lou Pi* (Pericarpium Trichosanthis).

PHARMACOLOGICAL EFFECTS

1. **Antitussive**: Administration of a *She Gan Ma Huang Tang* preparation at 0.4 mL/10g was associated with marked antitussive effects in mice with artificially-induced cough.[1]
2. **Expectorant**: Administration of *She Gan Ma Huang Tang* in mice was associated with marked expectorant effects at high doses, but not at low doses.[2]
3. **Antiasthmatic**: Administration of *She Gan Ma Huang Tang* has been shown to have a relaxant effect on the bronchial smooth muscle to relieve wheezing and dyspnea.[3]

CLINICAL STUDIES AND RESEARCH

1. **Bronchitis**: Use of modified *She Gan Ma Huang Tang* was associated with 90.75% effectiveness in treating bronchitis. The herbal treatment used *She Gan Ma Huang Tang* as the base formula, and added *Wu Gong* (Scolopendra) for spastic cough; *Shi Gao* (Gypsum Fibrosum) and *Huang Qin* (Radix Scutellariae) for fever; and *Che Qian Zi* (Semen Plantaginis) for diarrhea.[4]
2. **Bronchitis in children**: Use of modified *She Gan Ma Huang Tang* was associated with 94.7% effectiveness in treating dyspnea and bronchitis in 38 children. *She Gan Ma Huang Tang* was modified as follows: for the presence of excess heat, *Huang Qin* (Radix Scutellariae), *Yu Xing Cao* (Herba Houttuyniae), and *Shi Gao* (Gypsum Fibrosum) were added, and *Wu Wei Zi* (Fructus Schisandrae Chinensis), *Xi Xin* (Radix et Rhizoma Asari), and *Ban Xia* (Rhizoma Pinelliae) were removed; for dry cough without sputum, *Mai Dong* (Radix Ophiopogonis), *Pi Pa Ye* (Folium Eriobotryae), and *Bai Bu* (Radix Stemonae) were added; for cough with clear, watery sputum, *Zi Su Zi* (Fructus Perillae) and *Ku Xing Ren* (Semen Armeniacae Amarum) were added; for sticky, yellow sputum,

81

Chapter 1 – Exterior-Releasing Formulas   Section 1 – Acrid and Warm Exterior-Releasing Formulas

Xiǎo Qīng Lóng Tāng (Minor Bluegreen Dragon Decoction)

Gua Lou Pi (Pericarpium Trichosanthis) and Tian Zhu Huang (Concretio Silicea Bambusae) were added, and Xi Xin (Radix et Rhizoma Asari), Sheng Jiang (Rhizoma Zingiberis Recens), and Da Zao (Fructus Jujubae) were removed; for wheezing with chest congestion, Bai Jie Zi (Semen Sinapis), Zi Su Zi (Fructus Perillae), and Di Long (Pheretima) were added; and for Spleen and Lung qi deficiencies, Dang Shen (Radix Codonopsis) and Bai Zhu (Rhizoma Atractylodis Macrocephalae) were added. Of 38 patients, the study reported complete recovery in 34 cases, improvement in 2 cases, and no benefit in 2 cases.[5]

3. **Asthma**: Use of modified She Gan Ma Huang Tang was effective in treating asthma. The herbal treatment contained She Gan Ma Huang Tang plus Dan Nan Xing (Arisaema cum Bile) and Ku Xing Ren (Semen Armeniacae Amarum) as the base formula, with addition of Yin Yang Huo (Herba Epimedii), Fu Zi (Radix Aconiti Lateralis Praeparata), and Rou Gui (Cortex Cinnamomi) for cold-type asthma; Shi Gao (Gypsum Fibrosum), Sang Bai Pi (Cortex Mori), and Yu Xing Cao (Herba Houttuyniae) for heat-type asthma; and Bu Gu Zhi (Fructus Psoraleae), Zhong Ru Shi (Stalactitum), and Huang Qi (Radix Astragali) during remission of asthma. Wang Bu Liu Xing (Semen Vaccariae) seeds were applied topically to acupuncture points on the ear. Of 100 patients, the study reported significant improvement in 35 cases, moderate improvement in 57 cases, and no benefit in 8 cases. The overall rate of effectiveness was 92%.[6]

AUTHORS' COMMENTS

Xiao Qing Long Tang (Minor Bluegreen Dragon Decoction) and She Gan Ma Huang Tang both release exterior wind-cold and treat interior tan yin (phlegm retention).

• Xiao Qing Long Tang is indicated for severe wind-cold attack with constitutional water accumulation; it involves more severe symptoms of profuse, watery nasal discharge and sputum. It treats internal fluid accumulation with exterior excess, wind-cold invasion.

• She Gan Ma Huang Tang focuses less on wind-cold condition and more on phlegm stagnation causing symptoms of cough and dyspnea with sputum. It more strongly directs Lung qi downward and relieves dyspnea.[7]

References

1. Zhong Yi Fang Ji Xian Dai Yan Jiu (Modern Study of Medical Formulae in Traditional Chinese Medicine) 1997;66.
2. Zhong Yi Fang Ji Xian Dai Yan Jiu (Modern Study of Medical Formulae in Traditional Chinese Medicine) 1997;66-67.
3. Zhong Yi Yao Xue Bao (Report of Chinese Medicine and Herbology) 1990;3:36.
4. Nan Jing Zhong Yi Xue Yuan Xue Bao (Journal of Nanjing University of Traditional Chinese Medicine) 1993;4:46.
5. Shan Dong Zhong Yi Za Zhi (Shandong Journal of Chinese Medicine) 1996;11:499.
6. Shi Yong Zhong Yi Yao Za Zhi (Journal of Practical Chinese Medicine and Medicinals) 1997;5:14.
7. Wang MZ, et al. Zhong Yi Xue Wen Da Ti Ku (Questions and Answers on Traditional Chinese Medicine: Herbal Formulas).

Cāng Ěr Zǐ Sǎn (Xanthium Powder)

蒼耳子散
苍耳子散

Pinyin Name: Cang Er Zi San
Literal Name: Xanthium Powder
Alternate Names: Cang Er San, Tsang Erh San, Xanthium Formula
Original Source: Ji Sheng Fang (Formulas to Aid the Living) by Yan Yong-He in 1253

COMPOSITION

Cang Er Zi (Fructus Xanthii), chao (dry-fried)	7.5g
Xin Yi Hua (Flos Magnoliae)	15g
Bai Zhi (Radix Angelicae Dahuricae)	30g
Bo He (Herba Menthae)	1.5g

82

Cāng Ěr Zǐ Sǎn (Xanthium Powder)

DOSAGE / PREPARATION / ADMINISTRATION

Sun-dry the ingredients and then grind them into a fine powder. Take 6g per dose after meals with an herbal tea made from *Cong Bai* (Bulbus Allii Fistulosi) and *Cha Ye* (Folium Camelliae).

CHINESE THERAPEUTIC ACTIONS

1. Dispels wind
2. Opens the nasal orifices

CLINICAL MANIFESTATIONS

Nasal obstruction caused by wind: stuffy nose, thick, yellow nasal discharge, and frontal and temporal headaches.

CLINICAL APPLICATIONS

Acute or chronic sinusitis, and acute or chronic allergic rhinitis.

EXPLANATION

Cang Er Zi San (Xanthium Powder) treats wind attacking the exterior. Wind invasion is characterized by symptoms such as nasal discharge and frontal headache, while heat invasion is characterized by thick, yellow nasal discharge. Clinically, this formula may be used for patients suffering

from rhinitis, who exhibit symptoms such as stuffy nose, runny nose, and headache.

Cang Er Zi (Fructus Xanthii) and *Xin Yi Hua* (Flos Magnoliae), the two chief herbs, unblock the nasal passages and are commonly used together for their synergistic effect. *Bai Zhi* (Radix Angelicae Dahuricae) opens the nasal orifices, dispels wind, and discharges pus. *Bo He* (Herba Menthae) releases wind-heat from the exterior. *Bai Zhi* (Radix Angelicae Dahuricae) and *Bo He* (Herba Menthae) relieve headache caused by wind. *Cong Bai* (Bulbus Allii Fistulosi) and *Cha Ye* (Folium Camelliae) enhance the overall effects of the formula.

MODIFICATIONS

- If there is increased Lung heat, add *Di Gu Pi* (Cortex Lycii) and *Sang Bai Pi* (Cortex Mori).
- For copious, purulent nasal discharge, add *Jin Yin Hua* (Flos Lonicerae Japonicae) and *Lian Qiao* (Fructus Forsythiae).

AUTHORS' COMMENTS

Cang Er Zi San may slightly irritate the digestive system. To avoid this irritation, dry-fry *Cang Er Zi* (Fructus Xanthii) first before use, and take the formula after meals.

Cang Er Zi San (Xanthium Powder)

Diagnosis	Signs and Symptoms	Treatment	Herbs
Nasal obstruction due to wind	• Nasal obstruction and frontal headache: exterior wind • Runny nose with thick, yellow nasal discharge: wind condition	• Dispels wind • Opens the nasal orifices	• *Cang Er Zi* (Fructus Xanthii) and *Xin Yi Hua* (Flos Magnoliae) unblock the nasal passages. • *Bai Zhi* (Radix Angelicae Dahuricae) opens the nasal orifices, dispels wind, and discharges pus. • *Bo He* (Herba Menthae) releases wind-heat from the exterior. • *Cong Bai* (Bulbus Allii Fistulosi) and *Cha Ye* (Folium Camelliae) enhance the overall effects of the formula

EXTERIOR-RELEASING FORMULAS

Chapter 1 – Exterior-Releasing Formulas 　　　　*Section 1 – Acrid and Warm Exterior-Releasing Formulas*

Xīn Yí Săn (Magnolia Flower Powder)

辛夷散

Pinyin Name: Xin Yi San
Literal Name: Magnolia Flower Powder
Alternate Names: *Hsin I San*, Magnolia Flower Formula
Original Source: *Ji Sheng Fang* (Formulas to Aid the Living) by Yan Yong-He in 1253

COMPOSITION

Xin Yi Hua (Flos Magnoliae)

Sheng Ma (Rhizoma Cimicifugae)

Bai Zhi (Radix Angelicae Dahuricae)

Xi Xin (Radix et Rhizoma Asari)

Fang Feng (Radix Saposhnikoviae)

Qiang Huo (Rhizoma et Radix Notopterygii)

Gao Ben (Rhizoma et Radix Ligustici)

Chuan Xiong (Rhizoma Chuanxiong)

Mu Tong (Caulis Akebiae)

Zhi Gan Cao (Radix et Rhizoma Glycyrrhizae Praeparata cum Melle)

DOSAGE / PREPARATION / ADMINISTRATION

The source text states to grind equal amounts of the ingredients into powder. Take 6g of the powder per dose with tea after meals.

CHINESE THERAPEUTIC ACTIONS

1. Releases wind-cold from the exterior
2. Opens the nasal orifices

CLINICAL MANIFESTATIONS

Nasal obstruction caused by wind-cold: stuffy nose, profuse, clear or white nasal discharge, and headache.

CLINICAL APPLICATIONS

Allergy, allergic rhinitis, sinusitis, rhinitis, sinus congestion, and sinus headache.

EXPLANATION

Xin Yi San (Magnolia Flower Powder) is one of the most commonly used formulas for opening the nasal orifices.

Xin Yi San (Magnolia Flower Powder)

Diagnosis	Signs and Symptoms	Treatment	Herbs
Nasal obstruction caused by wind-cold	• Nasal obstruction and frontal headache: exterior wind • Runny nose with clear or white nasal discharge: wind-cold condition	• Releases wind-cold from the exterior • Opens the nasal orifices	• *Xin Yi Hua* (Flos Magnoliae), *Sheng Ma* (Rhizoma Cimicifugae), and *Bai Zhi* (Radix Angelicae Dahuricae) raise clear qi to the head to open the nasal orifices. • *Xi Xin* (Radix et Rhizoma Asari) warms the Lung to resolve phlegm and helps open the nasal orifices. • *Fang Feng* (Radix Saposhnikoviae) and *Qiang Huo* (Rhizoma et Radix Notopterygii) dispel wind-cold. • *Gao Ben* (Rhizoma et Radix Ligustici) and *Chuan Xiong* (Rhizoma Chuanxiong) relieve headache. • *Mu Tong* (Caulis Akebiae) opens obstruction in the nose, and drains dampness and eliminates water accumulation through urination. • *Zhi Gan Cao* (Radix et Rhizoma Glycyrrhizae Praeparata cum Melle) harmonizes the herbs.

84

Xīn Yí Sǎn (Magnolia Flower Powder)

Consisting of mostly warm exterior-releasing herbs, this formula is suitable for nasal problems caused by wind-cold. As wind-cold attacks the exterior of the body, it travels upward to affect the nose. Clinical presentations include stuffy nose with clear or white nasal discharge, and headache.

In this formula, the herbs of light quality – *Xin Yi Hua* (Flos Magnoliae), *Sheng Ma* (Rhizoma Cimicifugae), and *Bai Zhi* (Radix Angelicae Dahuricae) – raise clear qi to the head to open the nasal orifices. *Xin Yi Hua* (Flos Magnoliae) and *Bai Zhi* (Radix Angelicae Dahuricae) are two commonly used herbs for nasal problems. *Xi Xin* (Radix et Rhizoma Asari) warms the Lung to resolve phlegm and helps the previous two herbs open the nasal orifices. *Fang Feng* (Radix Saposhnikoviae) and *Qiang Huo* (Rhizoma et Radix Notopterygii) dispel wind-cold. *Gao Ben* (Rhizoma et Radix Ligustici) and *Chuan Xiong* (Rhizoma Chuanxiong) relieve headache. *Mu Tong* (Caulis Akebiae) opens obstruction in the nose, and drains dampness and eliminates water accumulation through urination. *Zhi Gan Cao* (Radix et Rhizoma Glycyrrhizae Praeparata cum Melle) harmonizes the formula.

MODIFICATIONS
- For clear nasal discharge from wind-cold invasion, add *Jing Jie* (Herba Schizonepetae) and *Qiang Huo* (Rhizoma et Radix Notopterygii).
- For abscess caused by accumulation of wind-dampness, add *Cang Zhu* (Rhizoma Atractylodis) and *Lian Qiao* (Fructus Forsythiae).
- With abscess and loss of smell, add *Pai Nong San* (Drain the Pus Powder).

CLINICAL STUDIES AND RESEARCH

Allergic rhinitis: Perennial allergic rhinitis was effectively treated with *Xin Yi San* 9g, *Xiao Qing Long Tang* (Minor Bluegreen Dragon Decoction) 3g, and *Xiang Sha Liu Jun Zi Tang* (Six-Gentlemen Decoction with Aucklandia and Amomum) 3g. The patients were given 15g (9+3+3) of herbal extract per day in three equal doses. The mechanism of action was attributed to the suppression of nasal mucosa inflammation by normalizing stimulatory effects of allergic nasal discharge in patients with H-IgE allergic rhinitis.[1]

RELATED FORMULAS
Xīn Yí Sǎn (Magnolia Flower Powder)
辛夷散
Pinyin Name: Xin Yi San
Literal Name: Magnolia Flower Powder
Original Source: *Yi Fang Ji Jie* (Analytical Collection of Medical Formulas) by Wang Ang in 1682

Xin Yi Hua (Flos Magnoliae)
Sheng Ma (Rhizoma Cimicifugae)
Bai Zhi (Radix Angelicae Dahuricae)
Xi Xin (Radix et Rhizoma Asari)
Fang Feng (Radix Saposhnikoviae)
Gao Ben (Rhizoma et Radix Ligustici)
Chuan Xiong (Rhizoma Chuanxiong)
Cha Ye (Folium Camelliae)
Mu Tong (Caulis Akebiae)
Gan Cao (Radix et Rhizoma Glycyrrhizae)

This formula is commonly used to treat nasal problems caused by wind-cold. Clinical presentations include stuffy nose with clear or white nasal discharge.

There are two variations of *Xin Yi San*:
- *Xin Yi San* from *Ji Sheng Fang* (Formulas to Aid the Living) contains *Qiang Huo* (Rhizoma et Radix Notopterygii), and is slightly better for treating headache.
- *Xin Yi San* from *Yi Fang Ji Jie* (Analytical Collection of Medical Formulas) uses *Gan Cao* (Radix et Rhizoma Glycyrrhizae) and *Cha Ye* (Folium Camelliae), and is slightly better for reducing swelling and nasal obstruction.

Jiā Wèi Xīn Yí Sǎn
(Augmented Magnolia Flower Powder)
加味辛夷散
Pinyin Name: Jia Wei Xin Yi San
Literal Name: Augmented Magnolia Flower Powder
Original Source: *Tian Jin Zhong Yi Xue Yuan* (Tianjin University of Chinese Medicine) in 1989

Xin Yi Hua (Flos Magnoliae)
Cang Er Zi (Fructus Xanthii)
Gao Ben (Rhizoma et Radix Ligustici)
Bai Zhi (Radix Angelicae Dahuricae)
Sheng Ma (Rhizoma Cimicifugae)
Chuan Xiong (Rhizoma Chuanxiong)
Ma Huang (Herba Ephedrae)
Fang Feng (Radix Saposhnikoviae)
Chuan Mu Tong (Caulis Clematidis Armandii)
Gan Cao (Radix et Rhizoma Glycyrrhizae)
Cha Ye (Folium Camelliae)
Zhi Shi (Fructus Aurantii Immaturus)
Gan Jiang (Rhizoma Zingiberis)
Jie Geng (Radix Platycodonis)
Wu Wei Zi (Fructus Schisandrae Chinensis)

Jia Wei Xin Yi San (Augmented Magnolia Flower Powder) releases wind-cold from the exterior, opens the nasal orifices, and relieves pain. Clinically, it treats sinusitis or rhinitis caused by wind-cold, with symptoms

Chapter 1 – Exterior-Releasing Formulas　　　　　*Section 1 – Acrid and Warm Exterior-Releasing Formulas*

Xīn Yí Săn (Magnolia Flower Powder)

such as nasal obstruction, pain in the sinus cavity, profuse, clear or white nasal discharge, and headache.

AUTHORS' COMMENTS

Xin Yi San is one of the most commonly used formulas today for treating nose allergies. The key symptoms include nasal congestion, clear, watery nasal discharge, loss of smell, and headache.

Reference

1. Yang SH, Hong CY, Yu CL. The stimulatory effects of nasal discharge from patients with perennial allergic rhinitis on normal human neutrophils are normalized after treatment with a new mixed formula of Chinese herbs. International Immunopharmacology 2002 Nov;2(12):1627-39.

Qīng Bí Tāng (Clear the Nose Decoction)

清鼻湯

清鼻汤

Pinyin Name: *Qing Bi Tang*
Literal Name: Clear the Nose Decoction
Alternate Name: Pueraria Nasal Combination
Original Source: *Yan Fang* (Time-Tested Formulas) of unknown author and date

COMPOSITION

Ge Gen (Radix Puerariae Lobatae)	12g
Ma Huang (Herba Ephedrae)	6g
Sheng Jiang (Rhizoma Zingiberis Recens)	3g
Yi Yi Ren (Semen Coicis)	10g
Jie Geng (Radix Platycodonis)	9g
Xin Yi Hua (Flos Magnoliae)	8g
Shi Gao (Gypsum Fibrosum)	2g
Da Huang (Radix et Rhizoma Rhei)	3g
Chuan Xiong (Rhizoma Chuanxiong)	3g
Rou Gui (Cortex Cinnamomi)	5g
Bai Shao (Radix Paeoniae Alba)	3g
Da Zao (Fructus Jujubae)	2g
Gan Cao (Radix et Rhizoma Glycyrrhizae)	2g

DOSAGE / PREPARATION / ADMINISTRATION

Prepare the ingredients as a decoction and take while warm with meals, to avoid possible digestive discomfort.

CHINESE THERAPEUTIC ACTIONS

1. Clears nasal obstruction
2. Releases the exterior

CLINICAL MANIFESTATIONS

Nasal obstruction caused by damp-heat: stuffy nose, yellow and sticky nasal discharge, sneezing, headache, itchy nose and throat, decreased sense of smell, decreased energy level, and fatigue.

CLINICAL APPLICATIONS

Acute and chronic sinusitis and rhinitis.

EXPLANATION

Qing Bi Tang (Clear the Nose Decoction) specifically treats nasal obstruction caused by damp-heat, with the diagnostic symptom of yellow and sticky discharge. This syndrome may occur secondary to an acute exterior attack or a chronic condition. If the nasal obstruction is the result of an exterior condition, other symptoms of an exterior attack may be present, such as sneezing, headache, aversion to cold, and itching of the nose and throat. If the nasal obstruction is chronic in nature, patients may

Qīng Bí Tāng (Clear the Nose Decoction)

Qing Bi Tang (Clear the Nose Decoction)

Diagnosis	Signs and Symptoms	Treatment	Herbs
Nasal obstruction caused by damp-heat	• Stuffy nose with yellow, sticky discharge: accumulation of damp-heat • Decreased sense of smell: damp-heat blocking the sensory orifices • Sneezing, headache, aversion to cold, and an itching sensation in the nose and throat: exterior condition	• Clears nasal obstruction • Releases the exterior	• *Ge Gen* (Radix Puerariae Lobatae), *Ma Huang* (Herba Ephedrae), and *Sheng Jiang* (Rhizoma Zingiberis Recens) release exterior pathogens. • *Yi Yi Ren* (Semen Coicis) and *Jie Geng* (Radix Platycodonis) drain dampness and eliminate pus. • *Xin Yi Hua* (Flos Magnoliae) opens the nasal passages and unblocks nasal obstruction. • *Shi Gao* (Gypsum Fibrosum) and *Da Huang* (Radix et Rhizoma Rhei) clear heat and reduce swelling. • *Chuan Xiong* (Rhizoma Chuanxiong) activates blood circulation and unblocks stagnation. • *Rou Gui* (Cortex Cinnamomi) warms the body and moderates the effects of the harsh and cold herbs. • *Bai Shao* (Radix Paeoniae Alba) balances the acrid and warm herbs. • *Da Zao* (Fructus Jujubae) and *Gan Cao* (Radix et Rhizoma Glycyrrhizae) harmonize the formula.

experience a decreased sense of smell, decreased energy level, fatigue, and other allergy symptoms.

Ge Gen (Radix Puerariae Lobatae), *Ma Huang* (Herba Ephedrae), and *Sheng Jiang* (Rhizoma Zingiberis Recens) release exterior pathogens. *Yi Yi Ren* (Semen Coicis) and *Jie Geng* (Radix Platycodonis) drain dampness and eliminate pus. *Xin Yi Hua* (Flos Magnoliae) opens the nasal passages and unblocks nasal obstruction. *Shi Gao* (Gypsum Fibrosum) and *Da Huang* (Radix et Rhizoma Rhei), both cold in nature, clear heat and reduce swelling. *Chuan Xiong* (Rhizoma Chuanxiong) activates blood circulation and relieves headaches associated with nasal symptoms. *Rou Gui* (Cortex Cinnamomi) warms the body, dispels cold, and moderates the harsh and cold properties of *Shi Gao* (Gypsum Fibrosum) and *Da Huang* (Radix et Rhizoma Rhei). *Bai Shao* (Radix Paeoniae Alba) harmonizes *ying* (nutritive) and *wei* (defensive) levels, and balances the acrid and warm herbs in this formula. *Da Zao* (Fructus Jujubae) and *Gan Cao* (Radix et Rhizoma Glycyrrhizae) harmonize the formula.

MODIFICATIONS
• If there is headache, add *Bai Zhi* (Radix Angelicae Dahuricae).
• For sinus infection, add *Huang Qin* (Radix Scutellariae) and *Huang Lian* (Rhizoma Coptidis).

RELATED FORMULA

Yóu Bí Tāng (Benefit the Nose Decoction)

優鼻湯
优鼻汤

Pinyin Name: *You Bi Tang*
Literal Name: Benefit the Nose Decoction
Original Source: *Yan Fang* (Time-Tested Formulas) of unknown author and date

Ma Huang (Herba Ephedrae)
Chuan Xiong (Rhizoma Chuanxiong)
Bai Shao (Radix Paeoniae Alba)
Gan Cao (Radix et Rhizoma Glycyrrhizae)
Da Zao (Fructus Jujubae)
Sheng Jiang (Rhizoma Zingiberis Recens)
Ge Gen (Radix Puerariae Lobatae)
Gui Zhi (Ramulus Cinnamomi)
Bai Zhi (Radix Angelicae Dahuricae)
Jie Geng (Radix Platycodonis)
Xin Yi Hua (Flos Magnoliae)
Da Huang (Radix et Rhizoma Rhei)
Huang Qin (Radix Scutellariae)
Shi Gao (Gypsum Fibrosum)

You Bi Tang (Benefit the Nose Decoction) clears nasal obstruction and releases the exterior. Clinically, this formula treats nasal obstruction caused by damp-heat,

Qīng Bí Tāng (Clear the Nose Decoction)

with key symptoms such as yellow, sticky nasal discharge, sneezing, and headache.

The original formulation of *Qing Bi Tang* contains *Rou Gui* (Cortex Cinnamomi), a Kidney yang tonic herb that warms the interior. Today, *Rou Gui* (Cortex Cinnamomi) is usually replaced with *Gui Zhi* (Ramulus Cinnamomi), which can release the exterior and warm the peripheral channels and collaterals.

Qing Bi Tang and *You Bi Tang* (Benefit the Nose Decoction) contain very similar ingredients, and have essentially the same clinical applications.
- *Qing Bi Tang* contains *Yi Yi Ren* (Semen Coicis) and drains dampness.
- *You Bi Tang* contains *Huang Qin* (Radix Scutellariae) and effectively clears heat.

AUTHORS' COMMENTS

Qing Bi Tang and *You Bi Tang* are formulated based on the clinical experience of past herbalists. These formulas have been refined after years of trial and error, and are very effective for treating sinusitis and rhinitis characterized by damp-heat. The original sources of these two formulas are unavailable because they have not been formally cited in any reference or textbook.

There are three formulas that commonly treat various types of sinusitis and rhinitis:
- *Cang Er Zi San* (Xanthium Powder) is best for wind-heat condition characterized by nasal obstruction with yellow discharge.
- *Xin Yi San* (Magnolia Flower Powder) is most effective for wind-cold condition characterized by nasal obstruction with clear, white discharge.
- *Qing Bi Tang* (Clear the Nose Decoction) targets damp-heat condition characterized by nasal obstruction with yellow, sticky nasal discharge that has a foul smell.

Chinese Herbal Formulas and Applications

Section 2

辛凉解表剂
— Acrid and Cold Exterior-Releasing Formulas

EXTERIOR-RELEASING FORMULAS

Sāng Jú Yǐn (Mulberry Leaf and Chrysanthemum Decoction)
桑菊飲
桑菊饮

Pinyin Name: *Sang Ju Yin*
Literal Name: Mulberry Leaf and Chrysanthemum Decoction
Alternate Names: *Sang Chu Yin*, Morus Leaves and Chrysanthemum Drink, Mulberry and Chrysanthemum Decoction, Morus and Chrysanthemum Combination
Original Source: *Wen Bing Tiao Bian* (Systematic Differentiation of Warm Disease) by Wu Ju-Tong in 1798

COMPOSITION

Sang Ye (Folium Mori)	7.5g
Ju Hua (Flos Chrysanthemi)	3g
Bo He (Herba Menthae)	2.4g
Lian Qiao (Fructus Forsythiae)	4.5g
Jie Geng (Radix Platycodonis)	6g
Ku Xing Ren (Semen Armeniacae Amarum)	6g
Lu Gen (Rhizoma Phragmitis)	6g
Gan Cao (Radix et Rhizoma Glycyrrhizae)	2.4g

DOSAGE / PREPARATION / ADMINISTRATION

Cook the ingredients with 2 cups of water until the liquid is reduced to 1 cup. Take the decoction twice daily.

CHINESE THERAPEUTIC ACTIONS

1. Dispels wind and clears heat
2. Ventilates the Lung and arrests coughing

CLINICAL MANIFESTATIONS

Early stage of wind-warmth syndrome: cough, mild fever, and slight thirst.

CLINICAL APPLICATIONS

Common cold, influenza, acute bronchitis, acute tonsillitis, coughing, and other upper respiratory infections.

EXPLANATION

Sang Ju Yin (Mulberry Leaf and Chrysanthemum Decoction) is a relatively mild formula that treats the early stage or mild case of wind-warmth syndrome, a condition that

is similar to, but less severe, than wind-heat syndrome. Coughing, the prominent symptom of this syndrome, arises when the wind-warmth factor affects the normal Lung qi flow. Since this wind-warmth syndrome is mild in nature, the fever and thirst will be slight.

Sang Ye (Folium Mori) and *Ju Hua* (Flos Chrysanthemi) expel the wind-warmth factor and clear Lung heat. *Bo He* (Herba Menthae) helps clear the wind-warmth from the upper *jiao*. *Jie Geng* (Radix Platycodonis), with its ascending tendency, and *Ku Xing Ren* (Semen Armeniacae Amarum), with its descending tendency, regulate Lung qi to relieve cough. *Lian Qiao* (Fructus Forsythiae) clears heat and eliminates toxins in the upper *jiao*. *Lu Gen* (Rhizoma Phragmitis) clears heat and promotes the generation of body fluids to relieve thirst. *Gan Cao* (Radix et Rhizoma Glycyrrhizae) harmonizes the herbs.

In this formula, *Sang Ye* (Folium Mori) and *Ju Hua* (Flos Chrysanthemi) are used as chief herbs to gently disperse

89

Sāng Jú Yǐn (Mulberry Leaf and Chrysanthemum Decoction)

Sang Ju Yin (Mulberry Leaf and Chrysanthemum Decoction)

Diagnosis	Signs and Symptoms	Treatment	Herbs
Early stage of wind-warmth syndrome	• Mild fever: exterior wind-warmth • Slight thirst: heat consuming body fluids • Cough: wind-warmth affecting Lung qi circulation	• Dispels wind and clears heat • Ventilates the Lung and arrests cough	• *Sang Ye* (Folium Mori) and *Ju Hua* (Flos Chrysanthemi) dispel exterior wind-warmth factor and clear interior Lung heat. • *Bo He* (Herba Menthae) clears wind-warmth factor from the upper *jiao*. • *Lian Qiao* (Fructus Forsythiae) clears heat and eliminates toxins in the upper *jiao*. • *Jie Geng* (Radix Platycodonis) and *Ku Xing Ren* (Semen Armeniacae Amarum) regulate Lung qi to relieve coughing. • *Lu Gen* (Rhizoma Phragmitis) clears heat and promotes the generation of body fluids to relieve thirst. • *Gan Cao* (Radix et Rhizoma Glycyrrhizae) harmonizes the herbs.

early-stage wind-warmth that is beginning to affect the Lung. Although *Bo He* (Herba Menthae) is colder, and has a stronger exterior-releasing effect, it is not suitable as the chief herb for two main reasons. First, its exterior-releasing effect is too strong, and may further damage body fluids, create heat phlegm and aggravate cough. Second, it does not clear Lung heat nor arrest the cough. Therefore, *Bo He* (Herba Menthae) is not suitable as the chief ingredient, but is used as the deputy herb to help *Sang Ye* (Folium Mori) and *Ju Hua* (Flos Chrysanthemi) release wind-warmth.

MODIFICATIONS

• For severe cough with yellow sputum caused by Lung heat, add *Huang Qin* (Radix Scutellariae) and *Sang Bai Pi* (Cortex Mori).

• For cough with sticky sputum that is difficult to expectorate, add *Gua Lou Pi* (Pericarpium Trichosanthis), *Dong Gua Zi* (Semen Benincasae), and *Zhe Bei Mu* (Bulbus Fritillariae Thunbergii).

• For cough with blood-streaked sputum, add *Bai Mao Gen* (Rhizoma Imperatae), *Ou Jie* (Nodus Nelumbinis Rhizomatis), and *Qian Cao* (Radix et Rhizoma Rubiae).

• If there is labored breathing or dyspnea characterized by more heat and dryness in the *qi* (energy) level, add *Shi Gao* (Gypsum Fibrosum) and *Zhi Mu* (Rhizoma Anemarrhenae) to clear the Lung.

• When there is more thirst, add *Tian Hua Fen* (Radix Trichosanthis) and *Zhi Mu* (Rhizoma Anemarrhenae).

• If accompanied by a sore throat, add *She Gan* (Rhizoma Belamcandae), *Shan Dou Gen* (Radix et Rhizoma Sophorae Tonkinensis), and *Niu Bang Zi* (Fructus Arctii).

• For eye disorders caused by wind-warmth invasion, add *Chan Tui* (Periostracum Cicadae).

• For eye disorders caused by Liver heat, add *Jue Ming Zi* (Semen Cassiae) and *Ji Li* (Fructus Tribuli).

CAUTIONS / CONTRAINDICATIONS

• *Sang Ju Yin* is an acrid and cold formula that treats wind-warmth condition. It is inappropriate for cough caused by wind-cold.

• This formula has only mild potency to treat cough caused by wind-warmth invasion. In cases of severe cough caused by Lung heat, the use of this formula alone will not be sufficient. Modification with additional herbs and doses, or selection of another formula is necessary for proper treatment.

PHARMACOLOGICAL EFFECTS

1. **Effect on temperature regulation**: Administration of *Sang Ju Yin* was associated with reduction of body temperature in rabbits with artificially-induced fever. The formula, however, has a slow onset of action, as the effect was not observed until 4 hours later. The researchers noted that the potency of this formula is similar to that of aspirin at 2 mg/kg.[1]

2. **Anti-inflammatory**: Administration of *Sang Ju Yin* was associated with marked anti-inflammatory effects in mice with swelling and inflammation. The mechanism of action is attributed to reversal of the increased capillary permeability. The minimum effective dose for anti-inflammatory effects was 0.307 g/kg. The pharmacokinetic parameters of *Sang Ju Yin* are: 4.83 hours for half life, 3.1

Sāng Jú Yǐn (Mulberry Leaf and Chrysanthemum Decoction)

hours for time to reach peak concentration, and 24.48 hours for duration of action.[2]

CLINICAL STUDIES AND RESEARCH

1. **Upper respiratory tract infection**: Patients with upper respiratory tract infection characterized by cough, fever, sticky sputum, and a dry mouth were treated with *Sang Ju Yin*. Out of 375 cases, the study reported satisfactory results in 359 cases (95.5%). No side effects were reported.[3]

2. **Cough**: Eighty pediatric patients with cough were treated with *Sang Ju Yin* plus *Ma Huang* (Herba Ephedrae) and *Gan Jiang* (Rhizoma Zingiberis) with 94% effectiveness. Modifications were made by adding *Shi Gao* (Gypsum Fibrosum) and *Huang Qin* (Radix Scutellariae) for Lung heat; *Ge Gen* (Radix Puerariae Lobatae) and *Tian Hua Fen* (Radix Trichosanthis) for thirst; *Bai Bu* (Radix Stemonae) and *Zi Wan* (Radix et Rhizoma Asteris) for severe cough; *Bai Guo* (Semen Ginkgo) and *Di Long* (Pheretima) for wheezing; *Xi Xin* (Radix et Rhizoma Asari) and *Fu Zi* (Radix Aconiti Lateralis Praeparata) for cold; *Chuan Bei Mu* (Bulbus Fritillariae Cirrhosae) and *Gua Lou Pi* (Pericarpium Trichosanthis) for profuse phlegm; *She Gan* (Rhizoma Belamcandae) and *Niu Bang Zi* (Fructus Arctii) for redness and swelling of the throat; *Bai Mao Gen* (Rhizoma Imperatae) and *Xian He Cao* (Herba Agrimoniae) for nosebleeds; and charred *Shan Zha* (Fructus Crataegi), charred *Shen Qu* (Massa Fermentata), and charred *Mai Ya* (Fructus Hordei Germinatus) for poor appetite. Of 80 cases, the study reported complete recovery in 64 cases after 2 packs of herbs, in 11 cases after 3-5 packs of herbs, and no benefit in 5 cases.[4]

3. **Influenza**: Use of modified *Sang Ju Yin* was associated with 86.5% effectiveness in treating 50 patients with influenza. The clinical presentations included signs and symptoms such as headache, stuffy nose, runny nose, cough, poor appetite, etc. The herbs were given in decoction daily. The study reported resolution of most symptoms within 2-4 days.[5]

4. **Epistaxis**: One study reported successful treatment of nosebleeds in all 60 patients within 2-7 days using *Sang Ju Yin* plus *Ce Bai Ye* (Cacumen Platycladi), *Xian He Cao* (Herba Agrimoniae), and others as needed. For modification, *Da Huang* (Radix et Rhizoma Rhei) was added if there was constipation.[6]

AUTHORS' COMMENTS

Sang Ju Yin is one of the most essential and effective formulas for treating <u>mild</u> cases of cough caused by wind-warmth invasion. This formula is also effective in treating dry cough, with scanty or no sputum, during the autumn. Because this formula is mild in nature, it is necessary to modify it to increase its potency and/or address associated complications. Please see the Modifications section for details.

Yin Qiao San (Honeysuckle and Forsythia Powder) and *Sang Ju Yin* are cool, acrid formulas used for the initial stages of warm febrile disorders. Both contain *Lian Qiao* (Fructus Forsythiae), *Jie Geng* (Radix Platycodonis), *Gan Cao* (Radix et Rhizoma Glycyrrhizae), *Bo He* (Herba Menthae), and *Lu Gen* (Rhizoma Phragmitis).

- *Yin Qiao San* has stronger heat-clearing and exterior-releasing effects.
- *Sang Ju Yin* more effectively ventilates the Lung to arrest coughing.

Sang Xing Tang (Mulberry Leaf and Apricot Kernel Decoction) and *Sang Ju Yin* both contain *Ku Xing Ren* (Semen Armeniacae Amarum) and *Sang Ye* (Folium Mori) to clear the Lung, relieve cough, and expel exterior factors.

- *Sang Xing Tang* is indicated for dryness and heat attacking the Lung. This formula contains moistening herbs, such as *Sha Shen* (Radix Glehniae seu Adenophorae) and *Zhe Bei Mu* (Bulbus Fritillariae Thunbergii), to treat dryness symptoms.
- *Sang Ju Yin* is indicated for wind-warmth attacking the Lung. It contains heat-clearing herbs, such as *Bo He* (Herba Menthae), *Lu Gen* (Rhizoma Phragmitis), and *Lian Qiao* (Fructus Forsythiae), to clear heat.[7]

According to Dr. Chang Wei-Yen, *Sang Ju Yin* can be combined with *Hu Yao Huang* (Herba Leucas Mollissimae), *Pao Zai Cao* (Herba Physalis Angulatae), and *Zhu Zi Cao* (Herba Euphorbiae Thymifoliae) to treat cough and dyspnea associated with wind-warmth invasion.

References

1. *Zhong Yao Tong Bao* (Journal of Chinese Herbology) 1986;11(1):51.
2. *Zhong Yao Yao Li Yu Ying Yong* (Pharmacology and Applications of Chinese Herbs) 1993;(1):1.
3. *Fu Jian Zhong Yi Yao* (Fujian Chinese Medicine and Herbology) 1957;2(6):25.
4. *Shi Yong Zhong Yi Yao Za Zhi* (Journal of Practical Chinese Medicine and Medicinals) 1999;7:16.
5. *Guang Dong Zhong Yi* (Guangdong Chinese Medicine) 1959;2:58.
6. *Xin Zhong Yi* (New Chinese Medicine) 1999;1:47.
7. Wang MZ, et al. *Zhong Yi Xue Wen Da Ti Ku* (Questions and Answers on Traditional Chinese Medicine: Herbal Formulas).

Chapter 1 – Exterior-Releasing Formulas　　　　　　　*Section 2 – Acrid and Cold Exterior-Releasing Formulas*

Yín Qiào Sǎn (Honeysuckle and Forsythia Powder)

銀翹散
银翘散

Pinyin Name: *Yin Qiao San*
Literal Name: Honeysuckle and Forsythia Powder
Alternate Names: *Yin Jiao San*, Lonicera and Forsythia Formula
Original Source: *Wen Bing Tiao Bian* (Systematic Differentiation of Warm Disease) by Wu Ju-Tong in 1798

COMPOSITION

Jin Yin Hua (Flos Lonicerae Japonicae)	30g [15g]
Lian Qiao (Fructus Forsythiae)	30g [15g]
Jing Jie Sui (Spica Schizonepetae)	12g [4g]
Dan Dou Chi (Semen Sojae Praeparatum)	15g [5g]
Jie Geng (Radix Platycodonis)	18g [6g]
Niu Bang Zi (Fructus Arctii)	18g [6g]
Bo He (Herba Menthae)	18g [6g]
Zhu Ye (Herba Phyllostachys)	12g [4g]
Gan Cao (Radix et Rhizoma Glycyrrhizae)	15g [5g]

DOSAGE / PREPARATION / ADMINISTRATION

Grind the ingredients into powder and take 18g of the powder with a decoction made from fresh *Lu Gen* (Rhizoma Phragmitis). The decoction of *Lu Gen* (Rhizoma Phragmitis) is prepared by cooking the herb in water until its aroma fills the air. Do not overcook the herb, since a light decoction (cooking for a short period of time) enters and treats the Lung, while a heavy decoction (cooking for long period of time) enters the middle *jiao*.

For patients with serious conditions, take the decoction three times during the day (2 hours apart) and one time at night. For patients with mild conditions, take the decoction twice during the day (3 hours apart) and one time at night. The treatment should be continued until the condition is resolved. Today, this formula may be prepared as a decoction with the doses suggested in brackets above.

CHINESE THERAPEUTIC ACTIONS

1. Releases the exterior with acrid and cold herbs
2. Clears heat and eliminates toxins

CLINICAL MANIFESTATIONS

Onset of *wen bing* (warm disease): fever, aversion to cold, slight aversion to wind, slight or absence of perspiration, headache, thirst, a sore throat, cough, a red tongue tip with a thin, white or thin, yellow tongue coating, and a superficial, rapid pulse.

CLINICAL APPLICATIONS

Common cold, influenza, high fever, pneumonia, acute upper respiratory infection, pharyngo-conjunctival fever, tonsillitis, parotitis, canker sores, viral myocarditis, epidemic encephalitis B, and drug-induced dermatitis.

EXPLANATION

Yin Qiao San (Honeysuckle and Forsythia Powder) treats the early stage of *wen bing* (warm disease), when heat enters through the nose and mouth and attacks the Lung. When heat attacks the *wei* (defensive) level of the skin, it produces symptoms of fever, aversion to cold, slight aversion to wind, and slight or absence of perspiration. When heat invades the Lung, it produces cough. Thirst and a red tongue tip are indications of heat damaging body fluids. A thin, white or thin, yellow tongue coating and a superficial, rapid pulse are signs of heat at the exterior.

Jin Yin Hua (Flos Lonicerae Japonicae) and *Lian Qiao* (Fructus Forsythiae) are the chief herbs in this formula. Acrid, aromatic and cold, they release exterior heat and eliminate toxins. *Jing Jie Sui* (Spica Schizonepetae) and *Dan Dou Chi* (Semen Sojae Praeparatum) open the skin pores to help expel exterior factors through mild perspiration. *Jie Geng* (Radix Platycodonis) regulates Lung qi and relieves the sore throat. *Bo He* (Herba Menthae) dispels wind-heat. *Zhu Ye* (Herba Phyllostachys) clears upper *jiao* heat, while *Niu Bang Zi* (Fructus Arctii) clears heat and eliminates toxins to relieve the sore throat. *Gan Cao* (Radix et Rhizoma Glycyrrhizae) clears heat and eliminates toxins. Finally, *Lu Gen* (Rhizoma Phragmitis) clears heat and promotes the generation of body fluids to relieve thirst.

Chinese Herbal Formulas and Applications

Yín Qiào Sǎn (Honeysuckle and Forsythia Powder)

Yin Qiao San (Honeysuckle and Forsythia Powder)

Diagnosis	Signs and Symptoms	Treatment	Herbs
Onset of *wen bing* (warm disease)	• Fever, aversion to cold, slight aversion to wind, slight or absence of perspiration: heat attacks the *wei* (defensive) level • Thirst, sore throat, and cough: heat enters the Lung through the mouth and nose • Thirst and a red tongue tip: body fluids damaged by heat • Thin, white or thin, yellow tongue coating and a superficial, rapid pulse: heat at the exterior	• Releases the exterior • Clears heat and eliminates toxins	• *Jin Yin Hua* (Flos Lonicerae Japonicae) and *Lian Qiao* (Fructus Forsythiae) release exterior heat and eliminate toxins. • *Jing Jie Sui* (Spica Schizonepetae) and *Dan Dou Chi* (Semen Sojae Praeparatum) open the skin pores to expel exterior factors via mild perspiration. • *Jie Geng* (Radix Platycodonis) regulates Lung qi and relieves sore throat. • *Niu Bang Zi* (Fructus Arctii) clears heat and eliminates toxins. • *Bo He* (Herba Menthae) dispels exterior wind-heat. • *Zhu Ye* (Herba Phyllostachys) clears interior heat from upper *jiao*. • *Lu Gen* (Rhizoma Phragmitis) clears heat and promotes the generation of body fluids. • *Gan Cao* (Radix et Rhizoma Glycyrrhizae) clears heat and eliminates toxins.

MODIFICATIONS

• For a sore and swollen throat, add *Ma Bo* (Lasiosphaera seu Calvatia), *She Gan* (Rhizoma Belamcandae), and *Xuan Shen* (Radix Scrophulariae); or *Pu Ji Xiao Du Yin* (Universal Benefit Decoction to Eliminate Toxin).

• If there is headache and aversion to wind, add *Fang Feng* (Radix Saposhnikoviae) and *Cong Bai* (Bulbus Allii Fistulosi).

• With irritability and thirst, add *Mai Dong* (Radix Ophiopogonis) and *Shi Gao* (Gypsum Fibrosum).

• If there is nausea, vomiting, and feeling of chest oppression, add *Huo Xiang* (Herba Agastaches) and *Zhi Qiao* (Fructus Aurantii).

• If there is thirst, add *Tian Hua Fen* (Radix Trichosanthis) or *Lu Gen* (Rhizoma Phragmitis).

• If there is cough, add *Ku Xing Ren* (Semen Armeniacae Amarum) and *Zhe Bei Mu* (Bulbus Fritillariae Thunbergii).

• For early stage of measles, add *Zi Cao* (Radix Arnebiae) and *Chan Tui* (Periostracum Cicadae).

• When there is more interior heat, add *Zhi Zi* (Fructus Gardeniae) and *Huang Qin* (Radix Scutellariae).

• When heat in the Lung has injured body fluids, add *Di Huang* (Radix Rehmanniae) and *Mai Dong* (Radix Ophiopogonis).

CAUTIONS / CONTRAINDICATIONS

• *Yin Qiao San* is contraindicated in cases of wind-cold invasion or in initial stages of damp-heat conditions.

• Wind-heat conditions can change rapidly. Optimal treatment requires close monitoring of clinical presentations and immediate adjustment of the herbal treatment.

• Avoid foods that are oily, greasy, raw, cold, or sour in nature while taking this herbal formula.[1]

PHARMACOLOGICAL EFFECTS

1. **Antibiotic**: According to *in vitro* studies, *Yin Qiao San* has broad spectrum of inhibitory effects against such pathogens as *Staphylococcus aureus*, *Bacillus subtilis*, *Bacillus proteus*, *Pseudomonas aeruginosa*, and *Candida albicans*. The minimum inhibitory concentration was 110 mg/mL (equivalent to 550 mg/mL of raw herb).[2]

2. **Effect on temperature regulation**: Administration of *Yin Qiao San* was effective in reducing body temperature in rabbits with artificially-induced fever. Oral ingestion of decoction at 3.8 mL/kg (equivalent to 8.8 g/kg of dried herbs) was effective in reducing body temperature by 1°C for up to six hours. In comparison with aspirin (0.2 mg/kg), the herbal formula and the drugs are approximately the same in their effect to reduce fever.[3]

3. **Anti-inflammatory**: Administration of various dosage forms of *Yin Qiao San* was effective in reducing swelling and inflammation in rats. The dosage forms tested include decoction, pills, and tea bags. It has been determined that to achieve an anti-inflammatory effect, the minimum effective dose is 1.5 g/kg. The pharmacokinetic parameters of *Yin Qiao San* are: 2.31 hours to reach peak therapeutic

93

Yín Qiào Sǎn (Honeysuckle and Forsythia Powder)

effect, 16.23 hours for duration of action, and 4.53 hours for half life.[4]

4. **Analgesic**: Administration of *Yin Qiao San* at doses of 50 mg/kg and 100 mg/kg via intraperitoneal injection was associated with mild analgesic effects in mice for up to one hour.[5]

CLINICAL STUDIES AND RESEARCH

1. **Common cold and influenza**: Three hundred patients with infectious viral infection were treated with *Yin Qiao San* with most reporting improvement after 1-2 doses.[6]

2. **High fever**: In one study, 102 children with high fever caused by infection were treated with 87.25% effectiveness using modified *Yin Qiao San*. Modifications included addition of *Shi Gao* (Gypsum Fibrosum), *Di Gu Pi* (Cortex Lycii), and *Zhi Mu* (Rhizoma Anemarrhenae) for persistent high fever; *Jiang Can* (Bombyx Batryticatus) and *Gou Teng* (Ramulus Uncariae cum Uncis) for spasms and cramps; *Ma Huang* (Herba Ephedrae), *Ku Xing Ren* (Semen Armeniacae Amarum), and *Qian Hu* (Radix Peucedani) for cough; *Chi Shao* (Radix Paeoniae Rubra), *Chan Tui* (Periostracum Cicadae), and *Ju Hua* (Flos Chrysanthemi) for red eyes; *Ban Xia* (Rhizoma Pinelliae) and *Sheng Jiang* (Rhizoma Zingiberis Recens) for nausea and vomiting; and *Yi Yi Ren* (Semen Coicis) and *Hua Shi* (Talcum) for diarrhea. After using 1-3 packs of the herbs, the study reported improvement in 89 of 102 patients.[7]

3. **Pneumonia**: One study reported recovery in all 25 children with pneumonia after they were treated with 3-5 packs of modified *Yin Qiao San* plus *Zhi Mu* (Rhizoma Anemarrhenae) and *Ku Xing Ren* (Semen Armeniacae Amarum). Additional modifications were made as needed. For irritability and thirst due to excess heat, *Tian Hua Fen* (Radix Trichosanthis) and *Huang Lian* (Rhizoma Coptidis) were added, and *Jing Jie Sui* (Spica Schizonepetae), *Bo He* (Herba Menthae) and *Niu Bang Zi* (Fructus Arctii) were removed. For severe cough with thick sputum, *Chuan Bei Mu* (Bulbus Fritillariae Cirrhosae) and *Gua Lou* (Fructus Trichosanthis) were added, and *Niu Bang Zi* (Fructus Arctii) and *Jing Jie Sui* (Spica Schizonepetae) were removed. For dry or foul-smelling stools, *Da Huang* (Radix et Rhizoma Rhei) was added, and *Jie Geng* (Radix Platycodonis) and *Bo He* (Herba Menthae) were removed. For reduced frequency and volume of urine with painful urination, *Che Qian Zi* (Semen Plantaginis) was added, and *Niu Bang Zi* (Fructus Arctii) and *Jing Jie Sui* (Spica Schizonepetae) were removed.[8]

4. **Acute upper respiratory infection**: In one report, 1150 patients with wind-heat exterior infection were treated with *Yin Qiao San* with relief of fever within an average of 2.7 days.[9]

5. **Tonsillitis**: Modified *Yin Qiao San* successfully treated 36 patients with acute tonsillitis. The base formula contained *Yin Qiao San* plus *Shan Dou Gen* (Radix et Rhizoma Sophorae Tonkinensis). *Ku Xing Ren* (Semen Armeniacae Amarum) and *Qian Hu* (Radix Peucedani) were added for cough; and *Shi Gao* (Gypsum Fibrosum) and *Zhi Mu* (Rhizoma Anemarrhenae) were added for high fever without aversion to cold. Of 36 patients, 24 had complete recovery and 12 had improvement. The average duration of treatment was 9 days.[10]

6. **Viral myocarditis**: Fifty-two patients with viral myocarditis were treated with 92.2% effectiveness using integrated treatment of herbs, rest, nutrition, and intravenous infusion of fluids and vitamin C. The herbal treatment contained *Yin Qiao San* plus *Dang Gui* (Radix Angelicae Sinensis), *Di Huang* (Radix Rehmanniae), and *Da Zao* (Fructus Jujubae) as the base formula, with the addition of *Ban Lan Gen* (Radix Isatidis) for sore throat; *Huang Qi* (Radix Astragali) and *Zhi Gan Cao* (Radix et Rhizoma Glycyrrhizae Praeparata cum Melle) for palpitations; and a larger dose of *Dang Gui* (Radix Angelicae Sinensis) for chest oppression and shortness of breath. Of 52 cases, complete recovery was reported in 38 cases, improvement in 10 cases, and no benefit in 4 cases.[11]

TOXICOLOGY

The LD_{50} for *Yin Qiao San* in mice via oral ingestion was 100 g/kg in decoction, and 75 g/kg in pills.[12]

RELATED FORMULAS

Yín Qiào Tāng (Honeysuckle and Forsythia Decoction)
銀翹湯
银翘汤
Pinyin Name: Yin Qiao Tang
Literal Name: Honeysuckle and Forsythia Decoction
Original Source: *Wen Bing Tiao Bian* (Systematic Differentiation of Warm Disease) by Wu Ju-Tong in 1798

Jin Yin Hua (Flos Lonicerae Japonicae)	15g
Lian Qiao (Fructus Forsythiae)	9g
Zhu Ye (Herba Phyllostachys)	6g
Gan Cao (Radix et Rhizoma Glycyrrhizae)	3g
Mai Dong (Radix Ophiopogonis)	12g
Di Huang (Radix Rehmanniae)	12g

The source text instructs to prepare the ingredients as a decoction. *Yin Qiao Tang* (Honeysuckle and Forsythia Decoction) treats mild *yangming* syndrome, which occurs as a result of the inappropriate use of downward draining herbs to treat an exterior condition. Consequently, the exterior pathogenic factors move to the interior and create heat. Furthermore, the improper use of downward

Yín Qiào Sǎn (Honeysuckle and Forsythia Powder)

draining herbs damages the body and causes qi and yin deficiencies.

To treat these types of cases, one must use exterior-releasing herbs in conjunction with yin-nourishing herbs. *Lian Qiao* (Fructus Forsythiae) and *Jin Yin Hua* (Flos Lonicerae Japonicae) release the exterior factors, while *Mai Dong* (Radix Ophiopogonis) and *Di Huang* (Radix Rehmanniae) nourish yin and clear heat. *Gan Cao* (Radix et Rhizoma Glycyrrhizae) tonify qi, and *Zhu Ye* (Herba Phyllostachys) clears any heat that may arise from yin deficiency. The three herbs, *Lian Qiao* (Fructus Forsythiae), *Jin Yin Hua* (Flos Lonicerae Japonicae), and *Zhu Ye* (Herba Phyllostachys) are selected particularly for their light quality, which allows them to clear heat without damaging yin.

Yín Qiào Jiě Dú Sǎn

(Honeysuckle and Forsythia Powder to Relieve Toxicity)

銀翹解毒散
银翘解毒散

Pinyin Name: *Yin Qiao Jie Du San*
Literal Name: Honeysuckle and Forsythia Powder to Relieve Toxicity
Original Source: *An Hui Zhong Yi Xue Yuan* (Anhui University School of Medicine) in 1990

Lian Qiao (Fructus Forsythiae)
Jin Yin Hua (Flos Lonicerae Japonicae)
Ban Lan Gen (Radix Isatidis)
Da Qing Ye (Folium Isatidis)
Pu Gong Ying (Herba Taraxaci)
Zi Hua Di Ding (Herba Violae)
Ye Ju Hua (Flos Chrysanthemi Indici)
Jie Geng (Radix Platycodonis)
Bo He (Herba Menthae)
Dan Zhu Ye (Herba Lophatheri)
Lu Gen (Rhizoma Phragmitis)
Jing Jie (Herba Schizonepetae)
Dan Dou Chi (Semen Sojae Praeparatum)
Niu Bang Zi (Fructus Arctii)
Gan Cao (Radix et Rhizoma Glycyrrhizae)
Huang Qin (Radix Scutellariae)
Sang Ye (Folium Mori)

Yin Qiao Jie Du San (Honeysuckle and Forsythia Powder to Relieve Toxicity) releases exterior wind-heat and eliminates heat and toxins. It treats the initial onset of *wen bing* (warm disease) with more severe signs and symptoms, such as high fever, severe sore and swollen throat, absence of perspiration or slight perspiration, aversion to wind, headache, thirst, coughing, a red tongue tip with a yellow tongue coating, and a superficial, rapid pulse.

AUTHORS' COMMENTS

Yin Qiao San is the representative formula for treating the initial stage of *wen bing* (warm disease), with chief manifestations of sore throat, fever, aversion to cold, slight aversion to wind, slight or absence of perspiration, thirst, and a superficial, rapid pulse. It is widely used in the treatment of various types of common cold and influenza, with sore throat as the key symptom. This formula is most effective when administered immediately after the warning signs and symptoms (such as throat discomfort) appear. Appropriate use of this formula will reduce the severity and duration of such viral infections.

Because this formula has been used for many centuries, some patients might have already developed some level of resistance to it. In such cases, herbs that clear heat and eliminate toxins should be added to enhance the overall effects, such as *Zi Hua Di Ding* (Herba Violae), *Ma Bian Cao* (Herba Verbenae), and *Chuan Xin Lian* (Herba Andrographis).

Yin Qiao San, a formula that releases wind-heat, contains *Jing Jie Sui* (Spica Schizonepetae), an herb that releases wind-cold, for two very important reasons. First, it encourages the yang qi of the body to move outward to the *wei* (defensive) level to produce sweating, and thereby release the wind-heat factor. Second, most of the herbs in *Yin Qiao San* are cold, and thus may constrict the skin pores and trap the pathogenic factors inside. *Jing Jie Sui* (Spica Schizonepetae), a warm herb that releases mild wind-cold, promotes the expelling of wind-heat toxins; it also offsets the possible negative effects of the cold herbs. Although *Jing Jie Sui* (Spica Schizonepetae) belongs to the wind-cold releasing category and has a slightly warm property, it is a relatively mild herb, and, at a low dose, will not injure yin.

Sang Ju Yin (Mulberry Leaf and Chrysanthemum Decoction) and *Yin Qiao San* both clear heat, eliminate toxins, disperse wind-heat, and ventilate the Lung. Both are suitable for wind-heat invasion with fever and cough. The differences between the two formulas are as follows:

- *Sang Ju Yin* contains *Sang Ye* (Folium Mori), *Ju Hua* (Flos Chrysanthemi), and *Ku Xing Ren* (Semen Armeniacae Amarum). This formula ventilates the Lung and arrests cough associated with initial stages of wind-heat invasion.
- *Yin Qiao San* contains *Jin Yin Hua* (Flos Lonicerae Japonicae), *Jing Jie* (Herba Schizonepetae), *Dan Dou Chi* (Semen Sojae Praeparatum), *Niu Bang Zi* (Fructus Arctii), and *Zhu Ye* (Herba Phyllostachys). This formula eliminates toxins to treat *wen bing* (warm disease) conditions with chief manifestations of sore throat and fever.

Chapter 1 – Exterior-Releasing Formulas   Section 2 – Acrid and Cold Exterior-Releasing Formulas

Yín Qiào Sǎn (Honeysuckle and Forsythia Powder)

References

1. *Zhong Yao Ming Fang Yao Li Yu Ying Yong* (Pharmacology and Applications of Famous Herbal Formulas) 1989;55-57.
2. *Zhong Cheng Yao* (Study of Chinese Patent Medicine) 1990;12(1):22.
3. *Zhong Yao Tong Bao* (Journal of Chinese Herbology) 1986;11(1):51.
4. *Zhong Yi Za Zhi* (Journal of Chinese Medicine) 1986;27(3):59.
5. *Zhong Cheng Yao* (Study of Chinese Patent Medicine) 1990;12(1):22.
6. *Hu Bei Zhong Yi Za Zhi* (Hubei Journal of Chinese Medicine) 1983;(2):19.
7. *Liao Ning Zhong Yi Za Zhi* (Liaoning Journal of Chinese Medicine) 1994;12:548.
8. *Hu Bei Zhong Yi Za Zhi* (Hubei Journal of Chinese Medicine) 1982;1:55.
9. *Zhong Cheng Yao Yan Jiu* (Research of Chinese Patent Medicine) 1986;(12):39.
10. *Hu Bei Zhong Yi Za Zhi* (Hubei Journal of Chinese Medicine) 1998;2:41.
11. *Hu Nan Zhong Yi Za Zhi* (Hunan Journal of Chinese Medicine) 1997;4:29.
12. *Zhong Yi Za Zhi* (Journal of Chinese Medicine) 1986;27(3):59.

Má Huáng Xìng Rén Gān Cǎo Shí Gāo Tāng
(Ephedra, Apricot Kernel, Licorice, and Gypsum Decoction)

麻黃杏仁甘草石膏湯
麻黄杏仁甘草石膏汤

Pinyin Name: *Ma Huang Xing Ren Gan Cao Shi Gao Tang*
Literal Name: Ephedra, Apricot Kernel, Licorice, and Gypsum Decoction
Alternate Names: *Ma Xing Gan Shi Tang, Ma Xing Shi Gan Tang, Ma Hsing Kan Shih Tang*, Ephedra, Apricot, Licorice and Gypsum Decoction; Ephedra, Apricot Kernel, Gypsum and Licorice Decoction; Ma-huang and Apricot Seed Decoction, Mahuang and Apricot Seed Combination
Original Source: *Shang Han Lun* (Discussion of Cold-Induced Disorders) by Zhang Zhong-Jing in the Eastern Han Dynasty

COMPOSITION

Ma Huang (Herba Ephedrae)	12g [5-9g]
Shi Gao (Gypsum Fibrosum), *fen sui* (pulverized)	24g [18g]
Ku Xing Ren (Semen Armeniacae Amarum)	50 kernels [9g]
Zhi Gan Cao (Radix et Rhizoma Glycyrrhizae Praeparata cum Melle)	6g

DOSAGE / PREPARATION / ADMINISTRATION

The source text states to cook *Ma Huang* (Herba Ephedrae) in 7 cups [1,400 mL] of water until it is reduced to 5 cups [1,000 mL]. Remove the foam from the top, add the other ingredients, and cook until the liquid reduces to 2 cups [400 mL]. Take 1 cup [200 mL] of the warm, strained decoction. Today, the decoction may be prepared using the doses suggested in brackets.

CHINESE THERAPEUTIC ACTIONS

1. Ventilates Lung qi
2. Clears Lung heat
3. Relieves cough and dyspnea

CLINICAL MANIFESTATIONS

Cough and dyspnea in Lung heat syndrome caused by exterior pathogenic factors: unremitting fever, thirst with a desire to drink, rhinalgia, coughing, dyspnea, with or without perspiration, a thin, white or thin, yellow tongue coating, and a slippery, rapid pulse.

CLINICAL APPLICATIONS

Upper respiratory tract infection, acute bronchitis, chronic bronchitis, pneumonia, whooping cough, influenza, cough and dyspnea, asthma, bronchial asthma, acute tracheitis, fever, acute pharyngitis, nasosinusitis, measles, diphtheria, and hemorrhoids.

EXPLANATION

Ma Huang Xing Ren Gan Cao Shi Gao Tang (Ephedra, Apricot Kernel, Licorice, and Gypsum Decoction) is indicated for Lung heat syndrome characterized by cough and dyspnea. This syndrome can be caused by an exterior wind-heat factor directly invading the Lung, or by an

Chinese Herbal Formulas and Applications

Má Huáng Xìng Rén Gān Căo Shí Gāo Tāng
(Ephedra, Apricot Kernel, Licorice, and Gypsum Decoction)

Ma Huang Xing Ren Gan Cao Shi Gao Tang (Ephedra, Apricot Kernel, Licorice, and Gypsum Decoction)

Diagnosis	Signs and Symptoms	Treatment	Herbs
Cough and dyspnea in Lung heat syndrome	• Coughing and dyspnea: heat affecting Lung qi circulation • Thirst with a desire to drink: heat damaging body fluids • Unremitting fever and rhinalgia: Lung heat • Thin, white or thin, yellow tongue coating: exterior heat • Rapid pulse: heat	• Releases exterior factors • Clears Lung heat • Corrects reversed flow of Lung qi	• *Ma Huang* (Herba Ephedrae) ventilates the Lung and directs Lung qi downward. • *Shi Gao* (Gypsum Fibrosum) clears Lung heat and restrains the warm property of *Ma Huang* (Herba Ephedrae). • *Ku Xing Ren* (Semen Armeniacae Amarum) corrects the reversed flow of Lung qi to relieve cough and dyspnea. • *Zhi Gan Cao* (Radix et Rhizoma Glycyrrhizae Praeparata cum Melle) generates body fluids and relieves thirst.

exterior wind-cold factor constricting the Lung. Both situations can create stagnation in the Lung that later transforms into heat.

Unremitting fever and rhinalgia occur as a result of heat trapped in the Lung. Coughing and dyspnea are the result of heat disrupting the proper descending flow of Lung qi. Heat damages body fluids, leading to thirst with a desire to drink. Heat also forces fluids out of the body, causing perspiration. However, this condition cannot be relieved by perspiration because it is no longer at the exterior level. If the heat damages body fluids extensively, there will be no perspiration.

Ma Huang (Herba Ephedrae), the chief herb, ventilates the Lung and directs Lung qi downward. *Shi Gao* (Gypsum Fibrosum) is the deputy herb, yet its dose is double the amount of the chief herb for two key reasons: to sedate Lung heat, and to prevent the warm property of *Ma Huang* (Herba Ephedrae) from creating more heat. *Ku Xing Ren* (Semen Armeniacae Amarum) helps *Ma Huang* (Herba Ephedrae) to correct the reversed flow of Lung qi and relieve cough and dyspnea. *Zhi Gan Cao* (Radix et Rhizoma Glycyrrhizae Praeparata cum Melle) helps *Shi Gao* (Gypsum Fibrosum) generate body fluids and relieve thirst. It also harmonizes the descending, dispersing, warm, and cold properties of all of the herbs in this formula.

MODIFICATIONS
• When there is more cough and dyspnea, add *Sang Bai Pi* (Cortex Mori) and *Di Gu Pi* (Cortex Lycii).
• For severe cough and dyspnea, add *Xie Bai San* (Drain the White Powder).
• If there is cough with sputum, add *Jie Geng* (Radix Platycodonis).

• If there is blood in the sputum, add *Bai Mao Gen* (Rhizoma Imperatae) and *Ce Bai Ye* (Cacumen Platycladi).
• For fever, accelerated respiration, a thin, yellow tongue coating, and a rapid pulse, add *Zi Su Ye* (Folium Perillae), *Sang Ye* (Folium Mori), *Di Long* (Pheretima) and *Sang Bai Pi* (Cortex Mori).
• If high fever is present, add *Jin Yin Hua* (Flos Lonicerae Japonicae) and *Lian Qiao* (Fructus Forsythiae).
• If accompanied by edema of the face and ankles, add *Ting Li Zi* (Semen Descurainiae seu Lepidii) and *Che Qian Zi* (Semen Plantaginis).
• For thick, profuse and yellow sputum, add *Huang Qin* (Radix Scutellariae), *Gua Lou* (Fructus Trichosanthis), and *Zhe Bei Mu* (Bulbus Fritillariae Thunbergii).
• When there is chest pain, add *Gua Lou Pi* (Pericarpium Trichosanthis) and *Si Gua Luo* (Retinervus Luffae Fructus).
• For unerupted measles or erupted measles with fever, thirst, cough, and labored breathing, add *Da Qing Ye* (Folium Isatidis), *Huang Qin* (Radix Scutellariae), and *Lian Qiao* (Fructus Forsythiae).

CAUTIONS / CONTRAINDICATIONS
• *Ma Huang Xing Ren Gan Cao Shi Gao Tang* should be used with caution in the following situations: patients with Spleen and Stomach qi deficiencies; children and elderly patients with general weakness; or individuals convalescing from chronic illnesses. When the use of this formula is necessary in such patients, it should be modified by adding *Sang Bai Pi* (Cortex Mori) and reducing the dose of *Shi Gao* (Gypsum Fibrosum).
• This formula is contraindicated for cough or dyspnea caused by wind-cold invasion or deficiency.
• According to one report, continuous use of over 10 packs of this formula in decoction has been associated with occasional incidents of poor appetite and abdominal distention.[1]

Chapter 1 – Exterior-Releasing Formulas   *Section 2 – Acrid and Cold Exterior-Releasing Formulas*

Má Huáng Xìng Rén Gān Cǎo Shí Gāo Tāng
(Ephedra, Apricot Kernel, Licorice, and Gypsum Decoction)

PHARMACOLOGICAL EFFECTS

1. **Antiasthmatic**: *Ma Huang Xing Ren Gan Cao Shi Gao Tang* demonstrated antiasthmatic effects to dilate the lung to treat asthma. The proposed mechanism of its antiasthmatic effects is its stimulation of beta2-adrenoceptors on bronchial smooth muscle and its anti-inflammatory ability to inhibit the neutrophil into the airway.[2] Though the individual component of *Ma Huang* (Herba Ephedrae) has effect to dilate the lung and treat cough and dyspnea, the effect is significantly less than the formula as a whole. It was pointed out that the maximum effect is achieved only when the four herbs are combined together. The stronger effect of the formula is attributed to the other three herbs, which not only help to treat the disorders, but also help to increase the extraction of ephedrine alkaloids by an additional 50%.[3]

2. **Antitussive**: Administration of *Ma Huang Xing Ren Gan Cao Shi Gao Tang* was associated with marked antitussive effects in mice and dogs with artificially-induced cough.[4]

3. **Effect on temperature regulation**: A group of rabbits with artificially-induced fever was divided into two groups to evaluate the effect of *Ma Huang Xing Ren Gan Cao Shi Gao Tang* on body temperature. Rabbits that received oral ingestion of the formula had an average of 1.27°C reduction of body temperature. Rabbits in the control group that did not receive any treatment had an average of 0.93°C increase of body temperature.[5]

4. **Mast cell stabilizer**: Administration of *Ma Huang Xing Ren Gan Cao Shi Gao Tang* and *Xiao Feng San* (Eliminate Wind Powder) at 4-40 mcg/mL was found to inhibit IgE-dependent histamine released from mouse cultured mast cells.[6]

CLINICAL STUDIES AND RESEARCH

1. **Acute bronchitis**: Use of *Ma Huang Xing Ren Gan Cao Shi Gao Tang* plus *Xiao Xian Xiong Tang* (Minor Sinking into the Chest Decoction) demonstrated a rate of effectiveness of 88% in treating acute bronchitis in 50 children. Additional modifications were made as deemed necessary. The herbs were cooked in water, and the resultant decoction (100 mL total) was taken in three to four equally-divided doses.[7]

2. **Chronic bronchitis**: Use of modified *Ma Huang Xing Ren Gan Cao Shi Gao Tang* produced good results in treating individuals with chronic bronchitis. The herbal treatment contained this formula plus *Huang Qin* (Radix Scutellariae), *Ban Xia* (Rhizoma Pinelliae) and *Yu Jin* (Radix Curcumae) as the base formula, plus *Yu Xing Cao* (Herba Houttuyniae) and *Jin Yin Hua* (Flos Lonicerae Japonicae) for presence of phlegm and heat; *Da Huang* (Radix et Rhizoma Rhei) and *Gua Lou* (Fructus Trichosanthis) for constipation; *Huang Qi* (Radix Astragali) and *Bai Zhu* (Rhizoma Atractylodis Macrocephalae) for qi deficiency; and *Tai Zi Shen* (Radix Pseudostellariae) and *Mai Dong* (Radix Ophiopogonis) for damaged yin. Of 46 cases, the study reported significant improvement in 34 cases, improvement in 8 cases, and no effect in 4 cases.[8]

3. **Pneumonia**: Use of *Ma Huang Xing Ren Gan Cao Shi Gao Tang* plus *Qing Dai* (Indigo Naturalis), *Huang Qin* (Radix Scutellariae) and others was associated with marked success in treating pneumonia in children. Modifications included addition of *Zi Su Zi* (Fructus Perillae), *Lai Fu Zi* (Semen Raphani) and *Di Long* (Pheretima) for hurried respiration with profuse sputum. The average duration of treatment was 6.2 days. Of 61 cases, the study reported complete recovery in 21 cases, near-recovery in 22 cases, improvement in 13 cases, and no effect in 5 cases.[9] According to another study, use of *Ma Huang Xing Ren Gan Cao Shi Gao Tang* plus *Ting Li Zi* (Semen Descurainiae seu Lepidii), *Da Qing Ye* (Folium Isatidis) and others was associated with 98.22% effectiveness in treating pneumonia in 56 children.[10] Lastly, 300 patients with pneumonia were treated with modified *Ma Huang Xing Ren Gan Cao Shi Gao Tang* with complete recovery in most patients within 2-3 days.[11]

4. **Whooping cough**: An effectiveness rate of 96.47% was reported for treating whooping cough using *Ma Huang Xing Ren Gan Cao Shi Gao Tang* plus *Bai Bu* (Radix Stemonae), *Ting Li Zi* (Semen Descurainiae seu Lepidii), *Da Zao* (Fructus Jujubae), and *Yi Tang* (Maltosum). The herbs were given in syrup form (10.5 g/mL) for 3-12 days. Of 228 patients, the study reported complete recovery in 195 patients and improvement in 25 patients.[12]

5. **Upper respiratory tract infection**: Good results were reported in treating patients with upper respiratory tract infection using *Ma Huang Xing Ren Gan Cao Shi Gao Tang*. The study reported that 69.8% of patients had improvement of cough, 75.9% had reduction of sputum, and 78.3% had improvement of cough and dyspnea.[13]

6. **Cough and dyspnea**: *Ma Huang Xing Ren Gan Cao Shi Gao Tang* plus *Ting Li Zi* (Semen Descurainiae seu Lepidii) and other herbs was effective in treating all 40 children with cough and dyspnea.[14] Another study reported 93.75% effectiveness in treating bronchial cough and dyspnea in 80 children using *Ma Huang Xing Ren Gan Cao Shi Gao Tang* plus *Zao Jiao Ci* (Spina Gleditsiae), *Sang Bai Pi* (Cortex Mori) and others as needed.[15] Lastly, use of *Ma Huang Xing Ren Gan Cao Shi Gao Tang* plus *Dan Nan Xing* (Arisaema cum Bile), *Qian Hu* (Radix Peucedani) and others was successful in treating 82 children with cough and dyspnea. The duration of treatment ranged from 10 to 13 days.[16]

7. **Asthma**: Use of modified *Ma Huang Xing Ren Gan Cao Shi Gao Tang* produced marked results in treating asthma.

98

Chinese Herbal Formulas and Applications

Má Huáng Xìng Rén Gān Cǎo Shí Gāo Tāng
(Ephedra, Apricot Kernel, Licorice, and Gypsum Decoction)

Of 47 cases, the study reported complete recovery in 17 cases, significant improvement in 13 cases, moderate improvement in 11 cases, and no benefit in 6 cases. The average duration of herbal treatment was 34 days.[17] In another study, use of modified *Ma Huang Xing Ren Gan Cao Shi Gao Tang* in 37 patients with asthma was associated with 91.9% effectiveness. The herbal treatment contained *Ma Huang Xing Ren Gan Cao Shi Gao Tang* plus *Yu Xing Cao* (Herba Houttuyniae), *Zi Su Zi* (Fructus Perillae) and others as the base formula. Furthermore, *Lai Fu Zi* (Semen Raphani), *She Gan* (Rhizoma Belamcandae) and *Di Long* (Pheretima) were added for severe asthma; *Huang Qin* (Radix Scutellariae) and *Tian Hua Fen* (Radix Trichosanthis) for heat; *Tian Zhu Huang* (Concretio Silicea Bambusae), *Dan Nan Xing* (Arisaema cum Bile) and *Zhu Ru* (Caulis Bambusae in Taenia) for phlegm; and *Sha Shen* (Radix Glehniae seu Adenophorae), *Mai Dong* (Radix Ophiopogonis) and *Yu Zhu* (Rhizoma Polygonati Odorati) for dry cough with little or no sputum.[18]

8. **Fever**: Use of modified *Ma Huang Xing Ren Gan Cao Shi Gao Tang* in decoction was effective in treating 40 children with fever caused by infection. The herbal treatment contained this formula plus *Jin Yin Hua* (Flos Lonicerae Japonicae), *Lian Qiao* (Fructus Forsythiae), and *Huang Qin* (Radix Scutellariae) for presence of heat and toxins; *Jie Geng* (Radix Platycodonis) for cough; and *Huang Lian* (Rhizoma Coptidis) for diarrhea. The study reported normal body temperature within 12 hours in 39 of 40 children.[19] Another report pointed out that while this formula is effective in reducing fever, it does not address the infection itself. Therefore, herbs with antibiotic effects should be added to increase the effectiveness of the treatment.[20]

9. **Acute pharyngitis**: One study involving 50 patients reported 94% effectiveness in treating acute pharyngitis using *Ma Huang Xing Ren Gan Cao Shi Gao Tang* plus *Ban Lan Gen* (Radix Isatidis), *Lian Qiao* (Fructus Forsythiae), and *Pu Gong Ying* (Herba Taraxaci).[21]

10. **Nasosinusitis**: In one study, 112 patients with acute nasosinusitis were treated with complete recovery in 90 patients, improvement in 19 patients, and no benefit in 3 patients. The overall rate of effectiveness was 97.4%. The herbal treatment contained *Ma Huang Xing Ren Gan Cao Shi Gao Tang* plus *Bai Zhi* (Radix Angelicae Dahuricae), *Cang Er Zi* (Fructus Xanthii), *Xin Yi Hua* (Flos Magnoliae), and others as needed. The duration of treatment ranged from 7-20 packs of herbs.[22]

RELATED FORMULA

Jiā Wèi Má Xìng Gān Shí Tāng (Augmented Ephedra, Apricot Kernel, Licorice, and Gypsum Decoction)

加味麻杏甘石湯
加味麻杏甘石汤

Pinyin Name: *Jia Wei Ma Xing Gan Shi Tang*
Literal Name: Augmented Ephedra, Apricot Kernel, Licorice, and Gypsum Decoction
Original Source: *Tian Jin Zhong Yi Xue Yuan* (Tianjin University of Chinese Medicine) in 1989

Ma Huang (Herba Ephedrae)
Ku Xing Ren (Semen Armeniacae Amarum)
Gan Cao (Radix et Rhizoma Glycyrrhizae)
Shi Gao (Gypsum Fibrosum)
Sang Bai Pi (Cortex Mori)
Di Gu Pi (Cortex Lycii)
Ting Li Zi (Semen Descurainiae seu Lepidii)
Gua Lou Pi (Pericarpium Trichosanthis)
Da Zao (Fructus Jujubae)
Lian Qiao (Fructus Forsythiae)
Pi Pa Ye (Folium Eriobotryae)
She Gan (Rhizoma Belamcandae)
Wu Wei Zi (Fructus Schisandrae Chinensis)

Jia Wei Ma Xing Gan Shi Tang (Augmented Ephedra, Apricot Kernel, Licorice, and Gypsum Decoction) treats Lung disorder characterized by the presence of heat and phlegm, with symptoms and signs such as coughing, dyspnea, wheezing, chest distention and congestion, fever and yellow sputum. Clinical applications include asthma, pneumonia, pertussis, or respiratory tract infections with heat manifestations.

AUTHORS' COMMENTS

Ma Huang Xing Ren Gan Cao Shi Gao Tang is one of the most popular and effective formulas for treating any respiratory disorders, in which the main diagnostic criterion is interior Lung heat. However, this formula is not recommended in the initial stages of wind-heat invasion with thirst and cough. The improper use of this formula will encourage the pathogenic factors to move more quickly into the Lung, instead of lingering at the *wei* (defensive) level.

Many modern disorders are not as simple as the symptoms described for this formula. For this reason, it is important to recognize when and how the patterns are different and to modify the formula accordingly to treat the complications. Depending on each individual case, this formula can be prescribed singularly, or used as a base formula with the addition of other herbs from the phlegm-eliminating, heat-clearing, cough-arresting and others categories. Please see the Modifications section for details.

Má Huáng Xìng Rén Gān Cǎo Shí Gāo Tāng
(Ephedra, Apricot Kernel, Licorice, and Gypsum Decoction)

Sang Ju Yin (Mulberry Leaf and Chrysanthemum Decoction) and *Ma Huang Xing Ren Gan Cao Shi Gao Tang* both arrest cough, but have the following differences:

- *Sang Ju Yin* is a mild formula that treats the initial attack of wind-heat manifesting in cough. Patients will not show severe symptoms, since the pathogenic factor still resides at the *wei* (defensive) level.
- *Ma Huang Xing Ren Gan Cao Shi Gao Tang* is a strong formula that clears and ventilates the Lung to arrest cough and dyspnea caused by Lung heat.

Da Qing Long Tang (Major Bluegreen Dragon Decoction) and *Ma Huang Xing Ren Gan Cao Shi Gao Tang* both expel the exterior and clear interior heat, but have the following differences:

- *Da Qing Long Tang*, derived from *Ma Huang Tang* (Ephedra Decoction) and has an increased dose of *Ma Huang* (Herba Ephedrae), strongly induces sweating. It is indicated for severe and acute wind-cold invasion at the exterior with moderate interior heat accumulation. Heat is trapped in the Lung and cannot be cleared as a result of the cold constriction at the exterior.
- *Ma Huang Xing Ren Gan Cao Shi Gao Tang* contains *Shi Gao* (Gypsum Fibrosum), which sedates excess Lung heat. This syndrome involves severe interior heat and a moderate exterior condition. In other words, wind-heat has progressed from the *wei* (defensive) level into the Lung and the *qi* (energy) level.

Ma Huang Xing Ren Gan Cao Shi Gao Tang and *Xie Bai San* (Drain the White Powder) both clear Lung heat to relieve cough and dyspnea, but have contrasting differences:

- *Ma Huang Xing Ren Gan Cao Shi Gao Tang* treats Lung heat syndrome following a wind-heat or wind-cold invasion. Besides addressing symptoms of cough and dyspnea, this formula also treats fever, thirst with a preference to drink, and a rapid, forceful pulse. It sedates Lung heat and ventilates Lung qi and primarily treats cases of excess pathogenic factors invading the Lung.
- *Xie Bai San* is designed for children who have hidden stagnant Lung heat that leads to qi reversal and gradual body fluid depletion. Aside from cough and dyspnea, accompanying symptoms include warm, steaming sensations on the skin, especially in the late afternoon, and a rapid, fine pulse. Because the *zang fu* organs in children are still tender, they are much more susceptible to damage. For this reason, the draining herbs in this formula, such as *Sang Bai Pi* (Cortex Mori), are milder in nature. *Di Gu Pi* (Cortex Lycii) clears deficiency heat, while *Geng Mi*

(Semen Oryzae) and *Gan Cao* (Radix et Rhizoma Glycyrrhizae) strengthen the Spleen and Stomach (earth element) in order to promote the Lung (metal element). Together, the herbs clear heat without injuring yin, and sedate the Lung without injuring *zheng* (upright) *qi*. In short, *Xie Bai San* cools and nourishes the Lung, and is indicated for chronic cases of cough or dyspnea in yin-deficient patients.[23]

References

1. *Zhong Xi Yi Jie He Za Zhi* (Journal of Integrated Chinese and Western Medicine) 1985;(9):540.
2. Kao ST, Yeh TJ, Hsieh CC, Shiau HB, Yeh FT, Lin JG. The effects of Ma-Xing-Gan-Shi-Tang on respiratory resistance and airway leukocyte infiltration in asthmatic guinea pigs. Immunopharmacol Immunotoxicol 2001 Aug;23(3):445-58.
3. *Zhong Yi Yao Yan Jiu Zi Liao* (Research and Resource of Chinese Medicine and Herbology) 1986;(1):31.
4. *Zhong Cheng Yao Yan Jiu* (Research of Chinese Patent Medicine) 1987;(4):47.
5. *Zhong Cheng Yao Yan Jiu* (Research of Chinese Patent Medicine) 1984;(6):21.
6. Shichijo K, Saito H. Effect of Chinese herbal medicines and disodium cromoglycate on IgE-dependent histamine release from mouse cultured mast cells. Int J Immunopharmacol 1997 Nov-Dec;19 (11-12):677-82.
7. *Shang Hai Zhong Yi Yao Za Zhi* (Shanghai Journal of Chinese Medicine and Herbology) 1986;1:26.
8. *Nan Jing Zhong Yi Yao Da Xue Xue Bao* (Journal of Nanjing University of Traditional Chinese Medicine and Medicinals) 1996;1:59.
9. *Zhe Jiang Zhong Yi Za Zhi* (Zhejiang Journal of Chinese Medicine) 1982;11-12:498.
10. *Hei Long Jiang Zhong Yi Yao* (Heilongjiang Chinese Medicine and Herbology) 1994;3:38.
11. *Zhong Yi Fang Ji Xian Dai Yan Jiu* (Modern Study of Medical Formulae in Traditional Chinese Medicine) 1997;(1):113.
12. *Jiang Xi Zhong Yi Yao* (Jiangxi Chinese Medicine and Herbology) 1960;10:25.
13. *Zhong Yi Fang Ji Xian Dai Yan Jiu* (Modern Study of Medical Formulae in Traditional Chinese Medicine) 1997;(1):113.
14. *Jiang Su Zhong Yi Za Zhi* (Jiangsu Journal of Chinese Medicine) 1965;11:15.
15. *Jiang Su Zhong Yi* (Jiangsu Chinese Medicine) 1988;7:11.
16. *Hu Bei Zhong Yi Za Zhi* (Hubei Journal of Chinese Medicine) 1992;3:16.
17. *Shi Yong Zhong Yi Nei Ke Za Zhi* (Journal of Practical Chinese Internal Medicine) 1989;4:23.
18. *Zhe Jiang Zhong Yi Xue Yuan Xue Bao* (Journal of Zhejiang University of Chinese Medicine) 1998;3:22.
19. *Hu Bei Zhong Yi Za Zhi* (Hubei Journal of Chinese Medicine) 1987;1:15.
20. *Hu Bei Zhong Yi Za Zhi* (Hubei Journal of Chinese Medicine) 1987;(1):15.
21. *Jiang Xi Zhong Yi Yao* (Jiangxi Chinese Medicine and Herbology) 1989;4:36.
22. *Zhong Yi Ming Fang Lin Chuang Xin Yong* (Contemporary Clinical Applications of Classic Chinese Formulas) 2001;646.
23. Wang MZ, et al. *Zhong Yi Xue Wen Da Ti Ku* (Questions and Answers on Traditional Chinese Medicine: Herbal Formulas).

Chinese Herbal Formulas and Applications

Yuè Bì Tāng (Maidservant from Yue Decoction)

越婢湯
越婢汤

Pinyin Name: *Yue Bi Tang*
Literal Name: Maidservant from Yue Decoction
Original Source: *Jin Gui Yao Lue* (Essentials from the Golden Cabinet) by Zhang Zhong-Jing in the Eastern Han Dynasty

COMPOSITION

Ma Huang (Herba Ephedrae)	18g [9g]
Shi Gao (Gypsum Fibrosum)	24g [18g]
Da Zao (Fructus Jujubae)	15 pieces [5 pieces]
Sheng Jiang (Rhizoma Zingiberis Recens)	9g [9g]
Gan Cao (Radix et Rhizoma Glycyrrhizae)	6g [5g]

DOSAGE / PREPARATION / ADMINISTRATION

The source text states to cook *Ma Huang* (Herba Ephedrae) with 6 cups [1,200 mL] of water. Remove the foam from the top, add the other ingredients, and cook until the liquid is reduced to 3 cups [600 mL]. Take the warm decoction in three equally-divided doses. Today, the decoction may be prepared using the doses suggested in brackets.

CHINESE THERAPEUTIC ACTIONS

1. Releases the exterior through diaphoresis
2. Eliminates water accumulation

CLINICAL MANIFESTATIONS

Wind at the exterior with water accumulation: generalized edema, aversion to wind, spontaneous sweating, absence of thirst, and a superficial pulse.

CLINICAL APPLICATIONS

Acute nephritis, edema due to nephritis, beriberi, rheumatoid arthritis, hydrocele, eczema, keratitis, and inguinal tinea.

EXPLANATION

Yue Bi Tang (Maidservant from Yue Decoction) treats wind at the exterior with water accumulation. Because of wind, there is spontaneous sweating, mild fever, aversion to wind, and a superficial pulse. Water accumulation at the exterior causes generalized edema throughout the body.

Ma Huang (Herba Ephedrae) releases the exterior, regulates water circulation, and relieves edema. *Shi Gao* (Gypsum Fibrosum) moderates the warm and acrid properties of *Ma Huang* (Herba Ephedrae). *Da Zao* (Fructus Jujubae) and *Sheng Jiang* (Rhizoma Zingiberis Recens) harmonize

Yue Bi Tang (Maidservant from Yue Decoction)

Diagnosis	Signs and Symptoms	Treatment	Herbs
Wind at the exterior with water accumulation	• Generalized edema: water accumulation at the exterior • Spontaneous sweating, mild fever, and aversion to wind: unresolved exterior wind condition • Superficial pulse: presence of exterior condition	• Releases the exterior through diaphoresis • Eliminates water accumulation	• *Ma Huang* (Herba Ephedrae) releases the exterior, regulates water circulation, and relieves edema. • *Shi Gao* (Gypsum Fibrosum) balances the warm and acrid properties of *Ma Huang* (Herba Ephedrae). • *Da Zao* (Fructus Jujubae) and *Sheng Jiang* (Rhizoma Zingiberis Recens) harmonize the *wei* (defensive) and *ying* (nutritive) levels, and prevent excessive loss of fluids through diaphoresis. • *Sheng Jiang* (Rhizoma Zingiberis Recens) disperses water accumulation from the muscles and exterior. • *Gan Cao* (Radix et Rhizoma Glycyrrhizae) harmonizes the herbs.

EXTERIOR-RELEASING FORMULAS

101

Yuè Bì Tāng (Maidservant from Yue Decoction)

the *wei* (defensive) and *ying* (nutritive) levels, and prevent the excessive loss of fluids through diaphoresis. *Sheng Jiang* (Rhizoma Zingiberis Recens) also helps *Ma Huang* (Herba Ephedrae) to disperse water accumulation from the muscles and exterior. *Gan Cao* (Radix et Rhizoma Glycyrrhizae) harmonizes the formula.

MODIFICATIONS

• If there is dysuria, add *Fu Ling* (Poria) and *Fang Ji* (Radix Stephaniae Tetrandrae).

• For edema throughout the body, add *Yin Chen* (Herba Artemisiae Scopariae) and *Fang Feng* (Radix Saposhnikoviae).

• When there is irritability, thirst and dryness, add *Zhi Mu* (Rhizoma Anemarrhenae) and *Huang Bo* (Cortex Phellodendri Chinensis).

• For cough and reversal of qi, add *Ban Xia* (Rhizoma Pinelliae).

RELATED FORMULA

Yuè Bì Jiā Zhú Tāng

(Maidservant from Yue Decoction plus Atractylodes)

越婢加术湯
越婢加术汤

Pinyin Name: *Yue Bi Jia Zhu Tang*
Literal Name: Maidservant from Yue Decoction plus Atractylodes
Alternate Names: *Yueh Pi Chia Shu Tang*, *Yue Bi Jia Shu Tang*, Spleen-Effusing plus Atractylodes Decoction, Atractylodes Combination
Original Source: *Jin Gui Yao Lue* (Essentials from the Golden Cabinet) by Zhang Zhong-Jing in the Eastern Han Dynasty

Ma Huang (Herba Ephedrae)	18g [9g]
Shi Gao (Gypsum Fibrosum)	24g [18g]
Sheng Jiang (Rhizoma Zingiberis Recens)	9g [9g]
Gan Cao (Radix et Rhizoma Glycyrrhizae)	6g [5g]
Da Zao (Fructus Jujubae)	15 pieces [5 pieces]
Bai Zhu (Rhizoma Atractylodis Macrocephalae)	12g [9g]

Yue Bi Jia Zhu Tang (Maidservant from Yue Decoction plus Atractylodes) treats water accumulation with the following signs and symptoms: generalized swelling and edema, a yellowish skin appearance, and dysuria. This formula releases the exterior and regulates water circulation.

This formula is a direct modification of *Yue Bi Tang*, with the addition of *Bai Zhu* (Rhizoma Atractylodis Macrocephalae), which strengthens the Spleen to regulate water and dry dampness. Overall, *Yue Bi Jia Zhu Tang* has a balanced exterior and interior approach to treating water accumulation, with *Yue Bi Tang* to release the exterior and induce diaphoresis, and *Bai Zhu* (Rhizoma Atractylodis Macrocephalae) to regulate water, dry dampness, and induce diuresis.

AUTHORS' COMMENTS

Ma Huang Xing Ren Gan Cao Shi Gao Tang (Ephedra, Apricot Kernel, Licorice, and Gypsum Decoction) and *Yue Bi Tang* both contain *Ma Huang* (Herba Ephedrae) and *Shi Gao* (Gypsum Fibrosum) to clear and ventilate the Lung.

• *Ma Huang Xing Ren Gan Cao Shi Gao Tang* strongly ventilates the Lung and clears heat to relieve cough, dyspnea, and wheezing.

• *Yue Bi Tang* effectively dispels water retention in the muscle level, because it contains a larger amount of *Ma Huang* (Herba Ephedrae), which, with the help of *Sheng Jiang* (Rhizoma Zingiberis Recens), expels water and reduces edema by inducing perspiration.

Chinese Herbal Formulas and Applications

Shēng Má Gě Gēn Tāng (Cimicifuga and Kudzu Decoction)

升麻葛根湯
升麻葛根汤

Pinyin Name: *Sheng Ma Ge Gen Tang*
Literal Name: Cimicifuga and Kudzu Decoction
Alternate Names: *Sheng Ma Ke Ken Tang*, Cimicifuga and Pueraria Decoction, Cimicifuga and Pueraria Combination
Original Source: *Xiao Er Yao Zheng Zhi Jue* (Craft of Medicinal Treatment for Childhood Disease Patterns) by Qian Yi in 1119

COMPOSITION

Sheng Ma (Rhizoma Cimicifugae)	[3-9g]
Ge Gen (Radix Puerariae Lobatae), *cuo* (grated)	[3-9g]
Chi Shao (Radix Paeoniae Rubra)	[6g]
Zhi Gan Cao (Radix et Rhizoma Glycyrrhizae Praeparata cum Melle), *cuo* (grated)	[3g]

Note: The original source text cites *Shao Yao* (Radix Paeonia), without specifying whether it is *Chi Shao* (Radix Paeoniae Rubra) or *Bai Shao* (Radix Paeoniae Alba). However, most clinicians agree that for purposes of treating measles (a disorder characterized by heat accumulation), *Chi Shao* (Radix Paeoniae Rubra) is a better choice, since it can clear heat and cool the blood. The use of *Bai Shao* (Radix Paeoniae Alba), sour in taste, carries the risk of retaining heat and toxins inside, and is therefore inappropriate under these circumstances.

DOSAGE / PREPARATION / ADMINISTRATION

Grind equal amounts of the ingredients into a fine powder. Cook 12g of the powder in 1.5 bowls of water until it is reduced to 1 bowl. Take the warm, strained decoction at any time during the day. Today, this formula may be prepared as a decoction with the doses suggested in brackets above.

CHINESE THERAPEUTIC ACTIONS

1. Dispels pathogenic factors from the muscle layer
2. Promotes the eruption of measles

CLINICAL MANIFESTATIONS

Measles: early stage of measles before or soon after the initial eruption, fever, and headache.

CLINICAL APPLICATIONS

Measles, influenza, common cold, herpes zoster, scarlet fever, boils, and tonsillitis.

EXPLANATION

Sheng Ma Ge Gen Tang (Cimicifuga and Kudzu Decoction) treats early stage of measles before or soon after the initial eruption. According to the theories of traditional Chinese medicine, measles is a disorder characterized by the presence of epidemic toxins at the exterior and heat accumulation in the Lung and Stomach. Since the Lung opens to the skin and the Spleen [Stomach] controls the

Sheng Ma Ge Gen Tang (Cimicifuga and Kudzu Decoction)

Diagnosis	Signs and Symptoms	Treatment	Herbs
Early stage of measles	• Measles: heat accumulation in the Lung and Stomach affecting the muscle layer • Fever and headache: heat at the exterior	• Dispels pathogenic factors from the muscle layer • Promotes the eruption of measles	• *Sheng Ma* (Rhizoma Cimicifugae) assists the ascension of clear yang, clears heat, and promotes the eruption of measles. • *Ge Gen* (Radix Puerariae Lobatae) relieves exterior heat from the muscle layer, promotes the eruption of measles, and generates body fluids. • *Chi Shao* (Radix Paeoniae Rubra) clears heat and cools the blood. • *Zhi Gan Cao* (Radix et Rhizoma Glycyrrhizae Praeparata cum Melle) harmonizes the herbs.

EXTERIOR-RELEASING FORMULAS

103

Chapter 1 – Exterior-Releasing Formulas　　　　　*Section 2 – Acrid and Cold Exterior-Releasing Formulas*

Shēng Má Gě Gēn Tāng (Cimicifuga and Kudzu Decoction)

muscles, the initial stage of measles involves faint marks underneath the skin in the muscles. The treatment strategy is to promote eruption and push the heat and toxins outward. For this reason, this formula uses herbs to relieve the exterior factors from the muscles, promote the eruption of measles, and clear heat and toxins.

Sheng Ma (Rhizoma Cimicifugae) assists the ascension of clear yang, clears heat, and promotes the eruption of measles. *Ge Gen* (Radix Puerariae Lobatae), the deputy herb, relieves exterior heat from the muscle layer, promotes the eruption of measles, and generates body fluids. *Chi Shao* (Radix Paeoniae Rubra) clears heat and cools the blood. *Zhi Gan Cao* (Radix et Rhizoma Glycyrrhizae Praeparata cum Melle) harmonizes the herbs and helps relieve aches and pains.

MODIFICATIONS

- For early stage of measles, add *Bo He* (Herba Menthae), *Jing Jie* (Herba Schizonepetae), *Chan Tui* (Periostracum Cicadae), *Niu Bang Zi* (Fructus Arctii), *Jin Yin Hua* (Flos Lonicerae Japonicae), and *Lian Qiao* (Fructus Forsythiae).
- For incomplete eruption of measles that are dark red in color, add *Xuan Shen* (Radix Scrophulariae), *Mu Dan Pi* (Cortex Moutan), *Zi Cao* (Radix Arnebiae), and *Da Qing Ye* (Folium Isatidis).
- If there is severe headache, add *Chuan Xiong* (Rhizoma Chuanxiong) and *Bai Zhi* (Radix Angelicae Dahuricae).
- For stiffness and pain of the back, add *Fang Feng* (Radix Saposhnikoviae) and *Qiang Huo* (Rhizoma et Radix Notopterygii).
- When there is persistent fever, add *Chai Hu* (Radix Bupleuri), *Huang Qin* (Radix Scutellariae), and *Fang Feng* (Radix Saposhnikoviae).
- If accompanied by severe itching, add *Chan Tui* (Periostracum Cicadae) and *Fang Feng* (Radix Saposhnikoviae).
- For sore and swollen throat, add *Huang Qin* (Radix Scutellariae) and *Jie Geng* (Radix Platycodonis).
- With thirst and irritability, add *Zhu Ye* (Herba Phyllostachys) and *Lu Gen* (Rhizoma Phragmitis).

CAUTIONS / CONTRAINDICATIONS

Sheng Ma Ge Gen Tang has tendencies to move outward and upward, and is contraindicated in the following situations: if the measles are fully erupted; or if the measles have already erupted and the heat has invaded a deeper level, manifesting in symptoms of accelerated respiration, dyspnea, and cough.

CLINICAL STUDIES AND RESEARCH

1. **Herpes zoster**: Twenty patients with herpes zoster were treated with satisfactory results using *Sheng Ma Ge Gen Tang* plus *Zi Cao* (Radix Arnebiae). Symptoms that

showed clinical improvement included itching, pain, fever, aversion to cold, and disturbed sleep.[1]

2. **Measles**: One study reported that use of *Sheng Ma Ge Gen Tang* for 8 days was associated with a marked inhibitory effect on measles virus. In addition, *Sheng Ma Ge Gen Tang* has a selective stimulation to the secretion of cytokine TNF-alpha.[2]

RELATED FORMULAS

Shēng Má Gě Gēn Tāng

(Cimicifuga and Kudzu Decoction)

升麻葛根湯
升麻葛根汤

Pinyin Name: *Sheng Ma Ge Gen Tang*
Literal Name: Cimicifuga and Kudzu Decoction
Original Source: *Yi Fang Ji Jie* (Analytical Collection of Medical Formulas) by Wang Ang in 1682

Sheng Ma (Rhizoma Cimicifugae)	[4.5-13.5g]
Ge Gen (Radix Puerariae Lobatae)	[3-9g]
Bai Shao (Radix Paeoniae Alba)	[3-9g]
Gan Cao (Radix et Rhizoma Glycyrrhizae)	[1.5-4.5g]
Sheng Jiang (Rhizoma Zingiberis Recens)	[1.5-4.5g]

This formula is designed to dispel wind, release the exterior, eliminate toxins, and promote the eruption of measles. It is generally used to treat early stage of measles before or soon after the initial eruption, with clinical manifestations of headache, dry nose, painful eyes, restless sleep, thirst, absence of perspiration, fever, and aversion to cold.

These two formulas have identical names, and very similar composition and functions.

- *Sheng Ma Ge Gen Tang* from *Xiao Er Yao Zheng Zhi Jue* (Craft of Medicinal Treatment for Childhood Disease Patterns) is a slightly cooler formula, as *Chi Shao* (Radix Paeoniae Rubra) is usually used to clear heat and cool blood.
- *Sheng Ma Ge Gen Tang* from *Yi Fang Ji Jie* (Analytical Collection of Medical Formulas) is a slightly warmer formula. It utilizes *Bai Shao* (Radix Paeoniae Alba) to harmonize *ying* (nutritive) level and *Sheng Jiang* (Rhizoma Zingiberis Recens) to release the exterior and balance the astringent effect of *Bai Shao* (Radix Paeoniae Alba).

Xuān Dú Fā Biǎo Tāng

(Dissipate Toxins and Release the Exterior Decoction)

宣毒發表湯
宣毒发表汤

Pinyin Name: *Xuan Du Fa Biao Tang*
Literal Name: Dissipate Toxins and Release the Exterior Decoction

104

Chinese Herbal Formulas and Applications

Shēng Má Gě Gēn Tāng (Cimicifuga and Kudzu Decoction)

Original Source: *Yi Zong Jin Jian* (Golden Mirror of the Medical Tradition) by Wu Qian in 1742

Sheng Ma (Rhizoma Cimicifugae)	[3g]
Ge Gen (Radix Puerariae Lobatae)	[3g]
Qian Hu (Radix Peucedani)	[5g]
Ku Xing Ren (Semen Armeniacae Amarum)	[6g]
Jie Geng (Radix Platycodonis)	[3g]
Zhi Qiao (Fructus Aurantii)	[3g]
Jing Jie (Herba Schizonepetae)	[3g]
Fang Feng (Radix Saposhnikoviae)	[3g]
Bo He (Herba Menthae)	[3g]
Mu Tong (Caulis Akebiae)	[3g]
Lian Qiao (Fructus Forsythiae)	[5g]
Niu Bang Zi (Fructus Arctii), *chao* (dry-fried)	[5g]
Dan Zhu Ye (Herba Lophatheri)	[2g]
Gan Cao (Radix et Rhizoma Glycyrrhizae)	[2g]

The source text states to prepare the ingredients as a decoction. Note: Doses of herbs are unavailable from the source text. Suggested doses are listed above in brackets.

Xuan Du Fa Biao Tang (Dissipate Toxins and Release the Exterior Decoction) is used at the beginning stage of measles to promote eruption; it releases the exterior, promotes the eruption of measles, stops coughing, and benefits the throat. *Sheng Ma* (Rhizoma Cimicifugae) and *Ge Gen* (Radix Puerariae Lobatae) clear heat and promote the eruption of measles. *Jing Jie* (Herba Schizonepetae), *Fang Feng* (Radix Saposhnikoviae), *Niu Bang Zi* (Fructus Arctii) and *Bo He* (Herba Menthae) clear heat and release exterior factors from the muscle layer. *Zhi Qiao* (Fructus Aurantii), *Jie Geng* (Radix Platycodonis), *Ku Xing Ren* (Semen Armeniacae Amarum) and *Qian Hu* (Radix Peucedani) regulate Lung qi, dispel phlegm, and stop cough. *Lian Qiao* (Fructus Forsythiae) clears heat and

eliminates toxins from the upper *jiao*; *Mu Tong* (Caulis Akebiae) drains heat downward; while *Dan Zhu Ye* (Herba Lophatheri) clears heat and relieves irritability. *Gan Cao* (Radix et Rhizoma Glycyrrhizae) eliminates toxins and harmonizes the herbs.

In comparison to *Sheng Ma Ge Gen Tang*, *Xuan Du Fa Biao Tang* more strongly vents the Lung, releases the exterior, clears heat, and eliminates toxins. Thus, *Xuan Du Fa Biao Tang* is used for individuals with early stage of measles with symptoms such as fever, no perspiration, cough, sore throat, irritability, thirst and dysuria.

AUTHORS' COMMENTS

Sheng Ma Ge Gen Tang is best for initial stages of measles with incomplete eruption, or absence of eruption due to heat trapped in the Lung and Stomach. This formula was originally used to treat smallpox. Today, however, its application has been extended to a wide variety of skin disorders, including measles, chickenpox, herpes simplex, and rashes.

To maximize the treatment results for skin disorders (e.g., measles, chickenpox, herpes simplex, and rashes), it is best to use herbs internally and topically. Internally, *Sheng Ma Ge Gen Tang* is given in decoction. Topically, *Xi He Liu* (Cacumen Tamaricis) or *Fu Ping* (Herba Spirodelae) is often used as a bath soak; alternatively, the decoction may be applied directly to the skin to help open the pores and induce the toxins to move outward.

References

1. *Xin Zhong Yi* (New Chinese Medicine) 1977;51.
2. Huang SP, Shieh GJ, Lee L, Teng HJ, Kao ST, Lin JG. Inhibition effect of shengma-gegen-tang on measles virus in Vero cells and human peripheral blood mononuclear cells. American Journal of Chinese Medicine 1997;25(1):89-96.

Chapter 1 – Exterior-Releasing Formulas　　　　　　　*Section 2 – Acrid and Cold Exterior-Releasing Formulas*

Zhú Yè Liǔ Báng Tāng
(Lophatherum, Tamarisk, and Arctium Decoction)

竹葉柳蒡湯
竹叶柳蒡汤

Pinyin Name: *Zhu Ye Liu Bang Tang*
Literal Name: Lophatherum, Tamarisk, and Arctium Decoction
Original Source: *Xian Xing Zhai Yi Xue Guang Bi Ji* (Wide-Ranging Medical Notes from the First-Awakened Studio) by Miao Xi-Yong in 1613

COMPOSITION

Xi He Liu (Cacumen Tamaricis)	15g [6g]
Niu Bang Zi (Fructus Arctii), *chao* (dry-fried)	4.5g
Jing Jie Sui (Spica Schizonepetae)	3g [4g]
Ge Gen (Radix Puerariae Lobatae)	4.5g
Zhi Mu (Rhizoma Anemarrhenae), *mi zhi* (fried with honey)	3g
Xuan Shen (Radix Scrophulariae)	6g
Mai Dong (Radix Ophiopogonis)	9g
Dan Zhu Ye (Herba Lophatheri)	30 leaves [1.5g]
Bo He (Herba Menthae)	3g
Chan Tui (Periostracum Cicadae)	3g
Gan Cao (Radix et Rhizoma Glycyrrhizae)	3g

DOSAGE / PREPARATION / ADMINISTRATION

The source text instructs to prepare the ingredients as a decoction. Today, the decoction may be prepared using the doses suggested in brackets.

CHINESE THERAPEUTIC ACTIONS

1. Releases the exterior and promotes the eruption of measles
2. Clears and sedates the Lung and Stomach

CLINICAL MANIFESTATIONS

Measles that fail to erupt: cough, irritability, a feeling of oppression, restlessness, soreness and pain of the throat.

CLINICAL APPLICATIONS

Measles.

EXPLANATION

Zhu Ye Liu Bang Tang (Lophatherum, Tamarisk and Arctium Decoction) treats conditions in which the measles fail to erupt, and are complicated by wind-cold at the exterior and heat in the interior. Because the wind-cold factor constricts the exterior, the measles cannot erupt. Moreover, interior Lung and Stomach heat cannot be released because the exterior is constricted, producing symptoms of high fever, absence of perspiration, cough, restlessness, a feeling of oppression, and soreness and pain of the throat.

The treatment plan is to release wind-cold from the exterior, clear interior heat, and promote the eruption of measles. *Xi He Liu* (Cacumen Tamaricis), the chief herb, promotes the eruption of measles. *Niu Bang Zi* (Fructus Arctii) dispels wind-heat and eliminates toxins. *Jing Jie Sui* (Spica Schizonepetae) and *Ge Gen* (Radix Puerariae Lobatae) release the exterior to facilitate the eruption of measles. *Zhi Mu* (Rhizoma Anemarrhenae) and *Xuan Shen* (Radix Scrophulariae) clear heat and promote generation of fluids. *Dan Zhu Ye* (Herba Lophatheri) clears heat from the upper *jiao* to relieve irritability and restlessness. *Bo He* (Herba Menthae) dispels wind-heat. *Chan Tui* (Periostracum Cicadae) drains Lung heat. *Mai Dong* (Radix Ophiopogonis) clears heat and promotes generation of fluids. *Gan Cao* (Radix et Rhizoma Glycyrrhizae) harmonizes the formula.

MODIFICATIONS

- If there is more heat in the interior, add *Shi Gao* (Gypsum Fibrosum) and *Geng Mi* (Semen Oryzae).
- When there is severe itching, add *Fang Feng* (Radix Saposhnikoviae) and increase the dose of *Chan Tui* (Periostracum Cicadae).

CAUTIONS / CONTRAINDICATIONS

Zhu Ye Liu Bang Tang has potent effects to release wind from the exterior and sedate heat in the interior. It should not be used for an extended period of time or at a large dose. Furthermore, it should be discontinued once the desired effects have been achieved.

106

Zhú Yè Liǔ Báng Tāng
(Lophatherum, Tamarisk, and Arctium Decoction)

Zhu Ye Liu Bang Tang (Lophatherum, Tamarisk and Arctium Decoction)

Diagnosis	Signs and Symptoms	Treatment	Herbs
Measles that fail to erupt	• Measles: exterior condition affecting the muscle layer • Irritability, restlessness, and a feeling of oppression: Lung and Stomach heat • Cough: heat affecting Lung qi circulation • Soreness and pain of the throat: heat and fire rising upward	• Releases the exterior • Promotes the eruption of measles • Clears and sedates Lung and Stomach heat	• *Xi He Liu* (Cacumen Tamaricis) promotes the eruption of measles. • *Niu Bang Zi* (Fructus Arctii) dispels wind-heat and eliminates toxins. • *Jing Jie Sui* (Spica Schizonepetae) and *Ge Gen* (Radix Puerariae Lobatae) release the exterior to facilitate the eruption of measles. • *Zhi Mu* (Rhizoma Anemarrhenae), *Xuan Shen* (Radix Scrophulariae), and *Mai Dong* (Radix Ophiopogonis) clear heat and promote generation of fluids. • *Dan Zhu Ye* (Herba Lophatheri) clears heat to relieve irritability and restlessness. • *Bo He* (Herba Menthae) dispels wind-heat. • *Chan Tui* (Periostracum Cicadae) drains Lung heat. • *Gan Cao* (Radix et Rhizoma Glycyrrhizae) harmonizes the formula.

Chái Gě Jiě Jī Tāng
(Bupleurum and Kudzu Decoction to Release the Muscle Layer)

柴葛解肌湯
柴葛解肌汤

Pinyin Name: *Chai Ge Jie Ji Tang*
Literal Name: Bupleurum and Kudzu Decoction to Release the Muscle Layer
Alternate Names: *Tsai Ko Chieh Chi Tang*, *Tao's Chai Ge Jie Ji Tang*, Bupleurum and Pueraria Decoction for Relieving Muscles, Tao's Bupleurum and Kudzu Decoction to Release the Muscle Layer, Bupleurum and Pueraria Combination
Original Source: *Shang Han Liu Shu* (Six Texts on Cold-Induced Disorders) by Tao Hua in 1445

COMPOSITION

Chai Hu (Radix Bupleuri)	[6g]
Ge Gen (Radix Puerariae Lobatae)	[9g]
Qiang Huo (Rhizoma et Radix Notopterygii)	[3g]
Bai Zhi (Radix Angelicae Dahuricae)	[3g]
Huang Qin (Radix Scutellariae)	[6g]
Jie Geng (Radix Platycodonis)	[3g]
Bai Shao (Radix Paeoniae Alba)	[6g]
Gan Cao (Radix et Rhizoma Glycyrrhizae)	[3g]

DOSAGE / PREPARATION / ADMINISTRATION

The source states to cook the herbs with 3 slices of *Sheng* *Jiang* (Rhizoma Zingiberis Recens), 2 pieces of *Da Zao* (Fructus Jujubae), and 3g [5g] of *Shi Gao* (Gypsum

Chái Gĕ Jiĕ Jī Tāng
(Bupleurum and Kudzu Decoction to Release the Muscle Layer)

Fibrosum) in 2 large bowls of water. Note: The herb doses are unavailable from the source text. Suggested doses are listed above in brackets.

CHINESE THERAPEUTIC ACTIONS

Clears heat and releases the muscles

CLINICAL MANIFESTATIONS

Wind-cold syndrome turning into heat: gradual decrease of aversion to cold with gradual increase of fever, headache, absence of perspiration, painful eyes and eye sockets, dry nose and throat, irritability, insomnia, a thin, yellow tongue coating, and a superficial and slightly surging pulse.

CLINICAL APPLICATIONS

Common cold and influenza, epidemic viral infection, upper respiratory tract infection, fever, high fever, tonsillitis, toothache, and trigeminal neuralgia.

EXPLANATION

Chai Ge Jie Ji Tang (Bupleurum and Kudzu Decoction to Release the Muscle Layer) treats the gradual transformation of *taiyang* wind-cold syndrome into *yangming* heat. Patients with the clinical manifestations described above generally start out with a wind-cold syndrome that, instead of being released, transforms into heat and moves into the interior. Since the *taiyang* syndrome is not resolved, symptoms such as headache, aversion to cold, absence of perspiration, and a superficial pulse remain. However, since heat is starting to form in the interior, patients may show irritability, insomnia, and a slightly surging pulse, which are all symptoms of *yangming* syndrome. Other

pathological symptoms of the Stomach and Large Intestine channels will manifest, including dry nose and throat, and painful eyes and eye sockets. The thin, yellow tongue coating suggests that the disease factor is transforming into heat.

The treatment approach is to release the muscles, and address *taiyang* and *yangming* syndromes concurrently. *Chai Hu* (Radix Bupleuri) and *Ge Gen* (Radix Puerariae Lobatae), the two chief herbs, dispel heat in the muscle layer and relieve various exterior symptoms. *Qiang Huo* (Rhizoma et Radix Notopterygii) enters the *taiyang* channel and *Bai Zhi* (Radix Angelicae Dahuricae) enters the *yangming* channel. Together, they dispel wind-cold, release the muscles, and relieve headache. *Huang Qin* (Radix Scutellariae) and *Shi Gao* (Gypsum Fibrosum) clear interior heat. *Jie Geng* (Radix Platycodonis) ventilates the Lung to dispel exterior factors. *Bai Shao* (Radix Paeoniae Alba) and *Gan Cao* (Radix et Rhizoma Glycyrrhizae) harmonize the *ying* (nutritive) level and prevent the drying herbs from damaging yin. *Sheng Jiang* (Rhizoma Zingiberis Recens) and *Da Zao* (Fructus Jujubae) harmonize the *ying* (nutritive) and *wei* (defensive) levels, as well as the exterior and interior. Since *Qiang Huo* (Rhizoma et Radix Notopterygii) enters the *taiyang* channel and *Ge Gen* (Radix Puerariae Lobatae) enters the *yangming* channel, there is no need to select additional guiding herbs.

Since this formula was developed by Dr. Tao, it is also referred to as *Tao's Chai Ge Jie Ji Tang* (Tao's Bupleurum

Chai Ge Jie Ji Tang (Bupleurum and Kudzu Decoction to Release the Muscle Layer)

Diagnosis	Signs and Symptoms	Treatment	Herbs
Wind-cold syndrome turning into heat	• Gradual decrease of aversion to cold and increase of fever: transformation of wind-cold into heat • Superficial and slightly surging pulse: presence of wind-cold and heat • Dry nose and throat, painful eyes and eye sockets, and irritability and insomnia: *yangming* interior heat	• Clears heat • Releases the muscle layer	• *Chai Hu* (Radix Bupleuri) and *Ge Gen* (Radix Puerariae Lobatae) dispel heat in the muscle layer. • *Qiang Huo* (Rhizoma et Radix Notopterygii) and *Bai Zhi* (Radix Angelicae Dahuricae) release exterior wind-cold. • *Huang Qin* (Radix Scutellariae) and *Shi Gao* (Gypsum Fibrosum) clear interior heat. • *Jie Geng* (Radix Platycodonis) ventilates the Lung. • *Bai Shao* (Radix Paeoniae Alba) and *Gan Cao* (Radix et Rhizoma Glycyrrhizae) harmonize the *ying* (nutritive) level and prevent the drying herbs from damaging yin. • *Sheng Jiang* (Rhizoma Zingiberis Recens) and *Da Zao* (Fructus Jujubae) harmonize the exterior and interior.

Chinese Herbal Formulas and Applications

Chái Gě Jiě Jī Tāng
(Bupleurum and Kudzu Decoction to Release the Muscle Layer)

and Kudzu Decoction to Release the Muscle Layer) to avoid confusion with *Cheng's Chai Ge Jie Ji Tang* (Cheng's Bupleurum and Kudzu Decoction to Release the Muscle Layer), discussed below in the Related Formula section.

MODIFICATIONS
- For headache caused by wind-cold, add *Fang Feng* (Radix Saposhnikoviae) and *Chuan Xiong* (Rhizoma Chuanxiong).
- If there is cough accompanied by sticky sputum, add *Gua Lou Zi* (Semen Trichosanthis) and *Chuan Bei Mu* (Bulbus Fritillariae Cirrhosae).
- With thirst, dry mouth and throat caused by heat drying body fluids, add *Zhi Mu* (Rhizoma Anemarrhenae) and *Tian Hua Fen* (Radix Trichosanthis).
- For vomiting and excessive amount of saliva and sputum, add *Ban Xia* (Rhizoma Pinelliae) and *Fu Ling* (Poria).

CAUTIONS / CONTRAINDICATIONS
- *Chai Ge Jie Ji Tang* is not suitable if the exterior cold has not moved into the deeper levels, and there is no interior heat. If this formula is used while the wind-cold factor is still at the superficial *taiyang* level, the disease will be encouraged to move into the deeper level and give rise to complications and deterioration.
- Do not use this formula if the heat has already attacked the *yangming* organs, producing symptoms such as abdominal pain and constipation.
- Avoid acrid, spicy, oily or greasy foods while taking this formula.[1]

CLINICAL STUDIES AND RESEARCH
1. **Epidemic viral infection**: Patients with epidemic viral infection were evaluated and treated with modified *Chai Ge Jie Ji Tang* with good results. Out of 393 patients, 240 had fever between 38-38.9°C / 100.4-102°F, 153 had fever between 39-40.5°C / 102.2-104.9°F; 188 were diagnosed as wind-cold, and 120 were diagnosed as wind-heat. The study reported that 48 hours after the treatment the temperature returned to normal in 378 cases (90%), with 95.2% effectiveness in the wind-cold group and 95.1% in the wind-heat group.[2]
2. **Upper respiratory tract infection**: In one study, 109 patients with upper respiratory tract infection were treated with *Chai Ge Jie Ji Tang* for 1-6 packs of herbs with complete recovery in all cases.[3]
3. **Fever**: Use of modified *Chai Ge Jie Ji Tang* in decoction was associated with 99.3% effectiveness in reducing body temperature in 874 infants and children (383 males and 491 females), all under 10 years of age, with fever of 38-40°C / 100.4-104°F and higher. The herbal treatment contained *Chai Hu* (Radix Bupleuri), *Ge Gen* (Radix Puerariae Lobatae), *Huang Qin* (Radix Scutellariae), *Qiang Huo* (Rhizoma et Radix Notopterygii), *Bai Zhi* (Radix Angelicae Dahuricae), *Bai Shao* (Radix Paeoniae Alba), *Jie Geng* (Radix Platycodonis), *Di Gu Pi* (Cortex Lycii), *Shi Gao* (Gypsum Fibrosum), and *Gan Cao* (Radix et Rhizoma Glycyrrhizae). *Gua Lou Pi* (Pericarpium Trichosanthis) and *Sang Bai Pi* (Cortex Mori) were added for cough; *Shan Dou Gen* (Radix et Rhizoma Sophorae Tonkinensis) and *Ban Lan Gen* (Radix Isatidis) for sore throat; *Bing Lang* (Semen Arecae) and *Ji Nei Jin* (Endothelium Corneum Gigeriae Galli) for food stagnation; *Huang Lian* (Rhizoma Coptidis) and *Che Qian Zi* (Semen Plantaginis) for diarrhea; and *Da Huang* (Radix et Rhizoma Rhei) and *Ku Xing Ren* (Semen Armeniacae Amarum) for dry stools. Of 874 patients, the study reported normalization of body temperature within one day in 492 patients, within 2 days in 277 patients, within 3 days in 99 patients, and no benefit in 6 patients.[4]
4. **High fever**: One hundred and ten patients with high fever were successfully treated with modified *Chai Ge Jie Ji Tang*. The herbal formula contained *Chai Hu* (Radix Bupleuri) 18g, *Ge Gen* (Radix Puerariae Lobatae) 20g, *Huang Qin* (Radix Scutellariae) 12g, *Qiang Huo* (Rhizoma et Radix Notopterygii) 10g, *Bai Zhi* (Radix Angelicae Dahuricae) 10g, *Jie Geng* (Radix Platycodonis) 10g, *Shi Gao* (Gypsum Fibrosum) 30g, *Bai Shao* (Radix Paeoniae Alba) 10g, *Gan Cao* (Radix et Rhizoma Glycyrrhizae) 3g, *Sheng Jiang* (Rhizoma Zingiberis Recens) 3 slices, and *Da Zao* (Fructus Jujubae) 2 pieces. The treatment protocol was to cook the herbs in 900 mL of water for 20 minutes to yield 500 mL of decoction, which was administered in three equally-divided doses within half a day. This entire process may be repeated up to three times (3 packs of herbs) per day if needed to induce perspiration and normalization of body temperature. Patients were instructed to avoid cold, raw, oily or greasy foods. Of 110 patients, the study reported normalization of body temperature in 37 patients after 1-2 packs of herbs, in 52 patients after 2-4 packs of herbs, and in 21 patients after 4-6 packs of herbs.[5]
5. **Tonsillitis**: Use of modified *Chai Ge Jie Ji Tang* to treat 48 patients with acute suppurative tonsillitis was associated with 95.8% effectiveness. The herbal treatment contained *Chai Hu* (Radix Bupleuri) 10g, *Bai Zhi* (Radix Angelicae Dahuricae) 10g, *Qiang Huo* (Rhizoma et Radix Notopterygii) 10g, *Huang Qin* (Radix Scutellariae) 10g, *Long Kui* (Herba Solanum Nigrum) 10g, *Bo He* (Herba Menthae) 10g (post-decocted), *Jie Geng* (Radix Platycodonis) 10g, *Ge Gen* (Radix Puerariae Lobatae) 15g, *He Ye* (Folium Nelumbinis) 15g, *Shi Gao* (Gypsum Fibrosum) 60g (pre-decocted), *Ma Bo* (Lasiosphaera seu Calvatia) 6g, and *Gan Cao* (Radix et Rhizoma Glycyrrhizae) 6g. The herbs

Chái Gě Jiě Jī Tāng
(Bupleurum and Kudzu Decoction to Release the Muscle Layer)

were given in decoction one time daily, for 3 packs of herbs per course of treatment. Of 48 cases, the study reported complete recovery in 17 cases, significant improvement in 29 cases, and no effect in 2 cases.[6]

RELATED FORMULA

Chái Gě Jiě Jī Tāng (Bupleurum and Kudzu Decoction to Release the Muscle Layer)

柴葛解肌湯
柴葛解肌汤

Pinyin Name: *Chai Ge Jie Ji Tang*
Literal Name: Bupleurum and Kudzu Decoction to Release the Muscle Layer
Alternate Name: *Cheng's Chai Ge Jie Ji Tang* (Cheng's Bupleurum and Kudzu Decoction to Release the Muscle Layer)
Original Source: *Yi Xue Xin Wu* (Medical Revelations) by Cheng Guo-Peng in 1732

Chai Hu (Radix Bupleuri)	3.6g [6g]
Ge Gen (Radix Puerariae Lobatae)	4.5g [9g]
Gan Cao (Radix et Rhizoma Glycyrrhizae)	1.5g [3g]
Chi Shao (Radix Paeoniae Rubra)	3g [6g]
Huang Qin (Radix Scutellariae)	4.5g [6g]
Zhi Mu (Rhizoma Anemarrhenae)	3g [5g]
Di Huang (Radix Rehmanniae)	6g [9g]
Mu Dan Pi (Cortex Moutan)	4.5g [3g]
Bei Mu (Bulbus Fritillariae)	3g [6g]

Note: The original source text cites *Shao Yao* (Radix Paeonia), without specifying whether it is *Chi Shao* (Radix Paeoniae Rubra) or *Bai Shao* (Radix Paeoniae Alba). However, most clinicians agree that *Chi Shao* (Radix Paeoniae Rubra) is more appropriate in this formula than *Bai Shao* (Radix Paeoniae Alba), since *Chi Shao* (Radix Paeoniae Rubra) can clear heat and cool the blood. The use of *Bai Shao* (Radix Paeoniae Alba), sour in taste, carries the risk of retaining heat and toxins inside, and is therefore inappropriate under these circumstances.

The source text states to prepare the ingredients as a decoction; and add 10 leaves of *Dan Zhu Ye* (Herba Lophatheri) for patients who exhibit irritability, and 9-18g of *Shi Gao* (Gypsum Fibrosum) for patients with incoherent speech. Today, this formula may be prepared as a decoction with the doses suggested in brackets above.

This formula treats exterior wind-cold that has turned into heat in the muscle layer and the interior. This syndrome is seen mostly in late spring and early summer when the weather starts to warm up. Clinically, patients may show fever, thirst, headache, and no aversion to cold.

Optimal treatment requires the use of herbs to release the exterior and clear the interior concurrently. *Chai Hu* (Radix Bupleuri) and *Ge Gen* (Radix Puerariae Lobatae) release the exterior and clear heat from the muscles. *Zhi Mu* (Rhizoma Anemarrhenae), *Huang Qin* (Radix Scutellariae), and *Bei Mu* (Bulbus Fritillariae) clear heat from the *qi* (energy) level. *Mu Dan Pi* (Cortex Moutan), *Di Huang* (Radix Rehmanniae), and *Chi Shao* (Radix Paeoniae Rubra) clear heat from the *xue* (blood) level. *Gan Cao* (Radix et Rhizoma Glycyrrhizae) harmonizes the formula.

These two formulas have identical names, but they are derived from different sources and have slightly different compositions and applications. Their differences are as follows:

- *Chai Ge Jie Ji Tang* from *Shang Han Liu Shu* (Six Texts on Cold-Induced Disorders) by Tao Hua has a focus on relieving the muscles. It has more exterior-releasing and muscle-relieving herbs than heat-clearing herbs.
- *Chai Ge Jie Ji Tang* from *Yi Xue Xin Wu* (Medical Revelations) by Cheng Guo-Peng emphasizes heat-clearing, rather than exterior-releasing or muscle-relieving actions. Thirst, rather than aversion to cold or aversion to wind, is the prominent symptom.

AUTHORS' COMMENTS

Chai Ge Jie Ji Tang from *Shang Han Liu Shu* (Six Texts on Cold-Induced Disorders) is the representative formula for treating lingering wind-cold that has moved to the interior, causing heat and affecting both *taiyang* and *yangming*. With more severe interior heat and less exterior cold, patients will show key symptoms of high fever with less aversion to cold, headache, body aches, orbital pain, dry nose, and a superficial and slightly surging pulse.

Gui Zhi Tang (Cinnamon Twig Decoction) and *Chai Ge Jie Ji Tang* are two representative formulas to relieve muscle aches and pains associated with external pathogenic invasion.

- *Gui Zhi Tang* is indicated for pain caused by wind-cold invasion.
- *Chai Ge Jie Ji Tang* is indicated for wind-cold invasion turning into heat that accumulates in the *yangming* channel.

References
1. *Zhong Yao Ming Fang Yao Li Yu Ying Yong* (Pharmacology and Applications of Famous Herbal Formulas) 1989;63-64.

Chái Gě Jiě Jī Tāng
(Bupleurum and Kudzu Decoction to Release the Muscle Layer)

2. *Hu Bei Zhong Yi Za Zhi* (Hubei Journal of Chinese Medicine) 1984;(3):34.

3. *He Nan Zhong Yi* (Henan Chinese Medicine) 1982;(4):37.

4. *Zhe Jiang Zhong Yi Za Zhi* (Zhejiang Journal of Chinese Medicine) 1990;5:206.

5. *Shi Yong Zhong Yi Nei Ke Za Zhi* (Journal of Practical Chinese Internal Medicine) 1997;1:24.

6. *Fu Jian Zhong Yi Yao* (Fujian Chinese Medicine and Herbology) 1999;4(3).

Cōng Chǐ Jié Gěng Tāng
(Scallion, Prepared Soybean, and Platycodon Decoction)

蔥鼓桔梗湯
葱鼓桔梗汤

Pinyin Name: *Cong Chi Jie Geng Tang*
Literal Name: Scallion, Prepared Soybean, and Platycodon Decoction
Original Source: *Tong Su Shang Han Lun* (Plain Version of Discussion of Cold-Induced Disorders) by Yu Gen-Chu in the Qing Dynasty

COMPOSITION

Cong Bai (Bulbus Allii Fistulosi), fresh	3-5 stalks
Dan Dou Chi (Semen Sojae Praeparatum)	9-15g
Bo He (Herba Menthae)	3-4.5g
Jie Geng (Radix Platycodonis)	3-4.5g
Lian Qiao (Fructus Forsythiae)	4.5-6g
Zhi Zi (Fructus Gardeniae), *chao jiao* (dry-fried to burnt)	6-9g
Dan Zhu Ye (Herba Lophatheri), fresh	30 leaves [3g]
Gan Cao (Radix et Rhizoma Glycyrrhizae)	1.8-2.4g

DOSAGE / PREPARATION / ADMINISTRATION
Prepare the ingredients as a decoction.

CHINESE THERAPEUTIC ACTIONS
1. Dispels wind and releases the exterior
2. Clears the Lung and purges heat

CLINICAL MANIFESTATIONS
Early stage of wind-warmth syndrome: headache, fever, aversion to cold, slight aversion to wind, coughing, sore throat, thirst, a red tongue tip with a thin, white tongue coating, and a superficial, rapid pulse.

CLINICAL APPLICATIONS
Common cold and influenza.

EXPLANATION
Cong Chi Jie Geng Tang (Scallion, Prepared Soybean, and Platycodon Decoction) is designed to treat the early stage of wind-warmth syndrome. Headache, fever, aversion to cold, and slight aversion to wind are the results of wind-warmth invading the exterior. Coughing, thirst, and sore throat are the results of wind-warmth affecting the Lung functioning.

Cong Bai (Bulbus Allii Fistulosi) activates yang and qi circulation. It is combined with *Dan Dou Chi* (Semen Sojae Praeparatum) to induce diaphoresis and release exterior symptoms. *Bo He* (Herba Menthae) dispels the exterior wind-warmth factor. *Jie Geng* (Radix Platycodonis) ventilates the Lung to regulate Lung qi. *Lian Qiao* (Fructus Forsythiae) clears heat in the upper *jiao*. *Zhi Zi* (Fructus Gardeniae) clears Lung and Heart heat. *Gan Cao* (Radix et Rhizoma Glycyrrhizae) and *Jie Geng* (Radix Platycodonis) soothe the throat and relieve throat pain. *Dan Zhu Ye* (Herba Lophatheri) clears heat.

Chapter 1 – Exterior-Releasing Formulas   *Section 2 – Acrid and Cold Exterior-Releasing Formulas*

Cōng Chǐ Jié Gěng Tāng
(Scallion, Prepared Soybean, and Platycodon Decoction)

Cong Chi Jie Geng Tang (Scallion, Prepared Soybean, and Platycodon Decoction)

Diagnosis	Signs and Symptoms	Treatment	Herbs
Early stage of wind-warmth syndrome	• Headache, fever, and slight aversion to cold: wind-warmth at the exterior • Coughing, thirst, and sore throat: wind-warmth damaging the Lung • Red tongue tip with thin, white tongue coat: exterior wind-warmth • Superficial, rapid pulse: exterior wind-warmth	• Dispels wind and releases the exterior • Clears the Lung and purges heat	• *Cong Bai* (Bulbus Allii Fistulosi) activates yang and qi circulation. • *Dan Dou Chi* (Semen Sojae Praeparatum) induces diaphoresis and releases exterior symptoms. • *Bo He* (Herba Menthae) dispels exterior wind-warmth. • *Jie Geng* (Radix Platycodonis) ventilates the Lung to regulate Lung qi. • *Lian Qiao* (Fructus Forsythiae), *Zhi Zi* (Fructus Gardeniae), and *Dan Zhu Ye* (Herba Lophatheri) clear heat from various parts of the body. • *Gan Cao* (Radix et Rhizoma Glycyrrhizae) and *Jie Geng* (Radix Platycodonis) soothe the throat and relieve throat pain.

MODIFICATIONS
• For more severe soreness and pain of the throat, add *Da Qing Ye* (Folium Isatidis).
• With cough and profuse sputum, add *Ku Xing Ren* (Semen Armeniacae Amarum) and *Ju Hong* (Exocarpium Citri Reticulatae).
• If there is a feeling of chest oppression, remove *Gan Cao* (Radix et Rhizoma Glycyrrhizae), and add *Zhi Qiao* (Fructus Aurantii) and *Dou Kou* (Fructus Amomi Rotundus).

CAUTIONS / CONTRAINDICATIONS
Cong Chi Jie Geng Tang should be used with caution in cases of wind-warmth conditions involving symptoms of fever and perspiration. In such conditions, *Cong Bai* (Bulbus Allii Fistulosi) and *Dan Dou Chi* (Semen Sojae Praeparatum) should be removed.

RELATED FORMULAS
Cōng Chǐ Tāng
(Scallion and Prepared Soybean Decoction)
蔥豉湯
葱豉汤
Pinyin Name: *Cong Chi Tang*
Literal Name: Scallion and Prepared Soybean Decoction
Original Source: *Zhou Hou Bei Ji Fang* (Emergency Formulas to Keep Up One's Sleeve) by Ge Hong in 341 A.D.

Cong Bai (Bulbus Allii Fistulosi)   1 handful [3 stalks]
Dan Dou Chi (Semen Sojae Praeparatum)   1 cup [6g]

The source text states to cook the ingredients with 3 cups [600 mL] of water until the liquid is reduced to 1 cup [200 mL]. Take the strained decoction immediately. If the patient does not sweat after taking the decoction, administer the formula again with the addition of *Ge Gen* (Radix Puerariae Lobatae) 6g and *Sheng Ma* (Rhizoma Cimicifugae) 6g. Decoct the herbs with 5 cups [1,000 mL] of water until the liquid is reduced to 2 cups [400 mL]. If the patient still does not sweat after taking this decoction, add *Ma Huang* (Herba Ephedrae) 6g, and administer the decoction again. Today, this formula may be prepared as a decoction with the doses suggested in brackets above.

Cong Chi Tang (Scallion and Prepared Soybean Decoction) treats early onset of a mild exterior syndrome through diaphoresis. Clinically, patients may show fever, aversion to cold, absence of perspiration, headache, stuffy or running nose, and sneezing.

This is a mild exterior-releasing formula. It has no cautions or contraindications, and is therefore suitable for most people with exterior syndromes.

Huó Rén Cōng Chǐ Tāng (Scallion and Prepared Soybean Decoction from the Book to Safeguard Life)
活人蔥豉湯
活人葱豉汤
Pinyin Name: *Huo Ren Cong Chi Tang*

112

Cōng Chǐ Jié Gěng Tāng
(Scallion, Prepared Soybean, and Platycodon Decoction)

Literal Name: Scallion and Prepared Soybean Decoction from the Book to Safeguard Life

Original Source: *Lei Zheng Huo Ren Shu* (Book to Safeguard Life Arranged According to Pattern) by Zhu Gong in 1108

Cong Bai (Bulbus Allii Fistulosi)	15 stalks [3g]
Dan Dou Chi (Semen Sojae Praeparatum)	2 large cups [6g]
Ma Huang (Herba Ephedrae)	1.2g [3g]
Ge Gen (Radix Puerariae Lobatae)	2.4g [6g]

The source text states to cook *Ma Huang* (Herba Ephedrae) first with 2 cups [400 mL] of water, and bring it to a boil 6 or 7 times. Remove the foam from the top, add *Ge Gen* (Radix Puerariae Lobatae), and bring to a boil 20 times or more. Finally, add *Dan Dou Chi* (Semen Sojae Praeparatum) and cook until the liquid is reduced to 0.8 cup [160 mL]. Take the warm, strained decoction in two equally-divided doses twice daily. To effectively promote sweating, prepare this formula with porridge and administer while warm to induce sweating. Today, this formula may be prepared as a decoction with the doses suggested in brackets above.

Huo Ren Cong Chi Tang (Scallion and Prepared Soybean Decoction from the Book to Safeguard Life) has a stronger exterior-releasing action, and is mainly used for treating exterior wind-cold syndrome that is one to two days past the initial onset. Clinically, patients will show headache, neck stiffness, back pain, aversion to cold, absence of perspiration, and a tight pulse.

AUTHORS' COMMENTS

Sang Ju Yin (Mulberry Leaf and Chrysanthemum Decoction) and *Cong Chi Jie Geng Tang* both treat early stages of wind-warmth.

- *Sang Ju Yin* ventilates Lung qi and relieves cough, and is more suitable for mild cases of wind-warmth.
- *Cong Chi Jie Geng Tang* clears the Lung and purges heat, and is more appropriate for moderate cases of wind-warmth invasion.

Níng Sòu Wán (Quiet the Cough Pill)

寧嗽丸
宁嗽丸

Pinyin Name: *Ning Sou Wan*

Literal Name: Quiet the Cough Pill

Alternate Names: Cough-Stopping Pill, Fritillaria and Platycodon Formula

Original Source: *Zhong Guo Guo Yao Gu You Cheng Fang Xuan Ji* (A Selection of Traditional Prescriptions of Chinese Medicine) by the Chinese Herbal Medicine Committee of the Ministry of the Interior in 1967

COMPOSITION

Zi Su Zi (Fructus Perillae)	60g
Ku Xing Ren (Semen Armeniacae Amarum)	45g
Jie Geng (Radix Platycodonis)	60g
Ban Xia (Rhizoma Pinelliae), *zhi* (prepared)	60g
Chuan Bei Mu (Bulbus Fritillariae Cirrhosae)	60g
Ju Hong (Exocarpium Citri Reticulatae)	30g
Bo He (Herba Menthae)	45g
Fu Ling (Poria)	60g
Gu Ya (Fructus Setariae Germinatus)	30g
Sang Bai Pi (Cortex Mori)	45g
Shi Hu (Caulis Dendrobii)	60g
Zhi Gan Cao (Radix et Rhizoma Glycyrrhizae Praeparata cum Melle)	15g

Chapter 1 – Exterior-Releasing Formulas   *Section 2 – Acrid and Cold Exterior-Releasing Formulas*

Níng Sòu Wán (Quiet the Cough Pill)

DOSAGE / PREPARATION / ADMINISTRATION

First cook *Sang Bai Pi* (Cortex Mori) and *Shi Hu* (Caulis Dendrobii) in water to obtain a decoction. Grind the rest of the ingredients into a fine powder. Mix the decoction and the powder together to form pills, which should resemble *Lu Dou* (Semen Phaseoli Radiati) in size. Take 4.5g of pills twice daily with warm water.

CHINESE THERAPEUTIC ACTIONS

1. Clears the Lung and disperses stagnation
2. Dissolves phlegm and relieves cough

CLINICAL MANIFESTATIONS

Exterior wind-heat: nasal obstruction, nasal discharge, headache, fever, cough with sputum, wheezing and dyspnea, sneezing, and aversion to wind.

CLINICAL APPLICATIONS

Cough, common cold with cough and phlegm, tracheitis, cough from acute and chronic bronchitis.

EXPLANATION

Ning Sou Wan (Quiet the Cough Pill) treats cases of exterior wind-heat attacking the body, with chief complaints of cough with sputum and fever. Since wind-heat can interfere with the normal functions of the Lung, symptoms and signs usually include cough, wheezing, dyspnea, nasal obstruction, nasal discharge, and headache.

Many herbs in this formula have distinct effects to dispel phlegm, clear the Lung, and arrest coughing; such herbs

include *Zi Su Zi* (Fructus Perillae), *Ku Xing Ren* (Semen Armeniacae Amarum), *Jie Geng* (Radix Platycodonis), *Ban Xia* (Rhizoma Pinelliae), *Chuan Bei Mu* (Bulbus Fritillariae Cirrhosae), and *Ju Hong* (Exocarpium Citri Reticulatae). *Bo He* (Herba Menthae) dispels exterior wind-heat. Its cooling property also helps restrict the other warm herbs from creating heat in the body. *Fu Ling* (Poria) and *Gu Ya* (Fructus Setariae Germinatus) strengthen the Spleen, transform water, and prevent further formation of dampness and phlegm. *Sang Bai Pi* (Cortex Mori) promotes urination and drains dampness from the body. *Shi Hu* (Caulis Dendrobii) moistens the Lung, relieves cough, and prevents the phlegm-eliminating herbs from injuring yin. *Zhi Gan Cao* (Radix et Rhizoma Glycyrrhizae Praeparata cum Melle) harmonizes the entire formula.

MODIFICATIONS

- For cough caused by common cold and influenza, add *Hua Gai San* (Canopy Powder).
- For cough caused by Lung heat, add *Xie Bai San* (Drain the White Powder).
- For cough caused by phlegm, add *Er Chen Tang* (Two-Cured Decoction).
- If there is a dry throat and thirst, add *Mai Dong* (Radix Ophiopogonis) and *Wu Wei Zi* (Fructus Schisandrae Chinensis).

Ning Sou Wan (Quiet the Cough Pill)

Diagnosis	Signs and Symptoms	Treatment	Herbs
Exterior wind-heat	• Headache, fever, and aversion to wind: exterior wind-heat condition • Nasal obstruction, nasal discharge, and sneezing: wind-heat affecting Lung qi circulation • Cough, wheezing and dyspnea: reversed flow of Lung qi • Sputum: presence of dampness and phlegm	• Clears the Lung and disperses stagnation • Dissolves phlegm and relieves cough	• *Zi Su Zi* (Fructus Perillae), *Ku Xing Ren* (Semen Armeniacae Amarum), *Jie Geng* (Radix Platycodonis), *Ban Xia* (Rhizoma Pinelliae), *Chuan Bei Mu* (Bulbus Fritillariae Cirrhosae), and *Ju Hong* (Exocarpium Citri Reticulatae) dispel phlegm, clear the Lung, and arrest cough. • *Bo He* (Herba Menthae) dispels exterior wind-heat. • *Fu Ling* (Poria) and *Gu Ya* (Fructus Setariae Germinatus) strengthen the Spleen and prevent the formation of dampness and phlegm. • *Sang Bai Pi* (Cortex Mori) promotes urination and drains dampness out of the body. • *Shi Hu* (Caulis Dendrobii) moistens the Lung, relieves cough, and prevents the phlegm-eliminating herbs from injuring yin. • *Zhi Gan Cao* (Radix et Rhizoma Glycyrrhizae Praeparata cum Melle) harmonizes the herbs.

Chinese Herbal Formulas and Applications

Dùn Sòu Săn (Long-Bout Cough Powder)

頓嗽散
顿嗽散

Pinyin Name: *Dun Sou San*
Literal Name: Long-Bout Cough Powder
Alternate Name: Morus and Platycodon Formula
Original Source: *Yan Fang* (Time-Tested Formulas) of unknown author and date

COMPOSITION

Chai Hu (Radix Bupleuri)	15g
Huang Qin (Radix Scutellariae)	9g
Sang Bai Pi (Cortex Mori)	9g
Jie Geng (Radix Platycodonis)	9g
Zhi Zi (Fructus Gardeniae)	7.5g
Shi Gao (Gypsum Fibrosum)	15g
Gan Cao (Radix et Rhizoma Glycyrrhizae)	3g

DOSAGE / PREPARATION / ADMINISTRATION

This formula is taken on an empty stomach with warm water.

CHINESE THERAPEUTIC ACTIONS

1. Arrests cough
2. Clears heat and dissolves phlegm

CLINICAL MANIFESTATIONS

Cough caused by heat: persistent or violent cough, cough with or without sputum.

CLINICAL APPLICATIONS

Cough, whooping cough, cough from common cold, influenza, or bronchitis.

EXPLANATION

Dun Sou San (Long-Bout Cough Powder) treats cough caused by heat. This formula uses *Chai Hu* (Radix Bupleuri) and *Huang Qin* (Radix Scutellariae) to clear heat from the chest to relieve the stifling sensation or the feeling of oppression and congestion. *Sang Bai Pi* (Cortex Mori) and *Jie Geng* (Radix Platycodonis) dissolve phlegm and relieve coughing. *Zhi Zi* (Fructus Gardeniae) clears heat from the Lung to relieve irritability. *Shi Gao* (Gypsum Fibrosum) clears heat from the Lung and lowers fever. *Gan Cao* (Radix et Rhizoma Glycyrrhizae) tonifies qi and harmonizes the formula.

AUTHORS' COMMENTS

Dun Sou San was originally developed in Japan for treating cough. Clinically, it treats cough secondary to pulmonary infections, such as common cold, bronchitis, or pertussis.

Dun Sou San (Long-Bout Cough Powder)

Diagnosis	Signs and Symptoms	Treatment	Herbs
Cough caused by heat	• Persistent or violent cough: heat disturbing Lung qi circulation • Cough with little sputum or no sputum: heat consuming body fluids	• Arrests cough • Clears heat and dissolves phlegm	• *Chai Hu* (Radix Bupleuri) and *Huang Qin* (Radix Scutellariae) clear heat from the chest and relieve the feeling of oppression or congestion. • *Sang Bai Pi* (Cortex Mori) and *Jie Geng* (Radix Platycodonis) dissolve phlegm and relieve coughing. • *Zhi Zi* (Fructus Gardeniae) clears heat and eliminates toxins. • *Shi Gao* (Gypsum Fibrosum) clears heat from the Lung and reduces fever. • *Gan Cao* (Radix et Rhizoma Glycyrrhizae) tonifies qi and harmonizes the herbs.

EXTERIOR-RELEASING FORMULAS

115

Chapter 1 – Exterior-Releasing Formulas   Section 2 – Acrid and Cold Exterior-Releasing Formulas

Zhǐ Sòu Sǎn (Stop Coughing Powder)

止嗽散

Pinyin Name: *Zhi Sou San*
Literal Name: Stop Coughing Powder
Alternate Names: *Chih Sou San*, Cough-Stopping Powder, Platycodon and Schizonepeta Formula, Citrus and Apricot Seed Formula
Original Source: *Yi Xue Xin Wu* (Medical Revelations) by Cheng Guo-Peng in 1732

COMPOSITION

Zi Wan (Radix et Rhizoma Asteris), *zheng* (steamed)	1,000g [9g]
Bai Qian (Rhizoma et Radix Cynanchi Stauntonii), *zheng* (steamed)	1,000g [9g]
Bai Bu (Radix Stemonae), *zheng* (steamed)	1,000g [9g]
Jie Geng (Radix Platycodonis), *chao* (dry-fried)	1,000g [9g]
Chen Pi (Pericarpium Citri Reticulatae)	500g [9g]
Jing Jie (Herba Schizonepetae)	1,000g [9g]
Gan Cao (Radix et Rhizoma Glycyrrhizae), *chao* (dry-fried)	375g [3g]

DOSAGE / PREPARATION / ADMINISTRATION

The source text instructions are to grind the ingredients into powder. Take 9g of the powder with boiled water after meals and before bedtime. This formula may be taken with a decoction of *Sheng Jiang* (Rhizoma Zingiberis Recens) if there are external wind-cold symptoms present. Today, this formula is generally administered by giving 6g of the powdered herbs with warm, boiled water or a decoction of *Sheng Jiang* (Rhizoma Zingiberis Recens). This formula may also be prepared as a decoction with the doses suggested in brackets above.

CHINESE THERAPEUTIC ACTIONS

1. Stops coughing and dissolves phlegm
2. Releases exterior factors and ventilates the Lung

CLINICAL MANIFESTATIONS

Wind invading the Lung: coughing, itchy throat, mild fever, aversion to cold, and a thin, white tongue coating.

CLINICAL APPLICATIONS

Cough, whooping cough, cough with exterior condition, respiratory tract infection, acute bronchitis, chronic bronchitis, interstitial pneumonia, and chronic prostatitis.

EXPLANATION

Zhi Sou San (Stop Coughing Powder) treats persistent coughing that cannot be alleviated after the administration of exterior-releasing herbs. In this situation, the exterior symptoms, such as headache, fever, aversion to cold, will be mostly resolved by the exterior-releasing method, but the abnormal Lung qi flow persists.

The treatment approach for this syndrome places more emphasis on arresting the cough, and less on releasing the exterior. *Zi Wan* (Radix et Rhizoma Asteris), *Bai Qian* (Rhizoma et Radix Cynanchi Stauntonii), and *Bai Bu* (Radix Stemonae) dissolve phlegm and stop cough. These three herbs have excellent synergistic effects to treat both

Zhi Sou San (Stop Coughing Powder)

Diagnosis	Signs and Symptoms	Treatment	Herbs
Wind invading the Lung	• Coughing and itchy throat: obstruction of Lung qi circulation • Headache, fever, and aversion to cold: exterior wind	• Stops coughing and dissolves phlegm • Releases exterior factors and ventilates the Lung	• *Zi Wan* (Radix et Rhizoma Asteris), *Bai Qian* (Rhizoma et Radix Cynanchi Stauntonii) and *Bai Bu* (Radix Stemonae) dissolve phlegm and stop cough. • *Jie Geng* (Radix Platycodonis) and *Chen Pi* (Pericarpium Citri Reticulatae) ventilate the Lung, cause the Lung qi to descend, and dissolve phlegm. • *Jing Jie* (Herba Schizonepetae) expels wind and relieves exterior symptoms. • *Gan Cao* (Radix et Rhizoma Glycyrrhizae) harmonizes the herbs.

116

Zhǐ Sòu Sǎn (Stop Coughing Powder)

acute and chronic cough. *Jie Geng* (Radix Platycodonis) and *Chen Pi* (Pericarpium Citri Reticulatae) ventilate the Lung, cause the Lung qi to descend, and dissolve phlegm. *Jing Jie* (Herba Schizonepetae) expels wind and relieves exterior symptoms. *Gan Cao* (Radix et Rhizoma Glycyrrhizae), besides harmonizing all of the herbs, works with *Jie Geng* (Radix Platycodonis) to relieve itchy throat.

MODIFICATIONS

- For cough caused by wind-heat, add *Sang Ye* (Folium Mori), *Ju Hua* (Flos Chrysanthemi), and *Bo He* (Herba Menthae).
- For cough with white sputum caused by a wind-cold invasion, add *Zi Su Ye* (Folium Perillae), *Fang Feng* (Radix Saposhnikoviae), and *Ku Xing Ren* (Semen Armeniacae Amarum).
- For dry cough with absence of sputum because of Lung dryness, add *Gua Lou* (Fructus Trichosanthis), *Bei Mu* (Bulbus Fritillariae), and *Zhi Mu* (Rhizoma Anemarrhenae).
- For dry cough with a sore throat, add *Sang Ye* (Folium Mori), *Sha Shen* (Radix Glehniae seu Adenophorae), and *She Gan* (Rhizoma Belamcandae).
- For cough and a greasy tongue coating caused by summer-dampness, add *Huo Xiang* (Herba Agastaches), *Pei Lan* (Herba Eupatorii), and *Xiang Ru* (Herba Moslae).
- For cough with profuse sputum, add *Ban Xia* (Rhizoma Pinelliae) and *Fu Ling* (Poria).
- For cough with profuse sputum and a stifling sensation in the chest due to phlegm-damp obstruction, add *Ban Xia* (Rhizoma Pinelliae), *Fu Ling* (Poria), and *Chen Pi* (Pericarpium Citri Reticulatae).
- For cough and fever in children, add *Jin Yin Hua* (Flos Lonicerae Japonicae), *Niu Bang Zi* (Fructus Arctii), *Huang Qin* (Radix Scutellariae), *Zi Su Zi* (Fructus Perillae), *Ku Xing Ren* (Semen Armeniacae Amarum), and *Chuan Bei Mu* (Bulbus Fritillariae Cirrhosae).
- If there are more exterior symptoms, add *Fang Feng* (Radix Saposhnikoviae), *Zi Su Ye* (Folium Perillae), and *Sheng Jiang* (Rhizoma Zingiberis Recens).
- With thirst, irritability, and dark yellow urine caused by interior heat, add *Zhi Zi* (Fructus Gardeniae), *Huang Qin* (Radix Scutellariae), and *Tian Hua Fen* (Radix Trichosanthis).

CAUTIONS / CONTRAINDICATIONS

- *Zhi Sou San* contains many herbs that are warm and drying in nature; thus, it is not suitable for chronic cough caused by yin deficiency, Lung heat, or phlegm heat.
- This formula should be used with extreme caution if the cough is accompanied by blood-streaked phlegm.[1]

CLINICAL STUDIES AND RESEARCH

1. **Cough**: Modified *Zhi Sou San* demonstrated 90% effectiveness in treating cough associated with various causes and conditions. In addition to *Zhi Sou San*, modifications were made as follows: for cough due to wind-cold, *Fang Feng* (Radix Saposhnikoviae), *Ku Xing Ren* (Semen Armeniacae Amarum), and *Qiang Huo* (Rhizoma et Radix Notopterygii) were added; for cough due to wind-heat, *Sang Ye* (Folium Mori) and *Ku Xing Ren* (Semen Armeniacae Amarum) were added and the dose of *Jing Jie* (Herba Schizonepetae) was reduced; for dampness and phlegm affecting the Lung, *Huang Qin* (Radix Scutellariae), *Jie Geng* (Radix Platycodonis), and *Ku Xing Ren* (Semen Armeniacae Amarum) were added, and *Jing Jie* (Herba Schizonepetae) was removed; for dryness affecting the Lung, *Sha Shen* (Radix Glehniae seu Adenophorae), *Xuan Shen* (Radix Scrophulariae), and *Zhi Mu* (Rhizoma Anemarrhenae) were added, and the doses were reduced for *Jing Jie* (Herba Schizonepetae), *Bai Qian* (Rhizoma et Radix Cynanchi Stauntonii), and *Chen Pi* (Pericarpium Citri Reticulatae).[2]

2. **Cough with exterior condition**: One study reported 94% effectiveness using modified *Zhi Sou San* to treat cough associated with an exterior condition. The herbal treatment contained *Zhi Sou San* plus *Mu Dan Pi* (Cortex Moutan) and *Dan Shen* (Radix et Rhizoma Salviae Miltiorrhizae) as the base formula. In addition, *Bai He* (Bulbus Lilii) and *Mai Dong* (Radix Ophiopogonis) were added for dry cough caused by dryness and heat damaging the Lung; *Yuan Zhi* (Radix Polygalae) and *Ban Xia* (Rhizoma Pinelliae) were added for cough with profuse, white sputum; and *Sang Bai Pi* (Cortex Mori) and *Huang Qin* (Radix Scutellariae) were added for cough with yellow sputum. Of 50 cases, the study reported complete recovery in 23 cases, improvement in 24 cases, and no benefit in 3 cases.[3]

3. **Whooping cough**: Modified *Zhi Sou San* was used to treat 40 patients with whooping cough with complete recovery in 33 patients and improvement in 7 patients. The herbal treatment was based on *Zhi Sou San*, with removal of *Bai Qian* (Rhizoma et Radix Cynanchi Stauntonii) and *Zi Wan* (Radix et Rhizoma Asteris) and the addition of *Qian Hu* (Radix Peucedani), *Tao Ren* (Semen Persicae), *Bei Mu* (Bulbus Fritillariae), *Jiang Can* (Bombyx Batryticatus), and *Di Long* (Pheretima). Additional modifications were made as follows: *Ban Xia* (Rhizoma Pinelliae) and *Gua Lou* (Fructus Trichosanthis) for cough with profuse phlegm; *Jin Yin Hua* (Flos Lonicerae Japonicae) and *Pu Gong Ying* (Herba Taraxaci) for fever; *Ban Xia* (Rhizoma Pinelliae) and *Zhe Shi* (Haematitum) for frequent nausea and vomiting; and *Mu Dan Pi* (Cortex

Chapter 1 - Exterior-Releasing Formulas　　　　　*Section 2 - Acrid and Cold Exterior-Releasing Formulas*

Zhǐ Sòu Săn (Stop Coughing Powder)

Moutan) and processed *Sang Bai Pi* (Cortex Mori) for blood in the sputum.[4]

4. **Respiratory tract infection**: Eighty patients with respiratory tract infections were divided into two groups and treated with herbs or drugs three times daily, for 3 days per course of treatment. Group one of 40 patients received *Zhi Sou San*, and group two of 40 patients received antibiotic drugs. For group one, the study reported complete recovery in 34 patients, moderate improvement in 5 patients, and no benefit in 1 case. For group two, the study reported complete recovery in 10 patients, moderate improvement in 12 patients, and no effect in 18 patients.[5]

5. **Acute bronchitis**: One hundred children with acute bronchitis were treated with complete recovery in 92 cases and improvement in 2 cases. The herbal treatment was based on *Zhi Sou San* with the addition of *Tian Zhu Huang* (Concretio Silicea Bambusae), *Gua Lou Pi* (Pericarpium Trichosanthis), *Huang Qi* (Radix Astragali), *Sang Bai Pi* (Cortex Mori), *Qian Hu* (Radix Peucedani), and *Jin Yin Hua* (Flos Lonicerae Japonicae). Most patients had complete recovery within 4-6 packs of herbs.[6] In another study, *Zhi Sou San* successfully treated 147 of 153 patients (91 males and 62 females) with bronchitis for 2-32 days. The duration of treatment was between 2 and 8 packs of herbs.[7]

6. **Chronic bronchitis**: One study reported marked effectiveness using modified *Zhi Sou San* to treat chronic bronchitis. Of 30 patients, 23 had significant improvement, 6 had improvement, and 1 had slight improvement. The herbal treatment was modified by removing *Jing Jie* (Herba Schizonepetae) and adding *Ku Xing Ren* (Semen Armeniacae Amarum) and *Dan Shen* (Radix et Rhizoma Salviae Miltiorrhizae) to *Zhi Sou San*. Furthermore, *Huang Qin* (Radix Scutellariae) and *Sang Bai Pi* (Cortex Mori) were added for hot phlegm; *Ma Huang* (Herba Ephedrae) and *Xi Xin* (Radix et Rhizoma Asari) for cold phlegm; *Sha Shen* (Radix Glehniae seu Adenophorae) and *Mai Dong* (Radix Ophiopogonis) for Lung dryness; and *Dang Shen* (Radix Codonopsis) and *Huang Qi* (Radix Astragali) for Lung and Spleen qi deficiencies.[8]

7. **Interstitial pneumonia**: Modified *Zhi Sou San* showed marked effectiveness in treating interstitial pneumonia. The base formula included *Zhi Sou San* plus *Tao Ren* (Semen Persicae) and *Ban Lan Gen* (Radix Isatidis). Other herbs were added as deemed necessary: *San Ao Tang* (Three-Unbinding Decoction) for wind-cold; *Ma Huang Xing Ren Gan Cao Shi Gao Tang* (Ephedra, Apricot Kernel, Licorice, and Gypsum Decoction), *Jin Yin Hua* (Flos Lonicerae Japonicae), and *Lian Qiao* (Fructus Forsythiae) for fever with cough; and *Ping Wei San* (Calm the Stomach Powder) for excessive dampness and phlegm. Each course of treatment was 6 days. The average duration of treatment was 1.6 courses.[9]

8. **Chronic prostatitis**: Concurrent use of *Ding Chuan Tang* (Arrest Wheezing Decoction) and *Zhi Sou San* demonstrated 94.29% effectiveness in treating chronic prostatitis. Modifications include addition of *Huang Bo* (Cortex Phellodendri Chinensis) and *Cang Zhu* (Rhizoma Atractylodis) for increased white blood cells in the prostatic fluids; addition of *Gou Ji* (Rhizoma Cibotii), *Xu Duan* (Radix Dipsaci), *Ba Ji Tian* (Radix Morindae Officinalis) and *Yin Yang Huo* (Herba Epimedii) for significant reduction of lecithin mass; addition of *Zhi Mu* (Rhizoma Anemarrhenae), *Huang Bo* (Cortex Phellodendri Chinensis) and *Di Huang* (Radix Rehmanniae) for yin deficiency; addition of *Huang Qi* (Radix Astragali), *Dang Shen* (Radix Codonopsis) and *Sheng Ma* (Rhizoma Cimicifugae) for yang deficiency; and addition of *Dan Shen* (Radix et Rhizoma Salviae Miltiorrhizae) and *Yan Hu Suo* (Rhizoma Corydalis) for blood stagnation. Of 70 patients, 29 had complete recovery, 37 had improvement, 3 had no results, and 1 discontinued treatment.[10]

RELATED FORMULA

Zhǐ Ké Tāng (Stop Coughing Decoction)

止咳湯
止咳汤

Pinyin Name: *Zhi Ke Tang*
Literal Name: Stop Coughing Decoction
Original Source: *Guang An Men Yi Yuan* (Guang An Men Hospital) in 1990

Zi Su Ye (Folium Perillae)
Sheng Jiang (Rhizoma Zingiberis Recens)
Bai Jie Zi (Semen Sinapis)
Mai Dong (Radix Ophiopogonis)
Gan Cao (Radix et Rhizoma Glycyrrhizae)
Ting Li Zi (Semen Descurainiae seu Lepidii)
Ku Xing Ren (Semen Armeniacae Amarum)
Zi Su Zi (Fructus Perillae)
Wu Mei (Fructus Mume)

Zhi Ke Tang (Stop Coughing Decoction) has been used primarily as a symptomatic treatment for cough arising from various causes. It contains herbs that release wind from the exterior, eliminate phlegm, nourish yin, and cause Lung qi to descend. Clinically, it may be used to treat cough due to external wind-heat or wind-cold, internal Lung yin deficiency, or other causes. However, although this is an effective formula for suppressing cough, it is necessary to identify the cause(s) of the cough and select treatment accordingly for optimal results.

Zhǐ Sòu Sǎn (Stop Coughing Powder)

AUTHORS' COMMENTS

Zhi Sou San ventilates the Lung, expels wind, and is widely used to treat cough due to various causes. It is especially effective in treating cough with lingering exterior pathogenic factors. Key symptoms include cough with a tickling sensation in the throat, slight aversion to wind, fever, and a thin, white tongue coating.

Jin Fei Cao San (Inula Powder) and *Zhi Sou San* are both commonly used to treat wind invading the Lung.

- *Jin Fei Cao San* is more suitable for the initial stages of wind invasion with cough and profuse sputum. It contains many herbs that release the exterior and ventilate the Lung, such as *Ma Huang* (Herba Ephedrae), *Jing Jie* (Herba Schizonepetae), and *Xuan Fu Hua* (Flos Inulae).
- *Zhi Sou San* treats wind attacking the Lung that leads to disruption of Lung qi and resulting in cough. The herbs in this formula are primarily from the cough-arresting category, such as *Zi Wan* (Radix et Rhizoma Asteris), *Bai Qian* (Rhizoma et Radix Cynanchi Stauntonii), *Bai Bu* (Radix Stemonae), and *Jie Geng* (Radix Platycodonis). *Zhi Sou San* does not contain many exterior wind-cold releasing herbs, since the focus of the formula is on directing Lung qi downward and arresting cough.

Ning Sou Wan (Quiet the Cough Pill), *Dun Sou San* (Long-Bout Cough Powder), and *Zhi Sou San* (Stop Coughing Powder) are three formulas that commonly treat cough. Their differences are as follows:

- *Ning Sou Wan* quiets cough caused by wind-heat.
- *Dun Sou San* settles cough caused by heat and phlegm in the interior.
- *Zhi Sou San* stops cough caused by wind at the exterior and phlegm in the interior.

References

1. *Zhong Yao Ming Fang Yao Li Yu Ying Yong* (Pharmacology and Applications of Famous Herbal Formulas) 1989;599-600.
2. *Yun Nan Zhong Yi Zhong Yao Za Zhi* (Yunnan Journal of Traditional Chinese Medicine and Herbal Medicine) 1999;4:15.
3. *Zhong Yi Ming Fang Lin Chuang Xin Yong* (Contemporary Clinical Applications of Classic Chinese Formulas) 2001;136.
4. *Shan Xi Zhong Yi* (Shanxi Chinese Medicine) 1994;8:368.
5. *Shi Zhen Guo Yao Yan Jiu* (Research of Shizhen Herbs) 1995;2:37.
6. *Shi Yong Zhong Xi Yi Jie He Za Zhi* (Practical Journal of Integrated Chinese and Western Medicines) 1995;10:634.
7. *Zhong Yi Ming Fang Lin Chuang Xin Yong* (Contemporary Clinical Applications of Classic Chinese Formulas) 2001;138.
8. *Zhong Yuan Yi Kan* (Resource Journal of Chinese Medicine) 1994;5:44.
9. *Shi Yong Zhong Xi Yi Jie He Za Zhi* (Practical Journal of Integrated Chinese and Western Medicines) 1995;3:152.
10. *Shi Yong Zhong Yi Nei Ke Za Zhi* (Journal of Practical Chinese Internal Medicine) 1997;1:21.

Chapter 1 – Exterior-Releasing Formulas　　　　　*Section 2 – Acrid and Cold Exterior-Releasing Formulas*

Jīng Jiè Lián Qiào Tāng (Schizonepeta and Forsythia Decoction)
荊芥連翹湯
荆芥连翘汤

Pinyin Name: *Jing Jie Lian Qiao Tang*
Literal Name: Schizonepeta and Forsythia Decoction
Alternate Names: *Ching Chieh Lien Chiao Tang, Jing Jie Lian Chiao Tang*, Schizonepeta and Forsythia Combination
Original Source: *Wan Bing Hui Chun* (Restoration of Health from the Myriad Diseases) by Gong Ting-Xian in 1587

COMPOSITION

Jing Jie (Herba Schizonepetae)
Fang Feng (Radix Saposhnikoviae)
Lian Qiao (Fructus Forsythiae)
Jie Geng (Radix Platycodonis)
Huang Qin (Radix Scutellariae)
Zhi Zi (Fructus Gardeniae)
Bai Zhi (Radix Angelicae Dahuricae)
Chai Hu (Radix Bupleuri)
Zhi Qiao (Fructus Citri Aurantii)
Dang Gui (Radix Angelicae Sinensis)
Chuan Xiong (Rhizoma Chuanxiong)
Bai Shao (Radix Paeoniae Alba)
Gan Cao (Radix et Rhizoma Glycyrrhizae)

DOSAGE / PREPARATION / ADMINISTRATION

Cook all of the ingredients in water, and take the decoction after meals. Note: Exact doses of the herbs are unavailable. The source text only states to use equal amounts of all the herbs, except for *Gan Cao* (Radix et Rhizoma Glycyrrhizae), which should be used at half the dose.

CHINESE THERAPEUTIC ACTIONS

1. Releases wind-heat from the exterior
2. Dispels heat, fire, and toxins

CLINICAL MANIFESTATIONS

Suppuration of the ears and nose due to wind-heat attacking the upper *jiao*: swelling, inflammation and infection of the ears and nose, abscess and suppuration of the affected area, dark brown discoloration of the skin, perspiration and an oily feeling on the palms and soles, and abdominal rigidity.

CLINICAL APPLICATIONS

Otitis media, sinusitis, rhinitis, suppuration of the ears and nose, tonsillitis, nosebleeds, and acne.

EXPLANATION

Jing Jie Lian Qiao Tang (Schizonepeta and Forsythia Decoction) treats inflammation and swelling of the ears and nose. The disease progression begins with wind-heat attacking the upper *jiao*. As wind-heat travels upward, it directly attacks the ears and nose, leading to inflammation and swelling. As heat accumulates in the affected area, suppuration develops, leading to the formation and discharge of pus.

Clinically, wind-heat attacking the ears is characterized by swelling and pain of the inner ear, abscess and discharge of pus, deafness, and tinnitus; and wind-heat attacking the nose is characterized by swelling and obstruction of the nasal passage, loss of smell, abscess, and yellow nasal discharge. According to the original text, patients with marked dark brown discoloration of the skin, perspiration, and an oily feeling on the palms and soles respond remarkably well to this herbal formula.

Jing Jie (Herba Schizonepetae) and *Fang Feng* (Radix Saposhnikoviae) release exterior wind. *Lian Qiao* (Fructus Forsythiae) and *Jie Geng* (Radix Platycodonis) reduce swelling and inflammation, as well as eliminate pus and toxins. *Huang Qin* (Radix Scutellariae) and *Zhi Zi* (Fructus Gardeniae) purge fire and reduce inflammation. *Bai Zhi* (Radix Angelicae Dahuricae) dispels wind and unblocks obstruction in the ears and nose. *Chai Hu* (Radix Bupleuri) dispels wind, and with *Zhi Qiao* (Fructus Aurantii), relieves the feeling of distention caused by qi stagnation. *Dang Gui* (Radix Angelicae Sinensis), *Chuan Xiong* (Rhizoma Chuanxiong), and *Bai Shao* (Radix Paeoniae Alba) tonify the blood and promote blood circulation. *Gan Cao* (Radix et Rhizoma Glycyrrhizae) harmonizes the formula.

120

Jīng Jiè Lián Qiào Tāng (Schizonepeta and Forsythia Decoction)

Jing Jie Lian Qiao Tang (Schizonepeta and Forsythia Decoction)

Diagnosis	Signs and Symptoms	Treatment	Herbs
Suppuration of the ears and nose	Swelling, inflammation and infection of the ears and nose: wind-heat attacking the upper body	• Releases wind-heat from the exterior • Dispels heat, fire, and toxins	• *Jing Jie* (Herba Schizonepetae) and *Fang Feng* (Radix Saposhnikoviae) release exterior wind and relieve itching. • *Lian Qiao* (Fructus Forsythiae) and *Jie Geng* (Radix Platycodonis) reduce swelling and inflammation and eliminate pus and abscesses. • *Huang Qin* (Radix Scutellariae) and *Zhi Zi* (Fructus Gardeniae) purge fire and reduce inflammation. • *Bai Zhi* (Radix Angelicae Dahuricae) dispels wind and unblocks obstruction in the ears and nose. • *Chai Hu* (Radix Bupleuri) dispels wind. • *Zhi Qiao* (Fructus Aurantii) activates qi circulation and relieves distention. • *Dang Gui* (Radix Angelicae Sinensis), *Chuan Xiong* (Rhizoma Chuanxiong), and *Bai Shao* (Radix Paeoniae Alba) tonify the blood and promote blood circulation. • *Gan Cao* (Radix et Rhizoma Glycyrrhizae) harmonizes the herbs.

MODIFICATIONS

- For hypertrophic sinusitis or rhinitis, add *Xin Yi Hua* (Flos Magnoliae) and *Cang Er Zi* (Fructus Xanthii).
- If there is swelling and pain caused by wind-heat, add *Jin Yin Hua* (Flos Lonicerae Japonicae) and *Huang Lian* (Rhizoma Coptidis).

- For nasal obstruction, combine with *Qing Bi Tang* (Clear the Nose Decoction).
- If there is loss of smell, combine with *Xin Yi San* (Magnolia Flower Powder).

121

Chapter 1 – Exterior-Releasing Formulas　　　　*Section 2 – Acrid and Cold Exterior-Releasing Formulas*

Xīn Yí Qīng Fèi Yǐn (Magnolia Decoction to Clear the Lung)

辛夷清肺飲
辛夷清肺饮

Pinyin Name: *Xin Yi Qing Fei Yin*
Literal Name: Magnolia Decoction to Clear the Lung
Alternate Names: *Hsin I Ching Fei Tang, Xin Yi Ching Fei Tang*, Magnolia Flower and Gypsum Decoction, Magnolia and Gypsum Combination
Original Source: *Wai Ke Zheng Zong* (True Lineage of External Medicine) by Chen Shi-Gong in 1617

COMPOSITION

Xin Yi Hua (Flos Magnoliae)	1.8g
Sheng Ma (Rhizoma Cimicifugae)	0.9g
Pi Pa Ye (Folium Eriobotryae)	3 leaves
Huang Qin (Radix Scutellariae)	3g
Zhi Zi (Fructus Gardeniae)	3g
Shi Gao (Gypsum Fibrosum)	3g
Zhi Mu (Rhizoma Anemarrhenae)	3g
Bai He (Bulbus Lilii)	3g
Mai Dong (Radix Ophiopogonis)	3g
Gan Cao (Radix et Rhizoma Glycyrrhizae)	1.5g

DOSAGE / PREPARATION / ADMINISTRATION

Cook the herbs in 2 bowls of water until the liquid is reduced to 80%. Take the warm, strained decoction after meals. Note: Before cooking the herbs, place *Xin Yi Hua* (Flos Magnoliae) in a cheese cloth, and remove the hair-like particles from *Pi Pa Ye* (Folium Eriobotryae), to prevent discomfort of the throat while drinking the decoction.

CHINESE THERAPEUTIC ACTIONS

1. Clears heat from the Lung
2. Disperses stagnation and unblocks nasal obstruction

CLINICAL MANIFESTATIONS

Nasal obstruction caused by Lung heat: stuffy nose, nasal obstruction, yellow nasal discharge that is thick and sticky, and a decreased sense of smell.

CLINICAL APPLICATIONS

Sinusitis, rhinitis, and nasal obstruction.

EXPLANATION

Xin Yi Qing Fei Yin (Magnolia Decoction to Clear the Lung) treats nasal obstruction caused by Lung heat. In addition to stuffy nose, other signs include visible swelling and congestion of the sinus cavity. The discharge is often thick, sticky and yellow in color, and the sense of smell is often impaired.

Xin Yi Hua (Flos Magnoliae), the chief herb, effectively unblocks stagnation of the nose to treat various types of nasal disorders. *Sheng Ma* (Rhizoma Cimicifugae) has an ascending function, bringing the effect of the formula to the head to open the orifices. *Pi Pa Ye* (Folium Eriobotryae), *Huang Qin* (Radix Scutellariae), and *Zhi Zi* (Fructus Gardeniae) clear damp-heat from the Lung, while *Shi Gao* (Gypsum Fibrosum) and *Zhi Mu* (Rhizoma Anemarrhenae) clear heat and fire from the Lung. *Bai He* (Bulbus Lilii) and *Mai Dong* (Radix Ophiopogonis) promote generation of fluids and moisten the Lung. They prevent the acrid herbs in this formula from damaging Lung yin. Lastly, *Gan Cao* (Radix et Rhizoma Glycyrrhizae) harmonizes the herbs.

MODIFICATIONS

- For exterior wind-cold conditions, add *Fang Feng* (Radix Saposhnikoviae) and *Qiang Huo* (Rhizoma et Radix Notopterygii).
- If there is pus and abscess caused by wind and dampness, add *Cang Zhu* (Rhizoma Atractylodis) and *Lian Qiao* (Fructus Forsythiae).
- For nasal congestion caused by wind-heat, add *Cang Er Zi* (Fructus Xanthii) and *Bo He* (Herba Menthae).
- When there is clear nasal discharge caused by wind-cold, add *Jing Jie* (Herba Schizonepetae) and *Qiang Huo* (Rhizoma et Radix Notopterygii).

Xīn Yí Qīng Fèi Yǐn (Magnolia Decoction to Clear the Lung)

Xin Yi Qing Fei Yin (Magnolia Decoction to Clear the Lung)

Diagnosis	Signs and Symptoms	Treatment	Herbs
Nasal obstruction caused by Lung heat	• Stuffy nose with swelling and congestion of the sinus cavity and impaired sense of smell: Lung heat affecting normal qi circulation • Thick, sticky and yellow nasal discharge: presence of heat	• Clears heat from the Lung • Disperses stagnation and unblocks nasal obstruction	• *Xin Yi Hua* (Flos Magnoliae) unblocks stagnation of the nose to treat nasal disorders. • *Sheng Ma* (Rhizoma Cimicifugae) has an lifting function to guide the formula to the head to open the sensory orifices. • *Pi Pa Ye* (Folium Eriobotryae), *Huang Qin* (Radix Scutellariae), and *Zhi Zi* (Fructus Gardeniae) clear damp-heat from the Lung. • *Shi Gao* (Gypsum Fibrosum) and *Zhi Mu* (Rhizoma Anemarrhenae) clear heat and fire from the Lung. • *Bai He* (Bulbus Lilii) and *Mai Dong* (Radix Ophiopogonis) promote generation of fluids and moisten the Lung. • *Gan Cao* (Radix et Rhizoma Glycyrrhizae) harmonizes the herbs.

Chapter 1 – Exterior-Releasing Formulas   **Section 3 – Supporting [the Upright] and Releasing [the Exterior] Formulas**

Section 3

扶正解表剂

Supporting [the Upright] and Releasing [the Exterior] Formulas

Bài Dú Săn (Overcome Pathogenic Influences Powder)

败毒散
败毒散

Pinyin Name: *Bai Du San*
Literal Name: Overcome Pathogenic Influences Powder
Alternate Names: *Ren Shen Bai Du San, Jen Shen Pai Tu San,* Ginseng Detoxifying Formula, Ginseng Antiphlogistic Powder, Ginseng Powder to Overcome Pathogenic Influences, Ginseng and Mentha Formula
Original Source: *Xiao Er Yao Zheng Zhi Jue* (Craft of Medicinal Treatment for Childhood Disease Patterns) by Qian Yi in 1119

COMPOSITION

Qiang Huo (Rhizoma et Radix Notopterygii)	30g [9g]
Du Huo (Radix Angelicae Pubescentis)	30g [9g]
Chuan Xiong (Rhizoma Chuanxiong)	30g [9g]
Zhi Qiao (Fructus Aurantii)	30g [9g]
Jie Geng (Radix Platycodonis), *chao* (dry-fried)	30g [9g]
Qian Hu (Radix Peucedani)	30g [9g]
Fu Ling (Poria)	30g [9g]
Chai Hu (Radix Bupleuri), *xi* (washed)	30g [9g]
Gan Cao (Radix et Rhizoma Glycyrrhizae)	15g [5g]
Ren Shen (Radix et Rhizoma Ginseng)	30g [9g]

DOSAGE / PREPARATION / ADMINISTRATION

The source text states to grind the ingredients into powder. Cook 6g of the powder with *Sheng Jiang* (Rhizoma Zingiberis Recens) and *Bo He* (Herba Menthae) in water to obtain a decoction. Today, this formula may be prepared as a decoction with the doses suggested in brackets above.

CHINESE THERAPEUTIC ACTIONS

1. Releases the exterior through diaphoresis
2. Dispels wind, cold, and dampness
3. Tonifies qi

CLINICAL MANIFESTATIONS

Exterior wind, cold and dampness with qi deficiency: aversion to cold, fever, headache, neck stiffness, joint pain, body ache, absence of perspiration, nasal obstruction, cough with sputum, a feeling of distension and fullness in the chest and diaphragm, a pale tongue with a white, greasy tongue coating, and a superficial, soggy or superficial, rapid pulse that is forceless upon pressure.

CLINICAL APPLICATIONS

Influenza, common cold, respiratory tract infection, infection with fever, cough, hoarseness of voice, nasal congestion, parotitis, urticaria, eczema, suppurative infection, rheumatism, dizziness, and acute viral hepatitis.

EXPLANATION

Bai Du San (Overcome Pathogenic Influences Powder) treats weak and deficient patients who suffer from an attack by exterior wind, cold and dampness. Aversion to cold, fever, absence of perspiration, neck stiffness, joint pain, and body aches are all indications of wind, cold and dampness attacking the exterior and muscles. Wind-cold

Bài Dú Săn (Overcome Pathogenic Influences Powder)

Bai Du San (Overcome Pathogenic Influences Powder)

Diagnosis	Signs and Symptoms	Treatment	Herbs
Exterior wind, cold and dampness with qi deficiency	• Aversion to cold, fever, absence of perspiration, neck stiffness, joint pain, and body aches: wind, cold and dampness attacking the exterior and the muscles • Nasal obstruction, cough with sputum, feeling of distention and fullness in the chest and diaphragm area: wind-cold invading the Lung • Pale tongue and a forceless pulse: qi deficiency	• Releases the exterior through diaphoresis • Dispels wind, cold and dampness • Tonifies yuan (source) qi	• Qiang Huo (Rhizoma et Radix Notopterygii) and Du Huo (Radix Angelicae Pubescentis) dispel wind, cold, and dampness from the body. • Chuan Xiong (Rhizoma Chuanxiong) activates blood circulation and dispels exterior wind-cold. • Zhi Qiao (Fructus Aurantii) regulates Lung qi to relieve distention and fullness. • Jie Geng (Radix Platycodonis) and Qian Hu (Radix Peucedani) dispel phlegm and relieve coughing. • Fu Ling (Poria) dispels dampness and tonifies the middle jiao. • Chai Hu (Radix Bupleuri), Bo He (Herba Menthae) and Sheng Jiang (Rhizoma Zingiberis Recens) release the exterior factors. • Gan Cao (Radix et Rhizoma Glycyrrhizae) harmonizes the herbs. • Ren Shen (Radix et Rhizoma Ginseng) tonifies yuan (source) qi.

may constrict the Lung, and cause nasal obstruction, cough with sputum, a feeling of distention and fullness in the chest and diaphragm. A greasy tongue coating and a soggy pulse are signs of dampness. A pale tongue and a pulse that is forceless upon pressure indicate underlying qi deficiency.

The treatment goals are to dispel wind, cold, and dampness and to tonify yuan (source) qi. Qiang Huo (Rhizoma et Radix Notopterygii) and Du Huo (Radix Angelicae Pubescentis) act as the chief herbs to dispel wind, cold, and dampness from the whole body. Chuan Xiong (Rhizoma Chuanxiong) activates blood circulation to relieve pain. It also dispels exterior wind and cold. Chai Hu (Radix Bupleuri) helps the chief herbs release the exterior. Zhi Qiao (Fructus Aurantii) regulates the qi flow of the Lung to relieve chest distention and fullness. Jie Geng (Radix Platycodonis) and Qian Hu (Radix Peucedani) relieve coughing and dispel phlegm. Fu Ling (Poria) dispels dampness through diuresis and tonifies the middle jiao. Bo He (Herba Menthae) and Sheng Jiang (Rhizoma Zingiberis Recens) help relieve exterior symptoms. Gan Cao (Radix et Rhizoma Glycyrrhizae) harmonizes the herbs.

To help a deficient body dispel exterior factors, the interior must also be strengthened; hence, a small amount of Ren Shen (Radix et Rhizoma Ginseng) is used to tonify yuan (source) qi, which strengthens the body to help expel the exterior factors. Moreover, Ren Shen (Radix et Rhizoma Ginseng) balances and prevents the acrid and strong properties of the exterior-releasing herbs from damaging the weak body. Lastly, by tonifying qi, this herb prevents future re-infections and reduces the susceptibility of the body to exterior pathogens.

MODIFICATIONS

- If there is itching or eczema, add Ku Shen (Radix Sophorae Flavescentis) and Chan Tui (Periostracum Cicadae).
- For rash or incomplete eruption of dermatological disorders caused by wind-heat and toxins, add Xiao Feng San (Eliminate Wind Powder).
- For the initial stages of skin lesions such as sores and carbuncles, remove Ren Shen (Radix et Rhizoma Ginseng) and add Jin Yin Hua (Flos Lonicerae Japonicae) and Lian Qiao (Fructus Forsythiae).
- For febrile diseases with thirst but no aversion to wind or cold, add Huang Qin (Radix Scutellariae).
- If there is no sign of dampness at the exterior, remove Qiang Huo (Rhizoma et Radix Notopterygii), Du Huo (Radix Angelicae Pubescentis) and Fu Ling (Poria).
- If there is no sign of coughing or sputum, remove Jie Geng (Radix Platycodonis) and Qian Hu (Radix Peucedani).

Chapter 1 – Exterior-Releasing Formulas   **Section 3 – Supporting [the Upright] and Releasing [the Exterior] Formulas**

Bài Dú Săn (Overcome Pathogenic Influences Powder)

CAUTIONS / CONTRAINDICATIONS

- The dose of *Ren Shen* (Radix et Rhizoma Ginseng) should be carefully adjusted according to each patient's condition. It should not constitute more than ten percent of the entire formula. *Bai Du San* was originally designed for children. For adults who do not have significant qi deficiency, the dose of *Ren Shen* (Radix et Rhizoma Ginseng) should be decreased.

- *Bai Du San* is a warm, acrid formula that is contraindicated in cases of exterior wind-heat invasion, interior heat, or yin deficiency with exterior invasion.

CLINICAL STUDIES AND RESEARCH

1. **Infection with fever**: In one study, 136 children with epidemic infection and fever were evaluated and treated. The ages of the children ranged from 6 months to 12 years, with length of illness between 1-7 days prior to the evaluation and herbal treatment. Out of 136 cases, 36 had been treated previously with antibiotic drugs without success, 79 were treated with herbs only, and 21 received concurrent herbal and drug treatment. The study reported complete recovery in 125 cases after 3 days. The other 11 cases continued to have fever and needed additional treatment.[1]

2. **Respiratory tract infection**: Use of *Bai Du San* in decoction was associated with 94% effectiveness in treating infants and young children with upper respiratory infection caused by virus. The herbal treatment contained 6g each of *Chai Hu* (Radix Bupleuri), *Qian Hu* (Radix Peucedani), *Tai Zi Shen* (Radix Pseudostellariae), *Chuan Xiong* (Rhizoma Chuanxiong), *Zhi Qiao* (Fructus Aurantii), *Fu Ling* (Poria), and *Jie Geng* (Radix Platycodonis); 5g each of *Qiang Huo* (Rhizoma et Radix Notopterygii) and *Du Huo* (Radix Angelicae Pubescentis); 3g of *Bo He* (Herba Menthae); and 3 pieces of *Sheng Jiang* (Rhizoma Zingiberis Recens). Of 37 cases, the study reported complete recovery in 17 cases, marked improvement in 18 cases, and no benefit in 2 cases.[2]

3. **Acute viral hepatitis**: Use of modified *Bai Du San* demonstrated good results in treating 152 patients (between 16 and 35 years of age) of acute viral hepatitis within 5-12 days from onset of illness. The herbal formula contained 9g each of *Dang Shen* (Radix Codonopsis), *Fu Ling* (Poria), *Zhi Qiao* (Fructus Aurantii), *Jie Geng* (Radix Platycodonis), *Chai Hu* (Radix Bupleuri), *Qian Hu* (Radix Peucedani), *Chuan Xiong* (Rhizoma Chuanxiong), *Qiang Huo* (Rhizoma et Radix Notopterygii), *Du Huo* (Radix Angelicae Pubescentis), and *Gan Cao* (Radix et Rhizoma Glycyrrhizae); 3g of *Bo He* (Herba Menthae); and 3 pieces of *Sheng Jiang* (Rhizoma Zingiberis Recens). *Yin Chen* (Herba Artemisiae Scopariae) and *Jin Qian Cao* (Herba Lysimachiae) were added for those with jaundice; and *Pu Gong Ying* (Herba Taraxaci) and *Bai Jiang Cao* (Herba cum

Radice Patriniae) were added for those without jaundice. The herbs were administered in decoction twice daily, for 4 weeks per course of treatment. The duration of treatment varied from 28-42 packs of herbs, with an average of 31.9 packs. Of 152 patients, the study reported complete recovery in 139 patients and no benefit in 13 patients. The overall rate of effectiveness was 91.4%.[3]

4. **Parotitis**: Use of modified *Bai Du San* showed good results in treating chronic suppurative parotitis in 36 patients. The herbal treatment contained *Ren Shen* (Radix et Rhizoma Ginseng) 30g, *Chai Hu* (Radix Bupleuri) 15g, *Qian Hu* (Radix Peucedani) 15g, *Qiang Huo* (Rhizoma et Radix Notopterygii) 12g, *Du Huo* (Radix Angelicae Pubescentis) 12g, *Jie Geng* (Radix Platycodonis) 12g, *Fu Ling* (Poria) 12g, *Bo He* (Herba Menthae) 9g, *Gan Cao* (Radix et Rhizoma Glycyrrhizae) 9g, *Kun Bu* (Thallus Eckloniae) 9g, *Tao Ren* (Semen Persicae) 9g, and *Zhi Qiao* (Fructus Aurantii) 9g. Furthermore, *Huang Qi* (Radix Astragali) 30g was added for severe qi deficiency; *Mu Li* (Concha Ostreae) 12g, *Xuan Shen* (Radix Scrophulariae) 12g and *Hong Hua* (Flos Carthami) 3g were added for severe swelling of the parotid glands; and *Bai Hua She She Cao* (Herba Hedyotis) 12g, and *Ban Zhi Lian* (Herba Scutellariae Barbatae) 9g were added for profuse abscesses and discharges. Of 36 patients, 25 had complete recovery and 11 had improvement.[4]

RELATED FORMULAS

Rén Shēn Bài Dú Săn
(Ginseng Powder to Overcome Pathogenic Influences)

人参败毒散
人參敗毒散

Pinyin Name: Ren Shen Bai Du San
Literal Name: Ginseng Powder to Overcome Pathogenic Influences
Original Source: *Tai Ping Hui Min He Ji Ju Fang* (Imperial Grace Formulary of the Tai Ping Era) by the Imperial Medical Department in 1078-85

Chai Hu (Radix Bupleuri)
Gan Cao (Radix et Rhizoma Glycyrrhizae)
Jie Geng (Radix Platycodonis)
Ren Shen (Radix et Rhizoma Ginseng)
Chuan Xiong (Rhizoma Chuanxiong)
Fu Ling (Poria), remove the peel
Zhi Qiao (Fructus Aurantii), *chao* (dry-fried) with bran
Qian Hu (Radix Peucedani)
Qiang Huo (Rhizoma et Radix Notopterygii)
Du Huo (Radix Angelicae Pubescentis)

The source text states to grind equal amounts of the ingredients into powder, and cook 6g of the powder with

126

Bài Dú Săn (Overcome Pathogenic Influences Powder)

Sheng Jiang (Rhizoma Zingiberis Recens) and *Bo He* (Herba Menthae) in water to obtain a decoction.

Bai Du San (Overcome Pathogenic Influences Powder) and *Ren Shen Bai Du San* (Ginseng Powder to Overcome Pathogenic Influences) are essentially the same formulas with the same indications. The minor differences between these two formulas are preparation of some of the ingredients, and the dose of *Gan Cao* (Radix et Rhizoma Glycyrrhizae). Because of their overwhelming similarities, the names "*Bai Du San*" and "*Ren Shen Bai Du San*" are sometimes used interchangeably.

Cāng Lǐn Săn (Old Rice Granary Powder)
倉廩散
仓廩散
Pinyin Name: *Cang Lin San*
Literal Name: Old Rice Granary Powder
Original Source: *Pu Ji Fang* (Formulas of Universal Benefit) by Teng Hong in the Ming Dynasty

Chai Hu (Radix Bupleuri)
Qian Hu (Radix Peucedani)
Chuan Xiong (Rhizoma Chuanxiong)
Zhi Qiao (Fructus Aurantii)
Qiang Huo (Rhizoma et Radix Notopterygii)
Du Huo (Radix Angelicae Pubescentis)
Fu Ling (Poria)
Jie Geng (Radix Platycodonis)
Ren Shen (Radix et Rhizoma Ginseng)
Gan Cao (Radix et Rhizoma Glycyrrhizae)
Geng Mi (Semen Oryzae)

The source text states to grind equal amounts of the ingredients into powder, and cook the powder as a decoction with *Sheng Jiang* (Rhizoma Zingiberis Recens) and *Bo He* (Herba Menthae). Take the strained decoction while warm.

Cang Lin San (Old Rice Granary Powder) treats fasting dysentery, a type of dysentery characterized by anorexia or inability to eat, or vomiting upon eating and drinking. The main actions of this formula are to release the exterior, tonify qi, eliminate toxins, and stop vomiting. Because fasting dysentery is caused by Stomach and Spleen deficiencies, *Geng Mi* (Semen Oryzae) serves as an important ingredient in this formula to nourish the Stomach and Spleen and dispel dampness.

AUTHORS' COMMENTS

Bai Du San was originally designed for children, whose *yuan* (source) *qi* is still insufficient. A small amount of *Ren Shen* (Radix et Rhizoma Ginseng) is added to boost the *yuan qi* to help push out the exterior pathogenic factors. Today, however, the clinical applications of *Bai Du San* have been vastly expanded. In addition to the traditional indications, this formula is now commonly used for various types of patients (children, the elderly, and patients who are convalescent, postpartum, nursing, or with deficiency) and for various conditions (common colds, bronchitis, allergic dermatitis, urticaria, eczema and other disorders with itching of the skin characterized by wind-cold with dampness).

Bai Du San and *Jing Fang Bai Du San* (Schizonepeta and Saposhnikovia Powder to Overcome Pathogenic Influences) both treat beginning stages of suppuration, characterized by sores and ulcerations with fever, aversion to cold, absence of sweating, a thin, white tongue coating, and a superficial pulse. The differences between these two formulas are as follows:

- *Bai Du San* primarily treats wind-cold with dampness attacking a constitutionally deficient body. Treating suppuration, sores, and ulceration is its secondary function, and this secondary function may not be listed in some texts. *Bai Du San* contains *Ren Shen* (Radix et Rhizoma Ginseng) to treat skin disorders characterized by the presence of wind and cold **with** underlying weakness and deficiency.

- *Jing Fang Bai Du San* primarily treats initial stages of dermatological disorders with wind, cold, and dampness accumulating in the muscle layer. Localized redness and swelling along with exterior signs of cough, body aches, headache, and absence of sweating are present. *Jing Fang Bai Du San* does not contain *Ren Shen* (Radix et Rhizoma Ginseng), and primarily treats skin disorders characterized by wind and cold **without** underlying weakness and deficiency.[5]

References
1. *Shan Xi Yi Kan* (Shanxi Journal of Medicine) 1994;15(8):347.
2. *Shan Xi Zhong Yi* (Shanxi Chinese Medicine) 1999;7:297.
3. *Zhong Yi Ming Fang Lin Chuang Xin Yong* (Contemporary Clinical Applications of Classic Chinese Formulas) 2001;458.
4. *Cheng Du Zhong Yi Yao Da Xue Xue Bao* (Journal of Chengdu University of Traditional Chinese Medicine and Medicinals) 1997;2:26.
5. Wang MZ, et al. *Zhong Yi Xue Wen Da Ti Ku* (Questions and Answers on Traditional Chinese Medicine: Herbal Formulas).

Chapter 1 – Exterior-Releasing Formulas **Section 3 – Supporting [the Upright] and Releasing [the Exterior] Formulas**

Shēn Sū Yǐn (Ginseng and Perilla Leaf Decoction)

參蘇飲
参苏饮

Pinyin Name: *Shen Su Yin*
Literal Name: Ginseng and Perilla Leaf Decoction
Alternate Names: Ginseng and Perilla Drink, Ginseng and Perilla Decoction, Ginseng and Perilla Combination
Original Source: *Tai Ping Hui Min He Ji Ju Fang* (Imperial Grace Formulary of the Tai Ping Era) by the Imperial Medical Department in 1078-85

COMPOSITION

Ge Gen (Radix Puerariae Lobatae)	22.5g [6g]
Zi Su Ye (Folium Perillae)	22.5g [6g]
Qian Hu (Radix Peucedani)	22.5g [6g]
Ban Xia (Rhizoma Pinelliae), *chao* (dry-fried with ginger juice)	22.5g [6g]
Jie Geng (Radix Platycodonis)	15g [4g]
Chen Pi (Pericarpium Citri Reticulatae)	15g [4g]
Zhi Qiao (Fructus Aurantii), *chao* (dry-fried) with bran	15g [4g]
Mu Xiang (Radix Aucklandiae)	15g [4g]
Ren Shen (Radix et Rhizoma Ginseng)	22.5g [6g]
Fu Ling (Poria)	22.5g [6g]
Gan Cao (Radix et Rhizoma Glycyrrhizae)	15g [4g]

DOSAGE / PREPARATION / ADMINISTRATION

Grind the ingredients coarsely and cook 12g of the powder with 7 slices of *Sheng Jiang* (Rhizoma Zingiberis Recens) and 1 piece of *Da Zao* (Fructus Jujubae) in 1.5 bowls of water until it is reduced to 60%. Take the warm, strained decoction any time during the day. This formula may also be prepared as a decoction with the doses suggested in brackets above.

CHINESE THERAPEUTIC ACTIONS

1. Tonifies qi and releases the exterior
2. Expels phlegm and stops cough

CLINICAL MANIFESTATIONS

Exterior wind-cold syndrome with interior *tan yin* (phlegm retention): aversion to cold, fever, headache, nasal obstruction, coughing with profuse sputum, fullness and distention in the chest and diaphragm, fatigue, lethargy, shortness of breath, no desire to speak, a white tongue coating, and a superficial pulse.

CLINICAL APPLICATIONS

Common cold, influenza, bronchitis, pneumonia, and upper respiratory tract infection.

EXPLANATION

Shen Su Yin (Ginseng and Perilla Leaf Decoction) tonifies qi, dispels exterior pathogenic factors, expels phlegm, and stops cough. Clinically, patients will manifest wind-cold at the exterior (aversion to cold, fever, headache, and nasal obstruction) and *tan yin* (phlegm retention) in the interior (coughing with profuse sputum, epigastric fullness and distention in the chest and diaphragm). In addition, patients will have qi deficiency, with symptoms such as fatigue, lethargy, shortness of breath, and no desire to speak.

Ge Gen (Radix Puerariae Lobatae) and *Zi Su Ye* (Folium Perillae), the chief herbs, release exterior wind-cold factor. *Qian Hu* (Radix Peucedani), *Ban Xia* (Rhizoma Pinelliae), and *Jie Geng* (Radix Platycodonis) arrest cough, dissolve phlegm, and ventilate Lung qi. *Chen Pi* (Pericarpium Citri Reticulatae) and *Zhi Qiao* (Fructus Aurantii) regulate qi and expand the chest. *Mu Xiang* (Radix Aucklandiae) regulates qi, dries dampness, and unblocks stagnation. *Ren Shen* (Radix et Rhizoma Ginseng) tonifies qi, while *Fu Ling* (Poria) strengthens the Spleen and drains dampness. *Gan Cao* (Radix et Rhizoma Glycyrrhizae) harmonizes the middle *jiao* and the entire formula.

Chinese Herbal Formulas and Applications

Shēn Sū Yǐn (Ginseng and Perilla Leaf Decoction)

Shen Su Yin (Ginseng and Perilla Leaf Decoction)

Diagnosis	Signs and Symptoms	Treatment	Herbs
Exterior wind-cold and interior *tan yin* (phlegm retention) with underlying qi deficiency	• Aversion to cold, fever, headache, and nasal obstruction: exterior wind-cold • Coughing with profuse sputum, epigastric fullness and distention in the chest and diaphragm: interior *tan yin* (phlegm retention) • Fatigue, lethargy, shortness of breath, and no desire to speak: qi deficiency	• Tonifies qi and releases the exterior • Expels phlegm and stops cough	• *Ge Gen* (Radix Puerariae Lobatae) and *Zi Su Ye* (Folium Perillae) release exterior wind-cold and regulate qi. • *Qian Hu* (Radix Peucedani), *Ban Xia* (Rhizoma Pinelliae), and *Jie Geng* (Radix Platycodonis) ventilate Lung qi, expel phlegm, and arrest cough. • *Chen Pi* (Pericarpium Citri Reticulatae) and *Zhi Qiao* (Fructus Aurantii) regulate qi and expand the chest. • *Mu Xiang* (Radix Aucklandiae) regulates qi and unblocks stagnation. • *Ren Shen* (Radix et Rhizoma Ginseng) tonifies Lung and Spleen qi. • *Fu Ling* (Poria) strengthens the Spleen and drains dampness. • *Gan Cao* (Radix et Rhizoma Glycyrrhizae) harmonizes the middle *jiao* and the entire formula.

MODIFICATIONS

• For cough, wheezing, aversion to cold, and absence of perspiration caused by wind-cold, add *Ma Huang* (Herba Ephedrae), *Ku Xing Ren* (Semen Armeniacae Amarum), and *Jin Fei Cao* (Herba Inulae).

• For cough, wheezing and hurried respiration caused by wind-heat, add *Zhi Mu* (Rhizoma Anemarrhenae) and *Bei Mu* (Bulbus Fritillariae).

• For cough caused by Lung cold, add *Wu Wei Zi* (Fructus Schisandrae Chinensis) and *Gan Jiang* (Rhizoma Zingiberis).

• For cough caused by Lung heat, add *Ku Xing Ren* (Semen Armeniacae Amarum), *Huang Qin* (Radix Scutellariae), and *Sang Bai Pi* (Cortex Mori).

• When there is chest fullness and profuse sputum, add *Gua Lou Zi* (Semen Trichosanthis).

• For headache, add *Xi Xin* (Radix et Rhizoma Asari) and *Chuan Xiong* (Rhizoma Chuanxiong).

• If there is abdominal pain and diarrhea, add *Huo Xiang* (Herba Agastaches) and *Sha Ren* (Fructus Amomi).

• For patients with less qi stagnation, remove *Mu Xiang* (Radix Aucklandiae).

PHARMACOLOGICAL EFFECTS

1. **Antipyretic**: Administration of *Shen Su Yin* at 0.54g/kg in rabbits was associated with marked antipyretic effects in rabbits with artificially-induced fever.[1]

2. **Antitussive and expectorant**: Use of *Shen Su Yin* was associated with both antitussive and expectorant effects in mice.[2]

CLINICAL STUDIES AND RESEARCH

1. **Upper respiratory tract infection**: One study reported good results using modified *Shen Su Yin* to treat 39 patients with upper respiratory tract infection arising from various causes (34 with viral infection and 5 with bacterial infection). In addition to *Shen Su Yin* as the base formula, modifications included addition of *Huang Qin* (Radix Scutellariae) and *Zhe Bei Mu* (Bulbus Fritillariae Thunbergii) for phlegm and heat obstructing the Lung; and *Gua Lou* (Fructus Trichosanthis) for constipation. Of 39 cases, the study reported recovery in 33 cases within 4-17 days, and 6 more cases in 18-20 days.[3]

2. **Infection**: Use of modified *Shen Su Yin* was associated with good results in treating 60 patients with frequent infection caused by qi deficiency. The herbal treatment included *Ren Shen* (Radix et Rhizoma Ginseng), *Fu Ling* (Poria), *Chen Pi* (Pericarpium Citri Reticulatae), *Ban Xia* (Rhizoma Pinelliae), *Zi Su Ye* (Folium Perillae), *Qian Hu* (Radix Peucedani), *Ge Gen* (Radix Puerariae Lobatae), *Jie Geng* (Radix Platycodonis), *Chai Hu* (Radix Bupleuri), *Zhi Qiao* (Fructus Aurantii), *Mu Xiang* (Radix Aucklandiae), and *Zhi Gan Cao* (Radix et Rhizoma Glycyrrhizae Praeparata cum Melle). *Bai Bu* (Radix Stemonae) and *Xian He Cao* (Herba Agrimoniae) were added for chronic and frequent cough; *Bai Qian* (Rhizoma et Radix Cynanchi Stauntonii) and *Zi Wan* (Radix et Rhizoma Asteris) were added for cough with profuse white sputum; and *Huang Qi* (Radix Astragali) was added for profuse perspiration with weakness and fatigue. Of 60 cases, the study reported complete

Chapter 1 – Exterior-Releasing Formulas   **Section 3 – Supporting [the Upright] and Releasing [the Exterior] Formulas**

Shēn Sū Yǐn (Ginseng and Perilla Leaf Decoction)

recovery in 38 cases within 3 packs of herbs, in 20 cases after 4-6 packs, and 2 cases after 7-10 packs.[4]

3. **Common cold**: *Shen Su Yin* was used to treat 100 geriatric patients with common cold with good results. The treatment protocol was to use this formula in suspension form, using 20g of the herbs per dose two times daily. Of cases patients, the study reported complete recovery in 49 cases, significant improvement in 33 cases, moderate improvement in 9 cases, and no benefit in 9 cases. The overall rate of effectiveness was 91%.[5]

AUTHORS' COMMENTS

Shen Su Yin was originally designed to treat wind-cold invasion with pre-existing damp and phlegm accumulation in the interior. Thus, *Shen Su Yin* contains the ingredients of *Er Chen Tang* (Two-Cured Decoction) to dispel dampness and phlegm.

Bai Du San (Overcome Pathogenic Influences Powder) and *Shen Su Yin* both contain *Ren Shen* (Radix et Rhizoma Ginseng), and are exterior-releasing formulas used to treat wind-cold invasion in individuals with qi deficiency.

The differences between these formulas are as follows:

- *Bai Du San* relieves dampness lodging in the channels, causing body aches, neck and shoulder stiffness, and headache. It is better at treating wind-cold and dampness at the superficial level.

- *Shen Su Yin* dispels dampness affecting the Lung, manifesting in white nasal discharge, white sputum, chest congestion, and a feeling of heaviness. It focuses on dispelling exterior wind and cold, harmonizing *ying* (nutritive) *qi* and *wei* (defensive) *qi*, dispelling phlegm, and stopping cough. It is suitable for wind-cold invasion in those patients, especially young children or the elderly, who are qi deficient and have damp accumulation.

References

1. *Zhong Yao Yao Li Yu Lin Chuang* (Pharmacology and Clinical Applications of Chinese Herbs) 1992;8(3):6.
2. *Zhong Yao Yao Li Yu Lin Chuang* (Pharmacology and Clinical Applications of Chinese Herbs) 1992;8(3):6.
3. *Liao Ning Zhong Yi Za Zhi* (Liaoning Journal of Chinese Medicine) 1987;12:48.
4. *Fu Jian Zhong Yi Yao* (Fujian Chinese Medicine and Herbology) 1996;6:49.
5. *Xin Zhong Yi* (New Chinese Medicine) 1987;8:54.

Zài Zào Sǎn (Renewal Powder)

再造散

Pinyin Name: *Zai Zao San*
Literal Name: Renewal Powder
Alternate Names: *Chai Chao San*, Renewal Formula
Original Source: *Shang Han Liu Shu* (Six Texts on Cold-Induced Disorders) by Tao Hua in 1445

COMPOSITION

Huang Qi (Radix Astragali)	[6g]
Ren Shen (Radix et Rhizoma Ginseng)	[3g]
Gui Zhi (Ramulus Cinnamomi)	[3g]
Fu Zi (Radix Aconiti Lateralis Praeparata)	[3g]
Xi Xin (Radix et Rhizoma Asari)	[2g]
Qiang Huo (Rhizoma et Radix Notopterygii)	[3g]
Fang Feng (Radix Saposhnikoviae)	[3g]
Chuan Xiong (Rhizoma Chuanxiong)	[3g]
Gan Cao (Radix et Rhizoma Glycyrrhizae)	[1.5g]
Sheng Jiang (Rhizoma Zingiberis Recens), *wei* (roasted)	[3g]

DOSAGE / PREPARATION / ADMINISTRATION

The source text states to cook the ingredients with 2 pieces of *Da Zao* (Fructus Jujubae) in 2 large bowls of

water until the liquid is reduced to 1 large bowl. Add a small amount [3g] of dry-fried *Chi Shao* (Radix Paeoniae Rubra) and bring the decoction to a boil 3 times. Take the

130

Zài Zào Săn (Renewal Powder)

strained decoction while warm. Note: The doses of herbs are unavailable from the source text. Suggested doses are listed above in brackets.

CHINESE THERAPEUTIC ACTIONS

1. Strengthens yang and benefits qi
2. Releases the exterior and induces diaphoresis

CLINICAL MANIFESTATIONS

Exterior wind-cold with yang qi deficiency: headache, severe aversion to cold, mild fever, absence of perspiration, cold limbs, lassitude, drowsiness, preference for resting, a pale face, a low voice, a pale tongue with a thin, white coating, and a deep and forceless, or superficial, big and forceless pulse.

CLINICAL APPLICATIONS

Common cold and influenza.

EXPLANATION

Zai Zao San (Renewal Powder) treats exterior wind-cold in patients with yang qi deficiency. Exterior wind-cold causes headache, fever, aversion to cold, and absence of perspiration. Yang qi deficiency in the interior causes cold limbs, lassitude, drowsiness, a pale face, a low voice, and a forceless pulse. The wind-cold factor in this case usually cannot be dispelled by using only exterior-releasing

herbs, because the body is too weak to expel any pathogenic factors. Even if the wind-cold can be dispelled by the exterior-releasing herbs, the patient's yang qi may collapse after perspiration. Because of the intertwined interior and exterior nature in this case, the treatment plan must focus on dispelling exterior wind-cold and tonifying yang qi at the same time.

Huang Qi (Radix Astragali) and Ren Shen (Radix et Rhizoma Ginseng), the chief herbs, tonify qi and consolidate the exterior. Together, they prevent yang qi from collapsing as a result of perspiration. Gui Zhi (Ramulus Cinnamomi), Fu Zi (Radix Aconiti Lateralis Praeparata), and Xi Xin (Radix et Rhizoma Asari) release the exterior, strengthen yang, and disperse cold. Qiang Huo (Rhizoma et Radix Notopterygii), Fang Feng (Radix Saposhnikoviae), and Chuan Xiong (Rhizoma Chuanxiong) dispel exterior wind-cold and disperse cold. Dry-fried Chi Shao (Radix Paeoniae Rubra) restrains the warm herbs of this formula from injuring the blood and body fluids, without impairing their ability to induce perspiration. Gan Cao (Radix et Rhizoma Glycyrrhizae) moderates the formula and prevents excessive and profuse sweating. Da Zao (Fructus Jujubae) and roasted Sheng Jiang (Rhizoma Zingiberis Recens) nourish and warm the Spleen and Stomach to increase the production of qi and body fluids.

Zai Zao San (Renewal Powder)

Diagnosis	Signs and Symptoms	Treatment	Herbs
Exterior wind-cold with yang qi deficiency	• Headache, severe aversion to cold and mild fever: exterior wind-cold • Cold limbs, lassitude, drowsiness, preference for resting, a pale face, and a low voice: yang qi deficiency • Pale tongue with a thin, white coating: yang qi deficiency with exterior wind-cold • A superficial, big and forceless pulse: exterior wind-cold with yang qi deficiency	• Strengthens yang and benefits qi • Releases the exterior and induces diaphoresis	• Huang Qi (Radix Astragali) and Ren Shen (Radix et Rhizoma Ginseng) tonify qi and consolidate the exterior. • Gui Zhi (Ramulus Cinnamomi), Fu Zi (Radix Aconiti Lateralis Praeparata), and Xi Xin (Radix et Rhizoma Asari) release the exterior, strengthen yang, and disperse cold. • Qiang Huo (Rhizoma et Radix Notopterygii), Fang Feng (Radix Saposhnikoviae), and Chuan Xiong (Rhizoma Chuanxiong) dispel exterior wind-cold and disperse cold. • Chi Shao (Radix Paeoniae Rubra) restrains the warm herbs from injuring the blood and body fluids. • Gan Cao (Radix et Rhizoma Glycyrrhizae) moderates the formula and prevents excessive and profuse sweating. • Da Zao (Fructus Jujubae) and Sheng Jiang (Rhizoma Zingiberis Recens) nourish and warm the Spleen and Stomach to increase the production of qi and body fluids.

Chapter 1 – Exterior-Releasing Formulas **Section 3 – Supporting [the Upright] and Releasing [the Exterior] Formulas**

Má Huáng Fù Zǐ Xì Xīn Tāng
(Ephedra, Asarum, and Prepared Aconite Decoction)

麻黃附子細辛湯
麻黄附子细辛汤

Pinyin Name: *Ma Huang Fu Zi Xi Xin Tang*
Literal Name: Ephedra, Asarum, and Prepared Aconite Decoction
Alternate Names: *Ma Huang Fu Tzu Hsi Hsin Tang*, Ma-huang and Asarum Decoction, Ma-huang, Aconite and Asarum Decoction; Mahuang, Aconite and Asarum Combination
Original Source: *Shang Han Lun* (Discussion of Cold-Induced Disorders) by Zhang Zhong-Jing in the Eastern Han Dynasty

COMPOSITION

Ma Huang (Herba Ephedrae)	6g [5-6g]
Fu Zi (Radix Aconiti Lateralis Praeparata), *pao* (blast-fried)	1 pieces [3-9g]
Xi Xin (Radix et Rhizoma Asari)	6g [3g]

DOSAGE / PREPARATION / ADMINISTRATION

The source text states to cook *Ma Huang* (Herba Ephedrae) first with 10 cups [2,000 mL] of water until the liquid is reduced by 2 cups [400 mL]. Remove the foam from the top, add the rest of the ingredients, and cook until the liquid is reduced to 3 cups [600 mL]. Take 1 cup [200 mL] of the warm, strained decoction three times a day. Today, the decoction may be prepared using the doses suggested in brackets.

CHINESE THERAPEUTIC ACTIONS

Strengthens yang and releases the exterior

CLINICAL MANIFESTATIONS

Shaoyin syndrome complicated with *taiyang* syndrome: severe aversion to cold, absence of perspiration, mild or no fever, and a deep pulse.

CLINICAL APPLICATIONS

Rheumatic arthritis, bronchitis, bronchial asthma, influenza, common cold in weak or elderly patients, trigeminal neuralgia, facial paralysis, headache, and sciatica.

EXPLANATION

Ma Huang Fu Zi Xi Xin Tang (Ephedra, Asarum, and Prepared Aconite Decoction) treats *shaoyin* syndrome complicated with *taiyang* syndrome. The patient in this case has both interior yang deficiency and exterior wind-cold. This condition is characterized by symptoms such as severe aversion to cold, absence of perspiration, mild or no fever, and a deep pulse.

Ma Huang (Herba Ephedrae) releases wind-cold from the exterior. *Fu Zi* (Radix Aconiti Lateralis Praeparata) strengthens yang and warms the body in the interior. *Xi Xin* (Radix et Rhizoma Asari) performs two functions:

it assists *Ma Huang* (Herba Ephedrae) to release exterior cold, and it helps *Fu Zi* (Radix Aconiti Lateralis Praeparata) to strengthen interior yang and warm the body. This formula is thoughtfully crafted to release exterior wind-cold without damaging yang, and tonify interior yang without drawing wind-cold from the exterior into the interior.

MODIFICATIONS

- If there is headache and a wiry, tight pulse caused by wind-cold, add *Chuan Xiong* (Rhizoma Chuanxiong).
- For *bi zheng* (painful obstruction syndrome) due to wind, cold and dampness, add *Qiang Huo* (Rhizoma et Radix Notopterygii), *Du Huo* (Radix Angelicae Pubescentis), *Wei Ling Xian* (Radix et Rhizoma Clematidis) and *Qi She* (Agkistrodon).
- For chronic bronchitis or wheezing and dyspnea due to cold, add *Ban Xia* (Rhizoma Pinelliae), *Fu Ling* (Poria), *Chen Pi* (Pericarpium Citri Reticulatae), and *Gan Cao* (Radix et Rhizoma Glycyrrhizae).

CAUTIONS / CONTRAINDICATIONS

- *Ma Huang Fu Zi Xi Xin Tang* is contraindicated in patients with yang deficiency without exterior condition (i.e., they present with clinical manifestations such as cold body and extremities, aversion to cold, diarrhea with watery stools and undigested foods, and a deep, faint and fine pulse). The use of this formula in such cases may induce profuse perspiration leading to collapse of yang.
- Use of this formula is contraindicated during pregnancy and nursing.
- This formula is contraindicated in conditions characterized by heat, excess, and/or dryness.
- This formula must be used with extreme caution because all three herbs are extremely warm or hot. Inappropriate use of this formula may cause consumption of yin and

132

Chinese Herbal Formulas and Applications

Má Huáng Fù Zǐ Xì Xīn Tāng
(Ephedra, Asarum, and Prepared Aconite Decoction)

Ma Huang Fu Zi Xi Xin Tang (Ephedra, Asarum, and Prepared Aconite Decoction)

Diagnosis	Signs and Symptoms	Treatment	Herbs
Shaoyin syndrome complicated with *taiyang* syndrome	• Severe aversion to cold, absence of perspiration, mild or no fever: exterior (*taiyang*) condition • Deep pulse: interior (*shaoyin*) condition	• Releases the exterior • Strengthens yang	• *Ma Huang* (Herba Ephedrae) releases wind-cold from the exterior. • *Fu Zi* (Radix Aconiti Lateralis Praeparata) tonifies yang and warms the body. • *Xi Xin* (Radix et Rhizoma Asari) helps to release exterior wind-cold and strengthen interior yang.

body fluids and create side effects such as thirst, dry mouth and throat, insomnia, irritability, and others.[1]

PHARMACOLOGICAL EFFECTS

1. **Antiallergic**: *Ma Huang Fu Zi Xi Xin Tang* was effective in treating type I allergy model in mice. The proposed mechanism of action was the inhibition of IL-4 production.[2] L-ephedrine, a compound of *Ma Huang* (Herba Ephedrae) in *Ma Huang Fu Zi Xi Xin Tang*, is one of the major active constituents.[3] Potential therapeutic applications include passive cutaneous anaphylaxis and allergic rhinitis.[4,5]

2. **Anti-inflammatory**: In mice and rats, *Ma Huang Fu Zi Xi Xin Tang* showed significant anti-inflammatory activities by significantly inhibiting the increase in vascular permeability induced by acetic acid, the ear edema induced by arachidonic acid and phorbol ester, and the cutaneous extravasation induced by bradykinin and histamine. The study stated that the anti-inflammatory effects were exerted through the underlying mechanisms of preventing mediator release from mast cells and macrophages.[6]

CLINICAL STUDIES AND RESEARCH

1. **Rheumatic arthritis**: Use of herbal treatment was associated with 97.6% effectiveness in 85 patients (48 males and 37 females) between 5 and 62 years of age, with 10 days to 1 month history of illness with rheumatic arthritis. The herbal treatment contained *Ma Huang Fu Zi Xi Xin Tang* plus *Qiang Huo* (Rhizoma et Radix Notopterygii), *Du Huo* (Radix Angelicae Pubescentis), *Wei Ling Xian* (Radix et Rhizoma Clematidis), and others as the base formula. Additional modifications were made as follows: for *xing bi* (mobile painful obstruction), *Fang Feng* (Radix Saposhnikoviae), *Bai Zhi* (Radix Angelicae Dahuricae), *Qin Jiao* (Radix Gentianae Macrophyllae), and *Hai Feng Teng* (Caulis Piperis Kadsurae) were added; for *tong bi* (extremely painful obstruction), *Gan Jiang* (Rhizoma Zingiberis) and *Rou Gui* (Cortex Cinnamomi) were added; for *zhuo bi* (fixed painful obstruction), *Yi Yi Ren*

(Semen Coicis), and *Cang Zhu* (Rhizoma Atractylodis) were added; for *re bi* (heat painful obstruction), *Jin Yin Hua* (Flos Lonicerae Japonicae) and *Lian Qiao* (Fructus Forsythiae) were added; for *wan bi* (stubborn painful obstruction), *Di Long* (Pheretima) and *Quan Xie* (Scorpio) were added; and for chronic *bi zheng* (painful obstruction syndrome) with deficiency, *Sang Ji Sheng* (Herba Taxilli) and *Du Zhong* (Cortex Eucommiae) were added. The average duration of treatment was 12.5 days. Of 85 cases, the study reported complete recovery in 62 cases, significant improvement in 10 cases, moderate improvement in 11 cases, and no benefit in 2 cases.[7]

2. **Xiong bi (painful obstruction of the chest)**: Use of *Ma Huang Fu Zi Xi Xin Tang* plus *Gua Lou* (Fructus Trichosanthis), *Xie Bai* (Bulbus Allii Macrostemonis), and others was shown to be effective in treating *xiong bi* (painful obstruction of the chest). The herbs were given in decoction daily for 15 days per course of treatment, for 1-3 courses in total. Of 81 patients, the study reported significant improvement in 36 patients, moderate improvement in 38 patients, and no benefit in 7 patients. No recurrences were reported among 61 patients who came back for follow-up exams 6 months after the conclusion of the treatment.[8]

3. **Facial paralysis**: Complete recovery was reported in 118 of 132 patients having facial paralysis using *Ma Huang Fu Zi Xi Xin Tang*.[9]

4. **Sciatica**: Complete recovery was reported in 31 of 40 sciatica patients using *Ma Huang Fu Zi Xi Xin Tang* plus *Niu Xi* (Radix Achyranthis Bidentatae), *Mu Gua* (Fructus Chaenomelis), and others. The duration of treatment ranged from 14-40 days.[10]

HERB-DRUG INTERACTION

• **Ofloxacin-resistant infection**: Seven elderly patients with fever caused by bacterial infection of unknown origin failed to respond to ofloxacin 300 mg/day for 3 days. These patients were subsequently treated with *Ma Huang Fu Zi Xi Xin Tang* for 7 days, and the body temperature fell to

Chapter 1 – Exterior-Releasing Formulas   **Section 3 – Supporting [the Upright] and Releasing [the Exterior] Formulas**

Má Huáng Fù Zǐ Xì Xīn Tāng
(Ephedra, Asarum, and Prepared Aconite Decoction)

under 37°C (98.6°F) in all seven cases. The dose of *Fu Zi* (Radix Aconiti Lateralis Praeparata), one of the ingredients in this formula, was decreased by half.[11]

- **Drug-resistant Pseudomonas aeruginosa infection:** Use of *Ma Huang Fu Zi Xi Xin Tang* for 7 days was associated with good results in treating one elderly patient with fever and positive C-reactive protein (CRP) levels suffering from drug-resistant *Pseudomonas aeruginosa*. The treatment protocol was to administer 1,200 mg/day of dried extract made from *Ma Huang* (Herba Ephedrae) 4g, *Xi Xin* (Radix et Rhizoma Asari) 3g and *Fu Zi* (Radix Aconiti Lateralis Praeparata) 1g. The fever and CRP level returned to normal after 7 days of herbal treatment. The study concluded that *Ma Huang Fu Zi Xi Xin Tang* is a possible alternative for treatment of fever that does not respond to antibiotics for at least 3 days, especially for elderly patients.[12]

RELATED FORMULA

Má Huáng Fù Zǐ Gān Cǎo Tāng
(Ephedra, Prepared Aconite, and Licorice Decoction)

麻黃附子甘草湯
麻黄附子甘草汤

Pinyin Name: *Ma Huang Fu Zi Gan Cao Tang*
Literal Name: Ephedra, Prepared Aconite, and Licorice Decoction
Original Source: *Shang Han Lun* (Discussion of Cold-Induced Disorder) by Zhang Zhong-Jing in the Eastern Han Dynasty

Ma Huang (Herba Ephedrae)	6g [5-6g]
Fu Zi (Radix Aconiti Lateralis Praeparata), *pao* (blast-fried)	1 piece [3-9g]
Zhi Gan Cao (Radix et Rhizoma Glycyrrhizae Praeparata cum Melle)	6g [5-6g]

The source text states to cook *Ma Huang* (Herba Ephedrae) first with 10 cups [2,000 mL] of water until the liquid is reduced by 2 cups [400 mL]. Remove the foam from the top, add the rest of the ingredients, and cook until the liquid is reduced to 3 cups [600 mL]. Take 1 cup [200 mL] of the warm, strained decoction three times daily. Today, this formula may be prepared as a decoction with the doses suggested in brackets above.

Ma Huang Fu Zi Gan Cao Tang (Ephedra, Prepared Aconite, and Licorice Decoction) also treats combined *shaoyin* and *taiyang* syndromes. It focuses more on tonifying yang, dispelling exterior wind-cold, and promoting urination. Clinically, patients may show aversion to cold, body aches, absence of perspiration, slight fever, general

edema, shortness of breath, dysuria, and a deep, small pulse.

Ma Huang Fu Zi Xi Xin Tang and *Ma Huang Fu Zi Gan Cao Tang* both treat combined *shaoyin* and *taiyang* syndromes.

- *Ma Huang Fu Zi Xi Xin Tang* contains *Xi Xin* (Radix et Rhizoma Asari) and strongly releases the exterior and warms the interior.
- *Ma Huang Fu Zi Gan Cao Tang* contains *Gan Cao* (Radix et Rhizoma Glycyrrhizae), and is a gentler formula. It is usually used for patients having concurrent *taiyang* and *shaoyin* syndromes two to three days after the initial onset of illness.

AUTHORS' COMMENTS

Ma Huang Fu Zi Xi Xin Tang is a unique formula that treats both *shaoyin* and *taiyang* syndromes simultaneously, by tonifying interior yang and releasing exterior wind-cold. The diagnostic symptoms include severe aversion to cold, mild fever, and a deep pulse. The patient is often described to have severe aversion to cold that cannot be relieved by wearing extra clothing, a condition caused by simultaneous interior yang deficiency and exterior wind-cold.

One note of caution for both *Ma Huang Fu Zi Xi Xin Tang* and *Ma Huang Fu Zi Gan Cao Tang*: *Ma Huang* (Herba Ephedrae) must be used with yang tonics at the same time. This is because *Ma Huang* (Herba Ephedrae) is a very strong exterior-releasing herb, and if no yang or qi-tonifying herbs are added to supplement the deficient interior, the strong acrid and warm properties of *Ma Huang* (Herba Ephedrae) may cause profuse perspiration and lead to damage of both yin and yang, or even yang collapse.

One note of contraindication for *Ma Huang Fu Zi Xi Xin Tang* and *Ma Huang Fu Zi Gan Cao Tang*: these two formulas have only mild yang-tonic action. Thus, if the patient shows serious yang deficiency symptoms, such as watery diarrhea and a faint, fine pulse, do **not** use these formulas. The reason is that the exterior-releasing action of these two formulas is very strong and may cause profuse perspiration, while the yang-tonic action is too weak to make any difference in the interior. The best treatment in this situation is to administer *Si Ni Tang* (Frigid Extremities Decoction) first to tonify yang and warm the interior, and then subsequently treat the exterior syndrome.

Zai Zao San (Renewal Powder) and *Ma Huang Fu Zi Xi Xin Tang* are both indicated for patients with yang deficiency who contract wind-cold.

Má Huáng Fù Zǐ Xì Xīn Tāng
(Ephedra, Asarum, and Prepared Aconite Decoction)

- *Zai Zao San* treats more severe wind-cold symptoms with constitutional qi and yang deficiencies. It tonifies Spleen and Stomach qi and harmonizes the *ying* (nutritive) and *wei* (defensive) levels; at the same time it also tonifies yang and benefits qi.
- *Ma Huang Fu Zi Xi Xin Tang* treats yang deficiency with mild wind-cold symptoms.[13]

References

1. *Zhong Yao Ming Fang Yao Li Yu Ying Yong* (Pharmacology and Applications of Famous Herbal Formulas) 1989;72-73.
2. Ikeda Y, Iizuka A, Amagaya S, Ishige A, Komatsu Y, Fujihira E. Anti-type I allergic mechanisms of mao-bushi-saishin-to in mice. Jpn J Pharmacol. 2000 Jan;82(1):29-33.
3. Shibata H, Nabe T, Yamamura H, Kohno S. l-Ephedrine is a major constituent of Mao-Bushi-Saishin-To, one of the formulas of Chinese medicine, which shows immediate inhibition after oral administration of passive cutaneous anaphylaxis in rats. Inflamm Res. 2000 Aug;49(8):398-403.
4. Shibata H, Kohno S, Ohata K. Effects of mao-bushi-saishin-to (MBST) on experimental allergic models in rats. Arerugi. 1995 Oct;44(10):1234-40.
5. Shibata H, Kohno S, Ohata K. Effect of mao-bushi-saishin-to (MBST), a formula of Chinese medicines, on 48 hr homologous passive cutaneous anaphylaxis in rats. Arerugi. 1995 Sep;44(9):1167-75.
6. Ikeda Y, Iijima OT, Iizuka A, Ishige A, Amagaya S, Komatsu Y, Okada M, Abe C, Fujihira E. Anti-inflammatory effects of mao-bushi-saishin-to in mice and rats. Am J Chin Med. 1998;26(2):171-9.
7. *Chong Qing Zhong Yi Yao Za Zi* (Chongching Journal of Chinese Medicine and Medicinals), 1988;4:7.
8. *Zhong Yi Ming Fang Lin Chuang Xin Yong* (Contemporary Clinical Applications of Classic Chinese Formulas), 2001;651.
9. *Si Chuan Zhong Yi* (Sichuan Chinese Medicine), 1985;11:38.
10. *Zhong Yi Ming Fang Lin Chuang Xin Yong* (Contemporary Clinical Applications of Classic Chinese Formulas), 2001;651.
11. Kamei T. Toriumi Y. Tomioka H. Effect of Mao-bushi-saishin-to on infection of ofloxacin resistant bacteria and of unknown origin. Complementary Therapies in Medicine. 2000 Dec;8(4):276-9.
12. Kamei T, Kondoh T, Nagura S, Toriumi Y, Kumano H, Tomioka H. Improvement of C-reactive protein levels and body temperature of an elderly patient infected with Pseudomonas aeruginosa on treatment with Mao-bushi-saishin-to. Journal of Alternative & Complementary Medicine. 2000 Jun;6(3):235-9.
13. Wang MZ, et al. *Zhong Yi Xue Wen Da Ti Ku* (Questions and Answers on Traditional Chinese Medicine: Herbal Formulas).

Cōng Bái Qī Wèi Yǐn (Scallion Decoction with Seven Ingredients)
蔥白七味飲
葱白七味饮

Pinyin Name: *Cong Bai Qi Wei Yin*
Literal Name: Scallion Decoction with Seven Ingredients
Original Source: *Wai Tai Mi Yao* (Arcane Essentials from the Imperial Library) by Wang Tao in 752 A.D.

COMPOSITION

Cong Bai (Bulbus Allii Fistulosi), *qie* (sliced)	1 cup [9g]
Ge Gen (Radix Puerariae Lobatae), *qie* (sliced)	0.6 cup [9g]
Dan Dou Chi (Semen Sojae Praeparatum)	0.1 cup [6g]
Sheng Jiang (Rhizoma Zingiberis Recens), *qie* (sliced)	0.2 cup [6g]
Mai Dong (Radix Ophiopogonis)	0.6 cup [9g]
Di Huang (Radix Rehmanniae)	0.6 cup [9g]
Lao Shui (Aerated Water)	8 cups

DOSAGE / PREPARATION / ADMINISTRATION

The source text specifies to cook the herbs with 8 cups of *Lao Shui* (Aerated Water), a special aerated water which is prepared by repeatedly ladling water one thousand times in and out of a pail until bubbles form on the surface. Cook the herbs in this water until the liquid is reduced to one-third. Take the warm, strained decoction in three equally-divided doses daily. Today, the decoction may be prepared using the doses suggested in brackets.

CHINESE THERAPEUTIC ACTIONS

1. Releases the exterior
2. Nourishes yin and blood

Cōng Bái Qī Wèi Yǐn (Scallion Decoction with Seven Ingredients)

CLINICAL MANIFESTATIONS

Exterior wind-cold with underlying yin and blood deficiencies: headache, fever, mild aversion to cold, and absence of perspiration.

CLINICAL APPLICATIONS

Common cold, influenza, and respiratory tract infections.

EXPLANATION

Cong Bai Qi Wei Yin (Scallion Decoction with Seven Ingredients) treats patients with yin and blood deficiencies who have been attacked by exterior wind-cold. This formula is also suitable for treating those who have just recovered from a major illness, or those who suffered from severe hemorrhage and are now being attacked by exterior wind-cold.

To dispel the exterior wind-cold factor in individuals with underlying yin and blood deficiencies, exterior-releasing and tonic herbs should be employed concurrently. According to the theories of traditional Chinese medicine, blood and sweat are of the same origin. Therefore, if only exterior-releasing herbs are used to induce perspiration in blood deficient patients, depletion of blood may occur after perspiration. If only tonic herbs are used, the exterior cold factor cannot be resolved. Therefore, optimal treatment requires the use of exterior-releasing and tonic herbs simultaneously.

This formula contains *Cong Bai* (Bulbus Allii Fistulosi), *Ge Gen* (Radix Puerariae Lobatae), *Dan Dou Chi* (Semen Sojae Praeparatum), and *Sheng Jiang* (Rhizoma Zingiberis Recens) to release the exterior wind-cold. *Mai Dong* (Radix Ophiopogonis) and *Di Huang* (Radix Rehmanniae) tonify yin and blood to prevent any excessive sweating from damaging the body.

MODIFICATIONS

- If the aversion to cold is severe, add *Zi Su Ye* (Folium Perillae) and *Jing Jie* (Herba Schizonepetae).
- If the fever is prominent, add *Jin Yin Hua* (Flos Lonicerae Japonicae), *Lian Qiao* (Fructus Forsythiae), and *Huang Qin* (Radix Scutellariae).
- If there is bleeding (hematemesis, epistaxis, hemoptysis, or hematochezia), add *E Jiao* (Colla Corii Asini), *Ou Jie* (Nodus Nelumbinis Rhizomatis), and *San Qi* (Radix et Rhizoma Notoginseng).
- For indigestion, add *Chen Pi* (Pericarpium Citri Reticulatae).

CAUTIONS / CONTRAINDICATIONS

The source text advises avoiding *Wu Yi* (Fructus Ulmi Praeparatus) while taking *Cong Bai Qi Wei Yin*.

AUTHORS' COMMENTS

Cong Bai Qi Wei Yin is best for treating wind-cold invasion in patients with underlying yin and blood deficiencies caused by chronic illness or acute loss of blood through bleeding. The qi and blood of recovering patients are not fully restored back to normal levels. These individuals are much more susceptible to catching exterior pathogenic factors than healthy people. This formula mildly expels exterior wind-cold invasion while at the same time nourishes yin and blood.

Cong Bai Qi Wei Yin (Scallion Decoction with Seven Ingredients)

Diagnosis	Signs and Symptoms	Treatment	Herbs
Exterior wind-cold with underlying yin and blood deficiencies	• Headache, fever, mild aversion to cold, and absence of perspiration: exterior wind-cold • Recent history of bleeding: yin and blood deficiencies	• Releases the exterior • Nourishes yin and blood	• *Cong Bai* (Bulbus Allii Fistulosi), *Ge Gen* (Radix Puerariae Lobatae), *Dan Dou Chi* (Semen Sojae Praeparatum), and *Sheng Jiang* (Rhizoma Zingiberis Recens) release exterior wind-cold. • *Mai Dong* (Radix Ophiopogonis) and *Di Huang* (Radix Rehmanniae) tonify yin and blood.

Chinese Herbal Formulas and Applications

Jiā Jiǎn Wēi Ruí Tāng (Modified Polygonatum Odoratum Decoction)

加減葳蕤湯
加减葳蕤汤

Pinyin Name: *Jia Jian Wei Rui Tang*
Literal Name: Modified Polygonatum Odoratum Decoction
Original Source: *Tong Su Shang Han Lun* (Plain Version of Discussion of Cold-Induced Disorders) by Yu Gen-Chu in the Qing Dynasty

COMPOSITION

Yu Zhu (Rhizoma Polygonati Odorati)	6-9g [9g]
Cong Bai (Bulbus Allii Fistulosi)	2-3 stalks [6g]
Dan Dou Chi (Semen Sojae Praeparatum)	9-12g [9g]
Bo He (Herba Menthae)	3-4.5g [5g]
Jie Geng (Radix Platycodonis)	3-4.5g [5g]
Bai Wei (Radix et Rhizoma Cynanchi Atrati)	1.5-3g [3g]
Zhi Gan Cao (Radix et Rhizoma Glycyrrhizae Praeparata cum Melle)	1.5g [1.5g]
Da Zao (Fructus Jujubae)	2 pieces

DOSAGE / PREPARATION / ADMINISTRATION

The source text states to prepare the ingredients as a decoction. Take the strained decoction while warm. Today, the decoction may be prepared using the doses suggested in brackets.

CHINESE THERAPEUTIC ACTIONS

1. Nourishes yin and clears heat
2. Releases the exterior and induces diaphoresis

CLINICAL MANIFESTATIONS

Exterior wind-heat with chronic yin deficiency: headache, fever, slight aversion to wind and cold, absence of or slight perspiration, coughing with thick sputum that is difficult to expectorate, irritability, thirst, a dry throat, a red tongue body, and a rapid pulse.

CLINICAL APPLICATIONS

Common cold and influenza.

EXPLANATION

Jia Jian Wei Rui Tang (Modified Polygonatum Odoratum Decoction) treats patients with chronic yin deficiency who contract exterior wind-heat. Yin deficiency may develop into deficiency fire in the interior, which, when accompanied by exterior wind-heat, gives rise to symptoms such as headache, fever, cough, thirst, a dry throat, and slight aversion to wind and cold. Since yin and body fluids are deficient, there is no perspiration or just a slight perspiration. A red tongue body and a rapid pulse suggest heat in the interior.

The combination of exterior wind-heat and interior yin deficiency presents a dilemma: herbs that induce diaphoresis and release the exterior to dispel wind-heat are likely to damage yin, and herbs that nourish yin may bring exterior wind-heat into the interior and further complicate the illness. Thus, optimal treatment requires the concurrent use of both groups of herbs to maximize therapeutic effect and minimize adverse reactions.

Yu Zhu (Rhizoma Polygonati Odorati), the chief herb, nourishes yin and body fluids to moisten Lung dryness. Unlike most yin tonics, *Yu Zhu* (Rhizoma Polygonati Odorati) tonifies yin, moistens dryness, and replenishes fluids without creating stagnation. *Cong Bai* (Bulbus Allii Fistulosi), *Dan Dou Chi* (Semen Sojae Praeparatum), *Bo He* (Herba Menthae), and *Jie Geng* (Radix Platycodonis) release the exterior, ventilate the Lung, and stop coughing. *Bai Wei* (Radix et Rhizoma Cynanchi Atrati) cools the blood and clears heat to relieve irritability and thirst. *Bai Wei* (Radix et Rhizoma Cynanchi Atrati) is selected instead of the usual Lung heat-clearing herbs such as *Huang Qin* (Radix Scutellariae), because it cools the blood and clears heat without consuming yin. *Zhi Gan Cao* (Radix et Rhizoma Glycyrrhizae Praeparata cum Melle) and *Da Zao* (Fructus Jujubae) nourish and harmonize the middle *jiao*. This formula can clear deficiency heat and relieve exterior symptoms simultaneously.

MODIFICATIONS

• If there are severe exterior symptoms and signs, add *Ge Gen* (Radix Puerariae Lobatae) and *Fang Feng* (Radix Saposhnikoviae).

137

Chapter 1 – Exterior-Releasing Formulas   Section 3 – Supporting [the Upright] and Releasing [the Exterior] Formulas

Jiā Jiǎn Wéi Ruí Tāng (Modified Polygonatum Odoratum Decoction)

Jia Jian Wei Rui Tang (Modified Polygonatum Odoratum Decoction)

Diagnosis	Signs and Symptoms	Treatment	Herbs
Chronic yin deficiency accompanied by exterior wind-heat invasion	• Headache, fever, aversion to wind, and slight aversion to cold: exterior wind-heat • Coughing, irritability, thirst, and a dry throat: wind-heat consuming yin and body fluids • Red tongue body and a rapid pulse: presence of heat	• Nourishes yin and clears heat • Releases the exterior and induces diaphoresis	• *Yu Zhu* (Rhizoma Polygonati Odorati) nourishes yin and body fluids to moisten Lung dryness. • *Cong Bai* (Bulbus Allii Fistulosi), *Dan Dou Chi* (Semen Sojae Praeparatum), *Bo He* (Herba Menthae), and *Jie Geng* (Radix Platycodonis) release the exterior, ventilate the Lung, and stop coughing. • *Bai Wei* (Radix et Rhizoma Cynanchi Atrati) cools the blood and clears heat. • *Zhi Gan Cao* (Radix et Rhizoma Glycyrrhizae Praeparata cum Melle) and *Da Zao* (Fructus Jujubae) nourish and harmonize the middle *jiao*.

• When accompanied by irritability and thirst, add *Zhu Ye* (Herba Phyllostachys), *Sha Shen* (Radix Glehniae seu Adenophorae), and *Tian Hua Fen* (Radix Trichosanthis).

• For cough with a dry throat and sputum that is difficult to expectorate, add *Niu Bang Zi* (Fructus Arctii) and *Gua Lou Pi* (Pericarpium Trichosanthis).

CAUTIONS / CONTRAINDICATIONS
Jia Jian Wei Rui Tang is not suitable for exterior conditions that do not have underlying yin deficiency.

RELATED FORMULA
Wéi Ruí Tāng (Polygonatum Odoratum Decoction)
葳蕤湯
葳蕤汤
Pinyin Name: *Wei Rui Tang*
Literal Name: Polygonatum Odoratum Decoction
Original Source: *Bei Ji Qian Jin Yao Fang* (Thousands of Golden Prescriptions for Emergencies) by Sun Si-Miao in the Tang Dynasty

Yu Zhu (Rhizoma Polygonati Odorati)	60g [6g]
Bai Wei (Radix et Rhizoma Cynanchi Atrati)	60g [6g]
Ma Huang (Herba Ephedrae)	60g [6g]
Du Huo (Radix Angelicae Pubescentis)	60g [6g]
Ku Xing Ren (Semen Armeniacae Amarum)	60g [6g]
Chuan Xiong (Rhizoma Chuanxiong)	60g [6g]
Gan Cao (Radix et Rhizoma Glycyrrhizae)	60g [6g]

Qing Mu Xiang (Radix Aristolochiae)	60g [6g]
Shi Gao (Gypsum Fibrosum)	90g [9g]

The source text states to grind the ingredients into powder. Cook the powder [doses not specified by the source text] in 8 cups of water until the liquid is reduced to 3 cups. Take the strained decoction in three equally-divided doses while warm to induce sweating. Today, this formula may be prepared as a decoction using the doses suggested in brackets above.

Wei Rui Tang (Polygonatum Odoratum Decoction) releases exterior wind-heat, ventilates the Lung, clears Lung heat, and regulates qi and blood. Clinically, patients may show symptoms such as perspiration, heaviness of the whole body, dyspnea, lethargy, and dysuria.

Wei Rui Tang is a modification of *Ma Huang Xing Ren Gan Cao Shi Gao Tang* (Ephedra, Apricot Kernel, Licorice, and Gypsum Decoction) with the addition of yin-nourishing, heat-clearing, blood-regulating, and qi-activating herbs.

AUTHORS' COMMENTS
Jia Jian Wei Rui Tang treats yin-deficient patients who suffer from wind-heat invasion. Thus, it may be used in elderly and postpartum patients, and those with tonsillitis, pharyngitis, and tuberculosis, because they are more likely to have yin deficiency.

138

Chinese Herbal Formulas and Applications

Chapter 1 — Summary

— Exterior-Releasing Formulas

Exterior-releasing formulas treat exterior syndromes that are caused by the six exterior pathogenic factors of wind, cold, heat, summer-heat, dampness, and dryness. These formulas are grouped into three separate categories according to their different actions.

SECTION 1: ACRID AND WARM EXTERIOR-RELEASING FORMULAS

Name	Similarities	Differences
Ma Huang Tang (Ephedra Decoction)	Release wind-cold in exterior-excess conditions	Ventilates the Lung and relieves dyspnea
Da Qing Long Tang (Major Bluegreen Dragon Decoction)		Clears interior heat and relieves irritability
Hua Gai San (Canopy Powder)	Release wind-cold, ventilate the Lung, direct Lung qi downward	Strongly dispels phlegm
Jin Fei Cao San (Inula Powder)		Strongly releases the exterior
Gui Zhi Tang (Cinnamon Twig Decoction)	Releases wind-cold in exterior-deficient conditions	Harmonizes _ying_ (nutritive) and _wei_ (defensive) levels
Ge Gen Tang (Kudzu Decoction)	Release exterior wind-cold, relieve muscle stiffness and pain	Relieves muscle stiffness and pain in the neck
Jiu Wei Qiang Huo Tang (Nine-Herb Decoction with Notopterygium)		Relieves muscle stiffness and pain throughout the body
Xiang Su San (Cyperus and Perilla Leaf Powder)	Release wind-cold, regulate qi circulation	Regulates qi circulation in the middle _jiao_
Xing Su Yin (Apricot Kernel and Perilla Leaf Decoction)		Dispels wind-cold, dissolves phlegm, regulates qi circulation in the upper _jiao_
Shi Shen Tang (Ten-Immortal Decoction)		Regulates qi circulation in the upper and middle _jiaos_
Xiao Qing Long Tang (Minor Bluegreen Dragon Decoction)	Release exterior wind-cold, eliminate interior phlegm	Relieves severe wind-cold attack
She Gan Ma Huang Tang (Belamcanda and Ephedra Decoction)		Relieves phlegm stagnation
Cang Er Zi San (Xanthium Powder)	Release exterior wind, open the nasal orifices	Treats nasal disorders caused by exterior wind
Xin Yi San (Magnolia Flower Powder)		Treats nasal disorders caused by wind-cold
Qing Bi Tang (Clear the Nose Decoction)		Treats nasal disorders caused by damp-heat

Ma Huang Tang (Ephedra Decoction) and _Da Qing Long Tang_ (Major Bluegreen Dragon Decoction), containing both _Ma Huang_ (Herba Ephedrae) and _Gui Zhi_ (Ramulus Cinnamomi), are strong exterior-releasing formulas that treat severe cold at the exterior.

- _Ma Huang Tang_ is suitable for exterior excess-cold syndrome characterized by aversion to cold, fever, no perspiration, a superficial, tight pulse, and some degree of dyspnea or shortness of breath.

139

Chapter 1 — Summary

- *Da Qing Long Tang* is used when severe constriction caused by exterior excess cold generates some interior heat. The symptoms include all those found in the *Ma Huang Tang* syndrome, plus irritability.

Hua Gai San (Canopy Powder) and *Jin Fei Cao San* (Inula Powder), containing *Ma Huang* (Herba Ephedrae) but not *Gui Zhi* (Ramulus Cinnamomi), are moderate exterior-releasing formulas that treat exterior wind-cold with Lung dysfunction.
- *Hua Gai San* treats wind-cold attacking the Lung, causing fullness and congestion of the chest with coughing, wheezing, and dyspnea.
- *Jin Fei Cao San* treats exterior wind-cold syndromes in which the functioning of the Lung is severely compromised.

Gui Zhi Tang (Cinnamon Twig Decoction), containing *Gui Zhi* (Ramulus Cinnamomi) but not *Ma Huang* (Herba Ephedrae), is weaker than *Ma Huang Tang* (Ephedra Decoction) in its exterior-releasing effects. However, because it contains *Bai Shao* (Radix Paeoniae Alba), it can harmonize the *ying* (nutritive) and *wei* (defensive) levels. It is suitable for exterior deficiency-cold syndromes.

Ge Gen Tang (Kudzu Decoction) and *Jiu Wei Qiang Huo Tang* (Nine-Herb Decoction with Notopterygium) both release exterior wind-cold and relieve muscle stiffness and pain.
- *Ge Gen Tang* treats exterior-excess, wind-cold syndromes accompanied by stiffness and pain of the neck.
- *Jiu Wei Qiang Huo Tang* dispels exterior wind, cold, and dampness. It relieves muscle stiffness and pain throughout the body.

Xiang Su San (Cyperus and Perilla Leaf Powder), *Xing Su Yin* (Apricot Kernel and Perilla Leaf Decoction), and *Shi Shen Tang* (Ten-Immortal Decoction) have mild-to-moderate abilities to release exterior wind-cold. All have functions to regulate qi circulation and relieve interior qi stagnation.
- *Xiang Su San* treats exterior wind-cold with qi stagnation in the middle *jiao*, with signs and symptoms such as fever, aversion to cold, no perspiration, and chest and abdominal fullness and rigidity.
- *Xing Su Yin* is designed specially for children who have wind-cold attacking the exterior parts of the body, with signs and symptoms such as headache, fever, aversion to cold, nausea, vomiting, drooling, sticky nasal discharge, sneezing, and cough.
- *Shi Shen Tang* treats exterior wind-cold with qi stagnation in the upper and middle *jiaos*, with signs and symptoms such as fever, cough, dyspnea, chest congestion, hypochondriac distention, aversion to cold, and no perspiration.

Xiao Qing Long Tang (Minor Bluegreen Dragon Decoction) and *She Gan Ma Huang Tang* (Belamcanda and Ephedra Decoction) both release exterior wind-cold and treat interior phlegm retention.
- *Xiao Qing Long Tang* emphasizes releasing severe cases of wind-cold attack and dispels *yin* (invisible phlegm).
- *She Gan Ma Huang Tang* focuses on restoring the appropriate flow of Lung qi, relieving dyspnea, and eliminating *tan yin* (phlegm retention).

Cang Er Zi San (Xanthium Powder), *Xin Yi San* (Magnolia Flower Powder), and *Qing Bi Tang* (Clear the Nose Decoction) treat nasal disorders, such as sinusitis and rhinitis.
- *Cang Er Zi San* treats nasal disorders caused by wind, with signs and symptoms such as stuffy nose, thick, yellow nasal discharge, and frontal and temporal headaches.
- *Xin Yi San* treats nasal disorders caused by wind-cold, with signs and symptoms such as stuffy nose, profuse, clear and white nasal discharge, and headache.

Chinese Herbal Formulas and Applications

Chapter 1 — Summary

- *Qing Bi Tang* treats nasal disorders that are changing from an exterior (wind-cold or wind-heat) to an interior (damp-heat) condition. Clinical manifestations include stuffy nose, yellow and sticky nasal discharge, sneezing, fatigue, headache, an itchy nose and throat, a decreased sense of smell, and decreased energy level.

SECTION 2: ACRID AND COLD EXTERIOR-RELEASING FORMULAS

Name	Similarities	Differences
Sang Ju Yin (Mulberry Leaf and Chrysanthemum Decoction)	Release exterior wind-heat	Stronger functions to ventilate the Lung to suppress cough
Yin Qiao San (Honeysuckle and Forsythia Powder)		Stronger functions to clear heat, relieve sore throat, and release the exterior
Ma Xing Gan Shi Tang (Ephedra, Apricot Kernel, Licorice, and Gypsum Decoction)	Release exterior wind-heat, clear Lung heat	Ventilates the Lung, clears Lung heat, and relieves cough and dyspnea.
Yue Bi Tang (Maidservant from Yue Decoction)		Eliminates water accumulation and relieves edema
Sheng Ma Ge Gen Tang (Cimicifuga and Kudzu Decoction)	Release exterior pathogenic factors from the muscle layer	Raises yang qi and promotes the eruption of measles
Zhu Ye Liu Bang Tang (Lophatherum, Tamarisk and Arctium Decoction)		Clears Lung and Stomach heat and promotes the eruption of measles
Chai Ge Jie Ji Tang (Bupleurum and Kudzu Decoction to Release the Muscle Layer)		Resolves the transformation of *taiyang* wind-cold into *yangming* heat
Cong Chi Jie Geng Tang (Scallion, Prepared Soybean, and Platycodon Decoction)		Releases wind-heat and clears Lung heat
Ning Sou Wan (Quiet the Cough Pill)	Clear Lung heat, suppress cough	Releases exterior wind-heat, clears Lungs heat
Dun Sou San (Long-Bout Cough Powder)		Clears heat and dissolves phlegm
Zhi Sou San (Stop Coughing Powder)		Releases exterior wind, dissolves phlegm
Jing Jie Lian Qiao Tang (Schizonepeta and Forsythia Decoction)	Dispel wind-heat from the upper parts of the body	Dispels heat, fire, and toxins, treats ear and nose disorders
Xin Yi Qing Fei Yin (Magnolia Decoction to Clear the Lung)		Clears Lung heat, treats lung and nose disorders

Sang Ju Yin (Mulberry Leaf and Chrysanthemum Decoction) and **Yin Qiao San** (Honeysuckle and Forsythia Powder) are cool, acrid formulas that release exterior wind-heat to treat the initial stages of warm febrile disorders.

- *Sang Ju Yin* has a stronger effect to ventilate the Lung to arrest cough. It treats exterior wind-warmth syndrome characterized by reversed flow of Lung qi and other mild exterior wind-heat symptoms.
- *Yin Qiao San* has stronger heat-clearing and exterior-releasing effects. It is suitable for severe wind-heat conditions or *wen bing* (warm disease) disorders, with symptoms of heat and toxicity, such as fever, thirst, and sore throat.

Ma Huang Xing Ren Gan Cao Shi Gao Tang (Ephedra, Apricot Kernel, Licorice, and Gypsum Decoction) and **Yue Bi Tang** (Maidservant from Yue Decoction) both release exterior wind-heat and clear Lung heat.

141

EXTERIOR-RELEASING FORMULAS

Chapter 1 — Summary

- *Ma Huang Xing Ren Gan Cao Shi Gao Tang* has stronger functions to clear Lung heat and ventilate the Lung. It treats Lung heat caused by exterior pathogenic factors, with symptoms such as unremitting fever, thirst with a desire to drink, coughing and dyspnea.
- *Yue Bi Tang* releases the exterior and eliminates water accumulation. It treats conditions in which there are signs and symptoms of aversion to wind, spontaneous sweating, absence of thirst, and generalized edema.

Sheng Ma Ge Gen Tang (Cimicifuga and Kudzu Decoction), **Zhu Ye Liu Bang Tang** (Lophatherum, Tamarisk and Arctium Decoction), **Chai Ge Jie Ji Tang** (Bupleurum and Kudzu Decoction to Release the Muscle Layer), and **Cong Chi Jie Geng Tang** (Scallion, Prepared Soybean, and Platycodon Decoction) have similar functions to release exterior pathogenic factors from the muscle layer.

- *Sheng Ma Ge Gen Tang* lifts yang qi, relieves the muscles, and enhances the eruption of measles. It treats incomplete eruption of measles with fever and absence of sweating.
- *Zhu Ye Liu Bang Tang* clears Lung and Stomach heat, eliminates toxins, and promotes the eruption of measles.
- *Chai Ge Jie Ji Tang* dispels exterior factors from the muscles and clears heat, and is indicated in conditions in which the disease factor is turning from wind-cold into wind-heat. It may be used to treat heat affecting the *yangming* channel, or heat affecting all three yang channels (*taiyang*, *yangming*, and *shaoyang*).
- *Cong Chi Jie Geng Tang* is a mild formula used to treat the early stage of wind-heat syndrome. It may be used for mild cases of Lung heat with thirst and a sore throat.

Ning Sou Wan (Quiet the Cough Pill), **Dun Sou San** (Long-Bout Cough Powder), and **Zhi Sou San** (Stop Coughing Powder) clear heat and suppress cough.

- *Ning Sou Wan* releases exterior wind-heat and clears Lung heat to relieve cough.
- *Dun Sou San* clears heat and dissolves phlegm to suppress cough.
- *Zhi Sou San* releases exterior wind and dissolves phlegm to stop cough.

Jing Jie Lian Qiao Tang (Schizonepeta and Forsythia Decoction) and **Xin Yi Qing Fei Yin** (Magnolia Decoction to Clear the Lung) both dispel wind-heat from the upper parts of the body.

- *Jing Jie Lian Qiao Tang* dispels heat, fire, and toxins to treat inflammation and swelling of the ears and nose.
- *Xin Yi Qing Fei Yin* clears Lung heat to treat obstruction and congestion of the nose.

Chinese Herbal Formulas and Applications

Chapter 1 — Summary

SECTION 3: SUPPORTING [THE UPRIGHT] AND RELEASING [THE EXTERIOR] FORMULAS

Name	Similarities	Differences
Bai Du San (Overcome Pathogenic Influences Powder)	Release exterior wind-cold, tonify qi	Tonifies qi, dispels wind, cold and dampness
Shen Su Yin (Ginseng and Perilla Leaf Decoction)		Tonifies Lung and Spleen qi, dispels phlegm, and stops cough
Zai Zao San (Renewal Powder)	Release exterior wind-cold, strengthen yang	Strengthens yang and qi
Ma Huang Fu Zi Xi Xin Tang (Ephedra, Asarum, and Prepared Aconite Decoction)		Strongly strengthens yang
Cong Bai Qi Wei Yin (Scallion Decoction with Seven Ingredients)	Releases exterior wind-cold	Nourishes yin and blood
Jia Jian Wei Rui Tang (Modified Polygonatum Odoratum Decoction)	Releases exterior wind-heat	Nourishes yin

Bai Du San (Overcome Pathogenic Influences Powder) and **Shen Su Yin** (Ginseng and Perilla Leaf Decoction) both release exterior wind-cold. They both contain *Ren Shen* (Radix et Rhizoma Ginseng) to tonify qi in individuals with underlying weakness and deficiency.

- *Bai Du San* relieves dampness lodged in the channels, causing body aches, neck and shoulder stiffness, and headache. It is better at treating wind-cold and dampness at the superficial level.
- *Shen Su Yin* focuses on dispelling dampness affecting the Lung, manifesting in white nasal discharge, white sputum, chest congestion, and a feeling of heaviness. It is stronger in regulating Lung qi and dissolving phlegm. It is better for treating invasion of wind-cold in individuals who are qi deficient and who also have interior *tan yin* (phlegm retention).

Zai Zao San (Renewal Powder), acrid and warm, strengthens yang and nourishes qi while inducing sweating. It is suitable for patients with yang qi deficiency in the interior and excess cold at the exterior.

Ma Huang Fu Zi Xi Xin Tang (Ephedra, Asarum, and Prepared Aconite Decoction) is a unique formula that treats both *shaoyin* (interior) and *taiyang* (exterior) syndromes simultaneously, by strengthening interior yang and releasing exterior wind-cold.

Cong Bai Qi Wei Yin (Scallion Decoction with Seven Ingredients) nourishes yin and blood and releases exterior pathogenic factors. It is suitable for exterior wind-cold syndrome in patients with constitutional yin and blood deficiencies.

Jia Jian Wei Rui Tang (Modified Polygonatum Odoratum Decoction) nourishes yin and releases exterior factors to treat exterior wind-heat syndrome accompanied by yin deficiency.

Chapter 2

— Downward Draining Formulas

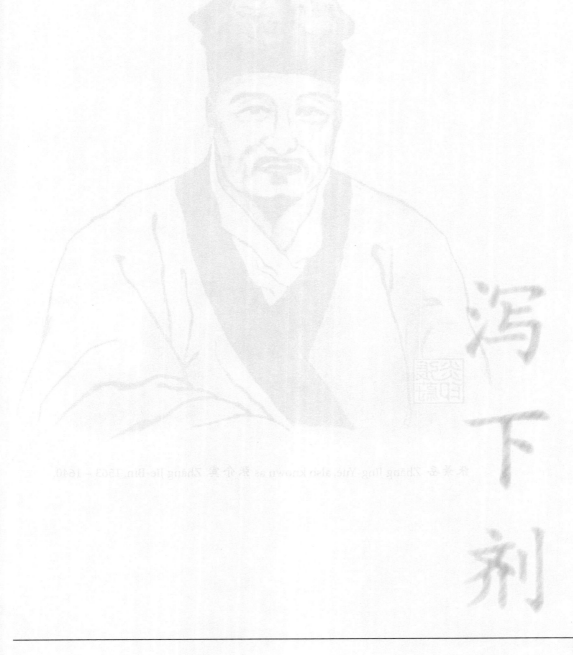

张景岳 Zhāng Jǐng-Yuè

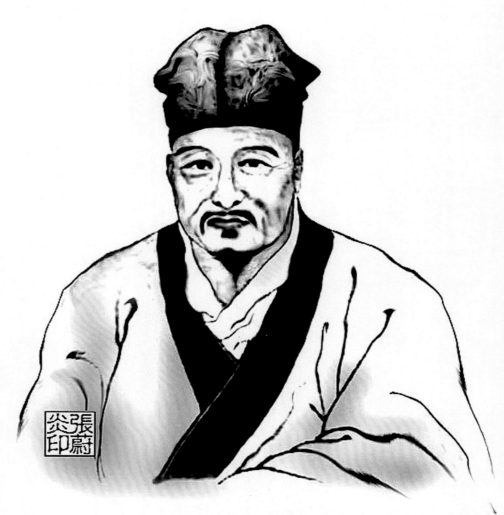

张景岳 Zhāng Jǐng-Yuè, also known as 张介宾 Zhāng Jiè-Bín, 1563 – 1640.

张景岳 Zhāng Jǐng-Yuè

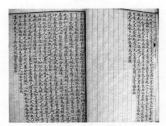

景岳全书 *Jing Yue Quan Shu* (Collected Treatises of [Zhang] Jing Yue) in 1624.

Born into a wealthy military family, Zhang Jing-Yue was intensely curious and could afford the time and money to explore many different interests. Zhang studied astrology, philosophy, music, medicine, and many other subjects. Of all the topics, Zhang was most interested in and excelled in medicine. He specialized in and studied the *Huang Di Nei Jing* (Yellow Emperor's Inner Classic) for 30 years.

During the Ming dynasty when Zhang practiced medicine, many physicians over-prescribed the use of herbs that were acrid, hot and drying, and consequently injured yin and body fluids. Zhang proposed and used tonic herbs to rescue damaged yin and body fluids, and significantly influenced the practice of Traditional Chinese Medicine. Many tonic formulas he used then are still frequently prescribed today.

Zhang published many texts in his lifetime, and is best known for 景岳全书 *Jing Yue Quan Shu* (Collected Treatises of [Zhang] Jing Yue) in 1624. This comprehensive text discussed many aspects of medicine, including theory, treatment strategies, herbs, formulas, gynecology, pediatrics, and more. Because of his military background, Zhang also proposed treatment strategies based on miliary tactics, such as 八阵 *Ba Zhen* (Eight Arrays of Formulas): 补 *bu* (tonic) formulas to treat deficiency, 和 *he* (harmonizing) formulas to treat disharmony, 攻 *gong* (attack) formulas to treat excess, 散 *san* (disperse) formulas to disperse exterior conditions, 寒 *han* (cold) formulas to clear heat, 热 *re* (hot) formulas to dispel cold, 固 *gu* (stabilize) formulas to stop loss (of body fluids), and 因 *yin* (pattern-specific) formulas to treat specific disorders.

As a great compliment, Zhang Jing-Yue is remembered by many as the reincarnation of Zhang Zhong-Jing.

Examples of formulas of Zhang Jing-Yue that are in common use today include:
- *Zhou Che Wan* (Vessel and Vehicle Pill)
- *Ji Chuan Jian* (Benefit the River [Flow] Decoction)
- *Chai Hu Shu Gan San* (Bupleurum Powder to Spread the Liver)
- *Tong Xie Yao Fang* (Important Formula for Painful Diarrhea)
- *Yu Nu Jian* (Jade Woman Decoction)
- *Zuo Gui Wan* (Restore the Left [Kidney] Pill)
- *You Gui Wan* (Restore the Right [Kidney] Pill)
- *Tai Shan Pan Shi San* (Powder that Gives the Stability of Mount Tai)

Dynasties & Kingdoms	Year
Xia Dynasty 夏	2100-1600 BCE
Shang Dynasty 商	1600-1100 BCE
Zhou Dynasty 周	1100-221 BCE
Qin Dynasty 秦	221-207 BCE
Han Dynasty 漢	206 BCE-220
Three Kingdoms 三國	220-280
Western Jin Dynasty 西晉	265-316
Eastern Jin Dynasty 東晉	317-420
Northern and Southern Dynasties 北南朝	420-581
Sui Dynasty 隋	581-618
Tang Dynasty 唐	618-907
Five Dynasties 五代	907-960
Song Dynasty 宋	960-1279
Liao Dynasty 遼	916-1125
Jin Dynasty 金	1115-1234
Yuan Dynasty 元	1271-1368
Ming Dynasty 明	**1368-1644**
Qing Dynasty 清	1644-1911
Republic of China 中華民國	1912-Present Day
People's Republic of China 中華人民共和國	1949-Present Day

Chapter 2 – Downward Draining Formulas

Table of Contents

Chapter 2. Downward Draining Formulas · **145**
Biography of Zhang Jing-Yue · 146

Section 1. Cold Purgatives · **152**
Da Cheng Qi Tang (Major Order the Qi Decoction) · 152
   Fu Fang Da Cheng Qi Tang (Revised Major Order the Qi Decoction) · · · · · · · · · · · · · · · · · 155
   Jia Jian Cheng Qi Tang (Modified Order the Qi Decoction) · 156
Xiao Cheng Qi Tang (Minor Order the Qi Decoction) · 158
Tiao Wei Cheng Qi Tang (Regulate the Stomach and Order the Qi Decoction) · · · · · · · · · · 160
Da Xian Xiong Tang (Major Sinking into the Chest Decoction) · 161
   Da Xian Xiong Wan (Major Sinking into the Chest Pill) · 163
Yi Zi Tang (Yi Word Decoction) · 164
   Qing Chang Tang (Clear the Intestines Decoction) · 165

Section 2. Warm Purgatives · **166**
Da Huang Fu Zi Tang (Rhubarb and Prepared Aconite Decoction) · 166
Wen Pi Tang (Warm the Spleen Decoction) · 169
San Wu Bei Ji Wan (Three-Substance Pill for Emergencies) · 171
   San Wu Bai San (Three-Substance White Powder) · 172

Section 3. Moist Laxatives · **174**
Ma Zi Ren Wan (Hemp Seed Pill) · 174
   Wu Ren Wan (Five-Seed Pill) · 176
Run Chang Wan (Moisten the Intestines Pill) · 177
   Run Chang Wan (Moisten the Intestines Pill) · 178
   Ma Zi Run Chang Wan (Hemp Seed Pill to Moisten the Intestines) · · · · · · · · · · · · · · · · · 178
Ji Chuan Jian (Benefit the River [Flow] Decoction) · 179

Section 4. Harsh Expellants (Cathartics) · **181**
Shi Zao Tang (Ten-Jujube Decoction) · 181
   Kong Xian Dan (Control Mucus Special Pill) · 182
Zhou Che Wan (Vessel and Vehicle Pill) · 184
Shu Zao Yin Zi (Spread and Unblock Decoction) · 185

Section 5: Purgative and Tonic Formulas · **187**
Huang Long Tang (Yellow Dragon Decoction) · 187
   Xin Jia Huang Long Tang (Newly-Augmented Yellow Dragon Decoction) · · · · · · · · · · · · 189
Zeng Ye Cheng Qi Tang (Increase the Fluids and Order the Qi Decoction) · · · · · · · · · · · · · 190
   Cheng Qi Yang Ying Tang (Order the Qi and Nourish the Nutritive Qi Decoction) · · · · · 192

Downward Draining Formulas (Summary) · **193**

Chapter 2 — Overview

— Downward Draining Formulas

Definition: Downward draining formulas consist mostly of purgative herbs, and function to pass stools, drain excess heat, dispel accumulation and stagnation from the Stomach and Intestines, and drastically eliminate water retention and cold stagnation. This method of treatment is known as *xia fa* (draining downward), one of the *ba fa* (eight treatment methods) described in the *Huang Di Nei Jing* (Yellow Emperor's Inner Classic) in the first or second century, A.D.

I n general, downward draining formulas treat interior excess syndromes characterized by constipation and water retention. Constipation may be hot or cold in nature, and the patients may be generally healthy or have pre-existing underlying deficiencies. To address varying disease characteristics and patient constitutions, these formulas have been designed with distinct functions, to be carefully prescribed. These formulas' complexities and distinctiveness are reflected in five subcategories of action.

"Interior excess syndrome" refers to a wide variety of disorders and illnesses, including qi stagnation, blood stagnation, phlegm retention, food stagnation, constipation, water retention, parasitic infestation, and others. This chapter primarily discusses downward draining formulas that treat interior excess syndromes characterized by constipation and water retention. Treatment of other interior excess conditions is discussed in other chapters.

SUBCATEGORIES OF ACTION

1. Cold Purgatives

These formulas eliminate interior excess conditions involving heat stagnation or accumulation. Common clinical manifestations include constipation, abdominal fullness, distention, or pain. In severe cases, there may be tidal fever, a yellow tongue coating, and an excess pulse.

Herbs commonly used to purge interior heat and excess include *Da Huang* (Radix et Rhizoma Rhei) and *Mang Xiao* (Natrii Sulfas). Formulas commonly used to purge interior heat and excess include *Da Cheng Qi Tang* (Major Order the Qi Decoction), *Xiao Cheng Qi Tang* (Minor Order the Qi Decoction) and *Da Xian Xiong Tang* (Major Sinking into the Chest Decoction).

2. Warm Purgatives

Warm purgative formulas address interior excess cold syndromes. Common clinical manifestations include constipation, epigastric and abdominal fullness and distention, abdominal pain alleviated by warmth, cold to icy extremities, a white, slippery tongue coating, and a deep, tight pulse.

Interior excess cold syndromes are treated with herbs that are warm or hot (to disperse cold) with downward draining functions (to dispel interior excess), such as *Fu Zi* (Radix Aconiti Lateralis Praeparata), *Gan Jiang* (Rhizoma Zingiberis), and *Ba Dou* (Semen Crotonis). Formulas commonly used to purge interior excess cold include *Da Huang Fu Zi Tang* (Rhubarb and Prepared Aconite Decoction), *Wen Pi Tang* (Warm the Spleen Decoction), and *San Wu Bei Ji Wan* (Three-Substance Pill for Emergencies). Interior-warming formulas may be added to these warm purgative formulas enhance the overall therapeutic impact.

Interior excess syndromes are characterized by constipation and water retention.

Chapter 2 – Downward Draining Formulas

Chapter 2 — Overview

3. Moist Laxatives

Moist laxative formulas treat constipation caused by heat and dryness in the Intestines, which damage yin. These formulas lubricate the Intestines to promote normal bowel movements. Most formulas in this subcategory are composed of moist laxatives and cold purgatives.

Representative herbs include *Huo Ma Ren* (Fructus Cannabis), *Ku Xing Ren* (Semen Armeniacae Amarum), *Tao Ren* (Semen Persicae), and *Yu Li Ren* (Semen Pruni). Representative formulas include *Ma Zi Ren Wan* (Hemp Seed Pill) and *Run Chang Wan* (Moisten the Intestines Pill).

Moist laxatives also treat constipation associated with chronic illness, in which there is Kidney yang deficiency or *ming men* (life gate) fire insufficiency. Exemplar herbs that warm and tonify the Kidney and lubricate the Intestines include *Rou Cong Rong* (Herba Cistanches) and *Dang Gui* (Radix Angelicae Sinensis). One representative formula is *Ji Chuan Jian* (Benefit the River [Flow] Decoction).

4. Harsh Expellants (Cathartics)

These formulas treat excess syndromes involving interior accumulation of water and heat. This group of downward draining formulas eliminates internal swelling and excess water accumulation through defecation and urination. Clinical applications of harsh expellants include treatment of hydrothorax, ascites, edema, and difficulties in urination and defecation. These formulas are potentially toxic and drastic in effect, and should be used with extreme caution, especially in individuals who have generalized deficiencies.

Harsh expellant formulas eliminate swelling and excess water through defecation and urination.

Herbs with potent action to eliminate excess syndromes of interior water accumulation include *Yuan Hua* (Flos Genkwa), *Gan Sui* (Radix Kansui), and *Qian Niu Zi* (Semen Pharbitidis). Exemplar formulas include *Shi Zao Tang* (Ten-Jujube Decoction) and *Zhou Che Wan* (Vessel and Vehicle Pill).

5. Purgative and Tonic Formulas

These formulas treat constipation characterized by concurrent internal excess and deficiency. This syndrome requires the use of both downward draining and tonifying methods to ensure that the stools are moved and the qi is not damaged. These two methods cannot be used individually if both conditions are present. If only the downward draining method is employed, the qi may consequently become more deficient. If only the tonifying method is used, then the constipated stool may become more stagnant.

Downward-draining formulas tend to consume Stomach qi: they should be discontinued immediately once the desired effects have been achieved.

Downward draining herbs commonly used to drain interior excess include *Da Huang* (Radix et Rhizoma Rhei) and *Mang Xiao* (Natrii Sulfas). Tonic herbs frequently used to tonify interior deficiency include *Ren Shen* (Radix et Rhizoma Ginseng), *Dang Gui* (Radix Angelicae Sinensis), *Di Huang* (Radix Rehmanniae), and *Xuan Shen* (Radix Scrophulariae). Exemplar formulas having both downward draining and tonic actions include *Xin Jia Huang Long Tang* (Newly-Augmented Yellow Dragon Decoction) and *Zeng Ye Cheng Qi Tang* (Increase the Fluids and Order the Qi Decoction).

CAUTIONS / CONTRAINDICATIONS

- Downward draining formulas are designed to treat interior excess syndromes. If patients have both exterior and interior excess symptoms, then one should dispel the exterior factor first, before eliminating the interior excess. In some cases, both exterior and interior factors may be dispelled at the same time.
- Downward draining formulas should be used with caution during pregnancy, in postpartum and nursing mothers, in the elderly and infants and children, or any individual with bleeding disorders, or underlying qi, blood, and/or body fluid deficiencies. In general, for these patients, use tonic herbs either after, or in conjunction with, the downward draining formulas.

Chinese Herbal Formulas and Applications

Chapter 2 — Overview

- Since most of the downward draining formulas have a tendency to consume Stomach qi, they should be discontinued immediately once the desired effects have been achieved.
- To prevent further consumption of Stomach qi, avoid foods that are oily, greasy, or hard to digest.

PROCESSING

Da Huang (Radix et Rhizoma Rhei) and *Mang Xiao* (Natrii Sulfas) are commonly used in downward draining formulas. To potentiate the downward draining effect, *Da Huang* (Radix et Rhizoma Rhei) is usually post-decocted, and *Mang Xiao* (Natrii Sulfas) is usually dissolved in the decoction immediately prior to ingestion. Cooking these two herbs in the decoction with the rest of the herbs compromises the overall potency and effectiveness of the formulas.

PHARMACOLOGICAL EFFECTS & CLINICAL APPLICATIONS

Downward draining formulas primarily treat gastrointestinal disorders, such as constipation, intestinal obstruction, and related imbalances.

> *Proper formula selection depends on the patient's overall constitution and the nature of the constipation.*

1. **Constipation**: Almost all downward draining formulas have purgative and/or laxative effects, and commonly treat constipation. Downward draining formulas have different potencies and mechanisms of action. Proper formula selection depends on the characteristics of the constipation and the overall constitution of the patient. *Da Cheng Qi Tang* (Major Order the Qi Decoction) and *Xiao Cheng Qi Tang* (Minor Order the Qi Decoction) have potent purgative actions to treat moderate to severe constipation. Their mechanism of action involves stimulating the intestines to increase contraction and peristalsis.[1,2] *Ma Zi Ren Wan* (Hemp Seed Pill) and *Run Chang Wan* (Moisten the Intestines Pill) have moderate laxative effects to treat mild to moderate constipation. Their mechanisms of action are lubrication of the intestines and promotion of bowel movement.[3]

2. **Intestinal obstruction**: Some potent downward draining formulas, such as *Da Cheng Qi Tang* (Major Order the Qi Decoction) and *Da Xian Xiong Tang* (Major Sinking into the Chest Decoction), treat intestinal obstruction by strongly stimulating the intestines to promote evacuation of the bowels.[4,5,6]

3. **Gastrointestinal disorders**: Downward draining formulas treat gastrointestinal disorders, such as acute abdominal pain,[7] chronic colitis,[8] chronic gastritis,[9] peptic ulcer disease,[10] acute gastroenteritis,[11] acute appendicitis,[12] and post-surgical constipation.[13]

References

1. *Zhong Guo Zhong Xi Yi Jie He Za Zhi* (Chinese Journal of Integrative Chinese and Western Medicine) 1993;(1):33.
2. *Zhong Yi Fang Ji Xian Dai Yan Jiu* (Modern Study of Medical Formulae in Traditional Chinese Medicine) 1997;146-147.
3. *Zhong Xi Yi Jie He Za Zhi* (Journal of Integrated Chinese and Western Medicine) 1990;(6):5.
4. *Zhong Guo Zhong Xi Yi Jie He Za Zhi* (Chinese Journal of Integrative Chinese and Western Medicine) 1993;(1):33.
5. *Zhong Guo Zhong Xi Yi Jie He Za Zhi* (Chinese Journal of Integrative Chinese and Western Medicine) 1989;5:282.
6. *Chi Jiao Yi Sheng Za Zhi* (Journal of Barefoot Doctors) 1975;(2):26.
7. *Zhong Yi Fang Ji Xian Dai Yan Jiu* (Modern Study of Medical Formulae in Traditional Chinese Medicine) 1997;4(1):20.
8. *Yun Nan Zhong Yi Za Zhi* (Yunan Journal of Chinese Medicine) 1993;2:10.
9. *Hu Bei Zhong Yi Za Zhi* (Hubei Journal of Chinese Medicine) 1988;6:8.
10. *Zhong Yi Za Zhi* (Journal of Chinese Medicine) 1985;8:52.
11. *Zhong Yi Ming Fang Lin Chuang Xin Yong* (Contemporary Clinical Applications of Classic Chinese Formulas) 2001;85-86.
12. *Xin Zhong Yi* (New Chinese Medicine) 1985;(11):22.
13. *Zhong Yi Za Zhi* (Journal of Chinese Medicine) 1965;10:40.

Chapter 2 – Downward Draining Formulas   Section 1 – Cold Purgatives

Section 1

寒下剂
— Cold Purgatives

Dà Chéng Qì Tāng (Major Order the Qi Decoction)

大承氣湯
大承气汤

Pinyin Name: *Da Cheng Qi Tang*
Literal Name: Major Order the Qi Decoction
Alternate Names: *Ta Cheng Chi Tang, Da Cheng Chi Tang,* Major Chi-Infusing Decoction, Major Purgative Decoction, Major Rhubarb Combination
Original Source: *Shang Han Lun* (Discussion of Cold-Induced Disorders) by Zhang Zhong-Jing in the Eastern Han Dynasty

COMPOSITION

Da Huang (Radix et Rhizoma Rhei), *xi* (washed) with liquor	12g
Mang Xiao (Natrii Sulfas)	0.3 cup [6-9g]
Hou Po (Cortex Magnoliae Officinalis), *zhi* (fried with liquid)	24g [15-24g]
Zhi Shi (Fructus Aurantii Immaturus)	5 pieces [12g]

DOSAGE / PREPARATION / ADMINISTRATION

The source text instructions are to first cook *Zhi Shi* (Fructus Aurantii Immaturus) and *Hou Po* (Cortex Magnoliae Officinalis) with 10 cups [2,000 mL] of water until 5 cups [1,000 mL] of the liquid remain. Discard the residue, add *Da Huang* (Radix et Rhizoma Rhei), and cook until the liquid is further reduced to 2 cups [400 mL]. Discard the residue, add *Mang Xiao* (Natrii Sulfas), and bring the decoction to a boil 1-2 times using only low intensity fire. Take half [1 cup] of the warm decoction twice daily. Discontinue the formula once bowel movement has been induced.

Today, this formula is prepared as a decoction using the doses suggested in brackets above, with *Da Huang* (Radix et Rhizoma Rhei) post-decocted only for a short period of time and *Mang Xiao* (Natrii Sulfas) dissolved into the warm, strained decoction immediately before ingestion.

CHINESE THERAPEUTIC ACTIONS

Drastically drains heat and accumulation downward

CLINICAL MANIFESTATIONS

1. Excess *yangming fu* (hollow organ) syndrome: constipation, fullness and distention of epigastrium and abdomen, abdominal pain aggravated by pressure, a feeling of hardness upon palpation, and, in severe cases, tidal fever, delirium, trembling and perspiration of the extremities, a dry, yellow prickly or dry, black tongue coating, and a deep, slippery, and excess pulse.

2. Impacted stools accompanied by watery fluids: blue-green, watery fluids with a foul smell, abdominal and periumbilical pain, abdominal rigidity resembling a solid mass when palpated, a dry tongue and mouth, and a slippery, excess pulse.

3. Interior excess heat causing *re jue* (heat reversal), convulsions, and mania.

CLINICAL APPLICATIONS

Severe constipation, habitual constipation, post-operative constipation, enteroparalysis, intestinal obstruction, cholecystitis, hepatitis, infection of gallbladder and bile duct, pancreatitis, acute pancreatitis, appendicitis, acute appendicitis, tetanus, urinary stones, acute eczema, food poisoning requiring purging of toxic substances, organophosphorus poisoning, and lead poisoning.

EXPLANATION

Da Cheng Qi Tang (Major Order the Qi Decoction) is representative of cold purgative formulas and has a wide

152

Dà Chéng Qì Tāng (Major Order the Qi Decoction)

Da Cheng Qi Tang (Major Order the Qi Decoction)

Diagnosis	Signs and Symptoms	Treatment	Herbs
Accumulation of excess heat in the Stomach and Intestines	• Constipation, fullness and distention in the epigastrium and abdomen, abdominal pain aggravated by pressure, and a feeling of hardness upon palpation: accumulation of excess heat in the Stomach and Intestines • Dry mouth and tongue: heat drying up body fluids • Dry, yellow prickly or dry, black tongue coating, and a deep, excess pulse: interior excess heat	Drastically drains heat and accumulation downward	• *Da Huang* (Radix et Rhizoma Rhei) clears heat and purges constipated stools. • *Mang Xiao* (Natrii Sulfas) clears heat, moistens dryness, and softens the stool. • *Hou Po* (Cortex Magnoliae Officinalis) activates qi circulation and disperses accumulation. • *Zhi Shi* (Fructus Aurantii Immaturus) relieves fullness and distention.

range of functions. This formula was first presented in *Shang Han Lun* (Discussion of Cold-Induced Disorders) for treating *yangming fu* (hollow organs) syndrome. This syndrome arises when the wind-cold factor is not dispelled at the exterior. It then travels into the interior *zang fu* organs, where it transforms into heat, and binds with the stools.

This *yangming fu* syndrome is a condition characterized by interior excess heat. Because the heat is bound up with the stool, the stool becomes hard, causing constipation. The dry stool may disturb qi circulation, causing fullness and distention of the epigastrium and abdomen. In severe cases, the heat disturbs the Heart and *shen* (spirit) and gives rise to delirium. Trembling and perspiration of the extremities are the consequences of interior excess heat forcing body fluids out of the body. The dry mouth and tongue signify heat drying up body fluids. The tongue and pulse conditions both suggest interior excess heat.

Some patients with interior excess heat may show slightly different clinical manifestations. Some may actually pass blue-green fluids rectally. The reason for this is that the heat and stools are so tightly interlocked that the turbid water in the intestines has nowhere to go but to be excreted rectally as watery fluids. The fetid smell is caused by heat and stagnation. Because the stools are so hard in the large intestine, they feel like a solid mass when palpated.

This formula can treat patients who have *re jue* (heat reversal), convulsions, and mania caused by interior excess heat. *Re jue* (heat reversal) is a morbid condition in which excess pathogenic heat consumes body fluids. Damaged body fluids impair the normal circulation of yang qi and give rise to cold extremities. The spasms and cramps seen in convulsions are caused by heat consuming yin and body fluids; the insufficient yin and body fluids

fail to nourish the tendons. Mania is caused by heat disturbing the *shen* (spirit) in extreme cases.

All of the above conditions have the same etiology: interior heat accumulates in the Stomach and Intestines, causing consumption of yin and body fluids. The four diagnostic signs associated with use of this formula are: *pi* (distention), *man* (fullness), *zao* (dryness), and *shi* (hardness), with a dry yellow or black tongue coating, and a deep, slippery and excess pulse. Treatment calls for the use of drastic purgative herbs to quickly dispel heat and accumulation. Immediate action must be taken in order to preserve yin and body fluids from being consumed further.

Da Huang (Radix et Rhizoma Rhei), the chief herb, clears the Stomach and Intestines by quickly purging heat and constipated stools. *Mang Xiao* (Natrii Sulfas), the deputy herb, clears heat, moistens dryness, and softens the stools. *Da Huang* (Radix et Rhizoma Rhei) and *Mang Xiao* (Natrii Sulfas) mutually enforce each other in their actions of dispelling heat and purging constipated stools. *Hou Po* (Cortex Magnoliae Officinalis) and *Zhi Shi* (Fructus Aurantii Immaturus) regulate qi flow to relieve fullness and distention, and activate qi circulation to help dispel heat and stagnant stools.

MODIFICATIONS
• If there is severe thirst as a result of dryness and heat, add *Shi Gao* (Gypsum Fibrosum) and *Zhi Mu* (Rhizoma Anemarrhenae).
• When there is qi and blood stagnation, add *Chi Shao* (Radix Paeoniae Rubra) and *Tao Ren* (Semen Persicae).
• If accompanied by qi deficiency, add *Ren Shen* (Radix et Rhizoma Ginseng).
• For yin or body fluid deficiencies, add *Xuan Shen* (Radix Scrophulariae) and *Di Huang* (Radix Rehmanniae).

Chapter 2 – Downward Draining Formulas　　　　　　　　　　　　*Section 1 – Cold Purgatives*

Dà Chéng Qì Tāng (Major Order the Qi Decoction)

- With a feeling of fullness, distention, and oppression in the abdomen, add *Lai Fu Zi* (Semen Raphani) and *Mu Xiang* (Radix Aucklandiae).
- For dry stools and pain, increase the dose of *Mang Xiao* (Natrii Sulfas) and add *Gua Lou Zi* (Semen Trichosanthis).
- For hemorrhoids, constipation, and painful defecation, add *Huang Qin* (Radix Scutellariae) and *Ru Xiang* (Gummi Olibanum).
- For ascites, add *Gan Sui* (Radix Kansui) and *Yuan Hua* (Flos Genkwa).

CAUTIONS / CONTRAINDICATIONS

- Do not use *Da Cheng Qi Tang* when the exterior syndrome is not yet resolved, or for mild to moderate cases of constipation.
- This is a drastic downward draining formula. This formula is contraindicated in pregnant women, and in geriatric or convalescing patients. It is also contraindicated in individuals with yin or qi deficiency, or generalized weakness.
- Discontinue this formula once the desired effects are achieved. Prolonged use may injure the qi.

PHARMACOLOGICAL EFFECTS

1. **Gastrointestinal**: Administration of *Da Cheng Qi Tang* in guinea pigs was been associated with increased contraction and peristalsis. The mechanism of action is attributed to the stimulating effect on the smooth muscles of the intestines.[1]
2. **Digestive**: The effect of *Da Cheng Qi Tang* on the organs associated with digestion was evaluated by administering the formula to rats. The study reported that the herbs had a stimulating effect on the gastrointestinal system and increased the production of gastric acid and pancreatic enzymes. The herbs, however, had little influence on the production and release of bile acid.[2]
3. **Antibiotic**: Administration of *Da Cheng Qi Tang* was associated with an inhibitory effect *in vitro* against *Staphylococcus aureus*, *Salmonella typhi*, *Bacillus dysenteriae*, and *Bacillus paratyphosus*.[3]
4. **Effect on atherosclerosis**: *Da Cheng Qi Tang* prevented arteriosclerosis by inhibiting the proliferation of vascular smooth muscle cells.[4]

CLINICAL STUDIES AND RESEARCH

1. **Intestinal obstruction**: Sixty-six patients with intestinal obstruction were treated with *Da Cheng Qi Tang* with 100% success rate. In follow-ups, 46 patients had no recurrence within 3 years. The 20 patients who had recurrences were treated with the same formula with complete recovery.[5] In another study, individuals with intestinal obstruction were divided into two groups and treated with herbs accordingly. Group one with 78 patients (42 males, 36 females, average of 43 years of age) was treated with *Da Cheng Qi Tang* plus *Lai Fu Zi* (Semen Raphani) and *Huang Qin* (Radix Scutellariae) in decoction one time daily for up to three days with 92.3% effectiveness. Group two with 92 patients (52 males, 40 females, average of 41 years of age) was treated with *Da Cheng Qi Tang* only in decoction one time daily for up to two days with 76.1% effectiveness.[6]

2. **Enteroparalysis**: Administration of modified *Da Cheng Qi Tang* was associated with good results in treating 40 patients with enteroparalysis. Clinical results include passage of gas, bowel movement, and relief of abdominal distention and pain within 2 to 6 hours.[7]

3. **Infection of gallbladder and bile duct**: A modification of *Da Cheng Qi Tang* was used to treat 128 patients with acute infection of the gallbladder or the bile duct with complete recovery in 81 patients, moderate improvement in 33 patients, and no benefit in 14 patients. The study concluded an overall rate of effectiveness of 89%.[8]

4. **Cholecystitis**: One study reported marked improvement using modified *Da Cheng Qi Tang* to treat 75 patients with acute inflammation of the gallbladder. The herbal treatment contained *Da Cheng Qi Tang* plus *Pu Gong Ying* (Herba Taraxaci), *Jin Qian Cao* (Herba Lysimachiae) and *San Qi* (Radix et Rhizoma Notoginseng) as the base formula. Modifications included addition of *Xiang Fu* (Rhizoma Cyperi) and *Yu Jin* (Radix Curcumae) for qi stagnation; *Jin Yin Hua* (Flos Lonicerae Japonicae) and *Lian Qiao* (Fructus Forsythiae) for excess heat; and *Yin Chen* (Herba Artemisiae Scopariae) and *Zhi Zi* (Fructus Gardeniae) for damp-heat. The herbs were given in decoction two times daily. The average duration of treatment was 8.34 days. The study reported recovery in 50 of 75 patients.[9]

5. **Acute appendicitis**: Modified *Da Cheng Qi Tang* was used to treat 150 patients with acute appendicitis with compete recovery in 147 patients, improvement in 2 patients, and referral to surgery in one patient. The patients received herbs for 3 to 6 days. The formula used included *Da Huang* (Radix et Rhizoma Rhei) 15 to 30g (post-decocted), *Hou Po* (Cortex Magnoliae Officinalis) 10g, *Zhi Qiao* (Fructus Aurantii) 10g, *Bai Jiang Cao* (Herba cum Radice Patriniae) 30g, *Bai Hua She She Cao* (Herba Hedyotis) 30g, *Da Xue Teng* (Caulis Sargentodoxae) 30g, *Hu Zhang* (Rhizoma et Radix Polygoni Cuspidati) 30g, *Dan Shen* (Radix et Rhizoma Salviae Miltiorrhizae) 25g, and *Tao Ren* (Semen Persicae) 12g.[10]

6. **Acute pancreatitis**: Modified *Da Cheng Qi Tang* has been shown to effectively treat acute pancreatitis. The study used *Da Cheng Qi Tang* plus *Huang Qin* (Radix Scutellariae), *Huang Bo* (Cortex Phellodendri Chinensis), and *Chai Hu* (Radix Bupleuri) as the base formula, with addition of

Dà Chéng Qì Tāng (Major Order the Qi Decoction)

Jin Yin Hua (Flos Lonicerae Japonicae) and *Lian Qiao* (Fructus Forsythiae) for excess heat in the Stomach and Intestines; *Yin Chen* (Herba Artemisiae Scopariae) and *Zhi Zi* (Fructus Gardeniae) for damp-heat jaundice; and *Ku Lian Pi* (Cortex Meliae), *Bing Lang* (Semen Arecae), and *Xi Xin* (Radix et Rhizoma Asari) for biliary ascariasis. The treatment protocol was to administer 500 mL of the decoction twice daily six hours apart. For those without constipation, *Mang Xiao* (Natrii Sulfas) and *Da Huang* (Radix et Rhizoma Rhei) were removed from the formula, and the decoction was given only one time per day. The study reported complete recovery in all 48 patients (20 males and 28 females) with an average of 8.34 days.[11]

7. **Tetanus**: An herbal treatment that contained *Da Cheng Qi Tang* plus *Chan Tui* (Periostracum Cicadae) was used successfully to treat mild to moderate cases of tetanus.[12]

8. **Urolithiasis**: An herbal formula that contained *Da Cheng Qi Tang* plus *Hai Jin Sha* (Spora Lygodii) and *Jin Qian Cao* (Herba Lysimachiae) demonstrated success in treating urinary stones. The study reported complete recovery in 134 of 138 patients (97.2%). The duration of treatment (for successful expulsion of the stones) ranged from 2 to 33 days.[13]

9. **Acute eczema**: Use of modified *Da Cheng Qi Tang* effectively treated acute eczema. The herbal treatment consisted of *Da Cheng Qi Tang* plus *Chan Tui* (Periostracum Cicadae), *Chi Shao* (Radix Paeoniae Rubra) and *Jin Yin Hua* (Flos Lonicerae Japonicae) as the base formula. Modifications included the addition of *Bai Xian Pi* (Cortex Dictamni) and *Ku Shen* (Radix Sophorae Flavescentis) for severe itching; the removal of *Mang Xiao* (Natrii Sulfas) and the addition of *Shan Yao* (Rhizoma Dioscoreae) for loose stools; *Pu Gong Ying* (Herba Taraxaci) and *Cang Zhu* (Rhizoma Atractylodis) for eczema with discharge; and *Di Long* (Pheretima) for elevated body temperature. The duration of treatment ranged from 10 to 20 days. Of 34 patients, the study reported complete recovery in 19 patients within 10 days, complete recovery in 13 patients within 20 days, and improvement in 2 patients within 20 days.[14]

10. **Organophosphorus poisoning**: Patients with acute organophosphorus poisoning were first treated with gastric lavage followed by administration of one dose of *Da Cheng Qi Tang* via gastric tube. Of 35 patients, the study reported complete recovery in 32 patients and fatality in 3 patients.[15]

11. **Lead poisoning**: One study reported complete recovery in all 30 patients suffering from chronic lead poisoning. The herbal formula used *Da Cheng Qi Tang* as the base formula, and added *Yan Hu Suo* (Rhizoma Corydalis) and *Wu Yao* (Radix Linderae) for acute and excruciating abdominal pain; *Qian Niu Zi* (Semen Pharbitidis) and *Yu Li Ren* (Semen Pruni) for chronic constipation; *Shan Zha* (Fructus Crataegi), *Lai Fu Zi* (Semen Raphani), and *Ji Nei Jin* (Endothelium Corneum Gigeriae Galli) for poor appetite; *Ren Shen* (Radix et Rhizoma Ginseng), *Huang Qi* (Radix Astragali), *Dang Gui* (Radix Angelicae Sinensis), and *Bai Shao* (Radix Paeoniae Alba) for qi and blood deficiencies.[16]

RELATED FORMULAS

Fù Fāng Dà Chéng Qì Tāng

(Revised Major Order the Qi Decoction)

複方大承氣湯
复方大承气汤

Pinyin Name: *Fu Fang Da Cheng Qi Tang*
Literal Name: Revised Major Order the Qi Decoction
Original Source: *Zhong Xi Yi Jie He Zhi Liao Ji Fu Zheng* (Combined Chinese and Western Medical Treatment of the Acute Abdomen) by Nankai Hospital of Tianjin in 1973

Hou Po (Cortex Magnoliae Officinalis)	15-30g
Lai Fu Zi (Semen Raphani), *chao* (dry-fried)	15-30g
Zhi Shi (Fructus Aurantii Immaturus)	15g
Tao Ren (Semen Persicae)	9g
Chi Shao (Radix Paeoniae Rubra)	15g
Da Huang (Radix et Rhizoma Rhei), post-decocted	15g
Mang Xiao (Natrii Sulfas), *chong fu* (taken drenched)	9-15g

Prepare this formula as a decoction and add *Da Huang* (Radix et Rhizoma Rhei) near the end of cooking. Dissolve *Mang Xiao* (Natrii Sulfas) in the strained decoction prior to ingestion. Today, for maximum effect in removing intestinal obstruction, the first dose may be administered by nasogastric tube, followed by rectal instillation in the form of an enema as the second dose 2-3 hours later.

Fu Fang Da Cheng Qi Tang (Revised Major Order the Qi Decoction) primarily treats intestinal obstruction by promoting defecation, while regulating qi and blood at the same time. It is indicated for *yangming fu* (hollow organs) excess syndrome with prominent abdominal fullness and bloating. Today, it commonly treats uncomplicated intestinal obstruction, and prevents post-surgical adhesions in the abdominal cavity.

This formula is a modification of *Da Cheng Qi Tang*. *Lai Fu Zi* (Semen Raphani), a digestive herb, helps *Hou Po* (Cortex Magnoliae Officinalis) regulate qi and relieve abdominal fullness. *Tao Ren* (Semen Persicae) and *Chi Shao* (Radix Paeoniae Rubra) activate blood circulation and dispel blood stagnation. They also lubricate the intestines to help promote defecation.

155

Dà Chéng Qì Tāng (Major Order the Qi Decoction)

Jiā Jiǎn Chéng Qì Tāng
(Modified Order the Qi Decoction)

加減承氣湯
加减承气汤

Pinyin Name: *Jia Jian Cheng Qi Tang*
Literal Name: Modified Order the Qi Decoction
Original Source: *An Hui Zhong Yi Xue Yuan* (Anhui University School of Medicine) in 1990

Da Huang (Radix et Rhizoma Rhei)
Hou Po (Cortex Magnoliae Officinalis)
Zhi Shi (Fructus Aurantii Immaturus)
Mang Xiao (Natrii Sulfas)
Huo Ma Ren (Fructus Cannabis)
Tao Ren (Semen Persicae)
Bai Shao (Radix Paeoniae Alba)

Jia Jian Cheng Qi Tang (Modified Order the Qi Decoction) drains stagnation and obstruction in the Intestines downward. It generally treats severe constipation characterized by heat. In addition to using herbs that clear heat and drain downward, this formula also contains herbs to gently moisten the Intestines and nourish yin, to prevent the bitter and cold herbs from consuming excessive amount of yin and body fluids.

AUTHORS' COMMENTS

Da Cheng Qi Tang is the standard downward draining formula in the treatment of excess *yangming fu* (hollow organs) syndrome. Traditionally, the four main diagnostic symptoms are *pi* (distention), *man* (fullness), *zao* (dryness) and *shi* (hardness).

- 痞 *Pi* (distention) is the feeling of oppression, obstruction, and increased pressure in the chest and epigastrium.
- 满 *Man* (fullness) is the feeling of bloating and fullness in the epigastric and abdominal regions.
- 燥 *Zao* (dryness) refers to the dry, compacted stool, which feels hard upon abdominal palpation.
- 实 *Shi* (hardness) signifies an excess condition in which the dry, hard stools are interlocked with heat, causing constipation and abdominal pain that intensifies with palpation.

The potency of *Da Cheng Qi Tang* is directly dependent on the preparation of two ingredients: *Da Huang* (Radix et Rhizoma Rhei) and *Mang Xiao* (Natrii Sulfas). *Da Huang* (Radix et Rhizoma Rhei) must be post-decocted to preserve its purgative functions; otherwise, it will lose much of its purgative effect if it is cooked together with the rest of the herbs. *Mang Xiao* (Natrii Sulfas) is also kept aside during the cooking process. When the cooking process is finished and the herb residue is filtered out, *Mang Xiao* (Natrii Sulfas) should be dissolved into the

warm decoction immediately before ingestion. The rationale for this preparation can also be explained from a biochemical perspective. *Da Huang* (Radix et Rhizoma Rhei) contains sennoside and emodin as the main active ingredients responsible for purgative and laxative actions. These two compounds are highly sensitive to heat, and will be deactivated with prolonged exposure if cooked for a long period of time. *Mang Xiao* (Natrii Sulfas), on the other hand, is a mineral substance that does not require extraction with cooking. If added to the decoction during the cooking process, it will only be lost when the decoction is filtered out and the herb residues discarded. For these reasons, it is important to following the specific instructions to ensure the efficacy of this formula.

This formula can also be used in postpartum patients who show no signs of exterior conditions but have lower abdominal pain and hardness with retention of lochia, constipation, irritability, fever, and delirious speech during the day but recovery at night. However, *Da Cheng Qi Tang* must be given carefully as most postpartum women are weak and deficient.

This formula can be used for any excess heat conditions, or for fire flaring upward accompanied by constipation or hardness of the stool, since it can purge out the excess. Three of the most effective outlets for clearing fire include inducing diaphoresis, promoting diuresis, and purging the bowels. Since this formula helps guide heat down and out of the body, it is extremely effective in enhancing the overall effect of other heat-clearing herbs.

Da Cheng Qi Tang (Major Order the Qi Decoction), *Xiao Cheng Qi Tang* (Minor Order the Qi Decoction), and *Tiao Wei Cheng Qi Tang* (Regulate the Stomach and Order the Qi Decoction) share many similarities, but have notable differences. All three formulas contain *Da Huang* (Radix et Rhizoma Rhei) to purge stagnation and heat in the Large Intestine to treat *yangming fu* (hollow organs) syndrome. Common symptoms include constipation and abdominal pain that worsens upon pressure. The differences are as follows:

- *Da Cheng Qi Tang* contains *Da Huang* (Radix et Rhizoma Rhei), *Mang Xiao* (Natrii Sulfas), *Zhi Shi* (Fructus Aurantii Immaturus), and *Hou Po* (Cortex Magnoliae Officinalis). The four ingredients together treat *pi* (distention), *man* (fullness), *zao* (dryness), and *shi* (hardness). The constipation is characterized by extremely hard stools.
- *Xiao Cheng Qi Tang* contains *Da Huang* (Radix et Rhizoma Rhei) and decreased doses of *Zhi Shi* (Fructus Aurantii Immaturus) and *Hou Po* (Cortex Magnoliae Officinalis) to treat qi stagnation signs and symptoms

156

Dà Chéng Qì Tāng (Major Order the Qi Decoction)

Comparison of Three "*Cheng Qi Tang* (Order the Qi Decoctions)"

Formula Names	*Pi* (Distention)	*Man* (Fullness)	*Zao* (Dryness)	*Shi* (Hardness)
Da Cheng Qi Tang (Major Order the Qi Decoction)	severe	severe	severe	severe
Xiao Cheng Qi Tang (Minor Order the Qi Decoction)	moderate	moderate		moderate
Tiao Wei Cheng Qi Tang (Regulate the Stomach and Order the Qi Decoction)			severe	severe

of *pi* (distention), *man* (fullness) and *shi* (hardness). The constipation is characterized by moderately hard stools.

- *Tiao Wei Cheng Qi Tang* contains *Da Huang* (Radix et Rhizoma Rhei), *Mang Xiao* (Natrii Sulfas), and *Gan Cao* (Radix et Rhizoma Glycyrrhizae), and is the mildest among the three formulas. It softens the stools rather than treating *pi* (distention) and *man* (fullness).[17]

Da Cheng Qi Tang and *Da Xian Xiong Tang* (Major Sinking into the Chest Decoction) are both downward draining formulas that contain *Mang Xiao* (Natrii Sulfas) and *Da Huang* (Radix et Rhizoma Rhei).

- *Da Cheng Qi Tang* specifically treats constipation characterized by *pi* (distention), *man* (fullness), *zao* (dryness), and *shi* (hardness). *Da Cheng Qi Tang* targets mainly symptoms in the lower abdomen, such as dry, hard stools stagnant in the Large Intestine. In this formula, *Da Huang* (Radix et Rhizoma Rhei) is post-decocted to ensure that it retains its purgative action and induces bowel movement.
- *Da Xian Xiong Tang* treats epigastric fullness, distention and pain accompanied by constipation. It treats symptoms manifesting mainly in the chest and epigastrium by dispelling water accumulation and purging heat. In this formula, *Da Huang* (Radix et Rhizoma Rhei) is pre-decocted to lessen its potent diarrhea-inducing effects.

References

1. *Zhong Guo Zhong Xi Yi Jie He Za Zhi* (Chinese Journal of Integrative Chinese and Western Medicine) 1993;(1):33.
2. *Zhong Xi Yi Jie He Za Zhi* (Journal of Integrated Chinese and Western Medicine) 1985;(6):338.
3. *Zhong Yao Yao Li Yu Ying Yong* (Pharmacology and Applications of Chinese Herbs) 1988;4(3):1.
4. Chung HJ, Kim DW, Maruyama I, Tani T. Effects of traditional Chinese formulations on rat carotid artery injured by balloon endothelial denudation. Am J Chin Med. 2003;31(2):201-12.
5. *Zhong Yi Yao Xin Xi* (Information on Chinese Medicine and Herbology) 1995;(3):46.
6. *Zhong Guo Zhong Xi Yi Jie He Za Zhi* (Chinese Journal of Integrative Chinese and Western Medicine) 1989;5:282.
7. *Zhong Guo Zhong Xi Yi Jie He Za Zhi* (Chinese Journal of Integrative Chinese and Western Medicine) 1992;11:695.
8. *Ji Lin Zhong Yi Yao* (Jilin Chinese Medicine and Herbology) 1988;(2):12.
9. *Fu Jian Zhong Yi Yao* (Fujian Chinese Medicine and Herbology) 1992;1:31.
10. *Xin Zhong Yi* (New Chinese Medicine) 1985;(11):22.
11. *Liao Ning Zhong Yi Za Zhi* (Liaoning Journal of Chinese Medicine) 1985;2:24.
12. *Zhong Yi Ming Fang Lin Chuang Xin Yong* (Contemporary Clinical Applications of Classic Chinese Formulas) 2001;55.
13. *Zhong Xi Yi Jie He Za Zhi* (Journal of Integrated Chinese and Western Medicine) 1989;11:692.
14. *Shan Dong Zhong Yi Za Zhi* (Shandong Journal of Chinese Medicine) 1996;6:261.
15. *Shi Yong Zhong Xi Yi Jie He Za Zhi* (Practical Journal of Integrated Chinese and Western Medicines) 1993;2:755.
16. *Jiang Xi Zhong Yi Yao* (Jiangxi Chinese Medicine and Herbology) 1993;1:17.
17. Wang MZ, et al. *Zhong Yi Xue Wen Da Ti Ku* (Questions and Answers on Traditional Chinese Medicine: Herbal Formulas).

Chapter 2 – Downward Draining Formulas   *Section 1 – Cold Purgatives*

Xiǎo Chéng Qì Tāng (Minor Order the Qi Decoction)

小承氣湯
小承气汤

Pinyin Name: *Xiao Cheng Qi Tang*
Literal Name: Minor Order the Qi Decoction
Alternate Names: *Hsiao Cheng Chi Tang*, Minor Qi-Infusing Decoction, Minor Purgative Decoction, Minor Rhubarb Combination
Original Source: *Shang Han Lun* (Discussion of Cold-Induced Disorders) by Zhang Zhong-Jing in the Eastern Han Dynasty

COMPOSITION

Da Huang (Radix et Rhizoma Rhei), *xi* (washed) with liquor	12g
Hou Po (Cortex Magnoliae Officinalis), *zhi* (fried with liquid)	6g
Zhi Shi (Fructus Aurantii Immaturus), *zhi* (fried with liquid)	3 large pieces [9g]

DOSAGE / PREPARATION / ADMINISTRATION

Cook the ingredients with 4 cups [800 mL] of water until reduced to 1.2 cups [240 mL]. Take the warm, strained decoction in two equally-divided doses twice daily.

CHINESE THERAPEUTIC ACTIONS

Gently drains heat and accumulation downward

CLINICAL MANIFESTATIONS

1. Excess *yangming fu* (hollow organs) syndrome: constipation, delirium, tidal fever, fullness and distention of the chest and abdomen, a yellow tongue coating that is old- and dirty-looking in appearance, and a rapid, slippery pulse.
2. Early stage of dysentery with rectal tenesmus, and epigastric and abdominal distention and pain.

CLINICAL APPLICATIONS

Constipation, post-operative constipation, acute simple intestinal obstruction, intestinal paralysis, absence of intestinal peristalsis, abdominal distention and pain, chronic gastritis, acute gastroenteritis, viral hepatitis, acute cholecystitis, acute appendicitis, acute febrile disease, hypertension, obesity, and food intoxication.

EXPLANATION

Xiao Cheng Qi Tang (Minor Order the Qi Decoction) treats *yangming fu* (hollow organs) syndrome of moderate severity, characterized by the presence of *pi* (distention), *man* (fullness), and *shi* (hardness). However, there is no *zao* (dryness). *Da Huang* (Radix et Rhizoma Rhei), the chief herb, clears heat in the Stomach and Intestines and purges constipated stools. *Hou Po* (Cortex Magnoliae Officinalis) and *Zhi Shi* (Fructus Aurantii Immaturus) regulate qi flow to relieve fullness and distention, and activate qi circulation to help dispel heat and stagnant stools.

Xiao Cheng Qi Tang is a variation of *Da Cheng Qi Tang* (Major Order the Qi Decoction), and basically has the same purgative effect, except that it is a milder formula for *yangming fu* (hollow organs) syndrome of moderate severity. Therefore, it is not necessary to post-decoct *Da Huang* (Radix et Rhizoma Rhei), as in *Da Cheng Qi Tang* (Major Order the Qi Decoction). Instead, *Da Huang* (Radix et Rhizoma Rhei) is fully cooked to moderate its potent downward draining effects. Additionally, the doses of *Hou Po* (Cortex Magnoliae Officinalis) and *Zhi Shi* (Fructus Aurantii Immaturus) are decreased, since the condition is not as severe. Lastly, *Mang Xiao* (Natrii Sulfas) is not used since there is an absence of *zao* (dryness).

MODIFICATIONS

- If there is generalized weakness and qi deficiency, add *Huang Qi* (Radix Astragali) and *Ren Shen* (Radix et Rhizoma Ginseng).
- If there is generalized weakness and blood deficiency, add *Dang Gui* (Radix Angelicae Sinensis) and *Chuan Xiong* (Rhizoma Chuanxiong).
- When there is irritability and restlessness as a result of Lung deficiency, add *Mai Dong* (Radix Ophiopogonis) and *Wu Wei Zi* (Fructus Schisandrae Chinensis).
- For tonsillitis, add *Shan Dou Gen* (Radix et Rhizoma Sophorae Tonkinensis) and *Jie Geng* (Radix Platycodonis).

CAUTIONS / CONTRAINDICATIONS

Refer to *Da Cheng Qi Tang* (Major Order the Qi Decoction).

PHARMACOLOGICAL EFFECTS

1. **Gastrointestinal:** Administration of *Xiao Cheng Qi Tang* was associated with increased contraction and peristalsis. The mechanism of action was attributed to the stimulating effect on the smooth muscles of the intestines.[1,2]
2. **Antibiotic:** Administration of *Xiao Cheng Qi Tang* was associated with an inhibitory effect *in vitro* against *Staphylococcus aureus* and *E. coli*. Also, the inhibitory effect of the formula was determined to be stronger than the individual ingredients.[3]

Xiăo Chéng Qi Tāng (Minor Order the Qi Decoction)

Xiao Cheng Qi Tang (Minor Order the Qi Decoction)

Diagnosis	Signs and Symptoms	Treatment	Herbs
Accumulation of excess heat in the Stomach and Intestines	• Constipation with fullness and distention of the chest and abdomen: accumulation of excess heat in the Stomach and Intestines • Yellow tongue coating: interior excess heat	Gently drains heat and accumulation downward	• Fully-cooked *Da Huang* (Radix et Rhizoma Rhei) gently clears heat and purges the constipated stools. • *Hou Po* (Cortex Magnoliae Officinalis) activates qi circulation and disperses accumulation. • *Zhi Shi* (Fructus Aurantii Immaturus) relieves fullness and distention.

CLINICAL STUDIES AND RESEARCH

1. **Gastrointestinal disorders**: *Xiao Cheng Qi Tang* has been shown in many studies to treat various types of gastrointestinal disorders, such as post-operative constipation, intestinal paralysis, absence of intestinal peristalsis, abdominal distention and pain, etc.[4]

2. **Post-operative constipation**: Eighty-six geriatric patients were treated with modified *Xiao Cheng Qi Tang* for prevention and treatment of post-operative constipation. The first dose of the formula was given 48 hours after the surgery, and the second dose was given 6 hours later (54 hours after the surgery) only if necessary. The study reported 100% success rate, with 53 patients showing gas or bowel movement after the first dose, and the remaining 33 patients after the second dose.[5]

3. **Chronic gastritis**: Use of modified *Xiao Cheng Qi Tang* was associated with 96.36% effectiveness in the treatment of chronic gastritis in 55 patients.[6]

4. **Acute gastroenteritis**: Modified *Xiao Cheng Qi Tang* effectively treated acute gastroenteritis in 91 patients (49 males and 42 females) between 1 and 5 years of age, with 1-3 days history of illness. The study reported immediate improvement in 16 cases, significant improvement in 42 cases, moderate improvement in 26 cases, and no benefit in 7 cases. The overall rate of effectiveness was 92.3%. The herbal treatment used *Xiao Cheng Qi Tang* plus charred *Shan Zha* (Fructus Crataegi) and charred *Shen Qu* (Massa Fermentata) as the base formula. *Mu Xiang* (Radix Aucklandiae) was added for abdominal pain; *Lian Qiao* (Fructus Forsythiae), and *Bo He* (Herba Menthae) were added for fever; *Sha Ren* (Fructus Amomi), *Huang Lian* (Rhizoma Coptidis), and *Ban Xia* (Rhizoma Pinelliae) were added for recurrent nausea and vomiting. The herbs were given one time daily in decoction.[7]

5. **Viral hepatitis**: Administration of modified *Xiao Cheng Qi Tang* effectively treated 39 of 40 patients with viral hepatitis. Of those who responded to the treatment, none had recurrence during the follow-up exam one year later. All patients received two courses of treatment, with 15 days per course. The herbal treatment contained *Xiao Cheng Qi Tang* plus *Gan Cao* (Radix et Rhizoma Glycyrrhizae) as the base formula. Additionally, *Cang Zhu* (Rhizoma Atractylodis) was added for dampness; and charred *Shan Zha* (Fructus Crataegi) and charred *Ji Nei Jin* (Endothelium Corneum Gigeriae Galli) were added for indigestion. Pharmaceutical drugs were added as supportive treatment when necessary.[8]

HERB-DRUG INTERACTION

Opioid-induced constipation and nausea: One study reported marked effectiveness using *Xiao Cheng Qi Tang* to relieve constipation and nausea caused by excessive use of opioid analgesics in 40 patients with terminal cancer. For constipation, the study reported complete recovery in 30 cases, improvement in 8 cases, and no benefit in 2 cases. For nausea, the study reported complete relief in 19 cases and improvement in 9 cases.[9]

AUTHORS' COMMENTS

Please refer to *Da Cheng Qi Tang* (Major Order the Qi Decoction) for a detailed comparison with *Xiao Cheng Qi Tang* and *Tiao Wei Cheng Qi Tang* (Regulate the Stomach and Order the Qi Decoction).

References

1. *Zhong Guo Zhong Xi Yi Jie He Za Zhi* (Chinese Journal of Integrative Chinese and Western Medicine) 1993;(1):33.
2. *Zhong Yi Fang Ji Xian Dai Yan Jiu* (Modern Study of Medical Formulae in Traditional Chinese Medicine) 1997;146-147.
3. *Zhong Yi Za Zhi* (Journal of Chinese Medicine) 1955;10:36.
4. *Zhong Yi Ming Fang Lin Chuang Xin Yong* (Contemporary Clinical Applications of Classic Chinese Formulas) 2001;85.
5. *Bei Jing Zhong Yi Za Zhi* (Beijing Journal of Chinese Medicine) 1991;(5):31.
6. *Hu Bei Zhong Yi Za Zhi* (Hubei Journal of Chinese Medicine) 1988;6:8.
7. *Zhong Yi Ming Fang Lin Chuang Xin Yong* (Contemporary Clinical Applications of Classic Chinese Formulas) 2001;85-86.
8. *Yun Nan Yi Yao* (Yunan Medicine and Herbology) 1982;3:102.
9. *Xin Zhong Yi* (New Chinese Medicine) 1996;2:52.

Chapter 2 – Downward Draining Formulas   *Section 1 – Cold Purgatives*

Tiáo Wèi Chéng Qì Tāng
(Regulate the Stomach and Order the Qi Decoction)

調胃承氣湯
调胃承气汤

Pinyin Name: *Tiao Wei Cheng Qi Tang*
Literal Name: Regulate the Stomach and Order the Qi Decoction
Alternate Names: *Tiao Wei Cheng Chi Tang*, Stomach-Regulating and Qi-Infusing Decoction, Stomach-Regulating and Purgative Decoction, Rhubarb and Mirabilitum Combination
Original Source: *Shang Han Lun* (Discussion of Cold-Induced Disorders) by Zhang Zhong-Jing in the Eastern Han Dynasty

COMPOSITION

Da Huang (Radix et Rhizoma Rhei), *xi* (washed) with liquor	12g
Mang Xiao (Natrii Sulfas)	0.5 cup [9-12g]
Zhi Gan Cao (Radix et Rhizoma Glycyrrhizae Praeparata cum Melle)	6g

DOSAGE / PREPARATION / ADMINISTRATION

Cook *Da Huang* (Radix et Rhizoma Rhei) and *Zhi Gan Cao* (Radix et Rhizoma Glycyrrhizae Praeparata cum Melle) in 3 cups [600 mL] of water and reduce the liquid to 1 cup [200 mL]. Filter and discard the residue, then add *Mang Xiao* (Natrii Sulfas) and bring the decoction to a boil 1-2 times using low intensity fire. Take the entire decoction while warm.

CHINESE THERAPEUTIC ACTIONS

Slowly drains heat and accumulation downward

CLINICAL MANIFESTATIONS

1. *Yangming fu* (hollow organs) syndrome characterized by dryness and heat in the Stomach and Intestines: constipation, thirst, irritability, fever, delirious speech, "steaming" sensations of the whole body, fullness and distention of the abdomen, a yellow tongue coating, and a slippery, rapid pulse.
2. Heat in the Stomach and Intestines causing maculae, hematemesis, epistaxis, toothache, and swelling and soreness of the mouth and throat.

CLINICAL APPLICATIONS

Food poisoning, acute gastroenteritis, acute simple intestinal obstruction, acute cholecystitis, acute appendicitis, and constipation.

EXPLANATION

Tiao Wei Cheng Qi Tang (Regulate the Stomach and Order the Qi Decoction) treats *yangming fu* (hollow organs) syndrome characterized by dryness and heat in the Stomach and Intestines. In this condition, *zao* (dryness) and *shi* (hardness) are present, but *pi* (distension) and *man* (fullness) are absent. *Da Huang* (Radix et Rhizoma Rhei) clears Stomach and Intestines heat and purges constipated stools. *Mang Xiao* (Natrii Sulfas) clears heat, moistens dryness, and softens the stools. *Gan Cao* (Radix et Rhizoma Glycyrrhizae) tonifies qi and harmonizes the formula.

Tiao Wei Cheng Qi Tang, a variation of *Da Cheng Qi Tang* (Major Order the Qi Decoction), is indicated for *yangming fu* (hollow organs) syndrome characterized by severe constipation and mild fullness of the epigastrium and abdomen. In this formula, *Da Huang* (Radix et

Tiao Wei Cheng Qi Tang (Regulate the Stomach and Order the Qi Decoction)

Diagnosis	Signs and Symptoms	Treatment	Herbs
Accumulation of excess heat in the Stomach and Intestines	• Constipation with fullness and distention of the chest and abdomen: accumulation of excess heat in the Stomach and Intestines • Thirst, irritability, fever, "steaming" sensations of the whole body: dryness and heat • Yellow tongue coating: interior excess heat	Slowly drains heat and accumulation downward	• Fully-cooked *Da Huang* (Radix et Rhizoma Rhei) slowly clears heat and purges the constipated stool. • *Mang Xiao* (Natrii Sulfas) clears heat, moistens dryness, and softens the stool. • *Gan Cao* (Radix et Rhizoma Glycyrrhizae) tonifies qi and harmonizes the formula.

160

Chinese Herbal Formulas and Applications

Tiáo Wèi Chéng Qì Tāng
(Regulate the Stomach and Order the Qi Decoction)

Rhizoma Rhei) is fully cooked to moderate its potent downward draining effects. *Mang Xiao* (Natrii Sulfas) is used at a slightly higher dose to address dryness and heat. *Hou Po* (Cortex Magnoliae Officinalis) and *Zhi Shi* (Fructus Aurantii Immaturus) are removed since *pi* (distention) and *man* (fullness) are absent in this condition. *Gan Cao* (Radix et Rhizoma Glycyrrhizae) is added to tonify qi and harmonize the formula. Overall, *Tiao Wei Cheng Qi Tang* has a stronger effect in treating "dry-heat" and a weaker effect in treating "fullness," in comparison to *Da Cheng Qi Tang*.

CAUTIONS / CONTRAINDICATIONS

Refer to *Da Cheng Qi Tang* (Major Order the Qi Decoction).

HERB-DRUG INTERACTION

Drug overdose: Use of *Tiao Wei Cheng Qi Tang* was associated with satisfactory results in treating 24 patients with overdose of illegal drugs. The herbal formula contained *Da Huang* (Radix et Rhizoma Rhei) 10g, *Gan Cao* (Radix et Rhizoma Glycyrrhizae) 10g, and *Mang Xiao* (Natrii Sulfas) 10g. The patients received gastric lavage first, followed by administration of the herbs via a gastric tube with warm water. Bowel movement was induced within 2.5 to 4.0 hours in all patients.[1]

AUTHORS' COMMENTS

Please refer to *Da Cheng Qi Tang* (Major Order the Qi Decoction) for a detailed comparison with *Xiao Cheng Qi Tang* (Minor Order the Qi Decoction) and *Tiao Wei Cheng Qi Tang*.

Reference

1. *Si Chuan Zhong Yi* (Sichuan Chinese Medicine) 1996;1:37.

Dà Xiàn Xiōng Tāng (Major Sinking into the Chest Decoction)
大陷胸湯
大陷胸汤

Pinyin Name: *Da Xian Xiong Tang*
Literal Name: Major Sinking into the Chest Decoction
Original Source: *Shang Han Lun* (Discussion of Cold-Induced Disorders) by Zhang Zhong-Jing in the Eastern Han Dynasty

COMPOSITION

Da Huang (Radix et Rhizoma Rhei)	18g [10g]
Mang Xiao (Natrii Sulfas)	1 cup [10g]
Gan Sui (Radix Kansui)	1 spoonful [1g]

DOSAGE / PREPARATION / ADMINISTRATION

First cook *Da Huang* (Radix et Rhizoma Rhei) in 6 cups [1,200 mL] of water until the liquid is reduced to 2 cups [400 mL]. Filter and discard the residue, then add *Mang Xiao* (Natrii Sulfas), and bring the decoction to a boil 1-2 times. Grind *Gan Sui* (Radix Kansui) into a fine powder, and add it to 1 cup [200 mL] of the warm, strained decoction before ingestion. The bowel movement should be induced quickly. Discontinue the use of this formula once bowel movement has been induced.

Today, this formula is prepared as a decoction using the doses suggested in brackets above. Dissolve *Mang Xiao*

(Natrii Sulfas) into the warm, strained decoction, and then mix the powder of *Gan Sui* (Radix Kansui) into the decoction.

CHINESE THERAPEUTIC ACTIONS

Purges heat and eliminates water accumulation

CLINICAL MANIFESTATIONS

Jie xiong (stagnant chest): hardness, constipation, afternoon or tidal fever, shortness of breath, irritability, restlessness, thirst, fullness and pain in the epigastrium to the lower abdomen that intensify with pressure, a dry tongue, and a deep, tight and forceful pulse.

DOWNWARD DRAINING FORMULAS 2

161

Chapter 2 – Downward Draining Formulas | Section 1 – Cold Purgatives

Dà Xiàn Xiōng Tāng (Major Sinking into the Chest Decoction)

Da Xian Xiong Tang (Major Sinking into the Chest Decoction)

Diagnosis	Signs and Symptoms	Treatment	Herbs
Jie xiong (stagnant chest)	• Constipation, afternoon or tidal fever, irritability, restlessness, thirst, and a dry tongue: heat consuming fluids • Hardness, fullness, and pain in the epigastrium and lower abdomen: qi stagnation from interlocked heat and water • Deep, tight and forceful pulse: interior-excess	• Purges heat • Eliminates water accumulation	• *Da Huang* (Radix et Rhizoma Rhei) and *Mang Xiao* (Natrii Sulfas) purge heat and drain accumulation. • *Gan Sui* (Radix Kansui) drastically eliminates water accumulation and purges heat.

CLINICAL APPLICATIONS

Acute intestinal obstruction, acute pancreatitis, acute cholecystitis.

EXPLANATION

Da Xian Xiong Tang (Major Sinking into the Chest Decoction) treats *jie xiong* (stagnant chest), a condition characterized by accumulation of heat and water in the chest and diaphragm. As heat and water interlock and become stagnant, they block the circulation of qi, resulting in hardness, fullness and pain in the epigastrium and lower abdomen. Since the water fluid is interlocked with and injured by heat, constipation, afternoon or tidal fever, shortness of breath, irritability, thirst, and a dry tongue manifest. A deep, tight and forceful pulse suggests that this is an excess interior condition and that the body is not yet deficient.

Da Huang (Radix et Rhizoma Rhei) and *Mang Xiao* (Natrii Sulfas) purge heat and drain accumulation. *Gan Sui* (Radix Kansui) drastically eliminates water accumulation and purges heat. All three herbs have potent effects to quickly purge and drain downward. Once the desired effects are achieved, discontinue the formula to avoid damaging *zheng* (upright) qi.

CAUTIONS / CONTRAINDICATIONS

• *Da Xian Xiong Tang* should be discontinued immediately once the desired effects are achieved. Prolonged use may injure the qi.
• This formula is contraindicated in pregnant women, weak patients, or those who have just recovered from major illnesses.
• According to *Shi Ba Fan* (Eighteen Incompatibles), *Gan Cao* (Radix et Rhizoma Glycyrrhizae) is incompatible with *Gan Sui* (Radix Kansui) and should not be added to this formula.

PHARMACOLOGICAL EFFECTS

1. **Diuretic**: Administration of *Da Xian Xiong Tang* in mice at 12.5 g/kg was associated with increased excretion of urine. The urine was also determined to have a higher concentration of sodium and potassium in comparison with urine of untreated mice.[1]

2. **Gastrointestinal**: Administration of *Da Xian Xiong Tang* was associated with a marked increase in intestinal peristalsis and bowel movement induction.[2]

CLINICAL STUDIES AND RESEARCH

1. **Acute intestinal obstruction**: Administration of modified *Da Xian Xiong Tang* was used in treating 30 cases of intestinal obstruction. Each dose contained *Gan Sui* (Radix Kansui) 0.9g, *Da Huang* (Radix et Rhizoma Rhei) 0.6g, and *Mang Xiao* (Natrii Sulfas) 0.3g in fine powder form. The patients were given two doses of herbs per day (at least 4 hours apart). Complete recovery was reported in 27 of 30 cases within 24-48 hours. The three patients who did not respond received surgical treatment.[3] In another report, 72 patients with intestinal obstruction were treated with either *Da Cheng Qi Tang* (Major Order the Qi Decoction) or *Da Xian Xiong Tang* with a 75% success rate. Most patients responded within 24 hours. The number of doses given ranged from 1-10.[4]

2. **Acute pancreatitis**: Twenty patients with acute pancreatitis were treated with both *Da Xian Xiong Tang* and *Da Cheng Qi Tang* (Major Order the Qi Decoction), with modifications as needed. The patients did not receive antibiotic or intravenous fluids, and were not prohibited from eating. After the herbal treatment, the patients reported relief of abdominal pain after 2-48 hours (average of 19.5 hours), with complete remission of pain after 24-96 hours (average of 68 hours).[5] Another study reported 95% effectiveness in the treatment of acute pancreatitis using acupuncture plus an herbal formula that contained *Da Xian Xiong Tang* plus *Chai Hu* (Radix Bupleuri), *Yan Hu Suo* (Rhizoma Corydalis) and other herbs.[6]

Dà Xiàn Xiōng Tāng (Major Sinking into the Chest Decoction)

3. **Acute peritonitis**: Use of *Da Xian Xiong Tang* to treat acute peritonitis resulted in a 95% success rate (38 out of 40 patients). Each dose contained *Gan Sui* (Radix Kansui) 0.9g, *Da Huang* (Radix et Rhizoma Rhei) 0.6g, and *Mang Xiao* (Natrii Sulfas) 0.3g in fine powder form. The patients were instructed to take the herbs orally on an empty stomach two to four times daily by dissolving the herbs in 200 mL of hot water. The frequency of dosing varied, depending on the severity of illness. The herbs were ingested orally, or if necessary, given via a gastric tube.[7]

TOXICOLOGY

The LD_{50} of *Da Xian Xiong Tang* in decoction given via oral ingestion is 232 g/kg in mice.[8]

RELATED FORMULA

Dà Xiàn Xiōng Wán (Major Sinking into the Chest Pill)
大陷胸丸
Pinyin Name: Da Xian Xiong Wan
Literal Name: Major Sinking into the Chest Pill
Original Source: *Shang Han Lun* (Discussion of Cold-Induced Disorders) by Zhang Zhong-Jing in the Eastern Han Dynasty

Da Huang (Radix et Rhizoma Rhei)	240g
Ting Li Zi (Semen Descurainiae seu Lepidii),	
ao (simmered)	0.5 cup [175g]
Mang Xiao (Natrii Sulfas)	0.5 cup [175g]
Ku Xing Ren (Semen Armeniacae Amarum),	
ao (simmered) to black	0.5 cup [175g]

The source text instructs to grind *Da Huang* (Radix et Rhizoma Rhei) and *Ting Li Zi* (Semen Descurainiae seu Lepidii) into powder and sift evenly. Add *Mang Xiao* (Natrii Sulfas) and *Ku Xing Ren* (Semen Armeniacae Amarum) to the powder, and then grind together and form into pills, with each pill resembling the size of a small bullet. Separately cook 1 spoonful [1g] of the powdered *Gan Sui* (Radix Kansui) and 0.2 cup [40 mL] of *Feng Mi* (Mel) in 2 cups [400 mL] of water until the liquid is reduced to 1 cup [200 mL]. Take 1 pill with 1 cup of the warm, strained decoction. Bowel movement should be induced within one night. If not, take additional doses until bowel movement is successfully induced.

Today, the formula is prepared by grinding all of the herbs into powder, using the doses suggested in brackets above, and then mixing the powder with 30g of powdered *Gan Sui* (Radix Kansui) and 250g of *Feng Mi* (Mel) to make pills. Take 5-10g of pills per dose with warm, boiled water.

Da Xian Xiong Wan (Major Sinking into the Chest Pill) treats *jie xiong* (stagnant chest) with accumulation of heat and water in the chest only. Clinically, patients may show such symptoms as fullness, hardness, and pain in the chest, and neck stiffness.

Da Xian Xiong Wan is a gentler formula in comparison to *Da Xian Xiong Tang*. The dose of *Mang Xiao* (Natrii Sulfas) is reduced because there is no abdominal pain or fullness. *Ting Li Zi* (Semen Descurainiae seu Lepidii) and *Ku Xing Ren* (Semen Armeniacae Amarum) are added to clear Lung heat and regulate Lung qi; they also help to move the water downward. Moreover, since this formula is taken in pill form rather than decoction, it has a gentler effect.

AUTHORS' COMMENTS

Although *Da Cheng Qi Tang* (Major Order the Qi Decoction) and *Da Xian Xiong Tang* are both cold, drastic purgative formulas, and both contain *Da Huang* (Radix et Rhizoma Rhei) and *Mang Xiao* (Natrii Sulfas), they are quite different in nature.

- *Da Cheng Qi Tang* treats heat and stagnation in the Large Intestine; *Zhi Zi* (Fructus Gardeniae) and *Hou Po* (Cortex Magnoliae Officinalis) activate qi flow and push the constipated stools out of the body. *Da Huang* is post-decocted in *Da Cheng Qi Tang*, indicating that its purgative effect is the key function.
- *Da Xian Xiong Tang*, on the other hand, treats interlocked water and heat in the chest; it uses *Gan Sui* (Radix Kansui) to break up and eliminate stagnant water. *Da Huang* (Radix et Rhizoma Rhei) is pre-decocted in *Da Xian Xiong Tang*, indicating that the purgative effect is not primary in this formula.

Da Xian Xiong Tang and *Xiao Xian Xiong Tang* (Minor Sinking into the Chest Decoction) both treat stagnation in the chest.

- *Da Xian Xiong Tang* is a downward draining formula that treats a more serious interior condition characterized by stagnation of heat and water in the chest. Clinical presentations include hardened epigastrium with sensations of fullness and severe pain upon pressure.
- *Xiao Xian Xiong Tang* is a phlegm-dispelling formula that treats a less serious respiratory condition characterized by stagnation of heat and phlegm in the chest. Clinical presentations include a feeling of fullness in the chest and epigastrium, and pain upon pressure.

References
1. *Zhong Yao Yao Li Yu Lin Chuang* (Pharmacology and Clinical Applications of Chinese Herbs) 1989;5(2):5.
2. *Zhong Yi Fang Ji Xian Dai Yan Jiu* (Modern Study of Medical Formulae in Traditional Chinese Medicine) 1997;(1):156.

Chapter 2 – Downward Draining Formulas   *Section 1 – Cold Purgatives*

Dà Xiàn Xiōng Tāng (Major Sinking into the Chest Decoction)

3. *Zhong Cao Yao Tong Xun* (Journal of Chinese Herbal Medicine) 1979;9:35.
4. *Chi Jiao Yi Sheng Za Zhi* (Journal of Barefoot Doctors) 1975;(2):26.
5. *Zhong Yi Fang Ji Xian Dai Yan Jiu* (Modern Study of Medical Formulae in Traditional Chinese Medicine) 1997;(1):156.

6. *Zhong Cheng Yao Yan Jiu* (Research of Chinese Patent Medicine) 1984;1:28.
7. *Zhong Guo Zhong Xi Yi Jie He Za Zhi* (Chinese Journal of Integrative Chinese and Western Medicine) 1977;1:7.
8. *Zhong Yao Yao Li Yu Lin Chuang* (Pharmacology and Clinical Applications of Chinese Herbs) 1989;5(2):5.

Yǐ Zì Tāng (Yi Word Decoction)

乙字湯
乙字汤

Pinyin Name: *Yi Zi Tang*
Literal Name: Yi Word Decoction
Alternate Names: *I Chi Tang*, I-Character Decoction, Cimicifuga Combination
Original Source: *Asada's Prescriptions* by Sohaku Asada

COMPOSITION

Chai Hu (Radix Bupleuri)	5g
Sheng Ma (Rhizoma Cimicifugae)	1g
Dang Gui (Radix Angelicae Sinensis)	6g
Gan Cao (Radix et Rhizoma Glycyrrhizae)	3g
Huang Qin (Radix Scutellariae)	3g
Da Huang (Radix et Rhizoma Rhei)	1g

DOSAGE / PREPARATION / ADMINISTRATION

The source text states to cook the ingredients in 1 bowl of water and reduce it to 50%. Take the warm decoction in two or three equally-divided doses daily. Today, this formula may be prepared as a decoction with higher doses of the ingredients, approximately two to three times higher.

CHINESE THERAPEUTIC ACTIONS

1. Clears heat and promotes bowel movement
2. Cools the blood and eliminates toxins
3. Raises yang qi

CLINICAL MANIFESTATIONS

Accumulation of dampness, heat and toxins in the lower *jiao*: hemorrhoids, constipation, severe local pain, and slight bleeding. It is also used for women with menstrual bleeding, vaginal bleeding, abdominal pain, and the presence of dark blood with clots.

CLINICAL APPLICATIONS

Hemorrhoids, constipation, prolapse of rectum, and vaginal itching.

EXPLANATION

Yi Zi Tang (Yi Word Decoction) primarily treats hemorrhoids and constipation caused by accumulation of dampness, heat, and toxins in the lower *jiao*. In addition to hemorrhoids, patients will often experience constipation, severe pain, and possible bleeding. Because this formula is indicated for accumulation of dampness, heat, and toxins in the lower *jiao*, it also treats the gynecological problems listed above.

Chai Hu (Radix Bupleuri) and *Sheng Ma* (Rhizoma Cimicifugae) together have lifting functions to raise qi and restore the normal position of the rectum. *Dang Gui* (Radix Angelicae Sinensis) and *Gan Cao* (Radix et Rhizoma Glycyrrhizae) nourish the blood and replenish lost blood. Additionally, these two herbs have effects to relieve pain. *Huang Qin* (Radix Scutellariae) and *Da Huang* (Radix et Rhizoma Rhei) clear damp-heat and toxins from the Large Intestine and promote intestinal peristalsis.

164

Yǐ Zì Tāng (Yi Word Decoction)

Yi Zi Tang (Yi Word Decoction)

Diagnosis	Signs and Symptoms	Treatment	Herbs
Accumulation of dampness, heat and toxins in the lower *jiao*	• Hemorrhoids and/or constipation with severe pain: accumulation of dampness, heat and toxins in the lower *jiao* • Menstrual or vaginal bleeding with dark blood and clots: accumulation of dampness, heat and toxins in the lower *jiao*	• Clears heat and promotes bowel movement • Cools the blood and eliminates toxins • Raises yang qi	• *Chai Hu* (Radix Bupleuri) and *Sheng Ma* (Rhizoma Cimicifugae) have lifting functions to raise qi. • *Dang Gui* (Radix Angelicae Sinensis) and *Gan Cao* (Radix et Rhizoma Glycyrrhizae) nourish the blood and replenish lost blood. • *Huang Qin* (Radix Scutellariae) and *Da Huang* (Radix et Rhizoma Rhei) clear damp-heat and toxins from the Large Intestine and promote intestinal peristalsis.

MODIFICATIONS

• If the constipation is severe, increase the dose of *Da Huang* (Radix et Rhizoma Rhei) and add *Zhi Shi* (Fructus Aurantii Immaturus).

• When there are dry stools, add *Yu Li Ren* (Semen Pruni) and *Huo Ma Ren* (Fructus Cannabis).

• If there is itching and pain in the genitalia, add *Jin Yin Hua* (Flos Lonicerae Japonicae) and *Lian Qiao* (Fructus Forsythiae).

• If accompanied by profuse bleeding, add charred *Di Yu* (Radix Sanguisorbae), *Di Huang* (Radix Rehmanniae), and *Huang Lian* (Rhizoma Coptidis).

• For severe hemorrhoidal pain, add *Ru Xiang* (Gummi Olibanum), *Wu Yao* (Radix Linderae), and *Xiang Fu* (Rhizoma Cyperi).

• For hemorrhoids with accumulation of stagnant blood in the abdomen, add *Gui Zhi Fu Ling Wan* (Cinnamon Twig and Poria Pill).

• For rectal prolapse arising from qi deficiency, add *Bu Zhong Yi Qi Tang* (Tonify the Middle and Augment the Qi Decoction).

• For rectal prolapse with excess bleeding, add *Huai Hua San* (Sophora Japonica Flower Powder) or charred *Di Yu* (Radix Sanguisorbae), *Di Huang* (Radix Rehmanniae), and *Huang Lian* (Rhizoma Coptidis).

RELATED FORMULA

Qīng Cháng Tāng (Clear the Intestines Decoction)

清腸湯
请肠汤

Pinyin Name: *Qing Chang Tang*
Literal Name: Clear the Intestines Decoction
Original Source: *Guang An Men Yi Yuan* (Guang An Men Hospital) in 1990

Jin Yin Hua (Flos Lonicerae Japonicae)
Lian Qiao (Fructus Forsythiae)
Huai Hua (Flos Sophorae)
Di Yu (Radix Sanguisorbae)
Pu Gong Ying (Herba Taraxaci)
Chun Pi (Cortex Ailanthi)
Huang Qin (Radix Scutellariae)
Xian He Cao (Herba Agrimoniae)
Dang Gui (Radix Angelicae Sinensis)
Yu Li Ren (Semen Pruni)
He Zi (Fructus Chebulae)
Wu Wei Zi (Fructus Schisandrae Chinensis)

Qing Chang Tang (Clear the Intestines Decoction) treats general hemorrhoids, including internal or external hemorrhoids, with or without swelling, inflammation, or bleeding. This formula contains herbs that clear damp-heat, eliminate toxins, stop bleeding, and regulate bowel movements.

165

Chapter 2 – Downward Draining Formulas

Section 2 – Warm Purgatives

Section 2

温下剂

— Warm Purgatives

Dà Huáng Fù Zǐ Tāng (Rhubarb and Prepared Aconite Decoction)

大黃附子湯
大黄附子汤

Pinyin Name: *Da Huang Fu Zi Tang*
Literal Name: Rhubarb and Prepared Aconite Decoction
Original Source: *Jin Gui Yao Lue* (Essentials from the Golden Cabinet) by Zhang Zhong-Jing in the Eastern Han Dynasty

COMPOSITION

Fu Zi (Radix Aconiti Lateralis Praeparata), *pao* (blast-fried)	3 pieces [9g]
Xi Xin (Radix et Rhizoma Asari)	6g [3g]
Da Huang (Radix et Rhizoma Rhei)	9g

DOSAGE / PREPARATION / ADMINISTRATION

Cook the ingredients in 5 cups [1,000 mL] of water and reduce it to 2 cups [400 mL]. Take the warm, strained decoction in three equally-divided doses. For individuals who are otherwise robust and healthy, cook the herbs in 5 cups [1,000 mL] of water and reduce it to 2.5 cups [500 mL]. Take the warm, strained decoction in three equally-divided doses. Today, the decoction may be prepared using the doses suggested in brackets.

CHINESE THERAPEUTIC ACTIONS

1. Warms yang and disperses cold
2. Drains accumulation and eliminates stagnation

CLINICAL MANIFESTATIONS

Excess cold accumulation in the interior: hypochondriac and abdominal pain, constipation, cold to icy extremities, a white, greasy tongue coating, and a tight and wiry pulse.

CLINICAL APPLICATIONS

Acute abdominal pain, cholecystitis, dysentery, chronic colitis, enteritis, chronic renal failure, and uremia.

EXPLANATION

Da Huang Fu Zi Tang (Rhubarb and Prepared Aconite Decoction) treats excess cold accumulation in the interior. Cold accumulation blocks yang qi circulation to the limbs, resulting in cold extremities. Cold accumulation

Da Huang Fu Zi Tang (Rhubarb and Prepared Aconite Decoction)

Diagnosis	Signs and Symptoms	Treatment	Herbs
Excess cold accumulation in the interior	• Constipation with hypochondriac and abdominal pain: cold accumulation with qi and blood stagnation • Cold extremities: blocked yang qi circulation • White, greasy tongue coating and a tight, wiry pulse: interior cold	• Warms yang and disperses cold • Drains accumulation and eliminates stagnation	• *Fu Zi* (Radix Aconiti Lateralis Praeparata) warms the interior of the body and disperses cold. • *Xi Xin* (Radix et Rhizoma Asari) disperses cold, stagnation, and accumulation. • *Da Huang* (Radix et Rhizoma Rhei) clears heat and drains downward.

166

Dà Huáng Fù Zǐ Tāng (Rhubarb and Prepared Aconite Decoction)

also causes qi and blood stagnation, resulting in constipation with hypochondriac and abdominal pain. The tongue and pulse conditions are indicative of an excess cold syndrome.

Fu Zi (Radix Aconiti Lateralis Praeparata) warms the interior of the body and disperses cold. *Xi Xin* (Radix et Rhizoma Asari) disperses cold, stagnation and accumulation. *Da Huang* (Radix et Rhizoma Rhei) clears the Stomach and Intestines and breaks up qi stagnation, thereby relieving constipation, and hypochondriac and abdominal pain.

MODIFICATIONS

- For abdominal pain that lessens with the application of warmth, add *Gui Zhi* (Ramulus Cinnamomi) and *Bai Shao* (Radix Paeoniae Alba).
- If there is abdominal distention, add *Zhi Shi* (Fructus Aurantii Immaturus) and *Shen Qu* (Massa Fermentata).
- For abdominal fullness, distention, and a greasy tongue coating from stagnation, add *Hou Po* (Cortex Magnoliae Officinalis) and *Mu Xiang* (Radix Aucklandiae).
- In cases of qi deficiency, add *Dang Shen* (Radix Codonopsis) and *Huang Qi* (Radix Astragali).
- For Spleen and Stomach yang deficiencies, add *Ren Shen* (Radix et Rhizoma Ginseng) and *Gan Cao* (Radix et Rhizoma Glycyrrhizae).
- For the elderly and those who are weak, add *Gui Zhi* (Ramulus Cinnamomi) and fully-cook *Da Huang* (Radix et Rhizoma Rhei).
- For cold-type hernia, add *Xiao Hui Xiang* (Fructus Foeniculi) and *Rou Gui* (Cortex Cinnamomi).
- When there is severe pain, add *Rou Gui* (Cortex Cinnamomi).

CAUTIONS / CONTRAINDICATIONS

Because *Da Huang Fu Zi Tang* mainly treats excess cold accumulation in the interior, the dose of *Da Huang* (Radix et Rhizoma Rhei) should never exceed that of *Fu Zi* (Radix Aconiti Lateralis Praeparata).

PHARMACOLOGICAL EFFECTS

Gastrointestinal effect: Administration of a small dose of *Da Huang Fu Zi Tang* in mice and rabbits was associated with a stimulating effect on the intestines with increased peristalsis. Increased dose has not been associated with increased stimulation or inhibition. The effect of the formula was not blocked by atropine, indicating that the herbs probably exerted their effects directly on the intestines.[1]

CLINICAL STUDIES AND RESEARCH

1. **Acute abdomen**: The effects of *Da Huang Fu Zi Tang* were evaluated for treatment of acute abdominal pain, with such diagnosis as acute cholecystitis, cholelithiasis, intestinal obstruction, acute gastritis, and acute pancreatitis. Of 20 cases, the report stated immediate improvement in 9 cases, significant improvement in 5 cases, moderate improvement in 4 cases, and no benefit in 2 cases. The overall rate of effectiveness was 90%.[2]

2. **Chronic colitis**: Use of modified *Da Huang Fu Zi Tang* had 92.5% effectiveness in treating 27 patients with chronic ulcerative colitis. The herbal treatment used *Da Huang Fu Zi Tang* as the base formula, with the following modifications: *Xiao Hui Xiang* (Fructus Foeniculi), *Gan Jiang* (Rhizoma Zingiberis), and *Wu Yao* (Radix Linderae) for damp-cold; *Huang Lian* (Rhizoma Coptidis) and *Bai Tou Weng* (Radix Pulsatillae) for damp-heat; *Rou Cong Rong* (Herba Cistanches), *Ba Ji Tian* (Radix Morindae Officinalis) and *Bu Gu Zhi* (Fructus Psoraleae) for Spleen and Kidney yang deficiencies; and *Chai Hu* (Radix Bupleuri), *Xiang Fu* (Rhizoma Cyperi), *He Huan Pi* (Cortex Albiziae) and dry-fried *Bai Zhu* (Rhizoma Atractylodis Macrocephalae) for Liver excess and Spleen deficiency.[3]

3. **Chronic renal failure**: *Da Huang Fu Zi Tang* plus *Yi Mu Cao* (Herba Leonuri), calcined *Mu Li* (Concha Ostreae), and other herbs given via rectal instillation one time daily for 20 days was beneficial in treating chronic renal failure in 20 of 21 patients.[4] In another study, rectal instillation of *Da Huang Fu Zi Tang* plus *Mu Li* (Concha Ostreae) improved the symptoms and the overall condition of 34 patients.[5]

4. **Uremia**: Use of modified *Da Huang Fu Zi Tang* was associated with marked success in treating 46 patients with uremia. The herbal treatment contained *Da Huang Fu Zi Tang* plus *Yi Mu Cao* (Herba Leonuri), *Huang Qi* (Radix Astragali), and *Mang Xiao* (Natrii Sulfas) as the base formula, with the addition of *Che Qian Zi* (Semen Plantaginis) and *Bai Mao Gen* (Rhizoma Imperatae) for severe edema. The herbs were given in decoction via oral ingestion twice daily for 10 days per course of treatment. Additionally, 150 mL of the herbs were also given via rectal instillation (same formula and preparation) one time daily. Effective treatment was defined as resolution of the symptoms, with improvement of kidney functions as shown by lab reports. Of 46 patients, the rate of effectiveness was 85.7% among 14 individuals who received herbs via oral ingestion only, and 87.5% among 32 individuals who received herbs via both oral ingestion and rectal instillation.[6]

AUTHORS' COMMENTS

Da Huang Fu Zi Tang is the representative formula for treating constipation caused by cold accumulation. This formula can be used for post-operative syndrome associated with gallbladder removal, pain associated with gallstones, chronic dysentery, and uremia.

Dà Huáng Fù Zǐ Tāng (Rhubarb and Prepared Aconite Decoction)

Most downward draining formulas contain both *Da Huang* (Radix et Rhizoma Rhei) and *Mang Xiao* (Natrii Sulfas) because of their synergistic effect in treating constipation. *Da Huang Fu Zi Tang*, however, contains only *Da Huang* (Radix et Rhizoma Rhei) and **not** *Mang Xiao* (Natrii Sulfas) because this formula treats constipation caused by cold accumulation, manifesting in symptoms of hypochondriac and abdominal pain. The formula employs hot herbs, such as *Fu Zi* (Radix Aconiti Lateralis Praeparata) and *Xi Xin* (Radix et Rhizoma Asari), to disperse cold and relieve pain, and a cold herb, such as *Da Huang* (Radix et Rhizoma Rhei), to balance the temperature of the formula and induce bowel movement. *Mang Xiao* (Natrii Sulfas) is not used in this formula because its presence will create a synergistic effect with *Da Huang* (Radix et Rhizoma Rhei), and change the nature of the formula from warm to cold, thereby making the constipation (from cold accumulation) worse.

The condition associated with this formula involves both excess and deficiency, namely excess cold accumulation and yang deficiency. This condition is different than the one seen in *Da Cheng Qi Tang* (Major Order the Qi Decoction), which involves a purely excess heat condition. If the constipation is relieved after taking *Da Huang Fu Zi Tang*, that means the condition is stabilized. If the constipation persists after administering the formula and other symptoms such as vomiting, cold limbs, and a fine pulse appear, this indicates that the condition is worsening quickly.

Da Huang Fu Zi Tang treats complicated cases of excess cold and yang deficiency. Therefore, the treatment approach requires careful use and balance of hot and cold herbs. Although *Da Huang* (Radix et Rhizoma Rhei) is cold in nature, its cold tendency is neutralized by the hot nature of *Fu Zi* (Radix Aconiti Lateralis Praeparata) and the warm nature of *Xi Xin* (Radix et Rhizoma Asari). Zhang Zhong-Jing often used *Fu Zi* (Radix Aconiti Lateralis Praeparata) and *Xi Xin* (Radix et Rhizoma Asari) to treat excess cold accumulation deep inside the body. The dose of *Fu Zi* (Radix Aconiti Lateralis Praeparata) is greater in this formula than in *Ma Huang Fu Zi Xi Xin Tang* (Ephedra, Asarum, and Prepared Aconite Decoction), because it has to neutralize the cold temperature of *Da Huang* (Radix et Rhizoma Rhei). Also note that the dose of *Da Huang* (Radix et Rhizoma Rhei) is much less in this formula than in *Da Cheng Qi Tang* (Major Order the Qi Decoction), a cold purgative formula, indicating that the interior-warming action is of greater importance than the purgative action in this formula.

Da Huang Fu Zi Tang, *Wen Pi Tang* (Warm the Spleen Decoction), and *San Wu Bei Ji Wan* (Three-Substance Pill for Emergencies) are warm purgative formulas that treat constipation caused by cold accumulation. All three formulas purge stagnation, warm the interior, and relieve pain. All three formulas contain *Da Huang* (Radix et Rhizoma Rhei), but for different purposes.

- *Da Huang Fu Zi Tang* warms Spleen and Kidney yang and treats excess cold accumulation in the interior. The dose of *Da Huang* (Radix et Rhizoma Rhei) is less than *Fu Zi* (Radix Aconiti Lateralis Praeparata) to achieve a purgative effect without inducing more coldness. Of the three formulas, *Da Huang Fu Zi Tang* has the most moderate and balanced approach to warming the interior and purging downward.

- *Wen Pi Tang* warms Spleen yang to treat cold accumulation. *Da Huang* (Radix et Rhizoma Rhei) is used with several warm and hot herbs that tonify qi and purge the contents of the Intestines without creating coldness. Of the three formulas, *Wen Pi Tang* has the most potent effect to warm and tonify.

- *San Wu Bei Ji Wan* drastically purges downward to treat excess cold accumulation in the interior. *Da Huang* (Radix et Rhizoma Rhei) enhances the purgative effect, and antagonizes the adverse effects of *Ba Dou* (Semen Crotonis) by offsetting the latter's hot and acrid properties, thus preventing damage to the body. Of the three formulas, *San Wu Bei Ji Wan* is the strongest formula for purging downward.[7]

References

1. *Jing Fang Yan Jiu* (Research of Experienced Formulas) 1989;95.
2. *Zhong Yi Fang Ji Xian Dai Yan Jiu* (Modern Study of Medical Formulae in Traditional Chinese Medicine) 1997;4(1):20.
3. *Yun Nan Zhong Yi Za Zhi* (Yunan Journal of Chinese Medicine) 1993;2:10.
4. *Shan Dong Zhong Yi Za Zhi* (Shandong Journal of Chinese Medicine) 1988;4:21.
5. *Nei Meng Gu Zhong Yi Yao* (Traditional Chinese Medicine and Medicinals of Inner Mongolia) 1988;2:23.
6. *Shan Xi Zhong Yi Za Zhi* (Shanxi Journal Chinese Medicine) 1983;1:11.
7. Wang MZ, et al. *Zhong Yi Xue Wen Da Ti Ku* (Questions and Answers on Traditional Chinese Medicine: Herbal Formulas).

Chinese Herbal Formulas and Applications

Wēn Pí Tāng (Warm the Spleen Decoction)

溫脾湯
温脾汤

Pinyin Name: *Wen Pi Tang*
Literal Name: Warm the Spleen Decoction
Original Source: *Bei Ji Qian Jin Yao Fang* (Thousands of Golden Prescriptions for Emergencies) by Sun Si-Miao in the Tang Dynasty

COMPOSITION

Da Huang (Radix et Rhizoma Rhei)	12g
Fu Zi (Radix Aconiti Lateralis Praeparata)	1 large piece [9g]
Gan Jiang (Rhizoma Zingiberis)	6g
Ren Shen (Radix et Rhizoma Ginseng)	6g
Gan Cao (Radix et Rhizoma Glycyrrhizae)	6g [3g]

DOSAGE / PREPARATION / ADMINISTRATION

The source text states to grind the ingredients coarsely, cook them in 8 cups [1,600 mL] of water, and reduce the liquid to 2.5 cups [500 mL]. *Da Huang* (Radix et Rhizoma Rhei) should be post-decocted near the end. Take the warm, strained decoction in three equally-divided doses. Today, it is normally prepared as a decoction with the doses suggested in brackets above, and with *Da Huang* (Radix et Rhizoma Rhei) post-decocted.

CHINESE THERAPEUTIC ACTIONS

1. Warms and tonifies Spleen yang
2. Drains interior cold and accumulation downward

CLINICAL MANIFESTATIONS

Spleen yang deficiency syndrome leading to cold accumulation: constipation, or chronic diarrhea with blood and mucus; abdominal pain that is relieved by warmth; epigastric rigidity; cold hands and feet; and a deep and wiry pulse.

CLINICAL APPLICATIONS

Peptic ulcer disease, biliary ascariasis, and chronic renal failure.

EXPLANATION

Wen Pi Tang (Warm the Spleen Decoction) treats Spleen yang deficiency with interior cold accumulation. This condition usually occurs in individuals who frequently ingest cold beverages or eat raw foods, and who have pre-existing Spleen yang deficiency. The cold and raw foods cannot be digested and become obstructed in the Intestines, causing constipation. However, if the Spleen is deficient and fails to lift qi and nutrients, diarrhea with blood and mucus may occur. The presence of blood is the result of a deficient Spleen not being able to hold blood in the vessels, while mucus is a direct reflection of the Spleen's failure to transform dampness. Interior cold causes qi obstruction, leading to abdominal pain and epigastric rigidity. Since cold is the pathogenic factor, the severity of the pain is usually lessened by warmth. The cold hands and feet are

Wen Pi Tang (Warm the Spleen Decoction)

Diagnosis	Signs and Symptoms	Treatment	Herbs
Spleen yang deficiency with cold accumulation	• Constipation with abdominal coldness and pain that lessen with warmth: cold accumulation in the interior • Chronic diarrhea with blood and mucus: Spleen yang deficiency • Cold hands and feet: Spleen yang unable to warm the extremities • Abdominal pain and epigastric rigidity: interior cold obstructing qi circulation • Deep, wiry pulse: excess cold in the interior	• Warms and tonifies Spleen yang • Drains interior cold and accumulation downward	• *Da Huang* (Radix et Rhizoma Rhei) drains and purges accumulation and stagnation. • *Fu Zi* (Radix Aconiti Lateralis Praeparata) and *Gan Jiang* (Rhizoma Zingiberis) tonify Spleen yang and disperse interior cold. • *Ren Shen* (Radix et Rhizoma Ginseng) and *Gan Cao* (Radix et Rhizoma Glycyrrhizae) tonify qi and nourish the Spleen.

Chapter 2 – Downward Draining Formulas

Section 2 – Warm Purgatives

Wēn Pí Tāng (Warm the Spleen Decoction)

manifestations of a deficient Spleen yang unable to warm the extremities. A deep, wiry pulse indicates excess cold in the interior.

In this situation, simply using purgative herbs will further injure the middle *jiao*. Simply tonifying yang will warm the interior but will not achieve the purpose of dispelling accumulation and stagnation. To effectively treat this syndrome, both purgative and Spleen yang-tonifying herbs must be used together. *Da Huang* (Radix et Rhizoma Rhei) drains and purges accumulation and stagnation. *Fu Zi* (Radix Aconiti Lateralis Praeparata) and *Gan Jiang* (Rhizoma Zingiberis) tonify Spleen yang and disperse interior cold. *Ren Shen* (Radix et Rhizoma Ginseng) and *Gan Cao* (Radix et Rhizoma Glycyrrhizae) tonify qi and nourish the Spleen.

MODIFICATIONS

- When there is severe abdominal pain caused by cold, add *Rou Gui* (Cortex Cinnamomi) and *Gao Liang Jiang* (Rhizoma Alpiniae Officinarum).
- If accompanied by abdominal fullness, add *Mu Xiang* (Radix Aucklandiae) and *Hou Po* (Cortex Magnoliae Officinalis).
- For nausea and vomiting, add *Ban Xia* (Rhizoma Pinelliae) and *Sha Ren* (Fructus Amomi).
- If there is food stagnation and indigestion, add *Shen Qu* (Massa Fermentata) and *Lai Fu Zi* (Semen Raphani).
- For chronic diarrhea with heat and cold accumulation, add charred *Jin Yin Hua* (Flos Lonicerae Japonicae) and charred *Huang Qin* (Radix Scutellariae).
- For chronic nephritis with uremia, remove *Gan Jiang* (Rhizoma Zingiberis) and *Gan Cao* (Radix et Rhizoma Glycyrrhizae), and add *Chen Pi* (Pericarpium Citri Reticulatae), *Fu Ling* (Poria), and *Hou Po* (Cortex Magnoliae Officinalis).

CAUTIONS / CONTRAINDICATIONS

Wen Pi Tang treats constipation or diarrhea caused by Spleen yang deficiency and cold accumulation. It should not be used in cases of constipation caused by excess heat or diarrhea caused by damp-heat.

PHARMACOLOGICAL EFFECTS

1. **Gastrointestinal**: Administration of *Wen Pi Tang* at 10 g/kg effectively induced bowel movement in mice with artificially-induced constipation characterized by deficiency and cold of the Spleen and Stomach.[1]
2. **Nephroprotective**: Administration of *Wen Pi Tang* was associated with a dose-dependent effect to prevent and treat renal injuries induced by 3-morpholinosydnonimine and peroxynitrite.[2,3] It was shown in another study that

Wen Pi Tang has nephroprotective effects against ischemia-reperfusion kidney injury.[4]

CLINICAL STUDIES AND RESEARCH

1. **Peptic ulcer disease**: Use of modified *Wen Pi Tang* for an average of 37.2 days was associated with complete recovery in 39 of 45 patients with peptic ulcer disease.[5]
2. **Biliary ascariasis**: Administration of modified *Wen Pi Tang* was associated with relief in all 63 patients with biliary ascariasis. The study reported complete relief in 59 cases after one pack of herbs, and in 4 cases after three days of treatment.[6]
3. **Chronic renal failure**: Administration of *Wen Pi Tang* was associated with beneficial effects on the progression of chronic renal failure in 8 patients (between 24 and 59 years of age). The causes of chronic renal failure were chronic glomerulonephritis in 7 patients and systemic lupus erythematosus in 1 patient. The duration of treatment ranged from 40 to 402 weeks (mean: 228.1 +/- 118.8 weeks). The study reported that *Wen Pi Tang* has a beneficial effect to significantly retard the progression of chronic renal failure and to delay the need for dialysis.[7]

AUTHORS' COMMENTS

The composition of *Wen Pi Tang* resembles the composition of two other formulas that strongly warm yang and tonify qi.

- It resembles *Da Huang Fu Zi Tang* (Rhubarb and Prepared Aconite Decoction), a warm purgative formula that treats cold accumulation and interior excess. However, *Wen Pi Tang* does not contain *Xi Xin* (Radix et Rhizoma Asari), but instead has *Ren Shen* (Radix et Rhizoma Ginseng), *Gan Jiang* (Rhizoma Zingiberis), and *Gan Cao* (Radix et Rhizoma Glycyrrhizae).
- It also resembles *Si Ni Tang* (Frigid Extremities Decoction), an interior-warming formula that treats *shaoyin* cold syndrome with depletion of yang. *Wen Pi Tang* contains all three ingredients of *Si Ni Tang*, plus *Ren Shen* (Radix et Rhizoma Ginseng) and *Da Huang* (Radix et Rhizoma Rhei).

Da Huang Fu Zi Tang (Rhubarb and Prepared Aconite Decoction) and *Wen Pi Tang* both warm the interior and disperse cold accumulation to treat constipation. Both formulas contain *Fu Zi* (Radix Aconiti Lateralis Praeparata) to warm the interior, and *Da Huang* (Radix et Rhizoma Rhei) to purge accumulation in the Intestines. The differences between these two formulas are as follows:

- *Da Huang Fu Zi Tang* contains *Xi Xin* (Radix et Rhizoma Asari) to relieve pain and to open the channels to relieve cold extremities. It is indicated for generalized yang deficiency.

170

Wēn Pí Tāng (Warm the Spleen Decoction)

- *Wen Pi Tang* contains *Gan Jiang* (Rhizoma Zingiberis), *Gan Cao* (Radix et Rhizoma Glycyrrhizae), and *Ren Shen* (Radix et Rhizoma Ginseng) to tonify and warm the middle *jiao*. It is indicated for yang qi deficiency in the middle *jiao*.

References

1. *Zhong Yao Tong Bao* (Journal of Chinese Herbology) 1988;13(8):43.
2. Yokozawa T, Rhyu DY, Cho EJ. Protection by the Chinese prescription Wen-Pi-Tang against renal tubular LLC-PK1 cell damage induced by 3-morpholinosydnonimine. J Pharm Pharmacol. 2003 Oct;55(10):1405-12.
3. Rhyu DY, Yokozawa T, Choa EJ, Park JC. Prevention of peroxynitrite-induced renal injury through modulation of peroxynitrite production by the Chinese prescription Wen-Pi-Tang. Free Radic Res. 2002 Dec;36(12):1261-9.
4. Yokozawa T, Dong E, Chen CP. Protection of the kidney by Wen-Pi-Tang against ischemia-reperfusion injury. Phytomedicine. 2000 Jun;7(3):185-9.
5. *Zhong Yi Za Zhi* (Journal of Chinese Medicine) 1985;8:52.
6. *Liao Ning Zhong Yi Za Zhi* (Liaoning Journal of Chinese Medicine) 1982;6:8.
7. Mitsuma T, Yokozawa T, Oura H, Terasawa K, Narita M. Clinical evaluation of kampo medication, mainly with wen-pi-tang, on the progression of chronic renal failure. Nippon Jinzo Gakkai Shi. 1999 Dec;41(8):769-77.

Sān Wù Bèi Jí Wán (Three-Substance Pill for Emergencies)
三物備急丸
三物备急丸

Pinyin Name: *San Wu Bei Ji Wan*
Literal Name: Three-Substance Pill for Emergencies
Original Source: *Jin Gui Yao Lue* (Essentials from the Golden Cabinet) by Zhang Zhong-Jing in the Eastern Han Dynasty

COMPOSITION

Ba Dou (Semen Crotonis), *ao* (simmered) and *yan* (ground) to small particles	30g
Gan Jiang (Rhizoma Zingiberis)	30g
Da Huang (Radix et Rhizoma Rhei)	30g

DOSAGE / PREPARATION / ADMINISTRATION

The source text instructions are to grind the ingredients into powder, and mix the powder with honey to form pills that resemble the size of large beans. Take 3-4 pills per dose with warm water or liquor. Today, this formula is usually given in powder form along with rice soup or warm water. The dose is 0.6-1.5g of the powder for adults, and less for children.

CHINESE THERAPEUTIC ACTIONS

Drastically purges cold and accumulation

CLINICAL MANIFESTATIONS

Excess cold accumulation in the interior: sudden onset of excruciating epigastric and abdominal fullness and pain, stabbing pain in the chest, cyanotic facial complexion, rapid breathing, lockjaw, constipation, and a deep, tight pulse. In severe cases, there may be unconsciousness.

CLINICAL APPLICATIONS

Intestinal obstruction and acute appendicitis.

EXPLANATION

San Wu Bei Ji Wan (Three-Substance Pill for Emergencies) treats emergency cases of acute excess cold accumulation in the interior, which is usually caused by the stagnation of cold food in the Stomach and Intestines. The stagnant cold food causes sudden qi blockage, which then leads to fullness and pain in the epigastrium and abdomen. Hot, acrid herbs must be used to dispel cold, and drastic purgative herbs must be used to drain accumulation and stagnation.

Ba Dou (Semen Crotonis), the acrid and warm chief herb, is an extremely potent cathartic herb for dispelling cold accumulation. *Gan Jiang* (Rhizoma Zingiberis), the acrid and warm deputy herb, warms the body to help *Ba Dou* (Semen Crotonis) dispel cold. It also protects and assists Spleen yang. *Da Huang* (Radix et Rhizoma Rhei), the assistant and envoy herb, is bitter and cold, and dispels stagnation in the Stomach and Intestines. Its cold nature moderates the extreme acrid and hot properties of *Ba Dou* (Semen Crotonis).

171

Chapter 2 – Downward Draining Formulas　　　　　　　　　　　*Section 2 – Warm Purgatives*

Sān Wù Bèi Jí Wán (Three-Substance Pill for Emergencies)

San Wu Bei Ji Wan (Three-Substance Pill for Emergencies)

Diagnosis	Signs and Symptoms	Treatment	Herbs
Excess cold accumulation in the interior	• Sudden onset of excruciating epigastric and abdominal fullness and pain, constipation, stabbing pain in the chest, cyanotic facial complexion: excess cold accumulation in the interior • Deep, tight pulse: interior cold accumulation	Drastically purges cold accumulation	• *Ba Dou* (Semen Crotonis) strongly drains excess and dispels cold accumulation. • *Gan Jiang* (Rhizoma Zingiberis) warms Spleen yang and dispels cold. • *Da Huang* (Radix et Rhizoma Rhei) eliminates stagnation in the Stomach and Intestines.

CAUTIONS / CONTRAINDICATIONS

- Because *Ba Dou* (Semen Crotonis) is toxic, use *San Wu Bei Ji Wan* with extreme caution and only when necessary during emergency or severe conditions.
- The use of this formula, which is extremely acrid, hot and toxic, is contraindicated in pregnant women, elderly or weak patients, or heat conditions in general.
- If persistent diarrhea occurs after taking this formula, administer room-temperature rice porridge to help stop the diarrhea.
- *San Wu Bei Ji Wan* is an extremely potent formula. It should only be used when absolutely necessary, and only for a short period of time. Do not use this formula at large doses or for a prolonged period of time, since such practices can easily lead to dehydration and electrolyte imbalance.[1]

CLINICAL STUDIES AND RESEARCH

Intestinal obstruction: Patients with intestinal obstruction were treated with modified *San Wu Bei Ji Wan*. The herbal formula was given in pills, which was made by mixing a fine powder of *Da Huang* (Radix et Rhizoma Rhei), *Gan Jiang* (Rhizoma Zingiberis) and *Ba Dou* (Semen Crotonis) in 3:2:1 proportions. The treatment protocol was to administer 1 pill (1g) to patients under 14 years of age, and 1-2 pills (1-2g) to patients 15 years or older. The herbs were given every four hours until the condition was resolved. Out of 39 patients, the study reported complete recovery in 35 patients, improvement in 3 patients, and no benefit in 1 patient. The overall rate of effectiveness was 97.4% and the average time needed was 6.2 hours.[2]

RELATED FORMULA

Sān Wù Bái Sǎn (Three-Substance White Powder)
三物白散
Pinyin Name: *San Wu Bai San*
Literal Name: Three-Substance White Powder
Alternate Name: *Bai San* (White Powder)

Original Source: *Shang Han Lun* (Discussion of Cold-Induced Disorders) by Zhang Zhong-Jing in the Eastern Han Dynasty

Jie Geng (Radix Platycodonis)	0.9g
Ba Dou (Semen Crotonis), *ao* (simmered) to black and *yan* (ground) to small particles	0.3g
Bei Mu (Bulbus Fritillariae)	0.9g

Grind the ingredients into powder, and take 0.5g of the powder with warm water.

San Wu Bai San (Three-Substance White Powder) mainly treats *jie xiong* (stagnant chest) characterized by cold and phlegm accumulation in the chest. Patients may show dyspnea, profuse sputum formation with difficulty in swallowing, and a deep and tight, or an excess and forceful pulse. Moreover, patients will have vomiting if the disease is above the diaphragm, and diarrhea if it is below the diaphragm. Clinically, this formula may treat patients diagnosed with diphtheria, acute laryngeal infection, and inflammation of the throat.

San Wu Bei Ji Wan and *San Wu Bai San* (Three-Substance White Powder) are two extremely potent formulas that treat excess cold accumulation in the interior.

- *San Wu Bei Ji Wan* is the stronger formula of the two. It is indicated for excess cold accumulation in the gastrointestinal tract of the middle and lower *jiaos*, which may be caused by food obstruction.
- *San Wu Bai San* is a gentler formula and better suited for excess cold with phlegm accumulation in the chest region.

AUTHORS' COMMENTS

San Wu Bei Ji Wan is an extremely potent formula that should be reserved for true emergencies. Immediate diarrhea or vomiting is the goal after administration, as they indicate successful removal of offending agents from

Chinese Herbal Formulas and Applications

Sān Wù Bèi Jǐ Wán (Three-Substance Pill for Emergencies)

the body. Traditionally, if the jaws are locked, the herbs are forced into the mouth by breaking the teeth. Today, the formula is given via nasogastric tube if patients are unable to open their mouth.

Cold (i.e., room temperature) and hot porridges are commonly served with *San Wu Bei Ji Wan,* for contrasting purposes. Consuming room-temperature porridge serves to decrease the frequency of bowel movement in those

who experience continuous diarrhea after taking this formula. Warm porridge, on the other hand, enhances the purgative effect and promote defecation.

References
1. *Zhong Yao Ming Fang Yao Li Yu Ying Yong* (Pharmacology and Applications of Famous Herbal Formulas) 1989;85-86.
2. *Yun Nan Zhong Yi Za Zhi* (Yunan Journal of Chinese Medicine) 1982;(2):27.

Section 3

润下剂
— Moist Laxatives

Má Zǐ Rén Wán (Hemp Seed Pill)
麻子仁丸

Pinyin Name: Ma Zi Ren Wan
Literal Name: Hemp Seed Pill
Alternate Name: Apricot Seed and Linum Formula
Original Source: *Shang Han Lun* (Discussion of Cold-Induced Disorders) by Zhang Zhong-Jing in the Eastern Han Dynasty

COMPOSITION

Huo Ma Ren (Fructus Cannabis)	2 cups (480g) [20g]
Ku Xing Ren (Semen Armeniacae Amarum), *ao* (simmered)	1 cup (240g) [10g]
Bai Shao (Radix Paeoniae Alba)	240g [9g]
Da Huang (Radix et Rhizoma Rhei)	480g [12g]
Hou Po (Cortex Magnoliae Officinalis), *zhi* (fried with liquid)	1 *chi* (240g) [9g]
Zhi Shi (Fructus Aurantii Immaturus)	240g [9g]

Note: The source text provides the doses of some of the herbs in volume (cup) and length (*chi*). One cup is approximately 200 mL, and one *chi* is about 23 centimeters or 9 inches. To facilitate preparation, these units have been converted to weight (grams).

DOSAGE / PREPARATION / ADMINISTRATION

Grind the ingredients into powder, and mix with *Feng Mi* (Mel) to form pills. The pills should resemble *Wu Tong Zi* (Semen Firmianae), a small seed approximately 5 mm in diameter. Take 10 pills per dose, three times daily. The dose may be increased until the desired effect is achieved. Today, this formula may be prepared in pills or decoction. For pills, grind the herbs into powder and mix with honey to form pills. Take 9g of pills one to two times daily with warm water. For decoction, use the doses suggested in brackets above.

CHINESE THERAPEUTIC ACTIONS

1. Lubricates the Intestines and drains heat
2. Activates qi circulation and promotes defecation

CLINICAL MANIFESTATIONS

Dryness and heat in the Stomach and Intestines accompanied by deficiency of body fluids: constipation with dry, hard stools, and frequent urination.

CLINICAL APPLICATIONS

Habitual constipation, post-surgical constipation, drug-induced constipation, and constipation in elderly individuals or postpartum women.

EXPLANATION

Ma Zi Ren Wan (Hemp Seed Pill) treats dryness and heat in the Stomach and Large Intestine. Dryness and heat may consume water and body fluids in these two organs, causing dry stools, constipation, and difficult defecation. Dryness and heat in the Stomach also affects the Spleen, limiting the latter's ability to distribute water to various parts of the body. As a result, water passes out through the Urinary Bladder in the form of frequent urination.

The chief herb, *Huo Ma Ren* (Fructus Cannabis), is sweet and neutral, and enters the Spleen, Stomach, and Large Intestine to moisten dryness and lubricate the Intestines to facilitate bowel movement. The deputy herb, *Ku Xing Ren* (Semen Armeniacae Amarum), enters two organs connected by their *zang fu* relationship: the Large Intestine to moisten dryness and the Lung to regulate and guide qi downward. *Bai Shao* (Radix Paeoniae Alba) nourishes yin and blood, preserves yin, and relieves abdominal and intestinal pain and spasms. *Da Huang* (Radix et Rhizoma Rhei) purges the constipated stool

Chinese Herbal Formulas and Applications

Má Zǐ Rén Wán (Hemp Seed Pill)

Ma Zi Ren Wan (Hemp Seed Pill)

Diagnosis	Signs and Symptoms	Treatment	Herbs
Dryness and heat in the Stomach and Intestines with deficiency of body fluids	• Constipation with dry, hard stools: dryness and heat consuming water and body fluids • Frequent urination: abnormal distribution of water	• Lubricates the Intestines and drains heat • Activates qi circulation and promotes defecation	• *Huo Ma Ren* (Fructus Cannabis) moistens dryness and lubricates the Intestines. • *Ku Xing Ren* (Semen Armeniacae Amarum) moistens dryness and regulates qi. • *Bai Shao* (Radix Paeoniae Alba) nourishes yin and blood. • *Da Huang* (Radix et Rhizoma Rhei) purges constipated stools and drains heat. • *Hou Po* (Cortex Magnoliae Officinalis) and *Zhi Shi* (Fructus Aurantii Immaturus) activate qi circulation. • *Feng Mi* (Mel) lubricates the Intestines and moistens dryness.

and drains heat. *Hou Po* (Cortex Magnoliae Officinalis) and *Zhi Shi* (Fructus Aurantii Immaturus) activate qi to relieve bloating and distention and to eliminate the constipated stool. *Feng Mi* (Mel) helps *Huo Ma Ren* (Fructus Cannabis) lubricate the Intestines and moisten dryness. It also moderates the harsh properties of *Da Huang* (Radix et Rhizoma Rhei).

MODIFICATIONS

• For habitual constipation with dry stools in geriatric patients, reduce the dose of *Da Huang* (Radix et Rhizoma Rhei) and add *Bai Zi Ren* (Semen Platycladi), *Rou Cong Rong* (Herba Cistanches), and *Dang Gui* (Radix Angelicae Sinensis).

• For hemorrhoids and constipation, add *Huang Lian* (Rhizoma Coptidis), *Sheng Ma* (Rhizoma Cimicifugae), *Tao Ren* (Semen Persicae), and *Dang Gui* (Radix Angelicae Sinensis).

• For bleeding hemorrhoids, add *Ce Bai Ye* (Cacumen Platycladi), *Di Yu* (Radix Sanguisorbae), and *Huai Hua* (Flos Sophorae).

• When there is thirst and increased water intake as a result of Stomach heat, add *Shi Gao* (Gypsum Fibrosum) and *Zhi Mu* (Rhizoma Anemarrhenae).

• If there is frequent urination, add *Qian Shi* (Semen Euryales), *Sang Piao Xiao* (Ootheca Mantidis), and *Yi Zhi* (Fructus Alpiniae Oxyphyllae).

CAUTIONS / CONTRAINDICATIONS

• Though *Ma Zi Ren Wan* is classified as a moist laxative formula, it nonetheless has a moderate purgative effect since it contains *Da Huang* (Radix et Rhizoma Rhei), *Zhi Shi* (Fructus Aurantii Immaturus) and *Hou Po* (Cortex Magnoliae Officinalis) to drain downward, activate qi

circulation, and purge constipated stools. Therefore, this formula is not recommended for very weak or deficient patients. Moreover, it should not be taken daily over a long period of time, since this may consume qi and body fluids.

• This formula should be used with caution during pregnancy.

PHARMACOLOGICAL EFFECTS

1. **Laxative**: According to various laboratory studies in mice, administration of *Ma Zi Ren Wan* was associated with increased bowel movement, usually within 12 hours.[1]

2. **Gastrointestinal**: Administration of *Ma Zi Ren Wan* was associated with increased intestinal peristalsis in anesthetized rabbits.[2]

CLINICAL STUDIES AND RESEARCH

1. **Constipation**: According to one study, 557 patients with different causes and various severity of constipation were treated with *Ma Zi Ren Wan* with complete recovery in 281 patients, significant improvement in 229 patients, moderate improvement in 25 patients, and no change in 22 patients. The overall rate of effectiveness was 96%.[3]

2. **Post-surgical constipation**: Use of *Ma Zi Ren Wan* was reported to have 95.8% effectiveness in preventing post-surgical constipation. Of 500 patients, the study reported normal bowel movements (without dryness, pain or bleeding) in 479 patients. Of 21 patients who did not respond, 16 had a history of habitual constipation.[4]

HERB-DRUG INTERACTION

Drug-induced constipation: Constipation caused by antipsychotic drugs in 80 individuals was treated with marked success using *Ma Zi Ren Wan*. The herbs were given at 9 to 15g per dose, three times daily. For those with severe constipation, the form was switched from

Chapter 2 – Downward Draining Formulas　　　　　　　　　　　　*Section 3 – Moist Laxatives*

Má Zǐ Rén Wán (Hemp Seed Pill)

pills to decoction. Of 80 cases, the study reported complete recovery in 62 cases, improvement in 13 cases, and no change in 5 cases.[5]

RELATED FORMULA

Wǔ Rén Wán (Five-Seed Pill)

五仁丸

Pinyin Name: *Wu Ren Wan*

Literal Name: Five-Seed Pill

Original Source: *Shi Yi De Xiao Fang* (Effective Formulas from Generations of Physicians) by Wei Yi-Lin in 1345

Tao Ren (Semen Persicae)	30g [15g]
Ku Xing Ren (Semen Armeniacae Amarum), *chao* (dry-fried)	30g [15g]
Bai Zi Ren (Semen Platycladi)	15g [9g]
Song Zi Ren (Semen Pini)	3.75g [5g]
Yu Li Ren (Semen Pruni), *chao* (dry-fried)	3g [5g]
Chen Pi (Pericarpium Citri Reticulatae), *yan* (ground) to powder	120g [15g]

Mash the five seeds into a paste. Add powdered *Chen Pi* (Pericarpium Citri Reticulatae) and blend thoroughly. Mix the powder with honey to form small pills that resemble the size of *Wu Tong Zi* (Semen Firmianae), a small seed approximately 5 mm in diameter. Take 50 pills with rice soup on an empty stomach. Today, this formula is prepared by grinding all of the ingredients into powder, mixing the powder with honey, and forming into pills. Take 12g of pills per dose with warm, boiled water on an empty stomach. This formula may also be prepared as a decoction with the doses suggested in brackets above.

Wu Ren Wan (Five-Seed Pill) is composed of five seeds rich in oil to lubricate the Intestines and facilitate bowel movement. It treats constipation and dry stool caused by severe body fluid deficiency. It may also be used for constipation in geriatric or postpartum patients with blood deficiency. Clinical manifestations include constipation, dry stool, a dry mouth, and thirst with a desire to drink.

Ku Xing Ren (Semen Armeniacae Amarum), the chief herb, nourishes and treats intestinal dryness. It also directs Lung qi downward to help the functioning of the Large Intestine, as these two organs are connected by their *zang fu* relationship. *Tao Ren* (Semen Persicae), the deputy herb, helps *Ku Xing Ren* (Semen Armeniacae Amarum) moisten dryness and lubricate the bowels. *Bai Zi Ren* (Semen Platycladi) and *Yu Li Ren* (Semen Pruni), rich in oil, are moist laxatives that further lubricate the bowels and relieve dryness and heat in the Stomach and Intestines. *Song*

Zi Ren (Semen Pini) moistens the five *zang* (solid) organs and treats constipation caused by deficiency. *Feng Mi* (Mel) lubricates the bowels. Finally, *Chen Pi* (Pericarpium Citri Reticulatae) regulates qi to promote circulation in the abdomen and relieve distention or bloating.

Wu Ren Wan should be taken with caution during pregnancy, since it contains *Tao Ren* (Semen Persicae), a blood-moving herb.

AUTHORS' COMMENTS

Ma Zi Ren Wan is commonly used today to treat habitual constipation, hemorrhoids with dry stools, or constipation in deficient and elderly patients. It can also be used as the base formula to treat intestinal obstruction caused by parasites, or constipation arising from heat and dryness after rectal or colon surgeries.

Xiao Cheng Qi Tang (Minor Order the Qi Decoction) and *Ma Zi Ren Wan* have three ingredients in common: *Da Huang* (Radix et Rhizoma Rhei), *Zhi Shi* (Fructus Aurantii Immaturus), and *Hou Po* (Cortex Magnoliae Officinalis). While *Xiao Cheng Qi Tang* (Minor Order the Qi Decoction) is classified as a cold purgative formula, *Ma Zi Ren Wan* is known as a moist laxative formula for the following reasons:

- *Xiao Cheng Qi Tang* (Minor Order the Qi Decoction) is administered as a decoction, which is absorbed quickly to provide a more immediate and potent effect to drain and purge downwards.
- *Ma Zi Ren Wan* is administered as honey pills, which are absorbed slowly over a long period of time. Consequently, its effects are gentle, and its potency is moderate. Furthermore, *Ma Zi Ren Wan* contains additional ingredients, such as *Huo Ma Ren* (Fructus Cannabis), *Ku Xing Ren* (Semen Armeniacae Amarum), *Bai Shao* (Radix Paeoniae Alba), and *Feng Mi* (Mel). Some of these herbs are rich in oil and can lubricate the Intestines to promote the passage of stools. Others are sweet and has a moderating effect to prevent *Da Huang* (Radix et Rhizoma Rhei) from injuring *zheng* (upright) *qi*. Because the overall focus of this formula is to lubricate the intestines and regulate bowel movement, not to purge downwards, it is considered as a moist laxative.

References

1. *Zhong Xi Yi Jie He Za Zhi* (Journal of Integrated Chinese and Western Medicine) 1990;(6):5.
2. *Zhong Xi Yi Jie He Za Zhi* (Journal of Integrated Chinese and Western Medicine) 1990;(6):5.
3. *Hu Nan Zhong Yi Za Zhi* (Hunan Journal of Chinese Medicine) 1994;10(4):55.
4. *Zhong Yi Za Zhi* (Journal of Chinese Medicine) 1965;10:40.
5. *Si Chuan Zhong Yi* (Sichuan Chinese Medicine) 1996;9:29.

Rùn Cháng Wán (Moisten the Intestines Pill)

潤腸丸
润肠丸

Pinyin Name: *Run Chang Wan*
Literal Name: Moisten the Intestines Pill
Original Source: *Pi Wei Lun* (Discussion of the Spleen and Stomach) by Li Gao in 1249

COMPOSITION

Da Huang (Radix et Rhizoma Rhei)	15g
Tao Ren (Semen Persicae), *jin* (soaked)	30g
Huo Ma Ren (Fructus Cannabis)	37.5g
Dang Gui (Radix Angelicae Sinensis)	15g
Qiang Huo (Rhizoma et Radix Notopterygii)	15g

DOSAGE / PREPARATION / ADMINISTRATION

The source text advises to separately grind *Huo Ma Ren* (Fructus Cannabis) into a paste, and pound all of the other ingredients into powder. Mix the paste and the powder with *Feng Mi* (Mel) and form into small pills that resemble the size of *Wu Tong Zi* (Semen Firmianae), a small seed approximately 5 mm in diameter. Take 50 pills with warm water on an empty stomach. Today, this formula is prepared by grinding all of the ingredients into powder and mixing with *Feng Mi* (Mel) to form into pills. Take 12g of pills per dose with warm water on an empty stomach.

CHINESE THERAPEUTIC ACTIONS

1. Lubricates the Intestines and promotes defecation
2. Tonifies blood circulation and dispels wind

CLINICAL MANIFESTATIONS

Constipation characterized by blood deficiency: habitual constipation, constipation in elderly or weak individuals, dry and hard stools, lack of appetite, lethargy, dizziness, and palpitations.

CLINICAL APPLICATIONS

Constipation in anemic or elderly persons.

EXPLANATION

Run Chang Wan (Moisten the Intestines Pill) is a moist-laxative formula that treats constipation characterized by blood deficiency, which may occur as a result of an inappropriate diet or overwork.

Da Huang (Radix et Rhizoma Rhei) purges the bowels and clears heat. *Tao Ren* (Semen Persicae), *Huo Ma Ren* (Fructus Cannabis), and *Feng Mi* (Mel) moisten the Intestines and promote defecation. *Dang Gui* (Radix Angelicae Sinensis) tonifies blood and yin to lubricate the bowels. *Qiang Huo* (Rhizoma et Radix Notopterygii) expels wind and relieves pain.

MODIFICATIONS

- If there is fever, add *Chai Hu* (Radix Bupleuri).
- When there is abdominal pain, add *Mu Xiang* (Radix Aucklandiae).
- For blood deficiency, increase the dose of *Dang Gui* (Radix Angelicae Sinensis) and *Tao Ren* (Semen Persicae) and add *Shu Di Huang* (Radix Rehmanniae Praeparata) and *Hong Hua* (Flos Carthami).

Run Chang Wan (Moisten the Intestines Pill)

Diagnosis	Signs and Symptoms	Treatment	Herbs
Constipation characterized by blood deficiency	Constipation with dry and hard stools accompanied by dizziness and palpitations: blood deficiency	• Lubricates the Intestines and promotes defecation • Tonifies blood circulation and dispels wind	• *Da Huang* (Radix et Rhizoma Rhei) purges the bowels and clears heat. • *Tao Ren* (Semen Persicae), *Huo Ma Ren* (Fructus Cannabis), and *Feng Mi* (Mel) moisten the Intestines and promote bowel movement. • *Dang Gui* (Radix Angelicae Sinensis) tonifies blood and yin to lubricate the bowels. • *Qiang Huo* (Rhizoma et Radix Notopterygii) expels wind and relieves pain.

Rùn Cháng Wán (Moisten the Intestines Pill)

- For wind and dryness, add *Yu Li Ren* (Semen Pruni), *Zao Jiao Ci* (Spina Gleditsiae), and increase the dose of *Qiang Huo* (Rhizoma et Radix Notopterygii).
- If accompanied by qi deficiency, add *Ren Shen* (Radix et Rhizoma Ginseng) and *Yu Li Ren* (Semen Pruni).
- If there is qi stagnation, add *Bing Lang* (Semen Arecae) and *Mu Xiang* (Radix Aucklandiae).
- For hot phlegm accumulation, add *Gua Lou* (Fructus Trichosanthis) and *Zhu Li* (Succus Bambusae).
- When there is body fluid deficiency, add *Ren Shen* (Radix et Rhizoma Ginseng) and *Mai Dong* (Radix Ophiopogonis).

CAUTIONS / CONTRAINDICATIONS

Run Chang Wan should be used with caution during pregnancy.

RELATED FORMULAS

Rùn Cháng Wán (Moisten the Intestines Pill)

潤腸丸
润肠丸

Pinyin Name: *Run Chang Wan*
Literal Name: Moisten the Intestines Pill
Alternate Names: *Jun Chang Tang*, Bowel-Nourishing Decoction, Linum and Rhubarb Formula
Original Source: *Wan Bing Hui Chun* (Restoration of Health from the Myriad Diseases) by Gong Ting-Xian in 1587

Dang Gui (Radix Angelicae Sinensis)
Shu Di Huang (Radix Rehmanniae Praeparata)
Di Huang (Radix Rehmanniae)
Huo Ma Ren (Fructus Cannabis)
Tao Ren (Semen Persicae)
Ku Xing Ren (Semen Armeniacae Amarum)
Zhi Qiao (Fructus Aurantii)
Huang Qin (Radix Scutellariae)
Hou Po (Cortex Magnoliae Officinalis)
Da Huang (Radix et Rhizoma Rhei)
Gan Cao (Radix et Rhizoma Glycyrrhizae)

The source text states to use an equal amount for all ingredients, and half the amount for *Gan Cao* (Radix et Rhizoma Glycyrrhizae). Grind the ingredients into powder, and mix with *Feng Mi* (Mel) and form into small pills that resemble the size of *Wu Tong Zi* (Semen Firmianae), a small seed approximately 5 mm in diameter. Take 50 pills with warm water on an empty stomach. This formula treats constipation due to dryness and heat in the Stomach and Large Intestine.

Má Zǐ Rùn Cháng Wán
(Hemp Seed Pill to Moisten the Intestines)

麻子潤腸丸
麻子润肠丸

Pinyin Name: *Ma Zi Run Chang Wan*
Literal Name: Hemp Seed Pill to Moisten the Intestines
Original Source: *Tian Jin Zhong Yi Xue Yuan* (Tianjin University of Chinese Medicine) in 1989

Huo Ma Ren (Fructus Cannabis)
Yu Li Ren (Semen Pruni)
Gua Lou Zi (Semen Trichosanthis)
Ku Xing Ren (Semen Armeniacae Amarum)
Bai Shao (Radix Paeoniae Alba)
Dang Gui (Radix Angelicae Sinensis)
He Shou Wu (Radix Polygoni Multiflori)
Tao Ren (Semen Persicae)
Mang Xiao (Natrii Sulfas)
Xuan Shen (Radix Scrophulariae)
Da Huang (Radix et Rhizoma Rhei)
Zhi Shi (Fructus Aurantii Immaturus)
Hou Po (Cortex Magnoliae Officinalis)

Ma Zi Run Chang Wan (Hemp Seed Pill to Moisten the Intestines) moistens the Intestines, drains heat, nourishes yin, and tonifies the blood. Clinically, this formula treats elderly patients with habitual constipation characterized by underlying weakness and deficiencies.

AUTHORS' COMMENTS

Run Chang Wan and *Ma Zi Ren Wan* (Hemp Seed Pill) are moist-laxative formulas that gently treat mild to moderate cases of constipation.

- *Run Chang Wan* treats constipation characterized by blood deficiency.
- *Ma Zi Ren Wan* treats constipation characterized by body fluid deficiency, with dryness and heat in the Stomach and Intestines.

Chinese Herbal Formulas and Applications

Ji Chuān Jiān (Benefit the River [Flow] Decoction)

濟川煎
济川煎

Pinyin Name: *Ji Chuan Jian*
Literal Name: Benefit the River [Flow] Decoction
Original Source: *Jing Yue Quan Shu* (Collected Treatises of [Zhang] Jing Yue) by Zhang Jie-Bin (Zhang Jing-Yue) in 1624

COMPOSITION

Rou Cong Rong (Herba Cistanches), *xi* (washed) with liquor	6-9g
Dang Gui (Radix Angelicae Sinensis)	9-15g
Niu Xi (Radix Achyranthis Bidentatae)	6g
Ze Xie (Rhizoma Alismatis)	4.5g
Zhi Qiao (Fructus Citri Aurantii)	3g
Sheng Ma (Rhizoma Cimicifugae)	1.5-3g

DOSAGE / PREPARATION / ADMINISTRATION

Cook the ingredients with 1.5 bowls of water until 0.7 to 0.8 bowl of liquid remains. Take the decoction before meals.

CHINESE THERAPEUTIC ACTIONS

1. Warms the Kidney and tonifies *jing* (essence)
2. Lubricates the Intestines and promotes defecation

CLINICAL MANIFESTATIONS

Constipation in the elderly caused by Kidney yang deficiency: constipation, polyuria with clear urine, dizziness, vertigo, soreness and weakness of the knees and low back, cold sensation of the lumbar region, intolerance to cold, and cold extremities.

CLINICAL APPLICATIONS

Constipation, habitual constipation, chronic constipation, and constipation in the elderly.

EXPLANATION

The Kidney controls water metabolism. If Kidney yang is deficient, however, it is unable to control water metabolism and water will be excreted out of the body in the form of copious, clear urine. As a result of body fluids being excreted as urine, the Intestines lack moisture, and constipation or dry stool occurs. Dizziness, weak knees, soreness in the lower back, intolerance to cold, and cold extremities all indicate Kidney yang deficiency.

Rou Cong Rong (Herba Cistanches), the chief herb, warms and tonifies Kidney yang and *jing* (essence) in addition to lubricating the Intestines. *Dang Gui* (Radix Angelicae Sinensis) nourishes and harmonizes the blood, as well as lubricates the Intestines. *Niu Xi* (Radix Achyranthis Bidentatae), having a downward-directing tendency, nourishes the Kidney and strengthens the lower parts of the body to treat soreness and weakness of the back and knees. *Ze Xie* (Rhizoma Alismatis) promotes urination

Ji Chuan Jian (Benefit the River [Flow] Decoction)

Diagnosis	Signs and Symptoms	Treatment	Herbs
Constipation caused by Kidney yang deficiency	• Clear and copious urine: Kidney yang deficiency fails to control water metabolism • Constipation with dry stool: dryness in the Intestines • Dizziness, weak knees, sore lower back, intolerance to cold, and cold extremities: Kidney yang deficiency	• Warms Kidney yang and tonifies *jing* (essence) • Lubricates the Intestines and promotes defecation	• *Rou Cong Rong* (Herba Cistanches) warms and tonifies Kidney yang and *jing* (essence), and lubricates the Intestines. • *Dang Gui* (Radix Angelicae Sinensis) nourishes and harmonizes the blood. • *Niu Xi* (Radix Achyranthis Bidentatae) nourishes the Kidney. • *Ze Xie* (Rhizoma Alismatis) promotes urination to excrete turbidity in the Kidney. • *Zhi Qiao* (Fructus Aurantii) activates qi flow to relieve constipation. • *Sheng Ma* (Rhizoma Cimicifugae) raises yang qi.

DOWNWARD DRAINING FORMULAS — 2

179

Ji Chuān Jiān (Benefit the River [Flow] Decoction)

to excrete turbidity from the Kidney. *Zhi Qiao* (Fructus Aurantii) activates qi flow to help relieve constipation. *Sheng Ma* (Rhizoma Cimicifugae) raises yang qi, while directing turbidity to the lower parts of the body to be excreted.

MODIFICATIONS

- If there is qi deficiency, remove *Zhi Qiao* (Fructus Aurantii) and add *Ren Shen* (Radix et Rhizoma Ginseng).
- When accompanied by fatigue, lack of energy, and no desire to speak, add *Dang Shen* (Radix Codonopsis) and *Huang Qi* (Radix Astragali).
- For Kidney yin deficiency, add *Shu Di Huang* (Radix Rehmanniae Praeparata) and *Tian Dong* (Radix Asparagi).
- For chronic habitual constipation with intestinal dryness

and coldness, remove *Ze Xie* (Rhizoma Alismatis) and add *Suo Yang* (Herba Cynomorii) and *Huo Ma Ren* (Fructus Cannabis).
- When there is increased frequency and volume of urine, add *Yi Zhi* (Fructus Alpiniae Oxyphyllae) and *Sang Piao Xiao* (Ootheca Mantidis).
- For soreness and pain of the lower back and knees, add *Du Zhong* (Cortex Eucommiae), *Sang Ji Sheng* (Herba Taxilli), and *Xu Duan* (Radix Dipsaci).

CAUTIONS / CONTRAINDICATIONS

Ji Chuan Jian (Benefit the River [Flow] Decoction) warms the Kidney to treat constipation caused by Kidney yang deficiency. It is contraindicated in cases of constipation caused by excess heat.

Chinese Herbal Formulas and Applications

Section 4

逐水剤

— Harsh Expellants (Cathartics)

DOWNWARD DRAINING FORMULAS

2

Shi Zǎo Tāng (Ten-Jujube Decoction)
十棗湯
十枣汤

Pinyin Name: *Shi Zao Tang*
Literal Name: Ten-Jujube Decoction
Alternate Name: *Shi Zao Wan* (Ten-Jujube Pill)
Original Source: *Shang Han Lun* (Discussion of Cold-Induced Disorders) by Zhang Zhong-Jing in the Eastern Han Dynasty

COMPOSITION

Yuan Hua (Flos Genkwa), *ao* (simmered)
Gan Sui (Radix Kansui)
Da Ji (Radix Euphorbiae seu Knoxiae)

DOSAGE / PREPARATION / ADMINISTRATION

The source text instructions are to separately grind equal amounts of each herb into powder. Cook 10 pieces of *Da Zao* (Fructus Jujubae) in 1.5 cups [300 mL] of water until the liquid is reduced to 0.8 cup [160 mL]. Discard the herb residue and add the powdered herbs to the warm, strained decoction before ingestion. The dose of the powdered herbs is 1g for patients with a strong body constitution, and 0.5g for those with a weak body constitution. If the condition is not resolved, increase the dose by 0.5g, and administer the formula again the following day. Once bowel movement is induced, discontinue the formula, and serve porridge to facilitate recovery from the use of strong purgative herbs.

Today, this formula is normally prepared and administered in powder or capsule forms, at a dose of 0.5-1g per dose one time daily, on an empty stomach in the early morning, with a decoction made from 10 pieces of *Da Zao* (Fructus Jujubae). Once bowel movement is induced, discontinue the formula and take porridge for nourishment.

CHINESE THERAPEUTIC ACTIONS

Drastically purges water accumulation

CLINICAL MANIFESTATIONS

1. *Xuan yin* (pleural effusion): water retention in the hypochondrium, coughing with sharp chest and hypochondriac pain, epigastric distention and hardness, shortness of breath, dyspnea caused by extreme chest and back pain, dry heaves, headache, dizziness, vertigo, and a deep, wiry pulse.
2. Excess water accumulation (in the lower half of the body): generalized edema that is more severe on the lower half of the body, abdominal fullness, dyspnea, and difficult defecation and urination.

CLINICAL APPLICATIONS

Pleural effusion, pleuritis, ascites, acute or chronic nephritis, and hyperacidity of the stomach.

EXPLANATION

Shi Zao Tang (Ten-Jujube Decoction) treats various clinical manifestations arising from excess water retention in the interior. If water is retained in the chest and hypochondrium, the functioning of the Lung will be compromised, as seen in symptoms of coughing with chest and hypochondriac pain, shortness of breath, and/or dyspnea. If the water retention affects Stomach qi, nausea and dry heaves result. Headache, dizziness, and vertigo are caused by water retention blocking yang qi circulation. A deep pulse suggests damp accumulation and interior syndrome, and

181

Chapter 2 – Downward Draining Formulas　　　　　　　　*Section 4 – Harsh Expellants (Cathartics)*

Shí Zǎo Tāng (Ten-Jujube Decoction)

Shi Zao Tang (Ten-Jujube Decoction)

Diagnosis	Signs and Symptoms	Treatment	Herbs
Excess water accumulation	• Coughing with sharp chest and hypochondriac pain, shortness of breath and dyspnea: water accumulation in the upper *jiao* affecting the Lung • Epigastric distention and hardness, nausea, and dry heaves: water accumulation in the middle *jiao* affecting the Stomach • Headache, dizziness and vertigo: yang qi unable to ascend because of water retention	Drastically purges water accumulation	• *Yuan Hua* (Flos Genkwa) eliminates water retention in the chest and hypochondrium. • *Gan Sui* (Radix Kansui) eliminates water retention in the channels and collaterals. • *Da Ji* (Radix Euphorbiae seu Knoxiae) eliminates water retention in the *zang fu* organs. • *Da Zao* (Fructus Jujubae) protects the Stomach and lessens the toxicity of the other herbs.

the wiry nature of the pulse signifies water retention and extreme pain. If water is retained mainly in the abdomen, then there will be edema of the abdomen and lower parts of the body.

Since this is a serious excess water retention syndrome, it is necessary to use drastic cathartic herbs. *Yuan Hua* (Flos Genkwa) enters the Lung and eliminates water retention in the chest and hypochondrium. *Gan Sui* (Radix Kansui) eliminates water retention in the channels and collaterals. *Da Ji* (Radix Euphorbiae seu Knoxiae) eliminates water retention in the *zang fu* organs. These three herbs are very drastic, and can quickly eliminate water retention and any fullness or stagnation in the body. However, since all three herbs are toxic and may easily injure the qi, *Da Zao* (Fructus Jujubae) is added to lessen their toxicity and to protect the Stomach.

CAUTIONS / CONTRAINDICATIONS

• *Shi Zao Tang* is a very strong cathartic formula that is potentially toxic if used inappropriately. Therapeutic effect is generally observed immediately after administration. If the condition is not resolved after taking this formula, continue taking the formula for another day. If the patient is deficient and has excess water retention, tonic herbs may also be used. Depending on the patient's condition, tonic herbs may be used before, during and/or after purgation. The dose should gradually be increased daily and stopped when the desired effects are achieved. If the patient does not have underlying deficiency, use of herbs that tonify and regulate the digestive system is still recommended.

• Since this is a drastic purgative formula, it should be used with caution in all patients. Moreover, this formula is contraindicated during pregnancy and in nursing mothers.[1]

• *Gan Cao* (Radix et Rhizoma Glycyrrhizae) should not be added to this formula, since it is incompatible with *Yuan*

Hua (Flos Genkwa), *Gan Sui* (Radix Kansui), and *Da Ji* (Radix Euphorbiae seu Knoxiae).

• Do **not** cook *Yuan Hua* (Flos Genkwa), *Gan Sui* (Radix Kansui), and *Da Ji* (Radix Euphorbiae seu Knoxiae) in water, since side effects such as abdominal pain, nausea, and vomiting have been associated with the use of this formula in decoction form.

CLINICAL STUDIES AND RESEARCH

1. **Pleuritis**: Administration of *Shi Zao Tang* showed 89.2% effectiveness in treating 28 patients with inflammation of the pleura surrounding the lungs. Those with tuberculosis or pneumonia were also treated with pharmaceuticals accordingly. Out of 28 cases, the study reported complete recovery in 16 cases, marked improvement in 7 cases, moderate improvement in 2 cases, and no benefit in 3 cases.[2]

2. **Hyperacidity**: Administration of *Shi Zao Tang* was effective in treating individuals with hyperacidity of the stomach. The study reported complete recovery in all 14 patients without relapse.[3]

RELATED FORMULA

Kòng Xián Dān (Control Mucus Special Pill)

控涎丹

Pinyin Name: *Kong Xian Dan*

Literal Name: Control Mucus Special Pill

Original Source: *San Yin Ji Yi Bing Zheng Fang Lun* (Discussion of Illnesses, Patterns, and Formulas Related to the Unification of the Three Etiologies) by Chen Yan in 1174

Gan Sui (Radix Kansui)

Da Ji (Radix Euphorbiae seu Knoxiae)

Bai Jie Zi (Semen Sinapis)

182

Shí Zǎo Tāng (Ten-Jujube Decoction)

Grind equal amounts of all three ingredients into powder and form into pills with water. Take 5-10 pills with a mild ginger soup and food at bedtime. The dose may be increased for patients with serious conditions characterized by excess phlegm and qi. Today, the herbs are normally ground into a fine powder, and formed with water into pills that resemble the size of *Lu Dou* (Semen Phaseoli Radiati). Take 1-3g of pills with warm, boiled water and food at bedtime.

Kong Xian Dan (Control Mucus Special Pill) treats phlegm stagnation and water retention in the chest and diaphragm, with sudden excruciating and migrating pain in the chest, back, neck, waist, and even inguinal region. There may also be lethargy, severe intolerable headache, coldness and pain in the hands and feet, a temporary loss of taste in the mouth, thick and sticky sputum, a rattling sound of sputum in the throat at night, and excess secretion of saliva.

Shi Zao Tang and *Kong Xian Dan* are two formulas commonly used for water accumulation.

- *Shi Zao Tang* treats severe water retention that affects the whole body.
- *Kong Xian Dan* is the gentler formula of the two and treats both water and phlegm retention. *Kong Xian Dan* is a gentler formula because it is administered as special pills (pellets), which are absorbed over a longer period of time and reach a lower peak concentration, when compared with the decoction form. Also, *Kong Xian Dan* addresses phlegm retention, since it has the addition of *Bai Jie Zi* (Semen Sinapis) to eliminate phlegm.

AUTHORS' COMMENTS

Shi Zao Tang has a drastic and potent effect to eliminate water retention in the interior. Therefore, it should be used with extreme caution and only when needed. The formula is taken in powder form with a decoction made from *Da Zao* (Fructus Jujubae). While loose stools and/or diarrhea is an expected side effect of this formula, patients should not have more than 5 to 6 bowel movements

per day while using this formula. If the condition is not resolved after the initial dose, it may be repeated if the patients are otherwise healthy and are not experiencing serious side effects. However, discontinue this formula if patients experience fatigue and lack of appetite, or suffer from serious side effects.

Shi Zao Tang literally translates as "Ten-Jujube Decoction." This name infers that a decoction made from 10 jujubes is used to serve this formula. However, it is important to keep in mind that the main herb is ***not*** jujube, and the formula is ***not*** given in decoction form. The three main active herbs are *Yuan Hua* (Flos Genkwa), *Gan Sui* (Radix Kansui), and *Da Ji* (Radix Euphorbiae seu Knoxiae), and they must be given in powder form. Cooking these three herbs in water and administering this formula in decoction will only cause more side effects, such as serious abdominal pain, nausea, and vomiting. Furthermore, *Gan Sui* (Radix Kansui) has poor water solubility, and therefore is not suitable for use in decoction. Lastly, although *Da Zao* (Fructus Jujubae) is not the key active ingredient, it is an important part of the formula because it controls and minimizes the toxicity of the three main ingredients.

Gan Cao (Radix et Rhizoma Glycyrrhizae) is generally the preferred envoy herb for harmonizing formulas and moderating herbs with drastic or toxic effects. However, according to *Shi Ba Fan* (Eighteen Incompatibles), *Gan Cao* (Radix et Rhizoma Glycyrrhizae) is incompatible with all three herbs in this formula – *Yuan Hua* (Flos Genkwa), *Gan Sui* (Radix Kansui) and *Da Ji* (Radix Euphorbiae seu Knoxiae). Thus, *Da Zao* (Fructus Jujubae) is chosen in this formula to protect the Spleen and Stomach, moderate the drastic effects, and minimize toxicities.

References

1. *Zhong Yao Ming Fang Yao Li Yu Ying Yong* (Pharmacology and Applications of Famous Herbal Formulas) 1989;88-89.
2. *Shan Xi Zhong Yi* (Shanxi Chinese Medicine) 1998;6:279.
3. *Fu Jian Zhong Yi Yao* (Fujian Chinese Medicine and Herbology) 1963;3:42.

Chapter 2 – Downward Draining Formulas　　　　　*Section 4 – Harsh Expellants (Cathartics)*

Zhōu Chē Wán (Vessel and Vehicle Pill)

舟車丸
舟车丸

Pinyin Name: *Zhou Che Wan*
Literal Name: Vessel and Vehicle Pill
Original Source: *Jing Yue Quan Shu* (Collected Treatises of [Zhang] Jing Yue) by Zhang Jie-Bin (Zhang Jing-Yue) in 1624

COMPOSITION

Da Ji (Radix Euphorbiae seu Knoxiae), *chao* (dry-fried) with vinegar	30g
Yuan Hua (Flos Genkwa)	30g
Gan Sui (Radix Kansui), *wei* (roasted)	30g
Qian Niu Zi (Semen Pharbitidis), *yan* (ground) to powder	120g
Da Huang (Radix et Rhizoma Rhei)	60g
Chen Pi (Pericarpium Citri Reticulatae)	15g
Qing Pi (Pericarpium Citri Reticulatae Viride)	15g
Mu Xiang (Radix Aucklandiae)	15g
Bing Lang (Semen Arecae)	15g
Qing Fen (Calomelas)	3g

Note: *Qing Fen* (Calomelas) is a potentially toxic heavy metal, and is rarely used as a medicinal substance today. Its discussion here is included primarily for academic purposes, to reflect the historical use of this substance in its original formulation. Most herbal products today do not contain it; or it has been replaced with substitutes with similar functions. For additional information on its toxicity, please refer to *Chinese Medical Herbology and Pharmacology* by John Chen and Tina Chen.

DOSAGE / PREPARATION / ADMINISTRATION

Grind the ingredients into powder, and mix with water to form into pills that resemble the size of small beans. Take 5 pills three times daily with warm water on an empty stomach. Discontinue the formula after urination and bowel movement have been induced. Today, the recommended dosage is: take 3-6g of pills per dose one time daily with warm water on an empty stomach in the morning.

CHINESE THERAPEUTIC ACTIONS

1. Promotes qi circulation
2. Eliminates water accumulation

CLINICAL MANIFESTATIONS

Water accumulation accompanied by heat formation and qi stagnation: watery distention, ascites, edema, thirst, coarse breathing, abdominal rigidity, anuria, constipation, and a deep, rapid and forceful pulse.

CLINICAL APPLICATIONS

Edema, ascites, and liver cirrhosis.

EXPLANATION

Zhou Che Wan (Vessel and Vehicle Pill) treats water accumulation accompanied by heat formation and qi stagnation. The water and heat accumulation, along with qi stagnation, leads to the improper distribution of water fluids, causing edema, ascites, anuria, constipation, and thirst. Qi stagnation leads to coarse breathing and abdominal rigidity. A deep, rapid and forceful pulse suggests excess heat/water in the interior and a condition characterized by excess, rather than deficiency.

Since this is an emergency case of interior excess syndrome, drastic cathartic herbs are used to quickly remove water retention and heat formation. The three chief herbs, *Da Ji* (Radix Euphorbiae seu Knoxiae), *Yuan Hua* (Flos Genkwa), and *Gan Sui* (Radix Kansui) drastically purge water in the chest and abdomen. *Qian Niu Zi* (Semen Pharbitidis) and *Da Huang* (Radix et Rhizoma Rhei) purge the Intestines and eliminate water and heat. *Chen Pi* (Pericarpium Citri Reticulatae) relieves coarse breathing or chest oppression by activating Lung and Spleen qi. *Qing Pi* (Pericarpium Citri Reticulatae Viride) smoothes Liver qi flow, break up qi stagnation, and relieve abdominal rigidity. *Mu Xiang* (Radix Aucklandiae) regulates qi and water circulation in all three *jiaos* to relieve edema and watery distention. *Bing Lang* (Semen Arecae) breaks up qi stagnation, promotes the movement of qi downward, and eliminates water retention. *Qing Fen* (Calomelas) enhances the qi-activating and water-eliminating functions of the other herbs in this formula.

184

Zhōu Chē Wán (Vessel and Vehicle Pill)

Zhou Che Wan (Vessel and Vehicle Pill)

Diagnosis	Signs and Symptoms	Treatment	Herbs
Water accumulation accompanied by heat formation and qi stagnation	• Edema, ascites, anuria, constipation, and thirst: water accumulation and heat formation • Coarse breathing and abdominal rigidity: water accumulation and qi stagnation • Deep, rapid and forceful pulse: excess condition in the interior	• Promotes qi circulation • Eliminates water accumulation	• *Da Ji* (Radix Euphorbiae seu Knoxiae), *Yuan Hua* (Flos Genkwa) and *Gan Sui* (Radix Kansui) drastically purge water in the chest and the abdomen. • *Qian Niu Zi* (Semen Pharbitidis) and *Da Huang* (Radix et Rhizoma Rhei) purge the Intestines and eliminate water and heat. • *Chen Pi* (Pericarpium Citri Reticulatae), *Qing Pi* (Pericarpium Citri Reticulatae Viride), *Mu Xiang* (Radix Aucklandiae), and *Bing Lang* (Semen Arecae) regulate qi circulation. • *Qing Fen* (Calomelas) enhances the qi-activating and water-eliminating functions of the other herbs.

CAUTIONS / CONTRAINDICATIONS

• Many herbs in *Zhou Che Wan* are toxic, such as *Qing Fen* (Calomelas), *Yuan Hua* (Flos Genkwa), *Da Ji* (Radix Euphorbiae seu Knoxiae), and *Gan Sui* (Radix Kansui). Therefore, the doses should be adjusted carefully according to the severity of the condition and the patient's constitution.

• Prolonged use of this formula is contraindicated.

• Use of this formula is prohibited in pregnant women and patients with a weak constitution.

AUTHORS' COMMENTS

This formula is based on *Shi Zao Tang* (Ten-Jujube Decoction), with the addition of very strong cathartic herbs to purge water through urination and defecation, and the removal of *Da Zao* (Fructus Jujubae) so that the downward draining herbs can fully exert their potent and drastic effects without moderation. Only patients with a strong constitution should take this formula, and they should take it every other day, each time decreasing the dose of intake. Discontinue the use of the formula when the desired effects are achieved.

Shū Záo Yǐn Zǐ (Spread and Unblock Decoction)
疏鑿飲子
疏凿饮子

Pinyin Name: *Shu Zao Yin Zi*
Literal Name: Spread and Unblock Decoction
Original Source: *Ji Sheng Fang* (Formulas to Aid the Living) by Yan Yong-He in 1253

COMPOSITION

Shang Lu (Radix Phytolaccae)	[6g]
Bing Lang (Semen Arecae)	[9g]
Da Fu Pi (Pericarpium Arecae)	[15g]
Fu Ling Pi (Cortex Poria)	[30g]
Ze Xie (Rhizoma Alismatis)	[12g]
Mu Tong (Caulis Akebiae)	[12g]
Jiao Mu (Semen Zanthoxyli Bungeani)	[9g]
Chi Xiao Dou (Semen Phaseoli), *chao* (dry-fried)	[15g]
Qiang Huo (Rhizoma et Radix Notopterygii)	[9g]
Qin Jiao (Radix Gentianae Macrophyllae)	[9g]

DOWNWARD DRAINING FORMULAS

2

Chapter 2 – Downward Draining Formulas　　　　　　　　*Section 4 – Harsh Expellants (Cathartics)*

Shū Záo Yǐn Zǐ (Spread and Unblock Decoction)

DOSAGE / PREPARATION / ADMINISTRATION
The source text states to grind equal amounts of the ingredients into a coarse powder. Cook 12g of the powder with 5 slices of *Sheng Jiang* (Rhizoma Zingiberis Recens) in 1.5 bowls of water until 70% of the liquid remains. Take the warm, strained decoction any time during the day. This formula may also be prepared as a decoction with the doses suggested in brackets above.

CHINESE THERAPEUTIC ACTIONS
1. Drains downward
2. Eliminates water accumulation
3. Dispels wind and releases the exterior

CLINICAL MANIFESTATIONS
Excess water and damp accumulation: generalized edema, wheezing, thirst, anuria, and constipation.

CLINICAL APPLICATIONS
Edema, ascites, and liver cirrhosis.

EXPLANATION
Shu Zao Yin Zi (Spread and Unblock Decoction) treats excess accumulation of water and dampness in the body,

which causes the water to flow to the exterior or the skin level, giving rise to generalized edema. Since water is retained inside the body, it interferes with the normal functioning of the *San Jiao*, causing anuria and constipation. Excess water and dampness also affect the Lung's functioning, causing wheezing. Lastly, when water fluid is not properly distributed inside the body, thirst ensues.

This formula eliminates water accumulation from the whole body by using herbs that address the exterior and interior, and the upper and lower parts of the body. *Shang Lu* (Radix Phytolaccae) purges excess water and damp accumulation via urination and defecation. *Bing Lang* (Semen Arecae) and *Da Fu Pi* (Pericarpium Arecae) activate qi and move water fluid downward and outward. *Fu Ling Pi* (Cortex Poria), *Ze Xie* (Rhizoma Alismatis), *Mu Tong* (Caulis Akebiae), *Jiao Mu* (Semen Zanthoxyli Bungeani), and *Chi Xiao Dou* (Semen Phaseoli) promote urination to eliminate water and damp accumulation. *Qiang Huo* (Rhizoma et Radix Notopterygii), *Qin Jiao* (Radix Gentianae Macrophyllae), and *Sheng Jiang* (Rhizoma Zingiberis Recens) promote perspiration to expel water and dampness from the skin level.

Shu Zao Yin Zi (Spread and Unblock Decoction)

Diagnosis	Signs and Symptoms	Treatment	Herbs
Excess water and damp accumulation	• Generalized edema: water and damp accumulation • Anuria and constipation: excess water and damp accumulation interfering with the normal functioning of the *San Jiao* • Wheezing: water and damp accumulation affecting the Lung	• Drains downward • Eliminates water accumulation • Dispels wind and releases the exterior	• *Shang Lu* (Radix Phytolaccae) purges excess water and damp accumulation. • *Bing Lang* (Semen Arecae) and *Da Fu Pi* (Pericarpium Arecae) activate qi and move water fluid downward and out of the body. • *Fu Ling Pi* (Cortex Poria), *Ze Xie* (Rhizoma Alismatis), *Mu Tong* (Caulis Akebiae), *Jiao Mu* (Semen Zanthoxyli Bungeani) and *Chi Xiao Dou* (Semen Phaseoli) promote urination to eliminate water and damp accumulation. • *Qiang Huo* (Rhizoma et Radix Notopterygii), *Qin Jiao* (Radix Gentianae Macrophyllae), and *Sheng Jiang* (Rhizoma Zingiberis Recens) promote perspiration to expel water and dampness from the skin level.

Chinese Herbal Formulas and Applications

Section 5

攻补兼施剂
— Purgative and Tonic Formulas

2

DOWNWARD DRAINING FORMULAS

Huáng Lóng Tāng (Yellow Dragon Decoction)
黃龍湯
黄龙汤

Pinyin Name: *Huang Long Tang*
Literal Name: Yellow Dragon Decoction
Original Source: *Shang Han Liu Shu* (Six Texts on Cold-Induced Disorders) by Tao Hua in 1445

COMPOSITION

Da Huang (Radix et Rhizoma Rhei)	[9-12g]
Mang Xiao (Natrii Sulfas)	[6-9g]
Hou Po (Cortex Magnoliae Officinalis)	[9-12g]
Zhi Shi (Fructus Aurantii Immaturus)	[9g]
Ren Shen (Radix et Rhizoma Ginseng)	[6g]
Dang Gui (Radix Angelicae Sinensis)	[9g]
Gan Cao (Radix et Rhizoma Glycyrrhizae)	[3g]

DOSAGE / PREPARATION / ADMINISTRATION

The source text instructions are to cook the ingredients in 2 large bowls of water with 3 slices of *Sheng Jiang* (Rhizoma Zingiberis Recens) and 2 pieces of *Da Zao* (Fructus Jujubae). Add a small amount of *Jie Geng* (Radix Platycodonis) at the end, and bring the decoction to a boil one time. Take the strained decoction while hot. Note: The herb doses are not provided in the source text.

Today, this formula can be prepared as a decoction using the herb doses suggested in brackets above, with the addition of 3 slices of *Sheng Jiang* (Rhizoma Zingiberis Recens), 2 pieces of *Da Zao* (Fructus Jujubae), and 3g of *Jie Geng* (Radix Platycodonis).

CHINESE THERAPEUTIC ACTIONS

1. Clears heat and promotes defecation
2. Tonifies qi and blood

CLINICAL MANIFESTATIONS

Interior excess heat accompanied by qi and blood deficiencies: constipation characterized by only clear, watery fluids upon defecation; epigastric and abdominal

hardness and pain, and abdominal pain that worsens upon pressure; altered consciousness, delirium, or carphology in severe cases; thirst, fever, a dry mouth and tongue; low energy and a weak voice; a dry, yellow or dry, black tongue coating, and a deficient pulse.

CLINICAL APPLICATIONS

Intestinal obstruction and post-operative recovery of gastrointestinal function.

EXPLANATION

Huang Long Tang (Yellow Dragon Decoction) treats *yangming fu* (hollow organs) syndrome with qi and blood deficiencies. *Yangming fu* syndrome is characterized by stagnant excess heat in the Stomach and Large Intestine. If the heat consumes too much fluids in the Large Intestine, constipation occurs. If the stools in the Large Intestine become too dry and impacted, intestinal fluids may not be able to moisten the stools and the fluids are excreted in the form of clear, watery diarrhea.

Abdominal pain that worsens upon pressure is a sign that this is an excess interior syndrome. Delirium and

187

Chapter 2 – Downward Draining Formulas Section 5 – *Purgative and Tonic Formulas*

Huáng Lóng Tāng (Yellow Dragon Decoction)

Huang Long Tang (Yellow Dragon Decoction)

Diagnosis	Signs and Symptoms	Treatment	Herbs
Yangming fu (hollow organs) syndrome with qi and blood deficiencies	• Constipation, epigastric and abdominal hardness and pain, abdominal pain that worsens with pressure: interior excess heat • Delirium and carphology: interior excess heat disturbing the *shen* (spirit) • Thirst, a dry mouth and tongue, and a dry, yellow or dry, black tongue coating: interior heat consuming body fluids • Low energy, weak voice, and a deficient pulse: qi and blood deficiencies	• Clears heat and promotes defecation • Tonifies qi and blood	• *Da Huang* (Radix et Rhizoma Rhei) clears the Stomach and Intestines by dispelling heat and constipated stools. • *Mang Xiao* (Natrii Sulfas) clears heat, moistens dryness, and softens the stool. • *Hou Po* (Cortex Magnoliae Officinalis) activates qi circulation and disperses accumulations. • *Zhi Shi* (Fructus Aurantii Immaturus) relieves fullness and distention. • *Ren Shen* (Radix et Rhizoma Ginseng), *Gan Cao* (Radix et Rhizoma Glycyrrhizae), *Da Zao* (Fructus Jujubae), and *Dang Gui* (Radix Angelicae Sinensis) tonify qi, blood, and body fluids. • *Jie Geng* (Radix Platycodonis) raises the sunken qi of the Lung and Large Intestine. • *Sheng Jiang* (Rhizoma Zingiberis Recens) and *Gan Cao* (Radix et Rhizoma Glycyrrhizae) nourish the Stomach and harmonize the middle *jiao*.

carphology are caused by excess heat in the interior disturbing the *shen* (spirit), with carphology being a more serious symptom than delirium. Thirst, fever, and a dry mouth and tongue are signs of interior heat consuming body fluids. Low energy and a weak voice suggest qi deficiency. The dry, yellow or dry, black tongue coating indicates interior heat and body fluid damage. A deficient pulse suggests qi and blood deficiencies.

The treatment of this syndrome requires the use of purgative as well as tonic herbs. *Da Huang* (Radix et Rhizoma Rhei), *Mang Xiao* (Natrii Sulfas), *Hou Po* (Cortex Magnoliae Officinalis) and *Zhi Shi* (Fructus Aurantii Immaturus), the four herbs of *Da Cheng Qi Tang* (Major Order the Qi Decoction), purge excess heat in the *yangming* organs and promote qi circulation to relieve constipation and epigastric and abdominal hardness and pain. *Ren Shen* (Radix et Rhizoma Ginseng), *Gan Cao* (Radix et Rhizoma Glycyrrhizae), *Da Zao* (Fructus Jujubae), and *Dang Gui* (Radix Angelicae Sinensis) tonify qi, blood, and body fluids. *Jie Geng* (Radix Platycodonis) raises the sunken qi of the Lung and Large Intestine, two organs connected by their *zang fu* relationship. *Sheng Jiang* (Rhizoma Zingiberis Recens) and *Gan Cao* (Radix et Rhizoma Glycyrrhizae) nourish the Stomach and harmonize the middle *jiao*.

MODIFICATIONS
• For constipation in elderly patients with weakness and deficiency, decrease the dose of *Mang Xiao* (Natrii Sulfas)

and increase the dose of *Ren Shen* (Radix et Rhizoma Ginseng) and *Dang Gui* (Radix Angelicae Sinensis).
• If there is a dry mouth and lips caused by heat damaging body fluids, add *Di Huang* (Radix Rehmanniae), *Xuan Shen* (Radix Scrophulariae), and *Mai Dong* (Radix Ophiopogonis).

CAUTIONS / CONTRAINDICATIONS
• While *Huang Long Tang* tonifies, it contains potent purgative herbs such as *Da Huang* (Radix et Rhizoma Rhei) and *Mang Xiao* (Natrii Sulfas), and should not be used to treat constipation that is caused only by deficiencies without any interior excess heat.
• Bowel movement consisting of only clear, watery fluids is caused by constipation arising from interior excess heat. Since the clear, watery fluids do not represent actual diarrhea, do not treat this condition with astringent herbs, which will only further trap the heat pathogenic factor inside.

CLINICAL STUDIES AND RESEARCH
Post-operative recovery: Administration of modified *Huang Long Tang* was evaluated for its effects in restoring normal gastrointestinal function in post-operative patients. The formula was given as decoction 12 hours after the surgery, and the second dose was given 24 hours later if necessary. The formula included 10g each of *Da Huang* (Radix et Rhizoma Rhei) (post-decocted), *Zhi Shi* (Fructus Aurantii Immaturus), *Hou Po* (Cortex

Huáng Lóng Tāng (Yellow Dragon Decoction)

Magnoliae Officinalis), *Mai Dong* (Radix Ophiopogonis), *Dang Gui* (Radix Angelicae Sinensis), and *Dang Shen* (Radix Codonopsis). The study reported 93% effectiveness within 48 hours.[1]

RELATED FORMULA

Xīn Jiā Huáng Lóng Tāng

(Newly-Augmented Yellow Dragon Decoction)

新加黃龍湯
新加黄龙汤

Pinyin Name: Xin Jia Huang Long Tang
Literal Name: Newly-Augmented Yellow Dragon Decoction
Original Source: *Wen Bing Tiao Bian* (Systematic Differentiation of Warm Disease) by Wu Ju-Tong in 1798

Di Huang (Radix Rehmanniae)	15g
Gan Cao (Radix et Rhizoma Glycyrrhizae)	6g
Ren Shen (Radix et Rhizoma Ginseng), decoct separately	4.5g
Da Huang (Radix et Rhizoma Rhei)	9g
Mang Xiao (Natrii Sulfas)	3g
Xuan Shen (Radix Scrophulariae)	15g
Mai Dong (Radix Ophiopogonis)	15g
Dang Gui (Radix Angelicae Sinensis)	4.5g
Hai Shen (Strichopus Japonicus), *xi* (washed)	2 pieces
Sheng Jiang (Rhizoma Zingiberis Recens)	6 spoonfuls of juice

Cook all of the ingredients, except *Ren Shen* (Radix et Rhizoma Ginseng), in 8 cups of water until 3 cups of liquid remain. Take 1 cup of the decoction with a half cup of separately decocted *Ren Shen* (Radix et Rhizoma Ginseng) and 2 spoonfuls of ginger juice. Bowel movement should be induced within 1-2 hours. If not, repeat the same process and administer the second dose. If bowel movement is not induced after 24 hours, repeat the same process and administer the third dose. Discontinue the formula after bowel movement is induced.

To recover from the strong purgative effects of this formula, patients should take one dose of *Yi Wei Tang* (Benefit the Stomach Decoction). Note: *Yi Wei Tang* (Benefit the Stomach Decoction) contains *Sha Shen* (Radix Glehniae seu Adenophorae), *Mai Dong* (Radix Ophiopogonis), *Di Huang* (Radix Rehmanniae), *Yu Zhu* (Rhizoma Polygonati Odorati), and rock sugar. *Ren Shen* (Radix et Rhizoma Ginseng) may be added if needed.

Xin Jia Huang Long Tang (Newly-Augmented Yellow Dragon Decoction) clears heat, purges the stools, tonifies qi, and nourishes yin. It treats excess heat in the interior, accompanied by depletion of qi and yin with the following symptoms and signs: constipation, a feeling of fullness, hardness and rigidity in the abdomen, lethargy, low energy, a weak voice, a dry mouth and tongue, dry or chapped lips, and a dry, yellow or dry, black fissured tongue coating.

This formula treats *yangming fu* (hollow organs) syndrome with qi and yin deficiencies. Constipation and abdominal fullness and hardness are typical clinical manifestations of *yangming fu* syndrome, in which excess heat stagnates in the *yangming* organs. Heat stagnation in the *yangming* organs injures qi, yin and blood, causing lethargy, low energy, and a weak voice. Dry mouth, dry lips, and dry tongue with black fissured tongue coating suggest interior heat consuming yin and body fluids.

Da Huang (Radix et Rhizoma Rhei) and *Mang Xiao* (Natrii Sulfas) purge heat stagnation and constipated stools. *Xuan Shen* (Radix Scrophulariae), *Di Huang* (Radix Rehmanniae), *Mai Dong* (Radix Ophiopogonis), and *Hai Shen* (Strichopus Japonicus) nourish yin and body fluids. *Ren Shen* (Radix et Rhizoma Ginseng), *Gan Cao* (Radix et Rhizoma Glycyrrhizae), and *Dang Gui* (Radix Angelicae Sinensis) tonify qi and blood to strengthen the body. The juice of *Sheng Jiang* (Rhizoma Zingiberis Recens) harmonizes the Stomach and prevents vomiting.

Huang Long Tang and *Xin Jia Huang Long Tang* (Newly-Augmented Yellow Dragon Decoction) both clear heat, purge stagnation, and tonify qi and blood. Both treat interior heat accumulation, an excess condition with underlying qi and blood deficiencies. Both formulas contain *Da Huang* (Radix et Rhizoma Rhei), *Mang Xiao* (Natrii Sulfas), *Ren Shen* (Radix et Rhizoma Ginseng), *Dang Gui* (Radix Angelicae Sinensis), and *Gan Cao* (Radix et Rhizoma Glycyrrhizae). The differences are as follows:

- *Huang Long Tang* is based on *Da Cheng Qi Tang* (Major Order the Qi Decoction), with the addition of *Ren Shen* (Radix et Rhizoma Ginseng), *Dang Gui* (Radix Angelicae Sinensis), *Gan Cao* (Radix et Rhizoma Glycyrrhizae), *Sheng Jiang* (Rhizoma Zingiberis Recens), and *Da Zao* (Fructus Jujubae). It treats excess condition characterized by greater heat and stagnation, and has a stronger purgative effect than *Xin Jia Huang Long Tang*.

- *Xin Jia Huang Long Tang* is based on *Tiao Wei Cheng Qi Tang* (Regulate the Stomach and Order the Qi Decoction), with the addition of *Xuan Shen* (Radix Scrophulariae), *Di Huang* (Radix Rehmanniae), *Mai Dong* (Radix Ophiopogonis), *Hai Shen* (Strichopus Japonicus), *Ren Shen* (Radix et Rhizoma Ginseng), and *Dang Gui* (Radix Angelicae Sinensis). It is better than *Huang Long Tang* in tonifying deficiencies.

Huáng Lóng Tāng (Yellow Dragon Decoction)

AUTHORS' COMMENTS

A typical *yangming fu* (hollow organs) syndrome is characterized by excess heat stagnant in the *yangming* organs without deficiencies of qi, yin, blood and/or body fluids. *Da Cheng Qi Tang* (Major Order the Qi Decoction) is usually the formula of choice to treat this excess heat condition. However, if the qi, yin and/or blood are deficient, heat stagnation and constipation must be eliminated by using both purgative and tonic herbs. If tonic herbs are not used in this syndrome, the patient may either be too weak to dispel the heat stagnation or may completely collapse after defecation. *Huang Long Tang* and *Xin Jia Huang Long Tang* (Newly-Augmented Yellow Dragon Decoction) both treat *yangming fu* syndrome with underlying deficiencies by simultaneously purging heat and stagnation and tonifying deficiencies.

Reference
1. *Fu Jian Zhong Yi Yao* (Fujian Chinese Medicine and Herbology) 1993;24(5):18.

Zēng Yè Chéng Qi Tāng
(Increase the Fluids and Order the Qi Decoction)

增液承氣湯
增液承气汤

Pinyin Name: *Zeng Ye Cheng Qi Tang*
Literal Name: Increase the Fluids and Order the Qi Decoction
Original Source: *Wen Bing Tiao Bian* (Systematic Differentiation of Warm Disease) by Wu Ju-Tong in 1798

COMPOSITION

Xuan Shen (Radix Scrophulariae)	30g
Mai Dong (Radix Ophiopogonis)	24g
Di Huang (Radix Rehmanniae)	24g
Da Huang (Radix et Rhizoma Rhei)	9g
Mang Xiao (Natrii Sulfas)	4.5g

DOSAGE / PREPARATION / ADMINISTRATION

Cook the ingredients in 8 cups of water until 2 cups of liquid remain. Take 1 cup of the decoction. If bowel movement is not induced after taking the formula, administer another cup.

CHINESE THERAPEUTIC ACTIONS

1. Nourishes yin and generates body fluids
2. Purges heat and promotes defecation

CLINICAL MANIFESTATIONS

Yangming fu (hollow organs) syndrome characterized by Stomach and Intestines heat damaging yin and body fluids: severe constipation that cannot be relieved by regular purgative method; dry, immobile stools; abdominal fullness; thirst; and a dry mouth and throat.

CLINICAL APPLICATIONS

Anal fissures, renal insufficiency, postpartum anuria, and epistaxis.

EXPLANATION

In *yangming fu* (hollow organs) syndrome, heat stagnates in the Stomach and Large Intestine and causes the stools to be impacted. If the heat persists, yin and body fluids will be so severely damaged that even normal purgative methods would not be able to remove the dry, constipated stools. In such cases, two kinds of herbs must be used: sweet, cold, and moistening herbs that nourish yin and moisten dryness; and bitter and salty herbs that clear heat and drain downward. Nourishing yin and replenishing body fluids are essential steps in successfully removing the constipated stools and clearing stagnant interior heat.

190

Zēng Yè Chéng Qì Tāng
(Increase the Fluids and Order the Qi Decoction)

Zeng Ye Cheng Qi Tang (Increase the Fluids and Order the Qi Decoction)

Diagnosis	Signs and Symptoms	Treatment	Herbs
Yangming syndrome characterized by heat in the Stomach and Intestines damaging yin and body fluids	• Severe constipation with abdominal fullness: heat in the Stomach and Large Intestine with hard and constipated stools • Dry, immobile stools, thirst, a dry mouth and throat: damage to yin and body fluids	• Nourishes yin and generates body fluids • Purges heat and promotes defecation	• *Xuan Shen* (Radix Scrophulariae), *Mai Dong* (Radix Ophiopogonis) and *Di Huang* (Radix Rehmanniae) nourish yin and body fluids, clear heat, and moisten dryness. • *Da Huang* (Radix et Rhizoma Rhei) and *Mang Xiao* (Natrii Sulfas) purge excess heat, soften hardness, and remove constipated stools.

Zeng Ye Cheng Qi Tang (Increase the Fluids and Order the Qi Decoction) contains *Xuan Shen* (Radix Scrophulariae), *Mai Dong* (Radix Ophiopogonis), and *Di Huang* (Radix Rehmanniae), the three herbs in *Zeng Ye Tang* (Increase the Fluids Decoction), to nourish yin and body fluids, and to moisten dryness. *Da Huang* (Radix et Rhizoma Rhei) and *Mang Xiao* (Natrii Sulfas) purge excess heat, soften hardness, and remove constipated stools.

This formula, besides treating *yangming fu* (hollow organs) syndrome, may also be used to treat chronic constipation characterized by yin deficiency and dry heat in the Large Intestine.

MODIFICATIONS
• For constipation characterized by qi deficiency, add *Tai Zi Shen* (Radix Pseudostellariae) or *Xi Yang Shen* (Radix Panacis Quinquefolii).
• For bleeding hemorrhoids, add *Di Yu* (Radix Sanguisorbae) and *Huai Hua* (Flos Sophorae).

CAUTIONS / CONTRAINDICATIONS
Zeng Ye Cheng Qi Tang treats constipation characterized by heat damaging yin and body fluids. It is not appropriate for postpartum constipation caused by blood deficiency, or habitual constipation in geriatric patients caused by Kidney deficiency.

CLINICAL STUDIES AND RESEARCH
1. **Anal fissures**: Administration of modified *Zeng Ye Cheng Qi Tang* in 31 patients with anal fissures was associated with complete recovery in 29 patients and improvement in 2 patients. The history of illness ranged from 7 days to 5 years. The herbal treatment contained the following ingredients: *Xuan Shen* (Radix Scrophulariae) 15g, *Di Huang* (Radix Rehmanniae) 15g, *Mai Dong* (Radix Ophiopogonis) 15g, post-decocted *Da Huang* (Radix

et Rhizoma Rhei) 5g, and *Mang Xiao* (Natrii Sulfas) 5g. Dry-fried *Di Yu* (Radix Sanguisorbae) and dry-fried *Huai Hua* (Flos Sophorae) were added for hematochezia; and *Zhi Qiao* (Fructus Aurantii) and *Yan Hu Suo* (Rhizoma Corydalis) for severe pain. For those who experience multiple bowel movements or loose stools after herbal treatment, *Da Huang* (Radix et Rhizoma Rhei) should be reduced in dose or pre-decocted. The herbs were cooked in water, and decoction given daily, for an average of 7 packs of herbs.[1]

2. **Renal insufficiency**: Administration of *Zeng Ye Cheng Qi Tang* was shown to have beneficial effects in treating acute renal insufficiency in one study. The study entailed the administration of 200 mL of herbal solution via rectal enema two to four times daily. Of 49 patients, the study reported recovery in 41 patients, improvement in 2 patients, and fatality in 6 patients.[2]

3. **Postpartum anuria**: Thirty-four women with postpartum anuria were treated with herbs, with complete recovery in 13 patients after 1 pack of herbs, 19 patients after 2 packs, and 2 patients after 3 packs. The herbal formula contained *Xuan Shen* (Radix Scrophulariae) 30g, *Di Huang* (Radix Rehmanniae) 20g, *Mai Dong* (Radix Ophiopogonis) 20g, *Da Huang* (Radix et Rhizoma Rhei) 6g, *Mang Xiao* (Natrii Sulfas) 6g, *Che Qian Zi* (Semen Plantaginis) 30g, and *Jie Geng* (Radix Platycodonis) 10g. Modifications were made by adding *Huang Bo* (Cortex Phellodendri Chinensis) 10g and *Pu Gong Ying* (Herba Taraxaci) 50g for the presence of fever caused by infection.[3]

4. **Epistaxis**: Twelve patients with severe nosebleeds were successfully treated using *Zeng Ye Cheng Qi Tang* plus *Mu Dan Pi* (Cortex Moutan), *Zhi Shi* (Fructus Aurantii Immaturus), and *Hou Po* (Cortex Magnoliae Officinalis).[4]

HERB-DRUG INTERACTION
Phenothiazine-induced constipation: Use of modified *Zeng Ye Cheng Qi Tang* was beneficial in alleviating the side

Chapter 2 – Downward Draining Formulas　　　　　　　　　*Section 5 – Purgative and Tonic Formulas*

Zēng Yè Chéng Qì Tāng
(Increase the Fluids and Order the Qi Decoction)

effects related to use of phenothiazine in 30 psychiatric patients. Phenothiazine-induced side effects include constipation, a dry mouth with a bitter taste, nausea, etc. The herbal formula contained *Xuan Shen* (Radix Scrophulariae), *Di Huang* (Radix Rehmanniae), *Mai Dong* (Radix Ophiopogonis), *Da Huang* (Radix et Rhizoma Rhei), *Zhi Shi* (Fructus Aurantii Immaturus), *Hou Po* (Cortex Magnoliae Officinalis), and *Tian Hua Fen* (Radix Trichosanthis). The herbs were given in decoction form one time daily. Patients were instructed to continue with phenothiazine and herbs concurrently for four weeks, while avoiding all other treatments. Of 30 patients, the study reported complete recovery in 14 patients, significant effect in 10 patients, moderate effect in 3 patients, and no change in 3 patients. The overall rate of effectiveness was 90%.[5]

RELATED FORMULA

Chéng Qì Yǎng Yíng Tāng

(Order the Qi and Nourish the Nutritive Qi Decoction)

承氣養營湯
承气养营汤

Pinyin Name: *Cheng Qi Yang Ying Tang*

Literal Name: Order the Qi and Nourish the Nutritive Qi Decoction

Original Source: *Wen Yi Lun* (Discussion of Epidemic Warm Disease) by Wu You-Xing in 1642

Zhi Mu (Rhizoma Anemarrhenae)	[9g]
Dang Gui (Radix Angelicae Sinensis)	[6g]
Di Huang (Radix Rehmanniae)	[12g]
Da Huang (Radix et Rhizoma Rhei)	[12g]
Zhi Shi (Fructus Aurantii Immaturus)	[9g]
Hou Po (Cortex Magnoliae Officinalis)	[9g]
Bai Shao (Radix Paeoniae Alba)	[15g]

This formula is normally prepared as a decoction. Note: The source text did not provide the herb doses. Use the doses listed above in brackets.

This formula clears heat, promotes defecation, nourishes yin, and moistens dryness. Clinically, patients may show

symptoms such as constipation, persistent fever, dry and chapped lips, a dry throat with a desire to drink, and abdominal fullness, hardness and pain.

Cheng Qi Yang Ying Tang (Order the Qi and Nourish the Nutritive Qi Decoction) employs the strategies of two formulas: *Xiao Cheng Qi Tang* (Minor Order the Qi Decoction) to clear heat, purge the Intestines, and relieve abdominal fullness and pain; and *Si Wu Tang* (Four-Substance Decoction) to nourish yin and tonify the blood. Although the strategies are the same, one small modification has been made: *Chuan Xiong* (Rhizoma Chuanxiong), which is acrid and dry, is replaced by *Zhi Mu* (Rhizoma Anemarrhenae), which is bitter and cold. This substitution enhances the overall ability of the formula to nourish yin and tonify the blood.

Zeng Ye Cheng Qi Tang and *Cheng Qi Yang Ying Tang* (Order the Qi and Nourish the Nutritive Qi Decoction) both nourish yin, purge heat, relieve constipation, and purge accumulation.

• *Zeng Ye Cheng Qi Tang* more strongly nourishes yin and generates body fluids, and moderately clears heat.

• *Cheng Qi Yang Ying Tang* drains downward, nourishes yin, and tonifies the blood, all with equal emphasis.

AUTHORS' COMMENTS

Zeng Ye Cheng Qi Tang treats febrile disorders with constipation characterized by heat stagnation and yin and body fluid deficiencies. This formula can also be used in cases of constipation caused by high fever that occurs in acute infectious diseases and leads to body fluid deficiency. Another popular use is for hemorrhoids with dry stools and yin deficiency.

References

1. *An Hui Zhong Yi Xue Yuan Xue Bao* (Journal of Anhui University School of Medicine) 1993;4:28.
2. *Zhong Yi Za Zhi* (Journal of Chinese Medicine) 1986;10:32.
3. *Liao Ning Zhong Yi Za Zhi* (Liaoning Journal of Chinese Medicine) 1992;1:30.
4. *Si Chuan Zhong Yi* (Sichuan Chinese Medicine) 1988;6:47.
5. *Xin Yi Xue* (New Medicine) 1997;7:24.

192

Chinese Herbal Formulas and Applications

Chapter 2 — Summary

— Downward Draining Formulas

SECTION 1: COLD PURGATIVES

Name	Similarities	Differences
Da Cheng Qi Tang (Major Order the Qi Decoction)	Drain heat and accumulation downward	Strongest potency
Xiao Cheng Qi Tang (Minor Order the Qi Decoction)		Moderate to strong potency
Tiao Wei Cheng Qi Tang (Regulate the Stomach and Order the Qi Decoction)		Mild to moderate potency
Da Xian Xiong Tang (Major Sinking into the Chest Decoction)	Purges heat and eliminates water accumulation	Treats accumulation of heat and water in the chest
Yi Zi Tang (Yi Word Decoction)	Clears heat and promotes bowel movement	Cools the blood, eliminates toxins, and raises yang qi

Da Cheng Qi Tang (Major Order the Qi Decoction), **Xiao Cheng Qi Tang** (Minor Order the Qi Decoction), and **Tiao Wei Cheng Qi Tang** (Regulate the Stomach and Order the Qi Decoction) all contain *Da Huang* (Radix et Rhizoma Rhei) to purge stagnation and heat in the Large Intestine to treat *yangming fu* (hollow organs) syndrome.

- *Da Cheng Qi Tang* is the strongest of these three formulas, and may be used to treat all four manifestations of *pi* (distention), *man* (fullness), *zao* (dryness), and *shi* (hardness). The constipation is characterized by extremely hard stools.
- *Xiao Cheng Qi Tang* has moderate to strong potency and is used to treat qi stagnation signs and symptoms of *pi* (distention), *man* (fullness) and *shi* (hardness). The constipation is characterized by moderately hard stools.
- *Tiao Wei Cheng Qi Tang* is the mildest among the three formulas, and mainly softens the stools in constipation characterized by *zao* (dryness) and *shi* (hardness).

Da Cheng Qi Tang (Major Order the Qi Decoction) and **Da Xian Xiong Tang** (Major Sinking into the Chest Decoction) both purge heat stagnation.

- *Da Cheng Qi Tang* drastically purges stagnant heat from the Stomach and removes constipated stools from the Intestines.
- *Da Xian Xiong Tang* purges stagnant heat and water from the chest, a condition known as *jie xiong* (stagnant chest). It is an important formula for treating hardness, fullness, and pain in the epigastrium and lower abdomen, caused by the interlocking of heat and water.

Yi Zi Tang (Yi Word Decoction) clears heat and eliminates toxins from the lower *jiao* to treat constipation. In addition, it cools the blood, stops bleeding, and raises yang qi to relieve hemorrhoids.

Chapter 2 – Downward Draining Formulas

Chapter 2 — Summary

SECTION 2: WARM PURGATIVES

Name	Similarities	Differences
Da Huang Fu Zi Tang (Rhubarb and Prepared Aconite Decoction)	Drain cold and accumulation downward	Moderate potency and balanced effect to warm the interior and purge downward
Wen Pi Tang (Warm the Spleen Decoction)		Strongest formula to purge downward
San Wu Bei Ji Wan (Three-Substance Pill for Emergencies)		Strongest potency to warm and tonify the interior

Da Huang Fu Zi Tang (Rhubarb and Prepared Aconite Decoction), **Wen Pi Tang** (Warm the Spleen Decoction), and **San Wu Bei Ji Wan** (Three-Substance Pill for Emergencies) are warm purgative formulas with similar functions to drain downward and eliminate cold accumulation.

- *Da Huang Fu Zi Tang* also warms the channels and disperses coldness. It is suitable for treating constipation characterized by interior excess, cold accumulation, and underlying yang deficiency.
- *Wen Pi Tang* also warms and tonifies Spleen yang. It treats constipation caused by Spleen yang deficiency and cold accumulation. It is also used to treat chronic dysentery with red (blood) and white (mucus) stools.
- *San Wu Bei Ji Wan* quickly removes excess cold stagnation in the interior. With a drastic purgative action, this formula is suitable for treating constipation with stagnation of interior cold causing sudden distending pain in the chest and abdomen.

SECTION 3: MOIST LAXATIVES

Name	Similarities	Differences
Ma Zi Ren Wan (Hemp Seed Pill)	Lubricate the Intestines to relieve constipation	Drains heat and activates qi circulation
Run Chang Wan (Moisten the Intestines Pill)		Regulates blood circulation and tonifies the blood.
Ji Chuan Jian (Benefit the River [Flow] Decoction)		Warms Kidney yang and tonifies *jing* (essence)

Ma Zi Ren Wan (Hemp Seed Pill), **Run Chang Wan** (Moisten the Intestines Pill), and **Ji Chuan Jian** (Benefit the River [Flow] Decoction) all lubricate the Intestines to relieve constipation.

- *Ma Zi Ren Wan* purges heat and activates qi circulation. It relieves constipation characterized by dry-heat in the Stomach and Large Intestine.
- *Run Chang Wan* nourishes the blood and activates blood circulation. It is used for constipation characterized by blood deficiency.
- *Ji Chuan Jian* warms Kidney yang and nourishes *jing* (essence). It is suitable for constipation caused by Kidney yang and *jing* deficiencies.

194

Chinese Herbal Formulas and Applications

Chapter 2 — Summary

SECTION 4: HARSH EXPELLANTS (CATHARTICS)

Name	Similarities	Differences
Shi Zao Tang (Ten-Jujube Decoction)	Harsh expellants that purge water stagnation	Strengthens the middle *jiao*
Zhou Che Wan (Vessel and Vehicle Pill)		Activates qi circulation
Shu Zao Yin Zi (Spread and Unblock Decoction)		Releases the exterior

Shi Zao Tang (Ten-Jujube Decoction), *Zhou Che Wan* (Vessel and Vehicle Pill), and *Su Zao Yin Zi* (Spread and Unblock Decoction) all purge water stagnation from the interior.

- *Shi Zao Tang* purges water stagnation and strengthens the middle *jiao* simultaneously. It may be used for water accumulation in the upper (pleural effusion), middle (ascites), or lower (edema) parts of the body.
- *Zhou Che Wan*, a stronger purgative formula, activates qi circulation and purges water stagnation simultaneously. It is generally used for water accumulation in the middle (ascites) and lower (edema) parts of the body.
- *Su Zao Yin Zi*, a weak purgative formula, purges water stagnation and releases the exterior. It is primarily used for water accumulation at the exterior or skin level, which results in generalized edema.

SECTION 5: PURGATIVE AND TONIC FORMULAS

Name	Similarities	Differences
Huang Long Tang (Yellow Dragon Decoction)	Clear heat and promote defecation	Tonifies qi and blood
Zeng Ye Cheng Qi Tang (Increase the Fluids and Order the Qi Decoction)		Nourishes yin and generates body fluids

Huang Long Tang (Yellow Dragon Decoction) and *Zeng Ye Cheng Qi Tang* (Increase the Fluids and Order the Qi Decoction) both purge heat stagnation and tonify the body.

- *Huang Long Tang* specifically tonifies qi and blood, and is indicated for *yangming fu* (hollow organs) syndrome with deficiency of qi and blood.
- *Zeng Ye Cheng Qi Tang* has a strong nourishing and moisturizing action, and is suitable for severe constipation accompanied by severe deficiency of yin and body fluids.

Chapter 3

— Harmonizing Formulas

和
解
剂

吴有性 Wū Yǒu-Xing

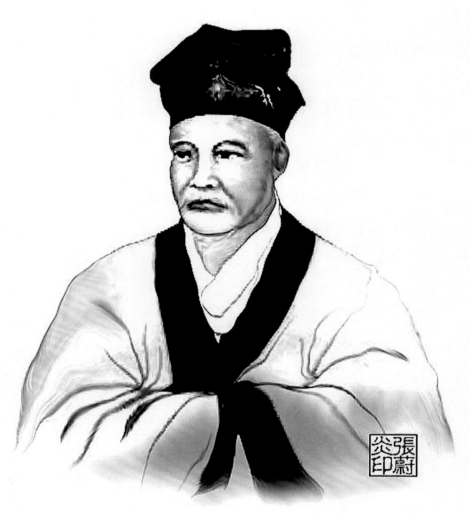

吴有性 Wū Yǒu-Xing, also known as 吴又可 Wū Yòu-Kě, 1580's – 1660's.[1]

吴有性 Wū Yǒu-Xīng

Wu You-Xing lived during the transition from the Ming dynasty to the Qing dynasty, a period dominated by war and characterized by extreme poverty and poor sanitary conditions. As a result, countless epidemics ravaged the country and killed millions of people. At the time, most physicians strictly followed the guidelines of 伤寒 *shang han* (cold damage), and achieved little or no success in treating 温疫 *wen yi* (warm epidemic). Wu observed that *wen yi* (warm epidemic) plagued everyone, starting "from one person to the entire household, from one household to the entire street, and from one street to the entire village." To better understand the patterns of this kind of disease, Wu risked his life by entering affected households and neighborhoods to personally observe and directly treat those who became ill. After years of clinical observation, Wu stated that epidemics such as *wen yi* (warm epidemic) are "**not** caused by wind, cold, summer-heat, nor dampness, but rather by 戾气 *li qi* (perverse qi)." He further elaborated that *li qi* (perverse qi) existed in the universe, but have "no sound nor smell, and no shape nor shadow." Furthermore, he observed that *li qi* (perverse qi) may be transmitted from one person to another via "heaven [air borne]" or "earth [direct contact]," and affect weak, deficient individuals (i.e., those with low immunity).

温疫论 *Wen Yi Lun* (Discussion of Epidemic Warm Disease) in 1642.

Based on these observations, Wu You-Xing wrote *Wen Yi Lun* (Discussion of Epidemic Warm Disease) in 1642, which was published approximately 200 years before the discovery of bacteria and other micro-organisms. It accurately described the origins and transmission of epidemic disease, and the importance of the immune system in relationship to the pathogens. Wu revolutionized and significantly influenced the theory and practice of traditional Chinese medicine, changes that persist even today.

Formulas originated by Wu You-Xing include:
- *Cheng Qi Yang Ying Tang* (Order the Qi and Nourish the Nutritive Qi Decoction)
- *Da Yuan Yin* (Reach the Membrane Source Decoction)

1. Exact dates of his birth and death are unknown.

Dynasties & Kingdoms	Year
Xia Dynasty 夏	2100-1600 BCE
Shang Dynasty 商	1600-1100 BCE
Zhou Dynasty 周	1100-221 BCE
Qin Dynasty 秦	221-207 BCE
Han Dynasty 漢	206 BCE-220
Three Kingdoms 三國	220-280
Western Jin Dynasty 西晉	265-316
Eastern Jin Dynasty 東晉	317-420
Northern and Southern Dynasties 北南朝	420-581
Sui Dynasty 隋	581-618
Tang Dynasty 唐	618-907
Five Dynasties 五代	907-960
Song Dynasty 宋	960-1279
Liao Dynasty 遼	916-1125
Jin Dynasty 金	1115-1234
Yuan Dynasty 元	1271-1368
Ming Dynasty 明	**1368-1644**
Qing Dynasty 清	1644-1911
Republic of China 中華民國	1912-Present Day
People's Republic of China 中華人民共和國	1949-Present Day

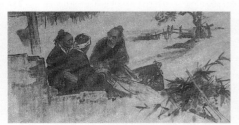

Wu personally entering the epidemic area to treat patients.

Chapter 3 – Harmonizing Formulas

Table of Contents

Chapter 3. Harmonizing Formulas ·· **197**
Biography of Wu You-Xing ··· 198

Section 1. *Shaoyang* Harmonizing Formulas ·· **206**
Xiao Chai Hu Tang (Minor Bupleurum Decoction) ·· 206
   Chai Hu Zhi Jie Tang (Bupleurum, Bitter Orange, and Platycodon Decoction) ····················· 215
   Chai Hu Jie Du Tang (Bupleurum Decoction to Relieve Toxicity) ··· 215
Chai Hu Gui Zhi Tang (Bupleurum and Cinnamon Twig Decoction) ·· 219
Chai Ling Tang (Bupleurum and Poria Decoction) ··· 222
Chai Xian Tang (Bupleurum Decoction to Raise the Sunken) ··· 226
Hao Qin Qing Dan Tang (Artemisia Annua and Scutellaria Decoction to Clear the Gallbladder) ···· 227
Chai Hu Da Yuan Yin (Bupleurum Decoction to Reach the Membrane Source) ······························· 230
   Da Yuan Yin (Reach the Membrane Source Decoction) ·· 231
   Qing Pi Yin (Clear the Spleen Decoction) ··· 231

Section 2. Liver and Spleen Harmonizing Formulas ··· **233**
Si Ni San (Frigid Extremities Powder) ·· 233
   Zhi Shi Shao Yao San (Immature Bitter Orange and Peony Powder) ···································· 236
Chai Hu Shu Gan San (Bupleurum Powder to Spread the Liver) ·· 238
Shu Gan Tang (Spread the Liver Decoction) ··· 241
Chai Hu Qing Gan Tang (Bupleurum Decoction to Clear the Liver) ·· 243
   Chai Hu Qing Gan Tang (Bupleurum Decoction to Clear the Liver) ····································· 244
   Zhi Zi Qing Gan Tang (Gardenia Decoction to Clear the Liver) ·· 245
Yi Gan San (Restrain the Liver Powder) ·· 245
Xiao Yao San (Rambling Powder) ··· 247
   Hei Xiao Yao San (Black Rambling Powder) ·· 252
Jia Wei Xiao Yao San (Augmented Rambling Powder) ··· 254
   Shi Wei Xiao Yao San (Ten-Ingredient Rambling Powder) ·· 256
Tong Xie Yao Fang (Important Formula for Painful Diarrhea) ·· 257

Section 3. Intestines and Stomach Harmonizing Formulas ··· **261**
Ban Xia Xie Xin Tang (Pinellia Decoction to Drain the Epigastrium) ··· 261
Sheng Jiang Xie Xin Tang (Fresh Ginger Decoction to Drain the Epigastrium) ································· 268
Gan Cao Xie Xin Tang (Licorice Decoction to Drain the Epigastrium) ··· 269
Huang Lian Tang (Coptis Decoction) ··· 271

Harmonizing Formulas (Summary) ··· **274**

Chinese Herbal Formulas and Applications

Chapter 3 — Overview

— Harmonizing Formulas

Definition: Harmonizing formulas treat complicated and co-existing but contrasting illness that cannot be addressed by one simple treatment method. This method of treatment is known as *he fa* (harmonizing), one of the *ba fa* (eight treatment methods) described in the *Huang Di Nei Jing* (Yellow Emperor's Inner Classic) in the first or second century, A.D.

The concept of complicated and co-existing but contrasting illness refers to disorders that affect more than one part of the body and often have opposite characteristics. For example, these disorders may affect the exterior and interior, upper and lower parts of the body, *ying* (nutritive) and *wei* (defensive) levels, or *qi* (energy) and *xue* (blood) levels. Moreover, the disorders can be characterized by both cold and heat, excess and deficiency. In such complex cases, it is inappropriate to solely release the exterior, drain the interior, tonify the deficiency, or clear the excess. Instead, it is more suitable to regulate and resolve these complex conditions through the use of harmonizing formulas.

Harmonizing formulas are frequently used to treat three main categories of disorders: *shaoyang* (half-interior, half-exterior) syndromes, Liver and Spleen disharmonies, and Intestine and Stomach disharmonies.

The characteristics of *shaoyang* syndrome is the presence of pathogens residing halfway between the exterior and interior. *Shaoyang* syndrome cannot be treated with only exterior-releasing formulas, since this would leave the interior pathogenic factor untreated. *Shaoyang* syndrome also cannot be addressed solely by targeting the interior with methods such as heat-clearing, downward draining, or emesis, since this would leave the exterior pathogenic factor untreated, or, worse, draw the pathogenic factor into the interior. Because *shaoyang* syndrome cannot be treated solely by releasing the exterior <u>or</u> resolving the interior, it must be harmonized by concurrently addressing the exterior and interior.

In addition to *shaoyang* syndrome, there are many other applications of harmonizing formulas. *Shaoyang* syndrome may also be characterized by heat in the Gallbladder channel. However, because the Gallbladder has a yin-yang relationship with the Liver, Gallbladder disorders easily result in Liver disorders. An unregulated Liver may then overact on the Spleen and Stomach, causing disorders such as Liver and Spleen disharmony, and Intestines and Stomach disharmony. Today, harmonizing methods are used to treat all of the above disorders.

> ~
> *Shaoyang* **disorders may be characterized by both cold and heat, or excess and deficiency.**
> ~

SUBCATEGORIES OF ACTION

Harmonizing formulas are organized into three subcategories to reflect the nature of the disharmony and the characteristics of relevant formulas.

1. *Shaoyang* Harmonizing Formulas

These formulas harmonize *shaoyang* (half-interior, half-exterior) syndrome. Common clinical manifestations include alternating spells of chills and fever, fullness and discomfort in the chest and hypochondrium, irritability, vomiting, lack of appetite, a bitter taste in the mouth, a dry throat, and vertigo.

Chapter 3 – Harmonizing Formulas

Chapter 3 — Overview

Herbs commonly used to harmonize *shaoyang* syndrome include *Huang Qin* (Radix Scutellariae) with *Chai Hu* (Radix Bupleuri), or *Huang Qin* (Radix Scutellariae) with *Qing Hao* (Herba Artemisiae Annuae). Representative formulas that harmonize *shaoyang* syndrome are *Xiao Chai Hu Tang* (Minor Bupleurum Decoction) and *Hao Qin Qing Dan Tang* (Artemisia Annua and Scutellaria Decoction to Clear the Gallbladder).

2. Liver and Spleen Harmonizing Formulas

~

***Shaoyang* syndromes cannot be treated with only exterior-releasing formulas.**

~

These formulas treat Liver qi stagnation (excess), which overacts on the Spleen (deficiency). Common clinical manifestations include a stifling sensation in the chest, hypochondriac pain, cold hands and feet; epigastric and abdominal fullness and pain, lack of appetite, diarrhea, rectal tenesmus; and breast distention and irregular menstruation in women.

Formulas that harmonize the Liver and Spleen generally include herbs that smooth Liver qi, strengthen the Spleen, regulate qi circulation, and nourish blood. Exemplar herbs include *Chai Hu* (Radix Bupleuri), *Zhi Qiao* (Fructus Aurantii), *Chen Pi* (Pericarpium Citri Reticulatae), *Xiang Fu* (Rhizoma Cyperi), *Dang Gui* (Radix Angelicae Sinensis), *Bai Shao* (Radix Paeoniae Alba), *Fu Ling* (Poria) and *Zhi Gan Cao* (Radix et Rhizoma Glycyrrhizae Praeparata cum Melle). Representative formulas include *Si Ni San* (Frigid Extremities Powder), *Xiao Yao San* (Rambling Powder), and *Tong Xie Yao Fang* (Important Formula for Painful Diarrhea).

3. Intestine and Stomach Harmonizing Formulas

These formulas treat accumulation of various pathogenic factors in the Stomach and Intestines. Such cases involve interlocking of heat and cold, which causes reversed qi flow in the Stomach and Intestines. Common clinical manifestations include nausea, vomiting, borborygmus, diarrhea, and epigastric and abdominal distention, fullness and pain.

Two types of herbs are commonly used to harmonize the Intestines and Stomach and treat the interlocking of heat and cold: acrid and warm herbs, such as *Gan Jiang* (Rhizoma Zingiberis) and *Sheng Jiang* (Rhizoma Zingiberis Recens); and bitter and cold herbs, such as *Huang Qin* (Radix Scutellariae) and *Huang Lian* (Rhizoma Coptidis). An exemplar formula is *Ban Xia Xie Xin Tang* (Pinellia Decoction to Drain the Epigastrium).

CAUTIONS / CONTRAINDICATIONS

- Harmonizing formulas do not have drastic or overtly powerful actions. Nevertheless, harmonizing formulas eliminate pathogenic factors from the body. Use of harmonizing formulas when not appropriate to the diagnosis may delay healing or even worsen the condition. For example, use of harmonizing formulas for an interior condition may lengthen the time required for healing; using them for an exterior syndrome may worsen the condition by drawing exterior pathogens inward.
- Harmonizing formulas should not be used in individuals with alternating fever and chills accompanied fatigue, weakness, irregular diet and lifestyle, and deficiency of qi or blood.

~

Solely targeting the interior with downward-draining formulas . . . [might] draw the pathogenic factor into the interior.

~

- Harmonizing formulas should not be used for conditions in which the exterior pathogenic factors have not yet entered *shaoyang*; for an interior condition that has progressed past *shaoyang*; or for *yangming* syndromes with excess heat.
- Historically, malaria has been diagnosed as a *shaoyang* disorder and treated with harmonizing formulas. But malaria may have various clinical manifestations: treatment with harmonizing formulas alone is no longer recommended.

PHARMACOLOGICAL EFFECTS & CLINICAL APPLICATIONS

Harmonizing formulas fall into three subcategories based on traditional therapeutic actions. These subcategories have distinct pharmacological effects and clinical applications.

1. ***Shaoyang* harmonizing formulas,** as the name implies, primarily relieve "half-interior, half-exterior" *shaoyang* syndromes. In allopathic medicine, such conditions are often characterized by

Chapter 3 — Overview

Chinese Herbal Formulas and Applications

chronic disease of internal organs. Clinically, *shaoyang* harmonizing formulas are most effective for chronic disease affecting the liver, gallbladder, pancreas, and kidneys.

- **Liver disorders**: *Shaoyang* harmonizing formulas have marked hepatoprotective effects and commonly treat liver disorder, including but not limited to chronic hepatitis,[1,2,3] liver fibrosis,[4] liver cancer,[5] and alcohol-induced liver disorders (hepatitis, fatty liver, and liver cirrhosis).[6] The mechanism of action differs among several formulas. *Xiao Chai Hu Tang* (Minor Bupleurum Decoction) protects the liver by augmenting the natural killer (NK) cell activity in the liver and increasing production of granulocyte colony-stimulating factor (G-CSF) in peripheral blood mononuclear cells.[7,8] *Si Ni San* (Frigid Extremities Powder) provides protective effects against liver injury through multiple mechanisms, such as protection of the hepatocyte membrane, enhancement of nitric oxide release, and dysfunction of liver-infiltrating cells, mainly by causing apoptosis.[9] *Chai Hu Gui Zhi Tang* (Bupleurum and Cinnamon Twig Decoction) protects the liver by inhibiting cell proliferation and induction of apoptosis in adjacent hepatocytes, in subjects with liver lesions induced by N-nitrosomorpholine.[10]

- **Gallbladder disorders**: Cholecystitis and cholelithiasis are gallbladder disorders commonly addressed by formulas that harmonize *shaoyang*, such as *Xiao Chai Hu Tang* (Minor Bupleurum Decoction),[11,12] and *Hao Qin Qing Dan Tang* (Artemisia Annua and Scutellaria Decoction to Clear the Gallbladder).[13] This action is attributed to their cholagogic effect to increase secretion of bile from the gallbladder, and facilitate its excretion into the intestines.[14]

- **Pancreatic disorders**: Some *shaoyang* harmonizing formulas have protective effects on the pancreas to treat various pancreatic disorders. For example, *Xiao Chai Hu Tang* (Minor Bupleurum Decoction) treats acute pancreatitis,[15] and *Chai Hu Gui Zhi Tang* (Bupleurum and Cinnamon Twig Decoction) treats chronic pancreatitis and pancreatic fibrosis.[16,17,18,19]

- **Kidney disorders**: *Xiao Chai Hu Tang* (Minor Bupleurum Decoction) has been shown effective in treatment of renal insufficiency,[20] and acute and chronic nephritis.[21] *Chai Ling Tang* (Bupleurum and Poria Decoction) has been used successfully to treat nephropathy,[22] diabetic nephropathy,[23] and steroid-dependent nephrotic syndrome.[24] The mechanisms of these nephroprotective effects have been attributed in part to the ability of the formulas to increase elimination of water,[25] and decrease serum albumin and total protein levels.[26]

2. **Liver and Spleen harmonizing formulas** treat a wide variety of disorders, including liver, gallbladder, gastrointestinal, mental, and sexual and reproductive disorders.

- **Liver disorders**: These formulas address liver disorders such as hepatitis,[27,28] chronic hepatitis,[29] and liver cirrhosis.[30,31] The hepatoprotective effects of these formulas include enhanced protection of the hepatocyte membrane, reduced damage to liver cells, decreased liver enzymes, and increased generation of new liver cells.[32,33,34] Exemplar formulas include *Si Ni San* (Frigid Extremities Powder), *Chai Hu Shu Gan San* (Bupleurum Powder to Spread the Liver), and *Xiao Yao San* (Rambling Powder).

- **Gallbladder disorders**: Cholecystitis and cholelithiasis are disorders commonly addressed by formulas such as *Si Ni San* (Frigid Extremities Powder),[35,36] *Chai Hu Shu Gan San* (Bupleurum Powder to Spread the Liver),[37,38] and *Xiao Yao San* (Rambling Powder).[39] The cholagogic effects of the formulas increase the production and secretion of bile acids.[40]

- **Gastrointestinal disorders**: These formulas treat a wide variety of gastrointestinal diseases, including superficial gastritis,[41] gastritis,[42] peptic ulcer,[43] chronic ulcerative colitis,[44] enteritis,[45,46] colitis,[47] ulcerative colitis,[48] and irritable bowel syndrome.[49,50] Exemplar formulas include *Si Ni San* (Frigid Extremities Powder), *Chai Hu Shu Gan San* (Bupleurum Powder to Spread the Liver), *Xiao Yao San* (Rambling Powder), and *Tong Xie Yao Fang* (Important Formula for Painful Diarrhea). The mechanism of action varies, depending on the disorder and the relevant formulas.

- **Mental disorders**: Many harmonizing formulas are used to treat various mental disorders. *Xiao Yao San* (Rambling Powder) has been used successfully for schizophrenia,[51] depression,[52] and neurosis.[53] *Jia Wei Xiao Yao San* (Augmented Rambling Powder) has been effective for affective and panic disorders.[54,55] *Chai Hu Shu Gan San* (Bupleurum Powder to Spread the Liver has been used

Chapter 3 — Overview

to treat insomnia.[56] The mechanism of action varies, depending on the disorder and the relevant formulas.

- **Sexual and reproductive disorders**: These formulas are effective in a wide variety of sexual and reproductive disorders in both men and women. *Si Ni San* (Frigid Extremities Powder) has been used effectively for impotence,[57] chronic adnexitis,[58] and infertility caused by blocked fallopian tubes.[59] *Chai Hu Shu Gan San* (Bupleurum Powder to Spread the Liver) has been used successfully for orchitis,[60] male sexual dysfunction (specifically, the inability to ejaculate),[61] and breast distention and pain.[62] Lastly, *Xiao Yao San* (Rambling Powder) is useful in cases of sexual dysfunction in men (impotence and inability to ejaculate),[63,64] and infertility in women.[65]

3. Unlike other harmonizing formulas that have a wide range of clinical applications, **Intestine and Stomach harmonizing formulas** target mainly gastrointestinal disorders.
- **Gastrointestinal disorders**: The conditions these formulas treat include superficial gastritis,[66] chronic gastritis,[67] atrophic gastritis,[68] peptic ulcer disease,[69] reflux esophagitis,[70] upper gastrointestinal bleeding,[71] indigestion,[72] gastroptosis,[73] gastroenteritis,[74] irritable bowel syndrome,[75] and ulcerative colitis.[76] Exemplar formulas include *Ban Xia Xie Xin Tang* (Pinellia Decoction to Drain the Epigastrium), *Sheng Jiang Xie Xin Tang* (Fresh Ginger Decoction to Drain the Epigastrium), and *Huang Lian Tang* (Coptis Decoction).

References

1. *Xin Yao Yu Lin Chuang* (New Medicine and the Clinical Application) 1982;4:651.
2. *Zhong Yi Fang Ji Xian Dai Yan Jiu* (Modern Study of Medical Formulae in Traditional Chinese Medicine) 1997;(1):199.
3. *Guo Wai Yi Xue Zhong Yi Zhong Yao Fen Ce* (Monograph of Chinese Herbology from Foreign Medicine) 1991;3:168.
4. Shimizu I. Sho-saiko-to: Japanese herbal medicine for protection against hepatic fibrosis and carcinoma. Journal of Gastroenterology & Hepatology 2000 Mar;15:D84-90.
5. Oka H, Yamamoto S, Kuroki T, Harihara S, Marumo T, Kim SR, Monna T, Kobayashi K, Tango T. Prospective study of chemoprevention of hepatocellular carcinoma with Sho-saiko-to (TJ-9). Cancer 1995 Sep 1;76(5):743-9.
6. *Guo Wai Yi Xue Zhong Yi Zhong Yao Fen Ce* (Monograph of Chinese Herbology from Foreign Medicine) 1991;13(6):31.
7. Kaneko M, Kawakita T, Tauchi Y, Saito Y, Suzuki A, Nomoto K. Augmentation of NK activity after oral administration of a traditional Chinese medicine, xiao-chai-hu-tang (shosaiko-to). Immunopharmacol Immunotoxicol 1994 Feb;16(1):41-53.
8. Yamashiki M, Asakawa M, Kayaba Y, Kosaka Y, Nishimura A. Herbal medicine "sho-saiko-to" induces in vitro granulocyte colony-stimulating factor production on peripheral blood mononuclear cells. J Clin Lab Immunol 1992;37(2):83-90.
9. Jiang J, Zhou C, Xu Q. Alleviating effects of Si-Ni-San, a traditional Chinese prescription, on experimental liver injury and its mechanisms. Biol Pharm Bull 2003 Aug;26(8):1089-94.
10. Tatsuta M, Iishi H, Baba M, Narahara H, Yano H, Sakai N. Suppression by Chai-hu-gui-zhi-tang of the development of liver lesions induced by N-nitrosomorpholine in Sprague-Dawley rats. Cancer Lett 2000 Apr 28;152(1):31-6.
11. *Fu Jian Zhong Yi Yao* (Fujian Chinese Medicine and Herbology) 1986;17(3):48.
12. *Shi Yong Zhong Xi Yi Jie He Za Zhi* (Practical Journal of Integrated Chinese and Western Medicines) 1993;4:218.
13. *Chang Chun Zhong Yi Xue Yuan Xue Bao* (Journal of Changchun University of Chinese Medicine) 1998;1:29.
14. *Guo Wai Yi Xue* (Foreign Medicine) 1991;13(4):46.
15. *Zhong Yi Za Zhi* (Journal of Chinese Medicine) 1982;9:40.
16. *Guo Wai Yi Xue* (Foreign Medicine) 1992;1:40.
17. Motoo Y, Su SB, Xie MJ, Taga H, Sawabu N. Effect of herbal medicine Saiko-keishi-to (TJ-10) on rat spontaneous chronic pancreatitis: comparison with other herbal medicines. Int J Pancreatol 2000 Apr;27(2):123-9.
18. Su SB, Motoo Y, Xie MJ, Sakai J, Taga H, Sawabu N. Expression of pancreatitis-associated protein (PAP) in rat spontaneous chronic pancreatitis: effect of herbal medicine Saiko-keishi-to (TJ-10). Pancreas 1999 Oct;19(3):239-47.
19. Su SB, Motoo Y, Xie MJ, Taga H, Sawabu N. Antifibrotic effect of the herbal medicine Saiko-keishi-to (TJ-10) on chronic pancreatitis in the WBN/Kob rat. Pancreas 2001 Jan;22(1):8-17.
20. *Shan Dong Zhong Yi Za Zhi* (Shandong Journal of Chinese Medicine) 1998;8:359.
21. *Zhong Yi Fang Ji Xian Dai Yan Jiu* (Modern Study of Medical Formulae in Traditional Chinese Medicine) 1997;190.
22. *Guo Wai Yi Xue Zhong Yi Zhong Yao Fen Ce* (Monograph of Chinese Herbology from Foreign Medicine) 1989;11(6):18.
23. *Guo Wai Yi Xue Zhong Yi Zhong Yao Fen Ce* (Monograph of Chinese Herbology from Foreign Medicine) 1990;(5):247.
24. Yoshikawa N, Ito H, Takekoshi Y, Honda M, Awazu M, Iijima K, Nakamura H, Seino Y, Takeda N, Hattori S, Matsuda I. Standard versus long-term prednisolone with sairei-to for initial therapy in childhood steroid-responsive nephrotic syndrome: a prospective controlled study. Nippon Jinzo Gakkai Shi 1998 Nov;40(8):587-90.
25. Fujitsuka N, Goto K, Takeda S, Aburada M. The diuretic effect of Sairei-to is mediated by nitric oxide production in pentobarbital-anesthetized rats. J Pharmacol Sci 2004 Feb;94(2):185-91.
26. Li P, Fujio S. Effects of chai ling tang on proteinuria in rat models. J Traditional Chinese Med 1995 Mar;15(1):48-52.

Chinese Herbal Formulas and Applications

Chapter 3 — Overview

27. *Shan Xi Xin Zhong Yi* (New Shanxi Chinese Medicine) 1987;(5):225.

28. *Hei Long Jiang Zhong Yi Yao* (Heilongjiang Chinese Medicine and Herbology) 1987;(1):25.

29. *Zhong Yi Yao Xue Bao* (Report of Chinese Medicine and Herbology) 1992;6:38.

30. *Liao Ning Zhong Yi Za Zhi* (Liaoning Journal of Chinese Medicine) 1996;4:169.

31. *Ji Lin Zhong Yi Yao* (Jilin Chinese Medicine and Herbology) 1986;(5):18.

32. Jiang J, Zhou C, Xu Q. Alleviating effects of Si-Ni-San, a traditional Chinese prescription, on experimental liver injury and its mechanisms. Biol Pharm Bull 2003 Aug;26(8):1089-94.

33. *Zhong Cao Yao* (Chinese Herbal Medicine) 1990;21(11):28.

34. *Zhong Cao Yao* (Chinese Herbal Medicine) 1990;21(11):28.

35. *Hu Nan Zhong Yi Za Zhi* (Hunan Journal of Chinese Medicine) 1989;4:39.

36. *An Hui Zhong Yi Xue Yuan Xue Bao* (Journal of Anhui University School of Medicine) 1995;4:32.

37. *Gan Su Zhong Yi Xue Yuan Xue Bao* (Journal of Gansu University of Chinese Medicine) 1995;2:37.

38. *Shi Yong Zhong Xi Yi Jie He Za Zhi* (Practical Journal of Integrated Chinese and Western Medicines) 1991;4(10):618.

39. am *Jiang Xi Zhong Yi Yao* (Jiangxi Chinese Medicine and Herbology) 1999;1:27.

40. *Shi Yong Zhong Yi Nei Ke Za Zhi* (Journal of Practical Chinese Internal Medicine) 1989;3(1):11.

41. *Zhe Jiang Zhong Yi Za Zhi* (Zhejiang Journal of Chinese Medicine) 1997;10:439.

42. *Bei Jing Zhong Yi Yao Da Xue Xue Bao* (Journal of Beijing University of Medicine and Medicinals) 1997;3:68.

43. *Zhe Jiang Zhong Yi Xue Yuan Xue Bao* (Journal of Zhejiang University of Chinese Medicine) 1997;2:53.

44. *Nei Meng Gu Zhong Yi Yao* (Traditional Chinese Medicine and Medicinals of Inner Mongolia) 1998;1:26.

45. *Hu Nan Zhong Yi Za Zhi* (Hunan Journal of Chinese Medicine) 1987;6:12.

46. *Ha Er Bing Zhong Yi* (Haerbing Chinese Medicine) 1964;4:25.

47. *Shan Xi Zhong Yi* (Shanxi Chinese Medicine) 1989;11:490.

48. *Shan Dong Zhong Yi Za Zhi* (Shandong Journal of Chinese Medicine) 1996;10:444.

49. *Si Chuan Zhong Yi* (Sichuan Chinese Medicine) 1997;11:25.

50. *Zhe Jiang Zhong Yi Za Zhi* (Zhejiang Journal of Chinese Medicine) 1996;11:502.

51. *Xin Zhong Yi* (New Chinese Medicine) 1983;(1):37.

52. *Bei Jing Zhong Yi* (Beijing Chinese Medicine) 1996;2:22.

53. *Fu Jian Zhong Yi Yao* (Fujian Chinese Medicine and Herbology) 1999;5:26.

54. Zhang LD, Zhang YL, Xu SH, Zhou G, Jin SB. Traditional Chinese medicine typing of affective disorders and treatment. American Journal of Chinese Medicine 1994;22(3-4):321-7.

55. Mantani N, Hisanaga A, Kogure T, Kita T, Shimada Y, Terasawa K. Four cases of panic disorder successfully treated with Kampo (Japanese herbal) medicines: Kami-shoyo-san and Hange-koboku-to. Psychiatry & Clinical Neurosciences 2002 Dec;56(6):617-20.

56. *Zhong Yi Ming Fang Lin Chuang Xin Yong* (Contemporary Clinical Applications of Classic Chinese Formulas) 2001;575.

57. *Hu Bei Zhong Yi Za Zhi* (Hubei Journal of Chinese Medicine) 1986;3:21.

58. *Chang Chun Zhong Yi Xue Yuan Xue Bao* (Journal of Changchun University of Chinese Medicine) 1995;1:43.

59. *Zhong Yi Ming Fang Lin Chuang Xin Yong* (Contemporary Clinical Applications of Classic Chinese Formulas) 2001;243.

60. *Shan Xi Zhong Yi* (Shanxi Chinese Medicine) 1993;14(2):54.

61. *Zhe Jiang Zhong Yi Za Zhi* (Zhejiang Journal of Chinese Medicine) 1990;25(6):253.

62. *Guang Xi Zhong Yi Yao* (Guangxi Chinese Medicine and Herbology) 1985;8(2):21.

63. *Ji Lin Zhong Yi Yao* (Jilin Chinese Medicine and Herbology) 1990;2:17.

64. *He Nan Zhong Yi* (Henan Chinese Medicine) 1997;3:174.

65. *Xin Zhong Yi* (New Chinese Medicine) 1995;5:38.

66. *Shan Xi Zhong Yi* (Shanxi Chinese Medicine) 1991;12(3):128.

67. *Tian Jin Zhong Yi* (Tianjin Chinese Medicine), 1997;1:15.

68. *Xin Zhong Yi* (New Chinese Medicine) 1988;7:35.

69. *Hei Long Jiang Zhong Yi Yao* (Heilongjiang Chinese Medicine and Herbology) 1996;5:27.

70. *Hei Long Jiang Zhong Yi Yao* (Heilongjiang Chinese Medicine and Herbology) 1998;3:30.

71. *Hu Bei Zhong Yi Za Zhi* (Hubei Journal of Chinese Medicine) 1987;3:22.

72. *Si Chuan Zhong Yi* (Sichuan Chinese Medicine) 1990;5:11.

73. *Shang Hai Zhong Yi Yao Za Zhi* (Shanghai Journal of Chinese Medicine and Herbology) 1998;4:30.

74. *Zhe Jiang Zhong Yi Za Zhi* (Zhejiang Journal of Chinese Medicine) 1985;4:155.

75. *Zhong Yi Ming Fang Lin Chuang Xin Yong* (Contemporary Clinical Applications of Classic Chinese Formulas) 2001;303.

76. *Xin Zhong Yi* (New Chinese Medicine) 1997;6:14.

Chapter 3 – Harmonizing Formulas   *Section 1 – Shaoyang Harmonizing Formulas*

Section 1

和解少阳剂

— Shaoyang Harmonizing Formulas

Xiǎo Chái Hú Tāng (Minor Bupleurum Decoction)

小柴胡湯
小柴胡汤

Pinyin Name: *Xiao Chai Hu Tang*
Literal Name: Minor Bupleurum Decoction
Alternate Names: *Hsiao Tsai Hu Tang*, Minor Bupleurum Combination
Original Source: *Shang Han Lun* (Discussion of Cold-Induced Disorders) by Zhang Zhong-Jing in the Eastern Han Dynasty

COMPOSITION

Chai Hu (Radix Bupleuri)	24g [12g]
Huang Qin (Radix Scutellariae)	9g [9g]
Ban Xia (Rhizoma Pinelliae), *xi* (washed)	0.5 cup [9g]
Sheng Jiang (Rhizoma Zingiberis Recens), *qie* (sliced)	9g [9g]
Ren Shen (Radix et Rhizoma Ginseng)	9g [6g]
Zhi Gan Cao (Radix et Rhizoma Glycyrrhizae Praeparata cum Melle)	9g [5g]
Da Zao (Fructus Jujubae), *bo* (opened)	12 pieces [4 pieces]

DOSAGE / PREPARATION / ADMINISTRATION

The source text specifies to cook the ingredients in 12 cups [2,400 mL] of water until 6 cups [1,200 mL] of the liquid remain. Discard the residue, and cook the strained decoction again until it is reduced to 3 cups [600 mL]. Take 1 cup [200 mL] of warm decoction per dose, three times daily. Today, the decoction may be prepared using the doses suggested in brackets.

CHINESE THERAPEUTIC ACTIONS

Harmonizes *shaoyang*

CLINICAL MANIFESTATIONS

1. *Shaoyang* syndrome: alternating spells of fever and chills, chest and hypochondriac fullness and discomfort, irritability, a bitter taste in the mouth, lack of appetite, nausea, vomiting, vertigo, a dry throat, a thin, white tongue coating, and a wiry pulse.
2. Any of the following disorders with *shaoyang* characteristics: gynecological disorders with heat in the uterus, Liver, or *chong* (thoroughfare) channel; malaria; jaundice; or any internal injury characterized by *shaoyang* syndrome.

CLINICAL APPLICATIONS

Hepatitis, viral hepatitis, chronic hepatitis, hepatic fibrosis and carcinoma, hepatocellular carcinomas, jaundice, cholecystitis, cholelithiasis, pancreatitis, fever, fever in cancer, nephritis, chronic renal insufficiency, acute tonsillitis, infectious parotitis, stomatitis, common cold, influenza, measles, bronchitis, pneumonia, pulmonary tuberculosis, cough, allergic rhinitis, bronchial asthma, reflux esophagitis, antral gastritis, gastritis, gastric pain, gastric prolapse, constipation, Meniere's syndrome, dizziness, seizures, migraine, angina, depression, chronic fatigue syndrome, morning sickness, postpartum infection, postpartum fever, dysmenorrhea, premenstrual syndrome, and malaria.

EXPLANATION

Xiao Chai Hu Tang (Minor Bupleurum Decoction) is the main formula for harmonizing *shaoyang* syndrome, one of the six stages of disease progression described in *Shang Han Lun* (Discussion of Cold-Induced Disorders). The *shaoyang* is situated between *yang* and *yin*, or between the exterior and interior; therefore, alternating spells of fever and chills may occur in *shaoyang* syndrome

206

Xiǎo Chái Hú Tāng (Minor Bupleurum Decoction)

Xiao Chai Hu Tang (Minor Bupleurum Decoction)

Diagnosis	Signs and Symptoms	Treatment	Herbs
Shaoyang syndrome	• Alternating spells of fever and chills: the location of the illness between exterior and interior • Chest and hypochondriac fullness and discomfort: qi stagnation • A bitter taste in the mouth, a dry throat, and irritability: heat in the *shaoyang* Gallbladder channel • Lack of appetite, nausea, and vomiting: Gallbladder heat invading the Stomach • Thin, white tongue coating: exterior condition • Wiry pulse: qi stagnation	Harmonizes *shaoyang*	• *Chai Hu* (Radix Bupleuri) releases the exterior, and *Huang Qin* (Radix Scutellariae) clears the interior. Together, they harmonize *shaoyang* disorders. • *Ban Xia* (Rhizoma Pinelliae) harmonizes the Stomach to relieve nausea and vomiting, and disperses stagnation. • *Sheng Jiang* (Rhizoma Zingiberis Recens) harmonizes the middle *jiao*. • *Ren Shen* (Radix et Rhizoma Ginseng), *Zhi Gan Cao* (Radix et Rhizoma Glycyrrhizae Praeparata cum Melle), and *Da Zao* (Fructus Jujubae) tonify Stomach qi, nourish body fluids, and harmonize the *ying* (nutritive) and *wei* (defensive) levels.

if the body is fighting both the pathogens outside and the disharmony inside.

Disorders in the *shaoyang* may cause qi stagnation and eventual heat formation in the Gallbladder channel (a *shaoyang* channel), giving rise to chest and hypochondriac fullness and discomfort, a bitter taste in the mouth, vertigo, a dry throat, and irritability. Lack of appetite, nausea, and vomiting are the results of Gallbladder heat invading the Stomach. The tongue coating is thin and white because the pathogenic factors have not yet transformed into internal heat. The wiry pulse is the result of qi stagnation in the *shaoyang* channel.

Because the disease resides between the exterior and the interior, it is not suitable to use only exterior-releasing herbs or only purgative herbs. Use of only exterior-releasing herbs will not treat the interior condition, and use of only heat-clearing or downward draining herbs will bring the pathogens from the exterior into the interior. Therefore, the harmonizing method is the most appropriate treatment approach in this condition.

Chai Hu (Radix Bupleuri) is the main herb for treating *shaoyang* disorders. The light quality of *Chai Hu* (Radix Bupleuri) lifts and disperses stagnation, as well as releases to the exterior. *Huang Qin* (Radix Scutellariae), a bitter and cold herb that enters the Gallbladder channel, is ideal for clearing *shaoyang* heat. Together, *Chai Hu* (Radix Bupleuri) disperses the exterior while *Huang Qin* (Radix Scutellariae) clears the interior to achieve the harmonizing effect. *Ban Xia* (Rhizoma Pinelliae), besides harmonizing

the Stomach to relieve nausea and vomiting, disperses stagnation in the body. *Sheng Jiang* (Rhizoma Zingiberis Recens) helps *Ban Xia* (Rhizoma Pinelliae) harmonize the middle *jiao*. It also reduces the toxicity of *Ban Xia* (Rhizoma Pinelliae). *Ren Shen* (Radix et Rhizoma Ginseng), *Zhi Gan Cao* (Radix et Rhizoma Glycyrrhizae Praeparata cum Melle), and *Da Zao* (Fructus Jujubae) tonify Stomach qi, nourish body fluids, and harmonize the *ying* (nutritive) and *wei* (defensive) levels. The combination of *Chai Hu* (Radix Bupleuri) and *Ren Shen* (Radix et Rhizoma Ginseng) also provides mutual check and balance for each others: *Chai Hu* (Radix Bupleuri) prevents the tonic effect of *Ren Shen* (Radix et Rhizoma Ginseng) from retaining the pathogens in the body, while *Ren Shen* (Radix et Rhizoma Ginseng) prevents the dispersing effect of *Chai Hu* (Radix Bupleuri) from damaging qi. Combined, these herbs expel the pathogens and strengthen bodily constitution.

Because the *shaoyang* stage is unstable and often short and transient, the symptoms listed above may not be clinically present all at the same time. Therefore, as suggested in *Shang Han Lun* (Discussion of Cold-Induced Disorders), this formula can be applied even if there is only one *shaoyang* symptom present clinically.

MODIFICATIONS
General Signs and Symptoms
• If accompanied by headache, add *Chuan Xiong* (Rhizoma Chuanxiong).
• If there is thirst, remove *Ban Xia* (Rhizoma Pinelliae) and add *Tian Hua Fen* (Radix Trichosanthis).

Xiǎo Chái Hú Tāng (Minor Bupleurum Decoction)

- With thirst and irritability from deficiency heat, add *Mai Dong* (Radix Ophiopogonis) and *Wu Wei Zi* (Fructus Schisandrae Chinensis).
- If there is no thirst, but a slight fever and exterior symptoms are present, remove *Ren Shen* (Radix et Rhizoma Ginseng) and add *Gui Zhi* (Ramulus Cinnamomi).
- With irritability, add *Dan Zhu Ye* (Herba Lophatheri) and *Geng Mi* (Semen Oryzae).
- With more irritability but absence of nausea or vomiting, remove *Ban Xia* (Rhizoma Pinelliae) and *Ren Shen* (Radix et Rhizoma Ginseng), and add *Gua Lou* (Fructus Trichosanthis).
- With abdominal pain, remove *Huang Qin* (Radix Scutellariae) and add *Bai Shao* (Radix Paeoniae Alba).
- With more vomiting or nausea, add *Sheng Jiang* (Rhizoma Zingiberis Recens) and *Chen Pi* (Pericarpium Citri Reticulatae).
- When there is indigestion in children, add *Bai Zhu* (Rhizoma Atractylodis Macrocephalae), *Chen Pi* (Pericarpium Citri Reticulatae), *Fu Ling* (Poria), and *Shan Zha* (Fructus Crataegi).
- If there is gum pain caused by yin deficiency, add *Shi Gao* (Gypsum Fibrosum).
- With palpitations and dysuria, remove *Huang Qin* (Radix Scutellariae) and add *Fu Ling* (Poria).
- With distention and hardness of the hypochondriac area caused by phlegm accumulation, remove *Da Zao* (Fructus Jujubae) and add *Mu Li* (Concha Ostreae).
- If the hypochondriac pain is severe, add *Qing Pi* (Pericarpium Citri Reticulatae Viride), *Bai Shao* (Radix Paeoniae Alba) and *Xiang Fu* (Rhizoma Cyperi).
- With a stifling sensation in the chest, add *Zhi Shi* (Fructus Aurantii Immaturus) and *Qing Pi* (Pericarpium Citri Reticulatae Viride).

Liver and Gallbladder Disorders

- For icteric jaundice and hepatitis, add *Zhi Shi* (Fructus Aurantii Immaturus), *Yin Chen* (Herba Artemisiae Scopariae), *Bai Shao* (Radix Paeoniae Alba), and *Jin Qian Cao* (Herba Lysimachiae).
- For damp-heat jaundice, add *Yin Chen* (Herba Artemisiae Scopariae), *Zhi Zi* (Fructus Gardeniae), and *Ban Lan Gen* (Radix Isatidis).
- For jaundice with more heat, add *Zhi Zi* (Fructus Gardeniae) and *Huang Bo* (Cortex Phellodendri Chinensis).

Infectious Disorders

- For common colds, add *Jing Jie* (Herba Schizonepetae), *Fang Feng* (Radix Saposhnikoviae), and *Ge Gen* (Radix Puerariae Lobatae).
- For influenza, add *Jin Yin Hua* (Flos Lonicerae Japonicae), *Lian Qiao* (Fructus Forsythiae), and *Ban Lan Gen* (Radix Isatidis).
- For acute bronchitis, add *Jie Geng* (Radix Platycodonis), *Zhi Qiao* (Fructus Aurantii), *Ku Xing Ren* (Semen Armeniacae Amarum), and *Bai Bu* (Radix Stemonae).
- For chronic bronchitis, add *Fu Ling* (Poria), *Chen Pi* (Pericarpium Citri Reticulatae), *Zi Wan* (Radix et Rhizoma Asteris), and *Kuan Dong Hua* (Flos Farfarae).
- For acute otitis media, add *Long Dan* (Radix et Rhizoma Gentianae) and *Zhi Zi* (Fructus Gardeniae).
- For urinary tract infection, add *Bian Xu* (Herba Polygoni Avicularis), *Che Qian Cao* (Herba Plantaginis), and *Hai Jin Sha* (Spora Lygodii).
- For malaria, add *Chang Shan* (Radix Dichroae), *Bing Lang* (Semen Arecae) and *Wu Mei* (Fructus Mume).

Gynecological Disorders

- For postpartum wind invasion with perspiration, remove *Chai Hu* (Radix Bupleuri).
- For postpartum wind invasion without fever, remove *Huang Qin* (Radix Scutellariae).
- For postpartum wind invasion with increased vomiting or nausea, increase the dose of *Sheng Jiang* (Rhizoma Zingiberis Recens).
- For postpartum wind invasion with marked deficiency, increase the dose of *Ren Shen* (Radix et Rhizoma Ginseng).
- When there is wind invasion during the menstrual period, add *Niu Xi* (Radix Achyranthis Bidentatae), *Tao Ren* (Semen Persicae), and *Mu Dan Pi* (Cortex Moutan).

CAUTIONS / CONTRAINDICATIONS

- *Xiao Chai Hu Tang* should be used with caution in patients with yin and/or blood deficiencies, in patients with upper excess and lower deficiency, or in patients with Liver fire. Inappropriate use of this formula may result in headache, dizziness, or bleeding gums.
- In general, there is no sweating associated with relief of symptoms, following the administration of *Xiao Chai Hu Tang*, since it harmonizes, rather than releases the exterior. However, some patients do show sweating prior to recovery. They should be monitored closely to prevent excessive sweating from injuring yin.
- Avoid cold, raw, pungent, and spicy foods while taking this formula.[1]

PHARMACOLOGICAL EFFECTS

1. **Hepatoprotective**: Administration of *Xiao Chai Hu Tang* was associated with preventive and beneficial effects against various types of drug- or chemical-induced liver damage. In one study, intraperitoneal injection of the formula in

Xiǎo Chái Hú Tāng (Minor Bupleurum Decoction)

Chinese Herbal Formulas and Applications

rats effectively controlled galactose-induced liver disorder in 65-70% of subjects by lowering the SGOT and SGPT.[2] Other studies have indicated that the formula is also effective against liver cirrhosis induced by carbon tetrachloride.[3] Yet another study reported that *Xiao Chai Hu Tang* was effective in treating liver inflammation and fibrosis.[4] One proposed mechanism of this hepatoprotective effect is the augmentation of natural killer (NK) cell activity in the liver.[5] Another proposed mechanism is a dose-dependent increase in the production of granulocyte colony-stimulating factor (G-CSF) on peripheral blood mononuclear cells.[6]

2. **Cholagogic**: Administration of *Xiao Chai Hu Tang* was associated with a marked effect of increasing the secretion of bile acid from the gallbladder and its excretion into the intestines in animals.[7]

3. **Immunostimulant**: Administration of *Xiao Chai Hu Tang* has marked effect on the immune system. In one study of mice, 100 mg/kg of the herb was associated with stimulating natural killer (NK) cells activities, while 200 mg/kg was associated with inhibition of NK cell activity.[8]

4. **Anti-inflammatory**: Intraperitoneal injection of the formula in rats at 200 mg/kg was associated with marked anti-inflammatory effects for up to 4 hours.[9] The anti-inflammatory effects were also present in rats whose adrenal glands had been surgically removed.[10]

5. **Effect on temperature regulation**: Administration of *Xiao Chai Hu Tang* was associated with effectiveness in reducing body temperature in rabbits with artificially-induced fever,[11] but it had little effect in rabbits with normal body temperature.[12]

6. **Gastrointestinal**: Administration of *Xiao Chai Hu Tang* was associated with inhibiting gastric acid production in rats. However, it had a stimulating effect on the intestines to increase peristalsis.[13]

7. **Effect on hypercholesterolemia and hyperlipidemia**: Administration of *Xiao Chai Hu Tang* and *Da Chai Hu Tang* (Major Bupleurum Decoction) was associated with beneficial effects in treating rats with cholesterol-induced hypercholesterolemia and aging-induced hyperlipidemia. Both formulas reduced total cholesterol in the liver and triglycerides in the liver and blood.[14]

8. **Antiallergic**: Administration of *Xiao Chai Hu Tang* had a dose-dependent effect to significantly inhibit histamine release to treat allergies. The proposed mechanism of this effect was attributed to the ability of *Xiao Chai Hu Tang* to inhibit IgE receptor-associated protein phosphorylation in the histamine release pathway.[15]

9. **Antiulcer**: *Xiao Chai Hu Tang* was effective in treating gastric ulcers in rats. *Xiao Chai Hu Tang* had a comparable effect to sucralfate in protecting the gastric mucosa, and had effects similar to cimetidine or atropine in inhibiting

gastric acid secretions.[16] *Xiao Chai Hu Tang* also showed an antiulcer effect against both water-immersion stress-induced gastric lesions and ethanol-induced gastric injury in a dose-dependent manner.[17]

10. **Antitumor**: Administration of *Xiao Chai Hu Tang* was associated with antitumor activity, presumably because it stimulates host-mediated factors such as the phagocytic function of the reticuloendothelial system and C3 cleavage producibility, and is closely related to TNF production. It is unclear whether *Xiao Chai Hu Tang* has a direct antitumor effect.[18]

11. **Antitumor and antimetastatic**: Administration of *Xiao Chai Hu Tang* in mice with malignant melanoma was associated with slowing tumor development and the transition to malignancy, decreasing incidence of distant metastasis to brain and kidney, and, at the malignant stage, prolonging life span.[19] The mechanism of this action was attributed to the ability of *Xiao Chai Hu Tang* to inhibit the growth of malignant melanoma cells by up-regulating Fas-mediated apoptosis and arresting the cell cycle through down-regulation of cyclin dependent kinases.[20] *Xiao Chai Hu Tang* also inhibited lung carcinoma growth and metastasis, with special reference to macrophage activation.[21]

12. **Radioprotective**: Administration of *Xiao Chai Hu Tang* and/or methylprednisolone was associated with protective effects against radiation-induced damage to lung tissues. The efficacy of radioprotective effect from the mildest to the most potent were *Xiao Chai Hu Tang*, methylprednisolone, and the combination of both (more effective than either alone).[22]

13. **Bioavailability**: Oral administration of *Xiao Chai Hu Tang* before or after meals did not show any significant difference in the maximum plasma concentration or the plasma concentration-time curve. The study concluded that timing of administration (before or after meals) did not affect the blood concentration (bioavailability) of *Xiao Chai Hu Tang*.[23]

CLINICAL STUDIES AND RESEARCH

1. **Chronic hepatitis**: In a double-blind multicenter clinical study involving 222 patients with chronic active hepatitis, use of *Xiao Chai Hu Tang* was associated with a decrease of HBeAg and an increase of anti-HBe antibodies. No remarkable side effects were noticed.[24] In another study, two groups of patients with chronic hepatitis were treated with modified *Xiao Chai Hu Tang* with good results. In one group of 41 patients with chronic infectious hepatitis, 26 patients had significant improvement and 13 patients had moderate improvement. In another group of 21 patients with chronic active hepatitis, 10 patients had significant improvement and 8 patients had moderate

Xiǎo Chái Hú Tāng (Minor Bupleurum Decoction)

improvement. The formula used contained *Chai Hu* (Radix Bupleuri) 12g, *Huang Qin* (Radix Scutellariae) 12g, *Tai Zi Shen* (Radix Pseudostellariae) 15g, *Ban Xia* (Rhizoma Pinelliae) 10g, *Gan Cao* (Radix et Rhizoma Glycyrrhizae) 6g, and dry-fried *Zhi Zi* (Fructus Gardeniae) 10g.[25] In another study, administration of *Xiao Chai Hu Tang* for 2-3 months was associated with marked symptomatic relief and improvement of liver function among 45 chronic hepatitis patients who did not respond to prednisone.[26]

2. **Viral hepatitis**: Use of *Xiao Chai Hu Tang* has been shown in many studies to effectively treat hepatitis. In one study, 307 patients with viral hepatitis were treated with 87.75% effectiveness using *Xiao Chai Hu Tang* plus *Zhi Zi* (Fructus Gardeniae) and *Hua Shi* (Talcum) as the base formula.[27] For 50 patients with chronic hepatitis B, one study reported 86.0% effectiveness using *Xiao Chai Hu Tang* plus *Zhu Ling* (Polyporus), *Huang Qi* (Radix Astragali), and *Zao Xiu* (Rhizoma Paridis) as the main herbal treatment.[28]

3. **Hepatitis C**: One study investigated the mechanism of action on the therapeutic effect of *Xiao Chai Hu Tang* to suppress liver cancer development. The study found that in hepatitis C patients, use of *Xiao Chai Hu Tang* could adjust the decreased IL-10 production and the increased IL-4 and IL-5 production of mononuclear cells, indicating that this moderate regulation of the cytokine production system may be useful in the prevention of disease progression.[29]

4. **Hepatic fibrosis and carcinoma**: *Xiao Chai Hu Tang* demonstrated chemopreventive and anti-carcinogenic effects against the development of hepatocellular carcinoma in cirrhotic patients. Evidence showed that *Xiao Chai Hu Tang* suppressed oxidative stress in hepatocytes and hepatic stellate cells, inhibited chemical hepatocarcinogenesis in animals, and acted as a biological response modifier by suppressing the proliferation of hepatoma cells by inducing apoptosis and arresting the cell cycle. Baicalin, baicalein, and saikosaponin-a are believed to be three of the main active compounds in *Xiao Chai Hu Tang* .[30] In another study, administration of *Xiao Chai Hu Tang* inhibited collagen production, while an increase in retinoid level inhibited activation of Ito cells, leading to inhibition and prevention of liver fibrosis.[31]

5. **Hepatocellular carcinomas**: In a prospective, randomized, non-blind controlled study, 260 patients with liver cirrhosis were randomly assigned to 2 groups: patients in the trial group were given 7.5 g/day of *Xiao Chai Hu Tang* orally in addition to the conventional drugs given to the control patients. After monitoring the patients for 60 months, the study reported that the incidence of hepatocellular carcinomas was lower and the survival rate was higher for the trial group compared with the control group. The researchers concluded that *Xiao Chai Hu Tang*

helped to prevent the development of hepatocellular carcinomas in patients with cirrhosis, particularly in patients without HBs antigen.[32]

6. **Cholecystitis and cholelithiasis**: One hundred patients with cholecystitis and cholelithiasis were treated with a combination of *Xiao Chai Hu Tang* and *Xiao Cheng Qi Tang* (Minor Order the Qi Decoction) with an 85% success rate of passing the stones.[33]

7. **Cholecystitis**: One study reported 98.9% effectiveness using *Xiao Chai Hu Tang* to treat cholecystitis. Of 285 patients (134 males, 151 females, average of 40.1 years of age, 2.7 years average duration of illness), 61 had acute cholecystitis and 224 had chronic cholecystitis. The treatment protocol was to administer the herbs in decoction one time daily for 15 days per course of treatment. The study reported complete recovery in 273 patients, improvement in 9 patients, and no effect in 3 patients.[34]

8. **Pancreatitis**: Fifty patients with acute pancreatitis were treated with marked improvement using acupuncture, modified *Xiao Chai Hu Tang,* and atropine. The average duration of treatment was 6.8 days, with most patients showing improvement after about 3 days.[35]

9. **Fever in cancer**: Thirty-two cancer patients with high fever were treated with good results using modified *Xiao Chai Hu Tang*. The treatment protocol was to use *Xiao Chai Hu Tang* plus *Bai Hua She She Cao* (Herba Hedyotis) and *Ban Zhi Lian* (Herba Scutellariae Barbatae) as the base formula. *Yu Ping Feng San* (Jade Windscreen Powder) and *Bie Jia* (Carapax Trionycis) were added for qi and yin deficiencies; *Yin Chen* (Herba Artemisiae Scopariae) and *Yi Yi Ren* (Semen Coicis) for damp-heat; and *Shi Gao* (Gypsum Fibrosum) and *Zhi Mu* (Rhizoma Anemarrhenae) for persistent high fever due to heat and toxins. Out of 32 patients, 17 had marked improvement, 13 had moderate improvement, and 2 had no improvement.[36]

10. **Fever**: Eighty-six patients with high fever (36 due to respiratory tract infection, 20 due to infection of the bile duct, 9 due to urinary tract infection, 4 due to postpartum infection, 2 due to toxemia, 3 due to hepatitis, 2 due to encephalitis, 2 due to influenza, 2 due to parotitis, 3 due to bacterial dysentery, and 3 due to unknown causes) were treated successfully. The study reported reduction of body temperature in 29 patients after 1-2 doses, 36 patients after 3-4 doses, and 21 patients after 4 doses.[37] According to another study, 128 patients with high fever were treated with *Xiao Chai Hu Tang* plus *Ban Lan Gen* (Radix Isatidis), *Mian Ma Guan Zhong* (Rhizoma Dryopteridis Crassirhizomatis), *Bai Wei* (Radix et Rhizoma Cynanchi Atrati) and others. *Ge Gen* (Radix Puerariae Lobatae) was added for body aches and pains; and *Mu Dan Pi* (Cortex Moutan) and *Di Huang* (Radix Rehmanniae) were added for red tongue body. Within 5 doses of herbs, the study

Xiǎo Chái Hú Tāng (Minor Bupleurum Decoction)

Chinese Herbal Formulas and Applications

reported normal temperature (37.2°C / 98.96°F or below) without recurrence of fever in 119 of 128 patients.[38]

11. **Nephritis**: Forty patients of acute and chronic nephritis were treated with electro-acupuncture and *Xiao Chai Hu Tang* with significant improvement. There were significant reductions of protein and cells in the urine.[39] Another study reported that the combination of *Xiao Chai Hu Tang* and *Ba Wei Di Huang Wan* (Eight-Ingredient Pill with Rehmannia) is beneficial in treating patients with chronic nephritis refractory to steroid therapy.[40]

12. **Chronic renal insufficiency**: Modified *Xiao Chai Hu Tang* was used with good results in treating 60 patients with chronic renal insufficiency. The herbal treatment included *Xiao Chai Hu Tang* plus *Dan Shen* (Radix et Rhizoma Salviae Miltiorrhizae), *Da Huang* (Radix et Rhizoma Rhei), *Yi Mu Cao* (Herba Leonuri), and other herbs as the base formula. *Tai Zi Shen* (Radix Pseudostellariae), *Di Huang* (Radix Rehmanniae), and *Gou Qi Zi* (Fructus Lycii) were added for qi and yin deficiencies with accumulation of dampness and toxins. *Fu Zi* (Radix Aconiti Lateralis Praeparata) and dry-fried *Bai Zhu* (Rhizoma Atractylodis Macrocephalae) were added for accumulation of water and dampness due to inability of Spleen and Kidney to regulate water circulation. The herbs were given for 3 months per course of treatment. Of 60 patients, the study reported significant improvement in 12 patients, moderate improvement in 24 patients, stabilization in 14 patients, and no benefit in 10 patients. The overall rate of effectiveness was 83.33%.[41]

13. **Cough**: *Xiao Chai Hu Tang* plus *Xi Xin* (Radix et Rhizoma Asari), *Gan Jiang* (Rhizoma Zingiberis), *Ku Xing Ren* (Semen Armeniacae Amarum), and others were used to treat 52 patients with chronic cough with marked improvement in 13 patients, moderate improvement in 35 patients, and no effect in 4 patients. The overall rate of effectiveness was 92.3%.[42]

14. **Bronchial asthma**: Use of *Xiao Chai Hu Tang* was reported to have a 64.3% effectiveness rate in treating chronic bronchial asthma dependent on steroid drugs for treatment. Of 28 patients, 4 had significant improvement and 14 had moderate improvement.[43]

15. **Reflux esophagitis**: Seventy-eight patients (40 males and 38 females) with reflux esophagitis for an average of 14 months (4 months to 3 years) were treated with modified *Xiao Chai Hu Tang* one time daily for 30 days. The base formula contained *Chai Hu* (Radix Bupleuri) 15g, *Huang Qin* (Radix Scutellariae) 10g, *Dang Shen* (Radix Codonopsis) 10g, *Ban Xia* (Rhizoma Pinelliae) 10g, *Gan Cao* (Radix et Rhizoma Glycyrrhizae) 6g, and *Da Zao* (Fructus Jujubae) 5 pieces. In addition, 30 grams of calcined *Wa Leng Zi* (Concha Arcae) were added for acid reflux; 20 grams of *Dan Shen* (Radix et Rhizoma Salviae Miltiorrhizae) were added for blood stagnation; and 30 grams each of *Wu Mei* (Fructus Mume) and *Bai Shao* (Radix Paeoniae Alba) were added for burning sensations and pain. The study reported complete recovery in 69 patients, moderate improvement in 6 patients, and no improvement in 3 patients. The overall success rate was 96.2%.[44]

16. **Antral gastritis**: *Xiao Chai Hu Tang* plus *Xuan Fu Hua* (Flos Inulae), *Tao Ren* (Semen Persicae), and others were used to treat 107 patients with antral gastritis with 90.70% effectiveness. The duration of treatment ranged from 1-3 courses, with 15 packs of herbs per course of treatment.[45]

17. **Gastritis**: Thirty-six patients with gastritis due to regurgitation of bile were treated with modified *Xiao Chai Hu Tang* for 30 days with marked results. Modifications of the herbs were as follows: *Dan Shen* (Radix et Rhizoma Salviae Miltiorrhizae) was added for chronic gastritis with blood stagnation; *Huang Lian* (Rhizoma Coptidis) for accumulation of heat; *Zhi Qiao* (Fructus Aurantii) for abdominal distention and fullness; *San Qi* (Radix et Rhizoma Notoginseng), *Hai Piao Xiao* (Endoconcha Sepiae) and *Bai Fan* (Alumen) for ulceration. Most patients reported complete recovery or resolution of all symptoms. Endoscopy also confirmed varying degrees of recovery.[46]

18. **Gastric pain**: Modified *Xiao Chai Hu Tang* was used to treat 151 patients with stomach pain with complete recovery reported in 84 patients, improvement in 49 patients, and no effect in 18 patients. Modifications included the addition of *Wu Mei* (Fructus Mume), *Dan Shen* (Radix et Rhizoma Salviae Miltiorrhizae), *Wu Ling Zhi* (Faeces Trogopteri), *Mu Dan Pi* (Cortex Moutan) and others as deemed necessary.[47]

19. **Gastric prolapse**: Administration of modified *Xiao Chai Hu Tang* for one month in 60 patients with gastric prolapse was associated with complete recovery in 29 patients, marked improvement in 22 patients, and slight improvement in 9 patients. The base formula contained *Xiao Chai Hu Tang* plus *Mai Ya* (Fructus Hordei Germinatus) and *Ji Nei Jin* (Endothelium Corneum Gigeriae Galli). *Xuan Fu Hua* (Flos Inulae) and *Zhe Shi* (Haematitum) were added for belching, distention, and pain. For epigastric pain, *Dang Shen* (Radix Codonopsis) was removed, and *Shi Xiao San* (Sudden Smile Powder) and *Da Huang* (Radix et Rhizoma Rhei) were added. For individuals with emotional disturbance, *Dang Gui* (Radix Angelicae Sinensis), *Bai Shao* (Radix Paeoniae Alba), and dry-fried *Xiang Fu* (Rhizoma Cyperi) were added. For feeling of coldness in the stomach region, *Wu Zhu Yu* (Fructus Evodiae) and *Gao Liang Jiang* (Rhizoma Alpiniae Officinarum) were added. For dampness affecting the Spleen, *Cang Zhu* (Rhizoma Atractylodis), *Zi Su Geng* (Caulis Perillae), and *Chen Pi* (Pericarpium Citri Reticulatae)

Xiǎo Chái Hú Tāng (Minor Bupleurum Decoction)

were added. For food stagnation, *Sha Ren* (Fructus Amomi) and *Jian Shen Qu* (Massa Fermentata Praeparata) were added. For yin deficiency, *Shi Hu* (Caulis Dendrobii) and *Sha Shen* (Radix Glehniae seu Adenophorae) were added.[48]

20.**Constipation**: Modified *Xiao Chai Hu Tang* was used successfully to treat constipation in geriatric patients. Of 48 patients, 30 had complete recovery, 16 had marked improvement, and 2 had slight improvement. The base formula included *Xiao Chai Hu Tang* plus *Tao Ren* (Semen Persicae), dry-fried *Lai Fu Zi* (Semen Raphani), and others. In addition, *Bai Jiang Cao* (Herba cum Radice Patriniae) and *Huang Qin* (Radix Scutellariae) were added for heat; *Yan Hu Suo* (Rhizoma Corydalis) and *Bai Shao* (Radix Paeoniae Alba) were given in larger doses for severe abdominal pain; and *Hou Po* (Cortex Magnoliae Officinalis) and *Da Fu Pi* (Pericarpium Arecae) were given for a feeling of heaviness and distention in the abdomen.[49]

21.**Acute tonsillitis**: Use of modified *Xiao Chai Hu Tang* was found to have 94% effectiveness (102 of 108 patients) in treating acute tonsillitis. The herbal treatment used *Xiao Chai Hu Tang* plus *She Gan* (Rhizoma Belamcandae) and *Xia Ku Cao* (Spica Prunellae) as the base formula, with the addition of *Ban Lan Gen* (Radix Isatidis) for severe sore throat; *Ma Bo* (Lasiosphaera seu Calvatia) and *Pu Gong Ying* (Herba Taraxaci) for abscesses; *Sang Bai Pi* (Cortex Mori) and *Gua Lou* (Fructus Trichosanthis) for coughing with profuse sputum; charred *Da Huang* (Radix et Rhizoma Rhei) for constipation; *Can Sha* (Faeces Bombycis) and *Che Qian Zi* (Semen Plantaginis) for loose stools; *Xin Yi Hua* (Flos Magnoliae) and *Cang Er Zi* (Fructus Xanthii) for profuse nasal discharge; and *Shi Gao* (Gypsum Fibrosum) and *Lu Gen* (Rhizoma Phragmitis) for thirst.[50]

22.**Infectious parotitis**: Modified *Xiao Chai Hu Tang* was effective in treating acute parotitis. The herbal treatment was based on *Xiao Chai Hu Tang*, with the addition of *Xia Ku Cao* (Spica Prunellae) and elimination of *Ren Shen* (Radix et Rhizoma Ginseng). *Jie Geng* (Radix Platycodonis) and *Niu Bang Zi* (Fructus Arctii) were added for early stages of infection; *Jing Jie* (Herba Schizonepetae) and *Fang Feng* (Radix Saposhnikoviae) for presence of exterior signs and symptoms; *Jiang Can* (Bombyx Batryticatus) and *Jin Yin Hua* (Flos Lonicerae Japonicae) for wind-heat and epidemic toxin; *Huo Xiang* (Herba Agastaches) and *Pei Lan* (Herba Eupatorii) for damp-heat in the interior; *Da Huang* (Radix et Rhizoma Rhei) for constipation; *Ju He* (Semen Citri Reticulatae) for mastitis; and *Li Zhi He* (Semen Litchi) for orchitis. Of 47 patients, 45 had complete recovery and 2 had no improvement.[51]

23.**Stomatitis**: Complete recovery was reported in all 40 patients with stomatitis using *Xiao Chai Hu Tang* plus *Huang Lian* (Rhizoma Coptidis) as a mouth gargle. The duration of treatment ranged from 3 to 15 doses of herbs.[52]

24.**Allergic rhinitis**: In one comparison study, patients with allergic rhinitis were treated with either herbs or drugs (antihistamine). In the herb group, *Xiao Chai Hu Tang* was used as the base formula, with the addition of *Xin Yi Hua* (Flos Magnoliae) and *Ju Hua* (Flos Chrysanthemi) for severe nose itching and sneezing; *Cang Zhu* (Rhizoma Atractylodis) and *Sheng Ma* (Rhizoma Cimicifugae) for profuse nasal discharge; *Bai Zhi* (Radix Angelicae Dahuricae) and *Bo He* (Herba Menthae) for severe sinus swelling and congestion; *Huang Qin* (Radix Scutellariae) and *Chuan Xiong* (Rhizoma Chuanxiong) for severe inflammation; *Tao Ren* (Semen Persicae) and *Ge Gen* (Radix Puerariae Lobatae) for nasal polyps; and other modifications as deemed necessary. The study reported 90.8% effectiveness for 65 patients in the herb group, and 76.9% effectiveness for 65 patients in the drug (antihistamine) group.[53]

25.**Meniere's syndrome**: One study involving 268 patients with Meniere's syndrome reported marked improvement in most of the patients when they were treated with modified *Xiao Chai Hu Tang*. The herbal treatment contained *Xiao Chai Hu Tang* with *Chuan Xiong* (Rhizoma Chuanxiong), *Ju Hua* (Flos Chrysanthemi), and others as needed. The overall rate of effectiveness was 97%.[54]

26.**Dizziness**: Administration of *Xiao Chai Hu Tang* plus *Fang Feng* (Radix Saposhnikoviae), *Huo Xiang* (Herba Agastaches), and others was effective within 24 hours in treating acute onset dizziness. Of 20 patients, 14 had complete recovery and 6 had slight to moderate improvement.[55]

27.**Migraine**: Administration of *Xiao Chai Hu Tang* plus *Chuan Xiong* (Rhizoma Chuanxiong), *Bai Zhi* (Radix Angelicae Dahuricae), and *Xi Xin* (Radix et Rhizoma Asari) in 50 patients with migraine headache was associated with complete recovery in 32 patients, improvement in 15 patients, and no effect in 3 patients. The overall rate of effectiveness was 94%.[56]

28.**Angina**: *Xiao Chai Hu Tang* demonstrated good results in treating 41 patients with angina. While 35 had resolution of symptoms, they showed varying degrees of improvement based on ECG reports. The herbal treatment used *Xiao Chai Hu Tang* plus *Dang Gui* (Radix Angelicae Sinensis), *Chuan Xiong* (Rhizoma Chuanxiong), and *Fu Zi* (Radix Aconiti Lateralis Praeparata) as the base formula. Larger doses of certain herbs were used depending on the differential diagnosis of the condition: *Ren Shen* (Radix et Rhizoma Ginseng) for severe qi deficiency; *Fu Zi* (Radix Aconiti Lateralis Praeparata) for severe yang deficiency;

Xiǎo Chái Hú Tāng (Minor Bupleurum Decoction)

Chai Hu (Radix Bupleuri), *Dang Gui* (Radix Angelicae Sinensis), and *Chuan Xiong* (Rhizoma Chuanxiong) for qi and blood stagnation; and *Ban Xia* (Rhizoma Pinelliae) and *Sheng Jiang* (Rhizoma Zingiberis Recens) for phlegm stagnation.[57]

29. **Depression**: One study reported 78.8% effectiveness using modified *Xiao Chai Hu Tang* to treat depression. Modifications to the formula included the addition of *Zeng Ye Tang* (Increase the Fluids Decoction) for yin-deficient heat; *Xiang Fu* (Rhizoma Cyperi), *Yu Jin* (Radix Curcumae), and *Zhi Qiao* (Fructus Aurantii) for Liver qi stagnation; and *Hou Po* (Cortex Magnoliae Officinalis), *Bai Zhu* (Rhizoma Atractylodis Macrocephalae) and *Fu Ling* (Poria) for damp and phlegm in the Spleen. Of 90 patients, the study reported complete recovery in 64 patients and improvement in 7 patients. Poor results were noted in 19 patients who were then treated with drugs.[58]

30. **Chronic fatigue syndrome**: Modified *Xiao Chai Hu Tang* was used to treat 36 patients with chronic fatigue syndrome characterized by low-grade fever, chills, depression, muscle aches and pains in the entire body, lack of energy, bitter taste in the mouth, poor appetite, etc. The herbal treatment used *Xiao Chai Hu Tang* plus *Ban Lan Gen* (Radix Isatidis) and *Gui Zhi* (Ramulus Cinnamomi) as the base formula, with more herbs added when necessary. Herbs were given for 10 days per course of treatment, for 1-4 courses. The study reported complete recovery in 26 patients, and improvement in 10 others.[59]

31. **Morning sickness**: One study reported 88% effectiveness using *Xiao Chai Hu Tang* to treat nausea and vomiting during pregnancy. Of 320 patients, the study reported complete relief in 180 patients, improvement in 100 patients, and no effect in 40 patients.[60]

32. **Postpartum infection**: Use of modified *Xiao Chai Hu Tang* had 96.6% effectiveness in treating 178 patients with postpartum viral infection (common cold or influenza). The herbal treatment contained *Xiao Chai Hu Tang* plus *Huang Qi* (Radix Astragali), *Yi Mu Cao* (Herba Leonuri) and *Dang Gui* (Radix Angelicae Sinensis) as the base formula. Modifications were made as needed. For dry mouth and stuffy or runny nose, *Sheng Jiang* (Rhizoma Zingiberis Recens) was removed and *Sang Ye* (Folium Mori), *Ju Hua* (Flos Chrysanthemi), *Bo He* (Herba Menthae), and *Lu Gen* (Rhizoma Phragmitis) were added. For nasal obstruction, *Zi Su Ye* (Folium Perillae) was added. For high fever without perspiration, *Qing Hao* (Herba Artemisiae Annuae) was added. For thick sticky sputum, *Zhi Mu* (Rhizoma Anemarrhenae) and *Zhe Bei Mu* (Bulbus Fritillariae Thunbergii) were added. For white foamy sputum, *Chen Pi* (Pericarpium Citri Reticulatae) and *Fu Ling* (Poria) were added. For sore throat, *Ban Lan Gen* (Radix Isatidis), *She Gan* (Rhizoma Belamcandae),

and *Ma Bo* (Lasiosphaera seu Calvatia) were added. For red tongue body with little tongue coating, *Yu Zhu* (Rhizoma Polygonati Odorati) was added. After 1-2 packs of herbal treatment, the study reported complete recovery in 154 patients, improvement in 18 patients, and no effect in 6 patients.[61]

33. **Postpartum fever**: Modified *Xiao Chai Hu Tang* effectively reduced body temperature within an average of 10 hours in all 60 postpartum women with fever. The herbal treatment contained *Xiao Chai Hu Tang* plus *Dang Gui* (Radix Angelicae Sinensis), *Yi Mu Cao* (Herba Leonuri), and others as the base formula. In addition, *Jin Yin Hua* (Flos Lonicerae Japonicae) and *Jing Jie* (Herba Schizonepetae) were added for sore throat; *Tao Ren* (Semen Persicae) and *Hong Hua* (Flos Carthami) for lower abdominal pain with spotting; and *Pu Gong Ying* (Herba Taraxaci) and dry-fried *Chuan Shan Jia* (Squama Manis) for breast distention and pain.[62]

34. **Dysmenorrhea**: Administration of *Xiao Chai Hu Tang* was associated with 96.5% effectiveness in relieving primary dysmenorrhea. The treatment protocol was to take the herbs starting the first day of the period for 10 days, for 3 months per course of treatment. Of 57 patients, the study reported complete recovery in 28 patients, significant improvement in 22 patients, slight improvement in 5 patients, and no effect in 2 patients.[63]

35. **Premenstrual syndrome (PMS)**: Use of modified *Xiao Chai Hu Tang* had 93.41% effectiveness in treating 167 women with PMS (complete relief in 77 patients, significant improvement in 57 patients, and moderate improvement in 22 patients). Modifications to the formula were made based on the condition of the patient. For breast distention and hypochondriac pain, *Chuan Lian Zi* (Fructus Toosendan), *Xia Ku Cao* (Spica Prunellae), and *Bai Shao* (Radix Paeoniae Alba) were added. For edema, *Fu Ling* (Poria), *Ze Xie* (Rhizoma Alismatis), and *Che Qian Zi* (Semen Plantaginis) were added. For irritability, restlessness, and elevated body temperature, *Ren Shen* (Radix et Rhizoma Ginseng) and *Ban Xia* (Rhizoma Pinelliae) were removed, and *Mu Dan Pi* (Cortex Moutan), *Zhi Zi* (Fructus Gardeniae) and *Di Huang* (Radix Rehmanniae) were added. For diarrhea, dry-fried *Bai Zhu* (Rhizoma Atractylodis Macrocephalae) and *Yi Yi Ren* (Semen Coicis) were added. For palpitations and insomnia, *Yuan Zhi* (Radix Polygalae), *Dang Gui* (Radix Angelicae Sinensis) and dry-fried *Suan Zao Ren* (Semen Ziziphi Spinosae) were added. For nausea and vomiting, *Gan Cao* (Radix et Rhizoma Glycyrrhizae) and *Da Zao* (Fructus Jujubae) were removed, and *Zhu Ru* (Caulis Bambusae in Taenia), and *Zi Su Geng* (Caulis Perillae) were added. For dizziness and headache, *Ju Hua* (Flos Chrysanthemi) and *Chuan Xiong* (Rhizoma Chuanxiong) were added.[64]

Chapter 3 – Harmonizing Formulas   *Section 1 – Shaoyang Harmonizing Formulas*

Xiǎo Chái Hú Tāng (Minor Bupleurum Decoction)

HERB-DRUG INTERACTION

- **Interferon**: Increased risk of acute pneumonitis may be associated with the use of interferon, *Xiao Chai Hu Tang*, or both in combination. Among patients with chronic hepatitis or liver cirrhosis, the frequency of drug-induced pneumonitis was 0.5% in those given only interferon-alpha, 0.7% in those given only *Xiao Chai Hu Tang*, and 4.0% in those given both interferon-alpha and *Xiao Chai Hu Tang*.[65] Many theories have been proposed on the mechanism of this interaction. One theory states that the herbs have not been shown to injure the lung tissues, but may over stimulate the neutrophils to release granulocytes, elastase and oxygen radicals, which subsequently damage lung tissue. The fibroblasts that repair the damaged tissue may increase the risk of pulmonary fibrosis.[66] Another theory states that acute pneumonitis associated with concurrent use of interferon and *Xiao Chai Hu Tang* may be due to allergic-immunological mechanisms.[67]

- **Interleukin 2**: Concurrent use of *Xiao Chai Hu Tang* and interleukin 2 showed a synergistic antitumor effect against murine renal cell carcinoma cell line in mice. The treatment protocol was to administer *Xiao Chai Hu Tang* at 2.5 g/kg daily over 30 days, and interleukin 2 at 10(4) U/subject by subcutaneous injection every other day for a total of 8 doses. The combination of these two substances inhibited growth of the tumor and prolonged survival significantly as compared with the untreated mice.[68]

- **Lamivudine (Epivir; 3TC)**: One study reported synergistic antiviral effect when *Xiao Chai Hu Tang* is combined with antiviral drugs such as zidovudine (AZT), lamivudine (3TC) or AZT plus 3TC. Used alone, *Xiao Chai Hu Tang* moderately inhibited HIV-1 replication at a concentration of 25 mcg/mL. Used together, *Xiao Chai Hu Tang* enhanced the anti-HIV-1 activity of 3TC. The researchers suggested that the combination of *Xiao Chai Hu Tang* and 3TC has potential as a chemotherapeutic modality for HIV-1 infection.[69]

- **5-fluorouracil (5-FU)**: The combination of 5-FU and *Xiao Chai Hu Tang* had a synergistic effect for treatment of cancer in mice by increasing the life span by 56% and alleviating side effects of 5-FU.[70]

- **Drug-induced liver damage**: Administration of *Xiao Chai Hu Tang* has been shown to have beneficial effects in preventing and/or treating damage induced by drugs, such as halothane, danazol, D-galactosamine, and carbon tetrachloride.[71,72,73,74]

- **Liver enzyme inhibition**: The effect of *Xiao Chai Hu Tang* on cytochrome P450 enzymes was evaluated in 26 healthy subjects. Use of this herbal formula (2.5g twice daily for 5 days) was associated with a decreased mean activity of CYP1A2 by 16% on both day 1 and day 5 compared with the baseline (P=0.001).[75] In another study on the metabolic activity of different cytochrome P450 (CYP) isoforms, *Xiao Chai Hu Tang* was reported to be a competitive inhibitor of CYP2C9, but not CYP2D6. The study concluded that because of this inhibitory effect on liver metabolism, care should be taken with concurrent use of *Xiao Chai Hu Tang* and drugs.[76]

- **Pentobarbital**: Administration of *Xiao Chai Hu Tang* was associated with significantly shortened pentobarbital-induced sleeping time in mice. The mechanism of this interaction was attributed to the up-regulation of the mRNA expression of CYP2B, CYP3A1, CYP2E1 and CYP4A1.[77]

- **Carbamazepine**: Administration of one dose of *Xiao Chai Hu Tang* was associated with decreased peak concentration, and the time needed to reach the peak concentration, of carbamazepine in rats. However, two-week repeated treatments of *Xiao Chai Hu Tang* did not affect plasma concentration-time profile or any pharmacokinetic parameter of carbamazepine, an indication that *Xiao Chai Hu Tang* did not affect the liver metabolism of carbamazepine. The study attributed the mechanism of this interaction to decreased gastrointestinal absorption of carbamazepine due to delayed gastric emptying.[78]

- **Tolbutamide**: *Xiao Chai Hu Tang* demonstrably reduced the bioavailability of tolbutamide after oral administration in rats. The formula was found to accelerate the initial absorption rate, reduce the area under the plasma concentration-time curve, and decrease the overall bioavailability of tolbutamide.[79] The mechanism of this interaction was attributed to the inhibitory effect of *Xiao Chai Hu Tang* on the function of gastric emptying, thereby decreasing gastrointestinal absorption of tolbutamide.[80]

- **Ofloxacin**: In an open, random-crossover investigation study with seven volunteers, a single dose of ofloxacin and a one-week dose of *Xiao Chai Hu Tang* were given concurrently. Using high-performance liquid chromatography to evaluate the bioavailability of ofloxacin, it was determined that there is no significant effect on the rate or extent of bioavailability of ofloxacin when given concurrently with *Xiao Chai Hu Tang*.[81]

TOXICOLOGY

- *Xiao Chai Hu Tang* has a very low toxicology profile. In one study, rats were given up to 640 mg/kg of the extract per day continuously for 6 months. At the end of the study, the animals were examined for body weight, general behavior, water and food intake, and function of vital organs. The study concluded that no abnormality could be observed.[82]

- **Interstitial pneumonia**: Over 200 patients of interstitial pneumonia have been associated with the use of *Xiao Chai Hu Tang* in Japan. While the exact mechanism of

214

Xiǎo Chái Hú Tāng (Minor Bupleurum Decoction)

this adverse reaction is not completely understood, it was suggested that phenolic compounds (lignans and flavonoids) present in this formula may induce apoptosis in human lung fibroblasts and peripheral blood mononuclear cells. Two phenolic compounds, baicalein and medicarpin, were found to significantly inhibit the growth and reduce the viability of lung fibroblasts. The researchers suggested that the phenolic compounds of *Xiao Chai Hu Tang* (especially baicalein and medicarpin) may have a direct effect on human lung fibroblasts and immune cells to induce apoptosis.[83] Note: *Xiao Chai Hu Tang* is one of the most commonly used herbal formulas in Japan. According to a study published in 1999, this formula has been administered to 1.5 million Japanese patients with chronic liver diseases.[84] In addition, there have been numerous other reports that document the safe and effective use of this formula. Thus, it is important to keep a proper perspective on the relative frequency of events, as well as risk-to-benefit analysis, in evaluating toxicology reports.

RELATED FORMULAS

Chái Hú Zhǐ Jié Tāng
(Bupleurum, Bitter Orange, and Platycodon Decoction)

柴胡枳桔湯
柴胡枳桔汤

Pinyin Name: *Chai Hu Zhi Jie Tang*
Literal Name: Bupleurum, Bitter Orange, and Platycodon Decoction
Original Source: *Chong Ding Tong Su Shang Han Lun* (Revised Popular Guide to the Discussion of Cold-Induced Disorders) by Yu Gen-Chu in the Qing Dynasty

Chai Hu (Radix Bupleuri)	3-4.5g
Zhi Qiao (Fructus Citri Aurantii)	4.5g
Ban Xia (Rhizoma Pinelliae), zhu (boiled) with ginger	4.5g
Sheng Jiang (Rhizoma Zingiberis Recens), fresh	3g
Huang Qin (Radix Scutellariae)	3-4.5g
Jie Geng (Radix Platycodonis)	3g
Chen Pi (Pericarpium Citri Reticulatae)	4.5g
Cha Ye (Folium Camelliae)	3g

Chai Hu Zhi Jie Tang (Bupleurum, Bitter Orange, and Platycodon Decoction) mainly harmonizes the *shaoyang*, releases the exterior, and regulates the chest and diaphragm. The main indication is *shaoyang* syndrome, with slightly greater emphasis on the exterior than the interior. Clinically, patients will show symptoms such as alternating fever and chills, headache (especially on the two corners of the forehead), deafness, vertigo, hypochondriac fullness and pain, a white, slippery tongue coating, a wiry, slippery

pulse on the right hand, and a wiry, superficial and big pulse on the left hand. This formula can be taken with *Cha Ye* (Folium Camelliae) to enhance the overall heat-clearing and damp-dispelling effects.

In comparison to *Xiao Chai Hu Tang*, which treats *shaoyang* syndrome with equal emphasis on both the exterior and interior, *Chai Hu Zhi Jie Tang* focuses on *shaoyang* syndromes in which there are more exterior symptoms than interior. For this reason, *Ren Shen* (Radix et Rhizoma Ginseng), *Zhi Gan Cao* (Radix et Rhizoma Glycyrrhizae Praeparata cum Melle), and *Da Zao* (Fructus Jujubae) are not used in this formula.

Chái Hú Jiě Dú Tāng
(Bupleurum Decoction to Relieve Toxicity)

柴胡解毒湯
柴胡解毒汤

Pinyin Name: *Chai Hu Jie Du Tang*
Literal Name: Bupleurum Decoction to Relieve Toxicity
Original Source: *An Hui Zhong Yi Xue Yuan* (Anhui University School of Medicine) in 1990

Chai Hu (Radix Bupleuri)
Huang Qin (Radix Scutellariae)
Yin Chen (Herba Artemisiae Scopariae)
Zhi Zi (Fructus Gardeniae)
Da Huang (Radix et Rhizoma Rhei)
Hu Zhang (Rhizoma et Radix Polygoni Cuspidati)
Yu Jin (Radix Curcumae)
Bai Shao (Radix Paeoniae Alba)
Fu Ling (Poria)
Ge Gen (Radix Puerariae Lobatae)
Ma Bian Cao (Herba Verbenae)
Qing Pi (Pericarpium Citri Reticulatae Viride)
Wu Wei Zi (Fructus Schisandrae Chinensis)
Nu Zhen Zi (Fructus Ligustri Lucidi)
Xia Ku Cao (Spica Prunellae)

Chai Hu Jie Du Tang (Bupleurum Decoction to Relieve Toxicity) treats *shaoyang* disorders characterized by chronic illness with heat and toxins accumulated in the body. This formula contains herbs that release the exterior, clear heat and eliminate toxins from the interior, and drain damp-heat from the Liver and Gallbladder. Clinically, it treats liver disorders, such as hepatitis, cirrhosis, and elevated liver enzyme levels.

AUTHORS' COMMENTS

Xiao Chai Hu Tang is traditionally used to treat alternating chills and fever, but can also be used for patients showing temperature differences in the body, such as cold

Xiǎo Chái Hú Tāng (Minor Bupleurum Decoction)

limbs but a warm body, or warm limbs and a cold body. Another condition that can also be treated with this formula is drastic temperature differences on the dorsal and palmar aspects of the hands, with the palmar aspect being cold and the dorsal aspect being warm.

Xiao Chai Hu Tang can be used for unremitting fever in children approximately one week after contracting an exterior condition. These patients exhibit fever that is not alleviated with antipyretic or antibiotic drugs. Though these drugs work well to temporarily bring down body temperature, the fever tends to return as soon as the therapeutic effect is over.

One unique application of *Xiao Chai Hu Tang* that requires additional explanation is the treatment of an exterior condition in women with blood deficiency. Loss of blood during menstruation and childbirth creates an emptiness in the uterus and the *chong* (thoroughfare) channel. Due to this void, pathogenic factors directly and easily invade into deeper levels of the body instead of lingering at the *wei* (defensive) level. The Liver stores blood, travels around the genital region, and traverses up the lower abdomen, and is closely related to the uterus and *chong* channel. If heat enters the uterus and *chong* channel, it affects the Liver, which in turn affects its paired organ, the Gallbladder. This stagnant heat creates disharmony in the *shaoyang* stage, leading to alternating chills and fever, hypochondriac fullness/discomfort, a bitter taste in the mouth, a dry throat, irritability, lack of appetite, nausea, and vomiting. *Xiao Chai Hu Tang* harmonizes the *shaoyang* and pushes the heat outward to relieve the heat trapped in the uterus and *chong* channel.[85]

Alternating chills and fever is a key symptom that can be treated with *Xiao Chai Hu Tang* or *Xiao Yao San* (Rambling Powder). However, the diagnostic criteria and clinical application guidelines are very different.

- *Xiao Chai Hu Tang* treats alternating chills and fever caused by exterior pathogenic factors that enter the *shaoyang* level and get trapped in the half-exterior and half-interior location. *Ren Shen* (Radix et Rhizoma Ginseng), *Da Zao* (Fructus Jujubae), and *Gan Cao* (Radix et Rhizoma Glycyrrhizae) strengthen the interior to push the pathogens outward and prevent them from invading further into the body, **not** to tonify the deficiencies. *Sheng Jiang* (Rhizoma Zingiberis Recens) is used with *Ban Xia* (Rhizoma Pinelliae) to treat nausea and irritability caused by Gallbladder heat invading the Stomach.
- *Xiao Yao San* treats alternating fever and chills caused by disharmony among the Liver, Spleen, and Gallbladder and accompanied by blood deficiency and Liver qi

stagnation; the chills and fever are **not** the result of an exterior invasion. *Dang Gui* (Radix Angelicae Sinensis), *Bai Shao* (Radix Paeoniae Alba), *Fu Ling* (Poria), and *Bai Zhu* (Rhizoma Atractylodis Macrocephalae) strengthen the Spleen to prevent the Liver from overacting. *Sheng Jiang* (Rhizoma Zingiberis Recens) warms the middle *jiao* to strengthen the Spleen.

Fever and chills (aversion to cold) are a common complaint in exterior conditions, but they must be differentiated correctly.

- In *taiyang* syndrome, fever and chills are present simultaneously.
- In *yangming* syndrome, there is high fever and absence of chills.
- In *shaoyang* syndrome, there are alternating spells of fever and chills.

Xiao Chai Hu Tang and *Xiao Yao San* (Rambling Powder) both contain *Chai Hu* (Radix Bupleuri) as the chief herb, but with different intent and at different doses:

- *Xiao Chai Hu Tang* treats *shaoyang* syndrome in which the pathogenic heat is trapped between the exterior and interior. In this case, signs of alternating chills and fever are more severe. As a result, a large dose of *Chai Hu* (Radix Bupleuri) is needed to harmonize *shaoyang* and clear the heat.
- *Xiao Yao San* (Rambling Powder) treats Liver qi stagnation accompanied by Spleen deficiency, manifesting in emotional complaints but involving less severe physical symptoms compared to that of *Xiao Chai Hu Tang*. Although *Chai Hu* (Radix Bupleuri) is also the chief herb, only a moderate dose is needed to regulate Liver qi. In this case, this herb serves more as a channel-guiding herb in this formula to address Liver qi stagnation. Using a large dose of *Chai Hu* (Radix Bupleuri) in *Xiao Yao San* is not appropriate because it shifts the effect of the formula from harmonizing to exterior-releasing. Moreover, patients with Liver qi stagnation often have underlying deficiencies, and using *Chai Hu* (Radix Bupleuri) at a large dose may exacerbate such deficiencies.

Xiao Chai Hu Tang and *Da Chai Hu Tang* (Major Bupleurum Decoction) both treat *shaoyang* disorders with alternating chills and fever, a bitter taste in the mouth, and chest and hypochondriac distention. Both formulas contain *Chai Hu* (Radix Bupleuri), *Huang Qin* (Radix Scutellariae), *Ban Xia* (Rhizoma Pinelliae), *Sheng Jiang* (Rhizoma Zingiberis Recens), and *Da Zao* (Fructus Jujubae). Despite the similarities, they have contrasting differences:

Xiăo Chái Hú Tāng (Minor Bupleurum Decoction)

- *Xiao Chai Hu Tang* contains *Chai Hu* (Radix Bupleuri) and *Huang Qin* (Radix Scutellariae) as chief herbs to harmonize the *shaoyang*. *Ren Shen* (Radix et Rhizoma Ginseng) strengthens the interior to prevent the pathogenic factors from moving further inward. This formula treats a variety of conditions, including exterior invasion in women during their menstruation, jaundice, and symptoms of malaria.

- *Da Chai Hu Tang* is mainly used for *yangming fu* (hollow organs) syndrome with excess heat in the body. *Da Huang* (Radix et Rhizoma Rhei), *Zhi Shi* (Fructus Aurantii Immaturus), and *Bai Shao* (Radix Paeoniae Alba) sedate heat in the *yangming* channel. The key sign for differential diagnosis is constipation with abdominal pain.[86]

Xiao Chai Hu Tang and *Hao Qin Qing Dan Tang* (Artemisia Annua and Scutellaria Decoction to Clear the Gallbladder) both harmonize *shaoyang* and treat chief manifestations of alternating chills and fever, as well as chest and hypochondriac distention and pain. Their main differences are as follows:

- *Xiao Chai Hu Tang* lifts clear yang qi and pushes pathogenic factors outward. Containing *Huang Qin* (Radix Scutellariae), *Ren Shen* (Radix et Rhizoma Ginseng), *Da Zao* (Fructus Jujubae), *Gan Cao* (Radix et Rhizoma Glycyrrhizae), *Ban Xia* (Rhizoma Pinelliae), and *Sheng Jiang* (Rhizoma Zingiberis Recens), this formula harmonizes *shaoyang*, dispels pathogenic factors, and restores *zheng* (upright) *qi* to treat alternating chills and fever, hypochondriac pain and distention, a bitter taste in the mouth, a dry throat, a thin, white tongue coating, and a wiry pulse.

- *Hao Qin Qing Dan Tang* clears damp-heat in the Stomach and Gallbladder, using *Qing Hao* (Herba Artemisiae Annuae) and *Huang Qin* (Radix Scutellariae) as the two main ingredients. The formula further contains *Zhu Ru* (Caulis Bambusae in Taenia), *Ban Xia* (Rhizoma Pinelliae), *Chi Fu Ling* (Poria Rubra), *Bi Yu San* (Jasper Powder), *Chen Pi* (Pericarpium Citri Reticulatae), and *Zhi Qiao* (Fructus Aurantii), to treat damp-heat with turbid phlegm accumulation in the *shaoyang* channel. Symptoms include alternating chills and fever with a greater degree of heat than cold, a bitter taste in the mouth, acid regurgitation, a thick, greasy tongue coating, and a slippery, rapid pulse on the right hand and a wiry, rapid pulse on the left hand.[87]

References

1. *Zhong Yao Ming Fang Yao Li Yu Ying Yong* (Pharmacology and Applications of Famous Herbal Formulas) 1989;92-96.
2. *Yao Xue Za Zhi* (Journal of Medicinals) 1984;104(7):798.
3. *Guo Wai Yi Xue* (Foreign Medicine) 1984;(5)279.
4. Kusunose M, Qiu B, Cui T, Hamada A, Yoshioka S, Ono M, Miyamura M, Kyotani S, Nishioka Y. Effect of Sho-saiko-to extract on hepatic inflammation and fibrosis in dimethylnitrosamine induced liver injury rats. Biol Pharm Bull 2002 Nov;25(11):1417-21.
5. Kaneko M, Kawakita T, Tauchi Y, Saito Y, Suzuki A, Nomoto K. Augmentation of NK activity after oral administration of a traditional Chinese medicine, xiao-chai-hu-tang (shosaiko-to). Immunopharmacol Immunotoxicol 1994 Feb;16(1):41-53.
6. Yamashiki M, Asakawa M, Kayaba Y, Kosaka Y, Nishimura A. Herbal medicine "sho-saiko-to" induces in vitro granulocyte colony-stimulating factor production on peripheral blood mononuclear cells. J Clin Lab Immunol 1992;37(2):83-90.
7. *Guo Wai Yi Xue* (Foreign Medicine) 1991;13(4):46.
8. *Guo Wai Yi Xue* (Foreign Medicine) 1991;13(4):43.
9. *Yao Xue Za Zhi* (Journal of Medicinals) 1984;104(5):509.
10. *Zhong Yi Fang Ji Xian Dai Yan Jiu* (Modern Study of Medical Formulae in Traditional Chinese Medicine) 1997;(1):184.
11. *Shan Xi Zhong Yi* (Shanxi Chinese Medicine) 1990;11(8):376.
12. *Gan Su Zhong Yi Xue Yuan Xue Bao* (Journal of Gansu University of Chinese Medicine) 1991;8(3):39.
13. *Zhong Yi Fang Ji Xian Dai Yan Jiu* (Modern Study of Medical Formulae in Traditional Chinese Medicine) 1997;(1):186.
14. Umeda M, Amagaya S, Ogihara Y. Effect of shosaikoto, daisaikoto and sannoshashinto (traditional Japanese and Chinese medicines) on experimental hyperlipidemia in rats. J Ethnopharmacol 1989 Oct;26(3):255-69.
15. Matsumoto T, Shibata T. The ex vivo effect of the herbal medicine sho-saiko-to on histamine release from rat mast cells. Eur Arch Otorhinolaryngol 1998;255(7):359-64.
16. Matsuta M, Kanita R, Tsutsui F, Yamashita A. Antiulcer properties of shosaiko-to. Nippon Yakurigaku Zasshi 1996 Oct;108(4):217-25.
17. Kase Y, Yuzurihara M, Iizuka S, Ishige A, Komatsu Y. The effects of hange-shashin-to on gastric function in comparison with sho-saiko-to. Biol Pharm Bull 1997 Nov;20(11):1155-9.
18. Ito H, Shimura K. Studies on the antitumor activity of traditional Chinese medicines. (II). The antitumor mechanism of traditional Chinese medicines. Gan To Kagaku Ryoho 1985 Nov;12(11):2149-54.
19. Kato M, Liu W, Yi H, Asai N, Hayakawa A, Kozaki K, Takahashi M, Nakashima I. The herbal medicine Sho-saiko-to inhibits growth and metastasis of malignant melanoma primarily developed in ret-transgenic mice. J Invest Dermatol 1998 Oct;111(4):640-4.
20. Liu W, Kato M, Akhand AA, Hayakawa A, Takemura M, Yoshida S, Suzuki H, Nakashima I. The herbal medicine sho-saiko-to inhibits the growth of malignant melanoma cells by upregulating Fas-mediated apoptosis and arresting cell cycle through downregulation of cyclin dependent kinases. Int J Oncol 1998 Jun;12(6):1321-6.
21. Ito H, Shimura K. Effects of a blended Chinese medicine, xiao-chai-hu-tang, on Lewis lung carcinoma growth and inhibition of lung metastasis, with special reference to macrophage activation. Jpn J Pharmacol 1986 Jul;41(3):307-14.
22. Kure F. The radioprotective effects of methylprednisolone and Sho-Saikoto on mouse lung. Nippon Igaku Hoshasen Gakkai Zasshi 1992 Jan 25;52(1):96-103.
23. Nishioka Y, Kyotani S, Miyamura M, Kusunose M. Influence of time of administration of a Shosaiko-to extract granule on blood concentration of its active constituents. Chem Pharm Bull (Tokyo) 1992 May;40(5):1335-7.
24. Hirayama C, Okumura M, Tanikawa K, Yano M, Mizuta M, Ogawa N. A multicenter randomized controlled clinical trial of Shosaiko-to in chronic active hepatitis. Gastroenterol Jpn 1989 Dec;24(6):715-9.
25. *Hu Nan Zhong Yi Za Zhi* (Hunan Journal of Chinese Medicine) 1989;5(3):5.

Xiăo Chái Hú Tāng (Minor Bupleurum Decoction)

26. *Xin Yao Yu Lin Chuang* (New Medicine and the Clinical Application) 1982;4:651.

27. *Hu Nan Zhong Yi Za Zhi* (Hunan Journal of Chinese Medicine) 1987;3:5.

28. *Zhe Jiang Zhong Yi Xue Yuan Xue Bao* (Journal of Zhejiang University of Chinese Medicine) 1999;3:36.

29. Yamashiki M, Nishimura A, Suzuki H, Sakaguchi S, Kosaka Y. Effects of the Japanese herbal medicine "Sho-saiko-to" (TJ-9) on in vitro interleukin-10 production by peripheral blood mononuclear cells of patients with chronic hepatitis C. Hepatology 1997 Jun;25(6):1390-7.

30. Shimizu I. Sho-saiko-to: Japanese herbal medicine for protection against hepatic fibrosis and carcinoma. Journal of Gastroenterology & Hepatology 2000 Mar;15 Suppl:D84-90.

31. Ono M, Miyamura M, Kyotani S, Saibara T, Ohnishi S, Nishioka Y. Effects of Sho-saiko-to extract on liver fibrosis in relation to the changes in hydroxyproline and retinoid levels of the liver in rats. J Pharm Pharmacol 1999 Sep;51(9):1079-84.

32. Oka H. Yamamoto S. Kuroki T. Harihara S. Marumo T. Kim SR. Monna T. Kobayashi K. Tango T. Prospective study of chemoprevention of hepatocellular carcinoma with Sho-saiko-to (TJ-9). Cancer 1995 Sep 1;76(5):743-9.

33. *Fu Jian Zhong Yi Yao* (Fujian Chinese Medicine and Herbology) 1986;17(3):48.

34. *Shi Yong Zhong Xi Yi Jie He Za Zhi* (Practical Journal of Integrated Chinese and Western Medicines) 1993;4:218.

35. *Zhong Yi Za Zhi* (Journal of Chinese Medicine) 1982;9:40.

36. *Shan Xi Zhong Yi* (Shanxi Chinese Medicine) 1995;2:57.

37. *Si Chuan Zhong Yi* (Sichuan Chinese Medicine) 1986;4(5):36.

38. *Hu Nan Zhong Yi Za Zhi* (Hunan Journal of Chinese Medicine) 1996;2:32.

39. *Zhong Yi Fang Ji Xian Dai Yan Jiu* (Modern Study of Medical Formulae in Traditional Chinese Medicine) 1997;(1):190.

40. *Zhong Yi Fang Ji Xian Dai Yan Jiu* (Modern Study of Medical Formulae in Traditional Chinese Medicine) 1997;(1):190.

41. *Shan Dong Zhong Yi Za Zhi* (Shandong Journal of Chinese Medicine) 1998;8:359.

42. *Shan Xi Zhong Yi* (Shanxi Chinese Medicine) 1995;6:12.

43. *Guo Wai Yi Xue Zhong Yi Zhong Yao Fen Ce* (Monograph of Chinese Herbology from Foreign Medicine) 1992;4:202.

44. *Zhong Guo Zhong Xi Yi Jie He Za Zhi* (Chinese Journal of Integrative Chinese and Western Medicine) 1992;12(11):686.

45. *Shi Yong Zhong Xi Yi Jie He Za Zhi* (Practical Journal of Integrated Chinese and Western Medicines) 1996;5:312.

46. *Zhong Yi Za Zhi* (Journal of Chinese Medicine) 1983;5:41.

47. *He Nan Zhong Yi* (Henan Chinese Medicine) 1995;4:212.

48. *Si Chuan Zhong Yi* (Sichuan Chinese Medicine) 1995;2:20.

49. *Shan Xi Zhong Yi* (Shanxi Chinese Medicine) 1996;5:33.

50. *Fu Jian Zhong Yi Yao* (Fujian Chinese Medicine and Herbology) 1996;3:36.

51. *An Hui Zhong Yi Xue Yuan Xue Bao* (Journal of Anhui University School of Medicine) 1995;2:35.

52. *Shan Xi Zhong Yi Xue Yuan Xue Bao* (Journal of Shanxi University School of Chinese Medicine) 1999;4:39.

53. *Shi Yong Zhong Yi Za Zhi* (Journal of Practical Chinese Medicine) 1995;2:27.

54. *Shi Yong Zhong Xi Yi Jie He Za Zhi* (Practical Journal of Integrated Chinese and Western Medicines) 1997;11:1054.

55. *Shi Yong Zhong Xi Yi Jie He Za Zhi* (Practical Journal of Integrated Chinese and Western Medicines) 1996;5:294.

56. *Guang Xi Zhong Yi Yao* (Guangxi Chinese Medicine and Herbology) 1996;3:3.

57. *He Nan Zhong Yi* (Henan Chinese Medicine) 1986;3:18.

58. *Shan Xi Zhong Yi* (Shanxi Chinese Medicine) 1996;2:10.

59. *He Bei Zhong Yi* (Hebei Chinese Medicine) 1998;6:375.

60. *Shan Xi Zhong Yi* (Shanxi Chinese Medicine) 1989;5:203.

61. *Si Chuan Zhong Yi* (Sichuan Chinese Medicine) 1996;10:41.

62. *Shi Yong Zhong Xi Yi Jie He Za Zhi* (Practical Journal of Integrated Chinese and Western Medicines) 1997;19:1927.

63. *Jiang Xi Zhong Yi Yao* (Jiangxi Chinese Medicine and Herbology) 1992;4:39.

64. *Bei Jing Zhong Yi* (Beijing Chinese Medicine) 1987;6:30.

65. Nakagawa A et al. Five patients of drug-induced pneumonitis due to Sho-saiko-to or interferon-alpha or both. Nihon Kyobu Shikkan Gakkai Zasshi. 1995 Dec; 33(12):1361-1366.

66. Murakami K, et al. A possible mechanism of interstitial pneumonia during interferon therapy with sho-saiko-to. Nihon Kyobu Shikkan Gakkai Zasshi 1995 Apr;33(4):389-94

67. Ishizaki T, Sasaki F, Ameshima S, Shiozaki K, Takahashi H, Abe Y, Ito S, Kuriyama M, Nakai T, Kitagawa M. Pneumonitis during interferon and/or herbal drug therapy in patients with chronic active hepatitis. European Respiratory Journal 1996 Dec;9(12):2691-6.

68. Huang Y, Marumo K, Murai M. Antitumor effects and pharma-cological interaction of xiao-chai-hu-tang (sho-saiko-to) and interleukin 2 in murine renal cell carcinoma. Keio J Med 1997 Sep; 46(3):132-7.

69. Piras G. Makino M. Baba M. Sho-saiko-to, a traditional Kampo medicine, enhances the anti-HIV-1 activity of lamivudine (3TC) in vitro. Microbiology & Immunology 1997;41(10):835-9.

70. Ohta T, Tawara M, Tatsuka M, Abe H, Odashima S. An approach to prolongation of survival rate in tumor bearing mice using 5-fluorouracil in combination with various kinds of herb medicine. Gan To Kagaku Ryoho 1983 Aug;10(8):1858-65.

71. Mitsukawa H, Ikeda K. Effect of sho-saiko-to (xiao-chai-hu-tang) on hepatic injury induced by halothane in rats. Masui 1991 May;40(5):794-800.

72. Yaginuma T, Okamura T, Takeuchi T, Nishii O, Fujimori R. Preventive effect of traditional herbal medicine, shosaiko-to, on danazol-induced hepatic damage. Int J Gynaecol Obstet 1989 Aug;29(4):337-41.

73. Ohta Y, Nishida K, Sasaki E, Kongo M, Hayashi T, Nagata M, Ishiguro I. Comparative study of oral and parenteral administration of sho-saiko-to (xiao-chaihu-tang) extract on D-galactosamine-induced liver injury in rats. Am J Chin Med 1997;25(3-4):333-42.

74. Amagaya S, Hayakawa M, Ogihara Y, Ohta Y, Fujiwara K, Oka H, Oshio H, Kishi T. Treatment of chronic liver injury in mice by oral administration of xiao-chai-hu-tang. J Ethnopharmacol 1989 Apr;25(2):181-7.

75. Saruwatari J, Nakagawa K, Shindo J, Nachi S, Echizen H, Ishizaki T. The in-vivo effects of sho-saiko-to, a traditional Chinese herbal medicine, on two cytochrome P450 enzymes (1A2 and 3A) and xanthine oxidase in man. Journal of Pharmacy & Pharmacology 2003 Nov;55(11):1553-9.

76. Takahashi K, Uejima E, Morisaki T, Takahashi K, Kurokawa N, Azu-ma J. In vitro inhibitory effects of Kampo medicines on metabolic reactions catalyzed by human liver microsomes. Journal of Clinical Pharmacy & Therapeutics 2003 Aug;28(4):319-27.

77. Nose M, Tamura M, Ryu N, Mizukami H, Ogihara Y.Sho-saiko-to and Saiko-keisi-to, the traditional Chinese and Japanese herbal medicines, altered hepatic drug-metabolizing enzymes in mice and rats when administered orally for a long time. J Pharm Pharmacol 2003 Oct;55(10):1419-26.

78. Ohnishi N, Okada K, Yoshioka M, Kuroda K, Nagasawa K, Takara K, Yokoyama T. Studies on interactions between traditional herbal and western medicines. V. effects of Sho-saiko-to (Xiao-Cai-hu-Tang) on the pharmacokinetics of carbamazepine in rats. Biol Pharm Bull 2002 Nov;25(11):1461-6.

Chinese Herbal Formulas and Applications

Xiǎo Chái Hú Tāng (Minor Bupleurum Decoction)

79. American Journal of Chinese Medicine 1999;27(3-4):355-63.
80. Nishimura N, Naora K, Hirano H, Iwamoto K. Effects of sho-saiko-to (xiao chai hu tang), a Chinese traditional medicine, on the gastric function and absorption of tolbutamide in rats. Yakugaku Zasshi 2001 Feb;121(2):153-9.
81. International Journal of Clinical Pharmacology and Therapeutics 1994 Feb;32(2):57-61.
82. *Yi Fang Xin Jie* (New Explanation for Medical Formulas) 1980;42.
83. Liu ZL, Tanaka S, Horigome H, Hirano T, Oka K. Induction of apoptosis in human lung fibroblasts and peripheral lymphocytes in vitro by Shosaiko-to derived phenolic metabolites. Biological & Pharmaceutical Bulletin 2002 Jan;25(1):37-41.

84. Yamashiki M, Nishimura A, Huang XX, Nobori T, Sakaguchi S, Suzuki H. Effects of the Japanese herbal medicine "Sho-saiko-to" (TJ-9) on interleukin-12 production in patients with HCV-positive liver cirrhosis. Developmental Immunology 1999;7(1):17-22.
85. Wang MZ, et al. *Zhong Yi Xue Wen Da Ti Ku* (Questions and Answers on Traditional Chinese Medicine: Herbal Formulas)
86. Wang MZ, et al. *Zhong Yi Xue Wen Da Ti Ku* (Questions and Answers on Traditional Chinese Medicine: Herbal Formulas)
87. Wang MZ, et al. *Zhong Yi Xue Wen Da Ti Ku* (Questions and Answers on Traditional Chinese Medicine: Herbal Formulas)

Chái Hú Guì Zhī Tāng (Bupleurum and Cinnamon Twig Decoction)

柴胡桂枝湯
柴胡桂枝汤

Pinyin Name: *Chai Hu Gui Zhi Tang*
Literal Name: Bupleurum and Cinnamon Twig Decoction
Alternate Names: *Tsai Hu Kuei Chih Tang, Cai Hu Gui Zhi Tang*, Bupleurum and Cinnamon Combination
Original Source: *Shang Han Lun* (Discussion of Cold-Induced Disorders) by Zhang Zhong-Jing in the Eastern Han Dynasty

COMPOSITION

Chai Hu (Radix Bupleuri)	12g
Huang Qin (Radix Scutellariae)	4.5g
Ren Shen (Radix et Rhizoma Ginseng)	4.5g
Ban Xia (Rhizoma Pinelliae), *xi* (washed)	0.25 cup [6-9g]
Gui Zhi (Ramulus Cinnamomi)	4.5g
Bai Shao (Radix Paeoniae Alba)	4.5g
Zhi Gan Cao (Radix et Rhizoma Glycyrrhizae Praeparata cum Melle)	3g
Sheng Jiang (Rhizoma Zingiberis Recens), *qie* (sliced)	4.5g
Da Zao (Fructus Jujubae), *bo* (opened)	6 pieces

DOSAGE / PREPARATION / ADMINISTRATION

The source text states to cook the herbs in 7 cups [1,400 mL] of water, and reduce the liquid to 3 cups [600 mL]. Take 1 cup [200 mL] of the strained decoction three times daily.

CHINESE THERAPEUTIC ACTIONS

1. Dispels pathogenic factors from *taiyang* and *shaoyang* stages
2. Harmonizes the exterior and interior

CLINICAL MANIFESTATIONS

Taiyang and *shaoyang* syndromes that appear six to seven days after the onset of illness: fever, chills, joint pain, nausea, a feeling of distention and obstruction beneath the heart, and abdominal pain.

CLINICAL APPLICATIONS

Common cold and influenza, fever, arrhythmia, chronic hepatitis, liver cirrhosis, jaundice, cholecystitis, cholelithiasis, gastric or duodenal ulcers, acid reflux, chronic pancreatitis, chronic appendicitis, peritonitis, nephritis, frozen shoulder, neurasthenia, seizures, epilepsy, and trigeminal neuralgia.

EXPLANATION

Chai Hu Gui Zhi Tang (Bupleurum and Cinnamon Twig Decoction) addresses disorders characterized by *shaoyang* and *taiyang* syndromes, with *shaoyang* symptoms predominating and *taiyang* symptoms lingering. *Shaoyang* syndrome is characterized by the feeling of distention and obstruction beneath the heart, and pain around the umbilical region or the lower abdomen. *Taiyang* syndrome is

219

Chapter 3 – Harmonizing Formulas   *Section 1 – Shaoyang Harmonizing Formulas*

Chái Hú Guì Zhī Tāng (Bupleurum and Cinnamon Twig Decoction)

Chai Hu Gui Zhi Tang (Bupleurum and Cinnamon Twig Decoction)

Diagnosis	Signs and Symptoms	Treatment	Herbs
Taiyang and *shaoyang* syndromes	• Headache, a feeling of heaviness in the head, joint pain, fever and chills: *taiyang* syndrome • Distention and obstruction beneath the heart, and pain around the umbilical region or the lower abdomen: *shaoyang* syndrome	• Dispels pathogenic factors from *taiyang* and *shaoyang* stages • Harmonizes the exterior and interior	• *Gui Zhi Tang* (Cinnamon Twig Decoction) treats *taiyang* syndrome by releasing the exterior. • *Xiao Chai Hu Tang* (Minor Bupleurum Decoction) treats *shaoyang* syndrome by harmonizing the exterior and interior.

characterized by headache, joint pain, fever, chills, and a feeling of heaviness in the head.

Chai Hu Gui Zhi Tang combines two formulas: *Xiao Chai Hu Tang* (Minor Bupleurum Decoction) and *Gui Zhi Tang* (Cinnamon Twig Decoction). *Xiao Chai Hu Tang* (Minor Bupleurum Decoction) treats *shaoyang* syndrome by harmonizing the exterior and interior. *Gui Zhi Tang* (Cinnamon Twig Decoction) treats *taiyang* syndrome by releasing the exterior. Combined, *Chai Hu Gui Zhi Tang* treats both *taiyang* and *shaoyang* syndromes.

Please refer to *Xiao Chai Hu Tang* (Minor Bupleurum Decoction) and *Gui Zhi Tang* (Cinnamon Twig Decoction) for additional information on these two formulas.

MODIFICATIONS
• With painful joints, add *Ge Gen* (Radix Puerariae Lobatae) and *Sheng Ma* (Rhizoma Cimicifugae).
• When there is a feeling of oppression and fullness in the epigastric region, add *Zhi Shi* (Fructus Aurantii Immaturus) and *Jie Geng* (Radix Platycodonis).

CAUTIONS / CONTRAINDICATIONS
Avoid cold, raw, oily, and greasy foods while taking *Chai Hu Gui Zhi Tang*.[1]

PHARMACOLOGICAL EFFECTS
1. **Antiulcer**: Administration of *Chai Hu Gui Zhi Tang* had a marked effect in preventing cysteamine-induced gastric ulcers in rats. The mechanism is attributed to decreased gastric acid production.[2]
2. **Immunostimulant**: Long-term administration of the formula was associated with an increase in lymphocytes in mice.[3]
3. **Anti-inflammatory**: Administration of *Chai Hu Gui Zhi Tang* was associated with marked anti-inflammatory effect in both acute and chronic inflammatory disorders in rats.[4]
4. **Analgesic**: *Chai Hu Gui Zhi Tang* was reported to be an effective treatment for trigeminal neuralgia in rats. This

mechanism of action was attributed to the ability of the formula to control pain in ligatured nerves by local effect, not by general analgesic effect.[5]

5. **Protective effect on the pancreas**: According to one study in rats, administration of *Chai Hu Gui Zhi Tang* was associated with inhibiting pancreatic fibrosis by suppressing transforming growth factor beta1 (TGF-beta1) expression.[6] Another study reported that *Chai Hu Gui Zhi Tang* effectively delayed the onset of chronic pancreatitis and suppressed pancreatitis-associated protein gene expression in rats.[7,8]

6. **Hepatoprotective**: Administration of *Chai Hu Gui Zhi Tang* was associated with treating liver lesions induced by N-nitrosomorpholine in rats. The mechanism of this hepatoprotective function was attributed to inhibition of cell proliferation and induction of apoptosis in adjacent hepatocytes.[9]

CLINICAL STUDIES AND RESEARCH
1. **Common cold and influenza**: Administration of modified *Chai Hu Gui Zhi Tang* was effective in treating common cold and influenza. Out of 2,650 patients, 2,220 were treated on an outpatient basis, and 430 were hospitalized. The study reported complete recovery in 2,405 patients, improvement in 208 patients, and no improvement in 37 patients. The overall rate effectiveness was 98.7%. The herbal treatment used *Chai Hu Gui Zhi Tang* as the base formula, and added *Ma Huang* (Herba Ephedrae) and *Xi Xin* (Radix et Rhizoma Asari) for more cold; *Qiang Huo* (Rhizoma et Radix Notopterygii) and *Fang Feng* (Radix Saposhnikoviae) for more wind; *Jin Yin Hua* (Flos Lonicerae Japonicae), *Lian Qiao* (Fructus Forsythiae), *Shi Gao* (Gypsum Fibrosum), and *Ban Lan Gen* (Radix Isatidis) for more heat; *Huo Xiang* (Herba Agastaches) and *Cang Zhu* (Rhizoma Atractylodis) for more damp; *Huang Qi* (Radix Astragali) or *Dang Shen* (Radix Codonopsis) for qi deficiency; *Fu Zi* (Radix Aconiti Lateralis Praeparata) and *Gan Jiang* (Rhizoma Zingiberis) for yang deficiency; *Mai Dong* (Radix Ophiopogonis), *Tian Hua Fen* (Radix Trichosanthis), and *Zhi Mu*

Chái Hú Guì Zhī Tāng (Bupleurum and Cinnamon Twig Decoction)

(Rhizoma Anemarrhenae) for yin deficiency; and *Long Gu* (Os Draconis) and *Mu Li* (Concha Ostreae) for profuse perspiration.[10]

2. **Fever**: Administration of 5 to 8 doses of modified *Chai Hu Gui Zhi Tang* was effective in treating patients with fever due to viral infection. Out of 112 patients, the study reported complete recovery in 85 patients, improvement in 13 patients, and no effect in 14 patients.[11]

3. **Arrhythmia**: Administration of modified *Chai Hu Gui Zhi Tang* effectively treated various types of arrhythmia. Out of 24 patients, the study reported complete recovery in 16 patients, improvement in 4 patients, and no benefit in 4 patients.[12]

4. **Neurasthenia**: One study reported satisfactory result using modified *Chai Hu Gui Zhi Tang* to treat 60 patients with neurasthenia. The herbal treatment protocol was to use this formula as the base, and add *Shan Zha* (Fructus Crataegi), *Shen Qu* (Massa Fermentata), and *Mai Ya* (Fructus Hordei Germinatus) for poor appetite and epigastric fullness and distention; *Ju Hua* (Flos Chrysanthemi) and *Bai Zhi* (Radix Angelicae Dahuricae) for dizziness and headache; *He Huan Hua* (Flos Albiziae) and *Mu Li* (Concha Ostreae) for insomnia; *Bai Zi Ren* (Semen Platycladi) and *Shi Chang Pu* (Rhizoma Acori Tatarinowii) for inability to concentrate; and *Chuan Lian Zi* (Fructus Toosendan) for chest oppression and discomfort.[13]

5. **Chronic hepatitis**: According to one study, 133 patients with chronic hepatitis were treated with this formula, and the study reported a rate of effectiveness of 62.3%. Significant effect was reported in 47 patients, moderate effect in 36 patients, mild effect in 9 patients, and no effect in 28 patients. Deterioration was reported in 13 patients.[14]

6. **Chronic pancreatitis**: Use of *Chai Hu Gui Zhi Tang* effectively treated chronic pancreatitis. Out of 21 patients who participated in the study, 10 were male, 11 were female, and the ages ranged between 15 to 84 years. The treatment protocol was to administer 7.5g of the formula daily in powdered extract for 8 weeks or more. Out of 21 patients, the study reported marked improvement in 8 patients, slight improvement in 7 patients, and no improvement in 6 patients. The overall rate effectiveness was 71%.[15]

7. **Frozen shoulder**: Administration of *Chai Hu Gui Zhi Tang* in 26 patients (2 males and 24 females) with frozen shoulder characterized by deficiency was associated with improvement in 22 patients and no effect in 4 patients.[16]

8. **Trigeminal neuralgia**: Use of *Chai Hu Gui Zhi Tang* effectively treated patients suffering from trigeminal neuralgia. This mechanism of action was attributed to the capacity of this formula to control the manifestation of pain in ligatured nerves by local effect, not by general analgesic effect.[17]

HERB-DRUG INTERACTION

- **Benzodiazepines**: Concurrent administration of *Chai Hu Gui Zhi Tang* and anticonvulsants, such as benzodiazepines, has been found to have a synergistic effect in treating epilepsy. *Chai Hu Gui Zhi Tang* acts as a partial agonist for the GABA-A receptor, and it activates the GABA-A receptor-mediated chloride current (Icl).[18]

- **Pentobarbital**: Administration of *Chai Hu Gui Zhi Tang* was associated with significantly shortened pentobarbital-induced sleeping time in mice. The mechanism of this interaction was attributed to the up-regulation of the mRNA expression of CYP2B, CYP3A1, and CYP4A1.[19]

TOXICOLOGY

Chai Hu Gui Zhi Tang has a relatively low toxicity. Continuous administration of the formula for four weeks in rats showed no abnormalities in the liver, spleen, kidney, or adrenal glands.[20]

References

1. *Zhong Yao Ming Fang Yao Li Yu Ying Yong* (Pharmacology and Applications of Famous Herbal Formulas) 1989;92-96.
2. *Guo Wai Yi Xue* (Foreign Medicine) 1985;7(6):35.
3. *Guo Wai Yi Xue* (Foreign Medicine) 1991;13(4):45.
4. *Yao Xue Za Zhi* (Journal of Medicinals) 1983;103(4):466.
5. Sunagawa M, Okada M, Guo SY, Hisamitsu T. Effectiveness of Saiko-Keishi-To (TJ-10, a Kampo herbal medicine) for trigeminal neuralgia in rats. Masui 2001 May;50(5):486-90.
6. Su SB, Motoo Y, Xie MJ, Taga H, Sawabu N. Antifibrotic effect of the herbal medicine Saiko-keishi-to (TJ-10) on chronic pancreatitis in the WBN/Kob rat. Pancreas 2001 Jan;22(1):8-17.
7. Motoo Y, Su SB, Xie MJ, Taga H, Sawabu N. Effect of herbal medicine Saiko-keishi-to (TJ-10) on rat spontaneous chronic pancreatitis: comparison with other herbal medicines. Int J Pancreatol 2000 Apr;27(2):123-9.
8. Su SB, Motoo Y, Xie MJ, Sakai J, Taga H, Sawabu N. Expression of pancreatitis-associated protein (PAP) in rat spontaneous chronic pancreatitis: effect of herbal medicine Saiko-keishi-to (TJ-10). Pancreas 1999 Oct;19(3):239-47.
9. Tatsuta M, Iishi H, Baba M, Narahara H, Yano H, Sakai N. Suppression by Chai-hu-gui-zhi-tang of the development of liver lesions induced by N-nitrosomorpholine in Sprague-Dawley rats. Cancer Lett 2000 Apr 28;152(1):31-6.
10. *Shi Zhen Guo Yi Guo Yao* (Shizhen National Herbs and Medicine) 1998;5:404.
11. *Shan Dong Zhong Yi Za Zhi* (Shandong Journal of Chinese Medicine) 1990;6:17.
12. *He Nan Zhong Yi* (Henan Chinese Medicine) 1991;4:11.
13. *Fu Jian Zhong Yi Yao* (Fujian Chinese Medicine and Herbology) 1986;4:28.
14. *Zhong Yi Fang Ji Xian Dai Yan Jiu* (Modern Study of Medical Formulae in Traditional Chinese Medicine) 1997;(1):199.
15. *Guo Wai Yi Xue* (Foreign Medicine) 1992;1:40.
16. *Guo Wai Yi Xue* (Foreign Medicine) 1992;2:105-106.
17. Sunagawa M, Okada M, Guo SY, Hisamitsu T. Effectiveness of Saiko-Keishi-To (TJ-10, a Kampo herbal medicine) for trigeminal neuralgia in rats. Masui 2001 May;50(5):486-90.

Chapter 3 – Harmonizing Formulas　　　　　　　　　　　*Section 1 – Shaoyang Harmonizing Formulas*

Chái Hú Guì Zhī Tāng (Bupleurum and Cinnamon Twig Decoction)

18. Sugiyama K, Kano T, Muteki T. Intravenous anesthetics, acting on the gamma-amino butric acid (GABA) A receptor, potentiate the herbal medicine "saiko-keishi-to"-induced chloride current. Masui 1997 Sep;46(9):1197-203.

19. Nose M, Tamura M, Ryu N, Mizukami H, Ogihara Y. Sho-saiko-to and Saiko-keisi-to, the traditional Chinese and Japanese herbal medicines, altered hepatic drug-metabolizing enzymes in mice and rats when administered orally for a long time. J Pharm Pharmacol 2003 Oct;55(10):1419-26.

20. *Yao Xue Za Zhi* (Journal of Medicinals) 1980;100(6):602.

Chái Líng Tāng (Bupleurum and Poria Decoction)

柴苓湯
柴苓汤

Pinyin Name: *Chai Ling Tang*
Literal Name: Bupleurum and Poria Decoction
Alternate Name: Bupleurum and Hoelen Combination
Original Source: *Shen Shi Zun Sheng Shu* (Master Shen's Book for Revering Life) by Shen Jin-Ao in 1773

COMPOSITION

Chai Hu (Radix Bupleuri)

Ban Xia (Rhizoma Pinelliae)

Huang Qin (Radix Scutellariae)

Ren Shen (Radix et Rhizoma Ginseng)

Gan Cao (Radix et Rhizoma Glycyrrhizae)

Bai Zhu (Rhizoma Atractylodis Macrocephalae)

Zhu Ling (Polyporus)

Fu Ling (Poria)

Ze Xie (Rhizoma Alismatis)

Gui Zhi (Ramulus Cinnamomi)

DOSAGE / PREPARATION / ADMINISTRATION

Chai Ling Tang is formulated by combining two formulas: *Xiao Chai Hu Tang* (Minor Bupleurum Decoction) and *Wu Ling San* (Five-Ingredient Powder with Poria). Please refer to these two formulas for additional information.

CHINESE THERAPEUTIC ACTIONS

1. Harmonizes the exterior and interior to relieve *shaoyang* syndrome
2. Dispels water stagnation and phlegm accumulation

CLINICAL MANIFESTATIONS

Shaoyang syndrome with water accumulation: alternating spells of chills and fever, thirst, a bitter taste in the mouth, anorexia, edema; a feeling of fullness and oppression in the chest and hypochondriac regions; vomiting and diarrhea with water intake; and a white tongue coating.

CLINICAL APPLICATIONS

Hepatitis, alcohol-induced liver damage, cholecystitis, edema, nephropathy, diabetic nephropathy, steroid-dependent nephrotic syndrome, rheumatoid arthritis, systemic lupus erythematosus, gastroenteritis, gastritis, enteritis, ulcerative colitis, otitis media, common cold, influenza, heat stroke, febrile disorders, recurrent miscarriages, and anovulation in polycystic ovary syndrome.

EXPLANATION

Chai Ling Tang (Bupleurum and Poria Decoction) treats *shaoyang* syndrome with water accumulation in the lower parts of the body. *Shaoyang* syndrome is characterized by alternating spells of chills and fever, a bitter taste in the mouth, and a feeling of fullness and oppression in the chest and hypochondriac regions; water accumulation is characterized by thirst, edema, and scanty urine. Vomiting and diarrhea are symptoms of malaria which can be alleviated with this formula.

222

Chinese Herbal Formulas and Applications

Chái Líng Tāng (Bupleurum and Poria Decoction)

Chai Ling Tang (Bupleurum and Poria Decoction)

Diagnosis	Signs and Symptoms	Treatment	Herbs
Shaoyang syndrome with water accumulation	• Alternating spells of chills and fever, a bitter taste in the mouth, and a feeling of fullness and oppression in the chest and hypochondriac region: *shaoyang* syndrome • Thirst, edema, and scanty urine: water accumulation	• Harmonizes the exterior and interior to relieve *shaoyang* syndrome • Dispels water stagnation and phlegm accumulation	• *Xiao Chai Hu Tang* (Minor Bupleurum Decoction) treats *shaoyang* syndrome. • *Wu Ling San* (Five-Ingredient Powder with Poria) treats water accumulation.

Chai Ling Tang is comprised of two formulas: *Xiao Chai Hu Tang* (Minor Bupleurum Decoction) which treats *shaoyang* syndrome by harmonizing the exterior and the interior; and *Wu Ling San* (Five-Ingredient Powder with Poria) which treats water accumulation in the lower parts of the body by resolving dampness and promoting the flow of yang qi.

Please refer to *Xiao Chai Hu Tang* (Minor Bupleurum Decoction) and *Wu Ling San* (Five-Ingredient Powder with Poria) for additional information on these two formulas.

MODIFICATIONS

- If accompanied by irritability and a dry mouth, add *Huang Lian* (Rhizoma Coptidis) and *Mai Dong* (Radix Ophiopogonis).
- With vomiting and thirst, add *Zhi Shi* (Fructus Aurantii Immaturus) and *Zhu Ru* (Caulis Bambusae in Taenia).
- With diarrhea and a dry mouth, add *Gan Jiang* (Rhizoma Zingiberis) and *Huang Bo* (Cortex Phellodendri Chinensis).
- When the vomiting and diarrhea is due to food stagnation, add *Ping Wei San* (Calm the Stomach Powder).
- When the vomiting and diarrhea is due to summer-heat accumulation, add *San Wu Xiang Ru Yin* (Mosla Three Decoction).
- When the vomiting and diarrhea is due to deficiency and cold, add *Wu Zhu Yu Tang* (Evodia Decoction).

PHARMACOLOGICAL EFFECTS

1. **Diuretic:** Administration of *Chai Ling Tang* at 10 times the normal dose to 10-month-old rats was associated with a marked increase in water and sodium excretion in the first 24-hour period. Continuous administration for 1 month was associated with weight reduction, but no abnormal reactions.[1] The mechanism of this diuretic action was attributed to the production of nitric oxide.[2]
2. **Endocrine:** Administration of 0.01-1.0 g/kg of *Chai Ling Tang* to male Wistar rats was associated with a stimulating effect on the endocrine system, as demonstrated by an increased plasma concentration of adrenocorticotropic hormone and a decreased level of corticotropin-releasing factor.[3]
3. **Nephroprotective:** Use of *Chai Ling Tang* was associated with beneficial effects in treating passive Heymann nephritis in rats, which is similar to human membranous nephropathy. The study reported that *Chai Ling Tang* significantly decreased serum albumin and total protein, and inhibited serum total cholesterol. The researchers concluded that proteinuria in passive Heymann nephritis can be significantly suppressed by *Chai Ling Tang*.[4]

CLINICAL STUDIES AND RESEARCH

1. **Hepatitis:** Use of *Chai Ling Tang* was associated with 55.3% effectiveness in treating chronic hepatitis. Of 48 patients, the study reported significant improvement in 4 patients, moderate improvement in 13 patients, slight improvement in 9 patients, and no benefit in 22 patients.[5]
2. **Alcohol-induced liver damages:** Twenty-seven patients with various types of alcohol-induced liver disorders (13 with hepatitis, 11 with fatty liver, and 3 with liver cirrhosis) were treated with good results using *Chai Ling Tang*. The treatment protocol was to administer 3g of the powdered extract three times daily before meals for at least 3 months. All patients were instructed to avoid consumption of alcohol. The study reported improved lab values of SGOT and LDH after one month, and improved lab values of SGOT, SGPT, LDH, gamma-GPT, and total bilirubin after three months. Of 27 patients, the study reported moderate improvement in 17 patients, slight improvement in 8 patients, no effect in 1 patient, and deterioration in 1 patient. The proposed mechanism of the hepatoprotective effects was attributed to ability of this formula to reduce inflammation, regulate the production and excretion of bile, and protect liver cell membrane.[6]
3. **Nephropathy:** Thirty-nine patients with nephropathy were divided into two groups, with both groups similar in age, severity of illness, and overall condition. Group one of 21 patients received herbal treatment, and group two of 18 patients received drug treatment. Patients in group one received *Chai Ling Tang* as the base formula, with

223

Chapter 3 – Harmonizing Formulas   *Section 1 – Shaoyang Harmonizing Formulas*

Chái Líng Tāng (Bupleurum and Poria Decoction)

minor modifications based on the four possible patterns (Lung and Kidney qi deficiencies, Spleen and Kidney yang deficiencies, Liver and Kidney yin deficiencies, and qi and yin deficiencies). Patients in group two received 1 mg/kg of prednisone daily in the morning with meals for eight weeks, followed by a gradual reduction in dose, and eventual discontinuation. The study reported that both groups responded well to the treatments, and group one showed faster relief of proteinuria.[7]

4. **Diabetic nephropathy**: Fifteen patients with diabetic nephropathy who were treated with *Chai Ling Tang* showed the following results: moderate improvement in 10 patients, slight improvement in 3 patients, and no improvement in 2 patients.[8]

5. **Steroid-dependent nephrotic syndrome**: Administration of *Chai Ling Tang* effectively treated 4 patients with steroid-dependent relapsing nephrotic syndrome associated with the use of prednisolone and immunosuppressive agents. After treatment with *Chai Ling Tang*, the study reported that relapse was markedly suppressed in three patients but not at all in the other. Based on this information, the researchers concluded that *Chai Ling Tang* was effective for steroid-dependent nephrotic syndrome.[9] Another study reported marked improvement in 37 children with steroid-dependent nephrotic syndrome treated with *Chai Ling Tang* while taking corticosteroids. After treatment with *Chai Ling Tang*, the study reported improvement with proteinuria, reduction of prednisone dose, and relief of side effects. The study indicated that *Chai Ling Tang* may be a useful steroid substitute for patients with steroid-dependent nephrotic syndrome who fail to respond to or manifest severe toxic effect from cytotoxic agents.[10] In one multicenter, randomized, controlled clinical trial, initial 8-week prednisolone and 2-year *Chai Ling Tang* was effective in 196 children with steroid-responsive nephrotic syndrome.[11]

6. **Rheumatoid arthritis**: Administration of 9g of *Chai Ling Tang* daily for 3 months was associated with marked improvements in 17 patients with rheumatoid arthritis.[12]

7. **Systemic lupus erythematosus (SLE)**: Daily administration of *Chai Ling Tang* in powdered extract (8.1 g/day in two to three equally-divided doses) for 6 to 12 months was effective in treating 69 patients with SLE. Patients with joint pain and increased sensitivity to light showed improvement after 9-12 months. Patients with proteinuria showed improvement after 6-12 months. Patients with decreased white blood cell counts showed improvement after 3 months. Patients with decreased CD4 and CD8 counts showed improvement after 12 months. Side effects were reported in 8 of 69 patients, and included thirst, nausea, palpitations, itching, and increased SGPT (in 1 case).[13] Another report concluded long-term

administration of *Chai Ling Tang* showed an inhibitory effect on SLE and was beneficial as a supportive treatment for patients with mild cases of SLE.[14]

8. **Ulcerative colitis**: Administration of *Chai Ling Tang* was effective in treating ulcerative colitis. In 3 patients, administration of this formula with 30mg of prednisolone and 4.0g of salicylazosulfapyridine effectively alleviated symptoms of ulcerative colitis. No recurrence was reported upon reduction and discontinuation of prednisolone.[15]

9. **Otitis media**: Use of *Chai Ling Tang* to treat suppurative otitis media in 35 children (with 46 affected ears) had a 78.3% rate of effectiveness.[16]

10. **Recurrent miscarriages**: Use of *Chai Ling Tang* to treat 10 of 12 women with a history of recurrent miscarriages who had shown positive antiphospholipid antibodies produced an 83.3% success rate. The 12 women had experienced a total of 27 spontaneous miscarriages in their previous pregnancies. The treatment protocol was to administer 9.0g daily of *Chai Ling Tang* before their next pregnancy. Of 12 patients, the study reported conversion of antiphospholipid antibodies from positive to negative in 9 patients, and successful pregnancy and delivery of a child in 10 patients. The study considered *Chai Ling Tang* to be an effective therapy for patients with recurrent miscarriages who were found to be positive for antiphospholipid antibodies.[17] In two other studies, use of *Chai Ling Tang* and *Dang Gui Shao Yao San* (Tangkuei and Peony Powder) helped to prevent autoimmunity-related recurrent miscarriages by correcting T helper-1/T helper-2 balance.[18,19]

11. **Anovulation in polycystic ovary syndrome**: Administration of *Chai Ling Tang* stimulated ovulation in 70.6% of anovulatory patients with polycystic ovary syndrome. Serum LH and the LH/FSH ratio significantly decreased, and serum testosterone levels did not significantly change during the treatment. The researchers concluded that *Chai Ling Tang* can be useful for the treatment of anovulation in polycystic ovary syndrome, especially because this condition does not respond well to clomiphene citrate or gonadotropin therapy.[20]

HERB-DRUG INTERACTION

• **Liver enzyme inhibition**: One study that examined the metabolic activity of different cytochrome P450 (CYP) isoforms reported *Chai Ling Tang* to be a competitive inhibitor of CYP3A4 (Ki value of 0.1 mg/mL), CYP2C9 (Ki value of 0.7-0.8 mg/mL), and CYP1A2 (inhibition > 68%), but not CYP2D6. The study concluded that because of this inhibitory effect on liver metabolism, care should be taken with concurrent use of *Chai Ling Tang* and drugs.[21]

224

Chái Líng Tāng (Bupleurum and Poria Decoction)

• **Ofloxacin**: In a study with 7 volunteers in an open, random, crossover fashion, no significant effect on the rate and extent of bioavailability of ofloxacin was noted with coadministrations of *Liu Jun Zi Tang* (Six-Gentlemen Decoction), *Xiao Chai Hu Tang* (Minor Bupleurum Decoction), or *Chai Ling Tang* (Bupleurum and Poria Decoction).[22]

References

1. *Guo Wai Yi Xue Zhong Yi Zhong Yao Fen Ce* (Monograph of Chinese Herbology from Foreign Medicine) 1981;2:57.
2. Fujitsuka N, Goto K, Takeda S, Aburada M. The diuretic effect of Sairei-to is mediated by nitric oxide production in pentobarbital-anesthetized rats. J Pharmacol Sci 2004 Feb;94(2):185-91.
3. *Guo Wai Yi Xue Zhong Yi Zhong Yao Fen Ce* (Monograph of Chinese Herbology from Foreign Medicine) 1993;15(2):31.
4. Li P, Fujio S. Effects of chai ling tang on proteinuria in rat models. J Tradit Chin Med 1995 Mar;15(1):48-52.
5. *Guo Wai Yi Xue Zhong Yi Zhong Yao Fen Ce* (Monograph of Chinese Herbology from Foreign Medicine) 1991;3:168.
6. *Guo Wai Yi Xue Zhong Yi Zhong Yao Fen Ce* (Monograph of Chinese Herbology from Foreign Medicine) 1991;13(6):31.
7. *Guo Wai Yi Xue Zhong Yi Zhong Yao Fen Ce* (Monograph of Chinese Herbology from Foreign Medicine) 1989;11(6):18.
8. *Guo Wai Yi Xue Zhong Yi Zhong Yao Fen Ce* (Monograph of Chinese Herbology from Foreign Medicine) 1990;(5):247.
9. Kimura K, Nanba S, Tojo A, Matsuoka H, Sugimoto T. Effects of sairei-to on the relapse of steroid-dependent nephrotic syndrome. Am J Chin Med 1990;18(1-2):45-50.
10. Liu XY. Therapeutic effect of chai-ling-tang (sairei-to) on the steroid-dependent nephrotic syndrome in children. American Journal of Chinese Medicine 1995;23(3-4):255-60.
11. Yoshikawa N, Ito H, Takekoshi Y, Honda M, Awazu M, Iijima K, Nakamura H, Seino Y, Takeda N, Hattori S, Matsuda I. Standard versus long-term prednisolone with sairei-to for initial therapy in childhood steroid-responsive nephrotic syndrome: a prospective controlled study. Nippon Jinzo Gakkai Shi 1998 Nov;40(8):587-90.
12. *Guo Wai Yi Xue Zhong Yi Zhong Yao Fen Ce* (Monograph of Chinese Herbology from Foreign Medicine) 1994;16(5):25.
13. *Guo Wai Yi Xue Zhong Yi Zhong Yao Fen Ce* (Monograph of Chinese Herbology from Foreign Medicine) 1994;16(5):25.
14. *Guo Wai Yi Xue Zhong Yi Zhong Yao Fen Ce* (Monograph of Chinese Herbology from Foreign Medicine) 1994;16(4):25.
15. *Guo Wai Yi Xue Zhong Yi Zhong Yao Fen Ce* (Monograph of Chinese Herbology from Foreign Medicine) 1993;15(4):22.
16. *Guo Wai Yi Xue Zhong Yi Zhong Yao Fen Ce* (Monograph of Chinese Herbology from Foreign Medicine) 1989;(5):285.
17. Takakuwa K. Yasuda M. Hataya I. Sekizuka N. Tamura M. Arakawa M. Higashino M. Hasegawa I. Tanaka K. Treatment for patients with recurrent abortion with positive antiphospholipid antibodies using a traditional Chinese herbal medicine. Journal of Perinatal Medicine 1996;24(5):489-94.
18. Fujii T, Kanai T, Kozuma S, Hamai Y, Hyodo H, Yamashita T, Miki A, Unno N, Taketani Y. Theoretical basis for herbal medicines, Tokishakuyaku-san and Sairei-to, in the treatment of autoimmunity-related recurrent abortion by correcting T helper-1/T helper-2 balance. American Journal of Reproductive Immunology 2000 Dec;44(6):342-6.
19. Fujii T. Herbal factors in the treatment of autoimmunity-related habitual abortion. Vitam Horm 2002;65:333-44.
20. Sakai A. Kondo Z. Kamei K. Izumi S. Sumi K. Induction of ovulation by Sairei-to for polycystic ovary syndrome patients. Endocrine Journal 1999 Feb;46(1):217-20.
21. Takahashi K. Uejima E. Morisaki T. Takahashi K. Kurokawa N. Azuma J. In vitro inhibitory effects of Kampo medicines on metabolic reactions catalyzed by human liver microsomes. Journal of Clinical Pharmacy & Therapeutics 2003 Aug;28(4):319-27.
22. Hasegawa T, Yamaki K, Nadai M, Muraoka I, Wang L, Takagi K, Nabeshima T. Lack of effect of Chinese medicines on bioavailability of ofloxacin in healthy volunteers. Int J Clin Pharmacol Ther 1994 Feb;32(2):57-61.

Chapter 3 – Harmonizing Formulas   *Section 1 – Shaoyang Harmonizing Formulas*

Chái Xiàn Tāng (Bupleurum Decoction to Raise the Sunken)

柴陷湯
柴陷汤

Pinyin Name: *Chai Xian Tang*
Literal Name: Bupleurum Decoction to Raise the Sunken
Alternate Names: *Tsai Hsien Tang, Cai Xian Tang*, Bupleurum Chest Bind Decoction, Bupleurum and Scute Combination
Original Source: *Shen Shi Zun Sheng Shu* (Master Shen's Book for Revering Life) by Shen Jin-Ao in 1773

COMPOSITION

Ban Xia (Rhizoma Pinelliae)
Sheng Jiang (Rhizoma Zingiberis Recens)
Huang Lian (Rhizoma Coptidis)
Huang Qin (Radix Scutellariae)
Chai Hu (Radix Bupleuri)
Gua Lou Zi (Semen Trichosanthis)
Ren Shen (Radix et Rhizoma Ginseng)
Gan Cao (Radix et Rhizoma Glycyrrhizae)
Da Zao (Fructus Jujubae)

DOSAGE / PREPARATION / ADMINISTRATION

Chai Xian Tang is formulated by combining two formulas: *Xiao Chai Hu Tang* (Minor Bupleurum Decoction) and *Xiao Xian Xiong Tang* (Minor Sinking into the Chest Decoction). Please refer to these two formulas for additional information.

CHINESE THERAPEUTIC ACTIONS

1. Harmonizes the exterior and interior to relieve *shaoyang* syndrome
2. Eliminates phlegm stagnation
3. Regulates qi circulation in the chest

CLINICAL MANIFESTATIONS

Shaoyang syndrome with phlegm stagnation: alternating spells of chills and fever, a bitter taste in the mouth, a feeling of fullness and oppression in the chest and hypochondriac region, chest pain with coughing or deep inhalation, thick and sticky phlegm that is difficult to expectorate, accelerated respiration, poor appetite, and a yellow tongue coating.

CLINICAL APPLICATIONS

Common cold and influenza, bronchitis, bronchial asthma, pneumonia, pleurisy, hepatitis, cholecystitis, and cholelithiasis.

EXPLANATION

Chai Xian Tang (Bupleurum Decoction to Raise the Sunken) treats *shaoyang* syndrome that is complicated by phlegm stagnation. Clinically, *shaoyang* syndrome is characterized by alternating spells of chills and fever, a bitter taste in the mouth, and a feeling of fullness and oppression in the chest and hypochondriac region. Phlegm stagnation is characterized by chest pain with

Chai Xian Tang (Bupleurum Decoction to Raise the Sunken)

Diagnosis	Signs and Symptoms	Treatment	Herbs
Shaoyang syndrome with phlegm stagnation	• Alternating spells of chills and fever, a bitter taste in the mouth, and fullness and oppression in the chest and hypochondriac region: *shaoyang* syndrome • Chest pain with coughing or deep inhalation, thick and sticky phlegm that is difficult to expectorate, accelerated respiration, and poor appetite: phlegm stagnation • Yellow tongue coating: internal heat	• Harmonizes the exterior and interior to relieve *shaoyang* syndrome • Eliminates phlegm stagnation • Regulates qi circulation in the chest	• *Xiao Chai Hu Tang* (Minor Bupleurum Decoction) treats *shaoyang* syndrome by harmonizing the exterior and interior. • *Xiao Xian Xiong Tang* (Minor Sinking into the Chest Decoction) dissolves phlegm, clears heat, and disperses stagnation.

226

Chái Xiàn Tāng (Bupleurum Decoction to Raise the Sunken)

coughing or deep inhalation, thick and sticky phlegm that is difficult to expectorate, accelerated respiration, and poor appetite. A yellow tongue coating indicates internal heat.

Chai Xian Tang is formulated by combining two formulas: *Xiao Chai Hu Tang* (Minor Bupleurum Decoction), which treats *shaoyang* syndrome by harmonizing the exterior and interior; and *Xiao Xian Xiong Tang* (Minor Sinking into the Chest Decoction) which dissolves phlegm, clears heat, and disperses stagnation.

Please refer to *Xiao Chai Hu Tang* (Minor Bupleurum Decoction) and *Xiao Xian Xiong Tang* (Minor Sinking into the Chest Decoction) for additional information on these two formulas.

MODIFICATIONS

- For increased phlegm, cough, and hypochondriac pain, add *Zhi Shi* (Fructus Aurantii Immaturus) and *Jie Geng* (Radix Platycodonis).
- With vomiting and chest pain, add *Zhu Ru* (Caulis Bambusae in Taenia) and *Chen Pi* (Pericarpium Citri Reticulatae).
- With palpitations, chest pain, and tightness in the lungs, combine with *Zhi Gan Cao Tang* (Honey-Fried Licorice Decoction).
- With sputum and cough with pain, add *Zhi Qiao* (Fructus Aurantii) and *Jie Geng* (Radix Platycodonis).
- With thirst and a sore throat, add *Shi Gao* (Gypsum Fibrosum) and *Zhi Mu* (Rhizoma Anemarrhenae).
- When there is excessive phlegm and pain during coughing, combine with *Wen Dan Tang* (Warm the Gallbladder Decoction).
- For stomatitis, oral sores, and sore throat, combine with *Qing Xin Li Ge Tang* (Clear the Epigastrium and Benefit the Diaphragm Decoction).

Hāo Qín Qīng Dǎn Tāng
(Artemisia Annua and Scutellaria Decoction to Clear the Gallbladder)

蒿芩清膽湯
蒿芩清胆汤

Pinyin Name: *Hao Qin Qing Dan Tang*
Literal Name: Artemisia Annua and Scutellaria Decoction to Clear the Gallbladder
Original Source: *Chong Ding Tong Su Shang Han Lun* (Revised Popular Guide to the Discussion of Cold-Induced Disorders) by Yu Gen-Chu in the Qing Dynasty

COMPOSITION

Qing Hao (Herba Artemisiae Annuae)	4.5-6g
Huang Qin (Radix Scutellariae)	4.5-9g
Zhu Ru (Caulis Bambusae in Taenia)	9g
Ban Xia (Rhizoma Pinelliae)	4.5g
Zhi Qiao (Fructus Aurantii)	4.5g
Chen Pi (Pericarpium Citri Reticulatae)	4.5g
Chi Fu Ling (Poria Rubra)	9g
Bi Yu San (Jasper Powder)	9g

DOSAGE / PREPARATION / ADMINISTRATION

Prepare the ingredients as a decoction. Note: *Bi Yu San* (Jasper Powder) is an herbal formula that contains *Hua Shi* (Talcum), *Gan Cao* (Radix et Rhizoma Glycyrrhizae), and *Qing Dai* (Indigo Naturalis). Please refer to *Liu Yi San* (Six-to-One Powder) under the Related Formula(s) section for additional information.

CHINESE THERAPEUTIC ACTIONS

1. Clears Gallbladder heat and dispels dampness
2. Harmonizes the Stomach and dissolves phlegm

CLINICAL MANIFESTATIONS

Gallbladder damp-heat: alternating spells of chills and fever (with fever being more prominent than chills), a

Hāo Qín Qīng Dǎn Tāng
(Artemisia Annua and Scutellaria Decoction to Clear the Gallbladder)

bitter taste in the mouth, dry heaves, hiccups; a stifling sensation in the chest, chest and hypochondriac pain and distention; regurgitation of yellow and sticky fluids that are bitter or sour in taste; a red tongue body with thick, white or yellowish tongue coating; and a slippery, rapid pulse on the right hand and a wiry, rapid pulse on the left hand.

CLINICAL APPLICATIONS
Cholelithiasis, gastritis, and fever.

EXPLANATION
Hao Qin Qing Dan Tang (Artemisia Annua and Scutellaria Decoction to Clear the Gallbladder) treats damp-heat in the Gallbladder and reversed flow of Stomach qi. Damp-heat in the Gallbladder causes alternating spells of fever and chills because the Gallbladder is a *shaoyang* organ, located between the exterior and the interior. Chest fullness and hypochondriac pain and distention arise as a result of heat in the Gallbladder and Liver channels; these channels travel through the chest and hypochondriac region. Because the wood element (Liver and Gallbladder) acts on the earth element (Spleen and Stomach), excess in the Gallbladder can negatively affect the Stomach, causing reversed flow of Stomach qi and damp obstruction, which manifest in dry heaves, nausea, hiccups, and regurgitation of yellow and sticky fluids that are bitter and sour in taste. A rapid pulse indicates heat. A slippery pulse on the right indicates damp obstruction produced by the Spleen,

while a wiry pulse on the left indicates qi stagnation in the Gallbladder.

Qing Hao (Herba Artemisiae Annuae) penetrates and clears heat in the *shaoyang* level. *Huang Qin* (Radix Scutellariae) purges and sedates heat in the Gallbladder. *Zhu Ru* (Caulis Bambusae in Taenia) clears heat and resolves phlegm. *Ban Xia* (Rhizoma Pinelliae) dries dampness and eliminates phlegm. *Zhi Qiao* (Fructus Aurantii) and *Chen Pi* (Pericarpium Citri Reticulatae) activate qi flow, expand the chest, and harmonize and regulate Stomach qi. *Chi Fu Ling* (Poria Rubra) and *Hua Shi* (Talcum) drain damp-heat out of the body through urination. *Qing Dai* (Indigo Naturalis) eliminates phlegm and interior heat. *Gan Cao* (Radix et Rhizoma Glycyrrhizae) harmonizes the Stomach and the formula.

MODIFICATIONS
- For tinnitus or diminished hearing from damp-heat accumulation, add *Shi Chang Pu* (Rhizoma Acori Tatarinowii), *Gou Teng* (Ramulus Uncariae cum Uncis), *Ju Hua* (Flos Chrysanthemi), and *Tong Cao* (Medulla Tetrapanacis).
- If there is excess vomiting, add *Zuo Jin Wan* (Left Metal Pill).
- With body aches and pains, add *Sang Zhi* (Ramulus Mori), *Yi Yi Ren* (Semen Coicis), and *Si Gua Luo* (Retinervus Luffae Fructus).
- For damp-heat jaundice, remove *Ban Xia* (Rhizoma Pinelliae) and *Chen Pi* (Pericarpium Citri Reticulatae);

Hao Qin Qing Dan Tang (Artemisia Annua and Scutellaria Decoction to Clear the Gallbladder)

Diagnosis	Signs and Symptoms	Treatment	Herbs
Gallbladder damp-heat	• Alternating spells of fever and chills: *shaoyang* level • A bitter taste in the mouth with chest fullness and hypochondriac pain and distention: heat in the Gallbladder and Liver channels • Dry heaves, nausea, hiccups, and regurgitation of fluids: reversed flow of Stomach qi • Red tongue body with a thick, white or yellowish tongue coating: heat condition • Slippery, rapid pulse on the right hand: damp obstruction • Wiry, rapid pulse on the left hand: qi stagnation	• Clears Gallbladder heat and dispels dampness • Harmonizes the Stomach and dissolves phlegm	• *Qing Hao* (Herba Artemisiae Annuae) penetrates and clears heat in the *shaoyang* level. • *Huang Qin* (Radix Scutellariae) purges and sedates heat in the Gallbladder. • *Zhu Ru* (Caulis Bambusae in Taenia) and *Ban Xia* (Rhizoma Pinelliae) clear heat, eliminate dampness and phlegm, and redirect Stomach qi downward. • *Zhi Qiao* (Fructus Aurantii) and *Chen Pi* (Pericarpium Citri Reticulatae) activate qi flow, expand the chest, and regulate Stomach qi. • *Chi Fu Ling* (Poria Rubra) and *Hua Shi* (Talcum) drain damp-heat out of the body through urination. • *Qing Dai* (Indigo Naturalis) eliminates phlegm and interior heat. • *Gan Cao* (Radix et Rhizoma Glycyrrhizae) harmonizes the Stomach and the formula.

Chinese Herbal Formulas and Applications

Hāo Qín Qīng Dǎn Tāng
(Artemisia Annua and Scutellaria Decoction to Clear the Gallbladder)

and add *Yin Chen* (Herba Artemisiae Scopariae) and *Zhi Zi* (Fructus Gardeniae).

- With dizziness and vertigo due to phlegm accumulation, add *Tian Ma* (Rhizoma Gastrodiae).
- With insomnia and palpitations, add *Hu Po* (Succinum) and *Huang Lian* (Rhizoma Coptidis).
- If there is coughing with yellow sputum, add *Yu Xing Cao* (Herba Houttuyniae), *Dong Gua Zi* (Semen Benincasae), and *Gua Lou Zi* (Semen Trichosanthis).
- For *lin zheng* (dysuria syndrome), add *Che Qian Zi* (Semen Plantaginis), *Mu Tong* (Caulis Akebiae), and *Ze Xie* (Rhizoma Alismatis).

CAUTIONS / CONTRAINDICATIONS

Avoid pungent, spicy, oily, or greasy foods while taking *Hao Qin Qing Dan Tang*.[1]

CLINICAL STUDIES AND RESEARCH

1. **Cholelithiasis**: Use of modified *Hao Qin Qing Dan Tang* demonstrated a success rate of 85% in eliminating gallstones. Of 60 cases involving gallstones, the study reported elimination of all stones in 46 cases, partial elimination of stones in 5 cases, no benefit in 5 cases, and surgical intervention in 4 cases. The herbal treatment contained this formula plus *Chai Hu* (Radix Bupleuri) for Liver qi stagnation; *Da Huang* (Radix et Rhizoma Rhei) for dry stools and constipation; and *Long Dan* (Radix et Rhizoma Gentianae), *Che Qian Zi* (Semen Plantaginis), and *Yin Chen* (Herba Artemisiae Scopariae) for severe jaundice. The duration of treatment ranged from 7 to 30 days of therapy.[2]

2. **Gastritis**: Good results were reported using modified *Hao Qin Qing Dan Tang* to treat gastritis caused by regurgitation of bile. In addition to this formula, modifications included the addition of *Chuan Lian Zi* (Fructus Toosendan) and *Wu Zhu Yu* (Fructus Evodiae) for severe pain; *Xiang Fu* (Rhizoma Cyperi) and *Zi Su Geng* (Caulis Perillae) for upper abdominal distention and pain; *Huang Lian* (Rhizoma Coptidis) and *Zhe Shi* (Haematitum) for increased acidity of the stomach; and other adjustments when deemed necessary. Of 52 cases, the study reported significant improvement in 43 cases and moderate improvement in 9 cases.[3]

3. **Fever**: Use of *Hao Qin Qing Dan Tang* was associated with 95% effectiveness in treating 100 patients with fever caused by an external infection. Clinical presentations included acute onset of fever (body temperature of 38.5°C / 101.3°F or higher), elevated body temperature especially in the evening and at night with or without perspiration; chills, sore throat, a dry mouth, a bitter taste in the mouth, cough, dysuria, a red tongue body with a thin, greasy white or yellow tongue coating, and a rapid pulse. The herbal treatment contained *Hao Qin Qing Dan Tang* plus *Bo He* (Herba Menthae) and *Ge Gen* (Radix Puerariae Lobatae). Of 100 cases, the study reported complete recovery in 37 cases, significant improvement in 58 cases, and no effect in 5 cases.[4] Another study reported 96.3% effectiveness using modified *Hao Qin Qing Dan Tang* to treat fever in 54 patients. Modifications included the addition of *Chai Hu* (Radix Bupleuri) for alternating spells of chills and fever; *Cang Zhu* (Rhizoma Atractylodis) and *Hou Po* (Cortex Magnoliae Officinalis) for chest fullness and distention; *Jie Geng* (Radix Platycodonis) for redness, swelling, and pain in the throat; and *Yu Jin* (Radix Curcumae) for a feeling of heaviness in the head.[5]

AUTHORS' COMMENTS

Hao Qin Qing Dan Tang is a commonly used formula for treating damp-heat with turbidity attacking the *shaoyang* level. This formula is indicated in the following conditions: jaundice with *lin zheng* (dysuria syndrome), vomiting caused by disharmony of the Liver and Stomach with turbidity in the Stomach, and dizziness and vertigo caused by phlegm obstruction.

Xiao Chai Hu Tang (Minor Bupleurum Decoction) and *Hao Qin Qing Dan Tang* both harmonize *shaoyang* syndrome, but have important differences:

- *Xiao Chai Hu Tang* harmonizes *shaoyang* syndrome that is caused initially by wind-cold invading the *taiyang* level, which then turns into heat, and moves deeper into the *shaoyang* level. The chief herb, *Chai Hu* (Radix Bupleuri), is an acrid, bitter, and cold herb that releases the exterior, lifts the clear yang, and disperses wind and heat.
- *Hao Qin Qing Dan Tang* harmonizes *shaoyang* syndrome that is caused by damp-heat invading the Gallbladder channel. The chief herb, *Qing Hao* (Herba Artemisiae Annuae), an acrid, bitter, and cold herb, works with other herbs to clear damp-heat from the *shaoyang*.

References

1. *Zhong Yao Ming Fang Yao Li Yu Ying Yong* (Pharmacology and Applications of Famous Herbal Formulas) 1989;92-96.
2. *Chang Chun Zhong Yi Xue Yuan Xue Bao* (Journal of Changchun University of Chinese Medicine) 1998;1:29.
3. *Si Chuan Zhong Yi* (Sichuan Chinese Medicine) 1996;6:28.
4. *Zhong Yi Ming Fang Lin Chuang Xin Yong* (Contemporary Clinical Applications of Classic Chinese Formulas) 2001;705.
5. *Shan Xi Zhong Yi* (Shanxi Chinese Medicine) 1999;2:81.

Chái Hú Dá Yuán Yǐn
(Bupleurum Decoction to Reach the Membrane Source)

柴胡達原飲
柴胡达原饮

Pinyin Name: *Chai Hu Da Yuan Yin*
Literal Name: Bupleurum Decoction to Reach the Membrane Source
Original Source: *Chong Ding Tong Su Shang Han Lun* (Revised Popular Guide to the Discussion of Cold-Induced Disorders) by Yu Gen-Chu in the Qing Dynasty

COMPOSITION

Chai Hu (Radix Bupleuri)	4.5g
Huang Qin (Radix Scutellariae)	4.5g
Zhi Qiao (Fructus Aurantii)	4.5g
Jie Geng (Radix Platycodonis)	3g
Hou Po (Cortex Magnoliae Officinalis)	4.5g
Cao Guo (Fructus Tsaoko)	1.8g
Qing Pi (Pericarpium Citri Reticulatae Viride)	4.5g
Bing Lang (Semen Arecae)	6g
He Ye Geng (Folium et Caulis Nelumbinis)	5 *cun* [9-15g]
Zhi Gan Cao (Radix et Rhizoma Glycyrrhizae Praeparata cum Melle)	2.1g

DOSAGE / PREPARATION / ADMINISTRATION

Prepare the ingredients as a decoction. Note: *Cun* is a Chinese measurement of length that is approximately equivalent to an inch. Today, the suggested dose of *He Ye Geng* (Folium et Caulis Nelumbinis) is between 9-15g.

CHINESE THERAPEUTIC ACTIONS

1. Dispels dampness and dissolves phlegm
2. Reaches and vents the *mo yuan* (membrane source)

CLINICAL MANIFESTATIONS

Damp and phlegm obstruction at the *mo yuan* (membrane source): a feeling of distention and fullness in the chest and diaphragm, irritability, heartburn, dizziness, a pasty sensation in the mouth, cough with sputum that is difficult to expectorate, intermittent fever and chills, a thick and greasy tongue coating, and a wiry, slippery pulse.

CLINICAL APPLICATIONS

Malaria

EXPLANATION

Chai Hu Da Yuan Yin (Bupleurum Decoction to Reach the Membrane Source) treats damp and phlegm obstruction at the *mo yuan* (membrane source). In traditional Chinese medicine, *mo yuan* (membrane source), situated midway

between the exterior and the interior of the body, is the doorway to the *San Jiao*. As dampness from the exterior enters the body through the nose and mouth, it settles and accumulates in the *mo yuan* to form phlegm. Damp and phlegm accumulation at the *mo yuan* causes disharmony between the exterior and interior, and obstructs the *San Jiao* qi flow, eventually producing symptoms such as a feeling of distention and fullness in the chest and diaphragm, irritability, heartburn, and dizziness. A greasy tongue coating and a slippery pulse are indications of dampness and phlegm.

Chai Hu (Radix Bupleuri) treats the exterior-interior nature of this condition. *Huang Qin* (Radix Scutellariae) clears damp-heat. Together, this pair of herbs treat the *shaoyang* syndrome of exterior and interior. *Zhi Qiao* (Fructus Aurantii) and *Jie Geng* (Radix Platycodonis) regulate qi in the upper *jiao*. *Hou Po* (Cortex Magnoliae Officinalis) and *Cao Guo* (Fructus Tsaoko) regulate qi in the middle *jiao*. *Qing Pi* (Pericarpium Citri Reticulatae Viride) and *Bing Lang* (Semen Arecae) regulate qi in the lower *jiao*. Together, these three pairs of herbs effectively regulate qi in the upper, middle, and lower *jiaos* to treat *San Jiao* disorders. *He Ye Geng* (Folium et Caulis Nelumbinis) regulates qi and relieves distention and fullness in the chest. *Zhi Gan Cao* (Radix et Rhizoma Glycyrrhizae Praeparata cum Melle) harmonizes the formula.

Chinese Herbal Formulas and Applications

Chái Hú Dá Yuán Yǐn
(Bupleurum Decoction to Reach the Membrane Source)

Chai Hu Da Yuan Yin (Bupleurum Decoction to Reach the Membrane Source)

Diagnosis	Signs and Symptoms	Treatment	Herbs
Obstruction of dampness and phlegm at the *mo yuan* (membrane source)	• Intermittent fever and chills, a feeling of distention and fullness in the chest and diaphragm, irritability, heartburn, and dizziness: damp and phlegm accumulation at the *mo yuan* • Greasy tongue coating and a slippery pulse: damp and phlegm accumulation	• Dispels dampness and dissolves phlegm • Reaches and vents the *mo yuan*	• *Chai Hu* (Radix Bupleuri) releases the exterior and *Huang Qin* (Radix Scutellariae) clears damp-heat from the interior. • *Zhi Qiao* (Fructus Aurantii) and *Jie Geng* (Radix Platycodonis) regulate qi in the upper *jiao*. • *Hou Po* (Cortex Magnoliae Officinalis) and *Cao Guo* (Fructus Tsaoko) regulate qi in the middle *jiao*. • *Qing Pi* (Pericarpium Citri Reticulatae Viride) and *Bing Lang* (Semen Arecae) regulate qi in the lower *jiao*. • *He Ye Geng* (Folium et Caulis Nelumbinis) regulates qi and relieves distention and fullness in the chest. • *Zhi Gan Cao* (Radix et Rhizoma Glycyrrhizae Praeparata cum Melle) harmonizes the formula.

RELATED FORMULAS

Dá Yuán Yǐn (Reach the Membrane Source Decoction)

達原飲
达原饮

Pinyin Name: *Da Yuan Yin*
Literal Name: Reach the Membrane Source Decoction
Original Source: *Wen Yi Lun* (Discussion of Epidemic Warm Disease) by Wu You-Xing in 1642

Bing Lang (Semen Arecae)	6g
Hou Po (Cortex Magnoliae Officinalis)	3g
Cao Guo (Fructus Tsaoko)	1.5g
Zhi Mu (Rhizoma Anemarrhenae)	3g
Bai Shao (Radix Paeoniae Alba)	3g
Huang Qin (Radix Scutellariae)	3g
Gan Cao (Radix et Rhizoma Glycyrrhizae)	1.5g

The source text states to cook the ingredients in 2 large bowls of water until 80% of the liquid remains. Take the warm decoction in the afternoon.

Da Yuan Yin (Reach the Membrane Source Decoction) vents the *mo yuan* (membrane source) and eliminates dampness and turbidity. The main indications include malaria and febrile disorders with pathogenic factors affecting the *mo yuan,* causing such symptoms as unpredictable patterns of alternating fever and chills (once every one to three days), chest oppression, nausea, vomiting, headache, irritability, restlessness, a wiry, rapid pulse, and a greasy tongue coating.

Qīng Pí Yǐn (Clear the Spleen Decoction)

清脾飲
请脾饮

Pinyin Name: *Qing Pi Yin*
Literal Name: Clear the Spleen Decoction
Alternate Name: *Qing Pi Tang*
Original Source: *Ji Sheng Fang* (Formulas to Aid the Living) by Yan Yong-He in 1253

Qing Pi (Pericarpium Citri Reticulatae Viride)
Hou Po (Cortex Magnoliae Officinalis),
    chao (dry-fried) and *zhi* (frying) with ginger juice
Bai Zhu (Rhizoma Atractylodis Macrocephalae)
Cao Guo (Fructus Tsaoko)
Chai Hu (Radix Bupleuri)
Fu Ling (Poria)
Huang Qin (Radix Scutellariae)
Ban Xia (Rhizoma Pinelliae),
    pao (blast-fried) in liquid 7 times
Zhi Gan Cao (Radix et Rhizoma
    Glycyrrhizae Praeparata cum Melle)

The source text specifies to coarsely grind equal amounts of the ingredients and cook 12g of the coarse powder with 5 slices of *Sheng Jiang* (Rhizoma Zingiberis Recens) in 1.5 bowls of water until 70% of the liquid remains. Take the strained decoction while warm.

Qing Pi Yin (Clear the Spleen Decoction) dries dampness, dissolves phlegm, purges heat, and clears the Spleen.

231

Chái Hú Dá Yuán Yǐn
(Bupleurum Decoction to Reach the Membrane Source)

Clinically, it treats malaria characterized by alternating spells of fever and chills (more fever and less chills), a bitter taste in the mouth, loss of appetite, dysuria, and a wiry, rapid pulse. This formula is called "Clear the Spleen Decoction," because it treats the cause of the illness, which is the inability of the Spleen to dry dampness and dissolve phlegm. As a result, dampness and phlegm obstruct the *mo yuan* (membrane source), eventually causing malaria with more fever than chills.

AUTHORS' COMMENTS

Hao Qin Qing Dan Tang (Artemisia Annua and Scutellaria Decoction to Clear the Gallbladder) and *Chai Hu Da Yuan Yin* both treat *shaoyang* conditions with alternating fever and chills.

- *Hao Qin Qing Dan Tang* is more appropriate for dampness and heat affecting the Gallbladder and Stomach, with heat being more prominent than dampness.
- *Chai Hu Da Yuan Yin* is more suitable for situations in which there is obstruction of dampness and phlegm at the *mo yuan* (membrane source), with dampness being more prominent than heat.

Chinese Herbal Formulas and Applications

Section 2

调和肝脾剂
— Liver and Spleen Harmonizing Formulas

Si Ni Săn (Frigid Extremities Powder)
四逆散

Pinyin Name: *Si Ni San*
Literal Name: Frigid Extremities Powder
Alternate Names: *Su Ni San*, Counterflow Cold Formula, Cold Limbs Powder, Bupleurum and Chih-shih Formula
Original Source: *Shang Han Lun* (Discussion of Cold-Induced Disorders) by Zhang Zhong-Jing in the Eastern Han Dynasty

COMPOSITION

Chai Hu (Radix Bupleuri)	[6g]
Zhi Shi (Fructus Aurantii Immaturus), *po* (opened) and *zhi* (fried with liquid)	[6g]
Bai Shao (Radix Paeoniae Alba)	[6g]
Zhi Gan Cao (Radix et Rhizoma Glycyrrhizae Praeparata cum Melle)	[6g]

DOSAGE / PREPARATION / ADMINISTRATION

The source text states to grind equal amounts of the ingredients into powder and sift evenly. Take one large spoonful of the powder (6-9g) with boiled water three times daily. Today, this formula may be prepared as a decoction with the doses suggested in brackets.

CHINESE THERAPEUTIC ACTIONS

1. Ventilates the pathogens outward and relieves constraint
2. Spreads Liver qi and harmonizes the Liver and Spleen

CLINICAL MANIFESTATIONS

1. *Shaoyin* syndrome with frigid extremities: cold hands and feet, a slight sensation of warmth in the body, dysuria, abdominal pain, diarrhea, and rectal tenesmus.
2. Disharmony of the Liver and Spleen: hypochondriac fullness and distention, epigastric and abdominal pain, and a wiry pulse.

CLINICAL APPLICATIONS

Syncope, hepatitis, cholecystitis, cholelithiasis, cirrhosis, biliary ascariasis, pancreatitis, superficial gastritis, acute and chronic gastritis, gastric neuralgia, peptic ulcer disease, epigastric pain, ulcerative colitis, intestinal obstruction, infertility, adnexitis, acute appendicitis, intercostal neuralgia, impotence, and hernia.

EXPLANATION

Si Ni San (Frigid Extremities Powder) treats *shaoyin* syndrome characterized by cold hands and feet. This condition begins with the progression of an exterior pathogenic factor from the *shaoyang* level into the more interior *shaoyin* level. As the disease migrates toward the interior, it blocks the circulation of Liver and Gallbladder qi to the extremities, resulting in coldness below the elbows and knees. In other words, the cold extremities in this case result from blocked circulation of qi, and not from yang deficiency. Also, the pulse is wiry and not weak, another indication that the condition is caused by qi stagnation and not by yang deficiency.

This formula also treats disharmony of the Liver and Spleen, with symptoms including hypochondriac fullness and distention, epigastric and abdominal pain, and a bitter taste in the mouth. Since the flow of Liver and Gallbladder qi to the exterior is blocked, it counterflows and overacts on the Spleen and Stomach, resulting in abdominal pain, diarrhea, and lack of appetite. Other symptoms and applications include breast distention, a short temper, irregular menstruation, and premenstrual syndrome.

To treat this syndrome, qi must be lifted and extended outward; the Liver and Spleen must also be harmonized and stagnant Liver qi smoothed. *Chai Hu* (Radix Bupleuri)

233

Chapter 3 – Harmonizing Formulas   *Section 2 – Liver and Spleen Harmonizing Formulas*

Si Ni Săn (Frigid Extremities Powder)

Si Ni San (Frigid Extremities Powder)

Diagnosis	Signs and Symptoms	Treatment	Herbs
Shaoyin syndrome characterized by frigid extremities	• Cold hands and feet: blocked qi circulation to the extremities • Hypochondriac fullness and distention and epigastric and abdominal pain: Liver and Spleen disharmony • Wiry pulse: excess condition	• Ventilates the pathogens outward and relieves constraint • Spreads Liver qi and harmonizes the Liver and Spleen	• *Chai Hu* (Radix Bupleuri) harmonizes the Liver and relieves Liver qi stagnation. • *Zhi Shi* (Fructus Aurantii Immaturus) activates qi and breaks up qi stagnation. • *Bai Shao* (Radix Paeoniae Alba) nourishes Liver blood and softens the Liver. • *Zhi Gan Cao* (Radix et Rhizoma Glycyrrhizae Praeparata cum Melle) tonifies qi and strengthens the middle *jiao*.

harmonizes and spreads the Liver and relieves Liver qi stagnation. *Zhi Shi* (Fructus Aurantii Immaturus) activates qi and breaks up qi stagnation. The lifting tendency of *Chai Hu* (Radix Bupleuri), coupled with the downward-directing action of *Zhi Shi* (Fructus Aurantii Immaturus), further facilitates the flow of qi to the extremities. *Bai Shao* (Radix Paeoniae Alba) nourishes Liver blood and softens the Liver. It helps *Zhi Shi* (Fructus Aurantii Immaturus) relieve pain in the hypochondriac area and treats other Liver qi stagnation symptoms. *Bai Shao* (Radix Paeoniae Alba) also prevents the drying nature of *Chai Hu* (Radix Bupleuri) from damaging yin. *Zhi Gan Cao* (Radix et Rhizoma Glycyrrhizae Praeparata cum Melle) tonifies qi and strengthens the middle *jiao*. It also harmonizes the formula and relieves gastrointestinal complaints arising when the Liver overacts on the Spleen and Stomach. Combined, these herbs lift the qi, smooth Liver qi, and restore the normal functioning of the Spleen.

Si Ni San is the basic formula for treating Liver qi stagnation. The cold extremities in this case do not suggest a cold syndrome, but rather constraint and stagnation of qi. In fact, if a patient with this condition is not treated in time, interior heat is likely to result.

MODIFICATIONS
• With severe Liver qi stagnation, add *Xiang Fu* (Rhizoma Cyperi) and *Yu Jin* (Radix Curcumae).
• If there is dysuria, add *Fu Ling* (Poria).
• If there is oliguria, add *Mu Tong* (Caulis Akebiae) and *Di Huang* (Radix Rehmanniae).
• With abdominal pain due to cold, add *Fu Zi* (Radix Aconiti Lateralis Praeparata).
• With acid regurgitation, add *Zuo Jin Wan* (Left Metal Pill).
• With nausea and vomiting, add *Huang Lian* (Rhizoma Coptidis) and *Sheng Jiang* (Rhizoma Zingiberis Recens).

• With diarrhea with tenesmus, add *Tong Xie Yao Fang* (Important Formula for Painful Diarrhea).
• With constipation, add *Da Huang* (Radix et Rhizoma Rhei) and *Mang Xiao* (Natrii Sulfas).
• When there is heat accumulation, add *Zhi Zi* (Fructus Gardeniae) and *Chuan Lian Zi* (Fructus Toosendan); or *Chai Hu Qing Gan Tang* (Bupleurum Decoction to Clear the Liver).
• With food stagnation or indigestion, add *Mai Ya* (Fructus Hordei Germinatus) and *Ji Nei Jin* (Endothelium Corneum Gigeriae Galli); or *Bao He Wan* (Preserve Harmony Pill).
• If there is Spleen deficiency, add *Dang Shen* (Radix Codonopsis) and *Bai Zhu* (Rhizoma Atractylodis Macrocephalae).
• If accompanied by hypertension, add *Zhe Shi* (Haematitum), *Long Gu* (Os Draconis), *Mu Li* (Concha Ostreae), and *Huang Qin* (Radix Scutellariae).
• With palpitations, add *Gui Zhi* (Ramulus Cinnamomi).
• With dysmenorrhea, add *Xiang Fu* (Rhizoma Cyperi), *Yan Hu Suo* (Rhizoma Corydalis), and *Shi Xiao San* (Sudden Smile Powder).
• For hepatic disorders, add *Yin Chen* (Herba Artemisiae Scopariae), *Jin Qian Cao* (Herba Lysimachiae), *Yu Jin* (Radix Curcumae), and *Dan Shen* (Radix et Rhizoma Salviae Miltiorrhizae).

CAUTIONS / CONTRAINDICATIONS
Frigid extremities is a symptom that may have various causes. *Si Ni San* must **not** be used indiscriminately as a symptomatic treatment for frigid extremities. Instead, it should only be used for cold hands and feet caused by blocked qi circulation failing to warm the extremities.

PHARMACOLOGICAL EFFECTS
1. **Gastrointestinal**: Alcohol extract of *Si Ni San* demonstrated an inhibitory effect on the gastrointestinal system and decreased the production of gastric acid.[1]

234

Si Ni Săn (Frigid Extremities Powder)

2. **Cardiovascular**: Administration of 60 mL of water extract of *Si Ni San* was associated with increased blood perfusion to the brain in patients with atherosclerosis and poor peripheral blood circulation. The same treatment had little effect on normal and healthy individuals.[2]

3. **Cardiotonic**: Intravenous injection of *Si Ni San* in dogs was associated with positive inotropic effects, positive chronotropic effects, and increased blood pressure.[3]

4. **Anti-arrhythmic**: Administration of *Si Ni San* was effective against arrhythmia induced by aconitine, epinephrine, and calcium chloride in rats and rabbits.[4,5]

5. **Hepatoprotective**: Administration of *Si Ni San* was associated with marked hepatoprotective effects against many substances, such as carbon tetrachloride (CCl4), Bacillus Calmette-Guerin (BCG), and picryl chloride (PCl-DTH). *Si Ni San* provided protective effects against liver injury through multiple mechanisms, such as protection of the hepatocyte membrane, enhancement of nitric oxide release, and dysfunction of liver-infiltrating cells, mainly by causing their apoptosis.[6]

CLINICAL STUDIES AND RESEARCH

1. **Hepatitis**: Thirty-three patients with hepatitis were treated with modified *Si Ni San* with significant improvement in 29 patients and moderate improvement in 4 patients. The herbal treatment contained *Si Ni San* plus *Yan Hu Suo* (Rhizoma Corydalis) 10g, *Hou Po* (Cortex Magnoliae Officinalis) 10g, *Yu Jin* (Radix Curcumae) 7g, and *Dan Shen* (Radix et Rhizoma Salviae Miltiorrhizae) 12g as the base formula. *Yin Chen* (Herba Artemisiae Scopariae) and *Zhi Zi* (Fructus Gardeniae) were added for jaundice; *Da Huang* (Radix et Rhizoma Rhei) was added for constipation; *Bai Zhu* (Rhizoma Atractylodis Macrocephalae), *Fu Ling* (Poria) and *Yi Yi Ren* (Semen Coicis) were added for diarrhea; *Mai Ya* (Fructus Hordei Germinatus), *Shan Zha* (Fructus Crataegi), and *Chen Pi* (Pericarpium Citri Reticulatae) were added for poor appetite; *Di Gu Pi* (Cortex Lycii) and *Qing Hao* (Herba Artemisiae Annuae) were added for low-grade fever; *Bie Jia* (Carapax Trionycis), *Mu Li* (Concha Ostreae) and *Qing Pi* (Pericarpium Citri Reticulatae Viride) were added for enlargement of the liver or spleen; and *Dang Shen* (Radix Codonopsis) was added for constant fatigue.[7]

2. **Hypochondriac pain due to hepatitis**: Administration of *Si Ni San* plus *Jin Ling Zi San* (Melia Toosendan Powder) in 65 patients with hypochondriac pain due to hepatitis was associated with complete relief in 38 patients, improvement in 16 patients, and no benefit in 11 patients.[8]

3. **Liver cirrhosis**: Use of modified *Si Ni San* to treat liver cirrhosis had beneficial effects. The herbal treatment contained *Si Ni San* plus *Huang Qi* (Radix Astragali), *Dan Shen* (Radix et Rhizoma Salviae Miltiorrhizae), *Bie*

Jia (Carapax Trionycis) and others as the base formula. Strategies for modifications included the addition of *Xiang Fu* (Rhizoma Cyperi) and *Yan Hu Suo* (Rhizoma Corydalis) for Liver qi stagnation; *Yu Jin* (Radix Curcumae) and *Huang Qin* (Radix Scutellariae) for heat; *Di Huang* (Radix Rehmanniae) and *Gou Qi Zi* (Fructus Lycii) for yin deficiency; *Dang Gui* (Radix Angelicae Sinensis) and *E Zhu* (Rhizoma Curcumae) for blood stagnation; and addition of *Fu Ling* (Poria) and *Yi Yi Ren* (Semen Coicis), and elimination of *Bie Jia* (Carapax Trionycis) for Spleen deficiency.[9]

4. **Cholecystitis**: Complete recovery was reported in 78 of 84 patients with chronic cholecystitis when treated with *Si Ni San* plus *Chuan Lian Zi* (Fructus Toosendan) and *Mu Xiang* (Radix Aucklandiae) as the base formula. Modifications included the addition of *Yu Jin* (Radix Curcumae) and *Yan Hu Suo* (Rhizoma Corydalis) for qi stagnation; *Jin Qian Cao* (Herba Lysimachiae) and *Da Huang* (Radix et Rhizoma Rhei) for gallstones; and *Huang Qin* (Radix Scutellariae) and *Jin Yin Hua* (Flos Lonicerae Japonicae) for damp-heat.[10]

5. **Cholelithiasis**: Forty-two patients with gallstones were treated with complete recovery in 31 patients, improvement in 10 patients, and no effect in 1 case. The herbal treatment included *Si Ni San* plus *Yu Jin* (Radix Curcumae), *Ji Nei Jin* (Endothelium Corneum Gigeriae Galli), *Jin Qian Cao* (Herba Lysimachiae), and others.[11]

6. **Biliary ascariasis**: Use of *Si Ni San* plus *Jin Ling Zi San* (Melia Toosendan Powder) was effective in treating biliary ascariasis in 40 patients (22 males and 18 females, between 6-45 years of age). The herbal treatment included *Chai Hu* (Radix Bupleuri) 10g, *Zhi Qiao* (Fructus Aurantii) 10g, *Chuan Lian Zi* (Fructus Toosendan) 10g, *Shi Jun Zi* (Fructus Quisqualis) 10g, *Bing Lang* (Semen Arecae) 10g, *Bai Shao* (Radix Paeoniae Alba) 18g, *Gan Cao* (Radix et Rhizoma Glycyrrhizae) 6g, and *Yan Hu Suo* (Rhizoma Corydalis) 12g. The study reported complete recovery in all 40 patients, with an average of 4.2 days of treatment.[12] In another study, successful expulsion of biliary ascariasis was reported in all 51 patients after treatment for 1 to 3 days with *Si Ni San* plus *Wu Mei* (Fructus Mume) and *Ku Lian Pi* (Cortex Meliae).[13]

7. **Superficial gastritis**: Thirty-five patients with superficial gastritis were treated with good results using modified *Si Ni San*. *Zhe Bei Mu* (Bulbus Fritillariae Thunbergii), *Huang Qin* (Radix Scutellariae) and *Xiang Fu* (Rhizoma Cyperi) were added for Liver and Stomach qi stagnation. *San Leng* (Rhizoma Sparganii), *E Zhu* (Rhizoma Curcumae), *Yan Hu Suo* (Rhizoma Corydalis), *San Qi* (Radix et Rhizoma Notoginseng), and *Chuan Lian Zi* (Fructus Toosendan) were added for stagnation in the Stomach channel.[14]

Chapter 3 – Harmonizing Formulas   *Section 2 – Liver and Spleen Harmonizing Formulas*

Si Ni Săn (Frigid Extremities Powder)

8. **Gastritis**: Use of modified *Si Ni San* demonstrated 93.3% effectiveness in treating 30 patients with gastritis caused by regurgitation of bile. The herbal treatment contained *Si Ni San* plus *Pu Gong Ying* (Herba Taraxaci), *Chen Pi* (Pericarpium Citri Reticulatae), *Huang Lian* (Rhizoma Coptidis) and others as the base formula. Modifications included the addition of *Chuan Lian Zi* (Fructus Toosendan) and *Yan Hu Suo* (Rhizoma Corydalis) for upper abdominal pain; and *Da Huang* (Radix et Rhizoma Rhei) for constipation. Of 30 patients, the study reported significant improvement in 16 patients, moderate improvement in 12 patients, and no effect in 2 patients.[15]

9. **Peptic ulcer disease**: One study of 70 peptic ulcer patients reported 93% effectiveness using *Si Ni San* plus *Hou Po* (Cortex Magnoliae Officinalis), *Shi Hu* (Caulis Dendrobii), *Mai Dong* (Radix Ophiopogonis), and others as needed. The duration of treatment was 30 days. Of 70 patients, the study reported complete recovery in 63 patients, improvement in 2 patients, and no improvement in 5 patients.[16]

10. **Epigastric pain**: One study reported marked success using herbs to treat 110 patients of epigastric pain arising from various causes (such as acute or chronic gastritis, gastric ulcer, duodenal ulcer). The herbal formula included *Si Ni San* plus *Yu Jin* (Radix Curcumae), *Mai Ya* (Fructus Hordei Germinatus), *Hou Po* (Cortex Magnoliae Officinalis), and others as needed. Of 110 patients, 55 had complete recovery, 33 had significant improvement, 20 had marked improvement, and 2 had no effect.[17]

11. **Ulcerative colitis**: One study reported significant improvement in 8 of 10 patients with chronic ulcerative colitis when treated with modified *Si Ni San*. Modifications were made by adding *Bai Jiang Cao* (Herba cum Radice Patriniae), *Da Xue Teng* (Caulis Sargentodoxae), and *Yi Yi Ren* (Semen Coicis) for damp-heat; *Dang Shen* (Radix Codonopsis), *Shan Yao* (Rhizoma Dioscoreae) and dry-fried *Bai Zhu* (Rhizoma Atractylodis Macrocephalae) for Spleen deficiency; and *Si Shen Wan* (Four-Miracle Pill) for Kidney yang deficiency.[18]

12. **Infertility**: Two hundred forty-six women with infertility due to blocked fallopian tubes were treated with 72.36% effectiveness (complete resolution in 136 patients, improvement in 42 patients, and no effect in 68 patients). The herbal treatment contained as the base formula *Chai Hu* (Radix Bupleuri) 10g, *Zhi Shi* (Fructus Aurantii Immaturus) 10g, *Chi Shao* (Radix Paeoniae Rubra) 10g, *Gan Cao* (Radix et Rhizoma Glycyrrhizae) 10g, *Dan Shen* (Radix et Rhizoma Salviae Miltiorrhizae) 10g and *Chuan Shan Jia* (Squama Manis) 15g. Modifications included addition of a larger dose of *Zhi Shi* (Fructus Aurantii Immaturus) for Liver stagnation, and *Shui Zhi* (Hirudo) for blood stagnation. The herbs were given in decoction daily for 3 months per course of treatment.[19]

13. **Adnexitis**: Administration of modified *Si Ni San* was associated with marked effect in all 48 patients with chronic adnexitis. In addition to the base formula, *Mu Tong* (Caulis Akebiae) and *Ze Xie* (Rhizoma Alismatis) were added for damp-heat; *Gui Zhi* (Ramulus Cinnamomi) and *Xiao Hui Xiang* (Fructus Foeniculi) were added for damp-cold; *Chuan Lian Zi* (Fructus Toosendan) and *Yan Hu Suo* (Rhizoma Corydalis) were added for severe pain; and *Hai Piao Xiao* (Endoconcha Sepiae) and *Tu Fu Ling* (Rhizoma Smilacis Glabrae) for profuse leukorrhea.[20]

14. **Impotence**: One study reported 88% effectiveness using modified *Si Ni San* to treat impotence in 25 men (between 25 and 47 years of age; with 3 months to 2 years history of illness). Of 25 men, the study reported complete recovery in 18 patients, significant improvement in 4 patients, and no improvement in 3 patients. The herbal treatment contained *Si Ni San* plus *Wu Gong* (Scolopendra) as the base formula. *Chuan Lian Zi* (Fructus Toosendan) was added for hypochondriac pain; *Zhi Zi* (Fructus Gardeniae) and *Mu Dan Pi* (Cortex Moutan) for dry mouth with bitter taste; *Yuan Zhi* (Radix Polygalae) and dry-fried *Suan Zao Ren* (Semen Ziziphi Spinosae) for insomnia and excessive dreams; *Ju Hua* (Flos Chrysanthemi) and *Tian Ma* (Rhizoma Gastrodiae) for dizziness, swelling and pain of the head; and *Gou Qi Zi* (Fructus Lycii), *Yi Zhi* (Fructus Alpiniae Oxyphyllae) and *Ba Ji Tian* (Radix Morindae Officinalis) for coldness and pain in the extremities and lower abdomen. The study noted that *Si Ni San* was selected as the herbal formula of choice because impotence in young men is often related to Liver qi stagnation overacting on the Spleen.[21]

TOXICOLOGY

In acute toxicology studies, the LD_{50} in mice was 413 g/kg via oral ingestion of decoction and 22.4 g/kg via intravenous injection. It was also noted that intravenous injection of the formula was associated with marked changes in electrocardiogram in rats and rabbits. In chronic toxicology studies, daily administration of the formula to rats in decoction at 15 g/kg for 20 days showed no abnormalities in either liver or kidney functions. The researchers also noted that the alcohol extract of the same formula showed more toxicity in both acute and chronic toxicology studies.[22]

RELATED FORMULA

Zhĭ Shí Sháo Yào Săn
(Immature Bitter Orange and Peony Powder)
枳實芍藥散
枳实芍药散
Pinyin Name: *Zhi Shi Shao Yao San*
Literal Name: Immature Bitter Orange and Peony Powder

Si Ni San (Frigid Extremities Powder)

Original Source: *Jin Gui Yao Lue* (Essentials from the Golden Cabinet) by Zhang Zhong-Jing in the Eastern Han Dynasty

Zhi Shi (Fructus Aurantii Immaturus),
   shao (burned) to black
Bai Shao (Radix Paeoniae Alba)

The source text states to grind equal amounts of the ingredients into powder. Take 1 large spoonful of the powder (6-9g) with porridge three times daily.

Zhi Shi Shao Yao San (Immature Bitter Orange and Peony Powder) is indicated for postpartum women with qi and blood stagnation. Clinically, patients may also have interior heat as a result of qi and blood stagnation. Some of the symptoms and signs include abdominal pain, irritability, and abscess or swelling.

Because women are often quite weak physically after delivery, they may not be able to withstand such strong treatment. Therefore, this formula has specific instructions on preparation and administration. *Zhi Shi* (Fructus Aurantii Immaturus) must be burned until brownish-black to temper its strong qi-activating and regulating functions. It is important to take this formula with wheat or rice porridge to nourish and strengthen the Spleen and Stomach to prevent the strong nature of *Zhi Shi* (Fructus Aurantii Immaturus) from injuring the middle *jiao*.

AUTHORS' COMMENTS

Si Ni San (Frigid Extremities Powder) is the foundation of many Liver qi-regulating formulas. Understanding the principles and uses of this formula will facilitate the understanding of other Liver qi-regulating formulas, such as *Zhi Shi Shao Yao San* (Immature Bitter Orange and Peony Powder), *Xiao Yao San* (Rambling Powder), *Jia Wei Xiao Yao San* (Augmented Rambling Powder), and *Chai Hu Shu Gan San* (Bupleurum Powder to Spread the Liver).

Si Ni San (Frigid Extremities Powder) and *Si Ni Tang* (Frigid Extremities Decoction) are two formulas with similar names that must **not** be confused. These two formulas treat different syndromes (qi stagnation vs. yang deficiency) that share similar symptoms (e.g., cold extremities/cold limbs).

- *Si Ni San*: Qi stagnation blocks and prevents yang qi from properly circulating to the extremities. Patients usually experience coldness below the knees and elbows, not in the entire limbs, as seen in patients of yang deficiency. In general, these patients also warm up faster when the extremities are exposed to heat. Other accompanying signs include abdominal discomfort and pain, and diarrhea. *Si Ni San* contains qi-regulating herbs to harmonize and smooth Liver qi flow and open channel circulation to the extremities. This condition is often seen when pathogenic factors invade from the outside and are trapped in the *shaoyang* channels, coupled with qi stagnation. When yang qi is no longer blocked by qi stagnation, the cold limbs will be resolved.

- *Si Ni Tang*: Yang deficiency with coldness manifests not only in cold extremities, but also in coldness of the whole limbs and all over the body. Comparatively speaking, this coldness is more severe and does not warm up when exposed to heat. Accompanying symptoms include a withered *shen* (spirit), desire to sleep, intolerance of cold, preference for lying in a fetal position, vomiting, abdominal pain, diarrhea with undigested food, and a faint, fine pulse. *Si Ni Tang* contains interior-warming herbs to boost Kidney yang to warm *ming men* (life gate) fire, thus warming the limbs.[23]

Si Ni San and *Yi Guan Jian* (Linking Decoction) both treat hypochondriac pain. The difference is as follows:

- *Si Ni San* treats epigastric, abdominal, or hypochondriac pain caused by Liver qi stagnation.
- *Yi Guan Jian* treats hypochondriac pain caused by Kidney and Liver yin deficiencies.[24]

References

1. *Tian Jin Zhong Yi* (Tianjin Chinese Medicine) 1987;(5):18.
2. *Zhong Yao Yao Li Yu Ying Yong* (Pharmacology and Applications of Chinese Herbs) 1991;7(1):29.
3. *Liao Ning Zhong Yi Za Zhi* (Liaoning Journal of Chinese Medicine) 1986;(7):40.
4. *Zhong Yao Yao Li Yu Ying Yong* (Pharmacology and Applications of Chinese Herbs) 1988;18.
5. *Zhong Yao Yao Li Yu Ying Yong* (Pharmacology and Applications of Chinese Herbs) 1992;8(4):37.
6. Jiang J, Zhou C, Xu Q. Alleviating effects of Si-Ni-San, a traditional Chinese prescription, on experimental liver injury and its mechanisms. Biol Pharm Bull 2003 Aug;26(8):1089-94.
7. *Shan Xi Xin Zhong Yi* (New Shanxi Chinese Medicine) 1987;(5):225.
8. *Zhong Yi Ming Fang Lin Chuang Xin Yong* (Contemporary Clinical Applications of Classic Chinese Formulas) 2001;244.
9. *Liao Ning Zhong Yi Za Zhi* (Liaoning Journal of Chinese Medicine) 1996;4:169.
10. *Hu Nan Zhong Yi Za Zhi* (Hunan Journal of Chinese Medicine) 1989;4:39.
11. *An Hui Zhong Yi Xue Yuan Xue Bao* (Journal of Anhui University School of Medicine) 1995;4:32.
12. *Guang Xi Zhong Yi Yao* (Guangxi Chinese Medicine and Herbology) 1985;1:14.
13. *Fu Jian Zhong Yi Yao* (Fujian Chinese Medicine and Herbology) 1962;2:37.
14. *Zhe Jiang Zhong Yi Za Zhi* (Zhejiang Journal of Chinese Medicine) 1997;10:439.

Chapter 3 – Harmonizing Formulas

Si Ni Săn (Frigid Extremities Powder)

15. *Bei Jing Zhong Yi Yao Da Xue Xue Bao* (Journal of Beijing University of Medicine and Medicinals) 1997;3:68.
16. *Zhe Jiang Zhong Yi Xue Yuan Xue Bao* (Journal of Zhejiang University of Chinese Medicine) 1997;2:53.
17. *Zhong Yi Ming Fang Lin Chuang Xin Yong* (Contemporary Clinical Applications of Classic Chinese Formulas) 2001;245.
18. *Nei Meng Gu Zhong Yi Yao* (Traditional Chinese Medicine and Medicinals of Inner Mongolia) 1998;1:26.
19. *Zhong Yi Ming Fang Lin Chuang Xin Yong* (Contemporary Clinical Applications of Classic Chinese Formulas) 2001;243.

20. *Chang Chun Zhong Yi Xue Yuan Xue Bao* (Journal of Changchun University of Chinese Medicine) 1995;1:43.
21. *Hu Bei Zhong Yi Za Zhi* (Hubei Journal of Chinese Medicine) 1986;3:21.
22. *Zhong Xi Yi Jie He Za Zhi* (Journal of Integrated Chinese and Western Medicine) 1988;8(10):601.
23. Wang MZ, et al. *Zhong Yi Xue Wen Da Ti Ku* (Questions and Answers on Traditional Chinese Medicine: Herbal Formulas).
24. Wang MZ, et al. *Zhong Yi Xue Wen Da Ti Ku* (Questions and Answers on Traditional Chinese Medicine: Herbal Formulas).

Chái Hú Shū Gān Săn (Bupleurum Powder to Spread the Liver)
柴胡疏肝散

Pinyin Name: *Chai Hu Shu Gan San*
Literal Name: Bupleurum Powder to Spread the Liver
Alternate Name: *Chai Hu Shu Gan Tang* (Bupleurum Decoction to Spread the Liver), Bupleurum and Cyperus Combination
Original Source: *Jing Yue Quan Shu* (Collected Treatises of [Zhang] Jing Yue) by Zhang Jie-Bin (Zhang Jing-Yue) in 1624

COMPOSITION

Chai Hu (Radix Bupleuri)	6g
Xiang Fu (Rhizoma Cyperi)	4.5g
Chen Pi (Pericarpium Citri Reticulatae), *chao* (dry-fried) with vinegar	6g
Zhi Qiao (Fructus Citri Aurantii), *chao* (dry-fried) with bran	4.5g
Bai Shao (Radix Paeoniae Alba)	4.5g
Chuan Xiong (Rhizoma Chuanxiong)	4.5g
Zhi Gan Cao (Radix et Rhizoma Glycyrrhizae Praeparata cum Melle)	1.5g

DOSAGE / PREPARATION / ADMINISTRATION

The source text states to cook the ingredients in 1.5 bowls of water until 80% of the liquid remains. Take the warm, strained decoction before meals.

CHINESE THERAPEUTIC ACTIONS

1. Regulates the Liver and promotes qi circulation
2. Harmonizes the blood and relieves pain

CLINICAL MANIFESTATIONS

Liver qi stagnation: hypochondriac fullness and pain, alternating spells of chills and fever, fidgeting, irritability, and abdominal pain and cramps. Female patients may experience swollen, painful breasts, dysmenorrhea, irregular menstrual cycle, and/or amenorrhea.

CLINICAL APPLICATIONS

Premenstrual syndrome, cholecystitis, cholelithiasis, hepatitis, gastritis, atrophic gastritis, peptic ulcer disease, irregular menstruation, dysmenorrhea, breast distention and pain, insomnia, emotional stress, depression, male sexual dysfunction, and orchitis.

EXPLANATION

Chai Hu Shu Gan San (Bupleurum Powder to Spread the Liver) treats Liver qi stagnation. The Liver is responsible for smoothing the qi flow in the body. If Liver qi is stagnant, pain may occur. Hypochondriac pain and chest fullness arise from Liver qi stagnation affecting the Liver channel, which runs through these regions of the body. The qi-smoothing function of the Liver is directly related to one's emotions. If Liver qi is stagnant, emotional disorders such as fidgeting and irritability occur. Liver qi stagnation may cause blood stagnation, resulting in irregular menstruation and dysmenorrhea in women. Pain and distention of the breasts are due to stagnation of Liver qi along the Liver channel. Stagnation of Liver qi (wood element) may also affect the Spleen and Stomach (earth element), causing abdominal pain and cramps.

238

Chái Hú Shū Gān Săn (Bupleurum Powder to Spread the Liver)

Chai Hu Shu Gan San (Bupleurum Powder to Spread the Liver)

Diagnosis	Signs and Symptoms	Treatment	Herbs
Liver qi stagnation	• Hypochondriac and chest fullness and pain: Liver qi stagnation along the Liver channel • Abdominal pain and cramps: Liver qi stagnation overacting on the Spleen and Stomach • Fidgeting, irritability: Liver qi stagnation affecting the emotions • Dysmenorrhea, irregular menstruation and/or amenorrhea: Liver qi stagnation affecting menstruation	• Regulates the Liver and promotes qi circulation • Harmonizes the blood and relieves pain	• *Chai Hu* (Radix Bupleuri) harmonizes and spreads the Liver and relieves Liver qi stagnation. • *Xiang Fu* (Rhizoma Cyperi) breaks up Liver qi stagnation and relieves pain. • *Chen Pi* (Pericarpium Citri Reticulatae) and *Zhi Qiao* (Fructus Aurantii) activate qi circulation and break up qi stagnation. • *Bai Shao* (Radix Paeoniae Alba) nourishes Liver blood to soften the Liver. • *Chuan Xiong* (Rhizoma Chuanxiong) activates blood circulation. • *Zhi Gan Cao* (Radix et Rhizoma Glycyrrhizae Praeparata cum Melle) harmonizes the herbs and relieves pain.

Chai Hu (Radix Bupleuri) harmonizes and spreads the Liver and relieves Liver qi stagnation. *Xiang Fu* (Rhizoma Cyperi) effectively breaks up Liver qi stagnation and relieve pain. *Chen Pi* (Pericarpium Citri Reticulatae) and *Zhi Qiao* (Fructus Aurantii) activate qi circulation and break up qi stagnation. *Bai Shao* (Radix Paeoniae Alba) nourishes the blood to the Liver to soften the Liver. *Chuan Xiong* (Rhizoma Chuanxiong) activates blood circulation. *Zhi Gan Cao* (Radix et Rhizoma Glycyrrhizae Praeparata cum Melle) harmonizes the herbs and relieves pain.

MODIFICATIONS

• With belching and acid reflux, add *Hai Piao Xiao* (Endoconcha Sepiae).
• If there is severe stomach pain, add *Yan Hu Suo* (Rhizoma Corydalis) and *Chuan Lian Zi* (Fructus Toosendan).
• With a burning sensation in the stomach and a bitter taste in the mouth, add *Huang Lian* (Rhizoma Coptidis) and *Huang Qin* (Radix Scutellariae).
• For breast distention and pain due to disharmony between the Stomach and Liver, add *Shen Ling Bai Zhu San* (Ginseng, Poria, and Atractylodes Macrocephala Powder).
• For liver spots, use *Chai Hu Shu Gan San* internally and apply *Bai Zhi* (Radix Angelicae Dahuricae) topically.
• If the hypochondriac pain is severe, add *Dang Gui* (Radix Angelicae Sinensis), *Yu Jin* (Radix Curcumae), and *Wu Yao* (Radix Linderae).
• For Liver qi stagnation that has turned into Liver fire, add *Zhi Zi* (Fructus Gardeniae) and *Chuan Lian Zi* (Fructus Toosendan).

CAUTIONS / CONTRAINDICATIONS

Chai Hu Shu Gan San is not recommended in patients with yin-deficient heat characterized by signs and symptoms such as a red tongue with little tongue coating, a dry mouth and throat, restlessness, and insomnia. Similarly, this formula should be discontinued in those who develop these symptoms after taking this formula.[1]

PHARMACOLOGICAL EFFECTS

1. **Cardiovascular**: Administration of *Chai Hu Shu Gan San* via intravenous injection in rabbits was associated with a marked improvement in blood circulation to various parts of the body, including the brain, heart, and liver.[2]
2. **Cholagogic**: Administration of *Chai Hu Shu Gan San* in rats was associated with increased production and release of bile acid after one hour.[3]

CLINICAL STUDIES AND RESEARCH

1. **Cholecystitis**: One study reported complete recovery in 25 of 30 patients with chronic cholecystitis when treated with *Chai Hu Shu Gan San* plus *Qing Pi* (Pericarpium Citri Reticulatae Viride), *Yu Jin* (Radix Curcumae), *Yan Hu Suo* (Rhizoma Corydalis), *Hou Po* (Cortex Magnoliae Officinalis), *Jin Qian Cao* (Herba Lysimachiae), and *Yin Chen* (Herba Artemisiae Scopariae).[4] In another study, 132 patients with chronic cholecystitis were treated with complete recovery in 39 patients, significant improvement in 46 patients, moderate improvement in 40 patients, and no effect in 7 patients. In addition to *Chai Hu Shu Gan San*, modifications were made by adding *Yu Jin* (Radix Curcumae) and *Jin Ling Zi San* (Melia Toosendan Powder)

Chái Hú Shū Gān Sǎn (Bupleurum Powder to Spread the Liver)

for qi stagnation; *Jin Qian Cao* (Herba Lysimachiae), *Hu Zhang* (Rhizoma et Radix Polygoni Cuspidati), and *Huang Qin* (Radix Scutellariae) for damp-heat. Electro-acupuncture and herbal injection at acupuncture points were performed, too.[5]

2. **Cholelithiasis and bile duct infection**: One hundred and sixteen patients with gallstones and infection of the bile duct were treated with complete recovery in 27 patients, significant improvement in 68 patients, moderate improvement in 16 patients, and no benefit in 5 patients. The herbal formula was modified from *Chai Hu Shu Gan San*, with addition of *Jin Qian Cao* (Herba Lysimachiae), *Da Huang* (Radix et Rhizoma Rhei), *Yu Jin* (Radix Curcumae), *Shan Zha* (Fructus Crataegi), *Huang Qin* (Radix Scutellariae), *Qing Pi* (Pericarpium Citri Reticulatae Viride), and *Ji Nei Jin* (Endothelium Corneum Gigeriae Galli), and elimination of *Chuan Xiong* (Rhizoma Chuanxiong).[6]

3. **Hepatitis B**: Sixty patients with chronic hepatitis B were treated with good results using modified *Chai Hu Shu Gan San*. The herbal formula contained *Chai Hu* (Radix Bupleuri) 10g, dry-fried *Bai Zhu* (Rhizoma Atractylodis Macrocephalae) 10g, *Zhi Shi* (Fructus Aurantii Immaturus) 10g, *Fu Ling* (Poria) 12g, *Yu Jin* (Radix Curcumae) 12g, *Bai Jiang Cao* (Herba cum Radice Patriniae) 12g, *Dan Shen* (Radix et Rhizoma Salviae Miltiorrhizae) 20g, *Bai Hua She She Cao* (Herba Hedyotis) 15g, *Chi Shao* (Radix Paeoniae Rubra) 15g, and others as needed. The herbs were given in decoction daily 1 to 2 hours after a meal. Of 60 patients, the study reported recovery in 12 patients, improvement in 46 patients, and no improvement in 2 patients. The overall rate of effectiveness was 96%.[7]

4. **Atrophic gastritis**: Thirty-nine patients with atrophic gastritis reported good results using modified *Chai Hu Shu Gan San*. The herbal formula contained *Chai Hu* (Radix Bupleuri) 12g, *Zhi Qiao* (Fructus Aurantii) 12g, *Xiang Fu* (Rhizoma Cyperi) 12g, *Bai Shao* (Radix Paeoniae Alba) 15g, *Chuan Xiong* (Rhizoma Chuanxiong) 10g, *Gan Cao* (Radix et Rhizoma Glycyrrhizae) 6g, *Yan Hu Suo* (Rhizoma Corydalis) 10g, *Chuan Lian Zi* (Fructus Toosendan) 6g, *Mu Xiang* (Radix Aucklandiae) 6g, *Dan Shen* (Radix et Rhizoma Salviae Miltiorrhizae) 15g, *Yu Jin* (Radix Curcumae) 15g, *Ban Xia* (Rhizoma Pinelliae) 10g, *Chen Pi* (Pericarpium Citri Reticulatae) 10g, charred *Shan Zha* (Fructus Crataegi) 15g, charred *Shen Qu* (Massa Fermentata) 15g, and charred *Mai Ya* (Fructus Hordei Germinatus) 15g. The study reported complete recovery in 23 of 39 patients.[8]

5. **Peptic ulcer disease**: Use of modified *Chai Hu Shu Gan San* was associated with beneficial effects in treating gastric or duodenal ulcers. The herbal formula was modified from *Chai Hu Shu Gan San*, with the removal of *Chuan Xiong* (Rhizoma Chuanxiong), and the addition of *Bai Ji* (Rhizoma Bletillae), *Sha Ren* (Fructus Amomi), *Xuan Shen* (Radix Scrophulariae), and *Pu Gong Ying* (Herba Taraxaci). The duration of treatment ranged from 3 to 12 packs of herbs.[9]

6. **Male sexual dysfunction**: Use of modified *Chai Hu Shu Gan San* was effective in treating 17 of 19 patients who were unable to ejaculate. The herbal treatment contained *Chai Hu Shu Gan San* plus *Ju He* (Semen Citri Reticulatae), *Shi Chang Pu* (Rhizoma Acori Tatarinowii), *Chuan Shan Jia* (Squama Manis), *Mu Tong* (Caulis Akebiae), *Hu Po* (Succinum), and others as needed.[10]

7. **Orchitis**: One study reported complete recovery in 32 of 37 patients with orchitis, when treated with an herbal formula that contained *Chai Hu Shu Gan San* plus *Huang Qin* (Radix Scutellariae), *Wu Yao* (Radix Linderae), *Tao Ren* (Semen Persicae), *Xiao Hui Xiang* (Fructus Foeniculi), *Ju He* (Semen Citri Reticulatae), *Bai Jiang Cao* (Herba cum Radice Patriniae), and others.[11]

8. **Breast distention and pain**: Complete relief of breast distention and pain was reported in 21 of 24 patients who were treated with modified *Chai Hu Shu Gan San*. The herbal formula contained *Chai Hu* (Radix Bupleuri) 12g, *Bai Shao* (Radix Paeoniae Alba) 12g, vinegar-fried *Chen Pi* (Pericarpium Citri Reticulatae) 10g, *Chuan Xiong* (Rhizoma Chuanxiong) 10g, *Xiang Fu* (Rhizoma Cyperi) 10g, dry-fried *Zhi Qiao* (Fructus Aurantii) 10g, *Yu Jin* (Radix Curcumae) 10g, *Tong Cao* (Medulla Tetrapanacis) 10g, *Bai Zhi* (Radix Angelicae Dahuricae) 10g, processed *Ru Xiang* (Gummi Olibanum) 10g, processed *Mo Yao* (Myrrha) 10g, *Pu Gong Ying* (Herba Taraxaci) 15g, and *Gan Cao* (Radix et Rhizoma Glycyrrhizae) 6g. The treatment protocol was to cook the herbs in water, and administer the decoction in three equally-divided doses daily, for 7 days per course of treatment.[12]

9. **Insomnia**: One study reported 96.7% effectiveness using modified *Chai Hu Shu Gan San* to treat patients with stubborn insomnia. The treatment protocol was to use this formula as the base, with the addition of *Chi Shao* (Radix Paeoniae Rubra) and *Dan Shen* (Radix et Rhizoma Salviae Miltiorrhizae) for blood stagnation; *Ju Hua* (Flos Chrysanthemi) and *Zhi Zi* (Fructus Gardeniae) for Liver excess; and *Dan Nan Xing* (Arisaema cum Bile) and *Shi Chang Pu* (Rhizoma Acori Tatarinowii) for phlegm accumulation. Of 30 patients, the study reported complete recovery in 26 patients, improvement in 3 patients, and no effect in one patient.[13]

AUTHORS' COMMENTS

Chai Hu Shu Gan San is one of the most commonly used formulas for treating Liver qi stagnation characterized by hypochondriac pain and alternating chills and fever. It

Chái Hú Shū Gān Sǎn (Bupleurum Powder to Spread the Liver)

also treats various types of menstrual disorders caused by Liver qi stagnation.

Chai Hu Shu Gan San is a variation of *Si Ni San* (Frigid Extremities Powder). Although the herbs in these two formulas are similar, their doses and emphases are different.

- *Si Ni San* treats both Spleen qi deficiency and obstructed circulation of Liver and Gallbladder qi. *Chai Hu* (Radix Bupleuri) and *Zhi Shi* (Fructus Aurantii Immaturus) are the only qi-moving herbs in this formula. *Zhi Gan Cao* (Radix et Rhizoma Glycyrrhizae Praeparata cum Melle) is used at a high dose to tonify qi and strengthen the Spleen.

- *Chai Hu Shu Gan San* mainly treats Liver qi stagnation, and contains many qi- and blood-moving herb, such as *Chai Hu* (Radix Bupleuri), *Zhi Qiao* (Fructus Aurantii), *Chen Pi* (Pericarpium Citri Reticulatae), *Chuan Xiong* (Rhizoma Chuanxiong), and *Xiang Fu* (Rhizoma Cyperi). *Zhi Gan Cao* (Radix et Rhizoma Glycyrrhizae Praeparata cum Melle) is used at a low dose for harmonizing purposes.

References

1. *Zhong Yao Ming Fang Yao Li Yu Ying Yong* (Pharmacology and Applications of Famous Herbal Formulas) 1989;112-113.
2. *Zhong Yao Yao Li Yu Lin Chuang* (Pharmacology and Clinical Applications of Chinese Herbs) 1987;4(4):17.
3. *Shi Yong Zhong Yi Nei Ke Za Zhi* (Journal of Practical Chinese Internal Medicine) 1989;3(1):11.
4. *Shan Xi Zhong Yi* (Shanxi Chinese Medicine) 1990;11(3):128.
5. *Gan Su Zhong Yi Xue Yuan Xue Bao* (Journal of Gansu University of Chinese Medicine) 1995;2:37.
6. *Shi Yong Zhong Xi Yi Jie He Za Zhi* (Practical Journal of Integrated Chinese and Western Medicines) 1991;4(10):618.
7. *Zhong Yi Yao Xue Bao* (Report of Chinese Medicine and Herbology) 1992;6:38.
8. *Shan Xi Zhong Yi* (Shanxi Chinese Medicine) 1995;16(1):28.
9. *Hei Long Jiang Zhong Yi Yao* (Heilongjiang Chinese Medicine and Herbology) 1987;1:41.
10. *Zhe Jiang Zhong Yi Za Zhi* (Zhejiang Journal of Chinese Medicine) 1990;25(6):253.
11. *Shan Xi Zhong Yi* (Shanxi Chinese Medicine) 1993;14(2):54.
12. *Guang Xi Zhong Yi Yao* (Guangxi Chinese Medicine and Herbology) 1985;8(2):21.
13. *Zhong Yi Ming Fang Lin Chuang Xin Yong* (Contemporary Clinical Applications of Classic Chinese Formulas) 2001;575.

Shū Gān Tāng (Spread the Liver Decoction)

疏肝湯
疏肝汤

Pinyin Name: *Shu Gan Tang*
Literal Name: Spread the Liver Decoction
Alternate Name: Bupleurum and Evodia Combination
Original Source: *Wan Bing Hui Chun* (Restoration of Health from the Myriad Diseases) by Gong Ting-Xian in 1587

COMPOSITION

Chai Hu (Radix Bupleuri)	3g
Qing Pi (Pericarpium Citri Reticulatae Viride)	3g
Zhi Qiao (Fructus Aurantii)	3g
Tao Ren (Semen Persicae)	3g
Hong Hua (Flos Carthami)	1.5g
Dang Gui (Radix Angelicae Sinensis)	3g
Chuan Xiong (Rhizoma Chuanxiong)	2.1g
Bai Shao (Radix Paeoniae Alba)	2.1g
Huang Lian (Rhizoma Coptidis), *chao* (dry-fried)	6g

DOSAGE / PREPARATION / ADMINISTRATION

The source text specifies to first dry-fry *Huang Lian* (Rhizoma Coptidis) with the juice of *Wu Zhu Yu* (Fructus Evodiae). Then grind all of the ingredients into powder and cook in water to make a decoction. Take the warm, strained decoction after meals.

CHINESE THERAPEUTIC ACTIONS

1. Regulates blood circulation and eliminates blood stasis
2. Opens the channels and collaterals and relieves pain

Shū Gān Tāng (Spread the Liver Decoction)

CLINICAL MANIFESTATIONS

Liver qi stagnation with blood stasis: hypochondriac fullness and pain, and alternating spells of fever and chills.

CLINICAL APPLICATIONS

Pain in the hypochondrium, intercostal neuralgia, intercostal pain, and pancreatitis.

EXPLANATION

Shu Gan Tang (Spread the Liver Decoction) treats hypochondriac pain caused by Liver qi stagnation with blood stasis. The classic text describes this condition as being characterized by fullness and pain in the hypochondrium. This condition may also occur secondary to internal or external injuries. Internal injuries include pancreatitis, and external injuries include trauma and contusion.

Because the fundamental disorder is Liver qi stagnation, *Chai Hu* (Radix Bupleuri) is used to treat the *shaoyang* syndrome and to spread Liver qi. *Qing Pi* (Pericarpium Citri Reticulatae Viride) and *Zhi Qiao* (Fructus Aurantii) regulate qi, and together with *Chai Hu* (Radix Bupleuri), relieve hypochondriac pain and fullness. Since qi and blood stagnations often occur together, blood movers are added to enhance the overall effect. *Tao Ren* (Semen Persicae) and *Hong Hua* (Flos Carthami) move the blood, eliminate blood stagnation, and relieve pain. *Dang Gui* (Radix Angelicae Sinensis) nourishes the blood and, with *Chuan Xiong* (Rhizoma Chuanxiong), moves the blood. *Dang Gui* (Radix Angelicae Sinensis) and *Bai Shao* (Radix Paeoniae Alba) soften the Liver by tonifying yin and blood. *Bai Shao* (Radix Paeoniae Alba) is one of the key herbs used to relax the muscles and relieve spasms and pain. Because Liver qi stagnation can easily turn into Liver heat and fire, *Huang Lian* (Rhizoma Coptidis) clears heat and fire. Lastly, *Wu Zhu Yu* (Fructus Evodiae) acts as a guiding herb to lead the therapeutic effect of the entire formula to the affected area.

AUTHORS' COMMENTS

Chai Hu Shu Gan San (Bupleurum Powder to Spread the Liver) and *Shu Gan Tang* both treat Liver qi stagnation with blood stasis.

- *Chai Hu Shu Gan San* places more emphasis on activating qi circulation.
- *Shu Gan Tang* focuses more on invigorating blood circulation and eliminating blood stasis.

Shu Gan Tang (Spread the Liver Decoction)

Diagnosis	Signs and Symptoms	Treatment	Herbs
Liver qi stagnation with blood stasis	• Hypochondriac fullness and pain: Liver qi stagnation with blood stasis • Alternating spells of fever and chills: *shaoyang* syndrome	• Regulates blood circulation and eliminates blood stasis • Opens the channels and collaterals and relieves pain	• *Chai Hu* (Radix Bupleuri) regulates Liver qi and spreads Liver qi stagnation. • *Qing Pi* (Pericarpium Citri Reticulatae Viride) and *Zhi Qiao* (Fructus Aurantii) regulate qi and relieve hypochondriac pain and fullness. • *Tao Ren* (Semen Persicae) and *Hong Hua* (Flos Carthami) move the blood, eliminate blood stagnation, and relieve pain. • *Dang Gui* (Radix Angelicae Sinensis) and *Chuan Xiong* (Rhizoma Chuanxiong) nourish the blood and regulate blood circulation. • *Dang Gui* (Radix Angelicae Sinensis) and *Bai Shao* (Radix Paeoniae Alba) tonify yin and blood to soften the Liver. • *Huang Lian* (Rhizoma Coptidis) clears heat and fire. • *Wu Zhu Yu* (Fructus Evodiae) guides the formula to the affected area.

Chái Hú Qīng Gān Tāng (Bupleurum Decoction to Clear the Liver)

柴胡清肝湯
柴胡清肝汤

Pinyin Name: *Chai Hu Qing Gan Tang*
Literal Name: Bupleurum Decoction to Clear the Liver
Alternate Names: *Tsai Hu Ching Kan Tang*, Bupleurum Liver-Clearing Decoction, Bupleurum and Rehmannia Combination
Original Source: *Yi Guan Tang* (Linking Clinic)

COMPOSITION

Huang Qin (Radix Scutellariae)	3g
Huang Lian (Rhizoma Coptidis)	3g
Huang Bo (Cortex Phellodendri Chinensis)	3g
Zhi Zi (Fructus Gardeniae)	4.5g
Di Huang (Radix Rehmanniae)	4.5g
Dang Gui (Radix Angelicae Sinensis)	6g
Bai Shao (Radix Paeoniae Alba)	4.5g
Chuan Xiong (Rhizoma Chuanxiong)	3g
Chai Hu (Radix Bupleuri)	4.5g
Jie Geng (Radix Platycodonis)	3g
Niu Bang Zi (Fructus Arctii)	4.5g
Lian Qiao (Fructus Forsythiae)	6g
Tian Hua Fen (Radix Trichosanthis)	3g
Bo He (Herba Menthae)	3g
Gan Cao (Radix et Rhizoma Glycyrrhizae)	3g

DOSAGE / PREPARATION / ADMINISTRATION

Prepare the ingredients as a decoction.

CHINESE THERAPEUTIC ACTIONS

Clears heat from the Liver, Gallbladder, and *San Jiao* channels

CLINICAL MANIFESTATIONS

Heat in the Liver, Gallbladder, and *San Jiao* channels: fever, chills, epistaxis, itching, loss of hearing, swelling of the lymph nodes, and formation of cellulitis.

CLINICAL APPLICATIONS

Lymphadenitis, adenoids, tonsillitis, measles, systemic lupus erythematosus, infectious viral hepatitis, dysmenorrhea, and chronic uteritis.

EXPLANATION

Chai Hu Qing Gan Tang (Bupleurum Decoction to Clear the Liver) clears heat in the Liver, Gallbladder, and *San Jiao* channels, characterized by symptoms such as fever, chills, epistaxis, loss of hearing, and swelling of the lymph nodes. Clinically, this formula is especially effective for infants and young children who are skinny, malnourished, and have a purplish-to-black facial complexion. Long-term use of this formula improves the physical condition of such patients and changes their underlying body constitution.

This formula is a modified combination of *Huang Lian Jie Du Tang* (Coptis Decoction to Relieve Toxicity) and *Si Wu Tang* (Four-Substance Decoction). *Huang Qin* (Radix Scutellariae), *Huang Lian* (Rhizoma Coptidis), *Huang Bo* (Cortex Phellodendri Chinensis), and *Zhi Zi* (Fructus Gardeniae), the four herbs in *Huang Lian Jie Du Tang* (Coptis Decoction to Relieve Toxicity), eliminate excess fire in the upper, middle, and lower *jiaos*. *Di Huang* (Radix Rehmanniae), *Dang Gui* (Radix Angelicae Sinensis), *Bai Shao* (Radix Paeoniae Alba), and *Chuan Xiong* (Rhizoma Chuanxiong), four herbs that follow the principles of *Si Wu Tang* (Four-Substance Decoction), cool the heat and moisten dryness in the blood. *Chai Hu* (Radix Bupleuri) is added as a channel-guiding herb to direct the formula to the Liver and Gallbladder. *Jie Geng* (Radix Platycodonis) clears heat from the head, eyes, throat, and chest. *Niu Bang Zi* (Fructus Arctii) and *Lian Qiao* (Fructus Forsythiae) clear heat from the Lung, benefit the throat, and dispel heat from the skin. *Tian Hua Fen* (Radix Trichosanthis) promotes the secretion of body fluids, reduces swelling, and discharges pus. *Bo He* (Herba Menthae) clears heat and relieves Liver qi stagnation. *Gan Cao* (Radix et Rhizoma Glycyrrhizae) harmonizes the formula.

Chapter 3 – Harmonizing Formulas   *Section 2 – Liver and Spleen Harmonizing Formulas*

Chái Hú Qīng Gān Tāng (Bupleurum Decoction to Clear the Liver)

Chai Hu Qing Gan Tang (Bupleurum Decoction to Clear the Liver)

Diagnosis	Signs and Symptoms	Treatment	Herbs
Heat in the Liver, Gallbladder, and *San Jiao* channels	Fever, chills, epistaxis, loss of hearing, and swelling of the lymph nodes: heat in the Liver, Gallbladder, and *San Jiao* channels	Clears heat from the Liver, Gallbladder, and *San Jiao* channels	• *Huang Qin* (Radix Scutellariae), *Huang Lian* (Rhizoma Coptidis), *Huang Bo* (Cortex Phellodendri Chinensis), and *Zhi Zi* (Fructus Gardeniae) clear heat and purge fire from the entire body. • *Di Huang* (Radix Rehmanniae), *Dang Gui* (Radix Angelicae Sinensis), *Bai Shao* (Radix Paeoniae Alba), and *Chuan Xiong* (Rhizoma Chuanxiong) tonify the blood and activate blood circulation. • *Chai Hu* (Radix Bupleuri) guides the formula to the Liver and Gallbladder. • *Jie Geng* (Radix Platycodonis) clears heat from the head, eyes, throat, and chest. • *Niu Bang Zi* (Fructus Arctii) and *Lian Qiao* (Fructus Forsythiae) clear heat from the Lung, benefit the throat, and dispel heat from the skin. • *Tian Hua Fen* (Radix Trichosanthis) promotes the secretion of body fluids, reduces swelling, and discharges pus. • *Bo He* (Herba Menthae) clears heat and relieves Liver qi stagnation. • *Gan Cao* (Radix et Rhizoma Glycyrrhizae) harmonizes the formula.

MODIFICATIONS

If accompanied by wind-heat symptoms, add *Qiang Huo* (Rhizoma et Radix Notopterygii) and *Jing Jie* (Herba Schizonepetae).

PHARMACOLOGICAL EFFECTS

Hepatoprotective and choleretic: Administration of *Chai Hu Qing Gan Tang* showed beneficial effects on the liver and gallbladder in rats. It had protective effects against experimental cholestasis induced by carbon tetrachloride or alpha-naphthylisothiocyanate, and a protective effect against the alterations of serum components, such as SGOT, SGPT, alkaline phosphatase and the concentration of serum bilirubin. The study concluded that *Chai Hu Qing Gan Tang* had choleretic effect to treat cholestasis and hepatoprotective effect to prevent liver parenchymal injury.[1]

RELATED FORMULAS

Chái Hú Qīng Gān Tāng
(Bupleurum Decoction to Clear the Liver)
柴胡清肝湯
柴胡清肝汤
Pinyin Name: *Chai Hu Qing Gan Tang*
Literal Name: Bupleurum Decoction to Clear the Liver
Original Source: *Wai Ke Zheng Zong* (True Lineage of External Medicine) by Chen Shi-Gong in 1617

Chai Hu (Radix Bupleuri)	4.5g
Di Huang (Radix Rehmanniae)	4.5g
Chi Shao (Radix Paeoniae Rubra)	4.5g
Niu Bang Zi (Fructus Arctii)	4.5g
Dang Gui (Radix Angelicae Sinensis)	6g
Lian Qiao (Fructus Forsythiae)	6g
Chuan Xiong (Rhizoma Chuanxiong)	3g
Huang Qin (Radix Scutellariae)	3g
Zhi Zi (Fructus Gardeniae)	3g
Tian Hua Fen (Radix Trichosanthis)	3g
Gan Cao (Radix et Rhizoma Glycyrrhizae)	3g
Fang Feng (Radix Saposhnikoviae)	3g

Cook the herbs in 2 cups of water until the liquid is reduced to 1.6 cups. Take the warm, strained decoction after meals. Note: Another source states to use *Bai Shao* (Radix Paeoniae Alba) in place of *Chi Shao* (Radix Paeoniae Rubra), and equal amounts (3g) of all the ingredients.

This formula treats Liver fire rising, causing the formation of sores and ulcers in the temple area of the head.

These two formulas have the exact same names and very similar functions, but are from different original sources.
• *Chai Hu Qing Gan Tang* from *Yi Guan Tang* (Linking Clinic) is a colder formula that strongly clears heat from the Liver, Gallbladder, and *San Jiao* channels.

Chinese Herbal Formulas and Applications

Chái Hú Qīng Gān Tāng (Bupleurum Decoction to Clear the Liver)

- *Chai Hu Qing Gan Tang* from *Wai Ke Zheng Zong* (True Lineage of External Medicine) is not as cold, and has been used historically for early-stage sores and ulcers in the temple area of the head.

Zhī Zǐ Qīng Gān Tāng

(Gardenia Decoction to Clear the Liver)

栀子清肝湯

栀子清肝汤

Pinyin Name: *Zhi Zi Qing Gan Tang*
Literal Name: Gardenia Decoction to Clear the Liver
Original Source: *An Hui Zhong Yi Xue Yuan* (Anhui University School of Medicine) in 1990

Zhi Zi (Fructus Gardeniae)

Xia Ku Cao (Spica Prunellae)

Xuan Shen (Radix Scrophulariae)

Zhi Mu (Rhizoma Anemarrhenae)

Zhe Bei Mu (Bulbus Fritillariae Thunbergii)

Mu Li (Concha Ostreae)

Zao Jiao Ci (Spina Gleditsiae)

Chuan Niu Xi (Radix Cyathulae)

Fang Feng (Radix Saposhnikoviae)

Huang Qi (Radix Astragali)

Yuan Zhi (Radix Polygalae)

Gan Cao (Radix et Rhizoma Glycyrrhizae)

Zhi Zi Qing Gan Tang (Gardenia Decoction to Clear the Liver) treats excess Liver fire accompanied by consumption of qi and yin. Clinically, it treats hyperthyroidism by clearing Liver fire, tonifying underlying qi and yin deficiencies, softening hardness and nodules, and calming the *shen* (spirit).

Reference

1. Sasaki T, Ohta S, Kamogawa A, Shinoda M. Protective effects of various Chinese traditional medicines against experimental cholestasis. Chem Pharm Bull (Tokyo) 1990 Feb;38(2):513-6.

Yì Gān Sǎn (Restrain the Liver Powder)

抑肝散

抑肝散

Pinyin Name: *Yi Gan San*
Literal Name: Restrain the Liver Powder
Alternate Names: *I Kan San,* Liver-Repressing Formula, Bupleurum Formula
Original Source: *Bao Ying Cuo Yao* (Synopsis of Caring for Infants) by Xue Kai in 1555

COMPOSITION

Chai Hu (Radix Bupleuri)	1.5g
Gou Teng (Ramulus Uncariae cum Uncis)	3g
Dang Gui (Radix Angelicae Sinensis)	3g
Chuan Xiong (Rhizoma Chuanxiong)	2.4g
Bai Zhu (Rhizoma Atractylodis Macrocephalae), *chao* (dry-fried)	3g
Fu Ling (Poria)	3g
Gan Cao (Radix et Rhizoma Glycyrrhizae)	1.5g

DOSAGE / PREPARATION / ADMINISTRATION

Prepare the ingredients as a decoction.

CHINESE THERAPEUTIC ACTIONS

1. Calms the Liver and clears Liver heat
2. Nourishes Liver blood and strengthens the Spleen

CLINICAL MANIFESTATIONS

Liver blood deficiency accompanied by Liver heat in infants and children: fever, being easily frightened and scared, muscle spasms and contraction, clenching of the teeth, nervousness, irritability, restlessness, insomnia, epilepsy, and alternating spells of fever and chills. Patients may also experience vomiting of saliva and sputum, and epigastric and abdominal fullness.

245

Chapter 3 – Harmonizing Formulas　　　　　　　　*Section 2 – Liver and Spleen Harmonizing Formulas*

Yī Gān Sǎn (Restrain the Liver Powder)

CLINICAL APPLICATIONS

Neurosis, neurasthenia, hysteria, insomnia, night crying in children, epilepsy, and menopausal disturbances.

EXPLANATION

Yi Gan San (Restrain the Liver Powder) treats Liver blood deficiency accompanied by Liver heat in infants and children. Liver heat rising leads to emotional instability, causing clinical manifestations such as irritability, bad temper, excitability, insomnia, nervousness, and epilepsy. Clinically, patients will show symptoms of deficiency and excess simultaneously. Liver blood deficiency is characterized by muscle spasms and contraction, clenching of the teeth, being easily frightened or scared; while the excess is characterized by nervousness, irritability, and restlessness. In addition, if the Liver overacts on the Spleen and Stomach, patients will show symptoms such as epigastric and abdominal fullness, lack of appetite, and vomiting of saliva and sputum.

To address the complicated situation of deficiency and excess, herbs are selected to nourish the blood, clear Liver fire, and harmonize the Liver, Spleen, and Stomach. The Liver must first be calmed and Liver heat cleared. Liver blood should also be nourished and the Spleen strengthened to prevent wood from overacting on earth. This formula contains *Chai Hu* (Radix Bupleuri) and *Gou Teng* (Ramulus Uncariae cum Uncis) to calm the Liver and clear Liver heat. *Dang Gui* (Radix Angelicae Sinensis) and *Chuan Xiong* (Rhizoma Chuanxiong) nourish Liver blood and soften the Liver. *Bai Zhu* (Rhizoma Atractylodis Macrocephalae) and *Fu Ling* (Poria) strengthen the Spleen. *Gan Cao* (Radix et Rhizoma Glycyrrhizae) harmonizes the herbs.

MODIFICATIONS

- With headache and dizziness, add *Bai Shao* (Radix Paeoniae Alba) and *Huang Lian* (Rhizoma Coptidis).
- For both qi and blood deficiencies, add *Ren Shen* (Radix et Rhizoma Ginseng), *Huang Qi* (Radix Astragali), *Bai Shao* (Radix Paeoniae Alba), *Shu Di Huang* (Radix Rehmanniae Praeparata), and *Di Huang* (Radix Rehmanniae).
- When there is a feeling of oppression and fullness in the abdomen, add *Zhi Shi* (Fructus Aurantii Immaturus) and *Hou Po* (Cortex Magnoliae Officinalis).
- With restless sleep, irritability and insomnia, add *Suan Zao Ren* (Semen Ziziphi Spinosae) and *Bai Zi Ren* (Semen Platycladi).
- With vomiting of sputum and saliva, add *Wen Dan Tang* (Warm the Gallbladder Decoction).
- If accompanied by dizziness, headache, and a disturbed *shen* (spirit), add *Bai Shao* (Radix Paeoniae Alba) and *Suan Zao Ren* (Semen Ziziphi Spinosae).

PHARMACOLOGICAL EFFECTS

Antidepressive and antinociceptive: Administration of *Yi Gan San*, *Bu Zhong Yi Qi Tang* (Tonify the Middle and Augment the Qi Decoction) and *Chai Hu Jia Long Gu Mu Li Tang* (Bupleurum plus Dragon Bone and Oyster Shell Decoction) for 14 consecutive days showed both antidepressive and antinociceptive properties in mice.[1]

AUTHORS' COMMENTS

Yi Gan San was originally formulated to treat Liver blood deficiency accompanied by Liver heat in infants and children. Today, it is commonly used to treat adults who lead stressful lifestyles, constantly thinking about work or other issues, and complaining of insomnia or difficulty in falling asleep. This formula can be served before bedtime to tranquilize the *shen* (spirit) and help patients fall asleep.

Yi Gan San (Restrain the Liver Powder)

Diagnosis	Signs and Symptoms	Treatment	Herbs
Liver blood deficiency accompanied by Liver heat rising	• Emotional instability, irritability, bad temper, excitability, insomnia and nervousness: Liver heat rising • Muscle spasms and contraction, clenching of teeth, easily frightened or scared: Liver blood deficiency • Epigastric and abdominal fullness, lack of appetite, and vomiting of saliva and sputum: Liver overacting on the Spleen and Stomach	• Calms the Liver and clears Liver heat • Nourishes Liver blood and strengthens the Spleen	• *Chai Hu* (Radix Bupleuri) and *Gou Teng* (Ramulus Uncariae cum Uncis) calm the Liver and clear Liver heat. • *Dang Gui* (Radix Angelicae Sinensis) and *Chuan Xiong* (Rhizoma Chuanxiong) nourish Liver blood and soften the Liver. • *Bai Zhu* (Rhizoma Atractylodis Macrocephalae) and *Fu Ling* (Poria) strengthen the Spleen. • *Gan Cao* (Radix et Rhizoma Glycyrrhizae) harmonizes the herbs.

246

Chinese Herbal Formulas and Applications

Yi Gān Sǎn (Restrain the Liver Powder)

According to Dr. Chang Wei-Yen, *Yi Gan San* can be used with *Yang Xin Tang* (Nourish the Heart Decoction), *Zhi Gan Cao Tang* (Honey-Fried Licorice Decoction), and *Tian Wang Bu Xin Dan* (Emperor of Heaven's Special Pill to Tonify the Heart) to treat palpitations and tachycardia.

Reference

1. Koshikawa N, Imai T, Takahashi I, Yamauchi M, Sawada S, Kansaku A. Effects of Hochu-ekki-to, Yoku-kan-san and Saiko-ka-ryukotsu-borei-to on behavioral despair and acetic acid-induced writhing in mice. Methods Find Exp Clin Pharmacol 1998 Jan-Feb;20(1):47-51.

Xiāo Yáo Sǎn (Rambling Powder)

逍遥散
逍遥散

Pinyin Name: *Xiao Yao San*
Literal Name: Rambling Powder
Alternate Names: *Hsiao Yao San*, Merry Life Powder, Bupleurum and Tang-kuei Formula, Tangkuei and Bupleurum Formula
Original Source: *Tai Ping Hui Min He Ji Ju Fang* (Imperial Grace Formulary of the Tai Ping Era) by the Imperial Medical Department in 1078-85

COMPOSITION

Chai Hu (Radix Bupleuri)	30g [9g]
Dang Gui (Radix Angelicae Sinensis), *cuo* (grated) and *chao* (dry-fried) slightly	30g [9g]
Bai Shao (Radix Paeoniae Alba)	30g [9g]
Bai Zhu (Rhizoma Atractylodis Macrocephalae)	30g [9g]
Fu Ling (Poria)	30g [9g]
Zhi Gan Cao (Radix et Rhizoma Glycyrrhizae Praeparata cum Melle)	15g [4.5g]

DOSAGE / PREPARATION / ADMINISTRATION

The source text instructs to grind the ingredients coarsely and then cook 6g of the powdered herbs with small amounts of roasted *Sheng Jiang* (Rhizoma Zingiberis Recens) and *Bo He* (Herba Menthae) in 1 large bowl of water until the liquid is reduced to 70%. Take the hot, strained decoction any time during the day. Today, this formula may be prepared as a decoction with the doses suggested in brackets, with 9g of roasted *Sheng Jiang* (Rhizoma Zingiberis Recens) and 4.5g of *Bo He* (Herba Menthae).

Note: There are two important notes on the preparation and dosing of herbs in this formula. *Sheng Jiang* (Rhizoma Zingiberis Recens) should be dry-roasted to decrease its acrid property and exterior-releasing effect. *Bo He* (Herba Menthae) should be kept at a low dose to clear Liver qi stagnation, since a high dose may produce an undesirable exterior-releasing effect. If not prepared properly, these two herbs will act as exterior-releasing herbs and further damage yin and blood.

CHINESE THERAPEUTIC ACTIONS

1. Soothes the Liver and relieves qi stagnation
2. Strengthens the Spleen
3. Nourishes the blood

CLINICAL MANIFESTATIONS

Liver qi stagnation with blood deficiency and Spleen deficiency: bilateral hypochondriac pain, alternating fever and chills, headache, vertigo, a dry mouth and throat, lassitude, lack of appetite, premenstrual syndrome (PMS) with breast distention, and a wiry, deficient pulse.

CLINICAL APPLICATIONS

Psychiatric disorders, emotional distress, anxiety, stress, neurasthenia, depression, neurosis, premenstrual syndrome, menstrual irregularity, menstrual disturbance, menstrual pain and cramps, functional uterine bleeding, menopause, hyperplasia of mammary glands, breast proliferation disease, fibrocystic breasts, lactation difficulties, oophoritic cyst, pelvic inflammatory disease, mastadenoma, gynecomastia, orchitis, prostatitis, sexual dysfunction,

247

Chapter 3 – Harmonizing Formulas   Section 2 – Liver and Spleen Harmonizing Formulas

Xiāo Yáo Sǎn (Rambling Powder)

infertility, impotence, hepatitis, liver cirrhosis, cholecystitis, anorexia, chronic gastritis, gastric ulcer, duodenal ulcer, irritable bowel syndrome, hyperlipidemia, pleurisy, optic nerve atrophy, central retinitis, and chloasma.

EXPLANATION

Xiao Yao San (Rambling Powder) treats Liver qi stagnation with blood deficiency and Spleen deficiency. The Liver stores blood and is responsible for dispersing and smoothing the qi flow of the body. Emotional distress, consumption of yin and blood, and malnourishment of the Liver can all cause Liver qi to become stagnant and impair the Liver's functioning. When Liver qi becomes stagnated, it will cause symptoms such as hypochondriac pain, headache, alternating spells of fever and chills, and vertigo. Liver qi stagnation contributes to yin and blood deficiencies, resulting in a dry mouth and dry throat. Liver qi stagnation overacts on a deficient Spleen, causing lassitude and lack of appetite. Lastly, Liver qi stagnation and blood deficiency affect menstruation, causing premenstrual syndrome (PMS) with breast distention.

In order to treat this syndrome, not only does Liver qi stagnation have to be dispersed, but it is also necessary to nourish Liver blood to soften the Liver. *Chai Hu* (Radix Bupleuri) smoothes Liver qi and disperses qi stagnation. However, *Chai Hu* (Radix Bupleuri) is drying in nature, and may further damage yin and blood. Therefore, herbs that nourish yin and tonify blood must be added. *Dang Gui* (Radix Angelicae Sinensis) is sweet, and tonifies the blood and relieves pain. *Bai Shao* (Radix Paeoniae Alba) nourishes the blood to soften the Liver to relieve distention and pain. *Bai Zhu* (Rhizoma Atractylodis Macrocephalae)

and *Fu Ling* (Poria) tonify the Spleen to help the generation of blood. *Zhi Gan Cao* (Radix et Rhizoma Glycyrrhizae Praeparata cum Melle) supplements qi and helps *Bai Shao* (Radix Paeoniae Alba) soften the Liver to relieve pain. Roasted *Sheng Jiang* (Rhizoma Zingiberis Recens) strongly warms and harmonizes the Stomach. A small amount of *Bo He* (Herba Menthae) helps *Chai Hu* (Radix Bupleuri) relieve Liver stagnation and clear any heat generated from qi stagnation.

MODIFICATIONS

- With irritability, a short-temper, and other signs of heat, add *Mu Dan Pi* (Cortex Moutan) and *Zhi Zi* (Fructus Gardeniae).
- When there is pain in the chest and hypochondriac region, add *San Leng* (Rhizoma Sparganii) and *E Zhu* (Rhizoma Curcumae).
- With poor appetite, add *Shen Qu* (Massa Fermentata) and *Ji Nei Jin* (Endothelium Corneum Gigeriae Galli).
- With vertigo and headache, add *Chuan Xiong* (Rhizoma Chuanxiong) and *Bai Zhi* (Radix Angelicae Dahuricae).
- If accompanied by qi deficiency, add *Huang Qi* (Radix Astragali) and *Ren Shen* (Radix et Rhizoma Ginseng).
- If accompanied by blood deficiency, add *Shu Di Huang* (Radix Rehmanniae Praeparata).
- With menstrual pain and cramps, add *Yan Hu Suo* (Rhizoma Corydalis), *Xiang Fu* (Rhizoma Cyperi) and *Mu Xiang* (Radix Aucklandiae).
- For irregular menstruation, add *Yi Mu Cao* (Herba Leonuri) and *Dan Shen* (Radix et Rhizoma Salviae Miltiorrhizae).
- When there is severe breast distention, add *Chai Hu Shu Gan San* (Buplerum Powder to Spread the Liver).

Xiao Yao San (Rambling Powder)

Diagnosis	Signs and Symptoms	Treatment	Herbs
Liver qi stagnation with blood deficiency and Spleen deficiency	• Bilateral hypochondriac pain, headache, vertigo, alternating spells of fever and chills: Liver qi stagnation • Dry mouth and dry throat: yin and blood deficiencies • Lassitude and lack of appetite: Spleen deficiency	• Soothes the Liver and relieves qi stagnation • Strengthens the Spleen • Nourishes the blood	• *Chai Hu* (Radix Bupleuri) smoothes the Liver qi and disperses the qi stagnation. • *Dang Gui* (Radix Angelicae Sinensis) and *Bai Shao* (Radix Paeoniae Alba) tonify blood, nourish yin, and soften the Liver. • *Bai Zhu* (Rhizoma Atractylodis Macrocephalae) and *Fu Ling* (Poria) tonify the Spleen to help the generation of blood. • Roasted *Sheng Jiang* (Rhizoma Zingiberis Recens) warms and harmonizes the Stomach. • *Bo He* (Herba Menthae) helps *Chai Hu* to relieve Liver qi stagnation and clear heat. • *Zhi Gan Cao* (Radix et Rhizoma Glycyrrhizae Praeparata cum Melle) harmonizes the herbs.

248

Xīāo Yáo Sǎn (Rambling Powder)

Chinese Herbal Formulas and Applications

- With insomnia due to stress and anxiety, add *Suan Zao Ren* (Semen Ziziphi Spinosae) and *Zhen Zhu Mu* (Concha Margaritiferae).
- With dizziness or vertigo, add *Gou Teng* (Ramulus Uncariae cum Uncis) and *Ju Hua* (Flos Chrysanthemi).

CAUTIONS / CONTRAINDICATIONS

- *Xiao Yao San* should be used with caution during pregnancy.
- This formula should be used with caution in cases of qi stagnation with underlying Liver and Kidney yin deficiencies, characterized by symptoms such as hypochondriac pain, chest and abdominal fullness and distention, a dry mouth and throat, a red tongue with little tongue coating, and a deep pulse.[1]

PHARMACOLOGICAL EFFECTS

1. **Central nervous system**: Administration of *Xiao Yao San* in mice and rats was associated with a mild inhibitory effect on the central nervous system to relieve pain and decrease the risk of seizures and epilepsy.[2]
2. **Hepatoprotective**: Administration of this formula was associated with marked hepatoprotective effect against carbon tetrachloride-induced liver damages. The formula reduced damage to liver cells, lowered liver enzymes, and promoted the generation of new liver cells.[3]
3. **Endocrine**: Administration of the formula was associated with an increase in weight of the uterus in laboratory animals. The effect was voided in animals whose ovaries had been surgically removed. The study suggested that the formula has an endocrine effect as it stimulated the ovary and increased the weight of the uterus.[4]
4. **Gastrointestinal**: Administration of the formula was associated with increased gastric acid production in mice and relaxation of the smooth muscles of the intestines in rabbits.[5]

CLINICAL STUDIES AND RESEARCH

1. **Schizophrenia**: Fourteen cases of schizophrenia characterized by Liver qi stagnation were treated with modified *Xiao Yao San* with satisfactory results.[6]
2. **Affective psychosis**: Twenty-six cases of affective psychosis were treated with modified *Xiao Yao San* with significant improvement in 16 cases, moderate improvement in 7 cases, and no benefit in 3 cases.[7]
3. **Depression**: One study reported 93.3% effectiveness using modified *Xiao Yao San* to treat depression in 60 patients. In addition to this formula, modifications included addition of *Qu Mai* (Herba Dianthi) and *Bian Xu* (Herba Polygoni Avicularis) for damp-heat in the lower *jiao*; *Zhi Mu* (Rhizoma Anemarrhenae) and *Huang Bo* (Cortex Phellodendri Chinensis) for Kidney yin

deficiency; *Shou Wu Teng* (Caulis Polygoni Multiflori) and *He Huan Pi* (Cortex Albiziae) for Heart yin deficiency; and *Xian Mao* (Rhizoma Curculiginis) and *Yin Yang Huo* (Herba Epimedii) for Kidney yang deficiency. The patients also received counseling. Of 60 patients, the study reported complete recovery in 32 patients, significant improvement in 16 patients, moderate improvement in 8 patients, and no improvement in 4 patients.[8]

4. **Neurosis**: One study reported 96% effectiveness using modified *Xiao Yao San* to treat 47 patients with neurosis. The herbal treatment contained *Xiao Yao San* plus *Yuan Zhi* (Radix Polygalae), *Shi Chang Pu* (Rhizoma Acori Tatarinowii) and others as the base formula. Modifications included addition of *Suan Zao Ren* (Semen Ziziphi Spinosae), *Bai Zi Ren* (Semen Platycladi) and *Shou Wu Teng* (Caulis Polygoni Multiflori) for palpitations and insomnia; *Zhe Shi* (Haematitum), *Jue Ming Zi* (Semen Cassiae) and *Di Long* (Pheretima) for Liver yang rising; *Sha Ren* (Fructus Amomi), *Shen Qu* (Massa Fermentata) and charred *Shan Zha* (Fructus Crataegi) for decreased food intake; *Gua Lou* (Fructus Trichosanthis), *Xie Bai* (Bulbus Allii Macrostemonis) and *Fo Shou* (Fructus Citri Sarcodactylis) for feeling of chest oppression; *Du Zhong* (Cortex Eucommiae), *Xu Duan* (Radix Dipsaci) and *Gou Qi Zi* (Fructus Lycii) for Kidney deficiency with low back soreness; *Huang Qi* (Radix Astragali), *Dang Shen* (Radix Codonopsis) and *Shu Di Huang* (Radix Rehmanniae Praeparata) for qi and blood deficiencies; *Dan Nan Xing* (Arisaema cum Bile), *Ban Xia* (Rhizoma Pinelliae) and *Chen Pi* (Pericarpium Citri Reticulatae) for more phlegm; and *Di Long* (Pheretima) and *Gui Zhi* (Ramulus Cinnamomi) for numbness of the fingers. Of 47 patients, the study reported complete recovery in 31 patients, improvement in 14 patients, and no improvement in 2 patients.[9]

5. **Premenstrual syndrome (PMS)**: *Xiao Yao San* has been confirmed in many studies to successfully treat PMS. Use of the formula in 32 women was associated with 96.88% effectiveness.[10] In another study, use of *Xiao Yao San* plus *Xiang Fu* (Rhizoma Cyperi) and *Yu Jin* (Radix Curcumae) was associated with 98% effectiveness in treating 62 women with PMS characterized by edema, breast distention, headache, and emotional disturbance.[11] Another study reported 93.3% effectiveness in treating PMS characterized by Liver stagnation turning into heat. The herbal treatment contained *Xiao Yao San* plus *Gou Teng* (Ramulus Uncariae cum Uncis), *Mu Dan Pi* (Cortex Moutan), *Qing Pi* (Pericarpium Citri Reticulatae Viride) and others.[12]

6. **Menstrual pain**: Forty-eight patients with menstrual pain were treated with modified *Xiao Yao San* with significant improvement in 30 patients, moderate improvement in 12 patients, and no effect in 6 patients. The overall effective rate reported was 87.5%. The ages of the patients

Chapter 3 – Harmonizing Formulas

Section 2 – Liver and Spleen Harmonizing Formulas

Xiāo Yáo Sǎn (Rambling Powder)

ranged from 15 to 45 years. The formula contained *Chai Hu* (Radix Bupleuri) 10g, *Ye Ju Hua* (Flos Chrysanthemi Indici) 10g, *Bo He* (Herba Menthae) 15g, *Dang Gui* (Radix Angelicae Sinensis) 15g, *Bai Zhu* (Rhizoma Atractylodis Macrocephalae) 15g, *Yan Hu Suo* (Rhizoma Corydalis) 15g, *Ba Ji Tian* (Radix Morindae Officinalis) 15g, *Fu Ling* (Poria) 20g, *Yi Mu Cao* (Herba Leonuri) 20g, *Liu Ji Nu* (Herba Artemisiae Anomalae) 20g, *Di Huang* (Radix Rehmanniae) 25g, *Bai Shao* (Radix Paeoniae Alba) 25g, *Mian Ma Guan Zhong* (Rhizoma Dryopteridis Crassirhizomatis) 60g, and *Gan Cao* (Radix et Rhizoma Glycyrrhizae) 5g.[13]

7. **Irregular menstruation**: One study reported 91.4% effectiveness using modified *Xiao Yao San* to treat various types of irregular menstruation. In addition to the base formula, *Mu Dan Pi* (Cortex Moutan) and *Zhi Zi* (Fructus Gardeniae) were added for early menstruation; *Xiang Fu* (Rhizoma Cyperi), *Dan Shen* (Radix et Rhizoma Salviae Miltiorrhizae) and *San Qi* (Radix et Rhizoma Notoginseng) were added for late menstruation; *Dan Shen* (Radix et Rhizoma Salviae Miltiorrhizae) and *Yi Mu Cao* (Herba Leonuri) were added for unpredictable (early or late) menstruation; charred *Pu Huang* (Pollen Typhae) and *Ze Lan* (Herba Lycopi) for hypermenorrhea; *Tao Ren* (Semen Persicae) and *Hong Hua* (Flos Carthami) for hypomenorrhea; and charred *Qian Cao* (Radix et Rhizoma Rubiae) and *Hai Piao Xiao* (Endoconcha Sepiae) for prolonged menstruation. Of 58 women, the study reported significant improvement in 45 patients, moderate improvement in 8 patients, and no improvement in 5 patients.[14]

8. **Menopause**: One hundred and fifty-eight patients with menopausal symptoms were treated with modified *Xiao Yao San* with significant improvement in 103 patients, moderate improvement in 51 patients, and no effect in 4 patients. The overall effectiveness was 97.5%. The formula contained *Xian Mao* (Rhizoma Curculiginis) 15g, *Yin Yang Huo* (Herba Epimedii) 10g, *Dang Gui* (Radix Angelicae Sinensis) 10g, *Ba Ji Tian* (Radix Morindae Officinalis) 10g, *Chai Hu* (Radix Bupleuri) 10g, *Fu Ling* (Poria) 10g, *Bai Shao* (Radix Paeoniae Alba) 10g, *Bai Zhu* (Rhizoma Atractylodis Macrocephalae) 10g, *Gui Zhi* (Ramulus Cinnamomi) 10g, *Zhi Mu* (Rhizoma Anemarrhenae) 3g, *Huang Bo* (Cortex Phellodendri Chinensis) 3g, *Bo He* (Herba Menthae) 3g, *Sheng Jiang* (Rhizoma Zingiberis Recens) 3g, *Gan Cao* (Radix et Rhizoma Glycyrrhizae) 6g, and *Da Zao* (Fructus Jujubae) 2 pieces.[15]

9. **Hyperplasia of mammary glands**: One hundred and thirty-two patients with hyperplasia of mammary glands were treated with modified *Xiao Yao San* with significant improvement in 103 patients, moderate improvement in 20 patients, mild improvement in 6 patients, and no effect in 3 patients. The overall effectiveness was 97.7%.

The treatment protocol was to administer 9g of herbs in pills twice daily for 20 days per course of treatment, for a total of 2 courses. The formula was modified depending on the condition of the patient. *Wang Bu Liu Xing* (Semen Vaccariae), *Ji Xue Teng* (Caulis Spatholobi), *Xiang Fu* (Rhizoma Cyperi), *Gua Lou* (Fructus Trichosanthis), and *Chi Shao* (Radix Paeoniae Rubra) were added for swelling and pain of the breast before menstruation. *Xia Ku Cao* (Spica Prunellae), *Tian Dong* (Radix Asparagi), *Ju He* (Semen Citri Reticulatae), *Zhe Bei Mu* (Bulbus Fritillariae Thunbergii), *Ru Xiang* (Gummi Olibanum), and *Mo Yao* (Myrrha) were added for swelling and pain of the breast after menstruation.[16]

10. **Breast proliferation disease**: One study reported 96.1% effectiveness in the treatment of breast proliferation disease in 51 patients using modified *Xiao Yao San* and *Er Chen Tang* (Two-Cured Decoction) for 3 months. This study demonstrated marked changes to the hormones as follows: very significant decline of saliva estradiol (P less than 0.001), significant decline of saliva progesterone (P less than 0.05), very significant decline of plasma prolactin (P less than 0.005), and insignificant changes of saliva testosterone. The researchers stated that these herbs could regulate the endocrine system to restore normal follicle function.[17]

11. **Mastadenoma**: One study reported marked success in the treatment of benign tumor of the breast in 174 women. The herbal prescription contained *Xiao Yao San* plus *San Leng* (Rhizoma Sparganii), *Gua Lou* (Fructus Trichosanthis), *Mu Li* (Concha Ostreae) and others. *Zhe Bei Mu* (Bulbus Fritillariae Thunbergii) and *Xia Ku Cao* (Spica Prunellae) were added for accumulation of heat and phlegm; *Zhi Zi* (Fructus Gardeniae) and *Zhi Mu* (Rhizoma Anemarrhenae) for restlessness and anger; *Yan Hu Suo* (Rhizoma Corydalis) and *Chuan Lian Zi* (Fructus Toosendan) for breast distention; *Huang Qi* (Radix Astragali) and *Dang Shen* (Radix Codonopsis) for qi deficiency; and *Shu Di Huang* (Radix Rehmanniae Praeparata) and *He Shou Wu* (Radix Polygoni Multiflori) for yin and blood deficiencies. Of 174 patients, the study reported recovery in 130 patients, marked improvement in 29 patients, moderate improvement in 10 patients, and no effect in 5 patients. The rate of effectiveness was 97.13%.[18]

12. **Lactation difficulties**: One study reported 93.3% effectiveness in promoting lactation among 30 postpartum women using *Xiao Yao San* plus *Tian Hua Fen* (Radix Trichosanthis), *Si Gua Luo* (Retinervus Luffae Fructus) and *Lou Lu* (Radix Rhapontici). The duration of treatment was 7 days per course of treatment.[19]

13. **Oophoritic cyst**: Use of modified *Xiao Yao San* was associated with marked effect to treat women with oophoritic cyst with pain, irregular menstruation and

250

Xīāo Yáo Sǎn (Rambling Powder)

Chinese Herbal Formulas and Applications

abnormal bleeding. The herbal treatment contained *Xiao Yao San* plus *Zao Jiao Ci* (Spina Gleditsiae), *Chuan Xiong* (Rhizoma Chuanxiong) and *Wa Leng Zi* (Concha Arcae) as the base formula, with addition of *Zhi Zi* (Fructus Gardeniae) and *Di Huang* (Radix Rehmanniae) for heat; *Rou Gui* (Cortex Cinnamomi) and *Pao Jiang* (Rhizoma Zingiberis Praeparatum) for cold; *Huang Qi* (Radix Astragali) and *Dang Shen* (Radix Codonopsis) for qi deficiency; charred *Di Huang* (Radix Rehmanniae) and charred *Huang Qin* (Radix Scutellariae) for yin deficiency; *Yu Jin* (Radix Curcumae) and *Zhi Qiao* (Fructus Aurantii) for qi and blood stagnation; and *Shu Di Huang* (Radix Rehmanniae Praeparata) and *Xu Duan* (Radix Dipsaci) for Kidney deficiency. Of 186 patients, the study reported complete recovery in 124 patients and improvement in 48 patients. The overall rate of effectiveness was 92%.[20]

14. **Orchitis**: One case of chronic orchitis was successfully treated with significant reduction of swelling and pain. The initial treatment was for 6 doses of a formula that contained *Xiao Yao San* plus *Sheng Ma* (Rhizoma Cimicifugae) 6g, *Huang Qi* (Radix Astragali) 15g, *Chen Pi* (Pericarpium Citri Reticulatae) 9g, *Ju He* (Semen Citri Reticulatae) 9g, and *Li Zhi He* (Semen Litchi) 9g. The follow-up treatment was for another 6 doses of the same formula, with addition of *Xia Ku Cao* (Spica Prunellae) 12g.[21]

15. **Prostatitis**: Eighteen patients of chronic prostatitis were treated with modified *Xiao Yao San* with complete recovery in 16 patients and moderate improvement in 2 patients.[22]

16. **Gynecomastia**: Administration of modified *Xiao Yao San* in 62 men with development of breasts was associated with complete recovery in 52 patients, significant improvement in 7 patients, and no effect in 3 patients. The duration of treatment was 30 days per course of treatment, for 1 to 5 courses total.[23] According to another study, use of *Xiao Yao San* was associated with 89% effectiveness in treating 35 men (between 17 and 73 years of age) who have had gynecomastia for 3 months to 5 years.[24]

17. **Infertility**: One study reported marked effectiveness using modified *Xiao Yao San* to treat infertility in 30 females (between 24-38 years of age). The herbal treatment contained *Xiao Yao San* plus *Yu Jin* (Radix Curcumae), *Xiang Fu* (Rhizoma Cyperi) and others as the base formula. Modifications included addition of *Fu Pen Zi* (Fructus Rubi) and *Tu Si Zi* (Semen Cuscutae) for Kidney deficiency; *Tao Ren* (Semen Persicae), *Chuan Niu Xi* (Radix Cyathulae) and *Yi Mu Cao* (Herba Leonuri) for blood stagnation; and *Chen Pi* (Pericarpium Citri Reticulatae) and *Ban Xia* (Rhizoma Pinelliae) for presence of dampness and phlegm. The herbs were given in decoction one time daily. The treatment protocol was to begin the herbal therapy for 7 days, starting on the fourth day after the end of the period, for 3 months per course of therapy, and 1-3 courses total. Of 30 patients at the end of the study, 20 were pregnant and 10 had varying degrees of improvement with menstruation.[25]

18. **Sexual dysfunction**: One study reported 96.6% effectiveness in treating 87 men with inability to ejaculate using modified *Xiao Yao San* and counseling. The herbal treatment contained *Xiao Yao San* plus *Long Gu* (Os Draconis), *Mu Li* (Concha Ostreae) and *Chuan Shan Jia* (Squama Manis) as the base formula. Modifications included addition of *Ban Xia* (Rhizoma Pinelliae), *Chen Pi* (Pericarpium Citri Reticulatae) and *Bai Jie Zi* (Semen Sinapis) for accumulation of dampness and phlegm; *Long Dan* (Radix et Rhizoma Gentianae), *Huang Qin* (Radix Scutellariae), *Mu Dan Pi* (Cortex Moutan) and *Zhi Zi* (Fructus Gardeniae) for damp-heat; *Xian Mao* (Rhizoma Curculiginis), *Yin Yang Huo* (Herba Epimedii) and *Jiu Cai Zi* (Semen Allii Tuberosi) for yang deficiency; and *Liu Wei Di Huang Wan* (Six-Ingredient Pill with Rehmannia) for yin deficiency with Liver excess. Of 87 patients, the study reported complete recovery in 76 patients, improvement in 8 patients, and no benefit in 3 patients.[26]

19. **Impotence**: Modified *Xiao Yao San* was reported in one study to be effective in treating impotence. Of 43 men, the study reported complete recovery in 31 patients, improvement in 9 patients and no improvement in 3 patients. The herbal treatment contained *Xiao Yao San* plus *Tu Si Zi* (Semen Cuscutae), *She Chuang Zi* (Fructus Cnidii), *Wu Wei Zi* (Fructus Schisandrae Chinensis) and *Wu Gong* (Scolopendra) as the base formula. Modifications included addition of *Ba Ji Tian* (Radix Morindae Officinalis), *Yin Yang Huo* (Herba Epimedii) and *Rou Cong Rong* (Herba Cistanches) for deficiency of *ming men* (life gate) fire; *Shou Wu Teng* (Caulis Polygoni Multiflori) and dry-fried *Suan Zao Ren* (Semen Ziziphi Spinosae) for deficiency and damage of Heart and Spleen; *Sheng Ma* (Rhizoma Cimicifugae) and dry-fried *Suan Zao Ren* (Semen Ziziphi Spinosae) for fear and fright damaging the Kidney; and *Che Qian Zi* (Semen Plantaginis) and *Ze Xie* (Rhizoma Alismatis) for damp-heat affecting the lower *jiao*. The patients were given the herbs for 15 days per course of treatment.[27]

20. **Hepatitis**: Thirty patients with hepatitis B were treated with this formula with moderate improvement in 29 patients. The formula was modified slightly depending on the condition of the patient.[28]

21. **Liver cirrhosis**: Seventeen patients with liver cirrhosis were treated with modified *Xiao Yao San* with significant improvement in 6 patients, moderate improvement in 9 patients, and no improvement in 2 patients.[29]

HARMONIZING FORMULAS

Chapter 3 – Harmonizing Formulas   Section 2 – Liver and Spleen Harmonizing Formulas

Xiāo Yáo Sǎn (Rambling Powder)

22. **Cholecystitis**: Administration of modified *Xiao Yao San* was associated with good results in treating 168 patients with cholecystitis (32 with acute and 136 with chronic cholecystitis). Of 168 patients, the study reported significant improvement in 79 patients and moderate improvement in 89 patients. Modifications to this formula included addition of *Yu Jin* (Radix Curcumae), *Chuan Lian Zi* (Fructus Toosendan), *Qing Pi* (Pericarpium Citri Reticulatae Viride) and *Zhi Qiao* (Fructus Aurantii) for hypochondriac pain radiating to the shoulder and back; *Hong Hua* (Flos Carthami) and *Dan Shen* (Radix et Rhizoma Salviae Miltiorrhizae) for fixed, stabbing pain in the hypochondrium with dark-colored tongue; *Sha Shen* (Radix Glehniae seu Adenophorae), *Shi Hu* (Caulis Dendrobii) and *Gou Qi Zi* (Fructus Lycii) for dry mouth with red tongue; *Da Huang* (Radix et Rhizoma Rhei), *Mang Xiao* (Natrii Sulfas), *Zhi Shi* (Fructus Aurantii Immaturus), and *Zhi Zi* (Fructus Gardeniae) for fever, nausea, vomiting and constipation; and *Jin Qian Cao* (Herba Lysimachiae) and *Hai Jin Sha* (Spora Lygodii) for presence of gallstones.[30]

23. **Anorexia**: Use of modified *Xiao Yao San* was associated with 100% effectiveness in improving appetite in 50 children with anorexia. The herbal treatment contained this formula plus dry-fried *Mai Ya* (Fructus Hordei Germinatus), *Ji Nei Jin* (Endothelium Corneum Gigeriae Galli), and others as needed. The average duration of treatment was 20.5 days. Of 50 children, 30 had complete recovery and 20 had improved appetite.[31]

24. **Irritable bowel syndrome (IBS)**: Administration of modified *Xiao Yao San* for 1-2 months in 52 patients with IBS was associated with complete recovery in 34 patients and improvement in 18 patients. The herbal treatment was based on *Xiao Yao San*, with addition of *Zhi Qiao* (Fructus Aurantii), *Mu Xiang* (Radix Aucklandiae) and *Yan Hu Suo* (Rhizoma Corydalis) for severe distention and pain; *Pao Jiang* (Rhizoma Zingiberis Praeparatum) and *Rou Gui* (Cortex Cinnamomi) for feeling of coldness in the abdomen; *Huang Qin* (Radix Scutellariae) and *Huang Lian* (Rhizoma Coptidis) for burning sensations and pain in the epigastric and abdominal regions; and addition of *Sha Ren* (Fructus Amomi) and *Bai Bian Dou* (Semen Lablab Album) and elimination of *Dang Gui* (Radix Angelicae Sinensis) for diarrhea.[32]

25. **Chloasma**: Use of *Xiao Yao San* for 15 packs of herbs per course of treatment was associated with effectiveness in treating excessive brown patches of irregular shape and size on the face or other parts of the body. Of 160 patients, the study reported complete recovery in 129 patients, significant recovery in 21 patients, improvement in 7 patients, and no effect in 3 patients.[33]

26. **Hyperlipidemia**: The effectiveness of using *Xiao Yao San* in treating hyperlipidemia was evaluated by dividing 126 patients into two groups. Group one received *Xiao Yao San* and group two received liquid extract of *Shan Zha* (Fructus Crataegi). There were 84 patients in group one, with an average age of 53 years (ranging from 35-73). There were 42 patients in group two, with an average age of 52 years (ranging from 37-72). Both groups were treated for 15 days per course of treatment, for a total of 3 courses. At the end, the study reported that both treatments were effective in reducing total cholesterol and triglyceride levels, with *Xiao Yao San* having 90.5% and 86.9% effectiveness, and the liquid extract of *Shan Zha* (Fructus Crataegi) having 78.5% and 76.2% effectiveness, respectively. The effectiveness rate was defined as greater than 10% reduction of total cholesterol and triglyceride levels.[34]

27. **Optic nerve atrophy**: Seventy patients (136 affected eyes) with atrophy of the optic nerve were treated with modified *Xiao Yao San* with satisfactory results.[35]

TOXICOLOGY

No fatality was observed following oral ingestion of the formula up to 200 g/kg (dried herb dose) in laboratory mice.[36]

RELATED FORMULA

Hēi Xiāo Yáo Sǎn (Black Rambling Powder)

黑逍遥散
黑逍遥散

Pinyin Name: Hei Xiao Yao San
Literal Name: Black Rambling Powder
Original Source: *Yi Lue Liu Shu* (Six Texts on the Essentials of Medicine)

Chai Hu (Radix Bupleuri)	1.5g
Gan Cao (Radix et Rhizoma Glycyrrhizae)	1.5g
Bai Shao (Radix Paeoniae Alba)	4.5g
Bai Zhu (Rhizoma Atractylodis Macrocephalae)	4.5g
Fu Ling (Poria)	4.5g
Dang Gui (Radix Angelicae Sinensis), chao (dry-fried)	9g [6g]
Di Huang (Radix Rehmanniae) or *Shu Di Huang* (Radix Rehmanniae Praeparata)	15g

The source text states to grind the ingredients coarsely and then cook 6g of the powdered herbs with one slice of *Sheng Jiang* (Rhizoma Zingiberis Recens) and a small amount of *Bo He* (Herba Menthae). Take the strained decoction while warm. Today, this formula may be prepared as a decoction using the doses suggested in brackets.

252

Xīāo Yáo Sǎn (Rambling Powder)

Hei Xiao Yao San (Black Rambling Powder) is formulated by adding *Di Huang* (Radix Rehmanniae) or *Shu Di Huang* (Radix Rehmanniae Praeparata) to *Xiao Yao San*. As the base, *Xiao Yao San* treats Liver qi stagnation. Add *Di Huang* (Radix Rehmanniae) if there are more heat symptoms, and add *Shu Di Huang* (Radix Rehmanniae Praeparata) if there is deficiency.

This formula regulates Liver qi, strengthens the Spleen, nourishes the blood, and regulates menstruation. Clinical manifestations include irregular menstruation with abdominal pain and a wiry, deficient pulse.

AUTHORS' COMMENTS

Xiao Yao San is often used as a base formula in treating many gynecological disorders or chronic hepatic disorders. Today, this formula commonly treats Liver qi stagnation caused by stress and a busy lifestyle. It is an excellent formula for treating emotional instability and other psycho-somatic disorders. It is a relatively mild formula that can be taken whenever necessary to help patients cope with their stressful life.

Chai Hu Shu Gan San (Bupleurum Powder to Spread the Liver) and *Xiao Yao San* are two of the most commonly used formulas to treat Liver qi stagnation.
- *Chai Hu Shu Gan San* focuses only on Liver qi stagnation, and is suitable for individuals with severe Liver qi stagnation.
- *Xiao Yao San* treats Liver qi stagnation with blood and Spleen deficiencies. It has a weaker qi-dispersing effect, but a stronger nourishing action. Thus, it is more suitable for deficient-type patients and/or for long-term use.

Xiao Yao San and *Si Ni San* (Frigid Extremities Powder) both harmonize the Liver (wood element) and Spleen (earth element) to treat such symptoms as hypochondriac or abdominal pain. Both formulas contain *Chai Hu* (Radix Bupleuri), *Bai Shao* (Radix Paeoniae Alba), and *Gan Cao* (Radix et Rhizoma Glycyrrhizae). The differences between these two formulas are as follows:
- *Xiao Yao San* regulates Liver qi, strengthens the Spleen, and nourishes the blood. It is more suitable for combined conditions of excess (Liver qi stagnation) and deficiency (blood and Spleen qi deficiencies). Chief manifestations of *Xiao Yao San* include hypochondriac pain, dizziness, headache, dry mouth and throat, listlessness, decreased dietary intake, irregular menstruation, and breast distention with a wiry, deficient pulse. It is also commonly used to treat emotional disturbances. *Xiao Yao San* contains *Bai Zhu* (Rhizoma Atractylodis Macrocephalae), *Fu Ling* (Poria), *Dang Gui* (Radix Angelicae Sinensis), *Sheng Jiang* (Rhizoma

Zingiberis Recens), *Bo He* (Herba Menthae), and *Zhi Gan Cao* (Radix et Rhizoma Glycyrrhizae Praeparata cum Melle) to strengthen the Spleen and nourish the blood.
- *Si Ni San* mainly treats an excess condition involving cold extremities caused by heat trapped in the body and blocking the qi from reaching the extremities. It uses *Chai Hu* (Radix Bupleuri) as the chief herb, and *Zhi Shi* (Fructus Aurantii Immaturus) to break up qi stagnation to allow qi to circulate to the extremities.

Xiao Yao San and *Yi Guan Jian* (Linking Decoction) both treat hypochondriac distention and pain, but the etiology of this condition and the focus of the formulas are quite different.
- *Xiao Yao San* addresses Liver qi stagnation accompanied by blood and Spleen deficiencies. It regulates Liver qi, spreads stagnation, strengthens the Spleen, and nourishes the blood. It is considered a harmonizing formula.
- *Yi Guan Jian* treats Liver and yin deficiencies with Liver qi stagnation. It is a tonic formula used to treat dry mouth and throat, acid regurgitation, mass accumulation, and hernia. It nourishes yin and regulates Liver qi.[37]

References

1. *Zhong Yao Ming Fang Yao Li Yu Ying Yong* (Pharmacology and Applications of Famous Herbal Formulas) 1989;114-115.
2. *Zhong Yao Yao Li Yu Ying Yong* (Pharmacology and Applications of Chinese Herbs) 1993;9(2):8.
3. *Zhong Cao Yao* (Chinese Herbal Medicine) 1990;21(11):28.
4. *Zhong Guo Yao Li Tong Xun* (Journal of Chinese Herbal Studies) 1988;(3):44.
5. *Zhong Guo Yao Li Tong Xun* (Journal of Chinese Herbal Studies) 1988;(3):44.
6. *Zhong Xi Yi Jie He Za Zhi* (Journal of Integrated Chinese and Western Medicine) 1982;(3):170.
7. *Xin Zhong Yi* (New Chinese Medicine) 1983;(1):37.
8. *Bei Jing Zhong Yi* (Beijing Chinese Medicine) 1996;2:22.
9. *Fu Jian Zhong Yi Yao* (Fujian Chinese Medicine and Herbology) 1999;5:26.
10. *Shi Zhen Guo Yao Yan Jiu* (Research of Shizhen Herbs) 1996;1:11.
11. *Shan Xi Zhong Yi* (Shanxi Chinese Medicine) 1997;6:242.
12. *Nan Jing Zhong Yi Yao Da Xue Xue Bao* (Journal of Nanjing University of Traditional Chinese Medicine and Medicinals) 1999;2:84.
13. *Shan Xi Zhong Yi* (Shanxi Chinese Medicine) 1995;16(6):244.
14. *Hu Nan Zhong Yi Xue Yuan Xue Bao* (Journal of Hunan University of Traditional Chinese Medicine) 1996;4:18.
15. *Shan Xi Yi Kan* (Shanxi Journal of Medicine) 1989;(8):343.
16. *Zhong Yi Za Zhi* (Journal of Chinese Medicine) 1993;(2):86.
17. Zhang GL. Treatment of breast proliferation disease with modified xiao yao san and er chen decoction. *Zhong Xi Yi Jie He Za Zhi* 1991 Jul; 11(7):400-2, 388.
18. *Jiang Su Zhong Yi* (Jiangsu Chinese Medicine) 1996;8:26.
19. *An Hui Zhong Yi Lin Chuang Za Zi* (Anhui Journal of Clinical Chinese Medicine) 1995;4:12.
20. *He Nan Zhong Yi* (Henan Chinese Medicine) 1999;3:46.
21. *Liao Ning Zhong Yi Za Zhi* (Liaoning Journal of Chinese Medicine) 1980;(2):36.
22. *Zhong Yi Za Zhi* (Journal of Chinese Medicine) 1990;(11):20.

Xiāo Yáo Sǎn (Rambling Powder)

23. *Gan Su Zhong Yi* (Gansu Chinese Medicine) 1994;6:35.
24. *Zhong Xi Yi Jie He Za Zhi* (Journal of Integrated Chinese and Western Medicine) 1988;2:86.
25. *Xin Zhong Yi* (New Chinese Medicine) 1995;5:38.
26. *He Nan Zhong Yi* (Henan Chinese Medicine) 1997;3:174.
27. *Ji Lin Zhong Yi Yao* (Jilin Chinese Medicine and Herbology) 1990;2:17.
28. *Hei Long Jiang Zhong Yi Yao* (Heilongjiang Chinese Medicine and Herbology) 1987;(1):25.
29. *Ji Lin Zhong Yi Yao* (Jilin Chinese Medicine and Herbology) 1986;(5):18.

30. *Jiang Xi Zhong Yi Yao* (Jiangxi Chinese Medicine and Herbology) 1999;1:27.
31. *Shan Xi Zhong Yi* (Shanxi Chinese Medicine) 1995;12:541.
32. *Si Chuan Zhong Yi* (Sichuan Chinese Medicine) 1997;11:25.
33. *Lin Chuang Pi Fu Ke Za Zhi* (Journal of Clinical Dermatology) 1992;6:30.
34. *Shan Xi Yi Kan* (Shanxi Journal of Medicine) 1995;16(3):109.
35. *Bei Jing Zhong Yi* (Beijing Chinese Medicine) 1986;(4):17.
36. *Zhong Guo Yao Li Tong Xun* (Journal of Chinese Herbal Studies) 1988;(3):44.
37. Wang MZ, et al. *Zhong Yi Xue Wen Da Ti Ku* (Questions and Answers on Traditional Chinese Medicine: Herbal Formulas).

Jiā Wèi Xiāo Yáo Sǎn (Augmented Rambling Powder)
加味逍遥散
加味逍遥散

Pinyin Name: *Jia Wei Xiao Yao San*
Literal Name: Augmented Rambling Powder
Alternate Names: *Dan Zhi Xiao Yao San* (Moutan and Gardenia Rambling Powder), *Ba Wei Xiao Yao San* (Eight-Ingredient Rambling Powder), *Chia Wei Hsiao Yao San*, Modified Merry Life Powder, Bupleurum and Peony Formula
Original Source: *Nei Ke Zhai Yao* (Summary of Internal Medicine) by Wen Sheng in the mid-19th century

COMPOSITION

Chai Hu (Radix Bupleuri)		30g [9g]
Dang Gui (Radix Angelicae Sinensis), *chao* (dry-fried) slightly		30g [9g]
Bai Shao (Radix Paeoniae Alba)		30g [9g]
Bai Zhu (Rhizoma Atractylodis Macrocephalae)		30g [9g]
Fu Ling (Poria)		30g [9g]
Zhi Gan Cao (Radix et Rhizoma Glycyrrhizae Praeparata cum Melle)		15g [4.5g]
Mu Dan Pi (Cortex Moutan)		30g [9g]
Zhi Zi (Fructus Gardeniae), *chao* (dry-fried)		30g [9g]

DOSAGE / PREPARATION / ADMINISTRATION

The source text instructs to grind the ingredients into powder, and cook 9g of the powdered herbs to make a decoction. Today, this formula is usually prepared as a decoction with the doses suggested in brackets.

CHINESE THERAPEUTIC ACTIONS

1. Soothes the Liver and relieves qi stagnation
2. Strengthens the Spleen
3. Nourishes the blood
4. Sedates heat and fire

CLINICAL MANIFESTATIONS

Liver qi stagnation accompanied by interior heat and underlying blood and Spleen deficiencies: irritability, restlessness, a short temper, hypochondriac pain, alternating spells of fever and chills, spontaneous perspiration, night sweats, headache, insomnia, vertigo, a dry mouth and throat, dry eyes, red cheeks, lassitude, lack of appetite, premenstrual or menstrual syndrome, and dysuria.

CLINICAL APPLICATIONS

Premenstrual syndrome, menstrual disturbance, menstrual pain and cramps, menopause, female infertility, emotional distress, emotional instability, anxiety, stress, neurasthenia, panic disorder, affective disorders, hepatitis, early stage of liver cirrhosis, hepatomegaly, stomatitis, inflammation and bleeding of the gums, cystitis, urinary tract infection, pelvic inflammatory disease, and fibrocystic breasts.

Chinese Herbal Formulas and Applications

Jiā Wèi Xiāo Yáo Sǎn (Augmented Rambling Powder)

EXPLANATION

Jia Wei Xiao Yao San (Augmented Rambling Powder) treats Liver qi stagnation accompanied by interior heat and underlying blood and Spleen deficiencies. As a result of deficiency in the interior (Spleen and blood), Liver qi stagnation is unrestrained and turns into heat and fire, leading to symptoms such as irritability, a short temper, spontaneous perspiration, night sweats, insomnia, headache, dry eyes, red cheeks, a dry mouth, irregular menstruation, lower abdominal pain, and dysuria.

Jia Wei Xiao Yao San is modified from *Xiao Yao San* (Rambling Powder), which resolves Liver qi stagnation, nourishes the blood, and strengthens the Spleen. The addition of *Mu Dan Pi* (Cortex Moutan) and *Zhi Zi* (Fructus Gardeniae) sedates interior heat arising from Spleen and blood deficiencies, and from Liver qi stagnation.

MODIFICATIONS

- For blood deficiency, fatigue, and low-grade fever, add *Chuan Xiong* (Rhizoma Chuanxiong) and *Shu Di Huang* (Radix Rehmanniae Praeparata).
- If the condition is marked by qi deficiency and fatigue, add *Huang Qi* (Radix Astragali) and *Ren Shen* (Radix et Rhizoma Ginseng).
- If accompanied by fidgeting, irritability, and thirst, add *Mai Dong* (Radix Ophiopogonis) and *Wu Wei Zi* (Fructus Schisandrae Chinensis).
- If there is painful urination, add *Che Qian Zi* (Semen Plantaginis).
- With alternating spells of chills and fever, combine with *Xiao Chai Hu Tang* (Minor Bupleurum Decoction).
- With cough and tidal fever, combine with *Wen Dan Tang* (Warm the Gallbladder Decoction).
- With fever and steaming bones sensations, combine with *Qing Hao Bie Jia Tang* (Artemisia Annua and Soft-Shelled Turtle Shell Decoction).

- For dermatological disorders in women, add *Chuan Xiong* (Rhizoma Chuanxiong) and *Di Huang* (Radix Rehmanniae).

CAUTIONS / CONTRAINDICATIONS

- *Jia Wei Xiao Yao San* should be used with caution during pregnancy.
- This formula is contraindicated in individuals with underlying deficiency and cold.[1]

PHARMACOLOGICAL EFFECTS

Anxiolytic: Use of *Jia Wei Xiao Yao San* showed anxiolytic effects through the neurosteroid synthesis followed by gamma-amino-butyric acidA/benzodiazepine (GABA(A)/BZP) receptor stimulations in male mice.[2]

CLINICAL STUDIES AND RESEARCH

1. **Menopause**: A randomized, controlled pilot study was performed to evaluate and compare the clinical effects of a 16-week treatment with *Jia Wei Xiao Yao San* and hormone replacement therapy (Premelle) in non-hysterectomized postmenopausal women. This study evaluated quality of life, and measured physiological parameters, such as follicle-stimulating hormone and estradiol levels. Both the herbs and drug effectively alleviated most of the menopausal symptoms with no significant differences. The formula demonstrated good compliance and safety, and was associated with a lower discontinuation rate due to lack of adverse side effects. The researchers concluded that *Jia Wei Xiao Yao San* is a safe and efficacious therapy and might be an alternative choice for relief of climacteric symptoms in postmenopausal women.[3]

2. **Affective disorders**: Administration of *Jia Wei Xiao Yao San* effectively treated affective disorders characterized by depressed Liver resulting in fire, mild yang deficiency and mild yin deficiency. Of 50 patients, the study reported marked improvement in 26 patients, improvement in 17 patients, and no improvement in 7 patients.[4]

Jia Wei Xiao Yao San (Augmented Rambling Powder)

Diagnosis	Signs and Symptoms	Treatment	Herbs
Liver qi stagnation accompanied by interior heat and underlying blood and Spleen deficiencies	• Bilateral hypochondriac pain, headache, vertigo, alternating spells of fever and chills: Liver qi stagnation • Irritability, a short temper, red cheeks, and dysuria: interior heat • Dry mouth and a dry throat: yin and blood deficiencies • Lassitude and lack of appetite: Spleen deficiency	• Soothes the Liver and relieves qi stagnation • Strengthens the Spleen • Nourishes the blood • Sedates heat and fire	• *Xiao Yao San* (Rambling Powder) treats Liver qi stagnation, nourishes the blood, and strengthens the Spleen. • *Mu Dan Pi* (Cortex Moutan) and *Zhi Zi* (Fructus Gardeniae) sedate interior heat and fire.

255

Chapter 3 – Harmonizing Formulas   *Section 2 – Liver and Spleen Harmonizing Formulas*

Jiā Wèi Xiāo Yáo Săn (Augmented Rambling Powder)

3. **Panic disorder**: Four patients diagnosed with panic disorder with agoraphobia, in accordance with the Diagnostic and Statistical Manual of Mental Disorders (DSM) criteria, were successfully treated with herbal medicine. Two patients were treated with *Jia Wei Xiao Yao San*, and 2 with *Ban Xia Hou Po Tang* (Pinellia and Magnolia Bark Decoction). Both formulas successfully relieved panic attacks, anticipatory anxiety and agoraphobia. The study concluded that these formulas may be useful as additional or alternative treatments for panic disorder.[5]

HERB-DRUG INTERACTION

• **Antipsychotic-induced Parkinsonism**: Use of *Jia Wei Xiao Yao San* was associated with statistically significant reduction ($P<0.01$) in tremors caused by antipsychotic-induced Parkinsonism in 8 patients. The tremors did not worsen in any of the patients, and there were no reports of side effects.[6]

• **Drug-induced menopause**: One study evaluated the therapeutic effects of certain herbal medicines on menopausal symptoms induced by gonadotropin-releasing hormone agonist therapy in Japanese women with endometriosis, adenomyosis, or leiomyoma. Menopausal symptoms induced by gonadotropin-releasing hormone agonist therapy in 13 patients were successfully treated with *Jia Wei Xiao Yao San*, *Dang Gui Shao Yao San* (Tangkuei and Peony Powder), *Shao Yao Gan Cao Tang* (Peony and Licorice Decoction), *Gui Zhi Fu Ling Wan* (Cinnamon Twig and Poria Pill), *Tao He Cheng Qi Tang* (Peach Pit Decoction to Order the Qi) or *Gui Zhi Tang* (Cinnamon Twig Decoction). Most importantly, there were no significant changes in serum estradiol levels after treatment with these herbal medicines. The researchers concluded that these herbal medicines can be recommended for menopausal symptoms induced by gonadotropin-releasing hormone agonists without a negative effect on serum estradiol levels.[7]

TOXICOLOGY

Use of *Jia Wei Xiao Yao San* was associated with one case of adult respiratory distress syndrome. After taking *Jia Wei Xiao Yao San* for treatment of seborrheic dermatitis, a 59-year-old female presented with a respiratory illness having clinical, radiologic and functional characteristics of adult respiratory distress syndrome, with increased number of lymphocytes, neutrophils, and eosinophils in the bronchoalveolar lavage fluid. The lymphocyte stimulation test with *Jia Wei Xiao Yao San* was positive.[8]

RELATED FORMULA

Shí Wèi Xiāo Yáo Săn (Ten-Ingredient Rambling Powder)
十味逍遥散
十味逍遥散
Pinyin Name: *Shi Wei Xiao Yao San*
Literal Name: Ten-Ingredient Rambling Powder
Original Source: *Nei Ke Zhai Yao* (Summary of Internal Medicine) by Wen Sheng in the mid-19th century

Chai Hu (Radix Bupleuri)
Dang Gui (Radix Angelicae Sinensis),
   chao (dry-fried) slightly
Bai Shao (Radix Paeoniae Alba)
Bai Zhu (Rhizoma Atractylodis Macrocephalae)
Fu Ling (Poria)
Zhi Gan Cao (Radix et Rhizoma Glycyrrhizae
   Praeparata cum Melle)
Sheng Jiang (Rhizoma Zingiberis Recens), *wei* (roasted)
Bo He (Herba Menthae)
Mu Dan Pi (Cortex Moutan)
Zhi Zi (Fructus Gardeniae), *chao* (dry-fried)

The source text instructs to grind the ingredients into powder, and cook 9g of the powdered herbs to make a decoction. Today, this formula is usually prepared as a decoction with the doses suggested in brackets.

Shi Wei Xiao Yao San (Ten-Ingredient Rambling Powder) treats Liver qi stagnation accompanied by interior heat and underlying blood and Spleen deficiencies. It is formulated by combining the ingredients from both *Xiao Yao San* (Rambling Powder) and *Jia Wei Xiao Yao San* (Augmented Rambling Powder).

• In comparison with *Xiao Yao San* (Rambling Powder), this formula has stronger effect to clear heat as it contains *Mu Dan Pi* (Cortex Moutan) and *Zhi Zi* (Fructus Gardeniae).

• In contrast with *Jia Wei Xiao Yao San* (Augmented Rambling Powder), it has better effect to regulate Liver qi circulation and harmonize the Stomach since it has *Bo He* (Herba Menthae) and roasted *Sheng Jiang* (Rhizoma Zingiberis Recens).

AUTHORS' COMMENTS

Jia Wei Xiao Yao San literally means "Augmented Rambling Powder." The augmentation refers to the addition of two herbs: *Mu Dan Pi* (Cortex Moutan) and *Zhi Zi* (Fructus Gardeniae). Thus, this formula is also known as *Dan Zhi Xiao Yao San* (Moutan and Gardenia Rambling Powder).

Jia Wei Xiao Yao San is one of the most commonly used formulas today, since stress is a major factor in the daily

256

Chinese Herbal Formulas and Applications

Jiā Wèi Xiāo Yáo Sǎn (Augmented Rambling Powder)

lives of many patients. As psychosomatic disorders increase, simply treating the symptoms and the physical discomforts may not be sufficient. This formula addresses the emotional aspects and treats the root of the condition in many cases. Although this formula contains strong heat-clearing and qi-regulating herbs that make it unsuitable for long-term use, many patients find it is impossible to change their lifestyle, or to reduce the stress factor that is the cause of their disorders. In those cases, a formula such as *Yi Guan Jian* (Linking Decoction) can be added to reduce the possibility of having these strong herbs create imbalances in the body.

References

1. *Zhong Yao Ming Fang Yao Li Yu Ying Yong* (Pharmacology and Applications of Famous Herbal Formulas) 1989;115-116.
2. Mizowaki M, Toriizuka K, Hanawa T. Anxiolytic effect of Kami-Shoyo-San (TJ-24) in mice: possible mediation of neurosteroid synthesis. Life Sci 2001 Sep 21;69(18):2167-77.
3. Chen LC, Tsao YT, Yen KY, Chen YF, Chou MH, Lin MF. A pilot study comparing the clinical effects of Jia-Wey Shiau-Yau San, a traditional Chinese herbal prescription, and a continuous combined hormone replacement therapy in postmenopausal women with climacteric symptoms. Maturitas 2003 Jan 30;44(1):55-62.
4. Zhang LD, Zhang YL, Xu SH, Zhou G, Jin SB. Traditional Chinese medicine typing of affective disorders and treatment. American Journal of Chinese Medicine 1994;22(3-4):321-7.
5. Mantani N, Hisanaga A, Kogure T, Kita T, Shimada Y, Terasawa K. Four cases of panic disorder successfully treated with Kampo (Japanese herbal) medicines: Kami-shoyo-san and Hange-koboku-to. Psychiatry & Clinical Neurosciences 2002 Dec;56(6):617-20.
6. Ishikawa T, Funahashi T, Kudo J. Effectiveness of the Kampo kami-shoyo-san (TJ-24) for tremor of antipsychotic-induced parkinsonism. Psychiatry Clin Neurosci 2000 Oct;54(5):579-82.
7. Tanaka T. Effects of herbal medicines on menopausal symptoms induced by gonadotropin-releasing hormone agonist therapy. Clin Exp Obstet Gynecol 2001;28(1):20-3.
8. Shiota Y, Wilson JG, Matsumoto H, Munemasa M, Okamura M, Hiyama J, Marukawa M, Ono T, Taniyama K, Mashiba H. Adult respiratory distress syndrome induced by a Chinese medicine, Kamisyoyo-san. Internal Medicine 1996 Jun;35(6):494-6.

Tòng Xiè Yào Fāng (Important Formula for Painful Diarrhea)

痛瀉要方
痛泻要方

Pinyin Name: *Tong Xie Yao Fang*
Literal Name: Important Formula for Painful Diarrhea
Alternate Names: *Bai Zhu Shao Yao San* (Atractylodes Macrocephala and Peony Powder), Important Formula for Painful Purging
Original Source: *Jing Yue Quan Shu* (Collected Treatises of [Zhang] Jing Yue) by Zhang Jie-Bin (Zhang Jing-Yue) in 1624

COMPOSITION

Bai Zhu (Rhizoma Atractylodis Macrocephalae), *chao* (dry-fried) with soil	90g [6g]
Bai Shao (Radix Paeoniae Alba), *chao* (dry-fried)	60g [6g]
Chen Pi (Pericarpium Citri Reticulatae), *chao* (dry-fried)	45g [4.5g]
Fang Feng (Radix Saposhnikoviae)	60g [3g]

DOSAGE / PREPARATION / ADMINISTRATION

The source text states that this formula may be prepared as a decoction, pills or powder. Today, this formula is usually prepared as a decoction with the doses suggested in brackets.

CHINESE THERAPEUTIC ACTIONS

1. Tonifies the Spleen and sedates the Liver
2. Dispels dampness and stops diarrhea

CLINICAL MANIFESTATIONS

Abdominal pain and diarrhea caused by Spleen deficiency and Liver excess: borborygmus, diarrhea, abdominal pain which persists after defecation, a thin, white tongue coating, and a wiry, moderate pulse at the *guan* position on both hands.

CLINICAL APPLICATIONS

Diarrhea, acute enteritis, chronic enteritis, chronic colitis, ulcerative colitis, irritable bowel syndrome, chronic cholecystitis, and various types of gastrointestinal disorders.

HARMONIZING FORMULAS

3

257

Chapter 3 – Harmonizing Formulas　　　　　*Section 2 – Liver and Spleen Harmonizing Formulas*

Tòng Xiè Yào Fāng (Important Formula for Painful Diarrhea)

EXPLANATION

Tong Xie Yao Fang (Important Formula for Painful Diarrhea) treats abdominal pain and diarrhea caused by the Liver overacting on the Spleen. The peculiarity of this syndrome is that the abdominal pain may persist after defecation; this is because the pain is not due to retention of food or other substances, and therefore cannot be alleviated by bowel evacuation. Rather, the pain is due to the Liver (excess) overacting on the Spleen (deficiency). Diarrhea is the direct reflection of digestive weakness secondary to an overactive Liver.

This formula contains *Bai Zhu* (Rhizoma Atractylodis Macrocephalae) as the chief herb to tonify the Spleen and dry dampness. *Bai Shao* (Radix Paeoniae Alba), the deputy herb, nourishes the blood and relieves pain by sedating the Liver and softening Liver qi. *Chen Pi* (Pericarpium Citri Reticulatae) regulates qi, dries dampness, awakens the Spleen, and harmonizes the middle *jiao*. *Fang Feng* (Radix Saposhnikoviae) disperses Liver qi to help stop the Liver from overacting on the Spleen, and directs the effects of the formula to the Spleen and Liver.

MODIFICATIONS

- For chronic diarrhea, add dry-fried *Sheng Ma* (Rhizoma Cimicifugae).
- If the diarrhea is caused by indigestion, chronic colitis or irritable bowel, add *Ge Gen* (Radix Puerariae Lobatae), and *Shan Zha* (Fructus Crataegi) and increase the dose of *Fang Feng* (Radix Saposhnikoviae).
- If the diarrhea is caused by acute gastroenteritis, tuberculosis of the colon, acute malaria or dysentery due to amoeba, add *Ge Gen Huang Qin Huang Lian Tang* (Kudzu, Coptis, and Scutellaria Decoction) and *Shan Zha* (Fructus Crataegi).
- If the diarrhea is caused by hyperthyroidism, add *Ge Gen* (Radix Puerariae Lobatae), *Mu Li* (Concha Ostreae), and *Xia Ku Cao* (Spica Prunellae), and increase the dose of

Bai Shao (Radix Paeoniae Alba) and *Fang Feng* (Radix Saposhnikoviae).

- For diarrhea in chronic hepatic diseases, add *Ge Gen* (Radix Puerariae Lobatae), *Shan Zha* (Fructus Crataegi), *Fu Ling* (Poria), and *Yi Yi Ren* (Semen Coicis).
- With chronic enteritis, add *Ge Gen* (Radix Puerariae Lobatae) and *Shan Zha* (Fructus Crataegi).
- When there is yang deficiency and cold, add *Gan Jiang* (Rhizoma Zingiberis) and *Fu Zi* (Radix Aconiti Lateralis Praeparata).
- With a greasy, yellow tongue coating, add *Huang Lian* (Rhizoma Coptidis).

CAUTIONS / CONTRAINDICATIONS

- *Fang Feng* (Radix Saposhnikoviae) is an important herb in this formula that serves two purposes: to disperse Liver qi stagnation and to guide the formula to the Spleen channel. However, its dose must not be arbitrarily increased or its function will shift to an exterior-releasing emphasis.
- Avoid cold, raw, oily or greasy foods while taking *Tong Xie Yao Fang*.[1]

PHARMACOLOGICAL EFFECTS

1. **Gastrointestinal**: This formula had a marked effect on the production of gastric acid in laboratory rats. At 25g/kg and 75g/kg (dose of dried herbs), it reduced gastric acid production by 59.1% and 64.1%, respectively.[2] The use of this formula was also associated with a marked inhibitory effect on intestinal peristalsis in rabbits.[3]
2. **Antibiotic**: This formula was associated with an inhibitory effect against *Bacillus dysenteriae*, *E. coli*, and *Staphylococcus aureus*.

CLINICAL STUDIES AND RESEARCH

1. **Diarrhea**: Use of *Tong Xie Yao Fang* was associated with recovery in 43 of 45 children with diarrhea.[4] Another study reported 93.8% effectiveness using modified *Tong Xie Yao Fang* to treat 32 patients with diarrhea.[5]

Tong Xie Yao Fang (Important Formula for Painful Diarrhea)

Diagnosis	Signs and Symptoms	Treatment	Herbs
Abdominal pain and diarrhea caused by Spleen deficiency and Liver excess	• Borborygmus, diarrhea, and abdominal pain that persists after diarrhea: Liver excess overacting on Spleen deficiency • Thin, white tongue coating and a wiry, moderate pulse: presence of deficient and excess conditions	• Tonifies the Spleen and sedates the Liver • Dispels dampness and stops diarrhea	• *Bai Zhu* (Rhizoma Atractylodis Macrocephalae) tonifies the Spleen and dries dampness. • *Bai Shao* (Radix Paeoniae Alba) nourishes the blood and relieves pain by sedating the Liver and softening Liver qi. • *Chen Pi* (Pericarpium Citri Reticulatae) regulates qi, dries dampness, and harmonizes the Stomach. • *Fang Feng* (Radix Saposhnikoviae) disperses Liver qi to help stop the Liver from overacting on the Spleen.

258

Tòng Xiè Yào Fāng (Important Formula for Painful Diarrhea)

2. **Acute enteritis**: Sixty patients with acute enteritis characterized by severe pain and diarrhea were treated with *Tong Xie Yao Fang* with a 90% overall rate of effectiveness. The patients received 1-2 packs of herbs for treatment. The study reported no side effects in most patients.[6]

3. **Chronic enteritis**: Thirty-five patients with chronic enteritis were treated with modified *Tong Xie Yao Fang* with complete recovery in 28 patients, moderate improvement in 5 patients, and no effect in 2 patients. The herbal treatment contained dry-fried *Bai Shao* (Radix Paeoniae Alba) 20-30g, dry-fried *Bai Zhu* (Rhizoma Atractylodis Macrocephalae) 15g, *Chen Pi* (Pericarpium Citri Reticulatae) 6g, and *Fang Feng* (Radix Saposhnikoviae) 10g. Modification included the addition of *Sheng Ma* (Rhizoma Cimicifugae) 6g for chronic diarrhea; increased dose of *Bai Shao* (Radix Paeoniae Alba), with the addition of *Mu Gua* (Fructus Chaenomelis) 6g, and *Mu Xiang* (Radix Aucklandiae) 6g for severe abdominal pain; and *Dang Shen* (Radix Codonopsis) 10g for fatigue.[7]

4. **Chronic colitis**: Twenty patients with chronic colitis were treated with modified *Tong Xie Yao Fang* for one and a half months with marked improvement in 14 patients, moderate improvement in 4 patients, and no effect in 2 patients. The treatment included *Fang Feng* (Radix Saposhnikoviae), *Bai Zhu* (Rhizoma Atractylodis Macrocephalae), *Chen Pi* (Pericarpium Citri Reticulatae), *Bai Shao* (Radix Paeoniae Alba), *Wu Mei* (Fructus Mume), *Mu Gua* (Fructus Chaenomelis), *Dang Shen* (Radix Codonopsis), *Shan Yao* (Rhizoma Dioscoreae), and *Shan Zha* (Fructus Crataegi).[8] Another study reported 93.55% effectiveness using modified *Tong Xie Yao Fang* to treat 124 patients with chronic colitis (25 with complete recovery, 68 with significant improvement, and 23 with moderate improvement). The herbal formula contained *Yi Yi Ren* (Semen Coicis) 20g, *Che Qian Zi* (Semen Plantaginis) 20g, *Huang Qi* (Radix Astragali) 15g, *Bai Jiang Cao* (Herba cum Radice Patriniae) 15g, *Bai Zhi* (Radix Angelicae Dahuricae) 15g, dry-fried *Bai Shao* (Radix Paeoniae Alba) 12g, *Hou Po* (Cortex Magnoliae Officinalis) 12g, *Fang Feng* (Radix Saposhnikoviae) 3g, *Bai Zhu* (Rhizoma Atractylodis Macrocephalae) 10g, *Ku Shen* (Radix Sophorae Flavescentis) 10g, dry-fried *Cang Zhu* (Rhizoma Atractylodis) 10g, *Mu Xiang* (Radix Aucklandiae) 5g, *Chen Pi* (Pericarpium Citri Reticulatae) 6g, and *Chai Hu* (Radix Bupleuri) 6g. The patients were given the herbs in decoction for 2 weeks per course of treatment, with duration of 1-6 courses total.[9]

5. **Ulcerative colitis**: Thirty-five patients with ulcerative colitis were treated with modified *Tong Xie Yao Fang* for 20 days with marked improvement in 30 patients and moderate improvement in 5 patients. The formula included *Bai Zhu* (Rhizoma Atractylodis Macrocephalae), *Bai Shao* (Radix Paeoniae Alba), *Chen Pi* (Pericarpium Citri Reticulatae), *Fang Feng* (Radix Saposhnikoviae), *Sheng Ma* (Rhizoma Cimicifugae), *Qin Pi* (Cortex Fraxini), and *Chi Shi Zhi* (Halloysitum Rubrum).[10] Another study reported 93.5% effectiveness for treatment of chronic colitis using *Tong Xie Yao Fang* plus *Shan Yao* (Rhizoma Dioscoreae), *Gu Ya* (Fructus Setariae Germinatus), *Mai Ya* (Fructus Hordei Germinatus), and other herbs as deemed necessary. Modifications included the addition of *Yan Hu Suo* (Rhizoma Corydalis) and a larger dose of *Bai Shao* (Radix Paeoniae Alba) for severe abdominal pain; *Mu Xiang* (Radix Aucklandiae), *Zhi Qiao* (Fructus Aurantii), and *Hou Po* (Cortex Magnoliae Officinalis) for Liver qi stagnation; *Chuan Lian Zi* (Fructus Toosendan) for qi stagnation turning into fire; *Da Huang* (Radix et Rhizoma Rhei), *Bing Lang* (Semen Arecae) and *Huang Lian* (Rhizoma Coptidis) for dampness in the Intestines; *Dang Shen* (Radix Codonopsis), *Huang Qi* (Radix Astragali) and *Yi Yi Ren* (Semen Coicis) for Spleen and qi deficiency; and *Si Shen Wan* (Four-Miracle Pill) for Spleen and Kidney deficiencies. Of 32 patients, the study reported complete recovery in 21 patients, improvement in 9 patients, and no benefit in 2 patients.[11]

6. **Irritable bowel syndrome (IBS)**: *Tong Xie Yao Fang* has been shown in many studies to effectively treat IBS. Fifty patients with IBS were treated with modified *Tong Xie Yao Fang* with complete recovery in 35 patients. The average length of treatment was 28.4 days, with a range of 23 to 120 days. Fifteen patients discontinued the treatment due to various reasons, with most showing some indications of improvement.[12] Another study reported 89.9% effectiveness using *Tong Xie Yao Fang* plus *Si Shen Wan* (Four-Miracle Pill) to treat 187 patients with IBS.[13] Lastly, one study reported 93.3% effectiveness using modified *Tong Xie Yao Fang* to treat 30 patients with IBS. The herbal treatment used *Tong Xie Yao Fang* as the base, with the addition of *Sheng Ma* (Rhizoma Cimicifugae) and *Chi Shi Zhi* (Halloysitum Rubrum) for chronic diarrhea; *Bu Gu Zhi* (Fructus Psoraleae) and *Rou Gui* (Cortex Cinnamomi) for Spleen and Kidney yang deficiencies; and *Chai Hu* (Radix Bupleuri) and *Dang Gui* (Radix Angelicae Sinensis) for Liver qi stagnation with blood deficiency. Each course of treatment lasted 1 month. Of 30 patients, the study reported significant improvement in 9 patients, improvement in 19 patients, and no improvement in 2 patients.[14]

AUTHORS' COMMENTS

Tong Xie Yao Fang was originally called *Bai Zhu Shao Yao San* (Atractylodes Macrocephala and Peony Powder), with the understanding that this was an "important formula for painful diarrhea," and that abdominal

Chapter 3 – Harmonizing Formulas   *Section 2 – Liver and Spleen Harmonizing Formulas*

Tòng Xiè Yào Fāng (Important Formula for Painful Diarrhea)

pain may persist after defecation. *Tong Xie Yao Fang* eventually became the "official" name of this formula, however, since this name meaningfully incorporates its primary function. Today, *Tong Xie Yao Fang* is commonly used as a foundational formula for treating various types of diarrhea.

Tong Xie Yao Fang treats abdominal pain and diarrhea caused by Spleen deficiency and Liver excess. Its formulation has a distinct rationale:

- *Bai Zhu* (Rhizoma Atractylodis Macrocephalae) and *Chen Pi* (Pericarpium Citri Reticulatae) strengthen the Spleen, dry dampness, and promote qi circulation. This formula does not use standard qi tonics, such as *Ren Shen* (Radix et Rhizoma Ginseng) and *Huang Qi* (Radix Astragali), because such herbs tonify qi and raise yang qi, but do not dry dampness and restore the normal transformation and transportation functions of the Spleen.
- *Fang Feng* (Radix Saposhnikoviae) is acrid, spreads Liver qi stagnation, awakens the Spleen, and dries dampness. It enters both the Liver and Spleen channels, raises yang, and stops diarrhea. When paired with *Bai Shao* (Radix Paeoniae Alba), it regulates Liver qi and relieves pain. When combined with *Bai Zhu* (Rhizoma Atractylodis Macrocephalae), it strengthens the Spleen and dispels dampness. *Chai Hu* (Radix Bupleuri), a standard Liver qi-regulating herb, is not used here because it does not strengthen the Spleen. In addition, *Chai Hu* (Radix Bupleuri) is slightly drying in nature, and may injure yin and contribute to more deficiency.[15]

Si Shen Wan (Four-Miracle Pill), *Shen Ling Bai Zhu San* (Ginseng, Poria, and Atractylodes Macrocephala Powder), and *Tong Xie Yao Fang* all treat diarrhea.

- *Si Shen Wan* warms and tonifies Spleen and Kidney yang to stop chronic diarrhea. It treats severe diarrhea that occurs in the early morning, and watery diarrhea that contains undigested food.

- *Shen Ling Bai Zhu San* treats diarrhea characterized by Spleen qi deficiency with damp accumulation, manifesting in fatigue, weakness of the limbs, and poor appetite.
- *Tong Xie Yao Fang* tonifies the Spleen and spreads Liver qi. This formula stops the type of diarrhea that accompanies stress-related abdominal pain. Patients will often complain of gas, bloating, or abdominal pain that is not relieved with diarrhea.[16]

References

1. *Zhong Yao Ming Fang Yao Li Yu Ying Yong* (Pharmacology and Applications of Famous Herbal Formulas) 1989;119-120.
2. *Zhong Yao Yao Li Yu Lin Chuang* (Pharmacology and Clinical Applications of Chinese Herbs) 1992;8:20.
3. *Hu Nan Zhong Yi Xue Yuan Xue Bao* (Journal of Hunan University of Traditional Chinese Medicine) 1987;7:42.
4. *Yun Nan Zhong Yi Za Zhi* (Yunan Journal of Chinese Medicine) 1986;4:24.
5. *Gan Su Zhong Yi* (Gansu Chinese Medicine) 1996;6:21.
6. *Ha Er Bing Zhong Yi* (Haerbing Chinese Medicine) 1964;4:25.
7. *Hu Nan Zhong Yi Za Zhi* (Hunan Journal of Chinese Medicine) 1987;6:12.
8. *Zhong Guo Gang Chang Za Zhi* (Chinese Journal of Anus and Intestines) 1987;4:27.
9. *Shan Xi Zhong Yi* (Shanxi Chinese Medicine) 1989;11:490.
10. *Hu Nan Zhong Yi Za Zhi* (Hunan Journal of Chinese Medicine) 1988;6:36.
11. *Shan Dong Zhong Yi Za Zhi* (Shandong Journal of Chinese Medicine) 1996;10:444.
12. *Shi Yong Zhong Yi Nei Ke Za Zhi* (Journal of Practical Chinese Internal Medicine) 1991;4:90.
13. *Hei Long Jiang Zhong Yi Yao* (Heilongjiang Chinese Medicine and Herbology) 1986;6:23.
14. *Zhe Jiang Zhong Yi Za Zhi* (Zhejiang Journal of Chinese Medicine) 1996;11:502.
15. Wang MZ, et al. *Zhong Yi Xue Wen Da Ti Ku* (Questions and Answers on Traditional Chinese Medicine: Herbal Formulas).
16. Wang MZ, et al. *Zhong Yi Xue Wen Da Ti Ku* (Questions and Answers on Traditional Chinese Medicine: Herbal Formulas).

Section 3

调和肠胃剂

— Intestines and Stomach Harmonizing Formulas

Bàn Xià Xiè Xīn Tāng (Pinellia Decoction to Drain the Epigastrium)

半夏瀉心湯
半夏泻心汤

Pinyin Name: *Ban Xia Xie Xin Tang*
Literal Name: Pinellia Decoction to Drain the Epigastrium
Alternate Names: *Pan Hsia Hsieh Hsin Tang, Ban Xia Xieh Xin Tang*, Pinellia Heart-Draining Decoction, Pinellia Combination
Original Source: *Shang Han Lun* (Discussion of Cold-Induced Disorders) by Zhang Zhong-Jing in the Eastern Han Dynasty

COMPOSITION

Ban Xia (Rhizoma Pinelliae), *xi* (washed)	0.5 cup [9g]
Gan Jiang (Rhizoma Zingiberis)	9g
Huang Qin (Radix Scutellariae)	9g
Huang Lian (Rhizoma Coptidis)	3g
Ren Shen (Radix et Rhizoma Ginseng)	9g
Da Zao (Fructus Jujubae), *bo* (opened)	12 pieces [4 pieces]
Zhi Gan Cao (Radix et Rhizoma Glycyrrhizae Praeparata cum Melle)	9g [6g]

Note: "*Xie xin*" literally means to "drain the Heart." However, the term is really used to indicate draining the area beneath the Heart, namely the epigastrium. Therefore, the literal name of the formula has been modified to reflect its actual applications.

DOSAGE / PREPARATION / ADMINISTRATION

The source text advises to cook the ingredients in 10 cups [2,000 mL] of water until 6 cups [1,200 mL] of liquid remain. Discard the residue, and cook the strained decoction again until it is reduced to 3 cups [600 mL]. Take 1 cup [200 mL] of the warm decoction three times daily. Today, the decoction may be prepared using the doses suggested in brackets.

CHINESE THERAPEUTIC ACTIONS

1. Harmonizes the Stomach and corrects the reversed flow of qi
2. Disperses the interlocking of heat and cold and relieves epigastric distention

CLINICAL MANIFESTATIONS

Stomach qi disharmony: epigastric fullness and distention without pain, dry heaves, vomiting with or without vomitus, borborygmus, diarrhea, a thin, yellow and greasy tongue coating, and a wiry, rapid pulse.

CLINICAL APPLICATIONS

Superficial gastritis, chronic gastritis, atrophic gastritis, gastritis, gastrectasis, peptic ulcer disease, hypersecretion of gastric acid, reflux esophagitis, stomatitis, upper gastrointestinal bleeding, gastroptosis, gastroenteritis, stomach pain, abdominal pain, irritable bowel syndrome, ulcerative colitis, diarrhea, nausea and vomiting due to motion sickness or pregnancy, infantile indigestion, cholecystitis and cholelithiasis, chronic hepatitis, liver cirrhosis, renal failure, stress, and depression.

EXPLANATION

Ban Xia Xie Xin Tang (Pinellia Decoction to Drain the Epigastrium), first cited in *Shang Han Lun* (Discussion of Cold-Induced Disorders), is designed to correct the improper treatment of *shaoyang* syndrome with downward

261

Bàn Xià Xiè Xīn Tāng (Pinellia Decoction to Drain the Epigastrium)

Ban Xia Xie Xin Tang (Pinellia Decoction to Drain the Epigastrium)

Diagnosis	Signs and Symptoms	Treatment	Herbs
Stomach qi disharmony	• Epigastric fullness and distention, borborygmus, diarrhea and vomiting: disharmony of the Stomach and Intestines with interlocking of heat and cold • Thin, yellow tongue coating: heat condition • Greasy tongue coating: damp accumulation • Wiry pulse: qi stagnation • Rapid pulse: interior heat	• Harmonizes the Stomach and corrects the reversed flow of qi • Disperses the interlocking of heat and cold and relieves epigastric distention	• *Ban Xia* (Rhizoma Pinelliae) disperses stagnation, relieves distention, directs reversed Stomach qi downward. • *Gan Jiang* (Rhizoma Zingiberis) warms the middle *jiao* and disperses cold accumulation. • *Huang Qin* (Radix Scutellariae) and *Huang Lian* (Rhizoma Coptidis) sedate heat and relieve distention. • *Ren Shen* (Radix et Rhizoma Ginseng), *Da Zao* (Fructus Jujubae) and *Zhi Gan Cao* (Radix et Rhizoma Glycyrrhizae Praeparata cum Melle) tonify the middle *jiao* and strengthen the Spleen.

draining herbs, which results in injury to the yang qi of the middle *jiao* and the drawing of exterior pathogens into the interior. By this stage of the improper treatment, heat usually forms in the interior, resulting in the interlocking of heat and cold factors. The interlocking of heat and cold affects the normal ascending functioning of the Spleen and the descending functioning of the Stomach, causing borborygmus, diarrhea, and vomiting. It also creates a feeling of epigastric distention that is not painful and is soft on palpation.

The thin, yellow tongue coating suggests heat formation inside the body, and the greasy nature of the coating is the result of qi stagnation and damp accumulation. A wiry pulse is the result of epigastric distention and qi stagnation, and a rapid pulse indicates interior heat. This condition involves simultaneous excess and deficiency, heat and cold.

The chief herb, *Ban Xia* (Rhizoma Pinelliae), disperses stagnation, relieves distention, and directs reversed Stomach qi downward to relieve nausea and vomiting. The assistant herb, *Gan Jiang* (Rhizoma Zingiberis), warms the middle *jiao* and disperses cold accumulation. *Huang Qin* (Radix Scutellariae) and *Huang Lian* (Rhizoma Coptidis) sedate heat and relieve distention. *Ren Shen* (Radix et Rhizoma Ginseng), *Da Zao* (Fructus Jujubae), and *Zhi Gan Cao* (Radix et Rhizoma Glycyrrhizae Praeparata cum Melle) tonify the middle *jiao* and strengthen the Spleen. *Zhi Gan Cao* also harmonizes the warm and cold properties of the other herbs in this formula. This formula simultaneously disperses and directs downward, tonifies and sedates, clears heat, and warms the interior to restore the proper functioning of the Spleen and Stomach.

MODIFICATIONS

• If there is a feeling of fullness and oppression in the chest and hypochondriac region, add *Zhi Shi* (Fructus Aurantii Immaturus) and *Jie Geng* (Radix Platycodonis).
• For diarrhea and abdominal pain, add *Mu Xiang* (Radix Aucklandiae) and *Bai Shao* (Radix Paeoniae Alba).
• With vomiting and belching, add *Chen Pi* (Pericarpium Citri Reticulatae) and *Fu Ling* (Poria).
• With vomiting and epigastric pain, combine with *San Huang Xie Xin Tang* (Three-Yellow Decoction to Sedate the Epigastrium).
• With vomiting and phlegm accumulation, combine with *Er Chen Tang* (Two-Cured Decoction).
• With vomiting of food particles, combine with *Ping Wei San* (Calm the Stomach Powder).
• When there is food stagnation, add charred *Shan Zha* (Fructus Crataegi) and *Shen Qu* (Massa Fermentata).
• If the tongue coating is thick, add *Hou Po* (Cortex Magnoliae Officinalis) and *Cang Zhu* (Rhizoma Atractylodis).
• If there is more deficiency, increase the dose of *Ren Shen* (Radix et Rhizoma Ginseng).

CAUTIONS / CONTRAINDICATIONS

• *Ban Xia Xie Xin Tang* is not suitable for epigastric distention and fullness or pain caused by accumulation of phlegm and heat, food stagnation, or qi stagnation.
• This formula should not be used in patients of nausea and vomiting caused by yin deficiency.[1]

PHARMACOLOGICAL EFFECTS

1. **Gastrointestinal**: *Ban Xia Xie Xin Tang* has been used to treat various types of gastrointestinal disorders. It has effects to normalize the upper and lower gastrointestinal system by raising the plasma levels of some hormones (somatostatin, motilin, and gastrin).[2]

262

Bàn Xià Xiè Xīn Tāng (Pinellia Decoction to Drain the Epigastrium)

Chinese Herbal Formulas and Applications

2. **Antiulcer**: Administration of the formula was associated with protective effects in rats with gastric or duodenal ulcer, especially against ethanol-induced gastric injury. The mechanism of the protective effect was attributed to the strengthening and regeneration of the gastric membrane and the increase in gastric mucin content.[3,4,5] In addition, the alcohol extract of the formula inhibits intestinal peristalsis in mice.[6]

3. **Analgesic**: Administration of an alcohol extract of this formula at 10 g/kg was associated with analgesic effects in mice.[7]

CLINICAL STUDIES AND RESEARCH

1. **Gastritis**: Modified *Ban Xia Xie Xin Tang* demonstrated 92.3% effectiveness in treating gastritis caused by bile acid regurgitation. The herbal treatment used *Ban Xia Xie Xin Tang* as the base formula, with elimination of *Da Zao* (Fructus Jujubae), substitution of *Tai Zi Shen* (Radix Pseudostellariae) for *Ren Shen* (Radix et Rhizoma Ginseng), and the addition of *Bai Shao* (Radix Paeoniae Alba) and *Zhi Qiao* (Fructus Aurantii). Furthermore, *Bai Zhu* (Rhizoma Atractylodis Macrocephalae) and *Fu Ling* (Poria) were added for poor appetite; *Shen Qu* (Massa Fermentata) and *Zhe Shi* (Haematitum) for frequent belching; *Qing Pi* (Pericarpium Citri Reticulatae Viride) for pain with needling sensations; substitution of *Pao Jiang* (Rhizoma Zingiberis Praeparatum) for *Gan Jiang* (Rhizoma Zingiberis) for loose stools; *Bai He* (Bulbus Lilii) for fatigue and shortness of breath; and addition of *Fu Zi* (Radix Aconiti Lateralis Praeparata) and removal of *Ban Xia* (Rhizoma Pinelliae), *Tai Zi Shen* (Radix Pseudostellariae), and *Gan Jiang* (Rhizoma Zingiberis) for pain, perspiration and chills. Of 52 patients, the study reported complete recovery in 16 patients, marked improvement in 18 patients, moderate improvement in 14 patients, and no improvement in 4 patients.[8]

2. **Superficial gastritis**: Thirty patients with superficial gastritis were treated with modified *Ban Xia Xie Xin Tang* with 90% effectiveness. The formula included *Ban Xia* (Rhizoma Pinelliae) 9g, *Huang Lian* (Rhizoma Coptidis) 9g, *Huang Qin* (Radix Scutellariae) 9g, *Wu Ling Zhi* (Faeces Trogopteri) 4.5g, *Pu Huang* (Pollen Typhae) 4.5g, *Gan Jiang* (Rhizoma Zingiberis) 6g, *Hou Po* (Cortex Magnoliae Officinalis) 6g, *Shi Chang Pu* (Rhizoma Acori Tatarinowii) 6g, *Dang Shen* (Radix Codonopsis) 15g, *Long Kui* (Herba Solanum Nigrum) 15g, *Dan Shen* (Radix et Rhizoma Salviae Miltiorrhizae) 15g, *Da Zao* (Fructus Jujubae) 5 pieces, and *Gan Cao* (Radix et Rhizoma Glycyrrhizae) 3g.[9] Another study reported 95% effectiveness in treating superficial gastritis in 60 patients using *Ban Xia Xie Xin Tang* plus *Yan Hu Suo* (Rhizoma Corydalis), *Mu Xiang* (Radix Aucklandiae), *Chai Hu* (Radix Bupleuri), *Wu Zhu Yu* (Fructus Evodiae), *Pei Lan* (Herba Eupatorii), charred *Shan Zha* (Fructus Crataegi), charred *Shen Qu* (Massa Fermentata), and charred *Mai Ya* (Fructus Hordei Germinatus).[10]

3. **Chronic gastritis**: Use of modified *Ban Xia Xie Xin Tang* was associated with 92.31% effectiveness in treating 52 patients with chronic gastritis. In addition to the formula, modifications included the addition of *Zhi Shi* (Fructus Aurantii Immaturus) and *Hou Po* (Cortex Magnoliae Officinalis) for gastric fullness and distention; *Zhu Ru* (Caulis Bambusae in Taenia) and *Chen Pi* (Pericarpium Citri Reticulatae) for nausea and vomiting; *Bai Zhu* (Rhizoma Atractylodis Macrocephalae) and *Fu Ling* (Poria) for loose stools; *Di Huang* (Radix Rehmanniae) and *Hei Zhi Ma* (Semen Sesami Nigrum) for dry stools; *Yan Hu Suo* (Rhizoma Corydalis) for epigastric pain; *Hai Piao Xiao* (Endoconcha Sepiae) and calcined *Wa Leng Zi* (Concha Arcae) for acid reflux; *Long Dan* (Radix et Rhizoma Gentianae) for bitter taste in the mouth; *Ji Nei Jin* (Endothelium Corneum Gigeriae Galli) and *Shen Qu* (Massa Fermentata) for poor appetite; and *Huang Qi* (Radix Astragali) for fatigue. Of 52 patients, 18 had complete recovery, 30 had marked improvement, and 4 had no improvement.[11]

4. **Atrophic gastritis**: Forty-nine patients with atrophic gastritis were diagnosed with Spleen and Stomach deficiencies and dampness with cold or heat. The patients were treated with modified *Ban Xia Xie Xin Tang* with marked improvement in 32 patients, moderate improvement in 16 patients and no benefit in one patient. The herbal treatment included the original formula with the addition of *Pu Gong Ying* (Herba Taraxaci), *Dan Shen* (Radix et Rhizoma Salviae Miltiorrhizae), and *Bai Shao* (Radix Paeoniae Alba).[12]

5. **Peptic ulcer disease**: One study reported marked success using modified *Ban Xia Xie Xin Tang* to treat peptic ulcer disease in 32 patients (18 with gastric and 14 with duodenal ulcers). In addition to the base formula, modifications included the addition of *Pao Jiang* (Rhizoma Zingiberis Praeparatum) to replace *Gan Jiang* (Rhizoma Zingiberis) in patients with bleeding; *Pao Jiang* (Rhizoma Zingiberis Praeparatum) and *Xiao Ji* (Herba Cirsii) for hematemesis; *Pao Jiang* (Rhizoma Zingiberis Praeparatum), *Xiao Ji* (Herba Cirsii), and *E Jiao* (Colla Corii Asini) for hematochezia; *Pao Jiang* (Rhizoma Zingiberis Praeparatum), *Xiao Ji* (Herba Cirsii), *E Jiao* (Colla Corii Asini) and *Bai Ji* (Rhizoma Bletillae) for hematochezia and hematemesis; and *Yan Hu Suo* (Rhizoma Corydalis) for abdominal pain. Of 32 patients, bleeding stopped in 21 patients after 4 packs of herbs, in 7 patients after 6 packs of herbs, and in 4 patients after 10 packs of herbs.[13]

Bàn Xià Xiè Xīn Tāng (Pinellia Decoction to Drain the Epigastrium)

6. **Reflux esophagitis**: An herbal formula that contained *Ban Xia Xie Xin Tang* plus *Zhu Ru* (Caulis Bambusae in Taenia), *Chen Xiang* (Lignum Aquilariae Resinatum) and *Zi Su Geng* (Caulis Perillae) was found to have good effect in treating 46 patients with reflux esophagitis. In addition to the base formula above, minor modifications were made by adding *Bai Shao* (Radix Paeoniae Alba) and *Wei Ling Xian* (Radix et Rhizoma Clematidis) for severe pain with difficulty swallowing; *Hai Piao Xiao* (Endoconcha Sepiae) and calcined *Wa Leng Zi* (Concha Arcae) for hyperacidity or duodenal ulcer; *Pu Gong Ying* (Herba Taraxaci) and *Zhi Zi* (Fructus Gardeniae) for burning in the stomach; *Chai Hu* (Radix Bupleuri) and *Jin Qian Cao* (Herba Lysimachiae) for cholecystitis or hypochondriac pain; and *Da Huang* (Radix et Rhizoma Rhei) and *Zhi Shi* (Fructus Aurantii Immaturus) for constipation. Of 46 patients, 8 had complete recovery, 34 had marked improvement, and 4 had no effect. The overall effectiveness was 91.3%.[14]

7. **Upper gastrointestinal bleeding**: According to one study, 39 patients with upper gastrointestinal bleeding were successfully treated with modified *Ban Xia Xie Xin Tang*. The average time needed to completely stop bleeding was 4.3 days, with a range of 3-6 days. The herbal treatment included the original formula with the addition of *Hua Rui Shi* (Ophicalcitum) 12g, *Ou Jie* (Nodus Nelumbinis Rhizomatis) 15g, and *Bai Ji* (Rhizoma Bletillae) 15g. Furthermore, *Mu Dan Pi* (Cortex Moutan), *Huang Qi* (Radix Astragali), *Dang Gui* (Radix Angelicae Sinensis), *Sha Shen* (Radix Glehniae seu Adenophorae), *Yu Zhu* (Rhizoma Polygonati Odorati), and others were added as needed.[15]

8. **Morning sickness**: In one report, 25 pregnant women with nausea and vomiting were treated with *Ban Xia Xie Xin Tang* for 6 doses with complete relief in 19 patients, and significant improvement in 6 patients.[16] In another report, 13 pregnant women with nausea and vomiting were treated with *Ban Xia Xie Xin Tang* plus *Zhu Ru* (Caulis Bambusae in Taenia) 15g. The study reported complete relief in 6 patients after 4 doses, and 7 patients after 6 doses.[17]

9. **Infantile indigestion**: Fifty-two infants with indigestion due to various reasons were treated with modified *Ban Xia Xie Xin Tang* with complete recovery in 1 to 4 doses. The base formula included *Ban Xia* (Rhizoma Pinelliae) 2g, *Huang Qin* (Radix Scutellariae) 2g, *Gan Jiang* (Rhizoma Zingiberis) 2g, *Dang Shen* (Radix Codonopsis) 2g, *Ge Gen* (Radix Puerariae Lobatae) 2g, *Fu Ling* (Poria) 2g, *Che Qian Zi* (Semen Plantaginis) 2g, *Huang Lian* (Rhizoma Coptidis) 1g, *Zhi Gan Cao* (Radix et Rhizoma Glycyrrhizae Praeparata cum Melle) 1g, and *Da Zao* (Fructus Jujubae) 6 pieces. Moreover, the following modifications were made: *Xuan Fu Hua* (Flos Inulae) 2g for severe nausea and vomiting; *Bai Zhu* (Rhizoma Atractylodis Macrocephalae) 3g, *Shan Yao* (Rhizoma Dioscoreae) 3g and *Qin Pi* (Cortex Fraxini) 2g for severe diarrhea; and charred *Shan Zha* (Fructus Crataegi) 2g, charred *Shen Qu* (Massa Fermentata) 2g and charred *Mai Ya* (Fructus Hordei Germinatus) 2g for food stagnation.[18]

10. **Gastroptosis**: One study reported 84.1% effectiveness using *Ban Xia Xie Xin Tang* plus *San Qi* (Radix et Rhizoma Notoginseng), *Huang Qi* (Radix Astragali), and *Sheng Ma* (Rhizoma Cimicifugae) to treat 38 patients with stomach prolapse characterized by Spleen deficiency and qi collapse (30 patients) and Stomach yin deficiency (8 patients). In addition to the base formula above, modifications were made by adding *Mai Ya* (Fructus Hordei Germinatus) and *Ji Nei Jin* (Endothelium Corneum Gigeriae Galli) for poor appetite; and *Sha Shen* (Radix Glehniae seu Adenophorae), *Mai Dong* (Radix Ophiopogonis), *Yu Zhu* (Rhizoma Polygonati Odorati), and *Di Huang* (Radix Rehmanniae) for Stomach yin deficiency. Of 38 patients, the study reported a marked effect in 20 patients, moderate effect in 12 patients, and no benefit in 6 patients.[19]

11. **Gastroenteritis**: One study reported good results using modified *Ban Xia Xie Xin Tang* to treat acute gastroenteritis. In addition to the base formula, modifications were made as follows: double the dose of *Huang Lian* (Rhizoma Coptidis) if there are more than five bowel movements (diarrhea) per day; *Ge Gen* (Radix Puerariae Lobatae) for presence of excessive heat; *Sheng Jiang* (Rhizoma Zingiberis Recens) for nausea, vomiting, or feeling of coldness in the abdomen; and *Mu Xiang* (Radix Aucklandiae) for abdominal fullness. Of 100 patients, 78 had complete recovery, 14 had improvement, and 8 had no effect. The overall rate of effectiveness was 92%.[20]

12. **Stomach pain**: One study reported 94% effectiveness using this formula to treat 100 geriatric patients (ages 60 and over) with stomach pain caused by gastritis, stomach ulcer and duodenal ulcer.[21] In another study, 294 of 300 patients with stomach pain (caused by gastritis, or gastric or duodenal ulcers) had complete recovery using modified *Ban Xia Xie Xin Tang*.[22]

13. **Abdominal pain**: Use of *Ban Xia Xie Xin Tang* plus *Yan Hu Suo* (Rhizoma Corydalis), *Zhi Qiao* (Fructus Aurantii), and others to treat 36 children with abdominal pain was associated with complete recovery in 34 patients and improvement in 2 patients. The overall rate of effectiveness was 94.4%.[23]

14. **Irritable bowel syndrome (IBS)**: Administration of *Ban Xia Xie Xin Tang* plus *Chai Hu* (Radix Bupleuri), *Mu Xiang* (Radix Aucklandiae), *Bai Shao* (Radix Paeoniae Alba), and *Yan Hu Suo* (Rhizoma Corydalis) daily for 4 weeks in 37 patients with IBS was associated with

Bàn Xià Xiè Xīn Tāng (Pinellia Decoction to Drain the Epigastrium)

complete recovery in 25 patients, improvement in 8 patients, and no effect in 4 patients. The overall effectiveness was 89.19%.[24] According to another study, 56 patients with IBS were treated with complete recovery in 35 patients (62.5%), improvement in 17 patients (30.36%), and no effect in 4 patients (7.14%). The herbal formula contained *Ban Xia Xie Xin Tang* plus *Bai Zhu* (Rhizoma Atractylodis Macrocephalae), *Mu Xiang* (Radix Aucklandiae) and *Bai Shao* (Radix Paeoniae Alba) as the base formula. Additional modifications included *Che Qian Zi* (Semen Plantaginis), *Bian Dou Yi* (Pericarpium Lablab Album), *Zhu Ling* (Polyporus) and *Ze Xie* (Rhizoma Alismatis) for loose stools; *Bai Tou Weng* (Radix Pulsatillae) and *Huang Bo* (Cortex Phellodendri Chinensis) for sticky stools with mucus; *Da Huang* (Radix et Rhizoma Rhei) for constipation; *Yi Yi Ren* (Semen Coicis) and *Huo Xiang* (Herba Agastaches) for dampness; *Bu Gu Zhi* (Fructus Psoraleae) for yang deficiency; *Sheng Jiang* (Rhizoma Zingiberis Recens) and *Zhu Ru* (Caulis Bambusae in Taenia) for nausea and vomiting; and the addition of *Hou Po* (Cortex Magnoliae Officinalis) and *Zhi Shi* (Fructus Aurantii Immaturus), and elimination of *Dang Shen* (Radix Codonopsis), *Bai Zhu* (Rhizoma Atractylodis Macrocephalae), and *Da Zao* (Fructus Jujubae) for abdominal distention, borborygmus, and pain that intensifies with pressure.[25]

15. **Ulcerative colitis**: Use of modified *Ban Xia Xie Xin Tang* was associated with 96.9% effectiveness in treating 33 patients with chronic ulcerative colitis. The base herbal formula contained this formula without *Da Zao* (Fructus Jujubae), and with the addition of *Da Huang* (Radix et Rhizoma Rhei). Furthermore, modifications based on individual conditions were made by adding *Mu Xiang* (Radix Aucklandiae), *Bai Shao* (Radix Paeoniae Alba), and *Dang Gui* (Radix Angelicae Sinensis) for abdominal pain; charred *Mu Dan Pi* (Cortex Moutan), charred *Di Huang* (Radix Rehmanniae), and charred *Huai Hua* (Flos Sophorae) for hematochezia; *Yi Yi Ren* (Semen Coicis) and *Ma Chi Xian* (Herba Portulacae) for severe diarrhea; *Sheng Ma* (Rhizoma Cimicifugae) for rectal tenesmus; *Chai Hu* (Radix Bupleuri) and *Zhi Qiao* (Fructus Aurantii) for hypochondriac fullness and pain; and the removal of *Huang Lian* (Rhizoma Coptidis) and the addition of *Bu Gu Zhi* (Fructus Psoraleae) and *Rou Gui* (Cortex Cinnamomi) for chronic diarrhea with soreness and coldness of the lower back and knees. Of 33 patients, 17 had complete recovery, 8 had marked improvement, 7 had moderate improvement, and 1 had no improvement.[26]

16. **Diarrhea**: Administration of 1 pack of *Ban Xia Xie Xin Tang* was effective in treating 20 of 25 patients with acute onset of diarrhea characterized by the presence of severe diarrhea, feeling of distention and oppression, and vomiting.[27]

17. **Cholecystitis and cholelithiasis**: Administration of modified *Ban Xia Xie Xin Tang* in 42 patients with chronic cholecystitis and cholelithiasis was associated with significant improvement in 25 patients, moderate improvement in 13 patients, and no improvement in 4 patients. The base formula included *Ban Xia Xie Xin Tang*, with the addition of *Hai Jin Sha* (Spora Lygodii), *Jin Qian Cao* (Herba Lysimachiae), and *Ji Nei Jin* (Endothelium Corneum Gigeriae Galli), and elimination of *Da Zao* (Fructus Jujubae). Furthermore, *Huang Qi* (Radix Astragali), *Bai Zhu* (Rhizoma Atractylodis Macrocephalae), and *Fu Ling* (Poria) were added for qi deficiency; *Da Huang* (Radix et Rhizoma Rhei) for constipation; and the addition of *Chuan Lian Zi* (Fructus Toosendan), *Pu Gong Ying* (Herba Taraxaci), *Hu Zhang* (Rhizoma et Radix Polygoni Cuspidati), and *Yin Chen* (Herba Artemisiae Scopariae) and elimination of *Dang Shen* (Radix Codonopsis) and *Gan Cao* (Radix et Rhizoma Glycyrrhizae) for a yellow, greasy tongue coating with a bitter taste in the mouth.[28]

18. **Hepatitis**: Administration of an herbal formula in 81 patients with chronic active hepatitis was associated with complete recovery in 46 patients (resolution of all symptoms and normalization of liver enzymes), improvement in 19 patients (improvement of symptoms and reduction of liver enzyme levels by 30% or more), and no effect in 16 patients. The herbal treatment contained *Ban Xia Xie Xin Tang* plus *Cang Zhu* (Rhizoma Atractylodis), *Bai Zhu* (Rhizoma Atractylodis Macrocephalae), *Fu Ling* (Poria), and *Yin Chen* (Herba Artemisiae Scopariae) as the base formula. Furthermore, *Zhi Zi* (Fructus Gardeniae) and *Che Qian Cao* (Herba Plantaginis) were added for dry mouth, yellow, greasy tongue coating, and yellow urine; *Hou Po* (Cortex Magnoliae Officinalis) and *Ji Nei Jin* (Endothelium Corneum Gigeriae Galli) for abdominal fullness and distention; *Di Huang* (Radix Rehmanniae), *Gou Qi Zi* (Fructus Lycii), and *Mai Dong* (Radix Ophiopogonis) for soreness and weakness of the lower back and knees; and *Yan Hu Suo* (Rhizoma Corydalis) and *Xiang Fu* (Rhizoma Cyperi) for hypochondriac fullness and pain.[29]

19. **Renal failure**: Fifty patients with chronic renal failure due to various causes showed improvement when treated with *Ban Xia Xie Xin Tang* plus *Fu Zi* (Radix Aconiti Lateralis Praeparata), *Rou Gui* (Cortex Cinnamomi), *Bai Zhu* (Rhizoma Atractylodis Macrocephalae), *Fu Ling* (Poria), and *Ze Xie* (Rhizoma Alismatis) as the base formula.[30]

20. **Stress and depression**: One study evaluated the clinical usefulness of herbal formulas in treating stress and depression by examining the modulatory effects of the

Bàn Xià Xiè Xīn Tāng (Pinellia Decoction to Drain the Epigastrium)

herbs on the hypothalamo-pituitary-adrenal axis and autonomic nervous function. Of several formulas tested, three were found to be effective on plasma ACTH and cortisol levels under stress. The study stated that the modulatory effects of these formulas might be beneficial in treating stress-related disease. Three formulas that were found to be effective were *Liu Jun Zi Tang* (Six-Gentlemen Decoction), *Ban Xia Xie Xin Tang,* and *Ban Xia Hou Po Tang* (Pinellia and Magnolia Bark Decoction).[31]

HERB-DRUG INTERACTION

- **Cisplatin- and irinotecan-induced diarrhea**: Diarrhea induced by cisplatin (Platinol) and irinotecan (Camptosar) was effectively controlled with *Ban Xia Xie Xin Tang* (7.5 g/day) in patients with advanced non-small-cell lung cancer. In comparison with the control group, patients who received *Ban Xia Xie Xin Tang* showed a significant improvement in diarrhea grades (P=0.044), as well as a reduced frequency of diarrhea grades 3 and 4 (one patient versus ten patients; P=0.018).[32] The mechanisms of this action was attributed to accelerated healing of the intestinal tract, improved colonic water absorption, and decreased levels of colonic prostaglandin E2 (PGE2).[33] In another study, use of *Ban Xia Xie Xin Tang* was also found to be effective in preventing and controlling diarrhea induced by cisplatin and irinotecan (CPT-11) in patients with non-small-cell lung cancer. In comparison with the 23 patients in the control group that did not receive any herbs, 18 patients in the herb group showed a significant improvement in diarrhea grades and reduced frequency of diarrhea grades. The therapeutic benefit of preventing and controlling diarrhea was attributed in part to baicalin, a beta-glucuronidase inhibitor.[34]
- **Irinotecan-induced diarrhea:** Numerous studies have shown that diarrhea induced by irinotecan (Camptosar) can be effectively controlled and treated with administration of *Ban Xia Xie Xin Tang*.[35,36,37]

TOXICOLOGY

Administration of *Ban Xia Xie Xin Tang* was associated with one case of pneumonitis in a 72-year-old woman. Upon admission to the hospital and discontinuation of the formula, the symptoms were relieved, and the X-ray findings improved markedly. This is believed to be the first case of pulmonary hypersensitivity induced by *Ban Xia Xie Xin Tang* in Japan.[38]

AUTHORS' COMMENTS

The original use of *Ban Xia Xie Xin Tang* aimed at treating Stomach qi disharmony caused by maltreatment of *shaoyang* syndrome with downward draining herbs. Today, the contemporary applications of this formula have been vastly expanded to include various gastrointestinal disorders characterized by the presence of hot and cold, exterior and interior, and disharmony of the Stomach and Intestines.

Ban Xia Xie Xin Tang is based on *Xiao Chai Hu Tang* (Minor Bupleurum Decoction) without *Chai Hu* (Radix Bupleuri) and *Sheng Jiang* (Rhizoma Zingiberis Recens), and with the addition of *Huang Lian* (Rhizoma Coptidis) and *Gan Jiang* (Rhizoma Zingiberis). This is the best formula to treat epigastric pain caused by various kinds of digestive dysfunctions.

A question is often raised as to why *Ban Xia Xie Xin Tang*, a formula that treats epigastric distention and fullness, would contain *Ren Shen* (Radix et Rhizoma Ginseng), *Gan Cao* (Radix et Rhizoma Glycyrrhizae), and *Da Zao* (Fructus Jujubae), three tonic herbs that could create more stagnation. The answer is that in *Ban Xia Xie Xin Tang*, epigastric distention and fullness are not caused by damp accumulation or stagnation, conditions that could be worsened with the use of tonic herbs. Instead, epigastric distention and fullness occur as a result of the misuse of herbs that injure the middle *jiao,* thus creating disruption of Stomach functioning in addition to heat and cold stagnation in the middle *jiao*. In this case, *Ren Shen* (Radix et Rhizoma Ginseng), *Gan Cao* (Radix et Rhizoma Glycyrrhizae), and *Da Zao* (Fructus Jujubae) serve to protect the Spleen, restore normal digestive functioning, and restore *zheng* (upright) *qi* which was damaged by the use of downward draining herbs.

There are three "*Xie Xin Tang* (Drain the Epigastrium)" formulas listed that treat epigastric fullness and distention. Even though the main symptoms are the same, the causes are different. Different causes in turn require different treatments. With minute changes in the composition and dosage of the formulas, their properties change as well.

- *Ban Xia Xie Xin Tang* treats epigastric distention caused by interlocking of heat and cold.
- *Sheng Jiang Xie Xin Tang* (Fresh Ginger Decoction to Drain the Epigastrium) treats epigastric distention caused by interlocking of heat and water.
- *Gan Cao Xie Xin Tang* (Licorice Decoction to Drain the Epigastrium) treats epigastric fullness caused by Stomach deficiency.

According to Dr. Chang Wei-Yen, *Huo Xiang Zheng Qi San* (Agastache Powder to Rectify the Qi) can be combined with *Ban Xia Xie Xin Tang* to treat vomiting, diarrhea, and epigastric pain caused by improper food intake or food poisoning. This combination is also effective in improving appetite in children.

Bàn Xià Xiè Xīn Tāng (Pinellia Decoction to Drain the Epigastrium)

References

1. *Zhong Yao Ming Fang Yao Li Yu Ying Yong* (Pharmacology and Applications of Famous Herbal Formulas) 1989;121-123.

2. Naito T, Itoh H, Yasunaga F, Takeyama M. Hange-shashin-to raises levels of somatostatin, motilin, and gastrin in the plasma of healthy subjects. Biol Pharm Bull 2002 Mar;25(3):327-31.

3. *Shan Xi Zhong Yi Xue Yuan Xue Bao* (Journal of Shanxi University School of Chinese Medicine) 1987;10(3):11.

4. Li J, Takeda H, Inazu M, Hayashi M, Tsuji M, Ikoshi H, Takada K, Matsumiya T. Protective effects of Hange-shashin-to on water-immersion restraint stress-induced gastric ulcers. Methods Find Exp Clin Pharmacol 1998 Jan-Feb;20(1):31-7.

5. Kase Y, Yuzurihara M, Iizuka S, Ishige A, Komatsu Y. The effects of hange-shashin-to on gastric function in comparison with sho-saiko-to. Biol Pharm Bull 1997 Nov;20(11):1155-9.

6. *Hu Nan Zhong Yi Za Zhi* (Hunan Journal of Chinese Medicine) 1986;5;21.

7. *Hu Nan Zhong Yi Za Zhi* (Hunan Journal of Chinese Medicine) 1986;5;21.

8. *Zhe Jiang Zhong Yi Xue Yuan Xue Bao* (Journal of Zhejiang University of Chinese Medicine) 1997;4;33.

9. *Fu Jian Zhong Yi Yao* (Fujian Chinese Medicine and Herbology) 1983;1;27.

10. *Shan Xi Zhong Yi* (Shanxi Chinese Medicine) 1991;12(3):128.

11. *Tian Jin Zhong Yi* (Tianjin Chinese Medicine) 1997;1:15.

12. *Xin Zhong Yi* (New Chinese Medicine) 1988;7:35.

13. *Hei Long Jiang Zhong Yi Yao* (Heilongjiang Chinese Medicine and Herbology) 1996;5:27.

14. *Hei Long Jiang Zhong Yi Yao* (Heilongjiang Chinese Medicine and Herbology) 1998;3:30.

15. *Hu Bei Zhong Yi Za Zhi* (Hubei Journal of Chinese Medicine) 1987;3:22.

16. *He Nan Zhong Yi* (Henan Chinese Medicine) 1992;3:10.

17. *Hei Long Jiang Zhong Yi Yao* (Heilongjiang Chinese Medicine and Herbology) 1988;1:24.

18. *Si Chuan Zhong Yi* (Sichuan Chinese Medicine) 1990;5:11.

19. *Shang Hai Zhong Yi Yao Za Zhi* (Shanghai Journal of Chinese Medicine and Herbology) 1998;4:30.

20. *Zhe Jiang Zhong Yi Za Zhi* (Zhejiang Journal of Chinese Medicine) 1985;4:155.

21. *Shang Hai Zhong Yi Yao Za Zhi* (Shanghai Journal of Chinese Medicine and Herbology) 1989;10:31.

22. *Shan Xi Zhong Yi* (Shanxi Chinese Medicine) 1997;7:299.

23. *Nei Meng Gu Zhong Yi Yao* (Traditional Chinese Medicine and Medicinals of Inner Mongolia) 1998;4:14.

24. *Zhe Jiang Zhong Yi Xue Yuan Xue Bao* (Journal of Zhejiang University of Chinese Medicine) 1997;3:29.

25. *Zhong Yi Ming Fang Lin Chuang Xin Yong* (Contemporary Clinical Applications of Classic Chinese Formulas) 2001;303.

26. *Xin Zhong Yi* (New Chinese Medicine) 1997;6:14.

27. *Si Chuan Zhong Yi* (Sichuan Chinese Medicine) 1989;5:35.

28. *Zhe Jiang Zhong Yi Xue Yuan Xue Bao* (Journal of Zhejiang University of Chinese Medicine) 1996;3:33.

29. *Xin Zhong Yi* (New Chinese Medicine) 1996;10:49.

30. *Zhong Yi Ming Fang Lin Chuang Xin Yong* (Contemporary Clinical Applications of Classic Chinese Formulas) 2001;304.

31. Naito T, Itoh H, Takeyama M. Some gastrointestinal function regulatory Kampo medicines have modulatory effects on human plasma adrenocorticotropic hormone and cortisol levels with continual stress exposure. Biological & Pharmaceutical Bulletin 2003 Jan;26(1):101-4.

32. Mori K, Kondo T, Kamiyama Y, Kano Y, Tominaga K. Preventive effect of Kampo medicine (Hangeshashin-to) against irinotecan-induced diarrhea in advanced non-small-cell lung cancer. Cancer Chemother Pharmacol 2003 May;51(5):403-6. Epub 2003 Apr 09.

33. Kase Y, Hayakawa T, Aburada M, Komatsu Y, Kamataki T. Preventive effects of Hange-shashin-to on irinotecan hydrochloride-caused diarrhea and its relevance to the colonic prostaglandin E2 and water absorption in the rat. Jpn J Pharmacol 1997 Dec;75(4):407-13.

34. Mori K, Kondo T, Kamiyama Y, Kano Y, Tominaga K. Preventive effect of Kampo medicine (Hangeshashin-to) against irinotecan-induced diarrhea in advanced non-small-cell lung cancer. Cancer Chemotherapy & Pharmacology 2003 May;51(5):403-6.

35. Takasuna K, Kasai Y, Kitano Y, Mori K, Kobayashi R, Hagiwara T, Kakihata K, Hirohashi M, Nomura M, Nagai E, et al. Protective effects of kampo medicines and baicalin against intestinal toxicity of a new anticancer camptothecin derivative, irinotecan hydrochloride (CPT-11), in rats. Jpn J Cancer Res 1995 Oct;86(10):978-84.

36. Sakata Y, Suzuki H, Kamataki T. Preventive effect of TJ-14, a kampo (Chinese herb) medicine, on diarrhea induced by irinotecan hydrochloride (CPT-11). Gan To Kagaku Ryoho 1994 Jul;21(8):1241-4.

37. Mori K, Hirose T, Machida S, Tominaga K. Kampo medicines for the prevention of irinotecan-induced diarrhea in advanced non-small cell lung cancer. Gan To Kagaku Ryoho 1998 Jul;25(8):1159-63.

38. Oketani N, Saito H, Ebe T. Pneumonitis due to Hangeshashin-to. Nihon Kyobu Shikkan Gakkai Zasshi 1996 Sep;34(9):983-8.

Shēng Jiāng Xiè Xīn Tāng
(Fresh Ginger Decoction to Drain the Epigastrium)

生薑瀉心湯
生姜泻心汤

Pinyin Name: *Sheng Jiang Xie Xin Tang*
Literal Name: Fresh Ginger Decoction to Drain the Epigastrium
Alternate Name: Pinellia and Ginger Combination
Original Source: *Shang Han Lun* (Discussion of Cold-Induced Disorders) by Zhang Zhong-Jing in the Eastern Han Dynasty

COMPOSITION

Ban Xia (Rhizoma Pinelliae), *xi* (washed)	0.5 cup [9g]
Sheng Jiang (Rhizoma Zingiberis Recens), *qie* (sliced)	12g [12g]
Gan Jiang (Rhizoma Zingiberis)	3g [3g]
Huang Qin (Radix Scutellariae)	9g [6g]
Huang Lian (Rhizoma Coptidis)	3g [3g]
Ren Shen (Radix et Rhizoma Ginseng)	9g [6g]
Da Zao (Fructus Jujubae), *bo* (opened)	12 pieces [4 pieces]
Zhi Gan Cao (Radix et Rhizoma Glycyrrhizae Praeparata cum Melle)	9g [6g]

Note: "*Xie xin*" literally means to "drain the Heart." However, the term is really used to indicate draining the area beneath the Heart, namely the epigastrium. Therefore, the literal name of the formula has been modified to reflect its actual applications.

DOSAGE / PREPARATION / ADMINISTRATION

The source text states to cook the ingredients in 10 cups [2,000 mL] of water until 6 cups [1,200 mL] of liquid remain. Discard the residue and cook the strained decoction again until it is reduced to 3 cups [600 mL]. Take 1 cup [200 mL] of the warm decoction three times daily. Today, the decoction may be prepared using the doses suggested in brackets.

CHINESE THERAPEUTIC ACTIONS

1. Harmonizes the Stomach and corrects the reversed flow of qi
2. Disperses the interlocking of heat and water and relieves epigastric distention

CLINICAL MANIFESTATIONS

Spleen and Stomach deficiencies with interlocking of heat and water in the interior: epigastric distention and hardness, belching, foul breath, borborygmus, and diarrhea.

CLINICAL APPLICATIONS

Acute gastroenteritis, peptic ulcer, epigastric distention, diarrhea, and dysentery.

EXPLANATION

Sheng Jiang Xie Xin Tang (Fresh Ginger Decoction to Drain the Epigastrium) was originally formulated for the following condition: individuals with exterior cold condition, who after inappropriate treatment with diaphoretic methods to release exterior cold, now suffers from damage to the middle *jiao*, deficiencies of the Spleen and Stomach, and interlocking of heat and water.

Sheng Jiang Xie Xin Tang aims at treating patients with Spleen and Stomach deficiencies, with the interlocking of heat and water in the interior. This formula is a modification of *Ban Xia Xie Xin Tang* (Pinellia Decoction to Drain the Epigastrium), with the addition of *Sheng Jiang* (Rhizoma Zingiberis Recens) and a reduction in the dose of *Gan Jiang* (Rhizoma Zingiberis). Because water and heat are interlocked, *Sheng Jiang* (Rhizoma Zingiberis Recens) warms the Stomach, stops nausea, and disperses water accumulation. *Gan Jiang* (Rhizoma Zingiberis) warms the Stomach, but the dose is reduced to avoid creating too much heat. Clinically, patients may show epigastric distention and hardness, belching, foul breath, borborygmus, and diarrhea.

MODIFICATIONS

- With nausea and vomiting of clear fluids, add *Zhi Shi* (Fructus Aurantii Immaturus) and *Hou Po* (Cortex Magnoliae Officinalis).
- If accompanied by thirst and a desire to drink, add *Fu Ling* (Poria) and *Ze Xie* (Rhizoma Alismatis).
- With diarrhea and abdominal pain, add *Bai Shao* (Radix Paeoniae Alba) and *Chen Pi* (Pericarpium Citri Reticulatae).
- If there is indigestion, add *Ping Wei San* (Calm the Stomach Powder).

Chinese Herbal Formulas and Applications

Shēng Jiāng Xiè Xīn Tāng
(Fresh Ginger Decoction to Drain the Epigastrium)

Sheng Jiang Xie Xin Tang (Fresh Ginger Decoction to Drain the Epigastrium)

Diagnosis	Signs and Symptoms	Treatment	Herbs
Spleen and Stomach deficiencies with the interlocking of heat and water in the interior	Epigastric distention and hardness, belching, foul breath, borborygmus and diarrhea	• Harmonizes the Stomach and corrects the reversed flow of qi • Disperses the interlocking of heat and water and relieves epigastric distention	• *Ban Xia* (Rhizoma Pinelliae) disperses stagnation, relieves distention, and directs reversed Stomach qi downward. • *Sheng Jiang* (Rhizoma Zingiberis Recens) warms the Stomach, stops nausea, and disperses water accumulation. • *Gan Jiang* (Rhizoma Zingiberis) warms the Stomach. • *Huang Qin* (Radix Scutellariae) and *Huang Lian* (Rhizoma Coptidis) sedate heat and relieve distention. • *Ren Shen* (Radix et Rhizoma Ginseng), *Da Zao* (Fructus Jujubae) and *Zhi Gan Cao* (Radix et Rhizoma Glycyrrhizae Praeparata cum Melle) tonify the middle *jiao* and strengthen the Spleen.

• With belching and water retention in the middle *jiao*, add *Wu Ling San* (Five-Ingredient Powder with Poria).

CLINICAL STUDIES AND RESEARCH

Epigastric distention: Use of modified *Sheng Jiang Xie Xin Tang* was effective in treating epigastric distention. Modifications included the elimination of *Sheng Jiang* (Rhizoma Zingiberis Recens) and *Ban Xia* (Rhizoma Pinelliae) for excess heat; and the elimination of *Huang*

Qin (Radix Scutellariae) and *Huang Lian* (Rhizoma Coptidis) for excess cold. Of 245 cases, the study reported complete recovery in 187 cases, improvement in 45 cases, and no effect in 13 cases.[1]

Reference
1. *Zhe Jiang Zhong Yi Za Zhi* (Zhejiang Journal of Chinese Medicine) 1988;2:75.

Gān Cǎo Xiè Xīn Tāng (Licorice Decoction to Drain the Epigastrium)

甘草瀉心湯
甘草泻心汤

Pinyin Name: *Gan Cao Xie Xin Tang*
Literal Name: Licorice Decoction to Drain the Epigastrium
Alternate Name: Pinellia and Licorice Combination
Original Source: *Shang Han Lun* (Discussion of Cold-Induced Disorders) by Zhang Zhong-Jing in the Eastern Han Dynasty

COMPOSITION

Ban Xia (Rhizoma Pinelliae), *xi* (washed)	0.5 cup [9g]
Gan Jiang (Rhizoma Zingiberis)	9g [6g]
Huang Qin (Radix Scutellariae)	9g [6g]
Huang Lian (Rhizoma Coptidis)	3g
Ren Shen (Radix et Rhizoma Ginseng)	9g [6g]
Da Zao (Fructus Jujubae), *bo* (opened)	12 pieces [4 pieces]
Zhi Gan Cao (Radix et Rhizoma Glycyrrhizae Praeparata cum Melle)	12g

HARMONIZING FORMULAS

269

Chapter 3 – Harmonizing Formulas   *Section 3 – Intestines and Stomach Harmonizing Formulas*

Gān Cǎo Xiè Xīn Tāng (Licorice Decoction to Drain the Epigastrium)

Note: According to *Shang Han Lun* (Discussion of Cold-Induced Disorders), this formula does not contain *Ren Shen* (Radix et Rhizoma Ginseng). However, *Ren Shen* (Radix et Rhizoma Ginseng) is listed as an ingredient in many subsequent texts, such as *Jin Gui Yao Lue* (Essentials from the Golden Cabinet) by Zhang Zhong-Jing in the Eastern Han Dynasty, *Qian Jin Yao Fang* (Thousand Ducat Prescriptions) by Sun Si-Miao in 581-685 A.D., and *Wai Tai Mi Yao* (Arcane Essentials from the Imperial Library) by Wang Tao in 752 A.D. Based on historical data and formulary analysis, most texts now include *Ren Shen* (Radix et Rhizoma Ginseng) as an ingredient.

"*Xie xin*" literally means to "drain the Heart." However, the term is really used to indicate draining the area beneath the Heart, namely the epigastrium. Therefore, the literal name of the formula has been modified to reflect its actual applications.

DOSAGE / PREPARATION / ADMINISTRATION

The source text instructs to cook the ingredients in 10 cups [2,000 mL] of water until 6 cups [1,200 mL] of liquid remain. Discard the residue and cook the strained decoction again until it is reduced to 3 cups [600 mL]. Take 1 cup [200 mL] of the warm decoction three times daily. Today, the decoction may be prepared using the doses suggested in brackets.

CHINESE THERAPEUTIC ACTIONS

1. Benefits qi and harmonizes the Stomach
2. Relieves epigastric distention and stops diarrhea

CLINICAL MANIFESTATIONS

Epigastric distention caused by Stomach deficiency and interlocking of heat and cold in the interior: epigastric fullness, distention and hardness, dry heaves, vomiting, irritability, borborygmus, and diarrhea with undigested food in the stools.

CLINICAL APPLICATIONS

Gastroenteritis, chronic gastritis, gastric or duodenal ulcers, hypersecretion of gastric acid, gastroptosis, chronic hepatitis, liver cirrhosis, motion sickness with nausea and vomiting, and stomatitis.

EXPLANATION

Gan Cao Xie Xin Tang (Licorice Decoction to Drain the Epigastrium) was originally formulated for the following condition: individuals with exterior cold condition, who after inappropriate treatment with downward draining herbs, now suffers from damage to the middle *jiao* and severe deficiencies of the Spleen and Stomach.

Gan Cao Xie Xin Tang is composed of *Ban Xia Xie Xin Tang* (Pinellia Decoction to Drain the Epigastrium), plus an extra 3g of *Zhi Gan Cao* (Radix et Rhizoma Glycyrrhizae Praeparata cum Melle), which is used in this formula to tonify the Stomach and treat diarrhea with undigested food in the stools. Please refer to *Ban Xia Xie Xin Tang* (Pinellia Decoction to Drain the Epigastrium) for the explanation of the etiology of this syndrome and the functions of the herbs in this formula.

Gan Cao Xie Xin Tang (Licorice Decoction to Drain the Epigastrium)

Diagnosis	Signs and Symptoms	Treatment	Herbs
Epigastric distention caused by Stomach deficiency	Epigastric fullness, distention and hardness, dry heaves, vomiting, irritability, borborygmus, and diarrhea with undigested food in the stools	• Benefits qi and harmonizes the Stomach • Relieves epigastric distention and stops diarrhea	• *Ban Xia* (Rhizoma Pinelliae) disperses stagnation, relieves distention, and directs reversed Stomach qi downward to relieve nausea and vomiting. • *Gan Jiang* (Rhizoma Zingiberis) warms the middle *jiao* and disperses cold accumulation. • *Huang Qin* (Radix Scutellariae) and *Huang Lian* (Rhizoma Coptidis) sedate heat and relieve distention. • *Ren Shen* (Radix et Rhizoma Ginseng) and *Da Zao* (Fructus Jujubae) tonify the middle *jiao* and strengthen the Spleen. • A larger dose of *Zhi Gan Cao* (Radix et Rhizoma Glycyrrhizae Praeparata cum Melle) greatly tonifies the Stomach and treats diarrhea with undigested food in the stools.

270

Chinese Herbal Formulas and Applications

Gān Cǎo Xiè Xīn Tāng (Licorice Decoction to Drain the Epigastrium)

MODIFICATIONS

- When there is a feeling of fullness and oppression in the chest and hypochondriac region, add *Zhi Shi* (Fructus Aurantii Immaturus) and *Jie Geng* (Radix Platycodonis).
- For diarrhea with abdominal pain, add *Mu Xiang* (Radix Aucklandiae) and *Bai Shao* (Radix Paeoniae Alba).
- With vomiting and belching, add *Chen Pi* (Pericarpium Citri Reticulatae) and *Fu Ling* (Poria).

- With vomiting and epigastric pain, combine with *San Huang Xie Xin Tang* (Three-Yellow Decoction to Sedate the Epigastrium).
- With vomiting with phlegm accumulation, combine with *Er Chen Tang* (Two-Cured Decoction).
- With vomiting of food particles, combine with *Ping Wei San* (Calm the Stomach Powder).

Huáng Lián Tāng (Coptis Decoction)

黃連湯
黄连汤

Pinyin Name: *Huang Lian Tang*
Literal Name: Coptis Decoction
Alternate Names: *Huang Lien Tang*, Coptis Combination
Original Source: *Shang Han Lun* (Discussion of Cold-Induced Disorders) by Zhang Zhong-Jing in the Eastern Han Dynasty

COMPOSITION

Huang Lian (Rhizoma Coptidis)	9g [6g]
Gan Jiang (Rhizoma Zingiberis)	9g [6g]
Gui Zhi (Ramulus Cinnamomi)	9g [6g]
Ban Xia (Rhizoma Pinelliae), *xi* (washed)	0.5 cup [9g]
Ren Shen (Radix et Rhizoma Ginseng)	6g [3g]
Da Zao (Fructus Jujubae), *bo* (opened)	12 pieces [4 pieces]
Zhi Gan Cao (Radix et Rhizoma Glycyrrhizae Praeparata cum Melle)	9g [6g]

DOSAGE / PREPARATION / ADMINISTRATION

The source text instructions are to cook the ingredients in 10 cups [2,000 mL] of water until 6 cups [1,200 mL] of liquid remain. Take 1 cup [200 mL] of the warm, strained decoction three times during the day, and two times at night. Today, the decoction may be prepared using the doses suggested in brackets.

CHINESE THERAPEUTIC ACTIONS

1. Regulates heat and cold imbalances
2. Harmonizes the Stomach and corrects the reversed flow of qi

CLINICAL MANIFESTATIONS

Heat in the chest and cold in the Stomach: irritability, a stifling sensation in the chest, nausea, abdominal pain, borborygmus, diarrhea, a white, slippery tongue coating, and a wiry pulse.

CLINICAL APPLICATIONS

Gastric ulcer, duodenal ulcer, atrophic gastritis, gastroenteritis, acid regurgitation, epigastric pain, stomatitis, acute food poisoning, and hangover.

EXPLANATION

Huang Lian Tang (Coptis Decoction) treats a condition complicated by both interlocking of heat and cold. The condition is commonly described as heat in the upper *jiao* (chest) and cold in the middle *jiao* (Stomach). Heat in the upper *jiao* directly affects the chest, leading to a stifling sensation, a feeling of oppression beneath the heart, and irritability. Cold in the middle *jiao* affects the flow of Stomach qi, causing nausea, vomiting, abdominal pain, borborygmus, and diarrhea.

Huang Lian (Rhizoma Coptidis) clears heat in the Stomach and upper *jiao*. *Gan Jiang* (Rhizoma Zingiberis) warms the middle and lower *jiaos*. *Gui Zhi* (Ramulus

3

HARMONIZING FORMULAS

271

Chapter 3 – Harmonizing Formulas   *Section 3 – Intestines and Stomach Harmonizing Formulas*

Huáng Lián Tāng (Coptis Decoction)

Huang Lian Tang (Coptis Decoction)

Diagnosis	Signs and Symptoms	Treatment	Herbs
Heat in the chest and cold in the Stomach	• Irritability with a stifling sensation in the chest: heat in the upper *jiao* • Nausea, vomiting, abdominal pain, borborygmus, and diarrhea: cold in the middle *jiao*	• Regulates heat and cold imbalances • Harmonizes the Stomach and corrects the reversed flow of qi	• *Huang Lian* (Rhizoma Coptidis) clears heat in the Stomach and the upper *jiao*. • *Gan Jiang* (Rhizoma Zingiberis) warms the middle and lower *jiaos*. • *Gui Zhi* (Ramulus Cinnamomi) disperses cold and warms the channels and collaterals. • *Ban Xia* (Rhizoma Pinelliae) harmonizes the Stomach and relieves nausea. • *Ren Shen* (Radix et Rhizoma Ginseng), *Da Zao* (Fructus Jujubae) and *Zhi Gan Cao* (Radix et Rhizoma Glycyrrhizae Praeparata cum Melle) tonify and harmonize the middle *jiao*. • *Zhi Gan Cao* (Radix et Rhizoma Glycyrrhizae Praeparata cum Melle) harmonizes the herbs.

Cinnamomi), acrid and warm, helps *Gan Jiang* (Rhizoma Zingiberis) disperse cold and also warms and opens the channels and collaterals. *Ban Xia* (Rhizoma Pinelliae) harmonizes the Stomach and relieves nausea. *Ren Shen* (Radix et Rhizoma Ginseng), *Da Zao* (Fructus Jujubae), and *Zhi Gan Cao* (Radix et Rhizoma Glycyrrhizae Praeparata cum Melle) tonify and harmonize the middle *jiao*. *Zhi Gan Cao* (Radix et Rhizoma Glycyrrhizae Praeparata cum Melle) also harmonizes the herbs.

MODIFICATIONS

• With constipation, add *Da Huang* (Radix et Rhizoma Rhei).
• With watery diarrhea and dysentery, add *Zhi Shi* (Fructus Aurantii Immaturus) and *Bai Zhu* (Rhizoma Atractylodis Macrocephalae).
• With nausea, vomiting, and diarrhea, add *Mu Xiang* (Radix Aucklandiae) and *Bai Shao* (Radix Paeoniae Alba).
• With nausea and a feeling of heat in the chest, add more *Huang Lian* (Rhizoma Coptidis) and *Zhu Ru* (Caulis Bambusae in Taenia).

CAUTIONS / CONTRAINDICATIONS

Huang Lian Tang should not be used in patients of nausea, vomiting, and stomach pain caused by yin deficiency.[1]

PHARMACOLOGICAL EFFECTS

Antitumor: One study reported that *Huang Lian Tang* had an antitumor effect on esophageal cancer cells (ECCs) *in vitro*, and may be useful as an alternative therapy. Berberine, a compound in *Huang Lian* (Rhizoma Coptidis), is believed to be one of the main active constituents in this formula.[2]

CLINICAL STUDIES AND RESEARCH

1. **Atrophic gastritis**: Ninety-eight patients with chronic atrophic gastritis were treated with 98.97% effectiveness using *Huang Lian Tang* plus *Chai Hu* (Radix Bupleuri) and *San Leng* (Rhizoma Sparganii) as the base formula. Modifications were made based on the condition of each person, and included *Ren Shen* (Radix et Rhizoma Ginseng) at a larger dose for gastric pain due to deficiency; *Huang Lian* (Rhizoma Coptidis) for gastric pain due to excess; *Zhi Shi* (Fructus Aurantii Immaturus) for a feeling of oppression in the epigastrium; *Huang Qi* (Radix Astragali) for fatigue; *Fu Zi* (Radix Aconiti Lateralis Praeparata) for chills; *Bai Zhu* (Rhizoma Atractylodis Macrocephalae) for qi deficiency and poor appetite; *Shen Qu* (Massa Fermentata) for food stagnation; *Fu Ling* (Poria) for loose stools; *Da Huang* (Radix et Rhizoma Rhei) for dry stools; *Huang Qin* (Radix Scutellariae) for bitter taste in the mouth; *Gui Zhi* (Ramulus Cinnamomi) at a larger dose for white, greasy tongue coat; and *Sheng Jiang* (Rhizoma Zingiberis Recens) to replace *Gan Jiang* (Rhizoma Zingiberis) for nausea and vomiting. Of the 98 patients, the study reported recovery in 16 patients, significant improvement in 64 patients, moderate improvement in 17 patients, and no effect in 1 patient.[3]

2. **Epigastric pain**: Use of modified *Huang Lian Tang* was associated with 95% effectiveness in treating epigastric pain in 40 patients (between 25-55 years of age, with 3 days to 5 years history of illness). The herbal treatment contained *Huang Lian* (Rhizoma Coptidis) 10g, *Zhi Gan Cao* (Radix et Rhizoma Glycyrrhizae Praeparata cum Melle) 10g, *Gan Jiang* (Rhizoma Zingiberis) 10g, *Ban Xia* (Rhizoma Pinelliae) 10g, *Ren Shen* (Radix et Rhizoma Ginseng) 6g, and *Da Zao* (Fructus Jujubae) 7 pieces. Modifications

272

Chinese Herbal Formulas and Applications

Huáng Lián Tāng (Coptis Decoction)

include *Dou Kou* (Fructus Amomi Rotundus) 6g, *Zhi Qiao* (Fructus Aurantii) 10g, and *Shen Qu* (Massa Fermentata) 10g for poor appetite and qi stagnation; *Dang Shen* (Radix Codonopsis) 15g and *Bai Zhu* (Rhizoma Atractylodis Macrocephalae) 10g for qi deficiency; *Chuan Lian Zi* (Fructus Toosendan) 10g and *Huang Qin* (Radix Scutellariae) 10g for Liver and Stomach heat; *Wu Zhu Yu* (Fructus Evodiae) 10g and calcined *Wa Leng Zi* (Concha Arcae) 15g for acid reflux and belching; and *Gui Zhi* (Ramulus Cinnamomi) and *Gan Jiang* (Rhizoma Zingiberis) for cold extremities. The treatment protocol was to cook the herbs in water and administer the decoction in three equally-divided doses daily. The average duration of treatment was 6 days. Of the 40 patients, the study reported complete relief in 22 patients, improvement in 16 patients, and no benefit in 2 patients.[4]

TOXICOLOGY

Huang Lian Tang has very little toxicity. According to one study, oral administration of this formula in powder form at 27g/kg for 7 days (equivalent to 400 times the normal therapeutic dose) did not cause any fatality in mice. All subjects showed no abnormalities with eating, drinking, or regular activities.[5]

AUTHORS' COMMENTS

Ban Xia Xie Xin Tang (Pinellia Decoction to Drain the Epigastrium) and *Huang Lian Tang* have similar composition. However, *Ban Xia Xie Xin Tang* contains a lower dose of *Huang Lian* (Rhizoma Coptidis), and has the addition of *Huang Qin* (Radix Scutellariae); while *Huang Lian Tang* contains a higher dose of *Huang Lian* (Rhizoma Coptidis), and has the addition of *Gui Zhi* (Ramulus Cinnamomi).

- *Ban Xia Xie Xin Tang* treats heat and cold accumulation in the chest and epigastric areas with predominant distention and nausea or vomiting. *Huang Qin* (Radix Scutellariae), *Sheng Jiang* (Rhizoma Zingiberis Recens), and *Ban Xia* (Rhizoma Pinelliae) open and direct stagnation downward.

- *Huang Lian Tang* treats epigastric distention with heat in the upper *jiao,* and cold in the middle *jiao.* The higher dose of *Huang Lian* is used to enhance the overall effect of the formula to clear heat from the upper *jiao,* while the addition of *Gui Zhi* (Ramulus Cinnamomi) helps *Gan Jiang* (Rhizoma Zingiberis) warm the Spleen, and opens and warms the channels and collaterals.

References

1. *Zhong Yao Ming Fang Yao Li Yu Ying Yong* (Pharmacology and Applications of Famous Herbal Formulas) 1989;123.
2. Iizuka N, Miyamoto K, Okita K, Tangoku A, Hayashi H, Yosino S, Abe T, Morioka T, Hazama S, Oka M. Inhibitory effect of Coptidis Rhizoma and berberine on the proliferation of human esophageal cancer cell lines. Cancer Lett 2000 Jan 1;148(1):19-25.
3. *Shi Yong Zhong Xi Yi Jie He Za Zhi* (Practical Journal of Integrated Chinese and Western Medicines) 1995;1:51.
4. *Zhe Jiang Zhong Yi Za Zhi* (Zhejiang Journal of Chinese Medicine) 1993;9:393.
5. *Zhong Guo Zhong Yao Za Zhi* (People's Republic of China Journal of Chinese Herbology) 1994;19(7):427.

HARMONIZING FORMULAS

3

Chapter 3 – Harmonizing Formulas

Chapter 3 — Summary

— Harmonizing Formulas

SECTION 1: *SHAOYANG* HARMONIZING FORMULAS

Name	Similarities	Differences
Xiao Chai Hu Tang (Minor Bupleurum Decoction)	Harmonize the exterior and interior to treat *shaoyang* syndrome	Standard formula to treat *shaoyang* syndrome: tonifies qi and strengthens the body
Chai Hu Gui Zhi Tang (Bupleurum and Cinnamon Twig Decoction)		Treats *taiyang* and *shaoyang* syndromes: dispels pathogenic factors from both stages
Chai Ling Tang (Bupleurum and Poria Decoction)		Treats *shaoyang* syndrome with water accumulation: dispels water stagnation, eliminates phlegm accumulation
Chai Xian Tang (Bupleurum Decoction to Raise the Sunken)		Treats *shaoyang* syndrome with phlegm stagnation: eliminates phlegm, regulates qi circulation in the chest
Hao Qin Qing Dan Tang (Artemisia Annua and Scutellaria Decoction to Clear the Gallbladder)		Treats damp-heat in the Gallbladder: dispels dampness, dissolves phlegm
Chai Hu Da Yuan Yin (Bupleurum Decoction to Reach the Membrane Source)		Treats damp and phlegm obstruction at the *mo yuan* (membrane source)

Xiao Chai Hu Tang (Minor Bupleurum Decoction) is the standard formula to harmonize *shaoyang* syndrome, a condition characterized by the presence of pathogenic factors located between the exterior and interior. In addition, this formula also tonifies qi and strengthens the body. Listed below are three variations of *Xiao Chai Hu Tang* that treat *shaoyang* syndrome with complications.

- *Chai Hu Gui Zhi Tang* (Bupleurum and Cinnamon Twig Decoction) treats both *taiyang* and *shaoyang* syndromes. It is formulated by combining two formulas together: *Xiao Chai Hu Tang* to treat *shaoyang* syndrome, and *Gui Zhi Tang* (Cinnamon Twig Decoction) to treat *taiyang* syndrome.
- *Chai Ling Tang* (Bupleurum and Poria Decoction) treats *shaoyang* syndrome with accumulation of water, dampness, and phlegm. It is formulated by combining two formulas together: *Xiao Chai Hu Tang* to treat the *shaoyang* syndrome, and *Wu Ling San* (Five-Ingredient Powder with Poria) to treat water accumulation.
- *Chai Xian Tang* (Bupleurum Decoction to Raise the Sunken) treats *shaoyang* syndrome with phlegm obstruction and qi stagnation in the chest. It is formulated by combining two formulas together: *Xiao Chai Hu Tang* to treat the *shaoyang* syndrome, and *Xiao Xian Xiong Tang* (Minor Sinking into the Chest Decoction) to treat phlegm obstruction and qi stagnation in the chest.

Hao Qin Qing Dan Tang (Artemisia Annua and Scutellaria Decoction to Clear the Gallbladder) and *Chai Hu Da Yuan Yin* (Bupleurum Decoction to Reach the Membrane Source) are two formulas that have similar functions to harmonize the exterior and interior to treat *shaoyang* syndrome.

- *Hao Qin Qing Dan Tang* cleanses the Gallbladder, harmonizes the Stomach, eliminates dampness, and dissolves phlegm. It is used to treat summer-heat invading the *shaoyang* with stagnation of dampness and phlegm. Hence, this formula is especially effective in treating *shaoyang* syndrome with severe interior heat accompanied by some dampness and phlegm.
- *Chai Hu Da Yuan Yin* eliminates obstruction of dampness and phlegm at the *mo yuan* (membrane source) and harmonizes the exterior and interior of the body.

Chinese Herbal Formulas and Applications

Chapter 3 — Summary

SECTION 2: LIVER AND SPLEEN HARMONIZING FORMULAS

Name	Similarities	Differences
Si Ni San (Frigid Extremities Powder)	Regulate Liver qi circulation, relieve Liver qi stagnation	Circulates yang qi to relieve *shaoyin* syndrome with frigid extremities
Chai Hu Shu Gan San (Bupleurum Powder to Spread the Liver)		Strongly activates qi circulation
Shu Gan Tang (Spread the Liver Decoction)		Strongly invigorates blood circulation
Chai Hu Qing Gan Tang (Bupleurum Decoction to Clear the Liver)		Clears heat from the Liver, Gallbladder, and *San Jiao* channels
Yi Gan San (Restrain the Liver Powder)		Clears Liver heat, nourishes Liver blood
Xiao Yao San (Rambling Powder)	Soothe the Liver and relieve qi stagnation, strengthen the Spleen, nourish blood	Treats Liver qi stagnation
Jia Wei Xiao Yao San (Augmented Rambling Powder)		Treats Liver qi stagnation with heat and fire
Tong Xie Yao Fang (Important Formula for Painful Diarrhea)	Sedates the Liver, tonifies the Spleen	Dispels dampness and stops diarrhea

Si Ni San (Frigid Extremities Powder) ventilates the pathogens outward, relieves constraint, spreads Liver qi, and harmonizes the Liver and Spleen. It treats *shaoyin* syndrome characterized by frigid extremities, or disharmony of the Liver and Spleen. Clinical manifestations include cold extremities, epigastric and abdominal pain, and diarrhea.

Chai Hu Shu Gan San (Bupleurum Powder to Spread the Liver) and *Shu Gan Tang* (Spread the Liver Decoction) both treat Liver qi stagnation with blood stasis characterized by hypochondriac fullness and pain with alternating fever and chills.
• *Chai Hu Shu Gan San* has stronger effect to activate qi circulation.
• *Shu Gan Tang* is more effective to invigorate blood circulation and eliminate blood stasis.

Chai Hu Qing Gan Tang (Bupleurum Decoction to Clear the Liver) is a potent formula that clears heat in the Liver, Gallbladder, and *San Jiao* channels. Clinical manifestations include fever, chills, epistaxis, loss of hearing, and swelling of the lymph nodes.

Yi Gan San (Restrain the Liver Powder) treats a complex condition of both excess (Liver heat) and deficiency (Liver blood). Clinical signs and symptoms include fever, easily frightened and scared, muscle spasms and contraction, clenching of the teeth, nervousness, irritability, restlessness, insomnia, epilepsy, and alternating spells of fever and chills.

Xiao Yao San (Rambling Powder) nourishes the blood, smoothes the Liver, and strengthens the Spleen. It treats Liver qi stagnation (often due to blood deficiency) and deficiency of the Spleen. Clinical manifestations include hypochondriac pain, alternating spells of fever and chills, headache, vertigo, a dry mouth and dry throat, low appetite, lassitude, irregular menstruation, and breast distention.

Jia Wei Xiao Yao San (Augmented Rambling Powder) is formulated by adding *Mu Dan Pi* (Cortex Moutan) and *Zhi Zi* (Fructus Gardeniae) to *Xiao Yao San* (Rambling Powder). In comparison to the base formula, *Jia Wei Xiao Yao San* (Augmented Rambling Powder) has an enhanced effect to clear heat and sedate fire, and is more suitable for cases in which Liver qi stagnation is turning into Liver heat and fire.

HARMONIZING FORMULAS

275

Chapter 3 – Harmonizing Formulas

Chapter 3 — Summary

Tong Xie Yao Fang (Important Formula for Painful Diarrhea) mainly treats abdominal pain and diarrhea caused by Liver overacting on the Spleen. The abdominal pain in this case usually persists after defecation.

SECTION 3: INTESTINE AND STOMACH HARMONIZING FORMULAS

Name	Similarities	Differences
Ban Xia Xie Xin Tang (Pinellia Decoction to Drain the Epigastrium)	"Drain the epigastrium" to relieve feeling of epigastric distention	Eliminates the interlocking of heat and cold
Sheng Jiang Xie Xin Tang (Fresh Ginger Decoction to Drain the Epigastrium)		Eliminates the interlocking of water and heat
Gan Cao Xie Xin Tang (Licorice Decoction to Drain the Epigastrium)		Tonifies Stomach deficiency
Huang Lian Tang (Coptis Decoction)	Regulates heat and cold imbalances	Treats heat in the upper *jiao* (chest) and cold in the middle *jiao* (Stomach)

Ban Xia Xie Xin Tang (Pinellia Decoction to Drain the Epigastrium), *Sheng Jiang Xie Xin Tang* (Fresh Ginger Decoction to Drain the Epigastrium), and *Gan Cao Xie Xin Tang* (Licorice Decoction to Drain the Epigastrium) are three formulas with similar names and functions: "*xie xin*" means "to drain the epigastrium."

- *Ban Xia Xie Xin Tang* treats epigastric distention caused by the interlocking of heat and cold. It activates qi stagnation, lowers the reversed flow of qi, and relieves epigastric distention and fullness.
- *Sheng Jiang Xie Xin Tang* treats epigastric distention caused by the interlocking of water and heat. It eliminates water accumulation, disperses nodules, harmonizes the Stomach, and relieves epigastric distention and hardness.
- *Gan Cao Xie Xin Tang* treats epigastric distention caused by Stomach deficiency. It tonifies qi, stops diarrhea, harmonizes the Stomach, and relieves epigastric distention, fullness and hardness.

Huang Lian Tang (Coptis Decoction) treats irritability and stifling sensations in the chest by resolving heat in the upper *jiao* and cold in the middle *jiao*. It regulates heat and cold imbalances, harmonizes the Stomach, and corrects the reversed flow of qi.

Chinese Herbal Formulas and Applications

Chapter 4

— Exterior- and Interior-Releasing Formulas

刘完素 Liǔ Yuǎn-Sù

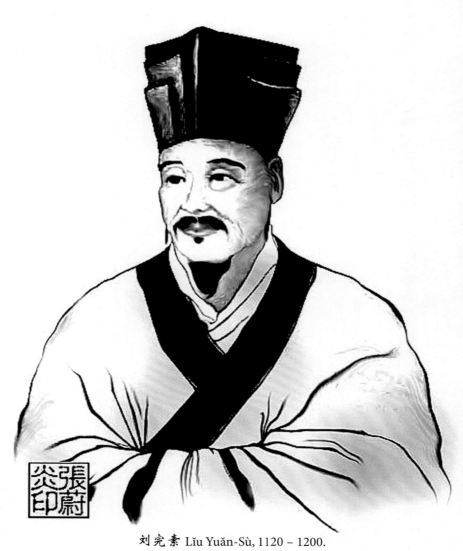

刘完素 Liǔ Yuǎn-Sù, 1120 – 1200.

刘完素 Liǔ Yuǎn-Sù

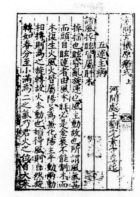

黄帝素问宣明论方 *Huang Di Su Wen Xuan Ming Lun Fang* (Formulas from the Discussion Illuminating the Yellow Emperor's Basic Questions) in 1172.

One of the most famous physicians of the Song and Jin dynasties, Liu Yuan-Su was born in the dry environment of northern China. People in the region primarily ate meat and cheese, foods that are warm and create dampness. Liu practiced medicine largely in times of war, thus his clinical practice was mainly concerned with injuries, subsequent infections, and death. Because of those geographic and historical influences, Liu developed 火热论 *huo re lun* (discussion of fire and heat), and proposed the use of cool and cold substances to treat heat and fire disorders. Liu believed that among *liu yin* (the six exogenous factors of wind, cold, summer-heat, dampness, dryness, and fire), heat (including summer-heat) and fire are the dominant factors in causing disorders. Liu's works are important because they introduced a concept significantly different from the classic theories of *shang han* (cold damage) by Zhang Zhong-Jing, which had been the main school of thought up to that time.

Liu Yuan-Su wrote many books in his lifetime, among the most famous are:
- 黄帝素问宣明论方 *Huang Di Su Wen Xuan Ming Lun Fang* (Formulas from the Discussion Illuminating the Yellow Emperor's Basic Questions)
- 宣明论方 *Xuan Ming Lun Fang* (Discussion of Dispersing and Brightening Formulas)
- 伤寒直格方论 *Shang Han Zhi Ge Fang Lun* (Direct Investigations of Formulas for Cold-Induced Disorders)

Some sample herbal formulas found in the wealth of clinical information in these texts are:
- *Fang Feng Tong Sheng San* (Saposhnikovia Powder that Sagely Unblocks)
- *Liu Yi San* (Six-to-One Powder)
- *Gui Ling Gan Lu Yin* (Cinnamon and Poria Sweet Dew Decoction)
- *Di Huang Yin Zi* (Rehmannia Decoction)

Dynasties & Kingdoms	Year
Xia Dynasty 夏	2100-1600 BCE
Shang Dynasty 商	1600-1100 BCE
Zhou Dynasty 周	1100-221 BCE
Qin Dynasty 秦	221-207 BCE
Han Dynasty 漢	206 BCE-220
Three Kingdoms 三國	220-280
Western Jin Dynasty 西晉	265-316
Eastern Jin Dynasty 東晉	317-420
Northern and Southern Dynasties 北南朝	420-581
Sui Dynasty 隋	581-618
Tang Dynasty 唐	618-907
Five Dynasties 五代	907-960
Song Dynasty 宋	960-1279
Liao Dynasty 潦	916-1125
Jin Dynasty 金	**1115-1234**
Yuan Dynasty 元	1271-1368
Ming Dynasty 明	1368-1644
Qing Dynasty 清	1644-1911
Republic of China 中華民國	1912-Present Day
People's Republic of China 中華人民共和國	1949-Present Day

Chapter 4 – Exterior- and Interior-Releasing Formulas

Table of Contents

Chapter 4. Exterior- and Interior-Releasing Formulas ·········· **277**
Biography of Liu Yuan-Su ·· 278

Section 1. Exterior-Releasing and Interior-Attacking Formulas ·········· **283**
Da Chai Hu Tang (Major Bupleurum Decoction) ·· 283
  Chai Hu Tang (Bupleurum Decoction) ··· 287
Hou Po Qi Wu Tang (Seven-Substance Decoction with Magnolia Bark) ········ 289
Fang Feng Tong Sheng San (Saposhnikovia Powder that Sagely Unblocks) ·········· 291
  Shuang Jie Tong Sheng San (Double Relieve Powder that Sagely Unblocks) ········ 294

Section 2. Exterior-Releasing and Interior-Clearing Formulas ·········· **295**
Ge Gen Huang Qin Huang Lian Tang (Kudzu, Coptis, and Scutellaria Decoction) ······ 295
  Ge Gen Huo Xiang Shao Yao Tang (Kudzu, Pogostemon, and Peony Decoction) ········ 298
Shi Gao Tang (Gypsum Decoction) ·· 299

Section 3. Exterior-Releasing and Interior-Warming Formulas ·········· **301**
Wu Ji San (Five-Accumulation Powder) ·· 301
  Wu Ji San (Five-Accumulation Powder) ·· 303
Chai Hu Gui Zhi Gan Jiang Tang (Bupleurum, Cinnamon Twig, and Ginger Decoction) ······ 304

Exterior- and Interior-Releasing Formulas (Summary) ·········· **306**

Chinese Herbal Formulas and Applications

Chapter 4 — Overview

— Exterior- and Interior-Releasing Formulas

Definition: Exterior- and interior-releasing formulas simultaneously treat exterior and interior syndromes. They incorporate strategies such as *han fa* (sweating), *xia fa* (draining downward), *qing fa* (clearing), and *wen fa* (warming). These methods first appeared as parts of *ba fa* (eight treatment methods), as described in the *Huang Di Nei Jing* (Yellow Emperor's Inner Classic) in the first or second century, A.D.

Exterior- and interior-releasing formulas treat the concurrent presence of exterior and interior conditions. Exterior conditions, usually characterized by wind-cold or wind-heat, are treated with exterior-releasing herbs. Interior conditions, generally characterized by excess or deficiency, and heat or cold, are treated with downward draining, heat-clearing or interior-warming herbs. In this complex condition, treating only the exterior syndrome will not relieve the interior syndrome, and treating only the interior syndrome will not release the exterior syndrome. Therefore, it is necessary to address and treat both at the same time.

Note: The condition of an (excess) exterior syndrome accompanied by interior deficiency is also addressed in Chapter 1: Exterior-Releasing Formulas.

SUBCATEGORIES OF ACTION

Exterior- and interior-releasing formulas are organized in three subcategories to reflect the nature of the disorders and characteristics of the formulas.

Exterior- and interior-releasing formulas treat concurrent exterior and interior conditions.

1. Exterior-Releasing and Interior-Attacking Formulas

These formulas are applicable when there are pathogenic factors present at both the exterior and the interior. Exterior conditions are usually characterized by wind-heat or wind-cold, while interior conditions are usually characterized by excess and accumulation of heat or cold. Clinical manifestations include aversion to cold, fever, abdominal fullness, constipation, and a red tongue with a yellow tongue coating.

Two types of herbs commonly address this condition: exterior-releasing herbs such as *Ma Huang* (Herba Ephedrae), *Gui Zhi* (Ramulus Cinnamomi), *Jing Jie* (Herba Schizonepetae), *Fang Feng* (Radix Saposhnikoviae), *Chai Hu* (Radix Bupleuri), and *Bo He* (Herba Menthae); and downward draining herbs such as *Da Huang* (Radix et Rhizoma Rhei) and *Mang Xiao* (Natrii Sulfas). Exemplar formulas include *Da Chai Hu Tang* (Major Bupleurum Decoction) and *Fang Feng Tong Sheng San* (Saposhnikovia Powder that Sagely Unblocks).

2. Exterior-Releasing and Interior-Clearing Formulas

These formulas treat wind-heat or wind-cold at the exterior co-existing with heat formation in the interior. Common signs and symptoms are aversion to cold, fever, irritability, restlessness, thirst, diarrhea, and dyspnea.

Two types of herbs commonly used to address this condition are: exterior-releasing herbs such as *Ma Huang* (Herba Ephedrae), *Dan Dou Chi* (Semen Sojae Praeparatum), and *Ge Gen* (Radix Puerariae Lobatae); and heat-clearing herbs such as *Huang Qin* (Radix Scutellariae), *Huang Lian* (Rhizoma Coptidis), *Huang Bo* (Cortex Phellodendri Chinensis), and *Shi Gao* (Gypsum Fibrosum). Representative formulas include *Ge Gen Huang Qin Huang Lian Tang* (Kudzu, Coptis, and Scutellaria Decoction) and *Shi Gao Tang* (Gypsum Decoction).

281

Chapter 4 – Exterior- and Interior-Releasing Formulas

Chapter 4 — Overview

3. **Exterior-Releasing and Interior-Warming Formulas**

When there is cold both at the exterior and in the interior, clinical manifestations include aversion to cold, fever, coldness and pain in the epigastrium and abdomen, a white tongue coating, and a slow pulse.

Two types of herbs are commonly used to address this condition: exterior-releasing herbs such as *Ma Huang* (Herba Ephedrae) and *Bai Zhi* (Radix Angelicae Dahuricae); and interior-warming herbs such as *Gan Jiang* (Rhizoma Zingiberis) and *Rou Gui* (Cortex Cinnamomi). An exemplar formula is *Wu Ji San* (Five-Accumulation Powder).

CAUTIONS / CONTRAINDICATIONS

~

Exterior- and interior-releasing formulas should be used <u>only</u> when both exterior and interior syndromes are present.

~

- Formulas that release both exterior and interior pathogens should be used only when both exterior and interior syndromes are present.
- Carefully differentiate exterior and interior syndromes on the basis of heat or cold, as well as excess or deficiency, and location of the differentiated pathogens, before applying any of these formulas.
- Carefully adjust the dosages of herbs in a formula according to the level of severity and balance of exterior and interior symptoms.

PHARMACOLOGICAL EFFECTS & CLINICAL APPLICATIONS

Similar to harmonizing formulas that treat *shaoyang* syndrome, exterior- and interior-releasing formulas treat both exterior and interior syndromes simultaneously. From allopathic perspectives, these formulas treat liver disorders (hepatitis and fatty liver),[1,2] gallbladder disorders (cholecystitis and cholelithiasis),[3] pancreatitis,[4] and gastrointestinal disorders (peptic ulcer, gastritis, gastric prolapse, diarrhea, dysentery, enteritis).[5,6,7,8,9,10] Exemplar formulas include *Da Chai Hu Tang* (Major Bupleurum Decoction) and *Ge Gen Huang Qin Huang Lian Tang* (Kudzu, Coptis, and Scutellaria Decoction).

References

1. *Shan Xi Zhong Yi* (Shanxi Chinese Medicine) 1989;5:223.
2. *Fu Jian Zhong Yi Yao* (Fujian Chinese Medicine and Herbology) 1995;6:43.
3. *Shan Dong Zhong Yi Za Zhi* (Shandong Journal of Chinese Medicine) 1987;3:18.
4. *Bei Jing Zhong Yi Xue Yuan Xue Bao* (Journal of Beijing University School of Medicine) 1991;14(4):12.
5. *Zhong Yi Fang Ji Xian Dai Yan Jiu* (Modern Study of Medical Formulae in Traditional Chinese Medicine) 1997;434.
6. *Guang Dong Yi Xue* (Guangdong Medicine) 1993;6:336.
7. *Zhe Jiang Zhong Yi Za Zhi* (Zhejiang Journal of Chinese Medicine) 1997;10:441.
8. *Jiang Xi Zhong Yi Yao* (Jiangxi Chinese Medicine and Herbology) 1959;6:28.
9. *Hu Bei Zhong Yi Za Zhi* (Hubei Journal of Chinese Medicine) 1983;2:24.
10. *He Nan Zhong Yi* (Henan Chinese Medicine) 1992;1:42.

282

Chinese Herbal Formulas and Applications

Section 1

解表攻里剂

— Exterior-Releasing and Interior-Attacking Formulas

EXTERIOR- AND INTERIOR-RELEASING FORMULAS

Dà Chái Hú Tāng (Major Bupleurum Decoction)
大柴胡湯
大柴胡汤

Pinyin Name: *Da Chai Hu Tang*
Literal Name: Major Bupleurum Decoction
Alternate Names: *Ta Tsai Hu Tang*, Major Bupleurum Combination
Original Source: *Jin Gui Yao Lue* (Essentials from the Golden Cabinet) by Zhang Zhong-Jing in the Eastern Han Dynasty

COMPOSITION

Chai Hu (Radix Bupleuri)	24g [15g]
Huang Qin (Radix Scutellariae)	9g
Da Huang (Radix et Rhizoma Rhei)	6g
Zhi Shi (Fructus Aurantii Immaturus), *zhi* (fried with liquid)	4 pieces [9g]
Bai Shao (Radix Paeoniae Alba)	9g
Ban Xia (Rhizoma Pinelliae), *xi* (washed)	0.5 cup [9g]
Sheng Jiang (Rhizoma Zingiberis Recens)	15g
Da Zao (Fructus Jujubae)	12 pieces [4 pieces]

DOSAGE / PREPARATION / ADMINISTRATION

The source text states to cook the ingredients in 12 cups [2,400 mL] of water until 6 cups [1,200 mL] of the liquid remain. Discard the residue and cook the strained decoction again to reduce it further. Take 1 cup [200 mL] of the warm decoction three times daily. Today, the decoction may be prepared using the doses suggested in brackets.

CHINESE THERAPEUTIC ACTIONS

1. Harmonizes *shaoyang* syndrome
2. Purges interior heat in *yangming* syndrome

CLINICAL MANIFESTATIONS

Shaoyang and *yangming* syndromes: alternate spells of chills and fever, fullness of chest and hypochondrium, continuous vomiting, a feeling of depression with slight fidgeting, fullness, distention and pain in the epigastrium, constipation or discharge of fluids rectally, a thick yellow tongue coating, and a wiry, forceful pulse.

CLINICAL APPLICATIONS

Gallbladder disorders, cholelithiasis, cholecystitis, biliary ascariasis, acute pancreatitis, hepatitis, fatty liver, hyperlipidemia, gastritis, gastric ulcer, duodenal ulcer, perforating ulcer, gastroenteritis, gastric prolapse, constipation, dysentery, acute tonsillitis, and obesity.

EXPLANATION

Da Chai Hu Tang (Major Bupleurum Decoction) treats *shaoyang* and *yangming* syndromes simultaneously by harmonizing the *shaoyang* stage and purging heat accumulation in the *yangming* stage. The clinical manifestations of alternating spells of chills and fever, fullness of the chest and hypochondrium, and continuous vomiting are all typical signs of a *shaoyang* pattern. A feeling of depression with slight fidgeting indicates a more severe form of *shaoyang* syndrome. Clinical manifestations indicating a *yangming* condition of excess heat include fullness and pain in the epigastrium and constipation. In severe cases, the stool may become so dry, hard and immobile, leading to discharge of fluids rectally. The yellow tongue coating indicates *yangming* heat in the body, and the wiry, forceful pulse indicates stagnation and the excess nature of this syndrome.

283

Dà Chái Hú Tāng (Major Bupleurum Decoction)

Da Chai Hu Tang (Major Bupleurum Decoction)

Diagnosis	Signs and Symptoms	Treatment	Herbs
Shaoyang and *yangming* syndromes	• Alternate spells of chills and fever, fullness of the chest and hypochondrium and continuous vomiting: *shaoyang* pattern • Fullness and pain in the epigastrium and constipation: *yangming* syndrome • Yellow tongue coating: heat in the body • Wiry, forceful pulse: stagnation and excess conditions	• Harmonizes *shaoyang* syndrome • Purges interior heat in *yangming* syndrome	• *Chai Hu* (Radix Bupleuri) and *Huang Qin* (Radix Scutellariae) harmonize *shaoyang* by releasing the exterior and clearing the interior. • *Da Huang* (Radix et Rhizoma Rhei) and *Zhi Shi* (Fructus Aurantii Immaturus) purge *yangming* Stomach heat and activate qi circulation. • *Bai Shao* (Radix Paeoniae Alba) harmonizes qi and blood. • *Ban Xia* (Rhizoma Pinelliae) and *Sheng Jiang* (Rhizoma Zingiberis Recens) direct the Stomach qi downward to relieve vomiting. • *Da Zao* (Fructus Jujubae) and *Sheng Jiang* (Rhizoma Zingiberis Recens) harmonize the herbs.

Normally, downward draining methods are prohibited in *shaoyang* syndrome, but unlike its typical manifestations, this is a combination of *shaoyang* and *yangming* syndromes. To effectively treat this set of symptoms, both harmonizing and downward draining methods must be used in order to treat the exterior and interior simultaneously.

Da Chai Hu Tang is designed following the principles of two formulas: *Xiao Chai Hu Tang* (Minor Bupleurum Decoction) to harmonize *shaoyang*, and *Da Cheng Qi Tang* (Major Order the Qi Decoction) to drain heat from *yangming*. *Chai Hu* (Radix Bupleuri), the chief herb, combines with *Huang Qin* (Radix Scutellariae) to harmonize the *shaoyang* and clear Gallbladder heat. *Da Huang* (Radix et Rhizoma Rhei) and *Zhi Shi* (Fructus Aurantii Immaturus) purge *yangming* Stomach heat and activate qi circulation to relieve fullness and dispel hardened stools. *Bai Shao* (Radix Paeoniae Alba) combines with *Da Huang* (Radix et Rhizoma Rhei) to relieve the abdominal pain from constipation; also, *Bai Shao* (Radix Paeoniae Alba) softens the Liver to relieve depression and fidgeting, and harmonizes qi and blood to help *Zhi Shi* (Fructus Aurantii Immaturus) relieve epigastric fullness and pain. *Ban Xia* (Rhizoma Pinelliae) and *Sheng Jiang* (Rhizoma Zingiberis Recens) direct Stomach qi downward to relieve vomiting. Finally, *Da Zao* (Fructus Jujubae) and *Sheng Jiang* (Rhizoma Zingiberis Recens) harmonize the *ying* (nutritive) and *wei* (defensive) levels, and all of the herbs.

For further explanation of the clinical manifestations of *shaoyang* and *yangming* patterns, please refer to *Xiao Chai Hu Tang* (Minor Bupleurum Decoction) and *Da Cheng Qi Tang* (Major Order the Qi Decoction).

MODIFICATIONS

• With excess dryness and heat in the *yangming* stage, add *Shi Gao* (Gypsum Fibrosum) and *Zhi Mu* (Rhizoma Anemarrhenae).
• With heat in the chest in the *shaoyang* stage, add *Huang Lian* (Rhizoma Coptidis).
• With excess heat and toxicity, add *Jin Yin Hua* (Flos Lonicerae Japonicae), *Lian Qiao* (Fructus Forsythiae), and *Pu Gong Ying* (Herba Taraxaci).
• With abdominal fullness and distention, add *Hou Po* (Cortex Magnoliae Officinalis), *Mu Xiang* (Radix Aucklandiae), and *Qing Pi* (Pericarpium Citri Reticulatae Viride).
• When there is severe pain, add *Yan Hu Suo* (Rhizoma Corydalis) and *Chuan Lian Zi* (Fructus Toosendan).
• For otitis media, add *Long Dan* (Radix et Rhizoma Gentianae).
• For parotitis, add *Bo He* (Herba Menthae) and *Ban Lan Gen* (Radix Isatidis).
• For gastroenteritis and fever, add *Zhu Ru* (Caulis Bambusae in Taenia), *Sha Ren* (Fructus Amomi), and *Chen Pi* (Pericarpium Citri Reticulatae).
• For jaundice, add *Yin Chen* (Herba Artemisiae Scopariae), *Zhi Zi* (Fructus Gardeniae), and *Jin Qian Cao* (Herba Lysimachiae); or *Yin Chen Hao Tang* (Artemisia Scoparia Decoction).
• For gallstones, add *Jin Qian Cao* (Herba Lysimachiae), *Hai Jin Sha* (Spora Lygodii), *Yu Jin* (Radix Curcumae), and *Ji Nei Jin* (Endothelium Corneum Gigeriae Galli).

CAUTIONS / CONTRAINDICATIONS

• *Da Chai Hu Tang* is contraindicated in patients with Spleen and Stomach deficiencies.

Dà Chái Hú Tāng (Major Bupleurum Decoction)

- *Da Huang* (Radix et Rhizoma Rhei) should be prescribed in moderation in this formula. Use of *Da Huang* (Radix et Rhizoma Rhei) in excessive amounts, or for a prolonged period of time may cause unnecessary depletion of body fluids, and can lead the disease deeper into the interior.
- Potential side effects associated with this formula include poor appetite, abdominal distention, diarrhea, and edema.
- Avoid cold or raw, pungent or spicy, and oily or greasy foods while taking this formula.[1]

PHARMACOLOGICAL EFFECTS

1. **Gastrointestinal**: Administration of *Da Chai Hu Tang* had marked antispasmodic and antiulcer effects on the gastrointestinal tract. According to laboratory experiments, the formula inhibited spasms and cramps of the smooth muscles of the intestines.[2] In addition, the herbs inhibited the production of gastric acid.[3] Lastly, administration of this formula in extract form at 250 mg/kg in rats was associated with a protective effect against damage to the stomach membrane induced by aspirin.[4]

2. **Hepatoprotective**: One study reported that *Da Chai Hu Tang* lowered elevated liver enzymes (SGPT and SGOT) and protected the liver from drug-induced damages.[5] Another study reported that *Da Chai Hu Tang* prevented the progression of acute liver injury induced by carbon tetrachloride by inhibiting enhanced lipid peroxidation and by improving disrupted active oxygen metabolism in the injured liver.[6]

3. **Cardiovascular**: The use of *Da Chai Hu Tang* has little or no impact on the cardiovascular system. There were minimal changes in blood pressure (both systolic and diastolic) and heart rate and rhythm.[7] There was, however, a slight drop of cholesterol and triglyceride levels.[8]

4. **Immunologic**: Administration of *Da Chai Hu Tang* enhanced the immune system. In mice with artificially suppressed immune systems, administration of the formula was associated with increased number of T-cells. There were, however, no significant changes with IgM and IgG.[9]

5. **Antibiotic**: *Da Chai Hu Tang* had a strong inhibitory effect *in vitro* against *Staphylococcus aureus* and *E. coli*.[10]

6. **Anti-inflammatory**: In mice with artificially-induced swelling and inflammation of the joints, the administration of *Da Chai Hu Tang* was determined to have an anti-inflammatory effect similar to aspirin.[11]

7. **Antihyperglycemic**: Administration of *Da Chai Hu Tang* was associated with a decreased blood glucose level at 30, 60, and 120 minutes after glucose loading in a tolerance test, and an increased serum insulin level at 120 minutes after glucose loading.

8. **Effect on lipid biosynthesis**: Administration of *Da Chai Hu Tang* was associated with decreased hepatic triglyceride biosynthesis and subsequent reduction in plasma VLDL

levels.[12] According to another study, administering *Da Chai Hu Tang* to subjects with diets high in cholesterol was associated with significantly lower plasma and hepatic cholesterol levels.[13] Another study showed *Da Chai Hu Tang* to beneficially affect lipid metabolism by significantly increasing high-density lipoprotein-cholesterol (HDL) with little antihypertensive effect.[14] Lastly, *Da Chai Hu Tang* significantly reduced plasma triglyceride levels.[15]

9. **Effect on atherosclerosis**: Administration of *Da Chai Hu Tang* prevented the formation of atherosclerotic lesions in rabbits. However, it did not improve hypercholesterolemia in these subjects. The mechanism of this preventative effect on the development of atheromatous plaque formation was attributed to the antioxidative activities of the formula.[16]

10. **Antihyperlipidemic**: Administration of *Xiao Chai Hu Tang* (Minor Bupleurum Decoction) and *Da Chai Hu Tang* was associated with beneficial effects in treating rats with cholesterol-induced hypercholesterolemia and aging-induced hyperlipidemia. Both formulas reduced total liver cholesterol and inhibited increases of serum and liver triglyceride.[17]

CLINICAL STUDIES AND RESEARCH

1. **Gallbladder disorders**: There have been numerous reports on the effect of *Da Chai Hu Tang* to treat gallbladder disorders, such as cholecystitis and cholelithiasis. In one report, 84 patients with gallbladder disorders (18 with cholecystitis and 73 with cholelithiasis) treated with modified *Da Chai Hu Tang* had complete recovery in 44 patients and improvement in 31 patients. The overall effectiveness was 89.28%.[18] In another report, 120 patients with cholelithiasis were treated with excellent results. The effectiveness was 88.2% for patients with stones in the bile duct, 78.5% for stones in the gallbladder, and 76.2% for stones in both the duct and the gallbladder.[19]

2. **Cholelithiasis**: *Da Chai Hu Tang* was used with good success to treat patients with gallstones after surgical removal of the gallbladder. The stones were successfully passed in 18 of 26 patients (69.2%). The duration of treatment ranged from 87-250 days.[20]

3. **Biliary ascariasis**: *Da Chai Hu Tang* has been shown in one study to effectively treat biliary ascariasis. Administration of modified *Da Chai Hu Tang* in decoction for an average of 15 days was associated with a 90.63% effectiveness in 32 patients. The researchers noted the formula to have marked anti-inflammatory, analgesic, cholagogic and antiparasitic effects. The herbal formula contained *Chai Hu* (Radix Bupleuri), *Huang Qin* (Radix Scutellariae), *Zhi Qiao* (Fructus Aurantii), *Ban Xia* (Rhizoma Pinelliae), *Bai Shao* (Radix Paeoniae Alba), *Sheng Jiang* (Rhizoma Zingiberis Recens), *Da Zao* (Fructus Jujubae),

Dà Chái Hú Tāng (Major Bupleurum Decoction)

Chapter 4 – Exterior- and Interior-Releasing Formulas Section 1 – Exterior-Releasing and Interior-Attacking Formulas

and *Da Huang* (Radix et Rhizoma Rhei). Strategies for modifications are as follows: for gallstones, add *Jin Qian Cao* (Herba Lysimachiae); and for jaundice, add *Yin Chen* (Herba Artemisiae Scopariae), *Zhi Zi* (Fructus Gardeniae), and *Da Huang* (Radix et Rhizoma Rhei) (post-decocted), and remove *Bai Shao* (Radix Paeoniae Alba), *Sheng Jiang* (Rhizoma Zingiberis Recens), and *Da Zao* (Fructus Jujubae).[21]

4. **Acute pancreatitis**: One study reported a pronounced effect using modified *Da Chai Hu Tang* to treat acute pancreatitis. The herbal treatment contained *Da Chai Hu Tang* plus *Xuan Ming Fen* (Natrii Sulfas Exsiccatus) 10g and *Zi Su Geng* (Caulis Perillae) 9g as the base formula. Modifications included addition of *Chuan Lian Zi* (Fructus Toosendan) 6g and *Da Fu Pi* (Pericarpium Arecae) 9g for qi stagnation; *Huang Lian* (Rhizoma Coptidis) 6g and *Da Fu Pi* (Pericarpium Arecae) 9g for damp-heat in the Liver and Gallbladder; addition of *Chuan Lian Zi* (Fructus Toosendan) 6g, *Huang Lian* (Rhizoma Coptidis) 6g, *Zhu Ru* (Caulis Bambusae in Taenia) 9g, and removal of *Zhi Shi* (Fructus Aurantii Immaturus) for excess heat in the Liver and Stomach; and addition of *Chi Shao* (Radix Paeoniae Rubra) 9g, *Tao Ren* (Semen Persicae) 9g, *Hong Hua* (Flos Carthami) 9g, and *Wu Ling Zhi* (Faeces Trogopteri) 9g, and removal of *Xuan Ming Fen* (Natrii Sulfas Exsiccatus) and *Ban Xia* (Rhizoma Pinelliae) in the case of qi and blood stagnation. The study showed 98.5% effectiveness among 216 patients.[22] In another report, 84 patients with acute pancreatitis were treated with modified *Da Chai Hu Tang* with good results. Most symptoms, such as abdominal pain, nausea, fever, and constipation, were resolved within 2-5 days. Laboratory results also confirmed the effectiveness of the treatment with blood amylase, urine amylase, and white blood cells returning to normal range in 2.9, 3.5, and 2 to 5 days, respectively.[23]

5. **Hepatitis**: In one study, 196 patients with acute icteric hepatitis treated with modified *Da Chai Hu Tang* recovered in 179 patients (asymptomatic with normal liver functions) and improved in 15 patients. The average duration of treatment was 25 days.[24]

6. **Fatty liver**: Use of modified *Da Chai Hu Tang* in 18 patients with fatty liver (6 months to 3 years history of illness) was associated with complete recovery in 5 patients, marked effect in 8 patients, slight improvement in 4 patients, and no effect in 1 case (94.4% effectiveness). The treatment protocol was to cook the herbs and drink the decoction in two equally-divided doses daily, for 30 days per course of treatment, with 7-10 days of rest in between courses, for a total of 2 courses. The base formula included *Chai Hu* (Radix Bupleuri) 12g, *Huang Qin* (Radix Scutellariae) 6-9g, *Ban Xia* (Rhizoma Pinelliae) 9g, *Bai Shao* (Radix Paeoniae Alba) 15g, *Zhi Shi* (Fructus Aurantii Immaturus) 6-9g, *Da Huang* (Radix et Rhizoma Rhei) 6-12g, *Dan Shen* (Radix et Rhizoma Salviae Miltiorrhizae) 15g, *Jue Ming Zi* (Semen Cassiae) 20g, and *Shan Zha* (Fructus Crataegi) 15g. Modifications included the addition of *Yu Jin* (Radix Curcumae) 10g and *Dan Shen* (Radix et Rhizoma Salviae Miltiorrhizae) 15g for chest and hypochondriac fullness and distention; *Fu Ling* (Poria) 15g and *Chen Pi* (Pericarpium Citri Reticulatae) 6g for nausea and vomiting; *Huang Jing* (Rhizoma Polygonati) 15g and *Shan Yao* (Rhizoma Dioscoreae) 20g for decreased intake of food and fatigue; *Da Huang* (Radix et Rhizoma Rhei) 12g and *Di Huang* (Radix Rehmanniae) 15g for constipation with dry mouth and bitter taste; *Chuan Lian Zi* (Fructus Toosendan) 10g and *Yan Hu Suo* (Rhizoma Corydalis) 10g for hypochondriac pain; and *Pu Huang* (Pollen Typhae) 9g and *Yin Chen* (Herba Artemisiae Scopariae) 15g for abnormal liver functions.[25]

7. **Hyperlipidemia**: Sixty-five patients with hyperlipidemia (49 had concurrent hypertension, 41 had concurrent diabetes) were treated with *Da Chai Hu Tang* with good results. The treatment protocol was to administer the herbs in granular extracts at 2.5g per dose, three times per day, for 16 weeks. At the conclusion of the study, the researchers stated that 71% of the patients had a moderate to significant reduction of serum cholesterol levels. Side effects reported in about 5% of the patients included poor appetite, abdominal distention, diarrhea, and edema.[26]

8. **Duodenal ulcer**: Thirty-four patients with duodenal ulcer were treated with *Da Chai Hu Tang* for 30 days with complete recovery in 23 patients, improvement in 9 patients, and no effect in 2 patients. The study reported an overall effectiveness rate of 94.1%.[27]

9. **Perforating ulcer**: In one study, 192 of 202 patients with acute perforating ulcer showed good response after treatment with *Da Chai Hu Tang*. Of 202 patients, only 20 still required surgery. The researchers were able to contact 75 of the patients for follow-up interviews 1-2 years later, and stated that there were no recurrences in 31 patients, significant improvement in 28 patients, and recurrence in 16 patients.[28]

10. **Gastric prolapse**: One study reported 97.4% effectiveness using modified *Da Chai Hu Tang* to treat gastric prolapse. Out of 228 patients with up to 21 years of prolapse, the study reported complete recovery in 120 patients, significant improvement in 84 patients, slight improvement in 18 patients, and no benefit in 6 patients. The treatment protocol was to cook the herbs and administer the decoction in multiple doses daily, for 15 days per course of treatment, followed by 3 days of rest, for a total of 3 courses. The herbal treatment contained *Chai Hu* (Radix Bupleuri) 10g, *Zhi Qiao* (Fructus Aurantii) 10g, *Huang Qin* (Radix

Dà Chái Hú Tāng (Major Bupleurum Decoction)

Scutellariae) 10g, *Ban Xia* (Rhizoma Pinelliae) 10g, *Cang Zhu* (Rhizoma Atractylodis) 10g, *Hou Po* (Cortex Magnoliae Officinalis) 10g, *Chen Pi* (Pericarpium Citri Reticulatae) 10g, *Bai Shao* (Radix Paeoniae Alba) 15g, *Da Huang* (Radix et Rhizoma Rhei) 6g, *Lu Gen* (Rhizoma Phragmitis) 30g, and *Gan Cao* (Radix et Rhizoma Glycyrrhizae) 5g. *Huang Lian* (Rhizoma Coptidis) was added for burning and heat sensation in the stomach; *Chuan Lian Zi* (Fructus Toosendan) for back swelling and hypochondriac pain; and *Sha Ren* (Fructus Amomi) for feelings of distention and prolapse in the lower abdomen.[29]

11. **Acute tonsillitis**: Modified *Da Chai Hu Tang* successfully treated 36 patients with acute tonsillitis. The base treatment included *Da Chai Hu Tang* plus *Jin Yin Hua* (Flos Lonicerae Japonicae) and *Lian Qiao* (Fructus Forsythiae). Modifications included addition of *Bai Zhi* (Radix Angelicae Dahuricae) for headache; *Ban Lan Gen* (Radix Isatidis) and *She Gan* (Rhizoma Belamcandae) for sore throat; and *Zhe Bei Mu* (Bulbus Fritillariae Thunbergii) for coughing. The treatment protocol was to give the herbs in decoction one time per day.[30]

HERB-DRUG INTERACTION

Aspirin- and ethanol-induced gastric lesions: Administration of *Da Chai Hu Tang* was associated with a notable effect to treat aspirin- and ethanol-induced gastric hemorrhagic lesions in rats. The gastroprotective effect of *Da Chai Hu Tang* was comparable to sucralfate (Carafate), cimetidine (Tagamet), and 16,16-dimethyl-prostaglandin E2 (DMPGE2).[31]

TOXICOLOGY

According to one case report in Japan, administration of *Dai-saiko-to* [*Da Chai Hu Tang*] was associated with one incidence of autoimmune hepatitis in one patient.[32] Note: Additional information on the medical history of this patient was unavailable at the time of publication.

RELATED FORMULA

Chái Hú Tāng (Bupleurum Decoction)

柴胡湯
柴胡汤

Pinyin Name: *Chai Hu Tang*
Literal Name: Bupleurum Decoction
Original Source: *Tian Jin Zhong Yi Xue Yuan* (Tianjin University of Chinese Medicine) in 1989

Chai Hu (Radix Bupleuri)
Huang Qin (Radix Scutellariae)
Bai Shao (Radix Paeoniae Alba)
Zao Jiao (Fructus Gleditsiae)
Da Huang (Radix et Rhizoma Rhei)

Sheng Jiang (Rhizoma Zingiberis Recens)
Da Zao (Fructus Jujubae)
Qing Pi (Pericarpium Citri Reticulatae Viride)
Huang Qi (Radix Astragali)
Ci Wu Jia (Radix et Rhizoma seu Caulis Acanthopanacis Senticosi)
Zhi Shi (Fructus Aurantii Immaturus)
Cha Ye (Folium Camelliae)
Ban Xia (Rhizoma Pinelliae)

Chai Hu Tang (Bupleurum Decoction) treats *shaoyang* disorder with accumulation of damp and phlegm. It clears heat in the interior, resolves dampness, eliminates phlegm, and tonifies qi. Clinically, this formula treats obese individuals who exhibit low energy, slow metabolism, and poor dietary habits.

AUTHORS' COMMENTS

A question is often raised as to how *Da Chai Hu Tang* can be used to treat both constipation and diarrhea. From a traditional Chinese medical perspective, the cause of constipation and diarrhea in this case is the same: excess heat in the Intestines that dries the stool and turns it into a hard, immobile mass. Accordingly, *Da Huang* (Radix et Rhizoma Rhei) and *Zhi Shi* (Fructus Aurantii Immaturus) are used to regulate qi and purge heat in the bowels. Because these two herbs dispel stagnation and heat in the Intestines, they can treat either constipation or diarrhea. Clearing or purging heat will resolve the root cause of the diarrhea. This is the same principle underlying *Da Cheng Qi Tang* (Major Order the Qi Decoction), in which a downward draining formula is used to purge watery diarrhea because fecal matter is still stagnant in the Intestines and has to be directed out. Note: Diarrhea in this case refers only to the passage of fluids rectally, and not the stool. This occurs because the stool is dry, hard and immobile, so the water in the intestines has nowhere to go but to be excreted rectally as watery fluids.[33]

Although *Da Cheng Qi Tang* (Major Order the Qi Decoction) and *Da Chai Hu Tang* share the same principle of using *Da Huang* to purge damp-heat in excess *yangming fu* (hollow organs) syndrome, there are contrasting differences:

- *Da Cheng Qi Tang* is used for <u>severe</u> *yangming fu* excess condition with constipation and the four symptoms of *pi* (distention), *man* (fullness), *zao* (dryness), and *shi* (hardness) with a dry, red tongue body with a yellow coating as well as abdominal pain that is worse with pressure.
- *Da Chai Hu Tang* treats *yangming fu* and *shaoyang* syndrome. One chief manifestation is focal distention and pain that does not increase when pressure is applied

Dà Chái Hú Tāng (Major Bupleurum Decoction)

to the abdomen. Therefore, the condition in *Da Chai Hu Tang* is not as severe as that seen in *Da Cheng Qi Tang*. Consequently, a smaller dose of *Da Huang* is used in *Da Chai Hu Tang* to purge excess heat and treat constipation. If *Da Cheng Qi Tang* is used, there is a hidden danger that *zheng* (upright) *qi* may be damaged, and the disease will progress from being in between *shaoyang* and *yangming* stages to moving deeper in the body.[34]

Xiao Chai Hu Tang (Minor Bupleurum Decoction) and *Da Chai Hu Tang* are both formulated to treat *shaoyang* stage disorder with alternating spells of chills and fever, a bitter taste in the mouth, and chest and hypochondriac distention. Both formulas contain *Chai Hu* (Radix Bupleuri), *Huang Qin* (Radix Scutellariae), *Ban Xia* (Rhizoma Pinelliae), *Sheng Jiang* (Rhizoma Zingiberis Recens), and *Da Zao* (Fructus Jujubae). Despite similarities, they have contrasting differences:

- *Xiao Chai Hu Tang* contains *Chai Hu* (Radix Bupleuri) and *Huang Qin* (Radix Scutellariae) as chief herbs to harmonize the *shaoyang* stage. *Ren Shen* (Radix et Rhizoma Ginseng) is used to support the underlying constitutional deficiency and to prevent the pathogenic factor from moving further inward. This formula can be used in a variety of patients, including women who catch colds during their periods, and individuals with malaria and/or jaundice.

- *Da Chai Hu Tang* is mainly used for *yangming fu* syndrome with excess heat accumulation in the body. *Da Huang* (Radix et Rhizoma Rhei) and *Zhi Shi* (Fructus Aurantii Immaturus) serve to sedate the heat in the *yangming* channel. The key differential diagnosis is constipation with abdominal pain.[35]

References

1. *Zhong Yao Ming Fang Yao Li Yu Ying Yong* (Pharmacology and Applications of Famous Herbal Formulas) 1989;92-96.
2. *Yao Xue Za Zhi* (Journal of Medicinals) 1982;102(4):371.
3. *Guo Wai Yi Xue* (Foreign Medicine) 1989;11(3):55.
4. *Guo Wai Yi Xue* (Foreign Medicine) 1988;10(5):36.
5. *Guo Wai Yi Xue Zhong Yi Zhong Yao Fen Ce* (Monograph of Chinese Herbology from Foreign Medicine) 1984;6(2):58.
6. Ohta Y, Sasaki E, Nishida K, Kobayashi T, Nagata M, Ishiguro I. Preventive effect of dai-saiko-to (da-chai-hu-tang) extract on disrupted hepatic active oxygen metabolism in rats with carbon tetrachloride-induced liver injury. Am J Chin Med 1995;23(1):53-64.
7. *Guo Wai Yi Xue Zhong Yi Zhong Yao Fen Ce* (Monograph of Chinese Herbology from Foreign Medicine) 1995;17(2):52.
8. *Zhong Yao Yao Li Yu Lin Chuang* (Pharmacology and Clinical Applications of Chinese Herbs) 1991;7:1.
9. *Zhong Yi Fang Ji Xian Dai Yan Jiu* (Modern Study of Medical Formulae in Traditional Chinese Medicine) 1997;432.
10. *Zhong Yi Za Zhi* (Journal of Chinese Medicine) 1955;10:36.
11. *Yao Xue Za Zhi* (Journal of Medicinals) 1983;103(4):466.
12. Yamamoto K, Ogawa Y, Yanagita T, Morito F, Fukushima N, Ozaki I, Mizuta T, Setoguchi Y, Sakai T. Pharmacological effects of dai-saiko-to on lipid biosynthesis in cultured human hepatocyte HepG2 cells. J Ethnopharmacol 1995 Apr;46(1):49-54.
13. Teramoto T, Matsushima T, Horie Y, Watanabe T. Production of apolipoprotein E-rich LDL by the liver. The effect of dietary cholesterol and some lipid lowering agents. Ann N Y Acad Sci 1990;598:301-7.
14. Saku K, Hirata K, Zhang B, Liu R, Ying H, Okura Y, Yoshinaga K, Arakawa K. Effects of Chinese herbal drugs on serum lipids, lipoproteins and apolipoproteins in mild to moderate essential hypertensive patients. J Hum Hypertens 1992 Oct;6(5):393-5.
15. Ying H, Saku K, Ando K, Okura Y, Yoshinaga K, Harada R, Hidaka K, Arakawa K. Effects of Chinese herbal drug, dai-saiko-to on plasma lipids, lipoproteins and liver lipid contents in guinea pig. Artery 1991;18(4):184-96.
16. Iizuka A, Iijima OT, Yoshie F, Makino B, Amagaya S, Komatsu Y, Kondo K, Matsumoto A, Itakura H. Inhibitory effects of Dai-saiko-to (Da-Chai-Hu-Tang) on the progression of atherosclerotic lesions in Kurosawa and Kusanagi-hypercholesterolemic rabbits. J Ethnopharmacol 1999 Apr;65(1):79.
17. Umeda M, Amagaya S, Ogihara Y. Effect of shosaikoto, daisaikoto and sannoshashinto (traditional Japanese and Chinese medicines) on experimental hyperlipidemia in rats. J Ethnopharmacol 1989 Oct;26(3):255-69.
18. *Yun Nan Zhong Yi Za Zhi* (Yunan Journal of Chinese Medicine) 1990;11(4):18.
19. *Shan Dong Zhong Yi Za Zhi* (Shandong Journal of Chinese Medicine) 1987;3:18.
20. *Zhong Yi Za Zhi* (Journal of Chinese Medicine) 1984;5:46.
21. *Zhong Yi Ming Fang Lin Chuang Xin Yong* (Contemporary Clinical Applications of Classic Chinese Formulas) 2001;61.
22. *Zhe Jiang Zhong Yi Za Zhi* (Zhejiang Journal of Chinese Medicine) 1988;6:252.
23. *Bei Jing Zhong Yi Xue Yuan Xue Bao* (Journal of Beijing University School of Medicine) 1991;14(4):12.
24. *Shan Xi Zhong Yi* (Shanxi Chinese Medicine) 1989;5:223.
25. *Fu Jian Zhong Yi Yao* (Fujian Chinese Medicine and Herbology) 1995;6:43.
26. *Xin Yao Yu Lin Chuang* (New Medicine and the Clinical Application) 1989;38(4):61.
27. *Zhong Yi Fang Ji Xian Dai Yan Jiu* (Modern Study of Medical Formulae in Traditional Chinese Medicine) 1997;434.
28. *Xin Yi Xue* (New Medicine) 1977;10-11:482.
29. *Zhe Jiang Zhong Yi Za Zhi* (Zhejiang Journal of Chinese Medicine) 1997;10:441.
30. *Si Chuan Zhong Yi* (Sichuan Chinese Medicine) 1987;5:44.
31. Takase H, Imanishi K, Miura O, Yumioka E, Watanabe H. Pharmacological studies on the effects of some traditional Chinese medicines on gastric functions. (3) The effects of oren-gedoku-to (OGT), san'o-syasin-to (SST), antyu-san (AS) and dai-saiko-to (DST) on ethanol- and aspirin-induced gastric lesions in rats. Nippon Yakurigaku Zasshi 1988 May;91(5):319-24.
32. Kamiyama T, Nouchi T, Kojima S, Murata N, Ikeda T, Sato C. Autoimmune hepatitis triggered by administration of an herbal medicine. American Journal of Gastroenterology 1997 Apr;92(4):703-4.
33. Wang MZ, et al. *Zhong Yi Xue Wen Da Ti Ku* (Questions and Answers on Traditional Chinese Medicine: Herbal Formulas).
34. Wang MZ, et al. *Zhong Yi Xue Wen Da Ti Ku* (Questions and Answers on Traditional Chinese Medicine: Herbal Formulas).
35. Wang MZ, et al. *Zhong Yi Xue Wen Da Ti Ku* (Questions and Answers on Traditional Chinese Medicine: Herbal Formulas).

Hòu Pò Qī Wù Tāng (Seven-Substance Decoction with Magnolia Bark)

厚樸七物湯
厚朴七物汤

Pinyin Name: *Hou Po Qi Wu Tang*
Literal Name: Seven-Substance Decoction with Magnolia Bark
Alternate Name: Magnolia Seven Combination
Original Source: *Jin Gui Yao Lue* (Essentials from the Golden Cabinet) by Zhang Zhong-Jing in the Eastern Han Dynasty

COMPOSITION

Hou Po (Cortex Magnoliae Officinalis)	24g [15g]
Zhi Shi (Fructus Aurantii Immaturus)	5 pieces [9g]
Da Huang (Radix et Rhizoma Rhei)	9g
Gui Zhi (Ramulus Cinnamomi)	6g
Da Zao (Fructus Jujubae)	10 pieces [4 pieces]
Sheng Jiang (Rhizoma Zingiberis Recens)	15g [12g]
Gan Cao (Radix et Rhizoma Glycyrrhizae)	9g

DOSAGE / PREPARATION / ADMINISTRATION

The source text states to cook the ingredients in 10 cups [2,000 mL] of water until 4 cups [800 mL] of the liquid remain. Take 0.8 cup [160 mL] of the warm, strained decoction three times daily. Today, the decoction may be prepared using the doses suggested in brackets.

CHINESE THERAPEUTIC ACTIONS

1. Expels the pathogenic factor from the exterior and muscle layer
2. Regulates qi
3. Promotes bowel movement

CLINICAL MANIFESTATIONS

Taiyang and *yangming* syndromes with interior excess: abdominal fullness, fever, constipation, and a superficial, rapid pulse.

CLINICAL APPLICATIONS

Acute febrile disorders, gastroenteritis, habitual constipation, and peritonitis.

EXPLANATION

Hou Po Qi Wu Tang (Seven-Substance Decoction with Magnolia Bark) treats *taiyang* and *yangming* syndromes complicated by interior excess. This condition develops as the result of improper treatment or lack of treatment, where, prior to resolution of the exterior condition, an interior excess develops. Fever with a superficial pulse indicates an exterior condition; while abdominal fullness with a rapid pulse indicates an interior condition. With such complications, the treatment must focus on expelling the pathogenic factors from both the exterior and interior.

This formula uses herbs that treat both interior and exterior conditions. *Hou Po* (Cortex Magnoliae Officinalis), *Zhi Shi* (Fructus Aurantii Immaturus), and *Da Huang* (Radix et Rhizoma Rhei) regulate qi and purge interior excess. *Gui Zhi* (Ramulus Cinnamomi), *Da Zao* (Fructus Jujubae), *Sheng Jiang* (Rhizoma Zingiberis Recens), and *Gan Cao* (Radix et Rhizoma Glycyrrhizae) release exterior pathogenic factors and harmonize *ying* (nutritive) and *wei* (defensive) levels.

Hou Po Qi Wu Tang (Seven-Substance Decoction with Magnolia Bark)

Diagnosis	Signs and Symptoms	Treatment	Herbs
Taiyang and *yangming* syndromes with interior excess	• Fever with superficial pulse: exterior (*taiyang*) condition • Abdominal fullness and constipation with rapid pulse: interior (*yangming*) condition	• Expels the pathogenic factor from the exterior and the muscle layer • Regulates qi • Promotes bowel movement	• *Hou Po* (Cortex Magnoliae Officinalis), *Zhi Shi* (Fructus Aurantii Immaturus) and *Da Huang* (Radix et Rhizoma Rhei) regulate qi and purge interior excess. • *Gui Zhi* (Ramulus Cinnamomi), *Da Zao* (Fructus Jujubae), *Sheng Jiang* (Rhizoma Zingiberis Recens) and *Gan Cao* (Radix et Rhizoma Glycyrrhizae) dispel exterior pathogenic factors and harmonize *ying* (nutritive) and *wei* (defensive) levels.

Hòu Pò Qī Wù Tāng (Seven-Substance Decoction with Magnolia Bark)

Hou Po Qi Wu Tang, similarly to *Da Chai Hu Tang* (Major Bupleurum Decoction), treats both interior and exterior syndromes at the same time. *Da Chai Hu Tang* treats the combination of *shaoyang* and *yangming* syndromes, while *Hou Po Qi Wu Tang* treats *taiyang* and *yangming* syndromes with interior excess.

MODIFICATION

With nausea, add *Ban Xia* (Rhizoma Pinelliae).

AUTHORS' COMMENTS

Hou Po Qi Wu Tang and *Da Chai Hu Tang* (Major Bupleurum Decoction) both treat *yangming* excess with abdominal pain and constipation. Both formulas have harmonizing and sedating functions, and contain *Da Huang* (Radix et Rhizoma Rhei), *Zhi Shi* (Fructus Aurantii Immaturus), *Sheng Jiang* (Rhizoma Zingiberis Recens), and *Da Zao* (Fructus Jujubae). The differences between these two formulas are as follows:

- *Da Chai Hu Tang* treats *shaoyang* and *yangming* disorders with alternating spells of chills and fever, a bitter taste in the mouth, chest and hypochondriac distention, abdominal fullness, constipation, a red tongue with a yellow coating, and a wiry, forceful pulse. *Chai Hu* (Radix Bupleuri) and

Huang Qin (Radix Scutellariae) are used to harmonize the *shaoyang*, while *Da Huang* (Radix et Rhizoma Rhei), *Zhi Shi* (Fructus Aurantii Immaturus), and *Bai Shao* (Radix Paeoniae Alba) purge *yangming* heat and relieve pain. *Sheng Jiang* (Rhizoma Zingiberis Recens), *Ban Xia* (Rhizoma Pinelliae), and *Da Zao* (Fructus Jujubae) harmonize the Stomach to relieve nausea and vomiting.

- *Hou Po Qi Wu Tang* treats *taiyang* and *yangming* disorders with exterior and interior conditions. Most of the signs and symptoms exhibited are of interior *yangming* origin, such as fever, abdominal fullness, and constipation. *Hou Po* (Cortex Magnoliae Officinalis) and *Zhi Shi* (Fructus Aurantii Immaturus) regulate qi and dispel fullness. When combined with *Da Huang* (Radix et Rhizoma Rhei), these herbs purge heat and clear the bowels. To relieve *taiyang* symptoms, *Gui Zhi* (Ramulus Cinnamomi), *Sheng Jiang* (Rhizoma Zingiberis Recens), *Gan Cao* (Radix et Rhizoma Glycyrrhizae), and *Da Zao* (Fructus Jujubae) are used. Because there is no abdominal pain, *Bai Shao* (Radix Paeoniae Alba) is not used.[1]

Reference

1. Wang MZ, et al. *Zhong Yi Xue Wen Da Ti Ku* (Questions and Answers on Traditional Chinese Medicine: Herbal Formulas).

Chinese Herbal Formulas and Applications

Fáng Fēng Tōng Shèng Sǎn
(Saposhnikovia Powder that Sagely Unblocks)

防風通聖散
防风通圣散

Pinyin Name: *Fang Feng Tong Sheng San*
Literal Name: Saposhnikovia Powder that Sagely Unblocks
Alternate Names: *Fang Feng Tung Sheng San*, Siler Sage-Inspired Formula, Siler and Platycodon Formula
Original Source: *Huang Di Su Wen Xuan Ming Lun Fang* (Formulas from the Discussion Illuminating the Yellow Emperor's Basic Questions) by Liu Yuan-Su in 1172

COMPOSITION

Fang Feng (Radix Saposhnikoviae)	15g [6g]
Jing Jie (Herba Schizonepetae)	7.5-15g [3-6g]
Ma Huang (Herba Ephedrae)	15g [6g]
Bo He (Herba Menthae)	15g [6g]
Da Huang (Radix et Rhizoma Rhei), *zheng* (steamed) with liquor	15g [6g]
Mang Xiao (Natrii Sulfas), post-decocted	15g [6g]
Shi Gao (Gypsum Fibrosum)	30g [12g]
Huang Qin (Radix Scutellariae)	30g [12g]
Lian Qiao (Fructus Forsythiae)	15g [6g]
Jie Geng (Radix Platycodonis)	30g [12g]
Zhi Zi (Fructus Gardeniae), *tan* (charred to ash)	7.5-15g [3-6g]
Hua Shi (Talcum)	90g [20g]
Dang Gui (Radix Angelicae Sinensis)	15g [6g]
Chuan Xiong (Rhizoma Chuanxiong)	15g [6g]
Bai Shao (Radix Paeoniae Alba), *chao* (dry-fried)	15g [6g]
Bai Zhu (Rhizoma Atractylodis Macrocephalae)	7.5-15g [3-6g]
Gan Cao (Radix et Rhizoma Glycyrrhizae)	60g [10g]

DOSAGE / PREPARATION / ADMINISTRATION

The source text instructs to grind the ingredients into powder, and cook 6g of the powder with 3 slices of *Sheng Jiang* (Rhizoma Zingiberis Recens) in 1 large bowl of water until the liquid is reduced to 60%. Take the strained decoction while warm. Today, this formula may also be prepared as pills. For pills, grind all the ingredients, except *Hua Shi* (Talcum), into a fine powder, and sift evenly. Mix the powder with water to form into pills. Coat the pills with finely-powdered *Hua Shi* (Talcum), and polish and dry the pills. Take 6g of pills twice daily. Alternatively, this formula may be prepared as a decoction using the doses suggested in brackets above. *Cong Bai* (Bulbus Allii Fistulosi) may be added to enhance the exterior-releasing effect of the formula.

Note: The exact doses of *Jing Jie* (Herba Schizonepetae), *Bai Zhu* (Rhizoma Atractylodis Macrocephalae) and *Zhi Zi* (Fructus Gardeniae) are unclear. One reference specifies 2.5 *qian* (7.5g), while another instructs 5 *qian* (15g). We list both for reference purposes.

CHINESE THERAPEUTIC ACTIONS

1. Expels wind and releases the exterior
2. Clears interior heat and promotes defecation

CLINICAL MANIFESTATIONS

Exterior wind-heat syndrome with accumulation of interior heat: severe aversion to cold and high fever, dizziness, vertigo, red and painful eyes, a bitter and dry mouth, throat discomfort or a sore throat, a feeling of distention and stifling sensation in the chest and diaphragm, coughing, dyspnea, thick and sticky nasal discharge and saliva, constipation, dark yellow-colored urine or dysuria. It also treats abscesses, sores, carbuncle, *chang feng* (intestinal wind), hemorrhoids, erysipelas, dermatitis, acne, and other conditions characterized by heat and toxins.

CLINICAL APPLICATIONS

Headache, migraine, acute mastitis, obesity, food poisoning, habitual constipation, hyperlipidemia, hypertension, arteriosclerosis, itching, acne, dermatitis, carbuncles, urticaria, acute conjunctivitis, influenza, and common cold.

4

EXTERIOR- AND INTERIOR-RELEASING FORMULAS

291

Chapter 4 – Exterior- and Interior-Releasing Formulas **Section 1** *– Exterior-Releasing and Interior-Attacking Formulas*

Fáng Fēng Tōng Shèng Sǎn
(Saposhnikovia Powder that Sagely Unblocks)

EXPLANATION

Fang Feng Tong Sheng San (Saposhnikovia Powder that Sagely Unblocks) has three main functions: it releases exterior wind-heat, clears interior heat, and drains downward. It is indicated for excess conditions at both the exterior (wind-heat) and interior (heat accumulation). Wind-heat at the exterior may cause exterior symptoms such as aversion to cold and fever. Because both wind and heat tend to ascend and attack the upper body, they may cause symptoms such as red and painful eyes, a dry mouth with a bitter taste, and a sore throat. And since the Lung is the organ that is most vulnerable to exterior pathogenic factors and heat, the wind-heat factor may also damage the Lung and cause symptoms such as a feeling of distention and a stifling sensation in the chest and diaphragm, coughing, and dyspnea. Thick, sticky nasal discharge and saliva indicate wind-heat damaging the exterior and the body fluids. Constipation and dysuria indicate excess heat in the interior damaging body fluids.

This formula uses *Fang Feng* (Radix Saposhnikoviae), *Jing Jie* (Herba Schizonepetae), *Ma Huang* (Herba Ephedrae), and *Bo He* (Herba Menthae) to clear the exterior wind-heat. *Da Huang* (Radix et Rhizoma Rhei) and *Mang Xiao* (Natrii Sulfas) purge interior heat and promote defecation. *Shi Gao* (Gypsum Fibrosum), *Huang Qin* (Radix Scutellariae), *Lian Qiao* (Fructus Forsythiae), *Jie Geng* (Radix Platycodonis), and *Zhi Zi* (Fructus Gardeniae) clear heat in the Lung and Stomach. *Hua Shi* (Talcum) dispels heat through urination and relieves dysuria. *Dang Gui* (Radix Angelicae Sinensis), *Chuan Xiong* (Rhizoma Chuanxiong), and *Bai Shao* (Radix Paeoniae Alba) nourish the blood and activate blood circulation. *Bai Zhu* (Rhizoma Atractylodis Macrocephalae) and *Gan Cao* (Radix et Rhizoma Glycyrrhizae) strengthen Spleen qi. These tonic herbs also prevent the heat-clearing and purgative herbs in this formula from injuring the body.

MODIFICATIONS

- For common cold or influenza caused by wind-cold, add *Qiang Huo* (Rhizoma et Radix Notopterygii).
- For common cold or influenza caused by wind-heat, add *Jin Yin Hua* (Flos Lonicerae Japonicae) and *Tian Hua Fen* (Radix Trichosanthis).
- When there is excess heat, add *Huang Lian* (Rhizoma Coptidis) and *Huang Bo* (Cortex Phellodendri Chinensis).
- With cough with excess phlegm, add *Ban Xia* (Rhizoma Pinelliae).
- For dermatological disorders without abscess and ulceration, combine with *Sheng Ma Ge Gen Tang* (Cimicifuga and Kudzu Decoction).
- For dermatological disorders with abscess and ulceration, combine with *Pai Nong San* (Drain the Pus Powder).

Fang Feng Tong Sheng San (Saposhnikovia Powder that Sagely Unblocks)

Diagnosis	Signs and Symptoms	Treatment	Herbs
Exterior wind-heat syndrome with accumulation of interior heat	• Aversion to cold and fever: exterior wind-heat • Red and painful eyes, bitter and dry mouth and sore throat: wind-heat attacking upper body • Thick and sticky nasal discharge and saliva: exterior wind-heat damaging the body fluids • Feeling of distention and a stifling sensation in the chest and diaphragm, coughing, and dyspnea: heat affecting the Lung • Constipation and dysuria: interior heat consuming body fluids	• Expels wind and releases the exterior • Clears interior heat and promotes defecation	• *Fang Feng* (Radix Saposhnikoviae), *Jing Jie* (Herba Schizonepetae), *Ma Huang* (Herba Ephedrae) and *Bo He* (Herba Menthae) clear the exterior wind-heat. • *Da Huang* (Radix et Rhizoma Rhei) and *Mang Xiao* (Natrii Sulfas) purge interior heat and promote defecation. • *Shi Gao* (Gypsum Fibrosum), *Huang Qin* (Radix Scutellariae), *Lian Qiao* (Fructus Forsythiae), *Jie Geng* (Radix Platycodonis) and *Zhi Zi* (Fructus Gardeniae) clear Lung and Stomach heat. • *Hua Shi* (Talcum) dispels heat through urination and relieves dysuria. • *Dang Gui* (Radix Angelicae Sinensis), *Chuan Xiong* (Rhizoma Chuanxiong) and *Bai Shao* (Radix Paeoniae Alba) nourish the blood and activate blood circulation. • *Bai Zhu* (Rhizoma Atractylodis Macrocephalae) and *Gan Cao* (Radix et Rhizoma Glycyrrhizae) strengthen Spleen qi.

Fáng Fēng Tōng Shèng Sǎn
(Saposhnikovia Powder that Sagely Unblocks)

- For erysipelas with faint skin lesions, add *Sheng Ma Ge Gen Tang* (Cimicifuga and Kudzu Decoction).
- For eczema, add *Xiao Feng San* (Eliminate Wind Powder).
- If there is no constipation, remove *Mang Xiao* (Natrii Sulfas) and *Da Huang* (Radix et Rhizoma Rhei).
- For hemorrhoids, add *Yi Zi Tang* (Yi Word Decoction).
- For high cholesterol, add *Jiao Gu Lan* (Rhizoma seu Herba Gynostemmatis) and *Jue Ming Zi* (Semen Cassiae).
- For obesity, add *He Ye* (Folium Nelumbinis) and *Yi Yi Ren* (Semen Coicis).
- If accompanied by qi deficiency, add *Ren Shen* (Radix et Rhizoma Ginseng).
- With summer-dampness with thirst, add *Yin Chen* (Herba Artemisiae Scopariae) and *Huang Lian* (Rhizoma Coptidis).
- For hangovers with fever and headache, add *Huang Lian* (Rhizoma Coptidis) and *Ge Hua* (Flos Puerariae).

CAUTIONS / CONTRAINDICATIONS

- *Fang Feng Tong Sheng San* is contraindicated in patients of deficiency or pregnancy.
- This formula should be used with caution in a patient having a sensitive gastrointestinal system because it contains strong downward draining herbs.

PHARMACOLOGICAL EFFECTS

1. **Cardiovascular**: According to laboratory experiments, administration of *Fang Feng Tong Sheng San* was associated with an inhibitory effect on the heart, reducing the heart rate, its contractile force, and blood pressure. It also has an anti-arrhythmic effect, as demonstrated in mice with aconitine-induced arrhythmia.[1]

2. **Metabolic**: Administration of *Fang Feng Tong Sheng San* in obese rats at 0.45 g/day for 11 weeks was effective in reducing cholesterol and triglycerides.[2]

3. **Thermogenic and anti-obesity**: Administration of *Fang Feng Tong Sheng San* suppressed body weight gain and prevented the elevation of serum triglyceride levels and body fat accumulation in female rats on a high fructose diet. The proposed mechanisms of actions included inhibition of triglyceride synthesis in the liver, enhancement of lipolysis in adipocytes and of thermogenesis in brown adipose tissue, and inhibition on the phosphodiesterase activity.[3,4]

CLINICAL STUDIES AND RESEARCH

1. **Headache**: In one study, *Fang Feng Tong Sheng San* was used to treat patients with stubborn headache arising from various causes, such as tension, migraine, hypertension, and sinus infection. Out of 27 patients, the study reported complete recovery in 19 patients (asymptomatic with no recurrence in 6 months), significant improvement in 5 patients (occasional recurrence with milder intensity), and no benefit in 3 patients.[5]

2. **Migraine**: One study reported 80% effectiveness using *Fang Feng Tong Sheng San* in pills, at dosages of 6 grams twice daily. The study reported that while many patients had recurrences, the frequency and severity were both reduced.[6]

3. **Acute mastitis**: In one report, modified *Fang Feng Tong Sheng San* was effective in treating 97 out of 113 patients with acute mastitis.[7]

4. **Obesity**: In one study, 147 patients who were overweight were treated with both ear acupuncture and *Fang Feng Tong Sheng San* for 2 months. The study reported significant results in 27 patients (6.57 kg average in weight reduction), improvement in 93 patients (3.03 kg average in weight reduction), and no improvement in 27 patients (1.06 kg average in weight reduction). The maximum weight reduction was 11.5 kg in one patient.[8]

5. **Hyperlipidemia**: One study reported 80.1% effectiveness using modified *Fang Feng Tong Sheng San* to treat hyperlipidemia in 121 patients (average age of 53.41, with range of 35-72 years old). Modifications to the original formula were made as follows: addition of *Ban Xia* (Rhizoma Pinelliae) for drooling of saliva; addition of *Shi Chang Pu* (Rhizoma Acori Tatarinowii) and elimination of *Mang Xiao* (Natrii Sulfas) for deafness; and elimination of *Ma Huang* (Herba Ephedrae) for spontaneous perspiration. Each course of treatment was 30 days. Of 121 patients, the study reported complete recovery in 69 patients, improvement in 28 patients, and no effect in 24 patients.[9] In another study, use of this formula was associated with 30% effectiveness in weight reduction in 68 patients. The study noted that the formula was most effective in female patients between 20 and 30 years of age.[10]

6. **Itching**: Use of modified *Fang Feng Tong Sheng San* in 40 geriatric patients with itching due to wind-heat was associated with great results. Of 40 patients, the study reported complete relief in 35 patients and no benefit in 5 patients. The duration of treatment was 2 weeks per course of treatment, for 2 courses total.[11]

7. **Acute conjunctivitis**: One study reported complete recovery of acute conjunctivitis in all 200 patients (74 unilateral, 126 bilateral) when treated with modified *Fang Feng Tong Sheng San*. Most patients showed improvements within 2-3 days, with duration of treatment ranging from 1 to 5 days. The herbal treatment contained this formula as the base, with the addition of *Hong Hua* (Flos Carthami) for red eyes; *Ji Li* (Fructus Tribuli), *Chan Tui* (Periostracum Cicadae), and *Man Jing Zi* (Fructus Viticis) for severe itching; *Bai Zhi* (Radix Angelicae

Fáng Fēng Tōng Shèng Sǎn
(Saposhnikovia Powder that Sagely Unblocks)

Dahuricae), *Qiang Huo*, (Rhizoma et Radix Notopterygii), and *Mo Yao* (Myrrha) for severe pain; *Che Qian Zi* (Semen Plantaginis) and *Ze Xie* (Rhizoma Alismatis) for profuse eye secretions; *Pu Gong Ying* (Herba Taraxaci), *Jin Yin Hua* (Flos Lonicerae Japonicae), and *Yu Xing Cao* (Herba Houttuyniae) for redness and swelling of the eyes; elimination of *Mang Xiao* (Natrii Sulfas) if there was no constipation; and elimination of *Ma Huang* (Herba Ephedrae) for spontaneous or night perspiration.[12]

TOXICOLOGY

Use of *Fang Feng Tong Sheng San* was associated with one incidence of pneumonitis in a 65-year-old man who complained of cough, fever, and dyspnea about one month after treatment with this formula. Upon discontinuation of this product, the patient recovered.[13]

RELATED FORMULA

Shuāng Jiě Tōng Shèng Sǎn
(Double Relieve Powder that Sagely Unblocks)

雙解通聖散
双解通圣散

Pinyin Name: *Shuang Jie Tong Sheng San*
Literal Name: Double Relieve Powder that Sagely Unblocks
Alternate Name: Siler and Platycodon Formula (Minus Rhubarb)
Original Source: *Yi Zong Jin Jian* (Golden Mirror of the Medical Tradition) by Wu Qian in 1742

Fang Feng (Radix Saposhnikoviae)	15g [6g]
Chuan Xiong (Rhizoma Chuanxiong)	15g [6g]
Dang Gui (Radix Angelicae Sinensis)	15g [6g]
Bai Shao (Radix Paeoniae Alba), *chao* (dry-fried)	15g [6g]
Bo He (Herba Menthae)	15g [6g]
Ma Huang (Herba Ephedrae)	15g [6g]
Lian Qiao (Fructus Forsythiae)	15g [6g]
Shi Gao (Gypsum Fibrosum)	30g [12g]
Huang Qin (Radix Scutellariae)	30g [12g]
Jie Geng (Radix Platycodonis)	30g [12g]
Hua Shi (Talcum)	90g [20g]
Gan Cao (Radix et Rhizoma Glycyrrhizae)	60g [10g]
Jing Jie (Herba Schizonepetae)	15g [3g]
Bai Zhu (Rhizoma Atractylodis Macrocephalae)	15g [3g]
Zhi Zi (Fructus Gardeniae), *tan* (charred to ash)	15g [3g]

The preparation and administration of this formula is the same as *Fang Feng Tong Sheng San*.

Shuang Jie Tong Sheng San (Double Relieve Powder that Sagely Unblocks) is essentially the same as *Fang Feng Tong Sheng San*. The main difference is the removal of two ingredients: *Mang Xiao* (Natrii Sulfas) and *Da Huang* (Radix et Rhizoma Rhei). This formula can be used for individuals having the same condition as described above, but without constipation.

AUTHORS' COMMENTS

Fang Feng Tong Sheng San is literally translated as "Saposhnikovia Powder that Sagely Unblocks" because this formula is known to induce perspiration without damaging the exterior and sedate heat without injuring the interior.

According to Dr. Chang Wei-Yen, dermatitis and skin rash can be treated effectively with *Fang Feng Tong Sheng San* and *Jing Fang Bai Du San* (Schizonepeta and Saposhnikovia Powder to Overcome Pathogenic Influences).

References

1. *Zhong Yao Yao Li Yu Lin Chuang* (Pharmacology and Clinical Applications of Chinese Herbs) 1989;5(3):3.
2. *Guo Wai Yi Xue* (Foreign Medicine) 1993;15(3):53.
3. Morimoto Y, Sakata M, Ohno A, Maegawa T, Tajima S. Effects of bofu-tsusho-san, a traditional Chinese medicine, on body fat accumulation in fructose-loaded rats. Nippon Yakurigaku Zasshi 2001 Jan;117(1):77-86.
4. Yoshida T, Sakane N, Wakabayashi Y, Umekawa T, Kondo M. Thermogenic, anti-obesity effects of bofu-tsusho-san in MSG-obese mice. Int J Obes Relat Metab Disord 1995 Oct;19(10):717-22.
5. *Tian Jin Yi Xue Za Zhi* (Journal of Tianjin Medicine and Herbology) 1977;2:82.
6. *Zhong Yi Za Zhi* (Journal of Chinese Medicine) 1989;6:17.
7. *Nei Meng Gu Zhong Yi Yao* (Traditional Chinese Medicine and Medicinals of Inner Mongolia) 1987;2:43.
8. *Si Chuan Zhong Yi* (Sichuan Chinese Medicine) 1988;2:26.
9. *Si Chuan Zhong Yi* (Sichuan Chinese Medicine) 1998;5:31.
10. *Zhong Cheng Yao Yan Jiu* (Research of Chinese Patent Medicine) 1984;4:36.
11. *Hei Long Jiang Zhong Yi Yao* (Heilongjiang Chinese Medicine and Herbology) 1992;1:33.
12. *Hu Bei Zhong Yi Za Zhi* (Hubei Journal of Chinese Medicine) 1988;5:29.
13. Matsushima H, Takayanagi N, Ubukata M, Tokunaga D, Mori S, Sato N, Kurashima K, Yanagisawa T, Sugita Y, Kawabata Y, Kanazawa M. A case of pneumonitis induced by Bofu-tsusho-san. Nihon Kokyuki Gakkai Zasshi 2002 Dec;40(12):955-9.

Chinese Herbal Formulas and Applications

Section 2

解表清里剂

— Exterior-Releasing and Interior-Clearing Formulas

4

EXTERIOR- AND INTERIOR-RELEASING FORMULAS

Gě Gēn Huáng Qín Huáng Lián Tāng

(Kudzu, Coptis, and Scutellaria Decoction)

葛根黃芩黃連湯

葛根黄芩黄连汤

Pinyin Name: *Ge Gen Huang Qin Huang Lian Tang*
Literal Name: Kudzu, Coptis, and Scutellaria Decoction
Alternate Names: *Ge Gen Qin Lian Tang, Ke Ken Huang Chin Huang Lien Tang,* Pueraria, Scute, and Coptis Decoction; Pueraria, Scutellaria and Coptis Decoction; Pueraria Coptis and Scute Combination
Original Source: *Shang Han Lun* (Discussion of Cold-Induced Disorders) by Zhang Zhong-Jing in the Eastern Han Dynasty

COMPOSITION

Ge Gen (Radix Puerariae Lobatae)	24g [15g]
Huang Qin (Radix Scutellariae)	9g
Huang Lian (Rhizoma Coptidis)	9g
Zhi Gan Cao (Radix et Rhizoma Glycyrrhizae Praeparata cum Melle)	6g

DOSAGE / PREPARATION / ADMINISTRATION

The source text states to cook *Ge Gen* (Radix Puerariae Lobatae) first in 8 cups [1,600 mL] of water until the liquid is reduced to 6 cups [1,200 mL]. Add the other ingredients and cook until the liquid is reduced to 2 cups [400 mL]. Take the warm, strained decoction in two equally-divided doses daily. Today, the decoction can be prepared using the dose of *Ge Gen* (Radix Puerariae Lobatae) suggested in brackets.

CHINESE THERAPEUTIC ACTIONS

1. Releases the exterior
2. Clears interior heat

CLINICAL MANIFESTATIONS

Wind-cold at the exterior with heat invading the interior: feverish sensation in the body, foul-smelling diarrhea, burning sensations of the anus after defecation, irritable and feverish sensation in the chest and epigastrium, a dry mouth, thirst, dyspnea with perspiration, a yellow tongue coating, and a rapid pulse.

CLINICAL APPLICATIONS

Diarrhea, dysentery, salmonella infection, amoebic dysentery, bacterial dysentery, gastritis, acute gastroenteritis, acute enteritis, ulcerative colitis, fever, influenza, common cold, measles, poliomyelitis, erysipelas, stomatitis, toothache, trachoma, conjunctivitis, inflammation of the lacrimal gland, and hangovers.

EXPLANATION

Ge Gen Huang Qin Huang Lian Tang (Kudzu, Coptis, and Scutellaria Decoction) was originally presented in *Shang Han Lun* (Discussion of Cold-Induced Disorders) for treating unresolved exterior wind-cold with heat invading the interior. This condition occurs when the exterior condition is incorrectly treated with downward draining herbs, leading to continued presence of exterior heat (minor condition) and its transformation into interior heat (major condition). Feverish sensations in the body indicate the presence of exterior heat. The interior heat may affect the Intestines and cause foul-smelling heat diarrhea. Interior heat may rise to attack the upper body and cause irritable and feverish sensations in the chest, a dry mouth, and thirst. The heat may damage the Lung to

295

Chapter 4 – Exterior- and Interior-Releasing Formulas   *Section 2 – Exterior-Releasing and Interior-Clearing Formulas*

Gě Gēn Huáng Qín Huáng Lián Tāng
(Kudzu, Coptis, and Scutellaria Decoction)

Ge Gen Huang Qin Huang Lian Tang (Kudzu, Coptis, and Scutellaria Decoction)

Diagnosis	Signs and Symptoms	Treatment	Herbs
Unresolved exterior wind-cold with heat invading the interior	• Feverish sensations in the body: presence of unresolved exterior wind-cold • Dyspnea: heat damaging the Lung • Irritability, a dry mouth, and thirst: interior heat consuming body fluids • Foul-smelling diarrhea with burning sensations: damp-heat in the Intestines • Yellow tongue coating and a rapid pulse: heat condition	• Releases the exterior • Clears interior heat	• *Ge Gen* (Radix Puerariae Lobatae) dispels the exterior factors and lifts Spleen qi to relieve diarrhea. • *Huang Qin* (Radix Scutellariae) and *Huang Lian* (Rhizoma Coptidis) clear heat and dry dampness to relieve diarrhea. • *Zhi Gan Cao* (Radix et Rhizoma Glycyrrhizae Praeparata cum Melle) harmonizes the herbs and calms the middle *jiao*.

cause dyspnea, and force body fluids out to the exterior, resulting in perspiration. A yellow tongue coating and a rapid pulse indicate a heat condition.

To properly treat this condition, exterior-releasing herbs must be used to treat the unresolved exterior condition, while interior heat-clearing herbs are used to sedate the interior. This formula contains *Ge Gen* (Radix Puerariae Lobatae) as the chief herb to dispel exterior factors, promote the production of body fluids to relieve the dry mouth and thirst, and direct Spleen qi upward to relieve diarrhea. *Huang Qin* (Radix Scutellariae) and *Huang Lian* (Rhizoma Coptidis) clear heat and dry dampness to relieve diarrhea. *Zhi Gan Cao* (Radix et Rhizoma Glycyrrhizae Praeparata cum Melle) harmonizes the herbs and calms the middle *jiao* to help relieve acute discomforts, such as burning sensations of the anus.

MODIFICATIONS
• When there is excess heat, add *Jin Yin Hua* (Flos Lonicerae Japonicae).
• With food stagnation, add *Mai Ya* (Fructus Hordei Germinatus), *Lai Fu Zi* (Semen Raphani), and *Shan Zha* (Fructus Crataegi).
• With vomiting, add *Ban Xia* (Rhizoma Pinelliae) and *Zhu Ru* (Caulis Bambusae in Taenia).
• With abdominal pain and cramps, add *Mu Xiang* (Radix Aucklandiae) and *Bai Shao* (Radix Paeoniae Alba).
• With abdominal pain and diarrhea, add *Bai Shao* (Radix Paeoniae Alba) and *Zhi Shi* (Fructus Aurantii Immaturus).
• For acute bacterial dysentery, add *Bai Tou Weng* (Radix Pulsatillae), *Mu Xiang* (Radix Aucklandiae), and *Qing Pi* (Pericarpium Citri Reticulatae Viride).
• If there is severe rectal tenesmus, add *Mu Xiang* (Radix Aucklandiae) and *Bing Lang* (Semen Arecae).

CAUTIONS / CONTRAINDICATIONS
Ge Gen Huang Qin Huang Lian Tang is contraindicated in diarrhea caused by cold and deficiency with deep, slow or weak pulse.

PHARMACOLOGICAL EFFECTS
1. **Antibacterial**: It has been demonstrated that decoction of *Ge Gen Huang Qin Huang Lian Tang* has an inhibitory effect *in vitro* against various microorganisms, especially *Staphylococcus aureus*, *Diplococcus pneumoniae*, and *Bacillus dysenteriae*.[1]
2. **Antipyretic**: In rabbits with artificially-induced fever, administration of *Ge Gen Huang Qin Huang Lian Tang* was associated with a marked effect to reduce fever, especially between 2-4 hours after ingestion. The treatment protocol was to administer 5 g/kg of the herbal decoction. In addition, the study noted that the effect of the herbs was comparable to 0.28 g/kg of aspirin.[2]
3. **Antiarrhythmic**: Intravenous injection of a *Ge Gen Huang Qin Huang Lian Tang* preparation was found to be effective in treating mice, rats, and rabbits with artificially-induced arrhythmia by injection of adrenaline and aconitine.[3]
4. **Gastrointestinal**: Administration of *Ge Gen Huang Qin Huang Lian Tang* in laboratory experiments has been associated with relieving diarrhea, slowing the peristalsis of the Intestines, and relieving spasms of the intestinal smooth muscles.[4]

CLINICAL STUDIES AND RESEARCH
1. **Diarrhea**: *Ge Gen Huang Qin Huang Lian Tang* has been shown via many studies to effectively treat diarrhea arising from various causes, such as acute or chronic enteritis, postpartum diarrhea, food poisoning, and infectious diarrhea.[5] In one study, 202 infants with acute diarrhea

Gě Gēn Huáng Qín Huáng Lián Tāng
(Kudzu, Coptis, and Scutellaria Decoction)

were treated with intravenous fluids and oral ingestion of *Ge Gen Huang Qin Huang Lian Tang* with an overall effectiveness of 88.6%. The average time needed to stop diarrhea was 3.5 days.[6] Another study reported satisfactory results using this formula to treat 513 infants and children with diarrhea in the summer.[7]

2. **Diarrhea during pregnancy**: Use of modified *Ge Gen Huang Qin Huang Lian Tang* in 30 pregnant women with diarrhea was associated with complete recovery in 25 patients, significant improvement in 4 patients, and no effect in 1 case. The herbal treatment contained this formula plus *Tu Si Zi* (Semen Cuscutae), *Sang Ji Sheng* (Herba Taxilli), and *Ai Ye* (Folium Artemisiae Argyi). Additional modifications included use of *Bai Shao* (Radix Paeoniae Alba) for restless fetus and *Shen Qu* (Massa Fermentata) for poor appetite. The herbs were given in decoction, in three equally-divided doses daily.[8]

3. **Salmonella infection**: Nineteen patients with acute salmonella infection were treated with complete recovery in 16 patients within 4 days, and 3 patients within 5 days.[9]

4. **Bacterial dysentery**: Forty patients with acute bacterial dysentery were treated with *Ge Gen Huang Qin Huang Lian Tang* with great success. The average recovery time was 1.15 days for reduction of fever, 4.51 days for relief of abdominal pain, 3.47 days for recovery of tenesmus, and 2.8 days for resolution of pus and blood in the stool. Overall, most patients reported stabilization of their condition within an average of 3.4 days.[10] Another study reported 96% effectiveness for treatment of acute bacterial dysentery in children using modified *Ge Gen Huang Qin Huang Lian Tang* via rectal enema. The treatment protocol was to cook the herbs in water to obtain 200 mL of herbal solution. Normal saline (300-500 mL) was used first to cleanse the intestines, prior to instilling 100 mL of the herbal solution. This procedure was repeated two times daily, for 3 days. Of 50 patients, the study reported significant improvement in 38 patients, improvement in 10 patients, and no benefit in 2 patients.[11]

5. **Amoebic dysentery**: One study reported 98.28% effectiveness using herbal therapy to treat 116 patients with amoebic dysentery. The herbal treatment contained *Ge Gen Huang Qin Huang Lian Tang* and *Bai Tou Weng Tang* (Pulsatilla Decoction), with addition of *Hou Po* (Cortex Magnoliae Officinalis) and *Huo Xiang* (Herba Agastaches), and removal of *Qin Pi* (Cortex Fraxini), as the base formula. Additional modifications included *Jin Yin Hua* (Flos Lonicerae Japonicae) for high fever; *Di Yu* (Radix Sanguisorbae) for the presence of blood in the stools; *Ban*

Xia (Rhizoma Pinelliae) for nausea and vomiting; and *Bai Shao* (Radix Paeoniae Alba) for abdominal pain. The herbs were given in decoction daily in two equally-divided doses. The study reported complete recovery in 114 of 116 patients.[12]

6. **Enteritis**: Use of this formula plus *Bai Tou Weng* (Radix Pulsatillae), *Chi Shao* (Radix Paeoniae Rubra) and *Lian Qiao* (Fructus Forsythiae) was effective in treating all 22 infants with enteritis. The herbs were given via rectal instillation, 40-50 mL rectally two times daily for 3-7 days.[13]

7. **Ulcerative colitis**: Thirty patients with chronic ulcerative colitis were treated with *Ge Gen Huang Qin Huang Lian Tang* with recovery in 10 patients, significant improvement in 12 patients, and slight improvement in 3 patients. The treatment protocol was to flood the colon with 250 mL of the decoction one time daily for 15 days per course of treatment, for a total of 1-3 courses of treatment.[14] Another study reported 87.5% effectiveness using modified *Ge Gen Huang Qin Huang Lian Tang* to treat 32 patients with chronic ulcerative colitis characterized by Large Intestine damp-heat and Spleen and Stomach weakness and deficiency.[15]

8. **Gastritis**: Sixty patients with chronic superficial gastritis were treated with good results using *Ge Gen Huang Qin Huang Lian Tang* plus *Xiang Fu* (Rhizoma Cyperi), *Bai Shao* (Radix Paeoniae Alba), and *Huo Xiang* (Herba Agastaches). Additional modifications included use of *Bai Hua She She Cao* (Herba Hedyotis) for constipation; *Mu Xiang* (Radix Aucklandiae) for loose stools; calcined *Wa Leng Zi* (Concha Arcae) for acid reflux; and *Zhu Ru* (Caulis Bambusae in Taenia) and *Ban Xia* (Rhizoma Pinelliae) for nausea and vomiting. Additionally, for abdominal distention, *Da Fu Pi* (Pericarpium Arecae) was added and *Bai Shao* (Radix Paeoniae Alba) was removed; and for food stagnation, dry-fried *Lai Fu Zi* (Semen Raphani), *Shan Zha* (Fructus Crataegi), and *Shen Qu* (Massa Fermentata) were added, and *Bai Shao* (Radix Paeoniae Alba) was removed. The study reported relief of gastric pain in all patients within 1-2 weeks of herbal treatment. Of 60 patients, 32 had significant improvement and 28 had moderate improvement.[16]

9. **Fever**: One study reported 97% effectiveness using modified *Ge Gen Huang Qin Huang Lian Tang* to treat 200 children with fever. Modifications to this formula included *Qing Hao* (Herba Artemisiae Annuae) for fever in spring, *Shi Gao* (Gypsum Fibrosum) in summer, *Jie Geng* (Radix Platycodonis) in fall, and *Ma Huang* (Herba Ephedrae) in winter. The study reported improvement in 197 of 200 patients.[17]

Chapter 4 – *Exterior- and Interior-Releasing Formulas*   Section 2 – *Exterior-Releasing and Interior-Clearing Formulas*

Gě Gēn Huáng Qín Huáng Lián Tāng
(Kudzu, Coptis, and Scutellaria Decoction)

TOXICOLOGY

The LD_{50} for alcohol extract of the formula via intravenous injection was 13.5 g/kg in mice. The cause of fatality was attributed to cardiovascular effects, with a decrease in heart rate and contractile force of the heart.[18]

RELATED FORMULA

Gě Gēn Huò Xiāng Sháo Yào Tāng

(Kudzu, Pogostemon, and Peony Decoction)

葛根藿香芍藥湯
葛根藿香芍药汤

Pinyin Name: *Ge Gen Huo Xiang Shao Yao Tang*
Literal Name: Kudzu, Pogostemon, and Peony Decoction
Original Source: *Jian Tai Zhen Suo Fang* (Herbal Prescriptions from *Jiantai* Clinic) by Chang Wei-Yen in 1981

Ge Gen (Radix Puerariae Lobatae)
Gan Cao (Radix et Rhizoma Glycyrrhizae)
Bai Shao (Radix Paeoniae Alba)
Huang Qin (Radix Scutellariae)
Huang Lian (Rhizoma Coptidis)
Da Huang (Radix et Rhizoma Rhei)
Rou Gui (Cortex Cinnamomi)
Xiang Fu (Rhizoma Cyperi)
Hou Po (Cortex Magnoliae Officinalis)
Guang Huo Xiang (Herba Pogostemonis)
Chen Pi (Pericarpium Citri Reticulatae)
Qing Pi (Pericarpium Citri Reticulatae Viride)
Zi Su Ye (Folium Perillae)
Fu Ling (Poria)
Bai Zhu (Rhizoma Atractylodis Macrocephalae)
Bai Zhi (Radix Angelicae Dahuricae)
Ban Xia (Rhizoma Pinelliae)
Zhi Qiao (Fructus Aurantii)
Sheng Jiang (Rhizoma Zingiberis Recens)
Da Zao (Fructus Jujubae)
Chun Pi (Cortex Ailanthi)
Wu Wei Zi (Fructus Schisandrae Chinensis)
Dang Gui (Radix Angelicae Sinensis)
Jie Geng (Radix Platycodonis)

Ge Gen Huo Xiang Shao Yao Tang (Kudzu, Pogostemon, and Peony Decoction) treats diarrhea characterized by the presence of damp-heat and toxins in the Intestines, accompanied by disharmony of the middle *jiao*. It is formulated following the principles of three classic formulas: *Ge Gen Huang Qin Huang Lian Tang* (Kudzu, Coptis, and Scutellaria Decoction) to clear heat in the interior; *Huo Xiang Zheng Qi San* (Agastache Powder to Rectify the Qi) to regulate qi and harmonize the middle *jiao*; and *Shao Yao Tang* (Peony Decoction) to clear heat

and eliminate toxins. Clinical applications of this formula include diarrhea, gastroenteritis, enteritis, dysentery, and food poisoning.

AUTHORS' COMMENTS

Clinically, *Ge Gen Huang Qin Huang Lian Tang* is safe for use in any condition involving heat in the Intestines, regardless of whether exterior symptoms are present or not. It is most important, however, **not** to use it in patients with deficiency and cold of the Spleen and Stomach.

Ge Gen Huang Qin Huang Lian Tang, Shao Yao Tang (Peony Decoction), and *Bai Tou Weng Tang* (Pulsatilla Decoction) are three commonly used formulas for diarrhea, each with a very different etiology and emphasis.

- *Ge Gen Huang Qin Huang Lian Tang* treats heat invading the interior as a result of the misuse of herbs while the pathogenic factor was still at the superficial level. Chief manifestations include foul-smelling diarrhea with burning sensations in the anus.
- *Shao Yao Tang* treats accumulation of damp-heat and toxins in the Large Intestine, leading to dysfunction and qi stagnation causing severe abdominal pain with blood and mucus in the stool and burning sensations in the anus. The key sign for the use of this formula is rectal tenesmus.
- *Bai Tou Weng Tang* treats accumulation of damp-heat and toxins in the Intestines at the *xue* (blood) level. The heat is more prominent than the dampness and is deep in the *xue* level, so more blood will be present in the stool. Other symptoms include abdominal pain, rectal tenesmus, mucus in the stool, and burning sensations in the anus.[19]

References

1. *Zhong Yi Fang Ji Xian Dai Yan Jiu* (Modern Study of Medical Formulae in Traditional Chinese Medicine) 1997;458.
2. *Zhong Yao Yao Li Yu Lin Chuang* (Pharmacology and Clinical Applications of Chinese Herbs) 1985;20.
3. *Ji Lin Zhong Yi Yao* (Jilin Chinese Medicine and Herbology) 1986;6:30.
4. *Zhong Yi Fang Ji Xian Dai Yan Jiu* (Modern Study of Medical Formulae in Traditional Chinese Medicine) 1997;460.
5. *Zhong Yi Fang Ji Xian Dai Yan Jiu* (Modern Study of Medical Formulae in Traditional Chinese Medicine) 1997;461.
6. *Zhong Cheng Yao* (Study of Chinese Patent Medicine) 1989;11(11):23.
7. *Jiang Xi Zhong Yi Yao* (Jiangxi Chinese Medicine and Herbology) 1959;6:28.
8. *Hu Bei Zhong Yi Za Zhi* (Hubei Journal of Chinese Medicine) 1995;5:33.
9. *Shi Yong Nei Ke Za Zhi* (Practical Journal of Internal Medicine) 1989;3(3):12.
10. *Hei Long Jiang Zhong Yi Yao* (Heilongjiang Chinese Medicine and Herbology) 1995;2:25.
11. *Zhe Jiang Zhong Yi Xue Yuan Xue Bao* (Journal of Zhejiang University of Chinese Medicine) 1998;4:16.

Gě Gēn Huáng Qín Huáng Lián Tāng
(Kudzu, Coptis, and Scutellaria Decoction)

12. *Hu Bei Zhong Yi Za Zhi* (Hubei Journal of Chinese Medicine) 1983;2:24.
13. *He Nan Zhong Yi* (Henan Chinese Medicine) 1992;1:42.
14. *Zhe Jiang Zhong Yi Za Zhi* (Zhejiang Journal of Chinese Medicine) 1992;6:279.
15. *Xin Zhong Yi* (New Chinese Medicine) 2000;10:19.

16. *Guang Dong Yi Xue* (Guangdong Medicine) 1993;6:336.
17. *Xin Zhong Yi* (New Chinese Medicine) 1997;9:45.
18. *Zhong Cheng Yao* (Study of Chinese Patent Medicine) 1992;14(4):38.
19. Wang MZ, et al. *Zhong Yi Xue Wen Da Ti Ku* (Questions and Answers on Traditional Chinese Medicine: Herbal Formulas).

Shí Gāo Tāng (Gypsum Decoction)
石膏湯
石膏汤

Pinyin Name: *Shi Gao Tang*
Literal Name: Gypsum Decoction
Original Source: *Wai Tai Mi Yao* (Arcane Essentials from the Imperial Library) by Wang Tao in 752 A.D.

COMPOSITION

Shi Gao (Gypsum Fibrosum)	6g
Ma Huang (Herba Ephedrae)	9g
Dan Dou Chi (Semen Sojae Praeparatum)	1 cup [9g]
Huang Qin (Radix Scutellariae)	6g
Huang Lian (Rhizoma Coptidis)	6g
Huang Bo (Cortex Phellodendri Chinensis)	6g
Zhi Zi (Fructus Gardeniae), *bo* (opened)	10 pieces [9g]

DOSAGE / PREPARATION / ADMINISTRATION

The source text instructs to cut the ingredients, cook them in 10 cups of water, and reduce the liquid to 3 cups. Take 1 cup of the warm, strained decoction three times daily. The source text advises to avoid consuming pork and coming into contact with cold water while taking this formula.

CHINESE THERAPEUTIC ACTIONS

1. Clears heat and eliminates toxins
2. Releases the exterior and induces perspiration

CLINICAL MANIFESTATIONS

Unresolved exterior syndrome with interior heat in all three *jiaos*: high fever, no perspiration, stiffness and a feeling of heaviness of the body and the extremities, dry nose, thirst, fidgeting, irritability, insomnia, delirium, incoherent speech, maculated skin, and a slippery, rapid pulse.

CLINICAL APPLICATIONS

Fever, irritability, and delirium.

EXPLANATION

Shi Gao Tang (Gypsum Decoction) treats unresolved exterior syndrome with interior excess heat in all three *jiaos*. This syndrome often originates from *taiyang* syndrome. If the excess exterior symptoms in a *taiyang* syndrome are not relieved over a period of time, heat and toxins are created in the three *jiaos*, or all over the body. High fever, no perspiration, stiffness of the body and the extremities, dry nose, thirst, fidgeting, irritability, insomnia, incoherent speech, and delirium all indicate excess at the exterior and heat in the interior. The heat and toxins may also cause maculated skin by forcing the blood out of the blood vessels.

To effectively treat this syndrome, both exterior-releasing and interior-clearing methods need to be used. This

EXTERIOR- AND INTERIOR-RELEASING FORMULAS

4

299

Chapter 4 – Exterior- and Interior-Releasing Formulas   *Section 2 – Exterior-Releasing and Interior-Clearing Formulas*

Shi Gāo Tāng (Gypsum Decoction)

Shi Gao Tang (Gypsum Decoction)

Diagnosis	Signs and Symptoms	Treatment	Herbs
Unresolved exterior syndrome with interior heat in all three *jiaos*	• High fever, no perspiration, stiffness and a feeling of heaviness of the body and the extremities: unreleased exterior condition • Dry nose and thirst: interior heat consuming body fluids • Fidgeting, irritability, insomnia incoherent speech, and delirium: interior heat disturbing *shen* (spirit) • Maculated skin: heat forcing blood outwards • Slippery, rapid pulse: interior heat	• Clears heat and eliminates toxins • Releases the exterior and induces perspiration	• *Shi Gao* (Gypsum Fibrosum) clears excessive heat and relieves irritability. • *Ma Huang* (Herba Ephedrae) and *Dan Dou Chi* (Semen Sojae Praeparatum) relieve exterior symptoms via diaphoresis. • *Huang Qin* (Radix Scutellariae), *Huang Lian* (Rhizoma Coptidis), *Huang Bo* (Cortex Phellodendri Chinensis) and *Zhi Zi* (Fructus Gardeniae) sedate the heat and dispel toxins from all three *jiaos*.

formula contains *Shi Gao* (Gypsum Fibrosum) as the chief herb to clear excess heat and relieve the irritability. *Ma Huang* (Herba Ephedrae) and *Dan Dou Chi* (Semen Sojae Praeparatum) relieve exterior symptoms by inducing sweating. *Huang Lian* (Rhizoma Coptidis), *Huang Qin* (Radix Scutellariae), *Huang Bo* (Cortex Phellodendri Chinensis), and *Zhi Zi* (Fructus Gardeniae), four herbs in *Huang Lian Jie Du Tang* (Coptis Decoction to Relieve Toxicity), sedate heat and dispel toxins from all three *jiaos*. These four herbs also counter the warm nature of *Ma Huang* (Herba Ephedrae) and prevent it from creating heat in the body.

AUTHORS' COMMENTS

Shi Gao Tang and *San Huang Shi Gao Tang* (Three-Yellow and Gypsum Decoction) both contain *Shi Gao* (Gypsum Fibrosum), *Huang Lian* (Rhizoma Coptidis), *Huang Qin* (Radix Scutellariae), *Huang Bo* (Cortex Phellodendri Chinensis) and *Zhi Zi* (Fructus Gardeniae) to sedate heat and dispel toxins from all three *jiaos*.

• *Shi Gao Tang* is an exterior- and interior-releasing formula; it treats exterior condition with interior heat.

• *San Huang Shi Gao Tang* is a heat-clearing formula; it only addresses the presence of heat and toxins in the interior.

Chinese Herbal Formulas and Applications

Section 3

解表溫里劑

— Exterior-Releasing and Interior-Warming Formulas

Wǔ Jī Sǎn (Five-Accumulation Powder)

五積散

五积散

Pinyin Name: *Wu Ji San*

Literal Name: Five-Accumulation Powder

Alternate Names: *Wu Chi San*, Five Accumulations Powder, Tangkuei and Magnolia Five Formula

Original Source: *Xian Shou Li Shang Xu Duan Mi Fang* (Secret Recipes for Treating Wounds and Bone-Setting Taught by Celestials) by Taoist Lin in 846 A.D.

COMPOSITION

Ma Huang (Herba Ephedrae)	180g
Bai Zhi (Radix Angelicae Dahuricae)	90g
Gan Jiang (Rhizoma Zingiberis)	120g
Rou Gui (Cortex Cinnamomi)	90g
Cang Zhu (Rhizoma Atractylodis)	600g
Hou Po (Cortex Magnoliae Officinalis)	120g
Chen Pi (Pericarpium Citri Reticulatae)	180g
Ban Xia (Rhizoma Pinelliae)	90g
Fu Ling (Poria)	90g
Dang Gui (Radix Angelicae Sinensis)	90g
Chuan Xiong (Rhizoma Chuanxiong)	90g
Bai Shao (Radix Paeoniae Alba)	90g
Jie Geng (Radix Platycodonis)	600g
Zhi Qiao (Fructus Citri Aurantii)	180g
Zhi Gan Cao (Radix et Rhizoma Glycyrrhizae Praeparata cum Melle)	90g

DOSAGE / PREPARATION / ADMINISTRATION

Source text instructions: grind the ingredients, except *Rou Gui* (Cortex Cinnamomi) and *Zhi Qiao* (Fructus Aurantii), into a coarse powder, dry-fry using low intensity fire until the color changes, and then remove from heat. Spread the powder and let it cool. Add the ground powder of *Rou Gui* (Cortex Cinnamomi) and *Zhi Qiao* (Fructus Aurantii), and mix them thoroughly. Cook 9g of this mixed powder with 3 slices of *Sheng Jiang* (Rhizoma Zingiberis Recens) in 1.5 bowls of water until 0.5 bowl of liquid remains. Take the strained decoction while warm.

CHINESE THERAPEUTIC ACTIONS

1. Releases the exterior
2. Warms the interior
3. Smoothes qi circulation and dissolves phlegm
4. Activates blood circulation and resolves accumulation

CLINICAL MANIFESTATIONS

Wind-cold at the exterior with five accumulations in the interior: fever, chills, no perspiration, headache, soreness of the body, neck stiffness, chest fullness, lack of appetite, nausea, vomiting, and abdominal pain. This formula is also used for women who have abdominal and chest pain caused by qi and blood disharmony, and menstrual irregularities that are cold in nature.

301

Chapter 4 – Exterior- and Interior-Releasing Formulas   **Section 3 –** *Exterior-Releasing and Interior-Warming Formulas*

Wŭ Jī Săn (Five-Accumulation Powder)

CLINICAL APPLICATIONS

Gastroenteritis, peptic ulcer, acid reflux, acute or chronic enteritis, hernia, sciatica, neuralgia, arthralgia, arthritis, headache, gout, trigeminal neuralgia, and irregular menstruation.

EXPLANATION

Wu Ji San (Five-Accumulation Powder) treats five types of accumulations: cold, dampness, qi, blood, and phlegm. This syndrome of multiple stagnations can be attributed to the presence of excess cold at both the exterior and interior. Excess cold constricting the exterior can cause fever, chills, no perspiration, and other exterior symptoms. Because cold is stagnant in nature, it may obstruct qi and blood flow to cause headache, soreness of the body, and neck stiffness. Excess cold in the interior is often the result of improper dietary intake of raw or cold food or beverages, which can obstruct qi and blood flow to cause accumulation of damp and phlegm. The phlegm may obstruct the Lung qi causing chest fullness. The presence of dampness and phlegm in the middle *jiao* damages the yang qi of the Spleen and Stomach; hence, appetite is affected. Various stagnations in the Stomach can cause the Stomach qi to rise abnormally, leading to nausea and vomiting. The abdominal and chest pains are caused by stagnation of both qi and blood.

To effectively treat this syndrome, the exterior cold has to be expelled with exterior-releasing herbs, and the interior cold removed with interior-warming herbs. In addition, aromatic and drying herbs should be used to dispel dampness and phlegm, and blood-activating herbs should be used to regulate the blood circulation.

Strong acrid and warm exterior-releasing herbs such as *Ma Huang* (Herba Ephedrae) and *Bai Zhi* (Radix Angelicae Dahuricae) release the exterior and induce perspiration. *Ma Huang* (Herba Ephedrae) also ventilates the Lung to relieve chest fullness. *Gan Jiang* (Rhizoma Zingiberis) and *Rou Gui* (Cortex Cinnamomi) warm the interior and relieve pain. Together, these four herbs can effectively treat exterior and interior cold. *Cang Zhu* (Rhizoma Atractylodis) and *Hou Po* (Cortex Magnoliae Officinalis), both aromatic in nature, dry dampness and strengthen the Spleen. *Chen Pi* (Pericarpium Citri Reticulatae), *Ban Xia* (Rhizoma Pinelliae), and *Fu Ling* (Poria) dissolve phlegm and regulate qi flow. *Dang Gui* (Radix Angelicae Sinensis), *Chuan Xiong* (Rhizoma Chuanxiong), and *Bai Shao* (Radix Paeoniae Alba) regulate blood circulation and help relieve pain. *Jie Geng* (Radix Platycodonis) and *Zhi Qiao* (Fructus Aurantii) regulate qi flow to help dissolve phlegm. *Zhi Gan Cao* (Radix et Rhizoma Glycyrrhizae Praeparata cum Melle)

Wu Ji San (Five-Accumulation Powder)

Diagnosis	Signs and Symptoms	Treatment	Herbs
Wind-cold at the exterior with five accumulations in the interior	• Fever, chills, no perspiration, headache, soreness of the body, and neck stiffness: qi and blood stagnation due to exterior-excess wind-cold • Chest fullness and lack of appetite: damp and phlegm stagnation • Nausea, and vomiting: reversed flow of Stomach qi due to stagnations • Abdominal and chest pain: qi and blood stagnation	• Releases the exterior • Warms the interior • Smoothes qi circulation and dissolves phlegm • Activates blood circulation and resolves accumulation	• *Ma Huang* (Herba Ephedrae) and *Bai Zhi* (Radix Angelicae Dahuricae) release the exterior and induce perspiration. • *Gan Jiang* (Rhizoma Zingiberis) and *Rou Gui* (Cortex Cinnamomi) warm the interior and relieve pain. • *Cang Zhu* (Rhizoma Atractylodis) and *Hou Po* (Cortex Magnoliae Officinalis) dry dampness and strengthen the Spleen. • *Chen Pi* (Pericarpium Citri Reticulatae), *Ban Xia* (Rhizoma Pinelliae) and *Fu Ling* (Poria) dissolve phlegm and regulate qi circulation. • *Dang Gui* (Radix Angelicae Sinensis), *Chuan Xiong* (Rhizoma Chuanxiong) and *Bai Shao* (Radix Paeoniae Alba) regulate blood circulation and relieve pain. • *Jie Geng* (Radix Platycodonis) and *Zhi Qiao* (Fructus Aurantii) regulate qi flow to dissolve phlegm. • *Zhi Gan Cao* (Radix et Rhizoma Glycyrrhizae Praeparata cum Melle) harmonizes the middle *jiao*, strengthens the Spleen, and harmonizes the herbs.

Wǔ Jī Sǎn (Five-Accumulation Powder)

harmonizes the middle *jiao*, strengthens the Spleen, and harmonizes the formula.

Because this formula activates qi and blood flow, warms the interior, and relieves pain, it is also effective in treating women with menstrual disorders and abdominal pain caused by cold stagnation.

MODIFICATIONS

- With abdominal pain due to food stagnation after meals, add *Shan Zha* (Fructus Crataegi) and *Mai Ya* (Fructus Hordei Germinatus).
- If accompanied by numbness and pain, add *Qiang Huo* (Rhizoma et Radix Notopterygii), *Du Huo* (Radix Angelicae Pubescentis), and *Fang Feng* (Radix Saposhnikoviae).
- With headache due to wind-cold, add *Sheng Ma* (Rhizoma Cimicifugae) and *Ge Gen* (Radix Puerariae Lobatae).
- When there is pain in the entire body, add *Ru Xiang* (Gummi Olibanum), *Mo Yao* (Myrrha), and *Xi Xin* (Radix et Rhizoma Asari).
- With cough, add *Sang Bai Pi* (Cortex Mori) and *Ku Xing Ren* (Semen Armeniacae Amarum).
- With low back pain, add *Niu Xi* (Radix Achyranthis Bidentatae), *Du Zhong* (Cortex Eucommiae), and *Xiao Hui Xiang* (Fructus Foeniculi).
- With edema of the legs, add *Wu Jia Pi* (Cortex Acanthopanacis) and *Da Fu Pi* (Pericarpium Arecae).
- With spasms of the hands and feet, add *Mu Gua* (Fructus Chaenomelis) and *Niu Xi* (Radix Achyranthis Bidentatae).
- If there is more interior cold, add *Wu Zhu Yu* (Fructus Evodiae).
- With painful menstruation, add *Xiang Fu* (Rhizoma Cyperi), *Yan Hu Suo* (Rhizoma Corydalis), and *Dan Shen* (Radix et Rhizoma Salviae Miltiorrhizae).
- With dry heaves from Stomach qi reversal, add *Wu Zhu Yu* (Fructus Evodiae), *Ren Shen* (Radix et Rhizoma Ginseng), *Bai Zhu* (Rhizoma Atractylodis Macrocephalae), *Xiang Fu* (Rhizoma Cyperi), and *Sha Ren* (Fructus Amomi).
- For *lin zheng* (dysuria syndrome) in women, add *Mu Tong* (Caulis Akebiae) and *Che Qian Zi* (Semen Plantaginis).

RELATED FORMULA

Wǔ Jī Sǎn (Five-Accumulation Powder)

五積散
五积散

Pinyin Name: *Wu Ji San*
Literal Name: Five-Accumulation Powder
Alternate Names: *Wu Chi San*, Five Accumulations Powder
Original Source: *Tai Ping Hui Min He Ji Ju Fang* (Imperial Grace Formulary of the Tai Ping Era) by the Imperial Medical Department in 1078-85

Ma Huang (Herba Ephedrae)	180g
Bai Zhi (Radix Angelicae Dahuricae)	90g
Gan Jiang (Rhizoma Zingiberis)	120g
Rou Gui (Cortex Cinnamomi)	90g
Cang Zhu (Rhizoma Atractylodis), *jin* (soaked) in rice water	720g
Hou Po (Cortex Magnoliae Officinalis)	120g
Chen Pi (Pericarpium Citri Reticulatae)	180g
Ban Xia (Rhizoma Pinelliae), *xi* (washed) 7 times	90g
Fu Ling (Poria)	90g
Dang Gui (Radix Angelicae Sinensis)	90g
Chuan Xiong (Rhizoma Chuanxiong)	90g
Bai Shao (Radix Paeoniae Alba)	90g
Jie Geng (Radix Platycodonis)	360g
Zhi Gan Cao (Radix et Rhizoma Glycyrrhizae Praeparata cum Melle)	90g
Zhi Qiao (Fructus Citri Aurantii), *chao* (dry-fried)	180g

These two formulas are essentially the same. Though they are derived from two different original sources, they have identical names, same composition, but they differ in the doses and preparation of the ingredients. Clinically, the functions of these two formulas are very similar and can be used interchangeably. According to the source texts, their differences are as follow:

- *Wu Ji San* from *Xian Shou Li Shang Xu Duan Mi Fang* (Secret Recipes for Treating Wounds and Bone-Setting Taught by Celestials) treats individuals with damages caused by five debilitation and seven damages (五劳七伤 *Wu Lao Qi Shang*).
- *Wu Ji San* from *Tai Ping Hui Min He Ji Ju Fang* (Imperial Grace Formulary of the Tai Ping Era) addresses external wind-cold due to exposure, and internal cold due to damages (外感风寒，内伤生冷 *Wai Gan Feng Han, Nei Shang Sheng Leng*).

AUTHORS' COMMENTS

Wu Ji San is literally named "five-accumulation powder" because it treats five types of accumulations: cold, dampness, qi, blood, and phlegm.

Chapter 4 – Exterior- and Interior-Releasing Formulas   Section 3 – Exterior-Releasing and Interior-Warming Formulas

Chái Hú Guì Zhī Gān Jiāng Tāng
(Bupleurum, Cinnamon Twig, and Ginger Decoction)

柴胡桂枝乾薑湯
柴胡桂枝干姜汤

Pinyin Name: *Chai Hu Gui Zhi Gan Jiang Tang*
Literal Name: Bupleurum, Cinnamon Twig, and Ginger Decoction
Alternate Name: Bupleurum Cinnamon and Ginger Combination
Original Source: *Shang Han Lun* (Discussion of Cold-Induced Disorders) by Zhang Zhong-Jing in the Eastern Han Dynasty

COMPOSITION

Chai Hu (Radix Bupleuri)	24g [15g]
Huang Qin (Radix Scutellariae)	9g
Tian Hua Fen (Radix Trichosanthis)	12g
Gui Zhi (Ramulus Cinnamomi)	9g [12g]
Gan Jiang (Rhizoma Zingiberis)	6g
Mu Li (Concha Ostreae), *ao* (simmered)	6g [20g]
Zhi Gan Cao (Radix et Rhizoma Glycyrrhizae Praeparata cum Melle)	6g [3g]

DOSAGE / PREPARATION / ADMINISTRATION

The source text states to cook the ingredients in 12 cups [2,400 mL] of water until the liquid is reduced to 6 cups [1,200 mL]. Discard the residue, and cook the strained decoction again until it is reduced to 3 cups [600 mL]. Take 1 cup [200 mL] of the warm decoction three times daily. Patients may feel slightly irritated after taking the first dose, but sweating is usually induced after taking the second dose, a sign that the condition is resolved. Today, the decoction may be prepared using the doses suggested in brackets.

CHINESE THERAPEUTIC ACTIONS

1. Harmonizes *shaoyang*
2. Warms interior and dispels water accumulation

CLINICAL MANIFESTATIONS

Shaoyang disorder with water accumulation in the interior: a feeling of fullness and clumping in the chest and hypochondrium, dysuria, thirst, absence of vomiting, perspiration of the head, alternating spells of chills and fever, and irritability.

CLINICAL APPLICATIONS

Common cold, influenza, pneumonia, bronchitis, hepatitis, cholecystitis, and malaria.

EXPLANATION

According to the source text, *Chai Hu Gui Zhi Gan Jiang Tang* (Bupleurum, Cinnamon Twig, and Ginger Decoction) treats patients who have had exterior condition for five to six days, and who have been treated unsuccessfully with exterior-releasing and downward draining methods. At this moment, the exterior condition is still unresolved, and the disease has moved interior. This condition is referred to as *shaoyang* disorder with water accumulation in the interior. *Shaoyang* disorders are typically described as "half-exterior and half-interior," with characteristic symptoms such as alternating spells of fever and chills, a feeling of fullness and clumping in the chest and hypochondrium, and irritability. In addition to *shaoyang* syndrome, water has accumulated in the interior. As normal water distribution becomes impaired, symptoms such as perspiration of the head, thirst, and dysuria occur.

Chai Hu (Radix Bupleuri) addresses the *shaoyang* stage of the disorder, harmonizing the "half-exterior and half-interior" condition and relieving alternating spells of fever and chills, and a feeling of fullness and clumping. *Huang Qin* (Radix Scutellariae) clears damp-heat and relieves feeling of fullness and clumping. *Tian Hua Fen* (Radix Trichosanthis) promotes generation of body fluids and relieves thirst, dry mouth, and dysuria. *Gui Zhi* (Ramulus Cinnamomi) eliminates the pathogenic factors that linger at the exterior, while *Gan Jiang* (Rhizoma Zingiberis) warms the interior to dispel cold. These two herbs also warm yang to dispel cold and eliminate water accumulation. *Mu Li* (Concha Ostreae) resolves phlegm and disperses the clumps. Lastly, *Zhi Gan Cao* (Radix et Rhizoma Glycyrrhizae Praeparata cum Melle) harmonizes the formula.

304

Chái Hú Guì Zhī Gān Jiāng Tāng

(Bupleurum, Cinnamon Twig, and Ginger Decoction)

Chai Hu Gui Zhi Gan Jiang Tang (Bupleurum, Cinnamon Twig, and Ginger Decoction)

Diagnosis	Signs and Symptoms	Treatment	Herbs
Shaoyang disorder with water accumulation in the interior	• Alternating spells of fever and chills, a feeling of fullness and clumping, and irritability: *shaoyang* disorder • Dysuria and thirst: damage of body fluids • Cold hands and feet and loose stools or diarrhea: cold condition	• Harmonizes and disperses clumps • Warms interior and dispels cold	• *Chai Hu* (Radix Bupleuri) harmonizes *shaoyang* condition of "half-exterior and half-interior." • *Huang Qin* (Radix Scutellariae) clears damp-heat and relieves the feeling of fullness and clumping. • *Tian Hua Fen* (Radix Trichosanthis) promotes generation of body fluids and relieves thirst, dry mouth and dysuria. • *Gui Zhi* (Ramulus Cinnamomi) eliminates the pathogenic factors that linger at the exterior. • *Gan Jiang* (Rhizoma Zingiberis) warms the interior to dispel cold. • *Mu Li* (Concha Ostreae) resolves phlegm and disperses the clumps. • *Zhi Gan Cao* (Radix et Rhizoma Glycyrrhizae Praeparata cum Melle) harmonizes the herbs.

MODIFICATIONS

- If there is difficulty with urination, add *Fu Ling* (Poria) and *Che Qian Zi* (Semen Plantaginis).
- With neck stiffness, add *Ge Gen* (Radix Puerariae Lobatae) and *Bai Shao* (Radix Paeoniae Alba).
- For anuria, add *Wu Zhu Yu* (Fructus Evodiae) and *Fu Ling* (Poria).
- For headache and perspiration of the head, add *Chuan Xiong* (Rhizoma Chuanxiong) and *Bai Zhi* (Radix Angelicae Dahuricae).
- For peritoneal tuberculosis, add *Bie Jia* (Carapax Trionycis) and *Bai Shao* (Radix Paeoniae Alba).
- For fever associated with tuberculosis, add *Huang Qi* (Radix Astragali) and *Bie Jia* (Carapax Trionycis).

TOXICOLOGY

One case of interstitial pneumonia was reported in a 57-year-old man who had taken Saikokeishikankyou-tou (*Chai Hu Gui Zhi Gan Jiang Tang*) for one month and *Lycium halimifolium Mil* (LHM) for two weeks. The diagnosis was confirmed when a lymphocyte stimulation test, skin test, and challenge test were all positive to these herbs. This was the first report on pneumonitis caused by this formula to be diagnosed by lymphocyte stimulation test, skin test, and challenge test.[1]

Reference

1. Heki U, Fujimura M, Ogawa H, Matsuda T, Kitagawa M. Pneumonitis caused by saikokeisikankyou-tou, an herbal drug. Internal Medicine 1997 Mar;36(3):214-7.

Chapter 4 – Exterior- and Interior-Releasing Formulas

Chapter 4 — Summary

— Exterior- and Interior-Releasing Formulas

SECTION 1: EXTERIOR-RELEASING AND INTERIOR-ATTACKING FORMULAS

Name	Similarities	Differences
Da Chai Hu Tang (Major Bupleurum Decoction)	Release the exterior and interior	Treats *shaoyang* and *yangming* syndromes
Hou Po Qi Wu Tang (Seven-Substance Decoction with Magnolia Bark)		Treats *taiyang* and *yangming* syndromes with interior excess
Fang Feng Tong Sheng San (Saposhnikovia Powder that Sagely Unblocks)		Treats exterior wind-heat syndrome with interior heat accumulation

Da Chai Hu Tang (Major Bupleurum Decoction) is the main formula to harmonize *shaoyang* and *yangming* syndromes. Key clinical manifestations include alternating spells of chills and fever, fullness and pain of the epigastrium, hot sensation in the hypochondriac region, constipation or diarrhea, a yellow tongue coating, and a wiry, forceful pulse.

Hou Po Qi Wu Tang (Seven-Substance Decoction with Magnolia Bark) treats *taiyang* and *yangming* syndromes with interior excess. Main signs and symptoms include abdominal fullness, fever, constipation, and a superficial, rapid pulse.

Fang Feng Tong Sheng San (Saposhnikovia Powder that Sagely Unblocks) treats concurrent exterior and interior excess heat syndrome. Clinical manifestations include chills, fever, constipation, red and painful eyes, dizziness, thick and sticky nasal discharge, sore throat, chest fullness, coughing, dyspnea, a bitter taste in the mouth, and a dry mouth.

SECTION 2: EXTERIOR-RELEASING AND INTERIOR-CLEARING FORMULAS

Name	Similarities	Differences
Ge Gen Huang Qin Huang Lian Tang (Kudzu, Coptis, and Scutellaria Decoction)	Release the exterior and clear the interior	Releases wind-cold from the exterior, clears heat from the interior
Shi Gao Tang (Gypsum Decoction)		Clears heat from the upper, middle, and lower *jiaos*

Ge Gen Huang Qin Huang Lian Tang (Kudzu, Coptis, and Scutellaria Decoction) releases wind-cold from the exterior and clears heat from in the interior. This formula mainly treats foul-smelling diarrhea or dysentery characterized by the presence of interior heat with an unresolved exterior condition. There is usually a burning sensation in the anus after defecation. The tongue coating is yellow and the pulse is rapid.

Shi Gao Tang (Gypsum Decoction) clears heat in all three *jiaos*, eliminates heat and toxins, and dispels exterior factors through perspiration. Clinical manifestations include high fever, chills with no perspiration, heaviness and stiffness of the body and the extremities, dry nose, thirst, fidgeting, and irritability.

Chinese Herbal Formulas and Applications

Chapter 4 — Summary

SECTION 3: EXTERIOR-RELEASING AND INTERIOR-WARMING FORMULAS

Name	Similarities	Differences
Wu Ji San (Five-Accumulation Powder)	Release the exterior and warm the interior	Releases wind-cold from the exterior and dispels accumulation of cold, dampness, qi, blood, and phlegm in the interior
Chai Hu Gui Zhi Gan Jiang Tang (Bupleurum, Cinnamon Twig, and Ginger Decoction)		Harmonizes *shaoyang*, dispels water accumulation

Wu Ji San (Five-Accumulation Powder) treats concurrent exterior and interior cold syndrome. Clinical manifestations include fever and chills without perspiration, soreness of the body, neck stiffness, chest fullness, nausea, vomiting, and abdominal pain. This formula can also be used for irregular menstruation caused by cold.

Chai Hu Gui Zhi Gan Jiang Tang (Bupleurum, Cinnamon Twig, and Ginger Decoction) treats *shaoyang* disorder with a feeling of fullness and clumping in the chest and hypochondrium. Key signs and symptoms include alternating spells of fever and chills, a feeling of fullness and clumping in the chest and hypochondrium, irritability, dysuria, thirst, cold hands and feet, and loose stools or diarrhea.

Chapter 5

— Heat-Clearing Formulas

清热剂

叶桂 Yè Guì

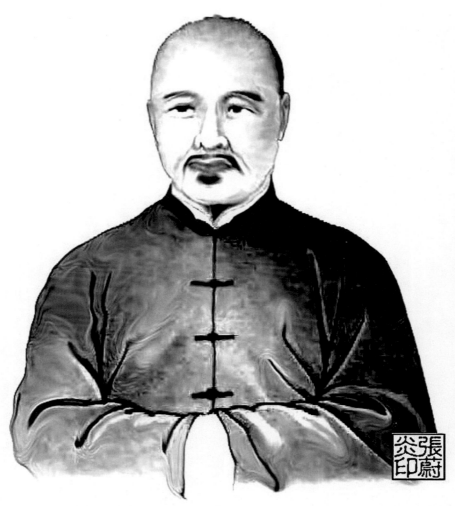

叶桂 Yè Guì, also known as 叶天士 Yè Tiān-Shì, 1666 – 1745.

叶桂 Yè Guì

Ye Gui, also known as Ye Tian-Shi, was born into a long family lineage of physicians. His father and grandfather were famous pediatricians. Ye began to learn medicine from his father at the age of twelve. When his father passed away two years later, Ye apprenticed with other teachers. Being very intelligent and extremely diligent, Ye absorbed and integrated knowledge from his family and seventeen other masters over the next ten years, and became one of the best physicians in the country.

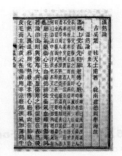

温热论 Wen Re Lun
(Discussion of Warm and Hot Disorders).[1]

Ye lived in southern China and practiced medicine during a time when epidemics plagued the country. At the time, most doctors still followed the principles of 伤寒 *shang han* (cold damage), and had little success in treating epidemic illnesses. Observing this, Ye proposed the theories of 温病 *wen bing* (warm disease), and developed additional theories of *Wei Qi Ying Xue Bian Zheng* (Defensive, Qi, Nutritive, Blood Differentiation) and their corresponding treatment strategies.[2]

Ye dedicated his entire life to clinical practice, and did not have time to write about his work. His extraordinary knowledge was organized and published by his apprentices. The most famous works attributed to Ye Gui include 温热论 *Wen Re Lun* (Discussion of Warm and Hot Disorders) and 临证指南医案 *Lin Zheng Zhi Nan Yi An* (Case Histories from the Compass of Clinical Patterns). The first text focused on theories and treatment principles, and the second text detailed case studies. Credited as one of the most influential physicians in establishing the framework of *wen bing* (warm disease), Ye Gui significantly influenced the practice of traditional Chinese medicine today.

1. Compiled and published between 1745 to 1766 by the apprentices of Ye Gui.
2. The diagnostic principles of *shang han* (cold damage) follow *Liu Jing Bian Zheng* (Six Stages Differentiation), from *taiyang*, through *yangming*, *shaoyang*, *taiyin*, and *shaoyin*, to *jueyin*. The diagnostic principles of *wen bing* (warm disease) follow *Wei Qi Ying Xue Bian Zheng* (Defensive, Qi, Nutritive, Blood Differentiation), from *wei* (defensive), *qi* (energy), and *ying* (nutritive) to *xue* (blood) levels. This latter set of diagnostic theories presented an alternative systematic perspective from which to evaluate the pathology of disease, and significantly expanded the practice of traditional Chinese medicine.

Dynasties & Kingdoms	Year
Xia Dynasty 夏	2100-1600 BCE
Shang Dynasty 商	1600-1100 BCE
Zhou Dynasty 周	1100-221 BCE
Qin Dynasty 秦	221-207 BCE
Han Dynasty 漢	206 BCE-220
Three Kingdoms 三國	220-280
Western Jin Dynasty 西晉	265-316
Eastern Jin Dynasty 東晉	317-420
Northern and Southern Dynasties 北南朝	420-581
Sui Dynasty 隋	581-618
Tang Dynasty 唐	618-907
Five Dynasties 五代	907-960
Song Dynasty 宋	960-1279
Liao Dynasty 遼	916-1125
Jin Dynasty 金	1115-1234
Yuan Dynasty 元	1271-1368
Ming Dynasty 明	1368-1644
Qing Dynasty 清	**1644-1911**
Republic of China 中華民國	1912-Present Day
People's Republic of China 中華人民共和國	1949-Present Day

Table of Contents

Chapter 5. Heat-Clearing Formulas ··· **309**
Biography of Ye Gui ··· 310

Section 1. *Qi* (Energy) Level-Clearing Formulas ··· **321**
Bai Hu Tang (White Tiger Decoction) ·· 321
   Bai Hu Jia Gui Zhi Tang (White Tiger plus Cinnamon Twig Decoction) ················· 323
   Bai Hu Jia Cang Zhu Tang (White Tiger plus Atractylodes Decoction) ··················· 323
Bai Hu Jia Ren Shen Tang (White Tiger plus Ginseng Decoction) ························· 325
Zhu Ye Shi Gao Tang (Bamboo Leaves and Gypsum Decoction) ·························· 326

Section 2. *Ying* (Nutritive) Level-Clearing and Blood-Cooling Formulas ·········· **330**
Qing Ying Tang (Clear the Nutritive Level Decoction) ·································· 330
Xi Jiao Di Huang Tang (Rhinoceros Horn and Rehmannia Decoction) ··················· 333
   Shen Xi Dan (Magical Rhinoceros Special Pill) ··· 335
   Qing Re Liang Xue Tang (Clear Heat and Cool the Blood Decoction) ·················· 335
   Fu Zheng Yi Yan Tang (Support the Upright and Suppress Cancer Decoction) ········· 336

Section 3. *Qi* (Energy) and *Xue* (Blood) Levels-Clearing Formulas ··············· **337**
Qing Wen Bai Du Yin (Clear Epidemics and Overcome Pathogenic Influences Decoction) ····· 337
   Hua Ban Tang (Transform Blotches Decoction) ·· 339

Section 4. Heat-Clearing and Toxin-Eliminating Formulas ·························· **341**
Huang Lian Jie Du Tang (Coptis Decoction to Relieve Toxicity) ························· 341
   Lian Qiao Jie Du Tang (Forsythia Decoction to Relieve Toxicity) ····················· 345
Huang Lian Shang Qing Wan (Coptis Pill to Clear the Upper) ·························· 347
Qing Shang Fang Feng Tang (Clear the Upper and Guard the Wind Decoction) ··········· 349
   Qing Re Jie Du Tang (Clear Heat and Relieve Toxicity Decoction) ····················· 350
Liang Ge San (Cool the Diaphragm Powder) ·· 351
Qing Liang Yin (Clearing and Cooling Decoction) ·· 354
Pu Ji Xiao Du Yin (Universal Benefit Decoction to Eliminate Toxin) ····················· 355
   Da Qing Tang (Isatis Decoction) ··· 358
San Huang Xie Xin Tang (Three-Yellow Decoction to Sedate the Epigastrium) ··········· 359
San Huang Shi Gao Tang (Three-Yellow and Gypsum Decoction) ······················· 361
   San Huang Shi Gao Tang (Three-Yellow and Gypsum Decoction) ······················· 362
Liu Shen Wan (Six-Miracle Pill) ··· 363

Table of Contents

Chinese Herbal Formulas and Applications

Section 5. *Zang Fu*-Clearing Formulas ⋯⋯⋯⋯⋯⋯⋯⋯⋯⋯⋯⋯⋯⋯⋯⋯⋯⋯ **365**
Dao Chi San (Guide Out the Red Powder) ⋯⋯⋯⋯⋯⋯⋯⋯⋯⋯⋯⋯⋯⋯⋯⋯⋯ 365
Qing Xin Lian Zi Yin (Lotus Seed Decoction to Clear the Heart) ⋯⋯⋯⋯⋯⋯⋯⋯ 368
Zhi Zi Chi Tang (Gardenia and Soja Decoction) ⋯⋯⋯⋯⋯⋯⋯⋯⋯⋯⋯⋯⋯⋯ 370
Long Dan Xie Gan Tang (Gentiana Decoction to Drain the Liver) ⋯⋯⋯⋯⋯⋯⋯⋯ 371
    Xie Qing Wan (Drain the Green Pill) ⋯⋯⋯⋯⋯⋯⋯⋯⋯⋯⋯⋯⋯⋯⋯⋯ 376
    Long Dan Jiang Ya Pian (Gentiana Pill to Lower [Blood] Pressure) ⋯⋯⋯⋯⋯ 376
    Long Dan Jie Du Tang (Gentiana Decoction to Relieve Toxicity) ⋯⋯⋯⋯⋯⋯ 376
    Zhi Zi Jiang Huo Tang (Gardenia Decoction to Descend Fire) ⋯⋯⋯⋯⋯⋯⋯ 377
Dang Gui Long Hui Wan (Tangkuei, Gentiana, and Aloe Pill) ⋯⋯⋯⋯⋯⋯⋯⋯⋯ 379
Xi Gan Ming Mu San (Wash the Liver and Brighten the Eyes Powder) ⋯⋯⋯⋯⋯⋯ 381
Xie Bai San (Drain the White Powder) ⋯⋯⋯⋯⋯⋯⋯⋯⋯⋯⋯⋯⋯⋯⋯⋯⋯⋯ 383
    Ting Li Da Zao Xie Fei Tang (Descurainia and Jujube Decoction to Drain the Lung) ⋯ 384
Qing Xin Li Ge Tang (Clear the Epigastrium and Benefit the Diaphragm Decoction) ⋯ 386
    Qing Xin Li Ge Tang (Clear the Epigastrium and Benefit the Diaphragm Decoction) ⋯ 387
Xiang Sheng Po Di San (Loud Sound Powder for a Broken Flute) ⋯⋯⋯⋯⋯⋯⋯⋯ 388
Zuo Jin Wan (Left Metal Pill) ⋯⋯⋯⋯⋯⋯⋯⋯⋯⋯⋯⋯⋯⋯⋯⋯⋯⋯⋯⋯⋯ 389
    Wu Ji Wan (Wu Ji Pill) ⋯⋯⋯⋯⋯⋯⋯⋯⋯⋯⋯⋯⋯⋯⋯⋯⋯⋯⋯⋯⋯ 391
    Xiang Lian Wan (Aucklandia and Coptis Pill) ⋯⋯⋯⋯⋯⋯⋯⋯⋯⋯⋯⋯ 391
    Qing Wei Tang (Clear the Stomach Decoction) ⋯⋯⋯⋯⋯⋯⋯⋯⋯⋯⋯ 392
Qing Wei San (Clear the Stomach Powder) ⋯⋯⋯⋯⋯⋯⋯⋯⋯⋯⋯⋯⋯⋯⋯⋯ 393
Xie Huang San (Drain the Yellow Powder) ⋯⋯⋯⋯⋯⋯⋯⋯⋯⋯⋯⋯⋯⋯⋯⋯ 396
Yu Nu Jian (Jade Woman Decoction) ⋯⋯⋯⋯⋯⋯⋯⋯⋯⋯⋯⋯⋯⋯⋯⋯⋯⋯ 398
Gan Lu Yin (Sweet Dew Decoction) ⋯⋯⋯⋯⋯⋯⋯⋯⋯⋯⋯⋯⋯⋯⋯⋯⋯⋯⋯ 401
Shao Yao Tang (Peony Decoction) ⋯⋯⋯⋯⋯⋯⋯⋯⋯⋯⋯⋯⋯⋯⋯⋯⋯⋯⋯ 402
    Shao Yao Yi Yi Ren Tang (Peony and Coicis Decoction) ⋯⋯⋯⋯⋯⋯⋯⋯ 405
    Shao Yao Hou Po Tang (Peony and Magnolia Bark Decoction) ⋯⋯⋯⋯⋯⋯ 405
Huang Qin Tang (Scutellaria Decoction) ⋯⋯⋯⋯⋯⋯⋯⋯⋯⋯⋯⋯⋯⋯⋯⋯⋯ 406
Bai Tou Weng Tang (Pulsatilla Decoction) ⋯⋯⋯⋯⋯⋯⋯⋯⋯⋯⋯⋯⋯⋯⋯⋯ 408
    Bai Tou Weng Jia Gan Cao E Jiao Tang (Pulsatilla Decoction plus Licorice and Ass-Hide Gelatin) ⋯⋯⋯ 410

Section 6. Deficiency-Heat Clearing Formulas ⋯⋯⋯⋯⋯⋯⋯⋯⋯⋯⋯⋯⋯⋯ **412**
Qing Hao Bie Jia Tang (Artemisia Annua and Soft-Shelled Turtle Shell Decoction) ⋯⋯ 412
    Zi Yin Qing Re Tang (Nourish Yin and Clear Heat Decoction) ⋯⋯⋯⋯⋯⋯ 414
Qin Jiao Bie Jia San (Gentiana Macrophylla and Soft-Shelled Turtle Shell Powder) ⋯⋯ 416
Qing Gu San (Cool the Bones Powder) ⋯⋯⋯⋯⋯⋯⋯⋯⋯⋯⋯⋯⋯⋯⋯⋯⋯⋯ 418
Dang Gui Liu Huang Tang (Tangkuei and Six-Yellow Decoction) ⋯⋯⋯⋯⋯⋯⋯⋯ 420
Zi Yin Jiang Huo Tang (Nourish Yin and Descend the Fire Decoction) ⋯⋯⋯⋯⋯⋯ 422

Heat-Clearing Formulas (Summary) ⋯⋯⋯⋯⋯⋯⋯⋯⋯⋯⋯⋯⋯⋯⋯⋯⋯⋯ **424**

HEAT-CLEARING FORMULAS

5

Chapter 5 — Overview

清热剂

— Heat-Clearing Formulas

Definition: Heat-clearing formulas clear heat, purge fire, cool the blood, eliminate toxins, nourish yin, and clear deficiency heat. This method of treatment is known as *qing fa* (clearing), one of the *ba fa* (eight treatment methods) described in the *Huang Di Nei Jing* (Yellow Emperor's Inner Classic) in the first or second century, A.D.

Heat-clearing formulas treat disorders characterized by warmth, heat, and fire. These three factors are actually the same pathogen, manifesting at different degrees of severity. For example, heat is actually a manifestation of extreme cases of warmth, and severe, intense heat is nothing other than fire. All three factors contribute to interior heat syndromes, which are treated by using cold herbs to clear heat.

~

Warmth, heat, and fire are the same pathogen manifesting at different degrees of severity.

~

Heat may be contracted externally or internally generated. External sources primarily refer to the *liu yin* (six exogenous factors). Internal sources may include emotional disturbances or imbalance of the *zang fu* organs. Once generated, heat may reside in differing levels of the body, affecting various *zang fu* organs. The different levels include *qi* (energy), *ying* (nutritive), and *xue* (blood). The *zang fu* organs most frequently affected by heat include the Heart, Liver, Gallbladder, Lung, Stomach, and Intestines.

SUBCATEGORIES OF ACTION

Due to the complex nature of heat, six sub-categories of heat-clearing formulas have been created to delineate the specificity of the heat, as it may be located in the *qi* (energy), *ying* (nutritive), and/or *xue* (blood) levels. It may affect different *zang* (solid) and *fu* (hollow) organs. Lastly, heat can have various intensities (warmth, heat, and fire) and characteristics (excess heat, deficiency heat, and heat toxins).

1. *Qi* (Energy) Level-Clearing Formulas

These formulas clear heat, reduce irritability, promote production of body fluids, and relieve thirst. They may be used to treat excess conditions (heat in the *qi* level), or complications of excess and deficiency conditions (heat in the *qi* level damaging qi, yin, and body fluids).

Heat attacking the *qi* level may produce signs and symptoms of high fever, sensations of warmth in the body, irritability, thirst, profuse sweating, aversion to heat, and a surging, big pulse. Herbs and formulas that commonly clear heat from the *qi* level include *Shi Gao* (Gypsum Fibrosum), *Zhi Mu* (Rhizoma Anemarrhenae), and *Bai Hu Tang* (White Tiger Decoction).

Heat in the *qi* level may damage qi, yin, and body fluids, causing signs and symptoms such as fever, profuse sweating, irritability and a stifling sensation in the chest, a dry mouth, and a red tongue body. Herbs and formulas that commonly clear heat, tonify qi, and/or nourish yin include *Shi Gao* (Gypsum Fibrosum), *Ren Shen* (Radix et Rhizoma Ginseng), *Mai Dong* (Radix Ophiopogonis), and *Zhu Ye Shi Gao Tang* (Bamboo Leaves and Gypsum Decoction).

2. *Ying* (Nutritive) Level-Clearing and Blood-Cooling Formulas

These formulas clear heat in the *ying* (nutritive) level, cool heat in the *xue* (blood) level, disperse blood stasis, and eliminate toxins.

Common clinical manifestations of heat in the *ying* level include: fever that increases in the evening, irritability, insomnia, absence of thirst, or thirst without a desire to drink, and occasionally,

Chinese Herbal Formulas and Applications

Chapter 5 — Overview

delirium or maculae. *Shui Niu Jiao* (Cornu Bubali) and *Di Huang* (Radix Rehmanniae) clear heat in the *ying* level. Moreover, because heat often attacks the *qi* (energy) level before it attacks the *ying* level, it is important to drive it outward, using herbs that clear heat from the *qi* level, such as *Jin Yin Hua* (Flos Lonicerae Japonicae), *Lian Qiao* (Fructus Forsythiae), and *Zhu Ye* (Herba Phyllostachys). An exemplar formula is *Qing Ying Tang* (Clear the Nutritive Level Decoction), which focuses on clearing heat from the *ying* level by ventilating heat from the *qi* level.

Common clinical manifestations of heat in the *xue* (blood) level include: various types of bleeding, maculae, delirium, mania, and a deep red tongue body with a prickly coating. *Shui Niu Jiao* (Cornu Bubali) and *Di Huang* (Radix Rehmanniae) are frequently used to clear heat and cool the blood. Additionally, because heat in the *xue* level is often complicated by bleeding and blood stasis, it is important to cool the blood, stop bleeding, and disperse blood stasis using herbs such as *Mu Dan Pi* (Cortex Moutan) and *Chi Shao* (Radix Paeoniae Rubra). An exemplar formula is *Xi Jiao Di Huang Tang* (Rhinoceros Horn and Rehmannia Decoction).

3. *Qi* (Energy) and *Xue* (Blood) Levels-Clearing Formula

These formulas clear heat in the *qi* (energy) level, cool heat in the *xue* (blood) level and purge fire and eliminate toxins. These formulas are suitable for treating excess heat and toxins, or epidemic toxins throughout the body affecting both *qi* and *xue* levels. Common clinical manifestations include high fever, irritability, strong thirst, epistaxis, hematemesis, maculae, and delirium. In these cases, use herbs and formulas to clear heat from the *qi* and *xue* levels simultaneously.

Herbs that clear heat from the *qi* (energy) level include *Shi Gao* (Gypsum Fibrosum) and *Zhi Mu* (Rhizoma Anemarrhenae). Herbs that clear heat from the *xue* (blood) level include *Shui Niu Jiao* (Cornu Bubali) and *Di Huang* (Radix Rehmanniae). An exemplar formula is *Qing Wen Bai Du Yin* (Clear Epidemics and Overcome Pathogenic Influences Decoction).

4. Heat-Clearing and Toxin-Eliminating Formulas

These formulas clear heat, purge fire, eliminate toxins, and generally treat three main conditions: excess heat, fire, and toxins in all three *jiaos*; heat stagnation in the chest and diaphragm; and wind-heat and epidemic toxins invading the head and facial regions.

> *Heat-clearing and toxin-eliminating formulas clear excess heat, fire, and toxins in all three jiaos.*

The presence of excess heat, fire, and toxins in all three *jiaos* is characterized by fever, irritability, delirium, epistaxis, maculae, boils, and sores. *Huang Lian* (Rhizoma Coptidis), *Huang Qin* (Radix Scutellariae), *Zhi Zi* (Fructus Gardeniae), and *Lian Qiao* (Fructus Forsythiae) commonly clear heat, purge fire, and eliminate toxins. An excellent formula that clears excess heat in all three *jiaos* is *Huang Lian Jie Du Tang* (Coptis Decoction to Relieve Toxicity) .

Stagnation of heat in the chest and diaphragm is characterized by fever, a red face, irritability and warm sensations in the chest and diaphragm, ulcerations of the mouth and tongue, constipation, and scanty, red urine. *Huang Lian* (Rhizoma Coptidis), *Huang Qin* (Radix Scutellariae), *Zhi Zi* (Fructus Gardeniae), and *Lian Qiao* (Fructus Forsythiae) clear heat, purge fire, and eliminate toxins. *Da Huang* (Radix et Rhizoma Rhei) and *Mang Xiao* (Natrii Sulfas) may be used to clear heat accumulated in the chest and diaphragm causing constipation and dysuria. An exemplar formula that guides and drains heat downward is *Liang Ge San* (Cool the Diaphragm Powder).

Wind-heat and epidemic toxins invading the head and facial regions are characterized by redness and painful swellings on the face, as well as by sore throat. *Niu Bang Zi* (Fructus Arctii), *Bo He* (Herba Menthae), and *Chan Tui* (Periostracum Cicadae) clear wind-heat and toxins affecting the upper parts of the body. *Pu Ji Xiao Du Yin* (Universal Benefit Decoction to Eliminate Toxin) is an excellent formula to dispel heat and toxins outward.

5. *Zang Fu*-Clearing Formulas

These formulas clear heat from the various *zang fu* organs and their associated channels and collaterals. Clinical manifestations vary, depending on the severity of the heat and the area affected.

315

Chapter 5 – Heat-Clearing Formulas

Chapter 5 — Overview

- Heat affecting the Heart is characterized by symptoms such as fidgeting, irritability and *shen* (spirit) disturbance. Herbs that clear heat from the Heart channel include *Huang Lian* (Rhizoma Coptidis), *Zhi Zi* (Fructus Gardeniae), *Lian Zi Xin* (Plumula Nelumbinis), and *Mu Tong* (Caulis Akebiae). The formula *Dao Chi San* (Guide Out the Red Powder) clears heat from the Heart.

- Liver and Gallbladder heat often presents with such symptoms as red eyes, hypochondriac pain, and a bitter taste in the mouth. Herbs that clear fire from the Liver and Gallbladder include *Long Dan* (Radix et Rhizoma Gentianae), *Xia Ku Cao* (Spica Prunellae), and *Qing Dai* (Indigo Naturalis). *Long Dan Xie Gan Tang* (Gentiana Decoction to Drain the Liver) is the primary formula that clears heat from Liver and Gallbladder.

- Lung heat is characterized by symptoms such as coughing, hurried respiration and dyspnea. Herbs that clear heat from the Lung include *Huang Qin* (Radix Scutellariae), *Sang Bai Pi* (Cortex Mori), *Shi Gao* (Gypsum Fibrosum), *Zhi Mu* (Rhizoma Anemarrhenae), and the formula *Xie Bai San* (Drain the White Powder).

- Stomach heat involves clinical manifestations of toothache, swelling and ulcerations of the gum, and foul breath. Herbs that clear heat from Spleen and Stomach include *Shi Gao* (Gypsum Fibrosum), and *Huang Lian* (Rhizoma Coptidis). *Xie Huang San* (Drain the Yellow Powder) and *Qing Wei San* (Clear the Stomach Powder) are key formulas that clear heat from the Stomach.

- Heat in the Intestines may cause symptoms such as abdominal pain, rectal tenesmus, and burning sensations of the anus. Herbs that clear heat from the Intestines include *Bai Tou Weng* (Radix Pulsatillae), *Huang Lian* (Rhizoma Coptidis), and *Huang Bo* (Cortex Phellodendri Chinensis). Two formulas that clear heat from the Intestines are *Bai Tou Weng Tang* (Pulsatilla Decoction) and *Shao Yao Tang* (Peony Decoction).

6. Deficiency-Heat Clearing Formulas

These formulas nourish yin, ventilate heat, and relieve steaming bones sensations. They mostly treat late stages of heat syndromes that involve damage to yin and body fluids. Common clinical manifestations include evening fever, morning chills, and a red tongue body with a scanty tongue coating. Sometimes chronic deficiency heat patients may experience chronic persistent fever, tidal fever, *wu xin re* (five-center heat), and steaming bones sensations.

Herbs that clear yin-deficient heat include *Bie Jia* (Carapax Trionycis), *Zhi Mu* (Rhizoma Anemarrhenae), *Di Huang* (Radix Rehmanniae), *Qing Hao* (Herba Artemisiae Annuae), and *Di Gu Pi* (Cortex Lycii). Exemplar formulas include *Qing Hao Bie Jia Tang* (Artemisia Annua and Soft-Shelled Turtle Shell Decoction), *Qin Jiao Bie Jia San* (Gentiana Macrophylla and Soft-Shelled Turtle Shell Powder), and *Qing Gu San* (Cool the Bones Powder).

CAUTIONS / CONTRAINDICATIONS

Generally speaking, heat-clearing formulas should only be used when there are no exterior symptoms or when exterior symptoms have been resolved, and heat is present at the interior. If there is heat at the exterior, then use exterior-releasing methods. If heat is located at both the exterior and interior, then use both exterior-releasing and heat-clearing methods. Heat-clearing formulas should not be used on their own if stagnation or hardness has formed in the interior. In these cases, use downward draining methods to eliminate stagnation. Timing and correct differentiation of syndromes are very important factors in using heat-clearing formulas.

The following notes and precautions apply when prescribing heat-clearing formulas:
- Examine carefully whether the heat syndrome is of deficiency or excess type.
- Examine carefully which *zang fu* organ is most involved in the heat syndrome.
- Examine carefully whether the symptoms indicate true heat or false heat.
- Heat-clearing herbs may damage the Stomach and consume yang, so it may be necessary to use Stomach-harmonizing herbs to prevent side effects.

Chinese Herbal Formulas and Applications

Chapter 5 — Overview

• Warm herbs are used as render milder the strong, bitter and cold formulas that clear heat. A small dose of these warm herbs will prevent the patient's body from rejecting the cold herbs, and improve the overall effectiveness of the formula.

PHARMACOLOGICAL EFFECTS & CLINICAL APPLICATIONS

Heat-clearing formulas, as stated earlier, are divided into six subcategories based on their traditional therapeutic actions. These six subcategories also have contrasting pharmacological effects and clinical applications.

Many heat-clearing formulas have antipyretic, anti-inflammatory and antibiotic effects.

1. **Qi (energy) level-clearing formulas** primarily treat fever with or without infection.
   • **Fever**: These formulas have marked antipyretic effects to treat fever with or without infection.[1] *Bai Hu Tang* (White Tiger Decoction) is the representative formula, and it has been used to lower temperature associated with viral infection,[2] encephalitis B,[3] and epidemic hemorrhagic fever.[4]
   • **Diabetes mellitus**: *Bai Hu Tang* (White Tiger Decoction) and *Bai Hu Jia Ren Shen Tang* (White Tiger plus Ginseng Decoction) both have marked hypoglycemic effects,[5,6] and have been used successfully to treat diabetes mellitus.[7,8]

2. **Ying (nutritive) level-clearing and blood-cooling formulas** are generally used to reduce fever and stop bleeding.
   • **Fever**: *Qing Ying Tang* (Clear the Nutritive Level Decoction) and *Xi Jiao Di Huang Tang* (Rhinoceros Horn and Rehmannia Decoction) have shown marked antipyretic effects to lower body temperature in subjects with artificially-induced fever.[9,10] Clinically, they have been used as adjunct treatment to lower body temperature.
   • **Bleeding**: *Xi Jiao Di Huang Tang* (Rhinoceros Horn and Rehmannia Decoction) stops bleeding and has been used successfully to treat thrombocytopenic purpura,[11,12] gastrointestinal bleeding,[13] epistaxis,[14] and other bleeding disorders.

3. **Formulas designed to clear heat from the qi (energy) and xue (blood) levels** treat fever and infection. For example, *Qing Wen Bai Du Yin* (Clear Epidemics and Overcome Pathogenic Influences Decoction) may be used to treat epidemic hemorrhagic fever,[15] pyogenic infection,[16] and leptospirosis.[17]

4. **Heat-clearing and toxin-eliminating formulas** have remarkable antibiotic effects, and are commonly used to treat a wide variety of diseases associated with infection and inflammation.
   • **Infection**: Many of these formulas have been used to treat various types of bacterial, viral, fungal, and other infections. These formulas have a wide range of clinical applications, including treatment of common cold and influenza,[18] otitis media,[19] pneumonia,[20] bronchiectasis,[21] respiratory tract infection,[22] infectious parotitis,[23] tonsillitis,[24,25,26] pharyngitis,[27] encephalitis B,[28] cerebrospinal meningitis,[29] and epidemic hemorrhagic fever.[30] Representative formulas include *Huang Lian Jie Du Tang* (Coptis Decoction to Relieve Toxicity), *Liang Ge San* (Cool the Diaphragm Powder), *Pu Ji Xiao Du Yin* (Universal Benefit Decoction to Eliminate Toxin), and *San Huang Xie Xin Tang* (Three-Yellow Decoction to Sedate the Epigastrium).
   • **Bleeding**: Some heat-clearing and toxin-eliminating formulas have hemostatic effects, and have been used successfully to stop bleeding. Clinical applications include upper and lower gastrointestinal bleeding,[31] and epistaxis.[32,33] Exemplar formulas include *San Huang Xie Xin Tang* (Three-Yellow Decoction to Sedate the Epigastrium) and *Liang Ge San* (Cool the Diaphragm Powder).

5. **Zang fu-clearing formulas** have excellent antibiotic and anti-inflammatory effects, and have been used to treat a wide range of localized disease characterized by infection and inflammation.
   • **Lung disorders**: The antibiotic effects of these formulas have been used successfully to treat lung disorders such as cough,[34] whooping cough,[35] and pneumonia.[36,37] Exemplar formulas include *Xie Bai San* (Drain the White Powder) and *Bai Tou Weng Tang* (Pulsatilla Decoction).

HEAT-CLEARING FORMULAS

5

317

- **Stomach disorders**: Formulas that clear heat from *zang fu* organs treat various types of stomach disorders, including but not limited to gastritis,[38,39] upper gastrointestinal bleeding,[40,41] erosive gastritis,[42] epigastric pain,[43] and gastroenteritis.[44] Exemplar formulas include *Zuo Jin Wan* (Left Metal Pill), *Long Dan Xie Gan Tang* (Gentiana Decoction to Drain the Liver), and *Yu Nu Jian* (Jade Woman Decoction).

- **Liver disorders** (hepatitis) and **gallbladder disorders** (cholecystitis) may be treated with *Long Dan Xie Gan Tang* (Gentiana Decoction to Drain the Liver).[45,46]

- **Intestinal disorders**: These formulas have been shown to treat various types of intestinal disorders characterized by infection and inflammation. Clinical applications include enteritis,[47] colitis,[48,49] ulcerative colitis,[50] dysentery,[51] bacterial dysentery,[52,53] and amoebic dysentery.[54] Representative formulas are *Shao Yao Tang* (Peony Decoction) and *Bai Tou Weng Tang* (Pulsatilla Decoction).

- **Kidney disorders**: *Qing Xin Lian Zi Yin* (Lotus Seed Decoction to Clear the Heart) successfully treats kidney disorders, such as glomerulonephritis,[55] pyelonephritis,[56] and nephrotic syndrome.[57]

- **Eye disorders** such as conjunctivitis may be treated with *Bai Tou Weng Tang* (Pulsatilla Decoction).[58]

- **Ear disorders** such as otitis media may be treated with *Long Dan Xie Gan Tang* (Gentiana Decoction to Drain the Liver).[59]

- **Nose disorders** such as epistaxis may be treated with *Xie Bai San* (Drain the White Powder) and *Yu Nu Jian* (Jade Woman Decoction).[60,61]

- **Mouth and throat disorders**, such as stomatitis,[62,63] gingivitis,[64] periodontitis,[65] periodontal disease,[66] halitosis,[67] infectious parotitis,[68] pharyngitis,[69] and other oral cavity disorders,[70] may be treated with *Dao Chi San* (Guide Out the Red Powder), *Qing Wei San* (Clear the Stomach Powder), *Xie Huang San* (Drain the Yellow Powder), and *Yu Nu Jian* (Jade Woman Decoction).

- **Male disorders** such as orchitis and prostatitis may be treated with *Long Dan Xie Gan Tang* (Gentiana Decoction to Drain the Liver).[71,72]

- **Female disorders** including mastitis, cervicitis, polycystic ovary syndrome, and pelvic inflammatory disease may be treated with *Long Dan Xie Gan Tang* (Gentiana Decoction to Drain the Liver) and *Bai Tou Weng Tang* (Pulsatilla Decoction).[73,74,75]

- **Urinary tract infection**: These formulas have a marked antibiotic activity, and have been used effectively to treat urinary tract infection. Three of these formulas are *Dao Chi San* (Guide Out the Red Powder),[76] *Long Dan Xie Gan Tang* (Gentiana Decoction to Drain the Liver),[77] and *Bai Tou Weng Tang* (Pulsatilla Decoction).[78]

- **Herpes**: *Dao Chi San* (Guide Out the Red Powder) and *Long Dan Xie Gan Tang* (Gentiana Decoction to Drain the Liver) have marked antiviral effects, used successfully to treat herpes infections (oral herpes, genital herpes, and herpes zoster).[79,80,81]

6. **Deficiency-heat clearing formulas** mainly treat fever, infection, and menopausal symptomology.

- **Fever**: Fever from various causes respond to these formulas; such as fever associated with cancer,[82,83] post-surgical fever,[84] and fever following bone fractures.[85] Representative formulas include *Qing Hao Bie Jia Tang* (Artemisia Annua and Soft-Shelled Turtle Shell Decoction) and *Dang Gui Liu Huang Tang* (Tangkuei and Six-Yellow Decoction).

- **Infection**: Some formulas with antibiotic activity have been used to treat viral infections of the respiratory tract[86,87] and pulmonary tuberculosis.[88,89] Two exemplar formulas are *Qing Hao Bie Jia Tang* (Artemisia Annua and Soft-Shelled Turtle Shell Decoction) and *Qin Jiao Bie Jia San* (Gentiana Macrophylla and Soft-Shelled Turtle Shell Powder).

- **Menopause**: Deficiency-heat clearing formulas are effective for symptoms of menopause, such as *Dang Gui Liu Huang Tang* (Tangkuei and Six-Yellow Decoction).[90]

References

1. *Yao Xue Tong Bao* (Report of Herbology) 1981;3:61.
2. *Liao Ning Zhong Yi Za Zhi* (Liaoning Journal of Chinese Medicine) 1984;4:54.
3. *Zhong Yi Za Zhi* (Journal of Chinese Medicine) 1958;4:246.
4. *Liao Ning Yi Yao* (Liaoning Medicine and Herbology) 1975;1:56.

Chinese Herbal Formulas and Applications

Chapter 5 — Overview

5. Morimoto Y, Sakata M, Ohno A, Maegawa T, Tajima S. Effects of Byakko-ka-ninjin-to, Bofu-tsusho-san and Gorei-san on blood glucose level, water intake and urine volume in KKAy mice. Yakugaku Zasshi 2002 Feb;122(2):163-8.

6. Kimura I, Nakashima N, Sugihara Y, Fu-jun C, Kimura M. The antihyperglycaemic blend effect of traditional chinese medicine byakko-ka-ninjin-to on alloxan and diabetic KK-CA(y) mice. Phytother Res 1999 Sep;13(6):484-8.

7. *He Nan Zhong Yi Xue Yuan Xue Bao* (Journal of University of Henan School of Medicine) 1976;3:34.

8. *He Nan Zhong Yi* (Henan Chinese Medicine) 1994;5:266.

9. *Cheng Du Zhong Yi Xue Yuan Xue Bao* (Journal of Chengdu University of Traditional Chinese Medicine) 1995;4:38.

10. *Zhong Yao Tong Bao* (Journal of Chinese Herbology) 1986;11(1):51.

11. *Zhong Yi Za Zhi* (Journal of Chinese Medicine) 1958;7:465.

12. *Zhong Yi Za Zhi* (Journal of Chinese Medicine) 1960;7:22.

13. *Zhong Yi Za Zhi* (Journal of Chinese Medicine) 1980;21(7):36.

14. *Shan Xi Zhong Yi* (Shanxi Chinese Medicine) 1989;10(4):163.

15. *Yi Xue Yan Jiu Tong Xun* (Report of Medical Studies) 1986;(5):3.

16. *Shan Xi Yi Kan* (Shanxi Journal of Medicine) 1983;4(4):13.

17. *Guang Xi Zhong Yi Yao* (Guangxi Chinese Medicine and Herbology) 1987;3:6.

18. *Shan Dong Zhong Yi Za Zhi* (Shandong Journal of Chinese Medicine) 1991;(2):37.

19. *Zhong Yi Za Zhi* (Journal of Chinese Medicine) 1994;35(10):608. 1988;10:67.

20. *Fu Jian Zhong Yi Yao* (Fujian Chinese Medicine and Herbology) 1985;(2):43.

21. *Zhong Xi Yi Jie He Za Zhi* (Journal of Integrated Chinese and Western Medicine) 1985;5:304.

22. *Guang Xi Zhong Yi Yao* (Guangxi Chinese Medicine and Herbology) 1989;(1):5.

23. *Zhong Yi Za Zhi* (Journal of Chinese Medicine) 1958;7:463.

24. *Shan Dong Zhong Yi Za Zhi* (Shandong Journal of Chinese Medicine) 1984;4:42.

25. *Jiang Su Zhong Yi* (Jiangsu Chinese Medicine) 1994;4:166.

26. *Xin Zhong Yi* (New Chinese Medicine) 1990;(3):23.

27. *Zhe Jiang Zhong Yi Xue Yuan Xue Bao* (Journal of Zhejiang University of Chinese Medicine) 1996;3:37.

28. *Fu Jian Zhong Yi Yao* (Fujian Chinese Medicine and Herbology) 1960;6:7.

29. *Guang Dong Zhong Yi* (Guangdong Chinese Medicine) 1960;6:296.

30. *Shan Xi Zhong Yi* (Shanxi Chinese Medicine) 1984;3:16.

31. *Xin Zhong Yi* (New Chinese Medicine) 1997;6:46.

32. *Yun Nan Zhong Yi Xue Yuan Xue Bao* (Journal of Yunnan University School of Medicine) 1996;4:38.

33. *Shi Yong Zhong Yi Yao Za Zhi* (Journal of Practical Chinese Medicine and Medicinals) 1993;3:21.

34. *Shi Yong Zhong Xi Yi Jie He Za Zhi* (Practical Journal of Integrated Chinese and Western Medicines) 1997;3:239.

35. *Yi Fang Xin Jie* (New Explanation for Medical Formulas) 1980;100.

36. *Shan Xi Zhong Yi* (Shanxi Chinese Medicine) 1995;16(8):362.

37. *Zhe Jiang Zhong Yi Za Zhi* (Zhejiang Journal of Chinese Medicine) 1986;12:551.

38. *Shang Hai Zhong Yi Za Zhi* (Shanghai Journal of Chinese Medicine) 1996;6:38.

39. *Shan Xi Zhong Yi* (Shanxi Chinese Medicine) 1997;4:14.

40. *Zhong Yi Fang Ji Xian Dai Yan Jiu* (Modern Study of Medical Formulae in Traditional Chinese Medicine) 1997;322.

41. *Zhong Yi Ming Fang Lin Chuang Xin Yong* (Contemporary Clinical Applications of Classic Chinese Formulas) 2001;186.

42. *Shi Yong Zhong Yi Za Zhi* (Journal of Practical Chinese Medicine) 1999;2:10.

43. *Hu Bei Zhong Yi Za Zhi* (Hubei Journal of Chinese Medicine) 1998;3:40.

44. *Hei Long Jiang Zhong Yi Yao* (Heilongjiang Chinese Medicine and Herbology) 1998;5:54.

45. *Jiang Xi Yi Xue Yuan Xue Bao* (Medical Journal of Jiangxi University of Medicine) 1998;3:123.

46. *Nei Meng Gu Zhong Yi Yao* (Traditional Chinese Medicine and Medicinals of Inner Mongolia) 1987;6(2):42.

47. *Shang Hai Zhong Yi Yao Za Zhi* (Shanghai Journal of Chinese Medicine and Herbology) 1960;6:254.

48. *Si Chuan Zhong Yi* (Sichuan Chinese Medicine) 1995;7:28.

49. *Xin Zhong Yi* (New Chinese Medicine) 1996;1:20.

50. *Si Chuan Zhong Yi* (Sichuan Chinese Medicine) 1995;3:33.

51. *Hei Long Jiang Zhong Yi Yao* (Heilongjiang Chinese Medicine and Herbology) 1989;6:29.

52. *Gan Su Zhong Yi* (Gansu Chinese Medicine) 1998;2:13.

53. *Nan Jing Zhong Yi Yao Da Xue Xue Bao* (Journal of Nanjing University of Traditional Chinese Medicine and Medicinals) 1997;5:311.

54. *Hu Bei Zhong Yi Za Zhi* (Hubei Journal of Chinese Medicine) 1983;2:24.

55. *Shan Xi Zhong Yi* (Shanxi Chinese Medicine) 1998;4:173.

56. *Shan Xi Zhong Yi* (Shanxi Chinese Medicine) 1998;4:173.

57. *Shan Xi Zhong Yi* (Shanxi Chinese Medicine) 1998;4:173.

58. *Zhong Yi Fang Ji Xian Dai Yan Jiu* (Modern Study of Medical Formulae in Traditional Chinese Medicine) 1997;346-47.

59. *Zhong Cheng Yao Yan Jiu* (Research of Chinese Patent Medicine) 1985;8:43.

60. *Hu Bei Zhong Yi Za Zhi* (Hubei Journal of Chinese Medicine) 1997;4:35.

61. *Jiang Xi Zhong Yi Yao* (Jiangxi Chinese Medicine and Herbology) 1986;5:18.

62. *Nei Meng Gu Zhong Yi Yao* (Traditional Chinese Medicine and Medicinals of Inner Mongolia) 1993;12(3):27.

63. *He Bei Zhong Yi* (Hebei Chinese Medicine) 1989;1:25.

64. *Shang Hai Zhong Yi Yao Za Zhi* (Shanghai Journal of Chinese Medicine and Herbology) 1994;6:31.

Chapter 5 — Overview

65. *Hu Nan Zhong Yi Za Zhi* (Hunan Journal of Chinese Medicine) 1997;5:36.
66. *Shan Dong Zhong Yi Za Zhi* (Shandong Journal of Chinese Medicine) 1996;9:402.
67. *Shan Xi Zhong Yi* (Shanxi Chinese Medicine) 1996;5:204.
68. *Shan Xi Zhong Yi* (Shanxi Chinese Medicine) 1991;(8):368.
69. *An Hui Zhong Yi Xue Yuan Xue Bao* (Journal of Anhui University School of Medicine) 1995;2:21.
70. *Zhong Xi Yi Jie He Za Zhi* (Journal of Integrated Chinese and Western Medicine) 1989;9(3):182.
71. *Zhong Yi Yao Yan Jiu* (Research of Chinese Medicine and Herbology) 1987;(4):39.
72. *Liao Ning Zhong Yi Za Zhi* (Liaoning Journal of Chinese Medicine) 1991;(6):32.
73. *Shi Yong Zhong Xi Yi Jie He Za Zhi* (Practical Journal of Integrated Chinese and Western Medicines) 1992;4:245.
74. *Zhong Yi Yao Xin Xi* (Information on Chinese Medicine and Herbology) 1989;(6):38.
75. *Shang Hai Zhong Yi Za Zhi* (Shanghai Journal of Chinese Medicine) 1982;12:17.
76. *Guang Xi Zhong Yi Yao* (Guangxi Chinese Medicine and Herbology) 1991;(3):104.
77. *Zhong Yi Fang Ji Xian Dai Yan Jiu* (Modern Study of Medical Formulae in Traditional Chinese Medicine) 1997;321.
78. *Hei Long Jiang Zhong Yi Yao* (Heilongjiang Chinese Medicine and Herbology) 1986;6:40.
79. *Nan Jing Zhong Yi Xue Yuan Xue Bao* (Journal of Nanjing University of Traditional Chinese Medicine) 1984;4(2):90.
80. *Zhong Yi Za Zhi* (Journal of Chinese Medicine) 1987;6:34.
81. *Jiang Su Zhong Yi* (Jiangsu Chinese Medicine) 1993;(3):22.
82. *Fu Jian Zhong Yi Yao* (Fujian Chinese Medicine and Herbology) 1996;1:21.
83. *Hu Nan Zhong Yi Za Zhi* (Hunan Journal of Chinese Medicine) 1997;5:27.
84. *Zhong Yi Yao Xue Bao* (Report of Chinese Medicine and Herbology) 1995;6:52.
85. *Zhe Jiang Zhong Yi Za Zhi* (Zhejiang Journal of Chinese Medicine) 1959;9:34.
86. *Zhong Yi Fang Ji Xian Dai Yan Jiu* (Modern Study of Medical Formulae in Traditional Chinese Medicine) 1997;351-52.
87. *Zhe Jiang Zhong Yi Za Zhi* (Zhejiang Journal of Chinese Medicine) 1992;27(6):251.
88. *Zhe Jiang Zhong Yi Za Zhi* (Zhejiang Journal of Chinese Medicine) 1993;28(5):206.
89. *Zhong Yi Fang Ji Xian Dai Yan Jiu* (Modern Study of Medical Formulae in Traditional Chinese Medicine) 1997;350-351.
90. *Jiang Su Zhong Yi* (Jiangsu Chinese Medicine) 1996;5:22.

Chinese Herbal Formulas and Applications

Section 1

清气分热剂
— Qi (Energy) Level-Clearing Formulas

Bái Hǔ Tāng (White Tiger Decoction)
白虎湯
白虎汤

Pinyin Name: *Bai Hu Tang*
Literal Name: White Tiger Decoction
Alternate Names: *Pai Hu Tang*, Gypsum Decoction, Gypsum Combination
Original Source: *Shang Han Lun* (Discussion of Cold-Induced Disorders) by Zhang Zhong-Jing in the Eastern Han Dynasty

COMPOSITION

Shi Gao (Gypsum Fibrosum), *fen sui* (pulverized)	48g [30g]
Zhi Mu (Rhizoma Anemarrhenae)	18g [9g]
Zhi Gan Cao (Radix et Rhizoma Glycyrrhizae Praeparata cum Melle)	6g [3g]
Geng Mi (Semen Oryzae)	0.6 cup [9g]

DOSAGE / PREPARATION / ADMINISTRATION

The source text recommends to cook the ingredients in 10 cups [2,000 mL] of water until *Geng Mi* (Semen Oryzae) is fully cooked. Take 1 cup [200 mL] of the warm, strained decoction three times daily. Today, the decoction may be prepared using the doses suggested in brackets above.

CHINESE THERAPEUTIC ACTIONS

Clears heat and generates body fluids

CLINICAL MANIFESTATIONS

Yangming jing (channel) syndrome; excess heat in the *yangming qi* (energy) level: high fever, flushed face, irritability, thirst with a strong desire to drink, profuse sweating, and aversion to heat. The pulse is either surging, big and forceful; or the pulse is slippery and rapid.

CLINICAL APPLICATIONS

High fever, bacterial or viral infections, common cold, influenza, encephalitis, meningitis, pneumonia, lobar pneumonia, epidemic hemorrhagic fever, heat stroke, periodontitis, gingivitis, rheumatism, and diabetes mellitus.

EXPLANATION

Bai Hu Tang (White Tiger Decoction) treats generalized excess interior heat with damage to body fluids. Excess

heat may form as a result of the migration of an exterior pathogen into the interior. A typical case is wind-cold traveling to the interior and transforming into heat. Because the disease location is in the interior and the factor is heat, there will be high fever without chills. Irritability is the result of heat attacking the *shen* (spirit). Heat in the interior may consume body fluids, causing thirst with a strong desire to drink. The interior heat may also force out body fluids, causing profuse sweating.

It is not appropriate to induce sweating to dispel the pathogenic factors because the heat is in the interior instead of the exterior. Neither is it suitable to approach this condition with purgative herbs because the heat has not yet attacked the *zang fu* and giving rise to constipation. Heat-clearing herbs that are acrid and drying in nature should not be used because they may damage yin even further. The most appropriate treatment strategy is to clear heat and generate fluids with the use of sweet and cold herbs.

Shi Gao (Gypsum Fibrosum) is the chief herb because it is the most effective herb for clearing heat in *yangming jing* (channel) syndrome or *qi* (energy) level, which manifests as Lung and Stomach fire. *Shi Gao* (Gypsum Fibrosum) reduces fever and relieves irritability, while *Zhi Mu*

321

Bái Hǔ Tāng (White Tiger Decoction)

Bai Hu Tang (White Tiger Decoction)

Diagnosis	Signs and Symptoms	Treatment	Herbs
Excess heat affecting *yangming jing* (channel) or *qi* (energy) level	• High fever with aversion to heat: excess heat in the interior • Thirst with a strong desire to drink: heat consuming body fluids • Profuse sweating: heat forcing body fluids outward • Surging, big and forceful pulse: excess heat in the interior	• Clears heat • Generates body fluids	• *Shi Gao* (Gypsum Fibrosum) clears heat in *yangming jing* (channel) and *qi* (energy) level. • *Zhi Mu* (Rhizoma Anemarrhenae) clears interior excess heat, nourishes yin and moistens dryness. • *Zhi Gan Cao* (Radix et Rhizoma Glycyrrhizae Praeparata cum Melle) and *Geng Mi* (Semen Oryzae) tonify and protect the Stomach, and prevent the extreme coldness of *Shi Gao* (Gypsum Fibrosum) from injuring the middle *jiao*.

(Rhizoma Anemarrhenae) helps to clear interior excess heat, as well as nourish yin and moisten dryness. Together, they relieve thirst and replenish fluids that are lost through perspiration. *Shi Gao* (Gypsum Fibrosum) is stronger in clearing heat, while *Zhi Mu* (Rhizoma Anemarrhenae) is more effective in moistening dryness. *Zhi Gan Cao* (Radix et Rhizoma Glycyrrhizae Praeparata cum Melle) and *Geng Mi* (Semen Oryzae) tonify and protect the Stomach, and prevent the extreme coldness of *Shi Gao* (Gypsum Fibrosum) from injuring the middle *jiao*.

MODIFICATIONS

• When there is excess heat in the body consuming yin and body fluids, add *Mai Dong* (Radix Ophiopogonis).
• For summer-heat invasion with thirst, add *San Wu Xiang Ru Yin* (Mosla Three Decoction).
• For gingivitis and toothache, add *Huang Lian* (Rhizoma Coptidis), *Huang Qin* (Radix Scutellariae) and *Bai Zhi* (Radix Angelicae Dahuricae).
• With constipation, thirst, and perspiration, add *Da Huang* (Radix et Rhizoma Rhei) and *Mang Xiao* (Natrii Sulfas).
• With belching and a feeling of oppression in the epigastric region, add *Ban Xia* (Rhizoma Pinelliae) and *Zhu Ru* (Caulis Bambusae in Taenia).
• When accompanied by alternating chills and fever, add *Chai Hu* (Radix Bupleuri) or *Xiao Chai Hu Tang* (Minor Bupleurum Decoction).
• For *qi* (energy) level *wen bing* (warm disease) with wind-heat invasion, add *Yin Qiao San* (Honeysuckle and Forsythia Powder).
• With high fever, thirst, irritability, delirium, and muscle twitching, add *Shui Niu Jiao* (Cornu Bubali) and *Gou Teng* (Ramulus Uncariae cum Uncis).
• With thirst due to *xiao ke* (wasting and thirsting) syndrome with Stomach heat, add *Tian Hua Fen* (Radix Trichosanthis), *Lu Gen* (Rhizoma Phragmitis), and *Mai Dong* (Radix Ophiopogonis).

• With swollen and painful gums with thirst and dry stools, add *Xuan Shen* (Radix Scrophulariae) and *Niu Xi* (Radix Achyranthis Bidentatae).
• If there is headache, add *Bai Zhi* (Radix Angelicae Dahuricae) and *Gao Ben* (Rhizoma et Radix Ligustici).
• For measles or toxic lesions on the skin, add *Sheng Ma Ge Gen Tang* (Cimicifuga and Kudzu Decoction).

CAUTIONS / CONTRAINDICATIONS

• *Bai Hu Tang* treats heat affecting *yangming jing* (channel), not *yangming fu* (hollow organs). *Yangming fu* (hollow organs) is treated with *Da Cheng Qi Tang* (Major Order the Qi Decoction).
• This formula is contraindicated in the following four situations: 1) fever and absence of sweating from an unresolved exterior condition; 2) a pulse that is fine or deep; 3) fever from blood deficiency evident by a surging pulse that feels empty upon pressure; and 4) a "true-cold, false-heat" condition in which the interior yin rejects and repels yang to the exterior.

PHARMACOLOGICAL EFFECTS

1. **Antipyretic**: According to *in vitro* studies, *Bai Hu Tang* and its ingredients all have varying degrees of antipyretic effects in rabbits. Administration of the herbal treatment was associated with reduction of body temperature by 1.3°C with *Bai Hu Tang*, 1.2°C with both *Shi Gao* (Gypsum Fibrosum) and *Zhi Mu* (Rhizoma Anemarrhenae), 0.7°C with *Zhi Mu* (Rhizoma Anemarrhenae), and 0.3°C with *Shi Gao* (Gypsum Fibrosum). It was also noted that while *Shi Gao* (Gypsum Fibrosum) had a faster onset, *Zhi Mu* (Rhizoma Anemarrhenae) had a longer overall duration.[1]

2. **Immunostimulant**: Injection of *Bai Hu Tang* in mice was associated with an increased phagocytic effect for up to 6 hours.[2]

Bái Hŭ Tāng (White Tiger Decoction)

Chinese Herbal Formulas and Applications

CLINICAL STUDIES AND RESEARCH

1. **High fever**: *Bai Hu Tang* is commonly used as the first choice for treatment of febrile conditions. In one report, 50 patients with high fever who were treated with decoction of the formula experienced a reduction of temperature to normal within two days.[3] In another study, 69 patients with fever caused by viral infection were treated with 87% effectiveness using modified *Bai Hu Tang*, with the removal of *Geng Mi* (Semen Oryzae) and *Gan Cao* (Radix et Rhizoma Glycyrrhizae), and the addition of *Ge Gen* (Radix Puerariae Lobatae) and *Chai Hu* (Radix Bupleuri).[4]

2. **Epidemic hemorrhagic fever**: Administration of modified *Bai Hu Tang* for 6-15 days was effective in reducing the duration of illness in all 40 patients with epidemic hemorrhagic fever.[5]

3. **Pneumonia**: Twenty patients with lobar pneumonia were treated with an injection of *Bai Hu Tang*; 13 patients had complete recovery, 4 patients had moderate improvement, and 3 patients experienced no change.[6]

4. **Encephalitis B**: One study of 78 patients with encephalitis B reported satisfactory results using *Bai Hu Tang* plus *Ban Lan Gen* (Radix Isatidis), *Lian Qiao* (Fructus Forsythiae), and *Ge Gen* (Radix Puerariae Lobatae). The patients were treated for 5 days per course of treatment. Of 78 patients, the study reported complete recovery in 69 patients, improvement in 4 patients, and fatality in 5 patients.[7] In another report, 31 patients with encephalitis B who were treated with a modification of the formula experienced a reduction of body temperature within the first day, resolution of most symptoms in the second day, and recovery in the third day.[8]

5. **Rheumatism**: Thirty-four patients with rheumatoid arthritis were treated with modified *Bai Hu Tang*. The rheumatism was characterized by redness, swelling, and pain, with duration of illness ranging from 2-36 days. Out of 34 patients, 8 had rheumatism in the upper extremities and 26 in the lower extremities. The treatment protocol was administration of the formula in decoction form one time daily. The study reported complete recovery in 23 patients, significant improvement in 7 patients, slight improvement in 2 patients, and no change in 2 patients.[9] Another study reported that administration of *Bai Hu Tang* plus *Zhi Chuan Wu* (Radix Aconiti Praeparata), *Ru Xiang* (Gummi Olibanum) and *Mo Yao* (Myrrha) was associated with complete relief in 22 of 28 patients with acute rheumatoid arthritis characterized by wind, dampness, and heat.[10]

6. **Diabetes mellitus**: Use of modified *Bai Hu Tang* in 268 patients was associated with recovery in 81 patients, significant effect in 58 patients, effectiveness in 110 patients, and no effect in 19 patients.[11] According to another study, 21 patients with diabetes mellitus were treated daily with an 800-1,000 mL decoction of *Bai Hu Tang* daily for approximately 6 months with 95% effectiveness. The dose of *Shi Gao* (Gypsum Fibrosum) may be increased to 120g if there is severe thirst.[12]

RELATED FORMULAS

Bái Hŭ Jiā Guì Zhī Tāng
(White Tiger plus Cinnamon Twig Decoction)

白虎加桂枝湯
白虎加桂枝汤

Pinyin Name: Bai Hu Jia Gui Zhi Tang
Literal Name: White Tiger plus Cinnamon Twig Decoction
Original Source: *Jin Gui Yao Lue* (Essentials from the Golden Cabinet) by Zhang Zhong-Jing in the Eastern Han Dynasty

Zhi Mu (Rhizoma Anemarrhenae)	18g [9g]
Zhi Gan Cao (Radix et Rhizoma Glycyrrhizae Praeparata cum Melle)	6g [3g]
Shi Gao (Gypsum Fibrosum)	48g [30g]
Geng Mi (Semen Oryzae)	0.2 cup [6g]
Gui Zhi (Ramulus Cinnamomi)	9g [5-9g]

The source text states to grind the ingredients into a coarse powder, and cook 15g of the powder in 1.5 large bowls of water until 80% of the liquid remains. Take the strained decoction while warm. Once sweating is induced, the condition will be resolved. Today, this formula may be prepared as a decoction using the doses suggested in brackets.

Bai Hu Jia Gui Zhi Tang (White Tiger plus Cinnamon Twig Decoction) is composed of *Bai Hu Tang* plus *Gui Zhi* (Ramulus Cinnamomi). With the addition of *Gui Zhi* (Ramulus Cinnamomi), this formula has the added functions to warm the channels and collaterals, and harmonize *ying* (nutritive) and *wei* (defensive) levels. It is often given to patients with *bi zheng* (painful obstruction syndrome) caused by wind, dampness, and heat. Chief complaints are joint swelling, burning pain, and/or muscle pain. Secondary symptoms include fever, loud breathing, irritability, thirst, and a wiry, rapid pulse. This formula can also be used for warm malarial disorders caused by heat manifesting in fever, no chills, joint pain, nausea, and vomiting.

Bái Hŭ Jiā Cāng Zhú Tāng
(White Tiger plus Atractylodes Decoction)

白虎加蒼朮湯
白虎加苍术汤

HEAT-CLEARING FORMULAS

5

323

Bái Hǔ Tāng (White Tiger Decoction)

Pinyin Name: *Bai Hu Jia Cang Zhu Tang*
Literal Name: White Tiger plus Atractylodes Decoction
Original Source: *Lei Zheng Huo Ren Shu* (Book to Safeguard Life Arranged According to Pattern) by Zhu Gong in 1108

Zhi Mu (Rhizoma Anemarrhenae)	18g [9g]
Zhi Gan Cao (Radix et Rhizoma Glycyrrhizae Praeparata cum Melle)	6g [3g]
Shi Gao (Gypsum Fibrosum)	48g [30g]
Geng Mi (Semen Oryzae)	9g [9g]
Cang Zhu (Rhizoma Atractylodis)	9g [9g]

The source text recommends to grind the ingredients into a coarse powder, and cook 15g of the powder in 1.5 large bowls of water until 80-90% of the liquid remains. Discard the herb residue, and take 60% of the warm, strained decoction per dose. Today, this formula may be prepared as a decoction using the doses suggested in brackets.

Bai Hu Jia Cang Zhu Tang (White Tiger plus Atractylodes Decoction) is composed of *Bai Hu Tang* plus *Cang Zhu* (Rhizoma Atractylodis). With the addition of *Cang Zhu* (Rhizoma Atractylodis), this formula can treat *yangming jing* (channel) syndrome accompanied by interior dampness. In addition to all the symptoms and signs found in *yangming jing* (channel) syndrome, other chief complaints include chest distention, profuse perspiration, warm sensations in the body, dyspnea, irritability, and a red tongue with a white, greasy tongue coating. It is used for *bi zheng* (painful obstruction syndrome) caused by wind, dampness, and heat.

AUTHORS' COMMENTS

Bai Hu Tang treats heat in *yangming jing* (channel) syndrome according to *Shang Han Lun* (Discussion of Cold-Induced Disorders), and treats heat in *yangming qi* (energy) level according to *wen bing* (warm disease)

theories. Although the names of the syndromes are different, they refer to the same condition: excess interior heat with damage to body fluids.

Bai Hu Tang is the representative formula for treating excess heat in *yangming jing* (channel) syndrome and *yangming qi* (energy) level, two conditions characterized by the "four bigs": "big fever" (high fever), "big sweating" (profuse sweating), "big thirst" (extreme thirst), and "big pulse" (surging, big, and forceful pulse). Clinically, this formula can be applied if the patient shows a surging, big, and forceful pulse, high fever, profuse perspiration, extreme thirst, and irritability.

According to Dr. Chang Wei-Yen, *Bai Hu Tang*, *Long Dan Xie Gan Tang* (Gentiana Decoction to Drain the Liver), and *Zhi Bai Di Huang Wan* (Anemarrhena, Phellodendron, and Rehmannia Pill) can be combined together to treat heat in the entire body, as these three formulas clear heat from the upper, middle, and lower *jiaos*, respectively.

References

1. *Yao Xue Tong Bao* (Report of Herbology) 1981;3:61.
2. *Zhong Guo Zhong Yao Za Zhi* (People's Republic of China Journal of Chinese Herbology) 1989;3:50.
3. *Jiang Su Zhong Yi Za Zhi* (Jiangsu Journal of Chinese Medicine) 1986;1:9.
4. *Liao Ning Zhong Yi Za Zhi* (Liaoning Journal of Chinese Medicine) 1984;4:54.
5. *Zhong Xi Yi Jie He Za Zhi* (Journal of Integrated Chinese and Western Medicine) 1987;5:300.
6. *Liao Ning Yi Yao* (Liaoning Medicine and Herbology) 1975;1:56.
7. *Tian Jin Yi Yao* (Tianjin Medicine and Herbology) 1980;7:422.
8. *Zhong Yi Za Zhi* (Journal of Chinese Medicine) 1958;4:246.
9. *Shang Hai Yi Yao Za Zhi* (Shanghai Journal of Medicine and Herbology) 1987;3:24.
10. *He Bei Zhong Yi* (Hebei Chinese Medicine) 1989;4:21.
11. *Shan Dong Zhong Yi Za Zhi* (Shandong Journal of Chinese Medicine) 1984;5:23.
12. *He Nan Zhong Yi Xue Yuan Xue Bao* (Journal of University of Henan School of Medicine) 1976;3:34.

Chinese Herbal Formulas and Applications

Bái Hǔ Jiā Rén Shēn Tāng (White Tiger plus Ginseng Decoction)

白虎加人参湯
白虎加人参汤

Pinyin Name: *Bai Hu Jia Ren Shen Tang*
Literal Name: White Tiger plus Ginseng Decoction
Alternate Names: *Pai Hu Chia Jen Shen Tang*, Ginseng plus White Tiger Decoction, Ginseng and Gypsum Combination
Original Source: *Shang Han Lun* (Discussion of Cold-Induced Disorders) by Zhang Zhong-Jing in the Eastern Han Dynasty

COMPOSITION

Shi Gao (Gypsum Fibrosum), *fen sui* (pulverized)	48g [30g]
Zhi Mu (Rhizoma Anemarrhenae)	18g [9g]
Zhi Gan Cao (Radix et Rhizoma Glycyrrhizae Praeparata cum Melle)	6g [3g]
Geng Mi (Semen Oryzae)	0.6 cup [9g]
Ren Shen (Radix et Rhizoma Ginseng)	9g [10g]

DOSAGE / PREPARATION / ADMINISTRATION

The source text states to cook the ingredients in 10 cups [2,000 mL] of water until *Geng Mi* (Semen Oryzae) is fully cooked. Take 1 cup [200 mL] of the warm, strained decoction three times daily. Today, the decoction may be prepared using the doses suggested in brackets.

CHINESE THERAPEUTIC ACTIONS

1. Clears heat
2. Tonifies qi and generates body fluids

CLINICAL MANIFESTATIONS

Yangming jing (channel) syndrome or excess heat in the *yangming qi* (energy) level with qi and body fluid deficiencies: high fever, flushed face, irritability, a dry mouth, thirst with a strong desire to drink, profuse sweating, aversion to cold in the upper back, and a big, forceless pulse.

CLINICAL APPLICATIONS

Bacterial or viral infections, influenza, encephalitis, meningitis, lobar pneumonia, febrile disorders, heat stroke, periodontitis, gingivitis, diabetes mellitus, and dry mouth and throat.

EXPLANATION

Bai Hu Jia Ren Shen Tang (White Tiger plus Ginseng Decoction) is composed of *Bai Hu Tang* (White Tiger Decoction) plus *Ren Shen* (Radix et Rhizoma Ginseng). It treats excess interior heat in *yangming jing* (channel) syndrome and qi (energy) level. Because heat may consume qi and dry up body fluids, corresponding symptoms such as thirst and profuse sweating will be present. Thus, in addition to using *Bai Hu Tang* (White Tiger Decoction) to clear heat and generate fluids, *Ren Shen* (Radix et Rhizoma Ginseng) is added to provide a stronger action to tonify qi and replenish body fluids.

MODIFICATIONS

- With fidgeting, irritability, and thirst, add *Mai Dong* (Radix Ophiopogonis) and *Wu Wei Zi* (Fructus Schisandrae Chinensis).
- For thirst during the summer, add *Xiang Fu* (Rhizoma Cyperi) and *Sha Shen* (Radix Glehniae seu Adenophorae).

PHARMACOLOGICAL EFFECTS

1. **Antidiabetic:** One study in mice confirmed that administration of *Bai Hu Jia Ren Shen Tang* was effective in treating polydipsia accompanied by diabetes mellitus. The herbs were given as food mixture for a total of 4 weeks.[1]
2. **Hypoglycemic:** Administration of *Bai Hu Jia Ren Shen Tang* was associated with marked effectiveness in reducing

Bai Hu Jia Ren Shen Tang (White Tiger plus Ginseng Decoction)

Diagnosis	Signs and Symptoms	Treatment	Herbs
Yangming heat with qi and fluids deficiencies	• High fever, profuse sweating, and extreme thirst: *yangming* syndrome • Thirst and a forceless pulse: excess heat consuming qi and body fluids	• Clears heat • Tonifies qi and generates body fluids	• *Bai Hu Tang* (White Tiger Decoction) clears excess heat to treat *yangming* syndrome. • *Ren Shen* (Radix et Rhizoma Ginseng) tonifies qi and replenishes body fluids.

5

HEAT-CLEARING FORMULAS

325

Chapter 5 – Heat-Clearing Formulas　　　　　　　　*Section 1 – Qi (Energy) Level-Clearing Formulas*

Bái Hǔ Jiā Rén Shēn Tāng (White Tiger plus Ginseng Decoction)

plasma glucose levels in both rabbits and mice.[2] Another study confirmed that both the individual ingredients and the formula had marked hypoglycemic effects in genetically obese diabetic mice.[3]

3. **Antipruritic**: Oral administration of *Bai Hu Jia Ren Shen Tang* (200 mg/kg) was associated with a marked effect to treat atopic dermatitis in mice. Therapeutic improvements included significantly reduced scratching frequency, and a decrease in skin temperature by 1.97°C. The study stated that this formula had an inhibitory effect on itching, and may be a useful antipruritic drug for atopic dermatitis.[4]

CLINICAL STUDIES AND RESEARCH

1. **Diabetes mellitus**: Use of *Bai Hu Jia Ren Shen Tang* lowered glucose levels in the blood and urine in patients with diabetes mellitus characterized by Stomach heat. This formula was effective in 56 of 64 patients (87.5% effectiveness).[5]

2. **Dry mouth and throat**: Administration of *Bai Hu Jia Ren Shen Tang* was effective in 12 of 15 patients in relieving dry mouth and throat.[6] Another study reported 80% effectiveness using *Bai Hu Jia Ren Shen Tang* to treat 30 patients with thirst caused by the use of antidepressant

drugs.[7] *Bai Hu Jia Ren Shen Tang* facilitated salivary secretion to relieve dry mouth and throat by stimulating efferent activity of the autonomic nerve fibers innervating the sublingual glands in a dose-dependent manner.[8]

References

1. Morimoto Y, Sakata M, Ohno A, Maegawa T, Tajima S. Effects of Byakko-ka-ninjin-to, Bofu-tsusho-san and Gorei-san on blood glucose level, water intake and urine volume in KKAy mice. Yakugaku Zasshi 2002 Feb;122(2):163-8.
2. *He Nan Zhong Yi* (Henan Chinese Medicine) 1994;5:266.
3. Kimura I, Nakashima N, Sugihara Y, Fu-jun C, Kimura M. The antihyperglycaemic blend effect of traditional chinese medicine byakko-ka-ninjin-to on alloxan and diabetic KK-CA(y) mice. Phytother Res 1999 Sep;13(6):484-8.
4. Tohda C, Sugahara H, Kuraishi Y, Komatsu K. Inhibitory effect of Byakko-ka-ninjin-to on itch in a mouse model of atopic dermatitis. Phytother Res 2000 May;14(3):192-4.
5. *He Nan Zhong Yi* (Henan Chinese Medicine) 1994;5:266.
6. *Guo Wai Yi Xue* (Foreign Medicine) 1992;2:106.
7. *Zhong Yi Fang Ji Xian Dai Yan Jiu* (Modern Study of Medical Formulae in Traditional Chinese Medicine) 1997;264.
8. Niijima A, Kubo M, Ichiki H, Komatsu Y, Maruno M, Okada M. Effect of byakko-ka-ninjin-to on the efferent activity of the autonomic nerve fibers innervating the sublingual gland of the rat. J Auton Nerv Syst 1997 Mar 19;63(1-2):46-50.

Zhú Yè Shí Gāo Tāng (Bamboo Leaves and Gypsum Decoction)
竹葉石膏湯
竹叶石膏汤

Pinyin Name: *Zhu Ye Shi Gao Tang*
Literal Name: Bamboo Leaves and Gypsum Decoction
Alternate Names: *Chu Yeh Shih Kao Tang*, Bamboo Leaves and Gypsum Combination
Original Source: *Shang Han Lun* (Discussion of Cold-Induced Disorders) by Zhang Zhong-Jing in the Eastern Han Dynasty

COMPOSITION

Zhu Ye (Herba Phyllostachys)	2 handfuls [15g]
Shi Gao (Gypsum Fibrosum)	48g [30g]
Ren Shen (Radix et Rhizoma Ginseng)	6g [5g]
Mai Dong (Radix Ophiopogonis)	1 cup [15g]
Ban Xia (Rhizoma Pinelliae), *xi* (washed)	0.5 cup [9g]
Zhi Gan Cao (Radix et Rhizoma Glycyrrhizae Praeparata cum Melle)	6g [3g]
Geng Mi (Semen Oryzae)	0.5 cup [15g]

Note: *Zhu Ye* (Herba Phyllostachys) and *Dan Zhu Ye* (Herba Lophatheri) have similar pinyin names and functions,

and are sometimes used interchangeably. According to the source text, *Zhu Ye* (Herba Phyllostachys) is used in

---

326

Zhú Yè Shí Gāo Tāng (Bamboo Leaves and Gypsum Decoction)

Zhu Ye Shi Gao Tang to clear heat and relieve irritability. Today, because *Zhu Ye* (Herba Phyllostachys) is not readily available, it is generally replaced with *Dan Zhu Ye* (Herba Lophatheri). In comparison, *Zhu Ye* (Herba Phyllostachys) is more effective in clearing Heart and Stomach heat, while *Dan Zhu Ye* (Herba Lophatheri) is better at clearing heat and promoting normal urination.

DOSAGE / PREPARATION / ADMINISTRATION

The source text states to cook all of the ingredients except *Geng Mi* (Semen Oryzae), in 10 cups [2,000 mL] of water until 6 cups [1,200 mL] of liquid remain. Discard the residue, add *Geng Mi* (Semen Oryzae) to the strained decoction and cook again until *Geng Mi* (Semen Oryzae) is fully cooked. Take 1 cup [200 mL] of the warm, strained decoction three times daily. Today, the decoction may be prepared using the doses suggested in brackets.

CHINESE THERAPEUTIC ACTIONS

1. Clears heat and generates body fluids
2. Tonifies qi and harmonizes the Stomach

CLINICAL MANIFESTATIONS

Lingering or residual heat resulting from *shang han* (cold damage), *wen bing* (warm disease) or summer-heat with both qi and yin damage: fever, profuse perspiration, a stifling sensation and distention in the chest or epigastrium, nausea, a dry mouth, thirst with a desire to drink, irritability, insomnia, a red tongue body with scanty coating, and a deficient, rapid pulse.

CLINICAL APPLICATIONS

Fever, common cold, influenza, pneumonia, measles, toothache, stomatitis, diabetes mellitus, gingivitis, summer-heat stroke, bronchitis, and bronchial asthma.

EXPLANATION

Zhu Ye Shi Gao Tang (Bamboo Leaves and Gypsum Decoction) is indicated in the late stage of *shang han* (cold damage), *wen bing* (warm disease), or febrile diseases in which the heat has diminished substantially, but the yin, body fluids, and qi are damaged. Irritability, a stifling sensation and distention in the chest or epigastrium, and fever that cannot be reduced with perspiration are indications that the heat has not been completely eliminated. Thirst, a dry mouth and lips, and a scanty tongue coating reflect consumption of yin and body fluids by heat.

This condition of lingering heat with underlying deficiencies must be treated carefully. Bitter and cold herbs that clear heat will not help generate body fluids and may further damage qi and yin. However, simply tonifying qi and yin will trap the residual heat inside. Therefore, the optimal treatment strategy is to sedate and tonify at the same time.

Zhu Ye (Herba Phyllostachys) and *Shi Gao* (Gypsum Fibrosum) clear interior heat to relieve fever and irritability. *Ren Shen* (Radix et Rhizoma Ginseng) and *Mai Dong* (Radix Ophiopogonis) tonify both qi and yin to promote generation of body fluids. *Ban Xia* (Rhizoma Pinelliae) corrects the reversed flow of Stomach qi to relieve nausea and vomiting. It also balances the tonic and cloying effects of *Ren Shen* (Radix et Rhizoma Ginseng) and *Mai Dong* (Radix Ophiopogonis). *Zhi Gan Cao* (Radix et Rhizoma Glycyrrhizae Praeparata cum Melle) and *Geng Mi* (Semen Oryzae) nourish the Stomach and harmonize the middle *jiao*.

Zhu Ye Shi Gao Tang (Bamboo Leaves and Gypsum Decoction)

Diagnosis	Signs and Symptoms	Treatment	Herbs
Lingering heat with qi and yin damage	• Irritability and insomnia: heat disturbing *shen* (spirit) • Fever, profuse perspiration: lingering heat not yet cleared • Dry mouth and thirst with a desire to drink: heat consuming body fluids • Chest or epigastric stuffiness and distention: heat injuring Lung and Stomach qi • Red tongue body with a scanty coating: heat damaging qi and body fluids • Deficient, rapid pulse: deficiency and excess conditions combined	• Clears heat and generates body fluids • Tonifies qi and harmonizes the Stomach	• *Zhu Ye* (Herba Phyllostachys) and *Shi Gao* (Gypsum Fibrosum) clear interior heat. • *Ren Shen* (Radix et Rhizoma Ginseng) and *Mai Dong* (Radix Ophiopogonis) tonify qi and yin. • *Ban Xia* (Rhizoma Pinelliae) corrects the reversed flow of Stomach qi. • *Zhi Gan Cao* (Radix et Rhizoma Glycyrrhizae Praeparata cum Melle) and *Geng Mi* (Semen Oryzae) nourish the Stomach and harmonize the middle *jiao*.

Zhú Yè Shí Gāo Tāng (Bamboo Leaves and Gypsum Decoction)

MODIFICATIONS

- With cough and dyspnea, add *Ku Xing Ren* (Semen Armeniacae Amarum).
- With cough and wheezing in pneumonia or bronchitis, add *Ma Huang* (Herba Ephedrae), *Ku Xing Ren* (Semen Armeniacae Amarum), *Huang Qin* (Radix Scutellariae), and *Yu Xing Cao* (Herba Houttuyniae).
- For deficiency condition with thirst, add *Huang Qi* (Radix Astragali) and *Wu Wei Zi* (Fructus Schisandrae Chinensis).
- For thirst during recovery stage of chronic illness, add *Bai Shao* (Radix Paeoniae Alba) and *Chai Hu* (Radix Bupleuri).
- With profuse sputum, add *Bei Mu* (Bulbus Fritillariae) and *Ju Hong* (Exocarpium Citri Reticulatae).
- With lingering heat after an exterior condition, add *Sheng Ma Ge Gen Tang* (Cimicifuga and Kudzu Decoction).
- With lingering heat in women, add *Si Wu Tang* (Four-Substance Decoction).
- When there is Stomach yin deficiency and flaring of Stomach fire manifesting in ulcerations in the mouth and a red tongue body, add *Shi Hu* (Caulis Dendrobii) and *Tian Hua Fen* (Radix Trichosanthis); or *Yu Nu Jian* (Jade Woman Decoction).
- With excess hunger caused by Stomach fire, add *Tian Hua Fen* (Radix Trichosanthis) and *Zhi Mu* (Rhizoma Anemarrhenae).

CAUTIONS / CONTRAINDICATIONS

Zhu Ye Shi Gao Tang is contraindicated in acute conditions of excess heat without underlying deficiencies. It is also contraindicated in individuals with fever, a stifling sensation in the chest, dry heaves, and a yellow, greasy tongue coating caused by damp accumulation.

PHARMACOLOGICAL EFFECTS

Hypoglycemic: Administration of a water extract of *Zhu Ye Shi Gao Tang* at 500 mg/kg via intraperitoneal injection was associated with reduction of blood glucose level in mice. However, the hypoglycemic effect was significant only during the fasting state, and not during the normal state.[1]

CLINICAL STUDIES AND RESEARCH

1. **Fever**: Forty-seven cases of fever (37.5-39.5°C / 99.5-103.1°F) with duration of illness from one week to three months and resistant to antibiotic therapy were treated with *Zhu Ye Shi Gao Tang*. The treatment protocol was daily administration of the formula as a decoction in three to five equally-divided doses for 1-5 days. Out of 47 cases, the study reported temperature of less than 37°C / 98.6°F in 40 cases.[2]

2. **Toothache**: In one report, 96 patients with toothache were divided into two groups and treated with modified *Zhu Ye Shi Gao Tang*. Group A of 60 patients received treatment within 3 days from the onset of illness, while Group B of 36 patients received treatment 4-6 days after the onset. The herbs were cooked twice to yield 2 batches of decoction, which were subsequently mixed together and taken before each meal. The study reported complete recovery in all 60 patients in group A, and only 30 out of 36 patients in group B. Complete recovery was defined as resolution of the symptoms, complete reduction of redness, swelling and pain, and normal chewing and eating without pain.[3]

AUTHORS' COMMENTS

Zhu Ye Shi Gao Tang is derived from *Bai Hu Tang* (White Tiger Decoction), with the addition of *Ren Shen* (Radix et Rhizoma Ginseng) to tonify qi, *Mai Dong* (Radix Ophiopogonis) to nourish yin, *Ban Xia* (Rhizoma Pinelliae) to harmonize the Stomach, and the replacement of *Zhi Mu* (Rhizoma Anemarrhenae) with *Zhu Ye* (Herba Phyllostachys) to clear heat and relieve irritability.

Bai Hu Tang (White Tiger Decoction) and *Zhu Ye Shi Gao Tang* both clear heat and generate body fluids to treat heat in the *qi* (energy) level. Both formulas contain *Shi Gao* (Gypsum Fibrosum), *Geng Mi* (Semen Oryzae), and *Gan Cao* (Radix et Rhizoma Glycyrrhizae). The differences are as follows:

- *Bai Hu Tang* is stronger for clearing heat as it has *Zhi Mu* (Rhizoma Anemarrhenae) as the deputy herb to enhance the heat-clearing effect of *Shi Gao* (Gypsum Fibrosum). It is best for excess heat in the *qi* (energy) level manifesting in symptoms of high fever, irritability, thirst, profuse perspiration, and a surging, big and forceful pulse. It treats excess heat and generate body fluids at the same time.
- *Zhu Ye Shi Gao Tang* also contains *Ren Shen* (Radix et Rhizoma Ginseng), *Mai Dong* (Radix Ophiopogonis), *Zhu Ye* (Herba Phyllostachys), and *Ban Xia* (Rhizoma Pinelliae), which make the formula weaker in clearing heat but stronger in tonifying qi and nourishing yin. It is best for the post-febrile stage of lingering heat with qi and yin damage. Symptoms include heat sensation, perspiration, thirst with a desire to drink, shortness of breath, red, dry tongue, and a deficient, rapid pulse.

Bai Hu Jia Ren Shen Tang (White Tiger plus Ginseng Decoction) and *Zhu Ye Shi Gao Tang* both treat individuals with heat and deficiency. The differences are as follows:

- *Bai Hu Jia Ren Shen Tang* is for <u>excess heat</u> in the *yangming jing* (channel) syndrome or *yangming qi* (energy) level with qi and fluid deficiencies.

Zhú Yè Shí Gāo Tāng (Bamboo Leaves and Gypsum Decoction)

- *Zhu Ye Shi Gao Tang* is for <u>lingering heat</u> from *shang han* (cold damage), *wen bing* (warm disease) or summer-heat, with injuries to both qi and yin.[4]

According to Dr. Richard Tan, *Zhu Ye Shi Gao Tang* can be used with *Zi Yin Jiang Huo Tang* (Nourish Yin and Descend the Fire Decoction) and *Bai Shao* (Radix Paeoniae Alba) to effectively treat hot flashes and other related heat symptoms associated with menopause.

References

1. *Han Fang Yi Xue* (Kampo Medicine) 1981;1:14.
2. *Yun Nan Zhong Yi Za Zhi* (Yunan Journal of Chinese Medicine) 1985;4:20.
3. *Si Chuan Zhong Yi* (Sichuan Chinese Medicine) 1994;10:52.
4. Wang MZ, et al. *Zhong Yi Xue Wen Da Ti Ku* (Questions and Answers on Traditional Chinese Medicine: Herbal Formulas).

Chapter 5 – Heat-Clearing Formulas   *Section 2 – Ying (Nutritive) Level-Clearing and Blood-Cooling Formulas*

Section 2

清营凉血剂

— Ying (Nutritive) Level-Clearing and Blood-Cooling Formulas

Qīng Yíng Tāng (Clear the Nutritive Level Decoction)
清營湯
清营汤

Pinyin Name: *Qing Ying Tang*
Literal Name: Clear the Nutritive Level Decoction
Original Source: *Wen Bing Tiao Bian* (Systematic Differentiation of Warm Disease) by Wu Ju-Tong in 1798

COMPOSITION

Xi Jiao (Cornu Rhinoceri), *chong fu* (taken drenched)	9g [2g]
Di Huang (Radix Rehmanniae)	15g [15-20g]
Mai Dong (Radix Ophiopogonis)	9g
Xuan Shen (Radix Scrophulariae)	9g
Jin Yin Hua (Flos Lonicerae Japonicae)	9g
Lian Qiao (Fructus Forsythiae)	6g
Huang Lian (Rhizoma Coptidis)	4.5g
Zhu Ye (Herba Phyllostachys)	3g [5g]
Dan Shen (Radix et Rhizoma Salviae Miltiorrhizae)	6g [9g]

Note: *Xi Jiao* (Cornu Rhinoceri) is derived from an endangered animal, and is rarely used as a medicinal substance today. Its discussion here is included primarily for academic purposes, to reflect the historical use of this substance in its original formulation. Most herbal products today have removed it completely, or replaced it with substitutes with similar functions.

Zhu Ye (Herba Phyllostachys) and *Dan Zhu Ye* (Herba Lophatheri) have similar pinyin names and functions, and are sometimes used interchangeably. According to the source text, *Zhu Ye* (Herba Phyllostachys) is used in *Qing Ying Tang* to clear Heart heat. Today, because *Zhu Ye* (Herba Phyllostachys) is not readily available, it is generally replaced with *Dan Zhu Ye* (Herba Lophatheri). In comparison, *Zhu Ye* (Herba Phyllostachys) is more effective in clearing Heart and Stomach heat, while *Dan Zhu Ye* (Herba Lophatheri) is better in clearing heat and promoting normal urination.

DOSAGE / PREPARATION / ADMINISTRATION

The source text states to cook the ingredients, except *Xi Jiao* (Cornu Rhinoceri), in 8 cups of water and reduce it down to 3 cups. Take 1 cup of the decoction three times daily with powdered *Xi Jiao* (Cornu Rhinoceri). Today, 2g of *Xi Jiao* (Cornu Rhinoceri) is generally replaced with 30g of *Shui Niu Jiao* (Cornu Bubali).

CHINESE THERAPEUTIC ACTIONS

1. Clears heat from the *ying* (nutritive) level
2. Nourishes yin and invigorates blood circulation

CLINICAL MANIFESTATIONS

Heat in the *ying* (nutritive) level: fever that worsens at night, irritability, occasional delirious speech, with or without thirst, insomnia, eyes that are open or closed for a prolonged period of time, subcutaneous maculopapular eruption, a dark, red and dry tongue, and a rapid pulse.

Chinese Herbal Formulas and Applications

Qīng Yíng Tāng (Clear the Nutritive Level Decoction)

Qing Ying Tang (Clear the Nutritive Level Decoction)

Diagnosis	Signs and Symptoms	Treatment	Herbs
Heat in the *ying* (nutritive) level	• Fever that worsens at night: interior heat damaging yin and *ying* (nutrition) • Irritability, delirious speech and insomnia: heat attacking the *ying* level and disturbing *shen* (spirit) • Thirst: heat consuming body fluids • Subcutaneous maculopapular eruption: heat in the *ying* level • A dark, red and dry tongue: interior heat damaging yin • Rapid pulse: heat condition	• Clears heat from the *ying* level • Nourishes yin	• *Xi Jiao* (Cornu Rhinoceri) clears heat in the *ying* level. • *Di Huang* (Radix Rehmanniae), *Mai Dong* (Radix Ophiopogonis) and *Xuan Shen* (Radix Scrophulariae) clear deficiency heat and nourish yin. • *Jin Yin Hua* (Flos Lonicerae Japonicae), *Lian Qiao* (Fructus Forsythiae), and *Huang Lian* (Rhizoma Coptidis) clear heat and eliminate toxins. • *Zhu Ye* (Herba Phyllostachys) clears the Heart and calms the *shen* to relieve irritability. • *Dan Shen* (Radix et Rhizoma Salviae Miltiorrhizae) invigorates blood circulation.

CLINICAL APPLICATIONS

Septicemia, Harada's syndrome, uveitis, optic neuritis, psoriasis, dermatitis, and purpura.

EXPLANATION

Qing Ying Tang (Clear the Nutritive Level Decoction) is the representative formula for treating heat in the *ying* (nutritive) level, the third stage of the *Wei Qi Ying Xue Bian Zheng* (Defensive, Qi, Nutritive, Blood Differentiation). In the *ying* level, heat damages yin and causes *shen* (spirit) disturbance. Hence, irritability and delirium are two key clinical manifestations of this syndrome. When yin is damaged, it gives rise to fever that worsens at night because yin cannot contain yang. Patients may have thirst or no thirst, depending on whether the heat has consumed body fluids or not. Signs of emerging subcutaneous maculopapular eruption suggest that the heat is in the *ying* level but has not yet progressed to the *xue* (blood) level. If the heat were to progress to the *xue* level, it will congeal the blood and create blood stagnation, giving rise to large patches of clearly visible purplish-red maculae. A dark, red and dry tongue and a rapid pulse suggest heat in the *ying* level damaging yin.

To treat this syndrome, first clear heat from the *ying* (nutritive) level. Second, nourish the damaged yin. Finally, activate blood circulation to dispel heat stagnation and prevent the heat from progressing further into the *xue* (blood) level.

Xi Jiao (Cornu Rhinoceri), the chief herb, clears heat in the *ying* (nutritive) level and cools blood in the *xue* (blood) level. *Di Huang* (Radix Rehmanniae), *Mai Dong* (Radix Ophiopogonis) and *Xuan Shen* (Radix Scrophulariae) clear deficiency heat and nourish yin and body fluids. *Jin Yin Hua* (Flos Lonicerae Japonicae), *Lian Qiao* (Fructus Forsythiae), and *Huang Lian* (Rhizoma Coptidis) clear heat and eliminate toxins. They assist the formula to bring heat and toxins from deeper aspects of the body (*ying* and *xue* levels) to the more superficial aspects (*qi* (energy) level) so that these toxins may be effectively cleared and eliminated. *Zhu Ye* (Herba Phyllostachys) clears the Heart and calms the *shen* (spirit) to relieve irritability. *Dan Shen* (Radix et Rhizoma Salviae Miltiorrhizae) invigorates blood circulation to remove blood stasis, and also assists the rest of the herbs in clearing heat.

MODIFICATIONS

• When there is a big, forceful pulse in the *chi* position and a dry tongue, remove *Huang Lian* (Rhizoma Coptidis).
• If accompanied by severe incoherence and delirious speech, add *An Gong Niu Huang Wan* (Calm the Palace Pill with Cattle Gallstone).
• With heat in both the *qi* (energy) and *ying* (nutritive) levels, add *Shi Gao* (Gypsum Fibrosum) and *Zhi Mu* (Rhizoma Anemarrhenae).

CAUTIONS / CONTRAINDICATIONS

Qing Ying Tang is contraindicated in cases of damp accumulation marked by a white, greasy tongue coating. Damp conditions cannot be treated with moistening and nourishing herbs.

HEAT-CLEARING FORMULAS

5

331

Chapter 5 – Heat-Clearing Formulas   ***Section 2*** *– Ying (Nutritive) Level-Clearing and Blood-Cooling Formulas*

Qīng Yíng Tāng (Clear the Nutritive Level Decoction)

PHARMACOLOGICAL EFFECTS

1. **Antipyretic**: In rabbits with artificially-induced fever, intraperitoneal injection of *Qing Ying Tang* at 5 mL/kg was associated with marked reduction of body temperature.[1]
2. **Antibiotic**: This formula exhibited an *in vitro* inhibitory effect against *Staphylococcus aureus, Staphylococcus albus, alpha-hemolytic streptococcus, beta-hemolytic streptococcus, Salmonella typhi, Bacillus paratyphosus,* and *Bacillus proteus.*[2]

CLINICAL STUDIES AND RESEARCH

1. **Septicemia**: Ten patients with septicemia were treated with modified *Qing Ying Tang* with good results. The study reported complete reduction of temperature in all cases after an average of 12.6 days. All patients were followed up one year after the completion of the treatment with no recurrence.[3]
2. **Harada's syndrome**: Seven patients with Harada's syndrome of uveitis were treated with concurrent Western and herbal treatment. Herbal treatment included modification of *Qing Ying Tang*. Following 3 months of treatment, the study reported improvement in 6 out of 7 patients.[4]
3. **Psoriasis**: Eighty-seven patients with psoriasis were treated with both oral and topical application of herbs with marked improvement reported in 90.8% of the patients. The herbal formula used orally was modified *Qing Ying Tang*, and the topical herbal preparation contained *Bi Ma Zi* (Semen Ricini) 50g, *Ku Xing Ren* (Semen Armeniacae Amarum) 50g, *Qing Fen* (Calomelas) 50g, *Duan Shi Gao* (Gypsum Fibrosum Praeparatum) 50g, *Bai Fan* (Alumen) 50g, and *Bing Pian* (Borneolum Syntheticum) 20g. The herbs were ground into a fine powder and mixed with petroleum jelly to make a paste. Clinical improvements after oral and topical treatments

included relief of itching, flaking, and restoration of normal skin color.[5] Another study of 5 psoriasis patients reported good results using the following formula in decoction form and administered daily: *Di Huang* (Radix Rehmanniae) 30g, *Huang Lian* (Rhizoma Coptidis) 20g, *Jin Yin Hua* (Flos Lonicerae Japonicae) 20g, *Lian Qiao* (Fructus Forsythiae) 20g, *Da Huang* (Radix et Rhizoma Rhei) 5g, *Zhu Ye* (Herba Phyllostachys) 15g, *Dan Shen* (Radix et Rhizoma Salviae Miltiorrhizae) 15g, *Xuan Shen* (Radix Scrophulariae) 15g, *Mu Tong* (Caulis Akebiae) 15g, *Shui Niu Jiao* (Cornu Bubali) 15g, and *Gan Cao* (Radix et Rhizoma Glycyrrhizae) 15g.[6]

4. **Optic neuritis**: One study reported good results using integrated treatments for 5 patients with acute optic neuritis. The herbal formula contained *Shui Niu Jiao* (Cornu Bubali), *Mu Dan Pi* (Cortex Moutan), *Dan Shen* (Radix et Rhizoma Salviae Miltiorrhizae), *Xuan Shen* (Radix Scrophulariae), *Huang Lian* (Rhizoma Coptidis), *Jin Yin Hua* (Flos Lonicerae Japonicae), *Lian Qiao* (Fructus Forsythiae), *Zhi Mu* (Rhizoma Anemarrhenae), *Bai Shao* (Radix Paeoniae Alba), *Jue Ming Zi* (Semen Cassiae), *Mai Dong* (Radix Ophiopogonis), *Dan Zhu Ye* (Herba Lophatheri), and others as needed. Dexamethasone 5mg was also given.[7]

References

1. *Cheng Du Zhong Yi Xue Yuan Xue Bao* (Journal of Chengdu University of Traditional Chinese Medicine) 1995;4:38.
2. *Zhong Yi Za Zhi* (Journal of Chinese Medicine) 1981;5:349.
3. *Zhong Yi Za Zhi* (Journal of Chinese Medicine) 1984;2:42.
4. *Tian Jin Zhong Yi* (Tianjin Chinese Medicine) 1993;3:38.
5. *Si Chuan Zhong Yi* (Sichuan Chinese Medicine) 1992;3:36.
6. *Zhong Yi Yao Xue Bao* (Report of Chinese Medicine and Herbology) 1996;6:42.
7. *Zhong Yi Ming Fang Lin Chuang Xin Yong* (Contemporary Clinical Applications of Classic Chinese Formulas) 2001;661.

Chinese Herbal Formulas and Applications

Xī Jiǎo Dì Huáng Tāng (Rhinoceros Horn and Rehmannia Decoction)

犀角地黄湯
犀角地黄汤

Pinyin Name: *Xi Jiao Di Huang Tang*
Literal Name: Rhinoceros Horn and Rehmannia Decoction
Original Source: *Bei Ji Qian Jin Yao Fang* (Thousands of Golden Prescriptions for Emergencies)

COMPOSITION

Xi Jiao (Cornu Rhinoceri)	3g [1.5-3g]
Di Huang (Radix Rehmanniae)	24g [30g]
Chi Shao (Radix Paeoniae Rubra)	9g [12g]
Mu Dan Pi (Cortex Moutan)	6g [9g]

Note: *Xi Jiao* (Cornu Rhinoceri) is derived from an endangered animal, and is rarely used as a medicinal substance today. Its discussion here is included primarily for academic purposes, to reflect the historical use of this substance in its original formulation. Most herbal products today have removed it completely, or replaced it with substitutes with similar functions.

The source text lists *Shao Yao* (Radix Paeoniae) as one of the ingredients, without specifying whether it is *Bai Shao* (Radix Paeoniae Alba) or *Chi Shao* (Radix Paeoniae Rubra). Today, most practitioners prefer to use *Chi Shao* (Radix Paeoniae Rubra) for its functions to clear heat and cool the blood.

DOSAGE / PREPARATION / ADMINISTRATION

The source text instructs to grind the ingredients coarsely. Cook the powdered herbs with 9 cups [1,800 mL] of water and reduce it to 3 cups [600 mL]. Take 1 cup [200 mL] of the decoction three times daily. Today, it is normally prepared as a decoction with the doses suggested in brackets. Moreover, the 1.5-3g of *Xi Jiao* (Cornu Rhinoceri) is generally replaced by 30g of *Shui Niu Jiao* (Cornu Bubali).

CHINESE THERAPEUTIC ACTIONS

1. Clears heat and eliminates toxins
2. Cools the blood and disperses blood stasis

CLINICAL MANIFESTATIONS

1. Heat in the *xue* (blood) level forcing blood out of the vessels: hematemesis, epistaxis, hematuria, hematochezia, etc.
2. Blood stasis: desire to rinse the mouth with water without swallowing it, forgetfulness, mania, irritability, chest pain, a feeling of abdominal fullness, and black, tarry stools.
3. Heat disturbing the Heart and *ying* (nutritive) level: mania, delirium, purplish-red or black maculae on the skin, and a red, prickly tongue.

CLINICAL APPLICATIONS

Hemorrhagic fever, encephalitis, meningitis, purulent meningitis, thrombocytopenic purpura, allergic purpura, leukocytic leukemia, septicemia, hepatitis, esophageal hemorrhage, upper gastrointestinal bleeding, and epistaxis.

EXPLANATION

Xi Jiao Di Huang Tang (Rhinoceros Horn and Rehmannia Decoction) clears interior heat, cools the blood, and disperses blood stasis to treat heat in the *xue* (blood) level. Heat in the blood may force the blood to move recklessly, often out of the vessels. When the yang channels are injured, bleeding occurs outside of the vessels and manifests upward and outward as hematemesis or epistaxis. When the yin channels are injured, blood moves downward, manifesting as hematuria and hematochezia. When the superficial channels are injured, there will be purpura or maculae on the skin.

The patient may desire to rinse their mouth with water because of heat, but will prefer not to swallow the water because heat has not damaged body fluids. If blood stasis invades the Heart, then chest pain, irritability, mania, or delirium may result. In addition, abdominal fullness and excretion of black, tarry stools may occur if blood stasis accumulates in the abdomen or the Intestines. If the tissues are severely attacked by heat, dark purplish maculae may appear on the skin.

Xi Jiao (Cornu Rhinoceri) enters directly into the *xue* (blood) level and clears heat in the Heart, cools the blood, and eliminates toxins. Combined, *Xi Jiao* (Cornu Rhinoceri) and *Di Huang* (Radix Rehmanniae) cool the blood and stop bleeding, as well as nourish yin and clear heat. *Chi Shao* (Radix Paeoniae Rubra) and *Mu Dan Pi* (Cortex Moutan) clear heat, cool the blood, and disperse blood stasis. This formula, therefore, cools the blood without causing blood stagnation.

HEAT-CLEARING FORMULAS

5

333

Chapter 5 – Heat-Clearing Formulas   *Section 2 – Ying (Nutritive) Level-Clearing and Blood-Cooling Formulas*

Xī Jiǎo Dì Huáng Tāng (Rhinoceros Horn and Rehmannia Decoction)

Xi Jiao Di Huang Tang (Rhinoceros Horn and Rehmannia Decoction)

Diagnosis	Signs and Symptoms	Treatment	Herbs
Heat in the *xue* (blood) level	• Bleeding: heat in the *xue* level forcing blood outward • Mania, delirium and irritability: heat disturbing the Heart and *shen* (spirit) • Chest pain and a feeling of abdominal fullness: blood stasis • Red, prickly tongue: heat damaging yin and blood	• Clears heat and eliminates toxins • Cools the blood and disperses blood stasis	• *Xi Jiao* (Cornu Rhinoceri) clears heat, cools the blood, and eliminates toxins from the *ying* (nutritive) and *xue* (blood) levels. • *Di Huang* (Radix Rehmanniae) cools the blood, stops bleeding, nourishes yin, and clears heat. • *Chi Shao* (Radix Paeoniae Rubra) and *Mu Dan Pi* (Cortex Moutan) cool the blood and disperse blood stasis.

MODIFICATIONS

- With more epistaxis or vomiting of blood, add *Bai Mao Gen* (Rhizoma Imperatae) and *Ce Bai Ye* (Cacumen Platycladi).
- With more hematochezia, add *Huai Hua* (Flos Sophorae) and *Di Yu* (Radix Sanguisorbae).
- With more hematuria, add *Bai Mao Gen* (Rhizoma Imperatae) and *Xiao Ji* (Herba Cirsii).
- When there is pent-up emotion or rage, add *Chai Hu* (Radix Bupleuri), *Huang Qin* (Radix Scutellariae), and *Zhi Zi* (Fructus Gardeniae).
- With delirium and mania with heat and blood stasis, add *Da Huang* (Radix et Rhizoma Rhei) and *Huang Qin* (Radix Scutellariae); or *Dang Gui Long Hui Wan* (Tangkuei, Gentiana, and Aloe Pill).

CAUTIONS / CONTRAINDICATIONS

Xi Jiao Di Huang Tang should be used to treat only bleeding caused by heat in the *xue* (blood) level leading to reckless movement of blood and bleeding from various parts of the body. It should <u>not</u> be used to treat bleeding caused by other reasons, such as constitutional deficiencies or external injuries.

PHARMACOLOGICAL EFFECTS

Antipyretic: In rabbits with artificially-induced fever, oral ingestion of *Xi Jiao Di Huang Tang* was effective in reducing the body temperature. The antipyretic effect has a slow onset of action (after 4 hours) but prolonged duration (up to 6 hours). The researchers characterized the antipyretic effect of *Xi Jiao Di Huang Tang* to be comparable to 0.2 mg/kg of aspirin.[1]

CLINICAL STUDIES AND RESEARCH

1. **Upper gastrointestinal bleeding**: In one report, 39 patients with upper gastrointestinal bleeding diagnosed with Stomach heat were treated with either *Xie Xin Tang* (Drain the Epigastrium Decoction) or modified *Xi Jiao Di Huang Tang* with 100% effectiveness. The report stated that most patients stopped bleeding within 24 hours after taking the herbs.[2]

2. **Epistaxis**: Sixty-one patients with chronic epistaxis were treated with *Xi Jiao Di Huang Tang* with good results. The bleeding stopped in 28 patients after treatment, with no recurrence within 6 months of follow-up. The bleeding was reduced significantly in 25 patients, with much less recurrence and severity. Slight improvement was reported in 7 other cases, and no benefit in 1 case. The overall rate of effectiveness was 98.49%.[3]

3. **Thrombocytopenic purpura**: In one clinical study, 11 patients with primary thrombocytopenic purpura were treated with *Xi Jiao Di Huang Tang* with complete recovery in 6 patients, marked effect in 4 patients, and no effect (and eventual fatality) in 1 patient. The study reported that after administration of the herbal treatment, there was a significant reduction of bleeding time and gradual increase in platelets. The effect of the herbal formula was attributed to an initial change in permeability of the blood vessels, followed by stimulation and increased production of platelets.[4] Other studies also confirmed that *Xi Jiao Di Huang Tang* in the original or slightly modified form had marked effect for treatment of thrombocytopenic purpura.[5,6]

4. **Hepatitis**: In one report, 13 patients with hepatitis (characterized by Gallbladder stagnation) were treated with modified *Xi Jiao Di Huang Tang* for one month with improvement reported in 12 patients. Most patients showed a decrease in skin itching and reduction of jaundice.[7]

HERB-DRUG INTERACTION

Drug-induced allergic dermatitis: Administration of modified *Xi Jiao Di Huang Tang* was associated with good results in treating 38 patients with drug-induced allergic

334

Xī Jiǎo Dì Huáng Tāng (Rhinoceros Horn and Rehmannia Decoction)

dermatitis. The treatment protocol was to administer the herbs in decoction form in two equally-divided doses daily in the morning and at night. The herbal formula used *Shui Niu Jiao* (Cornu Bubali) in place of *Xi Jiao* (Cornu Rhinoceri). Modifications were made by adding *Da Huang* (Radix et Rhizoma Rhei) for excess heat in the interior; and *Pu Gong Ying* (Herba Taraxaci), *Jin Yin Hua* (Flos Lonicerae Japonicae) and a larger dose of *Shui Niu Jiao* (Cornu Bubali) for toxins affecting the *ying* (nutritive) and *xue* (blood) levels. Of 38 cases, the study reported complete recovery in 33 cases and improvement in 5 cases.[8]

RELATED FORMULAS

Shén Xī Dān (Magical Rhinoceros Special Pill)

神犀丹

Pinyin Name: Shen Xi Dan
Literal Name: Magical Rhinoceros Special Pill
Original Source: *Wen Re Jing Wei* (Warp and Woof of Warm-Febrile Diseases) by Wang Meng-Ying in 1852

Xi Jiao (Cornu Rhinoceri)	180g
Shi Chang Pu (Rhizoma Acori Tatarinowii)	180g
Huang Qin (Radix Scutellariae)	180g
Di Huang (Radix Rehmanniae)	480g
Jin Yin Hua (Flos Lonicerae Japonicae)	480g
Jin Zhi (Excrementum Hominis)	300g
Lian Qiao (Fructus Forsythiae)	300g
Ban Lan Gen (Radix Isatidis)	270g
Dan Dou Chi (Semen Sojae Praeparatum)	240g
Xuan Shen (Radix Scrophulariae)	210g
Tian Hua Fen (Radix Trichosanthis)	120g
Zi Cao (Radix Arnebiae)	120g

Note: *Xi Jiao* (Cornu Rhinoceri) is derived from an endangered animal, and is rarely used as a medicinal substance today. Its discussion here is included primarily for academic purposes, to reflect the historical use of this substance in its original formulation. Most herbal products today have removed it completely, or replaced it with substitutes with similar functions.

The source text instructs to mix the liquids from *Xi Jiao* (Cornu Rhinoceri) and *Di Huang* (Radix Rehmanniae) with *Jin Zhi* (Excrementum Hominis). Then, add the powder from the rest of the ingredients to this mixture and form into pills. Take 1 pill (3g each) twice daily with boiled water that has been cooled to room temperature. Reduce the dose for children accordingly. Today, *Xi Jiao* (Cornu Rhinoceri) is generally replaced with *Shui Niu Jiao* (Cornu Bubali) [1,800g], and *Jin Zhi* (Excrementum Hominis) is removed from the formula.

Shen Xi Dan (Magical Rhinoceros Special Pill) clears heat, opens the sensory orifices, cools the blood, and eliminates toxins. It treats febrile disorders or epidemic summer-heat, in which the pathogens (heat and toxins) invade the *ying* (nutritive) and *xue* (blood) levels and cause depletion of yin and body fluids. Clinical presentations include high fever, delirium, eruptions of maculae on the skin, sores in the mouth and throat, red eyes, irritability, restlessness, and a scarlet tongue body.

Qīng Rè Liáng Xuè Tāng
(Clear Heat and Cool the Blood Decoction)

清熱涼血湯
清热凉血汤

Pinyin Name: Qing Re Liang Xue Tang
Literal Name: Clear Heat and Cool the Blood Decoction
Original Source: *Guang An Men Yi Yuan* (Guang An Men Hospital) in 1990

Di Huang (Radix Rehmanniae)
Xuan Shen (Radix Scrophulariae)
Chi Shao (Radix Paeoniae Rubra)
Zhi Mu (Rhizoma Anemarrhenae)
Mu Dan Pi (Cortex Moutan)
Tao Ren (Semen Persicae)
Hong Hua (Flos Carthami)
Ye Ju Hua (Flos Chrysanthemi Indici)
Jin Yin Hua (Flos Lonicerae Japonicae)
Lian Qiao (Fructus Forsythiae)
Zi Hua Di Ding (Herba Violae)
Ban Zhi Lian (Herba Scutellariae Barbatae)
Mo Han Lian (Herba Ecliptae)
Ling Zhi (Ganoderma)
Huang Bo (Cortex Phellodendri Chinensis)

Qing Re Liang Xue Tang (Clear Heat and Cool the Blood Decoction) is a contemporary formula developed specifically to treat systemic lupus erythematosus (SLE). The therapeutic effects of this formula are to clear heat, eliminate toxins, cool the blood and dispel blood stasis.

Because the clinical manifestations of lupus often vary from patient to patient, adjust the doses accordingly. Make modifications as needed, depending on the signs and symptoms as follows: add *Sang Zhi* (Ramulus Mori) and *Gua Lou Pi* (Pericarpium Trichosanthis) for coughing with phlegm; add *Sang Zhi* (Ramulus Mori) and *Qin Jiao* (Radix Gentianae Macrophyllae) for joint pain; add *Da Huang* (Radix et Rhizoma Rhei) for constipation; add *Bai Mao Gen* (Rhizoma Imperatae) for dysuria; add *Huang Bo* (Cortex Phellodendri Chinensis) and *Bai Zhi* (Radix

Xī Jiǎo Dì Huáng Tāng (Rhinoceros Horn and Rehmannia Decoction)

Angelicae Dahuricae) for leukorrhea; and add *Shi Gao* (Gypsum Fibrosum) for high fever.

Fǔ Zhèng Yì Yán Tāng
(Support the Upright and Suppress Cancer Decoction)

扶正抑癌湯
扶正抑癌汤

Pinyin Name: *Fu Zheng Yi Yan Tang*
Literal Name: Support the Upright and Suppress Cancer Decoction
Original Source: *Guang An Men Yi Yuan* (Guang An Men Hospital) in 1990

Huang Qi (Radix Astragali)
Dong Chong Xia Cao (Cordyceps)
Xi Yang Shen (Radix Panacis Quinquefolii)
E Zhu (Rhizoma Curcumae)
Bai Zhu (Rhizoma Atractylodis Macrocephalae)
Fu Ling (Poria)
Yi Yi Ren (Semen Coicis)
Ji Xue Teng (Caulis Spatholobi)
Zao Xiu (Rhizoma Paridis)
Ban Zhi Lian (Herba Scutellariae Barbatae)
Chuan Xin Lian (Herba Andrographis)
Huang Jing (Rhizoma Polygonati)

Fu Zheng Yi Yan Tang (Support the Upright and Suppress Cancer Decoction) treats excess conditions in individuals with underlying deficiencies. The excess, in the form of cancer, is often diagnosed as accumulation of phlegm, heat and toxins. The deficiencies represent the overall weakness, especially of *zheng* (upright) *qi*. Today, this formula is generally used to treat patients with cancer who are too weak to tolerate treatments such as chemotherapy and radiation.

AUTHORS' COMMENTS

Qing Ying Tang (Clear the Nutritive Level Decoction) and *Xi Jiao Di Huang Tang* both clear heat in the *ying* (nutritive) and *xue* (blood) levels and stop bleeding characterized by reckless movement of blood. Both formulas stop bleeding and contain blood-moving herbs to prevent the cold herbs from congealing the blood and creating further stagnation while clearing heat.

- *Qing Ying Tang* clears heat in the *ying* (nutritive) level and includes *Dan Shen* (Radix et Rhizoma Salviae Miltiorrhizae) to move blood and prevent the cold herbs from creating stagnation. It also helps to reduce maculopapular eruption that may be present on the skin, marked by bleeding that is just beginning. The condition in this case is not as severe as that seen in *Xi Jiao Di Huang Tang*.

- *Xi Jiao Di Huang Tang* clears heat in the *xue* (blood) level. It contains *Chi Shao* (Radix Paeoniae Rubra) and *Mu Dan Pi* (Cortex Moutan) to move blood and to prevent the cold herbs from creating stagnation. They also assist the other heat-clearing herbs to cool the blood. Bleeding is more prominent and severe in this condition.

Qing Ying Tang (Clear the Nutritive Level Decoction) and *Xi Jiao Di Huang Tang* both contain *Xi Jiao* (Cornu Rhinoceri) and *Di Huang* (Radix Rehmanniae) as chief herbs. The differences between these two formulas are as follows:

- *Qing Ying Tang* focuses on bringing the heat out from the *ying* (nutritive) level and clearing it through the *qi* (energy) level. It is suitable for initial stages of heat attacking the *ying* level, with symptoms of heat sensations at night, incoherent speech, and irritability.

- *Xi Jiao Di Huang Tang* treats more severe conditions of heat attacking the *ying* and *xue* levels and forcing blood out of the vessels, manifesting in various types of bleeding.

References

1. *Zhong Yao Tong Bao* (Journal of Chinese Herbology) 1986;11(1):51.
2. *Zhong Yi Za Zhi* (Journal of Chinese Medicine) 1980;21(7):36.
3. *Shan Xi Zhong Yi* (Shanxi Chinese Medicine) 1989;10(4):163.
4. *Zhong Yi Za Zhi* (Journal of Chinese Medicine) 1963;11:12.
5. *Zhong Yi Za Zhi* (Journal of Chinese Medicine) 1958;7:465.
6. *Zhong Yi Za Zhi* (Journal of Chinese Medicine) 1960;7:22.
7. *Zhong Yi Za Zhi* (Journal of Chinese Medicine) 1983;24(6):30.
8. *Hu Nan Zhong Yi Za Zhi* (Hunan Journal of Chinese Medicine) 1998;1:39.

Chinese Herbal Formulas and Applications

Section 3

气血两清剂

— Qi (Energy) and Xue (Blood) Levels-Clearing Formulas

Qīng Wēn Bài Dú Yǐn
(Clear Epidemics and Overcome Pathogenic Influences Decoction)

清瘟败毒飲
清瘟败毒饮

Pinyin Name: Qing Wen Bai Du Yin
Literal Name: Clear Epidemics and Overcome Pathogenic Influences Decoction
Original Source: *Yi Zhen Yi De* (Achievements Regarding Epidemic Rashes) by Yu Shi-Yu in 1794

COMPOSITION

Shi Gao (Gypsum Fibrosum)	24-36g; 60-120g; 180-240g
Zhi Mu (Rhizoma Anemarrhenae)	
Huang Lian (Rhizoma Coptidis)	3-4.5g; 6-12g;12-18g
Huang Qin (Radix Scutellariae)	
Zhi Zi (Fructus Gardeniae)	
Xi Jiao (Cornu Rhinoceri)	6-12g; 9-15g; 18-24g
Di Huang (Radix Rehmanniae)	6-12g; 9-15g; 18-30g
Chi Shao (Radix Paeoniae Rubra)	
Mu Dan Pi (Cortex Moutan)	
Lian Qiao (Fructus Forsythiae)	
Xuan Shen (Radix Scrophulariae)	
Zhu Ye (Herba Phyllostachys), fresh	
Jie Geng (Radix Platycodonis)	
Gan Cao (Radix et Rhizoma Glycyrrhizae)	

Note: *Xi Jiao* (Cornu Rhinoceri) is derived from an endangered animal, and is rarely used as a medicinal substance today. Its discussion here is included primarily for academic purposes, to reflect the historical use of this substance in its original formulation. Most herbal products today have removed it completely, or replaced it with substitutes with similar functions.

DOSAGE / PREPARATION / ADMINISTRATION

The source text states to first cook *Shi Gao* (Gypsum Fibrosum), bring it to a boil multiple times (more than ten), and then add the remaining ingredients. The three sets of doses correspond to small, medium and large doses for the four herbs listed, to treat mild, moderate and severe conditions. Doses for the other ten herbs are not available

in the original source. Today, *Xi Jiao* (Cornu Rhinoceri) is generally replaced with *Shui Niu Jiao* (Cornu Bubali) with the following doses: 60-120g; 90-150g; and 180-240g.

CHINESE THERAPEUTIC ACTIONS

1. Clears heat and eliminates toxins
2. Purges fire and cools the blood

CLINICAL MANIFESTATIONS

Wen yi (warm epidemics) characterized by excess heat and toxins in the *qi* (energy) and *xue* (blood) levels: high fever, extreme thirst, splitting headaches, dry heaves, mania, delirium, blurred vision, maculae, hematemesis, epistaxis, extreme coldness or convulsions of the four extremities, scorched lips, a dark red tongue body with

337

Chapter 5 – Heat-Clearing Formulas　　　　*Section 3 – Qi (Energy) and Xue (Blood) Levels-Clearing Formulas*

Qīng Wēn Bài Dú Yǐn
(Clear Epidemics and Overcome Pathogenic Influences Decoction)

dry or prickly tongue coating. The pulse may be any of the following: deep and rapid; deep, fine and rapid; or superficial, big and rapid.

CLINICAL APPLICATIONS

Epidemic hemorrhagic fever, encephalitis B, meningitis, pyogenic infection, leptospirosis, coxarthritis, viral pneumonia, acute icteric jaundice, nephritis, Behcet's syndrome, and dermatological disorders.

EXPLANATION

Wen yi (warm epidemics) are infectious or contagious diseases characterized by heat. In this case, excess heat and toxins affect the *qi* (energy) level and consume body fluids to cause high fever and extreme thirst. The heat and toxins may travel to the head and cause splitting headaches and blurred vision. If they travel to the Heart, mania and delirium occur. Eruptions of maculae on the skin, hematemesis, and epistaxis are all signs of heat in the *xue* (blood) level forcing the blood out of the vessels. In extreme cases when too much blood is lost, extreme coldness or convulsions of the four extremities may occur. Scorched lips, a dark red tongue body with dry or prickly coating are due to the presence of excess heat and toxins inside the body damaging body fluids. The pulse may be superficial, big and rapid, or deep and rapid, depending on whether the *qi* or *xue* level is more adversely affected.

Qing Wen Bai Du Yin (Clear Epidemics and Overcome Pathogenic Influences Decoction) contains *Shi Gao* (Gypsum Fibrosum) and *Zhi Mu* (Rhizoma Anemarrhenae) to clear excess heat in the *qi* (energy) level and protect against further loss of body fluids. *Huang Lian* (Rhizoma Coptidis), *Huang Qin* (Radix Scutellariae), and *Zhi Zi* (Fructus Gardeniae) clear heat and eliminate toxins in all three *jiaos*. *Xi Jiao* (Cornu Rhinoceri), *Di Huang* (Radix Rehmanniae), *Chi Shao* (Radix Paeoniae Rubra), and *Mu Dan Pi* (Cortex Moutan) clear heat from the *xue* (blood) level and disperse blood stagnation, which may form after the blood is forced out of the vessels. *Lian Qiao* (Fructus Forsythiae) and *Xuan Shen* (Radix Scrophulariae) clear heat and eliminate toxins. *Zhu Ye* (Herba Phyllostachys) clears the Heart and calms the *shen* (spirit). *Jie Geng* (Radix Platycodonis) directs the formula to the upper *jiao* and disperses heat from the body. Finally, *Gan Cao* (Radix et Rhizoma Glycyrrhizae) clears heat and harmonizes the formula.

MODIFICATIONS

- If there is Stomach qi reversal, add *Zhe Shi* (Haematitum) and *Zhu Ru* (Caulis Bambusae in Taenia).
- With constipation, add *Da Huang* (Radix et Rhizoma Rhei) and *Mang Xiao* (Natrii Sulfas).
- With dark or purplish maculae, add *Da Qing Ye* (Folium Isatidis) and *Zi Cao* (Radix Arnebiae).

Qing Wen Bai Du Yin (Clear Epidemics and Overcome Pathogenic Influences Decoction)

Diagnosis	Signs and Symptoms	Treatment	Herbs
Wen yi (warm epidemics) characterized by excess heat and toxins in the *qi* (energy) and *xue* (blood) levels	• High fever and extreme thirst: heat and toxins in the *qi* level consuming body fluids • Headache and blurred vision: heat and toxins traveling to the head • Mania and delirium: heat and toxins traveling to the Heart • Bleeding and eruptions of maculae on the skin: heat forcing the blood out of the vessels • Scorched lips, and a dark red tongue body with a dry or prickly tongue coating: excess heat and toxins in the interior	• Clears heat and eliminates toxins • Purges fire and cools the blood	• *Shi Gao* (Gypsum Fibrosum) and *Zhi Mu* (Rhizoma Anemarrhenae) clear excess heat from the *qi* level. • *Huang Lian* (Rhizoma Coptidis), *Huang Qin* (Radix Scutellariae), and *Zhi Zi* (Fructus Gardeniae) clear heat and eliminate toxins in all three *jiaos*. • *Xi Jiao* (Cornu Rhinoceri), *Di Huang* (Radix Rehmanniae), *Chi Shao* (Radix Paeoniae Rubra), and *Mu Dan Pi* (Cortex Moutan) clear heat from the *xue* level and disperse blood stagnation. • *Lian Qiao* (Fructus Forsythiae) and *Xuan Shen* (Radix Scrophulariae) clear heat and eliminate toxins. • *Zhu Ye* (Herba Phyllostachys) clears the Heart and calms the *shen* (spirit). • *Jie Geng* (Radix Platycodonis) directs the formula to the upper *jiao* and disperses heat out of the body. • *Gan Cao* (Radix et Rhizoma Glycyrrhizae) clears heat and harmonizes the herbs.

Qīng Wēn Bài Dú Yǐn
(Clear Epidemics and Overcome Pathogenic Influences Decoction)

- If accompanied by epistaxis, remove *Jie Geng* (Radix Platycodonis), and add *Bai Mao Gen* (Rhizoma Imperatae) and *Ce Bai Ye* (Cacumen Platycladi).
- When there are spasms, cramps and convulsions, add *Gou Teng* (Ramulus Uncariae cum Uncis) and *Di Long* (Pheretima).
- With swelling and pain of the throat, add *Shan Dou Gen* (Radix et Rhizoma Sophorae Tonkinensis) and *Niu Bang Zi* (Fructus Arctii).

CAUTIONS / CONTRAINDICATIONS

- *Qing Wen Bai Du Yin* contains many bitter and cold herbs, and should not be used if the condition is not characterized by the presence of heat, fire and toxins.
- This formula should be used with caution in cases of yang deficiency, or in individuals with deficiency and cold of the Spleen and Stomach.

CLINICAL STUDIES AND RESEARCH

1. **Epidemic hemorrhagic fever**: *Qing Wen Bai Du Yin* successfully treated 150 patients with epidemic hemorrhagic fever. The average time required to reduce fever to normal body temperature was 1.58 days. The mortality rate was less than 1%.[1]
2. **Pyogenic infection**: In one study, 113 patients with drug-resistent systemic pyogenic infection were treated with satisfactory results using modified *Qing Wen Bai Du Yin*. The study reported fatality in 20 of 113 patients.[2]
3. **Leptospirosis**: Use of modified *Qing Wen Bai Du Yin* was associated with 96% effectiveness in treating leptospirosis. The herbal formula contained *Shui Niu Jiao* (Cornu Bubali) 30g, *Shi Gao* (Gypsum Fibrosum) 30g, *Di Huang* (Radix Rehmanniae) 30g, *Tu Fu Ling* (Rhizoma Smilacis Glabrae) 30g, *Yi Yi Ren* (Semen Coicis) 30g, *Huang Lian* (Rhizoma Coptidis) 6g, *Zhi Mu* (Rhizoma Anemarrhenae) 10g, *Huang Qin* (Radix Scutellariae) 10g, *Zhi Zi* (Fructus Gardeniae) 10g, *Mu Dan Pi* (Cortex Moutan) 10g, and *Chi Shao* (Radix Paeoniae Rubra) 10g. One pack of herbs decocted in water was administered in two equally-divided doses. In severe cases, patients were given up to 2-3 packs of herbs per day. The study reported recovery in 65 of 68 patients using herbs, while the other three required additional drug treatment.[3]
4. **Coxarthritis**: One study reported effectiveness using modified *Qing Wen Bai Du Yin* to treat 13 patients with pyogenic coxarthritis. The patients were treated with up to 10 packs of herbs.[4]
5. **Behcet's syndrome**: Administration of modified *Qing Wen Bai Du Yin* was found to be effective in treating 11 patients with Behcet's syndrome. The study reported recovery in 6 cases after 15-20 packs of herbs, 3 cases after 25 packs, and 2 cases after 30-50 packs.[5]

RELATED FORMULA

Huà Bān Tāng (Transform Blotches Decoction)

化斑湯
化斑汤

Pinyin Name: Hua Ban Tang
Literal Name: Transform Blotches Decoction
Original Source: *Wen Bing Tiao Bian* (Systematic Differentiation of Warm Disease) by Wu Ju-Tong in 1798

Shi Gao (Gypsum Fibrosum)	30g
Zhi Mu (Rhizoma Anemarrhenae)	12g
Gan Cao (Radix et Rhizoma Glycyrrhizae)	9g
Xuan Shen (Radix Scrophulariae)	9g
Xi Jiao (Cornu Rhinoceri), *chong fu* (taken drenched)	6g [2-6g]
Geng Mi (Semen Oryzae)	1 scoop [9g]

Note: *Xi Jiao* (Cornu Rhinoceri) is derived from an endangered animal, and is rarely used as a medicinal substance today. Its discussion here is included primarily for academic purposes, to reflect the historical use of this substance in its original formulation. Most herbal products today have removed it completely, or replaced it with substitutes with similar functions.

The source text states to cook the ingredients in 8 cups of water and reduce it to 3 cups. Take the decoction [1 cup] three times daily. The herb residues are to be cooked again with one large bowl of water, and the resultant decoction should be taken at night. Today, *Xi Jiao* (Cornu Rhinoceri) is generally replaced with *Shui Niu Jiao* (Cornu Bubali) [60g]. Also, the decoction may be prepared using the doses suggested in brackets.

Hua Ban Tang (Transform Blotches Decoction) clears heat and cools the blood to treat conditions characterized by heat attacking the *qi* (energy) and *xue* (blood) levels. Clinical presentations include fever; warm body sensations, especially at night; presence of red blotches or maculae on the skin; and a rapid pulse.

Qing Wen Bai Du Yin and *Hua Ban Tang* (Transform Blotches Decoction) both clear heat and cool the blood. Their differences are as follows:

- *Qing Wen Bai Du Yin* contains large doses of herbs to treat severe cases of heat and toxins attacking the *qi* (energy) and *xue* (blood) levels.

Chapter 5 – Heat-Clearing Formulas   Section 3 – Qi (Energy) and Xue (Blood) Levels-Clearing Formulas

Qīng Wēn Bài Dú Yĭn
(Clear Epidemics and Overcome Pathogenic Influences Decoction)

• *Hua Ban Tang* uses moderate doses of herbs to treat mild to moderate cases of heat attacking the *qi* and *xue* levels.

AUTHORS' COMMENTS

Qing Wen Bai Du Yin has been used historically to treat *wen yi* (warm epidemics), conditions that correlate closely to biomedical disorders such as encephalitis B, meningitis, epidemic hemorrhagic fever, pyogenic infection, and other contagious diseases. Because these diseases vary drastically in severity, the ingredients of this formula differ in dose (up to 10 folds) dramatically.

The formulation of *Qing Wen Bai Du Yin* follows the principles of three formulas:

• *Bai Hu Tang* (White Tiger Decoction) to clear heat from the *qi* (energy) level.
• *Xi Jiao Di Huang Tang* (Rhinoceros Horn and Rehmannia Decoction) to clear heat from the *xue* (blood) level.
• *Huang Lian Jie Du Tang* (Coptis Decoction to Relieve Toxicity) to clear heat and eliminate toxins.

References

1. *Yi Xue Yan Jiu Tong Xun* (Report of Medical Studies) 1986;(5):3.
2. *Shan Xi Yi Kan* (Shanxi Journal of Medicine) 1983;4(4):13.
3. *Guang Xi Zhong Yi Yao* (Guangxi Chinese Medicine and Herbology) 1987;3:6.
4. *Shan Xi Zhong Yi* (Shanxi Chinese Medicine) 1988;4:152.
5. *He Nan Zhong Yi* (Henan Chinese Medicine) 1988;6:20.

340

Chinese Herbal Formulas and Applications

Section 4

清热解毒剂

— Heat-Clearing and Toxin-Eliminating Formulas

Huáng Lián Jiě Dú Tāng (Coptis Decoction to Relieve Toxicity)

黄連解毒湯
黄连解毒汤

Pinyin Name: *Huang Lian Jie Du Tang*
Literal Name: Coptis Decoction to Relieve Toxicity
Alternate Names: *Huang Lien Chieh Tu Tang*, Coptis and Scute Detoxifying Decoction, Coptis and Scute Combination
Original Source: *Wai Tai Mi Yao* (Arcane Essentials from the Imperial Library) by Wang Tao in 752 A.D.

COMPOSITION

Huang Qin (Radix Scutellariae)	6g
Huang Lian (Rhizoma Coptidis)	9g
Huang Bo (Cortex Phellodendri Chinensis)	6g
Zhi Zi (Fructus Gardeniae), *bo* (opened)	14 pieces [9g]

DOSAGE / PREPARATION / ADMINISTRATION

Coarsely cut the ingredients and cook the herbs in 6 cups [1,200 mL] of water until the liquid is reduced to 2 cups [400 mL]. Take the strained decoction in two equally-divided doses daily.

CHINESE THERAPEUTIC ACTIONS

Clears heat, purges fire and eliminates toxins

CLINICAL MANIFESTATIONS

Excess heat, fire and toxins in all three *jiaos*: high fever, fidgeting, irritability, a dry mouth and throat, delirium, insomnia; febrile diseases causing hematemesis, epistaxis, maculated skin; diarrhea, damp-heat jaundice; external abscesses, sores, cellulitis and boils with heat and toxins; yellow urine, a red tongue body with yellow tongue coating, and a rapid, forceful pulse.

CLINICAL APPLICATIONS

Encephalitis B, epidemic encephalitis, cerebrospinal meningitis, cerebrovascular accident, stroke, hypertension, post-ischemic brain injury, septicemia, pneumonia, otitis media, acute icteric jaundice, pelvic inflammatory disease, vaginitis, urinary tract infection, nephritis, acute enteritis, acute bacterial dysentery, bacterial dysentery, prophylactic treatment against post-surgical infection, sores, acne, impetigo herpetiformis, herpes, eczema of anus, cataract post-surgery, various bleeding disorders (hemoptysis, epistaxis, hematuria, rectal bleeding, etc.), and disorders with infection and inflammation.

EXPLANATION

Huang Lian Jie Du Tang (Coptis Decoction to Relieve Toxicity) commonly treats excess heat, fire, and toxins in all three *jiaos*. Fidgeting, irritability, and delirium are due to excess fire and toxins disturbing the *shen* (spirit). Hematemesis and epistaxis are due to heat forcing the blood to travel upward and out of the body. Maculated skin is due to heat injuring the channels and collaterals forcing the blood to travel outwards to the skin. Jaundice results when the stagnant damp-heat inside the body vaporizes out to the skin. External abscesses and sores are due to the stagnant heat in the muscles.

Although many clinical manifestations are indicated for this formula, the root cause for all of them is excess heat and fire in all three *jiaos*. This formula uses *Huang Lian* (Rhizoma Coptidis) to sedate fire in the Heart and middle *jiao*. *Huang Qin* (Radix Scutellariae) clears Lung heat and sedates fire in the upper *jiao*. *Huang Bo* (Cortex

341

Chapter 5 – Heat-Clearing Formulas   Section 4 – Heat-Clearing and Toxin-Eliminating Formulas

Huáng Lián Jiě Dú Tāng (Coptis Decoction to Relieve Toxicity)

Huang Lian Jie Du Tang (Coptis Decoction to Relieve Toxicity)

Diagnosis	Signs and Symptoms	Treatment	Herbs
Excess heat, fire and toxins in all three *jiaos*	• High fever: excess heat and fire • Fidgeting, irritability and delirium: excess fire and toxins disturbing the *shen* (spirit) • Dry mouth and throat: heat consuming body fluids • Hematemesis and epistaxis: heat forcing blood outward and upward • Maculated skin: heat injuring the channels and collaterals • Jaundice: stagnant damp-heat inside the body • External abscesses and sores: stagnant heat in the muscles • Yellow urine: heat attacking the lower *jiao* • Red tongue with a yellow tongue coating: heat and fire • Rapid, forceful pulse: excess condition of heat, fire and toxins	Clears heat, purges fire, and eliminates toxins	• *Huang Qin* (Radix Scutellariae) clears Lung heat and sedates fire in the upper *jiao*. • *Huang Lian* (Rhizoma Coptidis) sedates Heart fire and heat in the middle *jiao*. • *Huang Bo* (Cortex Phellodendri Chinensis) drains fire in the lower *jiao*. • *Zhi Zi* (Fructus Gardeniae) sedates fire in all three *jiaos* and guides heat downward.

Phellodendri Chinensis) sedates fire in the lower *jiao*. *Zhi Zi* (Fructus Gardeniae) sedates fire in all three *jiaos* and guides the heat downward.

MODIFICATIONS
- If there is constipation, add *Da Huang* (Radix et Rhizoma Rhei).
- With a dry mouth and throat, add *Mai Dong* (Radix Ophiopogonis) and *Wu Wei Zi* (Fructus Schisandrae Chinensis).
- With thirst and fever, add *Shi Gao* (Gypsum Fibrosum) and *Zhi Mu* (Rhizoma Anemarrhenae).
- With jaundice and fever, add *Da Huang* (Radix et Rhizoma Rhei) and *Yin Chen* (Herba Artemisiae Scopariae).
- With tenesmus and hematochezia, add *Mu Xiang* (Radix Aucklandiae) and *Bing Lang* (Semen Arecae).
- With frequent urination or oliguria, add *Che Qian Zi* (Semen Plantaginis) and *Mu Tong* (Caulis Akebiae).
- With cough accompanied by pus and blood, add *Jie Geng* (Radix Platycodonis) or *Jie Geng Tang* (Platycodon Decoction).
- For epistaxis, hematemesis, or purpura due to heat in the blood, add *Xuan Shen* (Radix Scrophulariae), *Di Huang* (Radix Rehmanniae), and *Mu Dan Pi* (Cortex Moutan).
- When there are abscesses and sores from accumulation of heat and toxins, add *Pu Gong Ying* (Herba Taraxaci) and *Zi Hua Di Ding* (Herba Violae); or *Wu Wei Xiao Du Yin* (Five-Ingredient Decoction to Eliminate Toxins).
- With ulceration of the skin accompanied by swelling and pain, combine with *Pai Nong San* (Drain the Pus Powder).

CAUTIONS / CONTRAINDICATIONS
- Prolonged use of this formula may injure the Spleen and Stomach. It is not suitable for someone with a weak constitution. Furthermore, this formula should be stopped immediately if the patient starts to show signs of yin deficiency.
- *Huang Lian Jie Du Tang* is contraindicated in patients with yin deficiency manifesting in a cracked tongue or mirror tongue, and in patients in which excess fire is not present.

PHARMACOLOGICAL EFFECTS
1. **Antipyretic**: Administration of *Huang Lian Jie Du Tang* was associated with a reduction in body temperature in numerous *in vitro* and *in vivo* experiments. In one study in rabbits with artificially-induced fever, use of the formula was found to have a slow onset but prolonged duration of antipyretic effect. The effect started at approximately 2 hours after the administration, peaked after 4 hours, and continued for 6 hours.[1] In another report, the antipyretic effect of the formula was described as similar to aspirin, following a laboratory study that compared the antipyretic effect of the formula with aspirin and normal saline.[2]

2. **Gastrointestinal**: Administration of water extract of *Huang Lian Jie Du Tang* at room temperature was associated with a marked inhibitory effect on the peristalsis of the intestines in mice. Similarly, it was found to be effective in treating spasms and cramps of the intestines.[3] Lastly, one study reported *Huang Lian Jie Du Tang* as a beneficial therapy for inflammatory bowel disease such as colitis, as the use of this formula was associated with quicker

342

Huáng Lián Jiě Dú Tāng (Coptis Decoction to Relieve Toxicity)

healing of lesions, and a reduction of inflammatory cell infiltration in rats.[4]

3. **Antiulcer**: One study reported that administration of *Huang Lian Jie Du Tang* was associated with a dose-dependent effect to prevent the development of stress-induced and ethanol-induced gastric lesions.[5,6,7] The report proposed two mechanisms for this gastroprotective effect: increased ability of the gastric mucosa to synthesize prostaglandin,[8] and decreased secretion of gastric acid.[9,10]

4. **Antidiarrheal**: Administration of water extract of *Huang Lian Jie Du Tang* at room temperature was associated with marked effect in treating diarrhea in mice.[11]

5. **Hepatoprotective**: Use of *Huang Lian Jie Du Tang* was associated with a protective effect on the liver.[12] In rats intoxicated with carbon tetrachloride, administration of *Huang Lian Jie Du Tang* prevented the progression of the liver injury in a dose-dependent manner by inhibiting the serum and hepatic triglyceride accumulation, and scavenging free radicals formed in the liver.[13,14]

6. **Antioxidant**: *Huang Lian Jie Du Tang* had an antioxidant effect to protect red blood cell membranes from free radicals. This antioxidant effect was dose-dependent at concentrations of 5 to 500 mcg/mL. Clinical use of this formula (7.5 g/day via oral ingestion) was associated with a significant decrease in susceptibility of red blood cells to hemolysis in humans.[15]

7. **Analgesic and anti-inflammatory**: Administration of a water extract of *Huang Lian Jie Du Tang* reduced pain and inflammation in mice.[16] The anti-inflammatory effects were exerted mainly in the early stages of inflammation, where increased capillary permeability and migration of leucocytes occurred.[17]

8. **Antihypertensive**: Administration of *Huang Lian Jie Du Tang* was associated with effectiveness in lowering blood pressure, as documented in numerous reports.[18] Water extract of the formula administered via intravenous injection in rats was associated with reduction of blood pressure and increase of heart rate in a dose-dependant fashion.[19] In another study, *Huang Lian Jie Du Tang* ameliorated hypertension caused by sympathetic system dominance in anesthetized rats.[20]

9. **Effect on arteriosclerosis**: *Huang Lian Jie Du Tang* prevented arteriosclerosis by inhibiting the proliferation of vascular smooth muscle cells.[21]

10. **Antihyperlipidemic**: Administration of *Huang Lian Jie Du Tang* was associated with decreased serum total cholesterol and low-density lipoprotein cholesterol levels. The mechanism of this antihyperlipidemic activity was attributed to the inhibition of HMG-CoA reductase. Of all the herbs in *Huang Lian Jie Du Tang*, *Huang Lian* (Rhizoma Coptidis) was believed to be the most potent inhibitor.[22]

11. **Metabolic**: Daily administration of *Huang Lian Jie Du Tang* in mice was associated with effectiveness in reducing blood glucose and cholesterol levels.[23]

12. **Ocular**: One study reported that administration of *Xi Gan Ming Mu San* (Wash the Liver and Brighten the Eyes Powder) and *Huang Lian Jie Du Tang* was associated with significantly suppressing (P < 0.001) the elevation of aqueous flares induced by lipopolysaccharides in rabbits.[24]

CLINICAL STUDIES AND RESEARCH

1. **Encephalitis B**: In one report, 56 patients with encephalitis B were treated with complete recovery in 51 patients and fatality in 4 patients. The average time for reduction of temperature was 4.9 days.[25]

2. **Cerebrospinal meningitis**: Twelve patients with infectious cerebrospinal meningitis were treated with complete recovery in 4 patients within 3 packs of herbs, in 2 patients after 4 packs, in 5 patients after 5 packs, and 1 patient after 6 packs. No long-term complications or sequelae were noted among all 12 patients.[26]

3. **Cerebrovascular accident**: One study stated that *Huang Lian Jie Du Tang* was useful in the treatment of cerebrovascular accident; this formula was found to improve microcirculation through lipid and protein metabolisms. Administration of the formula was associated with a significant decrease in plasma total cholesterol and triglyceride levels, and an increase in lipoprotein lipase mass. A considerable decline was also reported on plasma fibrinogen, an independent risk factor for cerebrovascular disease.[27]

4. **Stroke**: In one study, 120 patients with ischemic stroke confirmed with Western diagnosis were treated with modified *Huang Lian Jie Du Tang*. The treatment protocol was to administer the herbal decoction twice daily for 2-4 weeks in most patients, with some receiving treatment for up to 7 weeks. The study reported complete recovery in 48 patients, significant improvement in 38 patients, slight improvement in 29 patients, no change in 3 patients, and deterioration in 2 patients. The rate of effectiveness was 95.1%.[28]

5. **Post-ischemic brain injury**: Administration of 3 herbal formulas minimized post-ischemic brain injury by inhibiting production of free radicals and lipid peroxidation. Three formulas that were found to be effective, both *in vitro* and *in vivo*, were *Huang Lian Jie Du Tang*, *Chai Hu Jia Long Gu Mu Li Tang* (Bupleurum plus Dragon Bone and Oyster Shell Decoction), and *Gui Zhi Fu Ling Wan* (Cinnamon Twig and Poria Pill).[29]

6. **Transient cerebral ischemia**: Use of *Huang Lian Jie Du Tang* protected against the impairment of learning and memory induced by transient cerebral ischemia, because

Huáng Lián Jiě Dú Tāng (Coptis Decoction to Relieve Toxicity)

Huang Lian Jie Du Tang prevented the decrease in the acetylcholine content of the brain.[30]

7. **Pneumonia**: In one report, 35 pediatric patients with viral pneumonia were effectively treated with modified *Huang Lian Jie Du Tang*. Most patients had significant reduction of body temperature, cough, and other symptoms within 10-18 days.[31]

8. **Otitis media**: In one clinical study, 50 patients with otitis media were treated topically with a modified *Huang Lian Jie Du Tang* preparation, 4-5 drops in the affected ear(s) three to four times daily. Out of 50 patients, the study reported complete recovery in 32 patients, improvement in 9 patients, no change in 7 patients, and discontinuation of treatment in 2 patients.[32]

9. **Pelvic inflammatory disease**: In one study, 128 patients with pelvic inflammatory disease were treated with *Huang Lian Jie Du Tang* with 96.1% effectiveness. The treatment protocol was to cook the herbs in water to obtain 100 mL of herbal solution, which was administered at approximately 38°C / 100.4°F as a rectal enema one time daily for 10 days per course of treatment. Of 128 patients, the study reported complete recovery in 95 patients, significant improvement in 19 patients, moderate improvement in 9 patients, and no effect in 5 patients.[33]

10. **Vaginitis**: Topical application of a modified *Huang Lian Jie Du Tang* preparation one time daily for 5-7 days was successful in treating fungal or trichomonal vaginitis.[34]

11. **Bacterial dysentery**: In one report, 152 patients with bacterial dysentery characterized by the presence of mucus and blood in the stool were treated with rectal enema of a modified *Huang Lian Jie Du Tang* preparation which did not contain *Zhi Zi* (Fructus Gardeniae). Most patients exhibited marked reduction of temperature and other symptoms after just two procedures.[35]

12. **Prophylactic treatment against post-surgical infection**: *Huang Lian Jie Du Tang* has been used both before and after surgery with good success to prevent infection. Rectal instillation of the herbal solution prior to surgery on the colon effectively prevented infection and facilitated post-surgical recovery. The herbal formula contained *Huang Lian* (Rhizoma Coptidis) 30g, *Huang Qin* (Radix Scutellariae) 20g, *Huang Bo* (Cortex Phellodendri Chinensis) 20g, and *Zhi Zi* (Fructus Gardeniae) 30g. The treatment protocol was to cook the herbs in water twice, and the 2 resultant solutions mixed together (approximately 1,000 mL total), and instilled rectally while warm (35-40°C / 95-104°F).[36] In another study, administration of *Huang Lian Jie Du Tang* was associated with effectiveness in preventing infection in post-surgical patients. Of 50 patients who had various types of surgeries (primarily upper and lower extremities), use of herbs was successful in

preventing infection in 48 patients, with use of antibiotic drugs needed in 2 patients.[37]

13. **Abscesses and sores**: One study reported good results using herbs topically to treat abscesses and sores in the lower extremities. The herbal treatment contained *Huang Lian* (Rhizoma Coptidis) 10g, *Huang Bo* (Cortex Phellodendri Chinensis) 10g, *Huang Qin* (Radix Scutellariae) 10g, *Bai Zhi* (Radix Angelicae Dahuricae) 15g, and *Tu Fu Ling* (Rhizoma Smilacis Glabrae) 20g. The herbs were cooked in water, and the solution was used as an herbal wash topically on the affected area for 20 minutes, three times daily.[38]

14. **Acne**: According to a retrospective evaluation, *Huang Lian Jie Du Tang* was reported to be better than minocycline or erythromycin in the treatment against *Propionibacterium acnes*. Use of *Huang Lian Jie Du Tang* remained effective without significant increases in minimum inhibitory concentrations based on evaluations from 1990 to 1995. The efficacy of *Huang Lian Jie Du Tang* was attributed to *Huang Lian* (Rhizoma Coptidis) and *Huang Bo* (Cortex Phellodendri Chinensis), two herbs with strong antibacterial activity against *Propionibacterium acnes*.[39]

15. **Impetigo herpetiformis**: Use of modified *Huang Lian Jie Du Tang* was successful in treating 31 out of 31 patients with impetigo herpetiformis. The treatment protocol was to cook the herbs, and drink the decoction in two equally-divided doses daily. The herb residue was cooked again, and the resultant solution was used as an herbal wash on the affected area two to three times daily. The study reported complete recovery in all 31 patients, mostly within 10 days.[40]

16. **Eczema of anus**: One study reported marked success using modified *Huang Lian Jie Du Tang* to treat chronic eczema of anus. The herbal formula contained *Huang Lian* (Rhizoma Coptidis) 10g, *Huang Qin* (Radix Scutellariae) 8g, *Tu Fu Ling* (Rhizoma Smilacis Glabrae) 15g, and *Di Fu Zi* (Fructus Kochiae) 20g. The treatment protocol was to cook the herbs in water, then have the patient soak the affected area in the herbal solution 30 minutes, four times daily, for two weeks. No recurrences were reported in follow-up exams.[41]

17. **Lin zheng (dysuria syndrome)**: One study reported 96.9% effectiveness using modified *Huang Lian Jie Du Tang* to treat 32 patients with various types of *lin zheng* (dysuria syndrome). The herbal treatment contained *Huang Lian* (Rhizoma Coptidis) 12g, *Huang Qin* (Radix Scutellariae) 10g, *Huang Bo* (Cortex Phellodendri Chinensis) 10g, *Che Qian Zi* (Semen Plantaginis) 10g, *Da Huang* (Radix et Rhizoma Rhei) 10g, *Zhi Zi* (Fructus Gardeniae) 9g, *Bai Jiang Cao* (Herba cum Radice Patriniae) 15g, and *Fen Bi Xie* (Rhizoma Dioscoreae Hypoglaucae) 12g. The treatment protocol was to cook the herbs in water, and administer

Chinese Herbal Formulas and Applications

Huáng Lián Jiě Dú Tāng (Coptis Decoction to Relieve Toxicity)

the decoction in two equally-divided doses daily, for 7 days per course of treatment, for 1-2 courses total. During the herbal treatment, all patients were instructed to avoid foods that are pungent, hot, or sour. Of 32 patients, the study reported complete recovery in 22 patients, improvement in 9 patients, and no change in 1 patient.[42]

18. **Cataract surgery**: Use of *Huang Lian Jie Du Tang* and *Ge Gen Tang* (Kudzu Decoction) helped to reduce aqueous flare elevation after complicated cataract surgery. The treatment protocol was to administer *Huang Lian Jie Du Tang* (7.5 g/day) and *Ge Gen Tang* (Kudzu Decoction) (7.5 g/day) for 3 days before surgery, the day of surgery, and for 7 days after surgery. In comparison with the control group that did not receive herbs, oral administration of *Huang Lian Jie Du Tang* and *Ge Gen Tang* (Kudzu Decoction) decreases aqueous flare elevation after small-incision cataract surgery.[43]

HERB-DRUG INTERACTION

- **Drug-induced mucositis**: In 40 patients with acute leukemia treated with cytotoxic drugs, use of *Huang Lian Jie Du Tang* was associated with a marked effect to prevent iatrogenic mucositis, such as stomatitis and gastrointestinal mucosal injury. In the control group that did not receive herbs, the incidence was 71.6% for stomatitis, and 31.7% for diarrhea. In the herb group, the incidence was 27.9% for stomatitis, and 9.3% for diarrhea. The study concluded that *Huang Lian Jie Du Tang* had a significant preventive effect on mucositis caused by anticancer agents.[44]

- **Aspirin- and ethanol-induced gastric lesions**: Administration of *Huang Lian Jie Du Tang* was associated with success in treating aspirin- and ethanol-induced gastric hemorrhagic lesions in rats. The gastroprotective effect of *Huang Lian Jie Du Tang* was comparable to sucralfate (Carafate), cimetidine (Tagamet), and 16,16-dimethyl-prostaglandin E2 (DMPGE2).[45]

RELATED FORMULA

Lián Qiào Jiě Dú Tāng

(Forsythia Decoction to Relieve Toxicity)

連翹解毒湯
连翘解毒汤

Pinyin Name: Lian Qiao Jie Du Tang
Literal Name: Forsythia Decoction to Relieve Toxicity
Original Source: *Guang An Men Yi Yuan* (Guang An Men Hospital) in 1990

Lu Dou (Semen Phaseoli Radiati)

Gan Cao (Radix et Rhizoma Glycyrrhizae)

Dan Shen (Radix et Rhizoma Salviae Miltiorrhizae)

Lian Qiao (Fructus Forsythiae)

Jin Yin Hua (Flos Lonicerae Japonicae)

Bai Mao Gen (Rhizoma Imperatae)

Da Huang (Radix et Rhizoma Rhei)

Fang Feng (Radix Saposhnikoviae)

Lian Qiao Jie Du Tang (Forsythia Decoction to Relieve Toxicity) clears heat, eliminates toxins, and nourishes yin. Clinical applications of this formula include detoxification from chemical poisoning, food poisoning, and drug poisoning.

References

1. *Zhong Yao Tong Bao* (Journal of Chinese Herbology) 1986;1:5.
2. *Zhong Cheng Yao* (Study of Chinese Patent Medicine) 1993;8:29.
3. *Zhong Yi Fang Ji Xian Dai Yan Jiu* (Modern Study of Medical Formulae in Traditional Chinese Medicine) 1997;280-283.
4. Zhou H, Mineshita S. The effect of Oren-gedoku-to on experimental colitis in rats. J Pharm Pharmacol 1999 Sep;51(9):1065-74.
5. Ohta Y, Kobayashi T, Nishida K, Sasaki E, Ishiguro I. Preventive effect of Oren-gedoku-to (Huanglian-Jie-Du-Tang) extract on the development of stress-induced acute gastric mucosal lesions in rats. J Ethnopharmacol 1999 Nov 30;67(3):377-84.
6. Ohta Y, Kobayashi T, Nishida K, Nagata M, Ishiguro I. Therapeutic effect of Oren-gedoku-to extract on stress-induced acute gastric mucosal lesions in rats. Phytother Res 1999 Nov;13(7):588-92.
7. Takase H, Inoue O, Saito Y, Yumioka E, Suzuki A. Roles of sulfhydryl compounds in the gastric mucosal protection of the herb drugs composing oren-gedoku-to (a traditional herbal medicine). Jpn J Pharmacol 1991 Aug;56(4):433-9.
8. Suenaga T, Shirakawa T, Harada N, Tao C, Yamasaki M, Komatsu H, Matsumoto N, Kida M, Kawamoto Y, Murakami Y, et al. Mechanism of protective effects of ouren-gedoku-to and san'ou-syashin-to on the gastric mucosa. Nippon Yakurigaku Zasshi 1991 Oct;98(4):319-25.
9. Takase H, Tatsumi Y, Miura O, Yumioka E, Suzuki A. The mechanism of the inhibitory effects of oren-gedoku-to (OGT) on gastric acid secretion in rats. Nippon Yakurigaku Zasshi 1991 Feb;97(2):97-103.
10. *Guo Wai Yi Xue* (Foreign Medicine) 1988;5:36.
11. *Zhong Yi Fang Ji Xian Dai Yan Jiu* (Modern Study of Medical Formulae in Traditional Chinese Medicine) 1997;280-283.
12. *Zhong Yi Yao Yan Jiu Can Kao* (Research and Discussion of Chinese Medicine and Herbology) 1975;5:39.
13. Ohta Y, Sasaki E, Nishida K, Kongo M, Hayashi T, Nagata M, Ishiguro I. Inhibitory effect of Oren-gedoku-to (Huanglian-Jie-Du-Tang) extract on hepatic triglyceride accumulation with the progression of carbon tetrachloride-induced acute liver injury in rats. J Ethnopharmacol 1998 May;61(1):75-80.
14. Ohta Y, Sasaki E, Nishida K, Hayashi T, Nagata M, Ishiguro I. Preventive effect of oren-gedoku-to (huanglian-jie-du-tang) extract on progression of carbon tetrachloride-induced acute liver injury in rats. Am J Chin Med 1997;25(1):57-68.
15. Sekiya N, Shibahara N, Sakakibara I, Hattori N, Goto H, Terasawa K. Inhibitory effects of Oren-Gedoku-To (Huanglian-Jie-Du-Tang) on free radical-induced lysis of human red blood cells. Phytotherapy Research 2003 Feb;7(2):147-51.
16. *Zhong Yao Yao Li Yu Lin Chuang* (Pharmacology and Clinical Applications of Chinese Herbs) 1994;6:9.
17. Wang LM, Yamamoto T, Wang XX, Yang L, Koike Y, Shiba K, Mineshita S. Effects of oren-gedoku-to and unsei-in, Chinese traditional medicines, on interleukin-8 and superoxide dismutase in rats. J Pharm Pharmacol 1997 Jan;49(1):102-4.

HEAT-CLEARING FORMULAS

5

Huáng Lián Jiě Dú Tāng (Coptis Decoction to Relieve Toxicity)

18. *Zhong Yi Fang Ji Xian Dai Yan Jiu* (Modern Study of Medical Formulae in Traditional Chinese Medicine) 1997;280-281.

19. *Guo Wai Yi Xue* (Foreign Medicine) 1982;6:7.

20. Sanae F, Komatsu Y, Amagaya S, Chisaki K, Hayashi H. Effects of 9 Kampo medicines clinically used in hypertension on hemodynamic changes induced by theophylline in rats. Biol Pharm Bull 2000 Jun;23(6):762-5.

21. Chung HJ, Kim DW, Maruyama I, Tani T. Effects of traditional Chinese formulations on rat carotid artery injured by balloon endothelial denudation. Am J Chin Med 2003;31(2):201-12.

22. Kim YS, Jung EA, Shin JE, Chang JC, Yang HK, Kim NJ, Cho KH, Bae HS, Moon SK, Kim DH. Daio-Orengedokuto inhibits HMG-CoA reductase and pancreatic lipase. Biol Pharm Bull 2002 Nov;25(11):1442-5.

23. *Guo Wai Yi Xue* (Foreign Medicine) 1987;5:49.

24. Nagaki Y, Hayasaka S, Kadoi C, Matsumoto M, Nakamura N, Hayasaka Y. Effects of Orengedoku-to and Senkanmeimoku-to, traditional herbal medicines, on the experimental elevation of aqueous flare in pigmented rabbits. Am J Chin Med 2001;29(1):141-7.

25. *Fu Jian Zhong Yi Yao* (Fujian Chinese Medicine and Herbology) 1960;6:7.

26. *Guang Dong Zhong Yi* (Guangdong Chinese Medicine) 1960;6:296.

27. Sekiya N, Kogure T, Kita T, Kasahara Y, Sakakibara I, Goto H, Shibahara N, Shimada Y, Terasawa K. Reduction of plasma triglyceride level and enhancement of plasma albumin concentration by Orengedoku-to administration. Phytomedicine 2002 Jul;9(5):455-60.

28. *Zhong Yi Za Zhi* (Journal of Chinese Medicine) 1994;35(10):608.

29. Fushitani S, Minakuchi K, Tsuchiya K, Takasugi M, Murakami K. Studies on attenuation of post-ischemic brain injury by kampo medicines-inhibitory effects of free radical production. Yakugaku Zasshi 1995 Aug;115(8):611-7.

30. Xu J, Murakami Y, Matsumoto K, Tohda M, Watanabe H, Zhang S, Yu Q, Shen J. Protective effect of Oren-gedoku-to (Huang-Lian-Jie-Du-Tang) against impairment of learning and memory induced by transient cerebral ischemia in mice. J Ethnopharmacol 2000 Dec;73(3):405-13.

31. *Jiang Su Zhong Yi* (Jiangsu Chinese Medicine) 1996;2:3.

32. *Zhong Yi Za Zhi* (Journal of Chinese Medicine) 1994;35(10):608.

33. *Zhe Jiang Zhong Yi Xue Yuan Xue Bao* (Journal of Zhejiang University of Chinese Medicine) 1985;2:31.

34. *Xin Zhong Yi* (New Chinese Medicine) 1985;4:23.

35. *Tian Jin Yi Yao* (Tianjin Medicine and Herbology) 1976;6:294.

36. *Jiang Su Zhong Yi* (Jiangsu Chinese Medicine) 1998;3:30.

37. *Hu Bei Zhong Yi Za Zhi* (Hubei Journal of Chinese Medicine) 1981;4:30.

38. *Xin Zhong Yi* (New Chinese Medicine) 1998;1:52.

39. Higaki S, Nakamura M, Morohashi M, Hasegawa Y, Yamagishi T. Activity of eleven kampo formulations and eight kampo crude drugs against Propionibacterium acnes isolated from acne patients: retrospective evaluation in 1990 and 1995. J Dermatol 1996 Dec;23(12):871-5.

40. *An Hui Zhong Yi Xue Yuan Xue Bao* (Journal of Anhui University School of Medicine) 1987;3:16.

41. *Xin Zhong Yi* (New Chinese Medicine) 1998;1:52.

42. *Shi Yong Zhong Yi Yao Za Zhi* (Journal of Practical Chinese Medicine and Medicinals) 1998;12:19.

43. Ikeda N, Hayasaka S, Nagaki Y, Hayasaka Y, Kadoi C, Matsumoto M. Effects of traditional Sino-Japanese herbal medicines on aqueous flare elevation after small-incision cataract surgery. J Ocul Pharmacol Ther 2001 Feb;17(1):59-65.

44. Yuki F, Kawaguchi T, Hazemoto K, Asou N. Preventive effects of oren-gedoku-to (Huang-Lian-Jie-Du-Tang) on mucositis caused by anticancer agents in patients with acute leukemia. Gan To Kagaku Ryoho 2003 Sep;30(9):1303-7.

45. Takase H, Imanishi K, Miura O, Yumioka E, Watanabe H. Pharmacological studies on the effects of some traditional Chinese medicines on gastric functions. (3) The effects of oren-gedoku-to (OGT), san'o-syasin-to (SST), antyu-san (AS) and dai-saiko-to (DST) on ethanol- and aspirin-induced gastric lesions in rats. Nippon Yakurigaku Zasshi 1988 May;91(5):319-24.

Chinese Herbal Formulas and Applications

Huáng Lián Shàng Qīng Wán (Coptis Pill to Clear the Upper)

黃連上清丸
黄连上清丸

Pinyin Name: *Huang Lian Shang Qing Wan*
Literal Name: Coptis Pill to Clear the Upper
Alternate Names: *Huang Lien Shang Ching Wan*, Coptis Up-Clearing Pill, Coptis Phellodendron and Mint Formula
Original Source: *Si He Ting Ji Fang* (Collection of Formulas of Si He-Ting)

COMPOSITION

Huang Lian (Rhizoma Coptidis)	240g
Huang Qin (Radix Scutellariae)	240g
Huang Bo (Cortex Phellodendri Chinensis)	240g
Zhi Zi (Fructus Gardeniae)	240g
Da Huang (Radix et Rhizoma Rhei)	360g
Ju Hua (Flos Chrysanthemi)	120g
Jie Geng (Radix Platycodonis)	60g
Bo He (Herba Menthae)	120g
Jiang Huang (Rhizoma Curcumae Longae)	180g
Lian Qiao (Fructus Forsythiae)	180g
Xuan Shen (Radix Scrophulariae)	120g
Tian Hua Fen (Radix Trichosanthis)	60g
Ge Gen (Radix Puerariae Lobatae)	60g
Dang Gui (Radix Angelicae Sinensis)	120g
Chuan Xiong (Rhizoma Chuanxiong)	60g

DOSAGE / PREPARATION / ADMINISTRATION

Grind the ingredients into powder and mix with honey to form pills. Take 9g of pills with tea at bedtime.

CHINESE THERAPEUTIC ACTIONS

1. Clears heat and eliminates toxins
2. Purges fire and treats constipation

CLINICAL MANIFESTATIONS

Heat accumulation in all three *jiaos* with fire attacking the head: irritability, red eyes, a sore throat, pimples, ulcerations of the mouth and tongue, and pain and burning sensation during urination.

CLINICAL APPLICATIONS

Pneumonia, urinary tract infection, conjunctivitis, and febrile disorders.

EXPLANATION

Huang Lian Shang Qing Wan (Coptis Pill to Clear the Upper) has a wide range of clinical applications, but is most effective in treating heat and fire in the upper *jiao* attacking the head. Heat and fire in the three *jiaos* are characterized by fidgeting, irritability, and jaundice. As heat and fire move upward, they attack the head and the upper parts of the body, producing red eyes, a sore throat,

and ulcerations of the mouth and tongue. As heat and fire travel downward, they affect both bowel movement and urination, leading to constipation and pain, as well as burning sensations during urination.

Huang Lian (Rhizoma Coptidis), *Huang Qin* (Radix Scutellariae), *Huang Bo* (Cortex Phellodendri Chinensis), *Zhi Zi* (Fructus Gardeniae), and *Da Huang* (Radix et Rhizoma Rhei) are bitter and cold herbs that eliminate excess heat and fire in the upper, middle, and lower *jiaos*. *Huang Qin* (Radix Scutellariae) clears Lung heat and sedates fire in the upper *jiao*; *Huang Lian* (Rhizoma Coptidis) sedates fire in the Heart and middle *jiao*; *Huang Bo* (Cortex Phellodendri Chinensis) clears heat in the lower *jiao*; *Zhi Zi* (Fructus Gardeniae) sedates fire in all three *jiaos*; and *Da Huang* (Radix et Rhizoma Rhei) sedates fire and purges heat downward through defecation. *Ju Hua* (Flos Chrysanthemi), *Jie Geng* (Radix Platycodonis), *Bo He* (Herba Menthae), *Jiang Huang* (Rhizoma Curcumae Longae) and *Lian Qiao* (Fructus Forsythiae) dispel wind-heat and eliminate toxins from the exterior to relieve sore throat, red eyes, and ulcerations of the mouth and tongue. *Xuan Shen* (Radix Scrophulariae) and *Tian Hua Fen* (Radix Trichosanthis) clear heat and eliminate toxins. *Tian Hua Fen* (Radix Trichosanthis) and *Ge Gen* (Radix Puerariae Lobatae) promote generation of body fluids

5

HEAT-CLEARING FORMULAS

347

Chapter 5 – Heat-Clearing Formulas　　　　　*Section 4 – Heat-Clearing and Toxin-Eliminating Formulas*

Huáng Lián Shàng Qīng Wán (Coptis Pill to Clear the Upper)

Huang Lian Shang Qing Wan (Coptis Pill to Clear the Upper)

Diagnosis	Signs and Symptoms	Treatment	Herbs
Accumulation of heat in all three *jiaos* with fire attacking the head	• Red eyes, a sore throat and ulcerations of the mouth and tongue: heat and fire traveling to the head • Fidgeting and irritability: heat and fire affecting the upper body • Constipation and dysuria: heat and fire affecting the lower body	• Clears heat and eliminates toxins • Purges fire and treats constipation	• *Huang Lian* (Rhizoma Coptidis), *Huang Qin* (Radix Scutellariae), *Huang Bo* (Cortex Phellodendri Chinensis) and *Zhi Zi* (Fructus Gardeniae) eliminate excess heat and fire in the upper, middle, and lower *jiaos*. • *Da Huang* (Radix et Rhizoma Rhei) sedates fire and purges heat downward through defecation. • *Ju Hua* (Flos Chrysanthemi), *Jie Geng* (Radix Platycodonis), *Bo He* (Herba Menthae), *Jiang Huang* (Rhizoma Curcumae Longae), and *Lian Qiao* (Fructus Forsythiae) dispel heat and eliminate toxins from the exterior. • *Xuan Shen* (Radix Scrophulariae) and *Tian Hua Fen* (Radix Trichosanthis) clear heat and eliminate toxins. • *Tian Hua Fen* (Radix Trichosanthis) and *Ge Gen* (Radix Puerariae Lobatae) promote generation of body fluids and prevent the cold and bitter herbs from damaging yin. • *Dang Gui* (Radix Angelicae Sinensis) and *Chuan Xiong* (Rhizoma Chuanxiong) invigorate blood circulation, remove blood stasis, and relieve pain.

and prevent the cold and bitter herbs from damaging yin. *Dang Gui* (Radix Angelicae Sinensis) and *Chuan Xiong* (Rhizoma Chuanxiong) invigorate blood circulation, remove blood stasis, and relieve pain.

MODIFICATIONS

• With a dry mouth and throat, add *Mai Dong* (Radix Ophiopogonis) and *Wu Wei Zi* (Fructus Schisandrae Chinensis).

• With thirst and fever, add *Shi Gao* (Gypsum Fibrosum) and *Zhi Mu* (Rhizoma Anemarrhenae).

• With jaundice and fever, add *Da Huang* (Radix et Rhizoma Rhei) and *Yin Chen* (Herba Artemisiae Scopariae).

• With tenesmus and blood in the stool, add *Mu Xiang* (Radix Aucklandiae) and *Bing Lang* (Semen Arecae).

• With frequent urination and oliguria, add *Che Qian Zi* (Semen Plantaginis) and *Mu Tong* (Caulis Akebiae).

Qīng Shàng Fáng Fēng Tāng
(Clear the Upper and Guard the Wind Decoction)

清上防風湯

清上防风汤

Pinyin Name: *Qing Shang Fang Feng Tang*
Literal Name: Clear the Upper and Guard the Wind Decoction
Alternate Name: Siler Combination
Original Source: *Wan Bing Hui Chun* (Restoration of Health from the Myriad Diseases) by Gong Ting-Xian in 1587

COMPOSITION

Huang Lian (Rhizoma Coptidis)	1.5g
Huang Qin (Radix Scutellariae), *chao* (dry-fried) with liquor	2.1g
Zhi Zi (Fructus Gardeniae)	1.5g
Fang Feng (Radix Saposhnikoviae)	3g
Bo He (Herba Menthae)	1.5g
Jie Geng (Radix Platycodonis)	2.4g
Jing Jie (Herba Schizonepetae)	1.5g
Lian Qiao (Fructus Forsythiae)	2.4g
Zhi Qiao (Fructus Citri Aurantii)	1.5g
Bai Zhi (Radix Angelicae Dahuricae)	2.4g
Chuan Xiong (Rhizoma Chuanxiong)	2.1g
Gan Cao (Radix et Rhizoma Glycyrrhizae)	0.9g

DOSAGE / PREPARATION / ADMINISTRATION

Cook the herbs with a small amount of *Zhu Li* (Succus Bambusae) and take the warm, strained decoction after meals.

CHINESE THERAPEUTIC ACTIONS

1. Clears heat from the upper *jiao*
2. Clears heat and eliminates toxins

CLINICAL MANIFESTATIONS

Wind, heat, and toxins in the upper body: boils, acne, eczema, flushed face, and red eyes.

CLINICAL APPLICATIONS

Pimples, boils, eczema, conjunctivitis, otitis media, and gingivitis.

EXPLANATION

Qing Shang Fang Feng Tang (Clear the Upper and Guard the Wind Decoction) eliminates wind, heat and toxins from the upper parts of the body. The presentation of this condition is usually on the skin, evident as boils, acne, and eczema. Patients may also have red face and eyes. This is an effective formula for treating various upper body skin disorders characterized by heat and toxins.

Huang Lian (Rhizoma Coptidis), *Huang Qin* (Radix Scutellariae), and *Zhi Zi* (Fructus Gardeniae) synergistically clear heat from the upper parts of the body. In addition, these herbs also eliminate toxins. *Fang Feng* (Radix Saposhnikoviae), *Bo He* (Herba Menthae), *Jie Geng* (Radix Platycodonis), and *Jing Jie* (Herba Schizonepetae) enter the superficial layer of the body to eliminate wind, dispel phlegm, and eliminate toxins. *Lian Qiao* (Fructus Forsythiae) and *Zhi Qiao* (Fructus Aurantii) reduce swelling and drain pus. *Bai Zhi* (Radix Angelicae Dahuricae) and *Chuan Xiong* (Rhizoma Chuanxiong) travel upwards to guide the effects of the herbs to the upper body. *Gan Cao* (Radix et Rhizoma Glycyrrhizae) harmonizes the formula.

MODIFICATIONS

- With constipation, add *Da Huang* (Radix et Rhizoma Rhei).
- If there are sores that are itchy, add *Jin Yin Hua* (Flos Lonicerae Japonicae) and *Tu Fu Ling* (Rhizoma Smilacis Glabrae).
- With sores and swelling, add *Zhi Mu* (Rhizoma Anemarrhenae) and *Shi Gao* (Gypsum Fibrosum).
- When the acne is characterized by excessive pus, add a large dose of *Yi Yi Ren* (Semen Coicis).

Chapter 5 – Heat-Clearing Formulas   *Section 4 – Heat-Clearing and Toxin-Eliminating Formulas*

Qīng Shàng Fáng Fēng Tāng
(Clear the Upper and Guard the Wind Decoction)

Qing Shang Fang Feng Tang (Clear the Upper and Guard the Wind Decoction)

Diagnosis	Signs and Symptoms	Treatment	Herbs
Wind, heat, and toxins in the upper body	Boils, acne, eczema, and red face and eyes	• Clears heat from the upper *jiao* • Eliminates heat and toxins	• *Huang Lian* (Rhizoma Coptidis), *Huang Qin* (Radix Scutellariae) and *Zhi Zi* (Fructus Gardeniae) clear heat and eliminate toxins from the upper body. • *Fang Feng* (Radix Saposhnikoviae), *Bo He* (Herba Menthae), *Jie Geng* (Radix Platycodonis) and *Jing Jie* (Herba Schizonepetae) eliminate wind and toxins, and dispel phlegm. • *Lian Qiao* (Fructus Forsythiae) and *Zhi Qiao* (Fructus Aurantii) reduce swelling and drain pus. • *Bai Zhi* (Radix Angelicae Dahuricae) and *Chuan Xiong* (Rhizoma Chuanxiong) guide the herbs to the upper body. • *Gan Cao* (Radix et Rhizoma Glycyrrhizae) harmonizes the herbs.

RELATED FORMULA

Qīng Rè Jiě Dú Tāng

(Clear Heat and Relieve Toxicity Decoction)

清熱解毒湯
清热解毒汤

Pinyin Name: *Qing Re Jie Du Tang*
Literal Name: Clear Heat and Relieve Toxicity Decoction
Original Source: *Guang An Men Yi Yuan* (Guang An Men Hospital) in 1990

Huang Qin (Radix Scutellariae)
Huang Lian (Rhizoma Coptidis)
Ban Lan Gen (Radix Isatidis)
Lian Qiao (Fructus Forsythiae)
Niu Bang Zi (Fructus Arctii)

Ma Bo (Lasiosphaera seu Calvatia)
Xuan Shen (Radix Scrophulariae)
Bo He (Herba Menthae)
Chai Hu (Radix Bupleuri)
Zhe Bei Mu (Bulbus Fritillariae Thunbergii)
Jie Geng (Radix Platycodonis)
Chen Pi (Pericarpium Citri Reticulatae)
Gan Cao (Radix et Rhizoma Glycyrrhizae)

Qing Re Jie Du Tang (Clear Heat Relieve Toxicity Decoction) clears heat and eliminates toxins that affect the upper parts of the body. It is commonly used to treat infections that affect the ears, nose and throat. Clinical applications include ear infection, sinusitis and rhinitis, sore throat, and respiratory tract infection.

350

Liáng Gé Sǎn (Cool the Diaphragm Powder)

涼膈散
凉膈散

Pinyin Name: *Liang Ge San*
Literal Name: Cool the Diaphragm Powder
Alternate Names: *Lian Ke San*, Forsythia and Rhubarb Formula
Original Source: *Tai Ping Hui Min He Ji Ju Fang* (Imperial Grace Formulary of the Tai Ping Era) by the Imperial Medical Department in 1078-85

COMPOSITION

Lian Qiao (Fructus Forsythiae)	1,200g [18g]
Huang Qin (Radix Scutellariae)	300g [5g]
Zhi Zi (Fructus Gardeniae)	300g [5g]
Bo He (Herba Menthae)	300g [5g]
Po Xiao (Sal Glauberis)	600g [9g]
Da Huang (Radix et Rhizoma Rhei)	600g [9g]
Gan Cao (Radix et Rhizoma Glycyrrhizae)	600g [9g]

DOSAGE / PREPARATION / ADMINISTRATION

The source text states to grind the ingredients into a coarse powder. Cook 6g of the powder with 7 leaves of *Zhu Ye* (Herba Phyllostachys) and a small amount of *Feng Mi* (Mel) in one large bowl of water until it is reduced to 70%. Take the warm, strained decoction after meals. For young children, cook 1.5g of the powder per dose, or adjust it accordingly based on age. Once bowel movement has been induced, the formula should be discontinued. Today, this formula may be prepared as a decoction with the doses suggested in brackets and 3g of *Zhu Ye* (Herba Phyllostachys) and a small amount of *Feng Mi* (Mel).

CHINESE THERAPEUTIC ACTIONS

1. Purges fire and promotes defecation
2. Clears and purges heat from the upper and middle *jiaos*

CLINICAL MANIFESTATIONS

Accumulation of heat and fire in the upper and middle *jiaos*: irritability and a warm sensation in the chest and diaphragm, fever, thirst, red eyes, a warm face, extremely dry lips, ulcers on the mouth and tongue, a sore throat, epistaxis, hematemesis, constipation, dysuria with dark scanty urine, a red tongue body with a yellow tongue coating, and a slippery, rapid pulse.

CLINICAL APPLICATIONS

Infection, upper respiratory tract infection, pediatric pneumonia, lobar pneumonia, bronchiectasis, whooping cough, common cold and influenza, infectious parotitis, sore throat, bronchiectasis with hemoptysis, stomatitis, laryngitis, herpetic pharyngitis, tonsillitis, candidiasis, herpes labiales, gingivitis, epistaxis, cholecystitis, cholelithiasis, acute conjunctivitis, encephalitis, meningitis, diarrhea, and acute nephritis.

EXPLANATION

Liang Ge San (Cool the Diaphragm Powder) treats stagnation of heat and fire in the chest and diaphragm of the upper and middle *jiao*s. Heat accumulation in the upper and middle *jiao*s causes irritability, a warm sensation in the chest and diaphragm, fever, and thirst. If the heat travels upward to the head, then red eyes, a warm face, extremely dry lips, ulcers on the mouth and the tongue, and a sore throat manifest. Epistaxis and hematemesis occur in severe cases when heat travels upward and forces blood out of the blood vessels. If heat travels downward, constipation and dysuria occur. The yellow tongue coating and rapid pulse both suggest excess heat accumulation inside the body.

This formula uses heat-clearing herbs to clear heat in the upper *jiao*, and purgative herbs to sedate fire in the lower *jiao* through defecation. *Lian Qiao* (Fructus Forsythiae), used in a large amount in this formula, clears heat and eliminates toxins from the upper *jiao*. *Huang Qin* (Radix Scutellariae) and *Zhu Ye* (Herba Phyllostachys) clear heat from the Heart and upper *jiao* and relieve symptoms associated with the chest and diaphragm. *Zhi Zi* (Fructus Gardeniae) clears heat in all three *jiaos* and leads heat downward. *Bo He* (Herba Menthae) clears the head and benefits the throat. *Po Xiao* (Sal Glauberis) and *Da Huang* (Radix et Rhizoma Rhei), both purgative herbs, purge heat in the chest and diaphragm and eliminate it through defecation. *Feng Mi* (Mel) lubricates the bowels to facilitate the purgative effects of *Da Huang* (Radix et Rhizoma

351

Chapter 5 – Heat-Clearing Formulas   *Section 4 – Heat-Clearing and Toxin-Eliminating Formulas*

Liáng Gé Săn (Cool the Diaphragm Powder)

Liang Ge San (Cool the Diaphragm Powder)

Diagnosis	Signs and Symptoms	Treatment	Herbs
Accumulation of heat and fire in the upper and middle *jiao*s	• Irritability, a warm sensation in the chest and diaphragm, fever, and thirst: heat accumulated in the upper and middle *jiao*s • Red eyes, a warm face, extremely dry lips, ulcers on the mouth and tongue, and a sore throat: heat traveling upward to the head region • Constipation and dysuria: heat traveling downward • Epistaxis and hematemesis: heat travels upward forcing blood out of the vessels • Red tongue body with yellow tongue coating: excess heat • Rapid pulse: excess heat	• Purges fire and promotes defecation • Clears and purges heat from the upper and middle *jiao*s	• *Lian Qiao* (Fructus Forsythiae) clears heat and eliminates toxins in the upper *jiao*. • *Huang Qin* (Radix Scutellariae) and *Zhu Ye* (Herba Phyllostachys) clear heat from the Heart and upper *jiao*. • *Zhi Zi* (Fructus Gardeniae) clears heat in all three *jiao*s and leads heat downward. • *Bo He* (Herba Menthae) clears the head and benefits the throat. • *Po Xiao* (Sal Glauberis) and *Da Huang* (Radix et Rhizoma Rhei) purge heat in the chest and diaphragm and eliminate it through defecation. • *Feng Mi* (Mel) and *Gan Cao* (Radix et Rhizoma Glycyrrhizae) moisten, protect, and nourish Stomach yin.

Rhei) and *Po Xiao* (Sal Glauberis). *Gan Cao* (Radix et Rhizoma Glycyrrhizae) moderates the drastic effects of the purgative herbs. *Feng Mi* (Mel) and *Gan Cao* (Radix et Rhizoma Glycyrrhizae) also moisten, protect, and nourish Stomach yin.

MODIFICATIONS

• With cough, nausea, and vomiting, add *Ban Xia* (Rhizoma Pinelliae) and *Sheng Jiang* (Rhizoma Zingiberis Recens).
• With dysuria, add *Hua Shi* (Talcum) and *Fu Ling* (Poria).
• With dizziness and vertigo due to heat, add *Fang Feng* (Radix Saposhnikoviae), *Chuan Xiong* (Rhizoma Chuanxiong) and *Shi Gao* (Gypsum Fibrosum).
• With irritability and thirst, add *Tian Hua Fen* (Radix Trichosanthis).
• With a sore throat, add *Shan Dou Gen* (Radix et Rhizoma Sophorae Tonkinensis) and *Ban Lan Gen* (Radix Isatidis).
• When there is ulceration of the mouth and tongue, add *Huang Lian* (Rhizoma Coptidis) and *Di Gu Pi* (Cortex Lycii).
• If accompanied by chest pain, add *Chai Hu* (Radix Bupleuri), *Chuan Lian Zi* (Fructus Toosendan), and *Yan Hu Suo* (Rhizoma Corydalis).

CAUTIONS / CONTRAINDICATIONS

• Use this formula with caution during pregnancy. *Po Xiao* (Sal Glauberis) and *Da Huang* (Radix et Rhizoma Rhei) should be reduced in dose, or removed completely, during pregnancy.
• *Liang Ge San* is a strong formula that contains bitter and

cold herbs, and has heat-clearing and downward draining effects. Patients with a sensitive gastrointestinal tract may experience stomach pain and diarrhea, both of which are self-limiting with discontinuation of the formula. If such patients require this formula, remove *Da Huang* (Radix et Rhizoma Rhei) and administer the formula after meals.

CLINICAL STUDIES AND RESEARCH

1. **Common cold and influenza**: In a clinical trial, 257 patients with viral infections were divided into two groups, with 157 patients receiving herbal and 100 patients receiving drug treatment. The protocol for the herbal treatment was to administer modified *Liang Ge San* in decoction twice daily. The study reported complete recovery in 131 patients with 1-3 packs of herbs, and 26 patients with 4-6 packs. By comparison, patients who received antibiotic drug therapy all required at least 5 days to recover, with 63 needing more than 10 days. The researchers concluded that use of this formula may shorten the duration of illness for common cold and influenza.[1]

2. **Tonsillitis**: Modified *Liang Ge San* was used to treat 32 patients between the ages of 16 months and 12 years with acute tonsillitis with swelling, pain, and constipation. The treatment protocol was to administer the herbal decoction one time daily. The study reported complete recovery in 30 of 32 patients within a range of 4-8 days. Treatment was discontinued in two patients because of nausea and vomiting.[2]

3. **Pneumonia**: Modified *Liang Ge San* was used to treat 13 patients with lobar pneumonia with symptoms such as

Liáng Gé Săn (Cool the Diaphragm Powder)

aversion to cold, fever, cough, and chest pain. The treatment protocol was to administer the herbs in decoction one time daily for regular patients, and twice daily for severe cases. Of 13 patients with lobar pneumonia, the study reported complete recovery in 10 patients and improvement in 3 patients.[3]

4. **Bronchiectasis with hemoptysis**: Concurrent administration of antibiotic drugs and modified *Liang Ge San* was reported to be effective in the treatment of hemoptysis caused by bronchiectasis in 30 patients with a history of illness between 3 months to 15 years. The rationale of the treatment was to use antibiotic drugs to treat the infection, and herbs to stop bleeding. The herbal treatment contained *Da Huang* (Radix et Rhizoma Rhei) 6g, *Mang Xiao* (Natrii Sulfas) 6g, *Gan Cao* (Radix et Rhizoma Glycyrrhizae) 6g, *Bo He* (Herba Menthae) 6g, *Dan Zhu Ye* (Herba Lophatheri) 6g, *Lian Qiao* (Fructus Forsythiae) 9g, *Zhi Zi* (Fructus Gardeniae) 9g, *Huang Qin* (Radix Scutellariae) 9g, and *Feng Mi* (Mel) 18g. The herbs were cooked, and the decoction administered in two equally-divided doses. The duration of treatment was 10-15 packs of herbs per course of treatment, for up to two courses total. The average length of treatment was 7 days. Of 30 patients, the study reported significant effect in 22 patients, improvement in 6 patients, and no effect in 2 patients. The overall rate of effectiveness was 93.3%.[4]

5. **Herpetic pharyngitis**: One study reported marked success using modified *Liang Ge San* to treat herpetic pharyngitis in 28 children (17 males and 11 females). The herbal treatment contained *Chan Tui* (Periostracum Cicadae) 5g, *Bo He* (Herba Menthae) 5g (post-decocted), fresh *Lu Gen* (Rhizoma Phragmitis) 30g, *Niu Bang Zi* (Fructus Arctii) 6g, *Lian Qiao* (Fructus Forsythiae) 6g, *Xuan Shen* (Radix Scrophulariae) 6g, *Zhi Zi* (Fructus Gardeniae) 6g, *Da Huang* (Radix et Rhizoma Rhei) 5g (post-decocted), *Ban Lan Gen* (Radix Isatidis) 10g, *Gan Cao* (Radix et Rhizoma Glycyrrhizae) 10g, and *She Gan* (Rhizoma Belamcandae) 5g. Modifications were made as needed by adding *Jing Jie* (Herba Schizonepetae) for mild perspiration; *Shi Gao* (Gypsum Fibrosum) 30g (pre-decocted) for high fever; *Gou Teng* (Ramulus Uncariae cum Uncis) 6g or *Jiang Can* (Bombyx Batryticatus) 6g for high fever with seizure; and adding dry-fried *Zhi Qiao* (Fructus Aurantii) 5g and *Jue Ming Zi* (Semen Cassiae) 12g and removing *Da Huang* (Radix et Rhizoma Rhei) for dry stools in a constitutionally-deficient

person. The treatment protocol was to cook 1 pack of herbs and administer the decoction daily, for 3 days per course of treatment. The study reported 96.4% effectiveness after 2 courses of treatment, with improvements such as relief of irritability, sore throat, herpetic lesions, and constipation.[5]

6. **Epistaxis**: Twenty-four patients with epistaxis refractory to drug therapy were treated with 95.83% effectiveness using modified *Liang Ge San*. Modifications to the base formula included the addition of *San Qi* (Radix et Rhizoma Notoginseng) in powder for profuse bleeding; *E Jiao* (Colla Corii Asini) and *Bai Shao* (Radix Paeoniae Alba) for yin and blood deficiencies; *Huang Qi* (Radix Astragali) and *Tai Zi Shen* (Radix Pseudostellariae) for qi deficiency; *Long Dan* (Radix et Rhizoma Gentianae) for Liver fire rising; *Shi Gao* (Gypsum Fibrosum) and *Huang Lian* (Rhizoma Coptidis) for Stomach fire rising; and *Jing Jie* (Herba Schizonepetae) and *Ge Gen* (Radix Puerariae Lobatae) for presence of an exterior condition. Of 24 patients, the study reported complete recovery in 21 patients, improvement in 2 patients, and no change in 1 patient.[6]

AUTHORS' COMMENTS

Liang Ge San contains both heat-clearing and purgative herbs to eliminate accumulation of heat and fire in the upper and middle *jiao*s. Heat-clearing herbs are effective for clearing generalized non-stagnant heat in the body. However, in this syndrome in which heat stagnation is a factor, heat-clearing herbs alone may not be able to completely break up and eliminate the heat pathogen. Therefore, purgative herbs are also used to eliminate heat stagnation more effectively, even in cases in which the patient does not have constipation.

References

1. *Shan Dong Zhong Yi Za Zhi* (Shandong Journal of Chinese Medicine) 1991;(2):37.
2. *Xin Zhong Yi* (New Chinese Medicine) 1990;(3):23.
3. *Fu Jian Zhong Yi Yao* (Fujian Chinese Medicine and Herbology) 1985;(2):43.
4. *Zhong Xi Yi Jie He Za Zhi* (Journal of Integrated Chinese and Western Medicine) 1985;5:304.
5. *Zhe Jiang Zhong Yi Xue Yuan Xue Bao* (Journal of Zhejiang University of Chinese Medicine) 1996;3:37.
6. *Shi Yong Zhong Yi Yao Za Zhi* (Journal of Practical Chinese Medicine and Medicinals) 1993;3:21.

Chapter 5 – Heat-Clearing Formulas　　　　　*Section 4 – Heat-Clearing and Toxin-Eliminating Formulas*

Qīng Liáng Yǐn (Clearing and Cooling Decoction)

清凉飲
清凉饮

Pinyin Name: *Qing Liang Yin*
Literal Name: Clearing and Cooling Decoction
Alternate Name: Scute and Mentha Combination
Original Source: *Zheng Zhi Zhun Sheng* (Standards of Patterns and Treatments) by Wang Ken-Tang in 1602

COMPOSITION

Huang Qin (Radix Scutellariae)

Huang Lian (Rhizoma Coptidis)

Bo He (Herba Menthae)

Xuan Shen (Radix Scrophulariae)

Dang Gui (Radix Angelicae Sinensis)

Bai Shao (Radix Paeoniae Alba)

Gan Cao (Radix et Rhizoma Glycyrrhizae)

DOSAGE / PREPARATION / ADMINISTRATION

The doses of herbs and the instructions for preparation are unavailable from the original source. Today, this formula can be prepared and taken as a warm decoction any time during the day.

CHINESE THERAPEUTIC ACTIONS

Clears heat from the upper and middle *jiaos*

CLINICAL MANIFESTATIONS

Heat in the upper and middle *jiaos*: thirst, restlessness, foul breath, and a dry tongue and throat.

CLINICAL APPLICATIONS

Stomatitis, canker sores, and oral herpes.

EXPLANATION

Qing Liang Yin (Clearing and Cooling Decoction) treats heat attacking the upper and middle *jiaos,* leading to symptoms of both excess heat and deficiency of fluids. Excess heat is characterized by foul breath and restlessness, and deficiency of fluids is characterized by thirst, a dry tongue, and a dry throat.

This formula contains herbs that clear heat and moisten fluids. *Huang Qin* (Radix Scutellariae) and *Huang Lian* (Rhizoma Coptidis), two bitter and cold herbs, clear heat from the upper and middle *jiaos*. They address the excess component of this syndrome. *Bo He* (Herba Menthae) also clears heat. Although these three herbs clear heat exceedingly well, they carry the risk of drying up fluids and yin. Thus, *Xuan Shen* (Radix Scrophulariae) is added

Qing Liang Yin (Clearing and Cooling Decoction)

Diagnosis	Signs and Symptoms	Treatment	Herbs
Heat in the upper and middle *jiaos*	• Foul breath and restlessness: excess heat in the upper and middle *jiaos* • Thirst, and a dry tongue and throat: excess heat consuming body fluids	Clears heat from the upper and middle *jiaos*	• *Huang Qin* (Radix Scutellariae) and *Huang Lian* (Rhizoma Coptidis) clear heat from the upper and middle *jiaos*. • *Bo He* (Herba Menthae) clears heat. • *Xuan Shen* (Radix Scrophulariae) clears heat and replenishes yin and fluids. • *Dang Gui* (Radix Angelicae Sinensis) and *Bai Shao* (Radix Paeoniae Alba) nourish the blood and prevent the bitter and cold herbs from damaging the body. • *Gan Cao* (Radix et Rhizoma Glycyrrhizae) harmonizes the herbs.

354

Chinese Herbal Formulas and Applications

Qīng Liáng Yǐn (Clearing and Cooling Decoction)

because it both clears heat and replenishes yin and fluids. *Dang Gui* (Radix Angelicae Sinensis) and *Bai Shao* (Radix Paeoniae Alba) nourish the blood and prevent the bitter and cold herbs from damaging the body. Lastly, *Gan Cao* (Radix et Rhizoma Glycyrrhizae) harmonizes the herbs. The formula achieves its function of clearing heat from the upper and middle *jiaos* while protecting yin and body fluids.

MODIFICATIONS

With constipation caused by excess heat, add *Da Huang* (Radix et Rhizoma Rhei).

Pǔ Jì Xiāo Dú Yǐn (Universal Benefit Decoction to Eliminate Toxin)
普濟消毒飲
普济消毒饮

Pinyin Name: *Pu Ji Xiao Du Yin*
Literal Name: Universal Benefit Decoction to Eliminate Toxin
Alternate Names: *Pu Chi Hsiao Tu Yin*, Universal Salvation Detoxifying Drink, Everyone's Detoxifying Decoction, Scute and Cimicifuga Combination
Original Source: *Dong Heng Shi Xiao Fang* (Tested and Effective Formulas by Dong Heng) by Li Gao (also known as Li Dong-Heng) in 1266

COMPOSITION

Huang Qin (Radix Scutellariae), *chao* (dry-fried) with liquor	15g
Huang Lian (Rhizoma Coptidis), *chao* (dry-fried) with liquor	15g
Niu Bang Zi (Fructus Arctii)	3g
Lian Qiao (Fructus Forsythiae)	3g
Bo He (Herba Menthae)	3g
Jiang Can (Bombyx Batryticatus)	2.1g
Xuan Shen (Radix Scrophulariae)	6g
Ma Bo (Lasiosphaera seu Calvatia)	3g
Ban Lan Gen (Radix Isatidis)	3g
Jie Geng (Radix Platycodonis)	6g
Gan Cao (Radix et Rhizoma Glycyrrhizae)	6g
Chen Pi (Pericarpium Citri Reticulatae)	6g
Sheng Ma (Rhizoma Cimicifugae)	2.1g
Chai Hu (Radix Bupleuri)	6g
Ren Shen (Radix et Rhizoma Ginseng)	9g [3g]

DOSAGE / PREPARATION / ADMINISTRATION

The source text states to grind the ingredients into powder, cook it in water, and take the warm decoction frequently in small amounts. It may also be formed into pills with honey, and dissolved under the tongue before swallowing. For patients with constipation, add *Da Huang* (Radix et Rhizoma Rhei). Today, this formula may be prepared as a decoction with the dose of *Ren Shen* (Radix et Rhizoma Ginseng) suggested in brackets. Note: One variation of this formula contains 6g of *Bo He* (Herba Menthae) and omits *Ren Shen* (Radix et Rhizoma Ginseng).

CHINESE THERAPEUTIC ACTIONS

1. Clears heat and eliminates toxin
2. Dispels wind and disperses pathogenic factors

CLINICAL MANIFESTATIONS

Da tou wen (swollen head epidemic) with the presence of wind, heat, and toxin in the upper *jiao* and head: redness, swelling and pain of the face and head; red and swollen eyes, difficulty in opening the eyes; fever, aversion to cold, a sore throat, thirst, a dry, red tongue with a yellow tongue coating, and a rapid, forceful pulse.

355

Chapter 5 – Heat-Clearing Formulas　　　　　*Section 4 – Heat-Clearing and Toxin-Eliminating Formulas*

Pǔ Jì Xiāo Dú Yǐn (Universal Benefit Decoction to Eliminate Toxin)

CLINICAL APPLICATIONS

Epidemic hemorrhagic fever, respiratory tract infection, common cold, influenza, severe sore throat, infectious parotitis, acute tonsillitis, lymphadenitis, purulent inflammation and abscess of the face and head, erysipelas, herpes, carbuncles, boils, testitis, myocarditis, and conjunctivitis.

EXPLANATION

Pu Ji Xiao Du Yin (Universal Benefit Decoction to Eliminate Toxin) treats *da tou wen* (swollen head epidemic), an epidemic disease characterized by redness, swelling and pain of the face and head caused by wind, heat and toxin attacking the face and head. If the wind, heat, and toxin invade the head region, redness, swelling and pain of the face and head, difficulty in opening the eyes, sore throat, and thirst may result. Fever and aversion to cold suggest that the disease (wind-heat) is located at the exterior. The yellow tongue coating and rapid, forceful pulse suggest excess interior heat.

Huang Qin (Radix Scutellariae) and *Huang Lian* (Rhizoma Coptidis), the chief herbs of this formula, clear heat and eliminate toxin from the head. *Niu Bang Zi* (Fructus Arctii), *Lian Qiao* (Fructus Forsythiae), *Bo He* (Herba Menthae) and *Jiang Can* (Bombyx Batryticatus) disperse wind-heat accumulation in the head. *Xuan Shen* (Radix Scrophulariae), *Ma Bo* (Lasiosphaera seu Calvatia), and *Ban Lan Gen* (Radix Isatidis) clear heat and eliminate toxin. *Xuan Shen* (Radix Scrophulariae) also prevents the heat-clearing, damp-drying herbs from injuring yin. *Jie Geng* (Radix Platycodonis) and *Gan Cao* (Radix et Rhizoma Glycyrrhizae) synergistically relieve sore throat, thus helping the heat-clearing herbs. *Chen Pi* (Pericarpium Citri Reticulatae) regulates qi circulation to reduce swelling and inflammation. *Sheng Ma* (Rhizoma Cimicifugae) and *Chai Hu* (Radix Bupleuri), in addition to dispersing wind-heat, guide the other herbs upward to the head region where the condition is most critical. Finally, *Ren Shen* (Radix et Rhizoma Ginseng) tonifies qi, and prevents the bitter and cold heat-clearing herbs from damaging the body. Note: *Ren Shen* (Radix et Rhizoma Ginseng) may be removed from the formula when prescribed for individuals without underlying deficiencies.

MODIFICATIONS

- With constipation, add *Da Huang* (Radix et Rhizoma Rhei).
- If the heat and toxin are severe, add *Jin Yin Hua* (Flos Lonicerae Japonicae) and *Pu Gong Ying* (Herba Taraxaci).
- With headache, add *Qiang Huo* (Rhizoma et Radix Notopterygii).
- If there are more exterior symptoms, remove *Huang Qin* (Radix Scutellariae) and add *Jing Jie* (Herba Schizonepetae),

Pu Ji Xiao Du Yin (Universal Benefit Decoction to Eliminate Toxin)

Diagnosis	Signs and Symptoms	Treatment	Herbs
Da tou wen (swollen head epidemic)	• Fever and aversion to cold: exterior wind-heat • Redness, swelling and pain of the face and head, red and swollen eyes, difficulty in opening the eyes, and a sore throat: wind, heat and toxin invade the head region • Thirst: heat consuming body fluids • Dry, red tongue and yellow tongue coating: presence of heat and toxin • Rapid, forceful pulse: excess condition	• Clears heat and eliminates toxin • Dispels wind and disperses pathogenic factors	• *Huang Qin* (Radix Scutellariae) and *Huang Lian* (Rhizoma Coptidis) clear heat and eliminate toxin from the head. • *Niu Bang Zi* (Fructus Arctii), *Lian Qiao* (Fructus Forsythiae), *Bo He* (Herba Menthae), and *Jiang Can* (Bombyx Batryticatus) disperse wind-heat accumulation from the head. • *Xuan Shen* (Radix Scrophulariae), *Ma Bo* (Lasiosphaera seu Calvatia), and *Ban Lan Gen* (Radix Isatidis) clear heat and eliminate toxin. • *Jie Geng* (Radix Platycodonis) and *Gan Cao* (Radix et Rhizoma Glycyrrhizae) synergistically relieve sore throat. • *Chen Pi* (Pericarpium Citri Reticulatae) regulates qi circulation to reduce swelling and inflammation. • *Sheng Ma* (Rhizoma Cimicifugae) and *Chai Hu* (Radix Bupleuri) guide the other herbs upward to the head region. • *Ren Shen* (Radix et Rhizoma Ginseng) tonifies qi, and prevents the bitter and cold heat-clearing herbs from damaging the body.

Chinese Herbal Formulas and Applications

Pǔ Jì Xiāo Dú Yǐn (Universal Benefit Decoction to Eliminate Toxin)

Fang Feng (Radix Saposhnikoviae), *Chan Tui* (Periostracum Cicadae) and *Sang Ye* (Folium Mori).

- If the interior heat is severe, remove *Chai Hu* (Radix Bupleuri) and *Bo He* (Herba Menthae), and add *Jin Yin Hua* (Flos Lonicerae Japonicae) and *Qing Dai* (Indigo Naturalis), or *Shi Gao* (Gypsum Fibrosum) and *Huang Bo* (Cortex Phellodendri Chinensis).
- For nodules that are hard and difficult to reduce in size, add *Mu Dan Pi* (Cortex Moutan), *Bei Mu* (Bulbus Fritillariae), *Chi Shao* (Radix Paeoniae Rubra), *Si Gua Luo* (Retinervus Luffae Fructus) and *Xia Ku Cao* (Spica Prunellae).
- For patients who are unresponsive to antibiotic drugs or have a stubborn infection, add *Feng Wei Cao* (Herba Pteris), *Zi Hua Di Ding* (Herba Violae), *Hu Yao Huang* (Herba Leucas Mollissimae), and *Da Ding Huang* (Caulis Euonymi).

CAUTIONS / CONTRAINDICATIONS

- *Pu Ji Xiao Du Yin* should be used with caution in patients with deficiencies of yin or body fluids, because this formula is bitter, cold, acrid and dispersing in nature.
- Avoid foods that are pungent, spicy, oily or greasy while taking this formula.[1]

PHARMACOLOGICAL EFFECTS

Antibiotic: Numerous herbs in *Pu Ji Xiao Du Yin* have shown marked *in vitro* and *in vivo* antibacterial and antiviral effects.[2]

CLINICAL STUDIES AND RESEARCH

1. **Epidemic hemorrhagic fever**: Administration of *Pu Ji Xiao Du Yin* was associated with improving the condition of 435 patients with epidemic hemorrhagic fever. The formula was described to be effective in reducing fever, preventing shock, relieving dysuria and anuria, and improving the overall treatment outcome.[3]
2. **Infectious parotitis**: Modified *Pu Ji Xiao Du Yin* was used successfully in treating 90 children with infectious parotitis (21 cases were diagnosed as wind-heat and 69 as accumulation of heat and toxin). According to the study, the average time was 2.8 days for the reduction of fever (ranging from 1-8 days) and 3.7 days for swelling of the parotid glands (ranging from 2-9 days).[4] Another study reported good results using modified *Pu Ji Xiao Du Yin* to treat all 100 patients (64 males and 36 females) with infectious parotitis. The study reported that more than 77% of patients had complete recovery within 4 days. The herbal treatment reduced the average duration of illness by 3-5 days.[5]
3. **Respiratory tract infection**: Modified *Pu Ji Xiao Du Yin* was used as an herbal decoction one time daily to treat 35 children with respiratory tract infections and high fever (>39°C / 102.2°F). Within 96 hours, 30 out of 35 patients experienced reduction of fever and other symptoms. The rate of effectiveness was 85.7%. The herbal formula contained *Huang Qin* (Radix Scutellariae), *Huang Lian* (Rhizoma Coptidis), *Ban Lan Gen* (Radix Isatidis), *Lian Qiao* (Fructus Forsythiae), *Sheng Ma* (Rhizoma Cimicifugae), *Ma Bo* (Lasiosphaera seu Calvatia), *Jie Geng* (Radix Platycodonis), *Xuan Shen* (Radix Scrophulariae), *Bo He* (Herba Menthae), *Niu Bang Zi* (Fructus Arctii), *Jiang Can* (Bombyx Batryticatus), *Chai Hu* (Radix Bupleuri), *Chen Pi* (Pericarpium Citri Reticulatae) and *Gan Cao* (Radix et Rhizoma Glycyrrhizae).[6]
4. **Myocarditis**: Modified *Pu Ji Xiao Du Yin* was used to treat 48 patients with acute viral myocarditis characterized by chest pain, tachypnea, feeling of oppression in the chest, palpitations, fever, headache, cough, sore throat, abdominal pain and diarrhea. The herbal decoction was administered one time daily for 15 days per course of treatment. The study reported that out of 48 patients, 16 had complete recovery, 28 showed marked improvement, and 4 showed no change.[7]
5. **Tonsillitis**: Use of modified *Pu Ji Xiao Du Yin* in decoction successfully treated acute suppurative tonsillitis. The herbal formula contained the following ingredients: *Jin Yin Hua* (Flos Lonicerae Japonicae) 15g, *Lian Qiao* (Fructus Forsythiae) 9g, *Ge Gen* (Radix Puerariae Lobatae) 9g, *Ban Lan Gen* (Radix Isatidis) 12g, *Shan Dou Gen* (Radix et Rhizoma Sophorae Tonkinensis) 9g, *Ma Bo* (Lasiosphaera seu Calvatia) 9g, *Jie Geng* (Radix Platycodonis) 9g, *Xuan Shen* (Radix Scrophulariae) 12g, *Shi Gao* (Gypsum Fibrosum) 30g, *Zhu Ye* (Herba Phyllostachys) 9g, and *Gan Cao* (Radix et Rhizoma Glycyrrhizae) 3g. The dosage was one pack of herbs daily for children 6 years of age or younger, and 3 packs of herbs in two days for children 7 years or older. The herbs were cooked in water to obtain 150 mL of decoction, and taken in two to three equally-divided doses. Of 57 patients with acute suppurative tonsillitis, 88% had normal body temperature within 3 days along with resolution of other signs and symptoms.[8]
6. **Conjunctivitis**: One study reported good results using *Pu Ji Xiao Du Yin* to treat acute conjunctivitis in 164 patients (306 affected eyes). The herbal formula contained *Huang Qin* (Radix Scutellariae), *Huang Lian* (Rhizoma Coptidis), *Chen Pi* (Pericarpium Citri Reticulatae), *Xuan Shen* (Radix Scrophulariae), *Chai Hu* (Radix Bupleuri), *Lian Qiao* (Fructus Forsythiae), *Ban Lan Gen* (Radix Isatidis), *Ma Bo* (Lasiosphaera seu Calvatia), *Niu Bang Zi* (Fructus Arctii), *Bo He* (Herba Menthae), *Jiang Can* (Bombyx Batryticatus), and *Sheng Ma* (Rhizoma Cimicifugae). *Chi Shao* (Radix Paeoniae Rubra) and *Chuan Xiong* (Rhizoma Chuanxiong) were added for early-stage conjunctivitis,

HEAT-CLEARING FORMULAS

Chapter 5 – Heat-Clearing Formulas   *Section 4 – Heat-Clearing and Toxin-Eliminating Formulas*

Pŭ Jì Xiāo Dú Yĭn (Universal Benefit Decoction to Eliminate Toxin)

and *Di Huang* (Radix Rehmanniae) and *Mu Dan Pi* (Cortex Moutan) were added for ocular bleeding. The herbs were given in decoction form daily. The study reported 98.7% effectiveness among 164 patients, with an average of 2.5 days to recovery.[9]

7. **Erysipelas:** One study reported 94.2% effectiveness in treating 52 patients with erysipelas with 2 weeks to 3 years of history of illness. The herbs were decocted, and their residue was applied topically to the affected area. Of 52 cases, the study reported complete recovery in 41 cases, improvement in 8 cases, and no effect in 3 cases.[10]

RELATED FORMULA

Dà Qīng Tāng (Isatis Decoction)

大青湯
大青汤

Pinyin Name: *Da Qing Tang*
Literal Name: Isatis Decoction
Original Source: Guang An Men Yi Yuan (Guang An Men Hospital) in 1990

Da Qing Ye (Folium Isatidis)
Jin Yin Hua (Flos Lonicerae Japonicae)
Chuan Xin Lian (Herba Andrographis)
Pu Gong Ying (Herba Taraxaci)
Yu Xing Cao (Herba Houttuyniae)
Hu Zhang (Rhizoma et Radix Polygoni Cuspidati)
Huang Qin (Radix Scutellariae)
Huang Lian (Rhizoma Coptidis)
Huang Bo (Cortex Phellodendri Chinensis)
Zhi Zi (Fructus Gardeniae)
Da Huang (Radix et Rhizoma Rhei)

Da Qing Tang (Isatis Decoction) uses equal amounts of the ingredients to clear any type of heat and fire in the upper, middle, and lower *jiao*s. This contemporary formula may be used to treat many different types of infectious and inflammatory disorders throughout the body.

AUTHORS' COMMENTS

Pu Ji Xiao Du Yin is one of the best herbal antibiotic formulas to treat infectious and contagious diseases. The name *Pu Ji Xiao Du Yin* literally means "Universal Benefit Decoction to Eliminate Toxin," which implies that this formula treats everyone (universal benefit) with infectious diseases (heat and toxin).

Pu Ji Xiao Du Yin and *Xian Fang Huo Ming Yin* (Sublime Formula for Sustaining Life) both clear heat and eliminate toxin.

• *Pu Ji Xiao Du Yin* treats toxic heat affecting the upper *jiao* manifesting in symptoms such as redness, swelling, and pain of the face, difficulty in opening the eyes, a sore throat, thirst, and fever. It disperses wind-heat as well as toxin lodged in the head.

• *Xian Fang Huo Ming Yin* clears heat and eliminates toxin. It also moves qi and blood to eradicate nodules, swellings, carbuncles, and sores.

References

1. *Zhong Yao Ming Fang Yao Li Yu Ying Yong* (Pharmacology and Applications of Famous Herbal Formulas) 1989;143-145.
2. Chen J, Chen T. Chinese Medical Herbology and Pharmacology. City of Industry, CA: Art of Medicine Press, 2004.
3. *Shan Xi Zhong Yi* (Shanxi Chinese Medicine) 1984;3:16.
4. *Si Chuan Zhong Yi* (Sichuan Chinese Medicine) 1990;(5):25.
5. *Zhong Yi Za Zhi* (Journal of Chinese Medicine) 1958;7:463.
6. *Guang Xi Zhong Yi Yao* (Guangxi Chinese Medicine and Herbology) 1989;(1):5.
7. *Zhong Guo Zhong Xi Yi Jie He Za Zhi* (Chinese Journal of Integrative Chinese and Western Medicine) 1993;13(4):244.
8. *Shan Dong Zhong Yi Za Zhi* (Shandong Journal of Chinese Medicine) 1984;4:42.
9. *Hei Long Jiang Zhong Yi Yao* (Heilongjiang Chinese Medicine and Herbology) 1995;2:20.
10. *Hu Bei Zhong Yi Za Zhi* (Hubei Journal of Chinese Medicine) 1989;5:11.

358

Chinese Herbal Formulas and Applications

Sān Huáng Xiè Xīn Tāng
(Three-Yellow Decoction to Sedate the Epigastrium)

三黃瀉心湯
三黄泻心汤

Pinyin Name: *San Huang Xie Xin Tang*
Literal Name: Three-Yellow Decoction to Sedate the Epigastrium
Alternate Names: *Xie Xin Tang* (Drain the Epigastrium Decoction), *San Huang Hsieh Hsin Tang*, Three-Huang Heart-Draining Decoction, Coptis and Rhubarb Combination
Original Source: *Jin Gui Yao Lue* (Essentials from the Golden Cabinet) by Zhang Zhong-Jing in the Eastern Han Dynasty

COMPOSITION

Huang Qin (Radix Scutellariae)	3g [9g]
Huang Lian (Rhizoma Coptidis)	3g
Da Huang (Radix et Rhizoma Rhei)	6g

DOSAGE / PREPARATION / ADMINISTRATION

The source text states to cook the ingredients in 3 cups [600 mL] of water and reduce it to 1 cup [200 mL]. Take the warm, strained decoction immediately. Today, use the dose of *Huang Qin* (Radix Scutellariae) suggested in brackets.

CHINESE THERAPEUTIC ACTIONS

Purges fire and dries dampness

CLINICAL MANIFESTATIONS

Damp-heat in all three *jiaos*: hemoptysis, epistaxis, jaundice, chest oppression, irritability and restlessness, red eyes, swelling and pain of eyes, tongue and mouth ulcerations, external abscesses and sores, and constipation.

CLINICAL APPLICATIONS

1. Bleeding disorders (hemoptysis, epistaxis, hemorrhoidal bleeding, intestinal bleeding, gastrointestinal bleeding, hematuria, uterine bleeding, subcutaneous bleeding).
2. Gastrointestinal disorders (gastroenteritis, stomatitis, habitual constipation, dysentery, hemorrhoids).
3. Dermatological diseases (furuncles, carbuncles, urticaria).
4. Liver and gallbladder disorders (hepatitis, jaundice).
5. Others (sleep apnea, neurasthenia, neurosis, schizophrenia, conjunctivitis, trigeminal neuralgia, arteriosclerosis, cerebrovascular accident).

EXPLANATION

San Huang Xie Xin Tang (Three-Yellow Decoction to Sedate the Epigastrium) is one of the strongest formulas for treating damp-heat accumulation throughout the body, including in the upper, middle, and/or lower *jiaos*. Heat in the blood will cause reckless movement of the blood, leading to bleeding from various parts of the body, as in hemoptysis and epistaxis. Damp-heat accumulation in the upper *jiao* causes irritability, restlessness, and a feeling of oppression in the chest. Damp-heat accumulation in the Liver causes jaundice, as well as redness, swelling, and pain of the eyes. Damp-heat accumulation in the Stomach causes a sore throat and tongue and mouth ulcerations. Damp-heat accumulation in the lower *jiao* causes constipation. Damp-heat accumulation may also affect the skin, causing abscesses and sores. Clinically, damp-heat may affect many other parts of the body, manifesting in other signs and symptoms as well.

While damp-heat causes a wide variety of complications and disorders, the treatment strategy is rather simple. Only three herbs are required to manage and treat these conditions. *Huang Qin* (Radix Scutellariae), bitter and cold, enters the upper *jiao* to clear heat, purge fire, and dry dampness. *Huang Lian* (Rhizoma Coptidis), bitter and cold, enters the middle *jiao* to clear heat, purge fire, and dry dampness. *Da Huang* (Radix et Rhizoma Rhei), bitter and cold, enters the lower *jiao* to clear heat, purge fire, and eliminate toxins. All three herbs have a similar function of clearing damp-heat, yet they each focus on different parts of the body. The combination of these three herbs has a synergistic effect in relieving pain, stopping bleeding, reducing inflammation, and treating infection.

MODIFICATIONS

- With thirst due to dryness and heat, add *Shi Gao* (Gypsum Fibrosum) and *Zhi Mu* (Rhizoma Anemarrhenae).
- With delirium, add *Shi Chang Pu* (Rhizoma Acori Tatarinowii) and *Yu Jin* (Radix Curcumae).
- For icteric jaundice, add *Yin Chen* (Herba Artemisiae Scopariae), *Zhi Zi* (Fructus Gardeniae), and *Che Qian Cao* (Herba Plantaginis).
- With bleeding gums, add *Mang Xiao* (Natrii Sulfas).

HEAT-CLEARING FORMULAS 5

359

Sān Huáng Xiè Xīn Tāng
(Three-Yellow Decoction to Sedate the Epigastrium)

San Huang Xie Xin Tang (Three-Yellow Decoction to Sedate the Epigastrium)

Diagnosis	Signs and Symptoms	Treatment	Herbs
Damp-heat in the three *jiao*s	• Irritability, restlessness, and a feeling of chest oppression: damp-heat in the upper *jiao* • Jaundice with redness, swelling and pain of the eyes: damp-heat in the Liver (middle *jiao*) • Sore throat and ulcerations of the tongue and mouth: damp-heat in the Stomach (middle *jiao*) • Constipation: damp-heat in the lower *jiao*	Purges fire and dries dampness	• *Huang Qin* (Radix Scutellariae) enters the upper *jiao* to clear heat, purge fire, and dry dampness. • *Huang Lian* (Rhizoma Coptidis) enters the middle *jiao* to clear heat, purge fire, and dry dampness. • *Da Huang* (Radix et Rhizoma Rhei) enters the lower *jiao* to clear heat, purge fire, and eliminate toxins.

• For severe constipation, add *Mang Xiao* (Natrii Sulfas), *Zhi Shi* (Fructus Aurantii Immaturus), and *Hou Po* (Cortex Magnoliae Officinalis).

• With bleeding due to heat in the *xue* (blood) level, add *Mu Dan Pi* (Cortex Moutan) and *Di Huang* (Radix Rehmanniae).

• For severe abscesses and sores, add *Jin Yin Hua* (Flos Lonicerae Japonicae), *Lian Qiao* (Fructus Forsythiae), and *Zi Hua Di Ding* (Herba Violae).

CAUTIONS / CONTRAINDICATIONS

• *San Huang Xie Xin Tang* contains bitter and cold herbs that may damage the Spleen and Stomach. Thus, it should be discontinued when the desired effects are achieved. It should not be taken at large doses nor for a prolonged period of time.

• This formula is contraindicated during pregnancy and nursing, and in individuals with deficiency and cold of the Spleen and Stomach.[1]

PHARMACOLOGICAL EFFECTS

Gastroprotective: Use of *San Huang Xie Xin Tang* was found to have a protective effect on the gastrointestinal tract by inhibiting the gastric acid secretion via inhibition of H,K-ATPase activity. *San Huang Xie Xin Tang*, given 30 minutes earlier, has a protective effect on the gastric mucosa against drugs such as aspirin, HCL-aspirin, and ethanol. However, it was found to be ineffective against gastric lesions induced by indomethacin.[2,3]

CLINICAL STUDIES AND RESEARCH

1. **Gastrointestinal bleeding**: *San Huang Xie Xin Tang* was shown in many studies to effectively treat various types of gastrointestinal bleeding. In one study, administration of *San Huang Xie Xin Tang* in 60 patients (50 males and 10 females; between 14 and 70 years of age) was associated with treating gastrointestinal bleeding due to various causes (10 with gastritis, 35 with duodenal ulcer, 7 with gastric ulcer, and 8 with other causes). Of 60 cases, the study reported complete recovery in 50 cases, improvement in 9 cases, and voluntary discontinuation of treatment in 1 case (reason unknown).[4]

2. **Upper gastrointestinal bleeding**: Daily use of modified *San Huang Xie Xin Tang* in decoction was associated with complete recovery in 31 of 34 patients with acute and profuse bleeding from the upper gastrointestinal tract. The herbal formula contained *Da Huang* (Radix et Rhizoma Rhei) 10g, *Huang Lian* (Rhizoma Coptidis) 10g, *Huang Qin* (Radix Scutellariae) 12g, *Xian He Cao* (Herba Agrimoniae) 10g, *Ce Bai Ye* (Cacumen Platycladi) 15g, *Mu Dan Pi* (Cortex Moutan) 15g and *Xiao Ji* (Herba Cirsii) 15g. Individuals with severe loss of blood also received blood transfusions.[5]

3. **Lower gastrointestinal bleeding**: One study reported satisfactory results using modified *San Huang Xie Xin Tang* to treat 50 patients with hematochezia. The herbal formula contained *Da Huang* (Radix et Rhizoma Rhei) 15g, *Qian Cao* (Radix et Rhizoma Rubiae) 15g, *Zhi Zi* (Fructus Gardeniae) 10g, *Ou Jie* (Nodus Nelumbinis Rhizomatis) 10g, *Ce Bai Ye* (Cacumen Platycladi) 10g, *Huang Lian* (Rhizoma Coptidis) 10g, *Huang Qin* (Radix Scutellariae) 12g, and *Di Yu* (Radix Sanguisorbae) 12g. Furthermore, *Di Huang* (Radix Rehmanniae) and *Shi Hu* (Caulis Dendrobii) were added for individuals with a desire to drink water. Of 50 cases, the study reported complete recovery in 45 cases, improvement in 4 cases, and no change in 1 case.[6]

4. **Sleep apnea**: A 76-year-old male with obstructive sleep apnea syndrome was successfully treated with *San Huang Xie Xin Tang*. Polysomnography, performed before and after herbal treatment, showed a significant reduction in both the apnea index and the apnea plus hypopnea index.

Chinese Herbal Formulas and Applications

Sān Huáng Xiè Xīn Tāng
(Three-Yellow Decoction to Sedate the Epigastrium)

The mechanism for successful treatment of sleep apnea was attributed to alleviating upper airway resistance during sleep.[7]

AUTHORS' COMMENTS

Huang Lian Jie Du Tang (Coptis Decoction to Relieve Toxicity) and *San Huang Xie Xin Tang* both clear heat and eliminate toxins.

• *Huang Lian Jie Du Tang* clears heat and eliminates toxins from all three *jiaos*.

• *Xie Xin Tang*, with the addition of *Da Huang* (Radix et Rhizoma Rhei), has a purgative action in addition to its heat-clearing and detoxifying effects; therefore, it is more suitable for patients who have constipation caused by accumulation of heat and toxins.

References

1. *Zhong Yao Ming Fang Yao Li Yu Ying Yong* (Pharmacology and Applications of Famous Herbal Formulas) 1989;139-141.
2. Lin WC, Tan TW. The role of gastric muscle relaxation in cytoprotection induced by San-Huang-Xie-Xin-Tang in rats. J Ethnopharmacol 1994 Dec;44(3):171-9.
3. Satoh K, Nagai F, Seto T, Yamauchi H. The effects of kampo-formulation and the constituting crude drugs, prescribed for the treatment of peptic ulcer on H,K-ATPase activity. Yakugaku Zasshi 2001 Feb;121(2):173-8.
4. *Guang Xi Zhong Yi Yao* (Guangxi Chinese Medicine and Herbology) 1985;3(18).
5. *Yun Nan Zhong Yi Xue Yuan Xue Bao* (Journal of Yunnan University School of Medicine) 1996;4:38.
6. *Xin Zhong Yi* (New Chinese Medicine) 1997;6:46.
7. Hisanaga A, Saitoh O, Fukuda H, Kurokawa K, Okabe A, Tachibana H, Hagino H, Mita T, Yamashita I, Tsutsumi M, Kurachi M, Itoh T. Treatment of obstructive sleep apnea syndrome with a Kampo-formula, San'o-shashin-to: a case report. Psychiatry & Clinical Neurosciences 1999 Apr;53(2):303-5.

Sān Huáng Shí Gāo Tāng (Three-Yellow and Gypsum Decoction)
三黃石膏湯
三黄石膏汤

Pinyin Name: *San Huang Shi Gao Tang*
Literal Name: Three-Yellow and Gypsum Decoction
Alternate Name: Gypsum Coptis and Scute Combination
Original Source: *Wai Ke Zheng Zhi Zhun Sheng* (Standards of Patterns and Treatments in External Medicine) by Wang Ken-Tang in the Ming Dynasty

COMPOSITION

Huang Qin (Radix Scutellariae)	4.5g
Huang Lian (Rhizoma Coptidis)	6g
Huang Bo (Cortex Phellodendri Chinensis)	3g
Zhi Zi (Fructus Gardeniae)	3g
Shi Gao (Gypsum Fibrosum)	9g
Zhi Mu (Rhizoma Anemarrhenae)	4.5g
Xuan Shen (Radix Scrophulariae)	3g
Gan Cao (Radix et Rhizoma Glycyrrhizae)	2.1g

DOSAGE / PREPARATION / ADMINISTRATION

Prepare the ingredients as a decoction.

CHINESE THERAPEUTIC ACTIONS

Clears heat and eliminates toxins

CLINICAL MANIFESTATIONS

Interior heat and toxins: delirium, incoherent speech, irritability, thirst, constipation, and dysuria.

CLINICAL APPLICATIONS

Acute febrile diseases, measles, and various bleeding disorders.

EXPLANATION

San Huang Shi Gao Tang (Three-Yellow and Gypsum Decoction) treats heat and toxins located deep in the interior. When heat and toxins affect the Heart, they cause irritability. They may also affect the *shen* (spirit), leading

HEAT-CLEARING FORMULAS

5

361

Sān Huáng Shí Gāo Tāng (Three-Yellow and Gypsum Decoction)

San Huang Shi Gao Tang (Three-Yellow and Gypsum Decoction)

Diagnosis	Signs and Symptoms	Treatment	Herbs
Presence of heat and toxins in the interior	• Irritability, delirium and incoherent speech: heat and toxins affecting the Heart and disturbing the *shen* (spirit) • Thirst, constipation and dysuria: heat and toxins consuming body fluids	Clears heat and eliminates toxins	• *Huang Qin* (Radix Scutellariae), *Huang Lian* (Rhizoma Coptidis), *Huang Bo* (Cortex Phellodendri Chinensis) and *Zhi Zi* (Fructus Gardeniae) clear heat and eliminate toxins in all three *jiaos*. • *Shi Gao* (Gypsum Fibrosum) and *Zhi Mu* (Rhizoma Anemarrhenae) clear heat and promote the generation of fluids. • *Xuan Shen* (Radix Scrophulariae) clears deficiency heat from the *ying* (nutritive) and *xue* (blood) levels. • *Gan Cao* (Radix et Rhizoma Glycyrrhizae) harmonizes the herbs.

to delirium and incoherent speech. Finally, heat and toxins may consume body fluids, leading to thirst, constipation, and dysuria.

Huang Qin (Radix Scutellariae), *Huang Lian* (Rhizoma Coptidis), and *Huang Bo* (Cortex Phellodendri Chinensis) clear heat and eliminate toxins from the upper, middle, and lower *jiaos* respectively. *Zhi Zi* (Fructus Gardeniae) is added to ensure that heat and toxins are eliminated from all three *jiaos*. *Shi Gao* (Gypsum Fibrosum) and *Zhi Mu* (Rhizoma Anemarrhenae) clear heat and promote the generation of fluids, while *Xuan Shen* (Radix Scrophulariae) clears deficiency heat from the *ying* (nutritive) and *xue* (blood) levels. *Gan Cao* (Radix et Rhizoma Glycyrrhizae) harmonizes the formula.

MODIFICATIONS
- When the heat and toxins are more pronounced, add *Jin Yin Hua* (Flos Lonicerae Japonicae) and *Lian Qiao* (Fructus Forsythiae).
- With restlessness, irritability, and thirst, increase the doses of *Zhi Mu* (Rhizoma Anemarrhenae) and *Gan Cao* (Radix et Rhizoma Glycyrrhizae).
- With irritability and thirst as a result of summer-heat, add *Gan Lu Yin* (Sweet Dew Decoction).
- For acute hepatitis, add *Yin Chen* (Herba Artemisiae Scopariae) and *Long Dan* (Radix et Rhizoma Gentianae).

RELATED FORMULA
Sān Huáng Shí Gāo Tāng
(Three-Yellow and Gypsum Decoction)

三黄石膏湯
三黄石膏汤

Pinyin Name: *San Huang Shi Gao Tang*
Literal Name: Three-Yellow and Gypsum Decoction
Original Source: *Shang Han Liu Shu* (Six Texts on Cold-Induced Disorders) by Tao Hua in 1445

Huang Lian (Rhizoma Coptidis)	[3-6g]
Huang Qin (Radix Scutellariae)	[3-6g]
Huang Bo (Cortex Phellodendri Chinensis)	[3-6g]
Zhi Zi (Fructus Gardeniae)	[3-6g]
Ma Huang (Herba Ephedrae)	[3-6g]
Shi Gao (Gypsum Fibrosum)	[6-12g]
Dan Dou Chi (Semen Sojae Praeparatum)	[3-6g]
Sheng Jiang (Rhizoma Zingiberis Recens)	[3-6g]
Da Zao (Fructus Jujubae)	[2-5g]
Cha Ye (Folium Camelliae)	[2-5g]

This formula treats heat and toxins in the interior, with residual exterior conditions. Therefore, in addition to the heat-clearing herbs, this formula contains exterior-releasing herbs to dispel the exterior pathogenic factors, such as *Ma Huang* (Herba Ephedrae), *Dan Dou Chi* (Semen Sojae Praeparatum), *Sheng Jiang* (Rhizoma Zingiberis Recens), and *Cha Ye* (Folium Camelliae)

These two formulas have the exact same name, but are derived from different source texts and have slightly different herbs and functions.
- *San Huang Shi Gao Tang* from *Wai Ke Zheng Zhi Zhun Sheng* (Standards of Patterns and Treatments in External Medicine) treats heat and toxins located deep in the interior, without any exterior conditions.
- *San Huang Shi Gao Tang* from *Shang Han Liu Shu* (Six Texts on Cold-Induced Disorders) treats heat and toxins in the interior with residual exterior conditions.

AUTHORS' COMMENTS
According to Dr. Chang Wei-Yen, *San Huang Shi Gao Tang* can be combined with *Wen Qing Yin* (Warming and Clearing Decoction) to treat various dermatological disorders ranging from rashes or itching, to dermatitis and eczema caused by dryness.

Chinese Herbal Formulas and Applications

Liù Shén Wán (Six-Miracle Pill)

六神丸
六神丸

Pinyin Name: *Liu Shen Wan*
Literal Name: Six-Miracle Pill
Original Source: *Gu Jin Ming Fang* (Famous Classic and Contemporary Formulas) by Luo Mei in 1675

COMPOSITION

Chan Su (Venenum Bufonis)	3g
Niu Huang (Calculus Bovis)	4.5g
Xiong Huang (Realgar)	3g
She Xiang (Moschus)	4.5g
Bing Pian (Borneolum Syntheticum)	3g
Zhen Zhu (Margarita)	4.5g

Note: *Xiong Huang* (Realgar) is a potentially toxic heavy metal, and *She Xiang* (Moschus) is derived from an endangered animal. Both are rarely used as medicinal substances today. The discussion here is included primarily for academic purposes, to reflect the historical use of these substances in their original formulations. Most herbal products today have removed them completely, or replaced them with substitutes with similar functions. For additional information on the toxicity, please refer to *Chinese Medical Herbology and Pharmacology* by John Chen and Tina Chen.

DOSAGE / PREPARATION / ADMINISTRATION

The source text states to grind all substances into a fine powder. Dissolve *Chan Su* (Venenum Bufonis) in a grain-based liquor, and then add in the remaining powdered herbs to form pills. The pills should resemble *Bai Jie Zi* (Semen Sinapis) in size, and should be coated with *Bai Cao Shuang* (Pulvis Fumi Carbonisatus). Take 5-10 pills per day, two to three times daily. This formula may also be used topically.

CHINESE THERAPEUTIC ACTIONS

1. Clears heat and eliminates toxins
2. Reduces inflammation and relieves pain

CLINICAL MANIFESTATIONS

Presence of heat and toxins: unilateral or bilateral pustular tonsillitis, a sore and swollen throat and difficulty in swallowing, diphtheria, stomatitis, high fever with convulsions in infants, and throat cancer. It is also used for sores, abscesses, cellulitis, and various skin disorders.

CLINICAL APPLICATIONS

Herpes zoster, tonsillitis, pharyngitis, sore and swollen throat, throat cancer, diphtheria, stomatitis, chronic hepatitis, septicemia, angina, nephritis, leukemia, vaginitis, lymphangitis, mastitis, appendicitis, otitis media, periodontitis, and pulpitis.

EXPLANATION

Liu Shen Wan (Six-Miracle Pill) treats patterns of heat and toxins characterized by inflammation and pain. Internally, it is used for conditions such as tonsillitis, a sore and swollen throat, diphtheria, stomatitis, and throat cancer. Externally, it may be used to treat various types of dermatological disorders, such as sores, abscesses, cellulitis, and various skin disorders.

Chan Su (Venenum Bufonis), *Niu Huang* (Calculus Bovis), and *Xiong Huang* (Realgar) clear heat and eliminate toxins. *She Xiang* (Moschus) invigorates blood circulation and opens the channels and collaterals to assist the other herbs in clearing heat and eliminating toxins. *Bing Pian* (Borneolum Syntheticum) clears heat and relieves itching and pain. *She Xiang* (Moschus), *Chan Su* (Venenum Bufonis), and *Bing Pian* (Borneolum Syntheticum) also enhance the effects of the other herbs to clear heat and eliminate toxins. *Zhen Zhu* (Margarita) promotes healing and relieves itching.

CAUTIONS / CONTRAINDICATIONS

- *Liu Shen Wan* contains many potentially toxic herbs, such as *Chan Su* (Venenum Bufonis) and *Xiong Huang* (Realgar). Therefore, it is contraindicated during pregnancy and must be used with caution in individuals with underlying weakness and deficiency.
- While taking this herbal formula, refrain from smoking and drinking alcohol, and do not consume foods that are pungent or spicy.[1]

Chapter 5 – Heat-Clearing Formulas   *Section 4 – Heat-Clearing and Toxin-Eliminating Formulas*

Liù Shén Wán (Six-Miracle Pill)

Liu Shen Wan (Six-Miracle Pill)

Diagnosis	Signs and Symptoms	Treatment	Herbs
Presence of heat and toxins	• Tonsillitis, sore and swollen throat, diphtheria and stomatitis: presence of heat and toxins in the interior • Abscesses and sores: heat and toxins at the exterior	• Clears heat and eliminates toxins • Reduces inflammation and relieves pain	• *Chan Su* (Venenum Bufonis), *Niu Huang* (Calculus Bovis) and *Xiong Huang* (Realgar) clear heat and eliminate toxins. • *She Xiang* (Moschus) invigorates blood circulation and opens the channels and collaterals. • *Bing Pian* (Borneolum Syntheticum) clears heat and relieves itching and pain. • *Zhen Zhu* (Margarita) promotes healing and relieves itching.

CLINICAL STUDIES AND RESEARCH

1. **Herpes zoster**: Fifty-four patients with herpes zoster were successfully treated using topical application of *Liu Shen Wan*. The treatment protocol was to blend *Liu Shen Wan* with rice vinegar into an herbal paste, which was applied topically to the affected area three times daily. Of 54 patients, 31 had complete recovery within 1 day, 18 within 2 days, 4 within 3 days, and 1 after 4 days. None of the patients experienced post-herpetic neuralgia. No side effects were reported.[2] According to another study, *Liu Shen Wan* was used both internally and externally to treat 32 patients with herpes zoster. The treatment protocol was to ingest 10 pills twice daily for 6-8 days. The topical preparation was made by crushing the pills into a powder and then mixing it with essential oils to make an herbal paste. The herbal paste was applied to the affected area two to three times daily for 3-5 days. Lastly, vitamins B$_1$ and B$_{12}$ were also given via intramuscular injection. Of 32 cases, the study reported complete recovery in 18 cases within 3 days, 10 cases within 4 days, 3 cases within 5 days, and 1 case after 6 days.[3]

2. **Tonsillitis**: Topical application of a modified *Liu Shen Wan* was associated with 95.1% effectiveness in treating tonsillitis in 32 patients. The herbs were prepared by crushing 10 pills of *Liu Shen Wan* and one *Quan Xie* (Scorpio) into a powder, and then mixing it with rice vinegar to make a paste. The herbal paste was applied topically to the affected area for 12 hours per course of treatment. Of 32 patients, 23 had significant improvement within 24 hours, and 7 after 48 hours.[4]

3. **Others**: This formula has also been used to treat chronic hepatitis, septicemia, angina, nephritis, leukemia, cancer, vaginitis, pharyngitis, lymphangitis, mastitis, appendicitis, otitis media, diptheria, periodontitis, and pulpitis.

TOXICOLOGY

Use of *Liu Shen Wan* has been associated with itching, restlessness, irritability, pallor, nausea, vomiting, cold extremities, palpitations, sedation, dyspnea and chest congestion. Overdose may cause nausea, vomiting, diarrhea, abdominal pain, gastrointestinal irritation, dyspnea, respiratory depression, sedation, weak pulse, bradycardia, an irregular heartbeat, yellow discoloration of the skin, and general symptoms of dryness.[5] Note: These reactions are usually attributed to *Chan Su* (Venenum Bufonis) and *Xiong Huang* (Realgar), two substances that are considered potentially toxic.

References

1. *Zhong Yao Ming Fang Yao Li Yu Ying Yong* (Pharmacology and Applications of Famous Herbal Formulas) 1989;149-151.
2. *Xin Yi Xue* (New Medicine) 1991;1:598.
3. *Xin Jiang Zhong Yi Yao* (Xinjiang Chinese Medicine and Herbology) 1999;2:19.
4. *Jiang Su Zhong Yi* (Jiangsu Chinese Medicine) 1994;4:166.
5. *Zhong Yao Bu Liang Fan Ying Yu Zhi Liao* (Adverse Reactions and Treatment of Chinese Herbal Medicine) 1996;46.

Chinese Herbal Formulas and Applications

Section 5

清脏腑热剂
— Zang Fu-Clearing Formulas

HEAT-CLEARING FORMULAS

5

Dǎo Chi Sǎn (Guide Out the Red Powder)

導赤散
导赤散

Pinyin Name: *Dao Chi San*
Literal Name: Guide Out the Red Powder
Alternate Names: *Tao Chih San*, Fire-Inducing Powder, Rehmannia and Akebia Formula
Original Source: *Xiao Er Yao Zheng Zhi Jue* (Craft of Medicinal Treatment for Childhood Disease Patterns) by Qian Yi in 1119

COMPOSITION

Mu Tong (Caulis Akebiae)	[6g]
Di Huang (Radix Rehmanniae)	[6g]
Gan Cao (Radix et Rhizoma Glycyrrhizae)	[6g]

DOSAGE / PREPARATION / ADMINISTRATION

The source text recommends to grind equal amounts of the ingredients into powder. Cook 9g of the powder with *Zhu Ye* (Herba Phyllostachys) in one large bowl of water until half of the liquid remains. Take the warm decoction after meals. Today, this formula may be prepared as a decoction with the doses suggested in brackets.

CHINESE THERAPEUTIC ACTIONS

1. Clears the Heart and nourishes yin
2. Promotes urination and relieves *lin zheng* (dysuria syndrome)

CLINICAL MANIFESTATIONS

Excess fire in the Heart channel: fidgeting, irritability, warm sensations in the chest, thirst, a red face, a desire to drink cold water, and mouth and tongue ulcerations. If the heat migrates from the Heart to the Small Intestine channel, dark-colored urine, hematuria or dysuria will occur.

CLINICAL APPLICATIONS

Urinary tract infection, dysuria, urethritis, cystitis, glomerulonephritis, herpes zoster, oral herpes, stomatitis, oral cavity infection, infectious parotitis, and infertility.

EXPLANATION

Dao Chi San (Guide Out the Red Powder) is a representative formula for treating excess fire in the Heart and Small Intestine channels. The Heart is the organ that houses the mind. If the Heart is attacked by heat, fidgeting, irritability and warm sensations in the chest may occur. A red face and a desire to drink cold water result from an exuberance of heat traveling upwards. The tongue is the sensory organ of the Heart, therefore excess fire in the Heart channel may cause mouth and tongue ulcerations. The Small Intestine has a yin/yang, exterior/interior relationship with the Heart; consequently, heat in the Heart may migrate to and affect the Small Intestine. As a result, urination disorders such as dysuria, dark-colored urine, or hematuria occur.

To effectively treat this heat syndrome, the Heart fire must be cleared and urination promoted to guide the heat downward and out of the body. The chief herb in this formula, *Mu Tong* (Caulis Akebiae) sedates Heart fire, promotes urination to lead heat out of the body, and relieves dysuria. *Di Huang* (Radix Rehmanniae) clears heat and nourishes yin. Together, they clear heat without damaging yin, and nourish yin without retaining heat. *Zhu Ye* (Herba Phyllostachys) clears Heart fire and relieves

365

Dǎo Chì Sǎn (Guide Out the Red Powder)

Dao Chi San (Guide Out the Red Powder)

Diagnosis	Signs and Symptoms	Treatment	Herbs
Excess fire in the Heart and/or Small Intestine channels	• Fidgeting and irritability: heat attacking Heart and disturbing *shen* (spirit) • Thirst with a desire to drink cold water: heat consuming body fluids • Red face and mouth and tongue ulcerations: excess fire rising upward • Dysuria with dark-colored urine: excess fire affecting the Heart and Small Intestine	• Clears the Heart and nourishes yin • Promotes urination and relieves *lin zheng* (dysuria syndrome)	• *Mu Tong* (Caulis Akebiae) sedates fire from the Heart and Small Intestine. • *Di Huang* (Radix Rehmanniae) clears heat and nourishes yin. • *Zhu Ye* (Herba Phyllostachys) clears Heart fire and relieves fidgeting and irritability. • *Gan Cao* (Radix et Rhizoma Glycyrrhizae) clears heat and eliminates toxins

fidgeting and irritability. *Gan Cao* (Radix et Rhizoma Glycyrrhizae) clears heat, eliminates toxins, and prevents the cold tendency of *Di Huang* (Radix Rehmanniae) and *Mu Tong* (Caulis Akebiae) from injuring the Stomach.

MODIFICATIONS

• With irritability and heat in the chest, add *Huang Lian* (Rhizoma Coptidis) and *Huang Qin* (Radix Scutellariae).
• For *xue lin* (bloody dysuria), add *Mo Han Lian* (Herba Ecliptae), *Xiao Ji* (Herba Cirsii), *Hou Po* (Cortex Magnoliae Officinalis), and *Qu Mai* (Herba Dianthi).
• For *re lin* (heat dysuria) characterized by frequent and painful urination, add *Feng Wei Cao* (Herba Pteris), *Bai Mao Gen* (Rhizoma Imperatae), *Shi Wei* (Folium Pyrrosiae), *Che Qian Zi* (Semen Plantaginis), and *Chi Fu Ling* (Poria Rubra).
• With fever and thirst, add *Hua Shi* (Talcum) and *Shi Gao* (Gypsum Fibrosum).
• With stomatitis and ulcerations in the mouth, add *Jin Yin Hua* (Flos Lonicerae Japonicae), *Lian Qiao* (Fructus Forsythiae), and *Huang Lian* (Rhizoma Coptidis).
• When there is cystitis, add *Huang Qin* (Radix Scutellariae), *Deng Xin Cao* (Medulla Junci), and *Zhi Zi* (Fructus Gardeniae).
• For infants who cry and cannot sleep at night, add *Zhen Zhu Mu* (Concha Margaritiferae) and *Gou Teng* (Ramulus Uncariae cum Uncis).
• With severe edema, combine with *Wu Ling San* (Five-Ingredient Powder with Poria).
• For exanthema maculosum, add *Sheng Ma* (Rhizoma Cimicifugae), *Huang Lian* (Rhizoma Coptidis), and *Mu Dan Pi* (Cortex Moutan).

CAUTIONS / CONTRAINDICATIONS

• *Dao Chi San* should be used with caution in patients with Stomach and Spleen deficiencies because most herbs

in this formula are cold and may damage the digestive tract.
• This formula may not be appropriate for individuals with repetitive stomatitis.
• Avoid foods that are pungent, spicy, oily or greasy while taking this herbal formula.[1]

CLINICAL STUDIES AND RESEARCH

1. **Urinary tract infection**: In one clinical trial, 95 out of 100 patients with urinary tract infection were treated successfully with *Dao Chi San*. Five women who did not respond were later determined to have mycotic infection.[2]

2. ***Lin zheng* (dysuria syndrome)**: Administration of modified *Dao Chi San* to 14 patients with *lin zheng* (dysuria syndrome) was associated with complete recovery in 10 cases, improvement in 2 cases, and no effect in 2 cases. The herbal treatment contained *Dao Chi San* plus *Jin Yin Hua* (Flos Lonicerae Japonicae), *Tu Fu Ling* (Rhizoma Smilacis Glabrae), *Dan Zhu Ye* (Herba Lophatheri), and *Zhi Zi* (Fructus Gardeniae) as the base formula, with the addition of *Qing Hao* (Herba Artemisiae Annuae) and *Chai Hu* (Radix Bupleuri) for fever; *Huo Xiang* (Herba Agastaches) and *Ban Xia* (Rhizoma Pinelliae) for nausea and vomiting; *Bai Mao Gen* (Rhizoma Imperatae) and a larger dose of *Zhi Zi* (Fructus Gardeniae) for hematuria; and *Che Qian Zi* (Semen Plantaginis) for edema.[3]

3. **Oral herpes**: Thirty patients with stomatitis due to oral herpes were treated with modified *Dao Chi San* with marked success. The herbal treatment used *Dao Chi San* as the base formula, with the addition of *Huang Lian* (Rhizoma Coptidis) and *Mai Dong* (Radix Ophiopogonis) for irritability, thirst and red tongue tip; and *Da Huang* (Radix et Rhizoma Rhei) and *Huang Qin* (Radix Scutellariae) for constipation. Out of 30 cases, the study reported marked improvement in 20 cases (within 2 days), moderate improvement in 8 cases (within 3 days), and no improvement in 2 cases.[4]

Dǎo Chì Sǎn (Guide Out the Red Powder)

4. **Herpes zoster**: Use of modified *Dao Chi San* was associated with 100% effectiveness in treating all 12 patients with herpes zoster affecting various parts of the body (rib cage, hypochondrium, lower back, abdominal area, and legs). The herbal formula contained *Dao Chi San* plus *Xi Xin* (Radix et Rhizoma Asari), *Jin Yin Hua* (Flos Lonicerae Japonicae), and *Lian Qiao* (Fructus Forsythiae). Furthermore, *Chai Hu* (Radix Bupleuri) was added for herpes zoster affecting the upper body, and *Niu Xi* (Radix Achyranthis Bidentatae) for lower body. Of 12 patients, 5 patients recovered within 3-4 packs of herbs, and 7 after 6-8 packs of herbs.[5]

5. **Infectious parotitis**: Twenty-four patients with infectious parotitis (mumps) were treated with an herbal decoction with complete recovery in all cases. The herbal formula incorporated *Dao Chi San* with *Lian Qiao* (Fructus Forsythiae), *Huang Bo* (Cortex Phellodendri Chinensis), *Zhi Mu* (Rhizoma Anemarrhenae), *Hua Shi* (Talcum), *Ban Lan Gen* (Radix Isatidis), *Da Qing Ye* (Folium Isatidis), *Jin Yin Hua* (Flos Lonicerae Japonicae), *Dan Zhu Ye* (Herba Lophatheri), and *Zhi Zi* (Fructus Gardeniae). The duration of treatment ranged from 1 to 4 packs of herbs.[6]

6. **Infertility**: One study reported 93.35% effectiveness using modified *Dao Chi San* to treat 43 cases of male infertility caused by chronic prostatitis or seminal vesiculitis. The herbal formula contained *Di Huang* (Radix Rehmanniae) 30g, *Chi Shao* (Radix Paeoniae Rubra) 50g, *Fu Ling* (Poria) 15g, *Mu Tong* (Caulis Akebiae) 10g, *Ze Xie* (Rhizoma Alismatis) 10g, *Huang Bo* (Cortex Phellodendri Chinensis) 6g, *Dan Zhu Ye* (Herba Lophatheri) 10g, *Mu Dan Pi* (Cortex Moutan) 10g, *Dan Shen* (Radix et Rhizoma Salviae Miltiorrhizae) 15g, *Hong Hua* (Flos Carthami) 6g, *Jin Yin Hua* (Flos Lonicerae Japonicae) 30g, and *Yu Xing Cao* (Herba Houttuyniae) 30g. Modifications included addition of *Fen Bi Xie* (Rhizoma Dioscoreae Hypoglaucae) for cloudy urine; *Xu Duan* (Radix Dipsaci) for low back pain; *Bai Shao* (Radix Paeoniae Alba) for swelling of the genital area; *Nu Zhen Zi* (Fructus Ligustri Lucidi) and *Mo Han Lian* (Herba Ecliptae) for presence of a large number of white blood cells in the seminal fluids; *Pu Gong Ying* (Herba Taraxaci) and *Hua Shi* (Talcum) for presence of pus; and *He Shou Wu* (Radix Polygoni Multiflori) and *Gou Qi Zi* (Fructus Lycii) for decreased lecithin. The treatment protocol was to administer the herbs in decoction daily for 30 days per course of treatment. All patients were instructed to avoid smoking and alcohol during the treatment period. Of 43 cases, the study reported improved physical condition in 41 cases, and successful pregnancy in 19 cases.[7]

AUTHORS' COMMENTS

The key symptoms that indicate the use of *Dao Chi San* include burning urination that is dark colored and ulcerations or sores in the mouth, especially on the tongue. These two symptoms indicate that the heat in the Heart has transferred to the Small Intestine, thereby causing urinary dysfunction.

A question is sometimes raised that if *Dao Chi San* treats excess heat and fire in the Heart, why does the formula contain *Di Huang* (Radix Rehmanniae) but not *Huang Lian* (Rhizoma Coptidis)? According to Chinese medical history, *Dao Chi San* was originally designed in the Song Dynasty to treat children with Heart fire leading to bruxism. Because this formula was intended for children, whose patterns can easily alternate between heat and cold and excess and deficiency, *Di Huang* (Radix Rehmanniae) is used as a safe, yet effective herb to clear heat and nourish yin at the same time. *Huang Lian* (Rhizoma Coptidis), on the other hand, is not as suitable for children or for conditions with underlying constitutional deficiency, because this strong heat-clearing herb may further damage yin. *Huang Lian* (Rhizoma Coptidis) would be a good alternative to clear Heart fire only if it is used in relatively healthy adults or in conditions characterized by excess Heart fire. This is why in the original formulation for the treatment of excess Heart heat and fire in children, *Di Huang* (Radix Rehmanniae) was selected for its efficacy and safety.[8]

References

1. *Zhong Yao Ming Fang Yao Li Yu Ying Yong* (Pharmacology and Applications of Famous Herbal Formulas) 1989;185-186.
2. *Guang Xi Zhong Yi Yao* (Guangxi Chinese Medicine and Herbology) 1991;(3):104.
3. *Cheng Du Zhong Yi Xue Yuan Xue Bao* (Journal of Chengdu University of Traditional Chinese Medicine) 1989;2:29.
4. *Nan Jing Zhong Yi Xue Yuan Xue Bao* (Journal of Nanjing University of Traditional Chinese Medicine) 1984;4(2):90.
5. *Zhong Yi Za Zhi* (Journal of Chinese Medicine) 1987;6:34.
6. *Shan Xi Zhong Yi* (Shanxi Chinese Medicine) 1991;(8):368.
7. *Jiang Xi Yi Xue Yuan Xue Bao* (Medical Journal of Jiangxi University of Medicine) 1993;19.
8. Wang MZ, et al. *Zhong Yi Xue Wen Da Ti Ku* (Questions and Answers on Traditional Chinese Medicine: Herbal Formulas).

Chapter 5 – Heat-Clearing Formulas   *Section 5 – Zang Fu-Clearing Formulas*

Qīng Xīn Lián Zǐ Yǐn (Lotus Seed Decoction to Clear the Heart)
清心蓮子飲
清心莲子饮

Pinyin Name: *Qing Xin Lian Zi Yin*
Literal Name: Lotus Seed Decoction to Clear the Heart
Alternate Names: *Ching Hsin Lien Tzu Yin, Ching Xin Lian Zi Yin*, Lotus Seed Drink, Lotus Seed Combination
Original Source: *Tai Ping Hui Min He Ji Ju Fang* (Imperial Grace Formulary of the Tai Ping Era) by the Imperial Medical Department in 1078-85

COMPOSITION

Lian Zi (Semen Nelumbinis)	22.5g [15g]
Mai Dong (Radix Ophiopogonis)	15g [10g]
Huang Qin (Radix Scutellariae)	15g [10g]
Di Gu Pi (Cortex Lycii)	15g [10g]
Fu Ling (Poria)	22.5g [15g]
Che Qian Zi (Semen Plantaginis)	15g [10g]
Huang Qi (Radix Astragali), *mi zhi* (fried with honey)	22.5g [15g]
Ren Shen (Radix et Rhizoma Ginseng)	22.5g [15g]
Zhi Gan Cao (Radix et Rhizoma Glycyrrhizae Praeparata cum Melle)	15g [10g]

DOSAGE / PREPARATION / ADMINISTRATION

The source text states to grind the ingredients into powder. Cook 9g of the powder in 1.5 large bowl of water until 80% of the liquid remains. Cool the strained decoction and take it before meals on an empty stomach. Today, this formula may be prepared as a decoction with the doses suggested in brackets.

CHINESE THERAPEUTIC ACTIONS

1. Clears Heart fire
2. Tonifies qi and yin
3. Treats *lin zheng* (dysuria syndrome) with turbidity

CLINICAL MANIFESTATIONS

Heart fire with qi and yin deficiencies and damp-heat in the lower *jiao*: irritability, restlessness, a dry mouth and tongue, fever; depression, physical and mental overexertion; seminal emissions, turbid urine, abnormal uterine bleeding, and leukorrhea.

CLINICAL APPLICATIONS

Nephrotic syndrome, glomerulonephritis, pyelonephritis, pyelitis, nephritis, cystitis, inflammation of the urinary tract, urinary tract infection, prostatic hypertrophy, urolithiasis, nephrolithiasis, and diabetes mellitus.

EXPLANATION

Qing Xin Lian Zi Yin (Lotus Seed Decoction to Clear the Heart) treats Heart fire with qi and yin deficiencies and damp-heat in the lower *jiao*. This complicated condition is often due to excessive worry and thinking, or excessive indulgence in alcohol and sex. As a result of either mental or physical overexertion, there is excess heat and fire disturbing the Heart, leading to symptoms such as

Qing Xin Lian Zi Yin (Lotus Seed Decoction to Clear the Heart)

Diagnosis	Signs and Symptoms	Treatment	Herbs
Heart fire with qi and yin deficiencies and damp-heat in the lower *jiao*	• Irritability, restlessness, and depression: Heart fire • Abnormal genitourinary functions: Kidney yin deficiency	• Clears Heart fire • Tonifies qi and yin • Treats *lin zheng* (dysuria syndrome) with turbidity	• *Lian Zi* (Semen Nelumbinis) and *Mai Dong* (Radix Ophiopogonis) clear heat and fire from the Heart. • *Huang Qin* (Radix Scutellariae) and *Di Gu Pi* (Cortex Lycii) clear heat and relieve thirst. • *Fu Ling* (Poria) and *Che Qian Zi* (Semen Plantaginis) dispel damp-heat and promote normal urination. • *Huang Qi* (Radix Astragali), *Ren Shen* (Radix et Rhizoma Ginseng) and *Zhi Gan Cao* (Radix et Rhizoma Glycyrrhizae Praeparata cum Melle) tonify qi and facilitate recovery.

368

Qīng Xīn Lián Zǐ Yǐn (Lotus Seed Decoction to Clear the Heart)

irritability, restlessness, and depression. Overindulgence in sex or alcohol depletes Kidney yin, causing abnormal genitourinary functions.

Lian Zi (Semen Nelumbinis) and *Mai Dong* (Radix Ophiopogonis) clear heat and fire from the Heart. *Huang Qin* (Radix Scutellariae) and *Di Gu Pi* (Cortex Lycii) clear heat and relieve thirst. *Fu Ling* (Poria) and *Che Qian Zi* (Semen Plantaginis) dispel damp-heat and promote normal urination. *Huang Qi* (Radix Astragali), *Ren Shen* (Radix et Rhizoma Ginseng), and *Zhi Gan Cao* (Radix et Rhizoma Glycyrrhizae Praeparata cum Melle) tonify qi and facilitate recovery.

MODIFICATIONS
- With prominent fire and severe deficiency, add *Zhi Mu* (Rhizoma Anemarrhenae) and *Huang Bo* (Cortex Phellodendri Chinensis).
- With fever, add *Chai Hu* (Radix Bupleuri) and *Bo He* (Herba Menthae).

CAUTIONS / CONTRAINDICATIONS
Qing Xin Lian Zi Yin is contraindicated in *lin zheng* (dysuria syndrome) or leukorrhea caused by damp-heat in the Liver and Gallbladder.

PHARMACOLOGICAL EFFECTS
Hypoglycemic: According to a clinical study, administration of *Qing Xin Lian Zi Yin* was associated with a reduction of blood glucose level in patients with non-insulin dependant diabetes mellitus (NIDDM). Out of 20 patients who participated in the study, 84.2% showed a positive effect.[1]

CLINICAL STUDIES AND RESEARCH
1. **Diabetes mellitus**: Administration of *Qing Xin Lian Zi Yin* was shown to be effective in the treatment of type II diabetes mellitus. The treatment protocol was to administer 10g of this formula in pills three times daily before meals, for 30 days per course of treatment. Of 50 cases, the study reported significant results in 21 cases, moderate results in 18 cases, and no effect in 11 cases.[2]

2. **Nephrotic syndrome**: One study reported good results using modified *Qing Xin Lian Zi Yin* to treat patients with nephrotic syndrome characterized by Kidney yin deficiency, Lung and Spleen qi deficiencies, and deficiency fire. The herbal formula contained *Di Gu Pi* (Cortex Lycii) 25g, *Huang Qin* (Radix Scutellariae) 15g, *Di Huang* (Radix Rehmanniae) 15g, *Tai Zi Shen* (Radix Pseudostellariae) 15g, *Huang Qi* (Radix Astragali) 15g, *Che Qian Zi* (Semen Plantaginis) 15g, *Mai Dong* (Radix Ophiopogonis) 12g, *Fu Ling* (Poria) 12g, *Chai Hu* (Radix Bupleuri) 10g, *Shan Zhu Yu* (Fructus Corni) 10g, *Bai Mao Gen* (Rhizoma Imperatae)

30g, *Shi Wei* (Folium Pyrrosiae) 30g, and *Gan Cao* (Radix et Rhizoma Glycyrrhizae) 6g. Additional modifications were made as needed based on the condition of the patients. The herbs were given for approximately six months to stabilize the condition.[3]

3. **Glomerulonephritis**: Administration of modified *Qing Xin Lian Zi Yin* was found to be effective in treating acute glomerulonephritis, characterized by Kidney qi and yin deficiencies accompanied by yin-deficient fire. The herbal formula contained *Di Gu Pi* (Cortex Lycii) 15g, *Huang Qin* (Radix Scutellariae) 10g, *Mai Dong* (Radix Ophiopogonis) 10g, *Lian Zi Xin* (Plumula Nelumbinis) 6g, *Gan Cao* (Radix et Rhizoma Glycyrrhizae) 6g, *Bai Mao Gen* (Rhizoma Imperatae) 30g, *Huang Qi* (Radix Astragali) 12g, *Che Qian Zi* (Semen Plantaginis) 12g, *Shi Wei* (Folium Pyrrosiae) 20g, *Da Ji* (Herba Cirsii Japonici) 20g, and *Xiao Ji* (Herba Cirsii) 20g. The herbs were administered in decoction daily for approximately 5 months. Improvements were noted in most patients after about 15 packs of herbs. Clinical improvement included relief of night perspiration, improved appetite, improved sleeping pattern, and reduced number of cells in the urine. After the condition stabilized, the patients were then given *Liu Wei Di Huang Wan* (Six-Ingredient Pill with Rehmannia) for further consolidation.[4]

4. **Pyelonephritis**: One study reported success using modified *Qing Xin Lian Zi Yin* to treat pyelonephritis characterized by Heart and Kidney yin deficiencies with damp-heat affecting the Urinary Bladder. The herbal formula contained *Di Gu Pi* (Cortex Lycii) 15g, *Che Qian Zi* (Semen Plantaginis) 15g, *Bai He* (Bulbus Lilii) 15g, *Huang Qin* (Radix Scutellariae) 15g, *Mai Dong* (Radix Ophiopogonis) 12g, *Lian Zi* (Semen Nelumbinis) 12g, *Fu Ling* (Poria) 12g, *Bai Wei* (Radix et Rhizoma Cynanchi Atrati) 12g, *Pu Gong Ying* (Herba Taraxaci) 30g, *Huang Qi* (Radix Astragali) 20g, and *Yi Yuan San* (Benefit the Basal Powder) 18g. The above herbs were cooked in water and the decoction was taken daily, for 50 packs of herbs. The study reported normalization of all signs and symptoms, with no recurrence in follow-up exams.[5]

AUTHORS' COMMENTS
Qing Xin Lian Zi Yin can also be used for postpartum irritability, thirst, and heat caused by the sudden depletion of blood leading to yin-deficient heat.

References
1. *Guo Wai Yi Xue* (Foreign Medicine) 1993;(4):36.
2. *Shi Yong Zhong Xi Yi Jie He Za Zhi* (Practical Journal of Integrated Chinese and Western Medicines) 1998;6:523.
3. *Shan Xi Zhong Yi* (Shanxi Chinese Medicine) 1998;4:173.
4. *Shan Xi Zhong Yi* (Shanxi Chinese Medicine) 1998;4:173.
5. *Shan Xi Zhong Yi* (Shanxi Chinese Medicine) 1998;4:173.

Chapter 5 – Heat-Clearing Formulas   *Section 5 – Zang Fu-Clearing Formulas*

Zhī Zǐ Chǐ Tāng (Gardenia and Soja Decoction)

栀子豉湯
栀子豉汤

Pinyin Name: *Zhi Zi Chi Tang*
Literal Name: Gardenia and Soja Decoction
Alternate Names: *Chih Tzu Ku Tang*, *Zhi Zi Gu Tang*, Gardenia and Fermented Soybean Decoction, Cape Jasmine and Prepared Soybean Decoction, Gardenia and Soja Combination
Original Source: *Shang Han Lun* (Discussion of Cold-Induced Disorders) by Zhang Zhong-Jing in the Eastern Han Dynasty

COMPOSITION

Zhi Zi (Fructus Gardeniae)	14 pieces [9g]
Dan Dou Chi (Semen Sojae Praeparatum)	0.4 cup [9g]

DOSAGE / PREPARATION / ADMINISTRATION

First cook *Zhi Zi* (Fructus Gardeniae) in 4 cups [800 mL] of water, and reduce it to 2.5 cups [500 mL]. Add in *Dan Dou Chi* (Semen Sojae Praeparatum), and cook it until the liquid is reduced to 1.5 cups [300 mL]. Take the warm, strained decoction in two equally-divided doses.

CHINESE THERAPEUTIC ACTIONS

1. Clears heat and relieves irritability
2. Resolves congestion in the chest and epigastrium

CLINICAL MANIFESTATIONS

A general feeling of weakness and deficiency, irritability, insomnia, fullness and congestion in the chest and epigastrium, lack of appetite, and a yellow tongue coating.

CLINICAL APPLICATIONS

Insomnia, neurasthenia, acute cholecystitis, acute icteric jaundice, acute gastritis, and esophagitis.

EXPLANATION

Zhi Zi Chi Tang (Gardenia and Soja Decoction) is for patients who complain of weakness and irritability following inappropriate treatment of an exterior syndrome with *han fa* (sweating), *tu fa* (vomiting) or *xia fa* (draining downwards). These improper treatments result in a loss of body fluids and the patient will feel weak

and deficient. Moreover, the exterior factor moves inwards and transforms into heat in the chest and diaphragm and disturbs the Heart *shen* (spirit). As a result, patients have irritability, insomnia, and a sensation of fullness and congestion in the chest and diaphragm areas.

This simple formula contains only two herbs: *Zhi Zi* (Fructus Gardeniae) clears heat from the Heart and relieves irritability; and *Dan Dou Chi* (Semen Sojae Praeparatum) purges residual heat from the chest and diaphragm areas. These two herbs work synergistically to clear heat in the chest and epigastrium in a deficient patient.

MODIFICATIONS

• When accompanied by a dry mouth, a bitter taste, and a yellow tongue coating, add *Lian Qiao* (Fructus Forsythiae), *Huang Qin* (Radix Scutellariae), and *Lu Gen* (Rhizoma Phragmitis).
• With nausea and vomiting, add *Sheng Jiang* (Rhizoma Zingiberis Recens) and *Zhu Ru* (Caulis Bambusae in Taenia).

CAUTIONS / CONTRAINDICATIONS

Zhi Zi Chi Tang should be used with caution in cases of diarrhea caused by deficiency and cold of the Spleen and Stomach.

Zhi Zi Chi Tang (Gardenia and Soja Decoction)

Diagnosis	Signs and Symptoms	Treatment	Herbs
Heat in the chest and diaphragm	• Irritability, insomnia and a sensation of fullness and congestion in the chest and diaphragm areas: accumulation of heat in the chest and diaphragm disturbing the *shen* (spirit) • Generalized weakness and deficiency: loss of body fluids	• Clears heat and relieves irritability • Opens congestion in the chest and epigastrium	• *Zhi Zi* (Fructus Gardeniae) clears heat from the Heart and relieves irritability. • *Dan Dou Chi* (Semen Sojae Praeparatum) purges residual heat from the chest and epigastrium.

370

Chinese Herbal Formulas and Applications

Lóng Dăn Xiè Gān Tāng (Gentiana Decoction to Drain the Liver)

龍膽瀉肝湯
龙胆泻肝汤

Pinyin Name: *Long Dan Xie Gan Tang*
Literal Name: Gentiana Decoction to Drain the Liver
Alternate Names: *Lung Tan Hsieh Kan Tang*, Gentiana Liver-Draining Decoction (Pill), Gentiana Liver-Purging Decoction (Pill), Gentiana Combination
Original Source: *Yi Fang Ji Jie* (Analytical Collection of Medical Formulas) by Wang Ang in 1682

COMPOSITION

Long Dan (Radix et Rhizoma Gentianae), *chao* (dry-fried) with liquor	[6g]
Huang Qin (Radix Scutellariae), *chao* (dry-fried)	[9g]
Zhi Zi (Fructus Gardeniae), *chao* (dry-fried) with liquor	[9g]
Ze Xie (Rhizoma Alismatis)	[12g]
Mu Tong (Caulis Akebiae)	[9g]
Che Qian Zi (Semen Plantaginis)	[9g]
Di Huang (Radix Rehmanniae), *chao* (dry-fried) with liquor	[9g]
Dang Gui (Radix Angelicae Sinensis), *xi* (washed) with liquor	[3g]
Chai Hu (Radix Bupleuri)	[6g]
Gan Cao (Radix et Rhizoma Glycyrrhizae)	[6g]

DOSAGE / PREPARATION / ADMINISTRATION

The source text states to prepare the ingredients as a decoction. Note: Doses of herbs are unavailable from the source text. Suggested doses, however, are listed above in brackets.

CHINESE THERAPEUTIC ACTIONS

1. Sedates excess fire in the Liver and Gallbladder
2. Clears damp-heat in the lower *jiao*

CLINICAL MANIFESTATIONS

1. Flaring of excess fire in the Liver and Gallbladder: headache, red eyes, hypochondriac pain, a bitter taste in the mouth, deafness, and swollen or painful inner ears.
2. Damp-heat in the lower *jiao*: swelling and itching of the external genitalia, sweating in the groin, dysuria, turbid urine, and yellow, foul-smelling leukorrhea in women.

CLINICAL APPLICATIONS

Hypertension, hepatitis, hepatic cirrhosis, acute icteric hepatitis, acute cholecystitis, gastritis, upper gastrointestinal bleeding, erythematosis, urinary tract infection, urethritis, cystitis, nephritis, shingles, herpes zoster, chancre, gonorrhea, syphilis, leukemia, orchitis, prostatitis, male sexual dysfunction, bartholinitis, eczema of the scrotum, erysipelas, pelvic inflammatory disease, polycystic ovary syndrome, endometriosis, fallopian tube infection, ovaritis, prolapsed uterus, mastitis, cervicitis, abnormal vaginal discharge, Behcet's disease, acute conjunctivitis, acute otitis media, allergic rhinitis, oral lichen planus, hyperthyroidism, migraine, diabetes mellitus, and sciatica.

EXPLANATION

Long Dan Xie Gan Tang (Gentiana Decoction to Drain the Liver) treats excess fire in the Liver and Gallbladder. When excess fire in the Liver channel travels upward, it produces headache, painful eyes and ears, or deafness. When excess fire follows the channel to the hypochondriac region, hypochondriac pain and a bitter taste in the mouth occur. If it is the case of damp-heat, then the damp-heat follows the Liver channel downward to the lower *jiao* to cause swelling and itching of the external genitalia, sweating of the groin, dysuria with turbid urine, and, in the case of women, foul-smelling leukorrhea.

Long Dan (Radix et Rhizoma Gentianae), an extremely bitter and cold herb, sedates fire in the Liver and Gallbladder and clears damp-heat in the lower *jiao*. *Huang Qin* (Radix Scutellariae) and *Zhi Zi* (Fructus Gardeniae) help *Long Dan* (Radix et Rhizoma Gentianae) sedate fire and damp-heat in all three *jiaos*. To minimize the bitter and cold herbs in this formula from damaging the stomach, *Huang Qin* (Radix Scutellariae) is dry-fried, and *Long Dan* (Radix et Rhizoma Gentianae) and *Zhi Zi* (Fructus Gardeniae) are dry-fried with liquor. *Ze Xie* (Rhizoma Alismatis), *Mu Tong* (Caulis Akebiae), and *Che Qian Zi* (Semen Plantaginis) dispel damp-heat through the urine. In this syndrome, blood and yin may be consumed as a result of both the excess fire and the bitter cold herbs in this formula, so *Di Huang* (Radix Rehmanniae) and *Dang Gui* (Radix Angelicae Sinensis) are added to nourish and protect yin and blood. *Chai Hu* (Radix Bupleuri) regulates Liver qi and guides all of the herbs to the Liver. *Gan*

HEAT-CLEARING FORMULAS

5

371

Chapter 5 – Heat-Clearing Formulas   *Section 5 – Zang Fu-Clearing Formulas*

Lóng Dǎn Xiè Gān Tāng (Gentiana Decoction to Drain the Liver)

Long Dan Xie Gan Tang (Gentiana Decoction to Drain the Liver)

Diagnosis	Signs and Symptoms	Treatment	Herbs
Excess fire in the Liver and Gallbladder	• Headache, a bitter taste in the mouth, painful eyes and ears, or deafness: excess fire traveling upward along the Liver channel • Hypochondriac pain: excess fire traveling along the Liver channel • Swelling and itching of the external genitalia, sweating of the groin, dysuria, and leukorrhea in women: damp-heat traveling downward to the lower *jiao*	• Sedates excess fire in the Liver and Gallbladder • Clears damp-heat in the lower *jiao*	• *Long Dan* (Radix et Rhizoma Gentianae) sedates fire in the Liver and Gallbladder and clears damp-heat in the lower *jiao*. • *Huang Qin* (Radix Scutellariae) and *Zhi Zi* (Fructus Gardeniae) sedate fire and damp-heat in all three *jiaos*. • *Ze Xie* (Rhizoma Alismatis), *Mu Tong* (Caulis Akebiae) and *Che Qian Zi* (Semen Plantaginis) dispel damp-heat through the urine. • *Di Huang* (Radix Rehmanniae) and *Dang Gui* (Radix Angelicae Sinensis) nourish and protect yin and blood. • *Chai Hu* (Radix Bupleuri) regulates Liver qi and guides the herbs to the Liver. • *Gan Cao* (Radix et Rhizoma Glycyrrhizae) harmonizes the formula.

Cao (Radix et Rhizoma Glycyrrhizae) harmonizes the formula.

MODIFICATIONS
• With constipation, add *Da Huang* (Radix et Rhizoma Rhei) and *Mang Xiao* (Natrii Sulfas).
• With dysuria, add *Yin Chen* (Herba Artemisiae Scopariae) and *Fu Ling* (Poria).
• If there is acute glaucoma, add *Xuan Shen* (Radix Scrophulariae) and *Qiang Huo* (Rhizoma et Radix Notopterygii).
• With redness, swelling, and pain of the eyes, add *Chuan Xiong* (Rhizoma Chuanxiong) and *Ju Hua* (Flos Chrysanthemi).
• With urinary tract infection, add *Bian Xu* (Herba Polygoni Avicularis), *Qu Mai* (Herba Dianthi), *Bai Mao Gen* (Rhizoma Imperatae), and *Lian Qiao* (Fructus Forsythiae).
• When there is more visual disturbance, add *Ju Hua* (Flos Chrysanthemi) and *Jue Ming Zi* (Semen Cassiae); or *Xi Gan Ming Mu San* (Wash the Liver and Brighten the Eyes Powder).
• When there is more dampness, remove *Huang Qin* (Radix Scutellariae) and *Di Huang* (Radix Rehmanniae), and add *Hua Shi* (Talcum) and *Yi Yi Ren* (Semen Coicis); or *Ba Zheng San* (Eight-Herb Powder for Rectification).
• With redness and swelling of the scrotum or sores on the penis, remove *Chai Hu* (Radix Bupleuri) and add *Lian Qiao* (Fructus Forsythiae), *Huang Lian* (Rhizoma Coptidis), and *Da Huang* (Radix et Rhizoma Rhei).
• With itching in the genital regions, use *She Chuang Zi* (Fructus Cnidii) and *Ku Shen* (Radix Sophorae Flavescentis) topically as a wash on the affected area.

• For itchy nipples, add *Ju Ye* (Folium Citri Reticulatae) and *Fo Shou* (Fructus Citri Sarcodactylis).

CAUTIONS / CONTRAINDICATIONS
• *Long Dan Xie Gan Tang* should be used with caution in patients with deficiency and cold in the Spleen and Stomach, since this formula is cold and may injure the Spleen and Stomach to cause vomiting or diarrhea.
• This formula is contraindicated in patients with yang, yin, and/or blood deficiencies.
• This formula is contraindicated for prolonged use and should be discontinued once the desired effect is achieved.

PHARMACOLOGICAL EFFECTS
1. **Antibiotic**: Decoction of *Long Dan Xie Gan Tang* was associated with marked antibacterial effects, especially against beta-hemolytic streptococcus.[1]
2. **Anti-inflammatory**: Oral administration of *Long Dan Xie Gan Tang* in decoction was associated with marked anti-inflammatory effects in mice, with maximum effect observed 4 to 6 hours after ingestion. The mechanism of action is attributed to an inhibitive effect on blood vessel permeability.[2]
3. **Immunostimulant**: Oral administration of *Long Dan Xie Gan Tang* decoction at 50 g/kg was associated with increased phagocytic activity in mice within 3-6 hours.[3]
4. **Antiallergic**: Oral administration of *Long Dan Xie Gan Tang* decoction at 10 g/kg for 2 days was effective in minimizing shock and death caused by severe allergic reaction.[4]

372

Lóng Dǎn Xiè Gān Tāng (Gentiana Decoction to Drain the Liver)

5. **Cardiovascular**: *Long Dan Xie Gan Tang* was associated with marked hypotensive effects in anesthetized cats. The mechanisms of action were attributed to its effect of lowering heart rate, decreasing force of heart contraction, and dilation of blood vessels.[5]

CLINICAL STUDIES AND RESEARCH

1. **Hypertension**: In one study, modified *Long Dan Xie Gan Tang* was used to treat patients with hypertension with 88.89% effectiveness.[6] In another report, it was mentioned that *Long Dan Xie Gan Tang* is most effective for hypertension with headache, irritability, insomnia, thirst, a bitter taste in the mouth, dysuria, and a wiry, rapid pulse.[7] Lastly, 100 hypertensive patients characterized by Liver fire rising had good results when treated with a herbal formula that contained *Long Dan Xie Gan Tang* plus *Xia Ku Cao* (Spica Prunellae), *Jue Ming Zi* (Semen Cassiae), *Gou Teng* (Ramulus Uncariae cum Uncis), and others.[8]

2. **Hepatitis**: *Long Dan Xie Gan Tang* was shown in many studies to be effective in treating hepatitis. In one study, 32 patients with non-icteric hepatitis were treated with *Long Dan Xie Gan Tang* with complete recovery in 27 patients, some improvement in 4 patients, and no change in one patient.[9] In another study, 30 patients with icteric hepatitis were treated with *Long Dan Xie Gan Tang* with good results. The study reported improvement in most patients within 3-9 days, with jaundice resolving after 21.5 days and liver enzymes returning to normal after 30.8 days.[10] Lastly, one study of 40 patients with icteric jaundice reported 87.5% effectiveness using modified *Long Dan Xie Gan Tang* in decoction for 14 days per course of treatment.[11]

3. **Cholecystitis**: In one report, 8 patients with acute cholecystitis were treated with complete recovery in all patients using *Long Dǎn Xie Gan Tang* with the addition of *Ku Lian Pi* (Cortex Meliae) and *Da Huang* (Radix et Rhizoma Rhei).[12] Another study reported similar success using *Long Dan Xie Gan Tang* with the addition of *Yin Chen* (Herba Artemisiae Scopariae) and *Da Huang* (Radix et Rhizoma Rhei).[13] Lastly, 81 patients with acute cholecystitis were treated with 96.2% effectiveness using *Long Dan Xie Gan Tang* plus *Yin Chen* (Herba Artemisiae Scopariae), *Chuan Lian Zi* (Fructus Toosendan), and *Da Huang* (Radix et Rhizoma Rhei).[14]

4. **Gastritis**: Forty-seven patients with gastritis (characterized by damp-heat in the Spleen and Stomach, or Liver and Stomach heat) were treated with *Long Dan Xie Gan Tang* with significant improvement in 14 patients, moderate improvement in 31 patients, and no effect in 2 patients.[15]

5. **Upper gastrointestinal bleeding**: In one study, 200 patients with upper gastrointestinal bleeding were treated with modified *Long Dan Xie Gan Tang* with 98% effectiveness. The stools tested negative for the presence of blood within an average of 4 days.[16]

6. **Erythematosis**: Thirty-five patients with erythematosis were treated with good results using *Long Dan Xie Gan Tang* plus *Zhi Qiao* (Fructus Aurantii) and *Da Huang* (Radix et Rhizoma Rhei). Patients were given herbs three times daily, for 5 days (with 2 days of rest) per week, for 4 weeks per course of treatment, for 3 courses total. Of 35 patients, the study reported complete recovery in 24 patients, improvement in 8 patients and no benefit in 3 patients.[17]

7. **Urinary tract infection**: Eight patients with acute or chronic urinary tract infection were treated with *Long Dan Xie Gan Tang* with complete recovery in 6 patients and improvement in 2 patients.[18] In another report, 52 patients with acute or chronic pyelonephritis were treated with *Long Dan Xie Gan Tang* with complete recovery in 48 patients and improvement in 4 patients. The average time for recovery was 6.9 days.[19]

8. **Leukemia**: The effectiveness of *Long Dan Xie Gan Tang* was evaluated for treating acute leukemia characterized by damp-heat of the Liver and Gallbladder. Out of 26 patients with leukemia, 14 had significant improvement, 10 had moderate improvement, and 2 had no effect. The rate of effectiveness was 92.3% for the treatment. The herbal treatment included *Long Dan Xie Gan Tang* plus *Xia Ku Cao* (Spica Prunellae), *Ban Zhi Lian* (Herba Scutellariae Barbatae), and *Bai Hua She She Cao* (Herba Hedyotis) as the base formula. Modifications included addition of *Wu Wei Xiao Du Yin* (Five-Ingredient Decoction to Eliminate Toxins) and *Huang Lian Jie Du Tang* (Coptis Decoction to Relieve Toxicity) for excess heat; and *Xiang Sha Liu Jun Zi Tang* (Six-Gentlemen Decoction with Aucklandia and Amomum) for gastrointestinal disturbances.[20]

9. **Hyperthyroidism**: Eighteen hyperthyroid patients with elevated T3 and T4 were treated with *Long Dan Xie Gan Tang* with significant improvement in 6 patients, moderate improvement in 11 patients, and no change in 1 patient.[21]

10. **Migraine**: In one study, 20 patients with migraine were treated with modified *Long Dan Xie Gan Tang* with satisfactory results. The study reported that the addition of *Ju Hua* (Flos Chrysanthemi) and a large dose of *Bai Shao* (Radix Paeoniae Alba) were effective in enhancing the analgesic effect to relieve migraine.[22]

11. **Diabetes mellitus**: According to one study, 36 patients with diabetes mellitus characterized by obesity and elevated cholesterol and triglyceride levels were treated with modified *Long Dan Xie Gan Tang* with significant improvement in 28 patients, moderate improvement in 5 patients, and slight improvement in 3 patients. The treatment protocol was to administer the decoction twice

Lóng Dǎn Xiè Gān Tāng (Gentiana Decoction to Drain the Liver)

daily. The herbal treatment included *Huang Lian* (Rhizoma Coptidis), *Huang Qin* (Radix Scutellariae), *Long Dan* (Radix et Rhizoma Gentianae), *Zhi Zi* (Fructus Gardeniae), *Ze Xie* (Rhizoma Alismatis), *Mu Tong* (Caulis Akebiae), *Che Qian Zi* (Semen Plantaginis), *Di Huang* (Radix Rehmanniae), *Chai Hu* (Radix Bupleuri), *Fang Ji* (Radix Stephaniae Tetrandrae), *Can Sha* (Faeces Bombycis), and *Lian Zi Xin* (Plumula Nelumbinis).[23]

12. **Shingles**: *Long Dan Xie Gan Tang* was shown in many studies to be effective in treating herpes infection. In one report, 64 patients with shingles were treated with recovery in 49 patients, marked improvement in 12 patients, and moderate improvement in 3 patients. The treatment protocol was to administer *Long Dan Xie Gan Tang* plus *Sheng Ma* (Rhizoma Cimicifugae) for shingles above the waist, or instead add *Niu Xi* (Radix Achyranthis Bidentatae) for below the waist.[24] In another study, 318 of 336 patients had complete recovery from herpes zoster after using *Long Dan Xie Gan Tang* for 3-5 days.[25] In yet another study, 41 out of 45 patients with herpes zoster had complete recovery using modified *Long Dan Xie Gan Tang*. Treatment effects included healing of the lesions and pain relief.[26]

13. **Sciatica**: Administration of *Long Dan Xie Gan Tang* in 61 patients with sciatica was associated with significant relief in 23 patients, improvement in 36 patients, and no effect in 2 patients. The patients were instructed to cook the herbs in water, and drink the decoction in two equally-divided doses. Sciatica was characterized as damp-heat in the Liver channel leading to pain and discomfort. The herbal formula included *Long Dan Xie Gan Tang* plus *Hu Zhang* (Rhizoma et Radix Polygoni Cuspidati), *Di Long* (Pheretima), and others as deemed necessary.[27]

14. **Orchitis**: In one study using modified *Long Dan Xie Gan Tang*, 36 patients with acute orchitis were treated with significant improvement in all patients. Modifications were made based on the individual conditions. For swelling and pain of the testicles, *Yan Hu Suo* (Rhizoma Corydalis) and *Chuan Lian Zi* (Fructus Toosendan) were added. For swelling and hardening of the testicles, *Di Huang* (Radix Rehmanniae) was removed, and *Ju He* (Semen Citri Reticulatae), *Tao Ren* (Semen Persicae) and *Hong Hua* (Flos Carthami) were added. For hematuria, *Hu Zhang* (Rhizoma et Radix Polygoni Cuspidati) and *Bai Mao Gen* (Rhizoma Imperatae) were added. For frequent urination with burning sensation and pain, *Huang Bo* (Cortex Phellodendri Chinensis) and *Shi Wei* (Folium Pyrrosiae) were added. For orchitis with prostatitis, *Fen Bi Xie* (Rhizoma Dioscoreae Hypoglaucae) and *Li Zhi He* (Semen Litchi) were added. For those with concurrent *lin zheng* (dysuria syndrome) and urethritis, *Gan Cao* (Radix et Rhizoma Glycyrrhizae) was removed

and *Tu Fu Ling* (Rhizoma Smilacis Glabrae) and *Bi Yu San* (Jasper Powder) were added.[28] In another report, 12 patients with orchitis were treated with complete recovery in all patients using *Long Dan Xie Gan Tang* with *Chuan Lian Zi* (Fructus Toosendan), *Yan Hu Suo* (Rhizoma Corydalis), and *Li Zhi He* (Semen Litchi).[29]

15. **Prostatitis**: Forty-four patients with prostatitis characterized by damp-heat were treated with modified *Long Dan Xie Gan Tang* with complete recovery in 16 patients, significant improvement in 12 patients, moderate improvement in 13 patients, and no effect in 3 patients. The overall rate of effectiveness was 93.2%. The herbal treatment contained *Long Dan Xie Gan Tang* as the base formula, with the addition of *Bai Jiang Cao* (Herba cum Radice Patriniae), *Pu Gong Ying* (Herba Taraxaci) and a large dose of *Long Dan* (Radix et Rhizoma Gentianae) for damp-heat with a bitter taste in the mouth; *Ze Lan* (Herba Lycopi), *Ru Xiang* (Gummi Olibanum), *Tao Ren* (Semen Persicae) and *Chi Shao* (Radix Paeoniae Rubra) for hardening of the prostate; and *Yin Yang Huo* (Herba Epimedii) and *Fen Bi Xie* (Rhizoma Dioscoreae Hypoglaucae) for sexual dysfunction.[30] In another report, 30 patients with chronic prostatitis were treated with modified *Long Dan Xie Gan Tang* with complete recovery in 18 patients, significant improvement in 8 patients, moderate improvement in 2 patients, and no benefit in 2 patients. The overall rate of effectiveness was 93.3%.[31]

16. **Male sexual dysfunction**: According to one study on treatment of inability to ejaculate, the use of modified *Long Dan Xie Gan Tang* successfully treated all 9 men who experienced such sexual dysfunction. The base formula contained *Long Dan Xie Gan Tang* plus *Zhi Mu* (Rhizoma Anemarrhenae), *Hai Piao Xiao* (Endoconcha Sepiae), and *Qian Cao* (Radix et Rhizoma Rubiae). Modifications included addition of *Ze Xie* (Rhizoma Alismatis) and *Che Qian Zi* (Semen Plantaginis) for damp; larger doses of *Long Dan* (Radix et Rhizoma Gentianae), *Zhi Zi* (Fructus Gardeniae), and *Huang Bo* (Cortex Phellodendri Chinensis) for heat; *Er Zhi Wan* (Two-Ultimate Pill), *Bie Jia* (Carapax Trionycis), and a large dose of *Di Huang* (Radix Rehmanniae) for Liver and Kidney yin deficiencies; and *Dan Shen* (Radix et Rhizoma Salviae Miltiorrhizae), *Tu Fu Ling* (Rhizoma Smilacis Glabrae) and *Chuan Lian Zi* (Fructus Toosendan) for abnormally sticky sperm in nocturnal emissions.[32]

17. **Bartholinitis**: Concurrent use of herbs orally and topically in 35 patients with inflammation of the Bartholin's gland was associated with complete recovery in 23 patients, improvement in 10 patients, and no effect in 2 patients. The herbal treatment included *Long Dan Xie Gan Tang* plus *Pu Gong Ying* (Herba Taraxaci), *Zi Hua Di Ding* (Herba Violae), and *Ye Ju Hua* (Flos Chrysanthemi Indici)

Lóng Dăn Xiè Gān Tāng (Gentiana Decoction to Drain the Liver)

taken orally. Topical herbal treatment included *Da Huang* (Radix et Rhizoma Rhei), *Ye Ju Hua* (Flos Chrysanthemi Indici), *Pu Gong Ying* (Herba Taraxaci), and *Zi Hua Di Ding* (Herba Violae). For topical use, the herbs were cooked in water, and the patient was instructed to soak the affected area in the herbal solution. The duration of treatment was 7 days per course of treatment.[33]

18. **Eczema of the scrotum**: One study reports complete recovery in all 29 patients with acute eczema of the scrotum when treated with *Long Dan Xie Gan Tang* plus *Bai Xian Pi* (Cortex Dictamni), *Di Fu Zi* (Fructus Kochiae), and *Cang Zhu* (Rhizoma Atractylodis). The duration of treatment was 1 week per course of treatment, for 1-3 courses total.[34]

19. **Pelvic inflammatory disease**: Seven patients with acute pelvic inflammation were treated with a 100% success rate using *Long Dan Xie Gan Tang* for 6-9 doses. A laxative was used to relieve constipation if necessary.[35] Another study of 72 patients with chronic pelvic inflammation were treated with good results using *Long Dan Xie Gan Tang* plus *Huang Qi* (Radix Astragali) and *Xiang Fu* (Rhizoma Cyperi). The patients were instructed to begin taking the herbs after the last day of the period, and to stop taking the herbs when the period began. The duration of treatment was two menstrual cycles per course of treatment.[36]

20. **Polycystic ovary syndrome**: One study reported effectiveness using modified *Long Dan Xie Gan Tang* in treating polycystic ovary syndrome. Of 20 patients, 12 were diagnosed with Liver fire, 2 with damp and phlegm accumulation, and 6 with generalized deficiency. In addition to the base formula, *Da Huang* (Radix et Rhizoma Rhei) and *Mang Xiao* (Natrii Sulfas) were added for constipation. The treatment protocol was to administer 9 grams of herbs per day (in two doses daily) for 3 months. Herbal treatment was temporarily stopped during the periods. Of 20 patients, the study reported marked improvement in 8 patients and moderate improvement in 12 patients.[37]

21. **Prolapsed uterus**: In one report, 19 women with prolapsed uterus were treated with *Long Dan Xie Gan Tang* with complete recovery in 6 patients, improvement in 12 patients, and no change in 1 patient.[38]

22. **Mastitis**: Use of *Long Dan Xie Gan Tang* produced complete recovery in 92 of 100 patients with mastitis characterized by redness, swelling and pain. The treatment protocol was to cook the herbs in water, and drink the decoction in three equally-divided doses (approximately 50 mL per dose) daily for 7 days.[39]

23. **Cervicitis**: In one study, chronic cervicitis characterized by damp-heat in the Liver channel was treated effectively using oral and/or topical application of *Long Dan Xie Gan Tang* plus *Bai Jiang Cao* (Herba cum Radice Patriniae),

Huang Bo (Cortex Phellodendri Chinensis), and *Huang Qi* (Radix Astragali). The herbs were taken daily, for 20 days per course of treatment. The study reported 93.3% effectiveness among 356 patients.[40]

24. **Behcet's disease**: *Long Dan Xie Gan Tang* was shown in many studies to effectively treat Behcet's disease, a condition that affects the inner lining of the mouth and genitals, and the small blood vessels throughout the body. In one study of 21 patients (9 males and 12 females), duration of use ranging from 20 to 67 days was associated with complete recovery in 18 patients, improvement in 2 patients, and no change in 1 patient. The herbal treatment contained *Long Dan Xie Gan Tang* as the base formula, with addition of *Huang Qi* (Radix Astragali) and *Dang Shen* (Radix Codonopsis) for qi deficiency; *Mo Han Lian* (Herba Ecliptae) and *Nu Zhen Zi* (Fructus Ligustri Lucidi) for Liver and Kidney yin deficiencies; *Ku Shen* (Radix Sophorae Flavescentis) and *Bai Xian Pi* (Cortex Dictamni) for severe itching; *Da Huang* (Radix et Rhizoma Rhei) for constipation; and *Cang Zhu* (Rhizoma Atractylodis) for dampness.[41]

25. **Otitis media**: Eighty-five patients with chronic pyogenic otitis media were treated with an overall 89% success rate using *Long Dan Xie Gan Tang* with the addition of *Xin Yi Hua* (Flos Magnoliae) and *Cang Er Zi* (Fructus Xanthii).[42] In another report, 22 patients with acute pyogenic otitis media were treated with complete recovery in 14 patients, improvement in 6 patients, and no effect in 2 patients.[43] Lastly, one study of 20 patients with chronic otitis media due to damp-heat in the Liver and Gallbladder channels reported complete recovery in all patients using *Long Dan Xie Gan Tang*. The herbs were administered three times daily for 10 days per course of treatment, for 1-2 courses total.[44]

26. **Allergic rhinitis**: Thirteen patients with allergic rhinitis were treated with *Long Dan Xie Gan Tang* with complete recovery in 9 patients, improvement in 2 patients, and no effect in 2 patients. The overall rate of effectiveness was 84.62%. The duration of treatment averaged 24 days, with a range of 12-43 days.[45]

27. **Oral lichen planus**: Fifty-nine patients with oral lichen planus were treated with modified *Long Dan Xie Gan Tang* with complete recovery in 38 patients, improvement in 18 patients, and no effect in 3 patients. The overall rate of effectiveness was 94.92%.[46]

TOXICOLOGY

In acute toxicology studies, oral administration of the formula in mice at 26 g/kg showed no adverse reactions other than a short-term decrease in spontaneous physical activities (activities without a stimulus). No mortality was reported. With intravenous injection, the LD_{50} was determined to be 72g/kg.[47]

Chapter 5 – Heat-Clearing Formulas

Section 5 – Zang Fu-Clearing Formulas

Lóng Dǎn Xiè Gān Tāng (Gentiana Decoction to Drain the Liver)

RELATED FORMULAS

Xiè Qīng Wān (Drain the Green Pill)

瀉青丸
泻青丸

Pinyin Name: *Xie Qing Wan*
Literal Name: Drain the Green Pill
Original Source: *Xiao Er Yao Zheng Zhi Jue* (Craft of Medicinal Treatment for Childhood Disease Patterns) by Qian Yi in 1119

Dang Gui (Radix Angelicae Sinensis), *qie* (sliced) and *bei* (stone-baked)	[3g]
Long Dan (Radix et Rhizoma Gentianae), *bei* (stone-baked)	[3g]
Chuan Xiong (Rhizoma Chuanxiong)	[3g]
Zhi Zi (Fructus Gardeniae)	[3g]
Da Huang (Radix et Rhizoma Rhei), *wei* (roasted)	[3g]
Qiang Huo (Rhizoma et Radix Notopterygii)	[3g]
Fang Feng (Radix Saposhnikoviae), *qie* (sliced) and *bei* (stone-baked)	[3g]

The source text states to grind equal amounts of the ingredients into powder and form with honey into large pills (approximately the size of a chicken's head). Take 0.5-1 pill with brown sugar and a decoction made from *Zhu Ye* (Herba Phyllostachys). Today, the ingredients are normally ground into powder, and formed into small pills with boiled water that has been cooled to room temperature. Take 6g of pills twice daily with warm water that has been boiled or a decoction made from *Zhu Ye* (Herba Phyllostachys). Reduce the dose for children. This formula may be prepared as a decoction using the doses suggested in brackets above.

The main actions of *Xie Qing Wan* (Drain the Green Pill) are to clear Liver heat and purge Liver fire. Clinically, the patient may show red, swollen and painful eyes, fidgeting, irritability, restlessness, anger, insomnia, dark-colored urine, constipation, and a surging, excess pulse. In some patients, this formula may also be used for acute infantile convulsions, high fever, and muscle spasms.

Long Dan Xie Gan Tang and *Xie Qing Wan* (Drain the Green Pill) both clear Liver heat. *Xie Qing Wan* (Drain the Green Pill), however, is the weaker formula of the two in clearing Liver heat. In addition, it does not clear damp-heat from the lower *jiao*.

Lóng Dǎn Jiàng Yá Piàn

(Gentiana Pill to Lower [Blood] Pressure)

龍膽降壓片
龙胆降压片

Pinyin Name: *Long Dan Jiang Ya Pian*
Literal Name: Gentiana Pill to Lower [Blood] Pressure
Original Source: *An Hui Zhong Yi Xue Yuan* (Anhui University School of Medicine) in 1990

Long Dan (Radix et Rhizoma Gentianae)
Huang Qin (Radix Scutellariae)
Zhi Zi (Fructus Gardeniae)
Mu Li (Concha Ostreae)
Jue Ming Zi (Semen Cassiae)
Da Huang (Radix et Rhizoma Rhei)
Hua Shi (Talcum)
Ze Xie (Rhizoma Alismatis)
Chuan Mu Tong (Caulis Clematidis Armandii)
Che Qian Zi (Semen Plantaginis)
Di Huang (Radix Rehmanniae)
Dan Shen (Radix et Rhizoma Salviae Miltiorrhizae)
Ge Gen (Radix Puerariae Lobatae)
Niu Xi (Radix Achyranthis Bidentatae)

The main actions of *Long Dan Jiang Ya Pian* (Gentiana Pill to Lower [Blood] Pressure) are to clear heat and purge fire from the Liver and Gallbladder channels. Clinically, this formula may be used to treat various disorders characterized by heat and fire in the Liver and Gallbladder channels, such as hypertension, hepatitis, hepatic cirrhosis, acute icteric hepatitis, acute cholecystitis, urinary tract infection, urethritis, cystitis, nephritis, shingles, and herpes zoster.

Lóng Dǎn Jiě Dú Tāng

(Gentiana Decoction to Relieve Toxicity)

龍膽解毒湯
龙胆解毒汤

Pinyin Name: *Long Dan Jie Du Tang*
Literal Name: Gentiana Decoction to Relieve Toxicity
Original Source: *Guang An Men Yi Yuan* (Guang An Men Hospital) in 1990

Long Dan (Radix et Rhizoma Gentianae)
Jin Qian Cao (Herba Lysimachiae)
Niu Bang Zi (Fructus Arctii)
Jing Jie (Herba Schizonepetae)
Huang Lian (Rhizoma Coptidis)
Chi Shao (Radix Paeoniae Rubra)
Huang Qin (Radix Scutellariae)
Mu Dan Pi (Cortex Moutan)
Jin Yin Hua (Flos Lonicerae Japonicae)
Lian Qiao (Fructus Forsythiae)
Zi Hua Di Ding (Herba Violae)
Pu Gong Ying (Herba Taraxaci)
Jiang Huang (Rhizoma Curcumae Longae)

Lóng Dǎn Xiè Gān Tāng (Gentiana Decoction to Drain the Liver)

Zao Xiu (Rhizoma Paridis)

Huang Bo (Cortex Phellodendri Chinensis)

Zhi Zi (Fructus Gardeniae)

Di Huang (Radix Rehmanniae)

Gan Cao (Radix et Rhizoma Glycyrrhizae)

Long Dan Jie Du Tang (Gentiana Decoction to Relieve Toxicity) treats the rising of Liver fire and accumulation of damp-heat. It contains herbs that purge the Liver, clear heat, drain dampness, and promote urination. It is commonly used to treat shingles and herpes infection.

Zhī Zǐ Jiàng Huǒ Tāng

(Gardenia Decoction to Descend Fire)

栀子降火湯

栀子降火汤

Pinyin Name: *Zhi Zi Jiang Huo Tang*

Literal Name: Gardenia Decoction to Descend Fire

Original Source: *Jian Tai Yao Fang* (Herbal Prescriptions from *Jiantai* Clinic) by Chang Wei-Yen in 1981

Bian Xu (Herba Polygoni Avicularis)

Chai Hu (Radix Bupleuri)

Che Qian Zi (Semen Plantaginis)

Dang Gui (Radix Angelicae Sinensis)

Fu Ling (Poria)

Gan Cao (Radix et Rhizoma Glycyrrhizae)

Geng Mi (Semen Oryzae)

Huang Bo (Cortex Phellodendri Chinensis)

Huang Qin (Radix Scutellariae)

Long Dan (Radix et Rhizoma Gentianae)

Mu Dan Pi (Cortex Moutan)

Shan Yao (Rhizoma Dioscoreae)

Shan Zhu Yu (Fructus Corni)

Di Huang (Radix Rehmanniae)

Shi Gao (Gypsum Fibrosum)

Shu Di Huang (Radix Rehmanniae Praeparata)

Ze Xie (Rhizoma Alismatis)

Zhi Mu (Rhizoma Anemarrhenae)

Zhi Zi (Fructus Gardeniae)

Zhi Zi Jiang Huo Tang (Gardenia Decoction to Descend Fire) is a variation of *Long Dan Xie Gan Tang* (Gentiana Decoction to Drain the Liver) with the addition of *Bai Hu Tang* (White Tiger Decoction) and *Zhi Bai Di Huang Wan* (Anemarrhena, Phellodendron, and Rehmannia Pill). It treats heat in the upper, middle and lower *jiaos*. It clears excess heat in the Stomach, Lung, Liver and deficiency heat in the Kidney. It is a strong formula reserved only for those with severe excess fire signs.

AUTHORS' COMMENTS

Long Dan Xie Gan Tang is one of the most commonly used formulas today. It treats various conditions caused by excess fire in the Liver and Gallbladder, or damp-heat in the lower *jiao*.

Long Dan Xie Gan Tang, which drains damp-heat, contains blood-tonifying herbs such as *Di Huang* (Radix Rehmanniae) and *Dang Gui* (Radix Angelicae Sinensis) for three main reasons:

- First, this formula treats excess fire flaring upward in the Liver and Gallbladder channels, leading to headache, redness of the eyes, painful eyes, hypochondriac pain, a bitter taste in the mouth, tinnitus, and swelling of the ears. It contains *Long Dan* (Radix et Rhizoma Gentianae), *Huang Qin* (Radix Scutellariae), and *Zhi Zi* (Fructus Gardeniae) to sedate excess fire. Damp-drying herbs such as these are likely to injure yin and cause more flaring of excess heat and Liver fire. Therefore, *Di Huang* (Radix Rehmanniae) and *Dang Gui* (Radix Angelicae Sinensis) are needed to prevent the heat-clearing, damp-drying herbs from damaging yin and blood.
- Second, this formula contains *Che Qian Zi* (Semen Plantaginis), *Mu Tong* (Caulis Akebiae), and *Ze Xie* (Rhizoma Alismatis) to drain damp-heat in the lower *jiao* to treat genital itching, turbid urine, and yellow leukorrhea. To prevent these herbs from excessively draining dampness and injuring yin and blood, *Di Huang* (Radix Rehmanniae) and *Dang Gui* (Radix Angelicae Sinensis) are added.
- Third, *Chai Hu* (Radix Bupleuri) is used in this formula as a channel-guiding and qi-regulating herb to spread Liver qi. To prevent any possible excessive drying caused by *Chai Hu* (Radix Bupleuri), *Di Huang* (Radix Rehmanniae) and *Dang Gui* (Radix Angelicae Sinensis) are added.[48]

Long Dan Xie Gan Tang, *Xie Qing Wan* (Drain the Green Pill), and *Dang Gui Long Hui Wan* (Tangkuei, Gentiana, and Aloe Pill) all sedate excess fire in the Liver channel. The differences are as follows:

- *Long Dan Xie Gan Tang* sedates Liver fire, drains damp-heat, and protects and nourishes Liver blood. It is mostly used for Liver fire flaring with damp-heat accumulation in the lower *jiao*.
- *Xie Qing Wan* sedates Liver fire and disperses Liver qi stagnation with fire. It is most appropriate for Liver fire with stagnation.
- *Dang Gui Long Hui Wan* is the most bitter and cold formula of the three, and is designed to purge excess fire in the Liver through urination and defecation. It is an

Chapter 5 – Heat-Clearing Formulas

Section 5 – Zang Fu-Clearing Formulas

Lóng Dǎn Xiè Gān Tāng (Gentiana Decoction to Drain the Liver)

extremely strong formula reserved only for patients with excess fire accompanied by *shen* (spirit) disturbance and other severe symptoms.

According to Dr. Chang Wei-Yen, *Long Dan Xie Gan Tang* can be combined with other formulas for the following disorders:

- Migraines and headaches caused by Liver yang rising: use with *Tian Ma Gou Teng Yin* (Gastrodia and Uncaria Decoction).
- Headaches in menopausal women caused by flaring of Kidney fire: add *Bai Hu Tang* (White Tiger Decoction) and *Zhi Bai Di Huang Wan* (Anemarrhena, Phellodendron, and Rehmannia Pill).
- Various kinds of lower *jiao* infections, such as bladder infection, urinary tract infection, infection of the reproductive organs and chronic pelvic infection: add *Ba Zheng San* (Eight-Herb Powder for Rectification).
- Nephritis and glomerulonephritis: add *Ba Zheng San* (Eight-Herb Powder for Rectification), *Shui Ding Xiang* (Herba Ludwigiae Prostratae) and *Xian Feng Cao* (Herba Bidentis). For chronic nephritis, add *Ba Wei Di Huang Wan* (Eight-Ingredient Pill with Rehmannia).
- Glaucoma and increased pressure in the eyes: add *Ma Bian Cao* (Herba Verbenae), *Qian Li Guang* (Herba Senecionis Scandens), *Hu Zhang* (Rhizoma et Radix Polygoni Cuspidati), *Hu Yao Huang* (Herba Leucas Mollissimae), and *Ba Zheng San* (Eight-Herb Powder for Rectification).

References

1. *Zhong Yao Yao Li Du Li Yu Lin Chuang* (Pharmacology, Toxicology and Clinical Applications of Chinese Herbs) 1991;(1):5.
2. *Zhong Yi Fang Ji Xian Dai Yan Jiu* (Modern Study of Medical Formulae in Traditional Chinese Medicine) 1997;318-319.
3. *Zhong Yi Fang Ji Xian Dai Yan Jiu* (Modern Study of Medical Formulae in Traditional Chinese Medicine) 1997;318-319.
4. *Zhong Yao Yao Li Du Li Yu Lin Chuang* (Pharmacology, Toxicology and Clinical Applications of Chinese Herbs) 1991;(1):5.
5. *Zhong Yi Fang Ji Xian Dai Yan Jiu* (Modern Study of Medical Formulae in Traditional Chinese Medicine) 1997;320.
6. *Ke Yan Tong Xun* (Journal of Science and Research) 1983;(2):1.
7. *Jiang Xi Zhong Yi Yao* (Jiangxi Chinese Medicine and Herbology) 1959;(10):18.
8. *Nan Jing Zhong Yi Xue Yuan Xue Bao* (Journal of Nanjing University of Traditional Chinese Medicine) 1986;1:20.
9. *Xin Yi Yao Xue Za Zhi* (New Journal of Medicine and Herbology) 1978;10:49.
10. *Ke Yan Tong Xun* (Journal of Science and Research) 1983;(2):13.
11. *Jiang Xi Yi Xue Yuan Xue Bao* (Medical Journal of Jiangxi University of Medicine) 1998;3:123.
12. *Zhong Yi Fang Ji Xian Dai Yan Jiu* (Modern Study of Medical Formulae in Traditional Chinese Medicine) 1997;321.
13. *Nei Meng Gu Zhong Yi Yao* (Traditional Chinese Medicine and Medicinals of Inner Mongolia) 1987;6(2):42.
14. *Ji Lin Zhong Yi Yao* (Jilin Chinese Medicine and Herbology) 1997;2:32.
15. *Shang Hai Zhong Yi Za Zhi* (Shanghai Journal of Chinese Medicine) 1996;6:38.
16. *Zhong Yi Fang Ji Xian Dai Yan Jiu* (Modern Study of Medical Formulae in Traditional Chinese Medicine) 1997;322.
17. *Zhong Yi Za Zhi* (Journal of Chinese Medicine) 1982;4:269.
18. *Ke Yan Tong Xun* (Journal of Science and Research) 1983;(2):1.
19. *Zhong Yi Fang Ji Xian Dai Yan Jiu* (Modern Study of Medical Formulae in Traditional Chinese Medicine) 1997;321.
20. *Zhong Yi Za Zhi* (Journal of Chinese Medicine) 1980;21(4):276.
21. *Ke Yan Tong Xun* (Journal of Science and Research) 1983;(2):1.
22. *Zhong Yi Fang Ji Xian Dai Yan Jiu* (Modern Study of Medical Formulae in Traditional Chinese Medicine) 1997;321-322.
23. *Zhong Yi Yao Xue Bao* (Report of Chinese Medicine and Herbology) 1995;(4):45.
24. *Shan Xi Zhong Yi* (Shanxi Chinese Medicine) 1997;12:556.
25. *Zhong Yuan Yi Kan* (Resource Journal of Chinese Medicine) 1985;4:31.
26. *Jiang Su Zhong Yi* (Jiangsu Chinese Medicine) 1993;(3):22.
27. *Zhe Jiang Zhong Yi Xue Yuan Xue Bao* (Journal of Zhejiang University of Chinese Medicine) 1984;1:26.
28. *Hei Long Jiang Zhong Yi Yao* (Heilongjiang Chinese Medicine and Herbology) 1988;(6):44.
29. *Zhong Yi Yao Yan Jiu* (Research of Chinese Medicine and Herbology) 1987;(4):39.
30. *Fu Jian Zhong Yi Yao* (Fujian Chinese Medicine and Herbology) 1990;21(1):9.
31. *Liao Ning Zhong Yi Za Zhi* (Liaoning Journal of Chinese Medicine) 1991;(6):32.
32. *Jiang Xi Zhong Yi Yao* (Jiangxi Chinese Medicine and Herbology) 1990;4:16.
33. *Shan Xi Zhong Yi* (Shanxi Chinese Medicine) 1996;1:23.
34. *Guang Xi Zhong Yi Yao* (Guangxi Chinese Medicine and Herbology) 1998;1:37.
35. *Zhong Hua Fu Chan Ke Za Zhi* (Chinese Journal of Obstetrics and Gynecology) 1960;8(1):36.
36. *Hu Bei Zhong Yi Za Zhi* (Hubei Journal of Chinese Medicine) 1998;5:40.
37. *Shang Hai Zhong Yi Za Zhi* (Shanghai Journal of Chinese Medicine) 1982;12:17.
38. *Zhong Yi Yao Yan Jiu* (Research of Chinese Medicine and Herbology) 1993;(4):40.
39. *Shi Yong Zhong Xi Yi Jie He Za Zhi* (Practical Journal of Integrated Chinese and Western Medicines) 1992;4:245.
40. *Zhong Yi Yao Xin Xi* (Information on Chinese Medicine and Herbology) 1989;(6):38.
41. *Zhe Jiang Zhong Yi Za Zhi* (Zhejiang Journal of Chinese Medicine) 1988;5:220.
42. *Yi Xue Qing Kuang Jiao Liu* (Medical Information Exchange) 1975;(7):52.
43. *Shang Hai Yi Yao Za Zhi* (Shanghai Journal of Medicine and Herbology) 1985;(3):31.
44. *Zhong Cheng Yao Yan Jiu* (Research of Chinese Patent Medicine) 1985;8:43.
45. *Guang Xi Zhong Yi Yao* (Guangxi Chinese Medicine and Herbology) 1991;14(6):253.
46. *Si Chuan Zhong Yi* (Sichuan Chinese Medicine) 1993;(12):54.
47. *Zhong Yi Fang Ji Xian Dai Yan Jiu* (Modern Study of Medical Formulae in Traditional Chinese Medicine) 1997;320.
48. Wang MZ, et al. *Zhong Yi Xue Wen Da Ti Ku* (Questions and Answers on Traditional Chinese Medicine: Herbal Formulas).

Chinese Herbal Formulas and Applications

Dāng Guī Lóng Huì Wán (Tangkuei, Gentiana, and Aloe Pill)

當歸龍薈丸
当归龙荟丸

Pinyin Name: *Dang Gui Long Hui Wan*
Literal Name: Tangkuei, Gentiana, and Aloe Pill
Alternate Names: *Tang Kuei Lung Hui Wan*, Tang-kuei, Lung-tan, and Aloe Pill; Chinese Angelica, Gentiana and Aloe Pill; Tangkuei Gentiana and Aloe Formula
Original Source: *Dan Xi Xin Fa* (Teachings of [Zhu] Dan-Xi) by Zhu Zhen-Heng in 1481

COMPOSITION

Long Dan (Radix et Rhizoma Gentianae)	15g
Huang Qin (Radix Scutellariae)	30g
Huang Lian (Rhizoma Coptidis)	30g
Huang Bo (Cortex Phellodendri Chinensis)	30g
Zhi Zi (Fructus Gardeniae)	30g
Lu Hui (Aloe)	15g
Da Huang (Radix et Rhizoma Rhei)	15g
Mu Xiang (Radix Aucklandiae)	4.5g
Dang Gui (Radix Angelicae Sinensis)	30g
She Xiang (Moschus)	1.5g

DOSAGE / PREPARATION / ADMINISTRATION

The source text states to grind the ingredients into powder, mix with honey and form into small pills that resemble the size of small beans. Take 20 pills with a decoction made from *Sheng Jiang* (Rhizoma Zingiberis Recens). Today, the ingredients are normally ground into powder and formed into pills with water. Take 6g of pills per dose twice daily with warm, boiled water. Note: One variation of this formula contains 15g of *Qing Dai* (Indigo Naturalis) and 30g of *Long Dan* (Radix et Rhizoma Gentianae).

CHINESE THERAPEUTIC ACTIONS

Clears and purges excess fire from the Liver and Gallbladder channels

CLINICAL MANIFESTATIONS

Excess fire in the Liver and Gallbladder channels: dizziness, vertigo, tinnitus, loss of hearing, a sore throat, restlessness, constipation, dark, yellow urine, and dysuria. In severe cases, patients may have convulsions, epilepsy, semi-unconsciousness, delirium, restless *shen* (spirit), constipation, and mania.

CLINICAL APPLICATIONS

Hepatitis, cholecystitis, cholelithiasis, biliary ascariasis, gastritis, gastroenteritis, acute arthritis, pain with swelling and inflammation, pharyngitis, otitis media, cystitis, urethritis, vaginitis, chronic myelogenous leukemia, general inflammatory and febrile disorders, and acne.

EXPLANATION

The main action of *Dang Gui Long Hui Wan* (Tangkuei, Gentiana, and Aloe Pill) is to clear excess fire in the Liver and Gallbladder channels. Dizziness, vertigo, tinnitus, loss of hearing, sore throat, restlessness, constipation, dark yellow urine and dysuria are indications of excess fire in the Liver and Gallbladder channels. Epilepsy, semi-unconsciousness, delirium and mania are caused by excess fire disturbing the *shen* (spirit).

Long Dan (Radix et Rhizoma Gentianae), extremely bitter and cold, sedates excess fire in the Liver and Gallbladder and clears damp-heat in the lower *jiao*. *Huang Qin* (Radix Scutellariae), *Huang Lian* (Rhizoma Coptidis), *Huang Bo* (Cortex Phellodendri Chinensis), and *Zhi Zi* (Fructus Gardeniae) disperse fire and eliminate damp-heat from the upper, middle, and lower *jiaos*. These herbs clear damp-heat and have excellent anti-inflammatory functions to treat inflammation of various organs and tissues. *Lu Hui* (Aloe) and *Da Huang* (Radix et Rhizoma Rhei) drain downward, and eliminate excess heat and fire through defecation. *Mu Xiang* (Radix Aucklandiae) regulates qi circulation and relieves pain. Since both the excess fire and the bitter cold herbs in this formula have a tendency to consume yin and blood, *Dang Gui* (Radix Angelicae Sinensis) is used to nourish and protect yin and blood. Last, *She Xiang* (Moschus), an aromatic herb, is used to awaken patients who are unconscious or semi-unconscious.

5

HEAT-CLEARING FORMULAS

379

Chapter 5 – Heat-Clearing Formulas　　　　　　　　　　　*Section 5 – Zang Fu-Clearing Formulas*

Dāng Guī Lóng Huì Wán (Tangkuei, Gentiana, and Aloe Pill)

Dang Gui Long Hui Wan (Tangkuei, Gentiana, and Aloe Pill)

Diagnosis	Signs and Symptoms	Treatment	Herbs
Excess fire in the Liver and Gallbladder channels	• Dizziness, vertigo, tinnitus, loss of hearing, sore throat, restlessness, constipation, dark yellow urine and dysuria: excess fire in the Liver and Gallbladder channels • Epilepsy, semi-unconsciousness, delirium, and mania: excess fire disturbing the *shen* (spirit)	Clears and purges excess fire from the Liver and Gallbladder	• *Long Dan* (Radix et Rhizoma Gentianae) sedates excess fire in the Liver and Gallbladder and clears damp-heat in the lower *jiao*. • *Huang Qin* (Radix Scutellariae), *Huang Lian* (Rhizoma Coptidis), *Huang Bo* (Cortex Phellodendri Chinensis) and *Zhi Zi* (Fructus Gardeniae) disperse fire and eliminate damp-heat from all three *jiaos*. • *Lu Hui* (Aloe) and *Da Huang* (Radix et Rhizoma Rhei) drain downward, and eliminate heat and fire through defecation. • *Mu Xiang* (Radix Aucklandiae) regulates qi circulation and relieves pain. • *Dang Gui* (Radix Angelicae Sinensis) nourishes and protects yin and blood. • *She Xiang* (Moschus) awakens individuals who are unconscious or semi-unconscious.

MODIFICATIONS
• With irritability, thirst, and fever add *Mai Dong* (Radix Ophiopogonis) and *Wu Wei Zi* (Fructus Schisandrae Chinensis).
• With difficulty in urination, add *Mu Tong* (Caulis Akebiae) and *Di Huang* (Radix Rehmanniae).
• With constipation, add *Zhi Shi* (Fructus Aurantii Immaturus) and *Hou Po* (Cortex Magnoliae Officinalis).
• For chronic granulocytic leukemia, add *Qing Dai* (Indigo Naturalis).

CAUTIONS / CONTRAINDICATIONS
• *Dang Gui Long Hui Wan* is a very bitter and cold formula that may injure the Spleen and Stomach. It is contraindicated in patients with deficiency and cold in the middle *jiao*. Prolonged or heavy use is also contraindicated.
• *Dang Gui Long Hui Wan* should be reserved for a purely excess condition with no deficiency, since most herbs in the formula are sedating or moving in nature. This formula is contraindicated in cases of deficiency.
• This formula is contraindicated during pregnancy.[1]
• According to one report, use of this formula may cause side effects such as nausea, vomiting, diarrhea, abdominal pain, stomach discomfort, dizziness and fatigue.[2]

CLINICAL STUDIES AND RESEARCH
1. **Constipation**: One report involving 6 patients stated that *Dang Gui Long Hui Wan* was effective in treating constipation due to various causes.[3]
2. **Biliary ascariasis**: *Dang Gui Long Hui Wan* was effective in treating 15 patients with biliary ascariasis who did not respond to earlier treatment with *Wu Mei Wan* (Mume

Pill). No recurrence was found in follow-up exams 3-8 months later.[4]

3. **Acne**: One study reported 85% effectiveness using modified *Dang Gui Long Hui Wan* to treat acne in 20 women (between 17-30 years of age, with 7 months to 2 years of acne). The herbal formula contained *Dang Gui* (Radix Angelicae Sinensis), *Long Dan* (Radix et Rhizoma Gentianae), *Lu Hui* (Aloe), *Huang Qin* (Radix Scutellariae), *Mu Xiang* (Radix Aucklandiae), *Xiang Fu* (Rhizoma Cyperi), *Chai Hu* (Radix Bupleuri), and *Da Huang* (Radix et Rhizoma Rhei). Moreover, *Tao Ren* (Semen Persicae), *Hong Hua* (Flos Carthami), and *Dan Shen* (Radix et Rhizoma Salviae Miltiorrhizae) were added before menstruation to move blood and regulate menses; *Bai Shao* (Radix Paeoniae Alba), *Bai Zhu* (Rhizoma Atractylodis Macrocephalae), and *Dang Gui Wei* (Extremitas Radix Angelicae Sinensis) were added for individuals with scanty menstruation or amenorrhea; and *Huang Lian* (Rhizoma Coptidis) and *Zhi Zi* (Fructus Gardeniae) were added for irritability and constipation. The herbs were administered daily in decoction form for 1 month per course of treatment.[5]

References
1. *Zhong Yao Ming Fang Yao Li Yu Ying Yong* (Pharmacology and Applications of Famous Herbal Formulas) 1989;212-214.
2. *Si Chuan Zhong Cao Yao Tong Xun* (Sichuan Journal of Chinese Herbology) 1972;(3):25.
3. *Zhong Cheng Yao* (Study of Chinese Patent Medicine) 1988;10:25.
4. *Zhe Jiang Zhong Yi Za Zhi* (Zhejiang Journal of Chinese Medicine) 1965;7:20.
5. *Shang Hai Zhong Yi Za Zhi* (Shanghai Journal of Chinese Medicine) 1999;7:38.

380

Chinese Herbal Formulas and Applications

Xǐ Gān Míng Mù Sǎn (Wash the Liver and Brighten the Eyes Powder)

洗肝明目散

Pinyin Name: *Xi Gan Ming Mu San*
Literal Name: Wash the Liver and Brighten the Eyes Powder
Alternate Name: Gardenia and Vitex Combination
Original Source: *Wan Bing Hui Chun* (Restoration of Health from the Myriad Diseases) by Gong Ting-Xian in 1587

COMPOSITION

Dang Gui Wei (Extremitas Radix Angelicae Sinensis)

Chi Shao (Radix Paeoniae Rubra)

Chuan Xiong (Rhizoma Chuanxiong)

Di Huang (Radix Rehmanniae)

Huang Lian (Rhizoma Coptidis)

Huang Qin (Radix Scutellariae)

Zhi Zi (Fructus Gardeniae)

Shi Gao (Gypsum Fibrosum)

Qiang Huo (Rhizoma et Radix Notopterygii)

Fang Feng (Radix Saposhnikoviae)

Jie Geng (Radix Platycodonis)

Jing Jie (Herba Schizonepetae)

Bo He (Herba Menthae)

Jue Ming Zi (Semen Cassiae)

Lian Qiao (Fructus Forsythiae)

Man Jing Zi (Fructus Viticis)

Ji Li (Fructus Tribuli)

Ju Hua (Flos Chrysanthemi)

Gan Cao (Radix et Rhizoma Glycyrrhizae)

DOSAGE / PREPARATION / ADMINISTRATION

Grind equal amounts of the herbs into powder, cook in water, and take the warm, strained decoction after meals.

CHINESE THERAPEUTIC ACTIONS

1. Dispels wind-heat
2. Clears Liver heat and fire

CLINICAL MANIFESTATIONS

Wind-heat attacking the eyes: redness, swelling and pain of the eyes, dizziness, and headache.

CLINICAL APPLICATIONS

Sclerotic keratitis, keratitis, iritis, glaucoma, conjunctivitis, and eye infections.

EXPLANATION

Xi Gan Ming Mu San (Wash the Liver and Brighten the Eyes Powder) treats various types of eye problems characterized by wind-heat. The presence of wind-heat encourages the rise of Liver heat and fire. Because wind and heat tend to travel upward, they cause symptoms such as redness, swelling, and pain of the eyes.

Dang Gui Wei (Extremitas Radix Angelicae Sinensis), *Chi Shao* (Radix Paeoniae Rubra), *Chuan Xiong* (Rhizoma Chuanxiong), and *Di Huang* (Radix Rehmanniae) tonify the blood, as well as activate and promote the circulation of blood. *Huang Lian* (Rhizoma Coptidis), *Huang Qin* (Radix Scutellariae), *Zhi Zi* (Fructus Gardeniae), and *Shi Gao* (Gypsum Fibrosum) clear heat from the body. *Qiang Huo* (Rhizoma et Radix Notopterygii), *Fang Feng* (Radix Saposhnikoviae), *Jie Geng* (Radix Platycodonis), *Jing Jie* (Herba Schizonepetae) and *Bo He* (Herba Menthae) are all lifting herbs that clear wind and lead the effects of the other herbs to the head. *Jue Ming Zi* (Semen Cassiae), *Lian Qiao* (Fructus Forsythiae), *Man Jing Zi* (Fructus Viticis), *Ji Li* (Fructus Tribuli), and *Ju Hua* (Flos Chrysanthemi) clear heat from the Liver channel, and are excellent herbs for addressing various types of eye disorders. Lastly, *Gan Cao* (Radix et Rhizoma Glycyrrhizae) harmonizes the formula.

MODIFICATIONS

- If there is more tearing as a result of wind-heat, add *Xia Ku Cao* (Spica Prunellae) and *Xiang Fu* (Rhizoma Cyperi).

HEAT-CLEARING FORMULAS

5

381

Chapter 5 – Heat-Clearing Formulas　　　　　　　　　　　　*Section 5 – Zang Fu-Clearing Formulas*

Xǐ Gān Míng Mù Sǎn (Wash the Liver and Brighten the Eyes Powder)

Xi Gan Ming Mu San (Wash the Liver and Brighten the Eyes Powder)

Diagnosis	Signs and Symptoms	Treatment	Herbs
Wind-heat attacking the eyes	• Redness, swelling and pain of the eyes: wind-heat attacking the eyes • Dizziness and headache: wind-heat attacking the head	• Dispels wind-heat • Clears Liver heat and fire	• *Dang Gui Wei* (Extremitas Radix Angelicae Sinensis), *Chi Shao* (Radix Paeoniae Rubra), *Chuan Xiong* (Rhizoma Chuanxiong) and *Di Huang* (Radix Rehmanniae) tonify the blood and promote blood circulation. • *Huang Lian* (Rhizoma Coptidis), *Huang Qin* (Radix Scutellariae), *Zhi Zi* (Fructus Gardeniae) and *Shi Gao* (Gypsum Fibrosum) clear heat from the body. • *Qiang Huo* (Rhizoma et Radix Notopterygii), *Fang Feng* (Radix Saposhnikoviae), *Jie Geng* (Radix Platycodonis), *Jing Jie* (Herba Schizonepetae) and *Bo He* (Herba Menthae) dispel wind. • *Jue Ming Zi* (Semen Cassiae), *Lian Qiao* (Fructus Forsythiae), *Man Jing Zi* (Fructus Viticis), *Ji Li* (Fructus Tribuli) and *Ju Hua* (Flos Chrysanthemi) clear heat from the Liver channel. • *Gan Cao* (Radix et Rhizoma Glycyrrhizae) harmonizes the formula.

- With constipation, add *Da Huang* (Radix et Rhizoma Rhei).
- With Liver fire, add *Long Dan* (Radix et Rhizoma Gentianae) and *Chai Hu* (Radix Bupleuri), and remove *Bo He* (Herba Menthae).

PHARMACOLOGICAL EFFECTS

Ocular: One study reported that administration of *Xi Gan Ming Mu San* and *Huang Lian Jie Du Tang* (Coptis Decoction to Relieve Toxicity) was associated with significantly suppressed (P < 0.001) elevation of aqueous flare induced by lipopolysaccharides in rabbits.[1]

AUTHORS' COMMENTS

Xi Gan Ming Mu San and *Ming Mu Di Huang Wan* (Improve Vision Pill with Rehmannia) both improve and brighten vision.

- *Xi Gan Ming Mu San* is generally used for infection and inflammation of the eyes, characterized by wind-heat attacking the eyes.
- *Ming Mu Di Huang Wan* is more applicable for deterioration of the eyes due to aging, characterized by Liver and Kidney yin deficiencies.

Reference

1. Nagaki Y, Hayasaka S, Kadoi C, Matsumoto M, Nakamura N, Hayasaka Y. Effects of Orengedoku-to and Senkanmeimoku-to, traditional herbal medicines, on the experimental elevation of aqueous flare in pigmented rabbits. Am J Chin Med 2001;29(1):141-7.

Chinese Herbal Formulas and Applications

Xiè Bái Săn (Drain the White Powder)

瀉白散
泻白散

Pinyin Name: *Xie Bai San*
Literal Name: Drain the White Powder
Alternate Names: *Xie Fei San* (Drain the Lung Powder), White-Draining Formula, Morus and Lycium Formula
Original Source: *Xiao Er Yao Zheng Zhi Jue* (Craft of Medicinal Treatment for Childhood Disease Patterns) by Qian Yi in 1119

COMPOSITION

Sang Bai Pi (Cortex Mori), *chao* (dry-fried)	30g [15g]
Di Gu Pi (Cortex Lycii)	30g [15g]
Zhi Gan Cao (Radix et Rhizoma Glycyrrhizae Praeparata cum Melle)	3g [3g]

DOSAGE / PREPARATION / ADMINISTRATION

The source text states to grind the ingredients into powder. Cook the herbs with one pinch of *Geng Mi* (Semen Oryzae) in two small bowls of water until the liquid is reduced to 70%. Take the decoction before meals. Today, this formula may be prepared as a decoction with the doses suggested in brackets.

CHINESE THERAPEUTIC ACTIONS

1. Clears heat and sedates the Lung
2. Stops coughing and relieves dyspnea

CLINICAL MANIFESTATIONS

Lung heat: coughing, hurried respiration leading to dyspnea; a warm steaming sensation of the skin that is most prominent in the late afternoon; a red tongue body with a yellow coating; and a fine, rapid pulse.

CLINICAL APPLICATIONS

Pneumonia, bronchitis, epistaxis, cough, whooping cough, and asthma.

EXPLANATION

Xie Bai San (Drain the White Powder) treats Lung heat with reversed flow of Lung qi. As heat and fire accumulate in the Lung, they disturb the normal flow of Lung qi and cause it to rise abnormally, leading to coughing, hurried respiration and dyspnea. Warm steaming sensations (especially in the late afternoon) without measurable fever indicate that the yin is gradually being injured and deficiency fire is forming. A red tongue body with a yellow coating suggests accumulation of heat in the body, while a fine, rapid pulse suggests that the heat has damaged yin.

Sang Bai Pi (Cortex Mori) sedates Lung fire, clears Lung heat, and corrects the reversed flow of Lung qi. *Di Gu Pi* (Cortex Lycii) helps clear Lung heat and cools the warm, steaming sensations of the skin in the late afternoons. *Geng Mi* (Semen Oryzae) and *Zhi Gan Cao* (Radix et Rhizoma Glycyrrhizae Praeparata cum Melle) nourish and strengthen Lung and Stomach qi.

MODIFICATIONS

• For cough caused by dry heat, add *Bei Mu* (Bulbus Fritillariae), *Gua Lou Pi* (Pericarpium Trichosanthis),

Xie Bai San (Drain the White Powder)

Diagnosis	Signs and Symptoms	Treatment	Herbs
Coughing caused by Lung heat	• Coughing, hurried respiration and dyspnea: Lung heat causing reversed flow of Lung qi • Warm, steaming sensations of the skin (especially in the late afternoon): heat damaging yin with deficiency heat affecting the skin • Red tongue body and a yellow coating: heat in the body • Fine, rapid pulse: heat damaging yin	• Clears heat and sedates the Lung • Stops coughing and relieves dyspnea	• *Sang Bai Pi* (Cortex Mori) sedates Lung fire, clears stagnant heat, and corrects the reversed flow of Lung qi. • *Di Gu Pi* (Cortex Lycii) clears Lung heat and cools the warm steaming sensations of the skin. • *Geng Mi* (Semen Oryzae) and *Zhi Gan Cao* (Radix et Rhizoma Glycyrrhizae Praeparata cum Melle) nourish and strengthen Lung and Stomach qi.

383

Xiè Bái Sǎn (Drain the White Powder)

Sha Shen (Radix Glehniae seu Adenophorae), and *Ku Xing Ren* (Semen Armeniacae Amarum).

- If there is alternation of chills and fever, add *Chai Hu* (Radix Bupleuri) and *Bai Shao* (Radix Paeoniae Alba).
- With thirst with irritability, add *Mai Dong* (Radix Ophiopogonis) and *Wu Wei Zi* (Fructus Schisandrae Chinensis).
- With cough and wheezing, add *Ku Xing Ren* (Semen Armeniacae Amarum) and *Jie Geng* (Radix Platycodonis).
- With qi deficiency, add *Ren Shen* (Radix et Rhizoma Ginseng) and *Huang Qi* (Radix Astragali).
- With tidal fever due to yin deficiency, add *Qing Hao* (Herba Artemisiae Annuae), *Bie Jia* (Carapax Trionycis), and *Yin Chai Hu* (Radix Stellariae).
- When there is Lung abscess, add *Bei Mu* (Bulbus Fritillariae), *Zi Wan* (Radix et Rhizoma Asteris), *Jie Geng* (Radix Platycodonis), *Dang Gui* (Radix Angelicae Sinensis), and *Gua Lou Zi* (Semen Trichosanthis).
- With more heat in the Lung, add *Huang Qin* (Radix Scutellariae) and *Zhi Mu* (Rhizoma Anemarrhenae).

CAUTIONS / CONTRAINDICATIONS

Xie Bai San is contraindicated in cases of cough caused by wind-cold or deficiency and cold.

CLINICAL STUDIES AND RESEARCH

1. **Cough**: One study reported beneficial results using modified *Xie Bai San* to treat children with chronic cough. The herbal treatment used *Xie Bai San* as the base formula, and added *Zi Su Zi* (Fructus Perillae) and *Kuan Dong Hua* (Flos Farfarae) for individuals who have dyspnea; *Ban Xia* (Rhizoma Pinelliae) for profuse phlegm; *Shan Zha* (Fructus Crataegi) for poor appetite; and *Dong Gua Zi* (Semen Benincasae) for constipation.[1]
2. **Whooping cough**: Modified *Xie Bai San* was used to treat 63 patients with whooping cough with most reporting improved symptoms within 4-8 packs of herbs.[2]
3. **Pneumonia**: Fifty-eight children with pneumonia and cough were treated with modified *Xie Bai San* with 96.5% effectiveness. The study reported complete recovery in 48 cases, improvement in 8 cases, and no effect in 2 cases. The herbal treatment contained *Sang Bai Pi* (Cortex Mori) 6g, *Di Gu Pi* (Cortex Lycii) 6g, *Sha Shen* (Radix Glehniae seu Adenophorae) 6g, *Mai Dong* (Radix Ophiopogonis) 6g, *Huang Qin* (Radix Scutellariae) 3g, *Ku Xing Ren* (Semen Armeniacae Amarum) 3g, *Tao Ren* (Semen Persicae) 3g, *Bai Bu* (Radix Stemonae) 3g, *Chuan Bei Mu* (Bulbus Fritillariae Cirrhosae) 3g, *Bai Qian* (Rhizoma et Radix Cynanchi Stauntonii) 3g, *Ban Xia* (Rhizoma Pinelliae) 3g, *Gan Cao* (Radix et Rhizoma Glycyrrhizae) 1g, and *Shan Ci Gu* (Pseudobulbus Cremastrae seu Pleiones) 1-1.5g.[3]

4. **Epistaxis**: One study reported good results using modified *Xie Bai San* to treat 20 patients with nosebleeds. Modifications included the addition of *Sha Shen* (Radix Glehniae seu Adenophorae), *Yu Zhu* (Rhizoma Polygonati Odorati), *Mai Dong* (Radix Ophiopogonis), and *Sang Ye* (Folium Mori) for Lung dryness with yin deficiency; *Huang Qin* (Radix Scutellariae) and *Di Huang* (Radix Rehmanniae) for Lung heat; *Da Huang* (Radix et Rhizoma Rhei) and *Huang Lian* (Rhizoma Coptidis) for Stomach fire; and *Xi Yang Shen* (Radix Panacis Quinquefolii) and *Di Huang* (Radix Rehmanniae) for qi and yin deficiencies. Of 20 patients, 13 had complete recovery and 7 showed improvement.[4]

RELATED FORMULA

Tíng Lì Dà Zǎo Xiè Fèi Tāng
(Descurainia and Jujube Decoction to Drain the Lung)

葶藶大棗瀉肺湯
葶苈大枣泻肺汤

Pinyin Name: Ting Li Da Zao Xie Fei Tang
Literal Name: Descurainia and Jujube Decoction to Drain the Lung
Original Source: *Jin Gui Yao Lue* (Essentials from the Golden Cabinet) by Zhang Zhong-Jing in the Eastern Han Dynasty

Ting Li Zi (Semen Descurainiae seu Lepidii), *ao* (simmered) until yellow and *dao* (pounded) into the size of a bullet	[6-9g]
Da Zao (Fructus Jujubae)	12 pieces [4 pieces]

The source text instructs to first cook 12 pieces of *Da Zao* (Fructus Jujubae) in 3 cups [600 mL] of water and reduce it to 2 cups [400 mL]. Discard *Da Zao* (Fructus Jujubae), add *Ting Li Zi* (Semen Descurainiae seu Lepidii), and cook again until it is reduced to 1 cup [200 mL]. Take the decoction immediately. Today, the decoction may be prepared using the doses suggested in brackets.

Ting Li Da Zao Xie Fei Tang (Descurainia and Jujube Decoction to Drain the Lung) primarily sedates the Lung, regulates water, corrects the reversed flow of Lung qi, and relieves dyspnea. Clinically, it is commonly used for coughing and dyspnea with chest fullness and profuse phlegm and saliva.

Xie Bai San and *Ting Li Da Zao Xie Fei Tang* both drain the Lung.

- *Xie Bai San* drains the Lung to relieve coughing due to interior heat.
- *Ting Li Da Zao Xie Fei Tang* drains the Lung and relieves coughing due to the accumulation of phlegm and water.

Xiè Bái Săn (Drain the White Powder)

AUTHORS' COMMENTS

Xie Bai San, literally "Drain the White Powder," functions to drain heat from the Lung – the organ associated with the white color according to five elements theory.

Xie Bai San is a representative formula for treating cough caused by Lung heat. However, a question is sometimes raised that if *Xie Bai San* is formulated to sedate the Lung, why does the formula use *Sang Bai Pi* (Cortex Mori) and *Di Gu Pi* (Cortex Lycii), and not *Shi Gao* (Gypsum Fibrosum) and *Huang Qin* (Radix Scutellariae), to clear heat? Derived from *Xiao Er Yao Zheng Zhi Jue* (Craft of Medicinal Treatment for Childhood Disease Patterns), *Xie Bai San* was originally designed for children with Lung heat manifesting in both cough and dyspnea. *Huang Qin* (Radix Scutellariae) was not used because it can dry and damage yin in the process of clearing heat. *Shi Gao* (Gypsum Fibrosum) was also not selected because it is too strong for children's delicate internal organs. In contrast, *Sang Bai Pi* (Cortex Mori) and *Di Gu Pi* (Cortex Lycii) are more suitable, since they gently clear Lung heat and sedate Lung fire.[5]

Xie Bai San and *Ma Huang Xing Ren Gan Cao Shi Gao Tang* (Ephedra, Apricot Kernel, Licorice, and Gypsum Decoction) both clear Lung heat to relieve cough and wheezing, but have the following differences:

• *Xie Bai San* is designed for children who have accumulation of heat and fire in the Lung leading to qi reversal and gradual body fluid depletion. Aside from cough and wheezing, accompanying symptoms include warm, steaming sensations on the skin, especially in the late afternoon and a fine, rapid pulse. Because the *zang fu* organs in children are still tender, they are much more susceptible to damage. For that reason, the draining herbs

in this formula are milder in nature. *Sang Bai Pi* (Cortex Mori) and *Di Gu Pi* (Cortex Lycii) gently clears deficiency heat while *Geng Mi* (Semen Oryzae) and *Gan Cao* (Radix et Rhizoma Glycyrrhizae) strengthen the Spleen and Stomach (earth element) to support the Lung (metal element). Together, the herbs clear heat without injuring yin and sedate the Lung without injuring *zheng* (upright) *qi*. In summary, *Xie Bai San* cools and nourishes the Lung and is more for chronic cases of cough or wheezing with yin-deficient constitutions.

• *Ma Huang Xing Ren Gan Cao Shi Gao Tang* is designed for wind-heat or wind-cold invasion leading to Lung heat accumulation, which then causes reversed flow of Lung qi. Besides the symptoms of cough and wheezing, it also treats fever, thirst with a preference to drink, and a rapid pulse. *Ma Huang* (Herba Ephedrae) is used to disperse external pathogenic factors and is coupled with *Shi Gao* (Gypsum Fibrosum) to strongly sedate Lung and Stomach fire and also to generate body fluids. *Ku Xing Ren* (Semen Armeniacae Amarum) guides Lung qi downward, and further helps *Ma Huang* (Herba Ephedrae) regulate respiration. In summary, *Ma Huang Xing Ren Gan Cao Shi Gao Tang* sedates the Lung and ventilates qi, and is used mainly in cases of excess pathogenic factors invading the Lung.[6]

References

1. *Shi Yong Zhong Xi Yi Jie He Za Zhi* (Practical Journal of Integrated Chinese and Western Medicines) 1997;3:239.
2. *Yi Fang Xin Jie* (New Explanation for Medical Formulas) 1980;100.
3. *Shan Xi Zhong Yi* (Shanxi Chinese Medicine) 1995;16(8):362.
4. *Hu Bei Zhong Yi Za Zhi* (Hubei Journal of Chinese Medicine) 1997;4:35.
5. Wang MZ, et al. *Zhong Yi Xue Wen Da Ti Ku* (Questions and Answers on Traditional Chinese Medicine: Herbal Formulas).
6. Wang MZ, et al. *Zhong Yi Xue Wen Da Ti Ku* (Questions and Answers on Traditional Chinese Medicine: Herbal Formulas).

Chapter 5 – Heat-Clearing Formulas   *Section 5 – Zang Fu-Clearing Formulas*

Qīng Xīn Lì Gé Tāng
(Clear the Epigastrium and Benefit the Diaphragm Decoction)
清心利膈湯
清心利膈汤

Pinyin Name: *Qing Xin Li Ge Tang*
Literal Name: Clear the Epigastrium and Benefit the Diaphragm Decoction
Alternate Names: *Ching Hsin Li Ke Tang*, Heart-Clearing Diaphragm-Relieving Decoction, Arctium Combination
Original Source: *Zheng Zhi Zhun Sheng* (Standards of Patterns and Treatments) by Wang Ken-Tang in 1602

COMPOSITION

Fang Feng (Radix Saposhnikoviae)	4.5g
Jing Jie (Herba Schizonepetae)	4.5g
Bo He (Herba Menthae)	4.5g
Jie Geng (Radix Platycodonis)	4.5g
Huang Qin (Radix Scutellariae)	4.5g
Huang Lian (Rhizoma Coptidis)	4.5g
Zhi Zi (Fructus Gardeniae)	3g
Xuan Shen (Radix Scrophulariae)	2.1g
Niu Bang Zi (Fructus Arctii)	2.1g
Lian Qiao (Fructus Forsythiae)	3g
Da Huang (Radix et Rhizoma Rhei)	2.1g
Mang Xiao (Natrii Sulfas)	2.1g
Gan Cao (Radix et Rhizoma Glycyrrhizae)	2.1g

DOSAGE / PREPARATION / ADMINISTRATION

Cook the herbs in 2 bowls of water and reduce the liquid to 1 bowl. Take the warm, strained decoction after meals.

CHINESE THERAPEUTIC ACTIONS

1. Dispels wind and clears heat
2. Regulates qi and eliminates toxins

CLINICAL MANIFESTATIONS

Excess heat attacking the Lung and throat: severe pain and swelling of the throat, discomfort in the chest and epigastrium, fidgeting, irritability, preference for cold drinks, constipation, and dysuria.

CLINICAL APPLICATIONS

Sore throat, tonsillitis, strep throat, and parotitis.

EXPLANATION

Qing Xin Li Ge Tang (Clear the Epigastrium and Benefit the Diaphragm Decoction) treats cases of severe swelling and pain of the throat due to heat attacking the Lung and throat. Clinically, the sore throat is so severe that it is difficult to eat and swallow. In addition, heat in the Lung may lead to other symptoms, such as discomfort in the chest and epigastrium, fidgeting, irritability, and preference for cold drinks. Constipation and dysuria indicate excess heat traveling downward.

Fang Feng (Radix Saposhnikoviae), *Jing Jie* (Herba Schizonepetae), and *Bo He* (Herba Menthae) dispel the exterior pathogenic factors. *Jie Geng* (Radix Platycodonis) regulates Lung qi to eliminate phlegm and relieve chest discomfort. *Huang Qin* (Radix Scutellariae), *Huang Lian* (Rhizoma Coptidis) and *Zhi Zi* (Fructus Gardeniae) clear heat, purge fire, and eliminate toxins. Together, these herbs address the underlying cause of the illness. *Xuan Shen* (Radix Scrophulariae) benefits the throat as well as clears heat and preserves yin and body fluids by preventing their consumption by the bitter and cold herbs. *Niu Bang Zi* (Fructus Arctii) and *Lian Qiao* (Fructus Forsythiae) alleviate sore throat and eliminate heat and toxins. *Da Huang* (Radix et Rhizoma Rhei) and *Mang Xiao* (Natrii Sulfas) drain heat downward and relieve constipation. Lastly, *Gan Cao* (Radix et Rhizoma Glycyrrhizae) eliminates toxins and harmonizes the formula.

MODIFICATIONS

- With more soreness and swelling of the throat, add *Shan Dou Gen* (Radix et Rhizoma Sophorae Tonkinensis) and *She Gan* (Rhizoma Belamcandae).
- With drooling and thirst, add *Tian Hua Fen* (Radix Trichosanthis) and *Zhu Ru* (Caulis Bambusae in Taenia).
- With irritability and preference for cold drinks, add *Shi Gao* (Gypsum Fibrosum) and *Zhi Mu* (Rhizoma Anemarrhenae).

Qīng Xīn Lì Gé Tāng
(Clear the Epigastrium and Benefit the Diaphragm Decoction)

Qing Xin Li Ge Tang (Clear the Epigastrium and Benefit the Diaphragm Decoction)

Diagnosis	Signs and Symptoms	Treatment	Herbs
Excess heat attacking the Lung and throat	• Severe swelling and pain of the throat with difficulty in swallowing: heat attacking the throat • Chest and epigastric discomfort, fidgeting, irritability, and preference for cold drinks: heat affecting the Lung • Constipation and dysuria: excess heat traveling downward	• Dispels wind and clears heat • Regulates qi and eliminates toxins	• *Fang Feng* (Radix Saposhnikoviae), *Jing Jie* (Herba Schizonepetae) and *Bo He* (Herba Menthae) dispel the exterior pathogenic factors. • *Jie Geng* (Radix Platycodonis) eliminates phlegm and relieves chest discomfort. • *Huang Qin* (Radix Scutellariae), *Huang Lian* (Rhizoma Coptidis) and *Zhi Zi* (Fructus Gardeniae) clear heat, purge fire, and eliminate toxins. • *Xuan Shen* (Radix Scrophulariae) benefits the throat, clears heat and preserves yin and body fluids. • *Niu Bang Zi* (Fructus Arctii) and *Lian Qiao* (Fructus Forsythiae) clear heat and eliminate toxins to alleviate sore throat. • *Da Huang* (Radix et Rhizoma Rhei) and *Mang Xiao* (Natrii Sulfas) drain heat downward and relieve constipation. • *Gan Cao* (Radix et Rhizoma Glycyrrhizae) eliminates toxins and harmonizes the herbs.

RELATED FORMULA

Qīng Xīn Lì Gé Tāng (Clear the Epigastrium and Benefit the Diaphragm Decoction)

清心利膈湯
清心利膈汤

Pinyin Name: *Qing Xin Li Ge Tang*
Literal Name: Clear the Epigastrium and Benefit the Diaphragm Decoction
Original Source: *Zhong Guo Yi Xue Da Ci Dian* (Grand Dictionary of Chinese Medicine)

Dan Zhu Ye (Herba Lophatheri)	[6g]
Fang Feng (Radix Saposhnikoviae)	[4.5g]
Jing Jie (Herba Schizonepetae)	[4.5g]
Bo He (Herba Menthae)	[4.5g]
Jie Geng (Radix Platycodonis)	[4.5g]
Huang Qin (Radix Scutellariae)	[4.5g]
Huang Lian (Rhizoma Coptidis)	[4.5g]
Zhi Zi (Fructus Gardeniae)	[2.25g]
Lian Qiao (Fructus Forsythiae)	[2.25g]
Jin Yin Hua (Flos Lonicerae Japonicae)	[3g]
Xuan Shen (Radix Scrophulariae)	[2.25g]
Da Huang (Radix et Rhizoma Rhei)	[2.25g]
Mang Xiao (Natrii Sulfas)	[2.25g]
Niu Bang Zi (Fructus Arctii)	[2.25g]
Gan Cao (Radix et Rhizoma Glycyrrhizae)	[2.25g]

This formula dispels wind, clears heat, and eliminates toxins. It treats soreness and swelling of the throat and the surrounding glands. Other signs and symptoms may include irritability, restlessness, preference for cold drinks, constipation, and dysuria with yellow urine.

These two formulas have identical names, and very similar compositions and functions.

• *Qing Xin Li Ge Tang* from *Zheng Zhi Zhun Sheng* (Standards of Patterns and Treatments) is the classic formula designed to treat excess heat attacking the Lung and throat.

• *Qing Xin Li Ge Tang* from *Zhong Guo Yi Xue Da Ci Dian* (Grand Dictionary of Chinese Medicine) is the contemporary formula, with the addition of *Dan Zhu Ye* (Herba Lophatheri) and *Jin Yin Hua* (Flos Lonicerae Japonicae) to enhance the overall effects of clear heating and eliminating toxins.

Chapter 5 – Heat-Clearing Formulas   Section 5 – Zang Fu-Clearing Formulas

Xiǎng Shēng Pò Dí Sǎn (Loud Sound Powder for a Broken Flute)

響聲破笛散
响声破笛散

Pinyin Name: *Xiang Sheng Po Di San*
Literal Name: Loud Sound Powder for a Broken Flute
Alternate Names: *Tie Di Wan* (Iron Flute Pill), *Hsiang Sheng Po Ti Wan*, *Xiang Sheng Po Di Wan*, Loud Sound Resembling Broken Bamboo Powder, Gasping Formula
Original Source: *Wan Bing Hui Chun* (Restoration of Health from the Myriad Diseases) by Gong Ting-Xian in 1587

COMPOSITION

Lian Qiao (Fructus Forsythiae)	75g
Jie Geng (Radix Platycodonis)	75g
Chuan Xiong (Rhizoma Chuanxiong)	45g
He Zi (Fructus Chebulae), *wei* (roasted)	30g
Er Cha (Catechu)	60g
Sha Ren (Fructus Amomi)	30g
Bo He (Herba Menthae)	120g
Da Huang (Radix et Rhizoma Rhei), *zheng* (steamed) with liquor	30g
Gan Cao (Radix et Rhizoma Glycyrrhizae)	75g

DOSAGE / PREPARATION / ADMINISTRATION

Grind the ingredients into a fine powder, and mix with egg white to form pills. The pills should resemble a large bullet in size. Dissolve one pill under the tongue and swallow at bedtime.

CHINESE THERAPEUTIC ACTIONS

1. Clears Lung heat and dispels phlegm
2. Moistens dryness and nourishes yin

CLINICAL MANIFESTATIONS

Lung heat injuring yin and body fluids: hoarseness or loss of voice, a dry mouth and throat, and a scratchy throat.

CLINICAL APPLICATIONS

Hoarseness of voice, loss of voice, laryngitis, and discomfort of the throat.

EXPLANATION

Xiang Sheng Po Di San (Loud Sound Powder for a Broken Flute) is designed to treat hoarseness or loss of voice caused by excessive speaking or singing. The excessive use of the vocal cords produces an underlying yin deficiency with dryness and heat.

Lian Qiao (Fructus Forsythiae), *Jie Geng* (Radix Platy-codonis), and *Chuan Xiong* (Rhizoma Chuanxiong) reduce swelling and drain pus. *He Zi* (Fructus Chebulae) has a retaining and binding effect on the Lung to relieve cough, sore throat, and loss of voice. *Er Cha* (Catechu)

clears heat. *Sha Ren* (Fructus Amomi) moves qi and dispels dampness and phlegm. *Bo He* (Herba Menthae) releases the exterior and benefits the throat. *Da Huang* (Radix et Rhizoma Rhei) clears heat and reduces swelling. Lastly, *Gan Cao* (Radix et Rhizoma Glycyrrhizae) harmonizes the formula.

MODIFICATIONS

- With dryness of the mouth and throat, add *Mai Dong* (Radix Ophiopogonis) and *Tian Hua Fen* (Radix Trichosanthis).
- With loss of voice, add *Jin Yin Hua* (Flos Lonicerae Japonicae) and *She Gan* (Rhizoma Belamcandae).
- With difficulty in speaking, add *Huang Lian* (Rhizoma Coptidis) and *Huang Qin* (Radix Scutellariae).

AUTHORS' COMMENTS

This formula is designed specifically for individuals who have no voice or hoarseness of voice, caused by laryngitis, or excessive speaking or singing. In addition to taking this formula, they can facilitate recovery by drinking *Mu Hu Die* (Semen Oroxyli) and *Pang Da Hai* (Semen Sterculiae Lychnophorae) as tea throughout the day. Today, this formula is used most frequently by teachers, public speakers, musicians, and singers.

This formula is also known as 铁笛丸 *Tie Di Wan* (Iron Flute Pill), implying that one's vocal cord will be strong like an iron flute from the use of this formula.

388

Xiǎng Shēng Pò Dí Sǎn (Loud Sound Powder for a Broken Flute)

Xiang Sheng Po Di San (Loud Sound Powder for a Broken Flute)

Diagnosis	Signs and Symptoms	Treatment	Herbs
Lung heat damaging yin and body fluids	Hoarseness or loss of voice, laryngitis and discomfort of the throat	• Clears Lung heat and dispels phlegm • Moistens dryness and nourishes yin	• *Lian Qiao* (Fructus Forsythiae), *Jie Geng* (Radix Platycodonis) and *Chuan Xiong* (Rhizoma Chuanxiong) reduce swelling and drain pus. • *He Zi* (Fructus Chebulae) has a retaining and binding effect on the Lung to relieve cough, sore throat, and loss of voice. • *Er Cha* (Catechu) clears heat. • *Sha Ren* (Fructus Amomi) moves qi and dispels dampness and phlegm. • *Bo He* (Herba Menthae) releases the exterior and benefits the throat. • *Da Huang* (Radix et Rhizoma Rhei) clears heat and reduces swelling. • *Gan Cao* (Radix et Rhizoma Glycyrrhizae) harmonizes the herbs.

Zuǒ Jīn Wán (Left Metal Pill)

左金丸

Pinyin Name: *Zuo Jin Wan*
Literal Name: Left Metal Pill
Alternate Name: *Yu Lian Wan* (Evodia and Coptis Pill)
Original Source: *Dan Xi Xin Fa* (Teachings of [Zhu] Dan-Xi) by Zhu Zhen-Heng in 1481

COMPOSITION

Huang Lian (Rhizoma Coptidis)	180g [9g]
Wu Zhu Yu (Fructus Evodiae)	15-30g [1.5g]

DOSAGE / PREPARATION / ADMINISTRATION

The source text states to grind the ingredients into powder and form into pills with water. Take 50 pills [6g] with warm, boiled water. Today, this formula may be prepared as a decoction with the doses suggested in brackets.

CHINESE THERAPEUTIC ACTIONS

1. Clears the Liver and purges fire
2. Corrects the reversed flow of Stomach qi and stops vomiting

CLINICAL MANIFESTATIONS

Liver fire overacting on the Stomach: hypochondriac fullness and pain, epigastric distention, a bitter taste in the mouth, acid regurgitation, nausea, vomiting, belching, a red tongue body with a yellow tongue coating, and a wiry, rapid pulse.

CLINICAL APPLICATIONS

Acute and chronic gastritis, peptic ulcer disease, *H. pylori* infection, acid regurgitation, erosive gastritis, epigastric pain, and hepatitis.

EXPLANATION

Zuo Jin Wan (Left Metal Pill) treats Liver fire overacting on the Stomach. Liver fire results from Liver qi stagnation. Fire in the Liver channel leads to hypochondriac pain and a bitter taste in the mouth. Because wood is the

Zuǒ Jīn Wán (Left Metal Pill)

Zuo Jin Wan (Left Metal Pill)

Diagnosis	Signs and Symptoms	Treatment	Herbs
Liver fire overacting on the Stomach	• Hypochondriac fullness and pain and a bitter taste in the mouth: Liver fire • Epigastric distention, acid regurgitation, nausea, vomiting and belching: Liver fire overacting on the Stomach • Red tongue body and a yellow tongue coating: excess fire condition • Wiry, rapid pulse: Liver fire rising	• Clears the Liver and purges fire • Corrects Stomach heat and qi • Stops nausea and vomiting	• *Huang Lian* (Rhizoma Coptidis) sedates Liver fire and clears Stomach heat. • *Wu Zhu Yu* (Fructus Evodiae) corrects the reversed flow of Stomach qi to stop vomiting.

element that acts on earth, excess Liver fire overacts on the Stomach to cause Stomach heat and reversed flow of Stomach qi upwards. As a result, patients may experience epigastric pain, acid regurgitation, and/or vomiting.

Huang Lian (Rhizoma Coptidis) purges Liver fire and clears Stomach heat to treat both the cause and the symptoms. *Wu Zhu Yu* (Fructus Evodiae) corrects the reversed flow of Stomach qi to stop vomiting. The dose ratio of *Huang Lian* (Rhizoma Coptidis) to *Wu Zhu Yu* (Fructus Evodiae) is to be kept at 6:1 for two important reasons. First, *Huang Lian* (Rhizoma Coptidis) is the chief herb and must be used at a large dose to effectively clear Liver fire and Stomach heat. However, *Huang Lian* (Rhizoma Coptidis) is bitter and cold, and may damage the body when used at large doses. Therefore, a small dose of warm *Wu Zhu Yu* (Fructus Evodiae) is used to balance the bitter and cold properties of *Huang Lian* (Rhizoma Coptidis).

The rationale for the composition of this formula can also be explained using the mother and son relationship from Five-Element Theory, which states that excess condition of the mother element can be treated by sedating the son element. Thus, when the Liver [wood (mother) element] is in excess, the Heart [fire (son) element] can be sedated. So using *Huang Lian* (Rhizoma Coptidis) to sedate Heart fire indirectly treats Liver fire.

MODIFICATIONS
• With more severe acid regurgitation, add *Hai Piao Xiao* (Endoconcha Sepiae) and *Wa Leng Zi* (Concha Arcae).
• With more hypochondriac pain, add *Xiang Fu* (Rhizoma Cyperi) and *Fo Shou* (Fructus Citri Sarcodactylis); or *Si Ni San* (Frigid Extremities Powder).
• With abdominal pain, add *Bai Shao* (Radix Paeoniae Alba).
• For dysentery with abdominal pain and spasms, add *Bai Shao* (Radix Paeoniae Alba) and *Gan Cao* (Radix et Rhizoma Glycyrrhizae).

• If there are stress ulcers, add *Xiao Yao San* (Rambling Powder) or *Jia Wei Xiao Yao San* (Augmented Rambling Powder).
• For *H. pylori* infection, add *Bai Hua She She Cao* (Herba Hedyotis).

CAUTIONS / CONTRAINDICATIONS
• *Zuo Jin Wan* is contraindicated in cases of deficiency cold.
• This formula should not be used to treat hypochondriac pain caused by Liver, Gallbladder, and blood deficiencies.
• This formula is contraindicated during pregnancy.[1]
• Avoid cold or raw, pungent or spicy, and oily or greasy foods while taking this formula.[2]

PHARMACOLOGICAL EFFECTS
Gastrointestinal: Administration of a modified *Zuo Jin Wan* preparation was associated with protecting the stomach mucus membrane against sodium hydroxide, aspirin, and ethylamine hydrochloride in rats that have fasted for 24 hours. The dose of *Zuo Jin Wan* was 1 g/kg, and the formula was modified with the addition of one qi-regulating herb.[3]

CLINICAL STUDIES AND RESEARCH
1. **Gastritis**: *Zuo Jin Wan* was evaluated for its effectiveness in treating gastric ulcer due to reflux of bile to the stomach. Out of 24 patients, there were 10 males and 14 females, with ages ranging from 24 to 68 years of age. The history of illness ranged from 6 months to 7 years. Clinical presentations included stomach and gastric pain, nausea, vomiting, abdominal distention, and poor appetite. The basic formula used to treat these patients included *Huang Lian* (Rhizoma Coptidis) 5g, *Wu Zhu Yu* (Fructus Evodiae) 3g, *Jiang Xiang* (Lignum Dalbergiae Odoriferae) 10g, *Zhi Qiao* (Fructus Aurantii) 10g, *Niu Xi* (Radix Achyranthis Bidentatae) 10g, and *Da Huang* (Radix et Rhizoma Rhei) 10g. Minor modifications were made if necessary by adding *Chai Hu* (Radix Bupleuri), *Fo Shou* (Fructus Citri

Zuǒ Jīn Wán (Left Metal Pill)

Sarcodactylis), *Zhi Zi* (Fructus Gardeniae), *Yu Jin* (Radix Curcumae), and *Gan Cao* (Radix et Rhizoma Glycyrrhizae) for Liver fire overacting on the Stomach; *Dang Gui* (Radix Angelicae Sinensis), *Xiang Fu* (Rhizoma Cyperi), and *Qing Pi* (Pericarpium Citri Reticulatae Viride) for irregular menstruation with breast distention; *Chi Shao* (Radix Paeoniae Rubra), *Bai Shao* (Radix Paeoniae Alba), *San Qi* (Radix et Rhizoma Notoginseng), and *Shi Xiao San* (Sudden Smile Powder) for blood stagnation; and the addition of *Dang Shen* (Radix Codonopsis), dry-fried *Bai Zhu* (Rhizoma Atractylodis Macrocephalae), *Zhi Gan Cao* (Radix et Rhizoma Glycyrrhizae Praeparata cum Melle), and *Da Zao* (Fructus Jujubae), and the elimination of *Da Huang* (Radix et Rhizoma Rhei), for Spleen and Stomach deficiencies. The duration of treatment ranged from 15 to 56 days. The study reported effectiveness in 20 patients (complete resolution of symptoms with normal endoscopy), moderate effect in 3 patients (resolution of symptoms with minimal ulceration based on endoscopy), and no benefit in 1 patient. The overall rate of effectiveness was 95.8%.[4] Another study reported that gastritis due to regurgitation of bile acid can be treated effectively using *Zuo Jin Wan* plus *Bai Hua She She Cao* (Herba Hedyotis), *Zhi Shi* (Fructus Aurantii Immaturus), and *Cang Zhu* (Rhizoma Atractylodis). The duration of treatment was 15 days per course of treatment, for a total of 2 courses. Of 39 patients, 20 had complete recovery, 16 had significant improvement, and 3 had no change.[5]

2. **Erosive gastritis**: Use of modified *Zuo Jin Wan* to treat 44 patients with erosive gastritis was associated with 95.8% effectiveness. The herbs were decocted in water, and taken in two equally-divided doses daily. The duration of treatment was 20 days per course, for 2 courses. Modifications to the herbal treatment were made by adding herbs as follows: *Zhi Qiao* (Fructus Aurantii) and *Hou Po* (Cortex Magnoliae Officinalis) for fullness and distention in the upper abdominal area; *Tian Hua Fen* (Radix Trichosanthis) and *Shi Hu* (Caulis Dendrobii) for dry mouth and tongue with hunger but no desire to eat; *Hai Piao Xiao* (Endoconcha Sepiae) and calcined *Wa Leng Zi* (Concha Arcae) for acid reflux; *Shen Qu* (Massa Fermentata), *Mai Ya* (Fructus Hordei Germinatus), and *Ji Nei Jin* (Endothelium Corneum Gigeriae Galli) for anorexia; *Huo Ma Ren* (Fructus Cannabis) and *Yu Li Ren* (Semen Pruni) for constipation; and *Dang Shen* (Radix Codonopsis) and *Bai Zhu* (Rhizoma Atractylodis Macrocephalae) for Spleen and Stomach deficiencies. Of 44 cases, the study reported complete recovery in 31 cases, improvement in 11 cases, and no effect in 2 cases.[6]

3. **Epigastric pain**: One study reported 96.4% effectiveness using *Zuo Jin Wan* plus *Ban Xia* (Rhizoma Pinelliae) and *Chen Pi* (Pericarpium Citri Reticulatae) to treat epigastric pain. Of 110 patients, 19 had complete recovery, 56 had significant improvement, 31 had moderate improvement, and 4 had no effect.[7]

4. ***H. pylori* infection**: Use of *Zuo Jin Wan* was associated with successful treatment in 86 of 133 patients (64.7%) with *H. pylori* infection. The treatment protocol was to administer one pill twice daily for 2 weeks per course of treatment, for 2 courses total.[8]

HERB-DRUG INTERACTION

Aspirin: Administration of *Zuo Jin Wan* in rats was found to have marked protective effect against aspirin-induced damages to the stomach mucus membrane.[9]

RELATED FORMULAS

Wù Jǐ Wán (Wu Ji Pill)

戊己丸

Pinyin Name: *Wu Ji Wan*
Literal Name: Wu Ji Pill
Original Source: *Tai Ping Hui Min He Ji Ju Fang* (Imperial Grace Formulary of the Tai Ping Era) by the Imperial Medical Department in 1078-85

Huang Lian (Rhizoma Coptidis)	150g [10g]
Wu Zhu Yu (Fructus Evodiae), *chao* (dry-fried)	150g [10g]
Bai Shao (Radix Paeoniae Alba)	150g [10g]

The source text states to grind 150g of each ingredient into powder and form into pills with flour. The pills should resemble the size of *Wu Tong Zi* (Semen Firmianae), a small seed approximately 5 mm in diameter. Take 20 pills with rice soup three times daily on an empty stomach. This formula may be prepared as a decoction with the doses suggested in brackets.

Wu Ji Wan (Wu Ji Pill) treats disharmony of the Liver and Spleen with damp-heat dysentery. It clears the Liver, purges fire, and relieves pain. Clinically, the patient may show epigastric pain, abdominal pain, acid regurgitation, burning diarrhea, and dysentery.

Xiāng Lián Wán (Aucklandia and Coptis Pill)

香連丸
香连丸

Pinyin Name: *Xiang Lian Wan*
Literal Name: Aucklandia and Coptis Pill
Original Source: *Tai Ping Hui Min He Ji Ju Fang* (Imperial Grace Formulary of the Tai Ping Era) by the Imperial Medical Department in 1078-85

Zuǒ Jīn Wán (Left Metal Pill)

Huang Lian (Rhizoma Coptidis), *chao* (dry-fried) until
    red with 300g of *Wu Zhu Yu* (Fructus Evodiae)   600g
Mu Xiang (Radix Aucklandiae),
    do not expose to heat   144.2g

Dry-fry 600g of *Huang Lian* (Rhizoma Coptidis) with
300g of *Wu Zhu Yu* (Fructus Evodiae) first until *Huang
Lian* (Rhizoma Coptidis) turns red. Discard *Wu Zhu Yu*
(Fructus Evodiae). Grind the processed *Huang Lian*
(Rhizoma Coptidis) and *Mu Xiang* (Radix Aucklandiae)
into powder and form into pills with vinegar. The pills
should resemble the size of *Wu Tong Zi* (Semen Firmianae), a small seed approximately 5 mm in diameter.
Take 20 pills with rice.

Xiang Lian Wan (Aucklandia and Coptis Pill) clears heat,
dissolves dampness, regulate qi circulation, and stops
dysentery. Clinically, it may be used to treat damp-heat
dysentery with red (blood) or white (mucus) stools, rectal
tenesmus, abdominal pain, and a feeling of distention and
oppression in the chest and epigastrium.

Qīng Wèi Tāng (Clear the Stomach Decoction)
清胃湯
清胃汤
Pinyin Name: Qing Wei Tang
Literal Name: Clear the Stomach Decoction
Original Source: *An Hui Zhong Yi Xue Yuan* (Anhui
University School of Medicine) in 1990

Huang Lian (Rhizoma Coptidis)
Wu Zhu Yu (Fructus Evodiae)
Huang Qin (Radix Scutellariae)
Pu Gong Ying (Herba Taraxaci)
Ban Zhi Lian (Herba Scutellariae Barbatae)
Xian He Cao (Herba Agrimoniae)
Di Yu (Radix Sanguisorbae)
Mu Li (Concha Ostreae)
Zhe Bei Mu (Bulbus Fritillariae Thunbergii)
Chai Hu (Radix Bupleuri)
Xiang Fu (Rhizoma Cyperi)
Mai Ya (Fructus Hordei Germinatus)
Sha Ren (Fructus Amomi)
Huang Qi (Radix Astragali)

Bai Shao (Radix Paeoniae Alba)
Yan Hu Suo (Rhizoma Corydalis)

Qing Wei Tang (Clear the Stomach Decoction) clears
Stomach heat, corrects the reversed flow of Stomach qi,
stops bleeding, and relieves pain. Clinically, this formula
is used to treat various digestive problems, such as
gastrointestinal bleeding, stomach and duodenal ulcers,
and acid reflux.

AUTHORS' COMMENTS

Zuo Jin Wan treats Liver fire overacting on the Stomach.
There are two reasons why *Huang Lian* (Rhizoma
Coptidis) is a more suitable herb than *Long Dan* (Radix
et Rhizoma Gentianae) in this formula.

- *Huang Lian* (Rhizoma Coptidis) is better than *Long Dan*
(Radix et Rhizoma Gentianae) at sedating Heart fire.
Sedating the Heart will purge Liver fire according to the
mother-son relationship in Five-Element Theory.

- The chief complaints are upper gastrointestinal symptoms.
Huang Lian (Rhizoma Coptidis) is excellent at sedating
Stomach fire to treat acid regurgitation, burning pain,
nausea, and vomiting. *Long Dan* (Radix et Rhizoma
Gentianae) is an extremely bitter and cold herb, and
although it can sedate Liver fire, it may damage the
Stomach and cause more vomiting or nausea.[10]

References
1. *Zhong Yao Ming Fang Yao Li Yu Ying Yong* (Pharmacology and
Applications of Famous Herbal Formulas) 1989;189-191.
2. *Zhong Yao Ming Fang Yao Li Yu Ying Yong* (Pharmacology and
Applications of Famous Herbal Formulas) 1989;189-191.
3. *Zhong Yao Yao Li Yu Lin Chuang* (Pharmacology and Clinical
Applications of Chinese Herbs) 1993;9(4):9.
4. *Zhe Jiang Zhong Yi Za Zhi* (Zhejiang Journal of Chinese Medicine)
1993;28(9):394.
5. *Shan Xi Zhong Yi* (Shanxi Chinese Medicine) 1997;4:14.
6. *Shi Yong Zhong Yi Za Zhi* (Journal of Practical Chinese Medicine)
1999;2:10.
7. *Hu Bei Zhong Yi Za Zhi* (Hubei Journal of Chinese Medicine)
1998;3:40.
8. *Zhe Jiang Zhong Yi Za Zhi* (Zhejiang Journal of Chinese Medicine)
1997;10:437.
9. *Zhong Yao Yao Li Yu Lin Chuang* (Pharmacology and Clinical
Applications of Chinese Herbs) 1993;9(4):9.
10. Wang MZ, et al. *Zhong Yi Xue Wen Da Ti Ku* (Questions and
Answers on Traditional Chinese Medicine: Herbal Formulas).

Chinese Herbal Formulas and Applications

Qīng Wèi Sǎn (Clear the Stomach Powder)

清胃散

Pinyin Name: *Qing Wei San*
Literal Name: Clear the Stomach Powder
Alternate Names: *Ching Wei San*, Stomach-Clearing Powder, Coptis and Rehmannia Formula
Original Source: *Lan Shi Mi Cang* (Secrets from the Orchid Chamber) by Li Gao in 1336

COMPOSITION

Huang Lian (Rhizoma Coptidis)	0.9-1.8g [3-6g]
Di Huang (Radix Rehmanniae)	0.9g [6-12g]
Mu Dan Pi (Cortex Moutan)	1.5g [9g]
Dang Gui (Radix Angelicae Sinensis)	0.9g [6g]
Sheng Ma (Rhizoma Cimicifugae)	3g [6-9g]

DOSAGE / PREPARATION / ADMINISTRATION

The source text states to grind the ingredients into powder. Cook the herbs in 1.5 bowls of water until 70% of the liquid remains. Take the strained decoction after it has cooled. The dose of *Huang Lian* (Rhizoma Coptidis) may be increased in the summer. Today, this formula may be prepared as a decoction with the doses suggested in brackets.

CHINESE THERAPEUTIC ACTIONS

1. Clears Stomach heat
2. Cools the blood

CLINICAL MANIFESTATIONS

Heat accumulation in the Stomach: toothache with pain radiating to the temple leading to temporal headache; toothache that improves with coldness and worsens with heat; painful and swollen cheeks and oral cavity (lips and gum); swelling and ulcerations of the gum, bleeding gums; fever, foul breath, a dry mouth and tongue, a red tongue body with a yellow tongue coating, and a slippery, big and rapid pulse.

CLINICAL APPLICATIONS

Stomatitis, toothache, gingivitis, ulcerative gingivitis, periodontitis, periodontal disease, swelling of laryngo-pharynx, sore throat, trigeminal neuralgia, and halitosis.

EXPLANATION

Qing Wei San (Clear the Stomach Powder) clears Stomach heat. Since the Stomach channel travels to the cheeks and gum region, Stomach heat results in toothache and painful cheeks. The *yangming* Stomach is the organ that has an abundance of qi and blood. Thus, heat in the Stomach affects the blood and causes blood to flow out of its vessels, leading to swelling, ulceration and/or bleeding of the gums. Foul breath and a dry mouth are the results of Stomach heat rising.

Qing Wei San (Clear the Stomach Powder) uses *Huang Lian* (Rhizoma Coptidis) as the chief herb to clear heat in the Stomach. *Di Huang* (Radix Rehmanniae) cools the blood and nourishes yin. *Mu Dan Pi* (Cortex Moutan) clears heat and cools the blood. *Di Huang* (Radix Rehmanniae) and *Mu Dan Pi* (Cortex Moutan) also assist *Dang Gui* (Radix Angelicae Sinensis) to nourish and harmonize the blood. *Sheng Ma* (Rhizoma Cimicifugae) has two functions in this formula: it assists *Huang Lian* (Rhizoma Coptidis) to disperse rising Stomach heat and eliminate toxins, and it guides the other herbs in this formula to the *yangming* channel.

MODIFICATIONS

- With constipation, add *Da Huang* (Radix et Rhizoma Rhei) and *Mang Xiao* (Natrii Sulfas); or *Da Cheng Qi Tang* (Major Order the Qi Decoction).
- When there is swelling and pain of the gums, add *Huang Qin* (Radix Scutellariae) and *Xuan Shen* (Radix Scrophulariae).
- With swelling, inflammation and pain, add *Zhi Mu* (Rhizoma Anemarrhenae) and *Gan Cao* (Radix et Rhizoma Glycyrrhizae).
- With stomatitis, add *Jin Yin Hua* (Flos Lonicerae Japonicae) and *Lian Qiao* (Fructus Forsythiae).
- If there is toothache, add *Bai Hu Tang* (White Tiger Decoction).
- With toothache and headache, add *Xi Xin* (Radix et Rhizoma Asari) and *Bai Zhi* (Radix Angelicae Dahuricae).
- With thirst due to fluid deficiency, add *Xuan Shen* (Radix Scrophulariae) and *Tian Hua Fen* (Radix Trichosanthis).
- With thirst and preference for cold drinks due to more heat in the Stomach, add *Shi Gao* (Gypsum Fibrosum).
- With bleeding gums, add *Niu Xi* (Radix Achyranthis Bidentatae).
- With headache, add *Bai Zhi* (Radix Angelicae Dahuricae) and *Chuan Xiong* (Rhizoma Chuanxiong).

HEAT-CLEARING FORMULAS

5

393

Chapter 5 – Heat-Clearing Formulas　　　　　　　　　　*Section 5 – Zang Fu-Clearing Formulas*

Qīng Wèi Sǎn (Clear the Stomach Powder)

Qing Wei San (Clear the Stomach Powder)

Diagnosis	Signs and Symptoms	Treatment	Herbs
Stomach heat	• Toothache, painful cheeks, foul breath, painful and swollen cheeks and oral cavity: heat traveling up along the Stomach channel • Ulceration and/or bleeding of gums: heat forcing the blood to flow out of its vessels • Dry mouth and tongue: Stomach heat consuming body fluids • Red tongue body and a yellow tongue coating: heat condition • Slippery, big and rapid pulse: heat condition	• Clears Stomach heat • Cools blood	• *Huang Lian* (Rhizoma Coptidis) sedates excess heat in the Stomach. • *Di Huang* (Radix Rehmanniae) cools the blood and nourishes yin. • *Mu Dan Pi* (Cortex Moutan) clears heat and cools the blood. • *Dang Gui* (Radix Angelicae Sinensis) nourishes the blood. • *Sheng Ma* (Rhizoma Cimicifugae) clears heat, eliminates toxins, and guides the formula to the *yangming* channel.

• For burning diarrhea in children, remove *Di Huang* (Radix Rehmanniae), *Mu Dan Pi* (Cortex Moutan), and *Sheng Ma* (Rhizoma Cimicifugae); and add *Chuan Lian Zi* (Fructus Toosendan), *Huang Bo* (Cortex Phellodendri Chinensis), and *Di Yu* (Radix Sanguisorbae).

CAUTIONS / CONTRAINDICATIONS

Do not use *Qing Wei San* if the oral problems (toothache, swelling and pain of the gums, and gum bleeding) are caused by wind-cold, Kidney yin deficiency, or Kidney yin-deficient fire.

PHARMACOLOGICAL EFFECTS

1. **Anti-inflammatory**: In one laboratory study, injection of *Qing Wei San* was effective in reducing inflammation in rats. The injection given was a 5% solution with a dose of 10 mL/kg. Injection was given twice daily for 3 days.[1]

2. **Antibiotic**: Decoction of *Qing Wei San* was associated with mild inhibitory effects against *Staphylococcus aureus* and *Pseudomonas aeruginosa*, with a minimum inhibitory concentration (MIC) of 0.063 g/mL and 0.5 g/mL, respectively.[2]

3. **Immunostimulant**: In one experiment, oral ingestion of 0.5mL of a 0.5% solution of *Qing Wei San* for 3 days was associated with increased phagocytic activities by macrophages in mice.[3]

CLINICAL STUDIES AND RESEARCH

1. **Stomatitis**: In one clinical study, 75 patients with recurrent ulcerations were treated with *Qing Wei San* with good results in all patients. The patients were instructed to gargle and swallow the decoction three to five times daily. The patients recovered within an average of 6 days, with a range of 3-9 days.[4]

2. **Gingivitis**: In one report, patients with gingivitis were treated with satisfactory results using a combination of *Qing Wei San* and *Yu Nu Jian* (Jade Woman Decoction). Small modifications to the herbal formula were made as follows: *Da Huang* (Radix et Rhizoma Rhei) (post-decocted) for constipation; *Tian Hua Fen* (Radix Trichosanthis), *Lian Qiao* (Fructus Forsythiae), and *Zhu Ye* (Herba Phyllostachys) for severe gum swelling; and *Pu Huang* (Pollen Typhae), *Xian He Cao* (Herba Agrimoniae), *Bai Mao Gen* (Rhizoma Imperatae), and *Mo Han Lian* (Herba Ecliptae) for gum bleeding. Out of 103 cases, the study reported marked improvement in 94 cases (resolution of symptoms within 1 week) and moderate improvement in 9 cases (resolution of symptoms within 2 weeks).[5]

3. **Periodontitis**: Acute periodontitis in 56 patients was treated with marked success using *Qing Wei San* plus *Zhu Ye* (Herba Phyllostachys), *Lian Qiao* (Fructus Forsythiae), and *Tian Hua Fen* (Radix Trichosanthis). The herbs were given as decoction daily, and most patients experienced relief within 3-5 packs of herbs. Of 56 patients, the study reported complete relief in 32 cases, significant improvement in 19 cases, moderate improvement in 4 cases, and no effect in 1 case. The overall effectiveness was 98.2%.[6] Another study reported a marked effect using modified *Qing Wei San* to treat 52 patients with periodontitis. The herbal treatment contained *Qing Wei San* plus *Bai Hua She She Cao* (Herba Hedyotis) as the base formula, with addition of *Shi Gao* (Gypsum Fibrosum) and *Huang Lian* (Rhizoma Coptidis) for Stomach heat; *Bai Mao Gen* (Rhizoma Imperatae) and *Bai Ji* (Rhizoma Bletillae) for gum bleeding; *Sang Ji Sheng* (Herba Taxilli) and *Gou Ji* (Rhizoma Cibotii) for loose teeth; and *Da Huang* (Radix et Rhizoma Rhei) for constipation. After 7 days of herbal therapy, the study reported complete recovery in 41 cases,

394

Qīng Wèi Sǎn (Clear the Stomach Powder)

improvement in 8 cases, and no effect in 3 cases. The overall rate of effectiveness was 94%.[7]

4. **Periodontal disease**: Administration of *Qing Wei San* was associated with marked success in treating periodontal disease characterized by Stomach fire rising. The herbal treatment used *Qing Wei San* as the base formula, with the addition of *Da Huang* (Radix et Rhizoma Rhei) for constipation and *Yi Yi Ren* (Semen Coicis) and *Che Qian Zi* (Semen Plantaginis) for damp-heat. Of 58 cases, the study reported complete recovery in 38 cases, significant improvement in 15 cases, and slight improvement in 5 cases.[8]

5. **Halitosis**: One study reported good results using modified *Qing Wei San* to treat 32 patients with foul breath. In addition to the base formula, modifications were made as needed. For ulcerations of the mouth and tongue and redness, swelling, and pain of the gums, 30g of *Di Huang* (Radix Rehmanniae) was added, and the dose of *Huang Lian* (Rhizoma Coptidis) was increased to 15g. For abdominal distention and fullness, lack of appetite, belching and acid reflux, *Huang Qin* (Radix Scutellariae) and *Da Huang* (Radix et Rhizoma Rhei) were added, and *Dang Gui* (Radix Angelicae Sinensis) and *Sheng Ma* (Rhizoma Cimicifugae) were removed. For profuse, yellow sputum with chest and hypochondriac distention and pain, *Sheng Ma* (Rhizoma Cimicifugae) was removed, *Jin Yin Hua* (Flos Lonicerae Japonicae), *Di Gu Pi* (Cortex Lycii), and *Sang Bai Pi* (Cortex Mori) were added, and the dose of *Mu Dan Pi* (Cortex Moutan) was increased to 15g. The treatment protocol was to administer the herbs in decoction, for 6 packs of herbs per course of treatment, for 1-2 courses total. Of 32 cases, the study reported complete recovery in 31 cases and improvement in 1 case.[9]

TOXICOLOGY

In one acute toxicology study, no fatality was reported in mice following oral administration of a 100% solution of *Qing Wei San* at 0.4 mL per subject, a dose equivalent or greater than 150 times the normal adult dose in humans.[10]

AUTHORS' COMMENTS

Qing Wei San is commonly used for toothache caused by Stomach heat. The facial pain and toothache are located around the *yangming* channel on the face.

Qing Wei San, *Xie Huang San* (Drain the Yellow Powder), and *Yu Nu Jian* (Jade Woman Decoction) all clear heat, but have different underlying causes:

- *Qing Wei San* clears Stomach heat and cools the blood to treat toothache, bleeding gums, and/or swollen cheeks.
- *Xie Huang San* drains fire in the Spleen, which manifests in oral ulcers, foul breath, and a dry hot tongue.
- *Yu Nu Jian* nourishes Stomach yin and clears Stomach heat, treating both excess and deficiency. Symptoms include thirst, toothache, loose teeth, bleeding gums, and headache.

References

1. *Zhong Hua Kou Qiang Ke Za Zhi* (Chinese Journal of Stomatology) 1986;1:44.
2. *Zhong Hua Kou Qiang Ke Za Zhi* (Chinese Journal of Stomatology) 1986;1:44.
3. *Zhong Hua Kou Qiang Ke Za Zhi* (Chinese Journal of Stomatology) 1986;1:44.
4. *He Bei Zhong Yi* (Hebei Chinese Medicine) 1989;1:25.
5. *Shang Hai Zhong Yi Yao Za Zhi* (Shanghai Journal of Chinese Medicine and Herbology) 1994;6:31.
6. *Zhong Yi Za Zhi* (Journal of Chinese Medicine) 1985;7:65.
7. *Hu Nan Zhong Yi Za Zhi* (Hunan Journal of Chinese Medicine) 1997;5:36.
8. *Shan Dong Zhong Yi Za Zhi* (Shandong Journal of Chinese Medicine) 1996;9:402.
9. *Shan Xi Zhong Yi* (Shanxi Chinese Medicine) 1996;5:204.
10. *Zhong Hua Kou Qiang Ke Za Zhi* (Chinese Journal of Stomatology) 1986;1:44.

Chapter 5 – Heat-Clearing Formulas

Section 5 – Zang Fu-Clearing Formulas

Xiè Huáng Sǎn (Drain the Yellow Powder)

瀉黃散
泻黄散

Pinyin Name: *Xie Huang San*
Literal Name: Drain the Yellow Powder
Alternate Names: *Xie Pi San* (Drain the Spleen Powder), Siler and Licorice Formula
Original Source: *Xiao Er Yao Zheng Zhi Jue* (Craft of Medicinal Treatment for Childhood Disease Patterns) by Qian Yi in 1119

COMPOSITION

Shi Gao (Gypsum Fibrosum)	15g [5g]
Zhi Zi (Fructus Gardeniae)	3g [3g]
Fang Feng (Radix Saposhnikoviae), *qie* (sliced) and *bei* (stone-baked)	120g [12g]
Huo Xiang (Herba Agastaches)	21g [5g]
Gan Cao (Radix et Rhizoma Glycyrrhizae)	90g [9g]

Note: Please refer to the Authors' Comments for an explanation of the uncharacteristically high doses of *Fang Feng* (Radix Saposhnikoviae) and *Gan Cao* (Radix et Rhizoma Glycyrrhizae).

DOSAGE / PREPARATION / ADMINISTRATION

The source text states to grind the ingredients coarsely, dry-fry with honey-liquor until the aroma fills the air. Re-grind the coarse powder into a fine powder. Cook 3-6g of the powder in one large bowl of water until 50% of the liquid remains. Take the warm, strained decoction any time during the day. This formula may also be prepared as a decoction using the doses suggested in brackets.

CHINESE THERAPEUTIC ACTIONS

Purges latent fire in the Spleen and Stomach

CLINICAL MANIFESTATIONS

Latent fire in the Spleen and Stomach: mouth ulcerations, foul breath, a dry mouth and lips, irritability, thirst, frequent hunger, a red tongue body, and a rapid pulse.

CLINICAL APPLICATIONS

Stomatitis, epistaxis, halitosis, and fever.

EXPLANATION

Xie Huang San (Drain the Yellow Powder) treats latent fire of the Spleen and Stomach, a condition characterized by the presence of heat and fire hidden deep inside the body. According to traditional Chinese medicine principles, the sensory organ that belongs to the Spleen and Stomach is the mouth, and the condition of the Stomach and Spleen is manifested on the lips. Therefore, heat in the Spleen and Stomach travels upwards and results in mouth sores, foul breath, and a dry mouth and lips. Thirst and frequent hunger are the results of latent heat and fire in the Spleen

and Stomach damaging body fluids. Unlike excess Stomach fire, latent fire cannot be completely cleared if only heat-clearing herbs are used to sedate the heat. Because of the tendency of latent fire to stagnate and hide in the interior, it is necessary to use acrid herbs to disperse the heat outward.

Shi Gao (Gypsum Fibrosum) and *Zhi Zi* (Fructus Gardeniae) clear and sedate Spleen and Stomach fire. *Fang Feng* (Radix Saposhnikoviae) and *Huo Xiang* (Herba Agastaches) disperse and lift the latent fire so that the heat-clearing herbs can effectively clear the hidden heat. With its aromatic quality, *Huo Xiang* (Herba Agastaches) is also able to activate and restore the functioning of the Spleen and Stomach. *Gan Cao* (Radix et Rhizoma Glycyrrhizae) helps clear heat and protects Spleen and Stomach qi from being injured by the cold herbs in this formula. This formula uses dispersing/lifting and clearing/sedating methods to completely eliminate latent fire of the Spleen and Stomach.

MODIFICATIONS

- When there is a feeling of warmth in the body and extremities, add *Yin Chen* (Herba Artemisiae Scopariae) and *Huang Qin* (Radix Scutellariae).
- With irritability and thirst, add *Zhi Mu* (Rhizoma Anemarrhenae) and *Jie Geng* (Radix Platycodonis).
- With foul breath and mouth ulceration, add *Huang Lian* (Rhizoma Coptidis) and *Sheng Ma* (Rhizoma Cimicifugae).
- If the Stomach heat is severe, add *Huang Lian* (Rhizoma Coptidis).
- With irritability, add *Deng Xin Cao* (Medulla Junci) and *Chi Fu Ling* (Poria Rubra).
- With dysuria and dark urine, add *Hua Shi* (Talcum).

Chinese Herbal Formulas and Applications

Xiè Huáng Sǎn (Drain the Yellow Powder)

Xie Huang San (Drain the Yellow Powder)

Diagnosis	Signs and Symptoms	Treatment	Herbs
Latent fire of the Spleen and Stomach	• Mouth ulcerations and foul breath: rising of latent fire of the Spleen and Stomach • Thirst, a dry mouth and lips and frequent hunger: fire consuming body fluids • Red tongue body: heat condition • Rapid pulse: heat condition	Purges latent fire of the Spleen and Stomach	• *Shi Gao* (Gypsum Fibrosum) and *Zhi Zi* (Fructus Gardeniae) clear and sedate heat and fire from the Spleen and Stomach. • *Fang Feng* (Radix Saposhnikoviae) and *Huo Xiang* (Herba Agastaches) disperse and lift latent fire outward. • *Gan Cao* (Radix et Rhizoma Glycyrrhizae) clears heat and protects Spleen and Stomach qi.

CAUTIONS / CONTRAINDICATIONS

Do not use *Xie Huang San* in cases of Stomach yin deficiency.

CLINICAL STUDIES AND RESEARCH

1. **Stomatitis**: One study reported good results using modified *Xie Huang San* to treat stomatitis in 32 children. Modifications included the addition of *Huang Lian* (Rhizoma Coptidis) and *Zhu Ye* (Herba Phyllostachys) for stomatitis affecting a large surface area accompanied by severe pain; *Ji Su San* (Peppermint Powder) and *Che Qian Zi* (Semen Plantaginis) for foul breath and sticky tongue coating; *Da Huang* (Radix et Rhizoma Rhei) for constipation; and *Shan Zha* (Fructus Crataegi) and *Shen Qu* (Massa Fermentata) for poor appetite. The treatment protocol was to administer the herbs in decoction one time daily. According to the study, 23 children responded (72%) within 1-2 packs of herbs, 7 responded (22%) within 3-4 packs, and 2 responded after 6 packs. The average recovery time was approximately 5 days.[1] In another study, 31 adults with stomatitis were treated with herbs with complete recovery reported in 80% of patients. The herbal formula contained *Xie Huang San* plus *Fu Ling* (Poria), *Cang Zhu* (Rhizoma Atractylodis), *Ban Xia* (Rhizoma Pinelliae), *Yi Yi Ren* (Semen Coicis), *Huang Qin* (Radix Scutellariae), and *Chen Pi* (Pericarpium Citri Reticulatae). The treatment protocol was to cook the herbs in water, and drink the decoction in three equally-divided doses daily.[2]

2. **Fever**: One study reported good results using modified *Xie Huang San* to treat fever in 250 children. The body temperature ranged from 37.5-40°C / 99.5-104°F, and the duration of fever ranged from 1-6 days. The herbal treatment contained *Xie Huang San* plus *Qing Hao* (Herba Artemisiae Annuae), *Ku Xing Ren* (Semen Armeniacae Amarum), and others as needed. Of 250 cases, the study reported reduction of fever in 150 cases after 1 dose, and in 100 cases after 2 doses.[3]

AUTHORS' COMMENTS

According to the source text, *Xie Huang San* is formulated with significantly and uncharacteristically high doses of *Gan Cao* (Radix et Rhizoma Glycyrrhizae) and *Fang Feng* (Radix Saposhnikoviae). Many scholars argue that such high doses are inappropriate because these two herbs do not directly treat the latent fire in the Spleen and Stomach as indicated in *Xie Huang San*. In fact, *Gan Cao* (Radix et Rhizoma Glycyrrhizae) is a tonic herb and *Fang Feng* (Radix Saposhnikoviae) is an acrid and warm exterior-releasing herb, and use of these two herbs at high doses may exacerbate the latent fire condition.[4] This issue has been further scrutinized in several *in vitro* studies, in which it was found that the overall efficacy of the formula does not differ significantly whether *Fang Feng* (Radix Saposhnikoviae) was used at full or reduced doses (80% less). In fact, the studies reported that larger doses of *Fang Feng* (Radix Saposhnikoviae) decrease the anti-inflammatory effects of *Xie Huang San*.[5]

Please refer to *Qing Wei San* (Clear the Stomach Powder) for an examination of the contrasting differences between *Xie Huang San* and *Yu Nu Jian* (Jade Woman Decoction).

References

1. *Hu Bei Zhong Yi Za Zhi* (Hubei Journal of Chinese Medicine) 1989;1:24.
2. *Nei Meng Gu Zhong Yi Yao* (Traditional Chinese Medicine and Medicinals of Inner Mongolia) 1993;12(3):27.
3. *Si Chuan Zhong Yi* (Sichuan Chinese Medicine) 1985;31(6):36.
4. *Fang Ji Xue* (Chinese Herbal Formulas) 1995;163-165.
5. *Nan Jing Zhong Yi Xue Yuan Xue Bao* (Journal of Nanjing University of Traditional Chinese Medicine) 1986;(3):50.

HEAT-CLEARING FORMULAS

5

Chapter 5 – Heat-Clearing Formulas　　　　　　　　　　*Section 5 – Zang Fu-Clearing Formulas*

Yù Nǚ Jiān (Jade Woman Decoction)

玉女煎

Pinyin Name: Yu Nu Jian
Literal Name: Jade Woman Decoction
Alternate Names: *Yu Nu Chien*, Fairy Decoction, Rehmannia and Gypsum Decoction, Rehmannia and Gypsum Combination
Original Source: *Jing Yue Quan Shu* (Collected Treatises of [Zhang] Jing Yue) by Zhang Jie-Bin (Zhang Jing-Yue) in 1624

COMPOSITION

Shi Gao (Gypsum Fibrosum)	9-15g [15-30g]
Zhi Mu (Rhizoma Anemarrhenae)	4.5g
Shu Di Huang (Radix Rehmanniae Praeparata)	9-30g
Mai Dong (Radix Ophiopogonis)	6g
Chuan Niu Xi (Radix Cyathulae)	4.5g

DOSAGE / PREPARATION / ADMINISTRATION

Prepare the ingredients as a decoction with 1.5 bowls of water and cook until 70% of the liquid remains. The strained decoction may be taken warm or cool. The decoction may be prepared using the dose of *Shi Gao* (Gypsum Fibrosum) suggested in brackets.

CHINESE THERAPEUTIC ACTIONS

1. Clears Stomach heat
2. Nourishes yin

CLINICAL MANIFESTATIONS

1. Stomach heat accompanied by yin deficiency: irritability, warm sensations, thirst, a dry mouth, headache, toothache, gum bleeding, a red tongue body, and a yellow dry tongue coating.
2. *Xiao ke* (wasting and thirsting) syndrome with excess hunger and thirst.

CLINICAL APPLICATIONS

Gastrointestinal bleeding, epistaxis, recurrent ulceration of the oral cavity, oral cavity disorders, toothache, gingivitis, periodontitis, stomatitis, halitosis, periodontal disease, pharyngitis, diabetes mellitus, and trigeminal neuralgia.

EXPLANATION

Yu Nu Jian (Jade Woman Decoction) treats excess in the *yangming* channel with deficiency in the *shaoyin* channel—in other words, excess Stomach heat with underlying yin deficiency. The Stomach channel travels to the head region, so Stomach heat may travel upward along the channel to cause headache and toothache. If the heat forces blood out of the blood vessels, then gum bleeding may occur. Irritability, warm sensations, a dry mouth and thirst are common clinical manifestations of excess heat injuring yin and body fluids. A red tongue body with a dry, yellow coating implies excess heat damaging yin.

Shi Gao (Gypsum Fibrosum), the chief herb, is excellent for clearing Stomach heat. Its sweet taste promotes the production of body fluids and its acrid nature disperses heat. *Shu Di Huang* (Radix Rehmanniae Praeparata), the deputy herb, is used to nourish yin. Combined, these two herbs clear excess heat and nourish deficient yin. *Zhi Mu* (Rhizoma Anemarrhenae) helps *Shi Gao* (Gypsum Fibrosum) clear heat and moisten dryness. *Mai Dong* (Radix Ophiopogonis) helps *Shu Di Huang* (Radix Rehmanniae Praeparata) nourish yin. *Chuan Niu Xi* (Radix Cyathulae) leads heat downward to relieve bleeding and rising

Yu Nu Jian (Jade Woman Decoction)

Diagnosis	Signs and Symptoms	Treatment	Herbs
Stomach heat accompanied by yin deficiency	• Headache and toothache: Stomach heat traveling upward along the Stomach channel • Gum bleeding: Stomach heat forcing blood out of the blood vessels • Irritability, warm sensations, a dry mouth and thirst: excess heat injuring yin and body fluids • Red tongue body with a dry yellow coating: heat damaging yin	• Clears Stomach heat • Nourishes yin	• *Shi Gao* (Gypsum Fibrosum) and *Zhi Mu* (Rhizoma Anemarrhenae) clear heat, generate body fluids, and moisten dryness. • *Shu Di Huang* (Radix Rehmanniae Praeparata) and *Mai Dong* (Radix Ophiopogonis) nourish Stomach yin. • *Chuan Niu Xi* (Radix Cyathulae) leads heat downward to relieve bleeding and rising Stomach heat.

398

Yù Nǚ Jiān (Jade Woman Decoction)

Stomach heat. This formula is also commonly used for excessive hunger in middle (*jiao*) *xiao ke* (wasting and thirsting) syndrome.

MODIFICATIONS

- If the toothache is severe, add *Huang Lian* (Rhizoma Coptidis) and *Gan Cao* (Radix et Rhizoma Glycyrrhizae).
- With restlessness, irritability and thirst, add *Tian Dong* (Radix Asparagi) and *Di Huang* (Radix Rehmanniae).
- With vomiting of blood, add *Zhi Zi* (Fructus Gardeniae) and charred *Sheng Jiang* (Rhizoma Zingiberis Recens).
- If there is severe gum swelling and pain, add *Jin Yin Hua* (Flos Lonicerae Japonicae) and *Pu Gong Ying* (Herba Taraxaci); or *Gan Lu Yin* (Sweet Dew Decoction).
- When the bleeding gums are severe as a result of heat in the *xue* (blood) level, remove *Shu Di Huang* (Radix Rehmanniae Praeparata) and add *Di Huang* (Radix Rehmanniae), *Bai Mao Gen* (Rhizoma Imperatae), *Mo Han Lian* (Herba Ecliptae), and *Xuan Shen* (Radix Scrophulariae).
- With a sore throat, add *Ban Lan Gen* (Radix Isatidis) and *Da Qing Ye* (Folium Isatidis).
- With constipation, add *Da Huang* (Radix et Rhizoma Rhei) and *Mang Xiao* (Natrii Sulfas).
- With prominent yin deficiency, add *Bei Sha Shen* (Radix Glehniae) and *Shi Hu* (Caulis Dendrobii).
- When accompanied by insomnia, add *Suan Zao Ren* (Semen Ziziphi Spinosae) and *Shou Wu Teng* (Caulis Polygoni Multiflori).
- With stomatitis, add *Qing Wei San* (Clear the Stomach Powder).

CAUTIONS / CONTRAINDICATIONS

Yu Nu Jian is contraindicated in cases of loose stools due to deficiency and cold of the Spleen and Stomach.

PHARMACOLOGICAL EFFECTS

Hypoglycemic: In one experiment, oral administration of *Yu Nu Jian* at 5 mL/kg was associated with a gradual but sustained hypoglycemic effect in rabbits. The hypoglycemic effect was observed in these subjects between 3 to 9 hours after administration of the formula.[1]

CLINICAL STUDIES AND RESEARCH

1. **Gastrointestinal bleeding:** One study reported complete recovery in all 12 patients with upper gastrointestinal bleeding characterized by yin deficiency, with flushed face, dizziness, palpitations, poor sleeping patterns, warm sensations at the center of the palms and soles, hematemesis with profuse amount of bright red blood, a dry mouth with thirst, dark tarry stools, a red tongue body with little tongue coating, and a fine pulse. The herbal treatment contained *Yu Nu Jian* plus *Qian Cao* (Radix et Rhizoma Rubiae) as the base formula, with modifications as needed. For qi deficiency, *Dang Shen* (Radix Codonopsis) and *Tai Zi Shen* (Radix Pseudostellariae), or *Sheng Mai San* (Generate the Pulse Powder) were added. For severe bleeding, charred *Ce Bai Ye* (Cacumen Platycladi), *Mo Han Lian* (Herba Ecliptae), and *Zi Zhu* (Folium Callicarpae) were added.[2]

2. **Epistaxis:** Nosebleeds were successfully treated with an herbal formula containing *Yu Nu Jian* plus *Xian He Cao* (Herba Agrimoniae), *Ou Jie* (Nodus Nelumbinis Rhizomatis), *Di Huang* (Radix Rehmanniae), *Bai Mao Gen* (Rhizoma Imperatae) and *Qian Cao* (Radix et Rhizoma Rubiae). Of 55 patients with nosebleeds, 32 were diagnosed with Liver fire rising, 13 with Stomach fire, and 10 with yin-deficient heat. The herbs were given in decoction daily, for a total of 3-7 packs. The study reported complete recovery in 38 cases, marked effect in 14 cases, and no benefit in 3 cases.[3] In another study, 55 patients with nosebleeds were treated with complete recovery in 38 cases, improvement in 14 patients, and no effect in the rest. Most patients responded within 3-5 doses.[4]

3. **Recurrent ulceration of the oral cavity:** In one report, 32 patients with recurrent oral ulcerations were treated with modified *Yu Nu Jian* with satisfactory results. In addition to *Yu Nu Jian* as the base formula, modifications were made by adding: *Jin Yin Hua* (Flos Lonicerae Japonicae) and *Pu Gong Ying* (Herba Taraxaci) for gum swelling and pain; *Da Huang* (Radix et Rhizoma Rhei) and *Mang Xiao* (Natrii Sulfas) for constipation; *Zhi Zi* (Fructus Gardeniae) and *Huang Lian* (Rhizoma Coptidis) for Stomach fire; *Bei Sha Shen* (Radix Glehniae) and *Shi Hu* (Caulis Dendrobii) for yin deficiency; and *Suan Zao Ren* (Semen Ziziphi Spinosae) and *Shou Wu Teng* (Caulis Polygoni Multiflori) for poor sleeping patterns. Out of 32 patients, 15 showed complete recovery, 10 showed moderate improvement, and 7 showed no effect.[5]

4. **Oral cavity disorders:** Administration of *Yu Nu Jian* has been shown to effectively treat various types of oral cavity disorders. One report found *Yu Nu Jian* had a marked effect to treat swelling and pain of gums.[6] Modified *Yu Nu Jian* also showed marked success in treating 32 patients with recurrent stomatitis.[7] Lastly, use of this formula in 102 patients with toothache due to various causes was associated with complete relief in 68 cases and improvement in 34 cases.[8]

5. **Periodontal disease:** One study reported marked success using modified *Yu Nu Jian* to treat periodontal disease. Of 48 patients, the study reported complete recovery in 23 cases, marked effect in 20 cases, and slight improvement in 5 cases. The herbal treatment used *Yu Nu Jian* plus *Ku Shen* (Radix Sophorae Flavescentis) as the base formula,

Yù Nǚ Jiān (Jade Woman Decoction)

with addition of *Da Huang* (Radix et Rhizoma Rhei) for constipation and *Yi Yi Ren* (Semen Coicis) for damp-heat. The herbs were cooked in water, and the decoction was taken in two equally-divided doses.[9]

6. **Pharyngitis**: One study reported 93.44% effectiveness using modified *Yu Nu Jian* to treat 61 patients with chronic pharyngitis. In addition to using *Yu Nu Jian* as the base formula, modifications were made by adding *Huang Lian* (Rhizoma Coptidis) and *Zhi Zi* (Fructus Gardeniae) for irritability; *Bei Mu* (Bulbus Fritillariae) and *Tian Zhu Huang* (Concretio Silicea Bambusae) for cough with profuse phlegm; *Jin Yin Hua* (Flos Lonicerae Japonicae) and *Lian Qiao* (Fructus Forsythiae) for dry itchy throat with burning sensations; *Da Huang* (Radix et Rhizoma Rhei) for constipation; and *Chi Shao* (Radix Paeoniae Rubra) and *Mu Dan Pi* (Cortex Moutan) for swelling of the throat. The treatment protocol was to administer the herbs for 10 days per course of treatment, for 2-3 courses total. Of 61 cases, the study reported complete recovery in 9 cases, significant improvement in 23 cases, moderate improvement in 25 cases, and no effect in 4 cases.[10]

7. **Diabetes mellitus**: Use of modified *Yu Nu Jian* was associated with 86.5% effectiveness in treating 52 patients with adult-onset diabetes mellitus characterized by Stomach yin deficiency with dry heat. In addition to *Yu Nu Jian* as the base formula, *Zhi Bai Di Huang Wan* (Anemarrhena, Phellodendron, and Rehmannia Pill) was added for Kidney yin deficiency; *Sheng Mai San* (Generate the Pulse Powder) was added for qi and yin deficiencies; *Jin Gui Shen Qi Wan* (Kidney Qi Pill from the Golden Cabinet) was added for yin and yang deficiencies; *Ji Sheng Shen Qi Wan* (Kidney Qi Pill from Formulas that Aid the Living) was added for edema; and *Xiao Ke Fang* (Wasting and Thirsting Formula) for yin deficiency with dry heat.[11] Note: *Xiao Ke Fang* (Wasting and Thirsting Formula), as the name implies, is a formula that treats *xiao ke* (wasting and thirsting) syndrome. The exact composition of this formula was not available at the time of publication.

8. **Trigeminal neuralgia**: One study reported complete recovery in all 6 patients using herbs both orally and topically. The oral herbal formula contained *Yu Nu Jian* plus *Yan Hu Suo* (Rhizoma Corydalis), *Bai Zhi* (Radix Angelicae Dahuricae), *Fang Feng* (Radix Saposhnikoviae), and *Xi Xin* (Radix et Rhizoma Asari). The treatment protocol for topical application of herbs was to mix *Xiang Fu* (Rhizoma Cyperi) powder with egg white, and apply the paste to the center of the sole of the right foot at night. The duration of treatment ranged from 3-7 packs of herbs.[12]

AUTHORS' COMMENTS

Qing Wei San (Clear the Stomach Powder) and *Yu Nu Jian* both treat Stomach fire flaring upward causing toothache, gum bleeding, headache, thirst, a red tongue body and a yellow coating.

• *Qing Wei San* cools the blood and clears excess fire.

• *Yu Nu Jian* is indicated for Stomach fire with underlying Stomach and Kidney yin deficiencies. Consequently, the patient will feel more thirsty and dry, and the pulse will feel empty upon heavy pressure.

References

1. *Zhong Yao Tong Bao* (Journal of Chinese Herbology) 1984;6:33.
2. *Zhong Yi Ming Fang Lin Chuang Xin Yong* (Contemporary Clinical Applications of Classic Chinese Formulas) 2001;186.
3. *Shang Hai Zhong Yi Yao Za Zhi* (Shanghai Journal of Chinese Medicine and Herbology) 1985;19(6):39.
4. *Jiang Xi Zhong Yi Yao* (Jiangxi Chinese Medicine and Herbology) 1986;5:18.
5. *Fu Jian Zhong Yi Yao* (Fujian Chinese Medicine and Herbology) 1983;2:24.
6. *Zhong Yi Ming Fang Lin Chuang Xin Yong* (Contemporary Clinical Applications of Classic Chinese Formulas) 2001;184.
7. *Fu Jian Zhong Yi Yao* (Fujian Chinese Medicine and Herbology) 1983;14(2):24.
8. *Zhong Xi Yi Jie He Za Zhi* (Journal of Integrated Chinese and Western Medicine) 1989;9(3):182.
9. *An Hui Zhong Yi Xue Yuan Xue Bao* (Journal of Anhui University School of Medicine) 1999;6:37.
10. *An Hui Zhong Yi Xue Yuan Xue Bao* (Journal of Anhui University School of Medicine) 1995;2:21.
11. *Hu Bei Zhong Yi Za Zhi* (Hubei Journal of Chinese Medicine) 1984;6:33.
12. *Xin Yi Yao Xue Za Zhi* (New Journal of Medicine and Herbology) 1978;6:31.

Gān Lù Yǐn (Sweet Dew Decoction)

甘露飲
甘露饮

Pinyin Name: *Gan Lu Yin*
Literal Name: Sweet Dew Decoction
Alternate Names: *Kan Lu Yin*, Sweet Combination Drink, Sweet Combination
Original Source: *Tai Ping Hui Min He Ji Ju Fang* (Imperial Grace Formulary of the Tai Ping Era) by the Imperial Medical Department in 1078-85

COMPOSITION

Di Huang (Radix Rehmanniae)

Shu Di Huang (Radix Rehmanniae Praeparata)

Mai Dong (Radix Ophiopogonis)

Tian Dong (Radix Asparagi)

Pi Pa Ye (Folium Eriobotryae)

Shi Hu (Caulis Dendrobii)

Zhi Qiao (Fructus Aurantii), *chao* (dry-fried)

Yin Chen (Herba Artemisiae Scopariae)

Huang Qin (Radix Scutellariae)

Zhi Gan Cao (Radix et Rhizoma Glycyrrhizae Praeparata cum Melle)

DOSAGE / PREPARATION / ADMINISTRATION

Grind equal amounts of the ingredients coarsely, and cook 6g of the powder in 1 bowl of water and reduce it to 80%. Take the warm, strained decoction after meals. For treatment of loose teeth or swollen gums, swish and swallow the decoction.

CHINESE THERAPEUTIC ACTIONS

1. Clears damp-heat
2. Nourishes yin

CLINICAL MANIFESTATIONS

Damp-heat in the Spleen and Stomach: swelling, inflammation and suppuration in the gums, tongue and throat, sore throat with inflammation and pain, stomatitis, ulcerations of the tongue, and toothache. Jaundice with edema, fever, constipation, and dysuria.

CLINICAL APPLICATIONS

Stomatitis, ulcerative stomatitis, gingivitis, toothache, sore throat, conjunctivitis, and jaundice.

EXPLANATION

Gan Lu Yin (Sweet Dew Decoction) treats damp-heat in the Spleen and Stomach. When damp-heat travels up the gastrointestinal tract, patients exhibit signs and symptoms in the oral cavity, such as swelling and suppuration of the gums, tongue and throat, sore throat with inflammation and pain, stomatitis, and tongue ulcerations. If the damp-heat remains in the middle *jiao*, it may affect the adjacent organs, namely the Gallbladder, leading to jaundice, fever,

and mild edema of the extremities. If the damp-heat travels downward, it affects urination and bowel movement, leading to dysuria and constipation.

Di Huang (Radix Rehmanniae), *Shu Di Huang* (Radix Rehmanniae Praeparata), *Mai Dong* (Radix Ophiopogonis) and *Tian Dong* (Radix Asparagi) nourish yin and clear heat simultaneously. The heat-clearing function of these herbs addresses the underlying cause of the disease, while the yin-nourishing function prevents the cold herbs from damaging the body. *Pi Pa Ye* (Folium Eriobotryae) harmonizes the Stomach and clears Stomach heat. *Zhi Qiao* (Fructus Aurantii) breaks up stagnant qi, and promotes normal bowel movement and urination. *Shi Hu* (Caulis Dendrobii) clears deficiency heat from the Stomach. The combination of *Zhi Qiao* (Fructus Aurantii) and *Shi Hu* (Caulis Dendrobii) regulates the Stomach and Intestines to promote normal function of the gastrointestinal tract and relieve constipation. *Yin Chen* (Herba Artemisiae Scopariae) clears damp-heat, and is one of the most effective herbs for treating jaundice. *Huang Qin* (Radix Scutellariae) clears excess fire and damp-heat to reduce inflammation and relieve ulceration. Lastly, *Zhi Gan Cao* (Radix et Rhizoma Glycyrrhizae Praeparata cum Melle) harmonizes the herbs.

MODIFICATIONS

- With swelling and pain of the gums and teeth, add *Ge Gen* (Radix Puerariae Lobatae) and *Sheng Ma* (Rhizoma Cimicifugae).

Chapter 5 – Heat-Clearing Formulas   *Section 5 – Zang Fu-Clearing Formulas*

Gān Lù Yǐn (Sweet Dew Decoction)

Gan Lu Yin (Sweet Dew Decoction)

Diagnosis	Signs and Symptoms	Treatment	Herbs
Damp-heat in the Spleen and Stomach	• Swelling, inflammation, suppuration and pain of the oral cavity: damp-heat in the Spleen and Stomach traveling upward • Jaundice: damp-heat affecting the Gallbladder in the middle *jiao* • Dysuria and constipation: damp-heat traveling downward	• Clears damp-heat • Nourishes yin	• *Di Huang* (Radix Rehmanniae), *Shu Di Huang* (Radix Rehmanniae Praeparata), *Mai Dong* (Radix Ophiopogonis), *Tian Dong* (Radix Asparagi), *Pi Pa Ye* (Folium Eriobotryae) and *Shi Hu* (Caulis Dendrobii) nourish yin and clear heat. • *Zhi Qiao* (Fructus Aurantii) breaks up stagnant qi, and promotes normal bowel movement and urination. • *Yin Chen* (Herba Artemisiae Scopariae) clears damp-heat. • *Huang Qin* (Radix Scutellariae) clears excess fire and damp-heat. • *Zhi Gan Cao* (Radix et Rhizoma Glycyrrhizae Praeparata cum Melle) harmonizes the herbs.

• If accompanied by foul breath, add *Huang Lian* (Rhizoma Coptidis) and *Jie Geng* (Radix Platycodonis).
• With red eyes with swelling and pain, combine with *Liang Ge San* (Cool the Diaphragm Powder).
• With constipation, combine with *Da Cheng Qi Tang* (Major Order the Qi Decoction).

• If there are nosebleeds, add *Shui Niu Jiao* (Cornu Bubali).
• With stomatitis and oral lesions, add *Huang Lian* (Rhizoma Coptidis), *Jin Yin Hua* (Flos Lonicerae Japonicae), and *Lian Qiao* (Fructus Forsythiae).
• With a sore throat, add *Qing Wei San* (Clear the Stomach Powder).

Sháo Yào Tāng (Peony Decoction)
芍藥湯
芍药汤

Pinyin Name: *Shao Yao Tang*
Literal Name: Peony Decoction
Alternate Name: Peony Combination
Original Source: *Zheng Zhi Zhun Sheng* (Standards of Patterns and Treatments) by Wang Ken-Tang in 1602

COMPOSITION

Huang Lian (Rhizoma Coptidis)	15g [5-9g]
Huang Qin (Radix Scutellariae)	15g [9g]
Da Huang (Radix et Rhizoma Rhei)	9g [6g]
Dang Gui (Radix Angelicae Sinensis)	15g [9g]
Bai Shao (Radix Paeoniae Alba)	30g [15-20g]
Gan Cao (Radix et Rhizoma Glycyrrhizae), *chao* (dry-fried)	6g [5g]
Mu Xiang (Radix Aucklandiae)	6g [5g]
Bing Lang (Semen Arecae)	6g [5g]
Rou Gui (Cortex Cinnamomi)	7.5g [2-5g]

Chinese Herbal Formulas and Applications

Sháo Yào Tāng (Peony Decoction)

DOSAGE / PREPARATION / ADMINISTRATION

The source text states to grind the ingredients coarsely and cook 15g of the powder in two large bowls of water until one bowl of the liquid remains. Take the warm, strained decoction after meals. Today, this formula may be prepared as a decoction with the doses suggested in brackets.

CHINESE THERAPEUTIC ACTIONS

1. Harmonizes qi and blood
2. Clears heat and eliminates toxins

CLINICAL MANIFESTATIONS

Damp-heat dysentery: abdominal pain, rectal tenesmus, burning sensation of the anus, presence of white (mucus) and red (blood) stools, dark, scanty urine, and a greasy, yellow tongue coating.

CLINICAL APPLICATIONS

Bacterial dysentery, amoebic dysentery, acute enteritis, allergic colitis, acute colitis, and ulcerative colitis.

EXPLANATION

Shao Yao Tang (Peony Decoction) is the main formula used to treat dysentery characterized by damp-heat in the Intestines. In this syndrome, damp and heat stagnate in the Intestines, causing qi and blood stagnation. Qi and blood stagnation results in abdominal pain. Damp-heat injures the Intestines and causes the formation of mucus and blood in the stools, which, when defecated, appear white and red in color. Burning sensations of the anus, rectal tenesmus and dark, scanty urine are due to damp-heat traveling downward.

The treatment plan for this syndrome is first to harmonize qi and blood, and then to dispel damp-heat and eliminate toxins. A heavy dose of *Bai Shao* (Radix Paeoniae Alba) along with *Dang Gui* (Radix Angelicae Sinensis) is used to harmonize the *ying* (nutritive) and *xue* (blood) levels. *Bai Shao* (Radix Paeoniae Alba) also works with *Gan Cao* (Radix et Rhizoma Glycyrrhizae), as seen in the formula *Shao Yao Gan Cao Tang* (Peony and Licorice Decoction), to relieve pain and other urgent symptoms.

Huang Lian (Rhizoma Coptidis) and *Huang Qin* (Radix Scutellariae), both bitter and cold, clear heat and dry dampness. *Mu Xiang* (Radix Aucklandiae) and *Bing Lang* (Semen Arecae) move qi to relieve stagnation. *Da Huang* (Radix et Rhizoma Rhei), as a supplement to *Huang Lian* (Rhizoma Coptidis) and *Huang Qin* (Radix Scutellariae), purges and drains heat downward. *Da Huang* (Radix et Rhizoma Rhei) also quickly removes harmful retention or stagnation in the body via defecation, thereby supplementing the qi-moving effect of *Mu Xiang* (Radix Aucklandiae) and *Bing Lang* (Semen Arecae). Although it is a purgative herb, *Da Huang* (Radix et Rhizoma Rhei) is necessary in this formula to drain stagnation to treat diarrhea and dysentery. *Rou Gui* (Cortex Cinnamomi) restrains the bitter and cold herbs from injuring yin and prevents them from constricting damp-heat inside the body. This formula focuses on treating the cause of the diarrhea and dysentery rather than just relieving the symptoms.

MODIFICATIONS

- With more blood than pus in the stool, change *Dang Gui* (Radix Angelicae Sinensis) to *Dang Gui Wei* (Extremitas

Shao Yao Tang (Peony Decoction)

Diagnosis	Signs and Symptoms	Treatment	Herbs
Damp-heat dysentery	• Dysentery, burning sensations of the anus, rectal tenesmus and dark scanty urine: damp-heat traveling downward • Abdominal pain: qi and blood stagnation • Stools with mucus and blood: damp-heat damaging the blood vessels • Greasy, yellow tongue coating: accumulation of damp-heat	• Harmonizes qi and blood • Clears heat and eliminates toxins	• *Huang Lian* (Rhizoma Coptidis) and *Huang Qin* (Radix Scutellariae) clear heat, eliminate toxins, and dry dampness. • *Da Huang* (Radix et Rhizoma Rhei) purges heat and drains heat downward. • *Dang Gui* (Radix Angelicae Sinensis) and *Bai Shao* (Radix Paeoniae Alba) regulate and harmonize *ying* (nutritive) and *xue* (blood) levels. • *Bai Shao* (Radix Paeoniae Alba) and *Gan Cao* (Radix et Rhizoma Glycyrrhizae) relieve spasms, cramps and pain. • *Mu Xiang* (Radix Aucklandiae) and *Bing Lang* (Semen Arecae) regulate and harmonize qi. • *Rou Gui* (Cortex Cinnamomi) restrains the bitter and cold herbs from injuring yin.

HEAT-CLEARING FORMULAS

5

403

Sháo Yào Tāng (Peony Decoction)

Radix Angelicae Sinensis) and add *Mu Dan Pi* (Cortex Moutan).

- With a dry, yellow tongue coating and heat injuring the body fluids, remove *Rou Gui* (Cortex Cinnamomi).
- With food stagnation, remove *Gan Cao* (Radix et Rhizoma Glycyrrhizae), and add *Shan Zha* (Fructus Crataegi) and *Mai Ya* (Fructus Hordei Germinatus).
- With abdominal fullness and distention, remove *Rou Gui* (Cortex Cinnamomi) and *Gan Cao* (Radix et Rhizoma Glycyrrhizae), and add *Zhi Shi* (Fructus Aurantii Immaturus).
- With bloody diarrhea, increase the dose of *Da Huang* (Radix et Rhizoma Rhei).
- With cloudy and dark blood in the stool due to toxins in the *zang* (solid organ), add *Huang Bo* (Cortex Phellodendri Chinensis).

CAUTIONS / CONTRAINDICATIONS

- Do not use this formula if the dysentery is accompanied by exterior symptoms.
- This formula is not suitable for chronic dysentery or dysentery caused by deficiency and cold.

PHARMACOLOGICAL EFFECTS

1. **Gastrointestinal**: Administration of *Shao Yao Tang* was associated with stimulating the gastrointestinal tract and promoting expulsion of intestinal content. This effect was immediate and potent, with short duration. The potency of this action is directly proportional to the dose of the formula. It was noted that *Shao Yao Tang* did not have such an effect when *Bing Lang* (Semen Arecae) was removed from the formula.[1,2]

2. **Antibiotic**: Use of *Shao Yao Tang in vitro* was associated with an inhibiting effect on *Bacillus dysenteriae, E. coli, Pseudomonas aeruginosa, Bacillus proteus,* and *Staphylococcus aureus*. Interestingly, the formula has much less antibiotic effect without *Bing Lang* (Semen Arecae) even though when given individually, *Bing Lang* (Semen Arecae) does not have any antibiotic effect.[3]

3. **Anti-inflammatory**: Intraperitoneal injection of *Shao Yao Tang* in mice was associated with reducing swelling and inflammation.[4]

CLINICAL STUDIES AND RESEARCH

1. **Dysentery**: There have been many reports on the efficacy of *Shao Yao Tang* for the treatment of dysentery. In one report, modified *Shao Yao Tang* was effective in treating all 25 infants with dysentery characterized by damp-heat. Most patients had complete recovery within 2-4 packs, with some needing up to 6 packs of herbs. The herbal treatment contained *Shao Yao Tang*, with the addition of *Bai Zhu* (Rhizoma Atractylodis Macrocephalae) and *Tai*

Zi Shen (Radix Pseudostellariae) for chronic illness with qi deficiency; *Huo Xiang* (Herba Agastaches) and *Zhu Ru* (Caulis Bambusae in Taenia) for nausea and vomiting; and *Bai Tou Weng* (Radix Pulsatillae), *Pu Gong Ying* (Herba Taraxaci) and charred *Di Yu* (Radix Sanguisorbae) for severe bloody dysentery.[5]

2. **Bacterial dysentery**: *Shao Yao Tang* has been shown to be effective in treating bacterial dysentery in several studies. Modified *Shao Yao Tang* was effective in all 70 patients with bacterial dysentery.[6] According to another study, use of modified *Shao Yao Tang* was associated with 94% effectiveness in treating 50 patients with bacterial dysentery with high fever and bowel movements between 8-20 times per day.[7] Lastly, one study reported 98.9% effectiveness using modified *Shao Yao Tang* to treat 93 patients with bacterial dysentery. The herbal treatment contained *Shao Yao Tang* plus *Jin Yin Hua* (Flos Lonicerae Japonicae), *Di Yu* (Radix Sanguisorbae), *Bai Tou Weng* (Radix Pulsatillae), and *Yi Yi Ren* (Semen Coicis).[8]

3. **Colitis**: One study reported marked success using modified *Shao Yao Tang* to treat 48 patients with acute or chronic colitis. In addition to the base formula, the herbal treatment was modified by adding *Shan Zha* (Fructus Crataegi), *Gu Ya* (Fructus Setariae Germinatus), and *Mai Ya* (Fructus Hordei Germinatus) for undigested food in the stools; *Bai Zhu* (Rhizoma Atractylodis Macrocephalae), *Fu Ling* (Poria), *Shan Yao* (Rhizoma Dioscoreae), and *Bu Gu Zhi* (Fructus Psoraleae) for yang deficiency of the Spleen and Stomach; *Yi Yi Ren* (Semen Coicis) and *Bai Bian Dou* (Semen Lablab Album) for dampness; and eliminating *Rou Gui* (Cortex Cinnamomi) and adding *Zhi Shi* (Fructus Aurantii Immaturus) and *Hou Po* (Cortex Magnoliae Officinalis) for constipation with abdominal fullness. The duration of treatment was 5-10 packs of herbs for acute colitis, and 3-12 months for chronic colitis.[9]

4. **Ulcerative colitis**: Daily administration of modified *Shao Yao Tang* as rectal enema for one month was associated with resolution of all signs and symptoms in all 36 patients with ulcerative colitis. In addition to using *Shao Yao Tang* as the base formula, modifications included the addition of *Bai Tou Weng* (Radix Pulsatillae) and *Ma Chi Xian* (Herba Portulacae) for presence of pus and blood in the stools; *Huang Qi* (Radix Astragali), *Dang Shen* (Radix Codonopsis), and *E Jiao* (Colla Corii Asini) for qi and blood deficiencies; *Wu Mei* (Fructus Mume) and *Shi Liu Pi* (Pericarpium Granati) for chronic diarrhea; *Di Yu* (Radix Sanguisorbae) and *Bai Ji* (Rhizoma Bletillae) powder for severe hematochezia; a larger dose of *Bai Shao* (Radix Paeoniae Alba) for severe abdominal pain; and removal of *Mu Xiang* (Radix Aucklandiae) and *Bing Lang* (Semen Arecae) for absence of abdominal pain.[10]

Sháo Yào Tāng (Peony Decoction)

TOXICOLOGY

In one experiment on the acute toxicology of *Shao Yao Tang*, oral administration of 100 g/kg of the formula caused fatality in 11 out of 12 mice within 72 hours. However, when *Bing Lang* (Semen Arecae) was removed from the formula, no fatality was reported at the same dose. The researchers concluded that the toxicity of the formula is due in part to *Bing Lang* (Semen Arecae).[11]

RELATED FORMULAS

Sháo Yào Yì Yǐ Rén Tāng (Peony and Coicis Decoction)

芍藥薏苡仁湯
芍药薏苡仁汤

Pinyin Name: Shao Yao Yi Yi Ren Tang
Literal Name: Peony and Coicis Decoction
Original Source: *An Hui Zhong Yi Xue Yuan* (Anhui University School of Medicine) in 1990

Bai Shao (Radix Paeoniae Alba)
Yi Yi Ren (Semen Coicis)
Nan Sha Shen (Radix Adenophorae)
Shan Yao (Rhizoma Dioscoreae)
Shan Zha (Fructus Crataegi)
Hou Po (Cortex Magnoliae Officinalis)
Ma Chi Xian (Herba Portulacae)
Huang Lian (Rhizoma Coptidis)
Di Yu (Radix Sanguisorbae)
Shi Liu Pi (Pericarpium Granati)
Chun Pi (Cortex Ailanthi)
Fang Feng (Radix Saposhnikoviae)
Tao Ren (Semen Persicae)
Mu Li (Concha Ostreae)
Mai Ya (Fructus Hordei Germinatus)

Shao Yao Yi Yi Ren Tang (Peony and Coicis Decoction) treats intestinal disorders characterized by damp-heat. It contains herbs to drain damp-heat, eliminate toxins, and stop diarrhea. Clinical applications include ulcerative colitis, Crohn's disease, diarrhea, and dysentery with presence of mucus, pus, and blood in the stools.

Sháo Yào Hòu Pò Tāng

(Peony and Magnolia Bark Decoction)

芍藥厚樸湯
芍药厚朴汤

Pinyin Name: Shao Yao Hou Po Tang
Literal Name: Peony and Magnolia Bark Decoction
Original Source: *An Hui Zhong Yi Xue Yuan* (Anhui University School of Medicine) in 1990

Bai Shao (Radix Paeoniae Alba)
Hou Po (Cortex Magnoliae Officinalis)

Yin Chen (Herba Artemisiae Scopariae)
Bai Zhu (Rhizoma Atractylodis Macrocephalae)
Dang Shen (Radix Codonopsis)
Wu Wei Zi (Fructus Schisandrae Chinensis)
Yi Yi Ren (Semen Coicis)
Dang Gui (Radix Angelicae Sinensis)
Chai Hu (Radix Bupleuri)
Che Qian Zi (Semen Plantaginis)
Fu Ling (Poria)
Huang Bo (Cortex Phellodendri Chinensis)
Guang Huo Xiang (Herba Pogostemonis)
Pao Jiang (Rhizoma Zingiberis Praeparatum)
Qin Pi (Cortex Fraxini)
Zhi Gan Cao (Radix et Rhizoma Glycyrrhizae Praeparata cum Melle)
Chen Pi (Pericarpium Citri Reticulatae)
Fang Feng (Radix Saposhnikoviae)
Huang Lian (Rhizoma Coptidis)
Xiang Fu (Rhizoma Cyperi)
Bo He (Herba Menthae)
Bai Zhi (Radix Angelicae Dahuricae)

Shao Yao Hou Po Tang (Peony and Magnolia Bark Decoction) treats intestinal disorders characterized by damp-heat, Liver qi stagnation, and Spleen deficiency. This formula contains herbs that drain damp-heat, regulate qi circulation, strengthen the Spleen and stop diarrhea. It is mostly used to treat inflammatory bowel disorder with alternating diarrhea and constipation, abdominal bloating, pain or mucus, flatulence and a feeling of incomplete evacuation.

AUTHORS' COMMENTS

The source text states to use *Shao Yao* (Radix Paeoniae) without specifying whether it should be *Bai Shao* (Radix Paeoniae Alba) or *Chi Shao* (Radix Paeoniae Rubra). *Bai Shao* (Radix Paeoniae Alba) is better at relieving pain and harmonizing the *ying* (nutritive) and *xue* (blood) levels, while *Chi Shao* (Radix Paeoniae Rubra) is more effective for clearing heat and cooling the blood. Thus, most scholars and clinicians agree that *Bai Shao* (Radix Paeoniae Alba) is a more suitable herb in *Shao Yao Tang*.

Shao Yao Tang and *Bai Tou Weng Tang* (Pulsatilla Decoction) are both representative formulas for dysentery. Both formulas treat similar signs and symptoms, but have distinctive differences:

- *Shao Yao Tang* treats diarrhea with pus and blood (of equal amounts) in the stools caused by qi and blood stagnation with damp-heat accumulation. It harmonizes qi and blood while draining damp-heat accumulation.

Chapter 5 – Heat-Clearing Formulas   *Section 5 – Zang Fu-Clearing Formulas*

Sháo Yào Tāng (Peony Decoction)

- *Bai Tou Weng Tang* treats heat toxins invading the *xue* (blood) level leading to dysentery or diarrhea with burning sensation and the presence of pus and blood (with more blood than pus) in the stools. It has dual effects to bind the Intestines as well as to dispel toxins.[12]

Please refer to *Ge Gen Huang Qin Huang Lian Tang* (Kudzu, Coptis, and Scutellaria Decoction) for a discussion of the differences between *Shao Yao Tang* and *Bai Tou Weng Tang* (Pulsatilla Decoction) for treating diarrhea.

According to Dr. Chang Wei-Yen, *Shao Yao Tang* is often combined with *Ge Gen Huang Qin Huang Lian Tang* (Kudzu, Coptis, and Scutellaria Decoction) to treat acute burning diarrhea or enteritis caused by damp-heat accumulation with a feeling of rectal prolapse due to continuous diarrhea.

References

1. *Jiang Su Zhong Yi* (Jiangsu Chinese Medicine) 1988;9(6):34.
2. *Jiang Su Zhong Yi* (Jiangsu Chinese Medicine) 1959;3:22.
3. *Jiang Su Zhong Yi* (Jiangsu Chinese Medicine) 1988;9(6):34.
4. *Liao Ning Zhong Yi Za Zhi* (Liaoning Journal of Chinese Medicine) 1992;19(9):43.
5. *Hei Long Jiang Zhong Yi Yao* (Heilongjiang Chinese Medicine and Herbology) 1989;6:29.
6. *Liao Ning Yi Xue* (Liaoning Medicine) 1960;95:23.
7. *Shi Yong Zhong Xi Yi Jie He Za Zhi* (Practical Journal of Integrated Chinese and Western Medicines) 1992;12:764.
8. *Gan Su Zhong Yi* (Gansu Chinese Medicine) 1998;2:13.
9. *Si Chuan Zhong Yi* (Sichuan Chinese Medicine) 1995;7:28.
10. *Si Chuan Zhong Yi* (Sichuan Chinese Medicine) 1995;3:33.
11. *Jiang Su Zhong Yi* (Jiangsu Chinese Medicine) 1988;9(6):34.
12. Wang MZ, et al. *Zhong Yi Xue Wen Da Ti Ku* (Questions and Answers on Traditional Chinese Medicine: Herbal Formulas).

Huáng Qín Tāng (Scutellaria Decoction)

黃芩湯

黄芩汤

Pinyin Name: *Huang Qin Tang*
Literal Name: Scutellaria Decoction
Alternate Name: Scute and Licorice Combination
Original Source: *Shang Han Lun* (Discussion of Cold-Induced Disorders) by Zhang Zhong-Jing in the Eastern Han Dynasty

COMPOSITION

Huang Qin (Radix Scutellariae)	9g [9g]
Bai Shao (Radix Paeoniae Alba)	6g [9g]
Gan Cao (Radix et Rhizoma Glycyrrhizae)	6g [3g]
Da Zao (Fructus Jujubae)	12 pieces [4 pieces]

DOSAGE / PREPARATION / ADMINISTRATION

The source text states to cook the ingredients in 10 cups [2,000 mL] of water until 3 cups [600 mL] of the liquid remains. Take 1 cup [200 mL] of the warm, strained decoction twice during the day, and once at night. Today, the decoction may be prepared using the doses suggested in brackets.

CHINESE THERAPEUTIC ACTIONS

1. Clears heat and stops diarrhea
2. Harmonizes the middle *jiao* and relieves pain

CLINICAL MANIFESTATIONS

Damp-heat dysentery: mild fever, a bitter taste in the mouth, abdominal pain, diarrhea, dysentery, a red tongue with a yellow tongue coating, and a rapid pulse.

CLINICAL APPLICATIONS

Acute enteritis, colitis, tenesmus, dysentery, and traveler's diarrhea.

EXPLANATION

Huang Qin Tang (Scutellaria Decoction) treats damp-heat dysentery characterized by damp-heat in the Intestines.

406

Chinese Herbal Formulas and Applications

Huáng Qín Tāng (Scutellaria Decoction)

Huang Qin Tang (Scutellaria Decoction)

Diagnosis	Signs and Symptoms	Treatment	Herbs
Damp-heat dysentery	• Dysentery, mild fever, and abdominal pain: damp-heat in the Intestines • Red tongue with a yellow tongue coating and a rapid pulse: excess heat in the body	• Clears heat and stops diarrhea • Harmonizes the middle *jiao* and relieves pain	• *Huang Qin* (Radix Scutellariae) clears heat and dries dampness to relieve the dysentery. • *Bai Shao* (Radix Paeoniae Alba) and *Gan Cao* (Radix et Rhizoma Glycyrrhizae) relieve spasms and cramps. • *Gan Cao* (Radix et Rhizoma Glycyrrhizae) and *Da Zao* (Fructus Jujubae) nourish the Spleen and harmonize the middle *jiao*.

Damp-heat in the Intestines causes dysentery, mild fever, and abdominal pain. A yellow tongue coating and a rapid pulse suggest excess heat in the body.

This formula contains *Huang Qin* (Radix Scutellariae) to clear heat and dry dampness to relieve the dysentery. *Bai Shao* (Radix Paeoniae Alba) and *Gan Cao* (Radix et Rhizoma Glycyrrhizae) relieve spasms and cramps. *Gan Cao* (Radix et Rhizoma Glycyrrhizae) and *Da Zao* (Fructus Jujubae) nourish the Spleen and harmonize the middle *jiao*.

MODIFICATIONS

• With diarrhea and dysentery, combine with *Shao Yao Tang* (Peony Decoction).
• With tenesmus, epigastric distention, fever, and abdominal pain, add *Da Huang* (Radix et Rhizoma Rhei).
• With mucus and blood in the stool, add charred *Shan Zha* (Fructus Crataegi) and charred *Di Yu* (Radix Sanguisorbae).
• With dysentery and abdominal pain, add *Huang Lian* (Rhizoma Coptidis) and *Gan Jiang* (Rhizoma Zingiberis).
• With exterior pathogenic factors, add *Ge Gen* (Radix Puerariae Lobatae), *Jing Jie* (Herba Schizonepetae), *Lian Qiao* (Fructus Forsythiae), and *Jin Yin Hua* (Flos Lonicerae Japonicae).
• With thirst, dryness, and irritability, add *Zhi Shi* (Fructus Aurantii Immaturus) and *Chai Hu* (Radix Bupleuri).
• With nausea, vomiting, and abdominal pain, combine with *Huang Lian Tang* (Coptis Decoction).
• With nausea and vomiting caused by reversed flow of Stomach qi, add *Ban Xia* (Rhizoma Pinelliae) and *Sheng Jiang* (Rhizoma Zingiberis Recens).

CAUTIONS / CONTRAINDICATIONS

• *Huang Qin Tang* is contraindicated in dysentery or diarrhea caused by cold and dampness, and in patients with a dry mouth without thirst or a deep, slow pulse.
• Avoid foods that are pungent, spicy, oily or greasy while taking this herbal formula.[1]

CLINICAL STUDIES AND RESEARCH

Diarrhea: One study reported effectiveness using modified *Huang Qin Tang* to treat 120 children with diarrhea in autumn. The herbal treatment contained *Huang Qin* (Radix Scutellariae), *Bai Shao* (Radix Paeoniae Alba), *Gan Cao* (Radix et Rhizoma Glycyrrhizae), *Ge Gen* (Radix Puerariae Lobatae), *Fang Feng* (Radix Saposhnikoviae), *Bai Zhu* (Rhizoma Atractylodis Macrocephalae), *Mai Ya* (Fructus Hordei Germinatus), *Wu Mei* (Fructus Mume), *Chen Pi* (Pericarpium Citri Reticulatae), *Sheng Jiang* (Rhizoma Zingiberis Recens), and *Da Zao* (Fructus Jujubae). The treatment protocol was to cook the herbs in water, and administer the decoction daily. Of 120 cases, the study reported complete recovery in 93 cases and improvement in 27 cases within 3 days.[2]

AUTHORS' COMMENTS

The source text states to use *Shao Yao* (Radix Paeoniae) without specifying whether it should be *Bai Shao* (Radix Paeoniae Alba) or *Chi Shao* (Radix Paeoniae Rubra). *Bai Shao* (Radix Paeoniae Alba) has a better effect to relieve pain and harmonize the *ying* (nutritive) and *xue* (blood) levels, while *Chi Shao* (Radix Paeoniae Rubra) is more effective at clearing heat and cooling the blood. Thus, most scholars and clinicians agree that *Bai Shao* (Radix Paeoniae Alba) is a more suitable herb in *Huang Qin Tang*.

References

1. *Zhong Yao Ming Fang Yao Li Yu Ying Yong* (Pharmacology and Applications of Famous Herbal Formulas) 1989;197-198.
2. *Gan Su Zhong Yi* (Gansu Chinese Medicine) 1997;6:30.

Chapter 5 – Heat-Clearing Formulas   *Section 5 – Zang Fu-Clearing Formulas*

Bái Tóu Wēng Tāng (Pulsatilla Decoction)

白頭翁湯
白头翁汤

Pinyin Name: *Bai Tou Weng Tang*
Literal Name: Pulsatilla Decoction
Alternate Name: Anemone Combination
Original Source: *Shang Han Lun* (Discussion of Cold-Induced Disorders) by Zhang Zhong-Jing in the Eastern Han Dynasty

COMPOSITION

Bai Tou Weng (Radix Pulsatillae)	6g [15g]
Huang Lian (Rhizoma Coptidis)	9g [6g]
Huang Bo (Cortex Phellodendri Chinensis)	9g [12g]
Qin Pi (Cortex Fraxini)	9g [12g]

DOSAGE / PREPARATION / ADMINISTRATION

Cook the ingredients in 7 cups [1,400 mL] of water until 2 cups [400 mL] of the liquid remains. Take 1 cup [200 mL] of the warm, strained decoction. If the condition is not improved after the first dose, take another dose (1 cup or 200 mL). Today, the decoction may be prepared using the doses suggested in brackets.

CHINESE THERAPEUTIC ACTIONS

1. Clears heat and eliminates toxins
2. Cools the blood and stops dysentery

CLINICAL MANIFESTATIONS

Toxic heat dysentery: abdominal pain, rectal tenesmus, burning sensations of the anus, diarrhea that is more red (blood) than white (pus), thirst with a strong desire to drink, a red tongue body with a yellow tongue coating, and a wiry, rapid pulse.

CLINICAL APPLICATIONS

Bacterial dysentery, amoebic dysentery, acute or chronic enteritis, postpartum enteritis, colitis, ulcerative colitis, gastroenteritis, pneumonia, urinary tract infection, acute conjunctivitis, pelvic inflammatory disease, and leukorrhea.

EXPLANATION

Bai Tou Weng Tang (Pulsatilla Decoction) treats toxic heat dysentery, with toxic heat affecting the *jueyin* channel. If the toxic heat injures the qi and blood of the Stomach and Intestines, there will be abdominal pain, the presence of blood and pus in the stools, along with rectal tenesmus and burning sensations of the anus. Thirst with a strong desire to drink is caused by heat consuming body fluids as well as by body fluid depletion from the diarrhea.

Bai Tou Weng (Radix Pulsatillae) clears heat and eliminates toxins in the *xue* (blood) level. *Huang Lian* (Rhizoma Coptidis) helps *Bai Tou Weng* (Radix Pulsatillae) clear heat and eliminate toxins. *Huang Bo* (Cortex Phellodendri Chinensis) sedates damp-heat in the lower *jiao*. Together, they clear damp-heat, eliminate toxins, and stop diarrhea and dysentery. *Qin Pi* (Cortex Fraxini), a cold, astringent herb, clears heat, dries dampness, and relieves diarrhea and dysentery.

Bai Tou Weng Tang (Pulsatilla Decoction)

Diagnosis	Signs and Symptoms	Treatment	Herbs
Toxic heat dysentery	• Dysentery, abdominal pain, rectal tenesmus, burning sensations of the anus, and the presence of blood and pus in the stools: toxic heat in the Intestines • Thirst with a strong desire to drink: heat consuming body fluids • Red tongue body and a yellow tongue coating: excess heat • Wiry, rapid pulse: excess heat	• Clears heat and eliminates toxins • Cools the blood and stops dysentery	• *Bai Tou Weng* (Radix Pulsatillae) clears heat and eliminates toxins in the *xue* (blood) level. • *Huang Lian* (Rhizoma Coptidis) clears heat and eliminates toxins. • *Huang Bo* (Cortex Phellodendri Chinensis) clears damp-heat in the lower *jiao*. • *Qin Pi* (Cortex Fraxini) clears heat, dries dampness, and stops diarrhea and dysentery.

Chinese Herbal Formulas and Applications

Bái Tóu Wēng Tāng (Pulsatilla Decoction)

MODIFICATIONS

- With urinary urgency and pain, add *Mu Tong* (Caulis Akebiae), *Bai Mao Gen* (Rhizoma Imperatae), and *Jin Qian Cao* (Herba Lysimachiae).
- With chills and fever, add *Ge Gen* (Radix Puerariae Lobatae), *Jing Jie* (Herba Schizonepetae), *Jin Yin Hua* (Flos Lonicerae Japonicae), and *Lian Qiao* (Fructus Forsythiae).
- With severe abdominal pain and rectal tenesmus, add *Mu Xiang* (Radix Aucklandiae), *Bing Lang* (Semen Arecae), *Bai Shao* (Radix Paeoniae Alba), *Gan Cao* (Radix et Rhizoma Glycyrrhizae), and *Zhi Qiao* (Fructus Aurantii).
- For amoebic dysentery, add *Shi Liu Pi* (Pericarpium Granati).
- For bacterial dysentery, add *Di Yu* (Radix Sanguisorbae), *Xian He Cao* (Herba Agrimoniae), and *Mu Xiang* (Radix Aucklandiae).

CAUTIONS / CONTRAINDICATIONS

- *Bai Tou Weng Tang* treats heat-type dysentery, with toxic heat in the Intestines characterized by dark purplish blood. This formula is contraindicated in cases of chronic dysentery or diarrhea due to deficiency.
- This formula contains bitter and cold herbs which may injure the Spleen and Stomach. Therefore, it should not be taken at large doses or for a prolonged period of time.

PHARMACOLOGICAL EFFECTS

Antibiotic: Administration of *Bai Tou Weng Tang* in various doses was associated with an inhibitory effect *in vitro* against many different types of bacillus, staphylococcus, and other microorganisms.[1]

CLINICAL STUDIES AND RESEARCH

1. **Bacterial dysentery**: In one clinical study, 249 patients with bacterial dysentery were effectively treated, with an average of 1-5 days for reduction of body temperature and normal bowel movement within 3 days.[2] In another report, modified *Bai Tou Weng Tang* was used to treat 100 patients with bacterial dysentery with a 97% effectiveness rate and no reports of significant side effects.[3] Lastly, one study reported success using modified *Bai Tou Weng Tang* as a rectal enema to treat 87 patients with chronic bacterial dysentery. The treatment protocol was to cook the herbs in 1,000 mL of water to yield 200 mL of an herbal solution. The herbal solution was instilled into the rectum at bedtime for 5 days, followed by 2 days of rest. This cycle was repeated 1-4 times as needed. The study reported complete recovery in 65 of 87 patients.[4]
2. **Amoebic dysentery**: In one report, 22 out of 25 patients with amoebic dysentery were treated with complete recovery using modified *Bai Tou Weng Tang*. Out of 22

patients who had complete recovery, 5 responded within 11 doses, and 12 responded within 6-10 doses. The modifications included the addition of *Di Yu* (Radix Sanguisorbae) and *Ku Shen* (Radix Sophorae Flavescentis), and the removal of *Huang Lian* (Rhizoma Coptidis).[5] Another study reported complete recovery in 114 of 116 patients with amoebic dysentery using both *Bai Tou Weng Tang* and *Ge Gen Huang Qin Huang Lian Tang* (Kudzu, Coptis, and Scutellaria Decoction) with modifications. *Jin Yin Hua* (Flos Lonicerae Japonicae) was added for high fever with an aversion to cold. *Di Yu* (Radix Sanguisorbae) was added for blood in the stools. *Ban Xia* (Rhizoma Pinelliae) was added for nausea and vomiting. *Bai Shao* (Radix Paeoniae Alba) was added for abdominal pain.[6]
3. **Enteritis**: In one report, 144 patients with enteritis were treated with 95.8% effectiveness within 48 hours using *Bai Tou Weng Tang*.[7]
4. **Colitis**: One study reported 91.43% effectiveness using modified *Bai Tou Weng Tang* to treat 35 patients with colitis. In addition to using *Bai Tou Weng Tang* as the base formula, *Mu Dan Pi* (Cortex Moutan), *Dang Gui* (Radix Angelicae Sinensis) and charred *Jin Yin Hua* (Flos Lonicerae Japonicae) were added during acute episodes; and *Yan Hu Suo* (Rhizoma Corydalis), *Bai Zhu* (Rhizoma Atractylodis Macrocephalae), and *Tao Ren* (Semen Persicae) were added during remission. The treatment protocol was to administer the herbs twice daily, for 10 days per course of treatment, for 2 courses total. Of 35 cases, the study reported complete recovery in 14 cases, improvement in 18 cases, and no change in 3 cases.[8]
5. **Gastroenteritis**: One study reported complete recovery in 28 of 30 patients with gastroenteritis when treated with *Bai Tou Weng Tang*. The treatment protocol was to administer the herbs in capsule form three times daily, and relief was achieved in an average of 3 days.[9]
6. **Pneumonia**: In one report, 56 out of 67 patients with pneumonia were treated with complete recovery using modified *Bai Tou Weng Tang*. The 11 patients who did not respond, however, continued to deteriorate. In addition to *Bai Tou Weng Tang*, *Ku Xing Ren* (Semen Armeniacae Amarum), *Ma Huang* (Herba Ephedrae), *Yu Xing Cao* (Herba Houttuyniae), and *Da Qing Ye* (Folium Isatidis) were added for wind-heat attacking the Lung; *Di Huang* (Radix Rehmanniae), *Xuan Shen* (Radix Scrophulariae), *Di Gu Pi* (Cortex Lycii) and *Tian Hua Fen* (Radix Trichosanthis) for heat damaging the yin and body fluids; and *Di Huang* (Radix Rehmanniae), *Xuan Shen* (Radix Scrophulariae), *Sha Shen* (Radix Glehniae seu Adenophorae), *Dan Shen* (Radix et Rhizoma Salviae Miltiorrhizae), and *Bai Hua She She Cao* (Herba Hedyotis) for heat in the *qi* (energy) and *xue* (blood) levels.[10]

HEAT-CLEARING FORMULAS

5

409

Chapter 5 – Heat-Clearing Formulas   *Section 5 – Zang Fu-Clearing Formulas*

Bái Tóu Wēng Tāng (Pulsatilla Decoction)

7. **Urinary tract infection**: Modified *Bai Tou Weng Tang* was used to treat 63 patients with various types of urinary tract infections. Of all patients, 19 had acute infection, 44 had chronic infection; 12 had urethra infections, 33 had bladder infections, and 18 had kidney infections. The study reported marked improvement in 29 cases, moderate improvement in 24 cases, and no effect in 10 cases.[11]

8. **Pelvic inflammatory disease**: One study reported effectiveness using modified *Bai Tou Weng Tang* to treat acute pelvic inflammatory disease. In addition to the base formula, modifications were made by adding charred *Mian Ma Guan Zhong* (Rhizoma Dryopteridis Crassirhizomatis) and *Yi Mu Cao* (Herba Leonuri) for postpartum bleeding caused by presence of placental remnants; *Huang Qi* (Radix Astragali) and *Dang Shen* (Radix Codonopsis) for qi deficiency with spontaneous perspiration; *Jin Yin Hua* (Flos Lonicerae Japonicae) and *Pu Gong Ying* (Herba Taraxaci) for Stomach heat; *Xiang Fu* (Rhizoma Cyperi) and *Ju He* (Semen Citri Reticulatae) for lower abdominal pain; *Yi Yi Ren* (Semen Coicis) and *Qu Mai* (Herba Dianthi) for accumulation of fluid in the pelvic region; *Chen Pi* (Pericarpium Citri Reticulatae), *Fu Ling* (Poria), and *Sha Ren* (Fructus Amomi) for poor appetite; and *Da Huang* (Radix et Rhizoma Rhei) for dry stools. Of 107 cases, the study reported complete recovery in 67 cases after one course of treatment (10 days), and 40 cases after 2 courses (20 days).[12]

9. **Acute conjunctivitis**: Eighty-seven patients with acute conjunctivitis were treated with complete recovery within 1-3 doses. Out of 87 cases, 26 had complete recovery within 1 dose, 41 cases within 2 doses, and 20 cases within 3 doses. The herbal formula was modified by adding *Mu Zei* (Herba Equiseti Hiemalis).[13]

RELATED FORMULA

Bái Tóu Wēng Jiā Gān Cǎo Ē Jiāo Tāng

(Pulsatilla Decoction plus Licorice and Ass-Hide Gelatin)

白頭翁加甘草阿膠湯
白头翁加甘草阿胶汤

Pinyin Name: *Bai Tou Weng Jia Gan Cao E Jiao Tang*

Literal Name: Pulsatilla Decoction plus Licorice and Ass-Hide Gelatin

Original Source: *Jin Gui Yao Lue* (Essentials from the Golden Cabinet) by Zhang Zhong-Jing in the Eastern Han Dynasty

Bai Tou Weng (Radix Pulsatillae)	6g [15g]
Gan Cao (Radix et Rhizoma Glycyrrhizae)	6g [3g]
E Jiao (Colla Corii Asini)	6g [9g]
Qin Pi (Cortex Fraxini)	9g [12g]
Huang Lian (Rhizoma Coptidis)	9g [6g]
Huang Bo (Cortex Phellodendri Chinensis)	9g [12g]

The source text states to cook the ingredients in 7 cups [1,400 mL] of water until 2.5 cups [500 mL] of the liquid remain. Add *E Jiao* (Colla Corii Asini) to the strained decoction and stir until it is dissolved completely. Take the warm decoction in three equally-divided doses. Today, the decoction may be prepared using the doses suggested in brackets.

Bai Tou Weng Jia Gan Cao E Jiao Tang (Pulsatilla Decoction plus Licorice and Ass-Hide Gelatin) is composed of *Bai Tou Weng Tang* plus *Gan Cao* (Radix et Rhizoma Glycyrrhizae) and *E Jiao* (Colla Corii Asini). The main actions of this formula are to clear heat, eliminate toxins, tonify blood and nourish yin. The two additional herbs nourish blood and yin. This formula was originally designed for postpartum women with toxic heat dysentery accompanied by blood and yin deficiencies after delivery. Today, this formula is suitable for patients suffering from toxic heat dysentery who cannot tolerate solely sedating and draining herbs because of blood and yin deficiencies.

AUTHORS' COMMENTS

Shao Yao Tang (Peony Decoction) and *Bai Tou Weng Tang* both treat bacterial and amoebic dysentery.

• *Shao Yao Tang* treats damp-heat dysentery resulting from qi and blood stagnation. It contains moving and purging herbs and does not contain any astringent, binding herbs to stop diarrhea. Its treatment strategy is to harmonize the qi and blood as well as to clear damp-heat.

• *Bai Tou Weng Tang* is more suitable for treating heat dysentery in which the toxic heat has extensively injured the blood. The treatment plan for heat dysentery is to clear heat, eliminate heat toxins, and cool the blood to relieve the dysentery. The formula includes herbs that bind the Intestines and stop diarrhea.

Please refer to *Ge Gen Huang Qin Huang Lian Tang* (Kudzu, Coptis, and Scutellaria Decoction) for a comparative analysis with *Shao Yao Tang* (Peony Decoction) and *Bai Tou Weng Tang* in treating diarrhea.

References

1. *Ha Er Bing Zhong Yi* (Haerbing Chinese Medicine) 1965;8(3):34.
2. *Zhe Jiang Zhong Yi Za Zhi* (Zhejiang Journal of Chinese Medicine) 1957;6:242.
3. *Zhe Jiang Zhong Yi Za Zhi* (Zhejiang Journal of Chinese Medicine) 1986;4:178.
4. *Nan Jing Zhong Yi Yao Da Xue Xue Bao* (Journal of Nanjing University of Traditional Chinese Medicine and Medicinals) 1997;5:311.
5. *Zhong Yi Fang Ji Xian Dai Yan Jiu* (Modern Study of Medical Formulae in Traditional Chinese Medicine) 1997;344-345.
6. *Hu Bei Zhong Yi Za Zhi* (Hubei Journal of Chinese Medicine) 1983;2:24.
7. *Shang Hai Zhong Yi Yao Za Zhi* (Shanghai Journal of Chinese Medicine and Herbology) 1960;6:254.

Bái Tóu Wēng Tāng (Pulsatilla Decoction)

8. *Xin Zhong Yi* (New Chinese Medicine) 1996;1:20.
9. *Hei Long Jiang Zhong Yi Yao* (Heilongjiang Chinese Medicine and Herbology) 1998;5:54.
10. *Zhe Jiang Zhong Yi Za Zhi* (Zhejiang Journal of Chinese Medicine) 1986;12:551.

11. *Hei Long Jiang Zhong Yi Yao* (Heilongjiang Chinese Medicine and Herbology) 1986;6:40.
12. *He Nan Zhong Yi* (Henan Chinese Medicine) 1994;3:156.
13. *Zhong Yi Fang Ji Xian Dai Yan Jiu* (Modern Study of Medical Formulae in Traditional Chinese Medicine) 1997;346-347.

Section 6

清虚热剂
— Deficiency-Heat Clearing Formulas

Qīng Hāo Biē Jiǎ Tāng
(Artemisia Annua and Soft-Shelled Turtle Shell Decoction)

青蒿鱉甲湯
青蒿鳖甲汤

Pinyin Name: *Qing Hao Bie Jia Tang*
Literal Name: Artemisia Annua and Soft-Shelled Turtle Shell Decoction
Alternate Name: Artemisia Annua Decoction
Original Source: *Wen Bing Tiao Bian* (Systematic Differentiation of Warm Disease) by Wu Ju-Tong in 1798

COMPOSITION

Bie Jia (Carapax Trionycis)	15g
Qing Hao (Herba Artemisiae Annuae)	6g
Di Huang (Radix Rehmanniae)	12g
Zhi Mu (Rhizoma Anemarrhenae)	6g
Mu Dan Pi (Cortex Moutan)	9g

DOSAGE / PREPARATION / ADMINISTRATION

Cook the ingredients in 5 cups of water until it is reduced to 2 cups. Take 1 cup daily. Note: Cooking *Qing Hao* (Herba Artemisiae Annuae) at a high temperature for a prolonged period of time will destroy its active ingredients. Therefore, it should not be cooked with the rest of the herbs. Rather, for maximum effect, it should be steeped in hot water and served along with the decoction.

CHINESE THERAPEUTIC ACTIONS

Nourishes yin and vents interior deficiency heat

CLINICAL MANIFESTATIONS

Late-stage febrile diseases with extensive yin and body fluid deficiencies: a feeling of warmth at night and coolness in the morning, resolution of fever without perspiration, a red tongue body with a scanty tongue coating, and a fine, rapid pulse.

CLINICAL APPLICATIONS

Fever (from cancer, after surgery, and in children), common cold, vertigo, phthisis, chronic pyelonephritis, kidney tuberculosis, and menopausal symptoms.

EXPLANATION

Qing Hao Bie Jia Tang (Artemisia Annua and Soft-Shelled Turtle Shell Decoction) treats late-stage febrile diseases with extensive yin and body fluid deficiencies. Usually in late-stage febrile diseases, there is still some heat which has not been completely cleared, and now resides deep in the body. Moreover, yin and body fluids have been extensively injured and consumed by the heat pathogen, and produces a situation in which the insufficient yin fails to contain yang, resulting in the symptom of a feeling of warmth at night and coolness in the morning. Since the body fluids are already depleted, there is an absence of perspiration. A red tongue body with a scanty tongue coating, and a fine, rapid pulse suggest deficiency heat in the interior.

Because this is not a condition of excess heat in the *qi* (energy) level, strong heat-clearing herbs are not suitable. Neither are pure yin tonics called for, because pure tonification will trap the remaining heat inside the body. The best treatment plan is to clear and vent the heat while nourishing yin. *Bie Jia* (Carapax Trionycis) nourishes yin to clear heat; it has the unique function of entering deeply

Qīng Hāo Biē Jiǎ Tāng
(Artemisia Annua and Soft-Shelled Turtle Shell Decoction)

Qing Hao Bie Jia Tang (Artemisia Annua and Soft-Shelled Turtle Shell Decoction)

Diagnosis	Signs and Symptoms	Treatment	Herbs
Late-stage febrile diseases with extensive yin and body fluid deficiencies	• A feeling of warm sensations at night and cool sensations in the morning: late stage of febrile diseases in which heat resides deep in the body • Resolution of fever without perspiration and night fever that subsides in the daytime: extreme yin and body fluid deficiencies • Red tongue body, a scanty tongue coating, and a fine, rapid pulse: deficiency heat in the interior	Nourishes yin and vents interior deficiency heat	• *Bie Jia* (Carapax Trionycis) nourishes yin and clears heat deep in the body. • *Qing Hao* (Herba Artemisiae Annuae) vents deficiency heat and leads it out of the body. • *Di Huang* (Radix Rehmanniae), *Zhi Mu* (Rhizoma Anemarrhenae) and *Mu Dan Pi* (Cortex Moutan) nourish yin and clears deficiency heat.

into the *ying* (nutritive) and *xue* (blood) levels to search for and clear the remaining heat pathogen. *Qing Hao* (Herba Artemisiae Annuae), on the other hand, cannot enter into such a deep level. However, due to its aromatic property, it can vent the deficiency heat that *Bie Jia* (Carapax Trionycis) has cleared and guide it out of the body. *Di Huang* (Radix Rehmanniae) nourishes yin and clears heat. *Zhi Mu* (Rhizoma Anemarrhenae) moistens dryness and helps *Qing Hao* (Herba Artemisiae Annuae) and *Bie Jia* (Carapax Trionycis) clear deficiency heat. *Mu Dan Pi* (Cortex Moutan) is acrid and cold, and helps disperse and clear deficiency heat.

MODIFICATIONS

- With unremitting low-grade fever associated with tuberculosis of the kidney or chronic pyelonephritis, add *Bai Mao Gen* (Rhizoma Imperatae).
- With unremitting low-grade fever with unknown cause, add *Bai Wei* (Radix et Rhizoma Cynanchi Atrati), *Shi Hu* (Caulis Dendrobii) and *Di Gu Pi* (Cortex Lycii).
- With afternoon fever and cold sensations in the morning with thirst, remove *Di Huang* (Radix Rehmanniae) and add *Tian Hua Fen* (Radix Trichosanthis).
- For children with yin-deficient heat during the summer, add *Bai Wei* (Radix et Rhizoma Cynanchi Atrati) and *He Geng* (Caulis Nelumbinis).
- For steaming bones sensations caused by pulmonary tuberculosis, add *Bei Sha Shen* (Radix Glehniae) and *Mo Han Lian* (Herba Ecliptae).
- For pneumonia with measles and toxic heat lingering in the interior, add *Yin Chai Hu* (Radix Stellariae) and *Bai Wei* (Radix et Rhizoma Cynanchi Atrati).

CAUTIONS / CONTRAINDICATIONS

Qing Hao Bie Jia Tang is contraindicated in patients with yin deficiency and Liver wind rising.

CLINICAL STUDIES AND RESEARCH

1. **Fever in cancer**: Administration of modified *Qing Hao Bie Jia Tang* has been shown in many studies to effectively reduce body temperature in cancer patients with fever. In one study, use of the modified formula in 25 cancer patients with fever (15-60 days with fever) was associated with significant effect in 10 patients, moderate effect in 10 patients, and no effect in 5 patients. The herbs were given in decoction daily for 10 packs of herbs per course of treatment. The herbal formula contained *Qing Hao* (Herba Artemisiae Annuae) 15g, *Bie Jia* (Carapax Trionycis) 20g, *Di Huang* (Radix Rehmanniae) 10g, *Zhi Mu* (Rhizoma Anemarrhenae) 10g, *Mu Dan Pi* (Cortex Moutan) 15g, *Chai Hu* (Radix Bupleuri) 10g, *Bai Shao* (Radix Paeoniae Alba) 10g, *Gan Cao* (Radix et Rhizoma Glycyrrhizae) 3g, and *Bai Hua She She Cao* (Herba Hedyotis) 30g. Modifications were made by adding *Tai Zi Shen* (Radix Pseudostellariae) 10g, *Di Gu Pi* (Cortex Lycii) 10g, and *Tian Hua Fen* (Radix Trichosanthis) 15g for *wu xin re* (five-center heat); *Fo Shou* (Fructus Citri Sarcodactylis) 10g, *Yu Zhi Zi* (Fructus Akebiae) 10g, *Chen Pi* (Pericarpium Citri Reticulatae) 6g, *Gu Ya* (Fructus Setariae Germinatus) 10g, *Mai Ya* (Fructus Hordei Germinatus) 10g, and *Ji Nei Jin* (Endothelium Corneum Gigeriae Galli) 6g for poor appetite; *Fu Xiao Mai* (Fructus Tritici Levis) 30g and *Mu Li* (Concha Ostreae) 30g for night perspiration; *Yan Hu Suo* (Rhizoma Corydalis) 10g, *Wu Yao* (Radix Linderae) 10g, and *Xu Chang Qing* (Radix et Rhizoma Cynanchi Paniculati) 10g for severe pain; *Chuan Bei Mu* (Bulbus Fritillariae Cirrhosae) 10g, *Kuan Dong Hua* (Flos Farfarae) 10g, *Yu Zhu* (Rhizoma Polygonati Odorati) 10g, *Mai Dong*

Qīng Hāo Biē Jiǎ Tāng
(Artemisia Annua and Soft-Shelled Turtle Shell Decoction)

(Radix Ophiopogonis) 10g, *Jie Geng* (Radix Platycodonis) 5g, and *Pi Pa Ye* (Folium Eriobotryae) 10g for cough with scanty sputum that is hard to expectorate; and *Gua Lou* (Fructus Trichosanthis) 30g, *Huo Ma Ren* (Fructus Cannabis) 10g, and processed *Da Huang* (Radix et Rhizoma Rhei) 10g for constipation.[1]

2. **Fever in lung cancer**: Twenty patients with fever associated with lung cancer were treated with modified *Qing Hao Bie Jia Tang* with 90% effectiveness in reducing body temperature. The duration of fever prior to treatment ranged from 10-50 days, with temperature ranging from 38-39°C / 100.4-102.2°F or above. In addition to fever, other clinical presentations included cough, sputum with blood, a dry mouth and throat, *wu xin re* (five-center heat), tidal fever, a red tongue body with a scanty tongue coating, and a fine, rapid pulse. The herbal treatment contained *Qing Hao* (Herba Artemisiae Annuae) 15g, *Bie Jia* (Carapax Trionycis) 20g (pre-decocted), *Di Huang* (Radix Rehmanniae) 20g, *Zhi Mu* (Rhizoma Anemarrhenae) 10g, *Mu Dan Pi* (Cortex Moutan) 10g, *Tian Hua Fen* (Radix Trichosanthis) 15g, *Bai He* (Bulbus Lilii) 15g, *Zao Xiu* (Rhizoma Paridis) 30g, and *Bai Hua She She Cao* (Herba Hedyotis) 30g. Modifications were made by adding *Bai Mao Gen* (Rhizoma Imperatae) 30g and *Xian He Cao* (Herba Agrimoniae) 30g for coughing of blood; *Gua Lou* (Fructus Trichosanthis) 15g and *Yu Jin* (Radix Curcumae) 15g for feeling of oppression and pain in the chest; *Fu Xiao Mai* (Fructus Tritici Levis) 30g and *Mu Li* (Concha Ostreae) 15g (pre-decocted) for night sweats; *Huo Ma Ren* (Fructus Cannabis) 30g for constipation; dry-fried *Shan Zha* (Fructus Crataegi) 10g and dry-fried *Mai Ya* (Fructus Hordei Germinatus) 15g for poor appetite; and *Shi Gao* (Gypsum Fibrosum) 30g and *Di Gu Pi* (Cortex Lycii) 15g for high fever. The herbs were given in decoction for 10 days per course of treatment. Of 20 patients, the study reported significant improvement in 12 patients, moderate improvement in 6 patients, and no change in 2 patients.[2]

3. **Fever after surgery**: In one study, 100 women with persistent post-surgical low-grade fever (37.3-38°C / 99.1-100.4°F) refractory to antibiotic therapy were treated with modified *Qing Hao Bie Jia Tang* with good results. The herbal formula contained *Di Huang* (Radix Rehmanniae) 15g, processed *Bie Jia* (Carapax Trionycis) 12g, *Qing Hao* (Herba Artemisiae Annuae) 10g, *Zhi Mu* (Rhizoma Anemarrhenae) 10g, *Mu Dan Pi* (Cortex Moutan) 10g, *Bai Wei* (Radix et Rhizoma Cynanchi Atrati) 10g, *Yin Chai Hu* (Radix Stellariae) 10g, *Bai Shao* (Radix Paeoniae Alba) 10g, and *Gan Cao* (Radix et Rhizoma Glycyrrhizae) 5g. The herbs were given in decoction one time daily,

starting 5-10 days after surgery in 81 patients, and 11-15 days in 19 patients. Of 100 patients, 82 received only herbal therapy, and 18 received both herbal and antibiotic therapies. The study reported significant improvement in 70 patients, moderate improvement in 23 patients, and no effect in 7 patients.[3] In another study, 32 patients with post-surgical fever characterized by yin-deficient heat were treated with modified *Qing Hao Bie Jia Tang* with good results. Of 32 patients, the study reported normal body temperature in 8 patients after 1 day, 19 patients after 2 days, and 5 patients after 3 days.[4]

4. **Common cold**: Modified *Qing Hao Bie Jia Tang* was used with good results to treat common cold characterized by yin deficiency in 75 patients (48 males and 27 females, between 1 and 50 years of age, with 1-15 days of illness). The herbal formula contained *Qing Hao* (Herba Artemisiae Annuae) 10-15g, *Bie Jia* (Carapax Trionycis) 15-30g, *Sang Ye* (Folium Mori) 10-12g, *Tian Hua Fen* (Radix Trichosanthis) 10-12g, *Zhi Mu* (Rhizoma Anemarrhenae) 10-12g, and *Mu Dan Pi* (Cortex Moutan) 10-12g. Modifications were made as follows: *Tai Zi Shen* (Radix Pseudostellariae) for qi deficiency; *Bei Mu* (Bulbus Fritillariae) and *Bo He* (Herba Menthae) for cough, *Bai Wei* (Radix et Rhizoma Cynanchi Atrati) and *Mai Dong* (Radix Ophiopogonis) for severe yin deficiency; and *Ou Jie* (Nodus Nelumbinis Rhizomatis) and charred *Di Huang* (Radix Rehmanniae) for blood in the sputum. Out of 75 patients, 55 had complete recovery, 15 had significant improvement, and 5 had no benefit. The overall rate of effectiveness was 93.3%.[5]

5. **Vertigo**: Seventy-three patients with vertigo were treated with modified *Qing Hao Bie Jia Tang* with an overall effective rate of 93.2%. The herbal formula contained *Qing Hao* (Herba Artemisiae Annuae) 9g, *Bie Jia* (Carapax Trionycis) 12g (pre-decocted), *Zhi Mu* (Rhizoma Anemarrhenae) 9g, *Di Huang* (Radix Rehmanniae) 30g, *Mu Dan Pi* (Cortex Moutan) 9g, *Tian Ma* (Rhizoma Gastrodiae) 12g, *Ge Gen* (Radix Puerariae Lobatae) 30g, *Dan Shen* (Radix et Rhizoma Salviae Miltiorrhizae) 12g, and others as needed. Most patients had partial to complete resolution of vertigo within 7-14 days.[6]

RELATED FORMULA
Zī Yīn Qīng Rè Tāng
(Nourish Yin and Clear Heat Decoction)

滋陰清熱湯
滋阴清热汤

Pinyin Name: Zi Yin Qing Re Tang
Literal Name: Nourish Yin and Clear Heat Decoction
Original Source: *Tian Jin Zhong Yi Xue Yuan* (Tianjin University of Chinese Medicine) in 1989

Chinese Herbal Formulas and Applications

Qīng Hāo Biē Jiǎ Tāng
(Artemisia Annua and Soft-Shelled Turtle Shell Decoction)

Qing Hao (Herba Artemisiae Annuae)

Bai Wei (Radix et Rhizoma Cynanchi Atrati)

Di Huang (Radix Rehmanniae)

Zhi Mu (Rhizoma Anemarrhenae)

Mu Dan Pi (Cortex Moutan)

Gan Cao (Radix et Rhizoma Glycyrrhizae)

Suan Zao Ren (Semen Ziziphi Spinosae)

Da Zao (Fructus Jujubae)

Shou Wu Teng (Caulis Polygoni Multiflori)

Fu Xiao Mai (Fructus Tritici Levis)

Chai Hu (Radix Bupleuri)

Bai Shao (Radix Paeoniae Alba)

Di Gu Pi (Cortex Lycii)

Huang Bo (Cortex Phellodendri Chinensis)

Zi Yin Qing Re Tang (Nourish Yin and Clear Heat Decoction) follows the principles of two classic formulas: *Qing Hao Bie Jia Tang* (Artemisia Annua and Soft-Shelled Turtle Shell Decoction) to nourish yin and clear deficiency heat; and *Gan Mai Da Zao Tang* (Licorice, Wheat, and Jujube Decoction) to nourish the Heart and calm the *shen* (spirit). Clinical applications of this formula include menopause, hot flashes, night sweats, mood swings, irritability, and emotional instability.

AUTHORS' COMMENTS

Qing Hao Bie Jia Tang, *Qin Jiao Bie Jia San* (Gentiana Macrophylla and Soft-Shelled Turtle Shell Powder) and *Qing Gu San* (Cool the Bones Powder) all treat yin-deficient heat, but have the following differences:

- *Qing Hao Bie Jia Tang* nourishes yin through the use of *Bie Jia* (Carapax Trionycis) and vents heat through the aromatic property of *Qing Hao* (Herba Artemisiae Annuae). The formula emphasizes nourishing interior yin and dispersing deficiency heat to clear the deep, hidden heat. It is most suitable for late stages of febrile disorders with night fever and morning coolness.
- *Qin Jiao Bie Jia San* nourishes yin while dispersing residual lingering wind in the body due to improper

treatment of an exterior wind condition. It nourishes yin and blood and clears deficiency fire.

- *Qing Gu San* is the best formula for relieving steaming bones sensations and night fever because it contains the most herbs to clear deficiency heat. It emphasizes relieving steaming bones sensations by penetrating the heat and nourishing yin[7]

Qing Hao Bie Jia Tang and *Zhu Ye Shi Gao Tang* (Bamboo Leaves and Gypsum Decoction) both treat symptoms related to late-stage febrile disorders. Their differences are as follows:

- *Qing Hao Bie Jia Tang* more strongly nourishes yin and clears deficiency heat in the deeper parts of the body, and is more suitable for night fever, morning coolness, and absence of perspiration. It nourishes yin and vents heat.
- *Zhu Ye Shi Gao Tang* nourishes yin, benefits qi and harmonizes the Stomach. It is mainly used for late-stage febrile disorders with lingering fever, and qi and yin deficiencies, with symptoms such as perspiration, irritability, shortness of breath, thirst, and dry heaves or nausea. *Zhu Ye Shi Gao Tang* nourishes both yin and qi and harmonizes the Stomach.[8]

References

1. *Fu Jian Zhong Yi Yao* (Fujian Chinese Medicine and Herbology) 1996;1:21.
2. *Hu Nan Zhong Yi Za Zhi* (Hunan Journal of Chinese Medicine) 1997;5:27.
3. *Zhe Jiang Zhong Yi Za Zhi* (Zhejiang Journal of Chinese Medicine) 1981;11:509.
4. *Zhong Yi Yao Xue Bao* (Report of Chinese Medicine and Herbology) 1995;6:52.
5. *Zhong Yi Fang Ji Xian Dai Yan Jiu* (Modern Study of Medical Formulae in Traditional Chinese Medicine) 1997;351-352.
6. *Zhe Jiang Zhong Yi Xue Yuan Xue Bao* (Journal of Zhejiang University of Chinese Medicine) 1993;17(2):26.
7. Wang MZ, et al. *Zhong Yi Xue Wen Da Ti Ku* (Questions and Answers on Traditional Chinese Medicine: Herbal Formulas).
8. Wang MZ, et al. *Zhong Yi Xue Wen Da Ti Ku* (Questions and Answers on Traditional Chinese Medicine: Herbal Formulas).

HEAT-CLEARING FORMULAS

5

Qín Jiăo Biē Jiă Săn
(Gentiana Macrophylla and Soft-Shelled Turtle Shell Powder)

秦艽鱉甲散
秦艽鳖甲散

Pinyin Name: *Qin Jiao Bie Jia San*
Literal Name: Gentiana Macrophylla and Soft-Shelled Turtle Shell Powder
Alternate Names: *Chin Chiu Pieh Chia San, Chin Jiao Bie Jia San*, Chin-Chiu and Turtle Shell Formula, Large-Leaf Gentian and Turtle Shell Powder, Chin-chiu Formula
Original Source: *Wei Sheng Bao Jian* (Precious Mirror of Health) by Luo Tian-Yi in the Yuan Dynasty

COMPOSITION

Qin Jiao (Radix Gentianae Macrophyllae)	15g [5g]
Chai Hu (Radix Bupleuri)	30g [9g]
Bie Jia (Carapax Trionycis), *zhi* (fried with liquid) until crisp	30g [9g]
Zhi Mu (Rhizoma Anemarrhenae)	15g [5g]
Di Gu Pi (Cortex Lycii)	30g [9g]
Dang Gui (Radix Angelicae Sinensis)	15g [5g]

DOSAGE / PREPARATION / ADMINISTRATION

The source text instructs to grind the ingredients coarsely. Cook 15g of the powder with 5 pieces of *Qing Hao* (Herba Artemisiae Annuae) and 1 piece of *Wu Mei* (Fructus Mume) in one large bowl of water until 70% of the liquid remains. Take the warm, strained decoction on an empty stomach and again at bedtime. This formula may be prepared as a decoction using the doses suggested in brackets.

CHINESE THERAPEUTIC ACTIONS

1. Nourishes yin and blood
2. Clears deficiency heat and reduces steaming bones sensations

CLINICAL MANIFESTATIONS

Feng lao bing (wind consumption disease): steaming bones sensations, night sweats, tidal fever with warm sensations in the afternoon, red lips and cheeks, cough, lethargy, a dry mouth and throat, muscle emaciation, and a faint, rapid pulse.

CLINICAL APPLICATIONS

Recovery from chronic respiratory tract infection, such as pulmonary tuberculosis, chronic bronchitis, and pneumonia.

EXPLANATION

Qin Jiao Bie Jia San (Gentiana Macrophylla and Soft-Shelled Turtle Shell Powder) treats *feng lao bing* (wind consumption disease), a yin-deficient heat syndrome characterized by tidal fever and steaming bones sensations. This condition is caused by incorrect treatment of an exterior syndrome in which the exterior pathogenic factor travels to the interior and transforms into heat. The interior heat then consumes yin and blood to cause yin and blood deficiencies.

Two key clinical manifestations are tidal fever and steaming bones sensations, both of which are caused by yin-deficient heat in the interior. Other symptoms, such as night sweats and red lips and cheeks, are also typical of yin-deficient heat flaring upward. As a yin organ, the Lung is easily affected by heat. If the heat interferes with the qi flow of the Lung, coughing occurs. A dry mouth and throat are the direct results of lack of nourishment. Lethargy and emaciation of the muscles are due to heat extensively consuming the blood and due to lack of nourishment.

Qin Jiao (Radix Gentianae Macrophyllae) and *Chai Hu* (Radix Bupleuri) dispel wind and release the exterior. *Bie Jia* (Carapax Trionycis) and *Zhi Mu* (Rhizoma Anemarrhenae) nourish yin and clear heat. *Di Gu Pi* (Cortex Lycii) and *Qing Hao* (Herba Artemisiae Annuae) clear deficiency heat and relieve steaming bones sensations. *Dang Gui* (Radix Angelicae Sinensis) tonifies and harmonizes the blood. *Wu Mei* (Fructus Mume), an astringent herb, retains yin and body fluids and stops perspiration.

MODIFICATIONS

• With perspiration and aversion to wind, add *Huang Qi* (Radix Astragali) and *Bai Zhu* (Rhizoma Atractylodis Macrocephalae).

Chinese Herbal Formulas and Applications

Qín Jiǎo Biē Jiǎ Sǎn
(Gentiana Macrophylla and Soft-Shelled Turtle Shell Powder)

Qin Jiao Bie Jia San (Gentiana Macrophylla and Soft-Shelled Turtle Shell Powder)

Diagnosis	Signs and Symptoms	Treatment	Herbs
Feng lao bing (wind consumption disease)	• Tidal fever, steaming bones sensations, night sweats, and red lips and cheeks: deficiency heat rising upward • Dry mouth and throat: heat consuming body fluids in the Lung • Coughing: heat affecting Lung qi circulation • Lethargy and emaciation of the muscles: heat consuming the blood and hindering nourishment • Faint, rapid pulse: deficiency and heat condition	• Nourishes yin and blood • Clears deficiency heat and reduces steaming bones sensations	• *Qin Jiao* (Radix Gentianae Macrophyllae) and *Chai Hu* (Radix Bupleuri) dispel wind and release the exterior. • *Bie Jia* (Carapax Trionycis) and *Zhi Mu* (Rhizoma Anemarrhenae) nourish yin and clear heat. • *Di Gu Pi* (Cortex Lycii) and *Qing Hao* (Herba Artemisiae Annuae) clear deficiency heat and relieve steaming bones sensations. • *Dang Gui* (Radix Angelicae Sinensis) tonifies and harmonizes the blood. • *Wu Mei* (Fructus Mume) retains yin and body fluids and stops perspiration.

- If there is neck stiffness, add *Ge Gen* (Radix Puerariae Lobatae).
- With high fever and muscle spasms, add *Tian Ma* (Rhizoma Gastrodiae), *Gou Teng* (Ramulus Uncariae cum Uncis), and *Quan Xie* (Scorpio).
- When there is cough but no perspiration, add *Ma Huang* (Herba Ephedrae) and *Ku Xing Ren* (Semen Armeniacae Amarum).
- With cough and wheezing, add *Sang Bai Pi* (Cortex Mori) and *Zi Wan* (Radix et Rhizoma Asteris).
- With hot flashes, add *Bai Wei* (Radix et Rhizoma Cynanchi Atrati) and *Sha Shen* (Radix Glehniae seu Adenophorae).

CLINICAL STUDIES AND RESEARCH

1. **Pulmonary tuberculosis**: In one report, patients with pulmonary tuberculosis with tidal fever were treated with good results. Out of 24 patients, 21 had significant improvement and 3 had moderate improvement.[1]
2. **Viral infection**: In one report, 36 patients with viral infection of the respiratory tract were treated with modified *Qin Jiao Bie Jia San* with good results. Out of 36 patients, 9 had significant improvement, 24 had moderate improvement, and 3 had slight improvement. The modifications were as follows: *Huang Qi* (Radix Astragali) and *Bai Zhu* (Rhizoma Atractylodis Macrocephalae) were added for perspiration with aversion to wind; *Ge Gen* (Radix Puerariae Lobatae) was added for neck stiffness; *Tian Ma* (Rhizoma Gastrodiae), *Gou Teng* (Ramulus Uncariae cum Uncis), and *Quan Xie* (Scorpio) were added for high fever with convulsions; and *Ma*

Huang (Herba Ephedrae) and *Ku Xing Ren* (Semen Armeniacae Amarum) were added for cough and wheezing without perspiration.[2]

3. **Respiratory tract infection**: Recurrent respiratory tract infections in children were successfully treated with modified *Qin Jiao Bie Jia San*. The herbal treatment contained *Qin Jiao* (Radix Gentianae Macrophyllae) 5g, *Bie Jia* (Carapax Trionycis) 5g, *Tai Zi Shen* (Radix Pseudostellariae) 5g, *Bai Bu* (Radix Stemonae) 10g, *Di Gu Pi* (Cortex Lycii) 10g, *Zhi Mu* (Rhizoma Anemarrhenae) 6g, *Qing Hao* (Herba Artemisiae Annuae) 6g, *Chai Hu* (Radix Bupleuri) 6g, and *Wu Mei* (Fructus Mume) 6g. *Huang Qi* (Radix Astragali) 15g was added for qi deficiency; *Di Huang* (Radix Rehmanniae) 15g for yin deficiency; *Huang Qin* (Radix Scutellariae) 10g for phlegm and heat; and *Wu Wei Zi* (Fructus Schisandrae Chinensis) 5g for profuse perspiration. The treatment protocol was to administer the herbs in decoction form daily, for 7 days per course of treatment. Of 30 cases, the study reported complete recovery in 18 cases (complete resolution of all symptoms without recurrence for one year), significant improvement in 9 cases (resolution of symptoms), and no change in 3 cases. The overall rate of effectiveness was 90%.[3]

AUTHORS' COMMENTS

Qin Jiao Bie Jia San is commonly used for tidal fever or fluid-damage conditions in post febrile disorders and tuberculosis. It is also effective for chronic recurrent low-grade fever with no detectible medical cause.

Chapter 5 – Heat-Clearing Formulas　　　　　　　　　Section 6 – Deficiency-Heat Clearing Formulas

Qín Jiăo Biē Jiă Săn
(Gentiana Macrophylla and Soft-Shelled Turtle Shell Powder)

Please refer to *Qing Hao Bie Jia Tang* (Artemisia Annua and Soft-Shelled Turtle Shell Decoction), for a comparative analysis with *Qin Jiao Bie Jia San* and *Qing Gu San* (Cool the Bones Powder).

References

1. *Zhong Yi Yao Xin Xi* (Information on Chinese Medicine and Herbology) 1989;3:30.
2. *Zhe Jiang Zhong Yi Za Zhi* (Zhejiang Journal of Chinese Medicine) 1992;27(6):251.
3. *Zhe Jiang Zhong Yi Za Zhi* (Zhejiang Journal of Chinese Medicine) 1993;28(5):206.

Qīng Gŭ Săn (Cool the Bones Powder)
清骨散

Pinyin Name: *Qing Gu San*
Literal Name: Cool the Bones Powder
Original Source: *Zheng Zhi Zhun Sheng* (Standards of Patterns and Treatments) by Wang Ken-Tang in 1602

COMPOSITION

Yin Chai Hu (Radix Stellariae)	4.5g
Zhi Mu (Rhizoma Anemarrhenae)	3g
Hu Huang Lian (Rhizoma Picrorhizae)	3g
Di Gu Pi (Cortex Lycii)	3g
Qin Jiao (Radix Gentianae Macrophyllae)	3g
Qing Hao (Herba Artemisiae Annuae)	3g
Bie Jia (Carapax Trionycis), *zhi* (fried) with vinegar	3g
Gan Cao (Radix et Rhizoma Glycyrrhizae)	1.5g

DOSAGE / PREPARATION / ADMINISTRATION

Cook the ingredients in 2 large bowls of water until 80% of the liquid remain. Take the decoction between meals.

CHINESE THERAPEUTIC ACTIONS

1. Clears deficiency heat
2. Reduces tidal fever and steaming bones sensations

CLINICAL MANIFESTATIONS

Tidal fever and steaming bones sensations due to yin-deficient heat: tidal fever in late afternoon or at night, unremitting low-grade fever, night sweats, steaming bones sensations, irritability, emaciation, a dry throat, red cheeks, thirst, a red tongue body with a scanty tongue coating, and a fine, rapid pulse.

CLINICAL APPLICATIONS

Fever, pulmonary tuberculosis, and leukemia.

EXPLANATION

Qing Gu San (Cool the Bones Powder) treats chronic heat disorder leading to yin deficiency and deficiency heat. Deficiency heat in the interior consumes yin and body fluids, leading to tidal fever or unremitting low-grade fever

because yin is deficient relative to the yang of the body. Night sweats occur because yin, being deficient, is unable to contain yang when yang qi returns to the deeper levels of the body while one sleeps. Steaming bones sensations is an indication of yin deficiency with deficiency heat affecting the bone marrow. Emaciation and dry throat are the results of lack of yin nourishment. Irritability is the direct result of *shen* (spirit) disturbance, secondary to yin not being able to nourish the Heart, and also heat disturbing the *shen*. Red cheeks, a red tongue body with a scanty tongue coating, and a fine, rapid pulse are all clinical manifestations of yin deficiency with heat in the interior.

Yin Chai Hu (Radix Stellariae) clears deficiency heat in the deeper level and cools the blood without sedating the body. It is an essential herb for clearing heat deep in the bone marrow manifesting in steaming bones sensations. *Zhi Mu* (Rhizoma Anemarrhenae) nourishes yin and sedates deficiency fire. *Hu Huang Lian* (Rhizoma Picrorhizae) enters and clears heat in the *xue* (blood) level. *Di Gu Pi* (Cortex Lycii) clears deficiency heat in the Lung, Liver, and Kidney. *Qing Hao* (Herba Artemisiae Annuae) and *Qin Jiao* (Radix Gentianae Macrophyllae) penetrate

418

Qīng Gŭ Săn (Cool the Bones Powder)

Qing Gu San (Cool the Bones Powder)

Diagnosis	Signs and Symptoms	Treatment	Herbs
Tidal fever and steaming bones sensations	• Tidal fever, unremitting low-grade fever, and steaming bones sensations: deficiency heat consuming yin and body fluids • Night sweats: yang qi pushing yin outwards • Emaciation, thirst and a dry throat: lack of yin nourishment • Irritability: deficiency heat disturbing the *shen* (spirit) • Red cheeks, a red tongue body, scanty tongue coating, and a fine, rapid pulse: yin-deficient heat in the interior	• Clears deficiency heat • Reduces tidal fever and steaming bones sensations	• *Yin Chai Hu* (Radix Stellariae) clears deficiency heat and cools the blood without sedating the body. • *Zhi Mu* (Rhizoma Anemarrhenae) nourishes yin and sedates fire. • *Hu Huang Lian* (Rhizoma Picrorhizae) enters and clears heat in the *xue* (blood) level. • *Di Gu Pi* (Cortex Lycii) clears deficiency heat in the Lung, Liver and Kidney. • *Qing Hao* (Herba Artemisiae Annuae) and *Qin Jiao* (Radix Gentianae Macrophyllae) penetrate to the interior to clear heat in the deeper level by dispelling it outwards. • *Bie Jia* (Carapax Trionycis) nourishes yin and guides the other herbs deep into the interior to clear deficiency heat. • *Gan Cao* (Radix et Rhizoma Glycyrrhizae) harmonizes the herbs and protects the Stomach from the harsh properties of the heat-clearing herbs.

to the interior to clear heat in the deeper level by dispelling it outwards. *Bie Jia* (Carapax Trionycis) nourishes yin and guides the other herbs deep into the interior to clear deficiency heat. *Gan Cao* (Radix et Rhizoma Glycyrrhizae) harmonizes the formula and protects the Stomach from the harsh properties of the heat-clearing herbs.

MODIFICATIONS

• If there is more qi deficiency, add *Huang Qi* (Radix Astragali).
• If there is more yin deficiency, add *Di Huang* (Radix Rehmanniae) and *Mai Dong* (Radix Ophiopogonis).
• If there is more blood deficiency, add *Dang Gui* (Radix Angelicae Sinensis), *Bai Shao* (Radix Paeoniae Alba) and *Di Huang* (Radix Rehmanniae).
• With cough, add *E Jiao* (Colla Corii Asini), *Mai Dong* (Radix Ophiopogonis), and *Wu Wei Zi* (Fructus Schisandrae Chinensis).
• With Spleen qi deficiency manifesting as loose stools and poor appetite, remove *Hu Huang Lian* (Rhizoma Picrorhizae), *Qin Jiao* (Radix Gentianae Macrophyllae) and *Zhi Mu* (Rhizoma Anemarrhenae) and add *Bai Bian Dou* (Semen Lablab Album) and *Shan Yao* (Rhizoma Dioscoreae).

CAUTIONS / CONTRAINDICATIONS

Qing Gu San is inappropriate for severe cases of yin deficiency because its emphasis is to clear deficiency heat, not to nourish yin.

CLINICAL STUDIES AND RESEARCH

1. **Leukemia:** *Qing Gu San* was used to treat 59 patients (36 males and 23 females) with leukemia. The traditional Chinese medical diagnosis for these patients included toxic-fire in the Liver, heat in the blood, blood stagnation, yin-deficient fire, and deficiencies of qi, yin and blood. Modifications were made based on the exact condition of the patient. The study reported that out of 59 cases, 19 had significant improvement, 11 had moderate improvement, 20 had slight improvement, and 9 had no effect. The overall effectiveness rate reported by the study was 84.6%.[1]

2. **Tuberculosis:** *Qing Gu San* was given to 10 patients for constitutional support during active tuberculosis. Out of 10 cases, 8 had gradual improvement characterized by increased energy level and improved appetite within 1-3 weeks after the herbal therapy. The other 2 patients were transferred to another hospital and follow-up information was not available.[2]

3. **Fever:** Twenty out of 21 patients with persistent low-grade fever due to bone fractures were treated with good results using *Qing Gu San*. The body temperature was reduced within 1-2 doses.[3]

AUTHORS' COMMENTS

Qing Gu San is one of the best formulas for treating steaming bones sensations and tidal fever due to yin-deficient heat. Please refer to *Qing Hao Bie Jia Tang* (Artemisia Annua and

Chapter 5 – Heat-Clearing Formulas   Section 6 – Deficiency-Heat Clearing Formulas

Qīng Gǔ Sǎn (Cool the Bones Powder)

Soft-Shelled Turtle Shell Decoction), for a comparative analysis with *Qin Jiao Bie Jia San* (Gentiana Macrophylla and Soft-Shelled Turtle Shell Powder) and *Qing Gu San*.

References
1. *He Bei Zhong Yi* (Hebei Chinese Medicine) 1995;17(2):10.
2. *Zhong Yi Fang Ji Xian Dai Yan Jiu* (Modern Study of Medical Formulae in Traditional Chinese Medicine) 1997;350-351.
3. *Zhe Jiang Zhong Yi Za Zhi* (Zhejiang Journal of Chinese Medicine) 1959;9:34.

Dāng Guī Liù Huáng Tāng (Tangkuei and Six-Yellow Decoction)

當歸六黃湯
当归六黄汤

Pinyin Name: *Dang Gui Liu Huang Tang*
Literal Name: Tangkuei and Six-Yellow Decoction
Alternate Names: *Tang Kuei Liu Huang Tang*, Tang-kuei and Six Huang Decoction, Chinese Angelica and Six Yellow Herbs Decoction, Tangkuei and Six Yellow Combination
Original Source: *Lan Shi Mi Cang* (Secrets from the Orchid Chamber) by Li Gao in 1336

COMPOSITION

Dang Gui (Radix Angelicae Sinensis)	1 part [6g]
Di Huang (Radix Rehmanniae)	1 part [6g]
Shu Di Huang (Radix Rehmanniae Praeparata)	1 part [6g]
Huang Qin (Radix Scutellariae)	1 part [6g]
Huang Lian (Rhizoma Coptidis)	1 part [6g]
Huang Bo (Cortex Phellodendri Chinensis)	1 part [6g]
Huang Qi (Radix Astragali)	2 parts [12g]

DOSAGE / PREPARATION / ADMINISTRATION

Grind the ingredients coarsely. Cook 15g of the powder in 2 large bowls of water until it is reduced to 1 large bowl. Take the warm, strained decoction before meals. Reduce the dose by half for children. This formula may be prepared as a decoction using the doses suggested in brackets.

CHINESE THERAPEUTIC ACTIONS

1. Nourishes yin and sedates internal fire
2. Consolidates the exterior and stops perspiration

CLINICAL MANIFESTATIONS

Fever and night sweats due to yin-deficient heat and fire: a red face, irritability, dry mouth and lips, constipation, dark yellow urine, a red tongue body, and a rapid pulse.

CLINICAL APPLICATIONS

Pulmonary tuberculosis, silicosis, bronchitis, hepatitis, cholecystitis, nephritis, urinary tract infection, myocarditis, febrile disease, hyperthyroidism, thrombocytopenic purpura, abnormal perspiration, and menopause.

EXPLANATION

Dang Gui Liu Huang Tang (Tangkuei and Six-Yellow Decoction) treats fever and night sweats due to yin-deficient heat and fire, a condition that is characterized by a high level of yang and a low level of yin. Because of the dispersing characteristic of yang, yang easily surfaces to the exterior of the body when deficient yin can no longer retain it inside. When yang is dispersed to the exterior, body fluids may be carried out with the yang qi. Consequently, fever and night sweats occur. A red face and irritability are caused by heat and fire in the interior. Dry mouth and lips, constipation, and dark yellow urine are the results of fire consuming body fluids.

As the chief herbs, *Dang Gui* (Radix Angelicae Sinensis), *Di Huang* (Radix Rehmanniae) and *Shu Di Huang* (Radix Rehmanniae Praeparata) nourish yin and blood to control yang and fire. *Huang Qin* (Radix Scutellariae), *Huang Lian* (Rhizoma Coptidis), and *Huang Bo* (Cortex Phellodendri Chinensis) clear heat and sedate fire. Finally, *Huang Qi* (Radix Astragali) strengthen *wei* (defensive)

420

Chinese Herbal Formulas and Applications

Dāng Guī Liù Huáng Tāng (Tangkuei and Six-Yellow Decoction)

Dang Gui Liu Huang Tang (Tangkuei and Six-Yellow Decoction)

Diagnosis	Signs and Symptoms	Treatment	Herbs
Fever and night sweats due to yin-deficient heat and fire	• Fever and night sweats: yin-deficient heat and fire pushing body fluids outward • Red face and irritability: yin-deficient heat and fire • Dry mouth and lips, constipation and dark yellow urine: yin-deficient heat and fire consuming body fluids • Red tongue body and a rapid pulse: heat and fire conditions	• Nourishes yin and sedates internal fire • Consolidates the exterior and stops abnormal perspiration	• *Dang Gui* (Radix Angelicae Sinensis), *Di Huang* (Radix Rehmanniae) and *Shu Di Huang* (Radix Rehmanniae Praeparata) nourish yin and blood to control yang and fire. • *Huang Qin* (Radix Scutellariae), *Huang Lian* (Rhizoma Coptidis) and *Huang Bo* (Cortex Phellodendri Chinensis) clear heat and sedate fire. • *Huang Qi* (Radix Astragali) strengthens *wei* (defensive) *qi* to stop sweating.

qi to stop sweating, and works synergistically with *Dang Gui* (Radix Angelicae Sinensis) and *Shu Di Huang* (Radix Rehmanniae Praeparata) to promote the production of qi and blood.

MODIFICATIONS
• If there is more sweating, add *Fu Xiao Mai* (Fructus Tritici Levis) and *Ma Huang Gen* (Radix et Rhizoma Ephedrae).
• With a dry mouth and tidal fever due to Kidney yin-deficient fire, add *Zhi Mu* (Rhizoma Anemarrhenae) and *Gui Ban* (Plastrum Testudinis).
• For patients with yin deficiency but no internal fire, remove *Huang Qin* (Radix Scutellariae), *Huang Lian* (Rhizoma Coptidis), and *Huang Bo* (Cortex Phellodendri Chinensis) to prevent damage to the yin. Add *Xuan Shen* (Radix Scrophulariae) and *Mai Dong* (Radix Ophiopogonis) to clear deficiency heat and nourish yin.

CAUTIONS / CONTRAINDICATIONS
Dang Gui Liu Huang Tang is contraindicated in patients with loose stools due to Spleen and Stomach deficiencies.

CLINICAL STUDIES AND RESEARCH
1. **Perspiration**: *Dang Gui Liu Huang Tang* has been used successfully to treat abnormal perspiration due to various causes. In one study, 50 patients (32 males and 18 females, between 13 and 61 years of age) with spontaneous or night perspiration were treated with modified *Dang Gui Liu Huang Tang* with complete recovery in 43 patients, significant improvement in 5 patients, and no benefit in 2 patients. In addition to *Dang Gui Liu Huang Tang* as the base formula, modifications were made as follows: addition of *Gan Cao* (Radix et Rhizoma Glycyrrhizae) and a larger dose of *Huang Qi* (Radix Astragali) for qi and blood deficiencies; *Mai Dong* (Radix Ophiopogonis) and *Xi Yang Shen* (Radix Panacis Quinquefolii) for qi and yin deficiencies; and *Wu Wei Zi* (Fructus Schisandrae

Chinensis) and calcined *Long Gu* (Os Draconis) for profuse perspiration.[1]

2. **Menopause**: Thirty-three patients (between 44 and 56 years of age) with menopausal complaints were treated with modified *Dang Gui Liu Huang Tang* with significant improvement in 11 patients and moderate improvement in 22 patients. In addition to *Dang Gui Liu Huang Tang* as the base formula, modifications included addition of *Mu Dan Pi* (Cortex Moutan) and *Ze Xie* (Rhizoma Alismatis) for yin-deficient fire; *Bai Zhu* (Rhizoma Atractylodis Macrocephalae) and *Fang Feng* (Radix Saposhnikoviae) for profuse spontaneous sweating; *Er Zhi Wan* (Two-Ultimate Pill) and *Bai He* (Bulbus Lilii) for severe night sweats; and *Fu Shen* (Poria Paradicis) and *Wu Wei Zi* (Fructus Schisandrae Chinensis) for insomnia. The duration of treatment was 7 days per course of treatment.[2]

AUTHORS' COMMENTS
Dang Gui Liu Huang Tang and *Mu Li San* (Oyster Shell Powder) both nourish yin, clear heat, consolidate the exterior, and stop night sweats.
• *Dang Gui Liu Huang Tang* more strongly nourishes yin and clears heat. It is mainly used for night sweats, tidal fever, irritability, dryness of the mouth, lips, and stools, and other symptoms of yin-deficient heat.
• *Mu Li San* more strongly binds and stops sweating and is weaker at nourishing yin and clearing heat. It is mostly used to treat qi and yin deficiencies with spontaneous sweating occuring both day and night. Other symptoms include palpitations, being easily frightened, and shortness of breath.[3]

Huang Qi (Radix Astragali) is an important herb that is used in many formulas for different purposes. Below is a comparison of its functions in three important herbal formulas:

5

HEAT-CLEARING FORMULAS

421

Chapter 5 – Heat-Clearing Formulas   *Section 6 – Deficiency-Heat Clearing Formulas*

Dāng Guī Liù Huáng Tāng (Tangkuei and Six-Yellow Decoction)

- *Dang Gui Liu Huang Tang* contains *Huang Qi* (Radix Astragali) to tonify qi, consolidate *wei* (defensive) qi, and stop sweating. It mainly treats yin deficiency with flaring fire manifesting in fever, night sweats, thirst, and a red tongue body with a yellow coating.
- *Dang Gui Bu Xue Tang* (Tangkuei Decoction to Tonify the Blood) contains *Huang Qi* (Radix Astragali) at five times the amount of *Dang Gui* (Radix Angelicae Sinensis) to boost qi and generate blood. It is mainly used for blood deficiency with deficiency-heat signs of heat sensation, a flushed face, spontaneous sweating, and a surging, big and deficient pulse.
- *Bu Zhong Yi Qi Tang* (Tonify the Middle and Augment the Qi Decoction) contains *Huang Qi* (Radix Astragali)

to tonify qi and raise yang. It treats Spleen and Stomach qi deficiencies with prolapsed organs. Patients will also exhibit fatigue, poor appetite, decreased dietary intake, feverish sensations, chronic diarrhea, and spontaneous sweating.[4]

References
1. *Jiang Xi Zhong Yi Yao* (Jiangxi Chinese Medicine and Herbology) 1994;25(3):28.
2. *Jiang Su Zhong Yi* (Jiangsu Chinese Medicine) 1996;5:22.
3. Wang MZ, et al. *Zhong Yi Xue Wen Da Ti Ku* (Questions and Answers on Traditional Chinese Medicine: Herbal Formulas).
4. Wang MZ, et al. *Zhong Yi Xue Wen Da Ti Ku* (Questions and Answers on Traditional Chinese Medicine: Herbal Formulas).

Zī Yīn Jiàng Huǒ Tāng (Nourish Yin and Descend the Fire Decoction)

滋陰降火湯
滋阴降火汤

Pinyin Name: *Zi Yin Jiang Huo Tang*
Literal Name: Nourish Yin and Descend the Fire Decoction
Alternate Names: *Tzu Yin Chiang Huo Tang*, Phellodendron Decoction, Phellodendron Combination
Original Source: *Wan Bing Hui Chun* (Restoration of Health from the Myriad Diseases) by Gong Ting-Xian in 1587

COMPOSITION

Dang Gui (Radix Angelicae Sinensis), *xi* (washed) with liquor	3.6g
Bai Shao (Radix Paeoniae Alba), *xi* (washed) with liquor	6.9g
Shu Di Huang (Radix Rehmanniae Praeparata), *chao* (dry-fried) with ginger juice	3g
Tian Dong (Radix Asparagi)	3g
Mai Dong (Radix Ophiopogonis)	3g
Bai Zhu (Rhizoma Atractylodis Macrocephalae)	3g
Chen Pi (Pericarpium Citri Reticulatae)	2.1g
Zhi Gan Cao (Radix et Rhizoma Glycyrrhizae Praeparata cum Melle)	1.5g
Di Huang (Radix Rehmanniae)	2.4g
Zhi Mu (Rhizoma Anemarrhenae)	1.5g
Huang Bo (Cortex Phellodendri Chinensis), *chao* (dry-fried) with water and honey	1.5g

DOSAGE / PREPARATION / ADMINISTRATION

Cook the ingredients with 3 slices of *Sheng Jiang* (Rhizoma Zingiberis Recens) and 1 piece of *Da Zao* (Fructus Jujubae) in water to make a decoction. Add a small amount of *Zhu Li* (Succus Bambusae), *Tong Bian* (Infantis Urina) and the juice of *Sheng Jiang* (Rhizoma Zingiberis Recens) to the decoction prior to ingestion.

CHINESE THERAPEUTIC ACTIONS

1. Nourishes yin
2. Descends fire
3. Tonifies qi and blood

CLINICAL MANIFESTATIONS

Yin-deficient fire: fever, cough, sputum, dyspnea, night sweats, and a dry mouth.

422

Chinese Herbal Formulas and Applications

Zī Yīn Jiàng Huǒ Tāng (Nourish Yin and Descend the Fire Decoction)

Zi Yin Jiang Huo Tang (Nourish Yin and Descend the Fire Decoction)

Diagnosis	Signs and Symptoms	Treatment	Herbs
Yin-deficient fire	• Fever, cough with sputum and dyspnea: heat and fire rising upwards • Night sweats: yin-deficient fire • Dry mouth and constipation: heat consuming body fluids • Fine, rapid pulse: deficiency and heat conditions	• Nourishes yin • Descends fire • Tonifies qi and blood	• *Dang Gui* (Radix Angelicae Sinensis), *Bai Shao* (Radix Paeoniae Alba) and *Shu Di Huang* (Radix Rehmanniae Praeparata) tonify the blood. • *Tian Dong* (Radix Asparagi) and *Mai Dong* (Radix Ophiopogonis) tonify yin. • *Bai Zhu* (Rhizoma Atractylodis Macrocephalae), *Chen Pi* (Pericarpium Citri Reticulatae), *Zhi Gan Cao* (Radix et Rhizoma Glycyrrhizae Praeparata cum Melle) and *Da Zao* (Fructus Jujubae) tonify qi and activate qi circulation. • *Di Huang* (Radix Rehmanniae), *Zhi Mu* (Rhizoma Anemarrhenae) and *Huang Bo* (Cortex Phellodendri Chinensis) clear deficiency fire.

CLINICAL APPLICATIONS

Pulmonary tuberculosis, renal tuberculosis, chronic bronchitis, pneumonia, chronic nephritis, diabetes mellitus, nocturnal emissions, and spontaneous emissions.

EXPLANATION

Zi Yin Jiang Huo Tang (Nourish Yin and Descend the Fire Decoction) treats Kidney yin deficiency with Liver fire. Because of the underlying yin deficiency, the Kidney and Liver cannot be properly nourished and fire begins to rise upward. The fire usually disturbs the Stomach and Lung, leading to fever, cough, sputum, dyspnea, and a dry mouth. Night sweats are an indication of yin-deficient fire. Most patients with this condition will also have a dark complexion, constipation, and a fine, rapid pulse.

This formula aims to nourish the underlying deficiency and control the excess. *Dang Gui* (Radix Angelicae Sinensis), *Bai Shao* (Radix Paeoniae Alba), and *Shu Di Huang* (Radix Rehmanniae Praeparata) tonify the blood. *Tian Dong* (Radix Asparagi) and *Mai Dong* (Radix Ophiopogonis) tonify yin. *Bai Zhu* (Rhizoma Atractylodis Macrocephalae), *Chen Pi* (Pericarpium Citri Reticulatae),

Zhi Gan Cao (Radix et Rhizoma Glycyrrhizae Praeparata cum Melle), and *Da Zao* (Fructus Jujubae) tonify qi and activate qi circulation. *Di Huang* (Radix Rehmanniae), *Zhi Mu* (Rhizoma Anemarrhenae) and *Huang Bo* (Cortex Phellodendri Chinensis) are excellent herbs for descending fire in cases involving underlying deficiency.

MODIFICATIONS

• If the night sweats are severe, add *Huang Qi* (Radix Astragali) and *Suan Zao Ren* (Semen Ziziphi Spinosae).
• When there is steaming bones sensation, add *Di Gu Pi* (Cortex Lycii) and *Yin Chai Hu* (Radix Stellariae).
• With wheezing and dyspnea with phlegm, add *Sang Bai Pi* (Cortex Mori), *Zi Wan* (Radix et Rhizoma Asteris), *Huang Qin* (Radix Scutellariae), and *Zhu Li* (Succus Bambusae).
• With cough and profuse sputum, add *Bei Mu* (Bulbus Fritillariae), *Kuan Dong Hua* (Flos Farfarae), and *Sang Bai Pi* (Cortex Mori).
• With lower abdominal pain, add *Xiao Hui Xiang* (Fructus Foeniculi) and *Mu Xiang* (Radix Aucklandiae).
• With low-grade fever, add *Huang Lian* (Rhizoma Coptidis) and *Huang Qin* (Radix Scutellariae).

5

HEAT-CLEARING FORMULAS

Chapter 5 – Heat-Clearing Formulas

Chapter 5 — Summary

— Heat-Clearing Formulas

SECTION 1: *QI* (ENERGY) LEVEL-CLEARING FORMULAS

Name	Similarities	Differences
Bai Hu Tang (White Tiger Decoction)	Clear heat from the *qi* (energy) level	Generates body fluids
Bai Hu Jia Ren Shen Tang (White Tiger plus Ginseng Decoction)		Generates body fluids, tonifies qi
Zhu Ye Shi Gao Tang (Bamboo Leaves and Gypsum Decoction)		Generates body fluids, tonifies qi, harmonizes the Stomach

Bai Hu Tang (White Tiger Decoction) clears heat and promotes production of body fluids. It treats *yangming* (*qi* (energy) level) excessive heat with high fever, profuse perspiration, thirst, irritability, and a surging, big and forceful pulse.

Bai Hu Jia Ren Shen Tang (White Tiger plus Ginseng Decoction) is formulated by adding *Ren Shen* (Radix et Rhizoma Ginseng) to *Bai Hu Tang* (White Tiger Decoction), which enables the formula to tonify qi.

Zhu Ye Shi Gao Tang (Bamboo Leaves and Gypsum Decoction) clears heat and nourishes yin and qi to harmonize the Stomach. In comparison to *Bai Hu Tang* (White Tiger Decoction), this formula has a weaker heat-clearing effect, and therefore is used mostly to treat late-stage heat syndromes with damage to both qi and yin.

SECTION 2: *YING* (NUTRITIVE) LEVEL-CLEARING AND BLOOD-COOLING FORMULAS

Name	Similarities	Differences
Qing Ying Tang (Clear the Nutritive Level Decoction)	Clears heat from the *ying* (nutritive) level	Nourishes yin, invigorates blood circulation
Xi Jiao Di Huang Tang (Rhinoceros Horn and Rehmannia Decoction)	Clears heat and cools the blood in the *xue* (blood) level	Stops bleeding, disperses blood stasis

Qing Ying Tang (Clear the Nutritive Level Decoction) clears heat from the *ying* (nutritive) level, eliminates toxin, releases the heat, and nourishes yin. This formula is more appropriate for the initial stages of heat attacking the *ying* level, in which the patient manifests symptoms of heat sensations that worsen at night, incoherent speech and irritability.

Xi Jiao Di Huang Tang (Rhinoceros Horn and Rehmannia Decoction) clears heat, eliminates toxins, cools the blood, and disperses blood stagnation. This formula is suitable to treat more severe conditions of heat attacking the *xue* (blood) level forcing blood out of the vessels and manifesting in various types of bleeding.

Chinese Herbal Formulas and Applications

Chapter 5 — Summary

SECTION 3: *QI* (ENERGY) AND *XUE* (BLOOD) LEVELS-CLEARING FORMULA

Name	Actions
Qing Wen Bai Du Yin (Clear Epidemics and Overcome Pathogenic Influences Decoction)	Treats *wen yi* (warm epidemics) with heat and toxins in the *qi* (energy) and *xue* (blood) levels

Qing Wen Bai Du Yin (Clear Epidemics and Overcome Pathogenic Influences Decoction) clears heat, sedates fire, and eliminates toxins. It is a unique formula used to treat proliferation of heat toxins in both the *qi* and *xue* levels.

SECTION 4: HEAT-CLEARING AND TOXIN-ELIMINATING FORMULAS

Name	Similarities	Differences
Huang Lian Jie Du Tang (Coptis Decoction to Relieve Toxicity)		Treats upper, middle, and lower *jiaos*
Huang Lian Shang Qing Wan (Coptis Pill to Clear the Upper)		Treats upper, middle, and lower *jiaos*, and the head
Qing Shang Fang Feng Tang (Clear the Upper and Guard the Wind Decoction)		Treats upper *jiao* and upper parts of the body (face)
Liang Ge San (Cool the Diaphragm Powder)	Clear heat, sedate fire, and eliminate toxins	Treats upper and middle *jiaos*
Pu Ji Xiao Du Yin (Universal Benefit Decoction to Eliminate Toxin)		Treats upper *jiao* and the head
San Huang Xie Xin Tang (Three-Yellow Decoction to Sedate the Epigastrium)		Clears heat and fire, drains damp-heat from upper, middle, or lower *jiaos*
San Huang Shi Gao Tang (Three-Yellow and Gypsum Decoction)		Treats presence of heat and toxins deep inside the interior
Liu Shen Wan (Six-Miracle Pill)		Treats internal and external disorders due to heat and toxins

Huang Lian Jie Du Tang (Coptis Decoction to Relieve Toxicity) sedates fire and eliminates toxins. It is one of the most commonly used formulas to treat excess heat, fire, and toxins affecting all three *jiaos*.

Huang Lian Shang Qing Wan (Coptis Pill to Clear the Upper) and **Qing Shang Fang Feng Tang** (Clear the Upper and Guard the Wind Decoction) both clear heat, sedate fire, and eliminate toxins from the upper parts of the body.
- *Huang Lian Shang Qing Wan* is most effective for heat and fire attacking the upper body and head, but it may also be used to treat heat affecting the upper, middle, and lower *jiaos*, and the head.
- *Qing Shang Fang Feng Tang* is better for heat and toxins affecting the upper *jiao* and the upper parts of body (mostly the face), and it also dispels wind-heat.

Liang Ge San (Cool the Diaphragm Powder) sedates fire and induces bowel movements. It treats the presence of heat, fire, and toxins in the upper (chest) and middle (diaphragm) *jiaos* by clearing and venting the excess outward and draining it downward.

Pu Ji Xiao Du Yin (Universal Benefit Decoction to Eliminate Toxin) sedates fire and eliminates toxins in the upper *jiao* and head. It treats epidemic toxins in the head with a wind-heat diagnosis.

425

Chapter 5 – Heat-Clearing Formulas

Chapter 5 — Summary

San Huang Xie Xin Tang (Three-Yellow Decoction to Sedate the Epigastrium) and *San Huang Shi Gao Tang* (Three-Yellow and Gypsum Decoction) have similar names and functions. Both contain three "yellow" herbs to clear heat, purge fire, and eliminate toxins.

- *San Huang Xie Xin Tang* clears heat and fire, and drains damp-heat from the upper, middle or lower *jiao*s. The three "yellow" herbs are *Huang Qin* (Radix Scutellariae), *Huang Lian* (Rhizoma Coptidis), and *Da Huang* (Radix et Rhizoma Rhei).
- *San Huang Shi Gao Tang* treats heat and toxins deep inside the interior, such as heat and toxins affecting the Heart causing *shen* (spirit) disturbance, delirium, and incoherent speech. The three "yellow" herbs are *Huang Qin* (Radix Scutellariae), *Huang Lian* (Rhizoma Coptidis), and *Huang Bo* (Cortex Phellodendri Chinensis).

Liu Shen Wan (Six-Miracle Pill) is a potent formula that clears heat, eliminates toxins, reduces inflammation, and relieves pain. It may be taken internally or applied topically.

SECTION 5: *ZANG FU*-CLEARING FORMULAS

Name	Similarities	Differences
Dao Chi San (Guide Out the Red Powder)	Clear heat in the Heart and Small Intestine	Nourishes yin
Qing Xin Lian Zi Yin (Lotus Seed Decoction to Clear the Heart)		Tonifies qi and yin
Zhi Zi Chi Tang (Gardenia and Soja Decoction)	Clears heat in the Heart	Clears heat in the chest and diaphragm
Long Dan Xie Gan Tang (Gentiana Decoction to Drain the Liver)	Sedate excess fire in the Liver and Gallbladder	Clears damp-heat in the lower *jiao*
Dang Gui Long Hui Wan (Tangkuei, Gentiana, and Aloe Pill)		Use only in severe cases
Xi Gan Ming Mu San (Wash the Liver and Brighten the Eyes Powder)	Clears Liver heat, dispels wind-heat	Treats eye disorders due to wind-heat and Liver heat
Xie Bai San (Drain the White Powder)		Relieves coughing and dyspnea
Qing Xin Li Ge Tang (Clear the Epigastrium and Benefit the Diaphragm Decoction)	Clear Lung heat	Relieves sore throat
Xiang Sheng Po Di San (Loud Sound Powder for a Broken Flute)		Nourishes yin and restores voice functioning
Zuo Jin Wan (Left Metal Pill)	Clears Liver fire	Corrects the reversed flow of Stomach qi
Qing Wei San (Clear the Stomach Powder)		Cools the blood
Xie Huang San (Drain the Yellow Powder)	Clear Stomach heat and fire	Purges latent fire in the Spleen and Stomach
Yu Nu Jian (Jade Woman Decoction)		Nourishes yin
Gan Lu Yin (Sweet Dew Decoction)		Clears damp-heat in the Spleen and Stomach
Shao Yao Tang (Peony Decoction)	Clear damp-heat in the Intestines and stop dysentery	Harmonizes qi and blood
Huang Qin Tang (Scutellaria Decoction)		Harmonizes the middle *jiao* and relieves pain
Bai Tou Weng Tang (Pulsatilla Decoction)		Cools the blood

Dao Chi San (Guide Out the Red Powder) and *Qing Xin Lian Zi Yin* (Lotus Seed Decoction to Clear the Heart) both clear heat from the Heart organ and channel. Heat in the Heart organ is characterized

426

Chapter 5 — Summary

Chinese Herbal Formulas and Applications

by symptoms such as fidgeting, irritability, and restlessness. Heat in the Heart channel (and/or Small Intestines) is characterized by *lin zheng* (dysuria syndrome) with painful urination, cloudy urine, or blood-streaked urine.

* *Dao Chi San* calms Heart *shen* (spirit), cools the blood, promotes urination, and relieves dysuria. It treats heat in both the Heart and Small Intestine channels. It may be used for *lin zheng* (dysuria syndrome) with painful urination or blood-streaked urine.
* *Qing Xin Lian Zi Yin* clears heat in Heart (an excess condition in the upper *jiao*) and tonifies qi and Kidney yin (a deficient condition in the lower *jiao*). It may be used for *lin zheng* (dysuria syndrome) with turbid or cloudy urine.

Zhi Zi Chi Tang (Gardenia and Soja Decoction) clears heat in the Heart, chest and diaphragm to relieve irritability, insomnia, and a feeling of fullness and congestion in the chest.

Long Dan Xie Gan Tang (Gentiana Decoction to Drain the Liver) and *Dang Gui Long Hui Wan* (Tangkuei, Gentiana, and Aloe Pill) are two potent formulas that sedate excess fire in the Liver and Gallbladder channels.

* *Long Dan Xie Gan Tang* sedates Liver fire, drains damp-heat, and protects and nourishes Liver blood. It is mostly used for Liver fire flaring upward with damp-heat accumulation in the lower *jiao*.
* *Dang Gui Long Hui Wan* is an extremely bitter and cold formula designed to purge excess fire from the Liver through urination and defecation. It does not have any effect to protect or nourish Liver blood, and must be reserved only for cases of excess fire with severe symptoms.

Xi Gan Ming Mu San (Wash the Liver and Brighten the Eyes Powder) clears Liver heat and dispels wind-heat to treat various eye disorders.

Xie Bai San (Drain the White Powder), *Qing Xin Li Ge Tang* (Clear the Epigastrium and Benefit the Diaphragm Decoction) and *Xiang Sheng Po Di San* (Loud Sound Powder for a Broken Flute) clear Lung heat.

* *Xie Bai San* sedates Lung heat to relieve coughing, dyspnea, and coarse breathing.
* *Qing Xin Li Ge Tang* clears heat from the Lung and throat area to treat sore throat, tonsillitis, and parotitis.
* *Xiang Sheng Po Di San* clears heat, moistens dryness, and dispels phlegm. It is commonly used to treat hoarseness or loss of voice, dry mouth and throat, and ticklish or scratchy throat caused by Lung heat and Lung yin deficiency.

Zuo Jin Wan (Left Metal Pill), *Qing Wei San* (Clear the Stomach Powder), *Xie Huang San* (Drain the Yellow powder), *Yu Nu Jian* (Jade Woman Decoction), and *Gan Lu Yin* (Sweet Dew Decoction) all clear heat and treat stomach disorders.

* *Zuo Jin Wan* treats Liver fire overacting on the Stomach to address stomach disorders such as hypochondriac fullness and pain, epigastric distention, acid regurgitation, nausea, and vomiting.
* *Qing Wei San* clears Stomach heat and cools the blood. It treats rising Stomach fire manifesting in toothache, gum bleeding, and swollen cheeks.
* *Xie Huang San* drains latent fire of Spleen and Stomach invading the oral cavity. It may be used to treat oral ulcers, foul breath, and a dry, hot tongue.
* *Yu Nu Jian* nourishes Stomach yin and clears Stomach heat to manage both excess and deficiency conditions with symptoms such as thirst, toothache, loose teeth, bleeding gums, and headache.
* *Gan Lu Yin* clears damp-heat, cleanses the blood, and reduces inflammation. It treats damp-heat in the Spleen and Stomach with symptoms such as swelling, inflammation and suppuration of the gums and tongue, sore throat with inflammation and pain, stomatitis, tongue ulceration, and toothache.

Chapter 5 – Heat-Clearing Formulas

Chapter 5 — Summary

Shao Yao Tang (Peony Decoction), **Huang Qin Tang** (Scutellaria Decoction) and **Bai Tou Weng Tang** (Pulsatilla Decoction) all clear damp-heat in the Intestines to relieve diarrhea and dysentery.

- *Shao Yao Tang* (Peony Decoction) emphasizes harmonizing and activating qi and blood. It is more suitable for dysentery characterized by equal dampness and heat, with main signs and symptoms such as abdominal pain, rectal tenesmus, and presence of mucus and blood in the stools.
- *Bai Tou Weng Tang* (Pulsatilla Decoction) emphasizes cooling the blood to relieve dysentery. It is more suitable for treating dysentery characterized by more heat than dampness, with key signs and symptoms of rectal tenesmus, burning sensations of the anus, and presence of more blood than pus.
- *Huang Qin Tang* focuses on harmonizing the middle *jiao* and relieving pain. It is most suitable for dysentery characterized by disharmony between the Liver and Spleen, with key signs and symptoms such as mild fever, a bitter taste in the mouth, and abdominal pain.

SECTION 6: DEFICIENCY-HEAT CLEARING FORMULAS

Name	Similarities	Differences
Qing Hao Bie Jia Tang (Artemisia Annua and Soft-Shelled Turtle Shell Decoction)	Clear deficiency heat, nourish yin	Disperses deep-hidden deficiency heat
Qin Jiao Bie Jia San (Gentiana Macrophylla and Soft-Shelled Turtle Shell Powder)		Releases exterior wind
Qing Gu San (Cool the Bones Powder)		Relieves steaming bones sensation
Dang Gui Liu Huang Tang (Tangkuei and Six-Yellow Decoction)	Clear deficiency heat, tonify underlying deficiencies	Tonifies yin and qi
Zi Yin Jiang Huo Tang (Nourish Yin and Descend the Fire Decoction)		Tonifies yin, qi and blood
Qing Liang Yin (Clearing and Cooling Decoction)		Tonifies body fluids

Qing Hao Bie Jia Tang (Artemisia Annua and Soft-shelled Turtle Shell Decoction), **Qin Jiao Bie Jia San** (Gentiana Macrophylla and Soft-shelled Turtle Shell Powder), and **Qing Gu San** (Cool the Bones Powder) all nourish yin and clear deficiency-heat. They all treat deficiency-heat and deficiency-fire syndromes.

- *Qing Hao Bie Jia Tang* places equal emphasis on nourishing yin and releasing heat. It treats late stage heat syndromes (heat hidden in the yin) with night fever and morning coolness.
- *Qin Jiao Bie Jia San* mainly treats *feng lao bing* (wind consumption disease), which is due to transmission of an exterior pathogenic factor into the interior, thereby injuring yin. This formula consists of some wind-clearing and harmonizing herbs to dispel the pathogenic factors back out to the exterior.
- *Qing Gu San* mainly treats chronic deficiency-type of steaming bones sensation. This formula emphasizes clearing deficiency fire while nourishing yin.

Dang Gui Liu Huang Tang (Tangkuei and Six-Yellow Decoction) clears heat, nourishes yin, strengthens the exterior, and stops perspiration. It is used to treat yin deficiency with rising of fire.

Zi Yin Jiang Huo Tang (Nourish Yin and Descend the Fire Decoction) nourishes yin, tonifies qi and blood, and clears deficiency fire. It treats yin deficiency with fire from the Kidney and Liver.

Qing Liang Yin (Clearing and Cooling Decoction) clears heat and promotes the generation of body fluids. It treats heat attacking the upper and middle *jiaos* leading to excess heat and consumption of body fluids.

428

Chapter 6

— Summer-Heat-Dispelling Formulas

祛暑剂

吴塘 Wú Táng

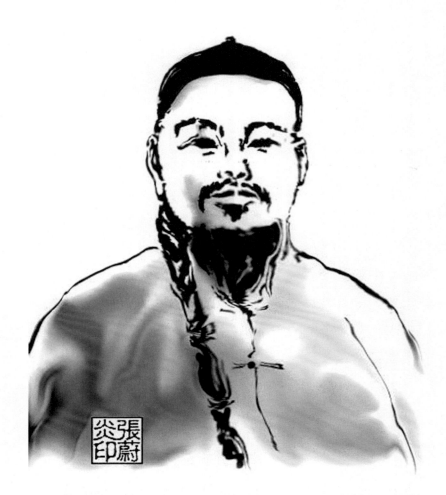

吴塘 Wú Táng, also known as 吴鞠通 Wú Jū-Tōng, 1758 – 1836.

吳塘 Wú Táng

Wu Tang was inspired to study medicine at nineteen years of age, when his father passed away from a warm disease epidemic. He was most influenced in his pursuit of medicine by Wu You-Xing's *Wen Yi Lun* (Discussion of Epidemic Warm Disease) and Ye Gui's *Wen Re Lun* (Discussion of Warm and Hot Disorders). Expanding beyond the theories of his predecessors, Wu proposed a new theory to treat *wen bing* (warm disease): *San Jiao Bian Zheng* (Triple Burner Differentiation). He stated that *wen bing* enters the body through the nose to affect the upper *jiao*, and the mouth to affect the middle *jiao*. If untreated, the disease will continue to deteriorate and affect the lower *jiao*.

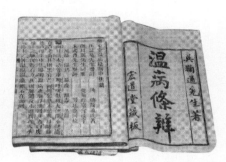

溫病條辨 *Wen Bing Tiao Bian* (Systematic Differentiation of Warm Disease) in 1798.

Wu Tang was also the first to recommend specific herbal treatments based on *Wei Qi Ying Xue Bian Zheng* (Defensive, Qi, Nutritive, Blood Differentiation). He recommended *Yin Qiao San* (Honeysuckle and Forsythia Powder) for *wen bing* (warm disease) affecting the *wei* (defensive) level, *Bai Hu Tang* (White Tiger Decoction) for *wen bing* affecting the *qi* (energy) level, *Qing Ying Tang* (Clear the Nutritive Level Decoction) for disease that has progressed to the *ying* (nutritive) level, and *Xi Jiao Di Huang Tang* (Rhinoceros Horn and Rehmannia Decoction) for treatment at the *xue* (blood) level. Furthermore, he observed that *wen bing* strongly consumes and damages yin and body fluids, and proposed using nourishing formulas to replenish the fluids and remedy the damage, such as *San Jia Fu Mai Tang* (Three-Shell Decoction to Restore the Pulse), *Da Ding Feng Zhu* (Major Arrest Wind Pearl) and *Xiao Ding Feng Zhu* (Minor Arrest Wind Pearl).

Wu Tang combined his academic and clinical experiences to publish *Wen Bing Tiao Bian* (Systematic Differentiation of Warm Disease) in 1798. His greatest contribution to *wen bing* (warm disease) is the integration of theories and treatment. While his predecessors (Wu You-Xing and Ye Gui) established the fundamental theories of *wen bing*, Wu Tang integrated the theories with clinically effective formulas, many of which are still in use today.

Many examples of formulas written by Wu Tang include:
- *Sang Ju Yin* (Mulberry Leaf and Chrysanthemum Decoction)
- *Yin Qiao San* (Honeysuckle and Forsythia Powder)
- *Zeng Ye Cheng Qi Tang* (Increase the Fluids and Order the Qi Decoction)
- *Qing Ying Tang* (Clear the Nutritive Level Decoction)
- *Qing Hao Bie Jia Tang* (Artemisia Annua and Soft-Shelled Turtle Shell Decoction)
- *Qing Luo Yin* (Clear the Collaterals Decoction)
- *Xin Jia Xiang Ru Yin* (Newly-Augmented Mosla Decoction)
- *An Gong Niu Huang Wan* (Calm the Palace Pill with Cattle Gallstone)
- *Xing Su San* (Apricot Kernel and Perilla Leaf Powder)
- *Sang Xing Tang* (Mulberry Leaf and Apricot Kernel Decoction)
- *Sha Shen Mai Dong Tang* (Glehnia and Ophiopogonis Decoction)
- *Zeng Ye Tang* (Increase the Fluids Decoction)

Dynasties & Kingdoms	Year
Xia Dynasty 夏	2100-1600 BCE
Shang Dynasty 商	1600-1100 BCE
Zhou Dynasty 周	1100-221 BCE
Qin Dynasty 秦	221-207 BCE
Han Dynasty 漢	206 BCE-220
Three Kingdoms 三國	220-280
Western Jin Dynasty 西晉	265-316
Eastern Jin Dynasty 東晉	317-420
Northern and Southern Dynasties 北南朝	420-581
Sui Dynasty 隋	581-618
Tang Dynasty 唐	618-907
Five Dynasties 五代	907-960
Song Dynasty 宋	960-1279
Liao Dynasty 遼	916-1125
Jin Dynasty 金	1115-1234
Yuan Dynasty 元	1271-1368
Ming Dynasty 明	1368-1644
Qing Dynasty 清	**1644-1911**
Republic of China 中華民國	1912-Present Day
People's Republic of China 中華人民共和國	1949-Present Day

Table of Contents

Chapter 6. Summer-Heat-Dispelling Formulas ·· **429**
  Biography of Wu Tang ·· 430

Qing Luo Yin (Clear the Collaterals Decoction) ·· 435
Xiang Ru San (Mosla Powder) ··· 436
  San Wu Xiang Ru Yin (Mosla Three Decoction) ·· 438
  Shi Wei Xiang Ru Yin (Ten-Ingredient Decoction with Mosla) ·· 438
Xin Jia Xiang Ru Yin (Newly-Augmented Mosla Decoction) ··· 439
Liu Yi San (Six-to-One Powder) ·· 441
  Liu Yi San (Six-to-One Powder) ·· 442
  Yi Yuan San (Benefit the Basal Powder) ·· 443
  Bi Yu San (Jasper Powder) ··· 443
  Ji Su San (Peppermint Powder) ·· 443
Gui Ling Gan Lu Yin (Cinnamon and Poria Sweet Dew Decoction) ·· 444
Qing Shu Yi Qi Tang (Clear Summer-Heat and Augment the Qi Decoction) ··· 446
  Qing Shu Yi Qi Tang (Clear Summer-Heat and Augment the Qi Decoction) ···························· 448

Summer-Heat-Dispelling Formulas (Summary) ··· **449**

Chinese Herbal Formulas and Applications

Chapter 6 — Overview

— Summer-Heat-Dispelling Formulas

Definition: Summer-heat-dispelling formulas, as the name implies, relieve summer-heat syndromes. Summer-heat, one of the *liu yin* (six exogenous factors), is the dominant exterior pathogenic factor during the hot and humid summer season. Summer-heat syndromes often occur in the summer, and are characterized by the presence of heat and dampness, as well as by consumption of and damage to qi and body fluids.

linical manifestations of summer-heat syndromes include fever, thirst, fidgeting, irritability, profuse perspiration, fatigue, heavy sensations of the body, dysuria, and a rapid pulse. As a result of high fever and profuse perspiration, qi and body fluids may be consumed and damaged. Therefore, optimal treatment of summer-heat syndromes requires the use of herbs that dispel summer-heat, tonify qi, and replenish body fluids.

> Summer-heat involves heat and dampness, consumption of qi, and damage to body fluids.

SUBCATEGORIES OF ACTION

Summer-heat-dispelling formulas are divided into four subcategories to reflect the nature of the disorder and characteristics of the formulas, as follows:

1. Summer-Heat-Dispelling and Heat-Clearing Formulas

These formulas are designed to treat summer-heat syndromes involving severe interior heat. Clinical manifestations include high fever, irritability, profuse perspiration, and thirst. Herbs commonly used to dispel summer-heat include *Xi Gua Cui Pi* (Exocarpium Citrulli), *Jin Yin Hua* (Flos Lonicerae Japonicae), and *He Ye* (Folium Nelumbinis). An exemplar formula is *Qing Luo Yin* (Clear the Collaterals Decoction).

2. Summer-Heat-Dispelling and Exterior-Releasing Formulas

These formulas are designed to relieve summer-heat in the interior and dispel any exterior factor(s) (usually wind-cold) at the skin and muscle levels. Summer-heat and wind-cold occur together when individuals try to cool down on hot summer days by drinking cold beverages and by wearing light clothing in the evening and at night. As a result, they contract both summer-heat and exterior wind-cold, and show signs and symptoms such as fever, aversion to cold, no perspiration, headache, irritability, and thirst. Commonly used herbs include *Huo Xiang* (Herba Agastaches), *Xiang Ru* (Herba Moslae) and *He Ye* (Folium Nelumbinis). An exemplar formula is *Xin Jia Xiang Ru Yin* (Newly-Augmented Mosla Decoction).

3. Summer-Heat-Dispelling and Dampness-Draining Formulas

These formulas are designed to relieve summer-heat and dispel internal dampness simultaneously. Summer-heat and dampness often occur together in eastern China because the east coast of China is generally very hot and humid during the summer. Common clinical manifestations include fever, irritability, thirst, chest and hypochondriac fullness/rigidity, and dysuria. This condition is treated by concurrent use of herbs that dispel summer-heat and drain dampness. Because internal dampness can be dispelled effectively through urination, herbs that regulate water and drain dampness

> Summer-heat and wind-cold occur together when people drink cold beverages on hot summer days and wear light clothing in the evening.

SUMMER-HEAT-DISPELLING FORMULAS

6

433

Chapter 6 – Summer-Heat-Dispelling Formulas

Chapter 6 — Overview

are commonly used, such as *Hua Shi* (Talcum), *Fu Ling* (Poria), and *Ze Xie* (Rhizoma Alismatis). Representative formulas include *Liu Yi San* (Six-to-One Powder) and *Gui Ling Gan Lu Yin* (Cinnamon and Poria Sweet Dew Decoction).

Herbs that clear heat and dispel dampness should be used simultaneously, and cautiously, to treat summer-heat.

4. Summer-Heat-Dispelling and Qi-Benefiting Formulas

These formulas are used when summer-heat has extensively damaged qi and body fluids. Common clinical manifestations include fever, warm sensations in the body, irritability, thirst, lassitude, weak breathing, profuse perspiration, and a deficient pulse. Herbs that benefit qi and nourish yin and body fluids are commonly used in these formulas, such as *Xi Yang Shen* (Radix Panacis Quinquefolii), *Ren Shen* (Radix et Rhizoma Ginseng), *Mai Dong* (Radix Ophiopogonis), *Shi Hu* (Caulis Dendrobii), and *Wu Wei Zi* (Fructus Schisandrae Chinensis). An exemplar formula is *Qing Shu Yi Qi Tang* (Clear Summer-Heat and Augment the Qi Decoction).

CAUTIONS / CONTRAINDICATIONS

As the name implies, summer-heat syndromes generally occur in the summer, and may be characterized by the presence of both heat and dampness. To properly treat this syndrome, herbs that clear heat and dispel dampness should be used simultaneously. However, use such herbs cautiously, because inappropriate use of heat-clearing herbs may damage yin, while inappropriate use of damp-resolving herbs may dry up needed body fluids.

PHARMACOLOGICAL EFFECTS & CLINICAL APPLICATIONS

Summer-heat-dispelling formulas primarily treat disorders of the respiratory and gastrointestinal tracts.

- **Respiratory disorders**: These formulas have been used effectively to treat various lung disorders, such as common cold or influenza,[1] pneumonia,[2] whooping cough,[3] and wheezing and dyspnea.[4] Representative formulas include *Xin Jia Xiang Ru Yin* (Newly-Augmented Mosla Decoction), *Liu Yi San* (Six-to-One Powder), and *Qing Shu Yi Qi Tang* (Clear Summer-Heat and Augment the Qi Decoction).

Summer-heat-dispelling formulas primarily treat infectious respiratory and gastrointestinal disorders.

- **Gastrointestinal disorders**: Diarrhea in infants, children and adults is frequently treated with good results using *Liu Yi San* (Six-to-One Powder) and *Gui Ling Gan Lu Yin* (Cinnamon and Poria Sweet Dew Decoction).[5,6]
- **Fever**: These formulas have been used effectively to treat fever in children and adults.[7,8,9] Exemplar formulas include *Xiang Ru San* (Mosla Powder) and *Xin Jia Xiang Ru Yin* (Newly-Augmented Mosla Decoction).

References

1. *Shang Hai Zhong Yi Yao Za Zhi* (Shanghai Journal of Chinese Medicine and Herbology) 1982;8:35.
2. *Zhe Jiang Zhong Yi Za Zhi* (Zhejiang Journal of Chinese Medicine) 1984;8:352.
3. *Shan Xi Zhong Yi* (Shanxi Chinese Medicine) 1986;10:441.
4. *Shan Xi Yi Kan* (Shanxi Journal of Medicine) 1992;3:104.
5. *Ji Lin Zhong Yi Yao* (Jilin Chinese Medicine and Herbology) 1987;6:24.
6. *Zhong Xi Yi Yi Jie He Za Zhi* (Journal of Integrated Chinese and Western Medicine) 1985;1:19.
7. *Fu Jian Zhong Yi Yao* (Fujian Chinese Medicine and Herbology) 1990;2:14.
8. *Zhong Yi Ming Fang Lin Chuang Xin Yong* (Contemporary Clinical Applications of Classic Chinese Formulas) 2001;708.
9. *Jiang Su Zhong Yi* (Jiangsu Chinese Medicine) 1999;7:28.

Chinese Herbal Formulas and Applications

Qīng Luò Yǐn (Clear the Collaterals Decoction)

清絡飲
清络饮

Pinyin Name: *Qing Luo Yin*
Literal Name: Clear the Collaterals Decoction
Original Source: *Wen Bing Tiao Bian* (Systematic Differentiation of Warm Disease) by Wu Ju-Tong in 1798

COMPOSITION

Jin Yin Hua (Flos Lonicerae Japonicae), fresh	6g
Bian Dou Hua (Flos Lablab Album), fresh	6g
Xi Gua Cui Pi (Exocarpium Citrulli)	6g
He Ye (Folium Nelumbinis), fresh	6g
Si Gua Pi (Pericarpium Luffae)	6g
Zhu Ye (Herba Phyllostachys), fresh	6g

DOSAGE / PREPARATION / ADMINISTRATION

Cook the ingredients in 2 cups of water and until 1 cup remains. Take the decoction twice daily.

CHINESE THERAPEUTIC ACTIONS

Clears heat and dispels summer-heat

CLINICAL MANIFESTATIONS

Summer-heat invading the Lung and *qi* (energy) level: fever, slight thirst, blurred vision, an unclear feeling and swelling sensation in the head, and a slight red tongue body with a thin, white tongue coating.

CLINICAL APPLICATIONS

Common cold or influenza in the summer and heat stroke.

EXPLANATION

This formula treats mild case of summer-heat affecting the Lung and *qi* (energy) level. This condition occurs when mild summer-heat directly attacks the Lung, or it can be a residual condition of summer-heat that has not been dispelled after using exterior-releasing herbs. Summer-heat may affect the Lung and consume fluids, leading to thirst. Summer-heat may attack the *qi* (energy) level to cause mild fever. Summer-heat may travel to the head and cause an unclear feeling and swelling sensation of the head. A slight red tongue body with a thin, white tongue coating suggests that this is a mild syndrome of heat.

Since the disorder is in the Lung and *qi* (energy) level, exterior-releasing herbs are not used. *Jin Yin Hua* (Flos Lonicerae Japonicae) and *Bian Dou Hua* (Flos Lablab Album), the chief herbs, are aromatic and can disperse and dispel summer-heat. *Xi Gua Cui Pi* (Exocarpium Citrulli) clears summer-heat. *Si Gua Pi* (Pericarpium Luffae) clears heat in the Lung and from its channel and collateral. *He Ye* (Folium Nelumbinis) disperses heat and dispels summer-heat. Because summer-heat can easily injure the Heart and disturb the *shen* (spirit), *Zhu Ye* (Herba Phyllostachys) is used to purge this heat through urination. Most of the herbs in this formula should be

Qing Luo Yin (Clear the Collaterals Decoction)

Diagnosis	Signs and Symptoms	Treatment	Herbs
Summer-heat invading the Lung and *qi* (energy) level	• Mild fever: summer-heat invading the *qi* (energy) level • Slight thirst: summer-heat consuming body fluids • Blurred vision, an unclear feeling and swelling sensation of the head: summer-heat blocking the sensory orifices • Slight red tongue body and a thin, white tongue coating: early stage of heat condition	Clears heat and dispels summer-heat	• *Jin Yin Hua* (Flos Lonicerae Japonicae), *Bian Dou Hua* (Flos Lablab Album), *Xi Gua Cui Pi* (Exocarpium Citrulli) and *He Ye* (Folium Nelumbinis) clear summer-heat. • *Si Gua Pi* (Pericarpium Luffae) clears heat in the Lung and its channel and collateral. • *Zhu Ye* (Herba Phyllostachys) clears the Heart and purges heat through urination.

6

SUMMER-HEAT-DISPELLING FORMULAS

435

Chapter 6 – Summer-Heat-Dispelling Formulas

Qīng Luò Yǐn (Clear the Collaterals Decoction)

used in the fresh and aromatic form to enhance the summer-heat dispersing action. Because this formula is intended to treat mild cases of summer-heat syndrome, it can be taken regularly as an herbal tea during the summer to prevent summer-heat invasion.

MODIFICATIONS

• With thirst, add *Tian Hua Fen* (Radix Trichosanthis), *Ge Gen* (Radix Puerariae Lobatae), and *Shi Hu* (Caulis Dendrobii).

• With fever, add *Shi Gao* (Gypsum Fibrosum) and *Zhi Mu* (Rhizoma Anemarrhenae).

• With summer-heat injuring the Lung manifesting in high-pitched cough with no sputum, add *Gan Cao* (Radix

et Rhizoma Glycyrrhizae), *Jie Geng* (Radix Platycodonis), *Ku Xing Ren* (Semen Armeniacae Amarum) and *Mai Dong* (Radix Ophiopogonis).

CAUTIONS / CONTRAINDICATIONS

Qing Luo Yin treats only mild to moderate cases of summer-heat. It is insufficient for severe cases of summer-heat.

AUTHORS' COMMENTS

Qing Luo Yin treats mild to moderate cases of summer-heat invading the Lung. This formula may be taken as a decoction for treatment, and it may also be taken in lower doses as a tea throughout the summer for prevention of heat strokes.

Xiāng Rú Sǎn (Mosla Powder)
香薷散

Pinyin Name: *Xiang Ru San*
Literal Name: Mosla Powder
Alternate Names: *Hsiang Ju Yin, Xiang Ru Yin*, Elsholtzia Drink, Elsholtzia Decoction
Original Source: *Tai Ping Hui Min He Ji Ju Fang* (Imperial Grace Formulary of the Tai Ping Era) by the Imperial Medical Department in 1078-85

COMPOSITION

Xiang Ru (Herba Moslae)	480g [9g]
Hou Po (Cortex Magnoliae Officinalis), *zhi* (fried with ginger juice)	240g [6g]
Bai Bian Dou (Semen Lablab Album), *chao* (dry-fried)	240g [6g]

Note: *Xiang Ru* (Herba Moslae) may be derived from two sources: *Mosla chinensis* and *Elsholtzia splendens*. Both herbs have similar functions, and have been used interchangeably in the history of Chinese herbal medicine. However, *Zhong Hua Ren Min Gong He Guo Yao Dian* (Pharmacopoeia of People's Republic of China) in 2005 identifies *Mosla chinensis* as the official source of *Xiang Ru*. Therefore, we have adopted mosla as the standard nomenclature for both single herbs and herbal formulas throughout this text.

DOSAGE / PREPARATION / ADMINISTRATION

The source text states to grind the ingredients into a coarse powder. Cook 9g of the powder with one large bowl of water and a small amount of grain-based liquor (approximately 10% of the total volume) until 70% of the liquid remains. Discard the residue, and cool the strained decoction before ingestion. Today, this formula may be prepared as a decoction with the doses suggested

in brackets, with or without the addition of grain-based liquor.

CHINESE THERAPEUTIC ACTIONS

1. Dispels summer-heat
2. Releases exterior cold
3. Resolves dampness and harmonizes the middle *jiao*

CLINICAL MANIFESTATIONS

Summer-heat syndrome with exterior cold and interior dampness: fever, aversion to cold, headache, lethargy; heavy sensations in the head and body, no perspiration, and stifling sensations in the chest; or nausea, vomiting, diarrhea, and abdominal pain with a white, greasy tongue coating and a superficial pulse.

CLINICAL APPLICATIONS

Common cold, heat stroke, gastroenteritis, bacterial dysentery, fever, and hypokalemia.

436

Chinese Herbal Formulas and Applications

Xiāng Rú Sǎn (Mosla Powder)

EXPLANATION

Xiang Ru San (Mosla Powder) treats summer-heat with exterior cold and interior dampness. More specifically, it treats exterior cold and interior dampness during the summer, a condition that often occurs when individuals try to cool down on hot summer days by drinking cold beverages and by wearing light clothing in the evening and at night. As a result, they contract both dampness in the interior (from drinking cold beverages) and wind-cold at the exterior (by wearing light clothing as the temperature cools down). Interior dampness blocks the qi flow to cause heaviness in the head, no perspiration, a stifling sensation in the chest, nausea, vomiting, diarrhea, lethargy, and abdominal pain. Fever, aversion to cold, and headache are common symptoms caused by exterior wind-cold. A white, greasy tongue coating indicates damp accumulation in the interior, and a superficial pulse is a sign of an exterior condition.

Xiang Ru (Herba Moslae), aromatic and warm, dispels the exterior cold factor and resolves interior dampness. Frequently used in the summer to treat exterior wind-cold, *Xiang Ru* (Herba Moslae) has been called the summer *Ma Huang* (Herba Ephedrae). *Hou Po* (Cortex Magnoliae Officinalis) activates qi flow and dries interior dampness to relieve the feeling of heaviness and the stifling sensation in the chest. *Bai Bian Dou* (Semen Lablab Album) tonifies qi, strengthens the Spleen, and dries dampness.

MODIFICATIONS

- With nasal obstruction or discharge, add *Cong Chi Tang* (Scallion and Prepared Soybean Decoction).
- With cramps and spasms, add *Mu Gua* (Fructus Chaenomelis).
- When there is more dampness, add *Fu Ling* (Poria) and *Gan Cao* (Radix et Rhizoma Glycyrrhizae).
- If there is Spleen deficiency with *zhong* (central) qi deficiency, add *Ren Shen* (Radix et Rhizoma Ginseng), *Huang Qi* (Radix Astragali), *Bai Zhu* (Rhizoma Atractylodis

Macrocephalae), and *Ju Hong* (Exocarpium Citri Reticulatae).
- With hypokalemia, combine with *Liu Yi San* (Six-to-One Powder) and *Bo He* (Herba Menthae).
- With aversion to cold and more superficial symptoms, add *Cong Bai* (Bulbus Allii Fistulosi) and *Dan Dou Chi* (Semen Sojae Praeparatum).

CAUTIONS / CONTRAINDICATIONS

- *Xiang Ru San* is not suitable for patients who suffer from summer-heat with perspiration, summer-heat with *wei* (defensive) qi deficiency with perspiration, or summer-heat with irritability and thirst.
- *Xiang Ru San* is not suitable for individuals with exterior wind-heat conditions.[1]

PHARMACOLOGICAL EFFECTS

Effect on temperature regulation: Administration of *Xiang Ru San* was associated with a temporary reduction of body temperature in rats with artificially-induced fever. The effectiveness of the formula was increased when a small amount of alcohol was added to the water during the cooking process to enhance the extraction of essential oils.[2]

CLINICAL STUDIES AND RESEARCH

1. **Fever:** Forty-five children with persistent fever (38-39°C / 100.4-102.2°F) longer than 10 days during the summer were treated with modified *Xiang Ru San* with success. Out of 45 cases, the study reported 14 cases with normal temperature after 1-3 days, 16 cases after 4-6 days, 12 cases after 7-9 days, and 3 cases with no effect after 10 days. *Xiang Ru San* was modified by adding *Ban Lan Gen* (Radix Isatidis), *Di Gu Pi* (Cortex Lycii), *Qing Hao* (Herba Artemisiae Annuae), and others as deemed necessary.[3]

2. **Hypokalemia:** Twenty-four patients with low potassium were treated with *Xiang Ru San* combined with *Liu Yi San* (Six-to-One Powder) and *Bo He* (Herba Menthae). After 2-4 doses, 19 returned to normal, 4 had some improvement, and 1 had no benefit.[4]

Xiang Ru San (Mosla Powder)

Diagnosis	Signs and Symptoms	Treatment	Herbs
Summer-heat syndrome with exterior cold and interior dampness	• Heavy sensation in the head, no perspiration, a stifling sensation in the chest, nausea, vomiting, diarrhea, lethargy, and abdominal pain: interior dampness • Fever, aversion to cold, and headache: exterior wind-cold • White, greasy tongue coating: damp accumulation • Superficial pulse: exterior condition	• Clears summer-heat • Releases exterior cold • Resolves dampness and harmonizes the middle *jiao*	• *Xiang Ru* (Herba Moslae) releases exterior cold. • *Hou Po* (Cortex Magnoliae Officinalis) activates qi flow and dries dampness. • *Bai Bian Dou* (Semen Lablab Album) tonifies qi, strengthens the Spleen, and dries dampness.

SUMMER-HEAT-DISPELLING FORMULAS

6

437

Chapter 6 – Summer-Heat-Dispelling Formulas

Xiāng Rú Sǎn (Mosla Powder)

RELATED FORMULAS

Sān Wù Xiāng Rú Yǐn (Mosla Three Decoction)

三物香薷飲
三物香薷饮

Pinyin Name: *San Wu Xiang Ru Yin*
Literal Name: Mosla Three Decoction
Original Source: *Zheng Zhi Zhun Sheng* (Standards of Patterns and Treatments) by Wang Ken-Tang in 1602

Xiang Ru (Herba Moslae)	[16g]
Hou Po (Cortex Magnoliae Officinalis)	[8g]
Bai Bian Dou (Semen Lablab Album)	[12g]

San Wu Xiang Ru Yin (Mosla Three Decoction) is taken as a decoction at room temperature because ingestion of warm decoction is sometimes associated with diarrhea. Note: Doses of herbs are unavailable from the source text. Suggested doses are listed above in brackets.

This formula primarily dispels summer-heat, eliminates toxins and stops diarrhea. It treats invasion of summer-heat with symptoms such as headache, fever, aversion to cold, irritability, abdominal pain, nausea and vomiting. Today, it may be used to treat enteritis, gastroenteritis, stomach flu, diarrhea, dysentery, and food poisoning.

This formula is used to treat sudden contraction of exterior condition during the summer. Because summer is characterized predominately by dampness and heat, the condition is defined as damp-heat affecting the exterior and the digestive tract. Damp-heat at the exterior causes headache, fever, and aversion to cold. Because damp-heat may be contracted via ingestion of cold or raw food, the patient may show abdominal pain, nausea, and vomiting.

This is a rather simple formula containing only three herbs. *Xiang Ru* (Herba Moslae) is regarded as one of the best herbs to release the exterior during the summer. It releases the exterior via diaphoresis, and drains dampness via urination. In addition, *Hou Po* (Cortex Magnoliae Officinalis) strengthens the Spleen, and *Bai Bian Dou* (Semen Lablab Album) relieves diarrhea. Altogether, this formula dispels summer-heat from the exterior and interior, while strengthening the Spleen and Stomach simultaneously.

Xiang Ru San and *San Wu Xiang Ru Yin* (Mosla Three Decoction) have the same ingredients, but are derived from different source texts. *Xiang Ru San* has specific doses and preparation methods for its ingredients, while the doses and preparation methods are unavailable for

San Wu Xiang Ru Yin. Because both formulas are used clinically, they are listed separately in this text.

Shí Wèi Xiāng Rú Yǐn
(Ten-Ingredient Decoction with Mosla)

十味香薷飲
十味香薷饮

Pinyin Name: *Shi Wei Xiang Ru Yin*
Literal Name: Ten-Ingredient Decoction with Mosla
Original Source: *Zhou Hou Bei Ji Fang* (Emergency Formulas to Keep Up One's Sleeve) by Ge Hong in 341 A.D.

Xiang Ru (Herba Moslae)	30g
Ren Shen (Radix et Rhizoma Ginseng)	15g
Bai Zhu (Rhizoma Atractylodis Macrocephalae)	15g
Chen Pi (Pericarpium Citri Reticulatae)	15g
Fu Ling (Poria)	15g
Huang Qi (Radix Astragali)	15g
Hou Po (Cortex Magnoliae Officinalis)	15g
Mu Gua (Fructus Chaenomelis)	15g
Bai Bian Dou (Semen Lablab Album)	15g
Zhi Gan Cao (Radix et Rhizoma Glycyrrhizae Praeparata cum Melle)	15g

Shi Wei Xiang Ru Yin (Ten-Ingredient Decoction with Mosla) disperses summer-heat, harmonizes the Spleen and Stomach, and benefits qi. It is used to treat summer-heat at the exterior with constitutional deficiency: exterior condition during the summer time, steaming sensations of the skin, heavy sensation of the head, heaviness and fatigue of the extremities and the body, headache, irritability, thirst, nausea, vomiting, diarrhea, and dizziness. There may also be perspiration with a deficient pulse. Today, it may be used to treat common cold, influenza, stomach flu, indigestion, and diarrhea.

This formula has herbs to clear summer-heat, harmonize the middle *jiao* and tonify qi. Aromatic and warm, *Xiang Ru* (Herba Moslae) disperses summer-heat from the exterior. *Hou Po* (Cortex Magnoliae Officinalis) resolves dampness and harmonizes the Stomach. *Bai Bian Dou* (Semen Lablab Album) resolves summer-heat and harmonizes the Spleen. *Ren Shen* (Radix et Rhizoma Ginseng) and *Huang Qi* (Radix Astragali) tonify qi and treat the underlying deficiency. *Huang Qi* (Radix Astragali) also strengthens *wei* (defensive) *qi* and stops perspiration. *Bai Zhu* (Rhizoma Atractylodis Macrocephalae), *Fu Ling* (Poria), and *Chen Pi* (Pericarpium Citri Reticulatae) strengthen the Spleen and Stomach, and relieve nausea, vomiting and diarrhea. *Mu Gua* (Fructus Chaenomelis) resolves dampness and promotes digestion. Lastly, *Gan Cao* (Radix et Rhizoma Glycyrrhizae) harmonizes the herbs.

Chinese Herbal Formulas and Applications

Xiāng Rú Sǎn (Mosla Powder)

AUTHORS' COMMENTS

Xiang Ru San is commonly used to treat acute enteritis, gastroenteritis, and bacterial dysentery characterized by wind, cold, and dampness. The key symptoms indicating use of this formula are aversion to cold, fever, a heavy sensation in the head, body aches, absence of perspiration, a stifling sensation in the chest, a white, greasy tongue coating, and a superficial pulse.

References

1. *Zhong Yao Ming Fang Yao Li Yu Ying Yong* (Pharmacology and Applications of Famous Herbal Formulas) 1989;50-51.
2. *Cheng Du Zhong Yi Xue Yuan Xue Bao* (Journal of Chengdu University of Traditional Chinese Medicine) 1992;12(2):39.
3. *Fu Jian Zhong Yi Yao* (Fujian Chinese Medicine and Herbology) 1990;2:14.
4. *Zhong Xi Yi Jie He Za Zhi* (Journal of Integrated Chinese and Western Medicine) 1988;1:19.

Xīn Jiā Xiāng Rú Yǐn (Newly-Augmented Mosla Decoction)
新加香薷飲
新加香薷饮

Pinyin Name: *Xin Jia Xiang Ru Yin*
Literal Name: Newly-Augmented Mosla Decoction
Original Source: *Wen Bing Tiao Bian* (Systematic Differentiation of Warm Disease) by Wu Ju-Tong in 1798

COMPOSITION

Xiang Ru (Herba Moslae)	6g
Bian Dou Hua (Flos Lablab Album), fresh	9g
Jin Yin Hua (Flos Lonicerae Japonicae)	9g
Lian Qiao (Fructus Forsythiae)	6g [9g]
Hou Po (Cortex Magnoliae Officinalis)	6g

Note: *Xiang Ru* (Herba Moslae) may be derived from two sources: *Mosla chinensis* and *Elsholtzia splendens*. Both herbs have similar functions, and have been used interchangeably in the history of Chinese herbal medicine. However, *Zhong Hua Ren Min Gong He Guo Yao Dian* (Pharmacopoeia of People's Republic of China) in 2005 identifies *Mosla chinensis* as the official source of *Xiang Ru*. Therefore, we have adopted mosla as the standard nomenclature for both single herbs and herbal formulas throughout this text.

DOSAGE / PREPARATION / ADMINISTRATION

The source text states to cook the ingredients in 5 cups of water until 2 cups remain. Take 1 cup of the strained decoction. Once sweating has been induced, the formula should be discontinued. If sweating does not occur, take another cup of the decoction. If there is still no sweating, repeat the steps above and administer another round of decoction. Today, the decoction may be prepared using the dose of *Lian Qiao* (Fructus Forsythiae) suggested in brackets.

CHINESE THERAPEUTIC ACTIONS

1. Dispels summer-heat
2. Releases exterior cold
3. Clears heat and resolves dampness

CLINICAL MANIFESTATIONS

Summer-heat disorders complicated by exterior cold and interior dampness: fever, slight aversion to cold, headache, no perspiration, thirst, a red face, a stifling sensation and discomfort in the chest, thick, white and greasy tongue coating, and a superficial, rapid pulse.

CLINICAL APPLICATIONS

Common cold, influenza, and febrile diseases in summer.

EXPLANATION

Xin Jia Xiang Ru Yin (Newly-Augmented Mosla Decoction), derived from *Xiang Ru San* (Mosla Powder), treats the type of summer-heat disorder that is complicated by exterior cold and interior damp factors. Patients who have this syndrome are usually first attacked by summer-heat.

SUMMER-HEAT-DISPELLING FORMULAS

6

439

Chapter 6 – Summer-Heat-Dispelling Formulas

Xīn Jiā Xiāng Rú Yǐn (Newly-Augmented Mosla Decoction)

Xin Jia Xiang Ru Yin (Newly-Augmented Mosla Decoction)

Diagnosis	Signs and Symptoms	Treatment	Herbs
Summer-heat disorders complicated by exterior cold and interior dampness	• Fever, slight aversion to cold, headache and no perspiration: exterior cold • Thirst and a red face: summer-heat consuming yin and body fluids • Stifling sensation and discomfort in the chest: dampness in the interior • White, greasy tongue coating: dampness in the interior • Superficial, rapid pulse: exterior cold and interior heat	• Dispels summer-heat • Releases the exterior • Clears heat and dampness	• *Xiang Ru* (Herba Moslae) releases the exterior cold factors and resolves interior dampness. • *Bian Dou Hua* (Flos Lablab Album), *Jin Yin Hua* (Flos Lonicerae Japonicae) and *Lian Qiao* (Fructus Forsythiae) clear summer-heat. • *Hou Po* (Cortex Magnoliae Officinalis) activates qi circulation and dries dampness.

Before it is relieved, however, they are further invaded by exterior cold factors as a result of lack of adequate clothing or other reasons. Because summer-heat is usually accompanied by dampness, interior dampness may arise as a result. Fever, slight aversion to cold, headache, and no perspiration are clinical manifestations associated with exterior cold. Thirst and a red face are the results of summer-heat damaging yin and body fluids. A stifling sensation and discomfort in the chest, along with a white, greasy tongue coating, indicate dampness in the interior. A superficial, rapid pulse is caused by exterior cold and summer-heat in the interior.

To effectively treat this syndrome, one should release exterior cold, dispel interior summer-heat, and resolve interior dampness. *Xiang Ru* (Herba Moslae), aromatic and warm, dispels the exterior cold factor and dissolves interior dampness. Frequently used in the summer to treat exterior wind-cold, *Xiang Ru* has been called the summer *Ma Huang* (Herba Ephedrae). *Bian Dou Hua* (Flos Lablab Album), *Jin Yin Hua* (Flos Lonicerae Japonicae), and *Lian Qiao* (Fructus Forsythiae) penetrate to the interior to clear summer-heat, especially in the upper *jiao* or the *qi* (energy) level. *Hou Po* (Cortex Magnoliae Officinalis) activates qi circulation and dries dampness to clear the thick tongue coating and relieve the chest stuffiness and discomfort.

CAUTIONS / CONTRAINDICATIONS

Xin Jia Xiang Ru Yin is generally given as a warm decoction. However, use of this formula as a warm decoction has been occasionally associated with nausea and vomiting. In such circumstances, the decoction should be given at room temperature.[1]

CLINICAL STUDIES AND RESEARCH

1. **Common cold or influenza in summer**: Modified *Xin Jia Xiang Ru Yin* was used to treat viral infection during the summer in 96 patients. The age of the patients ranged from 8-81 years of age, with average of 2.3 days of infection prior to receiving treatment. The study reported an average time of 1.77 days for reduction of fever, and 2.1 days for resolution of all other symptoms.[2]

2. **Fever**: Concurrent use of *Xin Jia Xiang Ru Yin* and *Hao Qin Qing Dan Tang* (Artemisia Annua and Scutellaria Decoction to Clear the Gallbladder) was reported to have 94% effectiveness in treating fever. Of 50 cases, the study reported complete recovery in 24 cases, significant improvement in 17 cases, moderate improvement in 6 cases, and no effect in 3 cases.[3]

3. **Febrile disease in summer**: Use of modified *Xin Jia Xiang Ru Yin* to treat 31 patients with febrile diseases in the summer demonstrated 93.5% effectiveness. The study reported complete recovery in 21 cases, near-recovery in 8 cases, and moderate improvement in 2 cases.[4]

AUTHORS' COMMENTS

Xiang Ru San (Mosla Powder) and *Xin Jia Xiang Ru Yin* both contain acrid and warm herbs such as *Xiang Ru* (Herba Moslae) and *Hou Po* (Cortex Magnoliae Officinalis) to expel exterior pathogenic factors, disperse cold and resolve dampness.

• *Xiang Ru San* is warmer in property, and is better for treating summer-heat disorders complicated by exterior cold and interior dampness.

• *Xin Jia Xiang Ru Yin* is slightly cooler in property, as it contains *Jin Yin Hua* (Flos Lonicerae Japonicae), *Bian Dou Hua* (Flos Lablab Album), and *Lian Qiao* (Fructus Forsythiae). It is better for summer-heat conditions with more heat, with symptoms such as thirst and a red face.

Chinese Herbal Formulas and Applications

Xīn Jiā Xiāng Rú Yǐn (Newly-Augmented Mosla Decoction)

References

1. *Hu Bei Zhong Yi Za Zhi* (Hubei Journal of Chinese Medicine) 1987;(5):44.
2. *Shang Hai Zhong Yi Yao Za Zhi* (Shanghai Journal of Chinese Medicine and Herbology) 1982;8:35.
3. *Zhong Yi Ming Fang Lin Chuang Xin Yong* (Contemporary Clinical Applications of Classic Chinese Formulas) 2001;708.
4. *Jiang Su Zhong Yi* (Jiangsu Chinese Medicine) 1999;7:28.

Liù Yī Sǎn (Six-to-One Powder)
六一散

Pinyin Name: *Liu Yi San*
Literal Name: Six-to-One Powder
Original Source: *Shang Han Zhi Ge Fang Lun* (Direct Investigations of Formulas for Cold-Induced Disorders) by Liu Yuan-Su in the Jin Dynasty

COMPOSITION

Hua Shi (Talcum)	180g [18g]
Gan Cao (Radix et Rhizoma Glycyrrhizae)	30g [3g]

Note: *Liu Yi San*, literally Six-to-One Powder, is so named to emphasize the 6:1 dose proportion of its two ingredients, *Hua Shi* (Talcum) and *Gan Cao* (Radix et Rhizoma Glycyrrhizae).

DOSAGE / PREPARATION / ADMINISTRATION

Grind the ingredients into a fine powder, and take 9g of the powder with warm water three times daily with a small amount of honey. This formula may also be taken cold with fresh well water. This formula may also be prepared as a decoction using the doses suggested in brackets above. Take the decoction two to three times daily.

CHINESE THERAPEUTIC ACTIONS

Dispels summer-heat and dampness

CLINICAL MANIFESTATIONS

Summer-heat and dampness: fever, irritability, thirst, dysuria, or diarrhea.

CLINICAL APPLICATIONS

Whooping cough, infantile diarrhea, nephrolithiasis, urolithiasis, urethritis, and allergy.

EXPLANATION

Liu Yi San (Six-to-One Powder) treats summer-heat syndrome accompanied by dampness. Fever and irritability are due to heat in the body affecting the *shen* (spirit). Thirst reflects the consumption of body fluids by summer-heat and dampness. The heat and dampness may obstruct the qi flow in the lower *jiao*, causing dysuria and diarrhea.

Hua Shi (Talcum) clears summer-heat and dampness through urination to treat irritability, thirst and dysuria. *Hua Shi* (Talcum) is cold in nature and bland in taste: cold clears heat from the *zang* (solid organs), and bland dispels dampness from the *fu* (hollow) organ (Urinary Bladder). However, the cold nature of *Hua Shi* (Talcum) may damage the Spleen and Stomach. Therefore, warm *Gan Cao* (Radix et Rhizoma Glycyrrhizae) is used to balance

Liu Yi San (Six-to-One Powder)

Diagnosis	Signs and Symptoms	Treatment	Herbs
Summer-heat with dampness	• Fever and irritability: heat disturbing the *shen* (spirit) • Thirst: consumption of body fluids by summer-heat and dampness • Dysuria: summer-heat and dampness affecting the lower *jiao*	Dispels summer-heat and dampness	• *Hua Shi* (Talcum) clears summer-heat and dampness through urination. • *Gan Cao* (Radix et Rhizoma Glycyrrhizae) clears heat and harmonizes the middle *jiao*.

6

SUMMER-HEAT-DISPELLING FORMULAS

Chapter 6 – Summer-Heat-Dispelling Formulas

Liù Yī Săn (Six-to-One Powder)

the coldness of *Hua Shi* (Talcum). In addition, *Gan Cao* (Radix et Rhizoma Glycyrrhizae) also clears heat and harmonizes the middle *jiao*.

Although *Liu Yi San* only has two herbs, it is well-formulated to maximize the overall effect and minimize the side effects. It clears heat without leaving dampness behind, and promotes diuresis without damaging yin.

MODIFICATIONS

• If there is urinary stone or dysuria, add *Jin Qian Cao* (Herba Lysimachiae) and *Hai Jin Sha* (Spora Lygodii).
• For diarrhea or dysentery with blood or pus, add charred *Shan Zha* (Fructus Crataegi) and *Gan Jiang* (Rhizoma Zingiberis).

CAUTIONS / CONTRAINDICATIONS

• *Liu Yi San* is not recommended in cases of summer-heat or dysuria without damp-heat accumulation, or in cases of polyuria caused by yang deficiency.
• This formula should be used with caution in patients with qi and yin deficiencies, and in individuals with Spleen and Stomach deficiencies.
• This formula is contraindicated during pregnancy.
• Direct contact between the powdered herbs and the mucous membranes should be avoided, as formation of granuloma has been reported.[1]

PHARMACOLOGICAL EFFECTS

1. **Diuretic**: Administration of *Liu Yi San* in mice was associated with a marked diuretic effect, with peak effect reached within the first hour after oral ingestion.[2]
2. **Protective**: Due to its small particles, large surface area, and binding property, *Hua Shi* (Talcum) has been used with good results to protect the skin and minimize irritation. One report stated that use of *Hua Shi* (Talcum) orally can block the absorption of toxins in the intestines.[3]

CLINICAL STUDIES AND RESEARCH

1. **Whooping cough**: Eighty patients with whooping cough were treated with modified *Liu Yi San* as decoction one time daily. Modifications were as follows: *Dang Shen* (Radix Codonopsis), *Bai Zhu* (Rhizoma Atractylodis Macrocephalae), and *Fu Ling* (Poria) were added for those who were overweight; and *Shu Di Huang* (Radix Rehmanniae Praeparata), *Dang Gui* (Radix Angelicae Sinensis), *Bai Shao* (Radix Paeoniae Alba), and *Chuan Xiong* (Rhizoma Chuanxiong) were added for those who were underweight. After 3-6 doses, the study reported 49 cases had complete recovery, 27 had marked improvement, and 4 discontinued treatment due to nausea and vomiting. The overall rate of effectiveness was 95%.[4]

2. **Infantile diarrhea**: Modified *Liu Yi San* demonstrated 96.6% effectiveness in the treatment of diarrhea in 150 infants. Additions were as follows: *Sha Ren* (Fructus Amomi) and *Huang Lian* (Rhizoma Coptidis) for infection; and *Bai Zhu* (Rhizoma Atractylodis Macrocephalae) and *Ren Shen* (Radix et Rhizoma Ginseng) for Spleen deficiency.[5]

3. **Nephrolithiasis and urolithiasis**: Thirty-six patients with kidney and bladder stones were treated with modified *Liu Yi San* with passage of stones in 30 patients and dissolution of stones in 6 patients. The base formula used included *Lou Gu* (Gryllotalpa) 5 pieces, *Hua Shi* (Talcum) 30g, and *Gan Cao* (Radix et Rhizoma Glycyrrhizae) 3g. The modifications were as follows: *Hai Jin Sha* (Spora Lygodii) 30g and *Jin Qian Cao* (Herba Lysimachiae) 30g for large stones; *Che Qian Zi* (Semen Plantaginis) 12g and *Shi Wei* (Folium Pyrrosiae) 12g for dysuria with burning sensations during urination; *Bai Mao Gen* (Rhizoma Imperatae) 30g, *Bian Xu* (Herba Polygoni Avicularis) 12g, and *Qu Mai* (Herba Dianthi) 12g for blood in the urine; and *Hu Po* (Succinum) 5g for colic pain.[6]

4. **Urethritis**: Ten patients with urethritis were treated with *Liu Yi San* twice daily. Most patients had complete recovery within 3-4 days, while some required 6 days of treatment.[7]

5. **Pesticide poisoning**: One study reported beneficial effect using *Liu Yi San* to treat individuals with organophosphorus pesticide poisoning. The treatment protocol was to take herbs with warm water in several divided doses.[8]

TOXICOLOGY

This formula is well-tolerated. However, it has been reported that granuloma may occur with direct contact between *Hua Shi* (Talcum) and mucous membranes.[9]

RELATED FORMULAS

Liù Yī Săn (Six-to-One Powder)

六一散

Pinyin Name: *Liu Yi San*
Literal Name: Six-to-One Powder
Original Source: *Xuan Ming Lun Fang* (Discussion of Dispersing and Brightening Formulas) by Liu Yuan-Su in the Jin and Yuan Dynasties

Hua Shi (Talcum)	180g [18g]
Zhi Gan Cao (Radix et Rhizoma Glycyrrhizae Praeparata cum Melle)	30g [3g]

The source text states to grind the ingredients into a fine powder, and take 9g of the powder with warm water three times daily with a small amount of honey. This formula may also be taken cold with fresh well water. To promote

442

Liù Yī Sǎn (Six-to-One Powder)

urination and induce sweating, take it with a decoction made from cooking 5 *cun* (approximately 5 inches) of *Cong Bai* (Bulbus Allii Fistulosi) and 50 pieces of *Dan Dou Chi* (Semen Sojae Praeparatum) in one large bowl of water and reducing it until 70% of the liquid remains. This formula may also be prepared as a decoction using the doses suggested in brackets above. Take the decoction two to three times daily.

These two formulas have the same names, ingredients (although they differ in processing method), indications, and are derived from the same time period (Jin Dynasty). Therefore, it is unclear which is the true original source for this formula. Both formulas are presented here to reflect their historical similarities and minor differences.

Yì Yuán Sǎn (Benefit the Basal Powder)
益元散
Pinyin Name: *Yi Yuan San*
Literal Name: Benefit the Basal Powder
Original Source: *Shang Han Zhi Ge Fang Lun* (Direct Investigations of Formulas for Cold-Induced Disorders) by Liu Yuan-Su in the Jin Dynasty

Hua Shi (Talcum)	180g
Gan Cao (Radix et Rhizoma Glycyrrhizae)	30g
Zhu Sha (Cinnabaris)	[9g]

Note: *Zhu Sha* (Cinnabaris) is a potentially toxic heavy metal, and is rarely used as a medicinal substance today. Its discussion here is included primarily for academic purposes, to reflect the historical use of this substance in its original formulation. Most herbal products today have removed it completely, or replaced it with substitutes with similar functions. For additional information on the toxicity, please refer to *Chinese Medical Herbology and Pharmacology* by John Chen and Tina Chen.

The source text states to grind the ingredients into a fine powder. Take 6g of the powdered formula with warm water or a decoction made from *Deng Xin Cao* (Medulla Junci).

Yi Yuan San (Benefit the Basal Powder) is composed of *Liu Yi San* plus *Zhu Sha* (Cinnabaris) and *Deng Xin Cao* (Medulla Junci). These two additional herbs help tranquilize the *shen* (spirit). Clinically, it treats the syndrome of summer-heat and dampness complicated by palpitations, insomnia, and excessive dreaming, as both *Zhu Sha* (Cinnabaris) and *Deng Xin Cao* (Medulla Junci) clear Heart fire and calm the *shen*.

Bì Yù Sǎn (Jasper Powder)
碧玉散
Pinyin Name: *Bi Yu San*
Literal Name: Jasper Powder
Original Source: *Shang Han Zhi Ge Fang Lun* (Direct Investigations of Formulas for Cold-Induced Disorders) by Liu Yuan-Su in the Jin Dynasty

Hua Shi (Talcum)	180g
Gan Cao (Radix et Rhizoma Glycyrrhizae)	30g
Qing Dai (Indigo Naturalis)	[9g]

Bi Yu San (Jasper Powder) treats the syndrome of summer-heat and dampness complicated by Liver and Gallbladder heat. Clinically, patients may show red eyes, a sore throat, and mouth and lips ulcerations in addition to all the symptoms listed under *Liu Yi San*.

Bi Yu San is composed of *Liu Yi San* plus *Qing Dai* (Indigo Naturalis). The original source, however, did not specify the dose of *Qing Dai* (Indigo Naturalis).

Jī Sū Sǎn (Peppermint Powder)
雞蘇散
鸡苏散
Pinyin Name: *Ji Su San*
Literal Name: Peppermint Powder
Original Source: *Shang Han Zhi Ge Fang Lun* (Direct Investigations of Formulas for Cold-Induced Disorders) by Liu Yuan-Su in the Jin Dynasty

Hua Shi (Talcum)	180g
Gan Cao (Radix et Rhizoma Glycyrrhizae)	30g
Bo He (Herba Menthae)	[7.5g]

Ji Su San (Peppermint Powder) is composed of *Liu Yi San* plus *Bo He* (Herba Menthae). It is commonly used to treat the syndrome of summer-heat and dampness complicated by exterior wind. Clinically, patients may have swelling sensations of the head, headache, coughing, and other symptoms of exterior wind.

AUTHORS' COMMENTS

Liu Yi San is mostly used for mild summer-heat with damp conditions. However, it is not a strong formula. If the condition is severe or acute, other appropriate formulas should be added to achieve maximum effect. It is mostly reserved as a foundation formula to which other herbs can be added.

Chapter 6 – Summer-Heat-Dispelling Formulas

Liù Yī Săn (Six-to-One Powder)

References

1. *Shan Dong Zhong Yi Xue Yuan Xue Bao* (Journal of Shandong University School of Chinese Medicine) 1976;78.
2. *Nan Jing Zhong Yi Xue Yuan Xue Bao* (Journal of Nanjing University of Traditional Chinese Medicine) 1985;169.
3. *Zhong Yao Yao Li Xue* (Study of Chinese Herbology) 1986;133.
4. *Shan Xi Zhong Yi* (Shanxi Chinese Medicine) 1986;10:441.
5. *Ji Lin Zhong Yi Yao* (Jilin Chinese Medicine and Herbology) 1987;6:24.
6. *Zhong Yi Za Zhi* (Journal of Chinese Medicine) 1979;7:34.
7. *Liao Ning Yi Yao* (Liaoning Medicine and Herbology) 1976;2:69.
8. *Shan Dong Zhong Yi Xue Yuan Xue Bao* (Journal of Shandong University School of Chinese Medicine) 1976;78.
9. *Si Chuan Zhong Yi* (Sichuan Chinese Medicine) 1991;12:12.

Guì Líng Gān Lù Yǐn (Cinnamon and Poria Sweet Dew Decoction)
桂苓甘露飲
桂苓甘露饮

Pinyin Name: *Gui Ling Gan Lu Yin*
Literal Name: Cinnamon and Poria Sweet Dew Decoction
Original Source: *Huang Di Su Wen Xuan Ming Lun Fang* (Formulas from the Discussion Illuminating the Yellow Emperor's Basic Questions) by Liu Yuan-Su in 1172

COMPOSITION

Hua Shi (Talcum)	120g
Gan Cao (Radix et Rhizoma Glycyrrhizae)	60g
Fu Ling (Poria)	30g
Zhu Ling (Polyporus)	15g
Ze Xie (Rhizoma Alismatis)	30g
Rou Gui (Cortex Cinnamomi)	60g
Bai Zhu (Rhizoma Atractylodis Macrocephalae), *zhi* (fried with liquid)	15g
Shi Gao (Gypsum Fibrosum)	60g
Han Shui Shi (Mirabilite)	60g

DOSAGE / PREPARATION / ADMINISTRATION

Grind the ingredients into powder and take 9g with warm water, fresh spring water, or preferably a decoction made from *Sheng Jiang* (Rhizoma Zingiberis Recens). For children, reduce the dose to 3g.

CHINESE THERAPEUTIC ACTIONS

1. Clears heat and dispels summer-heat
2. Regulates qi and dispels dampness

CLINICAL MANIFESTATIONS

Invasion of summer-heat and dampness: fever, headache, irritability, thirst, dysuria, and sudden turmoil disorder with vomiting or diarrhea.

CLINICAL APPLICATIONS

Dysentery, diarrhea, vomiting, infantile diarrhea, kidney stone, bladder stone, urethritis, and allergy.

EXPLANATION

Gui Ling Gan Lu Yin (Cinnamon and Poria Sweet Dew Decoction) treats summer-heat syndrome accompanied by interior damp accumulation. Summer-heat rising upwards in the body causes fever and headaches. Summer-heat may also disturb the *shen* (spirit), causing irritability. If heat consumes body fluids, thirst occurs. Summer-heat may travel downwards to the lower *jiao*, causing dysuria. Vomiting and diarrhea occur if the dampness stagnates in the middle *jiao* and impairs the Spleen and Stomach's ability to separate the clear from the turbid.

Gui Ling Gan Lu Yin is formulated following the principles of *Liu Yi San* (Six-to-One Powder) and *Wu Ling San* (Five-Ingredient Powder with Poria), with the addition of *Shi Gao* (Gypsum Fibrosum) and *Han Shui Shi* (Mirabilite).

According to the strategies of *Liu Yi San* (Six-to-One Powder), *Hua Shi* (Talcum) clears summer-heat and

444

Guì Líng Gān Lù Yǐn (Cinnamon and Poria Sweet Dew Decoction)

Gui Ling Gan Lu Yin (Cinnamon and Poria Sweet Dew Decoction)

Diagnosis	Signs and Symptoms	Treatment	Herbs
Summer-heat and dampness	• Fever and headaches: summer-heat rising upwards • Irritability and thirst: summer-heat consuming yin and disturbing the *shen* (spirit) • Dysuria: summer-heat travels downwards to the lower *jiao* • Vomiting and diarrhea: damp accumulation in the middle *jiao*	• Clears heat and dispels summer-heat • Regulates qi and dispels dampness	• *Hua Shi* (Talcum) and *Gan Cao* (Radix et Rhizoma Glycyrrhizae) dispel summer-heat and dampness. • *Fu Ling* (Poria), *Zhu Ling* (Polyporus), *Ze Xie* (Rhizoma Alismatis), *Rou Gui* (Cortex Cinnamomi) and *Bai Zhu* (Rhizoma Atractylodis Macrocephalae) regulate water circulation, dispel damp, and disperse water accumulation. • *Shi Gao* (Gypsum Fibrosum) and *Han Shui Shi* (Mirabilite) clear heat and dispel summer-heat.

dampness through urination; and *Gan Cao* (Radix et Rhizoma Glycyrrhizae) clears heat, harmonizes the Spleen and Stomach, and promotes the secretion of body fluids. Following the strategies of *Wu Ling San* (Five-Ingredient Powder with Poria), *Rou Gui* (Cortex Cinnamomi) warms yang qi and helps the urinary functioning of the lower *jiao*; *Fu Ling* (Poria), *Zhu Ling* (Polyporus) and *Ze Xie* (Rhizoma Alismatis) induce urination to dispel interior dampness and relieve dysuria; and *Bai Zhu* (Rhizoma Atractylodis Macrocephalae) strengthens the Spleen, dries dampness, and regulates qi flow. Lastly, *Shi Gao* (Gypsum Fibrosum) and *Han Shui Shi* (Mirabilite), both extremely cold, clear heat and dispel summer-heat.

CLINICAL STUDIES AND RESEARCH

Diarrhea: Administration of modified *Gui Ling Gan Lu Yin* along with adjustment in dietary habits showed 92.5% effectiveness in treating 80 children with diarrhea characterized by damp-heat. The herbal decoction contained *Fu Ling* (Poria), *Zhu Ling* (Polyporus), *Bai Zhu* (Rhizoma Atractylodis Macrocephalae), *Gan Cao* (Radix et Rhizoma Glycyrrhizae), *Gui Zhi* (Ramulus Cinnamomi), *Shi Gao* (Gypsum Fibrosum), *Han Shui Shi* (Mirabilite), and *Hua Shi* (Talcum) as the base formula. Modifications included the addition of *Ge Gen* (Radix Puerariae Lobatae) and *Jin Yin Hua* (Flos Lonicerae Japonicae) for the presence

of an exterior syndrome. Of 80 cases, the study reported complete recovery in 49 cases, significant improvement in 22 cases, moderate improvement in 3 cases, and no change in 6 cases. The overall success rate was 92.5%.[1]

AUTHORS' COMMENTS

Liu Yi San (Six-to-One Powder) and *Gui Ling Gan Lu Yin* both dispel summer-heat and dampness, but have the following differences:

• *Liu Yi San* contains only *Hua Shi* (Talcum) and *Gan Cao* (Radix et Rhizoma Glycyrrhizae), and its effect is thus weaker. It is mainly used as the base formula for summer-damp invasion with feverish sensations, thirst, irritability, and dysuria or diarrhea.

• *Gui Ling Gan Lu Yin* combines *Liu Yi San* (Six-to-One Powder) with *Wu Ling San* (Five-Ingredient Powder with Poria), *Shi Gao* (Gypsum Fibrosum), and *Han Shui Shi* (Mirabilite). Thus, it more strongly clears heat and dispels dampness. It is mainly used for summer-heat with dampness in patients who have interior water retention manifesting in fever, headache, thirst with a desire to drink, irritability, dysuria, vomiting, and/or diarrhea.[2]

References

1. *Zhong Xi Yi Jie He Za Zhi* (Journal of Integrated Chinese and Western Medicine) 1985;1:19.
2. Wang MZ, et al. *Zhong Yi Xue Wen Da Ti Ku* (Questions and Answers on Traditional Chinese Medicine: Herbal Formulas).

Chapter 6 – Summer-Heat-Dispelling Formulas

Qīng Shŭ Yì Qì Tāng
(Clear Summer-Heat and Augment the Qi Decoction)

清暑益氣湯
清暑益气汤

Pinyin Name: *Qing Shu Yi Qi Tang*
Literal Name: Clear Summer-Heat and Augment the Qi Decoction
Alternate Names: *Ching Shu I Chi Tang, Ching Shu Yi Chi Tang,* Summer-heat-clearing and Chi-tonifying Decoction, Astragalus and Atractylodes Combination
Original Source: *Wen Re Jing Wei* (Warp and Woof of Warm-Febrile Diseases) by Wang Meng-Ying in 1852

COMPOSITION

Xi Yang Shen (Radix Panacis Quinquefolii)	[5g]
Xi Gua Cui Pi (Exocarpium Citrulli)	[30g]
He Geng (Caulis Nelumbinis)	[15g]
Shi Hu (Caulis Dendrobii)	[15g]
Mai Dong (Radix Ophiopogonis)	[9g]
Zhi Mu (Rhizoma Anemarrhenae)	[6g]
Zhu Ye (Herba Phyllostachys)	[6g]
Huang Lian (Rhizoma Coptidis)	[3g]
Geng Mi (Semen Oryzae)	[15g]
Gan Cao (Radix et Rhizoma Glycyrrhizae)	[3g]

DOSAGE / PREPARATION / ADMINISTRATION

The herb doses are unavailable from the source text. Today, this formula may be prepared as a decoction with the doses suggested in brackets.

CHINESE THERAPEUTIC ACTIONS

1. Dispels summer-heat
2. Tonifies qi, nourishes yin, and generates body fluids

CLINICAL MANIFESTATIONS

Summer-heat damaging both qi and body fluids: fever, profuse perspiration, irritability, thirst, scanty, dark-colored urine, lethargy, shortness of breath, and a deficient, rapid pulse.

CLINICAL APPLICATIONS

Common cold in the summer, summer fever in children, heat stroke, febrile disorders, pneumonia, asthma, wheezing and dyspnea, chronic fatigue syndrome, lassitude of extremities, thirst, and loss of appetite.

EXPLANATION

Qing Shu Yi Qi Tang (Clear Summer-Heat and Augment the Qi Decoction) treats summer-heat syndromes with damage to both qi and body fluids. In this syndrome, excess heat forces body fluids out of the body, causing fever and profuse perspiration. The profuse perspiration may extensively consume and damage body fluids, leading to irritability, thirst, and dark, scanty urine. Qi travels with body fluids and may be lost and become deficient as a result of excess perspiration. Lethargy and shortness of breath are both signs of qi deficiency. A deficient, rapid pulse suggests qi deficiency and heat in the body.

Xi Yang Shen (Radix Panacis Quinquefolii), as a chief herb, clears heat and tonifies qi, yin and body fluids. *Xi Gua Cui Pi* (Exocarpium Citrulli), as the other chief herb of this formula, clears heat and resolves summer-heat. *He Geng* (Caulis Nelumbinis) helps *Xi Gua Cui Pi* (Exocarpium Citrulli) clear summer-heat. *Shi Hu* (Caulis Dendrobii) and *Mai Dong* (Radix Ophiopogonis) help *Xi Yang Shen* (Radix Panacis Quinquefolii) clear heat and nourish yin. *Zhi Mu* (Rhizoma Anemarrhenae) and *Zhu Ye* (Herba Phyllostachys) clear heat and relieve irritability. *Geng Mi* (Semen Oryzae) and *Gan Cao* (Radix et Rhizoma Glycyrrhizae) tonify qi and nourish the Stomach.

Although *Huang Lian* (Rhizoma Coptidis) is listed as an ingredient in this formula, use it cautiously as its bitter and cold nature may easily damage yin and body fluids. If the patient has only mild symptoms of summer-heat but severe symptoms of body fluids damage, omit *Huang Lian* (Rhizoma Coptidis) from the formula.

MODIFICATIONS

• When there is severe perspiration, add *Fu Xiao Mai* (Fructus Tritici Levis).

446

Qīng Shŭ Yì Qì Tāng
(Clear Summer-Heat and Augment the Qi Decoction)

Qing Shu Yi Qi Tang (Clear Summer-Heat and Augment the Qi Decoction)

Diagnosis	Signs and Symptoms	Treatment	Herbs
Summer-heat damaging both qi and body fluids	• Fever and profuse perspiration: summer-heat forcing body fluids out of the body • Irritability, thirst, and dark, scanty urine: summer-heat consuming body fluids • Lethargy and shortness of breath: summer-heat damaging qi • Deficient, rapid pulse: presence of deficiency and excess	• Dispels summer-heat • Tonifies qi, nourishes yin, and generates body fluids	• *Xi Yang Shen* (Radix Panacis Quinquefolii) tonifies qi, yin, and body fluids. • *Xi Gua Cui Pi* (Exocarpium Citrulli) and *He Geng* (Caulis Nelumbinis) strongly clear summer-heat. • *Shi Hu* (Caulis Dendrobii) and *Mai Dong* (Radix Ophiopogonis) nourish yin and body fluids. • *Zhi Mu* (Rhizoma Anemarrhenae) and *Zhu Ye* (Herba Phyllostachys) clear heat to relieve irritability. • *Geng Mi* (Semen Oryzae) and *Gan Cao* (Radix et Rhizoma Glycyrrhizae) tonify qi.

- With dysuria, add *Di Huang* (Radix Rehmanniae) and *Mu Tong* (Caulis Akebiae).
- With irritability, dryness and heat, add *Yin Chen* (Herba Artemisiae Scopariae) and *Zhi Zi* (Fructus Gardeniae).
- With deficiency of body fluids, add *Ge Gen* (Radix Puerariae Lobatae) and *Sha Shen* (Radix Glehniae seu Adenophorae).
- If there is qi deficiency, add *Ren Shen* (Radix et Rhizoma Ginseng) and *Huang Qi* (Radix Astragali).

CAUTIONS / CONTRAINDICATIONS

Qing Shu Yi Qi Tang is inappropriate in cases of summer-heat accompanied by dampness because it contains yin-tonic herbs such as *Mai Dong* (Radix Ophiopogonis) and *Zhi Mu* (Rhizoma Anemarrhenae).

CLINICAL STUDIES AND RESEARCH

1. **Wheezing and dyspnea**: In one clinical study, 76 patients with wheezing and dyspnea during the summer were treated with modified *Qing Shu Yi Qi Tang*. The formula included *Xi Yang Shen* (Radix Panacis Quinquefolii) 20g, *Di Long* (Pheretima) 20g, *Shi Hu* (Caulis Dendrobii) 15g, *Mai Dong* (Radix Ophiopogonis) 15g, *Zhu Ye* (Herba Phyllostachys) 15g, *Zhi Mu* (Rhizoma Anemarrhenae) 15g, *Di Huang* (Radix Rehmanniae) 10g, *Gan Cao* (Radix et Rhizoma Glycyrrhizae) 10g, *Xi Gua Cui Pi* (Exocarpium Citrulli) 10g, and addition of others as deemed necessary per condition of the patient. The treatment protocol was to boil the herbs in water, and ingest the decoction in two equal portions. Out of 76 cases, the study reported stabilization in 22 cases (no wheezing or dyspnea for the entire year), significant improvement in 34 cases (no wheezing or dyspnea for the current season), moderate improvement in 15 cases (still requiring other treatment), and no effect in 5 cases. The overall rate of effectiveness was 93.4%.[1]

2. **Pneumonia**: Fourteen patients with pneumonia were treated with modified *Qing Shu Yi Qi Tang* with complete recovery in 12 patients and no benefit in 2 patients. The formula used included fresh *He Ye* (Folium Nelumbinis) 30g, fresh *Xi Gua Cui Pi* (Exocarpium Citrulli) 60g, *Zhu Ye* (Herba Phyllostachys) 12g, *Shi Hu* (Caulis Dendrobii) 12g, *Mai Dong* (Radix Ophiopogonis) 12g, *Zhi Mu* (Rhizoma Anemarrhenae) 12g, *Jin Yin Hua* (Flos Lonicerae Japonicae) 18g, *Lian Qiao* (Fructus Forsythiae) 18g, *Huang Qin* (Radix Scutellariae) 15g, *Lu Gen* (Rhizoma Phragmitis) 15g, *Pi Pa Ye* (Folium Eriobotryae) 24g, *Ren Shen* (Radix et Rhizoma Ginseng) 9-12g, *Gan Cao* (Radix et Rhizoma Glycyrrhizae) 6g, and the addition of others as deemed necessary per condition of the patient. Complete recovery was defined as reduction of body temperature to normal within 12-72 hours with normal count of white blood cells within 24-72 hours.[2]

3. **Chronic fatigue syndrome**: Administration of modified *Qing Shu Yi Qi Tang* was effective in treating chronic fatigue syndrome characterized by Spleen qi deficiency with accumulation of dampness. The treatment protocol was to administer the herbs in decoction three times daily, for 7 days per course of treatment, for 2 courses total. The study reported 80% effectiveness.[3]

Chapter 6 – Summer-Heat-Dispelling Formulas

Qīng Shŭ Yì Qì Tāng
(Clear Summer-Heat and Augment the Qi Decoction)

RELATED FORMULA

Qīng Shŭ Yì Qì Tāng
(Clear Summer-Heat and Augment the Qi Decoction)

清暑益氣湯
清暑益气汤

Pinyin Name: *Qing Shu Yi Qi Tang*

Literal Name: Clear Summer-Heat and Augment the Qi Decoction

Original Source: *Pi Wei Lun* (Discussion of the Spleen and Stomach) by Li Gao in 1249

Huang Qi (Radix Astragali)	3g [6g]
Cang Zhu (Rhizoma Atractylodis), *jin* (soaked)	3g [3g]
Sheng Ma (Rhizoma Cimicifugae)	3g [3g]
Ren Shen (Radix et Rhizoma Ginseng)	1.5g [1.5g]
Ze Xie (Rhizoma Alismatis)	1.5g [3g]
Shen Qu (Massa Fermentata), *chao* (dry-fried)	1.5g [3g]
Chen Pi (Pericarpium Citri Reticulatae)	1.5g [1.5g]
Bai Zhu (Rhizoma Atractylodis Macrocephalae)	1.5g [3g]
Mai Dong (Radix Ophiopogonis)	0.9g [3g]
Dang Gui (Radix Angelicae Sinensis)	0.9g [1g]
Zhi Gan Cao (Radix et Rhizoma Glycyrrhizae Praeparata cum Melle)	0.9g [1g]
Qing Pi (Pericarpium Citri Reticulatae Viride)	0.75g [1g]
Huang Bo (Cortex Phellodendri Chinensis), *xi* (washed) with liquor	0.6-0.9g [3g]
Ge Gen (Radix Puerariae Lobatae)	0.6g [6g]
Wu Wei Zi (Fructus Schisandrae Chinensis)	9 pieces [1.5g]

The source text states to grind the herbs into powder, and cook it in 2 large bowls of water until it is reduced to 1 bowl. Take the warm, strained decoction on an empty stomach. Today, this formula may be prepared as a decoction with the doses suggested in brackets.

This formula has the identical name as the previous formula, but they are derived from different sources and have slightly different compositions and applications. Therefore, it is very important that the two are not confused or used interchangeably. A comparative analysis of these two formulas is provided in the Authors' Comments section.

This formula clears summer-heat, dries dampness, benefits qi, and strengthens the Spleen. Clinically, it is often used for patients with exterior summer-heat and underlying chronic qi deficiency. Patients may show symptoms such as a warm sensation throughout the body, headache, thirst, spontaneous perspiration, lethargy, lack of appetite, chest fullness, heaviness of the body, loose stools, dysuria, a greasy tongue coating, and a deficient pulse.

This formula has been used to treat chronic nonspecific colitis. According to one study, use of herbs was associated with good results in treating five patients with chronic nonspecific ulcerative colitis and seven with chronic nonspecific non-ulcerative colitis. The herbal formula was modified slightly, and contained the following ingredients: *Huang Qi* (Radix Astragali) 15g, *Dang Shen* (Radix Codonopsis) 15g, *Bai Zhu* (Rhizoma Atractylodis Macrocephalae) 8g, *Cang Zhu* (Rhizoma Atractylodis) 8g, *Dang Gui* (Radix Angelicae Sinensis) 8g, *Huang Bo* (Cortex Phellodendri Chinensis) 8g, *Ze Xie* (Rhizoma Alismatis) 8g, *Qing Pi* (Pericarpium Citri Reticulatae Viride) 5g, *Chen Pi* (Pericarpium Citri Reticulatae) 5g, *Sheng Ma* (Rhizoma Cimicifugae) 5g, *Ge Gen* (Radix Puerariae Lobatae) 24g, *Shen Qu* (Massa Fermentata) 6g, *Gan Cao* (Radix et Rhizoma Glycyrrhizae) 6g, *Mai Dong* (Radix Ophiopogonis) 10g, and *Wu Wei Zi* (Fructus Schisandrae Chinensis) 3g. Additional modifications were made as deemed necessary. The treatment protocol was to administer the herbs in decoction daily on an empty stomach, for two weeks per course of treatment. Of 12 cases, the study reported complete recovery in 2 cases, significant improvement in 6 cases, moderate improvement in 3 cases, and no benefit in 1 case. The overall rate of effectiveness was 91.67%.[4]

AUTHORS' COMMENTS

The primary and the related formulas have identical names: the former is also known as Wang's *Qing Shu Yi Qi Tang*, and the latter is referred to as Li's *Qing Shu Yi Qi Tang*.

Both formulas have the same name, and have similar compositions and functions to clear summer-heat and augment the qi. Their differences are as follows:

• *Qing Shu Yi Qi Tang* from *Wen Re Jing Wei* (Warp and Woof of Warm-Febrile Diseases) by Wang Meng-Ying, treats summer-heat damaging both qi and body fluids.

• *Qing Shu Yi Qi Tang* from *Pi Wei Lun* (Discussion of the Spleen and Stomach) by Li Gao, treats chronic qi deficiency complicated by exterior summer-heat.

References

1. *Shan Xi Yi Kan* (Shanxi Journal of Medicine) 1992;3:104.
2. *Zhe Jiang Zhong Yi Za Zhi* (Zhejiang Journal of Chinese Medicine) 1984;8:352.
3. *Yun Nan Zhong Yi Zhong Yao Za Zhi* (Yunan Journal of Chinese Medicine and Medicinals) 1997;6:4.
4. *Si Chuan Zhong Yi* (Sichuan Chinese Medicine) 1991;5:29.

Chinese Herbal Formulas and Applications

Chapter 6 — Summary

— Summer-Heat-Dispelling Formulas

Name	Similarities	Differences
Qing Luo Yin (Clear the Collaterals Decoction)	Dispels summer-heat, clears interior heat	Treats mild summer-heat syndromes
Xiang Ru San (Mosla Powder)	Dispel summer-heat, release the exterior	Treats summer-heat syndromes with cold and dampness
Xin Jia Xiang Ru Yin (Newly-Augmented Mosla Decoction)		Treats summer-heat syndromes with cold, dampness, and heat
Liu Yi San (Six-to-One Powder)	Dispel summer-heat, drain dampness	Mild in potency
Gui Ling Gan Lu Yin (Cinnamon and Poria Sweet Dew Decoction)		Moderate to strong in potency
Qing Shu Yi Qi Tang (Clear Summer-Heat and Augment the Qi Decoction)	Dispels summer-heat, tonifies qi, yin and body fluids	Treats summer-heat syndromes involving both excess and deficiency

Qing Luo Yin (Clear the Collaterals Decoction) relieves summer-heat and clears interior heat. The herbs in this formula are of light quality and are able to penetrate and clear interior heat. It is most suitable for treating mild summer-heat syndromes in which only the Lung is affected.

Xiang Ru San (Mosla Powder) and **Xin Jia Xiang Ru Yin** (Newly-Augmented Mosla Decoction) both relieve summer-heat and dispel exterior factors.
• *Xiang Ru San* is a warmer formula and is better for initial summer-heat syndromes with wind-cold and dampness.
• *Xin Jia Xiang Ru Yin* is a colder formula, and has a stronger effect to treat initial summer-heat syndromes with cold and dampness, but with indications of more heat.

Liu Yi San (Six-to-One Powder) and **Gui Ling Gan Lu Yin** (Cinnamon and Poria Sweet Dew Decoction) both relieve summer-heat and dispel dampness. Both treat summer-heat syndromes accompanied by dampness.
• *Liu Yi San* has mild potency and is considered a base formula for many other summer-heat-dispelling formulas.
• *Gui Ling Gan Lu Yin* is stronger and is more suitable for treating more serious cases.

Qing Shu Yi Qi Tang (Clear Summer-Heat and Augment the Qi Decoction) treats summer-heat syndromes with extensive damage to qi and body fluids.

Chapter 7

— Interior-Warming Formulas

王叔和 Wāng Shū-Hē

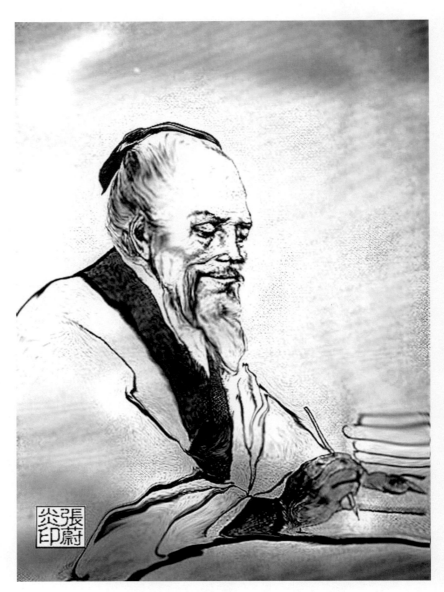

王叔和 Wāng Shū-Hē, third century.[1]

王叔和 Wāng Shū-Hē

Wang Shu-He is best known for preserving 伤寒杂病论 *Shang Han Za Bing Lun* (Discussion of Cold-Induced Disorders and Miscellaneous Diseases) by Zhang Zhong-Jing. Shortly after this text was published, it was lost during war time in the Eastern Han dynasty and the time of the Three Kingdoms. Realizing the tremendous importance of this text, Wang gathered bits and pieces of it wherever he could, re-organized it, and published it in two volumes:

- 伤寒论 *Shang Han Lun* (Discussion of Cold-Induced Disorders) emphasizes external disorders, classifying them according to *Liu Jing Bian Zheng* (Six Stages Differentiation).
- 金匮要略 *Jin Gui Yao Lue* (Essentials from the Golden Cabinet) focuses on internal and miscellaneous disease, classifying them according to *Ba Gang Bian Zheng* (Eight Principle Differentiation).

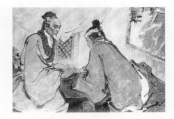

Wang Shu-He taking a patient's pulse.

Without Wang's effort, Zhang Zhong-Jing's work would have been lost altogether, or, at best, incomplete.

Wang also wrote one of the most significant texts on pulse diagnosis, 脉经 *Mai Jing* (Pulse Classics). Though there were many references to pulse and their indications in historical texts before his time, most references were scattered and disorganized. After studying the *Nei Jing* (Inner Classic), the *Nan Jing* (Classic of Difficult Issues), *Shang Han Za Bing Lun* (Discussion of Cold-Induced Disorders and Miscellaneous Diseases) and references from Hua Tuo, Wang published *Mai Jing* (Pulse Classics), the first comprehensive text that systemically stated the proper definitions of pulse-related terminology and techniques for pulse diagnosis. It established the proper positions for pulse assessment and their relationship to the *zang fu* organs. It also clearly defined 24 different pulse qualities and their meanings. Lastly, it emphasized the importance of correlating the pulse to the age, sex, height, weight, and disease pattern of the patient.

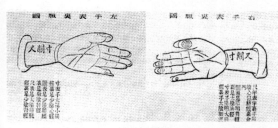

Pulse positions and definitions from 脉经 *Mai Jing* (Pulse Classics), third century.[2]

Dynasties & Kingdoms	Year
Xia Dynasty 夏	2100-1600 BCE
Shang Dynasty 商	1600-1100 BCE
Zhou Dynasty 周	1100-221 BCE
Qin Dynasty 秦	221-207 BCE
Han Dynasty 漢	206 BCE-220
Three Kingdoms 三國	**220-280**
Western Jin Dynasty 西晉	265-316
Eastern Jin Dynasty 東晉	317-420
Northern and Southern Dynasties 北南朝	420-581
Sui Dynasty 隋	581-618
Tang Dynasty 唐	618-907
Five Dynasties 五代	907-960
Song Dynasty 宋	960-1279
Liao Dynasty 遼	916-1125
Jin Dynasty 金	1115-1234
Yuan Dynasty 元	1271-1368
Ming Dynasty 明	1368-1644
Qing Dynasty 清	1644-1911
Republic of China 中華民國	1912-Present Day
People's Republic of China 中華人民共和國	1949-Present Day

1. Exact dates of birth and death are unknown.
2. Exact date of publication is unknown.

Chapter 7 – Interior-Warming Formulas

Table of Contents

Chapter 7. Interior-Warming Formulas ⸱⸱ **451**
Biography of Wang Shu-He ⸱⸱⸱ 452

Section 1. Middle-Warming and Cold-Dispelling Formulas ⸱⸱⸱⸱⸱⸱⸱⸱⸱⸱⸱⸱⸱⸱⸱⸱⸱⸱⸱ **459**
Li Zhong Wan (Regulate the Middle Pill) ⸱⸱⸱ 459
  Ren Shen Tang (Ginseng Decoction) ⸱⸱ 462
  Li Zhong Hua Tan Wan (Regulate the Middle and Transform Phlegm Pill) ⸱⸱⸱⸱⸱⸱ 462
Fu Zi Li Zhong Wan (Prepared Aconite Pill to Regulate the Middle) ⸱⸱⸱⸱⸱⸱⸱⸱⸱⸱⸱⸱⸱⸱⸱ 463
Gui Zhi Ren Shen Tang (Cinnamon Twig and Ginseng Decoction) ⸱⸱⸱⸱⸱⸱⸱⸱⸱⸱⸱⸱⸱⸱⸱⸱⸱⸱ 466
Wu Zhu Yu Tang (Evodia Decoction) ⸱⸱⸱ 467
Xiao Jian Zhong Tang (Minor Construct the Middle Decoction) ⸱⸱⸱⸱⸱⸱⸱⸱⸱⸱⸱⸱⸱⸱⸱⸱⸱⸱⸱⸱ 471
  Dang Gui Jian Zhong Tang (Tangkuei Decoction to Construct the Middle) ⸱⸱⸱⸱⸱⸱⸱⸱ 473
Huang Qi Jian Zhong Tang (Astragalus Decoction to Construct the Middle) ⸱⸱⸱⸱⸱⸱⸱⸱ 475
Gui Qi Jian Zhong Tang (Tangkuei and Astragalus Decoction to Construct the Middle) ⸱⸱⸱⸱ 479
Da Jian Zhong Tang (Major Construct the Middle Decoction) ⸱⸱⸱⸱⸱⸱⸱⸱⸱⸱⸱⸱⸱⸱⸱⸱⸱⸱⸱⸱⸱⸱⸱ 480
An Zhong San (Calm the Middle Powder) ⸱⸱⸱ 484

Section 2. Yang-Resuscitating Formulas ⸱⸱⸱⸱⸱⸱⸱⸱⸱⸱⸱⸱⸱⸱⸱⸱⸱⸱⸱⸱⸱⸱⸱⸱⸱⸱⸱⸱⸱⸱⸱⸱⸱ **486**
Si Ni Tang (Frigid Extremities Decoction) ⸱⸱⸱ 486
  Si Ni Jia Ren Shen Tang (Frigid Extremities Decoction plus Ginseng) ⸱⸱⸱⸱⸱⸱⸱⸱⸱⸱⸱⸱ 488
  Tong Mai Si Ni Tang (Unblock the Pulse Decoction for Frigid Extremities) ⸱⸱⸱⸱⸱⸱⸱⸱ 488
  Bai Tong Tang (White Penetrating Decoction) ⸱⸱⸱⸱⸱⸱⸱⸱⸱⸱⸱⸱⸱⸱⸱⸱⸱⸱⸱⸱⸱⸱⸱⸱⸱⸱⸱⸱⸱⸱⸱⸱⸱⸱ 489
  Shen Fu Tang (Ginseng and Prepared Aconite Decoction) ⸱⸱⸱⸱⸱⸱⸱⸱⸱⸱⸱⸱⸱⸱⸱⸱⸱⸱⸱⸱⸱⸱⸱ 489
Hui Yang Jiu Ji Tang (Restore and Revive the Yang Decoction) ⸱⸱⸱⸱⸱⸱⸱⸱⸱⸱⸱⸱⸱⸱⸱⸱⸱⸱⸱⸱ 490
Hei Xi Dan (Lead Special Pill) ⸱⸱ 492

Section 3. Channel-Warming and Cold-Dispersing Formulas ⸱⸱⸱⸱⸱⸱⸱⸱⸱⸱⸱⸱⸱⸱⸱⸱ **494**
Dang Gui Si Ni Tang (Tangkuei Decoction for Frigid Extremities) ⸱⸱⸱⸱⸱⸱⸱⸱⸱⸱⸱⸱⸱⸱⸱⸱⸱⸱ 494
  Dang Gui Si Ni Jia Wu Zhu Yu Sheng Jiang Tang (Tangkuei Decoction for Frigid Extremities plus Evodia and Fresh Ginger) ⸱⸱⸱⸱ 498
Huang Qi Gui Zhi Wu Wu Tang (Astragalus and Cinnamon Twig Five-Substance Decoction) ⸱⸱⸱⸱⸱⸱⸱⸱⸱⸱ 500

Interior-Warming Formulas (Summary) ⸱⸱⸱⸱⸱⸱⸱⸱⸱⸱⸱⸱⸱⸱⸱⸱⸱⸱⸱⸱⸱⸱⸱⸱⸱⸱⸱⸱⸱⸱⸱⸱⸱⸱⸱⸱⸱ **504**

Chinese Herbal Formulas and Applications

Chapter 7 — Overview

— Interior-Warming Formulas

Definition: Interior-warming formulas warm the interior, raise the yang, disperse cold, and dredge the channels and collaterals. This method of treatment is known as *wen fa* (warming), one of the *ba fa* (eight treatment methods) described in the *Huang Di Nei Jing* (Yellow Emperor's Inner Classic) in the first or second century, A.D.

Interior-warming formulas mainly treat interior cold syndromes affecting *zang fu* organs or various channels and collaterals. General signs and symptoms of interior cold include aversion to cold, preference for warmth, a bland taste in the mouth, the absence of thirst, and clear urine. There are many causes of interior cold syndromes, all of which can be summarized as either internally generated, externally contracted, or both. When an individual has constitutional yang deficiency, cold may be generated internally. If an individual is exposed to a cold factor, it may enter the interior and directly attack the *zang fu* organs. Additionally, cold syndromes may occur secondarily to inappropriate treatment. For example, excessive or prolonged use of cold formulas may lead to yang qi damage and the formation of interior cold. Incorrect (or lack of) treatment of exterior cold causes it to migrate to the interior, and results in accumulation of interior cold. Regardless of the etiological origin, interior cold must be treated with hot herbs that warm the interior.

Note: Cold, one of the *liu yin* (six exogenous factors), can attack either the exterior or interior of the body. The presence of cold at the exterior (such as wind-cold) is treated with exterior-releasing herbs, which is discussed in Chapter 1: Exterior-Releasing Formulas. The presence of cold in the interior (interior cold) is treated with interior-warming formulas, as discussed in this chapter.

SUBCATEGORIES OF ACTION

Because interior cold syndromes manifest with different severities and in different locations, interior warming formulas are differentiated into three sub-categories:

> Interior cold syndromes can be generated internally, contracted from the exterior, or both.

1. Middle-Warming and Cold-Dispelling Formulas

These formulas are designed to treat deficiency cold syndromes affecting the middle *jiao*. The Spleen and Stomach reside in the middle *jiao* and belong to the Earth element. Together, they are responsible for the transformation and transportation of food, sending clear *gu* (food) qi to the upper *jiao* and turbid food particles to the lower *jiao*. If the yang qi of the middle *jiao* is weakened as a result of cold, the functioning of the Spleen and Stomach will be impaired. Main clinical manifestations include epigastric and abdominal fullness and pain, relief of pain with pressure and warmth, lethargy, fatigue, vomiting of saliva, coldness of the extremities, acid regurgitation, nausea, vomiting, diarrhea, loss of appetite, no thirst, and a bland taste in the mouth. The tongue coating is usually white and slippery. The pulse is either deep and fine or deep and slow.

Commonly used herbs in the middle-warming and cold-dispelling formulas are *Gan Jiang* (Rhizoma Zingiberis), *Wu Zhu Yu* (Fructus Evodiae), and *Hua Jiao* (Pericarpium Zanthoxyli). In addition, herbs that tonify qi and strengthen the Spleen are usually added to increase the effectiveness of the formulas, such as *Ren Shen* (Radix et Rhizoma Ginseng), *Bai Zhu* (Rhizoma Atractylodis Macrocephalae), and *Yi Tang* (Maltosum). Exemplar formulas include *Li Zhong Wan* (Regulate the

455

Chapter 7 — Overview

Middle Pill), *Wu Zhu Yu Tang* (Evodia Decoction), *Xiao Jian Zhong Tang* (Minor Construct the Middle Decoction), and *Da Jian Zhong Tang* (Major Construct the Middle Decoction).

> Interior-warming formulas restore normal organ functioning in gastrointestinal and cardiovascular disorders.

2. Yang-Resuscitating Formulas

These formulas recuperate depleted Heart and Kidney yang and rescue patients from collapse. They are used to treat exhausted yang qi with cold affecting both the interior and the exterior. Because the preponderance of yin consumes yang, the following symptoms appear: extremely cold limbs, aversion to cold, desire to curl up the body when lying down, vomiting, abdominal pain, diarrhea with undigested foods, extreme fatigue, and, in severe cases, profuse perspiration of cold sweats. The pulse will be either deep and fine, or deep and faint.

In order to rescue yang from depletion, large doses of hot and acrid herbs must be used. Frequently used herbs in this category include *Fu Zi* (Radix Aconiti Lateralis Praeparata), *Gan Jiang* (Rhizoma Zingiberis), and *Rou Gui* (Cortex Cinnamomi). Representative formulas that resuscitate yang include *Si Ni Tang* (Frigid Extremities Decoction) and *Hui Yang Jiu Ji Tang* (Restore and Revive the Yang Decoction).

In extreme cases, the depletion of yang and abundance of cold in the interior will block the circulation of yang qi to the interior and redirect it to the exterior, giving rise to the condition of "true cold" (in the interior) and "false heat" (at the exterior). In addition to the signs and symptoms listed above, clinical manifestations of "false heat" may include warm body sensations, dry heaves, irritability, restlessness, and pale, red cheeks. These patients may reject the warm decoction or interior-warming herbs by vomiting. In such cases, administer the decoction at room temperature, or add a small amount of cold herbs to the interior-warming formulas; these modifications usually help the patient to better tolerate the decoction. One representative formula that treats "true cold" and "false heat" is *Bai Tong Tang* (White Penetrating Decoction), with the addition of bile from *Zhu Dan* (Fel Porcus).

3. Channel-Warming and Cold-Dispersing Formulas

These formulas treat exterior cold that is blocking and damaging the channels and collaterals in individuals with underlying deficiencies of yang qi, yin and blood. Common signs and symptoms include extremely cold hands and feet, numbness and pain of the extremities, reduced mobility of the joints, and formation of *yin* (deep-rooted) sores.

> Interior cold syndromes manifest with differing severities and locations.

Using only acrid and hot herbs will not effectively treat such conditions. Instead, it is more appropriate to combine them with herbs that dispel cold, tonify the blood, and warm and unblock the channels and collaterals. Herbs commonly used include *Gui Zhi* (Ramulus Cinnamomi), *Xi Xin* (Radix et Rhizoma Asari), *Dang Gui* (Radix Angelicae Sinensis), *Bai Shao* (Radix Paeoniae Alba), *Huang Qi* (Radix Astragali), and *Shu Di Huang* (Radix Rehmanniae Praeparata). Exemplar formulas include *Dang Gui Si Ni Tang* (Tangkuei Decoction for Frigid Extremities), *Huang Qi Gui Zhi Wu Wu Tang* (Astragalus and Cinnamon Twig Five-Substance Decoction), and *Yang He Tang* (Yang-Heartening Decoction).

CAUTIONS / CONTRAINDICATIONS

- Interior-warming formulas are designed to disperse cold in the interior. If the cold is located at the exterior level, then exterior-releasing formulas should be used.
- It is extremely important to correctly diagnose the presence of cold in the body. Severe consequences can result if interior-warming formulas are used to treat excess heat syndromes.
- Because interior warming formulas consist of acrid and warm herbs, they must be used carefully if the patient has yin deficiency or bleeding syndromes. Inappropriate use of interior warming herbs may easily create heat in the interior, further damaging yin and blood.
- Because a cold factor can easily damage yang and qi, it may be necessary to include yang- and qi-tonifying herbs in interior-warming formulas.

Chapter 7 — Overview

• External factors should also be considered when prescribing interior-warming formulas. These formulas must be used with more caution during the summer, or in hot climates, and they must be discontinued immediately when the desired effects are achieved. On the other hand, they can be used at slightly larger dosages or for longer periods of time during the winter, or in cold climates.

PHARMACOLOGICAL EFFECTS & CLINICAL APPLICATIONS

Interior-warming formulas are divided into three subcategories based on their traditional therapeutic actions. These subcategories also have contrasting pharmacological effects and clinical applications.

> Severe consequences can result if interior-warming formulas are used to treat excess heat syndromes.

1. **Middle-warming and cold-dispelling formulas** treat deficiency and cold of the middle *jiao* (Spleen and Stomach). From the perspective of allopathic medicine, these formulas are most effective in treating disorders of the gastrointestinal tract.

• **Gastrointestinal disorders**: These formulas treat a wide variety of gastrointestinal disorders, including but not limited to nausea,[1] vomiting,[2] anorexia,[3] diarrhea,[4] dysentery,[5] constipation,[6] peptic ulcer,[7,8,9] gastritis (atrophic gastritis, superficial gastritis, gastritis with ulcer),[10] enteritis,[11] ulcerative colitis,[12,13] irritable bowel syndrome,[14] obstructive bowel disease,[15] intestinal obstruction,[16] and post-operative ileus.[17] The mechanisms of action have been attributed in part to the antiulcer effects of these formulas to inhibit the production of gastric acid,[18] their analgesic effects to relieve pain,[19] and their antiemetic effects to relieve nausea and vomiting.[20] Specific pharmacological effects vary depending on the formula and the disease. Representative formulas include *Li Zhong Wan* (Regulate the Middle Pill), *Fu Zi Li Zhong Wan* (Prepared Aconite Pill to Regulate the Middle), *Xiao Jian Zhong Tang* (Minor Construct the Middle Decoction), and *Da Jian Zhong Tang* (Major Construct the Middle Decoction).

• **Others**: These formulas have also been used to treat other conditions that are associated with gastrointestinal disorders, such as stomatitis,[21] profuse salivation,[22] epigastric pain,[23] abdominal pain,[24,25] and a feeling of coldness in the abdomen.[26]

2. **Yang-resuscitating formulas** are used primarily to restore normal cardiovascular functions in patients who suffer acute heart attack.

• **Acute cardiac infarction**: *Si Ni Tang* (Frigid Extremities Decoction) has a marked effect on the cardiovascular system to increase the contractile force of the heart, increase blood pressure, and restore normal heart rhythm.[27] Clinically, it has been used to treat patients with acute cardiac infarction, with good success.[28]

3. **Channel-warming and cold-dispersing formulas** treat exterior cold that is blocking and damaging the channels and collaterals. From the perspective of allopathic medicine, these formulas are most effective in treating pain.

• **Pain**: These formulas are commonly used to treat many types and presentations of pain, such as headaches,[29] cancer pain,[30] sciatica,[31] frostbite,[32,33] peripheral neuritis,[34,35] diabetic neuropathy,[36] periarthritis of shoulder,[37,38] frozen shoulder,[39] neck and shoulder stiffness and pain,[40] and general aches and pains.[41] Exemplar formulas include *Dang Gui Si Ni Tang* (Tangkuei Decoction for Frigid Extremities) and *Huang Qi Gui Zhi Wu Wu Tang* (Astragalus and Cinnamon Twig Five-Substance Decoction).

References

1. *Zhong Cheng Yao Yan Jiu* (Research of Chinese Patent Medicine) 1985;1:46.
2. *Hu Nan Zhong Yi Za Zhi* (Hunan Journal of Chinese Medicine) 1998;2:42.
3. *He Nan Zhong Yi* (Henan Chinese Medicine) 1998;2:51.
4. *Gan Su Zhong Yi* (Gansu Chinese Medicine) 1993;2:22.
5. *Shan Dong Zhong Yi Za Zhi* (Shandong Journal of Chinese Medicine) 1983;2:21.
6. *Liao Ning Zhong Yi Za Zhi* (Liaoning Journal of Chinese Medicine) 1984;4:29.
7. *An Hui Zhong Yi Xue Yuan Xue Bao* (Journal of Anhui University School of Medicine) 1988;1:29.
8. *Zhe Jiang Zhong Yi Yao* (Zhejiang Chinese Medicine and Herbology) 1978;2:9.

Chapter 7 — Overview

9. *Ji Lin Zhong Yi Yao* (Jilin Chinese Medicine and Herbology) 1996;5:10.

10. *Jiang Xi Zhong Yi Yao* (Jiangxi Chinese Medicine and Herbology) 1981;3:32.

11. *Shang Hai Zhong Yi Yao Za Zhi* (Shanghai Journal of Chinese Medicine and Herbology) 1984;6:45.

12. *Zhong Yi Fang Ji Xian Dai Yan Jiu* (Modern Study of Medical Formulae in Traditional Chinese Medicine) 1997;1:14.

13. *Bei Jing Zhong Yi* (Beijing Chinese Medicine) 1997;1:19.

14. *Shi Yong Zhong Xi Yi Jie He Za Zhi* (Practical Journal of Integrated Chinese and Western Medicines) 1998;6:560.

15. Ohya T, Usui Y, Arii S, Iwai T, Susumu T. Effect of dai-kenchu-to on obstructive bowel disease in children. Am J Chin Med 2003;31(1):129-35.

16. *Guo Wai Yi Xue* (Foreign Medicine) 1993;15(5):39.

17. Hayakawa T, Kase Y, Saito K, Hashimoto K, Ishige A, Komatsu Y, Sasaki H. Effects of Dai-kenchu-to on intestinal obstruction following laparotomy. J Smooth Muscle Res 1999 Apr;35(2):47-54.

18. *Shan Dong Zhong Yi Za Zhi* (Shandong Journal of Chinese Medicine) 1984;2:22.

19. *Zhong Cheng Yao* (Study of Chinese Patent Medicine) 1990;5:25.

20. *Zhong Yi Fang Ji Xian Dai Yan Jiu* (Modern Study of Medical Formulae in Traditional Chinese Medicine) 1997; 378.

21. *Zhe Jiang Zhong Yi Za Zhi* (Zhejiang Journal of Chinese Medicine) 1992;10:474.

22. *Guang Xi Zhong Yi Yao* (Guangxi Chinese Medicine and Herbology) 1992;2:15.

23. *Shan Xi Zhong Yi* (Shanxi Chinese Medicine) 1984;5(1):13.

24. *Shan Xi Zhong Yi* (Shanxi Chinese Medicine) 1992;12:537.

25. *Ji Lin Zhong Yi Yao* (Jilin Chinese Medicine and Herbology) 1997;2:19.

26. Nagano T, Itoh H, Takeyama M. Effects of Dai-kenchu-to on levels of 5-hydroxytryptamine (serotonin) and vasoactive intestinal peptides in human plasma. Biol Pharm Bull 2000 Mar;23(3):352-3.

27. *Zhong Yi Fang Ji Xian Dai Yan Jiu* (Modern Study of Medical Formulae in Traditional Chinese Medicine) 1997;394-395.

28. *Tian Jin Yi Yao Tong Xun* (Publication of Tianjin Medicine and Herbology) 1972;11:1.

29. *Tian Jin Zhong Yi* (Tianjin Chinese Medicine) 1985;6:25.

30. *Zhong Yi Fang Ji Xian Dai Yan Jiu* (Modern Study of Medical Formulae in Traditional Chinese Medicine) 1997;424.

31. *Hu Nan Zhong Yi Za Zhi* (Hunan Journal of Chinese Medicine) 1997;2:48.

32. *Shan Dong Zhong Yi Za Zhi* (Shandong Journal of Chinese Medicine) 1984;2:37.

33. *Shan Dong Zhong Yi Za Zhi* (Shandong Journal of Chinese Medicine) 1990;3:49.

34. *Xin Zhong Yi* (New Chinese Medicine) 1996;2:46.

35. *Zhong Yi Yao Xin Xi* (Information on Chinese Medicine and Herbology) 1998;2:40.

36. *Hei Long Jiang Zhong Yi Yao* (Heilongjiang Chinese Medicine and Herbology) 1998;4:17.

37. *Xin Zhong Yi* (New Chinese Medicine) 1987;7:53.

38. *Si Chuan Zhong Yi* (Sichuan Chinese Medicine) 1993;1:40.

39. *Si Chuan Zhong Yi* (Sichuan Chinese Medicine) 1989;2:31.

40. *Shi Zhen Guo Yao Yan Jiu* (Research of Shizhen Herbs) 1999;5:362.

41. *Hu Nan Zhong Yi Za Zhi* (Hunan Journal of Chinese Medicine) 1997;6:29.

Chinese Herbal Formulas and Applications

Section 1

温中祛寒剂
— Middle-Warming and Cold-Dispelling Formulas

Lǐ Zhōng Wán (Regulate the Middle Pill)
理中丸

Pinyin Name: *Li Zhong Wan*
Literal Name: Regulate the Middle Pill
Alternate Name: Ginseng and Ginger Combination
Original Source: *Shang Han Lun* (Discussion of Cold-Induced Disorders) by Zhang Zhong-Jing in the Eastern Han Dynasty

COMPOSITION

Gan Jiang (Rhizoma Zingiberis)	9g
Ren Shen (Radix et Rhizoma Ginseng)	9g
Bai Zhu (Rhizoma Atractylodis Macrocephalae)	9g
Zhi Gan Cao (Radix et Rhizoma Glycyrrhizae Praeparata cum Melle)	9g

DOSAGE / PREPARATION / ADMINISTRATION

The source text recommends to grind the ingredients into powder and form into pills with honey. The pills should resemble egg yolk in size. Take 1 pill with warm water three times during the day and twice at night. If ingestion of the pills does not create a feeling of warmth in the abdomen, then this formula may also be given as a decoction.

CHINESE THERAPEUTIC ACTIONS

1. Warms the middle *jiao* and dispels cold
2. Tonifies qi and strengthens the Spleen and Stomach

CLINICAL MANIFESTATIONS

1. Deficiency and cold of the middle *jiao*: absence of thirst, vomiting, diarrhea, abdominal pain, lack of appetite, and *huo luan* (sudden turmoil disorder).
2. Bleeding due to yang deficiency: epistaxis, hematochezia, shortness of breath, lassitude, and a fine pulse or a deficient, big pulse with little force.
3. Others: chronic infantile convulsions; and recovery from illness with drooling of saliva or excessive production of foamy saliva.

CLINICAL APPLICATIONS

Acute or chonic gastritis, gastric or duodenal ulcers, epigastric pain, gastroptosis, stomatitis, irritable bowel syndrome, gastroenteritis, enteritis, bacterial dysentery, colitis, uterine bleeding, nephropathy, male infertility, and excessive salivation.

EXPLANATION

Li Zhong Wan (Regulate the Middle Pill) treats deficiency and cold of the middle *jiao*, where the Spleen and Stomach are located. The Spleen, responsible for transportation and transformation, raises the clear yang. The Stomach, responsible for accepting and digesting food, lowers the turbid yin. If the middle *jiao* is deficient as a result of coldness, the ascending and descending functions of the Spleen and Stomach may be impaired, causing diarrhea and vomiting. Abdominal pain is due to the presence of coldness. Lack of appetite is the result of deficiency of the middle *jiao* and impaired digestive functioning.

To treat this syndrome, use herbs to warm the middle *jiao*, dispel coldness, tonify Spleen qi, and invigorate the digestive function. *Gan Jiang* (Rhizoma Zingiberis), the chief herb, warms the middle *jiao* and dispels interior cold. *Ren Shen* (Radix et Rhizoma Ginseng) nourishes *yuan* (source) qi. *Bai Zhu* (Rhizoma Atractylodis Macrocephalae) strengthens the Spleen and dries dampness. *Zhi Gan Cao* (Radix et Rhizoma Glycyrrhizae Praeparata cum Melle) nourishes qi and harmonizes the middle *jiao*.

Li Zhong Wan can also be used to treat blood loss due to Spleen yang deficiency; a deficient Spleen fails to keep

459

Chapter 7 – Interior-Warming Formulas　　　　　　*Section 1 – Middle-Warming and Cold-Dispelling Formulas*

Lǐ Zhōng Wán (Regulate the Middle Pill)

Li Zhong Wan (Regulate the Middle Pill)

Diagnosis	Signs and Symptoms	Treatment	Herbs
Deficiency and cold of the middle *jiao*	• Diarrhea and vomiting: deficiency and cold of the middle *jiao* impairing the normal ascending and descending functions of the Spleen and Stomach • Abdominal pain: cold in the middle *jiao*	• Warms the middle *jiao* and dispels cold • Tonifies qi and strengthens the Spleen	• *Gan Jiang* (Rhizoma Zingiberis) warms the middle *jiao* and dispels interior cold. • *Ren Shen* (Radix et Rhizoma Ginseng) nourishes *yuan* (source) *qi*. • *Bai Zhu* (Rhizoma Atractylodis Macrocephalae) strengthens the Spleen and dries dampness. • *Zhi Gan Cao* (Radix et Rhizoma Glycyrrhizae Praeparata cum Melle) nourishes qi and harmonizes the middle *jiao*.

blood circulating within the vessels. Clinical manifestations include epistaxis, hematochezia, shortness of breath, lassitude, a pale face, and a fine pulse or a deficient, big pulse with little force. This syndrome of bleeding due to yang deficiency can be treated with *Li Zhong Wan*, with the addition of several other herbs such as *Huang Qi* (Radix Astragali), *Dang Gui* (Radix Angelicae Sinensis), and *E Jiao* (Colla Corii Asini); and the replacement of *Gan Jiang* (Rhizoma Zingiberis) with *Pao Jiang* (Rhizoma Zingiberis Praeparatum).

Li Zhong Wan may be used to treat chronic infantile convulsions if there are symptoms of yang deficiency of the middle *jiao*. Chronic infantile convulsions can be caused by congenital defects, malnutrition, excessive intake of cold food during the time of illness, or weakness after a major illness.

Drooling of saliva or excessive production of foamy saliva following recovery from illness occurs when Spleen qi deficiency with cold fails to metabolize water. Body fluids thus flow upwards in the form of profuse saliva. *Li Zhong Wan* can be taken at a low dose for a prolonged period of time.

MODIFICATIONS

• If there is severe abdominal pain due to deficiency and cold, add *Fu Zi* (Radix Aconiti Lateralis Praeparata) and *Rou Gui* (Cortex Cinnamomi).
• With abdominal fullness and decreased intake of food, add *Shen Qu* (Massa Fermentata) and *Hou Po* (Cortex Magnoliae Officinalis).
• With abdominal pain, diarrhea, acid regurgitation, and a red tongue body with a white coating, add *Huang Lian* (Rhizoma Coptidis).
• With fullness and distention in the middle *jiao*, add *Wu Zhu Yu* (Fructus Evodiae), *Ding Xiang* (Flos Caryophylli), and *Gao Liang Jiang* (Rhizoma Alpiniae Officinarum).

• With nausea and vomiting due to cold in the Stomach, add *Ding Xiang* (Flos Caryophylli) and *Shi Di* (Calyx Kaki).
• With vomiting due to phlegm accumulation, add *Ban Xia* (Rhizoma Pinelliae) and *Fu Ling* (Poria).
• If there is severe vomiting, remove *Bai Zhu* (Rhizoma Atractylodis Macrocephalae) and add *Sheng Jiang* (Rhizoma Zingiberis Recens) and *Wu Zhu Yu* (Fructus Evodiae).
• With qi stagnation, add *Zhi Shi* (Fructus Aurantii Immaturus) and *Fu Ling* (Poria).
• With deficiency, cold, and qi stagnation, add *Qing Pi* (Pericarpium Citri Reticulatae Viride) and *Chen Pi* (Pericarpium Citri Reticulatae).
• With frequent diarrhea, add *Rou Dou Kou* (Semen Myristicae) and *He Zi* (Fructus Chebulae).
• With severe edema, add *Fu Ling* (Poria), *Ze Xie* (Rhizoma Alismatis), and *Dong Gua Pi* (Exocarpium Benincasae).
• If there is bleeding due to yang deficiency, add *E Jiao* (Colla Corii Asini), *San Qi* (Radix et Rhizoma Notoginseng), and charred *Ce Bai Ye* (Cacumen Platycladi).

CAUTIONS / CONTRAINDICATIONS

• *Li Zhong Wan* is contraindicated in patients of exterior wind invasion with fever.
• This formula contains many herbs that are warm and drying, and therefore is contraindicated in conditions characterized by interior heat with yin deficiency.
• This formula must be used with caution during pregnancy, as it contains many herbs that are warm and hot in nature.[1]

PHARMACOLOGICAL EFFECTS

1. **Antiulcer**: *Li Zhong Wan* has been shown to be beneficial in facilitating the healing of stomach ulcers. In one experiment, rats with artificially-induced ulcer were divided into herb and placebo groups. After 10 days of treatment, the herb group had only 3.57 mm^2 of ulceration, while the placebo group had 11.72 mm^2 of ulceration.[2]

460

Lǐ Zhōng Wán (Regulate the Middle Pill)

2. **Adrenocortical**: The preliminary data showed that administration of *Li Zhong Wan* was associated with a regulating effect on the adrenal glands.[3]

3. **Effect on kidney function**: Administration of *Li Zhong Wan* was associated with a protective effect on kidney functions. In one study, continuous use of the formula for 1-3 months was effective in gradually reducing the amount of protein, cells, and blood urea nitrogen (BUN) in the urine.[4]

CLINICAL STUDIES AND RESEARCH

1. **Epigastric pain**: Use of modified *Li Zhong Wan* was associated with marked results in treating 30 patients with epigastric pain characterized by deficiency and cold. The herbal treatment contained this formula plus *Huang Qi* (Radix Astragali), *Fu Ling* (Poria), *Chen Pi* (Pericarpium Citri Reticulatae), and *Cao Dou Kou* (Semen Alpiniae Katsumadai). Additional modifications were made as follows: double the dose of *Huang Qi* (Radix Astragali) for qi deficiency; *Rou Gui* (Cortex Cinnamomi) and *Fu Zi* (Radix Aconiti Lateralis Praeparata) for presence of cold; *Cang Zhu* (Rhizoma Atractylodis) and *Bai Bian Dou* (Semen Lablab Album) for dampness; *Dan Shen* (Radix et Rhizoma Salviae Miltiorrhizae), *Yan Hu Suo* (Rhizoma Corydalis), and *Chuan Lian Zi* (Fructus Toosendan) for stagnation; and *Bei Sha Shen* (Radix Glehniae), *Bai Shao* (Radix Paeoniae Alba), and *Shan Yao* (Rhizoma Dioscoreae) for yin deficiency. Of 30 patients, the study reported complete recovery in 5 patients within one month, and complete recovery in 20 patients and improvement in 5 patients within three months.[5]

2. **Gastritis**: Thirty patients with various types of gastritis (atrophic gastritis, superficial gastritis, gastritis with ulcer) were treated with *Li Zhong Wan*. The study reported complete relief of pain in 25 patients and partial relief of pain in 5 patients. Seventeen showed improvement based on endoscopy, and 13 showed no significant changes.[6]

3. **Bacterial dysentery**: Eighteen patients with chronic bacterial dysentery were treated with modification of *Li Zhong Wan* with complete recovery in 16 and improvement in 2 patients. The average duration of treatment was 12 days. The modification included addition of *Huang Lian* (Rhizoma Coptidis) and *Fu Ling* (Poria).[7]

4. **Enteritis**: Thirty patients with acute or chronic enteritis with diarrhea were treated with *Li Zhong Wan* for 3-10 days with significant improvement in 18 patients, moderate improvement in 8 patients, and no effect in 4 patients. The study reported an overall effectiveness rate of 86.6%.[8]

5. **Renal insufficiency**: Herbs were used to treat 15 patients (6 males and 9 females) with compromised kidney function, which included 12 patients of glomerulonephritis, polycystic kidney, kidney tuberculosis, and diabetic nephropathy. The herbal treatment included in extract 1.7 grams of *Li Zhong Wan* and 2.5 grams *Da Huang Gan Cao Tang* (Rhubarb and Licorice Decoction), given three times daily 30 minutes before meals for 3 months. The study reported an effectiveness rate of 66.7% after the first month, which was subsequently dropped to 40%. No significant side effects were reported.[9] Note: *Da Huang Gan Cao Tang* (Rhubarb and Licorice Decoction) is not a commonly used formula, and is not discussed in detail in this text. The original source of this formula is *Shang Han Lun* (Discussion of Cold-Induced Disorders), with the following composition: *Da Huang* (Radix et Rhizoma Rhei) 12g and *Gan Cao* (Radix et Rhizoma Glycyrrhizae) 3g.

6. **Male infertility**: In one study, *Li Zhong Wan* and *Ba Wei Di Huang Wan* (Eight-Ingredient Pill with Rehmannia) were combined together to treat 10 patients with male infertility. The study reported an increased production of seminal fluid (from 2.73 mL to 3.28 mL), in sperm count (from 1170/mL to 2185/mL), and in sperm motility (from 29.0% to 35.5%).[10]

7. **Excessive salivation**: Forty-two children (38 males and 4 females) with excessive salivation (20 days to 3 years history of illness) due to Spleen yang deficiency were treated with satisfactory results using modified *Li Zhong Wan*. The average age was 5.8 years (ranges from 3-9 years), and the average length of treatment was 4.6 packs of herbs in decoction. The herbs included *Dang Shen* (Radix Codonopsis) 10-18g, *Yi Zhi* (Fructus Alpiniae Oxyphyllae) 5-10g, *Gan Jiang* (Rhizoma Zingiberis) 5-8g, *Gan Cao* (Radix et Rhizoma Glycyrrhizae) 4-6g, and *Bai Zhu* (Rhizoma Atractylodis Macrocephalae) 8-10g. Modifications were made by adding *Sha Ren* (Fructus Amomi) 4-6g and *Ji Nei Jin* (Endothelium Corneum Gigeriae Galli) 5-8g for poor appetite and loose stools accompanied by long-term excessive salivation; and the addition of *Wu Mei* (Fructus Mume) 10-18g, *Shi Jun Zi* (Fructus Quisqualis) 7-10g, and *Hua Jiao* (Pericarpium Zanthoxyli) 4-6g, and removal of *Gan Cao* (Radix et Rhizoma Glycyrrhizae), for intestinal parasites with abdominal pain. After the treatment, 40 out of 42 patients showed complete recovery without any recurrence within 3 months.[11]

8. **Stomatitis**: One study reported effectiveness using modified *Li Zhong Wan* to treat recurrent stomatitis in 106 patients (47 males and 59 females, between 1-72 years of age, with 3 months to 24 years history of illness). In addition to this formula, modifications were made as follows: replacing *Ren Shen* (Radix et Rhizoma Ginseng) with *Dang Shen* (Radix Codonopsis) for severe Spleen deficiency; addition of *Rou Gui* (Cortex Cinnamomi) for cold; and addition of *Huang Lian* (Rhizoma Coptidis) for heat. The study reported complete recovery in all 106 patients after 2-17 days of treatment.[12]

461

Chapter 7 – Interior-Warming Formulas   *Section 1 – Middle-Warming and Cold-Dispelling Formulas*

Lǐ Zhōng Wán (Regulate the Middle Pill)

RELATED FORMULAS

Rén Shēn Tāng (Ginseng Decoction)

人参汤
人参汤

Pinyin Name: *Ren Shen Tang*
Literal Name: Ginseng Decoction
Alternate Name: *Li Zhong Tang* (Regulate the Middle Decoction)
Original Source: *Jin Gui Yao Lue* (Essentials from the Golden Cabinet) by Zhang Zhong-Jing in the Eastern Han Dynasty

Ren Shen (Radix et Rhizoma Ginseng)	9g
Gan Cao (Radix et Rhizoma Glycyrrhizae)	9g
Gan Jiang (Rhizoma Zingiberis)	9g
Bai Zhu (Rhizoma Atractylodis Macrocephalae)	9g

The source text states to cook the ingredients in 8 cups [1,600 mL] of water and reduce it to 3 cups [600 mL]. Take 1 cup [200 mL] of the warm, strained decoction three times daily. The source text also recommends taking 1 cup of hot porridge and keeping the body covered with a blanket to induce a feeling of warmth.

Li Zhong Wan and *Ren Shen Tang* (Ginseng Decoction) have essentially the same ingredients at the same dosages.
- *Li Zhong Wan* is administered in pill form, which is absorbed slowly over a longer period of time to warm the middle *jiao*, dispel cold, and tonify Spleen and Stomach qi.
- *Ren Shen Tang* (Ginseng Decoction) is administered in decoction form, which is absorbed immediately to provide a faster onset of action. This formula is primarily used to treat a more urgent condition, such as *xiong bi* (painful obstruction of the chest) with symptoms such as cold extremities, fatigue, low energy, and feeble voice.

Lǐ Zhōng Huà Tán Wán

(Regulate the Middle and Transform Phlegm Pill)

理中化痰丸

Pinyin Name: *Li Zhong Hua Tan Wan*
Literal Name: Regulate the Middle and Transform Phlegm Pill
Original Source: *Ming Yi Za Zhu* (Miscellaneous Books of Ming Medicine) by Wang Lun in 1549 A.D.

Ren Shen (Radix et Rhizoma Ginseng)

Bai Zhu (Rhizoma Atractylodis Macrocephalae), *chao* (dry-fried)

Gan Jiang (Rhizoma Zingiberis)

Zhi Gan Cao (Radix et Rhizoma Glycyrrhizae Praeparata cum Melle)

Fu Ling (Poria)

Ban Xia (Rhizoma Pinelliae), *zhu* (boiled) with ginger

The source text states to grind the ingredients into a fine powder and form into small pills with water. Take 40-50 pills with warm, boiled water. Note: Herb doses are unavailable from the source text.

Li Zhong Hua Tan Wan (Regulate the Middle and Transform Phlegm Pill) is composed of *Li Zhong Wan* plus *Fu Ling* (Poria) and *Ban Xia* (Rhizoma Pinelliae), which are used in this formula to enhance the action of tonifying Spleen qi and dissolving phlegm. Clinically, the patient may show deficiency and cold of the Spleen and Stomach with stagnation of phlegm. The symptoms include nausea, vomiting, lack of appetite, loose stools, poor digestion, coughing with sputum, and drooling of saliva.

In comparison to *Li Zhong Wan*, *Li Zhong Hua Tan Wan* (Regulate the Middle and Transform Phlegm Pill) has a stronger action to dry dampness, strengthen the Spleen, and relieve nausea. Therefore, it is often used for patients who have deficiency and cold of the Spleen and Stomach, complicated by coughing with sputum and drooling of saliva.

AUTHORS' COMMENTS

Li Zhong Wan is one of the main formulas for treating deficiency and cold of the Spleen and Stomach. This formula was originally designed to be given as pills, which usually have a slower onset of action. When necessary in acute or severe cases, this formula may first be given in decoction form, and then followed by pills when the condition stabilizes.

Li Zhong Wan and *Si Jun Zi Tang* (Four-Gentlemen Decoction) both treat Spleen qi deficiency with poor appetite, diarrhea, and other signs and symptoms. Both formulas contain qi-tonifying herbs such as *Ren Shen* (Radix et Rhizoma Ginseng), *Bai Zhu* (Rhizoma Atractylodis Macrocephalae), and *Zhi Gan Cao* (Radix et Rhizoma Glycyrrhizae Praeparata cum Melle). Despite these similarities, the differences are as follows:
- *Li Zhong Wan* is for deficiency with cold of the middle *jiao* (Spleen and Stomach), characterized by abdominal pain, vomiting, diarrhea, polyuria, cold limbs, intolerance to cold, and a deep, fine pulse.
- *Si Jun Zi Tang* is for Spleen qi deficiency, characterized by a sallow complexion, poor appetite, decreased dietary intake, fatigue, a pale tongue body, and a fine, moderate pulse.[13]

462

Chinese Herbal Formulas and Applications

Lǐ Zhōng Wán (Regulate the Middle Pill)

References

1. *Zhong Yao Ming Fang Yao Li Yu Ying Yong* (Pharmacology and Applications of Famous Herbal Formulas) 1989;219-220.
2. *Shan Xi Yi Kan* (Shanxi Journal of Medicine) 1987;7:333.
3. *Jiang Xi Zhong Yi Yao* (Jiangxi Chinese Medicine and Herbology) 1981;3:32.
4. *Guo Wai Yi Xue* (Foreign Medicine) 1994;6:30.
5. *Shan Xi Zhong Yi* (Shanxi Chinese Medicine) 1984;5(1):13.
6. *Jiang Xi Zhong Yi Yao* (Jiangxi Chinese Medicine and Herbology) 1981;3:32.
7. *Shan Dong Zhong Yi Za Zhi* (*Shandong* Journal of Chinese Medicine) 1983;2:21.
8. *Shang Hai Zhong Yi Yao Za Zhi* (Shanghai Journal of Chinese Medicine and Herbology) 1984;6:45.
9. *Guo Wai Yi Xue* (Foreign Medicine) 1994;6:30.
10. *Zhong Yi Fang Ji Xian Dai Yan Jiu* (Modern Study of Medical Formulae in Traditional Chinese Medicine) 1997;371.
11. *Guang Xi Zhong Yi Yao* (Guangxi Chinese Medicine and Herbology) 1992;2:15.
12. *Zhe Jiang Zhong Yi Za Zhi* (Zhejiang Journal of Chinese Medicine) 1992;10:474.
13. Wang MZ, et al. *Zhong Yi Xue Wen Da Ti Ku* (Questions and Answers on Traditional Chinese Medicine: Herbal Formulas).

Fù Zǐ Lǐ Zhōng Wán (Prepared Aconite Pill to Regulate the Middle)
附子理中丸

Pinyin Name: *Fu Zi Li Zhong Wan*
Literal Name: Prepared Aconite Pill to Regulate the Middle
Alternate Names: *Fu Tzu Li Chung Tang* (*Wan*), *Fu Zi Li Zhong Tang* (*Wan*), Aconite, Ginseng and Ginger Decoction (Pill); Aconite Middle-Regulating Decoction (Pill); Aconite Ginseng and Ginger Combination
Original Source: *Tai Ping Hui Min He Ji Ju Fang* (Imperial Grace Formulary of the Tai Ping Era) by the Imperial Medical Department in 1078-85

COMPOSITION

Fu Zi (Radix Aconiti Lateralis Praeparata), *pao* (blast-fried)	90g [9g]
Gan Jiang (Rhizoma Zingiberis), *pao* (blast-fried)	90g [9g]
Ren Shen (Radix et Rhizoma Ginseng)	90g [9g]
Bai Zhu (Rhizoma Atractylodis Macrocephalae), *cuo* (grated)	90g [9g]
Zhi Gan Cao (Radix et Rhizoma Glycyrrhizae Praeparata cum Melle)	90g [9g]

DOSAGE / PREPARATION / ADMINISTRATION

The source text states to grind the ingredients into a fine powder and form into pills with honey. Each pill should weigh 3 grams. Place and disintegrate 1 pill in one bowl of water, then cook it until 70% of the liquid remains. Take the warm decoction before meals on an empty stomach. For children, divide the decoction into two to three separate doses. This formula may also be prepared as a decoction with the doses suggested in brackets.

CHINESE THERAPEUTIC ACTIONS

1. Warms yang and dispels cold
2. Tonifies qi and strengthens the Spleen

CLINICAL MANIFESTATIONS

Deficiency and cold of the Spleen and Stomach: extreme coldness of the body and the extremities, mild perspiration, indigestion, borborygmus, severe epigastric and abdominal fullness and pain, nausea, vomiting, diarrhea, and sudden turmoil disorder with muscle spasms.

CLINICAL APPLICATIONS

Gastroenteritis, gastritis, peptic ulcer disease, gastroatonia, prolapse of the stomach, ulcerative colitis, and infantile diarrhea.

EXPLANATION

Fu Zi Li Zhong Wan (Prepared Aconite Pill to Regulate the Middle) combines *Fu Zi* (Radix Aconiti Lateralis Praeparata) and *Li Zhong Wan* (Regulate the Middle Pill). It warms yang, dispels cold, benefits qi, and strengthens the Spleen. It is used for deficiency and cold secondary to yang deficiency of the Spleen and Stomach. Clinically, patients may show vomiting, diarrhea, muscle spasms, muscle stiffness in the extremities, and a white tongue coating.

INTERIOR-WARMING FORMULAS

7

463

Chapter 7 – Interior-Warming Formulas   *Section 1 – Middle-Warming and Cold-Dispelling Formulas*

Fù Zǐ Lǐ Zhōng Wán (Prepared Aconite Pill to Regulate the Middle)

Fu Zi Li Zhong Wan (Prepared Aconite Pill to Regulate the Middle)

Diagnosis	Signs and Symptoms	Treatment	Herbs
Deficiency and cold of the Spleen and Stomach	• Diarrhea and vomiting: deficiency and cold of the Spleen and Stomach affecting the normal ascending and descending functions • Abdominal pain and cold body and extremities: cold in the middle *jiao* affecting the body and extremities	• Warms yang and dispels cold • Tonifies qi and strengthens the Spleen	• *Fu Zi* (Radix Aconiti Lateralis Praeparata) dispels cold, tonifies yang and warms the entire body. • *Li Zhong Wan* (Regulate the Middle Pill) warms the middle *jiao*, tonifies qi and strengthens the Spleen and Stomach.

In comparison to *Li Zhong Wan* (Regulate the Middle Pill), *Fu Zi Li Zhong Wan* more strongly warms yang and dispels cold. In this formula, *Fu Zi* (Radix Aconiti Lateralis Praeparata) dispels cold, tonifies yang, and warms the entire body. *Gan Jiang* (Rhizoma Zingiberis) warms the middle *jiao* and dispels interior cold. *Ren Shen* (Radix et Rhizoma Ginseng) nourishes *yuan* (source) *qi*. *Bai Zhu* (Rhizoma Atractylodis Macrocephalae) strengthens the Spleen and dries dampness. *Zhi Gan Cao* (Radix et Rhizoma Glycyrrhizae Praeparata cum Melle) nourishes qi and harmonizes the middle *jiao*.

MODIFICATIONS
- With severe deficiency and cold, add *Rou Gui* (Cortex Cinnamomi) and *Cang Zhu* (Rhizoma Atractylodis).
- With nausea and vomiting of phlegm and saliva, add *Ban Xia* (Rhizoma Pinelliae) and *Fu Ling* (Poria).
- With tetanus-like vomiting and diarrhea, add *Huang Lian* (Rhizoma Coptidis) and *Zhi Shi* (Fructus Aurantii Immaturus).
- With stagnation of phlegm and food, add *Wei Ling Tang* (Calm the Stomach and Poria Decoction).

CAUTIONS / CONTRAINDICATIONS
- *Fu Zi Li Zhong Wan* should be used with extreme caution in patients who have yin deficiency because the hot and dry herbs can further damage yin.
- This formula is contraindicated during pregnancy.[1]

PHARMACOLOGICAL EFFECTS
Analgesic: In one study, injection of *Fu Zi Li Zhong Wan* was associated with analgesic effects in mice.[2]

CLINICAL STUDIES AND RESEARCH
1. **Peptic ulcer disease:** One study reported 91.5% effectiveness in the treatment of peptic ulcer characterized by deficiency and cold using *Fu Zi Li Zhong Wan*, *Huang Qi Jian Zhong Tang* (Astragalus Decoction to Construct the Middle), and others herbs as needed. Other herbs added included *Chai Hu* (Radix Bupleuri) and *Xiang Fu* (Rhizoma Cyperi) for a feeling of fullness and oppression in the chest and hypochondrium; *Yan Hu Suo* (Rhizoma Corydalis) and *Dan Shen* (Radix et Rhizoma Salviae Miltiorrhizae) for pain at a fixed location and purple tongue; *Chen Pi* (Pericarpium Citri Reticulatae) and *Fu Ling* (Poria) for fullness and distention of the epigastrium and a thick, greasy tongue coating; *Zhe Shi* (Haematitum) and *Xuan Fu Hua* (Flos Inulae) for nausea and vomiting; *Shen Qu* (Massa Fermentata), *Shan Zha* (Fructus Crataegi), *Gu Ya* (Fructus Setariae Germinatus) and *Mai Ya* (Fructus Hordei Germinatus) for poor appetite and indigestion. Of 59 patients, the study reported complete recovery in 37 patients, improvement in 17 patients, and no effect in 5 patients.[3]

2. **Ulcerative colitis:** Administration of modified *Fu Zi Li Zhong Wan* was effective in treating 78 patients with ulcerative colitis with a history of illness of 1-10 years. The herbal formula contained 12g each of *Fu Zi* (Radix Aconiti Lateralis Praeparata) (pre-decocted), *Gan Jiang* (Rhizoma Zingiberis), *Ren Shen* (Radix et Rhizoma Ginseng), *Zhi Gan Cao* (Radix et Rhizoma Glycyrrhizae Praeparata cum Melle), and *Bai Zhu* (Rhizoma Atractylodis Macrocephalae), and 8g each of *Chai Hu* (Radix Bupleuri) and *Sheng Ma* (Rhizoma Cimicifugae), and 20g of *He Zi* (Fructus Chebulae). For individuals with fever, abdominal pain, a yellow, greasy tongue coating and a slippery, rapid pulse, 30g of *Bai Tou Weng* (Radix Pulsatillae) and 10g of *Huang Bo* (Cortex Phellodendri Chinensis) were added, and *Gan Jiang* (Rhizoma Zingiberis) and *Fu Zi* (Radix Aconiti Lateralis Praeparata) were removed; for patients with poor appetite and abdominal distention, 20g each of charred *Shan Zha* (Fructus Crataegi), charred *Shen Qu* (Massa Fermentata), and charred *Mai Ya* (Fructus Hordei Germinatus) were added; and for severe early morning diarrhea, *Si Shen Wan* (Four-Miracle Pill) was added. The treatment protocol was to cook the herbs in decoction, and take the decoction in two equally-divided doses daily. The duration of treatment was between 7-40 packs of herbs. Of 78 patients, the study reported complete recovery in 34 patients, marked improvement in 35 patients, slight improvement in 7 patients, and no change in 2 patients.[4]

464

Fù Zǐ Lǐ Zhōng Wán (Prepared Aconite Pill to Regulate the Middle)

3. **Infantile diarrhea**: Thirty-six infants with ages ranging between under six months to three years with diarrhea refractory to drug treatment were treated with modified *Fu Zi Li Zhong Wan* with good results. The herbal formula included *Fu Zi* (Radix Aconiti Lateralis Praeparata) 3g, *Gan Jiang* (Rhizoma Zingiberis) 6g, *Dang Shen* (Radix Codonopsis) 10g, dry-fried *Bai Zhu* (Rhizoma Atractylodis Macrocephalae) 15g, *Fu Ling* (Poria) 15g, *Gui Zhi* (Ramulus Cinnamomi) 10g, *Zhu Ling* (Polyporus) 10g, *Ze Xie* (Rhizoma Alismatis) 6g, *Ying Su Ke* (Pericarpium Papaveris) 3g, *Cang Zhu* (Rhizoma Atractylodis) 6g, and *Chen Pi* (Pericarpium Citri Reticulatae) 6g. Modifications were made by adding 6g each of charred *Shan Zha* (Fructus Crataegi), charred *Shen Qu* (Massa Fermentata), and charred *Mai Ya* (Fructus Hordei Germinatus) for presence of undigested food in the stools; *Ge Gen* (Radix Puerariae Lobatae) 10g for fever; *Zhu Ru* (Caulis Bambusae in Taenia) 6g for nausea and vomiting; and *Mai Dong* (Radix Ophiopogonis) 6g and *Wu Wei Zi* (Fructus Schisandrae Chinensis) 6g for thirst. The treatment protocol was to cook the same herbs in water twice, mix the two batches of decoction together, and administer the decoction in four equally-divided doses. Of 36 patients, 25 had normal bowel movement within two packs of herbs, 9 within three packs, and 1 within four packs. However, one person required hospitalization because of continuous diarrhea and subsequent dehydration.[5]

AUTHORS' COMMENTS

Fu Zi Li Zhong Wan is formulated by combining *Fu Zi* (Radix Aconiti Lateralis Praeparata) and *Li Zhong Wan* (Regulate the Middle Pill). The addition of *Fu Zi* (Radix Aconiti Lateralis Praeparata) makes it a stronger formula to tonify both Spleen and Kidney yang. Therefore, *Fu Zi Li Zhong Wan* is reserved for more severe coldness.

Li Zhong Wan (Regulate the Middle Pill) and *Fu Zi Li Zhong Wan* have many similarities and differences:

- *Li Zhong Wan* is an interior-warming formula consisting of *Ren Shen* (Radix et Rhizoma Ginseng), *Gan Jiang* (Rhizoma Zingiberis), *Bai Zhu* (Rhizoma Atractylodis Macrocephalae), and *Zhi Gan Cao* (Radix et Rhizoma Glycyrrhizae Praeparata cum Melle). It warms the middle *jiao*, dispels cold, tonifies qi, and strengthens the Spleen. It is mainly used for digestive dysfunctions caused by deficiency and cold of the middle *jiao*, leading to symptoms of diarrhea, vomiting, abdominal pain, poor appetite, and no desire to drink. Also, it is used for yang deficiency with loss of blood, chronic infantile convulsions, and preference for sleep. It can also treat excessive salivation or *xiong bi* (painful obstruction of the chest) in convalescing patients with middle *jiao* deficiency and coldness.

- *Fu Zi Li Zhong Wan* is much more acrid and hot, as it contains *Fu Zi* (Radix Aconiti Lateralis Praeparata), one of the hottest herbs in the entire pharmacopeia. This formula warms and strengthens Spleen and Kidney yang. It is best for coldness and pain in the chest and abdomen, extreme coldness of the limbs and extremities, and muscle spasms and cramps. *Fu Zi Li Zhong Wan*, in comparison with *Li Zhong Wan*, is for more severe conditions of cold accumulation in the body.[6]

References

1. *Zhong Yao Ming Fang Yao Li Yu Ying Yong* (Pharmacology and Applications of Famous Herbal Formulas) 1989;220-221.
2. *Zhong Cheng Yao* (Study of Chinese Patent Medicine) 1990;5:25.
3. *An Hui Zhong Yi Xue Yuan Xue Bao* (Journal of Anhui University School of Medicine) 1988;1:29.
4. *Zhong Yi Fang Ji Xian Dai Yan Jiu* (Modern Study of Medical Formulae in Traditional Chinese Medicine) 1997;1:14.
5. *Gan Su Zhong Yi* (Gansu Chinese Medicine) 1993;2:22.
6. Wang MZ, et al. *Zhong Yi Xue Wen Da Ti Ku* (Questions and Answers on Traditional Chinese Medicine: Herbal Formulas)

Chapter 7 – Interior-Warming Formulas　　　　　*Section 1 – Middle-Warming and Cold-Dispelling Formulas*

Guì Zhī Rén Shēn Tāng (Cinnamon Twig and Ginseng Decoction)

桂枝人參湯
桂枝人参汤

Pinyin Name: *Gui Zhi Ren Shen Tang*
Literal Name: Cinnamon Twig and Ginseng Decoction
Alternate Name: Cinnamon and Ginseng Combination
Original Source: *Shang Han Lun* (Discussion of Cold-Induced Disorders) by Zhang Zhong-Jing in the Eastern Han Dynasty

COMPOSITION

Gui Zhi (Ramulus Cinnamomi)	12g
Ren Shen (Radix et Rhizoma Ginseng)	9g
Bai Zhu (Rhizoma Atractylodis Macrocephalae)	9g
Gan Jiang (Rhizoma Zingiberis)	9g
Zhi Gan Cao (Radix et Rhizoma Glycyrrhizae Praeparata cum Melle)	12g

DOSAGE / PREPARATION / ADMINISTRATION

The source text instructs to cook the ingredients, except *Gui Zhi* (Ramulus Cinnamomi), in 9 cups [1,800 mL] of water until 5 cups [1,000 mL] of liquid remain. Add *Gui Zhi* (Ramulus Cinnamomi) and cook until the liquid is reduced to 3 cups [600 mL]. Take 1 cup [200 mL] of the warm, strained decoction two times during the day and one time at night.

CHINESE THERAPEUTIC ACTIONS

1. Warms the interior and releases the exterior
2. Tonifies qi and relieves distention

CLINICAL MANIFESTATIONS

Exterior wind-cold and interior deficiency and cold: fever, aversion to cold, perspiration, constant diarrhea, distention and pain beneath the heart, and cold body and extremities.

CLINICAL APPLICATIONS

Influenza, common cold, gastric and duodenal ulcers, acute and chronic gastroenteritis, and prolapse of the stomach.

EXPLANATION

Gui Zhi Ren Shen Tang (Cinnamon Twig and Ginseng Decoction) originally appeared in *Shang Han Lun* (Discussion of Cold-Induced Disorders) as a treatment for patients with *taiyang* syndrome who have been treated improperly with downward draining methods. As a result of downward draining treatments, patients develop deficiency and cold in the interior. The overall condition then is complicated by exterior wind-cold and interior deficiency and cold. Clinically, fever, aversion to cold, and perspiration are representative of exterior wind-cold; and constant diarrhea, distention and pain beneath the heart,

and cold body and extremities are indicative of interior deficiency and cold. Effective treatment for this condition must focus on dispelling the exterior pathogenic factors as well as warming the interior cold.

Gui Zhi (Ramulus Cinnamomi) dispels wind and cold at the exterior and relieves body aches and pains. *Ren Shen* (Radix et Rhizoma Ginseng) and *Bai Zhu* (Rhizoma Atractylodis Macrocephalae) tonify qi, strengthen the Spleen, and stop diarrhea. *Gan Jiang* (Rhizoma Zingiberis) warms the interior and dispels cold. *Zhi Gan Cao* (Radix et Rhizoma Glycyrrhizae Praeparata cum Melle) relieves pain and harmonizes the formula.

MODIFICATIONS

- With epigastric fullness and oppression, add *Zhi Shi* (Fructus Aurantii Immaturus) and *Jie Geng* (Radix Platycodonis).
- With a feeling of distention and pain in the chest, add *Huang Lian* (Rhizoma Coptidis) and *Ban Xia* (Rhizoma Pinelliae).
- If there is constant diarrhea, add *Shan Yao* (Rhizoma Dioscoreae) and *Ge Gen* (Radix Puerariae Lobatae).

AUTHORS' COMMENTS

Gui Zhi Ren Shen Tang combines *Gui Zhi* (Ramulus Cinnamomi) and *Li Zhong Wan* (Regulate the Middle Pill). It is used mainly for patients who have deficiency and cold of the middle *jiao*, complicated by exterior symptoms. This condition results from improperly using downward draining methods to treat patients with exterior syndrome; the result is damage to the middle *jiao* in addition to unresolved exterior symptoms. Clinically, patients may show severe diarrhea, epigastric fullness and rigidity, and other exterior symptoms and signs. In this formula, it is important to note that *Gui Zhi* (Ramulus Cinnamomi) is purposely post-decocted to preserve its acrid and aromatic properties to release the exterior condition.

466

Guì Zhī Rén Shēn Tāng (Cinnamon Twig and Ginseng Decoction)

Gui Zhi Ren Shen Tang (Cinnamon Twig and Ginseng Decoction)

Diagnosis	Signs and Symptoms	Treatment	Herbs
Exterior wind-cold and interior deficiency and cold	• Fever, aversion to cold and perspiration: exterior wind-cold • Constant diarrhea, distention and pain beneath the heart and cold body and extremities: interior deficiency and cold	• Warms the interior and releases the exterior • Tonifies qi and relieves distention	• *Gui Zhi* (Ramulus Cinnamomi) dispels the wind-cold at the exterior and relieves body aches and pains. • *Ren Shen* (Radix et Rhizoma Ginseng) and *Bai Zhu* (Rhizoma Atractylodis Macrocephalae) tonify qi, strengthen the Spleen, and stop diarrhea. • *Gan Jiang* (Rhizoma Zingiberis) warms the interior and dispels cold. • *Zhi Gan Cao* (Radix et Rhizoma Glycyrrhizae Praeparata cum Melle) relieves pain and harmonizes the herbs.

Wú Zhū Yú Tāng (Evodia Decoction)

吳茱萸湯
吴茱萸汤

Pinyin Name: *Wu Zhu Yu Tang*
Literal Name: Evodia Decoction
Alternate Names: *Wu Chu Yu Tang*, Evodia Fruit Decoction, Evodia Combination
Original Source: *Shang Han Lun* (Discussion of Cold-Induced Disorders) by Zhang Zhong-Jing in the Eastern Han Dynasty

COMPOSITION

Wu Zhu Yu (Fructus Evodiae), *xi* (washed) in liquid 7 times	1 cup [3-9g]
Sheng Jiang (Rhizoma Zingiberis Recens), *qie* (sliced)	18g [18g]
Ren Shen (Radix et Rhizoma Ginseng)	9g [6g]
Da Zao (Fructus Jujubae), *bo* (opened)	12 pieces [4 pieces]

DOSAGE / PREPARATION / ADMINISTRATION

The source text states to cook the ingredients in 7 cups [1,400 mL] of water until 2 cups [400 mL] of liquid remain. Take 0.7 cup [140 mL] of the warm, strained decoction three times daily. Today, the decoction may be prepared using the doses suggested in brackets. Note: Some patients may experience exacerbation of the symptoms immediately after ingesting the herbs, which is a normal reaction and should abate in half an hour.

CHINESE THERAPEUTIC ACTIONS

1. Warms and tonifies the middle *jiao*
2. Corrects the reversed flow of qi and stops vomiting

CLINICAL MANIFESTATIONS

1. Vomiting due to deficiency and cold of the Stomach: vomiting sensations after eating, a feeling of fullness and distention in the chest and diaphragm, epigastric pain, belching, and acid regurgitation.
2. *Jueyin* headache with dry heaves (vomiting of saliva only).
3. *Shaoyin* vomiting and diarrhea with extremely cold hands and feet and severe fidgeting and irritability.

CLINICAL APPLICATIONS

Acute and chronic gastritis, gastroptosis, ulcerative colitis, vomiting, nausea, hiccup, food poisoning, acid reflux, morning sickness, headache, neurotic headache, migraine headache, habitual headache, Meniere's disease, trigeminal

Chapter 7 – Interior-Warming Formulas　　　　　*Section 1 – Middle-Warming and Cold-Dispelling Formulas*

Wú Zhū Yú Tāng (Evodia Decoction)

neuralgia, hypertension, and withdrawal reactions from drug addiction.

EXPLANATION

Wu Zhu Yu Tang (Evodia Decoction) treats vomiting due to deficiency and cold in the Stomach with rising of yin and cold upwards. This condition may be present in *yangming*, *shaoyin*, and *jueyin* disorders. In *yangming* disorder, deficiency and cold affect the Stomach and cause reversed flow of qi, leading to symptoms such as vomiting, belching, and acid regurgitation. In *jueyin* disorder, yin and cold rise upwards to cause vertex headache, dry heaves and vomiting of saliva. In *shaoyin* disorder, yin and cold rise upwards to cause vomiting, while yang is deficient and cannot reach upwards or outwards, resulting in diarrhea with extremely cold hands and feet.

Wu Zhu Yu (Fructus Evodiae), acrid, bitter, and very warm, is the chief herb in this formula. It warms the Stomach, dispels cold, harmonizes the middle *jiao*, and corrects the reversed flow of qi. *Sheng Jiang* (Rhizoma Zingiberis Recens) warms the Stomach and relieves nausea and vomiting. *Ren Shen* (Radix et Rhizoma Ginseng) tonifies *yuan* (source) *qi* and strengthens the Stomach. *Da Zao* (Fructus Jujubae) tonifies qi and harmonizes the middle *jiao*. *Sheng Jiang* (Rhizoma Zingiberis Recens) and *Da Zao* (Fructus Jujubae) also harmonize and regulate the *ying* (nutritive) and *wei* (defensive) levels.

MODIFICATIONS

- If there is severe nausea and vomiting, add *Ban Xia* (Rhizoma Pinelliae), *Sha Ren* (Fructus Amomi), and *Fu Ling* (Poria).
- For vomiting without cold extremities and severe fidgeting and irritability, use *Dang Shen* (Radix Codonopsis) instead of *Ren Shen* (Radix et Rhizoma Ginseng).
- With abdominal pain, add *Bai Shao* (Radix Paeoniae Alba).
- With abdominal pain and extreme coldness, add *Si Ni Tang* (Frigid Extremities Decoction).

- With fullness and distention in the abdominal region, add *Sha Ren* (Fructus Amomi) and *Hou Po* (Cortex Magnoliae Officinalis).
- With involuntary salivation, nausea or dry heaves, add *Gan Jiang* (Rhizoma Zingiberis) and *Rou Gui* (Cortex Cinnamomi).
- If there is frequent acid regurgitation, add *Hai Piao Xiao* (Endoconcha Sepiae) and *Wa Leng Zi* (Concha Arcae).
- With headache, add *Man Jing Zi* (Fructus Viticis), *Chuan Xiong* (Rhizoma Chuanxiong), *Dang Gui* (Radix Angelicae Sinensis), and *Ji Li* (Fructus Tribuli).
- With irritability and extreme coldness, add *Fu Zi* (Radix Aconiti Lateralis Praeparata) and *Xi Xin* (Radix et Rhizoma Asari).

CAUTIONS / CONTRAINDICATIONS

- *Wu Zhu Yu Tang* is contraindicated in individuals with vomiting and acid regurgitation caused by heat, and in patients with headaches caused by Liver yang rising.
- This formula may be served at room temperature, especially for individuals who cannot keep the warm decoction down because of vomiting.
- According to one reference, use of this formula in decoction is occasionally associated with chest discomfort, headache and dizziness. These side effects, however, are self-limiting and generally resolve within 30 minutes without intervention.[1]

PHARMACOLOGICAL EFFECTS

1. **Antiemetic**: In one experiment, the administration of *Wu Zhu Yu Tang* was found to be effective in suppressing vomiting in pigeons with artificially-induced vomiting. The researchers noted that while *Wu Zhu Yu* (Fructus Evodiae) and *Sheng Jiang* (Rhizoma Zingiberis Recens) each have antiemetic effects, the potency is not as strong as *Wu Zhu Yu Tang*.[2]

2. **Gastrointestinal**: Administration of *Wu Zhu Yu Tang* was associated with a general inhibitory effect on the gastrointestinal system. In one experiment of two groups

Wu Zhu Yu Tang (Evodia Decoction)

Diagnosis	Signs and Symptoms	Treatment	Herbs
Deficiency and cold of the Stomach	• Vomiting, belching, and acid regurgitation: reversed flow of qi due to deficiency and cold of the Stomach • Feeling of fullness and distention of the chest and diaphragm, and epigastric pain: presence of cold in the middle *jiao*	• Warms and tonifies the middle *jiao* • Corrects the reversed flow of qi and stops vomiting	• *Wu Zhu Yu* (Fructus Evodiae) warms the Stomach, dispels cold, harmonizes the middle *jiao*, corrects the reversed flow of qi. • *Sheng Jiang* (Rhizoma Zingiberis Recens) warms the Stomach and relieves nausea and vomiting. • *Ren Shen* (Radix et Rhizoma Ginseng) tonifies *yuan* (source) *qi* and strengthens the Stomach. • *Da Zao* (Fructus Jujubae) tonifies qi and harmonizes the middle *jiao*.

Wú Zhū Yú Tāng (Evodia Decoction)

of mice who were given the same amount of food, the group that received herbs had significantly more food remaining in the stomach than the group that received placebo.[3] In another experiment, administration of *Wu Zhu Yu Tang* inhibited the production of gastric acid, and increased the pH in the stomach.[4]

CLINICAL STUDIES AND RESEARCH

1. **Vomiting**: Use of *Wu Zhu Yu Tang* in 168 patients was associated with 91.7% effectiveness in relieving nausea and vomiting associated with cancer of the upper gastro-intestinal tract. The treatment protocol was to administer the herbs in decoction daily, for 6 packs of herbs per course of treatment.[5] In another study, use of modified *Wu Zhu Yu Tang* was associated with 100% effectiveness in treating neurogenic vomiting in 68 patients who have 3 months to 3 years history of illness. Modifications to this formula included the addition of *Huo Xiang* (Herba Agastaches) and *Pei Lan* (Herba Eupatorii) for dampness with a white, greasy tongue coating; *Chen Xiang* (Lignum Aquilariae Resinatum) and *Qing Pi* (Pericarpium Citri Reticulatae Viride) for chest and hypochondriac full-ness and pain; *Huang Lian* (Rhizoma Coptidis) and *Zhu Ru* (Caulis Bambusae in Taenia) for a red tongue body with irritability; and *Sha Ren* (Fructus Amomi) and *Mai Dong* (Radix Ophiopogonis) for chronic vomiting with Stomach yin deficiency. Of 68 patients, the study reported significant improvement in 53 patients and moderate improvement in 15 patients.[6]

2. **Nausea**: One study reported complete recovery in all 5 patients with nausea when treated with *Wu Zhu Yu Tang* plus *Shi Di* (Calyx Kaki), *Zhi Qiao* (Fructus Aurantii), and *Pi Pa Ye* (Folium Eriobotryae). The cause of nausea was determined to be weakness and deficiency of the Spleen and Stomach with accumulation of cold qi.[7]

3. **Headache**: Twenty-five patients (12 males and 13 females) with headaches were treated with 7.5g of extract of *Wu Zhu Yu Tang* daily. The study reported significant improvement in 9 patients, moderate improve-ment in 6 patients, slight improvement in 5 patients, and no change in 5 patients. The overall rate of effectiveness was 60%.[8]

4. **Meniere's syndrome**: Use of modified *Wu Zhu Yu Tang* was effective in treating Meniere's syndrome in 22 patients. The herbal treatment contained *Wu Zhu Yu Tang* plus *Gui Zhi* (Ramulus Cinnamomi) as the base formula, with addition of *Fu Zi* (Radix Aconiti Lateralis Praepa-rata) for chills and cold extremities; *Ban Xia* (Rhizoma Pinelliae) for nausea and vomiting; and *Huang Qi* (Radix Astragali) for qi deficiency. The herbal formula was given in decoction, with most patients reporting improvement within 3 packs of herbs. Of 22 patients, the study reported

complete recovery in 20 patients and improvement in 2 patients.[9]

5. **Ulcerative colitis**: Use of modified *Wu Zhu Yu Tang* was effective in treating chronic ulcerative colitis in 68 patients (between 20 and 58 years of age, with 1-12 years history of illness). In addition to the base formula, modifications were made as follows: *Chai Hu* (Radix Bupleuri) and *Ji Nei Jin* (Endothelium Corneum Gigeriae Galli) for Liver overacting on the Spleen; *Chuan Xiong* (Rhizoma Chuanxiong) and *Yan Hu Suo* (Rhizoma Corydalis) for a purple tongue with petechia spots and abdominal pain that worsens with pressure; *Bai Tou Weng* (Radix Pulsatillae) and *Qin Pi* (Cortex Fraxini) for damp-heat; *Xiao Hui Xiang* (Fructus Foeniculi) and *Fu Ling* (Poria) for damp-cold; *Shan Yao* (Rhizoma Dioscoreae) and dry-fried *Bai Bian Dou* (Semen Lablab Album) for Spleen and Stomach deficiencies; *Shen Qu* (Massa Fermentata) and dry-fried *Shan Zha* (Fructus Crataegi) for food stag-nation; *Ba Ji Tian* (Radix Morindae Officinalis) and *Bu Gu Zhi* (Fructus Psoraleae) for Spleen and Kidney yang deficiencies; *Dan Shen* (Radix et Rhizoma Salviae Miltior-rhizae), *Rou Dou Kou* (Semen Myristicae), charred *Qian Cao* (Radix et Rhizoma Rubiae), and charred *Pu Huang* (Pollen Typhae) for blood stagnation due to chronic illness. The treatment protocol was to administer the herbs in decoction twice daily, for 30 days per course of treatment, for 1-2 courses total. Of 68 patients, the study reported complete recovery in 42 patients, improvement in 23 patients, and no effect in 3 patients.[10]

6. **Hypertension**: Forty-four patients (11 males and 33 females) ages between 40-67 with hypertension were treated with modified *Wu Zhu Yu Tang* with good success. Clinical presentation of these patients included hyperten-sion with dizziness and vertigo, headache, and a feeling of swelling sensations and pain in the head. The treatment protocol was to administer the herbs in decoction twice daily. The formula included *Wu Zhu Yu* (Fructus Evodiae) 4g, *Ban Xia* (Rhizoma Pinelliae) 8g, *Dang Shen* (Radix Codonopsis) 10g, *Fu Ling* (Poria) 10g, *Fu Shen* (Poria Paradicis) 10g, *Bai Zhi* (Radix Angelicae Dahuricae) 10g, *Di Long* (Pheretima) 10g, *Jiang Can* (Bombyx Batryticatus) 10g, *Chai Hu* (Radix Bupleuri) 6g, *Qing Pi* (Pericarpium Citri Reticulatae Viride) 6g, *Chen Pi* (Pericarpium Citri Reticulatae) 6g, *Gou Teng* (Ramulus Uncariae cum Uncis) 30g, *Sheng Jiang* (Rhizoma Zingiberis Recens) 5-8 slices, *Da Zao* (Fructus Jujubae) 5-8 pieces, and *Zhi Gan Cao* (Radix et Rhizoma Glycyrrhizae Praeparata cum Melle) 4g. Other slight modifications were made as follows: addition of *Chuan Xiong* (Rhizoma Chuanxiong) 6g for a purple tongue; *Chan Tui* (Periostracum Cicadae) 5g for tinnitus; and removal of *Da Zao* (Fructus Jujubae) and addition of *Sha Ren* (Fructus Amomi) 3g and *Dou Kou*

INTERIOR-WARMING FORMULAS

7

Wú Zhū Yú Tāng (Evodia Decoction)

(Fructus Amomi Rotundus) 3g for a greasy tongue coating. Improvement was noted in most patients within 5 packs of herbs. Out of 44 patients, the study reported significant improvement in 34 patients, moderate improvement in 8 patients, and no effect in 2 patients. The overall rate of effectiveness was 95.45%.[11]

7. **Drug addiction**: Modified *Wu Zhu Yu Tang* was evaluated for its efficacy in treating 6 males with 4 months to 2 years history of drug addiction (both inhalation and injection of drugs). The exact herbal treatments varied depending on the clinical presentations. For individuals with withdrawal reactions characterized by severe headaches, extreme coldness of the extremities, salivation, a purple tongue with a moist tongue coating, and a wiry pulse, the corresponding herbal formula contained ingredients such as *Wu Zhu Yu* (Fructus Evodiae) 10g, *Ren Shen* (Radix et Rhizoma Ginseng) 15g, and *Sheng Jiang* (Rhizoma Zingiberis Recens) 15g. For individuals with withdrawal reactions characterized by irritability, palpitations, nausea, vomiting, foaming of the mouth, a pale face, extremely cold extremities, bone and joint pain, a blue and purple tongue with a white tongue coating, and a deep and fine pulse, the corresponding herbal formula contained *Wu Zhu Yu Tang* and *Li Zhong Tang* (Regulate the Middle Decoction), with *Fu Zi* (Radix Aconiti Lateralis Praeparata) 30g and *Fu Ling* (Poria) 30g. The study reported that after 2-4 weeks of continuous treatment, most of the withdrawal reactions are under good control, though some patients still experienced fatigue, poor appetite, and vomiting of clear fluids.[12]

AUTHORS' COMMENTS

Wu Zhu Yu Tang has a wide range of therapeutic actions, and may be used to treat *yangming*, *shaoyin*, and *jueyin* disorders. This formula is also extremely effective for women suffering from migraine headaches with nausea or vomiting, especially before the menstrual cycle.

Li Zhong Wan (Regulate the Middle Pill) and *Wu Zhu Yu Tang* both warm the middle *jiao* and dispel cold to treat abdominal pain, nausea, and diarrhea due to cold and deficiency of the middle *jiao*. Both formulas use *Ren Shen* (Radix et Rhizoma Ginseng) to tonify the Spleen and Stomach. Their differences are as follows:

- *Li Zhong Wan* warms the Stomach to dispel cold to treat vomiting, diarrhea, and excessive salivation. *Gan Jiang* (Rhizoma Zingiberis) and *Bai Zhu* (Rhizoma Atractylodis Macrocephalae) warm the Spleen and Stomach, and treat deficiency and cold of the middle *jiao*.

- *Wu Zhu Yu Tang* is specifically for deficiency and cold in the Liver and Stomach, with turbid yin rising causing headache, nausea, and vomiting of white foam. It uses *Wu Zhu Yu* (Fructus Evodiae) to warm the Liver channel and redirect rebellious Stomach qi. It uses a heavy dose of *Sheng Jiang* (Rhizoma Zingiberis Recens) to complement the effects of *Wu Zhu Yu* (Fructus Evodiae).[13]

References

1. *Zhong Yao Ming Fang Yao Li Yu Ying Yong* (Pharmacology and Applications of Famous Herbal Formulas) 1989;226-228.
2. *Zhong Yi Fang Ji Xian Dai Yan Jiu* (Modern Study of Medical Formulae in Traditional Chinese Medicine) 1997;378.
3. *Zhong Yi Fang Ji Xian Dai Yan Jiu* (Modern Study of Medical Formulae in Traditional Chinese Medicine) 1997;378.
4. *Zhong Yao Yao Li Yu Lin Chuang* (Pharmacology and Clinical Applications of Chinese Herbs) 1987;3:49.
5. *Shan Xi Zhong Yi* (Shanxi Chinese Medicine) 1997;1:9.
6. *Hu Nan Zhong Yi Za Zhi* (Hunan Journal of Chinese Medicine) 1998;2:42.
7. *Zhong Cheng Yao Yan Jiu* (Research of Chinese Patent Medicine) 1985;1:46.
8. *Guo Wai Yi Xue Zhong Yi Zhong Yao Fen Ce* (Monograph of Chinese Herbology from Foreign Medicine) 1982;4:18.
9. *Xin Zhong Yi* (New Chinese Medicine) 1990;4:18.
10. *Bei Jing Zhong Yi* (Beijing Chinese Medicine) 1997;1:19.
11. *Hei Long Jiang Zhong Yi Yao* (Heilongjiang Chinese Medicine and Herbology) 1995;6:9.
12. *Yun Nan Zhong Yi Xue Yuan Xue Bao* (Journal of Yunnan University School of Medicine) 1995;1:38.
13. Wang MZ, et al. *Zhong Yi Xue Wen Da Ti Ku* (Questions and Answers on Traditional Chinese Medicine: Herbal Formulas).

Xiǎo Jiàn Zhōng Tāng (Minor Construct the Middle Decoction)

小建中湯
小建中汤

Pinyin Name: Xiao Jian Zhong Tang
Literal Name: Minor Construct the Middle Decoction
Alternate Names: Hsiao Chien Chung Tang, Xiao Jian Zhung Tang, Minor Centre-Fortifying Decoction, Minor Middle-Strengthening Decoction, Minor Cinnamon and Peony Combination
Original Source: Shang Han Lun (Discussion of Cold-Induced Disorders) by Zhang Zhong-Jing in the Eastern Han Dynasty

COMPOSITION

Yi Tang (Maltosum)	1 cup [30g]
Gui Zhi (Ramulus Cinnamomi)	9g
Bai Shao (Radix Paeoniae Alba), chao (dry-fried) with liquor	18g
Zhi Gan Cao (Radix et Rhizoma Glycyrrhizae Praeparata cum Melle)	6g
Sheng Jiang (Rhizoma Zingiberis Recens), qie (sliced)	9g
Da Zao (Fructus Jujubae), bo (opened)	12 pieces [4 pieces]

DOSAGE / PREPARATION / ADMINISTRATION

Cook the ingredients, except Yi Tang (Maltosum), in 7 cups [1,400 mL] of water until 3 cups [600 mL] of liquid remain. Filter and discard the herb residue, add Yi Tang (Maltosum) to the strained liquid, and allow it to dissolve using low heat. Take 1 cup [200 mL] of the warm, strained decoction three times daily. Today, the decoction is prepared by using the doses suggested in brackets, and by cooking the herbs twice. Filter and discard the herb residue, and dissolve Yi Tang (Maltosum) in the strained decoction. Take the warm decoction in two equally-divided doses.

CHINESE THERAPEUTIC ACTIONS

1. Tonifies and warms the middle jiao
2. Harmonizes the interior and relieves pain

CLINICAL MANIFESTATIONS

Deficiency and cold of the middle jiao: abdominal pain that decreases with warmth and pressure, a pale tongue with a white tongue coating, and a fine, wiry and moderate pulse; palpitations, fidgeting, irritability, a sallow and dull complexion; sore limbs, warm extremities, and a dry mouth and throat.

CLINICAL APPLICATIONS

Debility and chronic illness in children, such as enuresis, frequent urination, constant crying, malnutrition, and low-grade fever; gastritis, peptic ulcer disease, epigastric pain, abdominal pain, habitual constipation, hepatitis B, chronic hepatitis, neurasthenia, anemia, and depression.

EXPLANATION

Xiao Jian Zhong Tang (Minor Construct the Middle Decoction) treats deficiency and cold of the middle jiao with three clinical manifestations. Deficiency of the middle jiao may give rise to interior cold, which then produces abdominal pain. The pain usually improves with warmth and pressure. Deficiency and cold of the middle jiao also compromises the generation of qi and blood, which results in palpitations, fidgeting, irritability, and a sallow and dull complexion. Lastly, deficiency and cold of the middle jiao results in the inability of the Spleen to produce qi and blood. An insufficiency of qi and blood disrupts the harmony between the ying (nutritive) and wei (defensive) levels. Sore limbs occur as ying (nutritive) cannot properly nourish the muscles and warm extremities; and a dry mouth and throat occur when wei (defensive) qi leaks outwards. A pale tongue with a white coating is a sign of deficiency, and a fine, wiry and moderate pulse suggests true deficiency and cold in the interior and pain.

Yi Tang (Maltosum), the chief herb, warms the middle jiao, tonifies Spleen qi, and nourishes Spleen yin. Furthermore, it softens the Liver to alleviate pain and moistens the Lung to relieve dryness. Gui Zhi (Ramulus Cinnamomi) warms yang and dispels cold. Bai Shao (Radix Paeoniae Alba) nourishes yin and blood and relieves pain. Zhi Gan Cao (Radix et Rhizoma Glycyrrhizae Praeparata cum Melle) tonifies qi and helps Yi Tang (Maltosum) and Gui Zhi (Ramulus Cinnamomi) warm the middle and benefit qi. Zhi Gan Cao (Radix et Rhizoma Glycyrrhizae Praeparata cum Melle) also helps Bai Shao (Radix Paeoniae Alba) nourish the Liver and alleviate pain. Sheng Jiang (Rhizoma Zingiberis Recens) warms the Stomach and Da Zao (Fructus Jujubae) tonifies the Spleen. These two herbs also harmonize the ying (nutritive) and wei (defensive) levels. In summary, this

Xiǎo Jiàn Zhōng Tāng (Minor Construct the Middle Decoction)

Xiao Jian Zhong Tang (Minor Construct the Middle Decoction)

Diagnosis	Signs and Symptoms	Treatment	Herbs
Deficiency and cold of the middle *jiao*	• Abdominal pain that decreases with warmth and pressure: cold and deficiency of the middle *jiao* • Palpitations and a dull and sallow complexion: qi and blood deficiencies • Sore limbs, warm extremities, and a dry mouth and throat: disharmony of *ying* (nutritive) and *wei* (defensive) levels • Pale tongue with a white coating: deficiency • Fine, wiry and moderate pulse: deficiency and cold in the interior	• Tonifies and warms the middle *jiao* • Harmonizes the interior and relieves pain	• *Yi Tang* (Maltosum) warms the middle *jiao*, tonifies Spleen qi, and nourishes Spleen yin. • *Gui Zhi* (Ramulus Cinnamomi) warms yang and dispels cold. • *Bai Shao* (Radix Paeoniae Alba) nourishes yin and blood. • *Zhi Gan Cao* (Radix et Rhizoma Glycyrrhizae Praeparata cum Melle) tonifies qi, warms the middle *jiao*, and alleviates pain. • *Sheng Jiang* (Rhizoma Zingiberis Recens) and *Da Zao* (Fructus Jujubae) warm the Stomach and tonify the Spleen.

formula warms and tonifies the middle *jiao*, which in turn alleviates the associated symptoms characterized by deficiency and cold.

MODIFICATIONS
• With fatigue due to qi deficiency, add *Huang Qi* (Radix Astragali) and *Ren Shen* (Radix et Rhizoma Ginseng).
• With fatigue due to blood deficiency, add *Dang Gui* (Radix Angelicae Sinensis) and *Chuan Xiong* (Rhizoma Chuanxiong).
• With a sallow complexion, fatigue and tiredness, remove *Yi Tang* (Maltosum) and add *Ren Shen* (Radix et Rhizoma Ginseng), *Huang Qi* (Radix Astragali) and *Dang Gui* (Radix Angelicae Sinensis).
• With irritability due to Lung deficiency, add *Mai Dong* (Radix Ophiopogonis) and *Wu Wei Zi* (Fructus Schisandrae Chinensis).
• If there is chronic weakness and deficiency in women, add *Si Wu Tang* (Four-Substance Decoction).
• If there is chronic weakness and deficiency in men, add *Si Jun Zi Tang* (Four-Gentlemen Decoction).

CAUTIONS / CONTRAINDICATIONS
• *Xiao Jian Zhong Tang* is contraindicated in cases of yin-deficient fire, and conditions characterized by middle *jiao* stagnation.
• This formula is not recommended for treating vomiting because the sweet herbs in this formula will create more stagnation and promote Stomach qi reversal.
• This formula is contraindicated in patients with intestinal parasites.

PHARMACOLOGICAL EFFECTS
1. **Antiulcer**: Administration of *Xiao Jian Zhong Tang* was associated with a protective effect on the stomach in rats. The beneficial effects are attributed to *Gui Zhi* (Ramulus Cinnamomi) for its effect to treat ulceration, *Bai Shao* (Radix Paeoniae Alba) for its effect to inhibit the production of gastric acid, and *Gan Cao* (Radix et Rhizoma Glycyrrhizae) and *Sheng Jiang* (Rhizoma Zingiberis Recens) for their effect to protect the mucous lining of the stomach.[1]
2. **Gastrointestinal**: Administration of *Xiao Jian Zhong Tang* was associated with a general inhibitory effect on the gastrointestinal system. According to a laboratory experiment, animals who received ingredients of *Xiao Jian Zhong Tang* responded with a decreased production of gastric acid and lowered rate of peristalsis.[2]

CLINICAL STUDIES AND RESEARCH
1. **Gastrointestinal disorders**: In one report, 21 patients with various types of gastrointestinal disorders (11 with peptic ulcers, 8 with superficial gastritis, and 2 with atrophic gastritis) were treated with modified *Xiao Jian Zhong Tang* for 15 consecutive doses. The formula included *Bai Shao* (Radix Paeoniae Alba) 15g, *Gui Zhi* (Ramulus Cinnamomi) 10g, *Gan Jiang* (Rhizoma Zingiberis) 5g, *Da Zao* (Fructus Jujubae) 5 pieces, *Zhi Gan Cao* (Radix et Rhizoma Glycyrrhizae Praeparata cum Melle) 5g, *Dang Shen* (Radix Codonopsis) 10g, *Bai Zhu* (Rhizoma Atractylodis Macrocephalae) 10g, *Fo Shou* (Fructus Citri Sarcodactylis) 10g, and *Yi Tang* (Maltosum) 30g. The study reported significant improvement in pain reduction in 20 out of 21 patients.[3]

Xiǎo Jiàn Zhōng Tāng (Minor Construct the Middle Decoction)

2. **Gastritis**: *Xiao Jian Zhong Tang* was reported in one study to have good effect to treat gastritis. Of 58 patients with chronic gastritis, 39 were diagnosed with atrophic gastritis and 19 with superficial gastritis. In addition to *Xiao Jian Zhong Tang*, modifications were made based on the individual conditions of the patients. For acid reflux, *Yi Tang* (Maltosum) was removed and *Wu Zhu Yu* (Fructus Evodiae), *Hai Piao Xiao* (Endoconcha Sepiae) and *Mu Li* (Concha Ostreae) were added. For pain at night, a purplish tongue with dark spots, *Yan Hu Suo* (Rhizoma Corydalis), *Chi Shao* (Radix Paeoniae Rubra), and *Dan Shen* (Radix et Rhizoma Salviae Miltiorrhizae) were added. For the presence of *H. pylori*, *Da Huang* (Radix et Rhizoma Rhei) and *Pu Huang* (Pollen Typhae) were added. For qi deficiency and generalized weakness, *Huang Qi* (Radix Astragali), *Fu Ling* (Poria), and *Bai Zhu* (Rhizoma Atractylodis Macrocephalae) were added. Out of 58 cases, the study reported complete recovery in 32 cases (55.5%), improvement in 18 cases (31.0%), and no benefit in 8 cases (13.8%). The overall rate of effectiveness was 86.2%.[4]

3. **Peptic ulcer disease**: Modified *Xiao Jian Zhong Tang* was used with good results in treating 31 of 35 patients with peptic ulcer and abdominal pain. No recurrence was noted amongst 31 patients in their one-year follow-up examination. The herbal treatment used *Xiao Jian Zhong Tang* plus *Gua Lou* (Fructus Trichosanthis), *Wu Zhu Yu* (Fructus Evodiae), and *Xie Bai* (Bulbus Allii Macrostemonis) as the base formula. For severe acid reflux, *Da Zao* (Fructus Jujubae) and *Yi Tang* (Maltosum) were removed and *Huang Lian* (Rhizoma Coptidis) and *Mu Li* (Concha Ostreae) were added. For nausea and vomiting, *Pao Jiang* (Rhizoma Zingiberis Praeparatum) was removed and *Ban Xia* (Rhizoma Pinelliae) and *Sheng Jiang* (Rhizoma Zingiberis Recens) were added. For frequent belching, *Xuan Fu Hua* (Flos Inulae), *Ban Xia* (Rhizoma Pinelliae), and *Zhe Shi* (Haematitum) were added. For feeling of chest and abdominal oppression and distention, *Da Zao* (Fructus Jujubae) was removed and *Hou Po* (Cortex Magnoliae Officinalis) and *Zhi Qiao* (Fructus Aurantii) were added. Lastly, *Fu Ling* (Poria) was added for palpitations and *Bai Zhu* (Rhizoma Atractylodis Macrocephalae) was added for loose stools.[5]

4. **Epigastric pain**: Numerous studies have shown that *Xiao Jian Zhong Tang* effectively treats epigastric pain due to various causes, including but not limited to chronic gastritis, gastric ulcer, duodenal ulcer, gastric prolapse, and others.[6,7]

5. **Abdominal pain**: *Xiao Jian Zhong Tang* was shown in two reports to effectively treat abdominal pain in infants and children between 3-10 years of age. Specific causes of abdominal pain were not stated in these reports.[8,9]

6. **Habitual constipation**: In one study, 11 patients with chronic habitual constipation were treated with modified *Xiao Jian Zhong Tang*. The formula included *Yi Tang* (Maltosum) 30g, *Bai Shao* (Radix Paeoniae Alba) 15g, *Gui Zhi* (Ramulus Cinnamomi) 6g, *Zhi Gan Cao* (Radix et Rhizoma Glycyrrhizae Praeparata cum Melle) 5g, and *Da Zao* (Fructus Jujubae) 5 pieces. The treatment protocol was to administer the herbs in decoction for seven days per course of treatment. The study reported success with all patients. Out of 11 patients, 4 responded within 1 course, 6 within 2 courses, and 1 after 5 courses. There were no recurrences in all patients in follow-up interviews 6 months after the termination of treatments.[10]

7. **Depression**: Twelve geriatric patients (over 65 years of age) with severe depression were treated daily with 7.5-15.0g of *Xiao Jian Zhong Tang* in extract form. Two weeks after the start of herbal therapy, 7 out of 12 patients reported improvement of mood. Four weeks after the start of herbal therapy, 10 out 12 patients reported improvement of mood. The study also reported that the patients who responded the most were ones who had feelings of guilt and constant suspicion. No significant side effects were reported.[11]

8. **Hepatitis B**: One study reported beneficial effect using modified *Xiao Jian Zhong Tang* to treat 68 patients with hepatitis B. The herbal treatment contained this formula plus *Sha Ren* (Fructus Amomi), *Ji Nei Jin* (Endothelium Corneum Gigeriae Galli), charred *Shan Zha* (Fructus Crataegi), charred *Shen Qu* (Massa Fermentata), and charred *Mai Ya* (Fructus Hordei Germinatus). Furthermore, modifications included addition of *Yin Chen* (Herba Artemisiae Scopariae), *Cang Zhu* (Rhizoma Atractylodis), *Pu Gong Ying* (Herba Taraxaci), and *Chui Pen Cao* (Herba Sedi) for damp-heat; *Dang Shen* (Radix Codonopsis), *Shan Yao* (Rhizoma Dioscoreae), *Bai Zhu* (Rhizoma Atractylodis Macrocephalae), and *Huang Qi* (Radix Astragali) for qi deficiency; *Bei Sha Shen* (Radix Glehniae), *Mai Dong* (Radix Ophiopogonis), *Gou Qi Zi* (Fructus Lycii), and *Yin Yang Huo* (Herba Epimedii) for yin deficiency; and other adjustments as needed. The duration of treatment was three months per course of treatment, for 1-2 courses. Of 68 cases, the study reported significant effect in 47 cases, moderate effect in 15 cases, and no effect in 6 cases. The overall rate of effectiveness was 91%.[12]

RELATED FORMULA

Dāng Guī Jiàn Zhōng Tāng
(Tangkuei Decoction to Construct the Middle)
當歸建中湯
当归建中汤

Chapter 7 – Interior-Warming Formulas　　　　　*Section 1 – Middle-Warming and Cold-Dispelling Formulas*

Xiǎo Jiàn Zhōng Tāng (Minor Construct the Middle Decoction)

Pinyin Name: *Dang Gui Jian Zhong Tang*
Literal Name: Tangkuei Decoction to Construct the Middle
Original Source: *Qian Jin Yi Fang* (Supplement to the Thousand Ducat Formulas) by Sun Si-Miao in 682 A.D.

Dang Gui (Radix Angelicae Sinensis)	12g
Gui Xin (Cortex Rasus Cinnamomi)	9g
Zhi Gan Cao (Radix et Rhizoma Glycyrrhizae Praeparata cum Melle)	6g
Bai Shao (Radix Paeoniae Alba), *chao* (dry-fried) with liquor	18g
Sheng Jiang (Rhizoma Zingiberis Recens), *qie* (sliced)	9g
Da Zao (Fructus Jujubae), *bo* (opened)	12 pieces [4 pieces]
Yi Tang (Maltosum)	18g

Cook the ingredients, except *Yi Tang* (Maltosum), in 10 cups [2,000 mL] of water until 3 cups [600 mL] of liquid remain. Filter and discard the herb residue, add *Yi Tang* (Maltosum) to the strained liquid, and allow it to dissolve over low intensity heat. Take 1 cup [200 mL] of the warm, strained decoction three times daily.

Dang Gui Jian Zhong Tang (Tangkuei Decoction to Construct the Middle) is composed of *Dang Gui* (Radix Angelicae Sinensis) and *Xiao Jian Zhong Tang*. It tonifies the blood, warms the middle *jiao*, and relieves pain. Clinically, patients may show abdominal pain, or lower abdominal pain that radiates to the lower back, in addition to all the symptoms listed in *Xiao Jian Zhong Tang*. This formula may also be used in postpartum women with generalized deficiency and weakness.

AUTHORS' COMMENTS

Abdominal pain may be caused by many different factors. Three potential causes and their diagnosis include pain that worsens with pressure is acute and excess in nature; pain that lessens with pressure is deficient and chronic in nature; and pain that worsens with cold and lessens with warmth is cold in nature. *Xiao Jian Zhong Tang* is designed to treat abdominal pain due to yang deficiency of the middle *jiao*, with key signs and symptoms of abdominal pain that lessens with pressure and warmth, a sallow and dull facial complexion, and a pale tongue with a white, slippery tongue coating.

There are four "*jian zhong tang* (construct the middle decoction)" formulas that have similar functions to warm and tonify the middle *jiao*.

- *Xiao Jian Zhong Tang* (Minor Construct the Middle Decoction) warms the yang of the middle *jiao*.

- *Huang Qi Jian Zhong Tang* (Astragalus Decoction to Construct the Middle) warms and tonifies qi of the middle *jiao*.
- *Dang Gui Jian Zhong Tang* (Tangkuei Decoction to Construct the Middle) harmonizes the blood and relieves pain.
- *Da Jian Zhong Tang* (Major Construct the Middle Decoction) redirects rising Stomach qi to treat nausea and vomiting.

Li Zhong Wan (Regulate the Middle Pill) and *Xiao Jian Zhong Tang* both warm the middle *jiao* and disperse cold to treat deficiency and cold of the middle *jiao* manifesting in abdominal and epigastric coldness and pain. Their differences are as follows:

- *Li Zhong Wan* treats Spleen yang deficiency with excess cold accumulation. This formula has a more qi tonic effect than *Xiao Jian Zhong Tang*. Manifestations include diarrhea, vomiting, abdominal pain, and poor appetite. It is also suitable for yang deficiency with sudden blood loss, chronic infantile convulsions, *xiong bi* (painful obstruction of the chest) syndrome, and excessive salivation in chronic diseases.
- *Xiao Jian Zhong Tang* warms the entire middle *jiao* and strengthens middle *jiao* yang qi. Patients usually also have yang deficiency of the middle *jiao* along with qi, blood, and yin deficiencies. The chief complaint is pain. Other symptoms include palpitations, irritability, a sallow complexion, warm sensations in the limbs, and a dry mouth and throat. It can also treat qi, yin, and blood deficiencies with fatigue, palpitations, and shortness of breath usually seen in postpartum women and in late stage diseases.[13]

Gui Zhi Tang (Cinnamon Twig Decoction) and *Xiao Jian Zhong Tang* are both from *Shang Han Lun* (Discussion of Cold-Induced Disorders). They have essentially the same ingredients except for one herb, yet the difference in doses significantly changes the functions and indications of these formulas.

- *Gui Zhi Tang* contains 9g each of *Bai Shao* (Radix Paeoniae Alba) and *Gui Zhi* (Ramulus Cinnamomi). At equal doses, the emphasis of these two herbs is to dispel wind-cold and harmonize the *ying* (nutritive) and *wei* (defensive) levels to treat an exterior condition lingering in the *taiyang* channel.
- *Xiao Jian Zhong Tang* was originally derived from *Gui Zhi Tang* (Cinnamon Twig Decoction) with the addition of *Yi Tang* (Maltosum). The rest of the ingredients are exactly the same. *Xiao Jian Zhong Tang* contains 30g of *Yi Tang* (Maltosum) and 18g of *Bai Shao* (Radix Paeoniae Alba);

474

Chinese Herbal Formulas and Applications

Xiǎo Jiàn Zhōng Tāng (Minor Construct the Middle Decoction)

whereas, there are only 9g in *Gui Zhi Tang* (Cinnamon Twig Decoction). With these two as the primary herbs used at higher doses, *Xiao Jian Zhong Tang* focuses on warming the middle *jiao*, tonifying deficiency, and relieving pain.[14]

References

1. *Guo Wai Yi Xue Zhong Yi Zhong Yao Fen Ce* (Monograph of Chinese Herbology from Foreign Medicine) 1983;6:45.
2. *Shan Dong Zhong Yi Za Zhi* (Shandong Journal of Chinese Medicine) 1984;2:22.
3. *Zhong Yi Za Zhi* (Journal of Chinese Medicine) 1981;11:657.
4. *Shi Yong Zhong Xi Yi Jie He Za Zhi* (Practical Journal of Integrated Chinese and Western Medicines) 1998;1:71.
5. *Zhe Jiang Zhong Yi Yao* (Zhejiang Chinese Medicine and Herbology) 1978;2:9.
6. *Fu Jian Zhong Yi Yao* (Fujian Chinese Medicine and Herbology) 1990;6:55.
7. *Zhong Yi Ming Fang Lin Chuang Xin Yong* (Contemporary Clinical Applications of Classic Chinese Formulas) 2001;87-88.
8. *Shan Xi Zhong Yi* (Shanxi Chinese Medicine) 1992;12:537.
9. *Ji Lin Zhong Yi Yao* (Jilin Chinese Medicine and Herbology) 1997;2:19.
10. *Liao Ning Zhong Yi Za Zhi* (Liaoning Journal of Chinese Medicine) 1984;4:29.
11. *Guo Wai Yi Xue Zhong Yi Zhong Yao Fen Ce* (Monograph of Chinese Herbology from Foreign Medicine) 1994;4:24.
12. *Zhong Yi Fang Ji Xian Dai Yan Jiu* (Modern Study of Medical Formulae in Traditional Chinese Medicine) 1997;385.
13. Wang MZ, et al. *Zhong Yi Xue Wen Da Ti Ku* (Questions and Answers on Traditional Chinese Medicine: Herbal Formulas).
14. Wang MZ, et al. *Zhong Yi Xue Wen Da Ti Ku* (Questions and Answers on Traditional Chinese Medicine: Herbal Formulas).

Huáng Qí Jiàn Zhōng Tāng
(Astragalus Decoction to Construct the Middle)

黃耆建中湯
黄芪建中汤

Pinyin Name: *Huang Qi Jian Zhong Tang*
Literal Name: Astragalus Decoction to Construct the Middle
Alternate Names: *Huang Chi Chien Chung Tang, Huang Qi Jian Zhung Tang*, Astragalus Centre-Fortifying Decoction, Astragalus Middle-Strengthening Decoction, Astragalus Combination
Original Source: *Jin Gui Yao Lue* (Essentials from the Golden Cabinet) by Zhang Zhong-Jing in the Eastern Han Dynasty

COMPOSITION

Yi Tang (Maltosum)	1 cup [30g]
Gui Zhi (Ramulus Cinnamomi)	9g
Bai Shao (Radix Paeoniae Alba), *chao* (dry-fried) with liquor	18g
Zhi Gan Cao (Radix et Rhizoma Glycyrrhizae Praeparata cum Melle)	6g
Sheng Jiang (Rhizoma Zingiberis Recens), *qie* (sliced)	9g
Da Zao (Fructus Jujubae), *bo* (opened)	12 pieces [4 pieces]
Huang Qi (Radix Astragali)	4.5g [12g]

DOSAGE / PREPARATION / ADMINISTRATION

Cook the ingredients, except *Yi Tang* (Maltosum), in 7 cups [1,400 mL] of water until 3 cups [600 mL] of liquid remain. Filter and discard the herb residue, add *Yi Tang* (Maltosum) to the strained liquid, and allow it to dissolve using low heat. Take 1 cup [200 mL] of the warm, strained decoction three times daily. Today, the decoction is prepared by using the doses suggested in brackets, and by cooking the herbs twice. Filter and discard the herb residue, and dissolve *Yi Tang* (Maltosum) in the strained decoction. Take the warm decoction in two equally-divided doses.

CHINESE THERAPEUTIC ACTIONS

1. Warms the middle *jiao* and tonifies qi
2. Harmonizes the interior and relieves pain

INTERIOR-WARMING FORMULAS

7

475

Huáng Qí Jiàn Zhōng Tāng
(Astragalus Decoction to Construct the Middle)

CLINICAL MANIFESTATIONS

Deficiency and cold of the middle *jiao* with severe qi deficiency: abdominal pain that decreases with warmth and pressure, a sallow and dull complexion, and a pale tongue with a white tongue coating. There might be palpitations, fidgeting, irritability, spontaneous perspiration, shortness of breath, lethargy, and a dry mouth and throat.

CLINICAL APPLICATIONS

Peptic ulcer disease, gastritis, antral gastritis, atrophic gastritis, gastric ulcer, duodenal ulcer, inflammatory bowel disease, irritable bowel syndrome, anorexia, constipation, allergic rhinitis, otitis media, leukopenia, lead poisoning, neurasthenia, pernicious anemia, hypoglycemia, chronic ulceration, delayed healing of wounds, and gangrene.

EXPLANATION

Huang Qi Jian Zhong Tang (Astragalus Decoction to Construct the Middle) is formulated by combining *Huang Qi* (Radix Astragali) and *Xiao Jian Zhong Tang* (Minor Construct the Middle Decoction). *Xiao Jian Zhong Tang* (Minor Construct the Middle Decoction) tonifies and warms the middle *jiao*, harmonizes the interior, and relieves pain. *Huang Qi* (Radix Astragali) tonifies qi to treat qi deficiency.

Please refer to *Xiao Jian Zhong Tang* (Minor Construct the Middle Decoction) for a complete explanation of this formula and its applications.

MODIFICATIONS

- For generalized weakness following an illness, combine with *Si Jun Zi Tang* (Four-Gentlemen Decoction).
- For generalized weakness in postpartum women, combine with *Si Wu Tang* (Four-Substance Decoction).

- For generalized weakness following a wind-cold disorder, combine with *Yu Ping Feng San* (Jade Windscreen Powder).
- With abdominal fullness, add *Hou Po* (Cortex Magnoliae Officinalis), *Sha Ren* (Fructus Amomi), and *Mu Xiang* (Radix Aucklandiae).
- With vomitus of clear fluids, add *Wu Zhu Yu* (Fructus Evodiae), *Ban Xia* (Rhizoma Pinelliae), and *Gan Jiang* (Rhizoma Zingiberis).
- With edema, add *Bai Zhu* (Rhizoma Atractylodis Macrocephalae), *Fu Ling* (Poria), and *Ze Xie* (Rhizoma Alismatis).

PHARMACOLOGICAL EFFECTS

1. **Gastrointestinal**: Administration of *Huang Qi Jian Zhong Tang* was effective in suppressing the production of gastric acid, thereby promoting the recovery from gastric ulcers in rats.[1]
2. **Immunostimulant**: One study reported an increase in IgG from 12.4-24.5 mg/mL to 12.4-30 mg/mL (an average increase of 1.59 mg/mL; $p<0.05$) following ingestion of *Huang Qi Jian Zhong Tang* for 20 doses while treating gastrointestinal disorders.[2]

CLINICAL STUDIES AND RESEARCH

1. **Peptic ulcer disease**: *Huang Qi Jian Zhong Tang* has been shown in many clinical studies to effectively treat gastric and duodenal ulcers. In one study, use of modified *Huang Qi Jian Zhong Tang* in 100 patients with peptic ulcer (gastric and duodenal ulcers) was associated with complete recovery in 85 patients, significant improvement in 13 patients, and no effect in 2 patients. The herbal treatment contained this formula plus *Hai Piao Xiao* (Endoconcha Sepiae) and *Bai Ji* (Rhizoma Bletillae). Additional modifications included *Yan Hu Suo* (Rhizoma Corydalis) for severe pain; *Zhi Qiao* (Fructus Aurantii) and *Chen Pi* (Pericarpium Citri Reticulatae) for fullness and distention in the chest and abdominal regions; *Wa Leng Zi* (Concha Arcae) and *Mai Ya* (Fructus Hordei Germinatus) for acid reflux; and *San Qi* (Radix et Rhizoma

Huang Qi Jian Zhong Tang (Astragalus Decoction to Construct the Middle)

Diagnosis	Signs and Symptoms	Treatment	Herbs
Deficiency and cold of the middle *jiao* with severe qi deficiency	• Abdominal pain that decreases with warmth and pressure, a sallow and dull complexion, a pale tongue with a white tongue coating, and fine, wiry and moderate pulse: deficiency and cold of the middle *jiao* • Spontaneous perspiration, shortness of breath and lethargy: qi deficiency	• Warms the middle *jiao* and tonifies qi • Harmonizes the interior and relieves pain	• *Xiao Jian Zhong Tang* (Minor Construct the Middle Decoction) tonifies and warms the middle *jiao*, harmonizes the interior, and relieves pain. • *Huang Qi* (Radix Astragali) tonifies qi.

Huáng Qí Jiàn Zhōng Tāng
(Astragalus Decoction to Construct the Middle)

Notoginseng) for bleeding.[3] According to another study, 12 patients (4 with gastric ulcer, 4 with duodenal ulcer, and 4 with both gastric and duodenal ulcers) were treated with modified *Huang Qi Jian Zhong Tang* with marked success. In addition to this formula, *Huang Lian* (Rhizoma Coptidis) and *Wu Zhu Yu* (Fructus Evodiae) were added for acid reflux; *Fan Xie Ye* (Folium Sennae) for constipation; and charred *Shan Zha* (Fructus Crataegi), charred *Shen Qu* (Massa Fermentata), and charred *Mai Ya* (Fructus Hordei Germinatus) for food stagnation. Of 12 patients, the study reported complete recovery in 9 patients, improvement in 2 patients, and no benefit in 1 patient.[4]

2. **Antral gastritis**: One study reported 92.6% effectiveness in the treatment of chronic antral gastritis using *Huang Qi Jian Zhong Tang* plus *Dan Shen* (Radix et Rhizoma Salviae Miltiorrhizae), *Tao Ren* (Semen Persicae), *Yan Hu Suo* (Rhizoma Corydalis), and minus *Yi Tang* (Maltosum). Additional modifications were made as need. For Stomach yin deficiency, *Sha Shen* (Radix Glehniae seu Adenophorae) and *Mai Dong* (Radix Ophiopogonis) were added, and *Gan Jiang* (Rhizoma Zingiberis) and *Gui Zhi* (Ramulus Cinnamomi) were removed. For disharmony of the Liver and Stomach, *Chai Hu* (Radix Bupleuri) and *Xiang Fu* (Rhizoma Cyperi) were added. For accumulation of phlegm in the middle *jiao*, *Ban Xia* (Rhizoma Pinelliae) and *Chen Pi* (Pericarpium Citri Reticulatae) were added. For food stagnation, *Shen Qu* (Massa Fermentata) and *Shan Zha* (Fructus Crataegi) were added. Of 41 patients, the study reported complete recovery in 23 patients, significant improvement in 9 patients, slight improvement in 6 patients, and no change in 3 patients.[5]

3. **Atrophic gastritis**: Use of modified *Huang Qi Jian Zhong Tang* was associated with 96% effectiveness in treating 101 patients with 1-20 years history of atrophic gastritis. In addition to this formula, modifications were made to include *Dang Shen* (Radix Codonopsis) for deficiency and cold of the Spleen and Stomach; *Dan Shen* (Radix et Rhizoma Salviae Miltiorrhizae) and *Chuan Lian Zi* (Fructus Toosendan) for Liver qi stagnation; and *Bai He* (Bulbus Lilii) for Spleen and Stomach yin deficiencies. The duration of treatment was four weeks per course of treatment, for a total of three courses. Of 101 patients, the study reported complete recovery in 59 patients, significant improvement in 24 patients, moderate improvement in 14 patients, and no effect in 4 patients.[6]

4. **Anorexia**: One study reported complete recovery in 26 of 32 children with anorexia using *Huang Qi Jian Zhong Tang* plus dry-fried *Gu Ya* (Fructus Setariae Germinatus) and *Sha Ren* (Fructus Amomi) in decoction for one week per course of treatment.[7]

5. **Constipation**: Fifty patients with constipation characterized by deficiency were treated with good results using *Huang Qi Jian Zhong Tang* plus *Nu Zhen Zi* (Fructus Ligustri Lucidi) and *Dang Gui* (Radix Angelicae Sinensis). Additional modifications were made as follows: a larger dose of *Huang Qi* (Radix Astragali) for constipation with qi deficiency; a larger dose of *Dang Gui* (Radix Angelicae Sinensis) for constipation with blood deficiency; *Fu Zi* (Radix Aconiti Lateralis Praeparata) and *Pao Jiang* (Rhizoma Zingiberis Praeparatum) for constipation with yang deficiency; *Rou Cong Rong* (Herba Cistanches), *Gou Qi Zi* (Fructus Lycii) and *Niu Xi* (Radix Achyranthis Bidentatae) for geriatric patients with soreness and weakness of the lower back and knees; and *Wu Wei Zi* (Fructus Schisandrae Chinensis) for presence of chloasma on the face. The treatment protocol was to administer the herbs in decoction form daily, for 10 days per course of treatment, for 1-2 courses total.[8]

6. **Irritable bowel syndrome (IBS)**: One study reported 92% effectiveness using modified *Huang Qi Jian Zhong Tang* to treat 50 patients with IBS. In addition to this formula, modifications were made by adding *Sha Ren* (Fructus Amomi) and *Lai Fu Zi* (Semen Raphani) for qi stagnation; *Huo Xiang* (Herba Agastaches), *Cang Zhu* (Rhizoma Atractylodis), and *Pei Lan* (Herba Eupatorii) for loose stools due to cold and dampness; *Sha Ren* (Fructus Amomi), *Gu Ya* (Fructus Setariae Germinatus) and *Ji Nei Jin* (Endothelium Corneum Gigeriae Galli) for food stagnation, poor appetite, and belching; *Chai Hu* (Radix Bupleuri) and *Fo Shou* (Fructus Citri Sarcodactylis) for Liver qi stagnation with hypochondriac pain; and *Fu Zi* (Radix Aconiti Lateralis Praeparata) and *Bu Gu Zhi* (Fructus Psoraleae) for soreness and weakness of the lower back and knees. The treatment protocol was to administer the herbs in decoction one time daily, for one month per course of treatment, for 1-4 courses total. Of 50 patients, the study reported complete recovery in 21 patients, significant improvement in 15 patients, moderate improvement in 10 patients, and no change in 4 patients.[9]

7. **Allergic rhinitis**: Sixty patients with allergic rhinitis were treated with significant improvement in 50 patients and moderate improvement in 10 patients. The herbal treatment contained *Huang Qi Jian Zhong Tang* plus *Ku Xing Ren* (Semen Armeniacae Amarum), *Gan Cao* (Radix et Rhizoma Glycyrrhizae), and *Ba Ji Tian* (Radix Morindae Officinalis). For individuals who showed presence of heat, *Huang Qin* (Radix Scutellariae) was added and *Ba Ji Tian* (Radix Morindae Officinalis) was removed. The herbs were given in decoction form one time daily, for between 7-20 days.[10]

Chapter 7 – Interior-Warming Formulas   *Section 1 – Middle-Warming and Cold-Dispelling Formulas*

Huáng Qí Jiàn Zhōng Tāng
(Astragalus Decoction to Construct the Middle)

8. **Otitis media**: One study reported good therapeutic effects using modified *Huang Qi Jian Zhong Tang* to treat chronic suppurative otitis media. In addition to this formula, modifications were made by adding *Long Dan* (Radix et Rhizoma Gentianae), *Che Qian Zi* (Semen Plantaginis), and *Jin Yin Hua* (Flos Lonicerae Japonicae) for profuse sticky ear discharge; *Huang Bo* (Cortex Phellodendri Chinensis), *Huang Lian* (Rhizoma Coptidis) and *Bai Jiang Cao* (Herba cum Radice Patriniae) for foul-smelling discharge; *Dang Gui* (Radix Angelicae Sinensis), *Yi Yi Ren* (Semen Coicis), *Bai Zhu* (Rhizoma Atractylodis Macrocephalae), and a large dose of *Jin Yin Hua* (Flos Lonicerae Japonicae) for profuse watery discharge; *Chuan Xiong* (Rhizoma Chuanxiong), *Man Jing Zi* (Fructus Viticis), *Bai Zhi* (Radix Angelicae Dahuricae) and *Pei Lan* (Herba Eupatorii) for severe headache; *Fang Feng* (Radix Saposhnikoviae), *Ji Li* (Fructus Tribuli), *Zhu Ru* (Caulis Bambusae in Taenia), and *Ban Xia* (Rhizoma Pinelliae) for nausea and dizziness. The treatment protocol was to cook the herbs in water and drink the decoction in two to three equally-divided doses. Of 30 patients, the study reported complete recovery in 10 patients, significant improvement in 14 patients, and no effect in 6 patients.[11]

9. **Leukopenia**: Twenty-six patients with decreased white blood cells count were effectively treated using *Huang Qi Jian Zhong Tang* plus *Huang Lian Jie Du Tang* (Coptis Decoction to Relieve Toxicity). In addition, *Bai Zhu* (Rhizoma Atractylodis Macrocephalae) and *Dang Gui* (Radix Angelicae Sinensis) were added for dizziness and fatigue; *Dang Shen* (Radix Codonopsis) and *Fu Ling* (Poria) for soreness and weakness of the extremities; *Shi Chang Pu* (Rhizoma Acori Tatarinowii) and *Yuan Zhi* (Radix Polygalae) for insomnia and palpitations; and *Huang Qi* (Radix Astragali) and *Huang Lian* (Rhizoma Coptidis) at large doses for frequent recurrences of infection. After 10-20 days of herbal therapy, the study reported complete recovery in 17 patients, improvement in 6 patients, and no benefit in 3 patients.[12]

10. **Athletic performance**: According to one study of 12 athletes randomly separated into a control group (treated with placebos) and the experimental group (treated with herbs), use of *Huang Qi Jian Zhong Tang* for 8 weeks was associated with effectively increasing time before exhaustion, positively influencing anaerobic threshold, and enhancing recovery from fatigue by increasing the uptake and the systemic utilization of oxygen.[13]

11. **Lead poisoning**: Use of this formula had a beneficial effect in treating 42 patients with chronic lead poisoning. Clinical improvements included relief of pain and reduced duration of treatment.[14]

TOXICOLOGY

According to one study on acute toxicology, the LD_{50} for subcutaneous injection of this formula in decoction form is 48 g/kg in mice.[15]

References

1. *Yao Xue Xue Bao* (Journal of Herbology) 1986;7:440.
2. *Shang Hai Zhong Yi Yao Za Zhi* (Shanghai Journal of Chinese Medicine and Herbology) 1983;2:28.
3. *Shan Xi Zhong Yi* (Shanxi Chinese Medicine) 1990;8:345.
4. *Ji Lin Zhong Yi Yao* (Jilin Chinese Medicine and Herbology) 1996;5:10.
5. *He Bei Zhong Yi* (Hebei Chinese Medicine) 1987;1:28.
6. *Hu Bei Zhong Yi Za Zhi* (Hubei Journal of Chinese Medicine) 1991;1:12.
7. *He Nan Zhong Yi* (Henan Chinese Medicine) 1998;2:51.
8. *Xin Zhong Yi* (New Chinese Medicine) 1996;3:30.
9. *Shi Yong Zhong Xi Yi Jie He Za Zhi* (Practical Journal of Integrated Chinese and Western Medicines) 1998;6:560.
10. *Liao Ning Zhong Yi Za Zhi* (Liaoning Journal of Chinese Medicine) 1990;5:39.
11. *Shan Xi Zhong Yi* (Shanxi Chinese Medicine) 1990;6:20.
12. *Zhe Jiang Zhong Yi Za Zhi* (Zhejiang Journal of Chinese Medicine) 1995;10:443.
13. Chen KT, Su CH, Hsin LH, Su YC, Su YP, Lin JG. Reducing fatigue of athletes following oral administration of huangqi jianzhong tang. Acta Pharmacologica Sinica 2002 Aug;23(8):757-61.
14. *Hu Nan Zhong Yi Za Zhi* (Hunan Journal of Chinese Medicine) 1989;3:22.
15. *Yao Xue Xue Bao* (Journal of Herbology) 1986;7:440.

Guī Qí Jiàn Zhōng Tāng
(Tangkuei and Astragalus Decoction to Construct the Middle)

歸耆建中湯
归芪建中汤

Pinyin Name: *Gui Qi Jian Zhong Tang*
Literal Name: Tangkuei and Astragalus Decoction to Construct the Middle
Alternate Name: Tangkuei, Astragalus and Peony Combination
Original Source: *Yi Fang Ji Jie* (Analytical Collection of Medical Formulas) by Wang Ang in 1682

COMPOSITION

Dang Gui (Radix Angelicae Sinensis)	12g
Huang Qi (Radix Astragali)	4.5g [12g]
Yi Tang (Maltosum)	1 cup [30g]
Bai Shao (Radix Paeoniae Alba), *chao* (dry-fried) with liquor	18g
Zhi Gan Cao (Radix et Rhizoma Glycyrrhizae Praeparata cum Melle)	6g
Gui Zhi (Ramulus Cinnamomi)	9g
Sheng Jiang (Rhizoma Zingiberis Recens), *qie* (sliced)	9g
Da Zao (Fructus Jujubae), *bo* (opened)	12 pieces [4 pieces]

DOSAGE / PREPARATION / ADMINISTRATION

Prepare the ingredients as a decoction. Today, the decoction may be prepared using the doses suggested in brackets.

CHINESE THERAPEUTIC ACTIONS

1. Tonifies qi and blood
2. Promotes generation of muscle tissues
3. Eases pain

CLINICAL MANIFESTATIONS

Abscesses and ulcerations with underlying qi and blood deficiencies: various types of abscesses and ulcerations, mild inflammation, small amounts of pus and discharge.

CLINICAL APPLICATIONS

Chronic abscess and ulceration of the skin, chronic otitis media, allergic rhinitis or sinusitis, spontaneous or night perspiration, and postpartum women with weakness, deficiency, and abdominal coldness and pain.

EXPLANATION

Gui Qi Jian Zhong Tang (Tangkuei and Astragalus Decoction to Construct the Middle) treats chronic abscesses and ulcerations with underlying qi and blood deficiencies. Chronic abscesses or ulcerations are often complicated by inflammation and formation and discharge of pus in the local area. Inflammation causes irritation to the nerve endings and results in pain and muscle spasms. Due to the chronic nature of the illness, most of these patients also have underlying qi and blood deficiencies. This formula tonifies the underlying qi and blood deficiencies, supplies nutrients to the affected area, and promotes generation of tissue to facilitate recovery.

Dang Gui (Radix Angelicae Sinensis) and *Huang Qi* (Radix Astragali) are the chief herbs; they tonify blood and qi to treat the underlying deficiencies and facilitate recovery. Moreover, *Dang Gui* (Radix Angelicae Sinensis) improves blood circulation to enhance healing and *Huang Qi* (Radix Astragali) promotes generation of flesh and new muscle tissues. Together, these two herbs effectively treat abscesses and ulcerations. *Yi Tang* (Maltosum) tonifies deficiency and strengthens the middle *jiao*. It supplies large amounts of essential nutrients to facilitate recovery from chronic illnesses. *Bai Shao* (Radix Paeoniae Alba) and *Zhi Gan Cao* (Radix et Rhizoma Glycyrrhizae Praeparata cum Melle), two herbs in *Shao Yao Gan Cao Tang* (Peony and Licorice Decoction), ease pain and relieve muscle spasms and cramps. Because patients with chronic qi and blood deficiencies may develop abdominal pain due to yang deficiency, warm herbs such as *Gui Zhi* (Ramulus Cinnamomi), *Sheng Jiang* (Rhizoma Zingiberis Recens), and *Da Zao* (Fructus Jujubae) are used to warm the middle *jiao* and relieve abdominal pain.

MODIFICATIONS

- If there are prominent signs of cold, add *Fu Zi* (Radix Aconiti Lateralis Praeparata) and *Xi Xin* (Radix et Rhizoma Asari).
- When there is infection of the abscesses and ulcerations, add *Wu Wei Xiao Du Yin* (Five-Ingredient Decoction to Eliminate Toxins).

Chapter 7 – Interior-Warming Formulas   *Section 1 – Middle-Warming and Cold-Dispelling Formulas*

Guī Qí Jiàn Zhōng Tāng
(Tangkuei and Astragalus Decoction to Construct the Middle)

Gui Qi Jian Zhong Tang (Tangkuei and Astragalus Decoction to Construct the Middle)

Diagnosis	Signs and Symptoms	Treatment	Herbs
Abscesses and ulcerations with qi and blood deficiencies	Chronic abscesses and ulcerations that do not heal: qi and blood deficiencies	• Tonifies qi and blood • Promotes generation of muscle tissues • Eases pain	• *Dang Gui* (Radix Angelicae Sinensis) and *Huang Qi* (Radix Astragali) tonify blood and qi to treat the underlying deficiencies and facilitate recovery. • *Yi Tang* (Maltosum) tonifies deficiency and strengthens the middle *jiao*. • *Bai Shao* (Radix Paeoniae Alba) and *Zhi Gan Cao* (Radix et Rhizoma Glycyrrhizae Praeparata cum Melle) ease pain and relieve muscle spasms and cramps. • *Gui Zhi* (Ramulus Cinnamomi), *Sheng Jiang* (Rhizoma Zingiberis Recens) and *Da Zao* (Fructus Jujubae) warm the middle *jiao* and relieve pain.

AUTHORS' COMMENTS

Gui Qi Jian Zhong Tang is a variation of *Xiao Jian Zhong Tang* (Minor Construct the Middle Decoction), but it has additional ingredients and significantly different applications.

• *Xiao Jian Zhong Tang* also warms and tonifies the middle, but primarily treats yang deficiency of the middle *jiao* with abdominal pain.

• *Gui Qi Jian Zhong Tang*, as the name implies, contains *Dang Gui* (Radix Angelicae Sinensis) and *Huang Qi* (Radix Astragali) to "construct the middle" by tonifying the blood and qi, which, in turn, strengthen the body and enhance recovery from abscesses and ulcerations.

Dà Jiàn Zhōng Tāng (Major Construct the Middle Decoction)
大建中湯
大建中汤

Pinyin Name: *Da Jian Zhong Tang*
Literal Name: Major Construct the Middle Decoction
Alternate Names: *Ta Chien Chung Tang, Da Jian Zhung Tang*, Major Centre-Fortifying Decoction, Major Middle-Strengthening Decoction, Major Zanthoxylum Combintion
Original Source: *Jin Gui Yao Lue* (Essentials from the Golden Cabinet) by Zhang Zhong-Jing in the Eastern Han Dynasty

COMPOSITION

Hua Jiao (Pericarpium Zanthoxyli), *chao* (dry-fried)	0.2 cup [3g]
Gan Jiang (Rhizoma Zingiberis)	12g [4.5g]
Ren Shen (Radix et Rhizoma Ginseng)	6g

DOSAGE / PREPARATION / ADMINISTRATION

Cook the ingredients in 4 cups [800 mL] of water until 2 cups [400 mL] of the liquid remain. Filter and discard the herb residue, add 1 cup [30g] of *Yi Tang* (Maltosum) to the strained liquid, and cook it over low heat until 1.5 cups [300 mL] of liquid remain. Take the warm, strained decoction in two equally-divided doses daily. The source text also recommends taking 2 cups [400 mL] of porridge

480

Dà Jiàn Zhōng Tāng (Major Construct the Middle Decoction)

between the two doses of herbs and throughout the day, and to cover the body with blankets. Today, the decoction is normally prepared by using the doses suggested in brackets and by cooking the herbs twice. Filter and discard the herb residue, and add 3g of *Yi Tang* (Maltosum) to the strained liquid. Take the warm decoction in two equally-divided doses.

CHINESE THERAPEUTIC ACTIONS

1. Tonifies and warms the middle *jiao*
2. Corrects the reversed flow of qi and relieves pain

CLINICAL MANIFESTATIONS

Yang deficiency of the middle *jiao* with proliferation of yin and cold: severe coldness and pain in the chest and epigastrium; vomiting with inability to eat; superficial skin pulsations throughout the abdomen; severe pain in the head and feet; a white, wet tongue coating; and a thin, tight pulse. In severe cases, cold limbs, a hidden pulse, or the type of irregular peristalsis that sounds like water movement in the abdominal cavity may be present.

CLINICAL APPLICATIONS

Gastritis, gastric ulcer, duodenal ulcer, slow motility of the intestines, intestinal spasms, uncomplicated intestinal obstruction, obstructive bowel disease, post-operative ileus, abdominal pain due to intestinal parasites, ascariasis, pancreatitis, cholecystitis, cholelithiasis, and urolithiasis.

EXPLANATION

Da Jian Zhong Tang (Major Construct the Middle Decoction) treats various pains/irregularities caused by yang deficiency and interior cold. Yang deficiency leads to yin excess, which then leads to proliferation of cold. Interior cold causes constriction and reversed flow of qi, resulting in severe coldness and pain in the chest and epigastrium, vomiting with inability to eat, and in some cases, superficial skin pulsations throughout the abdomen and severe

pain in the head and feet. The type of irregular peristalsis that sounds like water movement in the abdominal cavity is due to accumulation of water and cold in the abdomen. A white, wet tongue coating suggests that the amount of water in the body is higher than normal due to deficiency of yang and cold accumulation.

Da Jian Zhong Tang uses *Hua Jiao* (Pericarpium Zanthoxyli) as the chief herb. It is acrid and hot, and has functions to dispel cold and warm the Spleen and Stomach. *Gan Jiang* (Rhizoma Zingiberis) also warms the middle *jiao* and dispels cold. Together these two herbs raise the yang of the middle *jiao*, correct the reversed flow of qi, relieve pain, and stop vomiting. *Ren Shen* (Radix et Rhizoma Ginseng) and *Yi Tang* (Maltosum) both warm and tonify the Spleen and Stomach.

MODIFICATIONS

- With nausea and vomiting, add *Ban Xia* (Rhizoma Pinelliae) and *Sheng Jiang* (Rhizoma Zingiberis Recens).
- If there is severe coldness and pain in the chest and epigastric regions, add *Fu Zi* (Radix Aconiti Lateralis Praeparata) and *Xi Xin* (Radix et Rhizoma Asari).
- With coldness and pain in the abdominal region, combine with *Li Zhong Tang* (Regulate the Middle Decoction).
- With fullness and pain in the abdominal region, add *Hou Po* (Cortex Magnoliae Officinalis) and *Ku Xing Ren* (Semen Armeniacae Amarum).
- With nausea, vomiting, and severe abdominal pain, combine with *Ban Xia Xie Xin Tang* (Pinellia Decoction to Drain the Epigastrium).
- With headache due to cold, add *Wu Zhu Yu* (Fructus Evodiae).

CAUTIONS / CONTRAINDICATIONS

- *Da Jian Zhong Tang* contains many warm herbs, and should not be used to treat abdominal pain characterized by excess heat, damp-heat, or yin-deficient heat.

Da Jian Zhong Tang (Major Construct the Middle Decoction)

Diagnosis	Signs and Symptoms	Treatment	Herbs
Yang deficiency of the middle *jiao* with proliferation of yin and cold	• Severe coldness and pain in the chest, head and feet: proliferation of yin and cold causing constriction and stagnation • Vomiting with inability to eat: proliferation of yin and cold leading to reversed flow of qi upwards • White, wet tongue: water accumulation due to deficiency of yang and excess of cold • Thin, tight pulse: deficiency of yang and excess of cold	• Tonifies and warms the middle *jiao* • Corrects reversed flow of qi and relieves pain	• *Hua Jiao* (Pericarpium Zanthoxyli) and *Gan Jiang* (Rhizoma Zingiberis) warms the Spleen and Stomach and dispels cold. • *Ren Shen* (Radix et Rhizoma Ginseng) and *Yi Tang* (Maltosum) both warm and tonify the Spleen and Stomach.

481

Chapter 7 – Interior-Warming Formulas   *Section 1 – Middle-Warming and Cold-Dispelling Formulas*

Dà Jiàn Zhōng Tāng (Major Construct the Middle Decoction)

• Due to the warm nature of this formula, overdose may lead to such side effects as non-productive cough, edema, nausea, and vomiting.

PHARMACOLOGICAL EFFECTS

1. **Gastrointestinal:** Administration of *Da Jian Zhong Tang* was associated with accelerated movement of the small intestine.[1] Increased intestinal motility occurred as a result of *Da Jian Zhong Tang* stimulating the cholinergic and 5-hydroxytryptamine-3 receptors.[2,3] The stimulating effect can be blocked by atropine, spantide, tetrodotoxin or capsazepine.[4] Another study reported that administration of *Da Jian Zhong Tang* has a dose-dependent effect to increase intestinal blood flow without affecting the mean arterial blood pressure. These studies suggested that *Da Jian Zhong Tang* may be useful in the treatment of uncomplicated post-operative adhesive intestinal obstruction and intestinal ischemia-related diseases.[5,6]

2. **Effect on gallbladder:** According to laboratory studies in rats, administration of *Da Jian Zhong Tang* was associated with a stimulating effect on the production of bile acid, starting after 30 minutes and ending 4 hours after the administration.[7]

3. **Uterine:** Administration of *Da Jian Zhong Tang* via intra-duodenal or intravenous routes in anaesthetized rabbits was associated with intestinal motility but not the uterine motility. This suggests that *Da Jian Zhong Tang* has a selective stimulatory effect on the gastrointestinal tract, but not on the uterus. However, more studies are needed to determine whether *Da Jian Zhong Tang* could be administered during pregnancy.[8]

CLINICAL STUDIES AND RESEARCH

1. **Intestinal obstruction:** In one report, 10 patients (6 males and 4 females, between 59 and 75 years of age, average age of 64.4 years) with intestinal obstruction due to adhesion were treated with herbs for prevention of recurrent attack. Out of 10 patients, 6 received *Da Jian Zhong Tang*, 4 received concurrent *Da Jian Zhong Tang* and *Xiao Jian Zhong Tang* (Minor Construct the Middle Decoction). The study reported that 9 out of 10 patients responded well with no recurrent attacks in 8, 12, and 15 months follow-up exams. The other patient continued to take the herbs, but experienced nausea and vomiting.[9]

2. **Obstructive bowel disease:** One study used *Da Jian Zhong Tang* to treat 46 pediatric patients with various obstructive bowel diseases accompanied with chronic constipation (post-operative ileus, large abdominal surgery, ano-rectal anomaly, Hirschsprung's disease, functional bowel obstructions, and SMA syndrome). The treatment protocol was to mix 0.1-0.15 g/kg of the formula with 5-10 mL of warm water, and administer

orally two to three times a day. Of 46 cases, the study reported effective treatment in 39 cases (85%) and ineffective in 7 cases. No side effects were observed.[10]

3. **Post-operative ileus:** In one study, administration of *Da Jian Zhong Tang* was associated with marked effect to treat post-operative ileus, generally considered as an inevitable adverse consequence of abdominal surgical procedures. The treatment protocol was to administer 15g of *Da Jian Zhong Tang* orally daily for 14 days. Clinical improvements included reducing both the need for further surgery and the recurrence of post-operative ileus.[11] In another study, repeated administrations of *Da Jian Zhong Tang* (100 or 300 mg/kg) significantly inhibited the formation of intestinal obstruction, and prevented post-operative ileus following laparotomy. The mechanism of this effect was attributed to the gastroprokinetic and anti-inflammatory effects of the formula.[12]

4. **Post-surgical treatment:** In one study, *Da Jian Zhong Tang* was used to treat 23 patients with various types of complaints following an abdominal surgery. The study reported that the formula was effective in treating borborygmus, abdominal pain, and gastric distention associated with abdominal surgery.[13]

5. **Feelings of coldness in the abdomen:** *Da Jian Zhong Tang* has been used to treat yang deficiency and a feeling of coldness in the abdomen in traditional Chinese medicine. The pharmacological explanation of this application is attributed to the stimulatory effect of *Da Jian Zhong Tang* to increased 5-hydroxytryptamine (serotonin; 5-HT) levels and vasoactive intestinal peptide-immunoreactive substance secretion in the abdomen.[14]

6. **Ascariasis:** One report stated that administration of modified *Da Jian Zhong Tang* was effective in treating biliary ascariasis in 39 of 45 patients.[15] Another study reported successful treatment in all 8 patients with biliary ascariasis.[16]

HERB-DRUG INTERACTION

• **Antipsychotic drugs:** Eight patients with recurrent constipation and/or intestinal obstruction caused by use of antipsychotic drugs were treated with good success using *Da Jian Zhong Tang*. Of 8 cases, the study reported significant improvement in 4 cases, moderate improvement in 2 cases, and no change in 2 cases.[17]

• **Chlorpromazine-induced hypoperistalsis:** Chlorpromazine-induced hypoperistalsis can be treated effectively with *Da Jian Zhong Tang*, which has a dose-dependent effect to improve small intestinal peristalsis and distal colonic propulsion. *Hua Jiao* (Pericarpium Zanthoxyli) is believed to be the main ingredient that stimulates the cholinergic system, thereby enabling *Da Jian Zhong Tang* to improve chlorpromazine-induced hypoperistalsis.[18]

Chinese Herbal Formulas and Applications

Dà Jiàn Zhōng Tāng (Major Construct the Middle Decoction)

- **Morphine-induced constipation**: Administration of *Da Jian Zhong Tang* was found to be effective in alleviating severe constipation in cancer patients taking morphine to relieve pain. Use of *Da Jian Zhong Tang* did not alter the anti-nociceptive effect of morphine.[19]

AUTHORS' COMMENTS

In theory, sweet herbs should not be administered to patients experiencing vomiting. *Da Jian Zhong Tang*, however, contains a large amount of *Yi Tang* (Maltosum) but does not create additional disharmony because the vomiting described in this formula is not due to damp accumulation; rather, it is the result of cold accumulation disrupting the normal qi-lowering tendency of the Stomach. For that reason, *Yi Tang* (Maltosum) is used to harmonize the middle and relieve pain. Although it is sweet, it will not create more dampness and worsen the condition.

Xiao Jian Zhong Tang (Minor Construct the Middle Decoction) and *Da Jian Zhong Tang* both tonify and warm the middle to dispel cold and relieve pain. However, these two formulas have different compositions, functions, and indications.

- *Xiao Jian Zhong Tang* contains mainly sweet herbs to tonify, along with a large amount of the sour and slightly cold *Bai Shao* (Radix Paeoniae Alba) to relieve middle *jiao* pain. Its chief function is to tonify yang, qi, and blood, and warm the middle *jiao*.
- *Da Jian Zhong Tang* contains mainly acrid and sweet herbs to strengthen the middle *jiao*. It is weaker in harmonizing and tonifying but stronger in dispelling coldness. It is mainly used for middle *jiao* yang deficiency with excess cold accumulation.[20]

References

1. Satoh K, Kase Y, Hayakawa T, Murata P, Ishige A, Sasaki H. Dai-kenchu-to enhances accelerated small intestinal movement. Biol Pharm Bull 2001 Oct;24(10):1122-6.
2. Jin XL, Shibata C, Naito H, Ueno T, Funayama Y, Fukushima K, Matsuno S, Sasaki I. Intraduodenal and intrajejunal administration of the herbal medicine, dai-kenchu-tou, stimulates small intestinal motility via cholinergic receptors in conscious dogs. Dig Dis Sci 2001 Jun;46(6):1171-6.

3. Shibata C, Sasaki I, Naito H, Ueno T, Matsuno S. The herbal medicine Dai-Kenchu-Tou stimulates upper gut motility through cholinergic and 5-hydroxytryptamine 3 receptors in conscious dogs. Surgery 1999 Nov;126(5):918-24.
4. Satoh K, Hashimoto K, Hayakawa T, Ishige A, Kaneko M, Ogihara S, Kurosawa S, Yakabi K, Nakamura T. Mechanism of atropine-resistant contraction induced by Dai-kenchu-to in guinea pig ileum. Jpn J Pharmacol 2001 May;86(1):32-7.
5. Shibata C, Sasaki I, Naito H, Ueno T, Matsuno S. The herbal medicine Dai-Kenchu-Tou stimulates upper gut motility through cholinergic and 5-hydroxytryptamine 3 receptors in conscious dogs. Surgery 1999 Nov;126(5):918-24.
6. Murata P, Kase Y, Ishige A, Sasaki H, Kurosawa S, Nakamura T. The herbal medicine Dai-kenchu-to and one of its active components [6]-shogaol increase intestinal blood flow in rats. Life Sci 2002 Mar 15;70(17):2061-70.
7. *Zhong Xi Yi Jie He Za Zhi* (Journal of Integrated Chinese and Western Medicine) 1990;10:638.
8. Murata P, Hayakawa T, Satoh K, Kase Y, Ishige A, Sasaki H. Effects of Dai-kenchu-to, a herbal medicine, on uterine and intestinal motility. Phytother Res 2001 Jun;15(4):302-6.
9. *Guo Wai Yi Xue* (Foreign Medicine) 1993;15(5):39.
10. Ohya T, Usui Y, Arii S, Iwai T, Susumu T. Effect of dai-kenchu-to on obstructive bowel disease in children. Am J Chin Med 2003;31(1):129-35.
11. Itoh T, Yamakawa J, Mai M, Yamaguchi N, Kanda T. The effect of the herbal medicine dai-kenchu-to on post-operative ileus. J Int Med Res 2002 Jul-Aug;30(4):428-32.
12. Hayakawa T, Kase Y, Saito K, Hashimoto K, Ishige A, Komatsu Y, Sasaki H. Effects of Dai-kenchu-to on intestinal obstruction following laparotomy. J Smooth Muscle Res 1999 Apr;35(2):47-54.
13. *Guo Wai Yi Xue* (Foreign Medicine) 1993;15(5):39.
14. Nagano T, Itoh H, Takeyama M. Effects of Dai-kenchu-to on levels of 5-hydroxytryptamine (serotonin) and vasoactive intestinal peptides in human plasma. Biol Pharm Bull 2000 Mar;23(3):352-3.
15. *Zhe Jiang Zhong Yi Za Zhi* (Zhejiang Journal of Chinese Medicine) 1964;2:17.
16. *Zhong Xi Yi Jie He Za Zhi* (Journal of Integrated Chinese and Western Medicine) 1990;10:638.
17. *Guo Wai Yi Xue* (Foreign Medicine) 1994;16(2):28.
18. Satoh K, Kase Y, Yuzurihara M, Mizoguchi K, Kurauchi K, Ishige A. Effect of Dai-kenchu-to (Da-Jian-Zhong-Tang) on the delayed intestinal propulsion induced by chlorpromazine in mice. J Ethnopharmacol 2003 May;86(1):37-44.
19. Nakamura T, Sakai A, Isogami I, Noda K, Ueno K, Yano S. Abatement of morphine-induced slowing in gastrointestinal transit by Dai-kenchu-to, a traditional Japanese herbal medicine. Jpn J Pharmacol 2002 Feb;88(2):217-21.
20. Wang MZ, et al. *Zhong Yi Xue Wen Da Ti Ku* (Questions and Answers on Traditional Chinese Medicine: Herbal Formulas).

INTERIOR-WARMING FORMULAS

7

483

Chapter 7 – Interior-Warming Formulas   *Section 1 – Middle-Warming and Cold-Dispelling Formulas*

Ān Zhōng Sǎn (Calm the Middle Powder)
安中散

Pinyin Name: *An Zhong San*
Literal Name: Calm the Middle Powder
Alternate Names: *An Chung San, An Zhung San,* Interior Comforting Formula, Fennel and Galanga Formula
Original Source: *Tai Ping Hui Min He Ji Ju Fang* (Imperial Grace Formulary of the Tai Ping Era) by the Imperial Medical Department in 1078-85

COMPOSITION

Gan Cao (Radix et Rhizoma Glycyrrhizae), *chao* (dry-fried)	30g
Gao Liang Jiang (Rhizoma Alpiniae Officinarum), *chao* (dry-fried)	15g
Gan Jiang (Rhizoma Zingiberis), *pao* (blast-fried)	15g
Rou Gui (Cortex Cinnamomi)	15g
Xiao Hui Xiang (Fructus Foeniculi), *chao* (dry-fried)	15g
Yan Hu Suo (Rhizoma Corydalis)	15g
Mu Li (Concha Ostreae), *duan* (calcined)	12g

DOSAGE / PREPARATION / ADMINISTRATION

The source text states to grind the ingredients into powder, and take 6g of powder with a warm, grain-based liquor or lightly-salted water. Women should take this formula with water and a small amount of vinegar. Today, this formula is given in powder or decoction form. For powder, take 1-2g per dose two to three times daily. For decoction, cook the ingredients in water, and take the warm, strained decoction in two equally-divided doses daily.

Note: There are two variations of this formula. The standard formula is listed above, the variation contains *Sha Ren* (Fructus Amomi) in place of *Gan Jiang* (Rhizoma Zingiberis).

CHINESE THERAPEUTIC ACTIONS

1. Warms the Spleen and Stomach to disperse cold
2. Harmonizes the middle *jiao* to stop nausea
3. Regulates qi and blood circulation to relieve pain

CLINICAL MANIFESTATIONS

Deficiency and cold of the Spleen and Stomach with qi and blood stagnation: cramps and pain in the epigastric region, fullness and distention of the chest and hypochondriac region, acid reflux, nausea, vomiting, a sallow facial appearance, and fatigue.

CLINICAL APPLICATIONS

Generalized discomfort, cramping and pain in the epigastric region, stress-related gastric and duodenal ulcer, acid reflux, gastric prolapse, chronic gastritis, pyloric stenosis, menstrual pain and cramps, and dysmenorrhea.

EXPLANATION

An Zhong San (Calm the Middle Powder) treats deficiency and cold of the Spleen and Stomach with qi stagnation. Deficiency and cold of the middle *jiao* causes symptoms such as cramps and pain in the epigastric region, fullness and distention of the chest and hypochondriac region, a

An Zhong San (Calm the Middle Powder)

Diagnosis	Signs and Symptoms	Treatment	Herbs
Deficiency and cold of the Spleen and Stomach accompanied by qi and blood stagnation	• Cramps and pain, fullness and distention, a sallow facial appearance, and fatigue: deficiency and cold of the middle *jiao* • Acid reflux, nausea, and vomiting: reversed flow of qi	• Warms the Spleen and Stomach to disperse cold • Harmonizes the middle *jiao* • Regulates qi and blood circulation	• *Gan Cao* (Radix et Rhizoma Glycyrrhizae) tonifies the Spleen and relieves pain. • *Gao Liang Jiang* (Rhizoma Alpiniae Officinarum), *Gan Jiang* (Rhizoma Zingiberis) and *Rou Gui* (Cortex Cinnamomi) warm the middle *jiao* and dispel cold. • *Xiao Hui Xiang* (Fructus Foeniculi) and *Yan Hu Suo* (Rhizoma Corydalis) regulate qi and blood circulation to relieve pain. • *Mu Li* (Concha Ostreae) relieves pain in the stomach due to excessive amount of stomach acid.

484

Ān Zhōng Sǎn (Calm the Middle Powder)

sallow facial appearance, and fatigue. Deficiency and cold cause reversed flow of qi, resulting in acid reflux, nausea, and vomiting. Pain reflects the presence of cold with qi and blood stagnation.

Gan Cao (Radix et Rhizoma Glycyrrhizae) is used in a large dose to tonify the Spleen and moderate pain. *Gao Liang Jiang* (Rhizoma Alpiniae Officinarum), *Gan Jiang* (Rhizoma Zingiberis) and *Rou Gui* (Cortex Cinnamomi) warm the middle *jiao* and dispel cold. *Xiao Hui Xiang* (Fructus Foeniculi) and *Yan Hu Suo* (Rhizoma Corydalis) regulate qi and blood circulation to relieve pain. *Mu Li* (Concha Ostreae) relieves pain in the stomach due to excessive amount of stomach acid.

MODIFICATIONS

- With palpitations associated with mild physical exertion, add *Fu Ling* (Poria).
- With hyperacidity, add *Ping Wei San* (Calm the Stomach Powder) or *Ban Xia Xie Xin Tang* (Pinellia Decoction to Drain the Epigastrium).
- With food stagnation, add *Shen Qu* (Massa Fermentata), *Zhi Shi* (Fructus Aurantii Immaturus), and *Hou Po* (Cortex Magnoliae Officinalis).

- With nausea and vomiting, add *Ban Xia* (Rhizoma Pinelliae) and *Fu Ling* (Poria).
- For chronic stomach disorders, add *Liu Jun Zi Tang* (Six-Gentlemen Decoction).

CAUTIONS / CONTRAINDICATIONS

An Zhong San is not recommended for chest or abdominal pain caused by inflammation.

PHARMACOLOGICAL EFFECTS

1. **Gastrointestinal**: Administration of *An Zhong San* in powder or decoction form was associated with a decrease of gastric acid production, and a resultant increase of pH in the stomach.[1,2]
2. **Cholagogic**: Administration of alcohol extract of *An Zhong San* at 500 mg/kg in rats was associated with marked increase in the secretion of bile acid. The initial onset of action was 30 minutes, and the duration of action was approximately 4 hours.[3]

References
1. *Sheng Yao Xue Za Zhi* (Journal of Raw Herbology) 1986;2:123.
2. *Ri Ben Yao Li Xue Za Zhi* (Japanese Journal of Herbology) 1988;5:309.
3. *Sheng Yao Xue Za Zhi* (Journal of Raw Herbology) 1986;2:123.

Chapter 7 – Interior-Warming Formulas

Section 2 – Yang-Resuscitating Formulas

Section 2

回阳救逆剂
— Yang-Resuscitating Formulas

Si Ni Tang (Frigid Extremities Decoction)

四逆湯
四逆汤

Pinyin Name: *Si Ni Tang*
Literal Name: Frigid Extremities Decoction
Alternate Names: *Su Ni Tang*, Counterflow Cold Combination, Cold Limbs Decoction, Aconite Ginger and Licorice Combination
Original Source: *Shang Han Lun* (Discussion of Cold-Induced Disorders) by Zhang Zhong-Jing in the Eastern Han Dynasty

COMPOSITION

Sheng Fu Zi (Radix Aconiti Lateralis)	1 piece [6-9g]
Gan Jiang (Rhizoma Zingiberis)	4.5g [6-9g]
Zhi Gan Cao (Radix et Rhizoma Glycyrrhizae Praeparata cum Melle)	6g

DOSAGE / PREPARATION / ADMINISTRATION

Cook the ingredients in 3 cups [600 mL] of water until 1.2 cups [240 mL] of the liquid remain. Take the warm, strained decoction in two equally-divided doses daily. For patients with a strong constitution, a large piece (15g) of *Sheng Fu Zi* (Radix Aconiti Lateralis) and 9g of *Gan Jiang* (Rhizoma Zingiberis) may be used. Today, the decoction may be prepared using the doses suggested in brackets. *Sheng Fu Zi* (Radix Aconiti Lateralis) should be cooked first for one hour before adding and cooking the other herbs. The decoction should be taken while warm.

CHINESE THERAPEUTIC ACTIONS

1. Restores depleted yang
2. Rescues from counterflow cold

CLINICAL MANIFESTATIONS

1. *Shaoyin* syndrome: severely cold extremities, aversion to cold, preference to curl up the body when lying down, lassitude, drowsiness, vomiting, absence of thirst, abdominal pain, diarrhea, a white, slippery tongue coating, and a faint, fine pulse.
2. Depletion of yang due to excessive sweating in *taiyang* syndrome.

CLINICAL APPLICATIONS

Prostration, cardiac failure, cardiac infarction, shock, diarrhea, gastroenteritis, intoxication, and stomach prolapse.

EXPLANATION

Si Ni Tang (Frigid Extremities Decoction) is a standard formula used to treat *shaoyin* syndrome in which coldness has progressed to the *shaoyin* stage and Kidney yang is diminished and depleted. This extreme imbalance of yin and yang causes disharmony at the exterior (icy cold extremities, aversion to cold, preference to curl up the body when lying down, lassitude, and drowsiness) and in the interior (vomiting, absence of thirst, abdominal pain, and diarrhea with undigested food). A white, wet tongue coating and an indistinct faint and fine pulse suggest depletion of yang and proliferation of yin and coldness.

Proper treatment of this condition requires high doses of acrid and hot interior-warming herbs to restore yang and rescue from counterflow cold. *Sheng Fu Zi* (Radix Aconiti Lateralis), the chief herb, is an essential herb for warming *ming men* (life gate) fire and raising Kidney yang. It warms all twelve channels immediately and strongly dispels

486

Si Ni Tāng (Frigid Extremities Decoction)

Si Ni Tang (Frigid Extremities Decoction)

Diagnosis	Signs and Symptoms	Treatment	Herbs
Shaoyin syndrome	• Icy cold extremities, aversion to cold, preference to curl up the body when lying down, lassitude, and drowsiness: excess cold and yang deficiency at the exterior • Vomiting, absence of thirst, abdominal pain, and diarrhea with undigested food: excess cold and yang deficiency in the interior	• Recuperates depleted yang • Rescues from counterflow cold	• *Sheng Fu Zi* (Radix Aconiti Lateralis) warms *ming men* (life gate) fire, raises Kidney yang, and warms all twelve channels and dispels interior coldness. • *Gan Jiang* (Rhizoma Zingiberis) warms middle *jiao* yang and dispels interior cold. • *Zhi Gan Cao* (Radix et Rhizoma Glycyrrhizae Praeparata cum Melle) harmonizes the formula.

interior cold. The fresh, unprocessed form is used here because interior cold must be dispelled at once. Due to the urgency of the situation, the fresh, unprocessed *Sheng Fu Zi* (Radix Aconiti Lateralis) is selected for its potent and drastic effect over the processed *Fu Zi* (Radix Aconiti Lateralis Praeparata). *Gan Jiang* (Rhizoma Zingiberis), the deputy herb, warms middle *jiao* yang and dispels interior cold. The warmth of *Sheng Fu Zi* (Radix Aconiti Lateralis) is further enhanced by the addition of *Gan Jiang* (Rhizoma Zingiberis). Lastly, *Zhi Gan Cao* (Radix et Rhizoma Glycyrrhizae Praeparata cum Melle) reduces the toxicity of *Sheng Fu Zi* (Radix Aconiti Lateralis), and moderates the harsh and warm properties of *Gan Jiang* (Rhizoma Zingiberis) and *Sheng Fu Zi* (Radix Aconiti Lateralis).

MODIFICATIONS

• When there is extreme coldness of the extremities, add *Xi Xin* (Radix et Rhizoma Asari) and *Gui Zhi* (Ramulus Cinnamomi).
• If there is abdominal pain due to cold, add *Gui Zhi* (Ramulus Cinnamomi) and *Bai Shao* (Radix Paeoniae Alba).
• If there is abdominal pain due to blood deficiency, combine with *Si Wu Tang* (Four-Substance Decoction).
• With edema and palpitations, add *Ren Shen* (Radix et Rhizoma Ginseng) and *Fu Ling* (Poria).
• With edema or clear or white vaginal discharge from Spleen and Kidney yang deficiencies, add *Dang Shen* (Radix Codonopsis), *Fu Ling* (Poria), and *Ze Xie* (Rhizoma Alismatis).
• With nausea, vomiting, and a sore throat, add *Sheng Jiang* (Rhizoma Zingiberis Recens) and *Jie Geng* (Radix Platycodonis).
• With diarrhea accompanied by undigested food, combine with *Li Zhong Tang* (Regulate the Middle Decoction).
• With shortness of breath or accelerated respiration from qi deficiency, add *Ren Shen* (Radix et Rhizoma Ginseng).

CAUTIONS / CONTRAINDICATIONS

• *Si Ni Tang* is an extremely hot formula, and is contraindicated in cases of true-heat and false-cold conditions.
• *Si Ni Tang* should be stopped immediately after the hands and feet have warmed up.

PHARMACOLOGICAL EFFECTS

1. **Cardiovascular**: Administration of *Si Ni Tang* was associated with a marked influence on the cardiovascular system. In laboratory studies on rabbits, it increased the contractile force of the heart, increased blood pressure, and restored normal heart rhythm.[1]
2. **Immunostimulant**: Administration of *Si Ni Tang* was associated with an effect to enhance the immune system. In one experiment, the immune systems of rats were artificially suppressed with injection of hydrocortisone at 1.5 mg/100g/day for 7 days. The rats that also received the herbs in decoction were able to maintain their IgG count at a higher level in comparison to the rats that received only the hydrocortisone.[2]
3. **Analgesic and anti-inflammatory**: Intraperitoneal injection of *Si Ni Tang* was associated with marked analgesic and anti-inflammatory effects in rats.[3]
4. **Half-life**: According to pharmacokinetic studies using a two-compartment model, the half-life of *Si Ni Tang* is 5.8 hours.[4]

CLINICAL STUDIES AND RESEARCH

1. **Acute cardiac infarction**: In one report, 105 patients with acute cardiac infarction characterized by collapse of yang were treated with *Si Ni Tang* or with slight modification without a single case of fatality. Of 105 patients, 10 received concurrent herbal and drug treatments. The therapeutic benefit was attributed to the effect of the formula to increase blood pressure and the contractile force of the heart.[5]
2. **Diarrhea**: Seventy children with diarrhea characterized by watery stools, cold extremities, a weak pulse, and a thin, white tongue coating were treated with a decoction

Si Ni Tāng (Frigid Extremities Decoction)

of *Si Ni Tang* with the addition of *Huang Lian* (Rhizoma Coptidis). Out of 70 cases, the study reported complete recovery in 58 cases (less than 3 bowel movements per day), slight improvement in 8 cases (less than 5 bowel movements per day), and no change in 4 cases. The average length of treatment was 4 days, and ranged from 1-7 days.[6]

3. **Gastric prolapse**: Seven patients with stomach prolapse were treated with modified *Si Ni Tang* with marked improvement in all of the patients. The modification included addition of *Rou Gui* (Cortex Cinnamomi), *Zhang Mu Zi* (Fructus Camphora), and *Wu Zhu Yu* (Fructus Evodiae) for abdominal pain; *Zhi Zi* (Fructus Gardeniae), *Mu Xiang* (Radix Aucklandiae), and *Hou Po* (Cortex Magnoliae Officinalis) for abdominal distention; *Sha Ren* (Fructus Amomi) and *Ban Xia* (Rhizoma Pinelliae) for nausea; and *Shan Zha* (Fructus Crataegi) and *Mai Ya* (Fructus Hordei Germinatus) for belching.[7]

TOXICOLOGY

In a toxicology study, *Si Ni Tang* was prepared using the herbs in the proportion of *Sheng Fu Zi* (Radix Aconiti Lateralis) : *Gan Jiang* (Rhizoma Zingiberis) : *Gan Cao* (Radix et Rhizoma Glycyrrhizae) as 4:3:3. The LD_{50} of *Si Ni Tang* in mice is 5.821 g/kg via intraperitoneal injection and 71.78 g/kg via oral ingestion. The LD_{50} for *Sheng Fu Zi* (Radix Aconiti Lateralis) is 17.42 g/kg via oral ingestion. The subject was able to tolerate a larger dose of *Sheng Fu Zi* (Radix Aconiti Lateralis) when given in a combination, indicating that *Gan Cao* (Radix et Rhizoma Glycyrrhizae) and *Gan Jiang* (Rhizoma Zingiberis) can effectively reduce the toxicity of *Sheng Fu Zi* (Radix Aconiti Lateralis). The reduced toxicity of the formula was not associated with changes in concentration of the alkaloids.[8]

RELATED FORMULAS

Sì Nì Jiā Rén Shēn Tāng
(Frigid Extremities Decoction plus Ginseng)

四逆加人参汤
四逆加人参汤

Pinyin Name: Si Ni Jia Ren Shen Tang
Literal Name: Frigid Extremities Decoction plus Ginseng
Original Source: *Shang Han Lun* (Discussion of Cold-Induced Disorders) by Zhang Zhong-Jing in the Eastern Han Dynasty

Ren Shen (Radix et Rhizoma Ginseng)	3g
Sheng Fu Zi (Radix Aconiti Lateralis)	1 piece [6-9g]
Gan Jiang (Rhizoma Zingiberis)	4.5g [6-9g]
Zhi Gan Cao (Radix et Rhizoma Glycyrrhizae Praeparata cum Melle)	6g [9g]

Cook the ingredients in 3 cups [600 mL] of water until 1.2 cups [240 mL] of the liquid remain. Take the warm, strained decoction in two equally-divided doses daily. Today, the decoction may be prepared using the doses suggested in brackets

Si Ni Jia Ren Shen Tang (Frigid Extremities Decoction plus Ginseng) combines *Si Ni Tang* with *Ren Shen* (Radix et Rhizoma Ginseng). *Ren Shen* (Radix et Rhizoma Ginseng) is added in this case to tonify *yuan* (source) *qi* in patients with severe qi deficiency. This formula tonifies *yuan* (source) *qi*, recuperates depleted yang, and rescues the patient from collapse. Clinically, the patient may have shortness of breath and rapid breathing in addition to all the symptoms and signs listed in *Si Ni Tang*.

In comparison to *Si Ni Tang*, *Si Ni Jia Ren Shen Tang* (Frigid Extremities Decoction plus Ginseng) has a much stronger function to tonify *yuan* (source) *qi*. Therefore, it can be used on patients who have *shaoyin* cold syndrome complicated by shortness of breath and rapid breathing.

Tōng Mài Sì Nì Tāng
(Unblock the Pulse Decoction for Frigid Extremities)

通脉四逆汤
通脉四逆汤

Pinyin Name: Tong Mai Si Ni Tang
Literal Name: Unblock the Pulse Decoction for Frigid Extremities
Original Source: *Shang Han Lun* (Discussion of Cold-Induced Disorder) by Zhang Zhong-Jing in the Eastern Han Dynasty

Zhi Gan Cao (Radix et Rhizoma Glycyrrhizae Praeparata cum Melle)	6g
Sheng Fu Zi (Radix Aconiti Lateralis)	1 large piece [15g]
Gan Jiang (Rhizoma Zingiberis)	9g [9-12g]

Cook the ingredients in 3 cups [600 mL] of water until 1.2 cups [240 mL] of the liquid remain. Take the warm, strained decoction in two equally-divided doses daily. Today, the decoction may be prepared using the doses suggested in brackets.

Tong Mai Si Ni Tang (Unblock the Pulse Decoction for Frigid Extremities) treats *shaoyin* syndrome with severe yang deficiency, leading to yang on the verge of separating from yin. Clinically, the patient still has cold extremities, but now he or she will no longer have aversion to cold. Instead, there will be a red face, a cold sensation in the interior, and a warm sensation at the exterior, abdominal pain, sore throat, absence of diarrhea or diarrhea with

Si Ni Tāng (Frigid Extremities Decoction)

undigested food, and a fainting pulse. All these symptoms and signs point to the fact that yang is separating from yin and rushing out to the exterior, exemplified by signs of heat at the exterior and cold in the interior. This is a true-cold and false-heat syndrome, with presence of true cold in the interior and symptoms of false heat at the exterior. Thus, to stop yang from separating from yin, large doses of *Sheng Fu Zi* (Radix Aconiti Lateralis) and *Gan Jiang* (Rhizoma Zingiberis) are used to tonify yang.

In comparison to *Si Ni Tang*, *Tong Mai Si Ni Tang* (Unblock the Pulse Decoction for Frigid Extremities) is a stronger formula used for more serious cases of *shaoyin* syndrome with severe yang deficiency, in which yang is on the verge of separating from yin. Both formulas contain the same ingredients, but the doses are greater in the latter formula to address the true-cold, false-heat syndrome.

Bái Tōng Tāng (White Penetrating Decoction)

白通湯
白通汤

Pinyin Name: *Bai Tong Tang*
Literal Name: White Penetrating Decoction
Original Source: *Shang Han Lun* (Discussion of Cold-Induced Disorders) by Zhang Zhong-Jing in the Eastern Han Dynasty

Cong Bai (Bulbus Allii Fistulosi)	4 pieces
Gan Jiang (Rhizoma Zingiberis)	3g [3-5g]
Sheng Fu Zi (Radix Aconiti Lateralis)	1 piece [6-9g]

Cook the ingredients in 3 cups [600 mL] of water until 1 cup [200 mL] of the liquid remains. Take the warm, strained decoction in two equally-divided doses daily. Today, the decoction may be prepared using the doses suggested in brackets

Bai Tong Tang (White Penetrating Decoction) mainly treats *shaoyin* syndrome characterized by severe diarrhea and a fainting pulse. *Cong Bai* (Bulbus Allii Fistulosi) and *Sheng Fu Zi* (Radix Aconiti Lateralis) tonify yang qi and dispel cold. The dose of *Gan Jiang* (Rhizoma Zingiberis), which is acrid and drying, has been decreased to avoid further yin damage since patients with severe diarrhea may already have yin and body fluid deficiencies.

In comparison to *Si Ni Tang*, *Bai Tong Tang* (White Penetrating Decoction) emphasizes treating *shaoyin* syndrome with excess yin and cold affecting the lower *jiao*. Clinical manifestations include severe diarrhea in addition to all the symptoms and signs listed in *Si Ni Tang*.

Shēn Fù Tāng
(Ginseng and Prepared Aconite Decoction)

参附湯
参附汤

Pinyin Name: *Shen Fu Tang*
Literal Name: Ginseng and Prepared Aconite Decoction
Original Source: *Zheng Ti Lei Yao* (Catalogued Essentials for Correcting the Body) by Bi Li-Zhai (Ji) in 1529

Ren Shen (Radix et Rhizoma Ginseng)	12g [9g]
Fu Zi (Radix Aconiti Lateralis Praeparata), *pao* (blast-fried)	9g [6g]

Prepare the ingredients as a decoction. Today, the decoction may be prepared using the doses suggested in brackets.

This formula treats collapse of yang qi with profuse sweating, cold hands and feet, dizziness, shortness of breath, and even semi-unconsciousness. Collapse of yang qi occurs after severe illness with extreme deficiency, profuse bleeding in postpartum or *beng lou* (flooding and spotting) conditions, severe hemorrhage, and others.

Shen Fu Tang (Ginseng and Prepared Aconite Decoction) has only two ingredients. *Ren Shen* (Radix et Rhizoma Ginseng) tonifies *yuan* (source) *qi* and restore yang from collapse. *Fu Zi* (Radix Aconiti Lateralis Praeparata) warms yang qi and resuscitates the patient. This formula should be used only in emergency conditions. In severe instances, the doses listed above could be doubled. However, this formula only serves to quickly restore yang and should not be used once the patient has regained consciousness; otherwise, interior fire may be created.

AUTHORS' COMMENTS

Si Ni Tang is the representative formula for restoring depleted yang and rescuing patients from collapse. The original *Si Ni Tang* contains unprocessed *Sheng Fu Zi* (Radix Aconiti Lateralis) to utilize its potent effects to dispel cold and restore yang. However, *Sheng Fu Zi* (Radix Aconiti Lateralis) is rather toxic, and is generally unavailable. Therefore, 20-30 grams of processed *Fu Zi* (Radix Aconiti Lateralis Praeparata) may be used to replace 5-10 grams of *Sheng Fu Zi* (Radix Aconiti Lateralis).

Si Ni Tang (Frigid Extremities <u>Decoction</u>) and *Si Ni San* (Frigid Extremities <u>Powder</u>) are two formulas with similar names that must not be confused. These two formulas treat different syndromes (yang deficiency vs. qi stagnation) that share the same symptoms (cold limbs/extremities).

INTERIOR-WARMING FORMULAS

7

Chapter 7 – Interior-Warming Formulas

Section 2 – Yang-Resuscitating Formulas

Si Ni Tang (Frigid Extremities Decoction)

- *Si Ni Tang* (Frigid Extremities Decoction): Yang deficiency with coldness will manifest not only in icy cold limbs/extremities, but also cold sensations everywhere in the body. Comparatively speaking, this type of cold is more severe and will not warm up when exposed to heat because there is an underlying deficiency of *ming men* (life gate) fire. Accompanying symptoms include a withered *shen* (spirit), desire to sleep, intolerance to cold, preference to be in a fetal position, vomiting, abdominal pain, undigested food with diarrhea, and a deep, weak pulse. *Si Ni Tang* contains interior warming herbs to warm Kidney yang and boost *ming men* (life gate) fire in order to warm up the limbs/extremities.
- *Si Ni San* (Frigid Extremities Powder): Qi stagnation blocks and prevents yang qi from properly circulating to the extremities. Patients usually experience coldness below the knees and elbows instead of the entire limbs. In general, these patients warm up faster when the extremities are exposed to heat and blood circulation is restored. Other accompanying signs include abdominal pain and discomfort, diarrhea, and a wiry pulse. In summary, the coldness is due to qi blockage instead of yang deficiency. *Si*

Ni San is designed with qi-regulating herbs to harmonize and smooth Liver qi flow and open channel circulation to the extremities. This condition is often seen when pathogenic factors invade from the outside and get trapped in the *shaoyang* Liver/Gallbladder channels, coupled with qi stagnation. When yang qi is no longer blocked by qi stagnation, the symptom of cold limbs is relieved. [9]

References

1. *Zhong Yi Fang Ji Xian Dai Yan Jiu* (Modern Study of Medical Formulae in Traditional Chinese Medicine) 1997;394-395.
2. *Zhong Yi Za Zhi* (Journal of Chinese Medicine) 1988;10:59.
3. *Zhong Guo Zhong Yao Za Zhi* (People's Republic of China Journal of Chinese Herbology) 1992;2:104.
4. *Zhong Guo Yi Yuan Yao Xue Za Zhi* (Chinese Hospital Journal of Herbology) 1990;11:487.
5. *Tian Jin Yi Yao Tong Xun* (Publication of Tianjin Medicine and Herbology) 1972;11:1.
6. *Zhe Jiang Zhong Yi Za Zhi* (Zhejiang Journal of Chinese Medicine) 1981;10:422.
7. *Yun Nan Yi Xue Za Zhi* (Yunan Journal of Medicine) 1964;3:44.
8. *Zhe Jiang Zhong Yi Yao* (Zhejiang Chinese Medicine and Herbology) 1979;7:246.
9. Wang MZ, et al. *Zhong Yi Xue Wen Da Ti Ku* (Questions and Answers on Traditional Chinese Medicine: Herbal Formulas).

Hui Yáng Jiù Jí Tāng (Restore and Revive the Yang Decoction)

回陽救急湯
回阳救急汤

Pinyin Name: *Hui Yang Jiu Ji Tang*
Literal Name: Restore and Revive the Yang Decoction
Original Source: *Shang Han Liu Shu* (Six Texts on Cold-Induced Disorders) by Tao Hua in 1445

COMPOSITION

Fu Zi (Radix Aconiti Lateralis Praeparata)	[9g]
Gan Jiang (Rhizoma Zingiberis)	[6g]
Rou Gui (Cortex Cinnamomi)	[3g]
Ren Shen (Radix et Rhizoma Ginseng)	[6g]
Bai Zhu (Rhizoma Atractylodis Macrocephalae), *chao* (dry-fried)	[9g]
Fu Ling (Poria)	[9g]
Zhi Gan Cao (Radix et Rhizoma Glycyrrhizae Praeparata cum Melle)	[6g]
Chen Pi (Pericarpium Citri Reticulatae)	[6g]
Ban Xia (Rhizoma Pinelliae), *zhi* (prepared)	[9g]
Wu Wei Zi (Fructus Schisandrae Chinensis)	[3g]

DOSAGE / PREPARATION / ADMINISTRATION

Cook the ingredients with 3 slices of *Sheng Jiang* (Rhizoma Zingiberis Recens) in 2 large bowls of water.

Add 0.1g of *She Xiang* (Moschus) to the warm, strained decoction immediately before ingestion. Once the patient's hands and feet become warm, discontinue the formula.

490

Chinese Herbal Formulas and Applications

Huí Yáng Jiù Jí Tāng (Restore and Revive the Yang Decoction)

Note: Herb doses are unavailable from the source text. Suggested doses are listed above in brackets.

CHINESE THERAPEUTIC ACTIONS

1. Rescues yang from collapse in emergency situations
2. Strengthens qi and generates pulse

CLINICAL MANIFESTATIONS

Extreme yang deficiency with cold factor in *taiyin, shaoyin,* and *jueyin*: severe aversion to cold with the body curled up in a fetal position, icy cold extremities, vomiting, diarrhea, absence of thirst, abdominal pain, lack of energy with a constant desire to sleep, shivering, foaming of saliva at the mouth, purplish lips or nails, a pale tongue, a white tongue coating, and a deep and fine or impalpable pulse.

CLINICAL APPLICATIONS

Cardiac failure, cardiac infarction, shock, and prostration.

EXPLANATION

Hui Yang Jiu Ji Tang (Restore and Revive the Yang Decoction) treats severe yang deficiency with excess cold factor affecting *taiyin, shaoyin* and *jueyin* in the interior. The yang in this syndrome is extremely fragile and may become separated from yin at any time. Severe aversion to cold with the body curled up in a fetal position and cold extremities are all clinical manifestations of extreme cold of the body. Because the cold is stagnant in the middle *jiao*, the normal Spleen and Stomach functioning are disrupted, causing vomiting, diarrhea, and abdominal pain. The cold factor may cause severe contraction of the body and obstructed blood circulation, resulting in shivering of the body and purplish lips or nails.

Fu Zi (Radix Aconiti Lateralis Praeparata), *Gan Jiang* (Rhizoma Zingiberis), and *Rou Gui* (Cortex Cinnamomi) warm the interior, tonify yang, and dispel internal cold. *Ren Shen* (Radix et Rhizoma Ginseng), *Bai Zhu* (Rhizoma Atractylodis Macrocephalae), *Fu Ling* (Poria), and *Zhi Gan Cao* (Radix et Rhizoma Glycyrrhizae Praeparata cum Melle) tonify qi and strengthen the middle *jiao*. Because interior cold may lead to qi stagnation and damp accumulation, *Chen Pi* (Pericarpium Citri Reticulatae) and *Ban Xia* (Rhizoma Pinelliae) are used to activate qi circulation and eliminate dampness and phlegm that may accumulate as a result of a weak Spleen that is unable to metabolize water. *Wu Wei Zi* (Fructus Schisandrae Chinensis) combines with *Ren Shen* (Radix et Rhizoma Ginseng) to tonify qi and generate pulse, as in the formula *Sheng Mai San* (Generate the Pulse Powder). *She Xiang* (Moschus) opens all twelve channels to dispel cold and enhance the overall effect of the formula. The astringent effect of *Wu Wei Zi* (Fructus Schisandrae Chinensis) prevents the loss of qi by moderating the strong penetrating and dispersing effects of *She Xiang* (Moschus).

In summary, *Hui Yang Jiu Ji Tang* is formulated using the following strategies: *Si Ni Tang* (Frigid Extremities Decoction) and *Rou Gui* (Cortex Cinnamomi) to restore depleted yang, *Liu Jun Zi Tang* (Six-Gentlemen Decoction) to strengthen qi, *She Xiang* (Moschus) to open the

Hui Yang Jiu Ji Tang (Restore and Revive the Yang Decoction)

Diagnosis	Signs and Symptoms	Treatment	Herbs
Extreme yang deficiency with cold in the interior	• Severe aversion to cold, shivering, cold extremities and preference to curl up in a fetal position: extreme cold of the body with yang deficiency • Purplish lips or nails: obstructed blood circulation due to cold excess and yang deficiency • Vomiting, diarrhea, abdominal pain and foaming of saliva: cold stagnation in the middle *jiao* • Pale tongue with a white tongue coating, and a deep, fine or impalpable pulse: severe yang deficiency and cold	• Rescues yang from collapse in emergency situations • Strengthens qi, generates pulse	• *Fu Zi* (Radix Aconiti Lateralis Praeparata), *Gan Jiang* (Rhizoma Zingiberis) and *Rou Gui* (Cortex Cinnamomi) warm the interior, tonify yang, and dispel internal cold. • *Ren Shen* (Radix et Rhizoma Ginseng), *Bai Zhu* (Rhizoma Atractylodis Macrocephalae), *Fu Ling* (Poria) and *Zhi Gan Cao* (Radix et Rhizoma Glycyrrhizae Praeparata cum Melle) tonify qi and strengthen the middle *jiao*. • *Chen Pi* (Pericarpium Citri Reticulatae) and *Ban Xia* (Rhizoma Pinelliae) activate qi circulation and eliminate dampness and phlegm. • *She Xiang* (Moschus) opens all twelve channels to dispel cold and enhance the overall effect of the formula. • *Wu Wei Zi* (Fructus Schisandrae Chinensis) prevents loss of qi.

INTERIOR-WARMING FORMULAS

7

491

Chapter 7 – Interior-Warming Formulas　　　　　　　　　　*Section 2 – Yang-Resuscitating Formulas*

Huí Yáng Jiù Jí Tāng (Restore and Revive the Yang Decoction)

channels, and *Wu Wei Zi* (Fructus Schisandrae Chinensis) to balance the dispersing effect of *She Xiang* (Moschus).

MODIFICATIONS

- With vomiting or drooling of saliva, add salt-fried *Wu Zhu Yu* (Fructus Evodiae).
- If there is an impalpable pulse, add *Zhu Dan* (Fel Porcus).
- With constant diarrhea, add *Sheng Ma* (Rhizoma Cimicifugae) and *Huang Qi* (Radix Astragali).

- With constant vomiting, add the juice of *Sheng Jiang* (Rhizoma Zingiberis Recens).

CAUTIONS / CONTRAINDICATIONS

Hui Yang Jiu Ji Tang is an extremely hot and acrid formula, and should not be given at large doses or for a prolonged period of time. This formula should be discontinued immediately after the hands and feet have warmed up.

Hēi Xí Dān (Lead Special Pill)

黑錫丹
黑锡丹

Pinyin Name: *Hei Xi Dan*
Literal Name: Lead Special Pill
Original Source: *Tai Ping Hui Min He Ji Ju Fang* (Imperial Grace Formulary of the Tai Ping Era) by the Imperial Medical Department in 1078-85

COMPOSITION

Hei Xi (Lead), *jing* (cleaned)	60g
Liu Huang (Sulfur), use only the clear particles	60g
Fu Zi (Radix Aconiti Lateralis Praeparata), *pao* (blast-fried)	30g
Rou Gui (Cortex Cinnamomi), do not expose to heat	15g
Yang Qi Shi (Actinolitum), *shui fei* (refined with water) into fine particles	30g
Bu Gu Zhi (Fructus Psoraleae), *jin* (soaked) in liquor and *chao* (dry-fried)	30g
Hu Lu Ba (Semen Trigonellae), *jin* (soaked) in liquor and *chao* (dry-fried)	30g
Xiao Hui Xiang (Fructus Foeniculi), *chao* (dry-fried)	30g
Chen Xiang (Lignum Aquilariae Resinatum), do not expose to heat	30g
Mu Xiang (Radix Aucklandiae), do not expose to heat	30g
Rou Dou Kou (Semen Myristicae), *wei* (roasted)	30g
Chuan Lian Zi (Fructus Toosendan), *zheng* (steamed)	30g

Note: *Hei Xi* (Lead) is a potentially toxic heavy metal, and is rarely used as a medicinal substance today. Its discussion here is included primarily for academic purposes, to reflect the historical use of this substance in its original formulation. Most herbal products today have removed it completely, or replaced it with substitutes with similar functions. For additional information on the toxicity, please refer to *Chinese Medical Herbology and Pharmacology* by John Chen and Tina Chen.

pills should resemble the size of *Wu Tong Zi* (Semen Firmianae), a small seed approximately 5 mm in diameter. Take 30-40 pills per dose on an empty stomach. The source text advises that men should take the pills with a decoction made from *Da Zao* (Fructus Jujubae) or salt and *Sheng Jiang* (Rhizoma Zingiberis Recens), and women should take the pills with a decoction made from vinegar and *Ai Ye* (Folium Artemisiae Argyi). Today, this formula is given in pills, 3-9g of pills per dose with warm water.

DOSAGE / PREPARATION / ADMINISTRATION

The source text states to grind the ingredients into a fine powder and form into pills with a grain-based liquor. The

CHINESE THERAPEUTIC ACTIONS

1. Warms and tonifies true yang
2. Controls floating yang

492

Hēi Xī Dān (Lead Special Pill)

CLINICAL MANIFESTATIONS

1. Deficiency of Kidney yang with inability of the Kidney to grasp qi downward: excess condition of the upper body characterized by obstruction of phlegm in the chest with wheezing and dyspnea; and deficiency of the lower body characterized by extremely cold extremities, continuous perspiration with cold sweats, a pale tongue with a thin, white coating, and a deep, faint pulse.

2. *Ben tun* (running piglet): sensations of qi rushing upward from the lower abdomen to the chest, epigastrium and throat; distention and pain in the chest, hypochondrium, epigastrium, and abdomen.

3. Others: cold-type hernia with abdominal pain; borborygmus with loose stools; impotence and infertility in men due to yang deficiency; clear leukorrhea, irregular menstruation and infertility in women due to deficiency and cold of blood.

CLINICAL APPLICATIONS

Acute bronchial asthma, acute exacerbation of chronic bronchitis, and emphysema.

EXPLANATION

Hei Xi Dan (Lead Special Pill) treats severe cases of Kidney yang deficiency with excess in the upper body and deficiency in the lower body. Due to Kidney yang deficiency and its inability to grasp qi downward, there is excess condition in the upper body characterized by obstruction of phlegm in the chest with wheezing and dyspnea. Because Kidney yang deficiency fails to warm the body, there is deficiency of the lower body characterized by extremely cold extremities, continuous perspiration of cold sweats, a pale tongue with a thin, white coating, and a deep, faint pulse.

Hei Xi (Lead) anchors floating yang, guides qi downward, and relieve wheezing and dyspnea. *Liu Huang* (Sulfur) warms and tonifies *ming men* (life gate) fire to dispel cold. *Fu Zi* (Radix Aconiti Lateralis Praeparata) and *Rou Gui* (Cortex Cinnamomi) warm the Kidney and tonify Kidney yang to restore its normal functions. *Yang Qi Shi* (Actinolitum), *Bu Gu Zhi* (Fructus Psoraleae), and *Hu Lu Ba* (Semen Trigonellae) also warm *ming men* (life gate) and dispel cold. *Xiao Hui Xiang* (Fructus Foeniculi), *Chen Xiang* (Lignum Aquilariae Resinatum), *Mu Xiang* (Radix Aucklandiae) and *Rou Dou Kou* (Semen Myristicae) regulate qi, dissolve phlegm, and warm the Kidney. *Chuan Lian Zi* (Fructus Toosendan), a bitter and cold herb, is added to prevent the warm and drying herbs from injuring the body.

CAUTIONS / CONTRAINDICATIONS

- *Hei Xi Dan* is contraindicated during pregnancy.
- This formula is potentially toxic, and should only be used when absolutely necessary and only for a short period of time.

Hei Xi Dan (Lead Special Pill)

Diagnosis	Signs and Symptoms	Treatment	Herbs
Kidney yang deficiency with inability of the Kidney to grasp qi downwards	• Obstruction of phlegm in the chest with wheezing and dyspnea: excess in the upper body • Icy extremities, and continuous perspiration of cold sweats: deficiency of the lower body • Pale tongue with a thin, white coating: yang qi deficiency • Deep, faint pulse: deficiency and cold	• Warms and tonifies true yang • Controls floating yang	• *Hei Xi* (Lead) anchors floating yang, guides qi downward, and relieves wheezing and dyspnea. • *Liu Huang* (Sulfur) warms and tonifies *ming men* (life gate) fire to dispel cold. • *Fu Zi* (Radix Aconiti Lateralis Praeparata) and *Rou Gui* (Cortex Cinnamomi) warm and tonify Kidney yang to restore its normal functions. • *Yang Qi Shi* (Actinolitum), *Bu Gu Zhi* (Fructus Psoraleae) and *Hu Lu Ba* (Semen Trigonellae) warm *ming men* (life gate) fire and dispel cold. • *Xiao Hui Xiang* (Fructus Foeniculi), *Chen Xiang* (Lignum Aquilariae Resinatum), *Mu Xiang* (Radix Aucklandiae) and *Rou Dou Kou* (Semen Myristicae) regulate qi, dissolve phlegm, and warm the Kidney. • *Chuan Lian Zi* (Fructus Toosendan) prevents the warm and drying herbs from injuring the body.

Chapter 7 – Interior-Warming Formulas　　　　　*Section 3 – Channel-Warming and Cold-Dispersing Formulas*

Section 3

温经散寒剂

— Channel-Warming and Cold-Dispersing Formulas

Dāng Guī Sì Nì Tāng (Tangkuei Decoction for Frigid Extremities)

當歸四逆湯

当归四逆汤

Pinyin Name: *Dang Gui Si Ni Tang*

Literal Name: Tangkuei Decoction for Frigid Extremities

Alternate Names: *Tang Kuei Su Ni Tang, Tang Gui Si Ni Tang,* Tang-kuei and Counterflow Cold Decoction, Chinese Angelica Cold Limbs Decoction, Tangkuei and Jujube Combination

Original Source: *Shang Han Lun* (Discussion of Cold-Induced Disorders) by Zhang Zhong-Jing in the Eastern Han Dynasty

COMPOSITION

Dang Gui (Radix Angelicae Sinensis)	9g [12g]
Bai Shao (Radix Paeoniae Alba)	9g
Gui Zhi (Ramulus Cinnamomi)	9g
Xi Xin (Radix et Rhizoma Asari)	9g [1.5-3g]
Zhi Gan Cao (Radix et Rhizoma Glycyrrhizae Praeparata cum Melle)	6g
Da Zao (Fructus Jujubae), *bo* (opened)	25 pieces [8 pieces]
Mu Tong (Caulis Akebiae)	6g [3g]

DOSAGE / PREPARATION / ADMINISTRATION

Cook the ingredients in 8 cups [1,600 mL] of water until 3 cups [600 mL] of the liquid remain. Take 1 cup [200 mL] of the warm, strained decoction three times daily. Today, the decoction may be prepared using the doses suggested in brackets.

CHINESE THERAPEUTIC ACTIONS

1. Warms the channels and disperses cold
2. Nourishes the blood and opens the collaterals

CLINICAL MANIFESTATIONS

1. Invasion of cold with underlying deficiencies of yang qi and blood: icy cold hands and feet, a pale tongue, a white tongue coating, and a deep, thin pulse, or a thin pulse that is barely palpable.
2. Cold factor attacking the channels and collaterals causing pain at the waist, hips, legs, and feet.

CLINICAL APPLICATIONS

Pain, rheumatoid arthritis, fibromyalgia, sciatica, lumbago, headache, cancer pain, frostbite, periarthritis of shoulder, frozen shoulder, peripheral neuritis, Raynaud's disease, thromboangiitis obliterans, hypertrophic myelitis, prostatic hypertrophy, endometriosis, amenorrhea, pelvic inflammatory disease, peptic ulcer disease, post-surgical intestinal adhesion, intestinal colic, psoriasis, chronic urticaria, calluses and corns, allergic rhinitis, and benzene poisoning.

EXPLANATION

Dang Gui Si Ni Tang (Tangkuei Decoction for Frigid Extremities) treats invasion of cold with underlying deficiencies of yang qi and blood. The chief complaint in this syndrome is icy cold hands and feet, which may be caused by three factors. First, the yang qi is deficient, and therefore cannot warm the hands and feet. Second, blood is deficient and unable to nourish the hands and feet. Lastly, the cold factor itself makes the hands and feet more icy and cold. Invasion of cold also obstructs the channels and collaterals, leading to pain at the waist, hips, legs, and feet. A deep, thin pulse or a thin pulse that is

494

Chinese Herbal Formulas and Applications

Dāng Guī Sì Nì Tāng (Tangkuei Decoction for Frigid Extremities)

Dang Gui Si Ni Tang (Tangkuei Decoction for Frigid Extremities)

Diagnosis	Signs and Symptoms	Treatment	Herbs
Invasion of cold with underlying deficiencies of yang qi and blood	• Icy cold hands and feet: invasion of cold with underlying deficiencies of yang qi and blood • Pale tongue with a white tongue coating: presence of deficiency and cold • Deep, thin pulse or a thin pulse that is barely palpable: blood deficiency and invasion of cold	• Warms the channels and disperses cold • Nourishes the blood and opens the collaterals	• *Dang Gui* (Radix Angelicae Sinensis) and *Bai Shao* (Radix Paeoniae Alba) tonify and harmonize the blood. • *Gui Zhi* (Ramulus Cinnamomi) and *Xi Xin* (Radix et Rhizoma Asari) warm the channels, dispel exterior and interior cold, and restore yang qi. • *Zhi Gan Cao* (Radix et Rhizoma Glycyrrhizae Praeparata cum Melle) and *Da Zao* (Fructus Jujubae) strengthen the Spleen and tonify qi. • *Mu Tong* (Caulis Akebiae) opens the channels and collaterals to facilitate the circulation of qi and blood.

barely palpable indicates invasion of cold with underlying deficiencies.

This formula contains *Dang Gui* (Radix Angelicae Sinensis) and *Bai Shao* (Radix Paeoniae Alba) to tonify and harmonize the blood. *Gui Zhi* (Ramulus Cinnamomi) and *Xi Xin* (Radix et Rhizoma Asari) warm the channels, dispel exterior and interior cold, and restore yang qi. *Zhi Gan Cao* (Radix et Rhizoma Glycyrrhizae Praeparata cum Melle) and *Da Zao* (Fructus Jujubae) strengthen the Spleen, tonify qi, and assist *Bai Shao* (Radix Paeoniae Alba) and *Dang Gui* (Radix Angelicae Sinensis) in producing blood. Finally, *Mu Tong* (Caulis Akebiae) opens the channels and collaterals to facilitate the circulation of qi and blood.

MODIFICATIONS
• With nausea and vomiting due to cold and deficiency of the Stomach, add *Wu Zhu Yu* (Fructus Evodiae) and *Sheng Jiang* (Rhizoma Zingiberis Recens).
• With painful extremities due to wind and dampness, add *Sang Ji Sheng* (Herba Taxilli) and *Wei Ling Xian* (Radix et Rhizoma Clematidis).
• With soreness and pain of the lower back, add *Niu Xi* (Radix Achyranthis Bidentatae) and *Du Zhong* (Cortex Eucommiae).
• With dysmenorrhea due to coldness, add *Wu Yao* (Radix Linderae), *Xiao Hui Xiang* (Fructus Foeniculi), *Gao Liang Jiang* (Rhizoma Alpiniae Officinarum) and *Xiang Fu* (Rhizoma Cyperi).
• With severe deficiency and cold, add *Fu Zi* (Radix Aconiti Lateralis Praeparata), *Gan Jiang* (Rhizoma Zingiberis) and *Huang Qi* (Radix Astragali).
• For extreme cold after an illness, combine with *Xiao Chai Hu Tang* (Minor Bupleurum Decoction).

• With pain in the hips, back, legs and feet caused by blood deficiency and cold accumulation, add *Xu Duan* (Radix Dipsaci), *Niu Xi* (Radix Achyranthis Bidentatae), *Ji Xue Teng* (Caulis Spatholobi) and *Mu Gua* (Fructus Chaenomelis).
• For hernia due to cold, add *Wu Yao* (Radix Linderae), *Xiao Hui Xiang* (Fructus Foeniculi), and *Gao Liang Jiang* (Rhizoma Alpiniae Officinarum).

CAUTIONS / CONTRAINDICATIONS
Dang Gui Si Ni Tang is contraindicated in patients with yin-deficiency heat.

PHARMACOLOGICAL EFFECTS
Circulatory: Administration of *Dang Gui Si Ni Tang* in rabbits was associated with increased and improved blood perfusion to peripheral parts of the body with a relatively long duration of action.[1]

CLINICAL STUDIES AND RESEARCH
1. **Pain**: Use of *Dang Gui Si Ni Tang* has been shown to effectively treat pain in many parts of the body due to various causes. One study reported success in the treatment of 52 postpartum women with general aches and pains using *Dang Gui Si Ni Tang* plus *Huang Qi* (Radix Astragali) and *Sang Zhi* (Ramulus Mori) for 20 days to 3 months.[2] Another study also reported success using modified *Dang Gui Si Ni Tang* for 2-6 weeks to treat 33 patients with pain in the lower back and legs.[3] Lastly, one study reported 93.1% effectiveness in 116 patients with *tong bi* (extremely painful obstruction) using *Dang Gui Si Ni Tang* plus *Huang Qi* (Radix Astragali), *Ji Xue Teng* (Caulis Spatholobi) and others as needed. The treatment protocol was to administer herbs in decoction form daily, for 10 days per course of treatment, for 2-8 courses total.[4]

INTERIOR-WARMING FORMULAS

7

495

Dāng Guī Sì Nì Tāng (Tangkuei Decoction for Frigid Extremities)

2. **Headache**: Eighty-six patients with stubborn headache were treated with modified *Dang Gui Si Ni Tang* with satisfactory results. The herbal formula included *Dang Gui* (Radix Angelicae Sinensis) 15g, *Xi Xin* (Radix et Rhizoma Asari) 3g, *Tong Cao* (Medulla Tetrapanacis) 6g, *Wu Zhu Yu* (Fructus Evodiae) 5g, *Gui Zhi* (Ramulus Cinnamomi) 10g, *Bai Shao* (Radix Paeoniae Alba) 12g, *Zhi Gan Cao* (Radix et Rhizoma Glycyrrhizae Praeparata cum Melle) 10g, *Da Zao* (Fructus Jujubae) 10g, and *Sheng Jiang* (Rhizoma Zingiberis Recens) 12g. Treatment protocol was to administer the herbs in decoction one time daily for acute attack, and in pills (10 grams of the herbs total) two to three times daily for maintenance and prevention. Out of 86 patients, the study reported complete recovery in 31 patients (no recurrence within 6 months), significant improvement in 29 patients (no recurrence within 3 months), slight improvement in 21 patients, and no effect in 5 patients. The overall rate of effectiveness was 94.3%.[5]

3. **Cancer pain**: In one report, 50 patients with pain due to cancer were treated with modified *Dang Gui Si Ni Tang* with good results. The types of cancer included stomach (18 patients), esophageal (15 patients), lung (10 patients), and liver (7 patients). The formula included *Dang Gui* (Radix Angelicae Sinensis) 30-50g, *Bai Shao* (Radix Paeoniae Alba) 50-100g, *Gui Zhi* (Ramulus Cinnamomi) 10-30g, *Xi Xin* (Radix et Rhizoma Asari) 6-15g, *Mu Tong* (Caulis Akebiae) 10-15g, *Gan Cao* (Radix et Rhizoma Glycyrrhizae) 10-12g, and *Da Zao* (Fructus Jujubae) 5-10 pieces. The herbs were cooked in water for 30 minutes to yield 600 mL of decoction. The treatment protocol was to ingest 150 mL of the decoction every 6 hours for 3 days. Out of 50 patients, the study reported marked improvement in 18 patients, moderate improvement in 24 patients, slight improvement in 3 patients, and no effect in 8 patients. The overall rate of effectiveness was 84%.[6]

4. **Sciatica**: In one study, 18 out of 20 patients with sciatica reported complete recovery using modified *Dang Gui Si Ni Tang* for 6-20 days. Those who had complete recovery did not have a recurrence for 1 year following the initial treatment. The formula included *Dang Gui* (Radix Angelicae Sinensis) 15g, *Niu Xi* (Radix Achyranthis Bidentatae) 15g, *Bai Shao* (Radix Paeoniae Alba) 30g, *Wei Ling Xian* (Radix et Rhizoma Clematidis) 30g, *Ji Xue Teng* (Caulis Spatholobi) 30g, *Gui Zhi* (Ramulus Cinnamomi) 10g, *Zhi Chuan Wu* (Radix Aconiti Praeparata) 10g, *Zhi Cao Wu* (Radix Aconiti Kusnezoffii Praeparata) 10g, *Ru Xiang* (Gummi Olibanum) 10g, *Mo Yao* (Myrrha) 10g, *Gan Cao* (Radix et Rhizoma Glycyrrhizae) 10g, and *Xi Xin* (Radix et Rhizoma Asari) 3g. Furthermore, 6g of *San Qi* (Radix et Rhizoma Notoginseng) was added for severe pain.[7] Another study reported 95.5% effectiveness in 31 patients with sciatica using herbs daily for 30 days per course of treatment. The herbal formula contained *Dang Gui Si Ni Tang* plus *Niu Xi* (Radix Achyranthis Bidentatae), *Mu Tong* (Caulis Akebiae), *Wu Shao She* (Zaocys), *Ru Xiang* (Gummi Olibanum) and *Mo Yao* (Myrrha).[8]

5. **Frostbite**: One hundred patients with I-II degree frostbite were treated with topical applications of *Dang Gui Si Ni Tang*. The herbal formula included *Dang Gui* (Radix Angelicae Sinensis) 20g, *Gui Zhi* (Ramulus Cinnamomi) 15g, *Bai Shao* (Radix Paeoniae Alba) 20g, *Xi Xin* (Radix et Rhizoma Asari) 5g, *Zhi Gan Cao* (Radix et Rhizoma Glycyrrhizae Praeparata cum Melle) 5g, *Mu Tong* (Caulis Akebiae) 10g, and *Sheng Jiang* (Rhizoma Zingiberis Recens) 10g. The treatment protocol was to cook the herbs in 500 mL of water. During the cooking process, the affected area was placed in the direction of the vapor for steam therapy. In addition, following the steam therapy, the affected area was soaked in the herbal solution for 15-20 minutes. One pack of herbs may be used up to four times for such topical treatment. The treatment was repeated twice daily, for a total of 6-8 treatments. The study reported improvement in all patients, with reduction of swelling and pain.[9]

6. **Peripheral neuritis**: In one report, 12 patients with peripheral neuritis were treated with good results using modified *Dang Gui Si Ni Tang*. Out of 12 patients, 6 had bilateral neuritis of upper extremities, 4 had bilateral neuritis of lower extremities, and 2 had neuritis in all four extremities. The formula included *Dang Gui* (Radix Angelicae Sinensis) 15g, *Bai Shao* (Radix Paeoniae Alba) 15g, *Da Zao* (Fructus Jujubae) 15g, *Mu Tong* (Caulis Akebiae) 15g, *Gui Zhi* (Ramulus Cinnamomi) 10g, *Xi Xin* (Radix et Rhizoma Asari) 10g, and *Zhi Gan Cao* (Radix et Rhizoma Glycyrrhizae Praeparata cum Melle) 5g. Modifications were made as follow: *Ji Xue Teng* (Caulis Spatholobi) 30g, *Zhi Chuan Wu* (Radix Aconiti Praeparata) 10g, and *Zhi Cao Wu* (Radix Aconiti Kusnezoffii Praeparata) 10g were added for severe pain; and *Wu Gong* (Scolopendra) 2 pieces, *Quan Xie* (Scorpio) 6g, and *Huang Qi* (Radix Astragali) 20g were added for numbness. The preparation procedure was to cook the herbs in 300 mL of water to yield 100 mL of decoction. The treatment protocol was to administer 50 mL of the decoction twice daily. Those with chronic illness were also treated with topical application of herbs in the form of an herbal wash made by cooking the herb residue from the decoction in water. Out of 12 patients, the study reported complete recovery in 9 patients and improvement in 3 patients. The average length of treatment was 11 days, ranging from 6 to 25 days.[10]

7. **Periarthritis of shoulder**: Administration of modified *Dang Gui Si Ni Tang* in 20 patients with periarthritis of shoulder was associated with complete recovery in 10

Dāng Guī Sì Nì Tāng (Tangkuei Decoction for Frigid Extremities)

Chinese Herbal Formulas and Applications

patients, improvement in 8 patients, and no effect in 2 patients. The treatment protocol was to cook the herbs in water, and drink the decoction in equally-divided doses twice daily for 15 days per course of treatment, for 1-2 courses total. The herbal treatment contained *Dang Gui Si Ni Tang* as the base formula, and added *Huang Qi* (Radix Astragali) for qi deficiency; *Hei Lao Hu* (Radix Kadsurae Coccineae) for blood stagnation; and *Wu Shao She* (Zaocys) for migratory pain.[11]

8. **Frozen shoulder**: One study reported complete recovery in 30 of 32 patients with frozen shoulder when treated with *Dang Gui Si Ni Tang* plus *Ji Xue Teng* (Caulis Spatholobi). The treatment protocol was to administer the herbs in decoction daily, for 12 days per course of treatment, for 1-3 courses total.[12]

9. **Hypertrophic myelitis**: Use of modified *Dang Gui Si Ni Tang* was successful in treating 24 patients with hypertrophic myelitis affecting different areas of the spine. The duration of illness of the patients varied from 6 months to 4 years. Clinical presentations included pain, cold extremities, numbness, and weakness of the muscles. Of 24 patients, the study reported complete recovery in 12 patients, improvement in 11 patients, and no benefit in 1 patient. The overall rate of effectiveness was 95.8%.[13]

10. **Allergic rhinitis**: Sixty-five patients with allergic rhinitis were treated with *Dang Gui Si Ni Tang* plus *Huang Qi* (Radix Astragali) and *Dang Shen* (Radix Codonopsis) with 90% effectiveness. Modifications were made as follow: *Xian Mao* (Rhizoma Curculiginis) was added for Kidney yang deficiency; *Bai Zhu* (Rhizoma Atractylodis Macrocephalae) and *Fu Ling* (Poria) for Spleen qi deficiency; and *Mai Dong* (Radix Ophiopogonis), *Wu Mei* (Fructus Mume) and *Tai Zi Shen* (Radix Pseudostellariae) for qi and yin deficiencies. The treatment protocol was to administer the decoction daily in the morning and at night, for 30 days per course of treatment, for 1-2 courses. Patients were advised to discontinue all other medications, and avoid all spicy and pungent foods. Of 65 patients, the study reported complete recovery in 38 patients, improvement in 21 patients, and no effect in 6 patients.[14]

11. **Psoriasis**: In one study, 32 patients with psoriasis characterized by blood deficiency with exterior wind-cold were treated with herbs with complete recovery in 12 patients, improvement in 17 patients, and no effect in 3 patients. The effectiveness was 90.8%. The herbal treatment included *Dang Gui Si Ni Tang* plus *Fu Zi* (Radix Aconiti Lateralis Praeparata), *Quan Xie* (Scorpio), *Wu Gong* (Scolopendra) and *Mu Dan Pi* (Cortex Moutan). The duration of treatment was 1 month per course of treatment, for 2 courses total.[15]

12. **Prostatic hypertrophy**: Use of modified *Dang Gui Si Ni Tang* in 42 patients with prostatic hypertrophy was associated with complete recovery in 20 patients, improvement in 19 patients, and no change in 3 patients. The rate of effectiveness was 92.86%. The herbal treatment contained *Dang Gui Si Ni Tang* plus *Zhi Mu* (Rhizoma Anemarrhenae), *Huang Bo* (Cortex Phellodendri Chinensis), *Niu Xi* (Radix Achyranthis Bidentatae), *Che Qian Zi* (Semen Plantaginis), *Wang Bu Liu Xing* (Semen Vaccariae) and *Chuan Shan Jia* (Squama Manis). Each course of treatment was 10 days.[16]

13. **Endometriosis**: One study reported good results using modified *Dang Gui Si Ni Tang* to treat endometriosis in 10 women (between 21-52 years of age; 1 single, and 9 married with children). The base formula contained *Dang Gui Si Ni Tang* plus *E Zhu* (Rhizoma Curcumae), *Chuan Xiong* (Rhizoma Chuanxiong), *Pu Huang* (Pollen Typhae) and *Yi Mu Cao* (Herba Leonuri). *Huang Qi* (Radix Astragali) and *Dang Shen* (Radix Codonopsis) were added for qi deficiency; and smaller doses of *Dang Gui* (Radix Angelicae Sinensis), *Pu Huang* (Pollen Typhae) and *Chuan Xiong* (Rhizoma Chuanxiong) during the period. Herbs were given in decoction daily for 15 days per course of treatment. Of 10 patients, the study reported complete recovery in 2 patients, marked improvement in 6 patients, and no change in 2 patients.[17]

14. **Amenorrhea**: Forty-seven of 48 patients with amenorrhea were treated with good success using modified *Dang Gui Si Ni Tang*. The herbal formula contained *Dang Gui* (Radix Angelicae Sinensis), *Gui Zhi* (Ramulus Cinnamomi), *Bai Shao* (Radix Paeoniae Alba), *Xi Xin* (Radix et Rhizoma Asari), *Gan Cao* (Radix et Rhizoma Glycyrrhizae), *Tong Cao* (Medulla Tetrapanacis), *Da Zao* (Fructus Jujubae), *Yin Yang Huo* (Herba Epimedii), and processed *Huang Qi* (Radix Astragali). Modifications were made by adding *Chai Hu* (Radix Bupleuri), *Niu Xi* (Radix Achyranthis Bidentatae) and *Dan Shen* (Radix et Rhizoma Salviae Miltiorrhizae) for qi and blood stagnation; *Cang Zhu* (Rhizoma Atractylodis) and *Xiang Fu* (Rhizoma Cyperi) for overweight individuals with dampness and phlegm accumulation; *Shan Zha* (Fructus Crataegi) for poor appetite; *Yan Hu Suo* (Rhizoma Corydalis) and *Xiang Fu* (Rhizoma Cyperi) for abdominal pain; and *Che Qian Zi* (Semen Plantaginis) for profuse leukorrhea. The treatment protocol was to cook the herbs in water, and administer the decoction in two equally-divided doses, for 10 days per course of treatment, for 2-3 courses total.[18]

15. **Pelvic inflammatory disease**: Use of modified *Dang Gui Si Ni Tang* was associated with 94.7% effectiveness in treating 76 patients with pelvic inflammatory disease. The treatment contained this formula plus *Fen Bi Xie*

INTERIOR-WARMING FORMULAS

7

497

Dāng Guī Sì Nì Tāng (Tangkuei Decoction for Frigid Extremities)

(Rhizoma Dioscoreae Hypoglaucae), *Pu Gong Ying* (Herba Taraxaci) and *Jin Yin Hua* (Flos Lonicerae Japonicae) as the base. Additional modifications included *Yan Hu Suo* (Rhizoma Corydalis) and *Chuan Lian Zi* (Fructus Toosendan) for severe pain; *Di Yu* (Radix Sanguisorbae) and *Mian Ma Guan Zhong* (Rhizoma Dryopteridis Crassirhizomatis) for leukorrhea with blood and pus; *Li Zhi He* (Semen Litchi) and *Ju He* (Semen Citri Reticulatae) for lower abdominal swelling and pain; and *Du Zhong* (Cortex Eucommiae) and *Sang Ji Sheng* (Herba Taxilli) for soreness and weakness of the lower back and legs. The duration of treatment was 10 days per course of treatment, for 1-3 courses total. Of 76 patients, the study reported complete recovery in 52 patients, improvement in 20 patients, and no effect in 4 patients.[19]

16. **Post-surgical intestinal adhesion**: *Dang Gui Si Ni Tang* plus *Da Huang* (Radix et Rhizoma Rhei) was used to treat 108 patients with intestinal adhesion following such surgeries as removal of the appendix, gallbladder, and uterus. The herbs were cooked in 800 mL of water to yield 300 mL of decoction. The treatment protocol was to ingest 50 mL of decoction per dose, 5-6 times per day, for 5 days per course of treatment. Most patients were treated with 2-3 courses to control the pain and stabilize the condition. Out of 108 patients, the study reported complete recovery in 63 patients (asymptomatic for 3 months), significant improvement in 41 patients (mild pain only), and no change in 4 patients. The overall effectiveness rate was 96.3%.[20]

17. **Benzene poisoning**: One study reported effectiveness using *Dang Gui Si Ni Tang* to treat 20 patients with more than 24 hours of benzene poisoning. Clinical presentations included dark purple discoloration of the face, lips, extremities, and the entire body; cold extremities, weak respiration, a dull facial expression, abdominal pain, spasms, and cramps. In addition to herbal treatment, 8 patients also received oxygen and acupuncture treatments. The mechanism of action of this formula in treating benzene poisoning was attributed to its effect to increase blood perfusion to the brain, heart, and extremities.[21]

RELATED FORMULA

Dāng Guī Sì Nì Jiā Wú Zhū Yú Shēng Jiāng Tāng

(Tangkuei Decoction for Frigid Extremities plus Evodia and Fresh Ginger)

當歸四逆加吳茱萸生薑湯
当归四逆加吴茱萸生姜汤

Pinyin Name: Dang Gui Si Ni Jia Wu Zhu Yu Sheng Jiang Tang

Literal Name: Tangkuei Decoction for Frigid Extremities plus Evodia and Fresh Ginger

Original Source: *Shang Han Lun* (Discussion of Cold-Induced Disorders) by Zhang Zhong-Jing in the Eastern Han Dynasty

Dang Gui (Radix Angelicae Sinensis)	9g [12g]
Gui Zhi (Ramulus Cinnamomi)	9g
Bai Shao (Radix Paeoniae Alba)	9g
Xi Xin (Radix et Rhizoma Asari)	9g [1.5-3g]
Zhi Gan Cao (Radix et Rhizoma Glycyrrhizae Praeparata cum Melle)	6g
Mu Tong (Caulis Akebiae)	6g [3g]
Da Zao (Fructus Jujubae), *bo* (opened)	25 pieces [8 pieces]
Wu Zhu Yu (Fructus Evodiae)	2 cups [5g]
Sheng Jiang (Rhizoma Zingiberis Recens)	24g [15g]

The source text states to cook the ingredients in 6 cups [1,200 mL] of water and 6 cups [1,200 mL] of grain-based liquor until 5 cups [1,000 mL] of the liquid remain. Take the warm, strained decoction in five equally-divided doses. Today, the decoction may be prepared using the doses suggested in brackets.

Dang Gui Si Ni Jia Wu Zhu Yu Sheng Jiang Tang (Tangkuei Decoction for Frigid Extremities plus Evodia and Fresh Ginger) combines *Dang Gui Si Ni Tang* with *Wu Zhu Yu* (Fructus Evodiae) and *Sheng Jiang* (Rhizoma Zingiberis Recens). These two herbs are added to this formula to dispel chronic cold in the body in addition to tonifying blood and yang qi. Grain-based liquor is used to enhance the overall effect of dispelling cold and opening collaterals. Clinically, patients may show loose stools, vomiting, abdominal pain, a fine pulse that is barely palpable, and other symptoms related to chronic coldness.

In comparing the two formulas, *Dang Gui Si Ni Jia Wu Zhu Yu Sheng Jiang Tang* (Tangkuei Decoction for Frigid Extremities plus Evodia and Fresh Ginger) more strongly warms the channels and disperses cold than *Dang Gui Si Ni Tang*, and is therefore more suitable to treat patients with chronic coldness in addition to blood and yang qi deficiencies.

AUTHORS' COMMENTS

According to the source text, "*Tong Cao*" is stated as an ingredient in *Dang Gui Si Ni Tang*. The identity of this herb has been questioned, since "*Mu Tong*" and "*Tong Cao*" are two herbs with similar pinyin names and functions, and have been used interchangeably in the past. Both herbs have functions to promote urination and treat *lin zheng* (dysuria syndrome). However, *Mu Tong* (Caulis Akebiae) can open the channels and collaterals to treat pain, while *Tong Cao* (Medulla Tetrapanacis) can unblock

Dāng Guī Sī Nì Tāng (Tangkuei Decoction for Frigid Extremities)

Chinese Herbal Formulas and Applications

and promote lactation. Therefore, based on the indications of the formula and the functions of these two herbs, most scholars and clinicians agree that *Mu Tong* (Caulis Akebiae) is a more suitable herb than *Tong Cao* (Medulla Tetrapanacis) in *Dang Gui Si Ni Tang*.

There are three "*si ni* (frigid extremities)" formulas that are commonly used. Although they share similar names, they have distinct functions.

- *Si Ni San* (Frigid Extremities Powder) is a harmonizing formula that treats cold extremities caused by the advancement of exterior pathogenic factor into the interior. Its main function is to harmonize the exterior and interior and remove stagnation.
- *Si Ni Tang* (Frigid Extremities Decoction) is an interior-warming formula that resuscitates yang. It is an extremely hot formula that treats icy cold extremities caused by depletion of yang that is on the verge of collapse. The formula dispels cold, tonifies yang, and prevents collapse.
- *Dang Gui Si Ni Tang* (Tangkuei Decoction for Frigid Extremities) is an interior-warming formula to warm the channels and dispel cold. It treats cold extremities caused by cold with underlying deficiencies of yang qi and blood. It dispels cold, warms the yang, nourishes the blood, and opens the channels and collaterals.

According to Dr. Chang Wei-Yen, *Dang Gui Si Ni Tang* can be used in a small amount to treat angina or cardiac infarction, since it has the effect to open the vessels. Furthermore, *Dang Gui Si Ni Tang* can be combined with *Xue Fu Zhu Yu Tang* (Drive Out Stasis in the Mansion of Blood Decoction) for maximum effect.

References

1. *Zhong Hua Yi Xue Za Zhi* (Chinese Journal of Medicine) 1981;1:57.
2. *He Bei Zhong Yi* (Hebei Chinese Medicine) 1995;4:15.
3. *Zhong Yi Ming Fang Lin Chuang Xin Yong* (Contemporary Clinical Applications of Classic Chinese Formulas) 2001;336.
4. *Hu Nan Zhong Yi Za Zhi* (Hunan Journal of Chinese Medicine) 1997;6:29.
5. *Tian Jin Zhong Yi* (Tianjin Chinese Medicine) 1985;6:25.
6. *Zhong Yi Fang Ji Xian Dai Yan Jiu* (Modern Study of Medical Formulae in Traditional Chinese Medicine) 1997;424.
7. *Hu Bei Zhong Yi Za Zhi* (Hubei Journal of Chinese Medicine) 1986;2:39.
8. *Hu Nan Zhong Yi Za Zhi* (Hunan Journal of Chinese Medicine) 1997;2:48.
9. *Shan Dong Zhong Yi Za Zhi* (Shandong Journal of Chinese Medicine) 1984;2:37.
10. *Xin Zhong Yi* (New Chinese Medicine) 1996;2:46.
11. *Xin Zhong Yi* (New Chinese Medicine) 1987;7:53.
12. *Si Chuan Zhong Yi* (Sichuan Chinese Medicine) 1989;2:31.
13. *Hu Nan Zhong Yi Za Zhi* (Hunan Journal of Chinese Medicine) 1988;4:45.
14. *Yun Nan Zhong Yi Zhong Yao Za Zhi* (Yunan Journal of Chinese Medicine and Medicinals) 1999;4:29.
15. *Zhong Yi Ming Fang Lin Chuang Xin Yong* (Contemporary Clinical Applications of Classic Chinese Formulas) 2001;334.
16. *Yun Nan Zhong Yi Zhong Yao Za Zhi* (Yunan Journal of Chinese Medicine and Medicinals) 1998;4:15.
17. *Yun Nan Zhong Yi Za Zhi* (Yunan Journal of Chinese Medicine) 1993;6:14.
18. *Zhong Yi Fang Ji Xian Dai Yan Jiu* (Modern Study of Medical Formulae in Traditional Chinese Medicine) 1997;421.
19. *Shan Xi Zhong Yi* (Shanxi Chinese Medicine) 1995;12:533.
20. *Zhe Jiang Zhong Yi Za Zhi* (Zhejiang Journal of Chinese Medicine) 1995;3:107.
21. *Shang Hai Zhong Yi Yao Za Zhi* (Shanghai Journal of Chinese Medicine and Herbology) 1962;11:23.

Chapter 7 – Interior-Warming Formulas　　　　*Section 3 – Channel-Warming and Cold-Dispersing Formulas*

Huáng Qí Guì Zhī Wǔ Wù Tāng
(Astragalus and Cinnamon Twig Five-Substance Decoction)

黃耆桂枝五物湯
黄芪桂枝五物汤

Pinyin Name: *Huang Qi Gui Zhi Wu Wu Tang*
Literal Name: Astragalus and Cinnamon Twig Five-Substance Decoction
Alternate Names: *Huang Chi Wu Wu Tang, Huang Qi Wu Wu Tang*, Astragalus Five-Component Decoction, Astragalus Five-Herbs Decoction, Astragalus Five Decoction, Astragalus and Cinnamon Five Herb Combination
Original Source: *Jin Gui Yao Lue* (Essentials from the Golden Cabinet) by Zhang Zhong-Jing in the Eastern Han Dynasty

COMPOSITION

Huang Qi (Radix Astragali)	9g [12g]
Gui Zhi (Ramulus Cinnamomi)	9g
Bai Shao (Radix Paeoniae Alba)	9g
Sheng Jiang (Rhizoma Zingiberis Recens)	18g [12g]
Da Zao (Fructus Jujubae)	12 pieces [4 pieces]

DOSAGE / PREPARATION / ADMINISTRATION

Cook the herbs in 6 cups [1,200 mL] of water until it is reduced to 2 cups [400 mL]. Take 0.7 cup [140 mL] of the warm, strained decoction in three equally-divided doses. Today, the decoction may be prepared using the doses suggested in brackets.

CHINESE THERAPEUTIC ACTIONS

1. Tonifies qi and warms the channels
2. Harmonizes the *ying* (nutritive) level and unblocks obstruction

CLINICAL MANIFESTATIONS

Xue bi (blood painful obstruction): numbness of the extremities, and a slightly rough and tight pulse.

CLINICAL APPLICATIONS

Periarthritis of the shoulders, synovitis of the knees, neck and shoulder pain, peripheral neuritis, diabetic neuropathy, peripheral neuropathy, polyneuropathy, hemiplegia, muscle paralysis, facial paralysis, restless leg syndrome, beriberi, and frostbite.

EXPLANATION

Huang Qi Gui Zhi Wu Wu Tang (Astragalus and Cinnamon Twig Five-Substance Decoction) is designed to treat *xue bi* (blood painful obstruction). This condition begins in individuals with underlying weakness and deficiency. When the individuals are exposed to the wind, they experience obstruction of qi and blood circulation, which leads to localized numbness of the limbs and extremities. In severe cases, there may be muscle aches and pain. The slightly rough and tight pulse is representative of blood stasis.

Huang Qi (Radix Astragali) tonifies *wei* (defensive) qi and consolidates the exterior. *Gui Zhi* (Ramulus Cinnamomi) disperses wind-cold and opens the channels.

Huang Qi Gui Zhi Wu Wu Tang (Astragalus and Cinnamon Twig Five-Substance Decoction)

Diagnosis	Signs and Symptoms	Treatment	Herbs
Xue bi (blood painful obstruction)	• Numbness of the extremities: exterior wind blocking qi and blood circulation • Slightly rough and tight pulse: blood stasis	• Tonifies qi and warms the channels • Harmonizes the channels and unblocks obstructions	• *Huang Qi* (Radix Astragali) tonifies *wei* (defensive) *qi* and consolidates the exterior. • *Gui Zhi* (Ramulus Cinnamomi) disperses wind-cold and opens the channels. • *Bai Shao* (Radix Paeoniae Alba) nourishes the blood and harmonizes the *ying* (nutritive) and *wei* (defensive) levels. • *Sheng Jiang* (Rhizoma Zingiberis Recens) dispels wind-cold. • *Da Zao* (Fructus Jujubae) tonifies qi and blood.

500

Huáng Qí Gui Zhī Wǔ Wù Tāng
(Astragalus and Cinnamon Twig Five-Substance Decoction)

The combination of *Huang Qi* (Radix Astragali) and *Gui Zhi* (Ramulus Cinnamomi) tonifies qi, warms yang, harmonizes the blood, and opens the channels. *Bai Shao* (Radix Paeoniae Alba) nourishes the blood and harmonizes the *ying* (nutritive) level. The combination of *Gui Zhi* (Ramulus Cinnamomi) and *Bai Shao* (Radix Paeoniae Alba) also harmonizes the *ying* (nutritive) and *wei* (defensive) levels. *Sheng Jiang* (Rhizoma Zingiberis Recens) and *Gui Zhi* (Ramulus Cinnamomi) dispel wind-cold. *Da Zao* (Fructus Jujubae) tonifies qi and blood.

MODIFICATIONS

- With weak arms and hands, double the dose of *Gui Zhi* (Ramulus Cinnamomi).
- With weak knees and legs, add *Niu Xi* (Radix Achyranthis Bidentatae).
- With weak tendons, add *Mu Gua* (Fructus Chaenomelis).
- With deficiency of *yuan* (source) qi, add *Ren Shen* (Radix et Rhizoma Ginseng).
- With deficiency of yang, add *Fu Zi* (Radix Aconiti Lateralis Praeparata).
- With hemiparalysis affecting the left side, add *Dang Gui* (Radix Angelicae Sinensis).
- With hemiparalysis affecting the right side, double the dose of *Huang Qi* (Radix Astragali).
- With numbness of the body, add *Dang Gui* (Radix Angelicae Sinensis) and *Fang Feng* (Radix Saposhnikoviae).
- With painful extremities, add *Bai Zhu* (Rhizoma Atractylodis Macrocephalae) and *Fang Ji* (Radix Stephaniae Tetrandrae).
- With numbness and pain due to blood stagnation, combine with *Si Wu Tang* (Four-Substance Decoction).
- With numbness and pain due to wind obstruction, combine with *Xu Ming Tang* (Prolong Life Decoction).
- If there is more wind, add *Fang Feng* (Radix Saposhnikoviae) and *Fang Ji* (Radix Stephaniae Tetrandrae).
- If there is more blood stasis, add *Tao Ren* (Semen Persicae) and *Hong Hua* (Flos Carthami).
- When there is pain in postpartum women or after the menstrual cycles, add *Dang Gui* (Radix Angelicae Sinensis), *Chuan Xiong* (Rhizoma Chuanxiong) and *Ji Xue Teng* (Caulis Spatholobi).

CLINICAL STUDIES AND RESEARCH

1. **Periarthritis of the shoulders**: Integrative treatment using herbs and *tui-na* was effective in treating 63 patients with periarthritis of the shoulders. The herbal formula contained *Huang Qi* (Radix Astragali) 15g, *Gui Zhi* (Ramulus Cinnamomi) 5g, *Chi Shao* (Radix Paeoniae Rubra) 5g, *Bai Shao* (Radix Paeoniae Alba) 5g, *Da Zao* (Fructus Jujubae) 5g, *Qiang Huo* (Rhizoma et Radix Notopterygii)

5g, *Du Huo* (Radix Angelicae Pubescentis) 5g, *Fang Feng* (Radix Saposhnikoviae) 5g, *Dang Gui* (Radix Angelicae Sinensis) 5g, *Chuan Xiong* (Rhizoma Chuanxiong) 5g, *Xi Xin* (Radix et Rhizoma Asari) 5g, and *Sheng Jiang* (Rhizoma Zingiberis Recens) 5g. Modifications were made as follow: *Zhi Chuan Wu* (Radix Aconiti Praeparata) 3-6g and *Zhi Cao Wu* (Radix Aconiti Kusnezoffii Praeparata) 3-6g were added for severe pain characterized by cold; *Xu Duan* (Radix Dipsaci) 9g and *Du Zhong* (Cortex Eucommiae) 9g were added for elderly patients with Liver and Kidney deficiencies; *Sang Zhi* (Ramulus Mori) 15g and *Shen Jin Cao* (Herba Lycopodii) 12g were added for stiff joints with limited range of motion; and *Di Long* (Pheretima) 9g and *Wu Shao She* (Zaocys) 30g were added for chronic arthritis. Of 63 patients, the study reported complete recovery in 26 patients, significant improvement in 31 patients, and moderate improvement in 6 patients. The duration of treatment varied from 14-48 days, with an average of 29 days.[1]

2. **Synovitis of the knees**: Thirty-eight patients with synovitis of the knees responded well to herbal treatment and physical therapy. Herbal treatment contained *Huang Qi Gui Zhi Wu Wu Tang* plus *Dang Gui* (Radix Angelicae Sinensis). The herbs were given in decoction daily, for three weeks per course of treatment. The duration of treatment varied from 14-42 days. Of 38 patients, 32 had complete recovery and 6 had moderate improvement.[2]

3. **Neck and shoulder pain**: One study reported marked effect using modified *Huang Qi Gui Zhi Wu Wu Tang* to treat 48 patients with neck and shoulder stiffness and pain. In addition to *Huang Qi Gui Zhi Wu Wu Tang* as the base formula, *Mu Gua* (Fructus Chaenomelis) was added for stiff muscles with limited mobility; *Dang Gui* (Radix Angelicae Sinensis) and *Chuan Xiong* (Rhizoma Chuanxiong) were added for numbness; and *Ju Hua* (Flos Chrysanthemi) was added for dizziness. The herbs were given in decoction for 7 days per course of treatment. Of 48 patients, the study reported complete recovery in 20 patients, significant improvement in 18 patients and moderate improvement in 10 patients.[3]

4. ***Bi zheng* (painful obstruction syndrome)**: Use of *Huang Qi Gui Zhi Wu Wu Tang* was associated with good therapeutic effect to treat *bi zheng* (painful obstruction syndrome) characterized by yang deficiency and invasion cold and its subsequent obstruction of the channels and collaterals. The herbal treatment contained *Huang Qi Gui Zhi Wu Wu Tang* plus *Gu Sui Bu* (Rhizoma Drynariae), *Du Zhong* (Cortex Eucommiae), *Xu Duan* (Radix Dipsaci), and *Dang Gui* (Radix Angelicae Sinensis). Of 114 patients, the study reported significant improvement in 111 patients and no effect in 3 patients. The average

Huáng Qí Guì Zhī Wǔ Wù Tāng
(Astragalus and Cinnamon Twig Five-Substance Decoction)

duration of treatment was 5.4 packs of herbs, though the range was between 2 to 120 packs.[4]

5. **Peripheral neuritis**: *Huang Qi Gui Zhi Wu Wu Tang* was reported in several studies to effectively treat peripheral neuritis. According to one study, 51 patients with peripheral neuritis were effectively treated with *Huang Qi Gui Zhi Wu Wu Tang* plus *Sang Ji Sheng* (Herba Taxilli) and *Ji Xue Teng* (Caulis Spatholobi) as the base formula, with addition of *Mo Yao* (Myrrha) for severe pain; *Yi Yi Ren* (Semen Coicis) for swelling; *Tao Ren* (Semen Persicae) for dark purple skin appearance; *Jiang Huang* (Rhizoma Curcumae Longae) for neuritis in the upper limbs; and *Ren Shen Yang Ying Tang* (Ginseng Decoction to Nourish the Nutritive Qi) for neuritis in the lower limbs. Of 51 patients, the study reported complete recovery in 36 patients, improvement in 11 patients, and no effect in 4 patients.[5] According to another study, 198 patients with neuritis were treated with complete recovery in 195 patients, improvement in 2 patients, and no effect in 1 case. In addition to *Huang Qi Gui Zhi Wu Wu Tang*, *Sang Zhi* (Ramulus Mori), *Dang Gui* (Radix Angelicae Sinensis) and *Xi Xin* (Radix et Rhizoma Asari) were added for yang deficiency and cold obstruction; *Dang Gui* (Radix Angelicae Sinensis), *Ji Xue Teng* (Caulis Spatholobi) and *Sang Zhi* (Ramulus Mori) were added for blood deficiency; and *Ren Dong Teng* (Caulis Lonicerae Japonicae), *Tong Cao* (Medulla Tetrapanacis) and *Di Long* (Pheretima) were added, and *Gui Zhi* (Ramulus Cinnamomi) was removed for the presence of damp-heat.[6]

6. **Diabetic neuropathy**: One study reported 100% effectiveness using modified *Huang Qi Gui Zhi Wu Wu Tang* to treat diabetic neuropathy. The herbal treatment contained this formula plus *Jiang Can* (Bombyx Batryticatus), *Quan Xie* (Scorpio), *Wu Gong* (Scolopendra) and *Di Long* (Pheretima). Modifications included addition of *Sang Zhi* (Ramulus Mori) for burning sensations at the affected area; and *Fu Zi* (Radix Aconiti Lateralis Praeparata) for cold sensations. The herbs were given for 15 days per course of treatment. Of 30 patients, the study reported near-complete recovery in 13 patients, significant improvement in 10 patients, and moderate improvement in 7 patients.[7] Another study reported 85.71% effectiveness using modified *Huang Qi Gui Zhi Wu Wu Tang* to treat 42 patients with peripheral neuropathy. The herbal treatment contained *Huang Qi Gui Zhi Wu Wu Tang* plus *Dang Gui* (Radix Angelicae Sinensis), *Chi Shao* (Radix Paeoniae Rubra), *Ge Gen* (Radix Puerariae Lobatae), *Shan Yao* (Rhizoma Dioscoreae), *Shan Zhu Yu* (Fructus Corni), and *Ji Xue Teng* (Caulis Spatholobi) as the base formula. Additional modifications were made as needed to address complications of diabetes mellitus. The herbs were given for 10 days per course of

treatment. Of 42 patients, the study reported significant improvement in 24 patients, moderate improvement in 12 patients, and no effect in 6 patients.[8]

7. **Frostbite**: Modified *Huang Qi Gui Zhi Wu Wu Tang* was reported in one study to effectively treat 566 patients with frostbite. The herbal treatment contained *Huang Qi Gui Zhi Wu Wu Tang* plus *Ji Xue Teng* (Caulis Spatholobi) and *Fu Zi* (Radix Aconiti Lateralis Praeparata) as the base formula. Modifications were made based on the area affected, and included addition of *Bai Zhi* (Radix Angelicae Dahuricae) and *Chuan Xiong* (Rhizoma Chuanxiong) for the face; *Jiang Huang* (Rhizoma Curcumae Longae) and *Gui Zhi* (Ramulus Cinnamomi) for upper limbs; *Niu Xi* (Radix Achyranthis Bidentatae) and *Du Huo* (Radix Angelicae Pubescentis) for lower limbs; *Tao Ren* (Semen Persicae), *Chuan Shan Jia* (Squama Manis) and *Dang Gui* (Radix Angelicae Sinensis) for bruises and swelling; *Fu Ling* (Poria), *Wu Shao She* (Zaocys), *Cang Zhu* (Rhizoma Atractylodis) and *Yi Yi Ren* (Semen Coicis) for blisters; *Xi Xin* (Radix et Rhizoma Asari), *Ru Xiang* (Gummi Olibanum) and *Cong Bai* (Bulbus Allii Fistulosi) for severe pain; *Di Long* (Pheretima), *Hai Feng Teng* (Caulis Piperis Kadsurae) and *Quan Xie* (Scorpio) for numbness; and *Tu Fu Ling* (Rhizoma Smilacis Glabrae), *Da Xue Teng* (Caulis Sargentodoxae) and *Bai Jiang Cao* (Herba cum Radice Patriniae) for swelling, redness and pain. Of 566 patients, the study reported significant improvement in 453 patients and moderate improvement in 95 patients.[9]

8. **Restless leg syndrome**: Use of modified *Huang Qi Gui Zhi Wu Wu Tang* was associated with good results in treating 18 patients with restless leg syndrome. The herbal formula contained *Huang Qi* (Radix Astragali) 30g, *Gui Zhi* (Ramulus Cinnamomi) 12g, *Chuan Xiong* (Rhizoma Chuanxiong) 15g, *Dang Gui* (Radix Angelicae Sinensis) 12g, *Xi Xin* (Radix et Rhizoma Asari) 3g, *Di Long* (Pheretima) 12g, *Chuan Niu Xi* (Radix Cyathulae) 15g, *Bai Shao* (Radix Paeoniae Alba) 30g, and *Gan Cao* (Radix et Rhizoma Glycyrrhizae) 6g. Modifications were made by adding *Dan Shen* (Radix et Rhizoma Salviae Miltiorrhizae) 30g and *Ji Xue Teng* (Caulis Spatholobi) 30g for numbness and weakness of the extremities with qi and blood deficiencies; *Tao Ren* (Semen Persicae) 9g, *Hong Hua* (Flos Carthami) 9g, and *Huang Qi* (Radix Astragali) 60g for numbness and weakness of the extremities with qi deficiency and blood stagnation; and *Fu Zi* (Radix Aconiti Lateralis Praeparata) 12g and *Ma Huang* (Herba Ephedrae) 6g for cold extremities with yang deficiency. The herbs were given in decoction daily, with duration of treatment ranging from 6-25 packs of herbs. Of 18 patients, the study reported complete recovery in 12

Huáng Qí Guì Zhī Wǔ Wù Tāng
(Astragalus and Cinnamon Twig Five-Substance Decoction)

patients, significant improvement in 3 patients, moderate improvement in 2 patients, and no change in 1 patient.[10]

9. **Pulmonary heart disease**: One study reported marked success using *Huang Qi Gui Zhi Wu Wu Tang* to treat 70 patients with pulmonary heart disease. Use of the formula was associated with elevated plasma levels of prealbumin, transferrin and fibronectin, and lowered levels of C-reactive protein, ceruloplasmin, haptoglobin, alpha 1-antitrypsin and alpha 1-acid glycoprotein. In comparison, in the control group, which did not receive any herbs, only the levels of ceruloplasmin and C-reactive protein decreased significantly. The study stated that *Huang Qi Gui Zhi Wu Wu Tang* may enhance the therapeutic effects for pulmonary heart disease, regulate the metabolism of plasma proteins, and improve the quality of life of such patients.[11]

AUTHORS' COMMENTS

Dang Gui Si Ni Tang (Tangkuei Decoction for Frigid Extremities) and *Huang Qi Gui Zhi Wu Wu Tang* both warm the channels and dispel cold.

- *Dang Gui Si Ni Tang* is best at nourishing blood and opening the channels and collaterals.
- *Huang Qi Gui Zhi Wu Wu Tang* is mainly used for *bi zheng* (painful obstruction syndrome) in post-stroke patients, since it is better at tonifying qi and warming the channels and collaterals.

Huang Qi Gui Zhi Wu Wu Tang is a variation of *Gui Zhi Tang* (Cinnamon Twig Decoction), without *Gan Cao* (Radix et Rhizoma Glycyrrhizae), and with the addition of *Huang Qi* (Radix Astragali) and a higher dose of *Sheng Jiang* (Rhizoma Zingiberis Recens). Both formulas contain *Gui Zhi* (Ramulus Cinnamomi) to warm the channels and dispel cold.

References

1. *Si Chuan Zhong Yi* (Sichuan Chinese Medicine) 1993;1:40.
2. *Gan Su Zhong Yi* (Gansu Chinese Medicine) 1993;6:26.
3. *Shi Zhen Guo Yao Yan Jiu* (Research of Shizhen Herbs) 1999;5:362.
4. *Hu Bei Zhong Yi Za Zhi* (Hubei Journal of Chinese Medicine) 1995;6:11.
5. *Liao Ning Zhong Yi Za Zhi* (Liaoning Journal of Chinese Medicine) 1991;1:36.
6. *Zhong Yi Yao Xin Xi* (Information on Chinese Medicine and Herbology) 1998;2:40.
7. *He Bei Zhong Yi* (Hebei Chinese Medicine) 1998;5:301.
8. *Hei Long Jiang Zhong Yi Yao* (Heilongjiang Chinese Medicine and Herbology) 1998;4:17.
9. *Shan Dong Zhong Yi Za Zhi* (Shandong Journal of Chinese Medicine) 1990;3:49.
10. *Shi Yong Zhong Yi Nei Ke Za Zhi* (Journal of Practical Chinese Internal Medicine) 1993;3:43.
11. Che H, Luo K. Effects of huang qi wu wu decoction on plasma proteins in 70 patients of chronic pulmonary heart disease. Journal of Traditional Chinese Medicine 2000 Dec;20(4):254-7.

Chapter 7 – Interior-Warming Formulas

Chapter 7 — Summary

— Interior-Warming Formulas

SECTION 1: MIDDLE-WARMING AND COLD-DISPELLING FORMULAS

Name	Similarities	Differences
Li Zhong Wan (Regulate the Middle Pill)		Standard formula to treat deficiency and cold of the middle *jiao*
Fu Zi Li Zhong Wan (Prepared Aconite Pill to Regulate the Middle)	Warm the middle *jiao*, dispel cold, tonify qi	Stronger effect to tonify yang and dispel cold
Gui Zhi Ren Shen Tang (Cinnamon Twig and Ginseng Decoction)		Releases wind-cold from the exterior
Wu Zhu Yu Tang (Evodia Decoction)	Warms and tonifies the middle *jiao*, corrects the reversed flow of qi	Directs yin and cold downward
Xiao Jian Zhong Tang (Minor Construct the Middle Decoction)		Harmonizes the interior and relieves pain
Huang Qi Jian Zhong Tang (Astragalus Decoction to Construct the Middle)	Tonify and warm the middle *jiao*, dispel cold, relieve pain	Harmonizes the interior and relieves pain, tonifies qi
Gui Qi Jian Zhong Tang (Tangkuei and Astragalus Decoction to Construct the Middle)		Harmonizes the interior and relieves pain, tonifies qi and blood
Da Jian Zhong Tang (Major Construct the Middle Decoction)		Corrects the reversed flow of qi, strongly dispels cold and relieves pain
An Zhong San (Calm the Middle Powder)	Warms the Spleen and Stomach, dispels cold	Harmonizes the middle *jiao*, regulates qi and blood circulation

Li Zhong Wan (Regulate the Middle Pill), **Fu Zi Li Zhong Wan** (Prepared Aconite Pill to Regulate the Middle), and **Gui Zhi Ren Shen Tang** (Cinnamon Twig and Ginseng Decoction) are three formulas that warm the middle *jiao*, dispel cold, tonify qi, and strengthen the Spleen. They all treat deficiency and cold in the middle *jiao*.

- *Li Zhong Wan* is mainly used for digestive dysfunctions caused by deficiency and cold of the middle *jiao*, leading to symptoms of diarrhea, vomiting, abdominal pain, poor appetite, and no desire to drink. Other applications include bleeding due to yang deficiency, chronic infantile convulsions with drooling, and *xiong bi* (painful obstruction of the chest) due to deficiency and cold of the middle *jiao*.
- *Fu Zi Li Zhong Wan* contains *Fu Zi* (Radix Aconiti Lateralis Praeparata), and is a hotter and more acrid formula that warms and strengthens Spleen and Kidney yang. This formula is best for cold and pain in the chest and abdomen, extreme coldness of the limbs and extremities, and muscle spasms and cramps.
- *Gui Zhi Ren Shen Tang* contains *Gui Zhi* (Ramulus Cinnamomi), and has the added function to release exterior wind-cold. This formula is usually reserved for conditions characterized by deficiency and cold in the interior complicated by wind-cold at the exterior.

Wu Zhu Yu Tang (Evodia Decoction) warms and tonifies the middle *jiao*, corrects the reversed flow of qi, and stops vomiting. It mainly treats vomiting in the *yangming*, *shaoyin*, and *jueyin* levels. The focus is on deficiency and cold of the Stomach, accompanied by rising of yin and cold upward. Other clinical manifestations include fullness of the chest and gastralgia, *jueyin* headache, acid regurgitation, diarrhea, cold limbs, and irritability.

Chapter 7 — Summary

There are four "*jian zhong* (construct the middle)" formulas that warm and tonify the middle *jiao* to dispel cold and relieve pain.

• **Xiao Jian Zhong Tang** (Minor Construct the Middle Decoction) harmonizes and warms the middle *jiao* to relieve pain. The emphasis of this formula is on tonifying middle *jiao* yang deficiency.

• **Huang Qi Jian Zhong Tang** (Astragalus Decoction to Construct the Middle) has the addition of *Huang Qi* (Radix Astragali), which tonifies qi. This formula is more suitable for yang deficiency of the middle *jiao* complicated by qi deficiency.

• **Gui Qi Jian Zhong Tang** (Tangkuei and Astragalus Decoction to Construct the Middle) has the addition of both *Dang Gui* (Radix Angelicae Sinensis) and *Huang Qi* (Radix Astragali) to tonify the blood and qi. This is a good formula for treating chronic abscesses and ulcerations with underlying qi, blood, and yang deficiencies.

• **Da Jian Zhong Tang** (Major Construct the Middle Decoction) relieves pain, corrects the reversed flow of qi, dispels cold, and warms the middle *jiao*. The emphasis of this formula is on reducing the proliferation of yin and cold and tonifying yang deficiency of the middle *jiao*.

Xiao Jian Zhong Tang (Minor Construct the Middle Decoction) and **Da Jian Zhong Tang** (Major Construct the Middle Decoction) both tonify and warm the middle *jiao* to dispel cold and relieve pain.

• *Xiao Jian Zhong Tang* emphasizes tonifying yang, qi, and blood and warming the middle *jiao*.

• *Da Jian Zhong Tang* focuses mostly on dispelling cold and relieving pain.

An Zhong San (Calm the Middle Powder) strengthens and warms the Spleen and Stomach to disperse cold, and harmonizes the middle *jiao* to stop nausea and relieve pain. It is used primarily to treat deficiency and cold of the Spleen and Stomach accompanied by qi and blood stagnation.

SECTION 2: YANG-RESUSCITATING FORMULAS

Name	Similarities	Differences
Si Ni Tang (Frigid Extremities Decoction)		Restores depleted yang
Hui Yang Jiu Ji Tang (Restore and Revive the Yang Decoction)	Rescue yang from collapse	Strengthens qi, generates pulse
Hei Xi Dan (Lead Special Pill)		Controls floating yang, grasps qi downward

Si Ni Tang (Frigid Extremities Decoction) restores depleted yang and rescue from counterflow cold. This is the main formula to rescue and restore yang in the *shaoyin* stage. This Kidney yang depletion manifests in cold extremities, chills, preference to curl up when lying down, lassitude, drowsiness, vomiting, no thirst, abdominal pain, diarrhea, and a faint, fine pulse.

Hui Yang Jiu Ji Tang (Restore and Revive the Yang Decoction) is used in emergency situations when the yang is so depleted that there is danger of it separating from the yin at any time. This formula has the actions to rescue yang from collapse and strengthen qi to restore vitality. Because of the extreme yang deficiency with cold factor in *taiyin*, *shaoyin*, and *jueyin* stages, clinical manifestations will include severe chills, preference to curl up when lying down, icy extremities, vomiting, diarrhea, abdominal pain, lack of energy with constant desire to sleep, shivering, purplish lips or nails, a pale tongue, and a deep, fine pulse.

Hei Xi Dan (Lead Special Pill) treats severe cases of excess condition in the upper body (phlegm obstruction in the Lung) and deficient condition in the lower body (Kidney yang deficiency). Clinical manifestations include wheezing, dyspnea, extremely cold extremities, continuous perspiration with cold sweats, a pale tongue with a thin, white coating, and a deep, faint pulse.

Chapter 7 – Interior-Warming Formulas

Chapter 7 — Summary

SECTION 3: CHANNEL-WARMING AND COLD-DISPERSING FORMULAS

Name	Similarities	Differences
Dang Gui Si Ni Tang (Tangkuei Decoction for Frigid Extremities)	Warm the channels and collaterals, disperse cold	Stronger effect to nourish the blood
Huang Qi Gui Zhi Wu Wu Tang (Astragalus and Cinnamon Twig Five-Substance Decoction)		Better function to tonify qi

Dang Gui Si Ni Tang warms the channels and collaterals, disperses cold, and nourishes the blood. It is used for invasion of cold with deficiencies of blood and yang qi.

Huang Qi Gui Zhi Wu Wu Tang tonifies qi and warms the channels and collaterals. It treats *xue bi* (blood painful obstruction) due to exterior wind invading and blocking qi and blood circulation.

Chapter 8

— Tonic Formulas

补
益
剂

钱乙 Qīan Yǐ

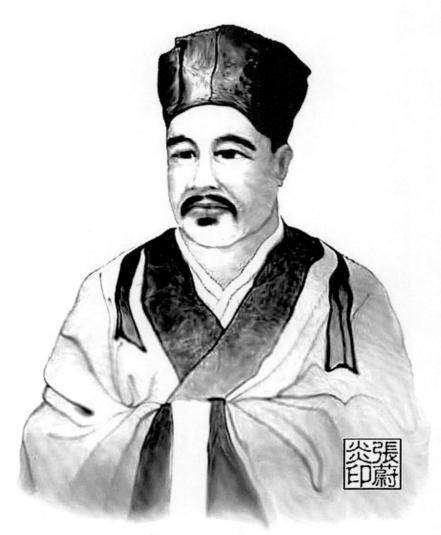

钱乙 Qīan Yǐ, 1032 – 1113.[1]

钱乙 Qián Yǐ

Qian Yi became an orphan at the age of three: his father left home and his mother passed away. Qian was adopted by his aunt, and studied medicine with his uncle. Qian treated his aunt and uncle as his real parents, even after he was told of his true family background.

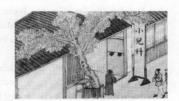

Painting of a pediatric clinic from the Song dynasty.

Qian studied and specialized in pediatrics for over 40 years. At one point, he successfully treated several children of the Imperial family, and was granted the position of 太医 the Supreme Physician. When he retired from the Imperial Palace and returned home, he began to compile his clinical experience. However, because he had *bi zheng* (painful obstruction syndrome) in his hands and could not write, his works were primarily organized by his apprentices. Finally in 1119, six years after his death, 小儿药症直决 *Xiao Er Yao Zheng Zhi Jue* (Craft of Medicinal Treatment for Childhood Disease Patterns) was published. This is considered to be the first and most authoritative text dedicated to pediatrics. In this text, Qian highlighted the importance of using "gentle and moistening" approaches to treat pediatric disorders, and opposed the use of potent herbs for drastic approaches such as attacking, purging, and even tonifying. Furthermore, he strongly emphasized the need to always balance the treatment with tonifying and sedating herbs simultaneously. This principle is reflected in one of his formulas that is among the most commonly used formulas today, *Liu Wei Di Huang Wan* (Six-Ingredient Pill with Rehmannia).[2]

Qian Yi is remembered as 儿科之圣 the Sage of Pediatrics.

Excellent formulas written by Qian Yi include:
- *Sheng Ma Ge Gen Tang* (Cimicifuga and Kudzu Decoction)
- *Xie Bai San* (Drain the White Powder)
- *Long Dan Xie Gan Tang* (Gentiana Decoction to Drain the Liver)
- *Dao Chi San* (Guide Out the Red Powder)
- *Xie Huang San* (Drain the Yellow Powder)
- *Liu Wei Di Huang Wan* (Six-Ingredient Pill with Rehmannia)
- *Bu Fei E Jiao Tang* (Tonify the Lung Decoction with Ass-Hide Gelatin)

1. Approximate year of birth.
2. The most famous herbal formula by Qian Yi, *Liu Wei Di Huang Wan* (Six-Ingredient Pill with Rehmannia), is also the one that gave him most trouble. When he first prescribed *Liu Wei Di Huang Wan* (Six-Ingredient Pill with Rehmannia), he was ridiculed by his colleagues for deviating from the gold standards established by Zhang Zhong-Jing and his original formulation – *Jin Gui Shen Qi Wan* (Kidney Qi Pill from the Golden Cabinet). Finally when questioned, he explained that "*Jin Gui Shen Qi Wan* is for adults. Children have abundant yang qi, and if given hot herbs such as *Gui Zhi* (Ramulus Cinnamomi) and *Fu Zi* (Radix Aconiti Lateralis Praeparata), may suffer from heat and nosebleeds." This explanation silenced his critics, as it showed that not only did Qian Yi understand Zhang Zhong-Jing's teaching, he was knowledgeable and flexible enough to improve upon it. Today, *Liu Wei Di Huang Wan* (Six-Ingredient Pill with Rehmannia) is frequently used for both pediatric and geriatric patients.

Dynasties & Kingdoms	Year
Xia Dynasty 夏	2100-1600 BCE
Shang Dynasty 商	1600-1100 BCE
Zhou Dynasty 周	1100-221 BCE
Qin Dynasty 秦	221-207 BCE
Han Dynasty 漢	206 BCE-220
Three Kingdoms 三國	220-280
Western Jin Dynasty 西晉	265-316
Eastern Jin Dynasty 東晉	317-420
Northern and Southern Dynasties 北南朝	420-581
Sui Dynasty 隋	581-618
Tang Dynasty 唐	618-907
Five Dynasties 五代	907-960
Song Dynasty 宋	960-1279
Liao Dynasty 潦	**916-1125**
Jin Dynasty 金	1115-1234
Yuan Dynasty 元	1271-1368
Ming Dynasty 明	1368-1644
Qing Dynasty 清	1644-1911
Republic of China 中華民國	1912-Present Day
People's Republic of China 中華人民共和國	1949-Present Day

Chapter 8 – Tonic Formulas

Table of Contents

Chapter 8. Tonic Formulas · 507
Biography of Qian Yi · 508

Section 1. Qi-Tonifying Formulas · 522
Si Jun Zi Tang (Four-Gentlemen Decoction) · 522
  Yi Gong San (Extraordinary Merit Powder) · 525
  Bao Yuan Tang (Preserve the Basal Decoction) · 525
Liu Jun Zi Tang (Six-Gentlemen Decoction) · 527
Xiang Sha Liu Jun Zi Tang (Six-Gentlemen Decoction with Aucklandia and Amomum) · 531
  Xiang Sha Liu Jun Zi Tang (Six-Gentlemen Decoction with Cyperus and Amomum) · 533
Xiang Sha Yang Wei Tang (Nourish the Stomach Decoction with Aucklandia and Amomum) · 534
Shen Ling Bai Zhu San (Ginseng, Poria, and Atractylodes Macrocephala Powder) · 535
  Qi Wei Bai Zhu San (Seven-Ingredient Powder with Atractylodes Macrocephala) · 539
  Shen Ling San (Ginseng and Poria Powder) · 539
Qi Pi Wan (Guide the Spleen Pill) · 540
Bu Zhong Yi Qi Tang (Tonify the Middle and Augment the Qi Decoction) · 542
  Ju Yuan Jian (Lift the Source Decoction) · 548
  Sheng Xian Tang (Raise the Sinking Decoction) · 549
Yi Qi Cong Ming Tang (Augment the Qi and Increase Acuity Decoction) · 551
Sheng Mai San (Generate the Pulse Powder) · 554
Ren Shen Ge Jie San (Ginseng and Gecko Powder) · 557
  Ren Shen Hu Tao Tang (Ginseng and Walnut Decoction) · 559
  Ren Shen Chong Cao Tang (Ginseng and Cordyceps Decoction) · 559
Bu Fei Tang (Tonify the Lung Decoction) · 560

Section 2. Blood-Tonifying Formulas · 562
Si Wu Tang (Four-Substance Decoction) · 562
  Sheng Yu Tang (Sage-Like Healing Decoction) · 567
  Sheng Yu Tang (Sage-Like Healing Decoction) · 567
  Jia Wei Si Wu Tang (Augmented Four-Substance Decoction) · 568
  Zhuang Jin Tang (Strengthen the Tendon Decoction) · 568
  Tiao Jing Yi Hao (Regulate Menses Formula One) · 568
  Tiao Jing Er Hao (Regulate Menses Formula Two) · 568
  Tiao Jing San Hao (Regulate Menses Formula Three) · 569
  Tiao Jing Si Hao (Regulate Menses Formula Four) · 569
Tao Hong Si Wu Tang (Four-Substance Decoction with Safflower and Peach Pit) · 571
Wen Qing Yin (Warming and Clearing Decoction) · 575
  Wen Qing Yin (Warming and Clearing Decoction) · 577
  Wen Qing Yin (Warming and Clearing Decoction) · 577
Guo Qi Yin (Delayed Menstruation Decoction) · 578
Dang Gui Bu Xue Tang (Tangkuei Decoction to Tonify the Blood) · 580
Gui Pi Tang (Restore the Spleen Decoction) · 583
  Gui Pi An Shen Tang (Restore the Spleen and Tranquilize the Spirit Decoction) · 587
Zhi Gan Cao Tang (Honey-Fried Licorice Decoction) · 589
  Jia Jian Fu Mai Tang (Modified Restore the Pulse Decoction) · 591
Nu Ke Bai Zi Ren Wan (Platycladus Seed Pill for Females) · 592
Dang Gui Shao Yao San (Tangkuei and Peony Powder) · 594
  Ren Shen Dang Shao San (Ginseng, Tangkuei, and Peony Powder) · 598
Shao Yao Gan Cao Tang (Peony and Licorice Decoction) · 599
  Jia Wei Shao Yao Gan Cao Tang (Augmented Peony and Licorice Decoction) · 603

Section 3. Qi- and Blood-Tonifying Formulas · 604
Ba Zhen Tang (Eight-Treasure Decoction) · 604
Shi Quan Da Bu Tang (All-Inclusive Great Tonifying Decoction) · 609
  Da Bu Tang (Great Tonifying Decoction) · 613
  Ren Shen Da Bu Tang (Ginseng Great Tonifying Decoction) · 613

Chinese Herbal Formulas and Applications

Table of Contents

Ren Shen Yang Ying Tang (Ginseng Decoction to Nourish the Nutritive Qi) ············· 615

Tai Shan Pan Shi San (Powder that Gives the Stability of Mount Tai) ················ 618

Bao Chan Wu You Fang (Preserve Pregnancy and Care-Free Decoction) ·············· 621

Dang Gui San (Tangkuei Powder) ·························· 623

Xiong Gui Tiao Xue Yin (Cnidium and Tangkuei Decoction to Regulate Blood) ········· 624

Section 4. Yin-Tonifying Formulas · 627

Liu Wei Di Huang Wan (Six-Ingredient Pill with Rehmannia) ················· 627

  Er Long Zuo Ci Wan (Pill for Deafness that Is Kind to the Left [Kidney]) ·········· 633

  Ming Mu Di Huang Wan (Improve Vision Pill with Rehmannia) ·············· 633

  Ming Mu Di Huang Wan (Improve Vision Pill with Rehmannia) ·············· 633

Zhi Bai Di Huang Wan (Anemarrhena, Phellodendron, and Rehmannia Pill) ········· 636

  Shi Wei Di Huang Wan (Ten-Ingredient Pill with Rehmannia) ·············· 639

Qi Ju Di Huang Wan (Lycium Fruit, Chrysanthemum, and Rehmannia Pill) ········· 640

Mai Wei Di Huang Wan (Ophiopogonis, Schisandra, and Rehmannia Pill) ·········· 642

Du Qi Wan (Capital Qi Pill) ···························· 644

Zuo Gui Wan (Restore the Left [Kidney] Pill) ····················· 645

  Zuo Gui Yin (Restore the Left [Kidney] Decoction) ·················· 647

  Jia Wei Zuo Gui Wan (Augmented Restore the Left [Kidney] Pill) ············ 647

Da Bu Yin Wan (Great Tonify the Yin Pill) ······················ 649

Hu Qian Wan (Hidden Tiger Pill) ·························· 651

  Hu Qian Wan (Hidden Tiger Pill) ························· 653

Er Zhi Wan (Two-Ultimate Pill) ··························· 654

  Sang Ma Wan (Mulberry Leaf and Sesame Seed Pill) ················· 656

Yi Guan Jian (Linking Decoction) ·························· 657

Shi Hu Ye Guang Wan (Dendrobium Pill for Night Vision) ················ 661

Zi Yin Di Huang Wan (Rehmannia Pill to Nourish Yin) ················· 663

Zi Shen Ming Mu Tang (Nourish the Kidney to Brighten the Eyes Decoction) ········ 664

Zi Shen Tong Er Tang (Nourish the Kidney to Unblock the Ears Decoction) ········· 666

Section 5. Yang-Tonifying Formulas · 668

Jin Gui Shen Qi Wan (Kidney Qi Pill from the Golden Cabinet) ·············· 668

  Shi Bu Wan (Ten-Tonic Pill) ··························· 671

Ba Wei Di Huang Wan (Eight-Ingredient Pill with Rehmannia) ·············· 672

Ji Sheng Shen Qi Wan (Kidney Qi Pill from Formulas that Aid the Living) ········· 675

You Gui Wan (Restore the Right [Kidney] Pill) ···················· 678

  You Gui Yin (Restore the Right [Kidney] Decoction) ················· 680

  Jia Wei You Gui Wan (Augmented Restore the Right [Kidney] Pill) ··········· 680

Huan Shao Dan (Return to Youth Pill) ························ 681

  Huan Shao Di Huang Wan (Rehmannia Pill to Return to Youth) ············ 683

  Bu Shen Tang (Tonify the Kidney Decoction) ···················· 683

Er Xian Tang (Two-Immortal Decoction) ······················ 684

  Er Xian Bu Shen Tang (Two-Immortal Decoction to Tonify the Kidney) ········· 686

Section 6. Yin- and Yang-Tonifying Formulas · 687

Gui Lu Er Xian Jiao (Tortoise Shell and Deer Antler Syrup) ··············· 687

  Bu Shen Wan (Tonify the Kidney Pill) ······················ 689

  Bu Gu Wan (Tonify the Bone Pill) ························ 689

Qi Bao Mei Ran Dan (Seven-Treasure Special Pill for Beautiful Whiskers) ········· 690

  Shou Wu Pian (Polygonum Pill) ························· 692

Di Huang Yin Zi (Rehmannia Decoction) ······················ 693

Tonic Formulas (Summary) · 696

TONIC FORMULAS

8

511

Chapter 8 – Tonic Formulas

Chapter 8 — Overview

— Tonic Formulas

Definition: Tonic formulas supplement qi, blood, yin, yang, *jing* (essence) and body fluids to treat various patterns of deficiency syndromes and damage to *zang fu* organs. This method of treatment is known as *bu fa* (tonifying), one of the *ba fa* (eight treatment methods) described in the *Huang Di Nei Jing* (Yellow Emperor's Inner Classic) in the first or second century, A.D.

~

Tonic formulas supplement qi, blood, yin, yang, *jing* and body fluids to treat deficiencies of prenatal or postnatal origin.

~

The term "deficiency syndromes" refers primarily to insufficiencies of qi, blood, yin, yang, *jing* (essence) and body fluids. Although there are many causes of deficiency, the causes can all be categorized as either of prenatal (genetic or gestational) or postnatal (inappropriate diet, overwork, emotional disturbances, or chronic illness) origin. Regardless of prenatal insufficiency or postnatal imbalance, these disorders are characterized by deficiencies of qi, blood, yin, yang, *jing* and body fluids in one or more of the five *zang* (solid organs).

In simple cases, herbs can be prescribed to directly treat the deficiency, such as qi-tonifying herbs to treat qi deficiency, and blood-tonifying herbs to treat blood deficiency. However, because qi, blood, yin and yang are mutually dependent, and the *zang* (solid) and *fu* (hollow) organs are closely connected to each other, deficiency syndromes usually do not occur independently. Rather, deficiency of one often affects the other, leading to deficiencies of multiple substances that affect more than one organ. Therefore, it is common to tonify qi and blood concurrently, or to supplement yin and yang simultaneously.

Besides directly tonifying the substance that is in deficiency, one could incorporate other supplemental strategies to enhance the overall tonifying effect. Examples are as follows:

- The Spleen and Stomach are both responsible for transformation and transportation of food and herbs. In chronic deficiency syndromes, these organs become deficient, which leads to compromised ability to digest and absorb the herbs. In such cases, it is beneficial to tonify the Spleen and Stomach to enhance the absorption of the entire formula, and maximize the overall therapeutic effect.

- In Five-Element theory, one treats deficiency syndromes by tonifying the "mother" organ to strengthen the "son" organ. For example, in the case of Liver deficiency, one can tonify the Kidney (water element, mother organ) to indirectly tonify the Liver (wood element, son organ). In the case of Lung deficiency, one can tonify the Spleen (earth element, mother organ) to indirectly tonify the Lung (metal element, son organ).

- Lastly, one theory posits the importance of tonifying the Kidney and Spleen to treat deficiency syndromes. The basis for this theory is that since Kidney *jing* (essence) is the source of prenatal health, and Spleen qi is the source of postnatal health, tonification of these organs will support the normal health and functioning of all the other organs.

~

Historically, qi and blood tonifying formulas have been used to treat pregnancy-related disorders.

~

SUBCATEGORIES OF ACTION

Tonic formulas are divided into six subcategories based on function:

1. Qi-Tonifying Formulas
These formulas primarily treat Spleen and Lung qi deficiencies. Common clinical manifestations of qi deficiency include lassitude, general weakness, weak extremities, shortness of breath, hurried respiration with mild physical exertion, a low voice, a pale

512

Chinese Herbal Formulas and Applications

Chapter 8 — Overview

face, loose stools, diarrhea, lack of appetite, spontaneous sweating, a pale tongue, and a weak or deficient, big pulse. In severe cases, there may be prolapse of organs such as the stomach, uterus, or rectum.

Qi-tonifying herbs, such as *Ren Shen* (Radix et Rhizoma Ginseng), *Dang Shen* (Radix Codonopsis), *Huang Qi* (Radix Astragali), *Bai Zhu* (Rhizoma Atractylodis Macrocephalae), and *Gan Cao* (Radix et Rhizoma Glycyrrhizae) are of primary importance in these formulas. Representative formulas include *Si Jun Zi Tang* (Four-Gentlemen Decoction), *Shen Ling Bai Zhu San* (Ginseng, Poria, and Atractylodes Macrocephala Powder), *Bu Zhong Yi Qi Tang* (Tonify the Middle and Augment the Qi Decoction), and *Sheng Mai San* (Generate the Pulse Powder).

2. Blood-Tonifying Formulas

These formulas contain blood-tonifying herbs to treat blood deficiency syndromes, which often affect the Heart and Liver. Common clinical manifestations of blood deficiency include dizziness, blurred vision, a pale face with sallow complexion, pale lips, dry and dull nails, palpitations, insomnia, dry stools, a pale and slightly red tongue with a slippery and/or dry tongue coating, and a pulse that is either fine and rapid or fine and rough. Women with blood deficiency may experience delayed menstruation, with pale, scanty menstrual discharge.

Herbs commonly used to tonify the blood include *Shu Di Huang* (Radix Rehmanniae Praeparata), *Dang Gui* (Radix Angelicae Sinensis), *Bai Shao* (Radix Paeoniae Alba), and *E Jiao* (Colla Corii Asini). Representative formulas include *Si Wu Tang* (Four-Substance Decoction), *Gui Pi Tang* (Restore the Spleen Decoction), and *Dang Gui Bu Xue Tang* (Tangkuei Decoction to Tonify the Blood).

> Because qi, blood, yin and yang are mutually dependent, and the *zang fu* closely connected, deficiencies usually do not occur independently: deficiency of one often affects another.

3. Qi- and Blood-Tonifying Formulas

These formulas use qi- and blood-tonifying herbs to treat qi and blood deficiencies simultaneously. Clinical manifestations of qi and blood deficiencies include dizziness, vertigo, palpitations, shortness of breath, poor appetite, fatigue, weak extremities, a pale face, a pale tongue with a thin, white tongue coating, and a deficient, fine pulse.

Qi- and blood-tonifying formulas incorporate both qi-tonifying herbs such as *Ren Shen* (Radix et Rhizoma Ginseng), *Huang Qi* (Radix Astragali), and *Bai Zhu* (Rhizoma Atractylodis Macrocephalae), and blood-tonifying herbs such as *Shu Di Huang* (Radix Rehmanniae Praeparata), *Dang Gui* (Radix Angelicae Sinensis), and *Bai Shao* (Radix Paeoniae Alba). Representative formulas include *Ba Zhen Tang* (Eight-Treasure Decoction), *Shi Quan Da Bu Tang* (All-Inclusive Great Tonifying Decoction), and *Ren Shen Yang Ying Tang* (Ginseng Decoction to Nourish the Nutritive Qi).

4. Yin-Tonifying Formulas

These formulas treat yin deficiency syndromes with yin-tonifying herbs. Yin deficiency is often associated with the Liver and Kidney, and involves common clinical manifestations such as emaciated appearance of the face and body, a dry throat and mouth, *wu xin re* (five-center heat), insomnia, dry stools, scanty and yellow urine, steaming bones sensation, night sweats, dry cough with no sputum, tidal fever, red cheeks, seminal emissions, soreness of the back and waist, a red tongue with a scanty and dry tongue coating, and a deep, fine and rapid pulse.

Herbs commonly used to treat yin deficiency include *Shu Di Huang* (Radix Rehmanniae Praeparata), *Mai Dong* (Radix Ophiopogonis), and *Tian Dong* (Radix Asparagi). Representative formulas include *Liu Wei Di Huang Wan* (Six-Ingredient Pill with Rehmannia), *Zuo Gui Wan* (Restore the Left [Kidney] Pill), *Da Bu Yin Wan* (Great Tonify the Yin Pill), and *Bu Fei E Jiao Tang* (Tonify the Lung Decoction with Ass-Hide Gelatin).

5. Yang-Tonifying Formulas

These formulas use yang-tonifying herbs to treat Kidney yang deficiency. Common clinical manifestations of Kidney yang deficiency include soreness and pain of the lower back and knees, weakness

TONIC FORMULAS

8

513

Chapter 8 – Tonic Formulas

Chapter 8 — Overview

and soreness of the extremities, a feeling of coldness and pain in the lower extremities, scanty or frequent urination, impotence or premature ejaculation in men, infertility in women, and a deep, fine or deep, hidden pulse at the *chi* position.

Herbs that are commonly used to tonify yang include *Fu Zi* (Radix Aconiti Lateralis Praeparata), *Rou Gui* (Cortex Cinnamomi), *Du Zhong* (Cortex Eucommiae), *Ba Ji Tian* (Radix Morindae Officinalis), and *Bu Gu Zhi* (Fructus Psoraleae). Representative formulas include *Jin Gui Shen Qi Wan* (Kidney Qi Pill from the Golden Cabinet) and *You Gui Wan* (Restore the Right [Kidney] Pill).

6. Yin- and Yang-Tonifying Formulas

These formulas treat concurrent yin and yang deficiencies. Clinical signs and symptoms include dizziness, vertigo, soreness and weakness of the lower back and knees, impotence, seminal emissions, aversion to cold, cold extremities, spontaneous or night sweats, and tidal fever.

Herbs that tonify yin include *Shu Di Huang* (Radix Rehmanniae Praeparata), *Mai Dong* (Radix Ophiopogonis), *Tian Dong* (Radix Asparagi), *Gui Ban* (Plastrum Testudinis), and *Zhi Mu* (Rhizoma Anemarrhenae). Herbs commonly used to tonify yang include *Fu Zi* (Radix Aconiti Lateralis Praeparata), *Rou Gui* (Cortex Cinnamomi), *Du Zhong* (Cortex Eucommiae), *Ba Ji Tian* (Radix Morindae Officinalis), and *Bu Gu Zhi* (Fructus Psoraleae). Representative formulas that tonify both yin and yang include *Di Huang Yin Zi* (Rehmannia Decoction) and *Gui Lu Er Xian Jiao* (Tortoise Shell and Deer Antler Syrup).

CAUTIONS / CONTRAINDICATIONS

- It is important to differentiate between deficient and excess conditions when considering the use of tonic herbs. While tonic herbs are prescribed to supplement deficiencies, clearing or draining herbs are used to eliminate excess conditions. Tonic herbs should *not* be used in excess conditions, as they will only worsen the condition. Clearing or draining herbs must *not* be used in cases of deficiency, as they will aggravate the condition by draining vital substances.

> **Most tonic formulas are cooked longer, at low temperatures, for complete extraction of ingredients.**

- Frequent or long-term use of tonic herbs may create stagnation. Therefore, tonic herbs should be combined with herbs that strengthen the Spleen, harmonize the Stomach, and move qi, and blood to ensure minimal side effects.
- Tonic formulas are most effective when taken on an empty stomach, or before meals, for better absorption.

PROCESSING

Most tonic herbs and formulas are cooked for a longer period of time than other types of herbs, at low temperatures, to ensure complete extraction of the active ingredients.

PHARMACOLOGICAL EFFECTS & CLINICAL APPLICATIONS

Tonic formulas are divided into six subcategories based on their traditional therapeutic actions. These six subcategories have contrasting pharmacological effects and clinical applications.

1. **Qi-tonifying formulas** mainly treat Spleen and Lung qi deficiencies. Although they are certainly effective, there is little clinical research on general symptoms of qi deficiency such as lassitude, general weakness, and weak extremities. Instead, most of the research focuses on treatment of specific biomedical disorders affecting the gastrointestinal system, such as gastritis, peptic ulcer, colitis, and irritable bowel syndrome.

   Many of these formulas are now used in cancer treatment, since they have demonstrated remarkable effects in alleviating the side effects associated with chemotherapy and radiation. Some formulas have antineoplastic effects based on performance during *in vitro* and *in vivo* studies.

   - **Gastrointestinal disorders**: Qi-tonifying formulas treat a wide variety of gastrointestinal disorders. Pharmacologically, they exert significant influence on the stomach and intestines, including but not limited to gastroprotective,[1] antiulcer,[2] a prokinetic action on gastric emptying,[3] and a regulatory effect on the intestines to either increase or decrease peristalsis.[4,5,6,7,8] Clinically, *Si Jun Zi*

514

Chinese Herbal Formulas and Applications

Chapter 8 — Overview

Tang (Four-Gentlemen Decoction) has been used to treat chronic gastritis,[9] peptic ulcer,[10,11] ulcerative colitis,[12] irritable bowel syndrome,[13] and epigastric or abdominal pain.[14] *Liu Jun Zi Tang* (Six-Gentlemen Decoction) has been used to treat abdominal pain,[15] gastritis,[16] duodenal ulcer,[17] indigestion,[18] and stomatitis.[19] *Shen Ling Bai Zhu San* (Ginseng, Poria, and Atractylodes Macrocephala Powder) has been used to address chronic colitis,[20] irritable bowel syndrome,[21] diarrhea,[22] and superficial gastritis.[23] Lastly, *Bu Zhong Yi Qi Tang* (Tonify the Middle and Augment the Qi Decoction) treats gastritis,[24] constipation,[25] and diarrhea.[26]

- **Morning sickness**: Three qi-tonifying formulas have been shown to treat nausea and vomiting. *Liu Jun Zi Tang* (Six-Gentlemen Decoction) is effective for morning sickness.[27] *Xiang Sha Liu Jun Zi Tang* (Six-Gentlemen Decoction with Aucklandia and Amomum) successfully treats morning sickness and anorexia.[28,29] *Bu Zhong Yi Qi Tang* (Tonify the Middle and Augment the Qi Decoction) relieves nausea and vomiting.[30]

> ~
> **Many tonic formulas alleviate side effects of chemotherapy and radiation. Others are antineoplastic.**
> ~

- **Chronic fatigue syndrome**: *Bu Zhong Yi Qi Tang* (Tonify the Middle and Augment the Qi Decoction) has been used successfully to treat chronic fatigue syndrome.[31]

- **Supportive treatment for chemoprotective and radioprotective effect**: Many qi-tonifying formulas demonstrate beneficial effects to alleviate the side effects associated with chemotherapy and radiation. For example, *Si Jun Zi Tang* (Four-Gentlemen Decoction) has a hematopoietic effect to increase both white and red blood cell counts in subjects treated with radiation.[32,33] *Liu Jun Zi Tang* (Six-Gentlemen Decoction) has shown *in vitro* antineoplastic effect by inhibiting the growth of cancer cells in mice.[34] *Shen Ling Bai Zhu San* (Ginseng, Poria, and Atractylodes Macrocephala Powder) has been used successfully to relieve nausea and vomiting associated with chemotherapy and radiation.[35,36] Lastly, *Bu Zhong Yi Qi Tang* (Tonify the Middle and Augment the Qi Decoction) treats immunosuppression induced by mitomycin C, and leukopenia induced by cyclophosphamide.[37,38]

- **Cancer**: Most qi-tonifying formulas are used as supportive therapy during chemotherapy and radiation, as discussed above. However, some formulas also have direct antineoplastic effects. *Si Jun Zi Tang* (Four-Gentlemen Decoction) has been shown to inhibit the growth of tumor cells in mice with esophageal and lung cancer.[39] *Liu Jun Zi Tang* (Six-Gentlemen Decoction) has been shown to inhibit the growth of cancer cells in mice by increasing macrophages and natural killer cells.[40] Lastly, *Bu Zhong Yi Qi Tang* (Tonify the Middle and Augment the Qi Decoction) exerts antineoplastic effects by enhancing natural killer cell activity, and suppressing the proliferation of certain cancer cells.[41,42]

2. **Blood-tonifying formulas** commonly treat a wide variety of disorders, including hematological, gynecological, obstetric, and dermatological disorders.

- **Hematological disorders**: As the name implies, blood-tonifying formulas treat blood-related disorders, such as anemia,[43,44] leucopenia,[45,46] and thrombopenic purpura.[47,48] The mechanism of these effects is attributed primarily to hematopoietic effects that increase blood cell production.[49,50] Formulas commonly used to treat hematological disorders include *Gui Pi Tang* (Restore the Spleen Decoction) and *Dang Gui Bu Xue Tang* (Tangkuei Decoction to Tonify the Blood).

- **Menstrual disorders**: Blood-tonifying formulas are very effective in treating a wide variety of menstrual disorders. *Si Wu Tang* (Four-Substance Decoction) has been shown to treat menstrual pain,[51] irregular menstruation,[52] and *beng lou* (flooding and spotting).[53] *Tao Hong Si Wu Tang* (Four-Substance Decoction with Safflower and Peach Pit) has been shown to treat dysmenorrhea.[54] *Dang Gui Bu Xue Tang* (Tangkuei Decoction to Tonify the Blood) has been used to treat amenorrhea.[55] *Gui Pi Tang* (Restore the Spleen Decoction) has been used to treat uterine bleeding,[56] *beng lou* (flooding and spotting),[57] and menopause.[58] Lastly, *Dang Gui Shao Yao San* (Tangkuei and Peony Powder) has been shown to treat uterine bleeding,[59] menopause,[60] and dysmenorrhea.[61,62] The general mechanisms of action are attributed to the regulatory effects on hormone production. The exact mechanisms, however, vary depending on the formulas and indications.

- **Gynecological disorders**: Blood-tonifying formulas address various gynecological disorders, including but not limited to endometriosis,[63] uterine myoma,[64] adnexitis,[65] pelvic inflammatory

TONIC FORMULAS

8

515

Chapter 8 — Overview

disease,[66,67] and dysmenorrhea in endometriotic and adenomyotic individuals.[68] Representative formulas include *Si Wu Tang* (Four-Substance Decoction) and *Dang Gui Shao Yao San* (Tangkuei and Peony Powder).

- **Obstetrics**: Several blood-tonifying formulas have been used to treat various pregnancy-related disorders and/or complications. For example, breech presentation may be corrected with *Si Wu Tang* (Four-Substance Decoction) and *Dang Gui Shao Yao San* (Tangkuei and Peony Powder).[69,70] Habitual miscarriage may be prevented with a combination of *Dang Gui Shao Yao San* (Tangkuei and Peony Powder) and *Chai Ling Tang* (Bupleurum and Poria Decoction).[71,72]
- **Infertility**: According to clinical studies, blood-tonifying formulas have been used successfully to treat infertility from various causes. Representative formulas include *Si Wu Tang* (Four-Substance Decoction),[73] *Tao Hong Si Wu Tang* (Four-Substance Decoction with Safflower and Peach Pit),[74] and *Dang Gui Shao Yao San* (Tangkuei and Peony Powder).[75]
- **Dermatological disorders**: Many skin disorders have been treated successfully with blood-tonifying formulas. The clinical applications include itching,[76,77] psoriasis,[78,79,80] urticaria,[81,82] eczema, acne,[83] and chloasma.[84] Furthermore, some formulas have also been shown to effectively treat dermatitis induced by cosmetics and penicillin.[85,86] Representative formulas include *Si Wu Tang* (Four-Substance Decoction), *Tao Hong Si Wu Tang* (Four-Substance Decoction with Safflower and Peach Pit), and *Dang Gui Shao Yao San* (Tangkuei and Peony Powder), as they have antipruritic and anti-inflammatory effects to relieve itching and inflammation of the skin.[87,88]
- **Headache**: Many blood-tonifying formulas have been shown to effectively treat various types of headache, such as neurogenic headache,[89] vascular headache,[90] and headache due to trauma.[91,92] Two representative formulas are *Si Wu Tang* (Four-Substance Decoction) and *Tao Hong Si Wu Tang* (Four-Substance Decoction with Safflower and Peach Pit).
- **Others**: Blood-tonifying formulas may also be used for other conditions, such as cardiovascular disease (arrhythmia, angina pectoris, and hypotension),[93,94,95] ophthalmic disorders (optic nerve atrophy, optic neuritis, and cataract),[96,97,98] hepatitis,[99] and many others.

3. **Qi- and blood-tonifying formulas** are composed of herbs that supplement qi and blood. The pharmacological effects of these formulas include those already mentioned above for qi-tonifying and blood-tonifying formulas, such as gastrointestinal disorders, hematological disorders, menstrual disorders, and gynecological disorders. Historically, these formulas have been used to treat pregnancy-related disorders, such as infertility,[100] habitual miscarriage,[101,102] morning sickness,[103] breech presentation,[104] and postpartum care.[105]

   Today, several of these formulas have been shown to have marked chemoprotective and radioprotective effects, and are now commonly used as supportive treatments for patients with cancer.[106,107] These, however, are just some of the many clinical applications of qi- and blood-tonifying formulas. Representative formulas include *Ba Zhen Tang* (Eight-Treasure Decoction), *Shi Quan Da Bu Tang* (All-Inclusive Great Tonifying Decoction), and *Ren Shen Yang Ying Tang* (Ginseng Decoction to Nourish the Nutritive Qi).

4. **Yin-tonifying formulas** tonify yin and generate body fluids; they primarily treat disorders associated with Kidney, Liver, Lung, and Stomach yin deficiencies. These formulas treat an extremely wide range and variety of disorders, and the summary below is only a brief attempt to identify the most common and significant applications.
- **Reproductive disorders**: Many yin-tonifying formulas have marked influence on the reproductive system, and have been used successfully to treat sexual and reproductive disorders, such as sexual dysfunction,[108,109] male infertility,[110,111] and female infertility.[112,113] The mechanisms of action vary, but have been attributed in part to the stimulation and regulation of both male and female sex hormones.[114,115] Exemplar formulas include *Liu Wei Di Huang Wan* (Six-Ingredient Pill with Rehmannia), *Zuo Gui Wan* (Restore the Left [Kidney] Pill), and *Er Xian Tang* (Two-Immortal Decoction).
- **Gynecological disorders**: Many yin-tonifying formulas have marked effects in treating gynecological disorders. For example, menopausal symptoms may be alleviated with *Liu Wei Di Huang Wan*

Chinese Herbal Formulas and Applications

Chapter 8 — Overview

(Six-Ingredient Pill with Rehmannia),[116] *Qi Ju Di Huang Wan* (Lycium Fruit, Chrysanthemum, and Rehmannia Pill),[117] and *Er Xian Tang* (Two-Immortal Decoction).[118] Premenstrual syndrome may be alleviated with *Yi Guan Jian* (Linking Decoction).[119] Uterine bleeding and amenorrhea may be treated with *Zuo Gui Wan* (Restore the Left [Kidney] Pill).[120,121]

- **Respiratory disorders**: Some yin-tonifying formulas have been used effectively to treat lung disorders. For example, *Liu Wei Di Huang Wan* (Six-Ingredient Pill with Rehmannia) has been used for bronchial asthma,[122] *Da Bu Yin Wan* (Great Tonify the Yin Pill) has been used for pulmonary tuberculosis,[123] and *Bu Fei E Jiao Tang* (Tonify the Lung Decoction with Ass-Hide Gelatin) has been used to treat cough due to various causes, such as asthma, bronchiectasis, bronchitis, pulmonary tuberculosis, and whooping cough.[124]

- **Gastrointestinal disorders**: Some yin-tonifying formulas have been used successfully to treat gastrointestinal disorders, such as atrophic gastritis,[125,126] peptic ulcer,[127] and chronic esophagitis.[128] The mechanism of action has been attributed in part to enhanced protection of the gastric mucosa.[129] Exemplar formulas include *Liu Wei Di Huang Wan* (Six-Ingredient Pill with Rehmannia) and *Yi Guan Jian* (Linking Decoction).

- **Diabetes mellitus**: Many yin-tonifying formulas successfully treat diabetes mellitus. Pharmacologically, these formulas effectively decrease plasma glucose levels.[130] Furthermore, some of these formulas continue to exert hypoglycemic effects in cases in which the pancreas has been surgically removed.[131] Clinically, formulas that have been used successfully in the treatment of diabetes mellitus include *Liu Wei Di Huang Wan* (Six-Ingredient Pill with Rehmannia),[132] *Zhi Bai Di Huang Wan* (Anemarrhena, Phellodendron, and Rehmannia Pill),[133] and *Mai Wei Di Huang Wan* (Ophiopogonis, Schisandra, and Rehmannia Pill).[134]

- **Hypertension**: Many yin-tonifying formulas have a marked influence on the cardiovascular system. Specifically, formulas that have been used to treat hypertension include *Liu Wei Di Huang Wan* (Six-Ingredient Pill with Rehmannia),[135] *Zhi Bai Di Huang Wan* (Anemarrhena, Phellodendron, and Rehmannia Pill),[136] *Qi Ju Di Huang Wan* (Lycium Fruit, Chrysanthemum, and Rehmannia Pill),[137,138] and *Yi Guan Jian* (Linking Decoction).[139]

- **Kidney disorders**: Some yin-tonifying formulas have shown nephroprotective effects, such as increasing blood perfusion to the kidneys, improving kidney function, and reducing the presence of protein and uric acid in the urine.[140] Clinically, *Liu Wei Di Huang Wan* (Six-Ingredient Pill with Rehmannia) has been used to treat chronic nephritis,[141] nephrotic syndrome,[142] chronic renal failure,[143] and periodic paralysis.[144] *Zhi Bai Di Huang Wan* (Anemarrhena, Phellodendron, and Rehmannia Pill) has been used to treat nephrotic syndrome.[145] *Qi Ju Di Huang Wan* (Lycium Fruit, Chrysanthemum, and Rehmannia Pill) has been used to treat chronic nephritis.[146]

- **Liver disorders**: Some yin-tonifying formulas have hepatoprotective effects against damage induced by such substances as carbon tetrachloride, thioacetamide, and prednisolone.[147,148,149] Clinically, *Liu Wei Di Huang Wan* (Six-Ingredient Pill with Rehmannia) has been used to treat chronic hepatitis,[150] *Er Zhi Wan* (Two-Ultimate Pill) for hepatitis B,[151] and *Yi Guan Jian* (Linking Decoction) for liver disease such as hepatitis, liver cirrhosis, and liver cancer.[152,153]

- **Thyroid disorders**: *Liu Wei Di Huang Wan* (Six-Ingredient Pill with Rehmannia) has been used successfully to treat hyperthyroidism and thyroid adenoma.[154,155] *Yi Guan Jian* (Linking Decoction) has been used to treat hyperthyroidism.[156]

5. **Yang-tonifying formulas** mainly treat sexual, reproductive, prostate, and kidney disorders.

- **Sexual and reproductive disorders**: Many yang-tonifying formulas have marked effects in treating sexual and reproductive disorders including sexual dysfunction,[157] male infertility,[158,159] and female infertility.[160,161] The pharmacological effects have been attributed in part to the stimulation and regulation of both male and female sex hormones.[162] Exemplar formulas include *Jin Gui Shen Qi Wan* (Kidney Qi Pill from the Golden Cabinet), *Ba Wei Di Huang Wan* (Eight-Ingredient Pill with Rehmannia), *Ji Sheng Shen Qi Wan* (Kidney Qi Pill from Formulas that Aid the Living), and *Zuo Gui Wan* (Restore the Left [Kidney] Pill).

Chapter 8 — Overview

- **Prostate disorders**: Prostatic hypertrophy has been treated successfully with Kidney yang tonic formulas, such as *Jin Gui Shen Qi Wan* (Kidney Qi Pill from the Golden Cabinet) and *Ba Wei Di Huang Wan* (Eight-Ingredient Pill with Rehmannia).[163,164,165]

- **Urinary disorders**: Yang-tonifying formulas are effective in treating urinary disorders (with or without enlarged prostate), such as dysuria,[166] frequent urination,[167] and urinary incontinence.[168] Representative formulas include *Jin Gui Shen Qi Wan* (Kidney Qi Pill from the Golden Cabinet) and *Ba Wei Di Huang Wan* (Eight-Ingredient Pill with Rehmannia).

- **Kidney disorders**: Some yang-tonifying formulas treat kidney disorders. *Jin Gui Shen Qi Wan* (Kidney Qi Pill from the Golden Cabinet) has been used to treat chronic glomerulonephritis.[169] *You Gui Dan* (Restore the Right [Kidney] Pill) and *Ji Sheng Shen Qi Wan* (Kidney Qi Pill from Formulas that Aid the Living) have been used to treat nephrotic syndrome.[170,171]

6. **Yin- and yang-tonifying formulas**, as the name implies, treat concurrent yin and yang deficiencies. Two exemplar formulas, *Gui Lu Er Xian Jiao* (Tortoise Shell and Deer Antler Syrup) and *Qi Bao Mei Ran Dan* (Seven-Treasure Special Pill for Beautiful Whiskers), treat a wide variety of disorders of yin and yang deficiencies, such as impotence,[172] male infertility,[173] and osteoporosis.[174,175]

References

1. Arakawa T, Higuchi K, Fujiwara Y, Watanabe T, Tominaga K, Hayakawa T, Kuroki T. Gastroprotection by Liu-Jun-Zi-Tang (TJ-43): possible mediation of nitric oxide but not prostaglandins or sulfhydryls. Drugs Under Experimental & Clinical Research 1999;25(5):207-10.
2. *Bei Jing Zhong Yi Yao Da Xue Xue Bao* (Journal of Beijing University of Medicine and Medicinals) 1994;17(5):57.
3. Tatsuta M, Iishi H. Effect of treatment with liu-jun-zi-tang (TJ-43) on gastric emptying and gastrointestinal symptoms in dyspeptic patients. Aliment Pharmacol Ther 1993 Aug;7(4):459-62.
4. *Xin Zhong Yi* (New Chinese Medicine) 1978;5:53.
5. *Nan Jing Zhong Yi Xue Yuan Xue Bao* (Journal of Nanjing University of Traditional Chinese Medicine) 1989;1:36.
6. *Zhong Yi Fang Ji Xian Dai Yan Jiu* (Modern Study of Medical Formulae in Traditional Chinese Medicine) 1997;499-500.
7. *Xin Yi Yao Xue Za Zhi* (New Journal of Medicine and Herbology) 1979;3:129.
8. *Zhong Yao Yao Li Yu Lin Chuang* (Pharmacology and Clinical Applications of Chinese Herbs) 1987;2:4.
9. *Zhong Yi Fang Ji Xian Dai Yan Jiu* (Modern Study of Medical Formulae in Traditional Chinese Medicine) 1997;480-81.
10. *Xin Zhong Yi* (New Chinese Medicine) 1982;11:12.
11. *Zhong Yi Za Zhi* (Journal of Chinese Medicine) 1980;21(12):947.
12. *Zhong Yi Za Zhi* (Journal of Chinese Medicine) 1987;10:28.
13. *Shang Hai Zhong Yi Za Zhi* (Shanghai Journal of Chinese Medicine) 1986;1:12.
14. *He Nan Zhong Yi* (Henan Chinese Medicine) 1986;3:1.
15. *Shan Xi Xin Zhong Yi* (New Shanxi Chinese Medicine) 1984;1:23.
16. *Zhong Yi Ming Fang Lin Chuang Xin Yong* (Contemporary Clinical Applications of Classic Chinese Formulas) 2001;160.
17. *Si Chuan Zhong Yi* (Sichuan Chinese Medicine) 1989;2:21.
18. *Zhong Yi Ming Fang Lin Chuang Xin Yong* (Contemporary Clinical Applications of Classic Chinese Formulas) 2001;161.
19. *Shi Yong Zhong Yi Za Zhi* (Journal of Practical Chinese Medicine) 1997;2:11.
20. *Shan Dong Zhong Yi Za Zhi* (Shandong Journal of Chinese Medicine) 1991;10(6):24.
21. *Shan Xi Zhong Yi* (Shanxi Chinese Medicine) 1998;7:312.
22. *Xin Yi Yao Xue Za Zhi* (New Journal of Medicine and Herbology) 1979;3:129.
23. *Zhong Yi Fang Ji Xian Dai Yan Jiu* (Modern Study of Medical Formulae in Traditional Chinese Medicine) 1997;509.
24. *Jiang Su Zhong Yi Za Zhi* (Jiangsu Journal of Chinese Medicine) 1997;11:514.
25. *Zhong Yi Fang Ji Xian Dai Yan Jiu* (Modern Study of Medical Formulae in Traditional Chinese Medicine) 1997;529.
26. *Shi Yong Zhong Xi Yi Jie He Za Zhi* (Practical Journal of Integrated Chinese and Western Medicines) 1998;3:262.
27. *Shang Hai Zhong Yi Yao Za Zhi* (Shanghai Journal of Chinese Medicine and Herbology) 1959;7:48.
28. *Zhong Hua Fu Chan Ke Za Zhi* (Chinese Journal of Obstetrics and Gynecology) 1960;8(1):33.
29. *Gan Su Zhong Yi Xue Yuan Xue Bao* (Journal of Gansu University of Chinese Medicine) 1995;2:26.
30. *He Bei Zhong Yi* (Hebei Chinese Medicine) 1986;6:13.
31. *Guo Wai Yi Xue Zhong Yi Zhong Yao Fen Ce* (Monograph of Chinese Herbology from Foreign Medicine) 1993;15(6):27.
32. *Zhong Yi Fang Ji Xian Dai Yan Jiu* (Modern Study of Medical Formulae in Traditional Chinese Medicine) 1997;477.
33. Hsu HY, Yang JJ, Lian SL, Ho YH, Lin CC. Recovery of the hematopoietic system by Si-Jun-Zi-Tang in whole body irradiated mice. J Ethnopharmacol 1996 Nov;54(2-3):69-75.
34. *Shi Yong Zhong Liu Xue Za Zhi* (Practical Journal of Cancer) 1987;1(4):6.
35. *Zhong Yi Yao Xin Xi* (Information on Chinese Medicine and Herbology) 1995;6:27.
36. *Gui Zhou Yi Yao* (Medicine and Medicinals from Guizhou) 1985;3:7.
37. Kido T, Mori K, Daikuhara H, Tsuchiya H, Ishige A, Sasaki H. The protective effect of hochu-ekki-to (TJ-41), a Japanese

Chinese Herbal Formulas and Applications

Chapter 8 — Overview

herbal medicine, against HSV-1 infection in mitomycin C-treated mice. Anticancer Res 2000 Nov-Dec;20(6A):4109-13.

38. Kaneko M, Kawakita T, Kumazawa Y, Takimoto H, Nomoto K, Yoshikawa T. Accelerated recovery from cyclophosphamide-induced leukopenia in mice administered a Japanese ethical herbal drug, Hochu-ekki-to. Immunopharmacology 1999 Nov;44(3):223-31.

39. *Shang Hai Zhong Yi Yao Za Zhi* (Shanghai Journal of Chinese Medicine and Herbology) 1984;1:2.

40. *Shi Yong Zhong Liu Xue Za Zhi* (Practical Journal of Cancer) 1987;1(4):6.

41. Kao ST, Yeh CC, Hsieh CC, Yang MD, Lee MR, Liu HS, Lin JG. The Chinese medicine Bu-Zhong-Yi-Qi-Tang inhibited proliferation of hepatoma cell lines by inducing apoptosis via G0/G1 arrest. Life Sciences 2001 Aug 17;69(13):1485-96.

42. Cho JM, Sato N, Kikuchi K. Prophylactic anti-tumor effect of Hochu-ekki-to (TJ41) by enhancing natural killer cell activity. In Vivo 1991 Jul-Aug;5(4):389-91.

43. *Shan Xi Zhong Yi Xue Yuan Xue Bao* (Journal of Shanxi University School of Chinese Medicine) 1988;1:29.

44. *Guo Wai Yi Yao Zhi Wu Yao Fen Ce* (Monograph of Foreign Botanical Medicine) 1993;15(3):44.

45. *An Hui Zhong Yi Xue Yuan Xue Bao* (Journal of Anhui University School of Medicine) 1987;6(3):43.

46. *Gan Su Zhong Yi* (Gansu Chinese Medicine) 1998;5:28.

47. *Zhong Yi Za Zhi* (Journal of Chinese Medicine) 1984;25(5):356.

48. *Bei Jing Zhong Yi Za Zhi* (Beijing Journal of Chinese Medicine) 1993;3:227.

49. *Zhong Yao Yao Li Yu Lin Chuang* (Pharmacology and Clinical Applications of Chinese Herbs) 1992;152.

50. *Hei Long Jiang Zhong Yi Yao* (Heilongjiang Chinese Medicine and Herbology) 1989;4:41.

51. *Shan Xi Zhong Yi* (Shanxi Chinese Medicine) 1982;3(2):21.

52. *Shang Hai Zhong Yi Yao Za Zhi* (Shanghai Journal of Chinese Medicine and Herbology) 1995;4:10.

53. *Nei Meng Gu Zhong Yi Yao* (Traditional Chinese Medicine and Medicinals of Inner Mongolia) 1989;1:27.

54. *Jiang Xi Zhong Yi Yao* (Jiangxi Chinese Medicine and Herbology) 1991;3:47.

55. *Shi Yong Zhong Xi Yi Jie He Za Zhi* (Practical Journal of Integrated Chinese and Western Medicines) 1991;8:477.

56. *Jiang Xi Zhong Yi Yao* (Jiangxi Chinese Medicine and Herbology) 1969;3:14.

57. *Nan Jing Zhong Yi Xue Yuan Xue Bao* (Journal of Nanjing University of Traditional Chinese Medicine) 1988;2:26.

58. *Shang Hai Zhong Yi Yao Za Zhi* (Shanghai Journal of Chinese Medicine and Herbology) 1985;5:31.

59. *Zhong Cheng Yao Yan Jiu* (Research of Chinese Patent Medicine) 1983;(9):17.

60. *Chang Yong Zhong Yao Cheng Fen Yu Yao Li Shou Ce* (A Handbook of the Composition and Pharmacology of Common Chinese Drugs) 1997;1:242.

61. Kotani N, Oyama T, Sakai I, Hashimoto H, Muraoka M, Ogawa Y, Matsuki A. Analgesic effect of a herbal medicine for treatment of primary dysmenorrhea--a double-blind study. American Journal of Chinese Medicine 1997;25(2):205-12.

62. Tanaka T. A novel anti-dysmenorrhea therapy with cyclic administration of two Japanese herbal medicines. Clinical & Experimental Obstetrics & Gynecology 2003;30(2-3):95-8.

63. *He Bei Zhong Yi* (Hebei Chinese Medicine) 1999;6:363.

64. Akase T, Akase T, Onodera S, Jobo T, Matsushita R, Kaneko M, Tashiro S. A comparative study of the usefulness of toki-shakuyaku-san and an oral iron preparation in the treatment of hypochromic anemia in cases of uterine myoma. Yakugaku Zasshi - Journal of the Pharmaceutical Society of Japan 2003 Sep;123(9):817-24.

65. *Hu Bei Zhong Yi Za Zhi* (Hubei Journal of Chinese Medicine) 1988;4:25.

66. *Shan Dong Zhong Yi Xue Yuan Xue Bao* (Journal of Shandong University School of Chinese Medicine) 1996;2:118.

67. *Hu Nan Yi Yao Za Zhi* (Hunan Journal of Medicine and Herbology) 1983;4:50.

68. Tanaka T. A novel anti-dysmenorrhea therapy with cyclic administration of two Japanese herbal medicines. Clinical & Experimental Obstetrics & Gynecology 2003;30(2-3):95-8.

69. *Shan Xi Zhong Yi* (Shanxi Chinese Medicine) 1991;7(3):22.

70. *Shan Xi Zhong Yi* (Shanxi Chinese Medicine) 1998;12:534.

71. Fujii T, Kanai T, Kozuma S, Hamai Y, Hyodo H, Yamashita T, Miki A, Unno N, Taketani Y. Theoretical basis for herbal medicines, Tokishakuyaku-san and Sairei-to, in the treatment of autoimmunity-related recurrent abortion by correcting T helper-1/T helper-2 balance. American Journal of Reproductive Immunology 2000 Dec;44(6):342-6.

72. Fujii T. Herbal factors in the treatment of autoimmunity-related habitual abortion. Vitam Horm 2002;65:333-44.

73. *Zhong Yi Za Zhi* (Journal of Chinese Medicine) 1986;10:35.

74. *He Bei Zhong Yi* (Hebei Chinese Medicine) 1998;15(2):26.

75. *Zhong Cheng Yao Yan Jiu* (Research of Chinese Patent Medicine) 1984;(10):30.

76. *Zhong Yi Za Zhi* (Journal of Chinese Medicine) 1988;8:608.

77. *Shi Yong Zhong Xi Yi Jie He Za Zhi* (Practical Journal of Integrated Chinese and Western Medicines) 1991;4:41.

78. *Yun Nan Zhong Yi Za Zhi* (Yunan Journal of Chinese Medicine) 1985;6:25.

79. *Shan Xi Zhong Yi* (Shanxi Chinese Medicine) 1990;11(2):106.

80. *Zhong Yi Za Zhi* (Journal of Chinese Medicine) 1988;29(5):366.

81. *Zhong Xi Yi Jie He Za Zhi* (Journal of Integrated Chinese and Western Medicine) 1991;4:242.

82. *He Bei Zhong Yi* (Hebei Chinese Medicine) 1995;17(4):47.

83. Higaki S, Toyomoto T, Morohashi M. Seijo-bofu-to, Jumi-haidoku-to and Toki-shakuyaku-san suppress rashes and incidental symptoms in acne patients. Drugs Exp Clin Res 2002;28(5):193-6.

84. *Bei Jing Zhong Yi Xue Yuan Xue Bao* (Journal of Beijing University School of Medicine) 1987;5:36.

85. *Zhong Yi Yao Xin Xi* (Information on Chinese Medicine and Herbology) 1992;9(5):36.

86. *Nei Meng Gu Zhong Yi Yao* (Traditional Chinese Medicine and Medicinals of Inner Mongolia) 1993;(3):1.

Chapter 8 — Overview

87. Dai Y, But PP, Chan YP, Matsuda H, Kubo M. Antipruritic and antiinflammatory effects of aqueous extract from Si-Wu-Tang. Biol Pharm Bull 2002 Sep;25(9):1175-8.

88. *Zhong Guo Zhong Yao Za Zhi* (People's Republic of China Journal of Chinese Herbology) 1994;19(11):680.

89. *Shan Xi Zhong Yi* (Shanxi Chinese Medicine) 1986;7(11):53.

90. *Zhong Cheng Yao Yan Jiu* (Research of Chinese Patent Medicine) 1994;2:16.

91. *Zhe Jiang Zhong Yi Xue Yuan Xue Bao* (Journal of Zhejiang University of Chinese Medicine) 1997;3:41.

92. *Zhong Yi Za Zhi* (Journal of Chinese Medicine) 1985;6:24.

93. *Shan Xi Yi Kan* (Shanxi Journal of Medicine) 1995;15(9):399.

94. *Tian Jin Yi Yao* (Tianjin Medicine and Herbology) 1972;26.

95. *Si Chuan Zhong Yi* (Sichuan Chinese Medicine) 1995;9:20.

96. *Yan Ke Tong Xun* (Journal of Ophthalmology) 1987;3:13.

97. *Zhong Yi Fang Ji Xian Dai Yan Jiu* (Modern Study of Medical Formulae in Traditional Chinese Medicine) 1997;1103.

98. *Zhong Yi Fang Ji Xian Dai Yan Jiu* (Modern Study of Medical Formulae in Traditional Chinese Medicine) 1997;1103.

99. *Zhong Yi Za Zhi* (Journal of Chinese Medicine) 1985;5:32.

100. *Zhong Yi Fang Ji Xian Dai Yan Jiu* (Modern Study of Medical Formulae in Traditional Chinese Medicine) 1997;639.

101. *Fu Jian Zhong Yi Yao* (Fujian Chinese Medicine and Herbology) 1960;10:3.

102. *He Bei Zhong Yi* (Hebei Chinese Medicine) 1991;13(3):24.

103. *Xin Jiang Zhong Yi Yao* (Xinjiang Chinese Medicine and Herbology) 1991;1:32.

104. *Shan Dong Zhong Yi Za Zhi* (Shandong Journal of Chinese Medicine) 1996;12:545.

105. Ushiroyama T, Sakuma K, Souen H, Nakai G, Morishima S, Yasuda K, Orino I, Ueki M. Therapeutic effects of Kyuki-chouketsu-in in restoring postpartum physical condition. American Journal of Chinese Medicine 2003;31(3):437-44.

106. Zee-Cheng RK. Shi-quan-da-bu-tang (ten significant tonic decoction), SQT. A potent Chinese biological response modifier in cancer immunotherapy, potentiation and detoxification of anticancer drugs. Methods Find Exp Clin Pharmacol 1992 Nov;14(9):725-36.

107. Miura S, Takimoto H, Yoshikai Y, Kumazawa Y, Yamada A, Nomoto K. Protective effect of Ren-Shen-Yang-Rong-Tang (Ninjin-youei-to) in mice with drug-induced leukopenia against Pseudomonas aeruginosa infection. Int J Immunopharmacol 1992 Oct;14(7):1249-57.

108. *Nan Jing Yi Xue Yuan Xue Bao* (Journal of Nanjing University of Medicine) 1988;4:331.

109. *Si Chuan Zhong Yi* (Sichuan Chinese Medicine) 1995;5:30.

110. *Hu Bei Zhong Yi Za Zhi* (Hubei Journal of Chinese Medicine) 1996;2:24.

111. *Guang Xi Zhong Yi Yao* (Guangxi Chinese Medicine and Herbology) 1996;2:43.

112. Chao SL, Huang LW, Yen HR. Pregnancy in premature ovarian failure after therapy using Chinese herbal medicine. Chang Gung Medical Journal 2003 Jun;26(6):449-52.

113. *Zhong Yi Fang Ji Xian Dai Yan Jiu* (Modern Study of Medical Formulae in Traditional Chinese Medicine) 1997;766.

114. *Zhong Yi Fang Ji Xian Dai Yan Jiu* (Modern Study of Medical Formulae in Traditional Chinese Medicine) 1997;709.

115. *Zhong Yi Ming Fang Lin Chuang Xin Yong* (Contemporary Clinical Applications of Classic Chinese Formulas) 2001;205.

116. *Zhong Xi Yi Jie He Za Zhi* (Journal of Integrated Chinese and Western Medicine) 1986;6:336.

117. *Shi Zhen Guo Yao Yan Jiu* (Research of Shizhen Herbs) 1998;1:11.

118. *He Bei Zhong Yi* (Hebei Chinese Medicine) 1995;17(4):14.

119. *Shan Xi Yi Kan* (Shanxi Journal of Medicine) 1992;5:201.

120. *Hu Nan Zhong Yi Za Zhi* (Hunan Journal of Chinese Medicine) 1997;3:57.

121. *Zhong Yi Za Zhi* (Journal of Chinese Medicine) 1984;7:35.

122. *Shen De Yan Jiu* (Research of Kidney) 1981;19.

123. *Xin Zhong Yi* (New Chinese Medicine) 1975;(4):40.

124. *Zhong Yi Fang Ji Xian Dai Yan Jiu* (Modern Study of Medical Formulae in Traditional Chinese Medicine) 1997;6:25.

125. *Shan Xi Zhong Yi* (Shanxi Chinese Medicine) 1999;4:161.

126. *Xin Jiang Zhong Yi Yao* (Xinjiang Chinese Medicine and Herbology) 1994;4:13.

127. *Gui Zhou Yi Yao* (Medicine and Medicinals from Guizhou) 1991;5:307.

128. *Zhong Yi Za Zhi* (Journal of Chinese Medicine) 1999;4:243.

129. *Gui Yang Yi Xue Yuan Xue Bao* (Journal of Guiyang Medical University) 1986;2:42.

130. *Guo Wai Yi Xue* (Foreign Medicine) 1986;4:11.

131. *Zhong Yi Fang Ji Xian Dai Yan Jiu* (Modern Study of Medical Formulae in Traditional Chinese Medicine) 1997;727.

132. *Hu Bei Zhong Yi Za Zhi* (Hubei Journal of Chinese Medicine) 1987;3:14.

133. *Shang Hai Zhong Yi Yao Za Zhi* (Shanghai Journal of Chinese Medicine and Herbology) 1991;10:23.

134. *Si Chuan Zhong Yi* (Sichuan Chinese Medicine) 1989;3:25.

135. *Hei Long Jiang Zhong Yi Yao* (Heilongjiang Chinese Medicine and Herbology) 1987;1:40.

136. *Zhong Cheng Yao* (Study of Chinese Patent Medicine) 1995;4:51.

137. *Zhong Yao Yao Li Yu Lin Chuang* (Pharmacology and Clinical Applications of Chinese Herbs) 1992;3:35.

138. *Xin Zhong Yi* (New Chinese Medicine) 1999;3:12.

139. *Zhong Yi Za Zhi* (Journal of Chinese Medicine) 1983;3:37.

140. *Zhong Yi Fang Ji Xian Dai Yan Jiu* (Modern Study of Medical Formulae in Traditional Chinese Medicine) 1997;710.

141. *Jiang Xi Zhong Yi Yao* (Jiangxi Chinese Medicine and Herbology) 1998;6:26.

142. *Zhe Jiang Zhong Yi Za Zhi* (Zhejiang Journal of Chinese Medicine) 1988;6:244.

Chapter 8 — Overview

143. *Shi Yong Zhong Yi Nei Ke Za Zhi* (Journal of Practical Chinese Internal Medicine) 1993;3:142.

144. *Zhong Yi Za Zhi* (Journal of Chinese Medicine) 1993;1:61.

145. *Shi Yong Zhong Yi Za Zhi* (Journal of Practical Chinese Medicine) 1995;6:10.

146. *Shi Yong Zhong Xi Yi Jie He Za Zhi* (Practical Journal of Integrated Chinese and Western Medicines) 1993;1:41.

147. *Zhong Guo Yao Ke Da Xue Xue Bao* (Journal of University of Chinese Herbology) 1989;6:951.

148. *Zhong Guo Zhong Yao Za Zhi* (People's Republic of China Journal of Chinese Herbology) 1992;(9):531.

149. *Zhong Yao Yao Li Yu Lin Chuang* (Pharmacology and Clinical Applications of Chinese Herbs) 1989;6:14.

150. *Nei Meng Gu Zhong Yi Yao* (Traditional Chinese Medicine and Medicinals of Inner Mongolia) 1998;1:4.

151. *Zhe Jiang Zhong Yi Xue Yuan Xue Bao* (Journal of Zhejiang University of Chinese Medicine) 1997;3:35.

152. *Shan Xi Yi Kan* (Shanxi Journal of Medicine) 1989;7:292.

153. *Fu Jian Zhong Yi Yao* (Fujian Chinese Medicine and Herbology) 1995;4:33.

154. *Zhong Yi Fang Ji Xian Dai Yan Jiu* (Modern Study of Medical Formulae in Traditional Chinese Medicine) 1997;712.

155. *Shan Xi Zhong Yi* (Shanxi Chinese Medicine) 1995;16(11):485.

156. *Hu Bei Zhong Yi Za Zhi* (Hubei Journal of Chinese Medicine) 1999;10:458.

157. *Guo Wai Yi Xue Zhong Yi Zhong Yao Fen Ce* (Monograph of Chinese Herbology from Foreign Medicine) 1991;13(1):47.

158. *Guo Wai Yi Yao Zhi Wu Yao Fen Ce* (Monograph of Foreign Botanical Medicine) 1991;1:45.

159. *Guo Wai Yi Xue Zhong Yi Zhong Yao Fen Ce* (Monograph of Chinese Herbology from Foreign Medicine) 1989;5:26.

160. *Guo Wai Yi Yao Zhi Wu Yao Fen Ce* (Monograph of Foreign Botanical Medicine) 1991;4:41.

161. Otani S, Usuki S, Iwasaki H, Inoue S, Yamashita K. Successful treatment of a infertile woman using hachimijiogan. Am J Chin Med 1991;19(2):145-54.

162. *Zhong Cheng Yao* (Study of Chinese Patent Medicine) 1993;11:24.

163. *Han Fang Yi Xue* (Kampo Medicine) 1983;5:14.

164. Sakamoto S, Kudo H, Kawasaki T, Kasahara N, Okamoto R. Effect of ba-wei-di-huang-wan (hachimi-jio-gan) on thymidine kinase and its isozyme activities in the prostate glands in rats. Am J Chin Med 1988;16(1-2):29-36.

165. Yoshimura K, Terai A, Arai Y. Two-week administration of low-dose Hachimi-jio-gan (Ba-Wei Di-Huang-Wan) for patients with benign prostatic hyperplasia. Hinyokika Kiyo 2003 Sep;49(9):509-14.

166. *Xin Zhong Yi* (New Chinese Medicine)1997;1:48.

167. *Zhong Yi Fang Ji Xian Dai Yan Jiu* (Modern Study of Medical Formulae in Traditional Chinese Medicine) 1997;680.

168. *Xin Zhong Yi* (New Chinese Medicine) 1995;27(1):50.

169. *Zhong Yi Za Zhi* (Journal of Chinese Medicine) 1956;12:635.

170. *Shan Xi Zhong Yi* (Shanxi Chinese Medicine) 1997;4:149.

171. *Shen De Yan Jiu* (Research of Kidney) 1981;93.

172. *Fu Jian Zhong Yi Yao* (Fujian Chinese Medicine and Herbology) 1995;26(3):59.

173. *Zhe Jiang Zhong Yi Za Zhi* (Zhejiang Journal of Chinese Medicine) 1995;9:400.

174. Hsu H. Effectiveness of Gui Lu Er Xian Jiao (Tortoise Shell and Deer Antler Syrup) on treatment of osteoporosis. Clinic Medline of Taiwan.

175. *Hu Nan Zhong Yi Za Zhi* (Hunan Journal of Chinese Medicine) 1999;2:26.

Chapter 8 – Tonic Formulas   *Section 1 – Qi-Tonifying Formulas*

Section 1

补气剂

— Qi-Tonifying Formulas

Si Jūn Zǐ Tang (Four-Gentlemen Decoction)

四君子湯
四君子汤

Pinyin Name: *Si Jun Zi Tang*
Literal Name: Four-Gentlemen Decoction
Alternate Names: *Szu Chun Tzu Tang, Si Jung Zi Tang,* Four Major Herb Decoction, Major Four Herb Combination
Original Source: *Tai Ping Hui Min He Ji Ju Fang* (Imperial Grace Formulary of the Tai Ping Era) by the Imperial Medical Department in 1078-85

COMPOSITION

Ren Shen (Radix et Rhizoma Ginseng)	[9g]
Bai Zhu (Rhizoma Atractylodis Macrocephalae)	[9g]
Fu Ling (Poria)	[9g]
Zhi Gan Cao (Radix et Rhizoma Glycyrrhizae Praeparata cum Melle)	[6g]

DOSAGE / PREPARATION / ADMINISTRATION

Grind equal amounts of the ingredients into a fine powder. Cook 6g of the powder in one large bowl of water until the liquid is reduced to 70%. The decoction may be taken any time during the day with an additional small pinch of salt. A small amount of *Sheng Jiang* (Rhizoma Zingiberis Recens) and *Da Zao* (Fructus Jujubae) may also be added to harmonize the formula.[1] Today, this formula may be prepared as a decoction with the doses suggested in brackets.

CHINESE THERAPEUTIC ACTIONS

1. Tonifies qi
2. Strengthens the Spleen

CLINICAL MANIFESTATIONS

Spleen and Stomach qi deficiencies: a pale face, a sallow complexion, a low voice, lassitude, weakness of the extremities, poor appetite, loose stools, a pale tongue, and a fine, moderate pulse.

CLINICAL APPLICATIONS

Chronic fatigue syndrome, chronic gastritis, peptic ulcer disease, gastroptosis, ulcerative colitis, irritable bowel syndrome, epigastric or abdominal pain, premenstrual syndrome, menstrual bleeding, chronic tonsillitis, and chronic hepatitis.

EXPLANATION

The Spleen and Stomach are the source of postnatal qi, as they are the most important organs for extracting nutrients and producing qi and blood. However, the Spleen and Stomach may be injured by an inappropriate diet or overwork. If these two organs become deficient and their digestive functions are affected, then the amount of qi produced would not be adequate. Lack of nourishment and qi deficiency render the face pale, produce a low voice, and bring about lassitude. Poor appetite is the result of an impaired digestive system. Loose stools are the result of the Spleen's inability to direct clear yang and water fluid to the upper *jiao*. Since the Spleen is related to the muscles, Spleen deficiency can result in weakness of the extremities. A pale tongue and a fine, moderate pulse are common signs of qi deficiency.

Si Jun Zi Tang (Four-Gentlemen Decoction) contains *Ren Shen* (Radix et Rhizoma Ginseng) as the chief herb because it greatly tonifies *yuan* (source) *qi*, strengthens the Spleen, and nourishes the Stomach. *Bai Zhu* (Rhizoma Atractylodis Macrocephalae), the deputy herb, tonifies

522

Si Jūn Zǐ Tāng (Four-Gentlemen Decoction)

Si Jun Zi Tang (Four-Gentlemen Decoction)

Diagnosis	Signs and Symptoms	Treatment	Herbs
Spleen and Stomach qi deficiencies	• Pale face, a sallow complexion, a low voice, and lassitude: Spleen and Stomach qi deficiencies and lack of nourishment • Loose stools: Spleen unable to guide clear yang upward • Pale tongue and a fine, moderate pulse: qi deficiency	• Tonifies qi • Strengthens the Spleen	• *Ren Shen* (Radix et Rhizoma Ginseng) greatly tonifies *yuan* (source) *qi*, strengthens the Spleen, and nourishes the Stomach. • *Bai Zhu* (Rhizoma Atractylodis Macrocephalae) tonifies Spleen qi and dries dampness in the middle *jiao*. • *Fu Ling* (Poria) tonifies the middle *jiao* and dispels dampness. • *Zhi Gan Cao* (Radix et Rhizoma Glycyrrhizae Praeparata cum Melle) tonifies Spleen qi and harmonizes the herbs.

Spleen qi and dries dampness in the middle *jiao*. *Fu Ling* (Poria), the assistant, tonifies the middle *jiao* and dispels dampness. *Zhi Gan Cao* (Radix et Rhizoma Glycyrrhizae Praeparata cum Melle), the envoy herb, tonifies Spleen qi and harmonizes the herbs.

Si Jun Zi Tang is a simple, yet extremely effective formula to tonify qi. It serves as the foundation for many qi-tonifying formulas that tonify the Spleen and nourish the Stomach to enable the production of qi and blood.

MODIFICATIONS

• For severe Spleen and Stomach qi deficiencies, add *Huang Qi* (Radix Astragali) and *Shan Yao* (Rhizoma Dioscoreae).
• If there is tidal fever due to Spleen deficiency, add *Chai Hu* (Radix Bupleuri) and *Bai Shao* (Radix Paeoniae Alba).
• With insomnia due to fear and fright, add *Sheng Jiang* (Rhizoma Zingiberis Recens) and *Suan Zao Ren* (Semen Ziziphi Spinosae).
• With constipation due to qi deficiency, add *Dang Gui* (Radix Angelicae Sinensis) and *Huo Ma Ren* (Fructus Cannabis).
• With diarrhea due to deficiency and cold in the middle *jiao*, add *Li Zhong Tang* (Regulate the Middle Decoction).
• With postpartum diarrhea, add *Wu Mei* (Fructus Mume) and *Chen Pi* (Pericarpium Citri Reticulatae).
• With constant loose stools or diarrhea, add *He Zi* (Fructus Chebulae).
• For hemorrhoids, add *Huang Qi* (Radix Astragali) and *Bai Bian Dou* (Semen Lablab Album).
• With low-grade fever due to chronic illness and deficiency, add *Gui Zhi* (Ramulus Cinnamomi) and *Fu Zi* (Radix Aconiti Lateralis Praeparata).
• With edema due to Spleen deficiency, add *Yi Yi Ren* (Semen Coicis), *Ze Xie* (Rhizoma Alismatis), and *Gui Zhi* (Ramulus Cinnamomi).

• With qi and blood deficiencies, combine with *Si Wu Tang* (Four-Substance Decoction).
• For *gan ji* (infantile malnutrition) caused by yin deficiency, add *Gou Qi Zi* (Fructus Lycii) and *Nu Zhen Zi* (Fructus Ligustri Lucidi).
• For *gan ji* (infantile malnutrition) caused by food stagnation, add *Mai Ya* (Fructus Hordei Germinatus).

CAUTIONS / CONTRAINDICATIONS

• *Si Jun Zi Tang*, while gentle, is slightly warm. Long-term use of this formula may cause a dry mouth, dry tongue, thirst, or irritability.
• This formula should be used with caution, or avoid in patients who have high fever, yin-deficient heat, excess heat, qi stagnation, body fluid deficiency, irritability, thirst, or constipation.

PHARMACOLOGICAL EFFECTS

1. **General**: Administration of *Si Jun Zi Tang* has been associated with a general effect to improve the health and well being of animal subjects. In mice with artificially-induced "Spleen deficiency" characterized by such symptoms as low body temperature, weight loss, decreased food intake, diarrhea, and inability to tolerate cold, ingestion of the formula reversed the symptoms and improved the overall health.[2]

2. **Gastrointestinal**: According to laboratory experiments in rabbits, administration of *Si Jun Zi Tang* was associated with a regulatory effect on the intestines. Depending on the condition of the subject, it either increased or decreased intestinal peristalsis.[3]

3. **Immunostimulant**: Administration of *Si Jun Zi Tang* was associated with an increase in T-lymphocytes, NK cells, and phagocytic activity of the macrophages.[4,5,6]

4. **Antineoplastic**: Administration of *Si Jun Zi Tang* was associated with an inhibitory effect on tumor cells in mice with esophageal and lung cancer.[7]

Chapter 8 – Tonic Formulas   Section 1 – Qi-Tonifying Formulas

Sī Jūn Zǐ Tāng (Four-Gentlemen Decoction)

5. **Hematopoietic**: Administration of *Si Jun Zi Tang* in decoction for one week was associated with an increase in both white and red blood cells in rats.[8]

6. **Radioprotective**: One study reported recovery of the hematopoietic system in whole-body irradiated mice using *Si Jun Zi Tang*. Specific beneficial effects included an increase of leukocytes, erythrocytes, thrombocytes, and hematocrit. Moreover, the radioprotective function was more effective for leukocytes and thrombocytes than other hematocytes.[9]

CLINICAL STUDIES AND RESEARCH

1. **Chronic gastritis**: In one clinical study, 32 patients with chronic superficial gastritis were treated with modified *Si Jun Zi Tang* with good results. Out of 32 patients, 24 reported resolution of symptoms within 10 days, and 8 within 20 days. The formula used included the addition of *Zhi Qiao* (Fructus Aurantii), *Ji Nei Jin* (Endothelium Corneum Gigeriae Galli), *Huang Qi* (Radix Astragali), and others as deemed necessary.[10]

2. **Peptic ulcer disease**: One study of 126 peptic ulcer patients reported 97.6% effectiveness using *Si Jun Zi Tang* plus *Huang Qi* (Radix Astragali), *San Leng* (Rhizoma Sparganii), and *Hai Piao Xiao* (Endoconcha Sepiae) as the base formula, with the addition of *Chai Hu* (Radix Bupleuri), *Bai Shao* (Radix Paeoniae Alba), and *Zhi Zi* (Fructus Gardeniae) for Liver stagnation with Spleen deficiency; and *Si Ni San* (Frigid Extremities Powder) for Liver and Stomach disharmony. The treatment protocol was to give the herbs in decoction twice daily for 4-8 weeks per course of treatment.[11] In another report, 115 patients with peptic ulcer characterized by Spleen deficiency were treated with *Si Jun Zi Tang* with satisfactory results. *Fu Long Gan* (Terra Flava Usta) and *Bai Ji* (Rhizoma Bletillae) were added for individuals with bleeding ulcer. The overall effectiveness was 92.8%.[12]

3. **Ulcerative colitis**: Sixty patients with chronic ulcerative colitis were treated with herbs with complete recovery in 40 patients, significant improvement in 13 patients, moderate improvement in 5 patients, and no effect in 2 patients. The herbal treatment included *Si Jun Zi Tang* plus *Huang Qi* (Radix Astragali), *Dang Gui* (Radix Angelicae Sinensis), *Yan Hu Suo* (Rhizoma Corydalis), and others as deemed necessary. The herbs were made into pills, and were given three times daily.[13]

4. **Irritable bowel syndrome (IBS)**: One study reported 92.9% effectiveness using modified *Si Jun Zi Tang* to treat irritable bowel syndrome. Of 57 patients, the study reported significant improvement in 39 patients, moderate improvement in 14 patients, and no change in 4 patients. The base herbal formula included *Si Jun Zi Tang* plus *Pao Jiang* (Rhizoma Zingiberis Praeparatum), *Qin Pi* (Cortex

Fraxini), and *Mu Xiang* (Radix Aucklandiae). Modifications were made by adding *Bai Shao* (Radix Paeoniae Alba) and *Yan Hu Suo* (Rhizoma Corydalis) for abdominal pain; *Chen Pi* (Pericarpium Citri Reticulatae) and dry-fried *Fang Feng* (Radix Saposhnikoviae) for abdominal pain causing urgent bowel movements; *Da Fu Pi* (Pericarpium Arecae) and *Zhi Qiao* (Fructus Aurantii) for feeling of incomplete evacuation after defecation; *Bai Tou Weng* (Radix Pulsatillae) and *Da Xue Teng* (Caulis Sargentodoxae) for mucus in the stools; *Cang Zhu* (Rhizoma Atractylodis) for profuse white mucus; *Di Yu* (Radix Sanguisorbae) and charred *Jin Yin Hua* (Flos Lonicerae Japonicae) for hematochezia; *Bu Gu Zhi* (Fructus Psoraleae) and *Rou Dou Kou* (Semen Myristicae) for 5 a.m. diarrhea; *Wu Bei Zi* (Galla Chinensis) and roasted *He Zi* (Fructus Chebulae) for frequent bowel movements with loose stools; *Rou Cong Rong* (Herba Cistanches) for constipation with yang deficiency; and *Shi Xiao San* (Sudden Smile Powder) for blood stagnation. The treatment protocol was to cook the herbs in water, and drink the decoction in three equally-divided doses daily.[14]

5. **Epigastric or abdominal pain**: Patients with epigastric or abdominal pain characterized by Spleen qi deficiency were treated with *Si Jun Zi Tang*. Out of 125 patients, the study reported recovery in 86 patients, significant improvement in 22 patients, and slight improvement in 17 patients.[15]

6. **Premenstrual syndrome (PMS)**: In one report, 50 patients with PMS were treated with modified *Si Jun Zi Tang* with significant results in 31 patients, moderate results in 15 patients, slight improvement in 2 patients, and no effect in 2 patients. The treatment protocol was to administer the herbs in decoction daily before and during menstruation. The formula included the addition of *Huang Qi* (Radix Astragali) and *Fu Zi* (Radix Aconiti Lateralis Praeparata).[16]

7. **Menstrual bleeding**: In one case report, a patient with a two-year history of profuse menstrual bleeding due to qi deficiency responded well to herbal treatment. The herbs included *Dang Shen* (Radix Codonopsis), *Bai Zhu* (Rhizoma Atractylodis Macrocephalae), *Fu Ling* (Poria), *Gan Cao* (Radix et Rhizoma Glycyrrhizae), and *Huang Qi* (Radix Astragali). *Dang Shen* (Radix Codonopsis) and *Huang Qi* (Radix Astragali) were used at a larger dose.[17]

8. **Chronic tonsillitis**: Twenty children with chronic tonsillitis were treated with modified *Si Jun Zi Tang* with recovery in 12 patients, significant improvement in 6 patients, slight improvement in 1 case, and no effect in 1 case. The average length of treatment was 5 days. The formula included the addition of *Huang Qi* (Radix Astragali) and *Fu Zi* (Radix Aconiti Lateralis Praeparata).[18]

9. **Chronic hepatitis**: One hundred patients with chronic hepatitis were treated with complete recovery in 61 patients,

524

Chinese Herbal Formulas and Applications

Sì Jūn Zǐ Tāng (Four-Gentlemen Decoction)

improvement in 31 patients, and no benefit in 8 patients. The treatment protocol was to administer 40-60 packs of herbs in decoction. The herbal formulas included *Si Jun Zi Tang* plus *Dang Gui* (Radix Angelicae Sinensis), *Bai Shao* (Radix Paeoniae Alba), *Chai Hu* (Radix Bupleuri), and others as follows: *Huang Qi* (Radix Astragali) for qi deficiency; *Ji Nei Jin* (Endothelium Corneum Gigeriae Galli) and charred *Mai Ya* (Fructus Hordei Germinatus) for indigestion and poor appetite; *Lian Zi* (Semen Nelumbinis), *Shan Yao* (Rhizoma Dioscoreae), and *Ze Xie* (Rhizoma Alismatis) for loose stools; *Yan Hu Suo* (Rhizoma Corydalis) and *Yu Jin* (Radix Curcumae) for hypochondriac pain; *San Leng* (Rhizoma Sparganii), *E Zhu* (Rhizoma Curcumae), and *Bie Jia* (Carapax Trionycis) for splenomegaly and hepatomegaly; *Tao Ren* (Semen Persicae), *Hong Hua* (Flos Carthami), and *Yi Mu Cao* (Herba Leonuri) for blood stagnation; *Fo Shou* (Fructus Citri Sarcodactylis) and *Xiang Yuan* (Fructus Citri) for qi stagnation; *Yin Chen* (Herba Artemisiae Scopariae) for jaundice; and *Shi Hu* (Caulis Dendrobii), *Yu Zhu* (Rhizoma Polygonati Odorati), and *Xuan Shen* (Radix Scrophulariae) for yin deficiency.[19]

RELATED FORMULAS

Yì Gōng Sǎn (Extraordinary Merit Powder)

異功散
异功散

Pinyin Name: *Yi Gong San*
Literal Name: Extraordinary Merit Powder
Original Source: *Xiao Er Yao Zheng Zhi Jue* (Craft of Medicinal Treatment for Childhood Disease Patterns) by Qian Yi in 1119

Ren Shen (Radix et Rhizoma Ginseng)	[6-9g]
Bai Zhu (Rhizoma Atractylodis Macrocephalae)	[6-9g]
Fu Ling (Poria)	[6-9g]
Gan Cao (Radix et Rhizoma Glycyrrhizae)	[3-6g]
Chen Pi (Pericarpium Citri Reticulatae)	[6-9g]

The source text states to grind equal amounts of the ingredients into a fine powder. Cook 6g of the powder with 5 slices of *Sheng Jiang* (Rhizoma Zingiberis Recens) and 2 pieces of *Da Zao* (Fructus Jujubae) in one large bowl of water until the liquid is reduced to 70%. Take the warm, strained decoction before meals. Today, this formula may be prepared as a decoction with the doses suggested in brackets.

Yi Gong San (Extraordinary Merit Powder) is composed of *Si Jun Zi Tang* plus *Chen Pi* (Pericarpium Citri Reticulatae). This formula tonifies and regulates qi, strengthens the Spleen, and harmonizes the Stomach. It is often used for patients with Spleen and Stomach deficiencies accompanied by qi stagnation, and characterized by such symptoms as poor appetite, fullness and discomfort of the chest and epigastrium, vomiting, and diarrhea.

Bǎo Yuán Tāng (Preserve the Basal Decoction)

保元湯
保元汤

Pinyin Name: *Bao Yuan Tang*
Literal Name: Preserve the Basal Decoction
Original Source: *Bo Ai Xin Jian* (Manual of Universal Lover from the Heart) by Wei Zhi in 1525

Huang Qi (Radix Astragali)	6-9g
Ren Shen (Radix et Rhizoma Ginseng)	6-9g
Rou Gui (Cortex Cinnamomi)	1.5-2.1g
Zhi Gan Cao (Radix et Rhizoma Glycyrrhizae Praeparata cum Melle)	3g

Cook the herbs with 1 slice of *Sheng Jiang* (Rhizoma Zingiberis Recens) in water. Take the strained decoction while warm.

Bao Yuan Tang (Preserve the Basal Decoction) tonifies qi and warms yang. This formula is generally used for patients with Spleen and Stomach qi deficiencies, accompanied by the presence of cold and insufficiency of yang. Clinically, this formula also may be prescribed for children with chicken pox characterized by yang and *yuan* (source) *qi* deficiencies, with symptoms such as lethargy, weakness, and intolerance to cold.

Bao Yuan Tang may be literally translated as "Preserve the Basal Decoction" or "Preserve the *Yuan* (Source) *Qi* Decoction." *Ren Shen* (Radix et Rhizoma Ginseng), *Huang Qi* (Radix Astragali) and *Zhi Gan Cao* (Radix et Rhizoma Glycyrrhizae Praeparata cum Melle) are used to effectively tonify *zhong* (central) *qi* and *yuan* (source) *qi*. *Rou Gui* (Cortex Cinnamomi) is added to warm yang, dispel cold, and enhance the overall qi-tonifying effect.

AUTHORS' COMMENTS

Si Jun Zi Tang is the representative formula for tonifying Spleen and Stomach qi deficiencies. It treats Spleen and Stomach qi deficiencies due to various causes or with various complications, as long as it is modified accordingly.

Si Jun Zi Tang tonifies qi to treat signs and symptoms such as pale and sallow complexion, feeble voice, weak extremities, and a weak pulse. This formula uses *Ren Shen* (Radix et Rhizoma Ginseng), a warm and sweet herb, to tonify Spleen and Stomach qi. *Bai Zhu* (Rhizoma Atractylodis

8

TONIC FORMULAS

525

Si Jūn Zǐ Tāng (Four-Gentlemen Decoction)

Macrocephalae) and *Fu Ling* (Poria) tonify Spleen and drains dampness. *Zhi Gan Cao* (Radix et Rhizoma Glycyrrhizae Praeparata cum Melle) is warm and sweet, and has functions to harmonize the middle *jiao* and tonify the qi. These four herbs have gentle properties, they are not too hot, not too dry, and are unlikely to create any side effects or adverse reactions, hence the name, Four Gentlemen.

Spleen and Stomach is the root of post-natal qi, and the origin of qi and blood genesis. Only if these two organs are strong with good digestive function, can all organs, and the rest of the body be nourished, healthy, and be free of illnesses. Therefore, *Si Jun Zi Tang* can be modified according to different conditions of cold, heat, excess or deficiency to tonify Spleen and Stomach qi, for the purpose of promoting overall bodily functions. Therefore, *Si Jun Zi Tang* is the basic formula for tonifying qi.

Si Jun Zi Tang and *Li Zhong Wan* (Regulate the Middle Pill) both treat Spleen qi deficiency with poor appetite, diarrhea, and other signs and symptoms. Both formulas contain qi-tonifying herbs such as *Ren Shen* (Radix et Rhizoma Ginseng), *Bai Zhu* (Rhizoma Atractylodis Macrocephalae), and *Zhi Gan Cao* (Radix et Rhizoma Glycyrrhizae Praeparata cum Melle). Although similar, their differences are as follows:

- *Si Jun Zi Tang* is indicated for <u>Spleen qi deficiency</u>, characterized by a sallow complexion, poor appetite, decreased food intake, fatigue, a pale tongue, and a fine, moderate pulse.
- *Li Zhong Wan* is for <u>deficiency and cold</u> of the middle *jiao* (Spleen and Stomach), characterized by abdominal pain,

vomiting, diarrhea, polyuria, cold limbs, intolerance to cold, and a deep and fine pulse.[20]

References

1. *Yi Fang Ji Jie* (Analytical Collection of Medical Formulas) 1682.
2. *Shang Hai Di Er Yi Ke Da Xue Xue Bao* (Journal of Second Shanghai University College of Medicine) 1984;3:7.
3. *Xin Zhong Yi* (New Chinese Medicine) 1978;5:53.
4. *Zhong Cheng Yao Yan Jiu* (Research of Chinese Patent Medicine) 1981;12:28.
5. *Zhong Yao Yao Li Yu Lin Chuang* (Pharmacology and Clinical Applications of Chinese Herbs) 1989;5(5):24.
6. *Zhong Xi Yi Jie He Za Zhi* (Journal of Integrated Chinese and Western Medicine) 1984;4(6):363.
7. *Shang Hai Zhong Yi Yao Za Zhi* (Shanghai Journal of Chinese Medicine and Herbology) 1984;1:2.
8. *Zhong Yi Fang Ji Xian Dai Yan Jiu* (Modern Study of Medical Formulae in Traditional Chinese Medicine) 1997;477.
9. Hsu HY, Yang JJ, Lian SL, Ho YH, Lin CC. Recovery of the hematopoietic system by Si-Jun-Zi-Tang in whole body irradiated mice. J Ethnopharmacol 1996 Nov;54(2-3):69-75.
10. *Zhong Yi Fang Ji Xian Dai Yan Jiu* (Modern Study of Medical Formulae in Traditional Chinese Medicine) 1997;480-481.
11. *Xin Zhong Yi* (New Chinese Medicine) 1982;11:12.
12. *Zhong Yi Za Zhi* (Journal of Chinese Medicine) 1980;21(12):947.
13. *Zhong Yi Za Zhi* (Journal of Chinese Medicine) 1987;10:28.
14. *Shang Hai Zhong Yi Za Zhi* (Shanghai Journal of Chinese Medicine) 1986;1:12.
15. *He Nan Zhong Yi* (Henan Chinese Medicine) 1986;3:1.
16. *Hu Bei Zhong Yi Za Zhi* (Hubei Journal of Chinese Medicine) 1989;2:6.
17. *Zhong Yi Yao Xue Bao* (Report of Chinese Medicine and Herbology) 1984;3:36.
18. *Guang Zhou Zhong Yi Xue Yuan Xue Bao* (Journal of Guangzhou University of Chinese Medicine) 1989;1:34.
19. *He Bei Zhong Yi* (Hebei Chinese Medicine) 1987;6:31.
20. Wang MZ, et al. *Zhong Yi Xue Wen Da Ti Ku* (Questions and Answers on Traditional Chinese Medicine: Herbal Formulas).

Chinese Herbal Formulas and Applications

Liù Jūn Zǐ Tāng (Six-Gentlemen Decoction)

六君子湯
六君子汤

Pinyin Name: *Liu Jun Zi Tang*
Literal Name: Six-Gentlemen Decoction
Alternate Names: *Liu Chun Tzu Tang* (*Wan*), Six Major Herb Decoction (Pill), Six Gentlemen Decoction (Pill), Major Six Herb Combination
Original Source: *Fu Ren Liang Fang* (Fine Formulas for Women) by Chen Zi-Ming in 1237

COMPOSITION

Ren Shen (Radix et Rhizoma Ginseng)	6g [9g]
Bai Zhu (Rhizoma Atractylodis Macrocephalae)	6g [9g]
Fu Ling (Poria)	6g [9g]
Zhi Gan Cao (Radix et Rhizoma Glycyrrhizae Praeparata cum Melle)	3g [6g]
Chen Pi (Pericarpium Citri Reticulatae)	3g [9g]
Ban Xia (Rhizoma Pinelliae)	3g [12g]

DOSAGE / PREPARATION / ADMINISTRATION

The source text states to prepare the ingredients as a decoction with the addition of small amounts of *Sheng Jiang* (Rhizoma Zingiberis Recens) (3 slices) and *Da Zao* (Fructus Jujubae) (2 pieces). Today, the decoction may be prepared using the doses suggested in brackets.

CHINESE THERAPEUTIC ACTIONS

1. Strengthens the Spleen and Stomach
2. Regulates qi and stops vomiting

CLINICAL MANIFESTATIONS

Spleen and Stomach qi deficiencies accompanied by dampness and phlegm: lack of appetite, loose stools, nausea, vomiting, a feeling of oppression and distention in the chest and epigastrium, coughing, and profuse, white, watery phlegm.

CLINICAL APPLICATIONS

Gastrointestinal disorders, abdominal pain, gastritis, chronic gastritis, gastric ulcer, duodenal ulcer, stomach prolapse, gastroptosis, indigestion, diarrhea, nausea, vomiting, morning sickness, stomach cancer, supportive treatment during chemotherapy, chronic bronchitis, stomatitis, pain in liver cancer, stress and depression, and neurasthenia.

EXPLANATION

Liu Jun Zi Tang (Six-Gentlemen Decoction) is derived from *Si Jun Zi Tang* (Four-Gentlemen Decoction) with the addition of *Ban Xia* (Rhizoma Pinelliae) and *Chen Pi* (Pericarpium Citri Reticulatae). It treats Spleen and Stomach deficiencies accompanied by damp and phlegm accumulation. Spleen and Stomach deficiencies may cause indigestion, leading to loss of appetite and loose stools.

Liu Jun Zi Tang (Six-Gentlemen Decoction)

Diagnosis	Signs and Symptoms	Treatment	Herbs
Spleen and Stomach qi deficiencies accompanied by dampness and phlegm	• Indigestion, loss of appetite, and loose stools: Spleen and Stomach deficiencies • Nausea and vomiting: reversed Stomach qi circulation due to damp accumulation • Coughing, and oppression and distention in the chest and epigastrium: obstructed Lung qi circulation due to damp accumulation • Profuse, white, watery phlegm: damp and phlegm accumulation	• Strengthens the Spleen and Stomach • Regulates qi and stops vomiting	• *Si Jun Zi Tang* (Four-Gentlemen Decoction) tonifies qi and strengthens the Spleen and Stomach. • *Chen Pi* (Pericarpium Citri Reticulatae) dries dampness and regulates Lung qi to reduce profuse phlegm. • *Ban Xia* (Rhizoma Pinelliae) breaks up qi stagnation to relieve chest stuffiness, and redirects rebellious Stomach qi to relieve nausea and vomiting.

TONIC FORMULAS

8

Chapter 8 – Tonic Formulas　　　　　　　　　　　　　　　　　*Section 1 – Qi-Tonifying Formulas*

Liù Jūn Zǐ Tāng (Six-Gentlemen Decoction)

Damp accumulation may block the normal descension of Stomach qi and cause qi reversal, manifesting as nausea and vomiting. When the Spleen produces dampness, it is stored in the Lung. If dampness stagnates in the chest and interrupts the flow of Lung qi, coughing and oppression and distention in the chest and epigastrium may occur. Profuse, white, watery phlegm indicates damp and phlegm accumulation inside the body.

Ren Shen (Radix et Rhizoma Ginseng), *Bai Zhu* (Rhizoma Atractylodis Macrocephalae), *Fu Ling* (Poria), and *Zhi Gan Cao* (Radix et Rhizoma Glycyrrhizae Praeparata cum Melle) tonify Spleen and Stomach qi, as explained in the section on *Si Jun Zi Tang* (Four-Gentlemen Decoction). *Chen Pi* (Pericarpium Citri Reticulatae) dries dampness and regulates Lung qi to reduce the profuse phlegm. *Ban Xia* (Rhizoma Pinelliae) breaks up qi stagnation to relieve chest stuffiness, and redirects rebellious Stomach qi to relieve nausea and vomiting.

MODIFICATIONS

- For deficiency and cold of the Spleen and Stomach, add *Wu Zhu Yu* (Fructus Evodiae), *Pao Jiang* (Rhizoma Zingiberis Praeparatum), and *Rou Gui* (Cortex Cinnamomi).
- If there is yang deficiency of the Spleen and Kidney, add *Bu Gu Zhi* (Fructus Psoraleae) and *Fu Zi* (Radix Aconiti Lateralis Praeparata).
- For diarrhea due to Spleen deficiency, add *Shan Yao* (Rhizoma Dioscoreae) and *Qian Shi* (Semen Euryales).
- For diarrhea caused by deficiency and cold in the middle *jiao*, add *Li Zhong Tang* (Regulate the Middle Decoction).
- For hemorrhoids, add *Huang Qi* (Radix Astragali) and *Bai Bian Dou* (Semen Lablab Album).
- With mucus in the stools, add *Ge Gen* (Radix Puerariae Lobatae), *Bai Shao* (Radix Paeoniae Alba), and *Mu Xiang* (Radix Aucklandiae).
- With abdominal pain and cramps due to Spleen deficiency, add *Chai Hu* (Radix Bupleuri), *Bai Shao* (Radix Paeoniae Alba), and *Dang Gui* (Radix Angelicae Sinensis).
- If there is lack of appetite, add *Shan Zha* (Fructus Crataegi), *Shen Qu* (Massa Fermentata), and *Mai Ya* (Fructus Hordei Germinatus).
- If there are exterior signs and symptoms, add *Fang Feng* (Radix Saposhnikoviae) and *Zi Su Ye* (Folium Perillae).
- With generalized blood deficiency in women, add *Si Wu Tang* (Four-Substance Decoction).
- With generalized deficiency after recovery from an illness, combine with *Xiao Chai Hu Tang* (Minor Bupleurum Decoction).
- For *gan ji* (infantile malnutrition) caused by yin deficiency, add *Gou Qi Zi* (Fructus Lycii) and *Nu Zhen Zi* (Fructus Ligustri Lucidi).

- For *gan ji* (infantile malnutrition) caused by food stagnation, add *Mai Ya* (Fructus Hordei Germinatus).

CAUTIONS / CONTRAINDICATIONS

- *Liu Jun Zi Tang*, although gentle, is slightly warm. Long-term use of this formula may cause dry mouth, dry tongue, thirst, or irritability.
- This formula should be used with caution, or avoid in patients who have high fever, yin-deficient heat, excess heat, qi stagnation, body fluid deficiency, irritability, thirst, or constipation.
- Avoid cold or raw, pungent or spicy, and oily or greasy foods while taking this formula.[1]

PHARMACOLOGICAL EFFECTS

1. **Gastrointestinal**: According to laboratory experiments in rabbits, administration of *Liu Jun Zi Tang* was associated with regulatory effects on the intestines. Depending on the condition of the subject, it will either increase or decrease intestinal peristalsis.[2] According to another study, *Liu Jun Zi Tang* promoted adaptive relaxation and provided symptom relief in patients with functional dyspepsia.[3] Lastly, one study reported *Liu Jun Zi Tang* to have a prokinetic action on gastric emptying to treat chronic dyspepsia.[4] In regards to plasma levels of gut-regulated peptide, administration of *Liu Jun Zi Tang* caused significant increases in plasma somatostatin and gastrin levels at 60 to 240 minutes compared with a placebo group.[5]

2. **Gastroprotective**: In one study in rats, use of *Liu Jun Zi Tang* had a dose-dependent effect and significantly inhibited gastric mucosal damage caused by absolute ethanol at doses over 500 mg/kg. The mechanism of this gastroprotective effect occurred partly through nitric oxide, not through prostaglandins or sulfhydryls.[6]

3. **Antineoplastic**: Subcutaneous injection of a modified *Liu Jun Zi Tang* preparation, followed by oral ingestion for 20 days was determined to have an inhibitory effect on the growth of cancer cells in mice. The mechanisms of action were attributed to an increase of macrophages and natural killer (NK) cells.[7]

CLINICAL STUDIES AND RESEARCH

1. **Abdominal pain**: Patients with abdominal pain were treated with modified *Liu Jun Zi Tang* for 20 days. The causes of abdominal pain included chronic gastritis, gastric ulcer, and duodenal ulcer. The formula included the addition of *Yan Hu Suo* (Rhizoma Corydalis) and *Bai Shao* (Radix Paeoniae Alba). Out of 123 patients, the study reported significant improvement in 49 patients, moderate improvement in 65 patients, and no effect in 9 patients. The overall efficacy rate reported was 92.7%.[8]

528

Liù Jūn Zǐ Tāng (Six-Gentlemen Decoction)

2. **Morning sickness**: In one report, 93 pregnant women with nausea and vomiting were treated with good results using *Liu Jun Zi Tang* with the addition of *Sheng Jiang* (Rhizoma Zingiberis Recens), *Zhu Ru* (Caulis Bambusae in Taenia), and *Zi Su Geng* (Caulis Perillae). Most patients experienced relief with 2-4 packs of herbs, with some needing up to 14 packs.[9]

3. **Gastritis**: According to one study, administration of *Liu Jun Zi Tang* to 207 patients with acute or chronic gastritis was associated with significant improvement in 62.9% and moderate improvement in 82.3% of patients. The treatment protocol was to administer 2.5g of the herbs in powder form, three times a day before meals.[10]

4. **Bitter taste in chronic gastritis**: Administration of *Liu Jun Zi Tang* was found to be effective in relieving a bitter taste in the mouth in patients diagnosed with chronic gastritis. The herbal therapy was very effective in 12 (80%) of 15 patients, with improvement noted in the other 3 patients. The average duration of treatment was 24.7 days for the 12 patients who responded. The study indicated that this formula may be a good remedy for the symptom of a bitter taste in the mouth in patients with chronic gastritis.[11]

5. **Duodenal ulcer**: Administration of modified *Liu Jun Zi Tang* was effective in treating 31 patients with duodenal ulcer. The herbal treatment contained *Liu Jun Zi Tang* plus *Yan Hu Suo* (Rhizoma Corydalis), *Hai Piao Xiao* (Endoconcha Sepiae), and *Bai Zhi* (Radix Angelicae Dahuricae) as the base formula. Additional modifications were made as follows: *Ru Xiang* (Gummi Olibanum) and *Mo Yao* (Myrrha) for severe pain; *Huang Lian* (Rhizoma Coptidis) for acid reflux and belching; *Zuo Jin Wan* (Left Metal Pill) for a bitter taste in the mouth, dry mouth, and acid reflux; *Si Ni San* (Frigid Extremities Powder) for hypochondriac pain; *Zhi Shi* (Fructus Aurantii Immaturus) for epigastric fullness and distention; and *Di Yu* (Radix Sanguisorbae) for hematochezia. The duration of treatment was 30 days per course of treatment. Of 31 patients, 9 had complete recovery, 11 had significant improvement, 8 had moderate improvement, and 3 had no improvement . The overall rate of effectiveness was 90.3%.[12]

6. **Stomatitis**: Administration of modified *Liu Jun Zi Tang* was associated with 96.16% effectiveness in treating 130 patients with stomatitis. The treatment protocol was to administer the herbs in decoction daily, with duration of treatment ranging from 6-30 packs of herbs. In addition to the base formula, the herbal formula was modified as follows: *Huang Qi* (Radix Astragali) and *Sha Shen* (Radix Glehniae seu Adenophorae) were added for Stomach yin deficiency; charred *Shan Zha* (Fructus Crataegi), charred *Shen Qu* (Massa Fermentata), charred *Mai Ya* (Fructus Hordei Germinatus), *Ji Nei Jin* (Endothelium Corneum Gigeriae Galli), and *Fo Shou* (Fructus Citri Sarcodactylis) for food stagnation in the middle *jiao* with acid reflux, nausea, and vomiting; *Bai Shao* (Radix Paeoniae Alba), *Wu Wei Zi* (Fructus Schisandrae Chinensis), and *Mu Li* (Concha Ostreae) for severe pain with a dry mouth and bad breath; *Dang Gui* (Radix Angelicae Sinensis), *Rou Cong Rong* (Herba Cistanches), and *Che Qian Zi* (Semen Plantaginis) for dysuria and constipation; and *Huang Lian* (Rhizoma Coptidis), *Jin Yin Hua* (Flos Lonicerae Japonicae), and *Xuan Shen* (Radix Scrophulariae) for Heart fire rising. Of 130 patients, the study reported complete recovery in 84 patients, improvement in 41 patients, and no change in 5 patients.[13]

7. **Indigestion**: One study reported 90.0% rate of effectiveness using modified *Liu Jun Zi Tang* to treat indigestion in 60 patients. In addition to the base formula, herbs were added as follows: *Wu Yao* (Radix Linderae), *Mu Xiang* (Radix Aucklandiae), and *Sha Ren* (Fructus Amomi) for qi stagnation; *Zhu Ru* (Caulis Bambusae in Taenia), *Huang Lian* (Rhizoma Coptidis), and *Pu Gong Ying* (Herba Taraxaci) for damp-heat; *Chi Shao* (Radix Paeoniae Rubra), *Dan Shen* (Radix et Rhizoma Salviae Miltiorrhizae), and *Dang Gui Wei* (Extremitas Radix Angelicae Sinensis) for chronic illness with blood stagnation, and processed *Huang Qi* (Radix Astragali) for qi deficiency. The duration of treatment was 30 days per course of treatment, for 2 courses total. Of 60 patients, the study reported complete recovery in 13 patients, significant improvement in 21 patients, moderate improvement in 14 patients, slight improvement in 6 patients, and no change in 6 patients.[14]

8. **Gastrointestinal disorder**: The use of *Liu Jun Zi Tang* has been associated with numerous benefits in treating gastrointestinal disorders, such as stomach prolapse, gastric pain, diarrhea, gastritis, and peptic ulcer.[15]

9. **Chronic bronchitis**: *Liu Jun Zi Tang* plus *Tu Si Zi* (Semen Cuscutae), *Wu Ling Zhi* (Faeces Trogopteri), and *Dan Shen* (Radix et Rhizoma Salviae Miltiorrhizae) effectively treated chronic bronchitis characterized by Spleen deficiency and phlegm obstruction in the Lung. The patients received 1 pack of herbs per day for a month, for a total of 30 packs. Of 30 patients, the study reported 93.3% rate of effectiveness.[16]

10. **Pain from liver cancer**: One study reported 87.7% effectiveness in relieving pain in 65 patients with liver cancer. The herbal formula contained *Liu Jun Zi Tang* plus *Hou Po* (Cortex Magnoliae Officinalis), *Dan Shen* (Radix et Rhizoma Salviae Miltiorrhizae), *Tu Bie Chong* (Eupolyphaga seu Steleophaga), *Shui Zhi* (Hirudo), *Wu Gong* (Scolopendra) and *Ma Qian Zi* (Semen Strychni).[17]

11. **Stress and depression**: One study evaluated the clinical usefulness of *Liu Jun Zi Tang* in the treatment of stress and depression by examining the modulatory effects of

Chapter 8 – Tonic Formulas   *Section 1 – Qi-Tonifying Formulas*

Liù Jūn Zǐ Tāng (Six-Gentlemen Decoction)

the herbs on the hypothalamo-pituitary-adrenal axis and autonomic nervous functions. Of several formulas tested, three were found to affect plasma ACTH and cortisol levels under stress. The study stated that the modulatory effects of these formulas might be beneficial in treating stress-related disease. The three formulas that were found to be effective were *Liu Jun Zi Tang, Ban Xia Xie Xin Tang* (Pinellia Decoction to Drain the Epigastrium), and *Ban Xia Hou Po Tang* (Pinellia and Magnolia Bark Decoction).[18]

HERB-DRUG INTERACTION

• **Chemotherapy-induced side effects**: Administration of *Liu Jun Zi Tang* showed effectiveness in alleviating gastrointestinal side effects associated with chemotherapy. The base formula included *Liu Jun Zi Tang* plus *Shen Qu* (Massa Fermentata), *Hou Po* (Cortex Magnoliae Officinalis), and *Shan Yao* (Rhizoma Dioscoreae). Modifications include the addition of *Huang Lian* (Rhizoma Coptidis), *Zhu Ru* (Caulis Bambusae in Taenia), and *Sheng Jiang* (Rhizoma Zingiberis Recens) for continuous nausea and vomiting; *Cang Zhu* (Rhizoma Atractylodis), *Pei Lan* (Herba Eupatorii), and *Zhi Qiao* (Fructus Aurantii) for a thick, greasy tongue coating; and *Huang Qi* (Radix Astragali), *Ji Xue Teng* (Caulis Spatholobi), and *Yin Yang Huo* (Herba Epimedii) for qi deficiency, fatigue, and low white blood cell count. Patients were given herbs three times daily until the end of their chemotherapy treatment. Of 74 patients, the study reported complete relief in 49 patients, improvement in 24 patients, and no effect in 1 case. The rate of effectiveness was 98.6%.[19] In another study involving 110 patients on chemotherapy, use of *Liu Jun Zi Tang* plus *Huang Qi* (Radix Astragali) and *Yi Yi Ren* (Semen Coicis) was associated with relieving nausea and vomiting, and increased white blood cell count.[20]

• **Levofloxacin**: In a study of 8 healthy subjects, co-administrations of levofloxacin and *Liu Jun Zi Tang* did not cause any significant differences in any pharmacokinetic parameters, urinary recovery and renal clearance of levofloxacin. The study concluded that *Liu Jun Zi Tang* did not have a significant effect on the rate and extent of bioavailability, or renal excretion of levofloxacin.[21]

• **Ofloxacin**: A study of 7 volunteers in an open, random crossover fashion found no significant effect on the rate and extent of bioavailability of ofloxacin with co-administrations of *Liu Jun Zi Tang, Xiao Chai Hu Tang* (Minor Bupleurum Decoction), or *Chai Ling Tang* (Bupleurum and Poria Decoction).[22]

TOXICOLOGY

Use of *Liu Jun Zi Tang* has been associated with one case of pneumonitis in a 79-year-old woman who complained

of dry cough and dyspnea on exertion after taking the herbs. At the time of publication, this is the only case of pulmonary hypersensitivity due to *Liu Jun Zi Tang* reported in the world.[23]

References

1. *Zhong Yao Ming Fang Yao Li Yu Ying Yong* (Pharmacology and Applications of Famous Herbal Formulas) 1989;249-251.

2. *Nan Jing Zhong Yi Xue Yuan Xue Bao* (Journal of Nanjing University of Traditional Chinese Medicine) 1989;1:36.

3. Hayakawa T, Arakawa T, Kase Y, Akiyama S, Ishige A, Takeda S, Sasaki H, Uno H, Fukuda T, Higuchi K, Kobayashi K. Liu-Jun-Zi-Tang, a kampo medicine, promotes adaptive relaxation in isolated guinea pig stomachs. Drugs Exp Clin Res 1999;25(5):211-8.

4. Tatsuta M, Iishi H. Effect of treatment with liu-jun-zi-tang (TJ-43) on gastric emptying and gastrointestinal symptoms in dyspeptic patients. Aliment Pharmacol Ther 1993 Aug;7(4):459-62.

5. Naito T, Itoh H, Yasunaga F, Takeyama M. Rikkunshi-to raises levels of somatostatin and gastrin in human plasma. Biol Pharm Bull 2001 Jul;24(7):841-3.

6. Arakawa T, Higuchi K, Fujiwara Y, Watanabe T, Tominaga K, Hayakawa T, Kuroki T. Gastroprotection by Liu-Jun-Zi-Tang (TJ-43): possible mediation of nitric oxide but not prostaglandins or sulfhydryls. Drugs Under Experimental & Clinical Research 1999;25(5):207-10.

7. *Shi Yong Zhong Liu Xue Za Zhi* (Practical Journal of Cancer) 1987;1(4):6.

8. *Shan Xi Xin Zhong Yi* (New Shanxi Chinese Medicine) 1984;1:23.

9. *Shang Hai Zhong Yi Yao Za Zhi* (Shanghai Journal of Chinese Medicine and Herbology) 1959;7:48.

10. *Zhong Yi Ming Fang Lin Chuang Xin Yong* (Contemporary Clinical Applications of Classic Chinese Formulas) 2001;160.

11. Motoo Y, Watanabe H, Okai T, Sawabu N. Effect of liu-junzi-tang on the symptom of bitter taste in patients with chronic gastritis. American Journal of Chinese Medicine 1995;23(2):153-7.

12. *Si Chuan Zhong Yi* (Sichuan Chinese Medicine) 1989;2:21.

13. *Shi Yong Zhong Yi Za Zhi* (Journal of Practical Chinese Medicine) 1997;2:11.

14. *Zhong Yi Ming Fang Lin Chuang Xin Yong* (Contemporary Clinical Applications of Classic Chinese Formulas) 2001;161.

15. *Zhong Yi Fang Ji Xian Dai Yan Jiu* (Modern Study of Medical Formulae in Traditional Chinese Medicine) 1997;493.

16. *Chong Qing Yi Yao* (Chongching Medicine and Herbology) 1994;5:309.

17. *Jiang Su Zhong Yi* (Jiangsu Chinese Medicine) 1997;6:23.

18. Naito T, Itoh H, Takeyama M. Some gastrointestinal function regulatory Kampo medicines have modulatory effects on human plasma adrenocorticotropic hormone and cortisol levels with continual stress exposure. Biological & Pharmaceutical Bulletin 2003 Jan;26(1):101-4.

19. *Shi Yong Zhong Xi Yi Jie He Za Zhi* (Practical Journal of Integrated Chinese and Western Medicines) 1992;9:528.

20. *Zhong Yi Yao Xin Xi* (Information on Chinese Medicine and Herbology) 1995;6:27.

21. Hasegawa T, Yamaki K, Muraoka I, Nadai M, Takagi K, Nabeshima T. Effects of traditional Chinese medicines on pharmacokinetics of levofloxacin. Antimicrobial Agents & Chemotherapy 1995 Sep;39(9):2135-7.

22. Hasegawa T, Yamaki K, Nadai M, Muraoka I, Wang L, Takagi K, Nabeshima T. Lack of effect of Chinese medicines on bioavailability of ofloxacin in healthy volunteers. Int J Clin Pharmacol Ther 1994 Feb;32(2):57-61.

23. Maruyama Y, Maruyama M, Takada T, Haraguchi M, Uno K. A case of pneumonitis due to Rikkunshi-to. Nihon Kyobu Shikkan Gakkai Zasshi 1994 Jan;32(1):84-9.

Chinese Herbal Formulas and Applications

Xiāng Shā Liù Jūn Zǐ Tāng
(Six-Gentlemen Decoction with Aucklandia and Amomum)

香砂六君子湯
香砂六君子汤

Pinyin Name: *Xiang Sha Liu Jun Zi Tang*
Literal Name: Six-Gentlemen Decoction with Aucklandia and Amomum
Alternate Names: *Hsiang Sha Liu Chun Tzu Tang*, Aucklandia and Amomum Gentlemen Decoction, Saussurea and Six-Major-Herb Decoction, Vladimiria and Cardamon Combination, Saussurea and Cardamon Combination
Original Source: *Gu Jin Ming Fang* (Famous Classic and Contemporary Formulas) by Luo Mei in 1675

COMPOSITION

Ren Shen (Radix et Rhizoma Ginseng)	3g
Bai Zhu (Rhizoma Atractylodis Macrocephalae)	6g
Fu Ling (Poria)	6g
Gan Cao (Radix et Rhizoma Glycyrrhizae)	2.1g
Ban Xia (Rhizoma Pinelliae)	3g
Chen Pi (Pericarpium Citri Reticulatae)	2.4g
Mu Xiang (Radix Aucklandiae)	2.1g
Sha Ren (Fructus Amomi)	2.4g

DOSAGE / PREPARATION / ADMINISTRATION

Prepare the ingredients as a decoction with 6g of *Sheng Jiang* (Rhizoma Zingiberis Recens).

CHINESE THERAPEUTIC ACTIONS

1. Tonifies qi, strengthens the Spleen, and harmonizes the Stomach
2. Regulates qi and warms the middle *jiao*

CLINICAL MANIFESTATIONS

Spleen and Stomach qi deficiencies accompanied by cold and damp stagnation in the middle *jiao*: loss of appetite, belching, fullness and/or pain of the abdomen and epigastrium, vomiting, and loose stools.

CLINICAL APPLICATIONS

Gastritis, chronic gastritis, gastric and duodenal ulcer, gastroenteritis, gastroptosis, chronic atrophic gastritis, irritable bowel syndrome, stomatitis, post-surgical diarrhea, morning sickness, anorexia, liver cirrhosis, bronchitis, and bronchiectasis.

EXPLANATION

Xiang Sha Liu Jun Zi Tang (Six-Gentlemen Decoction with Aucklandia and Amomum) combines *Liu Jun Zi Tang* (Six-Gentlemen Decoction) with *Mu Xiang* (Radix Aucklandiae) and *Sha Ren* (Fructus Amomi) to treat deficiency of the middle *jiao* with cold and damp stagnation. Spleen and Stomach deficiencies weaken the digestive system, causing loss of appetite, belching, and general weakness. Damp accumulation and cold stagnation cause fullness

and pain in the abdomen and epigastrium. In addition, dampness and cold block Stomach qi from descending properly, causing vomiting. Moreover, as a result of Spleen deficiency, the normally ascending qi of the Spleen actually descends, resulting in loose stools or diarrhea.

Ren Shen (Radix et Rhizoma Ginseng), *Bai Zhu* (Rhizoma Atractylodis Macrocephalae), *Fu Ling* (Poria), and *Gan Cao* (Radix et Rhizoma Glycyrrhizae), four herbs from *Si Jun Zi Tang* (Four-Gentlemen Decoction), tonify Spleen and Stomach qi. *Ban Xia* (Rhizoma Pinelliae) and *Chen Pi* (Pericarpium Citri Reticulatae) break up qi and damp stagnation, and correct the reversed flow of Stomach qi. *Mu Xiang* (Radix Aucklandiae) and *Sha Ren* (Fructus Amomi) warm the middle *jiao* and activate qi circulation to dissolve damp accumulation and relieve fullness and pain.

MODIFICATIONS

- With lack of appetite, add *Mai Ya* (Fructus Hordei Germinatus) and *Shan Zha* (Fructus Crataegi).
- If there is abdominal fullness due to deficiency and cold, add *Fu Zi* (Radix Aconiti Lateralis Praeparata) and *Gan Jiang* (Rhizoma Zingiberis).
- For Spleen and Stomach qi deficiencies, add *Huang Qi* (Radix Astragali) and *Shan Yao* (Rhizoma Dioscoreae).
- With nausea, vomiting, and food retention, add *Huo Xiang* (Herba Agastaches) and *Zhu Ru* (Caulis Bambusae in Taenia).
- With hot phlegm and qi deficiency, add ginger-processed *Huang Lian* (Rhizoma Coptidis).

8

TONIC FORMULAS

531

Chapter 8 – Tonic Formulas   *Section 1 – Qi-Tonifying Formulas*

Xiāng Shā Liù Jūn Zǐ Tāng
(Six-Gentlemen Decoction with Aucklandia and Amomum)

Xiang Sha Liu Jun Zi Tang (Six-Gentlemen Decoction with Aucklandia and Amomum)

Diagnosis	Signs and Symptoms	Treatment	Herbs
Spleen and Stomach qi deficiencies accompanied by cold and damp stagnation in the middle *jiao*	• Loss of appetite, belching, loose stools, and general weakness: Spleen and Stomach deficiencies • Chest pain and fullness: cold and damp accumulation in the Lung • Nausea and vomiting: cold and damp stagnation in the Stomach	• Tonifies qi, strengthens the Spleen, and harmonizes the Stomach • Regulates qi and warms the middle *jiao*	• *Ren Shen* (Radix et Rhizoma Ginseng), *Bai Zhu* (Rhizoma Atractylodis Macrocephalae), *Fu Ling* (Poria), and *Gan Cao* (Radix et Rhizoma Glycyrrhizae) tonify Spleen and Stomach qi. • *Ban Xia* (Rhizoma Pinelliae) and *Chen Pi* (Pericarpium Citri Reticulatae) break up qi and damp stagnation and correct the reversed flow of qi. • *Mu Xiang* (Radix Aucklandiae) and *Sha Ren* (Fructus Amomi) warm the middle *jiao*, activate qi circulation, and relieve fullness and pain.

• With cold phlegm and qi deficiency, add *Pao Jiang* (Rhizoma Zingiberis Praeparatum).

• With vomiting and diarrhea, combine with *Ping Wei San* (Calm the Stomach Powder).

• With vomiting and diarrhea due to summer-heat, combine with *San Huang Xie Xin Tang* (Three-Yellow Decoction to Sedate the Epigastrium).

• With vomiting and diarrhea due to deficiency and cold, combine with *Li Zhong Tang* (Regulate the Middle Decoction).

CAUTIONS / CONTRAINDICATIONS

Individuals taking *Xiang Sha Liu Jun Zi Tang* should avoid raw and cold foods.[1]

PHARMACOLOGICAL EFFECTS

1. **Gastrointestinal**: According to laboratory experiments in rabbits, administration of *Xiang Sha Liu Jun Zi Tang* was associated with a regulatory effect on the intestines. Depending on the condition of the subject, it either increased or decreased intestinal peristalsis.[2]

2. **Antiulcer**: Administration of *Xiang Sha Liu Jun Zi Tang* was associated with a marked effect in preventing and treating stomach ulcer in rats. The mechanisms of action were attributed to promotion of normal stomach mucosa, and decreased production of gastric acid.[3]

3. **Immunostimulant**: Administration of *Xiang Sha Liu Jun Zi Tang* was associated with an increase of IgM, IgA, and T cells.[4,5]

CLINICAL STUDIES AND RESEARCH

1. **Chronic atrophic gastritis**: *Xiang Sha Liu Jun Zi Tang* was used to treat patients with chronic atrophic gastritis characterized by deficiency and cold. Out of 25 cases, the study reported significant improvement with resolution of the symptoms in 18 cases, and moderate improvement

with slight pain in 7 cases.[6] In another study, use of *Xiang Sha Liu Jun Zi Tang* plus *Shan Yao* (Rhizoma Dioscoreae) daily was associated with complete recovery in 12 of 14 patients with chronic atrophic gastritis characterized by Spleen qi deficiency.[7]

2. **Gastritis**: Use of *Xiang Sha Liu Jun Zi Tang* daily for 4 weeks per course of treatment was associated with marked effect to treat chronic gastritis in elderly patients. Of 23 patients, the study reported complete recovery in 9 cases, marked improvement in 12 cases, and no effect in 2 cases. The overall effectiveness was 91.3%.[8]

3. **Irritable bowel syndrome (IBS)**: In one study, 40 patients with irritable bowel syndrome were treated with marked improvement in 18 cases, moderate improvement in 16 cases, and no effect in 6 cases. The herbal treatment included this formula plus *Yan Hu Suo* (Rhizoma Corydalis), *Ru Xiang* (Gummi Olibanum), and *Mo Yao* (Myrrha). Furthermore, *Xiang Fu* (Rhizoma Cyperi) and *Yu Jin* (Radix Curcumae) were added for emotional distress; and *Pu Huang* (Pollen Typhae) and *Wu Ling Zhi* (Faeces Trogopteri) were added for menstrual pain. The treatment protocol was to administer the herbs for 2 weeks per course of treatment, for 1-3 courses total.[9]

4. **Stomatitis**: In one report, 30 patients with recurrent stomatitis were treated with modified *Xiang Sha Liu Jun Zi Tang* in decoction with complete recovery in all patients. The length of treatment varied from 4-20 packs of herbs. The herbal treatment contained *Xiang Sha Liu Jun Zi Tang*, with the addition of *Zhi Zi* (Fructus Gardeniae) for diarrhea with preference for warm drinks; *Huang Lian* (Rhizoma Coptidis), *Zhu Ye* (Herba Phyllostachys), and *Di Huang* (Radix Rehmanniae) for red tongue tip from Heart fire rising; and the addition of *Mu Dan Pi* (Cortex Moutan) and removal of *Ren Shen* (Radix et Rhizoma Ginseng) for dry throat with a bitter taste in the mouth.[10]

532

Xiāng Shā Liù Jūn Zǐ Tāng

(Six-Gentlemen Decoction with Aucklandia and Amomum)

5. **Post-surgical diarrhea**: Administration of modified *Xiang Sha Liu Jun Zi Tang* was associated with 90.25% effectiveness in treating 113 patients with post-surgical diarrhea. The herbs were given in decoction daily for 2 weeks per course of treatment.[11]

6. **Morning sickness**: Modified *Xiang Sha Liu Jun Zi Tang* was used to treat pregnant women with nausea and vomiting with good results. Out of 52 cases, the study reported complete recovery in 42 cases, improvement in 9 cases, and no benefit in 1 case. Most patients responded within 1-3 days of herbal therapy.[12]

7. **Anorexia**: Modified *Xiang Sha Liu Jun Zi Tang* was used to treat 33 children with anorexia with 94% effectiveness. The herbal treatment included this formula plus *Bing Lang* (Semen Arecae), *Lai Fu Zi* (Semen Raphani), charred *Ji Nei Jin* (Endothelium Corneum Gigeriae Galli), and charred *Shan Zha* (Fructus Crataegi). The treatment protocol was to administer the herbs daily, with 8 packs of herbs per course of treatment, followed by 3-5 days of rest, and then a second 8-pack course. Of 33 patients, the study reported marked effectiveness in 19 cases, moderate effectiveness in 12 cases, and no effect in 2 cases.[13]

TOXICOLOGY

In an acute toxicology study, oral ingestion of *Xiang Sha Liu Jun Zi Tang* in decoction at 0.4 mL/10g (equivalent to 80 g/kg of raw herbs) twice daily for 7 days did not cause any abnormal behavior in animal subjects. In fact, some subjects had an increase in body weight. The dose given to the subjects was equivalent to 434 times the normal adult dose in humans.[14]

RELATED FORMULA

Xiāng Shā Liù Jūn Zǐ Tāng

(Six-Gentlemen Decoction with Cyperus and Amomum)

香砂六君子湯
香砂六君子汤

Pinyin Name: *Xiang Sha Liu Jun Zi Tang*

Literal Name: Six-Gentlemen Decoction with Cyperus and Amomum

Original Source: *Yi Fang Ji Jie* (Analytical Collection of Medical Formulas) by Wang Ang in 1682

Ren Shen (Radix et Rhizoma Ginseng)	6g
Bai Zhu (Rhizoma Atractylodis Macrocephalae)	6g
Fu Ling (Poria)	6g
Zhi Gan Cao (Radix et Rhizoma Glycyrrhizae Praeparata cum Melle)	3g
Chen Pi (Pericarpium Citri Reticulatae)	3g
Ban Xia (Rhizoma Pinelliae)	3g
Xiang Fu (Rhizoma Cyperi)	6g
Sha Ren (Fructus Amomi)	6g

This formula is composed by adding *Xiang Fu* (Rhizoma Cyperi) and *Sha Ren* (Fructus Amomi) to *Liu Jun Zi Tang* (Six-Gentlemen Decoction). This formula strengthens the Spleen, harmonizes the Stomach, regulates qi circulation, and stops pain. It treats Spleen and Stomach qi deficiencies accompanied by accumulation of cold and dampness in the middle *jiao*.

These two formulas above have identical Chinese characters and pinyin names. They also have very similar ingredients, doses, and functions.

- In the primary formula, "*Xiang*" refers to *Mu Xiang* (Radix Aucklandiae), a qi-regulating herb that treats qi stagnation of the Spleen and Stomach. *Gan Cao* (Radix et Rhizoma Glycyrrhizae) is used to tonify qi and harmonize the formula.

- In the related formula, "*Xiang*" refers to *Xiang Fu* (Rhizoma Cyperi), a qi-regulating herb that treats qi stagnation in the Liver and *San Jiao*. *Zhi Gan Cao* (Radix et Rhizoma Glycyrrhizae Praeparata cum Melle) is used to strongly tonify qi and harmonize the formula.

References

1. *Zhong Yao Ming Fang Yao Li Yu Ying Yong* (Pharmacology and Applications of Famous Herbal Formulas) 1989;405-406.
2. *Zhong Yi Fang Ji Xian Dai Yan Jiu* (Modern Study of Medical Formulae in Traditional Chinese Medicine) 1997;499-500.
3. *Bei Jing Zhong Yi Yao Da Xue Xue Bao* (Journal of Beijing University of Medicine and Medicinals) 1994;17(5):57.
4. *Liao Ning Zhong Yi Za Zhi* (Liaoning Journal of Chinese Medicine) 1982;7:4.
5. *Shan Dong Zhong Yi Za Zhi* (Shandong Journal of Chinese Medicine) 1986;27(11):53.
6. *Nan Jing Zhong Yi Xue Yuan Xue Bao* (Journal of Nanjing University of Traditional Chinese Medicine) 1987;4:23.
7. *Liao Ning Zhong Yi Za Zhi* (Liaoning Journal of Chinese Medicine) 1982;7:4.
8. *Shan Xi Zhong Yi Xue Yuan Xue Bao* (Journal of Shanxi University School of Chinese Medicine) 1999;3:44.
9. *Hu Bei Zhong Yi Za Zhi* (Hubei Journal of Chinese Medicine) 1997;3:15.
10. *Shan Dong Zhong Yi Za Zhi* (Shandong Journal of Chinese Medicine) 1991;10(5):32.
11. *Fu Jian Zhong Yi Yao* (Fujian Chinese Medicine and Herbology) 1996;3:34.
12. *Zhong Hua Fu Chan Ke Za Zhi* (Chinese Journal of Obstetrics and Gynecology) 1960;8(1):33.
13. *Gan Su Zhong Yi Xue Yuan Xue Bao* (Journal of Gansu University of Chinese Medicine) 1995;2:26.
14. *Zhong Yao Yao Li Yu Lin Chuang* (Pharmacology and Clinical Applications of Chinese Herbs) 1990;6(2):5.

Xiāng Shā Yǎng Wèi Tāng

(Nourish the Stomach Decoction with Aucklandia and Amomum)

香砂養胃湯
香砂养胃汤

Pinyin Name: *Xiang Sha Yang Wei Tang*
Literal Name: Nourish the Stomach Decoction with Aucklandia and Amomum
Alternate Name: Cyperus and Cluster Combination
Original Source: *Wan Bing Hui Chun* (Restoration of Health from the Myriad Diseases) by Gong Ting-Xian in 1587

COMPOSITION

Ren Shen (Radix et Rhizoma Ginseng)	1.5g
Bai Zhu (Rhizoma Atractylodis Macrocephalae)	3g
Fu Ling (Poria)	2.4g
Zhi Gan Cao (Radix et Rhizoma Glycyrrhizae Praeparata cum Melle), a small amount	[0.6g]
Cang Zhu (Rhizoma Atractylodis), *zhi* (prepared) with rice water and *chao* (dry-fried)	2.4g
Sha Ren (Fructus Amomi)	2.4g
Dou Kou (Fructus Amomi Rotundus)	2.1g
Xiang Fu (Rhizoma Cyperi), *chao* (dry-fried)	2.4g
Mu Xiang (Radix Aucklandiae)	1.5g
Hou Po (Cortex Magnoliae Officinalis), *chao* (dry-fried) with ginger juice	2.4g
Chen Pi (Pericarpium Citri Reticulatae)	2.4g

DOSAGE / PREPARATION / ADMINISTRATION

Grind the herbs into powder, and cook the powder with *Sheng Jiang* (Rhizoma Zingiberis Recens) and *Da Zao* (Fructus Jujubae) to make a decoction.

CHINESE THERAPEUTIC ACTIONS

1. Strengthens the Spleen and dispels dampness
2. Improves appetite

CLINICAL MANIFESTATIONS

Low appetite caused by Spleen deficiency: lack of appetite and epigastric discomfort or distention.

CLINICAL APPLICATIONS

Chronic gastritis, gastroenteritis, gastroptosis, and gastric and duodenal ulcer.

EXPLANATION

Spleen deficiency can lead to the formation of dampness, which causes loss of appetite because the transportation

Xiang Sha Yang Wei Tang (Nourish the Stomach Decoction with Aucklandia and Amomum)

Diagnosis	Signs and Symptoms	Treatment	Herbs
Low appetite caused by Spleen deficiency	• Lack of appetite: Spleen deficiency • Epigastric discomfort or distention: damp accumulation	• Strengthens the Spleen and dispels dampness • Improves appetite	• *Ren Shen* (Radix et Rhizoma Ginseng), *Bai Zhu* (Rhizoma Atractylodis Macrocephalae), *Fu Ling* (Poria), *Da Zao* (Fructus Jujubae), and *Zhi Gan Cao* (Radix et Rhizoma Glycyrrhizae Praeparata cum Melle) tonify Spleen qi. • *Cang Zhu* (Rhizoma Atractylodis), *Sha Ren* (Fructus Amomi), and *Dou Kou* (Fructus Amomi Rotundus) dry dampness and increase appetite. • *Xiang Fu* (Rhizoma Cyperi), *Mu Xiang* (Radix Aucklandiae), *Hou Po* (Cortex Magnoliae Officinalis), and *Chen Pi* (Pericarpium Citri Reticulatae) activate qi to dispel dampness. • *Sheng Jiang* (Rhizoma Zingiberis Recens) harmonizes the Stomach to increase appetite.

Chinese Herbal Formulas and Applications

Xiāng Shā Yǎng Wèi Tāng
(Nourish the Stomach Decoction with Aucklandia and Amomum)

and transformation functions of the Spleen are impaired. *Xiang Sha Yang Wei Tang* (Nourish the Stomach Decoction with Aucklandia and Amomum) tonifies Spleen qi, dispels dampness, and activates qi circulation.

Ren Shen (Radix et Rhizoma Ginseng), *Bai Zhu* (Rhizoma Atractylodis Macrocephalae), *Fu Ling* (Poria), *Da Zao* (Fructus Jujubae), and *Zhi Gan Cao* (Radix et Rhizoma Glycyrrhizae Praeparata cum Melle) tonify Spleen qi. *Cang Zhu* (Rhizoma Atractylodis), *Sha Ren* (Fructus Amomi), and *Dou Kou* (Fructus Amomi Rotundus) are aromatic herbs that dry dampness and increase appetite. *Xiang Fu*

(Rhizoma Cyperi), *Mu Xiang* (Radix Aucklandiae), *Hou Po* (Cortex Magnoliae Officinalis), and *Chen Pi* (Pericarpium Citri Reticulatae) activate qi to dispel dampness. *Sheng Jiang* (Rhizoma Zingiberis Recens) harmonizes the Stomach to improve appetite.

CAUTIONS / CONTRAINDICATIONS

Avoid raw and cold foods while taking *Xiang Sha Yang Wei Tang*.[1]

Reference
1. *Zhong Yao Ming Fang Yao Li Yu Ying Yong* (Pharmacology and Applications of Famous Herbal Formulas) 1989;622-623.

Shēn Líng Bái Zhú Sǎn
(Ginseng, Poria, and Atractylodes Macrocephala Powder)

参苓白术散
参苓白术散

Pinyin Name: *Shen Ling Bai Zhu San*
Literal Name: Ginseng, Poria, and Atractylodes Macrocephala Powder
Alternate Names: *Shen Ling Pai Chu San*, Ginseng, Poria and Bighead Atractylodes Powder; Ginseng and Atractylodes Formula
Original Source: *Tai Ping Hui Min He Ji Ju Fang* (Imperial Grace Formulary of the Tai Ping Era) by the Imperial Medical Department in 1078-85

COMPOSITION

Ren Shen (Radix et Rhizoma Ginseng)	960g [15g]
Bai Zhu (Rhizoma Atractylodis Macrocephalae)	960g [15g]
Fu Ling (Poria)	960g [15g]
Gan Cao (Radix et Rhizoma Glycyrrhizae), *chao* (dry-fried)	960g [9g]
Shan Yao (Rhizoma Dioscoreae)	960g [15g]
Lian Zi (Semen Nelumbinis)	480g [9g]
Bai Bian Dou (Semen Lablab Album), *jin* (soaked) in ginger juice and *chao* (dry-fried)	720g [12g]
Yi Yi Ren (Semen Coicis)	480g [9g]
Sha Ren (Fructus Amomi)	480g [6g]
Jie Geng (Radix Platycodonis), *chao* (dry-fried) to dark brown	480g [6g]

DOSAGE / PREPARATION / ADMINISTRATION

The source text states to grind the ingredients into a fine powder. Take 6g of the powder per dose with a decoction made from *Da Zao* (Fructus Jujubae). Adjust the dose accordingly for children. Today, this formula may be prepared as a decoction with the doses suggested in brackets.

CHINESE THERAPEUTIC ACTIONS

1. Tonifies qi and strengthens the Spleen
2. Resolves dampness and stops diarrhea

CLINICAL MANIFESTATIONS

Spleen and Stomach deficiencies with dampness: loose stools or diarrhea, vomiting, borborygmus, decreased

535

Chapter 8 – Tonic Formulas   *Section 1 – Qi-Tonifying Formulas*

Shēn Líng Bái Zhú Sǎn
(Ginseng, Poria, and Atractylodes Macrocephala Powder)

appetite, weak extremities, weight loss, a sallow facial appearance, epigastric or chest fullness and a stifling sensation, a pale red tongue with a white tongue coating, and a fine, moderate or deficient, moderate pulse.

CLINICAL APPLICATIONS

Superficial gastritis, chronic gastroenteritis, chronic diarrhea, infantile diarrhea, dyspepsia, duodenal ulcer, gastroptosis, chronic colitis, irritable bowel syndrome, proctitis, nephritis, hepatitis and liver cirrhosis, compromised immune system, supportive therapy for chemotherapy and radiation, debility after chronic illness, cognitive impairment, rhinitis, edema, and abnormal vaginal discharge.

EXPLANATION

Shen Ling Bai Zhu San (Ginseng, Poria, and Atractylodes Macrocephala Powder) treats Spleen and Stomach deficiencies with damp accumulation. The Spleen and Stomach are in charge of transforming and transporting nutrients; deficiency in these two organs weakens the digestive function. As a result, food travels quickly through the body without being properly digested or absorbed, hence giving rise to loose stools or diarrhea. A weak digestive system may result in decreased appetite, weak extremities, weight loss, and a sallow facial appearance. Spleen deficiency usually causes damp accumulation, which in turn obstructs Lung qi, causing epigastric or chest fullness

and distention. Dampness can also obstruct Stomach qi, causing nausea and vomiting. The tongue and pulse both suggest deficiency in the body.

Ren Shen (Radix et Rhizoma Ginseng), *Bai Zhu* (Rhizoma Atractylodis Macrocephalae), *Fu Ling* (Poria), and *Gan Cao* (Radix et Rhizoma Glycyrrhizae) tonify qi and strengthen the Spleen and Stomach. *Shan Yao* (Rhizoma Dioscoreae) and *Lian Zi* (Semen Nelumbinis) treat diarrhea by assisting *Ren Shen* (Radix et Rhizoma Ginseng) in strengthening the Spleen and tonifying qi. *Bai Bian Dou* (Semen Lablab Album) and *Yi Yi Ren* (Semen Coicis) help *Bai Zhu* (Rhizoma Atractylodis Macrocephalae) and *Fu Ling* (Poria) strengthen the Spleen and dispel dampness. *Sha Ren* (Fructus Amomi) awakens the Spleen and harmonizes the Stomach to regulate qi and resolve stagnation. *Jie Geng* (Radix Platycodonis) relieves chest fullness, and has an ascending function to help counteract diarrhea. *Gan Cao* (Radix et Rhizoma Glycyrrhizae) harmonizes both the middle *jiao* and the formula.

MODIFICATIONS

- For loose stools with abdominal pain due to cold, add *Gan Jiang* (Rhizoma Zingiberis) and *Rou Gui* (Cortex Cinnamomi).
- For loose stools with damp-heat, add *Huang Lian* (Rhizoma Coptidis), *Che Qian Zi* (Semen Plantaginis), and *Ze Xie* (Rhizoma Alismatis).

Shen Ling Bai Zhu San (Ginseng, Poria, and Atractylodes Macrocephala Powder)

Diagnosis	Signs and Symptoms	Treatment	Herbs
Spleen and Stomach deficiencies with dampness	• Diarrhea, borborygmus, decreased appetite, and a sallow facial appearance: Spleen and Stomach qi deficiencies • Weak extremities and weight loss: Spleen and Stomach qi deficiencies unable to nourish the body and limbs • Epigastric or chest fullness and distention: damp accumulation blocking Lung qi circulation • Nausea and vomiting: damp accumulation obstructing Stomach qi circulation • Pale tongue with white tongue coating: qi deficiency • Fine, moderate or deficient, moderate pulse: qi deficiency	• Tonifies qi and strengthens the Spleen • Resolves dampness and stops diarrhea	• *Ren Shen* (Radix et Rhizoma Ginseng), *Bai Zhu* (Rhizoma Atractylodis Macrocephalae), *Fu Ling* (Poria), and *Gan Cao* (Radix et Rhizoma Glycyrrhizae) tonify qi and strengthen the Spleen and Stomach. • *Shan Yao* (Rhizoma Dioscoreae) and *Lian Zi* (Semen Nelumbinis) strengthen the Spleen, tonify qi, and stop diarrhea. • *Bai Bian Dou* (Semen Lablab Album) and *Yi Yi Ren* (Semen Coicis) strengthen the Spleen and dispel dampness. • *Sha Ren* (Fructus Amomi) awakens the Spleen and harmonizes the Stomach to regulate qi and resolve stagnation. • *Jie Geng* (Radix Platycodonis) ventilates the Lung and relieves chest fullness. • *Gan Cao* (Radix et Rhizoma Glycyrrhizae) harmonizes the middle *jiao* and all the herbs.

536

Shēn Líng Bái Zhú Săn
(Ginseng, Poria, and Atractylodes Macrocephala Powder)

- With phlegm accumulation, add *Ban Xia* (Rhizoma Pinelliae) and *Chen Pi* (Pericarpium Citri Reticulatae).
- For constant diarrhea, add *Qian Shi* (Semen Euryales) and *Mu Xiang* (Radix Aucklandiae).
- With frequent urination, add *Yi Zhi* (Fructus Alpiniae Oxyphyllae).
- For food retention, vomiting, and diarrhea, combine with *Ping Wei San* (Calm the Stomach Powder).
- For indigestion in children, add dry-fried *Mai Ya* (Fructus Hordei Germinatus), *Shan Zha* (Fructus Crataegi), and *Shen Qu* (Massa Fermentata).

CAUTIONS / CONTRAINDICATIONS

- *Shen Ling Bai Zhu San* should be used with caution in the following conditions: yin-deficient fire and yin deficiency.
- Since this formula is slightly drying and warm in nature, it should be used with caution during pregnancy, and in patients with exterior or interior heat conditions.[1]

PHARMACOLOGICAL EFFECTS

Gastrointestinal: According to laboratory experiments in rabbits, administration of *Shen Ling Bai Zhu San* was associated with a regulatory effect on the intestines. Depending on the condition of the subject, it either increased or decreased the intestinal peristalsis.[2]

CLINICAL STUDIES AND RESEARCH

1. **Superficial gastritis**: Use of modified *Shen Ling Bai Zhu San* in 32 patients with superficial gastritis was associated with 96.7% effectiveness. The herbal treatment contained *Ren Shen* (Radix et Rhizoma Ginseng), *Bai Zhu* (Rhizoma Atractylodis Macrocephalae), *Fu Ling* (Poria), *Shan Yao* (Rhizoma Dioscoreae), *Gan Cao* (Radix et Rhizoma Glycyrrhizae), *Bai Bian Dou* (Semen Lablab Album), *Bai Shao* (Radix Paeoniae Alba), *Yan Hu Suo* (Rhizoma Corydalis), *Yi Yi Ren* (Semen Coicis), *Sha Ren* (Fructus Amomi), *Ying Su Ke* (Pericarpium Papaveris), and *Bai Ji* (Rhizoma Bletillae). Furthermore, modifications were made by adding *Wu Zhu Yu* (Fructus Evodiae) and *Gao Liang Jiang* (Rhizoma Alpiniae Officinarum) for cold; *Chai Hu* (Radix Bupleuri), *Huang Qin* (Radix Scutellariae), and *Huang Lian* (Rhizoma Coptidis) for Stomach heat; *Fu Zi* (Radix Aconiti Lateralis Praeparata) and *Rou Gui* (Cortex Cinnamomi) for deficiency and cold; *Shen Qu* (Massa Fermentata), *Shan Zha* (Fructus Crataegi) and *Mai Ya* (Fructus Hordei Germinatus) for food stagnation; *Chai Hu* (Radix Bupleuri), *Xiang Fu* (Rhizoma Cyperi) and *Dou Kou* (Fructus Amomi Rotundus) for qi stagnation; and *Dan Shen* (Radix et Rhizoma Salviae Miltiorrhizae), *Mo Yao* (Myrrha), and *E Zhu* (Rhizoma Curcumae) for blood stagnation. Of 32 cases, the study reported complete recovery in 15 cases, significant improvement in 9 cases, moderate improvement in 7 cases, and no effect in 1 case.[3]

2. **Diarrhea**: In one clinical study, 95 patients with diarrhea (negative for microorganism infection) were treated with modified *Shen Ling Bai Zhu San*. In addition to this formula, *Bu Zhong Yi Qi Tang* (Tonify the Middle and Augment the Qi Decoction) was given to patients with Spleen qi deficiency; *Fu Zi Li Zhong Wan* (Prepared Aconite Pill to Regulate the Middle) for Spleen yang deficiency; and *Si Shen Wan* (Four-Miracle Pill) for Spleen and Kidney yang deficiency. Out of 95 cases, the study reported significant improvement in 27 cases, moderate improvement in 41 cases, and no effect in 27 cases. The overall rate of effectiveness was 71.6%.[4]

3. **Chronic colitis**: Use of modified *Shen Ling Bai Zhu San* one time daily in decoction showed good results in treating chronic colitis characterized by Spleen deficiency and dampness. Modifications to the base formula included addition of *Mu Xiang* (Radix Aucklandiae), dry-fried *Zhi Qiao* (Fructus Aurantii), and dry-fried *Lai Fu Zi* (Semen Raphani) for qi stagnation; dry-fried *Gu Ya* (Fructus Setariae Germinatus), dry-fried *Mai Ya* (Fructus Hordei Germinatus), dry-fried *Shen Qu* (Massa Fermentata), and charred *Shan Zha* (Fructus Crataegi) for diarrhea; *Xiang Fu* (Rhizoma Cyperi), *Gao Liang Jiang* (Rhizoma Alpiniae Officinarum), and vinegar-fried *Yan Hu Suo* (Rhizoma Corydalis) for abdominal pain; *Bu Gu Zhi* (Fructus Psoraleae), roasted *Rou Dou Kou* (Semen Myristicae), and salt-fried *Wu Zhu Yu* (Fructus Evodiae) for deficiency and cold of the Spleen and Kidney; and *Huang Qi* (Radix Astragali), *Chai Hu* (Radix Bupleuri), and *Sheng Ma* (Rhizoma Cimicifugae) for diarrhea and rectal prolapse due to qi collapse. Out of 60 cases, the study reported complete recovery in 38 cases, significant improvement in 14 cases, slight improvement in 6 cases, and no effect in 2 cases. The overall rate of effectiveness was 97%.[5]

4. **Irritable bowel syndrome (IBS)**: Use of modified *Shen Ling Bai Zhu San* in 52 patients with irritable bowel syndrome was associated with 96.2% effectiveness. In addition to the base formula, modifications included addition of *Huang Qi* (Radix Astragali) and *He Zi* (Fructus Chebulae) for deficiency and weakness of the Spleen and Stomach; *Chai Hu* (Radix Bupleuri), *Yu Jin* (Radix Curcumae), and *Yan Hu Suo* (Rhizoma Corydalis) for Liver qi stagnation and Spleen deficiency; *Huang Lian* (Rhizoma Coptidis), *Pei Lan* (Herba Eupatorii), and *Bai Tou Weng* (Radix Pulsatillae) for Spleen deficiency with damp-heat; and *Bu Gu Zhi* (Fructus Psoraleae), *Rou Dou Kou* (Semen Myristicae), and *Wu Zhu Yu* (Fructus Evodiae)

Shēn Líng Bái Zhú Sǎn
(Ginseng, Poria, and Atractylodes Macrocephala Powder)

for Spleen and Kidney yang deficiency. The herbs were given in decoction daily, with duration of treatment ranging from 5-30 days (average of 18.1 days). Of 52 patients, the study reported complete recovery in 40 cases, improvement in 10 cases, and no effect in 2 cases.[6]

5. **Proctitis**: In one study, 12 patients with chronic proctitis were treated with *Shen Ling Bai Zhu San,* with complete recovery in 2 cases, remission in 4 cases, improvement in 5 cases, and no effect in 1 case. The overall rate of effectiveness was 91.67%. The herbal treatment contained *Shen Ling Bai Zhu San* plus *Sheng Ma* (Rhizoma Cimicifugae), *He Zi* (Fructus Chebulae), *Lian Zi* (Semen Nelumbinis), and *Wu Mei* (Fructus Mume). The treatment protocol was to cook the herbs and administer the decoction daily for 4 weeks.[7]

6. **Nephritis**: Administration of modified *Shen Ling Bai Zhu San* to 15 patients with nephritis was associated with significant improvement in 2 cases, moderate improvement in 4 cases, slight improvement in 2 cases, and no effect in 7 cases. Modifications to the original formula included the addition of *Di Huang* (Radix Rehmanniae), *Nu Zhen Zi* (Fructus Ligustri Lucidi), and *Gou Qi Zi* (Fructus Lycii) for nephritis characterized by Kidney yin deficiency; *Bai Mao Gen* (Rhizoma Imperatae), *Dan Shen* (Radix et Rhizoma Salviae Miltiorrhizae), *Chi Shao* (Radix Paeoniae Rubra), *Chuan Xiong* (Rhizoma Chuanxiong), and *Yi Mu Cao* (Herba Leonuri) for hematuria; and *Jin Yin Hua* (Flos Lonicerae Japonicae), *Huang Qin* (Radix Scutellariae), *Yu Xing Cao* (Herba Houttuyniae), *Pu Gong Ying* (Herba Taraxaci), and *Da Qing Ye* (Folium Isatidis) for upper respiratory tract infection characterized by damp-heat. The herbs were cooked in water, and the decoction taken in two equally-divided doses daily.[8]

7. **Compromised immune system**: One study reported good results using modified *Shen Ling Bai Zhu San* to treat 48 patients with compromised immunity. In addition to the base formula, *Huang Qi* (Radix Astragali) was added for qi deficiency, *Chen Pi* (Pericarpium Citri Reticulatae) for qi stagnation, and *Yin Chen* (Herba Artemisiae Scopariae) for damp-heat. The treatment protocol was to administer the herbs in decoction one time daily, delivering 20 packs of herbs per course of treatment, for 1-3 courses total. The study reported gradual improvement over the courses of treatment, based on better tongue coating and normal pulse.[9] (Note: Specific details were unavailable on rate of effectiveness, and subjective and objective improvements.)

8. **Cognitive impairment**: Use of modified *Shen Ling Bai Zhu San* was associated with improvement in 33 of 47 children (32 males and 15 females, between 1-5 years of age) with slow mental development. The herbal treatment contained this formula plus *Bu Gu Zhi* (Fructus Psoraleae),

Yi Zhi (Fructus Alpiniae Oxyphyllae), *He Shou Wu* (Radix Polygoni Multiflori), and *Rou Cong Rong* (Herba Cistanches). The treatment protocol was to cook the herbs in water and administer the decoction daily, for 4 packs of herbs per course of treatment, for 1-3 courses.[10]

9. **Rhinitis**: Administration of modified *Shen Ling Bai Zhu San* was associated with 92.7% effectiveness in treating 68 children with chronic rhinitis. The herbal treatment contained this formula plus *Huang Qi* (Radix Astragali), *Cang Er Zi* (Fructus Xanthii), and *Bai Zhi* (Radix Angelicae Dahuricae). Furthermore, modifications were made by adding *Huang Qi* (Radix Astragali) and *Jin Yin Hua* (Flos Lonicerae Japonicae) for profuse, yellow, and sticky nasal discharge; *Xin Yi Hua* (Flos Magnoliae) and *Shi Chang Pu* (Rhizoma Acori Tatarinowii) for severe nasal obstruction; *Tian Zhu Huang* (Concretio Silicea Bambusae), *Bai Jie Zi* (Semen Sinapis), and *Chen Pi* (Pericarpium Citri Reticulatae) for profuse sputum; *Fang Feng* (Radix Saposhnikoviae) for frequent infection; *Mai Ya* (Fructus Hordei Germinatus), *Gu Ya* (Fructus Setariae Germinatus), and *Shen Qu* (Massa Fermentata) for poor appetite and diarrhea; *Bai Mao Gen* (Rhizoma Imperatae), *Ce Bai Ye* (Cacumen Platycladi), and *Xian He Cao* (Herba Agrimoniae) for nosebleeds; and others as needed. Herbs were given in decoction daily for 10 days per course of treatment. Of 68 patients, the study reported complete recovery in 18 patients, marked improvement in 25 patients, moderate improvement in 20 patients, and no effect in 5 patients.[11]

10. *Xiao ke* (wasting and thirsting) syndrome: Administration of modified *Shen Ling Bai Zhu San* in 30 patients with *xiao ke* (wasting and thirsting) syndrome was associated with recovery in 11 patients, improvement in 17 patients, and no effect in 2 patients. In addition to the formula, modifications included the addition of *Shi Hu* (Caulis Dendrobii) for excessive thirst with a dry tongue and a white tongue coating; *Ze Xie* (Rhizoma Alismatis) and *Che Qian Zi* (Semen Plantaginis) for a white, greasy tongue coating and reduced frequency of urination; and *Shan Zhu Yu* (Fructus Corni) and *Wu Wei Zi* (Fructus Schisandrae Chinensis) for increased frequency of urination. The herbs were cooked in water, and the decoction was taken in two equally-divided doses daily for 1 month per course of treatment. All patients were instructed to control their diet. Those with a prescription for diabetes were instructed to continue using the drugs.[12]

11. **Edema**: Administration of *Shen Ling Bai Zhu San* was associated with complete recovery or significant improvement in 47 of 50 patients (10 males and 40 females, between 30-45 years of age) with edema. The treatment

Chinese Herbal Formulas and Applications

Shēn Líng Bái Zhú Sǎn
(Ginseng, Poria, and Atractylodes Macrocephala Powder)

protocol was to cook the herbs in water, and administer the decoction in three equally-divided doses daily for 1 week per course of treatment, for 1-2 courses total.[13]

HERB-DRUG INTERACTION

Supportive therapy for chemotherapy and radiation: *Shen Ling Bai Zhu San* alleviated gastrointestinal side effects associated with chemotherapy and radiation treatments among 96 patients with mid-to-severe stages of cancer. Of 96 cases, the study reported significant effect in 33 cases, moderate effect in 46 cases, and no effect in 17 cases.[14]

RELATED FORMULAS

Qī Wèi Bái Zhú Sǎn
(Seven-Ingredient Powder with Atractylodes Macrocephala)

七味白术散
七味白术散

Pinyin Name: *Qi Wei Bai Zhu San*
Literal Name: Seven-Ingredient Powder with Atractylodes Macrocephala
Alternate Name: *Bai Zhu San* (Atractylodes Macrocephala Powder)
Original Source: *Xiao Er Yao Zheng Zhi Jue* (Craft of Medicinal Treatment for Childhood Disease Patterns) by Qian Yi in 1119

Ren Shen (Radix et Rhizoma Ginseng)	7.5g
Fu Ling (Poria)	15g
Bai Zhu (Rhizoma Atractylodis Macrocephalae), chao (dry-fried)	15g
Huo Xiang (Herba Agastaches)	15g
Mu Xiang (Radix Aucklandiae)	6g
Gan Cao (Radix et Rhizoma Glycyrrhizae)	3g
Ge Gen (Radix Puerariae Lobatae)	15-30g

The source text states to grind the ingredients into powder, and cook 9g of the powder in water to make a decoction. This formula strengthens the Spleen, stops diarrhea, and resolves dampness.

Qi Wei Bai Zhu San (Seven-Ingredient Powder with Atractylodes Macrocephala) treats patients who have Spleen and Stomach deficiencies, with symptoms such as frequent and recurring diarrhea and vomiting, and abdominal fullness and pain.

Ren Shen (Radix et Rhizoma Ginseng), *Bai Zhu* (Rhizoma Atractylodis Macrocephalae), *Fu Ling* (Poria), and *Gan Cao* (Radix et Rhizoma Glycyrrhizae) tonify the Spleen and Stomach and dispel dampness. *Huo Xiang* (Herba

Agastaches) dispels dampness, harmonizes the middle *jiao*, and stops vomiting. *Mu Xiang* (Radix Aucklandiae) promotes qi circulation and relieves pain. *Ge Gen* (Radix Puerariae Lobatae) causes Stomach qi to ascend and stops diarrhea.

Shēn Líng Sǎn (Ginseng and Poria Powder)

参苓散
参苓散

Pinyin Name: *Shen Ling San*
Literal Name: Ginseng and Poria Powder
Original Source: *An Hui Zhong Yi Xue Yuan* (Anhui University School of Medicine) in 1990

Lian Zi (Semen Nelumbinis)
Yi Yi Ren (Semen Coicis)
Sha Ren (Fructus Amomi)
Jie Geng (Radix Platycodonis)
Bai Bian Dou (Semen Lablab Album)
Fu Ling (Poria)
Ren Shen (Radix et Rhizoma Ginseng)
Gan Cao (Radix et Rhizoma Glycyrrhizae)
Bai Zhu (Rhizoma Atractylodis Macrocephalae)
Shan Yao (Rhizoma Dioscoreae)
Huang Qi (Radix Astragali)

Shen Ling San (Ginseng and Poria Powder) tonifies the Spleen and Stomach and reinforces *wei* (defensive) qi. Individuals with chronic deficiencies often have *wei qi* deficiency, and are more susceptible to exterior wind-cold or wind-heat invasion. The addition of *Huang Qi* (Radix Astragali) to this formula helps tonify *wei qi* and increase protection against *liu yin* (six exogenous factors).

AUTHORS' COMMENTS

Shen Ling Bai Zhu San is based on *Si Jun Zi Tang* (Four-Gentlemen Decoction), with the addition of *Shan Yao* (Rhizoma Dioscoreae), *Bai Bian Dou* (Semen Lablab Album), *Lian Zi* (Semen Nelumbinis), *Yi Yi Ren* (Semen Coicis), *Sha Ren* (Fructus Amomi), and *Jie Geng* (Radix Platycodonis).

Shen Ling Bai Zhu San is a harmonious formula that is not too warm nor too dry; it tonifies without creating stagnation, and drains dampness without injuring qi. It tonifies both the Lung and the Spleen, illustrating the concept of tonifying the metal element by strengthening the earth element. The following are differences between *Si Jun Zi Tang* (Four-Gentlemen Decoction) and *Shen Ling Bai Zhu San*:

TONIC FORMULAS

8

539

Chapter 8 – Tonic Formulas   *Section 1 – Qi-Tonifying Formulas*

Shēn Líng Bái Zhú Sǎn
(Ginseng, Poria, and Atractylodes Macrocephala Powder)

- *Si Jun Zi Tang* has a moderate qi-tonifying effect, and treats Spleen and Stomach qi deficiencies.
- *Shen Ling Bai Zhu San* has a strong qi-tonifying effect, and also harmonizes digestion and dissolves stagnation. It treats Spleen and Stomach qi deficiencies with accumulation of dampness.[15]

Shen Ling Bai Zhu San, *Si Shen Wan* (Four-Miracle Pill), and *Tong Xie Yao Fang* (Important Formula for Painful Diarrhea) all bind the Intestines to treat diarrhea. The differences are as follows:

- *Shen Ling Bai Zhu San* is indicated for diarrhea characterized by Spleen qi deficiency with damp accumulation manifesting as fatigue, weakness of the limbs, and poor appetite.
- *Si Shen Wan* warms and tonifies Spleen and Kidney yang to stop chronic diarrhea. It is designed for severe diarrhea that occurs in the early morning and is watery or contains undigested food.
- *Tong Xie Yao Fang* tonifies the Spleen and spreads Liver qi. This formula stops stress-related diarrhea. Patients often complain of gas, bloating, or abdominal pain that is relieved with diarrhea.[16]

References

1. *Zhong Yao Ming Fang Yao Li Yu Ying Yong* (Pharmacology and Applications of Famous Herbal Formulas) 1989;251-252.
2. *Xin Yi Yao Xue Za Zhi* (New Journal of Medicine and Herbology) 1979;3:129.
3. *Zhong Yi Fang Ji Xian Dai Yan Jiu* (Modern Study of Medical Formulae in Traditional Chinese Medicine) 1997;509.
4. *Xin Yi Yao Xue Za Zhi* (New Journal of Medicine and Herbology) 1979;3:129.
5. *Shan Dong Zhong Yi Za Zhi* (Shandong Journal of Chinese Medicine) 1991;10(6):24.
6. *Shan Xi Zhong Yi* (Shanxi Chinese Medicine) 1998;7:312.
7. *Nan Jing Zhong Yi Yao Da Xue Xue Bao* (Journal of Nanjing University of Traditional Chinese Medicine and Medicinals) 1998;5:318.
8. *Zhong Xi Yi Jie He Za Zhi* (Journal of Integrated Chinese and Western Medicine) 1987;7:436.
9. *Ji Lin Zhong Yi Yao* (Jilin Chinese Medicine and Herbology) 1997;4:14.
10. *Shan Xi Zhong Yi* (Shanxi Chinese Medicine) 1997;8:348.
11. *Si Chuan Zhong Yi* (Sichuan Chinese Medicine) 1994;11:55.
12. *Zhong Yi Yao Xue Bao* (Report of Chinese Medicine and Herbology) 1999;4:23.
13. *Zhong Yi Yao Xue Bao* (Report of Chinese Medicine and Herbology) 1999;4:23.
14. *Gui Zhou Yi Yao* (Medicine and Medicinals from Guizhou) 1985;3:7.
15. Wang MZ, et al. *Zhong Yi Xue Wen Da Ti Ku* (Questions and Answers on Traditional Chinese Medicine: Herbal Formulas).
16. Wang MZ, et al. *Zhong Yi Xue Wen Da Ti Ku* (Questions and Answers on Traditional Chinese Medicine: Herbal Formulas).

Qǐ Pí Wán (Guide the Spleen Pill)
啟脾丸
启脾丸

Pinyin Name: *Qi Pi Wan*
Literal Name: Guide the Spleen Pill
Alternate Name: Lotus and Citrus Formula
Original Source: *Wan Bing Hui Chun* (Restoration of Health from the Myriad Diseases) by Gong Ting-Xian in 1587

COMPOSITION

Ren Shen (Radix et Rhizoma Ginseng)	30g
Fu Ling (Poria)	30g
Bai Zhu (Rhizoma Atractylodis Macrocephalae), *chao* (dry-fried)	30g
Zhi Gan Cao (Radix et Rhizoma Glycyrrhizae Praeparata cum Melle)	15g
Shan Zha (Fructus Crataegi)	15g
Chen Pi (Pericarpium Citri Reticulatae)	15g
Lian Zi (Semen Nelumbinis)	30g
Ze Xie (Rhizoma Alismatis)	15g
Shan Yao (Rhizoma Dioscoreae), *chao* (dry-fried)	30g

540

Chinese Herbal Formulas and Applications

Qì Pí Wán (Guide the Spleen Pill)

DOSAGE / PREPARATION / ADMINISTRATION

Grind the ingredients into powder, and mix with honey to form pills. The pills should resemble the size of *Wu Tong Zi* (Semen Firmianae), a small seed approximately 5 mm in diameter. Take 20-30 pills per dose with rice water on an empty stomach.

CHINESE THERAPEUTIC ACTIONS

1. Strengthens the Spleen and Stomach
2. Promotes normal digestion
3. Relieves diarrhea and vomiting

CLINICAL MANIFESTATIONS

Indigestion and food stagnation caused by Spleen and Stomach deficiencies: decreased appetite, diarrhea, abdominal pain, nausea, and vomiting.

CLINICAL APPLICATIONS

Indigestion, chronic gastroenteritis, chronic diarrhea, intestinal tuberculosis, and infantile malnutrition.

EXPLANATION

Qi Pi Wan (Guide the Spleen Pill) treats patients with chronic Spleen and Stomach deficiencies, giving rise to various complaints of the digestive system, such as decreased appetite, nausea and vomiting, indigestion, abdominal pain, and diarrhea. In addition to digestive

disorders, fatigue and lack of energy may be present due to poor absorption of nutrients.

Si Jun Zi Tang (Four-Gentlemen Decoction) is the foundation of this formula; its four constituents, *Ren Shen* (Radix et Rhizoma Ginseng), *Fu Ling* (Poria), *Bai Zhu* (Rhizoma Atractylodis Macrocephalae), and *Zhi Gan Cao* (Radix et Rhizoma Glycyrrhizae Praeparata cum Melle), strengthen the Spleen and Stomach and restore normal digestive functions. The addition of *Shan Zha* (Fructus Crataegi) and *Chen Pi* (Pericarpium Citri Reticulatae) regulate qi and promote normal appetite and digestion. *Lian Zi* (Semen Nelumbinis) strengthens the Spleen and relieves diarrhea. *Ze Xie* (Rhizoma Alismatis) resolves dampness. *Shan Yao* (Rhizoma Dioscoreae) tonifies the body and relieves thirst and diarrhea.

MODIFICATIONS

- For poor appetite, add *Mai Ya* (Fructus Hordei Germinatus) and *Shen Qu* (Massa Fermentata).
- With more nausea, vomiting, and epigastric fullness, add *Zhi Shi* (Fructus Aurantii Immaturus) and *Ban Xia* (Rhizoma Pinelliae).
- With more abdominal pain and diarrhea, add *Mu Xiang* (Radix Aucklandiae) and *Sha Ren* (Fructus Amomi).
- For diarrhea caused by wind-cold, add *Xiao Chai Hu Tang* (Minor Bupleurum Decoction).

Qi Pi Wan (Guide the Spleen Pill)

Diagnosis	Signs and Symptoms	Treatment	Herbs
Indigestion and food stagnation due to Spleen and Stomach deficiencies	• Nausea, vomiting and abdominal pain: food stagnation and indigestion • Decreased appetite, diarrhea, fatigue and lack of energy: Spleen and Stomach deficiencies	• Strengthens the Spleen and Stomach • Promotes normal digestion and relieves diarrhea	• *Ren Shen* (Radix et Rhizoma Ginseng), *Fu Ling* (Poria), *Bai Zhu* (Rhizoma Atractylodis Macrocephalae), and *Zhi Gan Cao* (Radix et Rhizoma Glycyrrhizae Praeparata cum Melle) strengthen the Spleen and Stomach and restore normal digestive functions. • *Shan Zha* (Fructus Crataegi) and *Chen Pi* (Pericarpium Citri Reticulatae) regulate qi and promote normal appetite and digestion. • *Lian Zi* (Semen Nelumbinis) strengthens the Spleen and relieves diarrhea. • *Ze Xie* (Rhizoma Alismatis) resolves dampness. • *Shan Yao* (Rhizoma Dioscoreae) tonifies the body and relieves thirst and diarrhea.

TONIC FORMULAS

8

541

Chapter 8 – Tonic Formulas   *Section 1 – Qi-Tonifying Formulas*

Bǔ Zhōng Yì Qì Tāng
(Tonify the Middle and Augment the Qi Decoction)

補中益氣湯
补中益气汤

Pinyin Name: *Bu Zhong Yi Qi Tang*
Literal Name: Tonify the Middle and Augment the Qi Decoction
Alternate Names: *Pu Chung I Chi Tang* (*Wan*), *Bu Zhong Yi Chi Tang* (*Wan*), Interior-Nourishing and Qi-Increasing Decoction (Pill), Middle-Reinforcing and Qi-Benefiting Decoction, Ginseng and Astragalus Combination
Original Source: *Pi Wei Lun* (Discussion of the Spleen and Stomach) by Li Gao in 1249

COMPOSITION

Huang Qi (Radix Astragali)	1.5-3g [15-30g]
Ren Shen (Radix et Rhizoma Ginseng)	0.9g [9g]
Bai Zhu (Rhizoma Atractylodis Macrocephalae)	0.9g [9g]
Zhi Gan Cao (Radix et Rhizoma Glycyrrhizae Praeparata cum Melle)	1.5g [15g]
Dang Gui (Radix Angelicae Sinensis), *bei* (stone-baked) with liquor	0.6g [6g]
Chen Pi (Pericarpium Citri Reticulatae)	0.6-0.9g [6-9g]
Chai Hu (Radix Bupleuri)	0.6-0.9g [6-9g]
Sheng Ma (Rhizoma Cimicifugae)	0.6-0.9g [6-9g]

DOSAGE / PREPARATION / ADMINISTRATION

Coarsely grind the ingredients into powder and cook it in 2 large bowls of water and reduce it to 1 large bowl. Take the warm, strained decoction between meals. Today, this formula may be prepared as a decoction with the doses suggested in brackets. It may also be administered as pills, by taking 10-15g of pills two to three times a day with warm, boiled water or ginger soup.

CHINESE THERAPEUTIC ACTIONS

1. Tonifies the middle *jiao* and benefits qi
2. Causes the yang qi to ascend and lifts prolapsed organs

CLINICAL MANIFESTATIONS

1. Spleen and Stomach qi deficiencies: a warm sensation in the body, spontaneous sweating, thirst with preference for warm drinks, shortness of breath, no desire to speak, fatigue, weakness of the extremities, a pale complexion, loose stools, a pale tongue with a thin, white coating, and a surging, forceless pulse.
2. Qi deficiency with prolapse of organs: prolapse of the rectum or uterus, chronic diarrhea or dysentery, *beng lou* (flooding and spotting), and conditions characterized by inability of yang qi to ascend.

CLINICAL APPLICATIONS

Weakness and debility after a severe illness, chronic fatigue syndrome, gastric prolapse, rectal prolapse, uterine prolapse, nephroptosis (renal ptosis), gastritis, nausea and vomiting, constipation, diarrhea, fever, leukopenia, compromised immunity, chronic bronchitis, common cold, dysuria, frequent urination, incontinence, seizure and epilepsy, myasthenia gravis, depression, uterine bleeding, excessive menstrual bleeding, leukorrhea, pernicious anemia, recurrent miscarriage, postpartum illnesses, postpartum anuria, male infertility, tinnitus, allergic rhinitis, cataract, chronic hepatitis, hepatoma, and hepatocellular carcinoma.

EXPLANATION

The Spleen and Stomach, which are responsible for the transformation and transportation of food, are the source of qi and blood production. When these two organs become deficient and cannot carry out their normal functions, there will be fatigue, weakness of the extremities, shortness of breath, lack of desire to speak, and a pale face and tongue. Because of qi deficiency, the clear yang cannot ascend, leading to loose stools, diarrhea, and dysentery.

In severe cases of Spleen and Stomach deficiencies, yang qi may be unable to hold the organs in their normal position, leading to prolapse of such internal organs as the stomach, uterus, and rectum. Furthermore, as yang qi, unable to ascend, sinks into yin, it causes feverish sensations, spontaneous sweating, and a surging, forceless pulse. Thirst is the result of qi deficiency not being able to transport fluids to the upper parts of the body. Thirst with preference for <u>warm</u> drinks indicates deficiency, which differentiates this condition from thirst caused by heat.

542

Chinese Herbal Formulas and Applications

Bǔ Zhōng Yì Qì Tāng
(Tonify the Middle and Augment the Qi Decoction)

Bu Zhong Yi Qi Tang (Tonify the Middle and Augment the Qi Decoction)

Diagnosis	Signs and Symptoms	Treatment	Herbs
Spleen and Stomach qi deficiencies with prolapse of yang qi	• Fatigue, weakness of the extremities, shortness of breath, lack of desire to speak, and a pale face and tongue: Spleen and Stomach qi deficiencies • Loose stools, diarrhea, and dysentery: qi deficiency with failure of clear yang qi to ascend • Prolapse of internal organs such as the stomach, uterus, and rectum: yang qi deficiency unable to lift internal organs • Pale complexion, a pale tongue with a thin, white coating: Spleen and Stomach qi deficiencies	• Tonifies the middle *jiao* and benefits qi • Causes yang qi to ascend and lifts prolapsed organs	• *Huang Qi* (Radix Astragali) tonifies *zhong* (central) *qi*, causes yang qi to ascend, and strengthens *wei* (defensive) *qi*. • *Ren Shen* (Radix et Rhizoma Ginseng), *Bai Zhu* (Rhizoma Atractylodis Macrocephalae), and *Zhi Gan Cao* (Radix et Rhizoma Glycyrrhizae Praeparata cum Melle) strengthen the Spleen, benefit qi, and tonify the middle *jiao*. • *Dang Gui* (Radix Angelicae Sinensis) tonifies the blood. • *Chen Pi* (Pericarpium Citri Reticulatae) regulates qi and harmonizes the Stomach. • *Chai Hu* (Radix Bupleuri) and *Sheng Ma* (Rhizoma Cimicifugae) cause yang qi to ascend and lift prolapsed organs.

Bu Zhong Yi Qi Tang (Tonify the Middle and Augment the Qi Decoction) uses *Huang Qi* (Radix Astragali) as the chief herb because it tonifies *zhong* (central) *qi* and causes the yang qi to ascend. It also strengthens *wei* (defensive) *qi* and protects the exterior. *Ren Shen* (Radix et Rhizoma Ginseng), *Bai Zhu* (Rhizoma Atractylodis Macrocephalae), and *Zhi Gan Cao* (Radix et Rhizoma Glycyrrhizae Praeparata cum Melle) strengthen the Spleen, benefit qi, and tonify the middle *jiao*. *Dang Gui* (Radix Angelicae Sinensis) tonifies the blood and enhances the production of qi. *Chen Pi* (Pericarpium Citri Reticulatae) regulates qi and harmonizes the Stomach. It also prevents the tonic herbs from creating stagnation in the middle *jiao*. *Chai Hu* (Radix Bupleuri) and *Sheng Ma* (Rhizoma Cimicifugae) cause yang qi to ascend and lift prolapsed organs.

MODIFICATIONS
• For chronic prolapse of the rectum or uterus, add *Chi Shi Zhi* (Halloysitum Rubrum).
• With headache and vertigo, add *Chuan Xiong* (Radix Chuanxiong) and *Man Jing Zi* (Fructus Viticis).
• With headache due to common cold or flu, add *Gao Ben* (Rhizoma et Radix Ligustici) and *Xi Xin* (Herba Cum Radice Asari).
• With abdominal fullness, distention, and pain, add *Huang Qin* (Radix Scutellariae Baicalensis) and *Bai Shao* (Radix Paeoniae Alba).
• With hypochondriac pain, add *Xiang Fu* (Rhizoma Cyperi).
• If there is a stifling sensation in the chest, add *Qing Pi* (Pericarpium Citri Reticulatae Viride).

• With pain in the extremities, add *Fang Feng* (Radix Saposhnikoviae) and *Qiang Huo* (Rhizoma et Radix Notopterygii).
• If there is more leukorrhea, add *Fu Ling* (Poria) and *Che Qian Zi* (Semen Plantaginis).
• With intolerance to cold and pain, add *Rou Gui* (Cortex Cinnamomi).
• With a heavy sensation in the body caused by dampness, add *Wu Ling San* (Five-Ingredient Powder with Poria).

CAUTIONS / CONTRAINDICATIONS
• *Bu Zhong Yi Qi Tang* is contraindicated in patients with yin deficiency or interior heat.
• As a general rule, the dose of this formula should be small. This formula consists of sweet and warm tonic herbs, which tend to be heavy and immobile in nature. Thus, a large dose of this formula may actually defeat the purpose of causing yang qi to ascend. For the individual ingredients, it is important keep the dose of *Huang Qi* (Radix Astragali) high to tonify qi, and the doses of *Chai Hu* (Radix Bupleuri) and *Sheng Ma* (Rhizoma Cimicifugae) should be just sufficient to raise yang qi.

PHARMACOLOGICAL EFFECTS
1. **Gastrointestinal**: According to laboratory experiments in rabbits, administration of *Bu Zhong Yi Qi Tang* was associated with a regulatory effect on the intestines. Depending on the condition of the subject, it will either increase or decrease intestinal peristalsis.[1]
2. **Influence on gastric acid secretion**: Administration of *Bu Zhong Yi Qi Tang* has a dose-dependent effect on the

8

TONIC FORMULAS

543

Chapter 8 – Tonic Formulas   *Section 1 – Qi-Tonifying Formulas*

Bǔ Zhōng Yi Qi Tāng
(Tonify the Middle and Augment the Qi Decoction)

secretion of gastric acid. A small dose of the herb has little or no benefit on the secretion of gastric acid, while a large dose will significantly increase both gastric acid production and release.[2]

3. **Adaptogenic**: Administration of *Bu Zhong Yi Qi Tang* has been shown to increase the ability of animals to adapt to physical stress. In one experiment, administration of herbs for seven days increased the ability of mice to tread water longer when threatened with drowning. It was also noted that the subjects responded better to decoction than to pills.[3]

4. **Antiaging**: Administration of *Bu Zhong Yi Qi Tang* in mice was associated with a dose-dependent effect to improve endurance, learning, memory, neuromuscular coordination, and changes in the levels of monoamines (dopamine and noradrenaline) in the brain.[4]

5. **Immunostimulant**: Administration of *Bu Zhong Yi Qi Tang* has been associated with an immune-enhancing effect. According to one study, use of the formula was linked with increased T-lymphocyte count, elevated levels of IFN and IL-2, and increased NK cells and macrophage activity.[5] According to another study, *Bu Zhong Yi Qi Tang* enhances interleukin-18-induced cell-mediated immunity and may enhance host defense mechanisms against pathogens.[6]

6. **Antiallergic**: Administration of *Bu Zhong Yi Qi Tang* was associated with good results in treating allergies by suppressing IgE antibody production and inhibiting histamine release in type I allergic reactions in mice immunized with ovalbumin.[7] According to another study, the antiallergic effect was attributed mainly to inhibition of Th2 cell responses.[8]

7. **Anticancer**: In one study, use of *Bu Zhong Yi Qi Tang* was associated with a dose-dependent effect to inhibit the proliferation of human hepatoma cell lines (Hep3B, HepG2, and HA22T), but not normal human hepatocytes (Chang liver, CCL-13). The mechanism of this anticancer effect was attributed to the formula's ability to suppress the proliferation of hepatoma cells by inducing apoptosis via G0/G1 arrest.[9] Another study reported a marked prophylactic antitumor effect by enhancing the natural killer cell activity.[10]

8. **Radioprotective**: One study reported marked protective effects using *Bu Zhong Yi Qi Tang* in mice irradiated with high and low doses of gamma-rays. *Bu Zhong Yi Qi Tang* protected the jejunal crypts ($p < 0.0001$), increased the formation of the endogenous spleen colony ($p < 0.05$), and reduced the frequency of radiation-induced apoptosis ($p < 0.05$). The study also noted that while the individual ingredients also have radioprotective effects, the formula as a whole is much more effective. The study concluded

that *Bu Zhong Yi Qi Tang* is a useful radioprotector, especially because it is a relatively non-toxic natural product.[11]

9. **Antibiotic**: Administration of *Bu Zhong Yi Qi Tang* was associated with marked effects to treat gastroduodenal diseases associated with *Helicobacter pylori* (*H. pylori*) infection. *Bu Zhong Yi Qi Tang* was found to be effective against *H. pylori* both *in vitro* and *in vivo*, and inhibited the growth of antibiotic-resistant strains of *H. pylori* as well as antibiotic-sensitive strains. In addition, concurrent use of *Bu Zhong Yi Qi Tang* and antibiotics completely eradicated the bacteria in mice. The antibiotic effect of *Bu Zhong Yi Qi Tang* was attributed partly to the induction of interferon.[12]

10. **Antiviral**: Administration of *Bu Zhong Yi Qi Tang* was associated with antiviral effects to treat mice infected with influenza virus. The mechanism of this antiviral effect was attributed to the enhancement of host immune responses, as the herbs do not have any inhibitory effect on the growth of influenza virus *in vitro*.[13]

11. **Effect on bone loss**: One study used *Bu Zhong Yi Qi Tang* and evaluated its effect on bone mass density in ovariectomized female rats at age 35 weeks. The subjects were given the formula by gastric tube for 8 weeks. The study reported that treatments using *Bu Zhong Yi Qi Tang* suppressed the ovariectomy-induced reduction of the bone mineral density in the whole and metaphysis of tibia. Furthermore, the study noted that there was a slight increase in serum levels of estradiol and progesterone maintaining bone mineral density values similar to that in the estradiol-treated ovariectomized rats, as well as the intact control rats. Based on this finding, the study suggested that *Bu Zhong Yi Qi Tang* prevented bone loss in ovariectomized rats because it elevated the serum levels of ovarian hormones slightly.[14]

12. **Antidepressive and antinociceptive**: Administration of *Bu Zhong Yi Qi Tang*, *Yi Gan San* (Restrain the Liver Powder), or *Chai Hu Jia Long Gu Mu Li Tang* (Bupleurum plus Dragon Bone and Oyster Shell Decoction) for 14 consecutive days showed both antidepressive and antinociceptive properties in mice.[15]

CLINICAL STUDIES AND RESEARCH

1. **Chronic fatigue syndrome**: *Bu Zhong Yi Qi Tang* was used to treat patients with chronic fatigue syndrome. Out of 50 patients, the study reported marked improvement in 2 patients, moderate improvement in 24 patients, and slight improvement in 24 patients.[16]

2. **Gastric prolapse**: In one study, 40 patients with stomach prolapse characterized by Spleen and Stomach deficiencies were treated with modified *Bu Zhong Yi Qi Tang* with

Bǔ Zhōng Yì Qì Tāng
(Tonify the Middle and Augment the Qi Decoction)

Chinese Herbal Formulas and Applications

complete recovery in 21 patients, marked improvement in 16 patients, and no benefit in 3 patients. The herbal treatment contained *Bu Zhong Yi Qi Tang* with modifications as needed. With Liver and qi stagnation, *Dang Shen* (Radix Codonopsis) was removed and *Fo Shou* (Fructus Citri Sarcodactylis), *Xiang Fu* (Rhizoma Cyperi), and *Zi Su Geng* (Caulis Perillae) were added. With food stagnation, *Dang Gui* (Radix Angelicae Sinensis) was removed, and charred *Shan Zha* (Fructus Crataegi), charred *Shen Qu* (Massa Fermentata), charred *Mai Ya* (Fructus Hordei Germinatus), *Ji Nei Jin* (Endothelium Corneum Gigeriae Galli), and dry-fried *Lai Fu Zi* (Semen Raphani) were added. With Stomach heat, *Dang Shen* (Radix Codonopsis) was removed, and dry-fried *Huang Lian* (Rhizoma Coptidis), *Pu Gong Ying* (Herba Taraxaci), and *Da Huang* (Radix et Rhizoma Rhei) were added. For Stomach cold, *Dang Gui* (Radix Angelicae Sinensis) was removed, and *Gan Jiang* (Rhizoma Zingiberis) and *Rou Gui* (Cortex Cinnamomi) were added. For Stomach yin deficiency, *Chai Hu* (Radix Bupleuri) and *Bai Zhu* (Rhizoma Atractylodis Macrocephalae) were removed, and *Sha Shen* (Radix Glehniae seu Adenophorae) and *Mai Dong* (Radix Ophiopogonis) were added. With blood stagnation, *Dang Shen* (Radix Codonopsis) and *Bai Zhu* (Rhizoma Atractylodis Macrocephalae) were removed, and *Tao Ren* (Semen Persicae), *Hong Hua* (Flos Carthami), and *Dan Shen* (Radix et Rhizoma Salviae Miltiorrhizae) were added.[17] In another study, modified *Bu Zhong Yi Qi Tang* was used to treat patients with stomach prolapse with good success. Out of 40 patients, the study reported complete recovery in 30 patients, improvement in 8 patients, and no benefit in 2 patients. The overall effectiveness rate was 95%.[18]

3. **Rectal prolapse**: Use of modified *Bu Zhong Yi Qi Tang* was successful in treating rectal prolapse in 68 patients with 3 months to 15 years history of illness. The herbal formula contained *Huang Qi* (Radix Astragali) 30g, *Ren Shen* (Radix et Rhizoma Ginseng) 20g, *Bai Zhu* (Rhizoma Atractylodis Macrocephalae) 5g, *Sheng Ma* (Rhizoma Cimicifugae) 5g, and *Chai Hu* (Radix Bupleuri) 5g. Modifications were made as follows: for frequent bowel movements with mucus and blood, add *Huang Lian* (Rhizoma Coptidis) 10g, *Chi Shi Zhi* (Halloysitum Rubrum) 10g, *Ying Su Ke* (Pericarpium Papaveris) 10g, and *Jin Ying Zi* (Fructus Rosae Laevigatae) 10g; for stubborn cough, add *Wu Wei Zi* (Fructus Schisandrae Chinensis) 15g, *Wu Bei Zi* (Galla Chinensis) 10g, and *Sang Bai Pi* (Cortex Mori) 10g; for constipation, add *Huo Ma Ren* (Fructus Cannabis) 15g and *Yu Li Ren* (Semen Pruni) 10g; for chronic illness with dry mouth and deficiency of body fluids, add *Shu Di Huang* (Radix Rehmanniae Praeparata) 15g, *Sha Shen* (Radix Glehniae seu Adenophorae)

15g, *Tian Dong* (Radix Asparagi) 15g, and *Yu Zhu* (Rhizoma Polygonati Odorati) 15g; and for profuse bleeding in the stools, add *Huai Hua* (Flos Sophorae) 10g, *Di Yu* (Radix Sanguisorbae) 15g, and *Ce Bai Ye* (Cacumen Platycladi) 15g.[19] Another study reported 94% effectiveness using modified *Bu Zhong Yi Qi Tang* to treat rectal prolapse. Modifications included the addition of *Wu Mei* (Fructus Mume), *Wu Bei Zi* (Galla Chinensis), and others as needed. Of 56 patients, the study reported significant improvement in 29 patients, moderate improvement in 24 patients, and no benefit in 3 patients.[20]

4. **Uterine prolapse**: One study reported good results using modified *Bu Zhong Yi Qi Tang* to treat 14 patients with prolapse of uterus. The herbal treatment contained *Bu Zhong Yi Qi Tang* as the base formula, with the addition of large doses of *Huang Qi* (Radix Astragali) and *Dang Shen* (Radix Codonopsis) for qi deficiency; *Xu Duan* (Radix Dipsaci) and *Du Zhong* (Cortex Eucommiae) for low back pain and frequent urination; and a large dose of *Zhi Qiao* (Fructus Aurantii) for those who did not respond well. After 9-18 packs of herbs, the study reported recovery in all 14 patients.[21]

5. **Nephroptosis (renal ptosis)**: Use of *Bu Zhong Yi Qi Tang* was effective in treating a 59-year-old woman with bilateral renal ptosis (a 6 cm decrease in position of the right kidney and a 5 cm decrease of the left kidney). The treatment protocol was to administer this formula at 7.5 g/day. The study reported relief of dull pain in the low back after 6 months, and improvement of nephroptosis (3 cm increase in the position of both kidneys) after 8 months. The study concluded that *Bu Zhong Yi Qi Tang* may be useful as a conservative therapy for nephroptosis.[22]

6. **Gastritis**: Gastritis due to regurgitation of bile acid in 89 patients was treated with complete recovery in 19 patients, marked improvement in 32 patients, moderate improvement in 30 patients, and no benefit in 8 patients. The overall effectiveness was 90%. In addition to *Bu Zhong Yi Qi Tang* as the base formula, modifications included addition of *Zuo Jin Wan* (Left Metal Pill) for acid reflux; *Ban Xia* (Rhizoma Pinelliae) for belching; *Fu Ling* (Poria) and *Shan Yao* (Rhizoma Dioscoreae) for loose stools; *Da Huang* (Radix et Rhizoma Rhei) for constipation; and *Bai Shao* (Radix Paeoniae Alba) for stomach pain.[23]

7. **Nausea and vomiting**: In one report, 26 out of 30 patients with nausea and vomiting were treated with good results using modified *Bu Zhong Yi Qi Tang*.[24]

8. **Constipation**: Modified *Bu Zhong Yi Qi Tang* successfully treated constipation in geriatric patients with qi deficiency, postpartum women with qi and blood deficiency, and pregnant women.[25]

TONIC FORMULAS

8

545

Bǔ Zhōng Yi Qi Tāng
(Tonify the Middle and Augment the Qi Decoction)

9. **Diarrhea**: One study reported good results using *Bu Zhong Yi Qi Tang* to treat geriatric patients with diarrhea characterized by Spleen deficiency. Out of the 33 patients, 16 were male and 17 were female, between 51-67 years of age, with 6 months to 15 years of illness. Patients were instructed to take herbs continuously for 1-1.5 months. The study reported complete recovery in 30 of 33 patients.[26]

10. **Fever**: Use of *Bu Zhong Yi Qi Tang* was effective in reducing fever secondary to chronic illness or postpartum weakness with qi and blood deficiencies. Of 20 patients treated, most reported a reduction of body temperature within 5 doses.[27] Another study on fever in 30 post-surgical patients reported 93.3% effectiveness using modified *Bu Zhong Yi Qi Tang* to reduce body temperature.[28]

11. **Leukopenia**: One study reported good results using modified *Bu Zhong Yi Qi Tang* in 80 patients (32 male, 48 female) with low white blood cell count due to various causes. In addition to the base formula, modifications included *Gu Ya* (Fructus Setariae Germinatus) and *Mai Ya* (Fructus Hordei Germinatus) for poor appetite; *Mai Dong* (Radix Ophiopogonis) and *Wu Wei Zi* (Fructus Schisandrae Chinensis) for palpitations; and *Cang Zhu* (Rhizoma Atractylodis) for damp. The herbs were cooked in water, and the decoction was taken in two equally-divided doses daily. Of 80 patients, the study reported a marked effect in 70 patients (> 2.0 x 10^9/L increase of WBC in 2 weeks); moderate improvement in 4 patients (1.0-1.9 x 10^9/L increase of WBC in 2 weeks), and no benefit in 6 patients (<0.9 x 10^9/L increase of WBC in 2 weeks).[29]

12. **Compromised immunity in elderly persons**: Administration of *Bu Zhong Yi Qi Tang* was effective in improving immunological capacity in a group of elderly patients. Clinical improvements included significantly enhanced natural killer (NK) activity and serum IFN-gamma level. The treatment protocol was to administer 7.5g of the formula daily for at least 120 days.[30]

13. **Common cold**: In one report, 50 geriatric patients with constitutional deficiencies and common cold were treated successfully with modified *Bu Zhong Yi Qi Tang*. The modifications were as follows: *Jing Jie* (Herba Schizonepetae) was added for aversion to cold; *Fang Feng* (Radix Saposhnikoviae) and *Qiang Huo* (Rhizoma et Radix Notopterygii) for body ache; *Bai Zhi* (Radix Angelicae Dahuricae) was added for headache; *Bo He* (Herba Menthae) for dizziness; *Ju Hua* (Flos Chrysanthemi) for blurred vision; and *Yu Ping Feng San* (Jade Windscreen Powder) after the resolution of exterior symptoms. The average length of treatment was 37.5 days. Out of 50 patients, the study reported complete recovery in 48 patients (complete resolution of all symptoms without recurrence for 1 year).[31]

14. **MRSA infection**: One study reported a marked effect using 5g per day of *Bu Zhong Yi Qi Tang* to treat 5 patients with MRSA infection. Prior to the herbal treatment, these 5 patients were bedridden with cerebrovascular disorder, dementia, and, in two patients, bed sores, and had resistance to several antibacterial drugs. After the herbal therapy, the study noted disappearance of MRSA, improvement in their general conditions, and no side effects. The study states that *Bu Zhong Yi Qi Tang* may be a useful drug for MRSA-infected patients.[32] According to another study, administration of *Bu Zhong Yi Qi Tang* in 34 patients with asymptomatic MRSA bacteriuria was associated with successful eradication of urine MRSA in 12 patients, and reduction of bacterial counts in urine culture to 10(2) CFU/mL or less in 10 patients. The treatment protocol was daily administration of 7.5g for at least 24 weeks.[33] Note: *Bu Zhong Yi Qi Tang* is not a "heat-clearing formula," nor has it shown antibiotic effects. There are two proposed theories on the successful use of this formula in treating MRSA infection. First, *Bu Zhong Yi Qi Tang* improves prognostic nutritional index, and subsequently assists the recovery of bio-defense function against these pathogens.[34] Second, *Bu Zhong Yi Qi Tang* helps to enhance defense against bacteria by up-regulating TLR4 (human toll-like receptor 4) surface expression in THP-1 cells (human monocytic cell line), both dose- and time-dependently. By enhancing their recognition, *Bu Zhong Yi Qi Tang* enhances defense against these gram-negative pathogens.[35]

15. **Hypertension**: One study used *Bu Zhong Yi Qi Tang* to treat hypertension characterized by qi deficiency. The background of the 15 patients were as follows: 9 males and 6 females; between 45-49 years of age, with 3-10 years history of illness. After continuous herbal treatment for 1-3 months, the study reported stabilization of blood pressure and relief of symptoms in 13 patients, and no benefit in 2 patients.[36]

16. **Dysuria**: Modified *Bu Zhong Yi Qi Tang* was used with good results in treating 27 patients with postpartum dysuria. The modification included the addition of *Dong Kui Zi* (Semen Malvae), *Fu Ling* (Poria), and *Che Qian Zi* (Semen Plantaginis). The treatment duration was 1-3 days.[37]

17. **Frequent urination**: In one report, pregnant women with frequent urination were treated with great success using *Bu Zhong Yi Qi Tang* with the addition of *Xu Duan* (Radix Dipsaci), dry-fried *Bai Shao* (Radix Paeoniae Alba), *Di Huang* (Radix Rehmanniae), *Huang Qin* (Radix Scutellariae), and *Shan Yao* (Rhizoma Dioscoreae). Pregnancy continued smoothly with no complications or side effects.[38]

Bǔ Zhōng Yi Qi Tāng
(Tonify the Middle and Augment the Qi Decoction)

18. **Incontinence**: Modified *Bu Zhong Yi Qi Tang* was used with good results in treating 57 patients with incontinence due to postpartum or post-surgical procedures. Modifications included the addition of a large dose of *Huang Qi* (Radix Astragali), as well as the addition of *Yi Zhi* (Fructus Alpiniae Oxyphyllae), *Wu Wei Zi* (Fructus Schisandrae Chinensis), *Fu Pen Zi* (Fructus Rubi), *Sang Piao Xiao* (Ootheca Mantidis), and calcined *Long Gu* (Os Draconis). Out of 57 patients, the study reported recovery in 45 patients and improvement in 12 patients.[39]

19. **Seizures and epilepsy**: In one report, 54 patients with seizures were treated with good results using concurrent herb and drug therapy. The treatment protocol was to administer modified *Bu Zhong Yi Qi Tang* daily, for a duration ranging from 6 to 112 packs of herbal decoctions. The drugs were discontinued or reduced in dose only when the patients were stabilized. During the follow-up interviews, 35 patients had no recurrence within 1 year, 11 patients had no recurrence within 2 years, and 16 had reduced number of seizures. There was no benefit in 2 patients.[40]

20. **Myasthenia gravis**: One hundred patients with myasthenia gravis were treated with an 86% effective rate using *Bu Zhong Yi Qi Tang* combined with general Kidney tonics.[41]

21. **Depression**: In one report, 50 patients with depression characterized by qi deficiency were treated with modified *Bu Zhong Yi Qi Tang*, with recovery in 28 patients, marked improvement in 17 patients, and slight improvement in 5 patients.[42]

22. **Menstrual bleeding**: Fifty patients with profuse menstrual bleeding treated with *Bu Zhong Yi Qi Tang* experienced 90% effectiveness.[43]

23. **Male infertility**: Use of *Bu Zhong Yi Qi Tang* was 51.1% effective in improving sperm count and motility in a group of 45 men.[44] In another study involving 55 men, the formula was 67.3% effective in improving the sperm count, and 74.5% effective in improving the sperm motility.[45] Furthermore, use of this formula showed improved semen quality in 22 idiopathic infertile patients.[46] Lastly, one study reported favorable results (higher sperm motility) using *Bu Zhong Yi Qi Tang* to treat 14 patients with unexplained male infertility.[47]

24. **Tinnitus**: Modified *Bu Zhong Yi Qi Tang* in decoction successfully treated 30 patients with tinnitus. Modifications included the addition of *Shu Di Huang* (Radix Rehmanniae Praeparata), *Dang Shen* (Radix Codonopsis), and *Huang Qi* (Radix Astragali) for qi and blood deficiencies; *Gou Qi Zi* (Fructus Lycii) and *Tu Si Zi* (Semen Cuscutae) for Kidney deficiency; *Bu Gu Zhi* (Fructus Psoraleae) and *Ba Ji Tian* (Radix Morindae Officinalis) for Kidney yang deficiency; *Long Dan* (Radix et Rhizoma Gentianae) and *Zhi Zi* (Fructus Gardeniae) for Liver and Gallbladder fire; and *Wu Ling Zhi* (Faeces Trogopteri), *Dan Shen* (Radix et Rhizoma Salviae Miltiorrhizae), and *Chi Shao* (Radix Paeoniae Rubra) for blood stagnation. The treatment protocol was to take the decoction one time daily for 5 days per course of treatment, for a total of 3 courses. Out of 30 patients, the study reported recovery in 23 patients, marked improvement in 2 patients, slight improvement in 3 patients, and no benefit in 2 patients.[48]

25. **Allergic rhinitis**: *Bu Zhong Yi Qi Tang* can be combined with *Yu Ping Feng San* (Jade Windscreen Powder) or *Xin Yi San* (Magnolia Flower Powder) to effectively treat allergic rhinitis within 2 months.[49]

26. **Cataract**: Use of modified *Bu Zhong Yi Qi Tang* to treat 18 geriatric patients with cataracts was associated with 90.6% effectiveness. The base formula contained *Bu Zhong Yi Qi Tang* plus *Gou Qi Zi* (Fructus Lycii) and *Shu Di Huang* (Radix Rehmanniae Praeparata). The treatment protocol was to administer the herbs in decoction daily, for 6 days per course of treatment, followed by 1 day of rest, for 1 month.[50]

27. **Chronic hepatitis**: In a clinical study, modified *Bu Zhong Yi Qi Tang* was used to treat patients with chronic hepatitis characterized by Spleen qi deficiency or accumulation of dampness affecting the Spleen. The modification included the addition of *Yin Chen* (Herba Artemisiae Scopariae), *Cang Zhu* (Rhizoma Atractylodis), *Zhi Zi* (Fructus Gardeniae), *Zhu Ling* (Polyporus), *Fu Ling* (Poria), *Ze Xie* (Rhizoma Alismatis), *Huang Lian* (Rhizoma Coptidis), and *Hua Shi* (Talcum). The study reported significant results in 80 patients and moderate results in 2 patients.[51]

28. **Hepatoma**: Administration of *Bu Zhong Yi Qi Tang* had a dose-dependent effect to inhibit the proliferation of human hepatoma cell lines (Hep3B, HepG2 and HA22T). The same formula, however, did not significantly inhibit the proliferation of normal human hepatocytes (Chang liver, CCL-13) at a concentration under 5,000 mcg/mL. The mechanism of this action was attributed to suppressed proliferation of hepatoma cells via G0/G1 cell cycle arrest and inhibition of DNA synthesis followed by apoptosis.[52]

29. **Hepatocellular carcinoma**: One study evaluated the cellular physiology of *Bu Zhong Yi Qi Tang* for the treatment of hepatocellular carcinoma. *In vitro* studies have shown that *Bu Zhong Yi Qi Tang* is capable of increasing granulocyte colony-stimulating-factor (G-CSF) and tumor necrosis factor-alpha (TNF-alpha) production by peripheral blood mononuclear cells. This effect was observed in both healthy volunteers and patients with hepatocellular carcinoma. Because of this unique effect to stimulate the production of TNF-alpha and G-CSF and activate the biological defensive mechanism, the researchers stated

Chapter 8 – Tonic Formulas   *Section 1 – Qi-Tonifying Formulas*

Bǔ Zhōng Yi Qi Tāng
(Tonify the Middle and Augment the Qi Decoction)

that *Bu Zhong Yi Qi Tang* may be beneficial for patients with hepatocellular carcinoma.[53]

HERB-DRUG INTERACTION

- **Mitomycin C-induced immunosuppression**: Administration of mitomycin C, a chemotherapy agent for cancer, is often associated with immunosuppression and infectious diseases. One study reported that *Bu Zhong Yi Qi Tang* had beneficial effects in mice, with improvements in spleen weight, number of colonies of granulocytes and macrophages forming in the bone-marrow cells, natural killer activity in splenocytes, and in susceptibility to lethal herpes simplex virus type-1 infection. The researchers concluded *Bu Zhong Yi Qi Tang* may be beneficial in immunocompromised patients receiving chemotherapeutic drugs.[54]

- **Cyclophosphamide-induced leukopenia**: Administration of *Bu Zhong Yi Qi Tang* (1,000 mg/kg) in mice treated with cyclophosphamide significantly prevented leukopenia. *Bu Zhong Yi Qi Tang* enhanced the production of hematopoietic lymphokines, stimulated the proliferation of hematopoietic progenitor cells, and consequently accelerated recovery from leukopenia. *Bu Zhong Yi Qi Tang* also contributed a protective effect against bacterial infection by activating phagocyte cells.[55]

- **Radiation-induced hypotension**: According to one study, 30 patients between 25-50 years of age, who had worked in areas with high exposure to radiation, were treated for hypotension. The average blood pressure was 25 mmHg below normal. The patients were divided into three groups according to diagnosis of Spleen qi deficiency, qi and yang deficiencies, and qi and yin deficiencies. Patients in all three groups received *Bu Zhong Yi Qi Tang* as the base formula. *Fu Zi* (Radix Aconiti Lateralis Praeparata) and *Yin Yang Huo* (Herba Epimedii) were added for those who had qi and yang deficiencies. *Sheng Mai San* (Generate the Pulse Powder) was added for those who had qi and yin deficiencies. After 5 days of treatment, the study reported marked improvement in 47% of patients, moderate improvement in 40%, and no improvement in 13%. Marked improvement was defined as subjective improvement of symptoms according to the patients with an objective increase in blood pressure of 15-24 mmHg, and moderate improvement was defined as no significant changes in subjective symptoms, but an increase of 15 mmHg of blood pressure.[56]

- **Liver metabolism**: One study on the metabolic activity of different cytochrome P450 (CYP) isoforms reported *Bu Zhong Yi Qi Tang* to be a competitive inhibitor of CYP3A4 (Ki value of 0.65 mg/mL) and CYP2C9 (Ki value of 0.7-0.8 mg/mL), but not CYP2D6. The study concluded

that because of this inhibitory effect on liver metabolism, care should be taken with concurrent use of *Bu Zhong Yi Qi Tang* and drugs.[57]

TOXICOLOGY

In an acute toxicology study, no fatality or abnormal reactions were noted in mice following oral ingestion of the formula at the dose of 166 g/kg twice daily for 3 days.[58]

RELATED FORMULAS

Jǔ Yuán Jiān (Lift the Source Decoction)
舉元煎
举元煎

Pinyin Name: *Ju Yuan Jian*
Literal Name: Lift the Source Decoction
Original Source: *Jing Yue Quan Shu* (Collected Treatises of [Zhang] Jing Yue) by Zhang Jie-Bin (Zhang Jing-Yue) in 1624

Ren Shen (Radix et Rhizoma Ginseng)	9-15g
Huang Qi (Radix Astragali), *zhi* (fried with liquid)	9-15g
Zhi Gan Cao (Radix et Rhizoma Glycyrrhizae Praeparata cum Melle)	3-6g
Sheng Ma (Rhizoma Cimicifugae), *chao* (dry-fried)	1.5-2.1g
Bai Zhu (Rhizoma Atractylodis Macrocephalae), *chao* (dry-fried)	3-6g

Prepare the ingredients by cooking the herbs in 1.5 large bowls of water until the liquid is reduced to 70-80%. Take the strained decoction while warm. This formula tonifies qi and causes yang to ascend. Clinically, it is used for patients who have severe qi deficiency with near-collapse of yang qi and profuse bleeding, with such symptoms as prolapsed organs, and continuous menstrual bleeding in women.

Ju Yuan Jian (Lift the Source Decoction) is modified from *Bu Zhong Yi Qi Tang*, with the removal of *Chen Pi* (Pericarpium Citri Reticulatae), *Dang Gui* (Radix Angelicae Sinensis), and *Chai Hu* (Radix Bupleuri). *Ju Yuan Jian* uses a higher dose of *Ren Shen* (Radix et Rhizoma Ginseng), and is thus more suitable than *Bu Zhong Yi Qi Tang* for patients with severe *yuan* (source) *qi* deficiency.

This formula may be modified as follows: for cold and yang qi deficiency, add *Rou Gui* (Cortex Cinnamomi), *Fu Zi* (Radix Aconiti Lateralis Praeparata), *Gan Jiang* (Rhizoma Zingiberis); and for loss of body fluids, add *Wu Mei* (Fructus Mume) or *Wen Ge* (Meretrix).

Chinese Herbal Formulas and Applications

Bǔ Zhōng Yì Qì Tāng
(Tonify the Middle and Augment the Qi Decoction)

Shēng Xiàn Tāng (Raise the Sinking Decoction)

升陷湯
升陷汤

Pinyin Name: *Sheng Xian Tang*
Literal Name: Raise the Sinking Decoction
Original Source: *Yi Xue Zhong Zhong Can Xi Lu* (Records of Heart-Felt Experiences in Medicine with Reference to the West) by Zhang Xi-Chun in 1918-34

Huang Qi (Radix Astragali)	18g
Zhi Mu (Rhizoma Anemarrhenae)	9g
Chai Hu (Radix Bupleuri)	4.5g
Jie Geng (Radix Platycodonis)	4.5g
Sheng Ma (Rhizoma Cimicifugae)	3g

The source text states to cook the herbs three times, and consume the decoction within one day. This formula tonifies qi, lifts prolapse, and raises sunken qi in the chest. Clinically, this formula is used for patients who have severe qi depression in the chest with symptoms such as rapid respiration, shortness of breath, severe dyspnea, and a deep, slow and weak pulse.

Sheng Xian Tang (Raise the Sinking Decoction) uses the same principles as *Bu Zhong Yi Qi Tang* to treat deficiency and sinking of qi in the chest. *Huang Qi* (Radix Astragali), the chief herb, tonifies Lung qi. *Jie Geng* (Radix Platycodonis) regulates Lung qi. *Sheng Ma* (Rhizoma Cimicifugae) and *Chai Hu* (Radix Bupleuri) ascend to lift sunken qi. *Zhi Mu* (Rhizoma Anemarrhenae) is bitter and cold, and neutralizes the warm tendency of *Huang Qi* (Radix Astragali) to prevent unwanted side effects.

AUTHORS' COMMENTS

It is often asked that if *Bu Zhong Yi Qi Tang* treats prolapsed organs, why are *Sheng Ma* (Rhizoma Cimicifugae) and *Chai Hu* (Radix Bupleuri) not used as chief herbs at larger doses to maximize the effects? There are two reasons why a large dose of these two herbs is inappropriate:

- First, the prolapse is caused by qi deficiency, so tonic herbs such as *Ren Shen* (Radix et Rhizoma Ginseng), *Bai Zhu* (Rhizoma Atractylodis Macrocephalae), and *Zhi Gan Cao* (Radix et Rhizoma Glycyrrhizae Praeparata cum Melle) must be used to treat the underlying deficiency, which is the root of the condition.

- Second, the primary function of *Chai Hu* (Radix Bupleuri) and *Sheng Ma* (Rhizoma Cimicifugae) is to release the exterior, and their secondary function is to lift prolapsed organs. If they are used at larger doses, their dispersing and

exterior-releasing functions would override their lifting effect and injure the *zheng* (upright) *qi* of the body.[59]

Huang Qi (Radix Astragali) is the main ingredient in three important formulas, but with slightly different purposes:

- *Bu Zhong Yi Qi Tang* contains *Huang Qi* (Radix Astragali) to tonify qi and cause yang to ascend. It treats Spleen and Stomach qi deficiencies with prolapsed organs. Patients will exhibit fatigue, poor appetite, decreased dietary intake, feverish sensation, chronic diarrhea, and spontaneous sweating.

- *Dang Gui Bu Xue Tang* (Tangkuei Decoction to Tonify the Blood) contains *Huang Qi* (Radix Astragali) at a dose five times higher than *Dang Gui* (Radix Angelicae Sinensis) to boost qi and generate blood. It is mainly used for blood deficiency with deficiency-heat signs of heat sensation, flushed face, spontaneous sweating, and a surging, big and deficient pulse.

- *Dang Gui Liu Huang Tang* (Tangkuei and Six-Yellow Decoction) uses *Huang Qi* (Radix Astragali) to tonify qi, consolidate *wei* (defensive) *qi*, and stop sweating. It mainly treats yin deficiency with flaring fire manifesting in spontaneous or night sweats, thirst, and a red tongue body with a yellow coating.[60]

References

1. *Zhong Yao Yao Li Yu Lin Chuang* (Pharmacology and Clinical Applications of Chinese Herbs) 1987;2:4.
2. *Zhong Yao Yao Li Yu Lin Chuang* (Pharmacology and Clinical Applications of Chinese Herbs) 1988;3:16.
3. *Zhong Yi Fang Ji Xian Dai Yan Jiu* (Modern Study of Medical Formulae in Traditional Chinese Medicine) 1997;524.
4. Shih HC, Chang KH, Chen FL, Chen CM, Chen SC, Lin YT, Shibuya A. Anti-aging effects of the traditional Chinese medicine bu-zhong-yi-qi-tang in mice. Am J Chin Med 2000;28(1):77-86.
5. *Zhong Yi Fang Ji Xian Dai Yan Jiu* (Modern Study of Medical Formulae in Traditional Chinese Medicine) 1997;520-521.
6. Tamura R, Takahashi HK, Xue D, Kubo S, Saito S, Nishibori M, Iwagaki H, Tanaka N. Enhanced effects of combined bu-zhong-yi-qi-tang (TJ-41) and interleukin-18 on the production of tumour necrosis factor-alpha and interferon-gamma in human peripheral blood mononuclear cells. J Int Med Res 2004 Jan-Feb;32(1):25-32.
7. Suzuki T, Takano I, Nagai F, Fujitani T, Ushiyama K, Okubo T, Seto T, Ikeda S, Kano I. Suppressive effects of Hochu-ekki-to, a traditional Chinese medicine, on IgE production and histamine release in mice immunized with ovalbumin. Biol Pharm Bull 1999 Nov;22(11):1180-4.
8. Kaneko M, Kawakita T, Nomoto K. Inhibition of eosinophil infiltration into the mouse peritoneal cavity by a traditional Chinese medicine, Bu-zhong-yi-qi-tang (Japanese name: Hochu-ekki-to). Immunopharmacol Immunotoxicol 1999 Feb;21(1):125-40.
9. Kao ST, Yeh CC, Hsieh CC, Yang MD, Lee MR, Liu HS, Lin JG. The Chinese medicine Bu-Zhong-Yi-Qi-Tang inhibited proliferation of hepatoma cell lines by inducing apoptosis via G0/G1 arrest. Life Sciences 2001 Aug 17;69(13):1485-96.

TONIC FORMULAS

8

549

Bǔ Zhōng Yì Qì Tāng
(Tonify the Middle and Augment the Qi Decoction)

10. Cho JM, Sato N, Kikuchi K. Prophylactic anti-tumor effect of Hochu-ekki-to (TJ41) by enhancing natural killer cell activity. In Vivo 1991 Jul-Aug;5(4):389-91.

11. Kim SH, Lee SE, Oh H, Kim SR, Yee ST, Yu YB, Byun MW, Jo SK. The radioprotective effects of bu-zhong-yi-qi-tang: a prescription of traditional Chinese medicine. Am J Chin Med 2002;30(1):127-37.

12. Yan XQ, Kita M, Minami M, Yamamoto T, Kuriyama H, Ohno T, Iwakura Y, Imanishi J. Antibacterial Effect of Kampo Herbal Formulation Hochu-Ekki-To (Bu-Zhong-Yi-Qi-Tang) on Helicobacter pylori Infection in Mice. Microbiol Immunol 2002;46(7):475-482.

13. Mori K, Kido T, Daikuhara H, Sakakibara I, Sakata T, Shimizu K, Amagaya S, Sasaki H, Komatsu Y. Effect of Hochu-ekki-to (TJ-41), a Japanese herbal medicine, on the survival of mice infected with influenza virus. Antiviral Res 1999 Dec 15;44(2):103-11.

14. Sassa S, Sakamoto S, Zhou YF, Mori T, Kikuchi T, Shinoda H. Preventive effects of a Chinese herbal medicine, hochu-ekki-to, on bone loss in ovariectomized rats. Medical Research Institute, Tokyo Medical and Dental University In Vivo 2001 Jan-Feb;15(1):25-8.

15. Koshikawa N, Imai T, Takahashi I, Yamauchi M, Sawada S, Kansaku A. Effects of Hochu-ekki-to, Yoku-kan-san and Saiko-ka-ryukotsu-borei-to on behavioral despair and acetic acid-induced writhing in mice. Methods Find Exp Clin Pharmacol 1998 Jan-Feb;20(1):47-51.

16. Guo Wai Yi Xue Zhong Yi Zhong Yao Fen Ce (Monograph of Chinese Herbology from Foreign Medicine) 1993;15(6):27.

17. Shi Yong Zhong Yi Za Zhi (Journal of Practical Chinese Medicine) 1998;8:20.

18. Shang Hai Zhong Yi Yao Za Zhi (Shanghai Journal of Chinese Medicine and Herbology) 1983;12:20.

19. Zhong Yi Yao Xue Bao (Report of Chinese Medicine and Herbology) 1995;3:42.

20. Hu Nan Zhong Yi Za Zhi (Hunan Journal of Chinese Medicine) 1997;3:48.

21. Shan Dong Yi Yao (Shandong Medicine and Herbology) 1979;4:43.

22. Ogawa Y, Fuji K, Shimada M, Yoshida H. A case of renal ptosis treated with hochu-ekki-to with improvement confirmed by excretory urography. Hinyokika Kiyo - Acta Urologica Japonica 2001 Sep;47(9):649-52.

23. Jiang Su Zhong Yi Za Zhi (Jiangsu Journal of Chinese Medicine) 1997;11:514.

24. He Bei Zhong Yi (Hebei Chinese Medicine) 1986;6:13.

25. Zhong Yi Fang Ji Xian Dai Yan Jiu (Modern Study of Medical Formulae in Traditional Chinese Medicine) 1997;529.

26. Shi Yong Zhong Xi Yi Jie He Za Zhi (Practical Journal of Integrated Chinese and Western Medicines) 1998;3:262.

27. Hunan Journal of Medicine and Herbology 1984;6:35.

28. Jiang Su Zhong Yi (Jiangsu Chinese Medicine) 1995;6:9.

29. Shi Yong Zhong Yi Yao Za Zhi (Journal of Practical Chinese Medicine and Medicinals) 1998;6:13.

30. Kuroiwa A, Liou S, Yan H, Eshita A, Naitoh S, Nagayama A. Effect of a traditional Japanese herbal medicine, Hochu-ekki-to (Bu-Zhong-Yi-Qi Tang), on immunity in elderly persons. Int Immunopharmacol 2004 Feb;4(2):317-24.

31. Zhe Jiang Zhong Yi Za Zhi (Zhejiang Journal of Chinese Medicine) 1992;10:444.

32. Itoh T, Itoh H, Kikuchi T. Five patients of MRSA-infected patients with cerebrovascular disorder and in a bedridden condition, for whom bu-zhong-yi-qi-tang (hochu-ekki-to) was useful. Shouseikai Ashiro Clinic, Ashiro Town, Iwate Pref., Japan. American Journal of Chinese Medicine 2000;28(3-4):401-8.

33. Nishida S. Effect of Hochu-ekki-to on asymptomatic MRSA bacteri-uria. Journal of Infection & Chemotherapy 2003 Mar;9(1):58-61.

34. Nishida S. Effect of Hochu-ekki-to on asymptomatic MRSA bacteri-uria. Journal of Infection & Chemotherapy 2003 Mar;9(1):58-61.

35. Mita Y, Dobashi K, Shimizu Y, Nakazawa T, Mori M. Surface expression of toll-like receptor 4 on THP-1 cells is modulated by Bu-Zhong-Yi-Qi-Tang and Shi-Quan-Da-Bu-Tang. Methods & Findings in Experimental & Clinical Pharmacology 2002 Mar; 24(2):67-70.

36. Shi Yong Zhong Yi Yao Za Zhi (Journal of Practical Chinese Medicine and Medicinals) 1998;3:262.

37. Shang Hai Zhong Yi Yao Za Zhi (Shanghai Journal of Chinese Medicine and Herbology) 1983;10:28.

38. Xin Zhong Yi (New Chinese Medicine) 1989;4:47.

39. Shan Xi Xin Zhong Yi (New Shanxi Chinese Medicine) 1988;6:258.

40. Zhong Yi Fang Ji Xian Dai Yan Jiu (Modern Study of Medical Formulae in Traditional Chinese Medicine) 1997;532.

41. Yi Xue Qing Kuang Jiao Liu (Medical Information Exchange) 1975;2:23.

42. Bei Jing Zhong Yi (Beijing Chinese Medicine) 1987;6:46.

43. Shan Xi Xin Zhong Yi (New Shanxi Chinese Medicine) 1986;8:340.

44. Zhong Xi Yi Jie He Za Zhi (Journal of Integrated Chinese and Western Medicine) 1989;4:242.

45. Guo Wai Yi Xue Zhong Yi Zhong Yao Fen Ce (Monograph of Chinese Herbology from Foreign Medicine) 1987;4:16.

46. Furuya Y, Akashi T, Fuse H. Effect of Bu-zhong-yi-qi-tang on seminal plasma cytokine levels in patients with idiopathic male infertility. Arch Androl 2004 Jan-Feb;50(1):11-4.

47. Amano T, Hirata A, Namiki M. Effects of Chinese herbal medicine on sperm motility and fluorescence spectra parameters. Archives of Andrology 1996 Nov-Dec;37(3):219-24.

48. Guang Xi Zhong Yi Yao (Guangxi Chinese Medicine and Herbology) 1989;2:12.

49. He Bei Zhong Yi (Hebei Chinese Medicine) 1989;4:9.

50. Fu Jian Zhong Yi Yao (Fujian Chinese Medicine and Herbology) 1995;2:12.

51. He Bei Zhong Yi (Hebei Chinese Medicine) 1984;3:24.

52. Kao ST, Yeh CC, Hsieh CC, Yang MD, Lee MR, Liu HS, Lin JG. The Chinese medicine Bu-Zhong-Yi-Qi-Tang inhibited proliferation of hepatoma cell lines by inducing apoptosis via G0/G1 arrest. China Medical College Hospital, China Medical College, Taichung, Taiwan. Life Sciences 2001 Aug 17;69(13):1485-96.

53. Kao ST, Yang SL, Hsieh CC, Yang MD, Wang TF, Lin JG. Immuno-modulation of Bu-Zhong-Yi-Qi-Tang on in vitro granulocyte colony-stimulating-factor and tumor necrosis factor-alpha production by peripheral blood mononuclear cells. Immunopharmacology & Immunotoxicology 2000 Nov;22(4):711-20.

54. Kido T, Mori K, Daikuhara H, Tsuchiya H, Ishige A, Sasaki H. The protective effect of hochu-ekki-to (TJ-41), a Japanese herbal medicine, against HSV-1 infection in mitomycin C-treated mice. Anticancer Res 2000 Nov-Dec;20(6A):4109-13.

55. Kaneko M, Kawakita T, Kumazawa Y, Takimoto H, Nomoto K, Yoshikawa T. Accelerated recovery from cyclophosphamide-induced leukopenia in mice administered a Japanese ethical herbal drug, Hochu-ekki-to. Immunopharmacology 1999 Nov;44(3):223-31.

56. Yun Nan Zhong Yi Za Zhi (Yunan Journal of Chinese Medicine) 1983;(3):28.

57. Takahashi K, Uejima E, Morisaki T, Takahashi K, Kurokawa N, Azuma J. In vitro inhibitory effects of Kampo medicines on metabolic reactions catalyzed by human liver microsomes. Journal of Clinical Pharmacy & Therapeutics 2003 Aug;28(4):319-27.

58. Xian Dai Shi Yong Yao Xue (Practical Applications of Modern Herbal Medicine) 1989;5:45.

Chinese Herbal Formulas and Applications

Bǔ Zhōng Yì Qì Tāng
(Tonify the Middle and Augment the Qi Decoction)

59. Wang MZ, et al. *Zhong Yi Xue Wen Da Ti Ku* (Questions and Answers on Traditional Chinese Medicine: Herbal Formulas).

60. Wang MZ, et al. *Zhong Yi Xue Wen Da Ti Ku* (Questions and Answers on Traditional Chinese Medicine: Herbal Formulas).

Yi Qì Cōng Míng Tāng (Augment the Qi and Increase Acuity Decoction)
益氣聰明湯
益气聪明汤

Pinyin Name: *Yi Qi Cong Ming Tang*
Literal Name: Augment the Qi and Increase Acuity Decoction
Alternate Names: *Yi Chi Cong Ming Tang, I Chi Chung Ming Tang*, Ginseng, Astragalus and Pueraria Decoction; Ginseng, Astragalus and Pueraria Combination
Original Source: *Dong Heng Shi Xiao Fang* (Tested and Effective Formulas by Dong Heng) by Li Gao (also known as Li Dong-Heng) in 1266

COMPOSITION

Ren Shen (Radix et Rhizoma Ginseng)	15g
Huang Qi (Radix Astragali)	15g
Ge Gen (Radix Puerariae Lobatae)	9g
Sheng Ma (Rhizoma Cimicifugae)	9g
Man Jing Zi (Fructus Viticis)	4.5g
Bai Shao (Radix Paeoniae Alba)	3g
Huang Bo (Cortex Phellodendri Chinensis), *zhi* (fried with liquor) and *chao* (dry-fried) till yellow	3g
Zhi Gan Cao (Radix et Rhizoma Glycyrrhizae Praeparata cum Melle)	15g

DOSAGE / PREPARATION / ADMINISTRATION

Grind the herbs into a coarse powder, and cook 9g in two bowls of water until it is reduced to one bowl. Take the strained decoction while warm.

CHINESE THERAPEUTIC ACTIONS

1. Tonifies qi and blood
2. Lifts yang qi and benefits the eyes and ears

CLINICAL MANIFESTATIONS

Compromised visual and auditory functions: diminished acuity of eyes and ears, blurred vision, dizziness, light-headedness, decreased appetite, spontaneous sweating, and chronic diarrhea.

CLINICAL APPLICATIONS

Cognitive dysfunction, cerebral arteriosclerosis, tinnitus, deafness, diminished vision, cataract, vertigo, otitis media, and ulcerative colitis.

EXPLANATION

Yi Qi Cong Ming Tang (Augment the Qi and Increase Acuity Decoction) treats compromised functioning and deterioration of the eyes and ears. It may be used to reverse deterioration, or preventively to maintain the acuity of both ears and eyes.

Ren Shen (Radix et Rhizoma Ginseng) and *Huang Qi* (Radix Astragali) tonify qi and strengthen the Spleen and Stomach. *Ge Gen* (Radix Puerariae Lobatae), *Sheng Ma* (Rhizoma Cimicifugae), and *Man Jing Zi* (Fructus Viticis) have an ascending function to lift yang qi and treat disorders of the upper parts of the body. When sufficient qi rises to the head, the normal functions of the eyes and ears will be restored. *Bai Shao* (Radix Paeoniae Alba) nourishes yin and harmonizes the blood. *Huang Bo* (Cortex Phellodendri Chinensis) controls deficiency fire. Lastly, *Zhi Gan Cao* (Radix et Rhizoma Glycyrrhizae Praeparata cum Melle) harmonizes the middle *jiao* and the other herbs in the formula.

8

TONIC FORMULAS

551

Chapter 8 – Tonic Formulas   Section 1 – Qi-Tonifying Formulas

Yi Qì Cōng Míng Tāng (Augment the Qi and Increase Acuity Decoction)

Yi Qi Cong Ming Tang (Augment the Qi and Increase Acuity Decoction)

Diagnosis	Signs and Symptoms	Treatment	Herbs
Deterioration of eye and ear functions	Diminished acuity of the eyes and ears, light-headedness, dizziness, decreased appetite, spontaneous sweating, and chronic diarrhea: qi and blood deficiencies	• Tonifies qi and blood • Lifts yang qi and benefits the eyes and ears	• *Ren Shen* (Radix et Rhizoma Ginseng) and *Huang Qi* (Radix Astragali) tonify qi and strengthen the Spleen and Stomach. • *Ge Gen* (Radix Puerariae Lobatae), *Sheng Ma* (Rhizoma Cimicifugae), and *Man Jing Zi* (Fructus Viticis) lift yang qi. • *Bai Shao* (Radix Paeoniae Alba) nourishes yin and harmonizes the blood. • *Huang Bo* (Cortex Phellodendri Chinensis) controls deficiency fire. • *Zhi Gan Cao* (Radix et Rhizoma Glycyrrhizae Praeparata cum Melle) harmonizes the herbs.

MODIFICATIONS

• With blurred vision and dizziness, add *Ju Hua* (Flos Chrysanthemi) and *Gou Qi Zi* (Fructus Lycii).

• With tinnitus due to Kidney deficiency, add *Zhi Bai Di Huang Wan* (Anemarrhena, Phellodendron, and Rehmannia Pill).

CAUTIONS / CONTRAINDICATIONS

• *Yi Qi Cong Ming Tang* is designed to treat compromised visual and auditory functions due to overall deterioration and deficiency. It should not be used if the eye and ear disorders are due to excess, such as Liver fire rising or damp-heat in the Liver and Gallbladder channels.[1]

• While taking this herbal formula, patients should avoid exposure to smoke and fire, and refrain from eating sour, cold, raw, oily or greasy foods.[2]

CLINICAL STUDIES AND RESEARCH

1. **Memory and cognition**: *Yi Qi Cong Ming Tang* has been used with satisfactory effect in treating geriatric patients with gradual deterioration of cognitive functions. In another study, use of modified *Yi Qi Cong Ming Tang* was associated with both subjective and objective improvements memory and cognitive performance in 30 geriatric patients with cerebral arteriosclerosis. The herbal treatment contained this formula plus *Tai Zi Shen* (Radix Pseudostellariae) and *Chi Shao* (Radix Paeoniae Rubra). The mechanism of action was attributed in part to the increased blood perfusion to the brain.[3]

2. **Tinnitus**: One study reported 96% effectiveness in the treatment of tinnitus characterized by Spleen deficiency using modified *Yi Qi Cong Ming Tang*. The herbal treatment contained the following ingredients: processed *Huang Qi* (Radix Astragali), *Dang Shen* (Radix Codonopsis),

dry-fried *Bai Zhu* (Rhizoma Atractylodis Macrocephalae), *Fu Ling* (Poria), *Sheng Ma* (Rhizoma Cimicifugae), *Ge Gen* (Radix Puerariae Lobatae), *Man Jing Zi* (Fructus Viticis), *Shi Chang Pu* (Rhizoma Acori Tatarinowii), *Sha Ren* (Fructus Amomi), dry-fried *Bai Shao* (Radix Paeoniae Alba), *Dan Shen* (Radix et Rhizoma Salviae Miltiorrhizae), dry-fried *Huang Bo* (Cortex Phellodendri Chinensis), and *Zhi Gan Cao* (Radix et Rhizoma Glycyrrhizae Praeparata cum Melle). Furthermore, modifications were made by adding dry-fried *Shan Yao* (Rhizoma Dioscoreae) and *Che Qian Zi* (Semen Plantaginis) for loose stools; and replacing *Dang Shen* (Radix Codonopsis) with *Ren Shen* (Radix et Rhizoma Ginseng) for *zhong* (central) *qi* deficiency. The treatment protocol was to cook the herbs 3 separate times, mix the 3 resulting decoctions together (the total amount should be approximately 450-600 mL), and administer in three equally-divided doses daily while warm, 2 hours after meals. The duration of treatment ranged from 1-7 days. Of 50 patients, the study reported complete recovery in 46 patients, improvement in 2 patients, and no benefit in 2 patients.[4]

3. **Vertigo**: Modified *Yi Qi Cong Ming Tang* was used to treat 52 geriatric patients with vertigo, with the history of illness ranging from 6 months to 3 years. The herbal treatment contained *Huang Qi* (Radix Astragali), *Dang Shen* (Radix Codonopsis), processed *Sheng Ma* (Rhizoma Cimicifugae), *Ge Gen* (Radix Puerariae Lobatae), *Man Jing Zi* (Fructus Viticis), *Huang Bo* (Cortex Phellodendri Chinensis), *Bai Shao* (Radix Paeoniae Alba), *Zhi Gan Cao* (Radix et Rhizoma Glycyrrhizae Praeparata cum Melle), *Tian Ma* (Rhizoma Gastrodiae), *Ban Xia* (Rhizoma Pinelliae), *Du Zhong* (Cortex Eucommiae), and *Niu Xi* (Radix Achyranthis Bidentatae). The treatment protocol was to cook the herbs in water, and administer the decoction in

552

Yi Qi Cōng Míng Tāng (Augment the Qi and Increase Acuity Decoction)

three equally-divided doses. Of 52 patients, the study reported complete recovery in 28 patients, improvement in 20 patients, and no benefit in 4 patients. The overall rate of effectiveness was 92.3%.[5]

4. **Otitis media**: One study reported good results for the treatment of suppurative otitis media using modified *Yi Qi Cong Ming Tang*. The herbal formula contained *Huang Qi* (Radix Astragali) 15g, *Ren Shen* (Radix et Rhizoma Ginseng) 15g, *Man Jing Zi* (Fructus Viticis) 9g, *Ge Gen* (Radix Puerariae Lobatae) 9g, *Bai Shao* (Radix Paeoniae Alba) 9g, *Huang Bo* (Cortex Phellodendri Chinensis) 6g, *Sheng Ma* (Rhizoma Cimicifugae) 6g, and *Zhi Gan Cao* (Radix et Rhizoma Glycyrrhizae Praeparata cum Melle) 6g. The herbs were given in decoction daily. Of 21 geriatric patients, the study reported complete recovery in 13 patients, moderate improvement in 6 patients, and no benefit in 2 patients.[6]

5. **Ulcerative colitis**: In a clinical trial on ulcerative colitis, patients were divided into two groups with one receiving herbs and the other receiving salicylazosulfapyridine. Patients in the herb group received the following formula: *Dang Shen* (Radix Codonopsis) 20-30g, *Ge Gen* (Radix Puerariae Lobatae) 20-30g, *Huang Qi* (Radix Astragali) 20-30g, dry-fried *Bai Shao* (Radix Paeoniae Alba) 12-18g, honey-fried *Sheng Ma* (Rhizoma Cimicifugae) 6-10g, dry-fried *Huang Bo* (Cortex Phellodendri Chinensis) 6-10g, *Man Jing Zi* (Fructus Viticis) 6-10g, and *Gan Cao* (Radix et Rhizoma Glycyrrhizae) 3-6g. Furthermore, *Shan Yao* (Rhizoma Dioscoreae) 30g and dry-fried *Bai Bian Dou* (Semen Lablab Album) 10g were added for Spleen and Stomach deficiencies; dry-fried *Cang Zhu* (Rhizoma Atractylodis) 10g and *Yi Yi Ren* (Semen Coicis) 20g were added for more damp; *Ma Chi Xian* (Herba Portulacae) 20g and *Huang Lian* (Rhizoma Coptidis) 6g were added

for heat; *Shen Qu* (Massa Fermentata) 10g and dry-fried *Shan Zha* (Fructus Crataegi) 10g were added for food stagnation; *Bu Gu Zhi* (Fructus Psoraleae) 10g and *Fu Zi* (Radix Aconiti Lateralis Praeparata) 10g were added for deficiency of *ming men* (life gate) fire; *Rou Dou Kou* (Semen Myristicae) 6-10g, *Ying Su Ke* (Pericarpium Papaveris) 6-10g, and dry-fried *Zhi Zi* (Fructus Gardeniae) 6-10g were added for constant diarrhea. Patients in the herb group received the herbs in decoction one time daily. Patients in the drug group received 4-6g of salicylazosulfapyridine daily. Corticosteroids were also given if needed. The duration of treatment was 1-2 months for both groups. At the end of treatment, the study reported that out of 45 patients in the herb group, there was marked improvement in 28 patients, moderate improvement in 10 patients, and no benefit in 7 patients. Out of 38 patients in the drug group, the study reported marked improvement in 7 patients, moderate improvement in 15 patients, and no benefit in 15 patients. The overall effectiveness rate was 84.4% in the herb group, and 60.6% in the drug group.[7]

References

1. *Zhong Yao Ming Fang Yao Li Yu Ying Yong* (Pharmacology and Applications of Famous Herbal Formulas) 1989;257-258.
2. *Zhong Yao Ming Fang Yao Li Yu Ying Yong* (Pharmacology and Applications of Famous Herbal Formulas) 1989;257-258.
3. *Shang Hai Zhong Yi Yao Za Zhi* (Shanghai Journal of Chinese Medicine and Herbology) 1991;5:41.
4. *Yun Nan Zhong Yi Za Zhi* (Yunan Journal of Chinese Medicine) 1993;3:25.
5. *Yun Nan Zhong Yi Xue Yuan Xue Bao* (Journal of Yunnan University School of Medicine) 1993;3:24.
6. *Shan Dong Yi Ke Da Xue Xue Bao* (Journal of Shandong University of Medicine) 1998;3:197.
7. *Zhe Jiang Zhong Yi Za Zhi* (Zhejiang Journal of Chinese Medicine) 1994;29(10):450.

Chapter 8 – Tonic Formulas   *Section 1 – Qi-Tonifying Formulas*

Shēng Mài Sǎn (Generate the Pulse Powder)

生脈散
生脉散

Pinyin Name: *Sheng Mai San*
Literal Name: Generate the Pulse Powder
Alternate Names: *Sheng Mai Yin* (Generate the Pulse Decoction), Ginseng and Ophiopogon Formula
Original Source: *Nei Wai Shang Bian Huo Lun* (Clarifying Doubts about Injury from Internal and External Causes) by Li Gao in 1247

COMPOSITION

Ren Shen (Radix et Rhizoma Ginseng)	1.5g [10g]
Mai Dong (Radix Ophiopogonis)	1.5g [10-15g]
Wu Wei Zi (Fructus Schisandrae Chinensis)	7 seeds [6g]

DOSAGE / PREPARATION / ADMINISTRATION

The source text states to prepare the ingredients as a decoction. It may be taken at any time of the day. Today, this formula is prepared by using larger doses of the ingredients, provided in brackets above, and cooking the herbs three times, and consuming the decoction within one day.

CHINESE THERAPEUTIC ACTIONS

1. Tonifies qi and promotes body fluid secretion
2. Astringes yin and stops perspiration

CLINICAL MANIFESTATIONS

1. Damaged qi and body fluids due to summer-heat and profuse sweating: a dry throat, thirst, irritability, lethargy, shortness of breath, and a fine, weak pulse.
2. Damaged qi and yin due to chronic coughing: coughing with scanty sputum, shortness of breath, spontaneous perspiration, a dry mouth and tongue with a dry, thin tongue coating, and a deficient, rapid or deficient, fine pulse.

CLINICAL APPLICATIONS

Shock, coronary artery disease, angina pectoris, myocardial infarction, cardiac failure, congestive heart failure,

arrhythmia, viral myocarditis, myocarditis, hypotension, cerebral infarction, Alzheimer's disease, leukopenia, chronic cough, pulmonary tuberculosis, chronic bronchitis, infertility, and diabetes mellitus.

EXPLANATION

Sheng Mai San (Generate the Pulse Powder) treats deficiencies of qi and yin, which may be caused by summer-heat inducing profuse sweating and damaging qi and body fluids. Damaged qi and yin may also occur from chronic coughing. Qi deficiency is characterized by spontaneous perspiration, lethargy, and shortness of breath. Yin deficiency is characterized by a dry mouth, thirst, irritability, coughing with scanty sputum, and a dry tongue with a thin, dry tongue coating.

Ren Shen (Radix et Rhizoma Ginseng), the chief herb, tonifies *yuan* (source) *qi* and strengthens the Lung. *Mai Dong* (Radix Ophiopogonis) nourishes yin, replenishes body fluids lost through perspiration, and relieves thirst and dry mouth. These two tonic herbs treat the root of the condition by replenishing what is lost and deficient. Lastly, *Wu Wei Zi* (Fructus Schisandrae Chinensis) astringes the Lung to stop sweating and arrest coughing.

Sheng Mai San (Generate the Pulse Powder)

Diagnosis	Signs and Symptoms	Treatment	Herbs
Damages to qi, yin, and body fluids	• Dry mouth, thirst, and irritability: yin and body fluid deficiencies • Profuse sweating or spontaneous perspiration, lethargy, and shortness of breath: qi deficiency • Dry tongue with a thin, dry tongue coating: yin and body fluid deficiencies • Deficient, rapid or deficient, fine pulse: qi and yin deficiencies	• Tonifies qi and promotes body fluid secretion • Astringes yin and stops perspiration	• *Ren Shen* (Radix et Rhizoma Ginseng) tonifies *yuan* (source) *qi* and strengthens the Lung. • *Mai Dong* (Radix Ophiopogonis) nourishes yin and replenishes body fluids. • *Wu Wei Zi* (Fructus Schisandrae Chinensis) astringes the Lung to stop sweating and coughing.

Shēng Mài Sǎn (Generate the Pulse Powder)

MODIFICATIONS

- If there is more yin deficiency, use *Xi Yang Shen* (Radix Panacis Quinquefolii) instead of *Ren Shen* (Radix et Rhizoma Ginseng).
- With irritability and insomnia due to neurasthenia, add *Suan Zao Ren* (Semen Ziziphi Spinosae) and *Bai Zi Ren* (Semen Platycladi).
- If there is a faint pulse and increased risk of shock, add a large dose of *Ren Shen* (Radix et Rhizoma Ginseng).
- For qi and yin deficiencies due to febrile disorder, add *Xuan Shen* (Radix Scrophulariae) and *Di Huang* (Radix Rehmanniae).
- For chronic respiratory disorder with cough, dyspnea, and sputum, add *Ku Xing Ren* (Semen Armeniacae Amarum) and *Chen Pi* (Pericarpium Citri Reticulatae).
- For chronic heart disorder with yin and yang deficiencies, add *Huang Qi* (Radix Astragali) and *Gan Cao* (Radix et Rhizoma Glycyrrhizae).
- For pulmonary tuberculosis, add *Shan Yao* (Rhizoma Dioscoreae) and *Bai Bu* (Radix Stemonae).

CAUTIONS / CONTRAINDICATIONS

- *Sheng Mai San* has an astringent action, and is contraindicated in patients with exterior syndromes or interior heat conditions.
- This formula is not recommended for chronic cough with Lung deficiency accompanied by an exterior syndrome.

PHARMACOLOGICAL EFFECTS

1. **Cardiovascular**: Administration of *Sheng Mai San* was associated with a marked effect on the cardiovascular system. In rabbits, it has a cardiotonic effect to increase the contractile force of heart tissues. It also prevents arrhythmia as demonstrated in laboratory experiments in rats. In addition, it increases blood perfusion to the coronary artery and the peripheral parts of the body.[1]
2. **Cardioprotective**: *Sheng Mai San* has a cardioprotective effect against post-ischemic myocardial dysfunction by opening the mitochondrial KATP channels.[2] It also reduces myocardial infarct size by activating protein kinase C and opening the mitochondrial KATP channel.[3] The lignan of *Wu Wei Zi* (Fructus Schisandrae Chinensis) is believed to be the major myocardial protective component in this formula.[4]
3. **Immunostimulant**: In mice, injection of *Sheng Mai San* at 0.4 mL per day for 5 days was associated with an increase in white blood cells and T-lymphocytes.[5]
4. **Central nervous system**: Administration of *Sheng Mai San* has a mild sedative effect on the central nervous system. It counters caffeine's stimulating effect.[6]
5. **Anti-inflammatory**: Administration of *Sheng Mai San* was associated with reduced swelling and inflammation

in rats. The effect was attributed to the increased gluco-corticoids production, because the formula had no benefit in subjects whose adrenal glands had been removed.[7]

CLINICAL STUDIES AND RESEARCH

1. **Coronary artery disease**: In one report, 41 patients with coronary artery disease were treated with *Sheng Mai San* with subjective improvement noted in 78% of patients, and ECG improvement in 14.5% of patients.[8] Another study reported 66.7% effectiveness in 35 patients with coronary artery disease using 20 mL of *Sheng Mai San* in liquid form three times daily for 3 weeks per course of treatment.[9]
2. **Angina pectoris**: Patients with angina characterized by qi and yin deficiencies were treated with intravenous injection of *Sheng Mai San* for 14 days per course of treatment with good results. Of 53 patients, the study reported marked effect in 12 patients, improvement in 35 patients, and no benefit in 6 patients. The overall rate of effectiveness was 88.6%.[10]
3. **Myocardial infarction**: Twelve patients with acute myocardial infarction were treated with oral ingestion of *Sheng Mai San* plus *Dang Gui* (Radix Angelicae Sinensis), *Yan Hu Suo* (Rhizoma Corydalis), *Chi Shao* (Radix Paeoniae Rubra), *Huang Qi* (Radix Astragali), *Bai Zhu* (Rhizoma Atractylodis Macrocephalae), *Fu Ling* (Poria), *Tao Ren* (Semen Persicae), and *Hong Hua* (Flos Carthami). Out of 12 patients, the study reported complete recovery in 4 patients, improvement in 6 patients, and no benefit in 2 patients.[11]
4. **Cerebral infarction**: Intravenous injection of *Sheng Mai San* was used to treat 96 patients with cerebral infarct (9 with complete paralysis, 72 with hemiparalysis, 16 with unconsciousness, 84 with deviation of the eyes and mouth, and 54 with speech difficulties). After treatment, the study reported complete recovery in 57 patients, marked improvement in 17 patients, moderate improvement in 14 patients, and no benefit in 8 patients. The overall rate of effectiveness was 91.7%.[12]
5. **Coronary heart disease**: One study reported marked results using *Sheng Mai San* to treat patients with coronary heart disease (30 with angina pectoris and 68 with acute myocardial infarction). The administration of the herbs was found to increase the levels of superoxide dismutase (SOD) and decreased glutathione peroxidase (GSH-Px) and malondialdehyde (MDA) in blood. By acting as an effective free radical scavenger in minimizing the lipid peroxidation damage, *Sheng Mai San* was considered effective for prevention and treatment of coronary heart disease.[13]
6. **Arrhythmia**: In one study, 36 patients with arrhythmia characterized by qi and yin deficiencies were treated first

Chapter 8 – Tonic Formulas   *Section 1 – Qi-Tonifying Formulas*

Shēng Mài Săn (Generate the Pulse Powder)

by intravenous injection, followed by oral ingestion, of *Sheng Mai San*. The study reported an overall effectiveness rate of 83.4%.[14] In another study, *Sheng Mai San* was associated with 85.7% effectiveness in treating 21 patients with chronic bradyarrhythmia.[15]

7. **Viral myocarditis**: Sixty-three patients with viral myocarditis were treated with good results using *Sheng Mai San* plus *Chi Shao* (Radix Paeoniae Rubra), *Long Gu* (Os Draconis), and *Mu Li* (Concha Ostreae). The treatment protocol was to administer the herbs in decoction daily for 15 days per course of treatment, for 1-2 courses total. The overall rate of effectiveness was 90%.[16]

8. **Myocarditis**: Twenty patients with myocarditis (15 were refractory to drug treatment) were treated with both *Sheng Mai San* and *Gan Mai Da Zao Tang* (Licorice, Wheat, and Jujube Decoction). Out of 20 patients, the study reported marked improvement in 6 patients, moderate improvement in 10 patients, and no benefit in 4 patients.[17]

9. **Hypotension**: One study reported 97.32% effectiveness using *Sheng Mai San* plus *Dang Gui* (Radix Angelicae Sinensis), *Gui Zhi* (Ramulus Cinnamomi), and *E Jiao* (Colla Corii Asini) to treat hypotension. Of 112 patients, the study reported complete recovery in 78 patients, marked improvement in 23 patients, and slight improvement in 8 patients. The treatment protocol was to cook the herbs in water and drink the decoction in three equally-divided doses. The duration of treatment was 3 courses, with 10 days per course.[18] According to another study, 15 patients with primary hypotension were treated with *Sheng Mai San*. The study noted that the blood pressure began to increase after one week. After 4 weeks of treatment, the average increase in blood pressure was 14 mmHg for systolic and 6.7 mmHg for diastolic.[19]

10. **Shock**: In one report, 17 patients with shock due to infection were treated with an injection of *Sheng Mai San* with an overall 88.2% effectiveness.[20] In another report, 8 patients with shock due to excessive loss of blood were treated with *Sheng Mai San* with excellent effect in 5 patients, improvement in 2 patients, and no benefit in 1 patient.[21]

11. **Alzheimer's disease**: One study reported good results in 14 patients with Alzheimer's disease using *Sheng Mai San* as a replacement for tea on a daily basis for 2 months.[27]

12. **Leukopenia**: Thirty-nine patients (21 males and 18 females, between 39-70 years of age) with leukopenia were treated with *Sheng Mai San* plus *Yu Zhu* (Rhizoma Polygonati Odorati), *Shi Hu* (Caulis Dendrobii), *Dang Gui* (Radix Angelicae Sinensis), and others as needed. The treatment protocol was to administer the herbs daily in decoction for 10 days per course of treatment, for 2-3 courses total. Of 39 patients, the study reported marked improvement in 14 patients, moderate improvement in 23

patients, and no benefit in 2 patients.[22]

13. **Infertility**: *Sheng Mai San* successfully treated infertility due to anovulation. The duration of treatment ranged from 1-6 months. Of 78 patients, the study reported pregnancy in 21 patients, normal ovulation in 17 patients, and no change in 40 patients.[23]

14. **Diabetes mellitus**: Twenty-one patients with diabetes were treated with 85.9% effectiveness using *Sheng Mai San* and *Liu Wei Di Huang Wan* (Six-Ingredient Pill with Rehmannia).[24]

TOXICOLOGY

In an acute toxicology study, no fatality or abnormal reactions were reported following intravenous injection at the dose of 0.4 g/20g. The LD_{50} was determined as 34.64 g/kg via injection.[25] In a chronic toxicology study, intravenous injection of the formula at 20 mL/kg/day for 15 days did not cause any abnormal reaction.[26]

AUTHORS' COMMENTS

Sheng Mai San consists of *Ren Shen* (Radix et Rhizoma Ginseng), *Mai Dong* (Radix Ophiopogonis), and *Wu Wei Zi* (Fructus Schisandrae Chinensis). Its primary functions are to tonify qi, generate fluids, astringe yin and generate pulse. *Ren Shen* (Radix et Rhizoma Ginseng) is the main and an essential ingredient in this formula because it is the most effective herb to warm the Heart, nourish *ying* (nutritive) level, and generate the pulse.

According to Dr. Chang Wei-Yen, *Sheng Mai San* can be combined with *Ba Zhen Tang* (Eight-Treasure Decoction) and *Tian Wang Bu Xin Dan* (Emperor of Heaven's Special Pill to Tonify the Heart) to treat headaches with dizziness, palpitations, frequent dreams, and coldness of the limbs caused by blood deficiency. In addition, *Sheng Mai San*, *Ren Shen Yang Ying Tang* (Ginseng Decoction to Nourish the Nutritive Qi), and *Yu Ping Feng San* (Jade Windscreen Powder) can be combined to enhance the immune system of those individuals who catch colds frequently.

Please refer to *Bu Fei E Jiao Tang* (Tonify the Lung Decoction with Ass-Hide Gelatin) for a comparison and contrast with *Da Bu Yin Wan* (Great Tonify the Yin Pill) and *Sheng Mai San*.

References

1. *Zhong Yi Fang Ji Xian Dai Yan Jiu* (Modern Study of Medical Formulae in Traditional Chinese Medicine) 1997;556-563.

2. Wang N, Minatoguchi S, Arai M, Uno Y, Nishida Y, Hashimoto K, Xue-Hai C, Fukuda K, Akao S, Takemura G, Fujiwara H. Sheng-Mai-San is protective against post-ischemic myocardial dysfunction in rats through its opening of the mitochondrial KATP channels. Circ J 2002 Aug;66(8):763-8.

Chinese Herbal Formulas and Applications

Shēng Mài Săn (Generate the Pulse Powder)

3. Wang N, Minatoguchi S, Uno Y, Arai M, Hashimoto K, Hashimoto Y, Yamaguchi K, Fukuda K, Akao S, Fujiwara H. Treatment with sheng-mai-san reduces myocardial infarct size through activation of protein kinase C and opening of mitochondrial KATP channel. Am J Chin Med 2001;29(2):367-75.

4. Li PC, Poon KT, Ko KM. Schisandra chinensis-dependent myocardial protective action of sheng-mai-san in rats. Am J Chin Med 1996;24(3-4):255-62.

5. *Zhong Guo Bing Li Sheng Li Za Zhi* (Chinese Journal of Pathology and Biology) 1987;3(1):38.

6. *Nei Meng Gu Zhong Yi Yao* (Traditional Chinese Medicine and Medicinals of Inner Mongolia) 1985;4:35.

7. *Yao Xue Tong Bao* (Report of Herbology) 1984;7:23.

8. *Zhe Jiang Zhong Yi Za Zhi* (Zhejiang Journal of Chinese Medicine) 1986;21(9):400.

9. *Zhong Hua Xin Xue Guan Bing Za Zhi* (Chinese Journal of Cardiology) 1987;3:144.

10. *Liao Ning Zhong Yi Za Zhi* (Liaoning Journal of Chinese Medicine) 1996;10:451.

11. *Chang Chun Zhong Yi Xue Yuan Xue Bao* (Journal of Changchun University of Chinese Medicine) 1997;2:13.

12. *Shi Yong Zhong Xi Yi Jie He Za Zhi* (Practical Journal of Integrated Chinese and Western Medicines) 1996;11:695.

13. Lu BJ, Rong YZ, Zhao MH. Effect of sheng mai san on lipid peroxidation in acute myocardial infarction patients. Zhongguo Zhong Xi Yi Jie He Za Zhi 1994 Dec;14(12):712-4.

14. *Tian Jin Yi Xue Za Zhi* (Journal of Tianjin Medicine and Herbology) 1983;1:43.

15. *Cheng Du Zhong Yi Xue Yuan Xue Bao* (Journal of Chengdu University of Traditional Chinese Medicine) 1981;2:52.

16. *Shan Dong Zhong Yi Za Zhi* (Shandong Journal of Chinese Medicine) 1995;5:207.

17. *Guang Zhou Zhong Yi Xue Yuan Xue Bao* (Journal of Guangzhou University of Chinese Medicine) 1984;2:51.

18. *He Bei Zhong Yi* (Hebei Chinese Medicine) 1993;2:11.

19. *Si Chuan Yi Xue* (Sichuan Medicine) 1981;2:100.

20. *Nei Meng Gu Zhong Yi Yao* (Traditional Chinese Medicine and Medicinals of Inner Mongolia) 1985;4:35.

21. *Zhong Hua Xin Xue Guan Bing Za Zhi* (Chinese Journal of Cardiology) 1980;8(2):90.

22. *Tian Jin Zhong Yi* (Tianjin Chinese Medicine) 1996;4:20.

23. *Zhong Yi Ming Fang Lin Chuang Xin Yong* (Contemporary Clinical Applications of Classic Chinese Formulas) 2001;260-261.

24. *Si Chuan Yi Xue* (Sichuan Medicine) 1989;7(12):20.

25. *Nei Meng Gu Zhong Yi Yao* (Traditional Chinese Medicine and Medicinals of Inner Mongolia) 1985;4:35.

26. *Zhong Yao Yao Li Yu Lin Chuang* (Pharmacology and Clinical Applications of Chinese Herbs) 1987;3(1):22.

27. *Zhong Yao Yao Li Yu Lin Chuang* (Pharmacology and Clinical Applications of Chinese Herbs) 1993;3:4.

Rén Shēn Gé Jiè Săn (Ginseng and Gecko Powder)

人参蛤蚧散

人参蛤蚧散

Pinyin Name: *Ren Shen Ge Jie San*
Literal Name: Ginseng and Gecko Powder
Alternate Name: Ginseng and Gecko Combination
Original Source: *Wei Sheng Bao Jian* (Precious Mirror of Health) by Luo Tian-Yi in the Yuan Dynasty

COMPOSITION

Ren Shen (Radix et Rhizoma Ginseng)	60g
Ge Jie (Gecko)	1 pair
Fu Ling (Poria)	60g
Sang Bai Pi (Cortex Mori)	60g
Ku Xing Ren (Semen Armeniacae Amarum), *chao* (dry-fried)	150g
Bei Mu (Bulbus Fritillariae)	60g
Zhi Mu (Rhizoma Anemarrhenae)	60g
Zhi Gan Cao (Radix et Rhizoma Glycyrrhizae Praeparata cum Melle)	150g

DOSAGE / PREPARATION / ADMINISTRATION

The source text instructs to grind the ingredients into a fine powder and store it in a porcelain container. Take the powdered formula with a small amount of water daily. Today, it is usually prepared as a powder. Take 6g with water on an empty stomach in the morning and evening.

Note: The source text specifies that *Ge Jie* (Gecko) should be processed first to remove its odor; this is done by soaking it in river water, and renewing the water daily, for five days. It is then fried until it turns yellow and crisp. Today, it is usually processed by washing and cleaning it with

Chapter 8 – Tonic Formulas   *Section 1 – Qi-Tonifying Formulas*

Rén Shēn Gé Jiè Sǎn (Ginseng and Gecko Powder)

liquor. Then, bake it using mild heat until it turns dry and crisp, and then grind it into a fine powder.

CHINESE THERAPEUTIC ACTIONS
1. Tonifies qi and clears the Lung
2. Arrests cough and relieves wheezing

CLINICAL MANIFESTATIONS
Chronic consumptive Lung disease due to deficiency heat: chronic cough, wheezing, dyspnea, thick, yellow sputum with or without blood and pus, a feeling of irritability and heat sensation in the chest, weight loss with or without facial edema, chronic lung atrophy, and a superficial, deficient pulse at the *cun* position.

CLINICAL APPLICATIONS
Chronic asthma, bronchial asthma, chronic bronchitis, tuberculosis, emphysema, and chronic respiratory tract infection.

EXPLANATION
Ren Shen Ge Jie San (Ginseng and Gecko Powder) treats chronic consumptive Lung disease due to deficiency heat. This syndrome usually originates from chronic coughing, which may weaken the qi and lead to weight loss. The Lung controls the distribution of water throughout the body. When the Lung is deficient and cannot properly distribute water, water stagnates, and dampness and phlegm begin to accumulate. Damp and phlegm accumulation causes facial edema and coughing with sputum. Chronic coughing and heat may also damage the blood

vessels, leading to bloody sputum. Damp and phlegm accumulation over time can create interior heat, which produces thick, yellow sputum and give rise to fidgeting. A superficial, deficient pulse at the *cun* position indicates severe Lung qi deficiency.

Ren Shen (Radix et Rhizoma Ginseng) tonifies *yuan* (source) *qi*, strengthens the Lung to improve respiration, and benefits the Spleen to eliminate dampness and phlegm. *Ge Jie* (Gecko), which enters the Lung and Kidney channels, tonifies the Lung to facilitate breathing, and benefits the Kidney to grasp qi downward. Tonifying the Lung and Kidney is absolutely necessary in chronic coughing syndromes, which involve deficiency of both organs. *Fu Ling* (Poria) strengthens the Spleen, dispels dampness and phlegm, and relieves facial edema. *Sang Bai Pi* (Cortex Mori) and *Ku Xing Ren* (Semen Armeniacae Amarum) correct the reversed flow of Lung qi to stop coughing and wheezing. *Bei Mu* (Bulbus Fritillariae) clears Lung heat, dispels phlegm, and stops coughing. *Zhi Mu* (Rhizoma Anemarrhenae) clears Lung heat and nourishes the Kidney to assist in grasping the qi downward. *Zhi Gan Cao* (Radix et Rhizoma Glycyrrhizae Praeparata cum Melle) tonifies qi and harmonizes the herbs.

MODIFICATIONS
- For more Lung and Kidney deficiencies, add *Dong Chong Xia Cao* (Cordyceps).
- With more phlegm accumulation, add *Lai Fu Zi* (Semen Raphani) and *Bai Jie Zi* (Semen Sinapis).
- With yin deficiency, add *Mai Dong* (Radix Ophiopogonis).

Ren Shen Ge Jie San (Ginseng and Gecko Powder)

Diagnosis	Signs and Symptoms	Treatment	Herbs
Chronic consumptive Lung disease	• Chronic coughing with thick, yellow sputum: damp and phlegm accumulation affecting Lung qi circulation • Facial edema: Lung deficiency unable to distribute water evenly • Bloody sputum: chronic coughing and heat damaging the blood vessels • Superficial, deficient pulse: Lung qi deficiency	• Tonifies qi and clears the Lung • Arrests cough and relieves wheezing	• *Ren Shen* (Radix et Rhizoma Ginseng) strengthens the Lung and tonifies *yuan* (source) *qi*. • *Ge Jie* (Gecko) tonifies the Lung and Kidney to improve breathing. • *Fu Ling* (Poria) strengthens the Spleen. • *Sang Bai Pi* (Cortex Mori) and *Ku Xing Ren* (Semen Armeniacae Amarum) correct the reversed flow of Lung qi to stop coughing and wheezing. • *Bei Mu* (Bulbus Fritillariae) clears Lung heat, dispels phlegm, and stops coughing. • *Zhi Mu* (Rhizoma Anemarrhenae) clears Lung heat and nourishes the Kidney. • *Zhi Gan Cao* (Radix et Rhizoma Glycyrrhizae Praeparata cum Melle) tonifies qi and harmonizes the herbs.

Chinese Herbal Formulas and Applications

Rén Shēn Gé Jiè Sǎn (Ginseng and Gecko Powder)

- With profuse bleeding with or without pus, add *Bai Mao Gen* (Rhizoma Imperatae), charred *Di Yu* (Radix Sanguisorbae) and charred *Ce Bai Ye* (Cacumen Platycladi).
- For acute asthma attack due to heat, combine with *Ma Huang Xing Ren Gan Cao Shi Gao Tang* (Ephedra, Apricot Kernel, Licorice, and Gypsum Decoction).
- For acute asthma attack due to cold, combine with *Xiao Qing Long Tang* (Minor Bluegreen Dragon Decoction).
- For chronic cough without heat signs, remove *Sang Bai Pi* (Cortex Mori) and *Zhi Mu* (Rhizoma Anemarrhenae).

CAUTIONS / CONTRAINDICATIONS

Ren Shen Ge Jie San is contraindicated in cases of cough and dyspnea caused by exterior conditions.

CLINICAL STUDIES AND RESEARCH

Respiratory disorders: In one report, 30 geriatric patients with chronic respiratory disorders (asthma, chronic bronchitis, bronchial asthma) characterized by deficiency and cold were treated with modified *Ren Shen Ge Jie San* with good results. The modified formula contained *Ren Shen* (Radix et Rhizoma Ginseng) 20g, *San Qi* (Radix et Rhizoma Notoginseng) 20g, *Chuan Bei Mu* (Bulbus Fritillariae Cirrhosae) 30g, and *Ge Jie* (Gecko) 2 pieces. The formula was given as a fine powder, 1.5-2.0g per dose, two to three times daily. The study noted that the herbs effectively reduced or prevented asthma attacks in these patients.[1]

RELATED FORMULAS

Rén Shēn Hú Táo Tāng (Ginseng and Walnut Decoction)

人参胡桃湯
人参胡桃汤

Pinyin Name: *Ren Shen Hu Tao Tang*
Literal Name: Ginseng and Walnut Decoction
Original Source: *Ji Sheng Fang* (Formulas to Aid the Living) by Yan Yong-He in 1253

Ren Shen (Radix et Rhizoma Ginseng), qie (sliced)	1 piece [9g]
Hu Tao Ren (Semen Juglandis)	5 nuts [9g]

The source text states to cook the ingredients with 5 slices of *Sheng Jiang* (Rhizoma Zingiberis Recens) in a small bowl of water until the liquid is reduced to 70%. Take the strained, warm decoction before bedtime. Today, cook the herbs and take the decoction in three equally-divided doses on an empty stomach three times a day in the morning, noon, and evening.

Ren Shen Hu Tao Tang (Ginseng and Walnut Decoction) tonifies Lung and Kidney and relieves wheezing and dyspnea. Clinically, this formula may be used to treat patients who cannot sleep due to coughing and wheezing characterized by Lung and Kidney deficiencies.

Rén Shēn Chóng Cǎo Tāng
(Ginseng and Cordyceps Decoction)

人参蟲草湯
人参虫草汤

Pinyin Name: *Ren Shen Chong Cao Tang*
Literal Name: Ginseng and Cordyceps Decoction
Original Source: *An Hui Zhong Yi Xue Yuan* (Anhui University School of Medicine) in 1990

Ren Shen (Radix et Rhizoma Ginseng)
Dong Chong Xia Cao (Cordyceps)
Huang Qi (Radix Astragali)

Ren Shen Chong Cao Tang (Ginseng and Cordyceps Decoction) tonifies Lung qi and Kidney yang, and is most effective in treating cough, wheezing, and dyspnea caused by Lung qi and Kidney yang deficiencies. This formula may also be taken on a long-term basis as a maintainance formula for asthma.

AUTHORS' COMMENTS

Ren Shen Ge Jie San and *Ren Shen Hu Tao Tang* (Ginseng and Walnut Decoction) both use *Ren Shen* (Radix et Rhizoma Ginseng) to tonify *yuan* (source) *qi* to treat asthma or cough due to deficiency. Their differences are:

- *Ren Shen Ge Jie San* is a stronger formula that is cold in nature, and is more suitable for prominent coughing and wheezing due to deficiency and heat. In this formula, *Ge Jie* (Gecko) and *Ren Shen* (Radix et Rhizoma Ginseng) tonify the Lung and Kidney to help the Kidney grasp the qi. *Sang Bai Pi* (Cortex Mori), *Bei Mu* (Bulbus Fritillariae), and *Ku Xing Ren* (Semen Armeniacae Amarum) clear and sedate the Lung to arrest wheezing and cough. *Fu Ling* (Poria) and *Gan Cao* (Radix et Rhizoma Glycyrrhizae) strengthen the Spleen, dispel dampness, and indirectly benefit Kidney qi. This formula is indicated for Kidney and Lung deficiencies, with dampness blocking the Kidney from grasping the qi downward.
- *Ren Shen Hu Tao Tang* is a gentler formula that is slightly warm in nature, and is more suitable for coughing and wheezing due to deficiency and cold. Warm herbs, such as *Ren Shen* (Radix et Rhizoma Ginseng), *Hu Tao Ren* (Semen Juglandis), and *Sheng Jiang* (Rhizoma Zingiberis Recens), tonify the Lung and Kidney.[2]

References
1. *Jiang Su Zhong Yi* (Jiangsu Chinese Medicine) 1988;(3):25.
2. Wang MZ, et al. *Zhong Yi Xue Wen Da Ti Ku* (Questions and Answers on Traditional Chinese Medicine: Herbal Formulas).

TONIC FORMULAS 8

559

Chapter 8 – Tonic Formulas　　　　　　　　　　　　　　*Section 1 – Qi-Tonifying Formulas*

Bǔ Fèi Tāng (Tonify the Lung Decoction)

補肺湯
补肺汤

Pinyin Name: *Bu Fei Tang*
Literal Name: Tonify the Lung Decoction
Alternate Name: Ginseng and Aster Combination
Original Source: *Yong Lei Qian Fang* (Everlasting Categorization of Seal Formulas)

COMPOSITION

Huang Qi (Radix Astragali)	24g
Ren Shen (Radix et Rhizoma Ginseng)	9g
Sang Bai Pi (Cortex Mori)	12g
Zi Wan (Radix et Rhizoma Asteris)	9g
Wu Wei Zi (Fructus Schisandrae Chinensis)	6g
Shu Di Huang (Radix Rehmanniae Praeparata)	24g

DOSAGE / PREPARATION / ADMINISTRATION

Prepare this formula as a decoction.

CHINESE THERAPEUTIC ACTIONS

1. Tonifies Lung qi
2. Strengthens *wei* (defensive) *qi*

CLINICAL MANIFESTATIONS

Lung qi deficiency: cough, dyspnea, wheezing, low energy, a low and weak voice, chills, intolerance of cold, spontaneous perspiration, a pale face, and a pale tongue with a thin, white coating.

CLINICAL APPLICATIONS

Chronic cough, asthma, and pulmonary tuberculosis.

EXPLANATION

Bu Fei Tang (Tonify the Lung Decoction) treats Lung qi deficiency characterized by wheezing and dyspnea.

Patients with weak Lung qi are unable to control rhythmic respiration, and thus they have symptoms such as wheezing, dyspnea, shortness of breath, and a low and weak voice. Wheezing and dyspnea may be due in part to Kidney deficiency, and its subsequent inability to grasp the qi. Deficient Lung qi is often accompanied by deficient *wei* (defensive) *qi*, which results in the body's inability to protect its exterior level. Consequently, patients usually present with chills, aversion to cold, and spontaneous perspiration. *Wei* (defensive) *qi* deficiency enables exterior cold factors to easily penetrate and constrict the Lung, causing cough, wheezing, and dyspnea. A pale face and a pale tongue with a thin, white coating are indicative of qi deficiency.

Huang Qi (Radix Astragali) and *Ren Shen* (Radix et Rhizoma Ginseng) address the root of the illness by tonifying qi and strengthening *wei* (defensive) *qi*. *Sang Bai Pi* (Cortex Mori) guides Lung qi downward to relieve

Bu Fei Tang (Tonify the Lung Decoction)

Diagnosis	Signs and Symptoms	Treatment	Herbs
Lung qi deficiency	• Wheezing, dyspnea, shortness of breath, and a low and weak voice: Lung qi deficiency • Chills, intolerance to cold, and spontaneous perspiration: *wei* (defensive) *qi* deficiency • Pale face and a pale tongue: qi deficiency	• Tonifies Lung qi • Strengthens *wei* (defensive) *qi*	• *Huang Qi* (Radix Astragali) and *Ren Shen* (Radix et Rhizoma Ginseng) tonify qi and strengthen *wei* (defensive) *qi*. • *Sang Bai Pi* (Cortex Mori) guides Lung qi downward to relieve wheezing and dyspnea. • *Zi Wan* (Radix et Rhizoma Asteris) moistens the Lung to relieve cough. • *Wu Wei Zi* (Fructus Schisandrae Chinensis) constricts Lung qi and stops spontaneous perspiration. • *Shu Di Huang* (Radix Rehmanniae Praeparata) tonifies the Kidney and enhances its function to grasp the qi downward to relieve

Bǔ Fèi Tāng (Tonify the Lung Decoction)

Chinese Herbal Formulas and Applications

wheezing and dyspnea. *Zi Wan* (Radix et Rhizoma Asteris) moistens the Lung to relieve cough. *Wu Wei Zi* (Fructus Schisandrae Chinensis) astringes Lung qi and stops spontaneous perspiration. *Wu Wei Zi* (Fructus Schisandrae Chinensis) and *Shu Di Huang* (Radix Rehmanniae Praeparata) tonify the Kidney and enhance its function of grasping qi downward.

MODIFICATIONS

- If there is severe qi deficiency, add *Si Jun Zi Tang* (Four-Gentlemen Decoction).
- With Kidney deficiency, add *Ren Shen Ge Jie San* (Ginseng and Gecko Powder).

CAUTIONS / CONTRAINDICATIONS

Avoid raw, uncooked, and cold types of foods while taking *Bu Fei Tang*.

Chapter 8 – Tonic Formulas　　　　　　　　　　　　　　　　　　*Section 2 – Blood-Tonifying Formulas*

Section 2

补血剂
— Blood-Tonifying Formulas

Sì Wù Tāng (Four-Substance Decoction)
四物湯
四物汤

Pinyin Name: *Si Wu Tang*
Literal Name: Four-Substance Decoction
Alternate Names: *Szu Wu Tang*, Four Component Decoction, Four Herbs Decoction, Tangkuei Four Combination
Original Source: *Tai Ping Hui Min He Ji Ju Fang* (Imperial Grace Formulary of the Tai Ping Era) by the Imperial Medical Department in 1078-85

COMPOSITION

Shu Di Huang (Radix Rehmanniae Praeparata), *zheng* (steamed) with liquor	[12g]
Dang Gui (Radix Angelicae Sinensis), *jin* (soaked) and *chao* (dry-fried) with liquor	[9-12g]
Bai Shao (Radix Paeoniae Alba)	[9-12g]
Chuan Xiong (Rhizoma Chuanxiong)	[6-9g]

DOSAGE / PREPARATION / ADMINISTRATION

The source text states to coarsely grind equal amounts of the ingredients. Cook 9g of the powder in 1.5 large bowls of water and reduce it to 80%. Take the warm, strained decoction on an empty stomach. The source text mentions that *Ai Ye* (Folium Artemisiae Argyi) and *E Jiao* (Colla Corii Asini) may be added for conditions such as restless fetus, lochioschesis, *beng lou* (flooding and spotting), and profuse menstrual bleeding. Today, it is usually prepared as a decoction with the doses suggested in brackets. Take the decoction in three equally-divided doses three times daily (morning, noon and evening).

CHINESE THERAPEUTIC ACTIONS

1. Nourishes the blood
2. Regulates blood circulation

CLINICAL MANIFESTATIONS

1. General blood deficiency: a pale face, pale lips, pale fingernails, a sallow appearance, dizziness, blurry vision, palpitations, insomnia, a pale tongue with a white tongue coating, and a fine, deficient or fine, wiry pulse.
2. Deficiency and injury of the *chong* (thoroughfare) and *ren* (conception) channels: irregular menstruation, hypomenorrhea or hypermenorrhea, delayed menstruation or

amenorrhea, trickling of blood with pale red color, hard abdominal mass from blood stasis, and pain around the umbilicus and lower abdomen.
3. Gestational and postpartum disorders: unstable fetus with bleeding, postpartum uterine bleeding with lower abdominal pain, chills and fever.

CLINICAL APPLICATIONS

Anemia, postpartum anemia, menstrual pain, irregular menstruation, abnormal vaginal discharge, breech presentation, threatened abortion, ectopic pregnancy, endometriosis, infertility, pelvic inflammatory disease, headache, neurogenic headache, vascular headache, headache due to trauma, insomnia, chronic nephritis, lumbago, sciatica, periarthritis of the shoulder, itching, dermatitis, psoriasis, urticaria, and allergic rhinitis.

EXPLANATION

Blood deficiency, which usually manifests in the areas of menstruation and pregnancy in women, may also manifest in other aspects. A pale face, pale lips, pale fingernails, and a sallow appearance are the results of the blood's inability to nourish the skin. The Liver stores blood; thus, insufficient blood in the Liver causes lack of nourishment in the upper body, leading to dizziness, blurry vision and

562

Sì Wù Tāng (Four-Substance Decoction)

Si Wu Tang (Four-Substance Decoction)

Diagnosis	Signs and Symptoms	Treatment	Herbs
Blood deficiency	• Pale face, pale lips, pale fingernails, a sallow appearance, dizziness, blurry vision, a pale tongue with a white tongue coating, and a fine, deficient pulse: blood deficiency • Palpitations and insomnia: blood deficiency unable to nourish the Heart • Irregular menstruation (hypomenorrhea, delayed menstruation, amenorrhea, hypermenorrhea and hard abdominal mass from blood stasis): deficiency and injury of the *chong* (thoroughfare) and *ren* (conception) channels	• Nourishes the blood • Regulates blood circulation	• *Shu Di Huang* (Radix Rehmanniae Praeparata) tonifies yin and promotes blood production. • *Dang Gui* (Radix Angelicae Sinensis) tonifies the blood, activates blood circulation, and regulates the menses. • *Bai Shao* (Radix Paeoniae Alba) nourishes the blood, consolidates yin, and harmonizes the blood. • *Chuan Xiong* (Rhizoma Chuanxiong) activates and regulates blood circulation.

tinnitus. The Heart dominates the blood, and deficiency of blood leads to lack of nourishment to the *shen* (spirit), causing palpitations and insomnia. A pale tongue with a white tongue coating is typical of blood deficiency, as is also the case with a fine pulse.

Si Wu Tang (Four-Substance Decoction) is indicated for deficiency or injury of the *chong* (thoroughfare) and *ren* (conception) channels with blood deficiency. The *chong* (thoroughfare) and *ren* (conception) channels are closely related to the blood and uterus, and deficiency of these two channels may cause delayed menstruation with scanty amount of blood (hypomenorrhea). Pale red menstruation suggests deficiency of blood. In severe cases, amenorrhea may occur. In addition to blood deficiency, there may be other complications. If the Spleen becomes very deficient and fails to keep the blood circulating within the vessels, hypermenorrhea may occur. If the Kidney becomes deficient, trickling of blood may occur. If there is coldness inside the body, qi and blood may stagnate, causing pain around the umbilicus and the lower abdomen. Since the *ren* (conception) channel dominates the uterus, deficiency or injury of the *ren* channel may result in lack of nourishment to the fetus, causing it to become unstable.

All of the herbs in this formula enter the *xue* (blood) level. *Shu Di Huang* (Radix Rehmanniae Praeparata), the chief herb, tonifies the blood. It also tonifies the Kidney, which generates the marrow necessary for increased blood production. When tonifying blood, it is essential to also move blood to prevent stagnation. *Dang Gui* (Radix Angelicae Sinensis) both tonifies blood and activates blood circulation. It nourishes the Liver and regulates

the menses. *Bai Shao* (Radix Paeoniae Alba) nourishes the blood and consolidates yin. It harmonizes the blood in the *ying* (nutritive) level. *Chuan Xiong* (Rhizoma Chuanxiong) activates and regulates blood circulation and prevents the tonic herbs from causing stagnation in the body.

MODIFICATIONS

• If there is profuse menstrual bleeding, add *Ai Ye* (Folium Artemisiae Argyi) and *E Jiao* (Colla Corii Asini).

• For irregular menstruation, add *E Jiao* (Colla Corii Asini), *Ai Ye* (Folium Artemisiae Argyi), and *Xiang Fu* (Rhizoma Cyperi).

• For dysmenorrhea due to qi stagnation and blood deficiency, add *Xiang Fu* (Rhizoma Cyperi) and *Yan Hu Suo* (Rhizoma Corydalis).

• For hypermenorrhea, add *Huang Qin* (Radix Scutellariae) and *Bai Zhu* (Rhizoma Atractylodis Macrocephalae).

• With qi deficiency, add *Ren Shen* (Radix et Rhizoma Ginseng) and *Huang Qi* (Radix Astragali).

• With severe qi deficiency, combine with *Si Jun Zi Tang* (Four-Gentlemen Decoction).

• With qi stagnation, add *Zhi Shi* (Fructus Aurantii Immaturus), *Hou Po* (Cortex Magnoliae Officinalis), *Xiang Fu* (Rhizoma Cyperi), and *Yu Jin* (Radix Curcumae).

• With tidal fever from blood deficiency, add *Mu Dan Pi* (Cortex Moutan) and *Di Gu Pi* (Cortex Lycii).

• With headache due to blood deficiency, add *Ju Hua* (Flos Chrysanthemi), *Gao Ben* (Rhizoma et Radix Ligustici), and *Gou Teng* (Ramulus Uncariae cum Uncis).

• With dizziness and vertigo, add *Qin Jiao* (Radix Gentianae Macrophyllae) and *Qiang Huo* (Rhizoma et Radix Notopterygii).

Sì Wù Tāng (Four-Substance Decoction)

- With vomiting of blood or nosebleeds, add *Ce Bai Ye* (Cacumen Platycladi) and *Qian Cao* (Radix et Rhizoma Rubiae).
- For the presence of phlegm in an overweight person, add *Ban Xia* (Rhizoma Pinelliae) and *Ju Hong* (Exocarpium Citri Reticulatae).
- For the presence of phlegm in an underweight person, add charred *Zhi Zi* (Fructus Gardeniae), *Zhi Mu* (Rhizoma Anemarrhenae), and *Huang Bo* (Cortex Phellodendri Chinensis).
- With abdominal pain, slight perspiration, and aversion to wind, add *Rou Gui* (Cortex Cinnamomi) and *Pao Jiang* (Rhizoma Zingiberis Praeparatum).
- If there is white or blood-streaked vaginal discharge, add *Xiang Fu* (Rhizoma Cyperi) and *Gui Zhi* (Ramulus Cinnamomi).

CAUTIONS / CONTRAINDICATIONS

- *Si Wu Tang* should be used with caution in patients with deficiency of the Spleen and Stomach, because the stagnating nature of *Shu Di Huang* (Radix Rehmanniae Praeparata) could affect digestion.
- Although this formula treats blood deficiency, it is not suitable for patients who suffer from blood or qi collapse, yin deficiency with heat, or those with middle *jiao* deficiency manifesting in diarrhea.
- This formula should be used with caution during pregnancy and at low doses in infants.[1]

PHARMACOLOGICAL EFFECTS

1. **Hematopoietic**: *Si Wu Tang*, *Si Jun Zi Tang* (Four-Gentlemen Decoction), and *Shi Quan Da Bu Tang* (All-Inclusive Great Tonifying Decoction), were given orally to mice to evaluate their effect for treatment of anemia. The study concluded that *Shi Quan Da Bu Tang* (All-Inclusive Great Tonifying Decoction) was most effective, followed by *Si Wu Tang*, and *Si Jun Zi Tang* (Four-Gentlemen Decoction).[2] The mechanism of action was attributed to increased activity of CSF.[3]

2. **Antiplatelet**: Administration of *Si Wu Tang* in mice was associated with a preventative effect on the formation of blood clots. The mechanism of action was attributed to its antiplatelet effect.[4,5]

3. **Radioprotective**: Administration of *Si Wu Tang* 5-120 minutes prior to exposure to X-ray was beneficial in minimizing the related side effects. Administration of the herbs afterwards, however, was not associated with any benefit. The protective effect of the herbs against radiation was attributed to its regulating effect on the immune system.[6] Another study reported significant protective effect against high and low dose of gamma-irradiation. Protective effects included reduced frequency of radia-

tion-induced apoptosis ($p < 0.05$) and increased formation of endogenous spleen colonies ($p < 0.05$).[7]

4. **Cognitive**: Administration of *Si Wu Tang* was associated with a dose dependant effect to improve memory and cognitive functions in rats. The dose given ranged from 0.5 to 1.0 g/kg of the dried herbs.[8]

5. **Antioxidant**: One study reports *Si Wu Tang* to have marked antioxidant and antiaging effects.[9]

6. **Cardiovascular**: According to one study on 7 healthy adult males (age, 22.3 +/- 1.8 years old), administration of *Si Wu Tang* induced an increase of diastolic blood pressure and mean blood pressure.[10]

7. **Antipruritic and anti-inflammatory**: One study reported *Si Wu Tang* to have marked antipruritic and anti-inflammatory effects for treatment of cutaneous pruritus, chronic inflammation, and other diseases. The mechanism of action was attributed to the inhibition of histamine release from mast cells in a concentration-dependent fashion.[11]

8. **Antitumor**: Administration of *Shi Quan Da Bu Tang* (All-Inclusive Great Tonifying Decoction) was associated with a preventive effect on endometrial carcinogenesis in mice. The antitumor effects of *Shi Quan Da Bu Tang* (All-Inclusive Great Tonifying Decoction) was attributed in part to the contents of *Si Wu Tang*, as the administration of these four herbs was found to have an inhibitory effect on estrogen-induced expression of c-fos, interleukin (IL)-1alpha and tumor necrosis factor (TNF)-alpha in uteri of ovariectomized mice.[12]

CLINICAL STUDIES AND RESEARCH

1. **Menstrual pain**: Many studies have shown that menstrual pain can be treated effectively with *Si Wu Tang*. In one study, 57 patients with menstrual pain were treated effectively using *Si Wu Tang* plus *Bai Zhi* (Radix Angelicae Dahuricae), *Mu Xiang* (Radix Aucklandiae), *Xiang Fu* (Rhizoma Cyperi), and others as the base formula. Further modifications were made as follows: for qi and blood stagnation, *Niu Xi* (Radix Achyranthis Bidentatae) and *Yi Mu Cao* (Herba Leonuri) were added; for stagnation of cold and dampness, *Ai Ye* (Folium Artemisiae Argyi) and *Rou Gui* (Cortex Cinnamomi) were added; for qi and blood deficiencies, *Huang Qi* (Radix Astragali) and *Dang Shen* (Radix Codonopsis) were added; for Liver qi stagnation, *Chai Hu* (Radix Bupleuri) and *Chuan Lian Zi* (Fructus Toosendan) were added; for Liver and Kidney yin deficiencies, *Gou Qi Zi* (Fructus Lycii) and *Nu Zhen Zi* (Fructus Ligustri Lucidi) were added; for severe menstrual pain, *Xue Jie* (Sanguis Draconis), *Su Mu* (Lignum Sappan), and *Tu Bie Chong* (Eupolyphaga seu Steleophaga) were added; and for abnormal development of the uterus, *Zi Shi Ying* (Fluoritum) and *Yin Yang Huo* (Herba Epimedii) were added. Of 57 patients, the study

Sì Wù Tāng (Four-Substance Decoction)

reported significant improvement in 25 patients, moderate improvement in 25 patients, and no improvement in 7 patients.[13] Another study of 62 patients with menstrual pain reported 95.1% effectiveness using an herbal formula that contained *Dang Gui* (Radix Angelicae Sinensis), *Chuan Xiong* (Rhizoma Chuanxiong), *Bai Shao* (Radix Paeoniae Alba), *Xiang Fu* (Rhizoma Cyperi), *Gan Cao* (Radix et Rhizoma Glycyrrhizae), and others. The treatment protocol was to take the herbs daily for approximately 7 days before the period, and discontinue when the period begins.[14] Lastly, in one report, patients with severe menstrual pain were treated successfully with *Si Wu Tang* with addition of *Shi Xiao San* (Sudden Smile Powder), *Dan Shen* (Radix et Rhizoma Salviae Miltiorrhizae), *Xiang Fu* (Rhizoma Cyperi), and *Yan Hu Suo* (Rhizoma Corydalis). The treatment protocol was to begin the herbal therapy for 3-5 days, starting 5-7 days prior to the menstruation, and continue for 3 months.[15]

2. **Irregular menstruation**: In one study, 174 of 180 women with irregular menstruation had complete recovery after herbal treatment. The base formula included *Si Wu Tang* plus *Xiang Fu* (Rhizoma Cyperi), *Fu Shen* (Poria Paradicis), and *Gan Cao* (Radix et Rhizoma Glycyrrhizae). *Huang Qin* (Radix Scutellariae) and *Zhi Zi* (Fructus Gardeniae) were added for heat in the *xue* (blood) level before the period; and *Huang Qi* (Radix Astragali) and *Gan Jiang* (Rhizoma Zingiberis) were added for cold in the *xue* (blood) level after the period. *Yan Hu Suo* (Rhizoma Corydalis) and *Qing Pi* (Pericarpium Citri Reticulatae Viride) were added for blood stagnation with scanty menstrual discharge; and *Huang Qi* (Radix Astragali) and *Bai Zhu* (Rhizoma Atractylodis Macrocephalae) were added for qi deficiency with profuse menstrual discharge.[16] According to another study, 40 women with irregular and painful menstruation were treated with modified *Si Wu Tang* with marked improvement in 24 patients, moderate improvement in 12 patients, and no benefit in 4 patients.[17]

3. *Beng lou* **(flooding and spotting)**: One study reported satisfactory results using modified *Si Wu Tang* to treat 27 women with *beng lou* (flooding and spotting). In addition to *Si Wu Tang* as the base formula, other herbs were added based on such differential diagnosis as heat in the *xue* (blood) level, qi deficiency, and Kidney deficiency.[18]

4. **Breech presentation**: Modified *Si Wu Tang* was used to treat 80 women with breech presentation. The herbal treatment was based on *Si Wu Tang*, with removal of *Shu Di Huang* (Radix Rehmanniae Praeparata) and addition of *Bai Zhu* (Rhizoma Atractylodis Macrocephalae) and *Fu Ling* (Poria). The herbs were given daily for 3 doses per course of treatment. The presentation was corrected in 20 out of 22 women who were between 7-8 months pregnant, and 55 out of 58 women who were more than 8 months

pregnant. The overall effectiveness rate was 93.75%.[19] Another study of 155 patients of breech presentation reported 78.2% effectiveness using an herbal formula that contained *Si Wu Tang* plus *Bai Zhu* (Rhizoma Atractylodis Macrocephalae), *Huang Qi* (Radix Astragali), and *Zhi Qiao* (Fructus Aurantii).[20]

5. **Endometriosis**: One study used modified *Si Wu Tang* to treat 51 women with endometriosis and reported complete recovery in 40 patients (79.4%) and improvement in 11 patients (21.6%). The treatment included *Si Wu Tang* plus *Chi Shao* (Radix Paeoniae Rubra), *Yi Mu Cao* (Herba Leonuri) and *Huang Qi* (Radix Astragali) as the base formula. Modifications were made by adding *Ze Lan* (Herba Lycopi) and *Shui Zhi* (Hirudo) for severe blood stagnation; *Di Gu Pi* (Cortex Lycii) and *Lian Qiao* (Fructus Forsythiae) for yin-deficient heat; *Bai Zhu* (Rhizoma Atractylodis Macrocephalae) and a large dose of *Huang Qi* (Radix Astragali) for qi deficiency; *He Shou Wu* (Radix Polygoni Multiflori) and *E Jiao* (Colla Corii Asini) for blood deficiency; *Ai Ye* (Folium Artemisiae Argyi) and *Rou Gui* (Cortex Cinnamomi) for cold in the uterus; and *Xia Ku Cao* (Spica Prunellae) and *Zhe Shi* (Haematitum) for Liver qi rising.[21]

6. **Infertility**: Use of modified *Si Wu Tang* was associated with good results to treat infertility. In addition to the base formula, *Zi Shi Ying* (Fluoritum), *Xian Mao* (Rhizoma Curculiginis), *Yin Yang Huo* (Herba Epimedii), *Tu Si Zi* (Semen Cuscutae), and *Fu Pen Zi* (Fructus Rubi) were added for Kidney yang deficiency; and *Nu Zhen Zi* (Fructus Ligustri Lucidi), *Mo Han Lian* (Herba Ecliptae), *Gou Qi Zi* (Fructus Lycii), *Wu Wei Zi* (Fructus Schisandrae Chinensis), *Xuan Shen* (Radix Scrophulariae), and *Mai Dong* (Radix Ophiopogonis) were added for Kidney yin deficiency. Each menstrual cycle was considered as one course of treatment (20 +/- 2 days). Herbs were not given during the period or if pregnancy was achieved. Successful pregnancy was reported once in 19 of 27 women. The average duration of treatment was 45 packs of herbs.[22]

7. **Pelvic inflammatory disease**: According to one study, 154 patients with pelvic inflammatory disease were treated with complete recovery in 89 patients, marked improvement in 46 patients, moderate improvement in 8 patients, and no benefit in 11 patients. The overall effectiveness was 92.9%. The herbal treatment contained *Si Wu Tang* plus *Chai Hu* (Radix Bupleuri), *Huang Qin* (Radix Scutellariae), and *Zi Hua Di Ding* (Herba Violae) as the base formula. Additional modifications were made when necessary. For fever, *Dang Gui* (Radix Angelicae Sinensis) was removed and *Jin Yin Hua* (Flos Lonicerae Japonicae) and *Lian Qiao* (Fructus Forsythiae) were added. For abdominal pain, *Yan Hu Suo* (Rhizoma Corydalis) and *Pu*

Sì Wù Tāng (Four-Substance Decoction)

Huang (Pollen Typhae) were added. For poor appetite and diarrhea, *Shu Di Huang* (Radix Rehmanniae Praeparata) was removed, and *Sha Ren* (Fructus Amomi) and *Mai Ya* (Fructus Hordei Germinatus) were added.[23]

8. **Insomnia**: Ten patients with insomnia were treated with herbs resulting in complete recovery in 6 patients (6-7 hours of sleep), moderate improvement in 3 patients (5-6 hours of sleep), and slight improvement in 1 patient. The herbal treatment combined *Si Wu Tang* with other herbs that invigorate blood circulation. The duration of treatment was one month or less.[24]

9. **Chronic nephritis**: It has been reported that patients with chronic nephritis characterized by proteinuria and hematuria responded well to the combination of *Si Wu Tang* and *Wu Ling San* (Five-Ingredient Powder with Poria). In a case report, two patients were successfully treated with herbs without recurrence for 5-7 years.[25]

10. **Lumbago**: In one study, 135 women with low back pain characterized by "deficiency" were treated with herbs resulting in complete recovery in 37 patients, marked improvement in 82 patients, and no benefit in 16 patients. The herbs used included *Si Wu Tang* and *Li Zhong Tang* (Regulate the Middle Decoction). The average duration of treatment was 6.52 days.[26]

11. **Sciatica**: Modified *Si Wu Tang* was used to treat 112 patients with sciatica (history of 6 months to 15 years) with significant improvement in 61 patients, moderate improvement in 44 patients, and no benefit in 7 patients. The overall effective rate was 93.8%. The base formula contained *Si Wu Tang* plus *Wu Gong* (Scolopendra) and *Wu Shao She* (Zaocys). Modifications included the addition of *Fu Zi* (Radix Aconiti Lateralis Praeparata) and *Rou Gui* (Cortex Cinnamomi) for *tong bi* (extremely painful obstruction); *Du Huo* (Radix Angelicae Pubescentis), *Qin Jiao* (Radix Gentianae Macrophyllae), and *Fang Feng* (Radix Saposhnikoviae) for *xing bi* (mobile painful obstruction); and *Fu Ling* (Poria), *Yi Yi Ren* (Semen Coicis) and *Cang Zhu* (Rhizoma Atractylodis) for *zhuo bi* (fixed painful obstruction).[27]

12. **Periarthritis of the shoulder**: One study reported marked effects in treating periarthritis of the shoulder using *Si Wu Tang* plus *Du Zhong* (Cortex Eucommiae), *Jiang Huang* (Rhizoma Curcumae Longae), *Xi Xin* (Radix et Rhizoma Asari), *Hu Zhang* (Rhizoma et Radix Polygoni Cuspidati), and others. Strategies for modifications included addition of *Fang Feng* (Radix Saposhnikoviae) for wind; *Zhi Chuan Wu* (Radix Aconiti Praeparata) for cold; *Dan Nan Xing* (Arisaema cum Bile) for dampness, and *Dang Shen* (Radix Codonopsis) for qi deficiency. Of 215 patients, the study reported complete recovery in 93 patients, improvement in 104 patients, and no benefit in 18 patients.[28]

13. **Neurogenic headache**: *Si Wu Tang* has been shown in numerous studies to effectively treat headache. According to one study, 44 patients with neurogenic headache were treated with modified *Si Wu Tang* with complete recovery in 23 patients, significant improvement in 13 patients, moderate improvement in 7 patients, and no benefit in 1 case. Modifications included addition of *Sang Ye* (Folium Mori) and *Ju Hua* (Flos Chrysanthemi) for dizziness due to Liver fire rising; *Tao Ren* (Semen Persicae) and *Hong Hua* (Flos Carthami) for sharp, stabbing headache; and *Gou Qi Zi* (Fructus Lycii) and *He Shou Wu* (Radix Polygoni Multiflori) for dizziness and pain.[29] According to another study, 20 of 24 patients with neurogenic headache had complete recovery after treatment with a formula that contained *Si Wu Tang* plus *Tian Ma* (Rhizoma Gastrodiae), *Jiang Can* (Bombyx Batryticatus), *Gan Cao* (Radix et Rhizoma Glycyrrhizae), *Da Zao* (Fructus Jujubae), *Shi Jue Ming* (Concha Haliotidis), and *Wu Gong* (Scolopendra).[30]

14. **Vascular headache**: One hundred and four patients with vascular headache were treated with modified *Si Wu Tang* with complete recovery in 80 patients, marked improvement in 16 patients, improvement in 6 patients, and no benefit in 2 patients. The base formula included *Si Wu Tang* plus *Yan Hu Suo* (Rhizoma Corydalis), *Xi Xin* (Radix et Rhizoma Asari) and *Shi Jue Ming* (Concha Haliotidis). Modifications included the addition of *Xia Ku Cao* (Spica Prunellae) and *Ju Hua* (Flos Chrysanthemi) for heat; *Gui Zhi* (Ramulus Cinnamomi) for cold; *Bai Zhi* (Radix Angelicae Dahuricae) for frontal headache; *Qiang Huo* (Rhizoma et Radix Notopterygii) for occipital headache; *Gao Ben* (Rhizoma et Radix Ligustici) for vertex headache; and others as needed. The duration of treatment was 7 days per course of treatment. The overall rate of effectiveness was 98%.[31]

15. **Headache due to trauma**: One study reported 96.2% effectiveness in treating 80 patients with headache due to trauma with an herbal formula that contained *Si Wu Tang*, *Huang Qi Gui Zhi Wu Wu Tang* (Astragalus and Cinnamon Twig Five-Substance Decoction), and others. Modifications included addition of *Xi Xin* (Radix et Rhizoma Asari) for severe pain; *Dang Shen* (Radix Codonopsis) for qi deficiency; *Bei Sha Shen* (Radix Glehniae) for yin deficiency; *Yin Yang Huo* (Herba Epimedii) for yang deficiency; and dry-fried *Shan Zha* (Fructus Crataegi) and *Ji Nei Jin* (Endothelium Corneum Gigeriae Galli) for poor appetite. Out of 80 patients, the study reported complete recovery in 48 patients, improvement in 29 patients, and no benefit in 3 patients.[32]

16. **Itching**: One study of 134 patients with skin itching reported 91.8% effectiveness when treated with *Si Wu*

Si Wù Tāng (Four-Substance Decoction)

Chinese Herbal Formulas and Applications

Tang plus *He Shou Wu* (Radix Polygoni Multiflori), *Wu Shao She* (Zaocys), and *Ji Li* (Fructus Tribuli).[33]

17. **Psoriasis**: One study consisting of 10 psoriasis patients reported successful results using as treatment *Si Wu Tang*, *Ma Huang Tang* (Ephedra Decoction), *Wu Shao She* (Zaocys), *Tu Bie Chong* (Eupolyphaga seu Steleophaga), *Qiang Huo* (Rhizoma et Radix Notopterygii), and others as needed.[34] According to another study, 13 patients with psoriasis were treated with complete recovery in 8 patients, improvement in 2 patients, and no benefit in 3 patients. The herbal formula included *Si Wu Tang* plus *Bai Xian Pi* (Cortex Dictamni), *Ku Shen* (Radix Sophorae Flavescentis), and *Da Zao* (Fructus Jujubae).[35]

18. **Urticaria**: Administration of a modified *Si Wu Tang* formula was found to be effective in treating both acute and chronic urticaria. The herbal formula contained *Si Wu Tang* plus *Chan Tui* (Periostracum Cicadae), *Gan Cao* (Radix et Rhizoma Glycyrrhizae), *Jiang Can* (Bombyx Batryticatus), and *Wu Shao She* (Zaocys). The treatment protocol was to administer the herbs in decoction, for 7-10 packs of herbs per course of treatment. Of 185 patients, the study reported complete recovery in 161 patients, improvement in 20 patients, and no benefit in 4 patients. Among 161 patients who had complete recovery, only 4 had recurrence within 1 year of follow-up.[36]

19. **Allergic rhinitis**: Forty-two patients with allergic rhinitis were treated with modified *Si Wu Tang* with good results. The herbs used included *Si Wu Tang* with additions such as *Cang Er Zi* (Fructus Xanthii), *Xin Yi Hua* (Flos Magnoliae), and *Xu Chang Qing* (Radix et Rhizoma Cynanchi Paniculati). *Ju Hua* (Flos Chrysanthemi) and *Bai Zhi* (Radix Angelicae Dahuricae) were added for headache; and *Yu Ping Feng San* (Jade Windscreen Powder) was added for *wei* (defensive) *qi* deficiency. The treatment protocol was to administer the herbs in decoction for 15 days per course of treatment, for a total of 2-4 courses. Out of 42 patients, the study reported complete recovery in 23 patients, marked improvement in 13 patients, and no benefit in 6 patients. The overall rate of effectiveness was 87.5%.[37]

HERB-DRUG INTERACTION

- **Penicillin-induced dermatitis**: Ten patients with dermatitis caused by penicillin were treated with herbs with complete recovery in 7 patients and improvement in 3 patients. The study also noted that the time required for recovery and improvement were shorter when treated with herbs in comparison with no treatment. The herbs used included *Si Wu Tang*, *Xie Bai San* (Drain the White Powder), and others as deemed necessary.[38]
- **Scopolamine-induced spatial cognitive deficits**: Administration of *Si Wu Tang* has a dose-dependent effect to

reverse scopolamine-induced impairments in radial maze performance in mice.[39]

TOXICOLOGY

In acute toxicology studies in mice, oral administration of water or methyl alcohol extract at 2 g/kg did not cause any fatality. No fatality was associated with intraperitoneal injection at 2 g/kg for the methyl alcohol extract, or 0.5 g/kg for the water extract. However, 60% fatality was reported with intraperitoneal injection at 1 g/kg for the water extract. The study concluded that the water extract of this formula is slightly more toxic than the alcohol extract.[40]

RELATED FORMULAS

Shèng Yù Tāng (Sage-Like Healing Decoction)

聖愈湯
圣愈汤

Pinyin Name: *Sheng Yu Tang*
Literal Name: Sage-Like Healing Decoction
Alternate Name: Tangkuei Four Plus Combination
Original Source: *Lan Shi Mi Cang* (Secrets from the Orchid Chamber) by Li Gao in 1336

Di Huang (Radix Rehmanniae)	0.9g
Shu Di Huang (Radix Rehmanniae Praeparata)	0.9g
Chuan Xiong (Rhizoma Chuanxiong)	0.9g
Ren Shen (Radix et Rhizoma Ginseng)	0.9g
Dang Gui (Radix Angelicae Sinensis)	1.5g
Huang Qi (Radix Astragali)	1.5g

The source text states to grind the herbs into a coarse powder, and cook it in two cups of water until it is reduced to one cup. Take the strained decoction while warm. *Sheng Yu Tang* (Sage-Like Healing Decoction) tonifies qi and blood. Clinical applications include sores and abscesses with hemorrhage, palpitations, restlessness, and insomnia.

Shèng Yù Tāng (Sage-Like Healing Decoction)

聖愈湯
圣愈汤

Pinyin Name: *Sheng Yu Tang*
Literal Name: Sage-Like Healing Decoction
Original Source: *Yi Zong Jin Jian* (Golden Mirror of the Medical Tradition) by Wu Qian in 1742

Shu Di Huang (Radix Rehmanniae Praeparata)	22.5g [8g]
Ren Shen (Radix et Rhizoma Ginseng)	22.5g [20g]
Dang Gui (Radix Angelicae Sinensis), *xi* (washed) with liquor	15g [15g]
Huang Qi (Radix Astragali), *zhi* (fried with liquid)	15g [18g]

8

TONIC FORMULAS

Sì Wù Tāng (Four-Substance Decoction)

The source text states to prepare this formula as a decoction. Today, *Ren Shen* (Radix et Rhizoma Ginseng) is usually replaced with 20g of *Dang Shen* (Radix Codonopsis), and this formula may be prepared as a decoction with the doses suggested indicated in brackets. This formula tonifies qi and blood, and is clinically applicable for female patients with symptoms of both qi and blood deficiencies, manifesting with early menstruation, excessive menstrual bleeding that is light in color, lethargy, weakness of the limbs, and low energy.

Jiā Wèi Sì Wù Tāng

(Augmented Four-Substance Decoction)

加味四物湯
加味四物汤

Pinyin Name: *Jia Wei Si Wu Tang*
Literal Name: Augmented Four-Substance Decoction
Original Source: *Yan Fang* (Time-Tested Formulas) from John H.F. Shen

Dang Gui (Radix Angelicae Sinensis)
Chuan Xiong (Rhizoma Chuanxiong)
Bai Shao (Radix Paeoniae Alba)
Shu Di Huang (Radix Rehmanniae Praeparata)
Bai Zhi (Radix Angelicae Dahuricae)
Ge Gen (Radix Puerariae Lobatae)
Ju Hua (Flos Chrysanthemi)
Ji Li (Fructus Tribuli)
Man Jing Zi (Fructus Viticis)
Sang Ji Sheng (Herba Taxilli)
Tian Ma (Rhizoma Gastrodiae)
Yu Jin (Radix Curcumae)

Jia Wei Si Wu Tang (Augmented Four-Substance Decoction) primarily treats stress, tension, or migraine headaches caused by Liver excess and blood deficiency. This formula tonifies the blood, nourishes yin, subdues hyperactive yang, extinguishes Liver wind, and relieves pain.

Zhuàng Jīn Tāng (Strengthen the Tendon Decoction)

壯筋湯
壮筋汤

Pinyin Name: *Zhuang Jin Tang*
Literal Name: Strengthen the Tendon Decoction
Original Source: *Tian Jin Zhong Yi Xue Yuan* (Tianjin University of Chinese Medicine) in 1989

Dang Gui (Radix Angelicae Sinensis)
Dang Shen (Radix Codonopsis)
Wu Jia Pi (Cortex Acanthopanacis)
Di Huang (Radix Rehmanniae)
Gu Sui Bu (Rhizoma Drynariae)

Chuan Niu Xi (Radix Cyathulae)
Bai Shao (Radix Paeoniae Alba)
He Shou Wu (Radix Polygoni Multiflori)
Qian Nian Jian (Rhizoma Homalomenae)
Xu Duan (Radix Dipsaci)

Zhuang Jin Tang (Strengthen the Tendon Decoction) treats chronic and long-term musculoskeletal disorders characterized by atrophy and wasting of muscles, tendons and ligaments, decreased range of motion and mobility of the joints, and generalized weakness, soreness and pain. The composition of this formula follows the general principles of *Si Wu Tang* (Four-Substance Decoction) to tonify the blood and activate blood circulation. In addition, it contains herbs that open the channels and collaterals and strengthen the muscles and tendons.

Tiáo Jīng Yī Hào (Regulate Menses Formula One)

調經一號
调经一号

Pinyin Name: *Tiao Jing Yi Hao*
Literal Name: Regulate Menses Formula One
Original Source: *Guang An Men Yi Yuan* (Guang An Men Hospital) in 1990

Dang Gui (Radix Angelicae Sinensis)
Ze Lan (Herba Lycopi)
Chong Wei Zi (Fructus Leonuri)
Bai Shao (Radix Paeoniae Alba)
Chi Shao (Radix Paeoniae Rubra)
Chuan Xiong (Rhizoma Chuanxiong)
Fu Ling (Poria)
Xiang Fu (Rhizoma Cyperi)

Tiáo Jīng Èr Hào (Regulate Menses Formula Two)

調經二號
调经二号

Pinyin Name: *Tiao Jing Er Hao*
Literal Name: Regulate Menses Formula Two
Original Source: *Guang An Men Yi Yuan* (Guang An Men Hospital) in 1990

Shu Di Huang (Radix Rehmanniae Praeparata)
Shan Yao (Rhizoma Dioscoreae)
Shan Zhu Yu (Fructus Corni)
Tu Si Zi (Semen Cuscutae)
Gou Qi Zi (Fructus Lycii)
Suo Yang (Herba Cynomorii)
Bai Zhu (Rhizoma Atractylodis Macrocephalae)
Dang Gui (Radix Angelicae Sinensis)
Bai Shao (Radix Paeoniae Alba)
Nu Zhen Zi (Fructus Ligustri Lucidi)

Sì Wù Tāng (Four-Substance Decoction)

Niu Xi (Radix Achyranthis Bidentatae)
Chong Wei Zi (Fructus Leonuri)
Chuan Xiong (Rhizoma Chuanxiong)
Fu Ling (Poria)
Mu Dan Pi (Cortex Moutan)
Wu Wei Zi (Fructus Schisandrae Chinensis)
Ze Xie (Rhizoma Alismatis)

Tiáo Jīng Sān Hào (Regulate Menses Formula Three)
調經三號
调经三号
Pinyin Name: *Tiao Jing San Hao*
Literal Name: Regulate Menses Formula Three
Original Source: *Guang An Men Yi Yuan* (Guang An Men Hospital) in 1990

Shan Zhu Yu (Fructus Corni)
Suo Yang (Herba Cynomorii)
Tu Si Zi (Semen Cuscutae)
Yi Mu Cao (Herba Leonuri)
Ba Ji Tian (Radix Morindae Officinalis)
Bai Shao (Radix Paeoniae Alba)
Dang Gui (Radix Angelicae Sinensis)
Gou Qi Zi (Fructus Lycii)
Du Zhong (Cortex Eucommiae)
Shu Di Huang (Radix Rehmanniae Praeparata)
Xu Duan (Radix Dipsaci)
Yin Yang Huo (Herba Epimedii)
Xiao Hui Xiang (Fructus Foeniculi)

Tiáo Jīng Sì Hào (Regulate Menses Formula Four)
調經四號
调经四号
Pinyin Name: *Tiao Jing Si Hao*
Literal Name: Regulate Menses Formula Four
Original Source: *Guang An Men Yi Yuan* (Guang An Men Hospital) in 1990

Yi Mu Cao (Herba Leonuri)
Bai Shao (Radix Paeoniae Alba)
Bai Zhu (Rhizoma Atractylodis Macrocephalae)
Chai Hu (Radix Bupleuri)
Chuan Niu Xi (Radix Cyathulae)
Chuan Xiong (Rhizoma Chuanxiong)
Dang Gui (Radix Angelicae Sinensis)
Fu Ling (Poria)
He Huan Pi (Cortex Albiziae)
Ju He (Semen Citri Reticulatae)
Xiang Fu (Rhizoma Cyperi)
Yu Jin (Radix Curcumae)
Gan Cao (Radix et Rhizoma Glycyrrhizae)
Lu Lu Tong (Fructus Liquidambaris)

These four formulas regulate menstruation and treat female infertility.

- *Tiao Jing Yi Hao* (Regulate Menses Formula One) addresses the menstrual phase of the cycle. It contains herbs to move qi and blood to ensure the smooth flow of the period.
- *Tiao Jing Er Hao* (Regulate Menses Formula Two) is used during the follicular phase. It contains herbs to tonify the blood to ensure that the essential nutrients and substances of the body are properly replenished so that the body is ready for conception.
- *Tiao Jing San Hao* (Regulate Menses Formula Three) is used during the ovulatory phase. It contains herbs to tonify Kidney yang to help the eggs mature and promote ovulation.
- *Tiao Jing Si Hao* (Regulate Menses Formula Four) is used during the luteal phase to address premenstrual syndrome. It contains herbs to regulate qi and calm the *shen* (spirit).

AUTHORS' COMMENTS

The ancient tradition observes the four seasons as a natural cycle of genesis (spring), growth (summer), harvest (autumn) and storing (winter), respectively. Similarly, *Si Wu Tang* is formulated following the same principles. *Dang Gui* (Radix Angelicae Sinensis), sweet, warm and nourishing, represents genesis of blood like the spring sun. *Chuan Xiong* (Rhizoma Chuanxiong), acrid, warm and dispersing, corresponds to the growth and prospering energy of summer. *Bai Shao* (Radix Paeoniae Alba), sour and astringent, represents harvest in the autumn. Lastly, *Shu Di Huang* (Radix Rehmanniae Praeparata), rich and tonifying, implies storage of blood in winter. These four substances balance each other similarly to the way that seasons are balanced in nature.

Si Wu Tang is considered to be the representative formula for tonifying the blood. Although the source text states to use equal amounts of all four ingredients, the doses may be modified depending on the condition of the individual patient. General guidelines for modifications are as follows:

- In patients with blood stagnation, *Bai Shao* (Radix Paeoniae Alba) should be replaced with *Chi Shao* (Radix Paeoniae Rubra).
- In patients with heat, *Shu Di Huang* (Radix Rehmanniae Praeparata) should be replaced with *Di Huang* (Radix Rehmanniae).
- In patients in which *Shu Di Huang* (Radix Rehmanniae Praeparata) is not used because of its cloying nature, the dose of *Bai Shao* (Radix Paeoniae Alba) should be higher than that of *Dang Gui* (Radix Angelicae Sinensis). This is

Sì Wù Tāng (Four-Substance Decoction)

the general principle in balancing tonics: adjust the individual dose of the herbs to balance the herbal temperature so that the formula is not too warm or cold.

Si Wu Tang is one of the most commonly used formulas to regulate menstruation. Modifications to enhance its efficacy in regulating menstruation are as follows:

- Presence of heat before the period: add *Mu Dan Pi* (Cortex Moutan) and *Huang Qin* (Radix Scutellariae).
- Yin deficiency before the period: add *Di Gu Pi* (Cortex Lycii), *Huang Bo* (Cortex Phellodendri Chinensis), and *Zhi Mu* (Rhizoma Anemarrhenae); and use *Di Huang* (Radix Rehmanniae) instead of *Shu Di Huang* (Radix Rehmanniae Praeparata).
- Cold stagnation after the period: use *Tao Hong Si Wu Tang* (Four-Substance Decoction with Safflower and Peach Pit) plus *Shi Xiao San* (Sudden Smile Powder).
- Scanty menstruation due to qi and blood stagnation: add *Tao Ren* (Semen Persicae), *Hong Hua* (Flos Carthami), and *Shi Xiao San* (Sudden Smile Powder).
- Scanty menstruation due to qi and blood deficiencies: add *Si Jun Zi Tang* (Four-Gentlemen Decoction), *Xiang Fu* (Rhizoma Cyperi), *Huang Qi* (Radix Astragali), and *Dan Shen* (Radix et Rhizoma Salviae Miltiorrhizae).
- Scanty menstruation due to Liver and Kidney yin deficiencies: add *Mai Dong* (Radix Ophiopogonis) and *He Shou Wu* (Radix Polygoni Multiflori).

References

1. *Zhong Yao Ming Fang Yao Li Yu Ying Yong* (Pharmacology and Applications of Famous Herbal Formulas) 1989;283-284.
2. *Shan Xi Zhong Yi Xue Yuan Xue Bao* (Journal of Shanxi University School of Chinese Medicine) 1986;2:40.
3. *Zhong Yao Yao Li Yu Lin Chuang* (Pharmacology and Clinical Applications of Chinese Herbs) 1992;152.
4. *Zhong Cheng Yao* (Study of Chinese Patent Medicine) 1993;15(1):44.
5. *Zhong Xi Yi Jie He Za Zhi* (Journal of Integrated Chinese and Western Medicine) 1981;7(2):100.
6. *Zhong Yi Fang Ji Xian Dai Yan Jiu* (Modern Study of Medical Formulae in Traditional Chinese Medicine) 1997;594.
7. Lee SE, Oh H, Yang JA, Jo SK, Byun MW, Yee ST, Kim SH. Radioprotective effects of two traditional Chinese medicine prescriptions: si-wu-tang and si-jun-zi-tang. Am J Chin Med 1999;27(3-4):387-96.
8. *Guo Wai Yi Xue Zhong Yi Zhong Yao Fen Ce* (Monograph of Chinese Herbology from Foreign Medicine) 1992;14(4):54.
9. *Liao Ning Zhong Yi Za Zhi* (Liaoning Journal of Chinese Medicine) 1992;8:45.
10. Xu FH, Uebaba K. Effect of Kampo formulations (traditional Chinese medicine) on circulatory parameters. Acupuncture & Electro-Therapeutics Research 1999;24(1):11-28.

11. Dai Y, But PP, Chan YP, Matsuda H, Kubo M. Antipruritic and antiinflammatory effects of aqueous extract from Si-Wu-Tang. Biol Pharm Bull 2002 Sep;25(9):1175-8.
12. Tagami K, Niwa K, Lian Z, Gao J, Mori H, Tamaya T. Preventive effect of Juzen-taiho-to on endometrial carcinogenesis in mice is based on Shimotsu-to constituent. Biol Pharm Bull 2004 Feb;27(2):156-61.
13. *Hu Bei Zhong Yi Za Zhi* (Hubei Journal of Chinese Medicine) 1990;2:16.
14. *Zhong Yi Za Zhi* (Journal of Chinese Medicine) 1988;5:41.
15. *Shan Xi Zhong Yi* (Shanxi Chinese Medicine) 1982;3(2):21.
16. *Hu Bei Zhong Yi Za Zhi* (Hubei Journal of Chinese Medicine) 1990;1:31.
17. *Shang Hai Zhong Yi Yao Za Zhi* (Shanghai Journal of Chinese Medicine and Herbology) 1995;4:10.
18. *Nei Meng Gu Zhong Yi Yao* (Traditional Chinese Medicine and Medicinals of Inner Mongolia) 1989;1:27.
19. *Shan Dong Zhong Yi Za Zhi* (Shandong Journal of Chinese Medicine) 1988;7(1):22.
20. *Shan Xi Zhong Yi* (Shanxi Chinese Medicine) 1991;7(3):22.
21. *He Bei Zhong Yi* (Hebei Chinese Medicine) 1999;6:363.
22. *Zhong Yi Za Zhi* (Journal of Chinese Medicine) 1986;10:35.
23. *Hu Nan Yi Yao Za Zhi* (Hunan Journal of Medicine and Herbology) 1983;4:50.
24. *Zhe Jiang Zhong Yi Za Zhi* (Zhejiang Journal of Chinese Medicine) 1988;2:70.
25. *Hu Bei Zhong Yi Za Zhi* (Hubei Journal of Chinese Medicine) 1982;4:32.
26. *Xin Zhong Yi* (New Chinese Medicine) 1986;18(8):41.
27. *Ji Lin Zhong Yi Yao* (Jilin Chinese Medicine and Herbology) 1991;(5):3.
28. *Zhe Jiang Zhong Yi Za Zhi* (Zhejiang Journal of Chinese Medicine) 1993;12:558.
29. *Shan Xi Yi Yao Za Zhi* (Shanxi Journal of Medicine and Herbology) 1975;6:47.
30. *Shan Xi Zhong Yi* (Shanxi Chinese Medicine) 1986;7(11):53.
31. *Zhong Cheng Yao Yan Jiu* (Research of Chinese Patent Medicine) 1994;2:16.
32. *Zhe Jiang Zhong Yi Xue Yuan Xue Bao* (Journal of Zhejiang University of Chinese Medicine) 1997;3:41.
33. *Zhong Yi Za Zhi* (Journal of Chinese Medicine) 1988;8:608.
34. *Zhe Jiang Zhong Yi Za Zhi* (Zhejiang Journal of Chinese Medicine) 1963;2:29.
35. *Yun Nan Zhong Yi Za Zhi* (Yunan Journal of Chinese Medicine) 1985;6:25.
36. *Zhong Xi Yi Jie He Za Zhi* (Journal of Integrated Chinese and Western Medicine) 1991;4:242.
37. *Hei Long Jiang Zhong Yi Yao* (Heilongjiang Chinese Medicine and Herbology) 1991;5:33.
38. *Nei Meng Gu Zhong Yi Yao* (Traditional Chinese Medicine and Medicinals of Inner Mongolia) 1993;(3):1.
39. Watanabe H, Ni JW, Ohta H, Ni XH, Matsumoto K. A kampo prescription, shimotsu-to, improves scopolamine-induced spatial cognitive deficits in rats. Yakubutsu Seishin Kodo 1991 Jun;11(3): 215-22.
40. *Guo Wai Yi Xue Zhong Yi Zhong Yao Fen Ce* (Monograph of Chinese Herbology from Foreign Medicine) 1984;5:305.

Chinese Herbal Formulas and Applications

Táo Hóng Sì Wù Tāng
(Four-Substance Decoction with Safflower and Peach Pit)

桃紅四物湯
桃红四物汤

Pinyin Name: *Tao Hong Si Wu Tang*
Literal Name: Four-Substance Decoction with Safflower and Peach Pit
Alternate Names: *Tao Hung Szu Wu Tang*, Persica, Carthamus and Tang-kuei Decoction; Peach Kernel and Safflower plus Four Herbs; Tangkuei Four and Persica Carthamus Combination
Original Source: *Yi Zong Jin Jian* (Golden Mirror of the Medical Tradition) by Wu Qian in 1742

COMPOSITION

Shu Di Huang (Radix Rehmanniae Praeparata)	6g [15g]
Dang Gui (Radix Angelicae Sinensis)	6g [12g]
Bai Shao (Radix Paeoniae Alba), *chao* (dry-fried)	6g [10g]
Chuan Xiong (Rhizoma Chuanxiong)	3g [8g]
Tao Ren (Semen Persicae)	6g [6g]
Hong Hua (Flos Carthami)	3g [4g]

DOSAGE / PREPARATION / ADMINISTRATION

Prepare this formula as a decoction, and take three times a day, making sure to finish within one day. Today, the decoction may be prepared using the doses suggested in brackets.

CHINESE THERAPEUTIC ACTIONS

1. Nourishes the blood
2. Regulates blood circulation
3. Eliminates blood stasis

CLINICAL MANIFESTATIONS

Blood deficiency with blood stagnation: early menstruation; excessive menstrual bleeding that is thick, sticky and purplish in color, or bleeding with blood clots; and abdominal fullness and pain.

CLINICAL APPLICATIONS

Dysmenorrhea, irregular menstruation, infertility, chronic pelvic inflammation, cerebral infarction, sequelae of stroke, hypertension, hyperlipidemia, diabetic neuropathy, headache, migraine, bone fractures, post-herpetic neuralgia, allergic rhinitis, optic nerve atrophy, optic neuritis, cataract, glaucoma, urticaria, itching, eczema, psoriasis, and chloasma.

EXPLANATION

Tao Hong Si Wu Tang (Four-Substance Decoction with Safflower and Peach Pit) contains *Si Wu Tang* (Four-Substance Decoction) plus *Tao Ren* (Semen Persicae) and *Hong Hua* (Flos Carthami). The addition of these two herbs enables this formula to dispel blood stagnation in addition to tonifying the blood and regulating blood circulation. Historically, it has been used for female patients who have early menstruation with excessive bleeding that is thick, sticky, and purplish in color, or bleeding with blood clots, and abdominal fullness and pain. Today, its clinical application has been extended to include many disorders characterized by both blood deficiency and blood stagnation.

Tao Hong Si Wu Tang is an ideal formula to tonify the blood, regulate blood circulation, and remove blood stagnation. It should be kept in mind, however, that

Tao Hong Si Wu Tang (Four-Substance Decoction with Safflower and Peach Pit)

Diagnosis	Signs and Symptoms	Treatment	Herbs
Blood deficiency with blood stagnation	• Pale face, pale lips, pale fingernails, a sallow appearance, and dizziness: blood deficiency • Abdominal fullness and pain, menstrual bleeding that is thick, sticky and purplish in color, or bleeding with blood clots: blood stagnation	• Nourishes the blood • Regulates blood circulation • Eliminates blood stasis	• *Si Wu Tang* (Four-Substance Decoction) tonifies the blood and regulates blood circulation. • *Tao Ren* (Semen Persicae) and *Hong Hua* (Flos Carthami) regulate blood circulation and eliminate blood stagnation.

TONIC FORMULAS

8

571

Chapter 8 – Tonic Formulas　　　　　　　　　　　　　　　*Section 2 – Blood-Tonifying Formulas*

Táo Hóng Sì Wù Tāng
(Four-Substance Decoction with Safflower and Peach Pit)

because it moves the blood, it could cause excessive menstrual bleeding in some patients if used too frequently or if used longer than necessary.

MODIFICATIONS

- If there are more signs of stagnation and heat, add *Mu Dan Pi* (Cortex Moutan) and *Zhi Zi* (Fructus Gardeniae).
- With abdominal distention and pain during menstruation, add *Xiang Fu* (Rhizoma Cyperi) and *Yan Hu Suo* (Rhizoma Corydalis).
- With more blood stasis, add *San Leng* (Rhizoma Sparganii) and *E Zhu* (Rhizoma Curcumae).
- For cerebrovascular accidents and complications, add *Huang Qi* (Radix Astragali), *Di Long* (Pheretima), *Niu Xi* (Radix Achyranthis Bidentatae), and *Gou Teng* (Ramulus Uncariae cum Uncis).
- For vascular headache, add *Gou Teng* (Ramulus Uncariae cum Uncis) and *Ji Li* (Fructus Tribuli).
- For optic nerve atrophy, add *Dan Shen* (Radix et Rhizoma Salviae Miltiorrhizae), *Chong Wei Zi* (Fructus Leonuri), *Xia Ku Cao* (Spica Prunellae), and *Gan Cao* (Radix et Rhizoma Glycyrrhizae).
- For amenorrhea, add *Yi Mu Cao* (Herba Leonuri), *Ze Lan* (Herba Lycopi), and *Zhi Gan Cao* (Radix et Rhizoma Glycyrrhizae Praeparata cum Melle).
- For psoriasis, add *Huang Qi* (Radix Astragali), *Fang Feng* (Radix Saposhnikoviae), *Bai Xian Pi* (Cortex Dictamni), *Chan Tui* (Periostracum Cicadae), and *Ku Shen* (Radix Sophorae Flavescentis).
- For injuries to tendons and ligaments, add *Ji Xue Teng* (Caulis Spatholobi) and *Niu Xi* (Radix Achyranthis Bidentatae).

CAUTIONS / CONTRAINDICATIONS

- *Tao Hong Si Wu Tang* should be used with caution in patients with digestive weakness.
- This formula should also be used with caution in anemic patients with coldness, since this formula is cool by nature.
- Since this formula has strong actions to regulate blood circulation and eliminate blood stasis, it should be discontinued once the desired effects are achieved to avoid profuse bleeding.
- This formula is contraindicated during pregnancy.
- This formula should be used with caution in menstrual disorders in women with underlying qi and blood deficiencies.[1]

PHARMACOLOGICAL EFFECTS

1. **Cardiovascular**: In an *in vitro* study, use of *Tao Hong Si Wu Tang* was shown to dilate the coronary artery and increase blood perfusion to cardiac muscles.[2]

2. **Antihyperlipidemic**: Administration of *Tao Hong Si Wu Tang* at 16 g/kg in rats was shown to decrease both total cholesterol and triglyceride levels.[3]

3. **Anti-inflammatory**: According to an *in vitro* study, oral administration of *Tao Hong Si Wu Tang* in rats at 8 g/kg and 16 g/kg was associated with marked anti-inflammatory effects similar to hydrocortisone 50 mg/kg. The study noted that the mechanisms of action of the herbs and the drug are very different. *Tao Hong Si Wu Tang* does not contribute to the negative feedback inhibition or the atrophy of the thymus or adrenal glands.[4]

CLINICAL STUDIES AND RESEARCH

1. **Dysmenorrhea**: The combination of *Tao Hong Si Wu Tang* plus *Shi Xiao San* (Sudden Smile Powder) was shown in one study to be effective in treating dysmenorrhea characterized by stagnation. In addition to these two formulas, *Chai Hu* (Radix Bupleuri), *Qing Pi* (Pericarpium Citri Reticulatae Viride), and *Xiang Fu* (Rhizoma Cyperi) were added for qi stagnation; *Xiao Hui Xiang* (Fructus Foeniculi), *Rou Gui* (Cortex Cinnamomi), and *Wu Zhu Yu* (Fructus Evodiae) for blood stagnation with interior cold; *Chuan Niu Xi* (Radix Cyathulae) and *Yan Hu Suo* (Rhizoma Corydalis) for severe pain. The herbs were given starting the fifth day of the menstrual cycle, for 20 days per course of treatment. Of 60 patients, the study reported complete recovery in 28 patients, improvement in 24 patients, and no benefit in 8 patients. The overall rate of effectiveness was 84.7%.[5]

2. **Infertility**: Use of modified *Tao Hong Si Wu Tang* was effective in treating female infertility caused by blocked fallopian tubes. The herbal treatment consisted of *Tao Hong Si Wu Tang* plus *Xiang Fu* (Rhizoma Cyperi), *Shui Zhi* (Hirudo), *Lu Lu Tong* (Fructus Liquidambaris), *Dan Shen* (Radix et Rhizoma Salviae Miltiorrhizae), *San Qi* (Radix et Rhizoma Notoginseng) powder, and others. For Kidney deficiency, *Sang Shen* (Fructus Mori) and *Xu Duan* (Radix Dipsaci) are added. For dampness and phlegm, *Cang Zhu* (Rhizoma Atractylodis), *Chen Pi* (Pericarpium Citri Reticulatae), and *Ban Xia* (Rhizoma Pinelliae) were added, and *Shu Di Huang* (Radix Rehmanniae Praeparata) was removed. For damp-heat, *Huang Bo* (Cortex Phellodendri Chinensis), *Yi Yi Ren* (Semen Coicis), *Tu Fu Ling* (Rhizoma Smilacis Glabrae), and *Pu Gong Ying* (Herba Taraxaci) were added, and *Shu Di Huang* (Radix Rehmanniae Praeparata) was removed. Of 60 women, the study reported successful pregnancy in 31 patients, normal flow of egg in the fallopian tubes in 7 patients, and ectopic pregnancy in 1 patient. The overall rate of effectiveness was 80%.[6]

572

Táo Hóng Sì Wù Tāng
(Four-Substance Decoction with Safflower and Peach Pit)

3. **Cerebral infarction**: Thirty-two patients with cerebral infarction were treated with complete recovery in 10 patients, significant improvement in 11 patients, moderate improvement in 9 patients, and no benefit in 2 patients. The herbal treatment contained *Tao Hong Si Wu Tang* plus *Ge Gen* (Radix Puerariae Lobatae), *Shui Zhi* (Hirudo) and *Huang Qi* (Radix Astragali).[7]

4. **Diabetic neuropathy**: Use of modified *Tao Hong Si Wu Tang* was associated with 96.4% effectiveness in treating peripheral neuropathy in 28 diabetic patients (22 with more than 5 years of illness, and 6 with less than 5 years of illness). The base formula contained *Tao Hong Si Wu Tang* plus *Huang Qi* (Radix Astragali), *Dang Shen* (Radix Codonopsis), *Huang Jing* (Rhizoma Polygonati) and *Gou Qi Zi* (Fructus Lycii). Additional modifications included *Xuan Shen* (Radix Scrophulariae) and *Huang Lian* (Rhizoma Coptidis) for irritability, thirst, polyphagia and polydypsia; and *Di Gu Pi* (Cortex Lycii) for *wu xin re* (five-center heat). Of 28 patients, the study reported complete recovery in 15 patients, moderate improvement in 9 patients, slight improvement in 3 patients, and no benefit in 1 patient.[8]

5. **Headache**: Vascular headache in 30 patients was treated with complete recovery in 13 patients and improvement in 17 patients using *Tao Hong Si Wu Tang* plus *Gao Ben* (Rhizoma et Radix Ligustici), *Bai Zhi* (Radix Angelicae Dahuricae), and *Xi Xin* (Radix et Rhizoma Asari).[9]

6. **Bone fractures**: Administration of an herbal formula was effective in reducing swelling and pain, and facilitating the recovery process. The herbal formula contained *Tao Hong Si Wu Tang* plus *Gu Sui Bu* (Rhizoma Drynariae), *Xu Duan* (Radix Dipsaci), *Zi Ran Tong* (Pyritum), *Tu Bie Chong* (Eupolyphaga seu Steleophaga), *Mu Xiang* (Radix Aucklandiae), and others as needed. Additional modifications included *Huang Bo* (Cortex Phellodendri Chinensis) for heat; unprocessed *Cao Wu* (Radix Aconiti Kusnezoffii) for cold; *Sang Zhi* (Ramulus Mori) for bone fractures in the upper extremities; and *Niu Xi* (Radix Achyranthis Bidentatae) for bone fractures in the lower extremities.[10]

7. **Allergic rhinitis**: Use of modified *Tao Hong Si Wu Tang* was shown to be effective in treating allergic rhinitis in 42 patients. The base formula contained *Tao Hong Si Wu Tang* plus *Cang Er Zi* (Fructus Xanthii), *Huang Qi* (Radix Astragali), *Fang Feng* (Radix Saposhnikoviae), and *Xin Yi Hua* (Flos Magnoliae). Modifications included addition of *Ma Huang* (Herba Ephedrae) and *Xi Xin* (Radix et Rhizoma Asari) for stuffy nose, frequent sneezing, and profuse watery nasal discharge; *Huang Qin* (Radix Scutellariae) and *Mu Dan Pi* (Cortex Moutan) for profuse yellow nasal discharge; *Fu Ling* (Poria), *Shan Yao* (Rhizoma Dioscoreae), and dry-fried *Bai Bian Dou* (Semen Lablab Album) for

Spleen deficiency with poor appetite; *Nu Zhen Zi* (Fructus Ligustri Lucidi) and *Wu Wei Zi* (Fructus Schisandrae Chinensis) for Kidney deficiency; and *Jing Jie* (Herba Schizonepetae) and *Chan Tui* (Periostracum Cicadae) for itchy nose. The duration of treatment ranged between 6-20 days. Of 42 patients, the study reported complete recovery in 31 patients, improvement in 9 patients, and no benefit in 2 patients.[11]

8. **Optic nerve atrophy**: Twenty-eight patients (34 affected eyes) with glaucoma and atrophy of the optic nerve were treated with good results using the combination of herbs and vasodilators. The herbal treatment contained *Tao Hong Si Wu Tang* plus *Gou Qi Zi* (Fructus Lycii), *Dan Shen* (Radix et Rhizoma Salviae Miltiorrhizae), *Ren Shen* (Radix et Rhizoma Ginseng), *Bai Zhu* (Rhizoma Atractylodis Macrocephalae), and *Ju Hua* (Flos Chrysanthemi). The average duration of treatment was 69 packs of herbs.[12]

9. **Optic neuritis**: One study reported beneficial effect in 32 patients with optic neuritis using *Tao Hong Si Wu Tang* plus *Dan Shen* (Radix et Rhizoma Salviae Miltiorrhizae), *Zhi Qiao* (Fructus Aurantii), *Fu Ling* (Poria), *Tong Cao* (Medulla Tetrapanacis), and *Gan Cao* (Radix et Rhizoma Glycyrrhizae). The herbs were given in decoction daily.[13]

10. **Cataract**: One study reported 98.4% effectiveness using modified *Tao Hong Si Wu Tang* to treat 200 patients (381 affected eyes) with cataract. The herbal treatment contained this formula plus *Dan Shen* (Radix et Rhizoma Salviae Miltiorrhizae), *Gou Qi Zi* (Fructus Lycii), *Ju Hua* (Flos Chrysanthemi), *Ji Li* (Fructus Tribuli), *Chan Tui* (Periostracum Cicadae), *Ye Ming Sha* (Faeces Vespertilionis Murini), *Qing Xiang Zi* (Semen Celosiae), *Jue Ming Zi* (Semen Cassiae), *Ci Shi* (Magnetitum), *Shen Qu* (Massa Fermentata), *Sang Shen* (Fructus Mori), and *Chen Pi* (Pericarpium Citri Reticulatae). Effectiveness was defined as improvement of visual acuity.[14]

11. **Glaucoma**: Twelve patients (19 affected eyes) with glaucoma characterized by Liver stagnation were treated with recovery in 7 eyes, significant improvement in 4 eyes, moderate improvement in 5 eyes, and no benefit in 3 eyes. The herbal formula contained *Tao Hong Si Wu Tang* plus *Su Mu* (Lignum Sappan), *Qiang Huo* (Rhizoma et Radix Notopterygii), *Bu Gu Zhi* (Fructus Psoraleae), *Hua Shi* (Talcum), *Jie Geng* (Radix Platycodonis), *Zhi Qiao* (Fructus Aurantii), *Da Huang* (Radix et Rhizoma Rhei), and *Gan Cao* (Radix et Rhizoma Glycyrrhizae).[15]

12. **Urticaria**: One study reported 85.8% effectiveness using modified *Tao Hong Si Wu Tang* to treat chronic urticaria. The herbal treatment contained this formula plus *Jing Jie* (Herba Schizonepetae), *He Shou Wu* (Radix Polygoni Multiflori), *Zao Jiao Ci* (Spina Gleditsiae), *Chan Tui* (Periostracum Cicadae), and others as needed. Of 42

Chapter 8 – Tonic Formulas   *Section 2 – Blood-Tonifying Formulas*

Táo Hóng Sì Wù Tāng
(Four-Substance Decoction with Safflower and Peach Pit)

patients, the study reported recovery in 20 patients, significant improvement in 10 patients, moderate improvement in 6 patients, and no benefit in 6 patients.[16] In another study, use of modified *Tao Hong Si Wu Tang* to treat 24 patients with stubborn urticaria was associated with complete recovery in all 24 patients. The herbal treatment contained this formula plus *Jiang Can* (Bombyx Batryticatus) and *Chan Tui* (Periostracum Cicadae) as the base formula, with addition of others as needed. The duration of treatment ranged from 7 to 15 packs of herbs.[17]

13.**Itching**: One study reported 93.5% effectiveness using modified *Tao Hong Si Wu Tang* to treat itching. The herbal treatment contained this formula plus *He Shou Wu* (Radix Polygoni Multiflori), *Di Fu Zi* (Fructus Kochiae), *Bai Xian Pi* (Cortex Dictamni), and *Ji Li* (Fructus Tribuli). Of 92 patients, the study reported complete recovery in 53 patients, moderate improvement in 33 patients, and no benefit in 6 patients.[18]

14.**Eczema**: Administration of *Tao Hong Si Wu Tang* plus *Dan Shen* (Radix et Rhizoma Salviae Miltiorrhizae), *Chi Shao* (Radix Paeoniae Rubra), and *Mu Dan Pi* (Cortex Moutan) in 64 patients with eczema was associated with complete recovery in 53 patients, significant improvement in 5 patients, and slight improvement in 6 patients.[19]

15.**Psoriasis**: Administration of modified *Tao Hong Si Wu Tang* was associated with 93.7% effectiveness in treating 32 patients with psoriasis. In addition to this formula, modifications were made by adding *Jin Yin Hua* (Flos Lonicerae Japonicae), *Lian Qiao* (Fructus Forsythiae), *Pu Gong Ying* (Herba Taraxaci), *Zi Cao* (Radix Arnebiae), *Xuan Shen* (Radix Scrophulariae), and *Ban Lan Gen* (Radix Isatidis) for damaged skin with spots; *Fu Ling* (Poria), *Che Qian Zi* (Semen Plantaginis), *Bai Xian Pi* (Cortex Dictamni) and *Ku Shen* (Radix Sophorae Flavescentis) for damaged skin with geographic appearance; *Jin Yin Hua* (Flos Lonicerae Japonicae), *Lian Qiao* (Fructus Forsythiae), *Pu Gong Ying* (Herba Taraxaci), *Zi Cao* (Radix Arnebiae), *Fu Ling* (Poria), *Che Qian Zi* (Semen Plantaginis), *Bai Xian Pi* (Cortex Dictamni), and *Yi Yi Ren* (Semen Coicis) for psoriatic arthritis; *Jin Yin Hua* (Flos Lonicerae Japonicae), *Pu Gong Ying* (Herba Taraxaci), *Zi Cao* (Radix Arnebiae), and *Xuan Shen* (Radix Scrophulariae) for psoriasis with sores; and *Xuan Shen* (Radix Scrophulariae), *Sha Shen* (Radix Glehniae seu Adenophorae), *Mai Dong* (Radix Ophiopogonis), *Mu Dan Pi* (Cortex Moutan), *Bai Xian Pi* (Cortex Dictamni), *Ku Shen* (Radix Sophorae Flavescentis), *Fang Feng* (Radix Saposhnikoviae), *Chan Tui* (Periostracum Cicadae), *Wu Shao She* (Zaocys) and *Quan Xie* (Scorpio) during the remission period. Of 32 patients, the study reported complete recovery in 23 patients, improvement in 7 patients, and no benefit in 2 patients.[20]

16.**Chloasma**: One study reported 73% effectiveness using modified *Tao Hong Si Wu Tang* to treat 30 women with irregular shape and size of brown patches on the face or other parts of the body. The base formula contained *Tao Hong Si Wu Tang* plus *Gui Zhi* (Ramulus Cinnamomi) and *Jiang Can* (Bombyx Batryticatus). Modifications were made as follows: *Yan Hu Suo* (Rhizoma Corydalis), *Wu Yao* (Radix Linderae), and *Chuan Lian Zi* (Fructus Toosendan) for painful menstruation; *San Leng* (Rhizoma Sparganii), *E Zhu* (Rhizoma Curcumae), *Dan Shen* (Radix et Rhizoma Salviae Miltiorrhizae), *Yi Mu Cao* (Herba Leonuri) and *Kun Bu* (Thallus Eckloniae) for amenorrhea or formation of nodules; *Cang Zhu* (Rhizoma Atractylodis), *Bai Zhu* (Rhizoma Atractylodis Macrocephalae), *Fu Ling* (Poria), and *Chun Pi* (Cortex Ailanthi) for profuse leukorrhea; *Chai Hu* (Radix Bupleuri), *Xiang Fu* (Rhizoma Cyperi), *Tu Si Zi* (Semen Cuscutae), and *Gou Qi Zi* (Fructus Lycii) for irregular menstruation; addition of *Mu Dan Pi* (Cortex Moutan) and *Huang Qi* (Radix Astragali) and removal of *Tao Ren* (Semen Persicae) and *Hong Hua* (Flos Carthami) before the period; and the addition of *Rou Gui* (Cortex Cinnamomi) and *Pao Jiang* (Rhizoma Zingiberis Praeparatum) after the period. The duration of treatment was 10 days per course, for 4-6 courses total. Of 30 patients, the study reported complete recovery in 7 patients, significant improvement in 11 patients, moderate improvement in 4 patients, and no benefit in 8 patients.[21]

HERB-DRUG INTERACTION

Cosmetics-induced dermatitis: One study reported good results in the treatment of dermatitis associated with the use of cosmetics using *Tao Hong Si Wu Tang* plus *Fang Feng* (Radix Saposhnikoviae), *Pu Gong Ying* (Herba Taraxaci), *Zi Hua Di Ding* (Herba Violae), and others. The herbs were given in decoction for 10 days per course of treatment. Most patients responded within 3-5 days, while some with severe conditions required up to 3 courses of treatment.[22]

AUTHORS' COMMENTS

Tao Hong Si Wu Tang is designed to treat gynecological disorders characterized by blood deficiency with blood stagnation. The emphasis of the formula is to tonify the blood and eliminate blood stasis. To potentiate the effects of the formula, *Bai Shao* (Radix Paeoniae Alba) can be replaced with *Chi Shao* (Radix Paeoniae Rubra) to enhance the blood-activating effect, and *Shu Di Huang* (Radix Rehmanniae Praeparata) can be replaced with *Di Huang* (Radix Rehmanniae) to nourish the blood without creating more stagnation.

Chinese Herbal Formulas and Applications

Táo Hóng Sì Wù Tāng
(Four-Substance Decoction with Safflower and Peach Pit)

References

1. *Zhong Yao Ming Fang Yao Li Yu Ying Yong* (Pharmacology and Applications of Famous Herbal Formulas) 1989;453-455.
2. *Jiang Su Zhong Yi Za Zhi* (Jiangsu Journal of Chinese Medicine) 1986;12:541.
3. *Zhong Xi Yi Jie He Za Zhi* (Journal of Integrated Chinese and Western Medicine) 1988;8(10):601.
4. *Zhong Guo Zhong Yao Za Zhi* (People's Republic of China Journal of Chinese Herbology) 1994;19(11):680.
5. *Jiang Xi Zhong Yi Yao* (Jiangxi Chinese Medicine and Herbology) 1991;3:47.
6. *He Bei Zhong Yi* (Hebei Chinese Medicine) 1995;15(2):26.
7. *Zhong Yi Han Shou Tong Xun* (Reports of Chinese Medicine) 1992;3:44.
8. *Shi Yong Zhong Yi Nei Ke Za Zhi* (Journal of Practical Chinese Internal Medicine) 1991;5(2):73.
9. *Zhong Yi Za Zhi* (Journal of Chinese Medicine) 1985;6:24.
10. *Gui Yang Yi Xue Yuan Xue Bao* (Journal of Guiyang Medical University) 1983;1:63.
11. *Zhong Yi Ming Fang Lin Chuang Xin Yong* (Contemporary Clinical Applications of Classic Chinese Formulas) 2001;1:29.
12. *Yan Ke Tong Xun* (Journal of Ophthalmology) 1987;3:13.
13. *Zhong Yi Fang Ji Xian Dai Yan Jiu* (Modern Study of Medical Formulae in Traditional Chinese Medicine) 1997;1103.
14. *Zhong Yi Fang Ji Xian Dai Yan Jiu* (Modern Study of Medical Formulae in Traditional Chinese Medicine) 1997;1103.
15. *Zhong Yi Za Zhi* (Journal of Chinese Medicine) 1983;24(1):34.
16. *Bei Jing Zhong Yi* (Beijing Chinese Medicine) 1997;5:31.
17. *He Bei Zhong Yi* (Hebei Chinese Medicine) 1995;17(4):47.
18. *Shi Yong Zhong Xi Yi Jie He Za Zhi* (Practical Journal of Integrated Chinese and Western Medicines) 1991;4:41.
19. *Zhong Yi Za Zhi* (Journal of Chinese Medicine) 1988;29(5):366.
20. *Shan Xi Zhong Yi* (Shanxi Chinese Medicine) 1990;11(2):106.
21. *Tian Jin Zhong Yi* (Tianjing Chinese Medicine) 1995;12(2):17.
22. *Zhong Yi Yao Xin Xi* (Information on Chinese Medicine and Herbology) 1992;9(5):36.

Wēn Qīng Yǐn (Warming and Clearing Decoction)
溫清飲
温清饮

Pinyin Name: *Wen Qing Yin*
Literal Name: Warming and Clearing Decoction
Alternate Names: *Wen Ching Yin* (Warming and Clearing Drink), *Wen Qing San* (Warming and Clearing Powder), Tangkuei and Gardenia Combination
Original Source: *Wan Bing Hui Chun* (Restoration of Health from the Myriad Diseases) by Gong Ting-Xian in 1587

COMPOSITION

Dang Gui (Radix Angelicae Sinensis)	4.5g
Shu Di Huang (Radix Rehmanniae Praeparata)	4.5g
Bai Shao (Radix Paeoniae Alba)	4.5g
Chuan Xiong (Rhizoma Chuanxiong)	4.5g
Huang Lian (Rhizoma Coptidis)	4.5g
Huang Qin (Radix Scutellariae)	4.5g
Huang Bo (Cortex Phellodendri Chinensis)	4.5g
Zhi Zi (Fructus Gardeniae)	4.5g

DOSAGE / PREPARATION / ADMINISTRATION

Grind the herbs into powder, and cook the powder in water to make a decoction. Take the warm, strained decoction on an empty stomach.

CHINESE THERAPEUTIC ACTIONS

1. Warms the menses
2. Cools the blood
3. Clears heat and eliminates toxins

CLINICAL MANIFESTATIONS

Gynecological disorders characterized by blood deficiency and heat: irregular menstruation with profuse bleeding, abdominal pain, fever, irritability, mood swings, thirst, a sallow facial appearance, alternating chills and fever, itchy skin, and emaciation.

8

TONIC FORMULAS

575

Chapter 8 – Tonic Formulas

Section 2 – Blood-Tonifying Formulas

Wēn Qīng Yǐn (Warming and Clearing Decoction)

CLINICAL APPLICATIONS

Uterine bleeding, excessive menstrual bleeding, leukorrhea, infertility, urinary tract infection, cystitis, uteritis, menopause and other gynecological disorders. Other uses include aphtha, neurodermatitis, lupus erythematosus, gastric ulcer, occult bleeding, pruritus, dermatitis, eczema, urticaria, and tinea.

EXPLANATION

Wen Qing Yin (Warming and Clearing Decoction) treats gynecological disorders complicated by both deficiency and excess. Irregular menstruation and profuse menstrual bleeding often indicate an underlying blood deficiency condition. Because the blood is deficient, many parts of the body cannot be nourished properly, leading to dry and itchy skin, a sallow facial appearance, and emaciation. Unfortunately, blood deficiency in this case is complicated by excess heat, as evident by symptoms such as fever, irritability, and mood swings. Lastly, due to the combination of both deficiency and excess, patients may also have alternating chills and fever.

This formula combines the principles of two formulas to address concurrent deficiency and excess. The herbs in *Si Wu Tang* (Four-Substance Decoction) - *Dang Gui* (Radix Angelicae Sinensis), *Shu Di Huang* (Radix Rehmanniae Praeparata), *Bai Shao* (Radix Paeoniae Alba), and *Chuan Xiong* (Rhizoma Chuanxiong) - tonify the blood and warm the menses. The herbs in *Huang Lian Jie Du Tang* (Coptis Decoction to Relieve Toxicity), *Huang Lian* (Rhizoma Coptidis), *Huang Qin* (Radix Scutellariae), *Huang Bo* (Cortex Phellodendri Chinensis), and *Zhi Zi* (Fructus Gardeniae) clear heat and eliminate toxins from the body. Because this formula has dual functions to "warm" the menses and "clear" heat, it is called "Warming and Clearing Decoction." This formula can also be used in men who have bleeding accompanied by a sallow facial appearance and emaciation.

MODIFICATIONS

- With profuse menstrual bleeding, add *E Jiao* (Colla Corii Asini) and *Ai Ye* (Folium Artemisiae Argyi).
- With leukorrhea and an itching sensation in the genital region, add *Jin Yin Hua* (Flos Lonicerae Japonicae), *Lian Qiao* (Fructus Forsythiae), and *Che Qian Zi* (Semen Plantaginis).
- If there is menstrual pain, add *Chen Pi* (Pericarpium Citri Reticulatae) and *Xiang Fu* (Rhizoma Cyperi).

PHARMACOLOGICAL EFFECTS

1. **Antiulcer**: Administration of *Wen Qing Yin* was associated with inhibiting the release of gastric acid in mice. Of two forms used, the decoction was associated with 51.8-65.9% effectiveness, and the capsule form was associated with 46.3-52.3% effectiveness.[1]

2. **Analgesic and anti-inflammatory**: Administration of *Wen Qing Yin* in both decoction and capsule forms was associated with relieving pain and reducing inflammation. The therapeutic effect was noted 30 minutes after administration, and lasted for 2-4 hours.[2] *Wen Qing Yin* is believed to exert its anti-inflammatory effects mainly on the early stages of inflammation, when increased capillary permeability and migration of leucocytes occur.[3]

3. **Antipruritic**: *Wen Qing Yin* has a marked antipruritic effect, and has been used successfully to inhibit substance P-induced scratching in mice. The mechanism of this antipruritic effect was attributed to the inhibition of cutaneous nitric oxide synthase 1 expression and nitric oxide production.[4]

4. **Dermatological**: One study reported *Wen Qing Yin* to be effective in treating acne vulgaris, by suppressing propionibacterium acnes lipase in seborrheic dermatitis.[5] *Wen Qing Yin* also has an inhibitory effect on rheologically-activated neutrophils, and has also been used successfully in treating other skin diseases, such as Behcet's disease, palmoplantar pustulosis and psoriasis vulgaris.[6]

5. **Immunosuppressant**: Administration of *Wen Qing Yin* was associated with inhibiting the induction phase of

Wen Qing Yin (Warming and Clearing Decoction)

Diagnosis	Signs and Symptoms	Treatment	Herbs
Gynecological disorders characterized by blood deficiency and heat	• Irregular menstruation and profuse menstrual bleeding: blood deficiency • Dry and itchy skin, a sallow facial appearance and emaciation: blood deficiency unable to nourish the tissues • Fever, irritability, and mood swings: heat condition	• Warms the menses • Cools the blood • Clears heat and eliminates toxins	• *Dang Gui* (Radix Angelicae Sinensis), *Shu Di Huang* (Radix Rehmanniae Praeparata), *Bai Shao* (Radix Paeoniae Alba) and *Chuan Xiong* (Rhizoma Chuanxiong) tonify the blood and warm the menses. • *Huang Lian* (Rhizoma Coptidis), *Huang Qin* (Radix Scutellariae), *Huang Bo* (Cortex Phellodendri Chinensis) and *Zhi Zi* (Fructus Gardeniae) clear heat and eliminate toxins from the body.

576

Wēn Qīng Yǐn (Warming and Clearing Decoction)

Chinese Herbal Formulas and Applications

various kinds of delayed hypersensitivity and local graft-versus-host reactions in experimental animals. Of the 8 herbs in this formula, *Huang Bo* (Cortex Phellodendri Chinensis) was determined to have the most potent suppressive effect on the cellular immune response.[7]

6. **Radioprotective**: Intraperitoneal injection of *Wen Qing Yin* was associated with a marked protective effect in mice against skin injury induced by irradiation.[8]

CLINICAL STUDIES AND RESEARCH

1. **Gynecological disorders**: *Wen Qing Yin* has been used to treat various types of gynecological disorders characterized by blood deficiency and heat. Clinically, *Da Huang* (Radix et Rhizoma Rhei) and *Mang Xiao* (Natrii Sulfas) were added to this formula in many cases. The duration of treatment was 1 month or more. Clinical applications included, but were not limited to, uterine bleeding, excessive menstrual bleeding, leukorrhea, infertility, urinary tract infection, cystitis, uteritis, and menopause.[9]

2. **Aphtha**: In one clinical study, 63 patients with aphtha were divided into two groups. Group one received *Wen Qing Yin* in decoction form and group two in capsules. Out of 19 patients in the decoction group, 15 showed a marked improvement and 4 showed no improvement (79% effectiveness). Out of 27 patients in the capsule group, 20 showed marked improvement and 7 showed no improvement (74% effectiveness).[10]

3. **Dermatological disorders**: *Wen Qing Yin* has been evaluated for its effectiveness in treating various dermatological disorders, including but not limited to psoriasis, pruritus, dermatitis, eczema, urticaria, and tinea. Most studies used *Wen Qing Yin* with minor modifications, with effectiveness ranging between 50-80%.[11,12,13]

TOXICOLOGY

In acute toxicology studies in mice, no abnormal reactions were observed following ingestion of *Wen Qing Yin*. The herbal formula was given in capsules at doses 50-100 times the normal adult human dose for 2 weeks.[14]

RELATED FORMULAS

Wēn Qīng Yǐn (Warming and Clearing Decoction)
溫清飲
温清饮
Pinyin Name: *Wen Qing Yin*
Literal Name: Warming and Clearing Decoction
Original Source: *Shen Shi Zun Sheng Shu* (Master Shen's Book for Revering Life) by Shen Jin-Ao in 1773

Dang Gui (Radix Angelicae Sinensis)
Chuan Xiong (Rhizoma Chuanxiong)
Bai Shao (Radix Paeoniae Alba)

Shu Di Huang (Radix Rehmanniae Praeparata)
Di Huang (Radix Rehmanniae)
Huang Lian (Rhizoma Coptidis)
Huang Qin (Radix Scutellariae)
Huang Bo (Cortex Phellodendri Chinensis)
Zhi Zi (Fructus Gardeniae)

This is a revised version of the original formulation, with the addition of *Di Huang* (Radix Rehmanniae). The doses are the same for all of the ingredients. The addition of *Di Huang* reinforces the original focus of nourishing blood and clearing heat.

Wēn Qīng Yǐn (Warming and Clearing Decoction)
溫清飲
温清饮
Pinyin Name: *Wen Qing Yin*
Literal Name: Warming and Clearing Decoction
Original Source: *He Han Yi Yao Xue Hui Zhi* (Hehan Journal of Medicine and Herbology)

Dang Gui (Radix Angelicae Sinensis)	10g
Chuan Xiong (Rhizoma Chuanxiong)	8g
Bai Shao (Radix Paeoniae Alba)	12g
Shu Di Huang (Radix Rehmanniae Praeparata)	12g
Huang Lian (Rhizoma Coptidis)	3-9g
Huang Qin (Radix Scutellariae)	6g
Huang Bo (Cortex Phellodendri Chinensis)	6g
Zhi Zi (Fructus Gardeniae)	9g

This is a revised version of the original formulation, with modified doses of each of the ingredients. This revised formula focuses more on tonifying the blood and less on clearing heat.

AUTHORS' COMMENTS

According to Dr. Chang Wei-Yen, *Wen Qing Yin* can be combined with *San Huang Shi Gao Tang* (Three-Yellow and Gypsum Decoction) to treat various types of dermatological disorders ranging from rashes or itchy skin, to dermatitis and eczema that are caused by dryness.

References

1. *Zhong Yi Fang Ji Xian Dai Yan Jiu* (Modern Study of Medical Formulae in Traditional Chinese Medicine) 1997;289.
2. *Zhong Yi Yao Xin Xi* (Information on Chinese Medicine and Herbology) 1986;4:12.
3. Wang LM, Yamamoto T, Wang XX, Yang L, Koike Y, Shiba K, Mineshita S. Effects of oren-gedoku-to and unsei-in, Chinese traditional medicines, on interleukin-8 and superoxide dismutase in rats. J Pharm Pharmacol 1997 Jan;49(1):102-4.
4. Andoh T, Al-Akeel A, Tsujii K, Nojima H, Kuraishi Y. Repeated treatment with the traditional medicine Unsei-in inhibits substance P-induced itch-associated responses through down regulation of the

Chapter 8 – Tonic Formulas *Section 2 – Blood-Tonifying Formulas*

Wēn Qīng Yǐn (Warming and Clearing Decoction)

expression of nitric oxide synthase 1 in mice. J Pharmacol Sci 2004 Feb;94(2):207-10.

5. Higaki S, Morohashi M. Propionibacterium acnes lipase in seborrheic dermatitis and other skin diseases and Unsei-in. Drugs Exp Clin Res 2003;29(4):157-9.

6. Iijima S, Otsuka F, Kikuchi Y. Unsei-in inhibits rheological activity of leukocytes: mechanism of action in neutrophil-related skin diseases. Am J Chin Med 1995;23(1):81-90.

7. Mori H, Fuchigami M, Inoue N, Nagai H, Koda A, Nishioka I. Principle of the bark of Phellodendron amurense to suppress the cellular immune response. Planta Med 1994 Oct;60(5):445-9.

8. Wang CM, Ohta S, Shinoda M. Studies on chemical protectors against radiation. XXIX. Protective effects of methanol extracts of

various Chinese traditional medicines on skin injury induced by X-irradiation. Yakugaku Zasshi 1990 Mar;110(3):218-24.

9. *Hei Long Jiang Zhong Yi Yao* (Heilongjiang Chinese Medicine and Herbology) 1980;5:35.

10. *Zhong Yi Yao Xin Xi* (Information on Chinese Medicine and Herbology) 1986;4:12.

11. *Yun Nan Zhong Yi Za Zhi* (Yunan Journal of Chinese Medicine) 1991;12(6):21.

12. *Zhong Cheng Yao* (Study of Chinese Patent Medicine) 1991;7:23.

13. *Yun Nan Zhong Yi Za Zhi* (Yunan Journal of Chinese Medicine) 1990;11(1):31.

14. *Zhong Yi Yao Xin Xi* (Information on Chinese Medicine and Herbology) 1986;4:12.

Guò Qí Yǐn (Delayed Menstruation Decoction)

過期飲
过期饮

Pinyin Name: *Guo Qi Yin*
Literal Name: Delayed Menstruation Decoction
Alternate Name: Cyperus and Carthamus Combination
Original Source: *Zheng Zhi Zhun Sheng* (Standards of Patterns and Treatments) by Wang Ken-Tang in 1602

COMPOSITION

Shu Di Huang (Radix Rehmanniae Praeparata)	6g
Dang Gui (Radix Angelicae Sinensis)	6g
Bai Shao (Radix Paeoniae Alba)	6g
Chuan Xiong (Rhizoma Chuanxiong)	3g
Tao Ren (Semen Persicae)	1.8g
Hong Hua (Flos Carthami)	2.1g
Xiang Fu (Rhizoma Cyperi)	6g
Mu Tong (Caulis Akebiae)	1.5g
E Zhu (Rhizoma Curcumae)	1.5g
Rou Gui (Cortex Cinnamomi)	1.2g
Zhi Gan Cao (Radix et Rhizoma Glycyrrhizae Praeparata cum Melle)	1.2g

DOSAGE / PREPARATION / ADMINISTRATION

Cook the ingredients in 2 bowls of water until it is reduced to 1 bowl. Take the warm, strained decoction before meals.

CHINESE THERAPEUTIC ACTIONS

1. Activates qi and blood circulation
2. Removes qi stagnation and blood stasis
3. Regulates the menstrual cycle

CLINICAL MANIFESTATIONS

Irregular menstruation caused by qi and blood stagnation: delayed menstruation or scanty menstruation, dark purplish menstrual flow with clots, distention and pain in the lower abdominal region that increase with pressure and decrease with the passage of clots, swelling and edema of the lower extremities, a feeling of oppression in the chest and epigastric region, a dry mouth, and a red or dark purple tongue body.

578

Chinese Herbal Formulas and Applications

Guò Qì Yǐn (Delayed Menstruation Decoction)

CLINICAL APPLICATIONS

Delayed menstruation, dysmenorrhea, scanty menstruation with dark purplish clots, pelvic inflammatory disease.

EXPLANATION

Guo Qi Yin (Delayed Menstruation Decoction) treats irregular menstruation characterized by qi and blood stagnation. Clinically, patients will have delayed menstruation or scanty menstruation. Since blood stagnation is the predominant factor in this case, the menstrual flow will be dark and purplish with blood clots. Additionally, blood stasis in the lower abdominal region will cause distention and pain, which increase with pressure and decrease with the passage of clots. Since blood stagnation often is accompanied by qi stagnation, patients may experience a feeling of oppression in the chest and epigastric region. Lastly, a dark purplish tongue body indicates blood stagnation.

This formula focuses on activating qi and blood circulation, removing blood stasis, and regulating the menstrual cycle. *Shu Di Huang* (Radix Rehmanniae Praeparata), *Dang Gui* (Radix Angelicae Sinensis), *Bai Shao* (Radix Paeoniae Alba) and *Chuan Xiong* (Rhizoma Chuanxiong), the four herbs in *Si Wu Tang* (Four-Substance Decoction),

tonify the blood, activate blood circulation, and regulate menstruation. *Tao Ren* (Semen Persicae) and *Hong Hua* (Flos Carthami) activate blood circulation and remove blood stasis. These two herbs have synergistic actions and are commonly used together. *Xiang Fu* (Rhizoma Cyperi), *Mu Tong* (Caulis Akebiae), and *E Zhu* (Rhizoma Curcumae) activate qi and blood circulation and eliminate qi and blood stagnation. *Rou Gui* (Cortex Cinnamomi) warms the Spleen and Kidney to dispel cold and relieve pain. *Zhi Gan Cao* (Radix et Rhizoma Glycyrrhizae Praeparata cum Melle) harmonizes the herbs.

MODIFICATIONS

- With irritability and thirst due to heat, add *Huang Lian* (Rhizoma Coptidis) and *Huang Qin* (Radix Scutellariae).
- With leukorrhea and abdominal pain, combine with *Ba Wei Dai Xia Fang* (Eight-Ingredient Formula for Leukorrhea).
- With itching and pain caused by dampness and heat, combine with *Huang Lian Jie Du Tang* (Coptis Decoction to Relieve Toxicity).
- If there is dizziness due to deficiency fire, combine with *Nu Ke Bai Zi Ren Wan* (Platycladus Seed Pill for Females).

CAUTIONS / CONTRAINDICATIONS

Guo Qi Yin is contraindicated during pregnancy.

Guo Qi Yin (Delayed Menstruation Decoction)

Diagnosis	Signs and Symptoms	Treatment	Herbs
Irregular menstruation caused by qi and blood stagnation	• Delayed menstruation or scanty menstruation with dark purplish blood clots: qi and blood stagnation • Distention and pain which increase with pressure and decrease with the passage of clots: blood stasis • A feeling of oppression in the chest and epigastric region: qi stagnation	• Activates qi and blood circulation • Removes qi stagnation and blood stasis • Regulates the menstrual cycle	• *Shu Di Huang* (Radix Rehmanniae Praeparata), *Dang Gui* (Radix Angelicae Sinensis), *Bai Shao* (Radix Paeoniae Alba) and *Chuan Xiong* (Rhizoma Chuanxiong) tonify the blood, activate blood circulation, and regulate menstruation. • *Tao Ren* (Semen Persicae) and *Hong Hua* (Flos Carthami) activate blood circulation and remove blood stasis. • *Xiang Fu* (Rhizoma Cyperi), *Mu Tong* (Caulis Akebiae), and *E Zhu* (Rhizoma Curcumae) activate qi and blood circulation and eliminate qi and blood stasis. • *Rou Gui* (Cortex Cinnamomi) warms the Spleen and Kidney to dispel cold and relieve pain. • *Zhi Gan Cao* (Radix et Rhizoma Glycyrrhizae Praeparata cum Melle) harmonizes the herbs.

TONIC FORMULAS 8

579

Chapter 8 – Tonic Formulas   *Section 2 – Blood-Tonifying Formulas*

Dāng Guī Bǔ Xuè Tāng (Tangkuei Decoction to Tonify the Blood)

當歸補血湯
当归补血汤

Pinyin Name: *Dang Gui Bu Xue Tang*
Literal Name: Tangkuei Decoction to Tonify the Blood
Alternate Names: *Tang Kuei Pu Hsieh Tang*, Tang-kuei Blood-Nourishing Decoction, Chinese Angelica Blood-Tonifying Decoction, Tangkuei and Astragalus Combination
Original Source: *Nei Wai Shang Bian Huo Lun* (Clarifying Doubts about Injury from Internal and External Causes) by Li Gao in 1247

COMPOSITION

Huang Qi (Radix Astragali)	30g
Dang Gui (Radix Angelicae Sinensis), *xi* (washed) with liquor	6g

DOSAGE / PREPARATION / ADMINISTRATION

The source text states to coarsely grind the ingredients and cook the powder in water to make a decoction. Take the warm, strained decoction before meals on an empty stomach. Today, it is usually prepared as a decoction by cooking the herbs three times. The decoction is taken in three equally-divided doses, three times daily in the morning, noon and evening.

CHINESE THERAPEUTIC ACTIONS

Tonifies qi and generates blood production

CLINICAL MANIFESTATIONS

Qi and blood deficiencies due to overexertion: warm sensations at the skin and muscle layers, a red face, irritability, thirst with a desire to drink warm water, slow healing of wounds, a pale tongue, and a surging, big and deficient pulse. In women during menstruation or after labor, there may be hypermenorrhea, excessive loss of blood after labor, a feverish sensation, and headache.

CLINICAL APPLICATIONS

Anemia, thrombopenic purpura, amenorrhea, functional uterine bleeding, leucopenia, supportive therapy during radiation treatment, ulcerative colitis, insufficient lactation, heel pain, arthritis, and neurasthenia.

EXPLANATION

Dang Gui Bu Xue Tang (Tangkuei Decoction to Tonify the Blood) is designed to treat exertion-induced qi and blood deficiencies. Over-exertion and overwork may damage qi and blood in the body, and lead to the floating of yang toward the exterior parts of the body. Clinical presentations include symptoms such as warm sensations at the skin and muscle layers, a red face, irritability, and thirst with a desire to drink warm water. Since qi is deficient and the body is exhausted, wound healing is slow and the tongue is pale. A surging, big and deficient pulse indicates floating of yang and deficiency of qi and blood. In women, there may be hypermenorrhea and excessive bleeding after labor, since qi is deficient and cannot properly control the blood.

The production of qi and blood is interdependent. Thus, both qi and blood tonics are used for optimal effect when treating deficiency. *Huang Qi* (Radix Astragali) and *Dang Gui* (Radix Angelicae Sinensis) tonify qi and blood. The dose of *Huang Qi* (Radix Astragali) is five times greater than *Dang Gui* (Radix Angelicae Sinensis) to greatly tonify *yuan* (source) *qi*, strengthen the Spleen, and ensure adequate production of blood. *Huang Qi* (Radix Astragali) also prevents the further leaking of yang and promotes the healing of wounds.

Dang Gui Bu Xue Tang (Tangkuei Decoction to Tonify the Blood)

Diagnosis	Signs and Symptoms	Treatment	Herbs
Qi and blood deficiencies due to over-exertion	• Irritability and thirst with a desire to drink warm water: deficiencies of qi, blood and body fluids • Slow wound healing: qi and blood deficiencies • Pale tongue and a surging, big and deficient pulse: qi and blood deficiencies with yang floating to the exterior	• Tonifies qi • Generates production of blood	• *Huang Qi* (Radix Astragali) tonifies qi. • *Dang Gui* (Radix Angelicae Sinensis) tonifies the blood.

Chinese Herbal Formulas and Applications

Dāng Guī Bǔ Xuè Tāng (Tangkuei Decoction to Tonify the Blood)

MODIFICATIONS

- For common cold or influenza with fever and headache during menstruation or postpartum, add *Cong Bai* (Bulbus Allii Fistulosi), *Dan Dou Chi* (Semen Sojae Praeparatum), *Sheng Jiang* (Rhizoma Zingiberis Recens), and *Da Zao* (Fructus Jujubae).
- For allergic purpura, add *Jiang Can* (Bombyx Batryticatus) and *Niu Xi* (Radix Achyranthis Bidentatae).
- For general blood deficiency, add *Shu Di Huang* (Radix Rehmanniae Praeparata), *He Shou Wu* (Radix Polygoni Multiflori), *Sang Ji Sheng* (Herba Taxilli), and *Bai Shao* (Radix Paeoniae Alba).
- If there is hypermenorrhea, add *Di Yu* (Radix Sanguisorbae), charred *Huang Qin* (Radix Scutellariae), and *Gan Cao* (Radix et Rhizoma Glycyrrhizae).
- For tachycardia, add *Sheng Mai San* (Generate the Pulse Powder).
- For ulcerated sores that do not heal, add *Jin Yin Hua* (Flos Lonicerae Japonicae), *Lian Qiao* (Fructus Forsythiae), and *Tian Hua Fen* (Radix Trichosanthis).
- For continuous bleeding, add calcined *Long Gu* (Os Draconis), *Shan Zhu Yu* (Fructus Corni), and *E Jiao* (Colla Corii Asini).

CAUTIONS / CONTRAINDICATIONS

Dang Gui Bu Xue Tang is contraindicated in patients with excess heat or yin-deficient heat with tidal fever.

PHARMACOLOGICAL EFFECTS

1. **Hematopoietic:** In experiments in mice, administration of *Dang Gui Bu Xue Tang* was associated with an increased red blood cell count.[1] It was noted that the formula was more effective than administering *Huang Qi* (Radix Astragali) or *Dang Gui* (Radix Angelicae Sinensis) individually with the same dose, implying that the formula has synergistic effect. Also, it was found that the herbs were more effective in increasing red blood cell count (but not white blood cells) when decocted for 90 minutes in comparison to 45 minutes.[2]
2. **Antiplatelet:** Use of *Dang Gui Bu Xue Tang* was found to be effective in blocking the aggregation of platelets and preventing the formation of blood clots.[3,4]
3. **Hepatoprotective:** Administration of *Dang Gui Bu Xue Tang* was associated with hepatoprotective effects against carbon tetrachloride in mice. The effects were attributed to increased blood circulation and increased regeneration of liver cells.[5]
4. **Immunostimulant:** In laboratory experiments in mice, the use of *Dang Gui Bu Xue Tang* was associated with an increase of phagocytic activities by macrophages. The effects of the herbs lasted up to 24 hours.[6]

CLINICAL STUDIES AND RESEARCH

1. **Thrombopenic purpura:** Twenty-four patients with thrombopenic purpura were treated with modified *Dang Gui Bu Xue Tang* with recovery in 7 patients, marked improvement in 12 patients, and slight improvement in 5 patients. The average length of treatment was 64 days. The herbal treatment contained *Dang Gui Bu Xue Tang* plus *Xue Yu Tan* (Crinis Carbonisatus), *Gan Cao* (Radix et Rhizoma Glycyrrhizae), and *Xian He Cao* (Herba Agrimoniae) as the base formula. Additional modifications were made accordingly for qi deficiency, blood deficiency, yin deficiency, and yang deficiency.[7]
2. **Amenorrhea:** Thirty-seven women with amenorrhea due to abnormal development of the uterus were treated with the following herbal prescription with 91.89% effectiveness. The herbal treatment contained *Dang Gui Bu Xue Tang* plus *San Leng* (Rhizoma Sparganii), *E Zhu* (Rhizoma Curcumae), and *Dan Shen* (Radix et Rhizoma Salviae Miltiorrhizae) as the base formula. Additional modifications were made if necessary. The duration of treatment was 6 months. Of 37 patients, the study reported marked improvement in 23 patients, moderate improvement in 11 patients, and no benefit in 3 patients.[8]
3. **Leucopenia:** Twenty patients with leucopenia were treated with modified *Dang Gui Bu Xue Tang* with marked effect in 8 patients, moderate effect in 11 patients, and no effect in 1 patient. The formula contained *Dang Gui* (Radix Angelicae Sinensis), *Huang Qi* (Radix Astragali), *San Leng* (Rhizoma Sparganii), and *Gan Cao* (Radix et Rhizoma Glycyrrhizae). The treatment protocol was to administer the herbs one time daily for 3-4 weeks.[9]
4. **Ulcerative colitis:** One study reported a 90% rate of effectiveness in 31 patients with chronic ulcerative colitis when treated with *Dang Gui Bu Xue Tang* plus *Jiao Gu Lan* (Rhizoma seu Herba Gynostemmatis), *Dan Shen* (Radix et Rhizoma Salviae Miltiorrhizae), *Chuan Xiong* (Rhizoma Chuanxiong), *Xiang Fu* (Rhizoma Cyperi), and others. In addition, *Bai Tou Weng* (Radix Pulsatillae) was added for damp-heat; *Gan Jiang* (Rhizoma Zingiberis) for Spleen deficiency; and *San Qi* (Radix et Rhizoma Notoginseng) for hematochezia.[10]
5. **Insufficient lactation:** Use of modified *Dang Gui Bu Xue Tang* was successful in promoting lactation in 96 women within 3 months after delivery. The herbal treatment contained this formula plus *Ren Shen* (Radix et Rhizoma Ginseng). Furthermore, *Shi Gao* (Gypsum Fibrosum) was added in summer and *Gui Zhi* (Cortex Rasus Cinnamomi) was added in winter. The study reported 100% effectiveness, with most noticeable success when treatment began within one month of delivery.[11]
6. **Heel pain:** One study reported good results using modified *Dang Gui Bu Xue Tang* to treat 30 patients with heel

TONIC FORMULAS

8

Chapter 8 – Tonic Formulas　　　　　　　　　　　　　　*Section 2 – Blood-Tonifying Formulas*

Dāng Guī Bǔ Xuè Tāng (Tangkuei Decoction to Tonify the Blood)

pain. The herbal formula contained *Dang Gui Bu Xue Tang* plus *Du Zhong* (Cortex Eucommiae), *Xu Duan* (Radix Dipsaci), and *Gou Ji* (Rhizoma Cibotii), with addition of other herbs as needed for Liver and Kidney yin deficiencies, or Spleen and Kidney yang deficiencies. Of 30 patients, the study reported significant improvement in 18 patients, moderate improvement in 9 patients, and slight improvement in 3 patients.[12]

7. **Arthritis**: In one study, 51 patients with various presentations of arthritis were treated with modified *Dang Gui Bu Xue Tang* with good results. The base formula included *Dang Gui* (Radix Angelicae Sinensis), *Huang Qi* (Radix Astragali), *Gui Zhi* (Ramulus Cinnamomi), *Hai Feng Teng* (Caulis Piperis Kadsurae), *Qin Jiao* (Radix Gentianae Macrophyllae), and *Zhi Chuan Wu* (Radix Aconiti Praeparata). The modifications included the addition of *Fang Feng* (Radix Saposhnikoviae) and *Qiang Huo* (Rhizoma et Radix Notopterygii) for *xing bi* (mobile painful obstruction); *Fang Ji* (Radix Stephaniae Tetrandrae) and *Yi Yi Ren* (Semen Coicis) for *zhuo bi* (fixed painful obstruction); *Zhi Mu* (Rhizoma Anemarrhenae), *Shi Gao* (Gypsum Fibrosum), and *Ren Dong Teng* (Caulis Lonicerae Japonicae) for *re bi* (heat painful obstruction); and *Xi Xin* (Radix et Rhizoma Asari) for *tong bi* (extremely painful obstruction). The treatment protocol was to administer the herbs on a daily basis for 10 days per course of treatment, for a duration of 10-45 days. Out of 51 patients, the study reported recovery in 36 patients, improvement in 10 patients, and no benefit in 5 patients. The study noted that the formula was most effective for *tong bi* (extremely painful obstruction) and *zhuo bi* (fixed painful obstruction), and less effective for *re bi* (heat painful obstruction).[13]

HERB-DRUG INTERACTION

Chemotherapy- and radiation-induced leucopenia: One study reported 90.2% effectiveness using modified *Dang Gui Bu Xue Tang* to treat 102 patients with leucopenia due to chemotherapy and radiation. The herbal treatment contained this formula plus *Gou Qi Zi* (Fructus Lycii) and *Gu Sui Bu* (Rhizoma Drynariae). The average increase in white blood cell count was 1.665×10^9/L, from 2.939×10^9/L before herbal treatment to 4.600×10^9/L after the treatment. Of 102 patients, the study reported significant improvement in 39 patients, moderate improvement in 53 patients, and no benefit in 10 patients.[14]

AUTHORS' COMMENTS

It is often asked that if *Dang Gui Bu Xue Tang* is a blood-tonifying formula, why is the dose of *Huang Qi* (Radix Astragali), which is a qi tonic, five times greater than that of *Dang Gui* (Radix Angelicae Sinensis), which is a blood

tonic? The answer is that the production of blood is directly dependent on an adequate supply of qi. In other words, to effectively tonify blood, qi must be tonified first. That is why *Huang Qi* (Radix Astragali) is used at a dose five times greater than *Dang Gui* (Radix Angelicae Sinensis).[15]

Heat sensation is a symptom that is ascribed to both *Bai Hu Tang* (White Tiger Decoction) and *Dang Gui Bu Xue Tang*. It is crucial to diagnose correctly the cause of this heat sensation, since in one condition the heat arises from excess and in the other is caused by deficiency. One key difference is that the patient for which *Bai Hu Tang* (White Tiger Decoction) is appropriate will be thirsty with a desire to drink <u>cold</u> beverages. This is an indication of excess heat. Moreover, the patient will exhibit high fever and profuse sweating. In *Dang Gui Bu Xue Tang* syndrome, thirst is also present but the patient prefers <u>warm</u> drinks. A feverish sensation is present, but there is no perspiration. The pulse is surging, big and <u>forceful</u> in *Bai Hu Tang* on all three levels of pressure, while in *Dang Gui Bu Xue Tang*, the pulse is surging, big and <u>deficient</u> and forceless upon pressure.

Huang Qi (Radix Astragali) is the main ingredient in three important formulas with slightly different purposes:

• *Bu Zhong Yi Qi Tang* (Tonify the Middle and Augment the Qi Decoction) uses *Huang Qi* (Radix Astragali) to tonify qi and lift yang. It treats Spleen and Stomach qi deficiencies with prolapsed organs. Patients will exhibit fatigue, poor appetite, decreased dietary intake, a feverish sensation, chronic diarrhea, and spontaneous sweating.

• *Dang Gui Bu Xue Tang* contains *Huang Qi* (Radix Astragali) at a dose five times greater than that of *Dang Gui* (Radix Angelicae Sinensis) to boost qi and generate blood. It treats blood deficiency with deficiency-heat signs of heat sensations, a flushed face, spontaneous sweating, and a surging, big and deficient pulse that is forceless upon pressure.

• *Dang Gui Liu Huang Tang* (Tangkuei and Six-Yellow Decoction) uses *Huang Qi* (Radix Astragali) to tonify qi, consolidate *wei* (defensive) *qi,* and stop sweating. It mainly treats yin deficiency with flaring fire manifesting in spontaneous or night sweating, thirst, and a red tongue with a yellow coating.[16]

References

1. *Hei Long Jiang Zhong Yi Yao* (Heilongjiang Chinese Medicine and Herbology) 1989;4:41.
2. *Zhong Cheng Yao* (Study of Chinese Patent Medicine) 1991;13(5):44.
3. *Zhong Yao Yao Li Yu Lin Chuang* (Pharmacology and Clinical Applications of Chinese Herbs) 1990;6(5):40.

582

Chinese Herbal Formulas and Applications

Dāng Guī Bǔ Xuè Tāng (Tangkuei Decoction to Tonify the Blood)

4. *Zhong Yao Yao Li Yu Lin Chuang* (Pharmacology and Clinical Applications of Chinese Herbs) 1993;1.
5. *Zhong Yao Yao Li Yu Lin Chuang* (Pharmacology and Clinical Applications of Chinese Herbs) 1993;9(4):4.
6. *Xin Yi Yao Xue Za Zhi* (New Journal of Medicine and Herbology) 1979;3(5):27.
7. *Zhong Yi Za Zhi* (Journal of Chinese Medicine) 1984;25(5):356.
8. *Shi Yong Zhong Xi Yi Jie He Za Zhi* (Practical Journal of Integrated Chinese and Western Medicines) 1991;8:477.
9. *An Hui Zhong Yi Xue Yuan Xue Bao* (Journal of Anhui University School of Medicine) 1987;6(3):43.
10. *Yun Nan Zhong Yi Za Zhi* (Yunan Journal of Chinese Medicine) 1994;5:13.

11. *Nei Meng Gu Zhong Yi Yao* (Traditional Chinese Medicine and Medicinals of Inner Mongolia) 1998;4:12.
12. *Shang Hai Zhong Yi Yao Za Zhi* (Shanghai Journal of Chinese Medicine and Herbology) 1984;11:31.
13. *He Bei Zhong Yi Za Zhi* (Hebei Journal of Chinese Medicine) 1986;1:46.
14. *Gan Su Zhong Yi* (Gansu Chinese Medicine) 1998;5:28.
15. Wang MZ, et al. *Zhong Yi Xue Wen Da Ti Ku* (Questions and Answers on Traditional Chinese Medicine: Herbal Formulas).
16. Wang MZ, et al. *Zhong Yi Xue Wen Da Ti Ku* (Questions and Answers on Traditional Chinese Medicine: Herbal Formulas).

Guī Pí Tāng (Restore the Spleen Decoction)

歸脾湯
归脾汤

Pinyin Name: Gui Pi Tang
Literal Name: Restore the Spleen Decoction
Alternate Names: *Kuei Pi Tang*, Back to the Spleen Decoction, Ginseng and Longan Decoction, Ginseng and Longan Combination
Original Source: *Ji Sheng Fang* (Formulas to Aid the Living) by Yan Yong-He in 1253

COMPOSITION

Ren Shen (Radix et Rhizoma Ginseng)	15g [6g]
Huang Qi (Radix Astragali)	30g [12g]
Bai Zhu (Rhizoma Atractylodis Macrocephalae)	30g [9g]
Zhi Gan Cao (Radix et Rhizoma Glycyrrhizae Praeparata cum Melle)	7.5g [3g]
Dang Gui (Radix Angelicae Sinensis)	3g [9g]
Long Yan Rou (Arillus Longan)	30g [12g]
Fu Shen (Poria Pararadicis)	30g [9g]
Yuan Zhi (Radix Polygalae), *mi zhi* (fried with honey)	3g [6g]
Suan Zao Ren (Semen Ziziphi Spinosae), *chao* (dry-fried)	30g [12g]
Mu Xiang (Radix Aucklandiae), do not expose to heat	15g [6g]

Note: *Dang Gui* (Radix Angelicae Sinensis) and *Yuan Zhi* (Radix Polygalae) were not listed in the source text; they were added by Bi Li-Zhai in the 16th century in *Jiao Zhu Fu Ren Liang Fang* (Revised Fine Formulas for Women).

DOSAGE / PREPARATION / ADMINISTRATION

The source text instructs to grind the ingredients coarsely. Cook 12g of the powder with 5 slices of *Sheng Jiang* (Rhizoma Zingiberis Recens) and 1 piece of *Da Zao* (Fructus Jujubae) in 1.5 large bowls of water until it is reduced to 70%. Take the warm, strained decoction at any time of the day. This formula may also be prepared as pills by mixing the powdered herbs with honey. Take 15g of pills per dose on an empty stomach three times daily with warm, boiled water. Today, this formula may be prepared as a decoction with the doses suggested in brackets.

CHINESE THERAPEUTIC ACTIONS

1. Tonifies qi and nourishes the blood
2. Strengthens the Spleen and nourishes the Heart

CLINICAL MANIFESTATIONS

1. Heart and Spleen deficiencies due to over-thinking and excessive worrying: palpitations, forgetfulness, insomnia, night sweats, deficiency heat, low appetite, lassitude, a sallow facial complexion, a pale tongue with a thin, white tongue coating, and a fine, moderate pulse.

583

Chapter 8 – Tonic Formulas   *Section 2 – Blood-Tonifying Formulas*

Guī Pí Tāng (Restore the Spleen Decoction)

2. A deficient Spleen unable to keep the blood circulating within the vessels: hematochezia, scanty or massive uterine bleeding, early menstruation, hypermenorrhea of pale blood, prolonged menstrual period, and thick, white vaginal discharge.

CLINICAL APPLICATIONS

Anemia, thrombocytopenia, thrombopenic purpura, allergic purpura, gastric and duodenal ulcer, myasthenia gravis, congestive heart disease, supraventricular tachy-cardia, insomnia, dizziness, headache, neurasthenia, personality disorders, neurological disorders, menopause, functional endometrorrhagia, uterine bleeding, menstrual bleeding, choroidopathy, hepatitis, addiction, and benzene poisoning.

EXPLANATION

Gui Pi Tang (Restore the Spleen Decoction) is renowned for treating Heart (blood) and Spleen (qi) deficiencies. The common cause of this syndrome is over-thinking or excessive worrying, which consumes the blood and injures qi. Symptoms of Heart (blood) deficiency include palpitations, forgetfulness, and insomnia. Symptoms of Spleen (qi) deficiency include low appetite, lassitude, and a sallow facial complexion. A pale tongue with a thin, white tongue coating and a fine, moderate pulse indicate qi and blood deficiencies.

This formula is also indicated for patients in which the Spleen fails to hold blood inside the vessels because of Spleen qi deficiency. Symptoms of bleeding, such as hema-tochezia, may occur. Women may have symptoms of uterine bleeding, early menstruation, and hypermenorrhea

with pale blood and no clots. If the Spleen is deficient and dampness ensues, then thick, white vaginal discharge may occur as a result of dampness descending to the lower parts of the body.

Ren Shen (Radix et Rhizoma Ginseng), *Huang Qi* (Radix Astragali), *Bai Zhu* (Rhizoma Atractylodis Macrocephalae), and *Zhi Gan Cao* (Radix et Rhizoma Glycyrrhizae Praeparata cum Melle) warm and tonify Spleen qi. *Dang Gui* (Radix Angelicae Sinensis) and *Long Yan Rou* (Arillus Longan) nourish the Liver, tonify Heart blood, and regu-late blood circulation. *Fu Shen* (Poria Paradicis), *Yuan Zhi* (Radix Polygalae) and *Suan Zao Ren* (Semen Ziziphi Spinosae) nourish the Heart and calm the *shen* (spirit). *Mu Xiang* (Radix Aucklandiae) moves qi and prevents the stagnating nature of the tonic herbs from impairing the Spleen and Stomach. *Sheng Jiang* (Rhizoma Zingib-eris Recens) and *Da Zao* (Fructus Jujubae) harmonize the middle *jiao*. In short, this formula nourishes the Heart, strengthens the Spleen, and tonifies qi and blood.

MODIFICATIONS

- If there is fever, add *Chai Hu* (Radix Bupleuri) and *Zhi Zi* (Fructus Gardeniae).
- For insomnia due to fear and fright, add *Gou Teng* (Ramulus Uncariae cum Uncis) and *Bai Zi Ren* (Semen Platycladi).
- With poor appetite, add *Chen Pi* (Pericarpium Citri Reticulatae) and *Ban Xia* (Rhizoma Pinelliae).
- With fatigue and decreased intake of food, add *Sha Ren* (Fructus Amomi) and *Cang Zhu* (Rhizoma Atractylodis).
- If there is cough, add *Zi Wan* (Radix et Rhizoma Asteris) and *Jie Geng* (Radix Platycodonis).

Gui Pi Tang (Restore the Spleen Decoction)

Diagnosis	Signs and Symptoms	Treatment	Herbs
Heart and Spleen deficiencies	• Palpitations, forgetfulness, and insomnia: Heart blood deficiency • Low appetite, lassitude, and a sallow facial complexion: Spleen qi deficiency • Pale tongue with a thin, white tongue coating: qi and blood deficiencies • Fine, moderate pulse: qi and blood deficiencies	• Tonifies qi and nourishes the blood • Strengthens the Spleen and nourishes the Heart	• *Ren Shen* (Radix et Rhizoma Ginseng), *Huang Qi* (Radix Astragali), *Bai Zhu* (Rhizoma Atractylodis Macrocephalae), and *Zhi Gan Cao* (Radix et Rhizoma Glycyrrhizae Praeparata cum Melle) warm and tonify Spleen qi. • *Dang Gui* (Radix Angelicae Sinensis) and *Long Yan Rou* (Arillus Longan) nourish the Liver, tonify Heart blood, and regulate blood circulation. • *Fu Shen* (Poria Paradicis), *Yuan Zhi* (Radix Polygalae) and *Suan Zao Ren* (Semen Ziziphi Spinosae) nourish the Heart to calm the *shen* (spirit). • *Mu Xiang* (Radix Aucklandiae) moves qi and moderates the stagnating nature of the tonic herbs. • *Sheng Jiang* (Rhizoma Zingiberis Recens) and *Da Zao* (Fructus Jujubae) harmonize the middle *jiao*.

584

Chinese Herbal Formulas and Applications

Guī Pí Tāng (Restore the Spleen Decoction)

- With the presence of blood during coughing, add *Xiao Ji* (Herba Cirsii) and *Ou Jie* (Nodus Nelumbinis Rhizomatis).
- For irregular amount of menstrual bleeding, add *Shan Zhu Yu* (Fructus Corni) and *Wu Wei Zi* (Fructus Schisandrae Chinensis).
- To tonify blood and stop bleeding, add *Shu Di Huang* (Radix Rehmanniae Praeparata) and *E Jiao* (Colla Corii Asini).
- For uterine bleeding, add *E Jiao* (Colla Corii Asini), *Ai Ye* (Folium Artemisiae Argyi), and *Bai Shao* (Radix Paeoniae Alba).
- If there is profuse menstrual bleeding, add *Di Yu* (Radix Sanguisorbae) and *E Jiao* (Colla Corii Asini).
- For *beng lou* (flooding and spotting) due to cold and deficiency, add *Ai Ye* (Folium Artemisiae Argyi), *Pao Jiang* (Rhizoma Zingiberis Praeparatum), *Xue Yu Tan* (Crinis Carbonisatus), and *Wu Wei Zi* (Fructus Schisandrae Chinensis).
- For *beng lou* (flooding and spotting) due to heat, add charred *Di Huang* (Radix Rehmanniae) and *E Jiao* (Colla Corii Asini).

CAUTIONS / CONTRAINDICATIONS
- *Gui Pi Tang* is contraindicated in cases of interior heat or yin deficiency with a rapid pulse.
- *Gui Pi Tang* is relatively neutral in property and usually does not produce side effects even with long-term use. However, should one feel dryness (e.g., a dry mouth, dry nose and constipation) after taking this formula, consume diluted salt water to offset the dryness.[1]
- While taking this formula, avoid excessive thinking and worrying, refrain from physical exhaustion, and cease eating foods that are raw and cold in nature.[2]

PHARMACOLOGICAL EFFECTS
1. **Antiulcer:** Use of *Gui Pi Tang* was effective in preventing stress-induced ulcer in mice. The mechanism of action was attributed to the regulatory effect of the herbs on the central nervous system to reduce the production and secretion of gastric acid.[3]
2. **Cognitive:** Use of *Gui Pi Tang* was effective in improving cognition in mice with impaired memory due to drugs, electric shock, or aging.[4]

CLINICAL STUDIES AND RESEARCH
1. **Hepatitis:** In one report, 9 patients with hepatitis and thrombopenia were treated with modified *Gui Pi Tang* with recovery in 5 patients (asymptomatic with no recurrence within 2 years), improvement in 2 patients, and no benefit in 2 patients. Most patients began to notice improvement within 14-21 days of treatment.[5]

2. **Headache and dizziness:** Modified *Gui Pi Tang* was used with good success to treat 22 patients with headache and dizziness due to intrathecal injection of anesthetics that did not respond to drug treatment. Complete relief of the symptoms was reported in 17 patients within 3 doses, 2 patients within 4-6 doses, and 3 patients within 8-10 doses.[6]
3. **Dizziness:** Twenty-five patients with dizziness were treated for an average of 30 days (ranges of 12-60 days) with complete recovery in 12 patients, marked improvement in 8 patients, slight improvement in 4 patients, and no benefit in 1 patient. The overall rate of effectiveness was 96%. The causes of dizziness included neurasthenia, menopause, anemia, and cervical hyperosteogeny.[7]
4. **Neurasthenia:** In one study, 200 patients with history of neurasthenia of 2-15 years were treated with modified *Gui Pi Tang* with good results. The formula used included *Chai Hu* (Radix Bupleuri), *Huang Qi* (Radix Astragali), *Dang Shen* (Radix Codonopsis), *Dang Gui* (Radix Angelicae Sinensis), dry-fried *Bai Shao* (Radix Paeoniae Alba), *Di Huang* (Radix Rehmanniae), *Yin Chen* (Herba Artemisiae Scopariae), dry-fried *Bai Zhu* (Rhizoma Atractylodis Macrocephalae), *Fu Ling* (Poria), *Mu Xiang* (Radix Aucklandiae), *Suan Zao Ren* (Semen Ziziphi Spinosae), processed *Yuan Zhi* (Radix Polygalae), *Wu Wei Zi* (Fructus Schisandrae Chinensis), *Shi Chang Pu* (Rhizoma Acori Tatarinowii), *She Xiang* (Moschus), *Bo He* (Herba Menthae), *Gan Cao* (Radix et Rhizoma Glycyrrhizae), and *Feng Mi* (Mel). The treatment protocol was to take 15g of herbs as pills three times daily for 20 days per course of treatment. Out of 200 patients, the study reported recovery in 128 patients (asymptomatic with no recurrence within 1 year), marked effect in 48 patients (asymptomatic with no recurrence within 6 months), slight improvement in 19 patients, and no benefit in 5 patients. The overall rate of effectiveness was 97.5%.[8] Another study involving 100 patients with neurasthenia reported 91% effectiveness, with improvement such as resolution of tinnitus, fatigue, and insomnia.[9]
5. **Insomnia:** In one study, 450 patients with histories of severe insomnia for 7 days to 5 years were treated with modified *Gui Pi Tang* and acupuncture with good results. The formula used included *Ren Shen* (Radix et Rhizoma Ginseng) 15g, *Huang Qi* (Radix Astragali) 15-30g, *Bai Zhu* (Rhizoma Atractylodis Macrocephalae) 10-20g, *Fu Ling* (Poria) 10-20g, *Suan Zao Ren* (Semen Ziziphi Spinosae) 15-25g, *Yuan Zhi* (Radix Polygalae) 15-25g, *Dang Gui* (Radix Angelicae Sinensis) 15-25g, *Gan Cao* (Radix et Rhizoma Glycyrrhizae) 10g, and *Mu Xiang* (Radix Aucklandiae) 10g. *Long Dan* (Radix et Rhizoma Gentianae), *Chai Hu* (Radix Bupleuri), and *Zhi Zi* (Fructus Gardeniae) were added for Liver fire; *Ban Xia* (Rhizoma

8

TONIC FORMULAS

585

Chapter 8 – Tonic Formulas   *Section 2 – Blood-Tonifying Formulas*

Guī Pí Tāng (Restore the Spleen Decoction)

Pinelliae) and *Chen Pi* (Pericarpium Citri Reticulatae) were added for hot phlegm; *Xuan Shen* (Radix Scrophulariae), *Zhi Mu* (Rhizoma Anemarrhenae), and *Mai Dong* (Radix Ophiopogonis) were added for yin-deficient heat. The herbs were given as a decoction one time daily. Out of 45 patients, the study reported recovery in 18 patients (over 6 hours of sleep for 2 weeks), marked effect in 10 patients (over 4 hours of sleep for 2 weeks), slight improvement in 7 patients, and no benefit in 5 patients. The overall rate of effectiveness was 87.5%.[10] In another study, modified *Gui Pi Tang* was used to treat 31 patients with insomnia with an 80.6% rate of effectiveness. In addition to the base formula, modifications included addition of *Bai Zi Ren* (Semen Platycladi) and *Shu Di Huang* (Radix Rehmanniae Praeparata) for Heart and Spleen deficiencies; *Huang Lian* (Rhizoma Coptidis), *Zhi Zi* (Fructus Gardeniae) and *Di Huang* (Radix Rehmanniae) for yin-deficient fire; and *Zhu Ru* (Caulis Bambusae in Taenia), *Huang Lian* (Rhizoma Coptidis), and *Chen Pi* (Pericarpium Citri Reticulatae) for Spleen deficiency with hot phlegm.[11]

6. **Anemia**: In one study, 19 patients with anemia due to iron deficiency were treated with 79% effectiveness within one month.[12] In another study, 20 patients with anemia due to hemorrhage were treated for an average of 24 doses (ranges from 5-49 doses) of decoction with good results.[13] Lastly, its effectiveness is documented in patients with compromised kidney function with anemia and leucopenia.[14]

7. **Thrombopenic purpura**: In one study, 46 patients with primary thrombopenic purpura were treated with modified *Gui Pi Tang* with good results. The formula included *Huang Qi* (Radix Astragali) 15-30g, *Dang Gui* (Radix Angelicae Sinensis) 10-15g, *Di Huang* (Radix Rehmanniae) 10-30g, *Ce Bai Ye* (Cacumen Platycladi) 15-30g, *He Ye* (Folium Nelumbinis) 10-15g, dry-fried *Huai Hua* (Flos Sophorae) 10-15g, *Shan Zhu Yu* (Fructus Corni) 10-30g, *San Qi* (Radix et Rhizoma Notoginseng) 2-6g given in powder separately, *Xian He Cao* (Herba Agrimoniae) 30g, *E Jiao* (Colla Corii Asini) 10-15g dissolved in decoction immediately before ingestion, and *Gan Cao* (Radix et Rhizoma Glycyrrhizae) 10g. The treatment protocol was to administer the herbs in decoction one time daily for one month per course of treatment. The average length of treatment was three courses. Out of 46 patients, the study reported marked effect in 11 patients (asymptomatic with normal platelet count for at least 3 months), improvement in 15 patients (asymptomatic with normal platelet count for at least 2 months), slight improvement in 11 patients (slight subjective and objective improvement) and no benefit in 9 patients. The overall rate of effectiveness was 80.4%.[15]

8. **Menopause**: Eighteen patients with menopausal symptoms were treated with excellent results using *Gui Pi Tang* with addition of *Long Gu* (Os Draconis) and *Mu Li* (Concha Ostreae). The duration of treatment was between 6-27 packs of herbs.[16]

9. **Uterine bleeding**: In one report, 11 patients with profuse uterine bleeding characterized by Spleen deficiency were treated with 3-9 doses. The study reported that bleeding stopped in all patients.[17] Another study of 135 patients with uterine bleeding reported marked results using *Gui Pi Tang*.[18]

10. **Beng lou (flooding and spotting)**: One study reported 91.3% effectiveness using modified *Gui Pi Tang* to treat 46 patients with *beng lou* (flooding and spotting). The modifications included removal of *Dang Gui* (Radix Angelicae Sinensis), *Yuan Zhi* (Radix Polygalae) and *Mu Xiang* (Radix Aucklandiae), and addition of *Xian He Cao* (Herba Agrimoniae), *Shu Di Huang* (Radix Rehmanniae Praeparata), and others as needed.[19]

11. **Choroidopathy**: Use of modified *Gui Pi Tang* in 57 patients with fluid accumulation under the retina was associated with complete recovery in 35 patients, improvement in 18 patients, and no benefit in 4 patients. The herbal treatment was based on *Gui Pi Tang*, with the removal of *Yuan Zhi* (Radix Polygalae) and *Long Yan Rou* (Arillus Longan), and the addition of *Gou Qi Zi* (Fructus Lycii), *Gu Jing Cao* (Flos Eriocauli), *Mi Meng Hua* (Flos Buddlejae), and others. Modifications were made as follows: for Liver and Kidney yin deficiencies, *Tai Zi Shen* (Radix Pseudostellariae), *Shan Zhu Yu* (Fructus Corni), *Di Huang* (Radix Rehmanniae), *Mu Dan Pi* (Cortex Moutan), and *Ju Hua* (Flos Chrysanthemi) were added, and *Dang Shen* (Radix Codonopsis) and *Mu Xiang* (Radix Aucklandiae) were removed; and for Liver qi stagnation, *Chai Hu* (Radix Bupleuri), *Yu Jin* (Radix Curcumae), *Bai Shao* (Radix Paeoniae Alba), and *Chuan Xiong* (Rhizoma Chuanxiong) were added, and *Dang Shen* (Radix Codonopsis) and *Huang Qi* (Radix Astragali) were removed.[20]

12. **Addiction**: One study reported good results using *Gui Pi Tang* as a supportive therapy in individuals with a recent history of substance abuse to control spontaneous perspiration, insomnia, and loss of appetite. The duration of herbal therapy was 3 months.[21]

13. **Benzene poisoning**: Twenty-seven patients with chronic benzene poisoning were treated with good results using modified *Gui Pi Tang* with the addition of such herbs as *Huang Qi* (Radix Astragali), *E Jiao* (Colla Corii Asini), *Dan Shen* (Radix et Rhizoma Salviae Miltiorrhizae), or *Bai Shao* (Radix Paeoniae Alba) as needed. Of 27 patients, the study reported recovery in 6 patients and improvement in 21 patients.[22]

586

Chinese Herbal Formulas and Applications

Guī Pí Tāng (Restore the Spleen Decoction)

RELATED FORMULA

Guī Pí Ān Shén Tāng

(Restore the Spleen and Tranquilize the Spirit Decoction)

歸脾安神湯
归脾安神汤

Pinyin Name: *Gui Pi An Shen Tang*
Literal Name: Restore the Spleen and Tranquilize the Spirit Decoction
Original Source: *Guang An Men Yi Yuan* (Guang An Men Hospital) in 1990

Bai Zhu (Rhizoma Atractylodis Macrocephalae)
Fu Ling (Poria)
Huang Qi (Radix Astragali)
Yuan Zhi (Radix Polygalae)
He Huan Pi (Cortex Albiziae)
Long Yan Rou (Arillus Longan)
Suan Zao Ren (Semen Ziziphi Spinosae)
Wu Wei Zi (Fructus Schisandrae Chinensis)
Ren Shen (Radix et Rhizoma Ginseng)
Xiang Fu (Rhizoma Cyperi)
Zhi Gan Cao (Radix et Rhizoma Glycyrrhizae Praeparata cum Melle)
Dang Gui (Radix Angelicae Sinensis)
Sheng Jiang (Rhizoma Zingiberis Recens)
Da Zao (Fructus Jujubae)

Gui Pi An Shen Tang (Restore the Spleen and Tranquilize the Spirit Decoction) tonifies qi, nourishes the blood, and calms the *shen* (spirit). It commonly treats insomnia due to Heart and Spleen deficiencies, which arise from over-thinking and excessive worrying.

AUTHORS' COMMENTS

Gui Pi Tang, literally "Restore the Spleen Decoction," has an important function to tonify qi, generate blood, and restore and normalize transportation and transformation functions of the Spleen. It is vital to ensure that Spleen functions properly, as it is the root of post-natal qi, and the origin of qi and blood.

Although *Dang Gui* (Radix Angelicae Sinensis) and *Yuan Zhi* (Radix Polygalae) were not used in the original formulation of *Gui Pi Tang*, they are generally used today as *Dang Gui* (Radix Angelicae Sinensis) greatly enhances the effect to tonify blood, and *Yuan Zhi* (Radix Polygalae) strongly increases the efficacy to nourish the Heart and tranquilize the mind.

Gui Pi Tang is one of the most commonly used formulas for treating Heart (blood) and Spleen (qi) deficiencies. *Gui Pi Tang* and *Si Wu Tang* (Four-Substance Decoction) both nourish and produce blood, as well as treat irregular menstruation, abnormal uterine bleeding, and other gynecological disorders. Their differences are as follows:

- *Gui Pi Tang* mainly strengthens the Spleen and tonifies qi. It also tonifies the blood and nourishes Heart *shen* (spirit) to treat Spleen and Heart deficiency patterns that manifest in symptoms such as forgetfulness, palpitations, insomnia, night sweats, hot flashes, poor appetite, fatigue, a sallow complexion, a pale tongue with a thin tongue coating, and a fine, moderate pulse. Because the Spleen is responsible for holding blood in the vessels, this formula is effective for uterine bleeding, early menstruation, profuse menstrual bleeding, or trickling of blood due to Spleen deficiency.

- *Si Wu Tang* tonifies and moves the blood at the same time. It also treats abdominal pain, restless fetus, postpartum bleeding, and mass accumulation.[23]

Gui Pi Tang and *Tian Wang Bu Xin Dan* (Emperor of Heaven's Special Pill to Tonify the Heart) both nourish the Heart and calm the *shen* (spirit) to treat palpitations, forgetfulness, and insomnia.

- *Gui Pi Tang* is designed for individuals who worry excessively, leading to qi and blood deficiencies of the Spleen and Heart. Other than *shen* disturbance signs, patients will exhibit poor appetite, decreased dietary intake, lassitude, shortness of breath, spontaneous sweating, and other Spleen deficiency signs. In addition to tranquilizing herbs such as *Suan Zao Ren* (Semen Ziziphi Spinosae), *Fu Shen* (Poria Paradicis), *Long Yan Rou* (Arillus Longan), and *Yuan Zhi* (Radix Polygalae), this formula contains Spleen tonic herbs, such as *Ren Shen* (Radix et Rhizoma Ginseng), *Huang Qi* (Radix Astragali), *Bai Zhu* (Rhizoma Atractylodis Macrocephalae), and *Gan Cao* (Radix et Rhizoma Glycyrrhizae).

- *Tian Wang Bu Xin Dan* is indicated for disharmony of the Heart and Kidney, with Kidney yin and blood deficiencies unable to nourish the Heart, leading to Heart fire. Besides blood deficiency signs of palpitations, forgetfulness and insomnia, there will be symptoms of Heart fire, such as irritability, night sweats, nocturnal emissions, ulcers on the tongue, and dry stools or constipation. This formula uses herbs that nourish yin and blood and have tranquilizing and calming effects, such as *Suan Zao Ren* (Semen Ziziphi Spinosae), *Bai Zi Ren* (Semen Platycladi), *Yuan Zhi* (Radix Polygalae), *Tian Dong* (Radix Asparagi), and *Mai Dong* (Radix Ophiopogonis).[24]

Gui Pi Tang, *Tian Wang Bu Xin Dan* (Emperor of Heaven's Special Pill to Tonify the Heart), and *Suan Zao Ren Tang* (Sour Jujube Decoction) all nourish and calm the *shen* (spirit) to treat palpitations, forgetfulness, insomnia, and associated symptoms and signs.

8

TONIC FORMULAS

587

Chapter 8 – Tonic Formulas   Section 2 – Blood-Tonifying Formulas

Guī Pí Tāng (Restore the Spleen Decoction)

- *Gui Pi Tang* tonifies qi and blood and strengthens the Spleen. The two organs involved are the Spleen and Heart. Symptoms include poor appetite, fatigue, lassitude, possible blood in the stool or uterine bleeding. *Gui Pi Tang* is suitable for individuals who think and worry excessively, and who have poor appetite.
- *Tian Wang Bu Xin Dan* nourishes yin and blood to tonify the Heart and calm the *shen*. Key organs involved are the Heart and Kidney. In addition to *shen* disturbance signs, symptoms of yin and blood deficiencies include dry stools, a red tongue body with a scanty coating, and a fine, rapid pulse. Most patients who suffer from Heart and Kidney deficiencies are usually older and have the key sign of forgetfulness.
- *Suan Zao Ren Tang* nourishes the blood, calms the *shen*, clears heat, and relieves irritability. It treats Liver blood deficiency with flaring of deficiency fire causing *shen* disturbance. The key organ involved is the Liver, with signs of dizziness, vertigo, irritability, and a fine, wiry pulse. Individuals who tend to have *Suan Zao Ren Tang* syndrome are mostly women who are under stress for a prolonged period of time and have depleted their Liver blood.[25]

Gui Pi Tang and *Gu Jing Wan* (Stabilize the Menses Pill) both treat hypermenorrhea and *beng lou* (flooding and spotting).

- *Gui Pi Tang* tonifies the Spleen and Heart, and treats menstrual bleeding that is light in color. It is most suitable for individuals with qi and blood deficiencies, with accompanying symptoms such as weakness, poor appetite, insomnia, and palpitations.
- *Gu Jing Wan* nourishes yin, clears heat, and treats excessive menstrual bleeding that is dark red in color, with or without clots. The tongue body is red and the pulse is wiry, rapid.[26]

Gui Pi Tang and *Bu Zhong Yi Qi Tang* (Tonify the Middle and Augment the Qi Decoction) both use *Ren Shen* (Radix et Rhizoma Ginseng), *Huang Qi* (Radix Astragali), *Bai Zhu* (Rhizoma Atractylodis Macrocephalae), and *Gan Cao* (Radix et Rhizoma Glycyrrhizae) to tonify qi and strengthen the Spleen. The difference is:

- The other herbs in *Gui Pi Tang* focus on nourishing the *shen* (spirit) and tonifying the blood. This formula is mainly used for *shen* disturbance or bleeding.
- The other herbs in *Bu Zhong Yi Qi Tang* lift yang and treat prolapse. This formula is mainly used for qi deficiency leading to organ prolapse.

References

1. *Zhong Yao Ming Fang Yao Li Yu Ying Yong* (Pharmacology and Applications of Famous Herbal Formulas) 1989;285-286.
2. *Zhong Yao Ming Fang Yao Li Yu Ying Yong* (Pharmacology and Applications of Famous Herbal Formulas) 1989;285-286.
3. *Tian Jin Zhong Yi* (Tianjin Chinese Medicine) 1995;4:28.
4. *Zhong Yao Yao Li Yu Lin Chuang* (Pharmacology and Clinical Applications of Chinese Herbs) 1990;6(5):2.
5. *Zhong Yi Za Zhi* (Journal of Chinese Medicine) 1985;5:32.
6. *Hu Bei Zhong Yi Za Zhi* (Hubei Journal of Chinese Medicine) 1984;2:19.
7. *Yun Nan Zhong Yi Za Zhi* (Yunan Journal of Chinese Medicine) 1994;15(1):21.
8. *Zhong Yi Yao Xin Xi* (Information on Chinese Medicine and Herbology) 1995;12(5):39.
9. *He Bei Zhong Yi* (Hebei Chinese Medicine) 1987;2:34.
10. *Zhong Yi Yao Xin Xi* (Information on Chinese Medicine and Herbology) 1995;12(4):39.
11. *Fu Jian Zhong Yi Yao* (Fujian Chinese Medicine and Herbology) 1996;6:16.
12. *Zhong Cheng Yao Yan Jiu* (Research of Chinese Patent Medicine) 1987;5:20.
13. *Shan Xi Zhong Yi Xue Yuan Xue Bao* (Journal of Shanxi University School of Chinese Medicine) 1988;1:29.
14. *Guo Wai Yi Yao Zhi Wu Yao Fen Ce* (Monograph of Foreign Botanical Medicine) 1993;15(3):44.
15. *Bei Jing Zhong Yi Za Zhi* (Beijing Journal of Chinese Medicine) 1993;3:227.
16. *Shang Hai Zhong Yi Yao Za Zhi* (Shanghai Journal of Chinese Medicine and Herbology) 1985;5:31.
17. *Jiang Xi Zhong Yi Yao* (Jiangxi Chinese Medicine and Herbology) 1959;3:14.
18. *Jiang Xi Zhong Yi Yao* (Jiangxi Chinese Medicine and Herbology) 1969;3:14.
19. *Nan Jing Zhong Yi Xue Yuan Xue Bao* (Journal of Nanjing University of Traditional Chinese Medicine) 1988;2:26.
20. *Shi Yong Zhong Yi Za Zhi* (Journal of Practical Chinese Medicine) 1997;6:5.
21. *Hu Nan Zhong Yi Za Zhi* (Hunan Journal of Chinese Medicine) 1998;3:25.
22. *Hu Bei Zhong Yi Za Zhi* (Hubei Journal of Chinese Medicine) 1987;6:18.
23. Wang MZ, et al. *Zhong Yi Xue Wen Da Ti Ku* (Questions and Answers on Traditional Chinese Medicine: Herbal Formulas).
24. Wang MZ, et al. *Zhong Yi Xue Wen Da Ti Ku* (Questions and Answers on Traditional Chinese Medicine: Herbal Formulas).
25. Wang MZ, et al. *Zhong Yi Xue Wen Da Ti Ku* (Questions and Answers on Traditional Chinese Medicine: Herbal Formulas).
26. Wang MZ, et al. *Zhong Yi Xue Wen Da Ti Ku* (Questions and Answers on Traditional Chinese Medicine: Herbal Formulas).

588

Chinese Herbal Formulas and Applications

Zhī Gān Cǎo Tāng (Honey-Fried Licorice Decoction)

炙甘草湯
炙甘草汤

Pinyin Name: *Zhi Gan Cao Tang*

Literal Name: Honey-Fried Licorice Decoction

Alternate Names: *Fu Mai Tang* (Restore the Pulse Decoction), *Chih Kan Tsao Tang*, Baked Licorice Decoction, Roasted Licorice Decoction, Licorice Combination

Original Source: *Shang Han Lun* (Discussion of Cold-Induced Disorders) by Zhang Zhong-Jing in the Eastern Han Dynasty

COMPOSITION

Zhi Gan Cao (Radix et Rhizoma Glycyrrhizae Praeparata cum Melle)	12g
Ren Shen (Radix et Rhizoma Ginseng)	6g
Da Zao (Fructus Jujubae), *bo* (opened)	30 pieces [5-10 pieces]
Di Huang (Radix Rehmanniae)	48g [30g]
Mai Dong (Radix Ophiopogonis)	0.5 cup [9g]
E Jiao (Colla Corii Asini)	6g
Huo Ma Ren (Fructus Cannabis)	0.5 cup [9g]
Sheng Jiang (Rhizoma Zingiberis Recens), *qie* (sliced)	9g
Gui Zhi (Ramulus Cinnamomi)	9g

DOSAGE / PREPARATION / ADMINISTRATION

Cook the ingredients, except *E Jiao* (Colla Corii Asini), in approximately 7 cups [1,400 mL] of grain-based liquor and 8 cups [1,600 mL] of water until it is reduced to 3 cups [600 mL]. Add *E Jiao* (Colla Corii Asini) to the warm, strained decoction and allow it to completely dissolve. Take 1 cup [200 mL] of the warm decoction three times a day. Today, this formula is usually prepared by cooking the ingredients in water to obtain a decoction. Use the doses suggested in brackets above. Add 10 mL of grain-based liquor to the warm, strained decoction. Separately dissolve *E Jiao* (Colla Corii Asini) in boiling water, and add it to the warm, strained decoction. Take the decoction in three equally-divided doses and finish it within one day.

CHINESE THERAPEUTIC ACTIONS

1. Tonifies qi and nourishes yin
2. Tonifies the blood and restores the pulse

CLINICAL MANIFESTATIONS

1. Qi and blood deficiencies: a bound or intermittent pulse, palpitations, arrhythmia, weak physical condition, shortness of breath, and a pale tongue with a mirror-like dry surface.
2. Lung atrophy due to deficiency and consumption: dry coughing with little or no sputum, bloody streaks in the sputum, shortness of breath, fidgeting, disturbed sleep, spontaneous perspiration or night sweats, a skinny appearance, an occasional feeling of warm sensation, a dry throat and tongue, difficult defecation, and a deficient, rapid pulse.

CLINICAL APPLICATIONS

Coronary heart disease, rheumatic heart disease, arrhythmia, angina pectoris, viral myocarditis, hypotension, endocarditis, hyperthyroidism, and hyperactivity of the sympathetic nervous system.

EXPLANATION

Zhi Gan Cao Tang (Honey-Fried Licorice Decoction) treats bound or intermittent pulse due to qi and blood deficiencies. In this condition, qi is deficient and cannot flow freely, and blood is deficient and cannot nourish the Heart. A weak physical condition, shortness of breath, spontaneous sweating, and a skinny appearance indicate qi deficiency. Palpitations, insomnia, and a dry, mirror-like tongue surface indicate yin and blood deficiencies. Dry coughing with little or no sputum, the presence of blood in the sputum, night sweats, and a dry throat and tongue suggest yin and body fluid deficiencies.

Zhi Gan Cao (Radix et Rhizoma Glycyrrhizae Praeparata cum Melle), *Ren Shen* (Radix et Rhizoma Ginseng), and *Da Zao* (Fructus Jujubae) tonify Heart and Spleen qi. *Di Huang* (Radix Rehmanniae), *Mai Dong* (Radix Ophiopogonis), *E Jiao* (Colla Corii Asini), and *Huo Ma Ren* (Fructus Cannabis) tonify Heart blood, nourish Lung yin, and replenish body fluids. *Sheng Jiang* (Rhizoma Zingiberis Recens), *Gui Zhi* (Ramulus Cinnamomi), and the grain-based alcohol activate yang and qi flow to restore the pulse.

8

TONIC FORMULAS

589

Chapter 8 – Tonic Formulas   *Section 2 – Blood-Tonifying Formulas*

Zhǐ Gān Cǎo Tāng (Honey-Fried Licorice Decoction)

Zhi Gan Cao Tang (Honey-Fried Licorice Decoction)

Diagnosis	Signs and Symptoms	Treatment	Herbs
Bound or intermittent pulse with qi and blood deficiencies	• Bound or intermittent pulse with palpitations and arrhythmia: qi deficiency unable to flow freely, and blood deficiency unable to nourish the Heart • Weak physical condition, shortness of breath, spontaneous sweating, and a skinny appearance: qi deficiency • Palpitations, insomnia, and a dry, mirror-like tongue surface: yin and blood deficiencies • Dry coughing with little or no sputum, the presence of blood in the sputum, night sweats, and a dry throat and tongue: yin and body fluid deficiencies	• Tonifies qi and nourishes yin • Tonifies the blood and restores the pulse	• *Zhi Gan Cao* (Radix et Rhizoma Glycyrrhizae Praeparata cum Melle), *Ren Shen* (Radix et Rhizoma Ginseng) and *Da Zao* (Fructus Jujubae) tonify Heart and Spleen qi. • *Di Huang* (Radix Rehmanniae), *Mai Dong* (Radix Ophiopogonis), *E Jiao* (Colla Corii Asini), and *Huo Ma Ren* (Fructus Cannabis) tonify Heart blood, nourish Lung yin, and replenish body fluids. • *Sheng Jiang* (Rhizoma Zingiberis Recens), *Gui Zhi* (Ramulus Cinnamomi), and grain-based alcohol activate yang and qi flow to restore the pulse.

This formula also can be used to treat Lung atrophy due to deficiency and consumption. This condition is characterized by Lung yin deficiency, with symptoms such as dry coughing with little or no sputum, fidgeting, and night sweats. However, if there are severe symptoms of yin deficiency, the doses of *Sheng Jiang* (Rhizoma Zingiberis Recens), *Gui Zhi* (Ramulus Cinnamomi) and grain-based alcohol should be decreased.

MODIFICATIONS
• If there is qi deficiency, add *Huang Qi* (Radix Astragali).
• If there is yang deficiency, add *Fu Zi* (Radix Aconiti Lateralis Praeparata).
• With insomnia, add *Suan Zao Ren* (Semen Ziziphi Spinosae) and *Bai Zi Ren* (Semen Platycladi).
• With generalized fatigue and deficiency, add *Tian Dong* (Radix Asparagi) and *Shu Di Huang* (Radix Rehmanniae Praeparata).
• With poor appetite, add *Chen Pi* (Pericarpium Citri Reticulatae) and *Ban Xia* (Rhizoma Pinelliae).
• With cough due to Lung atrophy, add *Jie Geng* (Radix Platycodonis) and *Zhi Shi* (Fructus Aurantii Immaturus).
• If there is a feeling of chest congestion and oppression, add *Fu Ling* (Poria) and *Ku Xing Ren* (Semen Armeniacae Amarum).
• With irritability and fright, add *Huang Qi* (Radix Astragali) and *Wu Wei Zi* (Fructus Schisandrae Chinensis).
• With nausea and vomiting, add *Wen Dan Tang* (Warm the Gallbladder Decoction).
• For edema, add *Fu Ling* (Poria) and *Che Qian Zi* (Semen Plantaginis).

CAUTIONS / CONTRAINDICATIONS
• *Zhi Gan Cao Tang* is not appropriate for individuals with severe edema or a fine pulse.
• This formula has a slight moistening and lubricating effect on the intestines. Therefore, it should be used with caution in patients with diarrhea and dysentery.[1]

PHARMACOLOGICAL EFFECTS
1. **Cardiovascular**: Injection of a preparation of *Zhi Gan Cao Tang* was associated with an inhibitory effect on the cardiac tissues to lower the heart rate, reduce the contractile force of the heart, and decrease the blood perfusion to the coronary artery. Its inhibitory effect also counters the stimulating effect of adrenalin.[2] Additionally, administration of this formula was shown to have a protective effect against ischemia of the cardiac muscles.[3]
2. **Antiarrhythmic**: *Zhi Gan Cao Tang* has been shown in many studies to be beneficial in treating arrhythmia due to various causes. In one report, administration of the formula in many different animal subjects was effective in treating arrhythmia induced by drugs such as aconitine, $CaCl_2$, and adrenalin.[4]

CLINICAL STUDIES AND RESEARCH
1. **Arrhythmia**: In a clinical study, patients with coronary heart disease and arrhythmia were divided into two groups. The first group of 23 patients received the normal dose of the herbs decocted in water and alcohol. The second group of 23 patients received only 25% the normal dose of the herbs decocted in water without alcohol. All patients were monitored for their signs (ECG) and symptoms (palpitations, shortness of breath, fatigue, and chest

590

Zhi Gān Cǎo Tāng (Honey-Fried Licorice Decoction)

Chinese Herbal Formulas and Applications

congestion). At the end of treatment, the study reported that out of 23 patients in the first group, 16 patients had complete recovery, 4 had marked improvement, and 3 showed no change. In comparison with the second group of 23 patients, 6 patients had complete recovery, 9 had marked improvement, and 8 showed no change. The overall rate of effectiveness was 87.1% in the first group, and 65.2% in the second group.[5]

2. **Angina pectoris**: One hundred and fifty patients with angina pectoris and coronary heart disease were treated with modified *Zhi Gan Cao Tang* with marked effect in 48 patients, improvement in 90 patients, and no change in 12 patients. The overall rate of effectiveness was 92%. Most patients began to notice improvement within 1-3 weeks. The herbal formula was based on *Zhi Gan Cao Tang*, with elimination of *Huo Ma Ren* (Fructus Cannabis) and *Sheng Jiang* (Rhizoma Zingiberis Recens), and the addition of *Gui Ban* (Plastrum Testudinis), *Wu Wei Zi* (Fructus Schisandrae Chinensis), and *Ji Xue Teng* (Caulis Spatholobi).[6]

3. **Viral myocarditis**: Use of *Zhi Gan Cao Tang* in 38 patients with viral myocarditis was associated with complete recovery in 30 patients, improvement in 4 patients, no change in 2 patients, and fatality in 2 patients.[7] Another report stated 87.5% effectiveness (21 of 24 patients) using this formula to treat viral myocarditis.[8]

4. **Hypotension**: Fifty patients with low blood pressure were treated with good results using modified *Zhi Gan Cao Tang*. Most patients responded within 1-2 weeks, while some needed up to 1 month of herbal therapy. The average length of treatment was 15.8 days.[9]

RELATED FORMULA

Jiā Jiǎn Fù Mài Tāng
(Modified Restore the Pulse Decoction)

加減復脈湯
加减复脉汤

Pinyin Name: Jia Jian Fu Mai Tang
Literal Name: Modified Restore the Pulse Decoction
Original Source: *Wen Bing Tiao Bian* (Systematic Differentiation of Warm Disease) by Wu Ju-Tong in 1798

Zhi Gan Cao (Radix et Rhizoma Glycyrrhizae Praeparata cum Melle)	18g
Di Huang (Radix Rehmanniae)	18g
Bai Shao (Radix Paeoniae Alba)	18g
Mai Dong (Radix Ophiopogonis)	15g
E Jiao (Colla Corii Asini)	9g
Huo Ma Ren (Fructus Cannabis)	9g

Cook the ingredients in 8 bowls of water until the liquid is reduced to 80%. Take the warm, strained decoction on an empty stomach in three equally-divided doses in the morning, afternoon, and at night. *E Jiao* (Colla Corii Asini) is prepared according to the same instructions specified in *Zhi Gan Cao Tang* (Honey-Fried Licorice Decoction).

Jia Jian Fu Mai Tang (Modified Restore the Pulse Decoction) nourishes the blood, astringes yin, generates body fluids, and moistens dryness. Clinically, this formula is often used for patients who have *yangming fu* (hollow organs) excess syndrome, in which the excess heat has been cleared, but the interior deficiency still persists. Patients may show a deficient, big pulse with warm palms and soles, which indicate yin deficiency and possibly some deficiency heat. Successful treatment in this case requires tonifying interior deficiencies without generating heat. Using *Zhi Gan Cao Tang* as a base formula, this formula adds *Bai Shao* (Radix Paeoniae Alba) to enhance the overall functions of tonifying blood, yin, and body fluids. On the other hand, *Ren Shen* (Radix et Rhizoma Ginseng), *Da Zao* (Fructus Jujubae), *Sheng Jiang* (Rhizoma Zingiberis Recens), and *Gui Zhi* (Ramulus Cinnamomi) are removed to prevent possible heat formation or other side effects.

AUTHORS' COMMENTS

Zhi Gan Cao Tang has excellent function to tonify qi, replenish blood, nourish yin and warm yang. Historically, it is considered to be the most effective formula to treat irregular heart beat characterized as a bound pulse (结脉 *jie mai*, also translated as a knotted pulse, is a slow pulse with pulses at irregular intervals) and intermittent pulse (代脉 *dai mai*, is a pulse interspersed with more relatively regular pauses). Because of its ability to restore normal rhythmic pulse, *Zhi Gan Cao Tang* is also known as *Fu Mai Tang* (Restore the Pulse Decoction).

Zhi Gan Cao Tang and *Sheng Mai San* (Generate the Pulse Powder) both treat "pulse" disorders, but have the following similarities and differences:

- *Zhi Gan Cao Tang* treats a bound and intermittent, or a deficient and rapid pulse caused by qi and blood deficiencies and their subsequent inability to nourish Heart *shen* (spirit). Additional signs and symptoms include palpitations, shortness of breath, and a pale tongue with a scanty tongue coating. *Zhi Gan Cao Tang* nourishes Heart blood and tonifies Heart yang to "restore pulse."

- *Sheng Mai San* treats a deficient, fine pulse caused by heat injuring qi and yin. Additional symptoms include profuse sweating, fatigue, shortness of breath, a dry throat, and thirst. *Sheng Mai San* tonifies qi, promotes the production of body fluids, and astringes yin to "generate pulse."[10]

8 TONIC FORMULAS

591

Chapter 8 – Tonic Formulas　　　　　　　　　　　　　　*Section 2 – Blood-Tonifying Formulas*

Zhì Gān Cǎo Tāng (Honey-Fried Licorice Decoction)

Zhi Gan Cao Tang and *Tian Wang Bu Xin Dan* (Emperor of Heaven's Special Pill to Tonify the Heart) both nourish yin and blood to treat palpitations, anxiety, insomnia, and dry stools.

• *Zhi Gan Cao Tang* involves qi and blood deficiencies. Insufficiency of blood fails to nourish the Heart. When qi is deficient, the yang is weak and cannot generate the pulse, which leads to a bound or intermittent pulse. Thus, qi tonics must be used in conjunction with yin and blood tonics to generate the pulse. *Shu Di Huang* (Radix Rehmanniae Praeparata), *Sheng Jiang* (Rhizoma Zingiberis Recens), *E Jiao* (Colla Corii Asini), *Mai Dong* (Radix Ophiopogonis), and *Da Zao* (Fructus Jujubae) nourish yin and blood. *Ren Shen* (Radix et Rhizoma Ginseng) and *Zhi Gan Cao* (Radix et Rhizoma Glycyrrhizae Praeparata cum Melle) warm and tonify qi. *Gui Zhi* (Ramulus Cinnamomi) and *Sheng Jiang* (Rhizoma Zingiberis Recens) assist Heart yang to restore the pulse.

• *Tian Wang Bu Xin Dan* is suitable for Heart yin and blood deficiencies, with excess Heart yang flaring. Anxiety, decreased sleep, palpitations, a withered *shen* (spirit),

nocturnal emissions, and nervousness are the results of the *shen* not being nourished. Thus, nourishing herbs and *shen*-calming herbs are used together.[11]

References
1. *Zhong Yao Ming Fang Yao Li Yu Ying Yong* (Pharmacology and Applications of Famous Herbal Formulas) 1989;299-300.
2. *Zhong Yao Yao Li Yu Lin Chuang* (Pharmacology and Clinical Applications of Chinese Herbs) 1994;6:1.
3. *Zhong Yao Yao Li Yu Lin Chuang* (Pharmacology and Clinical Applications of Chinese Herbs) 1994;4:5.
4. *Zhong Yi Fang Ji Xian Dai Yan Jiu* (Modern Study of Medical Formulae in Traditional Chinese Medicine) 1997;622.
5. *Shan Xi Yi Kan* (Shanxi Journal of Medicine) 1995;15(9):399.
6. *Tian Jin Yi Yao* (Tianjin Medicine and Herbology) 1972;26.
7. *Jiang Su Zhong Yi Za Zhi* (Jiangsu Journal of Chinese Medicine) 1984;5(1):25.
8. *Shang Hai Zhong Yi Yao Za Zhi* (Shanghai Journal of Chinese Medicine and Herbology) 1989;5:36.
9. *Si Chuan Zhong Yi* (Sichuan Chinese Medicine) 1995;9:20.
10. Wang MZ, et al. *Zhong Yi Xue Wen Da Ti Ku* (Questions and Answers on Traditional Chinese Medicine: Herbal Formulas).
11. Wang MZ, et al. *Zhong Yi Xue Wen Da Ti Ku* (Questions and Answers on Traditional Chinese Medicine: Herbal Formulas).

Nǔ Kē Bǎi Zǐ Rén Wán (Platycladus Seed Pill for Females)
女科柏子仁丸

Pinyin Name: *Nu Ke Bai Zi Ren Wan*
Literal Name: Platycladus Seed Pill for Females
Alternate Names: *Bai Zi Ren Wan* (Platycladus Seed Pill), Biota and Cyathula Formula
Original Source: *Fu Ren Liang Fang* (Fine Formulas for Women) by Chen Zi-Ming in 1237

COMPOSITION

Bai Zi Ren (Semen Platycladi), *cuo* (grated)	15g
Shu Di Huang (Radix Rehmanniae Praeparata)	90g
Xu Duan (Radix Dipsaci)	60g
Niu Xi (Radix Achyranthis Bidentatae)	15g
Juan Bai (Herba Selaginellae)	15g
Ze Lan (Herba Lycopi)	60g

DOSAGE / PREPARATION / ADMINISTRATION

Grind the ingredients into a fine powder and mix with honey to form pills. The pills should resemble the size of

Wu Tong Zi (Semen Firmianae), a small seed approximately 5 mm in diameter. Take 30 pills with rice water on an empty stomach.

592

Chinese Herbal Formulas and Applications

Nŭ Kē Băi Zĭ Rén Wán (Platycladus Seed Pill for Females)

CHINESE THERAPEUTIC ACTIONS

Tonifies the blood and nourishes yin

CLINICAL MANIFESTATIONS

Irregular menstruation and amenorrhea due to blood and yin deficiencies: anxiety, soreness and pain of the abdomen and lower back, dizziness and light-headedness, and tidal fever.

CLINICAL APPLICATIONS

Irregular menstruation, amenorrhea, and menstrual disorders.

EXPLANATION

Nu Ke Bai Zi Ren Wan (Platycladus Seed Pill for Females) is often prescribed in the treatment of irregular menstruation and amenorrhea due to blood and yin deficiencies. If untreated, chronic blood and yin deficiencies can lead to the complication of deficiency heat rising upward. Clinically, the symptoms and signs of underlying deficiency include soreness and pain of the abdomen and lower back, dizziness and light-headedness; and those of deficiency heat include anxiety and tidal fever.

The aim of this formula is to tonify the blood, nourish yin, and restore normal menstruation. *Bai Zi Ren* (Semen

Platycladi) nourishes the Heart and calms the *shen* (spirit) to relieve irritability and anxiety secondary to deficiency heat. *Shu Di Huang* (Radix Rehmanniae Praeparata), *Xu Duan* (Radix Dipsaci), and *Niu Xi* (Radix Achyranthis Bidentatae) tonify the Liver and Kidney and benefit the *chong* (thoroughfare) and *ren* (conception) channels. Together, they treat the underlying deficiencies of the body. *Juan Bai* (Herba Selaginellae) and *Ze Lan* (Herba Lycopi) restore normal menstruation by activating blood circulation and opening the channels and collaterals.

MODIFICATIONS

- With headache due to blood deficiency, add *Dang Gui* (Radix Angelicae Sinensis) and *Chuan Xiong* (Rhizoma Chuanxiong).
- If there is low back pain due to qi deficiency, add *Ren Shen* (Radix et Rhizoma Ginseng) and *Huang Qi* (Radix Astragali).
- With abdominal pain due to blood stagnation, add *Tao Ren* (Semen Persicae) and *Hong Hua* (Flos Carthami).
- For amenorrhea due to blood deficiency, add *Si Wu Tang* (Four-Substance Decoction).
- For amenorrhea due to blood stagnation, add *Tao Ren Cheng Qi Tang* (Peach Pit Decoction to Order the Qi).
- For amenorrhea due to overexertion, add *Xiao Chai Hu Tang* (Minor Bupleurum Decoction).

Nu Ke Bai Zi Ren Wan (Platycladus Seed Pill for Females)

Diagnosis	Signs and Symptoms	Treatment	Herbs
Irregular menstruation and amenorrhea due to blood and yin deficiencies	• Soreness and pain of the abdomen and lower back, dizziness and light-headedness: blood and yin deficiencies • Anxiety and tidal fever: deficiency heat	Tonifies the blood and nourishes yin	• *Bai Zi Ren* (Semen Platycladi) nourishes the Heart and calms the *shen* (spirit) to relieve irritability and anxiety. • *Shu Di Huang* (Radix Rehmanniae Praeparata), *Xu Duan* (Radix Dipsaci), and *Niu Xi* (Radix Achyranthis Bidentatae) tonify the Liver and Kidney and benefit the *chong* (thoroughfare) and *ren* (conception) channels. • *Juan Bai* (Herba Selaginellae) and *Ze Lan* (Herba Lycopi) restore normal menstruation by activating blood circulation and opening the channels and collaterals.

TONIC FORMULAS

8

593

Chapter 8 – Tonic Formulas

Section 2 – Blood-Tonifying Formulas

Dāng Guī Sháo Yào Sǎn (Tangkuei and Peony Powder)

當歸芍藥散
当归芍药散

Pinyin Name: *Dang Gui Shao Yao San*
Literal Name: Tangkuei and Peony Powder
Alternate Names: *Tang Kuei Shao Yao San*, Tang-kuei and Peony Formula, Tangkuei and Peony Formula
Original Source: *Jin Gui Yao Lue* (Essentials from the Golden Cabinet) by Zhang Zhong-Jing in the Eastern Han Dynasty

COMPOSITION

Dang Gui (Radix Angelicae Sinensis)	9g
Chuan Xiong (Rhizoma Chuanxiong)	24g [9g]
Bai Shao (Radix Paeoniae Alba)	48g
Bai Zhu (Rhizoma Atractylodis Macrocephalae)	12g
Fu Ling (Poria)	12g
Ze Xie (Rhizoma Alismatis)	24g

DOSAGE / PREPARATION / ADMINISTRATION

The source text states to grind the ingredients into a fine powder. Take 6g of powder per dose with a grain-based liquor three times daily. Today, this formula can also be given in decoction twice daily, with the dose of *Chuan Xiong* (Rhizoma Chuanxiong) suggested in brackets. Note: The source text states to use 24g of *Chuan Xiong* (Rhizoma Chuanxiong). Today, most practitioners and commercial products use only 9g.

CHINESE THERAPEUTIC ACTIONS

1. Nourishes the blood to soften the Liver
2. Strengthens the Spleen and resolves dampness

CLINICAL MANIFESTATIONS

Abdominal pain with edema during pregnancy due to blood deficiency and abnormal water circulation: continuous cramping pain in the abdomen, anemia, a pale face, palpitations, dizziness, vertigo, tinnitus, fatigue, lack of energy, sore back, extreme coldness of the hands and feet, and edema.

CLINICAL APPLICATIONS

Dysmenorrhea, menstrual irregularity, uterine bleeding, abdominal pain and cramps, leukorrhea, hypochromic anemia, luteal insufficiency, infertility, habitual miscarriage, unstable pregnancy, breech presentation, gestational hypertension, abdominal pain during pregnancy, adnexitis, pelvic inflammatory disease, menopause, anemia, dizziness, vertigo, palpitations, chloasma, acne, chronic nephritis, beriberi, and angina.

EXPLANATION

Dang Gui Shao Yao San (Tangkuei and Peony Powder) treats abdominal pain and edema during pregnancy characterized by blood deficiency and abnormal water circulation. Abdominal pain is generally considered to be the main indication for this formula. Due to the deficient nature of the illness, the abdominal pain is characterized as dull, cramping, and continuous but not severe. It is generally accompanied by a feeling of coldness in the body, hands, and feet. Since there is blood deficiency, patients could present with anemia, palpitations, dizziness, and vertigo. With abnormal water circulation, patients may experience edema and a heavy sensation. Edema, which occurs most frequently in the lower extremities, is a sign of water accumulation; and the heavy sensation, which is most prominent in the head, is a sign of damp accumulation.

Dang Gui (Radix Angelicae Sinensis) tonifies the blood and activates blood circulation. It regulates menstruation, treats anemia, and relieves abdominal pain. *Chuan Xiong* (Rhizoma Chuanxiong) activates and regulates blood circulation. *Bai Shao* (Radix Paeoniae Alba) nourishes the blood and consolidates yin. In addition, *Bai Shao* (Radix Paeoniae Alba) has an excellent effect to relieve spasms and cramps of both the skeletal and smooth muscles. It is commonly used in large quantities to relieve abdominal pain and cramps. *Bai Zhu* (Rhizoma Atractylodis Macrocephalae) and *Fu Ling* (Poria) strengthen the Spleen and resolve dampness. *Fu Ling* (Poria) and *Ze Xie* (Rhizoma Alismatis) have a diuretic action to relieve edema.

MODIFICATIONS

• For unstable pregnancy, add *Sha Ren* (Fructus Amomi), *Du Zhong* (Cortex Eucommiae), *Xu Duan* (Radix Dipsaci), *Ai Ye* (Folium Artemisiae Argyi), and *Huang Qin* (Radix Scutellariae).

Dāng Guī Sháo Yào Sǎn (Tangkuei and Peony Powder)

Dang Gui Shao Yao San (Tangkuei and Peony Powder)

Diagnosis	Signs and Symptoms	Treatment	Herbs
Abdominal pain with edema due to blood deficiency and abnormal water metabolism	• Anemia, palpitations, dizziness, vertigo and feeling of coldness in the body, hands, and feet: blood deficiency • Edema and a heavy sensation: abnormal water metabolism with damp accumulation	• Nourishes the blood to soften the Liver • Strengthens the Spleen to regulate water metabolism	• *Dang Gui* (Radix Angelicae Sinensis) tonifies the blood and activates blood circulation. • *Chuan Xiong* (Rhizoma Chuanxiong) activates and regulates blood circulation. • *Bai Shao* (Radix Paeoniae Alba) nourishes the blood and consolidates yin. • *Bai Zhu* (Rhizoma Atractylodis Macrocephalae) and *Fu Ling* (Poria) strengthen the Spleen and resolve dampness. • *Fu Ling* (Poria) and *Ze Xie* (Rhizoma Alismatis) relieve edema.

- For amenorrhea with severe edema due to dampness, combine with *Wu Ling San* (Five-Ingredient Powder with Poria).
- If there is severe abdominal pain, add *Xiang Fu* (Rhizoma Cyperi) and *Ai Ye* (Folium Artemisiae Argyi).
- With dizziness and headache, add *Bai Zhi* (Radix Angelicae Dahuricae), *Huang Qi* (Radix Astragali), and *Qiang Huo* (Rhizoma et Radix Notopterygii).
- With irritability and thirst, add *Huang Lian* (Rhizoma Coptidis) and *Huang Qin* (Radix Scutellariae).
- If there are more signs and symptoms of cold, add *Wu Zhu Yu* (Fructus Evodiae) and *Gui Zhi* (Ramulus Cinnamomi).

PHARMACOLOGICAL EFFECTS

1. **Endocrine**: Administration of *Dang Gui Shao Yao San* has a stimulating effect on the production and secretion of hormones.[1] One *in vitro* study reported that *Dang Gui Shao Yao San* stimulated preovulatory follicles before a luteinizing hormone (LH) surge to secrete progesterone, but it suppressed estradiol-17 beta secretion by growing preovulatory follicles before a LH surge.[2]

2. **Ovulatory**: Administration of *Dang Gui Shao Yao San* has marked effects on the endocrine system and the ovaries. In one experiment, the use of *Dang Gui Shao Yao San* at 0.5 g/kg successfully induced ovulation in 30% of the mice. In contrast, the use of gonadotropin-releasing hormone was associated with a 65% success rate in promoting ovulation. Lastly, the combination of herbs and drugs were 90% effective in inducing ovulation. The study suggested that the formula has either a direct or an indirect stimulating effect on the endocrine system.[3] Another study stated that *Dang Gui Shao Yao San* may treat ovulatory disorders by stimulating both steroidogenesis and the ovulatory process.[4]

3. **Effect on uterus**: Administration of *Dang Gui Shao Yao San* was associated with an increased uterine weight in rats. This effect is voided if the ovaries were surgically removed.[5] Other studies suggested that this formula is beneficial in fertility by promoting implantation and early growth.[6]

4. **Hemodynamic**: Administration of *Dang Gui Shao Yao San* was associated with a dual effect on the hemodynamics of the blood. In one study, continuous administration of the formula at 0.5 g/kg for 17 days was associated with decreased viscosity of the blood in pregnant rats. In another study, it was noted that the formula was effective at stopping bleeding in mice and reduces the amount of blood loss during an injury.[7]

5. **Immunostimulant**: Administration of *Dang Gui Shao Yao San* was associated with a significant increase in lymphocyte proliferation in aged rats. It also showed an antagonizing effect against the inhibition of isoprel on lymphocyte proliferation.[8]

6. **Radioprotective**: One study evaluated the protective effect of *Dang Gui Shao Yao San* in mice treated with single X-irradiation. The study found that this formula had a dose-dependent effect that protected mice and prevented hematopoietic injury from sublethal effects of radiation. *Dang Gui Shao Yao San* was given at doses of 10 and 20 mg/20g body weight, for 7 consecutive days before irradiation. Pretreatment of *Dang Gui Shao Yao San* increased the number of femoral spleen colony-forming units (CFU-S) that survived irradiation, and significantly ameliorated leukopenia, thrombocytopenia and the degression of hematocrits after irradiation.[9]

7. **Antioxidant**: In one study in rats, administration of *Dang Gui Shao Yao San* was associated with free radical scavenging activity, which contributed to its prophylactic effect against free radical-mediated neurological diseases associated with aging.[10]

Chapter 8 – Tonic Formulas   *Section 2 – Blood-Tonifying Formulas*

Dāng Guī Sháo Yào Săn (Tangkuei and Peony Powder)

CLINICAL STUDIES AND RESEARCH

1. **Abdominal pain during pregnancy**: One study reported 96.5% effectiveness using *Dang Gui Shao Yao San* to treat 86 pregnant women with abdominal pain. The duration of treatment ranged from 3-14 days.[11]

2. **Gestational hypertension**: Administration of *Dang Gui Shao Yao San* was effective in controlling gestational hypertension in 46 women. The herbal formula did not affect the normal development of the fetus, and did not contribute to excess bleeding during labor (loss of blood did not exceed 400 mL in all cases). In addition, the hypertension did not become permanent in any of the 46 women.[12] In another study, administration of modified *Dang Gui Shao Yao San* in 52 women with moderate severity of gestational hypertension showed excellent effects. Improvements included increased volume of urination, reduction of edema, and lowered blood pressure. Furthermore, there were no complications with labor or bleeding during delivery. There were no adverse reactions in any of the women or their babies.[13]

3. **Breech presentation**: In one study, 217 pregnant women with breech presentation were treated with *Dang Gui Shao Yao San* with excellent results. Breech presentation was corrected within 3-6 doses in all 87 women (100%) with first pregnancy, and 128 out of 130 women (98.5%) with previous pregnancy. The herbal formula contained *Dang Gui Shao Yao San* plus *Xu Duan* (Radix Dipsaci), *Sang Ji Sheng* (Herba Taxilli), and others.[14] According to another study, use of *Dang Gui Shao Yao San* was associated with successful correction of breech presentation in 217 of 239 patients (90.8% rate of success).[15]

4. **Infertility**: Twenty women with infertility were treated with *Dang Gui Shao Yao San* with a 100% success rate. All 20 women became pregnant and had normal pregnancy and delivery. According to other references, the success rate of the formula is approximately 55%.[16]

5. **Uterine bleeding**: Modified *Dang Gui Shao Yao San* showed 91.3% effectiveness in treating 437 patients with uterine bleeding due to various causes. Modifications included addition of *Di Yu* (Radix Sanguisorbae), *Hai Piao Xiao* (Endoconcha Sepiae), and dry-fried *Pu Huang* (Pollen Typhae) for profuse bleeding; *Dang Shen* (Radix Codonopsis) and *Huang Qi* (Radix Astragali) for qi deficiency; and *Qian Cao* (Radix et Rhizoma Rubiae) and *Wu Ling Zhi* (Faeces Trogopteri) for severe abdominal pain. The study reported relief for most patients within 1-3 packs of herbs.[17] According to another study, 99 patients with uterine bleeding due to various causes were treated with *Dang Gui Shao Yao San* with an overall effectiveness rate of 91%.[18]

6. **Habitual miscarriage**: Two studies reported that use of *Dang Gui Shao Yao San* and *Chai Ling Tang* (Bupleurum and Poria Decoction) helped to prevent autoimmunity-related recurrent miscarriage by correcting T helper-1/T helper-2 balance.[19,20]

7. **Luteal insufficiency**: Administration of *Dang Gui Shao Yao San* in women with luteal insufficiency was found to be effective in improving luteal insufficiency as determined by daily measurement of basal body temperature and plasma progesterone levels. In women with normal menstrual cycles, use of the formula did not cause any adverse effects on hormonal levels such as prolactin, gonadotropins, steroids, estrogens, pregnanediol and luteinizing hormone (LH). No side effects were reported. The researchers concluded that *Dang Gui Shao Yao San* improves luteal insufficiency in women but does not affect the hormonal levels of women with normal menstrual cycles.[21]

8. **Dysmenorrhea**: One double-blind study evaluated the therapeutic effect of *Dang Gui Shao Yao San* versus placebo for treatment of primary dysmenorrhea characterized by "a combination of 'deficiency of yin,' 'cold,' and 'stagnant blood' syndromes." The patients were treated with herbs or placebo during 2 menstrual cycles and were followed for 2 additional cycles. At the end of the study, it was noted that women who received *Dang Gui Shao Yao San* had a significant alleviation of dysmenorrhea in comparison to those treated with placebo.[22]

9. **Dysmenorrhea**: Seventeen patients with dysmenorrhea (including recurrent endometriotic and adenomyotic patients) obtained complete relief within three months when treated with the following cyclic therapy. The treatment protocol was to alternate giving *Dang Gui Shao Yao San* and *Shao Yao Gan Cao Tang* (Peony and Licorice Decoction) within the menstrual cycle. Clinical improvements included relief of pain, biphasic changes in basal body temperature patterns, improved level of estradiol, and successful pregnancy and delivery in one case. The study concluded that this cyclic therapy of two herbal formulas can be a conservative antidysmenorrhea therapy for endometriotic and adenomyotic patients who desire pregnancy.[23]

10. **Menopause**: Administration of *Dang Gui Shao Yao San* has been shown to have marked effects in alleviating menopausal symptoms. In one study involving 24 women, the formula was extremely effective in 2 cases, moderately effective in 16 cases, and not effective in 6 cases. The formula contained *Fu Ling* (Poria), *Cang Zhu* (Rhizoma Atractylodis), *Bai Shao* (Radix Paeoniae Alba), *Ze Xie* (Rhizoma Alismatis), *Dang Gui* (Radix Angelicae Sinensis), and *Chuan Xiong* (Rhizoma Chuanxiong). The herbs were given in extract form, 2.5g twice daily before meals for 2 months.[24] In another study involving 13 women with menopause induced by hysterectomy, the

596

Dāng Guī Sháo Yào Sǎn (Tangkuei and Peony Powder)

Chinese Herbal Formulas and Applications

formula was extremely effective in 4 women, moderately effective in 5 women, and had no effect in 4 women.[25]

11. **Hypochromic anemia in uterine myoma**: One study compared the therapeutic benefits of *Dang Gui Shao Yao San* and an oral iron preparation in the treatment of hypochromic anemia in cases of uterine myoma. Out of 25 patients, 10 were treated with herbs and 15 with iron, for a total of 8 weeks. The study reported that the iron group had improvement in blood counts and the laboratory parameters of anemia, while the herb group had improvement in the signs and symptoms of anemia, such as facial pallor, spoon-shaped nails and dizziness. Side effects were observed in 80% of the oral iron group, but no significant side effects were observed in the herb group. The study concluded that *Dang Gui Shao Yao San* may be useful in resolving the symptoms of mild or moderate anemia associated with uterine myoma.[26]

12. **Adnexitis**: Administration of modified *Dang Gui Shao Yao San* in 49 patients with adnexitis was associated with complete recovery in 34 patients, improvement in 11 patients, and no effect in 4 patients. The rate of effectiveness was 91.8%. The herbal treatment contained *Dang Gui* (Radix Angelicae Sinensis), *Bai Shao* (Radix Paeoniae Alba), *Fu Ling* (Poria), *Bai Zhu* (Rhizoma Atractylodis Macrocephalae), and *Ze Xie* (Rhizoma Alismatis) in the following ratios (1:5.6:2.7:1.3:1.3:2.7). The treatment protocol was to administer 5 capsules (0.4g of herb powder per capsule) three times daily for 15 days per course of treatment.[27]

13. **Pelvic inflammatory disease**: Use of modified *Dang Gui Shao Yao San* in 160 patients with chronic pelvic inflammatory disease was associated with complete recovery in 99 patients, significant improvement in 42 patients, moderate improvement in 15 patients, and no effect in 4 patients. The effectiveness was 97.50%. The herbal treatment contained *Dang Gui Shao Yao San* plus *Bai Hua She She Cao* (Herba Hedyotis), *Da Xue Teng* (Caulis Sargentodoxae), and *Yi Yi Ren* (Semen Coicis) as the base formula. *Di Huang* (Radix Rehmanniae) and *Mu Dan Pi* (Cortex Moutan) were added for the presence of damp-heat; *Tao Ren* (Semen Persicae) and *Dan Shen* (Radix et Rhizoma Salviae Miltiorrhizae) for qi and blood stagnation; and *Xiao Hui Xiang* (Fructus Foeniculi) and *Rou Gui* (Cortex Cinnamomi) for cold stagnation in the womb.[28]

14. **Chloasma**: Use of modified *Dang Gui Shao Yao San* was associated with 91.1% effectiveness in treating 235 patients with irregular brownish or blackish spots, especially on the face. The herbal treatment contained *Dang Gui Shao Yao San* plus *Yi Yi Ren* (Semen Coicis) and *Bai Zhi* (Radix Angelicae Dahuricae) as the base formula, with addition of *Chai Hu* (Radix Bupleuri) and *Xiang Fu* (Rhizoma Cyperi) for Liver qi stagnation; *Tao Ren* (Semen Persicae), *Hong Hua* (Flos Carthami), and *Ze Lan* (Herba Lycopi) for blood stagnation; *Mu Dan Pi* (Cortex Moutan) and dry-fried *Zhi Zi* (Fructus Gardeniae) for heat in the blood; processed *Huang Qi* (Radix Astragali) and *Dang Shen* (Radix Codonopsis) for qi deficiency; *E Jiao* (Colla Corii Asini) and *Ji Xue Teng* (Caulis Spatholobi) for blood deficiency; *Cang Zhu* (Rhizoma Atractylodis), *Zhu Ling* (Polyporus), and *Ze Xie* (Rhizoma Alismatis) for accumulation of dampness; *Fu Zi* (Radix Aconiti Lateralis Praeparata) and *Rou Gui* (Cortex Cinnamomi) for Kidney yang deficiency; and *Di Huang* (Radix Rehmanniae) and *Shi Hu* (Caulis Dendrobii) for Kidney yin deficiency. An herbal preparation was also applied topically to the affected area. Composition of the topical preparation was unavailable at the time of publication. Of 235 patients, the study reported complete recovery in 58 patients, significant improvement in 69 patients, moderate improvement in 87 patients, and no change in 21 patients.[29]

15. **Acne**: One study reported that *Dang Gui Shao Yao San* effectively suppressed acne rashes as well as incidental symptoms. In contrast, suppression of incidental symptoms could not be achieved with antimicrobial drugs, suggesting that the herbs may have other mechanisms of action.[30]

16. **Angina**: Ninety-six patients with angina due to decreased blood perfusion were treated with modified *Dang Gui Shao Yao San* with significant improvement in 27 patients, moderate improvement in 52 patients, mild improvement in 11 patients, and no effect in 6 patients. The treatment protocol was to administer the herbs in decoction twice daily, in the morning and at night. The base formula contained *Dang Gui* (Radix Angelicae Sinensis) 10-12g, *Chi Shao* (Radix Paeoniae Rubra) 10-12g, *Fu Ling* (Poria) 10-12g, *Bai Zhu* (Rhizoma Atractylodis Macrocephalae) 10-12g, *Ze Xie* (Rhizoma Alismatis) 10-12g, *Chuan Xiong* (Rhizoma Chuanxiong) 10-12g, *Tai Zi Shen* (Radix Pseudostellariae) 20-40g, *Dan Shen* (Radix et Rhizoma Salviae Miltiorrhizae) 10-30g, and *Shui Zhi* (Hirudo) 10-30g. Herbs were added based on the condition of the individual patient. *Ren Shen* (Radix et Rhizoma Ginseng) 10g was added for qi deficiency. *Bai Jie Zi* (Semen Sinapis) 10g, *Dan Nan Xing* (Arisaema cum Bile) 10g, and *Gua Lou* (Fructus Trichosanthis) 30g were added for phlegm stagnation. *Chuan Xiong* (Rhizoma Chuanxiong) 30-60g and *Shui Zhi* (Hirudo) 30-60g were added for severe blood stagnation.[31]

17. **Dizziness and vertigo**: Twenty patients with dizziness and vertigo were treated with *Dang Gui Shao Yao San* with complete recovery in 12 patients and moderate improvement in 8 patients.[32] It has been suggested that this formula has a marked regulating effect on blood pressure, and

8

TONIC FORMULAS

Chapter 8 – Tonic Formulas   Section 2 – Blood-Tonifying Formulas

Dāng Guī Sháo Yào Sǎn (Tangkuei and Peony Powder)

therefore could benefit patients with hypertension or hypotension characterized by deficiency.[33]

HERB-DRUG INTERACTION

- **Colchicine-induced learning impairment**: Concurrent administration of *Dang Gui Shao Yao San* and colchicine was associated with improvement in learning acquisition deficit induced by colchicine in rats. The action mechanism of *Dang Gui Shao Yao San* may be involved in the increase in the level of superoxide dismutase.[34]

- **Drug-induced menopause**: One study evaluated the therapeutic effects of certain herbal medicines on menopausal symptoms induced by gonadotropin-releasing hormone agonist therapy in Japanese women with endometriosis, adenomyosis, or leiomyoma. According to this study, menopausal symptoms induced by gonadotropin-releasing hormone agonist therapy in 13 patients were successfully treated with *Dang Gui Shao Yao San*, *Shao Yao Gan Cao Tang* (Peony and Licorice Decoction), *Gui Zhi Fu Ling Wan* (Cinnamon Twig and Poria Pill), *Jia Wei Xiao Yao San* (Augmented Rambling Powder), *Tao He Cheng Qi Tang* (Peach Pit Decoction to Order the Qi), or *Gui Zhi Tang* (Cinnamon Twig Decoction). Of 11 patients with hot flashes, *Dang Gui Shao Yao San* provided some relief in all 11 patients, and total relief in 4 patients. Most importantly, there were no significant changes in serum estradiol levels after treatment with these herbal medicines. The researchers concluded that these herbal medicines can be recommended for menopausal symptoms induced by gonadotropin-releasing hormone agonists without a negative effect on serum estradiol levels.[35]

TOXICOLOGY

This formula has little toxicity. No fatality was reported following oral ingestion of the formula at 8-10 g/kg in mice. Moreover, no abnormalities were observed in the fetus following oral administration of the formula at 8 g/kg/day for 7-17 days in pregnant rats.[36]

RELATED FORMULA

Rén Shēn Dāng Sháo Sǎn

(Ginseng, Tangkuei, and Peony Powder)

人參當芍散
人参当芍散

Pinyin Name: *Ren Shen Dang Shao San*
Literal Name: Ginseng, Tangkuei, and Peony Powder
Alternate Name: Ginseng and Tangkuei Formula
Original Source: *Yan Fang* (Time-Tested Formulas) of unknown author and date

Dang Gui (Radix Angelicae Sinensis)	9g
Bai Shao (Radix Paeoniae Alba)	48g

Fu Ling (Poria)	12g
Bai Zhu (Rhizoma Atractylodis Macrocephalae)	12g
Ze Xie (Rhizoma Alismatis)	24g
Chuan Xiong (Rhizoma Chuanxiong)	9g
Ren Shen (Radix et Rhizoma Ginseng)	90g
Rou Gui (Cortex Cinnamomi)	30g
Gan Cao (Radix et Rhizoma Glycyrrhizae)	30g

Ren Shen Dang Shao San (Ginseng, Tangkuei, and Peony Powder) is a modification of *Dang Gui Shao Yao San* with the addition of *Ren Shen* (Radix et Rhizoma Ginseng), *Gan Cao* (Radix et Rhizoma Glycyrrhizae), and *Rou Gui* (Cortex Cinnamomi). This formula tonifies qi and blood, strengthens the Spleen, and warms yang. Clinically, this formula is used to treat various disorders characterized by qi, blood and yang deficiencies, such as irregular menstruation, dysmenorrhea, infertility, unstable pregnancy, and postpartum care.

AUTHORS' COMMENTS

Dang Gui Shao Yao San was originally designed to treat abdominal pain with edema during pregnancy. Today, its clinical applications have been greatly expanded to include various menstrual, gestational and postpartum disorders characterized by blood deficiency and abnormal water circulation.

References

1. *Chang Yong Zhong Yao Cheng Fen Yu Yao Li Shou Ce* (A Handbook of the Composition and Pharmacology of Common Chinese Drugs) 1997;1:238.
2. Usuki S. Effects of hachimijiogan, tokishakuyakusan, keishibuku-ryogan, ninjinto and unkeito on estrogen and progesterone secretion in preovulatory follicles incubated in vitro. Am J Chin Med 1991;19(1):65-71.
3. *Guo Wai Yi Xue* (Foreign Medicine) 1988;10(4):44.
4. Irahara M, Yasui T, Tezuka M, Ushigoe K, Yamano S, Kamada M, Aono T. Evidence that Toki-shakuyaku-san and its ingredients enhance the secretion of a cytokine-induced neutrophil chemoattractant (CINC/gro) in the ovulatory process. Methods Find Exp Clin Pharmacol 2000 Dec; 22(10):725-30.
5. *Guo Wai Yi Xue* (Foreign Medicine) 1988;10(5):8.
6. *Zhong Yi Fang Ji Xian Dai Yan Jiu* (Modern Study of Medical Formulae in Traditional Chinese Medicine) 1997;(1):238.
7. *Zhong Yi Fang Ji Xian Dai Yan Jiu* (Modern Study of Medical Formulae in Traditional Chinese Medicine) 1997;(1):238.
8. He HW, Wang CE, Xie Y. Effect of supplemented danggui shaoyao powder and its disassembled prescriptions on lymphocytes proliferation in aged rats. Zhongguo Zhong Xi Yi Jie He Za Zhi 2003 Nov;23(11): 841-4.
9. Hsu HY, Lin CC. A preliminary study on the radioprotection of mouse hematopoiesis by dang-gui-shao-yao-san. J Ethnopharmacol 1996 Dec;55(1):43-8.
10. Ueda Y, Komatsu M, Hiramatsu M. Free radical scavenging activity of the Japanese herbal medicine toki-shakuyaku-san (TJ-23) and its effect on superoxide dismutase activity, lipid peroxides, glutamate,

Dāng Guī Sháo Yào Sǎn (Tangkuei and Peony Powder)

Chinese Herbal Formulas and Applications

and monoamine metabolites in aged rat brain. Neurochem Res 1996 Aug;21(8):909-14.

11. *Zhong Yuan Yi Kan* (Resource Journal of Chinese Medicine) 1992;5:36.

12. *Zhong Xi Yi Jie He Za Zhi* (Journal of Integrated Chinese and Western Medicine) 1986;6(12):714.

13. *Zhong Ji Yi Kan* (Medium Medical Journal) 1985;7:50.

14. *Fu Jian Zhong Yi Yao* (Fujian Chinese Medicine and Herbology) 1984;(4):18.

15. *Shan Xi Zhong Yi* (Shanxi Chinese Medicine) 1998;12:534.

16. *Zhong Cheng Yao Yan Jiu* (Research of Chinese Patent Medicine) 1984;(10):30.

17. *Hu Bei Zhong Yi Za Zhi* (Hubei Journal of Chinese Medicine) 1982;2:22.

18. *Zhong Cheng Yao Yan Jiu* (Research of Chinese Patent Medicine) 1983;(9):17.

19. Fujii T, Kanai T, Kozuma S, Hamai Y, Hyodo H, Yamashita T, Miki A, Unno N, Taketani Y. Theoretical basis for herbal medicines, Tokishakuyaku-san and Sairei-to, in the treatment of autoimmunity-related recurrent abortion by correcting T helper-1/T helper-2 balance. American Journal of Reproductive Immunology 2000 Dec;44(6):342-6.

20. Fujii T. Herbal factors in the treatment of autoimmunity-related habitual abortion. Vitam Horm 2002;65:333-44.

21. Usuki S, Higa TN, Soreya K. The improvement of luteal insufficiency in fecund women by tokishakuyakusan treatment. American Journal of Chinese Medicine 2002;30(2-3):327-38.

22. Kotani N, Oyama T, Sakai I, Hashimoto H, Muraoka M, Ogawa Y, Matsuki A. Analgesic effect of a herbal medicine for treatment of primary dysmenorrhea--a double-blind study. American Journal of Chinese Medicine 1997;25(2):205-12.

23. Tanaka T. A novel anti-dysmenorrhea therapy with cyclic administration of two Japanese herbal medicines. Clinical & Experimental Obstetrics & Gynecology 2003;30(2-3):95-8.

24. *Guo Wai Yi Xue* (Foreign Medicine) 1979;3:132.

25. *Chang Yong Zhong Yao Cheng Fen Yu Yao Li Shou Ce* (A Handbook of the Composition and Pharmacology of Common Chinese Drugs) 1997;1:242.

26. Akase T, Akase T, Onodera S, Jobo T, Matsushita R, Kaneko M, Tashiro S. A comparative study of the usefulness of toki-shakuyaku-san and an oral iron preparation in the treatment of hypochromic anemia in cases of uterine myoma. Yakugaku Zasshi - Journal of the Pharmaceutical Society of Japan 2003 Sep;123(9):817-24.

27. *Hu Bei Zhong Yi Za Zhi* (Hubei Journal of Chinese Medicine) 1988;4:25.

28. *Shan Dong Zhong Yi Xue Yuan Xue Bao* (Journal of Shandong University School of Chinese Medicine) 1996;2:118.

29. *Bei Jing Zhong Yi Xue Yuan Xue Bao* (Journal of Beijing University School of Medicine) 1987;5:36.

30. Higaki S, Toyomoto T, Morohashi M. Seijo-bofu-to, Jumi-haidoku-to and Toki-shakuyaku-san suppress rashes and incidental symptoms in acne patients. Drugs Exp Clin Res 2002;28(5):193-6.

31. *Zhe Jiang Zhong Yi Za Zhi* (Zhejiang Journal of Chinese Medicine) 1995;(12):542.

32. *Hu Bei Zhong Yi Za Zhi* (Hubei Journal of Chinese Medicine) 1982;(4):31.

33. *Nei Ke* (Internal Medicine) 1985;56(5):856.

34. Lu MC. Danggui shaoyao san improve colchichine-induced learning acquisition impairment in rats. Acta Pharmacol Sin 2001 Dec;22(12):1149-53.

35. Tanaka T. Effects of herbal medicines on menopausal symptoms induced by gonadotropin-releasing hormone agonist therapy. Clin Exp Obstet Gynecol 2001;28(1):20-3.

36. *Zhe Jiang Zhong Yi Za Zhi* (Zhejiang Journal of Chinese Medicine) 1987;22(8):345.

Sháo Yào Gān Cǎo Tāng (Peony and Licorice Decoction)
芍藥甘草湯
芍药甘草汤

Pinyin Name: *Shao Yao Gan Cao Tang*
Literal Name: Peony and Licorice Decoction
Alternate Names: *Shao Yao Kan Tsao Tang*, Peony and Licorice Combination
Original Source: *Shang Han Lun* (Discussion of Cold-Induced Disorders) by Zhang Zhong-Jing in the Eastern Han Dynasty

COMPOSITION

Bai Shao (Radix Paeoniae Alba)	12g
Zhi Gan Cao (Radix et Rhizoma Glycyrrhizae Praeparata cum Melle)	12g

DOSAGE / PREPARATION / ADMINISTRATION

Cook both herbs in 3 cups [600 mL] of water and reduce it to 1.5 cups [300 mL]. Take the warm, strained decoction in two equally-divided doses.

CHINESE THERAPEUTIC ACTIONS

1. Tonifies yin and blood
2. Replenishes body fluids

Chapter 8 – Tonic Formulas   *Section 2 – Blood-Tonifying Formulas*

Sháo Yào Gān Cǎo Tāng (Peony and Licorice Decoction)

CLINICAL MANIFESTATIONS

Spasms and cramps due to yin, blood and body fluid deficiencies: smooth or skeletal muscle spasms and cramps in various parts of the body, and tightness of the tendons and ligaments.

CLINICAL APPLICATIONS

Spasms, cramps, convulsions, stomach and intestinal cramps, trigeminal neuralgia, neuralgia, sciatica, frozen shoulder, systremma, restless leg syndrome, acute back pain, heel pain, chronic atrophic gastritis, peptic ulcer disease, gastric and abdominal pain, colitis, constipation, pain associated with cholelithiasis or urolithiasis, diabetes mellitus, hyperosteogeny, dysmenorrhea, perimenopause with uterine leiomyomas, and drug-induced menopause.

EXPLANATION

Shao Yao Gan Cao Tang (Peony and Licorice Decoction) can relieve various pains, spasms, or cramps due to deficiencies of yin, blood, and body fluids. This condition may arise as a result of excessive sweating, high fever, or excessive use of exterior-releasing herbs.

Bai Shao (Radix Paeoniae Alba) nourishes yin, tonifies the blood, and replenishes body fluids. *Zhi Gan Cao* (Radix et Rhizoma Glycyrrhizae Praeparata cum Melle) strengthens the Spleen and tonifies qi. Together, they relieve spasms and cramps due to deficiencies of yin, blood, and body fluids.

MODIFICATIONS

- For spasms and cramps of the extremities, add *Xi Xin* (Radix et Rhizoma Asari) and *Gan Jiang* (Rhizoma Zingiberis).
- If there is dysuria, add *Bai Zhu* (Rhizoma Atractylodis Macrocephalae) and *Fu Ling* (Poria).
- With back pain, add *Du Zhong* (Cortex Eucommiae), *Niu Xi* (Radix Achyranthis Bidentatae), and *Yan Hu Suo* (Rhizoma Corydalis).
- With neck and shoulder pain, add *Ge Gen* (Radix Puerariae Lobatae) or *Ge Gen Tang* (Kudzu Decoction).
- With severe pain, add *Yan Hu Suo* (Rhizoma Corydalis).

- For traumatic injuries involving bone fractures, add *Ru Xiang* (Gummi Olibanum) and *Mo Yao* (Myrrha), or *Zheng Gu Zi Jin Dan* (Purple and Gold Pill for Righteous Bones).
- For dysmenorrhea, add *Xiang Fu* (Rhizoma Cyperi) and *Shi Xiao San* (Sudden Smile Powder).
- For pain from kidney stones, add *Zhu Ling Tang* (Polyporus Decoction), *Hai Jin Sha* (Spora Lygodii), *Jin Qian Cao* (Herba Lysimachiae), and *Ji Nei Jin* (Endothelium Corneum Gigeriae Galli).

CAUTIONS / CONTRAINDICATIONS

- Use *Shao Yao Gan Cao Tang* with caution in patients with hypertension, since this formula contains a high dose of *Gan Cao* (Radix et Rhizoma Glycyrrhizae) and may cause water retention.
- Avoid cold or raw, pungent or spicy, and oily or greasy foods while taking this formula.[1]

PHARMACOLOGICAL EFFECTS

1. **Effect on the smooth muscles**: Administration of the formula had a marked inhibitory effect on the smooth muscles of the intestines in rabbits.[2]
2. **Effect on the skeletal muscles**: Administration of the formula had a marked effect to relax the skeletal muscles. Though the exact mechanism is not clear, part of the function is attributed to the lowered permeability of calcium and potassium across the cell membrane.[3]
3. **Analgesic**: In animal studies, *Shao Yao Gan Cao Tang* was very effective in relieving pain. In human studies, the formula was only slightly effective in relieving pain. The effectiveness increased significantly, however, when combined with acupuncture.[4]

CLINICAL STUDIES AND RESEARCH

1. **Trigeminal neuralgia**: In one study, 42 patients with trigeminal neuralgia were treated with modified *Shao Yao Gan Cao Tang* for 7-25 packs of herbs with relief of pain in all patients. In a follow up one year later, 30 patients experienced no recurrences, while 12 patients experienced a relapse of neuralgia six months after the conclusion of herbal treatment that was less frequent and less severe.

Shao Yao Gan Cao Tang (Peony and Licorice Decoction)

Diagnosis	Signs and Symptoms	Treatment	Herbs
Spasms and cramps	Spasms or cramps: deficiencies of yin, blood and body fluids	• Tonifies yin and blood • Replenishes body fluids	• *Bai Shao* (Radix Paeoniae Alba) nourishes yin, tonifies blood, and replenishes body fluids. • *Zhi Gan Cao* (Radix et Rhizoma Glycyrrhizae Praeparata cum Melle) strengthens the Spleen and tonifies qi.

600

Sháo Yào Gān Cǎo Tāng (Peony and Licorice Decoction)

The formula was modified by adding *Suan Zao Ren* (Semen Ziziphi Spinosae) and *Mu Gua* (Fructus Chaenomelis).[5]

2. **Neuralgia**: One study reported relief of neuralgia in all 59 patients when they were treated with *Shao Yao Gan Cao Tang* using *Bai Shao* (Radix Paeoniae Alba) 50g and *Gan Cao* (Radix et Rhizoma Glycyrrhizae) 30g. The duration of treatment ranged from 3-24 packs of herbs. In follow-up exams one year later, 42 of 59 patients did not have any recurrences. However, recurrences reported in the other 17 patients were at lower frequency and severity of pain.[6]

3. **Systremma**: Administration of *Shao Yao Gan Cao Tang* plus *Gui Zhi* (Ramulus Cinnamomi) and *Mu Gua* (Fructus Chaenomelis) was effective in treating all 85 patients with leg cramps in the calf characterized by Liver yin and blood deficiencies. The patients were given the herbs in decoction, for a total of 3-5 packs.[7]

4. **Restless leg syndrome**: In one study, 21 patients with restless leg syndrome were treated with modified *Shao Yao Gan Cao Tang* for 6-25 doses with complete recovery in all patients.[8] Another study reported 100% effectiveness among 54 patients (33 males and 21 females with 1 month to 11 years history of illness) with restless leg syndrome using *Shao Yao Gan Cao Tang* administered as tea three times daily for 2-9 packs of herbs. The herbal formula contained 15 grams each of *Bai Shao* (Radix Paeoniae Alba) and *Gan Cao* (Radix et Rhizoma Glycyrrhizae). The treatment protocol was to cook the herbs in 3 cups of water to yield 1 cup of decoction, which was then taken in two equally-divided doses.[9]

5. **Acute back pain**: In one study, 68 patients with acute back sprain were treated with *Shao Yao Gan Cao Tang* with complete recovery in 61 patients, moderate improvement in 6 patients, and no improvement in 1 patient. The herbal formula contained *Bai Shao* (Radix Paeoniae Alba) 20g, *Gan Cao* (Radix et Rhizoma Glycyrrhizae) 20g, and *San Qi* (Radix et Rhizoma Notoginseng) 6g. The herbs were given in decoction twice daily for 5 days.[10]

6. **Heel pain**: One study reported 98% effectiveness using *Shao Yao Gan Cao Tang* to treat heel pain. Of 300 patients with this condition, the study reported complete recovery in 165 patients within 3 packs of herbs, complete recovery in 108 patients within 6 packs of herbs, improvement in 21 patients after 7 packs of herbs, and no effect in 6 patients.[11]

7. **Muscle cramps in hemodialysis**: In a preliminary study, administration of *Shao Yao Gan Cao Tang* at 6 g/day for 4 weeks was effective in treating muscle cramps in maintenance hemodialysis patients. Of 5 patients, 2 had complete resolution of skeletal muscle cramps and 2 had decreased frequency and severity. No serious side effects were reported. The researchers concluded that *Shao Yao*

Gan Cao Tan is a safe, effective treatment for preventing muscle cramps in patients undergoing hemodialysis.[12]

8. **Chronic atrophic gastritis**: In one study, 82 patients with chronic atrophic gastritis were treated with 98.77% effectiveness using *Chi Shao* (Radix Paeoniae Rubra) 24g and *Gan Cao* (Radix et Rhizoma Glycyrrhizae) 6g as the base formula. Modifications were made by adding *Huang Lian* (Rhizoma Coptidis) and *Mu Dan Pi* (Cortex Moutan) for feelings of epigastric burning and pain; *Tian Hua Fen* (Radix Trichosanthis) for thirst; *Chai Hu* (Radix Bupleuri) and *Huang Qin* (Radix Scutellariae) for hypochondriac fullness and pain; *Pu Huang* (Pollen Typhae) and *Wu Ling Zhi* (Faeces Trogopteri) for distention and pain after meals; *Suan Zao Ren* (Semen Ziziphi Spinosae) and *Mu Dan Pi* (Cortex Moutan) for insomnia and irritability; and *Xuan Fu Hua* (Flos Inulae) and *Zhe Shi* (Haematitum) for belching. The average duration of treatment was approximately 60 days. Of 82 patients, the study reported complete recovery in 79 patients, improvement in 2 patients, and no change in 1 patient.[13] Another study reported 91.7% effectiveness using modified *Shao Yao Gan Cao Tang* to treat 36 patients with chronic atrophic gastritis.[14]

9. **Peptic ulcer disease**: In one study, 120 patients with peptic ulcer were treated with *Shao Yao Gan Cao Tang* with some success. The success rate was 63.5% for those diagnosed with deficiency and cold of the Spleen and Stomach, 74.4% for those diagnosed with Stomach yin deficiency, 84.6% for patients with qi and blood stagnation, and 66% for patients with Liver and Stomach disharmony.[15]

10. **Colitis**: One study reported 90.6% effectiveness in the treatment of chronic colitis using *Shao Yao Gan Cao Tang* as a base formula, plus *Hua Jiao* (Pericarpium Zanthoxyli), *Da Xue Teng* (Caulis Sargentodoxae) and others. Modifications included addition of *Wu Zhu Yu* (Fructus Evodiae) and *Pao Jiang* (Rhizoma Zingiberis Praeparatum) for damp-cold; *Huang Lian* (Rhizoma Coptidis) and *Yi Yi Ren* (Semen Coicis) for damp-heat; *Da Huang* (Radix et Rhizoma Rhei) for constipation; *Wu Mei* (Fructus Mume) for diarrhea; and *Huai Hua* (Flos Sophorae) for hematochezia. Of 32 patients, 17 had significant improvement, 12 had moderate improvement, and 3 had no benefit.[16]

11. **Constipation**: Sixty patients with habitual constipation were treated with modified *Shao Yao Gan Cao Tang* with good results. *Bai Zhu* (Rhizoma Atractylodis Macrocephalae) was added for qi deficiency. *Fu Zi* (Radix Aconiti Lateralis Praeparata) was added for cold.[17]

12. **Gastric and abdominal pain**: In one study, 171 patients with gastric and abdominal pain due to various causes were treated with injection of the formula that contained a 4:1 ratio of *Bai Shao* (Radix Paeoniae Alba) and *Gan*

Sháo Yào Gān Cǎo Tāng (Peony and Licorice Decoction)

Cao (Radix et Rhizoma Glycyrrhizae). The treatment was successful in 105 out of 120 patients with pain characterized by deficiency, and 26 out of 51 patients with pain characterized by excess.[18]

13. **Cholecystitis**: In one study, 36 patients with cholecystitis were treated with a large dose of *Shao Yao Gan Cao Tang* with good success. The formula contained 60-90g of *Bai Shao* (Radix Paeoniae Alba) and 15-30g of *Gan Cao* (Radix et Rhizoma Glycyrrhizae). *Chai Hu* (Radix Bupleuri), *Huang Qin* (Radix Scutellariae), and *Long Dan* (Radix et Rhizoma Gentianae) were added for alternation of fever and chills. *Da Huang* (Radix et Rhizoma Rhei), *Di Huang* (Radix Rehmanniae) and *Xuan Shen* (Radix Scrophulariae) were added for constipation. *Chuan Lian Zi* (Fructus Toosendan), *Yu Jin* (Radix Curcumae), and *Yan Hu Suo* (Rhizoma Corydalis) were added for pain. *Tian Hua Fen* (Radix Trichosanthis) and *Mu Dan Pi* (Cortex Moutan) were added if there was a bitter taste in the mouth. *Mai Ya* (Fructus Hordei Germinatus) and *Shan Zha* (Fructus Crataegi) were added for poor appetite. *Huo Xiang* (Herba Agastaches), *Zhu Ru* (Caulis Bambusae in Taenia), and *Ban Xia* (Rhizoma Pinelliae) were added for nausea and vomiting. *Hou Po* (Cortex Magnoliae Officinalis) and *Zhi Qiao* (Fructus Aurantii) were added for abdominal fullness. *Wu Mei Wan* (Mume Pill) was added for the presence of parasites. *Yin Chen* (Herba Artemisiae Scopariae) and *Zhi Zi* (Fructus Gardeniae) were added for jaundice. The treatment protocol was to cook the herbs in decoction, and administer the decoction one time daily for 5 days per course of treatment. Out of 36 patients, the study reported complete recovery in 26 patients, moderate improvement in 8 patients, and no change in 2 patients.[19]

14. **Urolithiasis**: One study reported moderate success in the treatment of urinary stones using *Shao Yao Gan Cao Tang* plus *Dong Kui Zi* (Semen Malvae), *Hua Shi* (Talcum), *Che Qian Zi* (Semen Plantaginis), and others as the base formula. Of the 30 patients, 19 had kidney stones, 1 had bladder stones, and 19 had stones in the ureter. The study reported complete recovery in 19 patients, effectiveness in 10 patients, and no effect in 1 patient.[20]

15. **Diabetes mellitus**: In one clinical study, 36 patients with diabetes mellitus were treated with the formula with marked effect in 15 patients, moderate effect in 10 patients, and no effect in 11 patients. The study also noted that the effectiveness increased with prolonged duration of the treatment.[21]

16. **Hyperosteogeny**: One hundred and sixty patients of hyperosteogeny were treated with varying degrees of success using *Shao Yao Gan Cao Tang* with the addition of *Ji Xue Teng* (Caulis Spatholobi) and *Wei Ling Xian* (Radix et Rhizoma Clematidis).[22]

17. **Menstrual pain**: Sixteen patients with severe menstrual pain were treated with complete recovery in 14 patients using *Shao Yao Gan Cao Tang* with addition of *Yan Hu Suo* (Rhizoma Corydalis) and *Xiang Fu* (Rhizoma Cyperi).[23]

18. **Perimenopause with uterine leiomyomas**: One study investigated the treatment of uterine leiomyomas in 30 perimenopausal women using Chinese herbal medicines and synthetic analogs of gonadotropin-releasing hormone. The Chinese herbs used included *Gui Zhi Fu Ling Wan* (Cinnamon Twig and Poria Pill) and *Shao Yao Gan Cao Tang*. The drugs used included buserelin and nafarelin given via intranasal administration. The study reported a reduction in leiomyomas (less than 60%) along with decreases in the serum levels of luteinizing hormone, follicle-stimulating hormone, estradiol, and the tumor marker CA-125. Side effects noted included slight bone loss, hypermenorrhea, and/or dysmenorrhea. The study concluded that this combination of drugs and herbs could be beneficial for treatment of uterine leiomyomas in perimenopausal patients.[24]

19. **Dysmenorrhea**: In one study, 17 patients with dysmenorrhea, including recurrent endometriotic and adenomyotic patients, obtained complete relief within three months when treated with the following cyclic therapy. The treatment protocol was to alternate giving *Dang Gui Shao Yao San* (Tangkuei and Peony Powder) and *Shao Yao Gan Cao Tang* within the menstrual cycle. Clinical improvements included relief of pain, biphasic changes in basal body temperature patterns, improved levels of estradiol, and successful pregnancy and delivery in one patient. The study concluded that cyclic therapy of these two herbal formulas can be a conservative antidysmenorrhea therapy for endometriotic and adenomyotic patients who desire pregnancy.[25]

HERB-DRUG INTERACTION

- **Neuroleptic-induced hyperprolactinemia**: According to a preliminary report, 11 schizophrenic patients with neuroleptic-induced hyperprolactinemia were treated with good success using *Shao Yao Gan Cao Tang*. After 4 weeks of herbal treatment, the mean plasma prolactin level decreased significantly from 28.9 +/- 14.5 ng/mL at baseline to 22.0 +/- 15.2 ng/mL. The potassium levels did not change significantly, and there were no adverse reactions or exacerbation of psychosis.[26]

- **Paclitaxel-induced myalgia/arthralgia**: Administration of both L-glutamine and *Shao Yao Gan Cao Tang* showed effects to decrease paclitaxel-induced myalgia/arthralgia.[27]

- **Drug-induced menopause**: One study evaluated the therapeutic effects of certain herbal medicines on menopausal symptoms induced by gonadotropin-releasing hormone

Sháo Yào Gān Cǎo Tāng (Peony and Licorice Decoction)

agonist therapy in Japanese women with endometriosis, adenomyosis, or leiomyoma. According to this study, menopausal symptoms induced by gonadotropin-releasing hormone agonist therapy in 13 patients were successfully treated using *Shao Yao Gan Cao Tang, Dang Gui Shao Yao San* (Tangkuei and Peony Powder), *Gui Zhi Fu Ling Wan* (Cinnamon Twig and Poria Pill), *Jia Wei Xiao Yao San* (Augmented Rambling Powder), *Tao He Cheng Qi Tang* (Peach Pit Decoction to Order the Qi) or *Gui Zhi Tang* (Cinnamon Twig Decoction). Most importantly, there were no significant change in serum estradiol levels after treatment with these herbal medicines. The researchers concluded that these herbal medicines can be recommended for menopausal symptoms induced by gonadotropin-releasing hormone agonists without a negative effect on serum estradiol levels.[28]

TOXICOLOGY

According to toxicology studies in mice, the use of the formula created less side effects than the use of the herbs individually.[29]

RELATED FORMULA

Jiā Wèi Sháo Yào Gān Cǎo Tāng

(Augmented Peony and Licorice Decoction)

加味芍藥甘草湯
加味芍药甘草汤

Pinyin Name: *Jia Wei Shao Yao Gan Cao Tang*
Literal Name: Augmented Peony and Licorice Decoction
Original Source: *Guang An Men Yi Yuan* (Guang An Men Hospital) in 1990

Bai Shao (Radix Paeoniae Alba)
Gan Cao (Radix et Rhizoma Glycyrrhizae)
Dang Gui (Radix Angelicae Sinensis)
Hua Jiao (Pericarpium Zanthoxyli)

Jia Wei Shao Yao Gan Cao Tang (Augmented Peony and Licorice Decoction) relieves spasms and cramps of both skeletal and smooth muscles. *Bai Shao* (Radix Paeoniae Alba) and *Gan Cao* (Radix et Rhizoma Glycyrrhizae) nourish yin, tonify qi, and replenish body fluids. *Dang Gui Wei* (Extremitas Radix Angelicae Sinensis) invigorates blood circulation. *Hua Jiao* (Pericarpium Zanthoxyli) dispels cold and relieves pain.

References

1. *Zhong Yao Ming Fang Yao Li Yu Ying Yong* (Pharmacology and Applications of Famous Herbal Formulas) 1989;289-92.
2. *Guo Wai Yi Xue* (Foreign Medicine) 1984;6(1):58.
3. *He Nan Zhong Yi* (Henan Chinese Medicine) 1986;(6):15.
4. *Guo Wai Yi Xue* (Foreign Medicine) 1984;6(1):58.
5. *Jiang Xi Yi Yao* (Jiangxi Medicine and Herbology) 1965;5(7):909.
6. *Zhong Yi Ming Fang Lin Chuang Xin Yong* (Contemporary Clinical Applications of Classic Chinese Formulas) 2001;313.
7. *Zhong Yi Za Zhi* (Journal of Chinese Medicine) 1985;6:450.
8. *Shan Dong Zhong Yi Za Zhi* (Shandong Journal of Chinese Medicine) 1986;(2):17.
9. *He Bei Zhong Yi* (Hebei Chinese Medicine) 1984;3:29.
10. *Zhe Jiang Zhong Yi Za Zhi* (Zhejiang Journal of Chinese Medicine) 1995;(11):524.
11. *Si Chuan Zhong Yi* (Sichuan Chinese Medicine) 1996;11:38.
12. Inoshita F, Ogura Y, Suzuki Y, Hara S, Yamada A, Tanaka N, Yamashita A, Marumo F. Effect of orally administered shao-yao-gan-cao-tang (Shakuyaku-kanzo-to) on muscle cramps in maintenance hemodialysis patients: a preliminary study. American Journal of Chinese Medicine 2003;31(3):445-53.
13. *Jiang Su Zhong Yi* (Jiangsu Chinese Medicine) 1998;1:29.
14. *Zhe Jiang Zhong Yi Xue Yuan Xue Bao* (Journal of Zhejiang University of Chinese Medicine) 1996;4:30.
15. *Chuan Dong Zhong Yi Za Zhi* (Chuandong Journal of Chinese Medicine) 1984;(2):22.
16. *Shang Hai Zhong Yi Yao Za Zhi* (Shanghai Journal of Chinese Medicine and Herbology) 1996;10:18.
17. *Yun Nan Zhong Yi Za Zhi* (Yunan Journal of Chinese Medicine) 1983;(8):79.
18. *Fu Jian Zhong Yi Yao* (Fujian Chinese Medicine and Herbology) 1961;9(4):44.
19. *Shi Yong Zhong Yi Za Zhi* (Journal of Practical Chinese Medicine) 1995;(4):10.
20. *Liao Ning Zhong Yi Za Zhi* (Liaoning Journal of Chinese Medicine) 1986;3:29.
21. *Liao Ning Zhong Yi Za Zhi* (Liaoning Journal of Chinese Medicine) 1980;(9):36.
22. *Zhong Yi Fang Ji Xian Dai Yan Jiu* (Modern Study of Medical Formulae in Traditional Chinese Medicine) 1997;(1):223.
23. *Bei Jing Zhong Yi* (Beijing Chinese Medicine) 1983;(1):33.
24. Sakamoto S, Mitamura T, Iwasawa M, Kitsunai H, Shindou K, Yagishita Y, Zhou YF, Sassa S. Conservative management for perimenopausal women with uterine leiomyomas using Chinese herbal medicines and synthetic analogs of gonadotropin-releasing hormone. In Vivo 1998 May-Jun;12(3):333-7.
25. Tanaka T. A novel anti-dysmenorrhea therapy with cyclic administration of two Japanese herbal medicines. Clinical & Experimental Obstetrics & Gynecology 2003;30(2-3):95-8.
26. Yamada K, Kanba S, Murata T, Fukuzawa M, Terashi B, Yagi G, Asai M. Effectiveness of shakuyaku-kanzo-to in neuroleptic-induced hyperprolactinemia: a preliminary report. Psychiatry & Clinical Neurosciences 1996 Dec;50(6):341-2.
27. Hasegawa K, Mizutani Y, Kuramoto H, Nagao S, Masuyama H, Hongo A, Kodama J, Yoshinouchi M, Hiramatsu Y, Kudo T, Okuda H. The effect of L-Glutamine and Shakuyaku-Kanzo-to for paclitaxel-induced myalgia/arthralgia. Gan To Kagaku Ryoho 2002 Apr;29(4):569-74.
28. Tanaka T. Effects of herbal medicines on menopausal symptoms induced by gonadotropin-releasing hormone agonist therapy. Clin Exp Obstet Gynecol 2001;28(1):20-3.
29. *Zhong Yi Fang Ji De Yao Li Yu Ying Yong* (Pharmacology and Applications of Chinese Herbal Formulas) 1990;296.

Chapter 8 – Tonic Formulas | Section 3 – Qi- and Blood-Tonifying Formulas

Section 3

气血两补剂
— Qi- and Blood-Tonifying Formulas

Bā Zhēn Tāng (Eight-Treasure Decoction)
八珍湯
八珍汤

Pinyin Name: *Ba Zhen Tang*
Literal Name: Eight-Treasure Decoction
Alternate Names: *Pa Chen Tang* (*Wan*), *Ba Zhen Tang* (*Wan*), Eight Jewel Decoction (Pill), Eight Treasures Decoction (Pill), Tangkuei and Ginseng Eight Combination
Original Source: *Zheng Ti Lei Yao* (Catalogued Essentials for Correcting the Body) by Bi Li-Zhai (Ji) in 1529

COMPOSITION

Ren Shen (Radix et Rhizoma Ginseng)	3g [3g]
Bai Zhu (Rhizoma Atractylodis Macrocephalae), *chao* (dry-fried)	3g [10g]
Fu Ling (Poria)	3g [8g]
Zhi Gan Cao (Radix et Rhizoma Glycyrrhizae Praeparata cum Melle), *chao* (dry-fried)	1.5g [5g]
Shu Di Huang (Radix Rehmanniae Praeparata), *ban* (blended) with liquor	3g [15g]
Dang Gui (Radix Angelicae Sinensis), *ban* (blended) with liquor	3g [10g]
Bai Shao (Radix Paeoniae Alba)	3g [8g]
Chuan Xiong (Rhizoma Chuanxiong)	3g [5g]

DOSAGE / PREPARATION / ADMINISTRATION

Cook the ingredients with 3 slices of *Sheng Jiang* (Rhizoma Zingiberis Recens) and 2 pieces of *Da Zao* (Fructus Jujubae) in 2 bowls of water until the liquid is reduced to 80%. Take the decoction before meals. Today, the decoction may be prepared using the doses suggested in brackets.

CHINESE THERAPEUTIC ACTIONS

Tonifies qi and blood

CLINICAL MANIFESTATIONS

Qi and blood deficiencies: a pale or sallow facial appearance, weakness of the limbs, shortness of breath, lack of desire to speak, poor appetite, palpitations, dizziness, a pale tongue with a thin, white coating, and a thin, deficient pulse.

CLINICAL APPLICATIONS

Anemia, thrombopenic purpura, headache, Sheehan's disease, atrophic gastritis, itching, orbital optic neuritis, peripheral neuritis, corneal ulcer, coronary artery disease, recovery from chronic illness, weakness during convalescence, post-surgical recovery, irregular menstruation, uterine bleeding, lumbago in women, prevention of miscarriage, and breech presentation.

EXPLANATION

Ba Zhen Tang (Eight-Treasure Decoction) was originally designed to treat qi and blood deficiencies caused by excessive bleeding. Today, however, this formula can be used in any condition involving qi and blood deficiencies, such as from chronic illnesses, or following the inappropriate use of clearing or draining herbs. A pale face and a sallow facial complexion are signs of blood deficiency. Weak limbs, shortness of breath, and low appetite are all due to qi deficiency. Palpitations and dizziness are signs of blood deficiency unable to nourish the *shen* (spirit). The tongue and pulse conditions described above indicate deficiencies of qi and blood.

604

Chinese Herbal Formulas and Applications

Bā Zhēn Tāng (Eight-Treasure Decoction)

Ba Zhen Tang (Eight-Treasure Decoction)

Diagnosis	Signs and Symptoms	Treatment	Herbs
Qi and blood deficiencies	• Weak limbs, shortness of breath, and low appetite: qi deficiency • Pale face, a sallow facial complexion, palpitations, and dizziness: blood deficiency • Pale tongue with a thin, white coating, and a thin, deficient pulse: deficiency condition	Tonifies qi and blood	• *Ren Shen* (Radix et Rhizoma Ginseng), *Bai Zhu* (Rhizoma Atractylodis Macrocephalae), *Fu Ling* (Poria) and *Zhi Gan Cao* (Radix et Rhizoma Glycyrrhizae Praeparata cum Melle) tonify qi. • *Shu Di Huang* (Radix Rehmanniae Praeparata), *Dang Gui* (Radix Angelicae Sinensis), *Bai Shao* (Radix Paeoniae Alba) and *Chuan Xiong* (Rhizoma Chuanxiong) nourish the blood. • *Sheng Jiang* (Rhizoma Zingiberis Recens) and *Da Zao* (Fructus Jujubae) harmonize the middle *jiao* to strengthen the Spleen and Stomach.

Ba Zhen Tang (Eight-Treasure Decoction) combines *Si Jun Zi Tang* (Four-Gentlemen Decoction) and *Si Wu Tang* (Four-Substance Decoction). *Ren Shen* (Radix et Rhizoma Ginseng), *Bai Zhu* (Rhizoma Atractylodis Macrocephalae), *Fu Ling* (Poria), and *Zhi Gan Cao* (Radix et Rhizoma Glycyrrhizae Praeparata cum Melle) tonify qi. *Shu Di Huang* (Radix Rehmanniae Praeparata), *Dang Gui* (Radix Angelicae Sinensis), *Bai Shao* (Radix Paeoniae Alba), and *Chuan Xiong* (Rhizoma Chuanxiong) nourish the blood. *Sheng Jiang* (Rhizoma Zingiberis Recens) and *Da Zao* (Fructus Jujubae) harmonize the middle *jiao* to strengthen the Spleen and Stomach and to counteract the potentially stagnating effect of the tonics.

Please refer to *Si Jun Zi Tang* (Four-Gentlemen Decoction) and *Si Wu Tang* (Four-Substance Decoction) for detailed explanations of these two formulas.

MODIFICATIONS

• With weakness and pain of the lower back, add *Niu Xi* (Radix Achyranthis Bidentatae) and *Du Zhong* (Cortex Eucommiae).
• For poor appetite, add *Shan Yao* (Rhizoma Dioscoreae), *Chen Pi* (Pericarpium Citri Reticulatae), and *Qian Shi* (Semen Euryales).
• For deficiencies of qi, blood, and yang, add *Huang Qi* (Radix Astragali) and *Rou Gui* (Cortex Cinnamomi).
• To regulate menstruation, add *Yi Mu Cao* (Herba Leonuri).
• For habitual miscarriage or to prevent miscarriage, add *Sha Ren* (Fructus Amomi) and *Zi Su Ye* (Folium Perillae).
• If there is abnormal uterine bleeding, add *E Jiao* (Colla Corii Asini) and *Ai Ye* (Folium Artemisiae Argyi).
• For constipation during pregnancy or vomiting and nausea, add *Xiao Chai Hu Tang* (Minor Bupleurum Decoction).

CAUTIONS / CONTRAINDICATIONS

• Avoid physical exhaustion and exposure to cold environments. Refrain from excessive sexual activity. Cease eating foods that are pungent and spicy.[1]
• *Ba Zhen Tang* is contraindicated in patients with heat or excess conditions.[2]

PHARMACOLOGICAL EFFECTS

1. **Hematopoietic**: In one experiment, it was determined that the administration of *Ba Zhen Tang* had a positive effect in treating mice with anemia due to profuse loss of blood. In comparison with the placebo group which did not receive any herbs, the mice that received the herbs for 10 days showed a significant increase of red blood cells. The study also noted that in normal subjects, use of *Ba Zhen Tang* caused only minor changes to the red blood cells and white blood cells.[3]
2. **Immunostimulant**: In one experiment, oral administration of *Ba Zhen Tang* daily for 7 days was associated with an increase in phagocytic activities by macrophages in mice.[4]
3. **Lymphatic**: In one laboratory experiment using mice, it was found that administration of *Ba Zhen Tang* was effective in countering the suppression of lymphocyte growth induced by hydrocortisone.[5]

CLINICAL STUDIES AND RESEARCH

1. **Anemia**: In a clinical study, 102 patients with anemia characterized by qi and blood deficiencies were treated with *Ba Zhen Tang* with recovery in 8 patients, marked improvement in 45 patients, moderate improvement in 42 patients, and no change in 7 patients. The overall effectiveness was 93.1%. The evaluation of effectiveness was based on both subjective and objective findings.[6] According to another study, anemia due to bleeding ulcer was effectively treated using *Ba Zhen Tang* plus *Zi He Che*

TONIC FORMULAS

8

605

Chapter 8 – Tonic Formulas   *Section 3 – Qi- and Blood-Tonifying Formulas*

Bā Zhēn Tāng (Eight-Treasure Decoction)

(Placenta Hominis), *E Jiao* (Colla Corii Asini), *Sha Ren* (Fructus Amomi), *Mu Xiang* (Radix Aucklandiae), and *Chen Pi* (Pericarpium Citri Reticulatae). Of 40 patients, the study reported complete recovery in 29 patients (72.5%), significant improvement in 10 patients (25%), and slight improvement in 1 patient (2.5%).[7]

2. **Thrombopenic purpura**: Modified *Ba Zhen Tang* was used to treat 42 patients (22 males and 20 females) with thrombopenic purpura. The causes of the illness included upper respiratory tract infection, enteritis, septicemia, and pyogenic otitis media. Out of 42 patients, the study reported recovery in 30 patients and improvement in 12 patients. Most patients responded within 5-6 days.[8]

3. **Post-surgical recovery**: In one study, 32 patients were divided into two groups for evaluation of post-surgical recovery. Group I received *Ba Zhen Tang*, and group II received standard antibiotic therapy. After treatment, the study reported the following findings: Patients in group I regained their appetite after approximately 24-28 hours, in comparison to the 48-52 hours for group II; and patients in group I felt normal 7-12 days after the surgery, in comparison to 8-25 days for patients in group II. In addition, all patients in group I had normal body temperature by day 5, but 3 patients in group II still had fever on the same date.[9]

4. **Prevention of miscarriage**: The effect of *Ba Zhen Tang* was evaluated for stabilization of pregnancy in 38 women (ages between 25-30 years) who had history of 2-5 miscarriages. The herbal formula included *Ba Zhen Tang* with addition of *Sha Ren* (Fructus Amomi) and *Zi Su Ye* (Folium Perillae). The study reported a 100% success rate in stabilizing the pregnancy to full term.[10]

5. **Breech presentation**: Modified *Ba Zhen Tang* was used to treat breech presentation in women who were more than 30 weeks pregnant. Modifications included addition of *Huang Qi* (Radix Astragali) and *Xu Duan* (Radix Dipsaci), and removal of *Fu Ling* (Poria). The herbs were given for 3-6 days. Out of 56 patients, the study reported corrected position in 45 patients (80.3% success rate).[11] In another study of 126 women with breech presentation, use of modified *Ba Zhen Tang* was associated with an 83.3% rate of effectiveness. The herbal formula given was modified by removing *Fu Ling* (Poria) and adding *Zhi Qiao* (Fructus Aurantii) and *Xu Duan* (Radix Dipsaci).[12]

6. **Sheehan's disease**: Satisfactory results were reported in 7 women who received modified *Ba Zhen Tang* for treatment of Sheehan's disease, a condition characterized by necrosis of the pituitary gland and hypopituitarism caused by postpartum hemorrhage. All 7 women were middle-aged, and had suffered profuse postpartum bleeding, hair loss in the axillary and genital areas, low libido, and general fatigue and weakness.[13]

7. **Headache**: One study evaluated *Ba Zhen Tang's* effectiveness in treating headache in 88 patients (29 males and 59 females). The age of the patients ranged from 16 to 79 years of age. The clinical presentations included headache, dizziness, fatigue, palpitations, and shortness of breath. *Ba Zhen Tang* was used as the base formula, with minor modifications if deemed necessary. The average duration of treatment was 20 packs of herbs given in decoction. Out of 88 patients, the study reported marked effect in 33 patients, improvement in 49 patients, and no change in 6 patients. The overall rate of effectiveness was 93.2%.[14]

8. **Atrophic gastritis**: Patients with chronic atrophic gastritis were treated with modified *Ba Zhen Tang* with 98.15% effectiveness. Herbal formulas were modified according to the condition of the patients. *Chai Hu* (Radix Bupleuri) and *Zhi Qiao* (Fructus Aurantii) were added for qi stagnation of the Liver and Stomach. *Huang Qi* (Radix Astragali) was added for qi deficiency of the Spleen and Stomach. *Sha Shen* (Radix Glehniae seu Adenophorae) and *Shi Hu* (Caulis Dendrobii) were added for yin deficiency with heat of the Stomach. *Bai Hua She She Cao* (Herba Hedyotis) and *Tu Fu Ling* (Rhizoma Smilacis Glabrae) were added for damp-heat accumulation in the middle *jiao*. The treatment protocol was to administer the herbs in decoction one time daily, for 6 months per course of treatment.[15]

9. **Itching**: Use of modified *Ba Zhen Tang* was effective in treating geriatric patients with constant skin itching. The formula contained *Ba Zhen Tang* with removal of *Ren Shen* (Radix et Rhizoma Ginseng), and addition of *Huang Qi* (Radix Astragali), *Chan Tui* (Periostracum Cicadae), *She Chuang Zi* (Fructus Cnidii), *Di Fu Zi* (Fructus Kochiae), *Bai Xian Pi* (Cortex Dictamni), and others as deemed necessary. Modifications included addition of *Nu Zhen Zi* (Fructus Ligustri Lucidi) for red tongue; *Dan Shen* (Radix et Rhizoma Salviae Miltiorrhizae) for chronic illness; and *Che Qian Zi* (Semen Plantaginis) for thick tongue coating. Of 36 patients, the study reported complete recovery in 20 patients (55.56%), improvement in 14 patients (38.89%) and no change in 2 patients (5.56%). The overall rate of effectiveness was 94.45%.[16]

10. **Coronary artery disease**: Administration of *Ba Zhen Tang* was associated with 95.8% effectiveness in 48 patients with coronary artery disease. Treatment was considered effective if there was either improvement of subjective symptoms or stabilization of ECG.[17]

11. **Corneal ulcer**: Thirty-six geriatric patients with corneal ulcer were treated with 88.9% effectiveness using modified *Ba Zhen Tang* plus antibiotic drugs. The herbal treatment used *Ba Zhen Tang* as the base, and added *Qian Shi* (Semen Euryales) and *Yi Yi Ren* (Semen Coicis) for Spleen qi deficiency; *He Shou Wu* (Radix Polygoni Multiflori),

606

Bā Zhēn Tāng (Eight-Treasure Decoction)

Gou Qi Zi (Fructus Lycii), *Shan Zhu Yu* (Fructus Corni), and *Shu Di Huang* (Radix Rehmanniae Praeparata) for Liver and Kidney deficiencies; and *Yi Zhi* (Fructus Alpiniae Oxyphyllae), *Ba Ji Tian* (Radix Morindae Officinalis), *Yin Yang Huo* (Herba Epimedii), and *Xian Mao* (Rhizoma Curculiginis) for Kidney qi deficiency. Antibiotic drugs were given locally and systemically. Of 36 patients, the study reported marked improvement in 12 patients, improvement in 20 patients, and no change in 4 patients.[18]

12. **Orbital optic neuritis**: *Ba Zhen Tang* effectively treated 14 patients with orbital optic neuritis. The average duration of treatment was 25.3 days.[19]

13. **Peripheral neuritis**: Thirteen patients with peripheral neuritis were treated with modified *Ba Zhen Tang*. The clinical presentation included numbness and pain of the upper and/or lower extremities. The modifications included addition of *Du Huo* (Radix Angelicae Pubescentis) and *Qiang Huo* (Rhizoma et Radix Notopterygii) for neuritis in the upper extremities; *Mu Gua* (Fructus Chaenomelis) and *Niu Xi* (Radix Achyranthis Bidentatae) for neuritis in the lower extremities; and elimination of *Shu Di Huang* (Radix Rehmanniae Praeparata) and *Gan Cao* (Radix et Rhizoma Glycyrrhizae) if there was fullness in the abdominal area with indigestion. Out of 13 patients, the study reported complete recovery in 11 patients and improvement in 2 patients. The average duration of treatment was 24 packs of the raw herbs in decoction (ranges from 12-36).[20]

14. **Organophosphorus-induced peripheral neuritis**: In one study, peripheral neuritis associated with acute organophosphorus poisoning was treated effectively using modified *Ba Zhen Tang*. The herbal treatment included *Ba Zhen Tang* plus *Gui Zhi* (Ramulus Cinnamomi) as the base formula. In addition, *Chi Shao* (Radix Paeoniae Rubra), *Dan Shen* (Radix et Rhizoma Salviae Miltiorrhizae), *Tao Ren* (Semen Persicae), and *Hong Hua* (Flos Carthami) were added for numbness of the extremities with dark blue/purple tongue; *Sang Zhi* (Ramulus Mori) for a feeling of heaviness in the upper extremities; *Niu Xi* (Radix Achyranthis Bidentatae) for a feeling of heaviness in the lower extremities; *Cang Zhu* (Rhizoma Atractylodis), *Fen Bi Xie* (Rhizoma Dioscoreae Hypoglaucae), *Huang Bo* (Cortex Phellodendri Chinensis), *Fang Ji* (Radix Stephaniae Tetrandrae), and *Mu Gua* (Fructus Chaenomelis) for a feeling of heaviness in the body and extremities; *Huang Bo* (Cortex Phellodendri Chinensis) and *Zhi Zi* (Fructus Gardeniae) for fever, a feeling of burning sensation and pain, irritability, and a red tongue; and *Gui Ban* (Plastrum Testudinis), *Mai Dong* (Radix Ophiopogonis), and *Zhi Mu* (Rhizoma Anemarrhenae) for tidal fever and night sweats. Out of 22 patients, 5 patients had complete recovery in 1 month, 5 patients had complete recovery in 2 months, 8 patients in 3 months, and 4 patients after 3 months.[21]

TOXICOLOGY

In an acute toxicology study, oral administration of the formula in decoction at 50 g/kg as a single dose did not cause any significant side effect in rats. In a chronic toxicology study, daily administration of the formula in decoction at 20 g/kg for 8 days did not cause any adverse reaction to the body weight, liver, adrenal glands, heart, uterus, or testicles. There was, however, a slight increase in the weight of the spleen.[22]

AUTHORS' COMMENTS

Ba Zhen Tang, *Shi Quan Da Bu Tang* (All-Inclusive Great Tonifying Decoction), and *Ren Shen Yang Ying Tang* (Ginseng Decoction to Nourish the Nutritive Qi) are three formulas that tonify qi and blood. All three formulas tonify Spleen qi with *Ren Shen* (Radix et Rhizoma Ginseng), *Fu Ling* (Poria), *Bai Zhu* (Rhizoma Atractylodis Macrocephalae), and *Gan Cao* (Radix et Rhizoma Glycyrrhizae), and nourish the blood with *Dang Gui* (Radix Angelicae Sinensis), *Shu Di Huang* (Radix Rehmanniae Praeparata), and *Bai Shao* (Radix Paeoniae Alba). Their differences are as follows:

- *Ba Zhen Tang* combines *Si Jun Zi Tang* (Four-Gentlemen Decoction) and *Si Wu Tang* (Four-Substance Decoction) with *Sheng Jiang* (Rhizoma Zingiberis Recens) and *Da Zao* (Fructus Jujubae). It is a neutral-temperature tonic that treats qi and blood deficiencies. Clinical manifestations include a sallow complexion, poor appetite, fatigue, shortness of breath, dizziness, blurred vision, palpitations, a pale tongue, and a thin, deficient pulse.

- *Shi Quan Da Bu Tang* combines *Ba Zhen Tang* with *Huang Qi* (Radix Astragali) and *Rou Gui* (Cortex Cinnamomi). The addition of these two single herbs changes the property of the formula from neutral to warm, making it more suitable for deficiency and cold conditions. Chief manifestations include qi and blood deficiencies with cough, poor appetite, seminal emissions, knee weakness, slow healing sores, and uterine bleeding.

- *Ren Shen Yang Ying Tang* is *Shi Quan Da Bu Tang* (All-Inclusive Great Tonifying Decoction) with the removal of *Chuan Xiong* (Rhizoma Chuanxiong), and the addition of *Chen Pi* (Pericarpium Citri Reticulatae), *Wu Wei Zi* (Fructus Schisandrae Chinensis), and *Yuan Zhi* (Radix Polygalae). *Wu Wei Zi* (Fructus Schisandrae Chinensis), *Ren Shen* (Radix et Rhizoma Ginseng), and *Huang Qi* (Radix Astragali) consolidate the exterior and prevent sweating. *Yuan Zhi* (Radix Polygalae) calms the *shen* (spirit), and resolves phlegm to benefit the production of

Bā Zhēn Tāng (Eight-Treasure Decoction)

qi and blood. This formula is more suitable for patients with qi and blood deficiencies with an unstable *shen*. Clinical manifestations include shortness of breath upon exertion, palpitations, a dry throat and lips. This formula does not create heat nor stagnation, when compared to other warm or heavy tonic formulas.[23]

According to Dr. Chang Wei-Yen, headaches with dizziness, palpitations, frequent dreams, and coldness of the limbs caused by blood deficiency can be treated effectively with *Ba Zhen Tang*, *Sheng Mai San* (Generate the Pulse Powder), and *Tian Wang Bu Xin Dan* (Emperor of Heaven's Special Pill to Tonify the Heart).

References

1. *Zhong Yao Ming Fang Yao Li Yu Ying Yong* (Pharmacology and Applications of Famous Herbal Formulas) 1989;296-297.
2. *Zhong Yao Ming Fang Yao Li Yu Ying Yong* (Pharmacology and Applications of Famous Herbal Formulas) 1989;296-297.
3. *Zhong Yi Fang Ji Xian Dai Yan Jiu* (Modern Study of Medical Formulae in Traditional Chinese Medicine) 1997;629.
4. *Hu Nan Zhong Yi Za Zhi* (Hunan Journal of Chinese Medicine) 1994;2:8.
5. *Zhong Guo Zhong Yao Za Zhi* (People's Republic of China Journal of Chinese Herbology) 1993;18(4):495.
6. *Hu Nan Zhong Yi Za Zhi* (Hunan Journal of Chinese Medicine) 1994;2:8.
7. *Jiang Xi Zhong Yi Yao* (Jiangxi Chinese Medicine and Herbology) 1997;6:24.
8. *Zhong Guo Zhong Xi Yi Jie He Za Zhi* (Chinese Journal of Integrative Chinese and Western Medicine) 1994;14(8):495.
9. *Zhong Xi Yi Jie He Za Zhi* (Journal of Integrated Chinese and Western Medicine) 1990;10(5):319.
10. *Fu Jian Zhong Yi Yao* (Fujian Chinese Medicine and Herbology) 1960;10:3.
11. *Zhong Yi Fang Ji Xian Dai Yan Jiu* (Modern Study of Medical Formulae in Traditional Chinese Medicine) 1997;632.
12. *Shan Dong Zhong Yi Za Zhi* (Shandong Journal of Chinese Medicine) 1996;12:545.
13. *Liao Ning Zhong Yi Za Zhi* (Liaoning Journal of Chinese Medicine) 1987;1:23.
14. *Liao Ning Zhong Yi Za Zhi* (Liaoning Journal of Chinese Medicine) 1992;19(12):20.
15. *He Bei Zhong Yi* (Hebei Chinese Medicine) 1987;9(6):16.
16. *Shi Yong Zhong Yi Za Zhi* (Journal of Practical Chinese Medicine) 1999;6:9.
17. *Zhong Yi Han Shou Tong Xun* (Reports of Chinese Medicine) 1991;6:48.
18. *Fu Jian Zhong Yi Yao* (Fujian Chinese Medicine and Herbology) 1995;4:57.
19. *Liao Ning Zhong Yi Za Zhi* (Liaoning Journal of Chinese Medicine) 1990;12:26.
20. *Zhe Jiang Zhong Yi Za Zhi* (Zhejiang Journal of Chinese Medicine) 1992;27(12):537.
21. *Zhong Yi Za Zhi* (Journal of Chinese Medicine) 1995;12:725.
22. *Zhong Yi Fang Ji Xian Dai Yan Jiu* (Modern Study of Medical Formulae in Traditional Chinese Medicine) 1997;630.
23. Wang MZ, et al. *Zhong Yi Xue Wen Da Ti Ku* (Questions and Answers on Traditional Chinese Medicine: Herbal Formulas).

Chinese Herbal Formulas and Applications

Shi Quán Dà Bǔ Tāng (All-Inclusive Great Tonifying Decoction)

十全大補湯
十全大补汤

Pinyin Name: *Shi Quan Da Bu Tang*
Literal Name: All-Inclusive Great Tonifying Decoction
Alternate Names: *Shih Chuan Ta Pu Tang* (*Wan*), *Shi Quan Da Bu Tang* (*Wan*), Complete Nourishment Decoction (Pill),
Ten Strong Tonic Herbs Decoction (Pill), Ginseng and Tangkuei Ten Combination
Original Source: *Tai Ping Hui Min He Ji Ju Fang* (Imperial Grace Formulary of the Tai Ping Era) by the Imperial Medical
Department in 1078-85

COMPOSITION

Ren Shen (Radix et Rhizoma Ginseng)	[8g]
Bai Zhu (Rhizoma Atractylodis Macrocephalae), *bei* (stone-baked)	[10g]
Fu Ling (Poria), *bei* (stone-baked)	[8g]
Zhi Gan Cao (Radix et Rhizoma Glycyrrhizae Praeparata cum Melle)	[5g]
Shu Di Huang (Radix Rehmanniae Praeparata),	
xi (washed) with liquor, *zheng* (steamed) and *bei* (stone-baked)	[8-15g]
Dang Gui (Radix Angelicae Sinensis), *xi* (washed)	[10g]
Bai Shao (Radix Paeoniae Alba)	[8g]
Chuan Xiong (Rhizoma Chuanxiong)	[5g]
Huang Qi (Radix Astragali)	[15g]
Rou Gui (Cortex Cinnamomi), do not expose to heat	[8g]

DOSAGE / PREPARATION / ADMINISTRATION

The source text states to grind equal amounts of the ingredients into a coarse powder. Cook 6g of the powder with 3 slices of *Sheng Jiang* (Rhizoma Zingiberis Recens) and 2 pieces of *Da Zao* (Fructus Jujubae) in 1 large bowl of water until the liquid is reduced to 70%. Take the warm decoction at any time during the day. Today, this formula may be prepared as a decoction with the doses suggested in brackets.

CHINESE THERAPEUTIC ACTIONS

Warms and tonifies qi and blood

CLINICAL MANIFESTATIONS

1. Deficiencies of qi and blood accompanied by yang deficiency and cold manifestations: lassitude, low appetite, a pale face, palpitations, insomnia, dizziness, intolerance to cold, and seminal emissions.
2. General deficiency of the body: deficient cough, poor appetite, a sallow appearance, weakness of the legs and knees, chronic ulcers or prolonged healing of wounds, and seminal emissions in men and *beng lou* (flooding and spotting) in women.

CLINICAL APPLICATIONS

Anemia, neutropenia, cancer, supportive therapy for chemotherapy and/or radiation, chronic atrophic gastritis, gastric prolapse, post-surgical recovery, Shwachman syndrome, Meniere's syndrome, and Sheehan's syndrome.

EXPLANATION

Shi Quan Da Bu Tang (All-Inclusive Great Tonifying Decoction) treats general deficiency and weakness of the body, conditions that may be caused by over-exertion, injuries, and chronic illnesses. The original text states that this formula has a wide range of effects and can be used to treat a variety of syndromes marked by qi and blood deficiencies.

This formula consists of *Si Jun Zi Tang* (Four-Gentlemen Decoction) and *Si Wu Tang* (Four-Substance Decoction), plus *Huang Qi* (Radix Astragali) and *Rou Gui* (Cortex Cinnamomi). *Ren Shen* (Radix et Rhizoma Ginseng), *Bai Zhu* (Rhizoma Atractylodis Macrocephalae), *Fu Ling* (Poria), and *Zhi Gan Cao* (Radix et Rhizoma Glycyrrhizae Praeparata cum Melle) tonify qi. *Shu Di Huang* (Radix Rehmanniae Praeparata), *Dang Gui* (Radix Angelicae Sinensis), *Bai Shao* (Radix Paeoniae Alba), and *Chuan Xiong* (Rhizoma Chuanxiong) nourish the blood. *Huang Qi* (Radix Astragali) tonifies qi and lifts yang qi to improve the general body condition. This herb also helps to speed the healing of wounds. *Rou Gui* (Cortex Cinnamomi) warms yang and dispels cold.

Please refer to *Si Jun Zi Tang* (Four-Gentlemen Decoction) and *Si Wu Tang* (Four-Substance Decoction) for detailed explanation of these two formulas.

8

TONIC FORMULAS

609

Chapter 8 – Tonic Formulas　　　　　　　　　　　　　　　*Section 3 – Qi- and Blood-Tonifying Formulas*

Shí Quán Dà Bŭ Tāng (All-Inclusive Great Tonifying Decoction)

Shi Quan Da Bu Tang (All-Inclusive Great Tonifying Decoction)

Diagnosis	Signs and Symptoms	Treatment	Herbs
Deficiencies of qi and blood accompanied by yang deficiency and cold manifestations	• Lassitude and low appetite: qi deficiency • Pale face, palpitations, insomnia, and dizziness: blood deficiency • Intolerance to cold: yang deficiency	Warms and tonifies qi and blood	• *Si Jun Zi Tang* (Four-Gentlemen Decoction) tonifies qi. • *Si Wu Tang* (Four-Substance Decoction) tonifies blood. • *Huang Qi* (Radix Astragali) tonifies qi and lifts yang. • *Rou Gui* (Cortex Cinnamomi) warms yang and dispels cold.

MODIFICATIONS

• For malnutrition, and emaciation with poor appetite: add *Shan Yao* (Rhizoma Dioscoreae) and *Qian Shi* (Semen Euryales).

• With sores and abscesses caused by qi and blood deficiencies, add *Zhi Qiao* (Fructus Aurantii), *Xiang Fu* (Rhizoma Cyperi), and *Lian Qiao* (Fructus Forsythiae).

• With spermatorrhea and nocturnal emissions, add *Shan Zhu Yu* (Fructus Corni), *Wu Wei Zi* (Fructus Schisandrae Chinensis), *Mai Dong* (Radix Ophiopogonis), and *Shan Yao* (Rhizoma Dioscoreae).

• If there is steaming bones sensation, add *Chai Hu* (Radix Bupleuri), *Yin Chai Hu* (Radix Stellariae), *Qing Hao* (Herba Artemisiae Annuae), and *Bie Jia* (Carapax Trionycis).

• With fatigue and general ache and pain, add *Gui Zhi* (Ramulus Cinnamomi) and *Ban Xia* (Rhizoma Pinelliae).

• With general weakness and deficiency, combine with *Xiao Jian Zhong Tang* (Minor Construct the Middle Decoction).

• With fatigue due to Spleen deficiency, combine with *Gui Pi Tang* (Restore the Spleen Decoction).

• With palpitations, fear, and fright, combine with *Yang Xin Tang* (Nourish the Heart Decoction).

• For menopause symptoms that do not respond to herbs that clear deficiency heat and nourish yin, add *Fu Zi* (Radix Aconiti Lateralis Praeparata).

• For *bi zheng* (painful obstruction syndrome), add *Niu Xi* (Radix Achyranthis Bidentatae) and *Xu Duan* (Radix Dipsaci).

CAUTIONS / CONTRAINDICATIONS

Because *Shi Quan Da Bu Tang* is a warm formula, it is contraindicated in patients with heat or excess conditions.

PHARMACOLOGICAL EFFECTS

1. **Immunostimulant**: Administration of *Shi Quan Da Bu Tang* was associated with immune-enhancing effects because it increases the number and/or the activities of the macrophages, B-lymphocytes, T-lymphocytes, and natural killer (NK) cells.[1]

2. **Hematopoietic**: In one study, the administration of *Shi Quan Da Bu Tang* for up to 10 days effectively treated mice with anemia caused by profuse blood loss. The use of this formula was associated with an increase in hemoglobin and red blood cells.[2] In another study, *Si Wu Tang* (Four-Substance Decoction), *Si Jun Zi Tang* (Four-Gentlemen Decoction) and *Shi Quan Da Bu Tang* were given orally to mice to evaluate their effect for treatment of anemia. The study concluded that *Shi Quan Da Bu Tang* was most effective, followed by *Si Wu Tang* and *Si Jun Zi Tang*.[3] The mechanism of action was attributed to increased activity of CSF.[4]

3. **Antineoplastic**: In one study in mice, the administration of *Shi Quan Da Bu Tang* was associated with an inhibitory effect on the growth of cancer cells. The mice that received the herbs survived longer in comparison with the control group. Also, it was noted that the use of herbs also minimized the side effects associated with chemotherapy treatments.[5]

4. **Antitumor and antimetastatic**: According to one *in vivo* study, use of *Shi Quan Da Bu Tang* was associated with marked antitumor and antimetastatic activities. Proposed mechanism of this action included enhancement of phagocytosis, cytokine induction, antibody production, and induction of the mitogenic activity of spleen cells. As a complement to western medical treatment, *Shi Quan Da Bu Tang* showed antitumor effects when combined with surgical excision, antitumor effects with or without other drugs, and protection against the deleterious effects of anticancer drugs as well as radiation-induced immunosuppression and bone marrow toxicity.[6] Specifically, in liver metastasis, one study reported that administration of *Shi Quan Da Bu Tang* had a dose-dependent inhibition of liver tumor colonies and significant enhancement of survival rate, without side effects, as compared with the untreated control.[7]

610

Chinese Herbal Formulas and Applications

Shí Quán Dà Bǔ Tāng (All-Inclusive Great Tonifying Decoction)

5. **Anticancer**: One study reported a promising preventative effect for endometrial cancers with use of *Shi Quan Da Bu Tang*. According to this study, this formula suppressed estradiol-17 beta (E2)-induced expression of c-fos/jun in uterine corpus and inhibited N-methyl-N-nitrosourea and E2-induced endometrial carcinogenesis in mice.[8] According to another study, *Shi Quan Da Bu Tang* suppressed primary melanocytic tumors through potentiation of T-cell-mediated antitumor cytotoxic immunity *in vivo*.[9]

6. **Antitumor**: Administration of *Shi Quan Da Bu Tang* was associated with a preventive effect on endometrial carcinogenesis in mice. The antitumor effect of *Shi Quan Da Bu Tang* was attributed in part to the contents of *Si Wu Tang*, as the administration of these four herbs was found to have an inhibitory effect on estrogen-induced expression of c-fos, interleukin (IL)-1alpha and tumor necrosis factor (TNF)-alpha in uteri of ovariectomized mice.[10]

7. **Antiaging**: One study found this formula to have marked anti-aging effects to prolong life expectancy in mice.[11]

8. **Effect on bone mass density**: Administration of *Shi Quan Da Bu Tang* for 19 weeks was effective in the prevention and treatment of osteoporosis in mice whose ovaries had been removed. In comparison with control groups (one receiving placebo and the other estradiol), *Shi Quan Da Bu Tang* was determined to be comparable in effect to estradiol, and significantly more effective than the placebo for prevention and treatment of osteoporosis.[12] This efficacy on prevention and treatment of osteoporosis was reproduced in another study that administered herbs for 49 days to rats with ovariectomy. In comparison with sham-operated rats, the bone mineral density (BMD) of tibia in ovariectomized rats decreased by 20%, but the BMD was unaffected in rats treated with *Shi Quan Da Bu Tang* or 17-beta-estradiol. The study concluded that *Shi Quan Da Bu Tang* is as effective as 17-beta-estradiol in preventing the development of bone loss induced by ovariectomy by preserving the fine particle surface of the bone.[13]

9. **Hepatoprotective**: Administration of *Shi Quan Da Bu Tang* was effective in treating N-nitrosomorpholine-induced hepatocarcinogenesis in male rats. The mechanism of action was attributed to the activation of the immune system.[14]

CLINICAL STUDIES AND RESEARCH

1. **Chronic atrophic gastritis**: Modified *Shi Quan Da Bu Tang* was used to treat 54 patients of chronic atrophic gastritis with good success. The formula included *Tai Zi Shen* (Radix Pseudostellariae), *Fu Ling* (Poria), *Bai Shao* (Radix Paeoniae Alba), *Dang Gui* (Radix Angelicae

Sinensis), *Shu Di Huang* (Radix Rehmanniae Praeparata), *Chuan Xiong* (Rhizoma Chuanxiong), *Ji Nei Jin* (Endothelium Corneum Gigeriae Galli), *Sha Ren* (Fructus Amomi), *San Leng* (Rhizoma Sparganii), *Mo Yao* (Myrrha), *Wu Yao* (Radix Linderae), and *Gan Cao* (Radix et Rhizoma Glycyrrhizae). In addition, *Huang Qi* (Radix Astragali) and *Bai Zhu* (Rhizoma Atractylodis Macrocephalae) were added for qi deficiency of the Spleen and Stomach. *Zhi Qiao* (Fructus Aurantii) and *Chai Hu* (Radix Bupleuri) were added for qi stagnation of the Spleen and Stomach. *Sha Shen* (Radix Glehniae seu Adenophorae) and *Shi Hu* (Caulis Dendrobii) were added for yin-deficient heat in the Stomach. *Bai Hua She She Cao* (Herba Hedyotis) and *Tu Fu Ling* (Rhizoma Smilacis Glabrae) were added for damp-heat accumulation in the middle *jiao*. The treatment protocol was to administer the herbs in decoction twice daily in the morning and at night. The treatment period was 6 months for one course of treatment. The overall effectiveness rate was 98.15%.[15]

2. **Gastric prolapse**: Concurrent treatment using acupuncture and herbs was found to be very effective in the treatment of gastric prolapse characterized by deficiencies of qi and blood with *zhong* (central) *qi* collapse. The treatment protocol for herbs was to administer *Shi Quan Da Bu Tang* for a total of 70 doses. Out of 15 patients, the study reported complete recovery in 4 patients, improvement in 10 patients, and no benefit in 1 patient.[16]

3. **Post-surgical recovery**: Administration of *Shi Quan Da Bu Tang* has marked beneficial effects on gastric cancer patients during the post-operative recovery by improving interleukin 2 reactivity, natural killer activity, nutritional index, and bone mineral indices.[17]

4. **Cancer**: According to one report that screened and evaluated 116 herbal formulas for treatment of cancer, *Shi Quan Da Bu Tang* was determined to be the most effective as a potent biological response modifier. Clinical benefits of *Shi Quan Da Bu Tang* included extremely low toxicity, self-regulatory and synergistic actions of its components in immunomodulatory and immunopotentiating effects, enhanced therapeutic activity in chemotherapy and radiotherapy, inhibited recurrence of malignancies, prolonged survival, and reduced adverse toxicities of many anticancer drugs.[18]

5. **Anemia**: Administration of *Shi Quan Da Bu Tang* effectively increased hemoglobin, red blood cells, and platelets in 41 patients with post-surgical proteinemia.[19]

6. **Meniere's syndrome**: In one study, 27 patients with Meniere's syndrome were treated with modified *Shi Quan Da Bu Tang* with good results. The formula included *Dang Shen* (Radix Codonopsis), *Bai Zhu* (Rhizoma Atractylodis Macrocephalae), *Fu Ling* (Poria), *Shu Di Huang* (Radix Rehmanniae Praeparata), *Huang Qi* (Radix Astragali), *Bai*

8

TONIC FORMULAS

611

Shí Quán Dà Bǔ Tāng (All-Inclusive Great Tonifying Decoction)

Shao (Radix Paeoniae Alba), *Dang Gui* (Radix Angelicae Sinensis), *Tian Ma* (Rhizoma Gastrodiae), *Ban Xia* (Rhizoma Pinelliae), *Chuan Xiong* (Rhizoma Chuanxiong), *Zhi Gan Cao* (Radix et Rhizoma Glycyrrhizae Praeparata cum Melle), and *Rou Gui* (Cortex Cinnamomi). The treatment protocol was to administer the herbs in decoction one time daily, for a total of 6-24 doses. Out of 27 patients, the study reported recovery in 23 patients (asymptomatic with no recurrences for 6 months), marked effect in 3 patients, and no benefit in 1 patient.[20]

7. **Sheehan's syndrome**: Continuous administration of modified *Shi Quan Da Bu Tang* for 2 months was effective in alleviating signs and symptoms in 7 patients with Sheehan's syndrome. The herbal treatment was based on *Shi Quan Da Bu Tang*, with addition of *Yi Mu Cao* (Herba Leonuri), *Yin Yang Huo* (Herba Epimedii) and *Zi He Che* (Placenta Hominis) and the removal of *Huang Qi* (Radix Astragali).[21]

8. **Shwachman syndrome**: Use of *Shi Quan Da Bu Tang* was associated with beneficial effects in patients with Shwachman syndrome, a rare disease characterized by decreased ability to digest food because the cells of the pancreas do not work properly.[22]

HERB-DRUG INTERACTION

- **Chemotherapy- and radiation-induced toxicities**: *Shi Quan Da Bu Tang* was shown in one study to have a marked protective effect against chemotherapy and radiation in cancer patients, including but not limited to such drugs as mitomycin, cisplatin, carboplatin, cyclophosphamide, and 5-fluorouracil.[23] Moreover, many journals reported that *Shi Quan Da Bu Tang* demonstrated effectiveness as a supportive therapy for cancer patients treated with chemotherapy and/or radiation. In one study, 50 patients with cancer (stomach, large intestine and breast) who were treated with chemotherapeutic agents (FT-207, 5-FU, UFT, MMC, CDDP, and ADM) and this herbal formula for one month showed good tolerance for the treatments. In another report, 30 women with malignant cancer of the uterus and ovaries were treated with the herbal formula with marked improvement such as more energy, better appetite, and warmer extremities. Use of the formula has also shown effect to reverse bone marrow suppression induced by such drugs as MMC, Ara-C, and MTX. In one study with 26 patients, the use of the herbal formula inhibited the reduction of white blood cells and red blood cells associated with the drugs. It was noted in another study that the use of the herbal formula had a protective effect for white blood cells, red blood cells, and platelets against radiation treatment in 15 cancer patients. Lastly, administration of *Shi Quan Da Bu Tang* starting one week before chemotherapy was associated with 88% effectiveness in alleviating nausea and vomiting associated with EAP treatment (adriamycin, cisplatin and etoposide) for stomach and pancreatic cancer.[24]

- **Chemotherapy-induced toxicities**: One study reported significant benefits using *Shi Quan Da Bu Tang* in cancer patients treated with chemotherapeutic agents. *Shi Quan Da Bu Tang* potentiates the therapeutic effect of many anticancer drugs, such as mitomycin, cisplatin, cyclophosphamide and fluorouracil. It also counteracts adverse side effects of these anticancer drugs, such as gastrointestinal disturbances such as anorexia, nausea, vomiting, hepatotoxicity, immunosuppression, leukopenia, thrombocytopenia, anemia, and nephropathy.[25]

- **Chemotherapy- and radiation-induced neutropenia**: One study reported 84.32% effectiveness using *Shi Quan Da Bu Tang* to treat decreased white blood cell count induced by chemotherapy and/or radiation in 134 patients (39 with stomach cancer, 28 with lung cancer, 17 with breast cancer, 13 with rectal cancer, 12 with lymphatic cancer, 12 with liver cancer, 7 with bladder cancer, and others).[26]

- **Cyclophosphamide- or prednisolone-induced immunosuppression**: One study demonstrated that use of *Shi Quan Da Bu Tang* and *Ren Shen Yang Ying Tang* (Ginseng Decoction to Nourish the Nutritive Qi) effectively prolonged survival rate and life span in mice with candida infection associated with immunosuppression induced by cyclophosphamide or prednisolone.[27]

- **Carboplatin- or cisplatin-induced myelosuppression**: One study reported that administration of *Shi Quan Da Bu Tang* was effective in mice to prevent myelosuppression induced by nine-times intraperitoneal administration of 15 mg/kg carboplatin or 3.0 mg/kg cisplatin, without affecting the antitumor activities of these agents.[28]

- **Cisplatin-induced toxicities**: According to another study, daily administration of *Shi Quan Da Bu Tang* in mice was effective to protect against nephrotoxicity, immunosuppression, hepatic toxicity, and gastrointestinal toxicity caused by intraperitoneal administration of 3.0 mg/kg cisplatin nine times (on days 3, 4, 5, 6, 7, 8, 10, 11, and 12). Furthermore, the antitumor effect of cisplatin was not reduced.[29]

- **Cis-diamminedichloroplatinum-induced nephrotoxicity and bone marrow toxicity**: Administration of *Shi Quan Da Bu Tang* was effective in treating nephrotoxicity and bone marrow toxicity caused by intraperitoneal administration of cis-diamminedichloroplatinum (CDDP), a chemotherapeutic agent. Furthermore, use of the herbs did not affect the antitumor activity of CDDP. This beneficial effect is attributed in part to *Dang Gui* (Radix Angelicae Sinensis) and its constituent sodium L-malate.[30]

- **Interferon-induced toxicities**: One study reported a synergistic effect to potentiate the antitumor effect and

Chinese Herbal Formulas and Applications

Shí Quán Dà Bǔ Tāng (All-Inclusive Great Tonifying Decoction)

decrease the toxicity using interferon-alpha and *Shi Quan Da Bu Tang* for treatment of lung metastasis of murine renal cell carcinoma. Interferon-alpha has been shown to significantly inhibit the metastasis of cancer cells, but is also associated with marked loss of body weight. This study demonstrated that the combination treatment of suboptimal doses of interferon-alpha and *Shi Quan Da Bu Tang* has marked effects to augment the antimetastatic effect without causing any loss of body weight, as compared to either treatment alone.[31]

- **Rifampin-induced neutropenia**: Administration of modified *Shi Quan Da Bu Tang* in 11 patients was effective in reversing neutropenia induced by rifampin within 7 days. The white blood cell count was below 3,000 cells/mcl in 4 patients, and between 3,000-4,000 cells/mcl in 7 patients.[32]

- **Levofloxacin**: In a study of 8 healthy volunteers in an open, random crossover fashion, co-administrations of levofloxacin and *Shi Quan Da Bu Tang* did not cause any significant differences in any pharmacokinetic parameters, urinary recovery and renal clearance of levofloxacin. The study concluded that *Shi Quan Da Bu Tang* does not have a significant effect on the rate and extent of bioavailability or renal excretion of levofloxacin.[33]

TOXICOLOGY

In a toxicology study, the LD_{50} for the oral administration of the formula in herbal extract was 15 g/kg in mice. The herbal extract was prepared by cooking 1.5g of *Gan Cao* (Radix et Rhizoma Glycyrrhizae) and 3.0g of the other 9 herbs in 285 mL of water for 1 hour to yield 2.3g of herbal extract. The study concluded that the formula has very little toxicity.[34]

RELATED FORMULAS

Dà Bǔ Tāng (Great Tonifying Decoction)

大補湯
大补汤

Pinyin Name: *Da Bu Tang*
Literal Name: Great Tonifying Decoction
Original Source: *An Hui Zhong Yi Xue Yuan* (Anhui University School of Medicine) in 1990

Xi Yang Shen (Radix Panacis Quinquefolii)
Bai Zhu (Rhizoma Atractylodis Macrocephalae)
Fu Ling (Poria)
Zhi Gan Cao (Radix et Rhizoma Glycyrrhizae Praeparata cum Melle)
Shu Di Huang (Radix Rehmanniae Praeparata)
Dang Gui (Radix Angelicae Sinensis)
Bai Shao (Radix Paeoniae Alba)

Chuan Xiong (Rhizoma Chuanxiong)
Rou Gui (Cortex Cinnamomi)
Huang Qi (Radix Astragali)
Shan Yao (Rhizoma Dioscoreae)
Wu Wei Zi (Fructus Schisandrae Chinensis)
Sheng Jiang (Rhizoma Zingiberis Recens)
Da Zao (Fructus Jujubae)

Da Bu Tang (Great Tonifying Decoction) tonifies qi, blood, yin, and yang. It is formulated using the general principles of *Si Jun Zi Tang* (Four-Gentlemen Decoction) to tonify qi, and *Si Wu Tang* (Four-Substance Decoction) to tonify blood. In addition, it contains the following herbs: *Gui Xin* (Cortex Rasus Cinnamomi) to warm yang, *Huang Qi* (Radix Astragali) to tonify qi, *Shan Yao* (Rhizoma Dioscoreae) to nourish yin, and *Wu Wei Zi* (Fructus Schisandrae Chinensis) to consolidate body fluids. *Sheng Jiang* (Rhizoma Zingiberis Recens) and *Da Zao* (Fructus Jujubae) strengthen the middle *jiao* and enhance the absorption of the tonic herbs. Clinically, this formula is used to treat generalized weakness and deficiency characterized by depletion of qi, blood, yin, and yang.

Rén Shēn Dà Bǔ Tāng
(Ginseng Great Tonifying Decoction)

人參大補湯
人参大补汤

Pinyin Name: *Ren Shen Da Bu Tang*
Literal Name: Ginseng Great Tonifying Decoction
Original Source: *An Hui Zhong Yi Xue Yuan* (Anhui University School of Medicine) in 1990

Ren Shen (Radix et Rhizoma Ginseng)
Bai Zhu (Rhizoma Atractylodis Macrocephalae)
Huang Qi (Radix Astragali)
Zhi Gan Cao (Radix et Rhizoma Glycyrrhizae Praeparata cum Melle)
Chen Pi (Pericarpium Citri Reticulatae)
Dang Gui (Radix Angelicae Sinensis)
Di Huang (Radix Rehmanniae)
Mai Dong (Radix Ophiopogonis)
Zhu Ru (Caulis Bambusae in Taenia)
Gou Qi Zi (Fructus Lycii)
Dong Chong Xia Cao (Cordyceps)
Ling Zhi (Ganoderma)
Shi Di (Calyx Kaki)

Ren Shen Da Bu Tang (Ginseng Great Tonifying Decoction) is a well-balanced formula to tonify qi, blood, yin, and yang. It treats individuals with extreme weakness and deficiency following chronic and debilitating illnesses.

TONIC FORMULAS

8

613

Chapter 8 – Tonic Formulas

Section 3 – Qi- and Blood-Tonifying Formulas

Shí Quán Dà Bǔ Tāng (All-Inclusive Great Tonifying Decoction)

Function	Composition	Si Jun Zi Tang	Si Wu Tang	Ba Zhen Tang	Shi Quan Da Bu Tang
Tonifies qi	*Ren Shen* (Radix et Rhizoma Ginseng)	✓		✓	✓
	Bai Zhu (Rhizoma Atractylodis Macrocephalae)	✓		✓	✓
	Fu Ling (Poria)	✓		✓	✓
	Zhi Gan Cao (Radix et Rhizoma Glycyrrhizae Praeparata cum Melle)	✓		✓	✓
Tonifies blood	*Dang Gui* (Radix Angelicae Sinensis)		✓	✓	✓
	Chuan Xiong (Rhizoma Chuanxiong)		✓	✓	✓
	Bai Shao (Radix Paeoniae Alba)		✓	✓	✓
	Shu Di Huang (Radix Rehmanniae Praeparata)		✓	✓	✓
Warms and lifts yang	*Huang Qi* (Radix Astragali)				✓
	Rou Gui (Cortex Cinnamomi)				✓

AUTHORS' COMMENTS

Si Jun Zi Tang (Four-Gentlemen Decoction), *Si Wu Tang* (Four-Substance Decoction), *Ba Zhen Tang* (Eight-Treasure Decoction), and *Shi Quan Da Bu Tang* (All-Inclusive Great Tonifying Decoction) illustrate the principles of combining formulas to treat various associated conditions.

References

1. *Zhong Yi Fang Ji Xian Dai Yan Jiu* (Modern Study of Medical Formulae in Traditional Chinese Medicine) 1997;652-654.
2. *Zhong Xi Yi Jie He Za Zhi* (Journal of Integrated Chinese and Western Medicine) 1989;9(10):622.
3. *Shan Xi Zhong Yi Xue Yuan Xue Bao* (Journal of Shanxi University School of Chinese Medicine) 1986;2:40.
4. *Zhong Yao Yao Li Yu Lin Chuang* (Pharmacology and Clinical Applications of Chinese Herbs) 1992;152.
5. *Zhong Yi Fang Ji Xian Dai Yan Jiu* (Modern Study of Medical Formulae in Traditional Chinese Medicine) 1997;655.
6. Saiki I. A Kampo medicine "Juzen-taiho-to"--prevention of malignant progression and metastasis of tumor cells and the mechanism of action. Biological & Pharmaceutical Bulletin 2000 Jun;23(6):677-88.
7. Ohnishi Y, Fujii H, Hayakawa Y, Sakukawa R, Yamaura T, Sakamoto T, Tsukada K, Fujimaki M, Nunome S, Komatsu Y, Saiki I. Oral administration of a Kampo (Japanese herbal) medicine Juzen-taiho-to inhibits liver metastasis of colon 26-L5 carcinoma cells. Jpn J Cancer Res 1998 Feb;89(2):206-13.
8. Mori H, Niwa K, Zheng Q, Yamada Y, Sakata K, Yoshimi N. Cell proliferation in cancer prevention; effects of preventive agents on estrogen-related endometrial carcinogenesis model and on an in vitro model in human colorectal cells. Mutation Research 2001 Sep 1;480-481:201-7.
9. Dai Y, Kato M, Takeda K, Kawamoto Y, Akhand AA, Hossain K, Suzuki H, Nakashima I. T-cell-immunity-based inhibitory effects of orally administered herbal medicine juzen-taiho-to on the growth of primarily developed melanocytic tumors in RET-transgenic mice. J Invest Dermatol 2001 Sep;117(3):694-701.
10. Tagami K, Niwa K, Lian Z, Gao J, Mori H, Tamaya T. Preventive effect of Juzen-taiho-to on endometrial carcinogenesis in mice is based on Shimotsu-to constituent. Biol Pharm Bull 2004 Feb;27(2):156-61.
11. *Zhong Cheng Yao* (Study of Chinese Patent Medicine) 1991;13(10):31.
12. *Guo Wai Yi Xue Zhong Yi Zhong Yao Fen Ce* (Monograph of Chinese Herbology from Foreign Medicine) 1991;13(4):42.
13. Hidaka S, Okamoto Y, Nakajima K, Suekawa M, Liu SY. Preventive effects of traditional Chinese (Kampo) medicines on experimental osteoporosis induced by ovariectomy in rats. Calcif Tissue Int 1997 Sep;61(3):239-46.
14. Tatsuta M, Iishi H, Baba M, Nakaizumi A, Uehara H. Inhibition by shi-quan-da-bu-tang (TJ-48) of experimental hepatocarcinogenesis induced by N-nitrosomorpholine in Sprague-Dawley rats. Eur J Cancer 1994;30A(1):74-8.
15. *He Bei Zhong Yi* (Hebei Chinese Medicine) 1987;6:16.
16. *Fu Jian Zhong Yi Yao* (Fujian Chinese Medicine and Herbology) 1985;3:19.
17. Horie Y, Kato K, Kameoka S, Hamano K. Bu ji (hozai) for treatment of postoperative gastric cancer patients. Am J Chin Med 1994;22(3-4):309-19.
18. Zee-Cheng RK. Shi-quan-da-bu-tang (ten significant tonic decoction), SQT. A potent Chinese biological response modifier in cancer immunotherapy, potentiation and detoxification of anticancer drugs. Methods Find Exp Clin Pharmacol 1992 Nov;14(9):725-36.
19. *Zhong Xi Yi Jie He Za Zhi* (Journal of Integrated Chinese and Western Medicine) 1989;10:622.
20. *Guang Xi Zhong Yi Yao* (Guangxi Chinese Medicine and Herbology) 1987;1:14.
21. *Liao Ning Zhong Yi Za Zhi* (Liaoning Journal of Chinese Medicine) 1987;1:22.
22. Hisha H, Kohdera U, Hirayama M, Yamada H, Iguchi-Uehira T, Fan TX, Cui YZ, Yang GX, Li Y, Sugiura K, Inaba M, Kobayashi Y, Ikehara S. Treatment of Shwachman syndrome by Japanese herbal medicine (Juzen-taiho-to): stimulatory effects of its fatty acids on hemopoiesis in patients. Stem Cells 2002;20(4):311-9.
23. Ikehara S, Kawamura H, Komatsu Y, Yamada H, Hisha H, Yasumizu R, Ohnishi-Inoue Y, Kiyohara H, Hirano M, Aburada M, et al. Effects of medicinal plants on hemopoietic cells. Adv Exp Med Biol 1992;319:319-30.
24. *Zhong Yi Fang Ji Xian Dai Yan Jiu* (Modern Study of Medical Formulae in Traditional Chinese Medicine) 1997;658-659.
25. Zee-Cheng RK. Shi-quan-da-bu-tang (ten significant tonic decoction), SQT. A potent Chinese biological response modifier in cancer immunotherapy, potentiation and detoxification of anticancer drugs. Methods Find Exp Clin Pharmacol 1992 Nov;14(9):725-36.
26. *Shi Yong Zhong Xi Yi Jie He Za Zhi* (Practical Journal of Integrated Chinese and Western Medicines) 1995;6:376.
27. Abe S, Ishibashi H, Tansho S, Hanazawa R, Komatsu Y, Yamaguchi H. Protective effect of oral administration of several traditional

614

Shí Quán Dà Bǔ Tāng (All-Inclusive Great Tonifying Decoction)

Kampo-medicines on lethal Candida infection in immunosuppressed mice. Nippon Ishinkin Gakkai Zasshi 2000;41(2):115-9.

28. Sugiyama K, Ueda H, Ichio Y. Protective effect of juzen-taiho-to against carboplatin-induced toxic side effects in mice. Biol Pharm Bull 1995 Apr;18(4):544-8.

29. Sugiyama K, Ueda H, Ichio Y, Yokota M. Improvement of cisplatin toxicity and lethality by juzen-taiho-to in mice. Biol Pharm Bull 1995 Jan;18(1):53-8.

30. Sugiyama K, Ueda H, Suhara Y, Kajima Y, Ichio Y, Yokota M. Protective effect of sodium L-malate, an active constituent isolated from Angelicae radix, on cis-diamminedichloroplatinum(II)-induced toxic side effect. Chem Pharm Bull (Tokyo) 1994 Dec;42(12):2565-8.

31. Muraishi Y, Mitani N, Yamaura T, Fuse H, Saiki I. Effect of interferon-alpha A/D in combination with the Japanese and Chinese traditional herbal medicine juzen-taiho-to on lung metastasis of murine renal cell carcinoma. Anticancer Res 2000 Sep-Oct;20(5A):2931-7.

32. *Hu Bei Zhong Yi Za Zhi* (Hubei Journal of Chinese Medicine) 1981;4:29.

33. Hasegawa T, Yamaki K, Muraoka I, Nadai M, Takagi K, Nabeshima T. Effects of traditional Chinese medicines on pharmacokinetics of levofloxacin. Antimicrobial Agents & Chemotherapy 1995 Sep; 39(9):2135-7.

34. *He Han Yi Yao Xue Hui Zhi* (Hehan Journal of Medicine and Herbology) 1984;1(1):68.

Rén Shēn Yǎng Yíng Tāng
(Ginseng Decoction to Nourish the Nutritive Qi)

人參養榮湯
人参养荣汤

Pinyin Name: *Ren Shen Yang Ying Tang*

Literal Name: Ginseng Decoction to Nourish the Nutritive Qi

Alternate Names: *Jen Shen Yang Yung Tang* (*Wan*), *Ren Shen Yang Rong Tang* (*Wan*), *Yang Ying Tang*, Ginseng Nutritive Decoction (Pill), Ginseng Nutrition Decoction (Pill), Nourish the Nutritive Qi Decoction, Ginseng and Rehmannia Combination

Original Source: *Tai Ping Hui Min He Ji Ju Fang* (Imperial Grace Formulary of the Tai Ping Era) by the Imperial Medical Department in 1078-85

COMPOSITION

Ren Shen (Radix et Rhizoma Ginseng)	30g [6g]
Huang Qi (Radix Astragali)	30g [12g]
Bai Zhu (Rhizoma Atractylodis Macrocephalae), *wei* (roasted)	30g [6g]
Shu Di Huang (Radix Rehmanniae Praeparata), *zhi* (prepared)	22.5g [9g]
Dang Gui (Radix Angelicae Sinensis)	30g [9g]
Bai Shao (Radix Paeoniae Alba)	90g [18g]
Wu Wei Zi (Fructus Schisandrae Chinensis)	22.5g [4g]
Fu Ling (Poria)	22.5g [4g]
Yuan Zhi (Radix Polygalae), *chao* (dry-fried)	15g [6g]
Chen Pi (Pericarpium Citri Reticulatae)	30g [6g]
Gui Xin (Cortex Rasus Cinnamomi)	30g [3g]
Zhi Gan Cao (Radix et Rhizoma Glycyrrhizae Praeparata cum Melle)	30g [3g]

DOSAGE / PREPARATION / ADMINISTRATION

Grind the ingredients into powder. Cook 12g of the powder with 3 slices of *Sheng Jiang* (Rhizoma Zingiberis Recens) and 2 pieces of *Da Zao* (Fructus Jujubae) in 1.5 bowls of water until the liquid is reduced to 70%. Take the strained decoction while warm. Today, the decoction may be prepared using the doses suggested in brackets.

CHINESE THERAPEUTIC ACTIONS

1. Tonifies both qi and blood
2. Nourishes the Heart and calms the *shen* (spirit)

CLINICAL MANIFESTATIONS

Exhaustion of the body due to consumptive diseases: lassitude, weakness, a sallow complexion, shortness of

Chapter 8 – Tonic Formulas   *Section 3 – Qi- and Blood-Tonifying Formulas*

Rén Shēn Yǎng Yíng Tāng
(Ginseng Decoction to Nourish the Nutritive Qi)

breath, dyspnea upon mild exertion, dizziness, palpitations, tendency to being easily frightened, insomnia, and a dry throat and lips.

CLINICAL APPLICATIONS

Anemia, chronic fatigue syndrome, emaciation, insomnia, connective tissue diseases, Raynaud's disease, micturition syncope, nephritis, male infertility, irregular menstruation, uterine bleeding, hepatitis C, cancer, and lung carcinoma.

EXPLANATION

Ren Shen Yang Ying Tang (Ginseng Decoction to Nourish the Nutritive Qi) treats qi and blood deficiencies accompanied by Heart instability. This syndrome usually follows exhaustion of the body from chronic consumptive diseases, in which both the qi and the blood are depleted. Qi deficiency may lead to lassitude, weakness, and shortness of breath. Blood deficiency leading to lack of nourishment to the Heart may cause dizziness, palpitations, and insomnia. Depletion of blood may lead to yin or blood deficiency, which causes the dry throat and lips.

Ren Shen (Radix et Rhizoma Ginseng), *Huang Qi* (Radix Astragali), and *Bai Zhu* (Rhizoma Atractylodis Macrocephalae) tonify qi. *Shu Di Huang* (Radix Rehmanniae Praeparata), *Dang Gui* (Radix Angelicae Sinensis), and *Bai Shao* (Radix Paeoniae Alba) tonify the blood. *Wu Wei Zi* (Fructus Schisandrae Chinensis), *Fu Ling* (Poria), and *Yuan Zhi* (Radix Polygalae) nourish the Heart and calm the *shen* (spirit). *Chen Pi* (Pericarpium Citri Reticulatae)

regulates qi flow and counteracts the stagnating properties of the tonic herbs. *Gui Xin* (Cortex Rasus Cinnamomi) tonifies yang and helps the regeneration of qi and blood. *Zhi Gan Cao* (Radix et Rhizoma Glycyrrhizae Praeparata cum Melle) tonifies qi and harmonizes the herbs. *Sheng Jiang* (Rhizoma Zingiberis Recens) and *Da Zao* (Fructus Jujubae) regulate the middle *jiao* and tonify qi and blood.

MODIFICATIONS

- With poor appetite, add *Cang Zhu* (Rhizoma Atractylodis) and *Hou Po* (Cortex Magnoliae Officinalis).
- With cough due to Lung deficiency, add *Chuan Bei Mu* (Bulbus Fritillariae Cirrhosae) and *Ku Xing Ren* (Semen Armeniacae Amarum).
- With a dry mouth and tongue, add *Mai Dong* (Radix Ophiopogonis) or *Tian Hua Fen* (Radix Trichosanthis).
- If there is spermatorrhea or nocturnal emissions, add *Long Gu* (Os Draconis) or *Jin Suo Gu Jing Wan* (Metal Lock Pill to Stabilize the Essence).
- With palpitations, fear, and fright, combine with *Yang Xin Tang* (Nourish the Heart Decoction).
- With fatigue due to Spleen deficiency, combine with *Gui Pi Tang* (Restore the Spleen Decoction).

PHARMACOLOGICAL EFFECTS

1. **Immunostimulant**: Administration of *Ren Shen Yang Ying Tang* in healthy male volunteers was associated with an increase in natural killer (NK) cells of up to 11% compared to the control group that did not receive any herbs.[1] In

Ren Shen Yang Ying Tang (Ginseng Decoction to Nourish the Nutritive Qi)

Diagnosis	Signs and Symptoms	Treatment	Herbs
Exhaustion of the body due to consumptive diseases	• Lassitude, weakness, and shortness of breath: qi deficiency • Dizziness, palpitations, and insomnia: blood deficiency • Dry throat and lips: yin and blood deficiencies	• Tonifies qi and blood • Nourishes the Heart and calms the *shen* (spirit)	• *Ren Shen* (Radix et Rhizoma Ginseng), *Huang Qi* (Radix Astragali) and *Bai Zhu* (Rhizoma Atractylodis Macrocephalae) tonify qi. • *Shu Di Huang* (Radix Rehmanniae Praeparata), *Dang Gui* (Radix Angelicae Sinensis) and *Bai Shao* (Radix Paeoniae Alba) tonify the blood. • *Wu Wei Zi* (Fructus Schisandrae Chinensis), *Fu Ling* (Poria) and *Yuan Zhi* (Radix Polygalae) nourish the Heart and calm the *shen*. • *Chen Pi* (Pericarpium Citri Reticulatae) regulates qi circulation. • *Gui Xin* (Cortex Rasus Cinnamomi) tonifies yang. • *Zhi Gan Cao* (Radix et Rhizoma Glycyrrhizae Praeparata cum Melle) harmonizes all of the herbs. • *Sheng Jiang* (Rhizoma Zingiberis Recens) and *Da Zao* (Fructus Jujubae) regulate the middle *jiao*.

616

Chinese Herbal Formulas and Applications

Rén Shēn Yǎng Yíng Tāng
(Ginseng Decoction to Nourish the Nutritive Qi)

another study, administration of this formula at 15g/day for one week to healthy people was associated with an increase of NK cells activity. This study suggested that *Ren Shen Yang Ying Tang* may be useful in the prevention of carcinogenesis.[2] It also significantly (P less than 0.01) augmented the production of granulocyte-macrophage colony-stimulating factor (GM-CSF).[3]

2. **Antihyperlipidemic**: Administration of *Ren Shen Yang Ying Tang* was associated with a reduction of plasma triglyceride levels.[4]

CLINICAL STUDIES AND RESEARCH

1. **Anemia**: In one study, 30 anemic patients (between age 30-55) were treated with iron supplements and *Ren Shen Yang Ying Tang* with satisfactory results.[5]

2. **Chronic fatigue syndrome**: *Ren Shen Yang Ying Tang* was used to treat 35 patients with chronic fatigue syndrome for over 6 months. The patients were treated for a total of 1-9 months. Out of 35 patients, the study reported improvement in 26 patients. No side effect or abnormal reactions were reported in the liver and kidneys.[6]

3. **Connective tissue diseases**: *Ren Shen Yang Ying Tang* was used to treat Raynaud's disease, scleroderma, mixed connective tissue disease (MCTD), and systemic lupus erythematosus (SLE). The treatment protocol was to administer 9g of the formula in extract daily for 4 weeks per course of treatment.[7]

4. **Raynaud's disease**: An extract of *Ren Shen Yang Ying Tang* successfully treated 39 patients with Raynaud's disease. Resolution of overall symptoms and increased temperature was reported in 16 patients, and alleviation of dryness in 2 patients. Five patients, however, experienced side effects, such as decreased appetite and abdominal pain.[8]

5. **Micturition syncope**: Administration of *Ren Shen Yang Ying Tang* was effective in treating micturition syncope. Of 25 patients, the study reported complete recovery in 20 patients, marked improvement in 3 patients, improvement in 1 patient, and no change in 1 patient.[9]

6. **Nephritis**: One study reported 74% effectiveness (71 out of 94 patients) in using *Ren Shen Yang Ying Tang* to treat nephritis. Improvements included the gradual resolution of symptoms such as edema, thirst, fever, and dysuria.[10]

7. **Male infertility**: Concurrent use of *Ren Shen Yang Ying Tang* and *Gui Zhi Fu Ling Wan* (Cinnamon Twig and Poria Pill) for 3 months effectively treated male infertility in 19 patients by increasing sperm count, concentration, and motility.[11]

8. **Hepatitis C**: One study reported *Ren Shen Yang Ying Tang* to be very effective in treating chronic hepatitis C. The mechanism of this effect was attributed to an inhibitory effect on hepatitis C virus infection, and also from the protective effect on immunological hepatopathy. *Wu Wei Zi* (Fructus Schisandrae Chinensis) contains gomisin A, which is believed to be the most active herbal component of this formula for this indication.[12]

9. **Cancer**: In one study, 35 patients with cancer of the genitourinary tract were treated with integrative medicine. Following surgery and/or chemotherapy, all patients were given a liquid extract of *Ren Shen Yang Ying Tang* for 4-12 weeks. The study reported that the herbs enhanced recovery and minimized the side effects of standard surgery and/or chemotherapy treatments.[13]

10. **Lung carcinoma**: Administration of *Ren Shen Yang Ying Tang* had a positive effect on life expectancy for patients with lung carcinoma. It decreased tumor marker levels (CEA and CA19-9), relieved cough, and improved appetite. The treatment protocol was to administer 15g of extract per day for 7 weeks.[14]

HERB-DRUG INTERACTION

• **Cyclophosphamide- or 5-fluorouracil-induced leukopenia**: One study compared the effect of *Ren Shen Yang Ying Tang* and recombinant human granulocyte-colony stimulating factor (rhuG-CSF) on leukopenia induced by cyclophosphamide (CY) or 5-fluorouracil (5-FU). Leukopenia was induced by subcutaneous injection of 200 mg/kg of CY or 5-FU, and severe reduction of leukocyte numbers in the peripheral blood was observed. Treatment protocol was daily administration of *Ren Shen Yang Ying Tang* (1 g/kg/day) and rhuG-CSF (2 mcg/mouse/day). The study reported that administration of *Ren Shen Yang Ying Tang* and rhuG-CSF decreased the number of colony-forming units in the spleen (CFU-S) in drug-treated mice. *Ren Shen Yang Ying Tang* was more effective for improving host resistance against 5-FU, and rhuG-CSF was more effective against CY.[15]

• **Cyclophosphamide- or prednisolone-induced immunosuppression**: One study demonstrated that *Shi Quan Da Bu Tang* (All-Inclusive Great Tonifying Decoction) and *Ren Shen Yang Ying Tang* effectively prolonged survival rate and life span in mice with candida infection associated with immunosuppression induced by cyclophosphamide or prednisolone.[16]

• **Scopolamine**: One study reported that *Ren Shen Yang Ying Tang* was associated with improvement in scopolamine-induced impairment of passive avoidance response in mice by enhancing the cholinergic system.[17]

AUTHORS' COMMENTS

Ren Shen Yang Ying Tang is one of the preferred tonic formulas for deficient patients, since its thermal nature is neutral and will not create heat nor cold in patients when

TONIC FORMULAS

8

Chapter 8 – Tonic Formulas | Section 3 – Qi- and Blood-Tonifying Formulas

Rén Shēn Yǎng Yíng Tāng
(Ginseng Decoction to Nourish the Nutritive Qi)

taken over a long period of time. Also, it does not cause stagnation like many heavy tonics.

Ren Shen Yang Ying Tang, *Sheng Mai San* (Generate the Pulse Powder), and *Yu Ping Feng San* (Jade Windscreen Powder) can be used together to enhance the immune system of individuals who catch colds frequently.

References

1. *Guo Wai Yi Xue Zhong Yi Zhong Yao Fen Ce* (Monograph of Chinese Herbology from Foreign Medicine) 1992;14(2):52.
2. Kamei T, Kumano H, Beppu K, Iwata K, Masumura S. Response of healthy individuals to ninjin-yoei-to extract--enhancement of natural killer cell activity. American Journal of Chinese Medicine 1998;26(1):91-5.
3. Okamura S, Shimoda K, Yu LX, Omori F, Niho Y. A traditional Chinese herbal medicine, ren-shen-yang-rong-tang (Japanese name: ninjin-yoei-to) augments the production of granulocyte-macrophage colony-stimulating factor from human peripheral blood mononuclear cells in vitro. Int J Immunopharmacol 1991;13(5):595-8.
4. *He Han Yi Yao Xue Hui Zhi* (Hehan Journal of Medicine and Herbology) 1994;44(5):207.
5. *Zhong Yi Fang Ji Xian Dai Yan Jiu* (Modern Study of Medical Formulae in Traditional Chinese Medicine) 1997;4(1):73.
6. *He Han Yi Yao Xue Hui Zhi* (Hehan Journal of Medicine and Herbology) 1991;8(3):414.
7. *Zhong Yi Fang Ji Xian Dai Yan Jiu* (Modern Study of Medical Formulae in Traditional Chinese Medicine) 1997;639.
8. *Guo Wai Yi Xue* (Foreign Medicine) 1992;2:107.
9. *Xin Zhong Yi* (New Chinese Medicine) 1991;9:33.
10. *Xin Zhong Yi Yao* (New Chinese Medicine and Medicinals) 1957;1:24.
11. *Zhong Yi Fang Ji Xian Dai Yan Jiu* (Modern Study of Medical Formulae in Traditional Chinese Medicine) 1997;639.
12. Cyong JC, Ki SM, Iijima K, Kobayashi T, Furuya M. Clinical and pharmacological studies on liver diseases treated with Kampo herbal medicine. American Journal of Chinese Medicine 2000;28 (3-4):351-60.
13. *Xin Yao Yu Lin Chuang* (New Medicine and the Clinical Application) 1993;42(4):91.
14. Kamei T, Kumano H, Iwata K, Nariai Y, Matsumoto T. The effect of a traditional Chinese prescription for a patient of lung carcinoma. Journal of Alternative & Complementary Medicine 2000 Dec;6(6):557-9.
15. Miura S, Takimoto H, Yoshikai Y, Kumazawa Y, Yamada A, Nomoto K. Protective effect of Ren-Shen-Yang-Rong-Tang (Ninjin-youei-to) in mice with drug-induced leukopenia against Pseudomonas aeruginosa infection. Int J Immunopharmacol 1992 Oct;14(7):1249-57.
16. Abe S, Ishibashi H, Tansho S, Hanazawa R, Komatsu Y, Yamaguchi H. Protective effect of oral administration of several traditional Kampo-medicines on lethal Candida infection in immunosuppressed mice. Nippon Ishinkin Gakkai Zasshi 2000;41(2):115-9.
17. Egashira N, Yuzurihara M, Hattori N, Sakakibara I, Ishige A. Ninjin-yoei-to (Ren-Shen-Yang-Rong-Tang) and Polygalae radix improves scopolamine-induced impairment of passive avoidance response in mice. Phytomedicine 2003;10(6-7):467-73.

Tài Shān Pán Shí Sǎn (Powder that Gives the Stability of Mount Tai)
泰山磐石散

Pinyin Name: *Tai Shan Pan Shi San*
Literal Name: Powder that Gives the Stability of Mount Tai
Original Source: *Jing Yue Quan Shu* (Collected Treatises of [Zhang] Jing Yue) by Zhang Jie-Bin (Zhang Jing-Yue) in 1624

COMPOSITION

Ren Shen (Radix et Rhizoma Ginseng)	3g [5g]
Huang Qi (Radix Astragali)	3g [15g]
Bai Zhu (Rhizoma Atractylodis Macrocephalae)	6g [10g]
Zhi Gan Cao (Radix et Rhizoma Glycyrrhizae Praeparata cum Melle)	1.5g [4g]
Shu Di Huang (Radix Rehmanniae Praeparata)	2.4g [10g]
Dang Gui (Radix Angelicae Sinensis)	3g [8g]
Bai Shao (Radix Paeoniae Alba)	2.4g [6g]
Xu Duan (Radix Dipsaci)	3g [5g]
Chuan Xiong (Rhizoma Chuanxiong)	2.4g [4g]
Huang Qin (Radix Scutellariae)	3g [5g]
Sha Ren (Fructus Amomi)	1.5g [4g]
Nuo Mi (Oryza Glutinosa)	a pinch [5g]

Chinese Herbal Formulas and Applications

Tài Shān Pán Shí Sǎn (Powder that Gives the Stability of Mount Tai)

DOSAGE / PREPARATION / ADMINISTRATION

The source text recommends to cook the ingredients in 1.5 bowls of water and reduce the liquid to 70%. Take the decoction between meals. During the first trimester of pregnancy, administer only one dose every 3 to 5 days. From the fourth months of pregnancy onward, this formula may be used safely without concerns. Today, the decoction may be prepared using the doses suggested in brackets. Take the decoction on an empty stomach in three equally-divided doses in the morning, afternoon, and at night.

CHINESE THERAPEUTIC ACTIONS

1. Tonifies qi and strengthens the Spleen
2. Nourishes the blood and stabilizes the fetus

CLINICAL MANIFESTATIONS

Qi and blood deficiencies during pregnancy: restless fetus, history of miscarriage or threatened miscarriage, a pale face, lassitude, general weakness, lack of appetite, a pale tongue with a thin, white tongue coating, and a slippery, forceless or deep, weak pulse.

CLINICAL APPLICATIONS

Pernicious vomiting, unstable pregnancy, painful menstruation, amenorrhea.

EXPLANATION

Tai Shan Pan Shi San (Powder that Gives the Stability of Mount Tai) treats instability of the fetus during pregnancy due to qi and blood deficiencies. A pale face, lassitude, general weakness, and lack of appetite are common signs of qi and blood deficiencies. A slippery, forceless pulse indicates pregnancy and underlying deficiency, and a deep, weak pulse indicates serious deficiency of qi and blood.

Ren Shen (Radix et Rhizoma Ginseng), *Huang Qi* (Radix Astragali), *Bai Zhu* (Rhizoma Atractylodis Macrocephalae), and *Zhi Gan Cao* (Radix et Rhizoma Glycyrrhizae Praeparata cum Melle) tonify qi and strengthen the Spleen. *Shu Di Huang* (Radix Rehmanniae Praeparata), *Dang Gui* (Radix Angelicae Sinensis), *Bai Shao* (Radix Paeoniae Alba), and *Xu Duan* (Radix Dipsaci) nourish the blood and tonify the Liver and Kidney. *Chuan Xiong* (Rhizoma Chuanxiong) regulates qi and blood circulation. *Huang Qin* (Radix Scutellariae) is combined with *Bai Zhu* (Rhizoma Atractylodis Macrocephalae) to clear heat, strengthen the Spleen, and stabilize the fetus. *Sha Ren* (Fructus Amomi) regulates qi, harmonizes the middle *jiao*, and stabilizes the fetus. *Nuo Mi* (Oryza Glutinosa) nourishes the Spleen and Stomach to ensure a healthy digestive system.

Tai Shan Pan Shi San is a modified version of *Shi Quan Da Bu Tang* (All-Inclusive Great Tonifying Decoction). *Rou Gui* (Cortex Cinnamomi) is removed because its warm property may disturb the fetus, and *Fu Ling* (Poria) is taken out because its downward draining effect is undesirable during pregnancy. *Xu Duan* (Radix Dipsaci), *Huang Qin* (Radix Scutellariae), *Sha Ren* (Fructus Amomi), and *Nuo Mi* (Oryza Glutinosa) are added as they all can stabilize the fetus.

Tai Shan Pan Shi San (Powder that Gives the Stability of Mount Tai)

Diagnosis	Signs and Symptoms	Treatment	Herbs
Qi and blood deficiencies during pregnancy	• Restless fetus: unstable pregnancy • Pale face, lassitude, general weakness, and lack of appetite: qi and blood deficiency • Pale tongue with a thin white tongue coating, and a slippery, forceless or deep, weak pulse: deficiency condition	• Tonifies qi and strengthens the Spleen • Nourishes the blood and stabilizes the fetus	• *Ren Shen* (Radix et Rhizoma Ginseng), *Huang Qi* (Radix Astragali), *Bai Zhu* (Rhizoma Atractylodis Macrocephalae) and *Zhi Gan Cao* (Radix et Rhizoma Glycyrrhizae Praeparata cum Melle) tonify qi and strengthen the Spleen. • *Shu Di Huang* (Radix Rehmanniae Praeparata), *Dang Gui* (Radix Angelicae Sinensis), *Bai Shao* (Radix Paeoniae Alba) and *Xu Duan* (Radix Dipsaci) nourish the blood and tonify the Liver and Kidney. • *Chuan Xiong* (Rhizoma Chuanxiong) regulates qi and blood circulation. • *Huang Qin* (Radix Scutellariae), *Bai Zhu* (Rhizoma Atractylodis Macrocephalae) and *Sha Ren* (Fructus Amomi) stabilize the fetus. • *Nuo Mi* (Oryza Glutinosa) nourishes the Spleen and Stomach.

TONIC FORMULAS

8

619

Chapter 8 – Tonic Formulas   Section 3 – Qi- and Blood-Tonifying Formulas

Tāi Shān Pán Shí Sǎn (Powder that Gives the Stability of Mount Tai)

MODIFICATIONS

- With severe vomiting, add *Zhu Ru* (Caulis Bambusae in Taenia), *Pi Pa Ye* (Folium Eriobotryae), *Ban Xia* (Rhizoma Pinelliae), and *Sheng Jiang* (Rhizoma Zingiberis Recens).
- With vomiting of yellow or green fluids, add *Huang Lian* (Rhizoma Coptidis).
- With depletion of body fluids, add *Xuan Shen* (Radix Scrophulariae) and *Mai Dong* (Radix Ophiopogonis).
- With unstable pregnancy, add *Du Zhong* (Cortex Eucommiae) and *E Jiao* (Colla Corii Asini).
- With more heat, increase the dose of *Huang Qin* (Radix Scutellariae) and decrease the dose of *Sha Ren* (Fructus Amomi).
- With Stomach deficiency, increase the dose of *Sha Ren* (Fructus Amomi) and decrease the dose of *Huang Qin* (Radix Scutellariae).
- With palpitations and insomnia, add *Suan Zao Ren* (Semen Ziziphi Spinosae), *Long Yan Rou* (Arillus Longan), and *Shou Wu Teng* (Caulis Polygoni Multiflori).
- With soreness and pain of the lower back, add *Du Zhong* (Cortex Eucommiae) and *Tu Si Zi* (Semen Cuscutae).
- When there are warning signs of miscarriage, such as vaginal bleeding and downward movement of the fetus, add *E Jiao* (Colla Corii Asini) and *Ai Ye* (Folium Artemisiae Argyi).

CAUTIONS / CONTRAINDICATIONS

While *Tai Shan Pan Shi San* is formulated specifically for pregnant women, it is not without risks. Herbs should be used for pregnant women only when the benefits outweigh the risks.

CLINICAL STUDIES AND RESEARCH

1. **Pernicious vomiting**: Modified *Tai Shan Pan Shi San* successfully treated vomiting during pregnancy. The formula included 7.5g each of *Dang Shen* (Radix Codonopsis), *Huang Qin* (Radix Scutellariae), *Bai Shao* (Radix Paeoniae Alba), and *Zhi Gan Cao* (Radix et Rhizoma Glycyrrhizae Praeparata cum Melle); 15g of *Huang Qi* (Radix Astragali); 10g each of *Dang Gui* (Radix Angelicae Sinensis), *Xu Duan* (Radix Dipsaci), and *Bai Zhu* (Rhizoma Atractylodis Macrocephalae); 5g each of *Chuan Xiong* (Rhizoma Chuanxiong), *Sha Ren* (Fructus Amomi), and *Geng Mi* (Semen Oryzae), and 20g of *Shu Di Huang* (Radix Rehmanniae Praeparata). *Zhu Ru* (Caulis Bambusae in Taenia), *Pi Pa Ye* (Folium Eriobotryae), *Ban Xia* (Rhizoma Pinelliae), and *Sheng Jiang* (Rhizoma Zingiberis Recens) were added for severe vomiting. *Huang Lian* (Rhizoma Coptidis) was added for vomiting of yellow or green fluids. *Xuan Shen* (Radix Scrophulariae) and *Mai Dong* (Radix Ophiopogonis) were added for depletion of body fluids. *Du Zhong* (Cortex Eucommiae) and *E Jiao*

(Colla Corii Asini) were added for unstable pregnancy. *Ren Shen* (Radix et Rhizoma Ginseng) and *Huang Qi* (Radix Astragali) were added for qi deficiency. The formulas were given as warm decoctions. Out of 88 patients, the study reported cessation of vomiting in 85 patients. Most patients responded within 1-6 doses of herbs.[1]

2. **Prevention of miscarriage**: Two studies have reported beneficial effects using *Tai Shan Pan Shi San* to prevent miscarriage in women with unstable pregnancy characterized by fatigue, poor appetite, abnormal bleeding, and other signs and symptoms of qi and blood deficiency.[2,3]

AUTHORS' COMMENTS

Today, *Tai Shan Pan Shi San* is used widely during pregnancy to prevent miscarriages. The standard protocol is to begin herbal therapy two months after conception. Take one dose of herbs in decoction form per week, for 2-3 months, for optimal effect.

Tai Shan Pan Shi San and *Ba Zhen Tang* (Eight-Treasure Decoction) both tonify qi and blood, but have the following differences:

- *Tai Shan Pan Shi San* is a qi and blood tonic that calms the fetus to treat unstable pregnancy and prevent habitual miscarriage due to deficiency.
- *Ba Zhen Tang* is a neutral-temperature tonic. It is mostly used for convalescing patients with qi and blood deficiencies, or those with sudden, profuse blood loss manifesting in dizziness, palpitations, shortness of breath, and lack of desire to speak.[4]

Tai Shan Pan Shi San and *Shi Quan Da Bu Tang* (All-Inclusive Great Tonifying Decoction) both use *Si Wu Tang* (Four-Substance Decoction) as the foundation to tonify the blood. They have the following differences:

- *Tai Shan Pan Shi San* is a qi and blood tonic that stabilizes the fetus; it contains *Xu Duan* (Radix Dipsaci), *Huang Qin* (Radix Scutellariae), *Bai Zhu* (Rhizoma Atractylodis Macrocephalae), and *Sha Ren* (Fructus Amomi). Clinical manifestations include qi and blood deficiencies with restless fetus or threatened miscarriage, a pale complexion, fatigue, poor appetite, a pale tongue, and a slippery, forceless or deep, weak pulse.
- *Shi Quan Da Bu Tang* is a warm tonic that replenishes qi and blood. Chief manifestations include chronic cough, poor appetite, weakness of the knees and back, non-healing ulcers, and chronic uterine bleeding, all due to qi and blood deficiencies.[5]

References
1. *Xin Jiang Zhong Yi Yao* (Xinjiang Chinese Medicine and Herbology) 1991;1:32.
2. *He Bei Zhong Yi* (Hebei Chinese Medicine) 1991;13(3):24.

620

Chinese Herbal Formulas and Applications

Tài Shān Pán Shí Săn (Powder that Gives the Stability of Mount Tai)

3. *Zhe Jiang Zhong Yi Xue Yuan Xue Bao* (Journal of Zhejiang University of Chinese Medicine) 1981;6:18.
4. Wang MZ, et al. *Zhong Yi Xue Wen Da Ti Ku* (Questions and Answers on Traditional Chinese Medicine: Herbal Formulas).
5. Wang MZ, et al. *Zhong Yi Xue Wen Da Ti Ku* (Questions and Answers on Traditional Chinese Medicine: Herbal Formulas).

Băo Chăn Wú Yōu Fāng
(Preserve Pregnancy and Care-Free Decoction)

保產無憂方
保产无忧方

Pinyin Name: *Bao Chan Wu You Fang*
Literal Name: Preserve Pregnancy and Care-Free Decoction
Alternate Names: *Pao Chan Wu You Fang*, Pregnancy Carefree Formula, Tangkuei and Parsley Combination
Original Source: *Fu Qing Zhu Nu Ke* (Women's Diseases According to Fu Qing-Zhu) by Fu Shan in 1827

COMPOSITION

Dang Gui (Radix Angelicae Sinensis), *xi* (washed) with liquor	4.5g
Chuan Xiong (Rhizoma Chuanxiong)	4.5g
Bai Shao (Radix Paeoniae Alba), *chao* (dry-fried) with liquor	3.6g
Hou Po (Cortex Magnoliae Officinalis), *chao* (dry-fried) with ginger	2.1g
Sheng Jiang (Rhizoma Zingiberis Recens)	3 slices
Zhi Qiao (Fructus Citri Aurantii), *chao* (dry-fried) with bran	1.8g
Chuan Bei Mu (Bulbus Fritillariae Cirrhosae)	3g
Huang Qi (Radix Astragali), *zhi* (fried with liquid)	2.4g
Ai Ye (Folium Artemisiae Argyi), *chao* (dry-fried)	2.1g
Jing Jie (Herba Schizonepetae), *chao* (dry-fried) till black	2.4g
Qiang Huo (Rhizoma et Radix Notopterygii)	1.5g
Tu Si Zi (Semen Cuscutae), *chao* (dry-fried) with liquor	4.2g
Gan Cao (Radix et Rhizoma Glycyrrhizae)	1.5g

DOSAGE / PREPARATION / ADMINISTRATION

Cook the ingredients in water to make a decoction. To preserve pregnancy, take the decoction while warm 3-5 times per month. To facilitate delivery, take the decoction while hot to induce labor.

CHINESE THERAPEUTIC ACTIONS

1. Benefits qi and nourishes the blood
2. Calms the fetus and stabilizes pregnancy
3. Induces labor before delivery

CLINICAL MANIFESTATIONS

Qi and blood deficiencies during pregnancy: nausea, vomiting, morning sickness, general weakness, soreness and pain of the lower back, abdominal pain, and general weakness. This formula can also be used to stabilize pregnancy in women with a prior history of miscarriage. It also facilitates labor and minimizes complications if taken immediately before delivery.

CLINICAL APPLICATIONS

Maintenance therapy during pregnancy, prevention of miscarriage, stabilization of pregnancy, and prevention of difficult labor.

EXPLANATION

Bao Chan Wu You Fang (Preserve Pregnancy and Care-Free Decoction) is designed specifically for women during pregnancy, with clinical applications such as stabilization of pregnancy, maintenance therapy during pregnancy, prevention of miscarriage, and facilitation of labor. Miscarriages or unstable pregnancies are generally caused

8

TONIC FORMULAS

621

Chapter 8 – Tonic Formulas   *Section 3 – Qi- and Blood-Tonifying Formulas*

Băo Chăn Wú Yōu Fāng
(Preserve Pregnancy and Care-Free Decoction)

Bao Chan Wu You Fang (Preserve Pregnancy and Care-Free Decoction)

Diagnosis	Signs and Symptoms	Treatment	Herbs
Qi and blood deficiencies during pregnancy	Nausea, vomiting, general weakness, soreness and pain of the lower back, abdominal pain, and general weakness: qi and blood deficiencies	• Benefits qi and nourishes the blood • Calms the fetus and stabilizes pregnancy	• *Dang Gui* (Radix Angelicae Sinensis), *Chuan Xiong* (Radix Ligustici) and *Bai Shao* (Radix Paeoniae Lactiflorae) nourish the blood. • *Hou Po* (Cortex Magnoliae Officinalis) regulates qi circulation. • *Sheng Jiang* (Rhizoma Zingiberis Officinalis Recens) harmonizes the middle *jiao* and warms the Spleen and Stomach. • *Zhi Qiao* (Fructus Citri Aurantii) and *Chuan Bei Mu* (Bulbus Fritillariae Cirrhosae) resolve stagnation and phlegm. • *Huang Qi* (Radix Astragali Membranacei) and *Ai Ye* (Folium Artemisiae Argyi) tonify qi and stop uterine bleeding. • *Jing Jie* (Herba Schizonepetae) stops bleeding. • *Qiang Huo* (Rhizoma et Radix Notopterygii) relieves pain. • *Tu Si Zi* (Semen Cuscutae Chinensis) tonifies Kidney yin and yang. • *Gan Cao* (Radix et Rhizoma Glycyrrhizae) harmonizes the herbs.

by qi and blood deficiencies. Deficiency of qi leads to the inability of the mother to hold the fetus in a safe and stable position, and deficiency of blood leads to inadequate nourishment of the fetus. This formula may also be used from the seventh month of pregnancy until labor to ensure a safe pregnancy and minimize complications. Finally, it can be used at the time of labor to induce contraction of the uterus and prevent difficult labor.

Dang Gui (Radix Angelicae Sinensis), *Chuan Xiong* (Radix Ligustici), and *Bai Shao* (Radix Paeoniae Lactiflorae) nourish the blood. *Hou Po* (Cortex Magnoliae Officinalis) regulates qi circulation. *Sheng Jiang* (Rhizoma Zingiberis Officinalis Recens) harmonizes the middle *jiao* and warms the Spleen and Stomach. Together, *Hou Po* (Cortex Magnoliae Officinalis) and *Sheng Jiang* (Rhizoma Zingiberis Recens) relieve nausea, vomiting, and morning sickness. *Zhi Qiao* (Fructus Citri Aurantii) and *Chuan Bei Mu* (Bulbus Fritillariae Cirrhosae) resolve stagnation and phlegm. *Huang Qi* (Radix Astragali Membranacei) and *Ai Ye* (Folium Artemisiae Argyi) treat unstable pregnancy by tonifying qi and stopping uterine bleeding. *Jing Jie* (Herba Schizonepetae) stops bleeding. *Qiang Huo* (Rhizoma et Radix Notopterygii) relieves pain. *Tu Si Zi* (Semen Cus-

cutae Chinensis) tonifies Kidney yin and yang. Lastly, *Gan Cao* (Radix et Rhizoma Glycyrrhizae) harmonizes the herbs.

MODIFICATIONS

• If there is restless fetus, add *Huang Qin* (Radix Scutellariae Baicalensis) and *Bai Zhu* (Rhizoma Atractylodis Macrocephalae).

• For unstable pregnancy with pain in the lower back, add *Xu Duan* (Radix Dipsaci Asperi) and *Du Zhong* (Cortex Eucommiae Ulmoidis).

• For unstable pregnancy with uterine bleeding, add *E Jiao* (Gelatinum Corii Asini), charred *Sheng Jiang* (Rhizoma Zingiberis Officinalis Recens), and *Di Huang* (Radix Rehmanniae Glutinosae).

• For unstable pregnancy with dizziness and vertigo, add *Ren Shen* (Radix et Rhizoma Ginseng) and *Bai Zhi* (Radix Angelicae Dahuricae).

CAUTIONS / CONTRAINDICATIONS

Although *Bao Chan Wu You Fang* is formulated specifically for pregnant women, it is not without risks. Herbs should be used for pregnant women only when the benefits outweigh the risks.

Chinese Herbal Formulas and Applications

Bǎo Chǎn Wú Yōu Fāng
(Preserve Pregnancy and Care-Free Decoction)

AUTHORS' COMMENTS

Tai Shan Pan Shi San (Powder that Gives the Stability of Mount Tai) and *Bao Chan Wu You Fang* both treat restless fetus and habitual miscarriage. The differences are as follows:

- *Tai Shan Pan Shi San* is stronger in tonifying qi and blood, strengthening the Spleen, and stabilizing pregnancy.
- *Bao Chan Wu You Fang* tonifies qi and blood, calms the fetus, and stabilizes pregnancy. It also promotes smooth delivery during labor.

Dāng Guī Sǎn (Tangkuei Powder)
當歸散
当归散

Pinyin Name: *Dang Gui San*
Literal Name: Tangkuei Powder
Alternate Name: Tangkuei Formula
Original Source: *Jin Gui Yao Lue* (Essentials from the Golden Cabinet) by Zhang Zhong-Jing in the Eastern Han Dynasty

COMPOSITION

Dang Gui (Radix Angelicae Sinensis)	48g
Bai Shao (Radix Paeoniae Alba)	48g
Chuan Xiong (Rhizoma Chuanxiong)	48g
Huang Qin (Radix Scutellariae)	48g
Bai Zhu (Rhizoma Atractylodis Macrocephalae)	24g

DOSAGE / PREPARATION / ADMINISTRATION

Grind the ingredients into a fine powder. Take 1 spoonful (6g) of powder per dose with a grain-based liquor two times daily.

CHINESE THERAPEUTIC ACTIONS

1. Nourishes the blood
2. Stabilizes pregnancy

CLINICAL MANIFESTATIONS

Blood deficiency during pregnancy: history of habitual miscarriage, unstable pregnancy, difficult labor, and postpartum weakness and anemia. Other indications of this formula include sore back and abdominal pain, hysteria, tidal fever with dryness, and thirst.

CLINICAL APPLICATIONS

Habitual miscarriage, unstable pregnancy, restless fetus, difficult labor, and general postpartum disorders.

EXPLANATION

Dang Gui San (Tangkuei Powder) treats general obstetric and gynecological problems associated with pregnancy.

Clinically, it is used to stabilize pregnancy and to prevent early labor and miscarriages. It can also treat postpartum disorders, such as weakness, anemia, sore back and abdominal pain, and tidal fever with dryness and thirst. The main diagnostic criterion, according to traditional Chinese medicine, is blood deficiency.

Dang Gui (Radix Angelicae Sinensis) tonifies the blood and activates blood circulation. *Bai Shao* (Radix Paeoniae Alba) nourishes the blood and consolidates yin. *Chuan Xiong* (Rhizoma Chuanxiong) regulates blood circulation. *Huang Qin* (Radix Scutellariae) clears heat and cools the blood to calm the fetus. *Bai Zhu* (Rhizoma Atractylodis Macrocephalae) strengthens the Spleen and benefits the blood. This is a well-balanced formula because it is neither stagnating nor drying in nature, and it is not cold in property.

MODIFICATIONS

- With headache due to wind-cold, add *Gui Zhi* (Ramulus Cinnamomi) and *Chai Hu* (Radix Bupleuri).
- With sore back and abdominal pain, add *Zhi Shi* (Fructus Aurantii Immaturus) and *Xiang Fu* (Rhizoma Cyperi).

TONIC FORMULAS

8

623

Chapter 8 – Tonic Formulas

Section 3 – Qi- and Blood-Tonifying Formulas

Dāng Guī Sǎn (Tangkuei Powder)

Dang Gui San (Tangkuei Powder)

Diagnosis	Signs and Symptoms	Treatment	Herbs
Blood deficiency during pregnancy	Habitual miscarriage, unstable pregnancy, difficult labor, and postpartum weakness and anemia	• Nourishes the blood • Stabilizes pregnancy	• *Dang Gui* (Radix Angelicae Sinensis) tonifies the blood. • *Bai Shao* (Radix Paeoniae Alba) nourishes the blood and consolidates yin. • *Chuan Xiong* (Rhizoma Chuanxiong) regulates blood circulation. • *Huang Qin* (Radix Scutellariae) clears heat and cools the blood to calm the fetus. • *Bai Zhu* (Rhizoma Atractylodis Macrocephalae) strengthens the Spleen and benefits the blood.

- With thirst due to dryness and heat, add *Huang Lian* (Rhizoma Coptidis) and *Zhi Mu* (Rhizoma Anemarrhenae).
- For postpartum care, combine with *Sheng Hua Tang* (Generation and Transformation Decoction).

CAUTIONS / CONTRAINDICATIONS

Although *Dang Gui San* is formulated specifically for pregnant women, it is not without risks. Herbs should be used for pregnant women only when the benefits outweigh the risks.

Xiōng Guī Tiáo Xuè Yǐn
(Cnidium and Tangkuei Decoction to Regulate Blood)

芎歸調血飲

芎归调血饮

Pinyin Name: *Xiong Gui Tiao Xue Yin*
Literal Name: Cnidium and Tangkuei Decoction to Regulate Blood
Alternate Names: *Xiong Gui Bu Xue Tang* (Cnidium and Tangkuei Decoction to Tonify Blood), Cnidium and Rehmannia Combination
Original Source: *Wan Bing Hui Chun* (Restoration of Health from the Myriad Diseases) by Gong Ting-Xian in 1587

COMPOSITION

Dang Gui (Radix Angelicae Sinensis)

Chuan Xiong (Rhizoma Chuanxiong)

Shu Di Huang (Radix Rehmanniae Praeparata)

Bai Zhu (Rhizoma Atractylodis Macrocephalae)

Fu Ling (Poria)

Gan Cao (Radix et Rhizoma Glycyrrhizae)

Chen Pi (Pericarpium Citri Reticulatae)

Wu Yao (Radix Linderae)

Xiang Fu (Rhizoma Cyperi), *chao* (dry-fried) with *Tong Bian* (Infantis Urina)

Mu Dan Pi (Cortex Moutan)

Yi Mu Cao (Herba Leonuri)

Gan Jiang (Rhizoma Zingiberis), *chao* (dry-fried) to black

Chinese Herbal Formulas and Applications

Xiōng Guī Tiáo Xuè Yǐn
(Cnidium and Tangkuei Decoction to Regulate Blood)

DOSAGE / PREPARATION / ADMINISTRATION

Cook the ingredients with 1 slice of *Sheng Jiang* (Rhizoma Zingiberis Recens) and 1 piece of *Da Zao* (Fructus Jujubae). Take the strained decoction while warm. For postpartum care, take this formula with a small amount of warm, grain-based liquor and *Tong Bian* (Infantis Urina). Note: The source text did not specify the doses of the herbs.

CHINESE THERAPEUTIC ACTIONS

1. Tonifies qi and blood
2. Harmonizes the Liver and Spleen
3. Regulates menstruation

CLINICAL MANIFESTATIONS

Postpartum complications: profuse bleeding, excessive loss of blood, spontaneous perspiration, a dry mouth, dizziness, light-headedness, tinnitus, emotional instability, fullness and distention of the hypochondrium, delirium, irritability, epigastric and abdominal pain, poor appetite, fever, and aversion to cold.

CLINICAL APPLICATIONS

Supportive treatment for various types of postpartum complications, such as anemia, retention of lochia, irregular menstruation, insufficient lactation, functional uterine bleeding, nausea, vomiting, and erratic behavior.

EXPLANATION

Xiong Gui Tiao Xue Yin (Cnidium and Tangkuei Decoction to Regulate Blood) treats various types of postpartum complications, including bleeding, qi and blood deficiencies, and disharmony of the Liver, Spleen, and Stomach. Due to postpartum bleeding, patients are likely to have both qi and blood deficiencies, with symptoms and signs such as spontaneous perspiration, a dry mouth, dizziness, light-headedness, and tinnitus. With Liver qi stagnation, patients experience emotional instability, fullness and distention of the hypochondrium, delirium, and irritability. If Liver qi overacts on the Spleen and Stomach, epigastric and abdominal pain and poor appetite will occur. Lastly, because the condition is both excess and deficient in nature, patients also may experience both fever and aversion to cold.

Dang Gui (Radix Angelicae Sinensis), *Chuan Xiong* (Rhizoma Chuanxiong), and *Shu Di Huang* (Radix Rehmanniae Praeparata) tonify the blood and regulate blood circulation. *Bai Zhu* (Rhizoma Atractylodis Macrocephalae), *Fu Ling* (Poria), and *Gan Cao* (Radix et Rhizoma Glycyrrhizae) strengthen the Spleen and tonify qi. Together, they nourish underlying qi and blood deficiencies in postpartum women. *Chen Pi* (Pericarpium Citri Reticulatae), *Wu Yao* (Radix Linderae), and *Xiang Fu* (Rhizoma Cyperi) regulate qi circulation and unblock

Xiong Gui Tiao Xue Yin (Cnidium and Tangkuei Decoction to Regulate Blood)

Diagnosis	Signs and Symptoms	Treatment	Herbs
Postpartum complications	• Postpartum bleeding with spontaneous perspiration, a dry mouth, dizziness, light-headedness and tinnitus: qi and blood deficiencies • Emotional instability, hypochondriac fullness and distention, delirium, and irritability: Liver qi stagnation • Epigastric and abdominal pain and poor appetite: Liver qi overacts on the Spleen and Stomach	• Tonifies qi and blood • Harmonizes the Liver and Spleen	• *Dang Gui* (Radix Angelicae Sinensis), *Chuan Xiong* (Rhizoma Chuanxiong) and *Shu Di Huang* (Radix Rehmanniae Praeparata) tonify the blood and regulate blood circulation. • *Bai Zhu* (Rhizoma Atractylodis Macrocephalae), *Fu Ling* (Poria) and *Gan Cao* (Radix et Rhizoma Glycyrrhizae) strengthen the Spleen and tonify qi. • *Chen Pi* (Pericarpium Citri Reticulatae), *Wu Yao* (Radix Linderae) and *Xiang Fu* (Rhizoma Cyperi) regulate qi circulation and unblock Liver qi stagnation. • *Mu Dan Pi* (Cortex Moutan) and *Yi Mu Cao* (Herba Leonuri) cool the blood and stop bleeding. • *Gan Jiang* (Rhizoma Zingiberis) warms the interior and dispels cold. • *Da Zao* (Fructus Jujubae), *Gan Cao* (Radix et Rhizoma Glycyrrhizae) and *Sheng Jiang* (Rhizoma Zingiberis Recens) strengthen the middle *jiao* and harmonize the herbs.

Chapter 8 – Tonic Formulas

Section 3 – Qi- and Blood-Tonifying Formulas

Xiōng Guī Tiáo Xuè Yǐn
(Cnidium and Tangkuei Decoction to Regulate Blood)

Liver qi stagnation. *Mu Dan Pi* (Cortex Moutan) and *Yi Mu Cao* (Herba Leonuri) cool the blood and stop bleeding. *Gan Jiang* (Rhizoma Zingiberis) warms the interior and dispels cold. *Da Zao* (Fructus Jujubae), *Gan Cao* (Radix et Rhizoma Glycyrrhizae), and *Sheng Jiang* (Rhizoma Zingiberis Recens) strengthen the middle *jiao* and harmonize the herbs. In short, this is an excellent formula for both treating and preventing various postpartum complications.

MODIFICATIONS

- With profuse and continuous bleeding, increase the dose of *Yi Mu Cao* (Herba Leonuri) and *Mu Dan Pi* (Cortex Moutan).
- With epigastric and abdominal fullness due to food stagnation, add *Zhi Shi* (Fructus Aurantii Immaturus), *Hou Po* (Cortex Magnoliae Officinalis), *Shan Zha* (Fructus Crataegi), and *Sha Ren* (Fructus Amomi).
- With pain in the lower abdomen, add *Yan Hu Suo* (Rhizoma Corydalis), *Tao Ren* (Semen Persicae), *Hong Hua* (Flos Carthami), and *Su Mu* (Lignum Sappan).
- With severe qi and blood deficiencies, add *Huang Qi* (Radix Astragali), or combine with *Dang Gui Bu Xue Tang* (Tangkuei Decoction to Tonify the Blood).
- With irritability, thirst, and dryness, add *Di Huang* (Radix Rehmanniae) and *Huang Qin* (Radix Scutellariae).

- With headache and vertigo, add *Bai Zhi* (Radix Angelicae Dahuricae) and *Huang Qi* (Radix Astragali).
- For *shen* (spirit) disturbance in which the patient becomes easily scared or frightened, add *Suan Zao Ren* (Semen Ziziphi Spinosae), *Yuan Zhi* (Radix Polygalae), and *Mai Dong* (Radix Ophiopogonis).

CLINICAL STUDIES AND RESEARCH

Postpartum recovery: One study compared the effects of herbs and drugs on postpartum recovery and healing. The study enrolled 171 women who had normal deliveries, and randomly assigned them to the following two groups: 85 women who received *Xiong Gui Tiao Xue Yin* at a dose of 6.0 g/day, and 86 women who received ergometrine (methylergometrine maleate) at a dose of 0.375 mg/day. Overall, the study reported marked beneficial effects of this formula on physical recovery in the postpartum period, although its biopharmacological properties are not known.[1]

Reference

1. Ushiroyama T, Sakuma K, Souen H, Nakai G, Morishima S, Yasuda K, Orino I, Ueki M. Therapeutic effects of Kyuki-chouketsu-in in restoring postpartum physical condition. American Journal of Chinese Medicine 2003;31(3):437-44.

Section 4

补阴剂
— Yin-Tonifying Formulas

Liù Wèi Dì Huáng Wán (Six-Ingredient Pill with Rehmannia)

六味地黃丸
六味地黃丸

Pinyin Name: *Liu Wei Di Huang Wan*
Literal Name: Six-Ingredient Pill with Rehmannia
Alternate Names: *Liu Wei Ti Huang Wan*, *Di Huang Wan*, Six-Flavour Rehmannia Pill, Rehmannia Bolus with Six Herbs, Rehmannia Six Pill, Rehmannia Six Formula
Original Source: *Xiao Er Yao Zheng Zhi Jue* (Craft of Medicinal Treatment for Childhood Disease Patterns) by Qian Yi in 1119

COMPOSITION

Shu Di Huang (Radix Rehmanniae Praeparata)	240g [24g]
Shan Zhu Yu (Fructus Corni)	120g [12g]
Shan Yao (Rhizoma Dioscoreae)	120g [12g]
Ze Xie (Rhizoma Alismatis)	90g [9g]
Mu Dan Pi (Cortex Moutan)	90g [9g]
Fu Ling (Poria)	90g [9g]

DOSAGE / PREPARATION / ADMINISTRATION

Grind the ingredients into powder and form into small pills with honey. The pills should resemble the size of *Wu Tong Zi* (Semen Firmianae), a small seed approximately 5 mm in diameter. Take the pills on an empty stomach three times daily with warm water. Today, it is usually prepared in pill form by mixing the powdered herbs with honey. Each pill should weigh approximately 15g. Take 1 pill three times daily on an empty stomach with warm, boiled water. This formula may also be prepared and administered in decoction form using the doses suggested in brackets.

CHINESE THERAPEUTIC ACTIONS

Nourishes Liver and Kidney yin

CLINICAL MANIFESTATIONS

1. Liver and Kidney yin deficiencies: dizziness, vertigo, tinnitus, deafness, blurred vision, soreness and weakness of the lower back and knees, seminal emissions, night sweats, and delayed closing or unclosed fontanel in infants.

2. Yin-deficient heat: steaming bones sensations, heat sensations in the palm and soles, tidal fever, thirst, toothache, a dry mouth and throat, a red tongue body with a scanty tongue coating, and a fine, rapid pulse. Can also be used for *xiao ke* (wasting and thirsting) syndrome.

CLINICAL APPLICATIONS

Diabetes mellitus, menopause, coronary heart disease, hypertension, hyperthyroidism, hypothyroidism, thyroid adenoma, bronchial asthma, atrophic gastritis, esophagitis, chronic nephritis, nephrotic syndrome, chronic renal failure, periodic paralysis, miscarriage, chronic hepatitis, stroke sequelae, chronic prostatitis, male or female infertility, impotence, frequent urination, galacturia, side effects of chemotherapy, heel pain, lumbago, retarded growth in children, optic neuritis, and central retinitis.

EXPLANATION

The Kidney dominates the bone and produces marrow, and because the brain is considered "the sea of the marrow," Kidney deficiency can affect the brain, causing dizziness

Chapter 8 – Tonic Formulas   *Section 4 – Yin-Tonifying Formulas*

Liù Wèi Dì Huáng Wán (Six-Ingredient Pill with Rehmannia)

Liu Wei Di Huang Wan (Six-Ingredient Pill with Rehmannia)

Diagnosis	Signs and Symptoms	Treatment	Herbs
Liver and Kidney yin deficiencies	• Soreness and weakness of the lower back and knees, dizziness, vertigo, tinnitus, deafness, and blurred vision: Liver and Kidney yin deficiencies • Tidal fever, heat sensations in the palms and soles, thirst, toothache, a dry mouth and throat: yin-deficient fire rising • Red tongue body with a scanty tongue coating and a fine, rapid pulse: yin-deficient fire	Nourishes Liver and Kidney yin	• *Shu Di Huang* (Radix Rehmanniae Praeparata) tonifies Kidney yin and *jing* (essence). • *Shan Zhu Yu* (Fructus Corni) nourishes the Liver and Kidney. • *Shan Yao* (Rhizoma Dioscoreae) tonifies the Spleen and Kidney. • *Ze Xie* (Rhizoma Alismatis) sedates the Kidney and causes turbidity to descend. • *Mu Dan Pi* (Cortex Moutan) sedates deficiency fire of the Liver. • *Fu Ling* (Poria) strengthens the Spleen and resolves dampness.

and vertigo. Weakness of the knees and lower back and loose teeth are due to Kidney yin deficiency, since the Kidney resides in the lower back and controls the bones. The ear is the sensory organ that belongs to the Kidney, and tinnitus and deafness may occur as a result of Kidney deficiency. Blurred vision is mainly caused by Liver deficiency, since the Liver opens into the eyes. The Kidney stores *jing* (essence), and when the Kidney becomes deficient, *jing* leaks out of the body causing seminal emissions. Deficiency fire resulting from yin deficiency causes symptoms such as tidal fever, night sweating, heat sensations in the palm and soles, thirst, toothache, and a dry mouth and throat. Delayed closing of the fontanel or unclosed fontanel in infants suggests a possible delay in development, which signifies prenatal *jing* deficiency and inadequate generation of marrow and bones. A red tongue body with a scanty coating suggests yin deficiency with fire. A fine, rapid pulse is typical of deficiency fire.

Liu Wei Di Huang Wan (Six-Ingredient Pill with Rehmannia) consists of three tonic and three sedative herbs. *Shu Di Huang* (Radix Rehmanniae Praeparata), the chief herb, tonifies Kidney yin and *jing* (essence), and fills the marrow. *Shan Zhu Yu* (Fructus Corni) nourishes the Liver and Kidney and astringes *jing. Shan Yao* (Rhizoma Dioscoreae) tonifies the Spleen and Kidney and consolidates *jing.* Together, these three tonic herbs address deficiencies in the Kidney, Liver, and Spleen. *Ze Xie* (Rhizoma Alismatis) sedates the Kidney, causes turbidity to descend, and controls the stagnating effect of *Shu Di Huang* (Radix Rehmanniae Praeparata). *Mu Dan Pi* (Cortex Moutan) sedates deficiency fire of the Liver, as well as balances the astringent property of *Shan Zhu Yu* (Fructus Corni). *Fu Ling* (Poria) strengthens the Spleen, resolves dampness, and balances *Shan Yao* (Rhizoma Dioscoreae).

One significant characteristic of this formula is that it sedates and tonifies at the same time. The purpose of sedation is to eradicate the turbidity and to prevent the stagnant properties of the tonic herbs from harming the body. The overall purpose of this formula, however, is to tonify, not to sedate. Therefore, the dose of the sedating herbs is less than that of the tonic herbs.

MODIFICATIONS
• With yin-deficient fire, add *Zhi Mu* (Rhizoma Anemarrhenae) and *Huang Bo* (Cortex Phellodendri Chinensis).
• With Spleen qi deficiency with qi stagnation, add dry-fried *Bai Zhu* (Rhizoma Atractylodis Macrocephalae), *Sha Ren* (Fructus Amomi), and *Chen Pi* (Pericarpium Citri Reticulatae).
• For *xiao ke* (wasting and thirsting) syndrome, add *Tian Hua Fen* (Radix Trichosanthis).
• For hypertension, add *Sang Ye* (Folium Mori), *Di Long* (Pheretima), and *Niu Xi* (Radix Achyranthis Bidentatae).
• For chronic nephritis, add *Yi Mu Cao* (Herba Leonuri), *Tian Hua Fen* (Radix Trichosanthis), and *Dan Zhu Ye* (Herba Lophatheri).
• For irregular menstruation, add *Xiang Fu* (Rhizoma Cyperi) and *Ai Ye* (Folium Artemisiae Argyi).
• With insomnia or neurasthenia, add *Suan Zao Ren* (Semen Ziziphi Spinosae) and *Bai Zi Ren* (Semen Platycladi).
• With weakness and pain of the lower back and knees, add *Niu Xi* (Radix Achyranthis Bidentatae) and *Du Zhong* (Cortex Eucommiae).
• With nocturnal emissions, combine with *Jin Suo Gu Jing Wan* (Metal Lock Pill to Stabilize the Essence).
• For tuberculosis of the kidney, add *Bai Ji* (Rhizoma Bletillae) and *San Qi* (Radix et Rhizoma Notoginseng).

628

Chinese Herbal Formulas and Applications

Liù Wèi Dì Huáng Wán (Six-Ingredient Pill with Rehmannia)

CAUTIONS / CONTRAINDICATIONS

- *Liu Wei Di Huang Wan* should be used with caution in humid areas where diseases are predominantly caused by dampness.
- Because this formula is greasy in nature, patients who have Spleen and Stomach deficiencies should use it with caution, as it may cause loose stools.
- This formula is contraindicated in patients of yang deficiency, exterior conditions, high fever, or alternating chills and fever.

PHARMACOLOGICAL EFFECTS

1. **Reproductive**: In laboratory experiments, the use of *Liu Wei Di Huang Wan* was associated with an increase in the weight of the sex organs, such as the ovaries, uterus, and testicles. There was also an increase in sperm counts in the male subjects. In addition, after ingestion of the herbs for 10 days, there was an increase in sexual activity by up to 40%.[1]

2. **Metabolic**: In laboratory experiments, the use of *Liu Wei Di Huang Wan* for 6 weeks lowered plasma cholesterol and triglycerides significantly in rats with elevated levels. In addition, there was an increase of HDL. However, the formula had little effect on plasma cholesterol and triglyceride levels in healthy rats.[2] It was noted that the three herbs with "sedating effects," namely *Ze Xie* (Rhizoma Alismatis), *Mu Dan Pi* (Cortex Moutan), and *Fu Ling* (Poria), were effective in reducing the cholesterol levels. On the other hand, the three herbs with "tonic effects," namely *Shu Di Huang* (Radix Rehmanniae Praeparata), *Shan Zhu Yu* (Fructus Corni), and *Shan Yao* (Rhizoma Dioscoreae), were not effective in reducing the cholesterol levels.[3]

3. **Hypoglycemic**: In rats with diabetes, the use of *Liu Wei Di Huang Wan* lowered plasma glucose levels.[4] In follow-up studies, it was determined that the formula was effective in reducing plasma glucose levels even if the pancreas was surgically removed. Therefore, it was concluded that the hypoglycemic effect of *Liu Wei Di Huang Wan* was not dependant on pancreas function.[5]

4. **Immunostimulant**: Use of *Liu Wei Di Huang Wan* was associated with an increase in white blood cell count and activity.[6] Moreover, use of this formula reversed the immune suppression induced by dexamethasone.[7]

5. **Adaptogenic**: Administration of *Liu Wei Di Huang Wan* improved the physical performances of mice. After ingesting the herbs orally for 2 weeks, the mice were able to swim for 14.9 minutes, compared to 11.5 minutes for the placebo group that did not receive herbs.[8]

6. **Hepatoprotective and nephroprotective**: Administration of *Liu Wei Di Huang Wan* had protective effects on both the liver and kidneys. It has a hepatoprotective effect against damages induced by such substances as carbon tetrachloride, thioacetamide, and prednisolone.[9] It also increased blood perfusion to the kidneys, improved the kidney function, and reduced protein and uric acid in the urine.[10]

7. **Antiarrhythmic**: In laboratory experiments in rats, an extract of *Liu Wei Di Huang Wan* was found to be effective in treating arrhythmia induced by chloroform, aconitine, ouabain, and adrenalin.[11]

8. **Hypotensive**: In anesthetized rats, intraduodenal administration of *Liu Wei Di Huang Wan* in decoction was effective in reducing blood pressure within 15 minutes. The mechanism of action was attributed to dilation of the blood vessels and reduction of peripheral resistance. The herbs did not affect the heart rate nor the contractile force of the heart.[12]

CLINICAL STUDIES AND RESEARCH

1. **Diabetes mellitus**: *Liu Wei Di Huang Wan* is one of the most effective formulas for treating diabetes mellitus. One study reported 93.55% effectiveness using modified *Liu Wei Di Huang Wan* to treat 62 patients with non-insulin dependant diabetes. The herbal treatment was based on *Liu Wei Di Huang Wan* plus *Ge Gen* (Radix Puerariae Lobatae) and *Li Zhi He* (Semen Litchi) as the base formula. Modifications varied depending on the presentation of diabetes and its complications, and were made as follows: for hunger and increased food intake, add *Shi Gao* (Gypsum Fibrosum) and *Yu Zhu* (Rhizoma Polygonati Odorati); for thirst and increased water intake, add *Sha Shen* (Radix Glehniae seu Adenophorae) and *Tian Hua Fen* (Radix Trichosanthis); for shortness of breath and spontaneous sweating, add *Huang Qi* (Radix Astragali) and *Tai Zi Shen* (Radix Pseudostellariae); for clear urine with increased volume, add *Sang Piao Xiao* (Ootheca Mantidis), *Ba Ji Tian* (Radix Morindae Officinalis), and *Rou Gui* (Cortex Cinnamomi); cloudy urine and night sweats, add *Zhi Mu* (Rhizoma Anemarrhenae) and *Huang Bo* (Cortex Phellodendri Chinensis); for dizziness and swelling of the head, add *Gou Teng* (Ramulus Uncariae cum Uncis), *Bai Shao* (Radix Paeoniae Alba), and *Niu Xi* (Radix Achyranthis Bidentatae); for chest oppression and palpitations, add *Dan Shen* (Radix et Rhizoma Salviae Miltiorrhizae), *Yu Jin* (Radix Curcumae), and *Shi Chang Pu* (Rhizoma Acori Tatarinowii); for obesity, add *Pei Lan* (Herba Eupatorii) and *He Ye* (Folium Nelumbinis); for blurred vision, add *Gu Jing Cao* (Flos Eriocauli) and *Qing Xiang Zi* (Semen Celosiae); and for severe blood stagnation, add *Tao Ren* (Semen Persicae), *Hong Hua* (Flos Carthami), and *Shui Zhi* (Hirudo). The patients were given the herbs for 30 days per course of treatment. Of 62 patients, the study reported complete recovery in 17 patients, improvement

TONIC FORMULAS

8

629

Liù Wèi Dì Huáng Wán (Six-Ingredient Pill with Rehmannia)

Chapter 8 – Tonic Formulas   *Section 4 – Yin-Tonifying Formulas*

in 41 patients, and no benefit in 4 patients.[13] In another study, 20 patients with adult-onset diabetes were treated with *Liu Wei Di Huang Wan* for 3-6 months with stabilization in 12 patients and improvement in 8 patients.[14] In another study, modified *Liu Wei Di Huang Wan* was used for 20 days to treat 53 patients with diabetes, with marked improvement in 46 patients, improvement in 5 patients, and no benefit in 2 patients.[15] In addition, the use of herbs stabilized blood glucose in conjunction with insulin injection.[16] Lastly, one study reported that use of modified *Liu Wei Di Huang Wan* was associated with 89.2% effectiveness in 65 patients with non-insulin dependant diabetes mellitus.[17]

2. **Menopause**: In one clinical study, 23 patients with menopausal symptoms were treated with *Liu Wei Di Huang Wan* and experienced marked improvement in 9 patients (39.1%), and moderate improvement in 14 patients (60.9%). The treatment protocol was to administer this formula in pills, 9 grams twice daily, in the morning and at night, for 3 months. Clinical improvements included relief of hot flashes, tidal fever, perspiration, palpitations, anxiety, restlessness, insomnia, forgetfulness, and others. In addition, after taking the herbs continuously for one year, it was noted that there was a decrease in FSH and an increase of estradiol. The mechanism of action was attributed to the formula's stimulating effect on the endocrine system.[18]

3. **Coronary heart disease**: Modified *Liu Wei Di Huang Wan* was used to treat patients with coronary heart disease characterized by Kidney deficiency with symptoms such as soreness of the lower back, weakness of the knees, and tinnitus. The formula used included the addition of *Bai Shao* (Radix Paeoniae Alba), *He Shou Wu* (Radix Polygoni Multiflori), and others. Out of 48 patients, the study reported symptomatic improvement in 24 patients, ECG improvement in 12 patients, and reduction of plasma cholesterol in 12 patients.[19]

4. **Hypertension**: Administration of 5-10 packs of *Liu Wei Di Huang Wan* effectively reduced blood pressure in all 31 patients with primary hypertension. In follow-up visits one year later, 23 patients had normal blood pressure, and 8 still had hypertension.[20] In one patient report, a patient with hypertension was treated with modified *Liu Wei Di Huang Wan* for 20 doses with good results. Blood pressure reduced from 160-180/110-120 mmHg to 140/90 mmHg. The patient continued to take the herbs for 6 months. The blood pressure did not elevate in any follow-up appointments up to 3 years later.[21]

5. **Hyperthyroidism**: Modified *Liu Wei Di Huang Wan* was used to treat patients with hyperthyroidism. Out of 31 patients, 28 had enlargement of the thyroid gland, 13 had protruding of the eyes, 29 had significant weight loss, and 28 had increased heart rate. After 15-20 doses

of herbal treatment, the study reported symptomatic improvement in most patients.[22]

6. **Thyroid adenoma**: In one study, 48 patients with a history of thyroid adenoma from 6 months to 8 years were treated with modified *Liu Wei Di Huang Wan* with good results. The base formula included *Shu Di Huang* (Radix Rehmanniae Praeparata) 30g, *Xuan Shen* (Radix Scrophulariae) 30g, *Mu Li* (Concha Ostreae) 30g pre-decocted, *Shan Yao* (Rhizoma Dioscoreae) 15g, *Fu Ling* (Poria) 15g, *Shan Zhu Yu* (Fructus Corni) 15g, *Xia Ku Cao* (Spica Prunellae) 15g, *Mu Dan Pi* (Cortex Moutan) 12g, *Ze Xie* (Rhizoma Alismatis) 12g, *Zhe Bei Mu* (Bulbus Fritillariae Thunbergii) 12g, and *Jiang Can* (Bombyx Batryticatus) 12g. Modifications included the addition of *Bie Jia* (Carapax Trionycis) for yin-deficient heat, *Tai Zi Shen* (Radix Pseudostellariae) for qi deficiency, *Chai Hu* (Radix Bupleuri) for qi stagnation, and *He Shou Wu* (Radix Polygoni Multiflori) for blood deficiency. The treatment protocol was to administer the herbs in decoction one time daily for 1-2 months. Out of 48 patients, the study reported recovery based on relief of symptoms in 26 patients, improvement in 21 patients, and no benefit in 1 patient. The overall effectiveness rate was 98%.[23]

7. **Bronchial asthma**: In one report, 64 patients with bronchial asthma characterized by Kidney deficiency were treated with *Liu Wei Di Huang Wan* with good results.[24]

8. **Atrophic gastritis**: Patients with a history of chronic atrophic gastritis for 6 months to 2 years were treated with modified *Liu Wei Di Huang Wan* for 6 months to 1 year with a 94% effectiveness rate. Out of 50 patients, the study reported recovery in 35 patients, moderate improvement in 10 patients, slight improvement in 2 patients, and no benefit in 3 patients.[25]

9. **Esophagitis**: Administration of large doses of *Liu Wei Di Huang Wan* in 98 patients with chronic esophagitis was associated with marked improvement in 86 patients and no benefit in 12 patients. The treatment protocol was to take 30 pills three times daily for 30 days per course of treatment, for 3-4 courses total.[26]

10. **Chronic nephritis**: Use of *Liu Wei Di Huang Wan* plus *Yu Mi Xu* (Stigma Maydis) was reported in one study to be effective in treating patients with chronic nephritis with hypertension and proteinuria.[27] The study found that administration of *Liu Wei Di Huang Wan* plus *Yu Mi Xu* (Stigma Maydis) in decoction daily for 3-24 months in 77 patients with chronic nephritis was associated with complete recovery in 22 patients, near-complete recovery in 36 patients, partial recovery in 13 patients, and no benefit in 6 patients. The study noted that most patients with chronic nephritis had underlying Kidney yin deficiency and damp-heat.[28]

630

Chinese Herbal Formulas and Applications

Liù Wèi Dì Huáng Wán (Six-Ingredient Pill with Rehmannia)

11. **Nephrotic syndrome**: Six patients with edema and proteinuria due to nephrotic syndrome were treated with modified *Liu Wei Di Huang Wan* for 50 days with good results. The study reported that edema and proteinuria were resolved in all patients.[29]

12. **Chronic renal failure**: In one study, 12 patients with chronic renal failure (8 with chronic nephritis, 2 with chronic glomerulonephritis, 1 with renal failure due to systemic lupus erythematosus, and 1 with renal failure due to atypical hemorrhagic fever) were treated with modified *Liu Wei Di Huang Wan* for 30-60 days with complete recovery in 8 patients, marked improvement in 3 patients, and slight improvement in 1 patient. A modification to the original formula used a higher dose of *Shan Zhu Yu* (Fructus Corni).[30]

13. **Periodic paralysis**: In one study, 58 patients (54 had hypokalemia) with periodic paralysis were effectively treated using *Liu Wei Di Huang Wan*. Of 58 patients, the study reported complete recovery in 46 patients, improvement in 10 patients, and no benefit in 2 patients. The treatment protocol was to administer the herbs in decoction daily for 15 days per course of treatment.[31]

14. **Miscarriage**: In one study, 55 women with history of miscarriage were treated with modified *Liu Wei Di Huang Wan* with great success. The formula included *Shu Di Huang* (Radix Rehmanniae Praeparata) 12g, *Shan Yao* (Rhizoma Dioscoreae) 15g, *Mu Dan Pi* (Cortex Moutan) 10g, *Shan Zhu Yu* (Fructus Corni) 10g, *Ze Xie* (Rhizoma Alismatis) 10g, and *Fu Ling* (Poria) 10g. Modifications included the addition of *Xian He Cao* (Herba Agrimoniae) 15g, *E Jiao* (Colla Corii Asini) 10g, and charred *Ai Ye* (Folium Artemisiae Argyi) 30g for bleeding; and *Du Zhong* (Cortex Eucommiae) 10g, *Sang Ji Sheng* (Herba Taxilli) 10g, and *Xu Duan* (Radix Dipsaci) 15g for soreness of the low back. The treatment was to administer the herbs in decoction one time daily for 7 days per course of treatment. The study reported full-term delivery in 53 out of 55 patients (96.4% success rate).[32]

15. **Chronic hepatitis**: Use of modified *Liu Wei Di Huang Wan* in 65 patients with chronic hepatitis was associated with significant effect in 12 patients, improvement in 49 patients, and no benefit in 4 patients. The treatment protocol was to use *Liu Wei Di Huang Wan* plus *Dang Gui* (Radix Angelicae Sinensis), *Bai Shao* (Radix Paeoniae Alba), and *Chuan Lian Zi* (Fructus Toosendan) as the base formula. For hypochondriac pain due to Liver qi stagnation, *Yan Hu Suo* (Rhizoma Corydalis), *Yu Jin* (Radix Curcumae), and *Chai Hu* (Radix Bupleuri) were added. For poor appetite, *Ji Nei Jin* (Endothelium Corneum Gigeriae Galli), *Shan Zha* (Fructus Crataegi), and *Shen Qu* (Massa Fermentata) were added. For a bitter taste in the mouth with a yellow tongue coating, *Zhi Zi* (Fructus

Gardeniae) and *Huang Qin* (Radix Scutellariae) were added. For a red tongue body with a dry mouth, *Xuan Shen* (Radix Scrophulariae) and *Shi Hu* (Caulis Dendrobii) were added. For soreness and weakness of the lower back and knees, *Gou Qi Zi* (Fructus Lycii) and *Du Zhong* (Cortex Eucommiae) were added. For enlargement of the Liver and/or Spleen, *Tao Ren* (Semen Persicae), *Hong Hua* (Flos Carthami), and *Bie Jia* (Carapax Trionycis) were added. Lastly, for accumulation of water in the abdomen, *Shu Di Huang* (Radix Rehmanniae Praeparata) was removed, and *Bai Mao Gen* (Rhizoma Imperatae) and *Da Fu Pi* (Pericarpium Arecae) were added.[33]

16. **Stroke sequelae**: Modified *Liu Wei Di Huang Wan* showed success in treating post-stroke patients in one study. The treatment protocol used this formula as the base, and added *Dang Gui Wei* (Extremitas Radix Angelicae Sinensis), *Huang Qi* (Radix Astragali), and *Di Long* (Pheretima) for qi deficiency and hemiplegia; *Du Zhong* (Cortex Eucommiae), *Sang Ji Sheng* (Herba Taxilli), and *Mai Dong* (Radix Ophiopogonis) for Liver and Kidney deficiencies; and *Tian Ma* (Rhizoma Gastrodiae), *Gou Teng* (Ramulus Uncariae cum Uncis), and *Shi Chang Pu* (Rhizoma Acori Tatarinowii) for wind-phlegm obstruction. Out of 20 patients, the study reported complete recovery in 6 patients, improvement in 12 patients, and no benefit in 2 patients. The overall rate of effectiveness was 90%.[34]

17. **Infertility**: Modified *Liu Wei Di Huang Wan* was used to treat infertility in 42 patients (16 males and 26 females between the ages of 22 to 37). The duration of marriage of the patients ranged from 1-14 years. The treatment included the addition of *Rou Cong Rong* (Herba Cistanches), *Dan Shen* (Radix et Rhizoma Salviae Miltiorrhizae), *Tu Si Zi* (Semen Cuscutae), *Fen Bi Xie* (Rhizoma Dioscoreae Hypoglaucae), and others as deemed necessary. After 3-6 months of herbal treatment, the study reported marked results in 31 patients, moderate results in 9 patients, and no benefit in 2 patients. (Note: Criteria for evaluation was not given.)[35]

18. **Male infertility**: One study reported 83.3% effectiveness using modified *Liu Wei Di Huang Wan* to treat 30 male patients with infertility. The herbal treatment included *Liu Wei Di Huang Wan* plus *Dang Gui* (Radix Angelicae Sinensis), *Tu Si Zi* (Semen Cuscutae), *Gou Qi Zi* (Fructus Lycii), and others as the base formula. *Bie Jia* (Carapax Trionycis), *He Shou Wu* (Radix Polygoni Multiflori), and a larger dose of *Shu Di Huang* (Radix Rehmanniae Praeparata) were used for severe Kidney deficiency; *Xian Mao* (Rhizoma Curculiginis), *Yin Yang Huo* (Herba Epimedii), and *Ba Ji Tian* (Radix Morindae Officinalis) were added for Kidney yang deficiency; *Hai Ma* (Hippocampus) and *Lu Jiao* (Cornu Cervi) were added for low sperm count; and *Huang Bo* (Cortex Phellodendri Chinensis), *Tao Ren*

8

TONIC FORMULAS

631

Chapter 8 – Tonic Formulas

Section 4 – Yin-Tonifying Formulas

Liù Wèi Dì Huáng Wán (Six-Ingredient Pill with Rehmannia)

(Semen Persicae), and *Ji Xue Teng* (Caulis Spatholobi) were added for semen that liquefied slowly. Other modifications were made if deemed necessary. The treatment protocol was to administer the herbs in decoction for 20 days per course of treatment, followed by 1 week of rest, and continuation of treatment if necessary. Of 30 patients, 19 had complete recovery (4 with 1 course of treatment, 6 after 2 courses, 9 after 3 courses), 6 had improvement, and 1 had no benefit. The overall rate of effectiveness was 83.3%.[36]

19. **Impotence**: One study of 18 impotent patients reported complete recovery in 12 patients, improvement in 4 patients, and no benefit in 2 patients using modified *Liu Wei Di Huang Wan*. The treatment protocol was to administer the herbs twice daily with 6g of salt in warm water. The duration of treatment ranged from 15-37 packs of herbs. The herbal treatment contained *Liu Wei Di Huang Wan* plus *Zhi Mu* (Rhizoma Anemarrhenae), *Rou Gui* (Cortex Cinnamomi), *Du Zhong* (Cortex Eucommiae), and *He Shou Wu* (Radix Polygoni Multiflori) as the base formula. In addition, a small amount of *Fu Zi* (Radix Aconiti Lateralis Praeparata) was added for cold extremities with frequent urination at night; *Qian Shi* (Semen Euryales) and *Jin Ying Zi* (Fructus Rosae Laevigatae) were added for spermatorrhea or nocturnal emissions; *Huang Qi* (Radix Astragali) and *Gou Qi Zi* (Fructus Lycii) were added for severe dizziness; *Long Gu* (Os Draconis) and *Mu Li* (Concha Ostreae) were added for palpitations and insomnia; and *Gui Ban* (Plastrum Testudinis) and *Huang Bo* (Cortex Phellodendri Chinensis) were added for tidal fever and red cheeks.[37]

20. **Chronic prostatitis**: In one study, 153 patients with chronic non-bacterial prostatitis were treated with modified *Liu Wei Di Huang Wan* with good results. In addition to this base formula, modifications were made as follows: for Kidney qi and *jing* (essence) deficiencies, *Rou Cong Rong* (Herba Cistanches), *Jin Ying Zi* (Fructus Rosae Laevigatae), and *Wu Wei Zi* (Fructus Schisandrae Chinensis) were added; for burning sensations and pain during urination, *Zhi Mu* (Rhizoma Anemarrhenae), *Che Qian Zi* (Semen Plantaginis), and *Bai Hua She She Cao* (Herba Hedyotis) were added; for burning sensations and pain during urination with seminal emissions and premature ejaculation, *Huang Bo* (Cortex Phellodendri Chinensis) and *Che Qian Zi* (Semen Plantaginis) were added; and for low back pain with dark tongue body and purple spots, *Wang Bu Liu Xing* (Semen Vaccariae), *Tao Ren* (Semen Persicae), and *Wu Gong* (Scolopendra) were added. The patients were given the herbs for 20 days per course of treatment. Out of 153 patients, the study reported complete recovery in 141 patients, improvement in 10 patients, and

no benefit in 2 patients.[38] In another study, administration of *Liu Wei Di Huang Wan* in 30 patients with chronic prostatitis was associated with complete recovery in 9 patients, marked improvement in 12 patients, slight improvement in 7 patients, and no benefit in 2 patients. The treatment protocol was to administer the herbs in decoction daily for 1 month per course of treatment, for 1-3 courses total. In addition, patients were instructed to sit in hot water for 15-20 minutes, twice daily, during the entire treatment period.[39]

21. **Frequent urination**: One study reported effectiveness in treating 46 of 47 children with frequent urination using modified *Liu Wei Di Huang Wan* as decoction one time daily. The duration of treatment ranged from 3-6 days.[40]

22. **Galacturia**: One study reported marked success using modified *Liu Wei Di Huang Wan* to treat 20 patients with galacturia. In addition to *Liu Wei Di Huang Wan*, *Dang Shen* (Radix Codonopsis), *Huang Qi* (Radix Astragali) and *Bai Zhu* (Rhizoma Atractylodis Macrocephalae) were added for Spleen deficiency; *Du Zhong* (Cortex Eucommiae) and *Niu Xi* (Radix Achyranthis Bidentatae) were added for soreness and pain of the lower back and knees; *Zhi Mu* (Rhizoma Anemarrhenae) and *Huang Bo* (Cortex Phellodendri Chinensis) for yin-deficient fire; *Mo Han Lian* (Herba Ecliptae) and *Xiao Ji* (Herba Cirsii) for hematuria; *Huang Bo* (Cortex Phellodendri Chinensis), *Bian Xu* (Herba Polygoni Avicularis), and *Qu Mai* (Herba Dianthi) for damp-heat in the lower *jiao*; *Shi Chang Pu* (Rhizoma Acori Tatarinowii) and *Ci Shi* (Magnetitum) for tinnitus, deafness, and vertigo; *Tu Si Zi* (Semen Cuscutae), *Yin Yang Huo* (Herba Epimedii), and *Ba Ji Tian* (Radix Morindae Officinalis) for Kidney yang deficiency; and the addition of *Yi Zhi* (Fructus Alpiniae Oxyphyllae) and *Sang Piao Xiao* (Ootheca Mantidis), and removal of *Ze Xie* (Rhizoma Alismatis), for frequent urination.[41]

23. **Heel pain**: One study reported 88.5% effectiveness using modified *Liu Wei Di Huang Wan* to treat 185 patients with heel pain. In addition to *Liu Wei Di Huang Wan*, modifications were made as follows: for Liver and Kidney deficiencies, *Gou Qi Zi* (Fructus Lycii) and *Gu Sui Bu* (Rhizoma Drynariae) were added; for qi and blood stagnation, *Tao Ren* (Semen Persicae), *Dan Shen* (Radix et Rhizoma Salviae Miltiorrhizae), and *Di Long* (Pheretima) were added; for obstruction of wind-cold, *Zhi Chuan Wu* (Radix Aconiti Praeparata) and *Wei Ling Xian* (Radix et Rhizoma Clematidis) were added; and for obstruction of damp-heat, *Huang Bo* (Cortex Phellodendri Chinensis), *Cang Zhu* (Rhizoma Atractylodis), and *Zhi Zi* (Fructus Gardeniae) were added. The duration of treatment ranged from 38 to 120 packs of herbs, with an average of 60 packs.[42]

Liù Wèi Dì Huáng Wán (Six-Ingredient Pill with Rehmannia)

HERB-DRUG INTERACTION

Chemotherapy-induced toxicities: One study reported marked improvement in patients treated with *Liu Wei Di Huang Wan* as an adjunct to chemotherapy. Clinical benefits included relief of nausea and vomiting, a decrease of hair loss and stomatitis, an improvement in appetite, and an increase in white blood cells, red blood cells, platelets, T-lymphocytes, and natural killer (NK) cells.[43]

TOXICOLOGY

According to one study, no abnormalities were noted in pregnant mice that received *Liu Wei Di Huang Wan* continuously throughout the third trimester.[44]

RELATED FORMULAS

Ěr Lóng Zuǒ Cí Wán

(Pill for Deafness that Is Kind to the Left [Kidney])

耳聾左慈丸
耳聾左慈丸

Pinyin Name: *Er Long Zuo Ci Wan*
Literal Name: Pill for Deafness that Is Kind to the Left [Kidney]
Original Source: *Guang Wen Yi Lun* (Discussion of Widespread Warm Epidemics) by Dai Tian-Zhang in 1722

Shu Di Huang (Radix Rehmanniae Praeparata)	240g
Shan Zhu Yu (Fructus Corni)	120g
Shan Yao (Rhizoma Dioscoreae)	120g
Fu Ling (Poria)	90g
Mu Dan Pi (Cortex Moutan)	90g
Ze Xie (Rhizoma Alismatis)	90g
Ci Shi (Magnetitum), *duan* (calcined)	60g
Shi Chang Pu (Rhizoma Acori Tatarinowii)	45g
Wu Wei Zi (Fructus Schisandrae Chinensis)	15g

Grind the herbs into a fine powder, and mix with honey to make pills. Take 9g of pills with lightly-salted water.

Er Long Zuo Ci Wan (Pill for Deafness that Is Kind to the Left [Kidney]) tonifies Liver and Kidney yin, and opens the sensory orifices (ear). It is based on *Liu Wei Di Huang Wan* with the addition of *Ci Shi* (Magnetitum), *Shi Chang Pu* (Rhizoma Acori Tatarinowii), and *Wu Wei Zi* (Fructus Schisandrae Chinensis). *Ci Shi* (Magnetitum) is commonly used to improve hearing. *Shi Chang Pu* (Rhizoma Acori Tatarinowii) opens the orifices and dispels phlegm that may be blocking the senses. *Wu Wei Zi* (Fructus Schisandrae Chinensis) prevents the leakage of *jing* (essence). Clinically, this formula treats tinnitus, impaired or diminished hearing, and deafness arising from Kidney deficiency. It also treats dizziness, red eyes, blurred vision, and a dry mouth and throat.

Míng Mù Dì Huáng Wán

(Improve Vision Pill with Rehmannia)

明目地黃丸
明目地黃丸

Pinyin Name: *Ming Mu Di Huang Wan*
Literal Name: Improve Vision Pill with Rehmannia
Alternate Name: Rehmannia Vision Formula
Original Source: *Shen Shi Yao Han* (Scrutiny of the Priceless Jade Patient) by Fu Ren-Yu in 1644

Shu Di Huang (Radix Rehmanniae Praeparata)	120g
Di Huang (Radix Rehmanniae), *xi* (washed) with liquor	60g
Shan Yao (Rhizoma Dioscoreae)	60g
Ze Xie (Rhizoma Alismatis)	60g
Shan Zhu Yu (Fructus Corni), *xi* (washed) with liquor	60g
Mu Dan Pi (Cortex Moutan), *xi* (washed) with liquor	60g
Chai Hu (Radix Bupleuri)	60g
Fu Shen (Poria Paradicis), *zheng* (steamed) with milk	60g
Dang Gui (Radix Angelicae Sinensis), *xi* (washed) with liquor	60g
Wu Wei Zi (Fructus Schisandrae Chinensis)	60g

Grind the herbs into a fine powder, and mix with honey to make pills. The pills should resemble the size of *Wu Tong Zi* (Semen Firmianae), a small seed approximately 5 mm in diameter. Take 9g of pills per dose on an empty stomach with lightly-salted water.

Ming Mu Di Huang Wan (Improve Vision Pill with Rehmannia) tonifies the Liver and Kidney and brightens vision. Clinically, it is used for blurred or diminished vision. This formula is based on *Liu Wei Di Huang Wan* with the addition of *Di Huang* (Radix Rehmanniae), *Chai Hu* (Radix Bupleuri), *Dang Gui* (Radix Angelicae Sinensis), *Fu Shen* (Poria Paradicis), and *Wu Wei Zi* (Fructus Schisandrae Chinensis). *Di Huang* (Radix Rehmanniae) clears deficiency heat caused by yin deficiency. *Chai Hu* (Radix Bupleuri) acts as a channel-guiding herb to the Liver, which opens to the eyes. *Dang Gui* (Radix Angelicae Sinensis) nourishes Liver blood to treat visual disorders. *Fu Shen* (Poria Paradicis) and *Wu Wei Zi* (Fructus Schisandrae Chinensis) calm the *shen* (spirit).

Míng Mù Dì Huáng Wán

(Improve Vision Pill with Rehmannia)

明目地黃丸
明目地黃丸

Pinyin Name: *Ming Mu Di Huang Wan*
Literal Name: Improve Vision Pill with Rehmannia
Alternate Name: Rehmannia Vision Formula

Chapter 8 – Tonic Formulas   *Section 4 – Yin-Tonifying Formulas*

Liù Wèi Dì Huáng Wán (Six-Ingredient Pill with Rehmannia)

Original Source: *Zhong Hua Ren Min Gong He Guo Yao Dian* (Pharmacopoeia of People's Republic of China) in 2005

Shu Di Huang (Radix Rehmanniae Praeparata)	160g
Mu Dan Pi (Cortex Moutan)	60g
Fu Ling (Poria)	60g
Gou Qi Zi (Fructus Lycii)	60g
Dang Gui (Radix Angelicae Sinensis)	60g
Ji Li (Fructus Tribuli)	60g
Shan Zhu Yu (Fructus Corni), *zhi* (fried with liquid)	80g
Shan Yao (Rhizoma Dioscoreae)	80g
Ze Xie (Rhizoma Alismatis)	60g
Ju Hua (Flos Chrysanthemi)	60g
Bai Shao (Radix Paeoniae Alba)	60g
Shi Jue Ming (Concha Haliotidis), *duan* (calcined)	80g

Grind the herbs into a fine powder, and mix with 35-50g of honey per 100g of powdered herbs to make pills. This is the contemporary version of *Ming Mu Di Huang Wan* (Improve Vision Pill with Rehmannia). It has functions to tonify Liver and Kidney yin, clear Liver heat, and brighten the eyes. It is generally used to treat blurred vision, photophobia, and excessive tearing with exposure to wind.

These two formulas have identical names, but are derived from different sources and have slightly different functions:

- *Ming Mu Di Huang Wan* from *Shen Shi Yao Han* (Scrutiny of the Priceless Jade Patient) by Fu Ren-Yu improves vision by tonifying Liver and Kidney yin.
- *Ming Mu Di Huang Wan* from *Zhong Hua Ren Min Gong He Guo Yao Dian* (Pharmacopoeia of People's Republic of China) improves vision by tonifying Liver and Kidney yin, and has added function to clear Liver heat.

AUTHORS' COMMENTS

Liu Wei Di Huang Wan is the representative formula to tonify Liver and Kidney yin, and is one of the most frequently prescribed formulas. Many herbal formulas that tonify Kidney yin are based on *Liu Wei Di Huang Wan*. Below are the key similarities and differences among these yin tonic formulas:

- *Liu Wei Di Huang Wan* is the most basic Kidney and Liver yin tonic formula.
- *Zhi Bai Di Huang Wan* (Anemarrhena, Phellodendron, and Rehmannia Pill) contains *Zhi Mu* (Rhizoma Anemarrhenae) and *Huang Bo* (Cortex Phellodendri Chinensis) to nourish yin and clear deficiency fire.
- *Mai Wei Di Huang Wan* (Ophiopogonis, Schisandra and Rehmannia Pill) is formulated with the addition of *Mai Dong* (Radix Ophiopogonis) and *Wu Wei Zi* (Fructus Schisandrae Chinensis). It nourishes yin, astringes the Lung, redirects the reversed flow of Lung qi, and arrests wheezing.
- *Qi Ju Di Huang Wan* (Lycium Fruit, Chrysanthemum, and Rehmannia Pill) has *Gou Qi Zi* (Fructus Lycii) and *Ju Hua* (Flos Chrysanthemi); it nourishes Kidney and Liver yin and benefits the eyes to brighten vision.[45]

There are many herbal formulas that tonify Liver and Kidney yin. Their similarities and differences are as follows:

- *Liu Wei Di Huang Wan* is the most representative formula for tonifying yin. It nourishes and tonifies the Liver, Kidney, and Spleen.
- *Zuo Gui Wan* (Restore the Left [Kidney] Pill) replenishes Kidney *jing* (essence) and treats depleted *jing* and marrow. It is a pure yin tonic formula without any sedating herbs to offset the heavy tonic effects. It has a stronger yin-tonifying effect than *Liu Wei Di Huang Wan*. However, because of its stagnating nature, it is usually not taken for a prolonged period of time.
- *Da Bu Yin Wan* (Great Tonify the Yin Pill) nourishes yin, sedates fire, anchors yang, and is best for Kidney water depletion with deficiency heat flaring that manifests in steaming bones sensation, tidal fever, cough with blood, and vomiting of blood.
- *Hu Qian Wan* (Hidden Tiger Pill) nourishes yin, sedates fire, and strengthens the bones and tendons. It is best for atrophy or degeneration of the bones and tendons caused by Kidney yin deficiency with heat.
- *Er Zhi Wan* (Two-Ultimate Pill) is a balanced yin tonic formula, not too warm or too cold, that mainly treats Kidney yin deficiency with dizziness and blurred vision.
- *Yi Guan Jian* (Linking Decoction) nourishes the middle jiao and smoothes Liver qi. It treats Liver and Kidney deficiencies with Liver qi stagnation causing chest and hypochondriac pain, acid regurgitation, a bitter taste in the mouth, and a dry mouth and throat.
- *Shi Hu Ye Guang Wan* (Dendrobium Pill for Night Vision) causes Liver yang and wind to descend, nourishes yin, and brightens the eyes. It is best for visual disorders caused by Liver and Kidney yin deficiencies with blood deficiency.
- *Gui Lu Er Xian Jiao* (Tortoise Shell and Deer Antler Syrup) tonifies Kidney yin and yang, *jing* (essence), and blood of the *du* (governing) and *ren* (conception) channels.
- *Qi Bao Mei Ran Dan* (Seven-Treasure Special Pill for Beautiful Whiskers) nourishes Kidney yin, tonifies Liver blood, and mainly treats hair disorders, such as hair loss, premature gray hair, and dry or brittle hair.[46]

Chinese Herbal Formulas and Applications

Liù Wèi Dì Huáng Wán (Six-Ingredient Pill with Rehmannia)

Function	Composition	Liu Wei Di Huang Wan	Zhi Bai Di Huang Wan	Du Qi Wan	Mai Wei Di Huang Wan	Qi Ju Di Huang Wan	Jin Gui Shen Qi Wan	Ba Wei Di Huang Wan
Tonifies Liver and Kidney yin	*Shu Di Huang* (Radix Rehmanniae Praeparata), *Shan Zhu Yu* (Fructus Corni) and *Shan Yao* (Rhizoma Dioscoreae)	✓	✓	✓	✓	✓	✓ *	✓
Lowers turbidity and resolves dampness	*Ze Xie* (Rhizoma Alismatis), *Mu Dan Pi* (Cortex Moutan) and *Fu Ling* (Poria)	✓	✓	✓	✓	✓	✓	✓
Clears deficiency fire	*Zhi Mu* (Rhizoma Anemarrhenae) and *Huang Bo* (Cortex Phellodendri Chinensis)		✓					
Astringes qi	*Wu Wei Zi* (Fructus Schisandrae Chinensis)			✓				
Tonifies and astringes Lung yin	*Wu Wei Zi* (Fructus Schisandrae Chinensis) and *Mai Dong* (Radix Ophiopogonis)				✓			
Nourishes and benefits the eyes	*Gou Qi Zi* (Fructus Lycii) and *Ju Hua* (Flos Chrysanthemi)					✓		
Warms Kidney yang	*Gui Zhi* (Ramulus Cinnamomi) and *Fu Zi* (Radix Aconiti Lateralis Praeparata)						✓	
Strongly warms Kidney yang	*Rou Gui* (Cortex Cinnamomi) and *Fu Zi* (Radix Aconiti Lateralis Praeparata)							✓

* *Di Huang* (Radix Rehmanniae) is used in place of *Shu Di Huang* (Radix Rehmanniae Praeparata).

References

1. *Zhong Yi Fang Ji Xian Dai Yan Jiu* (Modern Study of Medical Formulae in Traditional Chinese Medicine) 1997;709.
2. *Zhong Cheng Yao Yan Jiu* (Research of Chinese Patent Medicine) 1986;12:41.
3. *Zhong Guo Yao Ke Da Xue Xue Bao* (Journal of University of Chinese Herbology) 1990;4:241.
4. *Guo Wai Yi Xue* (Foreign Medicine) 1986;4:11.
5. *Zhong Cheng Yao Yan Jiu* (Research of Chinese Patent Medicine) 1984;11:25.
6. *Zhong Cheng Yao Yan Jiu* (Research of Chinese Patent Medicine) 1981;12:28.
7. *Zhong Guo Mian Yi Xue Za Zhi* (Chinese Journal of Immunology) 1987;5:296.
8. *Xin Yi Yao Xue Za Zhi* (New Journal of Medicine and Herbology) 1977;7:41.
9. *Zhong Guo Yao Ke Da Xue Xue Bao* (Journal of University of Chinese Herbology) 1989;6:951.
10. *Zhong Yi Fang Ji Xian Dai Yan Jiu* (Modern Study of Medical Formulae in Traditional Chinese Medicine) 1997;710.
11. *Zhong Yi Fang Ji Xian Dai Yan Jiu* (Modern Study of Medical Formulae in Traditional Chinese Medicine) 1997;704.
12. *Zhong Guo Yi Ke Da Xue Xue Bao* (Journal of University of Chinese Medicine) 1989;6:354.
13. *He Bei Zhong Yi* (Hebei Chinese Medicine) 1999;11:35.
14. *Yun Nan Yi Yao* (Yunan Medicine and Herbology) 1983;3:181.
15. *Hu Bei Zhong Yi Za Zhi* (Hubei Journal of Chinese Medicine) 1987;3:14.

Chapter 8 – Tonic Formulas　　　　　　　　　　　　　　　　*Section 4 – Yin-Tonifying Formulas*

Liù Wèi Dì Huáng Wán (Six-Ingredient Pill with Rehmannia)

16. *Zhong Hua Yi Xue Za Zhi* (Chinese Journal of Medicine) 1956;6:546.
17. *Hu Bei Zhong Yi Za Zhi* (Hubei Journal of Chinese Medicine) 1992;2:20.
18. *Zhong Xi Yi Jie He Za Zhi* (Journal of Integrated Chinese and Western Medicine) 1986;6:336.
19. *Shen De Yan Jiu* (Research of Kidney) 1981;19.
20. *Hei Long Jiang Zhong Yi Yao* (Heilongjiang Chinese Medicine and Herbology) 1987;1:40.
21. *Zhong Cheng Yao Yan Jiu* (Research of Chinese Patent Medicine) 1986;10:33.
22. *Zhong Yi Fang Ji Xian Dai Yan Jiu* (Modern Study of Medical Formulae in Traditional Chinese Medicine) 1997;712.
23. *Shan Xi Zhong Yi* (Shanxi Chinese Medicine) 1995;16(11):485.
24. *Shen De Yan Jiu* (Research of Kidney) 1981;19.
25. *Xin Jiang Zhong Yi Yao* (Xinjiang Chinese Medicine and Herbology) 1994;4:13.
26. *Zhong Yi Za Zhi* (Journal of Chinese Medicine) 1999;4:243.
27. *Hu Nan Yi Yao Za Zhi* (Hunan Journal of Medicine and Herbology) 1978;4:26.
28. *Jiang Xi Zhong Yi Yao* (Jiangxi Chinese Medicine and Herbology) 1998;6:26.
29. *Zhe Jiang Zhong Yi Za Zhi* (Zhejiang Journal of Chinese Medicine) 1988;6:244.
30. *Shi Yong Zhong Yi Nei Ke Za Zhi* (Journal of Practical Chinese Internal Medicine) 1993;3:142.
31. *Zhong Yi Za Zhi* (Journal of Chinese Medicine) 1993;1:61.
32. *Shan Xi Zhong Yi* (Shanxi Chinese Medicine) 1995;16(12):552.
33. *Nei Meng Gu Zhong Yi Yao* (Traditional Chinese Medicine and Medicinals of Inner Mongolia) 1998;1:4.
34. *Guang Ming Zhong Yi* (Guangming Chinese Medicine) 1998;5:28.
35. *Cheng Du Zhong Yi Xue Yuan Xue Bao* (Journal of Chengdu University of Traditional Chinese Medicine) 1993;1:20.
36. *Hu Bei Zhong Yi Za Zhi* (Hubei Journal of Chinese Medicine) 1996;2:24.
37. *Si Chuan Zhong Yi* (Sichuan Chinese Medicine) 1995;5:30.
38. *He Bei Zhong Yi* (Hebei Chinese Medicine) 1999;3:167.
39. *Shi Yong Zhong Yi Nei Ke Za Zhi* (Journal of Practical Chinese Internal Medicine) 1988;1:53.
40. *Shang Hai Zhong Yi Yao Za Zhi* (Shanghai Journal of Chinese Medicine and Herbology) 1998;6:31.
41. *Jiang Xi Yi Xue Yuan Xue Bao* (Medical Journal of Jiangxi University of Medicine) 1996;4:19.
42. *Chang Chun Zhong Yi Xue Yuan Xue Bao* (Journal of Changchun University of Chinese Medicine) 1998;4:21.
43. *Zhe Jiang Zhong Yi Xue Yuan Xue Bao* (Journal of Zhejiang University of Chinese Medicine) 1992;1:29.
44. *Zhong Yi Fang Ji Xian Dai Yan Jiu* (Modern Study of Medical Formulae in Traditional Chinese Medicine) 1997;710-711.
45. Wang MZ, et al. *Zhong Yi Xue Wen Da Ti Ku* (Questions and Answers on Traditional Chinese Medicine: Herbal Formulas).
46. Wang MZ, et al. *Zhong Yi Xue Wen Da Ti Ku* (Questions and Answers on Traditional Chinese Medicine: Herbal Formulas).

Zhī Bǎi Dì Huáng Wán

(Anemarrhena, Phellodendron, and Rehmannia Pill)

知柏地黃丸
知柏地黄丸

Pinyin Name: *Zhi Bai Di Huang Wan*
Literal Name: Anemarrhena, Phellodendron, and Rehmannia Pill
Alternate Names: *Zhi Bo Di Huang Wan, Zi Bo Di Huang Wan, Zhi Bai Ba Wei Wan, Chih Po Ti Huang Wan*, Eight-Ingredient Pill with Anemarrhena and Phellodendron, Anemarrhena, Phellodendron and Rehmannia Formula
Original Source: *Yi Zong Jin Jian* (Golden Mirror of the Medical Tradition) by Wu Qian in 1742

COMPOSITION

Shu Di Huang (Radix Rehmanniae Praeparata)	240g [24g]
Shan Zhu Yu (Fructus Corni)	120g [12g]
Shan Yao (Rhizoma Dioscoreae)	120g [12g]
Ze Xie (Rhizoma Alismatis)	90g [9g]
Mu Dan Pi (Cortex Moutan)	90g [9g]
Fu Ling (Poria)	90g [9g]
Zhi Mu (Rhizoma Anemarrhenae)	60g [6g]
Huang Bo (Cortex Phellodendri Chinensis)	60g [6g]

Zhī Bǎi Dì Huáng Wán
(Anemarrhena, Phellodendron, and Rehmannia Pill)

DOSAGE / PREPARATION / ADMINISTRATION

Prepare and administer this formula as honey pills or in decoction form. The instructions for preparation and administration for this formula are the same as *Liu Wei Di Huang Wan* (Six-Ingredient Pill with Rehmannia). For decoction, use the doses suggested in brackets.

CHINESE THERAPEUTIC ACTIONS

1. Nourishes Liver and Kidney yin
2. Clears yin-deficient fire

CLINICAL MANIFESTATIONS

Yin-deficient fire of the Liver and Kidney: steaming bones sensation, tidal fever, night sweats, irritability, soreness of the lower back and knees, and seminal emissions.

CLINICAL APPLICATIONS

Menopause, male infertility, hemospermia, diabetes mellitus, nephrotic syndrome, hypertension, tinnitus, epistaxis, dryness in geriatric patients, chronic neuritis, spontaneous perspiration, and gouty arthritis.

EXPLANATION

Zhi Bai Di Huang Wan (Anemarrhena, Phellodendron, and Rehmannia Pill) nourishes Liver and Kidney yin, and clears yin-deficient heat. This formula has similar actions as *Liu Wei Di Huang Wan* (Six-Ingredient Pill with Rehmannia) to tonify yin; however, it has a much stronger effect to clear yin-deficient fire of the Liver and Kidney, making it more effective for relieving steaming bones sensation, tidal fever, night sweats, and irritability.

This formula consists of the six herbs of *Liu Wei Di Huang Wan* (Six-Ingredient Pill with Rehmannia), which nourish Liver and Kidney yin, plus *Zhi Mu* (Rhizoma Anemarrhenae) and *Huang Bo* (Cortex Phellodendri Chinensis). *Zhi Mu* (Rhizoma Anemarrhenae) and *Huang Bo* (Cortex Phellodendri Chinensis) are excellent for

sedating yin-deficient fire of the Liver and Kidney. For a more detailed explanation of the clinical manifestations and the functions of each herb in this formula, please refer to *Liu Wei Di Huang Wan* (Six-Ingredient Pill with Rehmannia).

MODIFICATIONS

- With a dry mouth and sore throat, add *Xuan Shen* (Radix Scrophulariae) and *Jie Geng* (Radix Platycodonis).
- For thirst and irritability, add *Huang Qi* (Radix Astragali) and *Ren Shen* (Radix et Rhizoma Ginseng).
- If there is more soreness of the lower back, add *Niu Xi* (Radix Achyranthis Bidentatae) and *Du Zhong* (Cortex Eucommiae).

CAUTIONS / CONTRAINDICATIONS

Please refer to *Liu Wei Di Huang Wan* (Six-Ingredient Pill with Rehmannia).

CLINICAL STUDIES AND RESEARCH

1. **Male infertility**: Use of modified *Zhi Bai Di Huang Wan* was associated with 92.2% effectiveness in treating 220 men with infertility. The herbal treatment contained this formula plus *Bai Hua She She Cao* (Herba Hedyotis), *Pu Gong Ying* (Herba Taraxaci), *Dan Shen* (Radix et Rhizoma Salviae Miltiorrhizae), *Fen Bi Xie* (Rhizoma Dioscoreae Hypoglaucae), *Mu Li* (Concha Ostreae), *Niu Xi* (Radix Achyranthis Bidentatae), and *Shi Chang Pu* (Rhizoma Acori Tatarinowii) as the base formula. Additional modifications were made as necessary according to the condition of the patients. For Kidney yin deficiency, *Di Huang* (Radix Rehmanniae) and *Mu Dan Pi* (Cortex Moutan) were removed, and *Ba Ji Tian* (Radix Morindae Officinalis), *Rou Cong Rong* (Herba Cistanches), *Yin Yang Huo* (Herba Epimedii), *Huang Qi* (Radix Astragali), and *Gou Qi Zi* (Fructus Lycii) were added. For more damp-heat, *Da Huang* (Radix et Rhizoma Rhei) and *Mu Tong* (Caulis Akebiae) were added. For stagnation, *Wang Bu*

Zhi Bai Di Huang Wan (Anemarrhena, Phellodendron, and Rehmannia Pill)

Diagnosis	Signs and Symptoms	Treatment	Herbs
Yin-deficient fire of the Liver and Kidney	• Dizziness, vertigo, tinnitus, deafness, blurred vision, soreness and weakness of the lower back and knees, night sweats, seminal emissions, tidal fever, heat sensations in the palm and soles, thirst, and a dry mouth and throat: Liver and Kidney yin deficiency • Steaming bones sensation, tidal fever, and irritability: yin-deficient fire	• Nourishes Liver and Kidney yin • Clears yin-deficient fire	• *Liu Wei Di Huang Wan* (Six-Ingredient Pill with Rehmannia) nourishes Liver and Kidney yin. • *Zhi Mu* (Rhizoma Anemarrhenae) and *Huang Bo* (Cortex Phellodendri Chinensis) sedate yin-deficient fire of the Liver and Kidney.

Zhī Bǎi Dì Huáng Wán
(Anemarrhena, Phellodendron, and Rehmannia Pill)

Liu Xing (Semen Vaccariae), *Chi Shao* (Radix Paeoniae Rubra), and processed *Chuan Shan Jia* (Squama Manis) were added. For Liver qi stagnation, *Chai Hu* (Radix Bupleuri) and *Yu Jin* (Radix Curcumae) were added. Of 220 cases, the study reported pregnancy in their partners in 171 cases, improvement in 32 cases, and no benefit in 17 cases.[1]

2. **Hemospermia**: Administration of modified *Zhi Bai Di Huang Wan* was effective in treating blood in the semen in 108 patients. The herbal treatment contained the formula plus *Bai Mao Gen* (Rhizoma Imperatae), *Ou Jie* (Nodus Nelumbinis Rhizomatis), and *Mo Han Lian* (Herba Ecliptae) as the base formula. Additional modifications were made as needed. For more damp-heat causing a yellow, greasy tongue coating and painful urination, *Cang Zhu* (Rhizoma Atractylodis), *Hu Po* (Succinum), and *Liu Yi San* (Six-to-One Powder) were added, and *Shan Zhu Yu* (Fructus Corni) and *Shan Yao* (Rhizoma Dioscoreae) were removed. For heat and toxins in the interior leading to painful ejaculation, *Pu Gong Ying* (Herba Taraxaci) and *Bai Jiang Cao* (Herba cum Radice Patriniae) were added. For brown discoloration of the semen, *Da Huang* (Radix et Rhizoma Rhei) and *Chi Shao* (Radix Paeoniae Rubra) were added. For the presence of bright red blood in the semen, *Xian He Cao* (Herba Agrimoniae) and *Zi Zhu* (Folium Callicarpae) were added. For pale red blood in the semen with dizziness and fatigue, *Huang Qi* (Radix Astragali) and *Dang Shen* (Radix Codonopsis) were added, and *Bai Mao Gen* (Rhizoma Imperatae) and *Ze Xie* (Rhizoma Alismatis) were removed. Of 108 cases, the study reported complete recovery in 82 cases, improvement in 16 cases, and no benefit in 10 cases. The overall rate of effectiveness was 90.7%.[2]

3. **Diabetes mellitus**: Administration of modified *Zhi Bai Di Huang Wan* in 80 patients with type II diabetes mellitus was associated with normalization in 15 cases, significant improvement in 45 cases, slight improvement in 15 cases, and no benefit in 5 cases. The herbal formula contained *Zhi Bai Di Huang Wan*, with the elimination of *Fu Ling* (Poria) and *Ze Xie* (Rhizoma Alismatis), and the addition of *Jiao Gu Lan* (Rhizoma seu Herba Gynostemmatis), *Sha Shen* (Radix Glehniae seu Adenophorae), *Gou Qi Zi* (Fructus Lycii), *Shi Hu* (Caulis Dendrobii), *Shi Gao* (Gypsum Fibrosum), and others as needed.[3] In another study, 22 patients with diabetes were treated with modified *Zhi Bai Di Huang Wan*. In addition to diabetes, 8 patients had other complications, such as urinary tract infections, hypertension, coronary heart disease, and conjunctivitis. The patients were instructed to make dietary changes and take herbs on a daily basis. Out of 22 cases, the study

reported a marked effect in 15 cases, moderate improvement in 6 cases, and no benefit in 1 case.[4]

4. **Nephrotic syndrome**: In one study, 30 patients with nephrotic syndrome were treated with modified *Zhi Bai Di Huang Wan*. The age of the patients ranged from 15-61 years of age, with a history of kidney disorder from 3 days to 17 years. All patients received herbal treatment and dietary changes. Out of 30 cases, the study reported marked improvement in 18 cases, moderate improvement in 11 cases, and no benefit in 1 case. The herbal treatment contained this formula plus *Dan Shen* (Radix et Rhizoma Salviae Miltiorrhizae), *Yi Yi Ren* (Semen Coicis), *Xuan Shen* (Radix Scrophulariae), and *Yi Mu Cao* (Herba Leonuri). Additional modifications were made as needed. For Lung qi deficiency with frequent infection, *Yu Ping Feng San* (Jade Windscreen Powder) with a larger dose of *Huang Qi* (Radix Astragali) was added. For Spleen deficiency with dampness, *Dang Shen* (Radix Codonopsis), *Bai Zhu* (Rhizoma Atractylodis Macrocephalae), *Zhu Ling* (Polyporus), and *Che Qian Zi* (Semen Plantaginis) were added. For Liver yang rising, *Ju Hua* (Flos Chrysanthemi) and *Gou Teng* (Ramulus Uncariae cum Uncis) were added. For Liver and Kidney yin deficiencies, *Di Huang* (Radix Rehmanniae), *Gou Qi Zi* (Fructus Lycii), and *Mai Dong* (Radix Ophiopogonis) were added. For soreness and pain of the throat, *Shan Dou Gen* (Radix et Rhizoma Sophorae Tonkinensis) and *She Gan* (Rhizoma Belamcandae) were added. For severe hematuria, *Pu Huang* (Pollen Typhae), charred *Huang Qin* (Radix Scutellariae), charred *Da Huang* (Radix et Rhizoma Rhei), and a large dose of *Bai Mao Gen* (Rhizoma Imperatae) were added. For seminal emissions, calcined *Long Gu* (Os Draconis), *Qian Shi* (Semen Euryales), and *Jin Ying Zi* (Fructus Rosae Laevigatae) were added. For dry stools and constipation, *He Shou Wu* (Radix Polygoni Multiflori), *Dang Gui* (Radix Angelicae Sinensis), *Rou Cong Rong* (Herba Cistanches), *Sang Shen* (Fructus Mori), and *Da Huang* (Radix et Rhizoma Rhei) were added. For edema, *Da Fu Pi* (Pericarpium Arecae) and *Che Qian Zi* (Semen Plantaginis) were added.[5]

5. **Hypertension**: In one study, 40 patients with hypertension were diagnosed and treated with *Zhi Bai Di Huang Wan*. Out of 40 patients, 30 were diagnosed with secondary hypertension and 10 with primary hypertension. All patients were evaluated for both objective and subjective improvement, including blood pressure, headache, dizziness, feeling increased pressure in the head, insomnia, a bitter taste in the mouth, irritability, and a feeling of warmth in the palms and soles. Out of 10 patients with primary hypertension, the study reported improvement in 6 cases and no benefit in 4 cases after 8-9 weeks of treatment. Out of 30 cases of secondary hypertension, the study reported

Zhī Bǎi Dì Huáng Wán
(Anemarrhena, Phellodendron, and Rehmannia Pill)

improvement in 24 cases and no benefit in 6 cases after 4-5 weeks of treatment.[6]

6. **Epistaxis**: One study of 30 patients with stubborn nosebleeds reported good results using modified *Zhi Bai Di Huang Wan*. The herbal treatment contained the formula plus *Huang Qin* (Radix Scutellariae) and *Xiao Ji* (Herba Cirsii) as the base formula, with the addition of other herbs as needed. For wind-cold, *Fang Feng* (Radix Saposhnikoviae) and *Niu Xi* (Radix Achyranthis Bidentatae) were added. For wind-heat, *Sang Bai Pi* (Cortex Mori) and *Ju Hua* (Flos Chrysanthemi) were added. For Stomach fire rising, *Shi Hu* (Caulis Dendrobii) and *Mai Dong* (Radix Ophiopogonis) were added. For Liver fire rising, *Chai Hu* (Radix Bupleuri) and *Zi Wan* (Radix et Rhizoma Asteris) were added. For Liver and Kidney yin deficiencies with deficiency fire, *Gou Qi Zi* (Fructus Lycii) and *Di Gu Pi* (Cortex Lycii) were added. For Spleen deficiency and its inability to control blood circulation, *Huang Qi* (Radix Astragali) and *Tai Zi Shen* (Radix Pseudostellariae) were added. After 10 days of herbal treatment, the study reported complete recovery without recurrence for one year in 15 cases, improvement in 12 cases, and no benefit in 3 cases.[7]

7. **Dryness in geriatric patients**: Use of modified *Zhi Bai Di Huang Wan* showed good results in treating 24 geriatric patients with various complaints of dryness, such as a dry mouth, dry nose, constipation, etc.[8]

8. **Spontaneous perspiration**: Use of modified *Zhi Bai Di Huang Wan* in 16 patients with spontaneous perspiration was associated with recovery in 8 cases after 2 packs of herbs, in 3 cases after 3 packs of herbs, in another 3 cases after 4 packs of herbs, and 2 cases after 5 packs of herbs. The herbal treatment contained this formula plus *Gou Qi Zi* (Fructus Lycii), *Huang Qi* (Radix Astragali), and *Fu Xiao Mai* (Fructus Tritici Levis) as the base formula. Modifications include the addition of *Xia Ku Cao* (Spica Prunellae) and *Shi Jue Ming* (Concha Haliotidis) for hypertension; and *Suan Zao Ren* (Semen Ziziphi Spinosae) and *Bai Zi Ren* (Semen Platycladi) for palpitations. After the relief of spontaneous perspiration, the patients were switched to either *Liu Wei Di Huang Wan* (Six-Ingredient Pill with Rehmannia) or *Qi Ju Di Huang Wan* (Lycium Fruit, Chrysanthemum, and Rehmannia Pill) for consolidation.[9]

9. **Gouty arthritis**: Use of modified *Zhi Bai Di Huang Wan* plus topical application of an herbal paste was associated with recovery from gouty arthritis in 43 of 50 patients. The herbal formula contained *Zhi Bai Di Huang Wan* plus *Jin Qian Cao* (Herba Lysimachiae), *Che Qian Zi* (Semen Plantaginis), *Huang Qi* (Radix Astragali), *Niu Xi* (Radix

Achyranthis Bidentatae), and *Chi Shao* (Radix Paeoniae Rubra).[10]

HERB-DRUG INTERACTION

Streptomycin-induced toxicities: Administration of *Zhi Bai Di Huang Wan* showed effectiveness in treating streptomycin-induced toxicities in 39 patients between 10-73 years of age. Within 3-8 days following streptomycin injection, toxicities appeared, such as dizziness, tinnitus, deafness, muscle spasms and cramps, loss of balance when walking, nausea, vomiting, thirst, a dry mouth and throat, irritability, quick to anger, fatigue, poor appetite, night sweats, and dry stools. The treatment protocol was to administer modified *Zhi Bai Di Huang Wan* daily. The duration of treatment ranged from 10 to 116 days, with an average of 63 days. Of 39 cases, the study reported complete recovery in 30 cases, marked improvement in 6 cases, and moderate improvement in 3 cases. The study also noted that patients who responded the most were ones who sought treatment immediately after experiencing streptomycin toxicities.[11]

TOXICOLOGY

In an acute toxicology study, it was determined that the LD_{50} for a preparation of *Zhi Bai Di Huang Wan* was 13.31 g/kg via intraperitoneal injection in mice. The study concluded that the formula had very little toxicity.[12]

RELATED FORMULA

Shí Wèi Dì Huáng Wán
(Ten-Ingredient Pill with Rehmannia)
十味地黄丸
Pinyin Name: Shi Wei Di Huang Wan
Literal Name: Ten-Ingredient Pill with Rehmannia
Original Source: *Tian Jin Zhong Yi Xue Yuan* (Tianjin University of Chinese Medicine) in 1989

Shu Di Huang (Radix Rehmanniae Praeparata)
Shan Zhu Yu (Fructus Corni)
Shan Yao (Rhizoma Dioscoreae)
Ze Xie (Rhizoma Alismatis)
Fu Ling (Poria)
Mu Dan Pi (Cortex Moutan)
Gou Qi Zi (Fructus Lycii)
Ju Hua (Flos Chrysanthemi)
Zhi Mu (Rhizoma Anemarrhenae)
Huang Bo (Cortex Phellodendri Chinensis)

Shi Wei Di Huang Wan (Ten-Ingredient Pill with Rehmannia) tonifies Liver and Kidney yin and clears deficiency

Chapter 8 – Tonic Formulas   *Section 4 – Yin-Tonifying Formulas*

Zhī Bǎi Dì Huáng Wán
(Anemarrhena, Phellodendron, and Rehmannia Pill)

heat. It is commonly used in elderly patients who begin to experience deteriorating of ear and eye functions as a result of Liver and Kidney yin deficiencies and deficiency heat rising.

AUTHORS' COMMENTS

According to Dr. Chang Wei-Yen, *Bai Hu Tang* (White Tiger Decoction), *Long Dan Xie Gan Tang* (Gentiana Decoction to Drain the Liver), and *Zhi Bai Di Huang Wan* can be combined to treat headaches associated with flaring of Kidney fire, commonly seen in menopausal patients.

References

1. *Guang Xi Zhong Yi Yao* (Guangxi Chinese Medicine and Herbology) 1996;2:43.

2. *Liao Ning Zhong Yi Za Zhi* (Liaoning Journal of Chinese Medicine) 1996;11:504.
3. *Hu Nan Zhong Yi Za Zhi* (Hunan Journal of Chinese Medicine) 1997;6:7.
4. *Shang Hai Zhong Yi Yao Za Zhi* (Shanghai Journal of Chinese Medicine and Herbology) 1991;10:23.
5. *Shi Yong Zhong Yi Za Zhi* (Journal of Practical Chinese Medicine) 1995;6:10.
6. *Zhong Cheng Yao* (Study of Chinese Patent Medicine) 1995;4:51.
7. *He Bei Zhong Yi* (Hebei Chinese Medicine) 1995;4:46.
8. *Ji Lin Zhong Yi Yao* (Jilin Chinese Medicine and Herbology) 1993;3:24.
9. *Xin Zhong Yi* (New Chinese Medicine) 1999;11:44.
10. *He Bei Zhong Yi* (Hebei Chinese Medicine) 1997;2:39.
11. *He Nan Zhong Yi* (Henan Chinese Medicine) 1994;6:366.
12. *Zhong Yao Yao Li Yu Lin Chuang* (Pharmacology and Clinical Applications of Chinese Herbs) 1992;17:2.

Qǐ Jú Dì Huáng Wán
(Lycium Fruit, Chrysanthemum, and Rehmannia Pill)

杞菊地黄丸

杞菊地黄丸

Pinyin Name: *Qi Ju Di Huang Wan*
Literal Name: Lycium Fruit, Chrysanthemum, and Rehmannia Pill
Alternate Names: *Chi Chu Ti Huang Wan*, *Chi Ju Di Huang Wan*, Wolfberry, Chrysanthemum and Rehmannia Pill; Lycium, Chrysanthemum and Rehmannia Pill; Lycium, Chrysanthemum and Rehmannia Formula
Original Source: *Yi Ji* (Levels of Medicine)

COMPOSITION

Shu Di Huang (Radix Rehmanniae Praeparata)	240g [24g]
Shan Zhu Yu (Fructus Corni)	120g [12g]
Shan Yao (Rhizoma Dioscoreae)	120g [12g]
Ze Xie (Rhizoma Alismatis)	90g [9g]
Mu Dan Pi (Cortex Moutan)	90g [9g]
Fu Ling (Poria)	90g [9g]
Gou Qi Zi (Fructus Lycii)	90g [9g]
Ju Hua (Flos Chrysanthemi)	90g [9g]

DOSAGE / PREPARATION / ADMINISTRATION

Prepare and administer this formula as honey pills or in decoction form. The instructions for preparation and administration for this formula are the same as *Liu Wei Di Huang Wan* (Six-Ingredient Pill with Rehmannia). For decoction, use the doses suggested in brackets.

CHINESE THERAPEUTIC ACTIONS

Nourishes Liver and Kidney yin

CLINICAL MANIFESTATIONS

Liver and Kidney yin deficiencies with eye disorders: blurred vision, dry eyes, tearing of the eyes with exposure to wind; dizziness, vertigo, tinnitus, and soreness of the lower back and knees.

CLINICAL APPLICATIONS

Retrobulbar neuritis, retinitis, optic nerve atrophy, vitreous opacity, photosensitivity, photophobia, redness, swelling

640

Qǐ Jú Dì Huáng Wán
(Lycium Fruit, Chrysanthemum, and Rehmannia Pill)

and pain of eyes, blurry vision, excessive tearing with exposure to wind, chronic glaucoma, general visual disturbance, hypertension, diabetes mellitus, hyperemia, and menopause.

EXPLANATION

Qi Ju Di Huang Wan (Lycium Fruit, Chrysanthemum, and Rehmannia Pill), derived from *Liu Wei Di Huang Wan* (Six-Ingredient Pill with Rehmannia), tonifies Kidney and Liver yin, brightens the eyes, and improves vision. Compared to *Liu Wei Di Huang Wan*, this formula more strongly nourishes the Liver and benefits the eyes. The main clinical indication for this formula is deteriorated vision caused by Liver and Kidney yin deficiencies.

This formula consists of *Liu Wei Di Huang Wan* (Six-Ingredient Pill with Rehmannia) plus *Gou Qi Zi* (Fructus Lycii) and *Ju Hua* (Flos Chrysanthemi). *Liu Wei Di Huang Wan* (Six-Ingredient Pill with Rehmannia) tonifies Liver and Kidney yin. *Gou Qi Zi* (Fructus Lycii) and *Ju Hua* (Flos Chrysanthemi) improve vision and treat various eye disorders. For more information, please refer to *Liu Wei Di Huang Wan* (Six-Ingredient Pill with Rehmannia).

MODIFICATIONS

- For red eyes with swelling and pain, add *Zhi Mu* (Rhizoma Anemarrhenae) and *Huang Bo* (Cortex Phellodendri Chinensis).
- With diminished and dimmed vision, add *Dang Gui* (Radix Angelicae Sinensis) and *Huang Qi* (Radix Astragali).
- For more tearing with exposure to wind, add *Sheng Ma* (Rhizoma Cimicifugae) and *Ge Gen* (Radix Puerariae Lobatae).

CAUTIONS / CONTRAINDICATIONS

Please refer to *Liu Wei Di Huang Wan* (Six-Ingredient Pill with Rehmannia).

PHARMACOLOGICAL EFFECTS

1. **Immunostimulant**: One study reported a mild immuno-stimulant effect associated with the use of *Qi Ju Di Huang Wan* in mice. It increased phagocytic activities of macrophages.[1]
2. **Hypoglycemic**: Administration of *Qi Ju Di Huang Wan* was associated with reduced plasma glucose levels and decreased daily intake of water. The treatment protocol was to administer 2.5 g/kg and 5.0 g/kg of the formula via oral ingestion one time daily for 4 months.[2]

CLINICAL STUDIES AND RESEARCH

1. **Retinitis**: Use of *Qi Ju Di Huang Wan* in 140 patients with retinitis was associated with complete recovery in 22 patients, significant improvement in 21 patients, moderate improvement in 70 patients, and no benefit in 27 patients. The treatment protocol was to administer the herbs in decoction daily, for 3 weeks per course of treatment. The duration of treatment ranged from 30 to 118 days, with an average of 57 days.[3]
2. **Vitreous opacity**: One study reported success using modified *Qi Ju Di Huang Wan* to treat vitreous opacity in 34 patients (21 males and 13 females, between 38-76 years of age). The herbal formula contained *Gou Qi Zi* (Fructus Lycii) 15g, *Ju Hua* (Flos Chrysanthemi) 15g, *Shan Yao* (Rhizoma Dioscoreae) 15g, *Shan Zhu Yu* (Fructus Corni) 15g, *Shu Di Huang* (Radix Rehmanniae Praeparata) 20g, *Fu Ling* (Poria) 10g, *Ze Xie* (Rhizoma Alismatis) 10g, *Mu Dan Pi* (Cortex Moutan) 10g, *Tu Si Zi* (Semen Cuscutae) 10g, *Nu Zhen Zi* (Fructus Ligustri Lucidi) 10g, and *Jue Ming Zi* (Semen Cassiae) 10g. The treatment protocol was to cook the herbs in water, and administer the decoction in 2 equally-divided doses, two times daily for 30 days. Of 34 patients, the study reported significant improvement in 18 patients, moderate improvement in 11 patients, and no benefit in 5 patients. The overall rate of effectiveness was 85.29%.[4]

Qi Ju Di Huang Wan (Lycium Fruit, Chrysanthemum, and Rehmannia Pill)

Diagnosis	Signs and Symptoms	Treatment	Herbs
Liver and Kidney yin deficiencies with eye disorders	• Dizziness, vertigo, tinnitus, deafness, blurred vision, soreness and weakness of the lower back and knees, night sweats, seminal emissions, tidal fever, heat sensations in the palm and soles, thirst and a dry mouth and throat: Liver and Kidney yin deficiency • Blurred vision and dry eyes: Liver and Kidney yin deficiencies unable to nourish the eyes	• Nourishes Liver and Kidney yin • Nourishes the eyes and improve visual functions	• *Liu Wei Di Huang Wan* (Six-Ingredient Pill with Rehmannia) nourishes Liver and Kidney yin. • *Gou Qi Zi* (Fructus Lycii) and *Ju Hua* (Flos Chrysanthemi) improve vision and treat various visual disorders.

Chapter 8 – Tonic Formulas   *Section 4 – Yin-Tonifying Formulas*

Qǐ Jú Dì Huáng Wán
(Lycium Fruit, Chrysanthemum, and Rehmannia Pill)

3. **Hypertension**: Two studies have shown that administration of *Qi Ju Di Huang Wan* was effective in treating primary hypertension characterized by Kidney yin deficiency. The duration of treatment was 8-12 weeks per course of treatment. Clinical results included reduction of blood pressure and resolution of subjective symptoms.[5,6]

4. **Menopause**: In one study, 144 women with menopausal symptoms were treated effectively with *Qi Ju Di Huang Wan* as the base formula. Modifications were made by adding *Huang Lian* (Rhizoma Coptidis), *Bai Shao* (Radix Paeoniae Alba), and *Zhi Mu* (Rhizoma Anemarrhenae) for deficiency heat with a dry mouth and tongue, constipation, and irritability; *Fu Zi* (Radix Aconiti Lateralis Praeparata), *Dang Shen* (Radix Codonopsis), and *Dan Shen* (Radix et Rhizoma Salviae Miltiorrhizae) for Heart and Kidney yang deficiencies with palpitations and edema; and *Dang Shen* (Radix Codonopsis) and *Huang Qi* (Radix

Astragali) for Heart and Spleen deficiencies with poor appetite, excessive worries, and lack of desire to speak. Of 144 patients, the study reported complete recovery in 12 patients, significant improvement in 48 patients, moderate improvement in 32 patients, and no benefit in 52 patients.[7]

References
1. *Zhong Cheng Yao* (Study of Chinese Patent Medicine) 1990;10:28.
2. *Zhong Yao Yao Li Yu Lin Chuang* (Pharmacology and Clinical Applications of Chinese Herbs) 1993;9(4):2.
3. *An Hui Zhong Yi Xue Yuan Xue Bao* (Journal of Anhui University School of Medicine) 1989;4:18.
4. *Zhong Yi Yao Xue Bao* (Report of Chinese Medicine and Herbology) 1995;2:25.
5. *Zhong Yao Yao Li Yu Lin Chuang* (Pharmacology and Clinical Applications of Chinese Herbs) 1992;3:35.
6. *Xin Zhong Yi* (New Chinese Medicine) 1999;3:12.
7. *Shi Zhen Guo Yao Yan Jiu* (Research of Shizhen Herbs) 1998;1:11.

Mài Wèi Dì Huáng Wán
(Ophiopogonis, Schisandra, and Rehmannia Pill)

麥味地黃丸
麦味地黄丸

Pinyin Name: *Mai Wei Di Huang Wan*
Literal Name: Ophiopogonis, Schisandra, and Rehmannia Pill
Alternate Names: *Ba Xian Chang Shou Wan* (Eight-Immortal Pill for Longevity), *Mai Wei Ti Huang Wan* (Ophiopogon-Flavoured Rehmannia Pill)
Original Source: *Yi Ji* (Levels of Medicine)

COMPOSITION

Shu Di Huang (Radix Rehmanniae Praeparata)	240g [24g]
Shan Zhu Yu (Fructus Corni)	120g [12g]
Shan Yao (Rhizoma Dioscoreae)	120g [12g]
Ze Xie (Rhizoma Alismatis)	90g [9g]
Mu Dan Pi (Cortex Moutan)	90g [9g]
Fu Ling (Poria)	90g [9g]
Mai Dong (Radix Ophiopogonis)	90g [9g]
Wu Wei Zi (Fructus Schisandrae Chinensis)	60g [6g]

DOSAGE / PREPARATION / ADMINISTRATION

Prepare and administer this formula as honey pills or in decoction form. The instructions for preparation and administration for this formula are the same as *Liu Wei Di Huang Wan* (Six-Ingredient Pill with Rehmannia). For decoction, use the doses suggested in brackets.

642

Chinese Herbal Formulas and Applications

Mài Wèi Dì Huáng Wán
(Ophiopogonis, Schisandra, and Rehmannia Pill)

CHINESE THERAPEUTIC ACTIONS

1. Nourishes Liver and Kidney yin
2. Astringes Lung qi and nourishes Lung yin

CLINICAL MANIFESTATIONS

Kidney and Lung yin deficiencies: coughing, shortness of breath, tidal fever, night sweats, plus the clinical manifestations of yin deficiency found in *Liu Wei Di Huang Wan* (Six-Ingredient Pill with Rehmannia).

CLINICAL APPLICATIONS

Diabetes mellitus, asthma, tidal fever, and night perspiration.

EXPLANATION

Mai Wei Di Huang Wan (Ophiopogonis, Schisandra and Rehmannia Pill) is a variation of *Liu Wei Di Huang Wan* (Six-Ingredient Pill with Rehmannia), with the addition of *Mai Dong* (Radix Ophiopogonis) and *Wu Wei Zi* (Fructus Schisandrae Chinensis). *Liu Wei Di Huang Wan* (Six-Ingredient Pill with Rehmannia) tonifies Liver and Kidney yin. *Mai Dong* (Radix Ophiopogonis) and *Wu Wei Zi* (Fructus Schisandrae Chinensis) tonify Lung yin and stop coughing and shortness of breath.

PHARMACOLOGICAL EFFECTS

Hypoglycemic: In laboratory experiments, the use of *Mai Wei Di Huang Wan* had marked hypoglycemic effect if the plasma glucose level was between 180-350 mg/dL. However, it had little effect when the plasma glucose level was above 350 mg/dL.[1] While the exact mechanism of this hypoglycemic effect is not well understood, it has been determined that administration of this formula does not increase plasma insulin levels, and that it still had marked hypoglycemic effect in dogs whose pancreas had been surgically removed.[2]

CLINICAL STUDIES AND RESEARCH

1. **Diabetes mellitus**: One study reported satisfactory results using *Mai Wei Di Huang Wan* to treat 20 patients with diabetes mellitus with elevated blood glucose levels (180-410 mg/dL), glucose in the urine (++ to +++), and ketone in the urine (in 8 of 20 patients).[3]
2. **Tidal fever and night perspiration**: In one study, 150 patients with tidal fever and night sweats associated with pulmonary tuberculosis were treated with good results. The herbal treatment contained *Mai Wei Di Huang Wan* plus *Sha Shen* (Radix Glehniae seu Adenophorae), *Bai He* (Bulbus Lilii), and *Yu Zhu* (Rhizoma Polygonati Odorati) as the base formula. *Huang Qi* (Radix Astragali) was added for qi deficiency; *Zi Wan* (Radix et Rhizoma Asteris) was added for dry cough, and *Shan Zhu Yu* (Fructus Corni) for severe night sweats. Of 150 patients, the study reported resolution of tidal fever and night sweats in 146 patients, and no effect in 4 patients.[4]

References

1. *Zhong Yao Tong Bao* (Journal of Chinese Herbology) 1982;6:32.
2. *Zhong Yi Fang Ji Xian Dai Yan Jiu* (Modern Study of Medical Formulae in Traditional Chinese Medicine) 1997;727.
3. *Si Chuan Zhong Yi* (Sichuan Chinese Medicine) 1989;3:25.
4. *Zhong Yi Yan Jiu* (Research of Chinese Medicine) 1992;3:40.

Mai Wei Di Huang Wan (Ophiopogonis, Schisandra and Rehmannia Pill)

Diagnosis	Signs and Symptoms	Treatment	Herbs
Kidney and Lung yin deficiencies accompanied by coughing	• Dizziness, vertigo, tinnitus, deafness, blurred vision, soreness and weakness of the lower back and knees, night sweats, seminal emissions, tidal fever, heat sensations in the palm and soles, thirst and a dry mouth and throat: Liver and Kidney yin deficiencies • Coughing and shortness of breath: Lung yin deficiency	• Nourishes Liver and Kidney yin • Astringes and nourishes Lung yin to stop coughing	• *Liu Wei Di Huang Wan* (Six-Ingredient Pill with Rehmannia) nourishes Liver and Kidney yin. • *Mai Dong* (Radix Ophiopogonis) and *Wu Wei Zi* (Fructus Schisandrae Chinensis) tonify and astringe Lung yin.

643

Chapter 8 – Tonic Formulas　　　　　　　　　　　　*Section 4 – Yin-Tonifying Formulas*

Dū Qì Wán (Capital Qi Pill)

都氣丸
都气丸

Pinyin Name: *Du Qi Wan*
Literal Name: Capital Qi Pill
Original Source: *Yi Guan* (Thorough Knowledge of Medicine) by Zhao Xian-Ke in 1617

COMPOSITION

Shu Di Huang (Radix Rehmanniae Praeparata)	240g [24g]
Shan Zhu Yu (Fructus Corni)	120g [12g]
Shan Yao (Rhizoma Dioscoreae)	120g [12g]
Ze Xie (Rhizoma Alismatis)	90g [9g]
Mu Dan Pi (Cortex Moutan)	90g [9g]
Fu Ling (Poria)	90g [9g]
Wu Wei Zi (Fructus Schisandrae Chinensis)	60g [6g]

DOSAGE / PREPARATION / ADMINISTRATION

Prepare and administer this formula as honey pills or in decoction form. For decoction, use the doses suggested in brackets.

CHINESE THERAPEUTIC ACTIONS

1. Nourishes Kidney yin
2. Facilitates normal respiration

CLINICAL MANIFESTATIONS

Kidney yin deficiency accompanied by coughing and wheezing: dizziness, tinnitus, sore back, weak knees, coughing, and wheezing.

CLINICAL APPLICATIONS

Asthma, bronchial asthma, pulmonary emphysema, and pulmonary tuberculosis.

EXPLANATION

Du Qi Wan (Capital Qi Pill) is derived from *Liu Wei Di Huang Wan* (Six-Ingredient Pill with Rehmannia). Besides tonifying Kidney yin, this formula improves

respiration by invigorating Kidney qi. The Kidney assists Lung qi to descend in normal inspiration. If the Kidney is deficient, it is unable to grasp the qi and bring it down, giving rise to respiratory disorders. In addition to coughing and wheezing, other symptoms of Kidney yin deficiency, such as dizziness, tinnitus, sore back, and weak knees, might be present.

This formula consists of the six herbs of *Liu Wei Di Huang Wan* (Six-Ingredient Pill with Rehmannia) plus *Wu Wei Zi* (Fructus Schisandrae Chinensis). *Liu Wei Di Huang Wan* (Six-Ingredient Pill with Rehmannia) nourishes Liver and Kidney yin. *Wu Wei Zi* (Fructus Schisandrae Chinensis), a sour herb, tonifies the Kidney and astringes Lung qi to relieve coughing and wheezing. For more information on the functions of each individual herb in this formula, please refer to *Liu Wei Di Huang Wan* (Six-Ingredient Pill with Rehmannia).

CAUTIONS / CONTRAINDICATIONS

Please refer to *Liu Wei Di Huang Wan* (Six-Ingredient Pill with Rehmannia).

Du Qi Wan (Capital Qi Pill)

Diagnosis	Signs and Symptoms	Treatment	Herbs
Kidney yin deficiency accompanied by coughing and wheezing	• Dizziness, tinnitus, sore back, and weak knees: Kidney yin deficiency • Coughing and wheezing: Lung deficiency	• Nourishes Kidney yin • Facilitates normal respiration	• *Liu Wei Di Huang Wan* (Six-Ingredient Pill with Rehmannia) nourishes Liver and Kidney yin. • *Wu Wei Zi* (Fructus Schisandrae Chinensis) astringes Lung qi to relieve coughing and wheezing.

644

Chinese Herbal Formulas and Applications

Zuǒ Guī Wán (Restore the Left [Kidney] Pill)

左歸丸
左归丸

Pinyin Name: *Zuo Gui Wan*
Literal Name: Restore the Left [Kidney] Pill
Alternate Name: Cyathula and Rehmannia Formula
Original Source: *Jing Yue Quan Shu* (Collected Treatises of [Zhang] Jing Yue) by Zhang Jie-Bin (Zhang Jing-Yue) in 1624

COMPOSITION

Shu Di Huang (Radix Rehmanniae Praeparata)	240g [24g]
Gou Qi Zi (Fructus Lycii)	120g [12g]
Shan Zhu Yu (Fructus Corni)	120g [12g]
Gui Ban Jiao (Gelatinum Plastrum Testudinis), *chao* (dry-fried)	120g [12g]
Lu Jiao Jiao (Colla Cornus Cervi), *chao* (dry-fried)	120g [12g]
Tu Si Zi (Semen Cuscutae), *zhi* (prepared)	120g [12g]
Chuan Niu Xi (Radix Cyathulae), *xi* (washed) with liquor and *zheng* (steamed)	90g [9g]
Shan Yao (Rhizoma Dioscoreae), *chao* (dry-fried)	120g [12g]

DOSAGE / PREPARATION / ADMINISTRATION

The source text's instructions are to first steam *Shu Di Huang* (Radix Rehmanniae Praeparata) and smash it into a paste. Grind the other ingredients into powder, and mix it with the paste and honey to form small pills. Take one hundred or more pills with salted or boiled water before meals. Today, it is prepared by mixing the powdered herbs with honey to form pills, with each pill weighing about 15g. Take one pill on an empty stomach in the morning and at night with lightly-salted water. This formula may also be prepared as a decoction using the doses suggested in brackets.

CHINESE THERAPEUTIC ACTIONS

1. Nourishes yin and replenishes marrow and *jing* (essence)
2. Tonifies the Kidney

CLINICAL MANIFESTATIONS

Kidney yin deficiency with depletion of marrow and *jing* (essence): dizziness, vertigo, tinnitus, soreness and weakness of the lower back and knees, night and/or spontaneous sweating, seminal emissions and/or spermatorrhea, dribbling of urine, thirst with desire to drink, a dry mouth and throat, a mirror-like tongue surface with little coating, and a fine or rapid pulse.

CLINICAL APPLICATIONS

Male sexual dysfunction, impotence, seminal emissions, spermatorrhea, infertility due to premature ovarian failure, uterine bleeding, amenorrhea, multiple neuritis, and polyneuritis.

EXPLANATION

Zuo Gui Wan (Restore the Left [Kidney] Pill) is designed to tonify Kidney yin and replenish marrow and *jing* (essence). Because the brain is the sea of marrow, marrow deficiency may result in dizziness and vertigo. Kidney deficiency often causes deficiency of the lower body, leading to weak knees and sore back. Night and spontaneous sweating occur as deficiency heat forces body fluids outward, while a dry mouth and throat and thirst indicate general yin deficiency and insufficiency of body fluids. Seminal emissions and/or spermatorrhea are the result of deficiency fire causing the *jing* to leak out. A mirror-like tongue surface with little coating indicates severe yin deficiency. A fine pulse is a typical sign of yin deficiency.

This formula contains *Shu Di Huang* (Radix Rehmanniae Praeparata) to tonify the Kidney, nourish yin and replenish *jing* (essence). *Gou Qi Zi* (Fructus Lycii) nourishes the Liver, tonifies the Kidney, and improves vision. *Shan Zhu Yu* (Fructus Corni) has a sour taste, and astringes yin and body fluids to prevent further loss. *Gui Ban Jiao* (Gelatinum Plastrum Testudinis) and *Lu Jiao Jiao* (Colla Cornus Cervi) are two animal substances that have a very strong effect in nourishing the Kidney and tonifying the yin, yang and *jing* (essence). *Tu Si Zi* (Semen Cuscutae) combines with *Chuan Niu Xi* (Radix Cyathulae) to tonify the Kidney and strengthen the lower body to relieve sore low back and weak knees. *Shan Yao* (Rhizoma Dioscoreae) tonifies the Kidney and strengthens the Spleen.

TONIC FORMULAS

8

645

Chapter 8 – Tonic Formulas   *Section 4 – Yin-Tonifying Formulas*

Zuǒ Guī Wán (Restore the Left [Kidney] Pill)

Zuo Gui Wan (Restore the Left [Kidney] Pill)

Diagnosis	Signs and Symptoms	Treatment	Herbs
Kidney yin deficiency with depletion of marrow and *jing* (essence)	• Dizziness and vertigo: marrow deficiency of the brain • Weak knees, sore back, night sweats, a dry mouth and throat, and thirst: yin deficiency • Seminal emissions and/or spermatorrhea: deficiency fire pushing *jing* outward • Mirror-like tongue surface with little coating, and a fine pulse: severe yin deficiency	• Nourishes yin • Tonifies the Kidney	• *Shu Di Huang* (Radix Rehmanniae Praeparata) tonifies the Kidney, nourishes yin, and replenishes *jing*. • *Gou Qi Zi* (Fructus Lycii) nourishes the Liver, tonifies the Kidney, and improves vision. • *Shan Zhu Yu* (Fructus Corni) astringes yin and body fluids. • *Gui Ban Jiao* (Gelatinum Plastrum Testudinis) and *Lu Jiao Jiao* (Colla Cornus Cervi) nourish the Kidney and tonify yin, yang and *jing* (essence). • *Tu Si Zi* (Semen Cuscutae) and *Chuan Niu Xi* (Radix Cyathulae) tonify the Kidney and strengthen the lower body to relieve sore back and weak knees. • *Shan Yao* (Rhizoma Dioscoreae) tonifies the Kidney and strengthens the Spleen.

MODIFICATIONS

• For dry cough with scanty sputum, add *Bai He* (Bulbus Lilii).

• With tidal fever and steaming bones sensations, add *He Shou Wu* (Radix Polygoni Multiflori).

• With steaming bones sensations with fever at night, add *Di Gu Pi* (Cortex Lycii).

• With blood deficiency, add *He Shou Wu* (Radix Polygoni Multiflori) and *Huang Jing* (Rhizoma Polygonati).

• With qi deficiency, add *Ren Shen* (Radix et Rhizoma Ginseng) and *Huang Qi* (Radix Astragali).

• With flaring of deficiency fire, remove *Gou Qi Zi* (Fructus Lycii) and *Lu Jiao Jiao* (Colla Cornus Cervi), and add *Nu Zhen Zi* (Fructus Ligustri Lucidi) and *Mai Dong* (Radix Ophiopogonis).

• With dry stools, remove *Tu Si Zi* (Semen Cuscutae) and add *Rou Cong Rong* (Herba Cistanches).

• For irritability arising from Lung heat, add *Mai Dong* (Radix Ophiopogonis).

• If there is dryness caused by Heart heat, add *Xuan Shen* (Radix Scrophulariae).

CAUTIONS / CONTRAINDICATIONS

• *Zuo Gui Wan* mostly consists of stagnating herbs that could produce dampness inside the body, causing symptoms such as an uncomfortable sensation in the epigastrium, indigestion, and poor appetite. For patients with Spleen qi deficiency, qi-activating herbs such as *Sha Ren* (Fructus Amomi) and *Chen Pi* (Pericarpium Citri Reticulatae) can be added to prevent damp accumulation.

• This formula is not recommended for prolonged use, since most of the herbs are yin tonics that are stagnating in nature, and may impair Spleen and Stomach functions

and cause diarrhea or loose stools. *Liu Wei Di Huang Wan* (Six-Ingredient Pill with Rehmannia) is a more balanced and more suitable yin tonic for long-term use.

PHARMACOLOGICAL EFFECTS

Reproductive: Administration of *Zuo Gui Wan* in male mice had a dose-dependant effect to increase plasma testosterone levels and weight of the testicles.[1]

CLINICAL STUDIES AND RESEARCH

1. **Male sexual dysfunction**: Administration of *Zuo Gui Wan* effectively treated 7 men with sexual dysfunction characterized by Kidney deficiency with symptoms such as dizziness, tinnitus, soreness and weakness of the lower back and knees, night perspiration, seminal emissions, spermatorrhea, a dry mouth and tongue, a feeling of warmth at the center of the palms and soles, and decreased levels of testosterone. After herbal therapy, the study reported relief of signs and symptoms, and normalization of plasma testosterone levels.[2]

2. **Infertility due to premature ovarian failure**: According to one case report, a woman with premature ovarian failure and secondary amenorrhea for 8 years was treated with good results. The patient began to ovulate 3 months after treatment with modified *Zuo Gui Wan*. The patient then switched to clomiphene citrate. During the eight-month treatment with clomiphene citrate, there was no ovulation or conception, and the concentrations of follicle stimulating hormone and luteinizing hormone were still in the postmenopausal range. The patient then switched back to modified *Zuo Gui Wan*, and pregnancy was reported in one month. Based on this finding, the researchers suggested that *Zuo Gui Wan* may restore ovarian function

646

Zuǒ Guī Wán (Restore the Left [Kidney] Pill)

effectively and promptly, and offers another option for treating infertility in patients with premature ovarian failure. Note: Modified *Zuo Gui Wan* used in this report contained *Shu Di Huang* (Radix Rehmanniae Praeparata), *Shan Yao* (Rhizoma Dioscoreae), *Gou Qi Zi* (Fructus Lycii), *Shan Zhu Yu* (Fructus Corni), *Chuan Niu Xi* (Radix Cyathulae), *Tu Si Zi* (Semen Cuscutae), *Lu Jiao Jiao* (Colla Cornus Cervi), *Gui Ban Jiao* (Gelatinum Plastrum Testudinis), *Yin Yang Huo* (Herba Epimedii), and *Ba Ji Tian* (Radix Morindae Officinalis).[3]

3. **Uterine bleeding**: One study reported significant improvement in 17 of 22 patients using modified *Zuo Gui Wan* to treat uterine bleeding characterized by Kidney yin and/or yang deficiencies.[4] In another study, use of modified *Zuo Gui Wan* was associated with complete recovery in 38 of 45 patients with uterine bleeding. Modifications included the addition of *Er Zhi Wan* (Two-Ultimate Pill) for profuse bleeding due to yin deficiency and heat in the blood; *Bei Sha Shen* (Radix Glehniae) and *Huang Qi* (Radix Astragali) for qi deficiency; and the addition of *E Jiao* (Colla Corii Asini) and *Bai Shao* (Radix Paeoniae Alba), with the removal of *Lu Jiao Jiao* (Colla Cornus Cervi), for blood deficiency.[5]

4. **Amenorrhea**: Use of modified *Zuo Gui Wan* was effective in treating 9 of 14 patients with amenorrhea caused by Kidney yin deficiency. The duration of treatment was one month per course of treatment, for 2-3 courses.[6]

5. **Multiple neuritis**: In one study, 56 patients (between 15-58 years of age) with multiple neuritis were treated with modified *Zuo Gui Wan*. The history of illness ranged from 2 months to 1 year. The formula included *Shu Di Huang* (Radix Rehmanniae Praeparata) 20g, *Shan Yao* (Rhizoma Dioscoreae) 20g, *Sang Ji Sheng* (Herba Taxilli) 20g, *Shan Zhu Yu* (Fructus Corni) 15g, *Tu Si Zi* (Semen Cuscutae) 15g, *Gou Qi Zi* (Fructus Lycii) 15g, *Chuan Niu Xi* (Radix Cyathulae) 15g, *Du Zhong* (Cortex Eucommiae) 15g, *Wei Ling Xian* (Radix et Rhizoma Clematidis) 15g, *Qin Jiao* (Radix Gentianae Macrophyllae) 15g, *Dang Gui* (Radix Angelicae Sinensis) 15g, and *Chuan Xiong* (Rhizoma Chuanxiong) 10g. Other modifications were made if deemed necessary. The treatment protocol was to administer the herbs in decoction twice daily in the morning and at night. Out of 56 patients, the study reported recovery in 42 cases and improvement in 14 cases.[7]

6. **Polyneuritis**: Administration of modified *Zuo Gui Wan* in 56 patients with polyneuritis was associated with complete recovery in 42 cases and improvement in 14 cases. For Liver and Kidney deficiencies, *Dang Gui* (Radix Angelicae Sinensis) and *Chuan Xiong* (Rhizoma Chuanxiong) were removed, and *Zhi Mu* (Rhizoma Anemarrhenae) and *Gui Ban* (Plastrum Testudinis) were added. For Spleen and Stomach deficiencies, *Shu Di Huang* (Radix Rehmanniae

Praeparata) and *Shan Zhu Yu* (Fructus Corni) were removed, and *Dang Shen* (Radix Codonopsis), *Huang Qi* (Radix Astragali), and *Fu Ling* (Poria) were added.[8]

RELATED FORMULAS

Zuǒ Guī Yǐn (Restore the Left [Kidney] Decoction)

左歸飲
左归饮

Pinyin Name: *Zuo Gui Yin*

Literal Name: Restore the Left [Kidney] Decoction

Original Source: *Jing Yue Quan Shu* (Collected Treatises of [Zhang] Jing Yue) by Zhang Jie-Bin (Zhang Jing-Yue) in 1624

Shu Di Huang (Radix Rehmanniae Praeparata)	6-60g [9g]
Shan Yao (Rhizoma Dioscoreae)	6g
Gou Qi Zi (Fructus Lycii)	6g
Zhi Gan Cao (Radix et Rhizoma Glycyrrhizae Praeparata cum Melle)	3g
Fu Ling (Poria)	4.5g
Shan Zhu Yu (Fructus Corni)	3-6g [6g]

The source text states to cook the ingredients with two bowls of water until the liquid is reduced to 70%. Take the decoction between meals. Today, this formula may be prepared as a decoction with the doses suggested in brackets.

Zuo Gui Yin (Restore the Left [Kidney] Decoction) tonifies and benefits Kidney yin. Clinical manifestations include soreness of the lower back, seminal emissions and/or spermatorrhea, night sweats, a dry mouth and throat, thirst with desire to drink, a red tongue body with a mirror-like appearance, and a fine, rapid pulse.

Zuo Gui Wan (Restore the Left [Kidney] <u>Pill</u>) and *Zuo Gui Yin* (Restore the Left [Kidney] <u>Decoction</u>) have similar compositions and functions to treat Kidney yin deficiency.

• *Zuo Gui Wan* is a stronger formula, and is used for severe cases of Kidney yin deficiency.

• *Zuo Gui Yin* is less potent, and is used for mild to moderate cases of Kidney yin deficiency.

Jiā Wèi Zuǒ Guī Wán
(Augmented Restore the Left [Kidney] Pill)

加味左歸丸
加味左归丸

Pinyin Name: *Jia Wei Zuo Gui Wan*

Literal Name: Augmented Restore the Left [Kidney] Pill

Original Source: *Guang An Men Yi Yuan* (Guang An Men Hospital) in 1990

8

TONIC FORMULAS

647

Chapter 8 – Tonic Formulas   Section 4 – Yin-Tonifying Formulas

Zuǒ Guī Wán (Restore the Left [Kidney] Pill)

Shu Di Huang (Radix Rehmanniae Praeparata)

Shan Yao (Rhizoma Dioscoreae)

Gou Qi Zi (Fructus Lycii)

Shan Zhu Yu (Fructus Corni)

Fu Ling (Poria)

Niu Xi (Radix Achyranthis Bidentatae)

Tu Si Zi (Semen Cuscutae)

Mo Han Lian (Herba Ecliptae)

Sang Shen (Fructus Mori)

Huang Jing (Rhizoma Polygonati)

Nu Zhen Zi (Fructus Ligustri Lucidi)

Gan Cao (Radix et Rhizoma Glycyrrhizae)

Jia Wei Zuo Gui Wan (Augmented Restore the Left [Kidney] Pill) is a slight variation of the original Zuo Gui Wan (Restore the Left [Kidney] Pill). In addition to tonifying Kidney yin, Jia Wei Zuo Gui Wan (Augmented Restore the Left [Kidney] Pill) also nourishes Lung and Liver yin. This formula is most useful for patients with chronic illnesses who exhibit yin deficiency of the Kidney, Liver and Lung.

AUTHORS' COMMENTS

Liu Wei Di Huang Wan (Six-Ingredient Pill with Rehmannia) and Zuo Gui Wan are both designed to nourish yin, especially Kidney yin manifesting in soreness and weakness of the back and knees, dizziness, a dry mouth and dry throat, seminal emissions, night sweats, a red tongue body with a scanty tongue coating, and a fine pulse. Both formulas contain Shu Di Huang (Radix Rehmanniae Praeparata), Shan Yao (Rhizoma Dioscoreae), and Shan Zhu Yu (Fructus Corni) to nourish the Liver and strengthen the Spleen. Their differences are as follows:

• Liu Wei Di Huang Wan is a moderate Kidney yin tonic. It contains three tonic herbs, listed above, and three sedating herbs: Fu Ling (Poria), Ze Xie (Rhizoma Alismatis), and Mu Dan Pi (Cortex Moutan), which clear turbid water from the Kidney, promote water excretion, and clear heat respectively. They prevent the tonics from creating stagnating side effects. Liu Wei Di Huang Wan has a proper balance of tonifying and sedating herbs to prevent stagnation. This is a more harmonious and balanced formula that can be taken for a long period of time.

• Zuo Gui Wan is a very strong Kidney tonic, and is used for depletion of yin and jing (essence). It contains Shu Di Huang (Radix Rehmanniae Praeparata) at double the dose in Liu Wei Di Huang Wan (Six-Ingredient Pill with

Rehmannia), making Zuo Gui Wan richer. Most of the herbs in this formula are Kidney yin and jing tonics with no sedating herbs: Tu Si Zi (Semen Cuscutae), Chuan Niu Xi (Radix Cyathulae), Gou Qi Zi (Fructus Lycii), Lu Jiao Jiao (Colla Cornus Cervi), and Gui Ban Jiao (Gelatinum Plastrum Testudinis). Therefore, it should be used to immediately boost depleted yin and jing. However, this formula is not suitable for long-term use. [9]

Liu Wei Di Huang Wan (Six-Ingredient Pill with Rehmannia) differs from Zuo Gui Wan (Restore the Left [Kidney] Pill) in the same way Ba Wei Di Huang Wan (Eight-Ingredient Pill with Rehmannia) differs from You Gui Wan (Restore the Right [Kidney] Pill).

• Zuo Gui Wan and You Gui Wan both tonify the Kidney without sedation. Thus, they have a more potent and immediate tonifying effect, and are more suitable for treating acute and severe cases.

• Liu Wei Di Huang Wan and Ba Wei Di Huang Wan tonify and sedate the Kidney at the same time. They have a moderate tonifying effect, and are suitable for long-term use to treat chronic deficiency.

Zuo Gui Wan (Restore the Left [Kidney] Pill) and You Gui Wan (Restore the Right [Kidney] Pill) have similar names and functions. These formulas may be used singularly, or in combination.

• Zuo Gui Wan tonifies Kidney yin.

• You Gui Wan tonifies Kidney yang.

References

1. Zhong Yi Ming Fang Lin Chuang Xin Yong (Contemporary Clinical Applications of Classic Chinese Formulas) 2001;205.

2. Nan Jing Yi Xue Yuan Xue Bao (Journal of Nanjing University of Medicine) 1988;4:331.

3. Chao SL, Huang LW, Yen HR. Pregnancy in premature ovarian failure after therapy using Chinese herbal medicine. Chang Gung Medical Journal 2003 Jun;26(6):449-52.

4. Zhong Xi Yi Jie He Za Zhi (Journal of Integrated Chinese and Western Medicine) 1984;8:496.

5. Hu Nan Zhong Yi Za Zhi (Hunan Journal of Chinese Medicine) 1997;3:57.

6. Zhong Yi Za Zhi (Journal of Chinese Medicine) 1984;7:35.

7. Zhong Hua Ren Min Gong He Guo Yao Dian (Chinese Herbal Pharmacopoeia by People's Republic of China) 1995;348.

8. Zhong Yi Yao Xue Bao (Report of Chinese Medicine and Herbology) 1993;6:34.

9. Wang MZ, et al. Zhong Yi Xue Wen Da Ti Ku (Questions and Answers on Traditional Chinese Medicine: Herbal Formulas).

648

Chinese Herbal Formulas and Applications

Dà Bǔ Yīn Wán (Great Tonify the Yin Pill)

大補陰丸
大补阴丸

Pinyin Name: *Da Bu Yin Wan*
Literal Name: Great Tonify the Yin Pill
Alternate Names: *Da Bu Wan* (Great Tonify Pill), *Ta Pu Yin Wan*, Major Yin-Nourishing Pill, Rehmannia Combination
Original Source: *Dan Xi Xin Fa* (Teachings of [Zhu] Dan-Xi) by Zhu Zhen-Heng in 1481

COMPOSITION

Shu Di Huang (Radix Rehmanniae Praeparata), *zheng* (steamed) with liquor	180g [18g]
Gui Ban (Plastrum Testudinis), *zhi* (fried with liquid) till crisp	180g [18g]
Huang Bo (Cortex Phellodendri Chinensis), *chao* (dry-fried) to brown	120g [12g]
Zhi Mu (Rhizoma Anemarrhenae), *jin* (soaked) in liquor and *chao* (dry-fried)	120g [12g]

DOSAGE / PREPARATION / ADMINISTRATION

The source text instructs to grind the ingredients into powder, mix with honey and bone marrow from pigs' vertebrae, and form into pills. Take 70 pills with salted water on an empty stomach. Today, this formula is usually prepared by grinding all of the ingredients into a fine powder. Steam the bone marrow from the pigs' vertebrae until it is fully cooked, and then smash it into a paste. Mix the powdered herbs, marrow paste, and honey and form into pills. The pills should weigh 15g each. Take 1 pill in the morning and at night with lightly-salted water. Today, this formula may be prepared as a decoction using the doses suggested in brackets.

CHINESE THERAPEUTIC ACTIONS

Nourishes yin and clears deficiency fire

CLINICAL MANIFESTATIONS

Liver and Kidney yin deficiencies with deficiency fire rising upward: steaming bones sensation, tidal fever, night sweats, seminal emissions, atrophy and weakness of the knees and legs, coughing with or without blood, fidgeting, irritability, a short temper, decreased sleep with frequent dreams, nocturnal emissions, a red tongue body with a scanty coating, and a rapid, forceful pulse at the *chi* position.

CLINICAL APPLICATIONS

Diabetes mellitus, hyperthyroidism, bronchiectasis, seminal emissions, epididymitis, urinary tract infection, and tuberculosis of the lungs, kidneys, and bones.

EXPLANATION

Da Bu Yin Wan (Great Tonify the Yin Pill) is designed to treat Liver and Kidney yin deficiencies with deficiency fire rising upward. Yin deficiency may lead to deficiency fire rising, causing symptoms such as steaming bones sensation, tidal fever, night sweats, and seminal emissions. Atrophy and weakness of the knees and legs are caused by Liver and Kidney yin deficiencies. If deficiency fire flares

Da Bu Yin Wan (Great Tonify the Yin Pill)

Diagnosis	Signs and Symptoms	Treatment	Herbs
Liver and Kidney yin deficiencies with deficiency fire rising upward	• Steaming bones sensation, tidal fever, night sweats, and seminal emissions: yin-deficient fire rising • Atrophy and weakness of the knees and legs: Liver and Kidney yin deficiencies unable to nourish the bones and tendons • Fidgeting, irritability, a short temper, decreased sleep with frequent dreams: yin-deficient fire disturbing the Heart • Red tongue body with a scanty coating and a rapid, forceful pulse: yin-deficient fire rising	Nourishes yin and clears deficient fire	• *Shu Di Huang* (Radix Rehmanniae Praeparata) tonifies yin and replenishes *jing* (essence). • *Gui Ban* (Plastrum Testudinis) nourishes yin and anchors yang to control deficiency fire. • *Huang Bo* (Cortex Phellodendri Chinensis) strongly sedates deficiency fire. • *Zhi Mu* (Rhizoma Anemarrhenae) clears deficiency fire and moistens the Lung and Kidney.

TONIC FORMULAS

8

649

Chapter 8 – Tonic Formulas

Section 4 – Yin-Tonifying Formulas

Dà Bǔ Yīn Wán (Great Tonify the Yin Pill)

up to affect the Lung, coughing may occur. Bleeding can also accompany the cough if the deficiency fire damages the vessels. Similarly, if the deficiency fire flares up to affect the Heart, fidgeting, irritability and sleep disturbance may occur. A red tongue body with a scanty coating is representative of yin deficiency. A rapid, forceful pulse may be present if the deficiency fire flares up and causes acute symptoms. The rapid, forceful pulse at the *chi* position indicates the severity of the deficiency fire.

Shu Di Huang (Radix Rehmanniae Praeparata) tonifies yin and replenishes *jing* (essence). *Gui Ban* (Plastrum Testudinis) nourishes yin and anchors yang to control deficiency fire. Both greatly tonify the true yin of the body and thus help control the rising of deficiency fire. *Huang Bo* (Cortex Phellodendri Chinensis) strongly sedates deficiency fire. *Zhi Mu* (Rhizoma Anemarrhenae) clears deficiency fire and moistens the Lung and Kidney. Indeed, this formula consists of strong tonics to nourish Liver and Kidney yin, and sedating herbs to control the rising of deficiency fire. Bone marrow and honey nourish yin, replenish *jing*, and generate body fluids.

MODIFICATIONS
- If there is more yin deficiency, add *Mai Dong* (Radix Ophiopogonis) and *Tian Dong* (Radix Asparagi).
- With night sweats, add *Fu Xiao Mai* (Fructus Tritici Levis) and calcined *Mu Li* (Concha Ostreae).
- For spermatorrhea or nocturnal emissions, add *Jin Ying Zi* (Fructus Rosae Laevigatae), *Qian Shi* (Semen Euryales), and *Sang Piao Xiao* (Ootheca Mantidis).
- With sputum that is difficult to expectorate, add *Bai Bu* (Radix Stemonae) and *Kuan Dong Hua* (Flos Farfarae).
- With cough with sputum that is difficult to expectorate, add *Bai Bu* (Radix Stemonae) and *Chuan Bei Mu* (Bulbus Fritillariae Cirrhosae).
- With cough or vomiting with blood, add *Xian He Cao* (Herba Agrimoniae), *Bai Mao Gen* (Rhizoma Imperatae), and *Ce Bai Ye* (Cacumen Platycladi).

CAUTIONS / CONTRAINDICATIONS
- *Da Bu Yin Wan* is contraindicated in Spleen and/or Stomach deficiencies with loose stools and poor appetite.
- This formula is contraindicated in patients with excess heat and fire.
- Avoid foods that are pungent and spicy.[1]

CLINICAL STUDIES AND RESEARCH
1. **Pulmonary tuberculosis**: In one study, modified *Da Bu Yin Wan* was used to treat 10 patients with coughing of blood due to pulmonary tuberculosis. The diagnosis according to traditional Chinese medicine was Lung and

Kidney yin deficiencies leading to deficiency fire attacking the Lung. The herbal formula included *Di Huang* (Radix Rehmanniae) 12g, *Shu Di Huang* (Radix Rehmanniae Praeparata) 12g, charred *Zhi Zi* (Fructus Gardeniae) 6g, *Zhi Mu* (Rhizoma Anemarrhenae) 6g, *Gui Ban* (Plastrum Testudinis) 30g, *Mai Dong* (Radix Ophiopogonis) 15g, *Niu Xi* (Radix Achyranthis Bidentatae) 9g, *Pi Pa Ye* (Folium Eriobotryae) 9g, *Ce Bai Ye* (Cacumen Platycladi) 30g, and *Mo Han Lian* (Herba Ecliptae) 30g. Out of 10 patients, the study reported successful cessation of bleeding in 9 patients.[2]

2. **Epididymitis**: In one study, 18 patients with acute or chronic epididymitis were treated with modified *Da Bu Yin Wan* with good results. The formula included *Da Bu Yin Wan* with the addition of *Jin Yin Hua* (Flos Lonicerae Japonicae) 30g and *Li Zhi He* (Semen Litchi) 20g. In addition, *Xuan Shen* (Radix Scrophulariae) 30g, *Hai Zao* (Sargassum) 15g, and *Mu Dan Pi* (Cortex Moutan) 5g were added for swelling and pain of the testicles. *Chuan Lian Zi* (Fructus Toosendan) 6g and *Yan Hu Suo* (Rhizoma Corydalis) 6g were added for pain radiating to the abdomen and lower back. *Hai Zao* (Sargassum) 15g and *Chuan Lian Zi* (Fructus Toosendan) 20g were added for swelling, pain, and hardness in the affected area. Lastly, *Bai Jiang Cao* (Herba cum Radice Patriniae) 30g was added for fever. Treatment lasted from 5-55 days. The study reported recovery in all patients, with testicle size returning to normal. No recurrences were reported in any of the 10 patients who returned for a follow-up one year later.[3]

3. **Urinary tract infection**: In one study, modified *Da Bu Yin Wan* effectively treated urinary tract infection. Modifications to the formula included the addition of *Qu Mai* (Herba Dianthi) and *Che Qian Zi* (Semen Plantaginis) for painful urination; *Zhi Qiao* (Fructus Aurantii) for lower abdominal distention and urinary urgency; *Fen Bi Xie* (Rhizoma Dioscoreae Hypoglaucae) and *Yi Yi Ren* (Semen Coicis) for hematuria; *Xuan Shen* (Radix Scrophulariae) and *Shi Hu* (Caulis Dendrobii) for a red tongue body and lack of fluids; and injection of *Chai Hu* (Radix Bupleuri) for high fever. The study reported a 77.7% success rate (70 out of 90 patients) in treating urinary tract infection.[4]

AUTHORS' COMMENTS
Da Bu Yin Wan is an important formula that nourishes Liver and Kidney yin and clears deficiency fire. The key signs and symptoms include steaming bones sensation, tidal fever, night sweats, a red tongue body with a scanty coating, and a fine, rapid pulse.

Liu Wei Di Huang Wan (Six-Ingredient Pill with Rehmannia) and *Da Bu Yin Wan* both nourish yin.

650

Chinese Herbal Formulas and Applications

Dà Bǔ Yīn Wán (Great Tonify the Yin Pill)

- *Liu Wei Di Huang Wan* is a more neutral tonic to replenish Kidney yin.
- *Da Bu Yin Wan* strongly sedates deficiency fire with depletion of yin.[5]

Please refer to *Bu Fei E Jiao Tang* (Tonify the Lung Decoction with Ass-Hide Gelatin) for a comparative analysis with *Da Bu Yin Wan* and *Sheng Mai San* (Generate the Pulse Powder).

References

1. *Zhong Yao Ming Fang Yao Li Yu Ying Yong* (Pharmacology and Applications of Famous Herbal Formulas) 1989;313-14.
2. *Xin Zhong Yi* (New Chinese Medicine) 1975;(4):40.
3. *Zhe Jiang Zhong Yi Yao* (Zhejiang Chinese Medicine and Herbology) 1985;11-12:495.
4. *Ji Lin Zhong Yi Yao* (Jilin Chinese Medicine and Herbology) 1998;1:16.
5. Wang MZ, et al. *Zhong Yi Xue Wen Da Ti Ku* (Questions and Answers on Traditional Chinese Medicine: Herbal Formulas).

Hǔ Qián Wán (Hidden Tiger Pill)

虎潜丸
虎潛丸

Pinyin Name: *Hu Qian Wan*
Literal Name: Hidden Tiger Pill
Alternate Name: Phellodendron Formula
Original Source: *Dan Xi Xin Fa* (Teachings of [Zhu] Dan-Xi) by Zhu Zhen-Heng in 1481

COMPOSITION

Huang Bo (Cortex Phellodendri Chinensis), *chao* (dry-fried) with liquor	240g
Zhi Mu (Rhizoma Anemarrhenae), *chao* (dry-fried) with liquor	60g
Gui Ban (Plastrum Testudinis), *zhi* (fried) with liquor	120g
Shu Di Huang (Radix Rehmanniae Praeparata)	60g
Bai Shao (Radix Paeoniae Alba)	60g
Hu Gu (Os Tigris), *zhi* (fried) with liquid	30g
Suo Yang (Herba Cynomorii)	45g
Chen Pi (Pericarpium Citri Reticulatae)	60g
Gan Jiang (Rhizoma Zingiberis)	15g

Note: *Hu Gu* (Os Tigris) is derived from an endangered animal, and is rarely used as a medicinal substance today. Its discussion here is included primarily for academic purposes, to reflect the historical use of this substance in its original formulation. Most herbal products today have removed it completely, or replaced it with *Zhu Gu* (Os Porcus) which has similar functions.

DOSAGE / PREPARATION / ADMINISTRATION

Grind the ingredients into powder and form into pills with grain-based alcohol. Today, this formula is usually prepared by mixing the powdered herbs with honey to form pills, which should weigh 10g each. Take 1 pill in the morning and at night with lightly-salted water or warm water.

CHINESE THERAPEUTIC ACTIONS

1. Nourishes yin, and lowers and clears deficiency fire
2. Strengthens sinews and bones

CLINICAL MANIFESTATIONS

Weakness and atrophy of the bones and tendons associated with Liver and Kidney yin-deficient fire: weakness and soreness of the lower back, legs, and knees; weakness of the sinews and bones; atrophy of the muscles, sinews, and bones in the extremities; a red tongue body with little coating, and a fine, weak pulse.

CLINICAL APPLICATIONS

Sequelae of polio or stroke with numbness, weakness, and atrophy of the extremities; atrophy and degeneration of the nervous system, atrophy and degeneration of

8

TONIC FORMULAS

651

Chapter 8 – Tonic Formulas

Section 4 – Yin-Tonifying Formulas

Hŭ Qián Wán (Hidden Tiger Pill)

the reproductive system, lumbago, tuberculosis of the knee, muscle atrophy, flaccidity of muscles and bones, post-stroke complications, chronic arthritis, lateral spinal sclerosis, and hypocalcemia.

EXPLANATION

Hu Qian Wan (Hidden Tiger Pill) treats *wei zheng* (atrophy syndrome) with severe weakness and atrophy of the sinews and bones arising from Kidney yin deficiency, Liver blood deficiency, and yin-deficient fire. The Kidney controls the bones, and the Liver controls the sinews and tendons. If the Kidney and Liver are deficient, the bones and tendons may become weak and deficient as well. Deficiency fire dries yin and blood, causing malnourishment of the sinews. Prolonged lack of nourishment of the sinews leads to stiffness and spasms of the sinews, which can eventually progress to atrophy. Weak bones and tendons may lead to soreness of the lower back and knees, as well as weak legs and weakening of the leg muscles. A red tongue body with little coating indicates deficiency fire, and a fine, weak pulse suggests that the bones and tendons are becoming deficient.

Huang Bo (Cortex Phellodendri Chinensis) and *Zhi Mu* (Rhizoma Anemarrhenae) clear deficiency fire and strengthen yin of the lower *jiao*. *Gui Ban* (Plastrum Testudinis) nourishes Kidney yin, and replenishes *jing* (essence) and marrow. *Shu Di Huang* (Radix Rehmanniae Praeparata) and *Bai Shao* (Radix Paeoniae Alba) nourish yin and tonify the blood. *Hu Gu* (Os Tigris) strengthens the sinews and bones. *Suo Yang* (Herba Cynomorii) nourishes Kidney yang and *jing*. *Chen Pi* (Pericarpium Citri Reticulatae) and *Gan Jiang* (Rhizoma Zingiberis) strengthen the Spleen and harmonize the middle *jiao* to prevent the cold and stagnating herbs from damaging the digestive system.

MODIFICATIONS

- If there is more deficiency heat, use *Di Huang* (Radix Rehmanniae) instead of *Shu Di Huang* (Radix Rehmanniae Praeparata).
- With atrophy and weakness of the muscles due to blood deficiency, add *Chuan Xiong* (Rhizoma Chuanxiong) and *Du Zhong* (Cortex Eucommiae).
- With atrophy and weakness of the muscles due to qi deficiency, add *Ren Shen* (Radix et Rhizoma Ginseng) and *Huang Qi* (Radix Astragali).
- With atrophy and weakness of the muscles due to *jing* (essence) deficiency, add *Lu Jiao Shuang* (Cornu Cervi Degelatinatum) and *Rou Cong Rong* (Herba Cistanches).
- For seminal emissions, add *Long Gu* (Os Draconis) and *Mu Li* (Concha Ostreae).

CAUTIONS / CONTRAINDICATIONS

Hu Qian Wan is contraindicated in patients with atrophy caused by damp-heat invasion.

CLINICAL STUDIES AND RESEARCH

1. **Muscle atrophy and lateral spinal sclerosis**: It has been reported that *Hu Qian Wan* plus *Ren Shen* (Radix et Rhizoma Ginseng) and *Huang Qi* (Radix Astragali) is effective in treating muscle atrophy and lateral spinal sclerosis, especially if the conditions are characterized by yin and yang deficiencies.[1]

2. **Hypocalcemia**: Use of modified *Hu Qian Wan* was associated with good therapeutic effect in treating 15 patients with low plasma calcium levels following thyroidectomy. The formula contained *Huang Bo* (Cortex Phellodendri

Hu Qian Wan (Hidden Tiger Pill)

Diagnosis	Signs and Symptoms	Treatment	Herbs
Wei (atrophy) syndrome with Liver and Kidney yin-deficient fire	• Weakness and soreness of the lower back, legs and knees: Liver and Kidney yin deficiencies • Atrophy of the muscles, sinews and bones in the extremities: deficiency fire drying yin and blood, and causing malnourishment of soft tissues • Red tongue body with little coating and a fine, weak pulse: deficiency fire condition	• Nourishes yin and blood • Lowers and clears deficiency fire • Strengthens sinews and bones	• *Huang Bo* (Cortex Phellodendri Chinensis) and *Zhi Mu* (Rhizoma Anemarrhenae) clear deficiency fire. • *Gui Ban* (Plastrum Testudinis) nourishes Kidney yin, tonifies the blood, and replenishes *jing* (essence) and marrow. • *Shu Di Huang* (Radix Rehmanniae Praeparata) and *Bai Shao* (Radix Paeoniae Alba) nourish yin and tonify the blood. • *Hu Gu* (Os Tigris) strengthens the sinews and bones. • *Suo Yang* (Herba Cynomorii) nourishes Kidney yang and *jing*. • *Chen Pi* (Pericarpium Citri Reticulatae) and *Gan Jiang* (Rhizoma Zingiberis) strengthen the Spleen and harmonize the middle *jiao*.

652

Hǔ Qián Wán (Hidden Tiger Pill)

Chinensis) 12g, *Zhi Mu* (Rhizoma Anemarrhenae) 6g, *Suo Yang* (Herba Cynomorii) 6g, *Shu Di Huang* (Radix Rehmanniae Praeparata) 9g, *Bai Shao* (Radix Paeoniae Alba) 9g, *Gui Ban* (Plastrum Testudinis) 10g, *Chen Pi* (Pericarpium Citri Reticulatae) 10g, *Gan Jiang* (Rhizoma Zingiberis) 15g, *Long Gu* (Os Draconis) 18g, *Mu Li* (Concha Ostreae) 30g, *E Jiao* (Colla Corii Asini) 30g, and lamb 15g. Additional modifications were made if necessary. Of 15 cases, the study reported complete recovery in 8 cases, improvement in 4 cases, and no change in 3 cases.[2]

RELATED FORMULA

Hǔ Qián Wán (Hidden Tiger Pill)

虎潛丸
虎潜丸

Pinyin Name: Hu Qian Wan
Literal Name: Hidden Tiger Pill
Original Source: *Yi Fang Ji Jie* (Analytical Collection of Medical Formulas) by Wang Ang in 1682

Huang Bo (Cortex Phellodendri Chinensis)	[240g]
Gui Ban (Plastrum Testudinis)	[120g]
Zhi Mu (Rhizoma Anemarrhenae)	[60g]
Shu Di Huang (Radix Rehmanniae Praeparata)	[60g]
Niu Xi (Radix Achyranthis Bidentatae)	[60g]
Bai Shao (Radix Paeoniae Alba)	[60g]
Suo Yang (Herba Cynomorii)	[45g]
Chen Pi (Pericarpium Citri Reticulatae)	[60g]
Hu Gu (Os Tigris)	[30g]
Gan Jiang (Rhizoma Zingiberis)	[15g]
Dang Gui (Radix Angelicae Sinensis)	[45g]

Note: *Hu Gu* (Os Tigris) is derived from an endangered animal, and is rarely used as a medicinal substance today. Its discussion here is included primarily for academic purposes, to reflect the historical use of this substance in its original formulation. Most herbal products today have removed it completely, or replaced it with *Zhu Gu* (Os Porcus) which has similar functions.

The source text states to grind the ingredients into powder and form into pills with lamb. Take the pills with lightly-salted water. This formula nourishes yin, tonifies blood, and lowers and clears deficiency fire. It treats weakness and atrophy of the bones and tendons associated with Liver and Kidney yin-deficient fire.

Huang Bo (Cortex Phellodendri Chinensis) and *Zhi Mu* (Rhizoma Anemarrhenae) clear deficiency fire and strengthens yin of the lower *jiao*. *Gui Ban* (Plastrum Testudinis) nourishes yin and lamb strengthens yang.

Shu Di Huang (Radix Rehmanniae Praeparata) and *Bai Shao* (Radix Paeoniae Alba) nourish yin, and *Dang Gui* (Radix Angelicae Sinensis) tonifies blood. *Hu Gu* (Os Tigris) strengthens the sinews and bones. *Suo Yang* (Herba Cynomorii) nourishes Kidney yang and *jing* (essence). *Chen Pi* (Pericarpium Citri Reticulatae) and *Gan Jiang* (Rhizoma Zingiberis) strengthen the Spleen and harmonize the middle *jiao* to prevent the cold and stagnating herbs from damaging the digestive system. Lastly, *Niu Xi* (Radix Achyranthis Bidentatae) strengthens the tendons and bones, and guides the formula downwards to the affected areas.

These two formulas have the same names and similar ingredients.
- *Hu Qian Wan* from *Dan Xi Xin Fa* (Teachings of [Zhu] Dan-Xi) is considered to be the original formula, since it was formulated approximately 200 years earlier.
- *Hu Qian Wan* from *Yi Fang Ji Jie* (Analytical Collection of Medical Formulas) is more commonly used today, as it is a more balanced and more effective formula. It contains additional herbs, such as lamb to strengthen yang, *Dang Gui* (Radix Angelicae Sinensis) to tonify blood, and *Niu Xi* (Radix Achyranthis Bidentatae) to guide the formula to the affected areas.

AUTHORS' COMMENTS

Hu Qian Wan, a formula designed to treat Liver and Kidney yin deficiencies with weakness of the bones and tendons, uses *Gan Jiang* (Rhizoma Zingiberis) for three important reasons:
- *Gan Jiang* (Rhizoma Zingiberis) counters the bitter and cold effects of *Huang Bo* (Cortex Phellodendri Chinensis).
- *Gan Jiang* (Rhizoma Zingiberis) assists *Chen Pi* (Pericarpium Citri Reticulatae) in warming the middle *jiao*, strengthening the Spleen, regulating qi, and harmonizing the Stomach. Together, these two herbs prevent the yin tonics from creating stagnation in the middle *jiao*.
- *Gan Jiang* (Rhizoma Zingiberis) facilitates the generation of blood. According to Master Zhu Dan-Xi, it enters the Lung to benefit Lung qi, and enters the Liver channel to assist blood tonics in generating blood.[3]

Hu Qian Wan and *Da Bu Yin Wan* (Great Tonify the Yin Pill) both tonify Kidney yin, sedate fire, and contain *Shu Di Huang* (Radix Rehmanniae Praeparata), *Gui Ban* (Plastrum Testudinis), *Huang Bo* (Cortex Phellodendri Chinensis), and *Zhi Mu* (Rhizoma Anemarrhenae). Their differences are:
- *Hu Qian Wan* nourishes yin, sedates fire, and strengthens tendons and bones to treat yin-deficient heat in the Liver

Chapter 8 – Tonic Formulas

Hǔ Qián Wán (Hidden Tiger Pill)

and Kidney, with *jing* (essence) and blood deficiencies causing atrophy or degeneration of the bones, tendons, and connective tissues.

• *Da Bu Yin Wan* treats Liver and Kidney yin deficiencies with deficiency fire symptoms of steaming bones sensation, tidal fever, cough with blood, a red tongue body with a scanty tongue coating, and a rapid, forceful pulse.[4]

References
1. *Shang Hai Zhong Yi Yao Za Zhi* (Shanghai Journal of Chinese Medicine and Herbology) 1985;11:32.
2. *Zhe Jiang Zhong Yi Za Zhi* (Zhejiang Journal of Chinese Medicine) 1995;30(11):495.
3. Wang MZ, et al. *Zhong Yi Xue Wen Da Ti Ku* (Questions and Answers on Traditional Chinese Medicine: Herbal Formulas).
4. Wang MZ, et al. *Zhong Yi Xue Wen Da Ti Ku* (Questions and Answers on Traditional Chinese Medicine: Herbal Formulas).

Èr Zhì Wán (Two-Ultimate Pill)
二至丸

Pinyin Name: *Er Zhi Wan*
Literal Name: Two-Ultimate Pill
Alternate Name: Ligustrum and Eclipta Combination
Original Source: *Yi Fang Ji Jie* (Analytical Collection of Medical Formulas) by Wang Ang in 1682

COMPOSITION

Nu Zhen Zi (Fructus Ligustri Lucidi)	500g
Mo Han Lian (Herba Ecliptae)	500g

DOSAGE / PREPARATION / ADMINISTRATION

The source text specifies that *Nu Zhen Zi* (Fructus Ligustri Lucidi) should be picked at the winter solstice, and *Mo Han Lian* (Herba Ecliptae) at the summer solstice. Blend *Nu Zhen Zi* (Fructus Ligustri Lucidi) with honey and liquor and steam until it is fully cooked. Allow it to dry in a cool place without direct exposure to sunlight, then grind it into a fine powder, and filter it through a sieve. Cook *Mo Han Lian* (Herba Ecliptae) with *Sang Shen* (Fructus Mori) in water three times, discard the herb residue, and then cook the strained decoction further until it becomes a thick paste. Mix the *Nu Zhen Zi* (Fructus Ligustri Lucidi) powder and the *Mo Han Lian* (Herba Ecliptae) paste with honey to form pills, which should weigh 15g each. Take 1 pill in the morning and 1 at night with warm, boiled water.

CHINESE THERAPEUTIC ACTIONS

1. Tonifies the Kidney and nourishes the Liver
2. Nourishes yin and blood

CLINICAL MANIFESTATIONS

Kidney and Liver yin deficiencies: dizziness, blurred vision, a bitter taste in mouth, a dry throat, insomnia, excessive dreams, soreness and weakness of the lower back and knees, gradual atrophy of the lower limbs, nocturnal emissions, premature graying of hair, and hypermenorrhea.

CLINICAL APPLICATIONS

Chronic nephritis, aplastic anemia, hepatitis B, threatened miscarriage, neurasthenia, insomnia, palpitations, and bleeding disorders (hemoptysis, hematochezia, hematuria, and excessive menstrual bleeding).

EXPLANATION

Er Zhi Wan (Two-Ultimate Pill) treats Kidney and Liver yin deficiencies. Because the Liver opens to the eyes, Liver yin deficiency may cause dizziness and blurred vision. The Kidney channel reaches to the throat and tongue area, which may become dry as a result of Kidney yin and blood deficiencies. Kidney yin deficiency could lead to instability of yang, which would then affect the *shen* (spirit) to cause insomnia and excessive dreams. Yang instability could also give rise to leakage of essence, which manifests as nocturnal emissions. Since the Kidney is located in the lower back, Kidney deficiency may lead to weakness and soreness of the lower back and knees. Atrophy of the lower limbs is due to Kidney *jing* (essence) deficiency and lack of nourishment.

Nu Zhen Zi (Fructus Ligustri Lucidi) tonifies both Liver and Kidney yin and brightens the eyes. *Mo Han Lian* (Herba Ecliptae) is sweet, sour, and cold. It nourishes yin and consolidates *jing* (essence). *Sang Shen* (Fructus Mori)

Chinese Herbal Formulas and Applications

Èr Zhì Wán (Two-Ultimate Pill)

Er Zhi Wan (Two-Ultimate Pill)

Diagnosis	Signs and Symptoms	Treatment	Herbs
Kidney and Liver yin deficiencies	• Dizziness, blurred vision, premature gray hair, soreness and weakness of the lower back and knees, atrophy of the lower limbs: Kidney and Liver yin deficiencies • Insomnia and excessive dreaming: deficiency heat disturbing the *shen* (spirit) • Nocturnal emissions and hypermenorrhea: leakage of body fluids	• Tonifies the Kidney and nourishes the Liver • Nourishes yin and blood	• *Nu Zhen Zi* (Fructus Ligustri Lucidi) tonifies both Liver and Kidney yin. • *Mo Han Lian* (Herba Ecliptae) nourishes yin and consolidates *jing* (essence). • *Sang Shen* (Fructus Mori) nourishes yin and tonifies the blood.

nourishes yin and tonifies the blood, and strengthens the overall effect of the formula.

CAUTIONS / CONTRAINDICATIONS
• *Er Zhi Wan* is contraindicated in patients with atrophy caused by damp-heat invasion.
• This formula should be used with caution in individuals with diarrhea caused by deficiency and cold of the Spleen and Stomach.[1]

PHARMACOLOGICAL EFFECTS
1. **Immunostimulant**: Administration of *Er Zhi Wan* was associated with an immune-enhancing effect by increasing white blood cell and T-lymphocyte counts.[2] Use of the herbs was also effective in reversing immune-suppression induced by hydrocortisone.[3]
2. **Metabolic**: Administration of *Er Zhi Wan* at 20g per day for 60 days in rabbits was associated with a reduction in plasma cholesterol and triglyceride levels.[4]
3. **Antiplatelet and anticoagulant**: Administration of *Er Zhi Wan* in decoction was associated with both antiplatelet and anticoagulant effects in rabbits.[5]
4. **Hypoglycemic**: Administration of *Er Zhi Wan* was associated with a reduction in plasma glucose levels in mice. It significantly decreased the rise in plasma glucose levels associated with adrenalin.[6]
5. **Hepatoprotective**: Use of *Er Zhi Wan* was associated with marked hepatoprotective effects. In laboratory experiments in mice, it lowered liver enzyme levels and minimized liver damage induced by carbon tetrachloride.[7]

CLINICAL STUDIES AND RESEARCH
1. **Chronic nephritis**: Sixteen patients with chronic nephritis characterized by Liver and Kidney yin deficiencies with heat in the *xue* (blood) level were successfully treated with modified *Er Zhi Wan* and *Qi Ju Di Huang Wan* (Lycium Fruit, Chrysanthemum, and Rehmannia Pill). Modifications were made as follows: *Gui Ban* (Plastrum Testudinis)

and *Mai Dong* (Radix Ophiopogonis) for severe yin deficiency; *Long Dan* (Radix et Rhizoma Gentianae), *Xia Ku Cao* (Spica Prunellae), and *Huang Qin* (Radix Scutellariae) for Liver yang rising; and *Xian Mao* (Rhizoma Curculiginis) and *Yin Yang Huo* (Herba Epimedii) for yin and yang deficiencies. Out of 16 patients, the study reported recovery in 2 patients, improvement in 6 patients, slight improvement in 6 patients, and no improvement in 2 patients.[8]

2. **Aplastic anemia**: In one study, 74 patients with aplastic anemia were treated with modified *Er Zhi Wan* with a 71.7% rate of effectiveness. Treatments were modified as follows: *Ren Shen* (Radix et Rhizoma Ginseng), *E Jiao* (Colla Corii Asini), and *Huang Qi* (Radix Astragali) were added for qi and yin deficiencies; *Shu Di Huang* (Radix Rehmanniae Praeparata), *Tu Si Zi* (Semen Cuscutae), and *Dang Gui* (Radix Angelicae Sinensis) were added for Liver and Kidney yin deficiencies; and various herbs to tonify Spleen and Kidney yang were added if needed. In addition, pharmaceutical drugs were added for symptomatic treatment if necessary. Out of 74 patients, the study reported complete recovery in 11 patients, marked improvement in 27 patients, improvement in 15 patients, and no benefit in 21 patients.[9]

3. **Hepatitis B**: Modified *Er Zhi Wan* was used with good results to treat 80 patients with chronic hepatitis B characterized by Liver and Kidney yin deficiencies. The herbal treatments were modified as follows: *Yin Chen* (Herba Artemisiae Scopariae), *Chui Pen Cao* (Herba Sedi), and *Tu Fu Ling* (Rhizoma Smilacis Glabrae) were added for damp-heat; *Ban Lan Gen* (Radix Isatidis) and *Pu Gong Ying* (Herba Taraxaci) were added for heat; processed *Ji Nei Jin* (Endothelium Corneum Gigeriae Galli) and dry-fried *Gu Ya* (Fructus Setariae Germinatus) were added for poor appetite; and *Hu Zhang* (Rhizoma et Radix Polygoni Cuspidati) and processed *Da Huang* (Radix et Rhizoma Rhei) were added for constipation. At the conclusion of the study, 93.7% of patients had

TONIC FORMULAS 8

655

Chapter 8 – Tonic Formulas   *Section 4 – Yin-Tonifying Formulas*

Èr Zhì Wán (Two-Ultimate Pill)

symptomatic improvement and 91.2% showed improvement in liver function.[10]

4. **Threatened miscarriage**: Use of modified *Er Zhi Wan* successfully prevented miscarriages in 119 of 131 patients with threatened miscarriage. The base formula included *Er Zhi Wan* plus *Du Zhong* (Cortex Eucommiae), *Sang Ji Sheng* (Herba Taxilli), *Huo Xiang* (Herba Agastaches), *Zi Su Geng* (Caulis Perillae), and *Lu Jiao Shuang* (Cornu Cervi Degelatinatum). *Tai Zi Shen* (Radix Pseudostellariae) and *Huang Qi* (Radix Astragali) were added for qi deficiency; *Rou Cong Rong* (Herba Cistanches), *Ba Ji Tian* (Radix Morindae Officinalis), and *Zi He Che* (Placenta Hominis) were added for yang deficiency; *Di Huang* (Radix Rehmanniae), *Sang Ye* (Folium Mori), *Huang Qin* (Radix Scutellariae), and *Zhu Ru* (Caulis Bambusae in Taenia) were added for yin deficiency; *Gou Qi Zi* (Fructus Lycii) and *Lu Dou Yi* (Pericarpium Glycine Max) were added for blood deficiency; *Mu Xiang* (Radix Aucklandiae) and *Sha Ren* (Fructus Amomi) for qi stagnation; calcined *Long Gu* (Os Draconis) and *Mu Li* (Concha Ostreae) with *Xue Yu Tan* (Crinis Carbonisatus) for profuse bleeding; *Xuan Shen* (Radix Scrophulariae), *Huo Ma Ren* (Fructus Cannabis), and *Qian Hu* (Radix Peucedani) for constipation with dry stool; and others as needed. Out of 131 patients, 119 showed positive responses with alleviation of symptoms, termination of bleeding, and no reports of abnormal development of the fetus upon delivery.[11]

TOXICOLOGY

In a toxicology report, no fatality or poisoning was observed following oral administration of *Er Zhi Wan* at 80 g/kg in mice. Using intraperitoneal injection, the LD_{50} of the formula was 13.84 g/kg.[12]

RELATED FORMULA

Sāng Má Wán (Mulberry Leaf and Sesame Seed Pill)

桑麻丸

Pinyin Name: *Sang Ma Wan*
Literal Name: Mulberry Leaf and Sesame Seed Pill
Original Source: *Yi Fang Ji Jie* (Analytical Collection of Medical Formulas) by Wang Ang in 1682

Sang Ye (Folium Mori)	300g
Hei Zhi Ma (Semen Sesami Nigrum)	120g
Feng Mi (Mel)	300g

Crush *Hei Zhi Ma* (Semen Sesami Nigrum) open, and cook it with honey to obtain a thick paste. Grind *Sang Ye* (Folium Mori) into a fine powder. Mix the paste and the powder to form pills, which should weigh 10g each. Take 1 pill in the morning with salted water, and 1 pill in the evening with a grain-based liquor.

Sang Ma Wan (Mulberry Leaf and Sesame Seed Pill) nourishes Liver and Kidney yin, clears the head, and brightens the eyes. Clinically, patients might show yin and blood deficiencies, characterized by symptoms such as dizziness, blurred vision, chronic coughing, constipation, dry stools, dry skin and skin itching.

AUTHORS' COMMENTS

Most tonic formulas cannot be taken for long periods of time because of their stagnating character. However, *Er Zhi Wan* is a mild and non-stagnating tonic formula, and can be taken for a long period of time if necessary.

References

1. *Zhong Yao Ming Fang Yao Li Yu Ying Yong* (Pharmacology and Applications of Famous Herbal Formulas) 1989;315-316.
2. *Zhong Guo Zhong Yao Za Zhi* (People's Republic of China Journal of Chinese Herbology) 1992;(9):531.
3. *Zhong Yao Yao Li Yu Lin Chuang* (Pharmacology and Clinical Applications of Chinese Herbs) 1991;6:1.
4. *Zhong Yao Tong Bao* (Journal of Chinese Herbology) 1983;3:32.
5. *Xin Zhong Yi* (New Chinese Medicine) 1991;6:51.
6. *Bei Jing Zhong Yi* (Beijing Chinese Medicine) 1993;2:17.
7. *Zhong Guo Zhong Yao Za Zhi* (People's Republic of China Journal of Chinese Herbology) 1992;(9):531.
8. *Shi Yong Zhong Xi Yi Jie He Za Zhi* (Practical Journal of Integrated Chinese and Western Medicines) 1993;1:41.
9. *Hu Nan Yi Yao Za Zhi* (Hunan Journal of Medicine and Herbology) 1983;6:7.
10. *Zhe Jiang Zhong Yi Xue Yuan Xue Bao* (Journal of Zhejiang University of Chinese Medicine) 1997;3:35.
11. *Zhe Jiang Zhong Yi Za Zhi* (Zhejiang Journal of Chinese Medicine) 1998;4:161.
12. *Xin Zhong Yi* (New Chinese Medicine) 1990;11:51.

Chinese Herbal Formulas and Applications

Yī Guàn Jiān (Linking Decoction)

一貫煎
一贯煎

Pinyin Name: *Yi Guan Jian*

Literal Name: Linking Decoction

Original Source: *Xu Ming Yi Lei An* (Continuation of Famous Physicians' Patients Organized by Categories) in *Liu Zhou Yi Hua* (Medical Dialogues from Liuzhou) by Wei Zhi-Xiu in the mid-16th century

COMPOSITION

Di Huang (Radix Rehmanniae)	18-45 [30g]
Bei Sha Shen (Radix Glehniae)	9g [10g]
Mai Dong (Radix Ophiopogonis)	9g [10g]
Dang Gui (Radix Angelicae Sinensis)	9g [10g]
Gou Qi Zi (Fructus Lycii)	9-18g [12g]
Chuan Lian Zi (Fructus Toosendan)	4.5g [5g]

DOSAGE / PREPARATION / ADMINISTRATION

Prepare and administer this formula as a warm, strained decoction. Today, the decoction may be prepared using the doses suggested in brackets.

CHINESE THERAPEUTIC ACTIONS

1. Nourishes Kidney and Liver yin
2. Regulates Liver qi

CLINICAL MANIFESTATIONS

Liver and Kidney yin deficiencies accompanied by qi stagnation and blood dryness: pain in the chest, epigastric and hypochondriac regions, acid regurgitation, a sore throat, a dry mouth, a red tongue body with little moisture, and a pulse that is fine and weak or deficient and wiry. Occasionally, there may also be a hernia or mass.

CLINICAL APPLICATIONS

Atrophic gastritis, chronic gastritis, gastric and duodenal ulcers, gastric neurosis, premenstrual syndrome (PMS), ovarian dysfunction, gestational hypertension, hepatitis, liver cirrhosis, liver cancer, hypochondriac neuralgia, hyperthyroidism, and restless leg syndrome.

EXPLANATION

Yi Guan Jian (Linking Decoction) treats Kidney and Liver yin deficiencies accompanied by Liver qi stagnation and blood dryness. The Liver smoothes the qi flow and disperses stagnation in the body. Chronic illness, deficiency, excessive sexual activity, and frequent or prolonged intake of aromatic herbs may all cause yin deficiency and blood dryness. If Liver yin is deficient and the Liver becomes malnourished, Liver qi may become stagnant and invasive. Liver qi stagnation can lead to pain in the chest, epigastric and hypochondriac regions. If Liver qi overacts on the Stomach, acid reflux may occur. A sore throat, a dry mouth, and a red tongue body with little moisture are the results of yin deficiency and its inability to reach and moisten the upper parts of the body. Occasionally, there could be a hernia as a result of qi stagnation in the Liver

Yi Guan Jian (Linking Decoction)

Diagnosis	Signs and Symptoms	Treatment	Herbs
Liver and Kidney yin deficiencies accompanied by qi stagnation and blood dryness	• Chest and hypochondriac pain, hernia or mass: Liver qi stagnation • Acid regurgitation: Liver qi overacting on the Stomach • Sore throat, a dry mouth and a red tongue body with little moisture: yin deficiency unable to reach the upper parts of the body • Fine, weak pulse: yin deficiency • Deficient, wiry pulse: yin deficiency with pain	• Nourishes Kidney and Liver yin • Regulates Liver qi	• *Di Huang* (Radix Rehmanniae) tonifies Liver and Kidney yin and nourishes the blood. • *Bei Sha Shen* (Radix Glehniae), *Mai Dong* (Radix Ophiopogonis), *Dang Gui* (Radix Angelicae Sinensis) and *Gou Qi Zi* (Fructus Lycii) tonify yin, nourish the blood, generate body fluids, and soften the Liver. • *Chuan Lian Zi* (Fructus Toosendan) smoothes Liver qi and relieves pain.

Chapter 8 – Tonic Formulas   *Section 4 – Yin-Tonifying Formulas*

Yī Guàn Jiān (Linking Decoction)

channel, which passes through the inguinal region. In severe cases of stagnation, masses may form. A fine, weak pulse suggests yin deficiency, and a deficient, wiry pulse suggests yin deficiency and pain.

This formula contains *Di Huang* (Radix Rehmanniae) as the chief herb to tonify Liver and Kidney yin and nourish the blood. *Bei Sha Shen* (Radix Glehniae), *Mai Dong* (Radix Ophiopogonis), *Dang Gui* (Radix Angelicae Sinensis), and *Gou Qi Zi* (Fructus Lycii) are the deputy herbs that tonify yin, nourish the blood, generate body fluids, and soften the Liver. *Chuan Lian Zi* (Fructus Toosendan) serves as both assistant and envoy herb. It smoothes Liver qi circulation, and guides the rest of the herbs to the Liver channel. Since *Chuan Lian Zi* (Fructus Toosendan) is bitter and cold and may consume yin and blood, only a small amount is used.

MODIFICATIONS

- With a dry throat and a bitter taste in the mouth, add *Huang Lian* (Rhizoma Coptidis), *Huang Qin* (Radix Scutellariae), and *Tian Hua Fen* (Radix Trichosanthis).
- If there is constipation, add *Gua Lou Zi* (Semen Trichosanthis), *Huo Ma Ren* (Fructus Cannabis), and *Yu Li Ren* (Semen Pruni).
- With insomnia, add *Bai Zi Ren* (Semen Platycladi), *Suan Zao Ren* (Semen Ziziphi Spinosae), and *Wu Wei Zi* (Fructus Schisandrae Chinensis).
- With perspiration caused by deficiency heat, add *Shi Hu* (Caulis Dendrobii) and *Di Gu Pi* (Cortex Lycii).
- If there is more phlegm, add *Chuan Bei Mu* (Bulbus Fritillariae Cirrhosae) and *Gua Lou Zi* (Semen Trichosanthis).
- With abdominal pain, add *Bai Shao* (Radix Paeoniae Alba) and *Gan Cao* (Radix et Rhizoma Glycyrrhizae).
- With irritability and thirst, add *Zhi Mu* (Rhizoma Anemarrhenae) and *Shi Gao* (Gypsum Fibrosum).
- With weakness of the legs, add *Niu Xi* (Radix Achyranthis Bidentatae) and *Yi Yi Ren* (Semen Coicis).

CAUTIONS / CONTRAINDICATIONS

- *Yi Guan Jian* is contraindicated in individuals with hypochondriac pain caused by Liver fire rising without underlying deficiency.
- This formula is inappropriate for patients with qi and blood stagnation or phlegm accumulation, since it contains many tonics that can create more stagnation or produce more dampness and phlegm.

PHARMACOLOGICAL EFFECTS

1. **Hepatoprotective**: In laboratory experiments in mice, the use of *Yi Guan Jian* was effective in reducing liver damage caused by carbon tetrachloride.[1]

2. **Antiulcer**: According to laboratory experiments in mice, administration of *Yi Guan Jian* was associated with a marked effect for treating gastric and duodenal ulcer. The mechanism of action is attributed to enhancing the protective effect of the gastric mucosa, as the formula did not inhibit or neutralize the stomach acid.[2]

3. **Adaptogenic**: In one experiment, daily administration of *Yi Guan Jian* for 7 days was effective at significantly increasing physical performance in mice.[3]

CLINICAL STUDIES AND RESEARCH

1. **Atrophic gastritis**: In one study, 45 patients with atrophic gastritis were treated with *Yi Guan Jian* plus *Bai Hua She She Cao* (Herba Hedyotis). The age of the patients ranged from 28-64 years. The history of illness was between 6 months to 8 years. The traditional Chinese medicine diagnoses were Stomach yin deficiency (31 patients) and Liver and Stomach disharmony (14 patients). Out of 45 patients, the study reported marked improvement in 12 patients, improvement in 30 patients, and no benefit in 3 patients. Patients with Stomach yin deficiency responded better to the treatment.[4] Another study reported 94.92% effectiveness using modified *Yi Guan Jian* to treat atrophic gastritis characterized by Stomach yin deficiency. The herbal formula contained *Yi Guan Jian* plus *Bai Shao* (Radix Paeoniae Alba), *Wu Mei* (Fructus Mume), *E Zhu* (Rhizoma Curcumae), and others. Of 118 patients, the study reported significant improvement in 63 patients, moderate improvement in 49 patients, and no benefit in 6 patients.[5]

2. **Gastric and duodenal ulcers**: In one study, 18 patients with gastrointestinal disorders (10 with gastric ulcer and 8 with duodenal ulcer) were treated with modified *Yi Guan Jian* for 90 days with complete recovery in 8 patients, improvement in 7 patients, and no benefit in 3 patients. The overall effectiveness rate was 83.2%.[6]

3. **Premenstrual syndrome (PMS)**: Modified *Yi Guan Jian* was used to treat 36 women with PMS between ages of 25-40. The clinical presentations included irritability, anger, insomnia, dizziness, headache, breast distention and pain, joint soreness and pain, edema, and abdominal discomfort. Out of 36 patients, the study reported marked improvement in 26 patients and moderate improvement in 10 patients.[7]

4. **Ovarian dysfunction**: Modified *Yi Guan Jian* was used to treat women with abnormal ovarian functions. The base formula included *Yi Guan Jian* plus *Chai Hu* (Radix Bupleuri), *Bai Shao* (Radix Paeoniae Alba), *Nu Zhen Zi* (Fructus Ligustri Lucidi), and *Mu Dan Pi* (Cortex Moutan). In addition, *Da Huang* (Radix et Rhizoma Rhei), *Shui Zhi* (Hirudo), and *Niu Xi* (Radix Achyranthis Bidentatae) were added for amenorrhea; processed *He Shou Wu* (Radix

Yī Guàn Jiān (Linking Decoction)

Polygoni Multiflori) and *E Jiao* (Colla Corii Asini) were added for decreased menstrual discharge with insomnia; *Yi Mu Cao* (Herba Leonuri) and *Wu Yao* (Radix Linderae) for abdominal pain with menstruation; *Du Zhong* (Cortex Eucommiae) and *Xu Duan* (Radix Dipsaci) were added for low back pain; and *Shan Zha* (Fructus Crataegi), *Bai Zhu* (Rhizoma Atractylodis Macrocephalae), and *Shan Yao* (Rhizoma Dioscoreae) were added for lack of appetite due to Spleen deficiency. Out of 38 patients, the study reported complete recovery of ovarian function in 26 patients, marked improvement in 8 patients, improvement in 3 patients, and no benefit in one patient.[8]

5. **Gestational hypertension**: In one study, 74 pregnant women with hypertension were treated with modified *Yi Guan Jian*, with marked reduction in blood pressure and edema. The formula used *Yi Guan Jian* as the base formula. *Sang Ji Sheng* (Herba Taxilli), *Bai Shao* (Radix Paeoniae Alba), *Shi Jue Ming* (Concha Haliotidis), and *Dan Shen* (Radix et Rhizoma Salviae Miltiorrhizae) were added for Liver and Stomach yin deficiencies (70 patients). *Bai Zhu* (Rhizoma Atractylodis Macrocephalae), *Fu Ling Pi* (Cortex Poria), *Da Fu Pi* (Pericarpium Arecae), and *Chen Pi* (Pericarpium Citri Reticulatae) were added for Spleen deficiency with Liver excess (4 patients). Out of 74 patients, the study reported marked improvement in 47 patients, moderate improvement in 24 patients, and no benefit in 3 patients. Clinical improvements included marked reduction in blood pressure and edema. However, there was only slight improvement in proteinuria.[9]

6. **Liver diseases**: Modifications of *Yi Guan Jian* have been used in numerous studies to treat liver diseases, such as hepatitis, liver cirrhosis, and liver cancer. In one study, 50 patients with chronic hepatitis were treated with good results using modified *Yi Guan Jian* with the addition of *Bai Shao* (Radix Paeoniae Alba) and *Yu Jin* (Radix Curcumae).[10] In another study, 85 patients with liver cirrhosis were treated with modified *Yi Guan Jian* with 81.1% effectiveness.[11]

7. **Liver cancer**: In one study, 41 patients with liver cancer characterized by Liver and Kidney yin deficiencies were treated with good results using *Yi Guan Jian* plus *Zhi Mu* (Rhizoma Anemarrhenae) and *Gui Ban* (Plastrum Testudinis) as the base formula. In addition, *Du Zhong* (Cortex Eucommiae), *Sang Ji Sheng* (Herba Taxilli), and *He Shou Wu* (Radix Polygoni Multiflori) were added for dizziness and tinnitus; *Zhi Zi* (Fructus Gardeniae) and *Yin Chen* (Herba Artemisiae Scopariae) were added for jaundice; *Ze Xie* (Rhizoma Alismatis), *Dan Shen* (Radix et Rhizoma Salviae Miltiorrhizae,) and *Yu Jin* (Radix Curcumae) were added for ascites; and *Gu Ya* (Fructus Setariae Germinatus), *Mai Ya* (Fructus Hordei Germinatus), and *Shan Zha* (Fructus Crataegi) were added for poor appetite. Out of 41 patients, the study reported marked improvement in 7 patients, moderate improvement in 30 patients, and no improvement in 4 patients.[12]

8. **Fever during late-stage liver cancer**: Modified *Yi Guan Jian* showed effectiveness in treating liver cancer with fever. The formula was modified as follows: *Chai Hu* (Radix Bupleuri), *Bai Shao* (Radix Paeoniae Alba), and *Dan Shen* (Radix et Rhizoma Salviae Miltiorrhizae) were added for marked hypochondriac pain; *Che Qian Zi* (Semen Plantaginis), *Fu Ling* (Poria), and *Ze Xie* (Rhizoma Alismatis) were added for edema, ascites, and decreased urination; *Huang Qi* (Radix Astragali) and *Bai Zhu* (Rhizoma Atractylodis Macrocephalae) were added for nausea, poor appetite, and fatigue; and *Yin Chen* (Herba Artemisiae Scopariae) and *Che Qian Zi* (Semen Plantaginis) were added for jaundice. Out of 28 patients, the study reported a marked effect in 15 patients, moderate effect in 9 patients, and no effect in 4 patients.[13]

9. **Hyperthyroidism**: In one study, 40 patients with hyperthyroidism were treated with modified *Yi Guan Jian* with good results. The herbal treatment was modified as follows: *Hai Zao* (Sargassum), *Kun Bu* (Thallus Eckloniae), and *Niu Xi* (Radix Achyranthis Bidentatae) were added for thyroid gland enlargement; *Zhi Mu* (Rhizoma Anemarrhenae) and *Shi Gao* (Gypsum Fibrosum) were added for restlessness, irritability and a dry mouth; *Xuan Shen* (Radix Scrophulariae), charred *Shan Zha* (Fructus Crataegi), charred *Shen Qu* (Massa Fermentata), and charred *Mai Ya* (Fructus Hordei Germinatus) for poor appetite and abdominal pain; *Huang Qi* (Radix Astragali) and *Zhi Gan Cao* (Radix et Rhizoma Glycyrrhizae Praeparata cum Melle) were added for shortness of breath and profuse perspiration; and *Che Qian Zi* (Semen Plantaginis), *Ze Xie* (Rhizoma Alismatis), *Da Fu Pi* (Pericarpium Arecae), and *Gui Zhi* (Ramulus Cinnamomi) were added for edema and hypertension. Out of 40 patients, the study reported recovery in 20 patients, marked improvement in 12 patients, and slight improvement in 8 patients.[14]

10. **Restless leg syndrome**: In one study, 20 patients with restless legs were treated with an herbal formula for 15 days per course of treatment with good results. The formula contained *Yi Guan Jian* with *Gou Teng* (Ramulus Uncariae cum Uncis) and fresh *Mu Li* (Concha Ostreae). Out of 20 patients, the study reported complete recovery in 13 patients, improvement in 5 patients, and no benefit in 2 patients.[15]

TOXICOLOGY

No abnormal reaction was observed following oral ingestion at 50 g/kg of *Yi Guan Jian* as a bolus dose in mice.[16]

Chapter 8 – Tonic Formulas   *Section 4 – Yin-Tonifying Formulas*

Yī Guàn Jiān (Linking Decoction)

AUTHORS' COMMENTS

The following question is sometimes raised: if *Yi Guan Jian* treats chest, epigastric, and hypochondriac pain characterized by Liver qi stagnation, why are yin and blood tonics used instead of qi-regulating herbs such as *Zhi Shi* (Fructus Aurantii Immaturus) or *Chai Hu* (Radix Bupleuri)? The answer is that *Yi Guan Jian* is designed for individuals who have both Liver qi stagnation and Kidney and Liver yin deficiencies. Because there is yin deficiency, it is not suitable to use *Zhi Shi* (Fructus Aurantii Immaturus) or *Chai Hu* (Radix Bupleuri), since they are both drying herbs that deplete yin and will further exacerbate the yin deficiency.[17]

Yi Guan Jian, a yin tonic formula, uses *Chuan Lian Zi* (Fructus Toosendan), a bitter and cold herb that may damage yin, for the following reasons:

- *Chuan Lian Zi* (Fructus Toosendan) regulates Liver qi, sedates Liver heat, and prevents fire from forming. It prevents the yin and blood tonic herbs from causing stagnation in the middle *jiao*.
- While bitter and cold herbs, such as *Chuan Lian Zi* (Fructus Toosendan), can dry yin, this is not a concern in this patient because *Yi Guan Jian* contains many sweet and cold herbs, such as *Bei Sha Shen* (Radix Glehniae), *Mai Dong* (Radix Ophiopogonis), *Di Huang* (Radix Rehmanniae), *Gou Qi Zi* (Fructus Lycii), and *Dang Gui* (Radix Angelicae Sinensis). The sweet and cold herbs outnumber *Chuan Lian Zi* (Fructus Toosendan) and control its potentially adverse effects.[18]

Yi Guan Jian and *Xiao Yao San* (Rambling Powder) both treat hypochondriac distention and pain, but the etiologies contributing to this condition and the focus of the two formulas are quite different.

- *Yi Guan Jian* treats Liver and Kidney yin deficiencies with Liver qi stagnation. It nourishes yin and regulates Liver qi to treat a dry mouth, sore throat, acid regurgitation, mass accumulation, and hernias.
- *Xiao Yao San* addresses Liver qi stagnation with blood and Spleen deficiencies. It is considered a harmonizing formula. Symptoms include breast tenderness, headache, dizziness, alternating chills and fever, a dry mouth, irregular menstruation, stress, a withered *shen* (spirit), and decreased dietary intake. *Xiao Yao San* regulates Liver qi, spreads stagnation, strengthens the Spleen, and nourishes the blood.[19]

Yi Guan Jian and *Si Ni San* (Frigid Extremities Powder) both treat hypochondriac pain.

- *Yi Guan Jian* treats hypochondriac pain caused by Kidney and Liver yin deficiencies.
- *Si Ni San* treats epigastric, abdominal, or hypochondriac pain caused by Liver qi stagnation with yang qi pent up in the body.[20]

References

1. *Zhong Yao Yao Li Yu Lin Chuang* (Pharmacology and Clinical Applications of Chinese Herbs) 1989;6:14.
2. *Gui Yang Yi Xue Yuan Xue Bao* (Journal of Guiyang Medical University) 1986;2:42.
3. *Zhong Yi Fang Ji Xian Dai Yan Jiu* (Modern Study of Medical Formulae in Traditional Chinese Medicine) 1997;735.
4. *Si Chuan Zhong Yi* (Sichuan Chinese Medicine) 1987;1:33.
5. *Shan Xi Zhong Yi* (Shanxi Chinese Medicine) 1999;4:161.
6. *Gui Zhou Yi Yao* (Medicine and Medicinals from Guizhou) 1991;5:307.
7. *Shan Xi Yi Kan* (Shanxi Journal of Medicine) 1992;5:201.
8. *Gui Yang Zhong Yi Xue Yuan Xue Bao* (Journal of Guiyang University of Traditional Chinese Medicine) 1998;4:19.
9. *Zhong Yi Za Zhi* (Journal of Chinese Medicine) 1983;3:37.
10. *Hu Bei Zhong Yi Za Zhi* (Hubei Journal of Chinese Medicine) 1986;5:51.
11. *Shan Xi Yi Kan* (Shanxi Journal of Medicine) 1989;7:292.
12. *Fu Jian Zhong Yi Yao* (Fujian Chinese Medicine and Herbology) 1995;4:33.
13. *Fu Jian Zhong Yi Yao* (Fujian Chinese Medicine and Herbology) 1999;2:10.
14. *Hu Bei Zhong Yi Za Zhi* (Hubei Journal of Chinese Medicine) 1999;10:458.
15. *Liao Ning Zhong Yi Za Zhi* (Liaoning Journal of Chinese Medicine) 1991;4:40.
16. *Zhong Guo Zhong Yao Za Zhi* (People's Republic of China Journal of Chinese Herbology) 1989;9:42.
17. Wang MZ, et al. *Zhong Yi Xue Wen Da Ti Ku* (Questions and Answers on Traditional Chinese Medicine: Herbal Formulas).
18. Wang MZ, et al. *Zhong Yi Xue Wen Da Ti Ku* (Questions and Answers on Traditional Chinese Medicine: Herbal Formulas).
19. Wang MZ, et al. *Zhong Yi Xue Wen Da Ti Ku* (Questions and Answers on Traditional Chinese Medicine: Herbal Formulas).
20. Wang MZ, et al. *Zhong Yi Xue Wen Da Ti Ku* (Questions and Answers on Traditional Chinese Medicine: Herbal Formulas).

660

Chinese Herbal Formulas and Applications

Shí Hú Yè Guāng Wán (Dendrobium Pill for Night Vision)
石斛夜光丸

Pinyin Name: *Shi Hu Ye Guang Wan*
Literal Name: Dendrobium Pill for Night Vision
Alternate Name: Night Vision Formula
Original Source: *Yuan Ji Qi Wei* (Explanation of the Subtitles of the Original Mechanism) by Ni Wei-De in 1370

COMPOSITION

Shi Hu (Caulis Dendrobii)	15g
Mai Dong (Radix Ophiopogonis)	30g
Tian Dong (Radix Asparagi), *bei* (stone-baked)	60g
Di Huang (Radix Rehmanniae)	30g
Shu Di Huang (Radix Rehmanniae Praeparata)	30g
Wu Wei Zi (Fructus Schisandrae Chinensis), *chao* (dry-fried)	15g
Tu Si Zi (Semen Cuscutae), *jin* (soaked) in liquor	21g
Gou Qi Zi (Fructus Lycii)	21g
Niu Xi (Radix Achyranthis Bidentatae), *jin* (soaked) in liquor	23g
Rou Cong Rong (Herba Cistanches)	15g
Ren Shen (Radix et Rhizoma Ginseng)	60g
Fu Ling (Poria)	60g
Zhi Gan Cao (Radix et Rhizoma Glycyrrhizae Praeparata cum Melle)	15g
Shan Yao (Rhizoma Dioscoreae)	21g
Zhi Qiao (Fructus Citri Aurantii), *chao* (dry-fried) with bran	15g
Chuan Xiong (Rhizoma Chuanxiong)	15g
Ju Hua (Flos Chrysanthemi)	21g
Ku Xing Ren (Semen Armeniacae Amarum)	23g
Fang Feng (Radix Saposhnikoviae)	15g
Jue Ming Zi (Semen Cassiae)	24g
Ji Li (Fructus Tribuli)	15g
Qing Xiang Zi (Semen Celosiae)	15g
Huang Lian (Rhizoma Coptidis)	15g
Xi Jiao (Cornu Rhinoceri), thin slices	15g
Ling Yang Jiao (Cornu Saigae Tataricae), thin slices	15g

Note: *Xi Jiao* (Cornu Rhinoceri) and *Ling Yang Jiao* (Cornu Saigae Tataricae) are derived from endangered animals, and are rarely used as medicinal substances today. The discussion here is included primarily for academic purposes, to reflect the historical use of these substances in their original formulations. Most herbal products today have removed them completely, or replaced them with substitutes with similar functions.

DOSAGE / PREPARATION / ADMINISTRATION

Grind the ingredients into powder and filter it through a sieve. Mix the powdered herbs with honey to form pills. Take 30-50 pills with salted water or warm grain-based liquor. Today, this formula is prepared by mixing the powdered herbs with honey to form pills, each weighing 10g. Take 1 pill in the morning and at night with lightly-salted water.

CHINESE THERAPEUTIC ACTIONS

1. Soothes the Liver and calms Liver wind
2. Nourishes yin and brightens vision

CLINICAL MANIFESTATIONS

Liver and Kidney yin deficiencies leading to rising internal fire and wind: dilated pupils, blurred vision, photophobia, excess tearing with exposure to sunlight, dizziness, and vertigo.

CLINICAL APPLICATIONS

Glaucoma, cataract, retinitis, tinnitus, deafness, neurogenic headache, hypertension, and menopause.

EXPLANATION

Shi Hu Ye Guang Wan (Dendrobium Pill for Night Vision) treats Liver and Kidney yin deficiencies complicated by internal fire and wind. Liver and Kidney yin deficiencies

661

Chapter 8 – Tonic Formulas   *Section 4 – Yin-Tonifying Formulas*

Shí Hú Yè Guāng Wán (Dendrobium Pill for Night Vision)

Shi Hu Ye Guang Wan (Dendrobium Pill for Night Vision)

Diagnosis	Signs and Symptoms	Treatment	Herbs
Liver and Kidney yin deficiencies leading to rising internal fire and wind	• Dilated pupils and blurred vision: Liver and Kidney yin deficiencies unable to nourish the eyes • Photophobia and excessive tearing: Liver and Kidney yin deficiencies with rising of internal fire and wind	• Soothes the Liver and calms Liver wind • Nourishes yin and brightens vision	• *Shi Hu* (Caulis Dendrobii), *Mai Dong* (Radix Ophiopogonis), *Tian Dong* (Radix Asparagi), *Di Huang* (Radix Rehmanniae), *Shu Di Huang* (Radix Rehmanniae Praeparata) and *Wu Wei Zi* (Fructus Schisandrae Chinensis) nourish the blood and produce body fluids. • *Tu Si Zi* (Semen Cuscutae), *Gou Qi Zi* (Fructus Lycii), *Niu Xi* (Radix Achyranthis Bidentatae) and *Rou Cong Rong* (Herba Cistanches) nourish yin and tonify the Liver and Kidney. • *Ren Shen* (Radix et Rhizoma Ginseng), *Fu Ling* (Poria), *Zhi Gan Cao* (Radix et Rhizoma Glycyrrhizae Praeparata cum Melle) and *Shan Yao* (Rhizoma Dioscoreae) tonify the Spleen and Lung. • *Zhi Qiao* (Fructus Aurantii), *Chuan Xiong* (Rhizoma Chuanxiong), *Ju Hua* (Flos Chrysanthemi), *Ku Xing Ren* (Semen Armeniacae Amarum), *Fang Feng* (Radix Saposhnikoviae), *Jue Ming Zi* (Semen Cassiae), *Ji Li* (Fructus Tribuli) and *Qing Xiang Zi* (Semen Celosiae) clear heat and calm wind. • *Huang Lian* (Rhizoma Coptidis), *Xi Jiao* (Cornu Rhinoceri), and *Ling Yang Jiao* (Cornu Saigae Tataricae) soothe the Liver, purge the Heart, and cool the blood.

lead to an inability to nourish the eyes, resulting in dilated pupils and blurred vision. Liver and Kidney yin deficiencies are often accompanied by deficiency fire, which may cause photophobia and excessive tearing. Clinically, this formula can be used to treat various eye disorders, such as glaucoma, cataract, and retinitis.

This formula consists of 25 herbs, which may be grouped into five different categories of functions: nourish the blood and body fluids; tonify Liver and Kidney yin; tonify Lung and Spleen; calm wind and clear heat; and calm the Liver and purge the Heart. *Shi Hu* (Caulis Dendrobii), *Mai Dong* (Radix Ophiopogonis), *Tian Dong* (Radix Asparagi), *Di Huang* (Radix Rehmanniae), *Shu Di Huang* (Radix Rehmanniae Praeparata), and *Wu Wei Zi* (Fructus Schisandrae Chinensis) nourish the blood and generate body fluids. *Tu Si Zi* (Semen Cuscutae), *Gou Qi Zi* (Fructus Lycii), *Niu Xi* (Radix Achyranthis Bidentatae), and *Rou Cong Rong* (Herba Cistanches) nourish yin and tonify the Liver and Kidney. Because *gu* (food) *qi* constantly replenishes Kidney *jing* (essence), the Spleen and Lung should be tonified to ensure proper digestion and absorption.

The four herbs that tonify the Spleen and Lung are *Ren Shen* (Radix et Rhizoma Ginseng), *Fu Ling* (Poria), *Zhi Gan Cao* (Radix et Rhizoma Glycyrrhizae Praeparata cum Melle), and *Shan Yao* (Rhizoma Dioscoreae). Liver and Kidney yin and blood deficiencies can give rise to internal wind and heat. To sedate heat and clear wind, this formula uses *Zhi Qiao* (Fructus Aurantii), *Chuan Xiong* (Rhizoma Chuanxiong), *Ju Hua* (Flos Chrysanthemi), *Ku Xing Ren* (Semen Armeniacae Amarum), *Fang Feng* (Radix Saposhnikoviae), *Jue Ming Zi* (Semen Cassiae), *Ji Li* (Fructus Tribuli), and *Qing Xiang Zi* (Semen Celosiae). Finally, *Huang Lian* (Rhizoma Coptidis), *Xi Jiao* (Cornu Rhinoceri), and *Ling Yang Jiao* (Cornu Saigae Tataricae) soothe the Liver, purge the Heart, and cool the blood.

CAUTIONS / CONTRAINDICATIONS

Avoid pungent and spicy foods while taking *Shi Hu Ye Guang Wan*.[1]

Reference

1. *Zhong Yao Ming Fang Yao Li Yu Ying Yong* (Pharmacology and Applications of Famous Herbal Formulas) 1989;322-23.

Zī Yīn Dì Huáng Wán (Rehmannia Pill to Nourish Yin)

滋陰地黃丸
滋阴地黄丸

Pinyin Name: *Zi Yin Di Huang Wan*

Literal Name: Rehmannia Pill to Nourish Yin

Alternate Names: *Chih Yin Ti Huang Wan* (Yin-Nourishing Rehmannia Pill), *Shou Gan Di Huang Wan* (Cooked and Dried Rehmannia Pill); Rehmannia, Bupleurum and Scute Formula

Original Source: *Yi Fang Ji Jie* (Analytical Collection of Medical Formulas) by Wang Ang in 1682

COMPOSITION

Di Huang (Radix Rehmanniae)

Shu Di Huang (Radix Rehmanniae Praeparata)

Dang Gui (Radix Angelicae Sinensis)

Tian Dong (Radix Asparagi)

Ren Shen (Radix et Rhizoma Ginseng)

Gan Cao (Radix et Rhizoma Glycyrrhizae)

Huang Lian (Rhizoma Coptidis)

Huang Qin (Radix Scutellariae)

Di Gu Pi (Cortex Lycii)

Chai Hu (Radix Bupleuri)

Zhi Qiao (Fructus Aurantii)

Wu Wei Zi (Fructus Schisandrae Chinensis)

DOSAGE / PREPARATION / ADMINISTRATION

This formula is prepared and administered as pills.

CHINESE THERAPEUTIC ACTIONS

1. Nourishes yin
2. Tonifies qi and blood
3. Purges fire

CLINICAL MANIFESTATIONS

Blurred and impaired vision: blurred vision, red eyes, dilated pupils, and increased sensitivity to light.

EXPLANATION

Zi Yin Di Huang Wan (Rehmannia Pill to Nourish Yin) treats blurred and impaired vision caused by Liver fire

Zi Yin Di Huang Wan (Rehmannia Pill to Nourish Yin)

Diagnosis	Signs and Symptoms	Treatment	Herbs
Blurred and impaired vision	• Red eyes, dilated pupils, and increased sensitivity to light: Liver fire • Blurred vision and generalized weakness: qi, blood and yin deficiencies	• Nourishes yin • Tonifies qi and blood • Purges fire	• *Di Huang* (Radix Rehmanniae) and *Shu Di Huang* (Radix Rehmanniae Praeparata) nourish yin and tonify the blood. • *Dang Gui* (Radix Angelicae Sinensis) tonifies the blood. • *Tian Dong* (Radix Asparagi) nourishes yin. • *Ren Shen* (Radix et Rhizoma Ginseng) and *Gan Cao* (Radix et Rhizoma Glycyrrhizae) boost qi. • *Huang Lian* (Rhizoma Coptidis) and *Huang Qin* (Radix Scutellariae) clear excess Liver fire. • *Di Gu Pi* (Cortex Lycii) controls deficiency heat. • *Chai Hu* (Radix Bupleuri) and *Zhi Qiao* (Fructus Aurantii) dispel Liver qi stagnation. • *Wu Wei Zi* (Fructus Schisandrae Chinensis) tranquilizes the Heart and calms the *shen* (spirit).

Chapter 8 – Tonic Formulas

Section 4 – Yin-Tonifying Formulas

Zī Yīn Dì Huáng Wán (Rehmannia Pill to Nourish Yin)

rising with underlying qi, blood and yin deficiencies. When Liver fire rises upward, it causes red eyes, dilated pupils, and increased sensitivity to light. Blurred vision and generalized weakness can be attributed to the underlying qi, blood and yin deficiencies.

Di Huang (Radix Rehmanniae) and *Shu Di Huang* (Radix Rehmanniae Praeparata) together nourish yin and tonify the blood. *Dang Gui* (Radix Angelicae Sinensis) tonifies the blood, *Tian Dong* (Radix Asparagi) nourishes yin, and *Ren Shen* (Radix et Rhizoma Ginseng) and *Gan Cao*

(Radix et Rhizoma Glycyrrhizae) boost qi. *Huang Lian* (Rhizoma Coptidis) and *Huang Qin* (Radix Scutellariae) clear excess Liver fire, while *Di Gu Pi* (Cortex Lycii) controls deficiency heat. *Chai Hu* (Radix Bupleuri) and *Zhi Qiao* (Fructus Aurantii) dispel Liver qi stagnation. Lastly, *Wu Wei Zi* (Fructus Schisandrae Chinensis) tranquilizes the Heart and calms the *shen* (spirit).

CAUTIONS / CONTRAINDICATIONS

Patients with Liver fire should be advised to avoid hot and spicy foods while taking *Zi Yin Di Huang Wan*.

Zī Shèn Míng Mù Tāng
(Nourish the Kidney to Brighten the Eyes Decoction)

滋腎明目湯

滋肾明目汤

Pinyin Name: *Zi Shen Ming Mu Tang*
Literal Name: Nourish the Kidney to Brighten the Eyes Decoction
Alternate Name: Chrysanthemum Combination
Original Source: *Wan Bing Hui Chun* (Restoration of Health from the Myriad Diseases) by Gong Ting-Xian in 1587

COMPOSITION

Di Huang (Radix Rehmanniae)	2 parts
Shu Di Huang (Radix Rehmanniae Praeparata)	2 parts
Dang Gui (Radix Angelicae Sinensis)	2 parts
Bai Shao (Radix Paeoniae Alba)	2 parts
Chuan Xiong (Rhizoma Chuanxiong)	2 parts
Ren Shen (Radix et Rhizoma Ginseng)	2 parts
Gan Cao (Radix et Rhizoma Glycyrrhizae)	1 part
Ju Hua (Flos Chrysanthemi)	2 parts
Man Jing Zi (Fructus Viticis)	2 parts
Huang Lian (Rhizoma Coptidis)	2 parts
Zhi Zi (Fructus Gardeniae)	2 parts
Bai Zhi (Radix Angelicae Dahuricae)	2 parts
Jie Geng (Radix Platycodonis)	2 parts

DOSAGE / PREPARATION / ADMINISTRATION

The source text states to cook the ingredients with a small amount of *Cha Ye* (Folium Camelliae) and *Deng Xin Cao* (Medulla Junci) in water, and take the strained decoction while warm. Note: The source text only provided the proportions of the herbs, not the exact doses.

CHINESE THERAPEUTIC ACTIONS

1. Nourishes yin
2. Tonifies qi and blood
3. Clears heat

664

Chinese Herbal Formulas and Applications

Zī Shèn Míng Mù Tāng
(Nourish the Kidney to Brighten the Eyes Decoction)

CLINICAL MANIFESTATIONS

Blurred and impaired vision as a result of qi, blood and yin deficiencies: blurred vision, poor vision, eye strain, and excessive itching and tearing of the eyes.

CLINICAL APPLICATIONS

Deterioration of the eyes, impaired vision, blurred vision, cataract, and asthenopia.

EXPLANATION

Chronic qi, blood and yin deficiencies often result in malnourishment of the eyes and deterioration of their functions, producing symptoms such as blurred vision, poor vision, and eye strain.

Zi Shen Ming Mu Tang (Nourish the Kidney to Brighten the Eyes Decoction) tonifies qi and blood, nourishes yin, clears heat, and improves vision. *Di Huang* (Radix Rehmanniae) and *Shu Di Huang* (Radix Rehmanniae Praeparata) nourish yin. *Dang Gui* (Radix Angelicae Sinensis), *Bai Shao* (Radix Paeoniae Alba) and *Chuan Xiong* (Rhizoma Chuanxiong) tonify the blood and regulate blood circulation. *Ren Shen* (Radix et Rhizoma Ginseng) and *Gan Cao* (Radix et Rhizoma Glycyrrhizae) are added to tonify qi. Together, these seven herbs address the underlying

deficiencies. In addition, *Ju Hua* (Flos Chrysanthemi) and *Man Jing Zi* (Fructus Viticis) are added to clear the Liver and improve vision. *Huang Lian* (Rhizoma Coptidis) and *Zhi Zi* (Fructus Gardeniae) clear damp-heat, especially if there is redness and eye pain. *Bai Zhi* (Radix Angelicae Dahuricae) opens the orifices in the head. Moreover, *Bai Zhi* (Radix Angelicae Dahuricae) and *Jie Geng* (Radix Platycodonis) have ascending properties, and guide the therapeutic effects of the formula to the affected area. *Deng Xin Cao* (Medulla Junci) and *Cha Ye* (Folium Camelliae) eliminate excess water from the body.

MODIFICATIONS

- With vertigo and blacked-out vision, add *Huang Qi* (Radix Astragali) and *Gou Qi Zi* (Fructus Lycii).
- With excessive tearing and eye pain caused by wind-heat, add *Fang Feng* (Radix Saposhnikoviae) and *Jing Jie* (Herba Schizonepetae).
- With fatigue of the eyes, add *Fu Ling* (Poria) and *Bai Zhu* (Rhizoma Atractylodis Macrocephalae).
- For impaired vision or blurred vision caused by Kidney yin deficiency, add *Liu Wei Di Huang Wan* (Six-Ingredient Pill with Rehmannia).
- For cataract and blurred vision, add *Ba Wei Di Huang Wan* (Eight-Ingredient Pill with Rehmannia).

TONIC FORMULAS — 8

Zi Shen Ming Mu Tang (Nourish the Kidney to Brighten the Eyes Decoction)

Diagnosis	Signs and Symptoms	Treatment	Herbs
Impaired vision as a result of qi, blood and yin deficiencies	Blurred vision, poor vision, eye strain, and excessive itching and tearing of the eyes: qi, blood and yin deficiencies	• Nourishes yin • Tonifies qi and blood • Clears heat	• *Di Huang* (Radix Rehmanniae) and *Shu Di Huang* (Radix Rehmanniae Praeparata) nourish yin. • *Dang Gui* (Radix Angelicae Sinensis), *Bai Shao* (Radix Paeoniae Alba) and *Chuan Xiong* (Rhizoma Chuanxiong) tonify the blood and regulate blood circulation. • *Ren Shen* (Radix et Rhizoma Ginseng) and *Gan Cao* (Radix et Rhizoma Glycyrrhizae) tonify qi. • *Ju Hua* (Flos Chrysanthemi) and *Man Jing Zi* (Fructus Viticis) clear the Liver and improve vision. • *Huang Lian* (Rhizoma Coptidis) and *Zhi Zi* (Fructus Gardeniae) clear damp-heat and relieve redness and pain of the eyes. • *Bai Zhi* (Radix Angelicae Dahuricae) opens the orifices in the head. • *Jie Geng* (Radix Platycodonis) guides the formula upward to the affected area. • *Deng Xin Cao* (Medulla Junci) and *Cha Ye* (Folium Camelliae) promote the excretion of excess water from the body.

665

Chapter 8 – Tonic Formulas   *Section 4 – Yin-Tonifying Formulas*

Zī Shèn Tōng Ěr Tāng
(Nourish the Kidney to Unblock the Ears Decoction)

滋腎通耳湯
滋肾通耳汤

Pinyin Name: *Zi Shen Tong Er Tang*
Literal Name: Nourish the Kidney to Unblock the Ears Decoction
Alternate Name: Scute Combination
Original Source: *Wan Bing Hui Chun* (Restoration of Health from the Myriad Diseases) by Gong Ting-Xian in 1587

COMPOSITION

Di Huang (Radix Rehmanniae)
Dang Gui (Radix Angelicae Sinensis)
Chuan Xiong (Rhizoma Chuanxiong)
Bai Shao (Radix Paeoniae Alba)
Bai Zhi (Radix Angelicae Dahuricae)
Zhi Mu (Rhizoma Anemarrhenae), *chao* (dry-fried) with liquor
Huang Bo (Cortex Phellodendri Chinensis), *chao* (dry-fried) with liquor
Xiang Fu (Rhizoma Cyperi)
Chai Hu (Radix Bupleuri)
Huang Qin (Radix Scutellariae), *chao* (dry-fried) with liquor

DOSAGE / PREPARATION / ADMINISTRATION

Grate equal amounts of the herbs and cook them in water to make a decoction. Take the strained decoction while warm.

CHINESE THERAPEUTIC ACTIONS

1. Nourishes the Kidney
2. Tonifies the blood

CLINICAL MANIFESTATIONS

Impaired hearing: poor hearing and/or tinnitus.

CLINICAL APPLICATIONS

Deafness, tinnitus, and auditory depression.

EXPLANATION

Zi Shen Tong Er Tang (Nourish the Kidney to Unblock the Ears Decoction) treats hearing disorders caused by aging, infection, or accumulation of toxic substances. Common complaints include poor hearing and tinnitus. This formula is ideal for treating various types of hearing disorders, especially in elderly patients.

Zi Shen Tong Er Tang (Nourish the Kidney to Unblock the Ears Decoction)

Diagnosis	Signs and Symptoms	Treatment	Herbs
Impaired hearing	Poor hearing or tinnitus: Kidney and blood deficiencies unable to nourish the ears	• Nourishes the Kidney • Tonifies the blood	• *Di Huang* (Radix Rehmanniae) nourishes the Kidney. • *Dang Gui* (Radix Angelicae Sinensis), *Chuan Xiong* (Rhizoma Chuanxiong) and *Bai Shao* (Radix Paeoniae Alba) tonify the blood and regulate blood circulation. • *Bai Zhi* (Radix Angelicae Dahuricae) guides the formula to the upper parts of the body. • *Zhi Mu* (Rhizoma Anemarrhenae) and *Huang Bo* (Cortex Phellodendri Chinensis) nourish yin and clear deficiency heat. • *Xiang Fu* (Rhizoma Cyperi) and *Chai Hu* (Radix Bupleuri) unblock Liver qi stagnation. • *Huang Qin* (Radix Scutellariae) clears heat and reduces inflammation.

666

Chinese Herbal Formulas and Applications

Zī Shèn Tōng Ěr Tāng
(Nourish the Kidney to Unblock the Ears Decoction)

Di Huang (Radix Rehmanniae), the chief herb, nourishes the Kidney and treats the underlying deficiency. *Dang Gui* (Radix Angelicae Sinensis), *Chuan Xiong* (Rhizoma Chuanxiong), and *Bai Shao* (Radix Paeoniae Alba) tonify the blood and regulate blood circulation. *Bai Zhi* (Radix Angelicae Dahuricae) has an ascending function, and guides the formula to the upper parts of the body. *Zhi Mu* (Rhizoma Anemarrhenae) and *Huang Bo* (Cortex Phellodendri Chinensis) nourish yin and clear deficiency heat. *Xiang Fu* (Rhizoma Cyperi) and *Chai Hu* (Radix Bupleuri)

unblock Liver qi stagnation. *Huang Qin* (Radix Scutellariae) clears heat and reduces inflammation.

MODIFICATIONS

- For hearing disorders caused by toxicity of drugs, add *Huang Qi* (Radix Astragali) and *Lu Xian Cao* (Herba Pyrolae).
- If there is discomfort in the chest and diaphragm, add *Qing Pi* (Pericarpium Citri Reticulatae Viride) and *Zhi Qiao* (Fructus Aurantii).

667

Chapter 8 – Tonic Formulas   *Section 5 – Yang-Tonifying Formulas*

Section 5

补阳剂
— Yang-Tonifying Formulas

Jīn Gui Shèn Qì Wán (Kidney Qi Pill from the Golden Cabinet)
金匱腎氣丸
金匮肾气丸

Pinyin Name: *Jin Gui Shen Qi Wan*
Literal Name: Kidney Qi Pill from the Golden Cabinet
Alternate Names: *Shen Qi Wan* (Kidney Qi Pill), Kidney Qi Formula from the Golden Cabinet
Original Source: *Jin Gui Yao Lue* (Essentials from the Golden Cabinet) by Zhang Zhong-Jing in the Eastern Han Dynasty

COMPOSITION

Di Huang (Radix Rehmanniae)	24g
Shan Zhu Yu (Fructus Corni)	12g
Shan Yao (Rhizoma Dioscoreae)	12g
Fu Ling (Poria)	9g
Mu Dan Pi (Cortex Moutan)	9g
Ze Xie (Rhizoma Alismatis)	9g
Gui Zhi (Ramulus Cinnamomi)	3g
Fu Zi (Radix Aconiti Lateralis Praeparata), *pao* (blast-fried)	3g

DOSAGE / PREPARATION / ADMINISTRATION

Grind the ingredients into powder, mix the powder with honey and form into small pills resembling the size of *Wu Tong Zi* (Semen Firmianae), a small seed approximately 5 mm in diameter. Take 15-25 pills (6-10g) with a grain-based liquor twice daily.

CHINESE THERAPEUTIC ACTIONS

Warms and tonifies Kidney yang

CLINICAL MANIFESTATIONS

Kidney yang deficiency: lower back pain, weak legs, cold sensations in the lower body, pain and cramps in the lower abdomen, dysuria or polyuria, a pale, flabby tongue with a thin, white coating, and a deep, fine pulse at the *chi* position. It may also be used to treat leg *qi*, *tan yin* (phlegm retention), and *xiao ke* (wasting and thirsting) syndrome.

CLINICAL APPLICATIONS

Endocrine disorders (diabetes mellitus and insipidus, hyperaldosteronism, hypothyroidism); sexual and reproductive disorders (impotence, premature ejaculation, prostatic hypertrophy, male and female infertility, gynecomastia); genitourinary disorders (nephritis, nephrosclerosis, chronic glomerulonephritis, urolithiasis, renal tuberculosis, proteinuria, anuria, urinary incontinence, nocturia, vesical calculus, prostate disorders); cardiovascular disorders (coronary artery disease, arteriostenosis, hypertension, hypotension, post-stroke complications); respiratory disorders (chronic bronchitis, asthma, pulmonary emphysema); and other conditions such as lumbago and cataract.

EXPLANATION

Jin Gui Shen Qi Wan (Kidney Qi Pill from the Golden Cabinet) treats Kidney yang deficiency and/or deficiency of *ming men* (life gate) fire. Low back pain, weak legs, cold sensations in the lower back, and lower abdomenal pain and cramps are caused by Kidney yang deficiency and its inability to warm the lower parts of the body. Kidney yang is also responsible for regulating water circulation and metabolism, and its deficiency may cause water retention, which can give rise to dysuria, leg *qi*, and *tan yin* (phlegm retention). Polyuria may occur if there is Kidney

Jīn Guì Shèn Qì Wán (Kidney Qi Pill from the Golden Cabinet)

Jin Gui Shen Qi Wan (Kidney Qi Pill from the Golden Cabinet)

Diagnosis	Signs and Symptoms	Treatment	Herbs
Kidney yang deficiency	• Low back pain, weak legs, cold sensations in the lower back, and lower abdominal pain and cramps: Kidney yang deficiency unable to warm the lower parts of the body • Dysuria or polyuria: Kidney yang unable to regulate water circulation and metabolism • Deep, fine pulse at the *chi* position: Kidney yang deficiency	Warms and tonifies Kidney yang	• *Di Huang* (Radix Rehmanniae) tonifies Kidney yin and *jing* (essence). • *Shan Zhu Yu* (Fructus Corni) tonifies Kidney and Liver yin. • *Shan Yao* (Rhizoma Dioscoreae) tonifies the Kidney and Spleen. • *Fu Ling* (Poria), *Mu Dan Pi* (Cortex Moutan) and *Ze Xie* (Rhizoma Alismatis) sedate turbidity and prevent the greasiness of the tonic herbs from blocking the qi flow. • *Gui Zhi* (Ramulus Cinnamomi) and *Fu Zi* (Radix Aconiti Lateralis Praeparata) tonify Kidney yang.

deficiency in patients with *xiao ke* (wasting and thirsting) syndrome. A deep, fine pulse at the *chi* position is an indication of Kidney yang deficiency.

Jin Gui Shen Qi Wan is based on *Liu Wei Di Huang Wan* (Six-Ingredient Pill with Rehmannia), with the addition of *Gui Zhi* (Ramulus Cinnamomi) and *Fu Zi* (Radix Aconiti Lateralis Praeparata). The strategy behind this formula is to tonify Kidney yin to raise Kidney yang, since yin and yang are mutually dependent. This formula uses *Di Huang* (Radix Rehmanniae) to tonify Kidney yin and *jing* (essence), *Shan Zhu Yu* (Fructus Corni) to tonify Kidney and Liver yin, and *Shan Yao* (Rhizoma Dioscoreae) to tonify the Kidney and Spleen. To tonify Kidney yang, this formula uses a small amount of *Gui Zhi* (Ramulus Cinnamomi) and *Fu Zi* (Radix Aconiti Lateralis Praeparata). Only a small amount of these two warming herbs are needed to ignite the *ming men* (life gate) fire and raise Kidney yang. *Ze Xie* (Rhizoma Alismatis), *Fu Ling* (Poria), and *Mu Dan Pi* (Cortex Moutan) sedate turbidity and prevent the greasiness of the tonic herbs from blocking the qi flow.

MODIFICATIONS

• With dizziness and vertigo, add *Gou Qi Zi* (Fructus Lycii) and *Ju Hua* (Flos Chrysanthemi).
• For cataract and poor vision, add *Yi Qi Cong Ming Tang* (Augment the Qi and Increase Acuity Decoction).
• With leg *qi* and low back pain, add *Fang Ji Huang Qi Tang* (Stephania and Astragalus Decoction).
• For yin deficiency and generalized atrophy, add *Huang Qi Jian Zhong Tang* (Astragalus Decoction to Construct the Middle).
• For back pain and knee soreness, add *Niu Xi* (Radix Achyranthis Bidentatae) and *Du Zhong* (Cortex Eucommiae).

• For back pain, swelling of the legs, and dysuria, add *Niu Xi* (Radix Achyranthis Bidentatae) and *Che Qian Zi* (Semen Plantaginis).

CAUTIONS / CONTRAINDICATIONS

• *Jin Gui Shen Qi Wan* should be used with caution in patients who have poor appetite, loose stools, and chronic diarrhea caused by Spleen and Stomach deficiencies.
• This formula is contraindicated in patients with deficiency-heat rising, with symptoms such as a dry mouth and throat, and a red tongue with a scanty tongue coating.
• Possible side effects of the formula that have been reported include stomach discomfort, constipation, itching, rash, palpitations, and an irregular heart beat.[1]
• Use of this formula is contraindicated during pregnancy.[2]

PHARMACOLOGICAL EFFECTS

1. **Antiaging**: In numerous laboratory experiments, administration of *Jin Gui Shen Qi Wan* was associated with general improvements in the health and well-being of the subjects. The effects of the herbs include increased tolerance to cold weather, decreased risk of cancer formation, lower incidence of muscle atrophy, and decreased plasma cholesterol and triglyceride levels.[3]
2. **Immunostimulant**: Administration of *Jin Gui Shen Qi Wan* in mice at 0.3g each was associated with enhanced immunity by increasing the number of lymphocytes.[4]
3. **Endocrine**: Administration of *Jin Gui Shen Qi Wan* in 21-day-old mice for 28 days was associated with a stimulating effect on the endocrine system as evident in the increased weight of the pituitary glands, hypothalamus, and other glands. The dosage given to mice was equivalent to 10 times the human dose, according to weight calculation.[5]

Chapter 8 – Tonic Formulas   *Section 5 – Yang-Tonifying Formulas*

Jīn Guì Shèn Qì Wán (Kidney Qi Pill from the Golden Cabinet)

4. Reproductive: Administration of *Jin Gui Shen Qi Wan* in rats was associated with an increase in sperm count and sperm motility.[6]

CLINICAL STUDIES AND RESEARCH

1. **Diabetes mellitus**: In one study, 38 patients with type II diabetes mellitus for 3 months to 20 years were treated with modified *Jin Gui Shen Qi Wan*. The base formula included *Fu Zi* (Radix Aconiti Lateralis Praeparata) 9g, *Rou Gui* (Cortex Cinnamomi) 5g, *Di Huang* (Radix Rehmanniae) 15g, *Shan Zhu Yu* (Fructus Corni) 15g, *Dan Shen* (Radix et Rhizoma Salviae Miltiorrhizae) 15g, *Shan Yao* (Rhizoma Dioscoreae) 30g, *Long Gu* (Os Draconis) 30g, *Mu Dan Pi* (Cortex Moutan) 10g, *Huang Qi* (Radix Astragali) 20g, *Fu Ling* (Poria) 12g, *Ze Xie* (Rhizoma Alismatis) 12g, and *Wu Bei Zi* (Galla Chinensis) 12g. Other modifications were made based on the patients' clinical presentation. The treatment protocol was to administer the herbs in decoction one time daily for 30 days per course of treatment. Out of 38 patients, the study reported marked improvement in 8 patients, moderate improvement in 16 patients, slight improvement in 12 patients, and no benefit in 2 patients. The overall rate of effectiveness was 94.7%.[7]

2. **Hypertension**: Use of modified *Jin Gui Shen Qi Wan* in 40 patients with primary hypertension characterized by Spleen and Kidney yang deficiencies was associated with reduction of blood pressure in 82.5% of patients.[8]

3. **Coronary artery disease**: In one study, 60 geriatric patients with coronary artery disease were divided into two groups: 40 received herbs and 20 received vitamin E capsules. After 1 month of treatment, the study reported that in the herb group, 16 had marked improvement, 14 had moderate improvement, 8 had slight improvement, and 2 had no benefit. In the vitamin E group, 3 had marked improvement, 8 had moderate improvement, 4 had slight improvement, and 5 had no benefit. Overall, the effectiveness rate was 95% for the herb group and 75% for the vitamin E group.[9]

4. **Asthma**: In one study, 19 patients with asthma were treated with *Jin Gui Shen Qi Wan* as a maintenance therapy. The study indicated that up to 89.5% of the patients noted improvement after using the herbs.[10] According to another study, use of *Jin Gui Shen Qi Wan* three times daily for 6 months or more was associated with 89.5% effectiveness to prevent asthma attacks among 19 patients with asthma.[11]

5. **Lumbago**: In one report, 27 patients (aged 35-80 years) with low back pain due to various causes were treated with *Jin Gui Shen Qi Wan* for 4 weeks, with marked improvement in 6 patients, moderate improvement in 11 patients, and slight improvement in 3 patients. The overall rate of effectiveness was 70%.[12]

6. **Male infertility**: Administration of *Jin Gui Shen Qi Wan* plus *Ren Shen* (Radix et Rhizoma Ginseng) at 7.5 g/day for 12 weeks showed effectiveness in treating 10 male infertility patients between 28-36 years of age. The study noted that 90 days of herbal treatment was required for significant changes in sperm count and motility.[13] In another study, 51 men with infertility due to low sperm count and motility were treated with 7.5 g/day of *Jin Gui Shen Qi Wan*. Out of 51 men, pregnancy was reported in over 80% of couples within 3 months.[14]

7. **Female infertility**: In one study, 27 women with infertility caused by elevated prolactin levels (above 30 ng/mL) were treated with 2.5-10g of *Jin Gui Shen Qi Wan*. After 3 months of herbal therapy, prolactin levels decreased in 18 out of 27 patients. In addition, the level was < 30 ng/mL in 15 patients. In follow up interviews 6 months later, 12 women had become pregnant. No abnormalities were noted with the mothers or with the fetuses.[15]

8. **Impotence**: One study reported 43.2% effectiveness using *Jin Gui Shen Qi Wan* to treat 37 patients with impotence. The treatment protocol was to administer *Jin Gui Shen Qi Wan* in pills, 5g twice daily for 4 weeks.[16]

9. **Gynecomastia**: In one study, 32 men (21-69 years of age) with unilateral or bilateral gynecomastia for 2 months to 3 years were treated with modified *Jin Gui Shen Qi Wan*. The formula included *Rou Gui* (Cortex Cinnamomi) 6g, *Chi Shao* (Radix Paeoniae Rubra) 15g, *Bai Shao* (Radix Paeoniae Alba) 15g, *Dan Shen* (Radix et Rhizoma Salviae Miltiorrhizae) 15g, *Shu Di Huang* (Radix Rehmanniae Praeparata) 30g, and *Shan Yao* (Rhizoma Dioscoreae) 10g. In addition, *Xiang Fu* (Rhizoma Cyperi), *Chuan Lian Zi* (Fructus Toosendan), and *Yu Jin* (Radix Curcumae) were added for breast distention and pain. *Xia Ku Cao* (Spica Prunellae), *Zhe Bei Mu* (Bulbus Fritillariae Thunbergii), and *Xuan Shen* (Radix Scrophulariae) were added for swelling and hardness of the breast. *Lu Jiao Shuang* (Cornu Cervi Degelatinatum), *Xian Mao* (Rhizoma Curculiginis), and *Sang Ji Sheng* (Herba Taxilli) were added for soreness of the lower back and knees and lack of sexual desire. *Sha Ren* (Fructus Amomi), *Shen Qu* (Massa Fermentata), and *Bing Lang* (Semen Arecae) were added for poor appetite with a thick, greasy tongue coating. The treatment protocol was to administer the herbs one time daily for 20 days per course of treatment, for 3 courses total. Out of 32 patients, the study reported marked effect in 23 patients, moderate improvement in 7 patients, and no benefit in 2 patients. The overall rate of effectiveness was 93.7%.[17]

10. **Prostatic hypertrophy**: According to numerous reports, the use of *Jin Gui Shen Qi Wan* showed benefits in treating

Jīn Guì Shèn Qì Wán (Kidney Qi Pill from the Golden Cabinet)

patients with prostate-related disorders, such as dysuria, frequent urination, and prostate enlargement.[18] Complete recovery in 33 of 64 patients (51.5%) was reported in one study using modified *Jin Gui Shen Qi Wan* to treat prostatic hypertrophy with symptoms such as frequent urination (especially at night) and painful urination. The treatment protocol was to administer the herbs in decoction daily for 10 days per course of treatment until the resolution of symptoms, followed by maintainance therapy at 2 packs of herbs per week for 3 months.[19]

11. **Urinary incontinence**: In one study, 13 patients with 3 months to 1 year of incontinence were treated with *Jin Gui Shen Qi Wan* with salted water one time daily in the morning, for 10 days per course of treatment. The study reported that 6 patients had complete recovery after taking the herbs for 10-20 days, 4 had marked improvement after 20-30 days, 2 had slight improvement after 30-40 days, and 1 had no benefit.[20]

12. **Chronic glomerulonephritis**: One study of 12 patients with chronic glomerulonephritis characterized by yang deficiency reported success (recovery in 10 patients and no benefit in 2 patients) using modified *Jin Gui Shen Qi Wan*. *Wu Jia Pi* (Cortex Acanthopanacis) was added for individuals with edema in the legs. The duration of treatment was 21-90 days.[21]

13. **Cataract**: Use of *Jin Gui Shen Qi Wan* demonstrated effectiveness in treating geriatric patients with cataract. The study reported an overall effectiveness rate of 80%, with improvement in visual acuity noted in 60% of patients and stabilization of glaucoma in 20% of patients. The treatment protocol was to administer 3g of herbs in pills per day in two equally-divided doses. The study also noted that better prognosis was noted in individuals who began herbal therapy early.[22]

HERB-DRUG INTERACTION

Prednisone-induced adverse reactions: According to one report, use of *Jin Gui Shen Qi Wan* was effective in treating side effects and adverse reactions associated with long-term use of prednisone, such as dizziness, weight gain, perspiration, and emotional disturbance.[23]

TOXICOLOGY

According to a toxicology study, *Jin Gui Shen Qi Wan* was determined to have little toxicity. In rats, *Jin Gui Shen Qi Wan* in powder extract form was given at dosages of 40 mg/kg and 200 mg/kg in decoction one time daily for 6 months, and no abnormalities were noted in general signs and symptoms, complete blood count, urine analysis, and functions of the internal and reproductive organs.[24]

RELATED FORMULA

Shí Bǔ Wán (Ten-Tonic Pill)

十補丸

十补丸

Pinyin Name: *Shi Bu Wan*

Literal Name: Ten-Tonic Pill

Original Source: *Ji Sheng Fang* (Formulas to Aid the Living) by Yan Yong-He in 1253

Fu Zi (Radix Aconiti Lateralis Praeparata), pao (blast-fried)	60g [9g]
Wu Wei Zi (Fructus Schisandrae Chinensis)	60g [9g]
Shan Zhu Yu (Fructus Corni)	30g [9g]
Shan Yao (Rhizoma Dioscoreae), chao (dry-fried)	30g [9g]
Shu Di Huang (Radix Rehmanniae Praeparata), zheng (steamed) with liquor	30g [9g]
Lu Rong (Cornu Cervi Pantotrichum), zheng (steamed) with liquor	30g [3g]
Rou Gui (Cortex Cinnamomi), do not expose to heat	30g [3g]
Mu Dan Pi (Cortex Moutan)	30g [9g]
Ze Xie (Rhizoma Alismatis)	30g [6g]
Fu Ling (Poria)	30g [6g]

Grind the ingredients into a fine powder and form into small pills with honey. The pills should resemble *Wu Tong Zi* (Semen Firmianae), a small seed approximately 5 mm in diameter. Take 70 pills (9g) on an empty stomach with salted, grain-based liquor. Today, this formula may be prepared as a decoction with the doses suggested in brackets.

Shi Bu Wan (Ten-Tonic Pill) warms and tonifies Kidney yang. Clinically, patients may present with a dark facial complexion, cold feet, lower body edema, tinnitus, deafness, an emaciated complexion, weak knees, sore back, and dysuria.

Shi Bu Wan (Ten-Tonic Pill) is composed of *Liu Wei Di Huang Wan* (Six-Ingredient Pill with Rehmannia) and the addition of *Rou Gui* (Cortex Cinnamomi), *Fu Zi* (Radix Aconiti Lateralis Praeparata), *Lu Rong* (Cornu Cervi Pantotrichum), and *Wu Wei Zi* (Fructus Schisandrae Chinensis). *Liu Wei Di Huang Wan* (Six-Ingredient Pill with Rehmannia) tonifies Kidney yin. *Rou Gui* (Cortex Cinnamomi) and *Fu Zi* (Radix Aconiti Lateralis Praeparata) warm and tonify Kidney yang. *Lu Rong* (Cornu Cervi Pantotrichum) also warms and tonifies Kidney yang. *Wu Wei Zi* (Fructus Schisandrae Chinensis), an astringent herb, retains qi in the Kidney.

Chapter 8 – Tonic Formulas   *Section 5 – Yang-Tonifying Formulas*

Jīn Guì Shèn Qì Wán (Kidney Qi Pill from the Golden Cabinet)

AUTHORS' COMMENTS

Originally named "*Shen Qi Wan* (Kidney Qi Pill)" by Zhang Zhong-Jing in the Eastern Han Dynasty, this formula today is commonly referred to as *Jin Gui Shen Qi Wan* (Kidney Qi Pill from the Golden Cabinet). The reason for this change is to avoid confusion and errors, since there are at least 16 formulas with the identical name of "*Shen Qi Wan* (Kidney Qi Pill)" according to *Zhong Yi Fang Ji Da Ci Dian* (Grand Dictionary of Chinese Herbal Formulas).

Shen Qi Wan, literally Kidney Qi Pill, is so named because it uses only a small amount of *Gui Zhi* (Ramulus Cinnamomi) and *Fu Zi* (Radix Aconiti Lateralis Praeparata) to generate Kidney qi and ignite *ming men* (life gate) fire. Large doses of these two dry and hot herbs may not be appropriate because they may damage yin and consume fluids, leading to other adverse effects.

References

1. *Zhong Yi Fang Ji Xian Dai Yan Jiu* (Modern Study of Medical Formulae in Traditional Chinese Medicine) 1997;681-682.
2. *Zhong Yao Ming Fang Yao Li Yu Ying Yong* (Pharmacology and Applications of Famous Herbal Formulas) 1989;325-329.
3. *Zhong Yi Fang Ji Xian Dai Yan Jiu* (Modern Study of Medical Formulae in Traditional Chinese Medicine) 1997;669-670.
4. *Cheng Du Zhong Yi Xue Yuan Xue Bao* (Journal of Chengdu University of Traditional Chinese Medicine) 1985;4:40.
5. *Zhong Yi Fang Ji Xian Dai Yan Jiu* (Modern Study of Medical Formulae in Traditional Chinese Medicine) 1997;673.
6. *Zhong Cheng Yao* (Study of Chinese Patent Medicine) 1993;11:24.
7. *Xin Zhong Yi* (New Chinese Medicine) 1995;27(9):39.
8. *Yun Nan Zhong Yao Zhi* (Yunan Journal of Chinese Herbal Medicine) 1987;6:9.
9. *Zhe Jiang Zhong Yi Za Zhi* (Zhejiang Journal of Chinese Medicine) 1993;6:270.
10. *Yi Yao Wei Sheng* (Medicine, Medicinals, and Sanitation) 1977;6:33.
11. *Zhong Cheng Yao Yan Jiu* (Research of Chinese Patent Medicine) 1988;11:47.
12. *Han Fang Yi Xue* (Kampo Medicine) 1986;12:32.
13. *Guo Wai Yi Xue* (Foreign Medicine) 1985;1:46.
14. *Guo Wai Yi Yao Zhi Wu Yao Zhi Wu Yao Fen Ce* (Monograph of Foreign Botanical Medicine) 1991;1:45.
15. *Guo Wai Yi Yao Zhi Wu Yao Fen Ce* (Monograph of Foreign Botanical Medicine) 1991;4:41.
16. *Guo Wai Yi Xue Zhong Yi Zhong Yao Fen Ce* (Monograph of Chinese Herbology from Foreign Medicine) 1991;13(1):47.
17. *Xin Zhong Yi* (New Chinese Medicine) 1994;2:31.
18. *Zhong Yi Fang Ji Xian Dai Yan Jiu* (Modern Study of Medical Formulae in Traditional Chinese Medicine) 1997;680.
19. *Nan Jing Zhong Yi Yao Da Xue Xue Bao* (Journal of Nanjing University of Traditional Chinese Medicine and Medicinals) 1999;15(4):252.
20. *Xin Zhong Yi* (New Chinese Medicine) 1995;27(1):50.
21. *Zhong Yi Za Zhi* (Journal of Chinese Medicine) 1956;12:635.
22. *Zhong Cheng Yao* (Study of Chinese Patent Medicine) 1990;12:720.
23. *Zhong Yi Za Zhi* (Journal of Chinese Medicine) 1987;28(1):45.
24. *Han Fang Yi Xue* (Kampo Medicine) 1985;10:48.

Bā Wèi Dì Huáng Wán (Eight-Ingredient Pill with Rehmannia)
八味地黄丸
八味地黄丸

Pinyin Name: *Ba Wei Di Huang Wan*
Literal Name: Eight-Ingredient Pill with Rehmannia
Alternate Names: *Pa Wei Ti Huang Wan*, Eight-Flavour Rehmannia Pill, Rehmannia Bolus with Eight Herbs, Rehmannia Eight Formula
Original Source: *Yi Fang Ji Jie* (Analytical Collection of Medical Formulas) by Wang Ang in 1682

COMPOSITION

Shu Di Huang (Radix Rehmanniae Praeparata)	24g
Shan Zhu Yu (Fructus Corni)	12g
Shan Yao (Rhizoma Dioscoreae)	12g
Fu Ling (Poria)	9g
Mu Dan Pi (Cortex Moutan)	9g
Ze Xie (Rhizoma Alismatis)	9g
Rou Gui (Cortex Cinnamomi)	3g
Fu Zi (Radix Aconiti Lateralis Praeparata), *pao* (blast-fried)	3g

672

Bā Wèi Dì Huáng Wán (Eight-Ingredient Pill with Rehmannia)

DOSAGE / PREPARATION / ADMINISTRATION

Grind the ingredients into powder, and mix the powder with honey and form into small pills that resemble the size of *Wu Tong Zi* (Semen Firmianae), a small seed approximately 5 mm in diameter. Take 15-25 pills (6-10g) with a grain-based liquor twice daily.

CHINESE THERAPEUTIC ACTIONS

Warms and tonifies Kidney yang

CLINICAL MANIFESTATIONS

Kidney yang deficiency: low back pain, weak legs, cold sensations in the lower body, pain and cramps in the lower abdomen, dysuria or polyuria, a pale, flabby tongue with a thin, white tongue coating, and a deep, fine pulse at the *chi* position. It can also treat leg *qi*, *tan yin* (phlegm retention), and *xiao ke* (wasting and thirsting) syndrome.

CLINICAL APPLICATIONS

Endocrine disorders (diabetes mellitus and insipidus, hyperaldosteronism, hypothyroidism); sexual and reproductive disorders (impotence, premature ejaculation, male and female infertility, gynecomastia); genitourinary disorders (nephritis, nephrosclerosis, kidney stones, renal tuberculosis, proteinuria, anuria, incontinence, nocturia, vesical calculus, prostate disorders); cardiovascular disorders (coronary artery disease, arteriostenosis, hypertension, hypotension, post-stroke complications); and pulmonary disorders (chronic bronchitis, asthma, pulmonary emphysema). Other uses include lumbago, benign prostatic hyperplasia, cataract and other eye diseases.

EXPLANATION

Ba Wei Di Huang Wan (Eight-Ingredient Pill with Rehmannia) is a modification of *Jin Gui Shen Qi Wan* (Kidney Qi Pill from the Golden Cabinet). *Di Huang* (Radix Rehmanniae) is replaced with *Shu Di Huang* (Radix Rehmanniae Praeparata) to enhance the yin-tonic effect. *Gui Zhi* (Ramulus Cinnamomi) is substituted with *Rou Gui* (Cortex Cinnamomi) to increase the yang-tonic function. This slightly revised formula, *Ba Wei Di Huang Wan*, is a warmer and slightly stronger yang tonic than *Jin Gui Shen Qi Wan*.

For additional information, please refer to *Jin Gui Shen Qi Wan* (Kidney Qi Pill from the Golden Cabinet) and *Liu Wei Di Huang Wan* (Six-Ingredient Pill with Rehmannia).

MODIFICATIONS

Same as for *Jin Gui Shen Qi Wan* (Kidney Qi Pill from the Golden Cabinet).

CAUTIONS / CONTRAINDICATIONS

Same as for *Jin Gui Shen Qi Wan* (Kidney Qi Pill from the Golden Cabinet).

PHARMACOLOGICAL EFFECTS

1. **Immunosuppressant**: In one study, use of *Ba Wei Di Huang Wan* for 9 days was associated with suppressed development of MRL/lpr autoimmune diseases in mice.[1,2]

2. **Effect on the prostate**: *Ba Wei Di Huang Wan* has been used to treat various prostate disorders with great success. One study analyzed the mechanism of *Ba Wei Di Huang Wan* and found that this formula acts as a weak androgen and enhances prostatic thymidine kinase activity, but also acts as an anti-androgen and reduces prostatic thymidine kinase activity in the presence of androgen in immature rats.[3]

3. **Effect on bone mass density**: In one study on the prevention and treatment of osteoporosis, *Ba Wei Di Huang Wan*, *Wen Jing Tang* (Warm the Channels Decoction), and *Shi Quan Da Bu Tang* (All-Inclusive Great Tonifying Decoction) were administered for 49 days to rats with ovariectomy. Compared to sham-operated rats, the bone mineral density (BMD) of tibia in ovariectomized rats decreased by 20%, but the BMD was unaffected in rats treated with herbs or 17-beta-estradiol. The study concluded that these three formulas were as effective as 17-beta-estradiol in preventing the development of bone loss induced by ovariectomy by preserving the fine particle surface of the bone.[4]

4. **Antihypertensive and nephroprotective**: Administration of *Ba Wei Di Huang Wan* for 5 weeks dose-dependently decreased systolic blood pressure in rats fed with a high-salt (2% NaCl) diet. This blood pressure reduction was associated with a decrease in cardiac mass and thickness of the aortic wall, increased urinary excretion of prostaglandin E2, improved glomerular filtration rate, and improved glomerulosclerosis and arterial injury in the kidney. The study stated that *Ba Wei Di Huang Wan* had both antihypertensive and nephroprotective effects.[5]

5. **Endocrine**: Administration of *Ba Wei Di Huang Wan* was shown both *in vitro* and *in vivo* to stimulate the testes and increase the production of testosterone.[6] Use of this formula also stimulated the corpus luteum and increased secretion of progesterone.[7]

CLINICAL STUDIES AND RESEARCH

1. **Benign prostatic hyperplasia**: Use of *Ba Wei Di Huang Wan* for two weeks in 41 patients with benign prostatic hyperplasia was associated with significant improvements in emptying, weak stream, max flow rate, and total quality of life score, according to the International Prostate Symptom Score. Of 41 patients, 40% of patients responded well to

Chapter 8 – Tonic Formulas   *Section 5 – Yang-Tonifying Formulas*

Bā Wèi Dì Huáng Wán (Eight-Ingredient Pill with Rehmannia)

Ba Wei Di Huang Wan (Eight-Ingredient Pill with Rehmannia)

Diagnosis	Signs and Symptoms	Treatment	Herbs
Severe Kidney yang deficiency	• Low back pain, weak legs, cold sensations in the lower back, and lower abdominal pain and cramps: Kidney yang deficiency unable to warm the lower parts of the body • Dysuria or polyuria: Kidney yang unable to regulate water circulation and metabolism • Deep, fine pulse at the *chi* position: Kidney yang deficiency	Strongly warms and tonifies Kidney yang	• *Shu Di Huang* (Radix Rehmanniae Praeparata) strongly tonifies Kidney yin and *jing* (essence). • *Shan Zhu Yu* (Fructus Corni) tonifies Kidney and Liver yin. • *Shan Yao* (Rhizoma Dioscoreae) tonifies the Kidney and Spleen. • *Fu Ling* (Poria), *Mu Dan Pi* (Cortex Moutan) and *Ze Xie* (Rhizoma Alismatis) sedate turbidity and prevent the greasiness of the tonic herbs from blocking the qi flow. • *Rou Gui* (Cortex Cinnamomi) and *Fu Zi* (Radix Aconiti Lateralis Praeparata) strongly tonify Kidney yang.

Ba Wei Di Huang Wan therapy, although 2 did not finish administration as a result of epigastric discomfort.[8]

2. **Female infertility**: In one case report, use of bromocriptine was ineffective in treating one infertile hyperprolactinemic woman with a pituitary microadenoma. This woman was subsequently treated with *Ba Wei Di Huang Wan*, and succeeded in having a normal pregnancy and delivery.[9]

3. **Cataract and other eye diseases**: In one study, use of *Ba Wei Di Huang Wan* was associated with delaying cataract appearance by up to 13.9 years. The mechanism of this effect was attributed to inhibition of sodium-potassium ATPase activity and also the oxidation of lens protein.[10] According to another study in 12 healthy adults, administration of *Ba Wei Di Huang Wan* was associated with significant increase in the systolic flow velocity, diastolic flow velocity, and mean flow velocity in the central retinal artery. Because various eye diseases are associated with a decrease of blood flow in the central retinal artery, use of *Ba Wei Di Huang Wan* to increase blood flow provides positive effects for treatment of such eye diseases.[11]

AUTHORS' COMMENTS

According to *Zhong Yi Fang Ji Da Ci Dian* (Grand Dictionary of Chinese Herbal Formulas), there are seven different formulas with the same name of *Ba Wei Di Huang Wan* (Eight-Ingredient Pill with Rehmannia). All were written by different authors in various texts and references. The formula listed here is generally considered to be the most commonly used formulation today.

Jin Gui Shen Qi Wan (Kidney Qi Pill from the Golden Cabinet) and *Ba Wei Di Huang Wan* are essentially the same formulas, except for a few minor differences.

• *Jin Gui Shen Qi Wan* uses *Di Huang* (Radix Rehmanniae) to moderately nourish Kidney yin, and *Gui Zhi* (Ramulus Cinnamomi) to mildly warm Kidney yang. Overall, it is a milder formula that gently tonifies both Kidney yin and yang.

• *Ba Wei Di Huang Wan* uses *Shu Di Huang* (Radix Rehmanniae Praeparata) to strongly tonify Kidney yin, and *Rou Gui* (Cortex Cinnamomi) to strongly warm and tonify Kidney yang. Overall, it potently tonifies both Kidney yin and yang.

According to Dr. Chang Wei-Yen, chronic nephritis can be treated with a combination of *Ba Wei Di Huang Wan*, *Long Dan Xie Gan Tang* (Gentiana Decoction to Drain the Liver), *Ba Zheng San* (Eight-Herb Powder for Rectification), *Shui Ding Xiang* (Herba Ludwigiae Prostratae), and *Xian Feng Cao* (Herba Bidentis).

References

1. Furuya Y, Kawakita T, Nomoto K. Suppressive effect of a traditional Japanese medicine, Hachimi-jio-gan (Ba-Wei-Di-Huang-Wan), on the hyperresponsiveness to IL-18 in autoimmune MRL/MPJ-lpr/lpr mice. Int Immunopharmacol 2003 Mar;3(3):365-73.

2. Furuya Y, Kawakita T, Nomoto K. Immunomodulating effect of a traditional Japanese medicine, hachimi-jio-gan (ba-wei-di-huang-wan), on Th1 predominance in autoimmune MRL/MP-lpr/lpr mice. Int Immunopharmacol 2001 Mar;1(3):551-9.

3. Sakamoto S, Kudo H, Kawasaki T, Kasahara N, Okamoto R. Effect of ba-wei-di-huang-wan (hachimi-jio-gan) on thymidine kinase and its isozyme activities in the prostate glands in rats. Am J Chin Med 1988;16(1-2):29-36.

4. Hidaka S, Okamoto Y, Nakajima K, Suekawa M, Liu SY. Preventive effects of traditional Chinese (Kampo) medicines on experimental osteoporosis induced by ovariectomy in rats. Calcif Tissue Int 1997 Sep;61(3):239-46.

5. Hirawa N, Uehara Y, Kawabata Y, Numabe A, Takada S, Nagoshi H, Gomi T, Ikeda T, Omata M. Hachimi-jio-gan extract protects the

674

Chinese Herbal Formulas and Applications

Bā Wèi Dì Huáng Wán (Eight-Ingredient Pill with Rehmannia)

kidney from hypertensive injury in Dahl salt-sensitive rat. Am J Chin Med 1996;24(3-4):241-54.

6. Usuki S. Hachimijiogan produces testosterone in adult rat testes. Am J Chin Med 1988;16(3-4):93-105.

7. Usuki S. Effects of hachimijiogan, tokishakuyakusan and keishibu-kuryogan on progesterone secretions by corpus luteum. Am J Chin Med 1987;15(3-4):109-15.

8. Yoshimura K, Terai A, Arai Y. Two-week administration of low-dose Hachimi-jio-gan (Ba-Wei Di-Huang-Wan) for patients with benign prostatic hyperplasia. Hinyokika Kiyo 2003 Sep;49(9):509-14.

9. Otani S, Usuki S, Iwasaki H, Inoue S, Yamashita K. Successful treatment of a infertile woman using hachimijiogan. Am J Chin Med 1991;19(2):145-54.

10. Kamei A, Hisada T, Iwata S. The evaluation of therapeutic efficacy of hachimi-jio-gan (traditional Chinese medicine) to mouse hereditary cataract. J Ocul Pharmacol 1988 Winter;4(4):311-9.

11. Isobe H, Yamamoto K, Cyong JC. Effects of hachimi-jio-gan (ba-wei-di-huang-wan) on blood flow in the human central retinal artery. American Journal of Chinese Medicine 2003;31(3):425-35.

Jì Shēng Shèn Qì Wán

(Kidney Qi Pill from Formulas that Aid the Living)

濟生腎氣丸
济生肾气丸

Pinyin Name: *Ji Sheng Shen Qi Wan*

Literal Name: Kidney Qi Pill from Formulas that Aid the Living

Alternate Names: *Jia Wei Shen Qi Wan* (Augmented Kidney Qi Pill), *Chi Sheng Shen Qi Wan*, Life-Saving Renal Chi Pill, Life-Preserving Kidney-Qi Pill, Cyathula and Plantago Formula

Original Source: *Ji Sheng Fang* (Formulas to Aid the Living) by Yan Yong-He in 1253

COMPOSITION

Shu Di Huang (Radix Rehmanniae Praeparata)	15g [6g]
Shan Zhu Yu (Fructus Corni)	30g [6g]
Shan Yao (Rhizoma Dioscoreae), *chao* (dry-fried)	30g [6g]
Fu Ling (Poria)	30g [6g]
Mu Dan Pi (Cortex Moutan)	30g [6g]
Ze Xie (Rhizoma Alismatis)	30g [6g]
Fu Zi (Radix Aconiti Lateralis Praeparata), *pao* (blast-fried)	60g [9g]
Rou Gui (Cortex Cinnamomi), do not expose to heat	15g [3g]
Chuan Niu Xi (Radix Cyathulae), *jin* (soaked) with liquor	15g [6g]
Che Qian Zi (Semen Plantaginis), *zheng* (steamed) with liquor	30g [6g]

DOSAGE / PREPARATION / ADMINISTRATION

Grind the ingredients into a fine powder, mix with honey and form into small pills. The pills should resemble *Wu Tong Zi* (Semen Firmianae), a small seed approximately 5 mm in diameter. Take 70 pills (9g) with rice soup on an empty stomach. Today, this formula may be prepared as a decoction using the doses suggested in brackets.

CHINESE THERAPEUTIC ACTIONS

1. Warms and tonifies Kidney yang
2. Regulates water and relieves edema

CLINICAL MANIFESTATIONS

Kidney yang deficiency with water accumulation: severe pitting edema, cold sensations in the lower body, lumbago, fatigue, sensory numbness, and urinary difficulties.

CLINICAL APPLICATIONS

Diabetes mellitus, diabetic neuropathy, nephrotic syndrome, chronic nephritis, dysuria, oliguria, infertility, prostatic hypertrophy, and osteoporosis.

675

Chapter 8 – Tonic Formulas   *Section 5 – Yang-Tonifying Formulas*

Jì Shēng Shèn Qì Wán
(Kidney Qi Pill from Formulas that Aid the Living)

EXPLANATION

Ji Sheng Shen Qi Wan (Kidney Qi Pill from Formulas that Aid the Living) treats Kidney yang deficiency accompanied by water accumulation. Kidney yang deficiency is characterized by generalized decline in both physiological and physical functions as a result of insufficiency of *ming men* (life gate) fire to warm the Kidney, leading to compromises in endocrine, sexual, renal, cardiovascular, and pulmonary functions. Additionally, Kidney yang deficiency may lead to abnormal water circulation and metabolism, resulting in edema and urinary difficulties. Clinically, patients will exhibit symptoms and signs such as cold sensations in the lower body, lumbago, fatigue, sensory numbness, and urinary difficulties.

Ji Sheng Shen Qi Wan is comprised of *Liu Wei Di Huang Wan* (Six-Ingredient Pill with Rehmannia), plus *Rou Gui* (Cortex Cinnamomi), *Fu Zi* (Radix Aconiti Lateralis Praeparata), *Che Qian Zi* (Semen Plantaginis), and *Chuan Niu Xi* (Radix Cyathulae). *Liu Wei Di Huang Wan* (Six-Ingredient Pill with Rehmannia) tonifies the underlying Kidney yin deficiency. Hot in nature, *Fu Zi* (Radix Aconiti Lateralis Praeparata) and *Rou Gui* (Cortex Cinnamomi) tonify Kidney yang and warm the lower body. *Fu Zi* (Radix Aconiti Lateralis Praeparata) is an excellent herb to treat various chronic disorders with signs and symptoms of cold. *Rou Gui* (Cortex Cinnamomi) strengthens the Spleen and tonifies Kidney yang. It warms cold hands and feet, relieves abdominal cold and pain, and stops diarrhea. Lastly, *Chuan Niu Xi* (Radix Cyathulae) and *Che Qian Zi* (Semen Plantaginis) promote urination and relieve edema.

MODIFICATIONS
- With weakness and fatigue due to qi deficiency, add *Huang Qi* (Radix Astragali) and *Ren Shen* (Radix et Rhizoma Ginseng).

- For impotence and other sexual disorders, add *Gui Ban* (Plastrum Testudinis) and *Lu Jiao Shuang* (Cornu Cervi Degelatinatum).
- With soreness and pain in the upper and lower back, add *Du Zhong* (Cortex Eucommiae) and *Gou Qi Zi* (Fructus Lycii).
- With abdominal fullness and swelling, add *Huang Qi* (Radix Astragali) and *Fang Ji* (Radix Stephaniae Tetrandrae).

CAUTIONS / CONTRAINDICATIONS
- *Ji Sheng Shen Qi Wan* is contraindicated in the following situations: yin-deficient fire, excess fire and damaged body fluids, and the presence of an exterior condition.[1]
- Use of this formula is sometimes associated with gastrointestinal irritation. In one study, 5 out of 30 patients who took this formula reported gastrointestinal side effects. In another study, 4 out of 80 patients had similar reactions. In both studies, the gastrointestinal side effects were mild and self-limiting, and resolved spontaneously with discontinuation of the herbs.[2]

PHARMACOLOGICAL EFFECTS
Hypoglycemic: Administration of *Ji Sheng Shen Qi Wan* to 24 patients with diabetes mellitus with various complications was associated with a marked decrease in plasma glucose levels for two hours.[3]

CLINICAL STUDIES AND RESEARCH
1. **Diabetic neuropathy**: Administration of *Ji Sheng Shen Qi Wan* in 44 patients with diabetic neuropathy was associated with marked symptomatic improvement, such as relief of pain, numbness, perspiration, and weakness in the lower back and legs. The treatment protocol was to administer the herbs in extract, at doses of 7.5g daily in three equally-divided doses, for 12 weeks or more.[4]
2. **Nephrotic syndrome**: One study reported 94% effectiveness using modified *Ji Sheng Shen Qi Wan* to treat

Ji Sheng Shen Qi Wan (Kidney Qi Pill from Formulas that Aid the Living)

Diagnosis	Signs and Symptoms	Treatment	Herbs
Kidney yang deficiency with water accumulation	• General decline in physiological and physical functions: Kidney yang deficiency with insufficiency of *ming men* (life gate) fire • Edema and urinary difficulties: Kidney yang deficiency unable to regulate water circulation and metabolism • Cold sensations in the lower body, and sensory numbness: Kidney yang deficiency unable to warm the body	• Warms and tonifies Kidney yang • Regulates water and relieves edema	• *Liu Wei Di Huang Wan* (Six-Ingredient Pill with Rehmannia) nourishes Liver and Kidney yin. • *Fu Zi* (Radix Aconiti Lateralis Praeparata) and *Rou Gui* (Cortex Cinnamomi) tonify Kidney yang and warm the lower body. • *Chuan Niu Xi* (Radix Cyathulae) and *Che Qian Zi* (Semen Plantaginis) promote urination and relieve edema.

676

Chinese Herbal Formulas and Applications

Jì Shēng Shèn Qì Wán
(Kidney Qi Pill from Formulas that Aid the Living)

68 patients with nephrotic syndrome. Modifications included the addition of *Sang Bai Pi* (Cortex Mori) and *Bai Mao Gen* (Rhizoma Imperatae) for severe edema; *Yi Yi Ren* (Semen Coicis) and *Sha Ren* (Fructus Amomi) for abdominal fullness with poor appetite; *Zhi Mu* (Rhizoma Anemarrhenae) and *Huang Bo* (Cortex Phellodendri Chinensis) for Kidney yin-deficient fire; and *Wu Wei Xiao Du Yin* (Five-Ingredient Decoction to Eliminate Toxins) for red eyes and face with the presence of sores. Of 68 patients, the study reported complete recovery in 19 patients, improvement in 45 patients, and no change in 4 patients.[5]

3. **Infertility**: *Ji Sheng Shen Qi Wan* was reported in one study of 34 men to have a marked effect in treating male infertility by increasing sperm count and motility. The treatment protocol was to administer 7.5g per day of this formula for 3 months.[6] In another study, use of *Ji Sheng Shen Qi Wan* was associated with increased sperm count in 16 of 24 men with infertility.[7]

4. **Prostatic hypertrophy**: Administration of *Ji Sheng Shen Qi Wan* was beneficial in treating 23 patients with enlarged prostate who suffered from frequent and difficult urination. The treatment protocol was to administer 7.5 grams of the formula in extract form daily for 8 weeks. The study reported 84% effectiveness in treating frequent and difficult urination.[8]

5. **Osteoporosis**: Administration of 7.5g of *Ji Sheng Shen Qi Wan* daily for 6 months to 2 years in 50 patients (19 males and 31 females, between 61 to 84 years of age) with osteoporosis was associated with marked symptomatic improvements, such as relief of lower back pain and better quality of life.[9]

AUTHORS' COMMENTS

Originally named "*Jia Wei Shen Qi Wan* (Augmented Kidney Qi Pill)" by Yan Yong-He in 1253, this formula today is commonly referred to as *Ji Sheng Shen Qi Wan* (Kidney Qi Pill from Formulas that Aid the Living). The reason for this change is to avoid confusion and errors, since there are at many formulas with similar names according to *Zhong Yi Fang Ji Da Ci Dian* (Grand Dictionary of Chinese Herbal Formulas).

Jin Gui Shen Qi Wan (Kidney Qi Pill from the <u>Golden Cabinet</u>) and *Ji Sheng* Shen Qi Wan (Kidney Qi Pill from <u>Formulas that Aid the Living</u>) have similar names, but are derived from different sources and have slightly different functions:
- *Jin Gui Shen Qi Wan* has a balanced and stronger effect to tonify both Kidney yin and yang.
- *Ji Sheng Shen Qi Wan* has a stronger effect to tonify Kidney yang and promote urination.

References

1. *Zhong Yao Ming Fang Yao Li Yu Ying Yong* (Pharmacology and Applications of Famous Herbal Formulas) 1989;329-331.
2. *Zhong Yi Fang Ji Xian Dai Yan Jiu* (Modern Study of Medical Formulae in Traditional Chinese Medicine) 1997;688.
3. *Zhong Yi Fang Ji Xian Dai Yan Jiu* (Modern Study of Medical Formulae in Traditional Chinese Medicine) 1997;686-687.
4. *Guo Wai Yi Xue* (Foreign Medicine) 1992;1:44.
5. *Shan Xi Zhong Yi* (Shanxi Chinese Medicine) 1997;4:149.
6. *Guo Wai Yi Xue Zhong Yi Zhong Yao Fen Ce* (Monograph of Chinese Herbology from Foreign Medicine) 1995;6:27.
7. *Guo Wai Yi Xue Zhong Yi Zhong Yao Fen Ce* (Monograph of Chinese Herbology from Foreign Medicine) 1989;5:26.
8. *Han Fang Yi Xue* (Kampo Medicine) 1983;5:14.
9. *Zhong Yi Ming Fang Lin Chuang Xin Yong* (Contemporary Clinical Applications of Classic Chinese Formulas) 2001;310-311.

TONIC FORMULAS

8

677

Yòu Guī Wán (Restore the Right [Kidney] Pill)

右歸丸
右归丸

Pinyin Name: *You Gui Wan*
Literal Name: Restore the Right [Kidney] Pill
Alternate Name: Eucommia and Rehmannia Formula
Original Source: *Jing Yue Quan Shu* (Collected Treatises of [Zhang] Jing Yue) by Zhang Jie-Bin (Zhang Jing-Yue) in 1624

COMPOSITION

Rou Gui (Cortex Cinnamomi)	60-120g [6-12g]
Fu Zi (Radix Aconiti Lateralis Praeparata), *zhi* (prepared)	60-180g [6-18g]
Shu Di Huang (Radix Rehmanniae Praeparata)	240g [24g]
Shan Zhu Yu (Fructus Corni), *chao* (dry-fried)	90g [9g]
Shan Yao (Rhizoma Dioscoreae), *chao* (dry-fried)	120g [12g]
Gou Qi Zi (Fructus Lycii), *chao* (dry-fried)	120g [12g]
Lu Jiao Jiao (Colla Cornus Cervi), *chao* (dry-fried)	120g [12g]
Tu Si Zi (Semen Cuscutae), *zhi* (prepared)	120g [12g]
Du Zhong (Cortex Eucommiae), *chao* (dry-fried) with ginger juice	120g [12g]
Dang Gui (Radix Angelicae Sinensis)	90g [9g]

DOSAGE / PREPARATION / ADMINISTRATION

Grind the ingredients into powder and mix it with honey to form small pills. Take 100 or more pills with boiled water. Today, it is prepared by mixing the powdered herbs with honey to form pills, with each pill weighing about 15g. Take 1 pill on an empty stomach in the morning and at night with water. This formula may also be prepared as a decoction using the doses suggested in brackets.

CHINESE THERAPEUTIC ACTIONS

1. Warms and tonifies Kidney yang
2. Replenishes *jing* (essence) and tonifies the blood

CLINICAL MANIFESTATIONS

Kidney yang deficiency with diminished *ming men* (life gate) fire: low energy and lethargy as a result of chronic illness, aversion to cold, cold extremities, impotence, premature ejaculation, seminal emissions, low sperm count, urinary incontinence, loose stools with undigested food, weakness of the lower back and knees, and edema of the legs.

CLINICAL APPLICATIONS

Infertility, impotence, seminal emissions, frequent urination, nephrotic syndrome, chronic nephritis, diabetes mellitus, bronchial asthma, sciatica, lumbago, and hypertrophic myelitis.

EXPLANATION

You Gui Wan (Restore the Right [Kidney] Pill) treats Kidney yang deficiency with diminished *ming men* (life gate) fire. As the source of yang, when *ming men* (life gate) fire diminishes, the entire body will be affected. When Kidney yang is deficient, it is unable to warm the body, resulting in aversion to cold and cold extremities. Kidney yang deficiency may lead to Spleen and Stomach yang deficiencies, resulting in low energy, lethargy and loose stools with undigested food. In males, Kidney yang deficiency often leads to sexual and reproductive disorders, such as impotence, premature ejaculation, seminal emissions, and low sperm count. Kidney yang deficiency can affect urinary function and cause urinary disorders, such as urinary incontinence. It can also impair the body's ability to regulate water metabolism, giving rise to edema of the lower legs and loose stools. Because the Kidney resides in the low back area, Kidney deficiency may cause weakness of the lower back and knees. Chronic illness may consume the yang qi of the body, causing low energy and lethargy.

Rou Gui (Cortex Cinnamomi) and *Fu Zi* (Radix Aconiti Lateralis Praeparata) warm Kidney yang and raise *ming men* (life gate) fire. According to the yin-yang theory of mutual dependence, in order to effectively tonify Kidney yang, Kidney yin must also be nourished. Thus, this formula uses *Shu Di Huang* (Radix Rehmanniae Praeparata), *Shan Zhu Yu* (Fructus Corni), *Shan Yao* (Rhizoma Dioscoreae), and *Gou Qi Zi* (Fructus Lycii) to nourish Kidney yin and replenish *jing* (essence). *Lu Jiao Jiao* (Colla Cornus Cervi), *Tu Si Zi* (Semen Cuscutae), and *Du Zhong* (Cortex Eucommiae) warm Kidney yang, replenish *jing*, and tonify the Liver and Kidney to strengthen the bones and tendons. *Dang Gui* (Radix Angelicae Sinensis) tonifies the blood and nourishes the Liver.

Chinese Herbal Formulas and Applications

Yòu Guī Wán (Restore the Right [Kidney] Pill)

You Gui Wan (Restore the Right [Kidney] Pill)

Diagnosis	Signs and Symptoms	Treatment	Herbs
Kidney yang deficiency with diminished *ming men* (life gate) fire	• Low energy, lethargy, aversion to cold, and cold extremities: diminished *ming men* fire • Weakness of the lower back and knees, impotence, premature ejaculation, seminal emissions, low sperm count: Kidney yang deficiency • Urinary incontinence and edema of the legs: Kidney yang deficiency unable to regulate water circulation and metabolism	• Warms and tonifies Kidney yang • Replenishes *jing* (essence) and tonifies the blood	• *Rou Gui* (Cortex Cinnamomi) and *Fu Zi* (Radix Aconiti Lateralis Praeparata) warm Kidney yang and raise *ming men* fire. • *Shu Di Huang* (Radix Rehmanniae Praeparata), *Shan Zhu Yu* (Fructus Corni), *Shan Yao* (Rhizoma Dioscoreae) and *Gou Qi Zi* (Fructus Lycii) nourish Kidney yin and replenish *jing*. • *Lu Jiao Jiao* (Colla Cornus Cervi), *Tu Si Zi* (Semen Cuscutae), and *Du Zhong* (Cortex Eucommiae) warm Kidney yang, replenish *jing*, and tonify the Liver and Kidney. • *Dang Gui* (Radix Angelicae Sinensis) tonifies the blood and nourishes the Liver.

MODIFICATIONS

• For severe indigestion, acid regurgitation, or decreased dietary intake, add *Gan Jiang* (Rhizoma Zingiberis).
• With abdominal pain, add *Wu Zhu Yu* (Fructus Evodiae).
• With soreness and pain of the lower back and knees, add *Hu Tao Ren* (Semen Juglandis).
• For impotence as a result of yang deficiency, add *Ba Ji Tian* (Radix Morindae Officinalis) and *Rou Cong Rong* (Herba Cistanches Deserticolae).
• With seminal emissions or clear vaginal discharge, add *Bu Gu Zhi* (Fructus Psoraleae).
• For chronic diarrhea, add *Bu Gu Zhi* (Fructus Psoraleae), *Wu Wei Zi* (Fructus Schisandrae Chinensis), and *Rou Dou Kou* (Semen Myristicae).

CAUTIONS / CONTRAINDICATIONS

• *You Gui Wan* is contraindicated in cases of Kidney deficiency and damp accumulation.
• Avoid cold and raw foods while taking this formula.[1]

PHARMACOLOGICAL EFFECTS

1. **Immunostimulant**: In one experiment, daily administration of the formula at 30 g/kg orally for 5 days was associated with increased phagocytic activity of the macrophages in mice.[2]
2. **Adaptogenic**: Use of *You Gui Wan* was associated with improved physical performance in various laboratory studies. In one study, oral administration of the formula at 20-30 g/kg for 5 days increased the duration of swimming in mice (P<0.01).[3]
3. **Cognitive**: One study reported improved cognition (improved memory and decreased repetition of errors) in mice that were administered *You Gui Wan* at 30 g/kg and 20 g/kg (dose based on dried herbs) for 5 days.[4]

4. **Antiplatelet**: In one study, oral administration of the formula at 20 g/kg for 5 days was associated with a mild antiplatelet effect.[5]
5. **Hepatoprotective**: In a laboratory experiment, oral administration of the formula at 20-30 g/kg for 5 days was effective in protecting against liver damage induced by injection of 0.1% carbon tetrachloride.[6]

CLINICAL STUDIES AND RESEARCH

1. **Male infertility**: One study reported successful treatment in all 11 male patients with a history of infertility (the female partners became pregnant) using modified *You Gui Wan* in decoction.[7]
2. **Frequent urination**: Frequent urination in elderly patients was successfully treated using *You Gui Wan* plus *Suo Quan Wan* (Shut the Sluice Pill). In addition to these two formulas, others herbs were added as deemed necessary: *Dang Shen* (Radix Codonopsis) and *Huang Qi* (Radix Astragali) for Spleen and Lung qi deficiencies; *Chuan Xiong* (Rhizoma Chuanxiong) and *Dan Shen* (Radix et Rhizoma Salviae Miltiorrhizae) for blood stagnation; *Gui Ban* (Plastrum Testudinis), *Niu Xi* (Radix Achyranthis Bidentatae), and *Zhi Mu* (Rhizoma Anemarrhenae) for yin deficiency. *Gui Lu Er Xian Jiao* (Tortoise Shell and Deer Antler Syrup) was given at the end to consolidate the treatment effect. The treatment protocol was to administer the herbs in decoction daily for 3 weeks per course of treatment. Of 64 patients, 17 had complete recovery, 21 showed significant improvement, 21 showed slight improvement, and 5 showed no change.[8]
3. **Nephrotic syndrome**: In one report, 6 patients with nephrotic syndrome who were unresponsive to drug treatment (steroids) were treated with herbs with satisfactory results. General progress included symptomatic improvement and a reduction of protein in the urine.[9]

8

TONIC FORMULAS

679

Yòu Guī Wán (Restore the Right [Kidney] Pill)

4. **Bronchial asthma**: In a clinical study, long-term administration of *You Gui Wan* was successful in preventing asthma. The treatment protocol was to take the formula daily for 2 months prior to the seasonal changes starting in August. For patients who followed the protocol for 3 years, the success rate was between 83-95.5%. Moreover, 50% of the patients who were dependant on corticosteroids for prevention and treatment of asthma were able to discontinue the drugs.[10]

5. **Sciatica**: Use of modified *You Gui Wan* in 48 patients with sciatica was associated with complete recovery in 32 cases, significant improvement in 12 cases, and no benefit in 4 cases.[11]

6. **Hypertrophic myelitis**: Use of modified *You Gui Wan* successfully treated hypertrophic myelitis. The treatment protocol was to administer the herbs for 10-15 days per course of treatment, with duration ranging from 10-42 days. Of 48 patients, the study reported complete recovery in 31 cases and improvement in 17 cases. Most patients had relief of pain after 2-3 days, and resolution of all symptoms after 10 days.[12]

HERB-DRUG INTERACTION

Corticosteroid-induced immune suppression: One study found *You Gui Wan* to be effective in reversing corticosteroid-induced immune suppression in rats. The mechanism was attributed to the "yang-tonifying" effect of the formula, as subjects who use steroids for a long period of time often have "yang deficiency" signs and symptoms, such as edema, swelling, and immune-suppression.[13]

TOXICOLOGY

In an acute toxicology study, no fatality was reported in mice following oral ingestion of a bolus dose of 50 g/kg and 25 g/kg of raw herbs in decoction. No abnormalities were observed in follow-up observation for up to 7 days.[14]

RELATED FORMULAS

Yòu Guī Yǐn (Restore the Right [Kidney] Decoction)

右歸飲
右归饮

Pinyin Name: You Gui Yin
Literal Name: Restore the Right [Kidney] Decoction
Original Source: *Jing Yue Quan Shu* (Collected Treatises of [Zhang] Jing Yue) by Zhang Jie-Bin (Zhang Jing-Yue) in 1624

Shu Di Huang (Radix Rehmanniae Praeparata)	6-60g [6-30g]
Shan Yao (Rhizoma Dioscoreae), *chao* (dry-fried)	6g
Shan Zhu Yu (Fructus Corni)	3g
Gou Qi Zi (Fructus Lycii)	6g
Zhi Gan Cao (Radix et Rhizoma Glycyrrhizae Praeparata cum Melle)	3-6g [6g]
Du Zhong (Cortex Eucommiae), *zhi* (prepared) with fresh ginger	6g
Rou Gui (Cortex Cinnamomi)	3-6g [6g]
Fu Zi (Radix Aconiti Lateralis Praeparata), *zhi* (prepared)	3-9g [9g]

Cook the ingredients in two large bowls of water until the liquid is reduced to 70%. Take the warm decoction between meals. Today, the decoction may be prepared using the doses suggested in brackets.

You Gui Yin (Restore the Right [Kidney] Decoction) warms Kidney yang and tonifies Kidney *jing* (essence). Clinically, patients may have low energy, lethargy, abdominal pain, lower back soreness, cold extremities, and a fine pulse.

Jiā Wèi Yòu Guī Wán
(Augmented Restore the Right [Kidney] Pill)

加味右歸丸
加味右归丸

Pinyin Name: Jia Wei You Gui Wan
Literal Name: Augmented Restore the Right [Kidney] Pill
Original Source: *Guang An Men Yi Yuan* (Guang An Men Hospital) in 1990

Shu Di Huang (Radix Rehmanniae Praeparata)
Shan Yao (Rhizoma Dioscoreae)
Shan Zhu Yu (Fructus Corni)
Suo Yang (Herba Cynomorii)
Jiu Cai Zi (Semen Allii Tuberosi)
Niu Xi (Radix Achyranthis Bidentatae)
Tu Si Zi (Semen Cuscutae)
Du Zhong (Cortex Eucommiae)
Dang Gui (Radix Angelicae Sinensis)
Rou Gui (Cortex Cinnamomi)
Fu Zi (Radix Aconiti Lateralis Praeparata)
Zhi Gan Cao (Radix et Rhizoma Glycyrrhizae Praeparata cum Melle)

Jia Wei You Gui Wan (Augmented Restore the Right [Kidney] Pill) is a slight variation of the original *You Gui Wan*. In comparison to the original formulation, *Jia Wei You Gui Wan* (Augmented Restore the Right [Kidney] Pill) is slightly stronger, since it contains additional herbs to tonify Kidney yang and replenish Kidney *jing* (essence). This formula may be used for patients with primary Kidney yang deficiency accompanied by secondary Kidney yin and *jing* deficiencies.

Chinese Herbal Formulas and Applications

Yòu Guī Wán (Restore the Right [Kidney] Pill)

AUTHORS' COMMENTS

You Gui Wan (Restore the Right [Kidney] Pill) differs from *Ba Wei Di Huang Wan* (Eight-Ingredient Pill with Rehmannia) in the same way that *Zuo Gui Wan* (Restore the Left [Kidney] Pill) differs from *Liu Wei Di Huang Wan* (Six-Ingredient Pill with Rehmannia).

- *You Gui Wan* and *Zuo Gui Wan* tonify the Kidney without sedation. They have a more potent and immediate tonifying effect, and are more suitable for treating acute and severe cases.
- *Ba Wei Di Huang Wan* and *Liu Wei Di Huang Wan* tonify and sedate the Kidney at the same time. They have a moderate tonifying effect, and are suitable for long-term use to treat chronic deficiencies.

You Gui Wan (Restore the <u>Right</u> [Kidney] Pill) and *Zuo Gui Wan* (Restore the <u>Left</u> [Kidney] Pill) have similar names and functions. These formulas may be used singularly, or in combination.

- *You Gui Wan* tonifies Kidney yang.
- *Zuo Gui Wan* tonifies Kidney yin.

References

1. *Zhong Yao Ming Fang Yao Li Yu Ying Yong* (Pharmacology and Applications of Famous Herbal Formulas) 1989;339-342.
2. *Zhong Yao Yao Li Yu Lin Chuang* (Pharmacology and Clinical Applications of Chinese Herbs) 1990;6(4):6.
3. *Zhong Yao Yao Li Yu Lin Chuang* (Pharmacology and Clinical Applications of Chinese Herbs) 1990;6(4):6.
4. *Zhong Yao Yao Li Yu Lin Chuang* (Pharmacology and Clinical Applications of Chinese Herbs) 1990;6(4):6.
5. *Zhong Yao Yao Li Yu Lin Chuang* (Pharmacology and Clinical Applications of Chinese Herbs) 1990;6(4):6.
6. *Zhong Yao Yao Li Yu Lin Chuang* (Pharmacology and Clinical Applications of Chinese Herbs) 1990;6(4):6.
7. *He Bei Zhong Yi* (Hebei Chinese Medicine) 1988;4:31.
8. *Xin Zhong Yi* (New Chinese Medicine) 1997;1:48.
9. *Shen De Yan Jiu* (Research of Kidney) 1981;93.
10. *Zhong Yi Za Zhi* (Journal of Chinese Medicine) 1981;(5):341.
11. *Si Chuan Zhong Yi* (Sichuan Chinese Medicine) 1985;11:51.
12. *Hu Nan Zhong Yi Za Zhi* (Hunan Journal of Chinese Medicine) 1985;3:27.
13. *Shan Xi Zhong Yi* (Shanxi Chinese Medicine) 1989;6:277.
14. *Zhong Yao Yao Li Yu Lin Chuang* (Pharmacology and Clinical Applications of Chinese Herbs) 1990;6(4):6.

Huán Shào Dān (Return to Youth Pill)

還少丹
还少丹

Pinyin Name: *Huan Shao Dan*
Literal Name: Return to Youth Pill
Alternate Names: *Huan Shao Tan*, Youth-Returning Formula, Lycium Formula
Original Source: *Yang Shi Mi Fang* (Secret Formulas of the Yang Family)

COMPOSITION

Rou Cong Rong (Herba Cistanches)	30g
Ba Ji Tian (Radix Morindae Officinalis)	30g
Xiao Hui Xiang (Fructus Foeniculi)	30g
Shu Di Huang (Radix Rehmanniae Praeparata)	15g
Shan Zhu Yu (Fructus Corni), *jin* (soaked) in liquor for 1 night and *bei* (stone-baked)	30g
Gou Qi Zi (Fructus Lycii)	15g
Du Zhong (Cortex Eucommiae), *zhi* (fried) with liquor and the juice of fresh ginger	30g
Niu Xi (Radix Achyranthis Bidentatae), *jin* (soaked) in liquor for 1 night and *bei* (stone-baked)	45g
Fu Ling (Poria)	30g
Shan Yao (Rhizoma Dioscoreae)	45g
Wu Wei Zi (Fructus Schisandrae Chinensis)	30g
Yuan Zhi (Radix Polygalae)	30g
Shi Chang Pu (Rhizoma Acori Tatarinowii)	30g
Da Zao (Fructus Jujubae)	15g
Chu Shi Zi (Fructus Broussonetiae)	30g

Chapter 8 – Tonic Formulas　　　　　　　　　　　*Section 5 – Yang-Tonifying Formulas*

Huán Shào Dān (Return to Youth Pill)

DOSAGE / PREPARATION / ADMINISTRATION

Grind the ingredients into powder and mix with honey to form pills. The pills should resemble the size of *Wu Tong Zi* (Semen Firmianae), a small seed approximately 5 mm in diameter. Take 30 pills per dose three times daily on an empty stomach with a warm, grain-based liquor and/or warm, salted water. The source text states that improvement will be noted between 5 to 30 days of continuous use. It also states that this formula is safe for long-term use.

CHINESE THERAPEUTIC ACTIONS

1. Strengthens the Spleen, Stomach, Kidney and Heart
2. Tonifies qi, blood and *jing* (essence)
3. Warms yang

CLINICAL MANIFESTATIONS

Premature aging as a result of Spleen and Kidney deficiencies with insufficiency of qi, blood, yang and *jing* (essence): decreased libido, seminal emissions, generalized weakness and fatigue, anorexia, low-grade fever, forgetfulness, easily frightened, night sweats, toothache, and gum swelling.

CLINICAL APPLICATIONS

Spermatorrhea, seminal emissions, decreased libido, impotence, and premature aging.

EXPLANATION

Huan Shao Dan (Return to Youth Pill) treats premature aging in both men and women. Premature aging is commonly caused by excessive consumption of qi, blood, yang and *jing* (essence) with underlying deficiencies of the Spleen, Stomach, Heart and Kidney. Spleen and Stomach deficiencies result in an inadequate supply of qi, which manifests in symptoms such as generalized weakness, fatigue, and anorexia. Deficiencies of blood and Heart may lead to forgetfulness, being easily frightened, low-grade fever, and night sweats. Lastly, lack of *jing* is often accompanied by Kidney yang deficiency, leading to decreased libido, seminal emissions, and other sexual disorders.

Rou Cong Rong (Herba Cistanches), *Ba Ji Tian* (Radix Morindae Officinalis), and *Xiao Hui Xiang* (Fructus Foeniculi) strengthen Spleen qi and Kidney yang. *Shu Di Huang* (Radix Rehmanniae Praeparata), *Shan Zhu Yu* (Fructus Corni) and *Gou Qi Zi* (Fructus Lycii) nourish the Kidney and benefit qi. *Du Zhong* (Cortex Eucommiae) and *Niu Xi* (Radix Achyranthis Bidentatae) tonify the Kidney and strengthen the knees and lower back. *Fu Ling* (Poria) and *Shan Yao* (Rhizoma Dioscoreae) strengthen the Spleen and dissolve dampness. *Wu Wei Zi* (Fructus Schisandrae Chinensis) reduces the loss of fluids from the Kidney, namely seminal emissions. *Yuan Zhi* (Radix

Huan Shao Dan (Return to Youth Pill)

Diagnosis	Signs and Symptoms	Treatment	Herbs
Premature aging	• Generalized weakness, fatigue, and anorexia: deficiencies of qi, Spleen and Stomach • Forgetfulness, being easily frightened, low-grade fever, and night sweats: deficiencies of blood and Heart • Decreased libido, seminal emissions, and other sexual disorders: deficiencies of *jing* (essence) and Kidney	• Strengthens the Spleen, Stomach, Heart and Kidney • Tonifies the qi, blood, and *jing* • Warms yang	• *Rou Cong Rong* (Herba Cistanches), *Ba Ji Tian* (Radix Morindae Officinalis) and *Xiao Hui Xiang* (Fructus Foeniculi) strengthen the Spleen and Kidney. • *Shu Di Huang* (Radix Rehmanniae Praeparata), *Shan Zhu Yu* (Fructus Corni) and *Gou Qi Zi* (Fructus Lycii) nourish the Kidney and benefit qi. • *Du Zhong* (Cortex Eucommiae) and *Niu Xi* (Radix Achyranthis Bidentatae) tonify the Kidney and strengthen the knees and lower back. • *Fu Ling* (Poria) and *Shan Yao* (Rhizoma Dioscoreae) strengthen the Spleen and dissolve dampness. • *Wu Wei Zi* (Fructus Schisandrae Chinensis) reduces the loss of fluids from the Kidney. • *Yuan Zhi* (Radix Polygalae) tonifies the Heart and calms the *shen* (spirit). • *Shi Chang Pu* (Rhizoma Acori Tatarinowii) opens the sensory orifices. • *Da Zao* (Fructus Jujubae) tonifies qi and blood. • *Chu Shi Zi* (Fructus Broussonetiae) warms and tonifies yang to strengthen the muscles and bones.

Huán Shào Dān (Return to Youth Pill)

Polygalae) tonifies the Heart and calms the *shen* (spirit). *Shi Chang Pu* (Rhizoma Acori Tatarinowii) opens the sensory orifices and improves mental functions. *Da Zao* (Fructus Jujubae) tonifies qi and blood, and strengthens the Lung and Spleen. *Chu Shi Zi* (Fructus Broussonetiae) warms and tonifies yang to strengthen the muscles and bones. Taking the formula with salted water allows the salt to function as a channel-guiding substance to the Kidney, to enhance the Kidney tonifying effect of this formula.

MODIFICATIONS

- If there is lack of appetite, add *Lian Zi* (Semen Nelumbinis) and *Qian Shi* (Semen Euryales).
- With low-grade fever and night sweats, add *Mai Dong* (Radix Ophiopogonis) and *Ren Shen* (Radix et Rhizoma Ginseng).
- For fatigue and weakness, add *Ren Shen* (Radix et Rhizoma Ginseng), *Huang Qi* (Radix Astragali), and *Dang Gui* (Radix Angelicae Sinensis).

CAUTIONS / CONTRAINDICATIONS

- According to one report, use of *Huan Shao Dan* continuously for one month was associated with occasional side effects such as a dry mouth, constipation, and a feeling of warmth in the body. These reactions are self-limiting, and will resolve within 2 to 3 weeks. [1]
- Use of this formula is contraindicated during pregnancy. [2]

RELATED FORMULAS

Huán Shào Dì Huáng Wán
(Rehmannia Pill to Return to Youth)

還少地黃丸
还少地黄丸

Pinyin Name: Huan Shao Di Huang Wan
Literal Name: Rehmannia Pill to Return to Youth
Original Source: *Tian Jin Zhong Yi Xue Yuan* (Tianjin University of Chinese Medicine) in 1989

Shan Yao (Rhizoma Dioscoreae)
Niu Xi (Radix Achyranthis Bidentatae)
Shan Zhu Yu (Fructus Corni)
Fu Ling (Poria)
Wu Wei Zi (Fructus Schisandrae Chinensis)
Suo Yang (Herba Cynomorii)
Shi Chang Pu (Rhizoma Acori Tatarinowii)
Ba Ji Tian (Radix Morindae Officinalis)
Yuan Zhi (Radix Polygalae)
Du Zhong (Cortex Eucommiae)
He Shou Wu (Radix Polygoni Multiflori)
Xiao Hui Xiang (Fructus Foeniculi)
Gou Qi Zi (Fructus Lycii)

Shu Di Huang (Radix Rehmanniae Praeparata)
Da Zao (Fructus Jujubae)
Rou Gui (Cortex Cinnamomi)
Fu Zi (Radix Aconiti Lateralis Praeparata)
Ren Shen (Radix et Rhizoma Ginseng)
Zhi Gan Cao (Radix et Rhizoma Glycyrrhizae Praeparata cum Melle)
Mu Dan Pi (Cortex Moutan)
Ze Xie (Rhizoma Alismatis)

Huan Shao Di Huang Wan (Rehmannia Pill to Return to Youth) follows the principles of two classic formulas: *Huan Shao Dan* and *Ba Wei Di Huang Wan* (Eight-Ingredient Pill with Rehmannia). The combination of these two formulas enhances their overall synergy for tonifying Kidney yang and treating sexual, reproductive, endocrine, and musculoskeletal disorders. Clinical applications include premature aging with diminished sexual and physical functions.

Bǔ Shèn Tāng (Tonify the Kidney Decoction)

補腎湯
补肾汤

Pinyin Name: Bu Shen Tang
Literal Name: Tonify the Kidney Decoction
Original Source: *Tian Jin Zhong Yi Xue Yuan* (Tianjin University of Chinese Medicine) in 1989

Yin Yang Huo (Herba Epimedii)
Shu Di Huang (Radix Rehmanniae Praeparata)
Shan Yao (Rhizoma Dioscoreae)
Shan Zhu Yu (Fructus Corni)
Gou Qi Zi (Fructus Lycii)
Xian Mao (Rhizoma Curculiginis)
Tu Si Zi (Semen Cuscutae)
Du Zhong (Cortex Eucommiae)
Dang Gui (Radix Angelicae Sinensis)
Rou Gui (Cortex Cinnamomi)
Fu Zi (Radix Aconiti Lateralis Praeparata)
Ba Ji Tian (Radix Morindae Officinalis)
Suo Yang (Herba Cynomorii)
Ren Shen (Radix et Rhizoma Ginseng)
She Chuang Zi (Fructus Cnidii)

Bu Shen Tang (Tonify the Kidney Decoction) primarily treats sexual and reproductive disorders in both men and women by fortifying Kidney yang and *jing* (essence), tonifying qi, and nourishing the blood. Clinically, it treats disorders such as decreased libido, infertility, impotence, premature ejaculation, seminal emissions, and low sperm count.

683

Chapter 8 – Tonic Formulas   *Section 5 – Yang-Tonifying Formulas*

Huán Shào Dān (Return to Youth Pill)

References
1. *Zhong Guo Zhong Xi Yi Jie He Za Zhi* (Chinese Journal of Integrative Chinese and Western Medicine) 1992;12(1):20.
2. *Zhong Yao Ming Fang Yao Li Yu Ying Yong* (Pharmacology and Applications of Famous Herbal Formulas) 1989;345-346.

Èr Xiān Tāng (Two-Immortal Decoction)
二仙湯
二仙汤

Pinyin Name: *Er Xian Tang*
Literal Name: Two-Immortal Decoction
Alternate Name: Curculigo and Epimedium Combination
Original Source: *Zhong Yi Fang Ji Lin Chuan Shou Ce* (Clinical Handbook of Chinese Herbal Formulae)

COMPOSITION

Xian Mao (Rhizoma Curculiginis)	9-15g
Yin Yang Huo (Herba Epimedii)	9-15g
Ba Ji Tian (Radix Morindae Officinalis)	9g
Huang Bo (Cortex Phellodendri Chinensis)	4.5-9g
Zhi Mu (Rhizoma Anemarrhenae)	4.5-9g
Dang Gui (Radix Angelicae Sinensis)	9g

DOSAGE / PREPARATION / ADMINISTRATION

Prepare this formula as a decoction and take it in two equally-divided doses.

CHINESE THERAPEUTIC ACTIONS

1. Warms Kidney yang
2. Tonifies Kidney *jing* (essence)
3. Drains deficiency fire from the Kidney

CLINICAL MANIFESTATIONS

Kidney yin and yang deficiencies with fire rising: menstrual disturbances, amenorrhea, hot flashes, mood swings, night sweats, nervousness, irritability, insomnia, fatigue, lassitude, palpitations, and urinary frequency.

CLINICAL APPLICATIONS

Infertility, menopause, amenorrhea, essential hypertension, chronic glomerulonephritis, nephritis, nephropathy, chronic pyelonephritis, polycystic kidneys, aplastic anemia, and urinary tract infection.

EXPLANATION

Er Xian Tang (Two-Immortal Decoction) treats chronic and complicated disorders characterized by underlying Kidney yin and yang deficiencies, accompanied by deficiency fire rising. Because of Kidney yin deficiency, female patients may show symptoms such as menstrual disturbances, amenorrhea, hot flashes, and night sweats. Because of Kidney yang deficiency, patients will experience fatigue, lassitude, and urinary frequency. As a result of the chronic nature of the illness, Kidney yin and yang become ever more deficient and deficiency fire begins to rise to disturb the Heart, producing symptoms such as nervousness, irritability, mood swings, and insomnia.

The treatment strategy is to warm Kidney yang, tonify Kidney *jing* (essence), and drain deficiency fire. However, the selection of herbs and their doses is absolutely critical because herbs that tonify yang may contribute to more heat and fire, and herbs that clear fire may damage yin further. *Xian Mao* (Rhizoma Curculiginis), *Yin Yang Huo* (Herba Epimedii), and *Ba Ji Tian* (Radix Morindae Officinalis) warm Kidney yang and tonify Kidney *jing*. *Yin Yang Huo* (Herba Epimedii) tonifies both Kidney yin and yang. *Huang Bo* (Cortex Phellodendri Chinensis) and *Zhi Mu* (Rhizoma Anemarrhenae) nourish Kidney yin and clear deficiency fire. *Dang Gui* (Radix Angelicae Sinensis) nourishes the blood and regulates the *chong* (thoroughfare) and *ren* (conception) channels to treat menstrual disturbances.

Èr Xiān Tāng (Two-Immortal Decoction)

Er Xian Tang (Two-Immortal Decoction)

Diagnosis	Signs and Symptoms	Treatment	Herbs
Kidney yin and yang deficiencies with fire rising	• Menstrual disturbances, amenorrhea, hot flashes, and night sweats: Kidney yin deficiency • Fatigue, lassitude, and urinary frequency: Kidney yang deficiency • Nervousness, irritability, mood swings, and insomnia: deficiency fire rising to disturb the Heart	• Warms Kidney yang • Tonifies Kidney *jing* (essence) • Drains deficiency fire from the Kidney	• *Xian Mao* (Rhizoma Curculiginis), *Yin Yang Huo* (Herba Epimedii) and *Ba Ji Tian* (Radix Morindae Officinalis) warm Kidney yang and tonify Kidney *jing*. • *Huang Bo* (Cortex Phellodendri Chinensis) and *Zhi Mu* (Rhizoma Anemarrhenae) nourish Kidney yin and clear deficiency fire. • *Dang Gui* (Radix Angelicae Sinensis) nourishes the blood.

MODIFICATIONS

• For hypertension during menopause, add *Du Zhong* (Cortex Eucommiae).
• With hot flashes, add *Yin Chai Hu* (Radix Stellariae) and *Hu Huang Lian* (Rhizoma Picrorhizae).
• If there is insomnia, add *Yuan Zhi* (Radix Polygalae) and *Suan Zao Ren* (Semen Ziziphi Spinosae).

PHARMACOLOGICAL EFFECTS

1. **Endocrine**: One study evaluated the effect of *Er Xian Tang* and its components on sex hormones in rats. The rats were divided into four groups: group one was the control, group two received *Er Xian Tang*, group three received Kidney and blood-tonifying herbs [*Xian Mao* (Rhizoma Curculiginis), *Yin Yang Huo* (Herba Epimedii), *Dang Gui* (Radix Angelicae Sinensis), and *Ba Ji Tian* (Radix Morindae Officinalis)] and group four received herbs that clear yin-deficient fire [*Huang Bo* (Cortex Phellodendri Chinensis) and *Zhi Mu* (Rhizoma Anemarrhenae)]. The treatment protocol was to administer 10 times the normal dose daily for 10 days, followed by 3 days of rest, and repeat again for a total of 6 months of treatment. At the end of the treatment period, the study reported that in comparison with the control group, rats that received herbs had a statistically significant increase in testosterone in male rats and estradiol in female rats, and a decrease in luteinizing-releasing hormone in both sexes.[1] (Note: Information on comparisons among the three herb groups was unavailable at the time of publication.)

2. **Antihypertensive**: Administration of *Er Xian Tang* was associated with a marked reduction in blood pressure in various laboratory studies. In one study, administration of the formula at 10 g/kg for 2 weeks was associated with a 9-15% reduction in blood pressure in rats. In another study, administration of the formula to anesthetized cats at 6 g/kg was associated with a 30% reduction in blood pressure 2 hours after the treatment. The researchers noted that *Huang Bo* (Cortex Phellodendri Chinensis) and *Yin Yang Huo* (Herba Epimedii) were the main ingredients responsible for the antihypertensive effects of the formula.[2]

3. **Antioxidant**: Administration of *Er Xian Tang* was associated with an anti-aging effect, an antioxidant effect, and reduction of free radicals.[3]

CLINICAL STUDIES AND RESEARCH

1. **Infertility**: Administration of modified *Er Xian Tang* was successful in treating women with infertility due to irregular menstruation. Of the 26 women, 9 were between 25-27 years of age, 12 between 28-30 years of age, and 5 above 30 years of age. The treatment period ranged from 37 days to 1 year, with an average of 4-7 months. The study reported a success rate of 69.23% (18 pregnancies in 26 patients).[4]

2. **Menopause**: Many studies indicate that *Er Xian Tang* effectively treats menopausal signs and symptoms. In one study of 64 patients between the ages of 45-58, use of *Er Xian Tang* was deemed very effective. The formula contained 10g each of *Yin Yang Huo* (Herba Epimedii), *Xian Mao* (Rhizoma Curculiginis), *Ba Ji Tian* (Radix Morindae Officinalis), *Huang Bo* (Cortex Phellodendri Chinensis), *Zhi Mu* (Rhizoma Anemarrhenae), *Dang Gui* (Radix Angelicae Sinensis), and others if necessary. The treatment protocol was to administer the herbs in decoction daily for one month per course of treatment. Out of 64 patients, the study reported marked improvement in 41 patients, moderate improvement in 22 patients, and no change in 1 patient. The overall rate of effectiveness was 98%.[5]

3. **Nephropathy**: In one study, 60 children with a history of nephropathy from 3 days to 3 years were treated successfully with herbs. The children were divided into two groups: group one received prednisone, and group two received the prednisone with herbs. The herbal formula contained 10g of dry-fried *Bai Zhu* (Rhizoma Atractylodis Macrocephalae), and 6g each of *Xian Mao* (Rhizoma Curculiginis), *Yin Yang Huo* (Herba Epimedii), *Bu Gu*

Chapter 8 – Tonic Formulas　　　　　　　　　　　　　*Section 5 – Yang-Tonifying Formulas*

Èr Xiān Tāng (Two-Immortal Decoction)

Zhi (Fructus Psoraleae), *Huang Qi* (Radix Astragali), *Rou Cong Rong* (Herba Cistanches), *Dan Shen* (Radix et Rhizoma Salviae Miltiorrhizae), and *Fang Feng* (Radix Saposhnikoviae). The herbs were given as decoction daily. After one year of treatment, the study reported that individuals in group two (drug and herb group) responded much better than group one (drug group), with alleviation of signs and symptoms. Upon follow-up 3-6 months after the discontinuation of treatment, group two had only 6.6% recurrence, while group one had 36.6% recurrence.[6]

4. **Aplastic anemia**: In one study of 84 patients, use of *Er Xian Tang* to warm and tonify the Spleen and Kidney was associated with good results in treating aplastic anemia. Of 84 patients, the total effective rate was 84.5%, and the remission rate was 47.6%. The mechanism of action was attributed to the nourishing effect of the formula and stimulation of hemopoiesis stem cell. The experiment showed that use of *Er Xian Tang* was associated with an increase in CFU-S and GM-CFU in the bone marrow.[7]

RELATED FORMULA

Èr Xiān Bǔ Shèn Tāng

(Two-Immortal Decoction to Tonify the Kidney)

二仙補腎湯
二仙补肾汤

Pinyin Name: Er Xian Bu Shen Tang

Literal Name: Two-Immortal Decoction to Tonify the Kidney

Original Source: *Tian Jin Zhong Yi Xue Yuan* (Tianjin University of Chinese Medicine) in 1989

Xian Mao (Rhizoma Curculiginis)

Yin Yang Huo (Herba Epimedii)

Dang Gui (Radix Angelicae Sinensis)

Che Qian Zi (Semen Plantaginis)

Chuan Xiong (Rhizoma Chuanxiong)

Fu Ling (Poria)

Fu Pen Zi (Fructus Rubi)

Gou Qi Zi (Fructus Lycii)

He Shou Wu (Radix Polygoni Multiflori)

Huang Qi (Radix Astragali)

Jiu Cai Zi (Semen Allii Tuberosi)

Shu Di Huang (Radix Rehmanniae Praeparata)

Tu Si Zi (Semen Cuscutae)

Wu Wei Zi (Fructus Schisandrae Chinensis)

Er Xian Bu Shen Tang (Two-Immortal Decoction to Tonify the Kidney) tonifies Kidney yin, yang and *jing* (essence). It treats male infertility by enhancing the sexual and reproductive functions.

AUTHORS' COMMENTS

Er Xian Tang, literally "Two-Immortal Decoction," is aptly named for two reasons. First, the two chief herbs, *Xian Mao* (Rhizoma Curculiginis) and *Yin Yang Huo* (Herba Epimedii), effectively tonify the Kidney to prolong life. Second, it is called *Er Xian Tang* because the two chief herbs both contain "*Xian*" in their names: *Xian Mao* (Rhizoma Curculiginis) and *Xian Ling Pi* (Herba Epimedii). Note: *Xian Ling Pi* (Herba Epimedii) is an alternate name for *Yin Yang Huo* (Herba Epimedii).

References

1. *Zhong Guo Yi Yao Xue Bao* (Chinese Journal of Medicine and Herbology) 1992;7(5):24.
2. *Yi Xue Xue Bao* (Report of Medicine) 1962;9(5):287.
3. *Zhong Guo Zhong Xi Yi Jie He Za Zhi* (Chinese Journal of Integrative Chinese and Western Medicine) 1995;15(1):672.
4. *Zhong Yi Fang Ji Xian Dai Yan Jiu* (Modern Study of Medical Formulae in Traditional Chinese Medicine) 1997;766.
5. *He Bei Zhong Yi* (Hebei Chinese Medicine) 1995;17(4):14.
6. *Zhe Jiang Zhong Yi Za Zhi* (Zhejiang Journal of Chinese Medicine) 1994;29(8):379.
7. Lin L, Wu S, Tang J. Clinical observation and experimental study of the treatment of aplastic anemia by warming and tonifying the spleen and kidney. Zhong Xi Yi Jie He Za Zhi 1990 May;10(5):259,272-4.

Section 6

阴阳两补剂
— Yin- and Yang-Tonifying Formulas

GuĪ Lù Èr XiĀn JiĀo (Tortoise Shell and Deer Antler Syrup)

龜鹿二仙膠
龟鹿二仙胶

Pinyin Name: *Gui Lu Er Xian Jiao*
Literal Name: Tortoise Shell and Deer Antler Syrup
Alternate Names: *Gui Lu Er Xian Gao* (Tortoise Shell and Deer Antler Paste)
Original Source: *Yi Bian* (Ordinary Medicine) by Wang San-Cai in 1587

COMPOSITION

Gui Ban (Plastrum Testudinis)	2,400g
Mi Lu Jiao (Cornu Elaphuri)	4,800g
Ren Shen (Radix et Rhizoma Ginseng)	450g
Gou Qi Zi (Fructus Lycii)	900g

DOSAGE / PREPARATION / ADMINISTRATION

The source text states to use fresh deer horn from Pere David's deer (*Elaphurus davidianus*), and not from elk or red deer (*Cervus elaphus*). Cut *Mi Lu Jiao* (Cornu Elaphuri) and crush *Gui Ban* (Plastrum Testudinis) into small pieces, and soak them in running water for 3 days. Simmer these two substances for 7 days to obtain a condensed extract. Separately simmer *Ren Shen* (Radix et Rhizoma Ginseng) and *Gou Qi Zi* (Fructus Lycii) to obtain a condensed extract. Mix these two batches of condensed extracts together, and simmer it over low intensity fire to make a condensed syrup. The preparation is finished when drops of the syrup crystallize. Take 4.5-9g of the syrup on an empty stomach every morning with a grain-based alcohol or lightly-salted water.

CHINESE THERAPEUTIC ACTIONS

1. Replenishes yin and tonifies *jing* (essence)
2. Benefits qi and strengthens Kidney yang

CLINICAL MANIFESTATIONS

Kidney yin and yang deficiencies accompanied by blood and *jing* (essence) deficiencies of the *du* (governing) and *ren* (conception) channels: weight loss, seminal emissions, impotence, dizziness, blurred vision, and soreness and weakness of the lower back and knees.

CLINICAL APPLICATIONS

Osteoporosis, hypothyroidism, hypotension, impotence, nocturnal emissions, and lumbago.

EXPLANATION

Gui Lu Er Xian Jiao (Tortoise Shell and Deer Antler Syrup) treats Kidney yin and yang deficiencies, as well as deficiencies of *jing* (essence) and blood of the *du* (governing) and *ren* (conception) channels. Because of its wide range of functions, this formula can treat a variety of disorders.

Mi Lu Jiao (Cornu Elaphuri) enters the *du* (governing) channel and tonifies yang. *Gui Ban* (Plastrum Testudinis) enters the *ren* (conception) channel and tonifies yin. Together, these two animal substances have a synergistic effect to strongly tonify yin and yang, and to promote the generation of blood, *jing* (essence), and marrow. In addition, *Ren Shen* (Radix et Rhizoma Ginseng) tonifies *yuan* (source) qi, and *Gou Qi Zi* (Fructus Lycii) nourishes yin. Overall, this is an excellent and comprehensive formula that tonifies yin, yang, qi, blood, *jing*, and marrow.

MODIFICATIONS

• For frequent infections as a result of generalized weakness and deficiency, add *Huang Qi Jian Zhong Tang* (Astragalus Decoction to Construct the Middle) or *Bu*

TONIC FORMULAS

687

Chapter 8 – Tonic Formulas   *Section 6 – Yin- and Yang-Tonifying Formulas*

Guī Lù Èr Xiān Jiāo (Tortoise Shell and Deer Antler Syrup)

Gui Lu Er Xian Jiao (Tortoise Shell and Deer Antler Syrup)

Diagnosis	Signs and Symptoms	Treatment	Herbs
Kidney yin and yang deficiencies accompanied by insufficiencies of qi, blood and *jing* (essence)	• Weight loss, dizziness and blurred vision: qi and blood deficiencies • Seminal emissions and impotence: Kidney *jing* deficiency • Soreness and weakness of the lower back and knees: Kidney yin and yang deficiencies	• Replenishes yin and tonifies *jing* • Benefits qi and strengthens Kidney yang	• *Gui Ban* (Plastrum Testudinis) and *Mi Lu Jiao* (Cornu Elaphuri) tonify Kidney yin, yang, *jing*, and marrow. • *Ren Shen* (Radix et Rhizoma Ginseng) tonifies *yuan* (source) *qi*. • *Gou Qi Zi* (Fructus Lycii) nourishes yin and blood.

Zhong Yi Qi Tang (Tonify the Middle and Augment the Qi Decoction).

• For delayed menstruation accompanied by dizziness and abdominal pain, add *Si Wu Tang* (Four-Substance Decoction) or *Ba Zhen Tang* (Eight-Treasure Decoction).

• For atrophic arthritis, add *Ba Wei Di Huang Wan* (Eight-Ingredient Pill with Rehmannia) or *You Gui Wan* (Restore the Right [Kidney] Pill).

• For sciatica, add *Du Huo Ji Sheng Tang* (Angelica Pubescens and Taxillus Decoction) or *You Gui Wan* (Restore the Right [Kidney] Pill).

• For delayed healing of wounds, sores and abscesses, add *Ren Shen Yang Ying Tang* (Ginseng Decoction to Nourish the Nutritive Qi) or *Shi Quan Da Bu Tang* (All-Inclusive Great Tonifying Decoction).

• For infertility caused by low sperm count or abnormal ovulation, add *Dong Chong Xia Cao* (Cordyceps) and *Rou Gui* (Cortex Cinnamomi).

• For impotence, add *Yin Yang Huo* (Herba Epimedii) and *Du Zhong* (Cortex Eucommiae).

• For seminal emissions, add *Jin Ying Zi* (Fructus Rosae Laevigatae).

• If there is dizziness, add *Gou Qi Zi* (Fructus Lycii), *Ju Hua* (Flos Chrysanthemi), and *Tian Ma* (Rhizoma Gastrodiae).

CAUTIONS / CONTRAINDICATIONS

• *Gui Lu Er Xian Jiao* should be used with caution in cases of Spleen and/or Stomach deficiencies.

• This formula is contraindicated in patients with interior heat or yang rising.

PHARMACOLOGICAL EFFECTS

It has been reported that modified *Gui Lu Er Xian Jiao* has numerous valuable therapeutic effects, including but not limited to adaptogenic, antihyperlipidemic, and immunologic.[1]

CLINICAL STUDIES AND RESEARCH

1. **Osteoporosis**: In one clinical study, 28 women were given *Gui Lu Er Xian Jiao* to determine the effects of these herbs

in treatment of osteoporosis. The women's age ranged from 36 to 67, with an average age of 48.8 years. Osteoporosis was diagnosed and confirmed using bone mass density (BMD). The treatment protocol was to administer 5 grams of powdered extract of the herbal formula twice daily for one year. BMD was measured before and at the end of the trial. After one year of herbal therapy, there was an average increase of 3.4% BMD among the 28 women. The researchers concluded the herbs to be effective in the treatment of osteoporosis.[2]

2. **Impotence**: In one clinical study, modified *Gui Lu Er Xian Jiao* was used to treat 826 patients with impotence. The age of the patients ranged from 17-55, and the duration of the condition ranged from 6 months to 8 years. Out of 826 patients, 608 were married and 218 were single. The formula included *Gui Ban Jiao* (Gelatinum Plastrum Testudinis) 20g, *Lu Jiao Jiao* (Colla Cornus Cervi) 20g, *Yin Yang Huo* (Herba Epimedii) 30g, *Du Zhong* (Cortex Eucommiae) 10g, *Gou Qi Zi* (Fructus Lycii) 10g, *Shou Wu Teng* (Caulis Polygoni Multiflori) 30g, and others. Modifications included the addition of *Rou Gui* (Cortex Cinnamomi) and *Fu Zi* (Radix Aconiti Lateralis Praeparata) for feeling of coldness in the testicles, lower back, and legs; *Sha Ren* (Fructus Amomi), *Shan Yao* (Rhizoma Dioscoreae), and *Bai Zhu* (Rhizoma Atractylodis Macrocephalae) for poor appetite; *Suan Zao Ren* (Semen Ziziphi Spinosae), *Mai Dong* (Radix Ophiopogonis), and *Fu Shen* (Poria Paradicis) for excessive dreams at night; *Sang Shen* (Fructus Mori) and *Fu Pen Zi* (Fructus Rubi) for clear and profuse urination; and a larger dose of *Du Zhong* (Cortex Eucommiae) for incomplete erection. The formula was given orally as a decoction, and externally as steam therapy (by directing the steam to the penis). In addition, patients also received twice daily 30-50 mL of herbal wine made of *Ren Shen* (Radix et Rhizoma Ginseng) 20g and *Lu Rong* (Cornu Cervi Pantotrichum) 5g. Out of 826 cases, the study reported marked effects in 723 cases, improvement in 82 cases, and no effect in 21 cases. The overall effectiveness rate was 97.48%. The

688

Guī Lù Ér Xiān Jiāo (Tortoise Shell and Deer Antler Syrup)

Chinese Herbal Formulas and Applications

duration of treatment was between 3-16 packs of raw herbs as decoction.[3]

3. **Hypotension**: One study reported good results using modified *Gui Lu Er Xian Jiao* to raise blood pressure. The herbal formula contained *Gui Lu Er Xian Jiao* plus *Dang Gui* (Radix Angelicae Sinensis), *Tu Si Zi* (Semen Cuscutae), *Shu Di Huang* (Radix Rehmanniae Praeparata) and others. The herbs were given in decoction daily, for 20 days per course of treatment, with 2 courses for most patients. Of 62 cases, the study reported complete recovery in 35 cases, moderate improvement in 19 cases, slight improvement in 6 cases, and no benefit in 2 cases.[4]

RELATED FORMULAS

Bǔ Shèn Wán (Tonify the Kidney Pill)

補腎丸
补肾丸

Pinyin Name: *Bu Shen Wan*
Literal Name: Tonify the Kidney Pill
Original Source: *Guang An Men Yi Yuan* (Guang An Men Hospital) in 1990

Tu Si Zi (Semen Cuscutae)
Suo Yang (Herba Cynomorii)
Gou Qi Zi (Fructus Lycii)
Ren Shen (Radix et Rhizoma Ginseng)
Shu Di Huang (Radix Rehmanniae Praeparata)
Shan Yao (Rhizoma Dioscoreae)
Shan Zhu Yu (Fructus Corni)
Ze Xie (Rhizoma Alismatis)
Fu Ling (Poria)
Mu Dan Pi (Cortex Moutan)
Rou Gui (Cortex Cinnamomi)
Fu Zi (Radix Aconiti Lateralis Praeparata)
Hai Zao (Sargassum)
Kun Bu (Thallus Eckloniae)

Bu Shen Wan (Tonify the Kidney Pill) treats hypothyroidism characterized by Kidney yin, yang, and *jing* (essence) deficiency. This formula tonifies Kidney yin, yang and *jing* (essence), and warms the *ming men* (life gate) fire. In addition, *Hai Zao* (Sargassum) and *Kun Bu* (Thallus Eckloniae) dispel phlegm and soften nodules.

These two herbs are rich in iodine and are essential for the production of thyroid hormone.

Bǔ Gǔ Wán (Tonify the Bone Pill)

補骨丸
补骨丸

Pinyin Name: *Bu Gu Wan*
Literal Name: Tonify the Bone Pill
Original Source: *Guang An Men Yi Yuan* (Guang An Men Hospital) in 1990

Shu Di Huang (Radix Rehmanniae Praeparata)
Shan Yao (Rhizoma Dioscoreae)
Ren Shen (Radix et Rhizoma Ginseng)
Gou Qi Zi (Fructus Lycii)
Dang Gui (Radix Angelicae Sinensis)
Shan Zhu Yu (Fructus Corni)
Gu Sui Bu (Rhizoma Drynariae)
Xu Duan (Radix Dipsaci)

Bu Gu Wan (Tonify the Bone Pill) tonifies qi and blood, nourishes yin, strengthens yang, and replenishes *jing* (essence). Clinically, this formula treats bone disorders such as osteoporosis, and speeds recovery from bone fractures, because it incorporates *Gu Sui Bu* (Rhizoma Drynariae) and *Xu Duan* (Radix Dipsaci), which act as channel-guiding herbs to direct the effect of the formula to the affected area.

AUTHORS' COMMENTS

Mi Lu Jiao (Cornu Elaphuri) and *Lu Jiao* (Cornu Cervi) are both deer horns, and have similar functions. While the source text specifically uses *Mi Lu Jiao* (Cornu Elaphuri), many other references and herbal products use *Lu Jiao* (Cornu Cervi) as a substitute.

References

1. *Fang Ji Xue* (Chinese Herbal Formulas) 1995;284-286.
2. Hsu H. Effectiveness of Gui Lu Er Xian Jiao (Tortoise Shell and Deer Antler Syrup) on treatment of osteoporosis. Clinic Medline of Taiwan.
3. *Fu Jian Zhong Yi Yao* (Fujian Chinese Medicine and Herbology) 1995;26(3):59.
4. *Guang Xi Zhong Yi Yao* (Guangxi Chinese Medicine and Herbology) 1996;4:33.

8

TONIC FORMULAS

689

Chapter 8 – Tonic Formulas   *Section 6 – Yin- and Yang-Tonifying Formulas*

Qī Bǎo Měi Rán Dān

(Seven-Treasure Special Pill for Beautiful Whiskers)

七寶美髯丹
七宝美髯丹

Pinyin Name: *Qi Bao Mei Ran Dan*
Literal Name: Seven-Treasure Special Pill for Beautiful Whiskers
Alternate Names: *Chi Pao Mei Jan Tan*, *Qi Bao Mei Ran Wan*, Seven-Treasury Beard-Blackening Formula,
Seven-Treasure Pill for Beautiful Whiskers, Seven Treasures Formula
Original Source: *Yi Fang Ji Jie* (Analytical Collection of Medical Formulas) by Wang Ang in 1682

COMPOSITION

He Shou Wu (Radix Polygoni Multiflori), *zheng* (steamed) with *Hei Dou* (Semen Sojae) and sun-dried	480g [18g]
Gou Qi Zi (Fructus Lycii), *jin* (soaked) in liquor	240g [9g]
Tu Si Zi (Semen Cuscutae), *jin* (soaked) and *zheng* (steamed) in liquor	240g [9g]
Niu Xi (Radix Achyranthis Bidentatae), *jin* (soaked) in liquor	240g [9g]
Dang Gui (Radix Angelicae Sinensis), *xi* (washed) with liquor	240g [9g]
Bu Gu Zhi (Fructus Psoraleae), *ban* (blended) and *chao* (dry-fried) with *Hei Zhi Ma* (Semen Sesami Nigrum)	120g [6g]
Fu Ling (Poria), *ban* (blended) with milk	240g [18g]

DOSAGE / PREPARATION / ADMINISTRATION

The source text advises to prepare each herb as specified above. *He Shou Wu* (Radix Polygoni Multiflori) should be steamed and sun-dried nine times. Add *Fu Ling* (Poria) and *Niu Xi* (Radix Achyranthis Bidentatae) to *He Shou Wu* (Radix Polygoni Multiflori) on the seventh to ninth repetition of steaming and drying. Grind all seven herbs into powder and form into pills with honey. Take 1 pill (10g) in the morning and at night with a grain-based liquor or lightly-salted water. Today, this formula may be prepared as a decoction with the doses suggested in brackets.

CHINESE THERAPEUTIC ACTIONS

1. Nourishes Kidney *jing* (essence)
2. Nourishes Liver blood

CLINICAL MANIFESTATIONS

Liver and Kidney deficiencies: premature gray hair, loose teeth, seminal emissions, nocturnal emissions, and soreness and weakness of the lower back and knees.

CLINICAL APPLICATIONS

Alopecia, premature gray hair, premature aging, male infertility, nocturnal emissions, impotence, low sperm count, decreased sperm motility, lumbago, frequent urination, aplastic anemia, osteoporosis, chronic infectious hepatitis, and menopause.

EXPLANATION

Qi Bao Mei Ran Dan (Seven-Treasure Special Pill for Beautiful Whiskers) commonly treats premature aging

Qi Bao Mei Ran Dan (Seven-Treasure Special Pill for Beautiful Whiskers)

Diagnosis	Signs and Symptoms	Treatment	Herbs
Liver blood and Kidney *jing* (essence) deficiencies	• Premature gray hair: Kidney *jing* and Liver blood deficiencies • Loose teeth: marrow deficiency secondary to Kidney deficiency • Seminal emissions and nocturnal emissions: leaking of *jing* caused by Kidney deficiency • Soreness and weakness of the lower back and knees: Kidney deficiency	• Nourishes Kidney *jing* • Nourishes Liver blood	• *He Shou Wu* (Radix Polygoni Multiflori) tonifies the Kidney and Liver and replenishes blood and *jing*. • *Gou Qi Zi* (Fructus Lycii), *Tu Si Zi* (Semen Cuscutae) and *Hei Zhi Ma* (Semen Sesami Nigrum) nourish the Liver and Kidney. • *Niu Xi* (Radix Achyranthis Bidentatae) tonifies the Kidney and Liver. • *Dang Gui* (Radix Angelicae Sinensis) tonifies the blood. • *Bu Gu Zhi* (Fructus Psoraleae) warms the yang. • *Fu Ling* (Poria) prevents the tonics herbs from creating stagnation.

690

Chinese Herbal Formulas and Applications

Qī Bǎo Měi Rán Dān
(Seven-Treasure Special Pill for Beautiful Whiskers)

that is due to Kidney *jing* (essence) and Liver blood deficiencies. The Liver stores blood, and Liver blood deficiency causes malnourishment of the hair, leading to premature graying of the hair and hair loss. The Kidney produces marrow, which nourishes the bones and teeth. Thus, if the Kidney is deficient, the marrow may also become deficient and loose teeth may occur. Kidney deficiency may also lead to instability and leaking of *jing*, which results in seminal emissions and nocturnal emissions. Soreness and weakness of the lower back and knees are common clinical manifestations of Kidney deficiency.

He Shou Wu (Radix Polygoni Multiflori) is used heavily in this formula to tonify Kidney *jing* (essence). *Gou Qi Zi* (Fructus Lycii), *Tu Si Zi* (Semen Cuscutae), and *Hei Zhi Ma* (Semen Sesami Nigrum) nourish the Liver and Kidney to replenish Kidney *jing*. *Niu Xi* (Radix Achyranthis Bidentatae) tonifies the Kidney and Liver and strengthens the tendons and bones to relieve soreness and weakness of the lower back and knees. *Dang Gui* (Radix Angelicae Sinensis) tonifies the blood. Since yin and yang are mutually interdependent, *Bu Gu Zhi* (Fructus Psoraleae) is used to warm the yang and balance yin and yang. By adding a yang-tonifying herb to this formula, the yin-tonifying herbs may become more active, thus promoting harmony between yin and yang inside the body. *Fu Ling* (Poria) is added to promote urination, help the Spleen absorb the tonic herbs, and counter the greasy, stagnating properties of the tonic herbs.

MODIFICATIONS
- For premature gray hair without shine, add *Huang Qi* (Radix Astragali) and *Shu Di Huang* (Radix Rehmanniae Praeparata).
- To guide the effects of the herbs to the scalp, add *Ge Gen* (Radix Puerariae Lobatae).
- With soreness of the lower back, combine with *Du Zhong* (Cortex Eucommiae) and *Sang Ji Sheng* (Herba Taxilli).
- With tidal fever and night sweats, add *Di Gu Pi* (Cortex Lycii), *Nu Zhen Zi* (Fructus Ligustri Lucidi), and *Fu Xiao Mai* (Fructus Tritici Levis).
- With poor appetite and indigestion, add *Shan Yao* (Rhizoma Dioscoreae), *Bai Zhu* (Rhizoma Atractylodis Macrocephalae), *Shan Zha* (Fructus Crataegi), and *Mai Ya* (Fructus Hordei Germinatus).
- For yin deficiency and yang excess, add *Zhi Mu* (Rhizoma Anemarrhenae), *Huang Bo* (Cortex Phellodendri Chinensis), *Mai Dong* (Radix Ophiopogonis), and *Wu Wei Zi* (Fructus Schisandrae Chinensis).

- For yin and blood deficiencies, add *Nu Zhen Zi* (Fructus Ligustri Lucidi), *Mo Han Lian* (Herba Ecliptae), and *Fu Pen Zi* (Fructus Rubi).

CAUTIONS / CONTRAINDICATIONS
- *Qi Bao Mei Ran Dan* contains many tonic herbs, and should be used with caution in cases of Spleen and Stomach deficiencies or damp and phlegm accumulation.
- The processed form of *He Shou Wu* (Radix Polygoni Multiflori) should be used to maximize the tonic effect, and to minimize its downward draining effect. If the fresh, unprocessed form is used, patients may suffer from frequent episodes of loose stools and diarrhea.

PHARMACOLOGICAL EFFECTS
Cardiovascular: In one laboratory experiment, oral administration *Qi Bao Mei Ran Dan* in rabbits at 6 g/kg was associated with an antiplatelet effect two hours after the oral ingestion.[1]

CLINICAL STUDIES AND RESEARCH
1. **Alopecia**: In one study, 24 patients with alopecia were treated with oral and topical applications of herbs with good results. All patients received *Qi Bao Mei Ran Dan* as the base formula, with modifications as needed. For individuals with mixed white and yellow hair that appear malnourished, *Huang Qi* (Radix Astragali) and *Shu Di Huang* (Radix Rehmanniae Praeparata) were added to *Qi Bao Mei Ran Dan* for oral ingestion. In addition, they were treated with an herbal solution topically made of *Ce Bai Ye* (Cacumen Platycladi) 500g, *Sang Shen* (Fructus Mori) 500g, and *Mu Gua* (Fructus Chaenomelis) 250g. For individuals with yellow hair that is short and thin, *Zhi Mu* (Rhizoma Anemarrhenae), *Huang Bo* (Cortex Phellodendri Chinensis), *Mai Dong* (Radix Ophiopogonis), and *Wu Wei Zi* (Fructus Schisandrae Chinensis) were added to *Qi Bao Mei Ran Dan* for oral ingestion. They were also instructed to wash their hair with an herbal solution made from *Sang Ye* (Folium Mori) 60g and *Ma Ye* (Folium Cannabis) 60g. Lastly, for white hair that falls out easily, *Nu Zhen Zi* (Fructus Ligustri Lucidi) and *Mo Han Lian* (Herba Ecliptae) were added for oral ingestion. In addition, they were instructed to wash their hair with an herbal solution made from *He Zi* (Fructus Chebulae) 2 pieces, *Hu Tao Ren* (Semen Juglandis) 2 pieces, and fresh *Ce Bai Ye* (Cacumen Platycladi) 30g.[2]
2. **Male infertility**: In one study, 36 male patients with infertility were treated with modified *Qi Bao Mei Ran Dan* with good results. The ages of the patients ranged from 23-41 years, with the duration of marriage between 1-10 years. The formula included *Chuan Niu Xi* (Radix

TONIC FORMULAS 8

691

Qī Bǎo Měi Rán Dān
(Seven-Treasure Special Pill for Beautiful Whiskers)

Cyathulae) 9g, *Dang Gui* (Radix Angelicae Sinensis) 9g, *Bu Gu Zhi* (Fructus Psoraleae) 6g, *Fu Ling* (Poria) 6g, *He Shou Wu* (Radix Polygoni Multiflori) 12g, *Tu Si Zi* (Semen Cuscutae) 12g, *Gou Qi Zi* (Fructus Lycii) 12g, *Shu Di Huang* (Radix Rehmanniae Praeparata) 12g, and *Rou Gui* (Cortex Cinnamomi) 3g. In addition, *Du Zhong* (Cortex Eucommiae) 12g and *Sang Ji Sheng* (Herba Taxilli) 6g were added for soreness of the lower back and knees; *Zhi Mu* (Rhizoma Anemarrhenae) 6g and *Huang Bo* (Cortex Phellodendri Chinensis) 12g were added for irritability with a dry mouth. After continuous treatment for 20-30 days, pregnancy was reported within one year in 22 of 36 cases.[3]

3. **Aplastic anemia**: Use of modified *Qi Bao Mei Ran Dan* was effective in treating aplastic anemia. Of 38 patients, 15 were treated with herbs only and 23 were treated with herbs and drugs. Herbal treatment was based on *Qi Bao Mei Ran Dan*, and modifications varied depending on the differential diagnosis. For yin deficiency (20 cases), *Xuan Shen* (Radix Scrophulariae) 15g, *Mai Dong* (Radix Ophiopogonis) 15g, *Sang Shen* (Fructus Mori) 15g, *Can Sha* (Faeces Bombycis) 10g, *Shan Zhu Yu* (Fructus Corni) 10g, charred *Wu Mei* (Fructus Mume) 10g, charred *Zhi Zi* (Fructus Gardeniae) 10g, charred *Du Zhong* (Cortex Eucommiae) 10g, and charred *Zong Lu* (Petiolus Trachycarpi) were added. For yang deficiency (10 cases), *Xian Mao* (Rhizoma Curculiginis) 15g, *Rou Cong Rong* (Herba Cistanches) 15g, *Ba Ji Tian* (Radix Morindae Officinalis) 10g, *Yin Yang Huo* (Herba Epimedii) 10g, *Fu Zi* (Radix Aconiti Lateralis Praeparata) 6g, and *Lu Rong* (Cornu Cervi Pantotrichum) 6g were added. For yin and yang deficiency (8 cases), *Xiao Hui Xiang* (Fructus Foeniculi) 10g, *Xu Duan* (Radix Dipsaci) 10g, *Huang Jing* (Rhizoma Polygonati) 15g, and *Shan Yao* (Rhizoma Dioscoreae) 15g were added. The herbs were given in decoction daily, for 30 days per course of treatment, for a total of 3 courses. The study reported marked improvement in 20 of 38 patients.[4]

4. **Osteoporosis**: One study reported 90.8% effectiveness in using modified *Qi Bao Mei Ran Dan* to treat osteoporosis. The treatment protocol used this formula plus *Huang Qi* (Radix Astragali) and *Bai Zhu* (Rhizoma Atractylodis Macrocephalae) as the base formula, with the addition of *Gu Sui Bu* (Rhizoma Drynariae) and *San Qi* (Radix et Rhizoma Notoginseng) for bone fractures, and *Bai Shao* (Radix Paeoniae Alba) and *Gan Cao* (Radix et Rhizoma Glycyrrhizae) for severe pain. Out of 76 cases, the study reported significant improvement in 12 cases, moderate improvement in 57 cases, and no benefit in 7 cases.[5]

5. **Chronic infectious hepatitis**: In one study, 22 patients with chronic infectious hepatitis confirmed by Western medicine were treated successfully using modified *Qi Bao Mei Ran Dan*. The treatment protocol used this formula as the base, and added *Sha Ren* (Fructus Amomi) and *Hou Po* (Cortex Magnoliae Officinalis) for abdominal distention; *Huang Qi* (Radix Astragali) and *Dang Shen* (Radix Codonopsis) for fatigue; *Yan Hu Suo* (Rhizoma Corydalis) and *Chuan Lian Zi* (Fructus Toosendan) for hypochondriac pain; and *Bie Jia* (Carapax Trionycis) and *Mu Li* (Concha Ostreae) for hepatomegaly. The herbs were given daily for 2-3 months. Of 22 patients, the study reported complete recovery in 14 cases, improvement in 3 cases, and no effect in 5 cases. Complete recovery was defined as resolution of all symptoms with normal liver functions. Improvement included resolution of all symptoms with near normal liver functions.[6]

RELATED FORMULA

Shǒu Wū Piàn (Polygonum Pill)

首烏片
首乌片

Pinyin Name: Shou Wu Pian
Literal Name: Polygonum Pill
Original Source: *Guang An Men Yi Yuan* (Guang An Men Hospital) in 1990

He Shou Wu (Radix Polygoni Multiflori)
Hei Zhi Ma (Semen Sesami Nigrum)
Shu Di Huang (Radix Rehmanniae Praeparata)
Sang Shen (Fructus Mori)
Nu Zhen Zi (Fructus Ligustri Lucidi)
Mo Han Lian (Herba Ecliptae)
Bai Shao (Radix Paeoniae Alba)
Huang Qi (Radix Astragali)
Dang Gui (Radix Angelicae Sinensis)
Chuan Xiong (Rhizoma Chuanxiong)
Ge Gen (Radix Puerariae Lobatae)
Gui Zhi (Ramulus Cinnamomi)
Gan Cao (Radix et Rhizoma Glycyrrhizae)
Da Zao (Fructus Jujubae)

Shou Wu Pian (Polygonum Pill) is specifically designed to treat hair disorders by incorporating herbs to nourish yin, tonify the blood, and replenish *jing* (essence). Clinical applications include hair disorders such as premature gray hair and alopecia. This formula is also indicated for male infertility with signs of low sperm mobility, morphology and motility. The yin tonic herbs in this formula tonify the Kidney and restore *jing* and blood.

This formula is a variation of *Qi Bao Mei Ran Dan*. In comparison to the original formula, *Shou Wu Pian* (Polygonum

Chinese Herbal Formulas and Applications

Qī Bǎo Měi Rán Dān

(Seven-Treasure Special Pill for Beautiful Whiskers)

Pill) contains more yang tonic herbs to enhance *ming men* (life gate) fire and restore reproductive functions to treat low libido, spermatorrhea, and erectile dysfunction.

AUTHORS' COMMENTS

According to Dr. Wen-Qi Tsai, *Qi Bao Mei Ran Dan* not only nourishes the hair, but can be used for male infertility involving low sperm count and slow motility.

Gui Lu Er Xian Jiao (Tortoise Shell and Deer Antler Syrup) and *Qi Bao Mei Ran Dan* both tonify Liver and Kidney deficiencies.

- *Gui Lu Er Xian Jiao* treats deficiencies of yin, yang, qi, and blood of the *ren* (conception) and *du* (governing) channels. *Lu Jiao* (Cornu Cervi) tonifies yang, and *Gui Ban* (Plastrum Testudinis) tonifies yin, *Ren Shen* (Radix et Rhizoma Ginseng) boosts qi, and *Gou Qi Zi* (Fructus Lycii) nourishes the blood. All four herbs tonify; and this formula does not have any sedating nor draining effect. Today, the primary indication of *Gui Lu Er Xian Jiao* is treatment of bone disorders (osteoporosis, bone fractures, etc.).

- *Qi Bao Mei Ran Dan* tonifies Liver and Kidney blood and *jing* (essence) with tonic herbs such as *He Shou Wu* (Radix Polygoni Multiflori), *Gou Qi Zi* (Fructus Lycii), *Niu Xi* (Radix Achyranthis Bidentatae), *Tu Si Zi* (Semen Cuscutae), and *Dang Gui* (Radix Angelicae Sinensis). *Fu Ling* (Poria), a mild draining herb, helps to balance the stagnating side effects of the tonic herbs. Today, the main applications of *Qi Bao Mei Ran Dan* is treatment of hair disorders (alopecia, premature grey and white hair, etc.).[7]

References

1. *Zhong Yao Yao Li Yu Lin Chuang* (Pharmacology and Clinical Applications of Chinese Herbs) 1988;4(4):8.
2. *Fu Jian Zhong Yi Yao* (Fujian Chinese Medicine and Herbology) 1983;5:19.
3. *Zhe Jiang Zhong Yi Za Zhi* (Zhejiang Journal of Chinese Medicine) 1995;9:400.
4. *Zhong Xi Yi Jie He Za Zhi* (Journal of Integrated Chinese and Western Medicine) 1990;1:49.
5. *Hu Nan Zhong Yi Za Zhi* (Hunan Journal of Chinese Medicine) 1999;2:26.
6. *Zhe Jiang Zhong Yi Za Zhi* (Zhejiang Journal of Chinese Medicine) 1993;4:150.
7. Wang MZ, et al. *Zhong Yi Xue Wen Da Ti Ku* (Questions and Answers on Traditional Chinese Medicine: Herbal Formulas).

Di Huáng Yǐn Zǐ (Rehmannia Decoction)

地黄飲子
地黄饮子

Pinyin Name: *Di Huang Yin Zi*
Literal Name: Rehmannia Decoction
Original Source: *Huang Di Su Wen Xuan Ming Lun Fang* (Formulas from the Discussion Illuminating the Yellow Emperor's Basic Questions) by Liu Yuan-Su in 1172

COMPOSITION

Shu Di Huang (Radix Rehmanniae Praeparata)	[12g]
Shan Zhu Yu (Fructus Corni)	[9g]
Rou Cong Rong (Herba Cistanches), *jin* (soaked) in liquor and *bei* (stone-baked)	[9g]
Ba Ji Tian (Radix Morindae Officinalis)	[9g]
Fu Zi (Radix Aconiti Lateralis Praeparata), *pao* (blast-fried)	[6g]
Rou Gui (Cortex Cinnamomi)	[6g]
Mai Dong (Radix Ophiopogonis)	[6g]
Shi Hu (Caulis Dendrobii)	[9g]
Wu Wei Zi (Fructus Schisandrae Chinensis)	[6g]
Shi Chang Pu (Rhizoma Acori Tatarinowii)	[6g]
Yuan Zhi (Radix Polygalae)	[6g]
Fu Ling (Poria)	[6g]

8

TONIC FORMULAS

693

Chapter 8 – Tonic Formulas   *Section 6 – Yin- and Yang-Tonifying Formulas*

Dì Huáng Yǐn Zǐ (Rehmannia Decoction)

DOSAGE / PREPARATION / ADMINISTRATION

Grind equal amounts of the ingredients into powder. Cook 9g of the powder with 5 slices of *Sheng Jiang* (Rhizoma Zingiberis Recens), 1 piece of *Da Zao* (Fructus Jujubae), and 5-7 leaves of *Bo He* (Herba Menthae) in 1.5 bowls of water until the liquid is reduced to 80%. Take the decoction any time during the day. Today, this formula may be prepared as a decoction using the doses suggested in brackets.

CHINESE THERAPEUTIC ACTIONS

1. Tonifies Kidney yin and yang
2. Resolves phlegm and opens the orifices

CLINICAL MANIFESTATIONS

Aphasia and leg paralysis: aphasia caused by a stiff tongue, a dry mouth without desire to drink, leg paralysis, a pale tongue with a white, slippery, moist tongue coating, and a deep, fine and weak pulse.

CLINICAL APPLICATIONS

Cerebrovascular diseases, post-stroke sequelae, dementia, diabetes mellitus, itching, and myelanalosis.

EXPLANATION

Di Huang Yin Zi (Rehmannia Decoction) treats various symptoms of Kidney deficiency and deficiency yang rising. Kidney yin deficiency can lead to weakness of the bones and tendons, eventually resulting in leg paralysis. Kidney yin deficiency may also lead to rising of Kidney

yang, which can carry internal dampness and phlegm to the head, causing tongue stiffness, aphasia, and a dry mouth without desire to drink. Patient will have no desire to drink because there is no actual lack of body fluids. The tongue and pulse both indicate deficiency and dampness inside the body.

Shu Di Huang (Radix Rehmanniae Praeparata) and *Shan Zhu Yu* (Fructus Corni) nourish Kidney yin. *Rou Cong Rong* (Herba Cistanches) and *Ba Ji Tian* (Radix Morindae Officinalis) tonify and stabilize Kidney yang. *Fu Zi* (Radix Aconiti Lateralis Praeparata) and *Rou Gui* (Cortex Cinnamomi) warm the Kidney to cause floating yang to descend. *Mai Dong* (Radix Ophiopogonis), *Shi Hu* (Caulis Dendrobii), and *Wu Wei Zi* (Fructus Schisandrae Chinensis) nourish yin and body fluids. *Shi Chang Pu* (Rhizoma Acori Tatarinowii), *Yuan Zhi* (Radix Polygalae), and *Fu Ling* (Poria) connect and harmonize the Heart and Kidney, as well as dispel dampness and open the head orifices. *Bo He* (Herba Menthae) clears the head and opens the orifices. *Sheng Jiang* (Rhizoma Zingiberis Recens) and *Da Zao* (Fructus Jujubae) harmonize the herbs and enhance their tonic actions.

MODIFICATIONS

- If there is a hot sensation in the joints caused by Kidney yin deficiency, remove *Rou Gui* (Cortex Cinnamomi) and *Fu Zi* (Radix Aconiti Lateralis Praeparata), and add *Sang Zhi* (Ramulus Mori), *Di Gu Pi* (Cortex Lycii), and *Bie Jia* (Carapax Trionycis).

Di Huang Yin Zi (Rehmannia Decoction)

Diagnosis	Signs and Symptoms	Treatment	Herbs
Aphasia and leg paralysis with Kidney deficiency and deficient yang rising	• Leg paralysis: Kidney yin deficiency unable to nourish the bones and tendons • Tongue stiffness and aphasia: damp and phlegm accumulation in the head • Pale tongue with a white, slippery, moist tongue coating, and a deep, fine and weak pulse: deficiency and dampness	• Tonifies Kidney yin and yang • Resolves phlegm and opens the orifices	• *Shu Di Huang* (Radix Rehmanniae Praeparata) and *Shan Zhu Yu* (Fructus Corni) nourish Kidney yin. • *Rou Cong Rong* (Herba Cistanches) and *Ba Ji Tian* (Radix Morindae Officinalis) tonify and stabilize Kidney yang. • *Fu Zi* (Radix Aconiti Lateralis Praeparata) and *Rou Gui* (Cortex Cinnamomi) warm the Kidney. • *Mai Dong* (Radix Ophiopogonis), *Shi Hu* (Caulis Dendrobii) and *Wu Wei Zi* (Fructus Schisandrae Chinensis) nourish yin and body fluids. • *Shi Chang Pu* (Rhizoma Acori Tatarinowii), *Yuan Zhi* (Radix Polygalae) and *Fu Ling* (Poria) connect and harmonize the Heart and Kidney, dispel dampness, and open the head orifices. • *Bo He* (Herba Menthae) clears the head and opens the orifices. • *Sheng Jiang* (Rhizoma Zingiberis Recens) and *Da Zao* (Fructus Jujubae) harmonize the herbs.

Chinese Herbal Formulas and Applications

Di Huáng Yǐn Zǐ (Rehmannia Decoction)

- For Kidney yang deficiency with coldness and pain in the back and knees, add *Yin Yang Huo* (Herba Epimedii) and *Xian Mao* (Rhizoma Curculiginis).
- With qi deficiency, add *Huang Qi* (Radix Astragali) and *Ren Shen* (Radix et Rhizoma Ginseng).
- If there is no aphasia or a stiff tongue, remove *Shi Chang Pu* (Rhizoma Acori Tatarinowii), *Yuan Zhi* (Radix Polygalae), and *Bo He* (Herba Menthae).

CAUTIONS / CONTRAINDICATIONS

Di Huang Yin Zi is not recommended for individuals with Liver yang rising, since the formula is warm and tonifying, and may worsen the Liver yang condition.

CLINICAL STUDIES AND RESEARCH

1. **Cerebrovascular diseases**: It has been shown in many studies that the use of *Di Huang Yin Zi* is an effective supportive treatment for patients with various types of cerebrovascular diseases. One study reported beneficial effect using this formula to treat 240 patients with cerebral embolism.[1] Another study reported good results using this formula to treat 67 patients with cerebrovascular accident.[2]

2. **Post-stroke sequelae**: Modified *Di Huang Yin Zi* was successful in treating 24 patients with various types of post-stroke sequelae.[3]

3. **Dementia**: Use of *Di Huang Yin Zi* in 50 patients with dementia was associated with significant improvement in 24 patients, moderate improvement in 21 patients, and no effect in 5 patients.[4]

4. **Diabetes mellitus**: One study reported 80% effectiveness using modified *Di Huang Yin Zi* to treat 20 patients with diabetes mellitus characterized by qi and yin deficiencies.[5]

5. **Itching**: Use of *Di Huang Yin Zi* was associated with 80.5% effectiveness in 180 patients to treat itching caused by Liver and Kidney deficiencies. Of 180 patients, the study reported complete recovery in 103 patients, significant improvement in 42 patients, and no benefit in 35 patients.[6]

6. **Myelanalosis**: According to several studies, use of modified *Di Huang Yin Zi* was associated with beneficial effects in patients with pain in the spinal cord caused by neurosyphilis. One formula that reported good success contained *Di Huang Yin Zi* plus *Lu Jiao Shuang* (Cornu Cervi Degelatinatum), *Gui Ban Jiao* (Gelatinum Plastrum Testudinis), *Gou Qi Zi* (Fructus Lycii), *Suo Yang* (Herba Cynomorii), *Tian Ma* (Rhizoma Gastrodiae), and others.[7]

References

1. *He Bei Zhong Yi* (Hebei Chinese Medicine) 1986;1:12.
2. *Zhe Jiang Zhong Yi Xue Yuan Xue Bao* (Journal of Zhejiang University of Chinese Medicine) 1995;4:8.
3. *Hei Long Jiang Zhong Yi Yao* (Heilongjiang Chinese Medicine and Herbology) 1995;2:14.
4. *Bei Jing Zhong Yi* (Beijing Chinese Medicine) 1998;1:13.
5. *Shang Hai Zhong Yi Za Zhi* (Shanghai Journal of Chinese Medicine) 1995;8:28.
6. *Zhong Yi Za Zhi* (Journal of Chinese Medicine) 1983;5:27.
7. *Zhong Yi Fang Ji Xian Dai Yan Jiu* (Modern Study of Medical Formulae in Traditional Chinese Medicine) 1997;1265.

TONIC FORMULAS

8

695

Chapter 8 – Tonic Formulas

Chapter 8 — Summary

— Tonic Formulas

SECTION 1: QI-TONIFYING FORMULAS

Name	Similarities	Differences
Si Jun Zi Tang (Four-Gentlemen Decoction)		Base formula to tonify qi and strengthen the middle *jiao*
Liu Jun Zi Tang (Six-Gentlemen Decoction)	Tonify qi, strengthen the Spleen and Stomach	Eliminates dampness and phlegm
Xiang Sha Liu Jun Zi Tang (Six-Gentlemen Decoction with Aucklandia and Amomum)		Eliminates dampness and phlegm, regulates qi circulation, relieves pain
Xiang Sha Yang Wei Tang (Nourish the Stomach Decoction with Aucklandia and Amomum)		Regulates qi and dries dampness to increase appetite
Shen Ling Bai Zhu San (Ginseng, Poria, and Atractylodes Macrocephala Powder)	Tonify qi, strengthen the Spleen and Stomach, stop diarrhea	Resolves dampness
Qi Pi Wan (Guide the Spleen Pill)		Promotes digestion
Bu Zhong Yi Qi Tang (Tonify the Middle and Augment the Qi Decoction)	Tonify and raise qi, strengthen the Spleen and Stomach	Lifts yang qi and prolapsed organs
Yi Qi Cong Ming Tang (Augment the Qi and Increase Acuity Decoction)		Lifts yang qi and benefits the eyes and ears
Sheng Mai San (Generate the Pulse Powder)		Nourishes yin and body fluids
Ren Shen Ge Jie San (Ginseng and Gecko Powder)	Tonify Lung qi	Tonifies Lung and Kidney
Bu Fei Tang (Tonify the Lung Decoction)		Strengthens *wei* (defensive) *qi*

Si Jun Zi Tang (Four-Gentlemen Decoction) is the most commonly used and the most effective formula to tonify qi and strengthen the Spleen and Stomach. It treats Spleen and Stomach qi deficiencies arising from various causes or with various complications, and is often used as the base formula for many related conditions.

- *Liu Jun Zi Tang* (Six-Gentlemen Decoction) has the basic actions of *Si Jun Zi Tang* (Four-Gentlemen Decoction) but is stronger in dispelling dampness and phlegm.
- *Xiang Sha Liu Jun Zi Tang* (Six-Gentlemen Decoction with Aucklandia and Amomum) has the basic actions of *Liu Jun Zi Tang* (Six-Gentlemen Decoction) but is stronger in regulating qi, dispelling cold, and relieving pain.
- *Xiang Sha Yang Wei Tang* (Nourish the Stomach Decoction with Aucklandia and Amomum) primarily increases appetite in individuals with middle *jiao* deficiency.

Shen Ling Bai Zhu San (Ginseng, Poria, and Atractylodes Macrocephala Powder) and *Qi Pi Wan* (Guide the Spleen Pill) both tonify qi, strengthen the Spleen and Stomach, and stop diarrhea.

- *Shen Ling Bai Zhu San* strongly resolves dampness in cases of Spleen and Stomach qi deficiencies causing impairment in the transportation and transformation functions.
- *Qi Pi Wan* promotes digestion in cases of Spleen and Stomach qi deficiencies, in which there is an inability to properly digest and absorb foods.

Bu Zhong Yi Qi Tang (Tonify the Middle and Augment the Qi Decoction) and *Yi Qi Cong Ming Tang* (Augment the Qi and Increase Acuity Decoction) strengthen the Spleen and Stomach, and tonify and raise yang qi.

- *Bu Zhong Yi Qi Tang* not only treats the usual symptoms of Spleen qi deficiency, it also lifts yang qi and treats prolapse of internal organs.

Chinese Herbal Formulas and Applications

Chapter 8 — Summary

- *Yi Qi Cong Ming Tang* tonifies qi and blood, raises yang qi, and nourishes the Kidney and Liver. It tonifies underlying deficiencies and treats compromised visual and auditory functions.

Sheng Mai San (Generate the Pulse Powder), **Ren Shen Ge Jie San** (Ginseng and Gecko Powder) and **Bu Fei Tang** (Tonify the Lung Decoction) tonify Lung qi and treat lung disorders.

- *Sheng Mai San* tonifies qi, generates body fluids, astringes yin, and stops perspiration. It treats excess heat or chronic cough damaging qi and yin.
- *Ren Shen Ge Jie San* tonifies qi, clears Lung heat, stops cough, and relieves wheezing. Lung qi deficiency is the cause of cough and the excess sputum is due to the impairment of the transformation function of the Spleen. This formula can also be used for cough and dyspnea caused by the Kidney not being able to grasp the qi downward.
- *Bu Fei Tang* tonifies Lung qi to treat wheezing and dyspnea caused by Lung qi deficiency. It also strengthens *wei* (defensive) *qi* to relieve chills, intolerance to cold, and spontaneous perspiration.

SECTION 2: BLOOD-TONIFYING FORMULAS

Name	Similarities	Differences
Si Wu Tang (Four-Substance Decoction)	Tonify the blood, regulate blood circulation	Base formula to tonify the blood
Tao Hong Si Wu Tang (Four-Substance Decoction with Safflower and Peach Pit)		Eliminates blood stasis
Wen Qing Yin (Warming and Clearing Decoction)		Cools the blood, clears heat, eliminates toxins
Guo Qi Yin (Delayed Menstruation Decoction)		Activates qi and blood circulation
Dang Gui Bu Xue Tang (Tangkuei Decoction to Tonify the Blood)		Tonifies qi and promotes the generation of blood
Gui Pi Tang (Restore the Spleen Decoction)	Tonify qi and blood	Strengthens the Spleen, nourishes the Heart
Zhi Gan Cao Tang (Honey-Fried Licorice Decoction)		Nourishes yin, restores the pulse
Nu Ke Bai Zi Ren Wan (Platycladus Seed Pill for Females)	Tonify the blood	Nourishes yin
Dang Gui Shao Yao San (Tangkuei and Peony Powder)		Softens the Liver, strengthens the Spleen to regulate water metabolism
Shao Yao Gan Cao Tang (Peony and Licorice Decoction)	Replenishes body fluids	Harmonizes the *ying* (nutritive) and *wei* (defensive) levels

Si Wu Tang (Four-Substance Decoction) is the basic formula for tonifying and regulating the blood. It treats general blood deficiency with impairment of the *chong* (thoroughfare) and *ren* (conception) channels.

Tao Hong Si Wu Tang (Four-Substance Decoction with Safflower and Peach Pit) is formulated by adding *Tao Ren* (Semen Persicae) and *Hong Hua* (Flos Carthami) to *Si Wu Tang* (Four-Substance Decoction). The addition of these two herbs greatly enhances the effect in regulating blood circulation and eliminating blood stasis.

Wen Qing Yin (Warming and Clearing Decoction) is formulated by adding four heat-clearing herbs to *Si Wu Tang* (Four-Substance Decoction) to clear heat and cool the blood. The addition of these four herbs enables the formula to treat gynecological disorders caused by blood deficiency and heat.

Guo Qi Yin (Delayed Menstruation Decoction) tonifies blood, activates qi and blood circulation, and regulates menstrual cycles. It is used to treat irregular, delayed or scanty menstruation caused by qi and blood stagnation.

TONIC FORMULAS

8

697

Chapter 8 – Tonic Formulas

Chapter 8 — Summary

Dang Gui Bu Xue Tang (Tangkuei Decoction to Tonify the Blood) tonifies qi and blood in cases of over-exertion, which leads to the body's inability to retain the yang qi. Symptoms include warm skin, a feverish sensation, a red face, irritability, thirst with a strong desire to drink, slow healing of wounds, a full but deficient pulse may occur.

Gui Pi Tang (Restore the Spleen Decoction) tonifies qi, nourishes the blood, strengthens the Spleen, and nourishes the Heart. It treats Heart and Spleen deficiencies which manifest in palpitations, forgetfulness, insomnia, and night sweats. This formula can also be used for any type of bleeding caused by the Spleen not being able to hold the blood within the vessels.

Zhi Gan Cao Tang (Honey-Fried Licorice Decoction) treats a bound or intermittent pulse caused by qi and blood deficiencies. It can also treat Lung deficiency caused by over-exertion.

Nu Ke Bai Zi Ren Wan (Platycladus Seed Pill for Females) tonifies blood and nourishes yin to treat irregular menstruation and amenorrhea due to blood and yin deficiency.

Dang Gui Shao Yao San (Tangkuei and Peony Powder) nourishes the blood, softens the Liver, strengthens the Spleen, and regulates water metabolism. It treats abdominal pain with edema caused by blood deficiency and abnormal water metabolism.

Shao Yao Gan Cao Tang (Peony and Licorice Decoction) harmonizes the *ying* (nutritive) and *wei* (defensive) levels and replenishes body fluids. It is most effective for spasms and cramps caused by excessive sweating or deficiency of blood and body fluids.

SECTION 3: QI- AND BLOOD-TONIFYING FORMULAS

Name	Similarities	Differences
Ba Zhen Tang (Eight-Treasure Decoction)		Base formula to tonify qi and blood
Shi Quan Da Bu Tang (All-Inclusive Great Tonifying Decoction)	Tonify qi and blood	Tonifies qi, warms yang, dispels cold
Ren Shen Yang Ying Tang (Ginseng Decoction to Nourish the Nutritive Qi)		Nourishes the Heart and calms the *shen* (spirit)
Tai Shan Pan Shi San (Powder that Gives the Stability of Mount Tai)	Tonify qi and blood, stabilize pregnancy	Strengthens the Spleen
Bao Chan Wu You Fang (Preserve Pregnancy and Care-Free Decoction)		Treats complications associated with pregnancy and labor
Dang Gui San (Tangkuei Powder)		Treats complications associated with pregnancy and labor
Xiong Gui Tiao Xue Yin (Cnidium and Tangkuei Decoction to Regulate Blood)	Tonify qi and blood	Treats postpartum complications

Ba Zhen Tang (Eight-Treasure Decoction), ***Shi Quan Da Bu Tang*** (All-Inclusive Great Tonifying Decoction) and ***Ren Shen Yang Ying Tang*** (Ginseng Decoction to Nourish the Nutritive Qi) tonify qi and blood.
- *Ba Zhen Tang* is formulated by combining *Si Jun Zi Tang* (Four-Gentlemen Decoction) and *Si Wu Tang* (Four-Substance Decoction) to tonify qi and blood. It is neutral in thermal property, and will not warm nor cool the body.
- *Shi Quan Da Bu Tang* is formulated by adding *Huang Qi* (Radix Astragali) and *Rou Gui* (Cortex Cinnamomi) to *Ba Zhen Tang* (Eight-Treasure Decoction). The addition of these two herbs increases the overall warmth of the formula, and enhances the effects of benefiting qi, tonifying

698

Chinese Herbal Formulas and Applications

Chapter 8 — Summary

yang, and dispelling cold. This formula is suitable for qi and blood deficiencies accompanied by the presence of interior cold.

- *Ren Shen Yang Ying Tang* treats qi and blood deficiencies arising from chronic consumptive diseases. Chronic qi and blood deficiencies may lead to malnourishment and instability of the Heart. Thus, this formula contains herbs to nourish the Heart and calm the *shen* (spirit).

Tai Shan Pan Shi San (Powder that Gives the Stability of Mount Tai), **Bao Chan Wu You Fang** (Preserve Pregnancy and Care-Free Decoction), and **Dang Gui San** (Tangkuei Powder) all tonify qi and blood to treat restless fetus, habitual miscarriage, and spontaneous abortion.

- *Tai Shan Pan Shi San* strongly tonifies qi and blood, strengthens the Spleen, and stabilizes pregnancy. It calms the restless fetus and prevents habitual miscarriage or spontaneous abortion by tonifying the underlying deficiencies.
- *Bao Chan Wu You Fang* tonifies qi and blood and stabilizes pregnancy. It can treat pregnancy-related complications, such as restless fetus, morning sickness, general weakness, soreness and pain of the lower back, and abdominal pain. If taken immediately before delivery, it also can facilitate labor and minimize complications.
- *Dang Gui San* prevents and treats complications associated with pregnancy and labor due to blood deficiency.

Xiong Gui Tiao Xue Yin (Cnidium and Tangkuei Decoction to Regulate Blood) tonifies qi and blood, and treats postpartum complications such as uterine bleeding, anemia, retention of lochia, irregular menstruation, and insufficient lactation.

SECTION 4: YIN-TONIFYING FORMULAS

Name	Similarities	Differences
Liu Wei Di Huang Wan (Six-Ingredient Pill with Rehmannia)		Base formula to tonify Liver and Kidney yin
Zhi Bai Di Huang Wan (Anemarrhena, Phellodendron, and Rehmannia Pill)		Clears deficiency fire
Qi Ju Di Huang Wan (Lycium Fruit, Chrysanthemum, and Rehmannia Pill)	Tonify Liver, Spleen, and Kidney yin	Brightens the eyes, treats eye disorders
Mai Wei Di Huang Wan (Ophiopogonis, Schisandra and Rehmannia Pill)		Astringes the Lung, redirects Lung qi downward
Du Qi Wan (Capital Qi Pill)		Invigorates Kidney qi, grasps qi downward
Zuo Gui Wan (Restore the Left [Kidney] Pill)	Tonifies Kidney yin	Replenishes bone marrow and Kidney *jing* (essence)
Da Bu Yin Wan (Great Tonify the Yin Pill)	Tonify Liver and Kidney yin, clear deficiency fire	Clears deficiency fire
Hu Qian Wan (Hidden Tiger Pill)		Strengthens the sinews and bones
Er Zhi Wan (Two-Ultimate Pill)	Tonify Liver and Kidney yin	Nourishes the blood
Yi Guan Jian (Linking Decoction)		Regulates the Liver qi
Shi Hu Ye Guang Wan (Dendrobium Pill for Night Vision)		Calms Liver wind, treats eye disorders
Zi Yin Di Huang Wan (Rehmannia Pill to Nourish Yin)	Tonify Liver and Kidney yin, improve sensory functions	Clears Liver fire, treats eye disorders
Zi Shen Ming Mu Tang (Nourish the Kidney to Brighten the Eyes Decoction)		Tonifies qi and blood, treats eye disorders
Zi Shen Tong Er Tang (Nourish the Kidney to Unblock the Ears Decoction)		Tonifies the blood, treats ear disorders

8

TONIC FORMULAS

699

Chapter 8 – Tonic Formulas

Chapter 8 — Summary

Liu Wei Di Huang Wan (Six-Ingredient Pill with Rehmannia) is the representative formula in the yin-tonics category. It tonifies Liver and Kidney yin, and strengthens the water element while controlling wood. Kidney yin deficiency and deficiency fire may manifest as soreness and weakness of the lower back and knees, night sweats, heat sensations in the palms and soles, dizziness, vertigo, tinnitus, deafness, nocturnal emissions, tidal fever, and thirst. The tongue is red with a scanty coating, and the pulse is fine and rapid. Related formulas and their differential functions are as follows:

- *Zhi Bai Di Huang Wan* (Anemarrhena, Phellodendron, and Rehmannia Pill) is formulated by adding *Zhi Mu* (Rhizoma Anemarrhenae) and *Huang Bo* (Cortex Phellodendri Chinensis) to *Liu Wei Di Huang Wan* (Six-Ingredient Pill with Rehmannia). This formula nourishes yin and clears deficiency fire.
- *Qi Ju Di Huang Wan* (Lycium Fruit, Chrysanthemum, and Rehmannia Pill) is formulated by adding *Gou Qi Zi* (Fructus Lycii) and *Ju Hua* (Flos Chrysanthemi) to *Liu Wei Di Huang Wan* (Six-Ingredient Pill with Rehmannia). It nourishes Kidney and Liver yin and benefits the eyes to brighten vision.
- *Mai Wei Di Huang Wan* (Ophiopogonis, Schisandra and Rehmannia Pill) is formulated with the addition of *Mai Dong* (Radix Ophiopogonis) and *Wu Wei Zi* (Fructus Schisandrae Chinensis) to *Liu Wei Di Huang Wan* (Six-Ingredient Pill with Rehmannia). It nourishes yin, astringes the Lung, redirects Lung qi downward, and arrest wheezing.
- *Du Qi Wan* (Capital Qi Pill) tonifies Kidney yin and invigorates Kidney qi. It grasps qi downward to relieve wheezing and shortness of breath that arise from Kidney deficiency.

Zuo Gui Wan (Restore the Left [Kidney] Pill) is a potent formula that tonifies Kidney yin, fills bone marrow, and replenishes *jing* (essence). It contains primarily tonic herbs that are not balanced by sedating herbs. This is a strong tonic formula, and it is heavier and more stagnant in nature than *Liu Wei Di Huang Wan* (Six-Ingredient Pill with Rehmannia).

Da Bu Yin Wan (Great Tonify the Yin Pill) and *Hu Qian Wan* (Hidden Tiger Pill from the Analytic Collection) both tonify Liver and Kidney yin and clear deficiency fire.

- *Da Bu Yin Wan* treats yin deficiency of Liver and Kidney with flaring up of deficiency fire. Clinical manifestations include steaming bones sensation, tidal fever, night sweats, seminal emissions, weakness of knees and legs, a red tongue with a scanty coating, a rapid and forceful pulse at the *chi* position.
- *Hu Qian Wan* nourishes yin, clears deficiency-fire and strengthens bones and tendons. Weakness of bones and tendons are due to the lack of nourishment from Kidney yin. The clinical applications include soreness of lower back and knees, weakness of bones and tendons, and *wei zheng* (atrophy syndrome).

Er Zhi Wan (Two-Ultimate Pill) and *Yi Guan Jian* (Linking Decoction) tonify Liver and Kidney yin, nourish the blood, and moisten dryness.

- *Er Zhi Wan* tonifies Kidney and Liver yin deficiency and nourishes the blood. The key manifestations for this formula include a bitter taste in the mouth, dizziness, blurred vision, and premature graying of hair.
- *Yi Guan Jian* tonifies Liver and Kidney yin, regulates Liver qi, nourishes the blood, and moistens dryness. Clinical manifestations include chest and hypochondriac pain, acid regurgitation, a sore throat, and a dry mouth. Occasionally there may also be hernia.

Shi Hu Ye Guang Wan (Dendrobium Pill for Night Vision), *Zi Yin Di Huang Wan* (Rehmannia Pill to Nourish Yin), *Zi Shen Ming Mu Tang* (Nourish the Kidney to Brighten the Eyes Decoction), and *Zi Shen Tong Er Tang* (Nourish the Kidney to Unblock the Ears Decoction) all tonify Liver and Kidney yin, improve sensory (visual and auditory) functions, and treat eye and ear disorders.

700

Chinese Herbal Formulas and Applications

Chapter 8 — Summary

- *Shi Hu Ye Guang Wan* soothes the Liver, calms Liver wind, and nourishes yin to treat eye disorders.
- *Zi Yin Di Huang Wan* tonifies Liver and Kidney yin and clears Liver fire to treat eye disorders.
- *Zi Shen Ming Mu Tang* tonifies Liver and Kidney yin and supplements qi and blood to treat eye disorders.
- *Zi Shen Tong Er Tang* tonifies Liver and Kidney yin to treat ear disorders.

SECTION 5: YANG-TONIFYING FORMULAS

Name	Similarities	Differences
Jin Gui Shen Qi Wan (Kidney Qi Pill from the Golden Cabinet)	Tonify Kidney yang, warm *ming men* (life gate) fire	Base formula to tonify Kidney yang
Ba Wei Di Huang Wan (Eight-Ingredient Pill with Rehmannia)		Slightly stronger function to tonify Kidney yang
Ji Sheng Shen Qi Wan (Kidney Qi Pill from Formulas that Aid the Living)		Regulates water and relieves edema
You Gui Wan (Restore the Right [Kidney] Pill)	Tonify Kidney yang and *jing* (essence)	Tonifies the blood
Huan Shao Dan (Return to Youth Pill)		Tonifies qi and blood, strengthens the Spleen, Stomach, Kidney, and Heart
Er Xian Tang (Two-Immortal Decoction)		Clears deficiency fire

Jin Gui Shen Qi Wan (Kidney Qi Pill from the Golden Cabinet) tonifies Kidney yang and warms *ming men* (life gate) fire. Clinical applications of this formula include low back pain, weak legs, a cold sensation in the lower body, pain and cramps in the lower abdomen, and dysuria or polyuria.

Ba Wei Di Huang Wan (Eight-Ingredient Pill with Rehmannia) is a modified formula that is slightly stronger than the original *Jin Gui Shen Qi Wan* (Kidney Qi Pill from the Golden Cabinet) in tonifying Kidney yang and warming *ming men* (life gate) fire

Ji Sheng Shen Qi Wan (Kidney Qi Pill from Formulas that Aid the Living) tonifies Kidney yang and regulates water circulation. It treats water accumulation caused by Kidney yang deficiency, with signs and symptoms such as severe pitting edema, a cold sensation in the lower body, and dysuria or excessive urination.

You Gui Wan (Restore the Right [Kidney] Pill) tonifies Kidney yang, nourishes *jing* (essence), and nourishes the blood. This formula is indicated for chronic illness resulting in Kidney yang and *ming men* (life gate) fire deficiencies. This formula does not contain the "three sedative herbs"; hence, the tonifying action is stronger than that of *Jin Gui Shen Qi Wan* (Kidney Qi Pill from the Golden Cabinet).

Huan Shao Dan (Return to Youth Pill) is a comprehensive formula that tonifies qi, blood, Kidney yang and *jing* (essence). In addition, it strengthens the Spleen, Stomach, Kidney, and Heart. This formula is most effective for premature aging caused by generalized weakness and deficiencies.

Er Xian Tang (Two-Immortal Decoction) tonifies Kidney yang, replenishes Kidney *jing* (essence), and drains deficiency fire. This formula treats Kidney deficiency with deficiency fire rising, as seen in menopausal patients with hot flashes, mood swings, night sweats, nervousness, irritability, insomnia, and fatigue.

Chapter 8 – Tonic Formulas

Chapter 8 — Summary

SECTION 6: YIN- AND YANG-TONIFYING FORMULAS

Name	Similarities	Differences
Gui Lu Er Xian Jiao (Tortoise Shell and Deer Antler Syrup)	Tonify Kidney yin and yang	Tonifies qi and blood, replenishes *jing* (essence)
Qi Bao Mei Ran Dan (Seven-Treasure Special Pill for Beautiful Whiskers)		Tonifies Liver blood, replenishes *jing* (essence)
Di Huang Yin Zi (Rehmannia Decoction)		Dissolves phlegm, opens the orifices

Gui Lu Er Xian Jiao (Tortoise Shell and Deer Antler Syrup) tonifies qi and blood, supplements Kidney yin and yang, and replenishes *jing* (essence). Clinical applications of this formula include weight loss, seminal emissions, impotence, dizziness, and soreness and weakness of the lower back and knees.

Qi Bao Mei Ran Dan (Seven-Treasure Special Pill for Beautiful Whiskers) nourishes both Kidney *jing* (essence) and Liver blood to treat premature gray hair, loose teeth, seminal emissions, and soreness of the lower back and knees.

Di Huang Yin Zi (Rehmannia Decoction) tonifies Kidney yin and yang, dissolves phlegm, and opens the orifices. Clinical manifestations include aphasia caused by a stiff tongue, leg paralysis, a dry mouth without desire to drink, a pale tongue with a slippery, white and moist tongue coating, and a deep, fine and weak pulse.

702

Chapter 9

— Shen-Calming Formulas

安神剂

扁鹊 Biăn Què

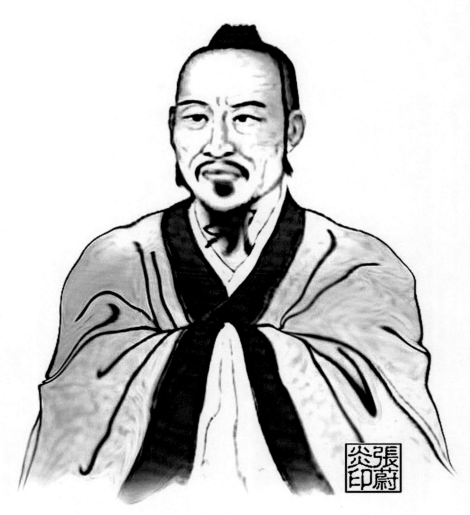

扁鹊 Biăn Què, also known as 秦越人 Qìn Yuè-Rēn, 407 – 310 BCE.[1]

扁鹊 Biǎn Què

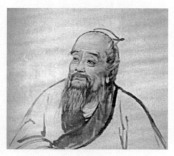

Bian Que.

So far as can be determined from recorded history, Bian Que is the founder of traditional Chinese medicine. The first physician spoken of in Chinese historical texts, Bian Que lived in the fifth century BCE. Bian Que understood all aspects of medicine, including herbs, acupuncture, internal and external medicine, gynecology, pediatrics, geriatrics, and disorders of the five senses. He was particularly skilled in the four diagnostic skills, including *wang* (inspection), *wen* (listening), *wen* (inquiry) and *qie* (palpation).

Bian Que authored two major texts during his life: 扁鹊内经 *Bian Que Nei Jing* (Internal Medicine according to Bian Que) and 扁鹊外经 *Bian Que Wai Jing* (External Medicine according to Bian Que). Physicians during the Han dynasty claimed to have studied the works of Bian Que. Unfortunately, both texts have been lost to history, and we are left with folklore and legends of his life and accomplishments.

There is one story that offers particular insight into the medical philosophy of Bian Que. King of Wei asked Bian Que one day, "You and your two brothers are all experts in medicine, which of you is the best?" Bian Que replied, "My eldest brother is the best, followed by my second brother, and I am the last." The king then asked, "Then why is it that you are the most famous?" Bian Que answered, "My eldest brother cures a disease before it shows any symptoms. Since people do not see the disease, they do not recognize his ability. My second brother terminates a disease in its early stages. People assume he is only capable of treating minor illnesses, so he is merely known within this locality and its neighborhood. As for me, I treat a disease when it is already very severe and serious. When I perform blood-letting by injecting needles into vessels, or apply medical ointment on the skin, people think I am well versed in medicine. Therefore, I have become well known all over the country." The king was quite satisfied with his answer and said, "You've spoken wisely."

Dynasties & Kingdoms	Year
Xia Dynasty 夏	2100-1600 BCE
Shang Dynasty 商	1600-1100 BCE
Zhou Dynasty 周	**1100-221 BCE**
Qin Dynasty 秦	221-207 BCE
Han Dynasty 漢	206 BCE-220
Three Kingdoms 三國	220-280
Western Jin Dynasty 西晉	265-316
Eastern Jin Dynasty 東晉	317-420
Northern and Southern Dynasties 北南朝	420-581
Sui Dynasty 隋	581-618
Tang Dynasty 唐	618-907
Five Dynasties 五代	907-960
Song Dynasty 宋	960-1279
Liao Dynasty 遼	916-1125
Jin Dynasty 金	1115-1234
Yuan Dynasty 元	1271-1368
Ming Dynasty 明	1368-1644
Qing Dynasty 清	1644-1911
Republic of China 中華民國	1912-Present Day
People's Republic of China 中華人民共和國	1949-Present Day

1. Approximate years of birth and death.

Table of Contents

Chapter 9. *Shen*-Calming Formulas · **703**
Biography of Bian Que · 704

Section 1. Sedative Formulas that Calm the *Shen* (Spirit) · **710**
Zhu Sha An Shen Wan (Cinnabar Pill to Tranquilize the Spirit) · 710
   Sheng Tie Luo Yin (Iron Filings Decoction) · 711
Zhen Zhu Mu Wan (Mother of Pearl Pill) · 712
Ci Zhu Wan (Magnetite and Cinnabar Pill) · 714
Chai Hu Jia Long Gu Mu Li Tang (Bupleurum plus Dragon Bone and Oyster Shell Decoction) · · · · · · · · · 715
   Chai Hu An Shen Tang (Bupleurum Decoction to Tranquilize the Spirit) · 720

Section 2. Nourishing Formulas that Calm the *Shen* (Spirit) · **722**
Suan Zao Ren Tang (Sour Jujube Decoction) · 722
   Ding Zhi Wan (Settle the Emotions Pill) · 723
Tian Wang Bu Xin Dan (Emperor of Heaven's Special Pill to Tonify the Heart) · 725
   Tian Wang Bu Xin Dan (Emperor of Heaven's Special Pill to Tonify the Heart) · 728
   Tian Wang Bu Xin Dan (Emperor of Heaven's Special Pill to Tonify the Heart) · 728
   Bai Zi Yang Xin Wan (Biota Seed Pill to Nourish the Heart) · 729
   Yang Xin Dan (Nourish the Heart Pill) · 729
   Zhen Zhong Dan (Pillow Special Pill) · 729
Gan Mai Da Zao Tang (Licorice, Wheat, and Jujube Decoction) · 731
   An Shen Tang (Tranquilize the Spirit Decoction) · 733
Yang Xin Tang (Nourish the Heart Decoction) · 735

***Shen*-Calming Formulas (Summary)** · **737**

Chinese Herbal Formulas and Applications

Chapter 9 — Overview

— Shen-Calming Formulas

Definition: *Shen*-calming formulas act to calm the *shen* (spirit) and tranquilize the mind. As such, they treat *shen* disturbance, a disorder characterized by palpitations, insomnia, irritability, restlessness, fear, fright, and other symptoms. *Shen* disturbance is associated with three *zang* (solid organs): the Heart, which stores the *shen*, the Liver, which stores the *hun* (ethereal soul), and the Kidney, which stores *zhi* (will-power). Therefore, imbalances of these organs contribute to *shen* disturbance.

W hile there are many causes of *shen* disturbance, the individual disturbances can nevertheless be categorized as either excess or deficient in nature.

In most cases, treating *shen* disturbance involves treating both cause and symptoms concurrently.

• **Excess**-type *shen* disturbance may be caused externally by fear and fright, and internally by Liver qi stagnation turning into fire. In either cases, these pathogens disturb the *shen*, leading to signs and symptoms such as irritability, fidgeting, restlessness, and abnormal levels of fear, fright, and anger. Because of the excess nature of the *shen* disturbance in these conditions, treatment usually involves herbs that clear heat and sedate the *shen*.

• **Deficient**-type *shen* disturbance may be caused by over-thinking and over-worrying, leading to Heart and Liver blood deficiencies, Heart yin deficiency, malnourishment of the *shen*, and rising of deficiency fire in the interior. Clinical signs and symptoms include palpitations, forgetfulness, deficiency-type irritability and restlessness, insomnia, and abnormal levels of fear. Because of the deficient nature of the *shen* disturbance, the treatment methods should be to nourish the Heart and calm the *shen*.

Although *shen* (spirit) disturbance is categorized as being either excess or deficient in nature, both may occur separately or together, and with or without complications. If both excess and deficiency symptoms are observed clinically, then both sedating and nourishing methods may be employed simultaneously. If complications are noted, select additional herbs accordingly. In most cases, treating *shen* disturbance will involve treating both the symptoms and the cause concurrently.

Shen (spirit) disturbance may also be complicated by internal heat, phlegm accumulation, and blood stasis. These conditions are discussed in Chapter 5: Heat-Clearing Formulas, Chapter 18: Phlegm-Dispelling Formulas, and Chapter 13: Blood-Regulating Formulas, respectively.

Shen-calming formulas are sedating and tranquilizing, to treat a wide variety of emotional, behavioral, and psychological disorders.

SUBCATEGORIES OF ACTION

Shen-calming formulas fall into two subcategories: **sedative** formulas to treat excess-type *shen* disturbance, and **nourishing** formulas that treat deficient-type *shen* disturbance.

1. **Sedative Formulas that Calm the *Shen* (Spirit)**

These formulas treat *shen* (spirit) disorders caused by hyperactivity of Heart yang and flaring upward of Heart fire. Common clinical manifestations include fidgeting, irritability, restlessness, insomnia, palpitations, epilepsy, and abnormal levels of fear, fright and anger.

Among the substances used to treat excess-type *shen* disturbance: *Ci Shi* (Magnetitum), *Long Chi* (Dens Draconis), and *Zhen Zhu Mu* (Concha Margaritiferae) sedate and calm the *shen*;

707

Chapter 9 – Shen-Calming Formulas

Chapter 9 — Overview

Di Huang (Radix Rehmanniae), *Shu Di Huang* (Radix Rehmanniae Praeparata), and *Dang Gui* (Radix Angelicae Sinensis) nourish yin and blood that may have been consumed by excess yang; and *Huang Lian* (Rhizoma Coptidis) may be added to clear excess heat and fire.

Exemplar formulas that sedate and calm the *shen* are *Zhu Sha An Shen Wan* (Cinnabar Pill to Tranquilize the Spirit), *Zhen Zhu Mu Wan* (Mother of Pearl Pill) and *Ci Zhu Wan* (Magnetite and Cinnabar Pill).

2. Nourishing Formulas that Calm the *Shen* (Spirit)

These formulas treat *shen* disturbance with deficiency fire rising upward, caused by yin and blood deficiencies. Common clinical manifestations include deficiency-type irritability and restlessness, insomnia, dream-disturbed sleep, palpitations, abnormal levels of fear, night sweats, forgetfulness, nocturnal emissions, a red tongue, and a scanty tongue coating.

> *Shen* disturbance may be complicated by interior heat, phlegm accumulation, and blood stasis.

Treatment simultaneously calms the *shen* and nourishes yin and blood. Herbs that calm the *shen* include *Suan Zao Ren* (Semen Ziziphi Spinosae), *Bai Zi Ren* (Semen Platycladi), *Wu Wei Zi* (Fructus Schisandrae Chinensis), and *Xiao Mai* (Fructus Tritici). Herbs that nourish yin and blood include *Di Huang* (Radix Rehmanniae), *Zhi Mu* (Rhizoma Anemarrhenae), *Mai Dong* (Radix Ophiopogonis), and *Dang Gui* (Radix Angelicae Sinensis).

Representative formulas include *Suan Zao Ren Tang* (Sour Jujube Decoction), *Tian Wang Bu Xin Dan* (Emperor of Heaven's Special Pill to Tonify the Heart), and *Gan Mai Da Zao Tang* (Licorice, Wheat, and Jujube Decoction).

CAUTIONS / CONTRAINDICATIONS

- Some sedative formulas that calm the *shen* (spirit) contain minerals or heavy metal substances. These formulas should not be taken for a long period of time, as they may injure the Spleen and Stomach. Furthermore, for *shen* disturbed patients who have constitutional Spleen and Stomach deficiencies, Spleen-tonifying and Stomach-harmonizing herbs should be added to prevent unwanted side effects of treatment.

- *Zhu Sha* (Cinnabaris), an ingredient traditionally found in some sedative formulas, is rarely used as a medicinal substance today. Its discussion here is included primarily for academic purposes, to reflect the historical use and influence of this substance.

PHARMACOLOGICAL EFFECTS & CLINICAL APPLICATIONS

> Heavy metal substances in *shen*-calming formulas are no longer used today, for safety reasons.

Shen-calming formulas calm the *shen* (spirit) and tranquilize the mind. From allopathic medicinal perspectives, these formulas primarily treat a wide variety of mental disorders. Note: The term "mental disorders" is used here loosely to describe a general and broad range of abnormal emotional, behavioral, and psychological conditions. It is not to be interpreted strictly as defined by any one diagnosis in the standard psychiatric *Diagnostic and Statistical Manual* (DSM).

- **Mental disorders**: *Shen*-calming herbs and formulas primarily treat a wide range of mental disorders. General pharmacological effects include sedative and hypnotic effects on the central nervous system to suppress both mental and physical activities.[1,2,3] One formula also demonstrated marked effectiveness in reducing elevated levels of serum corticosterone caused by emotional stress (psychological stress and conditioned-fear stress).[4] Clinically, *shen*-calming formulas have been used successfully to treat a wide variety of emotional, behavioral, and psychological disorders, including but not limited to insomnia,[5,6,7,8] neurasthenia,[9,10] neurosis,[11] schizophrenia,[12,13] depression,[14] and hysteria.[15] Formulas frequently used to calm the *shen* and treat mental disorders include *Suan Zao Ren Tang* (Sour Jujube Decoction), *Tian Wang Bu Xin Dan* (Emperor of Heaven's Special Pill to Tonify the Heart), *Yang Xin Tang* (Nourish the Heart Decoction), and *Gan Mai Da Zao Tang* (Licorice, Wheat, and Jujube Decoction).

- **Others**: *Shen*-calming formulas have also been used to treat seizures and epilepsy,[16] impotence,[17] nocturnal emissions,[18] enuresis,[19] and menopause.[20]

708

Chapter 9 — Overview

References

1. *Guo Wai Yi Xue* (Foreign Medicine) 1992;14(5):47.
2. *Zhong Yi Fang Ji Xian Dai Yan Jiu* (Modern Study of Medical Formulae in Traditional Chinese Medicine) 1997;849-850.
3. Journal of Ethnopharmacology 1986;15:289.
4. Sasaki K, Suzuki K, Yoshizaki F, Ando T. Effect of saiko-ka-ryukotsu-borei-to on the stress-induced increase of serum corticosterone in mice. Biol Pharm Bull 1995 Apr;18(4):563-5.
5. *Tian Jin Zhong Yi* (Tianjin Chinese Medicine) 1999;2:25.
6. *Shan Dong Yi Kan* (Shandong Medical Journal) 1965;27.
7. *He Nan Zhong Yi* (Henan Chinese Medicine) 1992;2:83.
8. *Zhe Jiang Zhong Yi Za Zhi* (Zhejiang Journal of Chinese Medicine) 1982;9:412.
9. *Zhong Xi Yi Jie He Yan Jiu Zi Liao* (Research Information on Integration of Chinese and Western Medicine) 1976;6:7.
10. *Jiang Su Yi Yao* (Jiangsu Journal of Medicine and Herbology) 1976;1:47.
11. *Han Fang Yi Xue* (Kampo Medicine) 1986;10(9):26.
12. *Shi Yong Zhong Xi Yi Jie He Za Zhi* (Practical Journal of Integrated Chinese and Western Medicines) 1998;2:170.
13. *Shang Hai Yi Yao Za Zhi* (Shanghai Journal of Medicine and Herbology) 1982;6:273.
14. *Liao Ning Zhong Yi Za Zhi* (Liaoning Journal of Chinese Medicine) 1984;12:34.
15. *Zhong Yi Za Zhi* (Journal of Chinese Medicine) 1960;2:32.
16. Hung-Ming W, Liu CS, Tsai JJ, Ko LY, Wei YH. Antioxidant and anticonvulsant effect of a modified formula of chaihu-longu-muli-tang. American Journal of Chinese Medicine 2002;30(2-3):339-46.
17. *Shan Xi Zhong Yi* (Shanxi Chinese Medicine) 1990;11(5):224.
18. *Shi Yong Zhong Xi Yi Jie He Za Zhi* (Practical Journal of Integrated Chinese and Western Medicines) 1991;12:729.
19. *Hu Bei Zhong Yi Za Zhi* (Hubei Journal of Chinese Medicine) 1986;1:19.
20. *Fu Jian Zhong Yi Yao* (Fujian Chinese Medicine and Herbology) 1960;10:17.

Section 1

重镇安神剂
— Sedative Formulas that Calm the Shen (Spirit)

Zhū Shā Ān Shén Wán (Cinnabar Pill to Tranquilize the Spirit)
朱砂安神丸

Pinyin Name: *Zhu Sha An Shen Wan*
Literal Name: Cinnabar Pill to Tranquilize the Spirit
Alternate Name: *An Shen Wan* (Tranquilize the Spirit Pill)
Original Source: *Yi Xue Fa Ming* (Medical Innovations) by Li Gao in the Jin Dynasty

COMPOSITION

Zhu Sha (Cinnabaris), *shui fei* (refined with water)	15g
Huang Lian (Rhizoma Coptidis), *xi* (washed) with liquor	18g
Dang Gui (Radix Angelicae Sinensis)	7.5g
Di Huang (Radix Rehmanniae)	7.5g
Zhi Gan Cao (Radix et Rhizoma Glycyrrhizae Praeparata cum Melle)	16.5g

Note: *Zhu Sha* (Cinnabaris) is a potentially toxic heavy metal, and is rarely used as a medicinal substance today. Its discussion here is included primarily for academic purposes, to reflect the historical use of this substance in its original formulation. Most herbal products today have removed it completely, or replaced it with substitutes with similar functions. For additional information on the toxicity, please refer to *Chinese Medical Herbology and Pharmacology* by John Chen and Tina Chen.

DOSAGE / PREPARATION / ADMINISTRATION

The source text states that all ingredients, except *Zhu Sha* (Cinnabaris), should be ground into a fine powder, steamed, and formed into small pills, about the size of corn kernels. Separately grind *Zhu Sha* (Cinnabaris) to fine powder, then refine it in water via *shui fei* (refining with water) technique, and allow it to dry in a cool place without direct exposure to sunlight. The *Zhu Sha* (Cinnabaris) powder is then used to coat the pills. The source text advises taking 15 pills after meals, swallowing them with saliva.

Today, this formula is usually prepared in pill form, with instructions to take 6-9g of pills before bedtime with water. This formula may also be prepared as a decoction with a proportionate adjustment in the doses of the herbs. *Zhu Sha* (Cinnabaris) should **not** be cooked in the decoction. Instead, it should be ground into powder and refined in water, and taken with the strained decoction.

CHINESE THERAPEUTIC ACTIONS
1. Tranquilizes the Heart and calms the *shen* (spirit)
2. Sedates fire and nourishes yin

CLINICAL MANIFESTATIONS
Heart fire rising with yin and blood deficiencies: irritability, anxiety, insomnia, frequent dreams, severe palpitations, desire to vomit but inability to do so, fear and fright, tongue ulcers, a red tongue body, and a fine, rapid pulse.

CLINICAL APPLICATIONS
Viral carditis, arrhythmia, night sweats, sleep-walking, neurasthenia, forgetfulness, anxiety, and depression.

EXPLANATION
Heart fire rising (excess) accompanied by yin and blood deficiencies may cause disturbances of the *shen* (spirit), which then lead to symptoms of irritability, insomnia, frequent dreams, severe palpitations, and fear and fright. Since the Heart opens to the tongue, Heart fire may produce tongue ulceration. The red tongue body and fine, rapid pulse are both signs of yin and blood deficiencies and heat in the Heart.

Chinese Herbal Formulas and Applications

Zhū Shā Ān Shén Wán (Cinnabar Pill to Tranquilize the Spirit)

Zhu Sha An Shen Wan (Cinnabar Pill to Tranquilize the Spirit)

Diagnosis	Signs and Symptoms	Treatment	Herbs
Heart fire rising with yin and blood deficiencies	• Irritability, insomnia, frequent dreams, severe palpitations, fear and fright: Heart fire disturbing the *shen* (spirit) • Tongue ulceration: Heart fire traveling upward to the tongue • Red tongue body and a fine, rapid pulse: yin and blood deficiencies and Heart fire rising	• Tranquilizes the Heart and calms the *shen* • Sedates fire • Nourishes yin	• *Zhu Sha* (Cinnabaris) tranquilizes the Heart and calms the *shen*. • *Huang Lian* (Rhizoma Coptidis) sedates Heart fire and relieves irritability. • *Dang Gui* (Radix Angelicae Sinensis) and *Di Huang* (Radix Rehmanniae) nourish the blood and yin. • *Zhi Gan Cao* (Radix et Rhizoma Glycyrrhizae Praeparata cum Melle) harmonizes all of the herbs.

Zhu Sha An Shen Wan (Cinnabar Pill to Tranquilize the Spirit) contains *Zhu Sha* (Cinnabaris) to tranquilize the Heart and calm the *shen* (spirit). *Huang Lian* (Rhizoma Coptidis) sedates Heart fire and relieves irritability. *Dang Gui* (Radix Angelicae Sinensis) and *Di Huang* (Radix Rehmanniae) nourish the blood and yin, which often become deficient in cases of heat and fire. *Zhi Gan Cao* (Radix et Rhizoma Glycyrrhizae Praeparata cum Melle) harmonizes all of the herbs.

MODIFICATIONS

• For neurasthenia causing insomnia, excessive dreams and forgetfulness, with phlegm and heat manifesting in a stifling sensation in the chest, and a greasy, yellow tongue coating, add *Gua Lou* (Fructus Trichosanthis) and *Zhu Ru* (Caulis Bambusae in Taenia).

• With palpitations and severe insomnia, add *Long Gu* (Os Draconis), *Mu Li* (Concha Ostreae), and *Ci Shi* (Magnetitum).

• With irritability and severe insomnia, add *Zhi Zi* (Fructus Gardeniae) and *Lian Zi Xin* (Plumula Nelumbinis).

CAUTIONS / CONTRAINDICATIONS

• *Zhu Sha An Shen Wan* is contraindicated in patients with yin deficiency. Also, it should not be used at a large dose or for a prolonged period of time.

• Because this formula contains *Zhu Sha* (Cinnabaris), it is contraindicated during pregnancy and in pediatric or geriatric patients.[1]

• Individuals who take this formula should avoid smoking and spicy, pungent, oily, and greasy foods.[2]

TOXICOLOGY

Because *Zhu Sha* (Cinnabaris) contains mercuric sulfide, it should never be processed with heat or cooked in decoction, as heat increases the toxicity of this substance. It should be used with extreme caution for those with compromised liver and kidney functions. Acute overdose of *Zhu Sha* (Cinnabaris) is characterized by disturbance of the central nervous system, nervousness, a metallic taste in the mouth, swollen gums, poor appetite, abdominal pain, diarrhea, tremors, sexual dysfunction, and liver and kidney damage.[3]

RELATED FORMULA

Shēng Tiě Luò Yǐn (Iron Filings Decoction)
生鐵落飲
生铁落饮
Pinyin Name: *Sheng Tie Luo Yin*
Literal Name: Iron Filings Decoction
Original Source: *Yi Xue Xin Wu* (Medical Revelations) by Cheng Guo-Peng in 1732

Tian Dong (Radix Asparagi)	9g
Mai Dong (Radix Ophiopogonis)	9g
Bei Mu (Bulbus Fritillariae)	9g
Dan Nan Xing (Arisaema cum Bile)	3g
Ju Hong (Exocarpium Citri Reticulatae)	3g
Yuan Zhi (Radix Polygalae)	3g
Shi Chang Pu (Rhizoma Acori Tatarinowii)	3g
Lian Qiao (Fructus Forsythiae)	3g
Fu Ling (Poria)	3g
Fu Shen (Poria Paradicis)	3g
Xuan Shen (Radix Scrophulariae)	4.5g
Gou Teng (Ramulus Uncariae cum Uncis)	4.5g
Dan Shen (Radix et Rhizoma Salviae Miltiorrhizae)	4.5g
Zhu Sha (Cinnabaris)	0.9g
Sheng Tie Luo (Frusta Ferri), *jian* (decocted) and *ao* (simmered)	[30g]

Note: *Zhu Sha* (Cinnabaris) is rarely used as a medicinal substance today. Its discussion here is included primarily for academic purposes, to reflect the historical use of

SHEN-CALMING FORMULAS

9

711

Chapter 9 – Shen-Calming Formulas   *Section 1 – Sedative Formulas that Calm the Shen (Spirit)*

Zhū Shā Ān Shén Wán (Cinnabar Pill to Tranquilize the Spirit)

this substance in its original formulation. Most herbal products today have removed it completely, or replaced it with substitutes with similar functions.

The source text states to first decoct and simmer *Sheng Tie Luo* (Frusta Ferri) in water for approximately 1.5 hours (the duration of time needed to burn 3 sticks of incense). Filter and discard the residue, and use this strained decoction to cook the other ingredients. Note: The source text does not specify the dose of *Sheng Tie Luo* (Frusta Ferri).

Sheng Tie Luo Yin (Iron Filings Decoction) treats *dian kuang* (mania and withdrawal) syndrome characterized by the rising of phlegm and fire. This formula tranquilizes the Heart, dispels phlegm, calms the *shen* (spirit), and anchors *zhi* (will-power).

Zhu Sha An Shen Wan and *Sheng Tie Luo Yin* both treat *shen* (spirit) disturbance.
• *Zhu Sha An Shen Wan* addresses *shen* disturbance caused by rising of Heart fire with yin and blood deficiencies.

This formula uses herbs to simultaneously purge fire and nourish yin.
• *Sheng Tie Luo Yi* treats *shen* disturbance caused by the rising of phlegm and fire, leading to *dian kuang* (mania and withdrawal). It does so by sedating the Heart and dispelling phlegm.

AUTHORS' COMMENTS

Zhu Sha (Cinnabaris) is rarely used as a medicinal substance today. It is discussed here and in other parts of this text primarily for academic purposes, to reflect the historical use of this substance. Most herbal manufacturers today either omit *Zhu Sha* (Cinnabaris) from formulas that historically specified its use, or substitute other medicinal substances with similar functions.

References
1. *Zhong Yao Ming Fang Yao Li Yu Ying Yong* (Pharmacology and Applications of Famous Herbal Formulas) 1989;368-369.
2. *Zhong Yao Ming Fang Yao Li Yu Ying Yong* (Pharmacology and Applications of Famous Herbal Formulas) 1989;368-369.
3. Chen J, Chen T. Chinese Medical Herbology and Pharmacology. City of Industry, CA: Art of Medicine Press, 2004.

Zhēn Zhū Mǔ Wán (Mother of Pearl Pill)
珍珠母丸

Pinyin Name: *Zhen Zhu Mu Wan*
Literal Name: Mother of Pearl Pill
Alternate Name: *Zhen Zhu Wan* (True Pearl Pill)
Original Source: *Pu Ji Ben Shi Fang* (Formulas of Universal Benefit from My Practice) by Xu Shu-Wei in 1132

COMPOSITION

Zhen Zhu Mu (Concha Margaritiferae), *yan* (ground) to powder	22.5g
Long Chi (Dens Draconis)	15g
Ren Shen (Radix et Rhizoma Ginseng)	30g
Dang Gui (Radix Angelicae Sinensis), *bei* (stone-baked)	45g
Shu Di Huang (Radix Rehmanniae Praeparata), *zheng* (steamed) with liquor	45g
Suan Zao Ren (Semen Ziziphi Spinosae), *chao* (dry-fried) and *yan* (ground) to small particles	30g
Bai Zi Ren (Semen Platycladi), *yan* (ground) to small particles	30g
Fu Shen (Poria Pararadicis)	15g
Xi Jiao (Cornu Rhinoceri), *bang* (scraped) into fine powder	15g
Chen Xiang (Lignum Aquilariae Resinatum)	15g

Note: *Xi Jiao* (Cornu Rhinoceri) is derived from an endangered animal, and *Zhu Sha* (Cinnabaris) is a potentially toxic heavy metal. Both are rarely used as medicinal substances

today. They are discussed here primarily for academic purposes, to reflect the historical use of these substances in its original formulation. Most herbal products today have

712

Zhēn Zhū Mǔ Wán (Mother of Pearl Pill)

removed them completely, or replaced them with substitutes with similar functions. For additional information on the toxicity, please refer to *Chinese Medical Herbology and Pharmacology* by John Chen and Tina Chen.

DOSAGE / PREPARATION / ADMINISTRATION

The source text states to grind the ingredients into powder, form into very small pills with honey, and coat the pills with *Zhu Sha* (Cinnabaris). The pills should resemble the size of *Wu Tong Zi* (Semen Firmianae), a small seed approximately 5 mm in diameter. Separately prepare a decoction of *Jin Bo* (gold foil), *Yin Bo* (silver foil), and *Bo He* (Herba Menthae). Take 40-50 pills with the strained decoction during the day and at bedtime.

CHINESE THERAPEUTIC ACTIONS

1. Tranquilizes the Heart and calms the *shen* (spirit)
2. Nourishes yin and blood

CLINICAL MANIFESTATIONS

Hyperactivity of Liver yang with yin and blood deficiencies: emotional instability, insomnia, fright, palpitations, dizziness, vertigo, and a fine, wiry pulse.

CLINICAL APPLICATIONS

Hypertension and neurasthenia.

EXPLANATION

Zhen Zhu Mu Wan (Mother of Pearl Pill) treats hyperactivity of Liver and Heart yang that is accompanied by underlying yin and blood deficiencies. The Heart is the organ that houses the mind. If yin and blood are deficient, then the *shen* (spirit) may become unstable, leading to insomnia and palpitations. Deficiency of yin with hyperactivity of yang may affect the brain, causing dizziness and vertigo.

Zhen Zhu Mu (Concha Margaritiferae) and *Long Chi* (Dens Draconis) subdue hyperactivity of Liver yang and calm Heart *shen* (spirit). *Zhen Zhu Mu* (Concha Margaritiferae) also enters the Heart and Liver channels, and guides the formula to these organs. *Ren Shen* (Radix et Rhizoma Ginseng), *Dang Gui* (Radix Angelicae Sinensis), and *Shu Di Huang* (Radix Rehmanniae Praeparata) nourish qi, yin, and blood. *Suan Zao Ren* (Semen Ziziphi Spinosae), *Bai Zi Ren* (Semen Platycladi), and *Fu Shen* (Poria Paradicis) calm the *shen* and anchor the *zhi* (will-power). They also help to promote restful sleep. *Xi Jiao* (Cornu Rhinoceri) enters the *xue* (blood) level to cool the blood and relieves fright and palpitations. *Chen Xiang* (Lignum Aquilariae Resinatum) lowers hyperactive yang to help calm the *shen*. *Zhu Sha* (Cinnabaris) calms the *shen* and guides the formula to the Heart. *Jin Bo* (gold foil) and *Yin Bo* (silver foil) calm the *shen*. *Bo He* (Herba Menthae) soothes Liver qi and clears Liver fire.

CAUTIONS / CONTRAINDICATIONS

Zhen Zhu Mu Wan contains rich tonics such as *Shu Di Huang* (Radix Rehmanniae Praeparata) and *Suan Zao Ren* (Semen Ziziphi Spinosae), and is not suitable for treating insomnia and *shen* (spirit) disturbance caused by phlegm and heat.

Zhen Zhu Mu Wan (Mother of Pearl Pill)

Diagnosis	Signs and Symptoms	Treatment	Herbs
Hyperactivity of Liver yang with yin and blood deficiencies	• Emotional instability, insomnia, and palpitations: yin and blood insufficient to nourish the *shen* (spirit) • Dizziness and vertigo: hyperactivity of yang due to deficiency of yin	• Nourishes yin and blood • Tranquilizes the Heart and calms the *shen*	• *Zhen Zhu Mu* (Concha Margaritiferae) and *Long Chi* (Dens Draconis) subdue hyperactivity of Liver yang and calm Heart *shen*. • *Ren Shen* (Radix et Rhizoma Ginseng), *Dang Gui* (Radix Angelicae Sinensis) and *Shu Di Huang* (Radix Rehmanniae Praeparata) nourish qi, yin and blood. • *Suan Zao Ren* (Semen Ziziphi Spinosae), *Bai Zi Ren* (Semen Platycladi), and *Fu Shen* (Poria Paradicis) calm the *shen* and anchor *zhi* (will-power). • *Xi Jiao* (Cornu Rhinoceri) enters the *xue* (blood) level and cools the blood. • *Chen Xiang* (Lignum Aquilariae Resinatum) lowers hyperactive yang to help calm the *shen*.

SHEN-CALMING FORMULAS

9

713

Chapter 9 – Shen-Calming Formulas   *Section 1 – Sedative Formulas that Calm the Shen (Spirit)*

Cí Zhū Wān (Magnetite and Cinnabar Pill)

磁朱丸

Pinyin Name: Ci Zhu Wan
Literal Name: Magnetite and Cinnabar Pill
Alternate Name: Shen Qu Wan (Medicated Leaven Pill)
Original Source: *Bei Ji Qian Jin Yao Fang* (Thousands of Golden Prescriptions for Emergencies) by Sun Si-Miao in the Tang Dynasty

COMPOSITION

Ci Shi (Magnetitum)	60g
Zhu Sha (Cinnabaris)	30g
Shen Qu (Massa Fermentata)	120g

Note: *Zhu Sha* (Cinnabaris) is a potentially toxic heavy metal, and is rarely used as a medicinal substance today. Its discussion here is included primarily for academic purposes, to reflect the historical use of this substance in its original formulation. Most herbal products today have removed it completely, or replaced it with substitutes with similar functions. For additional information on the toxicity, please refer to *Chinese Medical Herbology and Pharmacology* by John Chen and Tina Chen.

DOSAGE / PREPARATION / ADMINISTRATION

The source text instructs to grind the ingredients into powder and form into small pills with honey. The pills should resemble the size of *Wu Tong Zi* (Semen Firmianae), a small seed approximately 5 mm in diameter. Take 3 pills three times daily. Today this formula is prepared by grinding the ingredients into a powder and mixing it with honey to form pills. Take 6g of pills per dose, twice daily with water.

CHINESE THERAPEUTIC ACTIONS

1. Tranquilizes the mind and calms the *shen* (spirit)
2. Subdues hyperactive yang and brightens vision

CLINICAL MANIFESTATIONS

Heart and Kidney disharmony: palpitations, insomnia, dizziness, deafness, tinnitus, and blurred vision.

CLINICAL APPLICATIONS

Seizures, epilepsy, neurasthenia, insomnia, forgetfulness, psychiatric disorders, hypertension, tinnitus, cataract, and glaucoma.

EXPLANATION

Ci Zhu Wan (Magnetite and Cinnabar Pill) is indicated for disharmony of the Heart and Kidney (e.g., Heart yang excess and Kidney *jing* (essence) deficiency). Excess Heart yang may disturb the *shen* (spirit), leading to palpitations and insomnia. Deficiency of Kidney *jing* fails to nourish the sensory organs, causing dizziness, tinnitus, deafness, and blurred vision.

In this formula, *Ci Shi* (Magnetitum) subdues hyperactive yang and benefits Kidney yin. *Zhu Sha* (Cinnabaris) calms the *shen* (spirit) and anchors the *zhi* (will-power). Used together, these two herbs restore the harmonious relationship between the Heart and Kidney. *Shen Qu* (Massa Fermentata) protects the stomach from being injured by *Ci Shi* (Magnetitum) and *Zhu Sha* (Cinnabaris). *Shen Qu* (Massa Fermentata) can also increase digestion and absorption of nutrients to help replenish Kidney *jing* (essence).

MODIFICATIONS

• With a restless *shen* (spirit), dry eyes, or photophobia caused by Kidney yin deficiency, add *Liu Wei Di Huang Wan* (Six-Ingredient Pill with Rehmannia).

Ci Zhu Wan (Magnetite and Cinnabar Pill)

Diagnosis	Signs and Symptoms	Treatment	Herbs
Heart and Kidney disharmony	• Palpitations and insomnia: *shen* (spirit) disturbance caused by Heart yang excess • Dizziness, tinnitus, deafness, and blurred vision: Kidney *jing* (essence) unable to nourish the sensory organs	• Tranquilizes the mind and calms the *shen* • Sedates hyperactive yang and brightens vision	• *Ci Shi* (Magnetitum) subdues hyperactive yang and benefits Kidney yin. • *Zhu Sha* (Cinnabaris) calms the *shen* and anchors *zhi* (will-power). • *Shen Qu* (Massa Fermentata) protects the stomach from the harsh properties of the two mineral substances.

714

Ci Zhū Wān (Magnetite and Cinnabar Pill)

- For epilepsy and seizures with profuse phlegm, add *Dan Nan Xing* (Arisaema cum Bile), *Ban Xia* (Rhizoma Pinelliae), and *Tian Zhu Huang* (Concretio Silicea Bambusae).

CAUTIONS / CONTRAINDICATIONS

- *Ci Zhu Wan* is contraindicated in patients who do not show symptoms of Heart fire and Kidney and Liver yin deficiencies.
- Use with caution in patients with Spleen and Stomach deficiencies, as the mineral substances in this formula may be harsh on the digestive system.
- Because this formula contains *Zhu Sha* (Cinnabaris), it is contraindicated during pregnancy and in pediatric or geriatric patients.

AUTHORS' COMMENTS

Ci Zhu Wan has been found to be effective in treating various ocular disorders, such as cataract and glaucoma. For these applications, *Ci Zhu Wan* is often combined with *Qi Ju Di Huang Wan* (Lycium Fruit, Chrysanthemum, and Rehmannia Pill) or *Ming Mu Di Huang Wan* (Improve Vision Pill with Rehmannia).

Zhu Sha An Shen Wan (Cinnabar Pill to Tranquilize the Spirit) and *Ci Zhu Wan* are both tranquilizing formulas that treat restless *shen* (spirit), palpitations, and insomnia accompanied by frequent dreams.

- *Zhu Sha An Shen Wan* strongly sedates Heart fire to treat excess Heart fire that is injuring yin and blood, causing irritability, disorientation, insomnia, a feeling of misdirected qi flow in the chest with heat sensations, and occasional urges to vomit.
- *Ci Zhu Wan* settles the Heart, brightens vision, and anchors floating yang. It is best for Kidney *jing* (essence) deficiency with Heart yang rising. This disharmony between the Heart and Kidney causes insomnia, palpitations, tinnitus, blurred vision, and in severe cases, deafness and epilepsy.[1]

Reference

1. Wang MZ, et al. *Zhong Yi Xue Wen Da Ti Ku* (Questions and Answers on Traditional Chinese Medicine: Herbal Formulas).

Chái Hú Jiā Lóng Gǔ Mǔ Li Tāng
(Bupleurum plus Dragon Bone and Oyster Shell Decoction)

柴 胡 加 龍 骨 牡 蠣 湯

柴 胡 加 龙 骨 牡 蛎 汤

Pinyin Name: *Chai Hu Jia Long Gu Mu Li Tang*
Literal Name: Bupleurum plus Dragon Bone and Oyster Shell Decoction
Alternate Names: *Chai Hu Jia Long Mu Tang, Tsai Hu Chia Lung Ku Mu Li Tang*, Bupleurum and Dragon Bone Combination
Original Source: *Shang Han Lun* (Discussion of Cold-Induced Disorders) by Zhang Zhong-Jing in the Eastern Han Dynasty

COMPOSITION

Chai Hu (Radix Bupleuri)	12g
Huang Qin (Radix Scutellariae)	4.5g
Long Gu (Os Draconis)	4.5g
Mu Li (Concha Ostreae), *ao* (simmered)	4.5g
Qian Dan (Minium)	4.5g
Gui Zhi (Ramulus Cinnamomi)	4.5g
Da Huang (Radix et Rhizoma Rhei)	6g
Ban Xia (Rhizoma Pinelliae), *xi* (washed)	6-9g
Fu Ling (Poria)	4.5g
Ren Shen (Radix et Rhizoma Ginseng)	4.5g
Sheng Jiang (Rhizoma Zingiberis Recens), *qie* (sliced)	4.5g
Da Zao (Fructus Jujubae), *bo* (opened)	6 pieces

SHEN-CALMING FORMULAS

9

715

Chapter 9 – Shen-Calming Formulas   *Section 1 – Sedative Formulas that Calm the Shen (Spirit)*

Chái Hú Jiā Lóng Gǔ Mǔ Lì Tāng
(Bupleurum plus Dragon Bone and Oyster Shell Decoction)

Note: *Qian Dan* (Minium) is a potentially toxic heavy metal, and is rarely used as a medicinal substance today. Its discussion here is included primarily for academic purposes, to reflect the historical use of this substance in its original formulation. Most herbal products today have removed it completely, or replaced it with substitutes with similar functions. For additional information on the toxicity, please refer to *Chinese Medical Herbology and Pharmacology* by John Chen and Tina Chen.

DOSAGE / PREPARATION / ADMINISTRATION

Cook all of the ingredients, except *Da Huang* (Radix et Rhizoma Rhei), in 8 cups [1,600 mL] of water until the decoction is reduced to 4 cups [800 mL]. Add *Da Huang* (Radix et Rhizoma Rhei), and bring the decoction to a quick boil. Take 1 cup [200 mL] of the warm, strained decoction.

CHINESE THERAPEUTIC ACTIONS

1. Harmonizes the *shaoyang*
2. Unblocks the three yang stages
3. Calms the *shen* (spirit)

CLINICAL MANIFESTATIONS

1. Disorder in the three yang stages (*taiyang, yangming,* and *shaoyang*): fullness and distention in the chest, insomnia, anxiety, occasional palpitations, irritability, dysuria, delirium, feeling of heaviness in the entire body with inability to rotate the trunk, red tongue body, and a rapid, wiry pulse.
2. *Shaoyang* syndrome: chest fullness, irritability, excitability, dysuria, delirium, heaviness of the whole body, and difficulty in moving the body.

CLINICAL APPLICATIONS

Neurosis, neurotic palpitations, nervousness, anxiety, hysteria, neurasthenia, insomnia, depression, schizophrenia, menopausal disturbance, hypertension, valvular disease, angina pectoris, post-ischemic brain injury, hemiplegia, cerebral hemorrhage, hyperlipoproteinemia, atherosclerosis, seizure, epilepsy, pelvic inflammatory disease, hyperthyroidism, and Meniere's disease.

EXPLANATION

Chai Hu Jia Long Gu Mu Li Tang (Bupleurum plus Dragon Bone and Oyster Shell Decoction), first presented in *Shang Han Lun* (Discussion of Cold-Induced Disorders), was originally indicated for patients who receive improper downward draining treatment when their disorder is still at the exterior and has not yet entered the *yangming* stage.

As the result of improper downward draining treatment, the pathogenic factor travels inward to penetrate the *taiyang, yangming,* and *shaoyang* levels.

Clinically, patients usually exhibit a wide array of complex heat signs and symptoms. The presence of heat in the chest produces a feeling of fullness and distention; heat attacking the Heart causes insomnia, anxiety, and palpitations; heat in the *yangming* stage causes delirium; and heat in the *shaoyang* stage leads to a feeling of heaviness in the entire body with inability to rotate the trunk. The improper use of downward draining herbs may damage body fluids, thus causing constipation and urinary difficulties. A red tongue body and rapid, wiry pulse are also indicative of heat. While clinical presentations may vary between patients, the diagnostic feature is the *shen* (spirit) floating upward, as evident from symptoms such as anxiety, palpitations, and delirious speech.

The *shaoyang* syndrome discussed here is caused by the inappropriate use of downward draining methods instead of exterior-releasing methods for illnesses at the *taiyang* stage. Downward draining methods used inappropriately may result in penetration of the pathogenic factors into the interior of the body, causing a syndrome that is both exterior and interior, deficient and excess. Chest fullness, irritability, and excitability are caused by fire in the *shaoyang* channel. *Shaoyang* syndrome may affect the water passages, causing dysuria. Delirium is the result of Stomach heat and *shaoyang* fire disturbing the Heart. Heaviness of the body is the result of the disrupted flow of yang qi.

Chai Hu Jia Long Gu Mu Li Tang is based on *Xiao Chai Hu Tang* (Minor Bupleurum Decoction), which is the representative formula for harmonizing *shaoyang* syndrome. (Please refer to the section on *Xiao Chai Hu Tang* for complete details.) *Chai Hu* (Radix Bupleuri) and *Huang Qin* (Radix Scutellariae) clear heat from the *shaoyang* stage and harmonize the exterior and interior. *Long Gu* (Os Draconis), *Mu Li* (Concha Ostreae) and *Qian Dan* (Minium) calm the *shen* (spirit) to relieve anxiety, palpitations, and delirious speech. *Gui Zhi* (Ramulus Cinnamomi) dispels exterior pathogenic factors, while *Da Huang* (Radix et Rhizoma Rhei) drains internal heat. *Ban Xia* (Rhizoma Pinelliae) guides the qi downward, while *Fu Ling* (Poria) promotes normal urination. Furthermore, *Fu Ling* (Poria) and *Ren Shen* (Radix et Rhizoma Ginseng) strengthen the Spleen and calm the *shen*. *Sheng Jiang* (Rhizoma Zingiberis Recens) and *Da Zao* (Fructus Jujubae) harmonize the formula.

716

Chinese Herbal Formulas and Applications

Chái Hú Jiā Lóng Gǔ Mǔ Lì Tāng
(Bupleurum plus Dragon Bone and Oyster Shell Decoction)

Chai Hu Jia Long Gu Mu Li Tang (Bupleurum plus Dragon Bone and Oyster Shell Decoction)

Diagnosis	Signs and Symptoms	Treatment	Herbs
Disorder in the three yang stages	• A feeling of fullness and distention: heat in the chest • Insomnia, delirium, anxiety and palpitations: heat attacking the Heart and *shen* (spirit) • A feeling of heaviness in the entire body with inability to rotate the trunk: heat in the *shaoyang* stage • Constipation and urinary difficulties: heat damaging body fluids • A red tongue body and rapid, wiry pulse: interior heat	• Harmonizes the *shaoyang* • Unblocks the three yang stages • Calms the *shen* (spirit)	• *Chai Hu* (Radix Bupleuri) and *Huang Qin* (Radix Scutellariae) clear heat from the *shaoyang* stage and harmonize the exterior and interior. • *Long Gu* (Os Draconis), *Mu Li* (Concha Ostreae) and *Qian Dan* (Minium) calm the *shen* to relieve anxiety, palpitations, and delirious speech. • *Gui Zhi* (Ramulus Cinnamomi) dispels exterior pathogenic factors. • *Da Huang* (Radix et Rhizoma Rhei) drains internal heat. • *Ban Xia* (Rhizoma Pinelliae) causes qi to descend. • *Fu Ling* (Poria) promotes smooth urination. • *Ren Shen* (Radix et Rhizoma Ginseng) strengthens the Spleen and calms the *shen*. • *Sheng Jiang* (Rhizoma Zingiberis Recens) and *Da Zao* (Fructus Jujubae) harmonize all of the herbs.

MODIFICATIONS

- With palpitations and insomnia due to hypertension, add *Gou Teng* (Ramulus Uncariae cum Uncis) and *Du Zhong* (Cortex Eucommiae).
- With irritability and fullness in the chest, add *Huang Lian* (Rhizoma Coptidis) and *Tian Hua Fen* (Radix Trichosanthis).
- With delirious speech, add *Tian Ma* (Rhizoma Gastrodiae) and *Gou Teng* (Ramulus Uncariae cum Uncis).
- If there is dysuria, add *Mu Tong* (Caulis Akebiae) and *Fang Ji* (Radix Stephaniae Tetrandrae).
- With nightmares and vertigo, add *Long Dan* (Radix et Rhizoma Gentianae) and *Xia Ku Cao* (Spica Prunellae).
- When there is fatigue due to qi deficiency, add *Huang Qi* (Radix Astragali) and increase the dose of *Ren Shen* (Radix et Rhizoma Ginseng).
- With low back pain, add *Du Zhong* (Cortex Eucommiae) and *Niu Xi* (Radix Achyranthis Bidentatae).

CAUTIONS / CONTRAINDICATIONS

- For patients with a sensitive gastrointestinal system, remove *Da Huang* (Radix et Rhizoma Rhei), as this herb may cause loose stools.
- *Chai Hu Jia Long Gu Mu Li Tang* should be used cautiously in those with Spleen and Stomach deficiencies, as *Long Gu* (Os Draconis) and *Mu Li* (Concha Ostreae) are hard to digest.
- The original formula contains *Qian Dan* (Minium), commonly known as lead oxide red. Because *Qian Dan* (Minium) is toxic, there have been cases of anemia

associated with long-term use of this herbal formula.[1] Therefore, modern formulations generally omit this ingredient, or replace it with *Zhe Shi* (Haematitum), which also has a calming action.[2]

PHARMACOLOGICAL EFFECTS

1. **Central nervous system**: Continuous administration of this formula for seven days was associated with increased sleeping time, decreased body temperature, and decreased spontaneous activity in rats.[3]

2. **Antidepressant**: Administration of *Chai Hu Jia Long Gu Mu Li Tang* in mice successfully treated depression induced by chronic stress, by restoring the normal functioning of the hypothalamo-pituitary-adrenal system and the prefrontal cortex. Furthermore, studies have demonstrated that *Chai Hu Jia Long Gu Mu Li Tang* significantly prevented chronic stress-induced decreases in extracellular concentrations of dopamine and serotonin in the prefrontal cortex.[4,5] Lastly, administration of *Chai Hu Jia Long Gu Mu Li Tang*, *Yi Gan San* (Restrain the Liver Powder) and *Bu Zhong Yi Qi Tang* (Tonify the Middle and Augment the Qi Decoction) for 14 consecutive days showed both antidepressive and antinociceptive properties in mice.[6]

3. **Endocrine**: A study evaluated the relationship between *Chai Hu Jia Long Gu Mu Li Tang* and serum corticosterone in mice. The study found *Chai Hu Jia Long Gu Mu Li Tang* to be effective in reducing elevated corticosterone caused by emotional stress (psychological stress and conditioned-fear stress), but not physical stress (immobilized

9

SHEN-CALMING FORMULAS

717

Chapter 9 – Shen-Calming Formulas　　　　　　　*Section 1 – Sedative Formulas that Calm the Shen (Spirit)*

Chái Hú Jiā Lóng Gǔ Mǔ Lì Tāng
(Bupleurum plus Dragon Bone and Oyster Shell Decoction)

stress, forced-swim stress, and electric-shock stress). The researchers concluded that *Chai Hu Jia Long Gu Mu Li Tang* is more effective for stress associated with psychological changes, and less effective for stress caused by physical changes.[7]

4. **Sedative and hypnotic**: Administration of *Chai Hu Jia Long Gu Mu Li Tang* was associated with marked reduction in locomotor activity, and dose-dependent prolongation in the duration of drug-induced sleep time. The study suggested *Chai Hu Jia Long Gu Mu Li Tang* as a useful therapy against sleep disorder caused by excitation.[8]

5. **Antihypertensive**: *Chai Hu Jia Long Gu Mu Li Tang* has been used clinically in the treatment of hypertension. The mechanism of this antihypertensive effect was attributed to the antipressor effect (inhibition of vasoconstriction induced by nor-adrenaline).[9,10]

6. **Metabolic**: Administration of the extract of the formula to mice at 0.4 g/kg for 12 months was associated with reduction of total cholesterol and triglyceride levels in both the liver and blood vessels.[11]

7. **Effects on hypercholesterolemia and atherosclerosis**: Use of *Chai Hu Jia Long Gu Mu Li Tang* in rabbits was associated with prevention of hypercholesterolemia and protection against atheromatous lesions by affecting apoE and LDL receptor mRNA gene expression in the liver.[12] According to another study, *Chai Hu Jia Long Gu Mu Li Tang* prevented arteriosclerosis by inhibiting the proliferation of vascular smooth muscle cells.[13]

CLINICAL STUDIES AND RESEARCH

1. **Neurosis**: Thirty-two patients with neurosis were treated with this formula for two weeks, with significant improvement in 6 cases, moderate improvement in 6 cases, and slight improvement in 14 cases. The overall rate of effectiveness was 81.3%.[14]

2. **Depression**: Thirty-five patients (between 19-60 years of age) with depression were treated with *Chai Hu Jia Long Gu Mu Li Tang* plus *Sheng Tie Luo* (Frusta Ferri) with complete recovery in 15 cases, significant improvement in 10 cases, moderate improvement in 9 cases, and no improvement in 1 case. The formula was given in decoction daily for 30 days per course of treatment, and the duration of the treatment was between 14-90 days. The overall effectiveness rate was 97.1%.[15] According to another study, use of *Chai Hu Jia Long Gu Mu Li Tang* in 63 patients (15 males and 48 females) with depression was associated with recovery in 32 cases, improvement in 19 cases, and no effect in 12 cases.[16]

3. **Schizophrenia**: In one study, 67 patients with schizophrenia were divided into three groups. Group A contained 15

schizophrenic patients characterized by *shaoyang* disorder and treated with *Chai Hu Jia Long Gu Mu Li Tang*. Diazepam or chlordiazepoxide was given only if necessary to treat insomnia. Group B had 31 schizophrenic patients characterized by *shaoyang* disorder who were treated with *Chai Hu Jia Long Gu Mu Li Tang* as the primary treatment, with the addition of chlorpromazine or chlorprothixene at low doses (200mg per day or less). Group C had 21 schizophrenic patients characterized by *shaoyang* disorder with qi and blood stagnation; they were treated with modified *Chai Hu Jia Long Gu Mu Li Tang* as the primary treatment, with the addition of chlorpromazine or chlorprothixene at low doses (200mg per day or less). The modified formula used in Group C contained *Chai Hu* (Radix Bupleuri) 9g, *Huang Qin* (Radix Scutellariae) 9g, *Dang Gui* (Radix Angelicae Sinensis) 9g, *Chi Shao* (Radix Paeoniae Rubra) 9g, *Tao Ren* (Semen Persicae) 9g, *Hong Hua* (Flos Carthami) 9g, *Da Huang* (Radix et Rhizoma Rhei) 6-9g, *Chuan Xiong* (Rhizoma Chuanxiong) 6g, *Mu Li* (Concha Ostreae) 15g, *Sheng Jiang* (Rhizoma Zingiberis Recens) 6g, and *Da Zao* (Fructus Jujubae) 15g. The treatment protocol for herbs in all three groups was to cook the herbs in water, and administer the decoction daily for 30 days per course of treatment. Those who did not respond after the first course received a second course of treatment. Of 67 patients, the study reported complete recovery in 1 case, significant recovery in 35 cases, and improvement in 14 cases. The overall effectiveness was 76.1%.[17] Note: Comparative analysis of results among the three groups of patients was unavailable at the time of publication.

In another study, use of modified *Chai Hu Jia Long Gu Mu Li Tang* was associated with 86.67% effectiveness in treating 45 patients with schizophrenia. The herbal formula contained *Chai Hu* (Radix Bupleuri) 12g, *Long Gu* (Os Draconis) 20g, *Mu Li* (Concha Ostreae) 20g, *Dang Shen* (Radix Codonopsis) 15g, *Ban Xia* (Rhizoma Pinelliae) 12g, *Da Huang* (Radix et Rhizoma Rhei) 10g, *Fu Ling* (Poria) 12g, *Huang Qin* (Radix Scutellariae) 12g, *Gui Zhi* (Ramulus Cinnamomi) 6g, *Dan Shen* (Radix et Rhizoma Salviae Miltiorrhizae) 15g, *Sheng Jiang* (Rhizoma Zingiberis Recens) 3 slices, and *Da Zao* (Fructus Jujubae) 6 pieces. Most patients showed improvement after an average of 15 packs of herbs. Of 45 patients, the study reported significant improvement in 31 cases, moderate improvement in 8 cases, and no effect in 6 cases.[18]

4. **Hyperlipoproteinemia**: Modified *Chai Hu Jia Long Gu Mu Li Tang* showed marked effectiveness in treating hyperlipoproteinemia in 58 patients. The study divided all patients into three categories based on traditional

718

Chái Hú Jiā Lóng Gǔ Mǔ Lì Tāng
(Bupleurum plus Dragon Bone and Oyster Shell Decoction)

Chinese medical diagnoses. Hyperlipoproteinemia characterized by dampness and phlegm was treated with this formula plus *Fu Ling* (Poria), *Bai Zhu* (Rhizoma Atractylodis Macrocephalae), *Ban Xia* (Rhizoma Pinelliae), and others. Hyperlipoproteinemia characterized by Liver qi stagnation was treated with this formula plus *Zhi Qiao* (Fructus Aurantii), *Bai Shao* (Radix Paeoniae Alba), *Yu Jin* (Radix Curcumae) and others. Hyperlipoproteinemia characterized by Liver qi stagnation and Spleen deficiency was treated by this formula plus *Zhi Qiao* (Fructus Aurantii), *Yan Hu Suo* (Rhizoma Corydalis), *Fo Shou* (Fructus Citri Sarcodactylis), and others. The duration of treatment was 3 months per course of treatment. The study reported an overall rate of effectiveness of 87.9%.[19] In addition, another study stated that *Chai Hu Jia Long Gu Mu Li Tang* may prevent the development of vascular complications in hyperlipidemia patients, as use of the herbs was associated with reduction of triglycerides, total cholesterol, CD62P, PMPs, sE-selectin, and anti-oxidized LDL antibody.[20]

5. **Coronary restenosis** (accelerated atherosclerosis after percutaneous coronary intervention): Administration of *Chai Hu Jia Long Gu Mu Li Tang* had a marked effect to inhibit restenosis after percutaneous coronary intervention (PCI) in humans. The proposed mechanism of this effect is attributed to the inhibition of intimal smooth muscle cell proliferation, and reduction of serum total cholesterol and low-density lipoprotein cholesterol. The study also noted that *Chai Hu Jia Long Gu Mu Li Tang* maintained its therapeutic effect for up to 8 weeks after balloon injury. This study also stated that *Chai Hu Jia Long Gu Mu Li Tang* may prevent atherosclerosis, since restenosis after PCI is considered to be an accelerated atherosclerosis.[21,22]

6. **Pelvic inflammatory disease**: Chronic pelvic inflammatory disease was treated with marked success using modified *Chai Hu Jia Long Gu Mu Li Tang* plus *Jin Yin Hua* (Flos Lonicerae Japonicae) and *Pu Gong Ying* (Herba Taraxaci). In addition to the base formula, modifications were made by adding *Du Zhong* (Cortex Eucommiae), *Qian Shi* (Semen Euryales) and *Tu Si Zi* (Semen Cuscutae) for Kidney yang deficiency; *Er Zhi Wan* (Two-Ultimate Pill) for Kidney yin deficiency; *Yu Jin* (Radix Curcumae) and *Zhi Shi* (Fructus Aurantii Immaturus) for qi stagnation; and *Yi Yi Ren* (Semen Coicis) and *Cang Zhu* (Rhizoma Atractylodis) for dampness. The treatment protocol was to administer the herbs in decoction, for 6 packs of herbs per course of treatment, for a total of 2-6 courses. Of 323 patients, the study reported complete recovery in 178 cases, marked improvement in 112 cases, moderate improvement in 26 cases, and no effect in 7 cases. The overall rate of effectiveness was 94.7%.[23]

7. **Seizures and epilepsy**: A study reported 88% effectiveness using modified *Chai Hu Jia Long Gu Mu Li Tang* to treat 50 patients with epilepsy. The herbal treatment was based on *Chai Hu Jia Long Gu Mu Li Tang* without *Qian Dan* (Minium). Modifications included addition of *Shi Chang Pu* (Rhizoma Acori Tatarinowii), *Yuan Zhi* (Radix Polygalae) and *Dan Nan Xing* (Arisaema cum Bile) for the presence of excessive amounts of phlegm; *Suan Zao Ren* (Semen Ziziphi Spinosae), *Shou Wu Teng* (Caulis Polygoni Multiflori) and *He Huan Pi* (Cortex Albiziae) for insomnia due to deficiency and restlessness; *Shi Jue Ming* (Concha Haliotidis), *Gou Teng* (Ramulus Uncariae cum Uncis), *Sheng Tie Luo* (Frusta Ferri) and *Huang Lian* (Rhizoma Coptidis) for wind and yang rising; *Sha Shen* (Radix Glehniae seu Adenophorae), *Mai Dong* (Radix Ophiopogonis) and *Xuan Shen* (Radix Scrophulariae) for yin deficiency. Additional adjustments were also made, depending on the severity of the condition and age of the patients. Of 50 patients, the study reported near-recovery in 25 cases, improvement in 19 cases, and no effect in 6 cases.[24] Another study reported marked success using modified *Chai Hu Jia Long Gu Mu Li Tang* to treat 20 patients with seizures and epilepsy, reducing the seizure frequency from an average of 13.4 +/- 3.4 to 10.7 +/- 2.5 per month.[25]

8. **Insomnia**: Thirty-six patients with insomnia were treated with 88.9% effectiveness using modified *Chai Hu Jia Long Gu Mu Li Tang*. The herbal formula contained *Chai Hu* (Radix Bupleuri) 12-20g, *Long Gu* (Os Draconis) 20-30g, *Mu Li* (Concha Ostreae) 20-30g, *Huang Qin* (Radix Scutellariae) 10-15g, *Fu Ling* (Poria) 10-15g, *Ban Xia* (Rhizoma Pinelliae) 10-15g, *Da Huang* (Radix et Rhizoma Rhei) 6-10g, *He Huan Hua* (Flos Albiziae) 20g, *Da Zao* (Fructus Jujubae) 3-5 pieces, and *Sheng Jiang* (Rhizoma Zingiberis Recens) 3-5 slices. *Long Dan* (Radix et Rhizoma Gentianae) and *Zhi Zi* (Fructus Gardeniae) were added for Liver fire rising; *Shen Qu* (Massa Fermentata) and *Lai Fu Zi* (Semen Raphani) for Stomach disharmony; *Huang Lian* (Rhizoma Coptidis) and *E Jiao* (Colla Corii Asini) for yin-deficient fire; and *Dang Shen* (Radix Codonopsis) and *Dang Gui* (Radix Angelicae Sinensis) for Heart and Spleen deficiencies. Of 36 patients, the study reported significant improvement in 19 cases, moderate improvement in 13 cases, and no effect in 4 cases. The overall rate of effectiveness was 88.9%.[26]

9. **Postischemic brain injury**: Administration of three herbal formulas minimized postischemic brain injury by inhibiting production of free radicals and generation of

Chapter 9 – Shen-Calming Formulas   *Section 1 – Sedative Formulas that Calm the Shen (Spirit)*

Chái Hú Jiā Lóng Gǔ Mǔ Lì Tāng
(Bupleurum plus Dragon Bone and Oyster Shell Decoction)

lipid peroxidation. The three formulas found to be effective, both *in vitro* and *in vivo*, were *Chai Hu Jia Long Gu Mu Li Tang*, *Huang Lian Jie Du Tang* (Coptis Decoction to Relieve Toxicity), and *Gui Zhi Fu Ling Wan* (Cinnamon Twig and Poria Pill).[27]

HERB-DRUG INTERACTION

- **Carbamazepine**: Researchers evaluated the possibility of pharmacokinetic interactions between *Chai Hu Jia Long Gu Mu Li Tang* and carbamazepine. After extensive examination in rats, the researchers found no significant differences in the serum protein binding of carbamazepine and carbamazepine-10,11-epoxide, its active metabolite. Furthermore, one-week pretreatment with *Chai Hu Jia Long Gu Mu Li Tang* (1 g/kg/day) did not affect the plasma concentration-time profile or any pharmacokinetic parameter of carbamazepine or its metabolite. The researchers concluded that oral co-administration of *Chai Hu Jia Long Gu Mu Li Tang* with carbamazepine appears to be pharmacokinetically safe.[28]

- **Theophylline**: Administration of theophylline is often accompanied by side effects such as tachycardia and central nervous system stimulation. According to one study in rats and mice, administration of *Chai Hu Jia Long Gu Mu Li Tang* concurrent with theophylline successfully suppressed the cardiovascular and central nervous systems to alleviate theophylline-induced tachycardia, locomotion, and convulsions.[29]

TOXICOLOGY

Qian Dan (Minium), lead oxide red (Pb_3O_4), is a potentially toxic substance. Acute poisoning may occur following a bolus dose of 15 grams; chronic poisoning has been reported following daily ingestion of 2 mg of this mineral.[30] Two cases of anemia have been reported with the use of *Chai Hu Jia Long Gu Mu Li Tang* that contained *Qian Dan* (Minium). The cause of this toxicity was attributed to *Qian Dan* (Minium), as anemia is a potential consequence of lead poisoning.[31] Note: *Chai Hu Jia Long Gu Mu Li Tang* produced today do not contain *Qian Dan* (Minium), and should not cause these side effects.

RELATED FORMULA

Chái Hú Ān Shén Tāng
(Bupleurum Decoction to Tranquilize the Spirit)
柴胡安神湯
柴胡安神汤
Pinyin Name: *Chai Hu An Shen Tang*
Literal Name: Bupleurum Decoction to Tranquilize the Spirit

Original Source: *Tian Jin Zhong Yi Xue Yuan* (Tianjin University of Chinese Medicine) in 1989

Chai Hu (Radix Bupleuri)
Zhi Zi (Fructus Gardeniae)
Mu Li (Concha Ostreae)
Huang Qin (Radix Scutellariae)
Sheng Jiang (Rhizoma Zingiberis Recens)
Suan Zao Ren (Semen Ziziphi Spinosae)
Gou Teng (Ramulus Uncariae cum Uncis)
Xi Yang Shen (Radix Panacis Quinquefolii)
Shou Wu Teng (Caulis Polygoni Multiflori)
Bai Zhu (Rhizoma Atractylodis Macrocephalae)
Chuan Xiong (Rhizoma Chuanxiong)
Dang Gui (Radix Angelicae Sinensis)
Gui Zhi (Ramulus Cinnamomi)
Fu Ling (Poria)
Ban Xia (Rhizoma Pinelliae)
Da Huang (Radix et Rhizoma Rhei)
Da Zao (Fructus Jujubae)
Gan Cao (Radix et Rhizoma Glycyrrhizae)

Chai Hu An Shen Tang (Bupleurum Decoction to Tranquilize the Spirit) is a modified version of *Chai Hu Jia Long Gu Mu Li Tang*. The modifications include the removal of *Qian Dan* (Minium), which is generally deemed inappropriate for use today because of its potential toxicities. Furthermore, additional herbs are incorporated to enhance the effects of calming the *shen* (spirit), nourishing the blood, and tonifying qi. Common clinical applications of this formula include stress, anxiety, insomnia, emotional disturbances, and various types of mental disorders.

AUTHORS' COMMENTS

Chai Hu Jia Long Gu Mu Li Tang is one of today's most popular formulas for stress management. Similar to *Xiao Yao San* (Rambling Powder) which helps patients cope with daily stressful situations, this formula tranquilizes the *shen* (spirit), clears heat, and helps patients rest and fall asleep. Many psychosomatic disorders stem from Liver qi stagnation or Liver fire, which can be treated with the formulas mentioned above.

References

1. *Si Chuan Zhong Yi* (Sichuan Chinese Medicine) 1987;(12):30.
2. *Zhong Yao Ming Fang Yao Li Yu Ying Yong* (Pharmacology and Applications of Famous Herbal Formulas) 1989;372-373.
3. *Guo Wai Yi Xue* (Foreign Medicine) 1992;14(5):47.
4. Mizoguchi K, Yuzurihara M, Ishige A, Aburada M, Tabira T. Saiko-ka-ryukotsu-borei-to, a herbal medicine, ameliorates chronic stress-induced depressive state in rotarod performance. Pharmacol Biochem Behav 2003 May;75(2):419-25.

Chái Hú Jiā Lóng Gǔ Mǔ Lì Tāng
(Bupleurum plus Dragon Bone and Oyster Shell Decoction)

5. Mizoguchi K, Yuzurihara M, Ishige A, Sasaki H, Tabira T. Saiko-ka-ryukotsu-borei-to, an herbal medicine, prevents chronic stress-induced disruption of glucocorticoid negative feedback in rats. Life Sci 2002 Nov 22;72(1):67-77.

6. Koshikawa N, Imai T, Takahashi I, Yamauchi M, Sawada S, Kansaku A. Effects of Hochu-ekki-to, Yoku-kan-san and Saiko-ka-ryukotsu-borei-to on behavioral despair and acetic acid-induced writhing in mice. Methods Find Exp Clin Pharmacol 1998 Jan-Feb;20(1):47-51.

7. Sasaki K, Suzuki K, Yoshizaki F, Ando T. Effect of saiko-ka-ryukotsu-borei-to on the stress-induced increase of serum corticosterone in mice. Biol Pharm Bull 1995 Apr;18(4):563-5.

8. Iizuka S, Ishige A, Komatsu Y, Matsumiya T, Tsuji M, Takeda H. Effects of Saiko-ka-ryukotsu-borei-to on irritable characteristics in EI mice. Methods Find Exp Clin Pharmacol 1998 Jan-Feb;20(1):19-26.

9. Okano H, Ohkubo C. Anti-pressor effect of a Chinese-Japanese herbal medicine, saiko-ka-ryukotsu-borei-to on hemodynamics in rabbits. In Vivo 1999 Jul-Aug;13(4):333-7.

10. Wei MJ, Shintani F, Kanba S, Yagi G, Asai M, Kato R, Nakaki T. Endothelium-dependent and -independent vasoactive actions of a Japanese kampo medicine, Saiko-ka-ryukotsu-borei-to. Biomed Pharmacother 1997;51(1):38-43.

11. *Zhong Yi Fang Ji Xian Dai Yan Jiu* (Modern Study of Medical Formulae in Traditional Chinese Medicine) 1997;(1):203.

12. Yoshie F, Iizuka A, Kubo M, Komatsu Y, Matsumoto A, Itakura H, Takeda H, Matsumiya T, Kondo K. Protective effects of Saiko-ka-ryukotsu-borei-to (Chai-Hu-Jia-Long-Gu-Mu-Li-Tang) against atherosclerosis in Kurosawa and Kusanagi-hypercholesterolemic (KHC) rabbits. Pharmacol Res 2001 May;43(5):481-8.

13. Chung HJ, Kim DW, Maruyama I, Tani T. Effects of traditional Chinese formulations on rat carotid artery injured by balloon endothelial denudation. Am J Chin Med 2003;31(2):201-12.

14. *Han Fang Yi Xue* (Kampo Medicine) 1986;10(9):26.

15. *Shan Dong Zhong Yi Za Zhi* (Shandong Journal of Chinese Medicine) 1984;(3):24.

16. *Liao Ning Zhong Yi Za Zhi* (Liaoning Journal of Chinese Medicine) 1984;12:34.

17. *Zhong Xi Yi Jie He Za Zhi* (Journal of Integrated Chinese and Western Medicine) 1986;12:753.

18. *Shi Yong Zhong Xi Yi Jie He Za Zhi* (Practical Journal of Integrated Chinese and Western Medicines) 1998;2:170.

19. *Fu Jian Zhong Yi Yao* (Fujian Chinese Medicine and Herbology) 1997;4:12.

20. Nomura S, Hattori N, Sakakibara I, Fukuhara S. Effects of Saiko-ka-ryukotsu-borei-to in patients with hyperlipidemia. Phytomedicine 2001 May;8(3):165-73.

21. Kim DW, Chung HJ, Nose K, Maruyama I, Tani T. Preventive effects of a traditional Chinese formulation, Chaihu-jia-Longgu-Muli-tang, on intimal thickening of carotid artery injured by balloon endothelial denudation in rats. Journal of Pharmacy & Pharmacology 2002 Apr; 54(4):571-5.

22. Chung HJ, Maruyama I, Tani T. Saiko-ka-Ryukotsu-Borei-To inhibits intimal thickening in carotid artery after balloon endothelial denudation in cholesterol-fed rats. Biol Pharm Bull 2003 Jan;26(1):56-60.

23. *He Nan Zhong Yi* (Henan Chinese Medicine) 1999;1:18.

24. *Si Chuan Zhong Yi* (Sichuan Chinese Medicine) 1998;7:36.

25. Hung-Ming W, Liu CS, Tsai JJ, Ko LY, Wei YH. Antioxidant and anticonvulsant effect of a modified formula of chaihu-longu-muli-tang. American Journal of Chinese Medicine 2002;30(2-3):339-46.

26. *Tian Jin Zhong Yi* (Tianjin Chinese Medicine) 1999;2:25.

27. Fushitani S, Minakuchi K, Tsuchiya K, Takasugi M, Murakami K. Studies on attenuation of post-ischemic brain injury by kampo medicines-inhibitory effects of free radical production. Yakugaku Zasshi 1995 Aug;115(8):611-7.

28. Ohnishi N, Nakasako S, Okada K, Umehara S, Takara K, Nagasawa K, Yoshioka M, Kuroda K, Yokoyama T. Studies on interactions between traditional herbal and Western medicines. IV: lack of pharmacokinetic interactions between Saiko-ka-ryukotsu-borei-to and carbamazepine in rats. Eur J Drug Metab Pharmacokinet 2001 Jan-Jun;26(1-2):129-35.

29. Sanae F, Hayashi H, Chisaki K, Komatsu Y. Effects of Saiko-ka-ryukotsu-borei-to, a Japanese Kampo medicine, on tachycardia and central nervous system stimulation induced by theophylline in rats and mice. Jpn J Pharmacol 1999 Mar;79(3):283-8.

30. *Xian Dai Zhong Yao Yao Li Xue* (Contemporary Pharmacology of Chinese Herbs) 1997;1425.

31. *Si Chuan Zhong Yi* (Sichuan Chinese Medicine) 1987;5(12):30.

Chapter 9 – Shen-Calming Formulas *Section 2 – Nourishing Formulas that Calm the Shen (Spirit)*

Section 2

滋养安神剂
— Nourishing Formulas that Calm the Shen (Spirit)

Suān Zǎo Rén Tāng (Sour Jujube Decoction)
酸棗仁湯
酸枣仁汤

Pinyin Name: *Suan Zao Ren Tang*
Literal Name: Sour Jujube Decoction
Alternate Names: *Suan Zao Tang*, Zizyphus Combination
Original Source: *Jin Gui Yao Lue* (Essentials from the Golden Cabinet) by Zhang Zhong-Jing in the Eastern Han Dynasty

COMPOSITION

Suan Zao Ren (Semen Ziziphi Spinosae), *chao* (dry-fried)	2 cups [15-18g]
Chuan Xiong (Rhizoma Chuanxiong)	6g [3-5g]
Fu Ling (Poria)	6g [10g]
Zhi Mu (Rhizoma Anemarrhenae)	6g [8-10g]
Gan Cao (Radix et Rhizoma Glycyrrhizae)	3g

DOSAGE / PREPARATION / ADMINISTRATION

The source text states to first dry-fry *Suan Zao Ren* (Semen Ziziphi Spinosae), crack the seeds open, and then cook them with 8 cups [1,600 mL] of water until only 6 cups [1,200 mL] of the liquid remain. Add the other ingredients and cook until the liquid is further reduced to 3 cups [600 mL]. Take the warm, strained decoction in three equally-divided doses.

CHINESE THERAPEUTIC ACTIONS

1. Nourishes the blood and calms the *shen* (spirit)
2. Clears heat and relieves irritability

CLINICAL MANIFESTATIONS

Liver blood deficiency with deficiency-heat rising: irritability, insomnia, palpitations, night sweating, dizziness, vertigo, dry mouth and throat, and a fine, wiry pulse.

CLINICAL APPLICATIONS

Insomnia, nocturnal emissions, somnolence, neurasthenia, menopausal syndrome, and excessive worrying.

EXPLANATION

Suan Zao Ren Tang (Sour Jujube Decoction) treats insomnia characterized by Liver blood deficiency with deficiency heat rising, caused by over-exertion or chronic consumption. Palpitations and dry mouth and throat are due to blood deficiency and lack of adequate nourishment to the Heart. Patients with this syndrome may have yin deficiency and deficiency heat, which can cause irritability, insomnia, palpitations, and night sweats. Liver blood deficiency may contribute to hyperactivity of Liver yang, leading to dizziness and vertigo.

Suan Zao Ren (Semen Ziziphi Spinosae), the chief herb of this formula, nourishes Liver blood and calms Heart *shen* (spirit). *Chuan Xiong* (Rhizoma Chuanxiong) regulates Liver blood. *Fu Ling* (Poria) tranquilizes the mind and calms the *shen*. *Zhi Mu* (Rhizoma Anemarrhenae) nourishes yin and clears deficiency heat. *Gan Cao* (Radix et Rhizoma Glycyrrhizae) clears heat and harmonizes all of the herbs in this formula.

MODIFICATIONS

• If there is qi deficiency, add *Ren Shen* (Radix et Rhizoma Ginseng) and *Huang Qi* (Radix Astragali Membranacei).
• With night sweats, add *Ma Huang Gen* (Radix et Rhizoma Ephedrae) and *Wu Wei Zi* (Fructus Schisandrae Chinensis).
• With severe night sweats, add *Mu Li* (Concha Ostreae) and *Fu Xiao Mai* (Fructus Tritici Levis).

Chinese Herbal Formulas and Applications

Suān Zǎo Rén Tāng (Sour Jujube Decoction)

Suan Zao Ren Tang (Sour Jujube Decoction)

Diagnosis	Signs and Symptoms	Treatment	Herbs
Liver blood deficiency with deficiency-heat rising	• Insomnia, irritability, palpitations and night sweats: interior heat disturbing *shen* (spirit) and consuming yin • Palpitations, dry mouth and throat: blood deficiency unable to nourish the Heart • Dizziness and vertigo: Liver blood deficiency with hyperactivity of Liver yang	• Nourishes the blood and calms the *shen* • Clears heat and relieves irritability	• *Suan Zao Ren* (Semen Ziziphi Spinosae) nourishes Liver blood and calms Heart *shen*. • *Chuan Xiong* (Rhizoma Chuanxiong) regulates Liver blood. • *Fu Ling* (Poria) tranquilizes the mind and calms the *shen*. • *Zhi Mu* (Rhizoma Anemarrhenae) nourishes yin and clears deficiency heat. • *Gan Cao* (Radix et Rhizoma Glycyrrhizae) clears heat and harmonizes all of the herbs.

• With irritability, thirst, and insomnia, add *Mai Dong* (Tuber Ophiopogonis Japonici) and *Wu Wei Zi* (Fructus Schisandrae Chinensis).

• With irritability, restlessness, and insomnia, add *Wen Dan Tang* (Warm the Gallbladder Decoction).

• For insomnia due to blood deficiency, add *Dang Gui* (Radix Angelicae Sinensis), *Shu Di Huang* (Radix Rehmanniae Glutinosae Conquitae), and *He Shou Wu* (Radix Polygoni Multiflori).

• For insomnia due to heat, add *Mu Dan Pi* (Cortex Moutan Radicis), *Zhi Zi* (Fructus Gardeniae Jasminoidis), and *Dan Zhu Ye* (Herba Lophatheri).

• With fright and palpitations, add *Yuan Zhi* (Radix Polygalae Tenuifoliae) and *Shi Chang Pu* (Rhizoma Acori Graminei).

• With excessive thinking and insomnia, add *Yi Gan San* (Restrain the Liver Powder).

• With palpitations and excessive dreams, or waking up at night from nightmares due to Heart and Gallbladder deficiencies, add *Dang Shen* (Radix Codonopsis) and *Long Chi* (Dens Draconis).

• With deficiency fire flaring, remove *Chuan Xiong* (Rhizoma Chuanxiong) and add *Bai Shao* (Radix Paeoniae Alba), *Di Huang* (Radix Rehmanniae), and *Huang Lian* (Rhizoma Coptidis).

PHARMACOLOGICAL EFFECTS

Central nervous system: Administration of *Suan Zao Ren Tang* was associated with marked sedative and hypnotic effects. According to various experiments in mice, rats, guinea pigs, rabbits, dogs, and humans, administration of the formula decreased spontaneous physical activities, inhibited caffeine-induced stimulation, and potentiated the effects of sedative and hypnotic drugs.[1]

CLINICAL STUDIES AND RESEARCH

1. **Insomnia**: Use of modified *Suan Zao Ren Tang* was associated with 91.7% effectiveness in treating insomnia.

Modifications were made by adding *Long Dan* (Radix et Rhizoma Gentianae) and *Chai Hu* (Radix Bupleuri) for restlessness, irritability, anger, red eyes, a bitter taste in the mouth, red tongue, yellow tongue coating, and a wiry, rapid pulse; *Tao Ren* (Semen Persicae), *Hong Hua* (Flos Carthami), and *Shou Wu Teng* (Caulis Polygoni Multiflori) for blood stagnation; *E Jiao* (Colla Corii Asini), *Huang Bo* (Cortex Phellodendri Chinensis), and *Bie Jia* (Carapax Trionycis) for yin-deficient heat; *Dang Shen* (Radix Codonopsis), *Huang Qi* (Radix Astragali), and *He Huan Pi* (Cortex Albiziae) for qi and blood deficiencies; *Huang Qi* (Radix Astragali) and *Yuan Zhi* (Radix Polygalae) for Heart qi deficiency; and *Dan Nan Xing* (Arisaema cum Bile) and *Zhu Li* (Succus Bambusae) for profuse sputum. The herbs were given 30 minutes before bedtime. Of 72 patients, the study reported recovery in 47 cases, significant improvement in 12 cases, moderate improvement in 7 cases, and no effect in 6 cases.[2] In another study, 20 out of 31 patients (64.5%) reported improvement following ingestion of 2.5g of an extract preparation of *Suan Zao Ren Tang*. Improvement was defined as shorter time needed to fall asleep, better quality of sleep, and better energy during the following day.[3]

2. **Nocturnal emissions**: Modified *Suan Zao Ren Tang* was effective in treating 28 patients with nocturnal emissions. The modifications included the addition of *Huang Bo* (Cortex Phellodendri Chinensis) and others as deemed necessary. The duration of treatment ranged from 10 to 30 days. The overall effectiveness was 78.6%.[4]

RELATED FORMULA

Ding Zhi Wán (Settle the Emotions Pill)

定志丸

Pinyin Name: *Ding Zhi Wan*

Literal Name: Settle the Emotions Pill

Original Source: *Za Bing Yuan Liu Xi Zhu* (Wondrous Lantern for Peering into Origin and Development of Miscellaneous Diseases) by Shen Jin-Ao in 1773

SHEN-CALMING FORMULAS

9

723

Chapter 9 – Shen-Calming Formulas　　　　　　*Section 2 – Nourishing Formulas that Calm the Shen (Spirit)*

Suān Zǎo Rén Tāng (Sour Jujube Decoction)

Ren Shen (Radix et Rhizoma Ginseng)	90g
Fu Ling (Poria)	90g
Fu Shen (Poria Paradicis)	90g
Shi Chang Pu (Rhizoma Acori Tatarinowii)	60g
Yuan Zhi (Radix Polygalae),	
chao (dry-fried) with ginger	60g
Zhu Sha (Cinnabaris)	30g

Note: *Zhu Sha* (Cinnabaris) is a potentially toxic heavy metal, and is rarely used as a medicinal substance today. Its discussion here is included primarily for academic purposes, to reflect the historical use of this substance in its original formulation. Most herbal products today have removed it completely, or replaced it with substitutes with similar functions. For additional information on the toxicity, please refer to *Chinese Medical Herbology and Pharmacology* by John Chen and Tina Chen.

The source text states to grind all of the ingredients and only 15g of *Zhu Sha* (Cinnabaris) into powder and form into pills with honey. Use the other 15g of *Zhu Sha* (Cinnabaris) to coat the pills. Take 6g of pills with warm, boiled water, before bedtime.

The main actions of *Ding Zhi Wan* (Settle the Emotions Pill) are to tonify Heart qi, benefit cognitive functions, calm the *shen* (spirit), and ease fear and fright. It is generally indicated for individuals who have fear and fright, yet become easily angered, and have insomnia.

Suan Zao Ren Tang and *Ding Zhi Wan* (Settle the Emotions Pill) have functions to nourish and calm the *shen* (spirit).
- *Suan Zao Ren Tang* treats insomnia caused by blood deficiency and the inability of blood to nourish the Heart. The primary functions of the formula are to nourish the blood, clear heat, and calm the *shen*.
- *Ding Zhi Wan* treats insomnia with fear and fright caused by Heart qi deficiency. The main actions of the formula are to tonify Heart qi and calm the *shen*.

AUTHORS' COMMENTS

Suan Zao Ren Tang is one of the most commonly used formulas for treating insomnia. It is most effective for insomnia due to deficiency, irritability, and consumption, with such key signs and symptoms as irritability, palpitations, dry mouth and throat, and a fine, wiry pulse.

Proper processing of *Suan Zao Ren* (Semen Ziziphi Spinosae) is extremely important, as it will determine the overall effectiveness of this formula. According to the source text, *Suan Zao Ren* (Semen Ziziphi Spinosae) must be dry-fried first, then the seeds should be crushed open, before placing them in water for cooking. Dry-frying the seeds enhances the effects of tonifying Liver blood and treating insomnia; crushing them maximizes extraction of the active ingredients.[5]

Suan Zao Ren Tang, *Tian Wang Bu Xin Dan* (Emperor of Heaven's Special Pill to Tonify the Heart), and *Gan Mai Da Zao Tang* (Licorice, Wheat, and Jujube Decoction) all treat insomnia, palpitations, and anxiety caused by lack of nourishment to the Heart and leading to *shen* (spirit) disturbance.
- *Suan Zao Ren Tang* is best for nourishing Liver blood and clearing deficiency heat. Chief manifestations include irritability, restlessness, vertigo, night sweats, and dry mouth and throat.
- *Tian Wang Bu Xin Dan* is better for nourishing yin and blood caused by Kidney and Heart deficiencies. Chief manifestations include anxiety, decreased sleep, palpitations, and a withered *shen*.
- *Gan Mai Da Zao Tang* harmonizes the middle *jiao*, relieves pain, and treats yin deficiency of the *zang* organs with Liver qi stagnation and Heart deficiency. Chief manifestations include frequent crying urges, emotional mood swings, and absent-mindedness.[6]

Please refer to *Gui Pi Tang* (Restore the Spleen Decoction) for a comparison of the uses, similarities, and differences between *Tian Wang Bu Xin Dan* (Emperor of Heaven's Special Pill to Tonify the Heart) and *Suan Zao Ren Tang*.

References
1. *Zhong Yi Fang Ji Xian Dai Yan Jiu* (Modern Study of Medical Formulae in Traditional Chinese Medicine) 1997;849-850.
2. *He Nan Zhong Yi* (Henan Chinese Medicine) 1999;6:9.
3. *Shan Dong Yi Kan* (Shandong Medical Journal) 1965;27.
4. *Shi Yong Zhong Xi Yi Jie He Za Zhi* (Practical Journal of Integrated Chinese and Western Medicines) 1991;12:729.
5. *Zhe Jiang Zhong Yi Za Zhi* (Zhejiang Journal of Chinese Medicine) 1966;(1).
6. Wang MZ, et al. *Zhong Yi Xue Wen Da Ti Ku* (Questions and Answers on Traditional Chinese Medicine: Herbal Formulas).

724

Chinese Herbal Formulas and Applications

Tiān Wáng Bǔ Xīn Dān
(Emperor of Heaven's Special Pill to Tonify the Heart)

天王補心丹
天王补心丹

Pinyin Name: *Tian Wang Bu Xin Dan*
Literal Name: Emperor of Heaven's Special Pill to Tonify the Heart
Alternate Name: Ginseng and Zizyphus Formula
Original Source: *Jiao Zhu Fu Ren Liang Fang* (Revised Fine Formulas for Women) by Bi Li-Zhai in the 16th century

COMPOSITION

Di Huang (Radix Rehmanniae), *xi* (washed) with liquor	120g [12g]
Xuan Shen (Radix Scrophulariae)	15g [5g]
Tian Dong (Radix Asparagi)	30g [9g]
Mai Dong (Radix Ophiopogonis)	30g [9g]
Dan Shen (Radix et Rhizoma Salviae Miltiorrhizae)	15g [5g]
Dang Gui (Radix Angelicae Sinensis), *jin* (soaked) with liquor	30g [9g]
Ren Shen (Radix et Rhizoma Ginseng)	15g [5g]
Fu Ling (Poria)	15g [5g]
Suan Zao Ren (Semen Ziziphi Spinosae), *chao* (dry-fried)	30g [9g]
Wu Wei Zi (Fructus Schisandrae Chinensis)	30g [9g]
Bai Zi Ren (Semen Platycladi)	30g [9g]
Yuan Zhi (Radix Polygalae)	15g [5g]
Jie Geng (Radix Platycodonis)	15g [5g]

Note: *Zhu Sha* (Cinnabaris) is a potentially toxic heavy metal, and is rarely used as a medicinal substance today. Its discussion here is included primarily for academic purposes, to reflect the historical use of this substance in its original formulation. Most herbal products today have removed it completely, or replaced it with substitutes with similar functions. For additional information on the toxicity, please refer to *Chinese Medical Herbology and Pharmacology* by John Chen and Tina Chen.

DOSAGE / PREPARATION / ADMINISTRATION

Grind the ingredients into powder and form into small pills with honey. The pills should resemble the size of *Wu Tong Zi* (Semen Firmianae), a small seed approximately 5 mm in diameter. Coat the pills with *Zhu Sha* (Cinnabaris). Take 20-30 pills [9g] per dose on an empty stomach with either warm/hot boiled water or with a decoction of *Zhu Ye* (Herba Phyllostachys). Today, this formula may be prepared and administered as pills or decoction. For pills, take 9g per dose with warm/hot boiled water. For decoction, use the suggested doses in brackets above.

CHINESE THERAPEUTIC ACTIONS

1. Nourishes yin and tonifies the blood
2. Tonifies the Heart and Kidney
3. Calms the *shen* (spirit)

CLINICAL MANIFESTATIONS

Heart and Kidney deficiencies with yin and blood insufficiencies: generalized weakness and deficiency, forgetfulness, irritability, insomnia, palpitations, lassitude, nocturnal emissions, dry stools, tongue ulceration, a red tongue body with little coating, and a fine, rapid pulse.

CLINICAL APPLICATIONS

Coronary heart disease, angina, viral myocarditis, hypertension, hyperthyroidism, neurasthenia, mental instability, attention deficit disorder, insomnia, impotence, and hepatitis.

EXPLANATION

Tian Wang Bu Xin Dan (Emperor of Heaven's Special Pill to Tonify the Heart) is designed to treat Heart and Kidney deficiencies with yin and blood insufficiencies. Heart blood deficiency may lead to hyperactivity of yang, resulting in forgetfulness, irritability, insomnia, and palpitations. Deficiency of blood may cause malnourishment of the body, leading to lassitude. Kidney yin deficiency may lead to instability of the *jing* (essence) and nocturnal emissions. Dry stools indicate yin deficiency with insufficient nourishment to the bowels. Since the tongue is the sense organ that belongs to the Heart, Heart yin deficiency may lead to tongue ulcerations. A red tongue body with

SHEN-CALMING FORMULAS

9

725

Chapter 9 – Shen-Calming Formulas   *Section 2 – Nourishing Formulas that Calm the Shen (Spirit)*

Tiān Wáng Bǔ Xīn Dān
(Emperor of Heaven's Special Pill to Tonify the Heart)

Tian Wang Bu Xin Dan (Emperor of Heaven's Special Pill to Tonify the Heart)

Diagnosis	Signs and Symptoms	Treatment	Herbs
Heart and Kidney deficiencies with yin and blood insufficiencies	• Forgetfulness and palpitations: Heart blood deficiency • Irritability and insomnia: hyperactivity of yang due to Heart blood deficiency • Lassitude: malnourishment of the body due to blood deficiency • Dry stools: yin-deficient fire consuming body fluids • Tongue ulcerations: yin-deficient fire rising upward • Red tongue body with little coating and a fine, rapid pulse: yin-deficient fire	• Nourishes yin and tonifies the blood • Tonifies the Heart and Kidney • Calms the *shen* (spirit)	• *Di Huang* (Radix Rehmanniae) tonifies yin and blood, moistens dryness and helps to control hyperactivity of yang. • *Xuan Shen* (Radix Scrophulariae), *Tian Dong* (Radix Asparagi) and *Mai Dong* (Radix Ophiopogonis) tonify yin to clear deficiency fire. • *Dan Shen* (Radix et Rhizoma Salviae Miltiorrhizae) and *Dang Gui* (Radix Angelicae Sinensis) tonify blood and activate blood circulation. • *Ren Shen* (Radix et Rhizoma Ginseng) and *Fu Ling* (Poria) tonify qi and calm the *shen*. • *Suan Zao Ren* (Semen Ziziphi Spinosae) and *Wu Wei Zi* (Fructus Schisandrae Chinensis) astringe the Heart qi to calm the *shen*. • *Bai Zi Ren* (Semen Platycladi), *Yuan Zhi* (Radix Polygalae) and *Zhu Sha* (Cinnabaris) nourish the Heart to calm the *shen*. • *Jie Geng* (Radix Platycodonis) leads all of the herbs to the upper *jiao*. • *Zhu Sha* (Cinnabaris) and *Zhu Ye* (Herba Phyllostachys) calm the *shen* and guide the formula to the Heart.

little coating, and a fine, rapid pulse, both suggest yin deficiency.

Di Huang (Radix Rehmanniae) is the chief herb in this formula. It tonifies yin and blood, helps to control hyperactivity of yang, and moistens dryness. It also nourishes Kidney water, and helps to control Heart fire. *Xuan Shen* (Radix Scrophulariae), *Tian Dong* (Radix Asparagi), and *Mai Dong* (Radix Ophiopogonis) tonify yin to clear deficiency fire. *Dan Shen* (Radix et Rhizoma Salviae Miltiorrhizae) and *Dang Gui* (Radix Angelicae Sinensis) tonify blood and activate blood circulation. *Ren Shen* (Radix et Rhizoma Ginseng) and *Fu Ling* (Poria) tonify qi and calm the *shen* (spirit). *Suan Zao Ren* (Semen Ziziphi Spinosae) and *Wu Wei Zi* (Fructus Schisandrae Chinensis) astringe Heart qi to calm the *shen*. *Bai Zi Ren* (Semen Platycladi), *Yuan Zhi* (Radix Polygalae) and *Zhu Sha* (Cinnabaris) nourish the Heart to calm the *shen*. *Jie Geng* (Radix Platycodonis) is a channel-guiding herb that leads all of the herbs to the upper *jiao*. *Zhu Sha* (Cinnabaris) and *Zhu Ye* (Herba Phyllostachys) calm the *shen* and guide the formula to the Heart.

MODIFICATIONS
• With toothache, add *Qing Wei San* (Clear the Stomach Powder).

• With ulcerations of the mouth and tongue, add *Huang Lian* (Rhizoma Coptidis) and *Mu Dan Pi* (Cortex Moutan Radicis).

• With dry mouth and throat, add *Shi Hu* (Caulis Dendrobii) and *Yu Zhu* (Rhizoma Polygonati Odorati).

• If there is constipation, add *Zhi Shi* (Fructus Immaturus Citri Aurantii) and *Hou Po* (Cortex Magnoliae Officinalis).

• With severe palpitations, insomnia, or restless *shen* (spirit), add *Long Yan Rou* (Arillus Longanae Euphoriae) and *Shou Wu Teng* (Caulis Polygoni Multiflori).

• With inability to concentrate, forgetfulness, or to enhance memory, add *Yuan Zhi* (Radix Polygalae), *Shi Chang Pu* (Rhizoma Acori Tatarinowii), and *Yin Xing Ye* (Folium Ginkgo).

• For more severe insomnia, add *Long Gu* (Os Draconis) and *Ci Shi* (Magnetitum).

• For spermatorrhea or nocturnal emissions, add *Jin Ying Zi* (Fructus Rosae Laevigatae), *Qian Shi* (Semen Euryales), and *Mu Li* (Concha Ostreae).

726

Tiān Wáng Bǔ Xīn Dān
(Emperor of Heaven's Special Pill to Tonify the Heart)

- With dizziness and vertigo, add *Chuan Xiong* (Rhizoma Chuanxiong) and *Bai Zhi* (Radix Angelicae Dahuricae).
- With excessive thinking and worrying, add *Xiao Yao San* (Rambling Powder).
- For insomnia or restless sleep, add *Suan Zao Ren Tang* (Sour Jujube Decoction).

CAUTIONS / CONTRAINDICATIONS

- While taking *Tian Wang Bu Xin Dan*, avoid the following: cilantro, garlic, radishes, seafood, and liquor.
- This formula contains many rich tonics, which make it unsuitable for long-term use by patients who have Spleen and Stomach deficiencies, or those with damp or phlegm accumulation.
- According to one report, use of this formula may cause occasional side effects such as indigestion, epigastric fullness and distention, mild diarrhea, skin rashes, and itching.[1]

PHARMACOLOGICAL EFFECTS

1. **Central nervous system**: Many herbs in *Tian Wang Bu Xin Dan* have marked sedative and hypnotic effects, including *Dang Gui* (Radix Angelicae Sinensis), *Fu Ling* (Sclerotium Poriae Cocos), *Yuan Zhi* (Radix Polygalae Tenuifoliae), *Bai Zi Ren* (Semen Biotae Orientalis), and *Suan Zao Ren* (Semen Ziziphi Spinosae). Furthermore, some of the herbs also improve cognitive functions, such as *Ren Shen* (Radix et Rhizoma Ginseng) and *Wu Wei Zi* (Fructus Schisandrae Chinensis).[2]
2. **Cardiovascular**: Laboratory experiments in mice showed administration of the formula to be beneficial in cases of shock, angina, arrhythmia, and hypoxia. The mechanisms of action are attributed to increased blood perfusion to the heart and increased resistance to hypoxia.[3]

CLINICAL STUDIES AND RESEARCH

1. **Neurasthenia**: In one study, 218 patients with neurasthenia were treated with *Tian Wang Bu Xin Dan* with an overall 66.5% rate of effectiveness. The treatment protocol was to administer the herbs in pills, 10-15 pills (1 g/pill) three times daily before meals and at bedtime. The duration of treatment was 30 days per course.[4]
2. **Coronary heart disease**: *Tian Wang Bu Xin Dan* has beneficial effects in treating coronary heart disease, angina, hypotension, palpitations and insomnia. It was noted that the dose of *Ren Shen* (Radix et Rhizoma Ginseng) should be 15g or above to have significant impact.[5]
3. **Angina**: Use of modified *Tian Wang Bu Xin Dan* in 35 patients with angina was associated with complete recovery in 10 cases, improvement in 20 cases, and no effect in 5 cases. In addition to *Tian Wang Bu Xin Dan*

as the base formula, modifications were made as needed. For a feeling of severe oppression in the chest, *Fo Shou* (Fructus Citri Sarcodactylis), *Zhi Shi* (Fructus Aurantii Immaturus), and *Tan Xiang* (Lignum Santali Albi) were added. For severe angina pain, a preparation containing *Su He Xiang* (Styrax) and *Bing Pian* (Borneolum Syntheticum) was added. For Heart yin deficiency, *Dang Shen* (Radix Codonopsis) was added. For insomnia, *Shou Wu Teng* (Caulis Polygoni Multiflori) and *He Huan Pi* (Cortex Albiziae) were added. For a thick, greasy tongue coating, *Gua Lou* (Fructus Trichosanthis) was added. And, for irregular heartbeat, *Zhi Gan Cao* (Radix et Rhizoma Glycyrrhizae Praeparata cum Melle) was added.[6]

4. **Viral myocarditis**: In one study of 23 patients with viral myocarditis, use of modified *Tian Wang Bu Xin Dan* daily for 1-3 courses of treatment (10 days per course) was associated with 95.6% effectiveness. In addition to *Tian Wang Bu Xin Dan*, intravenous infusion of *Dan Shen* (Radix et Rhizoma Salviae Miltiorrhizae) was given for cases of severe blood stagnation. Of 23 cases, the study reported complete recovery in 16 cases, moderate improvement in 6 cases, and no effect in 1 case.[7]

5. **Insomnia**: Administration of *Tian Wang Bu Xin Dan* showed marked effectiveness in the treatment of insomnia. Depending on the dose and dosage form, the rate of success ranged from 87-96%.[8]

6. **Impotence**: Administration of modified *Tian Wang Bu Xin Dan* effectively treated 30 of 37 patients with impotence. The herbal treatment was based on *Tian Wang Bu Xin Dan*, with the addition of *Zhu Ye* (Herba Phyllostachys), *Mu Tong* (Caulis Akebiae), and *Zhu Sha* (Cinnabaris) for ulcerations of the mouth and tongue as well as burning sensations and pain in the penis; *Jin Ying Zi* (Fructus Rosae Laevigatae) and *Qian Shi* (Semen Euryales) for premature ejaculation and seminal emission; and *Gan Mai Da Zao Tang* (Licorice, Wheat, and Jujube Decoction) for palpitations with fear and fright. In addition to herbs, patients were advised to control their emotions, avoid spicy and pungent foods, and not to engage in excessive sexual activity.[9]

7. **Hepatitis**: In one study, modified *Tian Wang Bu Xin Dan* was used to treat 34 patients with chronic hepatitis characterized by yin deficiency. The patients presented with irritability, restlessness, insomnia, dizziness, vertigo, hypochondriac fullness, and pain. The treatment protocol was to administer the herbs in decoction one time daily, for 30 days per course of treatment. The average duration of treatment was 46.7 days. The study reported an overall effectiveness of 94.1%. Most patients reported improvement in signs and symptoms, reduced size of the spleen and liver, and decreased levels of liver enzymes.[10]

Chapter 9 – Shen-Calming Formulas　　　　　　　　*Section 2 – Nourishing Formulas that Calm the Shen (Spirit)*

Tiān Wáng Bǔ Xīn Dān
(Emperor of Heaven's Special Pill to Tonify the Heart)

TOXICOLOGY

Use of *Tian Wang Bu Xin Dan* has been associated with side effects such as a general feeling of warmth, thirst, rash and eczema of the entire body.[11] Note: These reactions are due to older formulations of the product containing *Zhu Sha* (Cinnabaris), a potentially toxic substance, in the coating of the pellets. Most products today do ***not*** contain *Zhu Sha* (Cinnabaris), and should not cause these side effects.

RELATED FORMULAS

Tiān Wáng Bǔ Xīn Dān

(Emperor of Heaven's Special Pill to Tonify the Heart)

天王補心丹
天王补心丹

Pinyin Name: *Tian Wang Bu Xin Dan*
Literal Name: Emperor of Heaven's Special Pill to Tonify the Heart
Original Source: *She Sheng Mi Pou* (Secrets Investigations into Obtaining Health) by Hong Ji in 1638

Di Huang (Radix Rehmanniae), *xi* (washed) with liquor	120g
Ren Shen (Radix et Rhizoma Ginseng)	15g
Dan Shen (Radix et Rhizoma Salviae Miltiorrhizae), *chao* (dry-fried) lightly	15g
Xuan Shen (Radix Scrophulariae), *chao* (dry-fried) lightly	15g
Fu Ling (Poria)	15g
Wu Wei Zi (Fructus Schisandrae Chinensis), *hong* (baked)	15g
Yuan Zhi (Radix Polygalae), *chao* (dry-fried)	15g
Jie Geng (Radix Platycodonis)	15g
Dang Gui (Radix Angelicae Sinensis), *xi* (washed) with liquor	60g
Tian Dong (Radix Asparagi)	60g
Mai Dong (Radix Ophiopogonis)	60g
Bai Zi Ren (Semen Platycladi), *chao* (dry-fried)	60g
Suan Zao Ren (Semen Ziziphi Spinosae)	60g

Grind the ingredients into powder and form into small pills with honey. The pills should resemble the size of *Wu Tong Zi* (Semen Firmianae), a small seed approximately 5 mm in diameter. Coat the pills with 9-15g of powdered *Zhu Sha* (Cinnabaris). Take 9g of pills per dose on an empty stomach with either warm/hot boiled water or with a decoction of *Long Yan Rou* (Arillus Longan). This formula has the same name and therapeutic actions as the primary formula, and they differ only in doses and preparation of the ingredients.

Tiān Wáng Bǔ Xīn Dān

(Emperor of Heaven's Special Pill to Tonify the Heart)

天王補心丹
天王补心丹

Pinyin Name: *Tian Wang Bu Xin Dan*
Literal Name: Emperor of Heaven's Special Pill to Tonify the Heart
Original Source: *Shi Yi De Xiao Fang* (Effective Formulas from Generations of Physicians) by Wei Yi-Lin in 1345

Di Huang (Radix Rehmanniae)	60g
Shu Di Huang (Radix Rehmanniae Praeparata)	60g
Fu Ling (Poria)	30g
Fu Shen (Poria Paradicis)	30g
Dang Gui (Radix Angelicae Sinensis)	30g
Yuan Zhi (Radix Polygalae)	30g
Shi Chang Pu (Rhizoma Acori Tatarinowii)	30g
Xuan Shen (Radix Scrophulariae)	30g
Ren Shen (Radix et Rhizoma Ginseng)	30g
Mai Dong (Radix Ophiopogonis)	30g
Tian Dong (Radix Asparagi)	30g
Jie Geng (Radix Platycodonis)	30g
Bai Bu (Radix Stemonae)	30g
Bai Zi Ren (Semen Platycladi)	30g
Du Zhong (Cortex Eucommiae)	30g
Zhi Gan Cao (Radix et Rhizoma Glycyrrhizae Praeparata cum Melle)	30g
Dan Shen (Radix et Rhizoma Salviae Miltiorrhizae)	30g
Suan Zao Ren (Semen Ziziphi Spinosae)	30g
Wu Wei Zi (Fructus Schisandrae Chinensis)	30g

The source text states to grind all ingredients into powder, and form into pills with honey. The pills are coated with *Jin Bo* (gold foil), and should weigh 3 grams each. Take one pill after meals and at bedtime with a decoction made from *Deng Xin Cao* (Medulla Junci) and *Da Zao* (Fructus Jujubae).

This formula has functions to moisten yin, nourish blood, tonify the Heart, and calm the *shen* (spirit). It is used to treat excessive worrying and over thinking, leading to symptoms such as dry mouth and throat, forgetfulness, nocturnal emission, ulcerations of the mouth and tongue, dry stools, a red tongue with thin tongue coating, and fine, rapid pulse.

Bǎi Zǐ Yǎng Xīn Wán

(Biota Seed Pill to Nourish the Heart)

柏子養心丸
柏子养心丸

728

Chinese Herbal Formulas and Applications

Tiān Wáng Bǔ Xīn Dān
(Emperor of Heaven's Special Pill to Tonify the Heart)

Pinyin Name: *Bai Zi Yang Xin Wan*
Literal Name: Biota Seed Pill to Nourish the Heart
Original Source: *Ti Ren Hui Bian* (Compilation of Materials of Benevolence for the Body) by Peng Yong-Guang in 1549

Bai Zi Ren (Semen Platycladi)	120g [12g]
Gou Qi Zi (Fructus Lycii)	90g [9g]
Mai Dong (Radix Ophiopogonis)	30g [5g]
Dang Gui (Radix Angelicae Sinensis)	30g [5g]
Shi Chang Pu (Rhizoma Acori Tatarinowii)	30g [5g]
Fu Shen (Poria Paradicis)	30g [5g]
Xuan Shen (Radix Scrophulariae)	60g [6g]
Shu Di Huang (Radix Rehmanniae Praeparata)	60g [6g]
Gan Cao (Radix et Rhizoma Glycyrrhizae)	15g [5g]

The source text states to grind the ingredients into powder and form into small pills with honey. The pills should resemble the size of *Wu Tong Zi* (Semen Firmianae), a small seed approximately 5 mm in diameter. Take 40-50 pills [6g] per dose. Today, this formula may be prepared as a decoction using the suggested doses in brackets.

The main actions of this formula are to nourish the Heart, calm the *shen* (spirit), tonify the Kidney, and nourish yin. *Bai Zi Yang Xin Wan* (Biota Seed Pill to Nourish the Heart) treats disharmony of the Heart and Kidney with deficiency of *ying* (nutrition) and blood, manifesting in symptoms such as disorientation, severe palpitations, excessive dreams, dream-disturbed sleep, forgetfulness, and night sweats.

Yǎng Xīn Dān (Nourish the Heart Pill)
養心丹
养心丹
Pinyin Name: *Yang Xin Dan*
Literal Name: Nourish the Heart Pill
Original Source: *Tian Jin Zhong Yi Xue Yuan* (Tianjin University of Chinese Medicine) in 1989

Di Huang (Radix Rehmanniae)
Ren Shen (Radix et Rhizoma Ginseng)
Dan Shen (Radix et Rhizoma Salviae Miltiorrhizae)
Xuan Shen (Radix Scrophulariae)
Fu Ling (Poria)
Wu Wei Zi (Fructus Schisandrae Chinensis)
Yuan Zhi (Radix Polygalae)
Jie Geng (Radix Platycodonis)
Dang Gui (Radix Angelicae Sinensis)
Tian Dong (Radix Asparagi)

Mai Dong (Radix Ophiopogonis)
Bai Zi Ren (Semen Platycladi)
Suan Zao Ren (Semen Ziziphi Spinosae)
Shi Chang Pu (Rhizoma Acori Tatarinowii)
Yin Xing Ye (Folium Ginkgo)

Yang Xin Dan (Nourish the Heart Pill) has essentially the same ingredients and functions as *Tian Wang Bu Xin Dan*. Minor modifications include the removal of *Zhu Sha* (Cinnabaris), which is deemed inappropriate for use today, and the addition of *Shi Chang Pu* (Rhizoma Acori Tatarinowii) and *Yin Xing Ye* (Folium Ginkgo) to help open the sensory orifices and improve the overall efficacy of the formula.

Zhěn Zhōng Dān (Pillow Special Pill)
枕中丹
Pinyin Name: *Zhen Zhong Dan*
Literal Name: Pillow Special Pill
Original Source: *Bei Ji Qian Jin Yao Fang* (Thousands of Golden Prescriptions for Emergencies) by Sun Si-Miao in the Tang Dynasty

Gui Ban (Plastrum Testudinis)
Long Gu (Os Draconis)
Yuan Zhi (Radix Polygalae)
Shi Chang Pu (Rhizoma Acori Tatarinowii)

Grind equal amounts of the ingredients into powder and form into pills with honey. Take 9g of pills per dose with grain-based liquor.

These herbs combine to calm the Heart, improve cognition, and sedate the *shen* (spirit). *Zhen Zhong Dan* (Pillow Special Pill) is generally used for individuals with forgetfulness and insomnia caused by a restless Heart and *shen* disturbance.

AUTHORS' COMMENTS
These three formulas have the same name, and similar functions and clinical applications.
- *Tian Wang Bu Xin Dan* from *Jiao Zhu Fu Ren Liang Fang* (Revised Fine Formulas for Women) is generally considered to be the representative formula, since this composition is most commonly used today.
- *Tian Wang Bu Xin Dan* from *She Sheng Mi Pou* (Secrets Investigations into Obtaining Health) is usually considered to be a related formula, but it was published approximately 200 years later. It has the same composition, but differ slightly in doses.

9

SHEN-CALMING FORMULAS

729

Chapter 9 – Shen-Calming Formulas   *Section 2 – Nourishing Formulas that Calm the Shen (Spirit)*

Tiān Wáng Bǔ Xīn Dān
(Emperor of Heaven's Special Pill to Tonify the Heart)

- *Tian Wang Bu Xin Dan* from *Shi Yi De Xiao Fang* (Effective Formulas from Generations of Physicians) is also considered to be a related formula. Though it was published first, this composition is not as frequently used today.

Tian Wang Bu Xin Dan, *Bai Zi Yang Xin Wan* (Biota Seed Pill to Nourish the Heart), and *Zhen Zhong Dan* (Pillow Special Pill) all treat insomnia. Their differences are as follows:

- *Tian Wang Bu Xin Dan* treats both the cause and the symptoms of insomnia by nourishing yin, tonifying blood, benefiting qi, and calming the Heart. It is one of the most commonly used formulas for treating insomnia arising from yin and blood deficiencies.
- *Bai Zi Yang Xin Wan* is primarily a tonic formula that treats insomnia caused by Heart and Kidney deficiencies.
- *Zhen Zhong Dan* is primarily a sedating formula that addresses forgetfulness and insomnia caused by a restless Heart and disturbed *shen* (spirit).

Tian Wang Bu Xin Dan and *Gui Pi Tang* (Restore the Spleen Decoction) both nourish the Heart and calm the *shen* (spirit) to treat palpitations, forgetfulness, and insomnia.

- *Tian Wang Bu Xin Dan* is indicated for patients with disharmony of the Heart and Kidney, in which a deficient Kidney yin is unable to nourish the Heart, and thus creates Heart fire. Besides blood deficiency signs of palpitations, forgetfulness, and insomnia, symptoms of Heart fire will also manifest such as that of irritability, night sweats, nocturnal emissions, ulcers on the tongue, and dry stools or constipation. This formula uses herbs that not only nourish yin and blood, but also have tranquilizing and calming effects, such as *Suan Zao Ren* (Semen Ziziphi Spinosae), *Bai Zi Ren* (Semen Platycladi), *Yuan Zhi* (Radix Polygalae), *Tian Dong* (Radix Asparagi), and *Mai Dong* (Radix Ophiopogonis).
- *Gui Pi Tang* is designed for individuals who worry excessively, resulting in qi and blood deficiencies of the Spleen and Heart. Other than *shen* (spirit) disturbance signs, they will exhibit poor appetite, decreased dietary intake, lassitude, shortness of breath, spontaneous sweating, and other Spleen deficiency signs. Therefore, besides tranquilizing herbs such as *Suan Zao Ren* (Semen Ziziphi Spinosae), *Fu Shen* (Poria Paradicis), *Long Yan Rou* (Arillus Longan), and *Yuan Zhi* (Radix Polygalae), this formula contains Spleen tonic herbs such as *Ren Shen* (Radix et Rhizoma Ginseng), *Huang Qi* (Radix Astragali), *Bai Zhu* (Rhizoma Atractylodis Macrocephalae), and

Gan Cao (Radix et Rhizoma Glycyrrhizae). *Mu Xiang* (Radix Aucklandiae) is added to regulate qi and awaken the Spleen. This formula can also be used for bleeding or bruising due to a deficient Spleen not being able to retain the blood inside the vessels.[12]

Tian Wang Bu Xin Dan and *Zhi Gan Cao Tang* (Honey-Fried Licorice Decoction) both nourish yin and blood, and thus address the palpitations, anxiety, insomnia, and dry stools.

- *Tian Wang Bu Xin Dan* is better for Heart yin and blood deficiencies with excess Heart yang flaring. Anxiety, decreased sleep, palpitations, withered *shen* (spirit), nocturnal emissions, and nervousness are the result of the *shen* not being nourished. Therefore, nourishing herbs as well as *shen*-calming herbs are used in this formula.
- *Zhi Gan Cao Tang* is mainly used for qi and blood deficiencies. Blood deficiency results in inability to nourish the Heart. With the qi being deficient, the yang is weak and cannot generate the pulse, leading to a bounding or intermittent pulse. Qi tonics, along with yin and blood tonics, are used to generate the pulse. *Shu Di Huang* (Radix Rehmanniae Praeparata), *Sheng Jiang* (Rhizoma Zingiberis Recens), *E Jiao* (Colla Corii Asini), *Mai Dong* (Radix Ophiopogonis), and *Da Zao* (Fructus Jujubae) nourish yin and blood. *Ren Shen* (Radix et Rhizoma Ginseng) and *Zhi Gan Cao* (Radix et Rhizoma Glycyrrhizae Praeparata cum Melle) warm and tonify qi. *Gui Zhi* (Ramulus Cinnamomi) and *Sheng Jiang* (Rhizoma Zingiberis Recens) assist Heart yang to generate the pulse. This formula can also be used for Lung qi and yin deficiencies, manifesting in emaciation, shortness of breath, anxiety, poor sleep, and spontaneous sweating.[13]

Tian Wang Bu Xin Dan is often used to treat forgetfulness or diminished mental acuity due to overwork or over-thinking. Today, this formula is used frequently by scholars and students preparing for exams, to help with their cognition.

According to Dr. Chang Wei-Yen, *Tian Wang Bu Xin Dan* can be combined with *Sheng Mai San* (Generate the Pulse Powder) and *Ba Zhen Tang* (Eight-Treasure Decoction) to treat those who suffer from headaches accompanied by dizziness, palpitations, frequent dreams, and cold limbs caused by blood deficiency. Also, the combination of *Tian Wang Bu Xin Dan* and *Sang Piao Xiao San* (Mantis Egg-Case Powder) effectively treats forgetfulness, bedwetting, enuresis, or seminal emissions.

730

Chinese Herbal Formulas and Applications

Tiān Wáng Bǔ Xīn Dān
(Emperor of Heaven's Special Pill to Tonify the Heart)

References

1. *Zhong Yao Ming Fang Yao Li Yu Ying Yong* (Pharmacology and Applications of Famous Herbal Formulas) 1989;318-319.
2. *Zhong Yi Fang Ji Xian Dai Yan Jiu* (Modern Study of Medical Formulae in Traditional Chinese Medicine) 1997;853-854.
3. *Zhong Xi Yi Jie He Yan Jiu Zi Liao* (Research Information on Integration of Chinese and Western Medicine) 1976;6:7.
4. *Zhong Xi Yi Jie He Yan Jiu Zi Liao* (Research Information on Integration of Chinese and Western Medicine) 1976;6:7.
5. *Si Chuan Zhong Yi* (Sichuan Chinese Medicine) 1986;1:48.
6. *Zhe Jiang Zhong Yi Za Zhi* (Zhejiang Journal of Chinese Medicine) 1998;11:513.
7. *Zhong Guo Yi Yao Xue Bao* (Chinese Journal of Medicine and Herbology) 1998;6:38.
8. *He Nan Zhong Yi* (Henan Chinese Medicine) 1992;2:83.
9. *Shan Xi Zhong Yi* (Shanxi Chinese Medicine) 1990;11(5):224.
10. *Shang Hai Yi Yao Za Zhi* (Shanghai Journal of Medicine and Herbology) 1982;5:8.
11. *Zhong Yao Bu Liang Fan Ying Yu Zhi Liao* (Adverse Reactions and Treatment of Chinese Herbal Medicine) 1996;60.
12. Wang MZ, et al. *Zhong Yi Xue Wen Da Ti Ku* (Questions and Answers on Traditional Chinese Medicine: Herbal Formulas).
13. Wang MZ, et al. *Zhong Yi Xue Wen Da Ti Ku* (Questions and Answers on Traditional Chinese Medicine: Herbal Formulas).

Gān Mài Dà Zǎo Tāng (Licorice, Wheat, and Jujube Decoction)
甘麥大棗湯
甘麦大枣汤

Pinyin Name: *Gan Mai Da Zao Tang*
Literal Name: Licorice, Wheat, and Jujube Decoction
Alternate Names: *Gan Cao Xiao Mai Da Zao Tang, Kan Mai Ta Tsao Tang, Kan Tsao Hsiao Mai Ta Tsao Tang, Gan Zao Xiao Mai Da Zao Tang*, Licorice, Wheat, and Date Decoction; Licorice and Jujube Combination
Original Source: *Jin Gui Yao Lue* (Essentials from the Golden Cabinet) by Zhang Zhong-Jing in the Eastern Han Dynasty

COMPOSITION

Gan Cao (Radix et Rhizoma Glycyrrhizae)	9g
Xiao Mai (Fructus Tritici)	1 cup [9-15g]
Da Zao (Fructus Jujubae)	10 pieces [5-7 pieces]

DOSAGE / PREPARATION / ADMINISTRATION

The source text states to prepare the ingredients as a decoction using 6 cups [1,200 mL] of water and reduce the liquid to 3 cups [600 mL]. Take the warm, strained decoction in three equally-divided doses daily. Today, the decoction may be prepared using the doses suggested in brackets.

CHINESE THERAPEUTIC ACTIONS

1. Nourishes the Heart and calms the *shen* (spirit)
2. Harmonizes the middle *jiao* and relieves acute conditions
3. Tonifies Spleen qi

CLINICAL MANIFESTATIONS

Zang zao (restless organ) disorder: absent-mindedness, frequent feelings of extreme sadness with the urge to cry, inability to control one's emotions, restless sleep, abnormal speech or behavior, disorientation, frequent yawning, and a red tongue body with scanty coating.

CLINICAL APPLICATIONS

Hysteria, neurosis, neurasthenia, autonomic dystonia, schizophrenia, menopause, enuresis, insomnia, sleep-walking, night-crying in infants, chorea, gastric cramping, uterine cramping, and coughing due to spasms of the trachea.

EXPLANATION

Gan Mai Da Zao Tang (Licorice, Wheat, and Jujube Decoction) specifically treats a Chinese medical condition called *zang zao* (restless organ) disorder; this condition is characterized by Heart blood deficiency and Liver qi stagnation. With Heart blood deficiency, the *shen* (spirit) becomes unstable and patients will show such symptoms as absent-mindedness, frequent feelings of extreme sadness with the urge to cry, inability to control one's emotions, and restless sleep. Because of Liver qi stagnation, the emotions of the patients become unstable. In mild cases, they may

9

SHEN-CALMING FORMULAS

731

Chapter 9 – Shen-Calming Formulas　　　　　　　　*Section 2 – Nourishing Formulas that Calm the Shen (Spirit)*

Gān Mài Dà Zǎo Tāng (Licorice, Wheat, and Jujube Decoction)

Gan Mai Da Zao Tang (Licorice, Wheat, and Jujube Decoction)

Diagnosis	Signs and Symptoms	Treatment	Herbs
Zang zao (restless organ) disorder	• Absent-mindedness, emotional instability, and restless sleep: Heart blood deficiency unable to nourish the *shen* (spirit) • Mood swings, irritability, and disorientation: Liver qi stagnation • Hysteria, neurosis, and abnormal speech or behavior: severe Liver qi stagnation • Frequent yawning and a red tongue body with scanty coating: dryness consuming yin	• Nourishes the Heart and calms the *shen* • Harmonizes the middle *jiao* and relieves acute conditions • Tonifies Spleen qi	• *Gan Cao* (Radix et Rhizoma Glycyrrhizae) harmonizes the middle *jiao* and nourishes the Heart. • *Xiao Mai* (Fructus Tritici) nourishes the Heart and calms the *shen*. • *Da Zao* (Fructus Jujubae) tonifies Spleen qi, relieves Liver stagnation, and nourishes the Heart.

experience mood swings, irritability, and disorientation. In severe cases, they may exhibit hysteria, neurosis, and abnormal speech or behavior. Clinically, this formula can be used to treat behavioral or emotional disorders characterized by deficiency.

Gan Cao (Radix et Rhizoma Glycyrrhizae) harmonizes the middle *jiao* and nourishes the Heart to relieve the acute condition. *Xiao Mai* (Fructus Tritici) nourishes the Heart and calms the *shen* (spirit). *Da Zao* (Fructus Jujubae) tonifies Spleen qi, relieves Liver qi stagnation, and nourishes the Heart. Combined, these three herbs tonify the Heart, relieve the acute condition, soften the Liver, relieve Liver qi stagnation, tranquilize the Heart, and calm the *shen*.

MODIFICATIONS

• When irritability and thirst are present, add *Mai Dong* (Radix Ophiopogonis) and *Wu Wei Zi* (Fructus Schisandrae Chinensis).

• With irritability, insomnia, a red tongue body with scanty coating, and other yin deficiency signs, add *Di Huang* (Radix Rehmanniae), *Bai Zi Ren* (Semen Platycladi), and *Bai He* (Bulbus Lilii).

• For insomnia, add *Bai He* (Bulbus Lilii), *Di Huang* (Radix Rehmanniae Glutinosae), and *Shou Wu Teng* (Caulis Polygoni Multiflori).

• With palpitations, fear, and fright, add *Ren Shen* (Radix et Rhizoma Ginseng) and *Huang Qi* (Radix Astragali).

• For infants who cry excessively at night, add *Chan Tui* (Periostracum Cicadae) and *Wu Zhu Yu* (Fructus Evodiae).

• For enuresis, add *Sang Piao Xiao* (Ootheca Mantidis), *Yi Zhi* (Fructus Alpinia Oxyphyllae), and *Tu Si Zi* (Semen Cuscutae Chinensis).

• With dizziness and a fine, wiry pulse due to Liver blood deficiency, add *Suan Zao Ren* (Semen Ziziphi Spinosae) and *Dang Gui* (Radix Angelicae Sinensis).

• With dry stools, add *Hei Zhi Ma* (Semen Sesami Nigrum) and *He Shou Wu* (Radix Polygoni Multiflori).

• For schizophrenia, add *Long Gu* (Os Draconis) and *Mu Li* (Concha Ostreae).

PHARMACOLOGICAL EFFECTS

1. **Central nervous system**: In one study, daily administration of the formula at 2-4 g/kg per day for 7 days was associated with increased sleeping time. The formula was also effective in treating and preventing artificially-induced seizures in mice.[1]

2. **Musculoskeletal**: In one experiment, administration of the formula effectively inhibited the contraction of the smooth muscles, such as the intestines and the uterus, in mice.[2]

CLINICAL STUDIES AND RESEARCH

1. ***Zang zao* (restless organ) disorder**: In one study of 38 patients (12 males and 26 females) with *zang zao* (restless organ) disorder, use of modified *Gan Mai Da Zao Tang* was associated with complete recovery in 28 cases, marked improvement in 7 cases, and no effect in 3 cases. The overall effectiveness was 92.1%. Modifications included the addition of *Bai He* (Bulbus Lilii) and *Di Huang* (Radix Rehmanniae) for restlessness, irritability, insomnia, dry mouth, and a red tongue body with little tongue coating; *Suan Zao Ren* (Semen Ziziphi Spinosae) and *Zhi Mu* (Rhizoma Anemarrhenae) for insomnia with excessive dreams, emotional instability, fidgeting, feeling of insecurity, and a wiry, rapid pulse; and *Huo Ma Ren* (Fructus Cannabis) and *Fu Ling* (Poria) for poor appetite and dry stools.[3]

2. **Menopause**: In one clinical study, 133 patients in menopause were treated with *Gan Mai Da Zao Tang* with good success. The effectiveness rate was 94.4% for tidal fever, 84.1% for perspiration, 92.7% for insomnia, 86.85% for headache, 67.8% for irritability and restlessness, and

Gān Mài Dà Zǎo Tāng (Licorice, Wheat, and Jujube Decoction)

70.2% for abdominal fullness.[4] According to another clinical study, use of the formula in 54 menopause patients was associated with complete relief in 35 cases, improvement in 14 cases, and no effect in 5 cases.[5] Lastly, 22 of 30 women (73.3%) with menopause experienced significant relief when treated with modified *Gan Mai Da Zao Tang*. Modifications included addition of *Suan Zao Ren* (Semen Ziziphi Spinosae) or *Fu Shen* (Poria Paradicis) for insomnia with restlessness and irritability, and larger dose and longer duration of treatment for severe conditions.[6]

3. **Insomnia**: In a clinical study, 110 patients with insomnia were treated with *Gan Mai Da Zao Tang* with the addition of *Bai He* (Bulbus Lilii), *Di Huang* (Radix Rehmanniae Glutinosae) and *Shou Wu Teng* (Caulis Polygoni Multiflori) with good success. The overall effectiveness reported was 74.2%.[7]

4. **Neurasthenia**: In one study, 92 out of 100 patients with neurasthenia, headache and insomnia were treated with complete recovery (28 cases) or marked improvement (64 cases) using *Gan Mai Da Zao Tang* with addition of *Bai He* (Bulbus Lilii) and *Zhi Mu* (Rhizoma Anemarrhenae).[8]

5. **Hysteria**: One study reported marked success using herbs and acupuncture to treat hysteria. The herbal formula was given in decoction, and contained *Gan Cao* (Radix et Rhizoma Glycyrrhizae) 20g, *Da Zao* (Fructus Jujubae) 30 pieces, *Xiao Mai* (Fructus Tritici) 60g and *Wu Wei Zi* (Fructus Schisandrae Chinensis) 12g. Acupuncture points selected included *Hegu* (LI 4), *Renzhong* (GV 26), *Neiguan* (PC 6), and others to regulate qi and emotions. Of 60 patients, the study reported stabilization and resolution of all clinical signs and symptoms, with no recurrence in follow-up visits 6 months after the conclusion of treatments.[9] According to another study, 27 patients with hysteria were treated with heavy doses of *Gan Mai Da Zao Tang* with recovery in 24 cases, marked improvement in 2 cases, slight improvement in 1 case, and no effect in 2 cases. The doses of the herbs used were *Gan Cao* (Radix et Rhizoma Glycyrrhizae) 24-45g, *Fu Xiao Mai* (Fructus Tritici Levis) 60g, and *Da Zao* (Fructus Zizyphi Jujubae) 10 pieces.[10] Lastly, 25 patients with hysteria were treated with *Gan Mai Da Zao Tang* plus electro-acupuncture (5 cases) with complete recovery in 22 cases, marked improvement in 2 cases, and slight improvement in 1 case.[11]

6. **Schizophrenia**: One report described *Gan Mai Da Zao Tang* with addition of *Long Gu* (Os Draconis) and *Mu Li* (Concha Ostreae) to be effective in treating 79 cases of schizophrenia. The duration of treatment was between 7-70 days. During the treatment period, 62 out of 79 patients were treated concurrently with a low dose of chlorpromazine (< 200mg per day). Out of 79 cases, the study reported recovery in 5 cases, marked effectiveness in 23 cases, moderate effects in 34 cases, and no effect in

17 cases.[12] According to another study, 146 schizophrenic patients were treated for 7-98 days with recovery in 11 cases, significant improvement in 44 cases, improvement in 64 cases, and no effect in 27 cases. The herbal treatment included *Gan Mai Da Zao Tang* plus wild-crafted *Bai He* (Bulbus Lilii) and *Di Huang* (Radix Rehmanniae). In addition, a small amount of chlorpromazine was given in 17 patients.[13]

7. **Enuresis**: A study of 28 children with bed-wetting characterized by deficiency and cold of the lower *jiao* treated with *Gan Mai Da Zao Tang* with addition of *Sang Piao Xiao* (Ootheca Mantidis), roasted *Yi Zhi* (Fructus Alpinia Oxyphyllae) and *Tu Si Zi* (Semen Cuscutae Chinensis) showed good results. After 10 days of herbal therapy, enuresis stopped in 13 cases. After 20 days of herbal therapy, enuresis stopped in all patients. In follow-up interviews 8-12 months later, only 2 out of 28 children had had any recurrence.[14]

8. **Chorea**: Fourteen children with chorea were treated with good success using *Gan Mai Da Zao Tang* plus *Gui Zhi Jia Long Gu Mu Li Tang* (Cinnamon Twig Decoction plus Dragon Bone and Oyster Shell) with modifications. The herbal formula contained the following ingredients: *Gan Cao* (Radix et Rhizoma Glycyrrhizae) 15g, *Fu Xiao Mai* (Fructus Tritici Levis) 30g, *Da Zao* (Fructus Jujubae) 10 pieces, *Gui Zhi* (Ramulus Cinnamomi) 12g, *Bai Shao* (Radix Paeoniae Alba) 15g, *Sheng Jiang* (Rhizoma Zingiberis Recens) 6g, *Long Gu* (Os Draconis) 30g, *Mu Li* (Concha Ostreae) 30g, *Yu Jin* (Radix Curcumae) 15g, *Gou Teng* (Ramulus Uncariae cum Uncis) 15g, *Qin Jiao* (Radix Gentianae Macrophyllae) 12g, and *Tian Ma* (Rhizoma Gastrodiae) 9g. The study reported recovery in 11 of 14 cases. The remaining three patients were also treated with drugs prior to recovery.[15]

RELATED FORMULA

Ān Shén Tāng (Tranquilize the Spirit Decoction)
安神湯
安神汤

Pinyin Name: *An Shen Tang*
Literal Name: Tranquilize the Spirit Decoction
Original Source: *Guang An Men Yi Yuan* (Guang An Men Hospital) in 1990

Gan Cao (Radix et Rhizoma Glycyrrhizae)
Fu Xiao Mai (Fructus Tritici Levis)
Da Zao (Fructus Jujubae)
Suan Zao Ren (Semen Ziziphi Spinosae)
Zhi Mu (Rhizoma Anemarrhenae)
Fu Ling (Poria)
Lian Zi Xin (Plumula Nelumbinis)
He Huan Hua (Flos Albiziae)

Gān Mài Dà Zǎo Tāng (Licorice, Wheat, and Jujube Decoction)

Shou Wu Teng (Caulis Polygoni Multiflori)

Chai Hu (Radix Bupleuri)

Gou Teng (Ramulus Uncariae cum Uncis)

Xiang Fu (Rhizoma Cyperi)

Bai Shao (Radix Paeoniae Alba)

An Shen Tang (Tranquilize the Spirit Decoction) is used primarily to treat emotional disorders characterized by *shen* (spirit) disturbance. It contains herbs that nourish the Heart, tranquilize the *shen*, regulate Liver qi circulation, sedate Liver fire, and tonify underlying deficiencies. Clinical applications of this formula include stress, irritability, anxiety, emotional instability, and insomnia.

AUTHORS' COMMENTS

Xiao Mai (Fructus Tritici) and *Fu Xiao Mai* (Fructus Tritici Levis) are derived from the same plant, and have similar characteristics and functions. When *Fu Xiao Mai* (Fructus Tritici Levis) and *Xiao Mai* (Fructus Tritici) are both placed in water, *Xiao Mai* (Fructus Tritici) sinks and *Fu Xiao Mai* (Fructus Tritici Levis) floats. *Fu Xiao Mai* (Fructus Tritici Levis) has astringent functions to stop sweating, while *Xiao Mai* (Fructus Tritici) can nourish the Heart and calm *shen*. The source text uses *Xiao Mai* (Fructus Tritici) to nourish the Heart to alleviate *shen* disturbance. Some contemporary texts recommend the use of *Fu Xiao Mai* (Fructus Tritici Levis) to treat yin-deficient heat and relieve spontaneous sweating and night sweats.

Gan Mai Da Zao Tang has also been used during pregnancy and after delivery to treat emotional instability and depression characterized by *zang zao* (restless organ) disorder.

References

1. Journal of Ethnopharmacology 1986;15:289.
2. *Guo Wai Yi Xue Zhong Yi Zhong Yao Fen Ce* (Monograph of Chinese Herbology from Foreign Medicine) 1983;3:53.
3. *Nan Jing Zhong Yi Yao Da Xue Xue Bao* (Journal of Nanjing University of Traditional Chinese Medicine and Medicinals) 1996;6:22.
4. *Fu Jian Zhong Yi Yao* (Fujian Chinese Medicine and Herbology) 1985;4:34.
5. *Xin Zhong Yi* (New Chinese Medicine) 1988;9:51.
6. *Fu Jian Zhong Yi Yao* (Fujian Chinese Medicine and Herbology) 1960;10:17.
7. *Zhe Jiang Zhong Yi Za Zhi* (Zhejiang Journal of Chinese Medicine) 1982;9:412.
8. *Jiang Su Yi Yao* (Jiangsu Journal of Medicine and Herbology) 1976;1:47.
9. *Shan Dong Zhong Yi Za Zhi* (Shandong Journal of Chinese Medicine) 1994;5:237.
10. *Jiang Su Yi Yao* (Jiangsu Journal of Medicine and Herbology) 1978;1:3.
11. *Zhong Yi Za Zhi* (Journal of Chinese Medicine) 1960;2:32.
12. *Zhe Jiang Zhong Yi Za Zhi* (Zhejiang Journal of Chinese Medicine) 1982;6:273.
13. *Shang Hai Yi Yao Za Zhi* (Shanghai Journal of Medicine and Herbology) 1982;6:273.
14. *Hu Bei Zhong Yi Za Zhi* (Hubei Journal of Chinese Medicine) 1986;1:19.
15. *Zhong Yi Za Zhi* (Journal of Chinese Medicine) 1986;5:26.

Chinese Herbal Formulas and Applications

Yǎng Xīn Tāng (Nourish the Heart Decoction)

養心湯
养心汤

Pinyin Name: *Yang Xin Tang*
Literal Name: Nourish the Heart Decoction
Alternate Names: *Yang Hsin Tang*, Heart-Nourishing Decoction, Astragalus and Zizyphus Combination
Original Source: *Ren Zhai Zhi Zhi* (Straight Directions of Benevolent Aid) by Yang Tu-Ying in 1264

COMPOSITION

Ren Shen (Radix et Rhizoma Ginseng)	0.3g
Huang Qi (Radix Astragali), *zhi* (fried with liquid)	15g
Bai Fu Ling (Poria Alba)	15g
Zhi Gan Cao (Radix et Rhizoma Glycyrrhizae Praeparata cum Melle)	12g
Dang Gui (Radix Angelicae Sinensis)	15g
Chuan Xiong (Rhizoma Chuanxiong)	15g
Fu Shen (Poria Paradicis)	15g
Yuan Zhi (Radix Polygalae), *yan* (drowned) in ginger juice and *bei* (stone-baked)	0.3g
Bai Zi Ren (Semen Platycladi)	0.3g
Wu Wei Zi (Fructus Schisandrae Chinensis)	0.3g
Suan Zao Ren (Semen Ziziphi Spinosae), *jin* (soaked) and *chao* (dry-fried) till aromatic	0.3g
Ban Xia Qu (Rhizoma Pinelliae Massa Fermentata)	15g
Rou Gui (Cortex Cinnamomi)	0.3g

DOSAGE / PREPARATION / ADMINISTRATION

The source text states to grind the ingredients into a coarse powder. Cook 9g of the powder with 5 slices of *Sheng Jiang* (Rhizoma Zingiberis Recens) and 2 pieces of *Da Zao* (Fructus Jujubae) in water, and take the warm, strained decoction before meals.

CHINESE THERAPEUTIC ACTIONS

1. Nourishes the Heart
2. Tonifies the blood

CLINICAL MANIFESTATIONS

Heart blood deficiency: palpitations, night sweats, insomnia, tendency towards being easily frightened, forgetfulness, restlessness, and mild fever.

CLINICAL APPLICATIONS

Anemia, neurasthenia, palpitations, absent-mindedness, and poor concentration.

EXPLANATION

Yang Xin Tang (Nourish the Heart Decoction) treats blood deficiency and the subsequent inability to nourish the Heart. Because it is malnourished, the Heart cannot carry out its normal functions. Thus, symptoms and signs of Heart blood deficiency such as palpitations, forgetfulness, insomnia, and night sweats may occur. Furthermore, Heart blood deficiency may contribute to *shen* (spirit)

disturbance, manifesting in symptoms such as being easily scared or frightened and restlessness.

This formula contains many tonic herbs and has a focus mainly on nourishing the Heart and replenishing the blood. Since production of blood requires an adequate amount of qi, this formula uses herbs to tonify qi and nourish blood concurrently. *Ren Shen* (Radix et Rhizoma Ginseng), *Huang Qi* (Radix Astragali), *Bai Fu Ling* (Poria Alba), and *Zhi Gan Cao* (Radix et Rhizoma Glycyrrhizae Praeparata cum Melle) tonify qi. *Dang Gui* (Radix Angelicae Sinensis) and *Chuan Xiong* (Rhizoma Chuanxiong) replenish and move the blood. *Fu Shen* (Poria Paradicis), *Yuan Zhi* (Radix Polygalae), *Bai Zi Ren* (Semen Platycladi), *Wu Wei Zi* (Fructus Schisandrae Chinensis), and *Suan Zao Ren* (Semen Ziziphi Spinosae) calm the *shen* (spirit). *Ban Xia Qu* (Rhizoma Pinelliae Massa Fermentata) dries dampness and eliminates phlegm, which may form from the use of tonic herbs. *Rou Gui* (Cortex Cinnamomi) acts as a guiding herb to direct the therapeutic effects of the herbs to the Heart channel. *Sheng Jiang* (Rhizoma Zingiberis Recens) and *Da Zao* (Fructus Jujubae) harmonize the herbs in the formula.

MODIFICATIONS

• With fever and thirst, add *Mai Dong* (Radix Ophiopogonis) and *Zhu Ru* (Caulis Bambusae in Taenia).

SHEN-CALMING FORMULAS

9

735

Chapter 9 – Shen-Calming Formulas   *Section 2 – Nourishing Formulas that Calm the Shen (Spirit)*

Yăng Xīn Tāng (Nourish the Heart Decoction)

Yang Xin Tang (Nourish the Heart Decoction)

Diagnosis	Signs and Symptoms	Treatment	Herbs
Heart blood deficiency	• Palpitations, forgetfulness, insomnia and night sweats: Heart blood deficiency • Fear, fright and restlessness: *shen* (spirit) disturbance	• Nourishes the Heart • Tonifies the blood	• *Ren Shen* (Radix et Rhizoma Ginseng), *Huang Qi* (Radix Astragali), *Bai Fu Ling* (Poria Alba) and *Zhi Gan Cao* (Radix et Rhizoma Glycyrrhizae Praeparata cum Melle) tonify qi. • *Dang Gui* (Radix Angelicae Sinensis) and *Chuan Xiong* (Rhizoma Chuanxiong) replenish and move blood. • *Fu Shen* (Poria Paradicis), *Yuan Zhi* (Radix Polygalae), *Bai Zi Ren* (Semen Platycladi), *Wu Wei Zi* (Fructus Schisandrae Chinensis) and *Suan Zao Ren* (Semen Ziziphi Spinosae) calm the *shen* (spirit). • *Ban Xia Qu* (Rhizoma Pinelliae Massa Fermentata) dries dampness and eliminates phlegm. • *Rou Gui* (Cortex Cinnamomi) guides the herbs to the Heart channel. • *Sheng Jiang* (Rhizoma Zingiberis Recens) and *Da Zao* (Fructus Jujubae) harmonize all of the herbs.

- With irritability, fever, and insomnia, add *Zhi Mu* (Rhizoma Anemarrhenae) and *Huang Bo* (Cortex Phellodendri Chinensis).
- If the patient is forgetful and easily frightened, add *Shi Chang Pu* (Rhizoma Acori Tatarinowii) and *Bai Shao* (Radix Paeoniae Alba).
- With palpitations, add *Bing Lang* (Semen Arecae) and *Chi Fu Ling* (Poria Rubra).

AUTHORS' COMMENTS

Yang Xin Tang, literally "Nourish the Heart Decoction," is a common generic name for a variety of formulas. There are at least 13 formulas with the exact same name documented in the history of Chinese herbal medicine, all with slightly different ingredients, doses, and indications.

736

Chinese Herbal Formulas and Applications

Chapter 9 — Summary

— Shen-Calming Formulas

SECTION 1: SEDATIVE FORMULAS THAT CALM THE *SHEN* (SPIRIT)

Name	Similarities	Differences
Zhu Sha An Shen Wan (Cinnabar Pill to Tranquilize the Spirit)	Tranquilize the mind and calm the *shen* (spirit)	Clears the Heart and purges fire
Zhen Zhu Mu Wan (Mother of Pearl Pill)		Calms the Heart and Liver yang
Ci Zhu Wan (Magnetite and Cinnabar Pill)		Harmonizes the Heart and Kidney, redirects ascending yang
Chai Hu Jia Long Gu Mu Li Tang (Bupleurum plus Dragon Bone and Oyster Shell Decoction)		Harmonizes the *shaoyang* and anchors the *shen*

Zhu Sha An Shen Wan (Cinnabar Pill to Tranquilize the Spirit), **Zhen Zhu Mu Wan** (Mother of Pearl Pill), **Ci Zhu Wan** (Magnetite and Cinnabar Pill), and **Chai Hu Jia Long Gu Mu Li Tang** (Bupleurum plus Dragon Bone and Oyster Shell Decoction) all tranquilize the mind and calm the *shen* (spirit). The common symptoms are irritability, insomnia, and palpitations.

• *Zhu Sha An Shen Wan* calms the Heart and purges fire. Excess Heart fire consumes yin and blood and creates symptoms of irritability, insomnia, frequent dreams, anxiety, and palpitations.

• *Zhen Zhu Mu Wan* controls hyperactivity of Liver and Heart yang in patients with yin and blood deficiencies. The key clinical manifestations include dizziness, vertigo, and a fine, wiry pulse.

• *Ci Zhu Wan* treats Heart and Kidney disharmony. By assisting the Kidney to restrain the hyperactivity of Heart yang, the herbs in the formula treat eye and ear disorders.

• *Chai Hu Jia Long Gu Mu Li Tang* harmonizes the *shaoyang*, calms and tranquilizes the body with heavy substances, dredges the yang, and purges heat. It is used for *shaoyang* stage in which the emotions are unstable.

SECTION 2: NOURISHING FORMULAS THAT CALM THE *SHEN* (SPIRIT)

Name	Similarities	Differences
Suan Zao Ren Tang (Sour Jujube Decoction)	Nourish the blood and yin, tonify the Heart, calm the *shen* (spirit)	Tonifies Liver blood and restrains Liver yang
Tian Wang Bu Xin Dan (Emperor of Heaven's Special Pill to Tonify the Heart)		Nourishes Heart and Kidney yin, calms the *shen*
Gan Mai Da Zao Tang (Licorice, Wheat, and Jujube Decoction)		Treats *zang zao* (restless organ) disorder, calms the *shen*
Yang Xin Tang (Nourish the Heart Decoction)		Tonifies Heart blood

Suan Zao Ren Tang (Sour Jujube Decoction), **Tian Wang Bu Xin Dan** (Emperor of Heaven's Special Pill to Tonify the Heart), **Gan Mai Da Zao Tang** (Licorice, Wheat, and Jujube Decoction), and **Yang Xin Tang** (Nourish the Heart Decoction) all have common functions of nourishing blood and yin, tonifying the Heart, and calming the *shen* (spirit).

• *Suan Zao Ren Tang* tonifies Liver blood to restrain hyperactive Liver yang, which can produce deficiency heat that disturbs the Heart and creates symptoms of irritability, insomnia, palpitations, night sweats, dizziness, and a dry mouth and throat. The pulse is usually fine, wiry.

Chapter 9 — Summary

- *Tian Wang Bu Xin Dan* tonifies blood, nourishes yin and calms the *shen*. The two deficient organs addressed by this formula are the Heart and Kidney. Key clinical manifestations include irritability, forgetfulness, and nocturnal emissions.
- *Gan Mai Da Zao Tang* is used for *zang zao* (restless organ) disorder and *shen* disturbance caused by Liver qi stagnation and Heart blood deficiency. Usually, this formula is used to harmonize and relieve acute conditions of emotional instability.
- *Yang Xin Tang* nourishes Heart blood deficiency to treat palpitations, night sweats, insomnia, fearfulness, forgetfulness, and restlessness.

Chinese Herbal Formulas and Applications

Chapter 10

— Orifice-Opening Formulas

开

窍

剂

华佗 Huǎ Tuǒ

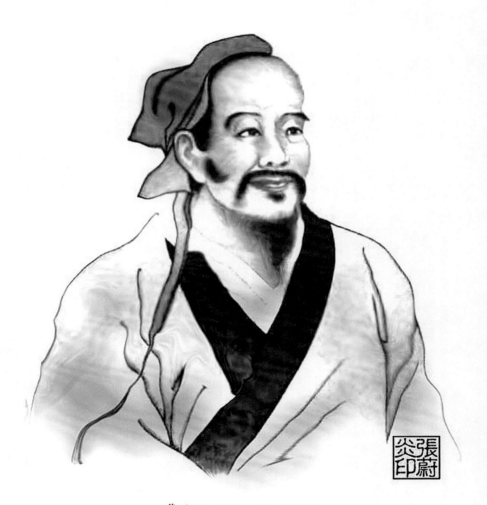

华佗 Huǎ Tuǒ, 110 – 207 CE.

华佗 Huǎ Tuǒ

Hua Tuo was born into a poor family. When Hua Tuo was seven years old, his father passed away, taking with him the only source of family income. Faced with financial hardship and poverty, Hua Tuo began to work in a local herbal pharmacy. While working there, Hua Tuo carefully observed the practice of medicine and pharmacy, and thus began the career of one of the best physicians in our profession.

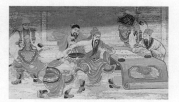

Hua Tuo performing arm surgery on 关羽 Guan Yu, one of the most famous generals in Chinese history.

Hua Tuo lived and practiced medicine during the end of the Eastern Han and beginning of the Three Kingdoms, a period of time characterized by political instability, with constant battles and turmoil. He sympathized with the common people whose lives were suppressed by the government, and dedicated his entire life to helping them. Therefore, Hua Tuo was also known as "the physician of the people." He preferred to treat the common folks of the world, and repeatedly refused to accept offers of the position of 太医 the Supreme Physician in the Imperial Palace.

Hua Tuo is respected for being the first surgeon and the inventor of anesthesia in Traditional Chinese Medicine. He believed that for diseases that could not be treated with acupuncture and herbs, the only solution was surgery to remove the cause. It is well-documented that Hua Tuo frequently performed surgery on various parts of the body by using an herbal formula called 麻沸散 *Ma Fei San* (Numbing and Boiling Powder) for systemic anesthesia.[1]

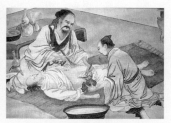

Hua Tuo performing abdominal surgery.

Despite his outstanding achievements, there were always more patients than Hua Tuo could possibly care for in his practice. Thus, he began to wonder why people were always sick, and what would make them healthier. He concluded that chronic illnesses were due, in part, to lack of physical activity, and proposed regular exercise as a remedy. As part of Hua Tuo's strong emphasis on the importance of physical activity, he developed 五禽戏 *Wu Qin Xi* (Five Animal Frolics), an exercise that imitates the physical movement of tigers, deers, monkeys, bears and birds.

In his later years, Hua Tuo was called by the emperor of the Wei Kingdom, 曹操 Cāo Cáo,[2] to treat his "head wind" [presumably migraine headache] that had not responded to any of the treatments by many other physicians. By the insertion of just one needle, the chronic headache was alleviated. Cao was so impressed that he insisted on having Hua Tuo as his personal physician. Hua Tuo tactfully refused, claiming that he needed to return home to attend to his sick wife. Shortly after returning home, he was called again, and subsequently forced by Cao to return to the Imperial Palace. Cao had another severe headache and wanted Hua Tuo to cure him, and would not let him leave the Imperial Palace. Hua Tuo stated that the headache was so severe that it could not be treated simply with herbs or acupuncture. The only cure would be to induce anesthesia, and surgically open the head to remove the cause of the headache. Cao thought Hua Tuo was making an attempt to assassinate him, and sentenced Hua Tuo to death. While in prison, Hua Tuo compiled all of his clinical experience in writing, and tried to give it to a prison guard for safe keeping. However, out of fear of Cao, the guard refused to do any favors or accept anything from Hua Tuo. In extreme anger and frustration, Hua Tuo burned his manuscripts, turning all his clinical knowledge to ashes. After Hua Tuo died, he was buried next to a flowing river of clear water – symbolizing that he was cleared from all wrong-doing.

1. The exact composition of *Ma Fei San* (Numbing and Boiling Powder), similar to all of Hua Tuo's clinical knowledge, was lost when his manuscripts were burned to ashes. Many physicians have attempted to re-create the same formulation based on historical records, but none achieved the same clinical efficacy as Hua Tuo's. This formula is believed to have contained *Yang Jin Hua* (Flos Daturae), *Cao Wu* (Radix Aconiti Kusnezoffii), *Bai Zhi* (Radix Angelicae Dahuricae), *Dang Gui* (Radix Angelicae Sinensis), and *Chuan Xiong* (Rhizoma Chuanxiong), among others.
2. 曹操 Cāo Cáo was the emperor of the Wei Kingdom during the period of the Three Kingdoms. Because these three kingdoms were at war constantly for approximately 60 years, Cao had many enemies and was always facing the threat of assassination. So when Hua Tuo offered to cure Cao's headache by "cutting his head open" to perform brain surgery, Cao naturally assumed he was using medicine as an excuse to kill him, and subsequently sentenced Huo Tuo to death. This story, however, is considered to be folklore, as there is no confirmed historical record of exact motive and circumstances associated with Hua Tuo's death.

Dynasties & Kingdoms	Year
Xia Dynasty 夏	2100-1600 BCE
Shang Dynasty 商	1600-1100 BCE
Zhou Dynasty 周	1100-221 BCE
Qin Dynasty 秦	221-207 BCE
Han Dynasty 漢	**206 BCE-220**
Three Kingdoms 三國	220-280
Western Jin Dynasty 西晉	265-316
Eastern Jin Dynasty 東晉	317-420
Northern and Southern Dynasties 北南朝	420-581
Sui Dynasty 隋	581-618
Tang Dynasty 唐	618-907
Five Dynasties 五代	907-960
Song Dynasty 宋	960-1279
Liao Dynasty 潦	916-1125
Jin Dynasty 金	1115-1234
Yuan Dynasty 元	1271-1368
Ming Dynasty 明	1368-1644
Qing Dynasty 清	1644-1911
Republic of China 中華民國	1912-Present Day
People's Republic of China 中華人民共和國	1949-Present Day

Chapter 10 – Orifice-Opening Formulas

Table of Contents

Chapter 10. Orifice-Opening Formulas **739**
Biography of Hua Tuo 740

Section 1. Cold Orifice-Opening Formulas **746**
An Gong Niu Huang Wan (Calm the Palace Pill with Cattle Gallstone) 746
   Niu Huang Qing Xin Wan (Cattle Gallstone Pill to Clear the Heart) 748
Zhi Bao Dan (Greatest Treasure Special Pill) 749
   Ju Fang Zhi Bao San (Greatest Treasure Powder from the Imperial Grace Formulary) ... 751
Zi Xue (Purple Snow) 752
Xiao Er Hui Chun Dan (Return of Spring Special Pill [Pediatric]) 754
Xing Jun San (Troop-Marching Powder) 756

Section 2. Warm Orifice-Opening Formulas **758**
Su He Xiang Wan (Liquid Styrax Pill) 758
   Guan Xin Su He Wan (Coronary Styrax Pill) 760
Zi Jin Ding (Purple Gold Special Pill) 760

Orifice-Opening Formulas (Summary) **762**

Chinese Herbal Formulas and Applications

Chapter 10 — Overview

— Orifice-Opening Formulas

Definition: Orifice-opening formulas are composed of aromatic herbs that open the sensory orifices, awaken the *shen* (spirit), and restore consciousness. Though "open the orifices" is not a specific treatment method listed in the *ba fa* (eight treatment methods) described in the *Huang Di Nei Jing* (Yellow Emperor's Inner Classic), cold orifice-opening formulas employ the *wen fa* (warming) method and warm orifice-opening formulas utilize the *qing fa* (clearing) method to treat corresponding disorders.

Unconsciousness with closed sensory orifices (described below) is a condition that is divided, for purposes of assessment and treatment, into two main diagnostic categories: excess and deficiency. It is very important to distinguish between excess and deficiency when treating unconsciousness with closed sensory orifices. Excess disorders, such as *bi zheng* (closed disorder), may be treated with orifice-opening formulas to open the sensory orifices, awaken the *shen* (spirit), and restore consciousness. Deficiency disorders, such as *tuo zheng* (abandoned syndrome), must be treated with herbs that tonify qi and restore yang.

- *Bi zheng* (closed disorder) is an excess disorder characterized by the following manifestations: unconsciousness, trismus, convulsions of the muscles, clenched fists, stiff limbs, and a forceful pulse. The nature of *bi zheng* (closed disorder) can be either hot or cold. Hot *bi zheng* (closed disorder) is due to heat toxins attacking the Pericardium, and is treated with cold orifice-opening formulas. Cold *bi zheng* (closed disorder) is due to cold-phlegm or qi stagnation causing turbidity to mist around the Heart. In this case, warm orifice-opening formulas are administered.

~

Orifice-opening formulas treat *bi zheng* (closed disorder), but are contraindicated for *bi zheng* (painful obstruction syndrome) and *tuo zheng* (abandoned syndrome).

~

- *Tuo zheng* (abandoned syndrome) is a deficiency disorder, with manifestations such as cold limbs, perspiration, extreme fatigue, open mouth, closed eyes, and enuresis. *Tuo zheng* (abandoned syndrome) should ***not*** be treated with herbs that open the orifices, as this will further accentuate the weakness and deficiency the individual is already experiencing. This deficient condition **must** be treated with herbs that tonify qi and restore yang.

Disorder	Primary Diagnosis	Secondary Diagnosis	Signs and Symptoms
Uncon-sciousness with closed sensory orifices	• *Bi zheng* (closed disorder)	• Hot *bi zheng* (closed disorder)	• High fever, unconsciousness, delirium, convulsions, and a forceful pulse
		• Cold *bi zheng* (closed disorder)	• Sudden unconsciousness, clenched jaw, pale face, cold extremities, white tongue coating, and a slow pulse
	• *Tuo zheng* (abandoned syndrome)		• Cold limbs, perspiration, extreme fatigue, open mouth, closed eyes, and enuresis

Note: The pinyin names are exactly the same for 闭证 *bi zheng* (closed disorder) and 痹证 *bi zheng* (painful obstruction syndrome), although the Chinese characters are different. These two disorders have very different symptomology, diagnoses, and treatments, and must be correctly identified to

743

Chapter 10 – Orifice-Opening Formulas

Chapter 10 — Overview

insure safe and effective treatment. To avoid confusion, the term *bi zheng* (closed disorder) will be displayed with its English translation throughout the entire text.

SUBCATEGORIES OF ACTION

Orifice-opening formulas are divided into two subcategories to reflect the differential diagnosis and treatment of hot and cold types of *bi zheng* (closed disorder).

1. **Cold Orifice-Opening Formulas**

These formulas treat hot *bi zheng* (closed disorder) caused by pathogenic heat toxins attacking the Pericardium and blocking the sensory orifices. The manifestations include high fever, unconsciousness, delirium, and convulsions. These formulas can also treat sudden unconsciousness due to *zhong feng* (wind stroke), or phlegm accumulation with heat signs and symptoms. In allopathic medical terminology, hot *bi zheng* (closed disorder) is often related to infectious diseases, meningitis, severe pneumonia, septicemia, heat stroke, liver diseases, or toxic uremia.

> *Orifice-opening formulas are generally for emergency use, and should be discontinued once the desired effects are achieved.*

Herbs commonly used to open the sensory orifices include *Bing Pian* (Borneolum Syntheticum), *Shi Chang Pu* (Rhizoma Acori Tatarinowii) and *Yu Jin* (Radix Curcumae). To enhance the opening of the sensory orifices, herbs are added to clear heat, purge fire, cool the blood, and eliminate toxins, such as *Niu Huang* (Calculus Bovis), *Huang Lian* (Rhizoma Coptidis), and *Shi Gao* (Gypsum Fibrosum). Representative formulas include *An Gong Niu Huang Wan* (Calm the Palace Pill with Cattle Gallstone), *Zi Xue* (Purple Snow), and *Zhi Bao Dan* (Greatest Treasure Special Pill).

2. **Warm Orifice-Opening Formulas**

These formulas are used to treat cold *bi zheng* (closed disorder) in which unconsciousness is due to *zhong feng* (wind stroke), cold stroke, and phlegm accumulation. The main clinical manifestations include sudden unconsciousness, clenched jaws, pale face, cold extremities, white tongue coating, and a slow pulse. In allopathic terminology, cold *bi zheng* (closed disorder) is usually caused by cerebrovascular accidents and poisoning.

Commonly used herbs include *Su He Xiang* (Styrax) and *Bing Pian* (Borneolum Syntheticum). They are usually combined with acrid, warm, qi-regulating herbs to enhance their effects, such as *Xiang Fu* (Rhizoma Cyperi), *Ding Xiang* (Flos Caryophylli), and *Bi Bo* (Fructus Piperis Longi). Exemplar formulas include *Su He Xiang Wan* (Liquid Styrax Pill) and *Zi Jin Ding* (Purple Gold Special Pill).

CAUTIONS / CONTRAINDICATIONS

> *Prolonged use of orifice-opening formulas will damage the yuan (source) qi.*

- *Tuo zheng* (abandoned syndrome), the deficiency disorder manifesting in cold limbs, unclenched fists, perspiration, extreme fatigue, open mouth, closed eyes, and enuresis, should be treated with herbs that tonify qi and restore yang. This condition must **not** be treated with orifice-opening formulas, which will only accentuate the underlying weakness and deficiency.

- Orifice-opening formulas are composed of acrid and aromatic herbs; therefore, prolonged use of these formulas will damage the *yuan* (source) *qi*. These formulas are generally reserved for emergency use only and should be discontinued once the desired effects are achieved.

- These formulas are contraindicated during pregnancy.

- *Yangming fu* (hollow organ) excess syndrome with altered consciousness and delirious speech should be treated with cold formulas that drain downward, rather than with orifice-opening formulas.

- *Yangming fu* (hollow organ) excess syndrome with pathogenic heat attacking the Pericardium should be treated with orifice-opening formulas first, followed by cold formulas that drain downward, or both methods of treatment together, depending on the urgency of the condition.

744

Chinese Herbal Formulas and Applications

Chapter 10 — Overview

PROCESSING

Orifice-opening formulas are usually prepared in pill form, powders, or injectables for two reasons. First, these herbs are aromatic in nature, and their effectiveness is destroyed when processed with heat (such as in decoction). Second, they must be available immediately during an emergency. Having these formulas in pills, powders, or injections ensures immediate access to them. Decoction is inappropriate because it requires too much time to prepare. Moreover, decoctions cannot be prepared in advance because of their short shelf life and the difficulty of storing them for any useful period of time.

PHARMACOLOGICAL EFFECTS & CLINICAL APPLICATIONS

Orifice-opening herbs and formulas are generally reserved for acute, emergent cases of sudden unconsciousness, which may have a wide variety of causes. The pharmacological effects observed vary: some have a stimulant effect on the central nervous system, such as *Zhang Nao* (Camphora), which awakens patients from unconsciousness;[1] others have a sedative effect on the central nervous system, such as *Shi Chang Pu* (Rhizoma Acori Tatarinowii), which suppresses seizures and epileptic activities.[2] Other pharmacological effects include antipyretic effects to reduce body temperature,[3] and hypotensive effects to lower blood pressure.[4] Clinical applications of orifice-opening formulas include unconsciousness from encephalitis B, meningitis, toxic uremia, hepatitis, acute icteric hepatitis, acute pancreatitis, cerebrovascular accident, seizures, and convulsions.[5]

> To be immediately available in emergency, orifice-opening formulas are prepared in pills, powder, or for injection.

However, because of the acute and urgent nature of these illnesses, there are very few controlled clinical research studies available for discussion. Exemplar formulas that open the sensory orifices include *An Gong Niu Huang Wan* (Calm the Palace Pill with Cattle Gallstone) and *Su He Xiang Wan* (Liquid Styrax Pill).

References

1. *Zhong Yao Xue* (Chinese Herbology) 1998;989-91.
2. *Zhong Yi Fang Ji Xian Dai Yan Jiu* (Modern Study of Medical Formulae in Traditional Chinese Medicine) 1997;870.
3. *Zhong Cheng Yao Yan Jiu* (Research of Chinese Patent Medicine) 1982;5:23.
4. *Zhong Yi Fang Ji Xian Dai Yan Jiu* (Modern Study of Medical Formulae in Traditional Chinese Medicine) 1997;871.
5. *Zhong Yi Fang Ji Xian Dai Yan Jiu* (Modern Study of Medical Formulae in Traditional Chinese Medicine) 1997;871-874.

ORIFICE-OPENING FORMULAS

10

Chapter 10 – Orifice-Opening Formulas　　　　　　　　*Section 1 – Cold Orifice-Opening Formulas*

Section 1

凉开剂
— Cold Orifice-Opening Formulas

Ān Gōng Niú Huáng Wán (Calm the Palace Pill with Cattle Gallstone)
安宮牛黃丸
安宫牛黄丸

Pinyin Name: *An Gong Niu Huang Wan*
Literal Name: Calm the Palace Pill with Cattle Gallstone
Alternate Name: *Niu Huang Wan* (Cattle Gallstone Pill)
Original Source: *Wen Bing Tiao Bian* (Systematic Differentiation of Warm Disease) by Wu Ju-Tong in 1798

COMPOSITION

Niu Huang (Calculus Bovis)	30g
She Xiang (Moschus)	7.5g
Xi Jiao (Cornu Rhinoceri)	30g
Huang Qin (Radix Scutellariae)	30g
Huang Lian (Rhizoma Coptidis)	30g
Zhi Zi (Fructus Gardeniae)	30g
Bing Pian (Borneolum Syntheticum)	7.5g
Yu Jin (Radix Curcumae)	30g
Zhu Sha (Cinnabaris)	30g
Zhen Zhu (Margarita)	15g
Xiong Huang (Realgar)	30g
Jin Bo (gold foil)	

Note: *Zhu Sha* (Cinnabaris) and *Xiong Huang* (Realgar) are potentially toxic heavy metals, and *Xi Jiao* (Cornu Rhinoceri) and *She Xiang* (Moschus) are derived from endangered animals. They are rarely used as medicinal substances today. The discussion of these substances here is included primarily for academic purposes, to reflect the historical use of these substances in its original formulation. Most herbal products today have removed them completely, or replaced them with substitutes with similar functions. For additional information on the toxicity of *Zhu Sha* (Cinnabaris) and *Xiong Huang* (Realgar), please refer to *Chinese Medical Herbology and Pharmacology* by John Chen and Tina Chen.

DOSAGE / PREPARATION / ADMINISTRATION

The source text states to grind the ingredients into a very fine powder and form into pills with honey. The pills should be 3g in weight, and are traditionally coated with *Jin Bo* (gold foil) and sealed with wax. For robust patients in severe condition, take 1 pill two to three times daily. For children, take one-half pill one time daily. If there is no response, a second dose may be given.

Today, this formula is prepared in four steps. First, process *Zhu Sha* (Cinnabaris), *Zhen Zhu* (Margarita), and *Xiong Huang* (Realgar) separately with the *shui fei* (refining with water) technique to obtain extremely fine powder. Second, grind *Niu Huang* (Calculus Bovis), *Xi Jiao* (Cornu Rhinoceri), *She Xiang* (Moschus), and *Bing Pian* (Borneolum Syntheticum) into a fine powder. Third, grind the remaining ingredients into powder. Finally, blend all of the herb powders together and mix with *Feng Mi* (Mel) and water to form large pills. Dry the pills in a cool place without direct exposure to sunlight. Take one pill daily.

746

Chinese Herbal Formulas and Applications

Ān Gōng Niú Huáng Wán (Calm the Palace Pill with Cattle Gallstone)

CHINESE THERAPEUTIC ACTIONS
1. Clears heat and opens the orifices
2. Dispels phlegm and eliminates toxins

CLINICAL MANIFESTATIONS
Febrile disorders with heat attacking the Pericardium and hot phlegm obstructing the orifices: high fever, fidgeting, irritability, delirium, coma, unconsciousness due to stroke, and infantile convulsions.

CLINICAL APPLICATIONS
Fever, encephalitis B, meningitis, dysentery, toxic uremia, hepatitis, acute icteric hepatitis, acute pancreatitis, cerebrovascular accident, seizures, and convulsions.

EXPLANATION
An Gong Niu Huang Wan (Calm the Palace Pill with Cattle Gallstone) is a representative formula for treating febrile disorders with heat attacking the Pericardium and hot phlegm obstructing the sensory orifices. The Heart, covered by the Pericardium, is the organ that houses the mind and controls the *shen* (spirit). If heat attacks the Pericardium, the patient may show *shen* disturbance, high fever, fidgeting, and irritability. If hot phlegm obstructs the sensory orifices and seizes the *shen,* the patient may lose consciousness, as in delirium and coma. Clinically, this formula is used to treat hot *bi zheng* (closed disorder) syndrome, as seen in stroke, coma, seizures, and epilepsy.

An Gong Niu Huang Wan uses *Niu Huang* (Calculus Bovis) to clear Heart heat, eliminate toxins, dispel phlegm, and open the orifices. *She Xiang* (Moschus) has a resuscitating function to open the sensory orifices and awaken the *shen* (spirit). Though *She Xiang* (Moschus) is a warm substance, it will not generate heat as the formula contains many cold herbs at large doses. *Xi Jiao* (Cornu Rhinoceri) clears heat, cools the blood, and eliminates toxins. *Huang Qin* (Radix Scutellariae), *Huang Lian* (Rhizoma Coptidis), and *Zhi Zi* (Fructus Gardeniae) clear heat, purge fire, and eliminate toxins. *Bing Pian* (Borneolum Syntheticum) and *Yu Jin* (Radix Curcumae) enhance the resuscitating function of *She Xiang* (Moschus) to open orifices and awaken the *shen*. *Zhu Sha* (Cinnabaris) and *Zhen Zhu* (Margarita) calm the *shen* and relieve fidgeting and irritability. *Xiong Huang* (Realgar) helps *Niu Huang* (Calculus Bovis) dispel phlegm and eliminate toxins. *Jin Bo* (gold foil) helps *Zhu Sha* (Cinnabaris) calm the *shen*. *Feng Mi* (Mel), as the envoy herb, regulates the middle *jiao* and strengthens the Stomach.

This formula can also be used to treat unconsciousness due to coma and infantile convulsions if the patient has the above clinical manifestations.

MODIFICATIONS
With heat entering the Pericardium and excess heat in the *fu* (hollow organs) manifesting in delirium, constipation,

An Gong Niu Huang Wan (Calm the Palace Pill with Cattle Gallstone)

Diagnosis	Signs and Symptoms	Treatment	Herbs
Febrile disorder with heat attacking the Pericardium and hot phlegm obstructing the orifices	• *Shen* (spirit) disturbance, high fever, fidgeting, and irritability: heat attacking the Pericardium • Delirium, coma and unconsciousness: hot phlegm obstructing the sensory orifices	• Clears heat and opens orifices • Dispels phlegm and eliminates toxins	• *Niu Huang* (Calculus Bovis) clears Heart heat, eliminates toxins, dispels phlegm, and opens orifices. • *She Xiang* (Moschus) opens sensory orifices and awakens the *shen*. • *Xi Jiao* (Cornu Rhinoceri) clears heat, cools the blood, and eliminates toxins. • *Huang Qin* (Radix Scutellariae), *Huang Lian* (Rhizoma Coptidis) and *Zhi Zi* (Fructus Gardeniae) clear heat, purge fire, and eliminate toxins. • *Bing Pian* (Borneolum Syntheticum) and *Yu Jin* (Radix Curcumae) open orifices and awaken the *shen*. • *Zhu Sha* (Cinnabaris), *Zhen Zhu* (Margarita), and *Jin Bo* (gold foil) calm the *shen* and relieve fidgeting and irritability. • *Xiong Huang* (Realgar) dispels phlegm and eliminates toxins. • *Feng Mi* (Mel) regulates the middle *jiao* and strengthens the Stomach.

ORIFICE-OPENING FORMULAS

10

Chapter 10 – Orifice-Opening Formulas　　　　　　　　　　*Section 1 – Cold Orifice-Opening Formulas*

Ān Gōng Niú Huáng Wán (Calm the Palace Pill with Cattle Gallstone)

and thirst that cannot be relieved by the intake of water, administer 2 pills of *An Gong Niu Huang Wan* plus 9g of powdered *Da Huang* (Radix et Rhizoma Rhei) in warm water.

CAUTIONS / CONTRAINDICATIONS

- *An Gong Niu Huang Wan* is contraindicated in cases of *zhong feng* (wind stroke) characterized by *tuo zheng* (abandoned syndrome).[1]
- Use of this formula is contraindicated during pregnancy.[2]

PHARMACOLOGICAL EFFECTS

1. **Central nervous system**: Laboratory experiments showed that administration of *An Gong Niu Huang Wan* had a sedative effect on the central nervous system by decreasing spontaneous physical activities and suppressing seizures.[3]
2. **Antipyretic**: Administration of the formula was effective in treating rabbits with artificially-induced fever. The antipyretic effect was observed one hour following ingestion, and lasted for 5-6 hours.[4]
3. **Anti-inflammatory**: In one study, the use of the formula was associated with marked effect to reduce swelling and inflammation. The effect was observed from 1 to 4.5 hours after administration.[5]
4. **Hypotensive**: In one experiment, intravenous injection of the formula was associated with an immediate drop of blood pressure of approximately 10-40 mmHg. The effect to lower blood pressure lasted for 3-5 minutes, with blood pressure returning to the previous level after 10 minutes.[6]

CLINICAL STUDIES AND RESEARCH

1. **Fever**: One report described 8 cancer patients with high fevers of 39.1-41.5°C (102.4-106.7°F) for an average of 5.6 days. They were treated with *An Gong Niu Huang Wan*, and all patients stopped using analgesic and anti-inflammatory drugs during the herbal therapy. The treatment protocol was to administer one pill of the formula twice daily for 3-5 days. The study reported that the temperature was reduced to below 38°C (100.4°F) within 4-72 hours (average of 27.2 hours). The study concluded the formula to be effective in treating fever in cancer patients.[7]
2. **Others**: *An Gong Niu Huang Wan* has been used to treat encephalitis B, meningitis, dysentery, toxic uremia, hepatitis, acute icteric hepatitis, acute pancreatitis, cerebrovascular accident, seizures, and convulsions.[8]

TOXICOLOGY

Use of *An Gong Niu Huang Wan* has been associated with side effects such as palpitations, dull pain in the upper abdominal area, fear, fright, restlessness, irritability, facial edema, rashes, and dark purple appearance that starts at the lips and then spreads to the rest of the body. Long-term use or gross overdose (over 60 pills per dose) has been associated with nephritis, with symptoms such as low back pain, decreased urination, red-colored urine, and the presence of protein and white blood cells in the urine.[9] Note: These reactions are usually attributed to *Zhu Sha* (Cinnabaris) and *Xiong Huang* (Realgar), two substances that are considered toxic.

RELATED FORMULA

Niú Huáng Qīng Xīn Wán
(Cattle Gallstone Pill to Clear the Heart)
牛黃清心丸
牛黃清心丸

Pinyin Name: *Niu Huang Qing Xin Wan*
Literal Name: Cattle Gallstone Pill to Clear the Heart
Original Source: *Dou Zhen Shi Yi Xin Fa* (Teachings of Generations of Physicians about Pox) by Wan Quan in 1568

Niu Huang (Calculus Bovis)	0.75g
Zhu Sha (Cinnabaris)	4.5g
Huang Lian (Rhizoma Coptidis)	15g
Huang Qin (Radix Scutellariae)	9g
Zhi Zi (Fructus Gardeniae)	9g
Yu Jin (Radix Curcumae)	6g

Note: *Zhu Sha* (Cinnabaris) is a potentially toxic heavy metal, and is rarely used as a medicinal substance today. Its discussion here is included primarily for academic purposes, to reflect the historical use of this substance in its original formulation. Most herbal products today have removed it completely, or replaced it with substitutes with similar functions. For additional information on the toxicity, please refer to *Chinese Medical Herbology and Pharmacology* by John Chen and Tina Chen.

Grind the ingredients into a fine powder, and form into pills with flour and water. The pills should resemble corn kernels in size. Take 7-8 pills with a decoction of *Deng Xin Cao* (Medulla Junci). Today, this formula is normally prepared by mixing the powdered herbs with honey to form pills. The pills should weigh 1.5g each. Take 2 pills per dose two to three times daily. Adjust the doses for children according to age and body weight.

Niu Huang Qing Xin Wan (Cattle Gallstone Pill to Clear the Heart) clears heat, eliminates toxins, opens the sensory orifices, and calms the *shen* (spirit). Clinically, this formula may be used for heat invading the Pericardium, leading

748

Chinese Herbal Formulas and Applications

Ān Gōng Niú Huáng Wán (Calm the Palace Pill with Cattle Gallstone)

to such symptoms as delirium, semi-unconsciousness, feverish sensations, fidgeting, and irritability. This formula may also be used for infantile convulsions in which there is constant muscle contraction, and for *zhong feng* (wind stroke) with closed sensory orifices.

An Gong Niu Huang Wan and *Niu Huang Qing Xin Wan* (Cattle Gallstone Pill to Clear the Heart) have similar compositions, actions, and indications.

• *An Gong Niu Huang Wan* has a stronger action to tranquilize the *shen* (spirit) and open the sensory orifices; hence, it is more suitable for such symptoms as high fever, semiconsciousness, and delirium.

• *Niu Huang Qing Xin Wan* functions more strongly to clear heat and eliminate toxins, and is more suitable for symptoms such as feverish sensations, fidgeting, and irritability.

AUTHORS' COMMENTS

An Gong Niu Huang Wan, *Zhi Bao Dan* (Greatest Treasure Special Pill), and *Zi Xue Dan* (Purple Snow Pill), are commonly referred to as "*San Bao* (Three Treasures)," as these are three of the most commonly used formulas to treat hot *bi zheng* (closed disorder).

• *An Gong Niu Huang Wan* is the coldest of the three formulas. It is most potent in clearing heat and eliminating toxins.
• *Zhi Bao Dan* is aromatic, and is the best for opening the sensory orifices to treat unconsciousness due to obstruction of phlegm and heat.
• *Zi Xue Dan* is most effective to calm Liver wind in treating seizures, epilepsy, and convulsions.

References

1. *Zhong Yao Ming Fang Yao Li Yu Ying Yong* (Pharmacology and Applications of Famous Herbal Formulas) 1989;379-381.
2. *Zhong Yao Ming Fang Yao Li Yu Ying Yong* (Pharmacology and Applications of Famous Herbal Formulas) 1989;379-381.
3. *Zhong Yi Fang Ji Xian Dai Yan Jiu* (Modern Study of Medical Formulae in Traditional Chinese Medicine) 1997;870.
4. *Zhong Cheng Yao Yan Jiu* (Research of Chinese Patent Medicine) 1982;5:23.
5. *Zhong Yi Fang Ji Xian Dai Yan Jiu* (Modern Study of Medical Formulae in Traditional Chinese Medicine) 1997;871.
6. *Zhong Yi Fang Ji Xian Dai Yan Jiu* (Modern Study of Medical Formulae in Traditional Chinese Medicine) 1997;871.
7. *Shi Yong Zhong Xi Yi Jie He Za Zhi* (Practical Journal of Integrated Chinese and Western Medicines) 1994;7(9):545.
8. *Zhong Yi Fang Ji Xian Dai Yan Jiu* (Modern Study of Medical Formulae in Traditional Chinese Medicine) 1997;871-874.
9. *Zhong Yao Bu Liang Fan Ying Yu Zhi Liao* (Adverse Reactions and Treatment of Chinese Herbal Medicine) 1996;74.

Zhì Bǎo Dān (Greatest Treasure Special Pill)
至寶丹
至宝丹

Pinyin Name: *Zhi Bao Dan*
Literal Name: Greatest Treasure Special Pill
Original Sources: *Tai Ping Hui Min He Ji Ju Fang* (Imperial Grace Formulary of the Tai Ping Era) by the Imperial Medical Department in 1078-85

COMPOSITION

She Xiang (Moschus), *yan* (ground) to small particles	0.3g [7.5g]
Bing Pian (Borneolum Syntheticum), *yan* (ground) to small particles	0.3g [7.5g]
An Xi Xiang (Benzoinum), *ao* (simmered) into paste	45g
Xi Jiao (Cornu Rhinoceri), *yan* (ground) to small particles	30g
Niu Huang (Calculus Bovis), *yan* (ground) to small particles	0.3g [7.5g]
Dai Mao (Carapax Eretmochelydis Imbricatae), *yan* (ground) to small particles	30g
Jin Bo (gold foil)	50 leaves
Yin Bo (silver foil), *yan* (ground) to small particles	50 leaves
Zhu Sha (Cinnabaris), *yan* (ground) and *shui fei* (refined with water)	30g
Hu Po (Succinum), *yan* (ground) to small particles	30g
Xiong Huang (Realgar), *yan* (ground) and *shui fei* (refined with water)	30g

ORIFICE-OPENING FORMULAS

10

749

Chapter 10 – Orifice-Opening Formulas   *Section 1 – Cold Orifice-Opening Formulas*

Zhì Bǎo Dān (Greatest Treasure Special Pill)

Note: *Zhu Sha* (Cinnabaris) and *Xiong Huang* (Realgar) are potentially toxic heavy metals, and *Xi Jiao* (Cornu Rhinoceri) and *She Xiang* (Moschus) are derived from endangered animals. They are rarely used as medicinal substances today. The discussion of these substances here is included primarily for academic purposes, to reflect the historical use of these substances in its original formulation. Most herbal products today have removed them completely, or replaced them with substitutes with similar functions. For additional information on the toxicity of *Zhu Sha* (Cinnabaris) and *Xiong Huang* (Realgar), please refer to *Chinese Medical Herbology and Pharmacology* by John Chen and Tina Chen.

DOSAGE / PREPARATION / ADMINISTRATION

Crush separately into fine powder *Xi Jiao* (Cornu Rhinoceri), *Dai Mao* (Carapax Eretmochelydis Imbricatae), *An Xi Xiang* (Benzoinum), and *Hu Po* (Succinum). *Zhu Sha* (Cinnabaris) and *Xiong Huang* (Realgar) are separately processed via the *shui fei* (refining with water) technique to obtain extremely fine powders. *Niu Huang* (Calculus Bovis), *She Xiang* (Moschus), and *Bing Pian* (Borneolum Syntheticum) are ground into powder. *Jin Bo* (gold foil) [25 leaves] and *Yin Bo* (silver foil) [50 leaves] are also ground into powder. Blend all the powders together, place them through a sieve, and mix with honey to form pills. Coat the pills with the remaining 25 leaves of *Jin Bo* (gold foil). The pills should weigh 3g each. Take 1 pill one time daily. Reduce the dose for children.

Note: The formulation today no longer uses *Jin Bo* (gold foil) or *Yin Bo* (silver foil), and has replaced *Xi Jiao* (Cornu Rhinoceri) with *Shui Niu Jiao* (Cornu Bubali). Please refer to the related formula *Ju Fang Zhi Bao San* (Greatest

Treasure Powder from the Imperial Grace Formulary) for additional information.

CHINESE THERAPEUTIC ACTIONS

1. Clears heat and opens the sensory orifices
2. Dissolves turbidity and eliminates toxins

CLINICAL MANIFESTATIONS

1. Heat stroke, *zhong feng* (wind stroke), *wen bing* (warm disease), and *bi zheng* (closed disorder) with obstruction of phlegm and heat: altered consciousness, delirium, feverish sensations, irritability, restlessness, hoarse voice with profuse sputum, red tongue body with a yellow, greasy tongue coating, and a slippery, rapid pulse.
2. Infantile seizures and epilepsy due to obstruction by phlegm and heat.

CLINICAL APPLICATIONS

Stroke, heat stroke, coma, seizures and epilepsy, and encephalitis B.

EXPLANATION

Zhi Bao Dan (Greatest Treasure Special Pill) treats various disorders characterized by obstruction of phlegm and heat in the interior. The phlegm and heat cover the Pericardium and block the sensory orifices. Due to the heat, there will be symptoms of feverish sensations, irritability, and restlessness. Phlegm, which covers the Pericardium and blocks the sensory orifices, causes symptoms such as altered consciousness and delirium.

This formula uses aromatic substances such as *She Xiang* (Moschus), *Bing Pian* (Borneolum Syntheticum), and *An Xi Xiang* (Benzoinum) to open the sensory orifices and

Zhi Bao Dan (Greatest Treasure Special Pill)

Diagnosis	Signs and Symptoms	Treatment	Herbs
Heat stroke, *zhong feng* (wind stroke), *wen bing* (warm disease), and *bi zheng* (closed disorder)	• Altered consciousness, delirium, feverish sensations, irritability, and restlessness: heat and phlegm covering the Pericardium and blocking the sensory orifices • Hoarse voice with profuse sputum: phlegm and heat in the interior • Red tongue body with a yellow, greasy tongue coating: phlegm and heat in the interior • Slippery, rapid pulse: phlegm and heat in the interior	• Clears heat and opens sensory orifices • Dissolves turbidity and eliminates toxins	• *She Xiang* (Moschus), *Bing Pian* (Borneolum Syntheticum), and *An Xi Xiang* (Benzoinum) open sensory orifices and dissolve turbidity. • *Xi Jiao* (Cornu Rhinoceri), *Niu Huang* (Calculus Bovis), and *Dai Mao* (Carapax Eretmochelydis Imbricatae) clear heat and eliminate toxins. • *Jin Bo* (gold foil), *Yin Bo* (silver foil), *Zhu Sha* (Cinnabaris), and *Hu Po* (Succinum) sedate the Heart and calm the *shen* (spirit). • *Xiong Huang* (Realgar) dispels phlegm and eliminates toxins.

750

Zhì Bǎo Dān (Greatest Treasure Special Pill)

dissolve turbidity. *Xi Jiao* (Cornu Rhinoceri), *Niu Huang* (Calculus Bovis), and *Dai Mao* (Carapax Eretmochelydis Imbricatae) clear heat and eliminate toxins. *Niu Huang* also treats seizures and epilepsy. *Jin Bo* (gold foil), *Yin Bo* (silver foil), *Zhu Sha* (Cinnabaris), and *Hu Po* (Succinum) sedate the Heart and calm the *shen* (spirit). *Xiong Huang* (Realgar) dispels phlegm and eliminates toxins.

MODIFICATIONS

For deficiency of *zheng* (upright) *qi*, administer *Zhi Bao Dan* with a decoction of *Ren Shen* (Radix et Rhizoma Ginseng).

CAUTIONS / CONTRAINDICATIONS

- *Zhi Bao Dan* is contraindicated in cases of yang excess and yin deficiency, as this formula has many acrid and drying herbs that may consume yin and body fluids.
- During pregnancy, this formula should only be used when absolutely necessary, and then, only with extreme caution.

RELATED FORMULA

Jú Fāng Zhì Bǎo Sǎn (Greatest Treasure Powder from the Imperial Grace Formulary)

局方至寶散
局方至宝散

Pinyin Name: Ju Fang Zhi Bao San
Literal Name: Greatest Treasure Powder from the Imperial Grace Formulary
Original Source: *Tai Ping Hui Min He Ji Ju Fang* (Imperial Grace Formulary of the Tai Ping Era) by the Imperial Medical Department in 1078-85

Shui Niu Jiao (Cornu Bubali)	240-300g
Zhu Sha (Cinnabaris)	30g

Xiong Huang (Realgar)	30g
Dai Mao (Carapax Eretmochelydis Imbricatae)	30g
Hu Po (Succinum)	30g
She Xiang (Moschus)	7.5g
Bing Pian (Borneolum Syntheticum)	7.5g
Niu Huang (Calculus Bovis)	15g
An Xi Xiang (Benzoinum)	45g

Note: *Zhu Sha* (Cinnabaris) and *Xiong Huang* (Realgar) are potentially toxic heavy metals, and *She Xiang* (Moschus) is derived from an endangered animal. They are rarely used as medicinal substances today. The discussion here is included primarily for academic purposes, to reflect the historical use of these substances in its original formulation. Most herbal products today have removed them completely, or replaced them with substitutes with similar functions. For additional information on the toxicity of *Zhu Sha* (Cinnabaris) and *Xiong Huang* (Realgar), please refer to *Chinese Medical Herbology and Pharmacology* by John Chen and Tina Chen.

Ju Fang Zhi Bao San (Greatest Treasure Powder from the Imperial Grace Formulary) is derived from *Zhi Bao Dan* (Greatest Treasure Special Pill), with two key changes. First, the dosage form has been changed from pills to powder. Second, three ingredients have been removed or replaced: *Jin Bo* (gold foil) and *Yin Bo* (silver foil) are no longer used today, and have been removed from this formula; while *Xi Jiao* (Cornu Rhinoceri) has been replaced by *Shui Niu Jiao* (Cornu Bubali). Note: The dose of *Shui Niu Jiao* (Cornu Bubali) was not available. However, the general consensus is 240-300g, since *Xi Jiao* (Cornu Rhinoceri) is approximately 8-10 times more potent than *Shui Niu Jiao* (Cornu Bubali).

10

ORIFICE-OPENING FORMULAS

751

Zǐ Xuě (Purple Snow)

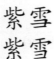

Pinyin Name: Zi Xue
Literal Name: Purple Snow
Alternate Name: Zi Xue Dan (Purple Snow Pill)
Original Source: Wai Tai Mi Yao (Arcane Essentials from the Imperial Library) by Wang Tao in 752 A.D.

COMPOSITION

Xi Jiao (Cornu Rhinoceri)	150g
Shi Gao (Gypsum Fibrosum)	1,500g
Han Shui Shi (Mirabilite)	1,500g
Hua Shi (Talcum)	1,500g
Xuan Shen (Radix Scrophulariae)	500g
Sheng Ma (Rhizoma Cimicifugae)	500g
She Xiang (Moschus), *yan* (ground) to small particles	1.5g
Mu Xiang (Radix Aucklandiae)	150g
Ding Xiang (Flos Caryophylli)	30g
Chen Xiang (Lignum Aquilariae Resinatum)	150g
Ling Yang Jiao (Cornu Saigae Tataricae)	150g
Zhu Sha (Cinnabaris), *shui fei* (refined with water) and *yan* (ground) to small particles	90g
Ci Shi (Magnetitum)	1,500g
Po Xiao (Sal Glauberis), *zhi* (prepared)	5,000g
Xiao Shi (Niter), *zhi* (prepared)	96g
Huang Jin (Gold)	3,000g
Zhi Gan Cao (Radix et Rhizoma Glycyrrhizae Praeparata cum Melle)	240g

Note: Zhu Sha (Cinnabaris) is a potentially toxic heavy metal, and Ling Yang Jiao (Cornu Saigae Tataricae), She Xiang (Moschus) and Xi Jiao (Cornu Rhinoceri) are derived from endangered animals. They are rarely used as a medicinal substance today. The discussion here is included primarily for academic purposes, to reflect the historical use of these substances in its original formulation. Most herbal products today have removed them completely, or replaced them with substitutes with similar functions. For additional information on the toxicity of Zhu Sha (Cinnabaris), please refer to *Chinese Medical Herbology and Pharmacology* by John Chen and Tina Chen.

DOSAGE / PREPARATION / ADMINISTRATION

Crush the mineral ingredients [Shi Gao (Gypsum Fibrosum), Huang Jin (Gold), Han Shui Shi (Mirabilite), Hua Shi (Talcum) and Ci Shi (Magnetitum)] into small particles and cook in water three times. Then add the herbal ingredients [Xuan Shen (Radix Scrophulariae), Mu Xiang (Radix Aucklandiae), Chen Xiang (Lignum Aquilariae Resinatum), Sheng Ma (Rhizoma Cimicifugae), Zhi Gan Cao (Radix et Rhizoma Glycyrrhizae Praeparata cum Melle) and Ding Xiang (Flos Caryophylli)] and cook in water three times. Filter and discard the residues, and cook the strained decoction and reduce it to a condensed paste.

Mix into this paste powdered Xiao Shi (Niter) and Po Xiao (Sal Glauberis), and blend thoroughly. Allow it to dry and then grind it into a fine powder. Grate and grind the horns [Xi Jiao (Cornu Rhinoceri) and Ling Yang Jiao (Cornu Saigae Tataricae)] into fine powder. Process Zhu Sha (Cinnabaris) via the *shui fei* (refining with water) technique to obtain an extremely fine powder. Grind She Xiang (Moschus) into powder. Mix these powders together, and place them through a sieve to obtain the final powdered formula. Take 1.5-3g of the powder per dose two times daily. Reduce the dose for children. As the literal name of the formula implies, the finished product resembles "purple snow."

Note: The source text state to use "Qing Mu Xiang" as one of the ingredients in this formula. However, it is believed that "Qing Mu Xiang" actually refers to Mu Xiang (Radix Aucklandiae) during that period. Therefore, most textbooks and clinicians now use Mu Xiang (Radix Aucklandiae) as the ingredient in this formula. Also, Po Xiao (Sal Glauberis) is usually replaced with Mang Xiao (Natrii Sulfas), which is more readily available. Huang

Zĭ Xuĕ (Purple Snow)

Jin (Gold) is replaced with *Jin Bo* (gold foil), or removed from the formula.

CHINESE THERAPEUTIC ACTIONS

1. Clears heat and opens the sensory orifices
2. Stops convulsions and calms the *shen* (spirit)

CLINICAL MANIFESTATIONS

Febrile disorders with heat attacking the Pericardium and rise of Liver wind: high fever, irritability, restlessness, altered consciousness, delirium, convulsions, thirst, dry lips, dysuria, constipation, infantile seizures, and epilepsy.

CLINICAL APPLICATIONS

Infantile seizures, epilepsy, and convulsions.

EXPLANATION

Zi Xue (Purple Snow) treats febrile disorders in which heat attacks the Pericardium and causes the rising of Liver wind. When heat attacks the Pericardium and disturbs the *shen* (spirit), there will be altered consciousness, delirium, irritability, and restlessness. The presence of heat in febrile disorders may also cause high fever, dysuria, and constipation. Heat may also stir Liver wind and cause it to rise

upward, leading to convulsions, seizures, and epilepsy. Lastly, heat may dry up body fluids, causing thirst and dry lips.

Xi Jiao (Cornu Rhinoceri) clears heat from the Heart and eliminates toxins. Sweet and cold, *Shi Gao* (Gypsum Fibrosum), *Han Shui Shi* (Mirabilite), and *Hua Shi* (Talcum) clear heat, purge fire, and preserve yin. *Xuan Shen* (Radix Scrophulariae) and *Sheng Ma* (Rhizoma Cimicifugae) clear heat and eliminate toxins. *She Xiang* (Moschus), *Mu Xiang* (Radix Aucklandiae), *Ding Xiang* (Flos Caryophylli), and *Chen Xiang* (Lignum Aquilariae Resinatum) activate qi circulation and open the sensory orifices. *Ling Yang Jiao* (Cornu Saigae Tataricae) clears the Liver, calms Liver wind, and relieves convulsions. *Zhu Sha* (Cinnabaris) and *Ci Shi* (Magnetitum) are heavy substances that anchor the *shen* (spirit) and relieve irritability and restlessness. *Huang Jin* (Gold) sedates the Heart, calms the *shen,* and eliminates toxins. *Po Xiao* (Sal Glauberis) and *Xiao Shi* (Niter) clear heat and drain it downward. Lastly, *Zhi Gan Cao* (Radix et Rhizoma Glycyrrhizae Praeparata cum Melle) harmonizes the formula.

Zi Xue (Purple Snow)

Diagnosis	Signs and Symptoms	Treatment	Herbs
Febrile disorders with heat attacking the Pericardium and rise of Liver wind	• High fever, altered consciousness, delirium, irritability, and restlessness: heat attacking the Pericardium and disturbing the *shen* (spirit) • Seizures and epilepsy: heat stirring Liver wind upwards • Thirst and dry lips: heat consuming body fluids in the upper body • Dysuria and constipation: heat damaging body fluids in the lower body	• Clears heat and opens sensory orifices • Stops convulsions and calms the *shen*	• *Xi Jiao* (Cornu Rhinoceri) clears heat from the Heart and eliminates toxins. • *Shi Gao* (Gypsum Fibrosum), *Han Shui Shi* (Mirabilite), and *Hua Shi* (Talcum) clear heat, purge fire, and preserve yin. • *Xuan Shen* (Radix Scrophulariae) and *Sheng Ma* (Rhizoma Cimicifugae) clear heat and eliminate toxins. • *She Xiang* (Moschus), *Mu Xiang* (Radix Aucklandiae), *Ding Xiang* (Flos Caryophylli) and *Chen Xiang* (Lignum Aquilariae Resinatum) activate qi circulation and open orifices. • *Ling Yang Jiao* (Cornu Saigae Tataricae) clears the Liver, calms Liver wind, and relieves convulsions. • *Zhu Sha* (Cinnabaris) and *Ci Shi* (Magnetitum) are heavy substances that anchor the *shen* and relieve irritability and restlessness. • *Po Xiao* (Sal Glauberis) and *Xiao Shi* (Niter) clear heat and drain it downward. • *Huang Jin* (Gold) sedates the Heart, calms the *shen,* and eliminates toxins. • *Zhi Gan Cao* (Radix et Rhizoma Glycyrrhizae Praeparata cum Melle) harmonizes the formula.

Chapter 10 – Orifice-Opening Formulas　　　　　　　　　　　　　　*Section 1 – Cold Orifice-Opening Formulas*

Zǐ Xuě (Purple Snow)

CAUTIONS / CONTRAINDICATIONS

- *Zi Xue* should be discontinued as soon as the desired effects are achieved. Prolonged use of this formula, or use at large doses, could cause such side effects as profuse sweating, nausea, vomiting, icy cold extremities, hurried respiration, palpitations, dizziness, and vertigo.
- Use of this formula is contraindicated during pregnancy.[1]
- Avoid spicy, pungent, oily, and greasy foods while taking this formula.[2]

AUTHORS' COMMENTS

Febrile disorders are often complicated by heat drying up body fluids. Therefore, it is important to note that this

formula uses sweet and cold herbs that clear heat and preserve body fluids [such as *Shi Gao* (Gypsum Fibrosum) and *Hua Shi* (Talcum)], instead of bitter and cold herbs that clear heat but damage yin and body fluids [such as *Huang Qin* (Radix Scutellariae) and *Huang Lian* (Rhizoma Coptidis)].

References
1. *Zhong Yao Ming Fang Yao Li Yu Ying Yong* (Pharmacology and Applications of Famous Herbal Formulas) 1989;385-386.
2. *Zhong Yao Ming Fang Yao Li Yu Ying Yong* (Pharmacology and Applications of Famous Herbal Formulas) 1989;385-386.

Xiǎo Ér Huí Chūn Dān (Return of Spring Special Pill [Pediatric])

小兒回春丹
小儿回春丹

Pinyin Name: *Xiao Er Hui Chun Dan*
Literal Name: Return of Spring Special Pill [Pediatric]
Alternate Name: *Hui Chun Dan* (Return of Spring Special Pill)
Original Source: *Jing Xiu Tang Yao Shuo* (Herbal Teachings from the Respectfully Decorated Hall) by Qian Shu-Tian

COMPOSITION

Niu Huang (Calculus Bovis)	12g
She Xiang (Moschus)	12g
Chuan Bei Mu (Bulbus Fritillariae Cirrhosae)	37.5g
Tian Zhu Huang (Concretio Silicea Bambusae)	37.5g
Dan Nan Xing (Arisaema cum Bile)	60g
Ban Xia (Rhizoma Pinelliae)	37.5g
Gou Teng (Ramulus Uncariae cum Uncis)	240g
Tian Ma (Rhizoma Gastrodiae)	37.5g
Quan Xie (Scorpio)	37.5g
Jiang Can (Bombyx Batryticatus)	37.5g
Zhu Sha (Cinnabaris)	sufficient amount
Da Huang (Radix et Rhizoma Rhei)	60g
Zhi Qiao (Fructus Citri Aurantii)	37.5g
Mu Xiang (Radix Aucklandiae)	37.5g
Chen Pi (Pericarpium Citri Reticulatae)	37.5g
Chen Xiang (Lignum Aquilariae Resinatum)	37.5g
Dou Kou (Fructus Amomi Rotundus)	37.5g
Tan Xiang (Lignum Santali Albi)	37.5g
Gan Cao (Radix et Rhizoma Glycyrrhizae)	26g

Note: *Zhu Sha* (Cinnabaris) is a potentially toxic heavy metal, and *She Xiang* (Moschus) is derived from an endangered animal. They are rarely used as medicinal substances today. The discussion here is included primarily for academic purposes, to reflect the historical use of these substances in its original formulation. Most

754

Xiǎo Ér Huì Chūn Dān (Return of Spring Special Pill [Pediatric])

herbal products today have removed them completely, or replaced them with substitutes with similar functions. For additional information on the toxicity of *Zhu Sha* (Cinnabaris), please refer to *Chinese Medical Herbology and Pharmacology* by John Chen and Tina Chen.

DOSAGE / PREPARATION / ADMINISTRATION

Grind the ingredients into powder and form into very small pills that weigh about 0.09g [90mg] each. *Zhu Sha* (Cinnabaris) is used to coat these pellets. For infants under 1 year of age, administer 1 pill, two to three times daily. For children between 1-2 years of age, administer 2 pills, two to three times daily.

CHINESE THERAPEUTIC ACTIONS

1. Opens the sensory orifices and stops convulsions
2. Clears heat and dissolves phlegm

CLINICAL MANIFESTATIONS

Infantile convulsions due to heat and phlegm: fever, fidgeting, irritability, restlessness, continuous crying at night, delirium, vomiting of milk, wheezing and dyspnea, coughing with sputum, abdominal pain, and diarrhea.

CLINICAL APPLICATIONS

Infantile seizures, epilepsy, and convulsions.

EXPLANATION

Xiao Er Hui Chun Dan (Return of Spring Special Pill [Pediatric]) is one of the most important and effective formulas for treating infantile seizures and epilepsy due to stagnation of interior heat and phlegm. Heat and phlegm can stagnate in the Heart and obstruct the *shen* (spirit), causing fidgeting, irritability, restlessness, continuous crying at night, and delirium. Heat and phlegm may accumulate in the Lung, leading to wheezing, dyspnea and cough with sputum. Heat and phlegm may affect the Stomach, causing vomiting, abdominal pain, and diarrhea. Finally, heat may stir internal wind and cause it to rise upward, producing convulsions.

This formula uses *Niu Huang* (Calculus Bovis) to clear heat, eliminate toxins, dispel phlegm, open the sensory orifices, calm Liver wind, and alleviate convulsions. The aromatic *She Xiang* (Moschus) can open the orifices and awaken *shen* (spirit). *Chuan Bei Mu* (Bulbus Fritillariae Cirrhosae), *Tian Zhu Huang* (Concretio Silicea

Xiao Er Hui Chun Dan (Return of Spring Special Pill [Pediatric])

Diagnosis	Signs and Symptoms	Treatment	Herbs
Infantile convulsions due to heat and phlegm	• Fidgeting, irritability, restlessness, continuous crying at night, and delirium: heat and phlegm stagnate in the Heart and obstruct the *shen* (spirit) • Vomiting, abdominal pain and diarrhea: heat and phlegm affecting the Stomach • Wheezing, dyspnea, and cough with sputum: heat and phlegm in the Lung • Convulsions: heat stirring internal wind upward	• Opens sensory orifices and stops convulsion • Clears heat and dissolves phlegm	• *Niu Huang* (Calculus Bovis) clears heat, eliminates toxins, dispels phlegm, calms Liver wind, and alleviates convulsions. • *She Xiang* (Moschus) opens the orifices and awakens *shen*. • *Chuan Bei Mu* (Bulbus Fritillariae Cirrhosae), *Tian Zhu Huang* (Concretio Silicea Bambusae), *Dan Nan Xing* (Arisaema cum Bile) and *Ban Xia* (Rhizoma Pinelliae) clear heat and dissolve phlegm. • *Gou Teng* (Ramulus Uncariae cum Uncis), *Tian Ma* (Rhizoma Gastrodiae), *Quan Xie* (Scorpio) and *Jiang Can* (Bombyx Batryticatus) calm internal wind and relieve convulsions. • *Zhu Sha* (Cinnabaris) quickly tranquilizes the mind and sedates Heart fire. • *Da Huang* (Radix et Rhizoma Rhei) purges fire and clears heat and phlegm stagnation. • *Zhi Qiao* (Fructus Aurantii), *Mu Xiang* (Radix Aucklandiae), *Chen Pi* (Pericarpium Citri Reticulatae), *Chen Xiang* (Lignum Aquilariae Resinatum), *Dou Kou* (Fructus Amomi Rotundus), and *Tan Xiang* (Lignum Santali Albi) regulate qi circulation to remove phlegm. • *Gan Cao* (Radix et Rhizoma Glycyrrhizae) harmonizes all of the herbs.

Chapter 10 – Orifice-Opening Formulas   *Section 1 – Cold Orifice-Opening Formulas*

Xiǎo Ér Huí Chūn Dān (Return of Spring Special Pill [Pediatric])

Bambusae), *Dan Nan Xing* (Arisaema cum Bile), and *Ban Xia* (Rhizoma Pinelliae) all clear heat and dissolve phlegm. *Gou Teng* (Ramulus Uncariae cum Uncis), *Tian Ma* (Rhizoma Gastrodiae), *Quan Xie* (Scorpio), and *Jiang Can* (Bombyx Batryticatus) calm Liver wind and relieve the convulsions. *Zhu Sha* (Cinnabaris) is a heavy substance that quickly tranquilizes the mind and helps sedate Heart fire. *Da Huang* (Radix et Rhizoma Rhei) purges fire and clears the stagnation of heat and phlegm. *Zhi Qiao* (Fructus Aurantii), *Mu Xiang* (Radix Aucklandiae), *Chen Pi* (Pericarpium Citri Reticulatae), *Chen Xiang* (Lignum Aquilariae Resinatum), *Dou Kou* (Fructus Amomi Rotundus), and *Tan Xiang* (Lignum Santali Albi)

regulate qi circulation to help remove the phlegm. *Gan Cao* (Radix et Rhizoma Glycyrrhizae) harmonizes all of the herbs.

CAUTIONS / CONTRAINDICATIONS

Xiao Er Hui Chun Dan is contraindicated in chronic convulsions with deficiency and cold of the Spleen and Kidney.

AUTHORS' COMMENTS

Xiao Er Hui Chun Dan is one of the best formulas to treat the acute onset of infantile convulsions. The four diagnostic keys are heat, phlegm, wind, and convulsions.

Xíng Jūn Sǎn (Troop-Marching Powder)
行軍散
行军散

Pinyin Name: *Xing Jun San*
Literal Name: Troop-Marching Powder
Original Source: *Huo Luan Lun* (Discussion of Sudden Turmoil Disorders) by Wan Shi-Xiong in 1862

COMPOSITION

She Xiang (Moschus)	3g
Bing Pian (Borneolum Syntheticum)	3g
Niu Huang (Calculus Bovis)	3g
Xiao Shi (Niter), *zhi* (prepared)	0.9g
Peng Sha (Borax)	3g
Xiong Huang (Realgar), *shui fei* (refined with water)	24g
Zhen Zhu (Margarita)	3g
Fei Jin (Gold)	20 leaves

Note: *Xiong Huang* (Realgar) is a potentially toxic heavy metal, and *She Xiang* (Moschus) is derived from an endangered animal. They are rarely used as medicinal substances today. The discussion here is included primarily for academic purposes, to reflect the historical use of these substances in its original formulation. Most herbal products today have removed them completely, or replaced them with substitutes with similar functions. For additional information on the toxicity of *Xiong Huang* (Realgar), please refer to *Chinese Medical Herbology and Pharmacology* by John Chen and Tina Chen.

DOSAGE / PREPARATION / ADMINISTRATION

The source text states to grind the ingredients separately into extremely fine powder. Mix these powders together and grind again. Place the powdered formula in a porcelain container and seal it with wax. Take 0.9-1.5g of the powdered formula per dose with boiled water at room temperature. Today, this formula is prepared by processing *Xiong Huang* (Realgar) and *Zhen Zhu* (Margarita) separately with the *shui fei* (refining with water) technique to obtain extremely fine powders. *Xiao Shi* (Niter), *Peng Sha* (Borax), *Niu Huang* (Calculus Bovis), *She Xiang*

756

Chinese Herbal Formulas and Applications

Xíng Jūn Sǎn (Troop-Marching Powder)

(Moschus) and *Bing Pian* (Borneolum Syntheticum) are ground into powder. All of these powders are blended and then sifted to produce the final powder. Take 0.3-0.9g of the powder per dose, two to three times daily.

CHINESE THERAPEUTIC ACTIONS

1. Opens the sensory orifices
2. Dispels filth and fetidness
3. Eliminates toxins

CLINICAL MANIFESTATIONS

1. *Sha zhang* (acute filthy disease) and sudden turmoil disorder in late summer and early fall: vomiting, diarrhea, abdominal pain, extreme irritability, chest oppression, and altered consciousness or unconsciousness.
2. Other uses: oral lesions, sore throat, and corneal opacity caused by wind-heat.

CLINICAL APPLICATIONS

Gastrointestinal infections and traveler's diarrhea.

EXPLANATION

Xing Jun San (Troop-Marching Powder) treats *sha zhang* (acute filthy disease) and sudden turmoil disorder, diseases contracted primarily via ingestion of raw, dirty, or filthy foods, leading to fever, chest oppression, abdominal distention, nausea, vomiting, and diarrhea. Ingestion of such unclean foods impairs normal digestion, leading to accumulation of dampness and phlegm, abnormal circulation of qi, and subsequent gastrointestinal symptoms such as abdominal distention, nausea, vomiting, and

diarrhea. Dampness and phlegm may also accumulate in the chest to cover the Pericardium, causing a feeling of chest oppression and altered consciousness.

This formula uses aromatic substances such as *She Xiang* (Moschus) and *Bing Pian* (Borneolum Syntheticum) as the chief agents to open the sensory orifices, active qi circulation, and dispel filth and fetidness. *Niu Huang* (Calculus Bovis) clears the Heart, eliminates toxins, dispels phlegm, and opens sensory orifices. *Xiao Shi* (Niter) purges heat and breaks stagnation. *Peng Sha* (Borax) clears heat and eliminates toxins. *Xiong Huang* (Realgar) is used at a large dose to dispel filth and fetidness and eliminate toxins. *Zhen Zhu* (Margarita) and *Fei Jin* (Gold) calm the *shen* (spirit).

CAUTIONS / CONTRAINDICATIONS

Use of *Xing Jun San* is contraindicated during pregnancy, since it contains many herbs that are acrid, aromatic, and dispersing.

AUTHORS' COMMENTS

This formula originally contained *Fei Jin* (Gold) to calm the *shen* (spirit). However, *Fei Jin* (Gold) is no longer used today, and has been replaced with *Sheng Jiang* (Rhizoma Zingiberis Recens), which relieves nausea and vomiting and harmonizes the middle *jiao*.

Xing Jun San, literally "Troop-Marching Powder", was originally used to ensure the health of military troops as they marched through different places and were exposed to environment and diet of poor sanitations.

Xing Jun San (Troop-Marching Powder)

Diagnosis	Signs and Symptoms	Treatment	Herbs
Sha zhang (acute filthy disease) and sudden turmoil disorder	• Abdominal distention, nausea, vomiting and diarrhea: damp and phlegm accumulation • A feeling of chest oppression and altered consciousness: damp and phlegm accumulation in the chest covering the Pericardium	• Opens the sensory orifices • Dispels filth and fetidness • Eliminates toxins	• *She Xiang* (Moschus) and *Bing Pian* (Borneolum Syntheticum) open the sensory orifices, activate qi circulation, and dispel filth and fetidness. • *Niu Huang* (Calculus Bovis) clears the Heart, eliminates toxins, dispels phlegm, and opens sensory orifices. • *Xiao Shi* (Niter) purges heat and breaks stagnation. • *Peng Sha* (Borax) clears heat and eliminates toxins. • *Xiong Huang* (Realgar) dispels filth and fetidness and eliminates toxins. • *Zhen Zhu* (Margarita) and *Fei Jin* (Gold) calm the *shen* (spirit).

ORIFICE-OPENING FORMULAS — 10

757

Section 2

温开剂

— Warm Orifice-Opening Formulas

Sū Hé Xiāng Wán (Liquid Styrax Pill)
蘇合香丸
苏合香丸

Pinyin Name: *Su He Xiang Wan*
Literal Name: Liquid Styrax Pill
Original Source: *Tai Ping Hui Min He Ji Ju Fang* (Imperial Grace Formulary of the Tai Ping Era) by the Imperial Medical Department in 1078-85

COMPOSITION

Su He Xiang (Styrax), *dun* (stewed)	30g
She Xiang (Moschus), *yan* (ground) to small particles	60g
Bing Pian (Borneolum Syntheticum), *yan* (ground) to small particles	30g
An Xi Xiang (Benzoinum), *ao* (simmered) the powder into paste	60g
Mu Xiang (Radix Aucklandiae)	60g
Tan Xiang (Lignum Santali Albi)	60g
Chen Xiang (Lignum Aquilariae Resinatum)	60g
Ru Xiang (Gummi Olibanum), *yan* (ground) to small particles	30g
Ding Xiang (Flos Caryophylli)	60g
Xiang Fu (Rhizoma Cyperi), *chao* (dry-fried)	60g
Bi Bo (Fructus Piperis Longi)	60g
Xi Jiao (Cornu Rhinoceri)	60g
Zhu Sha (Cinnabaris), *yan* (ground) and *shui fei* (refined with water)	60g
Bai Zhu (Rhizoma Atractylodis Macrocephalae)	60g
He Zi (Fructus Chebulae), *wei* (roasted)	60g

Note: *Zhu Sha* (Cinnabaris) is a potentially toxic heavy metal, and *Xi Jiao* (Cornu Rhinoceri) and *She Xiang* (Moschus) are derived from endangered animals. They are rarely used as medicinal substances today. The discussion here is included primarily for academic purposes, to reflect the historical use of these substances in its original formulation. Most herbal products today have removed them completely, or replaced them with substitutes with similar functions. For additional information on the toxicity of *Zhu Sha* (Cinnabaris), please refer to *Chinese Medical Herbology and Pharmacology* by John Chen and Tina Chen.

The source text states to use "*Qing Mu Xiang*" as one of the ingredients in this formula. However, it is believed that

"*Qing Mu Xiang*" actually refers to *Mu Xiang* (Radix Aucklandiae) during that period. Therefore, most textbooks and clinicians now use *Mu Xiang* (Radix Aucklandiae) as one of the ingredients in this formula.

DOSAGE / PREPARATION / ADMINISTRATION

Grind separately *She Xiang* (Moschus), *Bing Pian* (Borneolum Syntheticum) and *Xi Jiao* (Cornu Rhinoceri) into fine powder and sift all of these powders together. Process *Zhu Sha* (Cinnabaris) separately via the *shui fei* (refining with water) method to obtain an extremely fine powder. Grind and blend all the ingredients into powder. Separately simmer *An Xi Xiang* (Benzoinum) from powder into paste, and stew *Su He Xiang* (Styrax) from solid into liquid form, and then blend the paste and the

Sū Hé Xiāng Wán (Liquid Styrax Pill)

liquid together. Mix all of the ingredients (both powder and liquid) with honey to form large pills. Dry the pills in a cool place without direct exposure to sunlight. Take 1 pill one to two times daily.

CHINESE THERAPEUTIC ACTIONS

1. Opens the sensory orifices with aromatic herbs
2. Activates qi circulation and stops pain

CLINICAL MANIFESTATIONS

Cold *bi zheng* (closed disorder) syndrome caused by stagnation of cold, qi and phlegm: sudden unconsciousness, extreme pain in the chest and abdomen, lockjaw, pale face, blue lips, white tongue coating, and a slow pulse.

CLINICAL APPLICATIONS

Angina pectoris, coronary artery disease, and cerebrovascular accident.

EXPLANATION

Su He Xiang Wan (Liquid Styrax Pill) is the representative formula for treating cold *bi zheng* (closed disorder) syndrome caused by stagnation of cold, qi and phlegm. Interior cold or phlegm obstruction may suddenly block the qi flow and "seize" Heart *shen* (spirit). As a result, acute and serious symptoms such as sudden unconsciousness, lockjaw, and abdominal and chest pain occur.

To effectively treat this syndrome, all three methods of cold-dispersing, qi-regulating, and phlegm-dissolving must be employed. This formula uses aromatic substances such as *Su He Xiang* (Styrax), *She Xiang* (Moschus), *Bing Pian* (Borneolum Syntheticum), and *An Xi Xiang* (Benzoinum) to quickly open the sensory orifices. *Mu Xiang* (Radix Aucklandiae), *Tan Xiang* (Lignum Santali Albi), *Chen Xiang* (Lignum Aquilariae Resinatum), *Ru Xiang* (Gummi Olibanum), *Ding Xiang* (Flos Caryophylli), and *Xiang Fu* (Rhizoma Cyperi) activate qi circulation, dispel cold, and dissolve phlegm. *Bi Bo* (Fructus Piperis Longi) warms the interior and dispels cold. *Xi Jiao* (Cornu Rhinoceri) clears heat and eliminates toxins. *Zhu Sha* (Cinnabaris) quickly calms the *shen* (spirit) and stabilizes the mind. *Bai Zhu* (Rhizoma Atractylodis Macrocephalae) strengthens the Spleen and dispels dampness. *He Zi* (Fructus Chebulae) has a constricting effect to prevent the acrid and dispersing herbs of this formula from consuming too much *zheng* (upright) qi.

CAUTIONS / CONTRAINDICATIONS

- *Su He Xiang Wan* is contraindicated in cases of *tuo zheng* (abandoned syndrome) and hot *bi zheng* (closed disorder).
- Use of this formula is contraindicated during pregnancy.

Su He Xiang Wan (Liquid Styrax Pill)

Diagnosis	Signs and Symptoms	Treatment	Herbs
Cold *bi zheng* (closed disorder) syndrome due to stagnation of cold, qi and phlegm	• Sudden unconsciousness, lockjaw, and extreme pain in the chest and abdomen: cold *bi zheng* (closed disorder) • Pale face and blue lips: cold • Pain in the chest and abdomen: qi and blood stagnation	• Opens the sensory orifices with aromatic herbs • Activates qi circulation and stops pain	• *Su He Xiang* (Styrax), *She Xiang* (Moschus), *Bing Pian* (Borneolum Syntheticum) and *An Xi Xiang* (Benzoinum) quickly open the sensory orifices. • *Mu Xiang* (Radix Aucklandiae), *Tan Xiang* (Lignum Santali Albi), *Chen Xiang* (Lignum Aquilariae Resinatum), *Ru Xiang* (Gummi Olibanum), *Ding Xiang* (Flos Caryophylli) and *Xiang Fu* (Rhizoma Cyperi) activate qi circulation, dispel cold, and dissolve phlegm. • *Bi Bo* (Fructus Piperis Longi) warms the interior and dispels cold. • *Xi Jiao* (Cornu Rhinoceri) clears heat and eliminates toxins. • *Zhu Sha* (Cinnabaris) quickly calms the *shen* (spirit) and stabilizes the mind. • *Bai Zhu* (Rhizoma Atractylodis Macrocephalae) strengthens the Spleen and dispels dampness. • *He Zi* (Fructus Chebulae) prevents the acrid and dispersing herbs of this formula from consuming too much *zheng* (upright) qi.

Chapter 10 – Orifice-Opening Formulas

Section 2 – Warm Orifice-Opening Formulas

Sū Hé Xiāng Wán (Liquid Styrax Pill)

RELATED FORMULA

Guàn Xīn Sū Hé Wán (Coronary Styrax Pill)

冠心蘇合丸

冠心苏合丸

Pinyin Name: *Guan Xin Su He Wan*

Literal Name: Coronary Styrax Pill

Original Source: *Zhong Hua Ren Min Gong He Guo Yao Dian* (Pharmacopoeia of People's Republic of China) in 2005

Su He Xiang (Styrax)	50g
Bing Pian (Borneolum Syntheticum)	105g
Ru Xiang (Gummi Olibanum), *zhi* (prepared)	105g
Tan Xiang (Lignum Santali Albi)	210g
Tu Mu Xiang (Radix Inulae)	210g

Note: *Qing Mu Xiang* (Radix Aristolochiae) was used as one of the ingredients when this formulas was first cited in *Zhong Guo Yao Dian* (Dictionary of Chinese Medicine) in 1977. However, because *Qing Mu Xiang* (Radix Aristolochiae) contains aristolochic acid and is potentially toxic, most textbooks and clinicians have replaced it with *Tu Mu Xiang* (Radix Inulae).

The source text states to grind *Ru Xiang* (Gummi Olibanum), *Tan Xiang* (Lignum Santali Albi), and *Tu Mu Xiang* (Radix Inulae) into a fine powder. *Bing Pian* (Borneolum Syntheticum) is ground separately and then sifted together with the other herb powders. Heat up a sufficient amount of honey, add *Su He Xiang* (Styrax) and mix them together thoroughly. Then add the sifted herb powders and mix them together again. Form into 1,000 pills. Place 1 pill under the tongue or chew it before swallowing, one to three times daily. This formula may also be taken before bedtime or as needed.

The main actions of this formula are to open orifices with aromatic herbs, activate qi circulation, and relieve pain. Clinically, this formula is often used to treat angina pectoris characterized by stagnation of qi, phlegm, and turbidity.

Su He Xiang Wan and *Guan Xin Su He Wan* (Coronary Styrax Pill) both use warm herbs to open sensory orifices, regulate qi and blood circulation, and stop pain.

- *Su He Xiang Wan* has stronger effects to open sensory orifices, dispel cold, and regulate qi.
- *Guan Xin Su He Wan* has better function to relieve chest pain.

Zǐ Jīn Dìng (Purple Gold Special Pill)

紫金錠

紫金锭

Pinyin Name: *Zi Jin Ding*

Literal Name: Purple Gold Special Pill

Original Source: *Pian Yu Xin Shu* (Text from Heart of Jade) by Wu Quan in the mid-16th century

COMPOSITION

She Xiang (Moschus)	9g
Shan Ci Gu (Pseudobulbus Cremastrae seu Pleiones)	90g
Xiong Huang (Realgar)	30g
Qian Jin Zi (Semen Euphorbiae), frost	30g
Hong Da Ji (Radix Knoxiae)	45g
Zhu Sha (Cinnabaris)	30g
Wu Bei Zi (Galla Chinensis)	90g

Note: *Zhu Sha* (Cinnabaris) and *Xiong Huang* (Realgar) are potentially toxic heavy metals, and *She Xiang* (Moschus) is derived from an endangered animal. They are rarely used as medicinal substances today. The discussion here

is included primarily for academic purposes, to reflect the historical use of these substances in its original formulation. Most herbal products today have removed them completely, or replaced them with substitutes with

760

Zǐ Jīn Dǐng (Purple Gold Special Pill)

similar functions. For additional information on the toxicity, please refer to *Chinese Medical Herbology and Pharmacology* by John Chen and Tina Chen.

DOSAGE / PREPARATION / ADMINISTRATION

Grind the ingredients into powder and form into special pills with sticky rice paste. For topical application, crush the special pills and mix with water, and apply locally. Today, *Xiong Huang* (Realgar) and *Zhu Sha* (Cinnabaris) are processed with the *shui fei* (refining with water) technique to obtain extremely fine powder. *Shan Ci Gu* (Pseudobulbus Cremastrae seu Pleiones), *Wu Bei Zi* (Galla Chinensis) and *Hong Da Ji* (Radix Knoxiae) are crushed into powder. *She Xiang* (Moschus) is also crushed into powder. All of these powders are sifted together and mixed with the frost of *Qian Jin Zi* (Semen Euphorbiae). Mix sticky rice powder and water and form into a dough. Steam the dough, and mix with the herbal powder, and form into tablets. Dry the tablets in a cool place without direct exposure to sunlight. For internal use, take 0.6-1.5g of tablets twice daily. For topical use, crush the tablets, mix with vinegar, and apply to the affected area.

CHINESE THERAPEUTIC ACTIONS

1. Dissolves phlegm and opens the sensory orifices
2. Dispels filth and fetidness and eliminates toxins
3. Reduces swelling and relieves pain

CLINICAL MANIFESTATIONS

Accumulation of filth, fetidness, phlegm and turbidity: epigastric and abdominal distention, oppression and pain, nausea, vomiting, diarrhea, and phlegm syncope in children. This formula may be applied topically to treat abscesses and sores.

CLINICAL APPLICATIONS

Nausea and vomiting from gastrointestinal infections.

EXPLANATION

Zi Jin Ding (Purple Gold Special Pill) has a wide range of applications, and was used in the past to treat disorders characterized by accumulation of filth, fetidness, phlegm and turbidity leading to stagnation of qi. Clinical presentations include feeling of epigastric and abdominal distention, oppression and pain, nausea, vomiting, and diarrhea; phlegm syncope in children; and abscesses and sores when applied topically.

In this formula, *She Xiang* (Moschus) opens the sensory orifices, activates qi circulation and relieves pain. *Shan Ci Gu* (Pseudobulbus Cremastrae seu Pleiones) clears heat and reduces swellings. *Xiong Huang* (Realgar) dispels filth and fetidness and eliminates toxins. *Qian Jin Zi* (Semen Euphorbiae) and *Hong Da Ji* (Radix Knoxiae) eliminate phlegm and reduce swellings. *Zhu Sha* (Cinnabaris) calms the *shen* (spirit). *Wu Bei Zi* (Galla Chinensis) astringes the Intestines to relieve diarrhea. It also prevents the drastic and harsh herbs from damaging the body.

CAUTIONS / CONTRAINDICATIONS

- *Zi Jin Ding* should be used with caution during pregnancy, since *She Xiang* (Moschus) has potent dispersing effect.
- It should be used with caution and with reduced dose in children, since some ingredients in this formula are potentially toxic.

AUTHORS' COMMENTS

Zi Jin Ding can also be applied topically on abscesses and sores to reduce swelling and disperse nodules.

Zi Jin Ding (Purple Gold Special Pill)

Diagnosis	Signs and Symptoms	Treatment	Herbs
Accumulation of filth, fetidness, phlegm and turbidity	Epigastric and abdominal distention, oppression and pain, nausea, vomiting and diarrhea	• Dissolves phlegm and opens the sensory orifices • Dispels filth and fetidness and eliminates toxins • Reduces swellings and relieves pain	• *She Xiang* (Moschus) opens the sensory orifices, activates qi circulation, and relieves pain. • *Shan Ci Gu* (Pseudobulbus Cremastrae seu Pleiones) clears heat and reduces swellings. • *Xiong Huang* (Realgar) dispels filth and fetidness and eliminates toxins. • *Qian Jin Zi* (Semen Euphorbiae) and *Hong Da Ji* (Radix Knoxiae) eliminate phlegm and reduce swellings. • *Zhu Sha* (Cinnabaris) calms the *shen* (spirit). • *Wu Bei Zi* (Galla Chinensis) astringes the Intestines to relieve diarrhea.

Chapter 10 – Orifice-Opening Formulas

Chapter 10 — Summary

— Orifice-Opening Formulas

SECTION 1: COLD ORIFICE-OPENING FORMULAS

Name	Similarities	Differences
An Gong Niu Huang Wan (Calm the Palace Pill with Cattle Gallstone)	Open the sensory orifices, treat hot *bi zheng* (closed disorder)	Clears heat and eliminates toxins
Zhi Bao Dan (Greatest Treasure Special Pill)		Opens the sensory orifices, calms the *shen* (spirit)
Zi Xue (Purple Snow)		Calms Liver wind, relieves convulsions
Xiao Er Hui Chun Dan (Return of Spring Special Pill [Pediatric])	Open the sensory orifices	Treats infantile convulsions
Xing Jun San (Troop-Marching Powder)		Treats *sha zhang* (acute filthy disease)

An Gong Niu Huang Wan (Calm the Palace Pill with Cattle Gallstone), ***Zhi Bao Dan*** (Greatest Treasure Special Pill), and ***Zi Xue*** (Purple Snow) are generally considered to be the three representative formulas for treating hot *bi zheng* (closed disorder).

- *An Gong Niu Huang Wan* clears heat, eliminates toxins, opens the sensory orifices, and calms the *shen* (spirit). It mainly treats febrile disorders in which heat attacks the Pericardium and heat-phlegm obstructs the orifices.
- *Zhi Bao Dan* has potent functions to open the sensory orifices and calms the *shen* (spirit). It treats *bi zheng* (closed disorder) syndrome caused by heat-phlegm obstruction. It is also effective in treating infantile seizures, epilepsy, and convulsions caused by heat-phlegm obstruction.
- *Zi Xue* strongly calms Liver wind and stops convulsions, but is mild in clearing heat, eliminating toxins, opening the sensory orifices, and calming the *shen* (spirit). Thus, it is mostly used to treat febrile disorders in which heat attacks the Pericardium, giving rise to seizures, epilepsy, and convulsions.

Xiao Er Hui Chun Dan (Return of Spring Special Pill [Pediatric]) clears heat, dissolves phlegm, and opens the sensory orifices. As the name implies, it is designed for children to treat convulsions associated with heat and phlegm. The main clinical manifestations include fever, night crying, fright, delirium, irritability, and vomiting of milk.

Xing Jun San (Troop-Marching Powder) opens the sensory orifices, dispels filth and fetidness, and eliminates toxins. This formula was originally used to treat *sha zhang* (acute filthy disease), a gastrointestinal disease contracted primarily by ingestion of filthy (raw, dirty or unclean) foods. Clinical manifestations include fever, chest oppression, abdominal distention, nausea, vomiting, diarrhea, and in severe cases, altered consciousness.

Chinese Herbal Formulas and Applications

Chapter 10 — Summary

SECTION 2: WARM ORIFICE-OPENING FORMULAS

Name	Similarities	Differences
Su He Xiang Wan (Liquid Styrax Pill)	Open the sensory orifices, treat cold *bi zheng* (closed disorder)	Activates qi circulation, dispels cold, stops pain
Zi Jin Ding (Purple Gold Special Pill)		Dissolves phlegm, dispels filth and fetidness, eliminates toxins

Su He Xiang Wan (Liquid Styrax Pill) and ***Zi Jin Ding*** (Purple Gold Special Pill) are two warm formulas with similar functions to open the sensory orifices and treat cold *bi zheng* (closed disorder).

- *Su He Xiang Wan* has additional functions to activate qi circulation, dispel cold, and stop pain. It treats cases of altered consciousness due to cold *bi zheng* (closed disorder) with stagnation of cold, qi and phlegm. Clinical manifestations include sudden unconsciousness, locked jaws, and extreme pain in the chest and abdomen.
- *Zi Jin Ding* has additional functions to dissolve phlegm, dispel filth and fetidness, and eliminate toxins. It treats gastrointestinal disorders characterized by accumulation of filth, fetidness, phlegm, and turbidity. Clinical manifestations include feelings of epigastric and abdominal distention, oppression and pain, nausea, vomiting, and diarrhea.

Chapter 11

— Astringent Formulas

傅山 Fù Shān, also known as 傅青主 Fù Qīng-Zhǔ, 1607–1684.

固涩剂

Chapter 11 - Astringent Formulas

傅山 Fù Shán

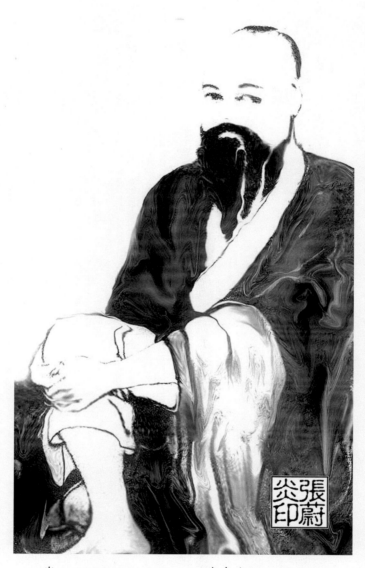

傅山 Fù Shán, also known as 傅青主 Fù Qíng-Zhǔ, 1607 – 1684.

傅山 Fù Shán

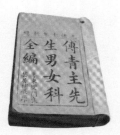

傅青主男科 *Fu Qing Zhu Nan Ke* (Men's Diseases According to Fu Qing-Zhu) and 傅青主女科 *Fu Qing Zhu Nu Ke* (Women's Diseases According to Fu Qing-Zhu), combined.

Fu Shan, also known as Fu Qing-Zhu,[1] is one of the most famous physicians from the Ming and Qing dynasties. He mastered the medical texts published before his time, and experimented with many *Yan Fang* (Time-Tested Formulas) from doctors during his own period of time. After many years of searching for and experimenting with regional remedies, Fu Shan discovered many unconventional, yet effective, herbal therapies. He concluded that it is extremely important to be completely open-minded when practicing medicine: "Do not be restricted to just one school of thought when making the diagnosis [whether *shang han* (cold damage) or *wen bing* (warm disease)], and do not be confined to a fixed formula when prescribing medicine." By this, he set a strong example for practitioners to modify and customize each treatment as needed.

Fu Shan is known for having cared for his patients above and beyond his duty as a physician. He would frequently treat the poor and homeless for free, pay for their herbal medicines, and even give them money for food and shelter. When he died at the age of 78, thousands of people came from near and far to attend his funeral, to show their appreciation for his compassion as a person and skills as a physician.

Fu Shan specialized in both men's and women's health, and significantly influenced the treatment of male and female disorders in Traditional Chinese Medicine. He wrote many books, and is best known for *Fu Qing Zhu Nan Ke* (Men's Diseases According to Fu Qing-Zhu) and *Fu Qing Zhu Nu Ke* (Women's Diseases According to Fu Qing-Zhu). Many of the formulas discussed in these texts are still in use today, such as *Wan Dai Tang* (End Discharge Decoction), *Bao Chan Wu You Fang* (Preserve Pregnancy and Care-Free Decoction), and *Sheng Hua Tang* (Generation and Transformation Decoction).

Dynasties & Kingdoms	Year
Xia Dynasty 夏	2100-1600 BCE
Shang Dynasty 商	1600-1100 BCE
Zhou Dynasty 周	1100-221 BCE
Qin Dynasty 秦	221-207 BCE
Han Dynasty 漢	206 BCE-220
Three Kingdoms 三國	220-280
Western Jin Dynasty 西晉	265-316
Eastern Jin Dynasty 東晉	317-420
Northern and Southern Dynasties 北南朝	420-581
Sui Dynasty 隋	581-618
Tang Dynasty 唐	618-907
Five Dynasties 五代	907-960
Song Dynasty 宋	960-1279
Liao Dynasty 遼	916-1125
Jin Dynasty 金	1115-1234
Yuan Dynasty 元	1271-1368
Ming Dynasty 明	**1368-1644**
Qing Dynasty 清	1644-1911
Republic of China 中華民國	1912-Present Day
People's Republic of China 中華人民共和國	1949-Present Day

---

1. Fu Shan was multi-talented. In addition to being an excellent physician, he was an expert in art, poetry, calligraphy, and martial arts. He was also a patriot in and soldier for the Ming dynasty, and led many revolts against the Qing dynasty. Eventually, when the Ming dynasty collapsed, he retreated to the mountains to quietly practice medicine. To avoid being tracked down and prosecuted, he changed his name to Fu Qing-Zhu, which is why all his publications carry this pseudonym.

Chapter 11 – Astringent Formulas

Table of Contents

Chapter 11. Astringent Formulas ⋯⋯⋯⋯⋯⋯⋯⋯⋯⋯⋯⋯⋯⋯⋯⋯⋯ **765**
Biography of Fu Shan ⋯⋯⋯⋯⋯⋯⋯⋯⋯⋯⋯⋯⋯⋯⋯⋯⋯⋯⋯⋯⋯⋯⋯⋯⋯ 766

Section 1. Exterior-Stabilizing Formulas to Stop Perspiration ⋯⋯⋯⋯⋯ **773**
Yu Ping Feng San (Jade Windscreen Powder) ⋯⋯⋯⋯⋯⋯⋯⋯⋯⋯⋯⋯⋯ 773
  Huang Qi Fang Feng Tang (Astragalus Decoction to Guard the Wind) ⋯⋯⋯⋯ 775
Mu Li San (Oyster Shell Powder) ⋯⋯⋯⋯⋯⋯⋯⋯⋯⋯⋯⋯⋯⋯⋯⋯⋯⋯ 776

Section 2. Lung-Restraining Formula to Relieve Cough ⋯⋯⋯⋯⋯⋯⋯ **779**
Jiu Xian San (Nine-Immortal Powder) ⋯⋯⋯⋯⋯⋯⋯⋯⋯⋯⋯⋯⋯⋯⋯⋯ 779

Section 3. Intestine-Binding Formulas to Stop Leakage ⋯⋯⋯⋯⋯⋯⋯ **781**
Zhen Ren Yang Zang Tang (True Man's Decoction for Nourishing the Organs) ⋯ 781
Si Shen Wan (Four-Miracle Pill) ⋯⋯⋯⋯⋯⋯⋯⋯⋯⋯⋯⋯⋯⋯⋯⋯⋯⋯ 784
Tao Hua Tang (Peach Blossom Decoction) ⋯⋯⋯⋯⋯⋯⋯⋯⋯⋯⋯⋯⋯⋯ 787
  Chi Shi Zhi Yu Yu Liang Tang (Halloysitum and Limonite Decoction) ⋯⋯⋯⋯ 788

Section 4. *Jing* (Essence)-Stabilizing Formulas to Stop Leakage ⋯⋯⋯ **789**
Jin Suo Gu Jing Wan (Metal Lock Pill to Stabilize the Essence) ⋯⋯⋯⋯⋯⋯ 789
  Shui Lu Er Xian Dan (Water and Earth Two Immortals Special Pill) ⋯⋯⋯⋯ 790
Liu Wei Gu Jing Wan (Rehmannia Six and Lotus Stamen Pill) ⋯⋯⋯⋯⋯⋯⋯ 791
Sang Piao Xiao San (Mantis Egg-Case Powder) ⋯⋯⋯⋯⋯⋯⋯⋯⋯⋯⋯⋯ 792
Suo Quan Wan (Shut the Sluice Pill) ⋯⋯⋯⋯⋯⋯⋯⋯⋯⋯⋯⋯⋯⋯⋯⋯ 795
Fu Tu Dan (Poria and Cuscuta Special Pill) ⋯⋯⋯⋯⋯⋯⋯⋯⋯⋯⋯⋯⋯ 797
Gui Zhi Jia Long Gu Mu Li Tang (Cinnamon Twig Decoction plus Dragon Bone and Oyster Shell) ⋯ 798
Zhi Zhuo Gu Ben Wan (Treat the Turbidity and Guard the Root Pill) ⋯⋯⋯⋯ 800

Section 5. Womb-Stabilizing Formulas to Stop Leakage ⋯⋯⋯⋯⋯⋯⋯ **802**
Gu Jing Wan (Stabilize the Menses Pill) ⋯⋯⋯⋯⋯⋯⋯⋯⋯⋯⋯⋯⋯⋯⋯ 802
  Gu Chong Tang (Stabilize *Chong* [Thoroughfare Channel] Decoction) ⋯⋯⋯⋯ 803
Zhen Ling Dan (Rouse the Spirits Special Pill) ⋯⋯⋯⋯⋯⋯⋯⋯⋯⋯⋯⋯ 805
Wan Dai Tang (End Discharge Decoction) ⋯⋯⋯⋯⋯⋯⋯⋯⋯⋯⋯⋯⋯⋯ 806
  Yi Huang Tang (Change the Yellow [Discharge] Decoction) ⋯⋯⋯⋯⋯⋯⋯⋯ 809
  Qing Dai Tang (Clear the Discharge Decoction) ⋯⋯⋯⋯⋯⋯⋯⋯⋯⋯⋯⋯ 809
Ba Wei Dai Xia Fang (Eight-Ingredient Formula for Leukorrhea) ⋯⋯⋯⋯⋯ 810

Astringent Formulas (Summary) ⋯⋯⋯⋯⋯⋯⋯⋯⋯⋯⋯⋯⋯⋯⋯⋯⋯ **812**

Chinese Herbal Formulas and Applications

Chapter 11 — Overview

— Astringent Formulas

固涩剂

Definition: Astringent formulas stabilize, bind, and stop the loss of qi, blood, *jing* (essence), and body fluids.

Qi, blood, *jing* (essence) and body fluids are vital substances of the body. These four substances are constantly being consumed and replaced, like the continuous flow of water in and out of a running river. It is this balance of consumption and replacement that helps to sustain health and life. However, in cases of over-consumption, lack of production, and/or continuous loss, disorders will surface. The loss of qi, blood, *jing*, or body fluids results in various clinical manifestations, such as spontaneous sweating, night sweats, chronic coughing, spermatorrhea, nocturnal emission, incontinence, chronic diarrhea, dysentery, leukorrhea and profuse menstrual bleeding. Clinical manifestations differ depending on the cause and location of the illness.

Astringent formulas treat disorders characterized by underlying deficiency with inability to produce qi, blood, *jing* (essence), or body fluids, and complicated by the continuous loss of these substances. In most cases, the cause and symptoms are treated concurrently by using tonic and astringent herbs. In cases of severe loss of qi, blood, *jing*, or body fluids, astringent herbs are used first to stop the immediate loss, followed by the use of tonic herbs to regenerate and replace these substances. In the case of qi and yang depletion, high doses of qi and yang-tonifying herbs should be used to restore qi and yang [*see* Chapter 6 Interior-Warming Formulas].

> Qi, blood, *jing* (essence) and body fluids are constantly being consumed and replaced, like the continuous flow of water in and out of a running river.

SUBCATEGORIES OF ACTION

Astringent formulas are divided into five subcategories according to their therapeutic actions and clinical applications.

1. **Exterior-Stabilizing Formulas to Stop Perspiration**
   These formulas are designed to treat spontaneous sweating due to *wei* (defensive) *qi* deficiency, or night sweating due to yin deficiency. *Huang Qi* (Radix Astragali) and *Bai Zhu* (Rhizoma Atractylodis Macrocephalae) tonify *wei* (defensive) *qi* to stop spontaneous sweating, while *Fu Xiao Mai* (Fructus Tritici Levis) and *Mu Li* (Concha Ostreae) benefit yin and relieve night sweats. One exemplar formula that treats spontaneous sweating is *Yu Ping Feng San* (Jade Windscreen Powder), while *Mu Li San* (Oyster Shell Powder) is an exemplar formula for treating night sweats.

2. **Lung-Restraining Formula to Relieve Cough**
   This formula is designed to treat chronic cough with Lung qi and yin deficiencies. The signs and symptoms of this condition include shortness of breath, spontaneous sweating, and a deficient, rapid pulse. In this case, astringent and tonic herbs are used together to treat the symptoms and the cause. For example, *Wu Wei Zi* (Fructus Schisandrae Chinensis) and *Wu Mei* (Fructus Mume) restrain the Lung and relieve cough, while *Ren Shen* (Radix et Rhizoma Ginseng) and *E Jiao* (Colla Corii Asini) tonify qi and nourish yin. A representative formula is *Jiu Xian San* (Nine-Immortal Powder).

ASTRINGENT FORMULAS

11

769

Chapter 11 – Astringent Formulas

Chapter 11 — Overview

~

Astringent herbs stop the immediate loss of qi, blood, *jing* (essence), or body fluids. Tonic herbs regenerate and replace them.

~

3. Intestine-Binding Formulas to Stop Leakage

These formulas treat diarrhea, dysentery, and in severe cases, rectal incontinence, characterized by chronic deficiency and cold of the Spleen and Kidney. Astringent herbs that bind the Intestines to stop diarrhea and dysentery include *Chi Shi Zhi* (Halloysitum Rubrum), *Rou Dou Kou* (Semen Myristicae), *He Zi* (Fructus Chebulae), and *Wu Wei Zi* (Fructus Schisandrae Chinensis). Tonic herbs that address deficiency and cold of the Spleen and Kidney include *Bu Gu Zhi* (Fructus Psoraleae), *Rou Gui* (Cortex Cinnamomi), *Gan Jiang* (Rhizoma Zingiberis), *Ren Shen* (Radix et Rhizoma Ginseng), and *Bai Zhu* (Rhizoma Atractylodis Macrocephalae). Exemplar formulas include *Zhen Ren Yang Zang Tang* (True Man's Decoction for Nourishing the Organs), *Si Shen Wan* (Four-Miracle Pill), and *Tao Hua Tang* (Peach Blossom Decoction).

4. *Jing* (Essence)-Stabilizing Formulas to Stop Leakage

Formulas in this subcategory treat problems such as spermatorrhea, nocturnal emission, urinary incontinence, or enuresis due to Kidney deficiency. Kidney deficiency, characterized by leakage of *jing* (essence) and manifested as spermatorrhea or nocturnal emission, is treated by herbs such as *Sha Yuan Zi* (Semen Astragali Complanati), *Lian Xu* (Stamen Nelumbinis), *Qian Shi* (Semen Euryales), and the formula *Jin Suo Gu Jing Wan* (Metal Lock Pill to Stabilize the Essence). Kidney deficiency characterized by leakage of urine with signs such as urinary incontinence or enuresis, may be treated with herbs and formulas such as *Sang Piao Xiao* (Ootheca Mantidis), *Sang Piao Xiao San* (Mantis Egg-Case Powder), and *Suo Quan Wan* (Shut the Sluice Pill).

5. Womb-Stabilizing Formulas to Stop Leakage

These formulas treat profuse menstrual bleeding, metrorrhagia, continuous leukorrhea, and various *beng lou* (flooding and spotting) disorders. Clinical manifestations include palpitations, shortness of breath, soreness and pain of the lower back, pale face, prolonged menstrual bleeding, continuous leukorrhea, pale tongue, and a deficient, weak and fine pulse. Commonly used herbs include calcined *Long Gu* (Os Draconis), calcined *Mu Li* (Concha Ostreae), *Hai Piao Xiao* (Endoconcha Sepiae), *Chun Pi* (Cortex Ailanthi) and *Wu Bei Zi* (Galla Chinensis). Representative formulas include *Gu Jing Wan* (Stabilize the Menses Pill), *Wan Dai Tang* (End Discharge Decoction), and *Yi Huang Tang* (Change the Yellow [Discharge] Decoction).

Though these conditions are generally characterized by Spleen and Kidney deficiencies with instability of *chong* (thoroughfare) and *ren* (conception) channels, the treatment needs to be modified accordingly, as these conditions often occur with complications.

- For *beng lou* (flooding and spotting) with additional signs and symptoms such as palpitations, shortness of breath, weakness and pain of the lower back, pale face, pale tongue, and a deficient, fine, and weak pulse, add *Chun Pi* (Cortex Ailanthi), *Long Gu* (Os Draconis), *Mu Li* (Concha Ostreae), and *Bai Guo* (Semen Ginkgo).
- For *beng lou* (flooding and spotting) characterized by weakness of Spleen qi or deficiency of *chong* (thoroughfare) and *ren* (conception) channels, add *Huang Qi* (Radix Astragali), *Bai Zhu* (Rhizoma Atractylodis Macrocephalae), and *Shan Zhu Yu* (Fructus Corni).
- For *beng lou* (flooding and spotting) accompanied by yin deficiency and heat in the blood, add *Gui Ban* (Plastrum Testudinis) and *Huang Bo* (Cortex Phellodendri Chinensis).
- For leukorrhea caused by damp-heat in the lower *jiao*, add *Che Qian Zi* (Semen Plantaginis).

~

In most cases, cause and symptoms are treated concurrently by using tonic and astringent herbs.

~

CAUTIONS / CONTRAINDICATIONS

- Astringent formulas are not suitable in disorders in which the loss of qi, blood, *jing* (essence), or body fluids is caused by excess syndromes with pathogenic factors residing in the interior. Examples include sweating due to heat, coughing due to phlegm retention, nocturnal emission due to fire, diarrhea and dysentery due to damp-heat, and metrorrhagia or leukorrhea due to heat in the blood. These are some of the syndromes not suitable

Chinese Herbal Formulas and Applications

Chapter 11 — Overview

with astringent formulas since the use of astringent herbs may trap the pathogenic factors inside the body, further aggravating the condition.

- Astringent formulas are primarily used to temporarily treat symptoms to stop the loss of qi, blood, *jing* (essence), or body fluids. It is important to also use tonic herbs to address the underlying deficiency.

PHARMACOLOGICAL EFFECTS & CLINICAL APPLICATIONS

Astringent formulas stop the loss of qi, blood, *jing* (essence), or body fluids from various parts of the body. From allopathic medical perspectives, these formulas treat respiratory, kidney, intestinal, genitourinary, menstrual, and gynecological disorders.

1. **Exterior-stabilizing formulas** that stop perspiration are designed to treat spontaneous or night sweating. They also address respiratory and kidney disorders.
   - **Sweating**: *Yu Ping Feng San* (Jade Windscreen Powder) and *Mu Li San* (Oyster Shell Powder) are formulas that have been used effectively to treat both spontaneous and night sweating.[1,2]
   - **Prevention of respiratory tract infection**: *Yu Ping Feng San* (Jade Windscreen Powder) is also frequently used for the prevention of respiratory tract infection,[3] as it has marked immunostimulant and antiviral effects.[4,5]
   - **Nephritis**: *Yu Ping Feng San* (Jade Windscreen Powder) has been shown to have nephroprotective effects,[6] and has been used to effectively treat nephritis.[7]

2. **The Lung-restraining formula** is used mainly to treat cough.
   - **Cough**: *Jiu Xian San* (Nine-Immortal Powder) effectively suppresses cough as many of its ingredients have antitussive and expectorant effects, such as *Ying Su Ke* (Pericarpium Papaveris),[8] *Kuan Dong Hua* (Flos Farfarae),[9] and *Jie Geng* (Radix Platycodonis).[10]

3. **Intestine-binding formulas** that stop leakage are used primarily to treat intestinal disorders marked by the loss of fluids, such as diarrhea and dysentery.
   - **Diarrhea and dysentery**: These formulas have been used with great success to treat diarrhea,[11,12,13] dysentery,[14,15] and colitis.[16,17] The mechanism of this antidiarrheal effect is attributed in part to the inhibition of intestinal peristalsis and increased reabsorption of water.[18] Exemplar formulas include *Zhen Ren Yang Zang Tang* (True Man's Decoction for Nourishing the Organs), *Si Shen Wan* (Four-Miracle Pill), and *Tao Hua Tang* (Peach Blossom Decoction).

> Astringent formulas are not suitable if the losses are caused by excess syndromes with pathogenic factors residing in the interior.

4. ***Jing* (essence)-stabilizing formulas** that stop leakage are primarily used to treat abnormalities of sperm (spermatorrhea and nocturnal emission) and urine (incontinence and enuresis).
   - **Spermatorrhea**: According to one report, *Jin Suo Gu Jing Wan* (Metal Lock Pill to Stabilize the Essence) demonstrated good results in treating severe spermatorrhea.[19]
   - **Urinary disorders**: These formulas are effective in the treatment of urinary disorders, such as enuresis,[20,21] frequent urination,[22,23] and urinary incontinence.[24] The mechanism of action is attributed in part to the antidiuretic effects of the formula.[25] Exemplar formulas include *Sang Piao Xiao San* (Mantis Egg-Case Powder) and *Suo Quan Wan* (Shut the Sluice Pill).

5. **Womb-stabilizing formulas** that stop leakage are mainly used to treat menstrual and gynecological disorders.
   - **Menstrual disorders**: *Gu Jing Wan* (Stabilize the Menses Pill) may be used to treat various menstrual disorders, such as irregular menstruation during puberty,[26] and *beng lou* (flooding and spotting) during the perimenopausal period.[27]
   - **Gynecological disorders**: *Wan Dai Tang* (End Discharge Decoction) is used to address many gynecological disorders, such as leukorrhea,[28] chronic cervicitis,[29] and acute or chronic vaginitis.[30]

Chapter 11 — Overview

References

1. *Zhe Jiang Zhong Yi Za Zhi* (Zhejiang Journal of Chinese Medicine) 1992;8:378.
2. *Fu Jian Zhong Yi Yao* (Fujian Chinese Medicine and Herbology) 1966;3:37.
3. *Zhong Yi Za Zhi* (Journal of Chinese Medicine) 1982;1:37.
4. *Zhong Yao Yao Li Yu Lin Chuang* (Pharmacology and Clinical Applications of Chinese Herbs) 1990;6(3):7.
5. *Jiang Xi Zhong Yi Yao* (Jiangxi Chinese Medicine and Herbology) 1989;6:40.
6. *Zhong Xi Yi Jie He Za Zhi* (Journal of Integrated Chinese and Western Medicine) 1986;4:299.
7. *Zhong Yi Za Zhi* (Journal of Chinese Medicine) 1992;33(5):24.
8. *Zhong Cao Yao Xue* (Study of Chinese Herbal Medicine) 1976;355.
9. *Zhong Yao Yao Li Yu Ying Yong* (Pharmacology and Applications of Chinese Herbs) 1983;1132.
10. *Zhong Yao Yao Li Yu Ying Yong* (Pharmacology and Applications of Chinese Herbs) 1983;866.
11. *Zhong Yi Fang Ji Xian Dai Yan Jiu* (Modern Study of Medical Formulae in Traditional Chinese Medicine) 1997;807-808.
12. *Zhe Jiang Zhong Yi Za Zhi* (Zhejiang Journal of Chinese Medicine) 1993;9:395.
13. *Shan Xi Zhong Yi* (Shanxi Chinese Medicine) 1990;1:30.
14. *Jiang Su Zhong Yi Za Zhi* (Jiangsu Journal of Chinese Medicine) 1987;5:17.
15. *Hu Nan Zhong Yi Za Zhi* (Hunan Journal of Chinese Medicine) 1994;4:38.
16. *Cheng Du Zhong Yi Xue Yuan Xue Bao* (Journal of Chengdu University of Traditional Chinese Medicine) 1989;4:27.
17. *Nei Meng Gu Zhong Yi Yao* (Traditional Chinese Medicine and Medicinals of Inner Mongolia) 1987;5:8.
18. *Zhong Cheng Yao Yan Jiu* (Research of Chinese Patent Medicine) 1981;9:31.
19. *Hu Nan Zhong Yi Za Zhi* (Hunan Journal of Chinese Medicine) 1987;3:46.
20. *Shan Xi Zhong Yi* (Shanxi Chinese Medicine) 1997;1:31.
21. *Jiang Su Zhong Yi* (Jiangsu Chinese Medicine) 1994;4:14.
22. *Fu Jian Zhong Yi Yao* (Fujian Chinese Medicine and Herbology) 1998;6:24.
23. *Hei Long Jiang Zhong Yi Yao* (Heilongjiang Chinese Medicine and Herbology) 1990;1:33.
24. *Bei Jing Zhong Yi* (Beijing Chinese Medicine) 1997;2:55.
25. *Zhong Yi Fang Ji Xian Dai Yan Jiu* (Modern Study of Medical Formulae in Traditional Chinese Medicine) 1997;823.
26. *Shang Hai Zhong Yi Yao Za Zhi* (Shanghai Journal of Chinese Medicine and Herbology) 1994;10:21.
27. *Shang Hai Zhong Yi Yao Za Zhi* (Shanghai Journal of Chinese Medicine and Herbology) 1994;10:21.
28. *Shang Hai Zhong Yi Yao Za Zhi* (Shanghai Journal of Chinese Medicine and Herbology) 1991;12:17.
29. *Jiang Su Zhong Yi* (Jiangsu Chinese Medicine) 1987;4:17.
30. *Xin Zhong Yi* (New Chinese Medicine) 1997;11:31.

Chinese Herbal Formulas and Applications

Section 1

固表止汗剂

— Exterior-Stabilizing Formulas to Stop Perspiration

Yù Píng Fēng Sǎn (Jade Windscreen Powder)
玉屏風散
玉屏风散

Pinyin Name: *Yu Ping Feng San*
Literal Name: Jade Windscreen Powder
Alternate Names: Jade Wind-Barrier Formula, Jade Screen Powder, Astragalus and Siler Formula
Original Source: *Dan Xi Xin Fa* (Teachings of [Zhu] Dan-Xi) by Zhu Zhen-Heng in 1481

COMPOSITION

Huang Qi (Radix Astragali)	30g [6g]
Bai Zhu (Rhizoma Atractylodis Macrocephalae)	60g [12g]
Fang Feng (Radix Saposhnikoviae)	30g [6g]

DOSAGE / PREPARATION / ADMINISTRATION

The source text states to grind the ingredients into powder. Cook 9g of the powdered herbs and 3 slices of *Sheng Jiang* (Rhizoma Zingiberis Recens) in 1.5 large bowls of water for decoction. Today, this formula may be prepared as a decoction with the doses suggested in brackets, with addition of 3 slices of *Sheng Jiang* (Rhizoma Zingiberis Recens) and 1 piece of *Da Zao* (Fructus Jujubae).[1]

CHINESE THERAPEUTIC ACTIONS

1. Tonifies *wei* (defensive) *qi*
2. Consolidates the exterior
3. Stops spontaneous sweating

CLINICAL MANIFESTATIONS

Wei (defensive) *qi* deficiency: spontaneous sweating, aversion to wind and cold, increased susceptibility to invasion of exterior pathogens, pale face, pale tongue, white tongue coating, and a floating, deficient pulse.

CLINICAL APPLICATIONS

Prevention of respiratory tract infection, allergic rhinitis, abnormal perspiration, nephritis, and facial paralysis.

EXPLANATION

Yu Ping Feng San (Jade Windscreen Powder) is commonly used to treat spontaneous sweating or increased susceptibility to invasion of exterior pathogens due to deficiency of *wei* (defensive) *qi*. *Wei qi* resides at the exterior of the body to regulate skin pores and protect the body from the invasion of exterior pathogenic factors. If *wei qi* becomes deficient, body fluids may leak out of the body through the open skin pores, resulting in spontaneous sweating. Deficiency of *wei qi* may lower the defensive function of the skin, increasing the patient's susceptibility to invasion of exterior pathogens. Pale face, pale tongue, and a deficient pulse all indicate qi deficiency.

This formula uses a large dose of *Huang Qi* (Radix Astragali) to strengthen *wei* (defensive) *qi* at the exterior and increase the body's defense against foreign pathogenic factors. *Bai Zhu* (Rhizoma Atractylodis Macrocephalae) assists *Huang Qi* (Radix Astragali) in strengthening the exterior to stop spontaneous sweating. *Fang Feng* (Radix Saposhnikoviae) dispels any exterior pathogenic factors, especially wind. This formula has a unique check and balance: the use of an exterior-releasing herb, *Fang Feng* (Radix Saposhnikoviae), prevents retention of pathogenic factors trapped by a qi-tonifying herb, *Huang Qi* (Radix

11

ASTRINGENT FORMULAS

773

Chapter 11 – Astringent Formulas   *Section 1 – Exterior-Stabilizing Formulas to Stop Perspiration*

Yù Píng Fēng Sǎn (Jade Windscreen Powder)

Yu Ping Feng San (Jade Windscreen Powder)

Diagnosis	Signs and Symptoms	Treatment	Herbs
Wei (defensive) *qi* deficiency	• Spontaneous sweating: leakage of body fluids due to deficiency of *wei qi* • Aversion to wind and cold and increased susceptibility to exterior conditions: deficiency of *wei qi* unable to protect the exterior • Pale face, pale tongue, white tongue coating and a deficient pulse: qi deficiency	• Tonifies *wei qi* • Protects the exterior • Stops spontaneous sweating	• *Huang Qi* (Radix Astragali) strengthens *wei qi* at the exterior and increases the body's defense. • *Bai Zhu* (Rhizoma Atractylodis Macrocephalae) strengthens the exterior and stops spontaneous sweating. • *Fang Feng* (Radix Saposhnikoviae) dispels any exterior pathogenic factors.

Astragali); and the use of a qi-tonifying herb prevents any damage to the body that may be induced by the use of an exterior-releasing herb. Thus, using an exterior-releasing herb in conjunction with a tonic herb prevents exterior pathogenic factors from being trapped in the interior and causing harm.

Yu Ping Feng San has functions to tonify *wei* (defensive) *qi*, protect the exterior, release exterior pathogenic factors, and stop perspiration. It is commonly used to treat individuals with spontaneous perspiration due to exterior deficiency, or individuals who frequently contract common colds and influenza.

MODIFICATIONS

• For common cold characterized by wind-cold, add *Cang Zhu* (Rhizoma Atractylodis) and *Qiang Huo* (Rhizoma et Radix Notopterygii).

• For common cold in a constitutionally deficient person, add *Jing Jie* (Herba Schizonepetae), *Zi Su Ye* (Folium Perillae), and *Dang Shen* (Radix Codonopsis).

• With dizziness due to blood deficiency, add *Dang Gui* (Radix Angelicae Sinensis) and *Chuan Xiong* (Rhizoma Chuanxiong).

• With skin eruptions, add *Dang Gui* (Radix Angelicae Sinensis) and *Bai Shao* (Radix Paeoniae Alba).

• With chronic or allergic sinusitis, add *Xin Yi Hua* (Flos Magnoliae) and *Cang Er Zi* (Fructus Xanthii).

• With spontaneous perspiration due to yang deficiency, add *Fu Zi* (Radix Aconiti Lateralis Praeparata).

• With severe spontaneous sweating, add *Fu Xiao Mai* (Fructus Tritici Levis), calcined *Mu Li* (Concha Ostreae), and *Ma Huang Gen* (Radix et Rhizoma Ephedrae).

• With fatigue due to qi deficiency, add *Ren Shen* (Radix et Rhizoma Ginseng) and *Gan Cao* (Radix et Rhizoma Glycyrrhizae).

• With generalized weakness and deficiency, add *Xiao Jian Zhong Tang* (Minor Construct the Middle Decoction).

CAUTIONS / CONTRAINDICATIONS

• *Yu Ping Feng San* is contraindicated in patients with exterior syndrome with spontaneous sweating. It should be used only for spontaneous sweating without exterior syndrome.

• This formula is inappropriate for individuals with night sweating caused by yin deficiency.

• Individuals who take this formula should avoid exposure to cold and wind, and refrain from raw, cold, oily and greasy foods.[2]

• According to one report, the use of this formula was associated with mild dry mouth in 8 out of 127 patients. Dry mouth appeared within the first 10 days of use, and was self-limiting and resolved between days 11 to 20. No other abnormalities were noted.[3]

PHARMACOLOGICAL EFFECTS

1. **Immunostimulant**: Administration of *Yu Ping Feng San* has been associated with increased immunity. According to one study, the use of this formula increased IgG and IgA in mice.[4] Another study reported that the use of this formula for 2 to 3 months increased NK cell count and activities.[5]

2. **Antiviral**: According to one *in vitro* study, *Yu Ping Feng San* has demonstrated inhibition on the replication of influenza A viruses.[6]

3. **Nephroprotective**: According to one study, administration of *Yu Ping Feng San* in rabbits was associated with marked reduction of creatinine in comparison with the control group which did not receive any herbs. *Yu Ping Feng San*, however, did not have any statistically-significant effect on proteinuria in the same subjects.[7]

CLINICAL STUDIES AND RESEARCH

1. **Prevention of respiratory tract infection**: According to one study, *Yu Ping Feng San* was evaluated for its effect in preventing recurrent respiratory tract infection in 32 children who have had a history of frequent infections.

774

Yù Píng Fēng Sǎn (Jade Windscreen Powder)

The treatment protocol was to administer *Yu Ping Feng San* for 14 weeks prior to winter. The study reported an overall effectiveness of 96.9%. Furthermore, the study noted that there was an increase in IgA, but no significant changes to IgG or IgM.[8]

2. **Allergic rhinitis**: According to one study, the use of modified *Yu Ping Feng San* was associated with good results to treat 495 patients with allergic rhinitis characterized by deficiency of the exterior. Of 495 patients, the study reported significant improvement in 293 cases, improvement in 120 cases, and no effect in 79 cases. The rate of effectiveness was 84%. Information was unavailable on 3 individuals who did not complete the study.[9]

3. **Perspiration**: In one study, 88 children with profuse perspiration were treated with satisfactory results using modified *Yu Ping Feng San*. Modifications were made based on traditional Chinese medical diagnosis. For qi deficiencies, *Da Zao* (Fructus Jujubae) 15g, *Nuo Mi Gen* (Radix Oryzae Glutinosae) 9g, calcined *Mu Li* (Concha Ostreae) 30g, and calcined *Long Gu* (Os Draconis) 30g were added. For qi and yin deficiencies, *Wu Wei Zi* (Fructus Schisandrae Chinensis) 4.5g and *Dang Gui* (Radix Angelicae Sinensis) 9g were added.[10]

4. **Nephritis**: According to one study, administration of modified *Yu Ping Feng San* was associated with beneficial effect in 29 of 33 patients. The treatment protocol was to administer the herbs in powder form, 9 grams three times daily for 3 consecutive days followed by 4 days of rest per week, for 6 months. The herbal formula contained *Huang Qi* (Radix Astragali) 20g, *Bai Zhu* (Rhizoma Atractylodis Macrocephalae) 15g, *Fang Feng* (Radix Saposhnikoviae) 12g, *Chen Pi* (Pericarpium Citri Reticulatae) 9g, *Lian Qiao* (Fructus Forsythiae) 40g, *Tu Fu Ling* (Rhizoma Smilacis Glabrae) 50g, and *Qiang Huo* (Rhizoma et Radix Notopterygii) 10g.[11]

5. **Facial paralysis**: According to one study, concurrent use of *Yu Ping Feng San* and *Bu Yang Huan Wu Tang* (Tonify the Yang to Restore Five Decoction) for treatment of facial paralysis in 49 patients was associated with complete recovery in 32 cases, significant improvement in 15 cases, and moderate improvement in 2 cases.[12]

TOXICOLOGY

Yu Ping Feng San has very little toxicity. According to one study on acute toxicology, administration of this formula at 100 g/kg in mice did not cause any abnormal reactions or fatalities.[13] According to another study on chronic toxicology in mice, oral administration of this formula at 15 g/kg/day for 14 days did not cause any abnormal reactions of the internal organs (heart, lung, liver, kidney, and stomach). However, some mild side effects were observed, such as diarrhea.[14]

RELATED FORMULA

Huáng Qí Fáng Fēng Tāng
(Astragalus Decoction to Guard the Wind)

黄耆防風湯
黄芪防风汤

Pinyin Name: *Huang Qi Fang Feng Tang*
Literal Name: Astragalus Decoction to Guard the Wind
Original Source: *Tian Jin Zhong Yi Da Xue* (Tianjin University of Chinese Medicine) in 1989

Huang Qi (Radix Astragali)
Fang Feng (Radix Saposhnikoviae)
Bai Zhu (Rhizoma Atractylodis Macrocephalae)
Dong Chong Xia Cao (Cordyceps)
Ling Zhi (Ganoderma)
Wu Wei Zi (Fructus Schisandrae Chinensis)

Huang Qi Fang Feng Tang (Astragalus Decoction to Guard the Wind) specifically tonifies *wei* (defensive) *qi* and prevents the invasion of *liu yin* (six exogenous factors). Clinically, it treats individuals with a compromised immune system, and can be used prophylactically to prevent infectious diseases by boosting the immune system.

AUTHORS' COMMENTS

Yu Ping Feng San is the key formula for tonifying and consolidating *wei* (defensive) *qi*. Key symptoms include spontaneous sweating, weakness, pale complexion, pale tongue, and a deficient pulse. These patients, due to *wei qi* deficiency, often catch infections more often than others. Today, this formula is commonly used to prevent infection in individuals who are weak, deficient, or have compromised immunity.

Yu Ping Feng San, *Sheng Mai San* (Generate the Pulse Powder), and *Ren Shen Yang Ying Tang* (Ginseng Decoction to Nourish the Nutritive Qi) can all be used to enhance the immune system of those individuals who frequently catch colds.

- *Yu Ping Feng San* tonifies *wei* (defensive) *qi*.
- *Sheng Mai San* (Generate the Pulse Powder) tonifies qi and generates body fluids.
- *Ren Shen Yang Ying Tang* tonifies qi and blood.

Yu Ping Feng San and *Gui Zhi Tang* (Cinnamon Twig Decoction) both treat spontaneous perspiration and aversion to wind, but have completely different clinical applications.

- *Yu Ping Feng San* is an astringent formula that treats spontaneous perspiration and aversion to wind. However, these symptoms are due to *wei* (defensive) *qi* deficiency with inability to consolidate the exterior. Besides leakage

11

ASTRINGENT FORMULAS

775

Chapter 11 – Astringent Formulas　　　　　　*Section 1 – Exterior-Stabilizing Formulas to Stop Perspiration*

Yù Píng Fēng Sǎn (Jade Windscreen Powder)

of body fluids, other symptoms include frequent catching of common colds, pale complexion, generalized weakness, and a deficient pulse. *Yu Ping Feng San* is designed for patients who have not yet contracted an exterior condition.

- *Gui Zhi Tang* is an exterior-releasing formula designed to treat wind-cold invasion with disharmony between the *ying* (nutritive) and *wei* (defensive) levels, causing symptoms such as fever, aversion to cold, perspiration, headache, stuffy nose, and a superficial pulse. *Gui Zhi Tang* is formulated to treat patients who are now suffering from an exterior wind-cold condition.[15]

References

1. Wei YL. *Shi Yi De Xiao Fang* (Effective Formulas from Generations of Physicians) 1345.
2. *Zhong Yao Ming Fang Yao Li Yu Ying Yong* (Pharmacology and Applications of Famous Herbal Formulas) 1989;349-350.
3. *Zhong Yao Ming Fang Yao Li Yu Ying Yong* (Pharmacology and Applications of Famous Herbal Formulas) 1989;349-350.
4. *Zhong Yao Yao Li Yu Lin Chuang* (Pharmacology and Clinical Applications of Chinese Herbs) 1990;6(3):7.
5. *Zhong Xi Yi Jie He Za Zhi* (Journal of Integrated Chinese and Western Medicine) 1990;12:22.
6. *Jiang Xi Zhong Yi Yao* (Jiangxi Chinese Medicine and Herbology) 1989;6:40.
7. *Zhong Xi Yi Jie He Za Zhi* (Journal of Integrated Chinese and Western Medicine) 1986;4:299.
8. *Zhong Yi Za Zhi* (Journal of Chinese Medicine) 1982;1:37.
9. *Zhong Yi Za Zhi* (Journal of Chinese Medicine) 1989;10:32.
10. *Zhe Jiang Zhong Yi Za Zhi* (Zhejiang Journal of Chinese Medicine) 1992;8:378.
11. *Zhong Yi Za Zhi* (Journal of Chinese Medicine) 1992;33(5):24.
12. *Shan Xi Zhong Yi* (Shanxi Chinese Medicine) 1989;11:496.
13. *Zhong Yi Fang Ji Xian Dai Yan Jiu* (Modern Study of Medical Formulae in Traditional Chinese Medicine) 1997;786.
14. *Zhong Yi Fang Ji Xian Dai Yan Jiu* (Modern Study of Medical Formulae in Traditional Chinese Medicine) 1997;1:5.
15. Wang MZ, et al. *Zhong Yi Xue Wen Da Ti Ku* (Questions and Answers on Traditional Chinese Medicine: Herbal Formulas).

Mǔ Lì Sǎn (Oyster Shell Powder)

牡蠣散
牡蛎散

Pinyin Name: *Mu Li San*
Literal Name: Oyster Shell Powder
Original Source: *Tai Ping Hui Min He Ji Ju Fang* (Imperial Grace Formulary of the Tai Ping Era) by the Imperial Medical Department in 1078-85

COMPOSITION

Mu Li (Concha Ostreae), *jin* (soaked) in rice water to remove soil and *shao* (burned) till red	30g
Huang Qi (Radix Astragali)	30g
Ma Huang Gen (Radix et Rhizoma Ephedrae), *xi* (washed)	30g

DOSAGE / PREPARATION / ADMINISTRATION

The source text states to grind the three ingredients into coarse powder. Cook 9g of the powder and approximately 100 pieces [15-30g] of *Xiao Mai* (Fructus Tritici) in 1.5 bowls of water until it is reduced down to 80%. Take the warm, strained decoction in two equally-divided doses at anytime during the day. Today this formula is prepared by cooking 9g of the coarsely-powdered herbs with 30g of *Xiao Mai* (Fructus Tritici) in water. It may also be prepared as a decoction with addition of *Xiao Mai* (Fructus Tritici) and proportional adjustment of doses of herbs.

CHINESE THERAPEUTIC ACTIONS

1. Protects the exterior
2. Stops spontaneous and night sweating

CLINICAL MANIFESTATIONS

Yin and qi deficiencies: spontaneous sweating, profuse and continuous sweating while sleeping at night, palpitations, irritability, shortness of breath, and lethargy.

CLINICAL APPLICATIONS

Post-surgical sweating, postpartum sweating, and sweating in pulmonary tuberculosis.

Mǔ Lì Sǎn (Oyster Shell Powder)

EXPLANATION

Mu Li San (Oyster Shell Powder) is designed to treat sweating due to deficiencies of yin and qi. Deficiency of yin may lead to sweating while sleeping, and deficiency of qi may lead to spontaneous sweating. Sweat is the body fluid that belongs to the Heart. Therefore, excessive sweating may cause Heart yin deficiency, leading to palpitations and irritability. Excessive sweating may also consume the qi since the qi travels with the sweat out of the body. Continuous consumption of qi in a qi-deficient individual would then lead to shortness of breath and lethargy.

The objectives of this formula are to tonify qi and yin to stop both spontaneous and night sweating. *Mu Li* (Concha Ostreae) benefits yin to stop night sweating, and anchors yang to relieve irritability. *Huang Qi* (Radix Astragali) tonifies qi, strengthens the exterior, and stops spontaneous sweating. *Ma Huang Gen* (Radix et Rhizoma Ephedrae) has an astringent effect to stop spontaneous and night sweating. *Xiao Mai* (Fructus Tritici) benefits Heart qi, nourishes Heart yin, stops sweating, and relieves irritability and palpitation. Indeed, this formula nourishes the qi and yin and strengthens the exterior to stop the abnormal sweating.

MODIFICATIONS

- With more qi deficiency, add *Ren Shen* (Radix et Rhizoma Ginseng) and *Bai Zhu* (Rhizoma Atractylodis Macrocephalae).
- With more yin deficiency, add *Shu Di Huang* (Radix Rehmanniae Praeparata) and *Bai Shao* (Radix Paeoniae Alba).
- With yang deficiency, add *Bai Zhu* (Rhizoma Atractylodis Macrocephalae) and *Fu Zi* (Radix Aconiti Lateralis Praeparata).
- With blood deficiency, add *Shu Di Huang* (Radix Rehmanniae Praeparata) and *He Shou Wu* (Radix Polygoni Multiflori).

- With Spleen deficiency, add *Bai Bian Dou* (Semen Lablab Album) and *Shan Yao* (Rhizoma Dioscoreae).
- With irritability and insomnia, add *Zhi Mu* (Rhizoma Anemarrhenae) and *Huang Bo* (Cortex Phellodendri Chinensis).
- With continuous sweating after ingestion of this formula, add *Wu Wei Zi* (Fructus Schisandrae Chinensis).

CAUTIONS / CONTRAINDICATIONS

Mu Li San is not suitable for night sweating caused by yin-deficient heat.

CLINICAL STUDIES AND RESEARCH

Perspiration: According to one study, the use of modified *Mu Li San* was effective in treating both spontaneous and night sweating in 28 patients (6 with spontaneous sweating, 15 with night sweating, and 7 with both). In addition to sweating, other complaints included poor appetite, dizziness, palpitations, fatigue and lack of energy. The study reported complete recovery in 20 cases, near-complete recovery in 5 cases, slight improvement in 1 case, and no effect in 2 cases. Most patients responded within 10 packs of herbs.[1]

AUTHORS' COMMENTS

Mu Li San is a commonly used formula in the treatment of sweating. The key signs and symptoms include spontaneous sweating (qi deficiency), night sweating (yin deficiency), shortness of breath, lethargy, pale tongue, and a fine, weak pulse. To further enhance the effect to stop sweating, *Fu Xiao Mai* (Fructus Tritici Levis) is used to replace *Xiao Mai* (Fructus Tritici).

Yu Ping Feng San and *Mu Li San* (Oyster Shell Powder) both treat sweating.

- *Yu Ping Feng San* is designed for exterior *wei* (defensive) *qi* deficiency with spontaneous sweating and aversion to wind, pale complexion, pale tongue, and a deficient pulse.

Mu Li San (Oyster Shell Powder)

Diagnosis	Signs and Symptoms	Treatment	Herbs
Yin and qi deficiencies	• Spontaneous sweating: qi deficiency • Night sweating: yin deficiency • Palpitation and irritability: Heart yin deficiency due to excessive sweating • Shortness of breath, lethargy: qi deficiency due to excessive sweating	• Protects the exterior • Stops spontaneous and night sweating	• *Mu Li* (Concha Ostreae) benefits yin to stop night sweating, and anchors yang to relieve irritability. • *Huang Qi* (Radix Astragali) tonifies qi, strengthens the exterior, and stops spontaneous sweating. • *Ma Huang Gen* (Radix et Rhizoma Ephedrae) has astringent effect to stop sweating. • *Xiao Mai* (Fructus Tritici) benefits Heart qi, nourishes Heart yin, stops sweating, and relieves irritability and palpitation.

Mǔ Lì Sǎn (Oyster Shell Powder)

Since this formula tonifies qi, consolidates the exterior, and stops sweating, it is indicated for individuals who frequently suffer from common colds.

- *Mu Li San* is indicated for general deficiency with profuse sweating, especially at night, palpitations, easily frightened, shortness of breath, irritability, and fatigue. It is more appropriate for individuals with yin and qi deficiencies with night sweating.[2]

Mu Li San and *Dang Gui Liu Huang Tang* (Tangkuei and Six-Yellow Decoction) both nourish yin, clear heat, consolidate the exterior, and stop night sweating.

- *Mu Li San* has a stronger effect to bind and stop sweating, and a weaker effect to nourish yin and clear heat. It is used mostly to treat qi and yin deficiencies with

sweating during the day and night. Other symptoms include palpitations, being easily frightened, and shortness of breath.

- *Dang Gui Liu Huang Tang* is stronger at nourishing yin and clearing heat. It is mainly used for night sweating with feverish sensation at night or tidal fever, irritability, dryness of the mouth, lips, and stools, and other signs of yin-deficient heat.[3]

References

1. *Fu Jian Zhong Yi Yao* (Fujian Chinese Medicine and Herbology) 1966;3:37.
2. Wang MZ, et al. *Zhong Yi Xue Wen Da Ti Ku* (Questions and Answers on Traditional Chinese Medicine: Herbal Formulas).
3. Wang MZ, et al. *Zhong Yi Xue Wen Da Ti Ku* (Questions and Answers on Traditional Chinese Medicine: Herbal Formulas).

Chinese Herbal Formulas and Applications

Section 2

敛肺止咳剂
— Lung-Restraining Formula to Relieve Cough

Jiǔ Xiān Sǎn (Nine-Immortal Powder)
九仙散

Pinyin Name: *Jiu Xian San*
Literal Name: Nine-Immortal Powder
Original Source: *Yi Xue Zheng Zhuan* (True Lineage of Medicine) by Yu Tian-Min in 1515

COMPOSITION

Ying Su Ke (Pericarpium Papaveris), *mi zhi* (fried with honey)	6g
Wu Wei Zi (Fructus Schisandrae Chinensis)	1.5g [3g]
Wu Mei (Fructus Mume)	1 piece [6g]
Ren Shen (Radix et Rhizoma Ginseng), *dun* (stewed) separately	1.5g [3g]
E Jiao (Colla Corii Asini)	1.5g [3g]
Kuan Dong Hua (Flos Farfarae)	1.5g [3g]
Bei Mu (Bulbus Fritillariae)	1.5g [3g]
Sang Bai Pi (Cortex Mori)	1.5g [3g]
Jie Geng (Radix Platycodonis)	1.5g [3g]

DOSAGE / PREPARATION / ADMINISTRATION

The source text states to grind all ingredients into powder. Cook the herbs with 3 slices of *Sheng Jiang* (Rhizoma Zingiberis Recens) in two large bowls of water until it is reduced down to one bowl. Take the warm, strained decoction. Today, this formula may be prepared as a decoction with the doses suggested in brackets.

CHINESE THERAPEUTIC ACTIONS

1. Restrains the Lung and stops coughing
2. Benefits qi and nourishes yin

CLINICAL MANIFESTATIONS

Chronic coughing with Lung yin and qi deficiencies: chronic, persistent coughing, severe coughing leading to wheezing, dyspnea and spontaneous sweating, and a deficient, rapid pulse.

CLINICAL APPLICATIONS

Pulmonary tuberculosis, chronic bronchitis, and coughing.

EXPLANATION

Jiu Xian San (Nine-Immortal Powder) is designed to treat chronic coughing with Lung yin and qi deficiencies. Chronic coughing injures the Lung, causing wheezing, dyspnea and shortness of breath. Chronic coughing also consumes qi and causes the inability of skin pores to close, leading to spontaneous sweating. Chronic coughing may also deplete yin, leading to deficiency heat, and manifesting in the form of a deficient, rapid pulse.

Ying Su Ke (Pericarpium Papaveris) in this formula is used to restrain the Lung and stop coughing. *Wu Wei Zi* (Fructus Schisandrae Chinensis) and *Wu Mei* (Fructus Mume) help restrain the Lung to stop coughing. *Ren Shen* (Radix et Rhizoma Ginseng) tonifies Lung qi. *Wu Wei Zi* (Fructus Schisandrae Chinensis) also assists *Ren Shen* (Radix et Rhizoma Ginseng) to tonify qi. *E Jiao* (Colla Corii Asini) nourishes Lung yin. *Kuan Dong Hua* (Flos Farfarae) and *Bei Mu* (Bulbus Fritillariae) descend Lung qi, stop coughing and wheezing, and dissolve phlegm. *Sang Bai Pi* (Cortex Mori) clears the Lung to stop coughing and wheezing. *Jie Geng* (Radix Platycodonis), besides relieving the coughing and dissolving the phlegm, guides all the other herbs upward to the Lung.

11

ASTRINGENT FORMULAS

779

Chapter 11 – Astringent Formulas

Section 2– Lung-Restraining Formula to Relieve Cough

Jiŭ Xiān Săn (Nine-Immortal Powder)

Jiu Xian San (Nine-Immortal Powder)

Diagnosis	Signs and Symptoms	Treatment	Herbs
Chronic coughing with damage of Lung yin and qi	• Chronic coughing, wheezing and shortness of breath: Lung yin and qi deficiencies • Spontaneous sweating: Lung qi deficiency unable to close skin pores • A deficient and rapid pulse: deficiency heat	• Restrains Lung and stops coughing • Benefits qi and nourishes yin	• *Ying Su Ke* (Pericarpium Papaveris) restrains the Lung and stops coughing. • *Wu Wei Zi* (Fructus Schisandrae Chinensis) and *Wu Mei* (Fructus Mume) restrain the Lung to stop coughing. • *Ren Shen* (Radix et Rhizoma Ginseng) tonifies the Lung qi. • *E Jiao* (Colla Corii Asini) nourishes the Lung yin. • *Kuan Dong Hua* (Flos Farfarae) and *Bei Mu* (Bulbus Fritillariae) descend Lung qi, stop coughing and wheezing, and dissolve phlegm. • *Sang Bai Pi* (Cortex Mori) clears the Lung to stop coughing and wheezing. • *Jie Geng* (Radix Platycodonis) relieves coughing and dissolves phlegm, and guides the other herbs upward to the Lung.

MODIFICATIONS

• With wheezing and dyspnea due to Lung and Kidney deficiencies, add *Shu Di Huang* (Radix Rehmanniae Praeparata), *Shan Zhu Yu* (Fructus Corni), *Shan Yao* (Rhizoma Dioscoreae), and *Hu Tao Ren* (Semen Juglandis).

• With loose stools and indigestion due to Spleen deficiency, add *Bai Zhu* (Rhizoma Atractylodis Macrocephalae), *Shan Yao* (Rhizoma Dioscoreae), and *Fu Ling* (Poria).

CAUTIONS / CONTRAINDICATIONS

• *Jiu Xian San* has a tonic effect, and as such, it is not appropriate for coughing due to exterior conditions with fever and aversion to cold. The use of tonic herbs may complicate the illness by drawing pathogenic factors from the exterior to the interior.

• Since this formula has a strong astringent action, it is not indicated for cases of coughing with profuse sputum, as the astringent effect may trap the pathogenic factors inside.

• Overdose or long-term usage of *Ying Su Ke* (Pericarpium Papaveris) may result in numerous side effects and adverse reactions, as this herb is potentially toxic and addictive.

780

Chinese Herbal Formulas and Applications

Section 3

涩肠固脱剂
— Intestines-Binding Formulas to Stop Leakage

Zhēn Rén Yăng Zàng Tāng
(True Man's Decoction for Nourishing the Organs)

真人養臟湯
真人养脏汤

Pinyin Name: *Zhen Ren Yang Zang Tang*
Literal Name: True Man's Decoction for Nourishing the Organs
Original Source: *Tai Ping Hui Min He Ji Ju Fang* (Imperial Grace Formulary of the Tai Ping Era) by the Imperial Medical Department in 1078-85

COMPOSITION

Ying Su Ke (Pericarpium Papaveris), *mi zhi* (fried with honey)	108g [15g]
Rou Dou Kou (Semen Myristicae), *wei* (roasted)	15g [6g]
He Zi (Fructus Chebulae)	36g [12g]
Rou Gui (Cortex Cinnamomi)	24g [3g]
Ren Shen (Radix et Rhizoma Ginseng)	18g [9g]
Bai Zhu (Rhizoma Atractylodis Macrocephalae), *bei* (stone baked)	18g [9g]
Dang Gui (Radix Angelicae Sinensis)	18g [6g]
Bai Shao (Radix Paeoniae Alba)	48g [15g]
Mu Xiang (Radix Aucklandiae), do not expose to heat	42g [4.5g]
Zhi Gan Cao (Radix et Rhizoma Glycyrrhizae Praeparata cum Melle)	24g [6g]

DOSAGE / PREPARATION / ADMINISTRATION

The source text states to grind the ingredients into coarse powder. Cook 6g of the powder in 1.5 bowls of water until it is reduced down to 80%. Take the warm, strained decoction before meal. Today, this formula may be prepared as a decoction with the doses suggested in brackets.

CHINESE THERAPEUTIC ACTIONS

1. Binds the intestines and stops diarrhea and dysentery
2. Warms and tonifies the Spleen and Kidney

CLINICAL MANIFESTATIONS

Chronic diarrhea or dysentery due to deficiency and cold of the Spleen and Kidney: uncontrollable bowel movement throughout the day and night, rectal tenesmus and prolapse, abdominal pain that is relieved by pressure and warmth, red or white dysentery, stools with pus or blood, lethargy, and loss of appetite.

CLINICAL APPLICATIONS

Chronic enteritis, chronic colitis, chronic diarrhea, chronic dysentery, and rectal prolapse.

EXPLANATION

Zhen Ren Yang Zang Tang (True Man's Decoction for Nourishing the Organs) is designed to treat chronic diarrhea or dysentery due to deficiency and cold of the Spleen and Kidney. Deficiency and cold of the Spleen and Kidney may cause the normally ascending qi of these two organs to descend, leading to diarrhea or dysentery. In severe cases, rectal prolapse may occur. Abdominal pain that is relieved by pressure and warmth indicates general deficiency and cold conditions. Presence of red [blood] or white [pus or mucus] stools and rectal tenesmus indicates disharmony of qi and blood. A chronic condition of diarrhea or dysentery may lead to generalized deficiency with lethargy and loss of appetite.

ASTRINGENT FORMULAS · 11

781

Chapter 11 – Astringent Formulas   *Section 3– Intestines-Binding Formulas to Stop Leakage*

Zhēn Rén Yǎng Zàng Tāng
(True Man's Decoction for Nourishing the Organs)

Zhen Ren Yang Zang Tang (True Man's Decoction for Nourishing the Organs)

Diagnosis	Signs and Symptoms	Treatment	Herbs
Chronic diarrhea or dysentery due to deficiency and cold of the Spleen and Kidney	• Uncontrollable bowel movement as diarrhea or dysentery: deficiency and cold of the Spleen and the Kidney unable to ascend qi • Abdominal pain that is minimized with pressure and warmth: deficiency and cold of the Spleen and the Kidney • Red [blood] or white [pus or mucus] dysentery and rectal tenesmus: disharmony of qi and blood	• Binds the intestines and stops diarrhea and dysentery • Warms and tonifies the Spleen and Kidney	• *Ying Su Ke* (Pericarpium Papaveris) binds the intestines to relieve diarrhea or dysentery. • *Rou Dou Kou* (Semen Myristicae) and *He Zi* (Fructus Chebulae) bind the Intestines and stop diarrhea. • *Rou Gui* (Cortex Cinnamomi) warms the Spleen and the Kidney to raise the yang. • *Ren Shen* (Radix et Rhizoma Ginseng) and *Bai Zhu* (Rhizoma Atractylodis Macrocephalae) warm the Spleen and tonify qi. • *Dang Gui* (Radix Angelicae Sinensis) and *Bai Shao* (Radix Paeoniae Alba) nourish the yin and the blood. • *Mu Xiang* (Radix Aucklandiae) regulates qi and relieves pain. • *Zhi Gan Cao* (Radix et Rhizoma Glycyrrhizae Praeparata cum Melle) harmonizes the herbs in this formula.

In general, diarrhea or dysentery due to deficiency and cold of the Spleen and Kidney should be treated with warm herbs that tonify these organs. However, in the case of severe diarrhea and dysentery with uncontrollable bowel movement and rectal prolapse, use of astringent herbs is necessary to quickly treat the symptoms.

This formula contains *Ying Su Ke* (Pericarpium Papaveris) to bind the Intestines to quickly relieve diarrhea or dysentery. *Rou Dou Kou* (Semen Myristicae) binds the intestines and warms the Spleen and Kidney. *He Zi* (Fructus Chebulae) helps to bind the Intestines and stop diarrhea. *Rou Gui* (Cortex Cinnamomi) warms the Spleen and Kidney to raise the yang. *Ren Shen* (Radix et Rhizoma Ginseng) and *Bai Zhu* (Rhizoma Atractylodis Macrocephalae) are used to warm the Spleen and tonify qi. Since chronic dysentery may damage the yin and blood, *Dang Gui* (Radix Angelicae Sinensis) and *Bai Shao* (Radix Paeoniae Alba) are used to nourish the yin and blood. *Mu Xiang* (Radix Aucklandiae) is employed in this formula for two reasons: to offset the rich tonics from causing stagnation and to regulate qi and relieve pain. *Zhi Gan Cao* (Radix et Rhizoma Glycyrrhizae Praeparata cum Melle) harmonizes the herbs in this formula. Also, the combination of *Zhi Gan Cao* (Radix et Rhizoma Glycyrrhizae Praeparata cum Melle) and *Bai Shao* (Radix Paeoniae Alba) has a good pain-relieving effect.

MODIFICATIONS

• For rectal prolapse, add *Sheng Ma* (Rhizoma Cimicifugae) and *Huang Qi* (Radix Astragali); or *Bu Zhong Yi Qi Tang* (Tonify the Middle and Augment the Qi Decoction).

• With cold extremities and diarrhea with undigested food due to Spleen and Kidney yang deficiencies, add *Fu Zi* (Radix Aconiti Lateralis Praeparata) and *Gan Jiang* (Rhizoma Zingiberis); or combine with *Fu Zi Li Zhong Wan* (Prepared Aconite Pill to Regulate the Middle).

CAUTIONS / CONTRAINDICATIONS

• *Zhen Ren Yang Zang Tang* contains astringent herbs, and is contraindicated for dysentery in which heat and toxins still remain in the body.

• This formula is designed for chronic diarrhea or dysentery with underlying deficiency and cold. It is inappropriate for acute cases of dysentery or diarrhea, which are often characterized by an excess condition.

• Avoid consumption of alcohol, fish, and foods that are raw, cold, oily, or greasy while taking this formula.

• Overdose or long-term usage of *Ying Su Ke* (Pericarpium Papaveris) may result in numerous side effects and adverse reactions, as this herb is potentially toxic and addictive.

782

Chinese Herbal Formulas and Applications

Zhēn Rén Yǎng Zàng Tāng
(True Man's Decoction for Nourishing the Organs)

CLINICAL STUDIES AND RESEARCH

1. **Chronic colitis**: According to one study, the use of modified *Zhen Ren Yang Zang Tang* was associated with 95.92% effectiveness in treating chronic colitis in 49 patients (37 males and 12 females, between 17-58 years of age, with 1-28 years history of illness). The herbal treatment contained the following ingredients: *Huang Qi* (Radix Astragali) 12-15g, *Dang Shen* (Radix Codonopsis) 12-30g, dry-fried *Bai Zhu* (Rhizoma Atractylodis Macrocephalae) 12-15g, *Dang Gui* (Radix Angelicae Sinensis) 9-12g, roasted *Rou Dou Kou* (Semen Myristicae) 9-15g, roasted *He Zi* (Fructus Chebulae) 9-15g, *Bai Shao* (Radix Paeoniae Alba) 9-15g, *Mu Xiang* (Radix Aucklandiae) 6-12g, *Rou Gui* (Cortex Cinnamomi) 3g [given in powder form], *Zhi Gan Cao* (Radix et Rhizoma Glycyrrhizae Praeparata cum Melle) 6-9g, *Chi Shi Zhi* (Halloysitum Rubrum) 15-30g, *Yan Hu Suo* (Rhizoma Corydalis) 9-15g, and *Wu Mei* (Fructus Mume) 9-15g as the base formula. Modifications included the addition of *Gan Jiang* (Rhizoma Zingiberis) for cold in the Stomach with cold extremities; *Sha Ren* (Fructus Amomi) and *Hou Po* (Cortex Magnoliae Officinalis) for poor appetite with abdominal distention; charred *Di Yu* (Radix Sanguisorbae) for yang deficiency with hematochezia; *Yin Yang Huo* (Herba Epimedii), *Du Zhong* (Cortex Eucommiae) and *Bu Gu Zhi* (Fructus Psoraleae) for Spleen and Kidney yang deficiencies; and *Er Cha* (Catechu) for ulceration of the intestinal mucous membrane. The treatment protocol was to administer the herbs in decoction one time per day, for 30 days per course of treatment. Patients were instructed to avoid all other medications (herbs and drugs) and refrain from eating greasy or oily foods. Of 49 patients, the study reported complete recovery in 29 cases, significant improvement in 10 cases, improvement in 8 cases, and no effect in 2 cases.[1]

2. **Chronic dysentery and rectal prolapse**: One study reported good results using modified *Zhen Ren Yang Zang Tang* to treat chronic dysentery and/or prolapsed rectum in 162 patients (108 with chronic dysentery and 54 with prolapse rectum). The herbal treatment contained *Ren Shen* (Radix et Rhizoma Ginseng) 5-20g, *Bai Zhu* (Rhizoma Atractylodis Macrocephalae) 5-20g, *Zhi Gan Cao* (Radix et Rhizoma Glycyrrhizae Praeparata cum Melle) 3-15g, *Rou Dou Kou* (Semen Myristicae) 5-30g, *Rou Gui* (Cortex Cinnamomi) 3-15g, *Fu Zi* (Radix Aconiti Lateralis Praeparata) 5-30g, *He Zi* (Fructus Chebulae) 5-30g, *Ying Su Ke* (Pericarpium Papaveris) 5-25g, *Bai Shao* (Radix Paeoniae Alba) 5-20g, *Dang Gui* (Radix Angelicae Sinensis) 5-10g, and *Mu Xiang* (Radix Aucklandiae) 3-10g. Furthermore, *Chi Shi Zhi* (Halloysitum Rubrum) 10-30g was added for those with chronic dysentery, and processed *Huang Qi* (Radix Astragali) was added for rectal prolapse. In addition, those with rectal prolapse were also treated with topical soaking of an herbal solution made from *Shi Liu Pi* (Pericarpium Granati), *Bai Fan* (Alumen) and *Wu Bei Zi* (Galla Chinensis). The treatment protocol was to cook the herbs and administer the decoction in three equally-divided doses daily, for 20 days per course of treatment, for up to 3 courses total. The study reported 91.7% effectiveness for treatment of chronic dysentery, and 87% for rectal prolapse.[2]

3. **Diarrhea**: Administration of modified *Zhen Ren Yang Zang Tang* was associated with good results in treating 78 patients with recurrent diarrhea and diabetes mellitus. The herbal treatment contained herbs such as *Ren Shen* (Radix et Rhizoma Ginseng) 5g [or *Dang Shen* (Radix Codonopsis) 30g], dry-fried *Bai Zhu* (Rhizoma Atractylodis Macrocephalae) 12g, *Rou Gui* (Cortex Cinnamomi) 12g, *Bai Shao* (Radix Paeoniae Alba) 12g, *Rou Dou Kou* (Semen Myristicae) 15g, *He Zi* (Fructus Chebulae) 15g, *Ying Su Ke* (Pericarpium Papaveris) 6g, *Mu Xiang* (Radix Aucklandiae) 6g, *Zhi Gan Cao* (Radix et Rhizoma Glycyrrhizae Praeparata cum Melle) 5g, and others as needed. For severe cold, *Fu Zi* (Radix Aconiti Lateralis Praeparata) 12g and *Gan Jiang* (Rhizoma Zingiberis) 10g were added. For diarrhea with clear watery stools, 5 a.m. diarrhea, or abdominal pain with preference of pressure, *Ba Ji Tian* (Radix Morindae Officinalis) 15g and *Bu Gu Zhi* (Fructus Psoraleae) 15g were added. For chronic diarrhea with stabbing pain in the abdomen with dark colored tongue with spots, *Wu Ling Zhi* (Faeces Trogopteri) 12g, *Pu Huang* (Pollen Typhae) 12g, and *Xi Xin* (Radix et Rhizoma Asari) 6g were added. The herbs were cooked in 800 mL of water, and the decoction was given for 5 days per course of treatment. Of 78 patients, the study reported complete control of bowel movement in 61 cases, improvement in 14 cases, and no effect in 3 cases. The overall rate of effectiveness was 96.2%.[3]

AUTHORS' COMMENTS

Zhen Ren Yang Zang Tang, *Ge Gen Huang Qin Huang Lian Tang* (Kudzu, Coptis, and Scutellaria Decoction), *Shao Yao Tang* (Peony Decoction) and *Bai Tou Weng Tang* (Pulsatilla Decoction) all treat diarrhea, but have different functions and indications.

• *Zhen Ren Yang Zang Tang* warms and tonifies the Spleen and Kidney to bind the Intestines to stop diarrhea. From a biomedical perspective, this formula is most effective for diarrhea due to inflammatory bowel condition, such as chronic colitis and enteritis.

11

ASTRINGENT FORMULAS

783

Chapter 11 – Astringent Formulas　　　　　　　　　　*Section 3– Intestines-Binding Formulas to Stop Leakage*

Zhēn Rén Yǎng Zàng Tāng
(True Man's Decoction for Nourishing the Organs)

- *Ge Gen Huang Qin Huang Lian Tang* treats damp-heat accumulation in the Intestines, which manifests in burning diarrhea, rectal tenesmus, and heat sensation. From a biomedical perspective, this formula is most effective for diarrhea due to various gastrointestinal infections.
- *Shao Yao Tang* regulates qi and blood, clears heat, and eliminates toxins to treat damp-heat accumulation and qi stagnation in the Intestines, causing abdominal pain, bloody stools with mucus, and rectal tenesmus. From a biomedical perspective, this formula is most effective for diarrhea due to various gastrointestinal infections.
- *Bai Tou Weng Tang* clears heat and eliminates toxins to treat toxic heat invading the *xue* (blood) level leading

to bloody diarrhea. From a biomedical perspective, this formula is most effective for diarrhea due to amoebic infection.[4]

References
1. *Cheng Du Zhong Yi Xue Yuan Xue Bao* (Journal of Chengdu University of Traditional Chinese Medicine) 1989;4:27.
2. *Gan Su Zhong Yi Xue Yuan Xue Bao* (Journal of Gansu University of Chinese Medicine) 1987;4:24.
3. *Zhe Jiang Zhong Yi Za Zhi* (Zhejiang Journal of Chinese Medicine) 1993;9:395.
4. Wang MZ, et al. *Zhong Yi Xue Wen Da Ti Ku* (Questions and Answers on Traditional Chinese Medicine: Herbal Formulas).

Si Shén Wán (Four-Miracle Pill)
四神丸

Pinyin Name: *Si Shen Wan*
Literal Name: Four-Miracle Pill
Original Source: *Zheng Zhi Zhun Sheng* (Standards of Patterns and Treatments) by Wang Ken-Tang in 1602

COMPOSITION

Bu Gu Zhi (Fructus Psoraleae)	120g [12g]
Rou Dou Kou (Semen Myristicae)	60g [6g]
Wu Zhu Yu (Fructus Evodiae), *jin* (soaked) and *chao* (dry-fried)	30g [3g]
Wu Wei Zi (Fructus Schisandrae Chinensis)	60g [6g]

DOSAGE / PREPARATION / ADMINISTRATION

The source text states to cook 100 pieces of *Da Zao* (Fructus Jujubae) with 240g of *Sheng Jiang* (Rhizoma Zingiberis Recens). Remove *Sheng Jiang* (Rhizoma Zingiberis Recens) and discard the seeds of *Da Zao* (Fructus Jujubae), and save the fruit. Separately grind the ingredients into powder. Blend the fruit of *Da Zao* (Fructus Jujubae) and the powder of ingredients to form small pills. The source text recommends to take 50-70 pills with water before meal or on an empty stomach. Today, this formula is usually prepared and administered in pills. Take 6-9g of pills once or twice daily. This formula may be prepared as a decoction with the doses suggested in brackets.

CHINESE THERAPEUTIC ACTIONS

1. Warms and tonifies the Spleen and Kidney
2. Binds the Intestines and stops diarrhea

CLINICAL MANIFESTATIONS

Deficiency and cold of the Spleen and Kidney: early morning diarrhea at around 5 a.m., chronic diarrhea, loss of appetite, soreness of the lower back, abdominal pain, cold limbs, lack of energy, and fatigue.

CLINICAL APPLICATIONS

Diarrhea, colitis with diarrhea, chronic colitis, dysentery, intestinal tuberculosis, constipation, enuresis, and spermatorrhea.

EXPLANATION

Si Shen Wan (Four-Miracle Pill) is particularly famous for treating early morning diarrhea at around 5 a.m. Early morning diarrhea is due to failure of the yang qi to ascend in the early morning. Soreness of the lower back indicates Kidney yang deficiency. Fatigue and loss of appetite

784

Si Shén Wán (Four-Miracle Pill)

Si Shen Wan (Four-Miracle Pill)

Diagnosis	Signs and Symptoms	Treatment	Herbs
Deficiency and cold of the Spleen and Kidney	• Early morning diarrhea: failure of the yang qi to ascend in the early morning • Soreness of the lower back: Kidney yang deficiency • Fatigue and loss of appetite: Spleen yang deficiency • Abdominal pain and cold extremities: accumulation of cold	• Warms and tonifies the Spleen and Kidney • Binds the Intestines and stops diarrhea	• *Bu Gu Zhi* (Fructus Psoraleae) warms the Kidney and invigorates *ming men* (life gate) fire. • *Rou Dou Kou* (Semen Myristicae) warms the Spleen and the Kidney and binds the intestines to stop diarrhea. • *Wu Zhu Yu* (Fructus Evodiae) warms the Spleen and the Stomach to relieve pain. • *Wu Wei Zi* (Fructus Schisandrae Chinensis) warms and binds the intestines to stop diarrhea. • *Sheng Jiang* (Rhizoma Zingiberis Recens) dispels cold and regulates water. • *Da Zao* (Fructus Jujubae) nourishes the Spleen and Stomach.

reflect Spleen yang deficiency. Abdominal pain and cold extremities are caused by accumulation of cold and inability of yang to warm the body.

Bu Gu Zhi (Fructus Psoraleae), the chief herb of this formula, warms the Kidney and invigorates *ming men* (life gate) fire. *Rou Dou Kou* (Semen Myristicae) warms the Spleen and Kidney and binds the intestines to stop diarrhea. *Wu Zhu Yu* (Fructus Evodiae) warms the Spleen and Stomach. It also disperses cold and relieves the abdominal pain. *Wu Wei Zi* (Fructus Schisandrae Chinensis) warms and binds the intestines. *Sheng Jiang* (Rhizoma Zingiberis Recens) dispels cold and regulates water. *Da Zao* (Fructus Jujubae) nourishes the Spleen and Stomach.

MODIFICATIONS

• For rectal prolapse, add *Huang Qi* (Radix Astragali) and *Sheng Ma* (Rhizoma Cimicifugae); or *Bu Zhong Yi Qi Tang* (Tonify the Middle and Augment the Qi Decoction).
• For pain of the back and coldness of the limbs, add *Rou Gui* (Cortex Cinnamomi) and *Fu Zi* (Radix Aconiti Lateralis Praeparata); or *You Gui Wan* (Restore the Right [Kidney] Pill).
• With lower abdominal pain, add *Xiao Hui Xiang* (Fructus Foeniculi) and *Mu Xiang* (Radix Aucklandiae).

CAUTIONS / CONTRAINDICATIONS

• *Si Shen Wan* contains tonic and astringent herbs to treat chronic diarrhea and dysentery due to deficiency. It is contraindicated in diarrhea caused by damp-heat accumulation or food stagnation.
• Avoid raw and cold foods while taking this formula.

PHARMACOLOGICAL EFFECTS

Antidiarrheal: *Si Shen Wan* has been shown to have marked antidiarrheal effect according to many studies and reports. The mechanism of this antidiarrheal effect has been attributed to its action to inhibit the intestinal peristalsis.[1]

CLINICAL STUDIES AND RESEARCH

1. **Diarrhea**: Many studies have shown *Si Shen Wan* to effectively treat diarrhea due to various reasons. One study reported complete recovery in 24 of 28 patients with 5 a.m. diarrhea when treated with *Si Shen Wan* plus *Pao Jiang* (Rhizoma Zingiberis Praeparatum), *Bai Zhu* (Rhizoma Atractylodis Macrocephalae), *Huang Qi* (Radix Astragali), *Fu Zi* (Radix Aconiti Lateralis Praeparata), and *Rou Gui* (Cortex Cinnamomi). The duration of treatment ranged from 12 to 36 packs of herbs.[2]

2. **Dysentery**: One study reported good results using *Si Shen Wan* plus *Tong Xie Yao Fang* (Important Formula for Painful Diarrhea) to treat dysentery characterized by Liver stagnation and Spleen deficiency. Clinical presentations included abdominal pain, hematochezia, rectal tenesmus, absence of fever and thirst, fatigue, aversion to cold, poor appetite, sallow facial appearance, emaciated complexion, white tongue coating, and a deep, fine pulse. The herbal formula contained *Bu Gu Zhi* (Fructus Psoraleae), *Wu Zhu Yu* (Fructus Evodiae), roasted *Rou Dou Kou* (Semen Myristicae), *Chen Pi* (Pericarpium Citri Reticulatae), *Fang Feng* (Radix Saposhnikoviae), *Mu Xiang* (Radix Aucklandiae), *Bai Shao* (Radix Paeoniae Alba), *Bai Zhu* (Rhizoma Atractylodis Macrocephalae), *Huang Lian* (Rhizoma Coptidis), *Gan Cao* (Radix et Rhizoma Glycyrrhizae), and *Wu Wei Zi* (Fructus Schisandrae

Chapter 11 – Astringent Formulas   *Section 3– Intestines-Binding Formulas to Stop Leakage*

Si Shén Wán (Four-Miracle Pill)

Chinensis). The study reported complete recovery in all 14 patients.[3]

3. **Irritable bowel syndrome**: One study reported a 93% success rate using *Si Shen Wan* and *Shen Ling Bai Zhu San* (Ginseng, Poria, and Atractylodes Macrocephala Powder) to treat alternation of diarrhea and constipation with abdominal pain in 30 patients with irritable bowel syndrome.[4]

4. **Colitis**: One study of colitis associated with diarrhea reported satisfactory results using modified *Si Shen Wan*. Patients were divided into early, middle and late stage of colitis with diarrhea. The formula for early stage contained *Wu Zhu Yu* (Fructus Evodiae) 10g, *Bu Gu Zhi* (Fructus Psoraleae) 20g, *Wu Wei Zi* (Fructus Schisandrae Chinensis) 10g, *Pao Jiang* (Rhizoma Zingiberis Praeparatum) 5g, *Da Huang* (Radix et Rhizoma Rhei) 12g, *Hou Po* (Cortex Magnoliae Officinalis) 15g, and *Fu Zi* (Radix Aconiti Lateralis Praeparata) 10g. The formula for middle stage contained *Si Shen Wan* plus *Huang Bo* (Cortex Phellodendri Chinensis) 12g, *Cang Zhu* (Rhizoma Atractylodis) 15g, and *Huang Lian* (Rhizoma Coptidis) 15g. The formula for late stage contained *Si Shen Wan* plus *He Zi* (Fructus Chebulae) 12g and *Ying Su Ke* (Pericarpium Papaveris) 10g. The study reported 96.6% effectiveness among 100 patients.[5]

5. **Enuresis**: One study reported complete recovery in all 20 patients with enuresis when treated with *Si Shen Wan* plus *Yi Zhi* (Fructus Alpiniae Oxyphyllae). The duration of treatment ranged from 1 to 4 packs of herbs, with an average of 2 to 3 packs. No recurrence was reported in all 20 patients during follow up interview one year later.[6]

6. **Seminal emission**: One study reported marked improvement using modified *Si Shen Wan* to treat all 15 patients with seminal emission characterized by Spleen and Kidney yang deficiencies. Clinical presentations include pale face, fatigue, lack of energy, dizziness, tinnitus, soreness and weakness of the lower back and knees, frequent seminal emission, white and greasy tongue coating, and a deep, weak pulse. The herbal treatment contained *Rou Dou Kou* (Semen Myristicae) 12g, *Wu Wei Zi* (Fructus Schisandrae Chinensis) 12g, *Bu Gu Zhi* (Fructus Psoraleae) 30g, *Da Zao* (Fructus Jujubae) 30g, *Shan Zhu Yu* (Fructus Corni) 30g, *Wu Zhu Yu* (Fructus Evodiae) 6g, *Sheng Jiang* (Rhizoma Zingiberis Recens) 10g, and *Bai Shao* (Radix Paeoniae Alba) 24g. The duration of treatment was 15 packs of herbs.[7]

7. **Constipation**: One study reported marked effect using *Si Shen Wan* plus *Hua Jiao* (Pericarpium Zanthoxyli) and *Liu Huang* (Sulfur) to treat constipation characterized by deficiency and cold. Of 62 patients, the study reported complete recovery in 18 cases, marked improvement in 32 cases, and no effect in 12 cases.[8]

AUTHORS' COMMENTS

Si Shen Wan is literally known as "Four-Miracle Pill" because the four herbs in the formula readily and miraculously treat early morning diarrhea due to Kidney yang deficiency.

Zhen Ren Yang Zang Tang (True Man's Decoction for Nourishing the Organs) and *Si Shen Wan* are warm astringent formulas that stop diarrhea and dysentery due to deficiency and cold of the Spleen and Kidney.

• *Zhen Ren Yang Zang Tang* has a stronger astringent effect to stop diarrhea and dysentery. The formula contains qi and blood tonics to address the underlying qi and blood deficiencies. It has excellent effect to treat uncontrollable bowel movement throughout the day and night.

• *Si Shen Wan* has a more potent function to warm and tonify the deficiency and cold of the Spleen and Kidney. This formula is more effective to treat early morning diarrhea with undigested food.[9]

Si Shen Wan, *Shen Ling Bai Zhu San* (Ginseng, Poria, and Atractylodes Macrocephala Powder), and *Tong Xie Yao Fang* (Important Formula for Painful Diarrhea) all bind the Intestines and treat diarrhea.

• *Si Shen Wan* warms and tonifies Spleen and Kidney yang to stop chronic diarrhea. It is designed for severe diarrhea that occurs in the early morning, characterized by watery diarrhea that contains undigested food.

• *Shen Ling Bai Zhu San* is for Spleen qi deficiency diarrhea with damp accumulation, accompanied by fatigue, weakness of the limbs, and poor appetite.

• *Tong Xie Yao Fang* tonifies the Spleen and spreads Liver qi. This formula stops stress-related diarrhea. Patients will often complain of gas, bloating, or abdominal pain that is relieved with diarrhea.[10]

References

1. *Zhong Cheng Yao Yan Jiu* (Research of Chinese Patent Medicine) 1981;9:31.
2. *Shan Xi Zhong Yi* (Shanxi Chinese Medicine) 1990;5:224.
3. *Hu Nan Zhong Yi Za Zhi* (Hunan Journal of Chinese Medicine) 1994;4:38.
4. *Shan Xi Zhong Yi* (Shanxi Chinese Medicine) 1990;1:30.
5. *Nei Meng Gu Zhong Yi Yao* (Traditional Chinese Medicine and Medicinals of Inner Mongolia) 1987;5:8.
6. *Zhong Yi Za Zhi* (Journal of Chinese Medicine) 1982;2:14.
7. *Cheng Du Zhong Yi Xue Yuan Xue Bao* (Journal of Chengdu University of Traditional Chinese Medicine) 1990;1:33.
8. *Zhong Cheng Yao* (Study of Chinese Patent Medicine) 1989;4:45.
9. Wang MZ, et al. *Zhong Yi Xue Wen Da Ti Ku* (Questions and Answers on Traditional Chinese Medicine: Herbal Formulas).
10. Wang MZ, et al. *Zhong Yi Xue Wen Da Ti Ku* (Questions and Answers on Traditional Chinese Medicine: Herbal Formulas).

Chinese Herbal Formulas and Applications

Táo Huā Tāng (Peach Blossom Decoction)

桃花湯
桃花汤

Pinyin Name: *Tao Hua Tang*
Literal Name: Peach Blossom Decoction
Original Source: *Shang Han Lun* (Discussion of Cold-Induced Disorders) by Zhang Zhong-Jing during the Eastern Han Dynasty

COMPOSITION

Chi Shi Zhi (Halloysitum Rubrum)	48g [30g]
Gan Jiang (Rhizoma Zingiberis)	3g [9g]
Geng Mi (Semen Oryzae)	1 cup [30g]

DOSAGE / PREPARATION / ADMINISTRATION

The source text states to cook *Gan Jiang* (Rhizoma Zingiberis), *Geng Mi* (Semen Oryzae), and half of the amount of *Chi Shi Zhi* (Halloysitum Rubrum) in 7 cups [1,400 mL] of water until *Geng Mi* (Semen Oryzae) is well cooked. Take the warm, strained decoction with 1 spoonful [1g] of powdered *Chi Shi Zhi* (Halloysitum Rubrum) three times daily. Discontinue this formula when the desired effect is achieved. Today, this formula may be prepared as a decoction with the doses suggested in brackets.

CHINESE THERAPEUTIC ACTIONS

Warms up the middle *jiao* and binds the Intestines

CLINICAL MANIFESTATIONS

Diarrhea or dysentery due to deficiency and cold of the middle *jiao*: chronic diarrhea or dysentery with dark blood and pus in the stools, dysuria, abdominal pain that is alleviated by pressure and warmth, pale tongue, white tongue coating, and a fine, slow and weak pulse.

CLINICAL APPLICATIONS

Bacterial dysentery, amoebic dysentery, enteritis, chronic colitis, and diarrhea.

EXPLANATION

Tao Hua Tang (Peach Blossom Decoction) is originally presented in *Shang Han Lun* (Discussion of Cold-Induced Disorders) for treating *shaoyin* disorder where there is diarrhea with the presence of pus and dark blood in the stools. More specifically, the chronic diarrhea here is due to deficiency and cold of the middle *jiao* and dysfunction of the Intestines. Consequently, there is pus and blood in the stools, and abdominal pain that is relieved by pressure and warmth.

Chi Shi Zhi (Halloysitum Rubrum), the chief substance of this formula, has a warm and astringent nature to bind the Intestines, relieve diarrhea, and prevent rectal prolapse. *Gan Jiang* (Rhizoma Zingiberis) warms the middle *jiao* and dispels interior cold. *Geng Mi* (Semen Oryzae) nourishes the Stomach and harmonizes the middle *jiao*. This formula is effective in treating chronic diarrhea due to deficiency and cold of the middle *jiao*.

MODIFICATIONS

• For yang deficiency with excess cold, add *Ren Shen* (Radix et Rhizoma Ginseng), *Fu Zi* (Radix Aconiti Lateralis Praeparata) and *Zhi Gan Cao* (Radix et Rhizoma Glycyrrhizae Praeparata cum Melle); or *Fu Zi Li Zhong Wan* (Prepared Aconite Pill to Regulate the Middle).

• For severe abdominal pain, add *Dang Gui* (Radix Angelicae Sinensis) and *Bai Shao* (Radix Paeoniae Alba).

• With *chang feng* (intestinal wind) and blood in the stools, substitute *Gan Jiang* (Rhizoma Zingiberis) with *Pao Jiang* (Rhizoma Zingiberis Praeparatum).

CAUTIONS / CONTRAINDICATIONS

Tao Hua Tang contains astringent herbs to treat chronic diarrhea and dysentery due to deficiency. It is contra-indicated in diarrhea and dysentery caused by damp-heat accumulation.

CLINICAL STUDIES AND RESEARCH

1. **Bacterial dysentery**: Use of modified *Tao Hua Tang* was shown in many studies to effectively stop diarrhea in patients with bacterial dysentery.[1] One study used *Tao Hua Tang* plus *Ren Shen* (Radix et Rhizoma Ginseng) and *Fu Zi* (Radix Aconiti Lateralis Praeparata) to treat bacterial dysentery characterized by the presence of pus and blood in the stools, abdominal pain that diminishes with pressure, absence of thirst, pale tongue with white tongue coating, and a deep, forceless pulse.[2] Another

11

ASTRINGENT FORMULAS

787

Chapter 11 – Astringent Formulas   *Section 3– Intestines-Binding Formulas to Stop Leakage*

Táo Huā Tāng (Peach Blossom Decoction)

Tao Hua Tang (Peach Blossom Decoction)

Diagnosis	Signs and Symptoms	Treatment	Herbs
Diarrhea or dysentery due to deficiency and cold of the middle *jiao*	• Diarrhea with pus and dark blood in the stools: deficiency and cold of the middle *jiao* • Abdominal pain that decreases with pressure and warmth: presence of deficiency and cold	Warms up the middle *jiao* and binds the Intestines	• *Chi Shi Zhi* (Halloysitum Rubrum) warms and binds the Intestines to relieve diarrhea. • *Gan Jiang* (Rhizoma Zingiberis) warms the middle *jiao* and dispels the interior cold. • *Geng Mi* (Semen Oryzae) nourishes the Stomach and harmonizes the middle *jiao*.

study used *Tao Hua Tang* to treat chronic bacterial dysentery with 5 to 7 bowel movements daily, rectal tenesmus, poor appetite, fatigue, pale tongue with white, greasy tongue coating, and a slow pulse.[3]

2. **Diarrhea**: According to one study, administration of *Tao Hua Tang* to stop diarrhea, and *Xiang Sha Liu Jun Zi Tang* (Six-Gentlemen Decoction with Aucklandia and Amomum) to consolidate the constitution, was effective in the treatment and management of diarrhea characterized by deficiency and cold.[4]

RELATED FORMULA

Chì Shí Zhī Yǔ Yú Liáng Tang
(Halloysitum and Limonite Decoction)
赤石脂禹餘糧湯
赤石脂禹余粮汤
Pinyin Name: *Chi Shi Zhi Yu Yu Liang Tang*
Literal Name: Halloysitum and Limonite Decoction
Alternate Name: *Chi Shi Zhi Yu Liang Shi Tang*
Original Source: *Shang Han Lun* (Discussion of Cold-Induced Disorders) by Zhang Zhong-Jing during the Eastern Han Dynasty

Chi Shi Zhi (Halloysitum Rubrum),
 fen sui (pulverized)   48g [30g]
Yu Yu Liang (Limonitum), *fen sui* (pulverized) 48g [30g]

The source text states to cook the ingredients in 6 cups [1,200 mL] of water until it is reduced to 2 cups (400 mL). Take the warm, strained decoction in three equally-divided doses. Today, this formula may be prepared as a decoction with the doses suggested in brackets.

The main actions of this formula are to bind the Intestines and stop diarrhea. Clinically, the patient may have chronic diarrhea with uncontrollable bowel movements. The interior-warming action of *Chi Shi Zhi Yu Yu Liang Tang* (Halloysitum and Limonite Decoction) is not as strong as *Tao Hua Tang*; however, since the astringent action of this formula is quite strong, it can be used as a short-term symptomatic treatment to quickly stop diarrhea.

AUTHORS' COMMENTS

Tao Hua Tang is literally named "Peach Blossom Decoction" to describe the appearance of this formula. The color of its principle ingredient, *Chi Shi Zhi* (Halloysitum Rubrum), is crimson, and the color of *Geng Mi* (Semen Oryzae) is white. The combination of these two colors results in the peach color, hence the name Peach Blossom.

Chi Shi Zhi (Halloysitum Rubrum) is a mineral substance that is poorly soluble in water, and its effect is limited when used in decoction. Therefore, the source text specifically states to cook half the amount of *Chi Shi Zhi* (Halloysitum Rubrum) in decoction, and take an additional amount in powder form with the decoction, to ensure therapeutic effectiveness.

References

1. *Zhong Yi Fang Ji Xian Dai Yan Jiu* (Modern Study of Medical Formulae in Traditional Chinese Medicine) 1997;807-808.
2. *Zhe Jiang Zhong Yi Za Zhi* (Zhejiang Journal of Chinese Medicine) 1982;8:378.
3. *Jiang Su Zhong Yi Za Zhi* (Jiangsu Journal of Chinese Medicine) 1987;5:17.
4. *Zhong Yi Fang Ji Xian Dai Yan Jiu* (Modern Study of Medical Formulae in Traditional Chinese Medicine) 1997;807-808.

Chinese Herbal Formulas and Applications

Section 4

涩精止遗剂

— Jing (Essence)-Stabilizing Formulas to Stop Leakage

Jīn Suǒ Gù Jīng Wán (Metal Lock Pill to Stabilize the Essence)
金鎖固精丸
金锁固精丸

Pinyin Name: Jin Suo Gu Jing Wan
Literal Name: Metal Lock Pill to Stabilize the Essence
Alternate Names: *Chin Suo Ku Ching Wan*, Golden Lock Essence-Securing Pill, Golden Lock Pill for Consolidating the Essence, Lotus Stamen Formula
Original Source: *Yi Fang Ji Jie* (Analytical Collection of Medical Formulas) by Wang Ang in 1682

COMPOSITION

Sha Yuan Zi (Semen Astragali Complanati), *chao* (dry-fried)	60g [12g]
Qian Shi (Semen Euryales), *zheng* (steamed)	60g [12g]
Lian Xu (Stamen Nelumbinis)	60g [12g]
Long Gu (Os Draconis), *zhi* (fried with liquid) till crisp	30g [10g]
Mu Li (Concha Ostreae), *zhu* (boiled) in lightly salted water for 24 hours and *duan* (calcined) into powder	30g [10g]

DOSAGE / PREPARATION / ADMINISTRATION

The source text states to grind the ingredients into powder and form into pills with powdered *Lian Zi* (Semen Nelumbinis). Take the pills with salted water. Today this formula may be given in pills or decoction. For pills, take 9g per dose once or twice daily with water or lightly salted water. For decoction, use the suggested doses in brackets.

CHINESE THERAPEUTIC ACTIONS

Tonifies the Kidney and stabilizes the *jing* (essence)

CLINICAL MANIFESTATIONS

Seminal emission and/or spermatorrhea due to Kidney deficiency: seminal emission, spermatorrhea, urinary incontinence, frequent urination, lack of energy, weak knees, soreness and weakness of the legs, lower back pain, and tinnitus.

CLINICAL APPLICATIONS

Spermatorrhea, nocturnal emission, sexual dysfunction, enuresis, nocturia, diarrhea, and myasthenia gravis.

EXPLANATION

Jin Suo Gu Jing Wan (Metal Lock Pill to Stabilize the Essence) is designed to treat spermatorrhea and/or nocturnal emission due to Kidney deficiency. Kidney is the organ that stores *jing* (essence). If the Kidney is deficient, then the *jing* may become unstable and leak out of the body, resulting in seminal emission and/or spermatorrhea. In addition to Kidney *jing* deficiency, Kidney yin and yang may be deficient as well, leading to the following clinical manifestations: lack of energy, weak knees, sore back, and tinnitus.

Sha Yuan Zi (Semen Astragali Complanati), the chief herb of this formula, is used to tonify the Kidney and stabilize *jing* (essence). *Lian Zi* (Semen Nelumbinis) and *Qian Shi* (Semen Euryales) help the chief herb tonify the Kidney and stabilize *jing*. *Lian Xu* (Stamen Nelumbinis), prepared *Long Gu* (Os Draconis), and calcined *Mu Li* (Concha Ostreae) are used mainly to stabilize the leaking *jing*.

Since this formula concentrates on consolidating the *jing* (essence), it may be used to temporarily stop the leaking symptoms of seminal emission or spermatorrhea. However, it lacks strength in tonifying the Kidney; hence, once the

ASTRINGENT FORMULAS

11

Chapter 11 – Astringent Formulas　　　　*Section 4– Jing (Essence)-Stabilizing Formulas to Stop Leakage*

Jīn Suǒ Gù Jīng Wán (Metal Lock Pill to Stabilize the Essence)

Jin Suo Gu Jing Wan (Metal Lock Pill to Stabilize the Essence)

Diagnosis	Signs and Symptoms	Treatment	Herbs
Seminal emission and/or spermator-rhea due to Kidney deficiency	• Seminal emission and/or spermatorrhea: loss of *jing* (essence) due to Kidney deficiency • Soreness and weakness of the knees and legs, lower back pain and tinnitus: Kidney yin and yang deficiencies	Tonifies the Kidney and stabilizes the *jing*	• *Sha Yuan Zi* (Semen Astragali Complanati) tonifies the Kidney and stabilize the *jing*. • *Lian Zi* (Semen Nelumbinis) and *Qian Shi* (Semen Euryales) tonify the Kidney and stabilize the *jing*. • *Lian Xu* (Stamen Nelumbinis), *Long Gu* (Os Draconis) and *Mu Li* (Concha Ostreae) stabilize and stop the leaking *jing*.

spermatorrhea and/or seminal emission is/are stopped, more Kidney-tonic herbs should be used.

MODIFICATIONS

• For severe spermatorrhea or nocturnal emission, add *Jin Ying Zi* (Fructus Rosae Laevigatae) and *Wu Wei Zi* (Fructus Schisandrae Chinensis).

• With Kidney yang deficiency, add *Bu Gu Zhi* (Fructus Psoraleae), *Rou Cong Rong* (Herba Cistanches), and *Fu Zi* (Radix Aconiti Lateralis Praeparata).

• With Kidney yin deficiency, add *Liu Wei Di Huang Wan* (Six-Ingredient Pill with Rehmannia).

• With yin-deficient fire, add *Zhi Mu* (Rhizoma Anemarrhenae) and *Huang Bo* (Cortex Phellodendri Chinensis).

• With irritability and insomnia, add *Suan Zao Ren* (Semen Ziziphi Spinosae) and *Bai Zi Ren* (Semen Platycladi).

• With irritability and thirst from yin deficiency, add *Mai Dong* (Radix Ophiopogonis) and *Ren Shen* (Radix et Rhizoma Ginseng).

• With cold signs and/or symptoms, add *Rou Gui* (Cortex Cinnamomi) and *Fu Zi* (Radix Aconiti Lateralis Praeparata).

• With dry stools, add *Rou Cong Rong* (Herba Cistanches) and *Dang Gui* (Radix Angelicae Sinensis).

• With loose stools, add *Wu Wei Zi* (Fructus Schisandrae Chinensis) and *Bu Gu Zhi* (Fructus Psoraleae).

• With soreness and pain of the back, add *Du Zhong* (Cortex Eucommiae) and *Xu Duan* (Radix Dipsaci); or *Du Huo Ji Sheng Tang* (Angelica Pubescens and Taxillus Decoction).

• With impotence, add *Yin Yang Huo* (Herba Epimedii) and *Suo Yang* (Herba Cynomorii); or *Huan Shao Dan* (Return to Youth Pill).

• With leukorrhea, add *Fu Ling* (Poria) and *Yi Yi Ren* (Semen Coicis).

• With white, cloudy discharge, add *Sang Piao Xiao* (Ootheca Mantidis) and *Fen Bi Xie* (Rhizoma Dioscoreae Hypoglaucae).

CAUTIONS / CONTRAINDICATIONS

Jin Suo Gu Jing Wan contains many astringent herbs, and is therefore contraindicated in seminal emission and/or spermatorrhea due to Heart fire, Liver fire, Kidney yin-deficient fire, or damp-heat in the lower *jiao*.

CLINICAL STUDIES AND RESEARCH

1. **Spermatorrhea**: According to one report, *Jin Suo Gu Jing Wan* was used with good results to treat one patient with a three-year history of severe spermatorrhea accompanied by night perspiration, fatigue, sore lower back, low libido, impotence, premature ejaculation, and nocturnal emission. The treatment protocol was to administer 15 pills of *Jin Suo Gu Jing Wan* three times daily for one month.[1]

2. **Diarrhea**: One report stated that *Jin Suo Gu Jing Wan* can effectively treat diarrhea associated with chronic enteritis characterized by Spleen and Kidney deficiencies.[2]

3. **Myasthenia gravis**: One study reported marked success using *Jin Suo Gu Jing Wan* to treat one person with myasthenia gravis. Clinical manifestations included drooping eyelids, fatigue, lack of power in all four limbs, difficulty with chewing, shortness of breath, insomnia, spermatorrhea, low back pain, feeling of coldness in the legs, and red tongue with scanty tongue coating. The treatment protocol was to administer 12 grams of *Jin Suo Gu Jing Wan* three times daily with lightly salted water. Improvement was noted after two weeks of herbal therapy.[3]

RELATED FORMULA

Shuǐ Lù Èr Xiān Dān

(Water and Earth Two Immortals Special Pill)

水陸二仙丹
水陆二仙丹

Pinyin Name: *Shui Lu Er Xian Dan*

Literal Name: Water and Earth Two Immortals Special Pill

Original Source: *Hong Shi Ji Yan Fang* (Time-Tested Formulas of the Hong Family)

790

Chinese Herbal Formulas and Applications

Jīn Suǒ Gù Jīng Wán (Metal Lock Pill to Stabilize the Essence)

Qian Shi (Semen Euryales) [12g]

Jin Ying Zi (Fructus Rosae Laevigatae) [12g]

The source text states to use equal amounts of these two ingredients. Simmer *Jin Ying Zi* (Fructus Rosae Laevigatae) in low heat and condense it into paste. Separately grind *Qian Shi* (Semen Euryales) into fine powder. Mix the paste of *Jin Ying Zi* (Fructus Rosae Laevigatae) and the powder of *Qian Shi* (Semen Euryales) together to form pills. Take 9g of pills twice daily before meals with warm grain-based liquor or lightly salted water. Today, this formula may be prepared as a decoction with the doses suggested in brackets.

The main actions of this formula are to tonify the Kidney and consolidate *jing* (essence). Clinically, it may be used for seminal emission in men, and leukorrhea of persistent, clear and thin discharge in women.

Shui Lu Er Xian Dan (Water and Earth Two Immortals Special Pill) has similar, but weaker astringent and tonic effects, when compared with *Jin Suo Gu Jing Wan*.

AUTHORS' COMMENTS

Jin Suo Gu Jing Wan is one of the most commonly used formulas for treating seminal emission and spermatorrhea. Other key signs include tinnitus, soreness and weakness of the back and knees. It can also be used for seminal emission and spermatorrhea caused by neurasthenia or chronic prostatitis.

References

1. *Hu Nan Zhong Yi Za Zhi* (Hunan Journal of Chinese Medicine) 1987;3:46.
2. *Hu Bei Zhong Yi Za Zhi* (Hubei Journal of Chinese Medicine) 1985;2:41.
3. *Xin Zhong Yi* (New Chinese Medicine) 1973;5:30.

Liù Wèi Gù Jīng Wán (Rehmannia Six and Lotus Stamen Pill)
六味固精丸

Pinyin Name: *Liu Wei Gu Jing Wan*
Literal Name: Rehmannia Six and Lotus Stamen Pill
Alternate Name: Rehmannia Six and Stamen Formula
Original Source: Unavailable

COMPOSITION

Jin Suo Gu Jing Wan (Metal Lock Pill to Stabilize the Essence)
Liu Wei Di Huang Wan (Six-Ingredient Pill with Rehmannia)

DOSAGE / PREPARATION / ADMINISTRATION

This formula is taken before meals with warm water or lightly-salted water.

CHINESE THERAPEUTIC ACTIONS

1. Stabilizes *jing* (essence) and stops leakage of sperm
2. Tonifies the Kidney and replenishes the *jing* (essence)

CLINICAL MANIFESTATIONS

Seminal emission and/or spermatorrhea due to Kidney deficiency: seminal emission and/or spermatorrhea in individuals who are mentally and physically drained, possibly with neurasthenia.

CLINICAL APPLICATIONS

Seminal emission and/or spermatorrhea due to mental and physical exhaustion.

EXPLANATION

Liu Wei Gu Jing Wan (Rehmannia Six and Lotus Stamen Pill) is made by combining *Jin Suo Gu Jing Wan* (Metal Lock Pill to Stabilize the Essence) with *Liu Wei Di Huang Wan* (Six-Ingredient Pill with Rehmannia). The purpose of *Jin Suo Gu Jing Wan* (Metal Lock Pill to Stabilize the Essence) is to address the symptoms, which is seminal emission and/or spermatorrhea; and the purpose of *Liu Wei Di Huang Wan* (Six-Ingredient Pill with Rehmannia) is to address the cause, which is Liver and Kidney yin

ASTRINGENT FORMULAS

11

791

Chapter 11 – Astringent Formulas   *Section 4– Jing (Essence)-Stabilizing Formulas to Stop Leakage*

Liù Wèi Gù Jīng Wán (Rehmannia Six and Lotus Stamen Pill)

deficiencies. The combination of these two formulas offers both immediate and long-term benefits as both the cause and the symptoms are addressed simultaneously.

For additional and detailed information, please refer to *Jin Suo Gu Jing Wan* (Metal Lock Pill to Stabilize the Essence) and *Liu Wei Di Huang Wan* (Six-Ingredient Pill with Rehmannia).

Liu Wei Gu Jing Wan (Rehmannia Six and Lotus Stamen Pill)

Diagnosis	Signs and Symptoms	Treatment	Herbs
Seminal emission and/or spermatorrhea due to Kidney deficiency	Seminal emission and/or spermatorrhea	• Stabilizes *jing* (essence) and stops leakage of sperm • Tonifies the Kidney and replenishes the *jing*	• *Jin Suo Gu Jing Wan* (Metal Lock Pill to Stabilize the Essence) stabilizes *jing* and treats seminal emission and/or spermatorrhea. • *Liu Wei Di Huang Wan* (Six-Ingredient Pill with Rehmannia) tonifies Liver and Kidney yin deficiency.

Sāng Piāo Xiāo Sǎn (Mantis Egg-Case Powder)
桑螵蛸散

Pinyin Name: *Sang Piao Xiao San*
Literal Name: Mantis Egg-Case Powder
Alternate Names: *Sang Piao Hsiao San*, Mantis Egg-Case Formula, Mantis Formula
Original Source: *Ben Cao Yan Yi* (Extension of the Materia Medica) by Kou Zong-Shi in 1116

COMPOSITION

Sang Piao Xiao (Ootheca Mantidis)	30g [9g]
Long Gu (Os Draconis)	30g [15g]
Gui Ban (Plastrum Testudinis), *chu zhi* (fried with vinegar)	30g [15g]
Ren Shen (Radix et Rhizoma Ginseng)	30g [9g]
Dang Gui (Radix Angelicae Sinensis)	30g [9g]
Yuan Zhi (Radix Polygalae)	30g [6g]
Shi Chang Pu (Rhizoma Acori Tatarinowii)	30g [6g]
Fu Shen (Poria Pararadicis)	30g [12g]

DOSAGE / PREPARATION / ADMINISTRATION

The source text states to grind the ingredients into powder and take 6g at bedtime with a decoction made from *Ren Shen* (Radix et Rhizoma Ginseng). Today, this formula is usually taken [6g at bedtime] with a decoction made from *Dang Shen* (Radix Codonopsis). This formula may also be prepared as a decoction with the doses suggested in brackets.

CHINESE THERAPEUTIC ACTIONS

1. Regulates and tonifies the Heart and Kidney
2. Stabilizes *jing* (essence) and stops seminal emission

CLINICAL MANIFESTATIONS

Heart and Kidney deficiencies: frequent urination, cloudy urine that resembles rice water, seminal emission, enuresis, trance, forgetfulness and poor appetite.

792

Chinese Herbal Formulas and Applications

Sāng Piāo Xiāo Sǎn (Mantis Egg-Case Powder)

CLINICAL APPLICATIONS

Chronic nephritis, cystitis, frequent urination, enuresis, seminal emission, diabetes mellitus, neurasthenia, and constipation.

EXPLANATION

Sang Piao Xiao San (Mantis Egg-Case Powder) is designed to treat the various clinical manifestations caused by Heart and Kidney deficiencies. According to five element theory, the Kidney belongs to the water element and the Heart belongs to the fire element. If the Kidney (water) and the Heart (fire) cannot exist in harmony, then both organs may exhaust themselves. Kidney deficiency would lead to leaking of *jing* (essence), and resulting in seminal emission. Since the Kidney has an important function in regulating urination, deficiency of the Kidney would lead to enuresis and frequent urination. Finally, deficiency of the Heart may cause instability of the *shen* (spirit), leading to trance and forgetfulness.

To effectively treat this syndrome, the Heart and Kidney should be tonified and their harmonious relationship be restored. *Sang Piao Xiao* (Ootheca Mantidis), the chief substance of this formula, tonifies the Kidney, nourishes *jing* (essence), and stops seminal emission. *Long Gu* (Os Draconis) calms the *shen* (spirit) and stabilizes *jing. Gui Ban* (Plastrum Testudinis) nourishes yin and tonifies the Heart and Kidney. *Ren Shen* (Radix et Rhizoma Ginseng) tonifies *yuan* (source) qi, and *Dang Gui* (Radix Angelicae Sinensis) nourishes blood. *Yuan Zhi* (Radix Polygalae) and *Shi Chang Pu* (Rhizoma Acori Tatarinowii) calm and anchor the *shen* to restore harmony between the Heart and Kidney. *Fu Shen* (Poria Paradicis) calms the *shen*.

MODIFICATIONS

- With generalized fatigue and deficiency, add *Huang Qi* (Radix Astragali).
- With more frequent urination, add *Bai Zhu* (Rhizoma Atractylodis Macrocephalae) and *Gan Cao* (Radix et Rhizoma Glycyrrhizae).
- With dense urine that feels sticky, add *Shan Yao* (Rhizoma Dioscoreae) and *Qian Shi* (Semen Euryales).
- For enuresis or urinary incontinence, add *Yi Zhi* (Fructus Alpiniae Oxyphyllae) and *Fu Pen Zi* (Fructus Rubi).
- With forgetfulness and inability to concentrate, add *Bai Zi Ren* (Semen Platycladi) and *Long Chi* (Dens Draconis).
- With insomnia and forgetfulness, add *Wu Wei Zi* (Fructus Schisandrae Chinensis) and *Suan Zao Ren* (Semen Ziziphi Spinosae); or *Tian Wang Bu Xin Dan* (Emperor of Heaven's Special Pill to Tonify the Heart).
- For spermatorrhea or seminal emission, add *Suo Yang* (Herba Cynomorii) and *Shan Zhu Yu* (Fructus Corni).
- For spermatorrhea with a weak pulse, add *Sha Yuan Zi* (Semen Astragali Complanati).
- With Kidney yang deficiency, add *Ba Ji Tian* (Radix Morindae Officinalis) and *Fu Zi* (Radix Aconiti Lateralis Praeparata).
- With Liver and Kidney yin deficiencies, add *Liu Wei Di Huang Wan* (Six-Ingredient Pill with Rehmannia).

CAUTIONS / CONTRAINDICATIONS

Sang Piao Xiao San contains many tonic and astringent herbs to treat loss of *jing* (essence) and body fluids due to Heart and Kidney deficiencies. This formula is not suitable for treating seminal emission and frequent urination due to damp-heat in the lower *jiao*.

11

ASTRINGENT FORMULAS

Sang Piao Xiao San (Mantis Egg-Case Powder)

Diagnosis	Signs and Symptoms	Treatment	Herbs
Heart and Kidney deficiencies	• Enuresis and frequent urination with cloudy urine: Kidney deficiency unable to control urination • Seminal emission: leaking of *jing* (essence) due to Kidney deficiency • Trance and forgetfulness: Heart deficiency unable to nourish *shen* (spirit)	• Regulates and tonifies the Heart and the Kidney • Stabilizes *jing* and stops seminal emission	• *Sang Piao Xiao* (Ootheca Mantidis) tonifies the Kidney, nourishes the *jing* and stops seminal emission. • *Long Gu* (Os Draconis) calms the *shen* and stabilizes the *jing*. • *Gui Ban* (Plastrum Testudinis) nourishes yin and tonifies the Heart and Kidney. • *Ren Shen* (Radix et Rhizoma Ginseng) and *Dang Gui* (Radix Angelicae Sinensis) tonify qi and blood. • *Yuan Zhi* (Radix Polygalae), *Shi Chang Pu* (Rhizoma Acori Tatarinowii) and *Fu Shen* (Poria Paradicis) calm the *shen* to restore harmony to the Heart and Kidney.

793

Sāng Piāo Xiāo Sǎn (Mantis Egg-Case Powder)

CLINICAL STUDIES AND RESEARCH

1. **Frequent urination**: According to one study, administration of Sang Piao Xiao San in decoction was associated with good results in treating frequent urination in 51 children (between 3 to 6 years of age, with 2 to 20 days history of illness). The clinical presentations included frequent urination with dripping, clear urine, no feelings of pain during urination, pale tongue with thin, white coating, and a fine, weak pulse. Of 51 patients, the study reported recovery in 2 cases after 2 days, 4 cases after 3 days, 14 cases after 4 days, 21 cases after 5 days, 6 cases after 6 days, and 2 cases after 7 days. Information was unavailable on individuals who did not complete the study.[1]

2. **Enuresis**: One study reported satisfactory results using modified Sang Piao Xiao San to treat bedwetting in 56 children (between 4 to 14 years of age, with 3 months to 10 years of history). The herbal formula contained processed Huang Qi (Radix Astragali) 10g, dry-fried Dang Shen (Radix Codonopsis) 10g, Sang Piao Xiao (Ootheca Mantidis) 15g, Long Gu (Os Draconis) 10g, dry-fried Sheng Ma (Rhizoma Cimicifugae) 10g, Yi Zhi (Fructus Alpiniae Oxyphyllae) 10g, and Shan Yao (Rhizoma Dioscoreae) 10g. The treatment protocol was to administer the herbs in decoction daily, for 10 days per course of treatment. The duration of treatment ranged from 7 to 23 days, with an average of 3 weeks. Of 56 children, the study reported complete recovery in 34 cases (no bedwetting for 3 months), significant improvement in 20 cases (reduced frequency of bedwetting within 3 months) and no effect in 2 cases. The overall effectiveness was 96.5%.[2]

3. **Constipation**: Use of Sang Piao Xiao San was associated with satisfactory results in treating constipation in 27 elderly patients (19 males and 8 females, between 56 to 86 years of age, with 10 months to 9 years history of illness). The clinical presentation included difficulty passing stools, with one bowel movement every 4 to 8 days. The herbal formula contained Sang Piao Xiao (Ootheca Mantidis) 12g, Long Gu (Os Draconis) 21g, Qian Shi (Semen Euryales) 15g, Dang Shen (Radix Codonopsis) 10g, Gui Ban (Plastrum Testudinis) 10g, Dang Gui (Radix Angelicae Sinensis) 10g, Shi Chang Pu (Rhizoma Acori Tatarinowii) 10g, and Yuan Zhi (Radix Polygalae) 10g. Furthermore, modifications were made by adding Huang Qi (Radix Astragali), Bai Zhu (Rhizoma Atractylodis Macrocephalae) and a larger dose of Dang Shen (Radix Codonopsis) for qi deficiency; Bie Jia (Carapax Trionycis) and a larger dose of Gui Ban (Plastrum Testudinis) for yin deficiency; E Jiao (Colla Corii Asini) and a larger dose of Dang Gui (Radix Angelicae Sinensis) for blood deficiency; Huang Bo (Cortex Phellodendri Chinensis) and Zhi Mu (Rhizoma Anemarrhenae) for frequent and painful urination with dark color urination; and Yi Zhi (Fructus Alpiniae Oxyphyllae), Jin Ying Zi (Fructus Rosae Laevigatae) and larger doses of Sang Piao Xiao (Ootheca Mantidis) and Qian Shi (Semen Euryales) for frequent urination with clear urine. The duration of treatment ranged from 7 to 25 days. Of 27 patients, the study reported complete recovery in 20 cases, improvement in 5 cases, and no effect in 2 cases.[3]

AUTHORS' COMMENTS

Sang Piao Xiao San is the representative formula for treating loss of jing (essence) and body fluids due to Heart and Kidney deficiencies. Key symptoms in choosing this formula include enuresis, frequent urges to urinate, forgetfulness and diminished mental acuity. This formula can also be used for urinary incontinence during pregnancy or bedwetting in children.

Jin Suo Gu Jing Wan (Metal Lock Pill to Stabilize the Essence) and Sang Piao Xiao San are both astringent formulas that consolidate the jing (essence) and stop spermatorrhea.

- Jin Suo Gu Jing Wan is stronger in astringing and treating the symptoms of spermatorrhea.
- Sang Piao Xiao San consolidates jing and tonifies the Kidney and Heart to treat spermatorrhea, forgetfulness, bedwetting, enuresis, and other signs of Heart and Kidney deficiencies.[4]

According to Dr. Chang Wei-Yen, Sang Piao Xiao San can be combined with Tian Wang Bu Xin Dan (Emperor of Heaven's Special Pill to Tonify the Heart) to more effectively treat forgetfulness, bedwetting, enuresis, or seminal emission.

References

1. Hei Long Jiang Zhong Yi Yao (Heilongjiang Chinese Medicine and Herbology) 1990;1:33.
2. Jiang Su Zhong Yi (Jiangsu Chinese Medicine) 1994;4:14.
3. Zhe Jiang Zhong Yi Xue Yuan Xue Bao (Journal of Zhejiang University of Chinese Medicine) 1993;2:27.
4. Wang MZ, et al. Zhong Yi Xue Wen Da Ti Ku (Questions and Answers on Traditional Chinese Medicine: Herbal Formulas).

Chinese Herbal Formulas and Applications

Suō Quán Wán (Shut the Sluice Pill)

縮泉丸
缩泉丸

Pinyin Name: *Suo Quan Wan*
Literal Name: Shut the Sluice Pill
Alternate Name: Shut the Sluice Formula
Original Source: *Fu Ren Liang Fang* (Fine Formulas for Women) by Chen Zi-Ming in 1237

COMPOSITION

Yi Zhi (Fructus Alpiniae Oxyphyllae)	[9g]
Wu Yao (Radix Linderae)	[6g]

DOSAGE / PREPARATION / ADMINISTRATION

The source text states to grind equal amounts of *Yi Zhi* (Fructus Alpiniae Oxyphyllae) and *Wu Yao* (Radix Linderae) into powder. Separately cook powdered *Shan Yao* (Rhizoma Dioscoreae) [9-15g] with grain-based liquor until it becomes an herbal paste. Combine the powder and the paste to form pills. Take 70 pills per dose with salted grain-based liquor or rice soup. Today, this formula is usually administered by giving 6g of pills per dose once or twice a day with water. This formula may also be prepared as a decoction with the doses suggested in brackets.

CHINESE THERAPEUTIC ACTIONS

1. Warms the Kidney and dispels cold
2. Controls frequent urination and stops enuresis

CLINICAL MANIFESTATIONS

Frequent urination and enuresis due to deficiency and cold of the lower *jiao*: frequent and prolonged urination, dripping of urine after urination, clear urine; and enuresis in children.

CLINICAL APPLICATIONS

Frequent urination, urinary incontinence, enuresis, spermatorrhea, leukorrhea, and lumbago.

EXPLANATION

Suo Quan Wan (Shut the Sluice Pill) is designed to treat urinary disorders due to deficiency and cold of the lower *jiao*. The Kidney has functions of regulating urination and dispelling turbid water out of the body. If Kidney qi is deficient and cold starts to accumulate in the Urinary Bladder, then urinary disorders such as frequent urination and enuresis may occur.

In this formula, *Yi Zhi* (Fructus Alpiniae Oxyphyllae) warms the Kidney and Spleen to stop frequent urination and enuresis. *Wu Yao* (Radix Linderae) warms the lower *jiao* and disperses cold to restore the normal urinary functions of the Kidney and Urinary Bladder. *Shan Yao* (Rhizoma Dioscoreae) strengthens the Spleen and tonifies the Kidney to treat the underlying deficiency. It also stabilizes the *jing* (essence). These herbs are warm but not drying, and work to treat deficiency and cold and restore normal urination.

Even though *Suo Quan Wan* is effective, it is only mild to moderate in potency. In severe cases of frequent urination and enuresis, additional tonic and astringent herbs are called for to ensure adequate treatment.

MODIFICATIONS

- For frequent urination, add *Jin Ying Zi* (Fructus Rosae Laevigatae) and *Huang Qi* (Radix Astragali).
- For enuresis, add *Sang Piao Xiao* (Ootheca Mantidis), *Long Gu* (Os Draconis), and *Mu Li* (Concha Ostreae).

CAUTIONS / CONTRAINDICATIONS

Individuals who take *Suo Quan Wan* should avoid spicy and pungent foods.[1]

PHARMACOLOGICAL EFFECTS

Antidiuretic: According to one study, use of *Suo Quan Wan* in healthy rats was associated with marked antidiuretic effect. Furthermore, there was a reduced concentration in the urine of sodium and chloride, but increased concentration of potassium.[2]

CLINICAL STUDIES AND RESEARCH

1. **Frequent urination:** *Suo Quan Wan* has been shown in many studies to effectively treat frequent urination in children. According to one study, administration of this formula in powder form was associated with 93.75% effectiveness. Of 32 children, the study reported complete recovery in 27 cases, improvement in 3 cases, and no effect in 2 cases.[3] Another study also reported good results for treatment of frequent urination using *Suo*

11

ASTRINGENT FORMULAS

795

Chapter 11 – Astringent Formulas　　　　　　　*Section 4– Jing (Essence)-Stabilizing Formulas to Stop Leakage*

Suō Quán Wán (Shut the Sluice Pill)

Suo Quan Wan (Shut the Sluice Pill)

Diagnosis	Signs and Symptoms	Treatment	Herbs
Frequent urination and enuresis	Frequent and prolonged urination, dripping of urine after urination, and enuresis: deficiency and cold of the lower *jiao*	• Warms up the Kidney and dispels cold • Controls frequent urination and stops enuresis	• *Yi Zhi* (Fructus Alpiniae Oxyphyllae) tonifies and warms the Kidney to stop frequent urination and enuresis. • *Wu Yao* (Radix Linderae) warms the lower *jiao* and disperses cold to restore the normal urinary function of Kidney and the Urinary Bladder. • *Shan Yao* (Rhizoma Dioscoreae) strengthens the Spleen and tonifies the Kidney to treat the underlying deficiencies.

Quan Wan plus *Jin Ying Zi* (Fructus Rosae Laevigatae) and *Huang Qi* (Radix Astragali) as the base formula.[4]

2. **Urinary incontinence**: The use of modified *Suo Quan Wan* was shown in one study to have good effect to treat urinary and bowel incontinence in post-stroke patients. The herbal treatment contained this formula plus *Sang Piao Xiao* (Ootheca Mantidis), *Shan Zhu Yu* (Fructus Corni), *Bu Gu Zhi* (Fructus Psoraleae), *Tu Si Zi* (Semen Cuscutae) and *Huang Qi* (Radix Astragali) as the base formula. Furthermore, *Rou Dou Kou* (Semen Myristicae), *Wu Zhu Yu* (Fructus Evodiae) and *Wu Wei Zi* (Fructus Schisandrae Chinensis) were added for bowel incontinence; *Shi Chang Pu* (Rhizoma Acori Tatarinowii), *Yu Jin* (Radix Curcumae), *Yuan Zhi* (Radix Polygalae) and *Dan Nan Xing* (Arisaema cum Bile) were added for speech difficulties; *Tao Ren* (Semen Persicae), *Hong Hua* (Flos Carthami), *Di Long* (Pheretima), *Chi Shao* (Radix Paeoniae Rubra) and a larger dose of *Huang Qi* (Radix Astragali) for sallow facial appearance, fatigue, and weakness and paralysis of the extremities.[5]

3. **Enuresis**: According to one study, the use of *Suo Quan Wan* plus *Sang Piao Xiao* (Ootheca Mantidis), *Long Gu* (Os Draconis) and other herbs was associated with 95% effectiveness in treating 20 children with enuresis. Of 20 patients, 12 had complete recovery, 7 had improvement, and 1 had no effect.[6]

TOXICOLOGY

According to one toxicology study, administration of *Suo Quan Wan* at 10 g/kg, 15 g/kg and 20 g/kg daily (proportionally 50, 75 and 100 times the normal dose in human adults) for 2 days did not cause any abnormal reactions within 7 days of the observation period.[7]

AUTHORS' COMMENTS

Sang Piao Xiao San (Mantis Egg-Case Powder) and *Suo Quan Wan* both treat frequent urination and enuresis.

• *Sang Piao Xiao San* tonifies but is not warm in property. It tonifies the Heart and Kidney to treat not only frequent urination and enuresis, but also seminal emission and forgetfulness.

• *Suo Quan Wan* warms the Kidney to treat frequent urination and enuresis due to deficiency and cold. This formula is warm but not drying and mild in effect. If the symptoms are severe, other herbs should be added to achieve maximum effect.[8]

References

1. *Zhong Yao Ming Fang Yao Li Yu Ying Yong* (Pharmacology and Applications of Famous Herbal Formulas) 1989;352-353.
2. *Zhong Yi Fang Ji Xian Dai Yan Jiu* (Modern Study of Medical Formulae in Traditional Chinese Medicine) 1997;823.
3. *Ji Lin Zhong Yi Yao* (Jilin Chinese Medicine and Herbology) 1998;2:28.
4. *Fu Jian Zhong Yi Yao* (Fujian Chinese Medicine and Herbology) 1998;6:24.
5. *Bei Jing Zhong Yi* (Beijing Chinese Medicine) 1997;2:55.
6. *Shan Xi Zhong Yi* (Shanxi Chinese Medicine) 1997;1:31.
7. *Xin Zhong Yi* (New Chinese Medicine) 1991;12:49.
8. Wang MZ, et al. *Zhong Yi Xue Wen Da Ti Ku* (Questions and Answers on Traditional Chinese Medicine: Herbal Formulas).

Chinese Herbal Formulas and Applications

Fú Tū Dān (Poria and Cuscuta Special Pill)

茯菟丹

Pinyin Name: *Fu Tu Dan*
Literal Name: Poria and Cuscuta Special Pill
Alternate Name: Hoelen and Cuscuta Formula
Original Source: *Tai Ping Hui Min He Ji Ju Fang* (Imperial Grace Formulary of the Tai Ping Era) by the Imperial Medical Department in 1078-85

COMPOSITION

Fu Ling (Poria)	150g
Tu Si Zi (Semen Cuscutae), *jin* (soaked) in liquor	300g
Shi Lian Zi (Herba Sinocrassulae Indicae)	90g
Wu Wei Zi (Fructus Schisandrae Chinensis), *jin* (soaked) in liquor	210g
Shan Yao (Rhizoma Dioscoreae), *zhu* (boiled) with liquor	180g

Note: There is one variation of this formula from the source text, which contains only three herbs: *Tu Si Zi* (Semen Cuscutae) 150g, *Fu Ling* (Poria) 90g, and *Shi Lian Zi* (Herba Sinocrassulae Indicae) 60g.

DOSAGE / PREPARATION / ADMINISTRATION

The source text states to grind all the ingredients [except *Shan Yao* (Rhizoma Dioscoreae)] into powder. Separately cook 180g of powdered *Shan Yao* (Rhizoma Dioscoreae) in grain-based liquor and reduce it to a thick paste. Mix the powdered herbs and the paste to form into pills. The pills should resemble the size of *Wu Tong Zi* (Semen Firmianae), a small seed approximately 5 mm in diameter. Take 30-50 pills per dose on an empty stomach with rice water or lightly-salted water.

CHINESE THERAPEUTIC ACTIONS

1. Strengthens the Spleen and drains dampness
2. Tonifies the Kidney and stabilizes the *jing* (essence)
3. Benefits the Heart and calms the *shen* (spirit)

CLINICAL MANIFESTATIONS

Disharmony of the Heart and Kidney: spermatorrhea, premature ejaculation, white, turbid urine, increased volume of urine, thirst, increased food intake, and restlessness.

CLINICAL APPLICATIONS

Spermatorrhea, premature ejaculation, leakage of seminal fluids, general sexual dysfunction, and diabetes mellitus.

EXPLANATION

Fu Tu Dan (Poria and Cuscuta Special Pill) specifically treats spermatorrhea or premature ejaculation due to disharmony of the Heart and Kidney. The fundamental illness is an underlying Kidney deficiency, which is characterized by symptoms such as spermatorrhea, premature ejaculation, white, turbid urine, and increased volume of urine. Kidney deficiency may give rise to deficiency fire, which travels upward to affect the Heart, resulting in restlessness and thirst.

In this formula, *Fu Ling* (Poria) strengthens the Spleen, drains dampness, and calms the *shen* (spirit). *Tu Si Zi* (Semen Cuscutae) tonifies the Kidney and stops the loss

11

ASTRINGENT FORMULAS

Fu Tu Dan (Poria and Cuscuta Special Pill)

Diagnosis	Signs and Symptoms	Treatment	Herbs
Disharmony of the Heart and the Kidney	• Spermatorrhea, premature ejaculation, white turbid urine and increased volume of urine: loss of *jing* (essence) and body fluids due to Spleen and Kidney deficiencies • Restlessness and thirst: deficiency heat rising disturbing the Heart	• Strengthens the Spleen and drains dampness • Tonifies the Kidney and stabilizes the *jing* • Benefits the Heart and calms the *shen* (spirit)	• *Fu Ling* (Poria) strengthens the Spleen, drains dampness, and calms the *shen*. • *Tu Si Zi* (Semen Cuscutae) tonifies the Kidney and stops the loss of *jing*. • *Shi Lian Zi* (Herba Sinocrassulae Indicae) clears the urine. • *Wu Wei Zi* (Fructus Schisandrae Chinensis) calms the Heart to relieve restlessness. • *Shan Yao* (Rhizoma Dioscoreae) tonifies the Spleen and Kidney.

797

Chapter 11 – Astringent Formulas　　　　*Section 4– Jing (Essence)-Stabilizing Formulas to Stop Leakage*

Fú Tù Dān (Poria and Cuscuta Special Pill)

of *jing* (essence) [spermatorrhea or premature ejaculation] and body fluids [increased volume of white, turbid urine]. *Shi Lian Zi* (Herba Sinocrassulae Indicae) clears the urine and relieves white, turbid urine. *Wu Wei Zi* (Fructus Schisandrae Chinensis) calms the Heart to relieve restlessness. *Shan Yao* (Rhizoma Dioscoreae) tonifies the Spleen and Kidney to address the underlying deficiencies.

MODIFICATIONS
- With more impotence and premature ejaculation, add *Long Gu* (Os Draconis) and *Mu Li* (Concha Ostreae).

- With polyuria and white, cloudy urine, add *Fen Bi Xie* (Rhizoma Dioscoreae Hypoglaucae) and *Sang Piao Xiao* (Ootheca Mantidis).
- With generalized deficiency and coldness of the body and extremities, add *Rou Gui* (Cortex Cinnamomi) and *Fu Zi* (Radix Aconiti Lateralis Praeparata).
- With yin-deficient fire, add *Zhi Mu* (Rhizoma Anemarrhenae) and *Huang Bo* (Cortex Phellodendri Chinensis).
- With increased thirst and hunger, add *Sha Shen* (Radix Glehniae seu Adenophorae) and *Mai Dong* (Radix Ophiopogonis).

Gui Zhī Jiā Lóng Gǔ Mǔ Lì Tāng
(Cinnamon Twig Decoction plus Dragon Bone and Oyster Shell)

桂枝加龍骨牡蠣湯
桂枝加龙骨牡蛎汤

Pinyin Name: *Gui Zhi Jia Long Gu Mu Li Tang*
Literal Name: Cinnamon Twig Decoction plus Dragon Bone and Oyster Shell
Alternate Names: *Gui Zhi Jia Long Mu Tang*, Cinnamon and Dragon Bone Combination
Original Source: *Jin Gui Yao Lue* (Essentials from the Golden Cabinet) by Zhang Zhong-Jing during the Eastern Han Dynasty

COMPOSITION

Gui Zhi (Ramulus Cinnamomi)	9g
Bai Shao (Radix Paeoniae Alba)	9g
Long Gu (Os Draconis)	9g
Mu Li (Concha Ostreae)	9g
Sheng Jiang (Rhizoma Zingiberis Recens)	9g
Da Zao (Fructus Jujubae)	12 pieces
Gan Cao (Radix et Rhizoma Glycyrrhizae)	6g

DOSAGE / PREPARATION / ADMINISTRATION
The source text states to cook all the ingredients in 7 cups [1,400 mL] of water until it is reduced down to 3 cups [600 mL]. Take the warm, strained decoction in three equally-divided doses.

CHINESE THERAPEUTIC ACTIONS
1. Tonifies yin and yang
2. Harmonizes the *ying* (nutritive) and *wei* (defensive) levels
3. Stabilizes *jing* (essence)

CLINICAL MANIFESTATIONS
Deficiency of yin and yang accompanied by disharmony of the *ying* (nutritive) and *wei* (defensive) levels: spermatorrhea (in men), dreams of sexual intercourse (in women), lower abdominal contraction and pain, cold sensation at the tip of the penis, premature hair loss, gradual decline in physical strength and condition, palpitations, and insomnia.

CLINICAL APPLICATIONS
Impotence, spermatorrhea, premature ejaculation, nocturnal emission and other male sexual disorders, neurosis, insomnia, forgetfulness, and enuresis.

798

Chinese Herbal Formulas and Applications

Guì Zhī Jiā Lóng Gǔ Mǔ Lì Tāng
(Cinnamon Twig Decoction plus Dragon Bone and Oyster Shell)

Gui Zhi Jia Long Gu Mu Li Tang (Cinnamon Twig Decoction plus Dragon Bone and Oyster Shell)

Diagnosis	Signs and Symptoms	Treatment	Herbs
Deficiency of the yin and yang accompanied by disharmony of the *ying* (nutritive) and *wei* (defensive) levels	• Generalized weakness in physical strength and condition: yin and yang deficiencies • Spontaneous sweating, night sweating and muscle aches: disharmony of the *ying* (nutritive) and *wei* (defensive) levels • Lower abdominal contraction and pain, and cold sensation at the tip of penis: cold in the body	• Tonifies yin and yang • Harmonizes *ying* (nutritive) and *wei* (defensive) levels • Stabilizes *jing* (essence)	• *Gui Zhi* (Ramulus Cinnamomi) and *Bai Shao* (Radix Paeoniae Alba) balance yin and yang, and harmonize *ying* (nutritive) and *wei* (defensive) levels. • *Long Gu* (Os Draconis) and *Mu Li* (Concha Ostreae) balance yin and yang from the interior, prevent the loss of *jing*, and calm down the *shen* (spirit). • *Sheng Jiang* (Rhizoma Zingiberis Recens) warms up yang and dispels cold. • *Da Zao* (Fructus Jujubae) tonifies the qi and replenishes body fluids. • *Gan Cao* (Radix et Rhizoma Glycyrrhizae) harmonizes all the herbs.

EXPLANATION

This formula is designed to treat patients who experience chronic and gradual decline in physical and sexual functions. The underlying cause of this condition is deficiency of yin and yang accompanied by disharmony of the *ying* (nutritive) and *wei* (defensive) levels. Deficiency of yin and yang is representative of aging, whereby the patients experience generalized weakness in physical strength and condition. Because yin and yang are deficient and out of balance, patients experience irregular fever, headache, and dizziness. Furthermore, disharmony of the *ying* (nutritive) and *wei* (defensive) levels is characterized by spontaneous sweating, night sweating, and muscle aches. Due to the chronic nature of the illness, cold begins to build up in the body as the patient experiences lower abdominal contraction and pain, and cold sensation at the tip of the penis. As the overall constitution of the body declines, other symptoms and signs of sexual dysfunction begin to appear, such as spermatorrhea, impotence, nocturnal emission, premature ejaculation in men, and dreams of sexual intercourse in women.

Gui Zhi Jia Long Gu Mu Li Tang (Cinnamon Twig Decoction plus Dragon Bone and Oyster Shell) is a modification of *Gui Zhi Tang* (Cinnamon Twig Decoction) with the addition of *Long Gu* (Os Draconis) and *Mu Li* (Concha Ostreae). *Gui Zhi Tang* (Cinnamon Twig Decoction) is used as the base formula because it tonifies yin and yang, and harmonizes the *ying* (nutritive) and *wei* (defensive) levels. *Gui Zhi* (Ramulus Cinnamomi), sweet, pungent, and warm in property, tonifies yang and relieves body aches and pain. *Bai Shao* (Radix Paeoniae Alba), sour and

cold in nature, tonifies yin and consolidates body fluids. Together, *Gui Zhi* (Ramulus Cinnamomi) and *Bai Shao* (Radix Paeoniae Alba) harmonize *ying* (nutritive) and *wei* (defensive) levels. In addition to the pairing of *Gui Zhi* (Ramulus Cinnamomi) and *Bai Shao* (Radix Paeoniae Alba), which balances yin and yang from the exterior, *Long Gu* (Os Draconis) and *Mu Li* (Concha Ostreae) are added to balance yin and yang from the interior. *Long Gu* (Os Draconis) calms yang and prevents the loss of yang from the body; *Mu Li* (Concha Ostreae) preserves yin and restrains yang. Used together, *Long Gu* (Os Draconis) and *Mu Li* (Concha Ostreae) balance yin and yang from the interior, prevent the loss of *jing* (essence), and calm down the *shen* (spirit). Additionally, *Sheng Jiang* (Rhizoma Zingiberis Recens) helps *Gui Zhi* (Ramulus Cinnamomi) to warm yang and dispel cold from the body. *Da Zao* (Fructus Jujubae) tonifies qi and replenishes body fluids, while *Gan Cao* (Radix et Rhizoma Glycyrrhizae) relieves aches and pains and promotes the production of body fluid. *Da Zao* (Fructus Jujubae) and *Gan Cao* (Radix et Rhizoma Glycyrrhizae) also function as envoys to harmonize all the herbs in this formula.

MODIFICATIONS

• With spermatorrhea and weakness, add *Lu Jiao Shuang* (Cornu Cervi Degelatinatum) and *Gui Ban* (Plastrum Testudinis).
• With fatigue and qi deficiency, add *Ren Shen* (Radix et Rhizoma Ginseng) and *Huang Qi* (Radix Astragali).
• With sore back and feeling of pain in the bone, add *Du Zhong* (Cortex Eucommiae) and *Niu Xi* (Radix Achyranthis Bidentatae).

11

ASTRINGENT FORMULAS

799

Chapter 11 – Astringent Formulas   *Section 4– Jing (Essence)-Stabilizing Formulas to Stop Leakage*

Zhì Zhuó Gù Bĕn Wán
(Treat the Turbidity and Guard the Root Pill)

治濁固本丸
治浊固本丸

Pinyin Name: *Zhi Zhuo Gu Ben Wan*
Literal Name: Treat the Turbidity and Guard the Root Pill
Alternate Names: *Chih Cho Ku Pen Wan*, Turbidity-Curing Body-Securing Pill, Hoelen and Polyporus Formula
Original Source: *Yi Fang Ji Jie* (Analytical Collection of Medical Formulas) by Wang Ang in 1682

COMPOSITION

Huang Lian (Rhizoma Coptidis), *chao* (dry-fried)	60g
Huang Bo (Cortex Phellodendri Chinensis), *chao* (dry-fried)	30g
Fu Ling (Poria)	30g
Zhu Ling (Polyporus)	75g
Sha Ren (Fructus Amomi)	30g
Ban Xia (Rhizoma Pinelliae), *pao* (blast-fried) in water 7 times	30g
Lian Xu (Stamen Nelumbinis)	60g
Yi Zhi (Fructus Alpiniae Oxyphyllae)	30g
Zhi Gan Cao (Radix et Rhizoma Glycyrrhizae Praeparata cum Melle)	90g

DOSAGE / PREPARATION / ADMINISTRATION

The source text states to grind the ingredients into a fine powder and form into small pills. Take 50 pills on an empty stomach with warm grain-based liquor.

CHINESE THERAPEUTIC ACTIONS

1. Protects qi and *jing* (essence)
2. Clears damp-heat

CLINICAL MANIFESTATIONS

Damp-heat in the Urinary Bladder: white, turbid urine, spermatorrhea, and polyuria.

CLINICAL APPLICATIONS

Prostatic hypertrophy, chronic cystitis, chronic urethritis, and urinary tract infection.

EXPLANATION

Zhi Zhuo Gu Ben Wan (Treat the Turbidity and Guard the Root Pill) is designed to treat damp-heat in the Urinary Bladder leading to abnormal genitourinary function. Symptoms of such conditions include white and turbid urine, excessive frequency and amount of urination, and spermatorrhea.

Zhi Zhuo Gu Ben Wan (Treat the Turbidity and Guard the Root Pill)

Diagnosis	Signs and Symptoms	Treatment	Herbs
Damp-heat in the Urinary Bladder	Increased frequency and amount of urination, white turbid urine and spermatorrhea: damp-heat in the Urinary Bladder	• Protects qi and *jing* (essence) • Clears damp-heat	• *Huang Lian* (Rhizoma Coptidis) and *Huang Bo* (Cortex Phellodendri Chinensis) effectively clear damp-heat. • *Fu Ling* (Poria) and *Zhu Ling* (Polyporus) regulate the circulation of water and promote normal urination. • *Sha Ren* (Fructus Amomi) and *Ban Xia* (Rhizoma Pinelliae) strengthen the Spleen and Stomach to eliminate and prevent production of dampness. • *Lian Xu* (Stamen Nelumbinis) and *Yi Zhi* (Fructus Alpiniae Oxyphyllae) consolidate the *jing* and stop spermatorrhea. • *Zhi Gan Cao* (Radix et Rhizoma Glycyrrhizae Praeparata cum Melle) harmonizes all the herbs.

800

Zhi Zhuó Gù Běn Wán
(Treat the Turbidity and Guard the Root Pill)

In this formula, herbs are used to control urination and resolve turbidity. Bitter and cold, *Huang Lian* (Rhizoma Coptidis) and *Huang Bo* (Cortex Phellodendri Chinensis) effectively purge damp-heat. *Fu Ling* (Poria) and *Zhu Ling* (Polyporus) regulate the circulation of water and promote normal urination. *Sha Ren* (Fructus Amomi) and *Ban Xia* (Rhizoma Pinelliae) strengthen the Spleen and Stomach to eliminate and prevent production of dampness. *Lian Xu* (Stamen Nelumbinis) and *Yi Zhi* (Fructus Alpiniae Oxyphyllae) consolidate the *jing* (essence) and stop spermatorrhea. *Zhi Gan Cao* (Radix et Rhizoma Glycyrrhizae Praeparata cum Melle) harmonizes all the herbs in the formula. In short, this formula is used to treat loss of fluids (urine and sperm) through consolidating *jing* and clearing damp-heat.

MODIFICATIONS

- With more spermatorrhea and urination, add *Long Gu* (Os Draconis) and *Mu Li* (Concha Ostreae).
- With more white, turbid urine, add *Hai Piao Xiao* (Endoconcha Sepiae) and *Sang Piao Xiao* (Ootheca Mantidis).
- With soreness and pain of the lower back and legs, add *Du Zhong* (Cortex Eucommiae) and *Xu Duan* (Radix Dipsaci).

Chapter 11 – Astringent Formulas   *Section 5– Womb-Stabilizing Formulas to Stop Leakage*

Section 5

固崩止带剂

— Womb-Stabilizing Formulas to Stop Leakage

Gù Jīng Wán (Stabilize the Menses Pill)

固經丸

固经丸

Pinyin Name: *Gu Jing Wan*
Literal Name: Stabilize the Menses Pill
Original Source: *Yi Xue Ru Men* (Introduction to Medicine) by Li Ting in 1575

COMPOSITION

Gui Ban (Plastrum Testudinis)	30g [15g]
Bai Shao (Radix Paeoniae Alba)	30g [15g]
Huang Qin (Radix Scutellariae)	30g [15g]
Huang Bo (Cortex Phellodendri Chinensis)	9g [6g]
Chun Pi (Cortex Ailanthi)	21g [12g]
Xiang Fu (Rhizoma Cyperi)	7.5g [6g]

DOSAGE / PREPARATION / ADMINISTRATION

The source text states to grind the ingredients into powder and form into small pills with grain-based liquor. The pills should resemble the size of *Wu Tong Zi* (Semen Firmianae), a small seed approximately 5 mm in diameter. Take 50 pills per dose with grain-based liquor. Today the instruction is usually to administer 9g of pills once or twice a day with warm water. This formula may also be prepared as a decoction with suggested dosages in brackets.

CHINESE THERAPEUTIC ACTIONS

1. Nourishes yin and clears deficiency heat
2. Stabilizes menses and stops bleeding

CLINICAL MANIFESTATIONS

Beng lou (flooding and spotting) and hypermenorrhea due to deficiency heat in the interior: continuous menstrual bleeding or incessant dripping of blood from the uterus, bleeding of dark red blood, sometimes bleeding with purplish-black blood clots, irritability, heat sensations in the chest, abdominal pain, dysuria, red tongue, and a wiry, rapid pulse.

CLINICAL APPLICATIONS

Irregular menstruation, menstrual bleeding, and gastrointestinal bleeding.

EXPLANATION

Gu Jing Wan (Stabilize the Menses Pill) is designed to treat menstrual disorders, such as *beng lou* (flooding and spotting) and hypermenorrhea characterized by yin deficiency complicated with Liver stagnation and heat. As the heat and fire rise, they disturb *chong* (thoroughfare) and *ren* (conception) channels and force reckless movement of blood, resulting in bleeding or incessant dripping of blood from the uterus. Irritability and abdominal pain are due to Liver qi stagnation and heat.

To effectively treat this syndrome, one must nourish yin, clear heat, and stop bleeding. This formula contains *Gui Ban* (Plastrum Testudinis) to benefit the Kidney, nourish yin, and clear heat. *Bai Shao* (Radix Paeoniae Alba) nourishes Liver blood to soften the Liver and relieve pain. *Huang Qin* (Radix Scutellariae) and *Huang Bo* (Cortex Phellodendri Chinensis) clear heat, purge fire, and stop the bleeding. *Chun Pi* (Cortex Ailanthi), a cold, astringent

802

Chinese Herbal Formulas and Applications

Gù Jīng Wán (Stabilize the Menses Pill)

Gu Jing Wan (Stabilize the Menses Pill)

Diagnosis	Signs and Symptoms	Treatment	Herbs
Beng lou (flooding and spotting) due to deficiency heat of the interior	• Continuous menstrual bleeding or incessant dripping of blood from the uterus: yin-deficient heat pushing blood outwards • Irritability and abdominal pain: Liver qi stagnation and heat • Red tongue and a wiry, rapid pulse: Liver qi stagnation and heat	• Nourishes yin and clears deficiency heat • Stops bleeding and stabilizes menstruation	• *Gui Ban* (Plastrum Testudinis) benefits the Kidney, nourishes yin and clears heat. • *Bai Shao* (Radix Paeoniae Alba) nourishes blood, softens the Liver and relieves pain. • *Huang Qin* (Radix Scutellariae) and *Huang Bo* (Cortex Phellodendri Chinensis) clear the heat, purge fire and stop the bleeding. • *Chun Pi* (Cortex Ailanthi) stabilizes the menstruation. • *Xiang Fu* (Rhizoma Cyperi) regulates Liver qi.

herb, stabilizes menstruation and stops bleeding. *Xiang Fu* (Rhizoma Cyperi) regulates Liver qi and harmonizes the blood.

MODIFICATIONS

With more yin-deficiency heat signs such as tidal fever, flushed cheeks, and *wu xin re* (five-center heat): remove *Huang Bo* (Cortex Phellodendri Chinensis) and *Xiang Fu* (Rhizoma Cyperi); and add *Di Huang* (Radix Rehmanniae), *Shan Zhu Yu* (Fructus Corni), and *Di Gu Pi* (Cortex Lycii); or *Zhi Bai Di Huang Wan* (Anemarrhena, Phellodendron, and Rehmannia Pill).

CAUTIONS / CONTRAINDICATIONS

Gu Jing Wan is contraindicated in cases of excess heat, blood stagnation, and/or qi deficiency.

CLINICAL STUDIES AND RESEARCH

1. **Irregular menstruation**: One study reported good results using modified *Gu Jing Wan* to treat irregular menstruation in women during puberty characterized by Kidney yin deficiency with deficiency heat. The formula contained *Bie Jia* (Carapax Trionycis) 10g, *Bai Shao* (Radix Paeoniae Alba) 10g, dry-fried *Huang Qin* (Radix Scutellariae) 10g, *Chun Pi* (Cortex Ailanthi) 10g, *Xiang Fu* (Rhizoma Cyperi) 10g, *Bai Wei* (Radix et Rhizoma Cynanchi Atrati) 10g, dry-fried *Bai Zhu* (Rhizoma Atractylodis Macrocephalae) 10g, dry-fried *Wu Mei* (Fructus Mume) 10g, dry-fried *Dang Shen* (Radix Codonopsis) 18g, *Nu Zhen Zi* (Fructus Ligustri Lucidi) 12g, *Mo Han Lian* (Herba Ecliptae) 12g, and *Zhi Gan Cao* (Radix et Rhizoma Glycyrrhizae Praeparata cum Melle) 5g.[1]

2. ***Beng lou* (flooding and spotting)**: According to one study, *beng lou* (flooding and spotting) in perimenopausal women characterized by yin deficiency and heat in the blood may be treated with modified *Gu Jing Wan*. The herbal formula contained *Bie Jia* (Carapax Trionycis) 9g, dry-fried *Huang Qin* (Radix Scutellariae) 9g, dry-fried *Bai Shao* (Radix Paeoniae Alba) 9g, dry-fried *Huang Bo* (Cortex Phellodendri Chinensis) 9g, charred *Qian Cao* (Radix et Rhizoma Rubiae) 9g, *Chun Pi* (Cortex Ailanthi) 12g, charred *Dang Gui* (Radix Angelicae Sinensis) 12g, charred *Xu Duan* (Radix Dipsaci) 12g, dry-fried *Dang Shen* (Radix Codonopsis) 18g, *Zhi Gan Cao* (Radix et Rhizoma Glycyrrhizae Praeparata cum Melle) 4.5g, processed *Huang Jing* (Rhizoma Polygonati) 30g, *Hai Piao Xiao* (Endoconcha Sepiae) 30g, and *Sang Ji Sheng* (Herba Taxilli) 12g.[2]

3. **Bleeding**: *Gu Jing Wan* has been shown to effectively stop bleeding due to various causes. According to one report, it was effective in treating gastrointestinal bleeding. According to another report, it was effective for treating uterine bleeding and profuse menstrual bleeding.[3,4]

RELATED FORMULA

Gù Chōng Tāng
(Stabilize *Chong* [Thoroughfare Channel] Decoction)
固沖湯
固沖汤
Pinyin Name: *Gu Chong Tang*
Literal Name: Stabilize *Chong* [Thoroughfare Channel] Decoction
Original Source: *Yi Xue Zhong Zhong Can Xi Lu* (Records of Heart-Felt Experiences in Medicine with Reference to the West) by Zhang Xi-Chun in 1918-34

11

ASTRINGENT FORMULAS

803

Chapter 11 – Astringent Formulas   *Section 5– Womb-Stabilizing Formulas to Stop Leakage*

Gù Jīng Wán (Stabilize the Menses Pill)

Bai Zhu (Rhizoma Atractylodis Macrocephalae),
   chao (dry-fried)   30g
Huang Qi (Radix Astragali)   18g
Long Gu (Os Draconis), duan (calcined)
   and dao (pounded) into fine particles   24g
Mu Li (Concha Ostreae), duan (calcined)
   and dao (pounded) into fine particles   24g
Shan Zhu Yu (Fructus Corni)   24g
Bai Shao (Radix Paeoniae Alba)   12g
Hai Piao Xiao (Endoconcha Sepiae),
   dao (pounded) into fine particles   12g
Qian Cao (Radix et Rhizoma Rubiae)   9g
Zong Lu (Petiolus Trachycarpi), tan (charred to ash)   6g
Wu Bei Zi (Galla Chinensis),
   ya (pressed) into fine particles   1.5g

The source text states to prepare the ingredients as a decoction. *Wu Bei Zi* (Galla Chinensis) should be mixed with the decoction immediately prior to ingestion.

Gu Chong Tang (Stabilize *Chong* [Thoroughfare Channel] Decoction) tonifies qi, strengthens the Spleen, stabilizes the *chong* (thoroughfare) channel, and stops menstrual bleeding. With Spleen qi deficiency and *chong* (thoroughfare) channel instability, blood cannot circulate within the vessels leading to *beng lou* (flooding and spotting) and hypermenorrhea. Bleeding is usually excessive, pale and quite diluted. Furthermore, because of the deficient nature of the illness, the patient may show palpitations, shortness of breath, pale tongue, and a fine, weak pulse.

Gu Jing Wan and *Gu Chong Tang* (Stabilize *Chong* [Thoroughfare Channel] Decoction) both treat excess menstrual bleeding.

- *Gu Jing Wan* is used for bleeding due to yin-deficient heat causing reckless movement of blood.
- *Gu Chong Tang* is used for bleeding due to Spleen qi deficiency and instability of *chong* (thoroughfare) channel, leading to inability of blood to circulate within the blood vessels.

AUTHORS' COMMENTS

Gu Jing Wan and *Gui Pi Tang* (Restore the Spleen Decoction) both treat hypermenorrhea and *beng lou* (flooding and spotting).

- *Gu Jing Wan* nourishes yin, clears heat, and treats profuse bleeding that is dark red in color and may also be accompanied by clots. The tongue is red and the pulse is wiry and rapid.
- *Gui Pi Tang* tonifies the Spleen and Heart and treats bleeding that is lighter in color. *Gui Pi Tang* is most suitable for individuals with qi and blood deficiencies, with accompanying symptoms such as weakness, poor appetite, insomnia, and palpitations.[5]

References

1. *Shang Hai Zhong Yi Yao Za Zhi* (Shanghai Journal of Chinese Medicine and Herbology) 1994;10:21.
2. *Shang Hai Zhong Yi Yao Za Zhi* (Shanghai Journal of Chinese Medicine and Herbology) 1994;10:21.
3. *Si Chuan Zhong Yi* (Sichuan Chinese Medicine) 1986;6:56.
4. *Gan Su Zhong Yi Xue Yuan Xue Bao* (Journal of Gansu University of Chinese Medicine) 1995;3:16.
5. Wang MZ, et al. *Zhong Yi Xue Wen Da Ti Ku* (Questions and Answers on Traditional Chinese Medicine: Herbal Formulas).

804

Chinese Herbal Formulas and Applications

Zhèn Líng Dān (Rouse the Spirits Special Pill)

震靈丹
震灵丹

Pinyin Name: *Zhen Ling Dan*
Literal Name: Rouse the Spirits Special Pill
Original Source: *Tai Ping Hui Min He Ji Ju Fang* (Imperial Grace Formulary of the Tai Ping Era) by the Imperial Medical Department in 1078-85

COMPOSITION

Chi Shi Zhi (Halloysitum Rubrum), *duan* (calcined) with fire and *cui* (quenched) with vinegar	120g
Yu Yu Liang (Limonitum), *duan* (calcined) with fire and *cui* (quenched) with vinegar	120g
Zi Shi Ying (Fluoritum), *duan* (calcined) with fire and *cui* (quenched) with vinegar	120g
Zhe Shi (Haematitum), *duan* (calcined) with fire and *cui* (quenched) with vinegar	120g
Ru Xiang (Gummi Olibanum), *yan* (ground) to small particles separately	60g
Mo Yao (Myrrha), *yan* (ground) to small particles	60g
Wu Ling Zhi (Faeces Trogopteri), *yan* (ground) to small particles	60g
Zhu Sha (Cinnabaris), *shui fei* (refined with water)	30g

Note: *Zhu Sha* (Cinnabaris) is a potentially toxic heavy metal, and is rarely used as a medicinal substance today. Its discussion here is included primarily for academic purposes, to reflect the historical use of this substance in its original formulation. Most herbal products today have removed it completely, or replaced it with substitutes with similar functions. For additional information on the toxicity, please refer to *Chinese Medical Herbology and Pharmacology* by John Chen and Tina Chen.

DOSAGE / PREPARATION / ADMINISTRATION

The source text states to grind the ingredients into powder. Separately cook *Nuo Mi* (Oryza Glutinosa) into a paste. Combine the powder and the paste to form large pills. The pills should resemble the head of a small chicken in size. Dry the pills under the sun. Take one pill on an empty stomach daily. The source text states that men should take the pill with warm grain-based liquor, and women should take it with vinegar.

CHINESE THERAPEUTIC ACTIONS

Stops bleeding and dissolves blood stasis

CLINICAL MANIFESTATIONS

Beng lou (flooding and spotting) caused by deficiency and cold of the *chong* (thoroughfare) and *ren* (conception) channels accompanied by blood stasis in the uterus: continuous menstrual bleeding that is purplish red or purplish black in color, bleeding with or without clots, abdominal pain worsened by pressure and relieved by the passing of blood clots, dark purplish tongue, and a deep, fine and wiry pulse.

CLINICAL APPLICATIONS

Leukorrhea, uterine bleeding, and chronic diarrhea.

EXPLANATION

Zhen Ling Dan (Rouse the Spirits Special Pill) is designed to treat *beng lou* (flooding and spotting) caused by deficiency and cold of the *chong* (thoroughfare) and *ren* (conception) channels accompanied by blood stasis in the uterus. With deficiency and cold, blood leaves the *chong* (thoroughfare) and *ren* (conception) channels resulting in continuous menstrual bleeding. Once blood travels to the outside of the blood vessels, blood stasis may form, hence bleeding with purplish blood clots. Blood stasis may cause abdominal pain that is worsened by pressure. And when the blood clots are passed out, the pain may become lessened due to reduced blood stasis. The tongue and pulse conditions should show interior deficiency and cold along with blood stagnation.

Optimal treatment requires the use of herbs to warm the uterus, stabilize the *chong* (thoroughfare) and *ren* (conception) channels, stop bleeding, and dissolve blood stasis. In this formula, *Chi Shi Zhi* (Halloysitum Rubrum), *Yu Yu Liang* (Limonitum), *Zi Shi Ying* (Fluoritum), and *Zhe Shi* (Haematitum) warm the uterus, stabilize *chong* (thoroughfare) and *ren* (conception) channels, and stop bleeding. These four herbs should all be calcined first to enhance their warming and astringent effects. *Ru Xiang* (Gummi Olibanum), *Mo Yao* (Myrrha), and *Wu Ling Zhi* (Faeces Trogopteri) activate blood circulation to eliminate blood stasis, and regulate qi circulation to relieve pain.

11

ASTRINGENT FORMULAS

Chapter 11 – Astringent Formulas *Section 5– Womb-Stabilizing Formulas to Stop Leakage*

Zhèn Líng Dān (Rouse the Spirits Special Pill)

Zhen Ling Dan (Rouse the Spirits Special Pill)

Diagnosis	Signs and Symptoms	Treatment	Herbs
Beng lou (flooding and spotting)	• Continuous menstrual bleeding: deficiency and cold of the *chong* (thoroughfare) and *ren* (conception) channels • Abdominal pain, purplish red or purplish black menstrual discharge and bleeding with clots: blood stasis in the uterus • Dark purplish tongue, and a deep, fine and wiry pulse: blood stasis	Stops bleeding and dissolves blood stasis	• *Chi Shi Zhi* (Halloysitum Rubrum), *Yu Yu Liang* (Limonitum), *Zi Shi Ying* (Fluoritum) and *Zhe Shi* (Haematitum) warm the uterus, stabilize *chong* (thoroughfare) and *ren* (conception) channels, and stop bleeding. • *Ru Xiang* (Gummi Olibanum), *Mo Yao* (Myrrha) and *Wu Ling Zhi* (Faeces Trogopteri) activate the blood circulation to eliminate the blood stasis, and regulate the qi circulation to relieve pain. • *Nuo Mi* (Oryza Glutinosa) warms the middle *jiao* and tonifies qi. • *Zhu Sha* (Cinnabaris) tranquilizes the mind and reduces pain.

Nuo Mi (Oryza Glutinosa) is used to warm the middle *jiao* and tonify the qi. *Zhu Sha* (Cinnabaris) tranquilizes the mind and reduces the pain. Lastly, vinegar enhances the effect to resolve blood stasis.

CAUTIONS / CONTRAINDICATIONS

Zhen Ling Dan emphasizes on stopping menstrual bleeding and dissolving the blood stasis. It is not suitable for deficiency and cold syndromes without blood stasis.

Wán Dài Tāng (End Discharge Decoction)
完帶湯
完带汤

Pinyin Name: *Wan Dai Tang*
Literal Name: End Discharge Decoction
Alternate Names: *Wan Tai Tang*, Treating Morbid Leukorrhea Decoction, Atractylodes and Dioscorea Combination
Original Source: *Fu Qing Zhu Nu Ke* (Women's Diseases According to Fu Qing-Zhu) by Fu Shan in 1827

COMPOSITION

Bai Zhu (Rhizoma Atractylodis Macrocephalae), *chao* (dry-fried) with soil	30g
Shan Yao (Rhizoma Dioscoreae), *chao* (dry-fried)	30g
Ren Shen (Radix et Rhizoma Ginseng)	6g
Cang Zhu (Rhizoma Atractylodis), *zhi* (prepared)	9g
Chen Pi (Pericarpium Citri Reticulatae)	1.5g
Che Qian Zi (Semen Plantaginis), *chao* (dry-fried) with liquor	9g
Bai Shao (Radix Paeoniae Alba), *chao* (dry-fried) with liquor	15g
Chai Hu (Radix Bupleuri)	1.8g
Jing Jie Sui Tan (Spica Schizonepetae Carbonisata)	1.5g
Gan Cao (Radix et Rhizoma Glycyrrhizae)	3g

DOSAGE / PREPARATION / ADMINISTRATION

The source text states to prepare the ingredients as a decoction.

CHINESE THERAPEUTIC ACTIONS

1. Tonifies middle *jiao* and strengthens the Spleen
2. Dissolves damp and stops leukorrhea

Wán Dài Tāng (End Discharge Decoction)

CLINICAL MANIFESTATIONS

Abnormal vaginal discharge due to Spleen deficiency and Liver qi stagnation accompanied by dampness and turbidity in the lower *jiao*: odorless, clear, and thin leukorrhea that is white or light yellow in color, pale face, lethargy, loose stools, pale tongue, white tongue coating, and a moderate or soggy and weak pulse.

CLINICAL APPLICATIONS

Leukorrhea, cervicitis, vaginitis, abnormal vaginal discharge, infertility, edema during pregnancy, chronic hepatitis, glomerulonephritis, diarrhea, and irritable bowel syndrome.

EXPLANATION

Wan Dai Tang (End Discharge Decoction) is designed to treat abnormal vaginal discharge caused by Spleen qi deficiency and Liver qi stagnation. Stagnation of Liver qi may lead to Liver overacting on the Spleen, causing Spleen deficiency. Deficiency of the Spleen may cause production and accumulation of dampness and turbidity, which usually travel to the lower *jiao* due to their heavy and descending character and result in leukorrhea. Since there is no heat or infection, the leukorrhea will be clear, thin, odorless, and white or light yellow in color. Pale face, lethargy, loose stools, pale tongue, and a moderate or soggy and weak pulse indicate qi deficiency and damp accumulation.

This formula uses dry-fried *Bai Zhu* (Rhizoma Atractylodis Macrocephalae) and *Shan Yao* (Rhizoma Dioscoreae)

in heavy dosages to carry out two important functions. First, these two herbs strengthen the Spleen and tonify qi to facilitate the water metabolism function. Second, both herbs dry dampness and help reduce leukorrhea. *Ren Shen* (Radix et Rhizoma Ginseng) tonifies qi. *Cang Zhu* (Rhizoma Atractylodis) and *Chen Pi* (Pericarpium Citri Reticulatae) activate the qi flow and dry dampness. These two herbs also prevent the tonifying herbs from creating additional dampness and stagnation. *Che Qian Zi* (Semen Plantaginis) resolves dampness through urination. *Bai Shao* (Radix Paeoniae Alba) softens the Liver. *Chai Hu* (Radix Bupleuri) ascends the yang and activates Liver qi flow. *Jing Jie Sui Tan* (Spica Schizonepetae Carbonisata) has the function to stop leukorrhea. *Gan Cao* (Radix et Rhizoma Glycyrrhizae) harmonizes all the herbs in this formula.

MODIFICATIONS

- For vaginal discharge characterized by cold, add *Li Zhong Tang* (Regulate the Middle Decoction).
- For yellow vaginal discharge characterized by heat, add *Huang Bo* (Cortex Phellodendri Chinensis) and *Long Dan* (Radix et Rhizoma Gentianae); or *Huang Lian Jie Du Tang* (Coptis Decoction to Relieve Toxicity).
- For vaginal discharge secondary to chronic illness and deficiency, add *Long Gu* (Os Draconis) and *Mu Li* (Concha Ostreae).
- For chronic vaginal discharge that is white or clear, add *Lu Jiao Shuang* (Cornu Cervi Degelatinatum).
- With Spleen deficiency, add *Huang Qi* (Radix Astragali) and *Bai Bian Dou* (Semen Lablab Album).

Wan Dai Tang (End Discharge Decoction)

Diagnosis	Signs and Symptoms	Treatment	Herbs
Abnormal vaginal discharge due to Spleen deficiency and Liver qi stagnation	• Leukorrhea (clear, thin, odorless and white or light yellowish in color): Spleen deficiency with dampness and turbidity • Pale face, pale tongue, white tongue coating, lethargy and loose stools: Spleen deficiency • A moderate or soggy and weak pulse: Spleen deficiency with dampness accumulation	• Tonifies middle *jiao* and strengthens the Spleen • Dissolves dampness and stops leukorrhea	• *Bai Zhu* (Rhizoma Atractylodis Macrocephalae) and *Shan Yao* (Rhizoma Dioscoreae) strengthen the Spleen and dry dampness. • *Ren Shen* (Radix et Rhizoma Ginseng) tonifies qi. • *Cang Zhu* (Rhizoma Atractylodis) and *Chen Pi* (Pericarpium Citri Reticulatae) activate the qi flow and dry dampness. • *Che Qian Zi* (Semen Plantaginis) resolves dampness through urination. • *Bai Shao* (Radix Paeoniae Alba) softens the Liver. • *Chai Hu* (Radix Bupleuri) ascends the yang and activates Liver qi flow. • *Jing Jie Sui Tan* (Spica Schizonepetae Carbonisata) stops leukorrhea. • *Gan Cao* (Radix et Rhizoma Glycyrrhizae) harmonizes all the herbs.

Chapter 11 – Astringent Formulas   *Section 5– Womb-Stabilizing Formulas to Stop Leakage*

Wán Dài Tāng (End Discharge Decoction)

- With blood deficiency, add *Shu Di Huang* (Radix Rehmanniae Praeparata) and *Dang Gui* (Radix Angelicae Sinensis).
- With Spleen and Kidney deficiencies, add *Tu Si Zi* (Semen Cuscutae) and *Ba Ji Tian* (Radix Morindae Officinalis).
- With lower abdominal pain, add *Wu Yao* (Radix Linderae) and *Xiao Hui Xiang* (Fructus Foeniculi).
- With lower abdominal pain with cold and dampness, add *Pao Jiang* (Rhizoma Zingiberis Praeparatum) and *Xiao Hui Xiang* (Fructus Foeniculi).
- With soreness and weakness of the lower back and knees, add *Du Zhong* (Cortex Eucommiae) and *Xu Duan* (Radix Dipsaci).
- With lower back pain, add *Du Zhong* (Cortex Eucommiae) and *Tu Si Zi* (Semen Cuscutae).
- With low libido, add *Huan Shao Dan* (Return to Youth Pill).

CAUTIONS / CONTRAINDICATIONS

Wan Dai Tang is contraindicated in yellow or foul-smelling vaginal discharge caused by damp-heat.

PHARMACOLOGICAL EFFECTS

Anti-inflammatory: One study reported marked effect in reducing inflammation using *Wan Dai Tang* in mice given via intraperitoneal injection.[1]

CLINICAL STUDIES AND RESEARCH

1. **Leukorrhea**: One study reported improvement to complete recovery using modified *Wan Dai Tang* to treat 50 women with leukorrhea. The herbal formula contained *Tai Zi Shen* (Radix Pseudostellariae) 10g, charred *Bai Zhu* (Rhizoma Atractylodis Macrocephalae) 15g, processed *Cang Zhu* (Rhizoma Atractylodis) 6g, *Che Qian Zi* (Semen Plantaginis) 10g, *Zhi Gan Cao* (Radix et Rhizoma Glycyrrhizae Praeparata cum Melle) 3g, *Chen Pi* (Pericarpium Citri Reticulatae) 6g, *Chai Hu* (Radix Bupleuri) 3g, charred *Jing Jie* (Herba Schizonepetae) 2g, alcohol-fried *Bai Shao* (Radix Paeoniae Alba) 12g, *Shan Yao* (Rhizoma Dioscoreae) 30g, *Qian Shi* (Semen Euryales) 12g, *Bai Guo* (Semen Ginkgo) 7 pieces, and others as deemed necessary. The duration of treatment ranged from 5 to 14 packs of herbs.[2]

2. **Cervicitis**: According to one study, administration of modified *Wan Dai Tang* in decoction daily for 15 to 46 packs of herbs was effective in treating chronic cervicitis. Of 47 women, the study reported complete recovery in 25 cases, improvement in 18 cases, and no effect in 4 cases.[3]

3. **Vaginitis**: According to one study, the use of modified *Wan Dai Tang* was associated with good effect to treat acute or chronic vaginitis caused by *Candida albicans*. Modifications to the original formula were made by adding *Di Fu Zi* (Fructus Kochiae) and *Bai Xian Pi* (Cortex Dictamni) for itching in the genital region; *Mu Tong* (Caulis Akebiae), *Zhi Zi* (Fructus Gardeniae) and *Zhi Mu* (Rhizoma Anemarrhenae) for burning sensations and pain; *Qu Mai* (Herba Dianthi) and *Hua Shi* (Talcum) for frequent urination with pain; *Yu Xing Cao* (Herba Houttuyniae) and *Huang Bo* (Cortex Phellodendri Chinensis) for yellow discharge; *Xu Duan* (Radix Dipsaci) and *Du Zhong* (Cortex Eucommiae) for low back pain; and *Bu Gu Zhi* (Fructus Psoraleae), *Wu Wei Zi* (Fructus Schisandrae Chinensis), *Rou Dou Kou* (Semen Myristicae) and *Wu Zhu Yu* (Fructus Evodiae) for chronic illness. Of 31 patients, the study reported complete recovery in 28 cases, significant improvement in 2 cases, and no effect in 1 case.[4]

4. **Colitis**: One study reported good effect using modified *Wan Dai Tang* to treat chronic colitis associated with diarrhea. Clinical manifestations include varying severities of diarrhea, abdominal pain, decreased intake of food, fatigue, and presence of sticky mucus in the stools. In addition to *Wan Dai Tang* as the base formula, *Huang Lian* (Rhizoma Coptidis), *Di Yu* (Radix Sanguisorbae) and *Huai Hua* (Flos Sophorae) were added for hematochezia; *Mu Xiang* (Radix Aucklandiae) for rectal tenesmus; *Hou Po* (Cortex Magnoliae Officinalis) and *Zhi Qiao* (Fructus Aurantii) for abdominal distention; *Shen Qu* (Massa Fermentata) and *Ji Nei Jin* (Endothelium Corneum Gigeriae Galli) for decreased food intake; and *Rou Dou Kou* (Semen Myristicae) and *Shi Liu Pi* (Pericarpium Granati) for chronic diarrhea. Of 49 patients, the study reported complete recovery in 10 cases, significant improvement in 14 cases, and no effect in 4 cases. Information was unavailable on individuals who did not complete the study.[5]

5. **Irritable bowel syndrome (IBS)**: One study reported 92% effectiveness using modified *Wan Dai Tang* to treat 24 patients with IBS. In addition to the base formula, *Cang Zhu* (Rhizoma Atractylodis) and *Pu Gong Ying* (Herba Taraxaci) were added for more damp-heat; *Wu Zhu Yu* (Fructus Evodiae) and *Rou Dou Kou* (Semen Myristicae) for more deficiency and cold; *Mu Xiang* (Radix Aucklandiae) and *Gua Lou* (Fructus Trichosanthis) for abdominal distention; *Sheng Ma* (Rhizoma Cimicifugae) and *Bai Zhi* (Radix Angelicae Dahuricae) for frequent diarrhea; *Da Huang* (Radix et Rhizoma Rhei) for constipation; *Mu Xiang* (Radix Aucklandiae) and *Bing Lang* (Semen Arecae) for feeling of incomplete evacuation after defecation; and *Yi Zhi* (Fructus Alpiniae Oxyphyllae) and *Bu Gu Zhi* (Fructus Psoraleae) for chronic illness. Of 24 patients, the study reported complete recovery in 17 cases, improvement in 5 cases, and no effect in 2 cases.[6]

Wán Dài Tāng (End Discharge Decoction)

Chinese Herbal Formulas and Applications

RELATED FORMULAS

Yì Huáng Tāng

(Change the Yellow [Discharge] Decoction)

易黃湯

易黄汤

Pinyin Name: *Yi Huang Tang*

Literal Name: Change the Yellow [Discharge] Decoction

Original Source: *Fu Qing Zhu Nu Ke* (Women's Diseases According to Fu Qing-Zhu) by Fu Shan in 1827

Shan Yao (Rhizoma Dioscoreae), *chao* (dry-fried)	30g
Qian Shi (Semen Euryales), *chao* (dry-fried)	30g
Huang Bo (Cortex Phellodendri Chinensis), *chao* (dry-fried) with salted water	6g
Che Qian Zi (Semen Plantaginis), *chao* (dry-fried) with liquor	3g
Bai Guo (Semen Ginkgo), *fen sui* (pulverized)	10 kernels

The source text states to prepare the ingredients as a decoction. The main actions of *Yi Huang Tang* (Change the Yellow [Discharge] Decoction) are to strengthen the Spleen, dry dampness, clear heat, and stop leukorrhea. Clinically, it may be used to treat Spleen deficiency with damp-heat, characterized by symptoms such as yellow or white vaginal discharge that is sticky with a foul odor, and weak knees and lower back.

Qīng Dài Tāng (Clear the Discharge Decoction)

清帶湯

清带汤

Pinyin Name: *Qing Dai Tang*

Literal Name: Clear the Discharge Decoction

Original Source: *Yi Xue Zhong Zhong Can Xi Lu* (Records of Heart-Felt Experiences in Medicine with Reference to the West) by Zhang Xi-Chun in 1918-34

Shan Yao (Rhizoma Dioscoreae)	30g
Long Gu (Os Draconis), *dao* (pounded) into fine particles	18g
Mu Li (Concha Ostreae), *dao* (pounded) into fine particles	18g
Hai Piao Xiao (Endoconcha Sepiae), *dao* (pounded)	12g
Qian Cao (Radix et Rhizoma Rubiae)	9g

The source text states to prepare the ingredients as a decoction. The main actions of *Qing Dai Tang* (Clear the Discharge Decoction) are to strengthen the Spleen and stop abnormal vaginal discharge. Clinically, the patient may show red or white discharge that is diluted and large in quantity, weak lower back, pale tongue with white tongue coating, and a fine, moderate and deep pulse.

AUTHORS' COMMENTS

Wan Dai Tang, *Yi Huang Tang* (Change the Yellow [Discharge] Decoction), and *Qing Dai Tang* (Clear Discharge Decoction) all treat leukorrhea with Spleen deficiency.

- *Wan Dai Tang* treats leukorrhea due to Spleen deficiency and Liver qi stagnation.
- *Yi Huang Tang* treats leukorrhea due to Spleen deficiency with damp-heat accumulation.
- *Qing Dai Tang* treats leukorrhea due to Spleen deficiency.

Wan Dai Tang and *Long Dan Xie Gan Tang* (Gentiana Decoction to Drain the Liver) both treat leukorrhea.

- *Wan Dai Tang* is reserved for leukorrhea that is white and odorless, due to Spleen deficiency, Liver qi stagnation, and accumulation of dampness.
- *Long Dan Xie Gan Tang* is used only for yellow, thick, and foul-smelling leukorrhea, due to damp-heat attacking the Liver channel.[7]

According to Dr. Richard Tan, *Wan Dai Tang* can be combined with *Xin Yi San* (Magnolia Flower Powder) to treat leukorrhea that is clear or white in color.

References

1. *Liao Ning Zhong Yi Za Zhi* (Liaoning Journal of Chinese Medicine) 1992;6:43.
2. *Shang Hai Zhong Yi Yao Za Zhi* (Shanghai Journal of Chinese Medicine and Herbology) 1991;12:17.
3. *Jiang Su Zhong Yi* (Jiangsu Chinese Medicine) 1987;4:17.
4. *Xin Zhong Yi* (New Chinese Medicine) 1997;11:31.
5. *Hu Bei Zhong Yi Za Zhi* (Hubei Journal of Chinese Medicine) 1995;2:18.
6. *Zhe Jiang Zhong Yi Za Zhi* (Zhejiang Journal of Chinese Medicine) 1996;10:445.
7. Wang MZ, et al. *Zhong Yi Xue Wen Da Ti Ku* (Questions and Answers on Traditional Chinese Medicine: Herbal Formulas).

11

ASTRINGENT FORMULAS

809

Chapter 11 – Astringent Formulas　　　　　　　　*Section 5– Womb-Stabilizing Formulas to Stop Leakage*

Bā Wèi Dài Xià Fāng (Eight-Ingredient Formula for Leukorrhea)

八味帶下方
八味帯下方

Pinyin Name: *Ba Wei Dai Xia Fang*
Literal Name: Eight-Ingredient Formula for Leukorrhea
Alternate Names: *Pa Wei Tai Hsia Fang*, Eight-Taste Discharging Formula, Tangkuei Eight Herb Formula
Original Source: *Meika Hosen* (A Selection of Famous Physicians' Prescriptions) by Yoshine Hirai

COMPOSITION

Tu Fu Ling (Rhizoma Smilacis Glabrae)	4g
Jin Yin Hua (Flos Lonicerae Japonicae)	2g
Fu Ling (Poria)	3g
Mu Tong (Caulis Akebiae)	3g
Chen Pi (Pericarpium Citri Reticulatae)	2g
Da Huang (Radix et Rhizoma Rhei)	0.5-1g
Dang Gui (Radix Angelicae Sinensis)	5g
Chuan Xiong (Rhizoma Chuanxiong)	3g

DOSAGE / PREPARATION / ADMINISTRATION

Unavailable.

CHINESE THERAPEUTIC ACTIONS

1. Clears heat and eliminates toxins
2. Dries damp and disperses stagnations

CLINICAL MANIFESTATIONS

Leukorrhea characterized by damp-heat in the lower *jiao*: leukorrhea with yellow, white, or red discharge, generalized itching and discomfort in the genital region, abdominal pain, soreness of the lower back, and slight anemia.

CLINICAL APPLICATIONS

Acute or chronic leukorrhea with yellow vaginal discharge, gonorrheal leukorrhea, trichomonal leukorrhea, uteritis, and generalized itching of the genital region.

EXPLANATION

Ba Wei Dai Xia Fang (Eight-Ingredient Formula for Leukorrhea) is designed to treat acute or chronic leukorrhea due to damp-heat and toxins in the lower *jiao*. Therefore, effective treatment must focus on clearing damp-heat and toxins from the affected area.

In this formula, *Tu Fu Ling* (Rhizoma Smilacis Glabrae) and *Jin Yin Hua* (Flos Lonicerae Japonicae) clear heat and remove toxins. *Fu Ling* (Poria), *Mu Tong* (Caulis Akebiae), and *Chen Pi* (Pericarpium Citri Reticulatae) clear damp-heat. *Da Huang* (Radix et Rhizoma Rhei) drains pathogenic heat from the body. *Dang Gui* (Radix Angelicae Sinensis) and *Chuan Xiong* (Rhizoma Chuanxiong) nourish the blood and prevent the drying and draining herbs from consuming yin.

Ba Wei Dai Xia Fang (Eight-Ingredient Formula for Leukorrhea)

Diagnosis	Signs and Symptoms	Treatment	Herbs
Leukorrhea	Leukorrhea with yellow, white or red discharge: damp-heat in the lower *jiao*	• Clears heat and eliminates toxins • Dries dampness and disperses stagnations	• *Tu Fu Ling* (Rhizoma Smilacis Glabrae) and *Jin Yin Hua* (Flos Lonicerae Japonicae) clear heat and remove toxin. • *Fu Ling* (Poria), *Mu Tong* (Caulis Akebiae) and *Chen Pi* (Pericarpium Citri Reticulatae) clear damp-heat. • *Da Huang* (Radix et Rhizoma Rhei) drains pathogenic heat from the body. • *Dang Gui* (Radix Angelicae Sinensis) and *Chuan Xiong* (Rhizoma Chuanxiong) nourish the blood and prevent the drying and draining herbs from consuming yin.

Chinese Herbal Formulas and Applications

Bā Wèi Dài Xià Fāng (Eight-Ingredient Formula for Leukorrhea)

MODIFICATIONS

- With itching and pain in the genital region due to damp-heat, add *Huang Lian Jie Du Tang* (Coptis Decoction to Relieve Toxicity).
- For gonorrhea or syphilis in men or women, combine with *Long Dan Xie Gan Tang* (Gentiana Decoction to Drain the Liver).
- With blood deficiency and generalized weakness, add *Si Wu Tang* (Four-Substance Decoction).

CAUTIONS / CONTRAINDICATIONS

Patients with a sensitive gastrointestinal tract may wish to take *Ba Wei Dai Xia Fang* without *Da Huang* (Radix et Rhizoma Rhei), as this herb may cause diarrhea and stomach discomfort.

11

ASTRINGENT FORMULAS

811

Chapter 11 – Astringent Formulas

Chapter 11 — Summary

— Astringent Formulas

SECTION 1: EXTERIOR-STABILIZING FORMULAS TO STOP PERSPIRATION

Name	Similarities	Differences
Yu Ping Feng San (Jade Windscreen Powder)	Stabilize the exterior, stop perspiration	Tonifies *wei* (defensive) *qi* to stop spontaneous sweating
Mu Li San (Oyster Shell Powder)		Nourishes yin to stop night sweating

Yu Ping Feng San (Jade Windscreen Powder) tonifies qi and strengthens the exterior *wei* (defensive) level. It is used for spontaneous sweating due to *wei* (defensive) *qi* deficiency. It is also effective in strengthening *wei qi* and preventing frequent contraction of exterior wind-cold.

Mu Li San (Oyster Shell Powder) has a strong function to nourish yin and stop night sweating due to yin deficiency. It also stabilizes the exterior, tonifies qi, and stops spontaneous sweating due to *wei* (defensive) *qi* deficiency.

SECTION 2: LUNG-RESTRAINING FORMULA TO RELIEVE COUGH

Name	Similarities	Differences
Jiu Xian San (Nine-Immortal Powder)	Restrains the Lung	Tonifies Lung qi and yin

Jiu Xian San (Nine-Immortal Powder) restrains the Lung, tonifies qi and yin, and stops coughing. It is used for chronic cough, shortness of breath, and spontaneous sweating due to Lung qi and yin deficiencies.

SECTION 3: INTESTINES-BINDING FORMULAS TO STOP LEAKAGE

Name	Similarities	Differences
Zhen Ren Yang Zang Tang (True Man's Decoction for Nourishing the Organs)	Bind the Intestines, stop diarrhea and dysentery	Warms and tonifies the Spleen and Kidney; stronger astringent effect
Si Shen Wan (Four-Miracle Pill)		Warms and tonifies the Spleen and Kidney; stronger warming and tonifying effect
Tao Hua Tang (Peach Blossom Decoction)		Warms the middle *jiao*

Zhen Ren Yang Zang Tang (True Man's Decoction for Nourishing the Organs) warms and tonifies the Spleen and Kidney to stop diarrhea. Clinical manifestations include uncontrollable bowel movements, abdominal pain alleviated by pressure and warmth, rectal tenesmus and prolapse, red or white dysentery, stools with pus or blood, lethargy, and loss of appetite.

Si Shen Wan (Four-Miracle Pill) also has the action to warm and tonify the Spleen and Kidney to stop diarrhea. This formula is especially effective for 5 a.m. diarrhea due to Kidney yang deficiency. The clinical manifestations include early morning diarrhea, loss of appetite, soreness of the lower back, abdominal pain, cold extremities, lack of energy, pale tongue, and a thin, white tongue coating.

Chinese Herbal Formulas and Applications

Chapter 11 — Summary

Tao Hua Tang (Peach Blossom Decoction) warms the middle *jiao* and binds the Intestines. It is used mainly for diarrhea due to deficiency and cold of the Spleen and Stomach. Clinical manifestations include diarrhea, stools with dark blood and pus, dysuria, abdominal pain which is alleviated by warmth and pressure.

SECTION 4: *JING* (ESSENCE)-STABILIZING FORMULAS TO STOP LEAKAGE

Name	Similarities	Differences
Jin Suo Gu Jing Wan (Metal Lock Pill to Stabilize the Essence)	Restrain and stop the leakage of *jing* (essence)	Tonifies the Kidney
Liu Wei Gu Jing Wan (Rehmannia Six and Lotus Stamen Pill)		Strongly tonifies Liver and Kidney yin
Sang Piao Xiao San (Mantis Egg-Case Powder)		Tonifies the Heart and Kidney
Suo Quan Wan (Shut the Sluice Pill)		Warms the Kidney and astringes the Urinary Bladder
Fu Tu Dan (Poria and Cuscuta Special Pill)		Harmonizes the Heart and Kidney, strengthens the Spleen
Gui Zhi Jia Long Gu Mu Li Tang (Cinnamon Twig Decoction plus Dragon Bone and Oyster Shell)		Tonifies yin and yang; harmonizes *ying* (nutritive) and *wei* (defensive) levels
Zhi Zhuo Gu Ben Wan (Treat the Turbidity and Guard the Root Pill)		Clears heat, resolves dampness

Jin Suo Gu Jing Wan (Metal Lock Pill to Stabilize the Essence) tonifies Kidney and stabilizes the *jing* (essence). It treats spermatorrhea and/or seminal emission due to Kidney deficiency with signs and symptoms such as lack of energy, soreness and weakness of the back and knees, and tinnitus.

Liu Wei Gu Jing Wan (Rehmannia Six and Lotus Stamen Pill) is formulated by combining two formulas together: *Liu Wei Di Huang Wan* (Six-Ingredient Pill with Rehmannia) to tonify Liver and Kidney yin, and *Jin Suo Gu Jing Wan* (Metal Lock Pill to Stabilize the Essence) to restrain and stop the leakage of *jing* (essence). It treats spermatorrhea and/or seminal emission due to Liver and Kidney yin deficiencies.

Sang Piao Xiao San (Mantis Egg-Case Powder) tonifies the Heart and Kidney. It is used to treat deficiency of both the Heart and Kidney with clinical manifestations such as seminal emission, enuresis, frequent urination, cloudy urine, trance, and forgetfulness.

Suo Quan Wan (Shut the Sluice Pill) warms the Kidney and astringes the Urinary Bladder. It is used for Kidney qi deficiency with accumulation of cold in the Urinary Bladder causing enuresis and frequent, clear and prolonged urination. This formula is also effective for bedwetting in children.

Fu Tu Dan (Poria and Cuscuta Special Pill) strengthens the Spleen and drains dampness, tonifies the Kidney and stabilizes the *jing* (essence), and benefits the Heart and calms the *shen* (spirit). It treats spermatorrhea or premature ejaculation due to disharmony of the Heart and Kidney.

Gui Zhi Jia Long Gu Mu Li Tang (Cinnamon Twig Decoction plus Dragon Bone and Oyster Shell) tonifies yin and yang, harmonizes *ying* (nutritive) and *wei* (defensive) levels, and astringes *jing* (essence). It treats chronic and gradual decline in physical and sexual functions due to deficiency of yin and yang, accompanied by disharmony of the *ying* (nutritive) and *wei* (defensive) levels.

Zhi Zhuo Gu Ben Wan (Treat the Turbidity and Guard the Root Pill) clears heat, resolves dampness, and prevents the loss of qi and *jing* (essence). It treats genitourinary disorders due to damp-heat in the Urinary Bladder. Clinical manifestations include white and turbid urine, frequent and excessive amount of urination, and spermatorrhea.

Chapter 11 – Astringent Formulas

Chapter 11 — Summary

SECTION 5: WOMB-STABILIZING FORMULAS TO STOP LEAKAGE

Name	Similarities	Differences
Gu Jing Wan (Stabilize the Menses Pill)	Stabilize menstruation, stop bleeding	Nourishes yin, clears deficiency heat
Zhen Ling Dan (Rouse the Spirits Special Pill)		Warms the interior, eliminates blood stagnation, relieves pain
Wan Dai Tang (End Discharge Decoction)	Resolve dampness, stop leukorrhea	Tonifies qi, strengthens the Spleen, regulates Liver qi
Ba Wei Dai Xia Fang (Eight-Ingredient Formula for Leukorrhea)		Clears damp-heat and toxins in the lower *jiao*

Gu Jing Wan (Stabilize the Menses Pill) nourishes yin, clears deficiency heat, and stops abnormal menstrual bleeding. It is used for deficiency heat in the interior causing abnormal menstrual bleeding with dark red blood or purplish-black blood clots, irritability, abdominal pain, dysuria, hematuria, red tongue, and a wiry, rapid pulse.

Zhen Ling Dan (Rouse the Spirits Special Pill) is used for deficiency and cold in the *chong* (thoroughfare) and *ren* (conception) channels resulting in menstrual bleeding with blood stagnation. Clinical manifestations include continuous menstrual bleeding that is purplish-red or purplish-black in color, abdominal pain worsened by pressure, reduced pain with the passing of blood clots, dark purplish tongue, and a deep, fine and wiry pulse.

Wan Dai Tang (End Discharge Decoction) stops leukorrhea due to Spleen deficiency and Liver qi stagnation. Clinical manifestations include odorless, clear, and thick leukorrhea that is white or light yellow in color, pale face, and lethargy.

Ba Wei Dai Xia Fang (Eight-Ingredient Formula for Leukorrhea) treats leukorrhea due to damp-heat and toxins in the lower *jiao*. Clinical manifestations include leukorrhea with yellow, white, or red discharge, generalized itching and discomfort in the genital region, abdominal pain, soreness of the lower back, and slight anemia.

Chapter 12

— Qi-Regulating Formulas

理气剂

李时珍 Lǐ Shí-Zhēn

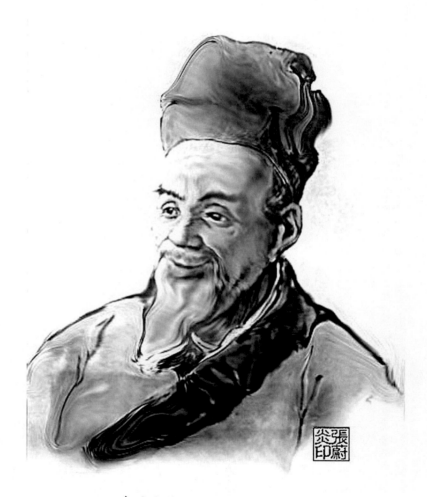

李时珍 Lǐ Shí-Zhēn, 1518 – 1593.

李时珍 Lǐ Shí-Zhēn

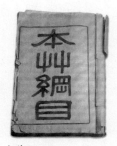

本草綱目 *Ben Cao Gang Mu*
(Materia Medica) in 1596.

Li Shi-Zhen was born into a long family lineage of physicians. However, his father refused to allow him to study medicine in his youth because at that time, physicians were held in low social esteem and had poor economic status. Li remained interested in medicine, and after years of insistence, his father finally agreed, and began to teach Li medicine when he was 23 years old. Li made tremendous advances in the next fifteen years. When he was 38, he was called to the Imperial Palace to become 太醫 the Supreme Physician. Three years later, he was promoted to Chief Supreme Physician. However, he disliked the politics of serving in the Imperial Palace, and resigned one year later to return home.

In Li's years of studying and practicing, he noticed many errors, omissions, and repetitions among herbal texts. Realizing that such errors create malpractice and jeopardize lives, he embarked on a life-long journey to research and rewrite the records of herbal medicine. During the research process, Li interviewed physicians and pharmacists, lived with hunters and farmers, and personally cultivated and tested many herbs, all to ensure accuracy of the information. In 1578, when Li Shi-Zhen was 60 years old, he finished the *Ben Cao Gang Mu* (Materia Medica) after 27 years of work. This was the most comprehensive of all herbal texts prior to the 17th century: it documented 1,892 medicinal substances (1,195 plants, 340 animals, and 357 mineral substances) classified into 6 sections, 52 scrolls, and 60 categories.

Ironically, Li spent his entire adult life in compiling the *Ben Cao Gang Mu* (Materia Medica), yet during his life time he found no one willing to invest the money to publish it. He eventually donated it to the Imperial Palace before he passed away, hoping that it would be preserved and passed on to future generations. Finally in 1596, three years after his death, it was published in Nanjing. Today, the *Ben Cao Gang Mu* (Materia Medica) is still considered one of the most important herbal texts, and has been translated into many languages, including English, Japanese, German, French and Russian.

Dynasties & Kingdoms	Year
Xia Dynasty 夏	2100-1600 BCE
Shang Dynasty 商	1600-1100 BCE
Zhou Dynasty 周	1100-221 BCE
Qin Dynasty 秦	221-207 BCE
Han Dynasty 漢	206 BCE-220
Three Kingdoms 三國	220-280
Western Jin Dynasty 西晉	265-316
Eastern Jin Dynasty 東晉	317-420
Northern and Southern Dynasties 北南朝	420-581
Sui Dynasty 隋	581-618
Tang Dynasty 唐	618-907
Five Dynasties 五代	907-960
Song Dynasty 宋	960-1279
Liao Dynasty 遼	916-1125
Jin Dynasty 金	1115-1234
Yuan Dynasty 元	1271-1368
Ming Dynasty 明	**1368-1644**
Qing Dynasty 清	1644-1911
Republic of China 中華民國	1912-Present Day
People's Republic of China 中華人民共和國	1949-Present Day

Table of Contents

Chapter 12. Qi-Regulating Formulas ·· **815**
Biography of Li Shi-Zhen ··· 816

Section 1. Qi-Moving Formulas ·· **822**
Yue Ju Wan (Escape Restraint Pill) ·· 822
  Xiang Fu Wan (Cyperus Pill) ··· 824
Jin Ling Zi San (Melia Toosendan Powder) ·· 825
  Yan Hu Suo San (Corydalis Powder) ··· 826
  Yan Hu Yi Hao (Corydalis Formula One) ·· 826
  Yan Hu Er Hao (Corydalis Formula Two) ·· 826
Ban Xia Hou Po Tang (Pinellia and Magnolia Bark Decoction) ·· 827
Zhi Shi Xie Bai Gui Zhi Tang (Immature Bitter Orange, Chinese Chive, and Cinnamon Twig Decoction) ········· 831
  Gua Lou Xie Bai Bai Jiu Tang (Trichosanthes Fruit, Chinese Chive, and Wine Decoction) ······················ 832
  Gua Lou Xie Bai Ban Xia Tang (Trichosanthes Fruit, Chinese Chive, and Pinellia Decoction) ··················· 832
  Jia Wei Gua Lou Xie Bai Tang (Augmented Trichosanthes Fruit and Chinese Chive Decoction) ················· 832
Ju He Wan (Tangerine Seed Pill) ··· 833
Tian Tai Wu Yao San (Top-Quality Lindera Powder) ·· 835
  San Ceng Hui Xiang Wan (Fennel Seed Pill with Three Levels) ··· 836
  Dao Qi Tang (Conduct the Qi Decoction) ·· 837
Nuan Gan Jian (Warm the Liver Decoction) ··· 838
Hou Po Wen Zhong Tang (Magnolia Bark Decoction for Warming the Middle) ·· 840
  Liang Fu Wan (Galangal and Cyperus Pill) ·· 841

Section 2. Qi-Descending Formulas ·· **842**
Su Zi Jiang Qi Tang (Perilla Fruit Decoction for Directing Qi Downward) ·· 842
  San Zi Jiang Qi Tang (Three-Seed Decoction for Directing Qi Downward) ··· 844
Ding Chuan Tang (Arrest Wheezing Decoction) ··· 845
Shen Mi Tang (Mysterious Decoction) ·· 847
Si Mo Tang (Four Milled-Herbs Decoction) ·· 849
  Wu Mo Yin Zi (Five Milled-Herbs Decoction) ·· 850
Xuan Fu Dai Zhe Shi Tang (Inula and Hematite Decoction) ··· 851
  Gan Jiang Ren Shen Ban Xia Wan (Ginger, Ginseng, and Pinellia Pill) ··· 853
Ju Pi Zhu Ru Tang (Tangerine Peel and Bamboo Shaving Decoction) ·· 854
  Ju Pi Zhu Ru Tang (Tangerine Peel and Bamboo Shaving Decoction) ··· 855
  Xin Zhi Ju Pi Zhu Ru Tang (Newly-Formulated Tangerine Peel and Bamboo Shaving Decoction) ··············· 856
Ding Xiang Shi Di Tang (Clove and Persimmon Calyx Decoction) ··· 856
  Shi Di Tang (Persimmon Calyx Decoction) ··· 858
Sheng Yang San Huo Tang (Raise the Yang and Disperse the Fire Decoction) ··· 858

Qi-Regulating Formulas (Summary) ··· **860**

Chinese Herbal Formulas and Applications

Chapter 12 — Overview

— Qi-Regulating Formulas

Definition: Qi-regulating formulas activate qi circulation to treat qi stagnation, and direct reversed flow of qi to descend.

Qi circulates throughout the body to provide warmth and protection, and ensures normal health and functioning in the interior (*zang fu* organs) and the exterior (the four extremities). Qi disorders result from excessive stress, overwork, emotional disturbances, inappropriate diet, or changes in the weather. Qi disorders are generally characterized by deficiency (qi deficiency) or excess (qi stagnation and reversed qi flow). These conditions may occur independently or concurrently. Qi deficiency is treated with qi-tonifying formulas (*see* Chapter 8: Tonic Formulas). Qi stagnation is smoothed with qi-moving formulas. Reversed flow of qi is corrected with qi-descending formulas. If the qi disorder is characterized by both qi stagnation and reversed qi flow, then qi-moving and qi-descending formulas must be prescribed together. Similarly, in patients with underlying qi deficiency, the use of qi-regulating formulas should be accompanied by qi-tonifying herbs/formulas to prevent further loss of qi.

SUBCATEGORIES OF ACTION

Qi-regulating formulas are divided into two subcategories.

1. Qi-Moving Formulas

These formulas activate qi circulation and disperse qi stagnation. Qi stagnation usually does not occur as an isolated condition or disorder. Qi stagnation is usually accompanied by stagnation of blood, phlegm, food, and other substances. Furthermore, qi stagnation in one organ may affect the normal functioning of other organs. Therefore, many qi-moving formulas are designed to treat qi stagnation with these complications. Qi stagnation is often seen among the Spleen/Stomach and Liver syndromes.

Spleen and Stomach qi stagnation result in epigastric and abdominal symptomology such as distention and fullness, poor appetite, nausea, vomiting, acid regurgitation, hiccups, belching, and constipation. Herbs commonly used to move Spleen and Stomach qi include *Chen Pi* (Pericarpium Citri Reticulatae), *Hou Po* (Cortex Magnoliae Officinalis), *Mu Xiang* (Radix Aucklandiae), *Zhi Shi* (Fructus Aurantii Immaturus), and *Sha Ren* (Fructus Amomi). Representative formulas for these purposes include *Yue Ju Wan* (Escape Restraint Pill) and *Hou Po Wen Zhong Tang* (Magnolia Bark Decoction for Warming the Middle).

Liver qi stagnation results in one or more disorders in the three *jiaos*: chest and hypochondriac distention and pain, hernia, irregular menstruation, and dysmenorrhea. Herbs commonly used to soothe Liver qi and unblock stagnation include *Xiang Fu* (Rhizoma Cyperi), *Wu Yao* (Radix Linderae), *Chuan Lian Zi* (Fructus Toosendan), *Qing Pi* (Pericarpium Citri Reticulatae Viride), and *Yu Jin* (Radix Curcumae). Representative formulas that move Liver qi include *Ban Xia Hou Po Tang* (Pinellia and Magnolia Bark Decoction) and *Ju He Wan* (Tangerine Seed Pill).

2. Qi-Descending Formulas

These formulas are designed to direct reversed flow of qi downward. Reversal of qi flow often occurs as a result of stagnation or obstruction (such as qi stagnation or phlegm obstruction). The Lung and Stomach are most likely to be affected by reversed qi flow.

---

*Qi circulates throughout the body to provide warmth and protection, and ensures normal health and functioning in the interior (*zang fu* organs) and the exterior (the four extremities).*

Qi stagnation is not an isolated condition – it is usually accompanied by stagnation of blood, phlegm, food, and other substances.

QI-REGULATING FORMULAS

12

819

Chapter 12 – Qi-Regulating Formulas

Chapter 12 — Overview

Reversed flow of Lung qi leads to coughing, wheezing, shortness of breath, and dyspnea. Herbs that help direct Lung qi downward include *Zi Su Zi* (Fructus Perillae), *Ku Xing Ren* (Semen Armeniacae Amarum), *Zi Wan* (Radix et Rhizoma Asteris), and *Hou Po* (Cortex Magnoliae Officinalis). Exemplar formulas include *Su Zi Jiang Qi Tang* (Perilla Fruit Decoction for Directing Qi Downward) and *Ding Chuan Tang* (Arrest Wheezing Decoction).

> Qi deficiency must not be treated with only qi-regulating herbs, which will further consume and injure the qi.

Reversed flow of Stomach qi may lead to acid regurgitation, nausea, vomiting, and hiccups. Herbs that redirect Stomach qi include *Xuan Fu Hua* (Flos Inulae), *Ban Xia* (Rhizoma Pinelliae), *Chen Pi* (Pericarpium Citri Reticulatae), *Ding Xiang* (Flos Caryophylli), *Zhe Shi* (Haematitum), *Shi Di* (Calyx Kaki), and *Zhu Ru* (Caulis Bambusae in Taenia). Exemplar formulas include *Xuan Fu Dai Zhe Shi Tang* (Inula and Hematite Decoction) and *Ju Pi Zhu Ru Tang* (Tangerine Peel and Bamboo Shaving Decoction).

CAUTIONS / CONTRAINDICATIONS

- Deficiency conditions, such as qi deficiency, must not be treated with qi-regulating herbs, which will further consume and injure the qi. These conditions must be treated with qi-tonifying herbs.
- Excess conditions, such as qi stagnation or reversed flow of qi, must not be treated with qi-tonifying formulas, which will only cause more stagnation. These conditions must be treated with qi-regulating herbs.
- Qi-regulating formulas often include acrid, drying, and aromatic herbs that consume qi and injure body fluids; thus, excessive or prolonged use is not recommended, especially for the pregnant women, elderly persons, individuals with yin-deficient fire, or those with a history of bleeding (such as excessive bleeding during menstrual periods and epistaxis).

PHARMACOLOGICAL EFFECTS & CLINICAL APPLICATIONS

Qi-regulating formulas are divided into subcategories based on differing traditional therapeutic actions: qi-moving and qi-descending. These appropriately have contrasting pharmacological effects and clinical applications.

> Qi-regulating formulas treat respiratory, gastrointestinal, and emotional disorders.

From a traditional Chinese medicine perspective, qi-moving formulas activate qi circulation and disperse qi stagnation to treat Spleen/Stomach and Liver imbalances. From allopathic medical perspectives, these formulas treat gastrointestinal disorders, emotional disorders, hernia, and globus hystericus.

- **Gastrointestinal disorders**: Qi-moving formulas treat gastrointestinal disorders, such as peptic ulcer disease,[1,2] enteritis,[3] and swallowing disorders.[4,5] Exemplar formulas include *Yue Ju Wan* (Escape Restraint Pill), *Jin Ling Zi San* (Melia Toosendan Powder), and *Ban Xia Hou Po Tang* (Pinellia and Magnolia Bark Decoction).
- **Emotional disorders**: Qi-moving formulas have been used successfully in treatment of various mental and psychiatric disorders, including depression,[6] schizophrenia,[7] neurosis,[8] hysteria,[9] stress and depression,[10] panic disorder,[11] and *dian kuang* (mania and withdrawal).[12] Exemplar formulas include *Yue Ju Wan* (Escape Restraint Pill) and *Ban Xia Hou Po Tang* (Pinellia and Magnolia Bark Decoction).
- **Hernia**: *Ju He Wan* (Tangerine Seed Pill) and *Nuan Gan Jian* (Warm the Liver Decoction) are two of the most effective formulas for treating hernia.[13]
- **Globus hystericus**: Known as *mei he qi* (plum-pit *qi*) in traditional Chinese medicine, this is a condition characterized by the feeling of having a foreign object obstructing the throat, that cannot be expectorated nor swallowed. Globus hystericus, and related conditions such as pharyngeal paraesthesia and swallowing disorders, can be treated effectively with formulas such as *Yue Ju Wan* (Escape Restraint Pill) and *Ban Xia Hou Po Tang* (Pinellia and Magnolia Bark Decoction).[14,15,16]

Qi-descending formulas are designed to correct reversed flow of Lung or Stomach qi by directing qi downward. From allopathic medical perspectives, these formulas treat respiratory and gastrointestinal disorders, and globus hystericus.

820

Chapter 12 — Overview

- **Respiratory disorders**: Many of these formulas exert marked influence on the respiratory tract. Pharmacological effects include antitussive,[17,18] antiallergic,[19] and antiasthmatic influences.[20] Clinically, these formulas have been successfully used to treat cough and wheezing,[21] asthma,[22,23] bronchopneumonia,[24] and bronchial asthma.[25] Exemplar formulas include *Su Zi Jiang Qi Tang* (Perilla Fruit Decoction for Directing Qi Downward), *Ding Chuan Tang* (Arrest Wheezing Decoction), and *Si Mo Tang* (Four Milled-Herbs Decoction).

- **Gastrointestinal disorders**: Clinical applications of qi-descending formulas include nausea and vomiting,[26,27,28] morning sickness,[29,30] peptic ulcer disease,[31] and gastritis.[32] Exemplar formulas include *Su Zi Jiang Qi Tang* (Perilla Fruit Decoction for Directing Qi Downward), *Xuan Fu Dai Zhe Shi Tang* (Inula and Hematite Decoction), and *Ding Xiang Shi Di Tang* (Clove and Persimmon Calyx Decoction).

- **Globus hystericus**: Qi-descending formulas also treat globus hystericus. Specifically, *Su Zi Jiang Qi Tang* (Perilla Fruit Decoction for Directing Qi Downward) treats *mei he qi* (plum-pit *qi*),[33] and *Xuan Fu Dai Zhe Shi Tang* (Inula and Hematite Decoction) is used for pharyngeal neurosis.[34]

References

1. *Hu Nan Zhong Yi Za Zhi* (Hunan Journal of Chinese Medicine) 1989;5(1):9.
2. *Shi Yong Zhong Yi Yao Za Zhi* (Journal of Practical Chinese Medicine and Medicinals) 1995;6:15.
3. *Fu Jian Zhong Yi Yao* (Fujian Chinese Medicine and Herbology) 1984;4:54.
4. Iwasaki K, Wang Q, Nakagawa T, Suzuki T, Sasaki H. The traditional Chinese Medicine Banxia Houpo Tang improves swallowing reflex. Phytomedicine 1999 May;6(2):103-6.
5. Iwasaki K, Wang Q, Seki H, Satoh K, Takeda A, Arai H, Sasaki H. The effects of the traditional chinese medicine, "Banxia Houpo Tang (Hange-Koboku To)" on the swallowing reflex in Parkinson's disease. Department of Geriatric Medicine, Tohoku University School of Medicine, Sendai, Japan. Phytomedicine 2000 Jul;7(4):259-63.
6. *Zhong Yi Fang Ji Xian Dai Yan Jiu* (Modern Study of Medical Formulae in Traditional Chinese Medicine) 1997;922-23.
7. *Jiang Su Zhong Yi* (Jiangsu Chinese Medicine) 1994;2:35.
8. *Si Chuan Zhong Yi* (Sichuan Chinese Medicine) 1986;4(5):18.
9. *Guo Wai Yi Xue Zhong Yi Zhong Yao Fen Ce* (Monograph of Chinese Herbology from Foreign Medicine) 1985;4:41.
10. Naito T, Itoh H, Takeyama M. Some gastrointestinal function regulatory Kampo medicines have modulatory effects on human plasma adrenocorticotropic hormone and cortisol levels with continual stress exposure. Biological & Pharmaceutical Bulletin 2003 Jan;26(1):101-4.
11. Mantani N, Hisanaga A, Kogure T, Kita T, Shimada Y, Terasawa K. Four cases of panic disorder successfully treated with Kampo (Japanese herbal) medicines: Kami-shoyo-san and Hange-koboku-to. Psychiatry & Clinical Neurosciences 2002 Dec;56(6):617-20.
12. *Jiang Xi Zhong Yi Yao* (Jiangxi Chinese Medicine and Herbology) 1989;20(4):34.
13. *Shan Xi Zhong Yi* (Shanxi Chinese Medicine) 1995;16(1):15.
14. *Zhong Guo Zhong Xi Yi Jie He Za Zhi* (Chinese Journal of Integrative Chinese and Western Medicine) 1993;3:11.
15. *Yun Nan Zhong Yi Za Zhi* (Yunan Journal of Chinese Medicine) 1992;13(5):16.
16. *Zhe Jiang Zhong Yi Za Zhi* (Zhejiang Journal of Chinese Medicine) 1983;8:345.
17. *Zhong Yao Yao Li Yu Lin Chuang* (Pharmacology and Clinical Applications of Chinese Herbs) 1992;8(5):13.
18. *Zhong Cheng Yao Yan Jiu* (Research of Chinese Patent Medicine) 1986;11:27.
19. Kao ST, Chang CH, Chen YS, Chiang SY, Lin JG. Effects of Ding-Chuan-Tang on bronchoconstriction and airway leucocyte infiltration in sensitized guinea pigs. Immunopharmacol Immunotoxicol 2004 Feb;26(1):113-24.
20. *Zhe Jiang Zhong Yi Za Zhi* (Zhejiang Journal of Chinese Medicine) 1989;24(3):123.
21. *Zhong Yi Za Zhi* (Journal of Chinese Medicine) 1964;10:32.
22. *Hu Bei Zhong Yi Za Zhi* (Hubei Journal of Chinese Medicine) 1997;19(2):17.
23. *Zhe Jiang Zhong Yi Za Zhi* (Zhejiang Journal of Chinese Medicine) 1987;22(1):508.
24. *Jiang Xi Zhong Yi Yao* (Jiangxi Chinese Medicine and Herbology) 1992;23(1):28.
25. *Xin Yi Xue* (New Medicine) 1972;9:14.
26. *Zhong Yi Yao Yan Jiu* (Research of Chinese Medicine and Herbology) 1995;2:31.
27. *Hei Long Jiang Zhong Yi Yao* (Heilongjiang Chinese Medicine and Herbology) 1991;3:19.
28. *Xin Zhong Yi* (New Chinese Medicine) 1995;7:48.
29. *Xin Jiang Zhong Yi Yao* (Xinjiang Chinese Medicine and Herbology) 1995;4:20.
30. *Tian Jin Zhong Yi* (Tianjin Chinese Medicine) 1989;3:5.
31. *Liao Ning Zhong Yi Za Zhi* (Liaoning Journal of Chinese Medicine) 1991;18(1):20.
32. *Shi Yong Zhong Xi Yi Jie He Za Zhi* (Practical Journal of Integrated Chinese and Western Medicines) 1990;3(31):152.
33. *Si Chuan Zhong Yi* (Sichuan Chinese Medicine) 1984;2(1):46.
34. *Shang Hai Zhong Yi Yao Za Zhi* (Shanghai Journal of Chinese Medicine and Herbology) 1984;4:18.

Chapter 12 – Qi-Regulating Formulas

Section 1 – Qi-Moving Formulas

Section 1

行气剂

— Qi-Moving Formulas

Yuè Jú Wán (Escape Restraint Pill)

越鞠丸

Pinyin Name: *Yue Ju Wan*
Literal Name: Escape Restraint Pill
Alternate Names: *Yue Chu Wan* (Stagnation-Relieving Pill), *Xiong Zhu Wan* (Cyperus and Atractylodes Pill), Ligusticum Chuanxiong and Atractylodes Pill, Cyperus and Atractylodes Combination
Original Source: *Dan Xi Xin Fa* (Teachings of [Zhu] Dan-Xi) by Zhu Zhen-Heng in 1481

COMPOSITION

Xiang Fu (Rhizoma Cyperi)	[6g]
Chuan Xiong (Rhizoma Chuanxiong)	[6g]
Zhi Zi (Fructus Gardeniae)	[6g]
Cang Zhu (Rhizoma Atractylodis)	[6g]
Shen Qu (Massa Fermentata)	[6g]

DOSAGE / PREPARATION / ADMINISTRATION

The source text instructions are to grind equal amounts of the ingredients into powder and form into pills with water. The pills should resemble *Lu Dou* (Semen Phaseoli Radiati) in size. Take 6-9g of pills with warm water. Today, this formula may be prepared as a decoction with the doses suggested in brackets above.

CHINESE THERAPEUTIC ACTIONS

Regulates qi and relieves constraint

CLINICAL MANIFESTATIONS

Qi stagnation: distention and oppression in the chest and diaphragm, epigastric and abdominal fullness and pain, acid regurgitation, indigestion, nausea, vomiting, and belching with a fetid odor.

CLINICAL APPLICATIONS

Psychiatric disorders (depression, schizophrenia and neurosis), *mei he qi* (plum-pit *qi*), gastritis, peptic ulcer disease, gastric neurosis, migraine, intercostal neuralgia, infectious hepatitis, cholecystitis, and cholelithiasis.

EXPLANATION

Yue Ju Wan (Escape Restraint Pill) treats mild to moderate cases of constraint in which qi stagnation has led to other complications, such as stagnation of blood, phlegm, heat, dampness, and food. If the qi is stagnant in the chest and abdomen, qi is not able to ascend or descend freely; chest distention and oppression as well as abdominal fullness and pain may occur. Qi stagnation of the Spleen and Stomach may lead to indigestion and reversed flow of Stomach qi, with symptoms such as acid regurgitation, nausea, and vomiting.

Since the underlying cause of these symptoms is qi stagnation, the primary focus of treatment is to relieve that stagnation. This formula has *Xiang Fu* (Rhizoma Cyperi) to activate qi circulation and relieve qi stagnation. *Chuan Xiong* (Rhizoma Chuanxiong) activates blood circulation to dispel blood stagnation. *Zhi Zi* (Fructus Gardeniae) clears heat and sedates fire. *Cang Zhu* (Rhizoma Atractylodis) dries dampness to clear damp and phlegm stagnation. *Shen Qu* (Massa Fermentata) promotes digestion and clears food stagnation.

This formula emphasizes the relief of qi stagnation. Once the qi can circulate smoothly, other stagnations will be resolved. However, if there are any complications or changes in condition, select additional herbs and adjust doses accordingly.

Chinese Herbal Formulas and Applications

Yuè Jú Wán (Escape Restraint Pill)

Yue Ju Wan (Escape Restraint Pill)

Diagnosis	Signs and Symptoms	Treatment	Herbs
Qi stagnation	• Chest distention/oppression and abdominal fullness/pain: qi stagnation in the chest and abdomen • Acid regurgitation, nausea and vomiting: reversed flow of Stomach qi due to qi stagnation	Regulates qi and relieves constraint	• *Xiang Fu* (Rhizoma Cyperi) activates qi circulation and relieves qi stagnation. • *Chuan Xiong* (Rhizoma Chuanxiong) activates blood circulation to dispel blood stagnation. • *Zhi Zi* (Fructus Gardeniae) clears heat and sedates fire. • *Cang Zhu* (Rhizoma Atractylodis) dries dampness to clear phlegm stagnation. • *Shen Qu* (Massa Fermentata) promotes digestion and clears food stagnation.

MODIFICATIONS

- For severe qi stagnation, bloating, distention, and sighing, add *Mu Xiang* (Radix Aucklandiae), *Zhi Qiao* (Fructus Aurantii), and *Hou Po* (Cortex Magnoliae Officinalis); or *Xiao Yao San* (Rambling Powder).
- When there is severe blood stagnation, add *Tao Ren* (Semen Persicae), *Hong Hua* (Flos Carthami), and *Chi Shao* (Radix Paeoniae Rubra); or the formula *Xue Fu Zhu Yu Tang* (Drive Out Stasis in the Mansion of Blood Decoction).
- With more dampness, add *Fu Ling* (Poria) and *Ze Xie* (Rhizoma Alismatis).
- With more phlegm, add *Ban Xia* (Rhizoma Pinelliae) and *Gua Lou* (Fructus Trichosanthis).
- With more food stagnation, add *Mai Ya* (Fructus Hordei Germinatus) and *Shan Zha* (Fructus Crataegi); or *Bao He Wan* (Preserve Harmony Pill).
- With more fire, add *Huang Qin* (Radix Scutellariae) and *Huang Lian* (Rhizoma Coptidis).
- With fullness, distention, and oppression, add *Hou Po* (Cortex Magnoliae Officinalis) and *Zhi Qiao* (Fructus Aurantii).

CAUTIONS / CONTRAINDICATIONS

Yue Ju Wan is contraindicated in cases of generalized weakness and deficiency with abdominal fullness, distention and oppression, loose stools and lack of appetite.

CLINICAL STUDIES AND RESEARCH

1. **Psychiatric disorders:** According to various reports, *Yue Ju Wan* has been used successfully to treat various psychiatric disorders, such as depression, schizophrenia, and neurosis. According to one study, use of *Yue Ju Wan* was associated with 94.4% effectiveness in treating 72 patients with psychiatric disorders. The treatment protocol was to administer 6g of this formula in pills, twice daily. For those who did not respond to initial treatment, the herbs were given in decoction, and the formulation was modified as follows: with more dampness, *Fu Ling* (Poria) and *Bai Zhi* (Radix Angelicae Dahuricae) were added; for more fire, *Qing Dai* (Indigo Naturalis) was added; for more phlegm, *Ban Xia* (Rhizoma Pinelliae) and *Dan Nan Xing* (Arisaema cum Bile) were added; for more blood stagnation, *Tao Ren* (Semen Persicae) and *Hong Hua* (Flos Carthami) were added; for more qi stagnation, *Mu Xiang* (Radix Aucklandiae) and *Bing Lang* (Semen Arecae) were added; and for more food stagnation, *Shan Zha* (Fructus Crataegi) and *Sha Ren* (Fructus Amomi) were added. Of 72 patients, the study reported complete recovery in 51 cases, improvement in 17 cases, and no benefit in 4 cases.[1,2,3]

2. **Mei he qi (plum-pit qi):** One study reported 95.45% effectiveness when using modified *Yue Ju Wan* to treat 44 patients with plum-pit qi. The herbal treatment contained *Chuan Xiong* (Rhizoma Chuanxiong) 10g, *Xiang Fu* (Rhizoma Cyperi) 15g, *Zhi Zi* (Fructus Gardeniae) 15g, *Shen Qu* (Massa Fermentata) 15g, and *Cang Zhu* (Rhizoma Atractylodis) 10g. Modifications were also made by adding *Er Chen Tang* (Two-Cured Decoction) for profuse phlegm; *Mai Dong* (Radix Ophiopogonis) and *Xuan Shen* (Radix Scrophulariae) for dry throat; *Ji Nei Jin* (Endothelium Corneum Gigeriae Galli) and *Mai Ya* (Fructus Hordei Germinatus) for decreased food intake; *Hou Po* (Cortex Magnoliae Officinalis) and *Zi Su Geng* (Caulis Perillae) for chest oppression; and *Dan Dou Chi* (Semen Sojae Praeparatum) and *Yu Jin* (Radix Curcumae) for irritability.[4]

3. **Peptic ulcer disease:** Use of modified *Yue Ju Wan* achieved an 88% rate of effectiveness in treating gastric and duodenal ulcers. The herbal formula contained *Cang*

QI-REGULATING FORMULAS

12

823

Chapter 12 – Qi-Regulating Formulas

Section 1 – Qi-Moving Formulas

Yuè Jú Wán (Escape Restraint Pill)

Zhu (Rhizoma Atractylodis) 10g, *Xiang Fu* (Rhizoma Cyperi) 10g, *Chuan Xiong* (Rhizoma Chuanxiong) 10g, dry-fried *Zhi Zi* (Fructus Gardeniae) 10g, *Chai Hu* (Radix Bupleuri) 10g, *Shen Qu* (Massa Fermentata) 15g, *Bai Shao* (Radix Paeoniae Alba) 20g, *Ying Su Ke* (Pericarpium Papaveris) 6g, and others as needed. The treatment protocols include giving the herbs in decoction daily, for 20 days per course of treatment, for 3 courses total (with a resting period of 5 days between courses). Of 50 patients, the study reported complete recovery in 19 cases, improvement in 25 cases, and no effect in 6 cases.[5]

4. **Migraine**: One study reported marked effectiveness using *Yue Ju Wan* to treat 50 patients with migraine headache (23 with unilateral symptoms, 17 with bilateral, and 10 with global headache). Clinical manifestations included recurrent headaches, dizziness, insomnia, poor appetite, nausea and/or vomiting, impaired vision and speech, and numb extremities. The herbal treatment used *Yue Ju Wan* as the base formula, and modifications were made as needed based on signs and symptoms. Of 50 cases, the study reported complete recovery in 45 cases and improvement in 5 cases. The duration of treatment ranged from 3 to 16 packs of herbs given in decoction form. In follow-up interviews one year later, 3 patients had experienced 1 recurrence and 2 patients had 2 recurrences.[6]

RELATED FORMULA

Xiàng Fù Wán (Cyperus Pill)

香附丸

Pinyin Name: *Xiang Fu Wan*

Literal Name: Cyperus Pill

Original Source: *An Hui Zhong Yi Xue Yuan* (Anhui University School of Medicine) in 1990

Chai Hu (Radix Bupleuri)

Xiang Fu (Rhizoma Cyperi)

Gou Teng (Ramulus Uncariae cum Uncis)

Mu Li (Concha Ostreae)

He Huan Pi (Cortex Albiziae)

Yuan Zhi (Radix Polygalae)

Chuan Xiong (Rhizoma Chuanxiong)

Yu Jin (Radix Curcumae)

Mai Ya (Fructus Hordei Germinatus)

Zhi Zi (Fructus Gardeniae)

Cha Ye (Folium Camelliae)

Shi Chang Pu (Rhizoma Acori Tatarinowii)

Da Zao (Fructus Jujubae)

Gan Cao (Radix et Rhizoma Glycyrrhizae)

Ci Wu Jia (Radix et Rhizoma seu Caulis Acanthopanacis Senticosi)

Xiang Fu Wan (Cyperus Pill) treats emotional disorders characterized by *shen* (spirit) disturbance accompanied by stagnation of qi, blood, dampness, phlegm, and food. Clinical applications include depression, schizophrenia, and neurosis.

AUTHORS' COMMENTS

Yue Ju Wan is the representative formula for all stagnations: qi, blood, phlegm, food, damp and fire. Today, it is commonly used to treat depression, manifested by fullness, stifling sensations and pain in the chest, hypochondriac, and abdominal areas. Indigestion and a feeling of obstruction in the body are also common complaints.

Yue Ju Wan can also be used for women who are overweight due to excessive accumulation of dampness and phlegm, and consequently experiencing infertility.

Yue Ju Wan is the basic formula for treating the six stagnations. In this syndrome, qi stagnation is the primary condition, and stagnation of blood, phlegm, food, dampness and fire stagnations is the secondary condition. "Yue ju," figuratively means "to overcome an obstacle," and thus refers to the ability of this formula to help the body escape the restrained qi. Once qi flows smoothly, other stagnations will slowly be resolved.

Yue Ju Wan contains five herbs to treat six stagnations: *Xiang Fu* (Rhizoma Cyperi) activates qi circulation, *Chuan Xiong* (Rhizoma Chuanxiong) invigorates blood circulation, *Zhi Zi* (Fructus Gardeniae) clears fire, *Cang Zhu* (Rhizoma Atractylodis) dries dampness, and *Shen Qu* (Massa Fermentata) eliminates food stagnation. Since phlegm is formed secondary to the stagnations of qi, blood, dampness and food, phlegm will also be resolved when other stagnations are eliminated. However, if needed for more acute or severe conditions, herbs that transform phlegm may be added, such as *Ban Xia* (Rhizoma Pinelliae).

References

1. *Zhong Yi Fang Ji Xian Dai Yan Jiu* (Modern Study of Medical Formulae in Traditional Chinese Medicine) 1997;922-923.
2. *Jiang Su Zhong Yi* (Jiangsu Chinese Medicine) 1994;2:35.
3. *Si Chuan Zhong Yi* (Sichuan Chinese Medicine) 1986;4(5):18.
4. *Yun Nan Zhong Yi Za Zhi* (Yunan Journal of Chinese Medicine) 1992;13(5):16.
5. *Hu Nan Zhong Yi Za Zhi* (Hunan Journal of Chinese Medicine) 1989;5(1):9.
6. *Shan Dong Zhong Yi Za Zhi* (Shandong Journal of Chinese Medicine) 1991;10(6):19.

Chinese Herbal Formulas and Applications

Jīn Líng Zǐ Sǎn (Melia Toosendan Powder)

金铃子散
金铃子散

Pinyin Name: *Jin Ling Zi San*
Literal Name: Melia Toosendan Powder
Original Source: *Su Wen Bing Ji Qi Yi Bao Ming Ji* (Collection of Writings on the Mechanisms of Illness, Suitability of Qi, and the Safeguarding of Life as Discussed in the Basic Questions) by Zhang Yuan-Su in 1186

COMPOSITION

Chuan Lian Zi (Fructus Toosendan)	30g [9g]
Yan Hu Suo (Rhizoma Corydalis)	30g [9g]

DOSAGE / PREPARATION / ADMINISTRATION

The source text recommends grinding the ingredients into a fine powder and taking 9g per dose with grain-based liquor. Today, this formula may be given in decoction with the doses suggested in brackets.

CHINESE THERAPEUTIC ACTIONS

1. Regulates qi and soothes the Liver
2. Activates blood circulation and stops pain

CLINICAL MANIFESTATIONS

Liver qi stagnation with interior heat: intermittent pain in the chest, abdominal, and hypochondriac areas, a bitter taste in the mouth, red tongue with yellow tongue coating, and a wiry, rapid pulse.

CLINICAL APPLICATIONS

Biliary ascariasis and peptic ulcer disease.

EXPLANATION

Jin Ling Zi San (Melia Toosendan Powder) is the basic formula for treatment of various types of pain caused by Liver qi stagnation that has led to the formation of heat. The Liver stores blood and smoothes the flow of qi in the body to disperse stagnation. If Liver qi is stagnant, various pains in the chest, abdomen, and hypochondrium occur, as the Liver channel passes through these regions. Many of these symptoms are intermittent in nature, as onset and

relief are closely associated with emotions. A bitter taste in the mouth, red tongue body, a yellow tongue coating, and a wiry, rapid pulse indicate that the qi stagnation has created interior heat.

Chuan Lian Zi (Fructus Toosendan) soothes Liver qi and sedates Liver fire. *Yan Hu Suo* (Rhizoma Corydalis) activates qi and blood circulation to relieve pain. Together, the two herbs soothe the Liver and activate qi and blood circulation to relieve pain.

MODIFICATIONS

- With hypochondriac distention and pain due to Liver qi stagnation or Liver fire rising, add *Chai Hu* (Radix Bupleuri), *Yu Jin* (Radix Curcumae), and *Zhi Zi* (Fructus Gardeniae).
- For dysmenorrhea, add *Xiang Fu* (Rhizoma Cyperi), *Yi Mu Cao* (Herba Leonuri), *Dan Shen* (Radix et Rhizoma Salviae Miltiorrhizae), and *Hong Hua* (Flos Carthami).
- With hernial pain from qi stagnation, add *Ju He* (Semen Citri Reticulatae) and *Li Zhi He* (Semen Litchi).
- When cold accumulation causes hernial pain, add *Wu Zhu Yu* (Fructus Evodiae) and *Xiao Hui Xiang* (Fructus Foeniculi).
- With gallstones or kidney stones, add *Jin Qian Cao* (Herba Lysimachiae), *Ji Nei Jin* (Endothelium Corneum Gigeriae Galli), *Yu Jin* (Radix Curcumae), and *Hai Jin Sha* (Spora Lygodii).

Jin Ling Zi San (Melia Toosendan Powder)

Diagnosis	Signs and Symptoms	Treatment	Herbs
Liver qi stagnation with interior heat	• Intermittent pain in the chest, abdomen and hypochondrium: Liver qi stagnation with blood stasis • Bitter taste in the mouth, a red tongue with yellow coating, and a wiry, rapid pulse: qi stagnation creating interior heat	• Regulates qi and soothes the Liver • Activates blood circulation and stops pain	• *Chuan Lian Zi* (Fructus Toosendan) soothes Liver qi and sedates Liver fire. • *Yan Hu Suo* (Rhizoma Corydalis) activates qi and blood circulation to relieve pain.

12

QI-REGULATING FORMULAS

825

Chapter 12 – Qi-Regulating Formulas

Section 1 – Qi-Moving Formulas

Jīn Líng Zǐ Sǎn (Melia Toosendan Powder)

CAUTIONS / CONTRAINDICATIONS

Jin Ling Zi San contains herbs that activate qi and blood circulation and should be used with caution during pregnancy.

CLINICAL STUDIES AND RESEARCH

1. **Biliary ascariasis**: All 40 patients in one study reported complete recovery from biliary ascariasis using *Jin Ling Zi San*, *Si Ni San* (Frigid Extremities Powder), *Bing Lang* (Semen Arecae), *Wu Mei* (Fructus Mume), *Huang Lian* (Rhizoma Coptidis), *Zi Su Ye* (Folium Perillae), and others as needed. The duration of treatment ranged from 1-10 days, with an average of 4.2 days.[1]

2. **Peptic ulcer disease**: One study reported marked effectiveness in relieving pain associated with gastric or duodenal ulcers using *Jin Ling Zi San*, *Shao Yao Gan Cao Tang* (Peony and Licorice Decoction), and other herbs as needed. The herbal formula contained *Yan Hu Suo* (Rhizoma Corydalis) 9g, *Chuan Lian Zi* (Fructus Toosendan) 9g, *Gan Cao* (Radix et Rhizoma Glycyrrhizae) 9g, *Hai Piao Xiao* (Endoconcha Sepiae) 9g, *Xiang Fu* (Rhizoma Cyperi) 9g, *Pu Gong Ying* (Herba Taraxaci) 15g, *Chen Xiang* (Lignum Aquilariae Resinatum) 12g, *Wu Yao* (Radix Linderae) 6g, and *Bai Ji* (Rhizoma Bletillae) 15g. Furthermore, *Dang Shen* (Radix Codonopsis) and *Huang Qi* (Radix Astragali) were added for qi deficiency; *Gao Liang Jiang* (Rhizoma Alpiniae Officinarum) and *Rou Gui* (Cortex Cinnamomi) for Stomach cold; *Sha Shen* (Radix Glehniae seu Adenophorae) and *Mai Dong* (Radix Ophiopogonis) for Stomach yin deficiency; and *E Jiao* (Colla Corii Asini), *Zi Zhu* (Folium Callicarpae), and *San Qi* (Radix et Rhizoma Notoginseng) for gastrointestinal bleeding. Of 46 patients, the study reported complete recovery in 29 cases, improvement in 12 cases, and no effect in 5 cases. The overall rate of effectiveness was 89%.[2]

RELATED FORMULAS

Yán Hú Suǒ Sǎn (Corydalis Powder)
延胡索散
Pinyin Name: *Yan Hu Suo San*
Literal Name: Corydalis Powder
Original Source: *Ji Sheng Fang* (Formulas to Aid the Living) by Yan Yong-He in 1253

Dang Gui (Radix Angelicae Sinensis), *jin* (soaked) in liquor, *cuo* (grated) and *chao* (dry-fried)	15g
Yan Hu Suo (Rhizoma Corydalis), *chao* (dry-fried)	15g
Pu Huang (Pollen Typhae), *chao* (dry-fried)	15g
Chi Shao (Radix Paeoniae Rubra)	15g
Rou Gui (Cortex Cinnamomi), do not expose to heat	15g
Jiang Huang (Rhizoma Curcumae Longae), *xi* (washed)	9g
Ru Xiang (Gummi Olibanum)	9g

Mo Yao (Myrrha)	9g
Mu Xiang (Radix Aucklandiae), do not expose to heat	9g
Zhi Gan Cao (Radix et Rhizoma Glycyrrhizae Praeparata cum Melle)	7.5g

The source text recommends: grind the ingredients into coarse powder, cook 12g of the powder and 7 slices of *Sheng Jiang* (Rhizoma Zingiberis Recens) in 1.5 large bowls of water until it is reduced to 70%. Take the warm, strained decoction before meals.

Yan Hu Suo San (Corydalis Powder) activates qi and blood circulation to regulate menstruation and relieve pain. Clinically, it may be used for menstrual pain caused by qi and blood stagnation, which is characterized by abdominal pain that radiates to the lower back or ribs. This formula can also be used for painful menstruation accompanied by emotional disturbances.

Jin Ling Zi San and *Yan Hu Suo San* (Corydalis Powder) both relieve pain due to qi and blood stagnation.

• *Jin Ling Zi San* is cold in nature, and thus is more suitable for qi and blood stagnation with interior heat.

• *Yan Hu Suo San* is warm in nature, and stronger in its overall action. It is therefore more suitable for patients with more severe qi and blood stagnation accompanied by interior cold.

Yán Hú Yī Haò (Corydalis Formula One)
延胡一號
延胡一号
Pinyin Name: *Yan Hu Yi Hao*
Literal Name: Corydalis Formula One
Original Source: *An Hui Zhong Yi Xue Yuan* (Anhui University School of Medicine) in 1990

Yan Hu Suo (Rhizoma Corydalis)
Dan Shen (Radix et Rhizoma Salviae Miltiorrhizae)
Chuan Xiong (Rhizoma Chuanxiong)
Bai Zhi (Radix Angelicae Dahuricae)
Ge Gen (Radix Puerariae Lobatae)

The main actions of this formula are to activate qi and blood circulation, and relieve pain. Clinically, it may be used for pain due to qi and blood stagnation, especially in the upper body, such as headaches and migraines.

Yán Hú Èr Haò (Corydalis Formula Two)
延胡二號
延胡二号
Pinyin Name: *Yan Hu Er Hao*
Literal Name: Corydalis Formula Two

826

Chinese Herbal Formulas and Applications

Jīn Líng Zǐ Sǎn (Melia Toosendan Powder)

Original Source: *An Hui Zhong Yi Xue Yuan* (Anhui University School of Medicine) in 1990

Yan Hu Suo (Rhizoma Corydalis)
San Leng (Rhizoma Sparganii)
E Zhu (Rhizoma Curcumae)
Gui Zhi (Ramulus Cinnamomi)
Dang Gui (Radix Angelicae Sinensis)

This formula activates qi and blood circulation and relieves pain. Clinically, it may be used for pain due to qi and blood stagnation, especially in the extremities, such as leg and arm pain.

AUTHORS' COMMENTS

This formula is named *Jin Ling Zi San* (Melia Toosendan Powder) because *Jin Ling Zi* (Fructus Toosendan) is the chief herb. *Jin Ling Zi* and *Chuan Lian Zi* both refer to the same herb: Fructus Toosendan. Today, the formula's name remains the same, but the standard herb name used today is *Chuan Lian Zi*.[3]

Jin Ling Zi San is the key formula used to treat hypochondriac pain caused by Liver qi stagnation turning into Liver fire. It is also an excellent formula for treating pain associated with duct obstruction, such as gallstones or kidney stones.

References
1. *Guang Xi Zhong Yi Yao* (Guangxi Chinese Medicine and Herbology) 1985;8(1):14.
2. *Shi Yong Zhong Yi Yao Za Zhi* (Journal of Practical Chinese Medicine and Medicinals) 1995;6:15.
3. *Zhong Hua Ren Min Gong He Guo Yao Dian* V1 (Chinese Herbal Pharmacopoeia by the People's Republic of China, Volume One), People's Republic of China, 2005.

Bàn Xià Hòu Pò Tāng (Pinellia and Magnolia Bark Decoction)
半夏厚樸湯
半夏厚朴汤

Pinyin Name: *Ban Xia Hou Po Tang*
Literal Name: Pinellia and Magnolia Bark Decoction
Alternate Names: *Pan Hsia Hou Pu Tang, Ban Xia Hou Pu Tang*, Pinellia and Magnolia Decoction, Pinellia and Magnolia Combination
Original Source: *Jin Gui Yao Lue* (Essentials from the Golden Cabinet) by Zhang Zhong-Jing in the Eastern Han Dynasty

COMPOSITION

Ban Xia (Rhizoma Pinelliae)	1 cup [12g]
Hou Po (Cortex Magnoliae Officinalis)	9g
Fu Ling (Poria)	12g
Sheng Jiang (Rhizoma Zingiberis Recens)	15g [9g]
Zi Su Ye (Folium Perillae)	6g

DOSAGE / PREPARATION / ADMINISTRATION

The source text states to cook the ingredients in 7 cups [1,400 mL] of water and reduce it to 4 cups [800 mL]. Take the warm, strained decoction in four equally-divided doses, three times during the day and one time at night. Today, the decoction may be prepared using the doses suggested in brackets.

CHINESE THERAPEUTIC ACTIONS

1. Activates qi and disperses stagnation
2. Directs reversed flow of qi downward
3. Dissolves phlegm

CLINICAL MANIFESTATIONS

Mei he qi (plum-pit qi): a sensation that a foreign object (such as a plum pit) is stuck in the throat and cannot be spit out or swallowed, difficulty in swallowing food, possible coughing or vomiting, and chest and hypochondriac fullness and oppression.

12

QI-REGULATING FORMULAS

827

Chapter 12 – Qi-Regulating Formulas

Section 1 – Qi-Moving Formulas

Bàn Xià Hòu Pò Tāng (Pinellia and Magnolia Bark Decoction)

CLINICAL APPLICATIONS

Globus hystericus, pharyngeal paraesthesia, swallowing disorder in aspiration pneumonia, sleep choking syndrome (sleep apnea and hypopnea), swallowing disorder in Parkinson's disease, hysteria, neurasthenia, nervousness, stress and depression, panic disorder, chronic laryngitis, tracheitis, enteritis, esophageal spasms, gastroptosis, and gastroatonia.

EXPLANATION

Mei he qi (plum-pit *qi*) is the feeling of having a foreign substance (such as a plum pit) obstructing the throat which cannot be expectorated nor swallowed. Since there is no physical obstruction, the feeling cannot be relieved by expectorating or swallowing. This condition usually begins with the formation of Liver qi stagnation caused by emotional disturbances. As Liver qi stagnates, it also interferes with qi flow in the Lung and Stomach. As a result of qi stagnation, body fluids accumulate and eventually lead to phlegm obstruction. This condition of qi stagnation and phlegm obstruction affects various parts of the body, including the throat (a feeling that there is a foreign object stuck in the throat), Lung (coughing and fullness of the chest and hypochondrium), and Stomach (vomiting).

Ban Xia Hou Po Tang (Pinellia and Magnolia Bark Decoction) contains *Ban Xia* (Rhizoma Pinelliae) as the chief herb to dissolve and disperse phlegm, and restore the descending function of the Stomach to relieve vomiting. *Hou Po* (Cortex Magnoliae Officinalis) activates qi to help *Ban Xia* (Rhizoma Pinelliae) clear the phlegm obstruction; it also directs the reversed flow of Lung and Stomach qi downward to relieve fullness, coughing and vomiting. *Fu Ling* (Poria) helps *Ban Xia* (Rhizoma Pinelliae) eliminate dampness and phlegm through diuresis. *Sheng Jiang* (Rhizoma Zingiberis Recens) disperses stagnation and

harmonizes the Stomach and relieves vomiting. Aromatic *Zi Su Ye* (Folium Perillae) regulates the Lung qi flow and smoothes Liver qi.

MODIFICATIONS

- With more phlegm and saliva, add *Chen Pi* (Pericarpium Citri Reticulatae) and *Gan Cao* (Radix et Rhizoma Glycyrrhizae).
- When there is cough and dyspnea, add *Bei Mu* (Bulbus Fritillariae) and *Ku Xing Ren* (Semen Armeniacae Amarum).
- With fullness and distention in the chest and hypochondriac region, add *Mu Xiang* (Radix Aucklandiae), *Qing Pi* (Pericarpium Citri Reticulatae Viride), and *Zhi Qiao* (Fructus Aurantii).
- If accompanied by a dry mouth and throat, add *Sha Shen* (Radix Glehniae seu Adenophorae), *Mai Dong* (Radix Ophiopogonis), and *Xuan Shen* (Radix Scrophulariae).
- With hoarseness of voice, add *Xuan Shen* (Radix Scrophulariae), *Mai Dong* (Radix Ophiopogonis), *Jie Geng* (Radix Platycodonis), and *Zi Wan* (Radix et Rhizoma Asteris); or *Xiang Sheng Po Di San* (Loud Sound Resembling Broken Flute Powder).
- For phlegm accumulation and stagnation, combine with *Er Chen Tang* (Two-Cured Decoction).
- For food stagnation, combine with *Liu He Tang* (Harmonize the Six Decoction).
- If there is depression, combine with *Yue Ju Wan* (Escape Restraint Pill).
- With palpitations and insomnia, combine with *Gan Mai Da Zao Tang* (Licorice, Wheat, and Jujube Decoction).
- When the qi stagnation is severe, add *Xiang Fu* (Rhizoma Cyperi) and *Yu Jin* (Radix Curcumae); or *Chai Hu Shu Gan San* (Bupleurum Powder to Spread the Liver).
- With hypochondriac pain, add *Chuan Lian Zi* (Fructus Toosendan) and *Yan Hu Suo* (Rhizoma Corydalis).

Ban Xia Hou Po Tang (Pinellia and Magnolia Bark Decoction)

Diagnosis	Signs and Symptoms	Treatment	Herbs
Mei he qi (plum-pit *qi*)	• Feeling of having a foreign substance obstructing the throat: qi stagnation and phlegm obstruction • Coughing, chest and hypochondrium fullness: phlegm accumulation in the Lung • Vomiting: phlegm accumulation in the Stomach	• Activates qi and disperses stagnation • Directs reversed flow of qi downward • Dissolves phlegm	• *Ban Xia* (Rhizoma Pinelliae) dissolves and disperses phlegm and restores the descending function of the Stomach. • *Hou Po* (Cortex Magnoliae Officinalis) activates qi to clear phlegm obstruction, and reverses ascending Lung and Stomach qi. • *Fu Ling* (Poria) eliminates dampness and phlegm through diuresis. • *Sheng Jiang* (Rhizoma Zingiberis Recens) harmonizes the Stomach. • *Zi Su Ye* (Folium Perillae) regulates Lung qi flow and smoothes Liver qi circulation.

828

Bàn Xià Hòu Pò Tāng (Pinellia and Magnolia Bark Decoction)

- If there is throat pain, add *Xuan Shen* (Radix Scrophulariae) and *Jie Geng* (Radix Platycodonis).
- With throat spasms and tightness, add *Zhi Shi* (Fructus Aurantii Immaturus) and *Jie Geng* (Radix Platycodonis).
- With deficiency and cold of the Stomach, add *Wu Zhu Yu* (Fructus Evodiae).
- With stress and anxiety due to Liver qi stagnation, add *Chai Hu* (Radix Bupleuri), *Yu Jin* (Radix Curcumae), *Xiang Fu* (Rhizoma Cyperi), and *Qing Pi* (Pericarpium Citri Reticulatae Viride).
- With snoring characterized by wind-cold, add *Xin Yi San* (Magnolia Flower Powder).
- With snoring characterized by wind-heat, add *Cang Er Zi San* (Xanthium Powder).

CAUTIONS / CONTRAINDICATIONS

- *Ban Xia Hou Po Tang* is not suitable for yin-deficient patients with red cheeks, red tongue, scanty tongue coating, and/or a bitter taste, because many herbs in this formula are acrid, bitter, warm, and drying.
- Patients with internal heat due to qi stagnation should not use this formula.

PHARMACOLOGICAL EFFECTS

1. **Sedative**: Administration of this formula in rats at 4 g/kg/day for 6 days was associated with a reduction of spontaneous physical activities. The effect was more obvious in a dark environment, and less in a bright one. The sedative effect lasted for approximately 2 days upon discontinuation of the herbal therapy. Another report states that the use of this formula at 2-4 g/kg prolonged sleeping time induced by phenobarbitals.[1]
2. **Antiallergic**: According to one report, use of *Ban Xia Hou Po Tang* was effective in treating contact dermatitis in mice.[2]
3. **Effect on the throat**: *Ban Xia Hou Po Tang* has been used with great success to treat various disorders of the throat, such as *mei he qi* (plum-pit *qi*), a hoarse voice, swallowing reflex, and others. The mechanism of this effect was attributed to stimulation of neuropeptidergic nerves locally.[3]
4. **Anxiolytic**: According to one study, administration of *Ban Xia Hou Po Tang* was associated with a marked anxiolytic effect in mice. The effect was attributed to the component honokiol from *Hou Po* (Cortex Magnoliae Officinalis), because administration of the formula without *Hou Po* did not have any anxiolytic effect.[4]

CLINICAL STUDIES AND RESEARCH

1. *Mei he qi* (**plum-pit *qi***): Administration of *Ban Xia Hou Po Tang* plus *Wu Zhu Yu* (Fructus Evodiae) and *Huang Lian* (Rhizoma Coptidis) in 74 patients with plum-pit *qi* was associated with complete recovery in 9 cases, improvement in 24 cases, and no effect in 41 cases.[5]
2. **Pharyngeal paraesthesia**: Use of modified *Ban Xia Hou Po Tang* was effective in treating pharyngeal paraesthesia. In addition to *Ban Xia Hou Po Tang* as the base formula, modifications were made by adding *Xiang Fu* (Rhizoma Cyperi), *Chen Pi* (Pericarpium Citri Reticulatae), and *Gua Lou* (Fructus Trichosanthis) for individuals with emotional stress and instability with a feeling of fullness and distention in the chest and hypochondrium; and *Huang Qi* (Radix Astragali), *Sha Shen* (Radix Glehniae seu Adenophorae), *Huang Lian* (Rhizoma Coptidis), *Huang Qin* (Radix Scutellariae), *Da Zao* (Fructus Jujubae), and *Mu Dan Pi* (Cortex Moutan) for individuals with qi and yin deficiencies due to chronic illness with fatigue, lack of energy, irritability, and insomnia. Of 34 patients, the study reported complete recovery in 8 cases, significant improvement in 20 cases, moderate improvement in 4 cases, and no effect in 2 cases. The overall effectiveness was 84.1%.[6]
3. **Sleep choking syndrome (sleep apnea and hypopnea)**: One case study reported success using *Ban Xia Hou Po Tang* to treat a 44-year-old Japanese male who suffered from multiple episodes of sleep choking syndrome (sleep apnea and hypopnea) almost every night. The patient had normal respiration during sleep with the exception of apnea episodes (0.92 events/h) and hypopnea episodes (2.77 events/hour). The patient had unsuccessful treatment using 500mg of acetazolamide prior to herbal therapy.[7]
4. **Swallowing disorder in aspiration pneumonia**: One study evaluated the therapeutic effect of *Ban Xia Hou Po Tang* for treatment of depressed swallowing reflex in patients with aspiration pneumonia. Of 32 geriatric patients (mean age 74.2 +/- 1.7 years), 24 were treated with herbs (7.5 g/day) and 12 with placebo. After 4 weeks of treatment, the herb group responded much better than the placebo group, using various measurements of swallowing reflex. The researchers suggested that *Ban Xia Hou Po Tang* improves the impaired swallowing reflex and may help to prevent aspiration pneumonia in the elderly.[8]
5. **Swallowing disorder in Parkinson's disease**: Use of *Ban Xia Hou Po Tang* was beneficial in treating 23 patients with Parkinson's disease (PD). After 4 weeks of herbal therapy, it was noted that this formula significantly improved the swallowing reflex in PD patients, and therefore can be a hopeful candidate for preventing aspiration pneumonia in PD.[9]
6. **Parkinson's disease**: According to one study, 8 patients with Parkinson's disease were treated with herbs for 2 years with significant improvement in 6 cases and

Bàn Xià Hòu Pò Tāng (Pinellia and Magnolia Bark Decoction)

moderate improvement in 2 cases. The herbal treatment contained 2 formulas: *Ban Xia Hou Po Tang* plus *Yi Gan San* (Restrain the Liver Powder).[10]

7. **Enteritis**: One study reported good results using *Ban Xia Hou Po Tang* plus *Ping Wei San* (Calm the Stomach Powder) to treat acute enteritis. The herbal formula contained *Zi Su Geng* (Caulis Perillae) 6g, *Ban Xia* (Rhizoma Pinelliae) 6g, *Hou Po* (Cortex Magnoliae Officinalis) 4-6g, *Cang Zhu* (Rhizoma Atractylodis) 4-6g, *Fu Ling* (Poria) 9g, and *Gan Cao* (Radix et Rhizoma Glycyrrhizae) 3g. Of 129 patients, the study reported complete recovery in 81 cases, significant improvement in 42 cases, and improvement in 6 cases.[11]

8. ***Dian kuang* (mania and withdrawal)**: One study reported good results using modified *Ban Xia Hou Po Tang* to treat 21 patients with *dian kuang* (mania and withdrawal). The herbal formula contained *Ban Xia* (Rhizoma Pinelliae) 10g, *Hou Po* (Cortex Magnoliae Officinalis) 10g, *Fu Ling* (Poria) 10g, *Zi Su Geng* (Caulis Perillae) 7g, *Zhen Zhu Mu* (Concha Margaritiferae) 10g, *He Huan Pi* (Cortex Albiziae) 10g, *Jiu Jie Chang Pu* (Rhizoma Anemones Altaicae) 10g, *Dan Zhu Ye* (Herba Lophatheri) 5g, *Lian Zi Xin* (Plumula Nelumbinis) 10g, and others as needed. The duration of treatment ranged from 10 to 45 days. The study reported recovery in 19 of 21 cases, with 2 cases needing chlorpromazine as addition therapy.[12]

9. **Hysteria**: One study reported successful treatment in 103 of 104 patients with hysteria characterized by phlegm stagnation using modified *Ban Xia Hou Po Tang*. The duration of treatment ranged from 5-27 days. During follow-up visits 7 years later, the study reported stabilization in 91 of 94 who returned.[13]

10. **Stress and depression**: One study evaluated the clinical usefulness of herbal formulas for the treatment of stress and depression by examining the modulatory effects of the herbs on the hypothalamo-pituitary-adrenal axis and autonomic nervous function. Of several formulas tested, three were found to be effective in lowering plasma ACTH and cortisol levels under stress. The study stated that the modulatory effects of these formulas might be beneficial in treating stress-related diseases. Three formulas found to be effective were *Liu Jun Zi Tang* (Six-Gentlemen Decoction), *Ban Xia Xie Xin Tang* (Pinellia Decoction to Drain the Epigastrium), and *Ban Xia Hou Po Tang*.[14]

11. **Panic disorder**: Four patients diagnosed with panic disorder with agoraphobia in accordance with the Diagnostic and Statistical Manual of Mental Disorders (DSM) criteria were successfully treated with herbal medicine. Two patients were treated with *Ban Xia Hou Po Tang*, and two with *Jia Wei Xiao Yao San* (Augmented Rambling Powder). Both formulas successfully relieved panic attacks, anticipatory anxiety, and agoraphobia. The study concluded that these formulas may be useful as additional or alternative treatments for panic disorder.[15]

AUTHORS' COMMENTS

Ban Xia Hou Po Tang is the most famous formula for treating the feeling of a foreign object stuck in the throat, commonly known as *mei he qi* (plum-pit *qi*) in traditional Chinese medicine, or globus hystericus in Western medicine.

References

1. *Zhong Yi Fang Ji Xian Dai Yan Jiu* (Modern Study of Medical Formulae in Traditional Chinese Medicine) 1997;934.

2. *Guo Wai Yi Xue Zhong Yi Zhong Yao Fen Ce* (Monograph of Chinese Herbology from Foreign Medicine) 1982;6:46.

3. Naito T, Itoh H, Takeyama M. Effects of Hange-koboku-to (Banxia-houpo-tang) on neuropeptide levels in human plasma and saliva. Biol Pharm Bull 2003 Nov;26(11):1609-13.

4. Kuribara H, Kishi E, Hattori N, Okada M, Maruyama Y. The anxiolytic effect of two oriental herbal drugs in Japan attributed to honokiol from magnolia bark. J Pharm Pharmacol 2000 Nov;52(11):1425-9.

5. *Zhe Jiang Zhong Yi Za Zhi* (Zhejiang Journal of Chinese Medicine) 1983;8:345.

6. *Zhong Guo Zhong Xi Yi Jie He Za Zhi* (Chinese Journal of Integrative Chinese and Western Medicine) 1993;3:11.

7. Hisanaga A, Itoh T, Hasegawa Y, Emori K, Kita T, Okabe A, Kurachi M. A case of sleep choking syndrome improved by the Kampo extract of Hange-koboku-to. Psychiatry Clin Neurosci 2002 Jun;56(3):325-7.

8. Iwasaki K, Wang Q, Nakagawa T, Suzuki T, Sasaki H. The traditional Chinese medicine banxia houpo tang improves swallowing reflex. Phytomedicine 1999 May;6(2):103-6.

9. Iwasaki K, Wang Q, Seki H, Satoh K, Takeda A, Arai H, Sasaki H. The effects of the traditional chinese medicine, "Banxia Houpo Tang (Hange-Koboku To)" on the swallowing reflex in Parkinson's disease. Department of Geriatric Medicine, Tohoku University School of Medicine, Sendai, Japan. Phytomedicine 2000 Jul;7(4):259-63.

10. *Zhong Yi Ming Fang Lin Chuang Xin Yong* (Contemporary Clinical Applications of Classic Chinese Formulas) 2001;309.

11. *Fu Jian Zhong Yi Yao* (Fujian Chinese Medicine and Herbology) 1984;4:54.

12. *Jiang Xi Zhong Yi Yao* (Jiangxi Chinese Medicine and Herbology) 1989;20(4):34.

13. *Guo Wai Yi Xue Zhong Yi Zhong Yao Fen Ce* (Monograph of Chinese Herbology from Foreign Medicine) 1985;4:41.

14. Naito T, Itoh H, Takeyama M. Some gastrointestinal function regulatory Kampo medicines have modulatory effects on human plasma adrenocorticotropic hormone and cortisol levels with continual stress exposure. Biological & Pharmaceutical Bulletin 2003 Jan;26(1):101-4.

15. Mantani N, Hisanaga A, Kogure T, Kita T, Shimada Y, Terasawa K. Four cases of panic disorder successfully treated with Kampo (Japanese herbal) medicines: Kami-shoyo-san and Hange-koboku-to. Psychiatry & Clinical Neurosciences 2002 Dec;56(6):617-20.

Chinese Herbal Formulas and Applications

Zhǐ Shí Xiè Bái Guì Zhī Tāng
(Immature Bitter Orange, Chinese Chive, and Cinnamon Twig Decoction)

枳實薤白桂枝湯
枳实薤白桂枝汤

Pinyin Name: Zhi Shi Xie Bai Gui Zhi Tang
Literal Name: Immature Bitter Orange, Chinese Chive, and Cinnamon Twig Decoction
Original Source: *Jin Gui Yao Lue* (Essentials from the Golden Cabinet) by Zhang Zhong-Jing in the Eastern Han Dynasty

COMPOSITION

Zhi Shi (Fructus Aurantii Immaturus)	4 pieces [12g]
Hou Po (Cortex Magnoliae Officinalis)	12g
Xie Bai (Bulbus Allii Macrostemonis)	0.5 cup [9-12g]
Gui Zhi (Ramulus Cinnamomi)	3g [6g]
Gua Lou (Fructus Trichosanthis), *dao* (pounded)	1 piece [12-24g]

DOSAGE / PREPARATION / ADMINISTRATION

The source text states to cook *Zhi Shi* (Fructus Aurantii Immaturus) and *Hou Po* (Cortex Magnoliae Officinalis) first in 5 cups [1,000 mL] of water and reduce it down to 2 cups [400 mL]. Discard the residue, add the rest of the ingredients to the strained decoction, and cook it again to bring it to a few boils. Take the warm, strained decoction in three equally-divided doses in one day. Today, the decoction may be prepared using the doses suggested in brackets above.

CHINESE THERAPEUTIC ACTIONS

1. Unblocks yang and disperses stagnations
2. Dispels phlegm and directs qi flow downward

CLINICAL MANIFESTATIONS

Xiong bi (painful obstruction of the chest): chest fullness and pain, chest pain radiating to the back, wheezing, coughing with sputum, shortness of breath, a sensation of qi rushing upward from the hypochondrium to the heart, a white and greasy tongue coating, and a deep, wiry pulse or tight pulse.

CLINICAL APPLICATIONS

Pleuritis, epigastric pain, hypochondriac pain, and cholecystitis.

EXPLANATION

Zhi Shi Xie Bai Gui Zhi Tang (Immature Bitter Orange, Chinese Chive, and Cinnamon Twig Decoction) is designed to treat *xiong bi* (painful obstruction of the chest) due to yang deficiency, phlegm accumulation and qi stagnation in the chest region. Chest yang deficiency may result in abnormal dispersion and distribution of fluids in the body, leading to phlegm accumulation. Accumulation of phlegm may further lead to qi stagnation, which then

Zhi Shi Xie Bai Gui Zhi Tang (Immature Bitter Orange, Chinese Chive, and Cinnamon Twig Decoction)

Diagnosis	Signs and Symptoms	Treatment	Herbs
Xiong bi (painful obstruction of the chest)	• Chest fullness and pain: qi stagnation in the chest • Coughing and wheezing: phlegm stagnation affecting Lung qi circulation • White and greasy tongue coating: phlegm and damp accumulation • A deep, wiry or tight pulse: cold in the interior	• Unblocks yang and disperses stagnations • Dispels phlegm and directs qi flow downward	• *Zhi Shi* (Fructus Aurantii Immaturus) activates qi circulation and breaks up qi stagnation to relieve chest fullness and pain. • *Hou Po* (Cortex Magnoliae Officinalis) redirects rising qi, dispels phlegm, and relieves fullness. • *Xie Bai* (Bulbus Allii Macrostemonis) warms and unblocks yang and disperses stagnation in the chest. • *Gui Zhi* (Ramulus Cinnamomi) activates yang to disperse cold. • *Gua Lou* (Fructus Trichosanthis) disperses stagnation and dispels phlegm.

QI-REGULATING FORMULAS

12

831

Chapter 12 – Qi-Regulating Formulas　　　　　　　　　　　*Section 1 – Qi-Moving Formulas*

Zhǐ Shí Xiè Bái Guì Zhī Tāng
(Immature Bitter Orange, Chinese Chive, and Cinnamon Twig Decoction)

causes chest fullness and pain. Qi stagnation may cause reversed flow of qi, resulting in radiating pain and a sensation of qi rushing upwards. If phlegm interferes with the flow of Lung qi, then symptoms such as coughing and wheezing will occur. A white, greasy tongue coating and a deep, wiry pulse or tight pulse suggest cold and dampness in the interior.

In this formula, *Zhi Shi* (Fructus Aurantii Immaturus) activates qi circulation and breaks up qi stagnation to relieve the feeling of fullness and pain. *Hou Po* (Cortex Magnoliae Officinalis) redirects rising qi, dispels phlegm, and relieves chest fullness. *Xie Bai* (Bulbus Allii Macrostemonis), acrid and warm, is able to warm and unblock yang and disperse stagnation in the chest. *Gui Zhi* (Ramulus Cinnamomi) activates yang to disperse cold. *Gua Lou* (Fructus Trichosanthis) disperses stagnation and dispels phlegm.

RELATED FORMULAS

Guā Lóu Xiè Bái Bái Jiǔ Tāng
(Trichosanthes Fruit, Chinese Chive, and Wine Decoction)

栝樓薤白白酒湯
瓜蒌薤白白酒汤

Pinyin Name: *Gua Lou Xie Bai Bai Jiu Tang*
Literal Name: Trichosanthes Fruit, Chinese Chive, and Wine Decoction
Original Source: *Jin Gui Yao Lue* (Essentials from the Golden Cabinet) by Zhang Zhong-Jing in the Eastern Han Dynasty

Gua Lou (Fructus Trichosanthis)	1 piece [12-24g]
Xie Bai (Bulbus Allii Macrostemonis)	0.5 cup [9-12g]
Grain-based liquor	7 cups [1,400 mL]

The source text recommends cooking the ingredients together in 7 cups of grain-based liquor, and reducing the combination to 2 cups. Take the warm, strained decoction twice daily. Today, this formula may be prepared as a decoction in a mixture of water and grain-based liquor, using the doses suggested in brackets above.

Gua Lou Xie Bai Bai Jiu Tang (Trichosanthes Fruit, Chinese Chive, and Wine Decoction) unblock yang to disperse stagnation, and activate qi to dispel phlegm. Clinically, this formula is used to treat *xiong bi* (painful obstruction of the chest) with symptoms such as chest fullness and pain, chest pain radiating to the back, dyspnea, shortness of breath, a white, greasy tongue coating, and a deep, wiry pulse or tight pulse.

Guā Lóu Xiè Bái Bàn Xià Tāng
(Trichosanthes Fruit, Chinese Chive, and Pinellia Decoction)

栝樓薤白半夏湯
瓜蒌薤白半夏汤

Pinyin Name: *Gua Lou Xie Bai Ban Xia Tang*
Literal Name: Trichosanthes Fruit, Chinese Chive, and Pinellia Decoction
Alternate Name: Trichosanthes Fruit Chinese Chive and Pinellia Combination
Original Source: *Jin Gui Yao Lue* (Essentials from the Golden Cabinet) by Zhang Zhong-Jing in the Eastern Han Dynasty

Gua Lou (Fructus Trichosanthis)	1 piece [12-24g]
Xie Bai (Bulbus Allii Macrostemonis)	9g
Ban Xia (Rhizoma Pinelliae)	0.5 cup [12g]
Grain-based liquor	10 cups [2,000 mL]

The source text recommends cooking all of the ingredients together in 10 cups [2,000 mL] of grain-based liquor, and reducing it by cooking down to 4 cups [800 mL]. Take 1 cup of the warm, strained decoction three times daily. Today, this formula may be prepared as a decoction in a mixture of water and grain-based liquor with the doses suggested in brackets.

Gua Lou Xie Bai Ban Xia Tang (Trichosanthes Fruit, Chinese Chive, and Pinellia Decoction) unblocks yang, disperses stagnation, dispels phlegm, and relieves chest fullness. Clinically, this formula is used to treat *xiong bi* (painful obstruction of the chest) caused by phlegm stagnation, in which severe chest fullness and pain radiate to the back and disturb sleep.

Jiā Wèi Guā Lóu Xiè Bái Tāng
(Augmented Trichosanthes Fruit and Chinese Chive Decoction)

加味栝樓薤白湯
加味瓜蒌薤白汤

Pinyin Name: *Jia Wei Gua Lou Xie Bai Tang*
Literal Name: Augmented Trichosanthes Fruit and Chinese Chive Decoction
Original Source: *An Hui Zhong Yi Xue Yuan* (Anhui University School of Medicine) in 1990

Gua Lou Pi (Pericarpium Trichosanthis)
Xie Bai (Bulbus Allii Macrostemonis)
Dan Shen (Radix et Rhizoma Salviae Miltiorrhizae)
Hong Hua (Flos Carthami)
Dang Gui (Radix Angelicae Sinensis)
Chuan Xiong (Rhizoma Chuanxiong)

832

Chinese Herbal Formulas and Applications

Zhǐ Shí Xiè Bái Guì Zhī Tāng
(Immature Bitter Orange, Chinese Chive, and Cinnamon Twig Decoction)

Ge Gen (Radix Puerariae Lobatae)

Gui Zhi (Ramulus Cinnamomi)

Zhi Shi (Fructus Aurantii Immaturus)

Hou Po (Cortex Magnoliae Officinalis)

Jiang Xiang (Lignum Dalbergiae Odoriferae)

Tao Ren (Semen Persicae)

Ren Shen (Radix et Rhizoma Ginseng)

Bai Shao (Radix Paeoniae Alba)

Jia Wei Gua Lou Xie Bai Tang (Augmented Trichosanthes Fruit and Chinese Chive Decoction) unblocks yang, activates qi and blood circulation, and dispels qi and blood stagnation. This formula may be used clinically to treat *xiong bi* (painful obstruction of the chest) with symptoms such as chest fullness and pain, chest pain radiating to the back, dyspnea, shortness of breath, and a dark purple tongue with prominent or red petechiae.

AUTHORS' COMMENTS

Zhi Shi Xie Bai Gui Zhi Tang, Gua Lou Xie Bai Bai Jiu Tang (Trichosanthes Fruit, Chinese Chive, and Wine Decoction) and *Gua Lou Xie Bai Ban Xia Tang* (Trichosanthes Fruit, Chinese Chive, and Pinellia Decoction) all relieve *xiong bi* (painful obstruction of the chest) by unblocking yang, dispersing stagnation, activating qi circulation, and dispelling phlegm.

- *Zhi Shi Xie Bai Gui Zhi Tang* more strongly unblocks yang and dispels interior cold. It is used primarily for severe cases of *xiong bi* caused by stagnation of qi and phlegm.
- *Gua Lou Xie Bai Bai Jiu Tang* has a milder function of activating yang and dispelling phlegm, and therefore is more suitable for mild *xiong bi*.
- *Gua Lou Xie Bai Ban Xia Tang* more strongly dispels phlegm and relieves stagnation, and therefore is more suitable for the treatment of *xiong bi* caused by severe phlegm stagnation.

Jú Hé Wán (Tangerine Seed Pill)
橘核丸

Pinyin Name: *Ju He Wan*

Literal Name: Tangerine Seed Pill

Alternate Names: *Chu He Pi (Wan), Ju He Pi (Wan)*, Tangerine Pip Pill, Citrus Seed Formula

Original Source: *Ji Sheng Fang* (Formulas to Aid the Living) by Yan Yong-He in 1253

COMPOSITION

Ju He (Semen Citri Reticulatae), *chao* (dry-fried)	30g [9g]
Chuan Lian Zi (Fructus Toosendan), *chao* (dry-fried)	30g [9g]
Mu Xiang (Radix Aucklandiae), do not expose to heat	15g [6g]
Hou Po (Cortex Magnoliae Officinalis), *chao* (dry-fried) with ginger juice	15g [6g]
Zhi Shi (Fructus Aurantii Immaturus), *chao* (dry-fried) with bran	15g [6g]
Tao Ren (Semen Persicae), *chao* (dry-fried) with bran	30g [9g]
Yan Hu Suo (Rhizoma Corydalis), *chao* (dry-fried)	15g [6g]
Gui Xin (Cortex Rasus Cinnamomi), do not expose to heat	15g [6g]
Mu Tong (Caulis Akebiae)	15g [6g]
Hai Zao (Sargassum), *xi* (washed)	30g [9g]
Kun Bu (Thallus Eckloniae), *xi* (washed)	30g [9g]
Hai Dai (Thallus Laminariae), *xi* (washed)	30g [9g]

DOSAGE / PREPARATION / ADMINISTRATION

The source text recommends grinding the ingredients into a fine powder and forming into small pills with grain-based liquor. Take 70 pills [9g] per dose with salted grain-based liquor or lightly-salted water on an empty stomach one to two times daily. Today, this formula may be prepared as a decoction with the doses suggested in brackets above.

12

QI-REGULATING FORMULAS

833

Chapter 12 – Qi-Regulating Formulas   *Section 1 – Qi-Moving Formulas*

Jú Hé Wán (Tangerine Seed Pill)

CHINESE THERAPEUTIC ACTIONS
1. Activates qi circulation and stops pain
2. Softens hardness and disperses nodules

CLINICAL MANIFESTATIONS
Hernia caused by damp-cold: swelling and enlargement of the testicles, hardening (like a rock) of the testicles, and pain radiating from the testes to the abdomen.

CLINICAL APPLICATIONS
Hernia, hydrocele, orchitis, epididymitis, testitis, and fallopian tube obstruction.

EXPLANATION
Ju He Wan (Tangerine Seed Pill) is designed to treat hernia with swelling and enlargement of the testicles from damp-cold invading the Liver channel. Because the *jueyin* channel of the Liver passes through the inguinal region, it is closely related to the external genitalia. In the early stage of damp-cold attacking the Liver channel, hernia may be characterized by swelling and enlargement of the testicles. In the later stage, when qi and blood become stagnant, the testicles may harden, with pain radiating from the testes to the lower abdomen.

Ju He (Semen Citri Reticulatae), which activates qi circulation and disperses qi stagnation, is indicated specifically for treating hernia. *Chuan Lian Zi* (Fructus Toosendan) and *Mu Xiang* (Radix Aucklandiae) assist *Ju He* (Semen Citri Reticulatae) in activating qi circulation and relieving pain. *Hou Po* (Cortex Magnoliae Officinalis) activates qi circulation to dry dampness. *Zhi Shi* (Fructus Aurantii Immaturus) activates qi and disperses any hardness or stagnation. *Tao Ren* (Semen Persicae) activates blood circulation and disperses blood stagnation. *Yan Hu Suo* (Rhizoma Corydalis) activates qi and blood circulation to stop pain. *Gui Xin* (Cortex Rasus Cinnamomi) warms the Kidney and Liver to disperse cold. *Mu Tong* (Caulis Akebiae) opens the blood vessels of the lower *jiao* and dispels dampness through diuresis. *Hai Zao* (Sargassum), *Kun Bu* (Thallus Eckloniae) and *Hai Dai* (Thallus Laminariae) soften hardness and disperse nodules.

MODIFICATIONS
- When there is severe pain due to blood stagnation, add *San Leng* (Rhizoma Sparganii) and *E Zhu* (Rhizoma Curcumae).
- When there is severe pain due to cold, add *Xiao Hui Xiang* (Fructus Foeniculi) and *Wu Zhu Yu* (Fructus Evodiae). The doses of *Gui Xin* (Cortex Rasus Cinnamomi) and *Mu Xiang* (Radix Aucklandiae) should also be increased.
- When there is severe pain due to heat, add *Huang Qin* (Radix Scutellariae), *Huang Bo* (Cortex Phellodendri Chinensis), and *Long Dan* (Radix et Rhizoma Gentianae).

Ju He Wan (Tangerine Seed Pill)

Diagnosis	Signs and Symptoms	Treatment	Herbs
Hernia caused by damp-cold	• Hernia with swelling and enlargement of the testicles: damp-cold attacking the Liver channel • Hardening of the testicles with pain radiating to the abdomen: qi and blood stagnation	• Activates qi circulation and stops pain • Softens hardness and disperses nodules	• *Ju He* (Semen Citri Reticulatae) activates qi circulation and disperses qi stagnation to treat hernia. • *Chuan Lian Zi* (Fructus Toosendan) and *Mu Xiang* (Radix Aucklandiae) activate qi circulation and stop pain. • *Hou Po* (Cortex Magnoliae Officinalis) activates qi circulation to dry dampness. • *Zhi Shi* (Fructus Aurantii Immaturus) activates qi and disperses any hardness or stagnation. • *Tao Ren* (Semen Persicae) activates blood circulation and disperses blood stagnation. • *Yan Hu Suo* (Rhizoma Corydalis) activates qi and blood circulation to stop pain. • *Gui Xin* (Cortex Rasus Cinnamomi) warms the Kidney and Liver to disperse coldness. • *Mu Tong* (Caulis Akebiae) opens the blood vessels of the lower *jiao* and dispels dampness through diuresis. • *Hai Zao* (Sargassum), *Kun Bu* (Thallus Eckloniae) and *Hai Dai* (Thallus Laminariae) soften hardness and disperse nodules.

834

Chinese Herbal Formulas and Applications

Jú Hé Wán (Tangerine Seed Pill)

- With redness, swelling, and itching of the scrotum, add *Huang Bo* (Cortex Phellodendri Chinensis), *Tu Fu Ling* (Rhizoma Smilacis Glabrae), and *Che Qian Zi* (Semen Plantaginis).

CLINICAL STUDIES AND RESEARCH

Female infertility due to obstructed fallopian tubes: According to one study, use of 9g of *Ju He Wan*, twice daily for 1-6 months, was effective in treating infertility due to blockage of the fallopian tubes. Of 96 patients, the study reported successful pregnancy in 39 cases, unblocked fallopian tubes in 25 cases, and improvement in 32 cases.[1]

AUTHORS' COMMENTS

Ju He Wan has been used historically to treat damp-cold hernia. Today, it has been found that this formula is also effective in treating female infertility arising from blockage of the fallopian tubes.

Ju He Wan, *Tian Tai Wu Yao San* (Top-Quality Lindera Powder) and *Nuan Gan Jian* (Warm the Liver Decoction) are three formulas commonly used to treat hernias caused by cold. The differences are as follows:

- *Ju He Wan* treats hernia caused by cold and dampness, in which the testicles are swollen, enlarged, and hardened.
- *Tian Tai Wu Yao San* treats intestinal hernia in which there is severe cold and qi stagnation.
- *Nuan Gan Jian* treats hernia characterized by Liver and Kidney deficiencies with cold accumulation and qi stagnation. Hernia is usually accompanied by lower abdominal pain without anatomical or physical changes.

Reference
1. *Shan Xi Zhong Yi* (Shanxi Chinese Medicine) 1992;8(4):17.

Tiān Tái Wū Yào Sǎn (Top-Quality Lindera Powder)

天臺烏藥散
天台乌药散

Pinyin Name: *Tian Tai Wu Yao San*
Literal Name: Top-Quality Lindera Powder
Original Source: *Yi Xue Fa Ming* (Medical Innovations) by Li Gao in the Jin Dynasty

COMPOSITION

Wu Yao (Radix Linderae)	15g [12g]
Mu Xiang (Radix Aucklandiae)	15g [6g]
Xiao Hui Xiang (Fructus Foeniculi)	15g [6g]
Qing Pi (Pericarpium Citri Reticulatae Viride)	15g [6g]
Gao Liang Jiang (Rhizoma Alpiniae Officinarum)	15g [9g]
Bing Lang (Semen Arecae)	2 pieces [9g]
Chuan Lian Zi (Fructus Toosendan)	10 pieces [12g]
Ba Dou (Semen Crotonis)	70 pieces [12g]

DOSAGE / PREPARATION / ADMINISTRATION

The source text recommends cracking open *Ba Dou* (Semen Crotonis) and dry-frying it with *Chuan Lian Zi* (Fructus Toosendan) and bran until the color turns from brown to black. Discard *Ba Dou* (Semen Crotonis) and the bran. Grind *Chuan Lian Zi* (Fructus Toosendan) and the other ingredients into powder. Take 3g of the powder per dose with warm grain-based liquor.

Today, this formula may be prepared as a decoction with the doses suggested in brackets above. First, dry-fry *Ba Dou* (Semen Crotonis) and *Chuan Lian Zi* (Fructus Toosendan) until their color turns from brown to black. Discard *Ba Dou* (Semen Crotonis), and cook *Chuan Lian Zi* (Fructus Toosendan) with the rest of the herbs in water. Take the warm, strained decoction with a small amount of grain-based liquor.

835

Chapter 12 – Qi-Regulating Formulas　　　　　　　　　　　　　　*Section 1 – Qi-Moving Formulas*

Tiān Tái Wū Yào Săn (Top-Quality Lindera Powder)

CHINESE THERAPEUTIC ACTIONS
1. Activates qi circulation and spreads Liver qi
2. Disperses cold and stops pain

CLINICAL MANIFESTATIONS
Hernia due to cold accumulation and qi stagnation: hernia of the small intestine, pain of the lower abdomen, and pain and swelling of the testicles.

CLINICAL APPLICATIONS
Hernia and leukorrhea.

EXPLANATION
The *jueyin* channel of the Liver passes through the inguinal region and the abdomen. Therefore, if cold stagnates along the pathway of the Liver channel, hernia could occur. *Tian Tai Wu Yao San* (Top-Quality Lindera Powder) is designed to treat hernia of the small intestine with pain and swelling of the testicles due to cold accumulation and qi stagnation.

This formula uses *Wu Yao* (Radix Linderae) to activate qi, spread Liver qi, and disperse cold to relieve pain. *Mu Xiang* (Radix Aucklandiae), *Xiao Hui Xiang* (Fructus Foeniculi), *Qing Pi* (Pericarpium Citri Reticulatae Viride), and *Gao Liang Jiang* (Rhizoma Alpiniae Officinarum) activate qi circulation, disperse stagnation, and dispel cold. *Bing Lang* (Semen Arecae) enters the lower *jiao* to activate qi circulation, dissolve stagnation, and disperse hardness. *Chuan Lian Zi* (Fructus Toosendan) activates qi circulation and disperses stagnation. Lastly, the hot nature of *Ba Dou* (Semen Crotonis) reduces the cold influence of *Chuan Lian Zi* (Fructus Toosendan) to enhance the overall benefit and minimize side effects. However, *Ba Dou* (Semen Crotonis) is discarded as its drastic purgative effect may adversely affect the patient.

MODIFICATIONS
- If there is severe cold, add *Wu Zhu Yu* (Fructus Evodiae) and *Rou Gui* (Cortex Cinnamomi).
- When there is blood stagnation, add *Tao Ren* (Semen Persicae) and *Hong Hua* (Flos Carthami).
- With severe pain, add *Chen Xiang* (Lignum Aquilariae Resinatum).
- To enhance the treatment of hernia, add *Ju He* (Semen Citri Reticulatae), *Li Zhi He* (Semen Litchi), *Chai Hu* (Radix Bupleuri), *Xiang Fu* (Rhizoma Cyperi), and *Yan Hu Suo* (Rhizoma Corydalis).
- With a feeling of prolapse and swelling, add *Li Zhi He* (Semen Litchi), *Ju He* (Semen Citri Reticulatae); or *Ju He Wan* (Tangerine Seed Pill).

CAUTIONS / CONTRAINDICATIONS
Tian Tai Wu Yao San is contraindicated when the hernia is caused by damp-heat in the lower *jiao*.

RELATED FORMULAS
Sān Céng Huí Xiāng Wán
(Fennel Seed Pill with Three Levels)
三層茴香丸
三层茴香丸
Pinyin Name: *San Ceng Hui Xiang Wan*
Literal Name: Fennel Seed Pill with Three Levels
Original Source: *Jing Yue Quan Shu* (Collected Treatises of [Zhang] Jing Yue) by Zhang Jie-Bin (Zhang Jing-Yue) in 1624

San Ceng Hui Xiang Wan (Fennel Seed Pill with Three Levels) actually consists of three formulas, or levels, to be used for different degrees of severity. The treatment protocol is to begin with the Level One formula, which should be sufficient for mild cases of hernial pain. If the

Tian Tai Wu Yao San (Top-Quality Lindera Powder)

Diagnosis	Signs and Symptoms	Treatment	Herbs
Hernia due to cold accumulation and qi stagnation	Hernia of the small intestine, lower abdominal pain, and testicular swelling and pain: cold accumulation and qi stagnation along the Liver channel	• Activates qi circulation and spreads Liver qi • Disperses cold and stops pain	• *Wu Yao* (Radix Linderae) activates qi, spreads Liver qi, and disperses cold to relieve pain. • *Mu Xiang* (Radix Aucklandiae), *Xiao Hui Xiang* (Fructus Foeniculi), *Qing Pi* (Pericarpium Citri Reticulatae Viride) and *Gao Liang Jiang* (Rhizoma Alpiniae Officinarum) activate qi circulation, disperse stagnation and dispel cold. • *Bing Lang* (Semen Arecae) enters the lower *jiao* to activate qi circulation, dissolve stagnation and disperse hardness. • *Chuan Lian Zi* (Fructus Toosendan) activates qi circulation and disperses stagnation.

836

Chinese Herbal Formulas and Applications

Tiān Tái Wū Yào Săn (Top-Quality Lindera Powder)

pain continues, Level Two and then Level Three formulas may be used.

Level One:

Xiao Hui Xiang (Fructus Foeniculi),	
chao (dry-fried) with salt till yellow	30g
Sha Shen (Radix Glehniae seu Adenophorae),	
xi (washed)	30g
Chuan Lian Zi (Fructus Toosendan), *pao* (blast-fried)	30g
Mu Xiang (Radix Aucklandiae)	30g

Level Two:

Xiao Hui Xiang (Fructus Foeniculi),	
chao (dry-fried) with salt till yellow	30g
Sha Shen (Radix Glehniae seu Adenophorae),	
xi (washed)	30g
Chuan Lian Zi (Fructus Toosendan), *pao* (blast-fried)	30g
Mu Xiang (Radix Aucklandiae)	30g
Bi Bo (Fructus Piperis Longi)	30g
Bing Lang (Semen Arecae)	15g

Level Three:

Xiao Hui Xiang (Fructus Foeniculi),	
chao (dry-fried) with salt till yellow	30g
Sha Shen (Radix Glehniae seu Adenophorae),	
xi (washed)	30g
Chuan Lian Zi (Fructus Toosendan), *pao* (blast-fried)	30g
Mu Xiang (Radix Aucklandiae)	30g
Bi Bo (Fructus Piperis Longi)	30g
Bing Lang (Semen Arecae)	15g
Fu Ling (Poria)	120g
Fu Zi (Radix Aconiti Lateralis Praeparata),	
pao (blast-fried)	15-30g

The source text recommends grinding all the ingredients into powder, and mixing with rice paste to form pills. The pills should resemble *Lu Dou* (Semen Phaseoli Radiati) in size. Take 20-30 pills per dose on an empty stomach, three times daily with warm grain-based liquor or salted water. The dose may be increased up to 30-40 pills depending on the severity of the condition.

The main actions of these three formula are to warm the Kidney, dispel cold, regulate Liver qi circulation, and relieve hernial pain. Clinically, the patient may have a "cold hernia" characterized by lower abdominal pain, cold testicles, enlargement and hardening of the testicles, and an enlarged scrotum that makes walking difficult.

Dǎo Qì Tāng (Conduct the Qi Decoction)
導氣湯
导气汤
Pinyin Name: *Dao Qi Tang*
Literal Name: Conduct the Qi Decoction
Original Source: *Shen Shi Zun Sheng Shu* (Master Shen's Book for Revering Life) by Shen Jin-Ao in 1773

Chuan Lian Zi (Fructus Toosendan)	12g
Mu Xiang (Radix Aucklandiae)	9g
Xiao Hui Xiang (Fructus Foeniculi)	6g
Wu Zhu Yu (Fructus Evodiae),	
pao (blast-fried) with liquid	3g

The source text recommends preparing the ingredients as a decoction. *Dao Qi Tang* (Conduct the Qi Decoction) activates qi circulation, spreads Liver qi, disperses cold, and relieves hernial pain. Clinically, this formula treats painful cold hernia.

AUTHORS' COMMENTS

Ju He Wan (Tangerine Seed Pill) and *Tian Tai Wu Yao San* both treat hernias caused by cold. The differences are as follows:

- *Ju He Wan* treats hernia caused by cold and damp accumulating in the body over a prolonged period of time, which causes the testicles to swell, enlarge, and harden.
- *Tian Tai Wu Yao San* treats hernia in which there is severe qi stagnation caused by Liver and Kidney deficiencies accompanied by coldness.

Tian Tai Wu Yao San, *San Ceng Hui Xiang Wan* (Fennel Seed Pill with Three Levels), and *Dao Qi Tang* (Conduct the Qi Decoction) all treat hernia characterized by qi and cold stagnation, but have the following differences:

- *Tian Tai Wu Yao San* more strongly regulates and spreads Liver qi.
- *San Ceng Hui Xiang Wan* more effectively disperses cold and warms the Kidney.
- *Dao Qi Tang* is similar in function to *Tian Tai Wu Yao San*, but is less potent.

12

QI-REGULATING FORMULAS

837

Chapter 12 – Qi-Regulating Formulas   *Section 1 – Qi-Moving Formulas*

Nuǎn Gān Jiān (Warm the Liver Decoction)

暖肝煎

Pinyin Name: *Nuan Gan Jian*
Literal Name: Warm the Liver Decoction
Original Source: *Jing Yue Quan Shu* (Collected Treatises of [Zhang] Jing Yue) by Zhang Jie-Bin (Zhang Jing-Yue) in 1624

COMPOSITION

Dang Gui (Radix Angelicae Sinensis)	6-9g
Gou Qi Zi (Fructus Lycii)	9g
Rou Gui (Cortex Cinnamomi)	3-6g
Xiao Hui Xiang (Fructus Foeniculi)	6g
Wu Yao (Radix Linderae)	6g
Chen Xiang (Lignum Aquilariae Resinatum)	3g
Fu Ling (Poria)	6g

DOSAGE / PREPARATION / ADMINISTRATION

The source text states to cook the ingredients with 3-5 slices of *Sheng Jiang* (Rhizoma Zingiberis Recens) in 1.5 bowls of water until it is reduced to 70%. Take the warm, strained decoction between meals. Note: If *Chen Xiang* (Lignum Aquilariae Resinatum) is unavailable, *Mu Xiang* (Radix Aucklandiae) may be used as a substitute.

CHINESE THERAPEUTIC ACTIONS

1. Warms the Liver and Kidney
2. Activates qi circulation, dispels cold, and stops pain

CLINICAL MANIFESTATIONS

Hernia due to cold in the Liver and Kidney channels: lower abdominal pain, hernia, and hardening of the testes.

CLINICAL APPLICATIONS

Hernia, chronic appendicitis, and urinary stones.

EXPLANATION

Nuan Gan Jian (Warm the Liver Decoction) is designed to treat hernia caused by cold of the Liver and Kidney.

Because both the Liver and Kidney channels pass through the lower abdomen, cold obstruction may lead to hernia and pain. Effective treatment of this syndrome requires warming the Liver and Kidney to address the cause, and activating qi circulation and dispelling cold to relieve the symptoms.

In this formula, *Dang Gui* (Radix Angelicae Sinensis) and *Gou Qi Zi* (Fructus Lycii) warm and tonify the Kidney and Liver. *Rou Gui* (Cortex Cinnamomi) and *Xiao Hui Xiang* (Fructus Foeniculi) warm the Kidney and Liver to dispel cold. *Wu Yao* (Radix Linderae) and *Chen Xiang* (Lignum Aquilariae Resinatum) activate qi to stop pain. *Fu Ling* (Poria) strengthens the Spleen and dispels dampness. *Sheng Jiang* (Rhizoma Zingiberis Recens) disperses cold and harmonizes the Stomach.

MODIFICATIONS

• With more cold, add *Wu Zhu Yu* (Fructus Evodiae), *Gan Jiang* (Rhizoma Zingiberis), and if necessary, *Fu Zi* (Radix Aconiti Lateralis Praeparata).

Nuan Gan Jian (Warm the Liver Decoction)

Diagnosis	Signs and Symptoms	Treatment	Herbs
Hernia due to cold in the Liver and Kidney channels	Hernia, hardening of testes, and lower abdominal pain: cold in the Liver and Kidney channels	• Warms the Liver and Kidney • Activates qi circulation, dispels cold, and stops pain	• *Dang Gui* (Radix Angelicae Sinensis) and *Gou Qi Zi* (Fructus Lycii) warm and tonify the Kidney and Liver. • *Rou Gui* (Cortex Cinnamomi) and *Xiao Hui Xiang* (Fructus Foeniculi) warm the Kidney and Liver to dispel cold. • *Wu Yao* (Radix Linderae) and *Chen Xiang* (Lignum Aquilariae Resinatum) activate qi to stop pain. • *Fu Ling* (Poria) strengthens the Spleen and dispels dampness. • *Sheng Jiang* (Rhizoma Zingiberis Recens) disperses cold and harmonizes the Stomach.

838

Nuǎn Gān Jiān (Warm the Liver Decoction)

- With more abdominal pain, add *Xiang Fu* (Rhizoma Cyperi).
- For testicular pain, add *Qing Pi* (Pericarpium Citri Reticulatae Viride) and *Ju He* (Semen Citri Reticulatae).

CAUTIONS / CONTRAINDICATIONS

Nuan Gan Jian is contraindicated in hernia with redness, swelling, and pain of the testicles caused by damp-heat in the lower *jiao*.

CLINICAL STUDIES AND RESEARCH

1. **Hernia**: Administration of modified *Nuan Gan Jian* successfully treated hernia in 251 patients between 1 and 70 years of age, with 1-3 year history of illness. The base formula contained *Gou Qi Zi* (Fructus Lycii) 15g, *Dang Gui* (Radix Angelicae Sinensis) 15g, *Fu Ling* (Poria) 15g, *Xiao Hui Xiang* (Fructus Foeniculi) 10g, *Wu Yao* (Radix Linderae) 10g, *Rou Gui* (Cortex Cinnamomi) 10g, and *Chen Xiang* (Lignum Aquilariae Resinatum) 5g. Additional modifications were made based on each patient's differential diagnosis. Herbs also were applied topically as an herbal paste when deemed necessary. The herbs were given in decoction daily for 7 days per course of treatment. Of 251 patients, the study reported resolution of symptoms in 195 cases, significant improvement in 22 cases, slight improvement in 16 cases, and no effect in 18 cases. The overall rate of effectiveness was 92.8%.[1]

2. **Chronic appendicitis**: One study reported good results treating chronic appendicitis using herbs both orally and topically. The herbal formula contained *Xiao Hui Xiang* (Fructus Foeniculi) 6g, *Rou Gui* (Cortex Cinnamomi) 6g, *Chen Xiang* (Lignum Aquilariae Resinatum) 6g, *Wu Yao* (Radix Linderae) 9g, *Dang Gui* (Radix Angelicae Sinensis) 9g, *Chuan Xiong* (Rhizoma Chuanxiong) 9g, and *Fu Ling* (Poria) 9g. Modifications were made as follows: *Shui Zhi* (Hirudo) 6g for pain upon palpation at lower right corner of the abdomen; and *Zhi Qiao* (Fructus Aurantii) 9g and *Bing Lang* (Semen Arecae) 9g for abdominal distention without pain upon palpation. The treatment protocol was to administer the herbs in decoction. The herb residue was put in a cloth bag while warm, and placed on the lower right corner of the lower abdomen for 30 minutes. The process (oral ingestion and topical application of herbs) was repeated one time per day for 10 days per course of treatment. Of 20 patients, the study reported complete recovery in 9 cases, significant improvement in 6 cases, moderate improvement in 4 cases, and no benefit in 1 case. The overall rate of effectiveness was 95%.[2]

AUTHORS' COMMENTS

Tian Tai Wu Yao San (Top-Quality Lindera Powder) and *Nuan Gan Jian* are two formulas commonly used in the treatment of hernia:

- *Tian Tai Wu Yao San* is better for hernias characterized more by qi stagnation than by cold.
- *Nuan Gan Jian* warms the Liver and is better for hernias characterized by more cold than qi stagnation.

References

1. *Shan Xi Zhong Yi* (Shanxi Chinese Medicine) 1995;16(1):15.
2. *Shi Yong Zhong Yi Nei Ke Za Zhi* (Journal of Practical Chinese Internal Medicine) 1994;8(2):29.

Chapter 12 – Qi-Regulating Formulas   *Section 1 – Qi-Moving Formulas*

Hòu Pò Wēn Zhōng Tāng
(Magnolia Bark Decoction for Warming the Middle)

厚楔溫中湯

厚朴温中汤

Pinyin Name: *Hou Po Wen Zhong Tang*
Literal Name: Magnolia Bark Decoction for Warming the Middle
Alternate Name: Magnolia Combination
Original Source: *Nei Wai Shang Bian Huo Lun* (Clarifying Doubts about Injury from Internal and External Causes) by Li Gao in 1247

COMPOSITION

Hou Po (Cortex Magnoliae Officinalis), *zhi* (prepared) with ginger	30g
Chen Pi (Pericarpium Citri Reticulatae)	30g
Mu Xiang (Radix Aucklandiae)	15g
Cao Dou Kou (Semen Alpiniae Katsumadai)	15g
Gan Jiang (Rhizoma Zingiberis)	2.1g
Fu Ling (Poria)	15g
Zhi Gan Cao (Radix et Rhizoma Glycyrrhizae Praeparata cum Melle)	15g

DOSAGE / PREPARATION / ADMINISTRATION

The source text recommends grinding the ingredients into a coarse powder. Cook 15g of the powder and 3 slices of *Sheng Jiang* (Rhizoma Zingiberis Recens) in 2 large bowls of water until it is reduced to one bowl. Take the warm, strained decoction before meals.

CHINESE THERAPEUTIC ACTIONS

1. Warms the middle *jiao* and activates qi circulation
2. Dries dampness and relieves abdominal fullness

CLINICAL MANIFESTATIONS

Damp-cold affecting the Spleen and Stomach: epigastric and abdominal distention, fullness and/or pain, low appetite, lethargy, white tongue coating, and a deep, wiry pulse.

CLINICAL APPLICATIONS

Peptic ulcer, chronic gastritis, chronic enteritis, chronic colitis, inflammatory bowel syndrome, chronic pancreatitis, and leukorrhea.

EXPLANATION

Hou Po Wen Zhong Tang (Magnolia Bark Decoction for Warming the Middle) treats various symptoms caused by damp-cold in the Spleen and Stomach. Dampness has a greasy and sticky character, while cold is constricting and stagnating by nature. Combined, these factors slow the circulation of qi and disrupt the ascending and descending functions of the Spleen and Stomach. As a result, abdominal fullness and pain, poor appetite, and lethargy manifest.

This formula contains *Hou Po* (Cortex Magnoliae Officinalis) to activate qi, dry dampness, and reduce distention and fullness. *Chen Pi* (Pericarpium Citri Reticulatae) and *Mu Xiang* (Radix Aucklandiae) activate qi and relieve pain. *Cao Dou Kou* (Semen Alpiniae Katsumadai) warms the middle *jiao*, dispels cold, dries dampness, and eliminates phlegm. *Gan Jiang* (Rhizoma Zingiberis) and *Sheng Jiang* (Rhizoma Zingiberis Recens) warm the Spleen and Stomach to dispel cold. *Fu Ling* (Poria) and *Zhi Gan Cao* (Radix et Rhizoma Glycyrrhizae Praeparata cum Melle) dispel dampness and strengthen the middle *jiao*.

Because the emphasis of this formula is on warming the middle *jiao*, it is also effective in treating nausea, vomiting, and epigastric pain resulting from cold invading the Stomach.

MODIFICATIONS

- With abdominal pain and diarrhea, add *Cang Zhu* (Rhizoma Atractylodis) and *Sha Ren* (Fructus Amomi).
- With nausea and vomiting of clear watery vomitus, add *Ban Xia* (Rhizoma Pinelliae) and *Bai Zhu* (Rhizoma Atractylodis Macrocephalae).
- For food stagnation, add *Shan Zha* (Fructus Crataegi) and *Shen Qu* (Massa Fermentata).
- When accompanied by a cold body and extremities due to deficiency and cold, add *Fu Zi* (Radix Aconiti Lateralis Praeparata) and *Rou Gui* (Cortex Cinnamomi).
- With edema and a feeling of heaviness in the body, add *Da Fu Pi* (Pericarpium Arecae).
- If there is severe pain, add *Rou Gui* (Cortex Cinnamomi) and *Gao Liang Jiang* (Rhizoma Alpiniae Officinarum).

840

Chinese Herbal Formulas and Applications

Hòu Pò Wēn Zhōng Tāng
(Magnolia Bark Decoction for Warming the Middle)

Hou Po Wen Zhong Tang (Magnolia Bark Decoction for Warming the Middle)

Diagnosis	Signs and Symptoms	Treatment	Herbs
Damp-cold affecting the Spleen and Stomach	• Epigastric and abdominal distention, fullness or pain: damp-cold in the Spleen and Stomach • Low appetite and lethargy: damp-cold accumulation affecting digestive functions	• Warms the middle *jiao* and activates qi circulation • Dries dampness and relieves abdominal fullness	• *Hou Po* (Cortex Magnoliae Officinalis) activates qi, dries dampness, and reduces distention and fullness. • *Chen Pi* (Pericarpium Citri Reticulatae) and *Mu Xiang* (Radix Aucklandiae) activate qi and relieve pain. • *Cao Dou Kou* (Semen Alpiniae Katsumadai) warms the middle *jiao*, dispels cold, dries dampness, and eliminates phlegm. • *Gan Jiang* (Rhizoma Zingiberis) and *Sheng Jiang* (Rhizoma Zingiberis Recens) warm the Spleen and Stomach to dispel cold. • *Fu Ling* (Poria) and *Zhi Gan Cao* (Radix et Rhizoma Glycyrrhizae Praeparata cum Melle) dispel dampness and strengthen the middle *jiao*.

CAUTIONS / CONTRAINDICATIONS

Avoid cold and raw foods while taking *Hou Po Wen Zhong Tang*.

RELATED FORMULA

Liáng Fù Wán (Galangal and Cyperus Pill)

良附丸

Pinyin Name: *Liang Fu Wan*
Literal Name: Galangal and Cyperus Pill
Original Source: *Liang Fang Yi Ye* (Small Collection of Fine Formulas) by Xie Yuan-Qing in 1842

Gao Liang Jiang (Rhizoma Alpiniae Officinarum),
    xi (washed) with liquor 7 times, *bei* (stone baked)
    and *yan* (ground) to small particles   [9g]
Xiang Fu (Rhizoma Cyperi), *xi* (washed) with
    vinegar 7 times, *bei* (stone baked) and
    yan (ground) to small particles   [9g]

The source text recommends using equal amounts of *Gao Liang Jiang* (Rhizoma Alpiniae Officinarum) and *Xiang Fu* (Rhizoma Cyperi). Wash *Gao Liang Jiang* (Rhizoma Alpiniae Officinarum) with a grain-based liquor, stone-bake it, and grind it into powder. Wash *Xiang Fu* (Rhizoma Cyperi) in vinegar, stone-bake it, and grind it into powder. The source text specifically instructs to prepare and store these two herbs separately. Immediately before serving, mix equal amounts of each powdered herb with a spoonful of ginger juice and a pinch of salt to form pills. Continue to take this formula until the condition is relieved.

Today, this formula is prepared by grinding the ingredients into powder. Take 6g (powder or pills) per dose one to two times daily with boiled water. This formula may also be prepared as a decoction with the doses suggested in brackets above.

Liang Fu Wan (Galangal and Cyperus Pill) activates qi circulation, soothes the Liver, dispels cold, and stops pain. It is designed to treat epigastric pain and vomiting caused by Liver qi or cold invading the Stomach. Clinical manifestations include epigastric pain, vomiting, and sometimes chest and hypochondriac pain.

In this formula *Gao Liang Jiang* (Rhizoma Alpiniae Officinarum) warms the Stomach, dispels cold, and relieves vomiting. *Xiang Fu* (Rhizoma Cyperi) soothes the Liver, activates qi circulation, and relieves pain.

Hou Po Wen Zhong Tang and *Liang Fu Wan* (Galangal and Cyperus Pill) both warm the middle *jiao*, regulate qi, and relieve pain.
- *Hou Po Wen Zhong Tang* emphasizes warming the middle *jiao*, dispelling cold, and drying dampness. This formula treats both Spleen and Stomach.
- *Liang Fu Wan* also warms the middle *jiao* and regulates qi, but focuses on treating the Spleen and Liver.

12

QI-REGULATING FORMULAS

841

Section 2

降气剂
— Qi-Descending Formulas

Sū Zǐ Jiàng Qì Tāng
(Perilla Fruit Decoction for Directing Qi Downward)

蘇子降氣湯
苏子降气汤

Pinyin Name: *Su Zi Jiang Qi Tang*
Literal Name: Perilla Fruit Decoction for Directing Qi Downward
Alternate Names: *Su Tzu Chiang Chi Tang, Su Zi Jiang Chi Tang,* Perilla Seed Decoction, Perilla Seed Combination
Original Source: *Tai Ping Hui Min He Ji Ju Fang* (Imperial Grace Formulary of the Tai Ping Era) by the Imperial Medical Department in 1078-85

COMPOSITION

Zi Su Zi (Fructus Perillae)	75g [9g]
Ban Xia (Rhizoma Pinelliae), *xi* (washed) with liquid 7 times	75g [9g]
Hou Po (Cortex Magnoliae Officinalis), *chao* (dry-fried) with ginger juice	30g [6g]
Qian Hu (Radix Peucedani)	30g [6g]
Rou Gui (Cortex Cinnamomi)	45g [3g]
Dang Gui (Radix Angelicae Sinensis)	45g [6g]
Gan Cao (Radix et Rhizoma Glycyrrhizae)	60g [6g]

DOSAGE / PREPARATION / ADMINISTRATION

The source text recommends grinding the ingredients into a fine powder. Cook 6g of the powder with 2 slices of *Sheng Jiang* (Rhizoma Zingiberis Recens), 1 piece of *Da Zao* (Fructus Jujubae) and 5 leaves [2g] of *Zi Su Ye* (Folium Perillae) in 1.5 large bowls of water until the liquid is reduced to 80% (1.2 large bowls). Take the hot strained liquid any time during the day. Today, this formula may be prepared as a decoction with the doses suggested in brackets.

CHINESE THERAPEUTIC ACTIONS

1. Directs Lung qi downward to relieve wheezing
2. Eliminates phlegm and stops coughing

CLINICAL MANIFESTATIONS

Upper excess with lower deficiency syndrome: abundant phlegm and watery sputum, wheezing, coughing, shortness of breath, dyspnea, abnormal respiration with more exhalation than inhalation, feeling of fullness and oppression in the chest and diaphragm; possible sore back and weak legs; possible lassitude, edema of the extremities; white, slippery or white, greasy tongue coating, and a weak pulse at the *chi* position.

CLINICAL APPLICATIONS

Bronchial asthma, chronic bronchitis, pulmonary emphysema, cough and wheezing, plum-pit *qi*, and morning sickness.

EXPLANATION

Su Zi Jiang Qi Tang (Perilla Fruit Decoction for Directing Qi Downward) is indicated for respiratory problems characterized by upper excess and lower deficiency. Upper excess refers to phlegm accumulation in the Lung, affecting the flow of Lung qi and causing feelings of fullness and oppression in the chest and diaphragm. Lower deficiency refers to deficiency of Kidney yang. Under normal conditions, the Kidney assists Lung qi to descend. However, when Kidney yang is deficient, the Lung qi may no longer

Sū Zǐ Jiàng Qì Tāng
(Perilla Fruit Decoction for Directing Qi Downward)

be able to descend properly, and wheezing or shortness of breath may occur. Clinically, inhalation will be shorter than exhalation. Also, Kidney deficiency may result in back pain and leg weakness. Moreover, edema may occur because Kidney yang is no longer able to regulate water metabolism, leaving the fluids to accumulate and form edema in the extremities, especially the lower limbs.

To treat upper excess, the reversed qi flow must be corrected and phlegm must be eliminated. To treat lower deficiency, Kidney yang must be reinforced. The chief herb of this formula, *Zi Su Zi* (Fructus Perillae), directs Lung qi downwards, eliminates phlegm, and relieves coughing and wheezing. *Ban Xia* (Rhizoma Pinelliae), *Hou Po* (Cortex Magnoliae Officinalis), and *Qian Hu* (Radix Peucedani) eliminate phlegm and relieve coughing and wheezing. Together, these four herbs treat the "upper excess." *Rou Gui* (Cortex Cinnamomi) warms Kidney yang to treat "lower deficiency." By warming and tonifying the Kidney, *Rou Gui* (Cortex Cinnamomi) enables the Kidney to grasp qi, pull it downward and facilitate inhalation. *Dang Gui* (Radix Angelicae Sinensis) nourishes blood to balance the acrid and drying herbs. *Sheng Jiang* (Rhizoma Zingiberis Recens) and *Zi Su Ye* (Folium Perillae) disperse cold and ventilate the Lung. *Gan Cao* (Radix et Rhizoma Glycyrrhizae) and *Da Zao* (Fructus Jujubae) harmonize the formula.

MODIFICATIONS

- For qi deficiency, add *Ren Shen* (Radix et Rhizoma Ginseng) and *Wu Wei Zi* (Fructus Schisandrae Chinensis).
- For deficiency and cold, add *Huang Qi* (Radix Astragali) and increase the dose of *Rou Gui* (Cortex Cinnamomi).
- With cough and dyspnea due to reversed flow of qi, add *Chen Xiang* (Lignum Aquilariae Resinatum).
- With cough and dyspnea accompanied by phlegm, add *Bei Mu* (Bulbus Fritillariae) and *Ku Xing Ren* (Semen Armeniacae Amarum); or *Er Chen Tang* (Two-Cured Decoction).
- With cough and dyspnea due to wind-cold, add *Ding Chuan Tang* (Arrest Wheezing Decoction).
- When there is nausea, add *Zhe Shi* (Haematitum).
- With nausea, vomiting, and drooling of saliva, add *Fu Ling* (Poria) and *Jie Geng* (Radix Platycodonis).
- With chest and epigastric fullness and oppression, add *Huang Qin* (Radix Scutellariae) and *Chai Hu* (Radix Bupleuri).

CAUTIONS / CONTRAINDICATIONS

- *Su Zi Jiang Qi Tang* is warm and drying, and is mainly used to reverse the flow of Lung qi and eliminate dampness and phlegm. It is not suitable for coughing or wheezing due to Lung deficiency, nor is it suitable for wheezing due to heat and phlegm accumulation in the Lung.
- Individuals who take this formula should avoid exposure to cold and wind, and refrain from eating raw, cold, oily and greasy foods.[1]

Su Zi Jiang Qi Tang (Perilla Fruit Decoction for Directing Qi Downward)

Diagnosis	Signs and Symptoms	Treatment	Herbs
Upper-excess, lower-deficiency syndrome	• Phlegm and sputum, wheezing, coughing, shortness of breath, dyspnea, and chest and hypochondriac fullness and oppression: phlegm accumulation [excess] in the Lung [upper] • Back soreness, weakness of lower extremities, lassitude, edema of lower extremities: yang deficiency of Kidney [lower]	• Directs Lung qi downward to relieve wheezing • Eliminates phlegm and stops coughing	• *Zi Su Zi* (Fructus Perillae) directs Lung qi downward, eliminates phlegm, and relieves coughing and wheezing. • *Ban Xia* (Rhizoma Pinelliae), *Hou Po* (Cortex Magnoliae Officinalis) and *Qian Hu* (Radix Peucedani) eliminate phlegm and relieve coughing and wheezing. • *Rou Gui* (Cortex Cinnamomi) warms Kidney yang to grasp qi downwards. • *Dang Gui* (Radix Angelicae Sinensis) nourishes blood to balance the acrid and drying herbs. • *Sheng Jiang* (Rhizoma Zingiberis Recens) and *Zi Su Ye* (Folium Perillae) disperse cold and ventilate the Lung. • *Gan Cao* (Radix et Rhizoma Glycyrrhizae) and *Da Zao* (Fructus Jujubae) harmonize the herbs.

Sū Zǐ Jiàng Qì Tāng
(Perilla Fruit Decoction for Directing Qi Downward)

PHARMACOLOGICAL EFFECTS

Respiratory: According to one study, administration of *Su Zi Jiang Qi Tang* in mice was associated with marked antitussive, antiasthmatic, and anti-inflammatory effects.[2]

CLINICAL STUDIES AND RESEARCH

1. **Cough and wheezing**: One study reported marked success using *Su Zi Jiang Qi Tang* to treat various respiratory disorders, such as bronchial asthma, chronic bronchitis, pulmonary emphysema, and others.[3]

2. ***Mei he qi* (plum-pit qi)**: According to one study, administration of *Su Zi Jiang Qi Tang* was effective in treating 55 of 60 patients who had plum-pit *qi* for 6 months to 2 years. The herbs were cooked in water, and the decoction was given in three equally-divided doses daily. The duration of treatment ranged from 6 to 10 packs of herbs.[4]

3. **Morning sickness**: Modified *Su Zi Jiang Qi Tang* was effective in treating nausea and vomiting in 94 of 96 pregnant women (between 21 and 30 years of age, mostly within the first 6-12 weeks of their first pregnancy). Clinical manifestations included nausea, vomiting (with clear fluids or saliva), nausea when smelling food and vomiting after eating food, feelings of fullness, distention and oppression in the chest. Dizziness and vertigo, fatigue, and a sallow facial appearance. The herbal formula contained *Zi Su Zi* (Fructus Perillae) 15g, *Ban Xia* (Rhizoma Pinelliae) 10g, *Chen Pi* (Pericarpium Citri Reticulatae) 10g, *Qian Hu* (Radix Peucedani) 10g, *Xuan Fu Hua* (Flos Inulae) 10g, *Huang Qin* (Radix Scutellariae) 10g, *Sha Ren* (Fructus Amomi) 10g, *Bai Zhu* (Rhizoma Atractylodis Macrocephalae) 10g, *Dang Gui* (Radix Angelicae Sinensis) 12g, *Xu Duan* (Radix Dipsaci) 12g, *Gan Cao* (Radix et Rhizoma Glycyrrhizae) 5g, and *Sheng Jiang* (Rhizoma Zingiberis Recens) 3 slices. *Zhu Ru* (Caulis Bambusae in Taenia) 12g, and *Bai Shao* (Radix Paeoniae Alba) 15g were added for Liver heat. *Fu Ling* (Poria) 10g was added and the dose of *Ban Xia* (Rhizoma Pinelliae) was increased for excess dampness and phlegm. Patients in the study reported improvement or complete relief within taking 5 packs of herbs.[5]

RELATED FORMULA

Sān Zǐ Jiàng Qì Tāng

(Three-Seed Decoction for Directing Qi Downward)

三子降氣湯
三子降气汤

Pinyin Name: *San Zi Jiang Qi Tang*

Literal Name: Three-Seed Decoction for Directing Qi Downward

Original Source: *Tian Jin Zhong Yi Xue Yuan* (Tianjin University of Chinese Medicine) in 1989

Bai Jie Zi (Semen Sinapis)

Zi Su Zi (Fructus Perillae)

Lai Fu Zi (Semen Raphani)

Ma Huang (Herba Ephedrae)

Pi Pa Ye (Folium Eriobotryae)

Ku Xing Ren (Semen Armeniacae Amarum)

Dang Gui (Radix Angelicae Sinensis)

Zhi Gan Cao (Radix et Rhizoma Glycyrrhizae Praeparata cum Melle)

Hou Po (Cortex Magnoliae Officinalis)

Rou Gui (Cortex Cinnamomi)

Zi Su Ye (Folium Perillae)

Ting Li Zi (Semen Descurainiae seu Lepidii)

Zao Jiao Ci (Spina Gleditsiae)

Chai Hu (Radix Bupleuri)

Chen Pi (Pericarpium Citri Reticulatae)

Wu Wei Zi (Fructus Schisandrae Chinensis)

San Zi Jiang Qi Tang (Three-Seed Decoction for Directing Qi Downward) is designed to treat wheezing and dyspnea characterized by phlegm in the Lung accompanied by underlying deficiency. Clinical applications include asthma, bronchitis, emphysema, and other chronic and debilitating respiratory disorders with wheezing and dyspnea. This formula is composed following the principles of two classic formulas: *San Zi Yang Qin Tang* (Three-Seed Decoction to Nourish One's Parents) and *Su Zi Jiang Qi Tang* (Perilla Fruit Decoction for Directing Qi Downward). The herbs in both formulas work synergistically to restore the correct downward flow of Lung qi to relieve wheezing and dyspnea, eliminate the storage of phlegm in the Lung, and restore the functioning of the Spleen.

AUTHORS' COMMENTS

Su Zi Jiang Qi Tang is indicated in classic textbooks for treating "upper excess, lower deficiency" syndrome. However, it is important to remember that the primary emphasis is upper excess (which is treated with four herbs), and the secondary focus is lower deficiency (which is addressed with only one herb).

References

1. *Zhong Yao Ming Fang Yao Li Yu Ying Yong* (Pharmacology and Applications of Famous Herbal Formulas) 1989;406-407.
2. *Zhong Yao Yao Li Yu Lin Chuang* (Pharmacology and Clinical Applications of Chinese Herbs) 1992;8(5):13.
3. *Zhong Yi Za Zhi* (Journal of Chinese Medicine) 1964;10:32.
4. *Si Chuan Zhong Yi* (Sichuan Chinese Medicine) 1984;2(1):46.
5. *Xin Jiang Zhong Yi Yao* (Xinjiang Chinese Medicine and Herbology) 1995;4:20.

Chinese Herbal Formulas and Applications

Dīng Chuǎn Tāng (Arrest Wheezing Decoction)

定喘湯
定喘汤

Pinyin Name: *Ding Chuan Tang*
Literal Name: Arrest Wheezing Decoction
Alternate Names: *Ting Chuen Tang, Din Chuan Tang*, Asthma-Stopping Decoction, Asthma-Relieving Decoction, Mahuang and Ginkgo Combination
Original Source: *She Sheng Zhong Miao Fang* (Marvelous Formulas for the Health of Multitudes) by Zhang Shi-Che in 1550

COMPOSITION

Ma Huang (Herba Ephedrae)	9g
Bai Guo (Semen Ginkgo), *zha* (crushed) and *chao* (dry-fried) till yellow 21 kernels [9g]	
Zi Su Zi (Fructus Perillae)	6g
Ku Xing Ren (Semen Armeniacae Amarum)	4.5g [9g]
Ban Xia (Rhizoma Pinelliae)	9g
Kuan Dong Hua (Flos Farfarae)	9g
Sang Bai Pi (Cortex Mori)	9g
Huang Qin (Radix Scutellariae)	4.5g [6g]
Gan Cao (Radix et Rhizoma Glycyrrhizae)	3g

DOSAGE / PREPARATION / ADMINISTRATION

The source text recommends decocting the ingredients in three bowls of water until two bowls of liquid remain. Take one bowl of decoction per dose twice daily at any time during the day. The source text prohibits the use of ginger in the decoction. Today, the decoction may be prepared with the doses suggested in brackets.

CHINESE THERAPEUTIC ACTIONS

1. Ventilates the Lung and directs Lung qi downwards
2. Dispels phlegm and relieves wheezing

CLINICAL MANIFESTATIONS

Wind-cold constricting the exterior and phlegm-heat accumulation in the interior: thick, sticky, yellow sputum that is difficult to expectorate, abundant phlegm, rapid breathing, coughing, wheezing, dyspnea; a yellow, greasy tongue coating, and a slippery, rapid pulse.

CLINICAL APPLICATIONS

Asthma, bronchial asthma, tracheitis, acute and chronic bronchitis, bronchiolitis, and bronchopneumonia.

EXPLANATION

Ding Chuan Tang (Arrest Wheezing Decoction) is one of the most commonly used formulas to treat wheezing and dyspnea due to exterior wind-cold and interior phlegm-heat. Patients suffering from this syndrome usually already have abundant phlegm that is thick, sticky and yellow. When the wind-cold factor attacks the exterior and

Ding Chuan Tang (Arrest Wheezing Decoction)

Diagnosis	Signs and Symptoms	Treatment	Herbs
Wind-cold at the exterior and phlegm-heat in the interior	• Abundant phlegm, rapid breathing, and thick, sticky yellow sputum: phlegm-heat accumulation in the interior • Coughing, wheezing and dyspnea: reversed flow of Lung qi • Yellow, greasy tongue coating and a slippery, rapid pulse: phlegm-heat accumulation in the interior	• Ventilates the Lung and redirects Lung qi • Dispels phlegm and relieves wheezing	• *Ma Huang* (Herba Ephedrae) releases the exterior wind-cold factor and ventilates the Lung. • *Bai Guo* (Semen Ginkgo) eliminates phlegm and astringes Lung qi. • *Zi Su Zi* (Fructus Perillae), *Ku Xing Ren* (Semen Armeniacae Amarum), *Ban Xia* (Rhizoma Pinelliae), and *Kuan Dong Hua* (Flos Farfarae) eliminate phlegm and direct the reversed flow of qi downwards. • *Sang Bai Pi* (Cortex Mori) and *Huang Qin* (Radix Scutellariae) clear Lung heat. • *Gan Cao* (Radix et Rhizoma Glycyrrhizae) harmonizes the herbs.

QI-REGULATING FORMULAS

12

845

Dìng Chuǎn Tāng (Arrest Wheezing Decoction)

constricts the Lung, the dispersing and descending functions of the Lung may be further inhibited, causing phlegm stagnation and heat. The tongue coating and pulse both indicate heat and phlegm accumulation in the body.

In this formula, *Ma Huang* (Herba Ephedrae) releases the exterior wind-cold factor and dilates the Lung to relieve wheezing and dyspnea. *Bai Guo* (Semen Ginkgo) eliminates phlegm and astringes Lung qi to relieve wheezing. The astringent effect of *Bai Guo* (Semen Ginkgo) also prevents *Ma Huang* (Herba Ephedrae) from over-venting the Lung and leading to the loss of Lung qi. The dispersing effect of *Ma Huang* (Herba Ephedrae) prevents *Bai Guo* (Semen Ginkgo) from retaining the disease in the body. *Zi Su Zi* (Fructus Perillae), *Ku Xing Ren* (Semen Armeniacae Amarum), *Ban Xia* (Rhizoma Pinelliae), and *Kuan Dong Hua* (Flos Farfarae) eliminate phlegm and direct the reversed flow of qi downwards to relieve wheezing and coughing. *Sang Bai Pi* (Cortex Mori) and *Huang Qin* (Radix Scutellariae) clear Lung heat and relieve wheezing and coughing. *Gan Cao* (Radix et Rhizoma Glycyrrhizae) harmonizes the formula.

MODIFICATIONS

- For wheezing and dyspnea due to wind-cold, combine with *Ma Huang Tang* (Ephedra Decoction).
- For wheezing and dyspnea due to damp-heat, combine with *Liang Ge San* (Cool the Diaphragm Powder).
- For wheezing and dyspnea due to excessive phlegm, combine with *Er Chen Tang* (Two-Cured Decoction).
- With feelings of oppression in the chest, add *Zhi Qiao* (Fructus Aurantii) and *Hou Po* (Cortex Magnoliae Officinalis).
- With irritability and thirst, add *Mai Dong* (Radix Ophiopogonis) and *Di Gu Pi* (Cortex Lycii).
- For sputum that is thick and difficult to expectorate, add *Gua Lou* (Fructus Trichosanthis), *Dan Nan Xing* (Arisaema cum Bile), and *Zhe Bei Mu* (Bulbus Fritillariae Thunbergii).
- With profuse sputum, add *Fu Hai Shi* (Pumice), *Ju Hong* (Exocarpium Citri Reticulatae), and *Gua Lou Pi* (Pericarpium Trichosanthis).
- When there is severe Lung heat with fever, add *Shi Gao* (Gypsum Fibrosum), *Yu Xing Cao* (Herba Houttuyniae), or *Ma Huang Xing Ren Gan Cao Shi Gao Tang* (Ephedra, Apricot Kernel, Licorice, and Gypsum Decoction).
- If accompanied by a severe stifling sensation in the chest, add *Zhi Qiao* (Fructus Aurantii) and *Zhu Ru* (Caulis Bambusae in Taenia).

CAUTIONS / CONTRAINDICATIONS

- *Ding Chuan Tang* should be used with caution during the very first stage of a wind invasion showing dyspnea without perspiration.
- This formula is contraindicated in chronic wheezing or cough caused by Lung and Kidney yin deficiencies.

PHARMACOLOGICAL EFFECTS

1. **Antiasthmatic**: Intraperitoneal injection of *Ding Chuan Tang* was shown to be effective in relieving asthma. The formula had no antiasthmatic effect when *Bai Guo* (Semen Ginkgo) was removed; but did have a significantly stronger antiasthmatic effect when the dose of *Bai Guo* was doubled. The study concluded that *Bai Guo* is an essential ingredient for this function.[1] The mechanism of its antiasthmatic effect was attributed to the formula's ability to blend histamine and acetylcholine, decrease contraction of external trachea smooth muscle, and promote secretion of phenol red in the respiratory tract.[2] Another study stated that *Ding Chuan Tang* may be used as a prophylactic treatment against allergen-induced asthma and airway inflammation via its bronchodilating influence and its ability to inhibit eosinophils in the airway.[3]

2. **Expectorant**: Intraperitoneal injection of *Ding Chuan Tang* in mice was shown to have a marked expectorant effect.[4]

3. **Antitussive**: According to one study, use of *Ding Chuan Tang* was associated with suppressing cough in mice.[5]

CLINICAL STUDIES AND RESEARCH

1. **Asthma**: Modified *Ding Chuan Tang* was effective in treating 36 patients with severe asthma. The herbal treatment contained *Ding Chuan Tang* plus *Dan Nan Xing* (Arisaema cum Bile), *Di Long* (Pheretima), *Yu Xing Cao* (Herba Houttuyniae), *Mian Hua Gen* (Radix Gossypii), *Fang Feng* (Radix Saposhnikoviae), and others. Antibiotic drugs were given in cases of severe infection. Of 36 patients, the study reported complete recovery in 24 cases, marked improvement in 10 cases, and no effect in 2 cases. The rate of effectiveness was 94.5%.[6]

2. **Asthma with bronchitis**: Use of modified *Ding Chuan Tang* showed good results in treating asthma associated with bronchitis in 63 infants (2 years of age or below, with more than 10 days of illness). The formula contained *Ma Huang* (Herba Ephedrae) 3g, *Huang Qin* (Radix Scutellariae) 4g, *Zi Su Zi* (Fructus Perillae) 4g, *Ku Xing Ren* (Semen Armeniacae Amarum) 4g, *Sang Bai Pi* (Cortex Mori) 4g, *Bai Guo* (Semen Ginkgo) 4g, *Ban Xia* (Rhizoma Pinelliae) 4g, *Kuan Dong Hua* (Flos Farfarae) 4g, *She Gan* (Rhizoma Belamcandae) 4g, *Jie Geng* (Radix Platycodonis) 4g, *Ban Lan Gen* (Radix Isatidis) 12g, and

Dìng Chuǎn Tāng (Arrest Wheezing Decoction)

Gan Cao (Radix et Rhizoma Glycyrrhizae) 2g. [The dose listed is for a 2 year old. Adjust the dose accordingly for infants under 2 years of age.] The herbs were given in decoction twice daily, for 7 days per course of treatment. Of 63 infants, the study reported complete recovery in 59 cases, improvement in 3 cases, and no benefit in 1 case. The rate of effectiveness was 98.4%.[7]

3. **Bronchopneumonia**: Administration of daily decoction of modified *Ding Chuan Tang* was effective in treating 34 patients with bronchopneumonia. The study reported resolution of cough and wheezing after an average of 4.61 days (range of 2.02 to 7.20 days) and complete recovery after 7.88 days (range of 4.66 to 11.70 days).[8]

4. **Bronchial asthma**: One study reported 97% effectiveness using modified *Ding Chuan Tang* to treat 100 patients with chronic bronchial asthma. The herbal formula contained *Ding Chuan Tang* plus *Yu Xing Cao* (Herba Houttuyniae), *Pu Gong Ying* (Herba Taraxaci), and others as needed. The treatment protocol was to administer the herbs in decoction form for 10 days per course of treatment. Of 100 patients, the study reported significant improvement in 83 cases and moderate improvement in 14 cases. The study described *Ding Chuan Tang* to have marked antiasthmatic, antitussive, and expectorant effects.[9]

TOXICOLOGY

According to one acute toxicology study, administration of *Ding Chuan Tang* at 150 g/kg in a bolus dose did not cause any abnormal reaction in dietary habits or physical activities.[10]

References

1. *Zhe Jiang Zhong Yi Za Zhi* (Zhejiang Journal of Chinese Medicine) 1989;24(3):123.
2. Li Z, Li T. Pharmacological study on asthma-relieving decoction (dingchuan tang) treating asthma. Zhong Yao Cai 1999 Aug;22(8):411-3.
3. Kao ST, Chang CH, Chen YS, Chiang SY, Lin JG. Effects of Ding-Chuan-Tang on bronchoconstriction and airway leucocyte infiltration in sensitized guinea pigs. Immunopharmacol Immunotoxicol 2004 Feb;26(1):113-24.
4. *Zhong Cheng Yao* (Study of Chinese Patent Medicine) 1986;11:27.
5. *Zhong Cheng Yao Yan Jiu* (Research of Chinese Patent Medicine) 1986;11:27.
6. *Hu Bei Zhong Yi Za Zhi* (Hubei Journal of Chinese Medicine) 1997;19(2):17.
7. *Zhe Jiang Zhong Yi Za Zhi* (Zhejiang Journal of Chinese Medicine) 1992;27(3):109.
8. *Jiang Xi Zhong Yi Yao* (Jiangxi Chinese Medicine and Herbology) 1992;23(1):28.
9. *Xin Yi Xue* (New Medicine) 1972;9:14.
10. *Zhe Jiang Zhong Yi Za Zhi* (Zhejiang Journal of Chinese Medicine) 1989;24(3):123.

Shén Mì Tāng (Mysterious Decoction)
神祕湯
神秘汤

Pinyin Name: *Shen Mi Tang*
Literal Name: Mysterious Decoction
Alternate Name: Mahuang and Magnolia Combination
Original Source: *Wai Tai Mi Yao* (Arcane Essentials from the Imperial Library) by Wang Tao in 752 A.D.

COMPOSITION

Ma Huang (Herba Ephedrae)	6g
Ku Xing Ren (Semen Armeniacae Amarum)	6g
Chen Pi (Pericarpium Citri Reticulatae)	3g
Hou Po (Cortex Magnoliae Officinalis)	6g
Zi Su Ye (Folium Perillae)	3g
Chai Hu (Radix Bupleuri)	3g
Gan Cao (Radix et Rhizoma Glycyrrhizae)	3g

Chapter 12 – Qi-Regulating Formulas   *Section 2 – Qi-Descending Formulas*

Shén Mì Tāng (Mysterious Decoction)

DOSAGE / PREPARATION / ADMINISTRATION
Prepare the ingredients as a decoction.

CHINESE THERAPEUTIC ACTIONS
1. Regulates qi
2. Eliminates phlegm

CLINICAL MANIFESTATIONS
Wheezing and dyspnea caused by stagnation of qi and phlegm: wheezing, dyspnea, sputum and phlegm, a rattling sound in the throat, and fullness and distention in the chest and hypochondrium.

CLINICAL APPLICATIONS
Asthma and bronchial asthma.

EXPLANATION
Shen Mi Tang (Mysterious Decoction) is designed to treat stagnation of qi and phlegm that affects the proper flow of Lung qi resulting in wheezing and dyspnea. Phlegm causes chest fullness and congestion, and an audible rattling sound in the throat accompanying breathing.

In this formula, *Ma Huang* (Herba Ephedrae) dilates the Lung to relieve wheezing and dyspnea. *Ku Xing Ren* (Semen Armeniacae Amarum) directs Lung qi downward to facilitate breathing. These two herbs are often combined to treat wheezing and dyspnea. *Chen Pi* (Pericarpium Citri Reticulatae) and *Hou Po* (Cortex Magnoliae Officinalis) both regulate qi and eliminate phlegm. *Zi Su Ye* (Folium Perillae) dispels wind-cold from the exterior. *Chai Hu* (Radix Bupleuri) clears heat from the exterior and interior, and eases distention in the chest and hypochondrium. Lastly, *Gan Cao* (Radix et Rhizoma Glycyrrhizae) harmonizes the formula. In short, this is a good formula for patients with wheezing and dyspnea caused by qi and phlegm stagnation.

Shen Mi Tang (Mysterious Decoction)

Diagnosis	Signs and Symptoms	Treatment	Herbs
Wheezing and dyspnea due to stagnation of qi and phlegm	• Wheezing and dyspnea: reversed flow of Lung qi • Sputum, chest fullness and congestion, and a rattling sound in the throat accompanying breathing: phlegm stagnation in the Lung	• Regulates qi • Eliminates phlegm	• *Ma Huang* (Herba Ephedrae) dilates the Lung to relieve wheezing and dyspnea. • *Ku Xing Ren* (Semen Armeniacae Amarum) directs Lung qi downward to facilitate breathing. • *Chen Pi* (Pericarpium Citri Reticulatae) and *Hou Po* (Cortex Magnoliae Officinalis) regulate qi and eliminate phlegm. • *Zi Su Ye* (Folium Perillae) dispels wind-cold from the exterior. • *Chai Hu* (Radix Bupleuri) clears heat from the exterior and interior, and eases distention in the chest and hypochondrium. • *Gan Cao* (Radix et Rhizoma Glycyrrhizae) harmonizes the formula.

848

Chinese Herbal Formulas and Applications

Si Mò Tāng (Four Milled-Herbs Decoction)

四蘑湯

四蘑汤

Pinyin Name: *Si Mo Tang*
Literal Name: Four Milled-Herbs Decoction
Original Source: *Ji Sheng Fang* (Formulas to Aid the Living) by Yan Yong-He in 1253

COMPOSITION

Wu Yao (Radix Linderae)	[9g]
Chen Xiang (Lignum Aquilariae Resinatum)	[3g]
Bing Lang (Semen Arecae)	[9g]
Ren Shen (Radix et Rhizoma Ginseng)	[3g]

DOSAGE / PREPARATION / ADMINISTRATION

The source text instructions are: mill equal amounts of the herbs, cook them with a small bowl of water, bring it to a boil three to five times, and take the decoction while warm. Today, the decoction may be prepared using the doses suggested in brackets.

CHINESE THERAPEUTIC ACTIONS

1. Activates qi circulation and redirects abnormal rising qi
2. Disperses stagnation and expands the chest

CLINICAL MANIFESTATIONS

Liver qi stagnation caused by instability of the seven emotions: irritability, a feeling of oppression in the chest and diaphragm, wheezing, hurried respiration, epigastric fullness and distention, and loss of appetite.

CLINICAL APPLICATIONS

Asthma and gynecomastia.

EXPLANATION

Si Mo Tang (Four Milled-Herbs Decoction) treats Liver qi stagnation caused by instability of the seven emotions (joy, anger, melancholy, over-thinking, grief, fear, and fright). When the Liver qi becomes stagnant, it fails to disperse smoothly in all directions, and may invade the Lung and Stomach. Irregular Lung qi flow leads to chest oppression and wheezing, while irregular Stomach qi flow leads to fullness and distention in the epigastrium, and loss of appetite. It is important to note that while the cause of the illness is Liver qi stagnation, the symptoms are associated with the Lung and Stomach. Optimal treatment requires a combination of herbs that simultaneously treats the cause and the symptoms.

In this formula, *Wu Yao* (Radix Linderae) spreads the Liver, activates qi circulation and disperses qi stagnation. *Chen Xiang* (Lignum Aquilariae Resinatum) regulates qi flow, corrects the reversed flow of qi, and relieves wheezing. *Bing Lang* (Semen Arecae) activates qi circulation and breaks down qi stagnation to relieve fullness of the epigastrium. If only qi-activating herbs were used, however, the qi of the body would be damaged or consumed. Therefore, *Ren Shen* (Radix et Rhizoma Ginseng) is added to tonify qi and strengthen the body.

MODIFICATIONS

- For strong patients experiencing anger and distended pain in the chest and abdomen, remove *Ren Shen* (Radix et Rhizoma Ginseng) and add *Mu Xiang* (Radix Aucklandiae) and *Zhi Shi* (Fructus Aurantii Immaturus).
- With constipation, belching, abdominal pain, and distention, add *Zhi Shi* (Fructus Aurantii Immaturus) and *Da Huang* (Radix et Rhizoma Rhei).

CLINICAL STUDIES AND RESEARCH

1. **Gynecomastia:** One study reported successful treatment of gynecomastia in 31 of 32 patients using modified *Si Mo Tang*. The herbal formula contained *E Zhu* (Rhizoma Curcumae) 9g, *Wu Yao* (Radix Linderae) 9g, *Bing Lang* (Semen Arecae) 9g, *Gua Lou Pi* (Pericarpium Trichosanthis) 9g, *Bei Mu* (Bulbus Fritillariae) 15g, *Dang Shen* (Radix Codonopsis) 15g, *Di Huang* (Radix Rehmanniae) 15g, dry-fried *Gu Ya* (Fructus Setariae Germinatus) 15g, *Yin Yang Huo* (Herba Epimedii) 12g, *Chen Xiang* (Lignum Aquilariae Resinatum) 2g, and others as needed. The herbs were given in decoction daily, for an average of 22 days (range from 10-42 days).[1]

2. **Asthma:** One study reported satisfactory results using modified *Si Mo Tang* to treat 12 patients with asthma. The herbal formula contained *Wu Yao* (Radix Linderae) 10g, *Ban Xia* (Rhizoma Pinelliae) 10g, *Dang Shen* (Radix Codonopsis) 10g, *Chen Xiang* (Lignum Aquilariae Resinatum) 6g, *Zhi Shi* (Fructus Aurantii Immaturus) 6g, *Bing Lang* (Semen Arecae) 6g, *Gan Cao* (Radix et Rhizoma Glycyrrhizae) 6g, *Zi Su Geng* (Caulis Perillae)

12

QI-REGULATING FORMULAS

849

Chapter 12 – Qi-Regulating Formulas   *Section 2 – Qi-Descending Formulas*

Sì Mò Tāng (Four Milled-Herbs Decoction)

Si Mo Tang (Four Milled-Herbs Decoction)

Diagnosis	Signs and Symptoms	Treatment	Herbs
Liver qi stagnation caused by instability of the seven emotions	• Emotional instability: Liver qi stagnation • Chest oppression, wheezing and hurried respiration: Liver qi stagnation affecting Lung qi circulation • Epigastric fullness and distention with no appetite: Liver qi stagnation affecting Stomach qi flow	• Activates qi circulation and corrects abnormal rising qi • Disperses stagnation and expands the chest	• *Wu Yao* (Radix Linderae) activates qi and disperses qi stagnation. • *Chen Xiang* (Lignum Aquilariae Resinatum) regulates qi flow and corrects the reversed flow of qi. • *Bing Lang* (Semen Arecae) activates qi circulation and breaks up qi stagnation. • *Ren Shen* (Radix et Rhizoma Ginseng) tonifies qi and strengthens the body.

12g, and *Bai Fu Ling* (Poria Alba) 15g. Furthermore, *Gua Lou* (Fructus Trichosanthis) 10g and *Huang Qin* (Radix Scutellariae) 10g were added for hot phlegm; and *Gan Jiang* (Rhizoma Zingiberis) 3g and *Gui Zhi* (Ramulus Cinnamomi) 3g were added for cold phlegm. Of 12 patients, the study reported significant improvement in 9 cases and moderate improvement in 3 cases.[2]

RELATED FORMULA

Wǔ Mò Yǐn Zǐ (Five Milled-Herbs Decoction)

五蘑飲子
五蘑饮子

Pinyin Name: Wu Mo Yin Zi
Literal Name: Five Milled-Herbs Decoction
Original Source: *Yi Bian* (Ordinary Medicine) by Wang San-Cai in 1587

Mu Xiang (Radix Aucklandiae)	[6g]
Chen Xiang (Lignum Aquilariae Resinatum)	[6g]
Bing Lang (Semen Arecae)	[9g]
Zhi Shi (Fructus Aurantii Immaturus)	[9g]
Wu Yao (Radix Linderae)	[9g]

The source text states to prepare this formula by grinding equal amounts of the ingredients and administer with a grain-based liquor. Today, this formula may be prepared as a decoction with the doses suggested in brackets.

Wu Mo Yin Zi (Five Milled-Herbs Decoction) is composed of *Si Mo Tang*, with the addition of *Zhi Shi* (Fructus Aurantii Immaturus) and *Mu Xiang* (Radix Aucklandiae), and the removal of *Ren Shen* (Radix et Rhizoma Ginseng). This change in composition gives the formula stronger

actions to activate qi and dispel qi stagnation. Clinically, the patient may show extreme anger, irritation, and fullness and pain in the chest and abdomen that radiate to other parts of the body.

Si Mo Tang and *Wu Mo Yin Zi* (Five Milled-Herbs Decoction) both treat qi stagnation and abnormal qi circulation. Their differences are as follows:

• *Si Mo Tang* simultaneously tonifies and regulates qi, making it more suitable for patients who are weak or deficient in nature.

• *Wu Mo Yin Zi* is a stronger formula for activating qi and dispelling stagnation, making it more suitable for patients who are strong or have pure excess conditions.

AUTHORS' COMMENTS

Si Mo Tang is used mainly for severe Liver qi stagnation with reversed flow of Lung and Stomach qi, manifesting in dyspnea, a stifling sensation and fullness in the chest and hypochondriac area, and distention and fullness in the epigastric area.

Si Mo Tang is prepared by milling the herbs and cooking them for a short period of time – just enough to bring the decoction to a few quick boils. The preparation is important because it retains the aromatic property of the qi-regulating herbs in this formula. Therefore, this formula is literally named "Four Milled-Herbs Decoction."

References
1. *Zhe Jiang Zhong Yi Za Zhi* (Zhejiang Journal of Chinese Medicine) 1992;27(12):538.
2. *Zhe Jiang Zhong Yi Za Zhi* (Zhejiang Journal of Chinese Medicine) 1987;22(12):508.

850

Chinese Herbal Formulas and Applications

Xuán Fù Dài Zhě Shí Tāng (Inula and Hematite Decoction)

旋覆代赭石湯
旋覆代赭石汤

Pinyin Name: *Xuan Fu Dai Zhe Shi Tang*
Literal Name: Inula and Hematite Decoction
Alternate Names: *Hsuan Fu Tai Che Shih Tang*, Inula and Red Ochre Decoction, Inula and Hematite Combination
Original Source: *Shang Han Lun* (Discussion of Cold-Induced Disorders) by Zhang Zhong-Jing in the Eastern Han Dynasty

COMPOSITION

Xuan Fu Hua (Flos Inulae)	9g
Zhe Shi (Haematitum)	3g [9g]
Sheng Jiang (Rhizoma Zingiberis Recens)	15g [10g]
Ban Xia (Rhizoma Pinelliae), *xi* (washed)	0.5 cup [9g]
Ren Shen (Radix et Rhizoma Ginseng)	6g
Zhi Gan Cao (Radix et Rhizoma Glycyrrhizae Praeparata cum Melle)	9g [6g]
Da Zao (Fructus Jujubae), *bo* (opened)	12 pieces [4 pieces]

DOSAGE / PREPARATION / ADMINISTRATION

The source text recommends cooking the herbs in 10 cups [2,000 mL] of water until it is reduced to 6 cups [1,200 mL]. Discard the herb residue, and cook the strained decoction again, reducing it to 3 cups [600 mL]. Take 1 cup [200 mL] of warm decoction three times daily. Today, this decoction may be prepared using the doses suggested in brackets.

CHINESE THERAPEUTIC ACTIONS

1. Dissolves phlegm and corrects abnormal rising qi
2. Benefits qi and harmonizes the Stomach

CLINICAL MANIFESTATIONS

Stomach qi deficiency with turbid phlegm stagnation: epigastric distention and hardness, unremitting belching, and hiccups.

CLINICAL APPLICATIONS

Morning sickness, nausea and vomiting, peptic ulcer disease, acid reflux, gastritis, pharyngoneurosis, gastrointestinal neurosis, gastrectasis, incomplete pyloric obstruction, vertigo, and Meniere's syndrome.

EXPLANATION

Xuan Fu Dai Zhe Shi Tang (Inula and Hematite Decoction) is formulated to treat Stomach qi deficiency with turbid phlegm stagnation. According to *Shang Han Lun* (Discussion of Cold-Induced Disorders), this condition occurs when patients with an exterior condition are treated with *han fa* (sweating), *tu fa* (vomiting), and *xia fa* (draining downward) methods. Though these treatments release the exterior condition, they damage *zhong* (central) *qi*, and lead to subsequent formation of phlegm and reversed flow of qi. Epigastric distention and hardness

Xuan Fu Dai Zhe Shi Tang (Inula and Hematite Decoction)

Diagnosis	Signs and Symptoms	Treatment	Herbs
Stomach qi deficiency with stagnation of turbid phlegm	• Epigastric distention and hardness: phlegm accumulation • Belching and hiccups: reversed flow of Stomach qi	• Dissolves phlegm and redirects abnormal rising qi • Benefits qi and harmonizes the Stomach	• *Xuan Fu Hua* (Flos Inulae) warms the Stomach, dissolves phlegm, and corrects the reversed flow of Stomach qi. • *Zhe Shi* (Haematitum) corrects the reversed flow of Stomach qi. • *Sheng Jiang* (Rhizoma Zingiberis Recens) warms the Stomach and redirects rising Stomach qi. • *Ban Xia* (Rhizoma Pinelliae) dries dampness, disperses phlegm, and harmonizes the Stomach. • *Ren Shen* (Radix et Rhizoma Ginseng), *Zhi Gan Cao* (Radix et Rhizoma Glycyrrhizae Praeparata cum Melle) and *Da Zao* (Fructus Jujubae) nourishes the Stomach and tonifies the Spleen.

12

QI-REGULATING FORMULAS

851

Chapter 12 – Qi-Regulating Formulas   *Section 2 – Qi-Descending Formulas*

Xuán Fù Dài Zhě Shí Tāng (Inula and Hematite Decoction)

indicate phlegm accumulation. Unremitting belching and hiccups indicate reversed flow of Stomach qi.

The chief herb of this formula, *Xuan Fu Hua* (Flos Inulae), warms the Stomach, dissolves phlegm, and corrects the reversed flow of Stomach qi to relieve belching and hiccups. *Zhe Shi* (Haematitum) is heavy and can guide Stomach qi downward to relieve belching. *Sheng Jiang* (Rhizoma Zingiberis Recens) warms the Stomach to dissolve phlegm and redirects the rising qi to relieve nausea and vomiting. *Ban Xia* (Rhizoma Pinelliae) dries dampness, disperses phlegm, and harmonizes the Stomach. It also assists *Xuan Fu Hua* (Flos Inulae) and *Zhe Shi* (Haematitum) to relieve belching and hiccups and reduce epigastric distention and hardness. *Ren Shen* (Radix et Rhizoma Ginseng) tonifies the Spleen and Stomach. *Zhi Gan Cao* (Radix et Rhizoma Glycyrrhizae Praeparata cum Melle) nourishes the middle *jiao*. *Da Zao* (Fructus Jujubae) nourishes the Stomach and tonifies the Spleen.

MODIFICATIONS

- When there is heat, add *Huang Lian* (Rhizoma Coptidis) and *Huang Qin* (Radix Scutellariae).
- With cough and drooling of phlegm, add *Fu Ling* (Poria) and *Chen Pi* (Pericarpium Citri Reticulatae).
- With epigastric fullness and oppression, add *Zhi Shi* (Fructus Aurantii Immaturus) and *Jie Geng* (Radix Platycodonis).
- For hiccups due to deficiency and cold, add *Ding Xiang* (Flos Caryophylli), *Shi Di* (Calyx Kaki), and *Wu Zhu Yu* (Fructus Evodiae).
- When there is Stomach yin deficiency, add *Mai Dong* (Radix Ophiopogonis) and *Shi Hu* (Caulis Dendrobii).
- For food stagnation, add *Ji Nei Jin* (Endothelium Corneum Gigeriae Galli) and *Shan Zha* (Fructus Crataegi).
- With profuse sputum, add *Fu Ling* (Poria) and *Chen Pi* (Pericarpium Citri Reticulatae).

CLINICAL STUDIES AND RESEARCH

1. **Morning sickness**: Administration of modified *Xuan Fu Dai Zhe Shi Tang* was shown in one study to effectively treat nausea and vomiting during pregnancy in 66 women. The herbal formula contained *Xuan Fu Hua* (Flos Inulae) 5g, *Zhe Shi* (Haematitum) 15-30g, *Dang Shen* (Radix Codonopsis) 10g, *Ban Xia* (Rhizoma Pinelliae) 10g, *Gan Cao* (Radix et Rhizoma Glycyrrhizae) 5g, *Da Zao* (Fructus Jujubae) 5 pieces, and *Sheng Jiang* (Rhizoma Zingiberis Recens) 3 slices. Furthermore, charred *Bai Zhu* (Rhizoma Atractylodis Macrocephalae), *Huang Jing* (Rhizoma Polygonati), *Shan Yao* (Rhizoma Dioscoreae), *Sha Ren* (Fructus Amomi), and *Mu Xiang* (Radix Aucklandiae) were added for Spleen and Stomach deficiency and

weakness; *Chuan Lian Zi* (Fructus Toosendan), *Huang Lian* (Rhizoma Coptidis), *Zhu Ru* (Caulis Bambusae in Taenia), and *Huang Qin* (Radix Scutellariae) for Liver and Stomach disharmony; *Fu Ling* (Poria), charred *Bai Zhu* (Rhizoma Atractylodis Macrocephalae), *Sha Ren* (Fructus Amomi), *Chen Pi* (Pericarpium Citri Reticulatae), and *Sheng Jiang* (Rhizoma Zingiberis Recens) for obstruction of dampness and phlegm; and *Xi Yang Shen* (Radix Panacis Quinquefolii), *Wu Mei* (Fructus Mume), *Wu Wei Zi* (Fructus Schisandrae Chinensis), *Xuan Shen* (Radix Scrophulariae), and *Mai Dong* (Radix Ophiopogonis) for yin and qi deficiencies. The study reported improvement or recovery in 65 of 66 women. The overall rate of effectiveness was 98.5%.[1]

2. **Nausea and vomiting**: Many studies have shown *Xuan Fu Dai Zhe Shi Tang* to effectively treat nausea and vomiting from various causes. One study of 60 patients reported good results for treating nausea and vomiting using modified *Xuan Fu Dai Zhe Shi Tang*. The herbal formula contained *Xuan Fu Hua* (Flos Inulae) 6g, *Zhe Shi* (Haematitum) 30g, *Ban Xia* (Rhizoma Pinelliae) 9g, *Shi Di* (Calyx Kaki) 6g, *Chen Pi* (Pericarpium Citri Reticulatae) 6g, *Gan Cao* (Radix et Rhizoma Glycyrrhizae) 9g, and others as needed. Of 60 patients, the study reported recovery in 4 cases after 2 packs of herbs, 46 cases after 4 packs, and 10 cases after 8 packs. No recurrence of nausea and vomiting were reported within 3 months of follow-ups.[2] According to another study involving 30 patients, use of this formula was associated with recovery in 17 cases within 3-6 packs of herbs, 10 cases within 12 packs of herbs, and no effect in 3 cases.[3]

3. **Peptic ulcer disease**: Administration of *Xuan Fu Dai Zhe Shi Tang* plus *Chuan Lian Zi* (Fructus Toosendan), *Yan Hu Suo* (Rhizoma Corydalis), and others was associated with satisfactory results in treating 30 patients with gastric and/or duodenal ulcers. Of 30 patients, the study reported complete recovery in 20 cases, improvement in 8 cases, and no effect in 2 cases. The overall rate of effectiveness was 93.4%.[4]

4. **Vertigo**: One study reported marked success using modified *Xuan Fu Dai Zhe Shi Tang* to treat vertigo characterized by Liver yang rising and accompanied by phlegm accumulation. The herbal formula contained *Xuan Fu Hua* (Flos Inulae), *Zhe Shi* (Haematitum), *Chen Pi* (Pericarpium Citri Reticulatae), *Fu Ling* (Poria), *Ban Xia* (Rhizoma Pinelliae), *Bai Zhu* (Rhizoma Atractylodis Macrocephalae), *Che Qian Zi* (Semen Plantaginis), *Gan Cao* (Radix et Rhizoma Glycyrrhizae), *Sang Ye* (Folium Mori), *Ju Hua* (Flos Chrysanthemi), and *Gou Teng* (Ramulus Uncariae cum Uncis). Modifications were made by adding *Shen Qu* (Massa Fermentata) for poor appetite, and *Niu Xi* (Radix Achyranthis Bidentatae) and

852

Xuán Fù Dài Zhě Shí Tāng (Inula and Hematite Decoction)

Dan Shen (Radix et Rhizoma Salviae Miltiorrhizae) for numbness of the extremities. The herbs were given in decoction daily, with most patients having improvement to recovery within 5-6 packs of herbs. Of 20 patients, the study reported complete recovery in 18 patients within 6 packs of herbs, and improvement in 2 cases.[5]

5. **Pharyngoneurosis**: One study reported marked success using *Xuan Fu Dai Zhe Shi Tang* to treat pharyngeal neurosis in 500 patients. The herbal formula contained *Xuan Fu Hua* (Flos Inulae) 15g, *Xiang Fu* (Rhizoma Cyperi) 15g, *Zhi Qiao* (Fructus Aurantii) 15g, *Zhe Shi* (Haematitum) 20g, *Ban Xia* (Rhizoma Pinelliae) 12g, *Jie Geng* (Radix Platycodonis) 12g, *Sheng Jiang* (Rhizoma Zingiberis Recens) 10g, *Zhi Gan Cao* (Radix et Rhizoma Glycyrrhizae Praeparata cum Melle) 5g, and others as needed. The duration of treatment ranged from 6 months to 3 years. The overall rate of effectiveness was 93%.[6]

RELATED FORMULA

Gān Jiāng Rén Shēn Bàn Xià Wán
(Ginger, Ginseng, and Pinellia Pill)

乾姜人參半夏丸
干姜人参半夏丸

Pinyin Name: *Gan Jiang Ren Shen Ban Xia Wan*
Literal Name: Ginger, Ginseng, and Pinellia Pill
Original Source: *Jin Gui Yao Lue* (Essentials from the Golden Cabinet) by Zhang Zhong-Jing in the Eastern Han Dynasty

Gan Jiang (Rhizoma Zingiberis)	3g [6g]
Ren Shen (Radix et Rhizoma Ginseng)	3g [6g]
Ban Xia (Rhizoma Pinelliae)	6g [9g]

The source text recommends grinding the ingredients into powder and forming into small pills with juice of *Sheng Jiang* (Rhizoma Zingiberis Recens). The pills should resemble the size of *Wu Tong Zi* (Semen Firmianae), a small seed approximately 5 mm in diameter. Take 10 pills three times daily. Today, the formula may be given in pills or decoction form. For pills, mix the powdered herbs with water and the juice of *Sheng Jiang* (Rhizoma Zingiberis Recens) to form pills. Take 3-6g of pills per dose. For decoction, use the doses suggested in brackets.

Gan Jiang Ren Shen Ban Xia Wan (Ginger, Ginseng, and Pinellia Pill) tonifies and warms the middle *jiao*, corrects the reversed flow of Lung qi, and stops vomiting. Clinically, it may be used for nausea and vomiting during pregnancy, or due to deficiency and cold of the Spleen and Stomach.

Xuan Fu Dai Zhe Shi Tang and *Gan Jiang Ren Shen Ban Xia Wan* (Ginger, Ginseng, and Pinellia Pill) both tonify the middle *jiao* and direct rising qi downward.

- *Xuan Fu Dai Zhe Shi Tang* is a potent formula that focuses primarily on correcting reversed flow of qi, secondarily on tonifying deficiency. It directly and potently suppresses nausea, vomiting, belching, hiccups, and other symptoms characterized by abnormally rising qi.
- *Gan Jiang Ren Shen Ban Xia Wan*, originally designed to treat morning sickness during pregnancy, uses small doses of herbs to gently warm the middle *jiao* to relieve nausea and vomiting. The formula is mild, and emphasizes on warming and tonifying more than countering the reversed flow of qi.

AUTHORS' COMMENTS

Xuan Fu Dai Zhe Shi Tang is effective for hiccups even if the cause is unknown. It usually is reserved as the last resort when all other treatments fail.

The dose of *Zhe Shi* (Haematitum) is intentionally low in order to prevent damage to Stomach qi. However, in patients with a strong stomach, the dose of *Zhe Shi* (Haematitum) can be increased and *Ren Shen* (Radix et Rhizoma Ginseng) and *Da Zao* (Fructus Jujubae) removed.

Xuan Fu Dai Zhe Shi Tang, *Ju Pi Zhu Ru Tang* (Tangerine Peel and Bamboo Shaving Decoction) and *Ding Xiang Shi Di Tang* (Clove and Persimmon Calyx Decoction) are three formulas that treat nausea, vomiting, and hiccups due to reversed flow of Stomach qi upwards.

- *Xuan Fu Dai Zhe Shi Tang* primarily treats reversed flow of Stomach qi due to Stomach deficiency with qi and phlegm stagnation.
- *Ju Pi Zhu Ru Tang* mainly addresses reversed flow of Stomach qi due to Stomach qi deficiency with Stomach heat.
- *Ding Xiang Shi Di Tang* is most effective for reversed flow of Stomach qi due to Stomach qi deficiency with Stomach cold.

References

1. *Tian Jin Zhong Yi* (Tianjin Chinese Medicine) 1989;3:5.
2. *He Bei Zhong Yi* (Hebei Chinese Medicine) 1990;12(4):3 .
3. *Zhong Yi Yao Yan Jiu* (Research of Chinese Medicine and Herbology) 1995;2:31.
4. *Liao Ning Zhong Yi Za Zhi* (Liaoning Journal of Chinese Medicine) 1991;18(1):20.
5. *Zhong Yi Yao Xue Bao* (Report of Chinese Medicine and Herbology) 1986;1:38.
6. *Shang Hai Zhong Yi Yao Za Zhi* (Shanghai Journal of Chinese Medicine and Herbology) 1984;4:18.

Chapter 12 – Qi-Regulating Formulas   *Section 2 – Qi-Descending Formulas*

Jú Pí Zhú Rú Tāng (Tangerine Peel and Bamboo Shaving Decoction)

橘皮竹茹湯
橘皮竹茹汤

Pinyin Name: Ju Pi Zhu Ru Tang
Literal Name: Tangerine Peel and Bamboo Shaving Decoction
Alternate Names: *Chu Pi Tsu Ju Tang*, *Ju Pi Zu Ru Tang*, Citrus and Bamboo Shaving Decoction, Citrus and Bamboo Combination
Original Source: *Jin Gui Yao Lue* (Essentials from the Golden Cabinet) by Zhang Zhong-Jing in the Eastern Han Dynasty

COMPOSITION

Chen Pi (Pericarpium Citri Reticulatae)	2 cups [12g]
Zhu Ru (Caulis Bambusae in Taenia)	2 cups [12g]
Ren Shen (Radix et Rhizoma Ginseng)	3g [3g]
Sheng Jiang (Rhizoma Zingiberis Recens)	24g [9g]
Da Zao (Fructus Jujubae)	30 pieces [5 pieces]
Gan Cao (Radix et Rhizoma Glycyrrhizae)	15g [6g]

DOSAGE / PREPARATION / ADMINISTRATION

The source text suggests cooking all of the ingredients in 10 cups [2,000 mL] of water until it is reduced to 3 cups [600 mL]. Take 1 cup of the warm decoction three times daily. Today, the decoction may be prepared using the doses suggested in brackets above.

CHINESE THERAPEUTIC ACTIONS

1. Counters reversed flow of qi to relieve hiccups
2. Benefits qi and clears heat

CLINICAL MANIFESTATIONS

Reversed flow of Stomach qi due to deficiency and heat: hiccups, dry heaves, and retching.

CLINICAL APPLICATIONS

Nausea, vomiting, hiccup, neurogenic nausea and vomiting, post-surgical nausea and vomiting, chemotherapy-induced nausea and vomiting, morning sickness, incomplete

pyloric obstruction, gastritis, erosive esophagitis, and vertigo.

EXPLANATION

Ju Pi Zhu Ru Tang (Tangerine Peel and Bamboo Shaving Decoction) treats hiccups, dry heaves or retching due to deficiency and heat of the Stomach. It contains herbs that tonify Stomach deficiency, clear heat, and correct reversed flow of Stomach qi.

In this formula, *Chen Pi* (Pericarpium Citri Reticulatae) regulates qi, harmonizes the Stomach, and relieves hiccups and retching. *Zhu Ru* (Caulis Bambusae in Taenia) clears Stomach heat and stops hiccups. *Ren Shen* (Radix et Rhizoma Ginseng) nourishes qi and strengthens the Stomach. Together with *Chen Pi* (Pericarpium Citri Reticulatae), *Ren Shen* (Radix et Rhizoma Ginseng) is able to tonify qi without causing stagnation. *Sheng Jiang* (Rhizoma Zingiberis Recens) harmonizes the Stomach to stop nausea

Ju Pi Zhu Ru Tang (Tangerine Peel and Bamboo Shaving Decoction)

Diagnosis	Signs and Symptoms	Treatment	Herbs
Reversed flow of Stomach qi due to deficiency and heat	Nausea, vomiting, hiccups or retching: Reversed flow of Stomach qi	• Corrects reversed flow of qi to relieve hiccups • Benefits qi and clears heat	• *Chen Pi* (Pericarpium Citri Reticulatae) regulates qi, and harmonizes the Stomach. • *Zhu Ru* (Caulis Bambusae in Taenia) clears Stomach heat. • *Ren Shen* (Radix et Rhizoma Ginseng) nourishes qi and strengthens the Stomach. • *Sheng Jiang* (Rhizoma Zingiberis Recens) harmonizes the Stomach. • *Da Zao* (Fructus Jujubae) and *Gan Cao* (Radix et Rhizoma Glycyrrhizae) tonify qi and harmonize the middle *jiao*.

854

Chinese Herbal Formulas and Applications

Jú Pí Zhú Rú Tāng (Tangerine Peel and Bamboo Shaving Decoction)

and vomiting. The warm nature of *Sheng Jiang* (Rhizoma Zingiberis Recens) also balances the cold influence of *Zhu Ru* (Caulis Bambusae in Taenia). *Da Zao* (Fructus Jujubae) and *Gan Cao* (Radix et Rhizoma Glycyrrhizae) help *Ren Shen* (Radix et Rhizoma Ginseng) to tonify qi and harmonize the middle *jiao*. This formula was formulated carefully to benefit qi without creating stagnation, and to clear deficiency heat without creating unnecessary cold in the body.

MODIFICATIONS

- For Stomach yin deficiency accompanied by thirst, add *Mai Dong* (Radix Ophiopogonis), *Shi Hu* (Caulis Dendrobii), or *Mai Men Dong Tang* (Ophiopogonis Decoction).
- For Stomach heat and Stomach qi and yin deficiencies, add *Mai Dong* (Radix Ophiopogonis), *Fu Ling* (Poria), *Ban Xia* (Rhizoma Pinelliae), and *Pi Pa Ye* (Folium Eriobotryae).
- When there is Stomach heat but no qi deficiency, add *Shi Di* (Calyx Kaki), and remove *Ren Shen* (Radix et Rhizoma Ginseng), *Gan Cao* (Radix et Rhizoma Glycyrrhizae), and *Da Zao* (Fructus Jujubae).
- For Stomach heat causing Stomach qi reversal, add *Huang Lian* (Rhizoma Coptidis).
- With phlegm, add *Ban Xia* (Rhizoma Pinelliae) and *Fu Ling* (Poria).

CAUTIONS / CONTRAINDICATIONS

Ju Pi Zhu Ru Tang is not suitable for hiccups and retching due to excess heat or deficiency cold.

CLINICAL STUDIES AND RESEARCH

1. **Vertigo**: One study reported success in treating 138 patients with vertigo characterized by wind and phlegm rising. The herbal formula was based on *Ju Pi Zhu Ru Tang* and *Xuan Fu Dai Zhe Shi Tang* (Inula and Hematite Decoction). This formula contained the following ingredients: *Xuan Fu Hua* (Flos Inulae) 10g, *Sheng Jiang* (Rhizoma Zingiberis Recens) 10g, *Ban Xia* (Rhizoma Pinelliae) 10g, *Fu Ling* (Poria) 10g, *Chen Pi* (Pericarpium Citri Reticulatae) 10g, *Pi Pa Ye* (Folium Eriobotryae) 10g, *Zhu Ru* (Caulis Bambusae in Taenia) 10g, *Zhe Shi* (Haematitum) 30g, *Dang Shen* (Radix Codonopsis) 15g, *Mai Dong* (Radix Ophiopogonis) 12g, *Gan Cao* (Radix et Rhizoma Glycyrrhizae) 6g, and *Da Zao* (Fructus Jujubae) 4 pieces. Additional modifications were made as necessary. Of 128 patients, the study reported complete recovery in 106 cases and improvement in 22 cases. No recurrences were reported in 6 months of follow-up.[1]
2. **Erosive esophagitis**: One study report 88.2% effectiveness using *Ju Pi Zhu Ru Tang* to treat patients with erosive esophagitis.[2]

HERB-DRUG INTERACTION

Chemotherapy-induced nausea and vomiting: One study reported a beneficial effect using modified *Ju Pi Zhu Ru Tang* to treat nausea and vomiting induced by chemotherapy. The herbal formula contained *Ren Shen* (Radix et Rhizoma Ginseng) 10g, *Dan Zhu Ye* (Herba Lophatheri) 30g, *Chen Pi* (Pericarpium Citri Reticulatae) 10g, *Sheng Jiang* (Rhizoma Zingiberis Recens) 20g, and *Da Zao* (Fructus Jujubae) 30g. The treatment protocol was to cook one pack of herbs in water to obtain 250 mL of decoction, which was administered in six to eight equally-divided doses daily. Five packs of herbs were given per course of treatment. Those with severe nausea and vomiting were also given 1g of charred salt to hold in the mouth to help to relieve nausea and vomiting.[3]

RELATED FORMULAS

Jú Pí Zhú Rú Tāng
(Tangerine Peel and Bamboo Shaving Decoction)

橘皮竹茹湯
橘皮竹茹汤

Pinyin Name: Ju Pi Zhu Ru Tang
Literal Name: Tangerine Peel and Bamboo Shaving Decoction
Original Source: *Ji Sheng Fang* (Formulas to Aid the Living) by Yan Yong-He in 1253

Chi Fu Ling (Poria Rubra)	30g
Chen Pi (Pericarpium Citri Reticulatae)	30g
Pi Pa Ye (Folium Eriobotryae)	30g
Mai Dong (Radix Ophiopogonis)	30g
Zhu Ru (Caulis Bambusae in Taenia)	30g
Ban Xia (Rhizoma Pinelliae),	
xi (washed) with liquid 7 times	30g
Ren Shen (Radix et Rhizoma Ginseng)	15g
Zhi Gan Cao (Radix et Rhizoma Glycyrrhizae	
Praeparata cum Melle)	15g

The source text states to grind the herbs into a coarse powder. Cook 12g of the powder and 5 slices of *Sheng Jiang* (Rhizoma Zingiberis Recens) with 1.5 large bowls of water until it is reduced to 80%. Take the warm, strained decoction at any time during the day.

The main actions of this formula are to correct reversed flow of qi, harmonize the Stomach, and clear heat. Clinically, the patient may have Stomach heat with such symptoms as hiccups, vomiting, thirst, and a low appetite.

This formula has the same name as the previous formula, but is derived from a different source and has a different composition and application. Therefore, it is important

12

QI-REGULATING FORMULAS

855

Chapter 12 – Qi-Regulating Formulas   Section 2 – Qi-Descending Formulas

Jú Pí Zhú Rú Tāng (Tangerine Peel and Bamboo Shaving Decoction)

that the two are not confused or used interchangeably. Contrasting aspects of these two formulas are discussed under Authors' Comments.

Xīn Zhì Jú Pí Zhú Rú Tāng (Newly-Formulated Tangerine Peel and Bamboo Shaving Decoction)
新制橘皮竹茹湯
新制橘皮竹茹汤
Pinyin Name: Xin Zhi Ju Pi Zhu Ru Tang
Literal Name: Newly-Formulated Tangerine Peel and Bamboo Shaving Decoction
Original Source: Wen Bing Tiao Bian (Systematic Differentiation of Warm Disease) by Wu Ju-Tong in 1798

Chen Pi (Pericarpium Citri Reticulatae)	9g
Zhu Ru (Caulis Bambusae in Taenia)	9g
Shi Di (Calyx Kaki)	7 pieces [9g]
Sheng Jiang (Rhizoma Zingiberis Recens),	
chong fu (taken drenched)	3 teaspoonfuls of juice

The source text recommends preparing the ingredients as a decoction. The dose of Sheng Jiang juice used in this formula is about 15 mL, mixed into the decoction immediately before administration.

Xin Zhi Ju Pi Zhu Ru Tang (Newly-Formulated Tangerine Peel and Bamboo Shaving Decoction) regulates qi, corrects the reversed flow of qi, and clears heat. Clinically,

the patient may show hiccups and vomiting due to Stomach heat, but with no signs of Stomach qi deficiency.

AUTHORS' COMMENTS

Ju Pi Zhu Ru Tang is often used for morning sickness, as it is a mild formula that will not harm the fetus. It also can be used for hiccups, nausea, and Stomach qi reversal signs caused by abdominal surgeries.

The formulas listed below regulate qi, harmonize the Stomach, clear heat, and stop hiccups. Their differences are as follows:

• *Ju Pi Zhu Ru Tang* from *Jin Gui Yao Lue* (Essentials from the Golden Cabinet) is indicated for hiccups due to Stomach heat accompanied by Stomach qi deficiency.
• *Ju Pi Zhu Ru Tang* from *Ji Sheng Fang* (Formulas to Aid the Living) treats hiccups due to Stomach heat, accompanied by qi and yin deficiencies.
• *Xin Zhi Ju Pi Zhu Ru Tang* (Newly-Formulated Tangerine Peel and Bamboo Shaving Decoction) treats hiccups due to Stomach heat with no underlying deficiency.

References
1. *Zhong Guo Nong Cun Yi Xue* (Chinese Agricultural Medicine) 1990;3:25.
2. *Zhong Yi Yao Xin Xi* (Information on Chinese Medicine and Herbology) 1988;5:19.
3. *Hei Long Jiang Zhong Yi Yao* (Heilongjiang Chinese Medicine and Herbology) 1991;3:19.

Dīng Xiāng Shì Dì Tāng (Clove and Persimmon Calyx Decoction)
丁香柿蒂湯
丁香柿蒂汤

Pinyin Name: Ding Xiang Shi Di Tang
Literal Name: Clove and Persimmon Calyx Decoction
Original Source: Zheng Yin Mai Zhi (Pattern, Cause, Pulse, and Treatment) by Qin Jing-Ming in 1702

COMPOSITION

Ding Xiang (Flos Caryophylli)	[6g]
Shi Di (Calyx Kaki)	[9g]
Ren Shen (Radix et Rhizoma Ginseng)	[3g]
Sheng Jiang (Rhizoma Zingiberis Recens)	[6g]

856

Dīng Xiāng Shì Dì Tāng (Clove and Persimmon Calyx Decoction)

DOSAGE / PREPARATION / ADMINISTRATION

The source text recommends preparing the ingredients as a decoction, but does not specify ingredient doses. Contemporary doses are indicated in brackets.

CHINESE THERAPEUTIC ACTIONS

1. Warms the middle *jiao* and benefits qi
2. Corrects reversed flow of qi to stop hiccups

CLINICAL MANIFESTATIONS

Deficiency and cold of the Stomach: constant hiccups, feelings of distention in the chest, and a slow pulse.

CLINICAL APPLICATIONS

Hiccups, nausea, vomiting, and gastritis.

EXPLANATION

Ding Xiang Shi Di Tang (Clove and Persimmon Calyx Decoction) is designed to treat hiccups due to deficiency and cold of the Stomach. Stomach qi deficiency may lead to cold accumulation, which block proper downward movement of qi. As qi flow reverses and rises upwards, it causes hiccups and a feeling of fullness and oppression in the chest. The slow pulse is indicative of Stomach cold.

This formula contains *Ding Xiang* (Flos Caryophylli) and *Shi Di* (Calyx Kaki) to warm the Stomach, dispel cold, and counter reversed flow of Stomach qi. These two herbs are essential for treating hiccups due to Stomach cold. *Ren Shen* (Radix et Rhizoma Ginseng) tonifies qi, and *Sheng Jiang* (Rhizoma Zingiberis Recens) warms and harmonizes the Stomach.

MODIFICATIONS

- When there is continuous vomiting, add *Ban Xia* (Rhizoma Pinelliae) and *Fu Ling* (Poria).
- If accompanied by heat signs, add *Huang Lian* (Rhizoma Coptidis) and *Zhu Ru* (Caulis Bambusae in Taenia).

- With stagnation of cold, qi, and phlegm, add *Ju Hong* (Exocarpium Citri Reticulatae), *Ban Xia* (Rhizoma Pinelliae), and *Chen Xiang* (Lignum Aquilariae Resinatum).
- With qi and phlegm stagnation, add *Ban Xia* (Rhizoma Pinelliae) and *Chen Pi* (Pericarpium Citri Reticulatae).
- When there are more cold signs, add *Rou Gui* (Cortex Cinnamomi) and *Wu Zhu Yu* (Fructus Evodiae).

CAUTIONS / CONTRAINDICATIONS

Ding Xiang Shi Di Tang is contraindicated in the treatment of hiccups caused by Stomach heat.

CLINICAL STUDIES AND RESEARCH

1. **Nausea and vomiting**: Administration of modified *Ding Xiang Shi Di Tang* was shown to have a marked effect in 18 patients to relieve nausea and vomiting from various causes (chronic gastritis, duodenal ulcer, cerebral embolism, and others). The herbal formula contained *Ding Xiang* (Flos Caryophylli), *Shi Di* (Calyx Kaki), *Ren Shen* (Radix et Rhizoma Ginseng), *Sheng Jiang* (Rhizoma Zingiberis Recens), *Zhi Qiao* (Fructus Aurantii), *Mu Xiang* (Radix Aucklandiae), *Chai Hu* (Radix Bupleuri), and others as needed. The treatment protocol was to cook the herbs in water to obtain 300 mL of decoction, which was taken in three equally-divided doses. In addition to herbs, the patients also were given acupuncture or acupressure treatments.[1]

2. **Gastritis**: According to one study, 53 patients with gastritis due to regurgitation of bile were successfully treated using *Ding Xiang Shi Di Tang* plus *Si Jun Zi Tang* (Four-Gentlemen Decoction). The herbal formula contained the following ingredients: *Ding Xiang* (Flos Caryophylli) 6g, *Shi Di* (Calyx Kaki) 6g, *Sheng Jiang* (Rhizoma Zingiberis Recens) 6g, *Dang Shen* (Radix Codonopsis) 12g, *Fu Ling* (Poria) 9g, *Bai Zhu* (Rhizoma Atractylodis Macrocephalae) 9g, and *Gan Cao* (Radix et Rhizoma Glycyrrhizae) 3g. The treatment protocol was to cook

Ding Xiang Shi Di Tang (Clove and Persimmon Calyx Decoction)

Diagnosis	Signs and Symptoms	Treatment	Herbs
Qi deficiency and cold of the Stomach	• Hiccups: reversed flow of Stomach qi • Feelings of distention in the chest: obstructed qi circulation • Slow pulse: cold condition	• Warms the middle *jiao* and benefits qi • Redirects reversed flow of qi and stops hiccups	• *Ding Xiang* (Flos Caryophylli) warms the Stomach, dispels cold, and redirects reversed flow of Stomach qi. • *Shi Di* (Calyx Kaki) reverses rising Stomach qi to relieve hiccups. • *Ren Shen* (Radix et Rhizoma Ginseng) tonifies qi. • *Sheng Jiang* (Rhizoma Zingiberis Recens) warms and harmonizes the Stomach.

Chapter 12 – Qi-Regulating Formulas

Section 2 – Qi-Descending Formulas

Dīng Xiāng Shì Dì Tāng (Clove and Persimmon Calyx Decoction)

the herbs in water, and administer the decoction in two equally-divided doses daily, for one month per course of treatment. Of 53 patients, the study reported significant improvement in 49 cases and moderate improvement in 4 cases.[2]

RELATED FORMULA

Shì Dì Tāng (Persimmon Calyx Decoction)

柿蒂湯

柿蒂汤

Pinyin Name: *Shi Di Tang*

Literal Name: Persimmon Calyx Decoction

Original Source: *Ji Sheng Fang* (Formulas to Aid the Living) by Yan Yong-He in 1253

Shi Di (Calyx Kaki)	30g [9g]
Ding Xiang (Flos Caryophylli)	30g [6g]

The source text instructions are: grind the herbs into powder, and cook 12g of the powder in 1.5 bowls of water with 5 slices of *Sheng Jiang* (Rhizoma Zingiberis Recens) until the liquid is reduced to 0.7 bowl. Take the strained decoction while warm at any time of the day. Today, this formula may be prepared as a decoction with the doses suggested in brackets.

Shi Di Tang (Persimmon Calyx Decoction) is composed of *Ding Xiang Shi Di Tang* without *Ren Shen* (Radix et Rhizoma Ginseng). The main actions of this formula are to warm the middle *jiao* and correct reversed flow of qi. Clinically, it may be used for patients who have unremitting hiccups due to cold in the Stomach, without underlying Stomach deficiency.

References

1. *Xin Zhong Yi* (New Chinese Medicine) 1995;7:48.
2. *Shi Yong Zhong Xi Yi Jie He Za Zhi* (Practical Journal of Integrated Chinese and Western Medicines) 1990;3(31):152.

Shēng Yáng Sàn Huǒ Tāng
(Raise the Yang and Disperse the Fire Decoction)

升陽散火湯

升阳散火汤

Pinyin Name: *Sheng Yang San Huo Tang*

Literal Name: Raise the Yang and Disperse the Fire Decoction

Alternate Name: Bupleurum and Ginseng Combination

Original Source: *Nei Wai Shang Bian Huo Lun* (Clarifying Doubts about Injury from Internal and External Causes) by Li Gao in 1247

COMPOSITION

Sheng Ma (Rhizoma Cimicifugae)	15g
Chai Hu (Radix Bupleuri)	24g
Qiang Huo (Rhizoma et Radix Notopterygii)	15g
Ge Gen (Radix Puerariae Lobatae)	15g
Du Huo (Radix Angelicae Pubescentis)	15g
Fang Feng (Radix Saposhnikoviae)	7.5g
Ren Shen (Radix et Rhizoma Ginseng)	15g
Bai Shao (Radix Paeoniae Alba)	15g
Gan Cao (Radix et Rhizoma Glycyrrhizae)	6g
Zhi Gan Cao (Radix et Rhizoma Glycyrrhizae Praeparata cum Melle)	9g

858

Shēng Yáng Sàn Huǒ Tāng
(Raise the Yang and Disperse the Fire Decoction)

DOSAGE / PREPARATION / ADMINISTRATION

The source text recommends grinding the ingredients into a coarse powder, and cooking 15g of the powder in 2 bowls of water until it is reduced to 1 bowl. Take the warm, strained decoction at any time of the day.

CHINESE THERAPEUTIC ACTIONS

1. Raises yang qi
2. Disperses stagnant heat and fire

CLINICAL MANIFESTATIONS

Cold obstruction and diversion of yang qi: feelings of heaviness and warmth in the extremities, and skin that is warm or hot to the touch.

CLINICAL APPLICATIONS

Influenza, tonsillitis, and sinusitis.

EXPLANATION

Sheng Yang San Huo Tang (Raise the Yang and Disperse the Fire Decoction) is designed to treat individuals with underlying Stomach deficiency, who after consuming cold foods, suffer from cold obstruction with diversion of yang qi to the four limbs. Because of the underlying deficiency, the Stomach is unable to process cold food, leading to stagnation of cold that blocks the normal ascension of yang. Consequently, the flow of yang is diverted to the exterior, and produces a feeling of warmth in the extremities, skin, and muscles.

This formula contains many warm and acrid herbs to properly address the condition of cold obstruction with diversion of yang qi. *Sheng Ma* (Rhizoma Cimicifugae) and *Chai Hu* (Radix Bupleuri) both have a general ascending action. *Qiang Huo* (Rhizoma et Radix Notopterygii) and *Ge Gen* (Radix Puerariae Lobatae) are particularly effective for the upper parts of the body, while *Du Huo* (Radix Angelicae Pubescentis) is effective for the lower parts. Lastly, *Fang Feng* (Radix Saposhnikoviae) has a generalized dispersing effect. To prevent the ascending and dispersing herbs from depleting qi and blood, *Ren Shen* (Radix et Rhizoma Ginseng) and *Bai Shao* (Radix Paeoniae Alba) tonify qi and nourish the blood. Fresh *Gan Cao* (Radix et Rhizoma Glycyrrhizae) purges stagnant fire from the Spleen, while honey-processed *Zhi Gan Cao* (Radix et Rhizoma Glycyrrhizae Praeparata cum Melle) strengthens the Spleen and Stomach.

CAUTIONS / CONTRAINDICATIONS

Avoid consumption of cold foods and beverages while taking *Sheng Yang San Huo Tang*.

Sheng Yang San Huo Tang (Raise the Yang and Disperse the Fire Decoction)

Diagnosis	Signs and Symptoms	Treatment	Herbs
Cold obstruction and diversion of yang qi	Feelings of heaviness and warmth in the extremities, skin that is warm or hot to the touch: diversion of yang qi to the exterior due to obstruction of cold in the interior	• Raises yang qi • Disperses stagnant heat and fire	• *Sheng Ma* (Rhizoma Cimicifugae) and *Chai Hu* (Radix Bupleuri) lift yang qi upward. • *Qiang Huo* (Rhizoma et Radix Notopterygii), *Ge Gen* (Radix Puerariae Lobatae), *Du Huo* (Radix Angelicae Pubescentis) and *Fang Feng* (Radix Saposhnikoviae) disperse cold from upper, lower and exterior parts of the body. • *Ren Shen* (Radix et Rhizoma Ginseng) and *Bai Shao* (Radix Paeoniae Alba) tonify qi and nourish blood. • *Gan Cao* (Radix et Rhizoma Glycyrrhizae) purges stagnant fire from the Spleen. • *Zhi Gan Cao* (Radix et Rhizoma Glycyrrhizae Praeparata cum Melle) strengthens the Spleen and Stomach.

Chapter 12 – Qi-Regulating Formulas

Chapter 12 — Summary

— Qi-Regulating Formulas

SECTION 1: QI-MOVING FORMULAS

Name	Similarities	Differences
Yue Ju Wan (Escape Restraint Pill)	Regulates qi circulation to relieve constraint	Treats qi, blood, phlegm, fire, damp, and food stagnation
Jin Ling Zi San (Melia Toosendan Powder)	Regulates qi circulation to relieve pain	Smoothes Liver qi, activates blood circulation
Ban Xia Hou Po Tang (Pinellia and Magnolia Bark Decoction)	Activate qi circulation, dissolve phlegm, direct reversed flow of qi downwards	Treats *mei he qi* (plum-pit *qi*) and phlegm stagnation
Zhi Shi Xie Bai Gui Zhi Tang (Immature Bitter Orange, Chinese Chive, and Cinnamon Twig Decoction)		Treats *xiong bi* (painful obstruction of the chest)
Ju He Wan (Tangerine Seed Pill)	Activate qi circulation, dispel cold, relieve pain, treat hernia	Stronger effect to soften hardness and disperse nodules
Tian Tai Wu Yao San (Top-Quality Lindera Powder)		Stronger effect to activate qi and dispel cold
Nuan Gan Jian (Warm the Liver Decoction)		Stronger effect to warm the Kidney and nourish the Liver
Hou Po Wen Zhong Tang (Magnolia Bark Decoction for Warming the Middle)	Activates qi circulation, warms the middle *jiao*	Dispels damp-cold in the Spleen and Stomach

Yue Ju Wan (Escape Restraint Pill) treats stagnation of qi, blood, phlegm, fire, dampness, and food. Because qi stagnation is the main cause of all the stagnations, this formula is categorized under the qi-regulating category. Clinical manifestations include chest fullness and rigidity, abdominal fullness and pain, acid regurgitation, nausea, vomiting, and indigestion.

Jin Ling Zi San (Melia Toosendan Powder) regulates qi circulation, smoothes the Liver, activates blood circulation, and stops pain. This formula is cold in nature, and thus is used for Liver qi stagnation with heat. It can also be used for menstrual pain due to stagnation of qi and blood, accompanied by heat. Other clinical manifestations include intermittent hypochondriac pain, chest and abdominal pain, a yellow tongue coating, and a wiry, rapid pulse.

Ban Xia Hou Po Tang (Pinellia and Magnolia Bark Decoction) activates qi, disperses stagnation, reverses the flow of ascending qi, and dissolves phlegm. It is used for *mei he qi* (plum-pit *qi*) caused by emotional disturbances. Other clinical manifestations include chest and hypochondriac pain.

Zhi Shi Xie Bai Gui Zhi Tang (Immature Bitter Orange, Chinese Chive, and Cinnamon Twig Decoction) activates yang, disperses stagnation, corrects the reversed flow of qi, and dispels phlegm. This formula is designed to treat *xiong bi* (painful obstruction of the chest) due to chest yang deficiency and stagnation of qi and phlegm. Clinical manifestations include fullness and pain, wheezing, coughing with sputum, shortness of breath, a white and greasy tongue coating, and a deep, wiry pulse or tight pulse.

Ju He Wan (Tangerine Seed Pill), *Tian Tai Wu Yao San* (Top-Quality Lindera Powder), and *Nuan Gan Jian* (Warm the Liver Decoction) are commonly used to treat hernia. They have similar actions to activate qi circulation, dispel cold, and relieve pain.

Chapter 12 — Summary

- *Ju He Wan* is best for damp-cold hernia, as it more strongly activates qi circulation, stops pain, softens hardness, and dissolves nodules. Clinical manifestations of this condition include swelling and enlargement or hardness of the testes, and pain radiating from the testes to the abdomen.
- *Tian Tai Wu Yao San* treats hernia of the small intestine, and pain and swelling in the testes due to qi stagnation and cold accumulation. Of the three formulas, this one has strongest actions to activate qi circulation, stop pain, disperse cold, and spread the Liver. Key signs and symptoms include lower abdominal pain radiating to the testicles, a pale tongue with white tongue coating, and a wiry pulse.
- *Nuan Gan Jian* treats hernial pain due to cold in the Liver and Kidney. Its primary actions are to warm the Liver and Kidney, activate qi circulation, and stop pain. Clinically, it is used for hernial pain with lower abdominal pain, a pale tongue with white tongue coating, and a deep, wiry pulse.

Hou Po Wen Zhong Tang (Magnolia Bark Decoction for Warming the Middle) mainly treats abdominal distention, fullness and pain due to qi stagnation and damp-cold in the Spleen and Stomach.

SECTION 2: QI-DESCENDING FORMULAS

Name	Similarities	Differences
Su Zi Jiang Qi Tang (Perilla Fruit Decoction for Directing Qi Downward)	Direct reversed flow of Lung qi downwards, relieve cough, wheezing, and dyspnea	Eliminates phlegm, warms the Kidney
Ding Chuan Tang (Arrest Wheezing Decoction)		Releases exterior wind-cold, eliminates interior hot phlegm
Shen Mi Tang (Mysterious Decoction)		Dispels qi and phlegm stagnation
Si Mo Tang (Four Milled-Herbs Decoction)		Unblocks Liver qi stagnation, directs Lung and Stomach qi downwards
Xuan Fu Dai Zhe Shi Tang (Inula and Hematite Decoction)	Direct reversed flow of Stomach qi downwards, relieve nausea, vomiting, and hiccups	Eliminates phlegm, warms the Stomach, dispels cold
Ju Pi Zhu Ru Tang (Tangerine Peel and Bamboo Shaving Decoction)		Tonifies Stomach qi, clears Stomach heat
Ding Xiang Shi Di Tang (Clove and Persimmon Calyx Decoction)		Warms and strengthens the Stomach, dispels cold
Sheng Yang San Huo Tang (Raise the Yang and Disperse the Fire Decoction)	Raises and regulates yang qi circulation	Disperses stagnant fire

Su Zi Jiang Qi Tang (Perilla Fruit Decoction for Directing Qi Downward) is used mainly for upper-excess and lower-deficiency syndrome. In this syndrome, upper excess refers to phlegm accumulation in the Lung, and lower deficiency refers to Kidney yang deficiency. Clinical manifestations include excess phlegm and sputum, wheezing, coughing, shortness of breath, chest and hypochondriac fullness, possible back soreness, lassitude, and a white, slippery tongue coating.

Ding Chuan Tang (Arrest Wheezing Decoction) ventilates the Lung, corrects the reversed flow of qi, relieves wheezing, and clears heat and phlegm. It is used for wheezing due to wind-cold constricting the exterior and phlegm-heat brewing in the interior. Clinical manifestations include rapid breathing, excess phlegm, thick, yellow sputum, coughing, wheezing, a yellow, greasy tongue coating, and a slippery, rapid pulse.

Shen Mi Tang (Mysterious Decoction) regulates Lung qi and eliminates phlegm to relieve cough, wheezing, and dyspnea. It is most effective for wheezing and dyspnea due to stagnation of qi and

Chapter 12 – Qi-Regulating Formulas

Chapter 12 — Summary

phlegm, with signs and symptoms such as shortness of breath, presence of sputum and phlegm in the lungs, a rattling sound in the throat, and fullness and distention in the chest and hypochondrium.

Si Mo Tang (Four Milled-Herbs Decoction) activates qi circulation, corrects the rising qi, disperses stagnation, and relieves chest oppression. It is used when there is irregular flow of Lung and Stomach qi as a result of Liver qi stagnation from emotional disturbances. Clinical manifestations include irritability, chest oppression, wheezing, fullness and oppression of the epigastrium, and lack of appetite.

Xuan Fu Dai Zhe Shi Tang (Inula and Hematite Decoction) dissolves phlegm, corrects the reversed flow of qi, and nourishes and harmonizes Stomach qi. It is used for Stomach qi deficiency with stagnation of phlegm and qi causing epigastric distention and hardness, with unremitting belching and hiccups.

Ju Pi Zhu Ru Tang (Tangerine Peel and Bamboo Shaving Decoction) nourishes qi, clears heat, and redirects Stomach qi to relieve hiccups and retching. This formula is used for hiccups, dry heaves and retching due to deficiency and heat of the Stomach.

Ding Xiang Shi Di Tang (Clove and Persimmon Calyx Decoction) warms and nourishes the middle *jiao*, corrects the reversed flow of qi, and stops hiccups. It is used for cold accumulation in the Stomach. Clinical manifestations include unremitting hiccups, distending sensation in the chest, and a slow pulse.

Sheng Yang San Huo Tang (Raise the Yang and Disperse the Fire Decoction) raises and regulates the circulation of yang qi to disperse stagnant fire and dissolve damp-heat. It treats obstruction of cold and diversion of yang qi characterized by feelings of heaviness and warmth in the extremities, and skin that is warm to the touch.

862

Chapter 13

— Blood-Regulating Formulas

理血剂

王清任 Wāng Qíng-Rèn

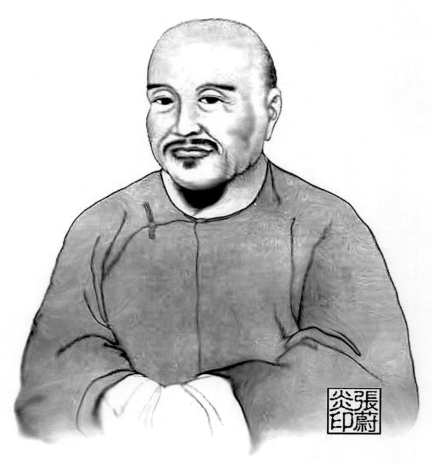

王清任 Wāng Qíng-Rèn, 1768 – 1831.

王清任 Wāng Qīng-Rèn

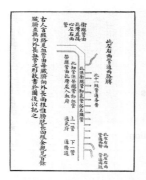 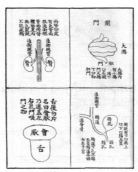

医林改错 *Yi Lin Gai Cuo* (Corrections of Errors Among Physicians)
in 1830, with illustrations and explanations of internal organs.

Wang Qing-Ren was born during the Qing dynasty. He grew up studying martial arts, and later pursued the study of traditional Chinese medicine. Because of his martial arts background, he had a good understanding of human anatomy.

Wang suspected many errors in the ancient texts.[1] He was the first person of his era to question traditional wisdom. To confirm his opinions, he personally observed the internal organs of corpses of executed convicts, and the deserted bodies of children who had died from epidemics.[2] After years of observation, Wang published *Yi Lin Gai Cuo* (Corrections of Errors Among Physicians) in 1830. In this text, he drew 25 precise illustrations of human anatomy from different angles and depth. Furthermore, based on his findings, he accurately pointed out many errors among medical texts at the time, such as the presence of the pancreas and diaphragm; corrected the mistaken notion that the liver was in the left hypochondrium; and stated that it is the brain that thinks (not the heart). Wang also said that "treating disease without knowing the internal organs is like a blind man walking in the dark." Wang was harshly criticized for his boldness, and his works were not recognized for a long time.

Wang parlayed his uncommon understanding of human anatomy to develop the use of blood-moving formulas to treat blood stasis disorders. His outstanding formulas for the treatment of blood stasis affecting different parts of the body include:

- *Tong Qiao Huo Xue Tang* (Unblock the Orifices and Invigorate the Blood Decoction)
- *Xue Fu Zhu Yu Tang* (Drive Out Stasis in the Mansion of Blood Decoction)
- *Ge Xia Zhu Yu Tang* (Drive Out Blood Stasis Below the Diaphragm Decoction)
- *Shao Fu Zhu Yu Tang* (Drive Out Blood Stasis in the Lower Abdomen Decoction)
- *Shen Tong Zhu Yu Tang* (Drive Out Blood Stasis from a Painful Body Decoction)
- *Bu Yang Huan Wu Tang* (Tonify the Yang to Restore Five Decoction)

1. In Chinese culture, it is extremely disrespectful to cut [dissect] the human body, which is considered a gift from heaven. Therefore, ancient Chinese physicians learned human anatomy from illustrations in the *Nei Jing* (Inner Classic), and accepted it as universal truth.
2. Wang claimed in his writing that he only observed, but did not cut or dissect, human bodies. The corpses were deserted bodies of executed convicts or dead children, whose bodies were torn open by wild animals. Therefore, he did not commit any act of disrespect to those dead individuals.

Dynasties & Kingdoms	Year
Xia Dynasty 夏	2100-1600 BCE
Shang Dynasty 商	1600-1100 BCE
Zhou Dynasty 周	1100-221 BCE
Qin Dynasty 秦	221-207 BCE
Han Dynasty 漢	206 BCE-220
Three Kingdoms 三國	220-280
Western Jin Dynasty 西晉	265-316
Eastern Jin Dynasty 東晉	317-420
Northern and Southern Dynasties 北南朝	420-581
Sui Dynasty 隋	581-618
Tang Dynasty 唐	618-907
Five Dynasties 五代	907-960
Song Dynasty 宋	960-1279
Liao Dynasty 遼	916-1125
Jin Dynasty 金	1115-1234
Yuan Dynasty 元	1271-1368
Ming Dynasty 明	1368-1644
Qing Dynasty 清	**1644-1911**
Republic of China 中華民國	1912-Present Day
People's Republic of China 中華人民共和國	1949-Present Day

Chapter 13 – Blood-Regulating Formulas

Table of Contents

Chapter 13. Blood-Regulating Formulas ·········· **863**
Biography of Wang Qing-Ren ··········· 864

Section 1. Blood-Invigorating and Stasis-Removing Formulas ·········· **873**
Tao He Cheng Qi Tang (Peach Pit Decoction to Order the Qi) ··········· 873
 Xia Yu Xue Tang (Drain Blood Stasis Decoction) ··········· 876
Tong Qiao Huo Xue Tang (Unblock the Orifices and Invigorate the Blood Decoction) ··········· 877
Xue Fu Zhu Yu Tang (Drive Out Stasis in the Mansion of Blood Decoction) ··········· 879
 San Jiao Zhu Yu Tang (Drive Out Blood Stasis in Three *Jiaos* Decoction) ··········· 883
Ge Xia Zhu Yu Tang (Drive Out Blood Stasis Below the Diaphragm Decoction) ··········· 885
Shao Fu Zhu Yu Tang (Drive Out Blood Stasis in the Lower Abdomen Decoction) ··········· 889
Shen Tong Zhu Yu Tang (Drive Out Blood Stasis from a Painful Body Decoction) ··········· 893
 Zhu Yu Tang (Drive Out Blood Stasis Decoction) ··········· 895
Fu Yuan Huo Xue Tang (Revive Health by Invigorating the Blood Decoction) ··········· 897
 Po Bu Zi Ye Tang (Cordia Decoction) ··········· 900
 Huo Xue Shun Qi Tang (Invigorate the Blood and Smooth the Qi Decoction) ··········· 900
Zheng Gu Zi Jin Dan (Purple and Gold Pill for Righteous Bones) ··········· 901
 Huo Xue Zhi Tong Tang (Invigorate the Blood and Stop Pain Decoction) ··········· 902
Qi Li San (Seven-Thousandths of a Tael Powder) ··········· 903
Bu Yang Huan Wu Tang (Tonify the Yang to Restore Five Decoction) ··········· 905
 Nao Wei Kang Wan (Benefit Brain Atrophy Pill) ··········· 909
Shi Xiao San (Sudden Smile Powder) ··········· 911
 Shou Nian San (Pinch Powder) ··········· 913
 Wen Jing Zhi Tong Tang (Warm the Channel and Stop Pain Decoction) ··········· 913
Huo Luo Xiao Ling Dan (Fantastically Effective Pill to Invigorate the Collaterals) ··········· 914
 Gong Wai Yun Fang (Ectopic Pregnancy Formula) ··········· 917
Dan Shen Yin (Salvia Decoction) ··········· 917
Wen Jing Tang (Warm the Channels Decoction) ··········· 919
Ai Fu Nuan Gong Wan (Mugwort and Cyperus Pill for Warming the Womb) ··········· 923
Sheng Hua Tang (Generation and Transformation Decoction) ··········· 925
 Tong Ru Wan (Unblock the Breast Pill) ··········· 927
Gui Zhi Fu Ling Wan (Cinnamon Twig and Poria Pill) ··········· 928
 Duo Ming Wan (Life-Taking Pill) ··········· 931
 Cui Sheng Tang (Birth-Hastening Decoction) ··········· 931
Zhe Chong Yin (Break the Conflict Decoction) ··········· 933
Bie Jia Jian Wan (Soft-Shelled Turtle Shell Pill) ··········· 935
Da Huang Zhe Chong Wan (Rhubarb and Eupolyphaga Pill) ··········· 937

Section 2. Stop-Bleeding Formulas ·········· **939**
Shi Hui San (Ten Partially-Charred Substances Powder) ··········· 939
 Zhi Xue Tang (Stop Bleeding Decoction) ··········· 941
Si Sheng Wan (Four-Fresh Pill) ··········· 942
Ke Xue Fang (Coughing of Blood Formula) ··········· 943
Huai Hua San (Sophora Japonica Flower Powder) ··········· 944
 Huai Jiao Wan (Sophora Japonica Fruit Pill) ··········· 946
Xiao Ji Yin Zi (Cirsium Decoction) ··········· 946
Huang Tu Tang (Yellow Earth Decoction) ··········· 948
Jiao Ai Tang (Ass-Hide Gelatin and Mugwort Decoction) ··········· 950

Blood-Regulating Formulas (Summary) ·········· **953**

Chinese Herbal Formulas and Applications

Chapter 13 — Overview

理血劑

— Blood-Regulating Formulas

Definition: Blood-regulating formulas invigorate blood circulation, remove blood stasis, and/or stop bleeding. They are used to treat blood stagnation and to stop bleeding.

B lood is a vital substance that continually circulates and nourishes both the inside (*zang fu* organs) and outside (extremities) of the body. Various etiologies contribute to disorders of blood deficiency, blood stagnation, and bleeding. These conditions may occur independently or concurrently. Blood deficiency is treated with blood-tonifying formulas (*see* Chapter 8: Tonic Formulas), blood stagnation is treated with blood-invigorating and stasis-removing formulas, and bleeding is treated with stop-bleeding formulas.

Differential diagnosis of blood disorders is extremely important for patient safety and for treatment success. One must determine whether the blood disorder is characterized by cold or heat, and whether it is of a deficient or excess nature. Furthermore, one needs to identify correctly the cause(s) of the blood disorder, and recognize whether the situation is severe or mild, and whether it is acute or chronic in nature. In emergency situations (e.g., acute and severe bleeding), it is more important to address the symptoms first (i.e., stop the bleeding). In non-emergent situations (e.g., chronic and mild blood disorders), one should concentrate on treating the cause, or address both the cause and the symptoms concurrently.

SUBCATEGORIES OF ACTION

Blood-regulating formulas are divided into two subcategories: blood-invigorating and stasis-removing formulas, and stop-bleeding formulas.

~

Blood-regulating formulas have distinct, opposite functions: to invigorate blood circulation and remove blood stasis, and to promote coagulation and stop bleeding.

~

1. **Blood-Invigorating and Stasis-Removing Formulas**

These formulas are suitable for treating blood stagnation, and are commonly used to treat the following conditions involving blood stagnation: acute trauma, chronic injuries, amenorrhea, dysmenorrhea, retention of lochia, hemiplegia, chest pain, epigastric pain, and initial onset of ulcerative diseases. Clinical manifestations of blood stagnation include sharp, stabbing pain at a fixed location, pain that intensifies with pressure, and stiffness and hardness at the affected area upon palpation. The tongue body is usually dark and purple in color, with prominent or pronounced petechiae.

Because conditions involving blood stagnation are often complex, other herbs are usually added to enhance the overall effectiveness of the treatment. If blood stasis is accompanied by qi stagnation, qi-regulating herbs are added to promote normal qi circulation. If blood stasis is generating heat, both blood-invigorating and heat-clearing herbs should be used at the same time. If blood stasis is caused by cold, herbs that warm the channels and disperse cold enhance the treatment effect. Finally, chronic stagnation may contribute to qi and blood deficiencies, thus requiring the use of qi- and blood-tonifying herbs.

Herbs commonly used to invigorate blood circulation and remove blood stasis include *Chuan Xiong* (Rhizoma Chuanxiong), *Tao Ren* (Semen Persicae), *Hong Hua* (Flos Carthami), *Chi Shao* (Radix Paeoniae Rubra), and *Dan Shen* (Radix et Rhizoma Salviae Miltiorrhizae). Exemplar formulas include *Tao He Cheng Qi Tang* (Peach Pit Decoction to Order the Qi), *Xue Fu Zhu Yu Tang* (Drive Out Stasis in the Mansion of Blood Decoction), *Fu Yuan Huo Xue Tang* (Revive Health by Invigorating the Blood Decoction), *Wen*

~

Differential diagnosis of blood disorders is extremely important for patient safety and for treatment success.

~

BLOOD-REGULATING FORMULAS

13

867

Chapter 13 – Blood-Regulating Formulas

Chapter 13 — Overview

Jing Tang (Warm the Channels Decoction), *Sheng Hua Tang* (Generation and Transformation Decoction), and *Shi Xiao San* (Sudden Smile Powder).

2. Stop-Bleeding Formulas

These formulas are used to treat various types of bleeding, such as epistaxis, hemoptysis, hematemesis, hematochezia, and abnormal menstrual bleeding.

Proper management of bleeding is rather complicated, as there are many factors that must be considered, such as its characteristics (cold or hot, deficiency or excess), location (upper or lower body), and urgency (acute or chronic). For example, bleeding due to heat in the *xue* (blood) level, causing reckless movement of blood, needs to be treated with herbs that cool the blood and stop bleeding; bleeding due to deficiency and damage to the *chong* (thoroughfare) and *ren* (conception) channels is treated with herbs that tonify blood and stop bleeding. In addition, bleeding in the upper body should be treated with an additional proportion of herbs that guide the blood downward; and bleeding in the lower parts of the body should be treated with herbs that lift upward. Furthermore, in acute and severe cases of bleeding, it is more important to treat the symptoms first and stop the bleeding than it is to initially address the underlying cause; while in chronic cases, it is more important to address the underlying cause. Lastly, profuse bleeding may contribute to collapse of qi, and this condition must be treated first by herbs that restore and rescue *yuan* (source) *qi* from collapse, before efforts to control the bleeding will succeed.

> In non-emergent situations, concentrate on treating the cause, or address both cause and symptoms concurrently.

Herbs commonly used to stop bleeding due to heat include *Ce Bai Ye* (Cacumen Platycladi), *Xiao Ji* (Herba Cirsii), *Bai Mao Gen* (Rhizoma Imperatae), and *Di Yu* (Radix Sanguisorbae). Herbs used to stop bleeding due to cold include *Pao Jiang* (Rhizoma Zingiberis Praeparatum), *Ai Ye* (Folium Artemisiae Argyi), and *Fu Long Gan* (Terra Flava Usta). Herbs commonly used to stop bleeding accompanied by blood stasis include *San Qi* (Radix et Rhizoma Notoginseng) and *Pu Huang* (Pollen Typhae). Furthermore, bleeding in the upper body should be treated with a small amount of herbs that guide the blood downward, such as *Niu Xi* (Radix Achyranthis Bidentatae) and *Da Huang* (Radix et Rhizoma Rhei); bleeding in the lower body should be treated with herbs that lift upward, such as charred *Jing Jie* (Herba Schizonepetae), charred *Sheng Ma* (Rhizoma Cimicifugae), and *Huang Qi* (Radix Astragali).

Exemplar formulas that stop bleeding include *Shi Hui San* (Ten Partially-Charred Substances Powder), *Huai Hua San* (Sophora Japonica Flower Powder), *Huang Tu Tang* (Yellow Earth Decoction), and *Jiao Ai Tang* (Ass-Hide Gelatin and Mugwort Decoction).

CAUTIONS / CONTRAINDICATIONS

- Use of blood-invigorating herbs may consume and damage the qi and blood, especially if used in large doses or for an extended period of time. Therefore, qi- and blood-tonifying herbs are often added to protect the body from adverse effects.
- Blood-regulating formulas have moving and dispersing characteristics, and should be used with extreme caution during pregnancy and in individuals with hypermenorrhea.
- Blood-activating herbs must be used cautiously, as overdose or prolonged use may contribute to more bleeding. If bleeding is accompanied by blood stasis (such as in a trauma situation), then blood-activating herbs should be used to clear any residual blood stagnation in the body, as well as taking appropriate stop-bleeding measures.

> In severe, acute bleeding, it is more important to treat the symptoms, stop the bleeding, than to initially address the underlying cause.

- Herbs that stop bleeding should not be given at large doses or for prolonged periods of time, as such uses may contribute to the development of blood stasis.
- Astringent herbs and formulas must be used with caution in cases of bleeding, as their binding and retaining effect may contribute to blood stasis.
- Bleeding in the upper body should ***not*** be treated with herbs that have ascending or lifting characteristics. Bleeding in the lower body should ***not*** be treated with herbs that have descending or sinking characteristics.

868

Chinese Herbal Formulas and Applications

Chapter 13 — Overview

PHARMACOLOGICAL EFFECTS & CLINICAL APPLICATIONS

Blood-regulating formulas are divided into two subcategories: 1) blood-invigorating and stasis-removing formulas, and 2) stop-bleeding formulas. These subcategories have distinct characteristics in Chinese herbal medicine; they also have contrasting Western pharmacology and clinical applications.

1. **Blood-invigorating and stasis-removing formulas** have a wide variety of pharmacological effects and clinical applications. The main applications are as follows:

   - **Clotting disorders**: Many blood-invigorating and stasis-removing herbs have been shown to have marked hematological effects. For example,
     - o *Dan Shen* (Radix et Rhizoma Salviae Miltiorrhizae) and *Chi Shao* (Radix Paeoniae Rubra) have anticoagulant effects,[1,2,3]
     - o *Dan Shen* (Radix et Rhizoma Salviae Miltiorrhizae), *Chuan Xiong* (Rhizoma Chuanxiong) and *Hong Hua* (Flos Carthami) have antiplatelet effects,[4,5,6] and
     - o *San Leng* (Rhizoma Sparganii) and *E Zhu* (Rhizoma Curcumae) have thrombolytic effects.[7,8]
   Similarly, blood-invigorating and stasis-removing formulas have marked anticoagulant, antiplatelet, and thrombolytic effects.[9,10,11,12,13,14] Clinical applications of these formulas include stroke,[15,16] ischemic stroke,[17] cerebral infarction,[18] post-stroke sequelae,[19] and deep vein thrombosis.[20] Exemplar formulas include *Xue Fu Zhu Yu Tang* (Drive Out Stasis in the Mansion of Blood Decoction) and *Bu Yang Huan Wu Tang* (Tonify the Yang to Restore Five Decoction).

   - **Cardiovascular disorders**: Many blood-invigorating and stasis-removing herbs and formulas have been shown to exert profound influence on the cardiovascular system. They dilate blood vessels, decrease blood pressure, and increase blood perfusion to smaller blood vessels.[21,22] Clinical applications include cardiac angina,[23] ischemia,[24] bradyarrhythmia,[25] and coronary heart disease.[26] Exemplar formulas include *Xue Fu Zhu Yu Tang* (Drive Out Stasis in the Mansion of Blood Decoction) and *Bu Yang Huan Wu Tang* (Tonify the Yang to Restore Five Decoction).

   - **Hyperlipidemia**: Many blood-invigorating and stasis-removing herbs and formulas have been shown to lower plasma cholesterol and triglyceride levels.[27,28,29] These formulas may be used to treat hyperlipidemia,[30] arteriosclerosis,[31] and atherosclerosis.[32,33] They also are used to treat associated clotting and cardiovascular disorders. Exemplar formulas include *Xue Fu Zhu Yu Tang* (Drive Out Stasis in the Mansion of Blood Decoction) and *Bu Yang Huan Wu Tang* (Tonify the Yang to Restore Five Decoction).

   - **Gynecological and obstetric disorders:** One of the most common and effective uses of blood-invigorating and stasis-removing formulas is in the treatment of gynecological and obstetric disorders. Clinical applications include uterine bleeding,[34,35] premenstrual syndrome,[36] dysmenorrhea,[37,38] amenorrhea,[39,40] anovulation,[41] infertility (male and female),[42,43,44,45] ectopic pregnancy,[46,47] endometriosis,[48,49,50] hysteromyoma,[51,52] uterine myomas,[53] uterine leiomyomas,[54] adnexitis,[55] oophoritic cyst,[56] hyperplasia of mammary glands,[57] and retention of lochia.[58] Exemplar formulas include *Shao Fu Zhu Yu Tang* (Drive Out Blood Stasis in the Lower Abdomen Decoction), *Shi Xiao San* (Sudden Smile Powder), *Wen Jing Tang* (Warm the Channels Decoction), *Ai Fu Nuan Gong Wan* (Mugwort and Cyperus Pill for Warming the Womb), *Sheng Hua Tang* (Generation and Transformation Decoction), and *Gui Zhi Fu Ling Wan* (Cinnamon Twig and Poria Pill).

   - **Pain**: Many blood-invigorating and stasis-removing herbs are well-documented for their analgesic and anti-inflammatory effects.[59,60,61,62,63] Clinical applications include headache,[64] sciatica,[65,66] arthritis,[67] rheumatoid arthritis,[68] lumbago,[69] and many others. Exemplar formulas include *Shen Tong Zhu Yu Tang* (Drive Out Blood Stasis from a Painful Body Decoction), *Fu Yuan Huo Xue Tang* (Revive Health by Invigorating the Blood Decoction), *Zheng Gu Zi Jin Dan* (Purple and Gold Pill for Righteous Bones), and *Huo Luo Xiao Ling Dan* (Fantastically Effective Pill to Invigorate the Collaterals).

   - **Traumatic injuries**: These formulas also treat traumatic injuries, such as concussion,[70,71,72] bone fractures,[73,74] and various external and sports injuries.[75] Exemplar formulas that treat traumatic injuries include *Tong Qiao Huo Xue Tang* (Unblock the Orifices and Invigorate the Blood

~
Blood-invigorating and stasis-removing herbs have anticoagulant, antiplatelet and thrombolytic effects.
~

BLOOD-REGULATING FORMULAS

13

869

Chapter 13 – Blood-Regulating Formulas

Chapter 13 — Overview

Decoction), *Fu Yuan Huo Xue Tang* (Revive Health by Invigorating the Blood Decoction), *Zheng Gu Zi Jin Dan* (Purple and Gold Pill for Righteous Bones), and *Qi Li San* (Seven-Thousandths of a Tael Powder).

- **Liver, gallbladder, and pancreatic disorders**: These formulas may be used for certain liver, gallbladder, and pancreatic disorders, such as hepatitis,[76,77,78] hepatic hemangioma,[79] liver abscess,[80] cholecystitis,[81] and pancreatitis.[82] Exemplar formulas include *Tao He Cheng Qi Tang* (Peach Pit Decoction to Order the Qi), *Ge Xia Zhu Yu Tang* (Drive Out Blood Stasis Below the Diaphragm Decoction), and *Fu Yuan Huo Xue Tang* (Revive Health by Invigorating the Blood Decoction).

- **Kidney disorders**: Some blood-invigorating and stasis-removing formulas have been successfully used to treat various kidney disorders, such as pyelonephritis,[83] renal insufficiency,[84] chronic nephritis,[85] and renal colic caused by stones.[86] Exemplar formulas include *Tao He Cheng Qi Tang* (Peach Pit Decoction to Order the Qi) and *Bu Yang Huan Wu Tang* (Tonify the Yang to Restore Five Decoction).

~

Stop-bleeding herbs are hemostatic: promote coagulation and stop bleeding.

~

2. **Stop-bleeding formulas** are used primarily for their hemostatic effect to stop bleeding.

- **Bleeding**: These formulas may be used to treat all types of bleeding disorders, including but not limited to epistaxis and hemoptysis in the upper body, hematemesis in the middle body, and hematochezia, hematuria, abnormal uterine bleeding, and bleeding hemorrhoids in the lower body.[87,88,89,90] Furthermore, they treat acute bleeding from external injuries such as trauma or sports injuries, or chronic bleeding from internal illnesses such as bleeding ulcers.[91,92] These hemostatic herbs and formulas increase platelets and facilitate the clotting cascade.[93] Representative formulas that stop bleeding include *Shi Hui San* (Ten Partially-Charred Substances Powder), *Huai Hua San* (Sophora Japonica Flower Powder), *Huang Tu Tang* (Yellow Earth Decoction), and *Jiao Ai Tang* (Ass-Hide Gelatin and Mugwort Decoction).

References

1. *Shang Hai Di Yi Xue Yuan Xue Bao* (Journal of First Shanghai Medical College), 1979; 6(3):144.
2. *Shang Hai Di Yi Xue Yuan Xue Bao* (Journal of First Shanghai Medical College), 1982; 9(1):14.
3. *Zhong Xi Yi Jie He Za Zhi* (Journal of Integrated Chinese and Western Medicine), 1984; 4(12):745.
4. *Shang Hai Di Yi Xue Yuan Xue Bao* (Journal of First Shanghai Medical College), 1979; 6(3):144.
5. *Shang Hai Di Yi Xue Yuan Xue Bao* (Journal of First Shanghai Medical College), 1982; 9(1):14.
6. *Hua Xi Yi Xue Za Zhi* (Huaxi Medical Journal), 1993; 8(3):170.
7. *Zhong Xi Yi Jie He Fang Zhi Yan Jiu Xue Guan Zhi Liao* (Research on Prevention and Treatment of Cardiovascular Disorders Using Integrated Chinese and Western Medicines), 1977; (3):47,50.
8. *Chang Yong Zhong Yao Cheng Fen Yu Yao Li Shou Ce* (A Handbook of the Composition and Pharmacology of Common Chinese Drugs), 1994; 175:176.
9. *Zhe Jiang Zhong Yi Za Zhi* (Zhejiang Journal of Chinese Medicine) 1988;23(7):319.
10. *Zhong Hua Nei Ke Xue Za Zhi* (Journal of Chinese Internal Medicine) 1977;2(2):79.
11. *Zhong Yi Ming Fang Lin Chuang Xin Yong* (Contemporary Clinical Applications of Classic Chinese Formulas) 2001;144.
12. *Zhong Cheng Yao Yan Jiu* (Research of Chinese Patent Medicine) 1983;8:31.
13. *Hu Nan Zhong Yi Xue Yuan Xue Bao* (Journal of Hunan University of Traditional Chinese Medicine) 1989;9:545.
14. *Yun Nan Zhong Yi Za Zhi* (Yunan Journal of Chinese Medicine) 1992;13(1):23.
15. Lin CC, Yen FL, Hsu FF, Lin JM. Anti-hypercholesterolaemia, antioxidant activity and free radical scavenger effects of traditional Chinese medicine prescriptions used for stroke. Journal of Pharmacy & Pharmacology 2000 Nov;52(11):1387-93.
16. *Liao Ning Zhong Yi Za Zhi* (Liaoning Journal of Chinese Medicine) 1984;9:26.
17. *Zhong Yi Za Zhi* (Journal of Chinese Medicine) 1984;9:45.
18. *Zhe Jiang Zhong Yi Za Zhi* (Zhejiang Journal of Chinese Medicine) 1997;7:317.
19. *Guang Dong Yi Xue* (Guangdong Medicine) 1992;13(1):39.
20. *Jiang Su Zhong Yi* (Jiangsu Chinese Medicine) 1998;2:33.
21. *Zhong Yao Yao Li Yu Lin Chuang* (Pharmacology and Clinical Applications of Chinese Herbs) 1993;9(1):8.
22. *Zhong Guo Yi Yao Xue Bao* (Chinese Journal of Medicine and Herbology) 1990;5(4):33.
23. *Xin Yi Yao Xue Za Zhi* (New Journal of Medicine and Herbology) 1976;5:41.
24. *Zhe Jiang Zhong Yi Za Zhi* (Zhejiang Journal of Chinese Medicine) 1997;10:445.
25. *Zhe Jiang Zhong Yi Xue Yuan Xue Bao* (Journal of Zhejiang University of Chinese Medicine) 1992;16(3):19.
26. *Tian Jin Zhong Yi* (Tianjin Chinese Medicine) 1993;5:22.
27. *Zhe Jiang Zhong Yi Za Zhi* (Zhejiang Journal of Chinese Medicine) 1988;23(7):319.
28. *Shan Xi Zhong Yi* (Shanxi Chinese Medicine) 1988;9(3):126.

870

Chapter 13 — Overview

29. *Zhong Xi Yi Jie He Za Zhi* (Journal of Integrated Chinese and Western Medicine) 1988;8(10):601.

30. *Zhong Xi Yi Jie He Za Zhi* (Journal of Integrated Chinese and Western Medicine) 1988;8(10):601.

31. *Shan Dong Zhong Yi Za Zhi* (Shandong Journal of Chinese Medicine) 1991;10(2):26.

32. *Hu Nan Zhong Yi Za Zhi* (Hunan Journal of Chinese Medicine) 1993;9(1):41.

33. *Jiang Su Zhong Yi* (Jiangsu Chinese Medicine) 1992;13(5):16.

34. *Shi Yong Zhong Xi Yi Jie He Za Zhi* (Practical Journal of Integrated Chinese and Western Medicines) 1993;6(6):380.

35. *Hu Bei Zhong Yi Za Zhi* (Hubei Journal of Chinese Medicine) 1990;4:17.

36. *Guo Wai Yi Xue* (Foreign Medicine) 1980;2(4):185.

37. *Zhe Jiang Zhong Yi Za Zhi* (Zhejiang Journal of Chinese Medicine) 1964;11:17.

38. *He Bei Zhong Yi* (Hebei Chinese Medicine) 1991;3:16.

39. *Shan Xi Zhong Yi* (Shanxi Chinese Medicine) 1991;12(5):200.

40. Ushiroyama T, Tsubokura S, Ikeda A, Ueki M. The effect of unkei-to on pituitary gonadotropin secretion and ovulation in anovulatory cycles of young women. Am J Chin Med 1995;23(3-4):223-30.

41. Ushiroyama T, Ikeda A, Sakai M, Hosotani T, Suzuki Y, Tsubokura S, Ueki M. Effects of unkei-to, an herbal medicine, on endocrine function and ovulation in women with high basal levels of luteinizing hormone secretion. Journal of Reproductive Medicine 2001 May;46(5):451-6.

42. *Hu Nan Yi Yao Za Zhi* (Hunan Journal of Medicine and Herbology) 1983;3:52.

43. *He Nan Zhong Yi* (Henan Chinese Medicine) 1985;3:29.

44. Yang CC, Chen JC, Chen GW, Chen YS, Chung JG. Effects of Shao-Fu-Zhu-Yu-Tang on motility of human sperm. American Journal of Chinese Medicine 2003;31(4):573-9.

45. *Shan Xi Zhong Yi* (Shanxi Chinese Medicine) 1995;11(5):20.

46. *Hu Bei Zhong Yi Za Zhi* (Hubei Journal of Chinese Medicine) 1982;16(5):48.

47. *Xin Zhong Yi* (New Chinese Medicine) 1984;11:33.

48. *Shang Hai Zhong Yi Yao Za Zhi* (Shanghai Journal of Chinese Medicine and Herbology) 1993;2:16.

49. *Zhong Xi Yi Jie He Za Zhi* (Journal of Integrated Chinese and Western Medicine) 1988;10:639.

50. *Jiang Su Zhong Yi* (Jiangsu Chinese Medicine) 1990;8:14.

51. *Bei Jing Zhong Yi* (Beijing Chinese Medicine) 1987;5:34.

52. *Shan Xi Zhong Yi* (Shanxi Chinese Medicine) 1997;11:508.

53. Sakamoto S, Yoshino H, Shirahata Y, Shimodairo K, Okamoto R. Pharmacotherapeutic effects of kuei-chih-fu-ling-wan (keishi-bukuryo-gan) on human uterine myomas. Am J Chin Med 1992;20(3-4):313-7.

54. Sakamoto S, Mitamura T, Iwasawa M, Kitsunai H, Shindou K, Yagishita Y, Zhou YF, Sassa S. Conservative management for perimenopausal women with uterine leiomyomas using Chinese herbal medicines and synthetic analogs of gonadotropin-releasing hormone. In Vivo 1998 May-Jun;12(3):333-7.

55. *Hu Bei Zhong Yi Za Zhi* (Hubei Journal of Chinese Medicine) 1987;5:14.

56. *Xin Zhong Yi* (New Chinese Medicine) 1995;8:40.

57. *Shan Xi Zhong Yi* (Shanxi Chinese Medicine) 1994;2:52.

58. *He Nan Zhong Yi* (Henan Chinese Medicine) 1993;4:35.

59. *Zhong Yao Yan Jiu* (Research of Chinese Herbology) 1993;6(4):15.

60. *Zhong Yao Yao Li Yu Lin* Chuang (Pharmacology and Clinical Applications of Chinese Herbs) 1987;37.

61. *Zhong Yao Yan Jiu* (Research of Chinese Herbology) 1993;6(4):15.

62. *Zhong Cheng Yao Yan Jiu* (Research of Chinese Patent Medicine) 1987;3:45.

63. *Shang Hai Zhong Yi Yao Za Zhi* (Shanghai Journal of Chinese Medicine and Herbology) 1985;10:29.

64. *Guang Xi Zhong Yi Yao* (Guangxi Chinese Medicine and Herbology) 1996;5:22.

65. *Si Chuan Zhong Yi* (Sichuan Chinese Medicine) 1985;11:50.

66. *Zhong Yi Fang Ji Xian Dai Yan Jiu* (Modern Study of Medical Formulae in Traditional Chinese Medicine) 1997;1012.

67. *Yun Nan Zhong Yao Zhi* (Yunan Journal of Chinese Herbal Medicine) 1989;3:46.

68. *Bei Jing Zhong Yi Za Zhi* (Beijing Journal of Chinese Medicine) 1988;6:35.

69. *Guang Xi Zhong Yi Yao* (Guangxi Chinese Medicine and Herbology) 1987;2:47.

70. *Shan Xi Zhong Yi* (Shanxi Chinese Medicine) 1991;12(11):511.

71. *Shan Xi Zhong Yi* (Shanxi Chinese Medicine) 1993;14(5):222.

72. *Zhe Jiang Zhong Yi Za Zhi* (Zhejiang Journal of Chinese Medicine) 1996;5:301.

73. *Zhong Yi Fang Ji Xian Dai Yan Jiu* (Modern Study of Medical Formulae in Traditional Chinese Medicine) 1997;999.

74. *Zhong Hua Wai Ke Za Zhi* (Chinese Journal of External Medicine) 1962;5:305.

75. *Jiang Su Zhong Yi* (Jiangsu Chinese Medicine) 1963;5:13.

76. *Zhong Yi Ming Fang Lin Chuang Xin Yong* (Contemporary Clinical Applications of Classic Chinese Formulas) 2001;561.

77. *Jiang Su Zhong Yi* (Jiangsu Chinese Medicine) 1995;7:10.

78. *Xin Yi Yao Xue Za Zhi* (New Journal of Medicine and Herbology) 1978;9:44.

79. *Jiang Su Zhong Yi* (Jiangsu Chinese Medicine) 1997;8:21.

80. *Zhong Guo Zhong Xi Yi Jie He Za Zhi* (Chinese Journal of Integrative Chinese and Western Medicine) 1993;8:491.

81. *Shan Dong Zhong Yi Za Zhi* (Shandong Journal of Chinese Medicine) 1993;12(3):28.

82. *Shi Yong Zhong Yi Yao Za Zhi* (Journal of Practical Chinese Medicine and Medicinals) 1994;10(4):27.

83. *Ji Lin Zhong Yi Yao* (Jilin Chinese Medicine and Herbology) 1986;4:10.

84. *Gan Su Zhong Yi* (Gansu Chinese Medicine) 1993;6(4):26.

Chapter 13 — Overview

85. *Shi Yong Zhong Yi Nei Ke Za Zhi* (Journal of Practical Chinese Internal Medicine) 1990;4(3):123.

86. *Hu Nan Yi Yao Za Zhi* (Hunan Journal of Medicine and Herbology) 1984;3:44.

87. *Fu Jian Zhong Yi Yao* (Fujian Chinese Medicine and Herbology) 1960;4:27.

88. *Hei Long Jiang Zhong Yi Yao* (Heilongjiang Chinese Medicine and Herbology) 1985;3:43.

89. *Zhong Hua Fu Chan Ke Za Zhi* (Chinese Journal of Obstetrics and Gynecology) 1959;5:413.

90. *Fu Jian Zhong Yi Yao* (Fujian Chinese Medicine and Herbology) 1991;22(3):12.

91. *Zhe Jiang Zhong Yi Za Zhi* (Zhejiang Journal of Chinese Medicine) 1958;7:21.

92. *Zhe Jiang Zhong Yi Yao* (Zhejiang Chinese Medicine and Herbology) 1963;7:4.

93. Chen J, Chen T. Chinese Medical Herbology and Pharmacology. City of Industry, CA: Art of Medicine Press, 2004.

Chinese Herbal Formulas and Applications

Section 1

活血祛瘀剂
— Blood-Invigorating and Stasis-Removing Formulas

Táo Hé Chéng Qì Tāng (Peach Pit Decoction to Order the Qi)
桃核承氣湯
桃核承气汤

Pinyin Name: *Tao He Cheng Qi Tang*
Literal Name: Peach Pit Decoction to Order the Qi
Alternate Names: *Tao He Cheng Chi Tang, Tao Ren Cheng Qi Tang, Tao Jen Cheng Chi Tang*, Persica Qi-Infusing Decoction, Peach Kernel Purgative Decoction, Persica and Rhubarb Combination
Original Source: *Shang Han Lun* (Discussion of Cold-Induced Disorders) by Zhang Zhong-Jing in the Eastern Han Dynasty

COMPOSITION

Tao Ren (Semen Persicae)	50 pieces [12g]
Da Huang (Radix et Rhizoma Rhei)	12g
Gui Zhi (Ramulus Cinnamomi)	6g
Mang Xiao (Natrii Sulfas)	6g
Zhi Gan Cao (Radix et Rhizoma Glycyrrhizae Praeparata cum Melle)	6g

DOSAGE / PREPARATION / ADMINISTRATION

The source text states to cook all the ingredients, except *Mang Xiao* (Natrii Sulfas), in 7 cups [1,400 mL] of water until the liquid is reduced to 2.5 cups [500 mL]. Discard the residue, add *Mang Xiao* (Natrii Sulfas), and bring the decoction to a slight boil. Take 0.5 cup [100 mL] of the warm, strained decoction three times daily after meals. This formula may cause loose stools.

CHINESE THERAPEUTIC ACTIONS

Breaks up blood stasis and drains it downward

CLINICAL MANIFESTATIONS

Blood accumulation in the lower *jiao*: acute lower abdominal pain with normal urination, delirium, irritability, thirst, fever at night, or mania in severe cases.

CLINICAL APPLICATIONS

Cholecystitis, hepatitis, enteroparalysis, pyelonephritis, renal insufficiency, renal colic, headache, pharyngitis, toothache, diabetes mellitus, schizophrenia, irregular menstruation, dysmenorrhea, amenorrhea, acute pelvic inflammation, and retention of lochia.

EXPLANATION

According to the *Shang Han Lun* (Discussion of Cold-Induced Disorders), *Tao He Cheng Qi Tang* (Peach Pit Decoction to Order the Qi) treats blood stagnation in the lower *jiao*. This condition occurs when a person suffering from a *taiyang* disorder is not relieved of the exterior pathogens, and the pathogens travel along the channel pathway and transform into heat in the interior. The heat then stagnates with the blood in the lower *jiao*, resulting in lower *jiao* blood stasis. Acute lower abdominal pain is due to blood stasis in the lower *jiao*. Delirium, irritability, thirst, fever at night, and mania are due to heat in the *xue* (blood) level. Because the water passages are not affected, urination is still normal.

Tao He Cheng Qi Tang consists of *Tiao Wei Cheng Qi Tang* (Regulate the Stomach and Order the Qi Decoction) plus *Tao Ren* (Semen Persicae) and *Gui Zhi* (Ramulus Cinnamomi). In this formula, *Tao Ren* (Semen Persicae) breaks up and dispels blood stagnation. *Da Huang* (Radix et Rhizoma Rhei) drains heat and blood stagnation downward. These two herbs, which together dispel blood stasis and heat, are the chief herbs in this formula. *Gui Zhi* (Ramulus Cinnamomi) opens the channels and collaterals to help

BLOOD-REGULATING FORMULAS

13

873

Chapter 13 – Blood-Regulating Formulas   *Section 1 – Blood-Invigorating and Stasis-Removing Formulas*

Táo Hé Chéng Qi Tāng (Peach Pit Decoction to Order the Qi)

Tao He Cheng Qi Tang (Peach Pit Decoction to Order the Qi)

Diagnosis	Signs and Symptoms	Treatment	Herbs
Accumulation of blood in the lower *jiao*	• Acute lower abdominal pain: blood stasis in the lower *jiao* • Delirium, irritability, and mania: heat disturbing the *shen* (spirit) • Thirst and fever at night: heat consuming yin and body fluids	Breaks up blood stasis and drains it downward	• *Tao Ren* (Semen Persicae) breaks up and dispels blood stagnation. • *Da Huang* (Radix et Rhizoma Rhei) drains heat and stagnation downward. • *Gui Zhi* (Ramulus Cinnamomi) opens the channels and collaterals to dispel blood stasis. • *Mang Xiao* (Natrii Sulfas) drains heat. • *Zhi Gan Cao* (Radix et Rhizoma Glycyrrhizae Praeparata cum Melle) supplements qi and regulates the middle *jiao*, and lessens the harsh effects of the other herbs.

Tao Ren (Semen Persicae) dispel blood stasis. *Mang Xiao* (Natrii Sulfas) drains heat and softens hardness to help *Da Huang* (Radix et Rhizoma Rhei) drain downwards. *Zhi Gan Cao* (Radix et Rhizoma Glycyrrhizae Praeparata cum Melle), besides supplementing qi and harmonizing the middle *jiao*, lessens the harsh effects of the other herbs to prevent injury to the qi.

MODIFICATIONS

• With blood deficiency, add *Dang Gui* (Radix Angelicae Sinensis) and *Bai Shao* (Radix Paeoniae Alba).
• With blood stagnation, add *San Qi* (Radix et Rhizoma Notoginseng) and *Chi Shao* (Radix Paeoniae Rubra).
• With qi stagnation, add *Xiang Fu* (Rhizoma Cyperi), *Wu Yao* (Radix Linderae), *Qing Pi* (Pericarpium Citri Reticulatae Viride), and *Mu Xiang* (Radix Aucklandiae).
• With constipation, add *Zhi Shi* (Fructus Aurantii Immaturus) and *Hou Po* (Cortex Magnoliae Officinalis).
• With restlessness and thirst, add *Huang Lian* (Rhizoma Coptidis) and *Huang Qin* (Radix Scutellariae).
• With oliguria, add *Che Qian Zi* (Semen Plantaginis), *Fu Ling* (Poria), and *Mu Tong* (Caulis Akebiae).
• With bleeding, add *Di Huang* (Radix Rehmanniae) and *Bai Mao Gen* (Rhizoma Imperatae).
• With distention and pain due to qi stagnation, add *Xiang Fu* (Rhizoma Cyperi) and *Zhi Qiao* (Fructus Aurantii).
• With trauma-related pain, add *Chi Shao* (Radix Paeoniae Rubra), *Dang Gui Wei* (Extremitas Radix Angelicae Sinensis), *Hong Hua* (Flos Carthami), and *Su Mu* (Lignum Sappan).
• With fire flaring upward manifesting in headache, distention in the head, red eyes and face, and vomiting of blood, add *Di Huang* (Radix Rehmanniae), *Mu Dan Pi* (Cortex Moutan), *Zhi Zi* (Fructus Gardeniae), and *Niu Xi* (Radix Achyranthis Bidentatae).

• For irregular menstruation or amenorrhea due to blood stasis, add *Dang Gui* (Radix Angelicae Sinensis) and *Hong Hua* (Flos Carthami).
• With gallstones, add *Jin Qian Cao* (Herba Lysimachiae), *Hai Jin Sha* (Spora Lygodii), *Yu Jin* (Radix Curcumae), and *Ji Nei Jin* (Endothelium Corneum Gigeriae Galli).

CAUTIONS / CONTRAINDICATIONS

• *Tao He Cheng Qi Tang* should be used only when the exterior pathogen is no longer present at the exterior. Therefore, if exterior symptoms are still present, exterior-releasing methods need to be employed before this formula can be given.
• Because this formula strongly breaks up blood stagnation and dispels heat, careful diagnosis should be made before applying this strong formula.
• This formula is contraindicated during pregnancy.
• Use of this formula is occasionally associated with side effects that include nausea, vomiting, and diarrhea.[1]

PHARMACOLOGICAL EFFECTS

1. **Purgative**: One study reported marked success using *Tao He Cheng Qi Tang* to induce bowel movements in constipated mice. The first bowel movement was generally reported within 4 hours after the administration of the herbs.[2]
2. **Antiplatelet and anticoagulant**: According to various *in vitro* studies, administration of *Tao He Cheng Qi Tang* has been associated with inhibiting platelet aggregation, inhibiting coagulation, and decreasing blood viscosity.[3,4]
3. **Antihyperlipidemic**: Administration of *Tao He Cheng Qi Tang* in animal subjects was associated with reduced plasma lipoprotein and triglyceride levels.[5]
4. **Hypoglycemic**: According to one study, administration of *Tao He Cheng Qi Tang* on an empty stomach to diabetic

874

Táo Hé Chéng Qì Tāng (Peach Pit Decoction to Order the Qi)

rats was associated with decreased plasma levels of glucose and insulin.[6]

5. **Anti-inflammatory**: Administration of *Tao He Cheng Qi Tang* in animal subjects was associated with reduced swelling and inflammation. The anti-inflammatory effect was attributed primarily to *Da Huang* (Radix et Rhizoma Rhei) and *Gan Cao* (Radix et Rhizoma Glycyrrhizae).[7,8]

CLINICAL STUDIES AND RESEARCH

1. **Cholecystitis**: Use of modified *Tao He Cheng Qi Tang* was associated with 94% effectiveness in treating cholecystitis in 100 patients (47 males and 53 females, between 19-54 years of age, with 1 day to 13 months history of illness). The herbal treatment contained *Tao Ren* (Semen Persicae), *Da Huang* (Radix et Rhizoma Rhei), *Gui Zhi* (Ramulus Cinnamomi), *Gan Cao* (Radix et Rhizoma Glycyrrhizae), *Huang Lian* (Rhizoma Coptidis), *Huang Qin* (Radix Scutellariae), and *Zhi Shi* (Fructus Aurantii Immaturus). The treatment protocol was to administer the decoction every 6 hours in acute cases, and twice daily in chronic cases. The duration of treatment ranged from 5-27 days. Of 100 patients, the study reported complete recovery in 23 cases, remission in 64 cases, improvement in 7 cases, and no effect in 6 cases.[9]

2. **Hepatitis**: Administration of *Tao He Cheng Qi Tang* and *Chai Ling Tang* (Bupleurum and Poria Decoction) in 10 patients with chronic active hepatitis was associated with significant reduction of liver enzymes and symptomatic improvements.[10]

3. **Enteroparalysis**: One study reported marked effectiveness using modified *Tao He Cheng Qi Tang* to treat 20 patients with enteroparalysis associated with traumatic injuries to the thoracic or lumbar spine. For patients with a severe condition, the formula was modified by removing *Gui Zhi* (Ramulus Cinnamomi) and adding *Zhi Shi* (Fructus Aurantii Immaturus), *Hou Po* (Cortex Magnoliae Officinalis), *Fan Xie Ye* (Folium Sennae), and others as needed. For those who did not have a bowel movement after the initial herbal treatment, 30 grams each of *Da Huang* (Radix et Rhizoma Rhei) and *Xuan Ming Fen* (Natrii Sulfas Exsiccatus) were added. The herbs were cooked in water, and the herbal solution (approximately 600 mL) was given via rectal enema. The study reported marked effect in most patients to induce bowel movement.[11]

4. **Pyelonephritis**: Use of modified *Tao He Cheng Qi Tang* was effective in treating 46 patients with chronic pyelonephritis. The formula was modified based on the condition of each individual patient. For individuals with diarrhea, *Mang Xiao* (Natrii Sulfas) was removed. For frequent and urgent urination, *Hua Shi* (Talcum) was added. For lower abdominal pain, a large dose of *Gui Zhi* (Ramulus Cinnamomi) or *Tian Tai Wu Yao San* (Top-Quality Lindera Powder) was added. Of 46 patients, the study reported significant improvement in 24 cases and improvement in 15 cases.[12]

5. **Renal insufficiency**: Administration of modified *Tao He Cheng Qi Tang* in 18 patients with renal insufficiency was associated with marked improvements in BUN, SCr, and CO_2CP. The herbal formula was given one time daily, and contained the following ingredients: *Tao Ren* (Semen Persicae), *Da Huang* (Radix et Rhizoma Rhei), *Gui Zhi* (Ramulus Cinnamomi), *Zhi Gan Cao* (Radix et Rhizoma Glycyrrhizae Praeparata cum Melle), *Huang Qi* (Radix Astragali), *Fu Zi* (Radix Aconiti Lateralis Praeparata), *Ze Xie* (Rhizoma Alismatis), *Yi Mu Cao* (Herba Leonuri), and *Nu Zhen Zi* (Fructus Ligustri Lucidi).[13]

6. **Renal colic**: One study reported pain relief using *Tao He Cheng Qi Tang* to treat renal colic caused by stones. The treatment protocol was to administer the herbs in decoction (1 pack per day, with decoction given in three equally-divided doses). The study reported relief of pain in all 11 patients within 2-3 days.[14]

7. **Headache**: One study reported marked results using modified *Tao He Cheng Qi Tang* to treat headache caused by physical trauma. Of 10 patients, the study reported significant relief of pain in 8 cases within 10 to 15 packs of herbs, and complete resolution of all symptoms after 40 to 90 packs of herbs.[15]

8. **Pharyngitis**: One clinical study evaluated the efficacy of modified *Tao He Cheng Qi Tang* in treating acute pharyngitis. The herbal treatment contained *Tao He Cheng Qi Tang* plus *Niu Xi* (Radix Achyranthis Bidentatae), *She Gan* (Rhizoma Belamcandae), *Jie Geng* (Radix Platycodonis), *Pang Da Hai* (Semen Sterculiae Lychnophorae), and others as needed. The average duration of treatment was 2.8 days. Of 47 patients, the study reported complete recovery in 21 cases within 2 packs of herbs, 24 cases within 3-4 packs of herbs, and 2 cases within 5 packs of herbs.[16]

9. **Toothache**: One study reported complete recovery in 94 of 100 patients with toothache using *Tao He Cheng Qi Tang* plus *Xia Ku Cao* (Spica Prunellae) and *Bai Zhi* (Radix Angelicae Dahuricae). Additional modifications were made as follows: *Fang Feng* (Radix Saposhnikoviae) and *Quan Xie* (Scorpio) for toothache due to wind and fire; *Shi Gao* (Gypsum Fibrosum) and *Sheng Ma* (Rhizoma Cimicifugae) for Stomach fire; *Di Huang* (Radix Rehmanniae) and *Bai Shao* (Radix Paeoniae Alba) for yin-deficient fire; *Lian Qiao* (Fructus Forsythiae) and *Bei Mu* (Bulbus Fritillariae) for abscesses; and *Feng Fang* (Nidus Vespae) and *Wei Ling Xian* (Radix et Rhizoma Clematidis) for pain due to dental caries.[17]

10. **Diabetes mellitus**: One study reported 79% effectiveness using *Tao He Cheng Qi Tang* to treat 106 patients with

Chapter 13 – Blood-Regulating Formulas   *Section 1 – Blood-Invigorating and Stasis-Removing Formulas*

Táo Hé Chéng Qi Tāng (Peach Pit Decoction to Order the Qi)

type II diabetes mellitus. The mechanism was attributed to the formula's ability to stimulate the beta-islet cells of the pancreas to produce more insulin.[18,19]

11. **Schizophrenia**: Use of *Tao He Cheng Qi Tang* was associated with beneficial effect in all 10 patients with schizophrenia that was characterized by blood stagnation in the lower *jiao*.[20]

HERB-DRUG INTERACTION

Drug-induced menopause: One study evaluated the therapeutic effects of certain herbal medicines on menopausal symptoms induced by gonadotropin-releasing hormone agonist therapy in Japanese women with endometriosis, adenomyosis, or leiomyoma. According to this study, 13 menopausal patients were successfully treated with *Tao He Cheng Qi Tang*, *Dang Gui Shao Yao San* (Tangkuei and Peony Powder), *Shao Yao Gan Cao Tang* (Peony and Licorice Decoction), *Gui Zhi Fu Ling Wan* (Cinnamon Twig and Poria Pill), *Jia Wei Xiao Yao San* (Augmented Rambling Powder), or *Gui Zhi Tang* (Cinnamon Twig Decoction). Most importantly, there were no significant changes in serum estradiol levels after treatment with these herbal medicines. The researchers concluded that these herbal medicines could be recommended for menopausal symptoms induced by gonadotropin-releasing hormone agonists without a negative effect on serum estradiol levels.[21]

RELATED FORMULA

Xià Yū Xuè Tāng (Drain Blood Stasis Decoction)

下瘀血湯
下瘀血汤

Pinyin Name: *Xia Yu Xue Tang*
Literal Name: Drain Blood Stasis Decoction
Original Source: *Jin Gui Yao Lue* (Essentials from the Golden Cabinet) by Zhang Zhong-Jing in the Eastern Han Dynasty

Da Huang (Radix et Rhizoma Rhei)	9g
Tao Ren (Semen Persicae)	20 pieces [9g]
Tu Bie Chong (Eupolyphaga seu Steleophaga), *ao* (simmered)	20 pieces [9g]

The source text states to prepare the ingredients as a decoction with the suggested dose in brackets. The main actions of *Xia Yu Xue Tang* (Drain Blood Stasis Decoction) are to break blood stasis and drain it downward. This formula is used primarily to treat postpartum women with abdominal pain due to stasis and hardening of blood in the umbilical region. The source text identifies this formula as treating "dried blood below the umbilicus."

Tao He Cheng Qi Tang and *Xia Yu Xue Tang* (Drain Blood Stasis Decoction) both treat blood stasis in the lower abdomen.

- *Tao He Cheng Qi Tang* treats lower abdominal pain due to heat accumulation and blood stasis. In addition to lower abdominal pain, there are also symptoms such as delirium, irritability, thirst, fever at night, or mania in severe cases.

- *Xia Yu Xue Tang* treats pain due to blood stasis in the umbilical region in postpartum women. The affected area (umbilical region) is painful and hard on palpation, but there are usually no systemic symptoms.

AUTHORS' COMMENTS

Tao He Cheng Qi Tang was used originally to treat blood stasis in the lower *jiao*. Today, its clinical application has been expanded, as this formula has been proven effective in treating various other conditions characterized by blood stasis, including:

- Sports injuries with bruises and severe pain that limit physical movements, accompanied by difficult defecation or urination.

- Headache, feelings of distention in the head, red eyes, or toothache caused by excessive fire rising.

- Epistaxis and hemoptysis (vomiting of purplish black blood) due to blood heat.

- Blood stagnation in women, such as amenorrhea, persistent bleeding after delivery, hardness and pain in the lower abdomen, and shortness of breath.

References

1. *Zhong Yao Ming Fang Yao Li Yu Ying Yong* (Pharmacology and Applications of Famous Herbal Formulas) 1989;451-453.
2. *Zhong Cheng Yao* (Study of Chinese Patent Medicine) 1990;11:24.
3. *Zhe Jiang Zhong Yi Za Zhi* (Zhejiang Journal of Chinese Medicine) 1988;23(7):319.
4. *Yao Xue Za Zhi* (Journal of Medicinals) 1983;103(7):313.
5. *Zhe Jiang Zhong Yi Za Zhi* (Zhejiang Journal of Chinese Medicine) 1988;23(7):319.
6. *Xin Zhong Yi* (New Chinese Medicine) 1988;20(4):53.
7. *Han Fang Yi Xue* (Kampo Medicine) 1984;1:11.
8. *Guo Wai Yi Xue* (Foreign Medicine) 1971;9(2):48.
9. *Shan Dong Zhong Yi Za Zhi* (Shandong Journal of Chinese Medicine) 1993;12(3):28.
10. *Zhong Yi Ming Fang Lin Chuang Xin Yong* (Contemporary Clinical Applications of Classic Chinese Formulas) 2001;561.
11. *Xin Zhong Yi* (New Chinese Medicine) 1984;2:34.
12. *Ji Lin Zhong Yi Yao* (Jilin Chinese Medicine and Herbology) 1986;4:10.
13. *Gan Su Zhong Yi* (Gansu Chinese Medicine) 1993;6(4):26.
14. *Hu Nan Yi Yao Za Zhi* (Hunan Journal of Medicine and Herbology) 1984;3:44.

876

Táo Hé Chéng Qì Tāng (Peach Pit Decoction to Order the Qì)

15. *He Nan Zhong Yi* (Henan Chinese Medicine) 1983;4:12.
16. *Guang Xi Zhong Yi Yao* (Guangxi Chinese Medicine and Herbology) 1989;12(2):21.
17. *Tian Jin Zhong Yi* (Tianjin Chinese Medicine) 1991;2:14.
18. *Zhong Guo Zhong Xi Yi Jie He Za Zhi* (Chinese Journal of Integrative Chinese and Western Medicine) 1992;12(2):74.
19. *Zhong Guo Zhong Yi Yao Xue Bao* (Chinese Journal of Chinese Medicine and Herbology) 1993;8(5):50.
20. *Shan Xi Zhong Yi* (Shanxi Chinese Medicine) 1983;3(3):14.
21. Tanaka T. Effects of herbal medicines on menopausal symptoms induced by gonadotropin-releasing hormone agonist therapy. Clin Exp Obstet Gynecol 2001;28(1):20-3.

Tōng Qiào Huó Xuè Tāng
(Unblock the Orifices and Invigorate the Blood Decoction)

通竅活血湯
通窍活血汤

Pinyin Name: *Tong Qiao Huo Xue Tang*
Literal Name: Unblock the Orifices and Invigorate the Blood Decoction
Original Source: *Yi Lin Gai Cuo* (Corrections of Errors Among Physicians) by Wang Qing-Ren in 1830

COMPOSITION

Chi Shao (Radix Paeoniae Rubra)	3g
Chuan Xiong (Rhizoma Chuanxiong)	3g
Tao Ren (Semen Persicae), *yan* (ground) till muddy	9g
Hong Hua (Flos Carthami)	9g
Lao Cong (Herba Allii Fistulosi), *qie* (sliced)	3 pieces [3-6g]
Sheng Jiang (Rhizoma Zingiberis Recens)	9g
She Xiang (Moschus)	0.15g
Da Zao (Fructus Jujubae)	7 pieces [5g]
Grain-based liquor	250g

Note: *She Xiang* (Moschus) is derived from an endangered animal, and is rarely used as a medicinal substance today. Its discussion here is included primarily for academic purposes, to reflect the historical use of this substance in its original formulation. Most herbal products today have removed it completely, or replaced it with substitutes with similar functions.

DOSAGE / PREPARATION / ADMINISTRATION

The source text states to cook all the ingredients, except *She Xiang* (Moschus), in a large bowl of water. Discard the residue, add *She Xiang* (Moschus) and a grain-based liquor to the strained decoction, and bring it to a boil twice. Take the warm decoction before bedtime. Today, this formula may be prepared as a decoction with the doses suggested in brackets, with the addition of a small amount of grain-based liquor.

CHINESE THERAPEUTIC ACTIONS

Activates blood circulation and opens the sensory orifices

CLINICAL MANIFESTATIONS

Blood stagnation in the head and face: headache, dizziness, chronic tinnitus and poor hearing, hair loss, facial appearance that is blue, green, or purple in color; with or without rosacea or vitiligo; emaciation in women due to blood disorders; *gan ji* (infantile malnutrition) with muscle wasting, enlarged abdomen, and tidal fever.

CLINICAL APPLICATIONS

Concussion, cerebrovascular accident, vascular headache, hypersomnia, rheumatoid arthritis, and carbon monoxide poisoning.

EXPLANATION

The main actions of *Tong Qiao Huo Xue Tang* (Unblock the Orifices and Invigorate the Blood Decoction) are to activate blood circulation and remove blood stagnation in the head and facial regions. It can be used for various conditions characterized by blood stagnation in the head and face.

Chapter 13 – Blood-Regulating Formulas   *Section 1 – Blood-Invigorating and Stasis-Removing Formulas*

Tōng Qiào Huó Xuè Tāng
(Unblock the Orifices and Invigorate the Blood Decoction)

Tong Qiao Huo Xue Tang (Unblock the Orifices and Invigorate the Blood Decoction)

Diagnosis	Signs and Symptoms	Treatment	Herbs
Blood stagnation in the head and face	• Headache with blue/green/purplish facial appearance: blood stagnation in the head • Chronic tinnitus and poor hearing: blood stagnation blocking the sensory orifices	• Activates blood circulation • Opens the sensory orifices	• *Chi Shao* (Radix Paeoniae Rubra), *Chuan Xiong* (Rhizoma Chuanxiong), *Tao Ren* (Semen Persicae), and *Hong Hua* (Flos Carthami) activate blood circulation and eliminate blood stasis. • *Lao Cong* (Herba Allii Fistulosi) unblocks stagnation and promotes the circulation of yang qi. • *She Xiang* (Moschus) opens the sensory orifices and restores their normal functions. • *Sheng Jiang* (Rhizoma Zingiberis Recens) and *Da Zao* (Fructus Jujubae) harmonize the herbs.

In this formula, *Chi Shao* (Radix Paeoniae Rubra), *Chuan Xiong* (Rhizoma Chuanxiong), *Tao Ren* (Semen Persicae), and *Hong Hua* (Flos Carthami) all activate blood circulation and eliminate blood stasis. *Lao Cong* (Herba Allii Fistulosi) unblocks stagnation and promotes the circulation of yang qi. *She Xiang* (Moschus) opens the sensory orifices and restores their normal functions. *Sheng Jiang* (Rhizoma Zingiberis Recens) and *Da Zao* (Fructus Jujubae) harmonize the herbs.

CLINICAL STUDIES AND RESEARCH

1. **Concussion**: One study reported a marked effect using modified *Tong Qiao Huo Xue Tang* to treat concussion. The herbal formula contained *Chuan Xiong* (Rhizoma Chuanxiong) 20g, *Niu Xi* (Radix Achyranthis Bidentatae) 20g, *Fu Ling* (Poria) 20g, *Huang Jing* (Rhizoma Polygonati) 20g, *Mu Dan Pi* (Cortex Moutan) 20g, *Tao Ren* (Semen Persicae) 10g, *Hong Hua* (Flos Carthami) 10g, *Tu Bie Chong* (Eupolyphaga seu Steleophaga) 10g, *Shi Chang Pu* (Rhizoma Acori Tatarinowii) 10g, *Bai Zhi* (Radix Angelicae Dahuricae) 6g, *Xi Xin* (Radix et Rhizoma Asari) 3g, and *Bo He* (Herba Menthae) 3g. Of 61 patients, the study reported complete recovery in 14 cases after 4-6 packs of herbs, and in 47 cases after 8-14 packs.[1]

2. **Carbon monoxide poisoning**: Use of modified *Tong Qiao Huo Xue Tang* was effective in treating 11 patients with carbon monoxide poisoning. The herbal formula contained *She Xiang* (Moschus) 6g, *Chi Shao* (Radix Paeoniae Rubra) 30g, *Chuan Xiong* (Rhizoma Chuanxiong) 30g, *Tao Ren* (Semen Persicae) 30g, *Hong Hua* (Flos Carthami) 30g, *Dan Shen* (Radix et Rhizoma Salviae Miltiorrhizae) 30g, *Yu Jin* (Radix Curcumae) 30g, *Huang Qi* (Radix Astragali) 50g, *Dang Gui* (Radix Angelicae Sinensis) 50g, *Shi Chang Pu* (Rhizoma Acori Tatarinowii) 20g, and others. The herbs were ground into a fine powder and placed into capsules. The treatment protocol was to administer 3g of herbs in capsules twice daily after meals with an herbal tea made by cooking 3 slices of *Sheng Jiang* (Rhizoma Zingiberis Recens), 3 pieces of *Cong Bai* (Bulbus Allii Fistulosi), and 7 pieces of *Da Zao* (Fructus Jujubae) in equal portions of water and grain-based liquor. The herbs were given for 1 month per course of treatment. Of 11 patients, the study reported significant improvement in 7 cases, moderate improvement in 3 cases, and no improvement in 1 case. No side effects were reported.[2]

References

1. *Shan Xi Zhong Yi* (Shanxi Chinese Medicine) 1991;12(11):511.
2. *Shan Xi Zhong Yi* (Shanxi Chinese Medicine) 1990;6(5):25.

Chinese Herbal Formulas and Applications

Xuè Fǔ Zhú Yū Tāng
(Drive Out Stasis in the Mansion of Blood Decoction)

血府逐瘀湯
血府逐瘀汤

Pinyin Name: *Xue Fu Zhu Yu Tang*
Literal Name: Drive Out Stasis in the Mansion of Blood Decoction
Alternate Names: *Hsieh Fu Chu Yu Tang*, Blood-House Blood Stasis-Dispelling Decoction, Persica and Carthamus Combination
Original Source: *Yi Lin Gai Cuo* (Corrections of Errors Among Physicians) by Wang Qing-Ren in 1830

COMPOSITION

Tao Ren (Semen Persicae)	12g
Hong Hua (Flos Carthami)	9g
Di Huang (Radix Rehmanniae)	9g
Dang Gui (Radix Angelicae Sinensis)	9g
Chi Shao (Radix Paeoniae Rubra)	6g
Chuan Xiong (Rhizoma Chuanxiong)	4.5g
Chai Hu (Radix Bupleuri)	3g
Zhi Qiao (Fructus Citri Aurantii)	6g
Jie Geng (Radix Platycodonis)	4.5g
Chuan Niu Xi (Radix Cyathulae)	9g
Gan Cao (Radix et Rhizoma Glycyrrhizae)	6g

DOSAGE / PREPARATION / ADMINISTRATION
Prepare as a decoction.

CHINESE THERAPEUTIC ACTIONS
1. Activates blood circulation and dispels blood stagnation
2. Activates qi circulation and relieves pain

CLINICAL MANIFESTATIONS
Blood stagnation in the chest and obstructed blood circulation: chronic stabbing pain at a fixed location in the chest and/or the head, hypochondriac pain, chronic and constant hiccups, dry heaves or vomiting after intake of water, palpitations, insomnia, restless sleep, fidgeting, bad temper, tidal fever in the evenings, dark red tongue body with petechiae spots on the top or the sides, dark lips, dark eyes, and a rough or wiry, tight pulse.

CLINICAL APPLICATIONS
Coronary heart disease, angina pectoris, hypertension, rheumatic heart disease, thrombosis, embolism, cardiac ischemia, bradyarrhythmia, stroke, concussion, post-concussion syndrome, cerebral atherosclerosis, hyperlipidemia, pneumothorax, physical injury to the chest, hepatitis, pancreatitis, headache, vascular headache, insomnia, phlebitis, mammary gland hyperplasia, pelvic inflammatory disease, schizophrenia, functional neurosis, endometriosis, and amenorrhea.

EXPLANATION
Xue Fu Zhu Yu Tang (Drive Out Stasis in the Mansion of Blood Decoction) treats various clinical manifestations induced by blood stagnation in the chest (the mansion of blood). Blood stagnation in the chest may cause stabbing pain at a fixed location in the chest and hypochondrium. Blood stagnation may cause pain in the body, which in turn may lead to restlessness, fidgeting, and bad temper. Chronic blood stagnation may contribute to Liver qi stagnation, which, when overacting on the Stomach, may cause hiccups, dry heaves and vomiting. Furthermore, chronic blood stasis contributes to heat formation, causing palpitations, insomnia, and tidal fever. A dark red tongue with petechiae indicates blood stagnation. A rough or wiry, tight pulse indicates blood stagnation with pain.

The design of this formula uses the principles of two formulas: *Tao Hong Si Wu Tang* (Four-Substance Decoction with Safflower and Peach Pit) to nourish blood, activate blood circulation, and eliminate blood stasis; and *Si Ni San* (Frigid Extremities Powder) to activate qi circulation, harmonize the blood, and smooth the Liver.

In this formula, *Tao Ren* (Semen Persicae) and *Hong Hua* (Flos Carthami) are used to break up blood stagnation and activate blood circulation. *Di Huang* (Radix Rehmanniae), *Dang Gui* (Radix Angelicae Sinensis), *Chi Shao*

BLOOD-REGULATING FORMULAS

13

879

Xuè Fǔ Zhú Yū Tāng
(Drive Out Stasis in the Mansion of Blood Decoction)

Xue Fu Zhu Yu Tang (Drive Out Stasis in the Mansion of Blood Decoction)

Diagnosis	Signs and Symptoms	Treatment	Herbs
Blood stagnation in the chest and obstructed blood circulation	• Chronic stabbing pain at a fixed location in the chest and head and hypochondriac pain: blood stagnation in the chest • Hiccups, dry heaves and vomiting: reversed flow of Stomach qi due to blood stagnation • Palpitations, insomnia, restless sleep, fidgeting, bad temper and tidal fever: *shen* (spirit) disturbance caused by blood stagnation • Dark lips and eyes: lack of nourishment due to blood stagnation • Dark red tongue with petechiae and rough or wiry, tight pulse: blood stagnation	• Activates blood circulation and dispels blood stagnation • Activates qi and relieves pain	• *Tao Ren* (Semen Persicae) and *Hong Hua* (Flos Carthami) break up blood stagnation and activate blood circulation. • *Di Huang* (Radix Rehmanniae), *Dang Gui* (Radix Angelicae Sinensis), *Chi Shao* (Radix Paeoniae Rubra), and *Chuan Xiong* (Rhizoma Chuanxiong) nourish blood, activate blood circulation, and clear heat. • *Chai Hu* (Radix Bupleuri) smoothes Liver qi and *Zhi Qiao* (Fructus Aurantii) regulates qi in the chest and the upper *jiao*. • *Jie Geng* (Radix Platycodonis) guides all of the herbs upward to the chest. • *Chuan Niu Xi* (Radix Cyathulae) unblocks stagnation in the blood vessels and guides blood downward. • *Gan Cao* (Radix et Rhizoma Glycyrrhizae) harmonizes the formula.

(Radix Paeoniae Rubra), and *Chuan Xiong* (Rhizoma Chuanxiong) nourish the blood, activate blood circulation, and clear heat. *Chai Hu* (Radix Bupleuri) smoothes Liver qi to relieve chest pain. *Zhi Qiao* (Fructus Aurantii) regulates qi in the chest and the upper *jiao*. *Jie Geng* (Radix Platycodonis) guides all of the herbs upward to the chest. *Chuan Niu Xi* (Radix Cyathulae) unblocks stagnation in the blood vessels and guides blood downwards. *Gan Cao* (Radix et Rhizoma Glycyrrhizae) harmonizes the formula. Overall, this formula has the unique and valuable attributes of activating blood circulation and dispelling blood stasis without injuring the blood, and soothing the Liver and relieving qi stagnation without consuming qi.

MODIFICATIONS

• With post-concussion complications, add *Quan Xie* (Scorpio) and *Gao Ben* (Rhizoma et Radix Ligustici).

• With allergic purpura, add *Ban Lan Gen* (Radix Isatidis) and *Qin Jiao* (Radix Gentianae Macrophyllae).

• With neck and shoulder stiffness and pain, add *Ge Gen* (Radix Puerariae Lobatae) and *Qiang Huo* (Rhizoma et Radix Notopterygii).

• With frontal headache due to heat and blood stagnation, add *Bai Zhi* (Radix Angelicae Dahuricae) and *Shi Gao* (Gypsum Fibrosum).

• With vertex headache due to wind, add *Qiang Huo* (Rhizoma et Radix Notopterygii) and *Gao Ben* (Rhizoma et Radix Ligustici).

• With headache accompanied by dizziness, vertigo, and tinnitus, add *Ju Hua* (Flos Chrysanthemi), *Gou Teng* (Ramulus Uncariae cum Uncis), and *Xia Ku Cao* (Spica Prunellae).

• With heat, add *Huang Qin* (Radix Scutellariae), *Long Dan* (Radix et Rhizoma Gentianae), and *Mu Dan Pi* (Cortex Moutan).

• With cold, add *Gui Zhi* (Ramulus Cinnamomi) and *Sheng Jiang* (Rhizoma Zingiberis Recens).

• With constipation, add *Da Huang* (Radix et Rhizoma Rhei).

• With blood stagnation and yin deficiency, add *Liu Wei Di Huang Wan* (Six-Ingredient Pill with Rehmannia).

• With blood stagnation and qi deficiency, add *Ren Shen* (Radix et Rhizoma Ginseng) and *Huang Qi* (Radix Astragali).

• With palpitations, add *Fu Shen* (Poria Paradicis) and *Bai Zi Ren* (Semen Platycladi).

• With angina, add *Dan Shen* (Radix et Rhizoma Salviae Miltiorrhizae) and *Jiang Xiang* (Lignum Dalbergiae Odoriferae).

• With feelings of distention, oppression, and pain in the chest, add *Chuan Lian Zi* (Fructus Toosendan) and *Yan Hu Suo* (Rhizoma Corydalis).

• With distention and the sensation of a mass or blockage in the hypochondriac area, add *Yu Jin* (Radix Curcumae) and *Dan Shen* (Radix et Rhizoma Salviae Miltiorrhizae).

• With insomnia and excessive dreams, add *Shou Wu Teng*

Xuè Fǔ Zhú Yū Tāng
(Drive Out Stasis in the Mansion of Blood Decoction)

(Caulis Polygoni Multiflori) and *He Huan Pi* (Cortex Albiziae).

- With amenorrhea and dysmenorrhea due to blood stasis, remove *Jie Geng* (Radix Platycodonis), and add *Xiang Fu* (Rhizoma Cyperi) and *Yi Mu Cao* (Herba Leonuri).
- To dissolve blood clots, add *Shui Zhi* (Hirudo), *Meng Chong* (Tabanus), *Da Huang* (Radix et Rhizoma Rhei), and *Tu Bie Chong* (Eupolyphaga seu Steleophaga).

CAUTIONS / CONTRAINDICATIONS

- *Xue Fu Zhu Yu Tang* is contraindicated in pregnancy, and in cases of hypermenorrhea, because this formula strongly activates blood circulation and removes blood stasis.
- If this formula is to be taken for a prolonged period of time, tonic herbs should be added accordingly.

PHARMACOLOGICAL EFFECTS

1. **Antiplatelet and anticoagulant**: Administration of *Xue Fu Zhu Yu Tang* was associated with a marked antiplatelet effect in animal subjects.[1,2] It also inhibits the formation of blood clots.[3] Lastly, it improves blood circulation by decreasing blood viscosity.[4]
2. **Cardiovascular**: Administration of *Xue Fu Zhu Yu Tang* was associated with reduced blood pressure, a response attributed to its effect to inhibit the rhythm and contractility of the heart. Furthermore, it has a regulatory effect on the blood vessels, causing them to relax or constrict.[5,6]
3. **Antihyperlipidemic**: Administration of *Xue Fu Zhu Yu Tang* in male rats at 16g/kg was associated with a reduction of plasma cholesterol levels. However, it did not affect the plasma glucose or triglyceride levels.[7]

CLINICAL STUDIES AND RESEARCH

1. **Cardiac ischemia**: One study reported 89.3% effectiveness using modified *Xue Fu Zhu Yu Tang* to treat elderly patients with cardiac ischemia. Of 84 patients, the study reported significant improvement in 29 cases, moderate improvement in 46 cases, and no effect in 9 cases. The duration ranged from 1-3 courses of treatment.[8]
2. **Bradyarrhythmia**: One study reported 92.8% effectiveness using modified *Xue Fu Zhu Yu Tang* in decoction daily to treat 28 patients with bradyarrhythmia. The herbal treatment contained *Tao Ren* (Semen Persicae) 10g, *Dang Gui* (Radix Angelicae Sinensis) 10g, *Chi Shao* (Radix Paeoniae Rubra) 10g, *Niu Xi* (Radix Achyranthis Bidentatae) 10g, *Fu Zi* (Radix Aconiti Lateralis Praeparata) 10g, *Gua Lou Pi* (Pericarpium Trichosanthis) 10g, *Hong Hua* (Flos Carthami) 5g, *Chuan Xiong* (Rhizoma Chuanxiong) 5g, *Jie Geng* (Radix Platycodonis) 5g, *Gan*

Cao (Radix et Rhizoma Glycyrrhizae) 3g, and *Huang Qi* (Radix Astragali) 15g. Of 28 patients, the study reported complete recovery in 14 cases, improvement in 12 cases, and no effect in 2 cases.[9]

3. **Pneumothorax**: One study reported complete recovery in all 12 patients with pneumothorax after 2-4 weeks of treatment with *Xue Fu Zhu Yu Tang*.[10]
4. **Hepatitis**: Administration of modified *Xue Fu Zhu Yu Tang* in decoction in 81 patients with chronic hepatitis was associated with complete recovery in 67 cases, improvement in 8 cases, and no effect in 6 cases. The overall effectiveness was 92.6%. In addition to the base formula, modifications were made as follows: *Huang Qin* (Radix Scutellariae) and *Zhi Zi* (Fructus Gardeniae) were added for dry mouth with bitter taste, yellow urine, and yellow greasy tongue coating; *Fu Ling* (Poria) and *Bai Zhu* (Rhizoma Atractylodis Macrocephalae) were added for abdominal fullness, loose stools, and a pale tongue body with a white coating; and *Shu Di Huang* (Radix Rehmanniae Praeparata) and *Gou Qi Zi* (Fructus Lycii) for *wu xin re* (five-center heat), soreness and weakness of the lower back and knees, and a red tongue body with a thin coating.[11]
5. **Pancreatitis**: One study reported complete recovery in 128 patients using integrated treatments of herbs and drugs. The herbal treatment included modified *Xue Fu Zhu Yu Tang* in decoction daily for 7 days per course of treatment. Western treatment included drugs and intravenous fluids (specific details were unavailable). Instructions were also given to follow a low-fat, high-protein, and high carbohydrate diet. The study reported complete recovery in all 128 patients within 3 courses of treatment.[12]
6. **Headache**: One study reported 93.33% effectiveness using modified *Xue Fu Zhu Yu Tang* to treat 15 patients with headache due to blood stagnation. Modifications to the formula included addition of *Shi Jue Ming* (Concha Haliotidis) and *Gou Teng* (Ramulus Uncariae cum Uncis) for Liver yang rising; *Shan Zhu Yu* (Fructus Corni) and *Gou Qi Zi* (Fructus Lycii) for Kidney deficiency; *Hou Po* (Cortex Magnoliae Officinalis) and *Bai Zhu* (Rhizoma Atractylodis Macrocephalae) for turbid dampness; and *Bai Zhi* (Radix Angelicae Dahuricae) and *Gao Ben* (Rhizoma et Radix Ligustici) for exterior wind-cold. Of 15 patients, 3 had complete recovery, 11 had marked improvement, and 1 had no response.[13]
7. **Vascular headache**: Fifty patients with vascular headaches responded well to modified *Xue Fu Zhu Yu Tang*. The herbal treatment contained *Tao Ren* (Semen Persicae) 12g, *Hong Hua* (Flos Carthami) 9g, *Dang Gui* (Radix Angelicae Sinensis) 9g, *Di Huang* (Radix Rehmanniae) 9g,

BLOOD-REGULATING FORMULAS

13

881

Chapter 13 – Blood-Regulating Formulas　　　　*Section 1 – Blood-Invigorating and Stasis-Removing Formulas*

Xuè Fǔ Zhú Yū Tāng
(Drive Out Stasis in the Mansion of Blood Decoction)

Chuan Xiong (Rhizoma Chuanxiong) 15g, *Chi Shao* (Radix Paeoniae Rubra) 6g, *Niu Xi* (Radix Achyranthis Bidentatae) 9g, *Jie Geng* (Radix Platycodonis) 5g, *Chai Hu* (Radix Bupleuri) 3g, *Zhi Qiao* (Fructus Aurantii) 6g, and *Gan Cao* (Radix et Rhizoma Glycyrrhizae) 3g. Additional modifications were made as follows: for frontal headache, *Bai Zhi* (Radix Angelicae Dahuricae), *Tian Ma* (Rhizoma Gastrodiae), and *Xi Xin* (Radix et Rhizoma Asari) were added; for occipital headache, *Qiang Huo* (Rhizoma et Radix Notopterygii) and *Du Huo* (Radix Angelicae Pubescentis) were used; for temporal headache, *Man Jing Zi* (Fructus Viticis), *Ju Hua* (Flos Chrysanthemi), and *Long Dan* (Radix et Rhizoma Gentianae) were included; and for vertex headache, *Gao Ben* (Rhizoma et Radix Ligustici) was added. The herbs were given in decoction daily, for 8 days per course of treatment. Of 50 patients, the study reported complete recovery in 34 cases, significant improvement in 11 cases, and no benefit in 5 cases. The overall effectiveness was 90%.[14]

8. **Insomnia**: Use of modified *Xue Fu Zhu Yu Tang* was associated with 93.5% effectiveness in treating 31 patients with stubborn insomnia. The base formula contained *Xue Fu Zhu Yu Tang*, with addition of *Shou Wu Teng* (Caulis Polygoni Multiflori) and *Hu Po* (Succinum), and elimination of *Chai Hu* (Radix Bupleuri) and *Chuan Xiong* (Rhizoma Chuanxiong). Modifications were made based on the condition of the patients. *Dang Shen* (Radix Codonopsis) and *Huang Qi* (Radix Astragali) were added for qi deficiency; *Shu Di Huang* (Radix Rehmanniae Praeparata) and *E Jiao* (Colla Corii Asini) were added for blood deficiency; *Gou Qi Zi* (Fructus Lycii) and *Shan Zhu Yu* (Fructus Corni) were added for yin deficiency; and *Chen Pi* (Pericarpium Citri Reticulatae) and *Ban Xia* (Rhizoma Pinelliae) were added to clear hot phlegm.[15]

9. **Phlebitis**: Administration of modified *Xue Fu Zhu Yu Tang* has been shown to effectively treat phlebitis. In addition to the base formula, *Mu Dan Pi* (Cortex Moutan) was added for redness and swelling associated with heat in the *xue* (blood) level; *San Qi* (Radix et Rhizoma Notoginseng) was added for blood vessel pain with swelling and inflammation; and *Huang Qi* (Radix Astragali) was added for a fine, weak pulse. Each course of treatment was 7 days. Of 38 patients, the study reported significant benefit in 8 cases, moderate improvement in 29 cases, and no effect in 1 case.[16] Another study reported marked effects using herbs orally and topically to treat phlebitis. The herbal formula for oral ingestion contained *Xue Fu Zhu Yu Tang* plus *Zhe Bei Mu* (Bulbus Fritillariae Thunbergii) and *Di Long* (Pheretima), and was given daily for 15 days per course of treatment. Herbs also were applied topically to the affected area twice daily

to relieve pain. Of 12 patients, the study reported complete recovery in 9 cases, improvement in 2 cases, and no effect in 1 case. The overall effectiveness was 92%.[17]

10. **Mammary gland hyperplasia**: According to one study, 104 patients with mammary gland hyperplasia were treated with complete recovery in 68 cases and moderate improvement in 27 cases (91.4% effectiveness). The herbal treatment contained *Xue Fu Zhu Yu Tang* as the base formula, with the addition of *San Leng* (Rhizoma Sparganii) and *E Zhu* (Rhizoma Curcumae), and removal of *Di Huang* (Radix Rehmanniae) and *Jie Geng* (Radix Platycodonis). Other herbs were added if deemed necessary.[18]

11. **Pelvic inflammatory disease**: One study reported 92% effectiveness using modified *Xue Fu Zhu Yu Tang* to treat 60 patients with chronic pelvic inflammatory disease. Modifications included the addition of *Xiao Hui Xiang* (Fructus Foeniculi) and *Pao Jiang* (Rhizoma Zingiberis Praeparatum) for cold sensations in the lower abdomen; *Pu Gong Ying* (Herba Taraxaci) and *Zi Hua Di Ding* (Herba Violae) for toxic heat; and *Yi Yi Ren* (Semen Coicis) for dampness. Of 60 patients, the study reported complete recovery in 24 cases, improvement in 31 cases, and no response in 5 cases.[19]

12. **Concussion**: One study reported 92.3% effectiveness for 12 patients with concussion using modified *Xue Fu Zhu Yu Tang*. The herbal treatment contained this formula plus *Shi Chang Pu* (Rhizoma Acori Tatarinowii) 10g, *Yuan Zhi* (Radix Polygalae) 15g, *Dan Shen* (Radix et Rhizoma Salviae Miltiorrhizae) 25g, *Mai Dong* (Radix Ophiopogonis) 16g, and *Suan Zao Ren* (Semen Ziziphi Spinosae) 13g. The herbs were given in decoction daily.[20]

13. **Stroke**: Benefit in the prevention and treatment of stroke and ischemia has been associated with many Chinese herbal formulas, including *Xue Fu Zhu Yu Tang*, *Bu Yang Huan Wu Tang* (Tonify the Yang to Restore Five Decoction), *Xiao Xu Ming Tang* (Minor Prolong-Life Decoction), and *Chai Hu Jia Long Gu Mu Li Tang* (Bupleurum plus Dragon Bone and Oyster Shell Decoction). The mechanisms of these beneficial effects were attributed to anti-hypercholesterolemia, antioxidant activity, and free radical scavenger effects of these formulas.[21]

14. **Cerebral atherosclerosis**: Sixty-three patients were treated with excellent results using modified *Xue Fu Zhu Yu Tang* plus ear acupuncture. The herbal treatment contained *Dang Gui* (Radix Angelicae Sinensis) 15-20g, *Di Huang* (Radix Rehmanniae) 5g, *Tian Ma* (Rhizoma Gastrodiae) 5g, *Tao Ren* (Semen Persicae) 9g, *Zhi Qiao* (Fructus Aurantii) 9g, *Chuan Xiong* (Rhizoma Chuanxiong) 9g, *Hong Hua* (Flos Carthami) 6g, *Chai*

882

Chinese Herbal Formulas and Applications

Xuè Fǔ Zhú Yū Tāng
(Drive Out Stasis in the Mansion of Blood Decoction)

Hu (Radix Bupleuri) 6g, *Gan Cao* (Radix et Rhizoma Glycyrrhizae) 6g, *Niu Xi* (Radix Achyranthis Bidentatae) 10g, *Chi Shao* (Radix Paeoniae Rubra) 10g, and *Dan Shen* (Radix et Rhizoma Salviae Miltiorrhizae) 15-30g. The duration of treatment ranged from 1-6 months. Of 63 patients, the study reported complete recovery in 42 cases, improvement in 13 cases, and no effect in 8 cases.[22]

15. **Hyperlipidemia**: Use of *Xue Fu Zhu Yu Tang* was associated with 95% effectiveness in reducing cholesterol and triglyceride levels. Of 20 patients, the study reported significant improvement in 11 cases, moderate improvement in 8 cases, and no effect in 1 case.[23]

16. **Schizophrenia**: According to one study of 66 schizophrenic patients with 3 months to 23 years history of illness, use of modified *Xue Fu Zhu Yu Tang* was associated with marked beneficial effects. The herbal treatment contained *Chai Hu* (Radix Bupleuri) 15g, *Hong Hua* (Flos Carthami) 10g, *Chi Shao* (Radix Paeoniae Rubra) 30g, *Chuan Xiong* (Rhizoma Chuanxiong) 15g, *Dan Shen* (Radix et Rhizoma Salviae Miltiorrhizae) 30g, and *Jiang Xiang* (Lignum Dalbergiae Odoriferae) 15g. Modifications were made by adding *Xiang Fu* (Rhizoma Cyperi) to regulate qi, *Da Huang* (Radix et Rhizoma Rhei) to clear heat, *Fu Ling* (Poria) and *Bai Zhu* (Rhizoma Atractylodis Macrocephalae) to strengthen the Spleen, and *Dang Shen* (Radix Codonopsis) and *Huang Qi* (Radix Astragali) to tonify qi. The treatment protocol was to cook the herbs in water and administer the decoction in two equally-divided doses daily for 8 weeks per course of treatment. In addition to Chinese herbs, a small dose of antipsychotic medication (selection depended on the condition of the patient) was given daily.[24]

17. **Endometriosis**: Use of *Xue Fu Zhu Yu Tang* was associated with 94% effectiveness in the treatment of 83 patients with endometriosis, using herbs orally and rectally. The herbal formula for oral ingestion contained *Dang Gui* (Radix Angelicae Sinensis) 9g, *Di Huang* (Radix Rehmanniae) 9g, *Hong Hua* (Flos Carthami) 9g, *Chi Shao* (Radix Paeoniae Rubra) 9g, *Niu Xi* (Radix Achyranthis Bidentatae) 9g, *Zhi Qiao* (Fructus Aurantii) 6g, *Jie Geng* (Radix Platycodonis) 6g, *Chuan Xiong* (Rhizoma Chuanxiong) 6g, *Gan Cao* (Radix et Rhizoma Glycyrrhizae) 6g, *Chai Hu* (Radix Bupleuri) 3g, and *Tao Ren* (Semen Persicae) 12g. Modifications were made by adding *Xi Xin* (Radix et Rhizoma Asari) and *Fu Zi* (Radix Aconiti Lateralis Praeparata) for blood stagnation with cold; *Chuan Lian Zi* (Fructus Toosendan), *Pu Huang* (Pollen Typhae), and *Wu Ling Zhi* (Faeces Trogopteri) for qi and blood stagnation; *Da Xue Teng* (Caulis Sargentodoxae) and *Bai Jiang Cao* (Herba cum Radice Patriniae) for blood stagnation with heat; *Huang*

Qi (Radix Astragali), *Dang Shen* (Radix Codonopsis), and *Mu Xiang* (Radix Aucklandiae) for blood stagnation with qi deficiency; *San Leng* (Rhizoma Sparganii) and *E Zhu* (Rhizoma Curcumae) for nodules and cysts; and *Yin Yang Huo* (Herba Epimedii), *Xian Mao* (Rhizoma Curculiginis) and *Tu Si Zi* (Semen Cuscutae) for infertility. The herbs were given as decoction in two equally-divided doses. Herbs also were given as rectal enema one time daily, with an herbal solution made from *San Leng* (Rhizoma Sparganii) 10g, *E Zhu* (Rhizoma Curcumae) 10g, *Da Xue Teng* (Caulis Sargentodoxae) 12g, *Zao Jiao Ci* (Spina Gleditsiae) 12g, *Feng Fang* (Nidus Vespae) 12g, *Chi Shao* (Radix Paeoniae Rubra) 12g, and *Tao Ren* (Semen Persicae) 6g. Of 83 patients, the study reported complete recovery in 41 cases, significant improvement in 27 cases, moderate improvement in 10 cases, and no improvement in 5 cases.[25]

18. **Amenorrhea**: One study reported marked success using modified *Xue Fu Zhu Yu Tang* in decoction daily to treat amenorrhea following miscarriage. The herbal formula contained *Niu Xi* (Radix Achyranthis Bidentatae) 12g, *Dang Gui* (Radix Angelicae Sinensis) 12g, *Di Huang* (Radix Rehmanniae) 12g, *Tao Ren* (Semen Persicae) 9g, *Hong Hua* (Flos Carthami) 9g, *Chi Shao* (Radix Paeoniae Rubra) 9g, *Chai Hu* (Radix Bupleuri) 9g, *Zhi Shi* (Fructus Aurantii Immaturus) 9g, *Chuan Xiong* (Rhizoma Chuanxiong) 6g, *Jie Geng* (Radix Platycodonis) 6g, and *Gan Cao* (Radix et Rhizoma Glycyrrhizae) 3g. Other modifications were made as needed based on the individual's condition. Of 33 patients, the study reported normal menstruation in 17 cases, significant improvement in 14 cases, and slight improvement in 2 cases. The duration of treatment ranged from 9-21 days.[26]

RELATED FORMULA

Sān Jiāo Zhú Yū Tāng
(Drive Out Blood Stasis in Three *Jiaos* Decoction)

三焦逐瘀湯
三焦逐瘀汤

Pinyin Name: San Jiao Zhu Yu Tang

Literal Name: Drive Out Blood Stasis in Three *Jiaos* Decoction

Original Source: *Jian Tai Yao Fang* (Herbal Prescriptions from *Jiantai* Clinic) by Chang Wei-Yen in 1981

Bai Shao (Radix Paeoniae Alba)	
Chai Hu (Radix Bupleuri)	
Chi Shao (Radix Paeoniae Rubra)	
Chuan Niu Xi (Radix Cyathulae)	
Chuan Xiong (Rhizoma Chuanxiong)	
Dang Gui (Radix Angelicae Sinensis)	

BLOOD-REGULATING FORMULAS

13

883

Chapter 13 – Blood-Regulating Formulas   *Section 1 – Blood-Invigorating and Stasis-Removing Formulas*

Xuè Fǔ Zhú Yū Tāng
(Drive Out Stasis in the Mansion of Blood Decoction)

Gan Cao (Radix et Rhizoma Glycyrrhizae)
Hong Hua (Flos Carthami)
Jie Geng (Radix Platycodonis)
San Leng (Rhizoma Sparganii)
Mu Dan Pi (Cortex Moutan)
Pu Huang (Pollen Typhae)
Rou Gui (Cortex Cinnamomi)
Di Huang (Radix Rehmanniae)
E Zhu (Rhizoma Curcumae)
Tao Ren (Semen Persicae)
Wu Yao (Radix Linderae)
Xiang Fu (Rhizoma Cyperi)
Yan Hu Suo (Rhizoma Corydalis)
Zhi Qiao (Fructus Aurantii)

San Jiao Zhu Yu Tang (Drive Out Blood Stasis in Three *Jiaos* Decoction) is a variation of *Xue Fu Zhu Yu Tang* (Drive Out Stasis in the Mansion of Blood Decoction) with the addition of blood moving herbs for the middle and lower *jiaos* and one of the strongest blood moving herbs, *Shui Zhi* (Hirudo). This formula is aimed at breaking up chronic or stubborn blood stasis from past injuries or blood clots with no outlet such as that seen in endometriosis. It is an extremely strong formula designed for short term use to quickly break up severe and chronic blood stasis to bring the body back to homeostasis.

AUTHORS' COMMENTS

There are four "*zhu yu tang* (drive out stasis decoction)" formulas that are commonly used for similar conditions. All four formulas contain *Chuan Xiong* (Rhizoma Chuanxiong), *Dang Gui* (Radix Angelicae Sinensis), *Tao Ren* (Semen Persicae), and *Hong Hua* (Flos Carthami) as key ingredients to activate blood, eliminate blood stasis, and relieve pain. Their main differences are as follows:

• *Xue Fu Zhu Yu Tang* (Drive Out Stasis in the Mansion of Blood Decoction) treats qi and blood stagnation in the upper *jiao* to alleviate pain in the chest and hypochondrium.
• *Ge Xia Zhu Yu Tang* (Drive Out Blood Stasis Below the Diaphragm Decoction) treats qi and blood stagnation in the middle *jiao* to alleviate pain below the diaphragm in areas such as the hypochondrium and the upper abdominal area.
• *Shao Fu Zhu Yu Tang* (Drive Out Blood Stasis in the Lower Abdomen Decoction) treats qi and blood stagnation with

cold in the lower *jiao* to address irregular menstruation, menstrual pain, and numerous gynecological disorders.
• *Shen Tong Zhu Yu Tang* (Drive Out Blood Stasis from a Painful Body Decoction) treats qi and blood stagnation with obstruction of the channels and collaterals in the extremities to relieve aches and pains.

References

1. *Zhong Yao Yao Li Yu Lin Chuang* (Pharmacology and Clinical Applications of Chinese Herbs) 1993;9(1):8.
2. *Zhong Hua Nei Ke Xue Za Zhi* (Journal of Chinese Internal Medicine) 1977;2(2):79.
3. *Zhong Yao Yao Li Yu Lin Chuang* (Pharmacology and Clinical Applications of Chinese Herbs) 1993;9(5):9.
4. *Zhong Guo Yi Yao Xue Bao* (Chinese Journal of Medicine and Herbology) 1990;5(4):33.
5. *Zhong Yao Yao Li Yu Lin Chuang* (Pharmacology and Clinical Applications of Chinese Herbs) 1993;9(1):8.
6. *Zhong Guo Yi Yao Xue Bao* (Chinese Journal of Medicine and Herbology) 1990;5(4):33.
7. *Shan Xi Zhong Yi* (Shanxi Chinese Medicine) 1988;9(3):126.
8. *Zhe Jiang Zhong Yi Za Zhi* (Zhejiang Journal of Chinese Medicine) 1997;10:445.
9. *Zhe Jiang Zhong Yi Xue Yuan Xue Bao* (Journal of Zhejiang University of Chinese Medicine) 1992;16(3):19.
10. *He Nan Zhong Yi* (Henan Chinese Medicine) 1990;10(1):33.
11. *Jiang Su Zhong Yi* (Jiangsu Chinese Medicine) 1995;7:10.
12. *Shi Yong Zhong Yi Yao Za Zhi* (Journal of Practical Chinese Medicine and Medicinals) 1994;10(4):27.
13. *Guang Xi Zhong Yi Yao* (Guangxi Chinese Medicine and Herbology) 1996;5:22.
14. *Zhong Guo Zhong Xi Yi Jie He Za Zhi* (Chinese Journal of Integrative Chinese and Western Medicine) 1995;15(7):438.
15. *Xin Zhong Yi* (New Chinese Medicine) 1996;8:32.
16. *Zhe Jiang Zhong Yi Za Zhi* (Zhejiang Journal of Chinese Medicine) 1997;4:157.
17. *Shi Yong Zhong Yi Nei Ke Za Zhi* (Journal of Practical Chinese Internal Medicine) 1992;6(3):21.
18. *Tian Jin Zhong Yi* (Tianjin Chinese Medicine) 1986;5:18.
19. *Gan Su Zhong Yi* (Gansu Chinese Medicine) 1995;4:34.
20. *Shan Xi Zhong Yi* (Shanxi Chinese Medicine) 1993;14(5):222.
21. Lin CC, Yen FL, Hsu FF, Lin JM. Anti-hypercholesterolaemia, antioxidant activity and free radical scavenger effects of traditional Chinese medicine prescriptions used for stroke. Journal of Pharmacy & Pharmacology 2000 Nov;52(11):1387-93.
22. *Hu Nan Zhong Yi Za Zhi* (Hunan Journal of Chinese Medicine) 1993;9(1):41.
23. *Zhong Xi Yi Jie He Za Zhi* (Journal of Integrated Chinese and Western Medicine) 1988;8(10):601.
24. *Zhong Guo Zhong Xi Yi Jie He Za Zhi* (Chinese Journal of Integrative Chinese and Western Medicine) 1993;13(7):397.
25. *Shang Hai Zhong Yi Yao Za Zhi* (Shanghai Journal of Chinese Medicine and Herbology) 1993;2:16.
26. *Shan Xi Zhong Yi* (Shanxi Chinese Medicine) 1991;12(5):200.

Chinese Herbal Formulas and Applications

Gé Xià Zhú Yū Tāng
(Drive Out Blood Stasis Below the Diaphragm Decoction)

膈下逐瘀湯
膈下逐瘀汤

Pinyin Name: *Ge Xia Zhu Yu Tang*
Literal Name: Drive Out Blood Stasis Below the Diaphragm Decoction
Alternate Name: Tangkuei and Corydalis Combination
Original Source: *Yi Lin Gai Cuo* (Corrections of Errors Among Physicians) by Wang Qing-Ren in 1830

COMPOSITION

Tao Ren (Semen Persicae), *yan* (ground) until muddy	9g
Hong Hua (Flos Carthami)	9g
Dang Gui (Radix Angelicae Sinensis)	9g
Chuan Xiong (Rhizoma Chuanxiong)	6g
Mu Dan Pi (Cortex Moutan)	6g
Chi Shao (Radix Paeoniae Rubra)	6g
Zhi Qiao (Fructus Citri Aurantii)	4.5g
Wu Yao (Radix Linderae)	6g
Xiang Fu (Rhizoma Cyperi)	4.5g
Wu Ling Zhi (Faeces Trogopteri), *chao* (dry-fried)	9g
Yan Hu Suo (Rhizoma Corydalis)	3g
Gan Cao (Radix et Rhizoma Glycyrrhizae)	9g

DOSAGE / PREPARATION / ADMINISTRATION

Prepare as a decoction.

CHINESE THERAPEUTIC ACTIONS

1. Activates blood circulation and dispels blood stagnation
2. Activates qi circulation and relieves pain

CLINICAL MANIFESTATIONS

Blood stagnation below the diaphragm: palpable mass in the abdomen due to blood stasis; formation of abdominal mass or hardness in children; and abdominal pain in a fixed area.

CLINICAL APPLICATIONS

Hematoporphyria, pleural adhesion, acute and chronic hepatitis, liver cirrhosis, hepatic hemangioma, cholecystitis, jaundice, splenomegaly, pelvic inflammatory disease, dysmenorrhea, amenorrhea, menopause, endometriosis, prostatic hypertrophy, chronic colitis, peptic ulcer disease, and tumors of the thyroid gland, uterus, and liver.

EXPLANATION

Ge Xia Zhu Yu Tang (Drive Out Blood Stasis Below the Diaphragm Decoction) activates qi and blood circulation, removes blood stagnation, and relieves pain in the region below the diaphragm. Because blood stagnation below the diaphragm is the underlying cause of the illness, the patient may experience severe pain and swelling.

Additionally, blood stagnation often presents as a mass or hardness in the abdominal region. Clinically, the patient may show symptoms such as fixed abdominal pain and a palpable mass in the abdomen.

Tao Ren (Semen Persicae) and *Hong Hua* (Flos Carthami) break up blood stagnation and activate blood circulation. These two herbs have synergistic effects and are often used together. *Dang Gui* (Radix Angelicae Sinensis) and *Chuan Xiong* (Rhizoma Chuanxiong) nourish the blood and activate blood circulation. The pairing of these herbs points to the fact that blood-tonifying herbs are commonly combined with blood-activating herbs to prevent tonification from turning into stagnation. *Mu Dan Pi* (Cortex Moutan) and *Chi Shao* (Radix Paeoniae Rubra) clear heat, cool the blood, and dispel blood stagnation. Because blood stagnation and qi stagnation often occur simultaneously, *Zhi Qiao* (Fructus Aurantii), *Wu Yao* (Radix Linderae), and *Xiang Fu* (Rhizoma Cyperi) are employed to activate and regulate qi circulation. *Zhi Qiao* (Fructus Aurantii) breaks down stagnation, *Wu Yao* (Radix Linderae) stimulates peristalsis of the intestines, and *Xiang Fu* (Rhizoma Cyperi) relieves pain. Because patients with blood stasis often experience severe pain, *Wu Ling Zhi* (Faeces Trogopteri) and *Yan Hu Suo* (Rhizoma Corydalis) are added to dispel blood stasis and relieve pain. Lastly, *Gan Cao* (Radix et Rhizoma Glycyrrhizae) tonifies qi and harmonizes the herbs in this formula.

BLOOD-REGULATING FORMULAS

13

885

Chapter 13 – Blood-Regulating Formulas   *Section 1 – Blood-Invigorating and Stasis-Removing Formulas*

Gé Xià Zhú Yū Tāng
(Drive Out Blood Stasis Below the Diaphragm Decoction)

Ge Xia Zhu Yu Tang (Drive Out Blood Stasis Below the Diaphragm Decoction)

Diagnosis	Signs and Symptoms	Treatment	Herbs
Blood stagnation below the diaphragm	Abdominal pain in a fixed location, presence of a mass or hardness in the abdomen: blood stagnation in the middle *jiao* area	• Activates blood circulation and dispels blood stagnation • Activates qi circulation and relieves pain	• *Tao Ren* (Semen Persicae) and *Hong Hua* (Flos Carthami) break up blood stagnation and activate blood circulation. • *Dang Gui* (Radix Angelicae Sinensis) and *Chuan Xiong* (Rhizoma Chuanxiong) nourish blood and activate blood circulation. • *Mu Dan Pi* (Cortex Moutan) and *Chi Shao* (Radix Paeoniae Rubra) clear heat, cool the blood, and dispel blood stagnation. • *Zhi Qiao* (Fructus Aurantii), *Wu Yao* (Radix Linderae), and *Xiang Fu* (Rhizoma Cyperi) regulate qi circulation and relieve pain. • *Wu Ling Zhi* (Faeces Trogopteri) and *Yan Hu Suo* (Rhizoma Corydalis) dispel blood stasis and relieve pain. • *Gan Cao* (Radix et Rhizoma Glycyrrhizae) tonifies qi and harmonizes all the herbs in this formula.

MODIFICATIONS

- With qi deficiency, add *Dang Shen* (Radix Codonopsis) and *Huang Qi* (Radix Astragali).
- With yin-deficient heat, add *Zhi Mu* (Rhizoma Anemarrhenae), *Sha Shen* (Radix Glehniae seu Adenophorae), and *Di Huang* (Radix Rehmanniae).
- With constipation, add *Da Huang* (Radix et Rhizoma Rhei).
- With blood in the vomitus or stools, add *Bai Ji* (Rhizoma Bletillae), *Huai Hua* (Flos Sophorae), and *Dan Shen* (Radix et Rhizoma Salviae Miltiorrhizae).
- With insomnia, add *Ci Shi* (Magnetitum).
- With allergic purpura, add large doses of *Gan Cao* (Radix et Rhizoma Glycyrrhizae), *Qin Jiao* (Radix Gentianae Macrophyllae), and *Ban Lan Gen* (Radix Isatidis).
- With menstrual pain and cramps, dysmenorrhea, and amenorrhea, combine with *Wen Jing Tang* (Warm the Channels Decoction), *Shao Yao Gan Cao Tang* (Peony and Licorice Decoction), and *Yan Hu Suo* (Rhizoma Corydalis).
- With emotional and behavioral changes during menopause, combine with *Ai Ye* (Folium Artemisiae Argyi), *Xiao Yao San* (Rambling Powder), and *Dang Gui Shao Yao San* (Tangkuei and Peony Powder).
- For chronic hepatitis and liver cirrhosis, combine with *Yin Chen Wu Ling San* (Artemisia Scoparia and Five-Ingredient Powder with Poria), *Jia Wei Xiao Yao San* (Augmented Rambling Powder), or *Xiao Chai Hu*

Tang (Minor Bupleurum Decoction). *San Qi* (Radix et Rhizoma Notoginseng), *E Zhu* (Rhizoma Curcumae), and *Bie Jia* (Carapax Trionycis) are also useful and can be added to these formulas.
- For liver cancer, add *Xiao Chai Hu Tang* (Minor Bupleurum Decoction), *Ban Zhi Lian* (Herba Scutellariae Barbatae), and *Bai Hua She She Cao* (Herba Hedyotis).
- For tumors on the thyroid gland, combine with *San Zhong Kui Jian Tang* (Disperse the Swelling and Break the Hardness Decoction), *Xiao Chai Hu Tang* (Minor Bupleurum Decoction), and *Xia Ku Cao* (Spica Prunellae).
- For chronic cholecystitis, combine with *Yin Chen Wu Ling San* (Artemisia Scoparia and Five-Ingredient Powder with Poria*)*, *Huang Lian Jie Du Tang* (Coptis Decoction to Relieve Toxicity), and *Jin Yin Hua* (Flos Lonicerae Japonicae).
- For uterine tumors, combine with *Gui Zhi Fu Ling Wan* (Cinnamon Twig and Poria Pill), *Bie Jia* (Carapax Trionycis), *E Zhu* (Rhizoma Curcumae), and *San Leng* (Rhizoma Sparganii).
- For jaundice and acute hepatitis, combine with *Jia Wei Xiao Yao San* (Augmented Rambling Powder).

CAUTIONS / CONTRAINDICATIONS

- *Ge Xia Zhu Yu Tang* should be used with caution during menstruation.
- Use of this formula is contraindicated during pregnancy.[1]

886

Chinese Herbal Formulas and Applications

Gé Xià Zhú Yū Tāng
(Drive Out Blood Stasis Below the Diaphragm Decoction)

CLINICAL STUDIES AND RESEARCH

1. **Hematoporphyria**: Use of *Ge Xia Zhu Yu Tang* was associated with complete recovery in all 8 patients with hematoporphyria characterized by qi and blood stagnation, with symptoms such as hypochondriac or upper abdominal pain that intensifies at night, and urine with red, yellow, or coffee-ground color.[2]

2. **Pleural adhesion**: Sixty patients with pleural adhesions were treated with complete recovery in 33 cases, significant improvement in 23 cases, moderate improvement in 2 cases, and no effect in 2 case. The herbal treatment used *Ge Xia Zhu Yu Tang* as the base formula, with the addition of *Gui Zhi* (Ramulus Cinnamomi), *Jing Jie* (Herba Schizonepetae), and *Fang Feng* (Radix Saposhnikoviae) for exterior wind-cold; *Jin Yin Hua* (Flos Lonicerae Japonicae), *Lian Qiao* (Fructus Forsythiae), and *Bo He* (Herba Menthae) for exterior wind-heat; *Huang Qin* (Radix Scutellariae), *Gua Lou* (Fructus Trichosanthis), and *Sang Bai Pi* (Cortex Mori) for Lung heat with cough; *Gan Jiang* (Rhizoma Zingiberis), *Xi Xin* (Radix et Rhizoma Asari), and *Wu Wei Zi* (Fructus Schisandrae Chinensis) for Lung cold with cough; and *Huang Qi* (Radix Astragali) and *Dang Shen* (Radix Codonopsis) for qi deficiency.[3]

3. **Hepatitis**: Use of *Ge Xia Zhu Yu Tang* in 25 patients with chronic active hepatitis was associated with alleviating pain, improving appetite, resolving jaundice, and relieving ascites.[4]

4. **Hepatic hemangioma**: Use of *Ge Xia Zhu Yu Tang* plus *Meng Chong* (Tabanus) and *San Leng* (Rhizoma Sparganii) was associated with 86% effectiveness in treating hepatic hemangioma. Modifications to the base formula were made as follows: *Huang Qi* (Radix Astragali), *Shan Yao* (Rhizoma Dioscoreae), and *Dan Shen* (Radix et Rhizoma Salviae Miltiorrhizae) for chronic hepatitis; *Bie Jia* (Carapax Trionycis) and *Mu Li* (Concha Ostreae) for liver cirrhosis; *Chai Hu* (Radix Bupleuri), *Huang Qin* (Radix Scutellariae), and *Yu Jin* (Radix Curcumae) for chronic cholecystitis; and *Jiang Xiang* (Lignum Dalbergiae Odoriferae), *Mu Xiang* (Radix Aucklandiae), and *Shan Zha* (Fructus Crataegi) for epigastric pain. Of 32 patients, the study reported complete recovery in 12 cases, significant improvement in 5 cases, moderate improvement in 12 cases, and no benefit in 3 cases.[5]

5. **Pelvic inflammatory disease**: Administration of modified *Ge Xia Zhu Yu Tang* was reported in one study to have 90.6% effectiveness in treating chronic pelvic inflammatory disease. The herbal treatment was based on this formula, with the addition of *Dan Shen* (Radix et Rhizoma Salviae Miltiorrhizae) and *Da Zao* (Fructus Jujubae), and the removal of *Wu Ling Zhi* (Faeces Trogopteri), *Zhi Qiao* (Fructus Aurantii), and *Wu Yao* (Radix Linderae). Furthermore, *Huang Qi* (Radix Astragali) and *Dang Shen* (Radix Codonopsis) were added for qi deficiency; *Shu Di Huang* (Radix Rehmanniae Praeparata) and *He Shou Wu* (Radix Polygoni Multiflori) were added for blood deficiency; *Mai Dong* (Radix Ophiopogonis) and *Sha Shen* (Radix Glehniae seu Adenophorae) were added for yin deficiency; *Fu Zi* (Radix Aconiti Lateralis Praeparata) and *Pao Jiang* (Rhizoma Zingiberis Praeparatum) were added for yang deficiency; *Huang Qin* (Radix Scutellariae) and *Ze Xie* (Rhizoma Alismatis) were added for damp-heat; and *Jin Yin Hua* (Flos Lonicerae Japonicae) and *Lian Qiao* (Fructus Forsythiae) were added for accumulation of heat and toxins. Of 64 patients, the study reported complete recovery in 21 cases, improvement in 37 cases, and no effect in 6 cases.[6]

6. **Ectopic pregnancy**: Use of modified *Ge Xia Zhu Yu Tang* was associated with successful termination of ectopic pregnancy in 19 of 20 patients (surgical intervention was needed in 1 case). The herbal treatment was based on this formula, with the addition of *Niu Xi* (Radix Achyranthis Bidentatae) and *Ru Xiang* (Gummi Olibanum) and removal of *Wu Ling Zhi* (Faeces Trogopteri), *Zhi Qiao* (Fructus Aurantii), *Chuan Xiong* (Rhizoma Chuanxiong), *Xiang Fu* (Rhizoma Cyperi), and others as deemed necessary.[7]

7. **Prostatic hypertrophy**: One study reported 90% effectiveness using modified *Ge Xia Zhu Yu Tang* to treat 22 patients with prostatic hypertrophy. The herbal treatment was based on this formula, with the addition of *Hua Shi* (Talcum) and the removal of *Wu Ling Zhi* (Faeces Trogopteri) and *Yan Hu Suo* (Rhizoma Corydalis). Furthermore, *Nu Zhen Zi* (Fructus Ligustri Lucidi), *Shan Zhu Yu* (Fructus Corni) and *Wu Wei Zi* (Fructus Schisandrae Chinensis) were added for Kidney yin deficiency; *Gui Zhi* (Ramulus Cinnamomi) and *Mu Hu Die* (Semen Oroxyli) were added for Kidney qi deficiency; and *Dang Shen* (Radix Codonopsis) and *Huang Qi* (Radix Astragali) were added for qi deficiency. Of 22 patients, the study reported recovery in 17 cases, improvement in 3 cases, and no effect in 2 cases.[8]

8. **Chronic colitis**: Use of modified *Ge Xia Zhu Yu Tang* in 75 patients with chronic colitis was associated with complete recovery in 63 cases, significant improvement in 9 cases, and improvement in 3 cases. The duration of treatment ranged from 3-9 days in most cases, with some cases requiring up to 40 days to resolve. The herbal formula contained *Dang Gui* (Radix Angelicae Sinensis) 9-12g, *Chi Shao* (Radix Paeoniae Rubra) 6-9g, *Xiang Fu*

BLOOD-REGULATING FORMULAS

13

887

Chapter 13 – Blood-Regulating Formulas   *Section 1 – Blood-Invigorating and Stasis-Removing Formulas*

Gé Xià Zhú Yū Tāng
(Drive Out Blood Stasis Below the Diaphragm Decoction)

(Rhizoma Cyperi) 6-9g, *Wu Yao* (Radix Linderae) 6-9g, *Wu Ling Zhi* (Faeces Trogopteri) 6-9g, *Zhi Qiao* (Fructus Aurantii) 6-9g, *Hong Hua* (Flos Carthami) 6g, and *Chuan Xiong* (Rhizoma Chuanxiong) 6g. Furthermore, modifications were made by adding *Dang Shen* (Radix Codonopsis) 9-12g and *Yi Yi Ren* (Semen Coicis) 12-15g for chronic illness; *Da Huang* (Radix et Rhizoma Rhei) 6-9g and *Huo Ma Ren* (Fructus Cannabis) 9-12g for difficulties with bowel movement; *Bai Jiang Cao* (Herba cum Radice Patriniae) 9-12g for deficiency heat; *Fu Zi* (Radix Aconiti Lateralis Praeparata) 3-5g for deficiency and cold; and *Da Huang* (Radix et Rhizoma Rhei), *Bai Tou Weng* (Radix Pulsatillae) and *Ma Chi Xian* (Herba Portulacae) for chronic ulcerative colitis with rectal tenesmus and mucous and blood in the stools.[9]

9. **Peptic ulcer disease**: One study reported that modified *Ge Xia Zhu Yu Tang* was effective in treating gastric or duodenal ulcer in 30 patients (24 males and 6 females, between 20-60 years of age, with 1-18 years history of illness). The herbal treatment contained *Dang Gui* (Radix Angelicae Sinensis) 10g, *Chi Shao* (Radix Paeoniae Rubra) 5g, *Wu Ling Zhi* (Faeces Trogopteri) 5g, *Chuan Xiong* (Rhizoma Chuanxiong) 4g, *Tao Ren* (Semen Persicae) 5g, *Mu Dan Pi* (Cortex Moutan) 5g, *Wu Yao* (Radix Linderae) 6g, *Yan Hu Suo* (Rhizoma Corydalis) 10g, *Gan Cao* (Radix et Rhizoma Glycyrrhizae) 8g, *Xiang Fu* (Rhizoma Cyperi) 10g, and *Zhi Qiao* (Fructus

Aurantii) 5g. After 3 months of herbal treatment in 30 patients, the study reported significant improvement in 18 cases, moderate improvement in 9 cases, and no effect in 3 cases.[10]

AUTHORS' COMMENTS

According to Dr. Chang Wei-Yen, *Ge Xia Zhu Yu Tang* can be combined with *Xue Fu Zhu Yu Tang* (Drive Out Stasis in the Mansion of Blood Decoction), *Zhe Chong Yin* (Break the Conflict Decoction), *Shui Zhi* (Hirudo), and *Yan Hu Suo* (Rhizoma Corydalis) to treat chronic blood stasis all over the body manifesting in pain and other complex, difficult-to-treat conditions.

References

1. *Zhong Yao Ming Fang Yao Li Yu Ying Yong* (Pharmacology and Applications of Famous Herbal Formulas) 1989;516-518.
2. *Xin Zhong Yi* (New Chinese Medicine) 1976;4:35.
3. *Bei Jing Zhong Yi* (Beijing Chinese Medicine) 1987;4:24.
4. *Xin Yi Yao Xue Za Zhi* (New Journal of Medicine and Herbology) 1978;9:44.
5. *Jiang Su Zhong Yi* (Jiangsu Chinese Medicine) 1997;8:21.
6. *Jiang Xi Zhong Yi Yao* (Jiangxi Chinese Medicine and Herbology) 1988;2:28.
7. *Hu Bei Zhong Yi Za Zhi* (Hubei Journal of Chinese Medicine) 1982;16(5):48.
8. *Si Chuan Zhong Yi* (Sichuan Chinese Medicine) 1998;1:36.
9. *Shan Xi Zhong Yi* (Shanxi Chinese Medicine) 1991;7(5):16.
10. *Xin Zhong Yi* (New Chinese Medicine) 1976;4:35.

888

Chinese Herbal Formulas and Applications

Shào Fù Zhú Yū Tāng
(Drive Out Blood Stasis in the Lower Abdomen Decoction)

少腹逐瘀湯
少腹逐瘀汤

Pinyin Name: *Shao Fu Zhu Yu Tang*
Literal Name: Drive Out Blood Stasis in the Lower Abdomen Decoction
Alternate Name: Fennel Seed and Corydalis Combination
Original Source: *Yi Lin Gai Cuo* (Corrections of Errors Among Physicians) by Wang Qing-Ren in 1830

COMPOSITION

Dang Gui (Radix Angelicae Sinensis)	9g
Chuan Xiong (Rhizoma Chuanxiong)	3g
Chi Shao (Radix Paeoniae Rubra)	6g
Wu Ling Zhi (Faeces Trogopteri), *chao* (dry-fried)	6g
Pu Huang (Pollen Typhae)	9g
Yan Hu Suo (Rhizoma Corydalis)	3g
Mo Yao (Myrrha)	6g
Gan Jiang (Rhizoma Zingiberis), *chao* (dry-fried)	0.6g [3g]
Xiao Hui Xiang (Fructus Foeniculi), *chao* (dry-fried)	7 pieces [1.5g]
Rou Gui (Cortex Cinnamomi)	3g

DOSAGE / PREPARATION / ADMINISTRATION

The source text states to prepare the ingredients as a decoction. Today, the decoction may be prepared using the doses suggested in brackets.

CHINESE THERAPEUTIC ACTIONS

1. Activates blood circulation and dispels blood stagnation
2. Warms and regulates menstruation to relieve pain

CLINICAL MANIFESTATIONS

Blood stagnation in the lower abdomen: pain and fullness in the lower abdominal region; formation of mass in the lower abdomen; multiple cycles of bleeding (between 3-5 times) within one period; menstrual pain, low back pain and lower abdominal fullness during the menstruation; excess menstrual bleeding that is black and/or purplish with blood clots; and *beng lou* (flooding and spotting) with lower abdominal pain.

CLINICAL APPLICATIONS

Female infertility, male infertility, amenorrhea, dysmenorrhea, painful menstruation, irregular menstruation, uterine bleeding, ectopic pregnancy, hysteromyoma, endometriosis, oophoritic cyst, ovarian cyst, pelvic inflammatory disease, hyperplastic tuberculosis of intestine, ulcerative colitis, and urinary stones.

EXPLANATION

Shao Fu Zhu Yu Tang (Drive Out Blood Stasis in the Lower Abdomen Decoction) is designed specifically for blood stagnation in the lower abdomen. It activates blood circulation to dispel blood stagnation, activates qi circulation to relieve pain, and warms the lower *jiao* to restore normal menstruation. Clinically, the patient may show pain and fullness in the lower abdominal region, menstrual pain, excess menstrual bleeding that is black and/or purplish with blood clots, and multiple cycles of bleeding (between 3-5 times) within one period.

In this formula, *Dang Gui* (Radix Angelicae Sinensis), *Chuan Xiong* (Rhizoma Chuanxiong), and *Chi Shao* (Radix Paeoniae Rubra) nourish the blood, activate blood circulation, and eliminate blood stasis. *Wu Ling Zhi* (Faeces Trogopteri) disperses blood stasis to relieve pain. *Pu Huang* (Pollen Typhae) regulates blood circulation. *Yan Hu Suo* (Rhizoma Corydalis) and *Mo Yao* (Myrrha) activate qi and blood circulation to relieve pain. *Gan Jiang* (Rhizoma Zingiberis) warms the menses and dispels cold. *Xiao Hui Xiang* (Fructus Foeniculi) and *Rou Gui* (Cortex Cinnamomi) warm the lower *jiao* to relieve pain.

MODIFICATIONS

- For amenorrhea or dysmenorrhea with blood stagnation accompanied by constipation, add *Da Huang* (Radix et Rhizoma Rhei) and *Mang Xiao* (Natrii Sulfas).

BLOOD-REGULATING FORMULAS

13

889

Shào Fù Zhú Yū Tāng
(Drive Out Blood Stasis in the Lower Abdomen Decoction)

Shao Fu Zhu Yu Tang (Drive Out Blood Stasis in the Lower Abdomen Decoction)

Diagnosis	Signs and Symptoms	Treatment	Herbs
Blood stagnation in the lower abdomen	• Pain and fullness in the lower abdominal region and formation of a mass in the lower abdomen: blood stagnation in the lower *jiao* area • Menstrual pain, multiple cycles of bleeding (between 3-5 times) within one period, excess menstrual bleeding that is black and purplish with blood clots: blood stagnation affecting menstruation	• Activates blood circulation and dispels blood stagnation • Warms and regulates menstruation to relieve pain	• *Dang Gui* (Radix Angelicae Sinensis), *Chuan Xiong* (Rhizoma Chuanxiong), and *Chi Shao* (Radix Paeoniae Rubra) nourish the blood, activate blood circulation, and eliminate blood stasis. • *Wu Ling Zhi* (Faeces Trogopteri) disperses blood stasis to relieve pain. • *Pu Huang* (Pollen Typhae) regulates blood circulation. • *Yan Hu Suo* (Rhizoma Corydalis) and *Mo Yao* (Myrrha) activate qi and blood circulation to relieve pain. • *Gan Jiang* (Rhizoma Zingiberis) warms the menses and dispels cold. • *Xiao Hui Xiang* (Fructus Foeniculi) and *Rou Gui* (Cortex Cinnamomi) warm the lower *jiao* to relieve pain.

• For infertility due to the absence of ovulation, add *Shan Yao* (Rhizoma Dioscoreae) or *Zi He Che* (Placenta Hominis).

• With early menstruation, add *Huang Qin* (Radix Scutellariae).

• With continuous and incessant menstrual bleeding due to heat, add *Huang Qin* (Radix Scutellariae) and *Huang Lian* (Rhizoma Coptidis).

• For cysts and fibroids in the lower abdominal area with pain and dark menstrual discharge, add *Hai Zao* (Sargassum), *Hai Dai* (Thallus Laminariae), *Kun Bu* (Thallus Eckloniae), *Xia Ku Cao* (Spica Prunellae), *Jin Yin Hua* (Flos Lonicerae Japonicae), *Zi Cao* (Radix Arnebiae), *Mu Li* (Concha Ostreae), *E Zhu* (Rhizoma Curcumae), *San Leng* (Rhizoma Sparganii), *Bie Jia* (Carapax Trionycis), and *Sang Ji Sheng* (Herba Taxilli).

• For chronic hepatitis, liver cirrhosis, and ascites, add *Chai Hu* (Radix Bupleuri), *Ban Lan Gen* (Radix Isatidis), *Huang Jing* (Rhizoma Polygonati), *Huang Qi* (Radix Astragali), *Gou Qi Zi* (Fructus Lycii), and *Ren Shen* (Radix et Rhizoma Ginseng).

CAUTIONS / CONTRAINDICATIONS

Shao Fu Zhu Yu Tang is contraindicated during pregnancy. Although useful for *beng lou* (flooding and spotting), this formula is **not** recommended in cases of *beng lou* with underlying qi deficiency.[1]

PHARMACOLOGICAL EFFECTS

Anti-inflammatory: According to one *in vitro* study, administration of *Shao Fu Zhu Yu Tang* at doses of 8g/kg or 16g/kg was associated with a marked anti-inflammatory effect in rats. The study noted that while *Shao Fu Zhu Yu Tang* and hydrocortisone both have marked anti-inflammatory effects, their mechanisms and side effects are quite different. The use of hydrocortisone was associated with the various side effects of the corticosteroid drugs, while *Shao Fu Zhu Yu Tang* did not have such side effects.[2]

CLINICAL STUDIES AND RESEARCH

1. **Female infertility:** According to one study, 45 of 46 patients successfully became pregnant after taking 3-5 packs of herbs per month starting at the beginning of the period, for 1-4 months. The causes of infertility included inflammation of the fallopian tubes, chronic pelvic inflammatory diseases, and anovulation. The standard herbal treatment was *Shao Fu Zhu Yu Tang*. Modifications included the addition of *Li Zhi He* (Semen Litchi), *Che Qian Zi* (Semen Plantaginis), *Jin Yin Hua* (Flos Lonicerae Japonicae), *Chuan Lian Zi* (Fructus Toosendan), *Pu Gong Ying* (Herba Taraxaci), and others specifically for inflammation of the fallopian tubes.[3] According to another study of 50 women with infertility (3-11 years) due to obstructed fallopian tubes, use of modified *Shao Fu Zhu Yu Tang* was associated with successful pregnancy in 51% of patients.[4]

Shào Fù Zhú Yū Tāng
(Drive Out Blood Stasis in the Lower Abdomen Decoction)

Chinese Herbal Formulas and Applications

2. **Male infertility**: One study reported successful treatment of male infertility in 17 of 20 patients using modified *Shao Fu Zhu Yu Tang*. The duration of treatment ranged from 20-40 days. In addition to the base formula, *Huang Jing* (Rhizoma Polygonati) was added for yang deficiency; *Fen Bi Xie* (Rhizoma Dioscoreae Hypoglaucae), *Shi Chang Pu* (Rhizoma Acori Tatarinowii), *Shi Wei* (Folium Pyrrosiae), and *Che Qian Zi* (Semen Plantaginis) were added for presence of pus in the sperm; *Huang Qi* (Radix Astragali) and *Yin Yang Huo* (Herba Epimedii) were added for poor sperm motility; and Kidney tonics for low sperm count.[5]

3. **Male infertility from sperm disorders**: Use of *Shao Fu Zhu Yu Tang* was associated with improvement in sperm mobility, quantity, and quality in 36 patients with chronic prostatitis after treatment for 60 days. The increase in sperm mobility was evaluated by computer-assisted semen analysis, and sperm quantity and quality with a high-powered intravital microscope. The mechanisms of this effect were attributed to increased sperm acrosin activity levels.[6]

4. **Ectopic pregnancy**: Use of modified *Shao Fu Zhu Yu Tang* successfully terminated pregnancy in all of 12 women with ectopic pregnancy. The herbal formula contained *Dan Shen* (Radix et Rhizoma Salviae Miltiorrhizae) 15g, dry-fried *Lai Fu Zi* (Semen Raphani) 15g, *Yi Mu Cao* (Herba Leonuri) 15g, *Chi Shao* (Radix Paeoniae Rubra) 10g, *Chuan Niu Xi* (Radix Cyathulae) 10g, *Hong Hua* (Flos Carthami) 6g, *Xiao Hui Xiang* (Fructus Foeniculi) 6g, *Tian Hua Fen* (Radix Trichosanthis) 15-30g, *Yi Yi Ren* (Semen Coicis) 20g, *Pu Huang* (Pollen Typhae) 17g, and *Gan Cao* (Radix et Rhizoma Glycyrrhizae) 5g. The treatment protocol was to cook the herbs in water, and administer the decoction in two to three equally-divided doses 1 hour before meals. In addition, anti-inflammatory drugs were given as adjunct therapy as needed. The duration of treatment ranged from 3 to 21 days.[7]

5. **Hysteromyoma**: Use of modified *Shao Fu Zhu Yu Tang* in 14 patients with hysteromyoma was associated with complete recovery in 8 cases, significant improvement in 4 cases, slight improvement in 1 case, and no effect in 1 case. The base formula was *Shao Fu Zhu Yu Tang* with the removal of *Gan Jiang* (Rhizoma Zingiberis) and *Chi Shao* (Radix Paeoniae Rubra), and addition of *Hong Hua* (Flos Carthami), *Tao Ren* (Semen Persicae), *San Leng* (Rhizoma Sparganii), *E Zhu* (Rhizoma Curcumae), *Juan Bai* (Herba Selaginellae), and *Yi Mu Cao* (Herba Leonuri). *Xiang Fu* (Rhizoma Cyperi), *Chuan Lian Zi* (Fructus Toosendan), and *Li Zhi He* (Semen Litchi) were added for severe qi stagnation; *Shui Zhi* (Hirudo), *Dan Shen* (Radix et Rhizoma Salviae Miltiorrhizae), and *Yi Mu Cao* (Herba Leonuri) were added for severe blood stagnation; and *Ba Zhen Tang* (Eight-Treasure Decoction) was given during the recovery period.[8]

6. **Endometriosis**: One study reported 97.5% effectiveness using modified *Shao Fu Zhu Yu Tang* to treat 40 women with endometriosis. For those with endometriosis characterized by cold obstruction and blood stagnation, unmodified *Shao Fu Zhu Yu Tang* was used for treatment. For those with endometriosis characterized by qi deficiency and blood stagnation, *Shao Fu Zhu Yu Tang* was modified by eliminating *Wu Ling Zhi* (Faeces Trogopteri) and adding *Huang Qi* (Radix Astragali), *Dang Shen* (Radix Codonopsis), *Sheng Ma* (Rhizoma Cimicifugae), and *Mu Xiang* (Radix Aucklandiae).[9]

7. **Oophoritic cyst**: Use of modified *Shao Fu Zhu Yu Tang* was associated with complete recovery in 46 of 50 patients. In addition to *Shao Fu Zhu Yu Tang*, modifications included the addition of *Nu Zhen Zi* (Fructus Ligustri Lucidi) and *Mo Han Lian* (Herba Ecliptae) for prolonged bleeding and increased menstrual discharge; *Huang Qi* (Radix Astragali) and *Dang Shen* (Radix Codonopsis) for qi deficiency; *Liu Wei Di Huang Wan* (Six-Ingredient Pill with Rehmannia) for yin deficiency; *San Qi* (Radix et Rhizoma Notoginseng) and *Yi Mu Cao* (Herba Leonuri) for severe abdominal pain caused by blood stagnation; and general tonic herbs when swelling and inflammation subsided. The duration of treatment ranged from 30-60 packs of herbs.[10]

8. **Dysmenorrhea**: Numerous studies have shown that *Shao Fu Zhu Yu Tang* treats dysmenorrhea. According to one study of 100 patients with dysmenorrhea characterized by cold and blood stagnation, administration of *Shao Fu Zhu Yu Tang* (starting 1 week before the period for 7-10 days) followed by *Wen Jing Tang* (Warm the Channels Decoction) (starting after the period for 2-3 months total) was associated with 100% effectiveness.[11] According to another study, use of modified *Shao Fu Zhu Yu Tang* for 1-8 packs was associated with marked success in 54 patients with dysmenorrhea. Of 46 patients who had complete recovery, no recurrences were reported within one year. Of 4 patients who had moderate improvement, no recurrences were reported within 3 months. Three had only symptomatic relief and 1 had no effect.[12]

9. **Uterine bleeding**: *Shao Fu Zhu Yu Tang* was shown to be effective in treating 32 women with uterine bleeding associated with functional disorder. In addition to this formula, modifications were made by adding *Bai Zhu* (Rhizoma Atractylodis Macrocephalae), *Dang Shen* (Radix Codonopsis), and *Huang Qi* (Radix Astragali)

BLOOD-REGULATING FORMULAS

13

Shào Fù Zhú Yū Tāng
(Drive Out Blood Stasis in the Lower Abdomen Decoction)

for qi deficiency; *Mu Dan Pi* (Cortex Moutan), *Ce Bai Ye* (Cacumen Platycladi), and *Di Huang* (Radix Rehmanniae) for heat in the blood; *Shu Di Huang* (Radix Rehmanniae Praeparata), *Xu Duan* (Radix Dipsaci), and *Tu Si Zi* (Semen Cuscutae) for Kidney deficiency. The treatment protocol was to administer the herbs in decoction starting on the first day of the period, for a total of 4 packs of herbs.[13]

10. **Pelvic inflammatory disease**: Forty-two women with pelvic inflammatory disease due to various causes (ligation, abortion, miscarriage, etc.) were treated with complete recovery in 26 cases, marked improvement in 9 cases, slight improvement in 4 cases, and no effect in 3 cases. The overall effectiveness was 92%. The herbal treatment contained *Shao Fu Zhu Yu Tang*, minus *Gan Jiang* (Rhizoma Zingiberis), plus *Bai Jiang Cao* (Herba cum Radice Patriniae) and *Huang Qi* (Radix Astragali). *Pu Gong Ying* (Herba Taraxaci), *Huang Bo* (Cortex Phellodendri Chinensis) and liquor-processed *Da Huang* (Radix et Rhizoma Rhei) were added for damp-heat; *Wu Zhu Yu* (Fructus Evodiae), *Wu Yao* (Radix Linderae), *Gan Jiang* (Rhizoma Zingiberis), and larger doses of *Xiao Hui Xiang* (Fructus Foeniculi) and *Rou Gui* (Cortex Cinnamomi) for qi stagnation with cold; and *San Leng* (Rhizoma Sparganii), and *E Zhu* (Rhizoma Curcumae) for qi and blood stagnation.[14]

11. **Hyperplastic tuberculosis of the intestine**: One study reported complete recovery in 70 of 76 patients with hyperplastic tuberculosis of the intestine using modified *Shao Fu Zhu Yu Tang*. The base formula contained *Shao Fu Zhu Yu Tang* plus *Bie Jia* (Carapax Trionycis) and *Gui Ban* (Plastrum Testudinis). Additional modifications were made as follows: *Huang Qi* (Radix Astragali) and *Dang Shen* (Radix Codonopsis) for qi deficiency; *Huo Ma Ren* (Fructus Cannabis) and *Rou Cong Rong* (Herba Cistanches) for yin deficiency and constipation; *Yin Chai Hu* (Radix Stellariae), *Zhi Mu* (Rhizoma Anemarrhenae), and *Mu Li* (Concha Ostreae) for tidal fever and night perspiration; *Bu Gu Zhi* (Fructus Psoraleae), *Rou Dou Kou* (Semen Myristicae), *Wu Wei Zi* (Fructus Schisandrae Chinensis), and *Wu Zhu Yu* (Fructus Evodiae) for "5 a.m. diarrhea;" *Lai Fu Zi* (Semen Raphani), *Hou Po* (Cortex Magnoliae Officinalis), and *Bing Lang* (Semen Arecae) for abdominal distention; *Ban Xia* (Rhizoma Pinelliae) and *Zhe Shi* (Haematitum) for severe nausea and vomiting; and *Cang Zhu* (Rhizoma Atractylodis) for dampness.[15]

12. **Ulcerative colitis**: One study reported 88.7% effectiveness using modified *Shao Fu Zhu Yu Tang* to treat 44 patients with ulcerative colitis.[16]

13. **Urinary stones**: One-hundred patients with urinary stones (16 in the kidneys, 81 in the ureters, and 3 in the bladder) treated with modified *Shao Fu Zhu Yu Tang* showed complete recovery in 65 cases, marked improvement in 22 cases, and no benefit in 13 cases. The overall effectiveness was 87%. In addition to the base formula, the herbal treatment was modified as follows: *Bai Shao* (Radix Paeoniae Alba) and *Gan Cao* (Radix et Rhizoma Glycyrrhizae) for soreness and pain of the lower back; *Bai Mao Gen* (Rhizoma Imperatae) and *Hu Po* (Succinum) for hematuria; *Huang Qi* (Radix Astragali) and *Dang Shen* (Radix Codonopsis) for qi deficiency; *Di Huang* (Radix Rehmanniae) and *Mo Han Lian* (Herba Ecliptae) for yin deficiency; *Jin Qian Cao* (Herba Lysimachiae) and *Shi Wei* (Folium Pyrrosiae) for painful urination; and removal of *Gan Jiang* (Rhizoma Zingiberis) and *Gui Zhi* (Ramulus Cinnamomi) for damp-heat.[17]

References

1. *Zhong Yao Ming Fang Yao Li Yu Ying Yong* (Pharmacology and Applications of Famous Herbal Formulas) 1989;461-463.
2. *Zhong Yao Yao Li Yu Lin Chuang* (Pharmacology and Clinical Applications of Chinese Herbs) 1987;37.
3. *Zhong Yi Za Zhi* (Journal of Chinese Medicine) 1985;1:36.
4. *Hu Nan Yi Yao Za Zhi* (Hunan Journal of Medicine and Herbology) 1983;3:52.
5. *He Nan Zhong Yi* (Henan Chinese Medicine) 1985;3:29.
6. Yang CC, Chen JC, Chen GW, Chen YS, Chung JG. Effects of Shao-Fu-Zhu-Yu-Tang on motility of human sperm. American Journal of Chinese Medicine 2003;31(4):573-9.
7. *Hu Bei Zhong Yi Za Zhi* (Hubei Journal of Chinese Medicine) 1991;7(5)17.
8. *Bei Jing Zhong Yi* (Beijing Chinese Medicine) 1987;5:34.
9. *Zhong Xi Yi Jie He Za Zhi* (Journal of Integrated Chinese and Western Medicine) 1988;10:639.
10. *Xin Zhong Yi* (New Chinese Medicine) 1995;8:40.
11. *He Nan Zhong Yi* (Henan Chinese Medicine) 1981;9:39.
12. *Zhe Jiang Zhong Yi Za Zhi* (Zhejiang Journal of Chinese Medicine) 1964;11:17.
13. *Shi Yong Zhong Xi Yi Jie He Za Zhi* (Practical Journal of Integrated Chinese and Western Medicines) 1993;6(6):380.
14. *Hu Bei Zhong Yi Za Zhi* (Hubei Journal of Chinese Medicine) 1993;15(3):23.
15. *Zhe Jiang Zhong Yi Za Zhi* (Zhejiang Journal of Chinese Medicine) 1989;1:9.
16. *Zhong Yi Yao Xin Xi* (Information on Chinese Medicine and Herbology) 1990;7(6):37.
17. *Zhong Xi Yi Jie He Za Zhi* (Journal of Integrated Chinese and Western Medicine) 1985;5:271.

Chinese Herbal Formulas and Applications

Shēn Tòng Zhú Yū Tāng
(Drive Out Blood Stasis from a Painful Body Decoction)

身痛逐瘀湯
身痛逐瘀汤

Pinyin Name: *Shen Tong Zhu Yu Tang*
Literal Name: Drive Out Blood Stasis from a Painful Body Decoction
Alternate Name: Cnidium and Notopterygium Combination
Original Source: *Yi Lin Gai Cuo* (Corrections of Errors Among Physicians) by Wang Qing-Ren in 1830

COMPOSITION

Tao Ren (Semen Persicae)	9g
Hong Hua (Flos Carthami)	9g
Dang Gui (Radix Angelicae Sinensis)	9g
Chuan Xiong (Rhizoma Chuanxiong)	6g
Mo Yao (Myrrha)	6g
Wu Ling Zhi (Faeces Trogopteri), *chao* (dry-fried)	6g
Di Long (Pheretima)	6g
Qin Jiao (Radix Gentianae Macrophyllae)	3g
Qiang Huo (Rhizoma et Radix Notopterygii)	3g
Xiang Fu (Rhizoma Cyperi)	3g
Niu Xi (Radix Achyranthis Bidentatae)	9g
Gan Cao (Radix et Rhizoma Glycyrrhizae)	6g

DOSAGE / PREPARATION / ADMINISTRATION
Prepare as a decoction.

CHINESE THERAPEUTIC ACTIONS
1. Activates qi and blood circulation
2. Dispels blood stagnation and opens the channels and collaterals
3. Unblocks *bi zheng* (painful obstruction syndrome) and relieves pain

CLINICAL MANIFESTATIONS
Pain due to qi and blood stagnation blocking the channels and collaterals: pain in the shoulder, elbow, waist and/or leg; and persistent, generalized pain throughout the whole body that does not respond to treatment.

CLINICAL APPLICATIONS
Arthritis, rheumatoid arthritis, sciatica, pain in the lower back and legs, lumbago, neuralgia, hyperosteogeny, and allergic purpura.

EXPLANATION
Shen Tong Zhu Yu Tang (Drive Out Blood Stasis from a Painful Body Decoction) activates qi and blood circulation, dispels blood stagnation, opens the channels and collaterals, and relieves pain. Clinically, it is often used for pain due to stagnation of qi and blood. Pain may be located in the shoulder, elbow, waist, leg, or throughout the whole body.

In this formula, *Tao Ren* (Semen Persicae) and *Hong Hua* (Flos Carthami) activate blood circulation and eliminate blood stasis. *Dang Gui* (Radix Angelicae Sinensis) and *Chuan Xiong* (Rhizoma Chuanxiong) nourish the blood and promote blood circulation. *Mo Yao* (Myrrha) relieves pain by invigorating blood circulation. *Wu Ling Zhi* (Faeces Trogopteri) and *Di Long* (Pheretima) dispel blood stasis and open the channels and collaterals. *Qin Jiao* (Radix Gentianae Macrophyllae) and *Qiang Huo* (Rhizoma et Radix Notopterygii) dispel wind-dampness to relieve pain. *Xiang Fu* (Rhizoma Cyperi) activates qi to relieve pain. *Niu Xi* (Radix Achyranthis Bidentatae) strengthens bones, tendons, and soft tissues. *Gan Cao* (Radix et Rhizoma Glycyrrhizae) harmonizes the herbs in the formula.

MODIFICATIONS
- With pain in the upper body, add *Ge Gen* (Radix Puerariae Lobatae).
- With pain the lower body, add *Du Huo* (Radix Angelicae Pubescentis).
- With pain in the extremities, add *Sang Zhi* (Ramulus Mori) and *Gui Zhi* (Ramulus Cinnamomi).

BLOOD-REGULATING FORMULAS

13

893

Chapter 13 – Blood-Regulating Formulas　　　　*Section 1 – Blood-Invigorating and Stasis-Removing Formulas*

Shēn Tòng Zhú Yū Tāng
(Drive Out Blood Stasis from a Painful Body Decoction)

Shen Tong Zhu Yu Tang (Drive Out Blood Stasis from a Painful Body Decoction)

Diagnosis	Signs and Symptoms	Treatment	Herbs
Pain due to qi and blood stagnation	Pain in the shoulder, elbow, waist, leg and/or the whole body: qi and blood stagnation blocking the channels and collaterals	• Activates qi and blood circulation • Dispels blood stagnation and opens the channels and collaterals • Unblocks *bi zheng* (painful obstruction syndrome) and relieves pain	• *Tao Ren* (Semen Persicae) and *Hong Hua* (Flos Carthami) activate blood circulation and eliminate blood stasis. • *Dang Gui* (Radix Angelicae Sinensis) and *Chuan Xiong* (Rhizoma Chuanxiong) nourish the blood and promote blood circulation. • *Mo Yao* (Myrrha) invigorates blood circulation and relieves pain. • *Wu Ling Zhi* (Faeces Trogopteri) and *Di Long* (Pheretima) dispel blood stasis and open the channels and collaterals. • *Qin Jiao* (Radix Gentianae Macrophyllae) and *Qiang Huo* (Rhizoma et Radix Notopterygii) dispel wind-dampness to relieve pain. • *Xiang Fu* (Rhizoma Cyperi) activates qi circulation to relieve pain. • *Niu Xi* (Radix Achyranthis Bidentatae) strengthens bones, tendons, and soft tissues. • *Gan Cao* (Radix et Rhizoma Glycyrrhizae) harmonizes the herbs.

CAUTIONS / CONTRAINDICATIONS

Use of *Shen Tong Zhu Yu Tang* is contraindicated during pregnancy.[1]

PHARMACOLOGICAL EFFECTS

Analgesic and anti-inflammatory: According to *in vitro* studies, administration of *Shen Tong Zhu Yu Tang* in tincture form was effective in relieving pain and reducing inflammation.[2]

CLINICAL STUDIES AND RESEARCH

1. *Bizheng* (painful obstruction syndrome): Administration of *Shen Tong Zhu Yu Tang* in 32 patients with *bi zheng* (painful obstruction syndrome) was associated with complete recovery in 12 cases, significant improvement in 10 cases, moderate improvement in 7 cases, and no improvement in 3 cases. The overall effectiveness was 90.6%. The herbal formula used *Shen Tong Zhu Yu Tang* as the base, with the addition of *Huang Qi* (Radix Astragali) and *Dang Shen* (Radix Codonopsis) for qi deficiency; *Fang Feng* (Radix Saposhnikoviae) and *Wei Ling Xian* (Radix et Rhizoma Clematidis) for wind; *Zhi Chuan Wu* (Radix Aconiti Praeparata) and *Xi Xin* (Radix et Rhizoma Asari) for cold; *Fu Ling* (Poria) and *Yi Yi Ren* (Semen Coicis) for damp; *Gui Zhi* (Ramulus Cinnamomi) and *Sang Zhi*

(Ramulus Mori) for pain in the upper limbs; *Sang Ji Sheng* (Herba Taxilli), *Xu Duan* (Radix Dipsaci), and *Gou Ji* (Rhizoma Cibotii) for pain in the lower limbs; *Ge Gen* (Radix Puerariae Lobatae) for pain in the neck; and *Feng Fang* (Nidus Vespae), *Wu Shao She* (Zaocys), *Quan Xie* (Scorpio), and dry-fried *Chuan Shan Jia* (Squama Manis) for stiff joints with deformation. For *re bi* (heat painful obstruction), *Jin Yin Hua* (Flos Lonicerae Japonicae), *Cang Zhu* (Rhizoma Atractylodis), and *Huang Bo* (Cortex Phellodendri Chinensis) were added, and *Qin Jiao* (Radix Gentianae Macrophyllae), *Qiang Huo* (Rhizoma et Radix Notopterygii), and *Chuan Xiong* (Rhizoma Chuanxiong) were removed. For *shi-re bi* (damp-heat painful obstruction), *Huang Lian* (Rhizoma Coptidis), *Jin Yin Hua* (Flos Lonicerae Japonicae), and *Yu Jin* (Radix Curcumae) were added, and *Niu Xi* (Radix Achyranthis Bidentatae), *Qin Jiao* (Radix Gentianae Macrophyllae), *Qiang Huo* (Rhizoma et Radix Notopterygii), and *Chuan Xiong* (Rhizoma Chuanxiong) were removed.[3]

2. **Arthritis**: Use of modified *Shen Tong Zhu Yu Tang* in 67 patients with arthritis was associated with complete recovery in 50 patients, significant improvement in 14 cases, and no effect in 3 cases. Modifications included the addition of *Fu Zi* (Radix Aconiti Lateralis Praeparata), *Xi Xin* (Radix et Rhizoma Asari), and *Wei Ling Xian*

Shēn Tòng Zhú Yū Tāng
(Drive Out Blood Stasis from a Painful Body Decoction)

(Radix et Rhizoma Clematidis) for arthritis due to cold; *Ren Dong Teng* (Caulis Lonicerae Japonicae), *Shi Gao* (Gypsum Fibrosum), *Huang Bo* (Cortex Phellodendri Chinensis), and *Yi Yi Ren* (Semen Coicis), and removal of *Qiang Huo* (Rhizoma et Radix Notopterygii), for arthritis due to heat; *Bai Shao* (Radix Paeoniae Alba) for stiffness of the tendons and ligaments; and *Jin Qian Bai Hua She* (Bungarus Parvus) and *Wu Shao She* (Zaocys) for "mobile" arthritis that affects multiple joints.[4]

3. **Rheumatoid arthritis**: One study of 46 patients with rheumatoid arthritis reported marked success using modified *Shen Tong Zhu Yu Tang*. Of 46 patients, the study reported recovery in 12 cases, improvement in 25 cases, slight improvement in 7 cases, and no effect in 2 cases. The duration of treatment was 2 months per course of treatment, for 3 courses total. The study also noted that the effect of the herbs was comparable to or better than that in the control group that received aspirin. The herbal formula contained *Shen Tong Zhu Yu Tang* as the base formula, and added *Gui Zhi* (Ramulus Cinnamomi), *Fang Feng* (Radix Saposhnikoviae), and *Wei Ling Xian* (Radix et Rhizoma Clematidis) for wind-dampness; *Gui Zhi* (Ramulus Cinnamomi), *Gan Jiang* (Rhizoma Zingiberis), and *Fu Ling* (Poria) for damp-cold; addition of *Cang Zhu* (Rhizoma Atractylodis), *Huang Bo* (Cortex Phellodendri Chinensis), and *Fang Feng* (Radix Saposhnikoviae), and removal of *Qiang Huo* (Rhizoma et Radix Notopterygii), for damp-heat; the addition of *Di Huang* (Radix Rehmanniae), *Gou Qi Zi* (Fructus Lycii), and *Nu Zhen Zi* (Fructus Ligustri Lucidi), and removal of *Qiang Huo* (Rhizoma et Radix Notopterygii) and *Qin Jiao* (Radix Gentianae Macrophyllae), for Kidney yin deficiency; and the addition of *Rou Gui* (Cortex Cinnamomi) and *Shan Zhu Yu* (Fructus Corni), and removal of *Qiang Huo* (Rhizoma et Radix Notopterygii) and *Qin Jiao* (Radix Gentianae Macrophyllae), for Kidney yang deficiency.[5]

4. **Sciatica**: Administration of *Shen Tong Zhu Yu Tang* for 7-45 days (average of 17.4 days) in 36 patients with sciatica was associated with complete recovery in 29 cases, significant improvement in 6 cases, and no effect in 1 case. The overall effectiveness was 97.2%. Furthermore, of 24 patients who returned for follow-up one year later, only 1 had recurrence.[6]

5. **Pain in the lower back and legs**: Administration of *Shen Tong Zhu Yu Tang* has been shown in 2 studies to effectively treat pain in the lower back and legs. Of 67 patients, the first study reported complete recovery in 53 cases, improvement in 9 cases, and no effect in 5 cases.[7] Of 52 patients in the second study, 12 had complete recovery, 26 had significant improvement, 9 had moderate improvement, and 5 had no effect.[8]

6. **Lumbago**: One study reported good results using modified *Shen Tong Zhu Yu Tang* to treat acute low back pain. Modifications included the addition of *Dang Shen* (Radix Codonopsis) and *Huang Qi* (Radix Astragali) for qi deficiency; and *Yan Hu Suo* (Rhizoma Corydalis) and *Qi Ye Lian* (Radix Schefflerae) for severe pain. The herbal treatment also was applied topically to the affected area. Of 15 patients, the study reported complete recovery in 8 cases, significant improvement in 3 cases, moderate improvement in 3 cases, and no benefit in 1 case.[9]

7. **Hyperosteogeny**: Hyperosteogeny of the lumbar spine was treated with modified *Shen Tong Zhu Yu Tang* with good results. Of 25 patients, the study reported complete relief in 18 cases, significant relief in 4 cases, and no effect in 3 cases.[10]

8. **Allergic purpura**: Use of modified *Shen Tong Zhu Yu Tang* for treatment of allergic purpura was associated with marked success in 30 patients (between 11-59 years of age with 2 days to 3 years history of illness). The herbal treatment contained *Dang Gui* (Radix Angelicae Sinensis) 15g, *Hong Hua* (Flos Carthami) 12g, *Mo Yao* (Myrrha) 12g, *Wu Ling Zhi* (Faeces Trogopteri) 12g, *Xiang Fu* (Rhizoma Cyperi) 12g, *Chuan Xiong* (Rhizoma Chuanxiong) 10g, *Tao Ren* (Semen Persicae) 10g, *Niu Xi* (Radix Achyranthis Bidentatae) 9g, *Qin Jiao* (Radix Gentianae Macrophyllae) 9g, *Di Long* (Pheretima) 9g, *Qiang Huo* (Rhizoma et Radix Notopterygii) 9g, and *Gan Cao* (Radix et Rhizoma Glycyrrhizae) 6g. Other modifications were made as needed based on the condition of the individual patients. The herbs were given in decoction daily for 5-32 days duration. Of 30 patients, the study reported complete recovery in 26 cases, significant improvement in 3 cases, and no benefit in one case.[11]

RELATED FORMULA

Zhú Yū Tāng (Drive Out Blood Stasis Decoction)

逐瘀湯
逐瘀汤

Pinyin Name: *Zhu Yu Tang*

Literal Name: Drive Out Blood Stasis Decoction

Original Source: *Jian Tai Zhen Suo Fang* (Herbal Prescriptions from *Jiantai* Clinic) by Chang Wei-Yen in 1981

Tao Ren (Semen Persicae)
Hong Hua (Flos Carthami)
San Leng (Rhizoma Sparganii)
E Zhu (Rhizoma Curcumae)
Chuan Xiong (Rhizoma Chuanxiong)

Chapter 13 – Blood-Regulating Formulas　　　　*Section 1 – Blood-Invigorating and Stasis-Removing Formulas*

Shēn Tòng Zhú Yū Tāng
(Drive Out Blood Stasis from a Painful Body Decoction)

Dan Shen (Radix et Rhizoma Salviae Miltiorrhizae)
Dang Gui (Radix Angelicae Sinensis)
Bai Shao (Radix Paeoniae Alba)
Fu Ling (Poria)
Er Cha (Catechu)
Ji Xue Teng (Caulis Spatholobi)
Xue Jie (Sanguis Draconis)
Gui Zhi (Ramulus Cinnamomi)
Sang Zhi (Ramulus Mori)
Sheng Ma (Rhizoma Cimicifugae)
Ding Xiang (Flos Caryophylli)
Qiang Huo (Rhizoma et Radix Notopterygii)
Qing Pi (Pericarpium Citri Reticulatae Viride)
Xiang Fu (Rhizoma Cyperi)
Gao Liang Jiang (Rhizoma Alpiniae Officinarum)
Lu Lu Tong (Fructus Liquidambaris)
Qin Jiao (Radix Gentianae Macrophyllae)
Yan Hu Suo (Rhizoma Corydalis)
Mu Dan Pi (Cortex Moutan)
Chuan Niu Xi (Radix Cyathulae)
Da Huang (Radix et Rhizoma Rhei)
Lian Zi (Semen Nelumbinis)
Da Zao (Fructus Jujubae)
Gan Cao (Radix et Rhizoma Glycyrrhizae)

Zhu Yu Tang (Drive Out Blood Stasis Decoction) is designed to treat pain in the extremities due to blood

stagnation. It is formulated based on the principles and ingredients of three classic formulas: *Shen Tong Zhu Yu Tang* (Drive Out Blood Stasis from a Painful Body Decoction) to eliminate blood stasis from the extremities; *Dang Gui Si Ni Tang* (Tangkuei Decoction for Frigid Extremities) to warm the channels and disperse cold; and *Zheng Gu Zi Jin Dan* (Purple and Gold Pill for Righteous Bones) to activate blood circulation and dispel blood stasis. Clinical applications include peripheral neuropathy, polyneuropathy, diabetic neuropathy, distal polyneuropathy, and neuralgia.

References

1. *Zhong Yao Ming Fang Yao Li Yu Ying Yong* (Pharmacology and Applications of Famous Herbal Formulas) 1989;466-468.
2. *Zhong Yao Yan Jiu* (Research of Chinese Herbology) 1993;6(4):15.
3. *Xin Zhong Yi* (New Chinese Medicine) 1995;9:42.
4. *Yun Nan Zhong Yao Zhi* (Yunan Journal of Chinese Herbal Medicine) 1989;3:46.
5. *Bei Jing Zhong Yi Za Zhi* (Beijing Journal of Chinese Medicine) 1988;6:35.
6. *Si Chuan Zhong Yi* (Sichuan Chinese Medicine) 1985;11:50.
7. *Hu Nan Zhong Yi Za Zhi* (Hunan Journal of Chinese Medicine) 1987;1:12.
8. *Zhe Jiang Zhong Yi Za Zhi* (Zhejiang Journal of Chinese Medicine) 1987;10:452.
9. *Guang Xi Zhong Yi Yao* (Guangxi Chinese Medicine and Herbology) 1987;2:47.
10. *Gan Su Zhong Yi* (Gansu Chinese Medicine) 1993;9:46.
11. *Bei Jing Zhong Yi* (Beijing Chinese Medicine) 1995;4:43.

Chinese Herbal Formulas and Applications

Fù Yuán Huó Xuè Tāng
(Revive Health by Invigorating the Blood Decoction)

復元活血湯
复元活血汤

Pinyin Name: *Fu Yuan Huo Xue Tang*
Literal Name: Revive Health by Invigorating the Blood Decoction
Alternate Names: *Shang Ke Fu Yuan Huo Xue Tang* (Revive Health by Invigorating the Blood Decoction from the Trauma Department), *Fu Yuan Huo Hsieh Tang, Fu Yuan Huo Xieh Tang*, Recovery and Blood Activating Decoction, Recovery Blood Activating Decoction, Tangkuei and Persica Combination
Original Source: *Yi Xue Fa Ming* (Medical Innovations) by Li Gao during the Jin Dynasty

COMPOSITION

Da Huang (Radix et Rhizoma Rhei), *jin* (soaked) in liquor	30g
Chai Hu (Radix Bupleuri)	15g
Dang Gui (Radix Angelicae Sinensis)	9g
Tao Ren (Semen Persicae), *jin* (soaked) in liquor and *yan* (ground) till muddy	50 pieces [9g]
Hong Hua (Flos Carthami)	6g
Tian Hua Fen (Radix Trichosanthis)	9g
Chuan Shan Jia (Squama Manis), *pao* (blast-fried)	6g
Gan Cao (Radix et Rhizoma Glycyrrhizae)	6g

DOSAGE / PREPARATION / ADMINISTRATION

Grind all of the ingredients into a coarse powder except for *Tao Ren* (Semen Persicae), which should be ground until muddy. Cook 30g of the herbs in 1.5 bowls of water and 0.5 bowl of grain-based liquor until the liquid is reduced to 70%. Take the warm, strained decoction before meals. Discontinue the formula once the pain is relieved.

CHINESE THERAPEUTIC ACTIONS

1. Activates blood circulation and dispels blood stasis
2. Soothes the Liver and opens the channels and collaterals

CLINICAL MANIFESTATIONS

Traumatic injuries with stagnation of qi and blood: traumatic or sports injuries, pain and swelling in the chest and hypochondriac region, musculoskeletal or soft tissue injuries, and severe, excruciating pain.

CLINICAL APPLICATIONS

Traumatic injuries, musculoskeletal or soft tissue injuries, concussion, scapulocostal syndrome, bone fractures, hepatic abscess, hypochondriac pain, costal chondritis, intercostal neuralgia, hyperplasia of mammary glands, ocular hemorrhage, asthma, and intestinal adhesion.

EXPLANATION

Fu Yuan Huo Xue Tang (Revive Health by Invigorating the Blood Decoction) was originally designed to treat traumatic and external injuries with blood stasis under the

hypochondrium. All traumatic and external injuries are characterized in part by qi and blood stagnation, regardless of the severity or area of injury. When there is an injury, the blood leaves the vessels and forms obstruction along the channels and collaterals. These obstructions block the smooth flow of qi, induce pain and numbness, and cause local swelling and inflammation. Moreover, since the Liver is the organ that stores blood, stagnation of blood in the peripheral parts of the body affects the normal functions of the Liver. If Liver qi becomes stagnant, the patient may experience hypochondriac pain and fullness. Although this formula is designed to treat injuries to the chest and hypochondriac regions, it is also effective for various other types of injuries.

In this formula, *Da Huang* (Radix et Rhizoma Rhei) drains heat and blood stasis to reduce pain and swelling. *Chai Hu* (Radix Bupleuri) smoothes Liver qi stagnation and relieves hypochondriac fullness and pain. It also guides *Da Huang* (Radix et Rhizoma Rhei) to the hypochondriac region to enhance its effect. *Dang Gui* (Radix Angelicae Sinensis), *Tao Ren* (Semen Persicae) and *Hong Hua* (Flos Carthami) activate blood circulation, remove blood stasis, reduce swelling and relieve pain. These herbs have a synergistic effect and are frequently used together. *Tian Hua Fen* (Radix Trichosanthis) clears heat and reduces swelling. It also promotes the generation of muscle tissues. *Chuan Shan Jia* (Squama Manis) is one of the most effective herbs for breaking up blood stasis and opening

BLOOD-REGULATING FORMULAS

13

897

Chapter 13 – Blood-Regulating Formulas　　　*Section 1 – Blood-Invigorating and Stasis-Removing Formulas*

Fù Yuán Huó Xuè Tāng
(Revive Health by Invigorating the Blood Decoction)

Fu Yuan Huo Xue Tang (Revive Health by Invigorating the Blood Decoction)

Diagnosis	Signs and Symptoms	Treatment	Herbs
Traumatic injuries with stagnation of qi and blood	• Swelling, inflammation, numbness, and pain: qi stagnation from traumatic injuries • Severe pain and bruises: blood stagnation from traumatic injuries • Chest and hypochondriac pain: Liver qi stagnation	• Activates blood circulation and dispels blood stasis • Soothes the Liver and opens the channels and collaterals	• *Da Huang* (Radix et Rhizoma Rhei) drains heat and blood stasis to reduce pain and swelling. • *Chai Hu* (Radix Bupleuri) regulates qi circulation and smoothes Liver qi stagnation. • *Dang Gui* (Radix Angelicae Sinensis), *Tao Ren* (Semen Persicae) and *Hong Hua* (Flos Carthami) activate blood circulation, remove blood stasis, reduce swelling and relieve pain. • *Tian Hua Fen* (Radix Trichosanthis) clears heat, reduces swelling, and promotes the generation of muscle tissue. • *Chuan Shan Jia* (Squama Manis) breaks up blood stasis and opens the channels and collaterals. • *Gan Cao* (Radix et Rhizoma Glycyrrhizae) relieves spasms and cramps, and harmonizes the herbs.

the channels and collaterals. Lastly, *Gan Cao* (Radix et Rhizoma Glycyrrhizae) not only relieves muscle spasms and cramps, but also harmonizes all of the herbs.

MODIFICATIONS

• With more qi stagnation, add *Mu Xiang* (Radix Aucklandiae), *Xiang Fu* (Rhizoma Cyperi), *Qing Pi* (Pericarpium Citri Reticulatae Viride), and *Zhi Qiao* (Fructus Aurantii).

• With more severe blood stasis, add *San Qi* (Radix et Rhizoma Notoginseng), *Ru Xiang* (Gummi Olibanum), and *Mo Yao* (Myrrha).

• With severe pain, add *Yan Hu Suo* (Rhizoma Corydalis).

• With insomnia, add *Yuan Zhi* (Radix Polygalae) and *Suan Zao Ren* (Semen Ziziphi Spinosae).

• With distention and pain in the chest and hypochondriac region, add *Qing Pi* (Pericarpium Citri Reticulatae Viride) and *Chuan Lian Zi* (Fructus Toosendan).

• With abdominal distention, add *Hou Po* (Cortex Magnoliae Officinalis) and *Zhi Qiao* (Fructus Aurantii).

• With upper back pain, add *Gui Zhi* (Ramulus Cinnamomi) and *Jiang Huang* (Rhizoma Curcumae Longae).

• With pain in the lower extremities, add *Chuan Niu Xi* (Radix Cyathulae) and *Mu Gua* (Fructus Chaenomelis).

CAUTIONS / CONTRAINDICATIONS

• *Fu Yuan Huo Xue Tang* is contraindicated during pregnancy, and in weak and deficient patients.

• This formula should be used with caution in patients with Spleen qi deficiency, as this formula may cause loose stools or diarrhea.

CLINICAL STUDIES AND RESEARCH

1. **Hepatic abscess**: Thirty-eight patients with hepatic abscess were divided into 5 diagnostic groups and treated accordingly with modified *Fu Yuan Huo Xue Tang*. Those diagnosed with liver abscess with qi and blood stagnation were treated with this formula without modification. Those with damp-heat in the Liver and Gallbladder accompanied by blood stagnation received this formula plus 10g each of *Long Dan* (Radix et Rhizoma Gentianae), *Chai Hu* (Radix Bupleuri), *Huang Qin* (Radix Scutellariae), *Zhi Zi* (Fructus Gardeniae), *Che Qian Zi* (Semen Plantaginis), *Mu Tong* (Caulis Akebiae), *Lian Qiao* (Fructus Forsythiae), *Shi Chang Pu* (Rhizoma Acori Tatarinowii), *Bai Bian Dou* (Semen Lablab Album), and *Huo Xiang* (Herba Agastaches). Those diagnosed with heat and toxins accompanied by qi and blood stagnation received this formula plus 15g each of *Ye Ju Hua* (Flos Chrysanthemi Indici), *Jin Yin Hua* (Flos Lonicerae Japonicae), *Zi Hua Di Ding* (Herba Violae), *Tu Fu Ling* (Rhizoma Smilacis Glabrae), *Pu Gong Ying* (Herba Taraxaci), and 10g of *Huang Qin* (Radix Scutellariae). Those diagnosed with cold accompanied by obstruction of the channels and collaterals received this formula plus 10g each of *Fu Zi* (Radix Aconiti Lateralis Praeparata), *Chuan Xiong* (Rhizoma Chuanxiong), and *Xiang Fu* (Rhizoma Cyperi), and 12g each of *Yi Yi Ren* (Semen Coicis), *Bai Jiang Cao* (Herba cum Radice Patriniae), and *Zao Jiao* (Fructus Gleditsiae). Lastly, those diagnosed with *zheng* (upright) *qi* deficiency with stagnation and toxins received this formula plus *Bai Zhu* (Rhizoma Atractylodis Macrocephalae) 10g, *Chuan Xiong* (Rhizoma

898

Fù Yuán Huó Xuè Tāng
(Revive Health by Invigorating the Blood Decoction)

Chuanxiong) 10g, *Shu Di Huang* (Radix Rehmanniae Praeparata) 12g, *Bai Shao* (Radix Paeoniae Alba) 12g, *Dang Shen* (Radix Codonopsis) 15g, and *Fu Ling* (Poria) 15g. The treatment protocol was to administer the herbs in decoction daily, with the duration of treatment ranging from 13-145 days (average of 34.7 days). Of 38 patients, the study reported complete recovery in 14 cases, near-complete recovery in 17 cases, and moderate improvement in 7 cases.[1]

2. **Hypochondriac pain**: Use of modified *Fu Yuan Huo Xue Tang* in 82 patients with hypochondriac pain characterized by Liver and blood stagnation was associated with remission in 25 cases, near-remission in 40 cases, improvement in 8 cases, and no effect in 9 cases.[2]

3. **Costal chondritis**: One study reported marked effectiveness using modified *Fu Yuan Huo Xue Tang* in treating 100 patients with costal chondritis with a history of illness between 15 days to 3.5 years. The herbs were given in decoction daily, for an average duration of 65 days of treatment.[3]

4. **Ocular hemorrhage**: One study reported 95.2% effectiveness using modified *Fu Yuan Huo Xue Tang* to treat 21 cases of internal eye bleeding associated with external trauma. The average duration of treatment was 6 days.[4]

5. ***Xiong bi*** **(painful obstruction of the chest)**: One study reported 82% effectiveness using *Fu Yuan Huo Xue Tang* to treat *xiong bi* (painful obstruction of the chest) in 48 patients. In addition to the original formula, the treatment was modified by adding *Yu Jin* (Radix Curcumae) and *Ge Gen* (Radix Puerariae Lobatae) for feeling of chest oppression and shortness of breath; *Gua Lou* (Fructus Trichosanthis) and *Zhi Zi* (Fructus Gardeniae) for irritability and dry mouth; *Yan Hu Suo* (Rhizoma Corydalis), *Xiang Fu* (Rhizoma Cyperi), and *Jiang Xiang* (Lignum Dalbergiae Odoriferae) for severe chest pain; *Dou Kou* (Fructus Amomi Rotundus) and *Shan Zha* (Fructus Crataegi) for food stagnation and poor appetite; *Fu Ling* (Poria), *Di Long* (Pheretima), and *Sheng Jiang* (Rhizoma Zingiberis Recens) for palpitations accompanied by edema in the lower legs; and *Fu Zi* (Radix Aconiti Lateralis Praeparata), *Gui Zhi* (Ramulus Cinnamomi), and *Ren Shen* (Radix et Rhizoma Ginseng) for perspiration accompanied by cold extremities.[5]

6. **Scapulocostal syndrome**: Use of *Fu Yuan Huo Xue Tang* was effective in treating 280 patients with stiffness and pain in the shoulder and scapula regions.[6]

7. **Bone fractures**: Concurrent use of *Fu Yuan Huo Xue Tang* plus *Qi Li San* (Seven-Thousandths of a Tael Powder) within the first 2 weeks of injury was shown to have a marked effect in reducing swelling and relieving pain in over 10,000 patients with bone fractures.[7]

8. **Concussion**: Use of modified *Fu Yuan Huo Xue Tang* was associated with 100% effectiveness in treating 53 patients with concussion. Modifications to the original formula included the addition of *Shi Chang Pu* (Rhizoma Acori Tatarinowii) and *Yuan Zhi* (Radix Polygalae) for unconsciousness; *Chuan Xiong* (Rhizoma Chuanxiong) and *Man Jing Zi* (Fructus Viticis) for headache and dizziness; *Zhe Shi* (Haematitum) and *Zhu Ru* (Caulis Bambusae in Taenia) for nausea and vomiting; *Ge Gen* (Radix Puerariae Lobatae) for neck stiffness; and *Suan Zao Ren* (Semen Ziziphi Spinosae) and *Yuan Zhi* (Radix Polygalae) for insomnia. Of 53 patients, the study reported complete recovery in 48 cases within 3-30 days, and improvement in 5 cases.[8]

9. **Intestinal adhesion**: Use of modified *Fu Yuan Huo Xue Tang* was associated with complete recovery in all 17 patients with intestinal adhesion, without recurrence for 6 months. The herbal treatment contained this formula with modifications such as the addition of *San Leng* (Rhizoma Sparganii), *E Zhu* (Rhizoma Curcumae), *Chi Shao* (Radix Paeoniae Rubra), and *Bai Shao* (Radix Paeoniae Alba) for severe abdominal pain; *Mu Xiang* (Radix Aucklandiae) and *Da Fu Pi* (Pericarpium Arecae) for severe abdominal distention; *Ban Xia* (Rhizoma Pinelliae) and *Zhe Shi* (Haematitum) for severe nausea and vomiting; *Zhi Shi* (Fructus Aurantii Immaturus) and *Xuan Ming Fen* (Natrii Sulfas Exsiccatus) for constipation accompanied by dry mouth and tongue.[9]

10. **Hyperplasia of mammary glands**: Use of modified *Fu Yuan Huo Xue Tang* was effective in treating uni- or bilateral hyperplasia of mammary glands in 80 women (between 20-50 years of age, with 0.5-5 years history of illness). The hyperplasia was characterized by swelling or stabbing pain, various sizes, and shapes of mobile nodules (0.5-3.5 cm) with defined borders. The herbal treatment contained vinegar-processed *Chai Hu* (Radix Bupleuri), *Chuan Shan Jia* (Squama Manis), *Rou Cong Rong* (Herba Cistanches), *He Shou Wu* (Radix Polygoni Multiflori), *Si Gua Luo* (Retinervus Luffae Fructus), *Gua Lou* (Fructus Trichosanthis), *Dang Gui* (Radix Angelicae Sinensis), *Tao Ren* (Semen Persicae), *Xiang Fu* (Rhizoma Cyperi), liquor-processed *Da Huang* (Radix et Rhizoma Rhei), *Hong Hua* (Flos Carthami), and *Gan Cao* (Radix et Rhizoma Glycyrrhizae). The herbs were administered in decoction daily for 20 days per course of treatment. Of 80 patients, 44 had complete recovery, 23 had significant improvement, 10 had moderate improvement, and 3 experienced no effect. The effectiveness rate was 96.25%.[10]

11. **Asthma**: One study reported good results using modified *Fu Yuan Huo Xue Tang* to treat asthma. The

Fù Yuán Huó Xuè Tāng
(Revive Health by Invigorating the Blood Decoction)

herbal treatment contained this formula plus *Ma Huang* (Herba Ephedrae), *Bai Shao* (Radix Paeoniae Alba), *Zhi Qiao* (Fructus Aurantii), and *Cang Er Zi* (Fructus Xanthii). Furthermore, *Gua Lou* (Fructus Trichosanthis), *Huang Qin* (Radix Scutellariae), and *Yu Xing Cao* (Herba Houttuyniae) were added for yellow, sticky sputum with a feeling of chest oppression; *Fu Zi* (Radix Aconiti Lateralis Praeparata), *Dang Shen* (Radix Codonopsis), and *Bai Zhu* (Rhizoma Atractylodis Macrocephalae) for Spleen and Kidney yang deficiencies; and *Ren Shen* (Radix et Rhizoma Ginseng) and *Ge Jie* (Gecko) for frequent asthma attacks. The study reported reduced frequency and severity of asthma attacks after 8-10 packs of herbs.[11]

RELATED FORMULAS

Pò Bò Zǐ Yè Tāng (Cordia Decoction)

破布子葉湯
破布子叶汤

Pinyin Name: *Po Bu Zi Ye Tang*
Literal Name: Cordia Decoction
Original Source: *Jian Tai Zhen Suo Fang* (Herbal Prescriptions from *Jiantai* Clinic) by Chang Wei-Yen in 1981

Po Bu Zi Ye (Folium Cordia Dichotoma)
Ru Xiang (Gummi Olibanum)
Mo Yao (Myrrha)
Huang Jin Gui (Caulis Vanieriae)
Liu Zhi Huang (Herba Solidaginis)
Mo Gu Xiao (Caulis Hyptis Capitatae)
Da Ding Huang (Caulis Euonymi)
Bai Zhi (Radix Angelicae Dahuricae)
Zhe Bei Mu (Bulbus Fritillariae Thunbergii)
Chen Pi (Pericarpium Citri Reticulatae)
Fang Feng (Radix Saposhnikoviae)
Jin Yin Hua (Flos Lonicerae Japonicae)
Tong Cao (Medulla Tetrapanacis)
Zao Jiao Ci (Spina Gleditsiae)
Tian Hua Fen (Radix Trichosanthis)
Dang Gui (Radix Angelicae Sinensis)
Gan Cao (Radix et Rhizoma Glycyrrhizae)

Po Bu Zi Ye Tang (Cordia Decoction) primarily treats bone spurs from chronic trauma, sports, and repetitive injuries. This formula contains herbs to activate qi and blood circulation, open the channels and collaterals, and eliminate stagnation.

RELATED FORMULA

Huó Xuè Shùn Qì Tāng
(Invigorate the Blood and Smooth the Qi Decoction)

活血順氣湯
活血顺气汤

Pinyin Name: *Huo Xue Shun Qi Tang*
Literal Name: Invigorate the Blood and Smooth the Qi Decoction
Original Source: *Guang An Men Yi Yuan* (Guang An Men Hospital) in 1990

Dang Gui (Radix Angelicae Sinensis)
Yu Jin (Radix Curcumae)
Zhi Qiao (Fructus Aurantii)
Chai Hu (Radix Bupleuri)
Xiang Fu (Rhizoma Cyperi)
Dan Shen (Radix et Rhizoma Salviae Miltiorrhizae)
Yan Hu Suo (Rhizoma Corydalis)
Chuan Xiong (Rhizoma Chuanxiong)
Tao Ren (Semen Persicae)
Hong Hua (Flos Carthami)
Fu Ling (Poria)
Si Gua Luo (Retinervus Luffae Fructus)
Jiang Xiang (Lignum Dalbergiae Odoriferae)

Huo Xue Shun Qi Tang (Invigorate the Blood and Smooth the Qi Decoction) is designed to treat traumatic injuries to the chest or upper back with sprain and strain, swelling, inflammation and pain. This formula contains herbs that activate qi and blood circulation, remove qi and blood stagnation, and relieve pain.

This formula can also be used to treat traumatic injuries to the extremities. For this application, *Chai Hu* (Radix Bupleuri) should be removed, and *Gui Zhi* (Ramulus Cinnamomi) and *Sang Zhi* (Ramulus Mori) should be added.

AUTHORS' COMMENTS

Fu Yuan Huo Xue Tang is one of the best formulas for treating physical injuries (trauma, sports, and external injuries) with pain, swelling, inflammation, bruising, and damage to the soft tissues. This formula originally was designed for trauma in the hypochondriac region, but is equally effective for injuries in the rest of the body.

Patients who suffer from chronic hypochondriac pain and distention, with raised rib cage when lying facing up, can benefit from the use of this formula.

This formula consists mainly of blood-activating herbs. To enhance the effect of this formula, some qi-activating herbs may be added since qi and blood stagnation often occur together.

Chinese Herbal Formulas and Applications

Fù Yuán Huó Xuè Tāng
(Revive Health by Invigorating the Blood Decoction)

References

1. *Zhong Guo Zhong Xi Yi Jie He Za Zhi* (Chinese Journal of Integrative Chinese and Western Medicine) 1993;8:491.
2. *Fu Jian Zhong Yi Yao* (Fujian Chinese Medicine and Herbology) 1994;1:33.
3. *Shan Dong Zhong Yi Za Zhi* (Shandong Journal of Chinese Medicine) 1994;1:42.
4. *Shi Yong Zhong Yi Yao Za Zhi* (Journal of Practical Chinese Medicine and Medicinals) 1999;8:11.
5. *Zhong Yi Yao Xin Xi* (Information on Chinese Medicine and Herbology) 1995;1:45.
6. *Yun Nan Zhong Yi Zhong Yao Za Zhi* (Yunan Journal of Chinese Medicine and Medicinals) 1997;1:23.
7. *Zhong Yi Fang Ji Xian Dai Yan Jiu* (Modern Study of Medical Formulae in Traditional Chinese Medicine) 1997;999.
8. *Zhe Jiang Zhong Yi Za Zhi* (Zhejiang Journal of Chinese Medicine) 1996;5:301.
9. *Jiang Su Zhong Yi* (Jiangsu Chinese Medicine) 1999;3:31.
10. *Shan Xi Zhong Yi* (Shanxi Chinese Medicine) 1994;2:52.
11. *Shang Hai Zhong Yi Yao Za Zhi* (Shanghai Journal of Chinese Medicine and Herbology) 1992;23(3):36.

Zhèng Gǔ Zǐ Jīn Dān (Purple and Gold Pill for Righteous Bones)
正骨紫金丹

Pinyin Name: *Zheng Gu Zi Jin Dan*
Literal Name: Purple and Gold Pill for Righteous Bones
Alternate Names: *Cheng Ku Tzu Chin Tan*, Rhubarb and Carthamus Formula
Original Source: *Yi Zong Jin Jian* (Golden Mirror of the Medical Tradition) by Wu Qian in 1742

COMPOSITION

Dang Gui (Radix Angelicae Sinensis)	60g
Bai Shao (Radix Paeoniae Alba)	60g
Xue Jie (Sanguis Draconis)	30g
Hong Hua (Flos Carthami)	30g
Er Cha (Catechu)	30g
Mu Dan Pi (Cortex Moutan)	15g
Da Huang (Radix et Rhizoma Rhei), prepared	30g
Mu Xiang (Radix Aucklandiae)	30g
Ding Xiang (Flos Caryophylli)	30g
Lian Zi (Semen Nelumbinis)	60g
Fu Ling (Poria)	60g
Gan Cao (Radix et Rhizoma Glycyrrhizae)	9g

DOSAGE / PREPARATION / ADMINISTRATION

The source text states to grind all the ingredients into a fine powder, then mix the powder with honey to form pills. Take 9g of the pills with a grain-based liquor or *Tong Bian* (Infantis Urina).

CHINESE THERAPEUTIC ACTIONS

1. Activates blood circulation and dispels blood stasis
2. Opens the channels and collaterals
3. Reduces swelling and bruising

CLINICAL MANIFESTATIONS

Traumatic injuries: various types of physical injuries with pain, swelling, inflammation, bruising, and damage to both soft tissues and bone.

CLINICAL APPLICATIONS

Bone fractures, joint dislocation, soft tissue injuries, sports injuries, and other external or traumatic injuries.

EXPLANATION

Zheng Gu Zi Jin Dan (Purple and Gold Pill for Righteous Bones) contains herbs to relieve pain, reduce swelling and bruises, and facilitate recovery of injuries to both soft tissues and bone. *Dang Gui* (Radix Angelicae Sinensis) and *Bai Shao* (Radix Paeoniae Alba) activate blood

BLOOD-REGULATING FORMULAS

13

901

Chapter 13 – Blood-Regulating Formulas　　*Section 1 – Blood-Invigorating and Stasis-Removing Formulas*

Zhèng Gǔ Zǐ Jīn Dān (Purple and Gold Pill for Righteous Bones)

Zheng Gu Zi Jin Dan (Purple and Gold Pill for Righteous Bones)

Diagnosis	Signs and Symptoms	Treatment	Herbs
Traumatic injuries	Physical injuries with pain, swelling, inflammation, and bruising: qi and blood stagnation with damage to soft tissues and bone	• Activates blood circulation and dispels blood stasis • Opens the channels and collaterals • Reduces swelling and bruising	• *Dang Gui* (Radix Angelicae Sinensis) and *Bai Shao* (Radix Paeoniae Alba) activate blood circulation, nourish blood, and replenish blood lost through injury. • *Xue Jie* (Sanguis Draconis) and *Hong Hua* (Flos Carthami) break up blood stagnation and facilitate the generation of new blood. • *Er Cha* (Catechu) and *Mu Dan Pi* (Cortex Moutan) cool the blood and clear heat. • *Da Huang* (Radix et Rhizoma Rhei) eliminates heat and drains blood stasis. • *Mu Xiang* (Radix Aucklandiae) and *Ding Xiang* (Flos Caryophylli) activate qi circulation and relieve pain. • *Lian Zi* (Semen Nelumbinis) and *Fu Ling* (Poria) tonify the Spleen and reduce swelling via urination. • *Gan Cao* (Radix et Rhizoma Glycyrrhizae) harmonizes the herbs.

circulation, nourish the blood, and replenish blood lost through injury. *Xue Jie* (Sanguis Draconis) and *Hong Hua* (Flos Carthami) break up blood stagnation and facilitate the generation of new blood. *Er Cha* (Catechu) and *Mu Dan Pi* (Cortex Moutan) cool the blood and clear the heat. *Da Huang* (Radix et Rhizoma Rhei) eliminates heat and drains blood stasis. *Mu Xiang* (Radix Aucklandiae) and *Ding Xiang* (Flos Caryophylli) activate qi circulation and relieve pain. *Lian Zi* (Semen Nelumbinis) and *Fu Ling* (Poria) tonify the Spleen and reduce swelling via urination. *Gan Cao* (Radix et Rhizoma Glycyrrhizae) harmonizes the herbs in the formula. In short, this is an excellent formula and is commonly used as the first choice for treating traumatic injuries to exterior parts of the body.

MODIFICATIONS

• With severe pain, add *Ru Xiang* (Gummi Olibanum) and *Mo Yao* (Myrrha).
• With bone fractures, add *You Gui Wan* (Restore the Right [Kidney] Pill).
• With prominent redness and swelling in bone fractures, add *You Gui Wan* (Restore the Right [Kidney] Pill) and *Huang Bo* (Cortex Phellodendri Chinensis).

RELATED FORMULA

Huó Xuè Zhǐ Tòng Tāng

(Invigorate the Blood and Stop Pain Decoction)
活血止痛湯
活血止痛汤
Pinyin Name: *Huo Xue Zhi Tong Tang*
Literal Name: Invigorate the Blood and Stop Pain Decoction
Original Source: *Tian Jin Zhong Yi Xue Yuan* (Tianjin University of Chinese Medicine) in 1989

Xiang Fu (Rhizoma Cyperi)
Xue Jie (Sanguis Draconis)
Er Cha (Catechu)
Da Huang (Radix et Rhizoma Rhei), prepared
Hong Hua (Flos Carthami)
Tao Ren (Semen Persicae)
Dang Gui (Radix Angelicae Sinensis)
Fu Ling (Poria)
Mu Dan Pi (Cortex Moutan)
E Zhu (Rhizoma Curcumae)
San Leng (Rhizoma Sparganii)
Su Mu (Lignum Sappan)
Bai Shao (Radix Paeoniae Alba)
Gan Cao (Radix et Rhizoma Glycyrrhizae)

Huo Xue Zhi Tong Tang (Invigorate the Blood and Stop Pain Decoction) activates blood circulation, dispels blood stasis, opens the channels and collaterals, reduces swelling

902

Chinese Herbal Formulas and Applications

Zhèng Gǔ Zǐ Jīn Dān (Purple and Gold Pill for Righteous Bones)

and bruising, and relieves pain. This formula contains *Ru Xiang* (Gummi Olibanum) and *Mo Yao* (Myrrha), and has a stronger pain-relieving effect for external or traumatic injuries in comparison to *Zheng Gu Zi Jin Dan* (Purple and Gold Pill for Righteous Bones).

AUTHORS' COMMENTS

It is important to note that *Zheng Gu Zi Jin Dan* specifically uses prepared *Da Huang* (Radix et Rhizoma Rhei) to clear heat and drain bruises. The use of unprepared *Da Huang* (Radix et Rhizoma Rhei) is inappropriate, as it will likely cause diarrhea due to its strong purgative and laxative effects.

Qī Lí Sǎn (Seven-Thousandths of a Tael Powder)
七厘散

Pinyin Name: *Qi Li San*
Literal Name: Seven-Thousandths of a Tael Powder
Original Source: *Liang Fang Yi Ye* (Small Collection of Fine Formulas) by Xie Yuan-Qing in 1842

COMPOSITION

Xue Jie (Sanguis Draconis)	30g
Hong Hua (Flos Carthami)	4.5g
Ru Xiang (Gummi Olibanum)	4.5g
Mo Yao (Myrrha)	4.5g
She Xiang (Moschus)	0.36g
Bing Pian (Borneolum Syntheticum)	0.36g
Er Cha (Catechu)	7.2g
Zhu Sha (Cinnabaris)	3.6g

Note: *Zhu Sha* (Cinnabaris) is a potentially toxic heavy metal, and *She Xiang* (Moschus) is derived from an endangered animal. They are rarely used as medicinal substances today. The discussion here is included primarily for academic purposes, to reflect the historical use of these substances in its original formulation. Most herbal products today have removed them completely, or replaced them with substitutes with similar functions. For additional information on the toxicity of *Zhu Sha* (Cinnabaris), please refer to *Chinese Medical Herbology and Pharmacology* by John Chen and Tina Chen.

DOSAGE / PREPARATION / ADMINISTRATION

The source text states to grind all the ingredients into a fine powder and store the powder in a porcelain container sealed with wax. For acute pain and/or bleeding, first take hot grain-based liquor with 0.22g of the powder for internal use. Then, make a paste for external application: mix the powdered herbs with hot grain-based liquor, and apply topically to the affected area.

Today this formula is prepared by grinding all ingredients into a fine powder and storing it in an airtight container. For internal use, take in 0.22-1.5g doses with a warm grain-based liquor or warm water. For external use, mix an adequate amount of the powder with a warm grain-based liquor and apply the herbal paste to the affected area. Note: In the title, a "*li*" is a unit of weight that equals 0.03124 gram. Seven "*li*" indicates the standard dose for this formula, which is 0.22 gram.

CHINESE THERAPEUTIC ACTIONS

1. Activates blood circulation and disperses blood stasis
2. Relieves pain and stops bleeding

CLINICAL MANIFESTATIONS

External injuries and traumas: blood stasis with swelling and pain due to injuries to soft tissue or bone; and bleeding due to cuts, burns, and other external traumas.

CLINICAL APPLICATIONS

External and traumatic injuries, bone fractures, herpes zoster, and infantile diarrhea.

BLOOD-REGULATING FORMULAS

13

903

Chapter 13 – Blood-Regulating Formulas   *Section 1 – Blood-Invigorating and Stasis-Removing Formulas*

Qī Lí Săn (Seven-Thousandths of a Tael Powder)

EXPLANATION

Qi Li San (Seven-Thousandths of a Tael Powder) is well-known for treating various symptoms due to traumatic injuries, such as broken or fractured bones, soft tissue injuries (muscles, ligaments, and tendons), swelling, pain, bruises, bleeding, or other blood stasis problems.

The treatment plan for this condition entails activating qi and blood circulation, dispelling blood stagnation, stopping bleeding, reducing swelling, and relieving pain. *Xue Jie* (Sanguis Draconis) dispels blood stagnation, relieves pain, and stops bleeding. *Hong Hua* (Flos Carthami) helps *Xue Jie* (Sanguis Draconis) to break up blood stasis and activate the blood. *Ru Xiang* (Gummi Olibanum) and *Mo Yao* (Myrrha) activate qi and blood circulation, break up blood stagnation, and relieve pain and swelling. *She Xiang* (Moschus) and *Bing Pian* (Borneolum Syntheticum) activate qi and blood circulation and open the channels and collaterals. Aromatic in nature, these two herbs dramatically enhance the overall effect to unblock the channels and collaterals and relieve pain. *Er Cha* (Catechu) clears heat. It also has an astringent effect to help *Xue Jie* (Sanguis Draconis) stop the bleeding and promote generation of new flesh. *Zhu Sha* (Cinnabaris) tranquilizes the *shen* (spirit), which is often unstable after traumatic injuries. Combined, these herbs activate circulation, remove stagnation, reduce swelling, relieve pain, stop bleeding, and promote healing.

MODIFICATIONS

With bone fractures or broken bones, add *San Qi* (Radix et Rhizoma Notoginseng), *Tu Bie Chong* (Eupolyphaga seu Steleophaga), and *Zi Ran Tong* (Pyritum).

CAUTIONS / CONTRAINDICATIONS

- *Qi Li San* is contraindicated during pregnancy because it contains many herbs that activate qi and blood circulation.
- It should not be taken for a prolonged period of time or at a high dose because the *Zhu Sha* (Cinnabaris) used in this formula is potentially toxic.
- Constipation is the most common side effect of *Qi Li San*.[1] Furthermore, allergic reactions (rash, itching, and urticaria) were reported in 2 of 200 patients who were given this formula for bone fractures.[2]

PHARMACOLOGICAL EFFECTS

1. **Anti-inflammatory**: *Qi Li San* has been shown to reduce inflammation and swelling in rats.[3]
2. **Analgesic**: According to one study, *Qi Li San* did not have a significant pain-relieving effect in mice.[4]

CLINICAL STUDIES AND RESEARCH

1. **Bone fractures**: Administration of *Qi Li San* in 26 patients with bone fractures showed promising results to speed up bone fusion.[5]
2. **Trauma**: Topical application of *Qi Li San* was effective in treating joint inflammation caused by external or traumatic injuries. The treatment protocol was to mix the powdered herbs with rubbing alcohol and apply the herbal paste to the affected area for 15-20 minutes. This treatment was performed daily or once every other day for 10-20 days per course of treatment. The duration of treatment was between 2-3 courses. Out of 7 patients, the study reported complete recovery in 3 cases, significant improvement in 2 cases, and slight improvement in 1 case.[6]

Qi Li San (Seven-Thousandths of a Tael Powder)

Diagnosis	Signs and Symptoms	Treatment	Herbs
External injuries and traumas	External trauma, such as broken or fractured bones, soft tissue injuries (muscles, ligaments and tendons), swelling, pain, bruises and bleeding: qi and blood stagnation	• Activates blood circulation and disperses blood stasis • Relieves pain and stops bleeding	• *Xue Jie* (Sanguis Draconis) dispels blood stagnation, relieves pain, and stops bleeding. • *Hong Hua* (Flos Carthami) breaks up blood stasis and activates the blood. • *Ru Xiang* (Gummi Olibanum) and *Mo Yao* (Myrrha) activate qi and blood circulation, break up blood stagnation, and relieve pain and swelling. • *She Xiang* (Moschus) and *Bing Pian* (Borneolum Syntheticum) activate qi and blood circulation and open the channels and collaterals. • *Er Cha* (Catechu) clears heat. • *Zhu Sha* (Cinnabaris) tranquilizes the *shen* (spirit).

904

Qī Lǐ Sǎn (Seven-Thousandths of a Tael Powder)

3. **Herpes zoster**: *Qi Li San* was used successfully in treating 46 patients with herpes zoster. The treatment protocol for adults was to administer 1.2g of the formula with warm water daily. Doses for children were adjusted accordingly. Out of 46 patients, the study reported complete recovery in 42 cases within 5 days, and 4 cases within 10 days.[7]

4. **Infantile diarrhea**: In one study, *Qi Li San* was used to treat 41 infants between the ages of 2-20 months who had 1-3 days of diarrhea in autumn. The treatment protocol was to administer 0.2g of the formula one time daily for mild to moderate diarrhea, and twice daily for severe diarrhea. Individuals with dehydration also received intravenous fluids. Those who responded to herbal treatment were instructed to continue taking the herbs for 2-3 days. Those who did not respond after 3 days discontinued herbal treatment, and were treated with other methods. Out of 41 cases, the study reported complete recovery in 19 cases within 48 hours, improvement in 9 cases within 72 hours, and no effect in 13 cases.[8]

TOXICOLOGY

Administration of *Qi Li San* has been associated with rare reports of rash, itching, and skin lesions.[9] (Note: These reactions are generally attributed to *Zhu Sha* (Cinnabaris), a potentially toxic substance, on the coating of the pellets.)

AUTHORS' COMMENTS

Qi Li San should ***not*** be prepared or taken in decoction form because many of its ingredients are aromatic and may lose their potency when cooked at a high temperature. Rather, the formula should be taken in powder or pill form with grain-based liquor and/or water. This formula, when applied topically, is also effective for relieving pain associated with herpes zoster.

References

1. *Zhong Hua Wai Ke Za Zhi* (Chinese Journal of External Medicine) 1962;10(5):305.
2. *Liao Ning Zhong Yi Za Zhi* (Liaoning Journal of Chinese Medicine) 1982;2:12.
3. *Zhong Cheng Yao Yan Jiu* (Research of Chinese Patent Medicine) 1987;3:45.
4. *Shang Hai Zhong Yi Yao Za Zhi* (Shanghai Journal of Chinese Medicine and Herbology) 1985;10:29.
5. *Zhong Hua Wai Ke Za Zhi* (Chinese Journal of External Medicine) 1962;5:305.
6. *Jiang Su Zhong Yi* (Jiangsu Chinese Medicine) 1963;5:13.
7. *Zhong Ji Yi Kan* (Medium Medical Journal) 1986;12:52.
8. *Shang Hai Zhong Yi Yao Za Zhi* (Shanghai Journal of Chinese Medicine and Herbology) 1985;10:29.
9. *Zhong Yao Bu Liang Fan Ying Yu Zhi Liao* (Adverse Reactions and Treatment of Chinese Herbal Medicine) 1996;92.

Bǔ Yáng Huán Wǔ Tāng (Tonify the Yang to Restore Five Decoction)

補陽還五湯
补阳还五汤

Pinyin Name: *Bu Yang Huan Wu Tang*
Literal Name: Tonify the Yang to Restore Five Decoction
Alternate Names: *Pu Yang Huan Wu Tang*, Yang Nourishing Five Returning Decoction, Invigorating Recuperation Decoction, Astragalus and Peony Combination
Original Source: *Yi Lin Gai Cuo* (Corrections of Errors Among Physicians) by Wang Qing-Ren in 1830

COMPOSITION

Huang Qi (Radix Astragali)	120g
Dang Gui Wei (Extremitas Radix Angelicae Sinensis)	6g
Chuan Xiong (Rhizoma Chuanxiong)	3g
Chi Shao (Radix Paeoniae Rubra)	4.5g
Hong Hua (Flos Carthami)	3g
Tao Ren (Semen Persicae)	3g
Di Long (Pheretima)	3g

Chapter 13 – Blood-Regulating Formulas　　　　　*Section 1 – Blood-Invigorating and Stasis-Removing Formulas*

Bǔ Yáng Huán Wǔ Tāng (Tonify the Yang to Restore Five Decoction)

DOSAGE / PREPARATION / ADMINISTRATION

Prepare as a decoction.

CHINESE THERAPEUTIC ACTIONS

1. Tonifies qi
2. Activates blood circulation
3. Opens the channels and collaterals

CLINICAL MANIFESTATIONS

Post-stroke sequelae: hemiplegia, deviation of the mouth and eyes, slurred speech, involuntary salivation, atrophy of the lower limbs, frequent urination or urinary incontinence, a white tongue coating, and a moderate pulse.

CLINICAL APPLICATIONS

Cerebrovascular disease, cerebral infarction, stroke, post-stroke sequelae, ischemic cerebrovascular disorder, paralysis, facial paralysis, brain trauma, cerebral atherosclerosis, coronary heart disease, arteriosclerosis obliterans, thromboangiitis obliterans, deep vein thrombosis, varicose veins, vascular headache, Raynaud's disease, acute myelitis, poliomyelitis, polyneuritis, chronic nephritis, chronic prostatitis, prostatic hypertrophy, sciatica, and numbness.

EXPLANATION

Bu Yang Huan Wu Tang (Tonify the Yang to Restore Five Decoction) is designed to treat various post-stroke symptoms. After a stroke, the qi may become deficient, the blood stagnant, and the channels and collaterals obstructed. As a result, the muscles and tendons become malnourished and the body cannot carry out normal physical functions, and symptoms such as hemiplegia, deviation of the mouth and eyes, slurred speech, involuntary salivation, and urinary incontinence may occur. Hemiplegia and deviation of the mouth and eyes indicate blood stagnation obstructing the channels and collaterals. Slurred speech, involuntary salivation, and urinary incontinence indicate qi deficiency with inability to control bodily functions.

This formula uses a large dose of *Huang Qi* (Radix Astragali) to greatly tonify *zheng* (upright) and *yuan* (source) *qi*. Abundance of qi promotes blood circulation, and allows elimination of blood stasis without damaging the body. *Dang Gui Wei* (Extremitas Radix Angelicae Sinensis), *Chuan Xiong* (Rhizoma Chuanxiong), *Chi Shao* (Radix Paeoniae Rubra), *Tao Ren* (Semen Persicae), and *Hong Hua* (Flos Carthami) activate the blood and eliminate blood stasis. *Di Long* (Pheretima) unblocks the channels and collaterals to restore normal physical functions. With sufficient qi, normal blood circulation, and unobstructed channels and collaterals, the body will gradually recover from all signs and symptoms of the previous injury or blockage.

MODIFICATIONS

- With slurred speech, add *Shi Chang Pu* (Rhizoma Acori Tatarinowii), *Yu Jin* (Radix Curcumae), and *Yuan Zhi* (Radix Polygalae).
- With facial paralysis and deviation of the eyes and mouth, add *Bai Fu Zi* (Rhizoma Typhonii), *Jiang Can* (Bombyx Batryticatus), and *Quan Xie* (Scorpio).
- For initial onset of hemiplegia, add *Fang Feng* (Radix Saposhnikoviae).
- For chronic hemiplegia without improvement, add *Shui Zhi* (Hirudo) and *Meng Chong* (Tabanus).
- With paralysis of the lower limbs, add *Du Zhong* (Cortex Eucommiae) and *Niu Xi* (Radix Achyranthis Bidentatae).
- With impaired mental functions, add *Shi Chang Pu* (Rhizoma Acori Tatarinowii), *Yin Xing Ye* (Folium Ginkgo), and *Jiu Ceng Ta* (Herba Ocimi Basilici).
- With epigastric distention and difficulty in breathing, add *Wu Yao* (Radix Linderae) and *Qing Pi* (Pericarpium Citri Reticulatae Viride).

Bu Yang Huan Wu Tang (Tonify the Yang to Restore Five Decoction)

Diagnosis	Signs and Symptoms	Treatment	Herbs
Post-stroke sequelae	• Hemiplegia and deviation of the mouth and eyes: blood stagnation obstructing the channels and collaterals • Slurred speech, involuntary salivation, and urinary incontinence: qi deficiency with inability to control body functions	• Tonifies qi • Activates blood circulation • Opens the channels and collaterals	• *Huang Qi* (Radix Astragali) greatly tonifies *zheng* (upright) and *yuan* (source) *qi*. • *Dang Gui Wei* (Extremitas Radix Angelicae Sinensis), *Chuan Xiong* (Rhizoma Chuanxiong), *Chi Shao* (Radix Paeoniae Rubra), *Tao Ren* (Semen Persicae), and *Hong Hua* (Flos Carthami) activate the blood and eliminate blood stasis. • *Di Long* (Pheretima) unblocks the channels and collaterals to restore normal physical functions.

Chinese Herbal Formulas and Applications

Bǔ Yáng Huán Wǔ Tāng (Tonify the Yang to Restore Five Decoction)

- With cold conditions, add *Fu Zi* (Radix Aconiti Lateralis Praeparata), *Rou Gui* (Cortex Cinnamomi), and *Ba Ji Tian* (Radix Morindae Officinalis).
- With Spleen and Stomach deficiencies, add *Dang Shen* (Radix Codonopsis) and *Bai Zhu* (Rhizoma Atractylodis Macrocephalae).
- With profuse phlegm, add *Ban Xia* (Rhizoma Pinelliae) and *Tian Zhu Huang* (Concretio Silicea Bambusae).
- With irritability and insomnia, and a wiry, deficient, rapid pulse, add *Zhi Zi* (Fructus Gardeniae) and *Suan Zao Ren* (Semen Ziziphi Spinosae).
- For coronary artery disorders, angina, and cardiac infarction, add *San Qi* (Radix et Rhizoma Notoginseng) and *Dan Shen* (Radix et Rhizoma Salviae Miltiorrhizae).

CAUTIONS / CONTRAINDICATIONS

- *Bu Yang Huan Wu Tang* is contraindicated in patients who have Liver wind rising, yin-deficient heat, or stagnation of phlegm.
- Because this formula contains strong blood-activating and blood-stasis removing herbs, it should not be used immediately after strokes caused by cerebral hemorrhage.
- This formula is contraindicated in post-stroke patients who have a forceful pulse, which indicates an excess condition. This formula contains a large dose of *Huang Qi* (Radix Astragali), a tonic with ascending properties, and may exacerbate excess conditions.

PHARMACOLOGICAL EFFECTS

1. **Effects on the central nervous system**: According to various *in vitro* studies, administration of *Bu Yang Huan Wu Tang* was associated with dilating blood vessels in the brain and improving blood perfusion to the brain.[1] The effect lasted for up to 1 hour following intravenous injection of this formula at 0.25-0.5 g/kg.[2] Furthermore, it was shown that use of *Bu Yang Huan Wu Tang* facilitated the healing and recovery of subjects who suffered from nervous system damage to the brain and spine.[3]
2. **Antiplatelet, anticoagulant and thrombolytic**: *Bu Yang Huan Wu Tang* has been shown to have antiplatelet, anticoagulant, and thrombolytic effects in both *in vitro* and *in vivo* studies.[4,5,6]
3. **Antihyperlipidemic**: According to various *in vitro* studies, administration of *Bu Yang Huan Wu Tang* was associated with a reduction in total cholesterol levels and triglyceride levels. No significant changes were noted in HDL.[7,8]
4. **Cardiovascular**: In one study of anesthetized rabbits, administration of *Bu Yang Huan Wu Tang* showed different effects at different doses. At 0.5 g/kg given via intravenous injection, no significant changes were noted to blood pressure and heart rate. At 1.0 to 2.0 g/kg given

via intravenous injection, blood pressure was reduced for up to 20 minutes with no changes to heart rate.[9]

CLINICAL STUDIES AND RESEARCH

1. **Cerebrovascular disease**: Use of *Bu Yang Huan Wu Tang* plus *Gui Zhi* (Ramulus Cinnamomi) and *Fu Zi* (Radix Aconiti Lateralis Praeparata) in 32 patients with cerebrovascular disease was associated with recovery in 12 cases, significant improvement in 17 cases, moderate improvement in 2 cases, and no effect in 1 case.[10]
2. **Cerebral infarction**: Fifty patients with cerebral infarction due to stenosis of the artery were treated with *Bu Yang Huan Wu Tang* with complete recovery in 31 cases, significant recovery in 9 cases, moderate improvement in 5 cases, and no effect in 5 cases.[11]
3. **Stroke**: According to one study, 150 patients with stroke characterized by qi deficiency and blood stagnation were treated with complete recovery in 64 cases, marked improvement in 40 cases, moderate improvement in 45 cases, and fatality in 1 case. Treatment included herbs, acupuncture, and *tui-na*. The herbal formula contained *Bu Yang Huan Wu Tang* plus *Dan Shen* (Radix et Rhizoma Salviae Miltiorrhizae) and *Ji Xue Teng* (Caulis Spatholobi).[12]
4. **Ischemic cerebrovascular disorder**: Administration of *Bu Yang Huan Wu Tang* has been shown in many studies to treat patients with ischemic stroke. According to one study, use of this formula plus *Chuan Shan Jia* (Squama Manis) and *Ji Xue Teng* (Caulis Spatholobi) for 2-3 months in 103 patients was associated with 96.3% effectiveness.[13] According to another study, concurrent treatment of herbs (*Bu Yang Huan Wu Tang* daily for 10 days per course of treatment) and acupuncture (every other day for 5 treatments per course) was associated with 97.7% effectiveness among 45 patients with ischemic cerebrovascular disorder.[14]
5. **Post-stroke sequelae**: Many studies of *Bu Yang Huan Wu Tang* have shown it to be one of the most effective herbal formulas for post-stroke sequelae. One study of 35 post-stroke patients reported 94% effectiveness when treated with modified *Bu Yang Huan Wu Tang*. The herbal formula contained *Huang Qi* (Radix Astragali) 30-120g, *Dang Gui* (Radix Angelicae Sinensis) 10g, *Chi Shao* (Radix Paeoniae Rubra) 10g, *Tao Ren* (Semen Persicae) 10g, *Hong Hua* (Flos Carthami) 10g, *Di Long* (Pheretima) 10g, *Dan Shen* (Radix et Rhizoma Salviae Miltiorrhizae) 30g, and *Chuan Xiong* (Rhizoma Chuanxiong) 6g. *Ban Xia* (Rhizoma Pinelliae) and *Chen Pi* (Pericarpium Citri Reticulatae) were added for phlegm and dampness; *Tian Ma* (Rhizoma Gastrodiae) and *Gou Teng* (Ramulus Uncariae cum Uncis) for Liver yang rising; *Dang Shen* (Radix Codonopsis) for qi and blood deficiencies; and

BLOOD-REGULATING FORMULAS

13

907

Bǔ Yáng Huán Wǔ Tāng (Tonify the Yang to Restore Five Decoction)

Da Huang (Radix et Rhizoma Rhei) and *Huo Ma Ren* (Fructus Cannabis) for constipation. The herbs were cooked in water, and the decoction was taken in two equally-divided doses in the afternoon and evening.[15]

6. **Paralysis**: Ninety-three patients with paralysis due to stroke were treated with *Bu Yang Huan Wu Tang* plus *Ji Xue Teng* (Caulis Spatholobi), *Niu Xi* (Radix Achyranthis Bidentatae), *Qian Nian Jian* (Rhizoma Homalomenae), and other herbs with good results (complete recovery in 40 cases, significant improvement in 31 cases, moderate improvement in 20 cases, and no effect in 2 cases).[16]

7. **Facial paralysis**: One study reported complete recovery in 18 of 20 patients with facial paralysis using *Bu Yang Huan Wu Tang* plus *Qian Zheng San* (Lead to Symmetry Powder).[17] Another study reported complete recovery in all 15 patients with facial paralysis using *Bu Yang Huan Wu Tang* plus *Wu Gong* (Scolopendra), *Fang Feng* (Radix Saposhnikoviae), *Jiang Can* (Bombyx Batryticatus), and others.[18]

8. **Brain trauma**: One study reported 97.2% effectiveness using *Bu Yang Huan Wu Tang* to treat brain trauma in 36 patients (between 8-62 years of age, 17 days to 11 years history of illness). Clinical improvements included relief of headache, dizziness, insomnia, excessive dreams, poor memory, speech difficulties, and paralysis. Of 36 patients, the study reported complete recovery in 26 cases, marked improvement in 9 cases, and no effect in 1 case. Each course of treatment was 30 days.[19]

9. **Cerebral atherosclerosis**: One study reported good results using modified *Bu Yang Huan Wu Tang* to treat 75 patients with cerebral atherosclerosis with hypertension. The herbal treatment contained this formula plus *Dan Shen* (Radix et Rhizoma Salviae Miltiorrhizae), *Ge Gen* (Radix Puerariae Lobatae), *Ji Xue Teng* (Caulis Spatholobi), *Shan Zha* (Fructus Crataegi), and *Gan Cao* (Radix et Rhizoma Glycyrrhizae).[20]

10. **Coronary heart disease**: *Bu Yang Huan Wu Tang* was reported in several studies to treat coronary heart disease. According to one study, use of modified *Bu Yang Huan Wu Tang* in decoction daily for 30 days per course of treatment was associated with 96.3% effectiveness for 82 patients.[21] According to another study, coronary heart disease characterized by qi deficiency and blood stagnation was treated with 83.7% effectiveness using *Bu Yang Huan Wu Tang* plus *Yu Jin* (Radix Curcumae) 10g, *Yi Mu Cao* (Herba Leonuri) 10g, *Gua Lou* (Fructus Trichosanthis) 10g, *Xie Bai* (Bulbus Allii Macrostemonis) 10g, and *Ban Xia* (Rhizoma Pinelliae) 10g. The herbs were given in decoction daily, for 10 days per course of treatment.[22]

11. **Arteriosclerosis obliterans**: Use of *Bu Yang Huan Wu Tang* plus *Ji Xue Teng* (Caulis Spatholobi), *Dang Shen* (Radix Codonopsis), *Gui Zhi* (Ramulus Cinnamomi), and *Gan Jiang* (Rhizoma Zingiberis) was associated with 87.7% effectiveness in treating early stage arteriosclerosis obliterans in 49 patients (between 40-82 years of age, with 15 days to 7 years history of illness).[23]

12. **Vascular headache**: One study of 26 patients with vascular headache reported complete recovery in 16 cases, improvement in 9 cases, and no effect in 1 case. The herbal treatment contained *Bu Yang Huan Wu Tang* plus *Niu Xi* (Radix Achyranthis Bidentatae), *Bai Zhi* (Radix Angelicae Dahuricae), and *Gan Cao* (Radix et Rhizoma Glycyrrhizae) as the base formula. Modifications included addition of *Shi Jue Ming* (Concha Haliotidis) and *Suan Zao Ren* (Semen Ziziphi Spinosae) for insomnia due to severe headache; and *Wu Wei Zi* (Fructus Schisandrae Chinensis) and *Long Chi* (Dens Draconis) for insomnia due to restlessness and irritability.[24]

13. **Raynaud's disease**: Use of *Bu Yang Huan Wu Tang* plus *Gui Zhi* (Ramulus Cinnamomi) in 31 patients with Raynaud's disease was associated with 90.3% effectiveness (18 with complete recovery, 10 with improvement, and 3 with no effect).[25]

14. **Poliomyelitis**: One study reported good results in treating poliomyelitis in young children using *Bu Yang Huan Wu Tang* plus *Yin Yang Huo* (Herba Epimedii) as the base formula, with modifications as needed. *Quan Xie* (Scorpio) and *Wu Gong* (Scolopendra) were added for treating the early stage of illness. *Qian Zheng San* (Lead to Symmetry Powder) was added for deviation of the eyes and mouth. *Sang Zhi* (Ramulus Mori) was added for paralysis of the arms, and *Niu Xi* (Radix Achyranthis Bidentatae) for paralysis of the legs. The study reported complete recovery in 37 of 42 patients.[26]

15. **Deep vein thrombosis**: One study reported good results using herbs and drugs to treat deep vein thrombosis in the legs. The herbal treatment contained *Bu Yang Huan Wu Tang* plus *Ji Xue Teng* (Caulis Spatholobi), *Niu Xi* (Radix Achyranthis Bidentatae), *Ren Dong Teng* (Caulis Lonicerae Japonicae) and others as needed. The drug was given via intravenous infusion (the name of the drug was not available). After 2-4 months of treatment in 18 patients, the study reported complete recovery in 14 cases and improvement in 4 cases.[27]

16. **Varicose veins**: One study reported good results using modified *Bu Yang Huan Wu Tang* to treat 30 patients with varicose veins (history of 4 to 20 years of illness). Of 30 patients, the study reported marked improvement in 21 cases and moderate improvement in 9 cases.[28]

17. **Polyneuritis**: Use of herbs topically as an herbal wash proved beneficial for treating polyneuritis. The warm herbal formula contained *Bu Yang Huan Wu Tang* plus *Dang Shen* (Radix Codonopsis), *Fu Ling* (Poria), *Bai Zhu*

Bǔ Yáng Huán Wǔ Tāng (Tonify the Yang to Restore Five Decoction)

(Rhizoma Atractylodis Macrocephalae), and others as needed. The treatment protocol was to cook the herbs in 1,500 mL of water to yield 1,000 mL of solution. (50g of ethanol was added to the final solution.) The herbal solution was applied topically to the affected area as an herbal wash. Of 19 patients, 13 had significant improvement and 6 had moderate improvement.[29]

18. **Chronic nephritis**: Use of *Bu Yang Huan Wu Tang* plus *Da Huang* (Radix et Rhizoma Rhei), *Ji Nei Jin* (Endothelium Corneum Gigeriae Galli), *Cang Zhu* (Rhizoma Atractylodis), and *Sang Ji Sheng* (Herba Taxilli) in 108 patients with chronic nephritis was associated with 96.3% effectiveness (73 with complete recovery, 16 with marked improvement, 15 with moderate improvement, and 4 with no effect).[30]

19. **Chronic prostatitis**: Sixty geriatric patients with chronic prostatitis were treated with herbs for 1 month with 95% effectiveness. The herbal treatment contained *Bu Yang Huan Wu Tang* plus *Ze Lan* (Herba Lycopi), *Yi Mu Cao* (Herba Leonuri), *Chuan Niu Xi* (Radix Cyathulae) and *Fu Ling* (Poria) as the base formula. Modifications included *Di Huang* (Radix Rehmanniae) for yin deficiency; *Yin Yang Huo* (Herba Epimedii) and *Ba Ji Tian* (Radix Morindae Officinalis) for yang deficiency; *Tian Ma* (Rhizoma Gastrodiae) for hypertension; *Wu Yao* (Radix Linderae), *Shui Zhi* (Hirudo), and *Tu Bie Chong* (Eupolyphaga seu Steleophaga) for qi stagnation; and others as needed.[31]

20. **Prostatic hypertrophy**: One study reported 93.78% effectiveness using modified *Bu Yang Huan Wu Tang* to treat 48 geriatric males with prostatic hypertrophy. The herbal treatment contained this formula plus *San Qi* (Radix et Rhizoma Notoginseng), *Wang Bu Liu Xing* (Semen Vaccariae), *Yu Xing Cao* (Herba Houttuyniae), and others as needed. The treatment protocol was to cook the herbs in water and drink 150 mL of decoction twice daily. Of 48 patients, the study reported significant improvement in 32 cases, moderate improvement in 13 cases, and no effect in 3 cases.[32]

21. **Sciatica**: Administration of *Bu Yang Huan Wu Tang* has been shown to be effective in treating sciatica. In one study of 100 patients with sciatica, 98% effectiveness was reported using *Bu Yang Huan Wu Tang* plus *Gui Zhi* (Ramulus Cinnamomi), *Gan Cao* (Radix et Rhizoma Glycyrrhizae), *Dang Shen* (Radix Codonopsis), and *Ji Xue Teng* (Caulis Spatholobi) for 8-25 packs of herbs.[33] Another study reported 92% effectiveness among 53 patients with sciatica using *Bu Yang Huan Wu Tang* plus *Fu Zi* (Radix Aconiti Lateralis Praeparata), *Rou Gui* (Cortex Cinnamomi), *Wu Gong* (Scolopendra), and *Quan Xie* (Scorpio).[34]

22. **Numbness**: Administration of *Bu Yang Huan Wu Tang* was associated with 98% effectiveness in treating 56 patients with numbness from various causes such as hyperlipidemia, post-stroke sequelae, or hypertension. The herbal formula contained *Huang Qi* (Radix Astragali) 60g, *Dang Gui* (Radix Angelicae Sinensis) 12g, *Chi Shao* (Radix Paeoniae Rubra) 12g, *Wu Gong* (Scolopendra) 12g, *Quan Xie* (Scorpio) 12g, *Hai Feng Teng* (Caulis Piperis Kadsurae) 12g, *Tao Ren* (Semen Persicae) 10g, *Hong Hua* (Flos Carthami) 10g, *Chuan Xiong* (Rhizoma Chuanxiong) 10g, *Di Long* (Pheretima) 10g, and *Fu Zi* (Radix Aconiti Lateralis Praeparata) 3g. Modifications were made by: adding *Dan Shen* (Radix et Rhizoma Salviae Miltiorrhizae) for blood stagnation; *He Shou Wu* (Radix Polygoni Multiflori) for blood deficiency; *Ban Xia* (Rhizoma Pinelliae) and *Fu Ling* (Poria) for dampness; and *Niu Xi* (Radix Achyranthis Bidentatae) and *Long Gu* (Os Draconis) for Liver yang rising. The herbs were given daily in decoction. Of 56 patients, the study reported complete recovery in 25 cases, improvement in 30 cases, and no effect in 1 case.[35]

TOXICOLOGY

Bu Yang Huan Wu Tang has very little toxicity. According to one acute toxicology study, the LD_{50} in mice via injection is equivalent to 149 g/kg of dried herbs.[36]

RELATED FORMULA

Nǎo Wěi Káng Wán (Benefit Brain Atrophy Pill)

脑萎康丸
脑萎康丸

Pinyin Name: *Nao Wei Kang Wan*
Literal Name: Benefit Brain Atrophy Pill
Original Source: *Tian Jin Bai Lou Yi Yuan* (Tianjin Bailou Hospital) in 1989

Dong Chong Xia Cao (Cordyceps)
Ren Shen (Radix et Rhizoma Ginseng)
Xi Yang Shen (Radix Panacis Quinquefolii)
San Qi (Radix et Rhizoma Notoginseng)
Yin Xing Ye (Folium Ginkgo)
Yi Mu Cao (Herba Leonuri)
Shan Zhu Yu (Fructus Corni)
Tian Ma (Rhizoma Gastrodiae)
Ba Ji Tian (Radix Morindae Officinalis)
Du Zhong (Cortex Eucommiae)
Gou Qi Zi (Fructus Lycii)
He Shou Wu (Radix Polygoni Multiflori)
Yi Zhi (Fructus Alpiniae Oxyphyllae)
Tu Si Zi (Semen Cuscutae)
Shan Yao (Rhizoma Dioscoreae)
Huang Qi (Radix Astragali)

BLOOD-REGULATING FORMULAS

13

Chapter 13 – Blood-Regulating Formulas   *Section 1 – Blood-Invigorating and Stasis-Removing Formulas*

Bŭ Yáng Huán Wŭ Tāng (Tonify the Yang to Restore Five Decoction)

Bai Zhu (Rhizoma Atractylodis Macrocephalae)

Fu Ling (Poria)

Shan Zha (Fructus Crataegi)

San Leng (Rhizoma Sparganii)

Dan Shen (Radix et Rhizoma Salviae Miltiorrhizae)

Hong Hua (Flos Carthami)

E Zhu (Rhizoma Curcumae)

Fen Bi Xie (Rhizoma Dioscoreae Hypoglaucae)

Di Huang (Radix Rehmanniae)

Shu Di Huang (Radix Rehmanniae Praeparata)

Gou Teng (Ramulus Uncariae cum Uncis)

Yuan Zhi (Radix Polygalae)

Shi Chang Pu (Rhizoma Acori Tatarinowii)

Bai Zhi (Radix Angelicae Dahuricae)

Nu Zhen Zi (Fructus Ligustri Lucidi)

Suo Yang (Herba Cynomorii)

Nao Wei Kang Wan (Benefit Brain Atrophy Pill) is designed specifically to treat individuals with compromised mental acuity and physical activity due to deterioration of the brain. Although the formula is rather complex, the main actions are to tonify Kidney yin, Kidney yang, and *jing* (essence); regulate qi and blood; remove blood stagnation; and open the sensory orifices to promote awareness and alertness. Clinically, this formula may be used for Parkinson's disease, Alzheimer's disease, dementia, and post-stroke patients with impaired mental and physical functions.

AUTHORS' COMMENTS

Bu Yang Huan Wu Tang is the representative formula for treating post-stroke patients with qi deficiency and blood stasis. It can be used any time after a stroke as long as the patient is showing signs of blood stasis with qi deficiency. The key symptoms include paralysis and a moderate pulse.

As the chief herb, *Huang Qi* (Radix Astragali) is used at a large dose to tonify qi and treat the underlying disorder. The dose of *Huang Qi* (Radix Astragali) may be started at approximately 30-60g, and increased gradually to obtain the desired effects. Upon recovery, it is important to continue taking the herbs for a period of time to consolidate the condition and prevent further strokes.

It has been debated whether it is appropriate to use *Bu Yang Huan Wu Tang* in patients with hypertension. The argument against is that *Huang Qi* (Radix Astragali), a warm tonic with ascending effect, may raise blood pressure. However, it has been shown that intravenous injection of *Huang Qi* (Radix Astragali) actually decreases blood pressure in anesthetized subjects via dilation of

peripheral blood vessels.[37] Furthermore, intravenous injection of *Bu Yang Huan Wu Tang* in anesthetized subjects did not have any significant effect on blood pressure.[38] Lastly, two clinical texts clearly state that *Bu Yang Huan Wu Tang* is not contraindicated in patients with hypertension.[39,40]

Bu Yang Huan Wu Tang treats sequelae of wind-stroke. This formula was composed by Dr. Wang Qing-Ren, who believed that one's qi, when healthy, is 100% functional, with an equal 50% bilateral distribution. In the case of hemiplegia, 50% of the qi is impaired. Since severe qi deficiency is the primary imbalance in this syndrome, *Huang Qi* (Radix Astragali) is used as the chief herb at very large dosage to strongly tonify *zheng* (upright) qi and *yuan* (source) qi, generate flesh, and improve atrophy. This herb also tonifies qi to move the blood and transform blood stasis. Qi deficiency leads to blood deficiency, which in turn impedes the circulation of *yuan* (source) qi and aggravates muscle atrophy. Therefore, small dosages of invigorating herbs such as *Chuan Xiong* (Rhizoma Chuanxiong), *Tao Ren* (Semen Persicae), *Hong Hua* (Flos Carthami), *Dang Gui* (Radix Angelicae Sinensis), *Chi Shao* (Radix Paeoniae Rubra) and *Di Long* (Pheretima) are added to enhance the blood-transforming function of this formula. In short, this formula is aimed at tonifying the yang qi, and nourishing the blood, muscles and sinews to restore bodily functions.

References

1. *Zhong Cheng Yao Yan Jiu* (Research of Chinese Patent Medicine) 1982;(7):34.

2. *Zhong Cheng Yao Yan Jiu* (Research of Chinese Patent Medicine) 1986;(12):29.

3. *Zhong Xi Yi Jie He Za Zhi* (Journal of Integrated Chinese and Western Medicine) 1984;8:491.

4. *Zhong Cheng Yao Yan Jiu* (Research of Chinese Patent Medicine) 1983;8:31.

5. *Hu Nan Zhong Yi Xue Yuan Xue Bao* (Journal of Hunan University of Traditional Chinese Medicine) 1989;9:545.

6. *Yun Nan Zhong Yi Za Zhi* (Yunan Journal of Chinese Medicine) 1992;13(1):23.

7. *Xin Zhong Yi* (New Chinese Medicine) 1984;1:46.

8. *Zhong Guo Zhong Yao Za Zhi* (People's Republic of China Journal of Chinese Herbology) 1995;20(11):685.

9. *Zhong Cheng Yao Yan Jiu* (Research of Chinese Patent Medicine) 1986;3:28.

10. *Gui Yang Zhong Yi Xue Yuan Xue Bao* (Journal of Guiyang University of Traditional Chinese Medicine) 1992;1:32.

11. *Zhe Jiang Zhong Yi Za Zhi* (Zhejiang Journal of Chinese Medicine) 1997;7:317.

12. *Liao Ning Zhong Yi Za Zhi* (Liaoning Journal of Chinese Medicine) 1984;9:26.

13. *Zhong Yi Za Zhi* (Journal of Chinese Medicine) 1984;9:45.

14. *Guang Xi Zhong Yi Yao* (Guangxi Chinese Medicine and Herbology) 1993;16(4):9.

15. *Guang Dong Yi Xue* (Guangdong Medicine) 1992;13(1):39.

910

Chinese Herbal Formulas and Applications

Bǔ Yáng Huán Wǔ Tāng (Tonify the Yang to Restore Five Decoction)

16. *He Bei Zhong Yi Za Zhi* (Hebei Journal of Chinese Medicine) 1986;6:17.
17. *Yun Nan Zhong Yi Za Zhi* (Yunan Journal of Chinese Medicine) 1985;5:64.
18. *Nei Meng Gu Zhong Yi Yao* (Traditional Chinese Medicine and Medicinals of Inner Mongolia) 1987;2:24.
19. *Shan Dong Zhong Yi Za Zhi* (Shandong Journal of Chinese Medicine) 1993;12(3):21.
20. *Jiang Su Zhong Yi* (Jiangsu Chinese Medicine) 1992;13(5):16.
21. *Hu Bei Zhong Yi Za Zhi* (Hubei Journal of Chinese Medicine) 1994;16(1):17.
22. *Tian Jin Zhong Yi* (Tianjin Chinese Medicine) 1993;5:22.
23. *Shan Dong Zhong Yi Za Zhi* (Shandong Journal of Chinese Medicine) 1991;10(2):26.
24. *Guang Xi Zhong Yi Yao* (Guangxi Chinese Medicine and Herbology) 1985;2:14.
25. *Shan Xi Zhong Yi* (Shanxi Chinese Medicine) 1996;11:494.
26. *Cheng Du Zhong Yi Xue Yuan Xue Bao* (Journal of Chengdu University of Traditional Chinese Medicine) 1991;2:27.
27. *Jiang Su Zhong Yi* (Jiangsu Chinese Medicine) 1998;2:33.
28. *Shang Hai Zhong Yi Yao Za Zhi* (Shanghai Journal of Chinese Medicine and Herbology) 1988;5:30.

29. *Si Chuan Zhong Yi* (Sichuan Chinese Medicine) 1996;2:22.
30. *Shi Yong Zhong Yi Nei Ke Za Zhi* (Journal of Practical Chinese Internal Medicine) 1990;4(3):123.
31. *Zhe Jiang Zhong Yi Xue Yuan Xue Bao* (Journal of Zhejiang University of Chinese Medicine) 1996;6:26.
32. *Xin Zhong Yi* (New Chinese Medicine) 1996;4:26.
33. *Guang Xi Zhong Yi Yao* (Guangxi Chinese Medicine and Herbology) 1980;2:6.
34. *Zhong Yi Fang Ji Xian Dai Yan Jiu* (Modern Study of Medical Formulae in Traditional Chinese Medicine) 1997;1012.
35. *Shan Xi Zhong Yi* (Shanxi Chinese Medicine) 1995;16(9):394.
36. *Xin Yi Yao Xue Za Zhi* (New Journal of Medicine and Herbology) 1977;9:40.
37. *Guo Wai Yi Xue Can Kao Za Zhi* (Foreign Journal of Medicine) 1977;4:231.
38. *Zhong Cheng Yao Yan Jiu* (Research of Chinese Patent Medicine) 1986;3:28.
39. *Zhong Yao Ming Fang Yao Li Yu Ying Yong* (Pharmacology and Applications of Famous Herbal Formulas) 1989;464-466.
40. *Zhong Yi Lin Chuan Fang Ji Xue* (Clinical Study of Chinese Herbal Formulas) 1995;167-169.

Shī Xiào Sǎn (Sudden Smile Powder)

失笑散

Pinyin Name: *Shi Xiao San*
Literal Name: Sudden Smile Powder
Alternate Name: Sudden Smile Formula
Original Source: *Tai Ping Hui Min He Ji Ju Fang* (Imperial Grace Formulary of the Tai Ping Era) by the Imperial Medical Department in 1078-85

COMPOSITION

Wu Ling Zhi (Faeces Trogopteri), *yan* (ground) to small particles with liquor	[6g]
Pu Huang (Pollen Typhae), *chao* (dry-fried) until aromatic	[6g]

DOSAGE / PREPARATION / ADMINISTRATION

The source text states to grind equal amount of both ingredients into a fine powder. Cook 6g of the powder with vinegar and condense it into a paste. Add 1 bowl of water and cook it again until the liquid is reduced to 70%, and take the warm decoction before meals. Today this formula is prepared by grinding the ingredients into a fine powder. Take 6g of the powder with a grain-based liquor or vinegar. This formula may also be prepared as a decoction with the doses suggested in brackets.

CHINESE THERAPEUTIC ACTIONS

1. Activates blood circulation and removes blood stasis
2. Disperses stagnation and stops pain

CLINICAL MANIFESTATIONS

Blood stasis in the body: sharp pain in the chest or abdomen, postpartum bleeding due to retention of lochia, irregular menstruation, and acute onset of pain in the lower abdomen.

CLINICAL APPLICATIONS

Dysmenorrhea, amenorrhea, irregular menstruation, endometriosis, infertility, uterine bleeding, uterine bleeding caused by abortion or miscarriage, ectopic pregnancy, postpartum abdominal pain, angina pectoris, coronary artery disease, viral hepatitis, and upper gastrointestinal bleeding.

BLOOD-REGULATING FORMULAS

13

911

Chapter 13 – Blood-Regulating Formulas   *Section 1 – Blood-Invigorating and Stasis-Removing Formulas*

Shī Xiào Sǎn (Sudden Smile Powder)

EXPLANATION

Shi Xiao San (Sudden Smile Powder) is a commonly used formula for treating various presentations of pain caused by blood stasis and obstruction of blood circulation. It is especially useful for treating blood stagnation in the Liver channel.

This formula combines *Wu Ling Zhi* (Faeces Trogopteri) with *Pu Huang* (Pollen Typhae) to activate blood circulation, remove blood stagnation, and relieve pain. This formula is prepared with grain-based liquor to enhance the effect to warm the channels and invigorate blood circulation. Furthermore, this formula is taken with vinegar to improve the function to disperse blood stasis and relieve pain.

MODIFICATIONS

- With more severe qi stagnation, add *Chuan Lian Zi* (Fructus Toosendan) and *Xiang Fu* (Rhizoma Cyperi).
- With more cold, add *Pao Jiang* (Rhizoma Zingiberis Praeparatum) and *Xiao Hui Xiang* (Fructus Foeniculi).
- With irregular menstruation due to blood stasis and blood deficiency, add *Si Wu Tang* (Four-Substance Decoction).

CAUTIONS / CONTRAINDICATIONS

- *Shi Xiao San* is contraindicated during pregnancy.
- This formula should be used with caution in patients with a weak or sensitive stomach.

PHARMACOLOGICAL EFFECTS

1. **Cardiovascular**: According to *in vitro* studies, use of *Shi Xiao San* was associated with reduced blood pressure and heart rate in both frogs and rabbits.[1,2]
2. **Antiplatelet**: According to an *in vitro* study in rats, administration of *Shi Xiao San* was associated with marked antiplatelet effect 4 hours after oral ingestion. The researchers noted that this formula has an antiplatelet effect comparable to aspirin.[3]
3. **Effect on the uterus**: According to clinical studies, *Shi Xiao San* has a marked regulatory effect on the uterus. It may stimulate contraction of the uterus to facilitate passage of placental remnants in postpartum women,

or relax smooth muscle to relieve menstrual cramps in women with dysmenorrhea or premenstrual syndrome.[4]

CLINICAL STUDIES AND RESEARCH

1. **Dysmenorrhea**: Many studies have reported success using *Shi Xiao San* to treat painful menstruation. According to one study, use of the formula in 108 women with dysmenorrhea was associated with significant relief in 72 cases, moderate improvement in 34 cases, and no effect in 2 cases. The treatment started herbal therapy 2-3 days prior to the period, for 5-7 packs of herbs per course of treatment.[5] Another study reported 97.5% effectiveness using this formula to treat 80 patients with dysmenorrhea. The treatment protocol was to administer one pack of herbs in decoction daily, starting 3 days before the period, for 6 packs of herbs per course of treatment, for a total of 3 menstrual cycles.[6]
2. **Endometriosis**: Thirty patients with endometriosis were treated with herbs, with complete recovery in 12 cases, marked improvement in 16 cases, and no effect in 2 cases. The herbal treatment contained dry-fried *Pu Huang* (Pollen Typhae) 8g, *Wu Ling Zhi* (Faeces Trogopteri) 12g, *Xue Jie* (Sanguis Draconis) 1.5g, and *San Qi* (Radix et Rhizoma Notoginseng) 1.5g.[7]
3. **Uterine bleeding**: According to one study, women with excessive uterine bleeding (in volume or duration) were treated with 84.7% effectiveness using *Dang Gui* (Radix Angelicae Sinensis) 9-12g, *Chuan Xiong* (Rhizoma Chuanxiong) 6-9g, *Pu Huang* (Pollen Typhae) 6-9g, dry-fried *Wu Ling Zhi* (Faeces Trogopteri) 10g, and *Tao Ren* (Semen Persicae) 10g. Of 59 patients, the study reported marked improvement in 43 cases, moderate improvement in 7 cases, and no effect in 9 cases.[8]
4. **Uterine bleeding caused by miscarriage**: *Shi Xiao San* has been shown to be effective in stopping bleeding in women with profuse bleeding following miscarriage. Most treatment protocols use *Shi Xiao San* as the base formula, with the addition of *Gui Zhi Fu Ling Wan* (Cinnamon Twig and Poria Pill) to discharge placental remnants, *Bu Zhong Yi Qi Tang* (Tonify the Middle and Augment the Qi Decoction) and/or *Gui Pi Tang* (Restore the Spleen Decoction) for qi and blood deficiencies, and heat-clearing herbs for infection.[9,10]

Shi Xiao San (Sudden Smile Powder)

Diagnosis	Signs and Symptoms	Treatment	Herbs
Blood stasis in the body	Abdominal pain, postpartum bleeding due to retention of lochia, irregular menstruation, and sharp pain in the lower abdomen: blood stasis with obstructed blood circulation	• Activates blood circulation and removes blood stasis • Disperses stagnation and stops pain	• *Wu Ling Zhi* (Faeces Trogopteri) activates blood circulation, removes blood stagnation, and relieves pain. • *Pu Huang* (Pollen Typhae) activates blood circulation, stops bleeding, and relieves pain.

912

Shī Xiào Sǎn (Sudden Smile Powder)

5. **Angina pectoris and coronary artery disease**: One study reported good results using *Shi Xiao San* to treat 46 patients with angina and coronary artery disease. The herbal formula contained 15g each of *Wu Ling Zhi* (Faeces Trogopteri), *Pu Huang* (Pollen Typhae), *Chuan Xiong* (Rhizoma Chuanxiong), *Tao Ren* (Semen Persicae), and *Hong Hua* (Flos Carthami). The treatment protocol was to administer the herbs in decoction daily, for 1 month per course of treatment, for 1-5 courses total. Of 44 patients, the study reported 88.6% effectiveness based on symptomatic evaluation, and 28.1% effectiveness based on EKG readings.[11]

6. **Viral hepatitis**: One study of 200 patients with viral hepatitis reported a 70% recovery rate using *Shi Xiao San* plus *Yin Chen Hao Tang* (Artemisia Scoparia Decoction). The base formula contained *Wu Ling Zhi* (Faeces Trogopteri) 10-15g, dry-fried *Pu Huang* (Pollen Typhae) 10-15g, *Yin Chen* (Herba Artemisiae Scopariae) 30-60g, *Zhi Zi* (Fructus Gardeniae) 10g, and *Da Huang* (Radix et Rhizoma Rhei) 10-30g. Other herbs were added depending on the condition of the individual. For acute hepatitis with jaundice, *Huang Bo* (Cortex Phellodendri Chinensis), *Yi Yi Ren* (Semen Coicis), *Fu Ling* (Poria), *Yu Jin* (Radix Curcumae), *Pu Gong Ying* (Herba Taraxaci), and *Jin Qian Cao* (Herba Lysimachiae) were added. For acute hepatitis without jaundice, *Long Dan* (Radix et Rhizoma Gentianae), *Mu Dan Pi* (Cortex Moutan), *Ze Xie* (Rhizoma Alismatis), *Fu Ling* (Poria), *Yi Yi Ren* (Semen Coicis), *Che Qian Zi* (Semen Plantaginis), *Mu Tong* (Caulis Akebiae), and *Chi Shao* (Radix Paeoniae Rubra) were added. For chronic infectious hepatitis, *Yu Jin* (Radix Curcumae), *Yan Hu Suo* (Rhizoma Corydalis), *Bai Shao* (Radix Paeoniae Alba), *Dang Gui* (Radix Angelicae Sinensis), *Chuan Xiong* (Rhizoma Chuanxiong), *Bai Zhu* (Rhizoma Atractylodis Macrocephalae), *Ji Nei Jin* (Endothelium Corneum Gigeriae Galli), and *Yi Yi Ren* (Semen Coicis) were added. For chronic active hepatitis, *Chi Shao* (Radix Paeoniae Rubra), *Mu Dan Pi* (Cortex Moutan), *Long Dan* (Radix et Rhizoma Gentianae), vinegar-processed *Chai Hu* (Radix Bupleuri), *Yu Jin* (Radix Curcumae), *Pu Gong Ying* (Herba Taraxaci), *Zhi Qiao* (Fructus Aurantii), *Yan Hu Suo* (Rhizoma Corydalis), and *Bai Hua She She Cao* (Herba Hedyotis) were added. With hepatomegaly or splenomegaly, *Dang Gui* (Radix Angelicae Sinensis), *Bai Shao* (Radix Paeoniae Alba), *Chuan Xiong* (Rhizoma Chuanxiong), *Yu Jin* (Radix Curcumae), *Yan Hu Suo* (Rhizoma Corydalis), *Zhi Qiao* (Fructus Aurantii), processed *Bie Jia* (Carapax Trionycis), *San Leng* (Rhizoma Sparganii), *E Zhu* (Rhizoma Curcumae), and *Bai Hua She She Cao* (Herba Hedyotis) were added. Of 139 patients with acute viral hepatitis, 112 experienced complete recovery. Of 61 patients with chronic viral hepatitis, 28 had recovered completely.[12]

RELATED FORMULAS

Shǒu Niān Sǎn (Pinch Powder)

手拈散

Pinyin Name: *Shou Nian San*
Literal Name: Pinch Powder
Original Source: *Qi Xiao Liang Fang* (Fine Formulas with Miraculous Results)

Yan Hu Suo (Rhizoma Corydalis)
Wu Ling Zhi (Faeces Trogopteri)
Cao Guo (Fructus Tsaoko)
Mo Yao (Myrrha)

The source text states to grind equal amounts of all the ingredients into a powder, and take 6g per dose with boiled water. This formula activates blood circulation, removes blood stagnation, activates qi circulation, and relieves pain. Clinically, it may be used for epigastric or abdominal pain due to qi and blood stagnation.

Shou Nian San (Pinch Powder) is a stronger and warmer formula than *Shi Xiao San*, and is more appropriate for treating pain characterized by cold and blood stagnation.

Wēn Jīng Zhǐ Tòng Tāng

(Warm the Channels and Stop Pain Decoction)

溫經止痛湯
温经止痛汤

Pinyin Name: *Wen Jing Zhi Tong Tang*
Literal Name: Warm the Channels and Stop Pain Decoction
Original Source: *Jian Tai Zhen Suo Fang* (Herbal Prescriptions from *Jiantai* Clinic) by Chang Wei-Yen in 1981

Pu Huang (Pollen Typhae)
Yan Hu Suo (Rhizoma Corydalis)
Ai Ye (Folium Artemisiae Argyi)
Gui Zhi (Ramulus Cinnamomi)
Wu Yao (Radix Linderae)
Xiang Fu (Rhizoma Cyperi)
Dang Gui (Radix Angelicae Sinensis)
Chuan Xiong (Rhizoma Chuanxiong)
Chi Shao (Radix Paeoniae Rubra)
Tao Ren (Semen Persicae)
Hong Hua (Flos Carthami)
Mu Dan Pi (Cortex Moutan)
Niu Xi (Radix Achyranthis Bidentatae)

Wen Jing Zhi Tong Tang (Warm the Channels and Stop Pain Decoction) is designed to treat menstrual disorders

BLOOD-REGULATING FORMULAS

13

913

Chapter 13 – Blood-Regulating Formulas　　　　*Section 1 – Blood-Invigorating and Stasis-Removing Formulas*

Shī Xiào Sǎn (Sudden Smile Powder)

characterized by qi stagnation and blood stasis. Clinical applications include dysmenorrhea with bloating, cramping, pain, and blood clots; endometriosis with severe menstrual cramping and pain; and pain associated with various gynecological disorders.

AUTHORS' COMMENTS

Shi Xiao San is one of the best formulas for dysmenorrhea. The main emphasis of this formula is to activate blood, dispel blood stasis, and relieve pain. It does not have a strong qi-activating function. Because blood and qi stagnation often occur together, this formula should be modified as needed.

The literal translation of *Shi Xiao San* on a word-for-word basis is *shi* (lose) *xiao* (smile) *san* (powder). However, this literal translation is misleading and does not convey the meaning of the formula. When *Shi Xiao San* is prescribed to treat severe pain associated with dysmenorrhea, the formula has such a strong and immediate effect to relieve pain that the patients break into a "sudden smile." They are often at a loss to know why the pain disappeared so quickly. So, while the literal translation of *Shi Xiao San* is

"lose a smile powder," the actual meaning is "at-a-loss and smile powder."

References

1. *Shan Xi Yi Yao Za Zhi* (Shanxi Journal of Medicine and Herbology) 1974;8:11.
2. *Shan Xi Yi Yao Za Zhi* (Shanxi Journal of Medicine and Herbology) 1974;8:17.
3. *Zhong Yao Xian Dai Yan Jiu Yu Ying Yong* (Modern Study of Traditional Chinese Medicine) 1997;1087.
4. *Shang Hai Zhong Yi Yao Za Zhi* (Shanghai Journal of Chinese Medicine and Herbology) 1963;9:1.
5. *Xin Jiang Zhong Yi Yao* (Xinjiang Chinese Medicine and Herbology) 1986;1:32.
6. *He Bei Zhong Yi* (Hebei Chinese Medicine) 1991;3:16.
7. *Jiang Su Zhong Yi* (Jiangsu Chinese Medicine) 1990;8:14.
8. *Hu Bei Zhong Yi Za Zhi* (Hubei Journal of Chinese Medicine) 1990;4:17.
9. *Zhe Jiang Zhong Yi Xue Yuan Xue Bao* (Journal of Zhejiang University of Chinese Medicine) 1985;2:20.
10. *Hu Bei Zhong Yi Za Zhi* (Hubei Journal of Chinese Medicine) 1986;2:42.
11. *Xin Yi Yao Xue Za Zhi* (New Journal of Medicine and Herbology) 1976;5:41.
12. *Hu Bei Zhong Yi Za Zhi* (Hubei Journal of Chinese Medicine) 1985;5:17.

Huó Luò Xiào Líng Dān

(Fantastically Effective Pill to Invigorate the Collaterals)

活絡效靈丹
活络效灵丹

Pinyin Name: *Huo Luo Xiao Ling Dan*
Literal Name: Fantastically Effective Pill to Invigorate the Collaterals
Original Source: *Yi Xue Zhong Zhong Can Xi Lu* (Records of Heart-Felt Experiences in Medicine With Reference to the West) by Zhang Xi-Chun in 1918-34

COMPOSITION

Dan Shen (Radix et Rhizoma Salviae Miltiorrhizae)	15g
Ru Xiang (Gummi Olibanum), fresh	15g
Mo Yao (Myrrha), fresh	15g
Dang Gui (Radix Angelicae Sinensis)	15g

DOSAGE / PREPARATION / ADMINISTRATION

Prepare as a decoction. This formula may also be administered in powder form. Grind the ingredients with the doses stated above into powder. Take the powder in four equally-divided doses with a warm, grain-based liquor.

CHINESE THERAPEUTIC ACTIONS

1. Activates blood circulation and dispels blood stasis
2. Unblocks the collaterals and relieves pain

Chinese Herbal Formulas and Applications

Huó Luò Xiào Líng Dān
(Fantastically Effective Pill to Invigorate the Collaterals)

CLINICAL MANIFESTATIONS

Qi and blood stagnation: heart and abdominal pain, pain of the arms and legs, bruises and swelling due to trauma, and other external disorders such as carbuncles, furuncles, multiple abscesses, scrofulae, and ulcers.

CLINICAL APPLICATIONS

Bi zheng (painful obstruction syndrome), heel pain, sciatica, ischemic stroke, coronary artery disease, angina pectoris, cerebrovascular accident, thromboangiitis obliterans, cervical spondylosis, ectopic pregnancy, and hysteromyoma.

EXPLANATION

Huo Luo Xiao Ling Dan (Fantastically Effective Pill to Invigorate the Collaterals) treats various types of pain and disorders, both external and internal, due to qi and blood stagnation. The formula uses *Dan Shen* (Radix et Rhizoma Salviae Miltiorrhizae) to invigorate blood circulation and remove blood stasis. *Ru Xiang* (Gummi Olibanum) and *Mo Yao* (Myrrha) activate qi and blood circulation to relieve pain. *Dang Gui* (Radix Angelicae Sinensis) nourishes the blood and activates blood circulation.

MODIFICATIONS

- With leg pain, add *Niu Xi* (Radix Achyranthis Bidentatae).
- With abdominal pain in women due to blood stagnation, add *Tao Ren* (Semen Persicae) and *Wu Ling Zhi* (Faeces Trogopteri).
- With yang-type sores with redness and swelling, add *Jin Yin Hua* (Flos Lonicerae Japonicae), *Lian Qiao* (Fructus Forsythiae), and *Zhi Mu* (Rhizoma Anemarrhenae).
- With yin-type sores that are hard, add *Rou Gui* (Cortex Cinnamomi) and *Lu Jiao Jiao* (Colla Cornus Cervi).
- With chronic sores that are slow to heal, add *Huang Qi* (Radix Astragali), *Zhi Mu* (Rhizoma Anemarrhenae), and *Gan Cao* (Radix et Rhizoma Glycyrrhizae).
- With abscesses of the internal organs, add *San Qi* (Radix

et Rhizoma Notoginseng) and *Niu Bang Zi* (Fructus Arctii).

CAUTIONS / CONTRAINDICATIONS

- *Huo Luo Xiao Ling Dan* is contraindicated during pregnancy and in the absence of blood stasis.[1]
- Use of this formula is sometimes associated with nausea, vomiting, and gastrointestinal discomfort. Under these circumstances, the doses of *Ru Xiang* (Gummi Olibanum) and *Mo Yao* (Myrrha) should be reduced to 6g to 9g from 15g.[2,3]

CLINICAL STUDIES AND RESEARCH

1. *Bi zheng* (painful obstruction syndrome): Administration of customized *Huo Luo Xiao Ling Dan* in 123 patients with *bi zheng* (painful obstruction syndrome) was associated with complete recovery in 102 cases, improvement in 17 cases, and no effect in 4 cases. The study stated that most patients began to notice an effect after 5 packs of herbs, improvement after 10 packs of herbs, and recovery between 20-40 packs of herbs.[4]

2. **Heel pain:** One study reported good results using modified *Huo Luo Xiao Ling Dan* to treat 60 patients with heel pain. Modifications to the formula included the addition of *Shi Hu* (Caulis Dendrobii) 15g, *Di Huang* (Radix Rehmanniae) 15g, and *Huang Bo* (Cortex Phellodendri Chinensis) 12g for yin deficiency; and *Dang Shen* (Radix Codonopsis) 12-15g and *Huang Qi* (Radix Astragali) 12-15g for qi deficiency. Of 60 patients, 45 recovered completely (able to resume normal physical activities without any restrictions), 14 experienced significant improvement (slight pain only after prolonged physical activities), and 1 had no benefit.[5]

3. **Sciatica:** *Huo Luo Xiao Ling Dan* has been shown in several studies to effectively treat sciatica. According to one study, 61 patients with sciatica were treated with good results using modified *Huo Luo Xiao Ling Dan*. Modifications to the formula included addition of *Du Huo* (Radix Angelicae Pubescentis) 10g, *Qin Jiao* (Radix

Huo Luo Xiao Ling Dan (Fantastically Effective Pill to Invigorate the Collaterals)

Diagnosis	Signs and Symptoms	Treatment	Herbs
Qi and blood stagnation	Heart and abdominal pain, pain of the arms and legs, and bruises and swelling due to trauma: qi and blood stagnation	• Activates blood and dispels blood stasis • Unblocks the collaterals and relieves pain	• *Dan Shen* (Radix et Rhizoma Salviae Miltiorrhizae) invigorates blood circulation and removes blood stasis. • *Ru Xiang* (Gummi Olibanum) and *Mo Yao* (Myrrha) activate the blood and qi to relieve pain. • *Dang Gui* (Radix Angelicae Sinensis) nourishes the blood and activates blood circulation.

BLOOD-REGULATING FORMULAS

13

915

Huó Luò Xiào Líng Dān
(Fantastically Effective Pill to Invigorate the Collaterals)

Gentianae Macrophyllae) 10g, and *Fang Feng* (Radix Saposhnikoviae) 10g for wind-cold; *Du Huo* (Radix Angelicae Pubescentis) 10g, *Ze Lan* (Herba Lycopi) 10g, and *Shen Jin Cao* (Herba Lycopodii) 20g for damp-cold; *Huang Bo* (Cortex Phellodendri Chinensis) 15g, *Zhi Mu* (Rhizoma Anemarrhenae) 10g, and *Mu Fang Ji* (Radix Cocculi Trilobi) 12g for damp-heat; and *Ma Qian Zi* (Semen Strychni) 0.3-0.9g and *Bai Zhi* (Radix Angelicae Dahuricae) 10g for severe pain. The treatment protocol was to cook the herbs in water, and administer the decoction in two equally-divided doses with a small amount of grain-based liquor daily, for 5 days per course of treatment, for 3-4 courses total. Of 61 patients, the study reported recovery in 43 cases, significant improvement in 12 cases, moderate improvement in 4 cases, and no effect in 2 cases.[6]

Another study reported 98% effectiveness using modified formulas to treat 119 patients with sciatica. The herbal treatment contained *Huo Luo Xiao Ling Dan* and *Shao Yao Gan Cao Tang* (Peony and Licorice Decoction) as the base formulas. Modifications included the addition of *Tao Ren* (Semen Persicae) and *Hong Hua* (Flos Carthami) for severe pain; *Zhi Chuan Wu* (Radix Aconiti Praeparata), *Zhi Cao Wu* (Radix Aconiti Kusnezoffii Praeparata), and *Cang Zhu* (Rhizoma Atractylodis) for severe pain during cold, rainy days; and *Wei Ling Xian* (Radix et Rhizoma Clematidis) and *Si Gua Luo* (Retinervus Luffae Fructus) for pain in the limbs. Of 119 patients, the study reported complete recovery in 89 cases, improvement in 29 cases, and no effect in 1 case.[7]

4. **Ischemic stroke**: One study reported good results when 77 patients with ischemic stroke were treated with large doses of modified *Huo Luo Xiao Ling Dan*. The herbal treatment contained 24 grams each of *Ru Xiang* (Gummi Olibanum), *Mo Yao* (Myrrha), *Dan Shen* (Radix et Rhizoma Salviae Miltiorrhizae), and *Dang Gui* (Radix Angelicae Sinensis). The duration of treatment was 10 days per course, for 3-5 courses total. Of 77 patients, the study reported near-complete recovery in 40 cases, significant improvement in 22 cases, moderate improvement in 12 cases, no effect in 2 cases, and fatality in 1 case.[8]

5. **Thromboangiitis obliterans**: Use of *Huo Luo Xiao Ling Dan* plus *Si Miao Yong An Tang* (Four-Valiant Decoction for Well-Being) in 17 patients with thromboangiitis obliterans was associated with complete recovery in 11 cases, significant improvement in 2 cases, and no effect in 4 cases. The treatment protocol was to cook the herbs in decoction, and administer the decoction in three to four equally-divided doses daily.[9]

6. **Cervical spondylosis**: One study reported good results treating cervical spondylosis using both oral and topical applications of herbs. For oral use, the herbal treatment contained *Huo Luo Xiao Ling Dan*, with the addition of *Gui Zhi* (Ramulus Cinnamomi) 5g, *Qiang Huo* (Rhizoma et Radix Notopterygii) 10g, and *Xi Xin* (Radix et Rhizoma Asari) 5g for cold; *Di Long* (Pheretima) 10g, *Ju Hua* (Flos Chrysanthemi) 10g, and *Sheng Ma* (Rhizoma Cimicifugae) 10g for heat; *Bai Jie Zi* (Semen Sinapis) 10g and *Fu Ling* (Poria) 10g for damp and phlegm; and *Qiang Huo* (Rhizoma et Radix Notopterygii) 10g and *Sang Zhi* (Ramulus Mori) 10g for numbness. The herbs were cooked in water, and the decoction was administered in three equally-divided doses, with a small amount of grain-based liquor. The herb residue (from the decoction) was combined with 50g of *Tou Gu Cao* (Caulis Impatientis) and a small amount of *Hua Jiao* (Pericarpium Zanthoxyli), cooked in water, and the resultant solution applied topically to the affected area. The duration was 5 packs of herbs per course of treatment, for 4-7 courses total. Of 50 patients, the study reported complete recovery in 23 cases, significant improvement in 17 cases, moderate improvement in 8 cases, and no effect in 2 cases.[10]

7. **Hysteromyoma**: Administration of modified *Huo Luo Xiao Ling Dan* to 29 patients with hysteromyoma was associated with complete recovery in 17 cases, significant improvement in 6 cases, moderate improvement in 4 cases, and no effect in 2 cases. The herbal treatment contained *Huo Luo Xiao Ling Dan* plus *Da Huang* (Radix et Rhizoma Rhei) and *Niu Xi* (Radix Achyranthis Bidentatae) as the base formula. Modifications were made as follows: *Fu Zi* (Radix Aconiti Lateralis Praeparata) and *Xi Xin* (Radix et Rhizoma Asari) for cold obstruction and blood stagnation; *Chuan Lian Zi* (Fructus Toosendan) and *Pu Huang* (Pollen Typhae) for qi and blood stagnation; *Bai Jiang Cao* (Herba cum Radice Patriniae) and *Pu Gong Ying* (Herba Taraxaci) for accumulation of heat and blood stagnation; *Huang Qi* (Radix Astragali) and *Dang Shen* (Radix Codonopsis) for qi deficiency and blood stagnation; *Du Zhong* (Cortex Eucommiae) and *Xu Duan* (Radix Dipsaci) for Spleen and Kidney deficiency; and *Ban Xia* (Rhizoma Pinelliae) and *Chen Pi* (Pericarpium Citri Reticulatae) for obese individuals with dampness and phlegm.[11]

8. **Ectopic pregnancy**: One study reported marked success in treating ectopic pregnancy using *Huo Luo Xiao Ling Dan* plus *Tian Hua Fen* (Radix Trichosanthis) and *Wu Gong* (Scolopendra) in decoction, two times daily for 7 days per course of treatment, for 2-3 courses. The study reported success in 46 of 50 patients.[12]

916

Huó Luò Xiào Líng Dān
(Fantastically Effective Pill to Invigorate the Collaterals)

RELATED FORMULA

Gōng Wài Yùn Fāng (Ectopic Pregnancy Formula)

宫外孕方

Pinyin Name: Gong Wai Yun Fang
Literal Name: Ectopic Pregnancy Formula
Original Source: *Shan Xi Yi Xue Yuan Yan Fang*
(Time-Tested Formulas from Shanxi Medical School)

Dan Shen (Radix et Rhizoma Salviae Miltiorrhizae)	15g
Chi Shao (Radix Paeoniae Rubra)	15g
Tao Ren (Semen Persicae)	9g

The source text states to prepare the ingredients as a decoction. *Gong Wai Yun Fang* (Ectopic Pregnancy Formula) is a time-tested formula specifically designed to treat ectopic pregnancy with symptoms such as profuse bleeding and acute onset of severe abdominal pain that starts in the lower abdomen and may extend to the entire abdomen. Please note that ectopic pregnancy is a serious, potentially life-threatening condition. Therefore, treatment of acute and emergency cases must be performed carefully, and only by qualified healthcare professionals.

References

1. *Zhong Yao Ming Fang Yao Li Yu Ying Yong* (Pharmacology and Applications of Famous Herbal Formulas) 1989;470-472.
2. *Shan Xi Xin Yi Yao* (New Medicine and Herbology of Shanxi) 1979;(11):47.
3. *Yun Nan Zhong Yi Za Zhi* (Yunan Journal of Chinese Medicine) 1983;(2):20.
4. *Hu Bei Zhong Yi Za Zhi* (Hubei Journal of Chinese Medicine) 1986;5:21.
5. *Zhe Jiang Zhong Yi Za Zhi* (Zhejiang Journal of Chinese Medicine) 1993;8:349.
6. *Si Chuan Zhong Yi* (Sichuan Chinese Medicine) 1993;9:23.
7. *Ji Lin Zhong Yi Yao* (Jilin Chinese Medicine and Herbology) 1997;2:10.
8. *Shan Xi Zhong Yi* (Shanxi Chinese Medicine) 1986;(6):152.
9. *Shan Dong Zhong Yi Za Zhi* (Shandong Journal of Chinese Medicine) 1991;5:24.
10. *Hu Bei Zhong Yi Za Zhi* (Hubei Journal of Chinese Medicine) 1993;5:14.
11. *Shan Xi Zhong Yi* (Shanxi Chinese Medicine) 1997;11:508.
12. *Bei Jing Yi Ke Da Xue Xue Bao* (Journal of Beijing University of Medicine) 1994;26(2):158.

Dān Shēn Yǐn (Salvia Decoction)

丹参饮

Pinyin Name: *Dan Shen Yin*
Literal Name: Salvia Decoction
Original Source: *Shi Fang Ge Kuo* (Collected Songs about Contemporary Formulas) by Chen Nian-Zi in 1801

COMPOSITION

Dan Shen (Radix et Rhizoma Salviae Miltiorrhizae)	30g
Tan Xiang (Lignum Santali Albi)	3-4.5g
Sha Ren (Fructus Amomi)	3-4.5g

DOSAGE / PREPARATION / ADMINISTRATION

The source text states to cook the herbs with one cup of water until the combination is reduced to 70% of its original volume. Take the strained decoction while it is warm.

CHINESE THERAPEUTIC ACTIONS

1. Activates blood circulation and removes blood stasis
2. Activates qi circulation and stops pain

CLINICAL MANIFESTATIONS

Heart [epigastric] and stomach pain due to qi and blood stagnation.

CLINICAL APPLICATIONS

Chronic atrophic gastritis, chronic gastritis, epigastric pain, and ulceration.

EXPLANATION

Dan Shen Yin (Salvia Decoction) is designed to treat heart [epigastric] and stomach pain due to qi and blood stagnation. The actual location of the pain is in the epigastrium, the area slightly below the heart. The pain is in a fixed location, and is worse with pressure upon palpation. Since this formula is slightly on the cold side, it is more suitable for epigastric pain caused by blood stagnation and heat.

Chapter 13 – Blood-Regulating Formulas   *Section 1 – Blood-Invigorating and Stasis-Removing Formulas*

Dān Shēn Yīn (Salvia Decoction)

Dan Shen Yin (Salvia Decoction)

Diagnosis	Signs and Symptoms	Treatment	Herbs
Heart [epigastric] and stomach pain due to qi and blood stagnation	Epigastric pain at a fixed location: qi and blood stagnation	• Activates blood circulation and removes blood stasis • Activates qi circulation and stops pain	• *Dan Shen* (Radix et Rhizoma Salviae Miltiorrhizae) activates blood circulation and removes blood stagnation. • *Tan Xiang* (Lignum Santali Albi) and *Sha Ren* (Fructus Amomi) activate qi circulation and relieve pain.

In this formula, a large dose of *Dan Shen* (Radix et Rhizoma Salviae Miltiorrhizae) is used to activate blood circulation and remove blood stagnation. *Tan Xiang* (Lignum Santali Albi) and *Sha Ren* (Fructus Amomi) activate qi circulation and relieve pain. Together, these three herbs activate qi and blood circulation and relieve pain.

MODIFICATIONS
• With nausea and vomiting, add *Ban Xia* (Rhizoma Pinelliae) and *Zhu Ru* (Caulis Bambusae in Taenia).
• With pain characterized by heat, add *Mu Dan Pi* (Cortex Moutan) and *Huang Qin* (Radix Scutellariae).

CAUTIONS / CONTRAINDICATIONS
Dan Shen Yin should be used with caution in patients who have bleeding disorders, because a large dose of *Dan Shen* (Radix et Rhizoma Salviae Miltiorrhizae) is used and may prolong bleeding.

PHARMACOLOGICAL EFFECTS
1. **Cardiovascular**: *Dan Shen Yin* has been shown to affect the cardiovascular system by dilating the coronary artery, increasing blood perfusion to the cardiac muscles, and reducing blood pressure.[1]
2. **Antiplatelet**: According to an *in vitro* study, administration of *Dan Shen Yin* was associated with a marked antiplatelet effect. Researchers noted the effect to be comparable to aspirin.[2]

CLINICAL STUDIES AND RESEARCH
1. **Ulceration**: According to one study, 106 patients with various types of ulcerations were treated with complete recovery in 70 cases, improvement in 31 cases, and no effect in 5 cases. The overall effectiveness was 95.3%. The herbal treatment included *Dan Shen Yin* plus *Chuan Lian Zi* (Fructus Toosendan) and *Yan Hu Suo* (Rhizoma Corydalis).[3]
2. **Chronic atrophic gastritis**: Continuous administration of modified *Dan Shen Yin* for 1-3 months was associated with a 92.7% success rate among 102 patients with chronic

atrophic gastritis characterized by blood stagnation with deficiency and cold.[4]
3. **Chronic gastritis**: Two studies reported marked effects using *Dan Shen Yin* to treat gastritis. One study reported 88.7% effectiveness in 106 patients with chronic gastritis using *Dan Shen Yin* plus *Dang Shen* (Radix Codonopsis), *Hong Hua* (Flos Carthami), and others as necessary.[5] Another study of 42 patients reported complete recovery in 20 cases and improvement in 22 cases using *Dan Shen Yin* plus *Pu Huang* (Pollen Typhae), vinegar-processed *Yan Hu Suo* (Rhizoma Corydalis), *Pu Gong Ying* (Herba Taraxaci), and others.[6]
4. **Epigastric pain**: One study of 58 patients with epigastric pain reported 98.3% effectiveness using modified *Dan Shen Yin*. The herbal treatment contained *Dan Shen Yin* plus *Fo Shou* (Fructus Citri Sarcodactylis), *Qian Nian Jian* (Rhizoma Homalomenae), *Zhi Gan Cao* (Radix et Rhizoma Glycyrrhizae Praeparata cum Melle), *Xiang Fu* (Rhizoma Cyperi), *Zi Wan* (Radix et Rhizoma Asteris), dry-fried *Bai Shao* (Radix Paeoniae Alba), processed *Da Huang* (Radix et Rhizoma Rhei), and others, depending on the pattern of disharmony. For severe qi stagnation with hypochondriac fullness and pain, *Yu Jin* (Radix Curcumae) and *Qing Pi* (Pericarpium Citri Reticulatae Viride) were added. For blood stagnation with chronic pain, *Yan Hu Suo* (Rhizoma Corydalis) and *E Zhu* (Rhizoma Curcumae) were added. For acid reflux and belching, *Zuo Jin Wan* (Left Metal Pill) and *Hai Piao Xiao* (Endoconcha Sepiae) were added. For food stagnation, charred *Shan Zha* (Fructus Crataegi), charred *Shen Qu* (Massa Fermentata), and charred *Mai Ya* (Fructus Hordei Germinatus) were added. For loose stools due to Spleen deficiency, *Dang Shen* (Radix Codonopsis) was added and *Da Huang* (Radix et Rhizoma Rhei) was removed.[7]

References
1. *Zhong Yi Ming Fang Lin Chuang Xin Yong* (Contemporary Clinical Applications of Classic Chinese Formulas) 2001;144.
2. *Zhong Yi Ming Fang Lin Chuang Xin Yong* (Contemporary Clinical Applications of Classic Chinese Formulas) 2001;144.
3. *Shan Dong Zhong Yi Za Zhi* (Shandong Journal of Chinese Medicine) 1986;2:21.

Dān Shēn Yín (Salvia Decoction)

4. *Zhong Yi Za Zhi* (Journal of Chinese Medicine) 1986;4:20.
5. *Zhong Xi Yi Jie He Za Zhi* (Journal of Integrated Chinese and Western Medicine) 1985;5:267.
6. *Guang Ming Zhong Yi* (Guangming Chinese Medicine) 1998;13(2):27.
7. *Zhe Jiang Zhong Yi Za Zhi* (Zhejiang Journal of Chinese Medicine) 1997;3:101.

Wēn Jīng Tāng (Warm the Channels Decoction)
溫經湯
温经汤

Pinyin Name: *Wen Jing Tang*
Literal Name: Warm the Channels Decoction
Alternate Names: *Wen Ching Tang*, Warm the Menses Decoction, Channel-Warming Decoction, Meridians-Warming Decoction, Tangkuei and Evodia Combination
Original Source: *Jin Gui Yao Lue* (Essentials from the Golden Cabinet) by Zhang Zhong-Jing in the Eastern Han Dynasty

COMPOSITION

Wu Zhu Yu (Fructus Evodiae)	9g
Gui Zhi (Ramulus Cinnamomi)	6g
Dang Gui (Radix Angelicae Sinensis)	6g
Chuan Xiong (Rhizoma Chuanxiong)	6g
Bai Shao (Radix Paeoniae Alba)	6g
Mu Dan Pi (Cortex Moutan)	6g
E Jiao (Colla Corii Asini)	6g
Mai Dong (Radix Ophiopogonis)	1 cup [9g]
Ren Shen (Radix et Rhizoma Ginseng)	6g
Gan Cao (Radix et Rhizoma Glycyrrhizae)	6g
Ban Xia (Rhizoma Pinelliae)	0.5 cup [6g]
Sheng Jiang (Rhizoma Zingiberis Recens)	6g

DOSAGE / PREPARATION / ADMINISTRATION

The source text states to cook the herbs in 10 cups [2,000 mL] of water until the liquid is reduced to 3 cups [600 mL]. Take the warm, strained decoction in three equally-divided doses.

CHINESE THERAPEUTIC ACTIONS

1. Warms the menses and disperses cold
2. Nourishes the blood and dispels blood stasis

CLINICAL MANIFESTATIONS

Deficiency and cold of the *chong* (thoroughfare) and *ren* (conception) channels with blood stagnation: irregular menstruation (early or delayed, prolonged or skipped menstruation, continuous menstrual bleeding, or amenorrhea), afternoon fever, irritability, hot palms and soles, dry mouth and lips, abdominal fullness, lower abdominal pain, and infertility in women.

CLINICAL APPLICATIONS

Irregular menstruation, dysmenorrhea, amenorrhea, anovulation, uterine bleeding, luteal phase defects, infertility in women, and vaginitis.

EXPLANATION

Wen Jing Tang (Warm the Channels Decoction) treats deficiency and cold of the *chong* (thoroughfare) and *ren* (conception) channels, accompanied by blood stagnation. The *chong* channel is the "sea of blood," and the *ren* channel dominates the uterus. Both of these channels originate in the lower abdomen, and are closely related to menstruation. Deficiency and cold of the *chong* and *ren* channels lead to qi and blood stagnation, causing irregular menstruation, continuous bleeding, coldness and pain in the lower abdomen, and infertility. Afternoon fever, irritability, hot palms and soles, and dry mouth and lips may occur as a result of blood deficiency and deficiency heat.

919

Chapter 13 – Blood-Regulating Formulas   *Section 1 – Blood-Invigorating and Stasis-Removing Formulas*

Wēn Jīng Tāng (Warm the Channels Decoction)

Wen Jing Tang (Warm the Channels Decoction)

Diagnosis	Signs and Symptoms	Treatment	Herbs
Deficiency and cold of the *chong* (thorough-fare) and *ren* (conception) channels with blood stagnation	• Irregular menstruation, continuous bleeding, cold-ness and pain in the lower abdomen and infertility: deficiency and cold of the *chong* (thoroughfare) and *ren* (conception) channels, accompanied by qi and blood stagnation • Afternoon fever, irritability, hot palms and soles, and dry mouth and lips: blood deficiency with deficiency heat • Abdominal fullness and lower abdominal pain: qi and blood stagnation	• Warms the menses and disperses cold • Nourishes the blood and dispels blood stasis	• *Wu Zhu Yu* (Fructus Evodiae) and *Gui Zhi* (Ramulus Cinnamomi) warm the channels, disperse cold, and open the blood vessels. • *Dang Gui* (Radix Angelicae Sinensis), *Chuan Xiong* (Rhizoma Chuanxiong) and *Bai Shao* (Radix Paeoniae Alba) nourish and activate the blood, dispel blood stasis, and regulate menstruation. • *Mu Dan Pi* (Cortex Moutan) activates blood circulation and relieves deficiency-heat symptoms. • *E Jiao* (Colla Corii Asini) and *Mai Dong* (Radix Ophiopogonis) nourish yin, moisten dryness and clear deficiency heat. • *Ren Shen* (Radix et Rhizoma Ginseng) and *Gan Cao* (Radix et Rhizoma Glycyrrhizae) tonify qi and strengthen the Spleen. • *Ban Xia* (Rhizoma Pinelliae) disperses hardness in the body to help remove blood stasis. • *Sheng Jiang* (Rhizoma Zingiberis Recens) harmonizes the herbs, warms the Stomach, and promotes digestion of food and absorption of nutrients.

This is a rather complicated syndrome characterized by deficiency and excess, and by heat and cold. Therefore, optimal treatment requires the use of herbs to warm the channels, dispel cold, nourish the blood, and dispel blood stasis. This formula uses *Wu Zhu Yu* (Fructus Evodiae) and *Gui Zhi* (Ramulus Cinnamomi) to warm the channels, disperse cold, and open the blood vessels. *Dang Gui* (Radix Angelicae Sinensis), *Chuan Xiong* (Rhizoma Chuanxiong), and *Bai Shao* (Radix Paeoniae Alba) nourish and activate the blood, dispel blood stasis, and regulate menstruation. *Mu Dan Pi* (Cortex Moutan) activates blood circulation and relieves deficiency-heat symptoms, such as afternoon fever and hot palms and soles. *E Jiao* (Colla Corii Asini) and *Mai Dong* (Radix Ophiopogonis) nourish yin, moisten dryness and clear deficiency heat. *Ren Shen* (Radix et Rhizoma Ginseng) and *Gan Cao* (Radix et Rhizoma Glycyrrhizae) tonify qi and strengthen the Spleen, which in turn produces blood and controls blood circulation. *Ban Xia* (Rhizoma Pinelliae) disperses any hardness in the body to help remove blood stasis. *Sheng Jiang* (Rhizoma Zingiberis Recens), besides harmonizing the herbs in this formula, also warms the Stomach to promote digestion of food and absorption of nutrients.

MODIFICATIONS

• With qi stagnation, add *Xiang Fu* (Rhizoma Cyperi) and *Wu Yao* (Radix Linderae).

• With qi deficiency, remove *Mu Dan Pi* (Cortex Moutan), *Chuan Xiong* (Rhizoma Chuanxiong), and *Wu Zhu Yu* (Fructus Evodiae), and add *Huang Qi* (Radix Astragali).

• With continuous, light-colored uterine bleeding, remove *Mu Dan Pi* (Cortex Moutan), and add *Ai Ye* (Folium Artemisiae Argyi) and *Shu Di Huang* (Radix Rehmanniae Praeparata).

• With *beng lou* (flooding and spotting), add *Ai Ye* (Folium Artemisiae Argyi) and increase the dose of *E Jiao* (Colla Corii Asini).

• With leukorrhea accompanied by itching, add *Jin Yin Hua* (Flos Lonicerae Japonicae), *Lian Qiao* (Fructus Forsythiae), and *Che Qian Zi* (Semen Plantaginis).

• With painful menstruation, add *Chen Pi* (Pericarpium Citri Reticulatae) and *Xiang Fu* (Rhizoma Cyperi).

• With feeling of coldness and pain in the lower abdomen, remove *Mu Dan Pi* (Cortex Moutan), *Mai Dong* (Radix Ophiopogonis), and add *Ai Ye* (Folium Artemisiae Argyi) and *Rou Gui* (Cortex Cinnamomi).

CAUTIONS / CONTRAINDICATIONS

Wen Jing Tang is contraindicated in cases characterized by excess, heat, and blood stasis.

PHARMACOLOGICAL EFFECTS

1. **Anti-inflammatory**: One study reported that *Wen Jing Tang* had an anti-inflammatory effect in treating dysmenorrhea,

920

Wēn Jīng Tāng (Warm the Channels Decoction)

Chinese Herbal Formulas and Applications

a common gynecological complaint. A preparation of *Wen Jing Tang* in rat uterine smooth muscle *in vitro* suppressed spontaneous contractions and prostaglandins F2alpha-induced contractions. *Wen Jing Tang* used in this study was extracted from a 50% alcohol solution and subsequently freeze-dried.[1]

2. **Endocrine**: According to an *in vivo* study in women with first- and second-grade amenorrhea, 8 weeks treatment with *Wen Jing Tang* induced a significant increase in plasma follicle-stimulating hormone, luteinizing hormone, and estradiol levels in both hyper- and hypo-functioning patients. The study reported that ovulation occurred in 61.3% and 66.7% of patients with first-grade amenorrhea, and in 27.3% and 22.4% of patients with second-grade amenorrhea, respectively. Based on these results, the study concluded that *Wen Jing Tang* was effective in improving gonadotropin and estradiol secretion in the treatment of either hyper- or hypo-functioning anovulatory women.[2] According to an *in vitro* study of female rats, administration of *Wen Jing Tang* at 5 or 500 mcg/mL increased luteinizing hormone release (60-95% increase) from the pituitary through hypothalamic LH-RH.[3] The study noted that *Wen Jing Tang* stimulated ovarian steroidogenesis and was attributed to stimulation of the hypothalamus-pituitary axis; increased secretion of sex steroid hormones (17-beta-estradiol and progesterone); cytokine-induced neutrophil chemoattractant with interleukin-1beta; and tumor necrosis factor alpha.[4]

3. **Effect on bone density**: According to one study on the prevention and treatment of osteoporosis, *Wen Jing Tang*, *Ba Wei Di Huang Wan* (Eight-Ingredient Pill with Rehmannia), and *Shi Quan Da Bu Tang* (All-Inclusive Great Tonifying Decoction) were administered for 49 days to rats with ovariectomy. In comparison with sham-operated rats, bone mineral density (BMD) of the tibias decreased by 20% in ovariectomized rats, but the BMD was unaffected in rats treated with herbs or 17-beta-estradiol. The study concluded that these three formulas are as effective as 17-beta-estradiol in preventing bone loss induced by ovariectomy by preserving the fine particle surface of the bone.[5]

CLINICAL STUDIES AND RESEARCH

1. **Uterine bleeding**: One study reported 96.2% effectiveness using modified *Wen Jing Tang* to treat 104 patients with uterine bleeding. The duration of treatment varied between 2-6 menstrual cycles. Of 104 patients, the study reported complete recovery in 38 cases, significant improvement in 40 cases, moderate improvement in 22 cases, and no effect in 4 cases.[6]

2. **Infertility**: Administration of modified *Wen Jing Tang* was associated with 88% effectiveness in treating 292 women with infertility. Modifications to the formula were made as follows: for early menstruation, *Tao Ren* (Semen Persicae) and *Hong Hua* (Flos Carthami) were added, and *Gui Zhi* (Ramulus Cinnamomi) and *Wu Zhu Yu* (Fructus Evodiae) were removed; for late menstruation, *Bu Gu Zhi* (Fructus Psoraleae), *Du Zhong* (Cortex Eucommiae), *Tao Ren* (Semen Persicae), and *Hong Hua* (Flos Carthami) were added, and *Mu Dan Pi* (Cortex Moutan) and *Mai Dong* (Radix Ophiopogonis) were removed; and for irregular menstruation (early or late), *Chai Hu* (Radix Bupleuri), *Yu Jin* (Radix Curcumae), and *Xiang Fu* (Rhizoma Cyperi) were added. For hypermenorrhea, *Xu Duan* (Radix Dipsaci), *Sang Ji Sheng* (Herba Taxilli), and *Lu Jiao Jiao* (Colla Cornus Cervi) were added; and for hypomenorrhea, *San Leng* (Rhizoma Sparganii), *Chuan Shan Jia* (Squama Manis), and *Yi Mu Cao* (Herba Leonuri) were added. The treatment protocol was to administer the herbs in decoction, starting on the first day of the period, continuously for 5 days.[7]

3. **Amenorrhea**: According to one study, use of *Wen Jing Tang* in 10 women between 20-28 years of age with amenorrhea was associated with complete recovery in 3 cases, improvement in 5 cases, and no effect in 2 cases. The treatment protocol was to administer the herbs starting at 5 g/day. The dosage was increased by 2.5 g/day for 4 weeks, to reach a final dosage of 15 g/day.[8] The mechanism of *Wen Jing Tang* to treat amenorrhea in anovulatory cycles in young women is attributed either to enhanced pituitary response to Gn-RH, or to improved pulsatile secretion of Gn-RH, which induces normalization of the diencephalon-pituitary-ovarian endocrine system in anovulatory patients.[9]

4. **Anovulation**: One study evaluated the efficacy of *Wen Jing Tang* for treating anovulation in women with high basal levels of luteinizing hormone. The study randomly divided 100 patients (38 with polycystic ovarian syndrome, and 62 with non-polycystic ovarian syndrome) into two groups: 52 were treated with *Wen Jing Tang* and 48 with placebo. The results showed that *Wen Jing Tang* induced significant decreases in plasma luteinizing hormone and significant increases in plasma estradiol levels (43.5%), in 8 weeks of herbal treatment. The rate of menstrual cycle improvement (including successful ovulation) was 50% in the polycystic ovarian syndrome group and 60% in the non-polycystic ovarian syndrome group.[10]

5. **Luteal phase defects**: One study evaluated the efficacy of *Wen Jing Tang* in treating luteal phase defects by comparing 103 subjects treated with herbs (7.5 g/day) and 94 control subjects. The study reported a 79.6% rate of correction of luteal phase defects in patients treated

BLOOD-REGULATING FORMULAS

13

921

Wēn Jīng Tāng (Warm the Channels Decoction)

with *Wen Jing Tang*, with clinical improvements such as decreased plasma luteinizing hormone, increased 17-beta-estradiol concentration in the follicular phase, increased progesterone (66.7%) in the mid-luteal phase (P < .05), development of the dominant follicle (P < .01) and endometrium (P < .001), and prolongation of the luteal phase (43%, P < .001) as measured by basal body temperature. Furthermore, the pregnancy rate in patients desiring pregnancy was 49.5% (41/83). The study concluded *Wen Jing Tang* to be an effective treatment for luteal phase defects.[11]

6. **Vaginitis**: According to one study, administration of *Wen Jing Tang* at 2.5g, three times daily for 2 weeks, was effective in treating 45 women with vaginitis due to various causes. Improvements included relief of sensations of burning, itching, discomfort, and pain. The study also noted that this formula may be used topically as an herbal wash or vaginal suppository.[12]

HERB-DRUG INTERACTION

Clomiphene citrate: According to one study, 16 infertile women who did not respond to clomiphene citrate alone were successfully treated with a combination of *Wen Jing Tang* and clomiphene citrate. The treatment protocol involved administration of *Wen Jing Tang* at a dose of 5 g/day every day from day 2 of the menstrual cycle, and clomiphene citrate at 150mg a day for 5 days from day 5 of the cycle. The study reported that ovulation occurred in 43.8% of the patients, and 48.6% of the cycles. No cases of ovarian hyperstimulation syndrome were observed. The researchers concluded that the combination of *Wen Jing Tang* and clomiphene citrate is an effective treatment for infertility due to anovulation, and should be used first before therapy with human menopausal gonadotropin.[13]

AUTHORS' COMMENTS

Depending on the context in which it is used, "*jing*" may be translated as "channels" (*jing mai*, channels and collaterals), or "menses" (*yue jing*, monthly menses). Therefore, *Wen Jing Tang* is translated in various texts as either "Warm the Channels Decoction" or "Warm the Menses Decoction."

Wen Jing Tang is literally known as "Warm the Channels Decoction" because it warms and tonifies cold and

deficiency in the *chong* (thoroughfare) and *ren* (conception) channels to treat disorders such as irregular menstruation, dysmenorrhea, and *beng lou* (flooding and spotting).

Wen Jing Tang is commonly used to treat *beng lou* (flooding and spotting). In this case, it is normal for patients to experience more bleeding initially. However, after the blood stasis is resolved, the bleeding gradually will cease.

References

1. Hsu CS, Yang JK, Yang LL. Effect of a dysmenorrhea Chinese medicinal prescription on uterus contractility in vitro. Phytother Res 2003 Aug;17(7):778-83.
2. Ushiroyama T, Hosotani T, Yamashita Y, Yamashita H, Ueki M. Effects of Unkei-to on FSH, LH and estradiol in anovulatory young women with hyper- or hypo-functioning conditions. Am J Chin Med 2003;31(5):763-71.
3. Miyake A, Lee JW, Tasaka K, Ohtsuka S, Aono T. Wen-jing-tang, a traditional Chinese herbal medicine increases luteinizing hormone release in vitro. Am J Chin Med 1986;14(3-4):157-60.
4. Yasui T, Matsuzaki T, Ogata R, Kiyokawa M, Ushigoe K, Uemura H, Kuwahara A, Ikawa H, Maegawa M, Furumoto H, Aono T, Irahara M. The herbal medicine Unkei-to stimulates the secretion of a cytokine-induced neutrophil chemoattractant, CINC/gro, in the rat ovarian cell culture. Am J Reprod Immunol 2003 Jan;49(1):14-20.
5. Hidaka S, Okamoto Y, Nakajima K, Suekawa M, Liu SY. Preventive effects of traditional Chinese (Kampo) medicines on experimental osteoporosis induced by ovariectomy in rats. Calcif Tissue Int 1997 Sep;61(3):239-46.
6. *Zhe Jiang Zhong Yi Za Zhi* (Zhejiang Journal of Chinese Medicine) 1993;28(7):299.
7. *Shan Xi Zhong Yi* (Shanxi Chinese Medicine) 1996;6:250.
8. *He Han Yi Yao Xue Hui Zhi* (Hehan Journal of Medicine and Herbology) 1986;3(3):233.
9. Ushiroyama T, Tsubokura S, Ikeda A, Ueki M. The effect of unkei-to on pituitary gonadotropin secretion and ovulation in anovulatory cycles of young women. Am J Chin Med 1995;23(3-4):223-30.
10. Ushiroyama T, Ikeda A, Sakai M, Hosotani T, Suzuki Y, Tsubokura S, Ueki M. Effects of unkei-to, an herbal medicine, on endocrine function and ovulation in women with high basal levels of luteinizing hormone secretion. Journal of Reproductive Medicine 2001 May;46(5):451-6.
11. Ushiroyama T, Ikeda A, Higashio S, Hosotani T, Yamashita H, Yamashita Y, Suzuki Y, Ueki M. Unkei-to for correcting luteal phase defects. Journal of Reproductive Medicine 2003 Sep;48(9):729-34.
12. *Zhong Cheng Yao* (Study of Chinese Patent Medicine) 1990;12(1):44.
13. Yoshimoto Y, Miyake A, Tasaka K, Aono T, Tanizawa O. Ovulation following combined therapy with wen-jing-tang and clomiphene citrate therapy in anovulatory women. Am J Chin Med 1989;17(3-4):243-4.

Chinese Herbal Formulas and Applications

Ài Fù Nuǎn Gōng Wán
(Mugwort and Cyperus Pill for Warming the Womb)

艾附暖宫丸
艾附暖宫丸

Pinyin Name: Ai Fu Nuan Gong Wan
Literal Name: Mugwort and Cyperus Pill for Warming the Womb
Alternate Name: Mugwort and Cyperus Combination
Original Source: *Ren Zhai Zhi Zhi* (Straight Directions of Benevolent Aid) by Yang Tu-Ying in 1264

COMPOSITION

Ai Ye (Folium Artemisiae Argyi), large leaves without twigs	90g [6g]
Xiang Fu (Rhizoma Cyperi), *zhu* (boiled) with vinegar, *dao* (pounded) into paste, and *bei* (stone baked) till dry in low heat	180g [12g]
Wu Zhu Yu (Fructus Evodiae), without twigs	90g [6g]
Rou Gui (Cortex Cinnamomi)	15g [5g]
Huang Qi (Radix Astragali)	90g [6g]
Dang Gui (Radix Angelicae Sinensis), *xi* (washed) with liquor	90g [6g]
Chuan Xiong (Rhizoma Chuanxiong)	90g [6g]
Bai Shao (Radix Paeoniae Alba), *chao* (dry-fried) with liquor	90g [6g]
Xu Duan (Radix Dipsaci)	45g [5g]
Di Huang (Radix Rehmanniae), *xi* (washed) with liquor and *bei* (stone baked) till dry	30g [6g]

DOSAGE / PREPARATION / ADMINISTRATION

The source text states to grind all of the ingredients into a fine powder and form into small pills with rice vinegar. The pills should resemble the size of *Wu Tong Zi* (Semen Firmianae), a small seed approximately 5 mm in diameter. Take 50-70 pills [6g] between meals with water mixed with a small amount of vinegar. Today, this formula may be prepared as a decoction with the doses suggested in brackets.

CHINESE THERAPEUTIC ACTIONS

1. Warms the uterus and the channels
2. Nourishes the blood and activates blood circulation

CLINICAL MANIFESTATIONS

Deficiency and cold of the uterus: leukorrhea, sallow and yellowish facial complexion, painful limbs, lethargy, low energy, decreased food intake, irregular menstruation, occasional lower abdominal pain, and infertility.

CLINICAL APPLICATIONS

Irregular menstruation and female infertility.

EXPLANATION

Ai Fu Nuan Gong Wan (Mugwort and Cyperus Pill for Warming the Womb) warms the uterus and channels [*chong* (thoroughfare) and *ren* (conception) channels], nourishes the blood, and activates blood circulation.

In this formula, *Ai Ye* (Folium Artemisiae Argyi) and *Xiang Fu* (Rhizoma Cyperi) are the chief herbs. *Ai Ye* (Folium Artemisiae Argyi) warms the channels, dispels cold, and relieves pain. *Xiang Fu* (Rhizoma Cyperi) regulates qi and relieves menstrual pain. *Wu Zhu Yu* (Fructus Evodiae) and *Rou Gui* (Cortex Cinnamomi) warm the channels, dispel cold, and activate the blood. *Huang Qi* (Radix Astragali) tonifies qi and lifts yang. *Dang Gui* (Radix Angelicae Sinensis), *Chuan Xiong* (Rhizoma Chuanxiong), and *Bai Shao* (Radix Paeoniae Alba) regulate menstruation by activating and nourishing the blood. *Xu Duan* (Radix Dipsaci) stops bleeding with its hemostatic action. *Di Huang* (Radix Rehmanniae) nourishes yin and promotes the secretion of body fluids.

CAUTIONS / CONTRAINDICATIONS

- The source text recommends avoiding raw or cold foods while taking *Ai Fu Nuan Gong Wan*.
- Patients should control their emotions, and avoid becoming angry or irritated.

CLINICAL STUDIES AND RESEARCH

Infertility: Use of modified *Ai Fu Nuan Gong Wan* was shown to have some effectiveness in treating 50 women with infertility. The herbal formula contained the original formula plus *Pu Huang* (Pollen Typhae), *Tu Si Zi* (Semen Cuscutae), and *Yi Mu Cao* (Herba Leonuri). The treatment protocol was to cook the herbs in water, and

Chapter 13 – Blood-Regulating Formulas 　　　　*Section 1 – Blood-Invigorating and Stasis-Removing Formulas*

Ài Fù Nuǎn Gōng Wán
(Mugwort and Cyperus Pill for Warming the Womb)

Ai Fu Nuan Gong Wan (Mugwort and Cyperus Pill for Warming the Womb)

Diagnosis	Signs and Symptoms	Treatment	Herbs
Deficiency and cold of the uterus	• Leukorrhea, sallow and yellowish facial complexion, irregular menstruation and infertility: deficiency and cold of the uterus • Lethargy, lack of energy, decreased food intake, and painful limbs: deficiency and cold	• Warms the uterus and channels • Nourishes and activates blood	• *Ai Ye* (Folium Artemisiae Argyi) warms the channels, dispels cold, and relieves pain. • *Xiang Fu* (Rhizoma Cyperi) regulates qi and relieves menstrual pain. • *Wu Zhu Yu* (Fructus Evodiae) and *Rou Gui* (Cortex Cinnamomi) warm the channels, dispel cold, and activate the blood. • *Huang Qi* (Radix Astragali) tonifies qi and lifts yang. • *Dang Gui* (Radix Angelicae Sinensis), *Chuan Xiong* (Rhizoma Chuanxiong), and *Bai Shao* (Radix Paeoniae Alba) regulate menstruation, and activate and nourish the blood. • *Xu Duan* (Radix Dipsaci) stops bleeding. • *Di Huang* (Radix Rehmanniae) nourishes yin and promotes the secretion of body fluids.

administer the decoction in three equally-divided doses daily. After 6 months of treatment, the study reported pregnancy in 25 cases, improved regularity of menstrual cycles (but not yet pregnant) in 19 cases, and no effect in 6 cases.[1] In another study, use of modified *Ai Fu Nuan Gong Wan* was effective in treating infertility due to such causes as irregular menstruation, blocked fallopian tubes, and abnormal development of the uterus. Of 72 patients, 65 successfully became pregnant, 4 had marked improvement of lower abdominal pain, and 3 had no benefit. The duration of treatment ranged from 1-12 months.[2]

AUTHORS' COMMENTS

Ai Fu Nuan Gong Wan and *Wen Jing Tang* (Warm the Channels Decoction) have similar functions in treating deficiency and cold of the uterus:

• *Ai Fu Nuan Gong Wan* more strongly nourishes the blood and warms the uterus. It treats conditions characterized by deficiency and cold of the uterus with more blood deficiency.

• *Wen Jing Tang* more strongly removes blood stagnation. It treats conditions characterized by deficiency and cold of the uterus, with both blood deficiency and blood stagnation.

References
1. *Jiang Xi Zhong Yi Yao* (Jiangxi Chinese Medicine and Herbology) 1993;6:45.
2. *Shan Xi Zhong Yi* (Shanxi Chinese Medicine) 1995;11(5):20.

Chinese Herbal Formulas and Applications

Shēng Huà Tāng (Generation and Transformation Decoction)

生化湯
生化汤

Pinyin Name: *Sheng Hua Tang*
Literal Name: Generation and Transformation Decoction
Alternate Names: Blood-Producing and Clotting-Cleaning Decoction, Blood-Regenerating and Stasis-Resolving Decoction, Tangkuei and Ginger Combination
Original Source: *Fu Qing Zhu Nu Ke* (Women's Diseases According to Fu Qing-Zhu) by Fu Shan in 1827

COMPOSITION

Dang Gui (Radix Angelicae Sinensis)	24g
Chuan Xiong (Rhizoma Chuanxiong)	9g
Tao Ren (Semen Persicae)	14 pieces [6g]
Pao Jiang (Rhizoma Zingiberis Praeparatum), *pao* (blast-fried) till black	1.5g
Zhi Gan Cao (Radix et Rhizoma Glycyrrhizae Praeparata cum Melle)	1.5g

DOSAGE / PREPARATION / ADMINISTRATION

The source text states to prepare the ingredients as a decoction by cooking the herbs in a liquid made of equal amounts of grain-based liquor and *Tong Bian* (Infantis Urina). Today the herbs are usually decocted with water, with or without the addition of a grain-based liquor.

CHINESE THERAPEUTIC ACTIONS

1. Activates blood circulation and dispels blood stasis
2. Warms the channels and relieves pain

CLINICAL MANIFESTATIONS

Postpartum blood deficiency with cold: retention of lochia causing bleeding, and a cold sensation with pain in the lower abdomen.

CLINICAL APPLICATIONS

Postpartum care to relieve pain and stop bleeding, end retention of lochia, resolve lower abdominal pain caused by blood stasis, hysteromyoma or metrypertrophia, ectopic pregnancy, and uterine bleeding caused by abortion or miscarriage.

EXPLANATION

Sheng Hua Tang (Generation and Transformation Decoction) is designed to treat postpartum blood deficiency complicated by cold invasion and blood stasis. After delivery, the mother's body is naturally blood deficient. Consequently, the deficient state of the body enables the cold pathogenic factor to invade the body and cause cold stagnation and blood stasis, producing clinical manifestations of continuous bleeding with a cold sensation and pain in the lower abdomen.

To successfully treat this syndrome, herbs need to be prescribed to tonify postpartum blood deficiency and eliminate blood stagnation. These two methods cannot be used separately because use of only blood tonics may

BLOOD-REGULATING FORMULAS

13

Sheng Hua Tang (Generation and Transformation Decoction)

Diagnosis	Signs and Symptoms	Treatment	Herbs
Postpartum blood deficiency with cold	• Postpartum bleeding: retention of lochia • Cold sensation with pain in the lower abdomen: cold accumulation and blood stagnation	• Activates blood circulation and dispels blood stasis • Warms the channels and stops pain	• *Dang Gui* (Radix Angelicae Sinensis) nourishes the blood and activates blood circulation. • *Chuan Xiong* (Rhizoma Chuanxiong) activates qi and blood circulation. • *Tao Ren* (Semen Persicae) activates the blood and breaks up blood stagnation. • *Pao Jiang* (Rhizoma Zingiberis Praeparatum) warms the channels, disperses cold, and relieves pain. • *Zhi Gan Cao* (Radix et Rhizoma Glycyrrhizae Praeparata cum Melle) harmonizes the herbs.

925

Chapter 13 – Blood-Regulating Formulas　　　*Section 1 – Blood-Invigorating and Stasis-Removing Formulas*

Shēng Huà Tāng (Generation and Transformation Decoction)

create more blood stasis, and use of only blood-invigorating herbs will exacerbate blood deficiency. Therefore, the optimal treatment is to incorporate both methods to generate blood production and transform blood stasis.

This formula has *Dang Gui* (Radix Angelicae Sinensis) to nourish the blood and activate blood circulation. *Chuan Xiong* (Rhizoma Chuanxiong) activates qi and blood circulation. *Tao Ren* (Semen Persicae) activates blood circulation and breaks up blood stagnation. *Pao Jiang* (Rhizoma Zingiberis Praeparatum) warms the channels, disperses cold, and relieves pain. *Zhi Gan Cao* (Radix et Rhizoma Glycyrrhizae Praeparata cum Melle) harmonizes the herbs in this formula. Lastly, the grain-based liquor warms and opens the channels and blood vessels, and potentiates the effects of the herbs. *Tong Bian* (Infantis Urina) benefits the yang and dissolves blood stasis. Overall, this formula tonifies blood, activates blood circulation, removes blood stasis, warms the channels, and relieves pain.

MODIFICATIONS

- With postpartum abdominal pain due to blood stagnation, add *Hong Hua* (Flos Carthami) and *Bai Shao* (Radix Paeoniae Alba).
- With severe postpartum abdominal pain due to blood stagnation, add *Pu Huang* (Pollen Typhae), *Wu Ling Zhi* (Faeces Trogopteri), and *Yan Hu Suo* (Rhizoma Corydalis).
- With postpartum lower abdominal coldness and pain, add *Rou Gui* (Cortex Cinnamomi) and *Xiao Hui Xiang* (Fructus Foeniculi).
- If the lower abdominal pain is not severe, remove *Tao Ren* (Semen Persicae).
- With postpartum fever, add *Chai Hu* (Radix Bupleuri) and *Huang Qin* (Radix Scutellariae).
- With postpartum qi deficiency and increased risk of qi collapse, wait until after all the placental remains have been fully discharged, then add *Ren Shen* (Radix et Rhizoma Ginseng) and *Huang Qi* (Radix Astragali).
- For postpartum constipation, add *Rou Cong Rong* (Herba Cistanches) and *Zhi Qiao* (Fructus Aurantii).

CAUTIONS / CONTRAINDICATIONS

- Use of this formula is contraindicated during pregnancy.
- Because many herbs in *Sheng Hua Tang* are warm in nature, this formula is not suitable for patients with blood stagnation accompanied by interior heat.
- Although this formula effectively treats retention of lochia, it is not necessary to use this formula for all postpartum women, as many are able to discharge placental remains smoothly. It should be used only when needed,

in cases of retention of lochia that are characterized by cold and blood stasis. [1]

PHARMACOLOGICAL EFFECTS

1. **Effect on the uterus**: According to an *in vitro* study, administration of *Sheng Hua Tang* was associated with increased uterine contractions in mice, especially pregnant ones. [2]
2. **Anticoagulant**: An *in vitro* study showed *Sheng Hua Tang* to have a marked anticoagulant effect. [3]

CLINICAL STUDIES AND RESEARCH

1. **Postpartum care**: *Sheng Hua Tang* has been used as the standard herbal therapy for postpartum care in traditional Chinese medicine, with its actions well-documented by clinical studies. It has been shown to effectively treat retention of lochia, [4] to facilitate return of the uterus to its normal position, [5] to relieve pain associated with uterine contractions, [6] and to address many postpartum complications. [7]
2. **Retention of lochia**: Retention of lochia was successfully treated in 32 of 34 patients using *Sheng Hua Tang* plus *Zhi Qiao* (Fructus Aurantii), and others as needed. [8]
3. **Hysteromyoma or metrypertrophia**: Hysteromyoma or metrypertrophia were treated successfully using *Sheng Hua Tang* plus dry-fried *Jing Jie* (Herba Schizonepetae) and *Yi Mu Cao* (Herba Leonuri) as the base formula, and the addition of *San Leng* (Rhizoma Sparganii), *E Zhu* (Rhizoma Curcumae), and *Rou Gui* (Cortex Cinnamomi) for hardness and nodules. Of 24 patients with hysteromyoma, the study reported complete recovery in 8 cases, improvement in 13 cases, and no effect in 3 cases, after 30 packs of herbs. Of 46 patients with metrypertrophia, the study reported complete recovery in 25 cases, improvement in 18 cases, and no effect in 3 cases, after 30 packs of herbs. [9]
4. **Ectopic pregnancy**: One study reported successful treatment in all 21 cases of ectopic pregnancy using modified *Sheng Hua Tang*, with the removal of *Gan Cao* (Radix et Rhizoma Glycyrrhizae) and *Pao Jiang* (Rhizoma Zingiberis Praeparatum), and the addition of *Gui Zhi* (Ramulus Cinnamomi), *Fu Ling* (Poria), *Chi Shao* (Radix Paeoniae Rubra), *Mu Dan Pi* (Cortex Moutan), and others as needed. [10]
5. **Uterine bleeding caused by abortion or miscarriage**: Many studies have reported a marked effect using modified *Sheng Hua Tang* to treat uterine bleeding due to various causes. In one study, use of *Sheng Hua Tang* and *Shi Xiao San* (Sudden Smile Powder) in 80 patients with uterine bleeding was associated with complete recovery in 72 cases, improvement in 6 cases, and no effect in 2 cases. [11] According to another report, 90 patients with

926

Chinese Herbal Formulas and Applications

Shēng Huà Tāng (Generation and Transformation Decoction)

uterine bleeding associated with abortion, miscarriage, or labor were treated with *Sheng Hua Tang* plus *Yi Mu Cao* (Herba Leonuri), *Pu Huang* (Pollen Typhae), and *Xue Yu Tan* (Crinis Carbonisatus) with good results. The duration of treatment was 5 packs of herbs per course of treatment, with most patients needing only one course of treatment.[12] Lastly, use of *Sheng Hua Tang* plus *Pu Gong Ying* (Herba Taraxaci), *Yi Mu Cao* (Herba Leonuri), and *E Jiao* (Colla Corii Asini) was associated with complete recovery in 31 of 36 patients with uterine bleeding caused by abortion. The duration of treatment ranged from 3-6 packs of herbs.[13]

RELATED FORMULA

Tōng Rú Wán (Unblock the Breast Pill)

通乳丸
通乳丸

Pinyin Name: *Tong Ru Wan*
Literal Name: Unblock the Breast Pill
Original Source: *Guang An Men Yi Yuan* (Guang An Men Hospital) in 1990

Xian Mao (Rhizoma Curculiginis)
Huang Qi (Radix Astragali)
Dang Gui (Radix Angelicae Sinensis)
Chuan Mu Tong (Caulis Clematidis Armandii)
Tong Cao (Medulla Tetrapanacis)
Bai Zhi (Radix Angelicae Dahuricae)
Wang Bu Liu Xing (Semen Vaccariae)
Yin Yang Huo (Herba Epimedii)

Tong Ru Wan (Unblock the Breast Pill) activates qi and blood circulation and unblocks stagnation in the breast.

Historically, this formula has been used primarily to promote lactation and facilitate nursing. Today, it may also be used to promote optimal growth and development of the breast.

AUTHORS' COMMENTS

Sheng Hua Tang dispels blood stasis and treats retention of lochia with lower abdominal coldness and pain. This widely-used formula is one of the most popular postpartum formulas in China today for clearing blood stasis. In certain parts of China, it is customary to give this formula immediately after delivery to ensure successful discharge of placental remnants.

References

1. *Zhong Yao Ming Fang Yao Li Yu Ying Yong* (Pharmacology and Applications of Famous Herbal Formulas) 1989.
2. *Shan Xi Yi Yao Za Zhi* (Shanxi Journal of Medicine and Herbology) 1980;9(3):6.
3. *Zhong Cheng Yao* (Study of Chinese Patent Medicine) 1993;15(1):44.
4. *Guang Dong Zhong Yi* (Guangdong Chinese Medicine) 1962;9:17.
5. *Xin Zhong Yi* (New Chinese Medicine) 1977;4:38.
6. *Zhong Yi Fang Ji Xian Dai Yan Jiu* (Modern Study of Medical Formulae in Traditional Chinese Medicine) 1997;1093-94.
7. *Jiang Xi Zhong Yi Yao* (Jiangxi Chinese Medicine and Herbology) 1960;6:25.
8. *He Nan Zhong Yi* (Henan Chinese Medicine) 1993;4:35.
9. *Shan Xi Yi Yao Za Zhi* (Shanxi Journal of Medicine and Herbology) 1980;6:21.
10. *Xin Zhong Yi* (New Chinese Medicine) 1984;11:33.
11. *Yun Nan Zhong Yi Za Zhi* (Yunan Journal of Chinese Medicine) 1988;3:43.
12. *Jiang Xi Zhong Yi Yao* (Jiangxi Chinese Medicine and Herbology) 1988;3:21.
13. *Shan Dong Zhong Yi Za Zhi* (Shandong Journal of Chinese Medicine) 1995;14(6):253.

BLOOD-REGULATING FORMULAS

13

Chapter 13 – Blood-Regulating Formulas   *Section 1 – Blood-Invigorating and Stasis-Removing Formulas*

Guì Zhī Fú Líng Wán (Cinnamon Twig and Poria Pill)

桂枝茯苓丸

Pinyin Name: *Gui Zhi Fu Ling Wan*
Literal Name: Cinnamon Twig and Poria Pill
Alternate Names: *Kuei Chih Fu Ling Wan, Qui Zhi Fu Ling Wang*, Cinnamon Twig and Hoelen Pill, Cinnamon and Hoelen Formula
Original Source: *Jin Gui Yao Lue* (Essentials from the Golden Cabinet) by Zhang Zhong-Jing in the Eastern Han Dynasty

COMPOSITION

Gui Zhi (Ramulus Cinnamomi)	[6g]
Fu Ling (Poria)	[6g]
Tao Ren (Semen Persicae)	[6g]
Mu Dan Pi (Cortex Moutan)	[6g]
Chi Shao (Radix Paeoniae Rubra)	[6g]

Note: The source text uses *Shao Yao* (Radix Paeoniae) in this formula, without specifying whether it is *Chi Shao* (Radix Paeoniae Rubra) or *Bai Shao* (Radix Paeoniae Alba). Today, *Chi Shao* (Radix Paeoniae Rubra) is usually used, as it has a better effect than *Bai Shao* (Radix Paeoniae Alba) to invigorate blood circulation and clear heat.

DOSAGE / PREPARATION / ADMINISTRATION

The source text states to grind equal amounts of the ingredients into powder and mix with honey to form into pills. The pills should resemble rabbit droppings in size. Take 1 pill before meals. If there is no response, increase to 3 pills per dose. Today this formula may be given in decoction with the doses suggested in brackets.

CHINESE THERAPEUTIC ACTIONS

1. Activates blood circulation and breaks up blood stasis
2. Disperses the formation of abnormal masses in the abdomen

CLINICAL MANIFESTATIONS

Blood stasis in the uterus (during pregnancy): instability of the fetus, continuous dripping of purplish-black blood, and abdominal pain that is worse with pressure.

CLINICAL APPLICATIONS

Hysteromyoma, oophoritic cyst, endometriosis, adnexitis, uterine myomas, uterine fibroids, ovarian cysts, lochioschesis, perimenopause with uterine leiomyomas, pelvic inflammatory disease, dysmenorrhea, amenorrhea, irregular menstruation, premenstrual syndrome, ectopic pregnancy, instability of the fetus, stillbirth, postpartum disorders, prostatic hypertrophy, male infertility with varicocele, post-ischemic brain injury, and scleroderma.

EXPLANATION

Gui Zhi Fu Ling Wan (Cinnamon Twig and Poria Pill) treats blood stasis in the womb during pregnancy. In such circumstances, blood stasis causes dripping of blood and instability of the fetus. If the blood stasis is not cleared, then the dripping of blood continues and the pregnancy will be adversely affected. However, blood-invigorating herbs must be used with extreme caution as they increase the risks of miscarriage. This formula is designed to gently and safely eliminate blood stasis and abdominal masses, without injuring the fetus or the mother.

In this formula, *Gui Zhi* (Ramulus Cinnamomi) warms the blood and opens the vessels to facilitate the smooth flow of blood. *Fu Ling* (Poria) has a draining effect, which guides blood stasis downward and eliminates it. *Fu Ling* (Poria) also strengthens the Heart and Spleen with its tonic effect, which helps to stabilize pregnancy and calm the fetus. *Tao Ren* (Semen Persicae) treats the underlying cause of the disorder by activating blood circulation and breaking up blood stasis. Blood stasis or masses in the abdomen may produce heat after an extended period; therefore, *Mu Dan Pi* (Cortex Moutan) and *Chi Shao* (Radix Paeoniae Rubra) are used to both activate blood circulation and clear the heat. The herbs are mixed with honey and administered as pills to moderate their potency and provide a gradual, gentle, and sustained effect over a long period of time.

MODIFICATIONS

- With menstrual pain and cramps, add *Xiang Fu* (Rhizoma Cyperi), *Chen Pi* (Pericarpium Citri Reticulatae), and *Yan Hu Suo* (Rhizoma Corydalis).
- With amenorrhea, add *Zhi Shi* (Fructus Aurantii Immaturus) and *Hong Hua* (Flos Carthami).
- With severe dysmenorrhea, add *Shi Xiao San* (Sudden Smile Powder) and *Yan Hu Suo* (Rhizoma Corydalis).

928

Guì Zhī Fú Líng Wán (Cinnamon Twig and Poria Pill)

Gui Zhi Fu Ling Wan (Cinnamon Twig and Poria Pill)

Diagnosis	Signs and Symptoms	Treatment	Herbs
Blood stasis in the uterus (during pregnancy)	Instability of the fetus, continuous uterine bleeding, and abdominal pain that worsens with pressure: blood stasis in the womb during pregnancy	• Activates blood circulation and breaks up blood stasis • Disperses abnormal masses formation in the abdomen	• *Gui Zhi* (Ramulus Cinnamomi) warms the blood and opens the vessels to facilitate blood circulation. • *Fu Ling* (Poria) eliminates and guides blood stasis downward. It also strengthens the Heart and Spleen to calm the fetus and stabilize pregnancy. • *Tao Ren* (Semen Persicae) activates blood circulation and breaks up blood stasis. • *Mu Dan Pi* (Cortex Moutan) and *Chi Shao* (Radix Paeoniae Rubra) activate blood circulation and clear heat.

• With severe blood stasis, add *San Leng* (Rhizoma Sparganii) and *E Zhu* (Rhizoma Curcumae).

CAUTIONS / CONTRAINDICATIONS

• *Gui Zhi Fu Ling Wan* gently treats blood stasis accompanied by minor presentation of heat. This formula is not suitable for serious conditions of blood stagnation, excess heat in the blood, and the absence of blood stasis.

• Patients with blood stasis and a deficient constitution should use *Dang Gui Shao Yao San* (Tangkuei and Peony Powder) instead of *Gui Zhi Fu Ling Wan*.

• Use of this formula has occasionally been associated with side effects such as abdominal distention and mild constipation.[1]

PHARMACOLOGICAL EFFECTS

1. **Antiplatelet**: According to clinical studies, administration of *Gui Zhi Fu Ling Wan* was associated with a marked antiplatelet effect, with potency similar to or greater than aspirin.[2] In addition, use of *Gui Zhi Fu Ling Wan* was associated with reduced blood viscosity. The onset of therapeutic action began 30 minutes after oral ingestion, and lasted up to 180 minutes.[3] This formula, however, does not seem to have a significant effect on prothrombin time (PT).[4]

2. **Anti-inflammatory**: A bolus dose of *Gui Zhi Fu Ling Wan* (60 g/kg via oral ingestion or 10 g/kg via intraperitonal injection) was associated with a marked anti-inflammatory effect in mice. The onset of action began approximately 30 minutes after administration, and lasted for up to 72 hours. It was proposed that the mechanism of this anti-inflammatory action is not related to the adrenal glands or glucocorticoids, because long-term use of this formula did not contribute to increased adrenal glands weight. Furthermore, in subjects whose adrenal glands had been surgically removed, *Gui Zhi Fu Ling Wan* had marked anti-inflammatory effect.[5]

3. **Endocrine**: Administration of *Gui Zhi Fu Ling Wan* to rats at 300 mg/kg for 14 days was associated with a marked reduction of LH and FSH.[6] *Gui Zhi Fu Ling Wan* has been shown to act as an LH-RH antagonist and/or as a weak anti-estrogen.[7]

4. **Nephroprotective**: One study reported a marked effect in retarding the progression of renal damage by administering *Gui Zhi Fu Ling Wan* to rats with diabetic nephropathy. The mechanism of this nephroprotective effect was attributed to its ability to improve metabolic abnormalities associated with diabetes.[8]

5. **Antioxidative**: Two studies reported that *Gui Zhi Fu Ling Wan* has a dose-dependent antioxidative effect to prevent the progression of atherosclerosis in cholesterol-fed rabbits.[9,10]

6. **Effect on uterine adenomyosis**: One study reported marked effects using *Gui Zhi Fu Ling Wan* to prevent and treat mice with uterine adenomyosis, a condition characterized by the abnormal growth of glands and stroma into and beyond the smooth muscle layers of the uterus. The study suggested *Gui Zhi Fu Ling Wan* to be a useful tool for the treatment of uterine adenomyosis in humans as well.[11]

CLINICAL STUDIES AND RESEARCH

1. **Pelvic inflammatory disease**: Administration of modified *Gui Zhi Fu Ling Wan* was associated with marked effectiveness in treating 200 patients with pelvic inflammatory disease. The herbal treatment contained this formula plus *Xiang Fu* (Rhizoma Cyperi), *Yan Hu Suo* (Rhizoma Corydalis), and *Dang Gui* (Radix Angelicae Sinensis).[12]

2. **Hysteromyoma**: One study reported 90% effectiveness using modified *Gui Zhi Fu Ling Wan* to treat hysteromyoma. The herbal formula contained *Gui Zhi Fu Ling Wan* plus *Chuan Shan Jia* (Squama Manis), *Gui Ban* (Plastrum Testudinis), *Bie Jia* (Carapax Trionycis), *E Zhu* (Rhizoma Curcumae), *San Leng* (Rhizoma Sparganii),

Chapter 13 – Blood-Regulating Formulas   *Section 1 – Blood-Invigorating and Stasis-Removing Formulas*

Guì Zhī Fú Líng Wán (Cinnamon Twig and Poria Pill)

and others. The treatment protocol was to begin herbal therapy starting three days after the last day of the period. The herbs were first cooked in water and concentrated to yield 100 mL of solution. This 100 mL was used as a rectal instillation. The same herbs were cooked again to yield 300 mL of herbal decoction, which was taken orally in two equally-divided doses, morning and night. Each course of treatment was 30 days. Of 40 patients, the study reported complete recovery in 4 cases, significant improvement in 14 cases, moderate improvement in 18 cases, and no effect in 4 cases.[13]

3. **Oophoritic cysts**: Use of herbs in 300 patients with oophoritic cysts was associated with a 95% rate of effectiveness. The herbal treatment contained *Gui Zhi Fu Ling Wan*, *Huang Yao Zi* (Herba Dioscoreae Bulbiferae), *Ji Nei Jin* (Endothelium Corneum Gigeriae Galli), *Shui Zhi* (Hirudo), *Li Zhi He* (Semen Litchi), and *Wu Yao* (Radix Linderae). The herbs were cooked in water, and the decoction was taken in four equally-divided doses daily. Also, *Da Huang Zhe Chong Wan* (Rhubarb and Eupolyphaga Pill) was given twice daily, morning and night. The duration of treatment ranged from 3-6 months. Of 300 patients, the study reported complete recovery in 225 cases, improvement in 30 cases, and no effect in 15 cases. Information was unavailable on 30 patients who did not complete the study.[14]

4. **Endometriosis**: One study reported marked success in treating endometriosis in 38 patients using *Gui Zhi Fu Ling Wan* plus *Da Huang* (Radix et Rhizoma Rhei) and *Gan Cao* (Radix et Rhizoma Glycyrrhizae). Modifications were made by adding *San Leng* (Rhizoma Sparganii), *E Zhu* (Rhizoma Curcumae), and *Chuan Shan Jia* (Squama Manis) in severe cases; *Ru Xiang* (Gummi Olibanum), *Mo Yao* (Myrrha) and *Lu Lu Tong* (Fructus Liquidambaris) for severe pain; large doses of *Da Huang* (Radix et Rhizoma Rhei) and *Tao Ren* (Semen Persicae) for constipation; *Huang Qi* (Radix Astragali) and *Dang Shen* (Radix Codonopsis) for generalized weakness and qi deficiency; and *Dang Gui* (Radix Angelicae Sinensis), *Xiang Fu* (Rhizoma Cyperi), and *Yi Mu Cao* (Herba Leonuri) for irregular menstruation.[15]

   According to a case report, use of *Gui Zhi Fu Ling Wan* in treating one endometriotic patient controlled the disorder and kept the patient symptom-free for more than 7 months. Furthermore, the study reported a decrease in specific IgM antibody titer without any suppression of serum CA-125 and estradiol levels.[16]

5. **Adnexitis**: Twenty patients with chronic adnexitis were treated with 90.3% effectiveness using modified *Gui Zhi Fu Ling Wan*. The duration of treatment ranged from 8-50 packs of herbs. Of 20 patients, the study reported

complete recovery in 6 cases, improvement in 12 cases, and no effect in 2 cases.[17]

6. **Uterine myomas**: Of 110 premenopausal patients with uterine myomas, administration of *Gui Zhi Fu Ling Wan* was associated with improving hypermenorrhea and dysmenorrhea in more than 90% of the cases, and shrinking uterine myomas in approximately 60% of the cases. The study proposed that *Gui Zhi Fu Ling Wan* might act as an LH-RH antagonist and a weak anti-estrogen on uterine DNA synthesis.[18]

7. **Premenstrual syndrome (PMS)**: Administration of *Gui Zhi Fu Ling Wan* in 20 patients with premenstrual syndrome was associated with 80% effectiveness. The herbs were given in powder form, with a dose of 5g per day. Of 20 patients, the study reported marked effectiveness in 6 cases, slight improvement in 10 cases, and no effect in 4 cases. The improvements were primarily associated with relief of pain in the low back and lower abdominal regions.[19]

8. **Amenorrhea**: According to one study, administration of *Gui Zhi Fu Ling Wan* was associated with a marked effect in treating amenorrhea in 20 patients with 2 months to 3 years history of illness. The study reported menstruation in 8 cases after 1-3 packs of herbs, in 7 cases after 4-6 packs of herbs, and no change in 5 cases.[20]

9. **Perimenopause with uterine leiomyomas**: One study investigated the treatment of uterine leiomyomas in 30 perimenopausal women using Chinese herbal medicines and synthetic analogs of gonadotropin-releasing hormone. The Chinese herbs used included *Gui Zhi Fu Ling Wan* and *Shao Yao Gan Cao Tang* (Peony and Licorice Decoction). The drugs used included buserelin and nafarelin given via intranasal administration. The study reported a reduction in leiomyomas (less than 60%), along with decreases in the serum levels of luteinizing hormone, follicle-stimulating hormone, estradiol, and the tumor marker CA-125. Side effects noted included slight bone loss and hypermenorrhea and/or dysmenorrhea. The study concluded that this combination of drugs and herbs could be beneficial in the treatment of uterine leiomyomas in patients a few years before menopause.[21]

10. **Prostatic hypertrophy**: According to one study, 31 patients with prostatic hypertrophy were treated with herbs resulting in recovery in 7 cases, improvement in 21 cases, and no effect in 3 cases. The herbal formula contained *Gui Zhi Fu Ling Wan* plus *Ju He* (Semen Citri Reticulatae), *Niu Xi* (Radix Achyranthis Bidentatae), *Hai Zao* (Sargassum), *Tu Bie Chong* (Eupolyphaga seu Steleophaga), *Huang Qi* (Radix Astragali), and others as needed.[22]

11. **Male infertility with varicocele**: According to one study, use of *Gui Zhi Fu Ling Wan* (7.5 g/day) for at least 3

930

Guì Zhī Fú Líng Wán (Cinnamon Twig and Poria Pill)

months was associated with marked success in treating male infertility with varicocele in 37 patients. The study reported an 80% disappearance rate (40 out of 50 varicoceles) for varicocele, 71.4% improvement in sperm concentration, and 62.1% improvement in sperm motility. The researchers considered *Gui Zhi Fu Ling Wan* to be an effective therapy for circulation disorders in varicocele as well as semen quality.[23]

12. **RBC (red blood cell) deformability**: Deterioration of RBC deformability and viscoelasticity is a condition often associated with the traditional Chinese diagnosis of "blood stasis syndrome." According to one study, the therapeutic effects of *Gui Zhi Fu Ling Wan* and pentoxifylline were compared in the treatment of multiple lacunar infarctions. Of 30 male patients, 18 were treated with 12g of *Gui Zhi Fu Ling Wan* daily for 4 weeks, and 12 were treated with pentoxifylline 300mg daily for 4 weeks. The study reported that *Gui Zhi Fu Ling Wan* had a significant effect on RBC deformability and increased intracellular ATP content, and was more effective than pentoxifylline for patients with more severe "blood stasis syndrome."[24]

13. **Post-ischemic brain injury**: According to one study, administration of three herbal formulas minimized post-ischemic brain injury by inhibiting free radicals and lipid peroxidation. The formulas that were found to be effective, both *in vitro* and *in vivo*, were *Gui Zhi Fu Ling Wan*, *Huang Lian Jie Du Tang* (Coptis Decoction to Relieve Toxicity), and *Chai Hu Jia Long Gu Mu Li Tang* (Bupleurum plus Dragon Bone and Oyster Shell Decoction).[25]

14. **Scleroderma**: According to one study that examined fibroblasts from 3 scleroderma patients and 2 normal controls, the use of *Gui Zhi Fu Ling Wan* significantly and selectively inhibited collagen synthesis in a dose-dependent manner, with a tendency for a stronger effect on scleroderma fibroblasts than on control cells.[26]

HERB-DRUG INTERACTION

Drug-induced menopause: One study evaluated the therapeutic effects of herbal medicines on menopausal symptoms induced by gonadotropin-releasing hormone-agonist therapy in Japanese women with endometriosis, adenomyosis, or leiomyoma. According to this study, menopausal symptoms induced by gonadotropin-releasing hormone-agonist therapy in 13 patients were successfully treated with *Gui Zhi Fu Ling Wan*, *Dang Gui Shao Yao San* (Tangkuei and Peony Powder), *Shao Yao Gan Cao Tang* (Peony and Licorice Decoction), *Jia Wei Xiao Yao San* (Augmented Rambling Powder), *Tao He Cheng Qi Tang* (Peach Pit Decoction to Order the Qi), or

Gui Zhi Tang (Cinnamon Twig Decoction). Most importantly, there were no significant changes in serum estradiol levels after treatment with these herbal medicines. The researchers concluded that these herbal medicines can be recommended for menopausal symptoms induced by gonadotropin-releasing hormone agonists without a negative effect on serum estradiol levels.[27]

TOXICOLOGY

Gui Zhi Fu Ling Wan has very little toxicity. Oral ingestion of this formula at 250 g/kg (maximum capacity of the stomach) in mice for one week did not cause any fatalities or abnormal reactions.[28]

RELATED FORMULAS

Duó Mìng Wán (Life-Taking Pill)
奪命丸
夺命丸

Pinyin Name: *Duo Ming Wan*
Literal Name: Life-Taking Pill
Original Source: *Fu Ren Liang Fang* (Fine Formulas for Women) by Chen Zi-Ming in 1237

Gui Zhi (Ramulus Cinnamomi)
Fu Ling (Poria)
Mu Dan Pi (Cortex Moutan)
Tao Ren (Semen Persicae)
Chi Shao (Radix Paeoniae Rubra)

Duo Ming Wan (Life-Taking Pill) has the same ingredients as *Gui Zhi Fu Ling Wan*, but in larger doses. The source text states to prepare this formula in pills, and administer 1 pill the size of a large bullet per dose with vinegar, for two consecutive doses.

This formula is used to treat cases in which a deceased fetus remains in the uterus, and the patient shows "fetus arresting the Heart" syndrome. This acute, serious condition is characterized by an extremely stuffy sensation in the chest, spontaneous cold sweating, and rapid and difficult breathing. This formula is taken with vinegar, which functions to constrict the body to relieve sweating and soften the stagnation to help eliminate the dead fetus.

Cuī Shēng Tāng (Birth-Hastening Decoction)
催生湯
催生汤

Pinyin Name: *Cui Sheng Tang*
Literal Name: Birth-Hastening Decoction
Original Source: *Ji Yin Gang Mu* (Materia Medica to Aid Yin) by Wu Zhi-Wang in 1620

BLOOD-REGULATING FORMULAS

13

931

Guì Zhī Fú Líng Wán (Cinnamon Twig and Poria Pill)

Gui Zhi (Ramulus Cinnamomi)

Fu Ling (Poria)

Mu Dan Pi (Cortex Moutan)

Tao Ren (Semen Persicae)

Chi Shao (Radix Paeoniae Rubra)

Cui Sheng Tang (Birth-Hastening Decoction) has the same ingredients as *Gui Zhi Fu Ling Wan*, but is given as a decoction.

This formula induces and facilitates delivery once the amniotic sac has been broken. However, it should be used only in patients with a strong, healthy constitution. It is given in decoction to provide a more immediate onset of action.

AUTHORS' COMMENTS

Gui Zhi Fu Ling Wan is commonly used to treat pregnant women with blood stasis in the uterus or lochia that manifests in dark black blood and low abdominal pain that worsens with pressure. Classic textbooks suggest that the dosage must be strictly followed, starting at one pill per dosage. If there is no response, the dosage may be increased up to three pills per dose. The dosage must never be drastically increased in an attempt to achieve an immediate effect. This condition can only be treated with low doses of herbs to gently dissolve and disperse blood stasis. Furthermore, this formula is prepared in honey pill form, as this dosage form slowly releases the ingredients for absorption to provide a gradual, gentle, and sustained effect for a long period of time.

Gui Zhi Fu Ling Wan treats blood stagnation in the womb, yet it is named after *Gui Zhi* (Ramulus Cinnamomi) and *Fu Ling* (Poria), but not any of the blood-invigorating herbs in this formula, such as *Tao Ren* (Semen Persicae), *Chi Shao* (Radix Paeoniae Rubra) or *Mu Dan Pi* (Cortex Moutan). This signifies that blood stagnation in the womb is a delicate situation that cannot simply be treated with herbs that activate blood circulation. Instead, *Gui Zhi* (Ramulus Cinnamomi) must be used to warm and open the blood vessels to create an "entry" for the blood-invigorating herbs to reach the affected area, and *Fu Ling* (Poria) needs to be used to provide an "exit" to guide and eliminate blood stasis downward. Furthermore, *Gui Zhi* (Ramulus Cinnamomi) and *Fu Ling* (Poria) are very gentle, and will not harm either the mother or the fetus.

In addition to the original clinical application (blood stasis during pregnancy), this formula is now used to treat various disorders characterized by blood stasis:

• This formula can also be used for irregular menstruation, post-menstrual abdominal pain, or continuous spotting of blood after delivery, with abdominal pain that is worse with pressure.

• This formula also is effective for amenorrhea due to blood stasis in which the patient experiences abdominal fullness and pain that increase with palpation and pressure. Immobile masses in the lower abdomen are indicative of blood stasis, with dark and purplish blood reflecting the same diagnosis. Furthermore, blood stasis is often accompanied by signs and symptoms such as flushed face, abdominal fullness and pain (pain increases with palpation or pressure), headache, shoulder stiffness, dizziness, and cold feet.

• This formula is also effective for dysmenorrhea due to blood stasis in the uterus, with symptoms such as blood stasis, uterine bleeding of dark purplish blood, abdominal fullness and pain (pain increases with pressure or palpation), immobile masses in the lower abdomen with pain and tenderness, and abdominal pain caused by abnormal abdominal masses or previous blood stasis in the uterus.

References

1. *Zhong Yao Ming Fang Yao Li Yu Ying Yong* (Pharmacology and Applications of Famous Herbal Formulas) 1989;455-457.

2. *Guo Wai Yi Xue* (Foreign Medicine) 1987;9(2):32.

3. *Zhong Yi Fang Ji Xian Dai Yan Jiu* (Modern Study of Medical Formulae in Traditional Chinese Medicine) 1997;1119.

4. *Guo Wai Yi Xue* (Foreign Medicine) 1983;4:206.

5. *Zhong Yao Yao Li Yu Lin Chuang* (Pharmacology and Clinical Applications of Chinese Herbs) 1985;13.

6. *Guo Wai Yi Xue* (Foreign Medicine) 1988;10(4):45.

7. Sakamoto S, Kudo H, Kawasaki T, Kuwa K, Kasahara N, Sassa S, Okamoto R. Effects of a Chinese herbal medicine, keishi-bukuryo-gan, on the gonadal system of rats. J Ethnopharmacol 1988 Jul-Aug;23(2-3):151-8.

8. Nakagawa T, Yokozawa T, Terasawa K, Nakanishi K. Therapeutic usefulness of Keishi-bukuryo-gan for diabetic nephropathy. J Pharm Pharmacol 2003 Feb;55(2):219-27.

9. Sekiya N, Goto H, Shimada Y, Terasawa K. Inhibitory effects of Keishi-bukuryo-gan on free radical induced lysis of rat red blood cells. Phytother Res 2002 Jun;16(4):373-6.

10. Tanaka T, Umesaki N, Mizuno K, Fujino Y, Ogita S. Anti-endometrial IgM autoantibodies in endometriotic patients: a preliminary study. Clin Exp Obstet Gynecol 2000;27(2):133-7.

11. Mori T, Sakamoto S, Singtripop T, Park MK, Kato T, Kawashima S, Nagasawa H. Suppression of spontaneous development of uterine adenomyosis by a Chinese herbal medicine, keishi-bukuryo-gan, in mice. Planta Med 1993 Aug;59(4):308-11.

12. *Xin Zhong Yi* (New Chinese Medicine) 1975;6:33.

13. *Shan Dong Zhong Yi Za Zhi* (Shandong Journal of Chinese Medicine) 1993;12(2)28.

14. *Zhong Yi Za Zhi* (Journal of Chinese Medicine) 1994;35(6):355.

15. *Shang Hai Zhong Yi Yao Za Zhi* (Shanghai Journal of Chinese Medicine and Herbology) 1996;6:32.

16. Tanaka T, Mizuno K, Umesaki N, Ogita S. A preliminary immunopharmacological study of an antiendometriotic herbal medicine, Keishi-bukuryo-gan. Osaka City Med J 1998 Jun;44(1):117-24.

17. *Hu Bei Zhong Yi Za Zhi* (Hubei Journal of Chinese Medicine) 1987;5:14.

Chinese Herbal Formulas and Applications

Guì Zhī Fú Líng Wán (Cinnamon Twig and Poria Pill)

18. Sakamoto S, Yoshino H, Shirahata Y, Shimodairo K, Okamoto R. Pharmacotherapeutic effects of kuei-chih-fu-ling-wan (kei-shi-bukuryo-gan) on human uterine myomas. Am J Chin Med 1992;20(3-4):313-7.

19. *Guo Wai Yi Xue* (Foreign Medicine) 1980;2(4):185.

20. *Gui Yang Zhong Yi Xue Yuan Xue Bao* (Journal of Guiyang Chinese Medical University) 1992;14(2):9.

21. Sakamoto S, Mitamura T, Iwasawa M, Kitsunai H, Shindou K, Yagishita Y, Zhou YF, Sassa S. Conservative management for perimenopausal women with uterine leiomyomas using Chinese herbal medicines and synthetic analogs of gonadotropin-releasing hormone. In Vivo 1998 May-Jun;12(3):333-7.

22. *Zhong Yi Fang Ji Xian Dai Yan Jiu* (Modern Study of Medical Formulae in Traditional Chinese Medicine) 1997;1123.

23. Ishikawa H, Ohashi M, Hayakawa K, Kaneko S. Hata M. Effects of guizhi-fuling-wan on male infertility with varicocele. American Journal of Chinese Medicine 1996;24(3-4):327-31.

24. Hikiami H, Goto H, Sekiya N, Hattori N, Sakakibara I, Shimada Y, Terasawa K. Comparative efficacy of Keishi-bukuryo-gan and pentoxifylline on RBC deformability in patients with "oketsu" syndrome. Phytomedicine 2003;10(6-7):459-66.

25. Fushitani S, Minakuchi K, Tsuchiya K, Takasugi M, Murakami K. Studies on attenuation of post-ischemic brain injury by kampo medicines-inhibitory effects of free radical production. Yakugaku Zasshi 1995 Aug;115(8):611-7.

26. Sheng FY, Ohta A, Yamaguchi M. Inhibition of collagen production by traditional Chinese herbal medicine in scleroderma fibroblast cultures. Intern Med 1994 Aug;33(8):466-71.

27. Tanaka T. Effects of herbal medicines on menopausal symptoms induced by gonadotropin-releasing hormone agonist therapy. Clin Exp Obstet Gynecol 2001;28(1):20-3.

28. *Zhong Yao Yao Li Yu Lin Chuang* (Pharmacology and Clinical Applications of Chinese Herbs) 1985;13.

Zhé Chōng Yǐn (Break the Conflict Decoction)

折衝飲
折冲饮

Pinyin Name: *Zhe Chong Yin*
Literal Name: Break the Conflict Decoction
Alternate Name: Cinnamon and Persica Combination
Original Source: *Fu Ke Chan Lun Fang* (Discussion of Formulas for Obstetrics and Gynecology)

COMPOSITION

Gui Zhi (Ramulus Cinnamomi)	3g
Tao Ren (Semen Persicae)	3g
Hong Hua (Flos Carthami)	1.5g
Mu Dan Pi (Cortex Moutan)	1.5g
Dang Gui (Radix Angelicae Sinensis)	2.4g
Bai Shao (Radix Paeoniae Alba)	3g
Chuan Xiong (Rhizoma Chuanxiong)	2.4g
Yan Hu Suo (Rhizoma Corydalis)	1.5g
Chuan Niu Xi (Radix Cyathulae)	2.4g
Gan Cao (Radix et Rhizoma Glycyrrhizae)	0.3g

DOSAGE / PREPARATION / ADMINISTRATION

The source text states to cook all ingredients in 2.5 bowls of water until reduced to 1.5 bowls. Take the strained decoction while warm.

CLINICAL MANIFESTATIONS

Blood stagnation in the lower *jiao*: acute or chronic pain in the lower abdominal region and lower back, vertigo, headache, irregular menstruation, dysmenorrhea, and amenorrhea.

CLINICAL APPLICATIONS

Irregular menstruation, dysmenorrhea, inflammation of the uterus or ovaries, endometriosis, and pelvic inflammatory disease.

EXPLANATION

Zhe Chong Yin (Break the Conflict Decoction) treats blood stagnation in the lower *jiao,* that interferes with normal menstruation and causes severe pain. Because of blood stagnation, patients may experience sharp, stabbing

933

Zhé Chōng Yǐn (Break the Conflict Decoction)

Zhe Chong Yin (Break the Conflict Decoction)

Diagnosis	Signs and Symptoms	Treatment	Herbs
Blood stagnation in the lower jiao	• Sharp, stabbing pain in a fixed location: blood stagnation in the lower jiao • Irregular menstruation, dysmenorrhea, and amenorrhea: blood stagnation affecting menstruation	• Activates blood circulation and dispels blood stasis • Disperses stagnation and clears obstruction	• *Gui Zhi* (Ramulus Cinnamomi) promotes circulation of yang qi and dispels stagnation in the lower *jiao*. • *Tao Ren* (Semen Persicae) and *Hong Hua* (Flos Carthami) activate blood, dispel blood stasis, and relieve pain. • *Mu Dan Pi* (Cortex Moutan) promotes both qi and blood circulation to disperse stagnation. • *Dang Gui* (Radix Angelicae Sinensis), *Bai Shao* (Radix Paeoniae Alba), and *Chuan Xiong* (Rhizoma Chuanxiong) tonify the blood, move blood circulation, and relieve pain. • *Yan Hu Suo* (Rhizoma Corydalis) and *Chuan Niu Xi* (Radix Cyathulae) activate qi and blood circulation and relieve pain. • *Gan Cao* (Radix et Rhizoma Glycyrrhizae) harmonizes the herbs.

pain in a fixed location. In addition, blood stagnation impairs the normal flow of blood, leading to irregular menstruation, dysmenorrhea, and amenorrhea. This formula also can be used to treat blood stagnation in the lower *jiao* following a miscarriage.

This formula contains many herbs that activate blood circulation, eliminate blood stasis, and disperse obstruction. *Gui Zhi* (Ramulus Cinnamomi) promotes the circulation of yang qi and dispels stagnation in the lower *jiao*. *Tao Ren* (Semen Persicae) and *Hong Hua* (Flos Carthami) activate blood circulation, dispel blood stasis, and relieve pain. *Mu Dan Pi* (Cortex Moutan) promotes both qi and blood circulation to disperse stagnation. *Dang Gui* (Radix Angelicae Sinensis), *Bai Shao* (Radix Paeoniae Alba), and *Chuan Xiong* (Rhizoma Chuanxiong) tonify the blood, move blood circulation, and relieve pain. *Yan Hu Suo* (Rhizoma Corydalis) and *Chuan Niu Xi* (Radix

Cyathulae), in addition to activating qi and blood circulation, also relieve pain. Lastly, *Gan Cao* (Radix et Rhizoma Glycyrrhizae) harmonizes the herbs. Overall, this is one of the best formulas for treating various obstetric and gynecological disorders characterized by blood stagnation in the lower *jiao*.

MODIFICATIONS
• With blood stagnation during menstruation, add *San Leng* (Rhizoma Sparganii) and *E Zhu* (Rhizoma Curcumae).
• With painful menstruation, add *Xiang Fu* (Rhizoma Cyperi) and *Ai Ye* (Folium Artemisiae Argyi).
• With dizziness and vertigo during menstruation, add *Ren Shen* (Radix et Rhizoma Ginseng) and *Huang Qi* (Radix Astragali).
• With painful menstruation due to wind and cold, add *Xiao Chai Hu Tang* (Minor Bupleurum Decoction).
• With abdominal pain after delivery, add *Sheng Hua Tang* (Generation and Transformation Decoction).

934

Chinese Herbal Formulas and Applications

Biē Jiǎ Jiān Wán (Soft-Shelled Turtle Shell Pill)

鱉甲煎丸
鱉甲煎丸

Pinyin Name: *Bie Jia Jian Wan*
Literal Name: Soft-Shelled Turtle Shell Pill
Original Source: *Jin Gui Yao Lue* (Essentials from the Golden Cabinet) by Zhang Zhong-Jing in the Eastern Han Dynasty

COMPOSITION

Bie Jia (Carapax Trionycis), *zhi* (fried with liquid)	90g
Da Huang (Radix et Rhizoma Rhei)	22.5g
Mang Xiao (Natrii Sulfas)	90g
Tu Bie Chong (Eupolyphaga seu Steleophaga), *ao* (simmered)	37g
Qiang Lang (Catharsium Molossus), *ao* (simmered)	45g
Shu Fu (Armadillidium Vulgare), *ao* (simmered)	22.5g
Chai Hu (Radix Bupleuri)	45g
Huang Qin (Radix Scutellariae)	22.5g
Bai Shao (Radix Paeoniae Alba)	37g
Hou Po (Cortex Magnoliae Officinalis)	22.5g
She Gan (Rhizoma Belamcandae), *pao* (blast-fried)	22.5g
Ting Li Zi (Semen Descurainiae seu Lepidii)	7.5g
Ban Xia (Rhizoma Pinelliae)	7.5g
Gan Jiang (Rhizoma Zingiberis)	22.5g
Gui Zhi (Ramulus Cinnamomi)	22.5g
Ren Shen (Radix et Rhizoma Ginseng)	7.5g
E Jiao (Colla Corii Asini)	22.5g
Tao Ren (Semen Persicae)	15g
Mu Dan Pi (Cortex Moutan)	37g
Ling Xiao Hua (Flos Campsis)	22.5g
Feng Fang (Nidus Vespae), *zhi* (fried with liquid)	30g
Qu Mai (Herba Dianthi)	22.5g
Shi Wei (Folium Pyrrosiae)	22.5g

DOSAGE / PREPARATION / ADMINISTRATION

The source text states to first mix 3kg (3,000 grams) of burnt ash with 10kg (10,000 grams) of grain-based liquor. Then filter out and discard the burnt ash. Add *Bie Jia* (Carapax Trionycis) to the strained liquid and cook it until the mixture becomes a thick paste. The remaining 22 herbs are ground into a fine powder, then mixed with this herbal paste and *Feng Mi* (Mel) to make small pills. Take 3g of pills three times daily.

CHINESE THERAPEUTIC ACTIONS

1. Activates qi and blood circulation
2. Dispels dampness and dissolves phlegm
3. Softens hardness and resolves masses

CLINICAL MANIFESTATIONS

Malaria with splenomegaly: chronic malaria with enlarged spleen, hypochondriac distention, immobile masses in the hypochondrium, abdominal pain, muscle wasting, decreased food intake, alternation of fever and chills, and amenorrhea.

CLINICAL APPLICATIONS

Splenomegaly, hepatomegaly, hepatitis, liver cirrhosis, and liver cancer.

EXPLANATION

Bie Jia Jian Wan (Soft-Shelled Turtle Shell Pill) historically was used to treat malaria with splenomegaly. Today, it is used to treat abdominal masses. Because of the chronic nature of this illness, there will be signs of qi and yang deficiencies, qi and blood stagnation, and damp and phlegm accumulation. The formation of masses may occur in the abdomen, hypochondrium, or in the form of splenomegaly.

In this formula, *Bie Jia* (Carapax Trionycis) softens nodules and resolves masses. The burnt ash and grain-

BLOOD-REGULATING FORMULAS

13

935

Chapter 13 – Blood-Regulating Formulas　　　*Section 1 – Blood-Invigorating and Stasis-Removing Formulas*

Biē Jiǎ Jiān Wán (Soft-Shelled Turtle Shell Pill)

Bie Jia Jian Wan (Soft-Shelled Turtle Shell Pill)

Diagnosis	Signs and Symptoms	Treatment	Herbs
Malaria with splenomegaly	• Alternation of fever and chills and hypochondriac distention: malaria • Immobile masses in the hypochondrium and abdominal pain: damp and phlegm accumulation • Muscle wasting and decreased food intake: underlying qi and blood deficiencies	• Activates qi and blood circulation • Dispels dampness and dissolves phlegm • Softens hardness and resolves masses	• *Bie Jia* (Carapax Trionycis) softens nodules and resolves masses. • *Da Huang* (Radix et Rhizoma Rhei), *Mang Xiao* (Natrii Sulfas), *Tu Bie Chong* (Eupolyphaga seu Steleophaga), *Qiang Lang* (Catharsium Molossus), and *Shu Fu* (Armadillidium Vulgare) break up blood stasis and resolve masses. • *Chai Hu* (Radix Bupleuri), *Huang Qin* (Radix Scutellariae), and *Bai Shao* (Radix Paeoniae Alba) harmonize the *shaoyang* and regulate Liver qi circulation. • *Hou Po* (Cortex Magnoliae Officinalis), *She Gan* (Rhizoma Belamcandae), *Ting Li Zi* (Semen Descurainiae seu Lepidii), and *Ban Xia* (Rhizoma Pinelliae) regulate qi and dispel phlegm. • *Gan Jiang* (Rhizoma Zingiberis) and *Gui Zhi* (Ramulus Cinnamomi) warm the body. • *Ren Shen* (Radix et Rhizoma Ginseng) and *E Jiao* (Colla Corii Asini) tonify qi and nourish blood. • *Tao Ren* (Semen Persicae), *Mu Dan Pi* (Cortex Moutan), *Ling Xiao Hua* (Flos Campsis) and *Feng Fang* (Nidus Vespae) activate blood circulation and remove blood stasis. • *Qu Mai* (Herba Dianthi) and *Shi Wei* (Folium Pyrrosiae) regulate water circulation and dispel dampness.

based liquor help *Bie Jia* (Carapax Trionycis) activate blood circulation, remove blood stasis, soften nodules, and resolve masses. *Da Huang* (Radix et Rhizoma Rhei), *Mang Xiao* (Natrii Sulfas), *Tu Bie Chong* (Eupolyphaga seu Steleophaga), *Qiang Lang* (Catharsium Molossus), and *Shu Fu* (Armadillidium Vulgare) break up blood stasis and resolve masses. *Chai Hu* (Radix Bupleuri), *Huang Qin* (Radix Scutellariae), and *Bai Shao* (Radix Paeoniae Alba) harmonize the *shaoyang* and regulate Liver qi circulation. *Hou Po* (Cortex Magnoliae Officinalis), *She Gan* (Rhizoma Belamcandae), *Ting Li Zi* (Semen Descurainiae seu Lepidii), and *Ban Xia* (Rhizoma Pinelliae) regulate qi and dispel phlegm. *Gan Jiang* (Rhizoma Zingiberis) and *Gui Zhi* (Ramulus Cinnamomi) warm the body. *Ren Shen* (Radix et Rhizoma Ginseng) and *E Jiao* (Colla Corii Asini) tonify qi and nourish the blood. *Tao Ren* (Semen Persicae), *Mu Dan Pi* (Cortex Moutan), *Ling Xiao Hua* (Flos Campsis), and *Feng Fang* (Nidus Vespae) activate blood circulation and remove blood stasis. *Qu Mai* (Herba Dianthi) and

Shi Wei (Folium Pyrrosiae) regulate water circulation and dispel dampness. Overall, this formula has a good balance of warm and cold, tonifying and sedating, and qi- and blood-activating herbs.

MODIFICATIONS

- With general weakness and deficiency, add *Huang Qi* (Radix Astragali), *Bai Zhu* (Rhizoma Atractylodis Macrocephalae), *Shu Di Huang* (Radix Rehmanniae Praeparata), and *Dang Gui* (Radix Angelicae Sinensis).
- With decreased food intake and indigestion, add *Shan Zha* (Fructus Crataegi), *Shen Qu* (Massa Fermentata), and *Ji Nei Jin* (Endothelium Corneum Gigeriae Galli).

CAUTIONS / CONTRAINDICATIONS

Bie Jia Jian Wan contains many herbs that strongly activate qi and blood circulation, dispel dampness, and dissolve phlegm. It should be used with caution in patients with *zheng* (upright) *qi* deficiency.

Chinese Herbal Formulas and Applications

Dà Huáng Zhè Chóng Wán (Rhubarb and Eupolyphaga Pill)

大黃蟅蟲丸
大黃蟅虫丸

Pinyin Name: *Da Huang Zhe Chong Wan*
Literal Name: Rhubarb and Eupolyphaga Pill
Original Source: *Jin Gui Yao Lue* (Essentials from the Golden Cabinet) by Zhang Zhong-Jing in the Eastern Han Dynasty

COMPOSITION

Da Huang (Radix et Rhizoma Rhei), *zheng* (steamed)	300g
Tu Bie Chong (Eupolyphaga seu Steleophaga)	0.5 cup [30g]
Tao Ren (Semen Persicae)	1 cup [60g]
Gan Qi (Resina Toxicodendri)	30g
Qi Cao (Holotrichia)	1 cup [60g]
Shui Zhi (Hirudo)	100 pieces [60g]
Meng Chong (Tabanus)	1 cup [60g]
Huang Qin (Radix Scutellariae)	60g
Ku Xing Ren (Semen Armeniacae Amarum)	1 cup [60g]
Di Huang (Radix Rehmanniae)	300g
Bai Shao (Radix Paeoniae Alba)	120g
Gan Cao (Radix et Rhizoma Glycyrrhizae)	90g

DOSAGE / PREPARATION / ADMINISTRATION

The source text states to grind all ingredients into a fine powder and form into pills with honey. The pills should resemble small beans in size. Take 5 pills with grain-based liquor three times daily. Today this formula is usually given in pills, 3g per dose, with warm water.

CHINESE THERAPEUTIC ACTIONS

1. Breaks up and dispels blood stasis
2. Generates new blood

CLINICAL MANIFESTATIONS

Extreme deficiency: emaciation, abdominal distention with an inability to eat, dry, rough and scaly skin, and dark appearance of the eyes with no spirit. These injuries result from the five consumptive lifestyles.

CLINICAL APPLICATIONS

Chronic hepatitis, liver fibrosis, liver cirrhosis, liver cancer, tubercular peritonitis, uterine leiomyoma, and esophageal varices.

EXPLANATION

Da Huang Zhe Chong Wan (Rhubarb and Eupolyphaga Pill) treats individuals with extreme deficiency and debility from the five consumptive lifestyles, including overeating, extreme hunger, depression, excessive drinking, and excessive sexual activity. Extreme deficiency and debility cause a condition known as "dried blood," which is characterized by heat drying up yin and blood leading to blood stasis. The condition is characterized by emaciation and weight loss because of extreme deficiency and debility. The "dried blood" is unable to nourish the skin and eyes; thus, the skin becomes dry, rough and scaly, and the eyes have a dark appearance with no spirit.

This condition requires herbs that break up and dispel blood stasis and promote the generation of new blood. In this formula, *Da Huang* (Radix et Rhizoma Rhei) and *Tu Bie Chong* (Eupolyphaga seu Steleophaga) act as the chief herbs to drain blood stasis, cool the blood, and clear heat. *Tao Ren* (Semen Persicae), *Gan Qi* (Resina Toxicodendri), *Qi Cao* (Holotrichia), *Shui Zhi* (Hirudo), and *Meng Chong* (Tabanus) assist the chief herbs to activate blood circulation and eliminate blood stasis in the channels and collaterals. *Huang Qin* (Radix Scutellariae) is paired with *Da Huang* (Radix et Rhizoma Rhei) to clear heat caused by stagnation. *Ku Xing Ren* (Semen Armeniacae Amarum) is paired with *Tao Ren* (Semen Persicae) to moisten dryness, remove blood stasis, and redirect qi. *Di Huang* (Radix Rehmanniae) and *Bai Shao* (Radix Paeoniae Alba) tonify blood and nourish yin. *Gan Cao* (Radix et Rhizoma Glycyrrhizae) harmonizes the herbs, and prevents the harsh herbs from further damaging the body.

BLOOD-REGULATING FORMULAS

13

Chapter 13 – Blood-Regulating Formulas   *Section 1 – Blood-Invigorating and Stasis-Removing Formulas*

Dà Huáng Zhè Chóng Wán (Rhubarb and Eupolyphaga Pill)

Da Huang Zhe Chong Wan (Rhubarb and Eupolyphaga Pill)

Diagnosis	Signs and Symptoms	Treatment	Herbs
Extreme deficiency due to the five consumptions	Emaciation, abdominal distention with an inability to eat, dry, rough and scaly skin, and dark appearance of the eyes: damages to yin and blood caused by "dried blood" and blood stagnation	• Breaks up and dispels blood stasis • Generates new blood	• *Da Huang* (Radix et Rhizoma Rhei) and *Tu Bie Chong* (Eupolyphaga seu Steleophaga) eliminate blood stasis, cool the blood, and clear heat. • *Tao Ren* (Semen Persicae), *Gan Qi* (Resina Toxicodendri), *Qi Cao* (Holotrichia), *Shui Zhi* (Hirudo), and *Meng Chong* (Tabanus) activate blood and eliminate blood stasis in the channels and collaterals. • *Huang Qin* (Radix Scutellariae) and *Da Huang* (Radix et Rhizoma Rhei) clear heat. • *Ku Xing Ren* (Semen Armeniacae Amarum) and *Tao Ren* (Semen Persicae) moisten dryness, remove blood stasis, and redirect qi. • *Di Huang* (Radix Rehmanniae) and *Bai Shao* (Radix Paeoniae Alba) tonify blood and nourish yin. • *Gan Cao* (Radix et Rhizoma Glycyrrhizae) harmonizes the herbs, and prevents the harsh herbs from further damaging the body.

CAUTIONS / CONTRAINDICATIONS

• Use of this formula may be associated with mild diarrhea. This side effect is self-limiting and does not require treatment or discontinuation of this formula. Another side effect associated with this formula is bleeding (mostly of the gums and nose). It may be necessary to discontinue this formula temporarily should bleeding become more profuse or if it lasts for a prolonged period of time.[1]

• *Da Huang Zhe Chong Wan* is contraindicated during pregnancy and in women with amenorrhea due to blood deficiency.[2]

AUTHORS' COMMENTS

Tu Bie Chong (Eupolyphaga seu Steleophaga) is known also as *Zhe Chong*, which explains the name of the formula, *Da Huang Zhe Chong Wan* (Rhubarb and Eupolyphaga Pill).

Although the condition this formula treats is characterized by both excess (blood stasis) and deficiency (qi and blood), the formula emphasizes eliminating blood stasis. Once this goal is accomplished, it is important to discontinue *Da Huang Zhe Chong Wan*, and treat the underlying deficiencies with a tonic formula.

This formula was originally designed to be given as pills, because blood stasis in an extremely deficient patient should be gradually softened, dispersed, and reduced. Aggressively attacking blood stasis by using potent blood-moving herbs in decoction will only create more deficiency and complications.

References
1. *Zhong Yao Ming Fang Yao Li Yu Ying Yong* (Pharmacology and Applications of Famous Herbal Formulas) 1989;469-70.
2. *Zhong Yao Ming Fang Yao Li Yu Ying Yong* (Pharmacology and Applications of Famous Herbal Formulas) 1989;469-70.

938

Section 2

Chinese Herbal Formulas and Applications

止血剂
— Stop-Bleeding Formulas

Shí Huī Săn (Ten Partially-Charred Substances Powder)
十灰散

Pinyin Name: *Shi Hui San*
Literal Name: Ten Partially-Charred Substances Powder
Original Source: *Shi Yao Shen Shu* (Miraculous Book of Ten Remedies) by Ge Qian-Sun in 1348

COMPOSITION

Da Ji (Radix Euphorbiae seu Knoxiae)	[9g]
Xiao Ji (Herba Cirsii)	[9g]
He Ye (Folium Nelumbinis)	[9g]
Qian Cao (Radix et Rhizoma Rubiae)	[9g]
Ce Bai Ye (Cacumen Platycladi)	[9g]
Bai Mao Gen (Rhizoma Imperatae)	[9g]
Zong Lu (Petiolus Trachycarpi)	[9g]
Zhi Zi (Fructus Gardeniae)	[9g]
Da Huang (Radix et Rhizoma Rhei)	[9g]
Mu Dan Pi (Cortex Moutan)	[9g]

DOSAGE / PREPARATION / ADMINISTRATION

The source text states to char to ashes equal amounts of the ingredients and grind into a fine powder. Separately pound *Ou Jie* (Nodus Nelumbinis Rhizomatis) or *Lai Fu Zi* (Semen Raphani) to obtain their juice. Take 15g of the powder per dose after meals with half a bowl of juice. Today, this formula may be prepared as a decoction with the doses suggested in brackets.

CHINESE THERAPEUTIC ACTIONS

Cools the blood and stops bleeding

CLINICAL MANIFESTATIONS

Bleeding due to heat in the *xue* (blood) level: hematemesis, hemoptysis, and other sudden onset bleeding symptoms.

CLINICAL APPLICATIONS

Hematemesis, hyphema, and gastrointestinal bleeding.

EXPLANATION

Shi Hui San (Ten Partially-Charred Substances Powder) treats bleeding due to heat in the *xue* (blood) level. Interior heat can invade the blood and force it out of the blood vessels, resulting in reckless movement of blood in various types of bleeding. Because of heat, bleeding is accompanied by bright red blood and a red or deep red tongue body.

In this formula, *Da Ji* (Radix Euphorbiae seu Knoxiae), *Xiao Ji* (Herba Cirsii), *He Ye* (Folium Nelumbinis), *Qian Cao* (Radix et Rhizoma Rubiae), *Ce Bai Ye* (Cacumen Platycladi), and *Bai Mao Gen* (Rhizoma Imperatae) cool the blood and stop bleeding. *Zong Lu* (Petiolus Trachycarpi) astringes the blood and provides immediate effect to stop bleeding. *Zhi Zi* (Fructus Gardeniae) clears heat and purges fire, while *Da Huang* (Radix et Rhizoma Rhei) drains heat and fire downwards. *Mu Dan Pi* (Cortex Moutan) has two functions in this formula: it clears heat to stop bleeding, and it activates blood circulation to prevent blood stasis. Blood activation is vital, because the sole use of stop-bleeding herbs in this case may lead to blood stagnation. The juice of *Ou Jie* (Nodus Nelumbinis Rhizomatis) or *Lai Fu Zi* (Semen Raphani) may be added to enhance the actions of clearing heat, cooling the blood, and stopping the bleeding.

BLOOD-REGULATING FORMULAS

13

939

Chapter 13 – Blood-Regulating Formulas *Section 2 – Stop-Bleeding Formulas*

Shi Huī Săn (Ten Partially-Charred Substances Powder)

Shi Hui San (Ten Partially-Charred Substances Powder)

Diagnosis	Signs and Symptoms	Treatment	Herbs
Bleeding due to heat in the *xue* (blood) level	Sudden onset bleeding: heat in the interior forcing blood out of the vessels	Cools the blood and stops bleeding	• *Da Ji* (Radix Euphorbiae seu Knoxiae), *Xiao Ji* (Herba Cirsii), *He Ye* (Folium Nelumbinis), *Qian Cao* (Radix et Rhizoma Rubiae), *Ce Bai Ye* (Cacumen Platycladi), and *Bai Mao Gen* (Rhizoma Imperatae) cool the blood and stop bleeding. • *Zong Lu* (Petiolus Trachycarpi) astringes the blood to stop bleeding immediately. • *Zhi Zi* (Fructus Gardeniae) clears heat and purges fire. • *Da Huang* (Radix et Rhizoma Rhei) drains heat and fire downwards. • *Mu Dan Pi* (Cortex Moutan) clears heat to stop bleeding, and activates blood circulation to prevent blood stasis. • *Ou Jie* (Nodus Nelumbinis Rhizomatis) or *Lai Fu Zi* (Semen Raphani) enhances the actions of clearing heat, cooling the blood, and stopping bleeding.

All of the herbs are charred to ashes to enhance their hemostatic effect. The formula is prepared and stored in powder form so it can be administered immediately as needed.

MODIFICATION

With acute bleeding due to heat flaring up, add *Niu Xi* (Radix Achyranthis Bidentatae) and *Zhe Shi* (Haematitum), and increase the doses of *Da Huang* (Radix et Rhizoma Rhei) and *Zhi Zi* (Fructus Gardeniae). Administer the formula in decoction form for faster results.

CAUTIONS / CONTRAINDICATIONS

• *Shi Hui San* should be used only as a short-term therapy to stop bleeding. Once the bleeding has stopped, the cause of bleeding must be identified and treated accordingly.

• This formula is designed for bleeding caused by an excess condition of heat in the *xue* (blood) level. It is contraindicated in bleeding conditions caused by deficiency and cold.

PHARMACOLOGICAL EFFECTS

Hemostatic: One study evaluated the hemostatic effect of *Shi Hui San* prepared by various methods. Method I was to char the herbs until the smoke turned from white to yellow in color, with the herbs appearing black on the outside and dark brown on the inside. Loss of herb weight on charring was 20%. Method II was to char the herbs until the smoke turned from white to yellow to bluegreen

in color, with the herbs appearing black on the outside and inside. Loss of herb weight on charring was 40%. Method III was to char the herbs until the smoke turned from white to yellow to bluegreen to clear in color, with the herbs appearing burnt on the outside and black on the inside. Loss of herb weight on charring was 60%. Method IV was to char the herbs until the smoke turned from white to yellow to bluegreen to clear in color, with the herbs appearing completely burnt throughout. Loss of herb weight on charring was 80%. These four preparations were then given to rabbits and their hemostatic effects were evaluated. Of the four preparations, the study concluded that the hemostatic effect was most potent in method I, followed by method II and method III. Method IV had no significant impact.[1]

CLINICAL STUDIES AND RESEARCH

1. **Hematemesis in pulmonary tuberculosis**: *Shi Hui San* was used to stop bleeding in pulmonary tuberculosis patients who were coughing blood. Herbal treatment effectively stopped bleeding in most patients within 4-6 days. Overall, the treatment was effective in 22 out of 27 patients.[2]

2. **Hematemesis in bronchiectasis**: Modified *Shi Hui San* given in decoction was effective in 8 bronchiectasis patients coughing blood. The treatment protocol was to combine *Shi Hui San* with *San Qi* (Radix et Rhizoma Notoginseng), *Chuan Bei Mu* (Bulbus Fritillariae Cirrhosae), and powdered *Bai Ji* (Rhizoma Bletillae).

940

Shǐ Huī Sǎn (Ten Partially-Charred Substances Powder)

The herbs were cooked in water, and the decoction given in three equally-divided doses daily. Bleeding stopped in most patients within 1-2 days, with complete recovery between 6-20 days. No recurrence was reported by patients in follow-up evaluations one year after treatment.[3]

3. **Hyphema**: Modified *Shi Hui San* was used to treat 10 patients with bleeding caused by external injuries to the anterior chamber of the eye. The treatment protocol was to administer *Shi Hui San* with 10g of *Hong Hua* (Flos Carthami) one time daily until the bleeding stopped. The patients were also treated with 1% atropine ophthalmic paste one time daily. The study reported that the bleeding stopped within 3-9 days. Upon discharge, 9 of 10 patients had restored normal visual acuity and all 10 had normal ocular pressure.[4]

4. **Gastrointestinal bleeding**: Administration of *Shi Hui San* and *Zuo Jin Wan* (Left Metal Pill) was shown to effectively treat upper gastrointestinal bleeding resulting from gastric or duodenal ulcers.[5]

RELATED FORMULA
Zhǐ Xuè Tāng (Stop Bleeding Decoction)

止血湯
止血汤

Pinyin Name: *Zhi Xue Tang*
Literal Name: Stop Bleeding Decoction
Original Source: *Guang An Men Yi Yuan* (Guang An Men Hospital) in 1990

San Qi (Radix et Rhizoma Notoginseng)
Jing Jie (Herba Schizonepetae)
Ai Ye (Folium Artemisiae Argyi)
Qian Cao (Radix et Rhizoma Rubiae)
Xian He Cao (Herba Agrimoniae)
Wu Wei Zi (Fructus Schisandrae Chinensis)
He Zi (Fructus Chebulae)
Ce Bai Ye (Cacumen Platycladi)
Di Yu (Radix Sanguisorbae)

Zhi Xue Tang (Stop Bleeding Decoction) has been used as an empirical formula to stop various types of bleeding, including internal bleeding (upper gastrointestinal, stomach, and/or duodenal bleeding, hemoptysis, hematuria, and excessive or irregular menstrual bleeding) and external bleeding (traumatic injuries). It is important to note that this formula treats only the symptom (bleeding), and not the cause. Therefore, after bleeding is stopped, it is necessary to identify and treat the cause.

AUTHORS' COMMENTS

Shi Hui San is designed to be an emergency herbal formula to quickly stop bleeding. It focuses primarily on treating the symptom (bleeding), and not the cause. Therefore, once the bleeding has stopped, the cause of bleeding should be determined and treated accordingly. *Shi Hui San* should not be taken for a prolonged period of time or in high doses.

In *Shi Hui San*, all ten herbs are partially charred to ash to enhance the astringent and hemostatic effects of the formula. Because of this unique processing, the formula is named appropriately "Ten Partially-Charred Substances Powder."

In contrast to the ten substances that are <u>charred to ashes</u> to stop bleeding, <u>fresh</u> *Ou Jie* (Nodus Nelumbinis Rhizomatis) or *Lai Fu Zi* (Semen Raphani) must be used to effectively clear heat and cool the blood.

References
1. *Nei Meng Gu Zhong Yi Yao* (Traditional Chinese Medicine and Medicinals of Inner Mongolia) 1984;3:46.
2. *Fu Jian Zhong Yi Yao* (Fujian Chinese Medicine and Herbology) 1960;4:27.
3. *Shi Zhen Guo Yao Yan Jiu* (Research of Shizhen Herbs) 1997;4:301.
4. *Zhong Guo Zhong Xi Yi Jie He Za Zhi* (Chinese Journal of Integrative Chinese and Western Medicine) 1987;3:175.
5. *Zhe Jiang Zhong Yi Yao* (Zhejiang Chinese Medicine and Herbology) 1963;7:4.

Chapter 13 – Blood-Regulating Formulas   Section 2 – Stop-Bleeding Formulas

Si Shēng Wán (Four-Fresh Pill)

四生丸

Pinyin Name: *Si Sheng Wan*
Literal Name: Four-Fresh Pill
Alternate Name: Rehmannia Four Formula
Original Source: *Fu Ren Liang Fang* (Fine Formulas for Women) by Chen Zi-Ming in 1237

COMPOSITION

Ce Bai Ye (Cacumen Platycladi), fresh	[12g]
Di Huang (Radix Rehmanniae), fresh	[15g]
He Ye (Folium Nelumbinis), fresh	[9g]
Ai Ye (Folium Artemisiae Argyi), fresh	[9g]

DOSAGE / PREPARATION / ADMINISTRATION

The source text states to grind equal amounts of the ingredients and form the powder into pills the size of egg yolks. Cook one pill with water and take the decoction. Today, this formula may be prepared as a decoction with the doses suggested in brackets.

CHINESE THERAPEUTIC ACTIONS

Cools the blood and stops bleeding

CLINICAL MANIFESTATIONS

Bleeding due to heat in the *xue* (blood) level: hematemesis and epistaxis with bright red blood, dry mouth and throat, red or deep red tongue body, and a wiry, rapid pulse.

CLINICAL APPLICATIONS

Gingivitis, peridonitis, hemoptysis, hematemesis, epistaxis, tuberculosis, and bronchiectasis.

EXPLANATION

Si Sheng Wan (Four-Fresh Pill) treats hematemesis or epistaxis due to heat in the *xue* (blood) level. If the heat factor invades the *xue* (blood) level and forces the blood out of their vessels, then symptoms of bleeding, such as hematemesis or epistaxis with bright red blood, may

occur. Dry mouth and throat are due to heat damaging the yin and body fluids. A red tongue body and a wiry, rapid pulse indicate excess heat in the interior.

This formula uses *Ce Bai Ye* (Cacumen Platycladi) to cool the blood and stop bleeding. *Di Huang* (Radix Rehmanniae) clears heat, cools the blood, and nourishes yin and body fluids. *He Ye* (Folium Nelumbinis) and *Ai Ye* (Folium Artemisiae Argyi) stop bleeding and disperse blood stagnation.

MODIFICATIONS

- With severe bleeding, add *Qian Cao* (Radix et Rhizoma Rubiae), *Mo Han Lian* (Herba Ecliptae), and *Ou Jie* (Nodus Nelumbinis Rhizomatis).
- With excessive uterine bleeding, add *Jiao Ai Tang* (Ass-Hide Gelatin and Mugwort Decoction).
- With bleeding ulcers, add *Huang Qin* (Radix Scutellariae), *Bai Zhu* (Rhizoma Atractylodis Macrocephalae), *Fu Zi* (Radix Aconiti Lateralis Praeparata), *E Jiao* (Colla Corii Asini), and *Gan Cao* (Radix et Rhizoma Glycyrrhizae).
- With constipation due to excess and heat, add *Qian Niu Zi* (Semen Pharbitidis), *Da Huang* (Radix et Rhizoma Rhei), *Zao Jiao* (Fructus Gleditsiae), and *Mang Xiao* (Natrii Sulfas).

Si Sheng Wan (Four-Fresh Pill)

Diagnosis	Signs and Symptoms	Treatment	Herbs
Bleeding due to heat in the *xue* (blood) level	• Hematemesis or epistaxis with bright red blood: heat in the *xue* (blood) level forcing blood out of the vessels • Dry mouth and throat: heat damaging yin and body fluids • Red tongue and a wiry, rapid pulse: excess heat in the interior	Cools the blood and stops bleeding	• *Ce Bai Ye* (Cacumen Platycladi) cools the blood and stops bleeding. • *Di Huang* (Radix Rehmanniae) clears heat, cools the blood, and nourishes yin and body fluids. • *He Ye* (Folium Nelumbinis) and *Ai Ye* (Folium Artemisiae Argyi) stop bleeding and disperse blood stagnation.

Chinese Herbal Formulas and Applications

Sì Shēng Wán (Four-Fresh Pill)

CAUTIONS / CONTRAINDICATIONS

Si Sheng Wan should be discontinued when the desired effect is achieved. Prolonged use or overdosing will result in cold accumulation, which may further aggravate the blood stasis.

AUTHORS' COMMENTS

For *Si Sheng Wan*, the original text specifically emphasized using the fresh, unprocessed form of all four herbs to maximize the heat-clearing and blood-cooling effects. Thus, this formula is appropriately named "Four-Fresh Pill." However, the fresh, unprocessed form of these four herbs may not be readily available. In that case, to enhance the hemostatic effect, herbs such as *Xiao Ji* (Herba Cirsii), *Bai Mao Gen* (Rhizoma Imperatae), *Ou Jie* (Nodus Nelumbinis Rhizomatis), and *Xian He Cao* (Herba Agrimoniae) can be added.

Ké Xuè Fāng (Coughing of Blood Formula)
咳血方

Pinyin Name: *Ke Xue Fang*
Literal Name: Coughing of Blood Formula
Original Source: *Dan Xi Xin Fa* (Teachings of [Zhu] Dan-Xi) by Zhu Zhen-Heng in 1481

COMPOSITION

Qing Dai (Indigo Naturalis), *shui fei* (refined with water)	[6g]
Zhi Zi (Fructus Gardeniae), *chao* (dry-fried) to black	[9g]
Gua Lou Zi (Semen Trichosanthis), oil removed	[9g]
Fu Hai Shi (Pumice)	[9g]
He Zi (Fructus Chebulae)	[6g]

DOSAGE / PREPARATION / ADMINISTRATION

The source text states to grind the ingredients into powder and form into pills with honey and the juice of *Sheng Jiang* (Rhizoma Zingiberis Recens). The pills should be dissolved in the mouth and then swallowed. Today, this formula may be prepared as a decoction with the doses suggested in brackets. Note: Original doses of herbs in pill form are unavailable from the source text.

CHINESE THERAPEUTIC ACTIONS

1. Clears fire and dissolves phlegm
2. Astringes the Lung and stops coughing

CLINICAL MANIFESTATIONS

Hemoptysis due to Liver fire invading the Lung: coughing with thick, sticky sputum and streaks of blood, a feeling of difficult-to-expectorate sputum stuck in the throat, irritability, fidgeting, short temper, stabbing pain in the chest and hypochondriac area, constipation, red cheeks, red tongue body with a yellow coating, and a wiry, rapid pulse.

CLINICAL APPLICATIONS

Hemoptysis, bronchiectasis, and pulmonary tuberculosis.

EXPLANATION

Ke Xue Fang (Coughing of Blood Formula) treats hemoptysis caused by Liver fire invading the Lung. As Liver fire rises upward, it dries Lung yin and fluids into a thick sputum, making it difficult to expectorate. Liver fire also affects Lung qi circulation, causing coughing and pain in the chest and hypochondriac area. Liver fire may damage the blood vessels, resulting in coughing with streaks of blood in the sputum. Other indications of excess Liver fire include irritability, fidgeting, constipation, red tongue body with a yellow coating, and a wiry, rapid pulse.

This formula aims to treat the cause (Liver fire invading the Lung), and not the symptom (bleeding), of hemoptysis. Therefore, it primarily uses herbs to clear Liver fire, dissolve phlegm, cool the blood, and stop coughing. The source text states that use of stop-bleeding herbs is not necessary because once the cause has been treated, hemoptysis will stop. In this formula, *Qing Dai* (Indigo Naturalis) and *Zhi Zi* (Fructus Gardeniae) sedate Liver fire and cool the blood. *Gua Lou Zi* (Semen Trichosanthis) and *Fu Hai Shi* (Pumice) clear heat, moisten dryness, and dissolve sputum. *He Zi* (Fructus Chebulae) astringes the Lung to relieve coughing.

BLOOD-REGULATING FORMULAS

13

943

Chapter 13 – Blood-Regulating Formulas　　　　　　　　　　　　　*Section 2 – Stop-Bleeding Formulas*

Ké Xuè Fāng (Coughing of Blood Formula)

Ke Xue Fang (Coughing of Blood Formula)

Diagnosis	Signs and Symptoms	Treatment	Herbs
Hemoptysis due to Liver fire invading the Lung	• Coughing: Liver fire affecting the Lung qi circulation • Thick, sticky sputum and streaks of blood, feeling of difficult-to-expectorate sputum stuck in the throat: Liver fire consuming Lung yin and fluids • Irritability and fidgeting: Liver fire disturbing the *shen* (spirit) • Constipation, red tongue body, yellow tongue coating, and a wiry, rapid pulse: excess Liver fire in the body	• Clears fire and dissolves phlegm • Astringes the Lung and stops coughing	• *Qing Dai* (Indigo Naturalis) and *Zhi Zi* (Fructus Gardeniae) sedate Liver fire and cool the blood. • *Gua Lou Zi* (Semen Trichosanthis) and *Fu Hai Shi* (Pumice) clear heat, moisten dryness, and dissolve the sputum. • *He Zi* (Fructus Chebulae) astringes the Lung to relieve coughing.

MODIFICATIONS
• With severe cough, add *Ku Xing Ren* (Semen Armeniacae Amarum).
• With coughing of profuse sputum, add *Bei Mu* (Bulbus Fritillariae), *Tian Zhu Huang* (Concretio Silicea Bambusae), and *Pi Pa Ye* (Folium Eriobotryae).
• With sputum and blood, and chest pain, add *Jiang Xiang* (Lignum Dalbergiae Odoriferae) and *Ju Luo* (Vascular Citri Reticulatae).
• With sputum that is scanty and difficult to expectorate due to heat injuring body fluids, add *Bei Sha Shen* (Radix Glehniae), *Mai Dong* (Radix Ophiopogonis), and *Pi Pa Ye* (Folium Eriobotryae).
• With epistaxis, remove *He Zi* (Fructus Chebulae) and *Fu Hai Shi* (Pumice); and add *Qing Hao* (Herba Artemisiae Annuae), *Mu Dan Pi* (Cortex Moutan), and *Bai Mao Gen* (Rhizoma Imperatae).

CAUTIONS / CONTRAINDICATIONS
• *Ke Xue Fang* is contraindicated in patients who have Lung and Kidney yin deficiencies, or Spleen qi deficiency with loose stools.
• This formula is contraindicated in cases of cough caused by Lung cold.

AUTHORS' COMMENTS
This formula is prepared as honey pills, and administered by dissolving the pills in the mouth. The purposes of this preparation and administration is to achieve gradual absorption and sustained effect of the formula. After the bleeding stops, the source text recommends using tonic formulas, such as *Ba Zhen Tang* (Eight-Treasure Decoction), to stabilize the condition and treat the underlying deficiencies.

Huái Huā Sǎn (Sophora Japonica Flower Powder)
槐花散

Pinyin Name: *Huai Hua San*
Literal Name: Sophora Japonica Flower Powder
Alternate Names: Sophora Flower Powder, Sophora Flower Formula
Original Source: *Pu Ji Ben Shi Fang* (Formulas of Universal Benefit from My Practice) by Xu Shu-Wei in 1132

COMPOSITION

Huai Hua (Flos Sophorae), *chao* (dry-fried)	[12g]
Ce Bai Ye (Cacumen Platycladi), *chu* (pestled) and *bei* (stone baked)	[12g]
Jing Jie Sui (Spica Schizonepetae)	[6g]
Zhi Qiao (Fructus Citri Aurantii), *chao* (dry-fried) with bran till yellow	[6g]

944

Chinese Herbal Formulas and Applications

Huái Huā Săn (Sophora Japonica Flower Powder)

DOSAGE / PREPARATION / ADMINISTRATION

The source text states to grind equal amounts of the ingredients into a fine powder and take 6g with rice soup on an empty stomach before meals. Today, this formula may be prepared as a decoction with the doses suggested in brackets. Note: Original doses of herbs are unavailable from the source text.

CHINESE THERAPEUTIC ACTIONS

1. Clears the Intestines and stops bleeding
2. Dispels wind and redirects qi

CLINICAL MANIFESTATIONS

Hematochezia due to *chang feng* (intestinal wind) and *zang du* (solid organ toxins): bleeding before or after defecation, blood in the stools, hemorrhoidal bleeding, and frank blood with bright red or dark black color.

CLINICAL APPLICATIONS

Rectal or intestinal bleeding, hemorrhoids, ulcerative colitis, and anal fissure.

EXPLANATION

Huai Hua San (Sophora Japonica Flower Powder) treats *chang feng* (intestinal wind) and *zang du* (solid organ toxins). *Chang feng* (intestinal wind) is caused by wind attacking the Intestines, leading to the discharge of bright red blood before defecation or in the stools. *Zang du* (solid organ toxins) is caused by toxins attacking the organ, leading to dysentery with dark black blood in the stools. Both conditions are characterized by wind, heat, and toxins attacking the Stomach and Intestines.

In this formula, *Huai Hua* (Flos Sophorae) clears damp-heat in the Intestines, cools the blood, and stops bleeding. *Ce Bai Ye* (Cacumen Platycladi) helps *Huai Hua* (Flos Sophorae) cool the blood and stop bleeding. *Jing Jie Sui* (Spica Schizonepetae) disperses wind from the Intestines.

It also enters the *xue* (blood) level and stops bleeding. *Zhi Qiao* (Fructus Aurantii) activates qi circulation in the Intestines to dispel toxins.

MODIFICATIONS

- With excessive bleeding, add *Di Yu* (Radix Sanguisorbae) and *Xiao Ji* (Herba Cirsii).
- With blood in the stools accompanied by abdominal pain, distention, and tenesmus, add *Mu Xiang* (Radix Aucklandiae) and *Hou Po* (Cortex Magnoliae Officinalis).
- With dry, hard stools accompanied by bleeding, add *Mang Xiao* (Natrii Sulfas) and *Huo Ma Ren* (Fructus Cannabis).
- With qi deficiency due to chronic bleeding, add *Huang Qi* (Radix Astragali), *Dang Shen* (Radix Codonopsis), and *Sheng Ma* (Rhizoma Cimicifugae).
- For bleeding hemorrhoids and prolapsed rectum, remove *Ce Bai Ye* (Cacumen Platycladi) and *Jing Jie* (Herba Schizonepetae), and add *Dang Gui* (Radix Angelicae Sinensis), *Huang Qin* (Radix Scutellariae), *Fang Feng* (Radix Saposhnikoviae), and *Di Yu* (Radix Sanguisorbae).
- For continuous and profuse bleeding leading to blood deficiency, add *Di Huang* (Radix Rehmanniae), *Dang Gui* (Radix Angelicae Sinensis), *Chuan Xiong* (Rhizoma Chuanxiong), and *Wu Mei* (Fructus Mume).
- With excess heat in the Intestines, add *Huang Lian* (Rhizoma Coptidis) and *Huang Bo* (Cortex Phellodendri Chinensis).

CAUTIONS / CONTRAINDICATIONS

- *Huai Hua San* is cold and thus is not suitable for long-term use.
- This formula is not suitable for chronic rectal bleeding or for hematochezia with symptoms of qi or yin deficiency.

Huai Hua San (Sophora Japonica Flower Powder)

Diagnosis	Signs and Symptoms	Treatment	Herbs
Hematochezia due to *chang feng* (intestinal wind) and *zang du* (solid organ toxins)	• Bright red blood in the stools: *chang feng* (intestinal wind) due to wind attacking the Intestines • Dysentery with dark black blood in the stools: *zang du* (solid organ toxins)	• Clears the intestines and stops bleeding • Dispels wind and descends qi	• *Huai Hua* (Flos Sophorae) clears damp-heat in the Intestines, cools the blood, and stops bleeding. • *Ce Bai Ye* (Cacumen Platycladi) cools the blood and stops bleeding. • *Jing Jie Sui* (Spica Schizonepetae) disperses wind and stops bleeding. • *Zhi Qiao* (Fructus Aurantii) activates qi circulation in the Intestines to dispel toxins.

BLOOD-REGULATING FORMULAS

13

945

Chapter 13 – Blood-Regulating Formulas

Section 2 – Stop-Bleeding Formulas

Huái Huā Sǎn (Sophora Japonica Flower Powder)

RELATED FORMULA

Huái Jiǎo Wán (Sophora Japonica Fruit Pill)

槐角丸

Pinyin Name: *Huai Jiao Wan*

Literal Name: Sophora Japonica Fruit Pill

Original Source: *Tai Ping Hui Min He Ji Ju Fang* (Imperial Grace Formulary of the Tai Ping Era) by the Imperial Medical Department in 1078-85

Huai Jiao (Fructus Sophorae), *chao* (dry-fried)	480g
Fang Feng (Radix Saposhnikoviae)	240g
Di Yu (Radix Sanguisorbae)	240g
Dang Gui (Radix Angelicae Sinensis), *jin* (soaked) in liquor for 1 night and *bei* (stone baked)	240g
Huang Qin (Radix Scutellariae)	240g
Zhi Qiao (Fructus Citri Aurantii), *chao* (dry-fried) with bran	240g

The source text states to grind all ingredients into a fine powder and mix it with a grain-based liquor to form pills.

The pills should resemble the size of *Wu Tong Zi* (Semen Firmianae), a small seed approximately 5 mm in diameter. Take 30 pills with rice soup any time during the day. Today, this formula is prepared by grinding the ingredients into a fine powder, then mixing it with water to form pills. Take 9g of pills daily with water.

Huai Jiao Wan (Sophora Japonica Fruit Pill) clears the Intestines to stop bleeding, dispels wind, and regulates qi. Clinically, it may be used to treat hematochezia, hemorrhoids, prolapsed rectum, and *chang feng* (intestinal wind) characterized by wind, heat, toxins, and damp-heat.

Huai Hua San and *Huai Jiao Wan* (Sophora Japonica Fruit Pill) both clear the Intestines and stop bleeding to treat hematochezia due to *chang feng* (intestinal wind).

- *Huai Hua San* has a stronger effect to cool the blood and stop bleeding.
- *Huai Jiao Wan* has a better effect to clear damp-heat, and an additional function to nourish the blood.

Xiǎo Jì Yǐn Zǐ (Cirsium Decoction)

小薊飲子

小蓟饮子

Pinyin Name: *Xiao Ji Yin Zi*

Literal Name: Cirsium Decoction

Alternate Name: Cephalanoplos Decoction

Original Source: *Dan Xi Xin Fa* (Teachings of [Zhu] Dan-Xi) by Zhu Zhen-Heng in 1481

COMPOSITION

Xiao Ji (Herba Cirsii)	15g [15g]
Ou Jie (Nodus Nelumbinis Rhizomatis)	15g [9g]
Pu Huang (Pollen Typhae), *chao* (dry-fried)	15g [9g]
Hua Shi (Talcum)	15g [15g]
Mu Tong (Caulis Akebiae)	15g [9g]
Dan Zhu Ye (Herba Lophatheri)	15g [9g]
Zhi Zi (Fructus Gardeniae)	15g [9g]
Di Huang (Radix Rehmanniae), *xi* (washed)	120g [30g]
Dang Gui (Radix Angelicae Sinensis), *jin* (soaked) in liquor	15g [6g]
Zhi Gan Cao (Radix et Rhizoma Glycyrrhizae Praeparata cum Melle)	15g [6g]

DOSAGE / PREPARATION / ADMINISTRATION

The source text states to coarsely grind all the ingredients. Cook 12g of the powder with 1.5 bowls of water until the liquid is reduced to 80%. Take the warm, strained decoction on an empty stomach before meals. Today, this formula may be prepared as a decoction with the doses suggested in brackets.

946

Chinese Herbal Formulas and Applications

Xiǎo Jì Yǐn Zǐ (Cirsium Decoction)

CHINESE THERAPEUTIC ACTIONS
1. Cools the blood and stops bleeding
2. Promotes urination and treats *lin zheng* (dysuria syndrome)

CLINICAL MANIFESTATIONS
Xue lin (bloody dysuria) caused by heat in the lower *jiao*: hematuria, frequent urination with a burning sensation and pain, red tongue body, and a rapid pulse.

CLINICAL APPLICATIONS
Acute urinary tract infection, proteinuria, hematuria, and acute glomerulonephritis.

EXPLANATION
Xiao Ji Yin Zi (Cirsium Decoction) treats *xue lin* (bloody dysuria) caused by heat in the lower *jiao*. In this syndrome, heat stagnates in the Urinary Bladder and damages the vessels, causing various urinary disorders such as hematuria and frequent urination with burning pain. A red tongue body and rapid pulse indicate heat.

The treatment plan for this syndrome is to cool the blood, stop bleeding, promote urination, and relieve pain. This formula contains *Xiao Ji* (Herba Cirsii) as the chief herb to cool the blood and stop bleeding. *Ou Jie* (Nodus Nelumbinis Rhizomatis) and *Pu Huang* (Pollen Typhae) cool the blood, stop bleeding, and resolve blood stasis. These two herbs effectively stop bleeding without creating blood stasis. *Hua Shi* (Talcum) clears heat and promotes

urination. *Mu Tong* (Caulis Akebiae), *Dan Zhu Ye* (Herba Lophatheri), and *Zhi Zi* (Fructus Gardeniae) drains fire from the Heart, Lung, and *San Jiao*. Since the presence of heat may damage yin and blood, *Di Huang* (Radix Rehmanniae) and *Dang Gui* (Radix Angelicae Sinensis) are added to clear heat, cool the blood, nourish yin and tonify blood. *Dang Gui* (Radix Angelicae Sinensis) also prevents the cold herbs in this formula from injuring the body. *Zhi Gan Cao* (Radix et Rhizoma Glycyrrhizae Praeparata cum Melle) harmonizes the herbs.

MODIFICATIONS
- With dysuria characterized by blood stagnation and heat, add *Shi Wei* (Folium Pyrrosiae), *Pu Gong Ying* (Herba Taraxaci) and *Huang Bo* (Cortex Phellodendri Chinensis).
- For chronic *xue lin* (bloody dysuria) with qi and blood deficiencies, reduce the doses of *Hua Shi* (Talcum) and *Mu Tong* (Caulis Akebiae), and add *Dang Shen* (Radix Codonopsis), *Huang Qi* (Radix Astragali), and *E Jiao* (Colla Corii Asini).
- With more heat, replace *Zhi Gan Cao* (Radix et Rhizoma Glycyrrhizae Praeparata cum Melle) with *Gan Cao* (Radix et Rhizoma Glycyrrhizae).
- With severe pain in the penis during urination, add *Hu Po* (Succinum).

CAUTIONS / CONTRAINDICATIONS
- *Xiao Ji Yin Zi* should only be used to treat excess *xue lin* (bloody dysuria), as it contains mostly cold and draining herbs.

BLOOD-REGULATING FORMULAS

13

Xiao Ji Yin Zi (Cirsium Decoction)

Diagnosis	Signs and Symptoms	Treatment	Herbs
Xue lin (bloody dysuria) caused by heat in the lower *jiao*	• Hematuria and frequent urination with burning pain: heat stagnates in the Urinary Bladder • Red tongue and rapid pulse: heat condition	• Cools the blood and stops bleeding • Promotes urination and treats *lin zheng* (dysuria syndrome)	• *Xiao Ji* (Herba Cirsii) cools the blood and stops the bleeding. • *Ou Jie* (Nodus Nelumbinis Rhizomatis) and *Pu Huang* (Pollen Typhae) cool the blood, stop bleeding, and resolve blood stasis. • *Hua Shi* (Talcum) clears heat and promotes urination to relieve pain. • *Mu Tong* (Caulis Akebiae), *Dan Zhu Ye* (Herba Lophatheri), and *Zhi Zi* (Fructus Gardeniae) drains fire from the Heart, Lung, and *San Jiao*. • *Di Huang* (Radix Rehmanniae) nourishes yin, cools the blood, and clears heat. • *Dang Gui* (Radix Angelicae Sinensis) nourishes blood and prevents the cold herbs in this formula from injuring the body. • *Zhi Gan Cao* (Radix et Rhizoma Glycyrrhizae Praeparata cum Melle) harmonizes the herbs.

947

Chapter 13 – Blood-Regulating Formulas

Section 2 – Stop-Bleeding Formulas

Xiǎo Jì Yǐn Zǐ (Cirsium Decoction)

- Chronic cases of *xue lin* (bloody dysuria) are often accompanied by underlying deficiencies, and must also be treated with tonifying herbs.

CLINICAL STUDIES AND RESEARCH

1. **Proteinuria**: Use of *Xiao Ji Yin Zi* plus *He Di* (Calyx Nelumbinis) in 35 patients with proteinuria was associated with 97% effectiveness (complete recovery in 19 cases, marked improvement in 9 cases, moderate improvement in 6 cases, and no improvement in 1 case). Patients were instructed to take the herbs daily, maintain a low-sodium diet, avoid exposure to wind and cold, and refrain from sexual activity during the treatment period.[1]

2. **Hematuria in urinary infection**: *Xiao Ji Yin Zi* and *Ba Zheng San* (Eight-Herb Powder for Rectification) were used to treat hematuria due to acute urinary infection. The treatment strategy was to use *Xiao Ji Yin Zi* as the main formula for *xue lin* (bloody dysuria), and *Ba Zheng San* (Eight-Herb Powder for Rectification) for *re lin* (heat dysuria). Furthermore, modifications were made by adding *Mu Dan Pi* (Cortex Moutan) and *Bai Mao Gen* (Rhizoma Imperatae) for excessive blood in the urine; and *Qu Mai* (Herba Dianthi) and *Che Qian Zi* (Semen Plantaginis) for burning sensations and pain in the urethra. Of 48 patients, the study reported complete recovery in 28 cases, significant improvement in 4 cases, moderate improvement in 10 cases, and no effect in 6 cases. The overall effectiveness was 87.5%. The duration of treatment ranged from 2-9 days.[2]

References

1. *Hu Nan Yi Yao Za Zhi* (Hunan Journal of Medicine and Herbology) 1984;6:14.
2. *Hei Long Jiang Zhong Yi Yao* (Heilongjiang Journal of Chinese Medicine and Herbology) 1985;3:43.

Huáng Tǔ Tāng (Yellow Earth Decoction)
黃土湯
黄土汤

Pinyin Name: *Huang Tu Tang*
Literal Name: Yellow Earth Decoction
Original Source: *Jin Gui Yao Lue* (Essentials from the Golden Cabinet) by Zhang Zhong-Jing in the Eastern Han Dynasty

COMPOSITION

Fu Long Gan (Terra Flava Usta)	24g [30g]
Bai Zhu (Rhizoma Atractylodis Macrocephalae)	9g
Fu Zi (Radix Aconiti Lateralis Praeparata), *pao* (blast-fried)	9g
Di Huang (Radix Rehmanniae)	9g
E Jiao (Colla Corii Asini)	9g
Huang Qin (Radix Scutellariae)	9g
Gan Cao (Radix et Rhizoma Glycyrrhizae)	9g

DOSAGE / PREPARATION / ADMINISTRATION

The source text states to cook the ingredients with 8 cups [1,600 mL] of water until the liquid is reduced to 3 cups [600 mL]. Take the warm decoction in two equally-divided doses. Today, it is recommended to cook *Fu Long Gan* (Terra Flava Usta) first, discard the residue, then cook the rest of the herbs in the strained decoction.

CHINESE THERAPEUTIC ACTIONS

1. Warms the yang and strengthens the Spleen
2. Nourishes the blood and stops bleeding

CLINICAL MANIFESTATIONS

Bleeding due to Spleen yang deficiency, accompanied by deficiency and cold in the middle *jiao*: various types of bleeding such as hematochezia, hematemesis, epistaxis, excessive menstrual bleeding, bleeding with pale-red or dull-red blood, cold extremities, sallow facial appearance, a pale tongue body with a white tongue coating, and a deep, fine, and forceless pulse.

948

Chinese Herbal Formulas and Applications

Huáng Tǔ Tāng (Yellow Earth Decoction)

CLINICAL APPLICATIONS

Upper gastrointestinal bleeding, epistaxis, hemorrhoidal bleeding, duodenal ulcers, and uterine bleeding.

EXPLANATION

Huang Tu Tang (Yellow Earth Decoction) treats bleeding due to Spleen yang deficiency and cold accumulation in the middle *jiao*. The Spleen keeps blood contained within the blood vessels. If Spleen yang is deficient, blood may leak out of the vessels, causing various types of bleeding. This inability to control the circulation of blood results in aimless movement of blood: hematemesis and epistaxis in the upper body, and hematochezia and excessive menstrual bleeding in the lower body. Cold extremities, sallow facial appearance, a pale tongue, and a deep, fine, and forceless pulse all suggest Spleen yang deficiency. The patient may become progressively weaker due to blood deficiency as blood is lost through gastrointestinal bleeding.

This formula contains *Fu Long Gan* (Terra Flava Usta) to warm the middle *jiao* and stop bleeding. *Bai Zhu* (Rhizoma Atractylodis Macrocephalae) and *Fu Zi* (Radix Aconiti Lateralis Praeparata) tonify and warm Spleen yang. These two acrid and warm herbs, however, tend to be moving and drying in nature and may consume blood in patients who are already deficient from bleeding. Therefore, *Di Huang* (Radix Rehmanniae) and *E Jiao* (Colla Corii Asini) are added to nourish yin, tonify the blood and stop bleeding. Furthermore, the warm property of *Bai Zhu* (Rhizoma Atractylodis Macrocephalae) and hot property of *Fu Zi* (Radix Aconiti Lateralis Praeparata) are moderated with the cold property of *Huang Qin* (Radix Scutellariae). Lastly, *Gan Cao* (Radix et Rhizoma Glycyrrhizae) harmonizes the herbs.

MODIFICATIONS

- With qi deficiency, add *Ren Shen* (Radix et Rhizoma Ginseng), *Dang Shen* (Radix Codonopsis), and *Huang Qi* (Radix Astragali).
- With profuse bleeding, add *San Qi* (Radix et Rhizoma Notoginseng) and *Bai Ji* (Rhizoma Bletillae).
- With diarrhea, use charred *Huang Qin* (Radix Scutellariae) and *Pao Jiang* (Rhizoma Zingiberis Praeparatum).
- With palpitations, remove *Huang Qin* (Radix Scutellariae), and add *Long Yan Rou* (Arillus Longan) and *Suan Zao Ren* (Semen Ziziphi Spinosae).

CAUTIONS / CONTRAINDICATIONS

- *Huang Tu Tang* should be used with caution in bleeding due to heat conditions.
- This formula is contraindicated in bleeding with an exterior condition.

CLINICAL STUDIES AND RESEARCH

1. **Upper gastrointestinal bleeding**: Upper gastrointestinal bleeding in 29 patients was treated with 89.6% effectiveness using *Huang Tu Tang* plus *Xian He Cao* (Herba Agrimoniae) and *Bai Ji* (Rhizoma Bletillae).[1]
2. **Duodenal bleeding**: One study reported complete recovery in 24 of 36 patients with duodenal ulcers and bleeding using *Huang Tu Tang* plus *Hua Rui Shi* (Ophicalcitum), *Bu Gu Zhi* (Fructus Psoraleae), and *Xian He Cao* (Herba Agrimoniae).[2]
3. **Hemorrhoidal bleeding**: One study reported successful treatment in all 16 patients with chronic hemorrhoidal bleeding using *Huang Tu Tang*.[3]

AUTHORS' COMMENTS

Huang Tu Tang is primarily used for hematochezia or *beng lou* (flooding and spotting) caused by Spleen yang

BLOOD-REGULATING FORMULAS

13

Huang Tu Tang (Yellow Earth Decoction)

Diagnosis	Signs and Symptoms	Treatment	Herbs
Bleeding due to Spleen yang deficiency and deficiency and cold in the middle *jiao*	• Hematemesis, epistaxis, hematochezia and menstrual bleeding: bleeding due to inability of yang qi to control the circulation of blood • Cold extremities, sallow facial appearance: cold accumulation and Spleen yang deficiency • Pale tongue and a deep, fine and forceless pulse: yang deficiency	• Warms the yang and strengthens the Spleen • Nourishes the blood and stops bleeding	• *Fu Long Gan* (Terra Flava Usta) warms the middle *jiao* and stops bleeding. • *Bai Zhu* (Rhizoma Atractylodis Macrocephalae) and *Fu Zi* (Radix Aconiti Lateralis Praeparata) warm Spleen yang. • *Di Huang* (Radix Rehmanniae) and *E Jiao* (Colla Corii Asini) nourish yin and tonify the blood. • *Huang Qin* (Radix Scutellariae) controls and balances the warm herbs. • *Gan Cao* (Radix et Rhizoma Glycyrrhizae) harmonizes the herbs.

949

Chapter 13 – Blood-Regulating Formulas   *Section 2 – Stop-Bleeding Formulas*

Huáng Tǔ Tāng (Yellow Earth Decoction)

deficiency. The blood is pale red or dull red in color. Patients usually exhibit a pale tongue body with a deep, fine, and forceless pulse. The two diagnostic criteria are "deficiency" and "cold."

Huang Tu, translated as "Yellow Earth," and literally describing the soot and ash from an enclosed fire pit, is the alternate or common name for *Fu Long Gan* (Terra Flava Usta). Thus, this formula is called *Huang Tu Tang* (Yellow Earth Decoction) because it contains *Huang Tu* as the chief herb. It is the chief herb because it represents the primary function of the formula to warm the middle *jiao* and stop bleeding.

Fu Long Gan (Terra Flava Usta) is not commonly used today. If it is unavailable, *Chi Shi Zhi* (Halloysitum Rubrum) may be used as a substitute.[4]

References

1. *Zhe Jiang Zhong Yi Za Zhi* (Zhejiang Journal of Chinese Medicine) 1958;7:21.
2. *Hei Long Jiang Zhong Yi Yao* (Heilongjiang Journal of Chinese Medicine and Herbology) 1996;3:16.
3. *Fu Jian Zhong Yi Yao* (Fujian Journal of Chinese Medicine and Herbology) 1991;22(3):12.
4. *Zhong Yao Ming Fang Yao Li Yu Ying Yong* (Pharmacology and Applications of Famous Herbal Formulas) 1989;519-520.

Jiāo Ài Tāng (Ass-Hide Gelatin and Mugwort Decoction)
膠艾湯
胶艾汤

Pinyin Name: *Jiao Ai Tang*
Literal Name: Ass-Hide Gelatin and Mugwort Decoction
Alternate Names: *Chiung Kuei Jiao Ai Tang, Qiong Gui Jiao Ai Tang, Xiong Gui Jiao Ai Tang*, Cnidium, Tang-kuei, Gelatin, and Mugwort Leaf Decoction; Cnidium, Tangkuei, Gelatin and Artemisia Decoction
Original Source: *Jin Gui Yao Lue* (Essentials from the Golden Cabinet) by Zhang Zhong-Jing in the Eastern Han Dynasty

COMPOSITION

E Jiao (Colla Corii Asini)	6g [6-9g]
Ai Ye (Folium Artemisiae Argyi)	9g
Dang Gui (Radix Angelicae Sinensis)	9g
Di Huang (Radix Rehmanniae)	18g [12-15g]
Bai Shao (Radix Paeoniae Alba)	12g
Chuan Xiong (Rhizoma Chuanxiong)	6g
Gan Cao (Radix et Rhizoma Glycyrrhizae)	6g

DOSAGE / PREPARATION / ADMINISTRATION

The source text states to cook the ingredients, except *E Jiao* (Colla Corii Asini), with 5 cups [1,000 mL] of water and 3 cups [600 mL] of grain-based liquor until the liquid is reduced to 3 cups [600 mL]. Discard the herbal residue. Dissolve *E Jiao* (Colla Corii Asini) into the warm, strained decoction until it melts completely. Take 1 cup [200 mL] of the warm decoction three times daily. The source text recommends taking the formula until the symptoms are resolved. Today, it is prepared as a decoction by cooking the herbs using the doses suggested in brackets in water, with or without a grain-based liquor. *E Jiao* (Colla Corii Asini) is dissolved into the warm, strained decoction immediately before serving.

CHINESE THERAPEUTIC ACTIONS

1. Tonifies the blood and stops bleeding
2. Regulates menses and calms the fetus

CLINICAL MANIFESTATIONS

Beng lou (flooding and spotting) due to deficiency and damage to the *chong* (thoroughfare) and *ren* (conception) channels in women: menstrual irregularity, menorrhagia, excessive and continuous menstrual bleeding and spotting, pale and thin blood without clots, and abdominal pain. It is also effective for unstable pregnancy with uterine pain and/or bleeding, and continuous bleeding after premature delivery or miscarriage.

950

Chinese Herbal Formulas and Applications

Jiāo Ài Tāng (Ass-Hide Gelatin and Mugwort Decoction)

CLINICAL APPLICATIONS

Uterine bleeding, endometriosis, prevention of spontaneous miscarriage, excessive menstrual bleeding, excessive bleeding during pregnancy, excessive postpartum bleeding, rectal bleeding, hemorrhoid bleeding, hematuria, hemoptysis, duodenal ulcers with bleeding, anemia, and thrombocytopenic purpura.

EXPLANATION

Jiao Ai Tang (Ass-Hide Gelatin and Mugwort Decoction) treats *beng lou* (flooding and spotting) due to deficiency and damage to the *chong* (thoroughfare) and *ren* (conception) channels. The *chong* channel is the sea of blood, and the *ren* channel dominates the uterus and fetus. If the *chong* and *ren* channels are damaged and become deficient, excessive and prolonged bleeding may occur. For pregnant women, this condition is characterized by unstable pregnancy, restless fetus, uterine bleeding, and abdominal pain.

The treatment plan for this syndrome is to tonify the blood, stop bleeding, regulate menstruation, and stabilize the fetus. In this formula *E Jiao* (Colla Corii Asini) nourishes the blood and stops bleeding. *Ai Ye* (Folium Artemisiae Argyi) warms the menses and stops bleeding. Combined, these two herbs regulate menstruation, treat *beng lou* (flooding and spotting), and stabilize the fetus. To tonify blood, regulate menstruation and move blood, this formula uses *Dang Gui* (Radix Angelicae Sinensis), *Di Huang* (Radix Rehmanniae), *Bai Shao* (Radix Paeoniae Alba), and *Chuan Xiong* (Rhizoma Chuanxiong), the four herbs in the blood-tonifying formula *Si Wu Tang* (Four-Substance Decoction). *Gan Cao* (Radix et Rhizoma Glycyrrhizae) also tonifies qi and harmonizes all the herbs in the formula. In addition, the combination of *Gan Cao* (Radix et Rhizoma Glycyrrhizae) and *E Jiao* (Colla Corii Asini) stops bleeding; and the combination of *Gan Cao* (Radix et Rhizoma Glycyrrhizae) and *Bai Shao* (Radix

Paeoniae Alba) relieves pain. Lastly, grain-based liquor increases the impact of the herbs and prevents the development of blood stasis.

MODIFICATIONS

- With qi deficiency, add *Ren Shen* (Radix et Rhizoma Ginseng) and *Huang Qi* (Radix Astragali).
- With pain in the abdomen and lower back, add *Zhi Shi* (Fructus Aurantii Immaturus) and *Hou Po* (Cortex Magnoliae Officinalis).
- With excessive bleeding, add *Xian He Cao* (Herba Agrimoniae) and *Di Yu* (Radix Sanguisorbae).
- With profuse bleeding, add charred *Di Yu* (Radix Sanguisorbae) and charred *Ai Ye* (Folium Artemisiae Argyi).
- With abdominal pain due to blood stagnation, add *Yan Hu Suo* (Rhizoma Corydalis) and *San Qi* (Radix et Rhizoma Notoginseng).
- With unstable pregnancy, add *Bao Chan Wu You Fang* (Preserve Pregnancy and Care-Free Decoction).
- With constant and restless movement of the fetus due to deficiency, add *Du Zhong* (Cortex Eucommiae), *Xu Duan* (Radix Dipsaci), and *Sang Ji Sheng* (Herba Taxilli).

CAUTIONS / CONTRAINDICATIONS

Jiao Ai Tang is contraindicated in cases of hypermenorrhea, or *beng lou* (flooding and spotting) caused by heat.

CLINICAL STUDIES AND RESEARCH

1. **Uterine bleeding**: Administration of *Jiao Ai Tang* effectively treated 25 patients with uterine bleeding due to functional disorders. The herbs were given in decoction once a day, with treatment duration varying from 4 to 8 packs of herbs.[1]
2. **Thrombocytopenic purpura**: Administration of modified *Jiao Ai Tang* was associated with 94% effectiveness in treating 17 patients with thrombocytopenic purpura. The herbal treatment contained this formula plus *Xuan Shen*

Jiao Ai Tang (Ass-Hide Gelatin and Mugwort Decoction)

Diagnosis	Signs and Symptoms	Treatment	Herbs
Beng lou (flooding and spotting)	Excessive and prolonged menstrual bleeding: deficiency of the *chong* (thoroughfare) and *ren* (conception) channels	• Tonifies blood and stops bleeding • Regulates menstruation and calms the fetus	• *E Jiao* (Colla Corii Asini) nourishes the blood and stops bleeding. • *Ai Ye* (Folium Artemisiae Argyi) warms the menses and stops bleeding. • *Dang Gui* (Radix Angelicae Sinensis), *Di Huang* (Radix Rehmanniae), *Bai Shao* (Radix Paeoniae Alba), and *Chuan Xiong* (Rhizoma Chuanxiong) tonify blood and regulate blood circulation. • *Gan Cao* (Radix et Rhizoma Glycyrrhizae) tonifies qi and harmonizes the herbs.

BLOOD-REGULATING FORMULAS

13

951

Jiāo Ài Tāng (Ass-Hide Gelatin and Mugwort Decoction)

(Radix Scrophulariae), *Mai Dong* (Radix Ophiopogonis), *Dan Shen* (Radix et Rhizoma Salviae Miltiorrhizae), and *Ren Shen* (Radix et Rhizoma Ginseng). Of 17 patients, the study reported significant improvement in 12 cases, moderate improvement in 4 cases, and no benefit in 1 case.[2]

3. **Duodenal ulcers and bleeding**: One study reported recovery in 49 of 50 patients with gastrointestinal bleeding caused by duodenal ulcers when treated with modified *Jiao Ai Tang* for 3-7 days. Recovery was confirmed by absence of blood in the stools and resolution of all symptoms.[3]

References

1. *Zhong Hua Fu Chan Ke Za Zhi* (Chinese Journal of Obstetrics and Gynecology) 1959;5:413.
2. *Hei Long Jiang Zhong Yi Yao* (Heilongjiang Journal of Chinese Medicine and Herbology) 1990;6:15.
3. *Zhong Yi Fang Ji Xian Dai Yan Jiu* (Modern Study of Medical Formulae in Traditional Chinese Medicine) 1997;1145.

Chinese Herbal Formulas and Applications

Chapter 13 — Summary

— Blood-Regulating Formulas

SECTION 1: BLOOD-INVIGORATING AND STASIS-REMOVING FORMULAS

Name	Similarities	Differences
Tao He Cheng Qi Tang (Peach Pit Decoction to Order the Qi)	Breaks up blood stasis and drains it downward	Treats blood stagnation in the lower *jiao*
Tong Qiao Huo Xue Tang (Unblock the Orifices and Invigorate the Blood Decoction)		Opens the sensory orifices in the head and face
Xue Fu Zhu Yu Tang (Drive Out Stasis in the Mansion of Blood Decoction)		Treats blood stagnation in the chest (upper *jiao*)
Ge Xia Zhu Yu Tang (Drive Out Blood Stasis Below the Diaphragm Decoction)	Activate blood circulation, dispel blood stagnation	Treats blood stagnation below the diaphragm (middle *jiao*)
Shao Fu Zhu Yu Tang (Drive Out Blood Stasis in the Lower Abdomen Decoction)		Treats blood stagnation in the lower abdomen (lower *jiao*)
Shen Tong Zhu Yu Tang (Drive Out Blood Stasis from a Painful Body Decoction)		Treats qi and blood stagnation throughout the body (extremities)
Fu Yuan Huo Xue Tang (Revive Health by Invigorating the Blood Decoction)		Traumatic injuries with pain and swelling in the chest and hypochondriac region
Zheng Gu Zi Jin Dan (Purple and Gold Pill for Righteous Bones)	Activate blood circulation, dispel blood stasis, treat traumatic injuries	Traumatic injuries of soft tissues and bones
Qi Li San (Seven-Thousandths of a Tael Powder)		Traumatic injuries of soft tissues and bones, stops bleeding
Bu Yang Huan Wu Tang (Tonify the Yang to Restore Five Decoction)	Activates blood circulation, opens the channels and collaterals	Tonifies qi, treats post-stroke sequelae
Shi Xiao San (Sudden Smile Powder)	Activate blood circulation, remove blood stasis, relieve chest and abdominal pain	Treats pain due to blood stagnation in the Liver channel
Huo Luo Xiao Ling Dan (Fantastically Effective Pill to Invigorate the Collaterals)		Treats swelling and pain due to blood stagnation from trauma
Dan Shen Yin (Salvia Decoction)		Treats pain in the epigastric and abdominal regions due to qi and blood stagnation
Wen Jing Tang (Warm the Channels Decoction)	Activate blood circulation, warm the channels/uterus, treat gynecological disorders	Warms the *chong* (thoroughfare) and *ren* (conception) channels, disperses cold, nourishes the blood
Ai Fu Nuan Gong Wan (Mugwort and Cyperus Pill for Warming the Womb)		Warms the uterus, nourishes the blood
Sheng Hua Tang (Generation and Transformation Decoction)		Warms the channels, stops pain
Gui Zhi Fu Ling Wan (Cinnamon Twig and Poria Pill)	Activate blood circulation, remove blood stasis, treat gynecological disorders	Gently activates blood circulation, gradually dissolves blood stagnation
Zhe Chong Yin (Break the Conflict Decoction)		Strongly activates blood circulation, dispels blood stasis, disperses stagnation
Bie Jia Jian Wan (Soft-Shelled Turtle Shell Pill)	Break up and eliminate stagnation, soften hardness and resolve masses	Activates qi and blood circulation, dispels dampness and phlegm
Da Huang Zhe Chong Wan (Rhubarb and Eupolyphaga Pill)		Promotes generation of new blood

BLOOD-REGULATING FORMULAS

13

953

Chapter 13 — Summary

Tao He Cheng Qi Tang (Peach Pit Decoction to Order the Qi) clears heat, and breaks up and dispels blood stasis. It is especially indicated for blood stagnation with heat in the lower *jiao* causing acute lower abdominal pain, delirium, irritability, thirst, fever at night, normal urination, or, in severe cases, mania.

There are five formulas that have similar functions to activate blood circulation and dispel blood stagnation. The difference between each of the five formulas is that they treat blood stagnation in different parts of the body.

- ***Tong Qiao Huo Xue Tang*** (Unblock the Orifices and Invigorate the Blood Decoction) activates blood circulation and opens the sensory orifices. It treats blood stagnation in the head and face, with signs and symptoms such as headache, dizziness, chronic tinnitus and poor hearing, and blue/green/purplish facial appearance.

- ***Xue Fu Zhu Yu Tang*** (Drive Out Stasis in the Mansion of Blood Decoction) activates qi and blood circulation, removes blood stagnation, and relieves pain. It is used to treat qi and blood stagnation in the chest, with prolonged and fixed stabbing pain in the chest.

- ***Ge Xia Zhu Yu Tang*** (Drive Out Blood Stasis Below the Diaphragm Decoction) activates qi and blood circulation, dispels blood stagnation, and relieves pain. It is most effective for blood stagnation below the diaphragm that is characterized by symptoms such as fixed abdominal pain, a feeling of an unmovable mass in the abdomen, and fullness and pain in the hypochondriac and abdominal regions.

- ***Shao Fu Zhu Yu Tang*** (Drive Out Blood Stasis in the Lower Abdomen Decoction) activates blood circulation, dispels blood stagnation, and warms and regulates menstruation. This formula is commonly used to treat blood stagnation in the lower abdomen, with signs and symptoms such as pain and fullness in the lower abdominal region, formation of a mass in the lower abdominal region, multiple cycles of bleeding (between 3-5 times) within one period, menstrual pain, low back pain and abdominal fullness during menstruation, and excessive menstrual bleeding that is black and purplish with blood clots.

- ***Shen Tong Zhu Yu Tang*** (Drive Out Blood Stasis from a Painful Body Decoction) activates qi and blood circulation, dispels blood stagnation, and opens the channels and collaterals. It is excellent in treating *bi zheng* (painful obstruction syndrome) due to qi and blood stagnation blocking the channels and collaterals. Clinical manifestations include pain in the shoulder, elbow, waist, leg, or the whole body.

Fu Yuan Huo Xue Tang (Revive Health by Invigorating the Blood Decoction), ***Zheng Gu Zi Jin Dan*** (Purple and Gold Pill for Righteous Bones), and ***Qi Li San*** (Seven-Thousandths of a Tael Powder) have excellent functions to treat traumatic injuries by activating blood circulation and dispelling blood stasis.

- *Fu Yuan Huo Xue Tang* treats severe stabbing pain in the hypochondriac region due to trauma. This formula activates blood circulation, removes blood stasis, soothes Liver qi, and dredges the collaterals.

- *Zheng Gu Zi Jin Dan* treats many different types of soft tissue and bone injuries, with symptoms such as pain, swelling, inflammation, and bruising. The main actions of this formula are to activate blood circulation, dispel blood stasis, open the channels and collaterals, and reduce swelling and bruises.

- *Qi Li San* treats severe cases of external or traumatic injuries with severe damage to soft tissues and bones, such as muscle sprain, tendon and ligament strain, or bone fracture. It is also very effective in stopping bleeding, reducing swelling, and relieving pain. This formula can be administered both externally and internally.

Chapter 13 — Summary

Bu Yang Huan Wu Tang (Tonify the Yang to Restore Five Decoction) tonifies qi, activates blood circulation, and invigorates the functions of the channels and collaterals. It is designed for post-stroke sequelae due to qi deficiency and blood stagnation, with symptoms such as hemiplegia, deviation of the mouth and eyes, difficulty in speech, involuntary leakage of saliva, atrophy of the lower extremities, and frequent urination or urinary incontinence.

Shi Xiao San (Sudden Smile Powder), ***Huo Luo Xiao Ling Dan*** (Fantastically Effective Pill to Invigorate the Collaterals), and ***Dan Shen Yin*** (Salvia Decoction) are formulas with similar functions to activate blood circulation, remove blood stasis, and relieve chest and abdominal pain. However, their clinical applications are rather different.

• *Shi Xiao San* activates blood circulation, removes blood stasis, disperses nodules, and stops pain. It is used mainly for sharp abdominal pain due to blood stagnation in irregular menstruation. It is also effective for postpartum bleeding due to residual placenta in the uterus.

• *Huo Luo Xiao Ling Dan* activates blood circulation, dispels blood stasis, and dredges the collaterals to relieve pain. This formula is effective for various types of pain and disorders due to qi and blood stagnation, such as chest and abdominal pain, pain of the arms and legs, and bruises and swelling due to trauma.

• *Dan Shen Yin* activates qi and blood circulation, removes blood stasis, and stops pain. It is used for heart (epigastric region) and stomach (upper abdominal area) pain due to qi and blood stagnation. The pain is fixed, and is intensified by pressure.

Wen Jing Tang (Warm the Channels Decoction), ***Ai Fu Nuan Gong Wan*** (Mugwort and Cyperus Pill for Warming the Womb), and ***Sheng Hua Tang*** (Generation and Transformation Decoction) are three formulas specifically designed for the treatment of gynecological disorders. All three have similar functions to activate blood circulation, remove blood stasis, and warm the channels/uterus.

• *Wen Jing Tang* treats blood stagnation due to deficiency cold in the *ren* (conception) and *chong* (thoroughfare) channels. This formula warms the channels, disperses cold, nourishes blood, and removes blood stasis. Clinical manifestations include irregular menstruation, afternoon fever, irritability, hot palms, dry mouth and lips, abdominal fullness, lower abdominal pain, and possible infertility in women.

• *Ai Fu Nuan Gong Wan* treats deficiency and cold of the uterus. It warms the uterus, nourishes the blood, and activates blood circulation. Clinical manifestations include leukorrhea, yellowish facial complexion, painful extremities, lethargy, lack of energy, low appetite, irregular menstruation, lower abdominal pain, and infertility.

• *Sheng Hua Tang* treats blood stagnation with interior cold and blood deficiency after delivery. It activates blood circulation, removes blood stasis, warms the channels, and stops pain. Clinical manifestations include continuous bleeding due to the placenta remaining in the uterus, and cold sensations with pain in the lower abdomen.

Gui Zhi Fu Ling Wan (Cinnamon Twig and Poria Pill) and ***Zhe Chong Yin*** (Break the Conflict Decoction) exert similar actions to activate blood circulation and remove blood stasis.

• *Gui Zhi Fu Ling Wan* is used traditionally during pregnancy to treat blood stagnation in the uterus. Clinical manifestations of this condition include instability of the fetus, continuous dripping of purplish black blood, and abdominal pain that is aggravated by pressure. Due to this delicate condition, this formula is composed carefully with herbs to gently activate blood circulation and gradually dissolve blood stagnation.

• *Zhe Chong Yin* treats irregular menstruation, dysmenorrhea, and amenorrhea due to blood stagnation in the lower *jiao* with severe pain in the lower abdominal region. It is potent in activating blood circulation, dispelling blood stasis, dissolving stagnation, and dispersing obstruction.

Chapter 13 – Blood-Regulating Formulas

Chapter 13 — Summary

Bie Jia Jian Wan (Soft-Shelled Turtle Shell Pill) and *Da Huang Zhe Chong Wan* (Rhubarb and Eupolyphaga Pill) break up and eliminate stagnation, soften hardness, and resolve masses.

- *Bie Jia Jian Wan* functions strongly to activate qi and blood circulation, dispel dampness and phlegm, and resolve hardness and masses. It is used primarily to treat chronic malaria with an enlarged spleen. Today, this formula may be used for splenomegaly, hepatomegaly, hepatitis, and liver cirrhosis.

- *Da Huang Zhe Chong Wan* has potent actions to break up and dispel blood stasis, and promote the generation of new blood. Historically, it was used to treat extreme deficiency and debility from consumptive lifestyles. Today, it may be used to treat hepatitis, liver fibrosis or cirrhosis, and uterine leiomyoma.

SECTION 2: STOP-BLEEDING FORMULAS

Name	Similarities	Differences
Shi Hui San (Ten Partially-Charred Substances Powder)	Cool the blood, stop bleeding	Stops bleeding from the upper parts of the body, such as hematemesis, hemoptysis, and gastrointestinal bleeding
Si Sheng Wan (Four-Fresh Pill)		Stops bleeding from the upper parts of the body, such as hematemesis and epistaxis
Ke Xue Fang (Coughing of Blood Formula)		Stops hemoptysis
Huai Hua San (Sophora Japonica Flower Powder)		Stops bleeding from the lower parts of the body, such as hematochezia
Xiao Ji Yin Zi (Cirsium Decoction)		Stops bleeding from the lower parts of the body, such as hematuria
Huang Tu Tang (Yellow Earth Decoction)	Tonify the blood, stop bleeding	Warms the yang and strengthens the Spleen
Jiao Ai Tang (Ass-Hide Gelatin and Mugwort Decoction)		Regulates menstruation and calms the fetus

Shi Hui San (Ten Partially-Charred Substances Powder) cools the blood and stops bleeding. It is used for hematemesis, hemoptysis, and other bleeding symptoms due to blood heat affecting the upper parts of the body. This is the most commonly used hemostatic formula for emergency cases of bleeding. Cease administration of this formula once the desired effect is achieved.

Si Sheng Wan (Four-Fresh Pill) cools the blood and stops bleeding. It is used for hematemesis and epistaxis with bright red blood, and dry mouth and throat due to blood heat affecting the upper parts of the body. Administration of this formula should be stopped once the desired effect is achieved.

Ke Xue Fang (Coughing of Blood Formula) clears fire, dissolves phlegm, astringes the Lung, and stops coughing. It is used for Liver fire invading the Lung, with manifestations such as coughing with thick sputum and streaks of blood.

Huai Hua San (Sophora Japonica Flower Powder) stops rectal bleeding, and clears wind, heat, and toxins in the Intestines. It is used for hematochezia and dysentery, with bleeding prior to or defecation, hemorrhoids, and bright or dark red blood in the stools.

Xiao Ji Yin Zi (Cirsium Decoction) cools the blood, stops bleeding, and promotes urination. It is used for *xue lin* (bloody dysuria) with heat causing hematuria, frequent urination with burning sensations and pain, a red tongue body, and a rapid pulse.

956

Chinese Herbal Formulas and Applications

Chapter 13 — Summary

Huang Tu Tang (Yellow Earth Decoction) warms yang, strengthens the Spleen, nourishes blood, and stops bleeding. It is used for deficiency and cold of the middle *jiao* causing bloody stools, hematemesis, epistaxis, excessive menstrual bleeding with pale red blood, cold extremities, and sallow facial appearance.

Jiao Ai Tang (Ass-Hide Gelatin and Mugwort Decoction) tonifies blood, stops bleeding, regulates menstruation, and stabilizes pregnancy. It is used to treat deficiency and damage to the *ren* (conception) and *chong* (thoroughfare) channels with clinical manifestations such as menorrhagia, excessive menstrual bleeding, or excessive bleeding during pregnancy or after delivery.

BLOOD-REGULATING FORMULAS

13

957

Chapter 13 — Summary

Huang Tu Tang (Yellow Earth Decoction) warms yang, strengthens the Spleen, nourishes blood, and stops bleeding. It is used for deficiency and cold of the middle jiao causing bloody stool, hematemesis, epistaxis, excessive menstrual bleeding with pale red blood, cold extremities, and sallow facial appearance.

Jiao Ai Tang (Ass-Hide Gelatin and Mugwort Decoction) tonifies blood, stops bleeding, regulates menstruation, and stabilizes pregnancy. It is used to treat deficiency and damage to the ren (conception) and chong (thoroughfare) channels with clinical manifestations such as menorrhagia, excessive menstrual bleeding, or excessive bleeding during pregnancy, or after delivery.

Chapter 14

— Wind-Expelling Formulas

治风剂

王燾 Wāng Táo

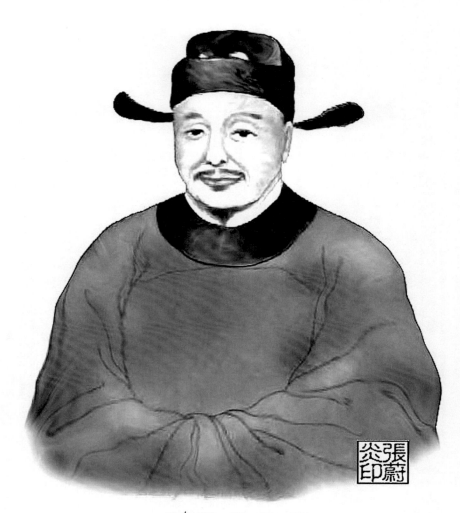

王燾 Wāng Táo, 670 – 755.

王燾 Wāng Táo

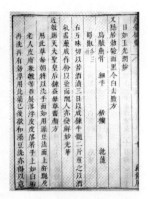

外台秘要 *Wai Tai Mi Yao* (Arcane Essentials from the Imperial Library) in 752.

Wang Tao was born into the Imperial family. Wang was the grandson of 唐太宗 Tang Tai-Zong, one of the most famous emperors in the Tang dynasty. Although Wang and his mother were privileged members of the Imperial family, they were always ill. Because of frequent contact with the best doctors in the entire country, Wang gradually developed an interest in medicine. With easy access to the best physicians in the Imperial Palace and the most comprehensive library in the country, the young scholar was in an excellent position to gain an overview of the field, and a discerning eye for the patterns and details in published works. Wang spent more than 20 years integrating all of the existing medical texts, filling in any omissions, and correcting errors. Published in 752 CE, *Wai Tai Mi Yao* (Arcane Essentials from the Imperial Library) was the most comprehensive text compiled during that era. It documented over 1,000 medical problems and over 6,900 herbal formulas for use in gynecology, obstetrics, pediatrics, psychiatry, dermatology, opthalmology, dentistry, and osteopathy. Carefully written and referenced in great detail, this text gave ordinary people a unique opportunity to gain deeper insight and understanding of medicine. Wang was credited as a great scholar of Traditional Chinese Medicine. *Wai Tai Mi Yao* (Arcane Essentials from the Imperial Library) was regarded by many as 世宝 a World Treasure.

Representative formulas from *Wai Tai Mi Yao* (Arcane Essentials from the Imperial Library) include:
- *Cong Bai Qi Wei Yin* (Scallion Decoction with Seven Ingredients)
- *Shi Gao Tang* (Gypsum Decoction)
- *Huang Lian Jie Du Tang* (Coptis Decoction to Relieve Toxicity)
- *Zi Xue Dan* (Purple Snow Pill)
- *Shen Mi Tang* (Mysterious Decoction)
- *Xu Ming Tang* (Prolong Life Decoction)

Dynasties & Kingdoms	Year
Xia Dynasty 夏	2100-1600 BCE
Shang Dynasty 商	1600-1100 BCE
Zhou Dynasty 周	1100-221 BCE
Qin Dynasty 秦	221-207 BCE
Han Dynasty 漢	206 BCE-220
Three Kingdoms 三國	220-280
Western Jin Dynasty 西晉	265-316
Eastern Jin Dynasty 東晉	317-420
Northern and Southern Dynasties 北南朝	420-581
Sui Dynasty 隋	581-618
Tang Dynasty 唐	**618-907**
Five Dynasties 五代	907-960
Song Dynasty 宋	960-1279
Liao Dynasty 遼	916-1125
Jin Dynasty 金	1115-1234
Yuan Dynasty 元	1271-1368
Ming Dynasty 明	1368-1644
Qing Dynasty 清	1644-1911
Republic of China 中華民國	1912-Present Day
People's Republic of China 中華人民共和國	1949-Present Day

Table of Contents

Chapter 14. Wind-Expelling Formulas ································ **959**

Biography of Wang Tao ·· 960

Section 1. External-Wind Releasing Formulas ············ **967**

Xiao Feng San (Eliminate Wind Powder) ··························· 967

    Qu Feng San (Dispel Wind Powder) ······························ 969

Dang Gui Yin Zi (Tangkuei Decoction) ··························· 970

Chuan Xiong Cha Tiao San (Ligusticum Chuanxiong Powder to be Taken with Green Tea) ··· 973

    Ju Hua Cha Tiao San (Chrysanthemum Powder to be Taken with Green Tea) ··· 976

Qian Zheng San (Lead to Symmetry Powder) ····················· 977

    Zhi Jing San (Stop Spasms Powder) ····························· 979

    Jia Wei Qian Zheng San (Augmented Lead to Symmetry Powder) ··· 980

Yu Zhen San (True Jade Powder) ································· 981

    Wu Hu Zhui Feng San (Five-Tiger Powder to Pursue Wind) ········ 982

Xiao Xu Ming Tang (Minor Prolong Life Decoction) ·············· 983

    Xiao Xu Ming Tang (Minor Prolong Life Decoction) ·············· 985

Xu Ming Tang (Prolong Life Decoction) ·························· 986

Da Qin Jiao Tang (Major Gentiana Macrophylla Decoction) ········ 988

Wu Yao Shun Qi San (Lindera Powder to Smooth the Flow of Qi) ··· 990

Section 2. Internal-Wind Extinguishing Formulas ········ **993**

Ling Jiao Gou Teng Tang (Antelope Horn and Uncaria Decoction) ··· 993

    Gou Teng Yin (Uncaria Decoction) ······························ 995

Gou Teng San (Uncaria Powder) ································· 996

Zhen Gan Xi Feng Tang (Sedate the Liver and Extinguish Wind Decoction) ··· 999

Jian Ling Tang (Construct Roof Tiles Decoction) ················· 1002

Tian Ma Gou Teng Yin (Gastrodia and Uncaria Decoction) ········ 1004

    Tian Ma Jiang Ya Pian (Gastrodia Pill to Lower [Blood] Pressure) ··· 1006

E Jiao Ji Zi Huang Tang (Ass-Hide Gelatin and Egg Yolk Decoction) ··· 1007

Da Ding Feng Zhu (Major Arrest Wind Pearl) ···················· 1009

    Xiao Ding Feng Zhu (Minor Arrest Wind Pearl) ················· 1011

    San Jia Fu Mai Tang (Three-Shell Decoction to Restore the Pulse) ··· 1011

    San Jia An Shen Wan (Three-Shell Pill to Tranquilize the Spirit) ··· 1011

Wind-Expelling Formulas (Summary) ······················· **1013**

Chinese Herbal Formulas and Applications

Chapter 14 — Overview

— Wind-Expelling Formulas

Definition: Wind-expelling formulas treat both external and internal wind. They disperse and release external wind with acrid herbs, and calm and extinguish internal wind with cold herbs.

External wind syndromes are those resulting from invasion of external wind at the exterior of the body, such as the muscles, joints, tendons, ligaments, bones, channels, and collaterals. Because external wind may combine with heat, cold, and damp, external wind syndromes are further classified into wind-heat, wind-cold, and wind-damp syndromes. The main clinical manifestations of external wind syndromes are headache, aversion to wind, itching of the skin, numbness of the extremities, painful joints, deviation of the mouth and eyes, and muscle convulsions.

Internal wind syndromes refer to Liver wind rising, as a manifestation of disorders of the *zang fu* organs. Common causes of internal wind rising include extreme heat, yin deficiency, and blood deficiency. Common clinical manifestations of internal wind syndromes are dizziness, vertigo, trembling, spasms and cramps of the four extremities, dysphasia, sudden unconsciousness, hemiplegia, and deviation of the mouth and eyes.

Proper treatment of wind disorders must begin with accurate differential diagnosis to determine the main characteristics: external or internal wind, deficiency or excess, and cold or hot. External wind must be treated with acrid and dispersing herbs that dispel external wind, and internal wind must be treated with cold herbs that extinguish internal wind. Furthermore, wind is often complicated by heat, cold, dampness, or phlegm, which must be addressed with the addition of appropriate herbs. External and internal wind may engender each other, or occur at the same time, leading to more complications. All these potential complications must be considered to ensure successful treatment.

SUBCATEGORIES OF ACTION

Wind-expelling formulas are thus divided into external-wind releasing formulas and internal-wind extinguishing formulas.

1. External-Wind Releasing Formulas

These formulas are suitable for treating various illnesses caused by external wind attacking the body. The external-wind releasing formulas are suitable for treating the invasion of external wind past the skin layer into the muscles, tendons, ligaments, bones, joints, channels, and collaterals. Commonly seen clinical manifestations include headache, dizziness, rubella, eczema, deviation of the mouth and eyes, dysphasia, joint pain, numbness, and limited movement. Tetanus is considered an external wind disorder, in which external wind enters the body via open wounds on the skin to cause symptoms such as lockjaw, spasms and cramps, and, in severe cases, kyphosis.

Herbs frequently used to disperse wind from the exterior include *Qiang Huo* (Rhizoma et Radix Notopterygii), *Du Huo* (Radix Angelicae Pubescentis), *Fang Feng* (Radix Saposhnikoviae), *Chuan Xiong* (Rhizoma Chuanxiong), *Bai Zhi* (Radix Angelicae Dahuricae), *Jing Jie* (Herba Schizonepetae), and *Bai Fu Zi* (Rhizoma Typhonii). Exemplar formulas include *Chuan Xiong Cha Tiao San* (Ligusticum Chuanxiong Powder to be Taken with Green Tea), *Qian Zheng San* (Lead to Symmetry Powder) and *Da Qin Jiao Tang* (Major Gentiana Macrophylla Decoction).

WIND-EXPELLING FORMULAS

14

~

External wind affects superficial aspects of the body, muscle and joints. Internal wind affects the *zang fu* organs in the interior.

~

963

Chapter 14 — Overview

Note: Two other chapters discuss formulas that treat external wind. Chapter 1: Exterior-Releasing Formulas, discusses the use of herbs that treat external wind invading only superficial parts of the body (e.g., the skin) causing various exterior symptoms, such as fever and aversion to cold. Chapter 17: Wind-Damp Dispelling Formulas, discusses the use of herbs to address external wind-dampness attacking the muscles and joints, such as found in *bi zheng* (painful obstruction syndrome).

2. Internal-Wind Extinguishing Formulas

These formulas are suitable for treating Liver wind rising associated with excess or deficiency conditions. Excess-type Liver wind is characterized by extreme heat or hyperactive Liver yang causing the wind to rise upward. Deficiency-type Liver wind is characterized by wind rising due to underlying yin and blood deficiencies.

> **Exterior and internal wind may engender each other, or occur at the same time, leading to more complications.**

Internal wind may rise upward as a result of extreme heat or hyperactive Liver yang. If the rising wind is caused by extreme heat, there may be persistent high fever, unconsciousness, and spasms and cramps of the four extremities. If the rising wind is caused by hyperactivity of Liver yang, there may be dizziness, vertigo, burning sensations and pain in the head, a rosy facial appearance (resembling that after alcohol consumption), sudden coma, deviation of the mouth, and hemiplegia.

Rising of wind caused by extreme heat or hyperactive Liver yang is considered an excess syndrome; therefore, the proper treatment plan is to sedate the Liver and extinguish wind. Herbs that sedate the Liver and calm wind include *Gou Teng* (Ramulus Uncariae cum Uncis), *Shi Jue Ming* (Concha Haliotidis), *Tian Ma* (Rhizoma Gastrodiae), *Ju Hua* (Flos Chrysanthemi), *Mu Li* (Concha Ostreae) and *Ji Li* (Fructus Tribuli). Exemplar formulas include *Tian Ma Gou Teng Yin* (Gastrodia and Uncaria Decoction), *Ling Jiao Gou Teng Tang* (Antelope Horn and Uncaria Decoction) and *Zhen Gan Xi Feng Tang* (Sedate the Liver and Extinguish Wind Decoction).

Internal wind may rise when there are underlying deficiencies. In cases of chronic *wen bing* (warm disease) damaging yin and/or blood, the rise of internal wind may lead to symptoms such as muscle spasms and cramps with peristalsis-like involuntary movements of the hands and feet. The proper treatment plan in this case would be to nourish yin and blood and extinguish internal wind. Herbs that nourish yin and blood to subdue rising wind include *Di Huang* (Radix Rehmanniae), *Bai Shao* (Radix Paeoniae Alba), *E Jiao* (Colla Corii Asini), and *Ji Zi Huang* (Galli Vitellus). Exemplar formulas include *Da Ding Feng Zhu* (Major Arrest Wind Pearl) and *E Jiao Ji Zi Huang Tang* (Ass-Hide Gelatin and Egg Yolk Decoction).

CAUTIONS / CONTRAINDICATIONS

- Proper diagnosis is crucial in the treatment of wind disorders. External wind must be released or dispersed outward, while Liver wind should be calmed and extinguished. Incorrect treatment of wind in the interior using external-wind releasing formulas that are acrid and dispersing in nature will worsen the condition by stimulating Liver yang and stirring Liver wind. Similarly, incorrect treatment of wind at the exterior using internal-wind extinguishing formulas will complicate the disorder by deepening the injury.
- Herbs that disperse external wind are often acrid, warm and drying. Therefore, they should be used with caution in individuals with underlying deficiencies of yin and/or body fluids.
- External wind is often accompanied by other pathogenic factors, such as heat, cold, dampness, or phlegm, which should also be addressed.
- External wind also may trigger the rise of Liver wind, leading to a complicated exterior / interior condition. In this case, both exterior and interior conditions must be addressed at the same time.
- Internal wind may be complicated by excess (extreme heat or Liver yang hyperactivity) or deficiency (yin and/or blood deficiencies), and must be diagnosed and treated accordingly.

Chinese Herbal Formulas and Applications

Chapter 14 — Overview

PHARMACOLOGICAL EFFECTS & CLINICAL APPLICATIONS

Wind is responsible for a wide variety of disorders. Accordingly, wind-expelling formulas are used to treat a broad spectrum of disease and illness.

1. **External-wind releasing formulas** generally treat conditions affecting the exterior of the body, such as the skin, muscles, tendons, ligaments, bones, joints, channels, and collaterals. Common clinical applications include:

   • **Skin disorders**: Pharmacologically, external-wind releasing formulas have mast cell stabilizing and antiallergic effects,[1,2] and are used to treat skin disorders such as itching,[3] urticaria,[4,5] eczema,[6] psoriasis,[7] and neurodermatitis.[8] *Xiao Feng San* (Eliminate Wind Powder) and *Dang Gui Yin Zi* (Tangkuei Decoction) are representative external-wind releasing formulas that treat dermatological disorders.

   • **Facial paralysis**: *Qian Zheng San* (Lead to Symmetry Powder) and *Yu Zhen San* (True Jade Powder) are external-wind releasing formulas frequently used to treat facial paralysis.[9,10,11,12]

   • **Pain**: Analgesic and anti-inflammatory effects are well documented among external-wind releasing formulas.[13,14] Clinically, these formulas treat headache,[15] migraine headache,[16] angioneurotic headache,[17] trigeminal pain,[18] and numbness and paralysis of the peripheral nerves.[19] Exemplar formulas include *Chuan Xiong Cha Tiao San* (Ligusticum Chuanxiong Powder to be Taken with Green Tea) and *Qian Zheng San* (Lead to Symmetry Powder).

> Exterior wind-releasing formulas are most effective for dermatological and musculoskeletal disorders.

2. **Internal-wind extinguishing formulas** usually treat cardiovascular disorders, such as hypertension, stroke, and post-stroke sequelae.

   • **Hypertension**: Internal-wind extinguishing formulas are well-documented for their antihypertensive effects to lower blood pressure.[20,21,22] Formulas that effectively treat hypertension include *Gou Teng San* (Uncaria Powder),[23] *Zhen Gan Xi Feng Tang* (Sedate the Liver and Extinguish Wind Decoction),[24] and *Tian Ma Gou Teng Yin* (Gastrodia and Uncaria Decoction).[25]

   • **Stroke and post-stroke sequelae**: Internal-wind extinguishing formulas have been shown to be effective in the prevention and treatment of stroke, and in management of post-stroke sequelae. The mechanisms of action are attributed in part to antiplatelet effects,[26] antihypertensive effects,[27] and the activation of nitric oxide synthase to improve cerebral circulation.[28] Formulas commonly used in the prevention and treatment of stroke include *Gou Teng San* (Uncaria Powder),[29] *Zhen Gan Xi Feng Tang* (Sedate the Liver and Extinguish Wind Decoction),[30] *Tian Ma Gou Teng Yin* (Gastrodia and Uncaria Decoction),[31] and *Di Huang Yin Zi* (Rehmannia Decoction).[32] Formulas frequently used to treat post-stroke sequelae include *Da Ding Feng Zhu* (Major Arrest Wind Pearl) and *Di Huang Yin Zi* (Rehmannia Decoction).[33,34]

> Internal-wind extinguishing formulas are most useful to treat cardiovascular disorders.

   • **Others**: Internal-wind extinguishing formulas may also treat other cardiovascular or circulatory disorders, including but not limited to dizziness,[35] vertigo,[36] tinnitus,[37] Alzheimer's disease,[38] vascular dementia,[39] and concussion.[40] Exemplar formulas include *Gou Teng San* (Uncaria Powder) and *Tian Ma Gou Teng Yin* (Gastrodia and Uncaria Decoction).

References

1. *Zhong Guo Yao Li Xue Bao* (Chinese Herbal Pharmacology Journal) 1990;5:34.
2. Shichijo K, Saito H. Effect of Chinese herbal medicines and disodium cromoglycate on IgE-dependent histamine release from mouse cultured mast cells. Int J Immunopharmacol 1997 Nov-Dec;19(11-12):677-82.
3. *Zhong Yi Yao Xue Bao* (Report of Chinese Medicine and Herbology) 1986;5:50.
4. *Ji Lin Zhong Yi Yao* (Jilin Chinese Medicine and Herbology) 1985;1:29.
5. *Tie Dao Yi Xue* (Tiedao Medicine) 1988;4:230.
6. *Xin Yi Yao Xue Za Zhi* (New Journal of Medicine and Herbology) 1976;8:15.
7. *Nei Meng Gu Zhong Yi Za Zi* (Inner Mongolia Journal of Traditional Chinese Medicine) 1992;1:14.
8. *Zhong Guo Zhong Xi Yi Jie He Za Zhi* (Chinese Journal of Integrative Chinese and Western Medicine) 1992;181.
9. *Nei Meng Gu Zhong Yi Yao* (Traditional Chinese Medicine and Medicinals of Inner Mongolia) 1990;9(4):18.
10. *He Bei Zhong Yi* (Hebei Chinese Medicine) 1985;4:30.
11. *Shi Zhen Guo Yao Yan Jiu* (Research of Shizhen Herbs) 1996;7(1):13.

WIND-EXPELLING FORMULAS

14

965

Chapter 14 — Overview

12. *Shan Xi Zhong Yi* (Shanxi Chinese Medicine) 1991;12(10):465.
13. *Zhong Yi Fang Ji Xian Dai Yan Jiu* (Modern Study of Medical Formulae in Traditional Chinese Medicine) 1997;1206.
14. *Zhong Yi Fang Ji Xian Dai Yan Jiu* (Modern Study of Medical Formulae in Traditional Chinese Medicine) 1997;1206.
15. *Jiang Xi Zhong Yi Yao* (Jiangxi Chinese Medicine and Herbology) 1992;6:47.
16. *Bei Jing Zhong Yi Yao Da Xue Xue Bao* (Journal of Beijing University of Medicine and Medicinals) 1994;17(4):36.
17. *Zhe Jiang Zhong Yi Za Zhi* (Zhejiang Journal of Chinese Medicine) 1998;2:61.
18. *Shan Dong Yi Yao* (Shandong Medicine and Herbology) 1994;12:55.
19. *Zhe Jiang Zhong Yi Za Zhi* (Zhejiang Journal of Chinese Medicine) 1989;6:255.
20. *Guo Wai Yi Xue* (Foreign Medicine) 1988;8:53.
21. *Xin Zhong Yi* (New Chinese Medicine) 1980;12:45.
22. *Zhong Yi Yao Yan Jiu Can Kao* (Research and Discussion of Chinese Medicine and Herbology) 1979;9:25.
23. *Guo Wai Yi Xue* (Foreign Medicine) 1979;2:35.
24. *Shi Yong Zhong Yi Nei Ke Za Zhi* (Journal of Practical Chinese Internal Medicine) 1990;1:26.
25. *Shi Yong Zhong Yi Nei Ke Za Zhi* (Journal of Practical Chinese Internal Medicine) 1990;1:26.
26. *Guo Wai Yi Xue* (Foreign Medicine) 1992;5:48.
27. *Guo Wai Yi Xue* (Foreign Medicine) 1988;8:53.
28. Sugimoto A, Goto K, Ishige A, Komatsu Y, Miyamoto KI. Effect of Choto-san, a Kampo medicine, on the cerebral blood flow autoregulation in spontaneously hypertensive rats. Japan J Pharmacol 2000 Jun;83(2):135-42.
29. Goto H, Yang Q, Kita T, Hikiami H, Shimada Y, Terasawa K. Effects of Choto-san on microcirculation, serum nitric oxide and lipid peroxides in patients with asymptomatic cerebral infarction. Am J Chin Med 2001;29(1):83-9.
30. *Zhe Jiang Zhong Yi Xue Yuan Xue Bao* (Journal of Zhejiang University of Chinese Medicine) 1988;5:18.
31. *Liao Ning Zhong Yi Za Zhi* (Liaoning Journal of Chinese Medicine) 1984;9:26.
32. *Zhe Jiang Zhong Yi Xue Yuan Xue Bao* (Journal of Zhejiang University of Chinese Medicine) 1995;4:8.
33. *Zhong Yi Han Shou Tong Xun* (Reports of Chinese Medicine) 1993;5:43.
34. *Hei Long Jiang Zhong Yi Yao* (Heilongjiang Chinese Medicine and Herbology) 1995;2:14.
35. *Shan Xi Zhong Yi Xue Yuan Xue Bao* (Journal of Shanxi University School of Chinese Medicine) 1996;19(4):28.
36. *Ji Lin Zhong Yi Yao* (Jilin Chinese Medicine and Herbology) 1995;5:34.
37. *Guo Wai Yi Xue* (Foreign Medicine) 1982;1:51.
38. *He Han Yi Yao Xue Hui Zhi* (Hehan Journal of Medicine and Herbology) 1989;3:454.
39. Itoh T, Shimada Y, Terasawa K. Efficacy of Choto-san on vascular dementia and the protective effect of the hooks and stems of Uncaria sinensis on glutamate-induced neuronal death. Mech Ageing Dev 1999 Nov;111(2-3):155-73.
40. *Nei Meng Gu Zhong Yi Yao* (Traditional Chinese Medicine and Medicinals of Inner Mongolia) 1990;1:2.

Chinese Herbal Formulas and Applications

Section 1

疏散外风剂
— External-Wind Releasing Formulas

Xiāo Fēng Sǎn (Eliminate Wind Powder)

消風散
消风散

Pinyin Name: *Xiao Feng San*
Literal Name: Eliminate Wind Powder
Alternate Names: *Hsiao Feng San*, Wind-Dispelling Formula, Wind-Dispelling Powder, Tangkuei and Arctium Formula
Original Source: *Wai Ke Zheng Zong* (True Lineage of External Medicine) by Chen Shi-Gong in 1617

COMPOSITION

Jing Jie (Herba Schizonepetae)	3g [6g]
Fang Feng (Radix Saposhnikoviae)	3g [6g]
Chan Tui (Periostracum Cicadae)	3g [6g]
Niu Bang Zi (Fructus Arctii)	3g [6g]
Cang Zhu (Rhizoma Atractylodis)	3g [6g]
Ku Shen (Radix Sophorae Flavescentis)	3g [6g]
Mu Tong (Caulis Akebiae)	1.5g [3g]
Shi Gao (Gypsum Fibrosum)	3g [6g]
Zhi Mu (Rhizoma Anemarrhenae)	3g [6g]
Di Huang (Radix Rehmanniae)	3g [6g]
Dang Gui (Radix Angelicae Sinensis)	3g [6g]
Hei Zhi Ma (Semen Sesami Nigrum)	3g [6g]
Gan Cao (Radix et Rhizoma Glycyrrhizae)	1.5g [3g]

DOSAGE / PREPARATION / ADMINISTRATION

The source text recommends cooking the ingredients with 2 bowls of water until the liquid is reduced to 80% (1.6 bowls). Take the strained decoction while warm. Today, the decoction can be prepared using the doses given in brackets above.

CHINESE THERAPEUTIC ACTIONS

1. Expels wind and nourishes the blood
2. Clears heat and dispels dampness

CLINICAL MANIFESTATIONS

Rashes: eczema and skin rashes with red discoloration affecting a large part of the body, severe itching and leakage of fluids upon scratching, a white or yellow tongue coating, and a superficial, rapid and forceful pulse.

CLINICAL APPLICATIONS

Eczema, urticaria, rashes, rubella, dermatitis, tinea capitis, psoriasis, and balanoposthitis.

EXPLANATION

Xiao Feng San (Eliminate Wind Powder) treats wind-dampness and wind-heat attacking the skin and muscle layers of the body, giving rise to rashes, eczema, severe itching, and leakage of fluids. The treatment approach for this syndrome is to dispel wind and dampness, clear heat, and cool the blood.

Jing Jie (Herba Schizonepetae), *Fang Feng* (Radix Saposhnikoviae), *Chan Tui* (Periostracum Cicadae), and *Niu Bang Zi* (Fructus Arctii) are the chief herbs that dispel wind from the exterior. *Cang Zhu* (Rhizoma Atractylodis)

WIND-EXPELLING FORMULAS

14

967

Xiāo Fēng Săn (Eliminate Wind Powder)

Xiao Feng San (Eliminate Wind Powder)

Diagnosis	Signs and Symptoms	Treatment	Herbs
Rashes	• Rashes or eczema with red discoloration, severe itching and discharge of fluids: wind-dampness and wind-heat attacking the skin and muscle layers of the body • White or yellow tongue coating, and a superficial, rapid and forceful pulse: wind-dampness or wind-heat condition	• Expels wind and nourishes the blood • Clears heat and dispels dampness	• *Jing Jie* (Herba Schizonepetae), *Fang Feng* (Radix Saposhnikoviae), *Chan Tui* (Periostracum Cicadae), and *Niu Bang Zi* (Fructus Arctii) dispel wind from the exterior. • *Cang Zhu* (Rhizoma Atractylodis) strengthens the Spleen and dries dampness. • *Ku Shen* (Radix Sophorae Flavescentis) clears heat and dries dampness. • *Mu Tong* (Caulis Akebiae) eliminates damp-heat through diuresis. • *Shi Gao* (Gypsum Fibrosum) and *Zhi Mu* (Rhizoma Anemarrhenae) clear heat and sedate fire. • *Di Huang* (Radix Rehmanniae), *Dang Gui* (Radix Angelicae Sinensis), and *Hei Zhi Ma* (Semen Sesami Nigrum) tonify blood, nourish yin, and moisten dryness. • *Gan Cao* (Radix et Rhizoma Glycyrrhizae) clears heat, eliminates toxins, and harmonizes the herbs.

strengthens the Spleen and dries dampness. *Ku Shen* (Radix Sophorae Flavescentis) clears heat and dries dampness. *Mu Tong* (Caulis Akebiae) eliminates damp-heat through diuresis. *Shi Gao* (Gypsum Fibrosum) and *Zhi Mu* (Rhizoma Anemarrhenae) clear heat and sedate fire. Since wind-dampness and wind-heat may injure yin and blood, *Di Huang* (Radix Rehmanniae), *Dang Gui* (Radix Angelicae Sinensis), and *Hei Zhi Ma* (Semen Sesami Nigrum) are added to tonify the blood, nourish yin, and moisten dryness. *Gan Cao* (Radix et Rhizoma Glycyrrhizae) clears heat, eliminates toxins, and harmonizes the formula.

MODIFICATIONS

• With more wind-heat, add *Jin Yin Hua* (Flos Lonicerae Japonicae) and *Lian Qiao* (Fructus Forsythiae).

• With more damp-heat, add *Di Fu Zi* (Fructus Kochiae) and *Che Qian Zi* (Semen Plantaginis).

• With heat in the *xue* (blood) level, add *Chi Shao* (Radix Paeoniae Rubra) and *Zi Cao* (Radix Arnebiae).

• For wet-type eczema with fluids in the lesions, add *Yi Yi Ren* (Semen Coicis).

• For allergic dermatitis with itching, add *Shi Wei Bai Du Tang* (Ten-Ingredient Decoction to Overcome Pathogenic Influences).

CAUTIONS / CONTRAINDICATIONS

• While taking *Xiao Feng San*, the following are contraindicated: spicy or greasy foods, seafood, cigarette smoking,

alcohol, and tea that is overly concentrated or steeped very long.

• Many herbs in this formula are acrid (exterior-releasing herbs) and drying (damp-dispelling herbs), and may damage yin and blood. Therefore, this formula should be used with caution in patients with qi and blood deficiencies.[1]

PHARMACOLOGICAL EFFECTS

1. **Antiallergic and immunosuppressive**: Administration of *Xiao Feng San* was associated with marked action to treat allergy and suppress the immune systems of mice.[2]

2. **Mast cell stabilizer**: Administration of *Xiao Feng San* and *Ma Huang Xing Ren Gan Cao Shi Gao Tang* (Ephedra, Apricot Kernel, Licorice, and Gypsum Decoction) at 4-40 mcg/mL was found to inhibit IgE-dependent histamine released from mouse-cultured mast cells.[3]

CLINICAL STUDIES AND RESEARCH

1. **Urticaria**: One study reported 97.6% effectiveness using modified *Xiao Feng San* to treat 124 patients with urticaria. Modifications to the formula included the addition of *Jin Yin Hua* (Flos Lonicerae Japonicae), *Wu Gong* (Scolopendra), *Zhi Zi* (Fructus Gardeniae), and *Huang Lian* (Rhizoma Coptidis) for wind-heat; *Ma Huang* (Herba Ephedrae) and *Gui Zhi* (Ramulus Cinnamomi) for wind-cold; and *He Shou Wu* (Radix Polygoni Multiflori), *Wu Wei Zi* (Fructus Schisandrae Chinensis), and *Wu Mei* (Fructus Mume) for yin deficiency. The herbs were given one time daily in decoction. Of 124 patients, the

Chinese Herbal Formulas and Applications

Xiāo Fēng Săn (Eliminate Wind Powder)

study reported complete recovery in 85 cases, significant improvement in 36 cases, and no effect in 3 cases.[4]

2. **Eczema**: Use of _Xiao Feng San_ in 44 patients with eczema was associated with complete recovery in 38 cases and near-complete recovery in 6 cases. The herbs were given on a daily basis, for an average of 20 days (ranging between 5 and 23 days). Those with severe eczema also received topical application of herbs, made by grinding fresh _Ma Chi Xian_ (Herba Portulacae) into an herbal paste. In addition to herbal treatment, all patients were instructed to maintain a bland diet and avoid spicy and pungent foods.[5]

3. **Balanoposthitis**: One study reported good results using modified _Xiao Feng San_ to treat inflammation of the foreskin and glans in uncircumcised males. The herbal formula contained _Jing Jie_ (Herba Schizonepetae) 10g, _Fang Feng_ (Radix Saposhnikoviae) 10g, _Tong Cao_ (Medulla Tetrapanacis) 10g, _Chan Tui_ (Periostracum Cicadae) 10g, _Ku Shen_ (Radix Sophorae Flavescentis) 10g, dry-fried _Cang Zhu_ (Rhizoma Atractylodis) 10g, _Dang Gui_ (Radix Angelicae Sinensis) 10g, _Zhi Mu_ (Rhizoma Anemarrhenae) 10g, _Di Huang_ (Radix Rehmanniae) 15g, _Shi Gao_ (Gypsum Fibrosum) 20g, _Jiang Can_ (Bombyx Batryticatus) 5g, and _Gan Cao_ (Radix et Rhizoma Glycyrrhizae) 5g. The treatment protocol was to cook the herbs in water, and administer the decoction in two equally-divided doses daily, for 5 days per course of treatment. Of 90 patients who had this condition (with a history of illness ranging from 14 days to 4 months), the study reported complete recovery in 82 cases within 1 course treatment, and 8 cases within 2 courses.[6]

4. **Psoriasis**: One study reported satisfactory results using modified _Xiao Feng San_ to treat psoriasis. The herbal treatment contained _Jin Yin Hua_ (Flos Lonicerae Japonicae) 15g, _Lian Qiao_ (Fructus Forsythiae) 15g, _Fang Feng_ (Radix Saposhnikoviae) 15g, _Dang Gui_ (Radix Angelicae Sinensis) 8g, _Qing Dai_ (Indigo Naturalis) 12g, _Jing Jie_ (Herba Schizonepetae) 10g, _Di Huang_ (Radix Rehmanniae) 12g, _Niu Bang Zi_ (Fructus Arctii) 10g, _Di Fu Zi_ (Fructus Kochiae) 10g, _Bai Xian Pi_ (Cortex Dictamni) 12g, _Cang Zhu_ (Rhizoma Atractylodis) 8g, _Chan Tui_ (Periostracum Cicadae) 10g, _Zi Cao_ (Radix Arnebiae) 10g, _Shi Gao_ (Gypsum Fibrosum) 12g, and _Gan Cao_ (Radix et Rhizoma Glycyrrhizae) 3g. The herbs were given in decoction daily.[7]

HERB-DRUG INTERACTION

Ampicillin-induced rash: Ampicillin-induced allergic rash in 68 patients was treated with herbs with 96% effectiveness, as reported in one study. The herbal treatment contained _Dang Gui_ (Radix Angelicae Sinensis) 9g, _Di Huang_ (Radix Rehmanniae) 9g, _Hei Zhi Ma_

(Semen Sesami Nigrum) 9g, _Jing Jie_ (Herba Schizonepetae) 9g, _Fang Feng_ (Radix Saposhnikoviae) 9g, _Niu Bang Zi_ (Fructus Arctii) 9g, _Chan Tui_ (Periostracum Cicadae) 9g, _Cang Zhu_ (Rhizoma Atractylodis) 9g, _Ku Shen_ (Radix Sophorae Flavescentis) 9g, _Duan Shi Gao_ (Gypsum Fibrosum Praeparatum) 9g, _Zhi Mu_ (Rhizoma Anemarrhenae) 9g, _Gan Cao_ (Radix et Rhizoma Glycyrrhizae) 4g, and _Mu Tong_ (Caulis Akebiae) 4g as the base formula. Modifications were made when necessary, with the addition of _Lian Qiao_ (Fructus Forsythiae) 6g for wind-heat; _Chi Shao_ (Radix Paeoniae Rubra) 9g for heat in the blood; _Da Huang_ (Radix et Rhizoma Rhei) 6g for heat and toxins; and the addition of _Che Qian Zi_ (Semen Plantaginis) 6g and elimination of _Cang Zhu_ (Rhizoma Atractylodis) for damp-heat. The study reported complete recovery in 65 of 68 patients within 1-4 packs of herbs given via herbal decoction.[8]

RELATED FORMULA

Qū Fēng Săn (Dispel Wind Powder)

祛風散
祛风散

Pinyin Name: _Qu Feng San_
Literal Name: Dispel Wind Powder
Original Source: _Guang An Men Yi Yuan_ (Guang An Men Hospital) in 1990

Jing Jie (Herba Schizonepetae)
Fang Feng (Radix Saposhnikoviae)
_Bo He_ (Herba Menthae)
Zhi Zi (Fructus Gardeniae)
Mu Dan Pi (Cortex Moutan)
Niu Bang Zi (Fructus Arctii)
Lian Qiao (Fructus Forsythiae)
Ku Shen (Radix Sophorae Flavescentis)
Yi Yi Ren (Semen Coicis)
_Di Fu Zi_ (Fructus Kochiae)
Bai Xian Pi (Cortex Dictamni)
Dang Gui (Radix Angelicae Sinensis)
Di Huang (Radix Rehmanniae)

Qu Feng San (Dispel Wind Powder) treats skin disorders by releasing wind, clearing heat, cooling the blood, and draining dampness. Clinical applications include rashes, itching, eczema, dermatitis, and skin allergies secondary to drugs, chemicals, or food.

AUTHORS' COMMENTS

In addition to using _Xiao Feng San_ internally to relieve itching, _Ku Shen_ (Radix Sophorae Flavescentis) and _She Chuang Zi_ (Fructus Cnidii) can be used as an external wash to enhance the overall effects. Furthermore,

WIND-EXPELLING FORMULAS

14

Chapter 14 – Wind-Expelling Formulas

Section 1 – External-Wind Releasing Formulas

Xiāo Fēng Sǎn (Eliminate Wind Powder)

topical application of *Ma Chi Xian* (Herba Portulacae) as an herbal paste also increases the overall effectiveness of *Xiao Feng San*.

From a traditional Chinese medical perspective, *Xiao Feng San* treats dermatological disorders caused by wind-dampness and wind-heat attacking the skin. In terms of anatomy and physiology, such dermatological disorders are similar in location and manifestation to allergic or hypersensitivity reactions.

References

1. *Zhong Yao Ming Fang Yao Li Yu Ying Yong* (Pharmacology and Applications of Famous Herbal Formulas) 1989;529-531.

2. *Zhong Guo Yao Li Xue Bao* (Chinese Herbal Pharmacology Journal) 1990;5:34.
3. Shichijo K, Saito H. Effect of Chinese herbal medicines and disodium cromoglycate on IgE-dependent histamine release from mouse cultured mast cells. Int J Immunopharmacol 1997 Nov-Dec;19(11-12):677-82.
4. *Ji Lin Zhong Yi Yao* (Jilin Chinese Medicine and Herbology) 1985;1:29.
5. *Xin Yi Yao Xue Za Zhi* (New Journal of Medicine and Herbology) 1976;8:15.
6. *Zhe Jiang Zhong Yi Za Zhi* (Zhejiang Journal of Chinese Medicine) 1993;5:212.
7. *Nei Meng Gu Zhong Yi Za Zi* (Inner Mongolia Journal of Traditional Chinese Medicine) 1992;1:14.
8. *Si Chuan Zhong Yi* (Sichuan Chinese Medicine) 1993;11(4):34.

Dāng Guī Yǐn Zǐ (Tangkuei Decoction)

當歸飲子
当归饮子

Pinyin Name: *Dang Gui Yin Zi*
Literal Name: Tangkuei Decoction
Alternate Names: *Tang Kuei Yin Tzu*, Tang-kuei Drink, Tangkuei and Tribulus Combination
Original Source: *Chong Ding Yan Shi Ji Sheng Fang* (Revised Formulas to Aid the Living from the Yan Family)

COMPOSITION

Di Huang (Radix Rehmanniae)	30g [9g]
Dang Gui (Radix Angelicae Sinensis)	30g [9g]
Bai Shao (Radix Paeoniae Alba)	30g [9g]
Chuan Xiong (Rhizoma Chuanxiong)	30g [9g]
Ji Li (Fructus Tribuli), *chao* (dry-fried)	30g [9g]
Jing Jie (Herba Schizonepetae)	30g [9g]
Fang Feng (Radix Saposhnikoviae)	30g [9g]
Huang Qi (Radix Astragali)	15g [6g]
He Shou Wu (Radix Polygoni Multiflori)	15g [6g]
Gan Cao (Radix et Rhizoma Glycyrrhizae)	15g [3g]

DOSAGE / PREPARATION / ADMINISTRATION

The source text recommends grinding the ingredients into a coarse powder. Cook 12g of the powder with 5 slices of *Sheng Jiang* (Rhizoma Zingiberis Recens) in 1.5 large bowls of water until the liquid is reduced to 80% (1.2 large bowls). Take the warm, strained decoction any time during the day. Today, this formula may be prepared as a decoction using the doses suggested in brackets above.

CHINESE THERAPEUTIC ACTIONS

1. Tonifies the blood and moistens dryness
2. Dispels wind and relieves itching

CLINICAL MANIFESTATIONS

Skin disorders caused by blood deficiency and exterior wind: anemia, dry and coarse skin, itching, swelling, abscesses, and ulceration.

CLINICAL APPLICATIONS

Eczema, rash, urticaria, neurodermatitis, ichthyosis, psoriasis, alopecia, carbuncles, furuncles, and atrophy of the sebaceous glands and sweat glands and skin tissue.

970

Chinese Herbal Formulas and Applications

Dāng Guī Yǐn Zǐ (Tangkuei Decoction)

EXPLANATION

Dang Gui Yin Zi (Tangkuei Decoction) treats skin disorders caused by blood deficiency and exterior wind. Blood deficiency can lead to malnourishment of the skin, characterized by dryness, coarseness, lack of moisture, and lack of skin tone. Patients with chronic blood deficiency accompanied by exterior wind and heat usually show more serious signs and symptoms of dermatological disorders, such as eczema and carbuncles, with or without abscesses and ulceration.

Dang Gui Yin Zi follows the principles of *Si Wu Tang* (Four-Substance Decoction) to tonify the blood, with the addition of herbs that treat wind and heat. *Di Huang* (Radix Rehmanniae) nourishes the blood and tonifies the Kidney. *Dang Gui* (Radix Angelicae Sinensis) both tonifies and activates blood circulation. *Bai Shao* (Radix Paeoniae Alba) nourishes the blood and consolidates yin. *Chuan Xiong* (Rhizoma Chuanxiong) activates and regulates blood circulation. *Ji Li* (Fructus Tribuli) dispels both internal and external wind to relieve itching, while *Jing Jie* (Herba Schizonepetae) and *Fang Feng* (Radix Saposhnikoviae) dispel exterior wind and treat various skin disorders. *Huang Qi* (Radix Astragali) tonifies *wei* (defensive) qi and strengthens the exterior. *He Shou Wu* (Radix Polygoni Multiflori) nourishes *jing* (essence) and blood. Lastly, *Gan Cao* (Radix et Rhizoma Glycyrrhizae) harmonizes the formula.

MODIFICATIONS

- For severe blood deficiency, add *Gou Qi Zi* (Fructus Lycii), *Huo Ma Ren* (Fructus Cannabis), and *Ji Xue Teng* (Caulis Spatholobi).
- For qi deficiency, add *Dang Shen* (Radix Codonopsis).
- With dry, scaly skin due to blood stasis, add *Dan Shen* (Radix et Rhizoma Salviae Miltiorrhizae) and *Hong Hua* (Flos Carthami).
- With itchy skin, combine with *Chan Tui* (Periostracum Cicadae), *Gou Teng* (Ramulus Uncariae cum Uncis), *Shou Wu Teng* (Caulis Polygoni Multiflori), and *He Huan Pi* (Cortex Albiziae).
- With dryness and atrophy of the skin due to lack of secretion from sebaceous and sweat glands, add *Shan Zhu Yu* (Fructus Corni) and *Huo Ma Ren* (Fructus Cannabis).
- To nourish the skin and slow the aging process of the skin, combine with *Liu Wei Di Huang Wan* (Six-Ingredient Pill with Rehmannia) or *Ba Wei Di Huang Wan* (Eight-Ingredient Pill with Rehmannia).
- For measles, add *Tu Fu Ling* (Rhizoma Smilacis Glabrae) and *Xuan Shen* (Radix Scrophulariae).
- With constipation, combine with *Ma Zi Ren Wan* (Hemp Seed Pill).

CAUTIONS / CONTRAINDICATIONS

While taking *Dang Gui Yin Zi*, patients should avoid alcohol and foods that are greasy, fatty, or deep-fried, as well as foods that are spicy, pungent, or stimulating in nature.

WIND-EXPELLING FORMULAS

14

Dang Gui Yin Zi (Tangkuei Decoction)

Diagnosis	Signs and Symptoms	Treatment	Herbs
Skin disorders caused by blood deficiency and wind	• Dry and coarse skin, lack of moisture and skin tone: blood unable to nourish the skin • Eczema and carbuncles with or without abscesses and ulceration: exterior wind and heat affecting the skin	• Tonifies blood and moistens dryness • Dispels wind and relieves itching	• *Di Huang* (Radix Rehmanniae) nourishes the blood and tonifies the Kidney. • *Dang Gui* (Radix Angelicae Sinensis) tonifies blood and regulates blood circulation. • *Bai Shao* (Radix Paeoniae Alba) nourishes the blood and consolidates yin. • *Chuan Xiong* (Rhizoma Chuanxiong) activates and regulates blood circulation. • *Ji Li* (Fructus Tribuli) dispels both internal and external wind to relieve itching. • *Jing Jie* (Herba Schizonepetae) and *Fang Feng* (Radix Saposhnikoviae) dispel exterior wind. • *Huang Qi* (Radix Astragali) tonifies *wei* (defensive) qi and strengthens the exterior. • *He Shou Wu* (Radix Polygoni Multiflori) nourishes *jing* (essence) and blood. • *Gan Cao* (Radix et Rhizoma Glycyrrhizae) harmonizes the herbs.

971

Dāng Guī Yǐn Zǐ (Tangkuei Decoction)

CLINICAL STUDIES AND RESEARCH

1. **Itching**: Administration of a modified *Dang Gui Yin Zi* formula was 96.15% effective in treating 78 geriatric patients with constant itching of the skin. The formula contained 12-15g of *Dang Gui* (Radix Angelicae Sinensis); 10-12 grams each of *Shu Di Huang* (Radix Rehmanniae Praeparata), *Huang Qi* (Radix Astragali), *Ji Li* (Fructus Tribuli), *Chuan Xiong* (Rhizoma Chuanxiong), *Jing Jie* (Herba Schizonepetae), and *Bai Shao* (Radix Paeoniae Alba); 30g of *He Shou Wu* (Radix Polygoni Multiflori); and 6g each of *Fang Feng* (Radix Saposhnikoviae) and *Gan Cao* (Radix et Rhizoma Glycyrrhizae). The treatment protocol was to cook the herbs in water, and drink the decoction in two to three equally-divided doses daily. The average duration of treatment was 26.5 packs of herbs. Out of 78 patients, the study reported complete recovery in 36 cases and improvement in 39 cases. Complete recovery was defined as relief of symptoms, with no recurrence 1-2 months after the termination of herbal treatment.[1]

2. **Urticaria**: Administration of *Dang Gui Yin Zi* had marked effectiveness in treating 56 patients with chronic urticaria that did not respond to drug treatment. The herbal treatment used *Dang Gui Yin Zi* as the base, and added *Dang Shen* (Radix Codonopsis) and *Bai Zhu* (Rhizoma Atractylodis Macrocephalae) for qi deficiency; *Mu Dan Pi* (Cortex Moutan) and *Xuan Shen* (Radix Scrophulariae) for yin deficiency; *Huang Qin* (Radix Scutellariae) and *Tu Fu Ling* (Rhizoma Smilacis Glabrae) for damp-heat; *Wu Zhu Yu* (Fructus Evodiae) and *Rou Gui* (Cortex Cinnamomi) for damp-cold; and *Chi Shao* (Radix Paeoniae Rubra) and *Dan Shen* (Radix et Rhizoma Salviae Miltiorrhizae) for blood stagnation. The treatment protocol was to cook the herbs in water, and drink the decoction in two to three equally-divided doses daily. The patients were instructed to discontinue the drugs during herbal treatment. Of 56 patients, the study reported complete recovery in 29 cases and moderate improvement in 16 cases after the first 5-day course of treatment. After the second course of treatment, the study reported complete recovery in 40 cases and moderate improvement in 12 cases. The rate of effectiveness was 80% after the first course, and 92.8% after the second course. The study noted that the group with qi and blood deficiencies was most responsive to the herbal treatment.[2]

3. **Neurodermatitis**: One report stated that administration of modified *Dang Gui Yin Zi,* plus topical application of steroids, was more effective (96.5% effectiveness in 86 patients) than topical application of steroids alone (65.4% effectiveness in 52 patients). The herbal formula contained 10g each of *Dang Gui* (Radix Angelicae Sinensis), *Chi Shao* (Radix Paeoniae Rubra), *Fang Feng* (Radix Saposhnikoviae), *Ji Li* (Fructus Tribuli), *Huang Qi* (Radix Astragali), *Hong Hua* (Flos Carthami), *Chan Tui* (Periostracum Cicadae), and *Di Fu Zi* (Fructus Kochiae); 15g of *Di Huang* (Radix Rehmanniae); 6g of *Chuan Xiong* (Rhizoma Chuanxiong); 30g of *He Shou Wu* (Radix Polygoni Multiflori), and others as deemed necessary.[3]

4. **Ichthyosis**: In one case report, a patient with a 10-year history of non-inflammatory scaling of the skin was treated successfully with 50 doses of *Dang Gui Yin Zi*, without recurrence during the 3 years of follow-up.[4] According to another report, a modified *Dang Gui Yin Zi* formula was found to have good effect in treating ichthyosis with rough, scale-like appearance of the skin all over the extremities, back, and chest. The herbal treatment contained *Dang Gui* (Radix Angelicae Sinensis) 10g, *Chuan Xiong* (Rhizoma Chuanxiong) 10g, *Bai Shao* (Radix Paeoniae Alba) 10g, *Gou Qi Zi* (Fructus Lycii) 10g, *Huang Qi* (Radix Astragali) 10g, *Bai Zhu* (Rhizoma Atractylodis Macrocephalae) 10g, *Di Fu Zi* (Fructus Kochiae) 10g, *Zi Cao* (Radix Arnebiae) 10g, *Ji Li* (Fructus Tribuli) 10g, *Chi Shao* (Radix Paeoniae Rubra) 6g, *He Shou Wu* (Radix Polygoni Multiflori) 10g, dry-fried *Jing Jie* (Herba Schizonepetae) 5g, *Fang Feng* (Radix Saposhnikoviae) 6g, and *Gan Cao* (Radix et Rhizoma Glycyrrhizae) 3g. The herbs were cooked in water, and the decoction administered in two equally-divided doses daily. The average duration of treatment was slightly over 6 months.[5]

5. **Alopecia**: Continuous administration of *Dang Gui Yin Zi* for 2-4 months was effective in treating 6 of 7 patients with alopecia. The hair was restored to normal quantity and color. In addition, no further hair loss was reported in these 6 patients upon follow-up, one year after the discontinuation of herbal treatment.[6]

AUTHORS' COMMENTS

From a traditional Chinese medical perspective, *Dang Gui Yin Zi* treats dermatological disorders caused by blood deficiency and exterior wind. In term of anatomy and physiology, such dermatological disorders are similar to atrophy of the skin tissue, sebaceous glands, and sweat glands.

Xiao Feng San (Eliminate Wind Powder) and *Dang Gui Yin Zi* both treat skin disorders characterized by wind at the exterior and blood deficiency in the interior.

- *Xiao Feng San* clears wind-dampness and wind-heat, and nourishes and cools the blood. It mainly treats rashes, eczema, and other skin disorders primarily caused by dampness and heat invading the exterior.
- *Dang Gui Yin Zi* tonifies blood, moistens dryness, and releases wind. It is more effective for eczema, rashes,

Chinese Herbal Formulas and Applications

Dāng Guī Yǐn Zǐ (Tangkuei Decoction)

urticaria, and other skin conditions complicated by both exterior (wind) and interior (dryness with blood deficiency) factors.

References

1. *Zhong Yi Yao Xue Bao* (Report of Chinese Medicine and Herbology) 1986;5:50.

2. *Tie Dao Yi Xue* (Tiedao Medicine) 1988;4:230.
3. *Zhong Guo Zhong Xi Yi Jie He Za Zhi* (Chinese Journal of Integrative Chinese and Western Medicine) 1992;181.
4. *Zhong Yi Za Zhi* (Journal of Chinese Medicine) 1985;6:442.
5. *Hu Nan Zhong Yi Za Zhi* (Hunan Journal of Chinese Medicine) 1989;5:33.
6. *Si Chuan Zhong Yi* (Sichuan Chinese Medicine) 1989;8:47.

Chuān Xiōng Chá Tiáo Sǎn

(Ligusticum Chuanxiong Powder to be Taken with Green Tea)

川芎茶調散
川芎茶调散

Pinyin Name: *Chuan Xiong Cha Tiao San*
Literal Name: Ligusticum Chuanxiong Powder to be Taken with Green Tea
Alternate Names: *Chuan Chiung Cha Tiao San*, Chuan Chiung and Tea-Regulating Formula, Tea-Blended Ligusticum Powder, Cnidium and Tea Formula
Original Source: *Tai Ping Hui Min He Ji Ju Fang* (Imperial Grace Formulary of the Tai Ping Era) by the Imperial Medical Department in 1078-85

COMPOSITION

Chuan Xiong (Rhizoma Chuanxiong)	120g [12g]
Bai Zhi (Radix Angelicae Dahuricae)	60g [6g]
Qiang Huo (Rhizoma et Radix Notopterygii)	60g [6g]
Xi Xin (Radix et Rhizoma Asari)	30g [3g]
Bo He (Herba Menthae), do not expose to heat	240g [12g]
Jing Jie (Herba Schizonepetae)	120g [12g]
Fang Feng (Radix Saposhnikoviae)	45g [4.5g]
Gan Cao (Radix et Rhizoma Glycyrrhizae)	60g [6g]

Note: There are two variations of this formula according to the source text. One contains 30g of *Xi Xin* (Radix et Rhizoma Asari) as stated above, the other contains instead 240g of dry-fried *Xiang Fu* (Rhizoma Cyperi).

DOSAGE / PREPARATION / ADMINISTRATION

The source text recommends grinding the ingredients into a fine powder. Take 6g per dose with green tea after meals. Today, this formula is usually given in powder or decoction form. For powder, take 6g of finely-ground powder with tea made from *Cha Ye* (Folium Camelliae) twice daily. For decoction, use the doses suggested in brackets.

CHINESE THERAPEUTIC ACTIONS

Clears wind and stops pain

CLINICAL MANIFESTATIONS

Headache caused by exterior wind attack: headache (frontal, temporal, occipital or vertex), aversion to cold, fever, vertigo, stuffy nose, a thin, white tongue coating, and a superficial pulse. Other key symptoms include nasal obstruction or discharge that is clear or white in color, sneezing, and body aches.

CLINICAL APPLICATIONS

Common cold, influenza, headache, migraine headache, angioneurotic headache, tension headache, neurogenic headache, trigeminal pain, peripheral nerve numbness and paralysis, nasal obstruction, rhinitis, sinusitis, and nasal polyps.

WIND-EXPELLING FORMULAS

14

973

Chuān Xiōng Chá Tiáo Săn
(Ligusticum Chuanxiong Powder to be Taken with Green Tea)

EXPLANATION

Chuan Xiong Cha Tiao San (Ligusticum Chuanxiong Powder to be Taken with Green Tea) treats headache caused by exterior wind attack. As the wind attacks the exterior, it travels along the channels to the head, causing headache and vertigo. Because wind is mobile in nature, the headache can manifest in irregular onset of pain, and may affect different parts of the head (frontal, temporal, occipital or vertex). Symptoms such as chills and fever indicate exterior wind affecting the superficial aspects of the body. Others signs and symptoms of exterior wind condition include stuffy nose, a thin, white tongue coating, and a superficial pulse.

This formula has *Chuan Xiong* (Rhizoma Chuanxiong), *Bai Zhi* (Radix Angelicae Dahuricae), and *Qiang Huo* (Rhizoma et Radix Notopterygii) to disperse wind and relieve headache. Among these herbs, *Chuan Xiong* (Rhizoma Chuanxiong) is especially effective in treating *shaoyang* (temporal) and *jueyin* (vertex) headaches; *Qiang Huo* (Rhizoma et Radix Notopterygii) is especially effective in treating *taiyang* (occipital) headaches; and *Bai Zhi* (Radix Angelicae Dahuricae) is effective in treating *yangming* (frontal) headaches. *Xi Xin* (Radix et Rhizoma Asari) dispels cold and relieves pain, especially from *shaoyin* headaches. It also opens sensory orifices to relieve nasal obstruction. *Bo He* (Herba Menthae) dispels wind, opens the orifices, and relieves headache. *Jing Jie* (Herba Schizonepetae) and *Fang Feng* (Radix Saposhnikoviae) are acrid and disperse wind from the upper parts of the body. *Gan Cao* (Radix et Rhizoma Glycyrrhizae) harmonizes the herbs. Finally, *Cha Ye* (Folium Camelliae), bitter and cold, is used for two main purposes: to clear the sensory orifices, and to prevent the warming, drying, and dispersing herbs from causing side effects.

MODIFICATIONS

- For headache or migraines caused by wind-heat, add *Ju Hua* (Flos Chrysanthemi) and *Jiang Can* (Bombyx Batryticatus).
- For headache caused by wind-cold, add *Sheng Jiang* (Rhizoma Zingiberis Recens) and *Zi Su Ye* (Folium Perillae).
- For headache caused by wind and phlegm, add *Ban Xia* (Rhizoma Pinelliae) and *Fu Ling* (Poria).
- For chronic, stubborn headache, add *Quan Xie* (Scorpio), *Jiang Can* (Bombyx Batryticatus), *Tao Ren* (Semen Persicae), and *Hong Hua* (Flos Carthami).
- For vertex headache, add *Gao Ben* (Rhizoma et Radix Ligustici).
- For headache with rhinitis and sinusitis, add *Cang Er Zi* (Fructus Xanthii) and *Xin Yi Hua* (Flos Magnoliae).
- For neurogenic headache, add *Man Jing Zi* (Fructus Viticis) and *Ji Li* (Fructus Tribuli).
- For headache from hypertension, remove *Qiang Huo* (Rhizoma et Radix Notopterygii), *Bai Zhi* (Radix Angelicae Dahuricae), and *Cha Ye* (Folium Camelliae); and add *Ju Hua* (Flos Chrysanthemi), *Bai Shao* (Radix Paeoniae Alba), *Ge Gen* (Radix Puerariae Lobatae), and *Gou Teng* (Ramulus Uncariae cum Uncis).

Chuan Xiong Cha Tiao San (Ligusticum Chuanxiong Powder to be Taken with Green Tea)

Diagnosis	Signs and Symptoms	Treatment	Herbs
Headache caused by exterior wind attack	• Headache, fever, aversion to cold, and vertigo: wind attacking the exterior and upper parts of the body • Stuffy nose, thin, white tongue coating, and a superficial pulse: exterior wind condition	• Clears wind • Stops pain	• *Chuan Xiong* (Rhizoma Chuanxiong), *Bai Zhi* (Radix Angelicae Dahuricae), and *Qiang Huo* (Rhizoma et Radix Notopterygii) disperse wind and relieve headache. • *Xi Xin* (Radix et Rhizoma Asari) dispels exterior wind and opens sensory orifices. • *Bo He* (Herba Menthae) dispels wind, opens the orifices, and relieves headache. • *Jing Jie* (Herba Schizonepetae) and *Fang Feng* (Radix Saposhnikoviae) disperse wind from the upper parts of the body. • *Gan Cao* (Radix et Rhizoma Glycyrrhizae) harmonizes the herbs. • *Cha Ye* (Folium Camelliae) clears the sensory orifices and prevents the warming, drying, and dispersing herbs from creating unwanted side effects.

Chinese Herbal Formulas and Applications

Chuān Xiōng Chá Tiáo Săn
(Ligusticum Chuanxiong Powder to be Taken with Green Tea)

CAUTIONS / CONTRAINDICATIONS
- Because many of the herbs in *Chuan Xiong Cha Tiao San* are warm in nature, cold herbs should be added if the headache is caused by wind-heat factors.
- Because this formula contains many acrid, warm, drying, and dispersing herbs, it is contraindicated in headaches caused by qi deficiency, blood deficiency, Kidney yin deficiency, Liver yin deficiency, Liver yang excess, or Liver wind rising.

PHARMACOLOGICAL EFFECTS
1. **Analgesic**: Administration of *Chuan Xiong Cha Tiao San* was associated with a marked analgesic effect in mice, with onset of action starting 15 minutes after oral ingestion, and lasting for approximately 3 hours.[1]
2. **Anti-inflammatory**: *Chuan Xiong Cha Tiao San* has been shown to have anti-inflammatory effects in mice and rats. The mechanism of this action is related to the adrenal cortex, as effectiveness was voided in subjects whose adrenal glands had been surgically removed.[2]
3. **Antipyretic**: Administration of *Chuan Xiong Cha Tiao San* has been shown to reduce fever in rats. The onset of action started approximately 30 minutes after oral ingestion, and duration of action was approximately 2 hours.[3]

CLINICAL STUDIES AND RESEARCH
1. **Headache**: One study showed that use of modified *Chuan Xiong Cha Tiao San* was very effective in treating headache. The herbal treatment contained this formula plus a higher dose of *Chuan Xiong* (Rhizoma Chuanxiong) as the base formula, with modifications as needed. For wind-heat headache, *Ge Gen* (Radix Puerariae Lobatae), *Ban Xia* (Rhizoma Pinelliae), *Wu Zhu Yu* (Fructus Evodiae), and *Gao Ben* (Rhizoma et Radix Ligustici) were added, and *Cha Ye* (Folium Camelliae) was removed. For wind-heat headache, *Cang Zhu* (Rhizoma Atractylodis) and *Gao Ben* (Rhizoma et Radix Ligustici) were added, and *Cha Ye* (Folium Camelliae) was removed. For Liver yang headache, *He Shou Wu* (Radix Polygoni Multiflori), *Sang Shen* (Fructus Mori), *Shi Jue Ming* (Concha Haliotidis), and *Zhen Zhu Mu* (Concha Margaritiferae) were added. For Kidney deficiency headache, *Gou Qi Zi* (Fructus Lycii), *Da Zao* (Fructus Jujubae), *Dang Gui* (Radix Angelicae Sinensis), *Shu Di Huang* (Radix Rehmanniae Praeparata), and *Du Zhong* (Cortex Eucommiae) were added. For qi deficiency headache, *Huang Qi* (Radix Astragali), *Dang Shen* (Radix Codonopsis), and *Dang Gui* (Radix Angelicae Sinensis) were added, and *Cha Ye* (Folium Camelliae) was removed. For blood deficiency headache, *Si Wu Tang* (Four-Substance Decoction) was added, and *Cha Ye* (Folium Camelliae) was removed. For headache due to

phlegm accumulation, *Bai Zhu* (Rhizoma Atractylodis Macrocephalae), *Tian Ma* (Rhizoma Gastrodiae), *Gou Teng* (Ramulus Uncariae cum Uncis), *Tu Bie Chong* (Eupolyphaga seu Steleophaga), and *Jiang Can* (Bombyx Batryticatus) were added. For blood stagnation headache, *Tao Ren* (Semen Persicae), *Hong Hua* (Flos Carthami), *Dan Shen* (Radix et Rhizoma Salviae Miltiorrhizae), and *Dang Gui* (Radix Angelicae Sinensis) were added. Of 150 patients, the study reported complete recovery in 142 cases, improvement in 6 cases, and no effect in 2 cases.[4]

2. **Migraine headache**: According to one clinical study, patients with migraine headache characterized by deficiency were divided into two groups for herbal treatment. In group one, modified *Chuan Xiong Cha Tiao San* was used as the base formula for treatment. *Dang Shen* (Radix Codonopsis) and *Bai Shao* (Radix Paeoniae Alba) were added for qi and blood deficiencies, and *Shu Di Huang* (Radix Rehmanniae Praeparata) and *Gou Qi Zi* (Fructus Lycii) were added for qi and yin deficiencies. In group two, patients were treated according to one of three diagnoses: *Ba Zhen Tang* (Eight-Treasure Decoction) for migraine headache due to qi and blood deficiencies; *Si Jun Zi Tang* (Four-Gentlemen Decoction) and *Liu Wei Di Huang Wan* (Six-Ingredient Pill with Rehmannia) for migraine headache due to qi and yin deficiencies; and *Qi Ju Di Huang Wan* (Lycium Fruit, Chrysanthemum, and Rehmannia Pill) for migraine headache due to Liver and Kidney yin deficiencies. The treatment protocol for both groups was to cook the herbs and administer the decoction in two equally-divided doses daily, for 7 days per course of treatment, for a total of 3 courses. In group one, the study reported complete recovery in 121 of 168 cases, improvement in 39 cases, and no effect in 8 cases (95.23% effectiveness). In group two involving 48 cases, the study reported complete recovery in 9 cases, improvement in 19 cases, and no effect in 20 cases (58.33% effectiveness).[5]

3. **Angioneurotic headache**: Modified *Chuan Xiong Cha Tiao San* successfully treated 52 patients with angioneurotic headache. In addition to the base formula, *Ban Xia Bai Zhu Tian Ma Tang* (Pinellia, Atractylodes Macrocephala, and Gastrodia Decoction) was added for more dampness and phlegm; *Xue Fu Zhu Yu Tang* (Drive Out Stasis in the Mansion of Blood Decoction) was added for blood stagnation; and *Jia Wei Xiao Yao San* (Augmented Rambling Powder) was added for Liver qi stagnation with heat. *Quan Xie* (Scorpio), *Wu Gong* (Scolopendra), and blood-moving herbs were added for those with chronic headache that required long-term treatment. Out of 52 patients, the study reported complete recovery in 16 cases, marked improvement in 19

WIND-EXPELLING FORMULAS

14

Chuān Xiōng Chá Tiáo Sǎn
(Ligusticum Chuanxiong Powder to be Taken with Green Tea)

cases, slight improvement in 12 cases, and no effect in 5 cases. The overall rate of effectiveness was 90.4%.[6]

4. **Trigeminal pain**: Use of *Chuan Xiong Cha Tiao San* was shown in one study to effectively treat trigeminal pain. Of 15 patients, the study reported complete recovery in 11 cases, and improvement in 4 cases. The duration of treatment ranged between 4 and 12 packs of herbs. The herbal treatment contained *Chuan Xiong* (Rhizoma Chuanxiong) 15g, *Bai Zhi* (Radix Angelicae Dahuricae) 15g, *Jing Jie* (Herba Schizonepetae) 12g, *Fang Feng* (Radix Saposhnikoviae) 12g, *Jiang Can* (Bombyx Batryticatus) 12g, *Man Jing Zi* (Fructus Viticis) 12g, *Xi Xin* (Radix et Rhizoma Asari) 6g, *Cha Ye* (Folium Camelliae) 6g, *Sheng Ma* (Rhizoma Cimicifugae) 6g, *Ye Ju Hua* (Flos Chrysanthemi Indici) 18g, *Bo He* (Herba Menthae) 10g, *Gan Cao* (Radix et Rhizoma Glycyrrhizae) 9g, and *Di Huang* (Radix Rehmanniae) 20g. Additional modifications were made as necessary.[7]

5. **Peripheral nerve numbness and paralysis**: Topical application of *Chuan Xiong Cha Tiao San* to acupuncture points was effective in treating numbness and paralysis of the peripheral nerves. The treatment protocol was to mix the powered formula with tea and apply it to the points daily for 5 days per course of treatment, followed by one day of rest, and then repeated with additional courses. The points selected included *Dicang* (ST 4), *Jiache* (ST 6), *Juliao* (ST 3), *Tinggong* (SI 19), and others. Duration of treatment varied between 5 and 36 days. Of 54 patients, the study reported complete recovery in 50 cases, marked improvement in 3 cases, and slight improvement in 1 case.[8]

6. **Sinusitis**: According to one report, 12 patients with sinusitis were treated with modified *Chuan Xiong Cha Tiao San* with complete recovery in 11 patients. The duration of treatment ranged from 3 to 9 doses of herbs, with an average of 6 doses. Herbal treatment was modified by removing *Xi Xin* (Radix et Rhizoma Asari), *Qiang Huo* (Rhizoma et Radix Notopterygii), and *Jing Jie* (Herba Schizonepetae), and adding *Huang Qin* (Radix Scutellariae), *Ju Hua* (Flos Chrysanthemi), *Xin Yi Hua* (Flos Magnoliae), *Cang Er Zi* (Fructus Xanthii), *Jin Yin Hua* (Flos Lonicerae Japonicae), and others if necessary.[9]

7. **Nasal polyps**: Twenty-one out of 23 patients with nasal polyps recovered completely by taking modified *Chuan Xiong Cha Tiao San*. The treatment protocol was to administer 10g of the formula in powder, three times daily for 21 days per course of treatment. The herbal treatment was modified by removing *Bo He* (Herba Menthae) and *Gan Cao* (Radix et Rhizoma Glycyrrhizae), and adding *Xin Yi Hua* (Flos Magnoliae), *Cang Er Zi* (Fructus Xanthii), *Shi Gao* (Gypsum Fibrosum), *Zao*

Jiao (Fructus Gleditsiae), *Zi Su Ye* (Folium Perillae), and others.[10]

TOXICOLOGY

In an acute toxicology study, administration of 50 g/kg of *Chuan Xiong Cha Tiao San* via gastric tube twice daily for 3 days was associated with reduced spontaneous activities in mice. In a chronic toxicology study, administration of 17 g/kg of this formula via gastric tube one time daily for 8 days was associated with an accelerated rate of growth and increased weight of the spleen. No other abnormalities were noted. The study concluded that this formula has little toxicity.[11]

RELATED FORMULA

Jú Huā Chá Tiáo Sǎn
(Chrysanthemum Powder to be Taken with Green Tea)

菊花茶調散
菊花茶调散

Pinyin Name: Ju Hua Cha Tiao San
Literal Name: Chrysanthemum Powder to be Taken with Green Tea
Original Source: *Yi Fang Ji Jie* (Analytical Collection of Medical Formulas) by Wang Ang in 1682

Bo He (Herba Menthae), do not expose to heat	24g
Chuan Xiong (Rhizoma Chuanxiong)	12g
Jing Jie (Herba Schizonepetae)	12g
Qiang Huo (Rhizoma et Radix Notopterygii)	3g
Bai Zhi (Radix Angelicae Dahuricae)	3g
Zhi Gan Cao (Radix et Rhizoma Glycyrrhizae Praeparata cum Melle)	3g
Fang Feng (Radix Saposhnikoviae)	4.5g
Xi Xin (Radix et Rhizoma Asari)	3g
Ju Hua (Flos Chrysanthemi)	3g
Jiang Can (Bombyx Batryticatus)	0.9g

The source recommends grinding the ingredients into a fine powder. Take 9g per dose after meals with tea made from *Cha Ye* (Folium Camelliae).

Ju Hua Cha Tiao San (Chrysanthemum Powder to be Taken with Green Tea) is composed of *Chuan Xiong Cha Tiao San* plus *Ju Hua* (Flos Chrysanthemi) and *Jiang Can* (Bombyx Batryticatus). *Ju Hua Cha Tiao San* dispels wind, relieves pain, and clears the eyes and head. Clinically, it treats wind-heat conditions with symptoms such as frontal or temporal headache, dizziness, and vertigo.

Chuan Xiong Cha Tiao San and *Ju Hua Cha Tiao San* both treat headache due to exterior wind.

Chinese Herbal Formulas and Applications

Chuān Xiōng Chá Tiáo Săn
(Ligusticum Chuanxiong Powder to be Taken with Green Tea)

- *Chuan Xiong Cha Tiao San* is more effective for wind-cold.
- *Ju Hua Cha Tiao San* is more effective for wind-heat.

AUTHORS' COMMENTS

Chuan Xiong Cha Tiao San is one of the most commonly used formulas for headache caused by exterior wind-cold invasion. This formula is also effective in treating migraines, vascular headaches, or sinus headaches that are cold in nature.

References

1. *Zhong Yi Fang Ji Xian Dai Yan Jiu* (Modern Study of Medical Formulae in Traditional Chinese Medicine) 1997;1206.
2. *Zhong Yi Fang Ji Xian Dai Yan Jiu* (Modern Study of Medical Formulae in Traditional Chinese Medicine) 1997;1206.
3. *Zhong Yi Fang Ji Xian Dai Yan Jiu* (Modern Study of Medical Formulae in Traditional Chinese Medicine) 1997;1207.
4. *Jiang Xi Zhong Yi Yao* (Jiangxi Chinese Medicine and Herbology) 1992;6:47.
5. *Bei Jing Zhong Yi Yao Da Xue Xue Bao* (Journal of Beijing University of Medicine and Medicinals) 1994;17(4):36.
6. *Zhe Jiang Zhong Yi Za Zhi* (Zhejiang Journal of Chinese Medicine) 1998;2:61.
7. *Shan Dong Yi Yao* (Shandong Medicine and Herbology) 1994;12:55.
8. *Zhe Jiang Zhong Yi Za Zhi* (Zhejiang Journal of Chinese Medicine) 1989;6:255.
9. *Zhe Jiang Zhong Yi Za Zhi* (Zhejiang Journal of Chinese Medicine) 1989;10:454.
10. *Fu Jian Zhong Yi Yao* (Fujian Chinese Medicine and Herbology) 1991;6:17.
11. *Zhong Yao Yao Li Yu Lin Chuang* (Pharmacology and Clinical Applications of Chinese Herbs) 1992;1:11.

Qiān Zhèng Săn (Lead to Symmetry Powder)

牵正散

牽正散

Pinyin Name: Qian Zheng San
Literal Name: Lead to Symmetry Powder
Alternate Name: Lead to Symmetry Formula
Original Source: *Yang Shi Jia Zang Fang* (Collected Formulas of the Yang Family) by Yang Tan in 1178

COMPOSITION

Bai Fu Zi (Rhizoma Typhonii)	[6g]
Jiang Can (Bombyx Batryticatus)	[6g]
Quan Xie (Scorpio), remove toxins	[3g]

DOSAGE / PREPARATION / ADMINISTRATION

The source text recommends grinding equal amounts of the fresh ingredients into powder. Take 3g per dose with a warm, grain-based liquor. Today, this formula may be prepared as a decoction with the doses suggested in brackets.

CHINESE THERAPEUTIC ACTIONS

1. Dispels wind
2. Resolves phlegm
3. Stops spasms

CLINICAL MANIFESTATIONS

Zhong feng (wind stroke) characterized by deviation of the eyes and mouth and facial spasms.

CLINICAL APPLICATIONS

Facial paralysis, trigeminal neuralgia, hemiplegia, and migraine headache.

EXPLANATION

According to traditional Chinese medicine, *zhong feng* (wind stroke) can affect either the channels and collaterals, or the *zang fu* organs. *Zhong feng* (wind stroke) affecting the channels and collaterals is characterized by deviation of the face and paralysis of the limbs. *Zhong feng* (wind stroke) affecting the *zang fu* organs involves loss of consciousness, hemiplegia, distortion of the face, dysphagia, and absence of urination and defecation during the attack.

WIND-EXPELLING FORMULAS

14

977

Qiān Zhèng Sǎn (Lead to Symmetry Powder)

Qian Zheng San (Lead to Symmetry Powder)

Diagnosis	Signs and Symptoms	Treatment	Herbs
Zhong feng (wind stroke)	Deviation of the eyes and mouth and facial spasms: obstruction of wind and phlegm in the channels and collaterals	• Dispels wind • Resolves phlegm • Stops spasms	• *Bai Fu Zi* (Rhizoma Typhonii) dispels wind and clears phlegm in the head and face. • *Jiang Can* (Bombyx Batryticatus) and *Quan Xie* (Scorpio) dispel wind and stop spasms.

Qian Zheng San (Lead to Symmetry Powder) is designed specifically for *zhong feng* (wind stroke) affecting the channels and collaterals, with obstruction of wind and phlegm in the face. The channels affected are foot *yangming* [Stomach] which encircles the mouth and lips, and foot *taiyang* [Urinary Bladder] which reaches the inner canthus of the eyes. When these two channels are attacked by wind and obstructed by phlegm, the wind and phlegm factors block the qi and blood circulation and cause malnourishment of the muscles and tendons, producing symptoms such as deviation of the eyes and mouth. Facial spasms may also occur.

To effectively treat this syndrome, wind and phlegm must be dispelled. At the same time, qi and blood circulation in the channels and collaterals have to be restored, and the spasms stopped. This formula uses *Bai Fu Zi* (Rhizoma Typhonii) to dispel wind and clear phlegm in the head. *Jiang Can* (Bombyx Batryticatus) and *Quan Xie* (Scorpio) dispel wind and stop spasms. In addition, *Jiang Can* (Bombyx Batryticatus) resolves phlegm, while *Quan Xie* (Scorpio) opens the channels and collaterals. These three herbs synergistically address the cause of *zhong feng* (wind stroke). Lastly, grain-based liquor enhances blood circulation and distribution of herbs to the affected areas.

MODIFICATIONS

- For facial paralysis caused by wind-cold, add *Qiang Huo* (Rhizoma et Radix Notopterygii) and *Fang Feng* (Radix Saposhnikoviae).
- For facial paralysis caused by wind-dampness, add *Wu Gong* (Scolopendra).
- For facial twitching, add *Wu Gong* (Scolopendra), *Tian Ma* (Rhizoma Gastrodiae), and *Di Long* (Pheretima).

CAUTIONS / CONTRAINDICATIONS

- *Qian Zheng San* is acrid, warm, and drying in nature, and should be reserved for *zhong feng* (wind stroke) characterized by cold, wind and phlegm.
- Because *Bai Fu Zi* (Rhizoma Typhonii) is acrid, warm, and drying in nature, *Qian Zheng San* is not recommended for treating deviation of the mouth or hemiplegia due to interior Liver wind rising, or due to qi deficiency and

blood stagnation. Modifications (such as listed above) are necessary to address the complications and associated conditions.

- Because *Bai Fu Zi* (Rhizoma Typhonii) and *Quan Xie* (Scorpio) are toxic, doses of these herbs should not exceed 6g when used in decoction.
- Use of this formula is contraindicated during pregnancy.[1]

PHARMACOLOGICAL EFFECTS

1. **Cardiovascular**: According to *in vitro* studies, administration of *Qian Zheng San* was associated with reduced peripheral vascular resistance in both rabbits and rats. The onset of action began approximately 10-20 minutes after administration, and reached maximal effect after 30 minutes.[2]
2. **Effect on the central nervous system**: Administration of *Qian Zheng San* has been shown to have both sedative and antiepileptic effects. Intraperitoneal injection, intravenous injection, and oral ingestion of this formula were associated with sedation in rabbits. Use of a *Qian Zheng San* preparation was effective in treating mice with artificially-induced seizures.[3]

CLINICAL STUDIES AND RESEARCH

1. **Facial paralysis**: *Qian Zheng San* has been shown in many studies to effectively treat facial paralysis. According to one study, 60 patients with facial paralysis were treated with integrative treatments (herbs and acupuncture) with complete recovery in 50 cases and significant improvement in 2 cases. The herbal treatment included *Qian Zheng San* plus *Wu Gong* (Scolopendra), *Tian Ma* (Rhizoma Gastrodiae), *Di Long* (Pheretima), and *Fang Feng* (Radix Saposhnikoviae). The treatment protocol consisted of grinding all the substances into a fine powder, and administering 5g of the powder two times daily with grain-based liquor. The patients also received electro-acupuncture treatments. The average duration of treatment to achieve recovery was 2 weeks, ranging from 3 to 30 days.[4]

According to another study, use of modified *Qian Zheng San* in 50 patients with facial paralysis was associated with 98% effectiveness (complete recovery in 44 cases, significant improvement in 3 cases, moderate improvement in 2

Chinese Herbal Formulas and Applications

Qiān Zhèng Sǎn (Lead to Symmetry Powder)

cases, and no effect in 1 case). The treatment protocol was to cook the herbs in water and administer the decoction in three equally-divided doses daily. The herbal treatment contained *Qian Zheng San* plus *Fang Feng* (Radix Saposhnikoviae), *Wu Gong* (Scolopendra), *Qiang Huo* (Rhizoma et Radix Notopterygii), *Ge Gen* (Radix Puerariae Lobatae), and *Gou Teng* (Ramulus Uncariae cum Uncis) as the base formula. Modifications included the addition of *Dan Nan Xing* (Arisaema cum Bile), *Shi Chang Pu* (Rhizoma Acori Tatarinowii), *Zhu Ru* (Caulis Bambusae in Taenia), and *Ban Xia* (Rhizoma Pinelliae) for excess conditions characterized by tongue stiffness and tremors with a yellow, greasy tongue coating; *Di Huang Yin Zi* (Rehmannia Decoction) for deficiency conditions characterized by weakness of the tongue with white tongue coating; *Huang Qi* (Radix Astragali), *Dang Shen* (Radix Codonopsis), *Tai Zi Shen* (Radix Pseudostellariae), and *Huang Jing* (Rhizoma Polygonati) for qi deficiency with shortness of breath; *Tao Ren* (Semen Persicae), *Hong Hua* (Flos Carthami), and *Chi Shao* (Radix Paeoniae Rubra) for blood stagnation with purplish discoloration of the lips; *Bai Zhu* (Rhizoma Atractylodis Macrocephalae) and *Fu Ling* (Poria) for excessive salivation; *Shi Gao* (Gypsum Fibrosum), *Jin Yin Hua* (Flos Lonicerae Japonicae), and *Lian Qiao* (Fructus Forsythiae) for red face and yellow tongue coating; and *Ju Hua* (Flos Chrysanthemi), *Bai Zhi* (Radix Angelicae Dahuricae), *Chai Hu* (Radix Bupleuri), and *Chuan Xiong* (Rhizoma Chuanxiong) for headache.[5]

Lastly, 88 patients with facial paralysis were treated with great success using herbs and/or acupuncture. The herbal treatment contained *Qian Zheng San* plus *Fang Feng* (Radix Saposhnikoviae), *Jin Yin Hua* (Flos Lonicerae Japonicae), *Tao Ren* (Semen Persicae), *Chuan Xiong* (Rhizoma Chuanxiong), *Huang Qin* (Radix Scutellariae), *Dan Shen* (Radix et Rhizoma Salviae Miltiorrhizae), *Chan Tui* (Periostracum Cicadae), *Bai Ji* (Rhizoma Bletillae), *Di Huang* (Radix Rehmanniae), *Wu Gong* (Scolopendra), and others as needed. *Ma Huang* (Herba Ephedrae) and *Xi Xin* (Radix et Rhizoma Asari) were added for exterior wind-cold; *Sang Ye* (Folium Mori) and *Bo He* (Herba Menthae) were added for exterior wind-heat; *Xi Yang Shen* (Radix Panacis Quinquefolii) for qi deficiency; *Dang Gui* (Radix Angelicae Sinensis) and *Bai Shao* (Radix Paeoniae Alba) for blood deficiency; *Tian Ma* (Rhizoma Gastrodiae) and *Meng Shi* (Lapis Micae seu Chloriti) for chronic illness with phlegm obstructing the channels and collaterals; and *Gou Teng* (Ramulus Uncariae cum Uncis), *Di Huang* (Radix Rehmanniae), and *Zhi Chuan Wu* (Radix Aconiti Praeparata) for wind and phlegm obstructing the channels and collaterals. Of 88 patients, 68 received concurrent herbs and acupuncture treatment, and 20 received acupuncture treatment only. The duration of

treatment ranged from 2 days to 1 year. The study reported a 95% rate of recovery.[6]

2. **Migraine headache:** One study reported good results using *Qian Zheng San* to treat patients with stubborn migraine headache. The dose varied depending on the severity of the headache. Furthermore, *Ba Zhen Tang* (Eight-Treasure Decoction) was given in decoction to patients with qi and blood deficiencies. The treatment protocol was to administer the herbs with warm water for 5 days per course of treatment, followed by 3 days of rest, and continuing with the next course of treatment. Of 25 patients, the study reported complete recovery in 8 cases, improvement in 15 cases, and no effect in 2 cases. The overall rate of effectiveness was 92%.[7]

3. **Trigeminal neuralgia**: Use of modified *Qian Zheng San* in 52 patients was associated with 94.2% effectiveness. The herbal treatment contained this formula plus *Dang Gui* (Radix Angelicae Sinensis), *Chan Tui* (Periostracum Cicadae), and others as the base formula. Furthermore, modifications included the addition of *Huang Qin* (Radix Scutellariae), *Gou Teng* (Ramulus Uncariae cum Uncis), and *Shi Gao* (Gypsum Fibrosum) for wind-heat; *Bai Fu Zi* (Rhizoma Typhonii), *Xi Xin* (Radix et Rhizoma Asari), and *Ma Huang* (Herba Ephedrae) for wind-cold; *Tao Ren* (Semen Persicae), *Hong Hua* (Flos Carthami), *Ban Xia* (Rhizoma Pinelliae), and *Dan Nan Xing* (Arisaema cum Bile) for blood stagnation and phlegm obstruction; and *Di Huang* (Radix Rehmanniae), *Mu Dan Pi* (Cortex Moutan), *Gui Ban* (Plastrum Testudinis), and *Nu Zhen Zi* (Fructus Ligustri Lucidi) for yin deficiency with blood heat. Of 52 patients, the study reported significant relief of pain in 32 cases, moderate improvement in 17 cases, and no benefit in 3 cases.[8]

RELATED FORMULAS

Zhǐ Jìng Sǎn (Stop Spasms Powder)

止痙散
止痙散

Pinyin Name: *Zhi Jing San*
Literal Name: Stop Spasms Powder
Original Source: *Shang Hai Zhong Yi Xue Yuan* (Shanghai University of Chinese Medicine)

Quan Xie (Scorpio)
Wu Gong (Scolopendra)

The source text states to grind equal amounts of the ingredients into a fine powder. Take 1-1.5g of powder with boiled water two to four times daily.

The main actions of this formula are to dispel wind and stop muscle spasms. Clinically, *Zhi Jing San* (Stop Spasms

WIND-EXPELLING FORMULAS

14

979

Chapter 14 – Wind-Expelling Formulas

Section 1 – External-Wind Releasing Formulas

Qiān Zhèng Sǎn (Lead to Symmetry Powder)

Powder) can treat muscle spasms, cramps, and convulsions. This formula also relieves pain, and is especially effective for stubborn headaches and joint pain.

Jiā Wèi Qiān Zhèng Sǎn
(Augmented Lead to Symmetry Powder)

加味牽正散
加味牽正散

Pinyin Name: Jia Wei Qian Zheng San
Literal Name: Augmented Lead to Symmetry Powder
Original Source: Guang An Men Yi Yuan (Guang An Men Hospital) in 1990

Bai Fu Zi (Rhizoma Typhonii)
Zhi Cao Wu (Radix Aconiti Kusnezoffii Praeparata)
Tian Nan Xing (Rhizoma Arisaematis)
Zhi Chuan Wu (Radix Aconiti Praeparata)
Bai Zhi (Radix Angelicae Dahuricae)
Fang Feng (Radix Saposhnikoviae)
Jing Jie (Herba Schizonepetae)
Chuan Xiong (Rhizoma Chuanxiong)
Dang Gui (Radix Angelicae Sinensis)
Si Gua Luo (Retinervus Luffae Fructus)
Yan Hu Suo (Rhizoma Corydalis)

Jia Wei Qian Zheng San (Augmented Lead to Symmetry Powder) treats exterior wind attacking the upper parts of the body, leading to obstruction in the channels and collaterals and stagnation of qi and blood. It contains herbs that release exterior wind, open the channels and collaterals, and activate qi and blood circulation. Clinical manifestations include deviation of the eyes and mouth, inability to completely close the eyes and mouth, facial paralysis, temporomandibular joint pain, and trigeminal neuralgia.

AUTHORS' COMMENTS

Qian Zheng San is the representative formula for treating zhong feng (wind stroke) characterized by deviation of the eyes and mouth and facial spasms. However, to obtain optimal results for facial paralysis (deviation of the eyes and mouth), herbs should be used both orally and topically at the same time. A topical formula that has been used successfully, contains Ban Xia (Rhizoma Pinelliae), Chen Pi (Pericarpium Citri Reticulatae), Wei Ling Xian (Radix et Rhizoma Clematidis), Zhi Chuan Wu (Radix Aconiti Praeparata), Zhi Cao Wu (Radix Aconiti Kusnezoffii Praeparata), and Bai Ji (Rhizoma Bletillae). This formula is prepared by grinding all of the herbs into powder, and making the powder into an herbal paste by mixing 9g of the powder with the juice from Sheng Jiang (Rhizoma Zingiberis Recens). The herbal paste is applied to the affected area(s) daily.

References

1. Zhong Yao Ming Fang Yao Li Yu Ying Yong (Pharmacology and Applications of Famous Herbal Formulas) 1989;532-533.
2. Zhong Yao Yao Li Yu Lin Chuang (Pharmacology and Clinical Applications of Chinese Herbs) 1987;3:332.
3. Zhong Yi Fang Ji Xian Dai Yan Jiu (Modern Study of Medical Formulae in Traditional Chinese Medicine) 1997;1170.
4. Nei Meng Gu Zhong Yi Yao (Traditional Chinese Medicine and Medicinals of Inner Mongolia) 1990;9(4):18.
5. He Bei Zhong Yi (Hebei Chinese Medicine) 1985;4:30.
6. Shi Zhen Guo Yao Yan Jiu (Research of Shizhen Herbs) 1996;7(1):13.
7. Shi Yong Zhong Yi Yao Za Zhi (Journal of Practical Chinese Medicine and Medicinals) 1997;2:5.
8. Si Chuan Zhong Yi (Sichuan Chinese Medicine) 1998;2:25.

980

Chinese Herbal Formulas and Applications

Yù Zhēn Sǎn (True Jade Powder)

玉真散

Pinyin Name: *Yu Zhen San*
Literal Name: True Jade Powder
Original Source: *Wai Ke Zheng Zong* (True Lineage of External Medicine) by Chen Shi-Gong in 1617

COMPOSITION

Bai Fu Zi (Rhizoma Typhonii)	[6g]
Tian Nan Xing (Rhizoma Arisaematis)	[6g]
Qiang Huo (Rhizoma et Radix Notopterygii)	[6g]
Fang Feng (Radix Saposhnikoviae)	[6g]
Bai Zhi (Radix Angelicae Dahuricae)	[6g]
Tian Ma (Rhizoma Gastrodiae)	[6g]

DOSAGE / PREPARATION / ADMINISTRATION

The source text recommends grinding equal amounts of the ingredients into powder. For internal use, take 6g with hot, grain-based liquor. For topical application, mix the powder with grain-based liquor and apply to the affected area. In cases of lockjaw and kyphosis, the source text advises to administer 9g of the powdered herbs with hot *Tong Bian* (Infantis Urina). The source text states that these methods will resolve cases of internal blood stagnation. In cases of dog bites, wash the wound with clean water and apply the powder to the affected area.

Today, equal amounts of the ingredients are ground into a fine powder, sifted, and taken in 3g doses with hot, grain-based liquor or *Tong Bian* (Infantis Urina). For external treatment, apply the powder to the affected area. This formula may be prepared as a decoction with the doses suggested in brackets above.

CHINESE THERAPEUTIC ACTIONS

1. Dispels wind and dissolves phlegm
2. Relieves spasms and stops convulsions

CLINICAL MANIFESTATIONS

Tetanus: lockjaw, tightly-closed mouth and lips, stiff body, muscle spasms, and kyphosis.

CLINICAL APPLICATIONS

Tetanus, facial paralysis, chorea, and external ulcerations.

EXPLANATION

Yu Zhen San (True Jade Powder) can treat tetanus, which according to traditional Chinese medicine theory, is due to wind invading the channels and collaterals through open wounds. The wind attacks the channels and collaterals, causes malnourishment of the muscles and tendons, and leads to spasms, convulsions and kyphosis.

To effectively treat this syndrome, wind must be dispelled and spasms and convulsions relieved. This formula contains *Bai Fu Zi* (Rhizoma Typhonii) and *Tian Nan Xing* (Rhizoma Arisaematis) to dispel wind, resolve phlegm, and relieve spasms and convulsions. *Qiang Huo* (Rhizoma et Radix Notopterygii), *Fang Feng* (Radix Saposhnikoviae), and *Bai Zhi* (Radix Angelicae Dahuricae) clear wind from the channels and collaterals. *Tian Ma* (Rhizoma Gastrodiae) extinguishes wind and relieves spasms. Lastly, *Tong Bian* (Infantis Urina) and grain-based liquor open the channels and collaterals, and activate qi and blood circulation.

MODIFICATIONS

• For severe convulsions and kyphosis, add *Quan Xie* (Scorpio), *Jiang Can* (Bombyx Batryticatus) and *Wu Gong* (Scolopendra).

CAUTIONS / CONTRAINDICATIONS

• Do not use this formula at high doses or for an extended period of time, since it contains unprocessed forms of *Bai Fu Zi* (Rhizoma Typhonii) and *Tian Nan Xing* (Rhizoma Arisaematis), which are both toxic.

• Although *Yu Zhen San* is intended to treat the acute phase of tetanus, it should be used with caution in the recovery phase if there is severe consumption of qi and body fluids. This formula is acrid and drying, and may further damage the qi and body fluids.[1]

• Use of this formula is contraindicated during pregnancy.[2]

CLINICAL STUDIES AND RESEARCH

1. **Facial paralysis**: One study reported 90% effectiveness using modified *Yu Zhen San* to treat facial paralysis. The herbal treatment contained 15g each of *Bai Fu Zi* (Rhizoma Typhonii), *Dan Nan Xing* (Arisaema cum Bile), *Qiang Huo* (Rhizoma et Radix Notopterygii), *Fang Feng* (Radix Saposhnikoviae), *Tian Ma* (Rhizoma Gastrodiae), and *Bai Zhi* (Radix Angelicae Dahuricae) as the base formula. *Huang Qi* (Radix Astragali) 50g was added

WIND-EXPELLING FORMULAS

14

981

Yù Zhēn Sǎn (True Jade Powder)

Yu Zhen San (True Jade Powder)

Diagnosis	Signs and Symptoms	Treatment	Herbs
Tetanus	Lockjaw, tightly closed mouth and lips, stiff body, muscle spasms and kyphosis: wind and phlegm attacking the channels and collaterals	• Dispels wind and dissolves phlegm • Relieves spasms and stops convulsions	• *Bai Fu Zi* (Rhizoma Typhonii) and *Tian Nan Xing* (Rhizoma Arisaematis) dispel wind, resolve phlegm, and relieve spasms and convulsions. • *Qiang Huo* (Rhizoma et Radix Notopterygii), *Fang Feng* (Radix Saposhnikoviae), and *Bai Zhi* (Radix Angelicae Dahuricae) clear wind from the channels and collaterals. • *Tian Ma* (Rhizoma Gastrodiae) extinguishes wind and relieves spasms.

for qi deficiency, and *Quan Xie* (Scorpio) 15g and *Jiang Can* (Bombyx Batryticatus) 15g for wind and phlegm obstructing the channels and collaterals. Of 43 patients, the study reported complete recovery in 17 cases, marked improvement in 22 cases, and no benefit in 4 cases.[3]

2. **Chorea**: One study reported beneficial effects using *Yu Zhen San* and *Ba Zhen Tang* (Eight-Treasure Decoction) to treat 29 patients with spasmodic, unco-ordinated movements of the limbs and facial muscles. The herbal treatment contained *Tian Nan Xing* (Rhizoma Arisaematis) 10g, *Bai Fu Zi* (Rhizoma Typhonii) 10g, *Tian Ma* (Rhizoma Gastrodiae) 10g, *Bai Zhi* (Radix Angelicae Dahuricae) 10g, *Qiang Huo* (Rhizoma et Radix Notopterygii) 10g, *Fang Feng* (Radix Saposhnikoviae) 10g, *Gou Teng* (Ramulus Uncariae cum Uncis) 20g, *Huang Qi* (Radix Astragali) 30g, *Dang Shen* (Radix Codonopsis) 30g, *Bai Shao* (Radix Paeoniae Alba) 15g, *Dang Gui* (Radix Angelicae Sinensis) 15g, *Chuan Xiong* (Rhizoma Chuanxiong) 15g, *Fu Ling* (Poria) 15g, *Bai Zhu* (Rhizoma Atractylodis Macrocephalae) 15g, and *Zhi Gan Cao* (Radix et Rhizoma Glycyrrhizae Praeparata cum Melle) 6g. Other modifications were made as needed. The duration of treatment ranged from 5 to 18 packs of herbs. Of 29 patients, the study reported significant improvement in 26 patients and no effect in 3 individuals.[4]

3. **External ulcerations**: According to one study, 46 of 50 patients with external ulcers were successfully treated with a topical application of *Yu Zhen San*. The treatment protocol was to cook the herbs in water, filter out the herb residues, and apply the filtered liquid solution to the affected area.[5]

TOXICOLOGY

• Use of this formula has been associated with side effects such as numbness of the mouth and tongue, burning sensations of the throat, ulcerations of the oral cavity, salivation, and edema. These side effects have been attrib-uted to the use of unprocessed *Tian Nan Xing* (Rhizoma Arisaematis).[6]

• According to two reports, gross overdose (9g) of this formula has been associated with symptoms such as numbness of the mouth and lips, nausea, vomiting, burn-ing sensations in the upper abdominal area, dizziness, irritability, restlessness, urinary and bowel incontinence, respiratory depression, and in one case, fatality.[7,8]

RELATED FORMULA

Wǔ Hǔ Zhūi Fēng Sǎn
(Five-Tiger Powder to Pursue Wind)

五虎追風散
五虎追风散

Pinyin Name: Wu Hu Zhui Feng San
Literal Name: Five-Tiger Powder to Pursue Wind
Original Source: *Shi Chuan En Jia Chuan Fang* (Family Formulas from Shi Chuan-En), published in *Zhong Yi Za Zhi* (Journal of Chinese Medicine) in 1955

Chan Tui (Periostracum Cicadae)	30g
Tian Nan Xing (Rhizoma Arisaematis), *zhi* (prepared)	6g
Tian Ma (Rhizoma Gastrodiae)	6g
Quan Xie (Scorpio)	7-9 pieces [3g]
Jiang Can (Bombyx Batryticatus), *chao* (dry-fried)	7-9 pieces [6g]

The source text states to cook the ingredients in water and take the strained decoction. Separately grind 1.5g of *Zhu Sha* (Cinnabaris) into a fine powder, and take it with 60 mL of grain-based liquor. The source text states that sweating from the palms and soles is an indication that the formula is effective. If sweating does not occur on the first day, the formula should be given again the next day, for a total of three consecutive days.

Note: *Zhu Sha* (Cinnabaris) is a potentially toxic heavy metal, and is rarely used as a medicinal substance today. Its discussion here is included primarily for academic purposes, to reflect the historical use of this substance in its original formulation. Most herbal products today have

Chinese Herbal Formulas and Applications

Yù Zhēn Sǎn (True Jade Powder)

removed it completely, or replaced it with substitutes with similar functions. For additional information on the toxicity, please refer to *Chinese Medical Herbology and Pharmacology* by John Chen and Tina Chen.

The main actions of this formula are to dispel wind, relieve muscle spasms, and alleviate pain. Clinically, it is often used for tetanus characterized by lockjaw, continuous spasms and cramps in the extremities, convulsions, and kyphosis.

Yu Zhen San and *Wu Hu Zhui Feng San* (Five-Tiger Powder to Pursue Wind) are two formulas commonly used to treat tetanus.
- *Yu Zhen San* has stronger actions to dispel wind and dissolve phlegm.
- *Wu Hu Zhui Feng San* is more potent to dispel wind and relieve muscle spasms, cramps, convulsions, and kyphosis.

AUTHORS' COMMENTS

Though *Yu Zhen San* is formulated specifically to treat tetanus, the standard practice in China today for treatment of tetanus is to integrate Western and traditional

Chinese medicine by coordinated administration of drug, herbal and acupuncture treatments.[9]

Qian Zheng San (Lead to Symmetry Powder) and *Yu Zhen San* are two formulas with similar effect to dispel wind.
- *Qian Zheng San* is most effective at dispelling wind from the face, and is commonly used to treat Bell's palsy with deviation of the eyes and mouth.
- *Yu Zhen San* is best at dispelling wind from the body, and is usually used for tetanus with severe muscle spasms and cramps throughout the body.

References
1. *Zhong Yao Ming Fang Yao Li Yu Ying Yong* (Pharmacology and Applications of Famous Herbal Formulas) 1989;533-534.
2. *Zhong Yao Ming Fang Yao Li Yu Ying Yong* (Pharmacology and Applications of Famous Herbal Formulas) 1989;533-534.
3. *Shan Xi Zhong Yi* (Shanxi Chinese Medicine) 1991;12(10):465.
4. *Hu Nan Zhong Yi Za Zhi* (Hunan Journal of Chinese Medicine) 1992;2:35.
5. *Shan Xi Zhong Yi* (Shanxi Chinese Medicine) 1989;10(12):551.
6. *Zhong Yao Ming Fang Yao Li Yu Ying Yong* (Pharmacology and Applications of Famous Herbal Formulas) 1989;533-534.
7. *Jiang Su Zhong Yi* (Jiangsu Chinese Medicine) 1986;1:42.
8. *Zhong Yi Fang Ji Xian Dai Yan Jiu* (Modern Study of Medical Formulae in Traditional Chinese Medicine) 1997;1166.
9. *Fang Ji Xue* (Chinese Herbal Formulas) 1995;434-435.

Xiǎo Xù Mìng Tāng (Minor Prolong Life Decoction)
小續命湯
小续命汤

Pinyin Name: *Xiao Xu Ming Tang*
Literal Name: Minor Prolong Life Decoction
Alternate Names: *Hsiao Hsu Ming Tang*, Ma-huang and Peony Decoction, Mahuang and Peony Combination, Mahuang and Ginseng Combination
Original Source: *Qian Jin Yao Fang* (Thousand Ducat Prescriptions) by Sun Si-Miao in 581-685 A.D.

COMPOSITION

Ma Huang (Herba Ephedrae)	30g [3-6g]
Fang Feng (Radix Saposhnikoviae)	45g [9-12g]
Ren Shen (Radix et Rhizoma Ginseng)	30g [3-6g]
Gan Cao (Radix et Rhizoma Glycyrrhizae)	30g [3-6g]
Bai Shao (Radix Paeoniae Alba)	30g [6-12g]
Chuan Xiong (Rhizoma Chuanxiong)	30g [3-6g]
Sheng Jiang (Rhizoma Zingiberis Recens)	150g [9-12 slices]
Fang Ji (Radix Stephaniae Tetrandrae)	30g [6-12g]
Fu Zi (Radix Aconiti Lateralis Praeparata)	1 piece [3-9g]
Gui Xin (Cortex Rasus Cinnamomi)	30g [3-6g]
Huang Qin (Radix Scutellariae)	30g [4.5-9g]
Ku Xing Ren (Semen Armeniacae Amarum)	30g [9-12g]

WIND-EXPELLING FORMULAS

14

983

Chapter 14 – Wind-Expelling Formulas   *Section 1 – External-Wind Releasing Formulas*

Xiǎo Xù Mìng Tāng (Minor Prolong Life Decoction)

DOSAGE / PREPARATION / ADMINISTRATION

The source text recommends grinding the ingredients into a coarse powder. First cook *Ma Huang* (Herba Ephedrae) in 12 cups of water, and bring it to a boil three times. Remove the foam from the top, add the rest of the herbs, and cook the decoction again until the liquid is reduced to 3 cups. Take the warm, strained decoction in three equally-divided doses. If the condition is not resolved, an additional 3-4 packs of herbs can be administered. Today, this formula may be prepared as a decoction, with the doses suggested in brackets above.

CHINESE THERAPEUTIC ACTIONS

1. Dispels wind and supports *zheng* (upright) *qi*
2. Warms the channels and opens yang

CLINICAL MANIFESTATIONS

Post-stroke complications with *zheng* (upright) *qi* deficiency: semi-unconsciousness or unconsciousness, hemiplegia, paralysis, muscle contractions and convulsions, deviation of the eyes and mouth, slurred speech, and low back pain.

CLINICAL APPLICATIONS

Stroke, paralysis, hemiplegia, migraine, arthritis, and post-stroke sequelae.

EXPLANATION

Xiao Xu Ming Tang (Minor Prolong Life Decoction) treats post-stroke complications manifesting in compromised

mental and/or physical functions. Affected mental functions include alteration of consciousness and slurred speech. Affected physical functions include hemiplegia, paralysis, muscle contractions and convulsions, and deviation of the eyes and mouth.

Because stroke is diagnosed as a wind disorder in traditional Chinese medicine, exterior-releasing herbs that dispel wind are used to treat post-stroke complications. As such, this formula employs *Ma Huang* (Herba Ephedrae) and *Fang Feng* (Radix Saposhnikoviae) to dispel wind and release the exterior. *Bai Shao* (Radix Paeoniae Alba) harmonizes the *wei* (defensive) and *ying* (nutritive) levels and prevents the exterior-releasing herbs from inducing excessive perspiration. Because of the underlying *zheng* (upright) *qi* deficiency, *Ren Shen* (Radix et Rhizoma Ginseng) and *Gan Cao* (Radix et Rhizoma Glycyrrhizae) are added to tonify qi; while *Bai Shao* (Radix Paeoniae Alba) and *Chuan Xiong* (Rhizoma Chuanxiong) tonify blood and regulate blood circulation. In addition, *Sheng Jiang* (Rhizoma Zingiberis Recens) dispels wind, *Fang Ji* (Radix Stephaniae Tetrandrae) dispels dampness, *Fu Zi* (Radix Aconiti Lateralis Praeparata) and *Gui Xin* (Cortex Rasus Cinnamomi) dispel cold, *Huang Qin* (Radix Scutellariae) clears heat, and *Ku Xing Ren* (Semen Armeniacae Amarum) regulates qi.

MODIFICATIONS

• With constipation, add *Zhi Shi* (Fructus Aurantii Immaturus) and *Da Huang* (Radix et Rhizoma Rhei).

Xiao Xu Ming Tang (Minor Prolong-Life Decoction)

Diagnosis	Signs and Symptoms	Treatment	Herbs
Post-stroke complications with *zheng* (upright) *qi* deficiency	Hemiplegia, paralysis, muscle contractions and convulsions, deviation of the eyes and mouth, slurred speech and low back pain: *zheng* (upright) *qi* deficiency leading to invasion of wind blocking the channels and collaterals	• Dispels wind and supports the *zheng* (upright) *qi* • Warms the channels and opens yang	• *Ma Huang* (Herba Ephedrae) and *Fang Feng* (Radix Saposhnikoviae) dispel wind and release the exterior. • *Ren Shen* (Radix et Rhizoma Ginseng) and *Gan Cao* (Radix et Rhizoma Glycyrrhizae) tonify qi. • *Bai Shao* (Radix Paeoniae Alba) and *Chuan Xiong* (Rhizoma Chuanxiong) tonify and regulate blood circulation. • *Sheng Jiang* (Rhizoma Zingiberis Recens) dispels wind. • *Fang Ji* (Radix Stephaniae Tetrandrae) dispels dampness. • *Fu Zi* (Radix Aconiti Lateralis Praeparata) and *Gui Xin* (Cortex Rasus Cinnamomi) dispel cold. • *Huang Qin* (Radix Scutellariae) clears heat. • *Ku Xing Ren* (Semen Armeniacae Amarum) regulates qi.

984

Chinese Herbal Formulas and Applications

Xiǎo Xù Mìng Tāng (Minor Prolong Life Decoction)

- When there is altered consciousness, add *Fu Ling* (Poria) and *Yuan Zhi* (Radix Polygalae).
- With spasms, pain, and numbness, add *Qiang Huo* (Rhizoma et Radix Notopterygii) and *Lian Qiao* (Fructus Forsythiae).
- With slurred speech, add *Shi Chang Pu* (Rhizoma Acori Tatarinowii) and *Zhu Li* (Succus Bambusae).
- With nausea, add *Ban Xia* (Rhizoma Pinelliae).
- With body aches and convulsions, add *Qiang Huo* (Rhizoma et Radix Notopterygii).
- If accompanied by a dry mouth and tongue, add *Shi Gao* (Gypsum Fibrosum) and *Zhi Mu* (Rhizoma Anemarrhenae).

PHARMACOLOGICAL EFFECTS

Radioprotective: According to one study in mice, administration of a methanol extract of *Xiao Xu Ming Tang* by intraperitoneal injection was shown to significantly increase the survival rate after a lethal dose of irradiation.[1]

RELATED FORMULA

Xiǎo Xù Mìng Tāng (Minor Prolong Life Decoction)
小續命湯
小续命汤
Pinyin Name: *Xiao Xu Ming Tang*
Literal Name: Minor Prolong Life Decoction
Alternate Names: *Hsiao Hsu Ming Tang*, Ma-huang and Peony Decoction
Original Source: *Yi Fang Ji Jie* (Analytical Collection of Medical Formulas) by Wang Ang in 1682

Ma Huang (Herba Ephedrae)	[3-6g]
Gui Zhi (Ramulus Cinnamomi)	[3-6g]
Gan Cao (Radix et Rhizoma Glycyrrhizae)	[3-6g]
Sheng Jiang (Rhizoma Zingiberis Recens)	[6-18g]
Ren Shen (Radix et Rhizoma Ginseng)	[3-6g]
Chuan Xiong (Rhizoma Chuanxiong)	[3-6g]
Ku Xing Ren (Semen Armeniacae Amarum)	[3-6g]
Fu Zi (Radix Aconiti Lateralis Praeparata)	[1.5-3g]
Fang Ji (Radix Stephaniae Tetrandrae)	[3-6g]
Bai Shao (Radix Paeoniae Alba)	[3-6g]
Huang Qin (Radix Scutellariae)	[3-6g]
Fang Feng (Radix Saposhnikoviae)	[1.5-9g]
Da Zao (Fructus Jujubae)	[1.5-3g]

This formula is designed to tonify qi, disperse cold, release wind and dispel dampness. It treats individuals with underlying qi deficiency complicated with wind-cold attacking the channels and collaterals. Clinical manifestations include hemiplegia, deviation of the eyes and mouth, speech difficulties, muscle spasms and cramps, convulsions, stiff muscles and headache.

These two formulas have the same names, and essentially the same ingredients and indications.

- *Xiao Xu Ming Tang* from *Qian Jin Yao Fang* (Thousand Ducat Prescriptions) contains *Gui Xin* (Cortex Rasus Cinnamomi), which has a stronger function to warm the interior.
- *Xiao Xu Ming Tang* from *Yi Fang Ji Jie* (Analytical Collection of Medical Formulas) utilizes *Gui Zhi* (Ramulus Cinnamomi), which has a better effect to dispel wind-cold and warm the channels and collaterals.

Reference
1. Wang CM, Ohta S, Shinoda M. Studies on chemical protectors against radiation. XXVII. Survival effects of methanol extracts of various Chinese traditional medicines on radiation injury. Yakugaku Zasshi 1989 Dec;109(12):949-53.

WIND-EXPELLING FORMULAS

14

Chapter 14 – Wind-Expelling Formulas　　　　*Section 1 – External-Wind Releasing Formulas*

Xù Míng Tāng (Prolong Life Decoction)

續命湯
续命汤

Pinyin Name: *Xu Ming Tang*
Literal Name: Prolong Life Decoction
Original Source: *Wai Tai Mi Yao* (Arcane Essentials from the Imperial Library) by Wang Tao in 752 A.D.

COMPOSITION

Ma Huang (Herba Ephedrae)	9g
Gui Xin (Cortex Rasus Cinnamomi)	9g
Gan Jiang (Rhizoma Zingiberis)	9g
Shi Gao (Gypsum Fibrosum), *fen sui* (pulverized)	9g
Ren Shen (Radix et Rhizoma Ginseng)	9g
Zhi Gan Cao (Radix et Rhizoma Glycyrrhizae Praeparata cum Melle)	9g
Ku Xing Ren (Semen Armeniacae Amarum)	9g
Dang Gui (Radix Angelicae Sinensis)	9g
Chuan Xiong (Rhizoma Chuanxiong)	4.5g

DOSAGE / PREPARATION / ADMINISTRATION

Grind the ingredients into a coarse powder, and cook it in 10 cups of water until the liquid is reduced to 4 cups. Take 1 cup of the warm, strained decoction per dose. Continue to administer the decoction until mild perspiration is achieved, then discontinue the formula.

CHINESE THERAPEUTIC ACTIONS

1. Dispels wind
2. Clears heat
3. Regulates qi
4. Nourishes the blood

CLINICAL MANIFESTATIONS

Post-stroke sequelae: hemiplegia, muscle paralysis, inability to turn the body, slurred speech, confusion, numbness and pain in the body, muscle stiffness, and cramps.

CLINICAL APPLICATIONS

Stroke sequelae, hemiplegia, paralysis, neuralgia, and arthritis.

EXPLANATION

Xu Ming Tang (Prolong Life Decoction) treats post-stroke complications with both mental and physical impairments. Mental impairments include slurred speech,

Xu Ming Tang (Prolong Life Decoction)

Diagnosis	Signs and Symptoms	Treatment	Herbs
Post-stroke sequelae	Hemiplegia, muscle paralysis, inability to turn the body, slurred speech, confusion, numbness and pain in the body, muscle stiffness and cramps: wind attacking the *wei* (defensive) and *ying* (nutritive) levels	• Dispels wind • Clears heat • Regulates qi • Nourishes blood	• *Ma Huang* (Herba Ephedrae) releases the exterior and dispels wind. • *Gui Xin* (Cortex Rasus Cinnamomi) and *Gan Jiang* (Rhizoma Zingiberis) warm and open the channels and collaterals. • *Shi Gao* (Gypsum Fibrosum) clears heat. • *Ren Shen* (Radix et Rhizoma Ginseng), *Zhi Gan Cao* (Radix et Rhizoma Glycyrrhizae Praeparata cum Melle) and *Ku Xing Ren* (Semen Armeniacae Amarum) tonify qi and regulate qi circulation. • *Dang Gui* (Radix Angelicae Sinensis) and *Chuan Xiong* (Rhizoma Chuanxiong) tonify blood and regulate blood circulation. • *Zhi Gan Cao* (Radix et Rhizoma Glycyrrhizae Praeparata cum Melle) harmonizes the herbs.

Chinese Herbal Formulas and Applications

Xù Mìng Tāng (Prolong Life Decoction)

confusion, and inability to think clearly. Physical impairments include hemiplegia, muscle paralysis, numbness, and pain.

In this formula, *Ma Huang* (Herba Ephedrae) releases the exterior and dispels wind from the *wei* (defensive) level. *Gui Xin* (Cortex Rasus Cinnamomi) and *Gan Jiang* (Rhizoma Zingiberis) warm and open the channels and collaterals. *Shi Gao* (Gypsum Fibrosum) clears heat, and balances the hot nature of *Gui Xin* (Cortex Rasus Cinnamomi) and *Gan Jiang* (Rhizoma Zingiberis). *Ren Shen* (Radix et Rhizoma Ginseng), *Zhi Gan Cao* (Radix et Rhizoma Glycyrrhizae Praeparata cum Melle) and *Ku Xing Ren* (Semen Armeniacae Amarum) tonify qi and regulate qi circulation. *Dang Gui* (Radix Angelicae Sinensis) and *Chuan Xiong* (Rhizoma Chuanxiong) tonify blood and regulate blood circulation. *Zhi Gan Cao* (Radix et Rhizoma Glycyrrhizae Praeparata cum Melle) harmonizes the herbs.

MODIFICATIONS

- With speech difficulty, add *Shi Chang Pu* (Rhizoma Acori Tatarinowii) and *Yuan Zhi* (Radix Polygalae).

- With numbness, add *Huang Qi* (Radix Astragali) and *Niu Xi* (Radix Achyranthis Bidentatae).
- With muscle spasms and cramps, add *Fang Feng* (Radix Saposhnikoviae) and *Fang Ji* (Radix Stephaniae Tetrandrae).

CAUTIONS / CONTRAINDICATIONS

According to the source text, *Hai Zao* (Sargassum) and *Cong Bai* (Herba Allii Fistulosi) should be avoided while taking *Xiao Xu Ming Tang*.

AUTHORS' COMMENTS

Xiao Xu Ming Tang (Minor Prolong-Life Decoction) and *Xu Ming Tang* (Prolong Life Decoction) have similar names and functions. Both formulas may prolong life in patients suffering from post-stroke complications with compromised mental and/or physical functions.

- *Xiao Xu Ming Tang* has stronger actions to warm yang and support *zheng* (upright) *qi*.
- *Xu Ming Tang* is better at dispelling wind and clearing heat.

WIND-EXPELLING FORMULAS

14

987

Chapter 14 – Wind-Expelling Formulas   *Section 1 – External-Wind Releasing Formulas*

Dà Qín Jiāo Tāng (Major Gentiana Macrophylla Decoction)

大秦艽湯
大秦艽汤

Pinyin Name: Da Qin Jiao Tang
Literal Name: Major Gentiana Macrophylla Decoction
Alternate Name: Major Chin-chiu Combination
Original Source: *Su Wen Bing Ji Qi Yi Bao Ming Ji* (Collection of Writings on the Mechanism of Illness, Suitability of Qi, and the Safeguarding of Life as Discussed in the Basic Questions) by Zhang Yuan-Su in 1186

COMPOSITION

Qin Jiao (Radix Gentianae Macrophyllae)	90g [9g]
Qiang Huo (Rhizoma et Radix Notopterygii)	30g [3g]
Du Huo (Radix Angelicae Pubescentis)	60g [6g]
Fang Feng (Radix Saposhnikoviae)	30g [3g]
Bai Zhi (Radix Angelicae Dahuricae)	30g [3g]
Xi Xin (Radix et Rhizoma Asari)	15g [2g]
Dang Gui (Radix Angelicae Sinensis)	60g [6g]
Bai Shao (Radix Paeoniae Alba)	60g [6g]
Shu Di Huang (Radix Rehmanniae Praeparata)	30g [3g]
Chuan Xiong (Rhizoma Chuanxiong)	60g [6g]
Bai Zhu (Rhizoma Atractylodis Macrocephalae)	30g [3g]
Fu Ling (Poria)	30g [3g]
Huang Qin (Radix Scutellariae)	30g [3g]
Shi Gao (Gypsum Fibrosum)	60g [6g]
Di Huang (Radix Rehmanniae)	30g [3g]
Gan Cao (Radix et Rhizoma Glycyrrhizae)	60g [6g]

DOSAGE / PREPARATION / ADMINISTRATION

The source text recommends grinding the ingredients into powder and cooking 30g of the powder in water to make a decoction. Take the warm, strained decoction any time during the day. The source text recommends adding 7 to 8 slices of *Sheng Jiang* (Rhizoma Zingiberis Recens) during cloudy days, and 3g of *Zhi Shi* (Fructus Aurantii Immaturus) for epigastric distention. Today, this formula may be prepared as a decoction with the doses suggested in brackets above.

CHINESE THERAPEUTIC ACTIONS

1. Dispels wind and clears heat
2. Nourishes the blood and activates blood circulation

CLINICAL MANIFESTATIONS

Early stage of *zhong feng* (wind stroke) with wind attacking the channels and collaterals: deviation of the eyes and mouth, stiff tongue and speech difficulties, numbness and difficulty in moving the extremities, a white tongue coating, and a superficial pulse.

CLINICAL APPLICATIONS

Cerebral embolism, cerebral hemorrhage, post-stroke sequelae (facial paralysis, hemiplegia, paralysis, deviation of the eyes and mouth, and speech difficulties), arthritis, fibromyalgia, and muscle atrophy.

EXPLANATION

Da Qin Jiao Tang (Major Gentiana Macrophylla Decoction) treats early-stage *zhong feng* (wind stroke), with wind attacking the channels and collaterals. This condition usually occurs when qi and blood are deficient and the body is vulnerable to attacks from external pathogens, especially wind. Wind is highly mobile and may suddenly attack the body and cause stagnation of qi and blood in the channels and collaterals. As a result of stagnation in the channels and collaterals, other symptoms develop, such as deviation of the eyes and mouth, stiff tongue, speech difficulties, and numbness and difficult movement of the extremities.

Qin Jiao (Radix Gentianae Macrophyllae), the chief herb of this formula, dispels wind and opens the channels and collaterals. The deputies, *Qiang Huo* (Rhizoma et Radix Notopterygii), *Du Huo* (Radix Angelicae Pubescentis), *Fang Feng* (Radix Saposhnikoviae), *Bai Zhi* (Radix Angelicae Dahuricae), and *Xi Xin* (Radix et Rhizoma

988

Chinese Herbal Formulas and Applications

Dà Qín Jiāo Tāng (Major Gentiana Macrophylla Decoction)

Da Qin Jiao Tang (Major Gentiana Macrophylla Decoction)

Diagnosis	Signs and Symptoms	Treatment	Herbs
Early stage of *zhong feng* (wind stroke), with wind attacking the channels and collaterals	Deviation of the eyes and mouth, stiff tongue, speech difficulties, and numbness and difficult movement of the extremities: stagnation of qi and blood in the channels and collaterals due to invasion of wind	• Dispels wind and clears heat • Nourishes the blood and activates blood circulation	• *Qin Jiao* (Radix Gentianae Macrophyllae) dispels wind and opens the channels and collaterals. • *Qiang Huo* (Rhizoma et Radix Notopterygii), *Du Huo* (Radix Angelicae Pubescentis), *Fang Feng* (Radix Saposhnikoviae), *Bai Zhi* (Radix Angelicae Dahuricae) and *Xi Xin* (Radix et Rhizoma Asari) dispel wind from the channels and collaterals. • *Dang Gui* (Radix Angelicae Sinensis), *Bai Shao* (Radix Paeoniae Alba), *Shu Di Huang* (Radix Rehmanniae Praeparata) and *Chuan Xiong* (Rhizoma Chuanxiong) nourish the blood and activate blood circulation. • *Bai Zhu* (Rhizoma Atractylodis Macrocephalae) and *Fu Ling* (Poria) tonify qi and strengthen the Spleen. • *Huang Qin* (Radix Scutellariae), *Shi Gao* (Gypsum Fibrosum) and *Di Huang* (Radix Rehmanniae) clear heat. • *Gan Cao* (Radix et Rhizoma Glycyrrhizae) harmonizes the herbs.

Asari), are warm and acrid and dispel wind from the channels and collaterals. More specifically, *Qiang Huo* (Rhizoma et Radix Notopterygii) dispels wind from the upper body, while *Du Huo* (Radix Angelicae Pubescentis) dispels wind from the lower body; *Qiang Huo* (Rhizoma et Radix Notopterygii) dispels wind from the *taiyang* level and *Bai Zhi* (Radix Angelicae Dahuricae) releases wind from the *yangming* level; and *Fang Feng* (Radix Saposhnikoviae) releases wind from the exterior and *Xi Xin* (Radix et Rhizoma Asari) opens the orifices. Together, these five deputy herbs help the chief herb to strongly dispel wind and open the channels and collaterals.

In addition to dispelling wind, *Dang Gui* (Radix Angelicae Sinensis), *Bai Shao* (Radix Paeoniae Alba), *Shu Di Huang* (Radix Rehmanniae Praeparata), and *Chuan Xiong* (Rhizoma Chuanxiong) nourish the blood, activate blood circulation, and neutralize the dryness caused by the wind-dispelling herbs in this formula; also, by nourishing Liver blood, the Liver may then smooth the qi flow to relieve numbness and spasms. *Bai Zhu* (Rhizoma Atractylodis Macrocephalae) and *Fu Ling* (Poria) tonify qi and strengthen the Spleen. Because qi and blood stagnation can easily create heat, heat-clearing herbs such as *Huang Qin* (Radix Scutellariae), *Shi Gao* (Gypsum Fibrosum), and *Di Huang* (Radix Rehmanniae) are also used in this formula. *Gan Cao* (Radix et Rhizoma Glycyrrhizae) harmonizes the formula.

MODIFICATIONS
• With severe deviation of the eyes and mouth, add *Quan Xie* (Scorpio) and *Wu Gong* (Scolopendra).
• With fullness and distention in the epigastrium, add *Zhi Shi* (Fructus Aurantii Immaturus).
• If there is no interior heat, remove *Huang Qin* (Radix Scutellariae), *Shi Gao* (Gypsum Fibrosum), and *Di Huang* (Radix Rehmanniae).
• If there are no prominent wind symptoms, reduce the number of exterior-wind-dispersing herbs in order to reduce the overall acrid nature of this formula.

CAUTIONS / CONTRAINDICATIONS
• *Da Qin Jiao Tang* treats external wind attacking the channels and collaterals, and is contraindicated in patients with internal wind.
• This formula is acrid and drying in nature, and should be used with extreme caution in cases of blood and/or yin deficiency.

CLINICAL STUDIES AND RESEARCH
1. **Cerebral embolism**: Administration of *Da Qin Jiao Tang* has been shown to be effective for treating acute cerebral embolism characterized by wind and phlegm obstructing the channels and collaterals. Of 240 patients, the study reported complete recovery in 98 patients (resolution of symptoms, with restored normal mental and physical functioning), significant improvement in 80 patients

WIND-EXPELLING FORMULAS

14

989

Chapter 14 – Wind-Expelling Formulas *Section 1 – External-Wind Releasing Formulas*

Dà Qín Jiāo Tāng (Major Gentiana Macrophylla Decoction)

(marked improvement of symptoms, with mild residual facial paralysis and speech difficulties), improvement in 56 cases (slight overall improvement of symptoms, but with continued difficulties in speech, swallowing, and physical activities) and no effect in 6 cases. The overall rate of effectiveness was 97.9%.[1]

2. **Cerebral hemorrhage**: Administration of modified *Da Qin Jiao Tang* was beneficial in treating 84 patients with cerebral hemorrhage in one study. The herbal formula contained *Qin Jiao* (Radix Gentianae Macrophyllae) 10g, *Di Huang* (Radix Rehmanniae) 15g, *Dang Gui* (Radix Angelicae Sinensis) 15g, *Chi Shao* (Radix Paeoniae Rubra) 12g, *Chuan Xiong* (Rhizoma Chuanxiong) 10g, *Niu Xi* (Radix Achyranthis Bidentatae) 15g, *Gui Zhi* (Ramulus Cinnamomi) 10g, *Shui Zhi* (Hirudo) 9g, and *Huang Qin* (Radix Scutellariae) 10g. The duration of treatment ranged from 30-50 days, with an average of 38 days. One pack of herbs was given in decoction daily. Of 84 patients, the study reported complete recovery in 40 cases, significant improvement in 16 cases, moderate improvement in 17 cases, and deterioration and eventual fatality in 11 cases.[2]

3. **Facial paralysis**: One study reported 94.2% effectiveness using modified *Da Qin Jiao Tang* to treat 52 patients with facial paralysis characterized by wind-cold. The herbal formula contained *Qin Jiao* (Radix Gentianae Macrophyllae) 12g, *Bai Fu Zi* (Rhizoma Typhonii) 12g, *Chuan Xiong* (Rhizoma Chuanxiong) 6g, *Gan Cao* (Radix et Rhizoma Glycyrrhizae) 6g, *Gui Zhi* (Ramulus Cinnamomi) 6g, *Qiang Huo* (Rhizoma et Radix Notopterygii), *Fang Feng* (Radix Saposhnikoviae), and *Dang Gui* (Radix Angelicae Sinensis). The dose of the last three herbs varied depending on the history and severity of illness. The herbs were given in decoction twice daily with meals in the morning and at night, for 12 days per course of treatment, for three courses total.[3]

AUTHORS' COMMENTS

Most of the herbs in this formula are acrid, warm, and dispersing in nature, and are suitable for the initial stages of wind attacking the channels and collaterals. However, because this formula is acrid and drying and may damage blood and body fluids, herbs that tonify the blood and generate body fluids should be used prophylactically.

References

1. *He Bei Zhong Yi* (Hebei Chinese Medicine) 1986;1:12.
2. *Zhong Yi Fang Ji Xian Dai Yan Jiu* (Modern Study of Medical Formulae in Traditional Chinese Medicine) 1997;1149.
3. *Si Chuan Zhong Yi* (Sichuan Chinese Medicine) 1994;4:28.

Wū Yào Shùn Qì Săn (Lindera Powder to Smooth the Flow of Qi)
烏藥順氣散
乌药顺气散

Pinyin Name: *Wu Yao Shun Qi San*

Literal Name: Lindera Powder to Smooth the Flow of Qi

Alternate Names: *Wu Yao Chun Chi San*, *Wu Yao Shun Chi San*, Lindera Chi-Regulating Formula, Lindera Chi-Regulating Powder, Lindera Formula

Original Source: *Tai Ping Hui Min He Ji Ju Fang* (Imperial Grace Formulary of the Tai Ping Era) by the Imperial Medical Department in 1078-85

COMPOSITION

Wu Yao (Radix Linderae)	60g
Chen Pi (Pericarpium Citri Reticulatae)	60g
Jiang Can (Bombyx Batryticatus), *chao* (dry-fried)	30g
Ma Huang (Herba Ephedrae)	60g
Chuan Xiong (Rhizoma Chuanxiong)	30g
Jie Geng (Radix Platycodonis)	30g
Pao Jiang (Rhizoma Zingiberis Praeparatum), *pao* (blast-fried)	15g
Zhi Qiao (Fructus Citri Aurantii), *chao* (dry-fried) with bran	30g
Bai Zhi (Radix Angelicae Dahuricae)	30g
Gan Cao (Radix et Rhizoma Glycyrrhizae), *chao* (dry-fried)	30g

990

Chinese Herbal Formulas and Applications

Wū Yào Shùn Qì Sǎn (Lindera Powder to Smooth the Flow of Qi)

DOSAGE / PREPARATION / ADMINISTRATION

The source text recommends grinding the ingredients into a fine powder. Cook 9g of the powder with 3 slices of *Sheng Jiang* (Rhizoma Zingiberis Recens) and 1 piece of *Da Zao* (Fructus Jujubae) in 1 bowl of water until the liquid is reduced to 70%. Take the strained decoction while warm.

CHINESE THERAPEUTIC ACTIONS

1. Dispels wind
2. Activates qi circulation and relieves pain
3. Eliminates phlegm

CLINICAL MANIFESTATIONS

1. *Zhong feng* (wind stroke): arthralgia, numbness and pain throughout the body, dysphasia, muscle and tendon stiffness, and paralysis.
2. Leg *qi* with leg weakness and difficulty walking.
3. Stabbing pain in the hypochondrium, epigastric and abdominal fullness, vomiting, diarrhea, and borborygmus.

CLINICAL APPLICATIONS

Syncope, cerebrovascular accident, cerebral hemorrhage, hemiplegia, trigeminal neuralgia, and Bell's palsy.

EXPLANATION

Wu Yao Shun Qi San (Lindera Powder to Smooth the Flow of Qi) treats *zhong feng* (wind stroke) and subsequent complications, such as muscle paralysis and limited mobility. In this case, the wind attacks the channels and collaterals in the extremities, causing numbness, stiffness, and pain throughout the body. This formula may also treat individuals with weak legs and difficulty walking. This formula is useful in the treatment of geriatric patients with internal wind and cold, or women with internal wind and blood deficiency. Clinical presentations include stabbing hypochondriac pain, epigastric and abdominal fullness, vomiting, diarrhea, and borborygmus.

Wu Yao (Radix Linderae) dispels wind, promotes qi circulation, and relieves pain. *Chen Pi* (Pericarpium Citri Reticulatae) regulates qi flow. *Jiang Can* (Bombyx Batryticatus) subdues wind and dispels phlegm. *Ma Huang* (Herba Ephedrae) dispels exterior wind-cold and regulates qi circulation. *Chuan Xiong* (Rhizoma Chuanxiong) dispels wind and activates blood circulation to relieve pain. *Jie Geng* (Radix Platycodonis) opens inhibited Lung qi and eliminates phlegm. *Pao Jiang* (Rhizoma Zingiberis Praeparatum) warms the Spleen and Lung to dissolve phlegm. *Zhi Qiao* (Fructus Aurantii) activates

Wu Yao Shun Qi San (Lindera Powder to Smooth the Flow of Qi)

Diagnosis	Signs and Symptoms	Treatment	Herbs
Zhong feng (wind stroke)	Numbness, stiffness and pain throughout the body, arthralgia, dysphasia and paralysis: wind attacking the channels and collaterals	• Dispels wind • Activates qi and relieves pain • Eliminates phlegm	• *Wu Yao* (Radix Linderae) dispels wind, promotes qi circulation and relieves pain. • *Chen Pi* (Pericarpium Citri Reticulatae) regulates qi flow. • *Jiang Can* (Bombyx Batryticatus) subdues wind and dispels phlegm. • *Ma Huang* (Herba Ephedrae) dispels exterior wind-cold and regulates qi circulation. • *Chuan Xiong* (Rhizoma Chuanxiong) dispels wind and activates blood circulation to relieve pain. • *Jie Geng* (Radix Platycodonis) opens inhibited Lung qi and eliminates phlegm. • *Pao Jiang* (Rhizoma Zingiberis Praeparatum) warms the Spleen and Lung to dissolve phlegm. • *Zhi Qiao* (Fructus Aurantii) activates qi flow and eliminates phlegm. • *Bai Zhi* (Radix Angelicae Dahuricae) dispels wind and activates qi flow to relieve pain. • *Gan Cao* (Radix et Rhizoma Glycyrrhizae), *Sheng Jiang* (Rhizoma Zingiberis Recens) and *Da Zao* (Fructus Jujubae) harmonize the herbs.

WIND-EXPELLING FORMULAS

14

991

Chapter 14 – Wind-Expelling Formulas   *Section 1 – External-Wind Releasing Formulas*

Wū Yào Shùn Qì Săn (Lindera Powder to Smooth the Flow of Qi)

qi flow and eliminates phlegm. *Bai Zhi* (Radix Angelicae Dahuricae) dispels wind and activates qi flow to relieve pain. *Gan Cao* (Radix et Rhizoma Glycyrrhizae), *Sheng Jiang* (Rhizoma Zingiberis Recens), and *Da Zao* (Fructus Jujubae) harmonize the formula.

MODIFICATIONS

- For post-stroke paralysis characterized by qi and blood deficiencies, add *Ren Shen* (Radix et Rhizoma Ginseng), *Bai Zhu* (Rhizoma Atractylodis Macrocephalae), *Dang Gui* (Radix Angelicae Sinensis), *Chuan Xiong* (Rhizoma Chuanxiong), and *Mai Dong* (Radix Ophiopogonis).
- If there is pain throughout the entire body, add *Dang Gui* (Radix Angelicae Sinensis), *Rou Gui* (Cortex Cinnamomi), *Ru Xiang* (Gummi Olibanum), and *Mo Yao* (Myrrha).
- With coldness and pain in the extremities, add *Fu Zi* (Radix Aconiti Lateralis Praeparata) and *Rou Gui* (Cortex Cinnamomi).
- With swelling and edema in the legs, add *Niu Xi* (Radix Achyranthis Bidentatae), *Du Huo* (Radix Angelicae Pubescentis), and *Wu Jia Pi* (Cortex Acanthopanacis).

- With soreness and pain in the lower back, add *Du Zhong* (Cortex Eucommiae) and *Niu Xi* (Radix Achyranthis Bidentatae).
- With body aches and bone pain, add *Niu Xi* (Radix Achyranthis Bidentatae) and *Sang Ji Sheng* (Herba Taxilli).
- If accompanied by spasms and cramps, add *Mu Gua* (Fructus Chaenomelis) and *Bai Shao* (Radix Paeoniae Alba).
- With numbness and pain in the body, add *Xiao Xu Ming Tang* (Minor Prolong Life Decoction).
- With slurred speech, add *Shi Chang Pu* (Rhizoma Acori Tatarinowii) and *Yuan Zhi* (Radix Polygalae).
- With severe breast distention, add *Chai Hu* (Radix Bupleuri), *Chuan Xiong* (Rhizoma Chuanxiong), and *Yu Jin* (Radix Curcumae).

CAUTIONS / CONTRAINDICATIONS

Use of *Wu Yao Shun Qi San* is contraindicated during pregnancy, and in patients with amenorrhea caused by blood deficiency.

Chinese Herbal Formulas and Applications

Section 2

平熄内风剂
— Internal-Wind Extinguishing Formulas

Líng Jiǎo Gōu Téng Tāng (Antelope Horn and Uncaria Decoction)
羚角鉤藤湯
羚角钩藤汤

Pinyin Name: *Ling Jiao Gou Teng Tang*
Literal Name: Antelope Horn and Uncaria Decoction
Original Source: *Tong Su Shang Han Lun* (Plain Version of Discussion of Cold-Induced Disorders) by Yu Gen-Chu in the Qing Dynasty

COMPOSITION

Ling Yang Jiao (Cornu Saigae Tataricae), pre-decocted	4.5g
Gou Teng (Ramulus Uncariae cum Uncis), post-decocted	9g
Sang Ye (Folium Mori)	6g
Ju Hua (Flos Chrysanthemi)	9g
Bai Shao (Radix Paeoniae Alba)	9g
Di Huang (Radix Rehmanniae)	15g
Chuan Bei Mu (Bulbus Fritillariae Cirrhosae)	12g
Zhu Ru (Caulis Bambusae in Taenia), fresh	15g
Fu Shen (Poria Pararadicis)	9g
Gan Cao (Radix et Rhizoma Glycyrrhizae)	2.4g

Note: *Ling Yang Jiao* (Cornu Saigae Tataricae) is derived from an endangered animal, and is rarely used as a medicinal substance today. Its discussion here is included primarily for academic purposes, to reflect the historical use of this substance in its original formulation. Most herbal products today have removed it completely, or replaced it with substitutes with similar functions.

DOSAGE / PREPARATION / ADMINISTRATION

The source text recommends cooking *Zhu Ru* (Caulis Bambusae in Taenia) with *Ling Yang Jiao* (Cornu Saigae Tataricae) before adding the rest of the ingredients. *Gou Teng* (Ramulus Uncariae cum Uncis) is to be post-decocted for only a short period of time. Note: If *Ling Yang Jiao* (Cornu Saigae Tataricae) is not available, it may be replaced with 20-30g of *Shan Yang Jiao* (Cornu Naemorhedis) for every 0.5-1.0g of *Ling Yang Jiao* (Cornu Saigae Tataricae) specified.

CHINESE THERAPEUTIC ACTIONS

1. Cools the Liver and extinguishes Liver wind
2. Generates fluids and relaxes tendons

CLINICAL MANIFESTATIONS

Excess heat in the Liver channel accompanied by Liver wind rising: persistent high fever, irritability, restlessness, muscle spasms in the extremities, convulsions, coma, dark red tongue body with a dry tongue coating, and a wiry, rapid pulse.

CLINICAL APPLICATIONS

Shingles, cerebral hemorrhage, stroke, post-stroke sequelae, and encephalitis B.

EXPLANATION

Ling Jiao Gou Teng Tang (Antelope Horn and Uncaria Decoction) treats excess heat in the Liver channel causing Liver wind rising. Due to excess pathogenic heat in the

WIND-EXPELLING FORMULAS

14

993

Chapter 14 – Wind-Expelling Formulas　　　　　*Section 2 – Internal-Wind Extinguishing Formulas*

Líng Jiǎo Gōu Téng Tāng (Antelope Horn and Uncaria Decoction)

Ling Jiao Gou Teng Tang (Antelope Horn and Uncaria Decoction)

Diagnosis	Signs and Symptoms	Treatment	Herbs
Excess heat in the Liver channel accompanied by Liver wind rising	• Persistent high fever: excess heat in the interior • Irritability, restlessness and coma: heat disturbing Heart *shen* (spirit) • Spasms and convulsions: Liver wind rising with deficiency of yin and fluids • Dark red tongue body with a dry tongue coating and a wiry, rapid pulse: excess Liver heat	• Cools the Liver and extinguishes Liver wind • Generates fluids and relaxes tendons	• *Ling Yang Jiao* (Cornu Saigae Tataricae) and *Gou Teng* (Ramulus Uncariae cum Uncis) cool the Liver, extinguish Liver wind, and clear heat. • *Sang Ye* (Folium Mori) and *Ju Hua* (Flos Chrysanthemi) clear Liver heat and extinguish Liver wind. • *Bai Shao* (Radix Paeoniae Alba) and *Di Huang* (Radix Rehmanniae) nourish yin and body fluids. • *Chuan Bei Mu* (Bulbus Fritillariae Cirrhosae) and *Zhu Ru* (Caulis Bambusae in Taenia) clear heat and resolve phlegm. • *Fu Shen* (Poria Paradicis) calms the *shen* (spirit) and stabilizes the Heart. • *Gan Cao* (Radix et Rhizoma Glycyrrhizae) harmonizes the herbs.

interior, persistent high fever occurs. The heat may disturb the *shen* (spirit), causing irritability, restlessness, and in severe cases unconsciousness. The heat may dry the body fluids and affect the muscles, causing spasms and convulsions. A dark red tongue body with a dry tongue coating and a wiry, rapid pulse indicate excess Liver heat and wind.

This formula has *Ling Yang Jiao* (Cornu Saigae Tataricae) and *Gou Teng* (Ramulus Uncariae cum Uncis) to cool the Liver, extinguish Liver wind, clear heat, and relieve spasms and convulsions. *Sang Ye* (Folium Mori) and *Ju Hua* (Flos Chrysanthemi) clear Liver heat and extinguish Liver wind. Because excess heat and wind may injure yin and dry body fluids, *Bai Shao* (Radix Paeoniae Alba) and *Di Huang* (Radix Rehmanniae) are added to nourish yin and body fluids. In addition, they soften the Liver and benefit the tendons. Since excess heat may dry body fluids and turn them into phlegm, *Chuan Bei Mu* (Bulbus Fritillariae Cirrhosae) and *Zhu Ru* (Caulis Bambusae in Taenia) are employed to clear heat and resolve phlegm. *Fu Shen* (Poria Paradicis) calms the *shen* (spirit) and stabilizes the Heart. *Gan Cao* (Radix et Rhizoma Glycyrrhizae) harmonizes the herbs in this formula. The combination of *Bai Shao* (Radix Paeoniae Alba) and *Gan Cao* (Radix et Rhizoma Glycyrrhizae) also relieves muscle spasms and cramps.

MODIFICATIONS
• With more interior heat, add *Da Qing Ye* (Folium Isatidis), *Xia Ku Cao* (Spica Prunellae), and *Jue Ming Zi* (Semen Cassiae).

• When phlegm accumulation alters consciousness, add *Tian Zhu Huang* (Concretio Silicea Bambusae) and *Zhu Li* (Succus Bambusae).
• With severe convulsions, add *Quan Xie* (Scorpio), *Wu Gong* (Scolopendra), and *Jiang Can* (Bombyx Batryticatus).
• When heat affects the *qi* (energy) level, add *Shi Gao* (Gypsum Fibrosum), and *Zhi Mu* (Rhizoma Anemarrhenae).
• When heat affects the *ying* (nutritive) and *xue* (blood) levels, add *Mu Dan Pi* (Cortex Moutan) and *Chi Shao* (Radix Paeoniae Rubra).
• With dizziness, vertigo, and hypertension caused by Liver heat rising, add *Niu Xi* (Radix Achyranthis Bidentatae) and *Ji Li* (Fructus Tribuli).
• For *bi zheng* (closed disorder) or unconsciousness caused by heat, combine with *An Gong Niu Huang Wan* (Calm the Palace Pill with Cattle Gallstone) or *Zi Xue Dan* (Purple Snow Pill).

CLINICAL STUDIES AND RESEARCH
Shingles: Use of modified *Ling Jiao Gou Teng Tang* was associated with good results in treating shingles affecting the face in 50 geriatric patients. Modifications included the addition of *Chai Hu* (Radix Bupleuri) and *Yan Hu Suo* (Rhizoma Corydalis) for severe pain; *Long Dan* (Radix et Rhizoma Gentianae), *Jin Qian Cao* (Herba Lysimachiae), and *Di Huang* (Radix Rehmanniae) for cholecystitis; *Tian Ma* (Rhizoma Gastrodiae), *Shi Jue Ming* (Concha Haliotidis), and *Niu Xi* (Radix Achyranthis Bidentatae) for elevated blood pressure; and *Dan Shen* (Radix et Rhizoma Salviae Miltiorrhizae) and *Yu Jin* (Radix Curcumae)

994

Chinese Herbal Formulas and Applications

Líng Jiǎo Gōu Téng Tāng (Antelope Horn and Uncaria Decoction)

for coronary artery disease. The duration of treatment ranged from 7 to 14 packs of herbs. Of 50 patients, the study reported complete recovery in 28 patients and improvement in 22 patients.[1]

RELATED FORMULA

Gōu Téng Yǐn (Uncaria Decoction)

鉤藤飲
钩藤饮

Pinyin Name: *Gou Teng Yin*

Literal Name: Uncaria Decoction

Original Source: *Yi Zong Jin Jian* (Golden Mirror of the Medical Tradition) by Wu Qian in 1742

Gou Teng (Ramulus Uncariae cum Uncis)	9g
Ling Yang Jiao (Cornu Saigae Tataricae), *chong fu* (taken drenched) in powder	0.3g
Quan Xie (Scorpio), remove toxins	0.9g
Ren Shen (Radix et Rhizoma Ginseng)	3g
Tian Ma (Rhizoma Gastrodiae)	6g
Zhi Gan Cao (Radix et Rhizoma Glycyrrhizae Praeparata cum Melle)	1.5g

Note: *Ling Yang Jiao* (Cornu Saigae Tataricae) is derived from an endangered animal, and is rarely used as a medicinal substance today. Its discussion here is included primarily for academic purposes, to reflect the historical use of this substance in its original formulation. Most herbal products today have removed it completely, or replaced it with substitutes with similar functions.

The source text states to prepare the ingredients as a decoction. This formula clears heat, extinguishes wind, tonifies qi, and relieves muscle spasms. Clinically, it treats infantile convulsions with upturned eyes, lockjaw, muscle spasms and convulsions, high fever, and other qi deficiency symptoms.

Ling Jiao Gou Teng Tang and *Gou Teng Yin* (Uncaria Decoction) both cool the Liver and extinguish Liver wind.

• *Ling Jiao Gou Teng Tang* has many actions, including calming Liver wind, nourishing yin and body fluids, and dispelling phlegm and heat. It treats patients with Liver heat excess and Liver wind rising, accompanied by deficiency of yin and body fluids and accumulation of phlegm.

• *Gou Teng Yin*, on the other hand, focuses on calming Liver wind and tonifying qi. It treats patients with Liver heat excess and Liver wind rising with underlying qi deficiency, as manifested in infantile convulsions.

Reference

1. *Jiang Su Zhong Yi* (Jiangsu Chinese Medicine) 1998;5:32.

14

WIND-EXPELLING FORMULAS

995

Chapter 14 – Wind-Expelling Formulas　　　　　　　　*Section 2 – Internal-Wind Extinguishing Formulas*

Gōu Téng Sǎn (Uncaria Powder)

鉤藤散
钩藤散

Pinyin Name: *Gou Teng San*
Literal Name: Uncaria Powder
Alternate Names: *Kou Teng San*, Gambir Formula
Original Source: *Pu Ji Ben Shi Fang* (Formulas of Universal Benefit from My Practice) by Xu Shu-Wei in 1132

COMPOSITION

Gou Teng (Ramulus Uncariae cum Uncis)	15g
Ren Shen (Radix et Rhizoma Ginseng)	15g
Fu Ling (Poria)	15g
Fu Shen (Poria Pararadicis)	15g
Mai Dong (Radix Ophiopogonis)	15g
Chen Pi (Pericarpium Citri Reticulatae)	15g
Ban Xia (Rhizoma Pinelliae), *jin* (soaked) in and *xi* (washed) with liquid	15g
Fang Feng (Radix Saposhnikoviae)	15g
Ju Hua (Flos Chrysanthemi)	15g
Shi Gao (Gypsum Fibrosum)	30g
Zhi Gan Cao (Radix et Rhizoma Glycyrrhizae Praeparata cum Melle)	3g

DOSAGE / PREPARATION / ADMINISTRATION

The source text recommends grinding the ingredients into powder, and cooking 12g of the powder with 7 slices of *Sheng Jiang* (Rhizoma Zingiberis Recens) in water. Take the strained decoction while warm.

CHINESE THERAPEUTIC ACTIONS

1. Clears heat from the Liver channel
2. Directs Liver yang downward and extinguishes Liver wind

CLINICAL MANIFESTATIONS

Liver excess: marked changes in emotions and behavior, irritability, feelings of qi rushing upward, feelings of oppression and distention beneath the heart, muscle spasms in the shoulders and back, red eyes, headache, dizziness, vertigo, tinnitus, palpitations, and insomnia. This syndrome is most commonly seen in middle-aged adults.

CLINICAL APPLICATIONS

Hypertension, headache, migraine, vertigo, dizziness, tinnitus, cerebral infarction, arteriosclerosis, atherosclerosis, hardening of the cranial arteries, Alzheimer's disease, dementia, Meniere's disease, neurosis, and chronic nephritis.

EXPLANATION

Gou Teng San (Uncaria Powder) treats Liver excess with severe vertigo. Clinically, patients mainly show excess heat in the Liver channel, Liver qi stagnation, and heat affecting the Heart. As heat travels upward along the Liver channel, patients experience symptoms such as a feeling of qi rushing upward, irritability, dizziness, vertigo, and headache. Heat in the Liver channel is often complicated by Liver qi stagnation, leading to symptoms such as marked changes in emotions and behavior, and feelings of oppression and distention beneath the heart. When heat travels upward and affects the Heart, patients will experience palpitations and insomnia. Moreover, patients with heat in the Liver channel may have Liver yin deficiency because heat damages yin. This condition often is seen in middle-aged adults who live and/or work in a high-stress, high-pressure environment. One diagnostic symptom is headache early in the morning or after resting, with the headache gradually diminishing upon walking or mild exercise.

Gou Teng (Ramulus Uncariae cum Uncis), the chief herb, regulates Liver qi, clears heat from the Liver channel, calms Liver wind, and relieves spasms. It effectively addresses all of the excess signs and symptoms in this condition. *Ren Shen* (Radix et Rhizoma Ginseng), *Fu Ling* (Poria) and *Fu Shen* (Poria Paradicis) tonify qi and tranquilize the *shen* (spirit). *Mai Dong* (Radix Ophiopogonis) nourishes yin. *Chen Pi* (Pericarpium Citri Reticulatae) and *Ban Xia* (Rhizoma Pinelliae) smooth the qi flow and direct qi downward. *Fang Feng* (Radix Saposhnikoviae) and *Ju Hua* (Flos Chrysanthemi) clear wind and heat from the eyes and head. *Shi Gao* (Gypsum Fibrosum) clears excess heat. *Sheng Jiang* (Rhizoma Zingiberis Recens) and *Gan Cao* (Radix et Rhizoma Glycyrrhizae) harmonize the herbs.

Gōu Téng Sǎn (Uncaria Powder)

Gou Teng San (Uncaria Powder)

Diagnosis	Signs and Symptoms	Treatment	Herbs
Liver excess	• Irritability, dizziness, vertigo, headache and feeling of qi rushing upward: heat traveling upwards along the Liver channel • Marked changes in emotions and behavior and feelings of oppression and distention beneath the heart: Liver qi stagnation with heat in the Liver channel • Palpitations and insomnia: Liver heat affecting the Heart	• Clears heat from the Liver channel • Directs Liver yang downward and extinguishes Liver wind	• *Gou Teng* (Ramulus Uncariae cum Uncis) regulates Liver qi, clears heat from the Liver channel, and calms Liver wind. • *Ren Shen* (Radix et Rhizoma Ginseng), *Fu Ling* (Poria) and *Fu Shen* (Poria Paradicis) tonify qi and tranquilize the *shen* (spirit). • *Mai Dong* (Radix Ophiopogonis) nourishes yin. • *Chen Pi* (Pericarpium Citri Reticulatae) and *Ban Xia* (Rhizoma Pinelliae) smooth qi flow and direct qi downward. • *Fang Feng* (Radix Saposhnikoviae) and *Ju Hua* (Flos Chrysanthemi) clear wind and heat from the eyes and head. • *Shi Gao* (Gypsum Fibrosum) clears excess heat. • *Sheng Jiang* (Rhizoma Zingiberis Recens) and *Gan Cao* (Radix et Rhizoma Glycyrrhizae) harmonize all of the herbs.

MODIFICATION

With headache and vertigo, add *Bai Zhi* (Radix Angelicae Dahuricae) and *Chuan Xiong* (Rhizoma Chuanxiong).

PHARMACOLOGICAL EFFECTS

1. **Cardiovascular**: Administration of *Gou Teng San* in rats was associated with a dose-dependant reduction of blood pressure and heartbeat.[1] It prevented stroke and prolonged life span in stroke-prone hypertensive rats.[2] The mechanisms for lowering blood pressure and preventing stroke were attributed to activation of nitric oxide synthase and improvement in cerebral circulation.[3]

2. **Antiplatelet**: According to *in vitro* studies in rats, *Gou Teng San* was shown to have marked antiplatelet effects. It improved blood circulation to the peripheral parts of the body and reduced mortality caused by embolism.[4]

3. **Neuroprotective**: Administration of *Gou Teng San* was associated with significantly delaying neuronal cell death in the hippocampal CA1 region after ischemia. The mechanism was attributed to its free-radical-scavenging activity.[5]

4. **Antioxidant**: *Gou Teng San* has been shown in several studies to have marked antioxidant and free-radical-scavenging effects, and may be used to treat radical-mediated diseases.[6,7]

5. **Anticonvulsant**: Administration of *Gou Teng San* was associated with a dose-dependent effect in treating mice with convulsions induced by picrotoxine, strychnine, and electroshock. *Gou Teng* (Ramulus Uncariae cum Uncis) is believed to be the main active ingredient in this mechanism, as the formula was ineffective without this herb. The active constituents of *Gou Teng* (Ramulus Uncariae cum Uncis) have been isolated and identified as geissoschizine methylether, hirsuteine, hirsutine, and isocorynoxeine.[8]

6. **Antidementia**: One study reported *Gou Teng San* to be effective in treating patients with vascular dementia. The antidementia effects were attributed to the anti-hypertensive, free-radical-scavenging, and anti-excitotoxic activities of this formula.[9] Furthermore, another study in mice reported that long-term administration of *Gou Teng San* could improve, to some extent, the impairment of memory caused by aging.[10]

7. **Antiamnestic**: According to one study in mice, administration of *Gou Teng San* was associated with antiamnestic effects based on the stimulation of serotonin 1A receptors.[11]

CLINICAL STUDIES AND RESEARCH

1. **Hypertension**: One study reported 91.7% effectiveness using modified *Gou Teng San* to treat high blood pressure in 182 patients (64 males, 118 females, mostly over 40 years of age). The herbal formula contained *Gou Teng* (Ramulus Uncariae cum Uncis) 3g, *Shi Gao* (Gypsum Fibrosum) 8g, *Chen Pi* (Pericarpium Citri Reticulatae) 3g, *Ban Xia* (Rhizoma Pinelliae) 4g, *Fu Ling* (Poria) 3.5g, *Ren Shen* (Radix et Rhizoma Ginseng) 2g, *Ju Hua* (Flos Chrysanthemi) 2g, *Gan Cao* (Radix et Rhizoma Glycyrrhizae) 1g, *Sheng Jiang* (Rhizoma Zingiberis Recens) 1.5g, *Mai Dong* (Radix Ophiopogonis) 4g, and *Fang Feng* (Radix Saposhnikoviae) 4g. The treatment

Gōu Téng Sǎn (Uncaria Powder)

protocol was to give the herbs in decoction, for an average of 7.4 months. Of 182 patients, the study reported a marked effect in 32 patients, moderate improvement in 60 patients, slight improvement in 75 patients, and no effect in 15 patients.[12]

2. **Cerebral infarction**: One study reported beneficial effects using *Gou Teng San* to treat 15 patients with asymptomatic cerebral infarction. Therapeutic benefits included improved microcirculation and decreased serum nitric oxide and lipid peroxides.[13]

3. **Alzheimer's disease**: One hundred and eighty patients with Alzheimer's disease were treated with beneficial effect using *Gou Teng San*. The treatment protocol was to use this formula in powder, at 7.5 g/day, for 8-12 weeks. Improvements included improved cognitive and physical activities, such as short-term memory, sleeping patterns, and speech patterns.[14]

4. **Dementia**: *Gou Teng San* was effective in the treatment of vascular dementia in two studies. According to one well-controlled but non-double blind study (60 patients), use of herbs was effective in global improvement rating, utility rating, and improvement of subjective symptoms, psychiatric symptoms, and disturbance in daily living activities. In the other study, a double-blind controlled study (139 patients), use of herbs was effective in global improvement rating, utility rating, and improvement of subjective symptoms, psychiatric symptoms, and disturbance in daily living activities.[15]

5. **Tinnitus**: Use of modified *Gou Teng San* was associated with good results in treating chronic tinnitus in 34 patients. The herbal treatment contained *Gou Teng* (Ramulus Uncariae cum Uncis), *Shi Gao* (Gypsum Fibrosum), *Chen Pi* (Pericarpium Citri Reticulatae), *Mai Dong* (Radix Ophiopogonis), *Ban Xia* (Rhizoma Pinelliae), *Fu Ling* (Poria), *Ren Shen* (Radix et Rhizoma Ginseng), *Fang Feng* (Radix Saposhnikoviae), *Sheng Jiang* (Rhizoma Zingiberis Recens), and *Ju Hua* (Flos Chrysanthemi). No side effects were noted.[16]

AUTHORS' COMMENTS

Gou Teng San (Uncaria Powder) and *Gou Teng Yin* (Uncaria Decoction) have similar names, but are different formulas.

- *Gou Teng San* treats Liver excess, with Liver heat, Liver yang, and Liver fire rising. It is frequently used to treat middle-aged adults with cardiovascular disorders.
- *Gou Teng Yin* treats Liver heat and wind rising with underlying deficiency. It is commonly used to treat infants with seizures and convulsions.

References

1. *Guo Wai Yi Xue* (Foreign Medicine) 1988;8:53.
2. Shimada Y, Yang Q, Yokoyama K, Goto H, Kasahara Y, Sekiya N, Hikiami H, Terasawa K. Choto-san prevents occurrence of stroke and prolongs life span in stroke-prone spontaneously hypertensive rats. Am J Chin Med 2003;31(1):79-85.
3. Sugimoto A, Goto K, Ishige A, Komatsu Y, Miyamoto KI. Effect of Choto-san, a Kampo medicine, on the cerebral blood flow auto-regulation in spontaneously hypertensive rats. Jpn J Pharmacol 2000 Jun;83(2):135-42.
4. *Guo Wai Yi Xue* (Foreign Medicine) 1992;5:48.
5. Dohi K, Satoh K, Ikeda Y, Ohtaki H, Shioda S, Aruga T. Neuroprotective effect from ischemia and direct free radical scavenging activity of Choto-san (kampo medicine). Acta Neurochir Suppl 2003;86:123-7.
6. Okayasu H, Suzuki F, Satoh K, Shioda S, Dohi K, Ikeda Y, Nakashima H, Komatsu N, Fujimaki M, Hashimoto K, Maki J, Sakagami H. Comparison of cytotoxicity and radical scavenging activity between tea extracts and Chinese medicines. In Vivo 2003 Nov-Dec;17(6):577-81.
7. Sekiya N, Shimada Y, Shibahara N, Takagi S, Yokoyama K, Kasahara Y, Sakakibara I, Terasawa K. Inhibitory effects of Choto-san (Diao-teng-san), and hooks and stems of Uncaria sinensis on free radical-induced lysis of rat red blood cells. Phytomedicine 2002 Oct;9(7):636-40.
8. Mimaki Y, Toshimizu N, Yamada K, Sashida Y. Anti-convulsion effects of choto-san and chotoko (Uncariae Uncis cam Ramlus) in mice, and identification of the active principles. Yakugaku Zasshi 1997 Dec;117(12):1011-21.
9. Watanabe H, Zhao Q, Matsumoto K, Tohda M, Murakami Y, Zhang SH, Kang TH, Mahakunakorn P, Maruyama Y, Sakakibara I, Aimi N, Takayama H. Pharmacological evidence for antidementia effect of Choto-san (Gouteng-san), a traditional Kampo medicine. Pharmacol Biochem Behav 2003 Jun;75(3):635-43.
10. Mizushima Y, Kan S, Yoshida S, Irie Y, Urata Y. Effect of Choto-san, a Kampo medicine, on impairment of passive avoidance performance in senescence accelerated mouse (SAM). Phytother Res 2003 May; 17(5):542-5.
11. Yuzurihara M, Goto K, Sugimoto A, Ishige A, Komatsu Y, Shimada Y, Terasawa K. Effect of Choto-san, a kampo medicine, on impairment of passive avoidance performance in mice. Phytother Res 1999 May;13(3):233-5.
12. *Guo Wai Yi Xue* (Foreign Medicine) 1979;2:35.
13. Goto H, Yang Q, Kita T, Hikiami H, Shimada Y, Terasawa K. Effects of Choto-san on microcirculation, serum nitric oxide and lipid peroxides in patients with asymptomatic cerebral infarction. Am J Chin Med 2001;29(1):83-9.
14. *He Han Yi Yao Xue Hui Zhi* (Hehan Journal of Medicine and Herbology) 1989;3:454.
15. Itoh T, Shimada Y, Terasawa K. Efficacy of Choto-san on vascular dementia and the protective effect of the hooks and stems of Uncaria sinensis on glutamate-induced neuronal death. Mech Ageing Dev 1999 Nov;111(2-3):155-73.
16. *Guo Wai Yi Xue* (Foreign Medicine) 1982;1:51.

Chinese Herbal Formulas and Applications

Zhèn Gān Xī Fēng Tāng
(Sedate the Liver and Extinguish Wind Decoction)

鎮肝熄風湯
镇肝熄风汤

Pinyin Name: *Zhen Gan Xi Feng Tang*
Literal Name: Sedate the Liver and Extinguish Wind Decoction
Alternate Name: Hematite and Scrophularia Combination
Original Source: *Yi Xue Zhong Zhong Can Xi Lu* (Records of Heart-Felt Experiences in Medicine with Reference to the West) by Zhang Xi-Chun in 1918-34

COMPOSITION

Niu Xi (Radix Achyranthis Bidentatae)	30g
Zhe Shi (Haematitum), *ya* (pressed) into fine particles	30g
Long Gu (Os Draconis), *dao* (pounded) into small particles	15g
Mu Li (Concha Ostreae), *dao* (pounded) into small particles	15g
Gui Ban (Plastrum Testudinis), *dao* (pounded) into small particles	15g
Xuan Shen (Radix Scrophulariae)	15g
Tian Dong (Radix Asparagi)	15g
Bai Shao (Radix Paeoniae Alba)	15g
Yin Chen (Herba Artemisiae Scopariae)	6g
Chuan Lian Zi (Fructus Toosendan), *dao* (pounded) into small particles	6g
Mai Ya (Fructus Hordei Germinatus)	6g
Gan Cao (Radix et Rhizoma Glycyrrhizae)	4.5g

DOSAGE / PREPARATION / ADMINISTRATION
Prepare the ingredients as a decoction.

CHINESE THERAPEUTIC ACTIONS
1. Sedates the Liver and extinguishes Liver wind
2. Nourishes yin and anchors yang

CLINICAL MANIFESTATIONS
Liver yang and wind rising due to Liver and Kidney yin deficiencies, with disrupted or reversed flow of qi and blood: dizziness, vertigo, headache with a warm sensation in the head, swelling of the eyes, tinnitus, irritability, a red face, gradually increasing difficulty moving the extremities, gradual worsening deviation of the mouth, belching, unconsciousness in some patients, and a wiry, long, forceful pulse.

CLINICAL APPLICATIONS
Stroke, cerebral hemorrhage, cerebral thrombosis, apoplexy, post-stroke sequelae, epilepsy, hypertension, vascular headache, concussion, chloasma (melasma), premenstrual syndrome, menopause, and hyperthyroidism.

EXPLANATION
Zhen Gan Xi Feng Tang (Sedate the Liver and Extinguish Wind Decoction) treats the various symptoms of Liver yang and wind rising, with underlying Kidney and Liver yin deficiencies. When Liver and Kidney yin are deficient, Liver yang and wind may rise uncontrollably. The hyperactive Liver yang and wind ascend and invade the head, causing dizziness, vertigo, and headache with a warm sensation in the head. Because the Liver and Kidney open to the eyes and ears respectively, hyperactive Liver yang and deficient Kidney yin may lead to swelling of the eyes and tinnitus. Irritability and a red face are due to hyperactivity of Liver yang, while difficulty in moving the extremities and deviation of the mouth are due to hyperactivity of Liver wind. The Liver in a state of excess may overact on the Stomach, causing belching. In severe cases, Liver yang may disturb qi and blood circulation and cause malnourishment, resulting in difficult movement of the extremities, hemiplegia, deviation of the eyes and mouth, and unconsciousness. A wiry, long, forceful pulse is an indication of Liver yang excess.

Niu Xi (Radix Achyranthis Bidentatae) is used as the chief herb in this formula. Bitter and sour, it enters the Liver and Kidney channels and nourishes these two organs. It also directs blood downwards to quickly correct the reversed flow of qi and blood. *Zhe Shi* (Haematitum), *Long Gu* (Os Draconis), and *Mu Li* (Concha Ostreae) sedate hyperactive Liver yang and calm Liver wind. *Gui Ban* (Plastrum Testudinis), *Xuan Shen* (Radix Scrophulariae), *Tian Dong* (Radix Asparagi), and *Bai Shao* (Radix

WIND-EXPELLING FORMULAS

14

999

Chapter 14 – Wind-Expelling Formulas   *Section 2 – Internal-Wind Extinguishing Formulas*

Zhèn Gān Xí Fēng Tāng
(Sedate the Liver and Extinguish Wind Decoction)

Zhen Gan Xi Feng Tang (Sedate the Liver and Extinguish Wind Decoction)

Diagnosis	Signs and Symptoms	Treatment	Herbs
Liver yang and wind rising due to Liver and Kidney yin deficiencies	• Dizziness, vertigo, tinnitus, and swelling of the eyes: Liver yang rising and Kidney yin deficiency • Irritability and red face: Liver yang rising • Difficulty in moving the extremities, and deviation of the mouth: Liver wind rising • Long, forceful pulse: Liver yang excess	• Sedates the Liver and extinguishes Liver wind • Nourishes yin and anchors yang	• *Niu Xi* (Radix Achyranthis Bidentatae) nourishes the Liver and Kidney and guides blood downwards. • *Zhe Shi* (Haematitum), *Long Gu* (Os Draconis) and *Mu Li* (Concha Ostreae) sedate hyperactive Liver yang and calm Liver wind. • *Gui Ban* (Plastrum Testudinis), *Xuan Shen* (Radix Scrophulariae), *Tian Dong* (Radix Asparagi) and *Bai Shao* (Radix Paeoniae Alba) nourish yin and body fluids to restrain hyperactive yang. • *Yin Chen* (Herba Artemisiae Scopariae), *Chuan Lian Zi* (Fructus Toosendan) and *Mai Ya* (Fructus Hordei Germinatus) smooth Liver qi circulation. • *Gan Cao* (Radix et Rhizoma Glycyrrhizae) harmonizes the herbs.

Paeoniae Alba) nourish yin and body fluids to restrain hyperactive yang. *Yin Chen* (Herba Artemisiae Scopariae), *Chuan Lian Zi* (Fructus Toosendan), and *Mai Ya* (Fructus Hordei Germinatus) smooth Liver qi circulation and prevent Liver qi stagnation. *Gan Cao* (Radix et Rhizoma Glycyrrhizae) harmonizes the herbs. The combination of *Mai Ya* (Fructus Hordei Germinatus) and *Gan Cao* (Radix et Rhizoma Glycyrrhizae) regulates Stomach qi and protects the stomach from the harsh mineral substances.

MODIFICATIONS
• If there is severe heat, add *Shi Gao* (Gypsum Fibrosum).
• If there is severe phlegm, add *Dan Nan Xing* (Arisaema cum Bile).
• With an empty or weak pulse upon pressure at the *chi* position, add *Shu Di Huang* (Radix Rehmanniae Praeparata) and *Shan Zhu Yu* (Fructus Corni).
• With headache, add *Xia Ku Cao* (Spica Prunellae), *Gou Teng* (Ramulus Uncariae cum Uncis), and *Ju Hua* (Flos Chrysanthemi).
• For stroke, add *Di Long* (Pheretima), *Dan Shen* (Radix et Rhizoma Salviae Miltiorrhizae), *Tao Ren* (Semen Persicae), and *Hong Hua* (Flos Carthami).
• For trigeminal neuralgia due to Liver yang or Liver fire rising, add *Long Dan* (Radix et Rhizoma Gentianae).
• For poorly formed stools, remove *Gui Ban* (Plastrum Testudinis) and *Zhe Shi* (Haematitum), and add *Chi Shi Zhi* (Halloysitum Rubrum).

CAUTIONS / CONTRAINDICATIONS
• *Zhen Gan Xi Feng Tang* is not recommended for dizziness and vertigo caused by blood deficiency, qi deficiency,

Kidney deficiency, or accumulation of dampness and phlegm.[1]
• This formula is not suitable for hypertension characterized by Kidney yin and yang deficiencies.[2]
• Occasional skin rashes have been reported following the use of this formula.[3]

PHARMACOLOGICAL EFFECTS
Antihypertensive: Administration of *Zhen Gan Xi Feng Tang* was associated with a marked reduction in blood pressure in anesthetized cats. The initial onset of action began 20 minutes after oral ingestion, and reduced the blood pressure by 29 mmHg for 40-100 minutes. Moreover, a greater antihypertensive effect was noted when *Zhen Gan Xi Feng Tang* was modified by eliminating *Gui Ban* (Plastrum Testudinis), *Mai Ya* (Fructus Hordei Germinatus), *Yin Chen* (Herba Artemisiae Scopariae), and *Gan Cao* (Radix et Rhizoma Glycyrrhizae); and adding *Xia Ku Cao* (Spica Prunellae), *Gou Teng* (Ramulus Uncariae cum Uncis), *He Shou Wu* (Radix Polygoni Multiflori), and *Shou Wu Teng* (Caulis Polygoni Multiflori). This modified *Zhen Gan Xi Feng Tang* was determined to have a more potent effect and a longer duration of action, reducing blood pressure by 43.5 mmHg for 80-110 minutes.[4]

CLINICAL STUDIES AND RESEARCH
1. **Stroke**: *Zhen Gan Xi Feng Tang* has been shown in many studies to effectively treat stroke. According to one study, use of modified *Zhen Gan Xi Feng Tang* was associated with 96% effectiveness in treating 50 patients with stroke.[5] In another study, use of modified *Zhen Gan Xi Feng Tang*

1000

Chinese Herbal Formulas and Applications

Zhèn Gān Xí Fēng Tāng
(Sedate the Liver and Extinguish Wind Decoction)

was associated with 92.75% effectiveness in treating 197 patients with stroke (144 caused by cerebral embolism, 42 by cerebral hemorrhage, and 11 by other causes).[6] Lastly, a study of 100 stroke patients reported 95% effectiveness using _Zhen Gan Xi Feng Tang_.[7]

2. **Cerebral hemorrhage**: Concurrent use of _Zhen Gan Xi Feng Tang_ and _An Gong Niu Huang Wan_ (Calm the Palace Pill with Cattle Gallstone) was associated with beneficial effects in treating cerebral hemorrhage. Of 84 patients, the study reported complete recovery in 40 patients, significant improvement in 16 patients, moderate improvement in 17 patients, and continued deterioration in 11 patients.[8]

3. **Cerebral thrombosis**: Seventy-one patients with cerebral thrombosis were treated with beneficial results using _Zhen Gan Xi Feng Tang_ and _Bu Yang Huan Wu Tang_ (Tonify the Yang to Restore Five Decoction). The exact herbal formula contained _Huang Qi_ (Radix Astragali) 30g, _Dan Shen_ (Radix et Rhizoma Salviae Miltiorrhizae) 30g, _Zhe Shi_ (Haematitum) 30g, _Long Gu_ (Os Draconis) 15g, _Mu Li_ (Concha Ostreae) 15g, _Niu Xi_ (Radix Achyranthis Bidentatae) 12g, _Dang Gui_ (Radix Angelicae Sinensis) 9g, _Chi Shao_ (Radix Paeoniae Rubra) 9g, _Chuan Xiong_ (Rhizoma Chuanxiong) 9g, _Di Long_ (Pheretima) 9g, _Tian Dong_ (Radix Asparagi) 9g, _Tao Ren_ (Semen Persicae) 6g, and _Hong Hua_ (Flos Carthami) 6g. The treatment protocol was to cook the herbs in water, and administer the decoction in two equally-divided doses in the morning and at night. Of 71 patients, the study reported recovery in 26 patients, improvement in 37 patients, and no benefit in 8 patients. The rate of effectiveness was 88.7%.[9]

4. **Hypertension**: One study reported good results for treatment of primary hypertension characterized by Liver yang rising, using modified _Zhen Gan Xi Feng Tang_ or _Tian Ma Gou Teng Yin_ (Gastrodia and Uncaria Decoction).[10]

5. **Vascular headache**: One study reported good results (91.4% effectiveness) using _Zhen Gan Xi Feng Tang_ to treat 70 patients with vascular headache. In addition to _Zhen Gan Xi Feng Tang_ as the base formula, modifications were made by adding _Gou Teng_ (Ramulus Uncariae cum Uncis) and _Bai Zhi_ (Radix Angelicae Dahuricae) for acute onset of severe headache; and _Dan Shen_ (Radix et Rhizoma Salviae Miltiorrhizae) and _Chuan Xiong_ (Rhizoma Chuanxiong) for chronic, unrelenting headache. One pack of herbs was given per day, for 15 days per course of treatment. Of 70 patients, the study reported near-complete recovery in 23 patients, improvement in 41 patients, and no change in 6 patients.[11]

6. **Concussion**: Use of _Zhen Gan Xi Feng Tang_ in 23 patients with concussion was associated with complete recovery in 18 patients, improvement in 4 patients, and discontinuation of treatment in 1 patient (reason unknown). In addition to this formula, _Shi Di_ (Calyx Kaki) and _Zhu Ru_ (Caulis Bambusae in Taenia) were added for nausea and vomiting; _San Qi_ (Radix et Rhizoma Notoginseng) was added for subdermal bleeding and bruises; and _Suan Zao Ren_ (Semen Ziziphi Spinosae) and _Zhen Zhu Mu_ (Concha Margaritiferae) for insomnia and palpitations.[12]

7. **Chloasma (Melasma)**: Use of modified _Zhen Gan Xi Feng Tang_ in 13 patients with blotchy, brownish pigmentation on the face was associated with complete recovery in 10 patients and significant improvement in 3 patients. The herbal treatment contained the following ingredients: _Niu Xi_ (Radix Achyranthis Bidentatae) 30g, _Zhe Shi_ (Haematitum) 30g, _Long Gu_ (Os Draconis) 15g, _Mu Li_ (Concha Ostreae) 15g, _Gui Ban_ (Plastrum Testudinis) 15g, _Bai Shao_ (Radix Paeoniae Alba) 15g, _Xuan Shen_ (Radix Scrophulariae) 15g, _Tian Dong_ (Radix Asparagi) 15g, _Chuan Lian Zi_ (Fructus Toosendan) 6g, _Mai Ya_ (Fructus Hordei Germinatus) 6g, _Yin Chen_ (Herba Artemisiae Scopariae) 6g, and _Gan Cao_ (Radix et Rhizoma Glycyrrhizae) 4.5g.[13]

8. **Menopause**: One study reported excellent results using modified _Zhen Gan Xi Feng Tang_ to treat 32 perimenopausal women with tidal fever and spontaneous perspiration. In addition to the base formula, modifications were made by including _Mo Han Lian_ (Herba Ecliptae) and _Sang Ji Sheng_ (Herba Taxilli) for tinnitus and low back pain; _Ji Li_ (Fructus Tribuli) and _Fo Shou_ (Fructus Citri Sarcodactylis) for breast distention; _Shi Hu_ (Caulis Dendrobii) and _Mai Dong_ (Radix Ophiopogonis) for a dry mouth and dry tongue; and other adjustments as needed. The study reported close to 100% effectiveness.[14]

AUTHORS' COMMENTS

Zhen Gan Xi Feng Tang is commonly used to treat stroke characterized by both excess (Liver yang and wind rising) and deficiency (Kidney and Liver yin deficiencies). It may be used before, during, and after stroke incidents. The key signs and symptoms include high blood pressure, dizziness, distended pain in the head, irritability, and a wiry, long, forceful pulse.

References

1. _Zhong Yao Ming Fang Yao Li Yu Ying Yong_ (Pharmacology and Applications of Famous Herbal Formulas) 1989;560-561.

2. _Zhong Yao Ming Fang Yao Li Yu Ying Yong_ (Pharmacology and Applications of Famous Herbal Formulas) 1989;560-561.

WIND-EXPELLING FORMULAS

14

1001

Chapter 14 – Wind-Expelling Formulas
Section 2 – Internal-Wind Extinguishing Formulas

Zhèn Gān Xī Fēng Tāng
(Sedate the Liver and Extinguish Wind Decoction)

3. *Zhong Yao Ming Fang Yao Li Yu Ying Yong* (Pharmacology and Applications of Famous Herbal Formulas) 1989;560-561.
4. *Xin Zhong Yi* (New Chinese Medicine) 1980;12:45.
5. *Shan Xi Zhong Yi* (Shanxi Chinese Medicine) 1995;9:410.
6. *Zhe Jiang Zhong Yi Xue Yuan Xue Bao* (Journal of Zhejiang University of Chinese Medicine) 1988;5:18.
7. *Zhe Jiang Zhong Yi Za Zhi* (Zhejiang Journal of Chinese Medicine) 1988;11:485.
8. *Zhong Yi Za Zhi* (Journal of Chinese Medicine) 1991;2:30.
9. *Zhe Jiang Zhong Yi Za Zhi* (Zhejiang Journal of Chinese Medicine) 1988;9:395.
10. *Shi Yong Zhong Yi Nei Ke Za Zhi* (Journal of Practical Chinese Internal Medicine) 1990;1:26.
11. *Zhong Xi Yi Jie He Za Zhi* (Journal of Integrated Chinese and Western Medicine) 1989;9:563.
12. *Nei Meng Gu Zhong Yi Yao* (Traditional Chinese Medicine and Medicinals of Inner Mongolia) 1990;1:2.
13. *Zhe Jiang Zhong Yi Za Zhi* (Zhejiang Journal of Chinese Medicine) 1992;4:160.
14. *Zhe Jiang Zhong Yi Xue Yuan Xue Bao* (Journal of Zhejiang University of Chinese Medicine) 1998;6:35.

Jiàn Líng Tāng (Construct Roof Tiles Decoction)
建瓴湯
建瓴汤

Pinyin Name: *Jian Ling Tang*
Literal Name: Construct Roof Tiles Decoction
Alternate Name: Dioscorea and Achyranthes Combination
Original Source: *Yi Xue Zhong Zhong Can Xi Lu* (Records of Heart-Felt Experiences in Medicine with Reference to the West) by Zhang Xi-Chun in 1918-34

COMPOSITION

Niu Xi (Radix Achyranthis Bidentatae)	30g
Zhe Shi (Haematitum), *ya* (pressed) into fine particles	24g
Long Gu (Os Draconis), *dao* (pounded) into fine particles	18g
Mu Li (Concha Ostreae), *dao* (pounded) into fine particles	18g
Shan Yao (Rhizoma Dioscoreae)	30g
Di Huang (Radix Rehmanniae)	18g
Bai Shao (Radix Paeoniae Alba)	12g
Bai Zi Ren (Semen Platycladi)	12g

DOSAGE / PREPARATION / ADMINISTRATION

The source text advises to prepare the ingredients as a decoction using water filled with iron rust. Today, the use of iron rust is generally omitted.

CHINESE THERAPEUTIC ACTIONS

1. Sedates the Liver and extinguishes Liver wind
2. Nourishes yin and calms the *shen* (spirit)

CLINICAL MANIFESTATIONS

Liver yang rising: dizziness, vertigo, tinnitus, swelling of the ears, palpitations, forgetfulness, irritability, restlessness, insomnia, excessive dreams, and a wiry, hard, and long pulse

CLINICAL APPLICATIONS

Hypertension, trigeminal neuralgia, headache, tinnitus, aphasia, and apraxia.

EXPLANATION

When Liver yang ascends, it affects the Heart and head. Disturbance of the Heart leads to disturbance of the *shen* (spirit); thus, patients usually experience palpitations, forgetfulness, insomnia, and excessive dreams. When Liver yang ascends to the head, patients exhibit signs and symptoms of dizziness, vertigo, tinnitus, and swelling of the ears. Liver yang excess leads to restlessness and irritability because the Liver controls emotions. A wiry, hard, and long pulse is indicative of Liver yang excess.

1002

Chinese Herbal Formulas and Applications

Jiàn Líng Tāng (Construct Roof Tiles Decoction)

Jian Ling Tang (Construct Roof Tiles Decoction)

Diagnosis	Signs and Symptoms	Treatment	Herbs
Liver yang rising	• Palpitations, forgetfulness, insomnia, excessive dreams, fidgeting and irritability: Liver yang affecting the Heart and disturbing the *shen* (spirit) • Dizziness, vertigo, tinnitus and swelling of the ears: Liver yang rising to the head • Wiry, hard, long pulse: Liver yang excess	• Sedates the Liver and extinguishes Liver wind • Nourishes yin and calms the *shen* (spirit)	• *Niu Xi* (Radix Achyranthis Bidentatae) nourishes the Liver and Kidney to calm wind and yang. • *Zhe Shi* (Haematitum), *Long Gu* (Os Draconis) and *Mu Li* (Concha Ostreae) sedate hyperactive Liver yang and calm Liver wind. • *Shan Yao* (Rhizoma Dioscoreae), *Di Huang* (Radix Rehmanniae) and *Bai Shao* (Radix Paeoniae Alba) nourish yin and generate fluids. • *Bai Zi Ren* (Semen Platycladi) nourishes the Heart and calms the *shen* (spirit) to relieve palpitations, insomnia, and excessive dreams.

Therapeutic functions of *Jian Ling Tang* (Construct Roof Tiles Decoction) include calming Liver yang, extinguishing Liver wind, tranquilizing the *shen* (spirit), and nourishing yin. *Niu Xi* (Radix Achyranthis Bidentatae) enters the Liver and Kidney and leads the blood downward to calm hyperactive yang and wind. Moreover, *Niu Xi* (Radix Achyranthis Bidentatae) nourishes the Liver and Kidney to calm the wind and yang. *Zhe Shi* (Haematitum), *Long Gu* (Os Draconis), and *Mu Li* (Concha Ostreae) sedate hyperactive Liver yang and calm Liver wind. *Shan Yao* (Rhizoma Dioscoreae) nourishes yin and strengthens the Spleen and Kidney, which are easily damaged by excess Liver yang. *Di Huang* (Radix Rehmanniae) clears heat, nourishes yin, and promotes generation of body fluids. *Bai Shao* (Radix Paeoniae Alba) nourishes yin and body fluids to restrain hyperactive yang. *Bai Zi Ren* (Semen Platycladi) nourishes the Heart and calms the *shen* to relieve palpitations, insomnia, and excessive dreams.

MODIFICATIONS

• For poorly formed stools, add *Lian Zi* (Semen Nelumbinis) from which *Lian Zi Xin* (Plumula Nelumbinis) has been removed.

• With aversion to cold, remove *Di Huang* (Radix Rehmanniae) and use *Shu Di Huang* (Radix Rehmanniae Praeparata).

• With trigeminal neuralgia caused by Liver fire and Liver yang, add *Long Dan* (Radix et Rhizoma Gentianae).

• With headache and vertigo, add *Xia Ku Cao* (Spica Prunellae).

• With excessive phlegm, add *Dan Nan Xing* (Arisaema cum Bile).

CLINICAL STUDIES AND RESEARCH

Hypertension: Numerous studies have shown *Jian Ling*

Tang to be effective in treating hypertension. According to one study, use of modified *Jian Ling Tang* was associated with 88.9% effectiveness in treating 90 patients with primary hypertension.[1] In another study, use of *Jian Ling Tang* was associated with 93.7% effectiveness in treating 66 patients with hypertension.[2]

AUTHORS' COMMENTS

Zhen Gan Xi Feng Tang (Sedate the Liver and Extinguish Wind Decoction) and *Jian Ling Tang* both treat Liver wind rising and yin deficiency.

• *Zhen Gan Xi Feng Tang* is stronger at extinguishing wind to treat excess conditions, but weaker at nourishing yin. Clinically, this formula is more effective in **treating** cerebral hemorrhage.

• *Jian Ling Tang* moderately sedates Liver yang, but strongly nourishes yin and tranquilizes the mind. Clinically, this formula is more effective in **preventing** cerebral hemorrhage.[3]

Jian Ling Tang is a contemporary formula specifically formulated to prevent cerebrovascular accident. It is prescribed when the following warning signs and symptoms are present:

• A wiry, hard and long pulse; or an excess pulse at the *cun* position and a deficient pulse at the *chi* position.

• Frequent experience of dizziness, vertigo, headache, forgetfulness, and tinnitus.

• Frequent feelings of qi rushing upwards from the stomach to obstruct eating and swallowing; or feelings of qi rushing upwards from the lower *jiao* to cause hiccups.

• Clinical manifestations of swollen tongue, speech difficulties, deviation of the eyes and mouth, numbness of the limbs, gradual loss of balance with walking difficulties, and feelings of heaviness on top (head) and lightness at the bottom (feet).

WIND-EXPELLING FORMULAS

14

1003

Chapter 14 – Wind-Expelling Formulas　　　　　　　　*Section 2 – Internal-Wind Extinguishing Formulas*

Jìàn Líng Tāng (Construct Roof Tiles Decoction)

References

1. *Liao Ning Zhong Ji Yi Kan* (Liaoning Journal of Medium Medicine) 1994;7:312.
2. *Xin Zhong Yi* (New Chinese Medicine) 1981;12:46.
3. *Fang Ji Xue* (Chinese Herbal Formulas) 1995;442-444.

Tiān Má Gōu Téng Yǐn (Gastrodia and Uncaria Decoction)
天麻鈎藤飲
天麻钩藤饮

Pinyin Name: *Tian Ma Gou Teng Yin*
Literal Name: Gastrodia and Uncaria Decoction
Alternate Name: Gambir Combination
Original Source: *Za Bing Zheng Zhi Xin Yi* (New Significance of Patterns and Treatment in Miscellaneous Diseases)

COMPOSITION

Tian Ma (Rhizoma Gastrodiae)	9g
Gou Teng (Ramulus Uncariae cum Uncis), post-decocted	12g
Zhi Zi (Fructus Gardeniae)	9g
Huang Qin (Radix Scutellariae)	9g
Shi Jue Ming (Concha Haliotidis), pre-decocted	18g
Yi Mu Cao (Herba Leonuri)	9g
Chuan Niu Xi (Radix Cyathulae)	12g
Du Zhong (Cortex Eucommiae)	9g
Sang Ji Sheng (Herba Taxilli)	9g
Shou Wu Teng (Caulis Polygoni Multiflori)	9g
Fu Shen (Poria Pararadicis), processed with *Zhu Sha* (Cinnabaris)	9g

Note: The source text directs the herbalist to process *Fu Shen* (Poria Paradicis) with *Zhu Sha* (Cinnabaris) to enhance the effect of calming the *shen* (spirit) and relieving insomnia. However, *Zhu Sha* (Cinnabaris) is rarely used as a medicinal substance today. Its discussion here is included primarily for academic purposes, to reflect the historical use of this substance in its original formulation. Most herbal products today have removed it completely, or replaced it with substitutes with similar functions. For additional information on the toxicity, please refer to *Chinese Medical Herbology and Pharmacology* by John Chen and Tina Chen.

DOSAGE / PREPARATION / ADMINISTRATION

Prepare the ingredients as a decoction.

CHINESE THERAPEUTIC ACTIONS

1. Calms Liver yang and extinguishes Liver wind
2. Clears heat
3. Activates blood circulation
4. Tonifies the Liver and Kidney

CLINICAL MANIFESTATIONS

Hyperactivity of Liver yang and Liver wind: headache, dizziness, vertigo, and insomnia.

CLINICAL APPLICATIONS

Hypertension, headache, trigeminal neuralgia, prevention and treatment of seizures and epilepsy, cerebral hemorrhage, cerebral embolism, stroke, cerebral infarction, ischemic stroke, hemiplegia, dizziness, vertigo, facial spasms, and neurasthenia.

EXPLANATION

Tian Ma Gou Teng Yin (Gastrodia and Uncaria Decoction) treats Liver yang hyperactivity and Liver wind rising. Excess Liver yang may lead to the rise of Liver wind, which then invades the head to cause headache, dizziness, and vertigo. Excess Liver yang may also affect the *shen* (spirit), causing insomnia, sleep disturbances, and excessive dreaming.

This formula contains *Tian Ma* (Rhizoma Gastrodiae) and *Gou Teng* (Ramulus Uncariae cum Uncis) to calm

1004

Chinese Herbal Formulas and Applications

Tiān Má Gōu Téng Yín (Gastrodia and Uncaria Decoction)

Tian Ma Gou Teng Yin (Gastrodia and Uncaria Decoction)

Diagnosis	Signs and Symptoms	Treatment	Herbs
Hyperactivity of Liver yang and Liver wind	• Headache, dizziness and vertigo: Liver yang and Liver wind rising • Insomnia and sleep disturbances: _shen_ (spirit) disturbance	• Calms Liver yang and extinguishes Liver wind • Clears heat • Activates blood circulation • Tonifies the Liver and Kidney	• _Tian Ma_ (Rhizoma Gastrodiae) and _Gou Teng_ (Ramulus Uncariae cum Uncis) calm Liver yang and extinguish Liver wind. • _Zhi Zi_ (Fructus Gardeniae) and _Huang Qin_ (Radix Scutellariae) clear heat, sedate fire, and prevent Liver yang from rising. • _Shi Jue Ming_ (Concha Haliotidis) clears heat and calms Liver yang. • _Yi Mu Cao_ (Herba Leonuri) activates blood circulation and regulates water circulation. • _Chuan Niu Xi_ (Radix Cyathulae) leads blood downward to calm the Liver. • _Du Zhong_ (Cortex Eucommiae) and _Sang Ji Sheng_ (Herba Taxilli) tonify the Liver and Kidney. • _Shou Wu Teng_ (Caulis Polygoni Multiflori) and _Fu Shen_ (Poria Paradicis) calm the _shen_ (spirit) and relieve insomnia.

Liver yang and extinguish Liver wind. _Zhi Zi_ (Fructus Gardeniae) and _Huang Qin_ (Radix Scutellariae) clear heat, sedate fire and prevent Liver yang from rising. _Shi Jue Ming_ (Concha Haliotidis) clears heat and calms Liver yang. _Yi Mu Cao_ (Herba Leonuri) activates blood circulation and regulates water circulation. _Chuan Niu Xi_ (Radix Cyathulae) leads the blood downward to calm the Liver. _Du Zhong_ (Cortex Eucommiae) and _Sang Ji Sheng_ (Herba Taxilli) tonify the Liver and Kidney. _Shou Wu Teng_ (Caulis Polygoni Multiflori) and _Fu Shen_ (Poria Paradicis) calm the _shen_ and relieve insomnia.

MODIFICATIONS

• With severe Liver yang rising, add _Zhe Shi_ (Haematitum), _Long Gu_ (Os Draconis), and _Mu Li_ (Concha Ostreae).

• With Liver yin deficiency, add _Bai Shao_ (Radix Paeoniae Alba) and _Gui Ban_ (Plastrum Testudinis).

• When there are post-stroke complications, add _Chi Shao_ (Radix Paeoniae Rubra), _Tao Ren_ (Semen Persicae), and _Hong Hua_ (Flos Carthami).

• With thirst and phlegm accumulation, add _Bei Mu_ (Bulbus Fritillariae) and _Zhu Ru_ (Caulis Bambusae in Taenia).

• For arteriosclerosis with hypertension, add _Huai Hua_ (Flos Sophorae) and _Hai Zao_ (Sargassum).

• For hypertension, add _Xia Ku Cao_ (Spica Prunellae), _Jue Ming Zi_ (Semen Cassiae) and _Zhen Zhu Mu_ (Concha Margaritiferae).

CAUTIONS / CONTRAINDICATIONS

Tian Ma Gou Teng Yin is contraindicated in conditions characterized by Liver wind rising because of yin deficiency, with symptoms such as a red tongue body, and a scanty or mirror-like tongue coating.[1]

PHARMACOLOGICAL EFFECTS

Antihypertensive: Use of _Tian Ma Gou Teng Yin_ markedly reduced blood pressure in dogs. However, it did not affect subjects with normal blood pressure. Based on this finding, the researchers suggest that this formula has a regulating effect on blood pressure.[2]

CLINICAL STUDIES AND RESEARCH

1. **Hypertension**: Administration of _Tian Ma Gou Teng Yin_ was effective in treating hypertension. In one study with 213 patients with primary hypertension, use of modified _Tian Ma Gou Teng Yin_ or _Zhen Gan Xi Feng Tang_ (Sedate the Liver and Extinguish Wind Decoction) was associated with marked effectiveness in reducing blood pressure in 156 patients, moderately reducing blood pressure in 19 patients, and no effect in 6 patients. The overall rate of effectiveness was 97.18%. Note: Information was unavailable on patients that did not complete the study.[3]

2. **Headache**: Use of _Tian Ma Gou Teng Yin_ was associated with complete recovery in 135 of 150 patients with headache characterized by Liver yang rising.[4]

3. **Epilepsy**: In one study, 15 children with epilepsy were treated with good results using modified _Tian Ma Gou Teng Yin_. The herbal formula contained _Tian Ma_

WIND-EXPELLING FORMULAS

14

1005

Chapter 14 – Wind-Expelling Formulas   *Section 2 – Internal-Wind Extinguishing Formulas*

Tiān Má Gōu Téng Yǐn (Gastrodia and Uncaria Decoction)

(Rhizoma Gastrodiae) 9g, *Gou Teng* (Ramulus Uncariae cum Uncis) 12g, *Shi Jue Ming* (Concha Haliotidis) 18g, *Huang Qin* (Radix Scutellariae) 9g, *Fu Ling* (Poria) 12g, *Shi Chang Pu* (Rhizoma Acori Tatarinowii) 8g, *Bai Shao* (Radix Paeoniae Alba) 12g, *Ju Hua* (Flos Chrysanthemi) 12g, *Nu Zhen Zi* (Fructus Ligustri Lucidi) 12g, *Dan Nan Xing* (Arisaema cum Bile) 9g, and others as needed. The herbs were given in decoction daily, for one month per course of treatment, for 1 to 6 courses total (average of 3 courses). Of 15 patients, the study reported significant improvement in 8 patients, moderate improvement in 4 patients, and no effect in 3 patients.[5]

4. **Ischemic stroke**: Use of modified *Tian Ma Gou Teng Yin* was associated with good success treating ischemic stroke in 243 patients. The study reported 68.42% effectiveness in 76 patients with stroke due to Liver fire and obstruction of channels and collaterals using this formula; 70% effectiveness in 150 patients with stroke due to qi deficiency and blood stagnation using this formula plus *Bu Yang Huan Wu Tang* (Tonify the Yang to Restore Five Decoction); and 53% effectiveness in 17 patients with stroke due to rising of yang and wind using this formula plus *Zhen Gan Xi Feng Tang* (Sedate the Liver and Extinguish Wind Decoction).[6]

5. **Dizziness**: Concurrent use of *Tian Ma Gou Teng Yin* and *Wen Dan Tang* (Warm the Gallbladder Decoction) was effective in treating all 24 patients with dizziness due to inner ear imbalance. The herbs were given in decoction daily.[7] According to another study, use of modified *Tian Ma Gou Teng Yin* was associated with 84.6% effectiveness in treating 78 patients with dizziness and vertigo. The herbal formula was based on *Tian Ma Gou Teng Yin*, with the addition of *Zhi Mu* (Rhizoma Anemarrhenae) and *Ju Hua* (Flos Chrysanthemi), and the elimination of *Yi Mu Cao* (Herba Leonuri). Additional modifications were made as needed.[8]

6. **Vertigo**: Use of modified *Tian Ma Gou Teng Yin* was associated with 97.06% effectiveness in treating vertigo. The herbal treatment contained *Tian Ma* (Rhizoma Gastrodiae) 30g, *Gou Teng* (Ramulus Uncariae cum Uncis) 30g, *Shi Jue Ming* (Concha Haliotidis) 40g, *Niu Xi* (Radix Achyranthis Bidentatae) 30g, *Sang Ji Sheng* (Herba Taxilli) 20g, *Du Zhong* (Cortex Eucommiae) 20g, *Zhi Zi* (Fructus Gardeniae) 30g, *Huang Qin* (Radix Scutellariae) 20g, *Fu Shen* (Poria Paradicis) 20g, *Yi Mu Cao* (Herba Leonuri) 30g, and *Shou Wu Teng* (Caulis Polygoni Multiflori) 30g. The herbs were given in decoction twice daily. The duration of treatment ranged from 3 to 4 weeks. Improvements included relief of blurred vision, dizziness, tinnitus, and vertigo. Of 98 patients, the study reported complete recovery in 65 patients, moderate improvement in 31 patients, and no effect in 2 patients.[9]

7. **Facial spasms**: Use of modified *Tian Ma Gou Teng Yin* in decoction daily for 7 to 14 days effectively treated 46 patients with facial spasms (32 with complete recovery, 8 with marked improvement, and 6 with slight improvement). The herbal formula was modified by removing *Shi Jue Ming* (Concha Haliotidis), *Zhi Zi* (Fructus Gardeniae), and *Shou Wu Teng* (Caulis Polygoni Multiflori), and adding *Bai Shao* (Radix Paeoniae Alba), *Dang Gui* (Radix Angelicae Sinensis), and *Gui Zhi* (Ramulus Cinnamomi). Furthermore, *Dang Shen* (Radix Codonopsis) was added for chronic deficiency; *Di Huang* (Radix Rehmanniae) and *Mai Dong* (Radix Ophiopogonis) were added for fluid deficiency; *Jue Ming Zi* (Semen Cassiae) and *Ju Hua* (Flos Chrysanthemi) were added for tinnitus and stuffy head due to Liver yang rising; *Mu Tong* (Caulis Akebiae) and *Che Qian Cao* (Herba Plantaginis) were added for dysuria; and *Da Huang* (Radix et Rhizoma Rhei) and *Feng Mi* (Mel) were added for constipation.[10]

8. **Neurasthenia**: Administration of modified *Tian Ma Gou Teng Yin* was associated with 97.2% effectiveness in 500 patients with neurasthenia (296 experienced complete recovery, 127 showed marked improvement, 64 had moderate improvement, and 13 had no effect). In addition to *Tian Ma Gou Teng Yin*, *Huang Lian Jie Du Tang* (Coptis Decoction to Relieve Toxicity) was added for Heart and Liver fire; *Huang Lian* (Rhizoma Coptidis) and *Wen Dan Tang* (Warm the Gallbladder Decoction) for hot phlegm; and *Tian Dong* (Radix Asparagi), *Bai Shao* (Radix Paeoniae Alba), and *Gui Ban* (Plastrum Testudinis) for yin deficiency.[11]

TOXICOLOGY

According to one study, administration of *Tian Ma Gou Teng Yin* in 168 adults was associated with thirst in 5 patients. No other abnormalities were noted.[12]

RELATED FORMULA

Tiān Má Jiàng Yá Piàn
(Gastrodia Pill to Lower [Blood] Pressure)

天麻降壓片
天麻降压片

Pinyin Name: Tian Ma Jiang Ya Pian
Literal Name: Gastrodia Pill to Lower [Blood] Pressure
Original Source: *Tian Jin Zhong Yi Xue Yuan* (Tianjin University of Chinese Medicine) in 1989

Tian Ma (Rhizoma Gastrodiae)
Gou Teng (Ramulus Uncariae cum Uncis)
Mu Li (Concha Ostreae)
Niu Xi (Radix Achyranthis Bidentatae)
Xia Ku Cao (Spica Prunellae)

Tiān Má Gōu Téng Yǐn (Gastrodia and Uncaria Decoction)

Jue Ming Zi (Semen Cassiae)
Du Zhong (Cortex Eucommiae)
Chuan Niu Xi (Radix Cyathulae)
Dan Shen (Radix et Rhizoma Salviae Miltiorrhizae)
Ge Gen (Radix Puerariae Lobatae)
Gou Qi Zi (Fructus Lycii)
Sha Yuan Zi (Semen Astragali Complanati)
Shan Zhu Yu (Fructus Corni)
Di Huang (Radix Rehmanniae)

Tian Ma Jiang Ya Pian (Gastrodia Pill to Lower [Blood] Pressure) calms Liver yang, subdues Liver wind, and nourishes yin. Clinically, it treats individuals with hypertension characterized by Liver yang and Liver wind rising, accompanied by underlying yin deficiency.

AUTHORS' COMMENTS

According to Dr. Chang Wei-Yen, *Tian Ma Gou Teng Yin* can be combined with *Long Dan Xie Gan Tang* (Gentiana Decoction to Drain the Liver) to treat migraines and headaches caused by Liver yang rising.

References

1. *Zhong Yi Lin Chuan Fang Ji Xue* (Clinical Study of Chinese Herbal Formulas) 1995;262-263.
2. *Zhong Yi Yao Yan Jiu Can Kao* (Research and Discussion of Chinese Medicine and Herbology) 1979;9:25.
3. *Shi Yong Zhong Yi Nei Ke Za Zhi* (Journal of Practical Chinese Internal Medicine) 1990;1:26.
4. *Shan Xi Zhong Yi* (Shanxi Chinese Medicine) 1990;7:297.
5. *Tian Jin Zhong Yi* (Tianjin Chinese Medicine) 1995;6:25.
6. *Liao Ning Zhong Yi Za Zhi* (Liaoning Journal of Chinese Medicine) 1984;9:26.
7. *Si Chuan Zhong Yi* (Sichuan Chinese Medicine) 1988;3:29.
8. *Shan Xi Zhong Yi Xue Yuan Xue Bao* (Journal of Shanxi University School of Chinese Medicine) 1996;19(4):28.
9. *Ji Lin Zhong Yi Yao* (Jilin Chinese Medicine and Herbology) 1995;5:34.
10. *Xin Zhong Yi* (New Chinese Medicine) 1993;10:28.
11. *He Nan Zhong Yi Xue Yuan Xue Bao* (Journal of University of Henan School of Medicine) 1998;13(4):52.
12. *Zhong Cheng Yao Yan Jiu* (Research of Chinese Patent Medicine) 1987;3:17.

Ē Jiāo Jī Zǐ Huáng Tāng (Ass-Hide Gelatin and Egg Yolk Decoction)

阿膠雞子黃湯
阿胶鸡子黄汤

Pinyin Name: E Jiao Ji Zi Huang Tang
Literal Name: Ass-Hide Gelatin and Egg Yolk Decoction
Original Source: *Tong Su Shang Han Lun* (Plain Version of Discussion of Cold-Induced Disorders) by Yu Gen-Chu in the Qing Dynasty

COMPOSITION

E Jiao (Colla Corii Asini), *yang* (melted) and *chong fu* (taken drenched)	6g
Ji Zi Huang (Galli Vitellus), pre-decocted	2 yolks
Di Huang (Radix Rehmanniae)	12g
Bai Shao (Radix Paeoniae Alba)	9g
Zhi Gan Cao (Radix et Rhizoma Glycyrrhizae Praeparata cum Melle)	1.8g
Gou Teng (Ramulus Uncariae cum Uncis)	6g
Shi Jue Ming (Concha Haliotidis), *chu* (pestled)	15g
Mu Li (Concha Ostreae), *chu* (pestled)	12g
Fu Shen (Poria Pararadicis)	12g
Luo Shi Teng (Caulis Trachelospermi)	9g

DOSAGE / PREPARATION / ADMINISTRATION

The source text recommends cooking *Ji Zi Huang* (Galli Vitellus) in water first, and use the liquid to prepare the other ingredients as a decoction.

CHINESE THERAPEUTIC ACTIONS

1. Nourishes yin and tonifies blood
2. Softens the Liver and extinguishes Liver wind

WIND-EXPELLING FORMULAS

14

Chapter 14 – Wind-Expelling Formulas   *Section 2 – Internal-Wind Extinguishing Formulas*

Ē Jiāo Jī Zǐ Huáng Tāng (Ass-Hide Gelatin and Egg Yolk Decoction)

CLINICAL MANIFESTATIONS

Liver wind rising due to pathogenic heat damaging yin and blood: muscle spasms and cramps, weakness and paralysis of the hands and feet, dizziness, vertigo, a deep red tongue body with a scanty tongue coating, and a fine, rapid pulse.

CLINICAL APPLICATIONS

Cerebral embolism and post-encephalitis complications.

EXPLANATION

E Jiao Ji Zi Huang Tang (Ass-Hide Gelatin and Egg Yolk Decoction) treats Liver wind rising due to pathogenic heat damaging yin and blood. This syndrome is commonly seen following *wen bing* (warm febrile diseases), in which the heat has damaged and consumed yin and blood. Yin and blood deficiencies cause malnourishment of the muscles and tendons, leading to spasms and cramps, difficulty in movement, and possible weakness and paralysis of the hands and feet. Yin and blood deficiencies may also contribute to Liver wind rising to the head, causing dizziness and vertigo. A deep red tongue body with a scanty tongue coating and a fine, rapid pulse suggest deficiency heat.

E Jiao (Colla Corii Asini) and *Ji Zi Huang* (Galli Vitellus), the chief herbs, nourish yin, tonify the blood, and sedate Liver wind and yang. *Di Huang* (Radix Rehmanniae), *Bai Shao* (Radix Paeoniae Alba), and *Zhi Gan Cao* (Radix et Rhizoma Glycyrrhizae Praeparata cum Melle) nourish yin and blood, soften the Liver, and extinguish Liver wind. Because yin and blood deficiencies may lead to Liver yang rising, *Gou Teng* (Ramulus Uncariae cum Uncis), *Shi Jue*

Ming (Concha Haliotidis), and *Mu Li* (Concha Ostreae) are added to sedate Liver yang and extinguish Liver wind. *Fu Shen* (Poria Paradicis) calms the *shen* (spirit). *Luo Shi Teng* (Caulis Trachelospermi) helps *Bai Shao* (Radix Paeoniae Alba) and *Gan Cao* (Radix et Rhizoma Glycyrrhizae) open the collaterals and relax the muscles and tendons to relieve spasms and cramps.

MODIFICATIONS

- With qi and yin deficiencies, add *Ren Shen* (Radix et Rhizoma Ginseng) and *Mai Dong* (Radix Ophiopogonis).
- If there is spontaneous sweating, add *Fu Xiao Mai* (Fructus Tritici Levis) and *Ma Huang Gen* (Radix et Rhizoma Ephedrae).

CAUTIONS / CONTRAINDICATIONS

E Jiao Ji Zi Huang Tang is contraindicated in cases of excess Liver fire in the absence of yin deficiency.

AUTHORS' COMMENTS

Ling Jiao Gou Teng Tang (Antelope Horn and Uncaria Decoction) and *E Jiao Ji Zi Huang Tang* both treat Liver yang and Liver wind conditions associated with *wen bing* (warm disease), but have the following differences:

- *Ling Jiao Gou Teng Tang* addresses Liver yang and Liver wind rising associated with early stages of *wen bing* (warm disease) in which the excess heat causes the Liver yang and wind to rise upwards. In addition, Liver yang and Liver wind intensify one another's severity, and worsen the condition. Therefore, this formula is composed primarily of herbs that clear heat, calm Liver yang and extinguish Liver wind.

E Jiao Ji Zi Huang Tang (Ass-Hide Gelatin and Egg Yolk Decoction)

Diagnosis	Signs and Symptoms	Treatment	Herbs
Liver wind rising with yin and blood deficiencies	• Spasms and cramps, difficulty in movement, and weakness and paralysis of the hands and feet: Liver wind rising with yin and blood deficiencies • Dizziness and vertigo: Liver wind rising • Deep red tongue body with scanty tongue coating and a fine-rapid pulse: deficiency-heat condition	• Nourishes yin and tonifies blood • Softens the Liver and extinguishes Liver wind	• *E Jiao* (Colla Corii Asini) and *Ji Zi Huang* (Galli Vitellus) nourish yin, tonify blood, and sedate Liver wind and yang. • *Di Huang* (Radix Rehmanniae), *Bai Shao* (Radix Paeoniae Alba) and *Zhi Gan Cao* (Radix et Rhizoma Glycyrrhizae Praeparata cum Melle) nourish yin and blood, soften the Liver, and extinguish Liver wind. • *Gou Teng* (Ramulus Uncariae cum Uncis), *Shi Jue Ming* (Concha Haliotidis), and *Mu Li* (Concha Ostreae) sedate Liver yang and extinguish Liver wind. • *Fu Shen* (Poria Paradicis) calms the *shen* (spirit). • *Luo Shi Teng* (Caulis Trachelospermi) relaxes the muscles and tendons.

1008

Chinese Herbal Formulas and Applications

Ē Jiāo Jī Zǐ Huáng Tāng (Ass-Hide Gelatin and Egg Yolk Decoction)

- *E Jiao Ji Zi Huang Tang* treats Liver yang rising and extinguishes Liver wind in chronic cases of *wen bing* (warm disease) in which heat has damaged yin and blood. When yin and blood become deficient, Liver yang and Liver wind begin to rise upwards. Therefore, this formula is composed of herbs that treat both excess (Liver yang and Liver wind rising) and deficiency (yin and blood deficiencies).

Dà Dìng Fēng Zhū (Major Arrest Wind Pearl)

大定風珠
大定风珠

Pinyin Name: *Da Ding Feng Zhu*
Literal Name: Major Arrest Wind Pearl
Original Source: *Wen Bing Tiao Bian* (Systematic Differentiation of Warm Disease) by Wu Ju-Tong in 1798

COMPOSITION

Ji Zi Huang (Galli Vitellus)	2 yolks
E Jiao (Colla Corii Asini)	9g
Di Huang (Radix Rehmanniae)	18g
Mai Dong (Radix Ophiopogonis)	18g
Bai Shao (Radix Paeoniae Alba)	18g
Gui Ban (Plastrum Testudinis)	12g
Bie Jia (Carapax Trionycis)	12g
Mu Li (Concha Ostreae)	12g
Huo Ma Ren (Fructus Cannabis)	6g
Wu Wei Zi (Fructus Schisandrae Chinensis)	6g
Zhi Gan Cao (Radix et Rhizoma Glycyrrhizae Praeparata cum Melle)	12g

DOSAGE / PREPARATION / ADMINISTRATION

The source text states to cook the ingredients with 8 cups of water until the decoction is reduced to 3 cups. Discard the residue. Blend *Ji Zi Huang* (Galli Vitellus) into the strained decoction, and take the resulting mixture in three equally-divided doses daily.

CHINESE THERAPEUTIC ACTIONS

1. Nourishes yin
2. Extinguishes Liver wind

CLINICAL MANIFESTATIONS

Severe yin deficiency with Liver wind rising: extreme lack of energy, clonic convulsions, a deep red tongue body with scanty tongue coating, and a deficient pulse.

CLINICAL APPLICATIONS

Stroke, spasms and cramps, convulsions, post-stroke insomnia, post-stroke paralysis, chorea minor, liver fibrosis, and encephalitis.

EXPLANATION

Da Ding Feng Zhu (Major Arrest Wind Pearl) treats severe yin deficiency with Liver wind rising. This condition may be caused by chronic *wen bing* (warm disease) disorders with heat consuming yin and fluids, or inappropriate use of herbs leading to damage of yin and loss of fluids. Severe yin deficiency may lead to depletion of energy and a deep red tongue with little coating. Severe yin deficiency also contributes to Liver wind rising, which may cause clonic convulsions. A deficient pulse suggests severe yin deficiency. Patients with this condition will have a strong tendency to go into shock.

This formula has *Ji Zi Huang* (Galli Vitellus) and *E Jiao* (Colla Corii Asini) to nourish yin and body fluids to extinguish Liver wind. *Di Huang* (Radix Rehmanniae), *Mai Dong* (Radix Ophiopogonis), and *Bai Shao* (Radix Paeoniae Alba) nourish yin and soften the Liver. *Gui Ban* (Plastrum Testudinis), *Bie Jia* (Carapax Trionycis) and *Mu Li* (Concha Ostreae) nourish yin and anchor the

WIND-EXPELLING FORMULAS

14

1009

Chapter 14 – Wind-Expelling Formulas　　　　　　　　*Section 2 – Internal-Wind Extinguishing Formulas*

Dà Dìng Fēng Zhū (Major Arrest Wind Pearl)

Da Ding Feng Zhu (Major Arrest Wind Pearl)

Diagnosis	Signs and Symptoms	Treatment	Herbs
Severe yin deficiency with Liver wind rising	• Depletion of energy and a deep red tongue with little coating: severe yin deficiency • Clonic convulsions: Liver wind rising • Deficient pulse: deficiency condition	• Nourishes yin • Extinguishes Liver wind	• *Ji Zi Huang* (Galli Vitellus) and *E Jiao* (Colla Corii Asini) nourish yin and body fluids to extinguish Liver wind. • *Di Huang* (Radix Rehmanniae), *Mai Dong* (Radix Ophiopogonis) and *Bai Shao* (Radix Paeoniae Alba) nourish yin and soften the Liver. • *Gui Ban* (Plastrum Testudinis), *Bie Jia* (Carapax Trionycis) and *Mu Li* (Concha Ostreae) nourish yin and anchor the yang. • *Huo Ma Ren* (Fructus Cannabis) nourishes yin and moistens dryness. • *Wu Wei Zi* (Fructus Schisandrae Chinensis) and *Zhi Gan Cao* (Radix et Rhizoma Glycyrrhizae Praeparata cum Melle) enhance the yin-tonifying action of the other herbs.

yang. *Huo Ma Ren* (Fructus Cannabis) nourishes yin and moistens dryness. *Wu Wei Zi* (Fructus Schisandrae Chinensis) and *Zhi Gan Cao* (Radix et Rhizoma Glycyrrhizae Praeparata cum Melle) are sour and sweet herbs that enhance the yin-tonifying action of the other herbs in this formula.

MODIFICATIONS
- With dyspnea due to qi deficiency, add *Ren Shen* (Radix et Rhizoma Ginseng).
- With spontaneous sweating, add *Huang Qi* (Radix Astragali), *Long Gu* (Os Draconis), and *Xiao Mai* (Fructus Tritici).
- With palpitations, add *Fu Shen* (Poria Paradicis), *Ren Shen* (Radix et Rhizoma Ginseng), and *Xiao Mai* (Fructus Tritici).
- With phlegm, add *Tian Zhu Huang* (Concretio Silicea Bambusae) and *Bei Mu* (Bulbus Fritillariae).
- With low-grade fever, add *Bai Wei* (Radix et Rhizoma Cynanchi Atrati) and *Di Gu Pi* (Cortex Lycii).

CAUTIONS / CONTRAINDICATIONS
Da Ding Feng Zhu should be used only for severe yin deficiency with no excess heat. It is **not** suitable for those who have both severe yin deficiency and excess interior heat.

CLINICAL STUDIES AND RESEARCH
1. **Post-stroke insomnia**: Thirty-six patients with post-stroke insomnia (an average of 3 months history of illness) were treated with marked effect using *Da Ding Feng Zhu*. The study reported an overall effectiveness of 94.4% (with at least 3 to 4 hours of sleep per night without the use of pharmaceutical drugs).[1]

2. **Post-stroke paralysis**: One hundred patients with post-stroke paralysis were treated with 98% effectiveness using both herbs and acupuncture. Herbal treatment varied depending on the diagnosis: modified *Da Ding Feng Zhu* was used for yin deficiency and yang excess; modified *Dao Tan Tang* (Guide Out Phlegm Decoction) was used for phlegm accumulation; modified *Bu Yang Huan Wu Tang* (Tonify the Yang to Restore Five Decoction) was used for qi deficiency and blood stagnation; and modified *Di Huang Yin Zi* (Rehmannia Decoction) was used for deficiency of *yuan* (source) qi. Acupuncture treatment included scalp or body acupuncture. The study noted that patients who received scalp acupuncture responded better than those who received body acupuncture.[2]

3. **Chorea minor**: In one study, modified *Da Ding Feng Zhu* was used in the treatment of chorea minor. The herbal formula contained *Da Ding Feng Zhu* with the removal of *Mai Dong* (Radix Ophiopogonis), *Huo Ma Ren* (Fructus Cannabis), and *Wu Wei Zi* (Fructus Schisandrae Chinensis) and the addition of *Gou Teng* (Ramulus Uncariae cum Uncis), *Jiang Can* (Bombyx Batryticatus), *Shi Jue Ming* (Concha Haliotidis), *Long Gu* (Os Draconis), *Shan Zhu Yu* (Fructus Corni), *Shan Yao* (Rhizoma Dioscoreae), and others as deemed necessary. Each course of treatment lasted one month. The study reported that most people began to show symptomatic improvement within 2 weeks, with marked improvement or complete recovery within 1-2 courses of treatments. Out of 12 cases, the study reported complete recovery in 4 cases, marked benefits in 6 cases, and no effect in 2 cases.[3]

4. **Liver fibrosis**: One study reported beneficial effects using *Da Ding Feng Zhu* to treat liver fibrosis. Of 56 patients,

1010

Dà Dìng Fēng Zhū (Major Arrest Wind Pearl)

30 were treated with herbs and 26 were treated with colchicine. After 3 months of treatment, the study reported that the herb group had significantly lowered levels of hyaluronic acid (HA), procollagen III (PC-III), IV collagen (IV-C), and laminin (LN), while the drug group only had lowered levels of HA. The study concluded that *Da Ding Feng Zhu* is effective in lowering serum indices in liver fibrosis.[4]

5. **Encephalitis**: Administration of *Da Ding Feng Zhu* was beneficial in treating complications of encephalitis during recovery in 8 children. Complications of encephalitis included cognitive and speech impairment. The average duration of treatment was approximately one month.[5]

RELATED FORMULAS

Xiǎo Dìng Fēng Zhū (Minor Arrest Wind Pearl)

小定風珠
小定风珠

Pinyin Name: *Xiao Ding Feng Zhu*
Literal Name: Minor Arrest Wind Pearl
Original Source: *Wen Bing Tiao Bian* (Systematic Differentiation of Warm Disease) by Wu Ju-Tong in 1798

Ji Zi Huang (Galli Vitellus), fresh	1 yolk
E Jiao (Colla Corii Asini)	6g
Gui Ban (Plastrum Testudinis)	18g
Tong Bian (Infantis Urina)	150 mL
Dan Cai (Mytilus Crassitesta)	9g

The source text states to first cook *Gui Ban* (Plastrum Testudinis) and *Dan Cai* (Mytilus Crassitesta) in 5 cups of water and reduce the decoction to 2 cups. Discard the residue, and dissolve *E Jiao* (Colla Corii Asini) in the strained liquid. Blend in *Ji Zi Huang* (Galli Vitellus), followed by *Tong Bian* (Infantis Urina), before ingestion.

This formula nourishes yin and extinguishes Liver wind. It can be used to treat chronic damp accumulation in the lower *jiao* accompanied by yin deficiency and Liver wind rising. *Xiao Ding Feng Zhu* (Minor Arrest Wind Pearl) has a similar, but milder effect in comparison to *Da Ding Feng Zhu* (Major Arrest Wind Pearl).

Sān Jiǎ Fù Mài Tāng

(Three-Shell Decoction to Restore the Pulse)

三甲復脈湯
三甲复脉汤

Pinyin Name: *San Jia Fu Mai Tang*
Literal Name: Three-Shell Decoction to Restore the Pulse
Original Source: *Wen Bing Tiao Bian* (Systematic Differentiation of Warm Disease) by Wu Ju-Tong in 1798

Zhi Gan Cao (Radix et Rhizoma Glycyrrhizae Praeparata cum Melle)	18g
Di Huang (Radix Rehmanniae)	18g
Bai Shao (Radix Paeoniae Alba)	18g
Mai Dong (Radix Ophiopogonis)	15g
E Jiao (Colla Corii Asini)	9g
Huo Ma Ren (Fructus Cannabis)	9g
Mu Li (Concha Ostreae)	15g
Bie Jia (Carapax Trionycis)	24g
Gui Ban (Plastrum Testudinis)	30g

Source text instructions are to prepare the ingredients as a decoction. *San Jia Fu Mai Tang* (Three-Shell Decoction to Restore the Pulse) was originally designed to nourish yin, restore the pulse, sedate Liver yang, and extinguish Liver wind. It has been used in the past to treat the late stages of febrile disorders, in which the heat is lodged deep in the lower *jiao,* and there is damage to yin. Clinically, patients may show symptoms such as spasms, altered consciousness, tremor, palpitations, a fine, skipping pulse, and, in severe cases, pain in the heart region.

Sān Jiǎ Ān Shén Wán

(Three-Shell Pill to Tranquilize the Spirit)

三甲安神丸
三甲安神丸

Pinyin Name: *San Jia An Shen Wan*
Literal Name: Three-Shell Pill to Tranquilize the Spirit
Original Source: *Shan Xi Zhong Yi* (Shanxi Chinese Medicine)

Zhi Gan Cao (Radix et Rhizoma Glycyrrhizae Praeparata cum Melle)
Di Huang (Radix Rehmanniae)
Bai Shao (Radix Paeoniae Alba)
Mai Dong (Radix Ophiopogonis)
Tian Dong (Radix Asparagi)
Mu Li (Concha Ostreae)
Zhi Zi (Fructus Gardeniae)
Mo Han Lian (Herba Ecliptae)
Tai Zi Shen (Radix Pseudostellariae)
Gou Teng (Ramulus Uncariae cum Uncis)
Shi Chang Pu (Rhizoma Acori Tatarinowii)
Yuan Zhi (Radix Polygalae)
Chuan Xiong (Rhizoma Chuanxiong)
Yu Jin (Radix Curcumae)

San Jia An Shen Wan (Three-Shell Pill to Tranquilize the Spirit) nourishes yin, sedates Liver yang, guides Liver wind downward, and calms the *shen* (spirit). It treats individuals with underlying yin deficiency, accompanied by Liver yang and Liver wind rising to disturb the

Dà Dìng Fēng Zhū (Major Arrest Wind Pearl)

shen. Clinical applications of this formula include forgetfulness, hyperactivity, and inability to concentrate.

AUTHORS' COMMENTS

E Jiao Ji Zi Huang Tang (Ass-Hide Gelatin and Egg Yolk Decoction) and *Da Ding Feng Zhu* both act to nourish yin and extinguish wind by utilizing herbs such as *E Jiao* (Colla Corii Asini), *Ji Zi Huang* (Galli Vitellus), *Bai Shao* (Radix Paeoniae Alba), *Zhi Gan Cao* (Radix et Rhizoma Glycyrrhizae Praeparata cum Melle) and *Mu Li* (Concha Ostreae). Their differences are as follows:

- *E Jiao Ji Zi Huang Tang* also has functions to sedate Liver yang and calm *shen* (spirit), as it contains herbs such as *Shi Jue Ming* (Concha Haliotidis), *Gou Teng* (Ramulus Uncariae cum Uncis), and *Fu Shen* (Poria Paradicis).

- *Da Ding Feng Zhu* has effects to astringe yin and sedate yang, with herbs such as *Bie Jia* (Carapax Trionycis), *Gui Ban* (Plastrum Testudinis) and *Wu Wei Zi* (Fructus Schisandrae Chinensis).

References

1. *Zhong Yi Han Shou Tong Xun* (Reports of Chinese Medicine) 1993;5:43.
2. *Shan Xi Zhong Yi* (Shanxi Chinese Medicine) 1987;1:19.
3. *Zhong Yi Yao Xin Xi* (Information on Chinese Medicine and Herbology) 1996;4:38.
4. Li W, Wang C, Zhang J. Effects of da ding feng zhu decoction in 30 cases of liver fibrosis. Journal of Traditional Chinese Medicine 2003 Dec;23(4):251-4.
5. *Hu Bei Zhong Yi Za Zhi* (Hubei Journal of Chinese Medicine) 1982;6:51.

Chinese Herbal Formulas and Applications

Chapter 14 — Summary

— Wind-Expelling Formulas

SECTION 1: EXTERNAL-WIND RELEASING FORMULAS

Name	Similarities	Differences
Xiao Feng San (Eliminate Wind Powder)	Expel wind, nourish the blood	Clears wind-dampness, dispels wind-heat
Dang Gui Yin Zi (Tangkuei Decoction)		Tonifies blood, moistens dryness
Chuan Xiong Cha Tiao San (Ligusticum Chuanxiong Powder to be Taken with Green Tea)	Expels wind, stops pain	Dispels wind from the upper body
Qian Zheng San (Lead to Symmetry Powder)	Dispel wind, dissolve phlegm	Dispels wind from the face, treats spasms, cramps, and deviation of the eyes and mouth
Yu Zhen San (True Jade Powder)		Dispels wind from the body, treats tetanus with spasms and cramps
Xiao Xu Ming Tang (Minor Prolong-Life Decoction)	Dispel wind, treat post-stroke sequelae	Tonifies *zheng* (upright) *qi*
Xu Ming Tang (Prolong Life Decoction)		Dispels wind, clears heat
Da Qin Jiao Tang (Major Gentiana Macrophylla Decoction)	Dispel wind, treat *zhong feng* (wind stroke)	Tonifies qi and blood
Wu Yao Shun Qi San (Lindera Powder to Smooth the Flow of Qi)		Activates qi circulation, relieves pain

Xiao Feng San (Eliminate Wind Powder) and *Dang Gui Yin Zi* (Tangkuei Decoction) treat skin disorders characterized by wind at the exterior and blood deficiency in the interior.
• *Xiao Feng San* treats rashes, eczema, and other skin disorders arising from wind, dampness, and heat invasion. It clears wind-dampness and wind-heat, and nourishes and cools the blood.
• *Dang Gui Yin Zi* treats eczema, rash, urticaria, and other skin conditions due to wind at the exterior and blood deficiency and dryness in the interior. It tonifies the blood, moistens dryness, and releases wind.

Chuan Xiong Cha Tiao San (Ligusticum Chuanxiong Powder to be Taken with Green Tea) dispels wind and stops pain in the head. It is used for headache, dizziness, chills, fever, stuffy nose, a thin, white tongue coating, and a superficial pulse.

Qian Zheng San (Lead to Symmetry Powder) and *Yu Zhen San* (True Jade Powder) both dispel wind and dissolve phlegm.
• *Qian Zheng San* treats wind attacking the face, characterized by facial spasms and deviation of the eyes and mouth. The cause is blockage of the channels and collaterals by wind and phlegm.
• *Yu Zhen San* treats wind attacking the body. It is indicated for tetanus with lockjaw, tightly-closed mouth and lips, a stiff body, muscle spasms, and kyphosis. It dispels wind, dissolves phlegm, relieves spasms, and stops pain.

Xiao Xu Ming Tang (Minor Prolong-Life Decoction) and *Xu Ming Tang* (Prolong Life Decoction) dispel wind and are commonly used to treat post-stroke sequelae.
• *Xiao Xu Ming Tang* dispels wind, warms yang, opens the channels, and supports *zheng* (upright) *qi*. It treats post-stroke complications with *zheng* (upright) *qi* deficiency, characterized by signs and symptoms such as hemiplegia, paralysis, muscle contraction and convulsions, deviation of the eyes and mouth, slurred speech, and low back pain.

WIND-EXPELLING FORMULAS

14

1013

Chapter 14 – Wind-Expelling Formulas

Chapter 14 — Summary

- *Xu Ming Tang* dispels wind, clears heat, regulates qi circulation, and nourishes the blood. It treats stroke due to wind attacking the *ying* (nutritive) and *wei* (defensive) levels, with post-stroke sequelae such as hemiplegia, muscle paralysis, inability to rotate the trunk, slurred speech, confusion, numbness and pain of the body, and muscle stiffness and cramps.

Da Qin Jiao Tang (Major Gentiana Macrophylla Decoction) and **Wu Yao Shun Qi San** (Lindera Powder to Smooth the Flow of Qi) dispel wind to treat *zhong feng* (wind stroke).

- *Da Qin Jiao Tang* dispels wind from the exterior and tonifies qi and blood in the interior. It treats early stages of *zhong feng* (wind stroke) with wind attacking the channels and collaterals in individuals with underlying qi and blood deficiencies. Clinical manifestations include deviation of the eyes and mouth, a stiff tongue and difficulty in speech, numbness and difficulty in moving the extremities, a white tongue coating, and a superficial pulse.
- *Wu Yao Shun Qi San* activates qi circulation and opens the channels and collaterals. It treats *zhong feng* (wind stroke) with complications such as arthralgia, numbness and pain throughout the body, dysphasia, stiffness of the muscles and tendons, and paralysis.

SECTION 2: INTERNAL-WIND EXTINGUISHING FORMULAS

Name	Similarities	Differences
Ling Jiao Gou Teng Tang (Antelope Horn and Uncaria Decoction)		Generates fluids, relaxes the tendons
Gou Teng San (Uncaria Powder)	Calm the Liver, extinguish Liver wind	Clears Liver heat, sedates Liver yang, extinguishes Liver wind
Zhen Gan Xi Feng Tang (Sedate the Liver and Extinguish Wind Decoction)		Nourishes Liver and Kidney yin
Jian Ling Tang (Construct Roof Tiles Decoction)		Nourishes yin, calms the *shen* (spirit)
Tian Ma Gou Teng Yin (Gastrodia and Uncaria Decoction)		Tonifies the Liver and Kidney
E Jiao Ji Zi Huang Tang (Ass-Hide Gelatin and Egg Yolk Decoction)	Extinguish Liver wind, nourish yin	Tonifies yin and blood
Da Ding Feng Zhu (Major Arrest Wind Pearl)		Strongly nourishes yin and tonifies blood

Ling Jiao Gou Teng Tang (Antelope Horn and Uncaria Decoction) is the strongest formula to clear heat and calm Liver wind. It is used for excess heat in the Liver channel accompanied by Liver wind rising. Clinical manifestations include persistent high fever, irritability, muscle spasms of the extremities, convulsions, coma, a dark red tongue with a dry tongue coating, and a wiry, rapid pulse.

Gou Teng San (Uncaria Powder) primarily treats Liver excess conditions characterized by Liver heat, Liver yang, and Liver wind rising. Clinical manifestations include severe vertigo, dizziness, headache, tinnitus, palpitations, a feeling of qi rushing upward, and marked changes in emotions and behavior.

Zhen Gan Xi Feng Tang (Sedate the Liver and Extinguish Wind Decoction) can be used for Liver yang and wind rising due to Liver and Kidney yin deficiencies. Clinical manifestations include dizziness, vertigo, headache with a warm sensation in the head, swelling of the eyes, itching of the skin, tinnitus, irritability, red face, numbness of the extremities, deviation of the mouth, belching, a long, forceful pulse, and in severe cases, unconsciousness.

Chinese Herbal Formulas and Applications

Chapter 14 — Summary

Jian Ling Tang (Construct Roof Tiles Decoction) treats mild to moderate cases of Liver yang rising with *shen* (spirit) disturbance. Clinical manifestations include dizziness, vertigo, tinnitus, swelling of the ears, palpitations, forgetfulness, irritability, fidgeting, insomnia, excessive dreams, and a wiry, hard, and long pulse.

Tian Ma Gou Teng Yin (Gastrodia and Uncaria Decoction) clears heat, activates the blood, and calms the *shen* (spirit). It is used for Liver yang and wind rising with symptoms such as headache, dizziness, and insomnia.

E Jiao Ji Zi Huang Tang (Ass-Hide Gelatin and Egg Yolk Decoction) calms Liver wind and nourishes yin and blood. Clinical manifestations include twitching of the hands and feet, dizziness, vertigo, a deep red tongue with a scanty tongue coating, and a fine, rapid pulse.

Da Ding Feng Zhu (Major Arrest Wind Pearl) calms Liver wind and nourishes yin and blood. Compared to *E Jiao Ji Zi Huang Tang* (Ass-Hide Gelatin and Egg Yolk Decoction), this formula is stronger at tonifying yin and blood. It is used for severe yin deficiency with Liver wind, and symptoms such as clonic convulsions, lack of energy, a deep red tongue with scanty tongue coating, and a deficient pulse.

WIND-EXPELLING FORMULAS

14

1015

Chapter 15

— Dryness-Relieving Formulas

治燥劑

陶弘景 Táo Hóng-Jǐng

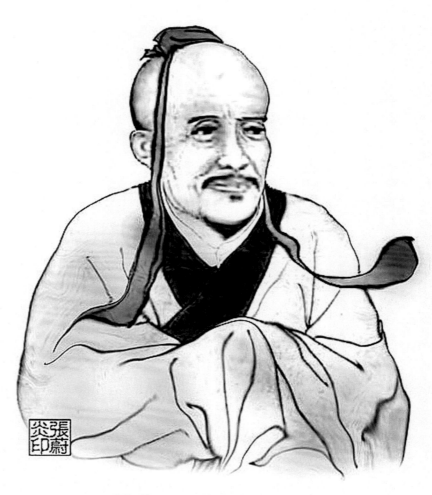

陶弘景 Táo Hóng-Jǐng, 456 – 536.

Chinese Herbal Formulas and Applications

陶弘景 Tāo Hóng-Jīng

The greatest contribution of Tao Hong-Jing to medicine was his revision of the 神农本草经 *Shen Nong Ben Cao Jing* (Divine Husbandman's Classic of the Materia Medica). A few hundred years after its publication in the second century CE, many parts of this text were missing. While many physicians attempted to restore the text to its original state, some filled the gaps with erroneous information, others inadvertently deleted parts of the original text, and none differentiated their personal input from the materials of the source text. As a result, this classic text became marred by errors, duplications and missing parts.

Tao embarked on a mission to restore and expand upon this classic text. In addition to the 365 medicinal substances listed in the original text, he added another 365 of the most useful medicinal substances of his time. He also expanded the contents to include subjects such as the processing of herbs, treatment of diseases, herbal antidotes for poisoning, cautions and contraindications, and herb-herb interactions. Furthermore, to distinguish the original work from his personal input, he marked the original work in red, and his own in black. Published in 480-498, 本草经集注 *Ben Cao Jing Ji Zhu* (Collection of Commentaries on the Classic of the Materia Medica) is a text of great historical importance. Not only did it restore and preserve one of the most important works in traditional Chinese medicine, it expanded the clinical usefulness of this work and had an incredible influence on later generations of practitioners.

Dynasties & Kingdoms	Year
Xia Dynasty 夏	2100-1600 BCE
Shang Dynasty 商	1600-1100 BCE
Zhou Dynasty 周	1100-221 BCE
Qin Dynasty 秦	221-207 BCE
Han Dynasty 漢	206 BCE-220
Three Kingdoms 三國	220-280
Western Jin Dynasty 西晉	265-316
Eastern Jin Dynasty 東晉	317-420
Northern and Southern Dynasties 北南朝	**420-581**
Sui Dynasty 隋	581-618
Tang Dynasty 唐	618-907
Five Dynasties 五代	907-960
Song Dynasty 宋	960-1279
Liao Dynasty 潦	916-1125
Jin Dynasty 金	1115-1234
Yuan Dynasty 元	1271-1368
Ming Dynasty 明	1368-1644
Qing Dynasty 清	1644-1911
Republic of China 中華民國	1912-Present Day
People's Republic of China 中華人民共和國	1949-Present Day

DRYNESS-RELIEVING FORMULAS

15

Chapter 15 – Dryness-Relieving Formulas

Table of Contents

Chapter 15. Dryness-Relieving Formulas **1017**
Biography of Tao Hong-Jing ··· 1018

Section 1. Dispersing and Moistening Formulas ········· **1025**
Xing Su San (Apricot Kernel and Perilla Leaf Powder) ······························ 1025
Sang Xing Tang (Mulberry Leaf and Apricot Kernel Decoction) ······················ 1027
　Qiao He Tang (Forsythia and Mint Decoction) ·································· 1028
Qing Zao Jiu Fei Tang (Eliminate Dryness and Rescue the Lung Decoction) ··········· 1029

Section 2. Nourishing and Moistening Formulas ········· **1033**
Yang Yin Qing Fei Tang (Nourish the Yin and Clear the Lung Decoction) ·············· 1033
Bai He Gu Jin Tang (Lily Bulb Decoction to Preserve the Metal) ···················· 1036
Bu Fei E Jiao Tang (Tonify the Lung Decoction with Ass-Hide Gelatin) ··············· 1039
　Yue Hua Wan (Moonlight Pill) ·· 1040
Qiong Yu Gao (Beautiful Jade Paste) ··· 1041
Mai Men Dong Tang (Ophiopogonis Decoction) ·································· 1043
　Mai Men Yang Yin Tang (Ophiopogonis Decoction to Nourish the Yin) ··········· 1045
Sha Shen Mai Dong Tang (Glehnia and Ophiopogonis Decoction) ···················· 1047
Yu Ye Tang (Jade Fluid Decoction) ·· 1049
　Xiao Ke Fang (Wasting and Thirsting Formula) ······························· 1051
Yu Quan Wan (Jade Spring Pill) ·· 1052
Zeng Ye Tang (Increase the Fluids Decoction) ···································· 1054

Dryness-Relieving Formulas (Summary) ················ **1057**

Chinese Herbal Formulas and Applications

Chapter 15 — Overview

— Dryness-Relieving Formulas

Definition: Dryness-relieving formulas disperse and moisten external dryness, and nourish and moisten internal dryness.

External dryness most often appears during the autumn, as summer dampness vanishes and autumn dryness appears. External dryness may affect the body, and cause the following signs and symptoms: fever, aversion to cold, dry mouth, sore throat, dry coughing, or coughing with scanty sputum. The treatment approach for external dryness is to ventilate and disperse dryness. External dryness is sometimes combined with coolness (which usually appears in late fall and early winter when the environment starts to turn cold) or warmth (which usually is present in late summer and early fall when the environment is still warm). In cases of dryness complicated by coolness or warmth, add herbs accordingly to treat the resultant conditions.

Internal dryness may occur as a result of chronic illness, excessive sexual activity, prolonged vomiting or diarrhea, or inappropriate use of acrid and warm herbs. All of these consume and damage *jing* (essence) and body fluids in the *zang fu* organs. Depending on which *zang fu* organs are most affected, internal dryness is classified as syndromes of: upper, middle, or lower *jiao* dryness. Upper *jiao* dryness affects the Lung and leads to dry coughing. Middle *jiao* dryness affects the Stomach and leads to vomiting and lack of appetite. Lower *jiao* dryness may affect the Kidney and leads to *xiao ke* (wasting and thirsting) syndrome. Lower *jiao* dryness may also affect the Large Intestine, causing dry stools and constipation. The treatment plan for internal dryness is to moisten the affected *zang fu* organ(s) in the affected *jiao(s)*.

SUBCATEGORIES OF ACTION

Dryness may affect the exterior and interior of the body. Similarly, dryness-relieving formulas are divided into dispersing and moistening formulas to treat dryness on the exterior, and nourishing and moistening formulas to treat dryness affecting the interior.

1. **Dispersing and Moistening Formulas**
   These formulas are designed to treat dryness on the exterior, which may be complicated by other *liu yin* (six exogenous factors) and become cool-dryness or warm-dryness.
   • Exterior cool-dryness is the result of the combination of cold and dry pathogenic factors that usually occur in late fall and early winter as the environment becomes increasingly cold and dry. As cool-dryness dominates the environment, it may attack the Lung and lead to signs and symptoms such as aversion to cold, headache, coughing, nasal congestion, dry mouth, and dry throat. Thus, exterior cool-dryness should be treated with warm herbs that gently disperse and moisten dryness, such as *Zi Su Ye* (Folium Perillae), *Jie Geng* (Radix Platycodonis), *Qian Hu* (Radix Peucedani), and *Xing Ren* (Semen Armeniacae Amarum). An exemplar formula is *Xing Su San* (Apricot Kernel and Perilla Leaf Powder).
   • Exterior warm-dryness is the result of the combination of heat and dry pathogenic factors that usually occur in late summer and early fall when the environment is still relatively warm and dry. When these pathogens attack the Lung, they cause signs and symptoms such as feverish sensations in the body, headache, dry coughing, dyspnea, hurried breathing, irritability, and thirst. This condition of warm-dryness should be treated with cold herbs that gently disperse and moisten dryness, such as *Sang Ye* (Folium Mori), *Xing Ren* (Semen Armeniacae Amarum), *Nan Sha Shen*

> From traditional Chinese medicine perspectives, these formulas treat dryness affecting the upper *jiao* (Lung), middle *jiao* (Stomach), and lower *jiao* (Large Intestine).

DRYNESS-RELIEVING FORMULAS

15

1021

Chapter 15 — Overview

(Radix Adenophorae), *Bei Sha Shen* (Radix Glehniae), and *Mai Dong* (Radix Ophiopogonis). Exemplar formulas include *Sang Xing Tang* (Mulberry Leaf and Apricot Kernel Decoction) and *Qing Zao Jiu Fei Tang* (Eliminate Dryness and Rescue the Lung Decoction).

Treatment for external dryness is to ventilate and disperse dryness. Treatment for internal dryness is to moisten the affected *zang fu*.

2. Nourishing and Moistening Formulas

These formulas treat dryness affecting the interior characterized by lack of body fluids in the *zang fu* organs. Clinical manifestations and treatment vary depending on the affected area.

- Upper *jiao* dryness affects the Lung and may cause dry coughing, scanty or no sputum, dry mouth and throat, and wheezing. This condition usually is treated with herbs and formulas that nourish and moisten the Lung, such as *Nan Sha Shen* (Radix Adenophorae), *Bei Sha Shen* (Radix Glehniae), *Tian Dong* (Radix Asparagi), *Mai Dong* (Radix Ophiopogonis), *Yang Yin Qing Fei Tang* (Nourish the Yin and Clear the Lung Decoction), and *Bai He Gu Jin Tang* (Lily Bulb Decoction to Preserve the Metal).

- Middle *jiao* dryness affects the Stomach and leads to vomiting, lack of appetite, thirst, dry mouth and throat, and persistent, indeterminate hunger. This condition usually is treated with herbs and formulas that nourish and moisten the Spleen and Stomach, such as *Shi Hu* (Caulis Dendrobii), *Yu Zhu* (Rhizoma Polygonati Odorati), *Mai Dong* (Radix Ophiopogonis), and *Mai Men Dong Tang* (Ophiopogonis Decoction).

- Lower *jiao* dryness affects the Kidney and leads to *xiao ke* (wasting and thirsting) syndrome. This condition is usually treated with herbs and formulas that nourish and moisten the Kidney, such as *Di Huang* (Radix Rehmanniae), *Shu Di Huang* (Radix Rehmanniae Praeparata), *Nu Zhen Zi* (Fructus Ligustri Lucidi), and *Yu Ye Tang* (Jade Fluid Decoction).

- Lower *jiao* dryness may also affect the Large Intestine and cause dry stools and constipation. This condition is usually treated with herbs and formulas that nourish and moisten the Large Intestine, such as *Xuan Shen* (Radix Scrophulariae) and *Zeng Ye Tang* (Increase the Fluids Decoction).

CAUTIONS / CONTRAINDICATIONS

- When treating dryness disorders, it is important to note that dryness can easily transform into heat and begin to damage yin and consume qi. Therefore, in addition to using dryness-relieving herbs, it is often necessary to add herbs to clear heat, purge fire, tonify qi, and promote generation of body fluids.

- Patients with dryness disorders should not be treated with acrid and aromatic herbs that consume qi, or bitter and drying herbs that injure yin, as the use of these herbs will only further deplete qi and yin.

- Dryness-relieving formulas have nourishing and moistening effects, and as such, are often heavy and greasy in nature. Prolonged or excessive use of these formulas would create internal dampness and stagnation of qi. Therefore, these formulas should be used with caution in the following conditions: Spleen qi deficiency with loose stools, qi stagnation, phlegm stagnation, and damp accumulation.

When treating dryness disorders, it is important to note that dryness can easily transform into heat and begin to damage yin and consume qi.

PHARMACOLOGICAL EFFECTS & CLINICAL APPLICATIONS

In traditional Chinese medicine, dryness-relieving formulas are generally used to treat imbalances of the Lung, Stomach, Kidney, and Large Intestine. From an allopathic medicine perspective, these formulas are most effective in treating chronic respiratory disorders, gastrointestinal (stomach and intestinal) disorders, and metabolic disorders.

- **Respiratory disorders**: Dryness-relieving formulas are very effective for treating chronic cases of respiratory disorders. Clinical indications include cough,[1,2,3,4] postinfectious cough,[5,6] dyspnea,[7] pneumonia,[8] chronic bronchitis,[9] bronchiectasis,[10] pneumothorax,[11] pulmonary tuberculosis,[12] and lung cancer.[13] The mechanisms of action for dryness-relieving formulas have been attributed in part to antitussive,[14] mucoactive,[15] and antibiotic effects of the herbs.[16] Exemplar formulas

1022

Chinese Herbal Formulas and Applications

Chapter 15 — Overview

include *Xing Su San* (Apricot Kernel and Perilla Leaf Powder), *Qing Zao Jiu Fei Tang* (Eliminate Dryness and Rescue the Lung Decoction), *Sha Shen Mai Dong Tang* (Glehnia and Ophiopogonis Decoction), *Bai He Gu Jin Tang* (Lily Bulb Decoction to Preserve the Metal), and *Mai Men Dong Tang* (Ophiopogonis Decoction).

- **Gastrointestinal disorders**: Dryness-relieving formulas are effective in treating chronic gastrointestinal disorders. Indications include, but are not limited to, atrophic gastritis,[17,18] chronic gastritis,[19] chronic atrophic gastritis,[20] chronic peptic ulcer disease,[21] and constipation.[22] Representative formulas include *Sha Shen Mai Dong Tang* (Glehnia and Ophiopogonis Decoction) and *Mai Men Dong Tang* (Ophiopogonis Decoction).

- **Diabetes mellitus**: Administration of certain dryness-relieving herbs and formulas has been shown to have a hypoglycemic effect to lower plasma glucose levels.[23,24,25,26] Formulas that have been shown to be effective in treating diabetes mellitus include *Sha Shen Mai Dong Tang* (Glehnia and Ophiopogonis Decoction),[27] *Bai He Gu Jin Tang* (Lily Bulb Decoction to Preserve the Metal),[28] *Yu Ye Tang* (Jade Fluid Decoction),[29] and *Zeng Ye Tang* (Increase the Fluids Decoction).[30]

- **Bleeding**: Dryness-relieving formulas do not have direct or potent action to stop bleeding. Rather, they are generally used to treat chronic cases of lung and stomach disorders accompanied by nosebleeds, and coughing or vomiting of blood. *Qing Zao Jiu Fei Tang* (Eliminate Dryness and Rescue the Lung Decoction) and *Yang Yin Qing Fei Tang* (Nourish the Yin and Clear the Lung Decoction) are commonly used to treat epistaxis, hemoptysis, and hematemesis.[31, 32,33]

- **Infection and inflammation**: Some dryness-relieving formulas have antibiotic and anti-inflammatory effects,[34,35] and have been used for conditions such as sore throat,[36] laryngitis,[37,38] tonsillitis,[39] pharyngitis,[40] and cheilitis.[41] Exemplar formulas include *Yang Yin Qing Fei Tang* (Nourish the Yin and Clear the Lung Decoction) and *Zeng Ye Tang* (Increase the Fluids Decoction).

> ~
> **From the allopathic perspective, dryness-relieving formulas are most effective in treating chronic respiratory, gastrointestinal and metabolic disorders.**
> ~

References

1. *Guang Xi Zhong Yi Yao* (Guangxi Chinese Medicine and Herbology) 1985;6:37.
2. *Shan Xi Zhong Yi* (Shanxi Chinese Medicine) 1992;11:492.
3. *Shan Xi Zhong Yi* (Shanxi Chinese *Medicine*) 1993;9:413.
4. Watanabe N, Gang C, Fukuda T. The effects of bakumondo-to (Mai-Men-Dong-Tang) on asthmatic and non-asthmatic patients with increased cough sensitivity. Nihon Kokyuki Gakkai Zasshi 2004 Jan;42(1):49-55.
5. Isohama Y, Kai H, Miyata T. Bakumondo-to, a traditional herbal medicine, stimulates phosphatidylcholine secretion, through the synergistic cross-talk between different signal transduction systems in alveolar type II cells. Nippon Yakurigaku Zasshi 1997 Oct;110(1):120P-125P.
6. Fujimori K, Suzuki E, Arakawa M. Clinical features of postinfectious chronic cough. Arerugi 1997 May;46(5):420-5.
7. *Si Chuan Zhong Yi* (Sichuan Chinese Medicine) 1989;2:19.
8. *He Bei Zhong Yi* (Hebei Chinese Medicine) 1998;1:40.
9. *Guo Wai Yi Xue* (Foreign Medicine) 1993;6:29.
10. *Hu Bei Zhong Yi Za Zhi* (Hubei Journal of Chinese Medicine) 1995;5:14.
11. *Xin Yi Xue* (New Medicine) 1977;(4-5):197.
12. *Zhong Guo Zhong Xi Yi Jie He Za Zhi* (Chinese Journal of Integrative Chinese and Western Medicine) 1991;2:119.
13. *Hei Long Jiang Zhong Yi Yao* (Heilongjiang Chinese Medicine and Herbology) 1982;4:25.
14. Kamei J, Nakamura R, Ichiki H, Kubo M. Antitussive principles of Glycyrrhizae radix, a main component of the Kampo preparations Bakumondo-to (Mai-men-dong-tang). Eur J Pharmacol 2003 May 23;469(1-3):159-63.
15. Miyata T. Novel approach to respiratory pharmacology--pharmacological basis of cough, sputum and airway clearance. Yakugaku Zasshi 2003 Dec;123(12):987-1006.
16. *Fu Jian Zhong Yi Yao* (Fujian Chinese Medicine and Herbology) 1964;9:1.
17. *Zhong Xi Yi Jie He Za Zhi* (Journal of Integrated Chinese and Western Medicine) 1986;6:342.
18. *Zhe Jiang Zhong Yi Za Zhi* (Zhejiang Journal of Chinese Medicine) 1990;10:437.
19. *An Hui Zhong Yi Xue Yuan Xue Bao* (Journal of Anhui University School of Medicine) 1994;2:25.
20. *Shi Yong Zhong Xi Yi Jie He Za Zhi* (Practical Journal of Integrated Chinese and Western Medicines) 1998;7:631.
21. *Zhong Yi Za Zhi* (Journal of Chinese Medicine) 1964;11:11.
22. *Zhong Yi Ming Fang Lin Chuang Xin Yong* (Contemporary Clinical Applications of Classic Chinese Formulas) 2001;723.
23. Miyata T. Novel approach to respiratory pharmacology--pharmacological basis of cough, sputum and airway clearance. Yakugaku Zasshi 2003 Dec;123(12):987-1006.
24. *Zhong Yao Tong Bao* (Journal of Chinese Herbology) 1994;4:33.
25. *Zhong Yao Yao Li Yu Lin Chuang* (Pharmacology and Clinical Applications of Chinese Herbs) 1992;21.
26. *Zhong Yao Tong Bao* (Journal of Chinese Herbology) 1982;6:32.
27. *Shan Xi Zhong Yi* (Shanxi Chinese Medicine) 1995;11:482.

DRYNESS-RELIEVING FORMULAS

15

1023

Chapter 15 — Overview

28. *Yun Nan Zhong Yi Za Zhi* (Yunan Journal of Chinese Medicine) 1995;4:22.
29. *Shan Xi Zhong Yi* (Shanxi Chinese Medicine) 1991;2:51.
30. *Zhong Yi Za Zhi* (Journal of Chinese Medicine) 1985;6:31.
31. *Gui Yang Zhong Yi Xue Yuan Xue Bao* (Journal of Guiyang Chinese Medical University) 1992;4:47.
32. *Bei Jing Zhong Yi* (Beijing Chinese Medicine) 1996;1:22.
33. *Nan Jing Zhong Yi Xue Yuan Xue Bao* (Journal of Nanjing University of Traditional Chinese Medicine) 1989;4:25.
34. *Zhong Guo Zhong Xi Yi Jie He Za Zhi* (Chinese Journal of Integrative Chinese and Western Medicine) 1982;2:153.
35. *Fu Jian Zhong Yi Yao* (Fujian Chinese Medicine and Herbology) 1964;9:1.
36. *Shi Yong Zhong Xi Yi Jie He Za Zhi* (Practical Journal of Integrated Chinese and Western Medicines) 1992;5(9):533.
37. *Zhong Yi Za Zhi* (Journal of Chinese Medicine) 1984;4:50.
38. *Shan Xi Zhong Yi* (Shanxi Chinese Medicine) 1995;5:203.
39. *Zhong Hua Er Bi Hou Ke Za Zhi* (Chinese Journal of Otolaryngology) 1958;6:445.
40. *Shan Xi Zhong Yi* (Shanxi Chinese Medicine) 1992;6:248.
41. *Si Chuan Zhong Yi* (Sichuan Chinese Medicine) 1986;12:48.

Section 1

轻宣润燥剂
— Dispersing and Moistening Formulas

Xing Sū Săn (Apricot Kernel and Perilla Leaf Powder)

杏蘇散
杏苏散

Pinyin Name: *Xing Su San*
Literal Name: Apricot Kernel and Perilla Leaf Powder
Alternate Names: *Hsing Su San*, Apricot and Perilla Powder, Apricot Seed and Perilla Formula
Original Source: *Wen Bing Tiao Bian* (Systematic Differentiation of Warm Disease) by Wu Ju-Tong in 1798

COMPOSITION

Zi Su Ye (Folium Perillae)	[6-9g]
Qian Hu (Radix Peucedani)	[6-9g]
Ku Xing Ren (Semen Armeniacae Amarum)	[6-9g]
Jie Geng (Radix Platycodonis)	[6g]
Ban Xia (Rhizoma Pinelliae)	[6-9g]
Fu Ling (Poria)	[6-9g]
Zhi Qiao (Fructus Citri Aurantii)	[6g]
Chen Pi (Pericarpium Citri Reticulatae)	[6g]
Sheng Jiang (Rhizoma Zingiberis Recens)	[6g]
Da Zao (Fructus Jujubae)	[6g]
Gan Cao (Radix et Rhizoma Glycyrrhizae)	[3-6g]

DOSAGE / PREPARATION / ADMINISTRATION

The source text lists the ingredients of this formula, but does not specify the doses and preparation. Today, this formula may be prepared as a decoction with the doses suggested in brackets.

CHINESE THERAPEUTIC ACTIONS

1. Dispels cool-dryness
2. Ventilates the Lung and dissolves phlegm

CLINICAL MANIFESTATIONS

Exterior syndrome of cool-dryness: mild headache, aversion to cold, absence of perspiration, coughing with thin sputum, stuffy nose, dry throat, a white tongue coating, and a wiry pulse.

CLINICAL APPLICATIONS

Influenza, bronchitis, nasal congestion, tracheitis, bronchiectasis, pulmonary emphysema, cough, and dyspnea.

EXPLANATION

Xing Su San (Apricot Kernel and Perilla Leaf Powder) dispels exterior cool-dryness and ventilates Lung qi. If the cool-dryness factors invade the exterior parts of the body, then symptoms such as mild headache and aversion to cold will occur, without perspiration. Cool-dryness factors also may invade the Lung, compromising its function of distributing water. As a result, water accumulates and turns into phlegm and causes symptoms such as coughing, stuffy nose, and dry throat.

In this formula, *Zi Su Ye* (Folium Perillae) and *Qian Hu* (Radix Peucedani) gently induce perspiration to release the exterior cool-dryness factors. *Ku Xing Ren* (Semen Armeniacae Amarum) and *Jie Geng* (Radix Platycodonis) ventilate the Lung and regulate Lung qi to relieve coughing. *Ban Xia* (Rhizoma Pinelliae) and *Fu Ling* (Poria) eliminate dampness and dissolve phlegm. *Zhi Qiao* (Fructus Aurantii) and *Chen Pi* (Pericarpium Citri Reticulatae) regulate

DRYNESS-RELIEVING FORMULAS

15

1025

Chapter 15 – Dryness-Relieving Formulas   *Section 1 – Dispersing and Moistening Formulas*

Xìng Sū Sǎn (Apricot Kernel and Perilla Leaf Powder)

Xing Su San (Apricot Kernel and Perilla Leaf Powder)

Diagnosis	Signs and Symptoms	Treatment	Herbs
Exterior cool-dryness	• Aversion to cold and absence of perspiration: exterior cool-dryness • Coughing with thin sputum and stuffy nose: obstructed Lung qi circulation • Mild headache: obstructed qi circulation • White tongue coating: exterior cool-dryness • Wiry pulse: interior phlegm	• Dispels cool-dryness • Ventilates the Lung and regulates Lung qi circulation • Dissolves phlegm	• *Zi Su Ye* (Folium Perillae) and *Qian Hu* (Radix Peucedani) release the exterior cool-dryness. • *Ku Xing Ren* (Semen Armeniacae Amarum) and *Jie Geng* (Radix Platycodonis) ventilate the Lung and regulate the Lung qi. • *Zhi Qiao* (Fructus Aurantii) and *Chen Pi* (Pericarpium Citri Reticulatae) regulate the Lung qi. • *Ban Xia* (Rhizoma Pinelliae) and *Fu Ling* (Poria) eliminate dampness and dissolve phlegm. • *Sheng Jiang* (Rhizoma Zingiberis Recens) and *Da Zao* (Fructus Jujubae) harmonize the *ying* (nutritive) and *wei* (defensive) levels. • *Gan Cao* (Radix et Rhizoma Glycyrrhizae) harmonizes all of the herbs.

Lung qi and expand the chest. *Sheng Jiang* (Rhizoma Zingiberis Recens), *Da Zao* (Fructus Jujubae), and *Gan Cao* (Radix et Rhizoma Glycyrrhizae) harmonize the *ying* (nutritive) and *wei* (defensive) levels.

MODIFICATIONS

• With headache, add *Gao Ben* (Rhizoma et Radix Ligustici) and *Fang Feng* (Radix Saposhnikoviae).

• With frontal headache, add *Bai Zhi* (Radix Angelicae Dahuricae).

• With more heat or fever, add *Chai Hu* (Radix Bupleuri) and *Huang Qin* (Radix Scutellariae).

• With thirst and dry mouth, add *Huang Qin* (Radix Scutellariae) and *Shi Gao* (Gypsum Fibrosum).

• With wind-cold at the exterior, add *Fang Feng* (Radix Saposhnikoviae) and *Jing Jie* (Herba Schizonepetae).

• For severe cough, add *Zi Wan* (Radix et Rhizoma Asteris) and *Kuan Dong Hua* (Flos Farfarae).

• For constant cough after perspiration, remove *Zi Su Ye* (Folium Perillae) and add *Zi Su Geng* (Caulis Perillae).

• For productive cough with phlegm, add *Er Chen Tang* (Two-Cured Decoction).

• For cough and dyspnea due to wind-cold invasion, add *Ding Chuan Tang* (Arrest Wheezing Decoction).

• With nausea and vomiting, add *Huo Xiang* (Herba Agastaches).

• With diarrhea and abdominal fullness, add *Cang Zhu* (Rhizoma Atractylodis) and *Hou Po* (Cortex Magnoliae Officinalis).

CAUTIONS/CONTRAINDICTIONS

• *Xing Su San* is an acrid and warm formula that treats exterior cool-dryness or wind-cold. It should not be used if the condition is characterized by warm-dryness or wind-heat.

• *Xing Su San* is gentle in nature and potency. It should only be used for mild-to-moderate cases of exterior cool-dryness or wind-cold conditions. Those with severe exterior conditions may require stronger acrid and warm exterior-releasing herbs, such as *Ma Huang* (Herba Ephedrae), *Gui Zhi* (Ramulus Cinnamomi) and *Qiang Huo* (Rhizoma et Radix Notopterygii).

CLINICAL STUDIES AND RESEARCH

1. **Cough:** Administration of modified *Xing Su San* was shown in numerous studies to effectively treat various types of cough. One study of 560 patients with cough due to an exterior condition reported complete recovery in 478 patients, significant improvement in 47 patients, moderate improvement in 16 patients, and no effect in 19 patients. The herbal formula contained *Ku Xing Ren* (Semen Armeniacae Amarum) 9g, *Zi Su Ye* (Folium Perillae) 9g, *Qian Hu* (Radix Peucedani) 12g, *Ban Xia* (Rhizoma Pinelliae) 9g, *Chen Pi* (Pericarpium Citri Reticulatae) 9g, *Sha Shen* (Radix Glehniae seu Adenophorae) 15g, *Gua Lou* (Fructus Trichosanthis) 12g, *Sang Bai Pi* (Cortex Mori) 12g, *Bei Mu* (Bulbus Fritillariae) 9g, *Jie Geng* (Radix Platycodonis) 9g, and *Gan Cao* (Radix et Rhizoma Glycyrrhizae) 6g. The herbs were cooked in water, and decoction taken in two equally-divided doses daily.[1]

1026

Xìng Sū Sǎn (Apricot Kernel and Perilla Leaf Powder)

2. **Coughing and dyspnea**: Use of modified *Xing Su San* was associated with a 95% rate of effectiveness in treating 57 children with coughing and dyspnea. The herbal formula contained *Ku Xing Ren* (Semen Armeniacae Amarum) 9g, *Qian Hu* (Radix Peucedani) 9g, *Fu Ling* (Poria) 9g, *Huang Qin* (Radix Scutellariae) 9g, *Jie Geng* (Radix Platycodonis) 6g, *Ban Xia* (Rhizoma Pinelliae) 6g, *Gan Cao* (Radix et Rhizoma Glycyrrhizae) 6g, *Chen Pi* (Pericarpium Citri Reticulatae) 6g, *Sang Bai Pi* (Cortex Mori) 6g, and *Bai Bu* (Radix Stemonae) 10g. The herbs were cooked in water, and decoction taken in three equally-divided doses daily. Of 57 patients, the study reported complete recovery in 38 patients, improvement in 16 patients, and no benefit in 3 patients. The duration of treatment ranged from 3 to 9 packs of herbs.[2]

AUTHORS' COMMENTS

Xing Su San is the representative formula for treating cough due to cool-dryness affecting the Lung. This type of cough occurs commonly in areas where the weather is cold and dry.

Xing Su San, *Sang Xing Tang* (Mulberry Leaf and Apricot Kernel Decoction), and *Qing Zao Jiu Fei Tang* (Eliminate Dryness and Rescue the Lungs Decoction) all treat dryness attacking the Lung.

- *Xing Su San* is specifically for cool-dryness attacking the Lung, when the chief complaints are cough with thin white sputum, headache, and nasal obstruction.
- *Sang Xing Tang* has moderate action to treat warm-dryness attacking the Lung. It treats mild to moderate cases of warm-dryness with symptoms of slight heat sensations in the body, and cough with scant or no sputum.
- *Qing Zao Jiu Fei Tang* has potent function to treat warm-dryness attacking the Lung. It is used for severe cases of warm-dryness attacking the Lung, with chief manifestations of fever, thirst, cough, dyspnea, and chest and hypochondriac pain.[3]

References

1. *Guang Xi Zhong Yi Yao* (Guangxi Chinese Medicine and Herbology) 1985;6:37.
2. *Si Chuan Zhong Yi* (Sichuan Chinese Medicine) 1989;2:19.
3. Wang MZ, et al. *Zhong Yi Xue Wen Da Ti Ku* (Questions and Answers on Traditional Chinese Medicine: Herbal Formulas).

Sāng Xìng Tāng (Mulberry Leaf and Apricot Kernel Decoction)

桑杏湯
桑杏汤

Pinyin Name: *Sang Xing Tang*
Literal Name: Mulberry Leaf and Apricot Kernel Decoction
Original Source: *Wen Bing Tiao Bian* (Systematic Differentiation of Warm Disease) by Wu Ju-Tong in 1798

COMPOSITION

Sang Ye (Folium Mori)	3g
Dan Dou Chi (Semen Sojae Praeparatum)	3g
Ku Xing Ren (Semen Armeniacae Amarum)	4.5g
Sha Shen (Radix Glehniae seu Adenophorae)	6g
Zhe Bei Mu (Bulbus Fritillariae Thunbergii)	3g
Li Pi (Pericarpium Pyri)	3g
Zhi Zi Pi (Pericarpium Gardeniae)	3g

DOSAGE / PREPARATION / ADMINISTRATION

The source text states to cook the ingredients with two cups of water until the decoction is reduced to one cup. Take the strained decoction while warm. Repeat this process if the condition is severe. The original source advises to cook *Sang Xing Tang* for only a short period of time. The rationale is that since this is a mild case of warm-dryness, a light decoction will be sufficient for treatment.

CHINESE THERAPEUTIC ACTIONS

Dispels and ventilates warm-dryness

DRYNESS-RELIEVING FORMULAS

15

1027

Chapter 15 – Dryness-Relieving Formulas   *Section 1 – Dispersing and Moistening Formulas*

Sāng Xíng Tāng (Mulberry Leaf and Apricot Kernel Decoction)

CLINICAL MANIFESTATIONS

Exterior warm-dryness affecting the Lung: feverish sensations, dry coughing without sputum, or with scanty, sticky sputum, thirst, dry throat, a red tongue with a thin, white and dry tongue coating, and a rapid, big pulse on the right hand.

CLINICAL APPLICATIONS

Whooping cough and coughing.

EXPLANATION

Sang Xing Tang (Mulberry Leaf and Apricot Kernel Decoction) is designed to treat mild cases of exterior warm-dryness invading the Lung. Warm-dryness is mild in nature and invades only the exterior of the body. Therefore, the patient may feel slightly warm but does not have high fever. Also, the warm-dryness may invade the Lung to disrupt qi circulation, dry up fluids, and cause symptoms such as dry coughing with or without sputum, thirst, dry throat, red tongue body, and a big, rapid pulse.

This formula uses *Sang Ye* (Folium Mori) and *Dan Dou Chi* (Semen Sojae Praeparatum) to ventilate the Lung and dispel warm-dryness. *Ku Xing Ren* (Semen Armeniacae Amarum) ventilates the Lung and regulates Lung qi. *Sha Shen* (Radix Glehniae seu Adenophorae) nourishes yin and moistens the Lung. *Zhe Bei Mu* (Bulbus Fritillariae Thunbergii) clears the Lung and dissolves phlegm. *Li Pi* (Pericarpium Pyri) moistens the Lung, generates fluids, and stops coughing. *Zhi Zi Pi* (Pericarpium Gardeniae) clears heat in the Lung and the diaphragm.

MODIFICATIONS

• With cough accompanied by thick, yellow sputum,

add *Tian Hua Fen* (Radix Trichosanthis) and *Gua Lou* (Fructus Trichosanthis).

• With heat and dryness injuring the Lung collaterals, leading to coughing of blood, add *Lu Gen* (Rhizoma Phragmitis), *Bai Mao Gen* (Rhizoma Imperatae), *Qing Dai* (Indigo Naturalis), and *Gua Lou* (Fructus Trichosanthis).

• If there is a dry, sore throat, add *Niu Bang Zi* (Fructus Arctii), *Bo He* (Herba Menthae), *Xuan Shen* (Radix Scrophulariae), and *Mai Dong* (Radix Ophiopogonis).

• With epistaxis, add *Mo Han Lian* (Herba Ecliptae) and *Bai Mao Gen* (Rhizoma Imperatae).

• With severe epistaxis due to heat, add *Qing Dai* (Indigo Naturalis), *Qing Hao* (Herba Artemisiae Annuae), *Mu Dan Pi* (Cortex Moutan), *Di Huang* (Radix Rehmanniae), and *Ce Bai Ye* (Cacumen Platycladi).

• With hemoptysis due to bronchiectasis, remove *Dan Dou Chi* (Semen Sojae Praeparatum), and add *Qing Dai* (Indigo Naturalis), *Gua Lou Pi* (Pericarpium Trichosanthis), and *He Zi* (Fructus Chebulae).

CAUTIONS / CONTRAINDICATIONS

• *Sang Xing Tang* should only be cooked for a short period of time to preserve its efficacy, as many herbs in this formula are aromatic.

• This formula is moderate in potency, and should only be used to treat lung disorders of mild to moderate severity.

RELATED FORMULA

Qiào Hé Tāng (Forsythia and Mint Decoction)
翹荷湯
翘荷汤
Pinyin Name: *Qiao He Tang*
Literal Name: Forsythia and Mint Decoction

Sang Xing Tang (Mulberry Leaf and Apricot Kernel Decoction)

Diagnosis	Signs and Symptoms	Treatment	Herbs
Exterior warm-dryness affecting the Lung	• Warm sensations: exterior warm-dryness • Thirst, dry throat, and dry coughing: warm-dryness damaging body fluids • Dry tongue coating and a rapid, big pulse: warm-dryness	• Dispels and ventilates warm-dryness • Clears Lung heat	• *Sang Ye* (Folium Mori) and *Dan Dou Chi* (Semen Sojae Praeparatum) ventilate the Lung and dispel the warm-dryness. • *Ku Xing Ren* (Semen Armeniacae Amarum) ventilates the Lung and regulates Lung qi. • *Sha Shen* (Radix Glehniae seu Adenophorae) nourishes yin and moistens the Lung. • *Zhe Bei Mu* (Bulbus Fritillariae Thunbergii) clears the Lung and dissolves phlegm. • *Li Pi* (Pericarpium Pyri) moistens the Lung, generates fluids, and stops the coughing. • *Zhi Zi Pi* (Pericarpium Gardeniae) clears heat in the Lung and diaphragm.

1028

Chinese Herbal Formulas and Applications

Sāng Xìng Tāng (Mulberry Leaf and Apricot Kernel Decoction)

Original Source: *Wen Bing Tiao Bian* (Systematic Differentiation of Warm Disease) by Wu Ju-Tong in 1798

Bo He (Herba Menthae)	4.5g
Lian Qiao (Fructus Forsythiae)	4.5g
Zhi Zi Pi (Pericarpium Gardeniae)	4.5g
Gan Cao (Radix et Rhizoma Glycyrrhizae)	3g
Jie Geng (Radix Platycodonis)	6g
Lu Dou Pi (Pericarpium Phaseoli Radiati)	6g

Cook the ingredients with 2 cups of water and cook until 1 cup of liquid remains. Take the strained decoction while warm. This formula should be given twice daily, and, in severe cases, three times daily.

Qiao He Tang (Forsythia and Mint Decoction) has actions to clear heat and dryness from the *qi* (energy) level in the upper *jiao*. Clinically, it treats tinnitus, red eyes, swollen gums, and sore throat due to heat and dryness attacking the upper parts of the body.

AUTHORS' COMMENTS

Xing Su San (Apricot Kernel and Perilla Leaf Powder) and *Sang Xing Tang* both treat cough caused by Lung dryness.

• *Xing Su San* treats cold-dryness attacking the Lung. Chief complaints include aversion to cold, absence of perspiration, and cough with thin, white sputum.

• *Sang Xing Tang* treats warm-dryness attacking the Lung. Chief complaints include warm sensations, dry cough with absence of sputum, thirst, and dry mouth and throat.[1]

Sang Xing Tang and *Sang Ju Yin* (Mulberry Leaf and Chrysanthemum Decoction) both contain *Ku Xing Ren* (Semen Armeniacae Amarum) and *Sang Ye* (Folium Mori) to clear the Lung, relieve cough, and expel exterior factor.

• *Sang Xing Tang* treats dryness with heat attacking the Lung. This formula contains moistening herbs such as *Sha Shen* (Radix Glehniae seu Adenophorae) and *Bei Mu* (Bulbus Fritillariae), to treat dryness symptoms.

• *Sang Ju Yin* treats wind-heat attacking the Lung. It contains heat-clearing herbs such as *Bo He* (Herba Menthae), *Lu Gen* (Rhizoma Phragmitis), and *Lian Qiao* (Fructus Forsythiae).[2]

References
1. Wang MZ, et al. *Zhong Yi Xue Wen Da Ti Ku* (Questions and Answers on Traditional Chinese Medicine: Herbal Formulas).
2. Wang MZ, et al. *Zhong Yi Xue Wen Da Ti Ku* (Questions and Answers on Traditional Chinese Medicine: Herbal Formulas).

Qīng Zào Jiù Fèi Tāng
(Eliminate Dryness and Rescue the Lung Decoction)

清燥救肺湯

清燥救肺汤

Pinyin Name: *Qing Zao Jiu Fei Tang*
Literal Name: Eliminate Dryness and Rescue the Lung Decoction
Alternate Names: *Ching Tsao Chiu Fei Tang*, *Ching Zao Jiu Fei Tang*, Dryness-Clearing and Lung-Rescuing Decoction, Eriobotrya and Ophiopogon Combination
Original Source: *Yi Men Fa Lu* (Precepts for Physicians) by Yu Chang in 1658

COMPOSITION

Sang Ye (Folium Mori)	9g
Shi Gao (Gypsum Fibrosum), *duan* (calcined)	7.5g
Mai Dong (Radix Ophiopogonis)	3.6g
Ku Xing Ren (Semen Armeniacae Amarum), *chao* (dry-fried) to yellow	2.1g
Pi Pa Ye (Folium Eriobotryae), *zhi* (fried with honey) to yellow	3g
E Jiao (Colla Corii Asini)	2.4g
Hei Zhi Ma (Semen Sesami Nigrum), *chao* (dry-fried) and *yan* (ground) to small particles	3g
Ren Shen (Radix et Rhizoma Ginseng)	2.1g
Gan Cao (Radix et Rhizoma Glycyrrhizae)	3g

DRYNESS-RELIEVING FORMULAS

15

1029

Chapter 15 – Dryness-Relieving Formulas

Section 1 – Dispersing and Moistening Formulas

Qīng Zào Jiù Fèi Tāng
(Eliminate Dryness and Rescue the Lung Decoction)

DOSAGE / PREPARATION / ADMINISTRATION

Cook the ingredients with 1 bowl of water until the liquid is reduced to 60% of the original volume. Take the warm, strained decoction two to three times daily.

CHINESE THERAPEUTIC ACTIONS

1. Clears dryness
2. Moistens the Lung

CLINICAL MANIFESTATIONS

Warm-dryness injuring the Lung: headache, fever, thirst, dry coughing with no sputum, shortness of breath, dyspnea, chest fullness, hypochondriac pain, irritability, dryness of the nose, mouth and throat; a dry tongue with no coating, and a big, rapid but deficient pulse.

CLINICAL APPLICATIONS

Cough, sore throat, laryngitis, pneumonia, bronchitis, bronchiectasis, pulmonary tuberculosis, influenza, asthma, upper respiratory tract infection, epistaxis, hemoptysis, itching, and alopecia areata.

EXPLANATION

Qing Zao Jiu Fei Tang (Eliminate Dryness and Rescue the Lung Decoction) is designed to treat severe cases of warm-dryness injuring the Lung. Warm-dryness may invade the exterior, causing headache and fever. If the warm-dryness invades the Lung and reverses the normal flow of Lung qi, then coughing, shortness of breath, dyspnea, chest and hypochondriac fullness and pain may occur. Because warm-dryness may easily damage Lung yin and body fluids, symptoms such as coughing with no sputum, dry nose and mouth, and thirst may be expected. The dry tongue with no coating and a big, rapid but deficient pulse indicate the presence of dryness and heat, and damage of qi and yin.

This formula contains Sang Ye (Folium Mori) to ventilate and moisten dryness and release pathogenic factors from the Lung. Shi Gao (Gypsum Fibrosum) and Mai Dong (Radix Ophiopogonis) clear the Lung heat and moisten the dryness. These three herbs form a good balance as they function to release the exterior, clear the warmth, and moisten the dryness. Furthermore, though Shi Gao (Gypsum Fibrosum) is heavy, sinking and cold in nature, prescribing it at a lower dose will not interfere with the releasing effect of Sang Ye (Folium Mori). Ku Xing Ren (Semen Armeniacae Amarum) and Pi Pa Ye (Folium Eriobotryae) benefit the Lung and regulate the flow of Lung qi. E Jiao (Colla Corii Asini) and Hei Zhi Ma (Semen Sesami Nigrum) moisten the Lung and nourish Lung yin. Ren Shen (Radix et Rhizoma Ginseng) and Gan Cao (Radix et Rhizoma Glycyrrhizae) tonify qi and the middle jiao, which, in turn, enhance the production of Lung qi.

MODIFICATIONS

- With profuse, difficult to expectorate sputum, add Chuan Bei Mu (Bulbus Fritillariae Cirrhosae) and Gua Lou Pi (Pericarpium Trichosanthis).
- With thirst and high fever due to excess heat, add Ling Yang Jiao (Cornu Saigae Tataricae) or Shui Niu Jiao (Cornu Bubali).

Qing Zao Jiu Fei Tang (Eliminate Dryness and Rescue the Lung Decoction)

Diagnosis	Signs and Symptoms	Treatment	Herbs
Warm-dryness injuring the Lung	• Headache and fever: warm-dryness at the exterior • Coughing, shortness of breath, dyspnea, chest and hypochondriac fullness and pain: reversed qi flow due to warm-dryness invading the Lung • Coughing with no sputum, dry nose and mouth, and thirst: warm-dryness damaging yin and body fluids • Dry tongue with no coating and a big, rapid but deficient pulse: warm-dryness damaging qi and yin	• Clears dryness • Moistens the Lung	• Sang Ye (Folium Mori) moistens dryness and releases pathogenic factors from the Lung. • Shi Gao (Gypsum Fibrosum) and Mai Dong (Radix Ophiopogonis) clear Lung heat and moisten dryness. • Ku Xing Ren (Semen Armeniacae Amarum) and Pi Pa Ye (Folium Eriobotryae) benefit the Lung and regulate the flow of Lung qi. • E Jiao (Colla Corii Asini) and Hei Zhi Ma (Semen Sesami Nigrum) moisten the Lung and nourish Lung yin. • Ren Shen (Radix et Rhizoma Ginseng) and Gan Cao (Radix et Rhizoma Glycyrrhizae) tonify qi.

1030

Chinese Herbal Formulas and Applications

Qīng Zào Jiù Fèi Tāng
(Eliminate Dryness and Rescue the Lung Decoction)

* With coughing of blood, add *Ce Bai Ye* (Cacumen Platycladi), *Xian He Cao* (Herba Agrimoniae) and *Bai Ji* (Rhizoma Bletillae).
* With hoarseness or loss of voice, add *He Zi* (Fructus Chebulae) and *Mu Hu Die* (Semen Oroxyli).
* For constipation, add *Huo Ma Ren* (Fructus Cannabis), *Rou Cong Rong* (Herba Cistanches), and *Tao Ren* (Semen Persicae).

CAUTIONS / CONTRAINDICATIONS

* *Qing Zao Jiu Fei Tang* contains many greasy tonics, and should be used with caution in cases of Spleen and Stomach deficiencies.
* Patients with warm-dryness injuring the Lung often have underlying deficiencies. Therefore, foods and herbs that are acrid, aromatic, bitter and drying should be avoided, as they will further damage qi and yin.

CLINICAL STUDIES AND RESEARCH

1. **Cough**: Administration of *Qing Zao Jiu Fei Tang* in 100 patients with cough due to Lung heat was associated with complete recovery in 50 patients, significant improvement in 40 patients, and moderate improvement in 10 patients. The patients were instructed to discontinue antibiotic drugs during herbal treatment.[1] In another study, 67 patients with a dry, non-productive cough refractory to antibiotic drug therapy were treated with good results using modified *Qing Zao Jiu Fei Tang*. The study reported that most patients began to feel improvement after 4 days of herbal therapy.[2]

2. **Sore throat**: One study reported good effect for treatment of sore throat using *Qing Zao Jiu Fei Tang* plus *Chan Tui* (Periostracum Cicadae), *Zi Wan* (Radix et Rhizoma Asteris), and *Bai Bu* (Radix Stemonae). Of 73 patients, the study reported complete recovery in 59 patients, improvement in 12 patients, and no improvement in 2 patients. The overall rate of effectiveness was 97.25%.[3]

3. **Laryngitis**: Administration of modified *Qing Zao Jiu Fei Tang* was reported in one study to be effective in treating 84 of 85 patients with loss of voice due to laryngitis. Modifications to the base formula included addition of *Jing Jie* (Herba Schizonepetae) and *Fang Feng* (Radix Saposhnikoviae) for wind-cold; *Chuan Bei Mu* (Bulbus Fritillariae Cirrhosae) and *Jie Geng* (Radix Platycodonis) for phlegm and heat; *Shi Gao* (Gypsum Fibrosum) for excess heat; and *Da Huang* (Radix et Rhizoma Rhei) for constipation. For individuals with Lung and Kidney deficiencies, *He Zi* (Fructus Chebulae) and *Huang Qi* (Radix Astragali) were added, *Sha Shen* (Radix Glehniae seu Adenophorae) was used in place of *Ren Shen* (Radix

et Rhizoma Ginseng), and *Shi Hu* (Caulis Dendrobii) was used in place of *Shi Gao* (Gypsum Fibrosum).[4]

4. **Pneumonia**: Administration of modified *Qing Zao Jiu Fei Tang* was associated with 85% effectiveness in treating 26 patients with pneumonia with symptoms such as frequent coughing, and scant sticky sputum that is difficult to expectorate. Modifications to the base formula included addition of *Wu Wei Zi* (Fructus Schisandrae Chinensis) and *Su Zi* (Fructus Perillae) for severe cough and dyspnea; *Di Huang* (Radix Rehmanniae) and charred *Zhi Zi* (Fructus Gardeniae) for constipation; and *Bai Shao* (Radix Paeoniae Alba) and *Yan Hu Suo* (Rhizoma Corydalis) for chest pain caused by cough. Of 26 patients, the study reported significant effects in 5 patients, moderate improvement in 17 patients, and no help in 4 patients.[5]

5. **Epistaxis**: One study reported successful termination of nosebleeds within 3 days in all of 24 patients using *Qing Zao Jiu Fei Tang* plus *Bai Mao Gen* (Rhizoma Imperatae), *Qian Cao* (Radix et Rhizoma Rubiae), and charred *Ou Jie* (Nodus Nelumbinis Rhizomatis).[6]

6. **Hemoptysis**: According to one study, use of modified *Qing Zao Jiu Fei Tang* was associated with good results to treat 38 patients with coughing of blood.[7]

7. **Itching**: Administration of modified *Qing Zao Jiu Fei Tang* was found to be effective in treating 18 geriatric patients with simple itching skin without other complications. Of 18 patients, the study reported complete recovery in 9 patients, improvement in 7 patients, and no benefit in 2 patients.[8]

8. **Alopecia areata**: Use of modified *Qing Zao Jiu Fei Tang* was associated with marked effect to treat 38 patients with alopecia areata. In addition to the base formula, modifications included the addition of *Ju Hua* (Flos Chrysanthemi) for headache; the removal of *Hei Zhi Ma* (Semen Sesami Nigrum) and the addition of *Huo Ma Ren* (Fructus Cannabis) and *Yu Li Ren* (Semen Pruni) for constipation. The study reported increased hair growth and resolution of other symptoms among 31 of 38 patients.[9]

AUTHORS' COMMENTS

Warm-dryness attacking the Lung is often accompanied by underlying deficiencies of qi, yin, and body fluids. Thus, to properly treat this syndrome, the warm-dryness must be cleared and the Lung must be moistened. It is important to note that this formula achieves this goal with the use of sweet and cold heat-clearing herbs such as *Shi Gao* (Gypsum Fibrosum), and not with bitter, cold and drying heat-clearing herbs such as *Huang Qin* (Radix Scutellariae).

DRYNESS-RELIEVING FORMULAS

15

Qīng Zào Jiù Fèi Tāng
(Eliminate Dryness and Rescue the Lung Decoction)

Qing Zao Jiu Fei Tang and *Sang Xing Tang* (Mulberry Leaf and Apricot Kernel Decoction) both effectively treat warm-dryness affecting the Lung.

- *Qing Zao Jiu Fei Tang* is generally reserved for <u>severe</u> cases of warm-dryness <u>injuring</u> the Lung, with such symptoms as high fever, cough, dyspnea, chest and hypochondrial fullness and pain, irritability, thirst, and dry mouth and throat.
- *Sang Xing Tang* is typically used for <u>mild</u> cases of warm-dryness <u>affecting</u> the Lung, with such symptoms as mild fever and mild cough.

Qing Zao Jiu Fei Tang and *Bai He Gu Jin Tang* (Lily Bulb Decoction to Preserve the Metal) both nourish yin and moisten dryness to treat dry cough with scanty sputum.

- *Qing Zao Jiu Fei Tang* treats dry cough due to exterior warm-dryness attacking the body with other symptoms of headache, fever, and dry throat and mouth.
- *Bai He Gu Jin Tang* treats dry cough from Kidney and Lung yin deficiencies with deficiency-heat rising. Besides

the dry cough, there are other yin-deficient symptoms such as night sweats, dry nose and throat, blood-streaked sputum, red tongue body, a scanty coating, and a fine, rapid pulse.

References

1. *Zhong Yi Han Shou Tong Xun* (Reports of Chinese Medicine) 1989;1:37.
2. *Shan Xi Zhong Yi* (Shanxi Chinese Medicine) 1992;11:492.
3. *Shi Yong Zhong Xi Yi Jie He Za Zhi* (Practical Journal of Integrated Chinese and Western Medicines) 1992;5(9):533.
4. *Zhong Yi Za Zhi* (Journal of Chinese Medicine) 1984;4:50.
5. *Shi Yong Zhong Xi Yi Jie He Za Zhi* (Practical Journal of Integrated Chinese and Western Medicines) 1998;12:1065.
6. *Gui Yang Zhong Yi Xue Yuan Xue Bao* (Journal of Guiyang Chinese Medical University) 1992;4:47.
7. *Bei Jing Zhong Yi* (Beijing Chinese Medicine) 1996;1:22.
8. *Shang Hai Yi Yao Za Zhi* (Shanghai Journal of Medicine and Herbology) 1996;10:19.
9. *Hu Nan Zhong Yi Za Zhi* (Hunan Journal of Chinese Medicine) 1989;2:43.

Chinese Herbal Formulas and Applications

Section 2

滋阴润燥剂
— Nourishing and Moistening Formulas

Yǎng Yīn Qīng Fèi Tāng
(Nourish the Yin and Clear the Lung Decoction)

養陰清肺湯
养阴清肺汤

Pinyin Name: Yang Yin Qing Fei Tang
Literal Name: Nourish the Yin and Clear the Lung Decoction
Alternate Name: Nourish the Yin and Clear the Lungs Combination
Original Source: Chong Lou Yu Yao (Jade Key to Many Towers) by Zheng Mei-Run in 1838

COMPOSITION

Di Huang (Radix Rehmanniae)	6g [12g]
Mai Dong (Radix Ophiopogonis)	3.6g [9g]
Xuan Shen (Radix Scrophulariae)	4.5g [9g]
Mu Dan Pi (Cortex Moutan)	2.4g [5g]
Bei Mu (Bulbus Fritillariae)	2.4g [5g]
Bai Shao (Radix Paeoniae Alba), chao (dry-fried)	2.4g [5g]
Bo He (Herba Menthae)	1.5g [3g]
Gan Cao (Radix et Rhizoma Glycyrrhizae)	1.5g [3g]

DOSAGE / PREPARATION / ADMINISTRATION

The source text states to prepare the ingredients as a decoction. Today, the decoction may be prepared using the doses suggested in brackets.

CHINESE THERAPEUTIC ACTIONS

Nourishes yin and clears the Lung

CLINICAL MANIFESTATIONS

Diphtheria: white curd-like spots that are hard to scrape off in the throat, swelling and pain in the throat, with or without fever, dry nose and lips, with or without coughing, and a wheezing sound when breathing.

CLINICAL APPLICATIONS

Diphtheria, chronic laryngitis, tuberculosis, tonsillitis, and epistaxis.

EXPLANATION

According to principles of traditional Chinese medicine,

diphtheria is caused by interior yin deficiency with heat, and is usually triggered by the attack of exterior epidemic toxins. According to the source text, this condition often affects individuals with underlying Lung and Kidney deficiencies, when they are exposed to dryness in the environment or consume acrid or spicy food. Because the Kidney channel passes through the throat and the throat connects the Lung with the exterior, Kidney and Lung yin deficiencies may contribute to yin-deficient heat. Furthermore, when yin-deficient heat is accompanied by attack of exterior epidemic toxins, the patient will experience swelling and pain in the throat, and dry nose and lips.

To treat this syndrome, it is most important to nourish yin, clear the Lung, and dispel toxins. In this formula, Di Huang (Radix Rehmanniae) nourishes Kidney yin, while Mai Dong (Radix Ophiopogonis) nourishes Lung yin. Xuan Shen (Radix Scrophulariae) clears deficiency fire and eliminates heat and toxins. Mu Dan Pi (Cortex Moutan) cools the blood and reduces swelling. Bei Mu (Bulbus

DRYNESS-RELIEVING FORMULAS

15

1033

Yǎng Yīn Qīng Fèi Tāng
(Nourish the Yin and Clear the Lung Decoction)

Yang Yin Qing Fei Tang (Nourish the Yin and Clear the Lung Decoction)

Diagnosis	Signs and Symptoms	Treatment	Herbs
Diphtheria	• Diphtheria: interior yin deficiency and exterior attack of epidemic toxins • White curd-like spots with swelling and pain in the throat: deficiency fire rising upward • Dry nose and lips: deficiency fire consuming body fluids • Coughing and wheezing sound: obstructed Lung qi circulation	• Nourishes yin • Clears the Lung	• *Di Huang* (Radix Rehmanniae) nourishes Kidney yin. • *Mai Dong* (Radix Ophiopogonis) nourishes Lung yin. • *Xuan Shen* (Radix Scrophulariae) clears deficiency fire and eliminates heat and toxins. • *Mu Dan Pi* (Cortex Moutan) cools the blood and reduces the swelling. • *Bei Mu* (Bulbus Fritillariae) moistens the Lung and dissolves phlegm. • *Bai Shao* (Radix Paeoniae Alba) nourishes yin. • *Bo He* (Herba Menthae) disperses dry heat and benefits the throat. • *Gan Cao* (Radix et Rhizoma Glycyrrhizae) harmonizes all of the herbs and eliminates toxins.

Fritillariae) moistens the Lung and dissolves phlegm. *Bai Shao* (Radix Paeoniae Alba) nourishes the yin and sedates the heat. *Bo He* (Herba Menthae) disperses dry heat and benefits the throat. *Gan Cao* (Radix et Rhizoma Glycyrrhizae) harmonizes the herbs and eliminates toxins.

MODIFICATIONS
• With severe dryness, add *Tian Dong* (Radix Asparagi) and *Shi Hu* (Caulis Dendrobii).
• For the initial stage of diphtheria, when exterior symptoms are still present, add *Sang Ye* (Folium Mori) and *Ge Gen* (Radix Puerariae Lobatae).
• When exterior signs and symptoms are prevalent, add *Sang Ye* (Folium Mori) and *Jin Yin Hua* (Flos Lonicerae Japonicae).
• With severe yin deficiency, add *Shu Di Huang* (Radix Rehmanniae Praeparata).

CAUTIONS / CONTRAINDICATIONS
Yang Yin Qing Fei Tang should be used with caution in patients who have loose stools due to Spleen deficiency.

PHARMACOLOGICAL EFFECTS
1. **Antibiotic**: *Yang Yin Qing Fei Tang* was shown to have marked effectiveness to suppress and kill *Corynebacterium diphtheriae*. The alcohol extract of the formula was shown to have a better antibiotic effect than water extract.[1]
2. **Immunostimulant**: Administration of *Yang Yin Qing Fei Tang* was shown to stimulate and increase the immune system in both normal and immune-compromised subjects.[2]

CLINICAL STUDIES AND RESEARCH
1. **Tonsillitis**: Use of modified *Yang Yin Qing Fei Tang* was effective in treating 50 patients with acute tonsillitis. Modifications included the addition of *Che Qian Zi* (Semen Plantaginis) for dysuria; and the addition of *Tian Hua Fen* (Radix Trichosanthis) for thirst. Most patients responded within 1 or 2 packs of herbs, with up to 4 packs in some patients. Of 50 patients, the study reported complete recovery in 45 patients, improvement in 3 patients, and no effect in 2 patients.[3] Another study evaluated the effectiveness of various modalities for treatment of acute tonsillitis. The rate of effectiveness and recovery are as follows: 94.1% and 90.3% in 104 patients for *Yang Yin Qing Fei Tang*, 91.8% and 51.3% in 74 patients for penicillin, and 70% and 45% in 40 patients for sulfonamide.[4]
2. **Laryngitis**: One study reported benefits using modified *Yang Yin Qing Fei Tang* to treat 345 patients with chronic laryngitis. Of 345 patients, the study reported complete recovery in 310 patients, improvement in 29 patients, and no change in 6 patients.[5]
3. **Epistaxis**: One study reported good results using modified *Yang Yin Qing Fei Tang* to treat 14 patients with nosebleeds. The herbal treatment contained *Di Huang* (Radix Rehmanniae), *Mai Dong* (Radix Ophiopogonis), *Xuan Shen* (Radix Scrophulariae), *Mu Dan Pi* (Cortex

Yǎng Yīn Qīng Fèi Tāng
(Nourish the Yin and Clear the Lung Decoction)

Moutan), *Bei Mu* (Bulbus Fritillariae), *Bo He* (Herba Menthae), *Bai Shao* (Radix Paeoniae Alba), and *Gan Cao* (Radix et Rhizoma Glycyrrhizae). Furthermore, *Shi Gao* (Gypsum Fibrosum), *Jin Yin Hua* (Flos Lonicerae Japonicae), and *Lian Qiao* (Fructus Forsythiae) were added for heat; *San Qi* (Radix et Rhizoma Notoginseng) for continuous and profuse bleeding; *Tian Hua Fen* (Radix Trichosanthis), *Sha Shen* (Radix Glehniae seu Adenophorae), *Shi Hu* (Caulis Dendrobii), and *Yu Zhu* (Rhizoma Polygonati Odorati) for dry mouth and throat; and *Huang Qi* (Radix Astragali) and *Dang Gui* (Radix Angelicae Sinensis) for qi and blood deficiencies. The patients were instructed to clean the nasal cavity with normal saline two to three times daily. The study reported complete recovery in all 14 patients. The duration of treatment was between 3 and 6 months. No recurrences were reported in follow-ups 6 to 12 months later.[6]

AUTHORS' COMMENTS

Yang Yin Qing Fei Tang and *Bai He Gu Jin Tang* (Lily Bulb Decoction to Preserve the Metal) both treat Lung and Kidney yin deficiencies. Both formulas contain *Di Huang* (Radix Rehmanniae), *Xuan Shen* (Radix Scrophulariae), *Mai Dong* (Radix Ophiopogonis), and *Bai Shao* (Radix Paeoniae Alba) to nourish Lung and Kidney yin. However, their differences are as follows:

* *Yang Yin Qing Fei Tang* also treats exterior invasion of heat and toxins manifesting in white curd-like spots that

are hard to scrape off in the throat, swelling and pain of the throat, dry nose and lips, and wheezing sounds when breathing. *Yang Yin Qing Fei Tang* also contains *Bo He* (Herba Menthae), *Bei Mu* (Bulbus Fritillariae), and *Mu Dan Pi* (Cortex Moutan) to expel pathogenic factors, resolve phlegm, and benefit the throat.

* *Bai He Gu Jin Tang* treats deficiency-heat rising and manifesting in cough with blood; sore, dry and painful throat, *wu xin re* (five-center heat), steaming bones sensations, night sweats, a red tongue body with scanty coating, and a fine and rapid pulse. *Bai He Gu Jin Tang* also contains *Bai He* (Bulbus Lilii), *Bei Mu* (Bulbus Fritillariae), and *Jie Geng* (Radix Platycodonis) to arrest cough and expel phlegm.[7]

References

1. *Fu Jian Zhong Yi Yao* (Fujian Chinese Medicine and Herbology) 1964;9:1.
2. *Zhong Cao Yao* (Chinese Herbal Medicine) 1991;9:409.
3. *Zhong Hua Yi Xue Za Zhi* (Chinese Journal of Medicine) 1962;3:169.
4. *Zhong Hua Er Bi Hou Ke Za Zhi* (Chinese Journal of Otolaryngology) 1958;6:445.
5. *Shan Xi Zhong Yi* (Shanxi Chinese Medicine) 1995;5:203.
6. *Nan Jing Zhong Yi Xue Yuan Xue Bao* (Journal of Nanjing University of Traditional Chinese Medicine) 1989;4:25.
7. Wang MZ, et al. *Zhong Yi Xue Wen Da Ti Ku* (Questions and Answers on Traditional Chinese Medicine: Herbal Formulas).

DRYNESS-RELIEVING FORMULAS

15

1035

Chapter 15 – Dryness-Relieving Formulas　　　　　　　　*Section 2 – Nourishing and Moistening Formulas*

Băi Hé Gù Jīn Tāng (Lily Bulb Decoction to Preserve the Metal)

百合固金湯
百合固金汤

Pinyin Name: *Bai He Gu Jin Tang*
Literal Name: Lily Bulb Decoction to Preserve the Metal
Alternate Names: *Pai Ho Ku Chin Tang (Wan)*, *Bei Ho Gu Jin Tang (Wan)*, Lily Gold-Firming Decoction (Pill), Lily Metal-Consolidation Decoction (Pill), Lily Combination
Original Source: *Yi Fang Ji Jie* (Analytical Collection of Medical Formulas) by Wang Ang in 1682

COMPOSITION

Di Huang (Radix Rehmanniae)	6g
Shu Di Huang (Radix Rehmanniae Praeparata)	9g
Mai Dong (Radix Ophiopogonis)	4.5g
Bai He (Bulbus Lilii)	3g
Bei Mu (Bulbus Fritillariae)	3g
Xuan Shen (Radix Scrophulariae)	2.4g
Dang Gui (Radix Angelicae Sinensis)	3g
Bai Shao (Radix Paeoniae Alba), *chao* (dry-fried)	3g
Jie Geng (Radix Platycodonis)	2.4g
Gan Cao (Radix et Rhizoma Glycyrrhizae)	3g

DOSAGE / PREPARATION / ADMINISTRATION

Prepare the ingredients as a decoction.

CHINESE THERAPEUTIC ACTIONS

1. Nourishes yin and moistens the Lung
2. Dissolves phlegm and stops coughing

CLINICAL MANIFESTATIONS

Yin deficiency of the Lung and Kidney: coughing with streaks of blood in the sputum, dry and sore throat, warm sensations in the palms and soles, steaming bones sensations, night sweats, red tongue body with little coating, and a fine, rapid pulse.

CLINICAL APPLICATIONS

Cough, bronchiectasis, chronic bronchitis, cor pulmonale, pneumothorax, pulmonary tuberculosis, lung cancer, pharyngitis, hemoptysis, coughing, asthma, and diabetes mellitus.

EXPLANATION

Bai He Gu Jin Tang (Lily Bulb Decoction to Preserve the Metal) is designed to treat Lung and Kidney yin deficiencies. Yin deficiency of the Lung and Kidney may lead to deficiency heat and injury of the blood vessels. Injury of the lung capillaries may lead to bleeding and coughing with streaks of blood. Dry and sore throat are due to deficiency heat drying up the body fluids. Warm palms and soles, steaming bones sensations,

night sweats, and fine, rapid pulse are all typical signs of yin-deficient heat.

Di Huang (Radix Rehmanniae) and *Shu Di Huang* (Radix Rehmanniae Praeparata) nourish yin and clear the deficiency fire. *Di Huang* (Radix Rehmanniae) further cools the blood and stops bleeding. *Mai Dong* (Radix Ophiopogonis), *Bai He* (Bulbus Lilii), and *Bei Mu* (Bulbus Fritillariae) nourish the yin, moisten the Lung, dissolve phlegm, and stop coughing. *Xuan Shen* (Radix Scrophulariae) cools the blood, clears the deficiency fire, and moistens dryness. *Dang Gui* (Radix Angelicae Sinensis) and *Bai Shao* (Radix Paeoniae Alba) nourish the yin and blood. *Jie Geng* (Radix Platycodonis) smoothes the Lung qi, relieves coughing, and dissolves phlegm. *Gan Cao* (Radix et Rhizoma Glycyrrhizae) harmonizes all the herbs in the formula. Lastly, the combination of *Gan Cao* (Radix et Rhizoma Glycyrrhizae) and *Jie Geng* (Radix Platycodonis) helps to relieve the sore throat.

MODIFICATIONS

- With fullness and distention of the chest and hypochondriac region, add *Zhi Shi* (Fructus Aurantii Immaturus) and *Chai Hu* (Radix Bupleuri).
- With sore throat and hoarse voice, add *Tian Dong* (Radix Asparagi) and *Zhi Mu* (Rhizoma Anemarrhenae).
- With more severe cough and dyspnea, add *Ku Xing Ren* (Semen Armeniacae Amarum), *Wu Wei Zi* (Fructus Schisandrae Chinensis), and *Kuan Dong Hua* (Flos Farfarae).

1036

Bǎi Hé Gù Jīn Tāng (Lily Bulb Decoction to Preserve the Metal)

Bai He Gu Jin Tang (Lily Bulb Decoction to Preserve the Metal)

Diagnosis	Signs and Symptoms	Treatment	Herbs
Lung and Kidney yin deficiencies	• Coughing with streaks of blood in the sputum: deficiency heat injuring the blood vessels • Dry and sore throat: deficiency heat consuming body fluids • Warm sensation in the palms and soles, steaming bones sensation, and night sweats: yin-deficient heat rising upward • Red tongue body with little coating and a fine, rapid pulse: yin-deficient heat	• Nourishes yin and moistens the Lung • Dissolves phlegm and stops coughing	• *Di Huang* (Radix Rehmanniae) and *Shu Di Huang* (Radix Rehmanniae Praeparata) nourish yin and clear deficiency fire. • *Di Huang* (Radix Rehmanniae) and *Xuan Shen* (Radix Scrophulariae) cool the blood, clear deficiency fire, and stops bleeding. • *Mai Dong* (Radix Ophiopogonis), *Bai He* (Bulbus Lilii) and *Bei Mu* (Bulbus Fritillariae) nourish yin, moisten the Lung, dissolve phlegm, and stop coughing. • *Dang Gui* (Radix Angelicae Sinensis) and *Bai Shao* (Radix Paeoniae Alba) nourish yin and tonify blood. • *Jie Geng* (Radix Platycodonis) smoothes Lung qi, relieves coughing, and dissolves phlegm. • *Gan Cao* (Radix et Rhizoma Glycyrrhizae) harmonizes all of the herbs.

- With thick, yellow sputum, add *Gua Lou* (Fructus Trichosanthis) and *Zhu Ru* (Caulis Bambusae in Taenia).
- With coughing of blood, remove *Jie Geng* (Radix Platycodonis), and add *Bai Mao Gen* (Rhizoma Imperatae), *Ce Bai Ye* (Cacumen Platycladi) and *Xian He Cao* (Herba Agrimoniae).
- With wheezing and dyspnea due to profuse phlegm, add *Xie Bai San* (Drain the White Powder).
- With wheezing and dyspnea due to heat, add *San Huang Xie Xin Tang* (Three-Yellow Decoction to Sedate the Epigastrium).
- If there are more heat signs, add *Zhi Mu* (Rhizoma Anemarrhenae) and *Yu Xing Cao* (Herba Houttuyniae).
- With severe night sweats, add *Wu Wei Zi* (Fructus Schisandrae Chinensis), *Fu Xiao Mai* (Fructus Tritici Levis), calcined *Mu Li* (Concha Ostreae), and *Ma Huang Gen* (Radix et Rhizoma Ephedrae).
- For pulmonary tuberculosis, add *Bai Ji* (Rhizoma Bletillae), *Bai Bu* (Radix Stemonae), and *Xia Ku Cao* (Spica Prunellae).

CAUTIONS / CONTRAINDICATIONS

- *Bai He Gu Jin Tang* is contraindicated in patients in whom coughing is characterized by excess conditions.
- Many herbs in this formula are hard to digest since they are cold, sweet, and heavy in nature. Therefore, patients with Spleen deficiency, characterized by loose stools, abdominal fullness and pain, and poor appetite, should use this formula with caution.

CLINICAL STUDIES AND RESEARCH

1. **Cough**: One study reported 90% effectiveness using modified *Bai He Gu Jin Tang* to treat 30 patients with cough characterized by dryness and heat. Modifications included addition of *Jin Yin Hua* (Flos Lonicerae Japonicae), *Ban Lan Gen* (Radix Isatidis), and *Niu Bang Zi* (Fructus Arctii) for sore throat; *Zi Su Ye* (Folium Perillae), *Huang Lian* (Rhizoma Coptidis), and *Gua Lou* (Fructus Trichosanthis) for feelings of oppression and pain in the chest; *Tian Zhu Huang* (Concretio Silicea Bambusae) for insomnia; and *Gua Lou Zi* (Semen Trichosanthis) for constipation.[1] Another study reported 97.6% effectiveness using *Bai He Gu Jin Tang* to treat 42 children with chronic cough.[2]

2. **Bronchiectasis**: One study reported good results using herbs to treat 50 patients with hemoptysis associated with bronchiectasis. The herbal formula contained *Di Huang* (Radix Rehmanniae) 15g, *Mai Dong* (Radix Ophiopogonis) 15g, *Bai He* (Bulbus Lilii) 15g, *Xian He Cao* (Herba Agrimoniae) 15g, *Bai Shao* (Radix Paeoniae Alba) 12g, *Dang Gui* (Radix Angelicae Sinensis) 12g, *Xuan Shen* (Radix Scrophulariae) 12g, *Bai Mao Gen* (Rhizoma Imperatae) 30g, *Bei Mu* (Bulbus Fritillariae) 6g, and *Gan Cao* (Radix et Rhizoma Glycyrrhizae) 6g. Additional modifications were made as needed. The treatment protocol was to administer one pack of herbs daily, for 15 to 20 packs continuously. The study reported marked improvements in most patients, with relief of symptoms such as cough and hemoptysis, and reduction of phlegm.[3]

DRYNESS-RELIEVING FORMULAS

15

1037

Chapter 15 – Dryness-Relieving Formulas　　　　*Section 2 – Nourishing and Moistening Formulas*

Băi Hé Gù Jīn Tāng (Lily Bulb Decoction to Preserve the Metal)

3. **Pneumothorax**: In one study, 30 patients with pneumothorax were divided into two groups and treated accordingly. Group one received *Bai He Gu Jin Tang*, one pack of herbs per day via decoction for 10 days per course, for a total of 3 to 4 courses of treatment. Group two received standard allopathic medical treatment (details of treatment were unavailable at the time of publication). The study noted that both treatments were effective. However, the average length of hospitalization was only 18.93 days for patients in the herb group, while the average was 27.85 days for the allopathic medicine group.[4] Another study reported marked success using the following formula to treat pneumothorax: *Bai He Gu Jin Tang* with the removal of *Dang Gui* (Radix Angelicae Sinensis) and *Shu Di Huang* (Radix Rehmanniae Praeparata) and the addition of *Sha Shen* (Radix Glehniae seu Adenophorae), *Pi Pa Ye* (Folium Eriobotryae), and *Gua Lou Pi* (Pericarpium Trichosanthis). Pneumothorax was resolved after an average of 11 days, with a range of 2 to 20 days.[5]

4. **Pulmonary tuberculosis**: In one study, 26 of 30 patients with pulmonary tuberculosis were treated with marked improvement using herbal medicine. The herbal treatment was *Bai He Gu Jin Tang* for yin deficiency, and *Bu Zhong Yi Qi Tang* (Tonify the Middle and Augment the Qi Decoction) for qi deficiency.[6]

5. **Lung cancer**: According to one study, administration of *Bai He Gu Jin Tang* was associated with symptomatic improvement in 22 of 38 patients with lung cancer characterized by Lung yin deficiency.[7]

6. **Diabetes mellitus**: Diabetes mellitus was treated effectively using modified *Bai He Gu Jin Tang* daily in decoction, for 20 days per course of treatment, for 4 courses total. Of 46 patients, the study reported improvement in 38 cases and no effect in 8 cases.[8]

AUTHORS' COMMENTS

Bai He Gu Jin Tang treats cough with blood-streaked sputum, yet it purposely excludes herbs that stop bleeding in its formulation. Bleeding in this case is caused by Kidney and Lung yin deficiencies with deficiency fire flaring upward and injuring the channels and collaterals, leading to symptoms such as dry and painful throat, *wu xin re* (five-center heat), steaming bones sensations, night sweats, and a red tongue with a scanty coating. The herbs used in this formula focus on nourishing yin and cooling deficiency fire. By treating the cause of the bleeding, there is no need to add additional herbs to stop bleeding. When yin is nourished, the bleeding will stop automatically.[9]

Bai He Gu Jin Tang and *Bu Fei E Jiao Tang* (Tonify the Lung Decoction with Ass-Hide Gelatin) both treat cough with blood-streaked sputum, a condition characterized by Lung yin deficiency with fire. Both formulas also nourish Lung yin and treat sore and dry throat, a red tongue body with a scanty coating, and a fine, rapid pulse.

- *Bai He Gu Jin Tang* treats Lung and Kidney yin deficiencies with deficiency-heat rising, and accompanying signs such as *wu xin re* (five-center heat), steaming bones sensations, and night sweats.
- *Bu Fei E Jiao Tang* is designed for Lung yin deficiency with fire, with chief complaints of cough with dyspnea and sputum that is not profuse in amount, and a superficial, fine and rapid pulse.[10]

Bai He Gu Jin Tang, *Qiong Yu Gao* (Beautiful Jade Paste), and *Mai Men Dong Tang* (Ophiopogonis Decoction) have similar effects to nourish yin and moisten the Lung. Their differences are as follows:

- *Bai He Gu Jin Tang* tonifies Lung and Kidney yin, and clears deficiency heat. It is most effective for cough with streaks of blood in the sputum.
- *Qiong Yu Gao* nourishes Lung yin and tonifies Spleen qi. It is primarily used to treat dry, non-productive cough caused by chronic deficiency and debility.
- *Mai Men Dong Tang* tonifies Lung and Stomach yin, and redirects abnormally rising qi downward. It is used to treat cough with difficult-to-expectorate sputum, and vomiting with lack of appetite.

References

1. *Fu Jian Zhong Yi Yao* (Fujian Chinese Medicine and Herbology) 1995;1:46.
2. *Shan Xi Zhong Yi* (Shanxi Chinese *Medicine*) 1993;9:413.
3. *Hu Bei Zhong Yi Za Zhi* (Hubei Journal of Chinese Medicine) 1995;5:14.
4. *Zhong Xi Yi Jie He Za Zhi* (Journal of Integrated Chinese and Western Medicine) 1986;5:280.
5. *Xin Yi Xue* (New Medicine) 1977;4-5:197.
6. *Zhong Guo Zhong Xi Yi Jie He Za Zhi* (Chinese Journal of Integrative Chinese and Western Medicine) 1991;2:119.
7. *Hei Long Jiang Zhong Yi Yao* (Heilongjiang Chinese Medicine and Herbology) 1982;4:25.
8. *Yun Nan Zhong Yi Za Zhi* (Yunan Journal of Chinese Medicine) 1995;4:22.
9. Wang MZ, et al. *Zhong Yi Xue Wen Da Ti Ku* (Questions and Answers on Traditional Chinese Medicine: Herbal Formulas).
10. Wang MZ, et al. *Zhong Yi Xue Wen Da Ti Ku* (Questions and Answers on Traditional Chinese Medicine: Herbal Formulas).

1038

Chinese Herbal Formulas and Applications

Bǔ Fèi Ē Jiāo Tāng (Tonify the Lung Decoction with Ass-Hide Gelatin)

補肺阿膠湯
补肺阿胶汤

Pinyin Name: *Bu Fei E Jiao Tang*
Literal Name: Tonify the Lung Decoction with Ass-Hide Gelatin
Alternate Names: *Bu Fei E Jiao San* (Tonify the Lung Powder with Ass-Hide Gelatin), *E Jiao San* (Ass-Hide Gelatin Powder), *Bu Fei San* (Tonify the Lung Powder)
Original Source: *Xiao Er Yao Zheng Zhi Jue* (Craft of Medicinal Treatment for Childhood Disease Patterns) by Qian Yi in 1119

COMPOSITION

E Jiao (Colla Corii Asini), *chao* (dry-fried) with bran	45g [9g]
Niu Bang Zi (Fructus Arctii), *chao* (dry-fried) till aromatic	7.5g [3g]
Ma Dou Ling (Fructus Aristolochiae), *bei* (stone-baked)	15g [6g]
Ku Xing Ren (Semen Armeniacae Amarum), *chao* (dry-fried)	7 kernels [6g]
Nuo Mi (Oryza Glutinosa), *chao* (dry-fried)	30g [6g]
Zhi Gan Cao (Radix et Rhizoma Glycyrrhizae Praeparata cum Melle)	7.5g [1.5g]

DOSAGE / PREPARATION / ADMINISTRATION

The source text states to dry-fry *E Jiao* (Colla Corii Asini) with bran, pound it into fine particles, and blend it with *Nuo Mi* (Oryza Glutinosa). This mixture is dry-fried again. Grind the other ingredients into powder, and mix everything together. Cook 3-6g of the powder in 1 large bowl of water until the liquid is reduced to 60% of the original volume. Take the warm decoction after meals.

Today, it is usually prepared as a decoction by cooking all of the herbs in water (using the suggested doses in brackets), except for *E Jiao* (Colla Corii Asini). Separately dissolve *E Jiao* (Colla Corii Asini) in boiling water, and mix it with the strained decoction before ingestion.

CHINESE THERAPEUTIC ACTIONS

1. Nourishes yin and tonifies the Lung
2. Arrests coughing and stops bleeding

CLINICAL MANIFESTATIONS

Lung yin deficiency further injured by excess heat invasion: coughing, wheezing, dry throat, scanty sputum, streaks of blood in the sputum, red tongue body with little coating, and a superficial, fine and rapid pulse.

CLINICAL APPLICATIONS

Pulmonary tuberculosis, pneumonia, bronchitis, asthma, bronchial asthma, tonsillitis, and coughing.

EXPLANATION

Bu Fei E Jiao Tang (Tonify the Lung Decoction with Ass-Hide Gelatin) treats excess heat invading a deficient Lung. Lung deficiency makes the body more vulnerable to attack by exterior pathogenic factors. Once these exterior pathogenic factors progress to the Lung and the interior and become stagnant, they can transform into excess heat. Excess heat disrupts the normal qi flow of the Lung, causing coughing and wheezing. Dry throat and coughing with bloody sputum indicate that the excess heat has injured the yin and body fluids, as well as the blood vessels. A red tongue body with little coating and a superficial, fine and rapid pulse indicate Lung heat and deficiency.

E Jiao (Colla Corii Asini) tonifies Lung yin, nourishes the blood, and stops bleeding. *Niu Bang Zi* (Fructus Arctii) disperses heat and relieves dry, sore throat. *Ma Dou Ling* (Fructus Aristolochiae) clears Lung heat, stops coughing, and dissolves phlegm. *Ku Xing Ren* (Semen Armeniacae Amarum) redirects the rising qi of the Lung downward to relieve coughing and wheezing. *Nuo Mi* (Oryza Glutinosa) and *Zhi Gan Cao* (Radix et Rhizoma Glycyrrhizae Praeparata cum Melle) nourish the Spleen.

MODIFICATIONS

- With a dry mouth, add *Sha Shen* (Radix Glehniae seu Adenophorae), *Mai Dong* (Radix Ophiopogonis), *Tian Dong* (Radix Asparagi), *Lu Gen* (Rhizoma Phragmitis), and *Bai He* (Bulbus Lilii).
- With sensations of chest oppression, add *Zhi Qiao* (Fructus Aurantii), *Gua Lou Pi* (Pericarpium Trichosanthis), and *Yu Jin* (Radix Curcumae).
- With sore throat, add *Jie Geng* (Radix Platycodonis) and *She Gan* (Rhizoma Belamcandae).
- With chest and hypochondriac pain during coughing, add *Zhi Shi* (Fructus Aurantii Immaturus), *Fo Shou* (Fructus Citri Sarcodactylis), and *Yu Jin* (Radix Curcumae).

DRYNESS-RELIEVING FORMULAS

15

1039

Chapter 15 – Dryness-Relieving Formulas   Section 2 – Nourishing and Moistening Formulas

Bǔ Fèi Ē Jiāo Tāng (Tonify the Lung Decoction with Ass-Hide Gelatin)

Bu Fei E Jiao Tang (Tonify the Lung Decoction with Ass-Hide Gelatin)

Diagnosis	Signs and Symptoms	Treatment	Herbs
Lung yin deficiency further injured by excess heat invasion	• Coughing and wheezing: excess heat disturbing Lung qi circulation • Dry throat, and scanty, blood-streaked sputum: excess heat consuming yin, drying body fluids, and damaging blood vessels • Red tongue body with little coating and a superficial, fine and rapid pulse: presence of heat and underlying deficiency	• Nourishes yin and tonifies the Lung • Arrests coughing and stops bleeding	• *E Jiao* (Colla Corii Asini) tonifies Lung yin, nourishes the blood, and stops bleeding. • *Niu Bang Zi* (Fructus Arctii) disperses heat and relieves the dry, sore throat. • *Ma Dou Ling* (Fructus Aristolochiae) clears Lung heat, stops coughing, and dissolves phlegm. • *Ku Xing Ren* (Semen Armeniacae Amarum) redirects Lung qi downward to relieve coughing and wheezing. • *Nuo Mi* (Oryza Glutinosa) and *Zhi Gan Cao* (Radix et Rhizoma Glycyrrhizae Praeparata cum Melle) nourish the Spleen and harmonize the herbs.

- With wheezing and dyspnea, add *Zi Su Zi* (Fructus Perillae) and *Qian Hu* (Radix Peucedani).
- If there is blood in the sputum, add *Bai Mao Gen* (Rhizoma Imperatae), *Bai Ji* (Rhizoma Bletillae), and *Bai He* (Bulbus Lilii).

CAUTIONS / CONTRAINDICATIONS

- *Bu Fei E Jiao Tang* contains many heavy tonics that are hard to digest, and is not recommended in cases of phlegm accumulation or Spleen and Stomach deficiencies.
- This formula is not appropriate for individuals with cough caused by wind-cold, or cough with profuse amounts of blood.

CLINICAL STUDIES AND RESEARCH

Cough: In one study, 84 patients with cough characterized by Lung yin deficiency due to various causes (bronchitis, bronchial asthma, bronchiectasis, pulmonary tuberculosis, and whooping cough) were treated with modified *Bu Fei E Jiao Tang* with good results. The formula included *E Jiao* (Colla Corii Asini) 15g, *Ma Dou Ling* (Fructus Aristolochiae) 10g, *Ku Xing Ren* (Semen Armeniacae Amarum) 10g, *Niu Bang Zi* (Fructus Arctii) 10g, *Gan Cao* (Radix et Rhizoma Glycyrrhizae) 6g, *Nuo Mi* (Oryza Glutinosa) 30g and other herbs if deemed necessary. Out of 84 patients, the study reported recovery in 65 cases, improvement in 17 cases, and no benefit in 2 cases.[1]

RELATED FORMULA

Yuè Huá Wán (Moonlight Pill)
月華丸
月华丸
Pinyin Name: *Yue Hua Wan*
Literal Name: Moonlight Pill

Original Source: *Yi Xue Xin Wu* (Medical Revelations) by Cheng Guo-Peng in 1732

Tian Dong (Radix Asparagi), *zheng* (steamed)	30g
Mai Dong (Radix Ophiopogonis), *zheng* (steamed)	30g
Di Huang (Radix Rehmanniae), *xi* (washed) with liquor	30g
Shu Di Huang (Radix Rehmanniae Praeparata), *zheng* (steamed) and sun-dried 9 times	30g
Shan Yao (Rhizoma Dioscoreae), *zheng* (steamed) with milk	30g
Bai Bu (Radix Stemonae), *zheng* (steamed)	30g
Sha Shen (Radix Glehniae seu Adenophorae), *zheng* (steamed)	30g
Chuan Bei Mu (Bulbus Fritillariae Cirrhosae), *zheng* (steamed)	30g
E Jiao (Colla Corii Asini)	30g
Fu Ling (Poria), *zheng* (steamed) with milk	15g
Ta Gan (Jecur Lutrae)	15g
San Qi (Radix et Rhizoma Notoginseng)	15g
Ju Hua (Flos Chrysanthemi)	60g
Sang Ye (Folium Mori), frost	60g

The source text states to cook and condense the herbs, except *E Jiao* (Colla Corii Asini), into an herbal paste. Then dissolve *E Jiao* (Colla Corii Asini) in the herbal paste, and mix the paste with honey to form pills. Each pill should weigh 15g. Take 1 pill three times daily by dissolving it under the tongue before swallowing the resultant liquid.

Yue Hua Wan (Moonlight Pill) tonifies the Lung, nourishes yin, arrests coughing, and stops bleeding. Clinically, it is often used for patients with Lung and Kidney yin

1040

Chinese Herbal Formulas and Applications

Bǔ Fèi Ē Jiāo Tāng (Tonify the Lung Decoction with Ass-Hide Gelatin)

deficiencies characterized by chronic coughing with sputum that may contain streaks of blood.

It may also be used in the middle or late stages of chronic tuberculosis, with symptoms such as tidal fever, dysphoria with feverish sensations in the chest, palms, and soles, emaciated complexion, dry coughing or productive coughing with streaks of blood in the phlegm, dry mouth, chest stuffiness, lack of appetite, lack of energy, obstructed bowel movements, and scanty urine.

AUTHORS' COMMENTS

Bu Fei E Jiao Tang and *Ren Shen Ge Jie San* (Ginseng and Gecko Powder) both treat coughing and relieve wheezing. Furthermore, both formulas have dual effects to tonify Lung deficiency and clear Lung heat. Their differences are as follows:

• *Bu Fei E Jiao Tang* mainly tonifies Lung yin to disperse heat. It is most suitable for patients with Lung yin-deficiency who suffer from heat invasion manifesting in cough, dyspnea, and wheezing. In comparison with *Ren Shen Ge Jie San*, *Bu Fei E Jiao Tang* is stronger for stopping bleeding, but does not assist the Kidney in grasping qi downward.

• *Ren Shen Ge Jie San* tonifies Lung qi deficiency, with additional functions of tonifying the Spleen, nourishing the Kidney, and helping the Kidney grasp the qi. It is most suitable for chronic cough with Kidney deficiency, resulting from an inability to grasp the qi and Spleen qi deficiency

producing dampness. In comparison with *Bu Fei E Jiao Tang*, *Ren Shen Ge Jie San* more strongly nourishes the Lung, but does not disperse wind-heat invasion.[2]

Bu Fei E Jiao Tang, *Da Bu Yin Wan* (Great Tonify the Yin Pill), and *Sheng Mai San* (Generate the Pulse Powder) all treat cough due to Lung deficiency. Their differences are as follows:

• *Bu Fei E Jiao Tang* treats Lung deficiency with excess heat. It is best for nourishing Lung yin, arresting cough, and stopping bleeding for patients with cough with dry throat, scanty sputum, red tongue body with scanty coating, and a superficial, fine and rapid pulse.

• *Da Bu Yin Wan* treats Lung and Kidney yin deficiencies with deficiency fire flaring. The symptoms include steaming bones sensation, tidal fever, red tongue body with scanty coating, and a rapid, forceful pulse.

• *Sheng Mai San* is best for Lung qi and yin deficiencies, as it benefits qi, generates body fluids, astringes yin, and stops sweating. It is best for patients with a weak constitution, who manifest shortness of breath, profuse sweating, thirst, and a deficient pulse.[3]

References

1. *Zhong Yi Fang Ji Xian Dai Yan Jiu* (Modern Study of Medical Formulae in Traditional Chinese Medicine) 1997;6:25.
2. Wang MZ, et al. *Zhong Yi Xue Wen Da Ti Ku* (Questions and Answers on Traditional Chinese Medicine: Herbal Formulas).
3. Wang MZ, et al. *Zhong Yi Xue Wen Da Ti Ku* (Questions and Answers on Traditional Chinese Medicine: Herbal Formulas).

Qióng Yù Gāo (Beautiful Jade Paste)

瓊玉膏
琼玉膏

Pinyin Name: *Qiong Yu Gao*
Literal Name: Beautiful Jade Paste
Original Source: *Hong Shi Ji Yan Fang* (Time-Tested Formulas of the Hong Family)

COMPOSITION

Di Huang (Radix Rehmanniae)	8,000g
Feng Mi (Mel)	5,000g
Ren Shen (Radix et Rhizoma Ginseng)	750g
Fu Ling (Poria)	1,500g

DOSAGE / PREPARATION / ADMINISTRATION

Grind *Ren Shen* (Radix et Rhizoma Ginseng) and *Fu Ling* (Poria) into a fine powder. Filter *Feng Mi* (Mel) to remove

impurities. Simmer *Di Huang* (Radix Rehmanniae) to obtain its juice and discard the herbal residue. Mix the powder, the honey and the juice, and cook them

Chapter 15 – Dryness-Relieving Formulas | Section 2 – Nourishing and Moistening Formulas

Qióng Yù Gāo (Beautiful Jade Paste)

together continuously over low heat for 3 days, until it is reduced to a thick paste. Store the paste in a container made from silver, stone, or porcelain. Avoid using iron during the processing or storage of this formula. Take 2 spoonfuls [6-9g] in the morning with hot water or warm, grain-based liquor.

CHINESE THERAPEUTIC ACTIONS

1. Nourishes yin and moistens the Lung
2. Tonifies qi and strengthens the Spleen

CLINICAL MANIFESTATIONS

Lung yin and Spleen qi deficiencies: generalized deficiency and debility, dry coughing with streaks of blood, dry throat, muscle wasting, shortness of breath, and fatigue.

CLINICAL APPLICATIONS

Diabetes mellitus, dermatitis, compromised immune system, and drug-induced cough.

EXPLANATION

Qiong Yu Gao (Beautiful Jade Paste) is designed to treat Lung disorders due to over-exertion, characterized by such symptoms as chronic, non-productive cough, dry mouth and throat, shortness of breath, and fatigue. This condition is characterized by Lung yin and Spleen qi deficiencies. Over-exertion and the chronic nature of the illness consume yin and qi, causing underlying deficiencies. Furthermore, deficiency of yin and qi contributes to rising of deficiency fire. As a result, the clinical manifestations of this condition include symptoms such as dry, non-productive cough with streaks of blood, dry throat, muscle wasting, shortness of breath, and fatigue.

In this formula, Di Huang (Radix Rehmanniae) nourishes yin, supplements body fluids, and clears deficiency fire. Feng Mi (Mel) nourishes the Lung and moistens dryness. Ren Shen (Radix et Rhizoma Ginseng) and Fu Ling (Poria) tonify Spleen qi and eliminate dampness and phlegm that accumulate in the Lung.

CAUTIONS / CONTRAINDICATIONS

Qiong Yu Gao is contraindicated in cases of coughing with blood caused by exterior conditions.

CLINICAL STUDIES AND RESEARCH

1. **Compromised immune system**: In one study of 16 geriatric patients with compromised immunity, administration of Qiong Yu Gao was associated with a general improvement in energy, appetite, and immunity. The treatment protocol was to administer 20-30 grams of the formula twice daily with meals. The herbal formula contained Di Huang (Radix Rehmanniae), Ren Shen (Radix et Rhizoma Ginseng), Fu Ling (Poria), Mai Dong (Radix Ophiopogonis), Tian Dong (Radix Asparagi), Di Gu Pi (Cortex Lycii), and Feng Mi (Mel).[1]

2. **Others**: Qiong Yu Gao has also been used to treat diabetes mellitus and dermatitis.

HERB-DRUG INTERACTION

Angiotensin-converting enzyme (ACE) inhibitors-induced cough: Administration of Qiong Yu Gao was found to be effective in preventing dry cough associated with ACE inhibitors.[2]

References
1. Guo Wai Yi Xue (Foreign Medicine) 1995;2:36.
2. Guo Wai Yi Xue (Foreign Medicine) 1995;2:36.

Qiong Yu Gao (Beautiful Jade Paste)

Diagnosis	Signs and Symptoms	Treatment	Herbs
Lung yin and Spleen qi deficiencies	• Dry, non-productive cough with streaks of blood and dry throat: Lung yin deficiency with deficiency fire • Generalized deficiency and debility, muscle wasting, fatigue and shortness of breath: Spleen qi deficiency	• Nourishes yin and moistens the Lung • Tonifies qi and strengthens the Spleen	• Di Huang (Radix Rehmanniae) nourishes yin, supplements body fluids, and clears deficiency fire. • Feng Mi (Mel) nourishes the Lung and moistens dryness. • Ren Shen (Radix et Rhizoma Ginseng) and Fu Ling (Poria) tonify Spleen qi and eliminate dampness and phlegm in the Lung.

1042

Chinese Herbal Formulas and Applications

Mài Mén Dōng Tāng (Ophiopogonis Decoction)

麥門冬湯
麦门冬汤

Pinyin Name: *Mai Men Dong Tang*
Literal Name: Ophiopogonis Decoction
Alternate Name: Ophiopogon Combination
Original Source: *Jin Gui Yao Lue* (Essentials from the Golden Cabinet) by Zhang Zhong-Jing in the Eastern Han Dynasty

COMPOSITION

Mai Dong (Radix Ophiopogonis)	7 cups [60-70g]
Ban Xia (Rhizoma Pinelliae)	1 cup [10-18g]
Ren Shen (Radix et Rhizoma Ginseng)	9g [6-9g]
Geng Mi (Semen Oryzae)	0.3 cup [6g]
Da Zao (Fructus Jujubae)	12 pieces [3-4 pieces]
Gan Cao (Radix et Rhizoma Glycyrrhizae)	6g [6g]

DOSAGE / PREPARATION / ADMINISTRATION

The source text states to cook the ingredients with 12 cups [2,400 mL] of water until the liquid is reduced to 6 cups [1,200 mL]. Take 1 cup [200 mL] of the warm, strained decoction three times during the day and once at night. Today, this formula may be prepared as a decoction with the doses suggested in brackets.

CHINESE THERAPEUTIC ACTIONS

1. Nourishes Lung and Stomach yin
2. Redirects reversed flow of qi and harmonizes the middle *jiao*

CLINICAL MANIFESTATIONS

1. Lung yin deficiency: coughing with difficult-to-expectorate sputum, coughing or spitting of saliva, dry mouth and throat, feelings of heat in the palms and soles, a red tongue body with scanty tongue coating, and a deficient, rapid pulse.

2. Stomach yin deficiency: nausea, vomiting, thirst, dry throat, a red tongue body with scanty tongue coating, and a deficient, rapid pulse.

CLINICAL APPLICATIONS

Nausea, vomiting, morning sickness, dry mouth and throat, stomach cramps, gastritis, peptic ulcer disease, chronic atrophic gastritis, bronchitis, cough, cough from interstitial pneumonia, postinfectious cough, and Sjogren's syndrome.

EXPLANATION

Mai Men Dong Tang (Ophiopogonis Decoction) is designed to treat Lung and/or Stomach yin deficiencies with deficiency fire rising. The deficiency fire disrupts normal flow of Lung qi, and causes it to move upward instead of downward, which produces cough. Moreover, deficiency fire damages body fluids, and as a result, patients experience sputum that cannot be easily expectorated, thirst

Mai Men Dong Tang (Ophiopogonis Decoction)

Diagnosis	Signs and Symptoms	Treatment	Herbs
Lung and/or Stomach yin deficiencies	• Coughing: reversed flow of Lung qi • Nausea and vomiting: reversed flow of Stomach qi • Difficult-to-expectorate sputum, thirst, dry mouth and throat, and sensations of heat in the palms and soles: deficiency fire • Red tongue with scanty tongue coating, and a deficient, rapid pulse: yin-deficient fire	• Nourishes Lung and Stomach yin • Corrects reversed flow of qi and harmonizes the middle *jiao*	• *Mai Dong* (Radix Ophiopogonis) nourishes yin and clears deficiency fire. • *Ban Xia* (Rhizoma Pinelliae) corrects the reversed flow of qi and dissolves phlegm. • *Ren Shen* (Radix et Rhizoma Ginseng) tonifies qi and generates body fluids. • *Geng Mi* (Semen Oryzae), *Da Zao* (Fructus Jujubae), and *Gan Cao* (Radix et Rhizoma Glycyrrhizae) nourish the Spleen and Stomach.

DRYNESS-RELIEVING FORMULAS

15

1043

Chapter 15 – Dryness-Relieving Formulas   Section 2 – Nourishing and Moistening Formulas

Mài Mén Dōng Tāng (Ophiopogonis Decoction)

and dry mouth and throat. Stomach yin deficiency may lead to reversed flow of qi upwards, causing nausea and vomiting. Sensations of heat in the palms and soles, a red tongue with a scanty tongue coating, and deficient, rapid pulse are typical signs of yin-deficient fire.

This formula contains *Mai Dong* (Radix Ophiopogonis) to nourish Lung and Stomach yin and clear deficiency fire. *Ban Xia* (Rhizoma Pinelliae) corrects the reversed flow of qi and dissolves phlegm. These two herbs also provide mutual checks and balances, as *Mai Dong* (Radix Ophiopogonis) controls the drying nature of *Ban Xia* (Rhizoma Pinelliae), while *Ban Xia* (Rhizoma Pinelliae) checks the cloying nature of *Mai Dong* (Radix Ophiopogonis). *Ren Shen* (Radix et Rhizoma Ginseng) combines with *Mai Dong* (Radix Ophiopogonis) to tonify the qi and generate body fluids. *Geng Mi* (Semen Oryzae), *Da Zao* (Fructus Jujubae), and *Gan Cao* (Radix et Rhizoma Glycyrrhizae) nourish the Spleen and Stomach and tonify *zhong* (central) *qi*.

MODIFICATIONS

- With tidal fever, add *Yin Chai Hu* (Radix Stellariae) and *Di Gu Pi* (Cortex Lycii).
- When there is severe damage to the body fluids, add *Bei Sha Shen* (Radix Glehniae) and *Yu Zhu* (Rhizoma Polygonati Odorati).
- With thirst and irritability, add *Shi Gao* (Gypsum Fibrosum) and *Zhi Mu* (Rhizoma Anemarrhenae).
- With burning epigastric pain or dry heaves caused by Stomach yin deficiency, add *Bai He* (Bulbus Lilii).

CAUTIONS / CONTRAINDICATIONS

Mai Men Dong Tang is not suitable for atrophy of the Lung characterized by deficiency and cold.[1]

PHARMACOLOGICAL EFFECTS

1. **Antitussive**: According to various *in vitro* studies, administration of *Mai Men Dong Tang* was associated with antitussive effects to stop cough.[2] The mechanism of this antitussive effect was attributed in part to *Gan Cao* (Radix et Rhizoma Glycyrrhizae), which contain a potent antitussive compound, liquilitin apioside.[3]

2. **Respiratory**: *Mai Men Dong Tang* has been shown to have mucoactive effect on the production or composition of airway secretions, resulting in increased effectiveness of mucociliary clearance. In addition, *Mai Men Dong Tang* also reduced airway hyper-responsiveness by inhibiting the release of acetylcholine from vagus nerve terminals. Clinically, it has been used with success to treat bronchitis and pharyngitis accompanying severe dry cough.[4,5]

3. **Hypoglycemic**: Administration of a water extract of *Mai Men Dong Tang* at 500 mg/kg given via intraperitoneal injection was shown to decrease blood glucose in mice with hereditary diabetes mellitus.[6]

4. **Beta-adrenergic**: According to a study in canines, administration of *Mai Men Dong Tang* potentiated beta-adrenergic functioning in airway smooth muscle, which reflects the efficacy of this formula to treat asthma and airway hyper-responsiveness.[7]

CLINICAL STUDIES AND RESEARCH

1. **Nausea and vomiting**: One study reported 92.8% effectiveness using modified *Mai Men Dong Tang* to treat stubborn nausea and vomiting characterized by Stomach yin deficiency. The duration of treatment ranged from 3 to 9 packs of herbs. The herbal formula contained *Mai Dong* (Radix Ophiopogonis), *Ban Xia* (Rhizoma Pinelliae), *Ren Shen* (Radix et Rhizoma Ginseng), *Zhi Gan Cao* (Radix et Rhizoma Glycyrrhizae Praeparata cum Melle), *Geng Mi* (Semen Oryzae), *Da Zao* (Fructus Jujubae), *Zhu Ru* (Caulis Bambusae in Taenia), *Shi Hu* (Caulis Dendrobii), and *Pi Pa Ye* (Folium Eriobotryae). Of 42 patients, the study reported complete recovery in 20 cases, significant improvement in 15 cases, moderate improvement in 4 cases, and no effect in 3 cases.[8]

2. **Morning sickness**: One study reported marked effectiveness in the treatment of nausea and vomiting in 20 women using *Mai Men Dong Tang* plus *Gou Qi Zi* (Fructus Lycii), *Zhu Ru* (Caulis Bambusae in Taenia), and *Sheng Jiang* (Rhizoma Zingiberis Recens). The herbs were given in decoction daily.[9]

3. **Dry mouth and throat**: Administration of *Mai Men Dong Tang* was associated with marked success in 258 patients with dry mouth and throat due to various causes (radiation treatment, pharyngitis, and others). The formula was given in extract form, at 9g per day, for 1 and 4 weeks.[10]

4. **Stomach cramps**: One study reported success using *Mai Men Dong Tang* to treat gastrointestinal cramps with nausea, vomiting, poor appetite, and other symptoms. A total of 3 packs of herbs were given in decoction.[11]

5. **Gastritis**: One study reported 78.57% effectiveness using modified *Mai Men Dong Tang* to treat 70 cases of chronic gastritis. Modifications to the base formula included the addition of *Si Ni San* (Frigid Extremities Powder) for Liver and Stomach disharmony; *Ban Xia Xie Xin Tang* (Pinellia Decoction to Drain the Epigastrium) for the presence of both cold and heat; *Li Zhong Tang* (Regulate the Middle Decoction) or *Xiao Jian Zhong Tang* (Minor Construct the Middle Decoction) for deficiency and cold of the Spleen and Stomach; and modifications of *Mai Men Dong Tang* for Stomach yin deficiency. The treatment

1044

Mài Mén Dōng Tāng (Ophiopogonis Decoction)

protocol was to administer one pack of herbs in decoction daily, for each 1 month course of treatment.[12]

6. **Chronic atrophic gastritis**: In one study, 30 patients with chronic atrophic gastritis were treated with good results using *Mai Men Dong Tang*. Clinical results include relief of symptoms, such as bloating, distention, and abdominal pain.[13]

7. **Peptic ulcer disease**: One study reported a 95% effectiveness using modified *Mai Men Dong Tang* to treat 19 patients with peptic ulcer with a history of 1-5 years of illness. Most patients reported relief of symptoms within an average of 9 packs of herbs.[14]

8. **Bronchitis**: According to one study, use of 9 grams per day of extract of *Mai Men Dong Tang* was associated with marked improvement for treatment of chronic bronchitis in 20 patients (5 males and 15 females). The study noted that 17 of 20 patients had a dry non-productive cough.[15]

9. **Cough**: According to one study, administration of *Mai Men Dong Tang* was associated with marked antitussive effects in both asthmatic and non-asthmatic patients. *Mai Men Dong Tang* was found to significantly improve the cough threshold value in 76% of patients with bronchial asthma, and in 82% without bronchial asthma. The study stated that *Mai Men Dong Tang* is an effective therapeutic preparation for cough hypersensitivity accompanying chronic diseases involving coughing, especially in cases of severe allergic inflammation.[16]

10. **Cough from interstitial pneumonia**: According to one case report, use of *Mai Men Dong Tang* was associated with dramatic relief of intractable dry cough within 10 days in a 50 year-old woman with progressive systemic sclerosis accompanied by interstitial pneumonia. Prior to herbal treatment, she was given a variety of antitussive agents over a one year period without success. The researchers stated that *Mai Men Dong Tang* may be a good antitussive agent for interstitial pneumonia associated with a dry cough that is resistant to other antitussives.[17]

11. **Postinfectious cough**: *Mai Men Dong Tang* was shown in many studies to be effective in the management of postinfectious cough.[18,19] According to one case study, use of *Mai Men Dong Tang* was associated with marked effects to suppress cough in a 63-year-old woman with interstitial lung disease and increased sensitivity of the cough reflex. Clinical improvements included subjective relief of cough, decreased cough scores, improved quality of life scores, and improved sensitivity of the cough reflex measured by inhalation of capsaicin.[20]

12. **Sjogren's syndrome**: According to one reports, *Mai Men Dong Tang* was used successfully to treat Sjogren's syndrome, a chronic inflammatory autoimmune disease characterized by dryness of mucous membranes. In this report, *Mai Men Dong Tang* significantly increased salivary secretion in 38 patients with Sjogren's syndrome.[21]

HERB-DRUG INTERACTION

- **Enalapril-induced cough**: Administration of *Mai Men Dong Tang* was found to be effective in treating 5 patients with dry cough induced by use of enalapril for 12 to 65 weeks. The treatment protocol was to administer the herbs in extract form, 9 grams per day in three equally-divided doses. Of 5 patients, the study reported significant improvement in 2 cases, moderate improvement in 2 cases, and no benefit in 1 case. Most patients responded within 2 to 4 days of herbal therapy, with no side effects noted.[22] The mechanisms were attributed to antitussive and mucoactive effects of *Mai Men Dong Tang*.[23]

- **Capsaicin-induced cough**: According to one study of 21 bronchial asthmatics with cough sensitivity to capsaicin, administration of 9 g/day of *Mai Men Dong Tang* significantly increased the cough threshold. The study noted that *Mai Men Dong Tang* was most effective in women, in asthmatic subjects with severe airway inflammation, and in patients having a disease duration of less than 1 year.[24]

TOXICOLOGY

Administration of *Mai Men Dong Tang* was associated with one case report of Stevens-Johnson syndrome. According to the report, after ingestion of this herbal formula, a 66-year-old female started to develop bullous and eroded lesions on the skin of her entire body and the mucous membranes of her oral cavity, conjunctiva, and cornea. A challenge test was done with a one hundredth dose, and it was positive at 72 hours. She was treated with methylprednisolone for a total of 5 days.[25]

RELATED FORMULA

Mài Mén Yǎng Yīn Tāng

(Ophiopogonis Decoction to Nourish the Yin)

麥門養陰湯
麦门养阴汤

Pinyin Name: *Mai Men Yang Yin Tang*

Literal Name: Ophiopogonis Decoction to Nourish the Yin

Original Source: *Guang An Men Yi Yuan* (Guang An Men Hospital) in 1990

Mai Dong (Radix Ophiopogonis)
Tian Dong (Radix Asparagi)
Bei Sha Shen (Radix Glehniae)
Nan Sha Shen (Radix Adenophorae)
Bai He (Bulbus Lilii)

Chapter 15 – Dryness-Relieving Formulas   *Section 2 – Nourishing and Moistening Formulas*

Mài Mén Dōng Tāng (Ophiopogonis Decoction)

Xi Yang Shen (Radix Panacis Quinquefolii)

Zhi Gan Cao (Radix et Rhizoma Glycyrrhizae Praeparata cum Melle)

Geng Mi (Semen Oryzae)

Da Zao (Fructus Jujubae)

Mai Men Yang Yin Tang (Ophiopogonis Decoction to Nourish the Yin) primarily treats chronic consumptive disorders characterized by the presence of dryness and deficiencies of yin and body fluids. Clinical manifestations include thirst, dry mouth, non-productive cough, constipation, dry stools, and general presentation of dryness in chronic consumptive disorders affecting the Lung and Stomach. This formula contains herbs that nourish Lung and Stomach yin, replenish body fluids, and harmonize the middle *jiao*.

AUTHORS' COMMENTS

Lung and/or Stomach yin deficiency(ies) with deficiency fire rising is a delicate condition that needs to be treated carefully. Strong heat-clearing herbs such as *Huang Lian* (Rhizoma Coptidis) and *Huang Qin* (Radix Scutellariae) are not appropriate, as they will consume yin and worsen the condition. Therefore, herbs such as *Mai Dong* (Radix Ophiopogonis) are used since they have gentle effects to nourish yin and clear deficiency fire. Because *Mai Dong* (Radix Ophiopogonis) is mild in potency, a large amount (60-70g) is needed or the effects will not be realized.

Mai Men Dong Tang and *Qing Zao Jiu Fei Tang* (Eliminate Dryness and Rescue the Lungs Decoction) both treat cough, dyspnea, and asthma caused by Lung yin deficiency.

• *Mai Men Dong Tang* moistens the Lung and replenishes Stomach yin to clear interior yin deficiency with heat.

• *Qing Zao Jiu Fei Tang* treats cough and Lung qi reversal caused by warm-dryness attacking from the exterior and injuring Lung yin.[26]

References

1. *Zhong Yao Ming Fang Yao Li Yu Ying Yong* (Pharmacology and Applications of Famous Herbal Formulas) 1989;614-615.
2. *Guo Wai Yi Xue* (Foreign Medicine) 1993;6:29.
3. Kamei J, Nakamura R, Ichiki H, Kubo M. Antitussive principles of Glycyrrhizae radix, a main component of the Kampo preparations Bakumondo-to (Mai-men-dong-tang). Eur J Pharmacol 2003 May 23;469(1-3):159-63.
4. Miyata T. Novel approach to respiratory pharmacology--pharmacological basis of cough, sputum and airway clearance. Yakugaku Zasshi 2003 Dec;123(12):987-1006.
5. Aizawa H, Yoshida M, Inoue H, Hara N. Traditional oriental herbal medicine, Bakumondo-to, suppresses vagal neuro-effector transmission in guinea pig trachea. J Asthma 2003;40(5):497-503.
6. *Guo Wai Yi Xue* (Foreign Medicine) 1981;6:10.
7. Tamaoki J, Chiyotani A, Takeyama K, Kanemura T, Sakai N, Konno K. Potentiation of beta-adrenergic function by saiboku-to and bakumondo-to in canine bronchial smooth muscle. Jpn J Pharmacol 1993 Jun;62(2):155-9.
8. *He Nan Zhong Yi* (Henan Chinese Medicine) 1990;1:21.
9. *Zhong Yi Yao Xue Bao* (Report of Chinese Medicine and Herbology) 1986;2:38.
10. *Guo Wai Yi Xue* (Foreign Medicine) 1995;3:30.
11. *Si Chuan Zhong Yi* (Sichuan Chinese Medicine) 1991;9:29.
12. *An Hui Zhong Yi Xue Yuan Xue Bao* (Journal of Anhui University School of Medicine) 1994;2:25.
13. *Shi Yong Zhong Xi Yi Jie He Za Zhi* (Practical Journal of Integrated Chinese and Western Medicines) 1998;7:631.
14. *Zhong Yi Za Zhi* (Journal of Chinese Medicine) 1964;11:11.
15. *Guo Wai Yi Xue* (Foreign Medicine) 1993;6:29.
16. Watanabe N, Gang C, Fukuda T. The effects of bakumondo-to (Mai-Men-Dong-Tang) on asthmatic and non-asthmatic patients with increased cough sensitivity. Nihon Kokyuki Gakkai Zasshi 2004 Jan;42(1):49-55.
17. Mizushima Y, Hirata A, Hori T, Sawazaki S, Sugiyama E, Kobayashi M. Antitussive effect of herbal medicine bakumondo-to: a case report. American Journal of Chinese Medicine 1996;24(3-4):321-5.
18. Isohama Y, Kai H, Miyata T. Bakumondo-to, a traditional herbal medicine, stimulates phosphatidylcholine secretion, through the synergistic cross-talk between different signal transduction systems in alveolar type II cells. Nippon Yakurigaku Zasshi 1997 Oct;110 Suppl 1:120P-125P.
19. Fujimori K, Suzuki E, Arakawa M. Clinical features of postinfectious chronic cough. Arerugi 1997 May;46(5):420-5.
20. Fujimori K, Suzuki E, Gejyo F. Effect of Bakumondo-to on increased sensitivity of the cough reflex in a Sjogren syndrome patient with interstitial lung disease. Arerugi 2001 Apr;50(4):407-13.
21. Ohno S, Suzuki T, Dohi Y. The effect of bakumondo-to on salivary secretion in Sjogren syndrome. Ryumachi 1990 Feb;30(1):10-6.
22. *Guo Wai Yi Xue* (Foreign Medicine) 1993;1:29.
23. Miyata T. Novel approach to respiratory pharmacology--pharmacological basis of cough, sputum and airway clearance. Yakugaku Zasshi 2003 Dec;123(12):987-1006.
24. Watanabe N, Cheng G, Fukuda T. Effects of Bakumondo-to (Mai-Men-Dong-Tang) on cough sensitivity to capsaicin in asthmatic patients with cough hypersensitivity. Arerugi 2003 May;52(5):485-91.
25. Mochitomi Y, Inoue A, Kawabata H, Ishida S, Kanzaki T. Stevens-Johnson syndrome caused by a health drink (Eberu) containing ophiopogonis tuber. Journal of Dermatology 1998 Oct;25(10):662-5.
26. Wang MZ, et al. *Zhong Yi Xue Wen Da Ti Ku* (Questions and Answers on Traditional Chinese Medicine: Herbal Formulas).

1046

Shā Shēn Mài Dōng Tāng (Glehnia and Ophiopogonis Decoction)

沙參麥冬湯
沙参麦冬汤

Pinyin Name: *Sha Shen Mai Dong Tang*
Literal Name: Glehnia and Ophiopogonis Decoction
Alternate Name: Glehnia and Ophiopogon Combination
Original Source: *Wen Bing Tiao Bian* (Systematic Differentiation of Warm Disease) by Wu Ju-Tong in 1798

COMPOSITION

Sha Shen (Radix Glehniae seu Adenophorae)	9g
Mai Dong (Radix Ophiopogonis)	9g
Yu Zhu (Rhizoma Polygonati Odorati)	6g
Tian Hua Fen (Radix Trichosanthis)	4.5g
Sang Ye (Folium Mori)	4.5g
Bai Bian Dou (Semen Lablab Album)	4.5g
Gan Cao (Radix et Rhizoma Glycyrrhizae)	3g

DOSAGE / PREPARATION / ADMINISTRATION

Cook the ingredients with 5 cups of water until the liquid is reduced to 2 cups. Take the decoction once daily.

CHINESE THERAPEUTIC ACTIONS

1. Clears and nourishes the Lung and Stomach
2. Promotes secretion of body fluids and moistens dryness

CLINICAL MANIFESTATIONS

Dryness damaging Lung and Stomach yin: dry throat, thirst, fever, dry coughing, and dry, sticky sputum.

CLINICAL APPLICATIONS

Atrophic gastritis, epigastric pain, lung cancer, pneumonia, bronchitis, dry cough, cough and wheezing in children, and diabetes mellitus.

EXPLANATION

Sha Shen Mai Dong Tang (Glehnia and Ophiopogonis Decoction) nourishes Lung and Stomach yin, promotes secretion of body fluids, and moistens dryness. It utilizes *Sha Shen* (Radix Glehniae seu Adenophorae) and *Mai Dong* (Radix Ophiopogonis) to promote generation of fluids, moisten dryness, and nourish Lung and Stomach yin. These two herbs also help to clear heat and dryness. *Yu Zhu* (Rhizoma Polygonati Odorati) and *Tian Hua Fen* (Radix Trichosanthis) promote generation of fluids and relieve thirst. *Sang Ye* (Folium Mori) releases warmth and dryness from the Lung. *Bai Bian Dou* (Semen Lablab Album) and *Gan Cao* (Radix et Rhizoma Glycyrrhizae) benefit qi, strengthen the middle *jiao*, and harmonize all of the herbs.

MODIFICATIONS

- With dry coughing and scanty sputum, add *Chuan Bei Mu* (Bulbus Fritillariae Cirrhosae) and *Gua Lou* (Fructus Trichosanthis).
- With chronic cough due to heat, add *Di Gu Pi* (Cortex Lycii) and *Jie Geng* (Radix Platycodonis).
- With constipation, add *Xuan Shen* (Radix Scrophulariae) and *Di Huang* (Radix Rehmanniae).

PHARMACOLOGICAL EFFECTS

Gastrointestinal: *Sha Shen Mai Dong Tang* has been shown to have various effects on the gastrointestinal system. It has protective effects against ethanol-induced stomach ulcers and bleeding in rats. It has a marked protective effect against drug-induced damage to the stomach and its mucous membrane. The mechanism of action is attributed in part to the increased generation of stomach mucous membrane and decreased production of stomach acid. Lastly, the formula is deemed to be more effective at higher dose (20 g/kg) than lower dose (10 g/kg).[1,2]

CLINICAL STUDIES AND RESEARCH

1. **Atrophic gastritis:** Administration of *Sha Shen Mai Dong Tang* was shown to effectively treat chronic atrophic gastritis. According to one study of 88 patients, improvement was seen in 97.7% of the patients, based on symptomatic evaluation, and improvement in 47.7% based on gastroscope evaluation.[3]

2. **Epigastric pain:** *Sha Shen Mai Dong Tang* was used in 40 patients to treat epigastric pain characterized by yin deficiency. Most patients had a history of between 7 and 20 years of illness. Clinical manifestations included dull or burning pain, especially on an empty stomach, a red tongue with little moisture and few fissures, and a fine,

Chapter 15 – Dryness-Relieving Formulas　　　　　　　　*Section 2 – Nourishing and Moistening Formulas*

Shā Shēn Mài Dōng Tāng (Glehnia and Ophiopogonis Decoction)

Sha Shen Mai Dong Tang (Glehnia and Ophiopogonis Decoction)

Diagnosis	Signs and Symptoms	Treatment	Herbs
Dryness damaging Lung and Stomach yin	• Dry coughing and dry, sticky sputum: dryness damaging Lung yin • Dry throat and thirst: dryness damaging Stomach yin	• Clears and nourishes the Lung and Stomach • Generates body fluids and moistens dryness	• *Sha Shen* (Radix Glehniae seu Adenophorae) and *Mai Dong* (Radix Ophiopogonis) promote the generation of fluids, moisten dryness, and nourish Lung and Stomach. • *Yu Zhu* (Rhizoma Polygonati Odorati) and *Tian Hua Fen* (Radix Trichosanthis) promote the generation of fluids and relieve thirst. • *Sang Ye* (Folium Mori) releases the warmth and dryness from the Lung. • *Bai Bian Dou* (Semen Lablab Album) and *Gan Cao* (Radix et Rhizoma Glycyrrhizae) benefit qi, strengthen the middle *jiao,* and harmonize all of the herbs.

rapid pulse. The herbal formula contained *Bei Sha Shen* (Radix Glehniae) 20g, *Mai Dong* (Radix Ophiopogonis) 12g, *Yu Zhu* (Rhizoma Polygonati Odorati) 10g, *Shi Hu* (Caulis Dendrobii) 15g, *Bai He* (Bulbus Lilii) 10g, *Shan Yao* (Rhizoma Dioscoreae) 15g, *Dan Shen* (Radix et Rhizoma Salviae Miltiorrhizae) 15g, and *Zhi Gan Cao* (Radix et Rhizoma Glycyrrhizae Praeparata cum Melle) 10g. The treatment protocol was to cook the herbs in water and administer the decoction in two to three equally-divided doses. Of 40 patients, the study reported complete recovery in 21 patients, marked improvement in 15 patients, moderate improvement in 3 patients, and no benefit in 1 patient. The overall effectiveness was 97.5%.[4]

3. **Lung cancer**: According to one study, administration of *Sha Shen Mai Dong Tang* plus a 10% *Ya Dan Zi* (Fructus Bruceae) preparation in 23 patients with lung cancer was associated with partial relief in 21.74%, stabilization in 39.13%, and no benefit in 39.13% of patients.[5]

4. **Pneumonia**: One study of 25 children with pneumonia reported complete recovery in 22 patients, significant improvement in 2 patients, and no benefit in 1 patient, after treatment with modified *Sha Shen Mai Dong Tang.*[6]

5. **Dry cough**: One study reported 96% effectiveness using modified *Sha Shen Mai Dong Tang* to treat 154 patients with dry cough. The herbal formula contained *Sha Shen* (Radix Glehniae seu Adenophorae), *Mai Dong* (Radix Ophiopogonis), *Yu Zhu* (Rhizoma Polygonati Odorati), *Tian Hua Fen* (Radix Trichosanthis), *Gan Cao* (Radix et Rhizoma Glycyrrhizae), *Sang Ye* (Folium Mori), *Bai Bian Dou* (Semen Lablab Album), and others. Furthermore, *Ge Gen* (Radix Puerariae Lobatae), *Bai Zhi* (Radix Angelicae Dahuricae), *Lian Qiao* (Fructus Forsythiae), *Chai Hu* (Radix Bupleuri), and *Ban Lan Gen* (Radix Isatidis) were added for cough with an exterior condition; and *Ku Xing Ren* (Semen Armeniacae Amarum), *Zhe Bei Mu*

(Bulbus Fritillariae Thunbergii), *Chuan Bei Mu* (Bulbus Fritillariae Cirrhosae), *Yu Xing Cao* (Herba Houttuyniae), and others were added for severe cough. The treatment protocol was to administer the herbs in decoction, for 2 to 5 days per treatment course. Of 154 patients, the study reported complete recovery in 76 patients, significant improvement in 54 patients, moderate improvement in 18 patients, and no benefit in 6 patients.[7]

6. **Cough and wheezing in children**: According to one study, 40 children with cough and wheezing were treated with good results using modified *Sha Shen Mai Dong Tang.* The herbal formula contained *Sha Shen* (Radix Glehniae seu Adenophorae), *Mai Dong* (Radix Ophiopogonis), *Tian Hua Fen* (Radix Trichosanthis), *Yu Zhu* (Rhizoma Polygonati Odorati), *Bai Bian Dou* (Semen Lablab Album), *Sang Ye* (Folium Mori), *Di Long* (Pheretima), *Jie Geng* (Radix Platycodonis), *Pi Pa Ye* (Folium Eriobotryae), and *Gan Cao* (Radix et Rhizoma Glycyrrhizae). Additional modifications were made by adding *Huang Qin* (Radix Scutellariae), and *Shi Gao* (Gypsum Fibrosum) for fever; and *Ma Huang* (Herba Ephedrae) and *Ku Xing Ren* (Semen Armeniacae Amarum) for severe wheezing. The dose of herbs varied depending on the age of the children. Of 40 patients, the study reported complete recovery in 29 patients, improvement in 9 patients, and no benefit in 2 patients.[8]

7. **Diabetes mellitus**: Administration of *Sha Shen Mai Dong Tang* in 186 patients with diabetes mellitus was associated with marked benefit in 106 patients, moderate effectiveness in 60 patients, and no benefit in 20 patients. The overall rate of effectiveness was 89.2%.[9]

AUTHORS' COMMENTS

The source text uses *Sha Shen* (Radix Glehniae seu Adenophorae) as the chief herb but does not specify

Chinese Herbal Formulas and Applications

Shā Shēn Mài Dōng Tāng (Glehnia and Ophiopogonis Decoction)

whether it is *Bei Sha Shen* (Radix Glehniae) or *Nan Sha Shen* (Radix Adenophorae). Both herbs have similar functions to moisten Lung yin, nourish the Stomach and generate body fluids. However, *Bei Sha Shen* (Radix Glehniae) is stronger in nourishing the yin and clearing heat, while *Nan Sha Shen* (Radix Adenophorae) is better to nourish yin and dispel phlegm. Therefore, *Bei Sha Shen* (Radix Glehniae) is generally considered more suitable for *Sha Shen Mai Dong Tang*.

Qing Zao Jiu Fei Tang (Eliminate Dryness and Rescue the Lungs Decoction) and *Sha Shen Mai Dong Tang* both contain *Sang Ye* (Folium Mori), *Mai Dong* (Radix Ophiopogonis), and *Gan Cao* (Radix et Rhizoma Glycyrrhizae) to moisten dryness.

• *Qing Zao Jiu Fei Tang* also contains *Shi Gao* (Gypsum Fibrosum), *Ren Shen* (Radix et Rhizoma Ginseng), *Hei Zhi Ma* (Semen Sesami Nigrum), *E Jiao* (Colla Corii Asini), *Ku Xing Ren* (Semen Armeniacae Amarum), and *Pi Pa Ye* (Folium Eriobotryae). *Qing Zao Jiu Fei Tang* has a stronger effect to ventilate the Lung, dispel external dryness, and clear heat. It strongly nourishes yin and benefits qi.

• *Sha Shen Mai Dong Tang* also contains *Sha Shen* (Radix Glehniae seu Adenophorae), *Yu Zhu* (Rhizoma Polygonati Odorati), *Bai Bian Dou* (Semen Lablab Album), and *Tian Hua Fen* (Radix Trichosanthis). *Sha Shen Mai Dong Tang* has weaker action to ventilate exterior heat-dryness, as its main effect is to moisten the Lung and Stomach and treat dryness with less exterior symptoms.[10]

Sang Xing Tang (Mulberry Leaf and Apricot Kernel Decoction) and *Sha Shen Mai Dong Tang* both treat heat and dryness.

• *Sang Xing Tang* treats heat and dryness injuring the Lung at the exterior level, with manifestations of slight heat sensations in the body, occasional cough, and slight thirst.

• *Sha Shen Mai Dong Tang* treats heat and dryness injuring yin, manifesting in Lung and Stomach yin-deficient symptoms of more severe thirst, dry cough with scanty sputum, nausea, and poor appetite.[11]

References

1. *Zhong Yi Fang Ji Xian Dai Yan Jiu* (Modern Study of Medical Formulae in Traditional Chinese Medicine) 1997.
2. *Bei Jing Zhong Yi Xue Yuan Xue Bao* (Journal of Beijing University School of Medicine) 1994;4:50.
3. *Zhong Xi Yi Jie He Za Zhi* (Journal of Integrated Chinese and Western Medicine) 1986;6:342.
4. *Hu Nan Zhong Yi Za Zhi* (Hunan Journal of Chinese Medicine) 1987;5:22.
5. *Ji Lin Zhong Yi Yao* (Jilin Chinese Medicine and Herbology) 1989;3:19.
6. *He Bei Zhong Yi* (Hebei Chinese Medicine) 1998;1:40.
7. *Si Chuan Zhong Yi* (Sichuan Chinese Medicine) 1987;4:25.
8. *Shang Hai Zhong Yi Yao Za Zhi* (Shanghai Journal of Chinese Medicine and Herbology) 1990;7:29.
9. *Shan Xi Zhong Yi* (Shanxi Chinese Medicine) 1995;11:482.
10. Wang MZ, et al. *Zhong Yi Xue Wen Da Ti Ku* (Questions and Answers on Traditional Chinese Medicine: Herbal Formulas).
11. Wang MZ, et al. *Zhong Yi Xue Wen Da Ti Ku* (Questions and Answers on Traditional Chinese Medicine: Herbal Formulas).

Yù Yè Tāng (Jade Fluid Decoction)

玉液湯

玉液汤

Pinyin Name: *Yu Ye Tang*
Literal Name: Jade Fluid Decoction
Original Source: *Yi Xue Zhong Zhong Can Xi Lu* (Records of Heart-Felt Experiences in Medicine with Reference to the West) by Zhang Xi-Chun in 1918-34

COMPOSITION

Huang Qi (Radix Astragali)	15g
Shan Yao (Rhizoma Dioscoreae)	30g
Ge Gen (Radix Puerariae Lobatae)	4.5g
Zhi Mu (Rhizoma Anemarrhenae)	18g
Tian Hua Fen (Radix Trichosanthis)	9g
Ji Nei Jin (Endothelium Corneum Gigeriae Galli)	6g
Wu Wei Zi (Fructus Schisandrae Chinensis)	9g

DRYNESS-RELIEVING FORMULAS

15

1049

Chapter 15 – Dryness-Relieving Formulas | *Section 2 – Nourishing and Moistening Formulas*

Yù Yè Tāng (Jade Fluid Decoction)

DOSAGE / PREPARATION / ADMINISTRATION
Prepare the ingredients as a decoction.

CHINESE THERAPEUTIC ACTIONS
1. Tonifies qi, nourishes yin and generates body fluids
2. Moistens dryness and relieves thirst

CLINICAL MANIFESTATIONS
Xiao ke (wasting and thirsting) syndrome: polydipsia with constant thirst, polyuria with increased volume and frequency of urination, turbid urine, lethargy, shortness of breath, and a deficient, fine and forceless pulse.

CLINICAL APPLICATIONS
Diabetes mellitus, chronic gastritis, and epigastric pain.

EXPLANATION
Yu Ye Tang (Jade Fluid Decoction) treats chronic *xiao ke* (wasting and thirsting) syndrome with qi and yin deficiencies with dryness and Kidney deficiency. When qi is deficient, water cannot be distributed properly to various parts of the body. With Lung and Stomach dryness, yin and body fluids become damaged. As a result, there is constant thirst and increased intake of water. Because of Kidney deficiency and abnormal water fluid distribution, there may be polyuria with an increase in both volume and frequency of urination, and turbid urine. Lastly, because of qi deficiency, there may be lethargy and shortness of breath. A pulse that is deficient, fine and forceless indicates exhaustion of qi and body fluids.

Huang Qi (Radix Astragali) and *Shan Yao* (Rhizoma Dioscoreae), the two chief herbs, tonify qi and yin

respectively. *Huang Qi* (Radix Astragali) tonifies Spleen qi, which in turn helps to regulate water circulation to relieve thirst. *Shan Yao* (Rhizoma Dioscoreae) relieves polyuria by tonifying the Spleen and consolidating the Kidney, and stops polydipsia by moistening the Lung and generating body fluids. *Ge Gen* (Radix Puerariae Lobatae) causes qi to ascend, which helps to distribute the fluids to the *zang* (solid organs). *Zhi Mu* (Rhizoma Anemarrhenae) and *Tian Hua Fen* (Radix Trichosanthis) nourish yin and moisten dryness to relieve thirst. *Ji Nei Jin* (Endothelium Corneum Gigeriae Galli) assists the Spleen to properly distribute the fluids; its enzymes especially help the Spleen and Stomach with digestion. *Wu Wei Zi* (Fructus Schisandrae Chinensis) astringes yin and consolidates Kidney *jing* (essence).

MODIFICATIONS
- With more qi deficiency, add *Ren Shen* (Radix et Rhizoma Ginseng) or *Xi Yang Shen* (Radix Panacis Quinquefolii).
- With more severe polyuria, add *Shan Zhu Yu* (Fructus Corni).

PHARMACOLOGICAL EFFECTS
Hypoglycemic: *Yu Ye Tang* has been shown in many studies to effectively reduce plasma glucose levels in rabbits and mice. The onset of the hypoglycemic action was observed after approximately 2 to 3 hours, and lasted until 6 to 7.5 hours after oral ingestion of this formula.[1,2,3]

CLINICAL STUDIES AND RESEARCH
1. **Diabetes mellitus**: *Yu Ye Tang* was shown in many studies to effectively treat diabetes mellitus. According to one study of 60 diabetic patients treated with modified *Yu Ye*

Yu Ye Tang (Jade Fluid Decoction)

Diagnosis	Signs and Symptoms	Treatment	Herbs
Xiao ke (wasting and thirsting) syndrome	• Thirst and increased intake of water: dryness damaging yin and body fluids • Polyuria with an increase in both volume and frequency of urination, and turbid urine: Kidney deficiency and abnormal water fluid distribution • Lethargy and shortness of breath: qi deficiency • A deficient, fine and forceless pulse: exhaustion of qi and body fluids.	• Tonifies qi and generates body fluids • Moistens dryness and relieves thirst	• *Huang Qi* (Radix Astragali) tonifies Spleen qi. • *Shan Yao* (Rhizoma Dioscoreae) tonifies the Spleen and Kidney to relieve polyuria and polydipsia. • *Ge Gen* (Radix Puerariae Lobatae) causes qi to ascend, and helps to distribute the fluids. • *Zhi Mu* (Rhizoma Anemarrhenae) and *Tian Hua Fen* (Radix Trichosanthis) nourish yin and moisten dryness to relieve the thirst. • *Ji Nei Jin* (Endothelium Corneum Gigeriae Galli) benefits the Spleen to improve distribution of water and digestion of food. • *Wu Wei Zi* (Fructus Schisandrae Chinensis) astringes yin and consolidates Kidney *jing* (essence).

Yù Yè Tāng (Jade Fluid Decoction)

Tang, 29 had marked improvement, 25 showed moderate improvement, and 6 had no effect. The herbal formula contained *Shan Yao* (Rhizoma Dioscoreae) 30g, *Tian Hua Fen* (Radix Trichosanthis) 30g, *Huang Qi* (Radix Astragali) 25g, *Zhi Mu* (Rhizoma Anemarrhenae) 15g, *Ji Nei Jin* (Endothelium Corneum Gigeriae Galli) 15g, *Ge Gen* (Radix Puerariae Lobatae) 15g, and *Wu Wei Zi* (Fructus Schisandrae Chinensis) 12g. Modifications included addition of *Shan Zhu Yu* (Fructus Corni) 15g, *Yi Zhi* (Fructus Alpiniae Oxyphyllae) 15g, *Fu Pen Zi* (Fructus Rubi) 20g, and *Sang Piao Xiao* (Ootheca Mantidis) 30g for soreness of the lower back and knees, fatigue, frequent urination, and cloudy urine.[4]

Another study reported 94.1% effectiveness using modified *Yu Ye Tang* to treat 51 patients with diabetes characterized by qi and yin deficiencies. The herbal formula was based on the modification of *Yu Ye Tang*, and contained *Ren Shen* (Radix et Rhizoma Ginseng), *Zhi Mu* (Rhizoma Anemarrhenae), *Ji Nei Jin* (Endothelium Corneum Gigeriae Galli), *Wu Wei Zi* (Fructus Schisandrae Chinensis), *Shan Yao* (Rhizoma Dioscoreae), *Huang Qi* (Radix Astragali), *Ge Gen* (Radix Puerariae Lobatae), and *Tian Hua Fen* (Radix Trichosanthis). The treatment protocol was to administer the formula in decoction daily, for 60 days per course of treatment, for a total of 3 to 6 courses. Of 51 patients, the study reported significant improvement in 22 cases, moderate improvement in 26 cases, and no effect in 3 cases.[5]

2. **Chronic gastritis**: One study reported a 69% success rate using modified *Yu Ye Tang* to treat chronic gastritis. Of 127 patients, the study reported complete recovery in 87 cases, improvement in 39 cases, and no effect in 1 case.[6]

3. **Epigastric pain**: Use of *Yu Ye Tang* was beneficial in treating 126 patients with epigastric pain characterized by Stomach yin deficiency. Western medical diagnoses included hypertrophic gastritis, gastric ulcer, duodenal ulcer, superficial gastritis, atrophic gastritis, and others. The herbal formula contained *Shan Yao* (Rhizoma Dioscoreae) 30g, *Huang Qi* (Radix Astragali) 15g, *Zhi Mu* (Rhizoma Anemarrhenae) 18g, *Ji Nei Jin* (Endothelium Corneum Gigeriae Galli) 6g, *Ge Gen* (Radix Puerariae Lobatae) 5g, *Wu Wei Zi* (Fructus Schisandrae Chinensis) 10g, and *Tian Hua Fen* (Radix Trichosanthis) 10g. Other modifications were made as needed. The herbs were cooked in water, and the decoction was administered in two to three equally-divided doses. Of 126 patients, the study reported complete recovery in 87 cases and improvement in 39 cases. The duration of treatment ranged from 30 to 100 packs of herbs.[7]

RELATED FORMULA

Xīao Kě Fāng (Wasting and Thirsting Formula)

消渴方

消渴方

Pinyin Name: *Xiao Ke Fang*
Literal Name: Wasting and Thirsting Formula
Original Source: *An Hui Zhong Yi Xue Yuan* (Anhui University School of Medicine) in 1990

Shan Yao (Rhizoma Dioscoreae)
Huang Qi (Radix Astragali)
Xi Yang Shen (Radix Panacis Quinquefolii)
Xuan Shen (Radix Scrophulariae)
Shi Gao (Gypsum Fibrosum)
Zhi Mu (Rhizoma Anemarrhenae)
Bai Zhu (Rhizoma Atractylodis Macrocephalae)
Cang Zhu (Rhizoma Atractylodis)
Dan Shen (Radix et Rhizoma Salviae Miltiorrhizae)
Hong Hua (Flos Carthami)
Lian Xu (Stamen Nelumbinis)
Lian Zi Xin (Plumula Nelumbinis)

The main actions of *Xiao Ke Fang* (Wasting and Thirsting Formula) are to tonify qi, nourish yin, clear heat, and invigorate the blood to dispel stagnation. It treats chronic *xiao ke* (wasting and thirsting) syndrome with underlying qi and yin deficiencies, accompanied by the rising of deficiency heat and stagnation of blood.

AUTHORS' COMMENTS

Yu Ye Tang is best for chronic *xiao ke* (wasting and thirsting) syndrome with damage to qi and yin. Chief complaints include constant thirst, hunger, and frequent urination.

Yu Ye Tang and *Liu Wei Di Huang Wan* (Six-Ingredient Pill with Rehmannia) both treat *xiao ke* (wasting and thirsting) syndrome. However, there are some differences:

- *Yu Ye Tang* treats *xiao ke* (wasting and thirsting) syndrome caused by dryness secondary to Kidney deficiency, and inability of the qi to properly disseminate fluids throughout the body. Besides thirst and desire to drink, other symptoms include frequent and profuse urination, fatigue, shortness of breath, and a deficient, fine and forceless pulse.

- *Liu Wei Di Huang Wan* treats *xiao ke* (wasting and thirsting) syndrome caused by Kidney and Liver yin deficiencies. Associated symptoms include soreness and weakness of the lower back and knees, dizziness, tinnitus, dry throat and mouth, red tongue with scanty coating, and a fine, rapid pulse.[8]

DRYNESS-RELIEVING FORMULAS

15

Chapter 15 – Dryness-Relieving Formulas　　　　　　　　　　　*Section 2 – Nourishing and Moistening Formulas*

Yù Yè Tāng (Jade Fluid Decoction)

References

1. *Zhong Yao Tong Bao* (Journal of Chinese Herbology) 1994;4:33.
2. *Zhong Yao Yao Li Yu Lin Chuang* (Pharmacology and Clinical Applications of Chinese Herbs) 1992;21.
3. *Zhong Yao Tong Bao* (Journal of Chinese Herbology) 1982;6:32.
4. *He Nan Zhong Yi* (Henan Chinese Medicine) 1990;6:22.
5. *Shan Xi Zhong Yi* (Shanxi Chinese Medicine) 1991;2:51.

6. *Zhe Jiang Zhong Yi Za Zhi* (Zhejiang Journal of Chinese Medicine) 1990;10:437.
7. *Hu Bei Zhong Yi Za Zhi* (Hubei Journal of Chinese Medicine) 1990;6:8.
8. Wang MZ, et al. *Zhong Yi Xue Wen Da Ti Ku* (Questions and Answers on Traditional Chinese Medicine: Herbal Formulas).

Yù Quán Wán (Jade Spring Pill)

玉泉丸

Pinyin Name: *Yu Quan Wan*
Literal Name: Jade Spring Pill
Alternate Names: *Yu Chuan Wan*, Jade-Spring Pill, Jade Source Combination
Original Source: *Za Bing Yuan Liu Xi Zhu* (Wondrous Lantern for Peering into Origin and Development of Miscellaneous Diseases) by Shen Jin-Ao in 1773

COMPOSITION

Tian Hua Fen (Radix Trichosanthis)	45g
Di Huang (Radix Rehmanniae)	30g
Ge Gen (Radix Puerariae Lobatae)	45g
Fu Ling (Poria)	30g
Mai Dong (Radix Ophiopogonis)	30g
Ren Shen (Radix et Rhizoma Ginseng)	30g
Huang Qi (Radix Astragali)	15g
Huang Qi (Radix Astragali), *mi zhi* (fried with honey)	15g
Wu Mei (Fructus Mume), *bei* (stone-baked)	30g
Wu Wei Zi (Fructus Schisandrae Chinensis)	30g
Gan Cao (Radix et Rhizoma Glycyrrhizae)	30g

DOSAGE / PREPARATION / ADMINISTRATION

The source text instructs to stone-bake *Wu Mei* (Fructus Mume), and fry 15g (which represents half of the total amount) of *Huang Qi* (Radix Astragali), with honey. Grind all of the ingredients into powder and form into pills with honey. The pills should resemble large bullets in size. Chew and swallow one pill per dose with warm water.

CHINESE THERAPEUTIC ACTIONS

1. Generates body fluids to relieve thirst
2. Nourishes yin to moisten dryness

CLINICAL MANIFESTATIONS

Xiao ke (wasting and thirsting) syndrome: irritability, thirst, increased intake of water, dry mouth and tongue, and increased urinary frequency. Patients may also have increased hunger, increased food intake, and turbid and sweet urine.

CLINICAL APPLICATIONS

Diabetes mellitus and diabetes insipidus.

EXPLANATION

Yu Quan Wan (Jade Spring Pill) treats *xiao ke* (wasting and thirsting) syndrome, a condition characterized by increased thirst and water intake, increased hunger with food intake, increased urination, and decreased body weight. The underlying etiology of *xiao ke* syndrome is yin deficiency with heat, especially in the Lung, Stomach, and Kidney. In addition to polydipsia, polyphagia, and polyuria, patients may also have irritability.

In this formula, *Tian Hua Fen* (Radix Trichosanthis) and *Di Huang* (Radix Rehmanniae) promote generation of body fluids and clear heat. *Ge Gen* (Radix Puerariae Lobatae) has an ascending function and disperses fluids to various parts of the body. These three herbs work synergistically to promote and disperse fluids, and treat

1052

Chinese Herbal Formulas and Applications

Yù Quán Wán (Jade Spring Pill)

Yu Quan Wan (Jade Spring Pill)

Diagnosis	Signs and Symptoms	Treatment	Herbs
Xiao ke (wasting and thirsting) syndrome	• Increased thirst and water intake with dry mouth and tongue: yin deficiency with Lung heat • Increased hunger and food intake: yin deficiency with Stomach heat • Increased urination: Kidney deficiency	• Generates body fluids to relieve thirst • Nourishes yin to moisten dryness	• *Tian Hua Fen* (Radix Trichosanthis) and *Di Huang* (Radix Rehmanniae) promote generation of body fluids and clear heat. • *Ge Gen* (Radix Puerariae Lobatae) has an ascending function and disperses fluids to various parts of the body. • *Fu Ling* (Poria) strengthens the Spleen and Stomach and promotes normal urination. • *Mai Dong* (Radix Ophiopogonis) nourishes the Lung and Stomach yin. • *Ren Shen* (Radix et Rhizoma Ginseng) and *Huang Qi* (Radix Astragali) tonify qi. • *Wu Mei* (Fructus Mume) and *Wu Wei Zi* (Fructus Schisandrae Chinensis) relieve thirst. • *Gan Cao* (Radix et Rhizoma Glycyrrhizae) harmonizes all of the herbs.

xiao ke (wasting and thirsting) syndrome. *Fu Ling* (Poria) strengthens the Spleen and Stomach and promotes normal urination. *Mai Dong* (Radix Ophiopogonis) nourishes the Lung and Stomach, and addresses the underlying yin deficiency. *Ren Shen* (Radix et Rhizoma Ginseng) and *Huang Qi* (Radix Astragali) tonify qi. *Wu Mei* (Fructus Mume) and *Wu Wei Zi* (Fructus Schisandrae Chinensis) relieve thirst. *Gan Cao* (Radix et Rhizoma Glycyrrhizae) harmonizes all of the herbs in the formula.

MODIFICATIONS

• With more yin deficiency and interior heat, add *Bie Jia* (Carapax Trionycis) and *Mu Dan Pi* (Cortex Moutan).
• With summer-dampness and heat, add *Bai Bian Dou* (Semen Lablab Album).
• With phlegm, add *Chen Pi* (Pericarpium Citri Reticulatae) and *Ban Xia* (Rhizoma Pinelliae).
• With Kidney yang deficiency, add *Tu Si Zi* (Semen Cuscutae), *Fu Zi* (Radix Aconiti Lateralis Praeparata), *Rou Gui* (Cortex Cinnamomi), and *Xian Mao* (Rhizoma Curculiginis).
• With Kidney yin deficiency, add *Xuan Shen* (Radix Scrophulariae), *Gou Qi Zi* (Fructus Lycii), and *Gui Ban* (Plastrum Testudinis).
• With excessive hunger, add *Di Huang* (Radix Rehmanniae) and *Shu Di Huang* (Radix Rehmanniae Praeparata).

CAUTIONS / CONTRAINDICATIONS

Avoid acrid and spicy foods while taking *Yu Quan Wan*.[1]

PHARMACOLOGICAL EFFECTS

Hypoglycemic: Administration of *Yu Quan Wan* in capsules or pills was associated with a reduction in plasma glucose levels in rabbits, with the action beginning approximately 3 hours after oral ingestion, and continuing for approximately 9 to 12 hours.[2]

CLINICAL STUDIES AND RESEARCH

1. **Diabetes mellitus**: Administration of *Yu Quan Wan* four times daily was associated with 86.35% effectiveness in treating 30 patients with type II diabetes mellitus.[3] Another study also reported good results using modified *Yu Quan Wan* four times daily to treat 18 patients with diabetes mellitus characterized by polydipsia, polyphagia, polyuria, and weight loss.[4]

2. **Rebound phenomenon**: One study reported that *Yu Quan Wan* helped to stabilize patients and prevented rebound phenomena as they tapered off hormone treatment for acute arthritis.[5]

TOXICOLOGY

In one acute toxicology study, administration of *Yu Quan Wan* in powder form at 12.5 g/kg/day in two equally-divided doses for two days did not cause any abnormal reactions within a 72 hour period of observation.[6]

AUTHORS' COMMENTS

Yu Ye Tang (Jade Fluid Decoction) and *Yu Quan Wan* are two formulas that treat *xiao ke* (wasting and thirsting)

DRYNESS-RELIEVING FORMULAS

15

1053

Chapter 15 – Dryness-Relieving Formulas   *Section 2 – Nourishing and Moistening Formulas*

Yù Quán Wán (Jade Spring Pill)

syndrome with therapeutic effects to tonify qi, nourish yin, generate body fluids, and moisten dryness.

- *Yu Ye Tang* uses *Huang Qi* (Radix Astragali) and *Shan Yao* (Rhizoma Dioscoreae) as chief herbs, and has a stronger function to tonify qi and yin.
- *Yu Quan Wan* uses *Tian Hua Fen* (Radix Trichosanthis) and *Di Huang* (Radix Rehmanniae) as chief herbs, and has a more potent effect to clear deficiency heat and generate body fluids.

References

1. *Zhong Yao Ming Fang Yao Li Yu Ying Yong* (Pharmacology and Applications of Famous Herbal Formulas) 1989;316-317.
2. *Zhong Cheng Yao* (Study of Chinese Patent Medicine) 1992;1:29.
3. *He Bei Zhong Yi* (Hebei Chinese Medicine) 1993;4:5.
4. *Zhong Yi Za Zhi* (Journal of Chinese Medicine) 1984;2:71.
5. *Ji Lin Zhong Yi Yao* (Jilin Chinese Medicine and Herbology) 1986;5:18.
6. *Zhong Cheng Yao Yan Jiu* (Research of Chinese Patent Medicine) 1982;4:27.

Zēng Yè Tāng (Increase the Fluids Decoction)

增液湯
增液汤

Pinyin Name: *Zeng Ye Tang*
Literal Name: Increase the Fluids Decoction
Original Source: *Wen Bing Tiao Bian* (Systematic Differentiation of Warm Disease) by Wu Ju-Tong in 1798

COMPOSITION

Xuan Shen (Radix Scrophulariae)	30g
Mai Dong (Radix Ophiopogonis)	24g
Di Huang (Radix Rehmanniae)	24g

DOSAGE / PREPARATION / ADMINISTRATION

Cook the ingredients with 8 cups of water and reduce it to 3 cups. For patients with dry mouth, take the entire decoction at once. Repeat this process if the patient does not have a bowel movement.

CHINESE THERAPEUTIC ACTIONS

1. Nourishes yin and clears heat
2. Moistens dryness and facilitates defecation

CLINICAL MANIFESTATIONS

Yangming fu (hollow organs) syndrome with yin and body fluid damage: lack of body fluids characterized by constipation, dry throat, thirst, and a deep, forceless pulse.

CLINICAL APPLICATIONS

Pharyngitis, cheilitis, rhinitis, stomatitis, constipation, hemorrhoids, morning sickness, post-surgical recovery, varicose veins, viral infection, and diabetes mellitus.

EXPLANATION

Zeng Ye Tang (Increase the Fluids Decoction) treats *yangming fu* (hollow organs) syndrome with severe damage

to yin and body fluids. Normally, *yangming fu* syndrome should be treated with downward draining herbs to quickly move stools in constipation. However, if yin and body fluids are already severely damaged due to heat and dryness, downward draining herbs could further damage the yin and body fluids. For this reason, yin-nourishing and dryness-moistening methods are employed in this condition, rather than downward draining herbs, to facilitate defecation.

Xuan Shen (Radix Scrophulariae), which is salty, bitter and cold, softens hardness, moistens dryness, and clears heat. *Mai Dong* (Radix Ophiopogonis) nourishes yin and body fluids. *Di Huang* (Radix Rehmanniae) nourishes yin and moistens dryness. All three herbs work synergistically to promote bowel movements by nourishing yin, moistening dryness, and clearing heat.

This formula is intended to promote defecation by nourishing yin and body fluids. Therefore, the dosage of this formula should be adjusted according to the severity of the constipation.

Zēng Yè Tāng (Increase the Fluids Decoction)

Zeng Ye Tang (Increase the Fluids Decoction)

Diagnosis	Signs and Symptoms	Treatment	Herbs
Yangming fu (hollow organs) syndrome	• Constipation with dry throat and thirst: heat severely damaging yin and body fluids in the Intestines • Deep, forceless pulse: deficiency condition	• Nourishes yin and clears heat • Moistens dryness and facilitates defecation	• *Xuan Shen* (Radix Scrophulariae) softens hardness, moistens dryness, and clears heat. • *Mai Dong* (Radix Ophiopogonis) nourishes yin and body fluids. • *Di Huang* (Radix Rehmanniae) nourishes yin and moistens dryness.

MODIFICATIONS

• For constipation that is unresolved after taking this formula, add a small amount of *Da Huang* (Radix et Rhizoma Rhei) and *Mang Xiao* (Natrii Sulfas) to soften and purge the stool.

• For Stomach yin deficiency with mirror-like tongue coating, and dry lips and throat, add *Sha Shen* (Radix Glehniae seu Adenophorae), *Yu Zhu* (Rhizoma Polygonati Odorati), and *Shi Hu* (Caulis Dendrobii).

CAUTIONS / CONTRAINDICATIONS

Zeng Ye Tang should only be used for constipation caused by heat and dryness severely damaging yin and body fluids. It should not be used indiscriminately to treat constipation, since it does not have any direct purgative or laxative effects.

PHARMACOLOGICAL EFFECTS

1. **Effect on body fluids**: Administration of *Zeng Ye Tang* in mice effectively minimized the loss of body fluids and electrolytes by relieving diarrhea induced by overdose of *Fan Xie Ye* (Folium Sennae).[1]

2. **Anti-inflammatory**: One study reported marked effectiveness in reducing inflammation in mice and rats using a preparation of *Zeng Ye Tang* given via intravenous injection at 25-30 mL/kg for 2 to 3 days.[2]

3. **Antipyretic**: One study reported that *Zeng Ye Tang* had a marked effect to reduce body temperature in rabbits with artificially-induced fever.[3]

CLINICAL STUDIES AND RESEARCH

1. **Pharyngitis**: One study reported 90.7% effectiveness using modified *Zeng Ye Tang* to treat 97 patients with chronic pharyngitis. The herbal formula contained *Xuan Shen* (Radix Scrophulariae), *Mai Dong* (Radix Ophiopogonis), *Jie Geng* (Radix Platycodonis), and *Gan Cao* (Radix et Rhizoma Glycyrrhizae). Of 97 patients, 63 had complete recovery, 25 had moderate improvement, and 9 received no benefit.[4]

2. **Cheilitis**: One study reported that use of modified *Zeng Ye Tang* was effective to treat inflammation of the lips. The herbal formula contained *Xuan Shen* (Radix Scrophulariae), *Di Huang* (Radix Rehmanniae), *Mai Dong* (Radix Ophiopogonis), *Jin Yin Hua* (Flos Lonicerae Japonicae), *Shi Hu* (Caulis Dendrobii), *Mu Dan Pi* (Cortex Moutan), and *Gan Cao* (Radix et Rhizoma Glycyrrhizae). Of 15 patients, the study reported complete recovery in 12 cases, significant improvement in 2 cases, and slight improvement in 1 case.[5]

3. **Rhinitis**: One study reported improvement in 54 of 65 patients with atrophic rhinitis when treated with *Zeng Ye Tang* plus *Ba Zhen Tang* (Eight-Treasure Decoction). In addition to these two formulas, modifications were made by using *Shi Hu* (Caulis Dendrobii) and *Yu Zhu* (Rhizoma Polygonati Odorati) for Stomach yin deficiency; *Mo Han Lian* (Herba Ecliptae) and *Xian He Cao* (Herba Agrimoniae) for nosebleeds; and *Huang Bo* (Cortex Phellodendri Chinensis) and *Zhi Mu* (Rhizoma Anemarrhenae) for foul smells in the nose. Lastly for individuals who suffer from severe rhinitis in fall and winter, *Chi Shao* (Radix Paeoniae Rubra) and larger doses of *Chuan Xiong* (Rhizoma Chuanxiong) and *Dang Gui* (Radix Angelicae Sinensis) were added to the formula.[6]

4. **Stomatitis caused by radiation treatment**: Use of *Zeng Ye Tang* was beneficial among 120 patients with nose cancer to alleviate stomatitis associated with radiation treatment. Clinical manifestations included thirst, dry mouth, thickened saliva, feeling of stickiness in the mouth, redness and swelling of gums, and ulcerations of the oral cavity with severe pain. The herbal formula contained *Di Huang* (Radix Rehmanniae) 12-25g, *Xuan Shen* (Radix Scrophulariae) 18g, *Mai Dong* (Radix Ophiopogonis) 15g, and others as needed. The herbs were cooked in water, and the decoction was administered in three to four equally-divided doses daily. The study reported that the herbs were effective in alleviating side effects associated with radiation treatment such as thirst, thickened saliva, red and swollen gums, ulcerations of the mouth, and pain. Of 120 patients, the study reported complete recovery in 41 cases, significant improvement in 65 cases, moderate improvement in 13 cases, and no effect in 1 case.[7]

Chapter 15 – Dryness-Relieving Formulas　　　　　　*Section 2 – Nourishing and Moistening Formulas*

Zēng Yè Tāng (Increase the Fluids Decoction)

5. **Viral infection**: Administration of modified *Zeng Ye Tang* in 50 children with viral infection was associated with complete recovery in 17 cases, significant improvement in 18 cases, moderate improvement in 13 cases, and no effect in 2 cases. The overall rate of effectiveness was 90%.[8]

6. **Constipation**: One study reported great success using *Zeng Ye Tang* to treat constipation. Of 50 patients, 41 had normal bowel movement within 3 days and 9 within 6 days.[9]

7. **Diabetes mellitus**: Administration of *Zeng Ye Tang* plus *Dang Shen* (Radix Codonopsis), *Shan Zhu Yu* (Fructus Corni) and others was shown in one study to reduce blood glucose levels in 102 patients with type II diabetes mellitus. Of 102 patients, the study reported significant effects in 30 cases, moderate effect in 57 cases, and no effect in 15 cases. The overall rate of effectiveness was 85.3%.[10]

8. **Morning sickness**: Intravenous infusion of 500-1,000 mL of *Zeng Ye Tang* was effective in treating nausea and vomiting in 44 of 45 pregnant women.[11]

9. **Post-surgical recovery**: One study reported good results using *Zeng Ye Tang* for 20 post-surgical patients. Improvements noted included faster recovery of intestinal peristalsis.[12]

10. **Varicose vein**: One study reported complete recovery in all 16 patients with varicose veins and associated sores of the legs, when treated with modified *Zeng Ye Tang*. Modifications included the addition of *Hai Zao* (Sargassum), *Kun Bu* (Thallus Eckloniae), and *Bie Jia* (Carapax Trionycis) for the presence of hardness and nodules in the legs; *Ze Xie* (Rhizoma Alismatis), *Fang Ji* (Radix Stephaniae Tetrandrae), and *Yi Yi Ren* (Semen Coicis) for sores and ulcerations with profuse discharge; *Chuan Lian Zi* (Fructus Toosendan) and *Yan Hu Suo* (Rhizoma Corydalis) for severe pain; and *Ji Xue Teng* (Caulis Spatholobi) and *Hong Hua* (Flos Carthami) for the presence of noticeable dark, purple spots on the legs. Herbs were also applied topically to treat sores and ulcerations.[13]

TOXICOLOGY

According to an acute toxicology study, the LD_{50} of *Zeng Ye Tang* given via intravenous injection is 84.1 g/kg in mice. In a chronic toxicology study in rabbits, administration of a 10% *Zeng Ye Tang* preparation given via intravenous injection daily for 30 days did not contribute to any significant changes in body weight, blood exam, or abnormalities of liver, kidney or heart.[14]

AUTHORS' COMMENTS

In classic texts, constipation characterized by yin and fluid deficiencies is compared to a boat stuck in the riverbed due to low water flow. In such cases, forcefully pushing the boat down the river will only further damage the boat. Instead, the ideal solution is to direct the boat to deeper water, so that it may float and flow smoothly. Similarly, constipation marked by yin and fluid deficiencies cannot be forcefully treated with drastic purgatives and laxatives, which will only further damage yin and consume fluids. Instead, herbs that nourish the yin and moisten dryness must be used to treat the underlying cause of this condition.

References

1. *Zhong Yi Fang Ji Xian Dai Yan Jiu* (Modern Study of Medical Formulae in Traditional Chinese Medicine) 1997;1306.
2. *Zhong Guo Zhong Xi Yi Jie He Za Zhi* (Chinese Journal of Integrative Chinese and Western Medicine) 1982;2:153.
3. *Zhong Yi Fang Ji Xian Dai Yan Jiu* (Modern Study of Medical Formulae in Traditional Chinese Medicine) 1997;1306-1307.
4. *Shan Xi Zhong Yi* (Shanxi Chinese Medicine) 1992;6:248.
5. *Si Chuan Zhong Yi* (Sichuan Chinese Medicine) 1986;12:48.
6. *Zhe Jiang Zhong Yi Za Zhi* (Zhejiang Journal of Chinese Medicine) 1980;5:220.
7. *Guang Xi Zhong Yi Yao* (Guangxi Chinese Medicine and Herbology) 1981;5:25.
8. *Zhong Yi Ming Fang Lin Chuang Xin Yong* (Contemporary Clinical Applications of Classic Chinese Formulas) 2001;723.
9. *Zhong Yi Ming Fang Lin Chuang Xin Yong* (Contemporary Clinical Applications of Classic Chinese Formulas) 2001;723.
10. *Zhong Yi Za Zhi* (Journal of Chinese Medicine) 1985;6:31.
11. *Zhong Yi Za Zhi* (Journal of Chinese Medicine) 1986;12:5.
12. *Zhong Xi Yi Jie He Za Zhi* (Journal of Integrated Chinese and Western Medicine) 1988;7:423.
13. *Xin Zhong Yi* (New Chinese Medicine) 1998;9:45.
14. *Zhong Yi Fang Ji Xian Dai Yan Jiu* (Modern Study of Medical Formulae in Traditional Chinese Medicine) 1997;1312.

Chinese Herbal Formulas and Applications

Chapter 15 — Summary

— Dryness-Relieving Formulas

SECTION 1: DISPERSING AND MOISTENING FORMULAS

Name	Similarities	Differences
Xing Su San (Apricot Kernel and Perilla Leaf Powder)	Relieves cool-dryness	Dispels cool-dryness, ventilates the Lung, dissolves phlegm
Sang Xing Tang (Mulberry Leaf and Apricot Kernel Decoction)	Relieve warm-dryness	Gently clears warm-dryness
Qing Zao Jiu Fei Tang (Eliminate Dryness and Rescue the Lung Decoction)		Strongly clears warm-dryness, nourishes yin, moistens dryness

Xing Su San (Apricot Kernel and Perilla Leaf Powder) dispels exterior cool-dryness, ventilates the Lung, and dissolves phlegm. It is used for exterior cool-dryness characterized by aversion to cold, absence of perspiration, coughing with thin and watery sputum, and headache with stuffy nose.

Sang Xing Tang (Mulberry Leaf and Apricot Kernel Decoction) and *Qing Zao Jiu Fei Tang* (Eliminate Dryness and Rescue the Lung Decoction) both treat warm-dryness affecting the Lung.
- *Sang Xing Tang* is used for <u>mild</u> cases of exterior warm-dryness attacking the Lung. It ventilates the Lung and dispels warm-dryness from the Lung. Clinical manifestations include slight fever, dry coughing with little or no sputum, thirst, and dry throat.
- *Qing Zao Jiu Fei Tang* is employed for <u>severe</u> warm-dryness attacking the Lung. It strongly moistens dryness and nourishes the Lung. The main clinical manifestations include fever, thirst, coughing with no sputum, shortness of breath, and fullness and pain in the chest and hypochondriac region.

SECTION 2: NOURISHING AND MOISTENING FORMULAS

Name	Similarities	Differences
Yang Yin Qing Fei Tang (Nourish the Yin and Clear the Lung Decoction)	Nourish and tonify Lung and Kidney yin	Clears Lung heat
Bai He Gu Jin Tang (Lily Bulb Decoction to Preserve the Metal)		Dissolves phlegm, stops coughing
Bu Fei E Jiao Tang (Tonify the Lung Decoction with Ass-Hide Gelatin)	Nourish Lung yin	Clears heat, stops bleeding, alleviates coughing
Qiong Yu Gao (Beautiful Jade Paste)		Tonifies qi and strengthens the Spleen
Mai Men Dong Tang (Ophiopogonis Decoction)	Nourish and tonify Lung and Stomach yin	Redirects the reversed flow of qi, harmonizes the middle *jiao*
Sha Shen Mai Dong Tang (Glehnia and Ophiopogonis Decoction)		Promotes secretion of body fluids, moistens dryness
Yu Ye Tang (Jade Fluid Decoction)	Nourish yin, generate body fluids, and moisten dryness	Strongly tonifies qi and nourishes yin
Yu Quan Wan (Jade Spring Pill)		Strongly clears deficiency heat and generates body fluids
Zeng Ye Tang (Increase the Fluids Decoction)	Generates body fluids in the Large Intestine, moistens dryness	Clears heat

DRYNESS-RELIEVING FORMULAS

15

1057

Chapter 15 — Summary

Yang Yin Qing Fei Tang (Nourish the Yin and Clear the Lung Decoction) nourishes Lung and Kidney yin and clears Lung heat. It is used mostly for diphtheria with swelling and pain in the throat, dry nose and lips, and a wheezing sound when breathing that resembles asthma conditions.

Bai He Gu Jin Tang (Lily Bulb Decoction to Preserve the Metal) nourishes Lung and Kidney yin, dissolves phlegm, and stops coughing. Due to Lung and Kidney yin-deficient fire, a sore throat and coughing with streaks of blood in the sputum may occur. Other clinical manifestations may include warm sensations in the palms and soles, steaming bones sensations, and night sweats.

Bu Fei E Jiao Tang (Tonify the Lung Decoction with Ass-Hide Gelatin) tonifies the Lung, nourishes yin, relieves coughing, and stops bleeding. Clinical manifestations include coughing, wheezing, dry throat, and bloody sputum.

Qiong Yu Gao (Beautiful Jade Paste) nourishes the Lung yin, benefits Spleen qi. This formula is used for prolonged, dry cough due to Lung yin deficiency. Because this is a chronic condition, qi-deficient signs of shortness of breath and lack of energy are also present.

Mai Men Dong Tang (Ophiopogonis Decoction) nourishes Lung and Stomach yin, corrects the reversed flow of qi, and harmonizes the middle *jiao*. It is used for Lung and Stomach yin deficiencies with manifestations of coughing, sputum that cannot be expectorated easily, vomiting, thirst, and a dry throat and mouth.

Sha Shen Mai Dong Tang (Glehnia and Ophiopogonis Decoction) nourishes the Lung and Stomach, promotes the secretion of body fluids, and moistens dryness. It is most effective for dryness damaging Lung and Stomach yin with signs and symptoms such as dry throat, thirst, fever, dry coughing, and dry, sticky sputum.

Yu Ye Tang (Jade Fluid Decoction) tonifies qi, nourishes yin, and generates body fluids. It is used for *xiao ke* (wasting and thirsting) syndrome with constant thirst, polyuria, turbid urine, lethargy, and shortness of breath.

Yu Quan Wan (Jade Spring Pill) generates body fluids to relieve thirst and nourishes yin to moisten dryness. It treats *xiao ke* (wasting and thirsting) syndrome with yin-deficient heat affecting the Lung, Stomach, and Kidney. Clinical manifestations include irritability, thirst, increased intake of water, dry mouth and tongue, and increased frequency of urination.

Zeng Ye Tang (Increase the Fluids Decoction) nourishes the yin, clears heat, moistens dryness, and promotes defecation. It is indicated for *yangming fu* (hollow organs) syndrome, in which yin has been damaged, resulting in constipation with dry stools.

Chapter 16

— Damp-Dispelling Formulas

王肯堂 Wāng Kěn-Tāng

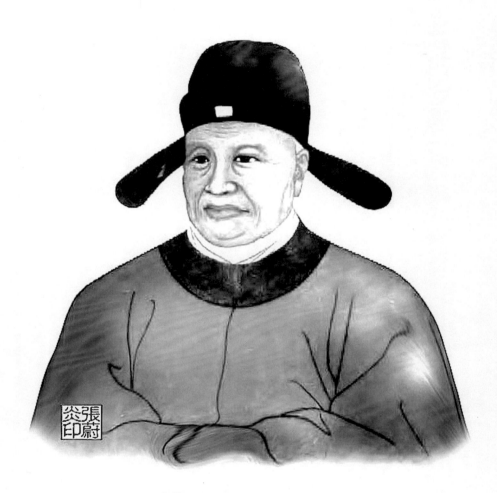

王肯堂 Wāng Kěn-Tāng, 1549 – 1613.

王肯堂 Wāng Kěn-Tāng

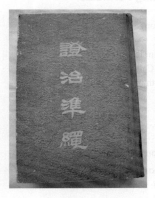

症治准绳 Zheng Zhi Zhun Sheng
(Standards of Patterns and Treatments)
in 1602.

Wang Ken-Tang was born during the Ming dynasty. When he was 17 years old, his mother became seriously ill. She was treated by many famous doctors who made differing diagnoses and prescribed various, sometimes conflicting, treatments. In the end, no one was able to cure her. Her condition slowly deteriorated, and she eventually passed away. Wang Ken-Tang was inspired to study medicine because of this tragic loss.

In his pursuit of medicine, Wang studied many texts and integrated the knowledge of all of the schools of thought that he encountered. In addition to being an excellent clinician, he dedicated the last ten years of his life to documenting his clinical experiences. Wang wrote many books to detail the pathology and treatment of many disorders, including internal medicine, gynecology, pediatrics, external medicine, the treatment of sores and abscesses, and other miscellaneous illnesses. Among his most famous works are:

- 症治准绳 Zheng Zhi Zhun Sheng (Standards of Patterns and Treatments)
- 妇症治准绳 Fu Ke Zheng Zhi Zhun Sheng (Standards of Patterns and Treatments in Gynecology)
- 儿科症治准绳 Er Ke Zheng Zhi Zhun Sheng (Standards of Patterns and Treatments in Pediatrics)
- 外科症治准绳 Wai Ke Zheng Zhi Zhun Sheng (Standards of Patterns and Treatments in External Medicine)
- 痈科症治准绳 Yong Ke Zheng Zhi Zhun Sheng (Standards of Patterns and Treatments in Sores and Abscesses)

Formulas written by Wang Ken-Tang include:
- *Shao Yao Tang* (Peony Decoction)
- *Qing Xin Li Ge Tang* (Clear the Epigastrium and Benefit the Diaphragm Decoction)
- *San Huang Shi Gao Tang* (Three-Yellow and Gypsum Decoction)
- *Qing Liang Yin* (Clearing and Cooling Decoction)
- *Qing Gu San* (Cool the Bones Powder)
- *Si Shen Wan* (Four-Miracle Pill)
- *Dao Shui Fu Ling Tang* (Poria Decoction to Drain Water)
- *Jian Pi Wan* (Strengthen the Spleen Pill)

Dynasties & Kingdoms	Year
Xia Dynasty 夏	2100-1600 BCE
Shang Dynasty 商	1600-1100 BCE
Zhou Dynasty 周	1100-221 BCE
Qin Dynasty 秦	221-207 BCE
Han Dynasty 漢	206 BCE-220
Three Kingdoms 三國	220-280
Western Jin Dynasty 西晉	265-316
Eastern Jin Dynasty 東晉	317-420
Northern and Southern Dynasties 北南朝	420-581
Sui Dynasty 隋	581-618
Tang Dynasty 唐	618-907
Five Dynasties 五代	907-960
Song Dynasty 宋	960-1279
Liao Dynasty 潦	916-1125
Jin Dynasty 金	1115-1234
Yuan Dynasty 元	1271-1368
Ming Dynasty 明	**1368-1644**
Qing Dynasty 清	1644-1911
Republic of China 中華民國	1912-Present Day
People's Republic of China 中華人民共和國	1949-Present Day

Table of Contents

Chapter 16. Damp-Dispelling Formulas ·· **1059**
Biography of Wang Ken-Tang ·· 1060

Section 1. Damp-Drying and Stomach-Harmonizing Formulas ···················· **1068**
Ping Wei San (Calm the Stomach Powder) ·· 1068
   Chai Ping Tang (Bupleurum and Calm the Stomach Decoction) ···················· 1071
Jia Wei Ping Wei San (Modified Calm the Stomach Powder) ···························· 1072
Xiang Sha Ping Wei San (Cyperus and Amomum Powder to Calm the Stomach) ···· 1073
   Xiang Sha Ping Wei San (Cyperus and Amomum Powder to Calm the Stomach) ···· 1075
Bu Huan Jin Zheng Qi San (Rectify the Qi Powder Worth More than Gold) ·········· 1075
Fu Ling Yin (Poria Decoction) ·· 1077
Huo Xiang Zheng Qi San (Agastache Powder to Rectify the Qi) ························ 1079
Liu He Tang (Harmonize the Six Decoction) ·· 1082
   Liu He Tang (Harmonize the Six Decoction) ·· 1083
Ge Hua Jie Cheng San (Pueraria Flower Powder for Detoxification and Awakening) ·· 1084

Section 2. Heat-Clearing and Damp-Dispelling Formulas ·························· **1086**
Yin Chen Hao Tang (Artemisia Scoparia Decoction) ·································· 1086
   Zhi Zi Bai Pi Tang (Gardenia and Phellodendron Decoction) ······················ 1089
   Yin Chen Si Ni Tang (Artemisia Scoparia Decoction for Frigid Extremities) ········ 1089
   Yin Chen Pai Shi Tang (Artemisia Scoparia Decoction to Expel Stone) ············ 1089
Yin Chen Wu Ling San (Artemisia Scoparia and Five-Ingredient Powder with Poria) ·· 1090
San Ren Tang (Three-Nut Decoction) ·· 1092
   Huo Po Xia Ling Tang (Agastache, Magnolia Bark, Pinellia, and Poria Decoction) ·· 1095
   Huang Qin Hua Shi Tang (Scutellaria and Talcum Decoction) ···················· 1095
Gan Lu Xiao Du Dan (Sweet Dew Special Pill to Eliminate Toxins) ·················· 1096
Lian Po Yin (Coptis and Magnolia Bark Decoction) ·································· 1099
Can Shi Tang (Silkworm Droppings Decoction) ······································ 1101
Ba Zheng San (Eight-Herb Powder for Rectification) ································ 1103
   Jia Wei Ba Zheng San (Augmented Eight Herb Powder for Rectification) ·········· 1105
   Fu Fang Ba Zheng San (Revised Eight-Herb Powder) ···························· 1105
   San Jin Pai Shi Tang (Three Gold Decoction to Expel Stone) ······················ 1106
Wu Lin San (Five-Ingredient Powder for Painful Urinary Dysfunction) ·············· 1107
   Huo Xue Tong Lin Tang (Invigorate the Blood to Unblock Dysuria Decoction) ······ 1107
   Qing Re Tong Lin Tang (Clear Heat to Unblock Dysuria Decoction) ················ 1108

Section 3. Water-Regulating and Damp-Resolving Formulas ······················ **1109**
Wu Ling San (Five-Ingredient Powder with Poria) ···································· 1109
   Si Ling San (Four-Ingredient Powder with Poria) ································ 1112
   Bai Mao Gen Tang (Imperata Decoction) ·· 1112
   Fu Ling Tang (Poria Decoction) ·· 1112
Wei Ling Tang (Calm the Stomach and Poria Decoction) ····························· 1113
Zhu Ling Tang (Polyporus Decoction) ·· 1115
Fang Ji Huang Qi Tang (Stephania and Astragalus Decoction) ······················ 1118
   Fang Ji Fu Ling Tang (Stephania and Poria Decoction) ·························· 1120
Wu Pi San (Five-Peel Powder) ·· 1121
   Wu Pi San (Five-Peel Powder) ·· 1123
Jiu Wei Bing Lang Jia Wu Fu Tang (Areca Nine Decoction plus Evodia and Poria) ·· 1123
Mu Fang Ji Tang (Cocculus Decoction) ·· 1125
Fen Xiao Tang (Separate and Reduce Decoction) ···································· 1127
Dao Shui Fu Ling Tang (Poria Decoction to Drain Water) ···························· 1129

Section 4. Warm Formulas that Dissolve Dampness ······························ **1131**
Ling Gui Zhu Gan Tang (Poria, Cinnamon Twig, Atractylodes Macrocephala, and Licorice Decoction) ·· 1131
Gan Cao Gan Jiang Fu Ling Bai Zhu Tang (Licorice, Ginger, Poria and Atractylodes Macrocephala Decoction) ·· 1133
Zhen Wu Tang (True Warrior Decoction) ·· 1135
   Fu Zi Tang (Prepared Aconite Decoction) ·· 1137
Shi Pi San (Bolster the Spleen Powder) ·· 1138
Bi Xie Fen Qing Yin (Dioscorea Hypoglauca Decoction to Separate the Clear) ········ 1140
   Bi Xie Fen Qing Yin (Dioscorea Hypoglauca Decoction to Separate the Clear) ······ 1141

Damp-Dispelling Formulas (Summary) ·· **1143**

Chinese Herbal Formulas and Applications

Chapter 16 — Overview

— Damp-Dispelling Formulas

Definition: Damp-dispelling formulas dry dampness, resolve turbidity, promote urination, and relieve dysuria. Damp-dispelling formulas are used primarily to treat disorders characterized by the accumulation of dampness and water.

Dampness is a yin pathogen that is heavy and stagnant. Damp syndromes are characterized by slow onset, but prolonged duration and frequent recurrence of symptoms. Damp disorders are classified as being either on the exterior (contracted externally) or in the interior (generated internally), but often dampness affects the interior and exterior concomitantly because the external channels and muscles are closely interrelated with the internal *zang fu* organs.

- Externally-contracted dampness occurs as a result of prolonged exposure to wet or damp environmental conditions, such as: rain or humid weather; repeated, direct exposure to water; and wearing sweat-soaked clothes. Externally-contracted dampness invades the exterior levels of the body (skin, muscles, channels, and collaterals) to cause fever, aversion to cold, heaviness of the head and body, painful joints, and edema of the face.
- Internally-generated dampness occurs as a result of inappropriate dietary habits, such as over-consumption of cold or raw foods, sweet or fatty foods, alcohol, and dairy products. These foods create dampness and turbidity, which injure Spleen qi and affect its normal transformation and transportation functions, causing symptoms such as chest and epigastric distention, and stifling sensations, nausea, vomiting, diarrhea, jaundice, edema of the lower limbs, and *lin zheng* (dysuria syndrome).

Damp disorders affect the functioning of the Spleen, Lung, and Kidney. The Spleen absorbs water, the Lung distributes water, and the Kidney eliminates water. Disorders in any of these organs cause abnormal circulation of water, leading to the accumulation of water and formation of dampness. Furthermore, obstruction of the *San Jiao* pathway can cause damp accumulation, and obstruction of the Urinary Bladder may cause dysuria. Because damp disorders are frequently associated with imbalances of the *zang fu* organs, accurate diagnosis is essential to successful treatment.

In addition, dampness may be complicated by other disorders and factors. It can combine with other environmental factors (wind, cold, heat, and summer-heat); it may affect different parts of the body (exterior or interior, upper or lower); and it may affect patients with various constitutions (deficiency or excess). Treatment methods vary, depending on the complications and patient conditions. Generally, if dampness is located in the upper or external parts of the body, exterior-releasing herbs are used to disperse dampness. If dampness is located in the lower or internal parts of the body, one may use aromatic, bitter, and drying herbs to resolve dampness, or sweet and bland diuretic herbs to dispel dampness. If dampness is combined with cold factors, the yang should be warmed and cold dispelled. If dampness is combined with heat, herbs that clear heat should be employed as well. If the body is deficient and the dampness is abundant, one needs to strengthen the body and dispel dampness. Lastly, if damp accumulation causes qi stagnation, herbs that invigorate qi circulation should be added. Note: Formulas that dispel wind-damp to treat *bi zheng* (painful obstruction syndrome) are discussed in Chapter 17: Wind-Damp Dispelling Formulas.

~
Damp-dispelling formulas treat accumulation of dampness and water at the exterior or in the interior.
~

DAMP-DISPELLING FORMULAS

16

Chapter 16 – Damp-Dispelling Formulas

Chapter 16 — Overview

SUBCATEGORIES OF ACTION

Because of the complexity of damp disorders, damp-dispelling formulas are divided into four sub-categories to reflect the nature of the disorders, and the corresponding characteristics of the formulas.

1. Damp-Drying and Stomach-Harmonizing Formulas

These formulas treat damp stagnation and turbidity that are accompanied by disharmony of the Spleen and Stomach. Typical clinical manifestations include epigastric and abdominal distention and fullness, belching, nausea, vomiting, acid regurgitation, diarrhea, decreased appetite, and fatigue.

Dampness in patterns of Spleen and Stomach disharmony is usually treated with bitter and warm herbs to dry dampness, or with aromatic herbs to resolve dampness, such as *Cang Zhu* (Rhizoma Atractylodis), *Bai Bian Dou* (Semen Lablab Album), *Huo Xiang* (Herba Agastaches), and *Hou Po* (Cortex Magnoliae Officinalis). Exemplar formulas include *Ping Wei San* (Calm the Stomach Powder) and *Huo Xiang Zheng Qi San* (Agastache Powder to Rectify the Qi).

2. Heat-Clearing and Damp-Dispelling Formulas

These formulas address either exterior damp-heat, interior damp-heat, or damp-heat in the lower *jiao*. Clinical applications include summer-heat, jaundice, *re lin* (heat dysuria), and *wei bi* (atrophic painful obstruction).

Herbs commonly used to clear heat and resolve dampness include *Yin Chen* (Herba Artemisiae Scopariae), *Yi Yi Ren* (Semen Coicis), and *Hua Shi* (Talcum). Herbs that clear heat and dry dampness include *Huang Lian* (Rhizoma Coptidis), *Huang Bo* (Cortex Phellodendri Chinensis), *Huang Qin* (Radix Scutellariae), and *Zhi Zi* (Fructus Gardeniae). Representative formulas are *Yin Chen Hao Tang* (Artemisia Scoparia Decoction), *San Ren Tang* (Three-Nut Decoction), and *Ba Zheng San* (Eight-Herb Powder for Rectification).

3. Water-Regulating and Damp-Resolving Formulas

These formulas treat excess damp accumulation blocking the water pathways, with clinical manifestations of edema, uroschesis, retention of urine, turbid urine, and diarrhea. In this case, herbs are used to dispel dampness and resolve water accumulation through urination.

Commonly used herbs include *Fu Ling* (Poria), *Ze Xie* (Rhizoma Alismatis), and *Zhu Ling* (Polyporus). Exemplar formulas that regulate water and resolve dampness include *Wu Ling San* (Five-Ingredient Powder with Poria) and *Wu Pi Yin* (Five-Peel Decoction).

4. Warm Formulas that Dissolve Dampness

These formulas treat cold-type damp disorders, in which yang fails to transform water. Clinical manifestations include edema of the body and legs, urinary difficulty, *tan yin* (phlegm retention), *bi zheng* (painful obstruction syndrome), and leg *qi* caused by damp-cold accumulation.

These disorders are treated with herbs that warm yang and regulate water, such as *Gui Zhi* (Ramulus Cinnamomi), *Bai Zhu* (Rhizoma Atractylodis Macrocephalae), *Fu Zi* (Radix Aconiti Lateralis Praeparata), and *Fu Ling* (Poria). Two representative formulas are *Ling Gui Zhu Gan Tang* (Poria, Cinnamon Twig, Atractylodes Macrocephala, and Licorice Decoction) and *Zhen Wu Tang* (True Warrior Decoction).

CAUTIONS / CONTRAINDICATIONS

Damp-dispelling formulas often incorporate two general categories of herbs: aromatic, acrid, and warm herbs that dry dampness; and sweet and bland herbs that resolve dampness. Although effective, both types of herbs easily damage yin and body fluids. Therefore, these formulas should be used with caution: during pregnancy; in patients with constitutional yin or body fluid deficiencies; and in individuals who have general weakness after a chronic illness.

~

The Spleen absorbs water, the Lung distributes water, and the Kidney eliminates water. Disorders in any of these organs may cause accumulation of water and formation of dampness.

~

1064

Chinese Herbal Formulas and Applications

Chapter 16 — Overview

PHARMACOLOGICAL EFFECTS & CLINICAL APPLICATIONS

From the traditional Chinese medical perspective, dampness is a complex disorder that may be complicated by other factors and affect different parts of the body. Correspondingly, damp-dispelling formulas have a wide range of pharmacological effects and clinical applications.

1. **Damp-drying and Stomach-harmonizing formulas** are primarily used to treat gastrointestinal disorders.

   • **Gastrointestinal disorders**: *Ping Wei San* (Calm the Stomach Powder) and *Huo Xiang Zheng Qi San* (Agastache Powder to Rectify the Qi) are two of the most commonly used and researched formulas for treating gastrointestinal disorders. *Ping Wei San* has been used to treat gastritis,[1] ulcerative colitis,[2] epigastric pain from gastritis,[3] peptic ulcer disease,[4] and anorexia.[5] *Huo Xiang Zheng Qi San* has been used to treat diarrhea,[6] gastroenteritis,[7] food poisoning,[8] and enteritis.[9]

2. **Heat-clearing and damp-dispelling formulas** clear damp-heat from the Liver, Gallbladder, and lower *jiao*. Pharmacologically, these formulas have antibiotic and anti-inflammatory effects, and have been used successfully to treat infections, as well as liver, gallbladder, kidney, and urinary disorders.

   • **Infection**: Many heat-clearing and damp-dispelling formulas have antibiotic effects, and have been successfully used to treat various types of infections. For example, *San Ren Tang* (Three-Nut Decoction) has been shown to treat pneumonia and otitis media,[10,11] *Gan Lu Xiao Du Dan* (Sweet Dew Special Pill to Eliminate Toxin) has been used to address encephalitis and laryngopharyngitis,[12,13] and *Ba Zheng San* (Eight-Herb Powder for Rectification) is effective for urethritis and urinary tract infection.[14,15]

   • **Liver disorders**: These formulas have hepatoprotective and antifibrotic effects.[16,17,18] Clinical applications include acute viral hepatitis,[19] acute icteric hepatitis,[20] acute infectious icteric hepatitis,[21] and hepatitis with hepatomegaly.[22] Exemplar formulas include *Yin Chen Hao Tang* (Artemisia Scoparia Decoction), *San Ren Tang* (Three-Nut Decoction), and *Gan Lu Xiao Du Dan* (Sweet Dew Special Pill to Eliminate Toxin).

   • **Gallbladder disorders**: These formulas have cholagogic and choleretic effects to stimulate and increase the production and release of bile acids to treat jaundice and cholestatic liver diseases.[23,24,25] Additional clinical applications include biliary atresia,[26] cholecystitis,[27] and icteric hepatitis.[28,29] Exemplar formulas include *Yin Chen Hao Tang* (Artemisia Scoparia Decoction) and *San Ren Tang* (Three-Nut Decoction).

   • **Kidney and urinary disorders**: These formulas have been used successfully to treat various kidney disorders (glomerulonephritis,[30] nephritis,[31] pyelonephritis,[32] and urinary stones[33]) and urinary disorders (urethritis and urinary tract infection).[34,35] Exemplar formulas include *San Ren Tang* (Three-Nut Decoction) and *Ba Zheng San* (Eight-Herb Powder for Rectifiation).

3. **Water-regulating and damp-resolving formulas** are used for excess damp accumulation that blocks the water pathways. From the perspectives of allopathic medicine, these formulas have a marked diuretic function, and are effective in treating various conditions characterized by water retention, such as cardiovascular, kidney, and urinary disorders.

   • **Edema**: Many of these formulas have a marked diuretic effect to increase the elimination of urine, sodium, chloride, potassium, and other electrolytes.[36] Clinically, *Wu Ling San* (Five-Ingredient Powder with Poria), *Zhu Ling Tang* (Polyporus Decoction), and *Wu Pi San* (Five-Peel Powder) are commonly used formulas for treating edema.[37,38,39]

   • **Cardiovascular disorders**: Many of these formulas have a direct or indirect effect in treating cardiovascular disorders. Some formulas have a diuretic effect to eliminate water and reduce cardiovascular stress.[40,41,42,43] Other formulas have vasodilative actions to reduce blood pressure.[44] Lastly, some formulas have positive chronotropic and inotropic effects on the heart.[45] Exemplar

> Dampness is a complex disorder, and correspondingly, damp-dispelling formulas have a wide range of pharmacological effects and clinical applications.

DAMP-DISPELLING FORMULAS

16

1065

Chapter 16 – Damp-Dispelling Formulas

Chapter 16 — Overview

formulas include *Wu Ling San* (Five-Ingredient Powder with Poria) and *Fang Ji Huang Qi Tang* (Stephania and Astragalus Decoction).

- **Kidney and urinary disorders**: Water-regulating and damp-resolving formulas have been successfully used to treat urinary disorders, such as nephritis,[46] acute nephritis,[47] renal failure,[48] urinary stones,[49,50] hydrocephalus,[51] uroschesis,[52] and hydronephrosis.[53,54] They can also be used for conditions such as hematuria,[55] galacturia,[56] and general urinary tract disorders.[57] The mechanisms of action are attributed in part to the diuretic effect of eliminating excess water retention,[58,59] and protecting the kidneys by decreasing plasma levels of blood urea nitrogen and creatinine.[60] Exemplar formulas include *Wu Ling San* (Five-Ingredient Powder with Poria), *Wei Ling Tang* (Calm the Stomach and Poria Decoction), *Zhu Ling Tang* (Polyporus Decoction), and *Fang Ji Huang Qi Tang* (Stephania and Astragalus Decoction).

4. **Warm formulas that resolve dampness** are commonly used to treat cardiovascular, kidney, and urinary disorders.

- **Cardiovascular disorders**: These formulas have been used successfully to treat cardiovascular disorders such as hypertension,[61] coronary artery disease,[62] and cardiac failure.[63,64] The pharmacological effects are attributed in part to circulatory improvements such as decreased resistance of blood flow, reduced blood viscosity, increased blood perfusion to internal organs, and decreased workload for the heart.[65] Exemplar formulas include *Ling Gui Zhu Gan Tang* (Poria, Cinnamon Twig, Atractylodes Macrocephala, and Licorice Decoction) and *Zhen Wu Tang* (True Warrior Decoction).

- **Kidney disorders**: These formulas have been effectively used to treat nephritis,[66] hydronephrosis,[67] nephrotic syndrome,[68] and chronic renal failure.[69] The mechanism of action is attributed to the nephroprotective effect which reduces the amount of protein and cells in the urine.[70] Exemplar formulas include *Ling Gui Zhu Gan Tang* (Poria, Cinnamon Twig, Atractylodes Macrocephala, and Licorice Decoction) and *Zhen Wu Tang* (True Warrior Decoction).

- **Urinary disorders**: Certain warm formulas that dispel dampness, such as *Bi Xie Fen Qing Yin* (Dioscorea Hypoglauca Decoction to Separate the Clear), have been successfully used to treat such urinary disorders as urethritis,[71] galacturia,[72] and *lin zheng* (dysuria syndrome).[73]

References

1. *Nan Jing Zhong Yi Yao Da Xue Xue Bao* (Journal of Nanjing University of Traditional Chinese Medicine and Medicinals) 1995;2:29.
2. *Shi Yong Zhong Yi Nei Ke Za Zhi* (Journal of Practical Chinese Internal Medicine) 1994;8(1):32.
3. *Xin Zhong Yi* (New Chinese Medicine) 1994;26(8):54.
4. *Liao Ning Zhong Yi Za Zhi* (Liaoning Journal of Chinese Medicine) 1990;14(11):20.
5. *Zhong Yi Yao Yan Jiu* (Research of Chinese Medicine and Herbology) 1994;1:20.
6. *Shan Dong Zhong Yi Xue Yuan Xue Bao* (Journal of Shandong University School of Chinese Medicine) 1993;1:39.
7. *Zhong Cao Yao* (Chinese Herbal Medicine) 1992;9:479.
8. *Shan Xi Zhong Yi* (Shanxi Chinese Medicine) 1990;5:224.
9. *Zhe Jiang Zhong Yi Xue Yuan Xue Bao* (Journal of Zhejiang University of Chinese Medicine) 1994;3:8.
10. *Hu Nan Zhong Yi Za Zhi* (Hunan Journal of Chinese Medicine) 1998;3:50.
11. *Zhe Jiang Zhong Yi Za Zhi* (Zhejiang Journal of Chinese Medicine) 1991;6:255.
12. *Jiang Su Zhong Yi* (Jiangsu Chinese Medicine) 1997;7:12.
13. *Xin Zhong Yi* (New Chinese Medicine) 1997;7:57.
14. *Guang Xi Zhong Yi Yao* (Guangxi Chinese Medicine and Herbology) 1992;4:9.
15. *Shan Xi Zhong Yi* (Shanxi Chinese Medicine) 1998;10:448.
16. Yamashiki M, Mase A, Arai I, Huang XX, Nobori T, Nishimura A, Sakaguchi S, Inoue K. Effects of the Japanese herbal medicine 'Inchinkoto' (TJ-135) on concanavalin A-induced hepatitis in mice. Clin Sci (Lond) 2000 Nov;99(5):421-31.
17. Iinuma Y, Kubota M, Yagi M, Kanada S, Yamazaki S, Kinoshita Y. Effects of the herbal medicine Inchinko-to on liver function in postoperative patients with biliary atresia--a pilot study. J Pediatr Surg 2003 Nov;38(11):1607-11.
18. Sakaida I, Tsuchiya M, Kawaguchi K, Kimura T, Terai S, Okita K. Herbal medicine Inchin-ko-to (TJ-135) prevents liver fibrosis and enzyme- altered lesions in rat liver cirrhosis induced by a choline-deficient L-amino acid-defined diet. J Hepatol 2003 Jun;38(6):762-9.
19. *Shan Xi Zhong Yi* (Shanxi Chinese Medicine) 1993;4:17.
20. *Zhong Yi Za Zhi* (Journal of Chinese Medicine) 1982;7:46.
21. *Shan Xi Zhong Yi* (Shanxi Chinese Medicine) 1998;3:19.

Chapter 16 — Overview

22. *Zhe Jiang Zhong Yi Za Zhi* (Zhejiang Journal of Chinese Medicine) 1980;10:462.

23. *Zhong Yi Za Zhi* (Journal of Chinese Medicine) 1982;7:72.

24. *Zhong Yi Ming Fang Lin Chuang Xin Yong* (Contemporary Clinical Applications of Classic Chinese Formulas) 2001;508

25. Shoda J, Miura T, Utsunomiya H, Oda K, Yamamoto M, Kano M, Ikegami T, Tanaka N, Akita H, Ito K, Suzuki H, Sugiyama Y. Genipin enhances Mrp2 (Abcc2)-mediated bile formation and organic anion transport in rat liver. Hepatology 2004 Jan;39(1):167-78.

26. Kobayashi H, Horikoshi K, Yamataka A, Lane GJ, Yamamoto M, Miyano T. Beneficial effect of a traditional herbal medicine (inchin-ko-to) in postoperative biliary atresia patients. Pediatric Surgery International 2001 Jul;17(5-6):386-9.

27. *Si Chuan Zhong Yi* (Sichuan Chinese Medicine) 1988;9:27.

28. *Zhong Yi Za Zhi* (Journal of Chinese Medicine) 1982;7:46.

29. *Shan Xi Zhong Yi* (Shanxi Chinese Medicine) 1998;3:19.

30. *Zhong Yi Fang Ji Xian Dai Yan Jiu* (Modern Study of Medical Formulae in Traditional Chinese Medicine) 1997;1355.

31. *Ha Er Bing Zhong Yi* (Haerbing Chinese Medicine) 1960;9:15.

32. *Liao Ning Zhong Yi Za Zhi* (Liaoning Journal of Chinese Medicine) 1986;1:19.

33. *Ji Lin Zhong Yi Yao* (Jilin Chinese Medicine and Herbology) 1983;5:19.

34. *Guang Xi Zhong Yi Yao* (Guangxi Chinese Medicine and Herbology) 1992;4:9.

35. *Shan Xi Zhong Yi* (Shanxi Chinese Medicine) 1998;10:448.

36. *Guo Wai Yi Xue Zhong Yi Zhong Yao Fen Ce* (Monograph of Chinese Herbology from Foreign Medicine) 1981;2:121.

37. *Zhong Yi Fang Ji Xian Dai Yan Jiu* (Modern Study of Medical Formulae in Traditional Chinese Medicine) 1997;1407.

38. *Guo Wai Yi Xue* (Foreign Medicine) 1983;5:292.

39. *Shan Xi Zhong Yi* (Shanxi Chinese Medicine) 1991;12(2):89.

40. *Zhong Hua Yi Xue Za Zhi* (Chinese Journal of Medicine) 1961;17(1):7.

41. *Guo Wai Yi Xue Zhong Yi Zhong Yao Fen Ce* (Monograph of Chinese Herbology from Foreign Medicine) 1983;6:24.

42. *Guo Wai Yi Xue Zhong Yi Zhong Yao Fen Ce* (Monograph of Chinese Herbology from Foreign Medicine) 1981;3:173.

43. *Guo Wai Yi Xue Zhong Yi Zhong Yao Fen Ce* (Monograph of Chinese Herbology from Foreign Medicine) 1984;5:78.

44. *Tian Jin Zhong Yi* (Tianjin Chinese Medicine) 1994;4:29.

45. Sugiyama A, Takahara A, Satoh Y, Yoneyama M, Saegusa Y, Hashimoto K. Cardiac effects of clinically available Kampo medicine assessed with canine isolated, blood-perfused heart preparations. Jpn J Pharmacol 2002 Mar;88(3):307-13.

46. *Guang Xi Zhong Yi Yao* (Guangxi Chinese Medicine and Herbology) 1984;4(10):16.

47. *Si Chuan Zhong Yi* (Sichuan Chinese Medicine) 1985;9:19.

48. *Zhong Yi Za Zhi* (Journal of Chinese Medicine) 1993;1:42.

49. *Zhong Yi Ming Fang Lin Chuang Xin Yong* (Contemporary Clinical Applications of Classic Chinese Formulas) 2001;133.

50. Takada M, Yano H, Kanbara N, Kurita T, Kohri K, Kato Y, Iguchi M. Effect of Chorei-to on spontaneous discharge of urinary stones after extracorporeal shock wave lithotripsy (ESWL). Hinyokika Kiyo 1997 Apr;43(4):311-4.

51. *Xin Yi Yao Xue Za Zhi* (New Journal of Medicine and Herbology) 1978;8:45.

52. *Si Chuan Zhong Yi* (Sichuan Chinese Medicine) 1997;4:26.

53. *Shan Xi Zhong Yi* (Shanxi Chinese Medicine) 1989;10(8):352.

54. *Shan Dong Zhong Yi Za Zhi* (Shandong Journal of Chinese Medicine) 1995;8:345.

55. *Zhong Yi Ming Fang Lin Chuang Xin Yong* (Contemporary Clinical Applications of Classic Chinese Formulas) 2001;636.

56. *Zhong Guo Nong Cun Yi Xue* (Chinese Agricultural Medicine) 1990;3:33.

57. Horii A, Maekawa M. Clinical evaluation of chorei-to and chorei-to-go-shimotsu-to in patients with lower urinary tract symptoms. Hinyokika Kiyo 1988 Dec;34(12):2237-41.

58. *Zhong Yi Fang Ji Xian Dai Yan Jiu* (Modern Study of Medical Formulae in Traditional Chinese Medicine) 1997;1407.

59. *Zhong Hua Yi Xue Za Zhi* (Chinese Journal of Medicine) 1961;17(1):7.

60. *Guo Wai Yi Xue Zhong Yi Zhong Yao Fen Ce* (Monograph of Chinese Herbology from Foreign Medicine) 1983;3:43.

61. *Shan Xi Zhong Yi* (Shanxi Chinese Medicine) 1983;2:6.

62. *Zhong Yi Han Shou Tong Xun* (Reports of Chinese Medicine) 1992;2:41.

63. *Tian Jin Yi Yao Za Zhi* (Journal of Tianjin Medicine and Herbology) 1967;8:503.

64. *Zhong Ji Yi Kan* (Medium Medical Journal) 1990;3:30.

65. *Zhong Xi Yi Jie He Za Zhi* (Journal of Integrated Chinese and Western Medicine) 1988;8(8):457.

66. *Zhong Yi Za Zhi* (Journal of Chinese Medicine) 1981;11:835.

67. *Shi Yong Zhong Yi Yao Za Zhi* (Journal of Practical Chinese Medicine and Medicinals) 1999;6:11.

68. *Shan Xi Zhong Yi* (Shanxi Chinese Medicine) 1987;2:70.

69. *Zhong Yi Ming Fang Lin Chuang Xin Yong* (Contemporary Clinical Applications of Classic Chinese Formulas) 2001;4:46.

70. *Zhong Yi Fang Ji Xian Dai Yan Jiu* (Modern Study of Medical Formulae in Traditional Chinese Medicine) 1997;1453.

71. *Xin Zhong Yi* (New Chinese Medicine) 1995;7:43.

72. *Shan Xi Zhong Yi* (Shanxi Chinese Medicine) 1994;6:273.

73. *Ji Lin Zhong Yi* (Jilin Chinese Medicine) 1990;2:16.

Chapter 16 – Damp-Dispelling Formulas | Section 1 – Damp-Drying and Stomach-Harmonizing Formulas

Section 1

燥湿和胃剂

— Damp-Drying and Stomach-Harmonizing Formulas

Píng Wèi Sǎn (Calm the Stomach Powder)

平胃散

Pinyin Name: Ping Wei San
Literal Name: Calm the Stomach Powder
Alternate Names: Ping Wei San (Wan), Stomach-Comforting Formula (Pill), Stomach-Calming Powder, Magnolia and Ginger Formula
Original Source: Tai Ping Hui Min He Ji Ju Fang (Imperial Grace Formulary of the Tai Ping Era) by the Imperial Medical Department in 1078-85

COMPOSITION

Cang Zhu (Rhizoma Atractylodis), *jin* (soaked) in rice water for 2 days	2,400g [15g]
Hou Po (Cortex Magnoliae Officinalis), *chao* (dry-fried) with ginger juice till aromatic	1,500g [9g]
Chen Pi (Pericarpium Citri Reticulatae)	1,500g [9g]
Gan Cao (Radix et Rhizoma Glycyrrhizae), *cuo* (grated) and *chao* (dry-fried)	900g [4g]

DOSAGE / PREPARATION / ADMINISTRATION

The source text instructions are to grind the ingredients into a fine powder. Cook 6g of the powder with 2 slices of *Sheng Jiang* (Rhizoma Zingiberis Recens) and 2 pieces of *Da Zao* (Fructus Jujubae) in 1 bowl of water until it is reduced to 70% volume. Take the hot, strained decoction on an empty stomach before meals with the optional addition of a pinch of salt. The source text states that frequent use of this formula regulates qi, harmonizes the Stomach, removes chronic food stagnation, dissolves phlegm, and prevents invasion of wind, cold, and dampness.

Today, this formula is commonly prepared and administered in powder or decoction form. For powder, grind the herbs into a fine powder and take 3-5g per dose with a decoction made from *Sheng Jiang* (Rhizoma Zingiberis Recens) and *Da Zao* (Fructus Jujubae). For decoction, use the doses suggested in brackets.

CHINESE THERAPEUTIC ACTIONS

1. Dries dampness and strengthens the Spleen
2. Activates qi circulation and harmonizes the Stomach

CLINICAL MANIFESTATIONS

Damp accumulation in the Spleen and Stomach: fullness and distention of the epigastrium and abdomen, decreased or loss of appetite, decreased sense of taste, nausea, vomiting, belching, acid regurgitation, a feeling of heaviness in the body and limbs, fatigue, lassitude, feeling lazy with preference of inactivity, diarrhea, a thick, white, greasy tongue coating, and a moderate pulse.

CLINICAL APPLICATIONS

Acute and chronic gastritis, gastric ulcer, duodenal ulcer, ulcerative colitis, epigastric pain caused by gastritis, gastric neurosis, gastroatonia, gastrectasia, anorexia, indigestion, and impotence.

EXPLANATION

Ping Wei San (Calm the Stomach Powder) is the basic formula for treating damp accumulation in the Spleen and Stomach. The Spleen, which is responsible for transportation and transformation, prefers a dry environment. If dampness accumulates and stagnates in the Spleen, impairing its transportation and transformation functions, then loss of appetite, decreased sense of taste, and diarrhea may occur. Damp accumulation also causes qi stagnation, resulting in fullness and distention of the epigastrium and abdomen. If dampness impairs the descending functions of the Stomach qi and causes disharmony, then nausea, vomiting, belching, and acid regurgitation may occur. Heavy-feeling body and limbs,

1068

Chinese Herbal Formulas and Applications

Píng Wèi Sǎn (Calm the Stomach Powder)

Ping Wei San (Calm the Stomach Powder)

Diagnosis	Signs and Symptoms	Treatment	Herbs
Damp accumulation in the Spleen and Stomach	• Loss of appetite, decreased sense of taste and diarrhea: damp accumulation affecting the Spleen and Stomach • Fullness and distention of the epigastrium and abdomen: qi stagnation and damp accumulation • Nausea, vomiting, belching and acid regurgitation: reversed flow of Stomach qi • Feeling of heavy body and limbs, constant fatigue, and lassitude: damp accumulation • White, greasy tongue coating and a moderate pulse: damp accumulation	• Dries dampness and strengthens the Spleen • Activates qi circulation and harmonizes the Stomach	• Cang Zhu (Rhizoma Atractylodis) dries dampness and strengthens the Spleen. • Hou Po (Cortex Magnoliae Officinalis) activates qi, dispels dampness, and relieves fullness and distention. • Chen Pi (Pericarpium Citri Reticulatae) regulates qi and relieves stagnation. • Sheng Jiang (Rhizoma Zingiberis Recens) and Da Zao (Fructus Jujubae) harmonize the Spleen and Stomach. • Gan Cao (Radix et Rhizoma Glycyrrhizae) harmonizes the middle jiao and the herbs.

constant fatigue, and lassitude are signs of damp accumulation. A white, greasy tongue coating and a moderate pulse are also indicators of dampness.

This formula's chief herb, *Cang Zhu* (Rhizoma Atractylodis), is bitter, dry, and warm, and dries dampness and strengthens the Spleen. The deputy herb, *Hou Po* (Cortex Magnoliae Officinalis), activates qi, dispels dampness, and relieves fullness and distention in the epigastrium and abdomen. *Chen Pi* (Pericarpium Citri Reticulatae) helps *Hou Po* (Cortex Magnoliae Officinalis) to regulate qi and relieve stagnation. *Sheng Jiang* (Rhizoma Zingiberis Recens) and *Da Zao* (Fructus Jujubae) harmonize the Spleen and Stomach. *Gan Cao* (Radix et Rhizoma Glycyrrhizae) harmonizes the middle jiao and all of the herbs in the formula.

MODIFICATIONS

• With damp-heat accumulation, add *Huang Lian* (Rhizoma Coptidis) and *Huang Qin* (Radix Scutellariae).
• With damp-cold accumulation, add *Gan Jiang* (Rhizoma Zingiberis), *Cao Dou Kou* (Semen Alpiniae Katsumadai) and *Rou Gui* (Cortex Cinnamomi).
• With fullness and feelings of oppression in the chest and abdomen, add *Mu Xiang* (Radix Aucklandiae) and *Zhi Qiao* (Fructus Aurantii).
• With epigastric and abdominal pain, add *Yan Hu Suo* (Rhizoma Corydalis) and *Xiang Fu* (Rhizoma Cyperi).
• With indigestion and poor appetite, add *Shan Zha* (Fructus Crataegi), *Mai Ya* (Fructus Hordei Germinatus), and *Shen Qu* (Massa Fermentata).
• With poor appetite due to Spleen deficiency, add *Ren*

Shen (Radix et Rhizoma Ginseng) and *Huang Qi* (Radix Astragali).
• For stomach flu, add *Huo Xiang* (Herba Agastaches) and *Ban Xia* (Rhizoma Pinelliae), or *Huo Xiang Zheng Qi San* (Agastache Powder to Rectify the Qi).
• For diarrhea, add *Bai Zhu* (Rhizoma Atractylodis Macrocephalae), *Yi Yi Ren* (Semen Coicis), and *Bai Bian Dou* (Semen Lablab Album).
• For diarrhea with blood due to heat, add *Huang Lian* (Rhizoma Coptidis).
• For diarrhea with mucus due to cold, add *Wu Zhu Yu* (Fructus Evodiae).
• For diarrhea due to dampness, add *Fu Ling* (Poria) and *Ze Xie* (Rhizoma Alismatis).
• For constipation, add *Da Huang* (Radix et Rhizoma Rhei) and *Mang Xiao* (Natrii Sulfas).
• For leukorrhea, add *Huang Qi* (Radix Astragali).
• For oliguria and dysuria, add *Fu Ling* (Poria) and *Ze Xie* (Rhizoma Alismatis).
• For edema and water retention, add *Sang Bai Pi* (Cortex Mori).

CAUTIONS / CONTRAINDICATIONS

Ping Wei San contains many bitter, acrid, warm and drying herbs that consume yin and blood. Therefore, use of this formula is contraindicated during pregnancy and in cases of yin or blood deficiency.[1]

CLINICAL STUDIES AND RESEARCH

1. **Gastritis:** According to one study of 46 patients (12 with chronic superficial gastritis, 26 with superficial atrophic gastritis, and 8 with atrophic gastritis), administration

DAMP-DISPELLING FORMULAS

16

1069

Píng Wèi Săn (Calm the Stomach Powder)

of modified *Ping Wei San* for one month per course of treatment was associated with complete recovery in 8 cases, significant improvement in 18 cases, moderate improvement in 16 cases, and no effect in 4 cases (all four had atrophic gastritis). The herbal formula contained *Ping Wei San* as the base formula, with the addition of *Ban Xia* (Rhizoma Pinelliae) and *Cao Guo* (Fructus Tsaoko) for more dampness; *Huang Lian* (Rhizoma Coptidis) and *Zhu Ru* (Caulis Bambusae in Taenia) for more damp-heat; dry-fried *Chai Hu* (Radix Bupleuri) and processed *Xiang Fu* (Rhizoma Cyperi) for qi stagnation; *Gao Liang Jiang* (Rhizoma Alpiniae Officinarum) for interior cold; and *Dang Shen* (Radix Codonopsis) and *Bai Zhu* (Rhizoma Atractylodis Macrocephalae) for deficiency of the middle *jiao*.[2]

2. **Ulcerative colitis**: Administration of modified *Ping Wei San* was associated with approximately 80% effectiveness in treating ulcerative colitis. The herbal formula contained *Cang Zhu* (Rhizoma Atractylodis), *Hou Po* (Cortex Magnoliae Officinalis), *Fang Feng* (Radix Saposhnikoviae), *Sheng Ma* (Rhizoma Cimicifugae), *Dang Shen* (Radix Codonopsis), and *Huang Qi* (Radix Astragali). In addition, charred *Da Huang* (Radix et Rhizoma Rhei), charred *Jin Yin Hua* (Flos Lonicerae Japonicae), and charred *Di Yu* (Radix Sanguisorbae) were added for hematochezia.[3]

3. **Epigastric pain caused by gastritis**: Use of modified *Ping Wei San* was effective in treating epigastric pain caused by gastritis (other causes were ruled out). The herbal formula contained *Xiang Fu* (Rhizoma Cyperi) 12-15g, *Gao Liang Jiang* (Rhizoma Alpiniae Officinarum) 4-8g, *Tan Xiang* (Lignum Santali Albi) 4-6g, *Dan Shen* (Radix et Rhizoma Salviae Miltiorrhizae) 15-30g, *Fo Shou* (Fructus Citri Sarcodactylis) 10g, *Wu Yao* (Radix Linderae) 10g, *Bai He* (Bulbus Lilii) 15-30g, *Huang Lian* (Rhizoma Coptidis) 3-4g, *Pu Gong Ying* (Herba Taraxaci) 30g, and *Gan Cao* (Radix et Rhizoma Glycyrrhizae) 6g. Furthermore, *Huang Qi* (Radix Astragali) and *Ren Shen* (Radix et Rhizoma Ginseng) were added for qi deficiency; *Gui Zhi* (Ramulus Cinnamomi) and *Bai Shao* (Radix Paeoniae Alba) were added, and *Huang Lian* (Rhizoma Coptidis) was removed, for the presence of cold; *Zi Su Geng* (Caulis Perillae) and *Xiang Yuan* (Fructus Citri) were added for epigastric fullness; *E Zhu* (Rhizoma Curcumae) or *Shi Xiao San* (Sudden Smile Powder) was added for blood stagnation; *Shi Hu* (Caulis Dendrobii) and a larger dose of *Bai Shao* (Radix Paeoniae Alba) were added and *Gao Liang Jiang* (Rhizoma Alpiniae Officinarum) removed, for yin deficiency. The treatment protocol was to give 1 pack of herbs in decoction daily, for 1 month per course of treatment, for 1-3 courses total. Of 56 patients, the study reported complete recovery in 33 cases, improvement in 20 cases, and no effect in 3 cases. The overall rate of effectiveness was approximately 95%.[4]

4. **Peptic ulcer disease**: One study reported complete recovery in 22 of 35 patients using modified *Ping Wei San* to treat gastric and/or duodenal ulcers. The herbal formula contained *Bai Shao* (Radix Paeoniae Alba) 25g, *Gan Cao* (Radix et Rhizoma Glycyrrhizae) 15g, *Chen Pi* (Pericarpium Citri Reticulatae) 15g, *Hou Po* (Cortex Magnoliae Officinalis) 15g, *Cang Zhu* (Rhizoma Atractylodis) 15g, *Huang Lian* (Rhizoma Coptidis) 5g, and *Wu Zhu Yu* (Fructus Evodiae) 5g. The duration of treatment ranged from 15-65 days, with an average of 45 days.[5]

5. **Anorexia**: One study reported success using modified *Ping Wei San* to treat 80 children with anorexia. The herbal formula contained *Cang Zhu* (Rhizoma Atractylodis) 7.5g, *Hou Po* (Cortex Magnoliae Officinalis) 6g, *Chen Pi* (Pericarpium Citri Reticulatae) 6g, *Fu Ling* (Poria) 6g, *Zhi Qiao* (Fructus Aurantii) 6g, *Ji Nei Jin* (Endothelium Corneum Gigeriae Galli) 9g, and *Gan Cao* (Radix et Rhizoma Glycyrrhizae) 5g. Additional modifications were made as needed. The duration of treatment ranged from 2-12 packs of herbs, with an average of 8 packs. The study reported improvement in appetite in all 80 children.[6]

6. **Impotence**: Administration of *Ping Wei San* was effective in treating impotence in 56 men (24 between 25-30 years of age; 27 between 31-40 years of age; and 5 between 41-45 years of age). The duration of illness ranged from 3 months to 10 years. The herbal formula contained *Cang Zhu* (Rhizoma Atractylodis) 20g, *Chen Pi* (Pericarpium Citri Reticulatae) 15g, *Hou Po* (Cortex Magnoliae Officinalis) 15g, *Shu Di Huang* (Radix Rehmanniae Praeparata) 25g, *Rou Gui* (Cortex Cinnamomi) 15g, *Fu Zi* (Radix Aconiti Lateralis Praeparata) 10g, *Jiu Cai Zi* (Semen Allii Tuberosi) 20g, and *Zhi Gan Cao* (Radix et Rhizoma Glycyrrhizae Praeparata cum Melle) 10g. Additional modifications were made as needed: *Yin Yang Huo* (Herba Epimedii) 15g was added for low sex drive; *Hong Hua* (Flos Carthami) 15g and *Wu Gong* (Scolopendra) 3 pieces for prolonged illness; *Fu Zi* (Radix Aconiti Lateralis Praeparata) 10g for yang deficiency; *Gou Qi Zi* (Fructus Lycii) 25g and *Dang Gui* (Radix Angelicae Sinensis) 15g for yin deficiency; *Long Gu* (Os Draconis) 20g and *Mu Li* (Concha Ostreae) 20g for spermatorrhea; *Huang Bo* (Cortex Phellodendri Chinensis) 25g for dampness in the genital area; *Suan Zao Ren* (Semen Ziziphi Spinosae) 15g for palpitations and insomnia; *Dang Shen* (Radix Codonopsis) 20g for poor appetite and lack of energy; *Xiang Fu* (Rhizoma Cyperi) 15g for chest congestion, hypochondriac pain, restlessness, and

Chinese Herbal Formulas and Applications

Píng Wèi Săn (Calm the Stomach Powder)

anger; and addition of *Huang Bo* (Cortex Phellodendri Chinensis) 15g and *Bai Mao Gen* (Rhizoma Imperatae) 20g, and removal of *Fu Zi* (Radix Aconiti Lateralis Praeparata) and *Rou Gui* (Cortex Cinnamomi), for dysuria. Of 56 men, the study reported complete recovery in 46 cases (82.1%), improvement in 7 cases (12.5%), and no effect in 3 cases (5.4%). Overall effectiveness was 94.6%.[7]

RELATED FORMULA

Chái Píng Tāng

(Bupleurum and Calm the Stomach Decoction)

柴平湯
柴平汤

Pinyin Name: *Chai Ping Tang*
Literal Name: Bupleurum and Calm the Stomach Decoction
Original Source: *Jing Yue Quan Shu* (Collected Treatises of [Zhang] Jing Yue) by Zhang Jie-Bin (Zhang Jing-Yue) in 1624

Chai Hu (Radix Bupleuri)	[6g]
Ren Shen (Radix et Rhizoma Ginseng)	[6g]
Ban Xia (Rhizoma Pinelliae)	[6g]
Huang Qin (Radix Scutellariae)	[6g]
Gan Cao (Radix et Rhizoma Glycyrrhizae)	[6g]
Chen Pi (Pericarpium Citri Reticulatae)	[6g]
Hou Po (Cortex Magnoliae Officinalis)	[6g]
Cang Zhu (Rhizoma Atractylodis)	[6g]

The source text states to prepare the ingredients with *Sheng Jiang* (Rhizoma Zingiberis Recens) and *Da Zao* (Fructus Jujubae) as a decoction. Note: The doses of the herbs were not given in the source text. Suggested doses are listed above in brackets.

Chai Ping Tang (Bupleurum and Calm the Stomach Decoction) is formulated by combining two formulas: *Xiao Chai Hu Tang* (Minor Bupleurum Decoction) and *Ping Wei San* (Calm the Stomach Powder). Thus, the main actions of this formula include harmonizing the *shaoyang*, harmonizing the Stomach, and dispelling dampness. Clinically, it may be used to treat patients with damp malaria characterized by intermittent chills and fever (more chills than fever), sensations of heaviness in the body and limbs, general body aches, distress in the epigastrium, nausea, a white, greasy tongue coating, and a soggy pulse.

References

1. *Zhong Yi Lin Chuan Fang Ji Xue* (Clinical Study of Chinese Herbal Formulas) 1995;217-218.
2. *Nan Jing Zhong Yi Yao Da Xue Xue Bao* (Journal of Nanjing University of Traditional Chinese Medicine and Medicinals) 1995;2:29.
3. *Shi Yong Zhong Yi Nei Ke Za Zhi* (Journal of Practical Chinese Internal Medicine) 1994;8(1):32.
4. *Xin Zhong Yi* (New Chinese Medicine) 1994;26(8):54.
5. *Liao Ning Zhong Yi Za Zhi* (Liaoning Journal of Chinese Medicine) 1990;14(11):20.
6. *Zhong Yi Yao Yan Jiu* (Research Journal of Chinese Medicine and Herbology) 1994;1:20.
7. *Shi Yong Zhong Yi Nei Ke Za Zhi* (Journal of Practical Chinese Internal Medicine) 1994;8(1):32.

DAMP-DISPELLING FORMULAS

16

1071

Chapter 16 – Damp-Dispelling Formulas　　*Section 1 – Damp-Drying and Stomach-Harmonizing Formulas*

Jiā Wèi Píng Wèi Sǎn (Modified Calm the Stomach Powder)

加味平胃散

Pinyin Name: *Jia Wei Ping Wei San*
Literal Name: Modified Calm the Stomach Powder
Alternate Name: Magnolia and Ginger Formula Modified
Original Source: *Yan Fang* (Time-Tested Formulas) of unknown author and date

COMPOSITION

Shan Zha (Fructus Crataegi)

Mai Ya (Fructus Hordei Germinatus)

Chen Pi (Pericarpium Citri Reticulatae)

Qing Pi (Pericarpium Citri Reticulatae Viride)

Chuan Xiong (Rhizoma Chuanxiong)

Cang Zhu (Rhizoma Atractylodis)

Hou Po (Cortex Magnoliae Officinalis)

Sha Ren (Fructus Amomi)

Xiang Fu (Rhizoma Cyperi)

Sheng Jiang (Rhizoma Zingiberis Recens)

Gan Cao (Radix et Rhizoma Glycyrrhizae)

DOSAGE / PREPARATION / ADMINISTRATION

Unavailable.

CHINESE THERAPEUTIC ACTIONS

1. Strengthens the Spleen and Stomach
2. Harmonizes the middle *jiao*
3. Relieves food stagnation

CLINICAL MANIFESTATIONS

Damp accumulation in the Spleen and Stomach: indigestion, sensations of oppression in the chest, abdominal pain, nausea, vomiting, diarrhea, postpartum abdominal fullness and distention with nausea and vomiting.

CLINICAL APPLICATIONS

Indigestion, gastric neurosis, gastric prolapse, and decreased or absent intestinal peristalsis.

EXPLANATION

Jia Wei Ping Wei San (Modified Calm the Stomach Powder) treats indigestion with damp accumulation in the Spleen and Stomach. Overindulgence in food commonly leads to food and qi stagnation. With food and qi stagnation, patients will likely experience indigestion, lack of appetite, nausea, vomiting, and fullness and distention of the epigastrium and abdomen. Long-term stagnation damages the Spleen and Stomach, leading to compromised transformation and transportation of food, characterized by loss of appetite, decreased tasting ability, and diarrhea. Lastly, dampness produces feelings of heaviness in the extremities, constant fatigue, and lassitude.

This formula has *Shan Zha* (Fructus Crataegi) to improve digestion, relieve abdominal fullness and distention, and effectively eliminate stagnation of fatty or greasy food. *Mai Ya* (Fructus Hordei Germinatus) improves digestion, increases appetite, and most effectively clears food stagnation from starch or carbohydrates. *Chen Pi* (Pericarpium Citri Reticulatae) and *Qing Pi* (Pericarpium Citri Reticulatae Viride) promote qi circulation, improve digestion, and dispel dampness.

Because qi stagnation is often accompanied by blood stagnation, *Chuan Xiong* (Rhizoma Chuanxiong) is added to promote blood circulation and prevent blood stasis. *Cang Zhu* (Rhizoma Atractylodis), *Hou Po* (Cortex Magnoliae Officinalis), and *Sha Ren* (Fructus Amomi) are commonly used together to dry dampness, strengthen the Spleen and Stomach, activate qi circulation, and relieve fullness and distention in the epigastrium and abdomen. *Xiang Fu* (Rhizoma Cyperi) regulates qi and relieves pain. *Sheng Jiang* (Rhizoma Zingiberis Recens) harmonizes the Spleen and Stomach. *Gan Cao* (Radix et Rhizoma Glycyrrhizae) harmonizes the herbs in the formula.

MODIFICATIONS

- For more severe food stagnation, add *Zhi Shi* (Fructus Aurantii Immaturus).
- With nausea, vomiting, and abdominal pain, combine with *Huang Lian Tang* (Coptis Decoction).
- With phlegm accumulation leading to fullness and feelings of oppression, combine with *Er Chen Tang* (Two-Cured Decoction).
- For Spleen and Stomach deficiencies, combine with *Si Jun Zi Tang* (Four-Gentlemen Decoction).

1072

Chinese Herbal Formulas and Applications

Jiā Wèi Píng Wèi Săn (Modified Calm the Stomach Powder)

Jia Wei Ping Wei San (Modified Calm the Stomach Powder)

Diagnosis	Signs and Symptoms	Treatment	Herbs
Damp accumulation in the Spleen and Stomach	• Indigestion, lack of appetite, nausea, vomiting, and fullness and distention of the epigastrium and the abdomen: food and qi stagnation • Feeling of heaviness in the extremities, constant fatigue and lassitude: accumulation of internal dampness	• Strengthens the Spleen and Stomach • Harmonizes the middle *jiao* • Relieves food stagnation	• *Shan Zha* (Fructus Crataegi) and *Mai Ya* (Fructus Hordei Germinatus) promote digestion and resolve food stagnation. • *Chen Pi* (Pericarpium Citri Reticulatae) and *Qing Pi* (Pericarpium Citri Reticulatae Viride) promote qi circulation, improve digestion, and dispel dampness. • *Chuan Xiong* (Rhizoma Chuanxiong) promotes blood circulation and prevents blood stasis. • *Cang Zhu* (Rhizoma Atractylodis), *Hou Po* (Cortex Magnoliae Officinalis) and *Sha Ren* (Fructus Amomi) dry dampness, strengthen the Spleen and Stomach, and activate qi circulation. • *Xiang Fu* (Rhizoma Cyperi) regulates qi and relieves pain. • *Sheng Jiang* (Rhizoma Zingiberis Recens) harmonizes the Spleen and Stomach. • *Gan Cao* (Radix et Rhizoma Glycyrrhizae) harmonizes the herbs.

AUTHORS' COMMENTS

Jia Wei Ping Wei San is modified from *Ping Wei San* (Calm the Stomach Powder) by adding herbs that promote digestion, dispel qi stagnation, and dry dampness.

Xiāng Shā Píng Wèi Săn
(Cyperus and Amomum Powder to Calm the Stomach)
香砂平胃散

Pinyin Name: *Xiang Sha Ping Wei San*
Literal Name: Cyperus and Amomum Powder to Calm the Stomach
Alternate Name: Cyperus Cardamon and Atractylodes Formula
Original Source: *Wan Bing Hui Chun* (Restoration of Health from the Myriad Diseases) by Gong Ting-Xian in 1587

COMPOSITION

Cang Zhu (Rhizoma Atractylodis), *zhi* (prepared) with rice water	6g
Hou Po (Cortex Magnoliae Officinalis), *chao* (dry-fried) with ginger juice	6g
Zhi Qiao (Fructus Citri Aurantii), *chao* (dry-fried) with bran	0.9g
Chen Pi (Pericarpium Citri Reticulatae)	6g
Sha Ren (Fructus Amomi)	1.5g
Xiang Fu (Rhizoma Cyperi), *chao* (dry-fried) with *Tong Bian* (Infantis Urina)	3g
Mu Xiang (Radix Aucklandiae)	1.5g
Shan Zha (Fructus Crataegi)	0.9g
Mai Ya (Fructus Hordei Germinatus), *chao* (dry-fried)	0.9g
Shen Qu (Massa Fermentata), *chao* (dry-fried)	0.9g
Gan Jiang (Rhizoma Zingiberis)	0.9g
Gan Cao (Radix et Rhizoma Glycyrrhizae)	0.9g

DAMP-DISPELLING FORMULAS

16

1073

Chapter 16 – Damp-Dispelling Formulas   *Section 1 – Damp-Drying and Stomach-Harmonizing Formulas*

Xiāng Shā Píng Wèi Sǎn
(Cyperus and Amomum Powder to Calm the Stomach)

DOSAGE / PREPARATION / ADMINISTRATION

The source text states to grind all of the ingredients except *Mu Xiang* (Radix Aucklandiae), into a fine powder, cook the powder with 3 slices of *Sheng Jiang* (Rhizoma Zingiberis Recens) and 1 snatch of *Lai Fu Zi* (Semen Raphani) in water. Take the warm, strained decoction with powdered *Mu Xiang* (Radix Aucklandiae).

CHINESE THERAPEUTIC ACTIONS

1. Harmonizes the middle *jiao* and resolves dampness
2. Regulates qi and reduces food stagnation

CLINICAL MANIFESTATIONS

Spleen and Stomach disharmony: nausea, vomiting, belching, chest fullness and distention, abdominal pain, diarrhea, and indigestion.

CLINICAL APPLICATIONS

Infantile malnutrition, indigestion, lack of appetite, diarrhea, and chronic disorders of the gastrointestinal tract.

EXPLANATION

Xiang Sha Ping Wei San (Cyperus and Amomum Powder to Calm the Stomach) treats disharmony of the Spleen and Stomach manifesting as impaired digestive functions. As a result, dampness accumulates in the middle *jiao*, causing reversed flow of qi upward. The resultant symptoms

include nausea, vomiting, and belching. Stagnation in the middle *jiao* causes indigestion, abdominal pain, distention, and fullness. Lastly, there may be diarrhea, as food cannot be digested and absorbed properly.

To properly address this condition, this formula has herbs that are aromatic, bitter, and warm to dry dampness, strengthen the Spleen, and harmonize the middle *jiao*. *Cang Zhu* (Rhizoma Atractylodis) dries dampness and strengthens the Spleen to relieve fullness and distention, treat poor appetite, and stop diarrhea. *Hou Po* (Cortex Magnoliae Officinalis) and *Zhi Qiao* (Fructus Aurantii) activate qi circulation to disperse stagnation. *Chen Pi* (Pericarpium Citri Reticulatae) and *Sha Ren* (Fructus Amomi) move qi, dry dampness, and eliminate phlegm. *Xiang Fu* (Rhizoma Cyperi) and *Mu Xiang* (Radix Aucklandiae) soothe Liver qi and relieve pain. *Shan Zha* (Fructus Crataegi), *Mai Ya* (Fructus Hordei Germinatus), and *Shen Qu* (Massa Fermentata) promote digestion and alleviate food stagnation. *Gan Jiang* (Rhizoma Zingiberis) warms the middle *jiao* and relieves nausea. *Gan Cao* (Radix et Rhizoma Glycyrrhizae) relieves abdominal pain, and harmonizes the herbs in the formula.

MODIFICATIONS

• With Spleen deficiency, add *Bai Zhu* (Rhizoma Atractylodis Macrocephalae) and *Dang Shen* (Radix Codonopsis).

Xiang Sha Ping Wei San (Cyperus and Amomum Powder to Calm the Stomach)

Diagnosis	Signs and Symptoms	Treatment	Herbs
Disharmony of the Spleen and Stomach	• Nausea, vomiting and belching: reversed flow of qi due to stagnation in the middle *jiao* • Indigestion, feelings of distention and fullness, abdominal pain and diarrhea: stagnation in the middle *jiao* with disharmony of the Spleen and Stomach	• Harmonizes the middle *jiao* and resolves dampness • Regulates qi and reduces food stagnation	• *Cang Zhu* (Rhizoma Atractylodis) dries dampness and strengthens the Spleen. • *Hou Po* (Cortex Magnoliae Officinalis) and *Zhi Qiao* (Fructus Aurantii) activate qi circulation to disperse stagnation. • *Chen Pi* (Pericarpium Citri Reticulatae) and *Sha Ren* (Fructus Amomi) move the qi, dry dampness, and eliminate phlegm. • *Xiang Fu* (Rhizoma Cyperi) and *Mu Xiang* (Radix Aucklandiae) soothe Liver qi circulation and relieve pain. • *Shan Zha* (Fructus Crataegi), *Mai Ya* (Fructus Hordei Germinatus) and *Shen Qu* (Massa Fermentata) promote digestion and alleviate food stagnation. • *Gan Jiang* (Rhizoma Zingiberis) warms and harmonizes the middle *jiao*. • *Gan Cao* (Radix et Rhizoma Glycyrrhizae) relieves abdominal pain and harmonizes the herbs.

1074

Chinese Herbal Formulas and Applications

Xiāng Shā Píng Wèi Sǎn
(Cyperus and Amomum Powder to Calm the Stomach)

- With Spleen and Stomach deficiencies, add *Huang Qi* (Radix Astragali) and *Shan Yao* (Rhizoma Dioscoreae).
- For nausea and vomiting caused by food stagnation, add *Huo Xiang* (Herba Agastaches) and *Zhu Ru* (Caulis Bambusae in Taenia).
- With long-term food stagnation, remove *Gan Jiang* (Rhizoma Zingiberis), and add *Da Huang* (Radix et Rhizoma Rhei).

RELATED FORMULA

Xiāng Shā Píng Wèi Sǎn

(Cyperus and Amomum Powder to Calm the Stomach)

香砂平胃散

Pinyin Name: *Xiang Sha Ping Wei San*

Literal Name: Cyperus and Amomum Powder to Calm the Stomach

Original Source: *Yi Zong Jin Jian* (Golden Mirror of the Medical Tradition) by Wu Qian in 1742

Cang Zhu (Rhizoma Atractylodis)	[6g]
Hou Po (Cortex Magnoliae Officinalis)	[4g]
Chen Pi (Pericarpium Citri Reticulatae)	[4g]
Xiang Fu (Rhizoma Cyperi)	[4g]
Sha Ren (Fructus Amomi)	[4g]
Zhi Qiao (Fructus Aurantii)	[4g]

Shan Zha (Fructus Crataegi)	[4g]
Mai Ya (Fructus Hordei Germinatus)	[4g]
Shen Qu (Massa Fermentata)	[4g]
Sheng Jiang (Rhizoma Zingiberis Recens)	[2g]
Bai Shao (Radix Paeoniae Alba)	[4g]
Gan Cao (Radix et Rhizoma Glycyrrhizae)	[2g]

This formula dries dampness, strengthens the Spleen, and promotes digestion. It is commonly used to treat food stagnation due to inappropriate dietary habits. Clinical manifestations include abdominal pain with food ingestion, lack of desire to eat, abdominal fullness, acid reflux, and preference for cold drinks.

These two formulas have identical names, and very similar composition and functions.

- *Xiang Sha Ping Wei San* from *Wan Bing Hui Chun* (Restoration of Health from the Myriad Diseases) has a slightly stronger effect to regulate qi circulation and relieve abdominal pain, as it contains both *Xiang Fu* (Rhizoma Cyperi) and *Mu Xiang* (Radix Aucklandiae).
- *Xiang Sha Ping Wei San* from *Yi Zong Jin Jian* (Golden Mirror of the Medical Tradition) has a slightly better effect to nourish yin and relieve abdominal spasms and cramps, as it has both *Bai Shao* (Radix Paeoniae Alba) and *Gan Cao* (Radix et Rhizoma Glycyrrhizae).

Bù Huàn Jīn Zhèng Qì Sǎn
(Rectify the Qi Powder Worth More than Gold)

不換金正氣散

不换金正气散

Pinyin Name: *Bu Huan Jin Zheng Qi San*

Literal Name: Rectify the Qi Powder Worth More than Gold

Alternate Names: *Pu Huan Chin Cheng Chi San*, Priceless Chi-Regulating Formula, Pinellia Atractylodes and Agastache Formula

Original Source: *Tai Ping Hui Min He Ji Ju Fang* (Imperial Grace Formulary of the Tai Ping Era) by the Imperial Medical Department in 1078-85

COMPOSITION

Cang Zhu (Rhizoma Atractylodis)

Hou Po (Cortex Magnoliae Officinalis)

Chen Pi (Pericarpium Citri Reticulatae)

Gan Cao (Radix et Rhizoma Glycyrrhizae)

Huo Xiang (Herba Agastaches)

Ban Xia (Rhizoma Pinelliae)

DAMP-DISPELLING FORMULAS

16

1075

Chapter 16 – Damp-Dispelling Formulas   *Section 1 – Damp-Drying and Stomach-Harmonizing Formulas*

Bù Huàn Jīn Zhèng Qì Sǎn
(Rectify the Qi Powder Worth More than Gold)

DOSAGE / PREPARATION / ADMINISTRATION

The source text states to grind equal amounts of the ingredients into a fine powder. Cook 9g of the powder with 3 slices of *Sheng Jiang* (Rhizoma Zingiberis Recens) and 2 pieces of *Da Zao* (Fructus Jujubae) in 1.5 bowls of water until it is reduced to 80% volume. Take the hot, strained decoction before meals.

Today, this formula is prepared by grinding all of the ingredients into a fine powder. Take 3-6g of the powder with a decoction made from *Sheng Jiang* (Rhizoma Zingiberis Recens) and *Da Zao* (Fructus Jujubae).

CHINESE THERAPEUTIC ACTIONS

1. Activates qi and resolves dampness
2. Harmonizes the Stomach and stops vomiting

CLINICAL MANIFESTATIONS

Damp accumulation in the middle *jiao*: vomiting, diarrhea, fever and chills, abdominal fullness and distention, and other urgent conditions such as sudden turmoil disorder.

CLINICAL APPLICATIONS

Acute or chronic gastroenteritis, gastric neurosis, food poisoning with nausea, vomiting, indigestion, poor appetite, belching, and acid reflux.

EXPLANATION

Bu Huan Jin Zheng Qi San (Rectify the Qi Powder Worth More than Gold) is often used in cases in which there are exorbitant damp accumulation symptoms, such as fever and chills, vomiting, diarrhea, abdominal distention and fullness, and other urgent symptoms associated with diseases such as malaria, dysentery, miasma and sudden turmoil disorder.

Bu Huan Jin Zheng Qi San is a modification of *Ping Wei San* (Calm the Stomach Powder), with the addition of *Huo Xiang* (Herba Agastaches) and *Ban Xia* (Rhizoma Pinelliae). The chief herb, *Cang Zhu* (Rhizoma Atractylodis), is bitter, drying, and warm and strongly dries dampness and strengthens the Spleen. The deputy herb *Hou Po* (Cortex Magnoliae Officinalis) activates qi, dispels dampness, and relieves fullness and distention in the epigastrium and abdomen. The assistant herb *Chen Pi* (Pericarpium Citri Reticulatae) regulates qi and relieves stagnation. Together, these three herbs dry dampness, strengthen the Spleen, and harmonize the Stomach. *Gan Cao* (Radix et Rhizoma Glycyrrhizae) harmonizes all of the herbs in the formula.

Adding *Huo Xiang* (Herba Agastaches) and *Ban Xia* (Rhizoma Pinelliae) to *Ping Wei San* (Calm the Stomach Powder) gives this formula a stronger ability to dispel dampness and regulate qi. *Huo Xiang* (Herba Agastaches), being strongly aromatic, activates qi, dispels dampness, harmonizes the Stomach to relieve nausea and vomiting, and eliminates exterior damp-heat. *Ban Xia* (Rhizoma Pinelliae) dries dampness and corrects reversed Stomach qi to relieve nausea and vomiting.

MODIFICATIONS

- With vomiting accompanied by excessive amount of sputum and saliva, add *Fu Ling* (Poria) and *Jie Geng* (Radix Platycodonis).

Bu Huan Jin Zheng Qi San (Rectify the Qi Powder Worth More than Gold)

Diagnosis	Signs and Symptoms	Treatment	Herbs
Accumulation of dampness in the middle *jiao*	Fever and chills, vomiting, diarrhea and abdominal distention and fullness: dampness accumulation	• Activates qi and resolves dampness • Harmonizes the Stomach and stops vomiting	• *Cang Zhu* (Rhizoma Atractylodis) strongly dries dampness and strengthens the Spleen. • *Hou Po* (Cortex Magnoliae Officinalis) activates qi, dispels dampness, and relieves fullness and distention of the epigastrium and abdomen. • *Chen Pi* (Pericarpium Citri Reticulatae) regulates qi and relieves stagnation. • *Gan Cao* (Radix et Rhizoma Glycyrrhizae) harmonizes the herbs. • *Huo Xiang* (Herba Agastaches) activates qi, dispels dampness, and harmonizes the Stomach. • *Ban Xia* (Rhizoma Pinelliae) dries dampness and redirects Stomach qi downward.

1076

Chinese Herbal Formulas and Applications

Bù Huàn Jīn Zhèng Qì Sǎn
(Rectify the Qi Powder Worth More than Gold)

- With severe diarrhea due to malaria, add *Huang Lian* (Rhizoma Coptidis) and *Huang Qin* (Radix Scutellariae).
- With wind-cold invasion, add *Fang Feng* (Radix Saposhnikoviae) and *Cong Bai* (Bulbus Allii Fistulosi).
- With severe diarrhea and vomiting, combine with *Huang Lian Tang* (Coptis Decoction).

CAUTIONS / CONTRAINDICATIONS

- Since many herbs in this formula are warm and drying in nature, patients with yin or blood deficiencies should use this formula with caution.

- Avoid foods that are raw, cold, oily, or greasy while taking *Bu Huan Jin Zheng Qi San.*

AUTHORS' COMMENTS

Bu Huan Jin Zheng Qi San was originally designed to treat urgent conditions such as malaria, miasma and sudden turmoil disorder. Although these conditions are uncommon today, this formula may still be used to address general gastrointestinal conditions such as vomiting, diarrhea, and abdominal fullness and distention.

Fú Líng Yǐn (Poria Decoction)
茯苓飲
茯苓饮

Pinyin Name: *Fu Ling Yin*
Literal Name: Poria Decoction
Alternate Name: Hoelen Combination
Original Source: *Jin Gui Yao Lue* (Essentials from the Golden Cabinet) by Zhang Zhong-Jing in the Eastern Han Dynasty

COMPOSITION

Fu Ling (Poria)	9g
Bai Zhu (Rhizoma Atractylodis Macrocephalae)	9g
Ren Shen (Radix et Rhizoma Ginseng)	6g
Chen Pi (Pericarpium Citri Reticulatae)	4.5g
Zhi Shi (Fructus Aurantii Immaturus)	6g
Sheng Jiang (Rhizoma Zingiberis Recens)	12g

DOSAGE / PREPARATION / ADMINISTRATION

The source text instructions are to cut the ingredients into small pieces, and cook them in 6 cups of water until the liquid is reduced to 1.8 cups. Take the strained decoction in three equally-divided doses.

CHINESE THERAPEUTIC ACTIONS

1. Strengthens the Spleen
2. Harmonizes the middle *jiao*
3. Resolves phlegm and dampness

CLINICAL MANIFESTATIONS

Stomach disorders including excessive gas and bloating, lack of appetite, inability to eat due to excessive gas in

the stomach, belching, or nausea; mild resistance in the epigastric region upon palpation.

CLINICAL APPLICATIONS

Gastritis, gastric prolapse, gastroptosis, acid reflux, gallstones, hiccups, and neurasthenia of the gastrointestinal tract.

EXPLANATION

Fu Ling Yin (Poria Decoction) treats phlegm and dampness in the chest, and is particularly indicated for patients who, after vomiting, experience symptoms such as excess gas in the stomach, a bloating sensation, and inability to eat. Patients may also experience other gastrointestinal symptoms such as belching and nausea.

DAMP-DISPELLING FORMULAS

16

1077

Chapter 16 – Damp-Dispelling Formulas   *Section 1 – Damp-Drying and Stomach-Harmonizing Formulas*

Fú Líng Yĭn (Poria Decoction)

Fu Ling Yin (Poria Decoction)

Diagnosis	Signs and Symptoms	Treatment	Herbs
Stomach disorders	Excessive gas and bloating, lack of appetite or inability to eat, belching, and nausea: stagnation of phlegm and dampness	• Strengthens the Spleen • Harmonizes the middle *jiao* • Resolves phlegm and dampness	• *Fu Ling* (Poria) and *Bai Zhu* (Rhizoma Atractylodis Macrocephalae) strengthen the Spleen and Stomach to dispel dampness in the middle *jiao*. • *Ren Shen* (Radix et Rhizoma Ginseng) tonifies qi and restores normal functioning of the Stomach. • *Chen Pi* (Pericarpium Citri Reticulatae) and *Zhi Shi* (Fructus Aurantii Immaturus) regulate qi circulation and strengthen the Spleen and Stomach. • *Sheng Jiang* (Rhizoma Zingiberis Recens) harmonizes the herbs.

In this formula, *Fu Ling* (Poria) and *Bai Zhu* (Rhizoma Atractylodis Macrocephalae) strengthen the Spleen and Stomach to dispel water stagnation in the middle *jiao*. *Ren Shen* (Radix et Rhizoma Ginseng) tonifies qi and restores the normal functions of the Stomach. *Chen Pi* (Pericarpium Citri Reticulatae) and *Zhi Shi* (Fructus Aurantii Immaturus) regulate qi circulation to relieve feelings of fullness and bloating. These two herbs also strengthen the Spleen and Stomach to increase appetite. *Sheng Jiang* (Rhizoma Zingiberis Recens) harmonizes the formula.

MODIFICATIONS

• With nausea and belching, add *Ban Xia* (Rhizoma Pinelliae).

• With indigestion, add *Mai Ya* (Fructus Hordei Germinatus) and *Shan Zha* (Fructus Crataegi).

• With stagnation of phlegm and water, add *Ban Xia* (Rhizoma Pinelliae) and *Jie Geng* (Radix Platycodonis).

• With inability to eat, add *Sha Ren* (Fructus Amomi) and *Shen Qu* (Massa Fermentata).

• For gallstones, add *Yin Chen* (Herba Artemisiae Scopariae) and *Ban Xia* (Rhizoma Pinelliae).

1078

Chinese Herbal Formulas and Applications

Huò Xiāng Zhèng Qì Sǎn (Agastache Powder to Rectify the Qi)

藿香正氣散
藿香正气散

Pinyin Name: *Huo Xiang Zheng Qi San*

Literal Name: Agastache Powder to Rectify the Qi

Alternate Names: *Huo Hsiang Cheng Qi San (Wan), Huo Xiang Zheng Qi San (Wan)*, Agastache Qi-Regulating Formula (Pill), Agastache Genuine-Qi Powder (Pill), Agastache Formula, Pogostemon Powder to Rectify the Qi, Pogostemon Formula

Original Source: *Tai Ping Hui Min He Ji Ju Fang* (Imperial Grace Formulary of the Tai Ping Era) by the Imperial Medical Department in 1078-85

COMPOSITION

Huo Xiang (Herba Agastaches)	90g [15g]
Zi Su Ye (Folium Perillae)	30g [5g]
Bai Zhi (Radix Angelicae Dahuricae)	30g [5g]
Ban Xia Qu (Rhizoma Pinelliae Massa Fermentata)	60g [10g]
Chen Pi (Pericarpium Citri Reticulatae)	60g [10g]
Bai Zhu (Rhizoma Atractylodis Macrocephalae)	60g [10g]
Fu Ling (Poria)	30g [5g]
Hou Po (Cortex Magnoliae Officinalis), *zhi* (fried with ginger juice)	60g [10g]
Da Fu Pi (Pericarpium Arecae)	30g [5g]
Jie Geng (Radix Platycodonis)	60g [10g]
Zhi Gan Cao (Radix et Rhizoma Glycyrrhizae Praeparata cum Melle)	75g [12g]

Note: Two types of "*Huo Xiang*" have commonly been used in the history of Chinese herbal medicine: *Guang Huo Xiang* (Herba Pogostemonis) and *Huo Xiang* (Herba Agastaches). Consulting the 2005 edition of *Zhong Hua Ren Min Gong He Guo Yao Dian* (Pharmacopoeia of People's Republic of China), *Guang Huo Xiang* (Herba Pogostemonis) is listed as an official entry, while *Huo Xiang* (Herba Agastaches) is not. Therefore, while many textbooks may still refer to "*Huo Xiang Zheng Qi San*" as "Agastache Powder to Rectify the Qi," most contemporary herbal products now use *Guang Huo Xiang* (Herba Pogostemonis) as the chief ingredient, and translate the formula as "Pogostemon Powder to Rectify the Qi."

DOSAGE / PREPARATION / ADMINISTRATION

The source text instructions are to grind the ingredients into a fine powder. Cook 6g of the powder with 3 slices of *Sheng Jiang* (Rhizoma Zingiberis Recens) and 1 piece of *Da Zao* (Fructus Jujubae) in 1 large bowl of water until it is reduced to 70%. Take the strained decoction while hot. Additionally, the source text recommends covering the body with blankets to promote sweating.

Today, this formula is generally prepared by grinding the herbs into a fine powder. Take 6g of the powder per dose with a decoction made from *Sheng Jiang* (Rhizoma Zingiberis Recens) and *Da Zao* (Fructus Jujubae). This formula may also be prepared as a decoction with the doses suggested in brackets.

CHINESE THERAPEUTIC ACTIONS

1. Releases the exterior and dispels dampness
2. Regulates qi and harmonizes the middle *jiao*

CLINICAL MANIFESTATIONS

Exterior wind-cold invasion accompanied by interior dampness: vomiting and diarrhea, fever, aversion to cold, headache, fullness and oppression in the chest and diaphragm, epigastric or abdominal pain, and a white, greasy tongue coating.

CLINICAL APPLICATIONS

Common cold or influenza in the summer, gastroenteritis, acute enteritis, acute colitis, diarrhea, food poisoning, heat stroke, fungal infection, and diaper rash.

EXPLANATION

Huo Xiang Zheng Qi San (Agastache Powder to Rectify the Qi) is commonly used to treat vomiting and diarrhea caused by an exterior wind-cold attack accompanied by interior dampness. Because of wind-cold at the exterior, headache, fever, and aversion to cold may be present. Damp stagnation and turbidity in the interior cause qi obstruction, leading to fullness and oppression in the chest and diaphragm, and epigastric or abdominal pain. Diarrhea and vomiting occur as dampness and turbidity accumulate in the Stomach and Intestines, which blocks clear qi from moving upward and turbid qi from moving

DAMP-DISPELLING FORMULAS

16

1079

Chapter 16 – Damp-Dispelling Formulas　　　*Section 1 – Damp-Drying and Stomach-Harmonizing Formulas*

Huò Xiāng Zhèng Qì Sǎn (Agastache Powder to Rectify the Qi)

Huo Xiang Zheng Qi San (Agastache Powder to Rectify the Qi)

Diagnosis	Signs and Symptoms	Treatment	Herbs
Exterior wind-cold accompanied by interior dampness	• Headache, fever and aversion to cold: exterior wind-cold • Fullness and oppression in the chest and diaphragm, and epigastric or abdominal pain: damp accumulation in the interior • Diarrhea and vomiting: dampness and turbidity affecting the Spleen and Stomach • White, greasy tongue coating: interior dampness	• Releases the exterior and dispels dampness • Regulates qi and harmonizes the middle *jiao*	• *Huo Xiang* (Herba Agastaches) releases exterior wind-cold and dispels dampness. • *Zi Su Ye* (Folium Perillae) and *Bai Zhi* (Radix Angelicae Dahuricae) release the exterior wind-cold and dispel interior dampness and turbidity. • *Ban Xia Qu* (Rhizoma Pinelliae Massa Fermentata) and *Chen Pi* (Pericarpium Citri Reticulatae) dry dampness, harmonize the Stomach, and lower reversed flow of qi. • *Bai Zhu* (Rhizoma Atractylodis Macrocephalae) and *Fu Ling* (Poria) strengthen the Spleen, dispel dampness, and harmonize the middle *jiao*. • *Hou Po* (Cortex Magnoliae Officinalis) and *Da Fu Pi* (Pericarpium Arecae) activate qi and dispel dampness. • *Jie Geng* (Radix Platycodonis) ventilates the Lung and resolves dampness. • *Sheng Jiang* (Rhizoma Zingiberis Recens), *Da Zao* (Fructus Jujubae), and *Zhi Gan Cao* (Radix et Rhizoma Glycyrrhizae Praeparata cum Melle) regulate the Spleen and Stomach and harmonize the herbs.

downward. A white, greasy tongue coating is a sign of dampness in the interior.

To treat this syndrome, not only must the exterior wind-cold be expelled, but the interior dampness and turbidity must be eliminated. Moreover, the qi should be regulated and the middle *jiao* harmonized. This formula has a large dose of *Huo Xiang* (Herba Agastaches) to release exterior wind-cold and dispel dampness. In addition, *Huo Xiang* (Herba Agastaches) treats nausea and vomiting by enabling the clear qi to ascend and turbid qi to descend. *Zi Su Ye* (Folium Perillae) and *Bai Zhi* (Radix Angelicae Dahuricae) help *Huo Xiang* (Herba Agastaches) release the exterior wind-cold and dispel interior dampness and turbidity. *Ban Xia Qu* (Rhizoma Pinelliae Massa Fermentata) and *Chen Pi* (Pericarpium Citri Reticulatae) dry dampness, harmonize the Stomach, lower reversed flow of qi, and relieve vomiting. *Bai Zhu* (Rhizoma Atractylodis Macrocephalae) and *Fu Ling* (Poria) strengthen the Spleen, dispel dampness, harmonize the middle *jiao*, and stop diarrhea. *Hou Po* (Cortex Magnoliae Officinalis) and *Da Fu Pi* (Pericarpium Arecae) activate qi to dispel dampness and relieve fullness. *Jie Geng* (Radix Platycodonis) ventilates the Lung to release exterior wind-cold and resolve dampness. *Sheng Jiang* (Rhizoma Zingiberis Recens),

Da Zao (Fructus Jujubae), and *Zhi Gan Cao* (Radix et Rhizoma Glycyrrhizae Praeparata cum Melle) regulate the Spleen and Stomach, and harmonize all of the herbs in this formula.

The emphasis of this formula is on dispelling dampness and harmonizing the Stomach. It has only a minor focus on expelling exterior wind-cold. It is best suited for treating exterior syndromes accompanied by internal dampness, causing disharmony in the middle *jiao* during the summer months. Historically, this formula has also been used to treat malaria and sudden turmoil disorder.

MODIFICATIONS

• With more heat, add *Huang Lian* (Rhizoma Coptidis) and *Huang Qin* (Radix Scutellariae).

• With more cold, add *Fu Zi* (Radix Aconiti Lateralis Praeparata) and *Gan Jiang* (Rhizoma Zingiberis).

• With more dampness, add *Yi Yi Ren* (Semen Coicis) and *Cang Zhu* (Rhizoma Atractylodis).

• With abdominal pain and diarrhea, add *Cang Zhu* (Rhizoma Atractylodis) and *Huang Lian* (Rhizoma Coptidis).

• With thirst, diarrhea, and oliguria, combine with *Wu Ling San* (Five-Ingredient Powder with Poria).

1080

Huò Xiāng Zhèng Qì Sǎn (Agastache Powder to Rectify the Qi)

- With scanty and difficult urination, add *Tong Cao* (Medulla Tetrapanacis), *Hua Shi* (Talcum), and *Ze Xie* (Rhizoma Alismatis).
- With tenesmus, add *Zhi Shi* (Fructus Aurantii Immaturus).
- With indigestion, add *Shen Qu* (Massa Fermentata) and *Shan Zha* (Fructus Crataegi).
- With epigastric and abdominal fullness and distention caused by qi stagnation, add *Mu Xiang* (Radix Aucklandiae) and *Yan Hu Suo* (Rhizoma Corydalis).

CAUTIONS / CONTRAINDICATIONS

- Most of the herbs in this formula are acrid and drying. Therefore, this formula is contraindicated in patients with yin and blood deficiencies.
- This formula should be used cautiously in patients with thirst and a yellow, greasy tongue coating due to damp-heat.
- Allergic reactions such as rashes, urticaria, and allergic purpura are sometimes associated with the use of *Huo Xiang Zheng Qi San*.[1]

PHARMACOLOGICAL EFFECTS

1. **Antispasmodic**: *Huo Xiang Zheng Qi San* was shown in many studies to effectively relax the smooth muscles of the gastrointestinal tract to relieve spasms and cramps.[2,3]
2. **Antiemetic**: One study reported that *Huo Xiang Zheng Qi San* was effective in relieving nausea and vomiting in pigeons with artificially-induced vomiting. The formula was given in liquid form, 11.64% concentration, at 20 mL/kg.[4]
3. **Antibacterial**: According to *in vitro* studies, administration of *Huo Xiang Zheng Qi San* was associated with an inhibitory effect against *Staphylococcus aureus*, *Salmonella typhi*, *Bacillus dysenteriae,* and *Bacillus proteus*.[5,6]

CLINICAL STUDIES AND RESEARCH

1. **Diarrhea**: Use of *Huo Xiang Zheng Qi San* effectively treated diarrhea in infants between 6 months and 3 years of age. Of 96 patients, the study reported complete recovery in 85 cases, improvement in 6 cases, and no improvement in 5 cases. The diarrhea generally stopped within 12-72 hours.[7]
2. **Gastroenteritis**: Administration of *Huo Xiang Zheng Qi San* was associated with effective treatment of acute gastroenteritis. Of 150 patients treated with this formula in powder form, 95 had complete recovery and 55 had improvement. Of 40 patients treated with this formula in decoction form, 39 had complete recovery.[8]
3. **Enteritis**: One study reported 95% effectiveness using *Huo Xiang Zheng Qi San* to treat 50 patients with acute enteritis during the summer and fall seasons.[9]

4. **Food poisoning**: Administration of modified *Huo Xiang Zheng Qi San* was associated with complete recovery within 52 hours in all 33 patients with acute food poisoning. Clinical improvements included resolution of symptoms such as headache, body aches and pains, and abdominal fullness and distention.[10]
5. **Fungal infection**: One study reported 86.6% effectiveness using *Huo Xiang Zheng Qi San* as an herbal wash to treat fungal infections of the skin (hands, feet, and body).[11]
6. **Diaper rash**: One study reported 95.8% effectiveness using *Huo Xiang Zheng Qi San* as an herbal wash to treat 48 babies with diaper rash. The treatment protocol was to apply the herbal solution to the affected area twice daily, for 7 days per course of treatment. Of 48 babies treated with one course of herbal therapy, 31 had significant improvement, 14 had moderate improvement, and 3 had no effect.[12]

TOXICOLOGY

No toxicity was reported in one acute toxicology study in laboratory animal subjects using *Huo Xiang Zheng Qi San* in powder extract form.[13] According to another study, oral administration of a 53.2% *Huo Xiang Zheng Qi San* solution at 25 mL/kg twice daily (approximately 583 times the normal human dose) for 7 days did not cause any abnormal reactions or fatality.[14]

AUTHORS' COMMENTS

Huo Xiang Zheng Qi San strongly transforms dampness and harmonizes the Stomach. Its action of releasing exterior wind-cold, however, is not as strong as other exterior-releasing formulas. This formula is appropriate for stomach flu symptoms such as aversion to cold, fever, vomiting, and diarrhea, and a thick, white tongue coating. The patient should be advised to cover up with a blanket to induce sweating.

According to Dr. Chang Wei-Yen, *Huo Xiang Zheng Qi San* combines well with *Ban Xia Xie Xin Tang* (Pinellia Decoction to Drain the Epigastrium) to treat vomiting, diarrhea, and epigastric pain caused by improper food intake. This combination is also effective for improving appetite in children.

Huo Xiang Zheng Qi San and *Liu He Tang* (Harmonize the Six Decoction) are two formulas that have been used to treat sudden turmoil disorder with vomiting and diarrhea.

- *Huo Xiang Zheng Qi San* contains *Huo Xiang* (Herba Agastaches) as the chief herb. The focus is to release exterior wind-cold and dispel interior dampness.

Chapter 16 – Damp-Dispelling Formulas *Section 1 – Damp-Drying and Stomach-Harmonizing Formulas*

Huò Xiāng Zhèng Qì Sǎn (Agastache Powder to Rectify the Qi)

• *Liu He Tang* contains *Ren Shen* (Radix et Rhizoma Ginseng) as the chief herb. Its main emphasis is on strengthening the Spleen.

References

1. *Zhong Cheng Yao* (Study of Chinese Patent Medicine) 1991;13(7):46.
2. *Zhong Cheng Yao Yan Jiu* (Research of Chinese Patent Medicine) 1984;6(5):15.
3. *Zhong Cao Yao* (Chinese Herbal Medicine) 1984;12:15.
4. *Zhong Cheng Yao* (Study of Chinese Patent Medicine) 1990;12(4):31.
5. *Zhong Cao Yao* (Chinese Herbal Medicine) 1984;12:15.
6. *Zhong Cheng Yao* (Study of Chinese Patent Medicine) 1990;12(4):31.
7. *Shan Dong Zhong Yi Xue Yuan Xue Bao* (Journal of Shandong University School of Chinese Medicine) 1993;1:39.
8. *Zhong Cao Yao* (Chinese Herbal Medicine) 1992;9:479.
9. *Zhe Jiang Zhong Yi Xue Yuan Xue Bao* (Journal of Zhejiang University of Chinese Medicine) 1994;3:8.
10. *Shan Xi Zhong Yi* (Shanxi Chinese Medicine) 1990;5:224.
11. *Lu Zhou Yi Xue Yuan Xue Bao* (Journal of Luzhou Institution of Medicine) 1992;3:192.
12. *Zhong Cheng Yao* (Study of Chinese Patent Medicine) 1995;17(2):49.
13. *Zhong Cao Yao* (Chinese Herbal Medicine) 1992;23(9):479.
14. *Zhong Cheng Yao* (Study of Chinese Patent Medicine) 1990;12(4):31.

Liù Hé Tāng (Harmonize the Six Decoction)

六和湯
六和汤

Pinyin Name: *Liu He Tang*
Literal Name: Harmonize the Six Decoction
Alternate Name: Cardamon Combination
Original Source: *Tai Ping Hui Min He Ji Ju Fang* (Imperial Grace Formulary of the Tai Ping Era) by the Imperial Medical Department in 1078-85

COMPOSITION

Ren Shen (Radix et Rhizoma Ginseng)	30g [3-5g]
Zhi Gan Cao (Radix et Rhizoma Glycyrrhizae Praeparata cum Melle)	30g [3-5g]
Huo Xiang (Herba Agastaches)	60g [6-10g]
Sha Ren (Fructus Amomi)	30g [3-5g]
Ban Xia (Rhizoma Pinelliae), *pao* (blast-fried) in liquid 7 times	30g [3-5g]
Hou Po (Cortex Magnoliae Officinalis), *zhi* (fried) with ginger juice	120g [12-15g]
Ku Xing Ren (Semen Armeniacae Amarum)	30g [3-5g]
Xiang Ru (Herba Moslae)	120g [12-15g]
Bai Bian Dou (Semen Lablab Album), *chao* (dry-fried) with ginger juice	60g [6-10g]
Mu Gua (Fructus Chaenomelis)	60g [6-10g]
Chi Fu Ling (Poria Rubra)	60g [6-10g]

DOSAGE / PREPARATION / ADMINISTRATION

The source text instructions are to grind the ingredients into powder. Cook 12g of the powder with 3 slices of *Sheng Jiang* (Rhizoma Zingiberis Recens) and 1 piece of *Da Zao* (Fructus Jujubae) in 1.5 bowls of water until it is reduced to 80% volume. Take the warm, strained decoction any time during the day. Today, this formula may be prepared as a decoction with the doses suggested in brackets.

CHINESE THERAPEUTIC ACTIONS

1. Strengthens the Spleen and harmonize the Stomach
2. Resolves dampness and dispels summer-heat

CLINICAL MANIFESTATIONS

Damp accumulation caused by an inappropriate diet, leading to Spleen and Stomach dysfunctioning: nausea, vomiting, diarrhea, fullness and distention in the chest and diaphragm, and a white, greasy tongue coating.

CLINICAL APPLICATIONS

Heat stroke, hangover, and disturbance of the gastro-intestinal system characterized by decreased appetite, vomiting, and diarrhea.

Chinese Herbal Formulas and Applications

Liù Hé Tāng (Harmonize the Six Decoction)

EXPLANATION

Liu He Tang (Harmonize the Six Decoction) is indicated for patients with dampness attacking and damaging the Spleen and Stomach caused by an inappropriate diet. This condition often arises on hot and humid summer days after eating raw, cold, or uncooked foods. Damp accumulation creates disharmony of the Spleen and Stomach, which causes such symptoms as nausea and vomiting. Fullness and distention in the chest and diaphragm result from dampness obstructing qi. Diarrhea is caused by dampness affecting the Spleen. Historically, this formula has been used to treat sudden turmoil disorder with vomiting and diarrhea.

The treatment plan for this syndrome is to dispel dampness, harmonize the Stomach, and strengthen the Spleen. In this formula, *Ren Shen* (Radix et Rhizoma Ginseng) and *Zhi Gan Cao* (Radix et Rhizoma Glycyrrhizae Praeparata cum Melle) strengthen the Spleen and dispel dampness. *Huo Xiang* (Herba Agastaches) and *Sha Ren* (Fructus Amomi) dispel dampness from the exterior and dry dampness in the interior. *Ban Xia* (Rhizoma Pinelliae), *Hou Po* (Cortex Magnoliae Officinalis), and *Ku Xing Ren* (Semen Armeniacae Amarum) regulate the qi flow and dispel dampness. *Xiang Ru* (Herba Moslae) and *Bai Bian Dou* (Semen Lablab Album) strengthen the Spleen and dispel dampness. *Mu Gua* (Fructus Chaenomelis) and *Chi Fu Ling* (Poria Rubra) dispel dampness, smooth the qi flow, and harmonize the middle *jiao*. *Zhi Gan Cao*

(Radix et Rhizoma Glycyrrhizae Praeparata cum Melle), *Sheng Jiang* (Rhizoma Zingiberis Recens) and *Da Zao* (Fructus Jujubae) harmonize the Spleen and Stomach, and harmonize the rest of the herbs in this formula.

MODIFICATIONS

- With exterior cold, add *Zi Su Ye* (Folium Perillae) and *Xiang Fu* (Rhizoma Cyperi).
- With severe exterior summer-dampness, increase the doses of *Xiang Ru* (Herba Moslae) and *Huo Xiang* (Herba Agastaches).
- With severe damp-heat accumulation, add *Yi Yi Ren* (Semen Coicis), *Hua Shi* (Talcum), *Che Qian Cao* (Herba Plantaginis), and *Huang Lian* (Rhizoma Coptidis).
- For excessive alcohol intake, add *Ge Hua* (Flos Puerariae) and *Shen Qu* (Massa Fermentata).

CAUTIONS / CONTRAINDICATIONS

Liu He Tang is dry and aromatic; therefore, it is not suitable for patients who have yin or body fluid deficiencies.

RELATED FORMULA

Liù Hé Tāng (Harmonize the Six Decoction)

六和湯
六和汤

Pinyin Name: *Liu He Tang*

Literal Name: Harmonize the Six Decoction

Original Source: *Yi Fang Kao* (Investigation of Medical Formulas) by Wu Kun in 1584

Liu He Tang (Harmonize the Six Decoction)

Diagnosis	Signs and Symptoms	Treatment	Herbs
Spleen and Stomach dysfunction with damp accumulation	• Nausea and vomiting: disharmony of the Spleen and Stomach caused by damp accumulation • Fullness and distention in the chest and diaphragm: dampness obstructing qi flow • Diarrhea: dampness affecting the Spleen	• Strengthens the Spleen and harmonizes the Stomach • Resolves dampness and dispels summer-heat	• *Ren Shen* (Radix et Rhizoma Ginseng) and *Zhi Gan Cao* (Radix et Rhizoma Glycyrrhizae Praeparata cum Melle) strengthen the Spleen and dispel dampness. • *Huo Xiang* (Herba Agastaches) and *Sha Ren* (Fructus Amomi) dispel dampness from the exterior and dry dampness in the interior. • *Ban Xia* (Rhizoma Pinelliae), *Hou Po* (Cortex Magnoliae Officinalis), and *Ku Xing Ren* (Semen Armeniacae Amarum) regulate the qi flow and dispel dampness. • *Xiang Ru* (Herba Moslae) and *Bai Bian Dou* (Semen Lablab Album) strengthen the Spleen and dispel dampness. • *Mu Gua* (Fructus Chaenomelis) and *Chi Fu Ling* (Poria Rubra) dispel dampness, regulate the qi flow, and harmonize the middle *jiao*. • *Sheng Jiang* (Rhizoma Zingiberis Recens) and *Da Zao* (Fructus Jujubae) harmonize the herbs.

DAMP-DISPELLING FORMULAS

16

1083

Liù Hé Tāng (Harmonize the Six Decoction)

Sha Ren (Fructus Amomi)	2.4g
Ban Xia (Rhizoma Pinelliae)	6g
Ku Xing Ren (Semen Armeniacae Amarum)	6g
Ren Shen (Radix et Rhizoma Ginseng)	6g
Bai Zhu (Rhizoma Atractylodis Macrocephalae)	6g
Huo Xiang (Herba Agastaches)	6g
Bai Bian Dou (Semen Lablab Album)	6g
Chi Fu Ling (Poria Rubra)	6g
Mu Gua (Fructus Chaenomelis)	4.5g
Hou Po (Cortex Magnoliae Officinalis)	2.4g
Gan Cao (Radix et Rhizoma Glycyrrhizae)	1.5g

This formula strengthens the Spleen, resolves dampness, lifts the clear and lowers the turbid. It is used to treat dampness injuring the Spleen and Stomach due to consumption of inappropriate foods during the summer. Clinical applications include sudden turmoil disorder, vomiting, diarrhea, feelings of fullness and distention in the chest and diaphragm, and a white slippery tongue coating.

These two formulas have the same name and very similar ingredients and indications.

- *Liu He Tang* from *Tai Ping Hui Min He Ji Ju Fang* (Imperial Grace Formulary of the Tai Ping Era) contains *Xiang Ru* (Herba Moslae), and is slightly stronger in resolving dampness and releasing the exterior.
- *Liu He Tang* from *Yi Fang Kao* (Investigation of Medical Formulas) contains *Bai Zhu* (Rhizoma Atractylodis Macrocephalae), and is better at strengthening the Spleen and Stomach.

AUTHORS' COMMENTS

Liu He Tang, literally "Harmonize the Six Decoction," refers to the purpose of harmonizing the Spleen and Stomach to ensure optimal absorption of the nutrients and proper nourishment of the "six" *fu* (hollow organs).

Gě Huā Jiě Chéng Săn

(Pueraria Flower Powder for Detoxification and Awakening)

葛花解醒散

Pinyin Name: *Ge Hua Jie Cheng San*
Literal Name: Pueraria Flower Powder for Detoxification and Awakening
Alternate Name: Pueraria Flower Formula
Original Source: *Yi Fang Ji Jie* (Analytical Collection of Medical Formulas) by Wang Ang in 1682

COMPOSITION

Ge Hua (Flos Puerariae)	15g
Dou Kou (Fructus Amomi Rotundus)	15g
Sha Ren (Fructus Amomi)	15g
Mu Xiang (Radix Aucklandiae)	1.5g
Qing Pi (Pericarpium Citri Reticulatae Viride)	1.5g
Chen Pi (Pericarpium Citri Reticulatae)	4.5g
Ren Shen (Radix et Rhizoma Ginseng)	4.5g
Bai Zhu (Rhizoma Atractylodis Macrocephalae)	6g
Fu Ling (Poria)	4.5g
Shen Qu (Massa Fermentata)	6g
Gan Jiang (Rhizoma Zingiberis)	6g
Zhu Ling (Polyporus)	4.5g
Ze Xie (Rhizoma Alismatis)	6g
Lian Hua (Flos Nelumbinis)	0.9g

DOSAGE / PREPARATION / ADMINISTRATION

The source text instructs to grind the ingredients into a fine powder. Take 9g of the powder with warm water.

The source text notes that this formula may induce mild sweating, an indication that the condition has resolved.

Chinese Herbal Formulas and Applications

Gě Huā Jiě Chéng Sǎn
(Pueraria Flower Powder for Detoxification and Awakening)

CHINESE THERAPEUTIC ACTIONS

1. Strengthens and harmonizes the Spleen and Stomach
2. Clears damp-heat

CLINICAL MANIFESTATIONS

Damp-heat in the Spleen and Stomach: nausea, vomiting, headache, dizziness, chest distention, lack of appetite, and fatigue.

CLINICAL APPLICATIONS

Intoxication from alcohol consumption, hangover, nausea, vomiting, and headache associated with the use of alcohol.

EXPLANATION

Ge Hua Jie Cheng San (Pueraria Flower Powder for Detoxification and Awakening) specifically treats damp-heat in the Spleen and Stomach caused by overindulgence and intoxication of alcohol. When damp-heat travels upward, it leads to nausea, vomiting, and headache. When damp-heat affects the middle *jiao*, it produces abdominal pain and cramps, as well as lack of appetite. When damp-heat travels downward, it leads to diarrhea and dysuria.

In this formula, *Ge Hua* (Flos Puerariae) is the chief herb because it facilitates the breakdown of alcohol and

relieves the side effects of alcohol intoxication. *Dou Kou* (Fructus Amomi Rotundus) and *Sha Ren* (Fructus Amomi) strengthen the Spleen and dry dampness. *Mu Xiang* (Radix Aucklandiae), *Qing Pi* (Pericarpium Citri Reticulatae Viride), and *Chen Pi* (Pericarpium Citri Reticulatae) regulate qi circulation, direct qi downward, and relieve nausea and vomiting. *Ren Shen* (Radix et Rhizoma Ginseng), *Bai Zhu* (Rhizoma Atractylodis Macrocephalae), and *Fu Ling* (Poria) strengthen the Spleen, tonify qi, and treat fatigue. *Shen Qu* (Massa Fermentata) facilitates the metabolism of alcohol in the stomach. *Gan Jiang* (Rhizoma Zingiberis) warms the middle *jiao* to relieve abdominal pain and cramps. *Zhu Ling* (Polyporus), *Ze Xie* (Rhizoma Alismatis), and *Lian Hua* (Flos Nelumbinis) drain dampness, regulate the water passages, and relieve dysuria.

MODIFICATIONS

- With headache, add *Chuan Xiong* (Rhizoma Chuanxiong) and *Bai Zhi* (Radix Angelicae Dahuricae).
- With severe nausea and vomiting, add *Sheng Jiang* (Rhizoma Zingiberis Recens) and *Hou Po* (Cortex Magnoliae Officinalis).

Ge Hua Jie Cheng San (Pueraria Flower Powder for Detoxification and Awakening)

Diagnosis	Signs and Symptoms	Treatment	Herbs
Damp-heat in the Spleen and Stomach	• Overindulgence and intoxication of alcohol: damp-heat accumulation in the Spleen and Stomach • Nausea, vomiting and headache: damp-heat traveling upwards • Abdominal pain and cramps and lack of appetite: damp-heat affecting the middle *jiao* • Diarrhea and dysuria: damp-heat traveling downward	• Strengthens and harmonizes the Spleen and Stomach • Clears damp-heat	• *Ge Hua* (Flos Puerariae) facilitates the breakdown of alcohol and relieves the side effects of alcohol intoxication. • *Dou Kou* (Fructus Amomi Rotundus) and *Sha Ren* (Fructus Amomi) strengthen the Spleen and dry dampness. • *Mu Xiang* (Radix Aucklandiae), *Qing Pi* (Pericarpium Citri Reticulatae Viride), and *Chen Pi* (Pericarpium Citri Reticulatae) regulate qi circulation, direct qi downward, and relieve nausea and vomiting. • *Ren Shen* (Radix et Rhizoma Ginseng), *Bai Zhu* (Rhizoma Atractylodis Macrocephalae), and *Fu Ling* (Poria) strengthen the Spleen and tonify qi. • *Shen Qu* (Massa Fermentata) facilitates the metabolism of alcohol in the stomach. • *Gan Jiang* (Rhizoma Zingiberis) warms the middle *jiao* to relieve abdominal pain and cramps. • *Zhu Ling* (Polyporus), *Ze Xie* (Rhizoma Alismatis), and *Lian Hua* (Flos Nelumbinis) regulate the water passages and relieve dysuria.

DAMP-DISPELLING FORMULAS

16

1085

Chapter 16 – Damp-Dispelling Formulas   *Section 2 – Heat-Clearing and Damp-Dispelling Formulas*

Section 2

清热祛湿剂

— Heat-Clearing and Damp-Dispelling Formulas

Yīn Chén Hāo Tāng (Artemisia Scoparia Decoction)

茵陳蒿湯
茵陈蒿汤

Pinyin Name: *Yin Chen Hao Tang*
Literal Name: Artemisia Scoparia Decoction
Alternate Name: Artemisia Combination
Original Source: *Shang Han Lun* (Discussion of Cold-Induced Disorders) by Zhang Zhong-Jing in the Eastern Han Dynasty

COMPOSITION

Yin Chen (Herba Artemisiae Scopariae)	18g
Zhi Zi (Fructus Gardeniae)	14 pieces [9g]
Da Huang (Radix et Rhizoma Rhei)	6g

DOSAGE / PREPARATION / ADMINISTRATION

The source text instructions are to first cook *Yin Chen* (Herba Artemisiae Scopariae) in 12 cups [2,400 mL] of water until the liquid is reduced to 6 cups [1,200 mL]. Add the other two herbs and cook the decoction until the liquid is reduced to 3 cups [600 mL]. Take the strained decoction in three equally-divided doses.

The source text states that use of the formula will induce normal urine that resembles the juice of *Zao Jiao* (Fructus Gleditsiae), which is pure red in color. After one night, the abdominal fullness will be relieved and the yellow discoloration of the eyes and skin will come out with the urine. Today, this formula is generally prepared as a decoction by cooking all three herbs at the same time.

CHINESE THERAPEUTIC ACTIONS

1. Clears heat
2. Resolves dampness
3. Relieves jaundice

CLINICAL MANIFESTATIONS

Damp-heat jaundice: bright yellow discoloration of the skin and sclera, slight abdominal fullness, dysuria, thirst, a yellow, greasy tongue coating, and a deep, rapid pulse.

CLINICAL APPLICATIONS

Hepatitis, infectious hepatitis, jaundice, biliary atresia, cholecystitis, cholelithiasis, hyperlipidemia, and seborrheic dermatitis.

EXPLANATION

Yin Chen Hao Tang (Artemisia Scoparia Decoction) is the formula of choice to treat damp-heat jaundice, a condition caused by stagnation of dampness and heat in the interior. This type of damp-heat jaundice, commonly referred to as yang jaundice, is characterized by a bright discoloration of the skin that resembles the color of fresh orange peel. The damp-heat can manifest outward to the muscles and skin, causing bright yellow discoloration of the skin and sclera. The damp-heat can also affect the lower *jiao*, producing slight abdominal fullness and dysuria. The heat may consume body fluids, causing thirst. A yellow, greasy tongue coating and a deep, rapid pulse both suggest damp-heat in the interior.

This formula contains *Yin Chen* (Herba Artemisiae Scopariae), the premier herb choice for clearing damp-heat jaundice. *Zhi Zi* (Fructus Gardeniae) clears damp-heat in the three *jiaos* and drains damp-heat out of the body through urination. *Da Huang* (Radix et Rhizoma Rhei) drains damp-heat through defecation. These three herbs

1086

Chinese Herbal Formulas and Applications

Yīn Chén Hāo Tāng (Artemisia Scoparia Decoction)

Yin Chen Hao Tang (Artemisia Scoparia Decoction)

Diagnosis	Signs and Symptoms	Treatment	Herbs
Damp-heat jaundice	• Bright yellow discoloration of the skin and sclera: damp-heat manifesting outward • Abdominal fullness and dysuria: damp-heat traveling downward • Thirst: damp-heat consuming body fluids • Yellow, greasy tongue coating and a deep, rapid pulse: damp-heat in the interior	• Clears heat • Resolves dampness • Relieves jaundice	• *Yin Chen* (Herba Artemisiae Scopariae) clears damp-heat from the Liver and Gallbladder. • *Zhi Zi* (Fructus Gardeniae) clears damp-heat in all three *jiaos* and drains it out of the body through urination. • *Da Huang* (Radix et Rhizoma Rhei) purges damp-heat through defecation.

have a synergistic effect to maximize the treatment result.

MODIFICATIONS

• For jaundice with more dampness, add *Fu Ling* (Poria), *Ze Xie* (Rhizoma Alismatis), and *Zhu Ling* (Polyporus).
• For jaundice with more heat, add *Huang Bo* (Cortex Phellodendri Chinensis) and *Long Dan* (Radix et Rhizoma Gentianae).
• For severe jaundice, add *Hu Zhang* (Rhizoma et Radix Polygoni Cuspidati) and *Pu Gong Ying* (Herba Taraxaci).
• With oliguria, add *Fu Ling* (Poria), *Ze Xie* (Rhizoma Alismatis), and *Hua Shi* (Talcum).
• With dysuria, add *Mu Tong* (Caulis Akebiae), *Hua Shi* (Talcum), and *Jin Qian Cao* (Herba Lysimachiae).
• With thirst and a feeling of fullness and oppression, add *Huang Lian* (Rhizoma Coptidis) and *Huang Qin* (Radix Scutellariae).
• With fever and chills, add *Chai Hu* (Radix Bupleuri) and *Huang Qin* (Radix Scutellariae).
• With scanty, yellow urine, add *Jin Qian Cao* (Herba Lysimachiae) and *Ze Xie* (Rhizoma Alismatis).
• With hypochondriac pain, add *Chai Hu* (Radix Bupleuri), *Chuan Lian Zi* (Fructus Toosendan), *Yu Jin* (Radix Curcumae), and *Xiang Fu* (Rhizoma Cyperi).
• With hypochondriac pain and abdominal fullness, add *Yu Jin* (Radix Curcumae), *Zhi Qiao* (Fructus Aurantii), and *Chuan Lian Zi* (Fructus Toosendan).
• With abdominal fullness and decreased food intake, add *Shan Zha* (Fructus Crataegi) and *Mai Ya* (Fructus Hordei Germinatus).
• With nausea and vomiting, add *Huang Lian* (Rhizoma Coptidis), *Bai Shao* (Radix Paeoniae Alba), and *Ban Xia* (Rhizoma Pinelliae).

CAUTIONS / CONTRAINDICATIONS

• *Yin Chen Hao Tang* should be used only for damp-heat jaundice and **not** damp-cold jaundice.

• The use of this formula is contraindicated during pregnancy.[1]

PHARMACOLOGICAL EFFECTS

1. **Cholagogic**: *Yin Chen Hao Tang* was associated with stimulating an increased production and release of bile acids. The alcohol extract of the formula was determined to be more effective than the water extract. In comparison with the control group that did not receive any herbs, administration of the alcohol extract increased the production of bile by 51.28%, while administration of the water extract increased the production of bile by 45.85%.[2] Some researchers have noted that to obtain the maximum cholagogic effect, a larger dose of *Da Huang* (Radix et Rhizoma Rhei) should be used in its fresh form or should be post-decocted. *Yin Chen* (Herba Artemisiae Scopariae) should also be post-decocted.[3]

2. **Choleretic**: One study reported *Yin Chen Hao Tang* to be a potent therapeutic agent for a number of cholestatic liver diseases by enhancing the bile acid-independent secretory capacity of hepatocytes. This therapeutic effect was attributed in part to genipin, an active compound of *Zhi Zi* (Fructus Gardeniae).[4]

3. **Hepatoprotective**: *Yin Chen Hao Tang* has been shown in many studies to effectively protect the liver from various drug- or chemical-induced hepatitis, including acetaminophen, carbon tetrachloride, alpha-naphthyliso-thiocyanate (ANIT), and concanavalin A.[5,6,7] This action was attributed to inhibited production of inflammatory cytokines and enhanced production of anti-inflammatory cytokines. The researchers also stated that administration of *Yin Chen Hao Tang* may be useful for treating severe acute hepatitis accompanying cholestasis in cases of autoimmune hepatitis.[8]

4. **Hepatoprotective and antifibrotic**: In 6 postoperative patients with biliary atresia, administration of *Yin Chen Hao Tang* was found to have a long-term protective and antifibrotic effect on the liver in patients with abnormal

DAMP-DISPELLING FORMULAS

16

1087

Chapter 16 – Damp-Dispelling Formulas　　　　*Section 2 – Heat-Clearing and Damp-Dispelling Formulas*

Yīn Chén Hāo Tāng (Artemisia Scoparia Decoction)

levels of liver enzyme and hyaluronic acid.[9] Another study showed that use of *Yin Chen Hao Tang* prevented artificially-induced liver fibrosis in rats.[10]

5. **Antihyperlipidemic**: Use of *Yin Chen Hao Tang* in mice was associated with a decrease in total cholesterol, LDL, and triglycerides levels, and an increase in HDL levels.[11]

CLINICAL STUDIES AND RESEARCH

1. **Hepatitis**: *Yin Chen Hao Tang* has been shown in many studies to be beneficial in treating hepatitis. Administration of modified *Yin Chen Hao Tang* to 247 patients with acute infectious icteric hepatitis was associated with recovery in 83 cases within 7 days, 158 cases within 15 days, and 6 cases within 20 days. The herbal treatment consisted of this formula plus *Bai Jiang Cao* (Herba cum Radice Patriniae), *Huang Bo* (Cortex Phellodendri Chinensis), *Long Dan* (Radix et Rhizoma Gentianae), *Yu Jin* (Radix Curcumae), and others.[12] Another study of 50 patients with acute icteric hepatitis who were treated with modified *Yin Chen Hao Tang* showed recovery in 47 cases, improvement in 2 cases, and no effect in 1 case (98% overall effectiveness). The herbal treatment contained this formula with the following modifications: *Huang Qin* (Radix Scutellariae), *Huang Lian* (Rhizoma Coptidis), and *Long Dan* (Radix et Rhizoma Gentianae) for more heat than dampness; *Cang Zhu* (Rhizoma Atractylodis), *Fu Ling* (Poria) and *Pei Lan* (Herba Eupatorii) for more dampness than heat; *Hou Po* (Cortex Magnoliae Officinalis) and *Lai Fu Zi* (Semen Raphani) for abdominal distention; *Zhu Ru* (Caulis Bambusae in Taenia), *Ban Xia* (Rhizoma Pinelliae) and *Sheng Jiang* (Rhizoma Zingiberis Recens) for nausea and vomiting; and *Yan Hu Suo* (Rhizoma Corydalis) and *Chuan Lian Zi* (Fructus Toosendan) for hypochondriac pain.[13] Lastly, one study reported good results using *Yin Chen Hao Tang* plus *Che Qian Zi* (Semen Plantaginis) and *Mu Tong* (Caulis Akebiae) to treat infants with acute viral hepatitis.[14]

2. **Jaundice**: It has been confirmed via numerous studies that *Yin Chen Hao Tang* is beneficial in treating jaundice. One study reported 90% effectiveness using modified *Yin Chen Hao Tang* to treat jaundice in 20 patients (16 with complete recovery, 2 with improvement, and 2 with no effect). The herbal treatment contained this formula plus *Bai Hua She She Cao* (Herba Hedyotis), *Da Qing Ye* (Folium Isatidis), *Ji Gu Cao* (Herba Abri), and others.[15] According to another study, use of modified *Yin Chen Hao Tang* was associated with 91% effectiveness to treat patients with persistent jaundice even after surgical removal of the gallbladder. The herbal treatment contained this formula, plus *Huang Qin* (Radix Scutellariae), *Yu Jin* (Radix Curcumae), *Jin Qian Cao* (Herba Lysimachiae),

and others. Of 12 patients in this study, 5 had significant improvement, 6 had moderate improvement, and 1 had no effect.[16] Lastly, 32 patients with jaundice associated with viral hepatitis were treated with large doses of *Yin Chen Hao Tang* with good results. In addition to the base formula, modifications included the addition of *Ban Xia* (Rhizoma Pinelliae) and *Zhu Ru* (Caulis Bambusae in Taenia) for nausea and vomiting; *Zhu Ling* (Polyporus), *Fu Ling* (Poria), and *Da Fu Pi* (Pericarpium Arecae) for accumulation of water; *Dan Shen* (Radix et Rhizoma Salviae Miltiorrhizae) and *Yu Jin* (Radix Curcumae) for hepatomegaly or splenomegaly; *Qin Jiao* (Radix Gentianae Macrophyllae) and *Qin Pi* (Cortex Fraxini) for itchy skin; and *Chai Hu* (Radix Bupleuri) and *Huang Qin* (Radix Scutellariae) for chills and fever. Of 32 patients, the study reported significant improvement in 23 cases and moderate improvement in 9 cases.[17]

3. **Biliary atresia**: Administration of *Yin Chen Hao Tang* was associated with beneficial effects in 18 postoperative biliary atresia patients between 3 and 23 years of age. Use of *Yin Chen Hao Tang* resulted in statistically significant improvements in glutamic oxaloacetic transaminase (GOT) (45%), glutamic pyruvic transaminase (GPT) (72%), gamma-glutamyl transpeptidase (gammaGTP) (72%), total bile acids (TBA) (72%), hyaluronic acid (HA) (67%), prolyl hydroxylase (PH) (40%), procollagen III peptide (PIIIP) (50%), and type IV collagen as markers of liver fibrosis (23%). The study concluded that long-term administration of *Yin Chen Hao Tang* in postoperative biliary atresia patients improved liver status as assessed by markers of liver function and fibrosis.[18]

4. **Hyperlipidemia**: Use of *Yin Chen Hao Tang* plus *Long Dan Xie Gan Tang* (Gentiana Decoction to Drain the Liver) to treat hyperlipidemia was associated with a reduction of cholesterol levels in 77 of 88 patients. The patients were instructed to discontinue all other herbal and drug treatment for hyperlipidemia throughout the study.[19]

5. **Seborrheic dermatitis**: One study reported 89.06% effectiveness using herbs orally and topically to treat seborrheic dermatitis. For oral use, the herbal formula contained *Yin Chen Hao Tang* plus *Bai Hua She She Cao* (Herba Hedyotis) 15g, *Ku Shen* (Radix Sophorae Flavescentis) 10g, *She Chuang Zi* (Fructus Cnidii) 10g, and *Di Fu Zi* (Fructus Kochiae) 10g. For topical application, the herbal formula contained *Ku Shen* (Radix Sophorae Flavescentis) 30g, *Ma Chi Xian* (Herba Portulacae) 30g, *Liu Huang* (Sulfur) 30g, *Ye Ju Hua* (Flos Chrysanthemi Indici) 20g, and *Bai Bu* (Radix Stemonae) 20g. Of 128 patients, the study reported complete recovery in 78 cases, significant improvement in 28 cases, moderate improvement in 8 cases, and no effect in 14 cases.[20]

1088

Chinese Herbal Formulas and Applications

Yīn Chén Hāo Tāng (Artemisia Scoparia Decoction)

RELATED FORMULAS

Zhī Zǐ Bǎi Pí Tāng
(Gardenia and Phellodendron Decoction)

栀子柏皮湯
栀子柏皮汤

Pinyin Name: Zhi Zi Bai Pi Tang
Literal Name: Gardenia and Phellodendron Decoction
Alternate Name: Zhi Zi Bo Pi Tang
Original Source: *Shang Han Lun* (Discussion of Cold-Induced Disorders) by Zhang Zhong-Jing in the Eastern Han Dynasty

Zhi Zi (Fructus Gardeniae)	15 pieces [9g]
Zhi Gan Cao (Radix et Rhizoma Glycyrrhizae Praeparata cum Melle)	3g
Huang Bo (Cortex Phellodendri Chinensis)	6g

The source text instructs to cook the herbs in 4 cups [800 mL] of water until the liquid is reduced to 1.5 cups [300 mL]. Take the strained decoction while warm.

Zhi Zi Bai Pi Tang (Gardenia and Phellodendron Decoction) clears heat and dispels dampness. It is used for patients with a recent history of an exterior syndrome that transformed into interior heat. Clinically, the patient may show symptoms of fever, yellow discoloration of the skin, irritability, heartburn, thirst, and a yellow tongue coating.

Yin Chen Hao Tang and *Zhi Zi Bai Pi Tang* (Gardenia and Phellodendron Decoction) both treat damp-heat jaundice.
- *Yin Chen Hao Tang* is generally considered the formula of choice for treating damp-heat jaundice.
- *Zhi Zi Bai Pi Tang* is more suitable for jaundice characterized by more heat than dampness. This formula has a stronger action to clear heat and a weaker action to dispel dampness.

Yīn Chén Sì Nì Tāng
(Artemisia Scoparia Decoction for Frigid Extremities)

茵陳四逆湯
茵陈四逆汤

Pinyin Name: Yin Chen Si Ni Tang
Literal Name: Artemisia Scoparia Decoction for Frigid Extremities
Original Source: *Wei Sheng Bao Jian* (Precious Mirror of Health) by Luo Tian-Yi in the Yuan Dynasty

Yin Chen (Herba Artemisiae Scopariae)	18g
Gan Jiang (Rhizoma Zingiberis)	4.5g
Zhi Gan Cao (Radix et Rhizoma Glycyrrhizae Praeparata cum Melle)	6g
Fu Zi (Radix Aconiti Lateralis Praeparata), pao (blast-fried)	1 piece [9g]

The source text instructs to prepare the ingredients as a decoction, and take the decoction after it is cooled to room temperature. The main actions of this formula are to tonify yang, warm the interior, dispel dampness, and relieve jaundice. Clinically, *Yin Chen Si Ni Tang* (Artemisia Scoparia Decoction for Frigid Extremities) may be used for patients with damp-cold (yin type) jaundice with symptoms such as dark, lusterless, and yellow discoloration of the skin, lethargy, withered *shen* (spirit), lack of appetite, cold extremities, and a deep, fine and forceless pulse.

Yin Chen Hao Tang and *Yin Chen Si Ni Tang* (Artemisia Scoparia Decoction for Frigid Extremities) both treat jaundice.
- *Yin Chen Hao Tang* is cold in nature, and more suitable for damp-heat (yang-type) jaundice with bright yellow discoloration.
- *Yin Chen Si Ni Tang* is warm in nature, and more suitable for damp-cold (yin-type) jaundice with dark yellow discoloration.

Yīn Chén Pái Shí Tāng
(Artemisia Scoparia Decoction to Expel Stone)

茵陳排石湯
茵陈排石汤

Pinyin Name: Yin Chen Pai Shi Tang
Literal Name: Artemisia Scoparia Decoction to Expel Stone
Original Source: *An Hui Zhong Yi Xue Yuan* (Anhui University School of Medicine) in 1990

Yin Chen (Herba Artemisiae Scopariae)
Da Huang (Radix et Rhizoma Rhei)
Jin Qian Cao (Herba Lysimachiae)
Long Dan (Radix et Rhizoma Gentianae)
Hai Jin Sha (Spora Lygodii)
Li Zhi He (Semen Litchi)
Zhi Qiao (Fructus Aurantii)
Wei Ling Xian (Radix et Rhizoma Clematidis)

Yin Chen Pai Shi Tang (Artemisia Scoparia Decoction to Expel Stone) clears heat and resolves dampness from the Liver and Gallbladder. Clinically, it is used to treat cholecystitis and cholelithiasis characterized by damp-heat.

DAMP-DISPELLING FORMULAS

16

1089

Chapter 16 – Damp-Dispelling Formulas   *Section 2 – Heat-Clearing and Damp-Dispelling Formulas*

Yīn Chén Hāo Tāng (Artemisia Scoparia Decoction)

AUTHORS' COMMENTS

According to Dr. Chang Wei-Yen, *Yin Chen Hao Tang* can be combined with *Da Chai Hu Tang* (Major Bupleurum Decoction) to treat cholecystitis, cholelithiasis, and fatty liver.

References

1. *Zhong Yao Ming Fang Yao Li Yu Ying Yong* (Pharmacology and Applications of Famous Herbal Formulas) 1989;423-425.
2. *Zhong Yao Yao Li Yu Lin Chuang* (Pharmacology and Clinical Applications of Chinese Herbs) 1987;3:52.
3. *Zhong Yi Za Zhi* (Journal of Chinese Medicine) 1982;7:72.
4. Shoda J, Miura T, Utsunomiya H, Oda K, Yamamoto M, Kano M, Ikegami T, Tanaka N, Akita H, Ito K, Suzuki H, Sugiyama Y. Genipin enhances Mrp2 (Abcc2)-mediated bile formation and organic anion transport in rat liver. Hepatology 2004 Jan;39(1):167-78.
5. *Zhong Yao Yao Li Yu Lin Chuang* (Pharmacology and Clinical Applications of Chinese Herbs) 1992;8:40.
6. *Shan Xi Yi Yao Za Zhi* (Shanxi Journal of Medicine and Herbology) 1975;3:79.
7. *Zhong Xi Yi Jie He Za Zhi* (Journal of Integrated Chinese and Western Medicine) 1985;6:56.
8. Yamashiki M, Mase A, Arai I, Huang XX, Nobori T, Nishimura A, Sakaguchi S, Inoue K. Effects of the Japanese herbal medicine

'Inchinko-to' (TJ-135) on concanavalin A-induced hepatitis in mice. Clin Sci (Lond) 2000 Nov;99(5):421-31.
9. Iinuma Y, Kubota M, Yagi M, Kanada S, Yamazaki S, Kinoshita Y. Effects of the herbal medicine Inchinko-to on liver function in post-operative patients with biliary atresia--a pilot study. J Pediatr Surg 2003 Nov;38(11):1607-11.
10. Sakaida I, Tsuchiya M, Kawaguchi K, Kimura T, Terai S, Okita K. Herbal medicine Inchin-ko-to (TJ-135) prevents liver fibrosis and enzyme-altered lesions in rat liver cirrhosis induced by a choline-deficient L-amino acid-defined diet. J Hepatol 2003 Jun;38(6):762-9.
11. *Zhong Cheng Yao* (Study of Chinese Patent Medicine) 1992;7:34.
12. *Zhong Yi Ming Fang Lin Chuang Xin Yong* (Contemporary Clinical Applications of Classic Chinese Formulas) 2001;507.
13. *Shan Xi Zhong Yi* (Shanxi Chinese Medicine) 1998;3:19.
14. *Shan Xi Zhong Yi* (Shanxi Chinese Medicine) 1993;4:17.
15. *Tian Jin Zhong Yi* (Tianjin Chinese Medicine) 1986;2:34.
16. *Jiang Su Zhong Yi* (Jiangsu Chinese Medicine) 1996;5:17.
17. *Zhong Yi Ming Fang Lin Chuang Xin Yong* (Contemporary Clinical Applications of Classic Chinese Formulas) 2001;508.
18. Kobayashi H, Horikoshi K, Yamataka A, Lane GJ, Yamamoto M, Miyano T. Beneficial effect of a traditional herbal medicine (inchin-ko-to) in postoperative biliary atresia patients. Pediatric Surgery International 2001 Jul;17(5-6):386-9.
19. *Shan Xi Zhong Yi* (Shanxi Chinese Medicine) 1997;5:220.
20. *Zhong Yi Yao Xue Bao* (Report of Chinese Medicine and Herbology) 1992;2:33.

Yīn Chén Wǔ Líng Sǎn

(Artemisia Scoparia and Five-Ingredient Powder with Poria)

茵陳五苓散
茵陈五苓散

Pinyin Name: *Yin Chen Wu Ling San*
Literal Name: Artemisia Scoparia and Five-Ingredient Powder with Poria
Alternate Names: Capillaries and Hoelen Five Formula, Artemisia and Hoelen Five Formula
Original Source: *Jin Gui Yao Lue* (Essentials from the Golden Cabinet) by Zhang Zhong-Jing in the Eastern Han Dynasty

COMPOSITION

Yin Chen (Herba Artemisiae Scopariae)	7.5g
Wu Ling San (Five-Ingredient Powder with Poria)	3.75g

DOSAGE / PREPARATION / ADMINISTRATION

The source text instructs to grind the ingredients into powder. Take one spoonful [6g] of the powder three times daily after meals.

CHINESE THERAPEUTIC ACTIONS

Dispels dampness and treats jaundice

CLINICAL MANIFESTATIONS

Damp-heat jaundice (more damp than heat) with dysuria.

CLINICAL APPLICATIONS

Jaundice, hepatitis, nephritis, renal cirrhosis, and hyper-lipoproteinemia.

Chinese Herbal Formulas and Applications

Yīn Chén Wǔ Líng Sǎn
(Artemisia Scoparia and Five-Ingredient Powder with Poria)

EXPLANATION

Yin Chen Wu Ling San (Artemisia Scoparia and Five-Ingredient Powder with Poria) is comprised of *Yin Chen* (Herba Artemisiae Scopariae) plus *Wu Ling San* (Five-Ingredient Powder with Poria). *Yin Chen* (Herba Artemisiae Scopariae) clears damp-heat and relieves jaundice. *Wu Ling San* (Five-Ingredient Powder with Poria) regulates water circulation, dispels dampness, and relieves dysuria. Clinically, this formula may be used to treat damp-heat jaundice (more damp than heat) with dysuria.

Please refer to *Wu Ling San* (Five-Ingredient Powder with Poria) for a detailed explanation of this formula.

MODIFICATIONS
- With fever and thirst, add *Shi Gao* (Gypsum Fibrosum) and *Zhi Mu* (Rhizoma Anemarrhenae).
- With dysuria, add *Mu Tong* (Caulis Akebiae) and *Di Huang* (Radix Rehmanniae).

PHARMACOLOGICAL EFFECTS
1. **Diuretic**: Administration of *Yin Chen Wu Ling San* at normal doses in adults did not significantly affect the urine output or concentration of electrolytes. However, at higher doses, it did increase the urine output without changing the concentration of the electrolytes.[1]
2. **Hepatoprotective**: One study reported that *Yin Chen Wu Ling San* had a protective effect against alcohol-induced liver damage in mice.[2]

CLINICAL STUDIES AND RESEARCH
1. **Yellow discoloration of the palms and soles**: Use of *Yin Chen Wu Ling San* plus *Bai Mao Gen* (Rhizoma Imperatae), *Dan Shen* (Radix et Rhizoma Salviae Miltiorrhizae) and *Hua Shi* (Talcum) was associated with a 100% success rate in treating 6 patients with yellow discoloration of the palms and soles. The cause of this illness was unrelated to jaundice, as confirmed by Western medicine. The traditional Chinese medical diagnosis was Spleen and blood deficiencies, with damp-heat accumulation.[3]
2. **Hyperlipoproteinemia**: Sixty patients with hyperlipoproteinemia were divided into two groups of 30 patients

each and treated with herbs. Group one received *Yin Chen Wu Ling San*, and group two received a preparation of *Jiao Gu Lan* (Rhizoma seu Herba Gynostemmatis). In group one, the study reported significant improvement in 19 cases, moderate improvement in 9 cases, and no effect in 2 cases (93% effectiveness). In group two, the study reported significant improvement in 6 cases, moderate improvement in 20 cases, and no effect in 4 cases (86.7% effectiveness).[4]

3. **Hepatitis and jaundice**: It has been shown in many studies that use of *Yin Chen Wu Ling San* with pharmaceuticals was associated with marked success in treating individuals with hepatitis and/or jaundice. One formula that successfully treated jaundice contained the following ingredients: *Yin Chen* (Herba Artemisiae Scopariae) 30g, dry-fried *Bai Zhu* (Rhizoma Atractylodis Macrocephalae) 30g, *Chi Fu Ling* (Poria Rubra) 30g, *Dan Shen* (Radix et Rhizoma Salviae Miltiorrhizae) 30g, *Fu Zi* (Radix Aconiti Lateralis Praeparata) 10-30g, *Ting Li Zi* (Semen Descurainiae seu Lepidii) 10-20g, *Ze Xie* (Rhizoma Alismatis) 15g, *Dang Shen* (Radix Codonopsis) 10g, *Gui Zhi* (Ramulus Cinnamomi) 10g, and *Zhi Gan Cao* (Radix et Rhizoma Glycyrrhizae Praeparata cum Melle) 10g.[5] For icteric hepatitis, one successful formula contained the following ingredients: *Yin Chen Wu Ling San* plus *Chuan Xiong* (Rhizoma Chuanxiong), *Dang Gui* (Radix Angelicae Sinensis), and *Da Huang* (Radix et Rhizoma Rhei).[6]

AUTHORS' COMMENTS
Yin Chen Hao Tang (Artemisia Scoparia Decoction), *Zhi Zi Bai Pi Tang* (Gardenia and Phellodendron Decoction) and *Yin Chen Wu Ling San* all treat damp-heat jaundice.
- *Yin Chen Hao Tang* is the most effective formula, and generally considered the first choice for damp-heat jaundice. Yellow discoloration of the skin and sclera and yellow urine are the diagnostic signs.
- *Zhi Zi Bai Pi Tang* is more suitable for jaundice characterized by more heat than dampness. In addition to yellow discoloration of the skin and sclera, there may be fever and irritability.

Yin Chen Wu Ling San (Artemisia Scoparia and Five-Ingredient Powder with Poria)

Diagnosis	Signs and Symptoms	Treatment	Herbs
Damp-heat jaundice	Jaundice with dysuria: damp-heat	Dispels dampness and treats jaundice	• *Yin Chen* (Herba Artemisiae Scopariae) clears damp-heat and relieves jaundice. • *Wu Ling San* (Five-Ingredient Powder with Poria) regulates water circulation, dispels dampness, and relieves dysuria.

DAMP-DISPELLING FORMULAS

16

1091

Chapter 16 – Damp-Dispelling Formulas   *Section 2 – Heat-Clearing and Damp-Dispelling Formulas*

Yīn Chén Wǔ Líng Sǎn
(Artemisia Scoparia and Five-Ingredient Powder with Poria)

- *Yin Chen Wu Ling San* is more appropriate for jaundice characterized by more dampness than heat. In addition to yellow discoloration of the skin and sclera, there may be dysuria.

References
1. *Guo Wai Yi Xue Zhong Yi Zhong Yao Fen Ce* (Monograph of Chinese Herbology from Foreign Medicine) 1983;6:24.

2. *Guo Wai Yi Xue Zhong Yi Zhong Yao Fen Ce* (Monograph of Chinese Herbology from Foreign Medicine) 1986;8(1):22.
3. *Bei Jing Zhong Yi* (Beijing Chinese Medicine) 1987;5:33.
4. *Zhong Guo Zhong Xi Yi Jie He Za Zhi* (Chinese Journal of Integrative Chinese and Western Medicine) 1996;8:470.
5. *Hu Bei Zhong Yi Za Zhi* (Hubei Journal of Chinese Medicine) 1986;3:50.
6. *Shang Hai Zhong Yi Yao Za Zhi* (Shanghai Journal of Chinese Medicine and Herbology) 1984;8:20.

Sān Rén Tāng (Three-Nut Decoction)
三仁湯
三仁汤

Pinyin Name: *San Ren Tang*
Literal Name: Three-Nut Decoction
Alternate Name: Triple Nut Combination
Original Source: *Wen Bing Tiao Bian* (Systematic Differentiation of Warm Disease) by Wu Ju-Tong in 1798

COMPOSITION

Ku Xing Ren (Semen Armeniacae Amarum)	15g [12g]
Dou Kou (Fructus Amomi Rotundus)	6g
Yi Yi Ren (Semen Coicis)	18g
Hua Shi (Talcum), *shui fei* (refined with water)	18g
Tong Cao (Medulla Tetrapanacis)	6g
Zhu Ye (Herba Phyllostachys)	6g
Ban Xia (Rhizoma Pinelliae)	15g [10g]
Hou Po (Cortex Magnoliae Officinalis)	6g

DOSAGE / PREPARATION / ADMINISTRATION

The source text instructs to cook the ingredients with 8 bowls of fresh spring water until it is reduced to 3 bowls. Take 1 bowl three times daily. Today, this formula may be prepared as a decoction with the doses suggested in brackets.

CHINESE THERAPEUTIC ACTIONS
1. Ventilates and smoothes the qi
2. Clears damp-heat

CLINICAL MANIFESTATIONS

Early stage of damp-warmth affecting the *qi* (energy) level: headache, aversion to cold, heaviness and pain of the body, chest oppression and discomfort, absence of hunger and thirst, a feeling of heat in the afternoon, pale, yellow face, pale tongue, and a wiry and fine or soggy pulse.

CLINICAL APPLICATIONS

Pneumonia, otitis media, fever, altitude stress, cardio-pulmonary diseases, hepatitis, cholecystitis, pyelone-phritis, glomerulonephritis, gastroenteritis, priapism, restless legs syndrome, arthritis, obesity with dizziness, and lymphadenitis.

EXPLANATION

San Ren Tang (Three-Nut Decoction) treats early stage damp-warmth (more dampness than heat) affecting the *qi* (energy) level. This condition usually occurs in late summer when there is an abundance of damp-warmth in the environment, and in those individuals with Spleen deficiency. Damp-warmth in the environment may affect the exterior of the body, causing headache and aversion to cold. Spleen deficiency may lead to damp production and subsequent formation of heat. The dampness and heat

1092

Chinese Herbal Formulas and Applications

Sān Rén Tāng (Three-Nut Decoction)

San Ren Tang (Three-Nut Decoction)

Diagnosis	Signs and Symptoms	Treatment	Herbs
Early stage of damp-warmth affecting the *qi* (energy) level	• Headache and aversion to cold: damp-warmth affecting the exterior • Heaviness and pain of the body, chest oppression and discomfort: accumulation of dampness obstructing qi circulation • Pale, yellow face: Spleen deficiency with damp accumulation • Pale tongue: qi deficiency	• Ventilates and smoothes qi • Clears damp-heat	• *Ku Xing Ren* (Semen Armeniacae Amarum) ventilates and regulates Lung qi and relieves chest oppression. • *Dou Kou* (Fructus Amomi Rotundus) dries dampness and activates the qi flow. • *Yi Yi Ren* (Semen Coicis) dispels dampness and strengthens the Spleen. • *Hua Shi* (Talcum), *Tong Cao* (Medulla Tetrapanacis) and *Zhu Ye* (Herba Phyllostachys) clear heat, dispel dampness and clear heat via urination. • *Ban Xia* (Rhizoma Pinelliae) and *Hou Po* (Cortex Magnoliae Officinalis) activate qi circulation, dispel dampness, and relieve distention.

may obstruct qi flow, causing pain, a feeling of heaviness, and chest oppression and discomfort. A pale, yellow face is a sign of Spleen deficiency with damp accumulation. A pale tongue is common for qi-deficient patients. A wiry, fine pulse may be present in patients suffering from pain and qi deficiency, while a soggy pulse may be present with severe damp accumulation.

This formula contains *Ku Xing Ren* (Semen Armeniacae Amarum) to ventilate and regulate the Lung qi and relieve chest oppression. Because the Lung is the organ that regulates water metabolism, restoring the normal flow of Lung qi helps to resolve dampness in the entire body. *Dou Kou* (Fructus Amomi Rotundus) is an acrid and aromatic herb that dries dampness and activates the qi flow. *Yi Yi Ren* (Semen Coicis) dispels dampness and strengthens the Spleen. *Hua Shi* (Talcum), *Tong Cao* (Medulla Tetrapanacis), and *Zhu Ye* (Herba Phyllostachys) clear heat, dispel dampness, and clear heat via urination. *Ban Xia* (Rhizoma Pinelliae) and *Hou Po* (Cortex Magnoliae Officinalis) activate qi circulation, dispel dampness, and relieve distention.

MODIFICATIONS
• For the initial stages of *wen bing* (warm disease) with dampness affecting the *wei* (defensive) level, add *Huo Xiang* (Herba Agastaches) and *Xiang Ru* (Herba Moslae).
• With alternating chills and fever, add *Qing Hao* (Herba Artemisiae Annuae) and *Cao Guo* (Fructus Tsaoko).
• With heat and a bitter taste in the mouth, add *Huang Lian* (Rhizoma Coptidis) and *Huang Qin* (Radix Scutellariae).

• With epigastric and abdominal fullness, distention, and a feeling of incomplete evacuation of stools, add *Lai Fu Zi* (Semen Raphani) and *Shen Qu* (Massa Fermentata).

CAUTIONS / CONTRAINDICATIONS
San Ren Tang treats conditions characterized by more dampness than heat. It is not suitable in cases characterized by more heat than dampness, or with the presence of dryness and heat.

CLINICAL STUDIES AND RESEARCH
1. **Pneumonia**: Forty patients with pneumonia were treated with *San Ren Tang* with complete recovery in 36 cases and improvement in 4 cases. The average duration of treatment was 4.8 days. The treatment used *San Ren Tang* as the base formula with the addition of *Da Qing Ye* (Folium Isatidis) for heat, *Sang Bai Pi* (Cortex Mori) for excessive perspiration, *Tai Zi Shen* (Radix Pseudostellariae) for weakness and deficiency, *Sha Shen* (Radix Glehniae seu Adenophorae) for damaged body fluids, and *Gua Lou Zi* (Semen Trichosanthis) for constipation.[1]
2. **Otitis media**: Modified *San Ren Tang* was used with good results for treatment of catarrhal otitis media. The modifications are as follows: *Ma Huang* (Herba Ephedrae) and *Shi Chang Pu* (Rhizoma Acori Tatarinowii) were added for nasal obstruction; and *Ze Xie* (Rhizoma Alismatis), *Che Qian Zi* (Semen Plantaginis), and *Ting Li Zi* (Semen Descurainiae seu Lepidii) were added for accumulation of fluids in the ear. Out of 110 patients, the study reported complete recovery in 66 cases, marked improvement in 17 cases, improvement in 19 cases, and no effect in 8 cases.[2]

DAMP-DISPELLING FORMULAS

16

1093

Sān Rén Tāng (Three-Nut Decoction)

3. **Cardiopulmonary diseases**: Thirty-two patients with chronic cardiopulmonary diseases were treated with modified *San Ren Tang* with complete recovery in 21 cases, marked effect in 7 cases, and slight improvement in 4 cases. Clinical presentations of the patients prior to herbal treatment included palpitations, shortness of breath, shallow and hurried respiration, dizziness, fatigue, white scanty sputum, a dark purple tongue with spots, a white greasy tongue coating, and a wiry, slippery or deep, rapid and fine pulse.[3]

4. **Hepatitis**: Use of modified *San Ren Tang* was associated with beneficially treating acute icteric hepatitis characterized by damp-heat affecting all three *jiaos*. The herbal treatment contained the following ingredients: *Yin Chen* (Herba Artemisiae Scopariae) 30g, *Tu Yin Chen* (Herba Origani), *Ku Xing Ren* (Semen Armeniacae Amarum) 5g, *Dou Kou* (Fructus Amomi Rotundus) 5g, *Yi Yi Ren* (Semen Coicis) 12g, *Hou Po* (Cortex Magnoliae Officinalis) 9g, *Dan Zhu Ye* (Herba Lophatheri) 6g, *Ban Xia* (Rhizoma Pinelliae) 9g, *Tong Cao* (Medulla Tetrapanacis) 5g, *Hua Shi* (Talcum) 18g, and *Zhi Zi* (Fructus Gardeniae) 12g. The herbs were administered in decoction form daily for 12 days.[4]

5. **Cholecystitis**: *San Ren Tang* was used to treat 38 patients with cholecystitis with complete recovery in 15 cases and improvement in 23 cases. The herbal formula used *San Ren Tang* as the base formula. *Chai Hu* (Radix Bupleuri) and *Huang Qin* (Radix Scutellariae) were added for aversion to cold and bitter taste in the mouth; *Yan Hu Suo* (Rhizoma Corydalis) and *Yu Jin* (Radix Curcumae) were added for hypochondriac pain; *Huo Xiang* (Herba Agastaches) and *Pei Lan* (Herba Eupatorii) were added for nausea, vomiting and abdominal distention; *Yin Chen* (Herba Artemisiae Scopariae) for jaundice; *Shan Zha* (Fructus Crataegi), *Mai Ya* (Fructus Hordei Germinatus), and *Shen Qu* (Massa Fermentata) were added for aversion to greasy, oily foods; and *Zhi Shi* (Fructus Aurantii Immaturus) was added for constipation.[5]

6. **Glomerulonephritis**: One hundred and twenty patients with glomerulonephritis (78 males and 42 females; between 6-45 years of age) were treated with complete recovery in 103 cases, significant improvement in 11 cases, and no effect in 6 cases. The herbal formula contained *Ku Xing Ren* (Semen Armeniacae Amarum) 15g, *Dou Kou* (Fructus Amomi Rotundus) 15g, *Yi Yi Ren* (Semen Coicis) 20g, *Hou Po* (Cortex Magnoliae Officinalis) 15g, *Ban Xia* (Rhizoma Pinelliae) 15g, *Tong Cao* (Medulla Tetrapanacis) 10g, *Hua Shi* (Talcum) 15g, *Zhu Ye* (Herba Phyllostachys) 20g, *Shi Wei* (Folium Pyrrosiae) 30g, *Bai Mao Gen* (Rhizoma Imperatae) 30g,

and others as needed. The duration of treatment ranged from 6-30 days, with an average of 12 days.[6]

7. **Gastroenteritis**: One study reported marked success using modified *San Ren Tang* to treat 300 patients with acute gastroenteritis. Clinical manifestations included edema, decreased urination, hematuria, proteinuria, elevated blood pressure, chest congestion with shortness of breath, cough with a small amount of foamy sputum, epigastric fullness, poor appetite, and nausea. The herbal formula contained *Ku Xing Ren* (Semen Armeniacae Amarum) 10g, *Dou Kou* (Fructus Amomi Rotundus) 10g, *Yi Yi Ren* (Semen Coicis) 30g, *Hua Shi* (Talcum) 15g, *Zhu Ye* (Herba Phyllostachys) 10g, *Hou Po* (Cortex Magnoliae Officinalis) 15g, *Tong Cao* (Medulla Tetrapanacis) 15g, *Ban Xia* (Rhizoma Pinelliae) 10g, charred *Shan Zha* (Fructus Crataegi) 15g, and *Gan Cao* (Radix et Rhizoma Glycyrrhizae) 5g. Additional modifications were made as needed. The herbs were cooked in water, and administered via decoction daily. The duration of treatment ranged from 2 to 8 packs of herbs. The study reported complete recovery or improvement in all 300 patients.[7]

8. **Priapism**: Use of modified *San Ren Tang* was effective in treating one case of priapism (prolonged, painful erection) and inability to ejaculate. The herbal formula contained *San Ren Tang* plus *Niu Xi* (Radix Achyranthis Bidentatae), *Wang Bu Liu Xing* (Semen Vaccariae), *Che Qian Zi* (Semen Plantaginis), *Pu Gong Ying* (Herba Taraxaci), and others. After 6 packs of herbal therapy, the priapism was resolved and the patient was able to ejaculate normally.[8] Interestingly, there are also case reports that *San Ren Tang* can effectively treat impotence.[9,10]

9. **Altitude stress**: Use of modified *San Ren Tang* was associated with good success in treating patients with acute altitude stress. The treatment protocol was to use *San Ren Tang* as the base formula. Modifications included *Chai Hu* (Radix Bupleuri) and *Fang Feng* (Radix Saposhnikoviae) for concurrent viral infection; *Wu Wei Zi* (Fructus Schisandrae Chinensis), *Dan Shen* (Radix et Rhizoma Salviae Miltiorrhizae), and *Shou Wu Teng* (Caulis Polygoni Multiflori) for insomnia and palpitations; *Ting Li Zi* (Semen Descurainiae seu Lepidii) and *Chuan Bei Mu* (Bulbus Fritillariae Cirrhosae) for severe cough; *Gua Lou* (Fructus Trichosanthis) for chest oppression; and the addition of *Bai Mao Gen* (Rhizoma Imperatae) and *Mo Han Lian* (Herba Ecliptae), with the removal of *Ban Xia* (Rhizoma Pinelliae), for epistaxis. Out of 50 patients, 39 had complete recovery, 6 had marked improvement, 2 had slight improvement, and 3 had no effect. The rate of complete recovery was 78%, and the overall effectiveness was 95%.[11]

Chinese Herbal Formulas and Applications

Sān Rén Tāng (Three-Nut Decoction)

RELATED FORMULAS

Huò Pò Xià Líng Tāng

(Agastache, Magnolia Bark, Pinellia, and Poria Decoction)

藿朴夏苓湯
藿朴夏苓汤

Pinyin Name: *Huo Po Xia Ling Tang*
Literal Name: Agastache, Magnolia Bark, Pinellia, and Poria Decoction
Original Source: *Gan Zheng Ji Yao* (Essential Compilation of Infectious Syndromes) by Yan Hong-Zhi in 1920

Huo Xiang (Herba Agastaches)	6g
Hou Po (Cortex Magnoliae Officinalis)	3g
Ban Xia (Rhizoma Pinelliae), zhu (boiled) with ginger	4.5g
Chi Fu Ling (Poria Rubra)	9g
Ku Xing Ren (Semen Armeniacae Amarum)	9g
Yi Yi Ren (Semen Coicis)	9g
Dou Kou (Fructus Amomi Rotundus)	9g
Zhu Ling (Polyporus)	4.5g
Dan Dou Chi (Semen Sojae Praeparatum)	9g
Ze Xie (Rhizoma Alismatis)	4.5g

The source text instructs to prepare the ingredients as a decoction. The main actions of this formula are to release the exterior and resolve dampness. Clinically, *Huo Po Xia Ling Tang* (Agastache, Magnolia Bark, Pinellia, and Poria Decoction) may be used for patients having an initial onset of damp-warmth invasion (more dampness than heat), characterized by symptoms such as fever, chills, lethargy, chest oppression, a thin, white tongue coating, and a soggy, moderate pulse.

Huáng Qín Huá Shí Tāng

(Scutellaria and Talcum Decoction)

黃芩滑石湯
黄芩滑石汤

Pinyin Name: *Huang Qin Hua Shi Tang*
Literal Name: Scutellaria and Talcum Decoction
Original Source: *Wen Bing Tiao Bian* (Systematic Differentiation of Warm Disease) by Wu Ju-Tong in 1798

Huang Qin (Radix Scutellariae)	9g
Hua Shi (Talcum)	9g
Fu Ling Pi (Cortex Poria)	9g
Da Fu Pi (Pericarpium Arecae)	6g
Dou Kou (Fructus Amomi Rotundus)	3g
Tong Cao (Medulla Tetrapanacis)	3g
Zhu Ling (Polyporus)	9g

The source text instructs to prepare the ingredients as a decoction. *Huang Qin Hua Shi Tang* (Scutellaria and Talcum Decoction) clears heat and dispels dampness. Clinically, it is often used for damp-warmth stagnation in the middle *jiao*, leading to such symptoms as persistent fever that temporarily decreases with perspiration but later rebounds, generalized body aches, thirst with little or no desire to drink water, a light yellow, slippery tongue coating, and a moderate pulse.

AUTHORS' COMMENTS

San Ren Tang, literally "Three-Nut Decoction," is so named because this formula contains three *ren* (seeds, nuts or fruits): *Ku Xing Ren* (Semen Armeniacae Amarum), *Yi Yi Ren* (Semen Coicis), and *Dou Kou* (Fructus Amomi Rotundus), which is also known as *Bai Dou Ren*.

San Ren Tang, *Huo Po Xia Ling Tang* (Agastache, Magnolia Bark, Pinellia and Poria Decoction), and *Huang Qin Hua Shi Tang* (Scutellaria and Talcum Decoction) all treat various presentations of damp-warmth. Their functions and indications vary, however.

- *San Ren Tang* clears heat and resolves dampness. It is generally used for the early stage of damp-warmth (more dampness than heat) affecting the *qi* (energy) level.
- *Huo Po Xia Ling Tang* resolves dampness and releases the exterior. It is appropriate for the early stage of damp-warmth invasion (more dampness than heat), with exterior signs and symptoms.
- *Huang Qin Hua Shi Tang* also clears heat and resolves dampness. It is used primarily for damp-warmth (with equal amounts of dampness and heat) affecting the middle *jiao*.

References

1. *Hu Nan Zhong Yi Za Zhi* (Hunan Journal of Chinese Medicine) 1998;3:50.
2. *Zhe Jiang Zhong Yi Za Zhi* (Zhejiang Journal of Chinese Medicine) 1991;6:255.
3. *Shan Dong Zhong Yi Za Zhi* (Shandong Journal of Chinese Medicine) 1997;11:504.
4. *Zhong Yi Za Zhi* (Journal of Chinese Medicine) 1982;7:46.
5. *Si Chuan Zhong Yi* (Sichuan Chinese Medicine) 1988;9:27.
6. *Zhong Yi Fang Ji Xian Dai Yan Jiu* (Modern Study of Medical Formulae in Traditional Chinese Medicine) 1997;1355.
7. *Shi Yong Zhong Yi Nei Ke Za Zhi* (Journal of Practical Chinese Internal Medicine) 1995;1:12.
8. *Shan Xi Zhong Yi* (Shanxi Chinese Medicine) 1995;4:178.
9. *Shang Hai Zhong Yi Yao Za Zhi* (Shanghai Journal of Chinese Medicine and Herbology) 1983;5:6.
10. *Zhong Yi Yao Xue Bao* (Report of Chinese Medicine and Herbology) 1993;4:30.
11. *Zhong Yi Za Zhi* (Journal of Chinese Medicine) 1988;3:211.

DAMP-DISPELLING FORMULAS

16

1095

Chapter 16 – Damp-Dispelling Formulas   *Section 2 – Heat-Clearing and Damp-Dispelling Formulas*

Gān Lù Xiāo Dú Dān (Sweet Dew Special Pill to Eliminate Toxin)

甘露消毒丹

Pinyin Name: *Gan Lu Xiao Du Dan*
Literal Name: Sweet Dew Special Pill to Eliminate Toxin
Alternate Names: *Kan Lu Hsiao Tu Tan*, *Pu Ji Xiao Du Dan*, Talc and Scute Formula, Sweet Dew Detoxication Pellet, Universal Benefit Special Pill to Eliminate Toxin, Forsythia and Acorus Formula
Original Source: *Xu Ming Yi Lei An* (Continuation of Famous Physicians' Cases Organized by Categories) by Wei Zhi-Xiu in 1770

COMPOSITION

Hua Shi (Talcum), *shui fei* (refined with water)	450g [15g]
Yin Chen (Herba Artemisiae Scopariae)	330g [11g]
Huang Qin (Radix Scutellariae)	300g [10g]
Shi Chang Pu (Rhizoma Acori Tatarinowii)	180g [6g]
Dou Kou (Fructus Amomi Rotundus)	120g [4g]
Huo Xiang (Herba Agastaches)	120g [4g]
She Gan (Rhizoma Belamcandae)	120g [4g]
Bo He (Herba Menthae)	120g [4g]
Chuan Bei Mu (Bulbus Fritillariae Cirrhosae)	150g [5g]
Mu Tong (Caulis Akebiae)	150g [5g]
Lian Qiao (Fructus Forsythiae)	120g [4g]

DOSAGE / PREPARATION / ADMINISTRATION

The source text instructs to sun-dry the ingredients and grind them into a fine powder. Take 9g of the powder per dose with boiled water. This formula is also given in pill form, and is prepared by mixing the powdered herbs with *Shen Qu* (Massa Fermentata) to form pills. Take 1 pill [9g] per dose with boiled water. Today, this formula may be prepared as a decoction with the doses suggested in brackets.

CHINESE THERAPEUTIC ACTIONS

1. Resolves dampness and dissolves turbidity
2. Clears heat and eliminates toxins

CLINICAL MANIFESTATIONS

Damp-warmth febrile disorder or epidemic diseases affecting the *qi* (energy) level: fever, lethargy, chest oppression, abdominal fullness, soreness of the extremities, sore throat, swelling of the lower cheeks, yellow discoloration of the skin, vomiting, diarrhea, thirst, scanty, dark, turbid urine, and a pale and white, a thick and greasy, or a dry and yellow tongue coating.

CLINICAL APPLICATIONS

Hepatitis, icteric infectious hepatitis, cholecystitis, jaundice, fever, enteric fever, encephalitis, gastritis, stomatitis, laryngopharyngitis, acute gastroenteritis, pyelonephritis, and leptospirosis.

EXPLANATION

Gan Lu Xiao Du Dan (Sweet Dew Special Pill to Eliminate Toxin) treats febrile disorder or epidemic diseases affecting the *qi* (energy) level. Warmth and dampness (equal amounts of each) may each intensify the severity of the other, causing fever, lethargy, and soreness of the extremities. Damp-warmth can cause qi stagnation, leading to chest oppression, abdominal fullness, vomiting or diarrhea. Furthermore, damp-warmth may rise upward and cause sore throat and swelling of the lower cheeks. It may also travel downward to produce scanty, dark, turbid urine; and travel outward to the skin to cause yellow discoloration. Lastly, a pale and white tongue coating may be apparent if the patient is weak and the qi is severely deficient; a thick and greasy tongue coating may be apparent if the patient has severe damp accumulation; and a dry and yellow tongue coating indicates of excess heat.

This formula contains *Hua Shi* (Talcum) to clear damp-heat, *Yin Chen* (Herba Artemisiae Scopariae) to dispel damp-heat and drain the yellow discoloration of the skin, and *Huang Qin* (Radix Scutellariae) to dry dampness and eliminate heat-toxins. *Shi Chang Pu* (Rhizoma Acori Tatarinowii), *Dou Kou* (Fructus Amomi Rotundus), and *Huo Xiang* (Herba Agastaches) are acrid and aromatic herbs that resolve dampness and turbidity and activate qi circulation. *She Gan* (Rhizoma Belamcandae), *Bo He*

1096

Gān Lù Xiāo Dú Dān (Sweet Dew Special Pill to Eliminate Toxin)

Gan Lu Xiao Du Dan (Sweet Dew Special Pill to Eliminate Toxin)

Diagnosis	Signs and Symptoms	Treatment	Herbs
Damp-warmth febrile disorder or epidemic diseases affecting the *qi* (energy) level	• Fever, lethargy, and soreness of the extremities: presence of damp-warmth • Chest oppression, abdominal fullness, vomiting or diarrhea: qi stagnation due to damp-warmth accumulation • Sore throat and swelling of the lower cheeks: damp-warmth traveling upward • Scanty, dark turbid urine: damp-warmth traveling downward • Yellow discoloration of the skin: damp-warmth traveling outward	• Resolves dampness and turbidity • Clears heat and eliminates toxins	• *Hua Shi* (Talcum), *Yin Chen* (Herba Artemisiae Scopariae), and *Huang Qin* (Radix Scutellariae) clear heat, dry dampness, and eliminate toxins. • *Shi Chang Pu* (Rhizoma Acori Tatarinowii), *Dou Kou* (Fructus Amomi Rotundus), and *Huo Xiang* (Herba Agastaches) resolve dampness and turbidity and activate qi circulation. • *She Gan* (Rhizoma Belamcandae), *Bo He* (Herba Menthae) and *Chuan Bei Mu* (Bulbus Fritillariae Cirrhosae) lower Lung qi and relieve soreness and swelling. • *Mu Tong* (Caulis Akebiae) clears damp-heat through diuresis. • *Lian Qiao* (Fructus Forsythiae) clears heat and eliminates toxins.

(Herba Menthae) and *Chuan Bei Mu* (Bulbus Fritillariae Cirrhosae) lower Lung qi and relieve sore throat. *Mu Tong* (Caulis Akebiae) helps *Hua Shi* (Talcum) and *Yin Chen* (Herba Artemisiae Scopariae) clear damp-heat through diuresis; and *Lian Qiao* (Fructus Forsythiae) helps *Huang Qin* (Radix Scutellariae) clear heat and eliminate toxins.

MODIFICATIONS

• With prominent signs of jaundice, add *Zhi Zi* (Fructus Gardeniae) and *Da Huang* (Radix et Rhizoma Rhei).
• With severe sore throat, add *Shan Dou Gen* (Radix et Rhizoma Sophorae Tonkinensis) and *Ban Lan Gen* (Radix Isatidis).
• With fever, add *Ku Shen* (Radix Sophorae Flavescentis) and *Huang Lian* (Rhizoma Coptidis).
• For cholecystitis, add *Jin Qian Cao* (Herba Lysimachiae).
• For pyelonephritis, add *Qu Mai* (Herba Dianthi), *Bian Xu* (Herba Polygoni Avicularis), *Bai Mao Gen* (Rhizoma Imperatae), *Da Ji* (Herba Cirsii Japonici), *Xiao Ji* (Herba Cirsii), and *Shi Wei* (Folium Pyrrosiae).
• For infectious hepatitis, increase the dose of *Yin Chen* (Herba Artemisiae Scopariae), add *Zhi Zi* (Fructus Gardeniae), *Huang Bo* (Cortex Phellodendri Chinensis), and *Da Huang* (Radix et Rhizoma Rhei).

CAUTIONS / CONTRAINDICATIONS

• *Gan Lu Xiao Du Dan* should be used with caution in cases of damp-heat with underlying yin and body fluid deficiencies.[1]
• Avoid eating foods that are raw, cold, spicy, pungent, oily, or greasy while taking this formula.[2]

PHARMACOLOGICAL EFFECTS

1. **Antipyretic**: Administration of *Gan Lu Xiao Du Dan* via oral ingestion in rats was associated with reduced body temperature in both normal subjects and those with artificially-induced fever. The duration of action was approximately 2 hours.[3]
2. **Hepatoprotective**: Use of *Gan Lu Xiao Du Dan* had protective effects against liver damage induced by carbon tetrachloride. The formula was administered as an oral decoction for a total of 12 days.[4]

CLINICAL STUDIES AND RESEARCH

1. **Gastritis**: Use of modified *Gan Lu Xiao Du Dan* was associated with 91% effectiveness in treating 66 patients with gastritis characterized by damp-heat. Of 66 patients, 51 had complete recovery, 5 had significant improvement, 4 had slight improvement, and 6 had no effect.[5]
2. **Laryngopharyngitis**: One study reported marked success using *Gan Lu Xiao Du Dan* to treat both acute and chronic laryngopharyngitis. Of 58 patients, the study reported complete recovery in 30 cases and significant improvement in 28 cases.[6]
3. **Stomatitis**: One study reported complete recovery from recurrent stomatitis using *Gan Lu Xiao Du Dan* to treat ulcers, and upon healing, using *Yu Ping Feng San* (Jade Windscreen Powder) to prevent recurrence.[7]
4. **Hepatitis**: According to one study, 26 infants with acute infectious hepatitis were treated with modified *Gan Lu Xiao Du Dan* with marked effects. The treatment protocol was to administer the herbs in decoction, with duration of treatment up to 5 weeks. Clinical improvement

Gān Lù Xiāo Dú Dān (Sweet Dew Special Pill to Eliminate Toxin)

included relief of jaundice, decrease of liver enzyme levels, reduction of hepatomegaly, and improved appetite.[8] Another study reported marked success treating 182 cases of acute icteric jaundice in children using *Gan Lu Xiao Du Dan* plus *Chai Hu* (Radix Bupleuri), *Fo Shou* (Fructus Citri Sarcodactylis), and *Yu Jin* (Radix Curcumae).[9]

5. **Fever**: One study reported 94.8% effectiveness using modified *Gan Lu Xiao Du Dan* to treat 78 patients with fever due to infectious disorders. Clinical manifestations included chills, fever, resolution of chills but not fever after perspiration, headache, feeling of heaviness in the head, fatigue, and loose stools. In addition to *Gan Lu Xiao Du Dan*, modifications included addition of *Yi Yi Ren* (Semen Coicis) and *Ban Xia* (Rhizoma Pinelliae) for excess dampness; and *Shi Gao* (Gypsum Fibrosum) for high fever. Of 78 patients, the study reported significant improvement in 31 cases, improvement in 43 cases, and no effect in 4 cases.[10]

6. **Encephalitis**: One study reported complete recovery from encephalitis in 13 of 16 patients using modified *Gan Lu Xiao Du Dan*. Modifications were made based on the individual condition of the patients. For early stage of encephalitis with fever, gradual onset of symptoms, presence of dampness, and greasy tongue coating, *She Gan* (Rhizoma Belamcandae) and *Lian Qiao* (Fructus Forsythiae) were removed, and *Dan Dou Chi* (Semen Sojae Praeparatum) and *Ku Xing Ren* (Semen Armeniacae Amarum) were added to the herbal formula. For middle stage of encephalitis with the disease migrating to the interior, and dampness turning into heat, with symptoms such as a bitter taste in the mouth, restlessness, and a red tongue body with yellow tongue coating, *Bo He* (Herba Menthae), *She Gan* (Rhizoma Belamcandae) and *Bei*

Mu (Bulbus Fritillariae) were removed, and *Huang Lian* (Rhizoma Coptidis), *Zhi Zi* (Fructus Gardeniae) and a larger dose of *Huang Qin* (Radix Scutellariae) were added. For late stage of encephalitis, with restlessness and muscle spasms, *She Gan* (Rhizoma Belamcandae), *Bo He* (Herba Menthae) and *Mu Tong* (Caulis Akebiae) were removed, and *Yu Jin* (Radix Curcumae) was added. Lastly, drugs such as dexamethasone were given if necessary.[11]

AUTHORS' COMMENTS

San Ren Tang (Three-Nut Decoction) and *Gan Lu Xiao Du Dan* both treat damp-warmth syndrome affecting the *qi* (energy) level.

- *San Ren Tang* treats early stage damp-warmth with more dampness than heat.
- *Gan Lu Xiao Du Dan* treats warmth and dampness (equal amounts of each) with the presence of heat-toxins.

References

1. *Zhong Yao Ming Fang Yao Li Yu Ying Yong* (Pharmacology and Applications of Famous Herbal Formulas) 1989;425-426.
2. *Zhong Yao Ming Fang Yao Li Yu Ying Yong* (Pharmacology and Applications of Famous Herbal Formulas) 1989;425-426.
3. *Zhong Guo Zhong Yao Za Zhi* (People's Republic of China Journal of Chinese Herbology) 1989;14(5):50.
4. *Zhong Guo Zhong Yao Za Zhi* (People's Republic of China Journal of Chinese Herbology) 1993;18(10):625.
5. *Zhe Jiang Zhong Yi Za Zhi* (Zhejiang Journal of Chinese Medicine) 1995;10:444.
6. *Xin Zhong Yi* (New Chinese Medicine) 1997;7:57.
7. *Zhong Cheng Yao* (Study of Chinese Patent Medicine) 1991;5:46.
8. *Zhe Jiang Zhong Yi Za Zhi* (Zhejiang Journal of Chinese Medicine) 1980;10:462.
9. *Si Chuan Zhong Yi* (Sichuan Chinese Medicine) 1986;3:31.
10. *Gan Su Zhong Yi* (Gansu Chinese Medicine) 1995;8(4):21.
11. *Jiang Su Zhong Yi* (Jiangsu Chinese Medicine) 1997;7:12.

Chinese Herbal Formulas and Applications

Lián Pò Yǐn (Coptis and Magnolia Bark Decoction)

連樸飲
连朴饮

Pinyin Name: *Lian Po Yin*
Literal Name: Coptis and Magnolia Bark Decoction
Alternate Name: Coptis and Magnolia Bark Combination
Original Source: *Huo Luan Lun* (Discussion of Sudden Turmoil Disorders) by Wan Shi-Xiong in 1862

COMPOSITION

Hou Po (Cortex Magnoliae Officinalis), *zhi* (prepared)	6g
Huang Lian (Rhizoma Coptidis), *chao* (dry-fried) with ginger juice	3g
Zhi Zi (Fructus Gardeniae), *chao jiao* (dry-fried to burnt)	9g
Dan Dou Chi (Semen Sojae Praeparatum), *chao* (dry-fried)	9g
Shi Chang Pu (Rhizoma Acori Tatarinowii)	3g
Ban Xia (Rhizoma Pinelliae), *zhi* (prepared)	3g
Lu Gen (Rhizoma Phragmitis)	60g

DOSAGE / PREPARATION / ADMINISTRATION

The source text instructs to prepare the ingredients as a decoction and take it while warm.

CHINESE THERAPEUTIC ACTIONS

1. Clears heat and resolves dampness
2. Regulates qi and harmonizes the middle *jiao*

CLINICAL MANIFESTATIONS

Accumulation of dampness and heat: excessive vomiting and diarrhea in sudden turmoil disorder, chest and epigastric distention and oppression, dark, scanty urine, and a yellow, greasy tongue coating.

CLINICAL APPLICATIONS

Gastrointestinal disorders, such as superficial gastritis, gastritis, duodenal ulcer, acute gastroenteritis, bacterial dysentery, and stomach influenza.

EXPLANATION

Lian Po Yin (Coptis and Magnolia Bark Decoction) was originally designed to treat severe vomiting and diarrhea associated with sudden turmoil disorder characterized by accumulation of dampness and heat. Dampness and heat affect the normal ascending and descending functions of the Spleen and Stomach, which causes vomiting and diarrhea. These two pathogens may also cause qi stagnation, resulting in feelings of distention and oppression in the chest and epigastric region. Dark, scanty urine and a yellow, greasy tongue coating indicate dampness and heat in the interior.

This formula contains *Hou Po* (Cortex Magnoliae Officinalis) to regulate qi and resolve dampness. *Huang Lian*

(Rhizoma Coptidis) clears heat and dries dampness. *Zhi Zi* (Fructus Gardeniae) and *Dan Dou Chi* (Semen Sojae Praeparatum) clear stagnant heat in the chest and epigastrium. *Shi Chang Pu* (Rhizoma Acori Tatarinowii), an aromatic herb, dissolves dampness to awaken the Spleen. *Ban Xia* (Rhizoma Pinelliae) dries dampness and lowers the reversed flow of Stomach qi downward. *Lu Gen* (Rhizoma Phragmitis), used at an exceptionally large dose, is especially effective for clearing heat, harmonizing the Stomach, and stopping vomiting.

MODIFICATIONS

* With severe diarrhea, add *Bai Bian Dou* (Semen Lablab Album) and *Yi Yi Ren* (Semen Coicis).
* With diarrhea and rectal tenesmus, add *Mu Xiang* (Radix Aucklandiae) and *Bing Lang* (Semen Arecae).
* With indigestion and food stagnation, add *Shan Zha* (Fructus Crataegi) and *Shen Qu* (Massa Fermentata).
* For conditions with more heat than dampness, add *Huang Qin* (Radix Scutellariae), *Jin Yin Hua* (Flos Lonicerae Japonicae), and *Lian Qiao* (Fructus Forsythiae).

CAUTIONS / CONTRAINDICATIONS

* *Lian Po Yin* treats vomiting and diarrhea caused by sudden turmoil disorder marked by accumulation of damp-heat. It should not be used if the condition is characterized by cold.
* Individuals with severe vomiting and diarrhea may experience dehydration from excessive loss of fluids. Electrolytes and fluids should be replenished accordingly.

CLINICAL STUDIES AND RESEARCH

Gastrointestinal disorders: Use of *Lian Po Yin* was reported effective in treating 39 patients with various

DAMP-DISPELLING FORMULAS

16

1099

Chapter 16 – Damp-Dispelling Formulas   *Section 2 – Heat-Clearing and Damp-Dispelling Formulas*

Lián Pò Yǐn (Coptis and Magnolia Bark Decoction)

Lian Po Yin (Coptis and Magnolia Bark Decoction)

Diagnosis	Signs and Symptoms	Treatment	Herbs
Accumulation of dampness and heat	• Excessive vomiting and diarrhea: accumulation of dampness and heat affecting the Spleen and Stomach • Chest and epigastric distention and oppression: qi stagnation due to accumulation of dampness and heat • Dark, scanty urine: dampness and heat traveling down to the lower *jiao* • Yellow, greasy tongue coating: dampness and heat in the interior	• Clears heat and resolves dampness • Regulates qi and harmonizes the middle *jiao*	• *Hou Po* (Cortex Magnoliae Officinalis) activates qi and resolves dampness. • *Huang Lian* (Rhizoma Coptidis) clears heat and dries dampness. • *Zhi Zi* (Fructus Gardeniae) and *Dan Dou Chi* (Semen Sojae Praeparatum) clear stagnant heat in the chest and epigastrium. • *Shi Chang Pu* (Rhizoma Acori Tatarinowii) dissolves dampness to awaken the Spleen. • *Ban Xia* (Rhizoma Pinelliae) dries dampness and guides the reversed flow of Stomach qi downward. • *Lu Gen* (Rhizoma Phragmitis) clears heat, harmonizes the Stomach, and stops vomiting.

types of gastrointestinal disorders (superficial gastritis, gastritis, duodenal ulcers, etc.) characterized by damp-heat affecting the Spleen and Stomach. Of 39 patients, the study reported significant improvement in 29 cases, moderate improvement in 9 cases, and no effect in 1 case. The overall effectiveness was 97.4%.[1]

AUTHORS' COMMENTS

Lian Po Yin is indicated for sudden turmoil disorder caused by accumulation of dampness and heat with symptoms such as excessive vomiting and diarrhea.

The main emphasis of the formula is to treat the cause (dampness and heat) by using herbs to clear heat, resolve dampness, regulate qi circulation, and harmonize the middle *jiao*. The formula does not focus on treating the symptoms (nausea and vomiting) because once dampness and heat are eliminated, all of the other symptoms will be resolved.

Reference

1. *Nan Jing Zhong Yi Xue Yuan Xue Bao* (Journal of Nanjing University of Traditional Chinese Medicine) 1990;4:24.

Chinese Herbal Formulas and Applications

Cán Shǐ Tāng (Silkworm Droppings Decoction)

蠶矢湯
蚕矢汤

Pinyin Name: *Can Shi Tang*
Literal Name: Silkworm Droppings Decoction
Original Source: *Huo Luan Lun* (Discussion of Sudden Turmoil Disorders) by Wan Shi-Xiong in 1862

COMPOSITION

Can Sha (Faeces Bombycis)	15g
Mu Gua (Fructus Chaenomelis)	9g
Da Dou Huang Juan (Semen Glycines Germinatum)	12g
Yi Yi Ren (Semen Coicis)	12g
Huang Qin (Radix Scutellariae), *chao* (dry-fried) with liquor	3g
Huang Lian (Rhizoma Coptidis), *chao* (dry-fried) with ginger juice	9g
Zhi Zi (Fructus Gardeniae), *chao jiao* (dry-fried till burnt)	5g
Ban Xia (Rhizoma Pinelliae), *zhi* (prepared)	3g
Tong Cao (Medulla Tetrapanacis)	3g
Wu Zhu Yu (Fructus Evodiae), *pao* (blast-fried)	0.9g

DOSAGE / PREPARATION / ADMINISTRATION

The source text instructs to cook the ingredients with "muddy water" or "yin yang water." Take the decoction in small sips after it cools down slightly. Today, it is normally prepared as a decoction. Note: "Muddy water" refers to fresh water from the well mixed with a small amount of soil. "Yin yang water" refers to the mixture of cold water from the well and hot water that has been boiled. These types of water had been described to have better effect to harmonize yin and yang, and normalize the ascending and descending qi.

CHINESE THERAPEUTIC ACTIONS

1. Clears heat and resolves dampness
2. Separates the clear (pure nutrients) from the turbid

CLINICAL MANIFESTATION

Spasms and cramps caused by sudden turmoil disorder due to damp-heat accumulation: abdominal pain, vomiting and diarrhea, thirst, irritability, restlessness, a yellow, thick, dry tongue coating, and a soggy, rapid pulse.

CLINICAL APPLICATIONS

Acute gastroenteritis, diarrhea, dysentery, and rheumatoid arthritis.

EXPLANATION

Can Shi Tang (Silkworm Droppings Decoction) treats spasms and cramps in sudden turmoil disorder due to damp-heat accumulation. According to traditional Chinese medicine, the Stomach is responsible for guiding the turbid qi downward, while the Spleen raises the clear qi upward. If damp-heat interferes with the normal ascending

and descending functions of the Spleen and Stomach, there will be abdominal pain, vomiting, and diarrhea. Furthermore, damp-heat rising upward leads to thirst and irritability. Lastly, as damp-heat consumes body fluids and excessive vomiting and diarrhea causes loss of body fluids, spasms and cramps occur due to severe loss of body fluids and malnourishment of the muscles. A yellow, thick, dry tongue coating indicates excess heat and loss of body fluids, while a soggy, rapid pulse suggests damp-heat in the interior.

As one of the most effective herbs for treating sudden turmoil disorder, *Can Sha* (Faeces Bombycis) treats vomiting and diarrhea by leading turbidity downward and guiding the pure nutrients upward. *Mu Gua* (Fructus Chaenomelis) dissolves dampness and harmonizes the middle *jiao*. Moreover, the combination of *Can Sha* (Faeces Bombycis) and *Mu Gua* (Fructus Chaenomelis) is effective in relieving muscle spasms and cramps in sudden turmoil disorder. *Da Dou Huang Juan* (Semen Glycines Germinatum) dissolves dampness and raises pure nutrients upward. *Yi Yi Ren* (Semen Coicis) dispels dampness and expels turbidity through urination. *Huang Qin* (Radix Scutellariae), *Huang Lian* (Rhizoma Coptidis), and *Zhi Zi* (Fructus Gardeniae) clear heat and dry dampness. *Ban Xia* (Rhizoma Pinelliae) dries dampness and corrects reversed flow of Stomach qi to stop vomiting. *Tong Cao* (Medulla Tetrapanacis) dispels turbidity through urination. *Wu Zhu Yu* (Fructus Evodiae) has a downward-guiding effect to help *Ban Xia* (Rhizoma Pinelliae) redirect the qi; it also assists *Huang Lian* (Rhizoma Coptidis) to clear heat and stop vomiting.

DAMP-DISPELLING FORMULAS

16

1101

Chapter 16 – Damp-Dispelling Formulas   *Section 2 – Heat-Clearing and Damp-Dispelling Formulas*

Cán Shǐ Tāng (Silkworm Droppings Decoction)

Can Shi Tang (Silkworm Droppings Decoction)

Diagnosis	Signs and Symptoms	Treatment	Herbs
Vomiting and diarrhea due to damp-heat accumulation	• Abdominal pain, vomiting, and diarrhea: damp-heat affecting the Spleen and Stomach • Thirst and irritability: damp-heat rising upwards • Spasms and cramps: loss of body fluids • Yellow, thick, dry tongue coating: heat consuming body fluids • Soggy, rapid pulse: damp-heat in the interior	• Clears heat and resolves dampness • Separates the clear (pure nutrients) from the turbid	• *Can Sha* (Faeces Bombycis) leads turbidity downward and guides the pure nutrients upward to treat vomiting and diarrhea. • *Mu Gua* (Fructus Chaenomelis) dissolves dampness and harmonizes the middle *jiao*. • *Da Dou Huang Juan* (Semen Glycines Germinatum) dissolves dampness and raises up pure nutrients. • *Yi Yi Ren* (Semen Coicis) dispels dampness and expels turbidity through urination. • *Huang Qin* (Radix Scutellariae), *Huang Lian* (Rhizoma Coptidis) and *Zhi Zi* (Fructus Gardeniae) clear heat and dry dampness. • *Ban Xia* (Rhizoma Pinelliae) dries dampness and stops vomiting. • *Tong Cao* (Medulla Tetrapanacis) dispels turbidity through urination. • *Wu Zhu Yu* (Fructus Evodiae) guides the formula downward.

CAUTIONS / CONTRAINDICATIONS

• *Can Shi Tang* treats vomiting and diarrhea in sudden turmoil disorder due to damp-heat accumulation. It should not be used if the condition is characterized by cold.

• Individuals with severe vomiting and diarrhea may experience dehydration from excessive loss of fluids. Electrolytes and fluids should be replenished accordingly.

• For individuals with nausea and vomiting, this formula may be given in room-temperature decoction to minimize symptoms.

AUTHORS' COMMENTS

Lian Po Yin (Coptis and Magnolia Bark Decoction) and *Can Shi Tang* both treat sudden turmoil disorder characterized by damp-heat accumulation.

• *Lian Po Yin* emphasizes harmonizing the Stomach and relieving vomiting and diarrhea.

• *Can Shi Tang* focuses more on alleviating severe spasms and cramps.

1102

Chinese Herbal Formulas and Applications

Bā Zhèng Sǎn (Eight-Herb Powder for Rectification)

八正散

Pinyin Name: *Ba Zheng San*
Literal Name: Eight-Herb Powder for Rectification
Alternate Names: *Pa Cheng San*, Dianthus Formula, Eight Corrections Powder
Original Source: *Tai Ping Hui Min He Ji Ju Fang* (Imperial Grace Formulary of the Tai Ping Era) by the Imperial Medical Department in 1078-85

COMPOSITION

Mu Tong (Caulis Akebiae)	480g [9g]
Qu Mai (Herba Dianthi)	480g [9g]
Bian Xu (Herba Polygoni Avicularis)	480g [9g]
Hua Shi (Talcum)	480g [9g]
Che Qian Zi (Semen Plantaginis)	480g [9g]
Zhi Zi (Fructus Gardeniae)	480g [9g]
Da Huang (Radix et Rhizoma Rhei), *wei* (roasted), *qie* (sliced) and *bei* (stone-baked)	480g [9g]
Zhi Gan Cao (Radix et Rhizoma Glycyrrhizae Praeparata cum Melle)	480g [9g]

DOSAGE / PREPARATION / ADMINISTRATION

The source text advises to grind equal amounts of the ingredients into a fine powder. Cook 6g of the powder with *Deng Xin Cao* (Medulla Junci) in 1 bowl of water until the liquid is reduced to 70% volume. Take the warm, strained decoction after meals and before bedtime. For children, reduce the dose accordingly. Today it is ground into powder and taken 6-9g per dose. This formula may be prepared as a decoction with the doses suggested in brackets.

CHINESE THERAPEUTIC ACTIONS

1. Clears heat and sedates fire
2. Regulates water circulation and relieves *lin zheng* (dysuria syndrome)

CLINICAL MANIFESTATIONS

Downward flow of damp-heat to the lower *jiao*: *re lin* (heat dysuria) syndrome, *xue lin* (bloody dysuria) syndrome, turbid and red-colored urine, painful sensation during urination, scanty drips of urine or anuria in severe cases, lower abdominal pain and fullness, dry mouth and throat, a yellow, greasy tongue coating, and a slippery, rapid pulse.

CLINICAL APPLICATIONS

Urinary tract infection, dysuria, urethritis, cystitis, pyelonephritis, nephritis, glomerulonephritis, pyonephritis, uroschesis, urolithiasis, prostatic hypertrophy, prostatitis, and gout.

EXPLANATION

Ba Zheng San (Eight-Herb Powder for Rectification) treats the downward flow of damp-heat to the lower *jiao*. Stagnant damp-heat in the Urinary Bladder causes various urinary disorders, such as *re lin* (heat dysuria), *xue lin* (bloody dysuria), uroschesis, and many others as listed above. Heat in the interior consumes body fluids and causes dry mouth and throat. The tongue and pulse presentations indicate damp-heat in the body.

In this formula, *Mu Tong* (Caulis Akebiae), *Qu Mai* (Herba Dianthi), *Bian Xu* (Herba Polygoni Avicularis), *Hua Shi* (Talcum), and *Che Qian Zi* (Semen Plantaginis) induce urination, relieve dysuria, and clear damp-heat. *Zhi Zi* (Fructus Gardeniae) sedates damp-heat in all three *jiaos*. *Da Huang* (Radix et Rhizoma Rhei) purges heat and sedates fire. *Deng Xin Cao* (Medulla Junci) leads the heat down and out through urination. *Zhi Gan Cao* (Radix et Rhizoma Glycyrrhizae Praeparata cum Melle) harmonizes the herbs and relieves pain.

MODIFICATIONS

- For *xue lin* (bloody dysuria), add *Xiao Ji* (Herba Cirsii) and *Bai Mao Gen* (Rhizoma Imperatae).
- For *shi lin* (stone dysuria), add *Jin Qian Cao* (Herba Lysimachiae) and *Hai Jin Sha* (Spora Lygodii).
- For *gao lin* (cloudy dysuria), add *Fen Bi Xie* (Rhizoma Dioscoreae Hypoglaucae) and *Shi Chang Pu* (Rhizoma Acori Tatarinowii).
- For *shi-re lin* (damp-heat dysuria) with severe burning sensations and dark yellow urine, add *Huang Bo* (Cortex Phellodendri Chinensis), *Jin Yin Hua* (Flos Lonicerae Japonicae), *Pu Gong Ying* (Herba Taraxaci), *Bai Hua She She Cao* (Herba Hedyotis), and *Zi Hua Di Ding* (Herba Violae).
- With oliguria, add *Yan Hu Suo* (Rhizoma Corydalis) and *Zhi Qiao* (Fructus Aurantii).

DAMP-DISPELLING FORMULAS

16

1103

Chapter 16 – Damp-Dispelling Formulas   *Section 2 – Heat-Clearing and Damp-Dispelling Formulas*

Bā Zhèng Sǎn (Eight-Herb Powder for Rectification)

Ba Zheng San (Eight-Herb Powder for Rectification)

Diagnosis	Signs and Symptoms	Treatment	Herbs
Downward flow of damp-heat to the lower *jiao*	• Dysuria or anuria, urination with burning sensations or pain, turbid and red-colored urine, or scanty drips of urine: damp-heat in the Urinary Bladder • Dry mouth and throat: damp-heat consuming body fluids • Yellow, greasy tongue coating and a slippery, rapid pulse: damp-heat in the interior	• Clears heat and sedates fire • Regulates water circulation and relieves *lin zheng* (dysuria syndrome)	• *Mu Tong* (Caulis Akebiae), *Qu Mai* (Herba Dianthi), *Bian Xu* (Herba Polygoni Avicularis), *Hua Shi* (Talcum), and *Che Qian Zi* (Semen Plantaginis) induce urination, relieve dysuria, and clear damp-heat. • *Zhi Zi* (Fructus Gardeniae) sedates damp-heat in all three *jiaos*. • *Da Huang* (Radix et Rhizoma Rhei) purges heat and sedates fire. • *Deng Xin Cao* (Medulla Junci) leads the heat down and out through urination. • *Zhi Gan Cao* (Radix et Rhizoma Glycyrrhizae Praeparata cum Melle) harmonizes the herbs and relieves pain.

- With more pain and burning sensations during urination, add *Huang Lian* (Rhizoma Coptidis) and *Di Huang* (Radix Rehmanniae).
- With more fullness and distention in the lower abdominal region, add *Wu Yao* (Radix Linderae) and *Chuan Lian Zi* (Fructus Toosendan).
- With edema, add *Fu Ling Pi* (Cortex Poria) and *Ze Xie* (Rhizoma Alismatis).

CAUTIONS / CONTRAINDICATIONS

- *Ba Zheng San* contains many strong herbs that are bitter and cold. It should be used with caution during pregnancy. It is not suitable for patients with weakness or generalized deficiencies since these herbs may cause weakness, light-headedness, and a decline in the overall constitution of the patient. This formula should be discontinued when the desired effects are achieved. Long-term use of this formula is contraindicated.
- Patients with a sensitive gastrointestinal tract may wish to take *Ba Zheng San* without *Da Huang* (Radix et Rhizoma Rhei) since *Da Huang* (Radix et Rhizoma Rhei) may cause diarrhea and discomfort.
- *Ba Zheng San* is formulated to treat *re lin* (heat dysuria), *xue lin* (bloody dysuria), and uroschesis. This formula should be modified accordingly (*see* Modifications) prior to its use for other types of *lin zheng* (dysuria syndrome). It is contraindicated in *gao lin* (cloudy dysuria), *qi lin* (qi dysuria), and *lao lin* (fatigue dysuria) unless modified accordingly.

PHARMACOLOGICAL EFFECTS

Antibacterial: *Ba Zheng San* has been shown in *in vitro* studies to have an inhibitory effect against *E. coli*, *Bacillus*

proteus, *Bacillus paratyphosus*, *Bacillus dysenteriae*, *Staphylococcus aureus*, and others.[1]

CLINICAL STUDIES AND RESEARCH

1. **Lin zheng (dysuria syndrome)**: Modified *Ba Zheng San* was used successfully to treat *lin zheng* (dysuria syndrome) infections transmitted via sexual intercourse. The herbal treatment included *Tu Fu Ling* (Rhizoma Smilacis Glabrae) 30g, *Hua Shi* (Talcum) 30g, *Fen Bi Xie* (Rhizoma Dioscoreae Hypoglaucae) 20g, *Cang Zhu* (Rhizoma Atractylodis) 15g, *Huang Bo* (Cortex Phellodendri Chinensis) 15g, *Che Qian Zi* (Semen Plantaginis) 15g, *Mu Tong* (Caulis Akebiae) 10g, *Bian Xu* (Herba Polygoni Avicularis) 10g, *Zhi Zi* (Fructus Gardeniae) 10g, *Da Huang* (Radix et Rhizoma Rhei) 10g, and *Gan Cao* (Radix et Rhizoma Glycyrrhizae) 3g. Additional modifications were made as needed. The treatment protocol was to administer the decoction in three equally-divided doses, for 3 days per course of treatment. Out of 32 patients, the study reported complete recovery in 18 cases, marked improvement in 13 cases, and no effect in 1 case.[2]

2. **Urethritis**: Administration of *Ba Zheng San* has been associated with marked effect in numerous studies. In one study, use of modified *Ba Zheng San* in 36 patients showed complete recovery in 20 cases, marked effect in 15 cases, and no effect in 1 case.[3] In another study, oral administration of modified *Ba Zheng San* in 48 patients resulted in complete recovery in 26 cases, marked improvement in 21 cases, and no effect in one case.[4]

3. **Urinary tract infection**: Ninety-seven patients with urinary tract infection were treated with good results using *Ba Zheng San*. Clinical presentations included frequent urination, urinary urgency, dysuria, low back

1104

Bā Zhèng Săn (Eight-Herb Powder for Rectification)

pain, and fever. The study reported 96.91% success, with complete recovery in 76 cases, moderate improvement in 18 cases, and no effect in 3 cases.[5]

4. **Pyelonephritis**: Administration of modified *Ba Zheng San* was associated with a 88.5% success in female patients with pyelonephritis. Out of 67 cases, the study reported complete recovery in 54 cases, improvement in 5 cases, and no effect in 8 cases.[6]

5. **Nephritis**: Administration of *Ba Zheng San* was shown to have therapeutic results when used to treat acute nephritis. Out of 11 cases, there was complete recovery in 4 cases, marked improvement in 5 cases, and slight improvement in 2 cases. Immediate improvements included alleviation of edema and proteinuria. Kidney function was restored to normal in most cases.[7]

6. **Urinary stones**: Administration of *Ba Zheng San* contributed to successful passage of urinary stones in 21 of 34 patients. The treatment protocol was to use a large dose of *Ba Zheng San* plus *Di Long* (Pheretima), *Ji Nei Jin* (Endothelium Corneum Gigeriae Galli), and *Hu Po* (Succinum). The patients were instructed to continue taking the herbs until the successful passage of stones. The duration of treatment varied from 3 to 108 days, with an average of 42.2 days.[8]

7. **Prostatic hypertrophy**: Administration of *Ba Zheng San* was associated with 89.3% effectiveness in treating geriatric men with prostatic hypertrophy. Out of 28 patients, the study showed recovery in 8 cases, marked effect in 12 cases, improvement in 5 cases, and no results in 3 cases.[9]

8. **Gout**: Modified *Ba Zheng San* was used to treat 15 patients with gout. For individuals with abnormal liver function, the herbal formula added *Yin Chen* (Herba Artemisiae Scopariae) 30g, *Chai Hu* (Radix Bupleuri) 10g, *Chi Shao* (Radix Paeoniae Rubra) 15g, *Bai Shao* (Radix Paeoniae Alba) 15g, and *Wu Wei Zi* (Fructus Schisandrae Chinensis) 10g. After one course of treatment, all patients showed varying decreases in plasma uric acid levels. Out of 15 patients, 9 had normal levels of uric acid and 6 had over 30% reduction. All patients had improvement of pain.[10]

9. **Edema during pregnancy**: Administration of modified *Ba Zheng San* for 14-50 days was effective in 33 out of 36 pregnant women with edema.[11] Note: *Ba Zheng San* must be used with caution during pregnancy as it contains many strong herbs that are bitter and cold.

RELATED FORMULAS

Jiā Wèi Bā Zhèng Săn
(Augmented Eight-Herb Powder for Rectification)
加味八正散

Pinyin Name: *Jia Wei Ba Zheng San*
Literal Name: Augmented Eight-Herb Powder for Rectification
Alternate Name: Dianthus Plus Formula
Original Source: *Tai Ping Hui Min He Ji Ju Fang* (Imperial Grace Formulary of the Tai Ping Era) by the Imperial Medical Department in 1078-85

Mu Tong (Caulis Akebiae)	500g
Qu Mai (Herba Dianthi)	500g
Bian Xu (Herba Polygoni Avicularis)	500g
Hua Shi (Talcum)	500g
Che Qian Zi (Semen Plantaginis)	500g
Zhi Zi (Fructus Gardeniae)	500g
Da Huang (Radix et Rhizoma Rhei)	500g
Zhi Gan Cao (Radix et Rhizoma Glycyrrhizae Praeparata cum Melle)	500g
Mu Xiang (Radix Aucklandiae)	500g

Jia Wei Ba Zheng San (Augmented Eight-Herb Powder for Rectification) is formulated by adding *Mu Xiang* (Radix Aucklandiae) to *Ba Zheng San* to enhance the qi-regulating and pain-relieving effects. *Jia Wei Ba Zheng San* can be used to treat swelling and pain in the testicles or scrotum in addition to all the functions and indications of *Ba Zheng San*.

Fù Fāng Bā Zhèng Săn (Revised Eight-Herb Powder)
複方八正散
复方八正散

Pinyin Name: *Fu Fang Ba Zheng San*
Literal Name: Revised Eight-Herb Powder
Original Source: *Jian Tai Zhen Suo Fang* (Herbal Prescriptions from *Jiantai* Clinic) by Chang Wei-Yen in 1981

Long Dan (Radix et Rhizoma Gentianae)
Zhi Zi (Fructus Gardeniae)
Da Huang (Radix et Rhizoma Rhei)
Huang Qin (Radix Scutellariae)
Huang Bo (Cortex Phellodendri Chinensis)
Bian Xu (Herba Polygoni Avicularis)
Hua Shi (Talcum)
Deng Xin Cao (Medulla Junci)
Ze Xie (Rhizoma Alismatis)
Che Qian Zi (Semen Plantaginis)
Qu Mai (Herba Dianthi)
Chai Hu (Radix Bupleuri)
Niu Xi (Radix Achyranthis Bidentatae)
Tao Ren (Semen Persicae)
Hong Hua (Flos Carthami)

DAMP-DISPELLING FORMULAS

16

1105

Bā Zhèng Săn (Eight-Herb Powder for Rectification)

Di Huang (Radix Rehmanniae)
Dang Gui (Radix Angelicae Sinensis)
Gan Cao (Radix et Rhizoma Glycyrrhizae)
Fu Ling (Poria)
Yi Yi Ren (Semen Coicis)
Ku Shen (Radix Sophorae Flavescentis)
Wu Yao (Radix Linderae)
She Chuang Zi (Fructus Cnidii)

Fu Fang Ba Zheng San (Revised Eight-Herb Powder) is based on the principles and ingredients of two classic formulas: *Ba Zheng San* (Eight-Herb Powder for Rectification) to clear heat and sedate fire in the lower *jiao*, and *Long Dan Xie Gan Tang* (Gentiana Decoction to Drain the Liver) to drain damp-heat in the Liver and Gallbladder channels. Clinically, this formula treats a wide variety of infectious and inflammatory conditions such as vaginitis, pelvic inflammatory disease, genito-urinary infections, pyelonephritis, urinary tract infection, and cystitis.

Sān Jín Pái Shí Tāng
(Three Gold Decoction to Expel Stone)

三金排石湯
三金排石汤

Pinyin Name: *San Jin Pai Shi Tang*
Literal Name: Three Gold Decoction to Expel Stone
Original Source: *An Hui Zhong Yi Xue Yuan* (Anhui University School of Medicine) in 1990

Hai Jin Sha (Spora Lygodii)
Jin Qian Cao (Herba Lysimachiae)
Shi Wei (Folium Pyrrosiae)
Chuan Lian Zi (Fructus Toosendan)
Yan Hu Suo (Rhizoma Corydalis)
Wei Ling Xian (Radix et Rhizoma Clematidis)
Zhi Qiao (Fructus Aurantii)
Fu Ling (Poria)
Zhu Ling (Polyporus)
Ze Xie (Rhizoma Alismatis)

San Jin Pai Shi Tang (Three Gold Decoction to Expel Stone) clears heat and promotes normal urination. It is most effective in treating *shi lin* (stone dysuria) with painful urination. Clinical applications include treatment of kidney and urinary stones.

AUTHORS' COMMENTS

Ba Zheng San is the representative formula for the treatment of damp-heat in the lower *jiao*. The key signs and symptoms include frequent urination, painful sensations during urination, turbid and dark urine, a red tongue body with a yellow, greasy coating, and a slippery, rapid pulse.

According to Dr. Chang Wei-Yen, *Ba Zheng San* can be combined with other formulas and herbs to treat different conditions:

- For nephritis and glomerulonephritis, combine *Ba Zheng San* with *Long Dan Xie Gan Tang* (Gentiana Decoction to Drain the Liver), *Shui Ding Xiang* (Herba Ludwigiae Prostratae), and *Xian Feng Cao* (Herba Bidentis). For chronic nephritis, add *Ba Wei Di Huang Wan* (Eight-Ingredient Pill with Rehmannia).

- For glaucoma and increased pressure in the eyes, combine *Ba Zheng San* with *Long Dan Xie Gan Tang* (Gentiana Decoction to Drain the Liver), *Ma Bian Cao* (Herba Verbenae), *Qian Li Guang* (Herba Senecionis Scandens), *Hu Zhang* (Rhizoma et Radix Polygoni Cuspidati), and *Hu Yao Huang* (Herba Leucas Mollissimae).

- For gout and high uric acid, combine *Ba Zheng San* with *Wan Dian Jin* (Radix Ilicis Asprellae), *Shan Pu Tao* (Radix Vitis Amurensis), and *Shui Ding Xiang* (Herba Ludwigiae Prostratae).

References

1. *Zhong Yi Yao Xin Xi* (Information on Chinese Medicine and Herbology) 1987;6:31.
2. *Guang Xi Zhong Yi Yao* (Guangxi Chinese Medicine and Herbology) 1992;4:9.
3. *An Hui Zhong Yi Xue Yuan Xue Bao* (Journal of Anhui University School of Medicine) 1994;4:30.
4. *Guang Xi Zhong Yi Yao* (Guangxi Chinese Medicine and Herbology) 1992;4:9.
5. *Shan Xi Zhong Yi* (Shanxi Chinese Medicine) 1998;10:448.
6. *Liao Ning Zhong Yi Za Zhi* (Liaoning Journal of Chinese Medicine) 1986;1:19.
7. *Ha Er Bing Zhong Yi* (Haerbing Chinese Medicine) 1960;9:15.
8. *Ji Lin Zhong Yi Yao* (Jilin Chinese Medicine and Herbology) 1983;5:19.
9. *Jiang Xi Zhong Yi Yao* (Jiangxi Chinese Medicine and Herbology) 1990;2:15.
10. *Shi Yong Zhong Xi Yi Jie He Za Zhi* (Practical Journal of Integrated Chinese and Western Medicines) 1995;4:244.
11. *Shan Xi Zhong Yi* (Shanxi Chinese Medicine) 1991;5:207.

Chinese Herbal Formulas and Applications

Wǔ Lín Sǎn (Five-Ingredient Powder for Painful Urinary Dysfunction)

五淋散

Pinyin Name: *Wu Lin San*
Literal Name: Five-Ingredient Powder for Painful Urinary Dysfunction
Alternate Names: Five-Strangury Formula, Gardenia and Hoelen Formula
Original Source: *Tai Ping Hui Min He Ji Ju Fang* (Imperial Grace Formulary of the Tai Ping Era) by the Imperial Medical Department in 1078-85

COMPOSITION

Chi Fu Ling (Poria Rubra)	180g [9g]
Dang Gui (Radix Angelicae Sinensis)	150g [7g]
Chi Shao (Radix Paeoniae Rubra)	600g [15g]
Zhi Zi (Fructus Gardeniae)	600g [15g]
Gan Cao (Radix et Rhizoma Glycyrrhizae)	150g [7g]

DOSAGE / PREPARATION / ADMINISTRATION

The source text instructs to grind the ingredients into a fine powder. Cook 6g of the powder with 1 bowl of water until the liquid is reduced to 80% volume. Take the decoction on an empty stomach before meals. Today, this formula may be prepared as a decoction with the doses suggested in brackets.

CHINESE THERAPEUTIC ACTIONS

1. Clears heat and cools the blood
2. Regulates water circulation and relieves *lin zheng* (dysuria syndrome)

CLINICAL MANIFESTATIONS

Heat in the Urinary Bladder: *xue lin* (bloody dysuria) with blood in the urine and severe pain upon urination; and cloudy urine with a feeling of sandy particles in the urine.

CLINICAL APPLICATIONS

Urethritis, cystitis, urolithiasis, and gonorrhea.

EXPLANATION

Wu Lin San (Five-Ingredient Powder for Painful Urinary Dysfunction) clears heat, cools the blood, and promotes normal urination. It treats *xue lin* (bloody dysuria) and *re lin* (heat dysuria) syndromes characterized by heat in the Urinary Bladder, with symptoms such as hematuria, dysuria, or cloudy urine.

In this formula, *Chi Fu Ling* (Poria Rubra) clears heat and promotes urination. *Dang Gui* (Radix Angelicae Sinensis) and *Chi Shao* (Radix Paeoniae Rubra) nourish the blood and moisten dryness. *Zhi Zi* (Fructus Gardeniae) clears heat and cools the blood. *Gan Cao* (Radix et Rhizoma Glycyrrhizae) relieves pain and harmonizes the formula.

MODIFICATIONS

- For *xue lin* (bloody dysuria), add *Xiao Ji* (Herba Cirsii), *Mo Han Lian* (Herba Ecliptae), and *Bai Mao Gen* (Rhizoma Imperatae).
- For *re lin* (heat dysuria), add *Huang Lian* (Rhizoma Coptidis).
- For *shi lin* (stone dysuria), add *Hai Jin Sha* (Spora Lygodii), *Jin Qian Cao* (Herba Lysimachiae), and *Shi Wei* (Folium Pyrrosiae).
- For *lin zheng* (dysuria syndrome) with qi deficiency in elderly patients, add *Ren Shen* (Radix et Rhizoma Ginseng), *Huang Qi* (Radix Astragali), and *Sheng Ma* (Rhizoma Cimicifugae).
- For *lin zheng* (dysuria syndrome) with blood stagnation, add *Tao Ren* (Semen Persicae), *Mu Dan Pi* (Cortex Moutan), *Yan Hu Suo* (Rhizoma Corydalis), and *Hu Po* (Succinum).
- With thirst due to heat and fire, add *Hua Shi* (Talcum) and *Shi Gao* (Gypsum Fibrosum).
- With jaundice, add *Yin Chen* (Herba Artemisiae Scopariae) and *Huang Qin* (Radix Scutellariae).

RELATED FORMULAS

Huó Xuè Tōng Lín Tāng

(Invigorate the Blood to Unblock Dysuria Decoction)

活血通淋湯
活血通淋汤

Pinyin Name: *Huo Xue Tong Lin Tang*
Literal Name: Invigorate the Blood to Unblock Dysuria Decoction
Original Source: *Guang An Men Yi Yuan* (Guang An Men Hospital) in 1990

Fu Ling (Poria)
Hua Shi (Talcum)
Tong Cao (Medulla Tetrapanacis)
Wang Bu Liu Xing (Semen Vaccariae)

DAMP-DISPELLING FORMULAS

16

1107

Chapter 16 – Damp-Dispelling Formulas   *Section 2 – Heat-Clearing and Damp-Dispelling Formulas*

Wŭ Lín Săn (Five-Ingredient Powder for Painful Urinary Dysfunction)

Wu Lin San (Five-Ingredient Powder for Painful Urinary Dysfunction)

Diagnosis	Signs and Symptoms	Treatment	Herbs
Heat in the Urinary Bladder	Hematuria, dysuria, and cloudy urine: heat in the Urinary Bladder	• Clears heat and cools the blood • Regulates water circulation and relieves *lin zheng* (dysuria syndrome)	• *Chi Fu Ling* (Poria Rubra) clears heat and promotes urination. • *Dang Gui* (Radix Angelicae Sinensis) and *Chi Shao* (Radix Paeoniae Rubra) nourish the blood and moisten dryness. • *Zhi Zi* (Fructus Gardeniae) clears heat and cools the blood. • *Gan Cao* (Radix et Rhizoma Glycyrrhizae) relieves pain and harmonizes all of the herbs.

Pu Gong Ying (Herba Taraxaci)
Huang Bo (Cortex Phellodendri Chinensis)
Qu Mai (Herba Dianthi)
Chi Shao (Radix Paeoniae Rubra)
Tao Ren (Semen Persicae)
San Leng (Rhizoma Sparganii)
E Zhu (Rhizoma Curcumae)
Yi Yi Ren (Semen Coicis)
Huang Qi (Radix Astragali)

Huo Xue Tong Lin Tang (Invigorate the Blood to Unblock Dysuria Decoction) treats *lin zheng* (dysuria syndrome) characterized by blood stagnation and heat. It contains herbs to promote normal urination, clear heat from the lower *jiao*, and activate blood circulation. Clinically, this formula is commonly used to treat enlarged prostate with incontinence, frequent urination, or painful urination.

Qīng Rè Tōng Lín Tāng
(Clear Heat to Unblock Dysuria Decoction)
清熱通淋湯
清热通淋汤
Pinyin Name: *Qing Re Tong Lin Tang*
Literal Name: Clear Heat to Unblock Dysuria Decoction
Original Source: *Guang An Men Yi Yuan* (Guang An Men Hospital) in 1990

Che Qian Zi (Semen Plantaginis)
San Leng (Rhizoma Sparganii)
E Zhu (Rhizoma Curcumae)
Huang Bo (Cortex Phellodendri Chinensis)
Jin Yin Hua (Flos Lonicerae Japonicae)
Tian Hua Fen (Radix Trichosanthis)
Zhe Bei Mu (Bulbus Fritillariae Thunbergii)
Chen Pi (Pericarpium Citri Reticulatae)

Dang Gui (Radix Angelicae Sinensis)
Fang Feng (Radix Saposhnikoviae)
Gan Cao (Radix et Rhizoma Glycyrrhizae)
Zao Jiao Ci (Spina Gleditsiae)
Wang Bu Liu Xing (Semen Vaccariae)

Qing Re Tong Lin Tang (Clear Heat to Unblock Dysuria Decoction) treats *lin zheng* (dysuria syndrome) characterized by heat, blood stagnation, and underlying deficiency and weakness. It contains herbs to promote normal urination, clear heat from the lower *jiao*, activate blood circulation, and tonify the blood. Clinically, this formula is commonly used to treat enlarged prostate with incontinence, frequent urination, or painful urination.

AUTHORS' COMMENTS
Ba Zheng San (Eight-Herb Powder for Rectification) and *Wu Lin San* both clear damp-heat from the Urinary Bladder to treat *re lin* (heat dysuria) and *xue lin* (bloody dysuria).
• *Ba Zheng San*, with its heat-clearing and damp-dispelling actions, is more suitable for treating *re lin* (heat dysuria) syndrome.
• *Wu Lin San*, stronger in clearing heat and cooling the blood, is more suitable for *xue lin* (bloody dysuria) syndrome.

Wu Lin San (Five-Ingredient Powder for Painful Urinary Dysfunction) and *Wu Ling San* (Five-Ingredient Powder with Poria) have similar pinyin names, but different functions.
• *Wu <u>Lin</u> San* contains five herbs to treat <u>*lin*</u> *zheng* (dysuria syndrome).
• *Wu <u>Ling</u> San* contains five herbs, with *Fu <u>Ling</u>* (Poria) as a main ingredients, to relieve water accumulation.

1108

Chinese Herbal Formulas and Applications

Section 3

利水渗湿剂
— Water-Regulating and Damp-Resolving Formulas

Wǔ Líng Sǎn (Five-Ingredient Powder with Poria)
五苓散

Pinyin Name: *Wu Ling San*
Literal Name: Five-Ingredient Powder with Poria
Alternate Names: Five-Ling Formula, Poria Powder with Five Herbs, Hoelen Five Herb Formula
Original Source: *Shang Han Lun* (Discussion of Cold-Induced Disorders) by Zhang Zhong-Jing in the Eastern Han Dynasty

COMPOSITION

Ze Xie (Rhizoma Alismatis)	3.75g [15g]
Zhu Ling (Polyporus)	2.25g [9g]
Fu Ling (Poria)	2.25g [9g]
Bai Zhu (Rhizoma Atractylodis Macrocephalae)	2.25g [9g]
Gui Zhi (Ramulus Cinnamomi)	1.5g [6g]

DOSAGE / PREPARATION / ADMINISTRATION

The source text instructs to grind the ingredients into powder and take 1 spoonful [6g] with boiled water three times daily. The source text recommends drinking plenty of warm water to promote sweating. Today, it is normally taken in powder form, 3-6g per dose. This formula may also be prepared as a decoction with the doses suggested in brackets.

CHINESE THERAPEUTIC ACTIONS

1. Regulates water circulation and dispels dampness
2. Warms yang and disperses water accumulation

CLINICAL MANIFESTATIONS

1. Exterior syndrome accompanied by accumulation of water and dampness in the interior: headache, fever, irritability, thirst with a strong desire to drink but vomiting immediately after drinking, urinary difficulty, white tongue coating, and a superficial pulse.
2. Accumulation of water and dampness in the interior: edema, loose stools, urinary difficulty, vomiting, and diarrhea due to sudden turmoil disorder.
3. *Tan yin* (phlegm retention): abdominal pulsation below the umbilicus, vomiting of foamy saliva, vertigo, shortness of breath, and possibly coughing.

CLINICAL APPLICATIONS

Acute and chronic nephritis, renal failure, gestational hypertension, urolithiasis, urinary tract infection, liver cirrhosis and ascites, acute enteritis with diarrhea, hydrocephalus, and Meniere's syndrome.

EXPLANATION

Wu Ling San (Five-Ingredient Powder with Poria), as originally used in *Shang Han Lun* (Discussion of Cold-Induced Disorders), treats water accumulation syndrome caused by disorders of both the *taiyang* channel and the *taiyang* organ. This syndrome begins with *taiyang* exterior (channel) syndrome, and, if left untreated, the pathogen may travel via the *taiyang* channel to affect the *taiyang* organ of the Urinary Bladder. At this point, the patient can be said to be suffering from both *taiyang* exterior (channel) and interior (organ) syndromes. Because the exterior condition has not been treated, there will still be exterior symptoms, such as headache and fever. Moreover, the pathogenic factors have moved interiorly to the *taiyang* organ of the Urinary Bladder to impair its water-dispersing function. Because fluids have accumulated in the lower *jiao* and are not being properly dispersed, irritability and a strong desire to drink are present. And since there is already fluid accumulation in the body, vomiting may occur after intake of water. The treatment

DAMP-DISPELLING FORMULAS

16

1109

Chapter 16 – Damp-Dispelling Formulas   *Section 3 – Water-Regulating and Damp-Resolving Formulas*

Wǔ Líng Sǎn (Five-Ingredient Powder with Poria)

Wu Ling San (Five-Ingredient Powder with Poria)

Diagnosis	Signs and Symptoms	Treatment	Herbs
Exterior syndrome accompanied by accumulation of water and dampness in the interior	• Headache and fever: exterior condition • Urinary difficulty, strong desire to drink with vomiting after drinking: accumulation of water and dampness in the interior • Superficial pulse: exterior condition	• Regulates water circulation and dispels dampness • Warms yang and disperses water accumulation	• *Ze Xie* (Rhizoma Alismatis) induces urination and eliminates water accumulation. • *Zhu Ling* (Polyporus) and *Fu Ling* (Poria) strengthen the Spleen, resolve dampness, and eliminate water accumulation. • *Bai Zhu* (Rhizoma Atractylodis Macrocephalae) strengthens the Spleen to dispel water and dampness. • *Gui Zhi* (Ramulus Cinnamomi) releases the exterior and promotes the flow of yang qi in the interior.

plan for this syndrome is to dispel water accumulation in the interior quickly through diuresis, and to release the *taiyang* syndrome at the exterior.

Ze Xie (Rhizoma Alismatis), the chief herb, directly enters the Urinary Bladder to induce urination and eliminate water accumulation. *Zhu Ling* (Polyporus) and *Fu Ling* (Poria) act as deputy herbs to strengthen the diuretic function of *Ze Xie* (Rhizoma Alismatis). *Bai Zhu* (Rhizoma Atractylodis Macrocephalae) strengthens the Spleen to dispel water and dampness. *Gui Zhi* (Ramulus Cinnamomi) relieves the *taiyang* syndrome with its exterior-releasing action, and promotes the flow of yang qi in the interior to help invigorate the function of the Urinary Bladder.

This formula can also be used to treat edema or urinary difficulty. In addition, since this formula can help the body excrete water through urination, it can also treat the type of diarrhea caused by excessive water or dampness traveling with the feces. The diarrhea stops once the water is separated from the feces and is directed out of the body through urination.

MODIFICATIONS

• With cold and dampness, add *Cang Zhu* (Rhizoma Atractylodis).
• With exterior symptoms, add *Yue Bi Tang* (Maidservant from Yue Decoction).
• With urinary incontinence and *zhong* (central) *qi* deficiency, add *Dang Shen* (Radix Codonopsis).
• With damp-heat jaundice, add *Yin Chen* (Herba Artemisiae Scopariae).
• With edema due to Spleen deficiency, add *Wu Pi Yin* (Five-Peel Decoction) and *Dang Shen* (Radix Codonopsis).

• With edema due to Kidney yang deficiency, add *Wu Pi Yin* (Five-Peel Decoction) and *Fu Zi* (Radix Aconiti Lateralis Praeparata).
• With edema due to Liver qi stagnation, add *Wu Pi Yin* (Five-Peel Decoction), *Qing Pi* (Pericarpium Citri Reticulatae Viride), and *Mu Xiang* (Radix Aucklandiae).
• With severe edema, add *Da Fu Pi* (Pericarpium Arecae), *Sang Bai Pi* (Cortex Mori), and *Chen Pi* (Pericarpium Citri Reticulatae).
• For diarrhea due to heat, remove *Gui Zhi* (Ramulus Cinnamomi) and add *Che Qian Zi* (Semen Plantaginis) and *Mu Tong* (Caulis Akebiae).
• For diarrhea due to damp-heat, add *Jin Yin Hua* (Flos Lonicerae Japonicae) and *Yin Chen* (Herba Artemisiae Scopariae).
• For diarrhea due to summer-dampness, add *Huo Xiang* (Herba Agastaches) and *Pei Lan* (Herba Eupatorii).
• For diarrhea due to summer-heat invasion, add *San Wu Xiang Ru Yin* (Mosla Three Decoction).
• With abdominal bloating and distention, add *Hou Po* (Cortex Magnoliae Officinalis) and *Chen Pi* (Pericarpium Citri Reticulatae).
• With thirst due to summer-heat, add *Bai Hu Tang* (White Tiger Decoction).
• With general thirst, add *Shi Gao* (Gypsum Fibrosum) and *Zhi Mu* (Rhizoma Anemarrhenae).
• With thirst and constipation, add *Gan Cao* (Radix et Rhizoma Glycyrrhizae), *Hua Shi* (Talcum), *Zhi Zi* (Fructus Gardeniae), and *Deng Xin Cao* (Medulla Junci).
• With body aches due to cold and damp accumulation, add *Qiang Huo* (Rhizoma et Radix Notopterygii).

CAUTIONS / CONTRAINDICATIONS

• Because this formula eliminates excess body fluids through the urine, it should not be used for a prolonged period of time.

1110

Chinese Herbal Formulas and Applications

Wǔ Líng Sǎn (Five-Ingredient Powder with Poria)

- This formula is contraindicated in individuals who have depleted body fluids from profuse perspiration or excessive vomiting or diarrhea, as its use could lead to further loss of body fluids
- _Wu Ling San_ is contraindicated in cases of damp-heat accumulation or urinary difficulty due to yin deficiency.
- In order to restore normal water metabolism, the Spleen and Kidney must be tonified if they are deficient, as these two organs regulate water circulation.

PHARMACOLOGICAL EFFECTS

1. **Diuretic**: _Wu Ling San_ had a marked diuretic effect in rats 1-2 hours after oral ingestion.[1] Another study reported that intravenous injection of _Wu Ling San_ in dogs was associated with increased elimination of urine, sodium, chloride, potassium, and other electrolytes.[2] Lastly, administration of _Wu Ling San_ in healthy adults was associated with 112% increase in urine output without any side effects.[3]

2. **Antihypertensive**: One study reported a significant and prolonged reduction in blood pressure using a _Wu Ling San_ preparation in rats. The mechanism of this antihypertensive effect was attributed to the diuretic and vasodilative actions of the formula. The herbal formula contained the following ingredients: _Zhu Ling_ (Polyporus) 9g, _Ze Xie_ (Rhizoma Alismatis) 15g, _Bai Zhu_ (Rhizoma Atractylodis Macrocephalae) 9g, _Fu Ling_ (Poria) 9g, and _Gui Zhi_ (Ramulus Cinnamomi) 6g.[4]

3. **Nephroprotective**: Administration of _Wu Ling San_ was associated with protecting the kidneys by decreasing plasma levels of blood urea nitrogen (BUN) and creatinine (Cr). This formula was found to also increase urine output, as well as elimination of electrolytes such as sodium, chloride, potassium, calcium, and magnesium.[5]

4. **Hepatoprotective**: _Wu Ling San_ has been shown to have a remarkable hepatoprotective effect in mice, especially against alcohol-induced liver damage.[6]

CLINICAL STUDIES AND RESEARCH

1. **Acute nephritis**: According to one study, 36 of 38 patients with acute nephritis had complete recovery using herbs in decoction. The herbal formula contained _Wu Ling San_, _Bai Mao Gen_ (Rhizoma Imperatae) and other herbs as deemed necessary. The study reported resolution of edema in 25 cases within 1-5 days, and 13 cases within 6-10 days. The duration of treatment was 15 days or less in 27 cases, 16-30 days in 9 cases, and over 1 month in 2 cases.[7]

2. **Renal failure**: Modified _Wu Ling San_ had good results in treating early stages of renal failure. Out of 20 patients, one study reported a marked improvement in 6 cases

and slight improvement in 14 cases.[8] Another study reported 87.5% effectiveness using modified _Wu Ling San_ to treat 24 patients with acute renal failure caused by chemotherapy treatments.[9]

3. **Gestational hypertension**: Use of modified _Wu Ling San_ was associated with a 75% success rate in treating hypertension during pregnancy. Of 209 patients, the study reported complete recovery in 156 cases. The treatment protocol was to administer the herbs in decoction daily for 10 days per course of treatment. The herbal formula included _Wu Ling San_ plus _Sang Ji Sheng_ (Herba Taxilli), _Da Fu Pi_ (Pericarpium Arecae), _Mu Gua_ (Fructus Chaenomelis), and _Sha Ren_ (Fructus Amomi).[10]

4. **Urolithiasis**: One study reported marked effect using modified _Wu Ling San_ to treat urinary stones. Of 53 patients, 33 successfully passed stones. The duration of treatment varied between 2-50 packs of herbs.[11]

5. **Liver cirrhosis and ascites**: Use of modified _Wu Ling San_ was associated with 89% effectiveness for treatment of 43 patients with liver cirrhosis and ascites. The herbal formula contained _Wu Ling San_ plus _Dan Shen_ (Radix et Rhizoma Salviae Miltiorrhizae), _Che Qian Zi_ (Semen Plantaginis), _Bai Mao Gen_ (Rhizoma Imperatae), _Da Fu Pi_ (Pericarpium Arecae), _Dang Gui_ (Radix Angelicae Sinensis), and _Chi Shao_ (Radix Paeoniae Rubra) given in decoction. 30g of _Da Huang_ (Radix et Rhizoma Rhei) were given via rectal enema. Of 43 patients, the study reported complete recovery in 23 cases, improvement in 13 cases, and no effect in 4 cases. The average duration of treatment was 31 days. Information was unavailable on 3 individuals who did not complete the study.[12]

6. **Hydrocephalus**: Use of modified _Wu Ling San_ was beneficial in 4 patients with hydrocephalus. The herbal formula was given in decoction, and contained _Fu Ling_ (Poria) 15g, _Da Fu Pi_ (Pericarpium Arecae) 15g, _Zhu Ling_ (Polyporus) 10g, _Ze Xie_ (Rhizoma Alismatis) 10g, _Niu Xi_ (Radix Achyranthis Bidentatae) 10g, _Che Qian Zi_ (Semen Plantaginis) 10g, _Bai Zhu_ (Rhizoma Atractylodis Macrocephalae) 5g, and _Gui Zhi_ (Ramulus Cinnamomi) 2g.[13]

7. **Meniere's syndrome**: One study reported success using modified _Wu Ling San_ to treat 61 patients with Meniere's syndrome. The herbal treatment contained _Wu Ling San_ plus _Dang Shen_ (Radix Codonopsis) and _Huang Qi_ (Radix Astragali), with additional modifications as needed. The overall effectiveness varied from 71.4-96.8%, depending on the traditional Chinese medical diagnosis. Those diagnosed with Spleen and Heart deficiencies were least responsive, while those with phlegm and damp accumulation were most responsive.[14]

DAMP-DISPELLING FORMULAS

16

1111

Chapter 16 – Damp-Dispelling Formulas   *Section 3 – Water-Regulating and Damp-Resolving Formulas*

Wŭ Líng Săn (Five-Ingredient Powder with Poria)

HERB-DRUG INTERACTION

Selective serotonin reuptake inhibitors (SSRIs): Use of *Wu Ling San* was beneficial in relieving adverse gastrointestinal events such as nausea and dyspepsia associated with the use of SSRIs in 20 patients (17 females and 3 males, between 21 to 74 years of age). After adding this formula to the previous drug regimen, the study reported complete disappearance of nausea and dyspepsia in 9 cases, improvement in 4 cases, slight improvement in 2 cases, and no change in 5 cases. Addition of *Wu Ling San* to SSRIs did not cause any adverse events in the 20 patients.[15]

RELATED FORMULAS

Sì Líng Săn (Four-Ingredient Powder with Poria)
四苓散
Pinyin Name: *Si Ling San*
Literal Name: Four-Ingredient Powder with Poria
Original Source: *Ming Yi Zhi Zhang* (Displays of Enlightened Physicians) by Huang Fu-Zhong in 16th century

Bai Zhu (Rhizoma Atractylodis Macrocephalae)	9g
Fu Ling (Poria)	9g
Zhu Ling (Polyporus)	9g
Ze Xie (Rhizoma Alismatis)	9g

The source text states to prepare the ingredients as a decoction. *Si Ling San* (Four-Ingredient Powder with Poria) is essentially *Wu Ling San* minus *Gui Zhi* (Ramulus Cinnamomi). Its main actions are to regulate water circulation and drain dampness. Clinically, this formula is used to treat interior dampness due to an inappropriate diet (such as excessive intake of dairy, greasy or deep-fried foods), resulting in such symptoms as scanty urine (oliguria) and loose stools.

Bái Máo Gēn Tāng (Imperata Decoction)
白茅根湯
白茅根汤
Pinyin Name: *Bai Mao Gen Tang*
Literal Name: Imperata Decoction
Original Source: *Guang An Men Yi Yuan* (Guang An Men Hospital) in 1990

Bai Mao Gen (Rhizoma Imperatae)
Huang Qi (Radix Astragali)
Lu Xian Cao (Herba Pyrolae)
Shan Zhu Yu (Fructus Corni)
Du Zhong (Cortex Eucommiae)
Huang Bo (Cortex Phellodendri Chinensis)
Fu Ling (Poria)

Mu Li (Concha Ostreae)
Jin Ying Zi (Fructus Rosae Laevigatae)
Shi Wei (Folium Pyrrosiae)

Bai Mao Gen Tang (Imperata Decoction) treats chronic *lin zheng* (dysuria syndrome) with urinary difficulty or anuria. It contains herbs that clear heat, promote normal urination, and eliminate water accumulation. Clinically, it is used to treat kidney disorders such as chronic nephritis, chronic nephrotic syndrome, and proteinuria.

Fú Líng Tāng (Poria Decoction)
茯苓湯
茯苓汤
Pinyin Name: *Fu Ling Tang*
Literal Name: Poria Decoction
Original Source: *Guang An Men Yi Yuan* (Guang An Men Hospital) in 1990

Fu Ling (Poria)
Zhu Ling (Polyporus)
Ze Xie (Rhizoma Alismatis)
Bai Zhu (Rhizoma Atractylodis Macrocephalae)
Sang Bai Pi (Cortex Mori)
Yi Yi Ren (Semen Coicis)
Gui Zhi (Ramulus Cinnamomi)
Hua Shi (Talcum)
Chen Pi (Pericarpium Citri Reticulatae)
Xiang Fu (Rhizoma Cyperi)
He Zi (Fructus Chebulae)
Wu Wei Zi (Fructus Schisandrae Chinensis)

Fu Ling Tang (Poria Decoction) treats edema and urinary difficulty caused by water accumulation. Clinical manifestations include edema, generalized swelling, feelings of heaviness or sluggishness in the body, fatigue, and hypersomnia. This formula contains herbs to strengthen the Spleen, resolve dampness, promote normal urination, and eliminate edema.

AUTHORS' COMMENTS

There are four formulas with similar compositions that regulate water and dispel dampness:
• *Wu Ling San* (Five-Ingredient Powder with Poria) is generally considered the standard formula. It has a dual function to release the exterior syndrome and dispel accumulation of water and dampness in the interior.
• *Si Ling San* (Four-Ingredient Powder with Poria) is formulated by removing *Gui Zhi* (Ramulus Cinnamomi) from *Wu Ling San*. It dispels accumulation of water and dampness in the interior, but does not release the exterior.

1112

Chinese Herbal Formulas and Applications

Wǔ Líng Sǎn (Five-Ingredient Powder with Poria)

- *Wei Ling Tang* (Calm the Stomach and Poria Decoction) combines *Ping Wei San* (Calm the Stomach Powder) and *Wu Ling San*. It dispels dampness and harmonizes the Stomach to treat accumulation of water and dampness in the interior causing abdominal distention and edema.
- *Yin Chen Wu Ling San* (Artemisia Scoparia and Five-Ingredient Powder with Poria) is formulated by adding *Yin Chen* (Herba Artemisiae Scopariae) to *Wu Ling San* to treat damp-heat jaundice (more heat than dampness) with urinary difficulty.

References

1. *Zhong Yi Fang Ji Xian Dai Yan Jiu* (Modern Study of Medical Formulae in Traditional Chinese Medicine) 1997;1407.
2. *Guo Wai Yi Xue Zhong Yi Zhong Yao Fen Ce* (Monograph of Chinese Herbology from Foreign Medicine) 1981;2:121.
3. *Zhong Hua Yi Xue Za Zhi* (Chinese Journal of Medicine) 1961;17(1):7.
4. *Tian Jin Zhong Yi* (Tianjin Chinese Medicine) 1994;4:29.
5. *Guo Wai Yi Xue Zhong Yi Zhong Yao Fen Ce* (Monograph of Chinese Herbology from Foreign Medicine) 1983;3:43.
6. *Guo Wai Yi Xue Zhong Yi Zhong Yao Fen Ce* (Monograph of Chinese Herbology from Foreign Medicine) 1986;1:22.
7. *Si Chuan Zhong Yi* (Sichuan Chinese Medicine) 1985;9:19.
8. *Xin Zhong Yi* (New Chinese Medicine) 1987;7:44.
9. *Zhong Yi Za Zhi* (Journal of Chinese Medicine) 1993;1:42.
10. *Shan Xi Zhong Yi* (Shanxi Chinese Medicine) 1993;12:534.
11. *Zhong Yi Ming Fang Lin Chuang Xin Yong* (Contemporary Clinical Applications of Classic Chinese Formulas) 2001;133.
12. *Shan Xi Zhong Yi* (Shanxi Chinese Medicine) 1989;7:295.
13. *Xin Yi Yao Xue Za Zhi* (New Journal of Medicine and Herbology) 1978;8:45.
14. *Zhe Jiang Zhong Yi Xue Yuan Xue Bao* (Journal of Zhejiang University of Chinese Medicine) 1995;3:30.
15. Yamada K, Yagi G, Kanba S. Effectiveness of Gorei-san (TJ-17) for treatment of SSRI-induced nausea and dyspepsia: preliminary observations. Clinical Neuropharmacology 2003 May-Jun;26(3):112-4.

Wèi Líng Tāng (Calm the Stomach and Poria Decoction)

胃苓湯
胃苓汤

Pinyin Name: *Wei Ling Tang*
Literal Name: Calm the Stomach and Poria Decoction
Alternate Names: Weiling Decoction, Stomach-Comforting with Five-Ling Decoction, Magnolia and Hoelen Combination
Original Source: *Dan Xi Xin Fa* (Teachings of [Zhu] Dan-Xi) by Zhu Zhen-Heng in 1481

COMPOSITION

Ping Wei San (Calm the Stomach Powder)	3g
Wu Ling San (Five-Ingredient Powder with Poria)	3g

DOSAGE / PREPARATION / ADMINISTRATION

The source text instructs to cook the ingredients with *Sheng Jiang* (Rhizoma Zingiberis Recens) and *Da Zao* (Fructus Jujubae). Take the decoction on an empty stomach.

CHINESE THERAPEUTIC ACTIONS

Dispels dampness and harmonizes the Stomach

CLINICAL MANIFESTATIONS

External cold damaging the Stomach and Spleen during the late summer and early fall: loose stools containing undigested food, continuous diarrhea, edema, fullness of the abdomen, and dysuria.

CLINICAL APPLICATIONS

Chronic gastritis, gastric neurosis, acute enteritis, diarrhea, ascites, nephritis, nephritic and cardiac edema, urinary retention, and Meniere's syndrome.

EXPLANATION

Wei Ling Tang (Calm the Stomach and Poria Decoction) is composed of *Ping Wei San* (Calm the Stomach Powder) plus *Wu Ling San* (Five-Ingredient Powder with Poria). Thus, this formula harmonizes the Stomach and dispels dampness. Clinically, it is often used for external cold damaging the Stomach and Spleen during the late summer and early fall. Patients in this case may have loose stools containing undigested food, continuous diarrhea, edema, abdominal fullness, and dysuria.

DAMP-DISPELLING FORMULAS

16

1113

Chapter 16 – Damp-Dispelling Formulas　　　*Section 3 – Water-Regulating and Damp-Resolving Formulas*

Wèi Líng Tāng (Calm the Stomach and Poria Decoction)

Wei Ling Tang (Calm the Stomach and Poria Decoction)

Diagnosis	Signs and Symptoms	Treatment	Herbs
External cold damaging the Stomach and Spleen	• Loose stools containing undigested food, thirst, and diarrhea: dampness affecting the Spleen and Stomach • Edema, fullness of the abdomen, and dysuria: obstructed water circulation	• Dispels dampness • Harmonizes the Stomach	• *Ping Wei San* (Calm the Stomach Powder) dries dampness, activates qi circulation, strengthens the Spleen, and harmonizes the Stomach. • *Wu Ling San* (Five-Ingredient Powder with Poria) warms yang, dispels dampness, and disperses water accumulation

Please refer to *Ping Wei San* (Calm the Stomach Powder) and *Wu Ling San* (Five-Ingredient Powder with Poria) for additional and detailed explanations of these two formulas.

MODIFICATIONS

• With exterior wind-cold, add *Bai Shao* (Radix Paeoniae Alba) and *Chai Hu* (Radix Bupleuri).
• With diarrhea, dysentery, and abdominal pain, add *Xiang Fu* (Rhizoma Cyperi) and *Sha Ren* (Fructus Amomi).
• With vomiting of phlegm and saliva, add *Jie Geng* (Radix Platycodonis) and *Ban Xia* (Rhizoma Pinelliae).

CLINICAL STUDIES AND RESEARCH

1. **Nephritis**: Twenty children with acute nephritis (duration of illness ranged from 5 to 63 days) were treated with marked improvement using modified *Wei Ling Tang*. Clinical presentation of the patients included edema and presence of red blood cells, white blood cells, and protein in the urine. The herbal formula contained *Cang Zhu* (Rhizoma Atractylodis) 6g, *Hou Po* (Cortex Magnoliae Officinalis) 9g, *Zhi Qiao* (Fructus Aurantii) 9g, *Zhu Ling* (Polyporus) 9g, *Ze Xie* (Rhizoma Alismatis) 9g, *Mu Tong* (Caulis Akebiae) 9g, *Che Qian Zi* (Semen Plantaginis) 9g, *Mu Xiang* (Radix Aucklandiae) 1g, *Chen Pi* (Pericarpium Citri Reticulatae) 3g, *Gan Cao* (Radix et Rhizoma Glycyrrhizae) 3g, and others as deemed necessary. The study reported satisfactory results in all 20 cases.[1]

2. **Meniere's syndrome**: Modified *Wei Ling Tang* was used in one clinical study to treat 32 patients with Meniere's syndrome with success. The herbal formula contained *Fu Ling* (Poria) 30g, *Gui Zhi* (Ramulus Cinnamomi) 15g, *Chen Pi* (Pericarpium Citri Reticulatae) 12g, *Cang Zhu* (Rhizoma Atractylodis) 10g, *Bai Zhu* (Rhizoma Atractylodis Macrocephalae) 10g, *Hou Po* (Cortex Magnoliae Officinalis) 10g, *Ze Xie* (Rhizoma Alismatis) 10g, *Zhu Ling* (Polyporus) 10g, *Ju Hua* (Flos Chrysanthemi) 10g, post-decocted *Gou Teng* (Ramulus Uncariae cum Uncis) 6g, and *Sheng Jiang* (Rhizoma Zingiberis Recens) 3 slices. Additional modifications were made if needed as follows: *Huang Qi* (Radix Astragali) 30g and *Dang Shen* (Radix Codonopsis) 10g for qi deficiency; *Bai Shao* (Radix Paeoniae Alba) 20g and *Dang Gui* (Radix Angelicae Sinensis) 15g for blood deficiency; *Ban Xia* (Rhizoma Pinelliae) 15g and *Zhu Li* (Succus Bambusae) 10 mL for damp and phlegm accumulation; *Fang Feng* (Radix Saposhnikoviae) 10g and *Jing Jie* (Herba Schizonepetae) 10g for aversion to wind; *Zhi Zi* (Fructus Gardeniae) 10g, *Dan Dou Chi* (Semen Sojae Praeparatum) 10g, *Huang Lian* (Rhizoma Coptidis) 10g, and *Long Dan* (Radix et Rhizoma Gentianae) 10g for excess fire. Of 32 patients, the study reported complete recovery in 28 cases and improvement in 4 cases. The duration of treatment ranged from 3 to 15 packs of herbs, with an average of 6 packs of herbs.[2]

3. **Diarrhea**: *Wei Ling Tang* has been shown in various studies to effectively treat diarrhea. According to one study, use of this formula was associated with 90% effectiveness in 31 children with acute diarrhea.[3] In another study, diarrhea due to acute enteritis in 125 patients was treated with complete recovery in 105 cases, significant improvement in 6 cases, moderate improvement in 4 cases, and no effect in 10 cases.[4]

References

1. *Guang Xi Zhong Yi Yao* (Guangxi Chinese Medicine and Herbology) 1984;4(10):16.
2. *Zhe Jiang Zhong Yi Za Zhi* (Zhejiang Journal of Chinese Medicine) 1994;3:13.
3. *Hu Nan Zhong Yi Za Zhi* (Hunan Journal of Chinese Medicine) 1990;2:48.
4. *Shan Xi Zhong Yi* (Shanxi Chinese Medicine) 1989;10(6):28.

Chinese Herbal Formulas and Applications

Zhū Líng Tāng (Polyporus Decoction)

豬苓湯
猪苓汤

Pinyin Name: *Zhu Ling Tang*
Literal Name: Polyporus Decoction
Alternate Names: *Chu Ling Tang*, Polyporus Combination
Original Source: *Shang Han Lun* (Discussion of Cold-Induced Disorders) by Zhang Zhong-Jing in the Eastern Han Dynasty

COMPOSITION

Zhu Ling (Polyporus)	3g [9g]
Fu Ling (Poria)	3g [9g]
Ze Xie (Rhizoma Alismatis)	3g [9g]
Hua Shi (Talcum), *fen sui* (pulverized)	3g [9g]
E Jiao (Colla Corii Asini)	3g [9g]

DOSAGE / PREPARATION / ADMINISTRATION

The source text instructs to cook all of the ingredients, except *E Jiao* (Colla Corii Asini), with 4 cups [800 mL] of water until the liquid is reduced to 2 cups [400 mL]. Discard the residue, and completely dissolve *E Jiao* (Colla Corii Asini) in the strained decoction. Take 0.7 cup [140 mL] of the warm decoction three times daily. Today, this formula may be prepared as a decoction with the doses suggested in brackets.

CHINESE THERAPEUTIC ACTIONS

1. Regulates water circulation
2. Clears heat and nourishes yin

CLINICAL MANIFESTATIONS

1. Interlocking of water and heat: dysuria, fever, thirst with a strong desire to drink, irritability, insomnia, with or without coughing, nausea, vomiting, and diarrhea.

2. *Xue lin* (bloody dysuria) syndrome: extreme painful urination, difficult urination with dripping of urine, and fullness and pain in the lower abdomen.

CLINICAL APPLICATIONS

Urinary tract infection, urethritis, dysuria, edema, nephritis, cystitis, hematuria, urolithiasis, uroschesis, hydronephrosis, galacturia, and prostatitis.

EXPLANATION

Zhu Ling Tang (Polyporus Decoction) was first introduced in *Shang Han Lun* (Discussion of Cold-Induced Disorders) for treating the condition of interlocking of water and heat. This condition starts as a *taiyang* syndrome at the exterior, and then transforms into a *yangming* or *shaoyang* syndrome and forms heat. This heat, when interlocked with water inside the body, impairs the proper distribution of water. Clinical presentations include

Zhu Ling Tang (Polyporus Decoction)

Diagnosis	Signs and Symptoms	Treatment	Herbs
Interlocking of water and heat	• Dysuria, difficult urination with dribbling of urine, painful urination, and blood in the urine: impaired distribution of water due to interlocking of water and heat • Desire to drink: heat consuming body fluids • Irritability and insomnia: heat disturbing the *shen* (spirit) • Coughing: interlocking of water and heat affecting the Lung • Nausea and vomiting: interlocking of water and heat affecting the Stomach • Diarrhea: interlocking of water and heat affecting the Large Intestine	• Regulates water circulation • Clears heat and nourishes yin	• *Zhu Ling* (Polyporus), *Fu Ling* (Poria) and *Ze Xie* (Rhizoma Alismatis) dispel water accumulation and dampness through urination. • *Hua Shi* (Talcum) clears heat and relieves dysuria. • *E Jiao* (Colla Corii Asini) nourishes yin and moistens dryness.

DAMP-DISPELLING FORMULAS

16

1115

Zhū Líng Tāng (Polyporus Decoction)

dysuria, difficult urination with dribbling of urine, painful urination, and blood in the urine. The interlocking of heat and water also injures the yin and causes thirst with a strong desire to drink, irritability, and insomnia. Lastly, interlocking of water and heat also affects the Lung to cause coughing, the Stomach to cause nausea and vomiting, and the Large Intestine to cause diarrhea.

The treatment plan is to regulate water circulation and dispel dampness through urination, as well as to clear heat and nourish yin. *Zhu Ling* (Polyporus), *Fu Ling* (Poria), and *Ze Xie* (Rhizoma Alismatis) dispel water accumulation and dampness through urination. *Hua Shi* (Talcum) clears heat and relieves dysuria. *E Jiao* (Colla Corii Asini) nourishes yin and moistens dryness. These five herbs have a proper balance to drain water without injuring yin, and to nourish yin without creating more stagnation.

MODIFICATIONS

- For *re lin* (heat dysuria), add *Zhi Zi* (Fructus Gardeniae) and *Che Qian Zi* (Semen Plantaginis), or *Ba Zheng San* (Eight-Herb Powder for Rectification).
- For *xue lin* (bloody dysuria), add *Bai Mao Gen* (Rhizoma Imperatae) and *Xiao Ji* (Herba Cirsii), or *Xiao Ji Yin Zi* (Cirsium Decoction).
- For *shi lin* (stone dysuria), add *Hai Jin Sha* (Spora Lygodii) and *Jin Qian Cao* (Herba Lysimachiae).
- For severe dysuria, add *Mu Tong* (Caulis Akebiae) and *Di Huang* (Radix Rehmanniae).
- With frequent urination, add *Cang Zhu* (Rhizoma Atractylodis) and *Bai Zhu* (Rhizoma Atractylodis Macrocephalae).
- With insomnia or irritability, add *Hu Po* (Succinum) and *Zhi Zi* (Fructus Gardeniae), or *Qing Xin Lian Zi Yin* (Lotus Seed Decoction to Clear the Heart).
- With restlessness, irritability, and thirst, add *Shi Gao* (Gypsum Fibrosum) and *Zhi Mu* (Rhizoma Anemarrhenae).

CAUTIONS / CONTRAINDICATIONS

Zhu Ling Tang primarily regulates water circulation and dispels water accumulation. Although it has a minor effect to nourish yin and moisten dryness, it should not be used in cases of extreme thirst due to severe damage of body fluids, such as from profuse perspiration.[1]

PHARMACOLOGICAL EFFECTS

1. **Diuretic**: Administration of *Zhu Ling Tang* at 10 times the normal dose for 1 month was associated with a marked diuretic effect in rats. The study noted that there were no noticeable changes to the electrolyte levels, such as calcium, magnesium, and potassium.[2,3]

2. **Nephroprotective**: One study reported that *Zhu Ling Tang* given via oral ingestion at 1 g/kg for 12 months was associated with protective and healing effects on the kidneys, and with prolonged life.[4]

3. **Effect on urinary stones**: One study reported that *in vitro* and *in vivo* administrations of *Zhu Ling Tang* corresponded with prevention of urinary stones by reducing struvite crystal formation and increasing the spontaneous discharge of stones in the urine.[5]

CLINICAL STUDIES AND RESEARCH

1. **Edema**: Administration of an herbal extract of *Zhu Ling Tang* to 11 patients at 2.5g per dose, twice daily for 1 month, was associated with marked increase in urination and reduction of edema. There were no significant changes to the blood levels of sodium and potassium.[6]

2. **Hematuria**: Use of modified *Zhu Ling Tang* was associated with 88.2% effectiveness in treating patients with blood in the urine due to various causes. Of 68 patients, the study reported complete recovery in 46 cases, improvement in 14 cases, and no effect in 8 cases.[7]

3. **Urolithiasis**: One study reported 97.1% effectiveness using modified *Zhu Ling Tang* to treat 35 patients with urinary stones. In addition to the base formula, modifications were made by adding *Pu Huang* (Pollen Typhae), *Da Ji* (Herba Cirsii Japonici), *Xiao Ji* (Herba Cirsii), and *Di Long* (Pheretima) for hematuria; and *Bai Shao* (Radix Paeoniae Alba) and *Mu Gua* (Fructus Chaenomelis) for severe colicky pain. The study reported relief of colicky pain within 20 minutes to 7 days. Stones were successfully expelled within 3 to 28 days in 31 of 35 patients.[8] According to another study, administration of *Zhu Ling Tang* was helpful in reducing the number of days (from an average of 21.5 days to 16.0 days) to successfully eliminate urinary stones.[9]

4. **Uroschesis**: One study reported a marked effect in treating 60 geriatric patients with uroschesis using modified *Zhu Ling Tang*. Modifications included addition of *Rou Gui* (Cortex Cinnamomi) and *Fu Zi* (Radix Aconiti Lateralis Praeparata) for aversion to cold, and soreness and weakness of the lower back and knees; *Ren Shen* (Radix et Rhizoma Ginseng) and *Huang Qi* (Radix Astragali) for soft, weak voice; *Chuan Shan Jia* (Squama Manis) and *Jin Qian Cao* (Herba Lysimachiae) for dysuria with lower abdominal fullness and distention; and *Ji Nei Jin* (Endothelium Corneum Gigeriae Galli) and *Jian Shen Qu* (Massa Fermentata Praeparata) for poor appetite. Most patients were able to resume normal urination within 3-6 packs of herbal treatment. Of 60 patients, the study reported complete recovery in 56 cases, improvement in 3 cases, and no effect in 1 case.[10]

Chinese Herbal Formulas and Applications

Zhū Líng Tāng (Polyporus Decoction)

5. **Hydronephrosis:** One study reported 91.1% effectiveness using modified *Zhu Ling Tang* to treat 45 patients with hydronephrosis. Modifications to the base formula included the addition of *Jin Qian Cao* (Herba Lysimachiae), *Hai Jin Sha* (Spora Lygodii), *Shi Wei* (Folium Pyrrosiae), *Wang Bu Liu Xing* (Semen Vaccariae), *Niu Xi* (Radix Achyranthis Bidentatae), and *Ji Nei Jin* (Endothelium Corneum Gigeriae Galli) for urinary stones; *Mu Tong* (Caulis Akebiae) and *Bian Xu* (Herba Polygoni Avicularis) for frequent, urgent, and painful urination; *Da Huang* (Radix et Rhizoma Rhei) for constipation; *Qian Cao* (Radix et Rhizoma Rubiae), *Mo Han Lian* (Herba Ecliptae), and *Bai Mao Gen* (Rhizoma Imperatae) for hematuria; and *Ze Lan* (Herba Lycopi), *Yi Mu Cao* (Herba Leonuri), *Gui Zhi* (Ramulus Cinnamomi), and others for prostatic hypertrophy. Of 45 patients, the study reported complete recovery in 38 cases, improvement in 3 cases, and no effect in 4 cases.[11]

6. **Galacturia:** All 10 patients with galacturia had complete recovery when treated using an herbal formula that contained *Zhu Ling Tang* plus *Huang Bo* (Cortex Phellodendri Chinensis), *Bai Mao Gen* (Rhizoma Imperatae), *Bian Xu* (Herba Polygoni Avicularis), and other herbs. The average duration of treatment was 8 packs of herbs, with some needing up to 21 packs.[12]

7. **Cystitis:** One study reported marked success in treating 107 patients with acute cystitis using 1-6 packs of modified *Zhu Ling Tang*.[13]

8. **Urinary tract disorder:** According to one study of 30 patients who complained of lower urinary tract symptoms without pyuria, administration of *Zhu Ling Tang* was associated with an efficacy rate of 92.9% for pollakisuria, 85.8% for miction pain, 85.7% for voiding discomfort, and 76.0% for total efficacy rate. No side effects were reported.[14]

AUTHORS' COMMENTS

Wu Ling San (Five-Ingredient Powder with Poria) and *Zhu Ling Tang* both regulate water circulation, dispel dampness, and treat urinary difficulty.

- *Wu Ling San* treats accumulation of water and dampness in the interior accompanied by exterior symptoms.
- *Zhu Ling Tang* treats accumulation of water and dampness with heat in the interior.

References

1. *Zhong Yi Lin Chuan Fang Ji Xue* (Clinical Study of Chinese Herbal Formulas) 1995;228-9.
2. *Guo Wai Yi Xue Zhong Yi Zhong Yao Fen Ce* (Monograph of Chinese Herbology from Foreign Medicine) 1981;3:173.
3. *Guo Wai Yi Xue Zhong Yi Zhong Yao Fen Ce* (Monograph of Chinese Herbology from Foreign Medicine) 1984;5:78.
4. *Guo Wai Yi Xue Zhong Yi Zhong Yao Fen Ce* (Monograph of Chinese Herbology from Foreign Medicine) 1984;5:78.
5. Koide T, Yamaguchi S, Utsunomiya M, Yoshioka T, Sugiyama K. The inhibitory effect of kampou extracts on in vitro calcium oxalate crystallization and in vivo stone formation in an animal model. Int J Urol 1995 May;2(2):81-6.
6. *Guo Wai Yi Xue* (Foreign Medicine) 1983;5:292.
7. *Zhong Yi Ming Fang Lin Chuang Xin Yong* (Contemporary Clinical Applications of Classic Chinese Formulas) 2001;636.
8. *Zhe Jiang Zhong Yi Xue Yuan Xue Bao* (Journal of Zhejiang University of Chinese Medicine) 1997;4:35.
9. Takada M, Yano H, Kanbara N, Kurita T, Kohri K, Kato Y, Iguchi M. Effect of Chorei-to on spontaneous discharge of urinary stones after extracorporeal shock wave lithotripsy (ESWL). Hinyokika Kiyo 1997 Apr;43(4):311-4.
10. *Si Chuan Zhong Yi* (Sichuan Chinese Medicine) 1997;4:26.
11. *Shan Dong Zhong Yi Za Zhi* (Shandong Journal of Chinese Medicine) 1995;8:345.
12. *Zhong Guo Nong Cun Yi Xue* (Chinese Agricultural Medicine) 1990;3:33.
13. *Zhe Jiang Zhong Yi Za Zhi* (Zhejiang Journal of Chinese Medicine) 1982;10:448.
14. Horii A, Maekawa M. Clinical evaluation of chorei-to and chorei-to-go-shimotsu-to in patients with lower urinary tract symptoms. Hinyokika Kiyo 1988 Dec;34(12):2237-41.

DAMP-DISPELLING FORMULAS

16

Chapter 16 – Damp-Dispelling Formulas　　　　*Section 3 – Water-Regulating and Damp-Resolving Formulas*

Fáng Jǐ Huáng Qi Tāng (Stephania and Astragalus Decoction)

防己黄耆湯
防己黄芪汤

Pinyin Name: *Fang Ji Huang Qi Tang*
Literal Name: Stephania and Astragalus Decoction
Alternate Name: Stephania and Astragalus Combination
Original Source: *Jin Gui Yao Lue* (Essentials from the Golden Cabinet) by Zhang Zhong-Jing in the Eastern Han Dynasty

COMPOSITION

Fang Ji (Radix Stephaniae Tetrandrae)	3g [6-12g]
Huang Qi (Radix Astragali)	3.75g [9-15g]
Bai Zhu (Rhizoma Atractylodis Macrocephalae)	2.25g [4.5-9g]
Gan Cao (Radix et Rhizoma Glycyrrhizae), *chao* (dry-fried)	1.5g [4.5-6g]

DOSAGE / PREPARATION / ADMINISTRATION

The source text instructions are to grind the ingredients into a coarse powder. Cook the powder [15g] with 4 slices of *Sheng Jiang* (Rhizoma Zingiberis Recens) and 1 piece of *Da Zao* (Fructus Jujubae) in 1.5 bowls of water until the liquid is reduced to 80% volume. After taking the warm, strained decoction, cover the body with blankets to promote mild sweating. Today, this formula may be prepared as a decoction with the doses suggested in brackets.

CHINESE THERAPEUTIC ACTIONS

1. Tonifies qi and dispels wind
2. Strengthens the Spleen and regulates water circulation

CLINICAL MANIFESTATIONS

Feng shui (wind water) or *feng shi* (wind damp) syndromes due to qi deficiency at the exterior: perspiration, aversion to wind, heaviness of the body, urinary difficulty, a pale tongue with a white tongue coating, and a superficial pulse.

CLINICAL APPLICATIONS

Arthritis, rheumatism, rheumatoid arthritis, periarthritis of shoulder, bone fractures, acute glomerulonephritis, chronic nephritis, hydronephrosis, idiopathic edema, edema in the legs, hydrocele, ascites, perspiration, and hircismus.

EXPLANATION

Fang Ji Huang Qi Tang (Stephania and Astragalus Decoction) treats *feng shui* (wind water) and *feng shi* (wind damp) syndromes at the exterior due to qi deficiency. *Feng shui* (wind water) syndrome is a condition caused by invasion of wind at the exterior parts of the body, leading to swelling and water accumulation. *Feng shi* (wind damp) syndrome is a condition caused by invasion of wind-damp, leading to pain and limited movements of the joints, muscles and bones. Both syndromes begin with qi deficiency at the exterior leading to invasion of wind, water and/or dampness at the exterior aspects of the body (skin, muscles, and joints). Perspiration and aversion to

Fang Ji Huang Qi Tang (Stephania and Astragalus Decoction)

Diagnosis	Signs and Symptoms	Treatment	Herbs
Feng shui (wind water) or *feng shi* (wind damp) syndromes due to qi deficiency	• Perspiration and aversion to wind: exterior wind and qi deficiency • Heaviness of the body and urinary difficulty: accumulation of water and dampness • Pale tongue with white coating: qi deficiency • Superficial pulse: exterior condition	• Tonifies qi and dispels wind • Strengthens the Spleen and regulates water circulation	• *Fang Ji* (Radix Stephaniae Tetrandrae) dispels wind and regulates water circulation. • *Huang Qi* (Radix Astragali) tonifies qi, consolidates the exterior, regulates water circulation, and reduces swelling. • *Bai Zhu* (Rhizoma Atractylodis Macrocephalae) tonifies qi, strengthens the Spleen, and dries dampness. • *Sheng Jiang* (Rhizoma Zingiberis Recens) and *Da Zao* (Fructus Jujubae) harmonize the *ying* (nutritive) and *wei* (defensive) levels. • *Gan Cao* (Radix et Rhizoma Glycyrrhizae) tonifies qi and harmonizes the herbs.

1118

Chinese Herbal Formulas and Applications

Fáng Jǐ Huáng Qí Tāng (Stephania and Astragalus Decoction)

wind are both due to exterior wind and qi deficiency. A sensation of heaviness of the body and urinary difficulty are the results of accumulation of water and dampness. A pale tongue with white coating suggests qi deficiency, and a superficial pulse indicates that the disease is located at the exterior.

Normally, an exterior syndrome should be treated with only exterior-releasing herbs. However, in the situation of an exterior condition complicated by qi deficiency and accompanied by water and damp accumulation, using only exterior-releasing herbs is both inappropriate and insufficient. It is inappropriate because herbs that release the exterior will only further deplete qi and invite more wind to attack the exterior. It is insufficient because exterior-releasing herbs cannot effectively dispel water and damp accumulation. Therefore, optimal treatment requires a balanced combination of exterior-releasing, qi-tonifying, and damp-dispelling herbs.

This formula contains *Fang Ji* (Radix Stephaniae Tetrandae) to dispel wind and regulate water circulation. *Huang Qi* (Radix Astragali) tonifies qi, consolidates the exterior, regulates water circulation, and reduces swelling. *Bai Zhu* (Rhizoma Atractylodis Macrocephalae) tonifies qi, strengthens the Spleen, and dries dampness. It also assists *Huang Qi* (Radix Astragali) to consolidate *wei* (defensive) *qi*. *Gan Cao* (Radix et Rhizoma Glycyrrhizae) tonifies qi and harmonizes all of the herbs in this formula. *Sheng Jiang* (Rhizoma Zingiberis Recens) and *Da Zao* (Fructus Jujubae) harmonize the *ying* (nutritive) and *wei* (defensive) levels.

MODIFICATIONS

- With edema, aversion to wind, and absence of sweating due to exterior wind attack, add *Ma Huang* (Herba Ephedrae), *Cang Zhu* (Rhizoma Atractylodis), *Fu Ling* (Poria), and *Yi Yi Ren* (Semen Coicis).
- With edema and swelling due to dampness, combine with *Wu Ling San* (Five-Ingredient Powder with Poria).
- With chest and abdominal fullness and distention, add *Chen Pi* (Pericarpium Citri Reticulatae) and *Hou Po* (Cortex Magnoliae Officinalis).
- With wheezing and dyspnea, add *Ma Huang* (Herba Ephedrae).
- With accelerated respiration and dyspnea, add *Ting Li Zi* (Semen Descurainiae seu Lepidii), *Hou Po* (Cortex Magnoliae Officinalis), and *Ku Xing Ren* (Semen Armeniacae Amarum).
- With abdominal pain due to Liver and Spleen disharmony, add *Bai Shao* (Radix Paeoniae Alba).

- With heaviness and pain of the joints, add *Cang Zhu* (Rhizoma Atractylodis), *Yi Yi Ren* (Semen Coicis), *Wei Ling Xian* (Radix et Rhizoma Clematidis), and *Mu Gua* (Fructus Chaenomelis).
- With numbness and pain in *bi zheng* (painful obstruction syndrome), add *Dang Gui* (Radix Angelicae Sinensis) and *Gui Zhi* (Ramulus Cinnamomi).

CAUTIONS / CONTRAINDICATIONS

- *Fang Ji Huang Qi Tang* treats edema characterized by qi deficiency and damp accumulation. It is contraindicated in edema caused by excess or heat conditions.
- Overdose of this formula has been associated with nausea and poor appetite.[1]

PHARMACOLOGICAL EFFECTS

Chronotropic and inotropic: *Fang Ji Huang Qi Tang* has positive chronotropic and inotropic effects via direct stimulation of the beta-adrenoceptor and/or the norepinephrine release from the postganglionic nerve terminals in the heart.[2]

CLINICAL STUDIES AND RESEARCH

1. **Perspiration**: Use of modified *Fang Ji Huang Qi Tang* was effective in treating profuse perspiration due to various reasons. In addition to the base formula, modifications were made as follows: a large amount of *Huang Qi* (Radix Astragali) was used for spontaneous perspiration due to yang deficiency; *Ma Huang Gen* (Radix et Rhizoma Ephedrae), *Fu Xiao Mai* (Fructus Tritici Levis), and calcined *Mu Li* (Concha Ostreae) for profuse perspiration; *Dang Gui* (Radix Angelicae Sinensis), *Shu Di Huang* (Radix Rehmanniae Praeparata), and *Di Huang* (Radix Rehmanniae) for yin-deficient fire; *Di Gu Pi* (Cortex Lycii), *Zhi Mu* (Rhizoma Anemarrhenae), and *Bie Jia* (Carapax Trionycis) for tidal fever.[3]

2. **Idiopathic edema**: One study reported 90.4% effectiveness using modified *Fang Ji Huang Qi Tang* to treat 52 patients with idiopathic edema. Modifications to the original formula were made based on the condition of each individual patient. For severe edema around the eyes, *Nu Zhen Zi* (Fructus Ligustri Lucidi), *Yi Mu Cao* (Herba Leonuri), and *Che Qian Zi* (Semen Plantaginis) were added. For emotional instability, *Chai Hu* (Radix Bupleuri), *Da Zao* (Fructus Jujubae), and *Yuan Zhi* (Radix Polygalae) were added. For hypotension, *Ren Shen* (Radix et Rhizoma Ginseng) was added. For edema during menstruation, *Xiang Fu* (Rhizoma Cyperi), *Yu Jin* (Radix Curcumae), and *Zhu Ling* (Polyporus) were added. Of 52 patients, the study reported complete recovery in 30 cases, improvement in 17 cases, and no effect in 5 cases.[4]

DAMP-DISPELLING FORMULAS

16

1119

Fáng Jǐ Huáng Qí Tāng (Stephania and Astragalus Decoction)

3. **Hydronephrosis**: Twenty-three patients with hydronephrosis were treated with complete recovery in 4 cases, improvement in 18 cases, and no effect in 1 case. The overall effectiveness was 95.6%. The herbal treatment contained *Fang Ji Huang Qi Tang* plus *Che Qian Zi* (Semen Plantaginis), *Jin Qian Cao* (Herba Lysimachiae), and others as needed.[5]

4. **Arthritis**: One study reported marked effect using modified *Fang Ji Huang Qi Tang* for 6 months to treat 200 cases of arthritis with various clinical presentations. In addition to the base formula, modifications were made based on the classification of arthritis. For arthritis due to damp-heat, *Jin Yin Hua* (Flos Lonicerae Japonicae), *Ye Ju Hua* (Flos Chrysanthemi Indici), *Lei Gong Teng* (Radix Tripterygii Wilfordii), and *Mu Dan Pi* (Cortex Moutan) were added. Of 65 patients with this diagnosis, 17 had resolution of all symptoms, 20 had marked improvement, 25 had moderate improvement, and 3 had no effect. For arthritis due to damp-cold, *Xi Xin* (Radix et Rhizoma Asari), *Gui Zhi* (Ramulus Cinnamomi), *Fu Zi* (Radix Aconiti Lateralis Praeparata), and *Zhi Chuan Wu* (Radix Aconiti Praeparata) were added. Of 135 patients with this diagnosis, 40 had resolution of all symptoms, 35 had marked improvement, 45 had moderate improvement, and 15 had no effect.[6]

5. **Rheumatoid arthritis**: Administration of *Fang Ji Huang Qi Tang* for 6 weeks showed good results in treating rheumatoid arthritis. Of 32 patients, the study reported significant improvement in 14 cases, moderate improvement in 5 cases, slight change in 9 cases, and deterioration in 4 cases.[7]

6. **Periarthritis of shoulder**: One study reported 96.6% effectiveness for treatment of periarthritis of the shoulder using acupuncture and herbs. The herbal formula contained *Fang Ji Huang Qi Tang* plus *Tao Ren* (Semen Persicae), *Hong Hua* (Flos Carthami) and *Chuan Xiong* (Rhizoma Chuanxiong). Of 30 patients, the study reported complete recovery in 22 cases, significant improvement in 5 cases, moderate improvement in 2 cases, and no effect in 1 case. Note: Details of the acupuncture treatment were unavailable at the time of publication.[8]

7. **Bone fractures**: Administration of modified *Fang Ji Huang Qi Tang* reduced swelling and inflammation among 97 patients with bone fractures. The herbal treatment contained this formula as the base, with the addition of *Gui Zhi* (Ramulus Cinnamomi) and *Ting Li Zi* (Semen Descurainiae seu Lepidii) for bone fractures in the arms; and *Fu Ling* (Poria) and *Ze Xie* (Rhizoma Alismatis) for fractures in the legs. Of 97 patients, the study reported complete recovery in 78 cases, improvement in 14 cases, and no effect in 5 cases. The overall effectiveness was 94.85%.[9]

8. **Hircismus**: Use of modified *Fang Ji Huang Qi Tang* was effective in treating 12 patients (3 males and 9 females; between 14-48 years of age; with 1 to 25 years history) with an offensive odor of the axillae. The herbal formula contained *Fang Ji* (Radix Stephaniae Tetrandrae) 30g, *Huang Qi* (Radix Astragali) 30g, dry-fried *Bai Zhu* (Rhizoma Atractylodis Macrocephalae) 15g, *Gan Cao* (Radix et Rhizoma Glycyrrhizae) 6g, *Sheng Jiang* (Rhizoma Zingiberis Recens) 9g, and *Da Zao* (Fructus Jujubae) 20g. Furthermore, *Bai Mao Gen* (Rhizoma Imperatae), *Che Qian Zi* (Semen Plantaginis), and *Che Qian Cao* (Herba Plantaginis) were added for excessive dampness; *Fu Ling Pi* (Cortex Poria) and *Ze Xie* (Rhizoma Alismatis) were added for Spleen deficiency; and *Yin Chen* (Herba Artemisiae Scopariae) and charred *Shan Zha* (Fructus Crataegi) were added for obesity. The study reported complete recovery in all 12 patients after a duration of 2 to 6.5 months of treatment.[10]

RELATED FORMULA

Fáng Jǐ Fú Líng Tāng (Stephania and Poria Decoction)

防己茯苓湯
防己茯苓汤

Pinyin Name: *Fang Ji Fu Ling Tang*
Literal Name: Stephania and Poria Decoction
Original Source: *Jin Gui Yao Lue* (Essentials from the Golden Cabinet) by Zhang Zhong-Jing in the Eastern Han Dynasty

Fang Ji (Radix Stephaniae Tetrandrae)	9g
Huang Qi (Radix Astragali)	9g
Gui Zhi (Ramulus Cinnamomi)	9g
Fu Ling (Poria)	18g
Gan Cao (Radix et Rhizoma Glycyrrhizae)	6g

The source text instructs to cook the herbs in 6 cups [1,200 mL] of water until it is reduced down to 2 cups [400 mL]. Take the warm, strained decoction in three equally-divided doses.

The main actions of this formula are to benefit the qi, promote the normal circulation of yang, and regulate water metabolism. Clinically, this formula is often used to treat edema of the extremities with a feeling of heaviness and urinary difficulty.

Fang Ji Huang Qi Tang and *Fang Ji Fu Ling Tang* (Stephania and Poria Decoction) both treat edema by tonifying qi and regulating water circulation.

- *Fang Ji Huang Qi Tang* is more suitable for edema due to qi deficiency with such symptoms as perspiration,

1120

Chinese Herbal Formulas and Applications

Fáng Jǐ Huáng Qí Tāng (Stephania and Astragalus Decoction)

aversion to wind, a feeling of heaviness in the body, and a superficial pulse.

• *Fang Ji Fu Ling Tang* is more suitable for edema with yang deficiency with such symptoms as general edema, edema of the extremities, and dysuria.

AUTHORS' COMMENTS

Fang Ji Huang Qi Tang is designed to treat accumulation of water and dampness due to qi deficiency. However, today this formula is used mainly for weight loss in patients with Spleen deficiency. Most of these patients do not have big appetite, but still gain weight regardless of how little they eat. They retain excessive amount of dampness and water because the transportation and water-metabolizing functions of the Spleen are impaired. Also, as the Spleen is the organ that controls the muscles, these patients often show flaccid or no muscle tone, in addition to obesity.

References

1. *Zhong Yao Ming Fang Yao Li Yu Ying Yong* (Pharmacology and Applications of Famous Herbal Formulas) 1989;434-5.
2. Sugiyama A, Takahara A, Satoh Y, Yoneyama M, Saegusa Y, Hashimoto K. Cardiac effects of clinically available Kampo medicine assessed with canine isolated, blood-perfused heart preparations. Jpn J Pharmacol 2002 Mar;88(3):307-13.
3. *Jiang Xi Yi Yao Za Zhi* (Jiangxi Journal of Medicine and Herbology) 1994;4:27.
4. *Shi Yong Zhong Xi Yi Jie He Za Zhi* (Practical Journal of Integrated Chinese and Western Medicines) 1997;11:1101.
5. *Shan Xi Zhong Yi* (Shanxi Chinese Medicine) 1989;10(8):352.
6. *Zhe Jiang Zhong Yi Za Zhi* (Zhejiang Journal of Chinese Medicine) 1989;2:59.
7. *Guo Wai Yi Xue* (Foreign Medicine) 1990;12(4):213.
8. *Zhong Yi Ming Fang Lin Chuang Xin Yong* (Contemporary Clinical Applications of Classic Chinese Formulas) 2001;382.
9. *Shi Yong Zhong Yi Yao Za Zhi* (Journal of Practical Chinese Medicine and Medicinals) 1996;4:9.
10. *Zhe Jiang Zhong Yi Za Zhi* (Zhejiang Journal of Chinese Medicine) 1994;4:177.

Wǔ Pí Sǎn (Five-Peel Powder)
五皮散

Pinyin Name: *Wu Pi San*
Literal Name: Five-Peel Powder
Alternate Names: *Wu Pi Yin*, Five-Pi Drink, Five Kinds of Peels Drink, Hoelen and Areca Combination
Original Source: *Zhong Zang Jing* (Treasury Classic) by Hua-Tuo in the Han Dynasty

COMPOSITION

Fu Ling Pi (Cortex Poria)	[9g]
Sheng Jiang Pi (Pericarpium Zingiberis Recens)	[9g]
Sang Bai Pi (Cortex Mori)	[9g]
Da Fu Pi (Pericarpium Arecae)	[9g]
Chen Pi (Pericarpium Citri Reticulatae)	[9g]

DOSAGE / PREPARATION / ADMINISTRATION

The source text instructs to grind equal amounts of the ingredients into a coarse powder. Cook 9g of the powder with 1.5 bowls of water until the liquid is reduced to 80% volume. Take the warm, strained decoction any time during the day. Today, this formula may be prepared as a decoction with the doses suggested in brackets.

CHINESE THERAPEUTIC ACTIONS

1. Dispels dampness and reduces swelling and edema
2. Regulates qi and strengthens the Spleen

CLINICAL MANIFESTATIONS

Pi shui (skin water) due to Spleen deficiency and damp accumulation: generalized edema of the whole body, heaviness of the body and extremities, epigastric and abdominal fullness or distention, shortness of breath, rapid breathing, urinary difficulty, edema during pregnancy, white, greasy tongue coating, and a deep, moderate pulse.

CLINICAL APPLICATIONS

Cardiac and nephritic edema, chronic nephritis, edema during pregnancy, generalized edema, and traumatic injuries.

DAMP-DISPELLING FORMULAS

16

1121

Wŭ Pí Săn (Five-Peel Powder)

EXPLANATION

When the Spleen is deficient, damp accumulates in the interior, which then overflows to the skin and muscles, causing generalized edema and swelling throughout the body and extremities. Damp accumulation can obstruct the flow of qi and cause epigastric and abdominal fullness and distention. If the damp accumulation affects the Lung, shortness of breath and rapid breathing may occur. Because water circulation is impaired, urinary difficulty may also occur.

Wu Pi San (Five-Peel Powder) uses Fu Ling Pi (Cortex Poria) to dispel dampness and relieve edema through diuresis. This herb also strengthens the Spleen and improves its transformation and transportation functions. Sheng Jiang Pi (Pericarpium Zingiberis Recens) disperses accumulation of water and dampness. Sang Bai Pi (Cortex Mori) redirects the rising Lung qi and restores normal water metabolism. Da Fu Pi (Pericarpium Arecae) activates qi circulation to disperse fluids and relieve fullness and distention. Chen Pi (Pericarpium Citri Reticulatae) harmonizes Stomach qi and disperses turbid dampness.

MODIFICATIONS

- With water accumulation above the waist, add Zi Su Ye (Folium Perillae), Jing Jie (Herba Schizonepetae), Fang Feng (Radix Saposhnikoviae), and Qin Jiao (Radix Gentianae Macrophyllae).
- With water accumulation below the waist, add Chi Xiao Dou (Semen Phaseoli), Fu Ling (Poria), Ze Xie (Rhizoma Alismatis), Fang Ji (Radix Stephaniae Tetrandrae), and Che Qian Zi (Semen Plantaginis).

- With severe edema, add Wu Ling San (Five-Ingredient Powder with Poria).
- With facial edema, add Chen Pi (Pericarpium Citri Reticulatae) and Sang Bai Pi (Cortex Mori).
- With edema during pregnancy, remove Sang Bai Pi (Cortex Mori), and add Bai Zhu (Rhizoma Atractylodis Macrocephalae).
- With generalized weakness and deficiency, add Dang Shen (Radix Codonopsis), Huang Qi (Radix Astragali), and Bai Zhu (Rhizoma Atractylodis Macrocephalae).
- With coldness, add Gan Jiang (Rhizoma Zingiberis) and Rou Gui (Cortex Cinnamomi).
- With abdominal fullness and distention, add Bai Zhu (Rhizoma Atractylodis Macrocephalae) and Cang Zhu (Rhizoma Atractylodis).

CAUTIONS / CONTRAINDICATIONS

Avoid foods that are raw, cold, oily, greasy or hard to digest while taking Wu Pi San.

CLINICAL STUDIES AND RESEARCH

1. **Edema**: Wu Pi San was shown in two studies to have satisfactory results in treating edema.[1]
2. **Traumatic injuries with swelling and inflammation**: Sixty-three patients with swelling and inflammation due to external trauma were effectively treated using Wu Pi San plus Bai Zhu (Rhizoma Atractylodis Macrocephalae) and San Qi (Radix et Rhizoma Notoginseng). Gui Zhi (Ramulus Cinnamomi) and Sang Zhi (Ramulus Mori) were added if the upper extremities were affected, and Chuan Niu Xi (Radix Cyathulae) was added for the lower extremities. The study reported marked effectiveness in all 63 patients, with swelling reduced in 18 cases after 2 days, 30 cases after 3 days, and 15 cases after 7 days.[2]

Wu Pi San (Five-Peel Powder)

Diagnosis	Signs and Symptoms	Treatment	Herbs
Pi shui (skin water) due to Spleen deficiency and damp accumulation	• Edema and swelling throughout the body and extremities: damp accumulation with Spleen deficiency • Epigastric and abdominal fullness and distention: damp accumulation obstructing qi circulation • Shortness of breath and rapid breathing: damp accumulation affecting the Lung • Urinary difficulty: damp accumulation affecting the Urinary Bladder	• Eliminates dampness and reduces swelling and edema • Regulates the qi and strengthens the Spleen	• Fu Ling Pi (Cortex Poria) dispels dampness and relieves edema through diuresis. • Sheng Jiang Pi (Pericarpium Zingiberis Recens) disperses accumulation of water and dampness. • Sang Bai Pi (Cortex Mori) redirects the rising Lung qi downward and restores normal water metabolism. • Da Fu Pi (Pericarpium Arecae) activates qi circulation and relieves fullness and distention. • Chen Pi (Pericarpium Citri Reticulatae) harmonizes Stomach qi and disperses dampness.

1122

Chinese Herbal Formulas and Applications

Wǔ Pí Sǎn (Five-Peel Powder)

RELATED FORMULA

Wǔ Pí Sǎn (Five-Peel Powder)

五皮散

Pinyin Name: *Wu Pi San*

Literal Name: Five-Peel Powder

Original Source: *Tai Ping Hui Min He Ji Ju Fang* (Imperial Grace Formulary of the Tai Ping Era) by the Imperial Medical Department in 1078-85

Sheng Jiang Pi (Pericarpium Zingiberis Recens)

Wu Jia Pi (Cortex Acanthopanacis)

Di Gu Pi (Cortex Lycii)

Da Fu Pi (Pericarpium Arecae)

Fu Ling Pi (Cortex Poria)

This formula treats edema by eliminating dampness, reducing swelling, dispelling wind-dampness, and opening the channels and collaterals.

Wu Pi San is the identical name of the main formula and the related formula; they have the same name, similar compositions, and essentially the same functions. Both formulas contain *Fu Ling Pi* (Cortex Poria), *Sheng Jiang Pi* (Pericarpium Zingiberis Recens), and *Da Fu Pi* (Pericarpium Arecae).

- *Wu Pi San*, from *Zhong Zang Jing* (Treasury Classic) by Hua-Tuo, contains *Sang Bai Pi* (Cortex Mori) and *Chen Pi* (Pericarpium Citri Reticulatae), and is better at regulating qi circulation.
- *Wu Pi San*, from *Tai Ping Hui Min He Ji Ju Fang* (Imperial Grace Formulary of the Tai Ping Era) by the Imperial Medical Department, contains *Wu Jia Pi* (Cortex Acanthopanacis) and *Di Gu Pi* (Cortex Lycii), and has a strong function to dispel wind-dampness and open the channels and collaterals.

References

1. *Shan Xi Zhong Yi* (Shanxi Chinese Medicine) 1991;12(2):89.
2. *Zhe Jiang Zhong Yi Za Zhi* (Zhejiang Journal of Chinese Medicine) 1994;11:511.

Jiǔ Wèi Bīng Láng Jiā Wú Fú Tāng

(Areca Nine Decoction plus Evodia and Poria)

九味檳榔加吳茯湯

九味槟榔加吴茯汤

Pinyin Name: *Jiu Wei Bing Lang Jia Wu Fu Tang*

Literal Name: Areca Nine Decoction plus Evodia and Poria

Alternate Name: Areca Seed Combination

Original Source: *Qian Tian Jia Fang* (Family Formulas of Qian Tian-Jia)

COMPOSITION

Bing Lang (Semen Arecae)

Chen Pi (Pericarpium Citri Reticulatae)

Hou Po (Cortex Magnoliae Officinalis)

Mu Xiang (Radix Aucklandiae)

Zi Su Ye (Folium Perillae)

Wu Zhu Yu (Fructus Evodiae)

Gui Zhi (Ramulus Cinnamomi)

Fu Ling (Poria)

Da Huang (Radix et Rhizoma Rhei)

Sheng Jiang (Rhizoma Zingiberis Recens)

Gan Cao (Radix et Rhizoma Glycyrrhizae)

DAMP-DISPELLING FORMULAS

16

1123

Chapter 16 – Damp-Dispelling Formulas　　　*Section 3 – Water-Regulating and Damp-Resolving Formulas*

Jiǔ Wèi Bīng Láng Jiā Wú Fú Tāng
(Areca Nine Decoction plus Evodia and Poria)

DOSAGE / PREPARATION / ADMINISTRATION

The source text instructs to prepare the ingredients as a decoction.

CHINESE THERAPEUTIC ACTIONS

1. Dispels water accumulation
2. Disperses qi and blood stagnation
3. Relieves constipation

CLINICAL MANIFESTATION

Water accumulation in the legs with qi and blood stagnation: beriberi, pitting edema, numbness, fatigue, and weakness of the legs, palpitations, distention beneath the heart, and constipation.

CLINICAL APPLICATIONS

Hypertension, myocarditis, congestive heart failure, beriberi, neurosis, and multiple neuritis.

EXPLANATION

Jiu Wei Bing Lang Jia Wu Fu Tang (Areca Nine Decoction plus Evodia and Poria) treats water accumulation in the legs accompanied by qi and blood stagnation. Pitting edema in the legs is diagnostic of water accumulation. As water accumulation affects the upper and middle *jiaos*, patients may experience palpitations, shortness of breath, and a feeling of distention beneath the heart. Water accumulation may also contribute to damp stagnation, leading to a feeling of fullness and distention. Furthermore, chronic water accumulation leads to qi and blood stagnation, which is characterized by numbness, fatigue, and weakness of the legs.

In this formula, *Bing Lang* (Semen Arecae) breaks up qi stagnation, eliminates water accumulation, and dispels phlegm. *Chen Pi* (Pericarpium Citri Reticulatae) regulates qi and dries dampness. *Hou Po* (Cortex Magnoliae Officinalis) dispels dampness, removes stagnation, and disperses distention. *Mu Xiang* (Radix Aucklandiae) promotes qi circulation and relieves pain and distention. *Zi Su Ye* (Folium Perillae), with its light and acrid properties, regulates qi circulation and harmonizes the middle *jiao*. *Wu Zhu Yu* (Fructus Evodiae) and *Gui Zhi* (Ramulus Cinnamomi) warm the yang to eliminate water and phlegm stagnation. *Fu Ling* (Poria) strengthens the Spleen, dispels dampness, and eliminates water accumulation. *Da Huang* (Radix et Rhizoma Rhei) relieves constipation. *Sheng Jiang* (Rhizoma Zingiberis Recens)

Jiu Wei Bing Lang Jia Wu Fu Tang (Areca Nine Decoction plus Evodia and Poria)

Diagnosis	Signs and Symptoms	Treatment	Herbs
Water accumulation in the legs with qi and blood stagnation	• Pitting edema in the legs: water accumulation in the extremities • Palpitations, shortness of breath and a feeling of distention beneath the heart: water accumulation in the upper and middle *jiaos* • Numbness, fatigue, and weakness of the legs: qi and blood stagnation secondary to water accumulation	• Dispels water accumulation • Disperses qi and blood stagnation • Relieves constipation	• *Bing Lang* (Semen Arecae) breaks up qi stagnation, eliminates water accumulation, and dispels phlegm. • *Chen Pi* (Pericarpium Citri Reticulatae) regulates qi and dries dampness. • *Hou Po* (Cortex Magnoliae Officinalis) dispels dampness, removes stagnation, and disperses distention. • *Mu Xiang* (Radix Aucklandiae) promotes qi circulation and relieves pain and distention. • *Zi Su Ye* (Folium Perillae) regulates qi circulation and harmonizes the middle *jiao*. • *Wu Zhu Yu* (Fructus Evodiae) and *Gui Zhi* (Ramulus Cinnamomi) warm the yang to eliminate water and phlegm stagnation. • *Fu Ling* (Poria) strengthens the Spleen, dispels dampness, and eliminates water accumulation. • *Da Huang* (Radix et Rhizoma Rhei) relieves constipation. • *Sheng Jiang* (Rhizoma Zingiberis Recens) and *Gan Cao* (Radix et Rhizoma Glycyrrhizae) harmonize the herbs in this formula.

1124

Chinese Herbal Formulas and Applications

Jiǔ Wèi Bīng Láng Jiā Wú Fú Tāng
(Areca Nine Decoction plus Evodia and Poria)

and *Gan Cao* (Radix et Rhizoma Glycyrrhizae) harmonize all of the herbs in this formula.

AUTHORS' COMMENTS

Jiu Wei Bing Lang Jia Wu Fu Tang can be combined with *Tian Ma Gou Teng Yin* (Gastrodia and Uncaria Decoction) to treat hypertension with edema and water retention. These formulas have a downward draining effect to guide fire down and out of the body.

Jiu Wei Bing Lang Jia Wu Fu Tang can be used with *Gua Lou Xie Bai Bai Jiu Tang* (Trichosanthes Fruit, Chinese Chive, and Wine Decoction) to treat hypertension complicated by high cholesterol and arteriosclerosis. Together, these two formulas eliminate accumulation of water and phlegm and dispel stagnation of qi and blood.

Mù Fáng Jǐ Tāng (Cocculus Decoction)
木防己湯
木防己汤

Pinyin Name: *Mu Fang Ji Tang*
Literal Name: Cocculus Decoction
Alternate Names: *Mu Fang Chi Tang*, Cocculus and Ginseng Combination
Original Source: *Jin Gui Yao Lue* (Essentials from the Golden Cabinet) by Zhang Zhong-Jing in the Eastern Han Dynasty

COMPOSITION

Mu Fang Ji (Radix Cocculi Trilobi)	9g
Shi Gao (Gypsum Fibrosum)	12 pieces [18g]
Ren Shen (Radix et Rhizoma Ginseng)	12g
Gui Zhi (Ramulus Cinnamomi)	6g

DOSAGE / PREPARATION / ADMINISTRATION

The source text instructs to cook the ingredients in 6 cups [1,200 mL] of water and reduce the liquid to 2 cups [400 mL]. Take the warm, strained decoction in two equally-divided doses.

CHINESE THERAPEUTIC ACTIONS

1. Activates water circulation to eliminate stagnation
2. Guides the reversed flow of qi downward

CLINICAL MANIFESTATIONS

Water accumulation in the upper *jiao*: shortness of breath, increased dyspnea when lying down, asthma, abdominal pain, fullness and distention in the epigastrium and chest, dark facial complexion, scanty urination, edema, and a deep, tight pulse.

CLINICAL APPLICATIONS

Congestive heart failure, cardiac asthma, edema due to nephritis, bronchial asthma, and pitting edema.

EXPLANATION

Mu Fang Ji Tang (Cocculus Decoction) treats water accumulation in the upper *jiao*, manifesting in an increase in pressure leading to chest distention and fullness, and abdominal pain. Water accumulation in the chest will directly affect the function of the Lungs, causing shortness of breath, dyspnea, and possibly asthma. Additionally, when the patient is in a horizontal position, the pressure in the lungs further increases, thereby aggravating the shortness of breath and dyspnea. Water accumulation also affects blood circulation, leading to palpitations, edema, and a dark facial complexion. Other symptoms and signs include scanty urination and a deep, tight pulse.

DAMP-DISPELLING FORMULAS

16

1125

Chapter 16 – Damp-Dispelling Formulas   Section 3 – Water-Regulating and Damp-Resolving Formulas

Mù Fáng Jǐ Tāng (Cocculus Decoction)

Mu Fang Ji Tang (Cocculus Decoction)

Diagnosis	Signs and Symptoms	Treatment	Herbs
Water accumulation in the upper *jiao*	• Chest distention and fullness, shortness of breath, and dyspnea: water accumulation affecting the Lung • Palpitations, edema, and a dark facial complexion: water accumulation affecting the Heart	• Activates water circulation to eliminate stagnation • Guides the reversed flow of qi downward	• *Mu Fang Ji* (Radix Cocculi Trilobi) promotes water circulation and eliminates water accumulation to relieve shortness of breath and dyspnea. • *Shi Gao* (Gypsum Fibrosum) clears Lung heat and relieves dyspnea. • *Ren Shen* (Radix et Rhizoma Ginseng) relieves dyspnea and facilitates the elimination of water accumulation in the chest and diaphragm. • *Gui Zhi* (Ramulus Cinnamomi) opens the channels and collaterals and prevents the reversed flow of qi from rising to the Lung.

In this prescription, herbs are formulated to activate water circulation and eliminate water accumulation. *Mu Fang Ji* (Radix Cocculi Trilobi), acrid and warm, relieves shortness of breath and dyspnea by promoting water circulation and eliminating water accumulation. *Shi Gao* (Gypsum Fibrosum), sweet and cold, clears Lung heat and relieves dyspnea. *Ren Shen* (Radix et Rhizoma Ginseng) relieves dyspnea and facilitates the elimination of water accumulation in the chest and diaphragm. *Gui Zhi* (Ramulus Cinnamomi) opens the channels and collaterals and prevents the reversed flow of qi from rising to the Lung. *Mu Fang Ji* (Radix Cocculi Trilobi) and *Gui Zhi* (Ramulus Cinnamomi) both have a diuretic effect to promote urination and eliminate water accumulation.

MODIFICATION

With wheezing and dyspnea due to congestive heart failure, add *Sang Bai Pi* (Cortex Mori), *Zi Su Zi* (Fructus Perillae), and *Sheng Jiang* (Rhizoma Zingiberis Recens).

CLINICAL STUDIES AND RESEARCH

Congestive heart failure: Administration of *Mu Fang Ji Tang* showed a protective effect against myocardial injury leading to congestive heart failure in an animal model.[1]

AUTHORS' COMMENTS

Because *Mu Fang Ji* (Radix Cocculi Trilobi) is not a commonly used herb and is sometimes difficult to obtain, it has been substituted in the past with *Fang Ji* (Radix Stephaniae Tetrandrae) (also known as *Han Fang Ji* or *Fen Fang Ji*) or *Guang Fang Ji* (Radix Aristolochia Westlandi). Although these three herbs function similarly as diuretics, they are, in fact, derived from different plant species, and should **not** be used interchangeably.

Reference

1. Wang WZ, Matsumori A, Matoba Y, Matsui S, Sato Y, Hirozane T, Shioi T, Sasayama S. Protective effects of Mu-Fang-Ji-Tang against myocardial injury in a murine model of congestive heart failure induced by viral myocarditis. Life Sci 1998;62(13):1139-46.

1126

Chinese Herbal Formulas and Applications

Fēn Xiāo Tāng (Separate and Reduce Decoction)

分消湯
分消汤

Pinyin Name: *Fen Xiao Tang*
Literal Name: Separate and Reduce Decoction
Alternate Name: Hoelen and Alisma Combination
Original Source: *Wan Bing Hui Chun* (Restoration of Health from the Myriad Diseases) by Gong Ting-Xian in 1587

COMPOSITION

Cang Zhu (Rhizoma Atractylodis), *jin* (soaked) in rice water and *chao* (dry-fried)	3g
Bai Zhu (Rhizoma Atractylodis Macrocephalae)	3g
Hou Po (Cortex Magnoliae Officinalis), *chao* (dry-fried) with ginger juice	3g
Chen Pi (Pericarpium Citri Reticulatae)	3g
Mu Xiang (Radix Aucklandiae)	0.9g
Xiang Fu (Rhizoma Cyperi)	2.4g
Zhi Shi (Fructus Aurantii Immaturus), *chao* (dry-fried) with bran	3g
Da Fu Pi (Pericarpium Arecae)	2.4g
Sha Ren (Fructus Amomi)	2.1g
Zhu Ling (Polyporus)	2.4g
Ze Xie (Rhizoma Alismatis)	2.4g
Fu Ling (Poria)	3g

DOSAGE / PREPARATION / ADMINISTRATION

The source text instructs to cook the ingredients with 1 slice of *Sheng Jiang* (Rhizoma Zingiberis Recens) and 1 piece of *Deng Xin Cao* (Medulla Junci) in water to make a decoction.

CHINESE THERAPEUTIC ACTIONS

1. Strengthens the Spleen
2. Regulates qi circulation to relieve fullness and distention
3. Regulates the water passages to eliminate water stagnation

CLINICAL MANIFESTATIONS

1. Severe abdominal fullness and distention due to Spleen deficiency: severe fullness and drum-like distention in the abdomen, decreased food intake, decreased appetite, acid regurgitation, dysuria, and scanty urine.
2. Water stagnation due to Spleen deficiency: feeling of fullness, distention, and oppression in the chest and abdomen, ascites, edema, belching, acid reflux, scanty urine, and constipation.

CLINICAL APPLICATIONS

Peritonitis, pitting edema, nephritis, and liver cirrhosis with ascites.

EXPLANATION

Fen Xiao Tang (Separate and Reduce Decoction) treats severe abdominal fullness with drum-like distention characterized by Spleen deficiency and damp accumulation.

Spleen deficiency, besides giving rise to damp accumulation, may cause inadequate transportation and transformation of nutrients. The dampness and untransformed nutrients usually accumulate in the abdomen, causing fullness and distention. Loss of appetite is the result of Spleen deficiency, and acid regurgitation arises from Stomach disharmony. Dysuria and scanty urine are the results of dampness and fluids being unable to pass out of the body through urination.

There are two major categories of herbs employed in this treatment strategy: herbs to strengthen the Spleen and Stomach, and herbs to eliminate dampness and water stagnation. *Cang Zhu* (Rhizoma Atractylodis) and *Bai Zhu* (Rhizoma Atractylodis Macrocephalae), both bitter, dry, and warm, resolve dampness and strengthen the Spleen. *Hou Po* (Cortex Magnoliae Officinalis) activates qi circulation, dispel dampness, and relieve fullness and distention in the epigastrium and abdomen. *Chen Pi* (Pericarpium Citri Reticulatae), *Mu Xiang* (Radix Aucklandiae), and *Xiang Fu* (Rhizoma Cyperi) regulate qi and relieve stagnation. *Zhi Shi* (Fructus Aurantii Immaturus), *Da Fu Pi* (Pericarpium Arecae), and *Sha Ren* (Fructus Amomi) strengthen the Spleen and Stomach to restore the normal food transformation and transportation. *Sheng Jiang* (Rhizoma Zingiberis Recens) harmonizes the Spleen and Stomach. *Zhu Ling* (Polyporus), *Ze Xie* (Rhizoma Alismatis), and *Fu Ling* (Poria) dispel water and dampness through diuresis. *Deng Xin Cao* (Medulla

DAMP-DISPELLING FORMULAS

16

1127

Chapter 16 – Damp-Dispelling Formulas   Section 3 – Water-Regulating and Damp-Resolving Formulas

Fēn Xiāo Tāng (Separate and Reduce Decoction)

Fen Xiao Tang (Separate and Reduce Decoction)

Diagnosis	Signs and Symptoms	Treatment	Herbs
Severe abdominal fullness and distention due to Spleen deficiency and damp accumulation	• Abdominal fullness and distention: accumulation of dampness in the abdomen • Loss of appetite: Spleen deficiency • Acid regurgitation: disharmony in the Stomach	• Strengthens the Spleen • Regulates qi circulation • Regulates water passages	• *Cang Zhu* (Rhizoma Atractylodis) and *Bai Zhu* (Rhizoma Atractylodis Macrocephalae) dry dampness and strengthen the Spleen. • *Hou Po* (Cortex Magnoliae Officinalis) activates qi circulation, dispels dampness, and relieves fullness and distention. • *Chen Pi* (Pericarpium Citri Reticulatae), *Mu Xiang* (Radix Aucklandiae), and *Xiang Fu* (Rhizoma Cyperi) regulate qi and relieve stagnation. • *Zhi Shi* (Fructus Aurantii Immaturus), *Da Fu Pi* (Pericarpium Arecae), and *Sha Ren* (Fructus Amomi) strengthen the Spleen and Stomach to restore the normal food transformation and transportation. • *Sheng Jiang* (Rhizoma Zingiberis Recens) harmonizes the Spleen and Stomach. • *Zhu Ling* (Polyporus), *Ze Xie* (Rhizoma Alismatis), and *Fu Ling* (Poria) dispel water and dampness through diuresis. • *Deng Xin Cao* (Medulla Junci) regulates qi, harmonizes the Spleen, induces diuresis, and clears heat.

Junci) has a wide variety of clinical functions, including regulating qi, harmonizing the Spleen, inducing diuresis, and clearing heat.

MODIFICATIONS

• With increased respiration rate, add *Chen Xiang* (Lignum Aquilariae Resinatum).

• With swelling and fullness in the abdomen due to food stagnation, add *Lai Fu Zi* (Semen Raphani).

• With a bitter taste in the mouth and hypochondriac fullness and distention, combine with *Xiao Chai Hu Tang* (Minor Bupleurum Decoction).

AUTHORS' COMMENTS

This formula is also used to treat severe cases of water accumulation (such as ascites and edema) caused by Spleen deficiency. Ascites is generally described as a drum-like distention in the abdomen, while edema is characterized by prolonged pits produced by pressure. Ascites and pitting edema are two diagnostic signs for prescribing this formula.

1128

Chinese Herbal Formulas and Applications

Dǎo Shuǐ Fú Líng Tāng (Poria Decoction to Drain Water)

導水茯苓湯
导水茯苓汤

Pinyin Name: *Dao Shui Fu Ling Tang*
Literal Name: Poria Decoction to Drain Water
Alternate Names: *Tao Shui Fu Ling Tang*, Hoelen, Atractylodes, and Areca Decoction
Original Source: *Zheng Zhi Zhun Sheng* (Standards of Patterns and Treatments) by Wang Ken-Tang in 1602

COMPOSITION

Chi Fu Ling (Poria Rubra)	90g
Ze Xie (Rhizoma Alismatis)	90g
Bai Zhu (Rhizoma Atractylodis Macrocephalae)	90g
Mu Gua (Fructus Chaenomelis)	30g
Bing Lang (Semen Arecae)	30g
Mai Dong (Radix Ophiopogonis)	90g
Zi Su Ye (Folium Perillae)	30g
Deng Xin Cao (Medulla Junci)	22.5g
Chen Pi (Pericarpium Citri Reticulatae)	22.5g
Mu Xiang (Radix Aucklandiae)	22.5g
Sha Ren (Fructus Amomi)	22.5g
Sang Bai Pi (Cortex Mori)	30g
Da Fu Pi (Pericarpium Arecae)	22.5g

DOSAGE / PREPARATION / ADMINISTRATION

The source text instructs to prepare the ingredients as a decoction.

CHINESE THERAPEUTIC ACTIONS

1. Dispels stagnant water and dries dampness
2. Eliminates water from the Lung
3. Harmonizes the Spleen

CLINICAL MANIFESTATIONS

Severe water accumulation: general edema of the body and extremities, dysuria, oliguria, and dyspnea.

CLINICAL APPLICATIONS

Nephrosclerosis, chronic nephritis, edema secondary to nephritis, edema and dyspnea secondary to congestive heart failure, beriberi, dysuria and ascites.

EXPLANATION

Dao Shui Fu Ling Tang (Poria Decoction to Drain Water) treats severe fluid accumulation affecting both urination and breathing. With fluid accumulation, patients often experience pitting edema, dysuria, and oliguria. This kind of edema in which the tissue shows prolonged pits produced by pressure is commonly described as "rotten melon." Dysuria and oliguria are characterized by sharp, cutting pain with very little volume of urine. Because the Lung regulates the water passages, excess water retention will affect its normal functions. The patient will experience wheezing and dyspnea, especially at night and when lying in a horizontal position.

To effectively treat this condition, this formula has herbs that dispel stagnant water from the body. *Chi Fu Ling* (Poria Rubra) and *Ze Xie* (Rhizoma Alismatis) are diuretic herbs that eliminate water accumulation through diuresis. *Chi Fu Ling* (Poria Rubra) and *Bai Zhu* (Rhizoma Atractylodis Macrocephalae) strengthen the Spleen and dry dampness. *Mu Gua* (Fructus Chaenomelis) dispels dampness from the lower body, and is especially effective in treating beriberi. *Bing Lang* (Semen Arecae) eliminates water and disperses stagnant qi in the chest. *Mai Dong* (Radix Ophiopogonis) nourishes the Lung, suppresses cough, and eliminates phlegm. *Zi Su Ye* (Folium Perillae) directs qi downward and relieves chest fullness. *Deng Xin Cao* (Medulla Junci) promotes normal urination and eliminates dampness and swelling. *Chen Pi* (Pericarpium Citri Reticulatae), *Mu Xiang* (Radix Aucklandiae), and *Sha Ren* (Fructus Amomi) regulate qi and reduce qi stagnation. *Sang Bai Pi* (Cortex Mori) regulates Lung qi to relieve wheezing and dyspnea. *Da Fu Pi* (Pericarpium Arecae) regulates water circulation and treats edema and abdominal fullness and distention.

DAMP-DISPELLING FORMULAS

16

1129

Chapter 16 – Damp-Dispelling Formulas　　　　*Section 3 – Water-Regulating and Damp-Resolving Formulas*

Dǎo Shǔi Fú Líng Tāng (Poria Decoction to Drain Water)

Dao Shui Fu Ling Tang (Poria Decoction to Drain Water)

Diagnosis	Signs and Symptoms	Treatment	Herbs
Severe water accumulation	• Pitting edema: severe water accumulation • Dysuria and oliguria with pain: water accumulation affecting urination • Wheezing and dyspnea: water accumulation affecting the Lung	• Dispels stagnant water and dries dampness • Eliminates water from the Lung	• *Chi Fu Ling* (Poria Rubra) and *Ze Xie* (Rhizoma Alismatis) eliminate water accumulation through diuresis. • *Chi Fu Ling* (Poria Rubra) and *Bai Zhu* (Rhizoma Atractylodis Macrocephalae) strengthen the Spleen and dry dampness. • *Mu Gua* (Fructus Chaenomelis) dispels dampness from the lower body. • *Bing Lang* (Semen Arecae) eliminates water and disperses stagnant qi in the chest. • *Mai Dong* (Radix Ophiopogonis) nourishes the Lung, suppresses cough, and eliminates phlegm. • *Zi Su Ye* (Folium Perillae) guides qi downward and relieves chest fullness. • *Deng Xin Cao* (Medulla Junci) promotes normal urination and eliminates dampness and swelling. • *Chen Pi* (Pericarpium Citri Reticulatae), *Mu Xiang* (Radix Aucklandiae), and *Sha Ren* (Fructus Amomi) regulate qi and reduce qi stagnation. • *Sang Bai Pi* (Cortex Mori) regulates Lung qi to relieve wheezing and dyspnea. • *Da Fu Pi* (Pericarpium Arecae) regulates water circulation and treats edema and abdominal fullness and distention.

MODIFICATIONS

• With oliguria, add *Mu Tong* (Caulis Akebiae), *Che Qian Zi* (Semen Plantaginis), and *Di Huang* (Radix Rehmanniae).

• With cough, dyspnea, and chest fullness, add *Hou Po* (Cortex Magnoliae Officinalis) and *Ku Xing Ren* (Semen Armeniacae Amarum).

1130

Chinese Herbal Formulas and Applications

Section 4

温化水湿剂
— Warm Formulas that Dissolve Dampness

Líng Guì Zhú Gān Tāng
(Poria, Cinnamon Twig, Atractylodes Macrocephala, and Licorice Decoction)

苓桂术甘湯
苓桂术甘汤

Pinyin Name: *Ling Gui Zhu Gan Tang*
Literal Name: Poria, Cinnamon Twig, Atractylodes Macrocephala, and Licorice Decoction
Alternate Names: *Fu Ling Gui Zhi Bai Zhu Gan Cao Tang, Ling Kuei Shu Kan Tang, Ling Gui Shu Gan Tang,* Hoelen, Cinnamon Twig, Atractylodes and Licorice Decoction; Poria, Cinnamon, Bighead Atractylodes and Licorice Decoction; Hoelen and Atractylodes Combination
Original Source: *Jin Gui Yao Lue* (Essentials from the Golden Cabinet) by Zhang Zhong-Jing in the Eastern Han Dynasty

COMPOSITION

Fu Ling (Poria)	12g
Gui Zhi (Ramulus Cinnamomi)	9g
Bai Zhu (Rhizoma Atractylodis Macrocephalae)	6g
Zhi Gan Cao (Radix et Rhizoma Glycyrrhizae Praeparata cum Melle)	6g

DOSAGE / PREPARATION / ADMINISTRATION

The source text instructions are to cook the ingredients with 6 cups [1,200 mL] of water until the liquid is reduced to 3 cups [600 mL]. Take the warm, strained decoction in three equally-divided doses.

CHINESE THERAPEUTIC ACTIONS

1. Warms and dissolves *tan yin* (phlegm retention)
2. Strengthens the Spleen and dispels dampness

CLINICAL MANIFESTATIONS

Tan yin (phlegm retention) syndrome caused by yang deficiency of the middle *jiao*: chest and hypochondriac fullness, dizziness, vertigo, palpitations, shortness of breath, coughing, white, slippery tongue coating, and a wiry, slippery pulse.

CLINICAL APPLICATIONS

Coronary artery disease, cardiac failure, Meniere's syndrome, motor dysfunction, dizziness and vertigo, nephrotic syndrome, chronic nephritis, hydronephrosis, edema, neurosis, anxiety, hysteria, polyhydramnios, Keshan disease, chronic bronchitis, and chronic gastritis.

EXPLANATION

According to the source text, *Ling Gui Zhu Gan Tang* (Poria, Cinnamon Twig, Atractylodes Macrocephala, and Licorice Decoction) was originally used to treat individuals who developed yang deficiency in the middle *jiao* after being incorrectly treated with emetic or downward draining methods for an exterior syndrome. As yang becomes deficient, the Spleen loses its ability to transform and transport food, resulting in water and dampness turning into *tan yin* (phlegm retention). If this phlegm becomes stagnated in the chest, fullness of the chest and epigastrium occurs. If the phlegm blocks the passage of the ascending yang qi, dizziness and vertigo occur. If it affects the Lung and disrupts the circulation of qi, coughing and shortness of breath occur. If it affects the circulation of qi around the Heart, palpitations occur.

In this formula, *Fu Ling* (Poria) acts as the chief herb to strengthen the Spleen, dispel dampness, and disperse

DAMP-DISPELLING FORMULAS

16

1131

Chapter 16 – Damp-Dispelling Formulas　　　　　　　　*Section 4 – Warm Formulas that Dissolve Dampness*

Líng Guì Zhú Gān Tāng
(Poria, Cinnamon Twig, Atractylodes Macrocephala, and Licorice Decoction)

Ling Gui Zhu Gan Tang (Poria, Cinnamon Twig, Atractylodes Macrocephala, and Licorice Decoction)

Diagnosis	Signs and Symptoms	Treatment	Herbs
Tan yin (phlegm retention) syndrome with yang deficiency of the middle *jiao*	• Chest and hypochondriac fullness: phlegm accumulation in the chest • Dizziness and vertigo: yang qi unable to ascend • Palpitations: phlegm accumulation affecting the Heart • Shortness of breath and coughing: phlegm accumulation affecting the Lung • White, slippery tongue coating and a wiry, slippery pulse: damp accumulation	• Warms and dissolves *tan yin* (phlegm retention) • Strengthens the Spleen and dispels dampness	• *Fu Ling* (Poria) strengthens the Spleen, dispels dampness, and disperses phlegm. • *Gui Zhi* (Ramulus Cinnamomi) disperses accumulated fluids and warms the body to dissolve phlegm. • *Bai Zhu* (Rhizoma Atractylodis Macrocephalae) strengthens the Spleen and dries dampness. • *Zhi Gan Cao* (Radix et Rhizoma Glycyrrhizae Praeparata cum Melle) tonifies the qi and harmonizes the herbs.

phlegm. *Gui Zhi* (Ramulus Cinnamomi) disperses accumulated fluids and warms the body to dissolve phlegm. *Bai Zhu* (Rhizoma Atractylodis Macrocephalae) strengthens the Spleen and dries dampness. *Zhi Gan Cao* (Radix et Rhizoma Glycyrrhizae Praeparata cum Melle) tonifies the qi and harmonizes the herbs.

MODIFICATIONS

• With nausea or vomiting from profuse phlegm accumulation, add *Er Chen Tang* (Two-Cured Decoction).

• With abdominal pain due to deficiency and cold, combine with *Li Zhong Tang* (Regulate the Middle Decoction).

• With diarrhea caused by Spleen qi deficiency and damp accumulation, add *Ping Wei San* (Calm the Stomach Powder).

• With generalized weakness and fatigue, combine with *Xiao Jian Zhong Tang* (Minor Construct the Middle Decoction).

• With epigastric distention or gurgling water sounds in the abdomen, add *Zhi Shi* (Fructus Aurantii Immaturus).

• With cough with profuse sputum, add *Ban Xia* (Rhizoma Pinelliae) and *Chen Pi* (Pericarpium Citri Reticulatae).

• With edema of the limbs and decreased urination, add *Zhu Ling* (Polyporus) and *Ze Xie* (Rhizoma Alismatis).

CAUTIONS / CONTRAINDICATIONS

Ling Gui Zhu Gan Tang contains many warm and drying herbs which may consume or injure body fluids. Therefore, it is contraindicated in cases of yin and/or body fluid deficiencies.

PHARMACOLOGICAL EFFECTS

1. **Cardiovascular**: Administration of *Ling Gui Zhu Gan Tang* via intraperitoneal injection at 20 mL/kg in mice was effective in preventing irregular heartbeat and increasing resistance against ischemia.[1]

2. **Sedative and hypnotic**: Administration of *Ling Gui Zhu Gan Tang* was associated with a sedative and hypnotic effect. It prolonged sleeping time induced by barbiturates and reduced spontaneous activities in mice.[2]

CLINICAL STUDIES AND RESEARCH

1. **Coronary artery disease**: Use of modified *Ling Gui Zhu Gan Tang* in 16 patients with coronary artery disease and angina was associated with marked improvement in 10 cases, moderate improvement in 5 cases, and no effect in 1 case.[3]

2. **Meniere's syndrome**: Use of *Ling Gui Zhu Gan Tang* plus *Ze Xie* (Rhizoma Alismatis) and *Zhe Shi* (Haematitum) in 53 patients with Meniere's syndrome was associated with significant recovery in 32 cases, improvement in 17 cases, and no effect in 4 cases (92.5% effectiveness).[4] According to another study, 72 patients with Meniere's syndrome were treated successfully using *Ling Gui Zhu Gan Tang* plus *Ze Xie* (Rhizoma Alismatis), *Dan Shen* (Radix et Rhizoma Salviae Miltiorrhizae), *Yuan Zhi* (Radix Polygalae), *Ge Gen* (Radix Puerariae Lobatae), and others as needed. Injection of dexamethasone into the tympanic cavity was given as an adjunct therapy.[5]

3. **Cardiac failure**: Ninety-six patients who were unresponsive to digitalis after long-term use or intolerant because of side effects were treated with *Ling Gui Zhu Gan Tang* plus *Sheng Mai San* (Generate the Pulse Powder) or *Zhi Gan Cao Tang* (Honey-Fried Licorice Decoction) with good results. Of 96 patients, the study reported significant improvement in 39 cases, moderate improvement in 36 cases, and no effect in 21 cases. The overall effectiveness was 77%.[6]

1132

Líng Guì Zhú Gān Tāng

(Poria, Cinnamon Twig, Atractylodes Macrocephala, and Licorice Decoction)

4. **Dizziness and vertigo**: Use of *Ling Gui Zhu Gan Tang* plus *Xiao Chai Hu Tang* (Minor Bupleurum Decoction) in 60 patients with dizziness and vertigo was associated with complete recovery in 52 cases, improvement in 6 cases, and no effect in 2 cases (96.7% effectiveness).[7]

5. **Nephrotic syndrome**: One study reported good results using both herbs and drugs to treat 17 patients with severe nephrotic syndrome. The herbal treatment contained *Ling Gui Zhu Gan Tang* plus *Yi Mu Cao* (Herba Leonuri), *Qian Shi* (Semen Euryales), *Ze Xie* (Rhizoma Alismatis), *Bai Mao Gen* (Rhizoma Imperatae), and others as needed. Hormonal drug treatment was given as needed. After 3 months of treatment, the study reported complete remission in 9 cases, near-complete remission in 5 cases, partial remission in 2 cases, and no effect in 1 case.[8]

6. **Hydronephrosis**: Use of modified *Ling Gui Zhu Gan Tang* in 33 patients with hydronephrosis was associated with significant improvement in 21 cases, moderate improvement in 9 cases, and no effect in 3 cases. Additions to the original formula included *Chuan Lian Zi* (Fructus Toosendan) and *Chi Shao* (Radix Paeoniae Rubra) for low back pain; *Shi Wei* (Folium Pyrrosiae) for painful urination; *Bai Mao Gen* (Rhizoma Imperatae) and *Hu Po* (Succinum) for hematuria; and *Ban Xia* (Rhizoma Pinelliae) for nausea and vomiting.[9]

7. **Polyhydramnios**: Thirty-two patients with acute excess amniotic fluids were treated with modified *Ling Gui Zhu Gan Tang*, with complete recovery in 22 cases, improvement in 7 cases, and no effect in 3 cases.[10]

8. **Keshan disease**: One study reported satisfactory results using modified *Ling Gui Zhu Gan Tang* to treat 16 patients with cardiomyopathy associated with selenium deficiency. The herbal formula contained *Ling Gui Zhu Gan Tang* plus *Yin Chen* (Herba Artemisiae Scopariae) and *Shan Zha* (Fructus Crataegi). Clinical improvements included relief of edema and swelling after 2 weeks, and increased force of heart contraction after one month.[11]

References

1. *Bei Jing Zhong Yi Xue Yuan Xue Bao* (Journal of Beijing University School of Medicine) 1990;13(4):47.
2. *Guo Wai Yi Xue Zhong Yi Zhong Yao Fen Ce* (Monograph of Chinese Herbology from Foreign Medicine) 1987;9(20):40.
3. *Zhong Yi Han Shou Tong Xun* (Reports of Chinese Medicine) 1992;2:41.
4. *Guang Dong Yi Xue* (Guangdong Medicine) 1993;3:151.
5. *Shi Yong Zhong Xi Yi Jie He Za Zhi* (Practical Journal of Integrated Chinese and Western Medicines) 1993;7:434.
6. *Tian Jin Yi Yao Za Zhi* (Journal of Tianjin Medicine and Herbology) 1967;8:503.
7. *Nei Meng Gu Zhong Yi Yao* (Traditional Chinese Medicine and Medicinals of Inner Mongolia) 1994;2:5.
8. *Shan Xi Zhong Yi* (Shanxi Chinese Medicine) 1987;2:70.
9. *Shi Yong Zhong Yi Yao Za Zhi* (Journal of Practical Chinese Medicine and Medicinals) 1999;6:11.
10. *Shang Hai Zhong Yi Yao Za Zhi* (Shanghai Journal of Chinese Medicine and Herbology) 1993;11:22.
11. *Zhong Yi Ming Fang Lin Chuang Xin Yong* (Contemporary Clinical Applications of Classic Chinese Formulas) 2001;447.

Gān Cǎo Gān Jiāng Fú Líng Bái Zhú Tāng

(Licorice, Ginger, Poria, and Atractylodes Macrocephala Decoction)

甘草乾姜茯苓白术湯
甘草干姜茯苓白术汤

Pinyin Name: *Gan Cao Gan Jiang Fu Ling Bai Zhu Tang*
Literal Name: Licorice, Ginger, Poria, and Atractylodes Macrocephala Decoction
Alternate Names: *Shen Chu Tang, Shen Zhu Tang, Shen Zhuo Tang*, Kidney Fixity Decoction
Original Source: *Jin Gui Yao Lue* (Essentials from the Golden Cabinet) by Zhang Zhong-Jing in the Eastern Han Dynasty

COMPOSITION

Gan Jiang (Rhizoma Zingiberis)	12g
Bai Zhu (Rhizoma Atractylodis Macrocephalae)	6g
Gan Cao (Radix et Rhizoma Glycyrrhizae)	6g
Fu Ling (Poria)	12g

Chapter 16 – Damp-Dispelling Formulas   *Section 4 – Warm Formulas that Dissolve Dampness*

Gān Cǎo Gān Jiāng Fú Líng Bái Zhú Tāng
(Licorice, Ginger, Poria, and Atractylodes Macrocephala Decoction)

DOSAGE / PREPARATION / ADMINISTRATION

The source text instructs to cook the ingredients with 5 cups [1,000 mL] of water until the liquid is reduced to 3 cups [600 mL]. Take the warm, strained decoction in three equally-divided doses. Today, it is normally prepared as a decoction.

CHINESE THERAPEUTIC ACTIONS

1. Warms yang and strengthens the Spleen
2. Dispels cold and dampness

CLINICAL MANIFESTATION

Cold and dampness in the lower body: coldness and pain of the lower back and body, feeling of extreme heavy sensation in the lower back, normal appetite and diet, absence of thirst, and normal urination.

CLINICAL APPLICATIONS

Low back pain, sciatica, lumbago, enuresis, superficial gastritis, duodenal ulcer, arthritis, impotence, gastritis, atrophic gastritis, and diarrhea.

EXPLANATION

Gan Cao Gan Jiang Fu Ling Bai Zhu Tang (Licorice, Ginger, Poria and Atractylodes Macrocephala Decoction) is often used for patients with cold and dampness in the lower half of the body, characterized by low back pain, extremely weak back, and cold sensations in the lower back. Because cold and dampness only affect the muscles, and not the interior *zang fu* organs, urination and diet are both normal.

Gan Jiang (Rhizoma Zingiberis), being acrid and warm, is used at a high dose to warm the Kidney and dispel cold fixed in the lower back. *Bai Zhu* (Rhizoma Atractylodis Macrocephalae) and *Gan Cao* (Radix et Rhizoma

Glycyrrhizae) strengthen the middle *jiao* and resolve dampness. *Fu Ling* (Poria), in addition to strengthening the middle *jiao*, also eliminates dampness through urination. In short, this formula focuses on both the Kidney and Spleen to address cold and dampness fixed in the lower body.

MODIFICATIONS

With severe pain, add *Fu Zi* (Radix Aconiti Lateralis Praeparata) and *Xi Xin* (Radix et Rhizoma Asari).

AUTHORS' COMMENTS

Because this formula treats cold and dampness located in the lower back around the kidney area, it is also known as 肾著汤 *Shen Zhuo Tang* (Kidney Fixity Decoction). It is important to note that this formula treats cold and dampness affecting the muscles near the kidney area. It does **not** address Kidney imbalance nor treat kidney diseases.

Ling Gui Zhu Gan Tang (Poria, Cinnamon Twig, Atractylodes Macrocephala, and Licorice Decoction) and *Gan Cao Gan Jiang Fu Ling Bai Zhu Tang* have similar ingredients and indications. They are both excellent formulas to strengthen the Spleen, warm yang, and dispel dampness.

- *Ling Gui Zhu Gan Tang* uses *Fu Ling* (Poria) as the chief herb and *Gui Zhi* (Ramulus Cinnamomi) as the deputy herb. The main emphasis of this formula is to warm yang and dispel dampness to resolve *tan yin* (phlegm retention).
- *Gan Cao Gan Jiang Fu Ling Bai Zhu Tang* uses *Gan Jiang* (Rhizoma Zingiberis) as the chief herb and *Fu Ling* (Poria) as the deputy herb. The main focus of this formula is to warm the middle *jiao*, dispel cold, and dispel dampness to treat cold and dampness in the lower back.

Gan Cao Gan Jiang Fu Ling Bai Zhu Tang (Licorice, Ginger, Poria and Atractylodes Macrocephala Decoction)

Diagnosis	Signs and Symptoms	Treatment	Herbs
Cold and dampness in the lower body	• Low back pain, extremely weak back, feeling of coldness and pain: cold accumulation • Heavy sensation in the lower back: damp accumulation	• Warms yang and strengthens the Spleen • Dispels cold and dampness	• *Gan Jiang* (Rhizoma Zingiberis) warms the Kidney and dispels cold fixed in the lower back. • *Bai Zhu* (Rhizoma Atractylodis Macrocephalae) and *Gan Cao* (Radix et Rhizoma Glycyrrhizae) strengthen the middle *jiao* and resolve dampness. • *Fu Ling* (Poria) strengthens the middle *jiao* and eliminates dampness through urination.

1134

Chinese Herbal Formulas and Applications

Zhēn Wŭ Tāng (True Warrior Decoction)

真武湯
真武汤

Pinyin Name: *Zhen Wu Tang*
Literal Name: True Warrior Decoction
Alternate Names: *Chen Wu Tang*, Ginger, Aconite, Hoelen and Peony Combination
Original Source: *Shang Han Lun* (Discussion of Cold-Induced Disorders) by Zhang Zhong-Jing in the Eastern Han Dynasty

COMPOSITION

Fu Zi (Radix Aconiti Lateralis Praeparata), *pao* (blast-fried)	1 piece [9g]
Fu Ling (Poria)	9g
Sheng Jiang (Rhizoma Zingiberis Recens)	9g
Bai Zhu (Rhizoma Atractylodis Macrocephalae)	6g
Bai Shao (Radix Paeoniae Alba)	9g

DOSAGE / PREPARATION / ADMINISTRATION

The source text instructs to cook the ingredients with 8 cups [1,600 mL] of water until the liquid is reduced to 3 cups [600 mL]. Take 0.7 cup [140 mL] of the warm, strained decoction three times daily.

CHINESE THERAPEUTIC ACTIONS

Warms yang and regulates water

CLINICAL MANIFESTATIONS

1. Spleen and Kidney yang deficiencies with water accumulation: urinary difficulty, heaviness and pain in the four limbs, abdominal pain, diarrhea, swelling and edema of the limbs, absence of thirst, white tongue coating, and a deep pulse.
2. *Taiyang* disorder: presence of exterior condition and fever unresolved after sweating, palpitations, vertigo and muscle twitching.

CLINICAL APPLICATIONS

Chronic renal failure, nephritis, chronic nephritis, edema, hypertension, amenorrhea, restless legs, rheumatoid arthritis, asthma, allergic sinusitis, Meniere's syndrome, leukorrhea, hypothyroidism, chronic enteritis, cardiac failure, arrhythmia, cough, cardiopulmonary diseases, insomnia, and dizziness.

EXPLANATION

Zhen Wu Tang (True Warrior Decoction) is the main formula for treating water accumulation caused by Spleen and Kidney yang deficiencies. The Spleen and Kidney are two very important organs involved in water metabolism. The Spleen is responsible for dispersing and distributing water, while the Kidney is responsible for eliminating water. If the yang of these two organs is deficient, the body cannot maintain normal water metabolism. If water and dampness accumulate in the body, they will overflow to the skin and muscles causing swelling, pain, and heavy

Zhen Wu Tang (True Warrior Decoction)

Diagnosis	Signs and Symptoms	Treatment	Herbs
Spleen and Kidney yang deficiencies with water accumulation	• Urinary difficulty: stagnant water circulation • Heaviness and pain and/or swelling and edema in the limbs: accumulation of damp and water • Abdominal pain, loose stools or diarrhea: Spleen and Kidney yang deficiencies • White tongue coating and a deep pulse: damp and cold condition	• Warms the yang and regulates water	• *Fu Zi* (Radix Aconiti Lateralis Praeparata) warms Spleen and Kidney yang. • *Fu Ling* (Poria) strengthens the Spleen, induces urination, and dispels water accumulation. • *Sheng Jiang* (Rhizoma Zingiberis Recens) warms the body, dispels cold, and disperses water accumulation. • *Bai Zhu* (Rhizoma Atractylodis Macrocephalae) strengthens the Spleen and dries dampness. • *Bai Shao* (Radix Paeoniae Alba) relieves pain, and balances and prevents the warm herbs from injuring yin.

DAMP-DISPELLING FORMULAS

16

1135

Chapter 16 – Damp-Dispelling Formulas   *Section 4 – Warm Formulas that Dissolve Dampness*

Zhēn Wŭ Tāng (True Warrior Decoction)

sensations in the limbs. If water and dampness block the normal rising of yang qi, vertigo will manifest. If water and dampness travel downward, loose stools or diarrhea may occur. Since the water circulation is stagnant, urinary difficulty also manifests.

Fu Zi (Radix Aconiti Lateralis Praeparata), the chief herb in this formula, warms the Spleen and Kidney to raise the yang. *Fu Ling* (Poria), the deputy herb, strengthens the Spleen, induces urination, and dispels water accumulation. *Sheng Jiang* (Rhizoma Zingiberis Recens) has two main functions: it helps *Fu Zi* (Radix Aconiti Lateralis Praeparata) warm the body to dispel cold, and it assists *Fu Ling* (Poria) to disperse and dispel water. *Bai Zhu* (Rhizoma Atractylodis Macrocephalae), the assistant herb, strengthens the Spleen and dries dampness to promote the Spleen's transformation functions. *Bai Shao* (Radix Paeoniae Alba), in addition to preventing the acrid, warm herbs in this formula from injuring yin, also relieves abdominal pain.

This formula may also be used to treat *taiyang* disorder where the exterior condition remains after sweating. As a result of sweating, yin and body fluids are both damaged, leading to palpitations, vertigo, and muscle twitching.

MODIFICATIONS

• Without urinary difficulty, remove *Fu Ling* (Poria) to prevent excessive loss of body fluids.
• With cough due to cold and water affecting the Lung, add *Gan Jiang* (Rhizoma Zingiberis), *Xi Xin* (Radix et Rhizoma Asari), and *Wu Wei Zi* (Fructus Schisandrae Chinensis).
• With severe edema, add *Wu Ling San* (Five-Ingredient Powder with Poria).
• For arthritis characterized by wind and dampness, add *Gui Zhi* (Ramulus Cinnamomi) and *Dang Shen* (Radix Codonopsis).
• With chronic and stubborn rashes and eczema, add *Ma Huang* (Herba Ephedrae), *Lian Qiao* (Fructus Forsythiae), and *Chi Xiao Dou* (Semen Phaseoli).
• With pain in the limbs, add *Ma Huang* (Herba Ephedrae) and *Xi Xin* (Radix et Rhizoma Asari).
• With diarrhea, remove *Bai Shao* (Radix Paeoniae Alba) and add *Gan Jiang* (Rhizoma Zingiberis).
• With vomiting, remove *Fu Zi* (Radix Aconiti Lateralis Praeparata) and add a large dose of *Sheng Jiang* (Rhizoma Zingiberis Recens).

CAUTIONS / CONTRAINDICATIONS

Zhen Wu Tang treats water accumulation caused by Spleen and Kidney yang deficiencies. Use of this formula is inappropriate if the water accumulation is caused only by excess condition.

PHARMACOLOGICAL EFFECTS

1. **Circulatory**: Administration of this formula for 22 days was associated with decreased resistance of blood flow, reduced blood viscosity, increased blood perfusion to internal organs, and decreased workload for the heart.[1]
2. **Nephroprotective**: Administration of *Zhen Wu Tang* was associated with beneficial effects in rats with chronic renal failure.[2] In one study of 18 patients with compromised renal functions, use of modified *Zhen Wu Tang* was associated with a reduction of IgA, IgG, IgM, and TF in the urine.[3]

CLINICAL STUDIES AND RESEARCH

1. **Cardiac failure**: Administration of modified *Zhen Wu Tang* has been shown to have a beneficial effect in treating cardiac failure. One study used *Zhen Wu Tang* plus *Wu Jia Pi* (Cortex Acanthopanacis), *Dan Shen* (Radix et Rhizoma Salviae Miltiorrhizae), and *Yi Mu Cao* (Herba Leonuri) as the base formula for treating heart failure.[4] Another study used *Zhen Wu Tang* plus *Tao Ren* (Semen Persicae) and *Hong Hua* (Flos Carthami) as the base formula to treat cardiopulmonary disorder with heart failure.[5]
2. **Hypertension**: One study reported 93% effectiveness using *Zhen Wu Tang* with *Fang Ji Fu Ling Tang* (Stephania and Poria Decoction) to treat 63 patients with hypertension characterized by yang deficiency.[6]
3. **Nephritis**: One study reported 80% effectiveness using modified *Zhen Wu Tang* to treat 30 patients with nephritis with edema. The study reported increased urination after an average of 17 days, and relief of edema after an average of 57 days.[7]
4. **Chronic renal failure**: *Zhen Wu Tang* has been reported in several studies to have beneficial effects in treating chronic renal failure. According to one study, use of modified *Zhen Wu Tang* in 12 patients with chronic renal failure was associated with remission in 3 cases, marked improvement in 5 cases, moderate improvement in 2 cases, and no effect in 2 cases.[8] In another study, use of modified *Zhen Wu Tang* was associated with 94.4% success in treating chronic renal disorder characterized by Kidney yang deficiency. Of 18 patients, the study reported remission of all symptoms in 8 cases, partial remission of symptoms in 9 cases, and no effect in 1 case.[9]
5. **Amenorrhea**: One study reported successful treatment of amenorrhea characterized by Kidney yang deficiency in 54 of 60 patients using modified *Zhen Wu Tang*.[10]

1136

Chinese Herbal Formulas and Applications

Zhēn Wŭ Tāng (True Warrior Decoction)

6. Restless legs: One study reported 90% success using modified *Zhen Wu Tang* to treat 25 patients with restless leg syndrome. Clinical presentations include unilateral or bilateral spasms and cramps of legs with feelings of soreness, numbness, swelling, and mild aches and pains.[11]

7. Asthma: Use of modified *Zhen Wu Tang* in 286 patients with bronchial asthma was associated with complete recovery in 92 cases, significant improvement in 134 cases, moderate improvement in 36 cases, and no effect in 24 cases.[12]

8. Allergic sinusitis: One study reported good results using modified *Zhen Wu Tang* to treat allergic sinusitis. In addition to the base formula, modifications included the addition of *Dang Shen* (Radix Codonopsis) and *Huang Qi* (Radix Astragali) for qi deficiency; and *Cang Er Zi* (Fructus Xanthii) and *Xin Yi Hua* (Flos Magnoliae) for nasal obstruction. Of 50 patients, the study reported complete recovery in 13 cases, significant improvement in 36 cases, and slight improvement in 1 case.[13]

9. Meniere's syndrome: *Zhen Wu Tang* has been shown to effectively treat dizziness and vertigo in many studies. According to one study of 42 patients with Meniere's syndrome, use of herbs was associated with complete recovery in 40 cases and improvement in 2 cases. In addition to *Zhen Wu Tang*, *Wu Zhu Yu* (Fructus Evodiae) and *Ban Xia* (Rhizoma Pinelliae) were added for frequent nausea and vomiting; *Ci Shi* (Magnetitum) for tinnitus; and *Long Gu* (Os Draconis) for Liver wind rising.[14]

RELATED FORMULA

Fù Zĭ Tāng (Prepared Aconite Decoction)

附子湯
附子汤

Pinyin Name: *Fu Zi Tang*

Literal Name: Prepared Aconite Decoction

Original Source: *Shang Han Lun* (Discussion of Cold-Induced Disorders) by Zhang Zhong-Jing in the Eastern Han Dynasty

Fu Zi (Radix Aconiti Lateralis Praeparata), pao (blast-fried)	2 pieces [12-18g]
Fu Ling (Poria)	9g
Ren Shen (Radix et Rhizoma Ginseng)	6g
Bai Zhu (Rhizoma Atractylodis Macrocephalae)	12g
Bai Shao (Radix Paeoniae Alba)	9g

The source text instructs to cook the ingredients with 8 cups [1,600 mL] of water until the liquid is reduced to 3 cups [600 mL]. Take 1 cup [200 mL] of the warm, strained decoction three times daily.

The main functions of this formula are to warm the channels, tonify yang, dispel cold, and resolve dampness. This formula is often used to relieve muscle aches and joint pain caused by yang deficiency accompanied by damp-cold invading the body. Clinically, the patient may show muscle aches, joint pain, cold limbs, aversion to cold, white, slippery tongue coating, and a deep, faint pulse.

Zhen Wu Tang and *Fu Zi Tang* (Prepared Aconite Decoction) both warm yang to dispel cold and dampness.

- *Zhen Wu Tang* contains *Sheng Jiang* (Rhizoma Zingiberis Recens), and is more suitable for relieving edema and water accumulation caused by yang deficiency.

- *Fu Zi Tang* contains *Ren Shen* (Radix et Rhizoma Ginseng) and larger doses of *Fu Zi* (Radix Aconiti Lateralis Praeparata) and *Bai Zhu* (Rhizoma Atractylodis Macrocephalae). Therefore, this formula is more suitable for treating joint and muscle pain caused by yang deficiency accompanied by cold and dampness in the body.

AUTHORS' COMMENTS

Zhen Wu Tang is one of the best formulas for treating edema or excess water retention due to Spleen and Kidney yang deficiencies. It effectively treats edema associated with hypothyroidism since the underlying cause of a low-functioning thyroid is Kidney yang deficiency. In addition to the signs and symptoms listed above, the patients often show cold hands and feet, aversion to cold, absence of thirst, white tongue coating, and a deep, slow or a deep, weak pulse.

References

1. *Zhong Xi Yi Jie He Za Zhi* (Journal of Integrated Chinese and Western Medicine) 1988;8(8):457.
2. *Zhong Guo Yi Yao Bao* (Chinese Journal of Medicine and Medicinals) 1991;6(4):46.
3. *Zhong Yi Fang Ji Xian Dai Yan Jiu* (Modern Study of Medical Formulae in Traditional Chinese Medicine) 1997;1453.
4. *Shi Yong Zhong Xi Yi Jie He Za Zhi* (Practical Journal of Integrated Chinese and Western Medicines) 1995;7:443.
5. *Zhong Ji Yi Kan* (Medium Medical Journal) 1990;3:30.
6. *Shan Xi Zhong Yi* (Shanxi Chinese Medicine) 1983;2:6.
7. *Zhong Yi Za Zhi* (Journal of Chinese Medicine) 1981;11:835
8. *Zhong Guo Zhong Yi Yao Xue Bao* (Chinese Journal of Chinese Medicine and Herbology) 1991;4:10.
9. *Zhong Yi Ming Fang Lin Chuang Xin Yong* (Contemporary Clinical Applications of Classic Chinese Formulas) 2001;4:46.
10. *Liao Ning Zhong Yi Za Zhi* (Liaoning Journal of Chinese Medicine) 1982;2:46.
11. *Shi Yong Zhong Yi Nei Ke Za Zhi* (Journal of Practical Chinese Internal Medicine) 1992;2:91.
12. *Si Chuan Zhong Yi* (Sichuan Chinese Medicine) 1992;11:34.
13. *Hei Long Jiang Zhong Yi Yao* (Heilongjiang Chinese Medicine and Herbology) 1992;3:34.
14. *Shan Xi Zhong Yi* (Shanxi Chinese Medicine) 1994;15(3):105.

DAMP-DISPELLING FORMULAS

16

1137

Chapter 16 – Damp-Dispelling Formulas　　　　　　　*Section 4 – Warm Formulas that Dissolve Dampness*

Shi Pi Săn (Bolster the Spleen Powder)

實脾散
实脾散

Pinyin Name: *Shi Pi San*
Literal Name: Bolster the Spleen Powder
Original Source: *Chong Ding Ji Sheng Fang* (Revised Formulas to Aid the Living)

COMPOSITION

Fu Zi (Radix Aconiti Lateralis Praeparata), *pao* (blast-fried)	30g [6g]
Gan Jiang (Rhizoma Zingiberis), *pao* (blast-fried)	30g [6g]
Fu Ling (Poria)	30g [6g]
Bai Zhu (Rhizoma Atractylodis Macrocephalae)	30g [6g]
Mu Gua (Fructus Chaenomelis)	30g [6g]
Hou Po (Cortex Magnoliae Officinalis), *chao* (dry-fried) with ginger	30g [6g]
Mu Xiang (Radix Aucklandiae), do not expose to heat	30g [6g]
Bing Lang (Semen Arecae)	30g [6g]
Cao Guo (Fructus Tsaoko)	30g [6g]
Zhi Gan Cao (Radix et Rhizoma Glycyrrhizae Praeparata cum Melle)	15g [3g]

DOSAGE / PREPARATION / ADMINISTRATION

The source text instructs to grind the ingredients into a coarse powder. Cook 12g of the powder with 5 slices of *Sheng Jiang* (Rhizoma Zingiberis Recens) and 1 piece of *Da Zao* (Fructus Jujubae) in 1.5 bowls of water until the liquid is reduced to 70% volume. Take the warm, strained decoction any time during the day. Today, this formula may be prepared as a decoction with the doses suggested in brackets.

CHINESE THERAPEUTIC ACTIONS

1. Warms yang and strengthens the Spleen
2. Activates qi and promotes water circulation

CLINICAL MANIFESTATIONS

Yin shui (yin edema) due to Spleen and Kidney yang deficiencies: severe edema in the lower half of the body, cold hands and feet, absence of thirst, chest and abdominal fullness and distention, loose stools, thick, greasy tongue coating, and a deep, slow pulse.

CLINICAL APPLICATIONS

Edema, hydramnios, chronic nephritis, and early stage liver cirrhosis and ascites.

EXPLANATION

Shi Pi San (Bolster the Spleen Powder) is commonly used to treat *yin shui* (yin edema) due to Spleen and Kidney yang deficiencies. According to traditional Chinese medicine theory, the Spleen transforms and transports water. If Spleen yang becomes deficient and cannot carry

out its normal functions, water and dampness accumulates, leading to edema in the lower limbs. Accumulation of water and dampness will affect qi circulation, leading to chest and abdominal fullness and distention. Moreover, the deficient Spleen yang will not be able to warm the body, causing cold hands and feet. Loose stools reflect Spleen and Kidney yang deficiencies and failure of yang to disperse the water upward. A thick, greasy tongue coating also indicates damp accumulation. A deep, slow pulse also indicates Spleen and Kidney yang deficiencies.

This formula has *Fu Zi* (Radix Aconiti Lateralis Praeparata) and *Gan Jiang* (Rhizoma Zingiberis) to warm Spleen and Kidney yang, activate water circulation and relieve edema. *Fu Ling* (Poria) and *Bai Zhu* (Rhizoma Atractylodis Macrocephalae) tonify the Spleen and dispel dampness via urination. *Mu Gua* (Fructus Chaenomelis) awakens the Spleen, dissolves dampness and eliminates water accumulation. *Hou Po* (Cortex Magnoliae Officinalis), *Mu Xiang* (Radix Aucklandiae), *Bing Lang* (Semen Arecae), and *Cao Guo* (Fructus Tsaoko) activate qi, regulate water circulation, and dissolve dampness. *Zhi Gan Cao* (Radix et Rhizoma Glycyrrhizae Praeparata cum Melle), *Sheng Jiang* (Rhizoma Zingiberis Recens), and *Da Zao* (Fructus Jujubae) tonify the Spleen and harmonize the herbs in this formula.

MODIFICATIONS

- With dysuria and severe edema, add *Zhu Ling* (Polyporus) and *Ze Xie* (Rhizoma Alismatis).
- With loose stools, add *Da Fu Pi* (Pericarpium Arecae).

1138

Chinese Herbal Formulas and Applications

Shi Pi San (Bolster the Spleen Powder)

Shi Pi San (Bolster the Spleen Powder)

Diagnosis	Signs and Symptoms	Treatment	Herbs
Yin shui (yin edema) due to Spleen and Kidney yang deficiencies	• Severe edema in the lower half of the body: yang deficiency unable to regulate water circulation • Loose stools: yang deficiency unable to disperse the water upward • Cold hands and feet: yang deficiency unable to warm the extremities • Thick greasy tongue coating: damp accumulation • Deep, slow pulse: Spleen and Kidney yang deficiencies	• Warms yang and strengthens the Spleen • Activates qi and promotes water circulation	• *Fu Zi* (Radix Aconiti Lateralis Praeparata) and *Gan Jiang* (Rhizoma Zingiberis) warm Spleen and Kidney yang. • *Fu Ling* (Poria) and *Bai Zhu* (Rhizoma Atractylodis Macrocephalae) tonify the Spleen and dispel dampness. • *Mu Gua* (Fructus Chaenomelis) awakens the Spleen, dissolves dampness and eliminates water accumulation. • *Hou Po* (Cortex Magnoliae Officinalis), *Mu Xiang* (Radix Aucklandiae), *Bing Lang* (Semen Arecae), and *Cao Guo* (Fructus Tsaoko) activate qi, regulate water circulation, and dissolve dampness. • *Zhi Gan Cao* (Radix et Rhizoma Glycyrrhizae Praeparata cum Melle), *Sheng Jiang* (Rhizoma Zingiberis Recens), and *Da Zao* (Fructus Jujubae) tonify the Spleen and harmonize the herbs.

• With lethargy due to qi deficiency, add *Dang Shen* (Radix Codonopsis), *Bai Zhu* (Rhizoma Atractylodis Macrocephalae), and *Huang Qi* (Radix Astragali).
• With severe swelling and edema, and decreased urinary output, add *Zhu Ling* (Polyporus) and *Ze Xie* (Rhizoma Alismatis).

CAUTIONS / CONTRAINDICATIONS

Shi Pi San treats edema due to deficiency. It is inappropriate for edema characterized by an excess condition.

CLINICAL STUDIES AND RESEARCH

Hydramnios: Use of *Shi Pi San* was associated with 93% effectiveness in treating hydramnios. Of 18 patients, the study reported complete recovery in 16 cases and no effect in 2 cases.[1]

AUTHORS' COMMENTS

Because the main emphasis of *Shi Pi San* is to strengthen the Spleen to activate qi and regulate water metabolism, it is named as "Bolster the Spleen Powder."

Zhen Wu Tang (True Warrior Decoction) and *Shi Pi San* have similar functions and compositions. Both formulas contain herbs that warm Spleen and Kidney yang to facilitate water circulation and elimination.
• *Zhen Wu Tang* is used primarily to treat water accumulation due to Kidney yang deficiency, with symptoms such as abdominal pain and swelling of the lower limbs.
• *Shi Pi San* is used mainly to treat water accumulation due to Spleen yang deficiency, with symptoms such as chest and abdominal fullness.

Reference
1. *Si Chuan Zhong Yi* (Sichuan Chinese Medicine) 1995;7:36.

DAMP-DISPELLING FORMULAS

16

1139

Chapter 16 – Damp-Dispelling Formulas   *Section 4 – Warm Formulas that Dissolve Dampness*

Bì Xiè Fēn Qīng Yǐn
(Dioscorea Hypoglauca Decoction to Separate the Clear)

萆薢分清飲
萆薢分清饮

Pinyin Name: *Bi Xie Fen Qing Yin*
Literal Name: Dioscorea Hypoglauca Decoction to Separate the Clear
Alternate Names: *Pi Hsieh Fen Ching Yin, Bi Xie Fen Ching Yin, Bie Xie Fen Qing Yin, Bei Xie Fen Qing Yin*, Tokoro Turbidity-Clearing Drink, Tokoro Combination
Original Source: *Dan Xi Xin Fa* (Teachings of [Zhu] Dan-Xi) by Zhu Zhen-Heng in 1481

COMPOSITION

Fen Bi Xie (Rhizoma Dioscoreae Hypoglaucae)	[9g]
Yi Zhi (Fructus Alpiniae Oxyphyllae)	[9g]
Wu Yao (Radix Linderae)	[9g]
Shi Chang Pu (Rhizoma Acori Tatarinowii)	[9g]

DOSAGE / PREPARATION / ADMINISTRATION

The source text instructs to grind the ingredients into a coarse powder and cook 15g in water with a pinch of salt. Take the warm, strained decoction before meals. Today, this formula may be prepared as a decoction with the doses suggested in brackets.

CHINESE THERAPEUTIC ACTIONS

1. Warms Kidney yang
2. Resolves dampness and dispels turbidity

CLINICAL MANIFESTATIONS

Deficiency and cold of the lower *jiao*: frequent urination with white, thick, turbid, and cloudy urine.

CLINICAL APPLICATIONS

Dysuria, galacturia, urethritis, cystitis, nephrotic syndrome, chronic pyelonephritis, chronic pelvic inflammatory disease, prostatitis, and impotence.

EXPLANATION

Bi Xie Fen Qing Yin (Dioscorea Hypoglauca Decoction to Separate the Clear) treats urinary disorders caused by deficiency and cold of the lower *jiao* accompanied by accumulation of dampness and turbidity. The Kidney is responsible for recycling fluids. When Kidney yang is deficient, the Kidney is unable to lift pure fluids to regulate urination, and frequent urination occurs. Because of accumulation of dampness and turbidity, the urine becomes white, thick, turbid, and cloudy.

This formula contains *Fen Bi Xie* (Rhizoma Dioscoreae Hypoglaucae) to resolve dampness and dispel turbidity. It is one of the most effective herbs to treat *gao lin* (cloudy dysuria) with white cloudy urine. *Yi Zhi* (Fructus Alpiniae Oxyphyllae) warms Kidney yang and binds the Kidney to stop frequent urination. *Wu Yao* (Radix Linderae) warms the Kidney and Urinary Bladder to relieve frequent urination. *Shi Chang Pu* (Rhizoma Acori Tatarinowii)

Bi Xie Fen Qing Yin (Dioscorea Hypoglauca Decoction to Separate the Clear)

Diagnosis	Signs and Symptoms	Treatment	Herbs
Deficiency and cold of the lower *jiao*	• Frequent urination: Kidney yang deficiency • White, thick, turbid, and cloudy urine: accumulation of dampness and turbidity	• Warms Kidney yang • Resolves dampness and turbidity	• *Fen Bi Xie* (Rhizoma Dioscoreae Hypoglaucae) dispels dampness and turbidity. • *Yi Zhi* (Fructus Alpiniae Oxyphyllae) warms Kidney yang and binds the Kidney to stop frequent urination. • *Wu Yao* (Radix Linderae) warms the Kidney and Urinary Bladder to relieve frequent urination. • *Shi Chang Pu* (Rhizoma Acori Tatarinowii) warms the Urinary Bladder and dispels deficiency and cold of the lower *jiao*.

1140

Chinese Herbal Formulas and Applications

Bì Xiè Fēn Qīng Yǐn
(Dioscorea Hypoglauca Decoction to Separate the Clear)

warms the Urinary Bladder and dispels deficiency and cold of the lower *jiao*. Finally, salt acts as an envoy to lead the herbs to the Kidney in the lower *jiao*.

MODIFICATIONS

- With more severe condition of white and turbid urine, add *Shan Yao* (Rhizoma Dioscoreae) and *Qian Shi* (Semen Euryales).
- With burning sensation during urination, add *Mu Tong* (Caulis Akebiae) and *Di Huang* (Radix Rehmanniae).
- With painful urination, add *Che Qian Zi* (Semen Plantaginis) and *Zhi Zi* (Fructus Gardeniae).
- With frequent urination, add *Yuan Zhi* (Radix Polygalae) and *Fu Shen* (Poria Paradicis).
- With abdominal pain caused by deficiency and cold, add *Rou Gui* (Cortex Cinnamomi) and *Xiao Hui Xiang* (Fructus Foeniculi).
- With lethargy and low back soreness, add *Ren Shen* (Radix et Rhizoma Ginseng) and *Lu Jiao Jiao* (Colla Cornus Cervi).
- With qi deficiency due to the chronic nature of this condition, add *Huang Qi* (Radix Astragali) and *Bai Zhu* (Rhizoma Atractylodis Macrocephalae).
- With profuse, white or clear vaginal discharge, add *Shan Yao* (Rhizoma Dioscoreae), *Bai Zhu* (Rhizoma Atractylodis Macrocephalae), *Fu Zi* (Radix Aconiti Lateralis Praeparata), and *Tu Si Zi* (Semen Cuscutae).

CAUTIONS / CONTRAINDICATIONS

Bi Xie Fen Qing Yin is contraindicated in patients with damp-heat in the Urinary Bladder characterized by frequent, painful urination, or burning sensation during urination.

CLINICAL STUDIES AND RESEARCH

1. *Lin zheng* (dysuria syndrome): One study of 62 males (between 21-50 years of age) with *lin zheng* (dysuria syndrome) reported 90.3% effectiveness when treated with 15 packs of *Bi Xie Fen Qing Yin*.[1]
2. **Galacturia**: Thirty-two patients with galacturia were treated with 96.9% rate of recovery using *Bi Xie Fen Qing Yin* plus *Ku Shen* (Radix Sophorae Flavescentis), *Gou Ji* (Rhizoma Cibotii), and *Tu Fu Ling* (Rhizoma Smilacis Glabrae). The duration of treatment varied between 6-18 packs of herbs.[2]
3. **Urethritis**: One study reported satisfactory results in 45 of 53 patients using *Bi Xie Fen Qing Yin* to treat non-bacterial urethritis.[3]
4. **Impotence**: Use of *Bi Xie Fen Qing Yin* was effective in treating impotence associated with prostatitis. In addition

to this formula, modifications were made by adding *Zhi Zi* (Fructus Gardeniae) and *Bai Hua She She Cao* (Herba Hedyotis) for urinary frequency, urgency, and pain; *Du Zhong* (Cortex Eucommiae) and *Chuan Niu Xi* (Radix Cyathulae) for low back soreness and pain; *Qian Shi* (Semen Euryales), *Tu Si Zi* (Semen Cuscutae), and *Wu Wei Zi* (Fructus Schisandrae Chinensis) for premature ejaculation; and *Shi Xian Tao* (Pseudobulbus Pholidotae Chinensis) for spermatorrhea or seminal emission. Of 108 patients, the study reported complete recovery in 21 cases, significant improvement in 32 cases, moderate improvement in 20 cases, and no effect in 35 cases.[4]

5. **Prostatitis**: One study reported good results using modified *Bi Xie Fen Qing Yin* to treat 46 patients with prostatitis. Modifications to this formula included the addition of *Bai Jiang Cao* (Herba cum Radice Patriniae), *Chi Xiao Dou* (Semen Phaseoli), and *Bian Xu* (Herba Polygoni Avicularis) for damp-heat; *Yin Yang Huo* (Herba Epimedii), *Shan Yao* (Rhizoma Dioscoreae), and *Rou Gui* (Cortex Cinnamomi) for Spleen and Kidney deficiencies; and *Tao Ren* (Semen Persicae), *Mo Yao* (Myrrha), and *Chi Shao* (Radix Paeoniae Rubra) for qi and blood stagnation. Of the 46 patients, the study reported recovery in 30 cases, improvement in 14 cases, and no effect in 2 cases. The overall effectiveness was 95.6%.[5]

RELATED FORMULA

Bì Xiè Fēn Qīng Yǐn

(Dioscorea Hypoglauca Decoction to Separate the Clear)

萆薢分清飲
萆薢分清饮

Pinyin Name: Bi Xie Fen Qing Yin
Literal Name: Dioscorea Hypoglauca Decoction to Separate the Clear
Original Source: *Yi Fang Ji Jie* (Analytical Collection of Medical Formulas) by Wang Ang in 1682

Yi Zhi (Fructus Alpiniae Oxyphyllae)	[9g]
Wu Yao (Radix Linderae)	[9g]
Fen Bi Xie (Rhizoma Dioscoreae Hypoglaucae)	[9g]
Shi Chang Pu (Rhizoma Acori Tatarinowii)	[9g]
Gan Cao (Radix et Rhizoma Glycyrrhizae)	[4.5g]
Fu Ling (Poria)	[4.5g]

This formula dispels dampness, promotes urination, and benefits qi. It is used to treat *gao lin* (cloudy dysuria) due to deficiency of *yuan* (source) *qi* and accumulation of dampness and turbidity in the lower *jiao*. Clinical manifestations include frequent urination with urine that appears white, cloudy and thick.

DAMP-DISPELLING FORMULAS

16

1141

Chapter 16 – Damp-Dispelling Formulas   *Section 4 – Warm Formulas that Dissolve Dampness*

Bì Xiè Fēn Qīng Yǐn
(Dioscorea Hypoglauca Decoction to Separate the Clear)

Bì Xiè Fēn Qīng Yǐn
(Dioscorea Hypoglauca Decoction to Separate the Clear)
草薢分清飲
草薢分清饮
Pinyin Name: *Bi Xie Fen Qing Yin*
Literal Name: Dioscorea Hypoglauca Decoction to Separate the Clear
Original Source: *Yi Xue Xin Wu* (Medical Revelations) by Cheng Guo-Peng in 1732

Fen Bi Xie (Rhizoma Dioscoreae Hypoglaucae)	6g [9g]
Huang Bo (Cortex Phellodendri Chinensis), *chao* (dry-fried) to brown	1.5g [3g]
Shi Chang Pu (Rhizoma Acori Tatarinowii)	1.5g [3g]
Fu Ling (Poria)	3g [6g]
Bai Zhu (Rhizoma Atractylodis Macrocephalae)	3g [6g]
Lian Zi Xin (Plumula Nelumbinis)	2.1g [4g]
Dan Shen (Radix et Rhizoma Salviae Miltiorrhizae)	4.5g [9g]
Che Qian Zi (Semen Plantaginis)	4.5g [9g]

The source text instructs to prepare the ingredients as a decoction. Today, the decoction may be prepared using with the doses suggested in brackets.

This formula clears heat, resolves dampness, separates the clear, and dissolves turbidity. It is generally used to treat damp-heat attacking the Urinary Bladder with white, cloudy urine and a yellow, greasy tongue coating. It may also be used to treat *gao lin* (cloudy dysuria).

AUTHORS' COMMENTS
Historically, *Bi Xie Fen Qing Yin* was used for patients whose urine resembles rice water. When the urine cools, it hardens into a thick paste or rice-like glue. Today,

this formula may be used for patients with proteinuria manifesting in turbid urine.

These three formulas have identical Chinese characters and pinyin names. They all contain *Fen Bi Xie* (Rhizoma Dioscoreae Hypoglaucae) and *Shi Chang Pu* (Rhizoma Acori Tatarinowii) to treat white, cloudy urine characterized by dampness and turbidity. Each has a slightly different composition and function, however.

- *Bi Xie Fen Qing Yin* from *Dan Xi Xin Fa* (Teachings of [Zhu] Dan-Xi) is a warmer formula, containing such herbs as *Wu Yao* (Radix Linderae) and *Yi Zhi* (Fructus Alpiniae Oxyphyllae). It is more effective for treating white, cloudy urine caused by deficiency and cold in the lower *jiao*.

- *Bi Xie Fen Qing Yin* from *Yi Fang Ji Jie* (Analytical Collection of Medical Formulas) is also a warm formula. In addition to *Wu Yao* (Radix Linderae) and *Yi Zhi* (Fructus Alpiniae Oxyphyllae), it also contains *Gan Cao* (Radix et Rhizoma Glycyrrhizae) and *Fu Ling* (Poria), to further enhance the effects to tonify qi and resolve dampness.

- *Bi Xie Fen Qing Yin* from *Yi Xue Xin Wu* (Medical Revelations) is a cooler formula, with *Huang Bo* (Cortex Phellodendri Chinensis) and *Che Qian Zi* (Semen Plantaginis). It is more appropriate for white, cloudy urine caused by damp-heat affecting the lower *jiao*.

References
1. *Ji Lin Zhong Yi* (Jilin Chinese Medicine) 1990;2:16.
2. *Shan Xi Zhong Yi* (Shanxi Chinese Medicine) 1994;6:273.
3. *Xin Zhong Yi* (New Chinese Medicine) 1995;7:43.
4. *Gui Yang Zhong Yi Xue Yuan Xue Bao* (Journal of Guiyang Chinese Medical University) 1996;4:62.
5. *Jiang Su Zhong Yi* (Jiangsu Chinese Medicine) 1997;12:20.

Chinese Herbal Formulas and Applications

Chapter 16 — Summary

— Damp-Dispelling Formulas

SECTION 1: DAMP-DRYING AND STOMACH-HARMONIZING FORMULAS

Name	Similarities	Differences
Ping Wei San (Calm the Stomach Powder)	Dry dampness, strengthen the Spleen and Stomach	Base formula that dries dampness in the middle *jiao*
Jia Wei Ping Wei San (Modified Calm the Stomach Powder)		Stronger effect to promote digestion and activate qi and blood circulation
Xiang Sha Ping Wei San (Cyperus and Amomum Powder to Calm the Stomach)		Stronger effect to activate qi circulation and unblock qi stagnation
Bu Huan Jin Zheng Qi San (Rectify the Qi Powder Worth More than Gold)		Stronger effect to dispel dampness and regulate qi
Fu Ling Yin (Poria Decoction)		Dispels dampness and phlegm
Huo Xiang Zheng Qi San (Agastache Powder to Rectify the Qi)	Dispel interior dampness, relieve acute onset of nausea and vomiting	Releases exterior wind-cold
Liu He Tang (Harmonize the Six Decoction)		Strengthens the Spleen and Stomach, harmonizes the middle *jiao*
Ge Hua Jie Cheng San (Pueraria Flower Powder for Detoxification and Awakening)		Treats over-indulgence and intoxication of alcohol

Ping Wei San (Calm the Stomach Powder) dries dampness, strengthens the Spleen, activates qi circulation, and harmonizes the Stomach. This is the main formula for treating accumulation of dampness in the Spleen and Stomach. The main clinical manifestations include epigastric and abdominal fullness and distention, and a white, thick, greasy tongue coating.

Jia Wei Ping Wei San (Modified Calm the Stomach Powder), *Xiang Sha Ping Wei San* (Cyperus and Amomum Powder to Calm the Stomach), and *Bu Huan Jin Zheng Qi San* (Rectify the Qi Powder Worth More than Gold) are all modifications of *Ping Wei San* (Calm the Stomach Powder). These three formulas have similar functions to dry dampness, strengthen the Spleen and Stomach, activate qi and blood circulation, and promote digestion. All have excellent functions to treat damp accumulation in the Spleen and Stomach with symptoms such as indigestion, abdominal pain, nausea, vomiting, and diarrhea.

• *Jia Wei Ping Wei San* has a slightly better effect to promote digestion and activate qi and blood circulation.
• *Xiang Sha Ping Wei San* has a stronger function to activate qi circulation and unblock qi stagnation.
• *Bu Huan Jin Zheng Qi San* has a stronger effect to dispel dampness and regulate qi.

Fu Ling Yin (Poria Decoction) strengthens the Spleen and Stomach, harmonizes the middle *jiao*, and dispels phlegm and dampness. It treats stomach disorders with excessive gas and bloating, no appetite, inability to eat due to excessive gas in the stomach, belching, nausea, and mild resistance in the epigastric region upon palpation.

Huo Xiang Zheng Qi San (Agastache Powder to Rectify the Qi), *Liu He Tang* (Harmonize the Six Decoction) and *Ge Hua Jie Cheng San* (Pueraria Flower Powder for Detoxification and Awakening) have similar functions of treating acute cases of dampness affecting the interior, with acute onset of nausea and vomiting.

DAMP-DISPELLING FORMULAS

16

1143

Chapter 16 – Damp-Dispelling Formulas

Chapter 16 — Summary

- *Huo Xiang Zheng Qi San* releases exterior wind-cold, dispels dampness, regulates qi, and harmonizes the middle *jiao*. It treats exterior wind-cold with interior dampness causing symptoms such as fever, chills, headache, fullness and oppression in the chest and diaphragm, vomiting, diarrhea, and epigastric or abdominal pain.
- *Liu He Tang* dissolves summer-dampness, strengthens the Spleen, and harmonizes the middle *jiao*. It mainly treats improper diet consumed during the summertime, leading to damp accumulation in the middle *jiao* affecting the normal transportation and transformation functions of the Spleen and Stomach. Clinical manifestations include chills, fever, headache, fullness and oppression in the chest and diaphragm, nausea, vomiting, borborygmus, and diarrhea.
- *Ge Hua Jie Cheng San* clears damp-heat and strengthens and harmonizes the Spleen and Stomach. It is most commonly used to prevent and treat alcohol intoxication.

SECTION 2: HEAT-CLEARING AND DAMP-DISPELLING FORMULAS

Name	Similarities	Differences
Yin Chen Hao Tang (Artemisia Scoparia Decoction)	Clear damp-heat, relieve jaundice	Principal formula for damp-heat jaundice
Yin Chen Wu Ling San (Artemisia Scoparia and Five-Ingredient Powder with Poria)		Relieves urinary difficulty
San Ren Tang (Three-Nut Decoction)	Clear damp-heat	Stronger effect to dispel dampness
Gan Lu Xiao Du Dan (Sweet Dew Special Pill to Eliminate Toxin)		Stronger effect to clear heat and eliminate toxins
Lian Po Yin (Coptis and Magnolia Bark Decoction)	Clear heat, dispel dampness, resolve turbidity	Harmonizes the Stomach and stops vomiting
Can Shi Tang (Silkworm Droppings Decoction)		Relieves spasms and cramps
Ba Zheng San (Eight-Herb Powder for Rectification)	Clear damp-heat in the lower *jiao*	Clears heat and sedates fire
Wu Lin San (Five-Ingredient Powder for Painful Urinary Dysfunction)		Clears heat and cools the blood

Yin Chen Hao Tang (Artemisia Scoparia Decoction) is the principal formula for treating jaundice caused by damp-heat. It clears heat, dissolves dampness, and relieves jaundice. Clinical manifestations include yellow discoloration of the skin and sclera, slight abdominal fullness, dysuria, thirst, yellow, greasy tongue coating, and a deep, rapid pulse.

Yin Chen Wu Ling San (Artemisia Scoparia and Five-Ingredient Powder with Poria) is formulated by adding *Yin Chen* (Herba Artemisiae Scopariae) to *Wu Ling San* (Five-Ingredient Powder with Poria). This formula treats damp-heat jaundice (more heat than dampness) with dysuria.

San Ren Tang (Three-Nut Decoction) and *Gan Lu Xiao Du Dan* (Sweet Dew Special Pill to Eliminate Toxin) have similar functions to treat warm-damp affecting the *qi* (energy) level.
- *San Ren Tang* has a stronger action to dispel dampness than to clear heat. It is mainly used in the beginning stage [*qi* (energy) level] of summer febrile syndrome with dampness being more predominant than heat. Clinical manifestations include headache, aversion to cold, heaviness and pain of the body, chest stuffiness, reduced appetite, and no thirst.
- *Gan Lu Xiao Du Dan* has more potent effects to dissolve dampness and turbidity, clear heat, and eliminate toxins. This formula treats damp-warmth febrile disorders or epidemic diseases in the beginning stage [*qi* (energy) level] with equal amounts of dampness and heat. Clinical manifestations include fever, lethargy, thirst, scanty, turbid urine, sore throat, yellow discoloration of the skin, chest stuffiness, vomiting, and diarrhea.

1144

Chinese Herbal Formulas and Applications

Chapter 16 — Summary

Lian Po Yin (Coptis and Magnolia Bark Decoction) and ***Can Shi Tang*** (Silkworm Droppings Decoction) both clear heat, dispel dampness, and resolve turbidity. Both can be used to treat sudden turmoil disorder with nausea and vomiting.

• *Lian Po Yin* is most effective in harmonizing the Stomach and stopping vomiting. It clears heat, dispels dampness, resolves turbidity, regulates qi, and harmonizes the middle *jiao*. It treats sudden turmoil disorder characterized by dampness and heat. Clinical manifestations include vomiting, diarrhea, fullness of the chest and hypochondrium, dark, scanty urine, and a yellow, greasy tongue coating.

• *Can Shi Tang* is best at relieving spasms and cramps. It clears heat, dispels dampness, and resolves turbidity. It has been used for sudden turmoil disorder characterized by dampness and heat. Clinical manifestations include abdominal pain, cramps, vomiting, diarrhea, thirst, irritability, and a thick, dry, yellow tongue coating.

Ba Zheng San (Eight-Herb Powder for Rectification) and ***Wu Lin San*** (Five-Ingredient Powder for Painful Urinary Dysfunction) are two formulas that clear damp-heat in the lower *jiao* to treat *lin zheng* (dysuria syndrome).

• *Ba Zheng San* clears heat, sedates fire, induces urination, and relieves *re lin* (heat dysuria). This is the main formula for *re lin* (heat dysuria) with damp-heat entangling in the lower *jiao*, causing symptoms of turbid and dark urine, painful urination, lower abdominal pain and distention, dry mouth and throat, scanty drips of urine, or anuria in severe cases.

• *Wu Lin San* clears heat, cools the blood, induces urination, and relieves *xue lin* (bloody dysuria). It is commonly used to treat heat in the Urinary Bladder leading to urinary difficulty, presence of blood in the urine, severe pain upon urination, and cloudy urine with a feeling of sandy particles in the urine.

SECTION 3: WATER-REGULATING AND DAMP-RESOLVING FORMULAS

Name	Similarities	Differences
Wu Ling San (Five-Ingredient Powder with Poria)	Regulate water circulation, dispel dampness	Warms yang, releases the exterior
Wei Ling Tang (Calm the Stomach and Poria Decoction)		Harmonizes the Stomach
Zhu Ling Tang (Polyporus Decoction)		Clears heat, nourishes yin
Fang Ji Huang Qi Tang (Stephania and Astragalus Decoction)	Regulates water circulation, releases exterior wind	Strengthens the Spleen, tonifies *wei* (defensive) *qi*
Wu Pi San (Five-Peel Powder)	Regulates water circulation, reduces edema	Strengthens the Spleen, regulates qi circulation
Jiu Wei Bing Lang Jia Wu Fu Tang (Areca Nine Decoction plus Evodia and Poria)	Regulate water circulation, eliminate water accumulation	Disperses qi and blood stagnation, treats water accumulation in the legs
Mu Fang Ji Tang (Cocculus Decoction)		Lowers abnormal rising of yin and fluids, treats water accumulation in the upper *jiao*
Fen Xiao Tang (Separate and Reduce Decoction)		Strengthens the Spleen, treats water accumulation in the abdomen and lower legs
Dao Shui Fu Ling Tang (Poria Decoction to Drain Water)		Strongly drains water accumulation, treats severe water accumulation throughout the body

DAMP-DISPELLING FORMULAS

16

1145

Chapter 16 – Damp-Dispelling Formulas

Chapter 16 — Summary

Wu Ling San (Five-Ingredient Powder with Poria) dispels dampness through diuresis, warms yang, and disperses water fluids. It can be used for any of the following three diagnoses: exterior syndrome accompanied by accumulation of water and dampness in the interior (*taiyang fu* [hollow organ] syndrome), interior accumulation of water and dampness, and *tan yin* (phlegm retention).

Wei Ling Tang (Calm the Stomach and Poria Decoction) combines *Ping Wei San* (Calm the Stomach Powder) with *Wu Ling San* (Five-Ingredient Powder with Poria). It dispels dampness and harmonizes the Stomach to treat accumulation of water and dampness in the interior causing abdominal distention and edema.

Zhu Ling Tang (Polyporus Decoction) induces diuresis, clears heat, and nourishes yin. It is used for yin deficiency with interlocking of water and heat in the Urinary Bladder with symptoms such as dysuria, fever, thirst with a strong desire to drink, irritability, and insomnia. This formula can also be used for *xue lin* (bloody dysuria) with characteristics of extremely painful urination with blood, and fullness and pain in the lower abdomen.

Fang Ji Huang Qi Tang (Stephania and Astragalus Decoction) expels external wind pathogens, tonifies *wei* (defensive) *qi*, strengthens the Spleen, and dispels dampness through urination. It is used for *wei* (defensive) *qi* deficiency with accumulation of water and dampness. Clinical manifestations include perspiration, aversion to wind, heaviness of the body, and urinary difficulty.

Wu Pi San (Five-Peel Powder) is the principal formula used to treat edema of the whole body caused by Spleen deficiency and damp accumulation. This formula eliminates dampness and water, regulates qi, and strengthens the Spleen. Clinical manifestations include edema of the whole body, heaviness of the limbs, no aversion to wind, epigastric and abdominal fullness or distention, shortness of breath, rapid breathing, and dysuria.

Jiu Wei Bing Lang Jia Wu Fu Tang (Areca Nine Decoction plus Evodia and Poria) dispels water accumulation and disperses qi and blood stagnation. It primarily treats qi and blood stagnation accompanied by water accumulation in the legs (beriberi and pitting edema) and in the chest (congestive heart failure). Clinical manifestations include edema, numbness and weakness of the legs, fatigue, palpitations, and a feeling of distention beneath the heart.

Mu Fang Ji Tang (Cocculus Decoction) activates water circulation to eliminate stagnation, and guides abnormally rising qi downward. It may be used to treat accumulation of water in the upper *jiao* (e.g., congestive heart failure). Clinical manifestations include shortness of breath, increased dyspnea when lying down, abdominal pain, and fullness and distention in the epigastrium and chest.

Fen Xiao Tang (Separate and Reduce Decoction) strengthens the Spleen, activates qi circulation, and regulates water circulation. It is mainly used to treat Spleen deficiency accompanied by severe cases of water accumulation in the abdomen (ascites with drum-like distention in the abdomen) and lower legs (pitting edema with prolonged presence of pits produced by pressure).

Dao Shui Fu Ling Tang (Poria Decoction to Drain Water) dispels stagnant water, dries dampness, eliminates water from the Lung, and harmonizes the Spleen. It treats severe water accumulation, as seen in cases of nephritis, ascites, edema, congestive heart failure, and dysuria.

1146

Chinese Herbal Formulas and Applications

Chapter 16 — Summary

SECTION 4: WARM FORMULAS THAT DISSOLVE DAMPNESS

Name	Similarities	Differences
Ling Gui Zhu Gan Tang (Poria, Cinnamon Twig, Atractylodes Macrocephala, and Licorice Decoction)	Warm yang in the middle *jiao*, dispel dampness and phlegm	Warms yang, dispels dampness, resolves *tan yin* (phlegm retention)
Gan Cao Gan Jiang Fu Ling Bai Zhu Tang (Licorice, Ginger, Poria and Atractylodes Macrocephala Decoction)		Warms the middle *jiao* and dispels cold and dampness in the lower back
Zhen Wu Tang (True Warrior Decoction)	Invigorate the yang, regulate water circulation	Strongly tonifies Kidney yang
Shi Pi San (Bolster the Spleen Powder)		Strongly tonifies Spleen yang
Bi Xie Fen Qing Yin (Dioscorea Hypoglauca Decoction to Separate the Clear)	Dissolves dampness, clears turbidity	Warms and tonifies Kidney yang

Ling Gui Zhu Gan Tang (Poria, Cinnamon Twig, Atractylodes Macrocephala, and Licorice Decoction) is the main formula for treating *tan yin* (phlegm retention) syndrome. It invigorates yang to disperse phlegm retention, strengthens the Spleen, and dispels dampness. Main clinical manifestations include fullness of the chest and hypochondriac region, dizziness, shortness of breath, coughing, palpitations, and a white, slippery tongue coating.

Gan Cao Gan Jiang Fu Ling Bai Zhu Tang (Licorice, Ginger, Poria and Atractylodes Macrocephala Decoction) warms yang, strengthens the Spleen, and dispels cold and dampness. It mostly treats cold and dampness in the lower back (kidney area). Clinical manifestations include coldness and pain of the lower back and lower body, heavy sensations of the body, normal appetite and diet, absence of thirst, and normal urination.

Zhen Wu Tang (True Warrior Decoction) and ***Shi Pi San*** (Bolster the Spleen Powder) warm the Spleen and Kidney, invigorate yang qi, and regulate water circulation. Both formulas treat edema due to yang deficiency.
• *Zhen Wu Tang* is more effective at tonifying Kidney yang with water accumulation. It warms Spleen and Kidney yang to treat symptoms of heaviness and pain of the limbs, abdominal pain, diarrhea, edema of the limbs, urinary difficulty, no thirst, vertigo, white tongue coating, and a deep pulse.
• *Shi Pi San* is stronger at warming the Spleen and activating qi circulation. It is used for *yin shui* (yin edema), and chest and abdominal fullness and pain caused by Spleen yang deficiency.

Bi Xie Fen Qing Yin (Dioscorea Hypoglauca Decoction to Separate the Clear) warms Kidney yang, dissolves dampness, and clears turbidity. It is used for frequent urination, with white, thick, turbid and cloudy urine due to deficiency cold of the lower *jiao*.

DAMP-DISPELLING FORMULAS

16

1147

Chapter 17

— Wind-Damp Dispelling Formulas

祛风湿剂

孙思邈 Sún Sí-Miǎo

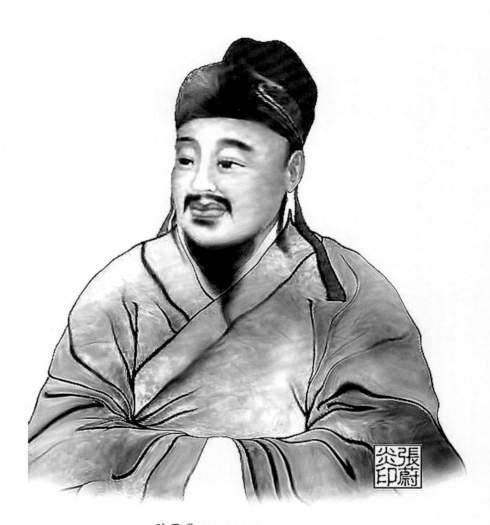

孙思邈 Sún Sí-Miǎo, 581 – 682.

孙思邈 Sún Sī-Miǎo

Born into a family mired in poverty and growing up as a chronically ill child, Sun Si-Miao realized the importance of health. He spent over 80 years of his life studying and practicing Traditional Chinese Medicine. Because Sun grew up as a peasant, he treated every patient equally, without regard for or inquiry into their background (whether they were royalty or peasants). Due to his own childhood illness, Sun strongly emphasized the importance of prevention, stating that "superior medicine **prevents** disease, and inferior medicine **treats** disease." Most importantly, Sun believed that every human life is worth more than a thousand pieces of gold, and expressed his dedication to this concept by incorporating it in naming all of his publications.

备急千金要方 *Bei Ji Qian Jin Yao Fang* (Thousands of Golden Prescriptions for Emergencies) is considered to be the first encyclopedia of Traditional Chinese Medicine. It addresses a wide variety of topics, such as internal and external medicine, gynecology, pediatrics, toxicology, diet, *tui-na*, pulse diagnosis, acupuncture, and more. Examples of his remedies include the use of oxen or sheep liver to treat night blindness, and sheep or deer thyroid glands and seaweed to treat goiter. 千金要方 *Qian Jin Yao Fang* (Thousand Ducat Prescriptions) and 千金翼方 *Qian Jin Yi Fang* (Supplement to the Thousand Ducat Formulas) elaborated upon and discussed in great detail all aspects of herbs and herbal formulas, including growing, harvesting, processing and storage of herbs and their uses in treatment. These two texts not only discussed herbal medicine in great detail, but offered great insights in acupuncture as well. Sun documented over 200 extraordinary points, including the discovery of *Shixuan* points and the naming of the *ah shi* point.[1] Sun strongly emphasized the importance of integrating acupuncture and herbs, and stated "[use of] acupuncture without herbs, or herbs without acupuncture, is not an act of a fine physician."

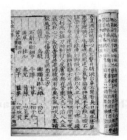

备急千金要方
Bei Ji Qian Jin Yao Fang (Thousands of Golden Prescriptions for Emergencies) in the middle of the 7th century.

Sun treated many patients in his lifetime, and was most famous for one incident, a story known as "opening the casket to revive the dead." According to legend, Sun encountered a funeral when he was traveling one day. As the family prepared to bury the deceased, Sun looked on and suddenly shouted: "Stop! Stop! This person may still be alive!" The family answered: "She is dead. Do not speak nonsense." Sun replied: "If she is really dead, her blood should clot. However, if you look carefully, there are drops of blood slowly seeping out from the casket. How can you be certain she is dead?" Upon inquiry with the husband, Sun found out that the presumed deceased was a middle-aged woman who was having a difficult labor trying to deliver her first child. Sun immediately lifted the casket lid to treat her with both acupuncture and herbs. After Sun inserted three needles, in *Renzhong* (GV 26), *Zhongwan* (CV 12) and *Zhongji* (CV 3), the woman promptly awakened. After taking an herbal decoction, she safely delivered a healthy baby.

Sun Si-Miao has made enormous contributions to all aspects of medicine and medicinal substances, and is remembered as 药王 the King of Medicine.

Exemplar formulas formulated Sun Si-Miao include:
- *Wei Rui Tang* (Polygonatum Odoratum Decoction)
- *Wen Pi Tang* (Warm the Spleen Decoction)
- *Dang Gui Jian Zhong Tang* (Tangkuei Decoction to Construct the Middle)
- *Ci Zhu Wan* (Magnetite and Cinnabar Pill)
- *Zhen Zhong Dan* (Pillow Special Pill)
- *Xiao Xu Ming Tang* (Minor Prolong Life Decoction)
- *Du Huo Ji Sheng Tang* (Angelica Pubescens and Taxillus Decoction)
- *Yan Tang Tan Tu Fang* (Salt Decoction to Induce Vomiting)
- *Wei Jing Tang* (Reed Decoction)

Dynasties & Kingdoms	Year
Xia Dynasty 夏	2100-1600 BCE
Shang Dynasty 商	1600-1100 BCE
Zhou Dynasty 周	1100-221 BCE
Qin Dynasty 秦	221-207 BCE
Han Dynasty 漢	206 BCE-220
Three Kingdoms 三國	220-280
Western Jin Dynasty 西晋	265-316
Eastern Jin Dynasty 東晋	317-420
Northern and Southern Dynasties 北南朝	420-581
Sui Dynasty 隋	**581-618**
Tang Dynasty 唐	618-907
Five Dynasties 五代	907-960
Song Dynasty 宋	960-1279
Liao Dynasty 遼	916-1125
Jin Dynasty 金	1115-1234
Yuan Dynasty 元	1271-1368
Ming Dynasty 明	1368-1644
Qing Dynasty 清	1644-1911
Republic of China 中華民國	1912-Present Day
People's Republic of China 中華人民共和國	1949-Present Day

---

1. When the practitioner palpates a point and the patient exclaims 'ah!' in pain, the "*ah shi* point" has been located.

Chapter 17 – Wind-Damp Dispelling Formulas

Table of Contents

Chapter 17. Wind-Damp Dispelling Formulas ⋯⋯⋯⋯ **1149**
Biography of Sun Si-Miao ⋯⋯⋯⋯⋯⋯⋯⋯⋯⋯⋯⋯⋯⋯⋯⋯ 1150

Section 1. Wind-Damp Dispelling Formulas ⋯⋯⋯⋯⋯⋯ **1156**
Qiang Huo Sheng Shi Tang (Notopterygium Decoction to Overcome Dampness) ⋯⋯⋯⋯ 1156
Juan Bi Tang (Remove Painful Obstruction Decoction) ⋯⋯⋯⋯⋯⋯⋯⋯⋯⋯⋯⋯⋯ 1158
  Jian Bi Tang (Remove Painful Obstruction in the Shoulders Decoction) ⋯⋯⋯⋯⋯ 1160
Du Huo Ji Sheng Tang (Angelica Pubescens and Taxillus Decoction) ⋯⋯⋯⋯⋯⋯⋯ 1161
  Yao Tong Fang Yi Hao (Low Back Pain Formula One) ⋯⋯⋯⋯⋯⋯⋯⋯⋯⋯⋯⋯ 1164
  Yao Tong Fang Er Hao (Low Back Pain Formula Two) ⋯⋯⋯⋯⋯⋯⋯⋯⋯⋯⋯⋯ 1164
  Xi Tong Fang Yi Hao (Knee Pain Formula One) ⋯⋯⋯⋯⋯⋯⋯⋯⋯⋯⋯⋯⋯⋯ 1165
  Xi Tong Fang Er Hao (Knee Pain Formula Two) ⋯⋯⋯⋯⋯⋯⋯⋯⋯⋯⋯⋯⋯⋯ 1165
  Ji Tong Tang (Spine Pain Decoction) ⋯⋯⋯⋯⋯⋯⋯⋯⋯⋯⋯⋯⋯⋯⋯⋯⋯⋯ 1165
San Bi Tang (Three-Painful Obstruction Decoction) ⋯⋯⋯⋯⋯⋯⋯⋯⋯⋯⋯⋯⋯⋯ 1167
Shu Jing Huo Xue Tang (Relax the Channels and Invigorate the Blood Decoction) ⋯⋯⋯ 1169
Shu Jin Li An San (Relax the Tendons and Instill Peace Powder) ⋯⋯⋯⋯⋯⋯⋯⋯⋯ 1171
Yi Yi Ren Tang (Coicis Decoction) ⋯⋯⋯⋯⋯⋯⋯⋯⋯⋯⋯⋯⋯⋯⋯⋯⋯⋯⋯⋯ 1173
Shang Zhong Xia Tong Yong Tong Feng Wan (Upper, Middle, and Lower General Use Pill for Wind-Pain) ⋯⋯⋯ 1175
  Tong Feng Wan (Wind-Pain Pill) ⋯⋯⋯⋯⋯⋯⋯⋯⋯⋯⋯⋯⋯⋯⋯⋯⋯⋯⋯⋯ 1176

Section 2. Damp-Cold Dispelling Formulas ⋯⋯⋯⋯⋯⋯ **1177**
Xiao Huo Luo Dan (Minor Invigorate the Collaterals Special Pill) ⋯⋯⋯⋯⋯⋯⋯⋯⋯ 1177
  Da Huo Luo Dan (Major Invigorate the Collaterals Special Pill) ⋯⋯⋯⋯⋯⋯⋯⋯ 1179
  Jia Wei Huo Luo Dan (Augmented Invigorate the Collaterals Special Pill) ⋯⋯⋯⋯ 1180
Da Fang Feng Tang (Major Saposhnikovia Decoction) ⋯⋯⋯⋯⋯⋯⋯⋯⋯⋯⋯⋯⋯ 1181
Ji Ming San (Powder to Take at Cock's Crow) ⋯⋯⋯⋯⋯⋯⋯⋯⋯⋯⋯⋯⋯⋯⋯⋯ 1183

Section 3. Damp-Heat Dispelling Formulas ⋯⋯⋯⋯⋯⋯ **1186**
Gui Zhi Shao Yao Zhi Mu Tang (Cinnamon Twig, Peony, and Anemarrhena Decoction) ⋯⋯ 1186
  Sang Zhi Shi Gao Zhi Mu Tang (Mulberry Twig, Gypsum, and Anemarrhena Decoction) ⋯⋯ 1187
Er Miao San (Two-Marvel Powder) ⋯⋯⋯⋯⋯⋯⋯⋯⋯⋯⋯⋯⋯⋯⋯⋯⋯⋯⋯⋯ 1188
  San Miao Wan (Three-Marvel Pill) ⋯⋯⋯⋯⋯⋯⋯⋯⋯⋯⋯⋯⋯⋯⋯⋯⋯⋯⋯ 1190
  Si Miao Wan (Four-Marvel Pill) ⋯⋯⋯⋯⋯⋯⋯⋯⋯⋯⋯⋯⋯⋯⋯⋯⋯⋯⋯⋯ 1190
Dang Gui Nian Tong Tang (Tangkuei Decoction to Lift the Pain) ⋯⋯⋯⋯⋯⋯⋯⋯⋯ 1191
  Nian Tong Tang (Lift the Pain Decoction) ⋯⋯⋯⋯⋯⋯⋯⋯⋯⋯⋯⋯⋯⋯⋯⋯⋯ 1193

Section 4. Damp-Phlegm Dispelling Formula ⋯⋯⋯⋯⋯ **1195**
Er Zhu Tang (Two-Atractylodes Decoction) ⋯⋯⋯⋯⋯⋯⋯⋯⋯⋯⋯⋯⋯⋯⋯⋯⋯ 1195

Wind-Damp Dispelling Formulas (Summary) ⋯⋯⋯⋯⋯⋯ **1197**

Chinese Herbal Formulas and Applications

Chapter 17 — Overview

— Wind-Damp Dispelling Formulas

Definition: Wind-damp dispelling formulas target exterior factors (wind-dampness, damp-heat, damp-cold, or damp-phlegm) that attack the superficial parts of the body, block the channels and collaterals, and cause swelling, inflammation, and pain. In addition to dispelling exterior factors, these formulas open the channels and collaterals, relax the tendons and ligaments, and relieve pain. Wind-damp disorders are characterized by symptoms such as headache, body aches, pain and numbness in the back and knees, and edema of the legs.

Wind-damp dispelling formulas are frequently used to treat *bi zheng* (painful obstruction syndrome), a condition characterized by stagnation and obstruction that may affect any tissue or organ, causing pain in the muscles, joints, tendons, or bones. In addition to affecting any part of the body, exterior wind-damp disorders may be complicated by cold or heat, leading to damp-cold or damp-heat disorders at the exterior. Since exterior wind-damp disorders are frequently associated with stagnation in the channels and collaterals, this condition should be treated by adding blood-activating herbs to wind-damp dispelling formulas. Chronic exterior wind-damp disorders may cause patients to become deficient; so adding qi-tonifying herbs to these formulas may be necessary in these situations. Furthermore, different types of *bi zheng* (painful obstruction syndrome) do not necessarily occur independently; rather, several types may occur together. Because there are multiple causes and complications, accurate diagnosis of *bi zheng* (painful obstruction syndrome) is essential to successful treatment.

- *Xing bi* (mobile painful obstruction) is caused by wind attacking the body. Like wind, which is light and mobile, *xing bi* (mobile painful obstruction) is characterized by pain in the upper body, and specifically, pain that travels from one area to another.
- *Tong bi* (extremely painful obstruction) is characterized by cold. Like cold, which is stationary and constricting, *tong bi* (extremely painful obstruction) is distinguished by severe pain at a fixed location. This type of pain intensifies with exposure to cold, and is relieved by exposure to warmth.
- *Zhuo bi* (fixed painful obstruction) often occurs when dampness affects specific, fixed areas. Like dampness, which is heavy and sinking, *zhuo bi* (fixed painful obstruction) is characterized by pain and swelling in the lower extremities.
- *Re bi* (heat painful obstruction) is characterized by local redness, swelling, burning, and pain. The heat results often from prolonged obstruction of the channels and collaterals by wind, cold, or dampness.
- *Wan bi* (stubborn painful obstruction) generally occurs after chronic or repetitive injuries to the same area, leading to stiffness, numbness, and reduced mobility.
- *Wei bi* (atrophic painful obstruction) is caused by Liver and Kidney deficiencies, characterized by atrophy, and by weakness and pain of the muscles and bones.
- *Xue bi* (blood painful obstruction) involves blood disorders, characterized by dull or sharp pain. Dull pain may be caused by deficiency of the blood needed to nourish the tendons and bones. Sharp pain, on the other hand, is often related to blood stagnation blocking the channels and collaterals.
- *Zhou bi* (generalized painful obstruction) is characterized by generalized pain in the bones and joints.

> **Wind-damp dispelling formulas are mainly used to treat *bi zheng* (painful obstruction syndrome) caused by exterior factors attacking the superficial parts of the body.**

WIND-DAMP DISPELLING FORMULAS

17

1153

Chapter 17 – Wind-Damp Dispelling Formulas

Chapter 17 — Overview

SUBCATEGORIES OF ACTION

Wind-damp disorders have multiple causes and complications. Therefore, wind-damp dispelling formulas are divided into four subcategories to delineate the nature of the disorders, and the characteristics of the formulas.

1. **Wind-Damp Dispelling Formulas**

   These formulas primarily dispel wind, cold, and dampness at the exterior causing symptoms such as headache, feelings of heaviness in the body, and pain in the extremities.

   Commonly used herbs that dispel wind-dampness include *Qiang Huo* (Rhizoma et Radix Notopterygii), *Du Huo* (Radix Angelicae Pubescentis), and *Fang Feng* (Radix Saposhnikoviae). Exemplar formulas are *Qiang Huo Sheng Shi Tang* (Notopterygium Decoction to Overcome Dampness) and *Du Huo Ji Sheng Tang* (Angelica Pubescens and Taxillus Decoction).

2. **Damp-Cold Dispelling Formulas**

   These formulas mainly warm yang and dispel cold and dampness from the exterior to treat *bi zheng* (painful obstruction syndrome) characterized by cold, dampness, and pain.

   Commonly used herbs include *Zhi Chuan Wu* (Radix Aconiti Praeparata), *Zhi Cao Wu* (Radix Aconiti Kusnezoffii Praeparata), *Fu Zi* (Radix Aconiti Lateralis Praeparata), *Gui Zhi* (Ramulus Cinnamomi), *Ma Huang* (Herba Ephedrae), *Cang Zhu* (Rhizoma Atractylodis), and *Bai Zhu* (Rhizoma Atractylodis Macrocephalae). Exemplar formulas include *Xiao Huo Luo Dan* (Minor Invigorate the Collaterals Special Pill) and *San Bi Tang* (Three-Painful Obstruction Decoction).

3. **Damp-Heat Dispelling Formulas**

   These formulas treat *bi zheng* (painful obstruction syndrome) characterized by heat and dampness, by clearing heat and dispelling dampness at external parts of the body.

   Commonly used herbs include *Cang Zhu* (Rhizoma Atractylodis), *Yi Yi Ren* (Semen Coicis), *Zhi Mu* (Rhizoma Anemarrhenae), and *Huang Bo* (Cortex Phellodendri Chinensis). Representative formulas include *Gui Zhi Shao Yao Zhi Mu Tang* (Cinnamon Twig, Peony, and Anemarrhena Decoction) and *Er Miao San* (Two-Marvel Powder).

4. **Damp-Phlegm Dispelling Formula**

   This formula dries dampness and eliminates phlegm obstructing the channels and collaterals. Commonly used herbs include *Cang Zhu* (Rhizoma Atractylodis), *Bai Zhu* (Rhizoma Atractylodis Macrocephalae), *Ban Xia* (Rhizoma Pinelliae), and *Tian Nan Xing* (Rhizoma Arisaematis). One exemplar formula is *Er Zhu Tang* (Two-Atractylodes Decoction).

CAUTIONS / CONTRAINDICATIONS

- Many wind-damp dispelling herbs and formulas are acrid, warm, and drying in nature, and may consume yin and blood. Therefore, they should be used with caution in patients with yin and/or blood deficiency.
- Wind-damp dispelling formulas are contraindicated in cases of Liver wind rising. Use of wind-damp dispelling formulas that are acrid, warm, and drying only exacerbates Liver wind conditions.
- Some herbs used in wind-damp dispelling formulas, such as *Zhi Chuan Wu* (Radix Aconiti Praeparata) and *Zhi Cao Wu* (Radix Aconiti Kusnezoffii Praeparata), are extremely hot and potentially toxic, and must be used with great caution to avoid unwanted or adverse effects.

~

Wind-damp dispelling formulas have remarkable analgesic and anti-inflammatory effects, and treat musculoskeletal disorders throughout the body.

~

PHARMACOLOGICAL EFFECTS & CLINICAL APPLICATIONS

Wind-damp dispelling formulas primarily treat musculoskeletal disorders. Pharmacologically, these formulas demonstrate remarkable analgesic and anti-inflammatory effects.[1,2,3] Clinical applications include presentations of swelling, inflammation, and pain at various locations throughout the body.

1154

Chinese Herbal Formulas and Applications

Chapter 17 — Overview

- **Arthritis**: Wind-damp dispelling formulas have been used successfully to treat many different types of arthritis, including, but not limited to osteoarthritis,[4] rheumatic arthritis,[5] gout,[6,7] periarthritis of the shoulders,[8] and many others.[9,10] Exemplar formulas include *Du Huo Ji Sheng Tang* (Angelica Pubescens and Taxillus Decoction), *Xiao Huo Luo Dan* (Minor Invigorate the Collaterals Special Pill), *Er Miao San* (Two-Marvel Powder), and *Juan Bi Tang* (Remove Painful Obstruction Decoction).

- **Neck pain**: According to clinical studies, neck pain can be treated effectively with *Qiang Huo Sheng Shi Tang* (Notopterygium Decoction to Overcome Dampness),[11] *Du Huo Ji Sheng Tang* (Angelica Pubescens and Taxillus Decoction),[12] and *Juan Bi Tang* (Remove Painful Obstruction Decoction).[13]

- **Sciatica**: *Du Huo Ji Sheng Tang* (Angelica Pubescens and Taxillus Decoction) and *Xiao Huo Luo Dan* (Minor Invigorate the Collaterals Special Pill) have been shown to successfully treat sciatica in several clinical studies.[14,15,16]

- **Neurodermatitis**: *Er Miao San* (Two-Marvel Powder) and *Dang Gui Nian Tong Tang* (Tangkuei Decoction to Lift the Pain) have been shown to effectively treat neurodermatitis.[17,18]

- **Musculoskeletal disorders**: Wind-damp dispelling formulas may also be used to treat other conditions characterized by swelling, inflammation, and pain. Clinical applications include hyperosteogeny,[19] prolapse of lumbar intervertebral disks,[20] ankylosing spondylitis,[21,22] and soft-tissue injuries.[23]

References

1. *Zhong Yi Fang Ji Xian Dai Yan Jiu* (Modern Study of Medical Formulae in Traditional Chinese Medicine) 1997;1466.
2. Lin CC, Chen MF, Chen CF. The anti-inflammatory effects of Chinese crude drug prescriptions on experimental arthritis. Am J Chin Med 1995;23(2):145-52.
3. *Zhong Guo Zhong Yao Za Zhi* (People's Republic of China Journal of Chinese Herbology) 1995;3:159.
4. *Ji Lin Zhong Yi Yao* (Jilin Chinese Medicine and Herbology) 1998;4:15.
5. *Si Chuan Zhong Yi* (Sichuan Chinese Medicine) 1996;14(10):38.
6. Chou CT, Kuo SC. The anti-inflammatory and anti-hyperuricemic effects of Chinese herbal formula danggui-nian-tong-tang on acute gouty arthritis: a comparative study with indomethacin and allopurinol. American Journal of Chinese Medicine 1995;23(3-4):261-71.
7. *Si Chuan Zhong Yi* (Sichuan Chinese Medicine) 1997;11:47.
8. *Yun Nan Zhong Yi Za Zhi* (Yunan Journal of Chinese Medicine) 1984;5(6):63.
9. *Hu Bei Zhong Yi Xue Yuan Xue Bao* (Journal of Hubei University of Medicine) 1993;2:56.
10. *Shi Yong Zhong Yi Nei Ke Za Zhi* (Journal of Practical Chinese Internal Medicine) 1997;2:36.
11. *Hu Nan Zhong Yi Za Zhi* (Hunan Journal of Chinese Medicine) 1997;2:13.
12. *An Hui Zhong Yi Xue Yuan Xue Bao* (Journal of Anhui University School of Medicine) 1995;14(1):37.
13. *Xin Zhong Yi* (New Chinese Medicine) 1994;26(10):51.
14. *Zhong Yi Han Shou Tong Xun* (Reports of Chinese Medicine) 1989;2:42.
15. *Shi Yong Zhong Yi Yao Za Zhi* (Journal of Practical Chinese Medicine and Medicinals) 1996;2:18.
16. *Nei Meng Gu Zhong Yi Yao* (Traditional Chinese Medicine and Medicinals of Inner Mongolia) 1992;3:24.
17. *Zhong Yuan Yi Kan* (Resource Journal of Chinese Medicine) 1990;4:12.
18. *Hu Nan Zhong Yi Za Zhi* (Hunan Journal of Chinese Medicine) 1992;8(4):42.
19. *Guang Xi Zhong Yi Yao* (Guangxi Chinese Medicine and Herbology) 1990;13(3):38.
20. *Yun Nan Zhong Yi Za Zhi* (Yunan Journal of Chinese Medicine) 1997;18(6):7.
21. *Shi Yong Zhong Yi Yao Za Zhi* (Journal of Practical Chinese Medicine and Medicinals) 1996;1:6.
22. *Xin Zhong Yi* (New Chinese Medicine) 1994;7:24.
23. *Hu Bei Zhong Yi Za Zhi* (Hubei Journal of Chinese Medicine) 1990;4:44.

WIND-DAMP DISPELLING FORMULAS

17

Chapter 17 – Wind-Damp Dispelling Formulas

Section 1 – Wind-Damp Dispelling Formulas

Section 1

祛风胜湿剂
— Wind-Damp Dispelling Formulas

Qiāng Huó Shèng Shī Tāng
(Notopterygium Decoction to Overcome Dampness)

羌活勝濕湯
羌活胜湿汤

Pinyin Name: *Qiang Huo Sheng Shi Tang*
Literal Name: Notopterygium Decoction to Overcome Dampness
Alternate Names: *Chiang Huo Sheng Shih Tang*, Chiang-huo Dampness-Overcoming Decoction, Notopterygium Damp-Expelling Decoction, Notopterygium and Tuhuo Combination
Original Source: *Nei Wai Shang Bian Huo Lun* (Clarifying Doubts about Injury from Internal and External Causes) by Li Gao in 1247

COMPOSITION

Qiang Huo (Rhizoma et Radix Notopterygii)	3g [6g]
Du Huo (Radix Angelicae Pubescentis)	3g [6g]
Fang Feng (Radix Saposhnikoviae)	1.5g [3g]
Gao Ben (Rhizoma et Radix Ligustici)	1.5g [3g]
Chuan Xiong (Rhizoma Chuanxiong)	1.5g [3g]
Man Jing Zi (Fructus Viticis)	0.9g [2g]
Zhi Gan Cao (Radix et Rhizoma Glycyrrhizae Praeparata cum Melle)	1.5g [3g]

DOSAGE / PREPARATION / ADMINISTRATION

The source text instructions are to grind the ingredients into a coarse powder, and cook it with 2 bowls of water until the liquid is reduced to 1 bowl. Take the hot strained decoction before meals on an empty stomach. Today, this formula may be prepared as a decoction with the doses suggested in brackets.

CHINESE THERAPEUTIC ACTIONS

Dispels wind and eliminates dampness

CLINICAL MANIFESTATIONS

Wind-dampness at the exterior: pain, stiffness and immobility of the shoulder and back, low back pain with difficulty of movement, heaviness of the body, headache, a white tongue coating, and a superficial pulse.

CLINICAL APPLICATIONS

Common cold, influenza, rhinitis, headache, cervical disorders, rheumatoid arthritis, and edema.

EXPLANATION

Qiang Huo Sheng Shi Tang (Notopterygium Decoction to Overcome Dampness) treats wind-dampness at the exterior affecting the muscles. This syndrome may occur when a patient is attacked by wind pathogen while sweating, or if the patient has lived in a damp and humid environment for a long period of time. The wind-damp factor may attack the *taiyang* channels and cause immobility and pain of the shoulders and back. Wind-dampness blocks the circulation and causes qi and blood stagnation, which, in turn, leads to headache, heaviness of the body, and low back pain.

This formula has *Qiang Huo* (Rhizoma et Radix Notopterygii) and *Du Huo* (Radix Angelicae Pubescentis) to dispel wind-dampness from both the upper and lower body, respectively. *Fang Feng* (Radix Saposhnikoviae) and *Gao Ben* (Rhizoma et Radix Ligustici) dispel wind-dampness from the *taiyang* channels and relieve the headache. *Chuan Xiong* (Rhizoma Chuanxiong) activates

1156

Chinese Herbal Formulas and Applications

Qiāng Huó Shèng Shī Tāng
(Notopterygium Decoction to Overcome Dampness)

Qiang Huo Sheng Shi Tang (Notopterygium Decoction to Overcome Dampness)

Diagnosis	Signs and Symptoms	Treatment	Herbs
Wind-dampness at the exterior	• Stiffness and pain in the shoulders and back: wind-damp factor attacking the *taiyang* channels • Headache, heaviness of the body, and low back pain: wind-dampness obstructing qi and blood circulation	Dispels wind and eliminates dampness	• *Qiang Huo* (Rhizoma et Radix Notopterygii) and *Du Huo* (Radix Angelicae Pubescentis) dispel wind-dampness from both the upper and lower body. • *Fang Feng* (Radix Saposhnikoviae) and *Gao Ben* (Rhizoma et Radix Ligustici) dispel wind-dampness from the *taiyang* channels and relieve the headache. • *Chuan Xiong* (Rhizoma Chuanxiong) activates blood circulation and relieves pain. • *Man Jing Zi* (Fructus Viticis) dispels wind and relieves pain. • *Zhi Gan Cao* (Radix et Rhizoma Glycyrrhizae Praeparata cum Melle) harmonizes the herbs.

blood circulation and relieves pain. *Man Jing Zi* (Fructus Viticis) dispels wind and relieves pain, especially headache. *Zhi Gan Cao* (Radix et Rhizoma Glycyrrhizae Praeparata cum Melle) harmonizes the herbs in the formula.

MODIFICATIONS
• For migraines, add *Chai Hu* (Radix Bupleuri) and *Huang Qin* (Radix Scutellariae).
• With stiffness and pain in the head and shoulders, add *Ge Gen* (Radix Puerariae Lobatae) and *Chi Shao* (Radix Paeoniae Rubra).
• With heavy sensations of the extremities and low back, add *Fang Ji* (Radix Stephaniae Tetrandrae) and *Fu Zi* (Radix Aconiti Lateralis Praeparata).
• With joint inflammation and pain, add *Cang Zhu* (Rhizoma Atractylodis), *Huang Bo* (Cortex Phellodendri Chinensis), and *Yi Yi Ren* (Semen Coicis).
• For arthritis, add *Chuan Xiong* (Rhizoma Chuanxiong), *Wei Ling Xian* (Radix et Rhizoma Clematidis), and *Wu Shao She* (Zaocys).

CAUTIONS / CONTRAINDICATIONS
• *Qiang Huo Sheng Shi Tang* contains exterior-releasing herbs to dispel wind-dampness from the exterior. While it is normal to experience mild sweating when taking this formula, profuse perspiration will damage both yin and yang and should be avoided.
• This formula is contraindicated for aches and pains due to *re bi* (heat painful obstruction), or in individuals with underlying yin deficiency.

PHARMACOLOGICAL EFFECTS
1. **Anti-inflammatory**: *Qiang Huo Sheng Shi Tang* given at doses

of 2.5 g/kg had marked effect to reduce inflammation.[1]
2. **Antipyretic**: Essential oils of *Qiang Huo Sheng Shi Tang* were shown to have antipyretic effects in mice.[2]

CLINICAL STUDIES AND RESEARCH
1. **Edema**: One study reported good results using *Qiang Huo Sheng Shi Tang* to treat edema, with modifications as follows: *Dang Shen* (Radix Codonopsis) and dry-fried *Bai Zhu* (Rhizoma Atractylodis Macrocephalae) for qi deficiency; *Fu Ling Pi* (Cortex Poria), *Ze Xie* (Rhizoma Alismatis), *Che Qian Zi* (Semen Plantaginis), and *Mu Tong* (Caulis Akebiae) for decreased volume and frequency of urination; *Gu Ya* (Fructus Setariae Germinatus), *Mai Ya* (Fructus Hordei Germinatus), dry-fried *Lai Fu Zi* (Semen Raphani), and *Shan Zha* (Fructus Crataegi) for food stagnation; and *Ba Ji Tian* (Radix Morindae Officinalis) and *Yin Yang Huo* (Herba Epimedii) for Kidney yang deficiency. Of 25 patients, urination was increased in all 25 cases within 2 packs of herbs. The edema was resolved in 4 cases within 6 packs of herbs, and in 6 cases within 10-15 packs.[3]

2. **Cervical disorders**: Use of *Qiang Huo Sheng Shi Tang* effectively treated 28 patients with cervical disorders with various clinical presentations. Modifications included the addition of *Gou Qi Zi* (Fructus Lycii) and *Sha Yuan Zi* (Semen Astragali Complanati) for blurred vision; *Qin Jiao* (Radix Gentianae Macrophyllae), *Quan Xie* (Scorpio), and *Wu Gong* (Scolopendra) for muscle stiffness in the face; *Hou Po* (Cortex Magnoliae Officinalis) and *Zi Su Geng* (Caulis Perillae) for difficulties with swallowing; *Dan Shen* (Radix et Rhizoma Salviae Miltiorrhizae), *Jiang Can* (Bombyx Batryticatus), and *Quan Xie* (Scorpio) for numbness of the tongue; *Ren*

WIND-DAMP DISPELLING FORMULAS

17

1157

Chapter 17 – Wind-Damp Dispelling Formulas   *Section 1 – Wind-Damp Dispelling Formulas*

Qiāng Huó Shèng Shī Tāng
(Notopterygium Decoction to Overcome Dampness)

Shen (Radix et Rhizoma Ginseng), *Huang Qi* (Radix Astragali), and *Sheng Ma* (Rhizoma Cimicifugae) for headache with hypotension; and *Fu Ling* (Poria), *Ze Xie* (Rhizoma Alismatis), *Che Qian Zi* (Semen Plantaginis), and *Niu Xi* (Radix Achyranthis Bidentatae) for headache with hypertension. Of 28 patients, the study reported complete recovery in 19 cases, marked effect in 5 cases, and no effect in 4 cases.[4]

AUTHORS' COMMENTS

Qiang Huo Sheng Shi Tang and *Jiu Wei Qiang Huo Tang* (Nine-Herb Decoction with Notopterygium) both contain *Qiang Huo* (Rhizoma et Radix Notopterygii) as the main ingredient, and both treat the presence of wind-dampness at the exterior. Their differences are as follows:

- *Qiang Huo Sheng Shi Tang* dispels wind-dampness and primarily treats heaviness, immobility, and pain in the shoulder and back.
- *Jiu Wei Qiang Huo Tang* dispels wind, cold, and dampness from the exterior, and clears heat from the interior. It mainly treats individuals with both exterior and interior conditions, with such symptoms as fever, chills, mild aches and pains, a bitter taste in the mouth, and slight thirst.

References

1. *Zhong Yi Fang Ji Xian Dai Yan Jiu* (Modern Study of Medical Formulae in Traditional Chinese Medicine) 1997;1466.
2. *Zhong Yao Yao Li Yu Lin Chuang* (Pharmacology and Clinical Applications of Chinese Herbs) 1995;11(4):1.
3. *Zhe Jiang Zhong Yi Za Zhi* (Zhejiang Journal of Chinese Medicine) 1997;5:206.
4. *Hu Nan Zhong Yi Za Zhi* (Hunan Journal of Chinese Medicine) 1997;2:13.

Juān Bì Tāng (Remove Painful Obstruction Decoction)
蠲痹湯
蠲痹汤

Pinyin Name: *Juan Bi Tang*
Literal Name: Remove Painful Obstruction Decoction
Alternate Names: *Chuan Pi Tang*, Impediment-Alleviating Decoction, Blockage-Relieving Decoction, Notopterygium and Turmeric Combination
Original Source: *Bai Yi Xuan Fang* (Selected Formulas)

COMPOSITION

Qiang Huo (Rhizoma et Radix Notopterygii)	45g [9g]
Fang Feng (Radix Saposhnikoviae)	45g [9g]
Chi Shao (Radix Paeoniae Rubra)	45g [9g]
Jiang Huang (Rhizoma Curcumae Longae)	45g [9g]
Huang Qi (Radix Astragali), *mi zhi* (fried with honey)	45g [9g]
Dang Gui (Radix Angelicae Sinensis)	45g [9g]
Zhi Gan Cao (Radix et Rhizoma Glycyrrhizae Praeparata cum Melle)	15g [3g]

DOSAGE / PREPARATION / ADMINISTRATION

The source text instructs to grind the ingredients into a coarse powder. Cook 15g of the powder with 5 slices of *Sheng Jiang* (Rhizoma Zingiberis Recens) in 2 bowls of water until the liquid is reduced to 1 bowl. Take the strained decoction while warm. Today, this formula may be prepared as a decoction with the doses suggested in brackets.

CHINESE THERAPEUTIC ACTIONS

1. Tonifies qi
2. Harmonizes the *ying* (nutritive) and *wei* (defensive) levels
3. Dispels wind and dampness

CLINICAL MANIFESTATIONS

Bi zheng (painful obstruction syndrome) caused by wind-dampness and accompanied by deficiencies of *ying*

1158

Chinese Herbal Formulas and Applications

Juān Bì Tāng (Remove Painful Obstruction Decoction)

Juan Bi Tang (Remove Painful Obstruction Decoction)

Diagnosis	Signs and Symptoms	Treatment	Herbs
Bi zheng (painful obstruction syndrome) with exterior excess and interior deficiency	• Pain in the neck, shoulder, and arm, and heaviness of the body and extremities: wind-dampness at the exterior • Numbness and weakness: deficiencies of *ying* (nutritive) and *wei* (defensive) *qi* in the interior	• Tonifies qi and harmonizes the *ying* (nutritive) and *wei* (defensive) levels • Dispels wind and dampness	• *Qiang Huo* (Rhizoma et Radix Notopterygii) and *Fang Feng* (Radix Saposhnikoviae) dispel wind-dampness and relieve pain. • *Chi Shao* (Radix Paeoniae Rubra) and *Jiang Huang* (Rhizoma Curcumae Longae) activate qi and blood circulation. • *Huang Qi* (Radix Astragali) and *Dang Gui* (Radix Angelicae Sinensis) tonify qi and blood, and harmonize the *ying* (nutritive) and *wei* (defensive) levels. • *Zhi Gan Cao* (Radix et Rhizoma Glycyrrhizae Praeparata cum Melle) and *Sheng Jiang* (Rhizoma Zingiberis Recens) harmonize the herbs in the formula.

(nutritive) and *wei* (defensive) *qi*: pain in the neck, shoulder, and arm, and numbness of the extremities.

CLINICAL APPLICATIONS

Osteoarthritis, rheumatoid arthritis, gouty arthritis, bursitis, frozen shoulder, periarthritis of the shoulders, tennis elbow, lumbago, and neck pain.

EXPLANATION

Juan Bi Tang (Remove Painful Obstruction Decoction) treats *bi zheng* (painful obstruction syndrome) due to deficiencies of *ying* (nutritive) and *wei* (defensive) *qi* with concurrent attack by wind-dampness. It is most effective for pain located in the upper parts of the body, such as the neck, shoulders, arms, and elbows. As a result of the underlying deficiencies in *ying* (nutritive) and *wei* (defensive) *qi*, patients experience numbness in the extremities, and general weakness and heaviness of the body. Moreover, deficiency of *ying* (nutritive) and *wei* (defensive) *qi* leaves patients more vulnerable to attacks by wind-dampness, a condition characterized by muscle stiffness, aches and pains, muscle spasms and cramps, and difficulty in moving.

In this formula, *Qiang Huo* (Rhizoma et Radix Notopterygii) and *Fang Feng* (Radix Saposhnikoviae) dispel wind-dampness and relieve pain. *Chi Shao* (Radix Paeoniae Rubra) and *Jiang Huang* (Rhizoma Curcumae Longae) activate qi and blood circulation. *Huang Qi* (Radix Astragali) and *Dang Gui* (Radix Angelicae Sinensis) tonify qi and blood, and harmonize the *ying* (nutritive) and *wei* (defensive) levels. *Zhi Gan Cao* (Radix et Rhizoma Glycyrrhizae Praeparata cum Melle) and *Sheng Jiang* (Rhizoma Zingiberis Recens) harmonize the herbs in the formula.

MODIFICATIONS

• With muscle aches and pains in the upper extremities due to wind-cold-dampness, add *Gui Zhi* (Ramulus Cinnamomi) and *Wei Ling Xian* (Radix et Rhizoma Clematidis).

• With muscle aches and pains in the lower extremities, add *Du Zhong* (Cortex Eucommiae), *Niu Xi* (Radix Achyranthis Bidentatae), and *Du Huo* (Radix Angelicae Pubescentis).

• With excessive dampness, add *Cang Zhu* (Rhizoma Atractylodis), *Fang Ji* (Radix Stephaniae Tetrandrae), and *Yi Yi Ren* (Semen Coicis).

• With severe pain due to cold, add *Fu Zi* (Radix Aconiti Lateralis Praeparata).

PHARMACOLOGICAL EFFECTS

Anti-inflammatory: One study reported marked effect using *Juan Bi Tang* at 4-8 g/kg to reduce swelling and inflammation. *Juan Bi Tang*, however, did not show analgesic effect at doses of 4, 8 and 16 g/kg.[1]

CLINICAL STUDIES AND RESEARCH

1. **Periarthritis of the shoulders**: In one study of 50 patients with periarthritis of the shoulders, the use of herbs was associated with complete recovery in 34 cases, significant improvement in 10 cases, and moderate improvement in 6 cases. The base formula contained *Juan Bi Tang* plus *Gui Zhi* (Ramulus Cinnamomi) and *Tou Gu Cao* (Caulis Impatientis) as guiding herbs. Modifications were made by adding a larger dose of *Huang Qi* (Radix Astragali) or *Si Jun Zi Tang* (Four-Gentlemen Decoction) for pain affecting the right shoulder; *Dang Gui* (Radix Angelicae Sinensis) or *Si Wu Tang* (Four-Substance Decoction) for pain affecting the left shoulder; *Ge Gen Tang* (Kudzu

WIND-DAMP DISPELLING FORMULAS

17

1159

Chapter 17 – Wind-Damp Dispelling Formulas　　　　　　　*Section 1 – Wind-Damp Dispelling Formulas*

Juān Bì Tāng (Remove Painful Obstruction Decoction)

Decoction) for pain in both the neck and shoulders; *Xiao Chai Hu Tang* (Minor Bupleurum Decoction) for concurrent neck pain and temporal headaches; *Huang Qi Gui Zhi Wu Wu Tang* (Astragalus and Cinnamon Twig Five-Substance Decoction) for numbness and weakness of the arms; *Ban Xia Bai Zhu Tian Ma Tang* (Pinellia, Atractylodes Macrocephala, and Gastrodia Decoction) for headaches; and others. The herbs were given in decoction, and most patients had complete recovery after approximately 10-20 packs of herbs.[2]

2. **Neck pain**: Forty-eight patients with neck pain were treated successfully using modified *Juan Bi Tang*. The herbal formula contained *Qiang Huo* (Rhizoma et Radix Notopterygii) 12g, *Fang Feng* (Radix Saposhnikoviae) 12g, *Jiang Huang* (Rhizoma Curcumae Longae) 12g, *Dang Gui* (Radix Angelicae Sinensis) 10g, *Chi Shao* (Radix Paeoniae Rubra) 15g, honey-processed *Huang Qi* (Radix Astragali), and *Zhi Gan Cao* (Radix et Rhizoma Glycyrrhizae Praeparata cum Melle) 8g. Additional modifications were made as needed. The treatment protocol was to cook the herbs in water, and administer the decoction in three equally-divided doses for 20 days per course of treatment. Of 48 patients, the study reported complete recovery in 36 cases, significant improvement in 11 cases, and no effect in 1 case.[3]

RELATED FORMULA

Jiān Bì Tāng

(Remove Painful Obstruction in the Shoulders Decoction)

肩痹湯

肩痹汤

Pinyin Name: *Jian Bi Tang*

Literal Name: Remove Painful Obstruction in the Shoulders Decoction

Original Source: *Tian Jin Zhong Yi Xue Yuan* (Tianjin University of Chinese Medicine) in 1989

Shan Zha (Fructus Crataegi)
Sang Shen (Fructus Mori)
Ji Xue Teng (Caulis Spatholobi)
Ge Gen (Radix Puerariae Lobatae)
Gui Zhi (Ramulus Cinnamomi)
Sang Zhi (Ramulus Mori)
Xi Xian Cao (Herba Siegesbeckiae)
Jiang Huang (Rhizoma Curcumae Longae)
Wu Jia Pi (Cortex Acanthopanacis)
Luo Shi Teng (Caulis Trachelospermi)
Dan Shen (Radix et Rhizoma Salviae Miltiorrhizae)
E Zhu (Rhizoma Curcumae)
Yan Hu Suo (Rhizoma Corydalis)
Bai Shao (Radix Paeoniae Alba)

Jian Bi Tang (Remove Painful Obstruction in the Shoulders Decoction) treats *bi zheng* (painful obstruction syndrome) affecting the upper extremities, including the shoulders, elbows, and wrists. Clinical manifestations include numbness, swelling, pain, decreased mobility and range of motion of the joints, and in severe cases, atrophy of the muscles. This formula contains herbs that tonify the Liver and Kidney, activate qi and blood circulation, and dispel wind-dampness.

References

1. *Zhong Yao Yao Li Yu Lin Chuang* (Pharmacology and Clinical Applications of Chinese Herbs) 1995;11:20.
2. *Yun Nan Zhong Yi Za Zhi* (Yunan Journal of Chinese Medicine) 1984;5(6):63.
3. *Xin Zhong Yi* (New Chinese Medicine) 1994;26(10):51.

1160

Chinese Herbal Formulas and Applications

Dú Huó Jì Shēng Tāng (Angelica Pubescens and Taxillus Decoction)

獨活寄生湯
独活寄生汤

Pinyin Name: *Du Huo Ji Sheng Tang*

Literal Name: Angelica Pubescens and Taxillus Decoction

Alternate Names: *Tu Huo Chi Sheng Tang*, Tu-huo and Loranthus Decoction, Pubescent Angelica and Loranthus Decoction, Tuhuo and Taxillus Combination

Original Source: *Bei Ji Qian Jin Yao Fang* (Thousands of Golden Prescriptions for Emergencies) by Sun Si-Miao in the Tang Dynasty

COMPOSITION

Du Huo (Radix Angelicae Pubescentis)	9g
Xi Xin (Radix et Rhizoma Asari)	6g
Fang Feng (Radix Saposhnikoviae)	6g
Qin Jiao (Radix Gentianae Macrophyllae)	6g
Sang Ji Sheng (Herba Taxilli)	6g
Du Zhong (Cortex Eucommiae)	6g
Chuan Niu Xi (Radix Cyathulae)	6g
Dang Gui (Radix Angelicae Sinensis)	6g
Chuan Xiong (Rhizoma Chuanxiong)	6g
Di Huang (Radix Rehmanniae)	6g
Bai Shao (Radix Paeoniae Alba)	6g
Ren Shen (Radix et Rhizoma Ginseng)	6g
Fu Ling (Poria)	6g
Gui Xin (Cortex Rasus Cinnamomi)	6g
Gan Cao (Radix et Rhizoma Glycyrrhizae)	6g

DOSAGE / PREPARATION / ADMINISTRATION

The source text instructs to grind the ingredients into a coarse powder, and cook it in 10 cups of water until the liquid is reduced to 3 cups. Take the warm, strained decoction in three equally-divided doses. The source text also advises to keep the body warm and to avoid exposure to cold.

CHINESE THERAPEUTIC ACTIONS

1. Dispels wind-dampness
2. Relieves *bi zheng* (painful obstruction syndrome)
3. Nourishes the Liver and Kidney
4. Tonifies qi and blood

CLINICAL MANIFESTATIONS

Chronic *bi zheng* (painful obstruction syndrome) with Liver and Kidney insufficiencies and qi and blood deficiencies: soreness and pain in the lower back and knees, numbness with difficult and limited range of motion in the limbs and extremities, aversion to cold and preference for warmth, palpitations, shortness of breath, pale tongue, white tongue coating, and a fine, weak pulse.

CLINICAL APPLICATIONS

Neck pain, low back pain, sciatica, hyperosteogeny, osteoarthritis, rheumatic arthritis, ankylosing spondylitis, prolapse of lumbar intervertebral disk, and postpartum aches and pains.

EXPLANATION

Du Huo Ji Sheng Tang (Angelica Pubescens and Taxillus Decoction) treats *bi zheng* (painful obstruction syndrome) characterized by chronic accumulation of wind, cold, and dampness with Liver and Kidney insufficiencies and qi and blood deficiencies. This syndrome begins with accumulation of wind, cold, and dampness in the channels and collaterals. As they obstruct qi and blood circulation, malnourishment of the Liver and Kidney occur. If this condition becomes chronic, qi, blood, Liver, and Kidney all become deficient. Thus, besides having aches and pains, the patient may also experience weakness of the knees and lower back, as well as difficulty in moving the limbs and extremities.

Since this condition is complicated by both excess (accumulation of wind, cold, and dampness) and deficiency (of Liver, Kidney, qi, and blood), optimal treatment requires the use of herbs that concurrently dispel wind, cold, and dampness, as well as herbs that nourish the Liver and Kidney; tonify qi and blood; and relieve pain.

WIND-DAMP DISPELLING FORMULAS

17

1161

Chapter 17 – Wind-Damp Dispelling Formulas　　　　　*Section 1 – Wind-Damp Dispelling Formulas*

Dú Huó Ji Shēng Tāng (Angelica Pubescens and Taxillus Decoction)

Du Huo Ji Sheng Tang (Angelica Pubescens and Taxillus Decoction)

Diagnosis	Signs and Symptoms	Treatment	Herbs
Chronic *bi zheng* (painful obstruction syndrome) with excess and deficiency	• Soreness and pain in the lower back and knees: wind-dampness affecting the muscles • Numbness with difficult and limited range of motion in the limbs and extremities, aversion to cold and preference for warmth, palpitations and shortness of breath: qi, blood, and Liver and Kidney deficiencies	• Dispels wind-dampness and stops pain • Nourishes the Liver and Kidney • Tonifies qi and blood	• *Du Huo* (Radix Angelicae Pubescentis) and *Xi Xin* (Radix et Rhizoma Asari) dispel wind, cold, and dampness. • *Fang Feng* (Radix Saposhnikoviae) and *Qin Jiao* (Radix Gentianae Macrophyllae) dispel wind-dampness. • *Sang Ji Sheng* (Herba Taxilli), *Du Zhong* (Cortex Eucommiae), and *Chuan Niu Xi* (Radix Cyathulae) dispel wind and dampness and tonify the Liver and Kidney. • *Dang Gui* (Radix Angelicae Sinensis), *Chuan Xiong* (Rhizoma Chuanxiong), *Di Huang* (Radix Rehmanniae), and *Bai Shao* (Radix Paeoniae Alba) tonify and activate blood circulation. • *Ren Shen* (Radix et Rhizoma Ginseng) and *Fu Ling* (Poria) strengthen the Spleen and tonify qi. • *Gui Xin* (Cortex Rasus Cinnamomi) warms the channels and opens the blood vessels. • *Gan Cao* (Radix et Rhizoma Glycyrrhizae) harmonizes the herbs.

In this formula, a large dose of *Du Huo* (Radix Angelicae Pubescentis) is used to dispel wind, cold, and dampness in the lower parts of the body. *Xi Xin* (Radix et Rhizoma Asari) disperses wind, cold, and dampness and relieves pain. *Fang Feng* (Radix Saposhnikoviae) dispels wind and dampness. *Qin Jiao* (Radix Gentianae Macrophyllae) dispels wind and dampness and soothes the tendons. *Sang Ji Sheng* (Herba Taxilli), *Du Zhong* (Cortex Eucommiae), and *Chuan Niu Xi* (Radix Cyathulae) dispel wind and dampness and also tonify the Liver and Kidney. *Dang Gui* (Radix Angelicae Sinensis), *Chuan Xiong* (Rhizoma Chuanxiong), *Di Huang* (Radix Rehmanniae), and *Bai Shao* (Radix Paeoniae Alba) tonify blood and activate blood circulation. *Ren Shen* (Radix et Rhizoma Ginseng) and *Fu Ling* (Poria) strengthen the Spleen and tonify qi. *Gui Xin* (Cortex Rasus Cinnamomi) warms the channels and opens the blood vessels. *Gan Cao* (Radix et Rhizoma Glycyrrhizae) harmonizes the herbs in the formula.

MODIFICATIONS

• For *tong bi* (extremely painful obstruction) with more cold, add *Fu Zi* (Radix Aconiti Lateralis Praeparata) and *Gan Jiang* (Rhizoma Zingiberis).
• For *zhuo bi* (fixed painful obstruction) with more dampness, remove *Shu Di Huang* (Radix Rehmanniae

Praeparata) and add *Fang Ji* (Radix Stephaniae Tetrandrae), *Yi Yi Ren* (Semen Coicis), and *Cang Zhu* (Rhizoma Atractylodis).
• For *xue bi* (blood painful obstruction) with blood stagnation, add *Hong Hua* (Flos Carthami) and *Tao Ren* (Semen Persicae).
• With sore back and painful knees, add *Qiang Huo* (Rhizoma et Radix Notopterygii) and *Xu Duan* (Radix Dipsaci).
• With severe pain, add *Zhi Chuan Wu* (Radix Aconiti Praeparata), *Zhi Cao Wu* (Radix Aconiti Kusnezoffii Praeparata), *Jin Qian Bai Hua She* (Bungarus Parvus), *Di Long* (Pheretima), and *Hong Hua* (Flos Carthami).
• With muscle weakness, add *Huang Qi* (Radix Astragali) and *Bai Zhu* (Rhizoma Atractylodis Macrocephalae).
• If there is no deficiency of *zheng* (upright) *qi*, remove *Ren Shen* (Radix et Rhizoma Ginseng) and *Shu Di Huang* (Radix Rehmanniae Praeparata).

CAUTIONS / CONTRAINDICATIONS

• *Du Huo Ji Sheng Tang* should be used with caution during pregnancy.
• This formula is contraindicated in *bi zheng* (painful obstruction syndrome) caused by excess heat or damp-heat.

1162

Chinese Herbal Formulas and Applications

Dú Huó Jì Shēng Tāng (Angelica Pubescens and Taxillus Decoction)

PHARMACOLOGICAL EFFECTS

1. **Analgesic and anti-inflammatory**: *Du Huo Ji Sheng Tang* has been shown to relieve pain and reduce inflammation in both rats and mice.[1,2]

2. **Anti-inflammatory**: Administration of *Du Huo Ji Sheng Tang* or *Dang Gui Nian Tong Tang* (Tangkuei Decoction to Lift the Pain) was associated with marked anti-inflammatory effects in suppressing the development of chronic arthritis induced by carrageenan or complete Freund's adjuvant. The researchers suggested that these herbal formulas may be considered as alternatives for non-steroidal anti-inflammatory drugs (NSAID).[3]

3. **Circulatory**: One study reported decreased vascular resistance and increased blood perfusion to the brain using *Du Huo Ji Sheng Tang* administered orally or via injection.[4]

4. **Antiplatelet**: *Du Huo Ji Sheng Tang* was shown to have a significant antiplatelet effect in rabbits.[5]

CLINICAL STUDIES AND RESEARCH

1. **Neck pain**: Use of modified *Du Huo Ji Sheng Tang* in one study for 1-4 courses of treatment was associated with 97% effectiveness. Of 69 patients, the study reported complete recovery in 41 cases, significant improvement in 20 cases, moderate improvement in 6 cases, and no effect in 2 cases.[6] In another neck pain study, modified *Du Huo Ji Sheng Tang* in 43 patients was associated with significant improvement in 31 cases, improvement in 8 cases, and slight improvement in 4 cases. The herbal treatment contained *Du Huo* (Radix Angelicae Pubescentis), *Dang Shen* (Radix Codonopsis), *Du Zhong* (Cortex Eucommiae), *Sang Ji Sheng* (Herba Taxilli), *Shu Di Huang* (Radix Rehmanniae Praeparata), *Fu Ling* (Poria), *Bai Shao* (Radix Paeoniae Alba), *Qin Jiao* (Radix Gentianae Macrophyllae), *Fang Feng* (Radix Saposhnikoviae), *Gui Zhi* (Ramulus Cinnamomi), *Chuan Niu Xi* (Radix Cyathulae), *Niu Xi* (Radix Achyranthis Bidentatae), *Dang Gui* (Radix Angelicae Sinensis), *Chuan Xiong* (Rhizoma Chuanxiong), *Hong Hua* (Flos Carthami), *Tao Ren* (Semen Persicae), *Yan Hu Suo* (Rhizoma Corydalis), *Xi Xin* (Radix et Rhizoma Asari), and *Gan Cao* (Radix et Rhizoma Glycyrrhizae). In addition, 16 mL of a *Dan Shen* (Radix et Rhizoma Salviae Miltiorrhizae) preparation was given via injection one time daily.[7]

2. **Sciatica**: In one study, use of modified *Du Huo Ji Sheng Tang* in 100 patients with sciatica was associated with recovery in 87 cases, significant improvement in 7 cases, moderate improvement in 3 cases, and no effect in 3 cases.[8] Another study reported significant relief of numbness and pain within 5 packs of modified *Du Huo Ji Sheng Tang* in 65 of 80 patients.[9] Additionally, use of modified *Du Huo Ji Sheng Tang* was associated with complete recovery in 85 of 105 patients who suffered from sciatica due to various causes. The herbal treatment contained this formula plus *Fang Ji* (Radix Stephaniae Tetrandrae), *Hai Tong Pi* (Cortex Erythrinae), *Ru Xiang* (Gummi Olibanum), *Mo Yao* (Myrrha), and others as needed.[10]

3. **Hyperosteogeny**: Thirty patients with hyperosteogeny of the knees were treated with complete recovery in 14 cases, significant improvement in 9 cases, moderate improvement in 4 cases, and no effect in 3 cases. The herbal treatment used *Du Huo Ji Sheng Tang* as the base formula, with the addition of *Fu Zi* (Radix Aconiti Lateralis Praeparata) 10g for increased severity of pain with exposure to cold; and *Jin Qian Bai Hua She* (Bungarus Parvus) 15g and *Wu Shao She* (Zaocys) 15g for chronic illness with limited mobility and altered physical appearance of the joints. The duration of treatment ranged from 2 months to 10 years.[11]

4. **Osteoarthritis**: Use of modified *Du Huo Ji Sheng Tang* in 24 patients with osteoarthritis for 1 week to 3 months was associated with complete recovery in 14 cases, significant improvement in 4 cases, moderate improvement in 3 cases, and no effect in 3 cases. The overall effectiveness was 87.5%.[12] Another study of 262 patients with osteoarthritis of the knees reported 94.7% effectiveness when treated with modified *Du Huo Ji Sheng Tang*. The clinical presentations included swelling, inflammation, and pain of the knees, with occasional deformation of the joint. The herbal treatment contained this formula plus *Wu Gong* (Scolopendra), *Mu Li* (Concha Ostreae), and others. In addition, an herbal paste was also applied topically to the affected areas. Of 262 patients, the study reported significant improvement in 77 cases, moderate improvement in 118 cases, moderate improvement in 55 cases, and no effect in 12 cases.[13]

5. **Rheumatic arthritis**: One study reported a marked effect using *Du Huo Ji Sheng Tang* plus *Si Miao San* (Four-Marvel Powder) to treat rheumatic arthritis of the knees characterized by pain, swelling, inflammation, numbness, decreased range of motion, and difficulty in walking. Of 104 patients, the study reported complete recovery in 84 cases, improvement in 11 cases, and no effect in 9 cases. The overall effectiveness was 91.3%.[14]

6. **Ankylosing spondylitis**: Use of modified *Du Huo Ji Sheng Tang* showed good results in treating 22 patients with a history of 3 months or more of ankylosing spondylitis characterized by stiffness and pain of the lower back. Modifications included the addition of *Gou Ji* (Rhizoma Cibotii) 10g, *Tu Si Zi* (Semen Cuscutae) 10g, and larger doses for *Sang Ji Sheng* (Herba Taxilli), *Du Zhong* (Cortex Eucommiae), and *Xu Duan* (Radix Dipsaci) for severe low back pain; *Bai Jie Zi* (Semen Sinapis) 6g, *San Leng* (Rhizoma Sparganii) 10g, and *E Zhu* (Rhizoma

WIND-DAMP DISPELLING FORMULAS

17

1163

Chapter 17 – Wind-Damp Dispelling Formulas　　　　　　　　*Section 1 – Wind-Damp Dispelling Formulas*

Dú Huó Ji Shēng Tāng (Angelica Pubescens and Taxillus Decoction)

Curcumae) 10g were added for chronic illness with phlegm accumulation. The duration of treatment was 2 months per course of treatment. Of 22 patients, the study reported significant improvement in 6 cases, moderate improvement in 14 cases, and no effect in 2 cases. The overall effectiveness was 90.9%.[15]

7. **Bizheng (painful obstruction syndrome):** Administration of *Du Huo Ji Sheng Tang* three times daily for 60-90 days in 52 patients was associated with significant improvement in 35 cases, moderate improvement in 15 cases, and no effect in 2 cases.[16] Another study reported marked effect using modified *Du Huo Ji Sheng Tang* to treat various types of *bi zheng* (painful obstruction syndrome). The herbal treatment used this formula as the base formula, with the following modifications: *Qiang Huo* (Rhizoma et Radix Notopterygii), *Sang Zhi* (Ramulus Mori), and *Ge Gen* (Radix Puerariae Lobatae) for wind; *Ma Huang* (Herba Ephedrae) and *Xi Xin* (Radix et Rhizoma Asari) for cold; *Yi Yi Ren* (Semen Coicis), *Cang Zhu* (Rhizoma Atractylodis), and *Mu Gua* (Fructus Chaenomelis) for dampness; *Quan Xie* (Scorpio), *Wu Gong* (Scolopendra), and *Jin Qian Bai Hua She* (Bungarus Parvus) for stubborn pain; *Chuan Shan Jia* (Squama Manis), *Tao Ren* (Semen Persicae), and *Hong Hua* (Flos Carthami) for blood stagnation; and *Ren Shen* (Radix et Rhizoma Ginseng) for generalized deficiency due to chronic illness. Of 55 patients, the study reported recovery in 22 cases, improvement in 30 cases, and no effect in 3 cases.[17]

8. **Prolapse of lumbar intervertebral disk:** Use of modified *Du Huo Ji Sheng Tang* was associated with improvement in 46 of 50 patients with prolapse of lumbar intervertebral disk confirmed by physical exam and CT scan. The herbal treatment contained this formula with modifications based on clinical presentations. For dampness and cold, *Fu Zi* (Radix Aconiti Lateralis Praeparata) 20g was added. For damp-heat, *Huang Bo* (Cortex Phellodendri Chinensis) 15g, *Huang Qin* (Radix Scutellariae) 12g, and *Cang Zhu* (Rhizoma Atractylodis) 15g were added, while *Gui Zhi* (Ramulus Cinnamomi), *Xi Xin* (Radix et Rhizoma Asari), and *Di Huang* (Radix Rehmanniae) were removed. For chronic pain with blood stagnation, *Dan Shen* (Radix et Rhizoma Salviae Miltiorrhizae) 20g was added.[18]

9. **Postpartum aches and pains:** One study reported marked results using modified *Du Huo Ji Sheng Tang* to treat 80 women with aches and pains after labor. In addition to this formula, modifications were made by adding *Fu Zi* (Radix Aconiti Lateralis Praeparata), larger doses of *Gui Zhi* (Ramulus Cinnamomi) and *Fang Ji* (Radix Stephaniae Tetrandrae) for wind-cold; *Mu Gua* (Fructus Chaenomelis) and *Cang Zhu* (Rhizoma Atractylodis) for

dampness; *Sang Zhi* (Ramulus Mori) and *Jiang Huang* (Rhizoma Curcumae Longae) for pain in the arms and shoulders; and *Niu Xi* (Radix Achyranthis Bidentatae) for pain in the lower body. Of 80 patients, the study reported complete recovery in 58 cases, significant improvement in 14 cases, moderate improvement in 6 cases, and no effect in 2 cases.[19] Note: Information is unavailable regarding whether these individuals were nursing while on the herbal treatment. Please consult additional information on the safety status of each individual herb prior to using them for nursing mothers.

RELATED FORMULAS

Yāo Tòng Fāng Yī Haò (Low Back Pain Formula One)

腰痛方一號
腰痛方一号

Pinyin Name: *Yao Tong Fang Yi Hao*
Literal Name: Low Back Pain Formula One
Original Source: *Tian Jin Zhong Yi Xue Yuan* (Tianjin University of Chinese Medicine) in 1989

Bai Shao (Radix Paeoniae Alba)
Ge Gen (Radix Puerariae Lobatae)
Xu Duan (Radix Dipsaci)
Gui Zhi (Ramulus Cinnamomi)
Xue Jie (Sanguis Draconis)
Ji Xue Teng (Caulis Spatholobi)
Du Huo (Radix Angelicae Pubescentis)
Mu Dan Pi (Cortex Moutan)
Mu Gua (Fructus Chaenomelis)
Chuan Niu Xi (Radix Cyathulae)
Wei Ling Xian (Radix et Rhizoma Clematidis)
Yan Hu Suo (Rhizoma Corydalis)
Zhi Gan Cao (Radix et Rhizoma Glycyrrhizae Praeparata cum Melle)

This contemporary formula treats acute and severe back pain caused by external injuries. This formula dispels wind-dampness, opens the channels and collaterals, and relieves low back pain.

Yāo Tòng Fāng Èr Haò (Low Back Pain Formula Two)

腰痛方二號
腰痛方二号

Pinyin Name: *Yao Tong Fang Er Hao*
Literal Name: Low Back Pain Formula Two
Original Source: *Tian Jin Zhong Yi Xue Yuan* (Tianjin University of Chinese Medicine) in 1989

Du Huo (Radix Angelicae Pubescentis)
Sang Ji Sheng (Herba Taxilli)

Chinese Herbal Formulas and Applications

Dú Huó Jì Shēng Tāng (Angelica Pubescens and Taxillus Decoction)

Bai Shao (Radix Paeoniae Alba)

Zhi Gan Cao (Radix et Rhizoma Glycyrrhizae Praeparata cum Melle)

Di Huang (Radix Rehmanniae)

Qian Nian Jian (Rhizoma Homalomenae)

Du Zhong (Cortex Eucommiae)

Wei Ling Xian (Radix et Rhizoma Clematidis)

Ji Xue Teng (Caulis Spatholobi)

Mu Gua (Fructus Chaenomelis)

Chuan Niu Xi (Radix Cyathulae)

This contemporary formula is designed to treat chronic back pain by strengthening the soft tissues to facilitate recovery. This formula dispels wind-dampness, nourishes the Liver and Kidney, and tonifies qi and blood.

Xī Tòng Fāng Yī Haò (Knee Pain Formula One)
膝痛方一號

Pinyin Name: *Xi Tong Fang Yi Hao*
Literal Name: Knee Pain Formula One
Original Source: *Tian Jin Zhong Yi Xue Yuan* (Tianjin University of Chinese Medicine) in 1989

Dang Gui (Radix Angelicae Sinensis)

Chuan Xiong (Rhizoma Chuanxiong)

Chi Shao (Radix Paeoniae Rubra)

Di Huang (Radix Rehmanniae)

Xu Duan (Radix Dipsaci)

Xiang Fu (Rhizoma Cyperi)

Hong Hua (Flos Carthami)

San Qi (Radix et Rhizoma Notoginseng)

Ze Lan (Herba Lycopi)

Su Mu (Lignum Sappan)

Tao Ren (Semen Persicae)

Wu Yao (Radix Linderae)

Da Huang (Radix et Rhizoma Rhei)

Chuan Niu Xi (Radix Cyathulae)

Yan Hu Suo (Rhizoma Corydalis)

Mu Gua (Fructus Chaenomelis)

Niu Xi (Radix Achyranthis Bidentatae)

Du Huo (Radix Angelicae Pubescentis)

Gan Cao (Radix et Rhizoma Glycyrrhizae)

This formula treats acute external or traumatic injuries to the lower limbs, including the legs, knees, and ankles. Clinical applications include acute injuries leading to broken bones, bone fractures, joint dislocation, soft tissue injuries, and generalized swelling and pain. This formula contains herbs that activate qi and blood circulation, remove qi and blood stagnation, clear heat, and drain fluids.

Xī Tòng Fāng Èr Haò (Knee Pain Formula Two)
膝痛方二號

Pinyin Name: *Xi Tong Fang Er Hao*
Literal Name: Knee Pain Formula Two
Original Source: *Tian Jin Zhong Yi Xue Yuan* (Tianjin University of Chinese Medicine) in 1989

Dang Gui (Radix Angelicae Sinensis)

Bai Shao (Radix Paeoniae Alba)

Di Huang (Radix Rehmanniae)

Shu Di Huang (Radix Rehmanniae Praeparata)

Dang Shen (Radix Codonopsis)

Bai Zhu (Rhizoma Atractylodis Macrocephalae)

Mu Dan Pi (Cortex Moutan)

Ze Xie (Rhizoma Alismatis)

Fu Ling (Poria)

Shan Yao (Rhizoma Dioscoreae)

Niu Xi (Radix Achyranthis Bidentatae)

Zhi Mu (Rhizoma Anemarrhenae)

Huang Bo (Cortex Phellodendri Chinensis)

Wu Jia Pi (Cortex Acanthopanacis)

Du Zhong (Cortex Eucommiae)

Qian Nian Jian (Rhizoma Homalomenae)

Shen Jin Cao (Herba Lycopodii)

Dan Shen (Radix et Rhizoma Salviae Miltiorrhizae)

Ji Xue Teng (Caulis Spatholobi)

Gan Cao (Radix et Rhizoma Glycyrrhizae)

Sheng Jiang (Rhizoma Zingiberis Recens)

Da Zao (Fructus Jujubae)

This formula treats chronic and degenerative disorders affecting the lower limbs, including the legs, knees and ankles. Historically, this formula has been used to treat *he xi feng* (crane's knee wind). Today, it is commonly used to treat chronic disorders of the leg, such as atrophy and degeneration of the soft tissues, weakness of the muscles and joints, and stiffness and decreased range of motion of the joints. This formula contains herbs that activate qi and blood circulation, remove qi and blood stagnation, tonify the Liver and Kidney, and strengthen the soft tissues.

Jí Tòng Tāng (Spine Pain Decoction)
脊痛湯
脊痛汤

Pinyin Name: *Ji Tong Tang*
Literal Name: Spine Pain Decoction
Original Source: *Tian Jin Zhong Yi Xue Yuan* (Tianjin University of Chinese Medicine) in 1989

Bai Shao (Radix Paeoniae Alba)

Dang Gui (Radix Angelicae Sinensis)

Chuan Xiong (Rhizoma Chuanxiong)

WIND-DAMP DISPELLING FORMULAS

17

1165

Dú Huó Ji Shēng Tāng (Angelica Pubescens and Taxillus Decoction)

Dan Shen (Radix et Rhizoma Salviae Miltiorrhizae)

Du Zhong (Cortex Eucommiae)

Chuan Niu Xi (Radix Cyathulae)

Yan Hu Suo (Rhizoma Corydalis)

San Leng (Rhizoma Sparganii)

E Zhu (Rhizoma Curcumae)

Ze Xie (Rhizoma Alismatis)

Yi Yi Ren (Semen Coicis)

Che Qian Zi (Semen Plantaginis)

Shen Jin Cao (Herba Lycopodii)

Gui Zhi (Ramulus Cinnamomi)

Gan Cao (Radix et Rhizoma Glycyrrhizae)

Ji Tong Tang (Spine Pain Decoction) treats spine disorders characterized by localized or radiating pain. It contains herbs to activate qi and blood circulation, reduce swelling and inflammation, and relieve pain. It is most effective for acute injuries of mild to moderate severity affecting the spine. It is less effective for chronic injuries in which the soft tissues have already stiffened or calcified.

AUTHORS' COMMENTS

Du Huo Ji Sheng Tang is one of the most commonly used formulas to treat muscle aches and pains due to both excess and deficiency. This formula is indicated for chronic *bi zheng* (painful obstruction syndrome) with obstruction of wind, cold, and dampness, accompanied by Liver and Kidney insufficiencies and qi and blood deficiencies. Today, *Du Huo Ji Sheng Tang* is commonly used for degeneration of bones, tendons, and ligaments due to aging. It is also one of the most effective formulas for treating low back pain.

References

1. *Zhong Cheng Yao Yan Jiu* (Research of Chinese Patent Medicine) 1988;5:28.
2. *Zhong Cao Yao* (Chinese Herbal Medicine) 1992;23(3):133.
3. Lin CC, Chen MF, Chen CF. The anti-inflammatory effects of Chinese crude drug prescriptions on experimental arthritis. Am J Chin Med 1995;23(2):145-52.
4. *Zhong Yi Fang Ji Xian Dai Yan Jiu* (Modern Study of Medical Formulae in Traditional Chinese Medicine) 1997;1469.
5. *Zhong Yao Yao Li Yu Lin Chuang* (Pharmacology and Clinical Applications of Chinese Herbs) 1990;6(6):7.
6. *Zhe Jiang Zhong Yi Za Zhi* (Zhejiang Journal of Chinese Medicine) 1993;3:134.
7. *An Hui Zhong Yi Xue Yuan Xue Bao* (Journal of Anhui University School of Medicine) 1995;14(1):37.
8. *Zhong Yi Han Shou Tong Xun* (Reports of Chinese Medicine) 1989;2:42.
9. *Gui Yang Yi Xue Yuan Xue Bao* (Journal of Guiyang Medical University) 1987;4:31.
10. *Shi Yong Zhong Yi Yao Za Zhi* (Journal of Practical Chinese Medicine and Medicinals) 1996;2:18.
11. *Guang Xi Zhong Yi Yao* (Guangxi Chinese Medicine and Herbology) 1990;13(3):38.
12. *Jiang Su Zhong Yi* (Jiangsu Chinese Medicine) 1993;3:11.
13. *Ji Lin Zhong Yi Yao* (Jilin Chinese Medicine and Herbology) 1998;4:15.
14. *Si Chuan Zhong Yi* (Sichuan Chinese Medicine) 1996;14(10):38.
15. *Shi Yong Zhong Yi Yao Za Zhi* (Journal of Practical Chinese Medicine and Medicinals) 1996;1:6.
16. *Shan Xi Zhong Yi* (Shanxi Chinese Medicine) 1989;3:10.
17. *Zhe Jiang Zhong Yi Za Zhi* (Zhejiang Journal of Chinese Medicine) 1998;4:165.
18. *Yun Nan Zhong Yi Za Zhi* (Yunan Journal of Chinese Medicine) 1997;18(6):7.
19. *Shi Yong Zhong Yi Yao Za Zhi* (Journal of Practical Chinese Medicine and Medicinals) 1998;14(4):11.

Chinese Herbal Formulas and Applications

Sān Bì Tāng (Three-Painful Obstruction Decoction)

三痹湯
三痹汤

Pinyin Name: *San Bi Tang*
Literal Name: Three-Painful Obstruction Decoction
Alternate Names: *San Pi Tang*, Chin-chiu and Tu-huo Decoction, Three Blockage Syndrome Decoction, Tuhuo and Astragalus Combination
Original Source: *Fu Ren Liang Fang* (Fine Formulas for Women) by Chen Zi-Ming in 1237

COMPOSITION

Du Huo (Radix Angelicae Pubescentis)	15g [3g]
Xi Xin (Radix et Rhizoma Asari)	30g [6g]
Qin Jiao (Radix Gentianae Macrophyllae)	15g [3g]
Fang Feng (Radix Saposhnikoviae)	30g [6g]
Gui Xin (Cortex Rasus Cinnamomi)	30g [6g]
Du Zhong (Cortex Eucommiae), *chao* (dry-fried) with ginger juice	30g [6g]
Xu Duan (Radix Dipsaci)	30g [6g]
Niu Xi (Radix Achyranthis Bidentatae)	30g [6g]
Dang Gui (Radix Angelicae Sinensis)	30g [6g]
Chuan Xiong (Rhizoma Chuanxiong)	15g [3g]
Bai Shao (Radix Paeoniae Alba)	30g [6g]
Di Huang (Radix Rehmanniae)	15g [3g]
Huang Qi (Radix Astragali)	30g [6g]
Ren Shen (Radix et Rhizoma Ginseng)	30g [6g]
Fu Ling (Poria)	30g [6g]
Gan Cao (Radix et Rhizoma Glycyrrhizae)	30g [6g]

DOSAGE / PREPARATION / ADMINISTRATION

The source text instructs to grind the ingredients into powder. Cook 15g of the powder with 3 slices of *Sheng Jiang* (Rhizoma Zingiberis Recens) and 1 piece of *Da Zao* (Fructus Jujubae) in 2 bowls of water until it is reduced to 1 bowl. Take the strained decoction while warm on an empty stomach. Today, this formula may be prepared as a decoction with the doses suggested in brackets.

CHINESE THERAPEUTIC ACTIONS

1. Tonifies qi and nourishes the blood
2. Dispels wind, cold, and dampness

CLINICAL MANIFESTATIONS

Joint pain due to stagnation of wind, cold, and dampness with underlying qi and blood deficiencies: numbness and pain of the muscles and joints, decreased range of motion, pain that worsens with exposure to cold and damp weather.

CLINICAL APPLICATIONS

Arthritis, rheumatism, and general aches and pains in the muscles and joints.

EXPLANATION

San Bi Tang (Three-Painful Obstruction Decoction) treats *bi zheng* (painful obstruction syndrome) characterized by accumulation of wind, cold, and dampness with qi and blood deficiencies. This condition begins with accumulation of wind, cold, and dampness in the channels and collaterals. As these pathogens block qi and blood circulation, they cause malnourishment to the muscles and tendons in the limbs, resulting in numbness and pain with decreased range of motion. The pain is intensified with exposure to cold and damp weather.

This formula contains *Du Huo* (Radix Angelicae Pubescentis) and *Xi Xin* (Radix et Rhizoma Asari) to dispel wind, eliminate dampness, relieve pain, and alleviate *bi zheng* (painful obstruction syndrome). *Qin Jiao* (Radix Gentianae Macrophyllae) and *Fang Feng* (Radix Saposhnikoviae) dispel wind and eliminate dampness. *Gui Xin* (Cortex Rasus Cinnamomi) warms the body and dispels cold. *Du Zhong* (Cortex Eucommiae), *Xu Duan* (Radix Dipsaci), and *Niu Xi* (Radix Achyranthis Bidentatae) tonify the Kidney and strengthen bones and tendons. *Dang Gui* (Radix Angelicae Sinensis), *Chuan Xiong* (Rhizoma Chuanxiong), *Bai Shao* (Radix Paeoniae Alba) and

WIND-DAMP DISPELLING FORMULAS

17

1167

Chapter 17 – Wind-Damp Dispelling Formulas   *Section 1 – Wind-Damp Dispelling Formulas*

Sān Bì Tāng (Three-Painful Obstruction Decoction)

San Bi Tang (Three-Painful Obstruction Decoction)

Diagnosis	Signs and Symptoms	Treatment	Herbs
Joint pain due to stagnation of wind, cold, and dampness with underlying qi and blood deficiencies	• Numbness and pain of the muscles and joints, and decreased range of motion: qi and blood deficiencies • Pain that worsens with exposure to cold and damp weather: accumulation of wind, cold, and dampness	• Tonifies qi and nourishes the blood • Dispels wind, cold, and dampness	• *Du Huo* (Radix Angelicae Pubescentis) and *Xi Xin* (Radix et Rhizoma Asari) dispel wind, eliminate dampness, relieve pain, and alleviate *bi zheng* (painful obstruction syndrome). • *Qin Jiao* (Radix Gentianae Macrophyllae) and *Fang Feng* (Radix Saposhnikoviae) dispel wind and eliminate dampness. • *Du Zhong* (Cortex Eucommiae), *Xu Duan* (Radix Dipsaci) and *Niu Xi* (Radix Achyranthis Bidentatae) tonify the Kidney and strengthen bones and tendons. • *Gui Xin* (Cortex Rasus Cinnamomi) warms the body and dispels cold. • *Dang Gui* (Radix Angelicae Sinensis), *Chuan Xiong* (Rhizoma Chuanxiong), *Bai Shao* (Radix Paeoniae Alba), and *Di Huang* (Radix Rehmanniae) nourish yin, tonify the blood, and activate blood circulation. • *Huang Qi* (Radix Astragali), *Ren Shen* (Radix et Rhizoma Ginseng), *Fu Ling* (Poria), and *Gan Cao* (Radix et Rhizoma Glycyrrhizae) tonify qi and strengthen the Spleen.

Di Huang (Radix Rehmanniae) nourish yin, tonify the blood, and activate blood circulation. *Huang Qi* (Radix Astragali), *Ren Shen* (Radix et Rhizoma Ginseng), *Fu Ling* (Poria), and *Gan Cao* (Radix et Rhizoma Glycyrrhizae) tonify qi and strengthen the Spleen.

MODIFICATIONS

• For *bi zheng* (painful obstruction syndrome) with more wind, add *Qiang Huo* (Rhizoma et Radix Notopterygii) and *Gui Zhi* (Ramulus Cinnamomi).

• For *bi zheng* (painful obstruction syndrome) with more cold, add *Ma Huang* (Herba Ephedrae) and *Fu Zi* (Radix Aconiti Lateralis Praeparata).

• For *bi zheng* (painful obstruction syndrome) with more dampness, add *Cang Zhu* (Rhizoma Atractylodis) and *Yin Chen* (Herba Artemisiae Scopariae).

AUTHORS' COMMENTS

San Bi Tang, literally "Three-Painful Obstruction Decoction," is so named because it has an excellent effect to dispel wind, cold, and dampness, the three most common factors leading to *bi zheng* (painful obstruction syndrome).

Du Huo Ji Sheng Tang (Angelica Pubescens and Taxillus Decoction) and *San Bi Tang* have similar effects to treat *bi zheng* (painful obstruction syndrome) with exterior excess and interior deficiency.

• *Du Huo Ji Sheng Tang* focuses on *bi zheng* (painful obstruction syndrome) with exterior excess (wind-cold-damp) and interior deficiency (Liver and Kidney). It is most effective for *bi zheng* (painful obstruction syndrome) affecting the lower body, including the lower back and knees.

• *San Bi Tang* emphasizes on *bi zheng* (painful obstruction syndrome) with exterior excess (wind-cold-damp) and interior deficiency (qi and blood). It is most suitable for *bi zheng* (painful obstruction syndrome) characterized by numbness, pain, and decreased range of motion in the arms and legs.

1168

Chinese Herbal Formulas and Applications

Shū Jīng Huó Xuè Tāng
(Relax the Channels and Invigorate the Blood Decoction)

疏經活血湯
疏经活血汤

Pinyin Name: *Shu Jing Huo Xue Tang*
Literal Name: Relax the Channels and Invigorate the Blood Decoction
Alternate Names: *Shu Ching Huo Hsieh Tang*, Clematis and Stephania Blood-Activating Decoction, Clematis and Stephania Combination
Original Source: *Wan Bing Hui Chun* (Restoration of Health from the Myriad Diseases) by Gong Ting-Xian in 1587

COMPOSITION

Dang Gui (Radix Angelicae Sinensis), *xi* (washed) with liquor	3.6g
Bai Shao (Radix Paeoniae Alba), *chao* (dry-fried) with liquor	4.5g
Di Huang (Radix Rehmanniae), *xi* (washed) with liquor	3g
Chuan Xiong (Rhizoma Chuanxiong)	1.8g
Tao Ren (Semen Persicae), *jian* (decocted) and *chao* (dry-fried)	3g
Fu Ling (Poria)	2.1g
Cang Zhu (Rhizoma Atractylodis), *jin* (soaked) in rice water	3g
Chen Pi (Pericarpium Citri Reticulatae)	3g
Qiang Huo (Rhizoma et Radix Notopterygii)	1.8g
Bai Zhi (Radix Angelicae Dahuricae)	1.8g
Wei Ling Xian (Radix et Rhizoma Clematidis), *xi* (washed) in liquor	3g
Fang Ji (Radix Stephaniae Tetrandrae), *xi* (washed) with liquor	1.8g
Fang Feng (Radix Saposhnikoviae)	1.8g
Long Dan (Radix et Rhizoma Gentianae)	1.8g
Chuan Niu Xi (Radix Cyathulae), *xi* (washed) with liquor	3g
Gan Cao (Radix et Rhizoma Glycyrrhizae)	1.2g

DOSAGE / PREPARATION / ADMINISTRATION

The source text instructs to cook the ingredients with 3 slices of *Sheng Jiang* (Rhizoma Zingiberis Recens) in water. Take the warm, strained decoction on an empty stomach. The source text recommends avoiding foods that are raw, cold, or damp in nature.

CHINESE THERAPEUTIC ACTIONS

1. Dredges the channels and collaterals
2. Invigorates blood circulation
3. Dispels dampness

CLINICAL MANIFESTATIONS

Body aches caused by exterior pathogens attacking the body with underlying deficiency: severe muscle aches, painful joints, radiating pain and numbness in the legs, and pain in the trunk.

CLINICAL APPLICATIONS

Arthritis, arthralgia, neuralgia, gout, lumbago, sciatica, purpura, hemiplegia, numbness and pain of the legs, and postpartum pain due to thrombosis.

EXPLANATION

Shu Jing Huo Xue Tang (Relax the Channels and Invigorate the Blood Decoction) treats *bi zheng* (painful obstruction syndrome) characterized by deficiency in the interior and excess at the exterior. The deficiency arises as a result of excessive sexual activity or over-consumption of alcohol, leading to emptiness of the channels and collaterals. As a result, wind, cold, and dampness can more easily attack the exterior, cause qi and blood stagnation, and produce pain all over the body.

The first four herbs in this formula, *Dang Gui* (Radix Angelicae Sinensis), *Bai Shao* (Radix Paeoniae Alba), *Di Huang* (Radix Rehmanniae), and *Chuan Xiong* (Rhizoma Chuanxiong), tonify the blood and activate blood circulation. *Tao Ren* (Semen Persicae) breaks up blood stagnation. *Fu Ling* (Poria) dispels dampness through diuresis, while *Cang Zhu* (Rhizoma Atractylodis) dries dampness. *Chen Pi* (Pericarpium Citri Reticulatae) regulates qi flow and dries dampness. *Qiang Huo* (Rhizoma et Radix Notopterygii), *Bai Zhi* (Radix Angelicae Dahuricae), *Wei Ling Xian* (Radix et Rhizoma Clematidis), *Fang Ji* (Radix Stephaniae Tetrandrae), and *Fang Feng* (Radix

WIND-DAMP DISPELLING FORMULAS

17

1169

Chapter 17 – Wind-Damp Dispelling Formulas

Section 1 – Wind-Damp Dispelling Formulas

Shū Jīng Huó Xuè Tāng
(Relax the Channels and Invigorate the Blood Decoction)

Shu Jing Huo Xue Tang (Relax the Channels and Invigorate the Blood Decoction)

Diagnosis	Signs and Symptoms	Treatment	Herbs
Body aches due to exterior excess with interior deficiency	Numbness and pain of the muscles and joints: deficiency of the channels and collaterals leading to invasion of wind, cold and dampness	• Dredges the channels and collaterals • Invigorates blood circulation • Dispels dampness	• *Dang Gui* (Radix Angelicae Sinensis), *Bai Shao* (Radix Paeoniae Alba), *Di Huang* (Radix Rehmanniae), and *Chuan Xiong* (Rhizoma Chuanxiong) tonify blood and activate blood circulation. • *Tao Ren* (Semen Persicae) breaks up blood stagnation. • *Fu Ling* (Poria) dispels dampness through diuresis. • *Cang Zhu* (Rhizoma Atractylodis) dries dampness. • *Chen Pi* (Pericarpium Citri Reticulatae) regulates qi flow and dries dampness. • *Qiang Huo* (Rhizoma et Radix Notopterygii), *Bai Zhi* (Radix Angelicae Dahuricae), *Wei Ling Xian* (Radix et Rhizoma Clematidis), *Fang Ji* (Radix Stephaniae Tetrandrae), and *Fang Feng* (Radix Saposhnikoviae) activate qi circulation, dispel wind and dampness, and relieve pain. • *Long Dan* (Radix et Rhizoma Gentianae) drains heat and dampness. • *Chuan Niu Xi* (Radix Cyathulae) activates blood circulation and tonifies the body. • *Gan Cao* (Radix et Rhizoma Glycyrrhizae) harmonizes the herbs.

Saposhnikoviae) activate qi circulation, dispel wind and dampness, and relieve pain. *Long Dan* (Radix et Rhizoma Gentianae) drains heat and dampness. *Chuan Niu Xi* (Radix Cyathulae) activates blood circulation and tonifies the body. *Gan Cao* (Radix et Rhizoma Glycyrrhizae) harmonizes the herbs.

MODIFICATIONS

• With pain in the upper body, add *Bo He* (Herba Menthae) and *Gui Zhi* (Ramulus Cinnamomi).

• With pain in the lower body, add *Mu Gua* (Fructus Chaenomelis), *Mu Tong* (Caulis Akebiae), *Huang Bo* (Cortex Phellodendri Chinensis), and *Yi Yi Ren* (Semen Coicis).

• With qi deficiency, add *Ren Shen* (Radix et Rhizoma Ginseng) and *Bai Zhu* (Rhizoma Atractylodis Macrocephalae).

• With blood deficiency, increase the doses of *Dang Gui* (Radix Angelicae Sinensis), *Bai Shao* (Radix Paeoniae Alba), *Shu Di Huang* (Radix Rehmanniae Praeparata), and *Chuan Xiong* (Rhizoma Chuanxiong).

• With phlegm, add *Tian Nan Xing* (Rhizoma Arisaematis) and *Ban Xia* (Rhizoma Pinelliae).

• With weakness and pain of the muscles and tendons, add *Huang Qi* (Radix Astragali) and *Bai Zhu* (Rhizoma Atractylodis Macrocephalae).

• With soreness and pain of the lower back and legs, add *Xu Duan* (Radix Dipsaci) and *Hong Hua* (Flos Carthami).

• With severe pain or paralysis of the legs, add *Mu Gua* (Fructus Chaenomelis), *Mu Tong* (Caulis Akebiae), *Huang Bo* (Cortex Phellodendri Chinensis), and *Yi Yi Ren* (Semen Coicis).

CAUTIONS / CONTRAINDICATIONS

Avoid foods that are raw, cold or damp in nature while taking *Shu Jing Huo Xue Tang*.

PHARMACOLOGICAL EFFECTS

Analgesic and anti-inflammatory: Administration of *Shu Jing Huo Xue Tang* was associated with reduction of pain and inflammation in adjuvant arthritic rats. The mechanism of action was attributed primarily to increased blood circulation.[1]

AUTHORS' COMMENTS

According to Dr. Chang Wei-Yen, *Shu Jing Huo Xue Tang* can be combined with *Shen Jin Cao* (Herba Lycopodii)

Chinese Herbal Formulas and Applications

Shū Jīng Huó Xuè Tāng
(Relax the Channels and Invigorate the Blood Decoction)

and *Tou Gu Cao* (Caulis Impatientis) to treat *xing bi* (mobile painful obstruction). Moreover, adding *Si Ni Tang* (Frigid Extremities Decoction) to this combination can help treat *zhuo bi* (fixed painful obstruction).

Reference

1. Kanai S, Taniguchi N, Higashino H. Study of sokei-kakketu-to (shu-jing-huo-xue-tang) in adjuvant arthritis rats. Am J Chin Med 2003;31(6):879-84.

Shū Jīn Lì Ān Sǎn (Relax the Tendons and Instill Peace Powder)
舒筋立安散

Pinyin Name: *Shu Jin Li An San*
Literal Name: Relax the Tendons and Instill Peace Powder
Alternate Name: Clematis and Carthamus Combination
Original Source: *Wan Bing Hui Chun* (Restoration of Health from the Myriad Diseases) by Gong Ting-Xian in 1587

COMPOSITION

Fang Feng (Radix Saposhnikoviae)
Qiang Huo (Rhizoma et Radix Notopterygii)
Wei Ling Xian (Radix et Rhizoma Clematidis)
Tian Nan Xing (Rhizoma Arisaematis), *chao* (dry-fried) with ginger
Cang Zhu (Rhizoma Atractylodis), *jin* (soaked) in rice water
Du Huo (Radix Angelicae Pubescentis)
Fu Ling (Poria)
Bai Zhu (Rhizoma Atractylodis Macrocephalae)
Fang Ji (Radix Stephaniae Tetrandrae)
Huang Qin (Radix Scutellariae), processed with liquor
Long Dan (Radix et Rhizoma Gentianae)
Lian Qiao (Fructus Forsythiae)
Mu Tong (Caulis Akebiae)
Ban Xia (Rhizoma Pinelliae), *chao* (dry-fried) with ginger
Chen Pi (Pericarpium Citri Reticulatae)
Tao Ren (Semen Persicae)
Hong Hua (Flos Carthami)
Niu Xi (Radix Achyranthis Bidentatae)
Di Huang (Radix Rehmanniae)
Fu Zi (Radix Aconiti Lateralis Praeparata), a small amount
Chuan Xiong (Rhizoma Chuanxiong)
Bai Zhi (Radix Angelicae Dahuricae)
Mu Gua (Fructus Chaenomelis)
Gan Cao (Radix et Rhizoma Glycyrrhizae)

DOSAGE / PREPARATION / ADMINISTRATION

The source text instructions are to cook the ingredients with juices from *Zhu Li* (Succus Bambusae) and *Sheng Jiang* (Rhizoma Zingiberis Recens). Take the strained decoction while warm. Note: The source text does not specify the doses for the ingredients.

CHINESE THERAPEUTIC ACTIONS

1. Disperses wind, cold, dampness, and heat
2. Activates blood circulation
3. Unblocks the channels and collaterals

CLINICAL MANIFESTATIONS

Bi zheng (painful obstruction syndrome): severe pain in the muscles and joints of the arms and legs.

WIND-DAMP DISPELLING FORMULAS

17

1171

Shū Jīn Lì Ān Săn (Relax the Tendons and Instill Peace Powder)

CLINICAL APPLICATIONS

Arthritis, arthralgia, neuralgia, hemiplegia, numbness and pain in the legs, and chronic vitamin B deficiency.

EXPLANATION

Shu Jin Li An San (Relax the Tendons and Instill Peace Powder) focuses on dispersing multiple pathogenic factors (wind, cold, dampness, and heat), activating blood circulation, and unblocking the channels and collaterals. The source text designated this relatively large formula for the treatment of joint pain with intensity and severity

similar to a "tiger's bite." This joint pain may occur in the arms or legs, or in various joints.

Fang Feng (Radix Saposhnikoviae) and *Qiang Huo* (Rhizoma et Radix Notopterygii) dispel wind to relieve numbness and stiffness of the joints. *Wei Ling Xian* (Radix et Rhizoma Clematidis), *Tian Nan Xing* (Rhizoma Arisaematis), *Cang Zhu* (Rhizoma Atractylodis), and *Du Huo* (Radix Angelicae Pubescentis) dispel wind and dampness, thereby relieving joint pain. *Fu Ling* (Poria) and *Bai Zhu* (Rhizoma Atractylodis Macrocephalae) warm the middle

Shu Jin Li An San (Relax the Tendons and Instill Peace Powder)

Diagnosis	Signs and Symptoms	Treatment	Herbs
Bi zheng (painful obstruction syndrome)	Severe pain in the muscles and joints of the arms and legs: wind, cold, dampness and/or heat blocking the channels and collaterals	• Disperses wind, cold, dampness, and heat • Activates blood circulation • Unblocks the channels and collaterals	• *Fang Feng* (Radix Saposhnikoviae) and *Qiang Huo* (Rhizoma et Radix Notopterygii) dispel wind to relieve numbness and stiffness of the joints. • *Wei Ling Xian* (Radix et Rhizoma Clematidis), *Tian Nan Xing* (Rhizoma Arisaematis), *Cang Zhu* (Rhizoma Atractylodis) and *Du Huo* (Radix Angelicae Pubescentis) dispel wind and dampness and relieve joint pain. • *Fu Ling* (Poria) and *Bai Zhu* (Rhizoma Atractylodis Macrocephalae) warm the middle *jiao* and tonify qi. • *Fang Ji* (Radix Stephaniae Tetrandrae), *Huang Qin* (Radix Scutellariae), *Long Dan* (Radix et Rhizoma Gentianae), *Lian Qiao* (Fructus Forsythiae), *Mu Tong* (Caulis Akebiae) and *Zhu Li* (Succus Bambusae) clear heat, purge fire, and reduce inflammation. • *Cang Zhu* (Rhizoma Atractylodis) and *Ban Xia* (Rhizoma Pinelliae) dry dampness and eliminate phlegm. • *Chen Pi* (Pericarpium Citri Reticulatae) regulates qi and resolves stagnation. • *Tao Ren* (Semen Persicae), *Hong Hua* (Flos Carthami), and *Niu Xi* (Radix Achyranthis Bidentatae) activate blood circulation, eliminate blood stasis, and relieve pain. • *Niu Xi* and *Di Huang* (Radix Rehmanniae) cool heat in the blood and nourish the body. • *Fu Zi* (Radix Aconiti Lateralis Praeparata), *Chuan Xiong* (Rhizoma Chuanxiong), and *Bai Zhi* (Radix Angelicae Dahuricae) dispel the wind-cold from the channels and collaterals to relieve pain. • *Mu Gua* (Fructus Chaenomelis) dispels wind and dampness to relieve pain. • *Gan Cao* (Radix et Rhizoma Glycyrrhizae) harmonizes the herbs within the formula.

1172

Shū Jīn Lì Ān Sǎn (Relax the Tendons and Instill Peace Powder)

jiao and tonify qi. *Fang Ji* (Radix Stephaniae Tetrandrae), *Huang Qin* (Radix Scutellariae), *Long Dan* (Radix et Rhizoma Gentianae), *Lian Qiao* (Fructus Forsythiae), *Mu Tong* (Caulis Akebiae), and *Zhu Li* (Succus Bambusae) clear heat, purge fire, and reduce inflammation. *Cang Zhu* (Rhizoma Atractylodis) and *Ban Xia* (Rhizoma Pinelliae) dry dampness and eliminate phlegm. *Chen Pi* (Pericarpium Citri Reticulatae) regulates qi and resolves stagnation. *Tao Ren* (Semen Persicae), *Hong Hua* (Flos Carthami), and *Niu Xi* (Radix Achyranthis Bidentatae) activate blood circulation, eliminate blood stasis, and relieve pain. *Niu Xi* (Radix Achyranthis Bidentatae) and *Di Huang* (Radix

Rehmanniae) cool heat in the blood and nourish the body. *Fu Zi* (Radix Aconiti Lateralis Praeparata), *Chuan Xiong* (Rhizoma Chuanxiong), and *Bai Zhi* (Radix Angelicae Dahuricae) dispel the wind-cold from the channels and collaterals to relieve pain. *Mu Gua* (Fructus Chaenomelis) dispels wind and dampness to relieve pain. *Gan Cao* (Radix et Rhizoma Glycyrrhizae) harmonizes the herbs within the formula.

MODIFICATIONS

With severe abdominal pain, add *Ru Xiang* (Gummi Olibanum) and *Mo Yao* (Myrrha).

Yì Yǐ Rén Tāng (Coicis Decoction)
薏苡仁湯
薏苡仁汤

Pinyin Name: *Yi Yi Ren Tang*
Literal Name: Coicis Decoction
Alternate Name: Coix Combination
Original Source: *Zhang Shi Yi Tong* (Comprehensive Medicine According to Master Zhang) by Zhang Lu-Xuan in 1695

COMPOSITION

Ma Huang (Herba Ephedrae)	2.4g
Gui Zhi (Ramulus Cinnamomi)	2.4g
Dang Gui (Radix Angelicae Sinensis)	4.5g
Bai Shao (Radix Paeoniae Alba), *xi* (washed) with liquor	4.5g
Cang Zhu (Rhizoma Atractylodis), *ban* (blended) and *chao* (dry-fried) with *Hei Zhi Ma* (Semen Sesami Nigrum)	3g
Yi Yi Ren (Semen Coicis), *pao* (blast-fried) with ginger	30g
Zhi Gan Cao (Radix et Rhizoma Glycyrrhizae Praeparata cum Melle)	2.1g
Sheng Jiang (Rhizoma Zingiberis Recens)	7 slices [4.5g]

DOSAGE / PREPARATION / ADMINISTRATION

The source text instructs to prepare the formula as a decoction.

CHINESE THERAPEUTIC ACTIONS

1. Dispels wind and dampness
2. Benefits qi
3. Activates blood circulation

CLINICAL MANIFESTATIONS

Bi zheng (painful obstruction syndrome) caused by wind-dampness: numbness and pain of the extremities, swelling, inflammation, decreased mobility and limited range of motion in the joints.

CLINICAL APPLICATIONS

Arthritis, arthralgia, rheumatoid arthritis, beriberi, nephritis, pulmonary edema, and pleurisy.

WIND-DAMP DISPELLING FORMULAS

17

1173

Chapter 17 – Wind-Damp Dispelling Formulas   *Section 1 – Wind-Damp Dispelling Formulas*

Yi Yǐ Rén Tāng (Coicis Decoction)

Yi Yi Ren Tang (Coicis Decoction)

Diagnosis	Signs and Symptoms	Treatment	Herbs
Bi zheng (painful obstruction syndrome) due to wind, cold, and dampness	Numbness and pain of the extremities, swelling, inflammation, decreased mobility, and limited range of motion in joints: wind, cold, and dampness attacking the muscles and joints	• Dispels wind and dampness • Benefits qi • Activates blood circulation	• *Ma Huang* (Herba Ephedrae) and *Gui Zhi* (Ramulus Cinnamomi) dispel wind-cold from the exterior, and drain dampness through urination. • *Gui Zhi* (Ramulus Cinnamomi) opens the channels and collaterals in the extremities to relieve pain. • *Dang Gui* (Radix Angelicae Sinensis) and *Bai Shao* (Radix Paeoniae Alba) activate blood circulation, harmonize the *ying* (nutritive) and *wei* (defensive) levels and relieve pain. • *Cang Zhu* (Rhizoma Atractylodis) and *Yi Yi Ren* (Semen Coicis) drain dampness. • *Zhi Gan Cao* (Radix et Rhizoma Glycyrrhizae Praeparata cum Melle) harmonizes the herbs.

EXPLANATION

Yi Yi Ren Tang (Coicis Decoction) was originally designed to treat *bi zheng* (painful obstruction syndrome) caused by wind-dampness. This condition, however, often occurs with complications, as wind-dampness may combine with cold and attack the muscles and joints, leading to such symptoms as numbness, pain, swelling, and inflammation.

The primary goals of this formula are to dispel wind, cold, and dampness, activate qi and blood circulation, and relieve pain. *Ma Huang* (Herba Ephedrae) and *Gui Zhi* (Ramulus Cinnamomi) are two of the strongest herbs for dispelling wind-cold from the exterior. They both also have a diuretic effect to drain dampness through urination. *Gui Zhi* (Ramulus Cinnamomi) also opens the channels and collaterals in the extremities to relieve pain. *Dang Gui* (Radix Angelicae Sinensis) and *Bai Shao* (Radix Paeoniae Alba) activate blood circulation, harmonize the *ying* (nutritive) and *wei* (defensive) levels, and relieve pain. *Cang Zhu* (Rhizoma Atractylodis) and *Yi Yi Ren* (Semen Coicis) drain dampness through urination. *Zhi Gan Cao* (Radix et Rhizoma Glycyrrhizae Praeparata cum Melle) harmonizes the herbs in the formula.

MODIFICATIONS
• With sweating, add *Shi Gao* (Gypsum Fibrosum).
• With heat, add *Huang Bo* (Cortex Phellodendri Chinensis).
• With cold, add *Fu Zi* (Radix Aconiti Lateralis Praeparata).

AUTHORS' COMMENTS
The two formulas with the same name that are discussed in this text are differentiated as follows. Though they have identical names, their compositions and clinical applications are different, and must not be confused with each others.
• *Yi Yi Ren Tang* (Coicis Decoction) from *Zhang Shi Yi Tong* (Comprehensive Medicine According to Master Zhang) by Zhang Lu-Xuan in 1695 dispels wind-dampness from the exterior to treat *bi zheng* (painful obstruction syndrome).
• *Yi Yi Ren Tang* (Coicis Decoction) from *Zheng Zhi Zhun Sheng* (Standards of Patterns and Treatments) by Wang Ken-Tang in 1602 dispels dampness from the Intestines to treat intestinal abscess. Note: Please refer to the discussion of this formula in *Yi Yi Fu Zi Bai Jiang San* (Coicis, Prepared Aconite, and Patrinia Powder), under the section titled Related Formula(s).

1174

Chinese Herbal Formulas and Applications

Shàng Zhōng Xià Tōng Yòng Tòng Fēng Wán
(Upper, Middle, and Lower General-Use Pill for Wind-Pain)

上中下通用痛風丸
上中下通用痛风丸

Pinyin Name: *Shang Zhong Xia Tong Yong Tong Feng Wan*
Literal Name: Upper, Middle, and Lower General-Use Pill for Wind-Pain
Alternate Names: *Shang Chung Hsia Tung Yung Tung Feng Wan*, Cinnamon and Angelica Pill, Cinnamon and Angelica
Formula
Original Source: *Dan Xi Xin Fa* (Teachings of [Zhu] Dan-Xi) by Zhu Zhen-Heng in 1481

COMPOSITION

Gui Zhi (Ramulus Cinnamomi)	[3g]
Qiang Huo (Rhizoma et Radix Notopterygii)	[3g]
Fang Ji (Radix Stephaniae Tetrandrae)	[9g]
Wei Ling Xian (Radix et Rhizoma Clematidis)	[3g]
Chuan Xiong (Rhizoma Chuanxiong)	[9g]
Tao Ren (Semen Persicae)	[9g]
Hong Hua (Flos Carthami)	[3g]
Bai Zhi (Radix Angelicae Dahuricae)	[9g]
Long Dan (Radix et Rhizoma Gentianae)	[9g]
Huang Bo (Cortex Phellodendri Chinensis)	[21g]
Cang Zhu (Rhizoma Atractylodis)	[21g]
Tian Nan Xing (Rhizoma Arisaematis)	[21g]
Shen Qu (Massa Fermentata)	[9g]

DOSAGE / PREPARATION / ADMINISTRATION

This formula is prepared and administered as pills with
warm water using the doses suggested in brackets.

CHINESE THERAPEUTIC ACTIONS

1. Dispels wind and dissolves dampness
2. Activates blood circulation and eliminates bruising

CLINICAL MANIFESTATIONS

Generalized *bi zheng* (painful obstruction syndrome):
aches and pains in the arms, legs, and throughout the
body.

CLINICAL APPLICATIONS

Arthritis, arthralgia, rheumatism, and gout.

EXPLANATION

Shang Zhong Xia Tong Yong Tong Feng Wan (Upper,
Middle, and Lower General-Use Pill for Wind-Pain) is a
generalized formula that treats aches and pains due to
various causes in varied locations in the body. *Bi zheng*
(painful obstruction syndrome) can be a complicated
disorder because the causes include cold, heat, dampness,
phlegm, and stagnation. This formula simplifies the
diagnostic procedure by focusing on relieving pain.
Therefore, it can be used for aches and pains throughout the body (upper, middle, and lower) due to various
causes.

This formula contains herbs with numerous functions:
reduce swelling, relieve pain, disperse stagnation, and
open the channels and collaterals. *Gui Zhi* (Ramulus
Cinnamomi), *Qiang Huo* (Rhizoma et Radix Notopterygii), *Fang Ji* (Radix Stephaniae Tetrandrae), and *Wei
Ling Xian* (Radix et Rhizoma Clematidis) reduce swelling
and relieve pain. *Chuan Xiong* (Rhizoma Chuanxiong),
Tao Ren (Semen Persicae), and *Hong Hua* (Flos Carthami)
activate blood circulation and relieve pain. *Bai Zhi*
(Radix Angelicae Dahuricae) dispels wind from the
exterior and relieves pain in the head region. *Long Dan*
(Radix et Rhizoma Gentianae) and *Huang Bo* (Cortex
Phellodendri Chinensis) clear heat and reduce swelling
and inflammation. *Cang Zhu* (Rhizoma Atractylodis)
dries dampness and *Tian Nan Xing* (Rhizoma Arisaematis) eliminates phlegm. *Shen Qu* (Massa Fermentata)
harmonizes and protects the middle *jiao*.

WIND-DAMP DISPELLING FORMULAS

17

1175

Shàng Zhōng Xià Tōng Yòng Tòng Fēng Wán
(Upper, Middle, and Lower General-Use Pill for Wind-Pain)

Shang Zhong Xia Tong Yong Tong Feng Wan (Upper, Middle and Lower General-Use Pill for Wind-Pain)

Diagnosis	Signs and Symptoms	Treatment	Herbs
Generalized *bi zheng* (painful obstruction syndrome)	Aches and pains in the arms, legs, and throughout the body: stagnation of cold, heat, dampness, and phlegm	• Dispels wind and dissolves dampness • Activates blood circulation and eliminates bruising	• *Gui Zhi* (Ramulus Cinnamomi), *Qiang Huo* (Rhizoma et Radix Notopterygii), *Fang Ji* (Radix Stephaniae Tetrandrae), and *Wei Ling Xian* (Radix et Rhizoma Clematidis) reduce swelling and relieve pain. • *Chuan Xiong* (Rhizoma Chuanxiong), *Tao Ren* (Semen Persicae), and *Hong Hua* (Flos Carthami) activate blood circulation and relieve pain. • *Bai Zhi* (Radix Angelicae Dahuricae) dispels wind from the exterior and relieves pain in the head region. • *Long Dan* (Radix et Rhizoma Gentianae) and *Huang Bo* (Cortex Phellodendri Chinensis) clear heat and reduce swelling and inflammation. • *Cang Zhu* (Rhizoma Atractylodis) dries dampness and *Tian Nan Xing* (Rhizoma Arisaematis) eliminates phlegm. • *Shen Qu* (Massa Fermentata) harmonizes and protects the middle *jiao*.

MODIFICATIONS
- For *bi zheng* (painful obstruction syndrome) caused by wind, cold, and dampness, add *Fang Feng* (Radix Saposhnikoviae) and *Du Huo* (Radix Angelicae Pubescentis).
- For *bi zheng* (painful obstruction syndrome) caused by blood deficiency, add *Dang Gui* (Radix Angelicae Sinensis) and *Bai Shao* (Radix Paeoniae Alba).
- For *bi zheng* (painful obstruction syndrome) caused by qi deficiency, add *Ren Shen* (Radix et Rhizoma Ginseng) and *Huang Qi* (Radix Astragali).
- For *bi zheng* (painful obstruction syndrome) caused by wind-cold, add *Ma Huang Tang* (Ephedra Decoction).
- For *bi zheng* (painful obstruction syndrome) caused by dampness and phlegm, add *Er Chen Tang* (Two-Cured Decoction).

RELATED FORMULA
Tòng Fēng Wán (Wind-Pain Pill)
痛風丸
痛風丸

Pinyin Name: Tong Feng Wan
Literal Name: Wind-Pain Pill

Original Source: *Tian Jin Zhong Yi Xue Yuan* (Tianjin University of Chinese Medicine) in 1989

Jin Qian Cao (Herba Lysimachiae)

Ze Xie (Rhizoma Alismatis)

Che Qian Zi (Semen Plantaginis)

Yi Yi Ren (Semen Coicis)

Shi Gao (Gypsum Fibrosum)

Zhi Mu (Rhizoma Anemarrhenae)

Huang Bo (Cortex Phellodendri Chinensis)

Cang Zhu (Rhizoma Atractylodis)

Chi Shao (Radix Paeoniae Rubra)

Ji Xue Teng (Caulis Spatholobi)

Di Huang (Radix Rehmanniae)

He Zi (Fructus Chebulae)

Wu Wei Zi (Fructus Schisandrae Chinensis)

Tong Feng Wan (Wind-Pain Pill) treats *tong feng* (wind-pain), a condition that is characterized by swelling, inflammation and pain with burning sensations of the joints. This formula contains herbs to clear heat, resolve dampness, activate blood circulation, and relieve pain. Today, this formula is used primarily to treat gout.

Chinese Herbal Formulas and Applications

Section 2

温散寒湿剂
— Damp-Cold Dispelling Formulas

Xiǎo Huó Luò Dān (Minor Invigorate the Collaterals Special Pill)
小活絡丹
小活络丹

Pinyin Name: *Xiao Huo Luo Dan*
Literal Name: Minor Invigorate the Collaterals Special Pill
Alternate Names: *Huo Luo Dan* (Invigorate the Collaterals Special Pill), Myrrh and Aconite Formula
Original Source: *Tai Ping Hui Min He Ji Ju Fang* (Imperial Grace Formulary of the Tai Ping Era) by the Imperial Medical Department in 1078-85

COMPOSITION

Zhi Chuan Wu (Radix Aconiti Praeparata), *pao* (blast-fried)	180g [6g]
Zhi Cao Wu (Radix Aconiti Kusnezoffii Praeparata), *pao* (blast-fried)	180g [6g]
Tian Nan Xing (Rhizoma Arisaematis), *pao* (blast-fried)	180g [6g]
Ru Xiang (Gummi Olibanum), *yan* (ground) to small particles	66g [5g]
Mo Yao (Myrrha), *yan* (ground) to small particles	66g [5g]
Di Long (Pheretima)	180g [6g]

DOSAGE / PREPARATION / ADMINISTRATION

The source text instructs to first blast-fry *Zhi Cao Wu* (Radix Aconiti Kusnezoffii Praeparata), *Zhi Chuan Wu* (Radix Aconiti Praeparata), and *Tian Nan Xing* (Rhizoma Arisaematis) to eliminate toxicity. Then, grind the ingredients into a fine powder and mix with grain-based liquor to form into small pills. The pills should resemble the size of *Wu Tong Zi* (Semen Firmianae), a small seed approximately 5 mm in diameter. Take 20 pills on an empty stomach at noon with cold, grain-based liquor or tea made from *Jing Jie* (Herba Schizonepetae).

Today, the ingredients are ground into a fine powder, sifted together, and formed into pills with honey. Take 1 pill [3g] twice daily, with aged, grain-based liquor or warm, boiled water. This formula may also be prepared as a decoction with the doses suggested in brackets.

CHINESE THERAPEUTIC ACTIONS

1. Dispels wind and dampness
2. Resolves phlegm and dredges the channels
3. Activates blood circulation and stops pain

CLINICAL MANIFESTATIONS

1. Obstruction of wind, cold, and dampness in the channels and collaterals: muscle spasms and cramps, limited mobility and difficult movement of the joints, painful extremities, and migratory pain.
2. *Zhong feng* (wind stroke) with obstruction of dampness, phlegm, and blood stasis in the channels and collaterals: numbness and pain in the extremities, and heaviness and pain in the lower back and legs.

CLINICAL APPLICATIONS

Arthritis, periarthritis of the shoulders, soft tissue injuries, sciatica, post-stroke sequelae, hemiplegia, and paralysis.

EXPLANATION

Xiao Huo Luo Dan (Minor Invigorate the Collaterals Special Pill) treats blocked qi and blood circulation caused by obstruction of wind, cold, and dampness in the channels and collaterals. The formula may be used for muscle and joint disorders with such symptoms such as spasms and cramps, limited mobility, difficult movement, and painful extremities. It may also be used for *zhong feng* (wind stroke) caused by obstruction of dampness, phlegm,

WIND-DAMP DISPELLING FORMULAS

17

1177

Chapter 17 – Wind-Damp Dispelling Formulas   *Section 2 – Damp-Cold Dispelling Formulas*

Xiǎo Huó Luò Dān (Minor Invigorate the Collaterals Special Pill)

Xiao Huo Luo Dan (Minor Invigorate the Collaterals Special Pill)

Diagnosis	Signs and Symptoms	Treatment	Herbs
Obstruction of wind, cold, and dampness in the channels and collaterals	• Spasms and cramps, limited mobility, difficult movement and painful extremities: obstruction of wind, cold, and dampness in the channels and collaterals • Numbness and pain of the extremities: dampness and phlegm obstruction with blood stasis in the channels and collaterals	• Dispels wind, cold, and dampness • Resolves phlegm and dredges the channels • Activates blood circulation and stops pain	• *Zhi Chuan Wu* (Radix Aconiti Praeparata) and *Zhi Cao Wu* (Radix Aconiti Kusnezoffii Praeparata) dispel wind-cold, warm and dredge the collaterals, and relieve pain. • *Tian Nan Xing* (Rhizoma Arisaematis) dries dampness and resolves phlegm. • *Ru Xiang* (Gummi Olibanum) and *Mo Yao* (Myrrha) activate qi and blood circulation and remove blood stasis. • *Di Long* (Pheretima) opens the channels and collaterals.

and blood stasis in the channels and collaterals, leading to numbness and pain of the extremities.

In this formula, *Zhi Chuan Wu* (Radix Aconiti Praeparata) and *Zhi Cao Wu* (Radix Aconiti Kusnezoffii Praeparata) dispel wind and dampness, and also warm and dredge the channels and collaterals. These two herbs also have a strong effect to dispel cold and relieve pain. *Tian Nan Xing* (Rhizoma Arisaematis) dries dampness and resolves phlegm in the channels and collaterals to relieve pain. *Ru Xiang* (Gummi Olibanum) and *Mo Yao* (Myrrha) activate qi and blood circulation and remove blood stasis. *Di Long* (Pheretima) opens the channels and collaterals. When taken with grain-based liquor, the herbs have a more powerful effect to dispel wind and cold, resolve dampness and phlegm, eliminate qi and blood stagnation, and open the channels and collaterals.

MODIFICATIONS

• For neuralgia or sciatica, add *Chi Shao* (Radix Paeoniae Rubra), *Wei Ling Xian* (Radix et Rhizoma Clematidis), and *Chuan Xiong* (Rhizoma Chuanxiong).
• For post-stroke complications, add *Dan Shen* (Radix et Rhizoma Salviae Miltiorrhizae) and *San Qi* (Radix et Rhizoma Notoginseng).
• For arthritis, add *Qiang Huo* (Rhizoma et Radix Notopterygii) and *Yi Tiao Gen* (Radix Moghaniae).
• If there is more wind, add *Da Qin Jiao Tang* (Major Gentiana Macrophylla Decoction).
• With Liver and Kidney yin deficiencies manifesting in weakness of the joints, add *Du Huo Ji Sheng Tang* (Angelica Pubescens and Taxillus Decoction).
• With severe pain, add *Yan Hu Suo* (Rhizoma Corydalis) and increase the doses of *Ru Xiang* (Gummi Olibanum) and *Mo Yao* (Myrrha).

CAUTIONS / CONTRAINDICATIONS

• *Xiao Huo Luo Dan* is a potent formula designed for individuals who have a strong constitution and who are generally healthy. It should be used with caution in individuals with blood deficiency or yin-deficient heat.
• The use of this formula is contraindicated during pregnancy.

PHARMACOLOGICAL EFFECTS

1. **Analgesic**: Administration of *Xiao Huo Luo Dan* at 20-100 mg/kg was associated with a marked analgesic effect in mice.[1]
2. **Sedative**: One study reported a dose-dependant sedative effect in mice.[2]
3. **Pharmacokinetic**: One study reported *Xiao Huo Luo Dan* to have a two-compartment model of distribution, with an average half-life of 13.16 hours.[3]

CLINICAL STUDIES AND RESEARCH

1. **Soft-tissue injuries**: Topical application of *Xiao Huo Luo Dan* was associated with excellent results in treating 50 patients with soft-tissue injuries. The topical preparation was made by soaking the pills in 75% ethanol then crushing the pills into paste. The herbal paste was applied to the affected area every other day for intact skin. If the wound was open, it was thoroughly cleaned and disinfected prior to application of the herbal paste. The study reported complete recovery in 49 of 50 patients within 3-5 applications of the herbal paste.[4]
2. **Sciatica**: Concurrent use of modified *Xiao Huo Luo Dan* via oral ingestion and topical application was associated with marked relief of sciatica. The treatment protocol was to cook the herbs in water and drink the decoction in two equally-divided doses daily. The herb residue was applied topically to the affected area. Each course of treatment was 20 days. Out of 32 patients, 20 had complete recovery,

1178

Xiǎo Huó Luò Dān (Minor Invigorate the Collaterals Special Pill)

Chinese Herbal Formulas and Applications

7 had significant improvement, 3 had slight improvement, and 2 had no change. The overall effectiveness was 93.75%.[5]

3. **Arthritis**: *Topical* application of modified *Xiao Huo Luo Dan* was effective in relieving pain in all 50 patients. The herbal formula contained unprocessed *Chuan Wu* (Radix Aconiti), unprocessed *Cao Wu* (Radix Aconiti Kusnezoffii), *Di Long* (Pheretima), unprocessed *Tian Nan Xing* (Rhizoma Arisaematis), *Ru Xiang* (Gummi Olibanum), *Mo Yao* (Myrrha), *Ma Qian Zi* (Semen Strychni), *Hong Hua* (Flos Carthami), *Shui Zhi* (Hirudo), and *Mu Gua* (Fructus Chaenomelis), all in equal portions. The herbs were ground into a fine powder, mixed with water to make a paste, and applied topically to the affected area. Of 50 patients, the study reported complete relief in 8 cases, significant improvement in 27 cases, and moderate improvement in 5 cases.[6] Note: The treatment protocol for this study was to apply the herbs *topically* since unprocessed forms of *Chuan Wu* (Radix Aconiti), *Cao Wu* (Radix Aconiti Kusnezoffii), and *Tian Nan Xing* (Rhizoma Arisaematis) can be extremely toxic if ingested orally.

TOXICOLOGY

Overdose of *Xiao Huo Luo Dan* (Minor Invigorate the Collaterals Special Pill) has been associated with occasional toxicity. Reported side effects include numbness in the hands and feet, stiff tongue, dizziness, pale face, cold extremities, perspiration, nausea, vomiting, diarrhea, palpitations, arrhythmia, and loss of consciousness. Allergy and acute gastrointestinal bleeding have been reported as well. The toxicity is attributed to *Zhi Chuan Wu* (Radix Aconiti Praeparata), *Zhi Cao Wu* (Radix Aconiti Kusnezoffii Praeparata), and *Tian Nan Xing* (Rhizoma Arisaematis).[7,8,9]

Toxicity associated with the use of this formula may be treated initially with gastric lavage. Use of an herbal decoction with *Gan Cao* (Radix et Rhizoma Glycyrrhizae) and *Lu Dou* (Semen Phaseoli Radiati) has also shown beneficial effects. Administration of intravenous fluids with dexamethasone (10mg twice daily) is also helpful.[10]

RELATED FORMULAS

Dà Huó Luò Dān

(Major Invigorate the Collaterals Special Pill)

大活络丹
大活络丹

Pinyin Name: Da Huo Luo Dan
Literal Name: Major Invigorate the Collaterals Special Pill
Original Source: *Lan Tai Gui Fan* (Guidelines from Lan-Tai) by Xu Da-Chun in 1764

Jin Qian Bai Hua She (Bungarus Parvus), *jin* (soaked) in liquor	60g
Wu Shao She (Zaocys), *jin* (soaked) in liquor	60g
Wei Ling Xian (Radix et Rhizoma Clematidis), *jin* (soaked) in liquor	60g
Zhu Jie Xiang Fu (Rhizoma Anemones Raddeanae), *jin* (soaked) in liquor	60g
Zhi Cao Wu (Radix Aconiti Kusnezoffii Praeparata)	60g
Tian Ma (Rhizoma Gastrodiae), *wei* (roasted)	60g
Quan Xie (Scorpio)	60g
He Shou Wu (Radix Polygoni Multiflori), *jin* (soaked) in a decoction of *Hei Dou* (Semen Sojae)	60g
Gui Ban (Plastrum Testudinis), *zhi* (fried with liquid)	60g
Ma Huang (Herba Ephedrae)	60g
Mian Ma Guan Zhong (Rhizoma Dryopteridis Crassirhizomatis)	60g
Zhi Gan Cao (Radix et Rhizoma Glycyrrhizae Praeparata cum Melle)	60g
Qiang Huo (Rhizoma et Radix Notopterygii)	60g
Rou Gui (Cortex Cinnamomi)	60g
Huo Xiang (Herba Agastaches)	60g
Wu Yao (Radix Linderae)	60g
Huang Lian (Rhizoma Coptidis)	60g
Shu Di Huang (Radix Rehmanniae Praeparata)	60g
Da Huang (Radix et Rhizoma Rhei), *zheng* (steamed)	60g
Mu Xiang (Radix Aucklandiae)	60g
Chen Xiang (Lignum Aquilariae Resinatum)	60g
Xi Xin (Radix et Rhizoma Asari)	30g
Chi Shao (Radix Paeoniae Rubra), oil removed	30g
Ding Xiang (Flos Caryophylli)	30g
Ru Xiang (Gummi Olibanum), oil removed	30g
Mo Yao (Myrrha), oil removed	30g
Jiang Can (Bombyx Batryticatus)	30g
Tian Nan Xing (Rhizoma Arisaematis), *zhi* (prepared) with ginger	30g
Qing Pi (Pericarpium Citri Reticulatae Viride)	30g
Gu Sui Bu (Rhizoma Drynariae)	30g
Dou Kou (Fructus Amomi Rotundus)	30g
An Xi Xiang (Benzoinum), *ao* (simmered) with liquor	30g
Fu Zi (Radix Aconiti Lateralis Praeparata), *zhi* (prepared) till black	30g
Huang Qin (Radix Scutellariae), *zheng* (steamed)	30g
Fu Ling (Poria)	30g
Xiang Fu (Rhizoma Cyperi), *jin* (soaked) in liquor and *bei* (stone-baked)	30g
Xuan Shen (Radix Scrophulariae)	30g
Bai Zhu (Rhizoma Atractylodis Macrocephalae)	30g
Fang Feng (Radix Saposhnikoviae)	75g
Ge Gen (Radix Puerariae Lobatae)	45g
Hu Gu (Os Tigris), *zhi* (fried with liquid)	45g
Dang Gui (Radix Angelicae Sinensis)	45g
Xue Jie (Sanguis Draconis)	21g

WIND-DAMP DISPELLING FORMULAS

17

1179

Chapter 17 – Wind-Damp Dispelling Formulas   *Section 2 – Damp-Cold Dispelling Formulas*

Xiǎo Huó Luò Dān (Minor Invigorate the Collaterals Special Pill)

Di Long (Pheretima), *zhi* (fried with liquid)	15g
Xi Jiao (Cornu Rhinoceri)	15g
She Xiang (Moschus)	15g
Song Xiang (Colophonium)	15g
Niu Huang (Calculus Bovis)	4.5g
Bing Pian (Borneolum Syntheticum)	4.5g
Ren Shen (Radix et Rhizoma Ginseng)	90g

Ren Shen (Radix et Rhizoma Ginseng)
Dang Gui (Radix Angelicae Sinensis)
Bai Shao (Radix Paeoniae Alba)
Chuan Xiong (Rhizoma Chuanxiong)
Di Huang (Radix Rehmanniae)
Du Zhong (Cortex Eucommiae)
Fang Feng (Radix Saposhnikoviae)

Note: *Xi Jiao* (Cornu Rhinoceri), *Hu Gu* (Os Tigris) and *She Xiang* (Moschus) are derived from endangered animals, and are rarely used as medicinal substances today. The discussion of this formula here is included primarily for academic purposes, and to reflect upon the historical use of these substances in its original formulation. In most herbal products today, these endangered substances have been removed completely, or have been replaced with substitutes having similar functions.

The source text states to grind all of the ingredients into powder, and form into pills with honey. The pills are coated with *Jin Bo* (gold foil), and should resemble *Long Yan He* (Semen Longan) in size. Take one pill with aged, grain-based liquor two times daily.

Da Huo Luo Dan (Major Invigorate the Collaterals Special Pill) dispels wind, tonifies qi and blood, opens the channels and collaterals, and relieves pain. Clinical applications include paralysis or hemiplegia in post-stroke patients, *wei bi* (atrophic painful obstruction), phlegm syncope, deep-rooted sores, and multiple abscesses.

Jiā Wèi Huó Luò Dān

(Augmented Invigorate the Collaterals Special Pill)

加味活絡丹
加味活絡丹

Pinyin Name: *Jia Wei Huo Luo Dan*
Literal Name: Augmented Invigorate the Collaterals Special Pill
Original Source: *An Hui Zhong Yi Xue Yuan* (Anhui University School of Medicine) in 1990

Zhi Chuan Wu (Radix Aconiti Praeparata)
Zhi Cao Wu (Radix Aconiti Kusnezoffii Praeparata)
Gui Zhi (Ramulus Cinnamomi)
Sang Zhi (Ramulus Mori)
Du Huo (Radix Angelicae Pubescentis)
Sang Ji Sheng (Herba Taxilli)
Ji Xue Teng (Caulis Spatholobi)
Chuan Niu Xi (Radix Cyathulae)
Yan Hu Suo (Rhizoma Corydalis)
Qin Jiao (Radix Gentianae Macrophyllae)
Wei Ling Xian (Radix et Rhizoma Clematidis)

Jia Wei Huo Luo Dan (Augmented Invigorate the Collaterals Special Pill) treats *bi zheng* (painful obstruction syndrome) characterized by cold and dampness. Its main actions are to warm and open the channels and collaterals, dispel cold and dampness, activate qi and blood circulation, and relieve pain. Clinical applications include arthritis, arthralgia, lumbago, sciatica, and general aches and pains characterized by cold.

AUTHORS' COMMENTS

Xiao Huo Luo Dan contains many warm and acrid herbs, making it suitable for cold *bi zheng* (painful obstruction syndrome) with tightness and cramping of the tendons, sinews, and joints. Patients may also experience numbness of the limbs. The tongue will be slightly purple with a white coating. This formula can also be used for post-stroke hemiplegia exhibiting excess signs. Key diagnostic symptoms include numbness, pain, and limited mobility.

Although wind and dampness are the pathogens that initially invade the muscles and joints, they often create other complications, such as qi, blood and phlegm stagnation. Therefore, treatment of *bi zheng* (painful obstruction syndrome) requires use of herbs that treat these associated conditions and complications. In this formula, strong herbs such as *Zhi Chuan Wu* (Radix Aconiti Praeparata) and *Zhi Cao Wu* (Radix Aconiti Kusnezoffii Praeparata) warm and dredge the collaterals, dispel cold and relieve pain. *Tian Nan Xing* (Rhizoma Arisaematis) dries dampness and resolves phlegm. *Ru Xiang* (Gummi Olibanum) and *Mo Yao* (Myrrha) are aromatic substances that activate qi and blood circulation and remove blood stasis. Lastly, *Di Long* (Pheretima) is used as a guiding herb to open the channels and collaterals

Xiao Huo Luo Dan and *Da Huo Luo Dan* both treat the blockages of wind, cold and damp pathogens in the channels and collaterals. Hence they are named Minor Invigorate the Collaterals Special Pill and Major Invigorate the Collaterals Special Pill, respectively.

As the names imply, <u>*Xiao*</u> *Huo Luo Dan* (<u>Minor</u> Invigorate the Collaterals Special Pill) and <u>*Da*</u> *Huo Luo Dan* (<u>Major</u>

Chinese Herbal Formulas and Applications

Xiǎo Huó Luò Dān (Minor Invigorate the Collaterals Special Pill)

Invigorate the Collaterals Special Pill) both invigorate and unblock the collaterals.

- *Xiao Huo Luo Dan* is more suitable for obstruction of wind, cold, and dampness, accumulation of phlegm, and stagnation of blood in the channels and collaterals (an excess condition) in individuals who are otherwise healthy. All of the herbs are aimed at such excess conditions.
- *Da Huo Luo Dan* treats obstruction of the collaterals (an excess condition) in individuals with underlying qi and blood deficiencies (a deficient condition). This formula uses qi and blood-tonifying herbs to support the underlying deficiencies, along with herbs to dispel wind and open the channels and collaterals.

References

1. *Zhong Guo Zhong Yao Za Zhi* (People's Republic of China Journal of Chinese Herbology) 1995;3:159.
2. *Zhong Yi Yao Xue Bao* (Report of Chinese Medicine and Herbology) 1995;6:13.
3. *Zhong Cheng Yao* (Study of Chinese Patent Medicine) 1994;3:34.
4. *Hu Bei Zhong Yi Za Zhi* (Hubei Journal of Chinese Medicine) 1990;4:44.
5. *Nei Meng Gu Zhong Yi Yao* (Traditional Chinese Medicine and Medicinals of Inner Mongolia) 1992;3:24.
6. *Hu Bei Zhong Yi Xue Yuan Xue Bao* (Journal of Hubei University of Medicine) 1993;2:56.
7. *Zhong Yuan Yi Kan* (Resource Journal of Chinese Medicine) 1986;5:43.
8. *Zhong Hua Yi Xue Za Zhi* (Chinese Journal of Medicine) 1979;2:123.
9. *Zhong Yao Ming Fang Yao Li Yu Ying Yong* (Pharmacology and Applications of Famous Herbal Formulas) 1989;539-41.
10. *Zhong Guo Zhong Yao Za Zhi* (People's Republic of China Journal of Chinese Herbology) 1995;6:375.

Dà Fáng Fēng Tāng (Major Saposhnikovia Decoction)
大防風湯
大防风汤

Pinyin Name: *Da Fang Feng Tang*
Literal Name: Major Saposhnikovia Decoction
Alternate Name: Major Siler Combination
Original Source: *Tai Ping Hui Min He Ji Ju Fang* (Imperial Grace Formulary of the Tai Ping Era) by the Imperial Medical Department in 1078-85

COMPOSITION

Dang Gui (Radix Angelicae Sinensis), *xi* (washed), *jin* (soaked) in liquor, and *chao* (dry-fried)	60g
Shu Di Huang (Radix Rehmanniae Praeparata), *xi* (washed)	60g
Bai Shao (Radix Paeoniae Alba)	60g
Chuan Xiong (Rhizoma Chuanxiong)	45g
Ren Shen (Radix et Rhizoma Ginseng)	30g
Bai Zhu (Rhizoma Atractylodis Macrocephalae)	60g
Huang Qi (Radix Astragali), *chao* (dry-fried)	60g
Niu Xi (Radix Achyranthis Bidentatae), *jin* (soaked) in liquor and *chao* (dry-fried)	30g
Du Zhong (Cortex Eucommiae), *chao* (dry-fried)	60g
Fang Feng (Radix Saposhnikoviae)	60g
Qiang Huo (Rhizoma et Radix Notopterygii)	30g
Fu Zi (Radix Aconiti Lateralis Praeparata), *pao* (blast-fried)	45g
Zhi Gan Cao (Radix et Rhizoma Glycyrrhizae Praeparata cum Melle)	30g

DOSAGE / PREPARATION / ADMINISTRATION

The source text instructs to grind the ingredients into powder. Cook 15g of the powder with 7 slices of *Sheng Jiang* (Rhizoma Zingiberis Recens) and 1 piece of *Da Zao* (Fructus Jujubae) in 1.5 bowls of water until the liquid is reduced to 80% volume. Take the warm, strained decoction on an empty stomach before meals.

WIND-DAMP DISPELLING FORMULAS

17

1181

Chapter 17 – Wind-Damp Dispelling Formulas | Section 2 – Damp-Cold Dispelling Formulas

Dà Fáng Fēng Tāng (Major Saposhnikovia Decoction)

CHINESE THERAPEUTIC ACTIONS

1. Tonifies qi and blood
2. Strengthens the muscles and tendons
3. Dispels wind, cold, and dampness

CLINICAL MANIFESTATIONS

Weakness and paralysis of the lower extremities caused by deficiency of qi and blood: generalized pain and numbness in the legs, weak knees, atrophy of the leg muscles, difficult movement, hemiplegia, and neuralgia.

CLINICAL APPLICATIONS

Arthritis, rheumatoid arthritis, paralysis of the lower extremities, hemiplegia, muscle atrophy, and neuralgia.

EXPLANATION

Da Fang Feng Tang (Major Saposhnikovia Decoction) was designed originally to treat conditions called *li feng* (dysenteric wind) and *he xi feng* (crane's knee wind). Both conditions are characterized by severe qi and blood deficiencies with wind, cold, and dampness at the exterior. *Li feng* (dysenteric wind) is a condition that occurs after dysentery, in which patients have trouble walking due to severe pain and atrophy of the leg muscles. *He xi feng* (crane's knee wind) is a condition in which there is such severe atrophy of the leg muscles that the legs appear to be covered only by skin, resembling the knees of a crane.

Patients with *he xi feng* (crane's knee wind) suffer from severe pain and swelling of the knees, and have difficulty in knee flexion and extension.

This formula contains herbs that tonify qi and blood, nourish the muscles and tendons, and dispel wind, cold, and dampness. *Dang Gui* (Radix Angelicae Sinensis), *Shu Di Huang* (Radix Rehmanniae Praeparata), *Bai Shao* (Radix Paeoniae Alba), and *Chuan Xiong* (Rhizoma Chuanxiong) tonify the blood and activate blood circulation. *Ren Shen* (Radix et Rhizoma Ginseng), *Bai Zhu* (Rhizoma Atractylodis Macrocephalae), and *Huang Qi* (Radix Astragali) tonify qi and strengthen the Spleen. *Niu Xi* (Radix Achyranthis Bidentatae) and *Du Zhong* (Cortex Eucommiae) tonify the Kidney, nourish tendons and muscles, and relieve pain. *Fang Feng* (Radix Saposhnikoviae) and *Qiang Huo* (Rhizoma et Radix Notopterygii) dispel wind and relieve numbness and joint pain. *Fu Zi* (Radix Aconiti Lateralis Praeparata), a hot herb, dispels cold and dampness. *Zhi Gan Cao* (Radix et Rhizoma Glycyrrhizae Praeparata cum Melle) and *Sheng Jiang* (Rhizoma Zingiberis Recens) harmonize the herbs in this formula. Overall, this formula effectively treats *bi zheng* (painful obstruction syndrome) with a constitutional deficiency of qi and blood, wind attacking the muscles and joints, and atrophy and impairment of the skeletal muscles.

Da Fang Feng Tang (Major Saposhnikovia Decoction)

Diagnosis	Signs and Symptoms	Treatment	Herbs
Li feng (dysenteric wind) and *he xi feng* (crane's knee wind)	• Trouble walking due to severe pain and atrophy of the leg muscles: *li feng* (dysenteric wind) characterized by severe deficiency of qi and blood • Severe atrophy of the leg muscles, severe pain and swelling of the knees with difficulty in knee flexion and extension: *he xi feng* (crane's knee wind) characterized by severe deficiency of qi and blood	• Tonifies qi and blood • Strengthens muscles and tendons • Dispels wind, cold, and dampness	• *Dang Gui* (Radix Angelicae Sinensis), *Shu Di Huang* (Radix Rehmanniae Praeparata), *Bai Shao* (Radix Paeoniae Alba), and *Chuan Xiong* (Rhizoma Chuanxiong) tonify the blood and activate blood circulation. • *Ren Shen* (Radix et Rhizoma Ginseng), *Bai Zhu* (Rhizoma Atractylodis Macrocephalae), and *Huang Qi* (Radix Astragali) tonify qi and strengthen the Spleen. • *Niu Xi* (Radix Achyranthis Bidentatae) and *Du Zhong* (Cortex Eucommiae) tonify the Kidney, nourish tendons and muscles, and relieve pain. • *Fang Feng* (Radix Saposhnikoviae) and *Qiang Huo* (Rhizoma et Radix Notopterygii) dispel wind and relieve numbness and joint pain. • *Fu Zi* (Radix Aconiti Lateralis Praeparata) dispels cold and dampness. • *Zhi Gan Cao* (Radix et Rhizoma Glycyrrhizae Praeparata cum Melle) and *Sheng Jiang* (Rhizoma Zingiberis Recens) harmonize the herbs.

1182

Chinese Herbal Formulas and Applications

Dà Fáng Fēng Tāng (Major Saposhnikovia Decoction)

MODIFICATIONS

For pain with blood stagnation, add *Tao Ren* (Semen Persicae) and *Hong Hua* (Flos Carthami).

CAUTIONS / CONTRAINDICATIONS

Da Fang Feng Tang is designed for musculoskeletal disorders caused by severe qi and blood deficiencies. Arthritis or musculoskeletal disorders characterized by excess without deficiency should not be treated with this formula as the warm and hot herbs may worsen the excessive condition.

PHARMACOLOGICAL EFFECTS

Antirheumatic: According to studies in mice, administration of *Da Fang Feng Tang* was associated with inhibiting iNOS expression and decreasing anti-collagen IgG antibody. The researchers suggested that *Da Fang Feng Tang* may be effective in treating rheumatoid arthritis in humans.[1,2]

References

1. Wang LR, Ishiguro N, Yamada E, Nishida Y, Sato K, Iwata H. The effect of da-fang-feng-tang on treatment of type II collagen-induced arthritis in DBA/1 mice. Am J Chin Med 1999;27(2):205-15.
2. Joe SM, Lee IS, Lee YT, Lee JH, Choi BT. Suppression of collagen-induced arthritis in rats by continuous administration of dae-bang-poong-tang (da-fang-feng-tang). Am J Chin Med 2001;29(2):355-65.

Jī Míng Sǎn (Powder to Take at Cock's Crow)

雞鳴散
鸡鸣散

Pinyin Name: *Ji Ming San*
Literal Name: Powder to Take at Cock's Crow
Alternate Names: *Chi Ming San*, Cock's Crow Powder, Areca Seed and Chaenomeles Formula
Original Source: *Lei Bian Zhu Shi Ji Yan Yi Fang* (Effective Medical Formulas Arranged by Category by Doctor Zhu) by Zhu Zuo in 1266

COMPOSITION

Bing Lang (Semen Arecae)	7 pieces [35g]
Mu Gua (Fructus Chaenomelis)	30g
Chen Pi (Pericarpium Citri Reticulatae)	30g
Zi Su Ye (Folium Perillae), including the twigs	9g
Jie Geng (Radix Platycodonis)	15g
Wu Zhu Yu (Fructus Evodiae)	6g
Sheng Jiang (Rhizoma Zingiberis Recens), including the peel	15g

DOSAGE / PREPARATION / ADMINISTRATION

The source text instructs to grind the ingredients into a coarse powder and cook it with 3 large bowls of water until it is reduced to 1.5 large bowls. Filter out the herbal residue and save the strained decoction. Cook the herbal residue again in 2 bowls of water until it is reduced to 1 bowl. Mix the two batches of strained decoction together, and take it at room temperature upon waking at 5 a.m. The decoction may be given warm during the winter. According to the source text, ingestion of this formula may induce black, watery stools, an indication of successful elimination of damp-cold from the Kidney.

Today, this formula is prepared as a decoction by cooking the ingredients twice, and mixing the two batches of decoction together. Take the decoction at room temperature on an empty stomach in the early morning.

CHINESE THERAPEUTIC ACTIONS

1. Activates qi circulation and causes turbidity to descend
2. Dispels cold and resolves dampness

CLINICAL MANIFESTATIONS

Leg *qi* characterized by dampness and cold: feeling of swelling, heaviness, weakness, numbness, coldness and

WIND-DAMP DISPELLING FORMULAS

17

1183

Chapter 17 – Wind-Damp Dispelling Formulas   *Section 2 – Damp-Cold Dispelling Formulas*

Jī Míng Sǎn (Powder to Take at Cock's Crow)

pain in the legs, fever, aversion to cold, spasms, chest stuffiness, and nausea.

CLINICAL APPLICATIONS

Beriberi, restless leg syndrome, filariasis, and edema.

EXPLANATION

Ji Ming San (Powder to Take at Cock's Crow) treats leg *qi* characterized by dampness and cold attacking the lower extremities. Leg *qi* usually originates from an invasion of exterior wind-cold, manifesting as irregularity in fluid metabolism and the formation of dampness and cold in the interior. The damp-cold factor then attacks the legs and obstructs the flow of qi and blood, causing swelling, heaviness, weakness, numbness, and pain in the lower legs. Fever and aversion to cold are symptoms deriving from exterior wind-cold attack. Chest stuffiness and nausea are the result of dampness obstructing the qi flow in the upper *jiao* and epigastrium.

Bing Lang (Semen Arecae), the chief herb of this formula, activates qi and dispels dampness. *Mu Gua* (Fructus Chaenomelis), the deputy herb, eliminates dampness and relaxes the muscles and tendons. *Chen Pi* (Pericarpium Citri Reticulatae), the other deputy herb, strengthens the Spleen, activates qi, and dispels dampness. *Zi Su Ye* (Folium Perillae) and *Jie Geng* (Radix Platycodonis) dispel exterior wind-cold and disperse interior qi stagnation. *Wu Zhu Yu* (Fructus Evodiae) and *Sheng Jiang* (Rhizoma Zingiberis Recens) warm and dissolve damp-cold to relieve nausea and chest stuffiness.

MODIFICATIONS

• With more exterior signs and symptoms, add *Gui Zhi* (Ramulus Cinnamomi) and *Fang Feng* (Radix Saposhnikoviae).

• With more cold and dampness in the interior, add *Rou Gui* (Cortex Cinnamomi) and *Fu Zi* (Radix Aconiti Lateralis Praeparata).

• With stifling sensations in the chest, lack of appetite, heavy sensations in the body, and a greasy tongue coating due to more dampness, add *Cang Zhu* (Rhizoma Atractylodis), *Fu Ling* (Poria), and *Hou Po* (Cortex Magnoliae Officinalis).

CAUTIONS / CONTRAINDICATIONS

• *Ji Ming San* treats leg *qi* characterized by damp-cold. It should not be used if the leg *qi* is caused by damp-heat.

• Use of this formula is contraindicated during pregnancy.[1]

• Use of this formula has been associated with such side effects as abdominal discomfort, nausea, vomiting, salivation, diarrhea, dizziness, and itching.[2]

CLINICAL STUDIES AND RESEARCH

1. **Edema**: According to one report, 27 patients with edema were treated with complete recovery in 22 cases and improvement in 5 cases. The herbal treatment contained *Ji Ming San* as the base formula, with the addition of *Fang Ji* (Radix Stephaniae Tetrandrae) and *Niu Xi* (Radix Achyranthis Bidentatae) for chronic illness; *Huang Qi* (Radix Astragali) for qi deficiency; and *Fu Zi* (Radix Aconiti Lateralis Praeparata) for yang deficiency.[3]

2. **Restless leg syndrome**: Use of *Ji Ming San* plus *Ji Xue Teng* (Caulis Spatholobi) was effective in treating all 27 patients with restless leg syndrome. The duration of treatment ranged from 3 to 12 days. Clinical improvements

Ji Ming San (Powder to Take at Cock's Crow)

Diagnosis	Signs and Symptoms	Treatment	Herbs
Leg *qi* characterized by dampness and cold	• Swelling, heaviness, weakness, numbness, and pain in the lower legs: damp-cold factor attacking the legs and obstructing qi and blood circulation • Fever and aversion to cold: exterior wind-cold • Chest stuffiness and nausea: dampness obstructing the qi flow in the upper *jiao* and epigastrium	• Activates qi circulation and causes turbidity to descend • Eliminates cold and dampness	• *Bing Lang* (Semen Arecae) activates qi and dispels dampness. • *Mu Gua* (Fructus Chaenomelis) eliminates dampness and relaxes the muscles and tendons. • *Chen Pi* (Pericarpium Citri Reticulatae) strengthens the Spleen, activates qi, and dispels dampness. • *Zi Su Ye* (Folium Perillae) and *Jie Geng* (Radix Platycodonis) dispel exterior wind-cold and disperse interior qi stagnation. • *Wu Zhu Yu* (Fructus Evodiae) and *Sheng Jiang* (Rhizoma Zingiberis Recens) warm and dissolve damp-cold.

1184

Jī Míng Sǎn (Powder to Take at Cock's Crow)

included resolution of all symptoms for at least 3 months on later follow-up.[4]

AUTHORS' COMMENTS

Ji Ming San, literally translated as "Powder to Take at Cock's Crow" is so named because this formula is most effective if taken early in the morning when the cock crows. When taken in early morning on an empty stomach, there is optimal absorption and fast onset of action. Furthermore, since yang qi begins to rise in the early morning, the effect of the herbs will follow yang qi and together dispel cold and dampness from the body.

References

1. *Zhong Yao Ming Fang Yao Li Yu Ying Yong* (Pharmacology and Applications of Famous Herbal Formulas) 1989;443-4.
2. *Zhong Yao Ming Fang Yao Li Yu Ying Yong* (Pharmacology and Applications of Famous Herbal Formulas) 1989;443-4.
3. *He Bei Zhong Yi* (Hebei Chinese Medicine) 1985;3:27.
4. *Liao Ning Zhong Yi Za Zhi* (Liaoning Journal of Chinese Medicine) 1994;5:27.

Chapter 17 – Wind-Damp Dispelling Formulas — *Section 3 – Damp-Heat Dispelling Formulas*

Section 3

燥湿清热剂
— Damp-Heat Dispelling Formulas

Gui Zhī Sháo Yào Zhī Mǔ Tāng
(Cinnamon Twig, Peony, and Anemarrhena Decoction)

桂枝芍藥知母湯
桂枝芍药知母汤

Pinyin Name: *Gui Zhi Shao Yao Zhi Mu Tang*
Literal Name: Cinnamon Twig, Peony, and Anemarrhena Decoction
Alternate Names: *Kuei Chih Shao Yao Chih Mu Tang*, Cinnamon and Anemarrhena Combination
Original Source: *Jin Gui Yao Lue* (Essentials from the Golden Cabinet) by Zhang Zhong-Jing in the Eastern Han Dynasty

COMPOSITION

Gui Zhi (Ramulus Cinnamomi)	12g
Ma Huang (Herba Ephedrae)	6g
Fang Feng (Radix Saposhnikoviae)	12g
Fu Zi (Radix Aconiti Lateralis Praeparata), *pao* (blast-fried)	6g
Bai Shao (Radix Paeoniae Alba)	9g
Zhi Mu (Rhizoma Anemarrhenae)	12g
Gan Cao (Radix et Rhizoma Glycyrrhizae)	6g
Bai Zhu (Rhizoma Atractylodis Macrocephalae)	15g
Sheng Jiang (Rhizoma Zingiberis Recens)	15g

DOSAGE / PREPARATION / ADMINISTRATION

The source text instructs to cook the ingredients in 7 cups [1,400 mL] of water until the liquid is reduced to 2 cups [400 mL]. Take 0.7 cup [210 mL] of the warm, strained decoction three times daily.

CHINESE THERAPEUTIC ACTIONS

1. Dispels wind-dampness
2. Clears heat
3. Unblocks the channels and collaterals

CLINICAL MANIFESTATIONS

Bi zheng (painful obstruction syndrome) caused by obstruction of wind-dampness and formation of heat: swollen and painful joints, emaciation, swollen feet, dizziness, shortness of breath, atrophy of the muscle, numbness of the extremities, and difficulty in walking and moving.

CLINICAL APPLICATIONS

Arthritis, rheumatoid arthritis, gouty arthritis, periarthritis of the shoulders, sciatica, and connective tissue disorders.

EXPLANATION

Gui Zhi Shao Yao Zhi Mu Tang (Cinnamon Twig, Peony, and Anemarrhena Decoction) treats *bi zheng* (painful obstruction syndrome) caused by accumulation of wind-dampness. Obstruction of wind-dampness in the joints leads to the formation of heat, manifesting as joint swelling and pain. The obstruction also blocks the supply of blood and nutrients to the area, thus contributing to the gradual atrophy of the muscles and numbness of the extremities. The muscle atrophy is sometimes so severe that *he xi feng* (crane's knee wind) is used to describe the condition in which the joint appears to be covered by nothing but the skin. Swelling, pain, and muscle atrophy all contribute to difficulty in walking and moving. In patients with chronic *bi zheng* (painful obstruction syndrome), dampness may

1186

Chinese Herbal Formulas and Applications

Guī Zhī Sháo Yào Zhī Mǔ Tāng
(Cinnamon Twig, Peony, and Anemarrhena Decoction)

Gui Zhi Shao Yao Zhi Mu Tang (Cinnamon Twig, Peony, and Anemarrhena Decoction)

Diagnosis	Signs and Symptoms	Treatment	Herbs
Bi zheng (painful obstruction syndrome) caused by wind-damp-ness and heat	• Joint swelling and pain: obstruction of wind-dampness with formation of heat • Atrophy of the muscles and numbness of the extremities with difficulty in walking and moving: lack of nourishment due to obstructions • Edema, decreased appetite, weight loss, emaciation, shortness of breath, and dizziness: accumulation of dampness in various parts of the body	• Dispels wind-dampness • Clears heat • Unblocks the channels and collaterals	• *Gui Zhi* (Ramulus Cinnamomi), *Ma Huang* (Herba Ephedrae) and *Fang Feng* (Radix Saposhnikoviae) dispel wind from the exterior. • *Fu Zi* (Radix Aconiti Lateralis Praeparata) warms the body and joints and relieves pain. • *Zhi Mu* (Rhizoma Anemarrhenae) clears heat and reduces swelling. • *Bai Shao* (Radix Paeoniae Alba) and *Gan Cao* (Radix et Rhizoma Glycyrrhizae) relieve muscle spasms and cramps. • *Bai Zhu* (Rhizoma Atractylodis Macrocephalae) strengthens the Spleen, dries dampness, and relieves edema. • *Sheng Jiang* (Rhizoma Zingiberis Recens) warms the middle *jiao* to improve appetite and increase food intake.

affect other parts of the body. Damp accumulation in the lower extremities leads to edema; damp stagnation in the middle *jiao* leads to decreased appetite, weight loss and emaciation; and dampness obstructs the normal flow of qi, leading to shortness of breath and dizziness.

In this formula, *Gui Zhi* (Ramulus Cinnamomi) and *Ma Huang* (Herba Ephedrae) warm and unblock the channels and collaterals. These two herbs, along with *Fang Feng* (Radix Saposhnikoviae), also dispel wind from the exterior parts of the body. *Fu Zi* (Radix Aconiti Lateralis Praeparata) warms the body and joints and relieves pain. Because *Fu Zi* (Radix Aconiti Lateralis Praeparata) is an extremely hot herb, cold herbs such as *Bai Shao* (Radix Paeoniae Alba) and *Zhi Mu* (Rhizoma Anemarrhenae) are used to balance the temperature of the formula and reduce any side effects that might be caused by *Fu Zi* (Radix Aconiti Lateralis Praeparata). Additionally, *Zhi Mu* (Rhizoma Anemarrhenae) clears heat and reduces swelling. *Bai Shao* (Radix Paeoniae Alba) and *Gan Cao* (Radix et Rhizoma Glycyrrhizae) synergistically relieve pain and treat muscle spasms and cramps. *Bai Zhu* (Rhizoma Atractylodis Macrocephalae) strengthens the Spleen, dries dampness, and relieves edema. *Sheng Jiang* (Rhizoma Zingiberis Recens) warms the middle *jiao* to improve appetite and increase food intake.

MODIFICATIONS

• With stiffness and pain of the joints that lessen with heat, increase the dose of *Gui Zhi* (Ramulus Cinnamomi), *Ma Huang* (Herba Ephedrae), and *Fu Zi* (Radix Aconiti Lateralis Praeparata).

• With body aches, numbness, and joint swelling that worsen in rainy, cold weather, add more *Bai Zhu* (Rhizoma Atractylodis Macrocephalae) and *Fu Zi* (Radix Aconiti Lateralis Praeparata).

• With burning joint pain that lessens during the day and worsens at night, add more *Zhi Mu* (Rhizoma Anemarrhenae), *Bai Shao* (Radix Paeoniae Alba), and *Gan Cao* (Radix et Rhizoma Glycyrrhizae).

• For *bi zheng* (painful obstruction syndrome) with more damp accumulation, add *Fu Ling* (Poria), *Yi Yi Ren* (Semen Coicis), and *Cang Zhu* (Rhizoma Atractylodis).

• With frequent recurrence of pain due to qi deficiency, add *Huang Qi* (Radix Astragali).

RELATED FORMULA

Sāng Zhī Shí Gāo Zhī Mǔ Tāng

(Mulberry Twig, Gypsum, and Anemarrhena Decoction)

桑枝石膏知母湯
桑枝石膏知母汤

Pinyin Name: *Sang Zhi Shi Gao Zhi Mu Tang*

Literal Name: Mulberry Twig, Gypsum, and Anemarrhena Decoction

Original Source: *An Hui Zhong Yi Xue Yuan* (Anhui University School of Medicine) in 1990

WIND-DAMP DISPELLING FORMULAS

17

1187

Chapter 17 – Wind-Damp Dispelling Formulas   Section 3 – Damp-Heat Dispelling Formulas

Guì Zhī Sháo Yào Zhī Mǔ Tāng
(Cinnamon Twig, Peony, and Anemarrhena Decoction)

Sang Zhi (Ramulus Mori)

Zhi Mu (Rhizoma Anemarrhenae)

Cang Zhu (Rhizoma Atractylodis)

Huang Bo (Cortex Phellodendri Chinensis)

Dang Gui (Radix Angelicae Sinensis)

Qiang Huo (Rhizoma et Radix Notopterygii)

Shi Gao (Gypsum Fibrosum)

Du Huo (Radix Angelicae Pubescentis)

Wei Ling Xian (Radix et Rhizoma Clematidis)

Fang Ji (Radix Stephaniae Tetrandrae)

Yi Yi Ren (Semen Coicis)

Luo Shi Teng (Caulis Trachelospermi)

Wu Jia Pi (Cortex Acanthopanacis)

Chi Shao (Radix Paeoniae Rubra)

Qin Jiao (Radix Gentianae Macrophyllae)

Huang Qin (Radix Scutellariae)

Sang Zhi Shi Gao Zhi Mu Tang (Mulberry Twig, Gypsum, and Anemarrhena Decoction) treats *bi zheng* (painful obstruction syndrome) caused by wind, heat, and dampness. This formula dispels wind-dampness, clears heat, unblocks the channels and collaterals, and relieves pain. Clinical applications include rheumatic heat disorders, arthritis, arthralgia, gout, fibromyalgia, and other joint disorders with heat manifestations of swelling, burning sensations, and inflammation.

Èr Miào Sǎn (Two-Marvel Powder)
二妙散

Pinyin Name: *Er Miao San*

Literal Name: Two-Marvel Powder

Original Source: *Dan Xi Xin Fa* (Teachings of [Zhu] Dan-Xi) by Zhu Zhen-Heng in 1481

COMPOSITION

Huang Bo (Cortex Phellodendri Chinensis), *chao* (dry-fried)	15g
Cang Zhu (Rhizoma Atractylodis), *jin* (soaked) in rice water and *chao* (dry-fried)	15g

DOSAGE / PREPARATION / ADMINISTRATION

The source text instructions are to soak *Cang Zhu* (Rhizoma Atractylodis) in rice water first. Dry-fry equal amounts of both herbs, and then grind them into powder. Take the powder with boiled water and fresh juice of *Sheng Jiang* (Rhizoma Zingiberis Recens). Today, this formula is prepared by grinding equal amounts of the ingredients into powder. Take 6g per dose two to three times daily. It may also be prepared as a decoction with the doses suggested in brackets.

CHINESE THERAPEUTIC ACTIONS

Clears heat and dries dampness

CLINICAL MANIFESTATIONS

Damp-heat attacking the lower half of the body: aches and pains in the bones and tendons; leg weakness and atrophy; redness, swelling, and pain of the knees with burning sensations; leukorrhea characterized by damp-heat; sores in the lower body characterized by damp-heat; scanty, yellow urine; and a yellow, greasy tongue coating.

CLINICAL APPLICATIONS

Arthritis, gouty arthritis, ankylosing spondylitis, neurodermatitis, eczema, erythromelalgia, and fungal infection.

EXPLANATION

Er Miao San (Two-Marvel Powder) treats *bi zheng* (painful obstruction syndrome) in the lower half of the body due to damp-heat. Damp-heat may attack the bones and tendons, causing aches and pains with redness, swelling, and burning sensations. Chronic cases of damp-heat may contribute to weakness and atrophy of the leg muscles. Damp-heat may also affect the *dai* (girdle) channel and genital region, causing leukorrhea and sores. Lastly, damp-heat may also interfere with the urinary system, causing scanty, yellow urine. A yellow, greasy tongue coating is a sign of damp-heat in the body.

Huang Bo (Cortex Phellodendri Chinensis), with its tendency to travel to the lower body, clears heat and dries dampness. *Cang Zhu* (Rhizoma Atractylodis), bitter and

1188

Chinese Herbal Formulas and Applications

Èr Miào Sǎn (Two-Marvel Powder)

Er Miao San (Two-Marvel Powder)

Diagnosis	Signs and Symptoms	Treatment	Herbs
Damp-heat attacking the lower body	• Aches and pains with redness, swelling, and burning sensations: damp-heat attacking the bones and tendons • Weakness and atrophy of the leg muscles: damp-heat accumulation blocking nourishment to the muscles • Leukorrhea and scanty, yellow urine: damp-heat affecting the lower body • Yellow, greasy tongue coating: damp-heat in the body	Clears heat and dries dampness	• *Huang Bo* (Cortex Phellodendri Chinensis) clears heat and dries dampness in the lower *jiao*. • *Cang Zhu* (Rhizoma Atractylodis) strengthens the Spleen and dries dampness.

warm, also dries dampness. *Er Miao San* contains only two herbs, yet it achieves marvelous results, which is why it is named "Two-Marvel Powder."

MODIFICATIONS

- For *bi zheng* (painful obstruction syndrome) with more heat than dampness, add *Huang Lian* (Rhizoma Coptidis), *Long Dan* (Radix et Rhizoma Gentianae), and *Ku Shen* (Radix Sophorae Flavescentis).
- For *bi zheng* (painful obstruction syndrome) with more dampness than heat, add *Hua Shi* (Talcum), *Fang Ji* (Radix Stephaniae Tetrandrae), and *Tong Cao* (Medulla Tetrapanacis).
- For *wei zheng* (atrophy syndrome) caused by damp-heat, add *Xi Xian Cao* (Herba Siegesbeckiae), *Wu Jia Pi* (Cortex Acanthopanacis), and *Lu Xian Cao* (Herba Pyrolae).
- For leg *qi* caused by damp-heat, add *Yi Yi Ren* (Semen Coicis), *Mu Gua* (Fructus Chaenomelis), and *Bing Lang* (Semen Arecae).
- With redness and swelling of the joints, add *Ren Dong Teng* (Caulis Lonicerae Japonicae), *Mu Gua* (Fructus Chaenomelis), and *Qin Jiao* (Radix Gentianae Macrophyllae).

CAUTIONS / CONTRAINDICATIONS

- *Er Miao San* is indicated for *bi zheng* (painful obstruction syndrome) with equal amounts of heat and dampness. Modification is needed if the amount of heat and dampness are not the same.
- This formula is contraindicated in patients with Liver and Kidney yin deficiencies, or with body fluids consumed by Lung heat.
- Avoid foods that are sweet, fatty, or greasy.[1]

CLINICAL STUDIES AND RESEARCH

1. **Arthritis**: Modified *Er Miao San* was used to treat 278 patients with various types of arthritis. Modifications

included: *Jin Yin Hua* (Flos Lonicerae Japonicae), *Pu Gong Ying* (Herba Taraxaci), *Zi Hua Di Ding* (Herba Violae), and *Tu Fu Ling* (Rhizoma Smilacis Glabrae) were added for arthritis with heat characterized by redness, inflammation, swelling, and pain; *Yi Yi Ren* (Semen Coicis), *Bai Hua She She Cao* (Herba Hedyotis), and larger doses of *Tu Fu Ling* (Rhizoma Smilacis Glabrae) and *Huang Bo* (Cortex Phellodendri Chinensis) were added for arthritis with damp-heat and toxins characterized by red spots; *Di Huang* (Radix Rehmanniae) and *Mu Dan Pi* (Cortex Moutan) were added for arthritis with yin-deficient heat characterized by a red tongue and a fine, rapid pulse; *Che Qian Cao* (Herba Plantaginis), *Fang Ji* (Radix Stephaniae Tetrandrae), and *Yi Yi Ren* (Semen Coicis) were added for accumulation of fluids in the joints. Out of 278 patients, the study reported complete recovery in 160 cases, significant improvement in 62 cases, moderate improvement in 44 cases, and no effect in 12 cases.[2]

2. **Gouty arthritis**: Use of modified *Er Miao San* topically and *San Miao Wan* (Three-Marvel Pill) orally was effective in treating acute gouty arthritis. The treatment protocol was to apply *Er Miao San* plus *Du Huo* (Radix Angelicae Pubescentis) and *Fu Rong Ye* (Folium Hibisci) topically to the affected area, and ingest *San Miao Wan* (Three-Marvel Pill) orally. The study reported that most people experienced a reduction of the symptoms (redness, swelling, and pain of the joints) within 1-2 days, and complete recovery within 5 days.[3]

3. **Ankylosing spondylitis**: Sixteen patients with ankylosing spondylitis characterized by damp-heat were effectively treated with an integrative approach using non-steroidal anti-inflammatory drugs, acupuncture, massage, and modified *Er Miao San*. The herbal formula contained *Cang Zhu* (Rhizoma Atractylodis), *Huang Bo* (Cortex Phellodendri Chinensis), *Sang Ji Sheng* (Herba Taxilli), *Gan Cao* (Radix et Rhizoma Glycyrrhizae), *Qin Jiao* (Radix

WIND-DAMP DISPELLING FORMULAS

17

1189

Èr Miào Sǎn (Two-Marvel Powder)

Gentianae Macrophyllae), *Fang Ji* (Radix Stephaniae Tetrandrae), *Gou Ji* (Rhizoma Cibotii), *Shi Nan Teng* (Ramulus Piper), and *Xu Chang Qing* (Radix et Rhizoma Cynanchi Paniculati). The researchers noted that the integrative treatment was better than any one treatment alone.[4] Note: Details of the integrative treatment were not available at the time of publication.

4. **Neurodermatitis**: An integrative treatment effectively treated 65 patients with neurodermatitis within an average of 7 days. The treatment protocol used modified *Er Miao San* as a topical herbal wash, followed by topical application of a mixture of dexamethasone, chloramphenicol, and rubbing alcohol. This treatment was repeated every other day.[5]

5. **Eczema**: In one study of 68 eczema patients, the use of *Er Miao San* was associated with a 47.06% rate of complete recovery and a 33.8% rate of improvement. The overall effectiveness was 80.86%.[6]

6. **Erythromelalgia**: Use of modified *Er Miao San* for 6 days was associated with 92.67% effectiveness in treating 176 patients with paroxysmal vasodilation with burning pain, increased skin temperature, and redness of the feet and hands. The herbal formula contained *Huang Bo* (Cortex Phellodendri Chinensis), *Cang Zhu* (Rhizoma Atractylodis), *Chuan Niu Xi* (Radix Cyathulae), *Fang Ji* (Radix Stephaniae Tetrandrae), and *Bai Zhi* (Radix Angelicae Dahuricae).[7]

7. **Fungal infection**: One study reported satisfactory results using modified *Er Miao San* topically to treat fungal infection on the feet. The herbal formula contained *Ku Shen* (Radix Sophorae Flavescentis), *Bai Fan* (Alumen), *Zi Cao* (Radix Arnebiae), and *Xu Chang Qing* (Radix et Rhizoma Cynanchi Paniculati). The herbs were cooked in water, and the resultant solution was used as an herbal soak. The patients were instructed to soak the affected area in the herbal solution for 20-30 minutes twice daily in the morning and at night.[8]

RELATED FORMULAS

Sān Miào Wán (Three-Marvel Pill)

三妙丸

Pinyin Name: San Miao Wan
Literal Name: Three-Marvel Pill
Alternate Names: *San Miao San* (Three-Marvel Powder), Atractylodes and Phellodendron Formula
Original Source: *Yi Xue Zheng Zhuan* (True Lineage of Medicine) by Yu Tian-Min in 1515

Huang Bo (Cortex Phellodendri Chinensis), *ban* (blended) with liquor and *chao* (dry-fried)   120g [12g]

Cang Zhu (Rhizoma Atractylodis), *jin* (soaked) in rice water for 1-2 nights and *bei* (stone-baked) to dry	180g [18g]
Chuan Niu Xi (Radix Cyathulae)	60g [6g]

The source text instructs to grind the ingredients into powder and form into small pills with flour. The pills should resemble the size of *Wu Tong Zi* (Semen Firmianae), a small seed approximately 5 mm in diameter. Take 50-70 pills on an empty stomach with a decoction made from salt and *Sheng Jiang* (Rhizoma Zingiberis Recens). Today, this formula may be prepared as a decoction with the doses suggested in brackets.

San Miao Wan (Three-Marvel Pill) clears heat and dries dampness, and is indicated for damp-heat affecting the lower half of the body. Patients may have joint pain, leg numbness, and burning sensations. Clinical applications include rheumatism, arthritis, beriberi, rashes, and eczema.

Sì Miào Wán (Four-Marvel Pill)

四妙丸

Pinyin Name: Si Miao Wan
Literal Name: Four-Marvel Pill
Alternate Name: *Si Miao San* (Four-Marvel Powder)
Original Source: *Cheng Fang Bian Du* (Convenient Reader of Established Formulas) by Zhang Bing-Cheng in 1904

Huang Bo (Cortex Phellodendri Chinensis)	[12g]
Yi Yi Ren (Semen Coicis)	[12g]
Cang Zhu (Rhizoma Atractylodis)	[12g]
Niu Xi (Radix Achyranthis Bidentatae)	[12g]

The source text instructs to grind the ingredients into powder and form into small pills with water. Take 6-9g of pills per dose with warm water. Today, this formula may be prepared as a decoction with the doses suggested in brackets.

Si Miao Wan (Four-Marvel Pill) clears heat and dissolves dampness, and is good for treating damp-heat affecting the lower half of the body. Patients may show pain and swelling of the joints, muscle atrophy, and leg numbness.

AUTHORS' COMMENTS

Er Miao San (Two-Marvel Powder), *San Miao Wan* (Three-Marvel Pill), and *Si Miao Wan* (Four-Marvel Pill) all treat musculoskeletal disorders characterized by damp-heat attacking the lower half of the body.

Chinese Herbal Formulas and Applications

Èr Miào Săn (Two-Marvel Powder)

- *Er Miao San* is the original formula that contains two herbs with equal emphasis on eliminating both dampness and heat.
- *San Miao Wan* is formulated with the addition of *Chuan Niu Xi* (Radix Cyathulae), which guides the formula to the lower parts of the body and tonifies the Liver and Kidney.
- *Si Miao Wan* is formulated with the addition of *Niu Xi* (Radix Achyranthis Bidentatae) and *Yi Yi Ren* (Semen Coicis), to tonify the Liver and Kidney and dry dampness. Of the three, this formula is most suitable for chronic cases of damp-heat affecting the lower half of the body, causing numbness and atrophy.

References

1. *Zhong Yao Ming Fang Yao Li Yu Ying Yong* (Pharmacology and Applications of Famous Herbal Formulas) 1989;416-7.
2. *Shi Yong Zhong Yi Nei Ke Za Zhi* (Journal of Practical Chinese Internal Medicine) 1997;2:36.
3. *Si Chuan Zhong Yi* (Sichuan Chinese Medicine) 1997;11:47.
4. *Xin Zhong Yi* (New Chinese Medicine) 1994;7:24.
5. *Zhong Yuan Yi Kan* (Resource Journal of Chinese Medicine) 1990;4:12.
6. *Zhe Jiang Zhong Yi Za Zhi* (Zhejiang Journal of Chinese Medicine) 1983;10:468.
7. *Hu Nan Zhong Yi Za Zhi* (Hunan Journal of Chinese Medicine) 1987;5:24.
8. *Shan Dong Zhong Yi Za Zhi* (Shandong Journal of Chinese Medicine) 1989;8(4):50.

Dāng Guī Niăn Tòng Tāng (Tangkuei Decoction to Lift the Pain)

當歸拈痛湯
当归拈痛汤

Pinyin Name: *Dang Gui Nian Tong Tang*
Literal Name: Tangkuei Decoction to Lift the Pain
Alternate Names: *Tang Kuei Nien Tung Tang*, Tang-kuei and Pain-Assuaging Decoction, Tangkuei and Anemarrhena Combination
Original Source: *Lan Shi Mi Cang* (Secrets from the Orchid Chamber) by Li Gao in 1336

COMPOSITION

Qiang Huo (Rhizoma et Radix Notopterygii)	15g
Ge Gen (Radix Puerariae Lobatae)	6g
Fang Feng (Radix Saposhnikoviae)	9g
Sheng Ma (Rhizoma Cimicifugae)	6g
Huang Qin (Radix Scutellariae), *xi* (washed) with liquor	9g
Ku Shen (Radix Sophorae Flavescentis), *chao* (dry-fried) in liquor	6g
Zhi Mu (Rhizoma Anemarrhenae), *xi* (washed) with liquor	9g
Yin Chen (Herba Artemisiae Scopariae), *xi* (washed) with liquor	15g
Ze Xie (Rhizoma Alismatis)	9g
Zhu Ling (Polyporus)	9g
Bai Zhu (Rhizoma Atractylodis Macrocephalae)	4.5g
Cang Zhu (Rhizoma Atractylodis)	6g
Ren Shen (Radix et Rhizoma Ginseng)	6g
Dang Gui (Radix Angelicae Sinensis)	9g
Zhi Gan Cao (Radix et Rhizoma Glycyrrhizae Praeparata cum Melle)	15g

DOSAGE / PREPARATION / ADMINISTRATION

The source text instructs to grind the ingredients into a coarse powder. Cook 30g of the powder in 2.5 bowls of water until the liquid is reduced to 1 bowl. Take the strained decoction while warm.

CHINESE THERAPEUTIC ACTIONS

1. Dispels wind and dampness
2. Clears heat and relieves pain

WIND-DAMP DISPELLING FORMULAS

17

1191

Chapter 17 – Wind-Damp Dispelling Formulas   Section 3 – Damp-Heat Dispelling Formulas

Dāng Guī Niǎn Tòng Tāng (Tangkuei Decoction to Lift the Pain)

CLINICAL MANIFESTATIONS

Dampness and heat affecting the joints and extremities: joint or musculoskeletal pain with redness, swelling, and inflammation; heavy sensation in the shoulders and back; fullness in the chest and epigastrium; dermatological disorders in the lower extremities with itching and pain; skin ulceration and abscess; and a deep, tight pulse.

CLINICAL APPLICATIONS

Arthritis and arthralgia with inflammation and swelling, gout, generalized joint and musculoskeletal pain, neurodermatitis, dermatitis in the lower extremities, genital itching, gonorrhea, dysuria, hematuria, sciatica, trigeminal nerve pain, neuritis, polyneuritis, neuralgia, and impetigo herpetiformis.

EXPLANATION

Dang Gui Nian Tong Tang (Tangkuei Decoction to Lift the Pain) is one of the most effective formulas for treating damp-heat joint and musculoskeletal disorders with pain, redness, swelling, and inflammation. Due to the damp nature of the illness, patients may experience heavy sensations in the shoulders and back and fullness in the chest and epigastrium. Due to the nature of heat, patients may experience redness, swelling, and inflammation in the joints and muscles. Moreover, as dampness and heat travel downward, patients may feel itching and pain in the lower extremities. In severe cases, there may also be ulceration and abscess of the skin.

In this formula, *Qiang Huo* (Rhizoma et Radix Notopterygii), *Ge Gen* (Radix Puerariae Lobatae), *Fang Feng* (Radix Saposhnikoviae), and *Sheng Ma* (Rhizoma Cimicifugae) dispel wind and dampness to relieve pain. *Huang Qin* (Radix Scutellariae), *Ku Shen* (Radix Sophorae Flavescentis), *Zhi Mu* (Rhizoma Anemarrhenae), and *Yin Chen* (Herba Artemisiae Scopariae) eliminate damp-heat from the body. *Ze Xie* (Rhizoma Alismatis) and *Zhu Ling* (Polyporus) resolve dampness and promote diuresis. *Bai Zhu* (Rhizoma Atractylodis Macrocephalae) and *Cang Zhu* (Rhizoma Atractylodis) strengthen the Spleen and dry dampness. *Ren Shen* (Radix et Rhizoma Ginseng) and *Dang Gui* (Radix Angelicae Sinensis) tonify qi and blood to facilitate recovery. *Zhi Gan Cao* (Radix et Rhizoma Glycyrrhizae Praeparata cum Melle) harmonizes the herbs in this formula.

MODIFICATIONS

- With redness, swelling, and inflammation, add *Huang Lian* (Rhizoma Coptidis) and *Shi Gao* (Gypsum Fibrosum).
- With severe pain in the joints and extremities, add *Gui Zhi* (Ramulus Cinnamomi) and *Bai Shao* (Radix Paeoniae Alba).
- With itching and pain of the skin, add *Jin Yin Hua* (Flos Lonicerae Japonicae) and *Lian Qiao* (Fructus Forsythiae).
- With severe swelling of the knees and legs, add *Fang Ji* (Radix Stephaniae Tetrandrae) and *Mu Gua* (Fructus Chaenomelis).

Dang Gui Nian Tong Tang (Tangkuei Decoction to Lift the Pain)

Diagnosis	Signs and Symptoms	Treatment	Herbs
Dampness and heat affecting the joints and extremities	• Feeling of heaviness and fullness: damp accumulation in the body • Redness, swelling, and inflammation in the joints and muscles: heat affecting the joints and muscles • Itching and pain in the lower extremities: damp-heat traveling downward • Skin ulceration and abscess: damp-heat traveling outward • Deep, tight pulse: damp-heat condition	• Dispels wind and dampness • Clears heat and relieves pain	• *Qiang Huo* (Rhizoma et Radix Notopterygii), *Ge Gen* (Radix Puerariae Lobatae), *Fang Feng* (Radix Saposhnikoviae), and *Sheng Ma* (Rhizoma Cimicifugae) dispel wind and dampness to relieve pain. • *Huang Qin* (Radix Scutellariae), *Ku Shen* (Radix Sophorae Flavescentis), *Zhi Mu* (Rhizoma Anemarrhenae), and *Yin Chen* (Herba Artemisiae Scopariae) eliminate damp-heat from the body. • *Ze Xie* (Rhizoma Alismatis) and *Zhu Ling* (Polyporus) resolve dampness. • *Bai Zhu* (Rhizoma Atractylodis Macrocephalae) and *Cang Zhu* (Rhizoma Atractylodis) strengthen the Spleen and dry dampness. • *Ren Shen* (Radix et Rhizoma Ginseng) and *Dang Gui* (Radix Angelicae Sinensis) tonify qi and blood. • *Zhi Gan Cao* (Radix et Rhizoma Glycyrrhizae Praeparata cum Melle) harmonizes the herbs.

1192

Dāng Guī Niǎn Tòng Tāng (Tangkuei Decoction to Lift the Pain)

- With body aches, add *Jiang Huang* (Rhizoma Curcumae Longae) and *Hai Tong Pi* (Cortex Erythrinae).
- With severe swelling and pain due to damp-heat, combine with *Huang Lian Jie Du Tang* (Coptis Decoction to Relieve Toxicity).
- With skin ulceration and abscess, combine with *Tuo Li Xiao Du Yin* (Drain the Interior and Detoxify Decoction).

CAUTIONS / CONTRAINDICATIONS

Avoid foods that are spicy, pungent, oily, or greasy.[1]

PHARMACOLOGICAL EFFECTS

Anti-inflammatory: Administration of *Dang Gui Nian Tong Tang* or *Du Huo Ji Sheng Tang* (Angelica Pubescens and Taxillus Decoction) was associated with a marked anti-inflammatory effect to suppress the development of chronic arthritis induced by carrageenan or complete Freund's adjuvant. The researchers suggested that these herbal formulas may be considered as alternatives for non-steroid anti-inflammatory drugs (NSAIDS).[2]

CLINICAL STUDIES AND RESEARCH

1. **Neurodermatitis**: Use of modified *Dang Gui Nian Tong Tang* in 30 patients was associated with complete recovery in 22 cases, improvement in 7 cases, and no effect in 1 case.[3]
2. **Impetigo herpetiformis**: One study of 86 patients with impetigo herpetiformis reported good results using modified *Dang Gui Nian Tong Tang* both internally and topically. The herbal treatment had the following modifications: for early-stage, during the eruption of lesions, *Bai Zhi* (Radix Angelicae Dahuricae) and *Dang Shen* (Radix Codonopsis) were removed, and *Tu Fu Ling* (Rhizoma Smilacis Glabrae), *Zi Hua Di Ding* (Herba Violae), *Ye Ju Hua* (Flos Chrysanthemi Indici), and *Jin Yin Hua* (Flos Lonicerae Japonicae) were added; during healing, *Di Fu Zi* (Fructus Kochiae) and *Chan Tui* (Periostracum Cicadae) were added to relieve itching. The treatment protocol was to cook the herbs in water two separate times and drink the decoction orally. The herb residue was cooked in water a third time and the resultant solution used as an herbal wash to the affected area. The study reported complete recovery in all 86 patients within 12 packs of herbs.[4]
3. **Rash**: Use of modified *Dang Gui Nian Tong Tang* in 47 patients with rash was associated with complete recovery in 38 cases, significant improvement in 5 cases, moderate improvement in 2 cases, and no effect in 2 cases. The duration of treatment ranged from 5 to 32 packs of herbs.[5]

4. **Gout**: One study reported 90% effectiveness using modified *Dang Gui Nian Tong Tang* to treat gout in 40 patients. The herbal formula contained *Dang Gui Nian Tong Tang* plus *Hu Zhang* (Rhizoma et Radix Polygoni Cuspidati), *Song Jie* (Lignum Pini Nodi), *Mu Gua* (Fructus Chaenomelis), and *Ren Dong Teng* (Caulis Lonicerae Japonicae). The duration of treatment ranged from 20-98 days, with most showing symptomatic improvements after 33-40 days and normalization of plasma uric acid levels after 90 days. Of 40 patients, the study reported complete recovery in 7 cases, improvement in 29 cases, and no response in 4 cases.[6]
5. *Bi zheng* **(painful obstruction syndrome)**: *Dang Gui Nian Tong Tang* has been shown to effectively treat musculoskeletal pain affecting various parts of the body, including shoulders, arms, and legs.[7,8,9,10]

RELATED FORMULA

Niǎn Tòng Tāng (Lift the Pain Decoction)

拈痛湯
拈痛汤

Pinyin Name: *Nian Tong Tang*
Literal Name: Lift the Pain Decoction
Original Source: *Yi Xue Qi Yuan* (Origins of the Medicine) by Zhang Yuan-Su in the Yuan Dynasty

Qiang Huo (Rhizoma et Radix Notopterygii)	15g
Gan Cao (Radix et Rhizoma Glycyrrhizae)	15g
Yin Chen (Herba Artemisiae Scopariae), *chao* (dry-fried) with liquor	15g
Fang Feng (Radix Saposhnikoviae)	9g
Cang Zhu (Rhizoma Atractylodis)	9g
Dang Gui (Radix Angelicae Sinensis)	9g
Zhi Mu (Rhizoma Anemarrhenae), *xi* (washed) with liquor	9g
Zhu Ling (Polyporus)	9g
Ze Xie (Rhizoma Alismatis)	9g
Sheng Ma (Rhizoma Cimicifugae)	3g
Bai Zhu (Rhizoma Atractylodis Macrocephalae)	3g
Huang Qin (Radix Scutellariae), *chao* (dry-fried)	3g
Ge Gen (Radix Puerariae Lobatae)	6g
Ren Shen (Radix et Rhizoma Ginseng)	6g
Ku Shen (Radix Sophorae Flavescentis), *jin* (soaked) in liquor	6g

The source text instructs to grind the herbs into powder. Cook 30g of the powder in water, and take the strained decoction while warm. *Nian Tong Tang* (Lift the Pain Decoction) is designed to treat damp-heat affecting the limbs and joints, with clinical manifestations such as swelling and pain in the limbs, heavy sensations in the shoulders and back, and discomfort in the chest and diaphragm.

Dāng Guī Niǎn Tòng Tāng (Tangkuei Decoction to Lift the Pain)

These two formulas have similar names and ingredients, and essentially have the same clinical applications. They are listed here to reflect both source texts that cited these two formulas.

AUTHORS' COMMENTS

According to Dr. Chang Wei-Yen, *re bi* (heat painful obstruction) can be effectively treated with *Dang Gui Nian Tong Tang*, and the addition of *Da Ding Huang* (Caulis Euonymi), *Shen Jin Cao* (Herba Lycopodii), and *Tou Gu Cao* (Caulis Impatientis).

References

1. *Zhong Yao Ming Fang Yao Li Yu Ying Yong* (Pharmacology and Applications of Famous Herbal Formulas) 1989;426-8.

2. Lin CC, Chen MF, Chen CF. The anti-inflammatory effects of Chinese crude drug prescriptions on experimental arthritis. Am J Chin Med 1995;23(2):145-52.

3. *Hu Nan Zhong Yi Za Zhi* (Hunan Journal of Chinese Medicine) 1992;8(4):42.

4. *Hu Nan Zhong Yi Za Zhi* (Hunan Journal of Chinese Medicine) 1990;6(6):42.

5. *Hu Bei Zhong Yi Za Zhi* (Hubei Journal of Chinese Medicine) 1986;1:21.

6. *Zhong Yi Za Zhi* (Journal of Chinese Medicine) 1987;28(2):60.

7. *Si Chuan Zhong Yi* (Sichuan Chinese Medicine) 1986;4(1):44.

8. *Ji Lin Zhong Yi Yao* (Jilin Chinese Medicine and Herbology) 1989;2:33.

9. *Hei Long Jiang Zhong Yi Yao* (Heilongjiang Chinese Medicine and Herbology) 1986;6:43.

10. *He Bei Zhong Yi* (Hebei Chinese Medicine) 1993;15(5):33.

Chinese Herbal Formulas and Applications

Section 4

燥湿祛痰剂
— Damp-Phlegm Dispelling Formula

Èr Zhú Tāng (Two-Atractylodes Decoction)

二术湯
二术汤

Pinyin Name: *Er Zhu Tang*
Literal Name: Two-Atractylodes Decoction
Alternate Name: Atractylodes and Arisaema Combination
Original Source: *Wan Bing Hui Chun* (Restoration of Health from the Myriad Diseases) by Gong Ting-Xian in 1587

COMPOSITION

Ban Xia (Rhizoma Pinelliae), *zhi* (prepared) with ginger	6g
Tian Nan Xing (Rhizoma Arisaematis)	3g
Bai Zhu (Rhizoma Atractylodis Macrocephalae)	3g
Cang Zhu (Rhizoma Atractylodis), *xi* (washed) in rice water and *chao* (dry-fried)	4.5g
Fu Ling (Poria)	3g
Qiang Huo (Rhizoma et Radix Notopterygii)	3g
Xiang Fu (Rhizoma Cyperi)	3g
Wei Ling Xian (Radix et Rhizoma Clematidis)	3g
Chen Pi (Pericarpium Citri Reticulatae)	3g
Huang Qin (Radix Scutellariae), *zhi* (prepared) with liquor	3g
Gan Cao (Radix et Rhizoma Glycyrrhizae)	3g

DOSAGE / PREPARATION / ADMINISTRATION

The source text instructs to cook the ingredients with *Sheng Jiang* (Rhizoma Zingiberis Recens). Take the strained decoction while warm.

CHINESE THERAPEUTIC ACTIONS

1. Dispels dampness and eliminates phlegm
2. Opens the channels and collaterals to relieve pain

CLINICAL MANIFESTATIONS

Musculoskeletal disorders of the arms and shoulders due to phlegm stagnation: aches and pains in the wrist, forearm, elbow, and shoulder; bursitis; tendonitis; and frozen shoulder.

CLINICAL APPLICATIONS

Frozen shoulder, bursitis, tendonitis, and neuralgia of the forearm.

EXPLANATION

Er Zhu Tang (Two-Atractylodes Decoction) treats musculoskeletal aches and pains due to damp and phlegm accumulation in the upper body. Dampness initially arises as a result of the inability of the Spleen to transport and transform water and food. Thus, patients may experience gastrointestinal weakness as a result of Spleen deficiency. Over time, dampness turns into phlegm and the phlegm accumulates in the muscles, causing aches and pains and other musculoskeletal disorders.

In this formula, *Ban Xia* (Rhizoma Pinelliae) and *Tian Nan Xing* (Rhizoma Arisaematis) dry dampness and eliminate phlegm. *Bai Zhu* (Rhizoma Atractylodis Macrocephalae), *Cang Zhu* (Rhizoma Atractylodis), and *Fu Ling* (Poria) strengthen the Spleen and Stomach and dry dampness. *Qiang Huo* (Rhizoma et Radix Notopterygii) dispels wind and dries dampness; and together with *Xiang Fu* (Rhizoma

WIND-DAMP DISPELLING FORMULAS

17

1195

Chapter 17 – Wind-Damp Dispelling Formulas　　　　*Section 4 – Damp-Phlegm Dispelling Formula*

Èr Zhú Tāng (Two-Atractylodes Decoction)

Er Zhu Tang (Two-Atractylodes Decoction)

Diagnosis	Signs and Symptoms	Treatment	Herbs
• Aches and pains due to damp and phlegm accumulation	• Aches and pains in the wrist, forearm, elbow, and shoulders: damp and phlegm accumulation in the upper body	• Dispels dampness and eliminates phlegm • Opens the channels and collaterals to relieve pain	• *Ban Xia* (Rhizoma Pinelliae) and *Tian Nan Xing* (Rhizoma Arisaematis) dry dampness and eliminate phlegm. • *Bai Zhu* (Rhizoma Atractylodis Macrocephalae), *Cang Zhu* (Rhizoma Atractylodis), and *Fu Ling* (Poria) strengthen the Spleen and Stomach and dry dampness. • *Qiang Huo* (Rhizoma et Radix Notopterygii) dispels wind and dries dampness. • *Xiang Fu* (Rhizoma Cyperi), *Wei Ling Xian* (Radix et Rhizoma Clematidis), and *Chen Pi* (Pericarpium Citri Reticulatae) regulate qi circulation. • *Huang Qin* (Radix Scutellariae) clears damp-heat and reduces swelling and inflammation. • *Sheng Jiang* (Rhizoma Zingiberis Recens) relieves nausea and vomiting by redirecting Stomach qi downward. • *Gan Cao* (Radix et Rhizoma Glycyrrhizae) harmonizes the herbs.

Cyperi) and *Wei Ling Xian* (Radix et Rhizoma Clematidis), these three herbs regulate qi circulation, open up the peripheral channels and collaterals, benefit the joints, and relieve muscle aches and pains. *Chen Pi* (Pericarpium Citri Reticulatae) activates and regulates the qi flow to remove the residual phlegm and dampness. *Huang Qin* (Radix Scutellariae) clears damp-heat and reduces swelling and inflammation. *Sheng Jiang* (Rhizoma Zingiberis Recens) relieves nausea and vomiting by redirecting Stomach qi downward; it also reduces the toxicity of *Ban Xia* (Rhizoma Pinelliae). *Gan Cao* (Radix et Rhizoma Glycyrrhizae) harmonizes the herbs in this formula.

MODIFICATIONS

• With neck stiffness, add *Ge Gen* (Radix Puerariae Lobatae) and *Gan Cao* (Radix et Rhizoma Glycyrrhizae).

• With headache and edema, add *Wu Ling San* (Five-Ingredient Powder with Poria).

• With soreness and pain of the joints, add *Niu Xi* (Radix Achyranthis Bidentatae), *Xu Duan* (Radix Dipsaci), and *Mu Fang Ji* (Radix Cocculi Trilobi).

• With phlegm in the Lung, add *Jie Geng* (Radix Platycodonis) and *Chai Hu* (Radix Bupleuri).

• For sciatica, add *Shu Jing Huo Xue Tang* (Relax the Channels and Invigorate the Blood Decoction).

1196

Chinese Herbal Formulas and Applications

Chapter 17 — Summary

— Wind-Damp Dispelling Formulas

SECTION 1: WIND-DAMP DISPELLING FORMULAS

Name	Similarities	Differences
Qiang Huo Sheng Shi Tang (Notopterygium Decoction to Overcome Dampness)		Treats soreness and pain of the neck, shoulders, and back
Juan Bi Tang (Remove Painful Obstruction Decoction)		Treats soreness and pain of the upper body with underlying *ying* (nutritive) and *wei* (defensive) *qi* deficiencies
Du Huo Ji Sheng Tang (Angelica Pubescens and Taxillus Decoction)		Treats soreness and pain of the lower back and knees with qi, blood, and yin deficiencies
San Bi Tang (Three-Painful Obstruction Decoction)	Dispel wind and damp-ness, treat *bi zheng* (painful obstruction syndrome)	Treats soreness and pain with qi and blood deficiencies
Shu Jing Huo Xue Tang (Relax the Channels and Invigorate the Blood Decoction)		Treats aches and pains due to damp accumulation and blood stagnation with underlying deficiencies
Shu Jin Li An San (Relax the Tendons and Instill Peace Powder)		Treats severe aches and pains with wind-cold from the exterior and clears damp-heat from the interior
Yi Yi Ren Tang (Coicis Decoction)		Treats numbness, swelling, and pain of the extremities due to wind-dampness
Shang Zhong Xia Tong Yong Tong Feng Wan (Upper, Middle, and Lower General Use Pill for Wind-Pain)		Treats aches and pains throughout the entire body

Qiang Huo Sheng Shi Tang (Notopterygium Decoction to Overcome Dampness) dispels wind and eliminates dampness. It is most effective for wind-dampness at the exterior affecting the neck, shoulder and back. Clinical manifestations include symptoms such as stiffness and immobility of the neck and shoulders, headache, heaviness of the body, low back pain with difficulty of movement, white tongue coating, and a superficial pulse.

Juan Bi Tang (Remove Painful Obstruction Decoction) dispels wind-dampness, tonifies qi, and harmonizes *ying* (nutritive) and *wei* (defensive) levels. This formula is most effective for *bi zheng* (painful obstruction syndrome) due to wind-dampness with underlying *ying* (nutritive) and *wei* (defensive) *qi* deficiencies. Clinical manifestations include neck pain, shoulder pain, and numbness of the extremities.

Du Huo Ji Sheng Tang (Angelica Pubescens and Taxillus Decoction) dispels wind-dampness, nourishes the Liver and Kidney, and tonifies qi and blood. It is generally used to treat chronic *bi zheng* (painful obstruction syndrome) with qi and blood, and Liver and Kidney deficiencies. Clinical manifestations include painful joints, lumbago, difficult movement of the extremities, aversion to cold and preference for warmth, palpitations, and shortness of breath.

San Bi Tang (Three-Painful Obstruction Decoction) dispels wind-cold-dampness, tonifies qi, and nourishes blood. It treats *bi zheng* (painful obstruction syndrome) due to stagnation of wind-cold-dampness with underlying qi and blood deficiencies. Clinical manifestations include numbness and pain of the muscles and joints, decreased range of motion, and pain exaggerated with exposure to cold and damp weather.

WIND-DAMP DISPELLING FORMULAS

17

1197

Chapter 17 – Wind-Damp Dispelling Formulas

Chapter 17 — Summary

Shu Jing Huo Xue Tang (Relax the Channels and Invigorate the Blood Decoction) dispels dampness, activates blood circulation, and opens the channels and collaterals. It is an excellent formula to treat *bi zheng* (painful obstruction syndrome) characterized by damp accumulation and blood stagnation blocking the channels and collaterals. Clinical signs and symptoms include severe muscle ache, painful joints, radiating pain in the leg, numbness in the lower extremities, and pain in the trunk and extremities.

Shu Jin Li An San (Relax the Tendons and Instill Peace Powder) activates blood circulation, eliminates wind-cold from the exterior, and clears damp-heat from the interior. It opens the channels and collaterals to relieve severe muscle and joint pain in the arms and legs.

Yi Yi Ren Tang (Coicis Decoction) dispels wind-dampness, activates blood circulation, and tonifies qi. It treats *bi zheng* (painful obstruction syndrome) characterized by wind-dampness with numbness and pain of the extremities, decreased mobility and range of motion of the joints with swelling and inflammation, and a lingering sensation of warmth or mild fever.

Shang Zhong Xia Tong Yong Tong Feng Wan (Upper, Middle, and Lower General Use Pill for Wind-Pain) dispels wind, dissolves dampness, activates blood circulation, and eliminates blood stasis. It is designed to treat generalized *bi zheng* (painful obstruction syndrome) that affects the entire body (upper, middle, and lower).

SECTION 2: DAMP-COLD DISPELLING FORMULAS

Name	Similarities	Differences
Xiao Huo Luo Dan (Minor Invigorate the Collaterals Special Pill)	Dispel damp-cold, treat *bi zheng* (painful obstruction syndrome)	Opens the channels and collaterals, dispels dampness and phlegm
Da Fang Feng Tang (Major Saposhnikovia Decoction)		Tonifies qi and blood, strengthens the muscles and tendons
Ji Ming San (Powder to Take at Cock's Crow)	Eliminates damp-cold, treats leg *qi*	Activates qi circulation, drains turbidity

Xiao Huo Luo Dan (Minor Invigorate the Collaterals Special Pill) dispels wind-cold-dampness, dissolves phlegm and dredges the channels, activates blood circulation, and stops pain. Stagnation of wind, cold, dampness, phlegm, and blood may produce clinical manifestations of difficult movement of the joints, pain and numbness in the extremities, migratory pain, and heaviness of the lower back and legs.

Da Fang Feng Tang (Major Saposhnikovia Decoction) dispels wind, cold and dampness, tonifies qi and blood, and strengthens muscles and tendons. It is used to treat weakness and paralysis of the lower extremities due to deficiencies of qi and blood. Clinical manifestations include generalized pain and numbness in the legs, weak knees, atrophy of the leg muscles, difficulty of movement, hemiplegia, and neuralgia.

Ji Ming San (Powder to Take at Cock's Crow) eliminates cold and dampness, drains turbidity, and activates qi circulation. It is mainly used for leg *qi* characterized by dampness and cold, with signs and symptoms such as aversion to cold, chest stuffiness, and feelings of swelling, heaviness, weakness, numbness, and pain of the legs.

1198

Chapter 17 — Summary

Chinese Herbal Formulas and Applications

SECTION 3: DAMP-HEAT DISPELLING FORMULAS

Name	Similarities	Differences
Gui Zhi Shao Yao Zhi Mu Tang (Cinnamon Twig, Peony, and Anemarrhena Decoction)	Dispels wind-dampness, clears heat	Reduces swelling, inflammation, and pain in the joints
Er Miao San (Two-Marvel Powder)	Dispel damp-heat, treat *bi zheng* (painful obstruction syndrome)	Clears damp-heat affecting the lower body
Dang Gui Nian Tong Tang (Tangkuei Decoction to Lift the Pain)		Treats damp-heat affecting the joints and extremities

Gui Zhi Shao Yao Zhi Mu Tang (Cinnamon Twig, Peony, and Anemarrhena Decoction) dispels wind-dampness, clears heat, and unblocks the channels and collaterals. It is primarily used to treat *bi zheng* (painful obstruction syndrome) characterized by invasion of wind-dampness and accumulation of heat, with symptoms and signs such as swollen and painful joints, emaciation, swollen feet, dizziness, shortness of breath, atrophy of the muscle, numbness of the extremities, and difficulty with walking and movement.

Er Miao San (Two-Marvel Powder) clears heat and dries dampness. It is used for mild damp-heat attacking the lower half of the body. Clinical manifestations include pain in the lower body, weak legs, redness, swelling, weakness, pain, and heat sensation in the knees, scanty, yellow urine, and leukorrhea.

Dang Gui Nian Tong Tang (Tangkuei Decoction to Lift the Pain) dispels wind, resolves dampness, clears heat, and relieves pain. It is one of the most effective formulas for treating damp-heat type of joint and musculoskeletal disorders with pain, redness, swelling and inflammation. Clinical manifestations include joint or musculoskeletal pain with redness, swelling and inflammation, heavy sensations in the shoulders and back, fullness in the chest and epigastric region, dermatological disorders in the lower extremities with itching and pain, ulceration and abscess of the skin, and a deep, tight pulse.

SECTION 4: DAMP-PHLEGM DISPELLING FORMULA

Name	Similarities	Differences
Er Zhu Tang (Two-Atractylodes Decoction)	Dispels dampness, eliminates phlegm	Opens up the channels and collaterals

Er Zhu Tang (Two-Atractylodes Decoction) dispels dampness, eliminates phlegm, opens up the channels and collaterals, and relieves pain. It treats musculoskeletal disorders of the arms and shoulders due to damp and phlegm stagnation. Clinical manifestations include aches and pains in the wrist, forearm, elbow, and shoulder, bursitis, tendinitis, and frozen shoulder.

WIND-DAMP DISPELLING FORMULAS

17

Chapter 18

— Phlegm-Dispelling Formulas

祛痰剂

朱震亨 Zhú Zhèn-Héng

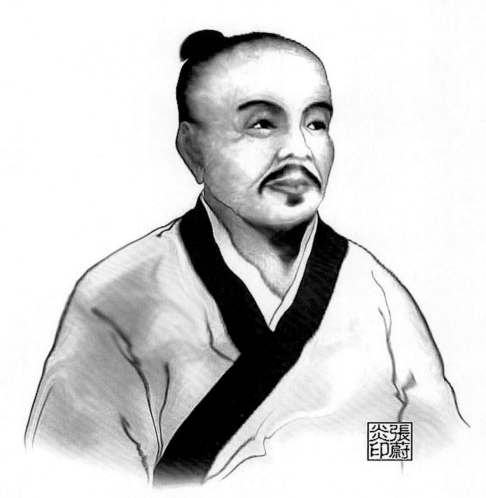

朱震亨 Zhú Zhèn-Héng, also known as
朱丹溪 Zhú Dán-Xí, 1281 – 1358.

朱震亨 Zhú Zhèn-Héng

Known as a wonder child, Zhu Zhen-Heng excelled in academia, rapidly passing his peers. He was able to recite thousands of verses by the time he was six years old. Because of his outstanding achievements at such a young age, Zhu's family had great hopes for him. Unfortunately, Zhu's father died when the boy was 15, and his mother was forced to raise three children on her own. With three young children and no man in the family, Zhu's family was repeatedly harassed and robbed by local bandits. Nevertheless, Zhu's mother maintained high spirits, and successfully raised all three children.

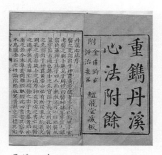

丹溪心法 *Dan Xi Xin Fa* (Teachings of [Zhu] Dan-Xi), published in 1481.

When Zhu was 30 years old, his mother became chronically ill and did not respond to treatment by any of the local physicians. Having been heavily influenced by her throughout his life, Zhu decided to undertake her treatment himself. He began to study medicine on his own, and five years later, successfully cured his mother's condition. This success ignited his interest, and he continued his pursuit of medicine. However, he improved little in the next ten years of studying on his own. Finally, at age 44, he bid farewell to his family, to go in search of a teacher. After a cross-country journey, he learned of 罗知悌 Luo Zhi-Ti, one of the best physicians of the time. However, Luo refused to accept any apprentices. To show his dedication, Zhu waited outside Luo's residence every day, without exception, for three months. Finally, touched by Zhu's dedication and sincerity, Luo accepted him as an apprentice. In the next three years, Zhu studied diligently and tirelessly. According to his biography, one of the most important lessons Zhu learned was to not rigidly follow only one school of thought, but to master and integrate all of them.

Zhu is most famous for one of his adages: "阳常有余，阴常不足. Yang is often in excess, yin is often insufficient." He observed this problem because many physicians during this era prescribed formulas from *Tai Ping Hui Min He Ji Ju Fang* (Imperial Grace Formulary of the Tai Ping Era). These formulas were warm and drying and often damaged yin and created fire. To correct this problem, he proposed many theories and formulas to nourish yin and purge fire. Today, he is credited as the founder of 滋阴派 the Yin-Nourishing Style.

Though Zhu did not begin his formal training in medicine until 44 years of age, he excelled in his later years as he did in his youth, and became known as one of the best physicians of his time. When he died at 77, he left volumes of drafts of his clinical experiences. His writings were later organized and published by his apprentices. Among the most famous of his works was the 丹溪心法 *Dan Xi Xin Fa* (Teachings of [Zhu] Dan-Xi) 1481.

Zhu Zhen-Heng is remembered by many as "one-dose Zhu," for his outstanding ability to cure disease with just one dose of herbs.

Some of the formulas written by Zhu Zhen-Heng are:
- *Dang Gui Long Hui Wan* (Tangkuei, Gentiana, and Aloe Pill)
- *Zuo Jin Wan* (Left Metal Pill)
- *Da Bu Yin Wan* (Great Tonify the Yin Pill)
- *Hu Qian Wan* (Hidden Tiger Pill)
- *Yu Ping Feng San* (Jade Windscreen Powder)
- *Yue Ju Wan* (Escape Restraint Pill)
- *Wei Ling Tang* (Calm the Stomach and Poria Decoction)
- *Bi Xie Fen Qing Yin* (Dioscorea Hypoglauca Decoction to Separate the Clear)
- *Er Miao San* (Two-Marvel Powder)
- *Gun Tan Wan* (Vaporize Phlegm Pill)
- *Bao He Wan* (Preserve Harmony Pill)

Dynasties & Kingdoms	Year
Xia Dynasty 夏	2100-1600 BCE
Shang Dynasty 商	1600-1100 BCE
Zhou Dynasty 周	1100-221 BCE
Qin Dynasty 秦	221-207 BCE
Han Dynasty 漢	206 BCE-220
Three Kingdoms 三國	220-280
Western Jin Dynasty 西晉	265-316
Eastern Jin Dynasty 東晉	317-420
Northern and Southern Dynasties 北南朝	420-581
Sui Dynasty 隋	581-618
Tang Dynasty 唐	618-907
Five Dynasties 五代	907-960
Song Dynasty 宋	960-1279
Liao Dynasty 遼	916-1125
Jin Dynasty 金	1115-1234
Yuan Dynasty 元	**1271-1368**
Ming Dynasty 明	1368-1644
Qing Dynasty 清	1644-1911
Republic of China 中華民國	1912-Present Day
People's Republic of China 中華人民共和國	1949-Present Day

Chapter 18 – Phlegm-Dispelling Formulas

Table of Contents

Chapter 18. Phlegm-Dispelling Formulas ································ **1201**
Biography of Zhu Zhen-Heng ··· 1202

Section 1. Damp-Drying and Phlegm-Dissolving Formulas ························ **1209**
Er Chen Tang (Two-Cured Decoction) ·· 1209
  Dao Tan Tang (Guide Out Phlegm Decoction) ·· 1211
  Di Tan Tang (Scour Phlegm Decoction) ·· 1212
  Zhi Suo Er Chen Tang (Two-Cured Decoction with Aurantium and Cardamon) ······· 1212
Wen Dan Tang (Warm the Gallbladder Decoction) ·· 1213
  Shi Wei Wen Dan Tang (Ten-Ingredient Decoction to Warm the Gallbladder) ········· 1216
Zhu Ru Wen Dan Tang (Bamboo Decoction to Warm the Gallbladder) ·················· 1217
Fu Ling Wan (Poria Pill) ··· 1219
Xiao Ban Xia Jia Fu Ling Tang (Minor Pinellia and Poria Decoction) ·················· 1220

Section 2. Heat-Clearing and Phlegm-Dissolving Formulas ······················ **1222**
Qing Qi Hua Tan Wan (Clear the Qi and Transform Phlegm Pill) ······················· 1222
  Hua Tan Wan (Transform Phlegm Pill) ·· 1223
Qing Fei Yin (Clear the Lung Drink) ·· 1224
Qing Fei Tang (Clear the Lung Decoction) ··· 1225
  Qing Fei Tang (Clear the Lung Decoction) ··· 1227
Zi Wan Tang (Aster Decoction) ·· 1229
Jie Geng Tang (Platycodon Decoction) ·· 1230
Ren Shen Xie Fei Tang (Ginseng Decoction to Sedate the Lung) ························· 1231
Gua Lou Zhi Shi Tang (Trichosanthes Fruit and Immature Bitter Orange Decoction) ··· 1233
Xiao Xian Xiong Tang (Minor Sinking into the Chest Decoction) ······················· 1235
  Chai Hu Xian Xiong Tang (Bupleurum Decoction for Sinking into the Chest) ·········· 1237
Gun Tan Wan (Vaporize Phlegm Pill) ··· 1238

Section 3. Dryness-Moistening and Phlegm-Dissolving Formula ·················· **1240**
Bei Mu Gua Lou San (Fritillaria and Trichosanthes Fruit Powder) ····················· 1240

Section 4. Warm Formulas that Dissolve Cold Phlegm ···························· **1242**
Ling Gan Wu Wei Jiang Xin Tang (Poria, Licorice, Schisandra, Ginger, and Asarum Decoction) ··· 1242
  Leng Xiao Wan (Cold Wheezing Pill) ··· 1243
  San Jian Gao (Three Constructive Paste) ··· 1244
San Zi Yang Qin Tang (Three-Seed Decoction to Nourish One's Parents) ··············· 1245

Section 5. Wind-Expelling and Phlegm-Dissolving Formulas ······················ **1247**
Ban Xia Bai Zhu Tian Ma Tang (Pinellia, Atractylodes Macrocephala, and Gastrodia Decoction) ··· 1247
  Ban Xia Bai Zhu Tian Ma Tang (Pinellia, Atractylodes Macrocephala, and Gastrodia Decoction) ·· 1250
Ding Xian Wan (Arrest Seizures Pill) ·· 1251
  He Che Wan Fang (Placenta Pill Formula) ··· 1253

Phlegm-Dispelling Formulas (Summary) ·· **1254**

Chinese Herbal Formulas and Applications

Chapter 18 — Overview

— Phlegm-Dispelling Formulas

Definition: Phlegm-dispelling formulas dissolve and dispel phlegm. According to traditional Chinese medical theory, there are two types of phlegm: *tan* (visible phlegm) and *yin* (invisible phlegm). *Tan* (visible phlegm) is the thick phlegm that travels in the channel and collateral pathways and affects different parts of the body. *Yin* (invisible phlegm) is the thin, watery phlegm that generally remains in the area where it was formed. Both *tan* (visible phlegm) and *yin* (invisible phlegm) are formed primarily by accumulation of water and dampness.

Phlegm [*tan* (visible phlegm) and *yin* (invisible phlegm)] disorders are closely related to the functions of the organs that control water: the Spleen, Lung, and Kidney. The Spleen transforms water, the Lung distributes water, and the Kidney eliminates water. Disorders in any of these three organs will lead to the accumulation of water and dampness, and eventually, the formation of phlegm. Once phlegm is formed, it may affect virtually any part of the body, including but not limited to the chest, diaphragm, stomach, intestines, all four extremities, and every channel and collateral. Presentations of phlegm disorders include symptoms and signs such as cough, wheezing, hurried respiration, dizziness, vertigo, nausea, vomiting, seizures, epilepsy, *dian kuang* (mania and withdrawal), and various types of hardness and nodule formation.

Successful treatment of phlegm disorders requires accurate determination of the cause. Generally speaking, for phlegm caused by deficiency of the Spleen, the treatment approach is to strengthen the Spleen, dry dampness, and dissolve phlegm. For phlegm caused by internal fire drying the body fluids and turning them into phlegm, it is best to clear heat and dispel phlegm. For phlegm caused by deficiency heat in the Lung consuming the body fluids and turning them into phlegm, the treatment approach is to moisten the Lung and dissolve phlegm. If the phlegm is produced by coldness in the Lung or by deficiency and cold of the Spleen and Kidney, the strategy involves warming yang and dissolving phlegm. For phlegm due to invasion of exterior factors affecting the qi flow of the Lung, it is necessary to ventilate the Lung and dissolve phlegm. In short, because phlegm disorders are complex in nature, optimal treatment requires the use of herbs to treat both the cause and the symptoms.

Additionally, phlegm disorders may be associated with various complications. Because the Lung is the organ that stores phlegm, it is often affected by phlegm disorders. Thus, treatment of phlegm disorders often requires the addition of herbs to dispel phlegm from the Lung. In patients with Liver wind, phlegm travels to the upper parts of the body, so it is necessary to use herbs to calm wind and dissolve phlegm. Moreover, phlegm stagnation affects qi circulation, while obstructed qi circulation contributes to phlegm stagnation. Because of this close relationship, phlegm-dispelling formulas often contain qi-regulating herbs to activate and regulate qi circulation. Lastly, if stagnant phlegm in the channels and collaterals causes the formation of hardness and nodules, one needs to use appropriate herbs to open the channels and collaterals, soften hardness, and disperse stagnation.

> **"Phlegm is the mother of hundreds of disorders,"** causing disorders in the *zang fu* as well as obstructions of the channels and collaterals.
> ∼

PHLEGM-DISPELLING FORMULAS

18

1205

Chapter 18 – Phlegm-Dispelling Formulas

Chapter 18 — Overview

SUBCATEGORIES OF ACTION

Phlegm-dispelling formulas are divided into five subcategories to accurately differentiate the nature of the disorders and characteristics of the corresponding formulas.

1. **Damp-Drying and Phlegm-Dissolving Formulas**

   These formulas are designed to treat damp-phlegm. The main signs and symptoms of damp-phlegm are coughing with profuse sputum that can be easily expectorated, feelings of distention with a stifling sensation in the chest and epigastrium, nausea, vomiting, and lassitude. The tongue coating is usually white and greasy, or slippery. The pulse is either moderate, or wiry and slippery.

   Herbs commonly used to dry dampness and dissolve phlegm include *Ban Xia* (Rhizoma Pinelliae) and *Tian Nan Xing* (Rhizoma Arisaematis). Furthermore, to prevent accumulation of dampness and phlegm, herbs are commonly used to strengthen the Spleen and regulate qi, such as *Chen Pi* (Pericarpium Citri Reticulatae) and *Bai Zhu* (Rhizoma Atractylodis Macrocephalae). Exemplar formulas that dry dampness and dissolve phlegm include *Er Chen Tang* (Two-Cured Decoction) and *Wen Dan Tang* (Warm the Gallbladder Decoction).

2. **Heat-Clearing and Phlegm-Dissolving Formulas**

   These formulas treat heat-phlegm syndromes, with common manifestations of coughing, chest pain, dizziness, thick, yellow sputum that is difficult to expectorate, a red tongue body with a greasy, yellow coating, and a slippery, rapid pulse.

   Herbs that clear heat and dissolve phlegm include *Gua Lou* (Fructus Trichosanthis) and *Dan Nan Xing* (Arisaema cum Bile). Representative formulas include *Qing Qi Hua Tan Wan* (Clear the Qi and Transform Phlegm Pill) and *Xiao Xian Xiong Tang* (Minor Sinking into the Chest Decoction).

   In severe cases of heat-phlegm syndromes, the sensory orifices may be blocked, leading to unconsciousness, seizures, epilepsy and convulsions. Such critical conditions must be treated with strong formulas that clear heat and open the sensory orifices, such as *An Gong Niu Huang Wan* (Calm the Palace Pill with Cattle Gallstone) and *Zi Xue* (Purple Snow) [*see* Chapter 10: Orifice-Opening Formulas].

3. **Dryness-Moistening and Phlegm-Dissolving Formula**

   > *Phlegm stagnation affects qi circulation, while obstructed qi circulation contributes to phlegm stagnation.*

   This formula treats dry phlegm that manifests as thick, sticky sputum that cannot be easily expectorated, a feeling of residual phlegm in the chest after expectoration, dryness and soreness of the throat, and a hoarse and raspy voice.

   Herbs and formulas commonly used to moisten dryness and dissolve phlegm are *Chuan Bei Mu* (Bulbus Fritillariae Cirrhosae), *Zhe Bei Mu* (Bulbus Fritillariae Thunbergii) and *Gua Lou* (Fructus Trichosanthis). One exemplar formula is *Bei Mu Gua Lou San* (Fritillaria and Trichosanthes Fruit Powder).

4. **Warm Formulas that Dissolve Cold Phlegm**

   These formulas treat cold-phlegm syndromes with common clinical manifestations of coughing with white, watery sputum, and a greasy, white tongue coating.

   Herbs that warm and dissolve phlegm include *Xi Xin* (Radix et Rhizoma Asari) and *Gan Jiang* (Rhizoma Zingiberis). Exemplar formulas include *San Zi Yang Qin Tang* (Three-Seed Decoction to Nourish One's Parents) and *Ling Gan Wu Wei Jiang Xin Tang* (Poria, Licorice, Schisandra, Ginger, and Asarum Decoction).

5. **Wind-Expelling and Phlegm-Dissolving Formulas**

   These formulas treat wind-phlegm in the interior, which arises when internal phlegm is accompanied by Liver wind rising, causing symptoms of headache, dizziness, vertigo, seizures, epilepsy, and loss of consciousness. In this case, herbs that dispel phlegm should be combined with herbs that

1206

Chinese Herbal Formulas and Applications

Chapter 18 — Overview

extinguish Liver wind. Representative formulas include *Ban Xia Bai Zhu Tian Ma Tang* (Pinellia, Atractylodes Macrocephala, and Gastrodia Decoction) and *Ding Xian Wan* (Arrest Seizures Pill).

Note: External wind-phlegm is a condition in which the pathogenic wind attacks the Lung and impairs its descending and dispersing functions. Consequently, turbid phlegm is created. Clinically, the signs and symptoms of this condition include aversion to wind, fever, and cough with profuse sputum. This condition is treated with herbs that release wind from the exterior and dispel phlegm from the interior. *Zhi Sou San* (Stop Coughing Powder) is one exemplar formula. For additional information, please refer to Chapter 1: Exterior-Releasing Formulas.

CAUTIONS / CONTRAINDICATIONS

- Phlegm-dispelling formulas should be used with caution in patients with hemoptysis, as many of these formulas are very drying in nature and may promote more coughing and bleeding.
- Phlegm-dispelling formulas generally have strong moving and dispersing effects. They should be used as needed, and discontinued when the desired effects are achieved.

> **Many of these formulas that are very drying in nature may promote more coughing and bleeding in patients with hemoptysis.**

PHARMACOLOGICAL EFFECTS & CLINICAL APPLICATIONS

It is commonly stated in traditional Chinese medicine texts that "phlegm is the mother of hundreds of disorders."[1] As such, phlegm-dispelling formulas can treat a wide variety of diseases. From an allopathic medical perspective, phlegm-dispelling formulas have an extremely wide range of pharmacological effects and clinical applications. The most common applications include respiratory disorders, gastrointestinal disorders, seizures, epilepsy, stroke, and others.

- **Respiratory disorders**: Phlegm-dispelling formulas have a marked influence on the respiratory tract, and have been used to treat a wide variety of respiratory tract disorders. Pharmacologically, these formulas have demonstrated expectorant,[2] antitussive,[3] and antiasthmatic effects.[4] Clinically, these formulas have been used successfully to treat diseases such as acute bronchitis,[5,6] chronic bronchitis,[7] aspiration pneumonia,[8] interstitial pneumonia,[9] tuberculous pleurisy,[10] exudative pleurisy,[11] bronchial asthma,[12] cough,[13] and silicosis.[14] Exemplar formulas that treat bronchitis include *Er Chen Tang* (Two-Cured Decoction), *Xiao Xian Xiong Tang* (Minor Sinking into the Chest Decoction), and *San Zi Yang Qin Tang* (Three-Seed Decoction to Nourish One's Parents). Exemplar formulas that treat pneumonia include *Qing Fei Tang* (Clear the Lung Decoction) and *Qing Qi Hua Tan Wan* (Clear the Qi and Transform Phlegm Pill). *Xiao Xian Xiong Tang* (Minor Sinking into the Chest Decoction) may be used to treat pleurisy and silicosis. *Zhi Sou San* (Stop Coughing Powder) may be used for cough.
- **Gastrointestinal disorders**: Phlegm-dispelling formulas have a marked effect on the gastrointestinal tract, and may be used to treat many gastrointestinal disorders, such as gastritis,[15] epigastric pain,[16] erosive gastritis,[17] and reflux esophagitis.[18] The pharmacological effects are attributed in part to the inhibition of gastric acid production.[19,20] Exemplar formulas include *Er Chen Tang* (Two-Cured Decoction), *Wen Dan Tang* (Warm the Gallbladder Decoction), and *Xiao Xian Xiong Tang* (Minor Sinking into the Chest Decoction).
- **Seizures and epilepsy**: *Er Chen Tang* (Two-Cured Decoction) and *Gun Tan Wan* (Vaporize Phlegm Pill) are two phlegm-dispelling formulas that have demonstrated effectiveness in treating seizures and epilepsy.[21,22]
- **Stroke**: *Wen Dan Tang* (Warm the Gallbladder Decoction) and *Gun Tan Wan* (Vaporize Phlegm Pill) are two formulas that have been used effectively to treat stroke.[23,24] *Ban Xia Bai Zhu Tian Ma Tang* (Pinellia, Atractylodes Macrocephala, and Gastrodia Decoction) may be used to treat facial paralysis that follows as a post-stroke sequelae.[25]
- **Meniere's syndrome**: *Wen Dan Tang* (Warm the Gallbladder Decoction) and *Ban Xia Bai Zhu Tian Ma Tang* (Pinellia, Atractylodes Macrocephala, and Gastrodia Decoction) are two formulas that have shown marked success in treating Meniere's syndrome.[26,27]

> **Phlegm-dispelling formulas have an extremely wide range of clinical applications, including respiratory disorders, gastrointestinal disorders, seizures, epilepsy, stroke, and others.**

PHLEGM-DISPELLING FORMULAS

18

1207

Chapter 18 – Phlegm-Dispelling Formulas

Chapter 18 — Overview

References

1. Wang GC, Yuan Dynasty.
2. *Zhong Yi Fang Ji Xian Dai Yan Jiu* (Modern Study of Medical Formulae in Traditional Chinese Medicine) 1997.
3. *Zhong Cheng Yao* (Study of Chinese Patent Medicine) 1988;9:27.
4. *Zhong Yao Yao Li Yu Lin Chuang* (Pharmacology and Clinical Applications of Chinese Herbs) 1992;8(3):15.
5. *Zhong Ji Yi Kan* (Medium Medical Journal) 1994;12:45.
6. *Zhong Yi Ming Fang Lin Chuang Xin Yong* (Contemporary Clinical Applications of Classic Chinese Formulas) 2001;138.
7. *Zhong Yuan Yi Kan* (Resource Journal of Chinese Medicine) 1994;5:44.
8. Mantani N, Kasahara Y, Kamata T, Sekiya N, Shimada Y, Usuda K, Sakakibara I, Hattori N, Terasawa K. Effect of Seihai-to, a Kampo medicine, in relapsing aspiration pneumonia--an open-label pilot study. Phytomedicine 2002 Apr;9(3):195-201.
9. *Shi Yong Zhong Xi Yi Jie He Za Zhi* (Practical Journal of Integrated Chinese and Western Medicines) 1995;3:152.
10. *Shang Hai Yi Yao Za Zhi* (Shanghai Journal of Medicine and Herbology) 1986;1:36.
11. *Shan Xi Zhong Yi* (Shanxi Chinese Medicine) 1994;15(8):368.
12. *Shan Xi Zhong Yi* (Shanxi Chinese Medicine) 1995;4:148.
13. *Yun Nan Zhong Yi Zhong Yao Za Zhi* (Yunnan Journal of Traditional Chinese Medicine and Herbal Medicine) 1999;4:15.
14. *Bei Jing Zhong Yi Yao Da Xue Xue Bao* (Journal of Beijing University of Medicine and Medicinals) 1994;17(1):37.
15. *Bei Jing Zhong Yi* (Beijing Chinese Medicine) 1990;1:5.
16. *Nei Meng Gu Zhong Yi Yao* (Traditional Chinese Medicine and Medicinals of Inner Mongolia) 1998;3:19.
17. *Jiang Xi Zhong Yi Yao* (Jiangxi Chinese Medicine and Herbology) 1998;6:22.
18. *Hu Bei Zhong Yi Za Zhi* (Hubei Journal of Chinese Medicine) 1997;3:20.
19. *Zhong Yao Xian Dai Yan Jiu Yu Ying Yong* (Modern Study of Traditional Chinese Medicine) 1993;165, 199, 388, 490.
20. *Zhong Cheng Yao Yan Jiu* (Research of Chinese Patent Medicine) 1985;8:23.
21. *Shi Yong Zhong Yi Nei Ke Za Zhi* (Journal of Practical Chinese Internal Medicine) 1994;2:17.
22. *An Hui Zhong Yi Xue Yuan Xue Bao* (Journal of Anhui University School of Medicine) 1988;3:33.
23. *Shan Xi Zhong Yi* (Shanxi Chinese Medicine) 1995;16(9):393.
24. *Si Chuan Zhong Yi* (Sichuan Chinese Medicine) 1995;2:20.
25. *Bei Jing Zhong Yi* (Beijing Chinese Medicine) 1991;6:31.
26. *Zhe Jiang Zhong Yi Xue Yuan Xue Bao* (Journal of Zhejiang University of Chinese Medicine) 1998;3:25.
27. *Shi Yong Zhong Yi Za Zhi* (Journal of Practical Chinese Medicine) 1998;7:22.

Chinese Herbal Formulas and Applications

Section 1

燥湿化痰剂
— Damp-Drying and Phlegm-Dissolving Formulas

Èr Chén Tāng (Two-Cured Decoction)
二陳湯
二陈汤

Pinyin Name: *Er Chen Tang*
Literal Name: Two-Cured Decoction
Alternate Names: *Er Chen Wan, Erh Chen Tang (Wan)*, Two-Chen Decoction (Pill), Two Vintage Herbs Decoction, Citrus and Pinellia Combination
Original Source: *Tai Ping Hui Min He Ji Ju Fang* (Imperial Grace Formulary of the Tai Ping Era) by the Imperial Medical Department in 1078-85

COMPOSITION

Ban Xia (Rhizoma Pinelliae), *xi* (washed) with liquid 7 times	15g
Ju Hong (Exocarpium Citri Reticulatae)	15g
Fu Ling (Poria)	9g
Zhi Gan Cao (Radix et Rhizoma Glycyrrhizae Praeparata cum Melle)	4.5g

DOSAGE / PREPARATION / ADMINISTRATION

The source text states to grind all of the ingredients into a coarse powder. Cook 12g of the powder with 7 slices of *Sheng Jiang* (Rhizoma Zingiberis Recens) and 1 piece of *Wu Mei* (Fructus Mume) in one large bowl of water until the liquid is reduced to 60%. Take the hot, strained decoction any time during the day. Today, this formula may be prepared as a decoction with 3g of *Sheng Jiang* (Rhizoma Zingiberis Recens) and 1 piece of *Wu Mei* (Fructus Mume).

CHINESE THERAPEUTIC ACTIONS

1. Dries dampness and dissolves phlegm
2. Regulates qi and harmonizes the middle *jiao*

CLINICAL MANIFESTATIONS

Damp-phlegm accumulation: profuse, white sputum that can be easily expectorated, a feeling of distention and a stifling sensation in the chest and epigastrium, nausea, vomiting, lassitude, weak extremities, possible vertigo, palpitations, white, moist tongue coating, and a slippery pulse.

CLINICAL APPLICATIONS

Upper respiratory tract infection, bronchitis, tracheitis, emphysema, gastritis, peptic ulcer disease, gastrointestinal neurosis, nausea, vomiting, goiter, Meniere's disease, seizures, and hangovers.

EXPLANATION

Er Chen Tang (Two-Cured Decoction) is the basic formula for treating damp-phlegm. According to traditional Chinese medicine theory, the Spleen sends up clear fluids to the upper *jiao*. If this function is impaired, dampness may accumulate in the Spleen and create phlegm. Thus, damp-phlegm syndromes usually result from Spleen deficiency or dysfunction. If the Spleen is deficient and full of dampness, its functions of transportation and transformation will be impaired, which will lead to insufficient supply of nutrients to the body and the extremities. The result will be lassitude and weak extremities.

The Lung, on the other hand, stores phlegm. Phlegm accumulation in the Lung manifests as coughing with profuse sputum. A feeling of distention and oppression in the chest and epigastrium arises as a result of damp-phlegm obstructing the chest. Nausea and vomiting are due to damp-phlegm obstructing Stomach qi and causing

PHLEGM-DISPELLING FORMULAS

18

1209

Chapter 18 – Phlegm-Dispelling Formulas   *Section 1 – Damp-Drying and Phlegm-Dissolving Formulas*

Èr Chén Tāng (Two-Cured Decoction)

Er Chen Tang (Two-Cured Decoction)

Diagnosis	Signs and Symptoms	Treatment	Herbs
Damp-phlegm accumulation	• Coughing with profuse sputum, distention and a stifling sensation in the chest and epigastrium: damp-phlegm affecting the Lung • Nausea and vomiting: reversed flow of Stomach qi due to damp-phlegm accumulation • Lassitude and weak extremities: damp-phlegm affecting the Spleen • Palpitations and vertigo: yang qi unable to ascend due to damp-phlegm accumulation • White, moist tongue coating, and a slippery pulse: damp-phlegm condition	• Dries dampness and dissolves phlegm • Regulates qi and harmonizes the middle *jiao*	• *Ban Xia* (Rhizoma Pinelliae) breaks up and dissolves phlegm and dries dampness. • *Ju Hong* (Exocarpium Citri Reticulatae) activates and regulates qi. • *Fu Ling* (Poria) strengthens the Spleen and dispels dampness. • *Sheng Jiang* (Rhizoma Zingiberis Recens) relieves nausea and vomiting by guiding Stomach qi downward. • *Wu Mei* (Fructus Mume) astringes the Lung to prevent qi loss. • *Zhi Gan Cao* (Radix et Rhizoma Glycyrrhizae Praeparata cum Melle) harmonizes all of the herbs.

it to rise abnormally. If damp-phlegm affects the ascent of yang qi, then palpitations and vertigo can occur.

Ban Xia (Rhizoma Pinelliae) acts as the chief herb in this formula because it is the best herb to break up and dissolve phlegm stagnation. Its acrid and warm properties can dissolve phlegm, dry dampness, and open pathways for the qi to flow. In addition, it corrects the reversed flow of Stomach qi to relieve nausea and vomiting. *Ju Hong* (Exocarpium Citri Reticulatae) activates and regulates qi to remove residual phlegm and dampness. *Fu Ling* (Poria) strengthens the Spleen and dispels dampness. *Sheng Jiang* (Rhizoma Zingiberis Recens) relieves nausea and vomiting by guiding Stomach qi downward, and helps to detoxify *Ban Xia* (Rhizoma Pinelliae). Since patients with this syndrome already have qi deficiency, a very small amount of *Wu Mei* (Fructus Mume) is used to astringe the Lung to prevent qi loss. The restraining effect of *Wu Mei* (Fructus Mume) also balances the dispersing nature of *Ban Xia* (Rhizoma Pinelliae), thereby minimizing the potential side effects of both herbs. *Zhi Gan Cao* (Radix et Rhizoma Glycyrrhizae Praeparata cum Melle) harmonizes all of the herbs and regulates the Lung and Spleen.

MODIFICATIONS

• For wind-phlegm characterized by bluish-green and shiny sputum, add *Dan Nan Xing* (Arisaema cum Bile), *Bai Fu Zi* (Rhizoma Typhonii), *Zao Jiao* (Fructus Gleditsiae), and *Zhu Li* (Succus Bambusae).

• For cold-phlegm characterized by clear sputum, add the juice of *Sheng Jiang* (Rhizoma Zingiberis Recens) and increase the dose of *Ban Xia* (Rhizoma Pinelliae).

• For heat-phlegm characterized by yellow sputum, add *Huang Qin* (Radix Scutellariae), *Gua Lou* (Fructus Trichosanthis), *Huang Lian* (Rhizoma Coptidis), *Zhu Ru* (Caulis Bambusae in Taenia), and *Dan Nan Xing* (Arisaema cum Bile).

• For damp-phlegm characterized by white sputum, add *Cang Zhu* (Rhizoma Atractylodis), *Bai Zhu* (Rhizoma Atractylodis Macrocephalae), and *Hou Po* (Cortex Magnoliae Officinalis).

• For dry-phlegm characterized by sputum that is yellow, thick and difficult to expectorate, add *Gua Lou* (Fructus Trichosanthis), *Ku Xing Ren* (Semen Armeniacae Amarum), and *Bei Mu* (Bulbus Fritillariae).

• For qi stagnation and phlegm accumulation, add *Hou Po* (Cortex Magnoliae Officinalis) and *Zhi Shi* (Fructus Aurantii Immaturus).

• For phlegm produced by food stagnation, add *Shan Zha* (Fructus Crataegi), *Mai Ya* (Fructus Hordei Germinatus), and *Shen Qu* (Massa Fermentata).

• For stubborn phlegm (chronic), add *Zhi Shi* (Fructus Aurantii Immaturus), *Dan Nan Xing* (Arisaema cum Bile), *Fu Hai Shi* (Pumice), and *Mang Xiao* (Natrii Sulfas).

• With nausea and vomiting due to alcohol consumption or hangover, add *Ge Hua Jie Cheng San* (Pueraria Flower Powder for Detoxification and Awakening).

• With nausea and vomiting due to cold in the Stomach and a deficient body constitution, add *Mu Xiang* (Radix Aucklandiae) and *Sha Ren* (Fructus Amomi).

• With vomiting with abdominal pain due to heat, combine with *Huang Lian Tang* (Coptis Decoction).

1210

Chinese Herbal Formulas and Applications

Èr Chén Tāng (Two-Cured Decoction)

- With morning sickness, add *Sha Ren* (Fructus Amomi), *Lian Qiao* (Fructus Forsythiae), and *Huang Qin* (Radix Scutellariae).
- If there is drooling of saliva in children, add *Yi Zhi* (Fructus Alpiniae Oxyphyllae) and brown sugar.
- If accompanied by depression, add *Yue Ju Wan* (Escape Restraint Pill).
- For pulmonary emphysema in the elderly, add *Kuan Dong Hua* (Flos Farfarae), *Zi Wan* (Radix et Rhizoma Asteris), and *Sha Ren* (Fructus Amomi).
- For asthma in children caused by heat, add *Ma Huang* (Herba Ephedrae), *Ku Xing Ren* (Semen Armeniacae Amarum), *Shi Gao* (Gypsum Fibrosum), and *Sang Bai Pi* (Cortex Mori).
- For nodules caused by phlegm obstructing the channels, add *Mu Li* (Concha Ostreae), *Xuan Shen* (Radix Scrophulariae), *Ge Qiao* (Concha Meretricis seu Cyclinae), *Mang Xiao* (Natrii Sulfas), *Hai Zao* (Sargassum), and *Kun Bu* (Thallus Eckloniae).

CAUTIONS / CONTRAINDICATIONS

- *Er Chen Tang* is acrid and drying and is not suitable for cough caused by Lung yin deficiency or Lung dryness. Similarly, this formula should not be used if the patient has scanty sputum, blood-streaked sputum, or coughing with blood.
- This formula is acrid, warm, and drying. Short-term use of this formula may be associated with dry mouth and thirst. Long-term use may cause consumption of yin and body fluids.[1]

PHARMACOLOGICAL EFFECTS

1. **Respiratory**: Ingredients of *Er Chen Tang* have been shown to have antitussive, expectorant, and antiasthmatic effects.[2]
2. **Gastrointestinal**: Ingredients of *Er Chen Tang* may inhibit the production of gastric acid.[3]

CLINICAL STUDIES AND RESEARCH

1. **Bronchitis**: Use of modified *Er Chen Tang* showed marked effectiveness in treating bronchitis. Out of 109 patients who had uncomplicated bronchitis, marked improvement was reported in 105 cases; and out of 66 who had bronchitis with wheezing and dyspnea, marked improvement was reported in 59 cases.[4]
2. **Bronchiolitis**: According to one study, 80 patients with bronchiolitis were treated with marked improvement in 48 cases, moderate improvement in 31 cases, and no effect in 1 case. The herbal treatment contained *Er Chen Tang* plus *Zi Su Zi* (Fructus Perillae), *Wu Wei Zi* (Fructus Schisandrae Chinensis), and *Jie Geng* (Radix Platycodonis).[5]

3. **Atrophic gastritis**: Use of modified *Er Chen Tang* was associated with 71% effectiveness in treating 128 patients with chronic atrophic gastritis. The herbal treatment included *Er Chen Tang* with *Bai Zhu* (Rhizoma Atractylodis Macrocephalae), *Sha Ren* (Fructus Amomi), and others as deemed necessary.[6]
4. **Diabetes mellitus**: Use of modified *Er Chen Tang* was effective in treating diabetes mellitus characterized by damp-heat. The herbal treatment included *Er Chen Tang* with *Cang Zhu* (Rhizoma Atractylodis), *Bai Zhu* (Rhizoma Atractylodis Macrocephalae), *Jue Ming Zi* (Semen Cassiae), *Dan Shen* (Radix et Rhizoma Salviae Miltiorrhizae), and *Ge Gen* (Radix Puerariae Lobatae) as the base formula. Out of 32 patients, the study reported complete recovery in 4 cases, marked effectiveness in 16 cases, slight improvement in 10 cases, and no effect in 2 cases. The overall effectiveness was 93.8%.[7]
5. **Seizures**: Use of modified *Er Chen Tang* was associated with 76.92% effectiveness in treating seizures. Out of 52 patients, the study reported marked effect in 12 cases, moderate effect in 28 cases, and no effect in 12 cases. Modifications were made on an individual basis.[8]
6. **Goiter**: In one report, use of *Er Chen Tang* effectively reduced the size of thyroid enlargement in 5 out of 7 patients. All patients received the classic formula without modifications or any other treatments.[9]

RELATED FORMULAS

Dǎo Tán Tāng (Guide Out Phlegm Decoction)

導痰湯
导痰汤

Pinyin Name: *Dao Tan Tang*
Literal Name: Guide Out Phlegm Decoction
Original Source: *Ji Sheng Fang* (Formulas to Aid the Living) by Yan Yong-He in 1253

Ban Xia (Rhizoma Pinelliae),	
xi (washed) with liquid 7 times	120g [12g]
Tian Nan Xing (Rhizoma Arisaematis),	
pao (blast-fried)	30g [6g]
Ju Hong (Exocarpium Citri Reticulatae)	30g [6g]
Zhi Shi (Fructus Aurantii Immaturus),	
chao (dry-fried) with bran	30g [6g]
Chi Fu Ling (Poria Rubra)	30g [6g]
Zhi Gan Cao (Radix et Rhizoma Glycyrrhizae	
Praeparata cum Melle)	15g [3g]

The source text states to grind the herbs into powder. Cook 12g of the powder with 10 slices of *Sheng Jiang* (Rhizoma Zingiberis Recens) in 2 bowls of water until it is reduced to 80%. Take the warm, strained decoction after meals.

PHLEGM-DISPELLING FORMULAS

18

1211

Èr Chén Tāng (Two-Cured Decoction)

Today, this formula may be prepared as a decoction with the doses suggested in brackets.

Dao Tan Tang (Guide Out Phlegm Decoction) dries dampness, dispels phlegm, activates qi circulation, and unblocks stagnation. Clinically, it treats phlegm stagnation in the chest and diaphragm with symptoms such as a feeling of fullness and distention in the chest and hypochondrium, coughing, nausea, and poor appetite. This formula also can be used for Liver wind rising with phlegm, with symptoms such as inability to eat due to nausea and vomiting, headache, and vertigo.

Dí Tán Tāng (Scour Phlegm Decoction)
滌痰湯
涤痰汤
Pinyin Name: *Di Tan Tang*
Literal Name: Scour Phlegm Decoction
Original Source: *Zheng Zhi Zhun Sheng* (Standards of Patterns and Treatments) by Wang Ken-Tang in 1602

Dan Nan Xing (Arisaema cum Bile),	
zhi (prepared) with ginger	7.5g [12g]
Ban Xia (Rhizoma Pinelliae),	
xi (washed) with liquid 7 times	7.5g [12g]
Zhi Shi (Fructus Aurantii Immaturus),	
chao (dry-fried) with bran	6g [10g]
Fu Ling (Poria)	6g [10g]
Ju Hong (Exocarpium Citri Reticulatae)	4.5g [7.5g]
Shi Chang Pu (Rhizoma Acori Tatarinowii)	3g [5g]
Ren Shen (Radix et Rhizoma Ginseng)	3g [5g]
Zhu Ru (Caulis Bambusae in Taenia)	2.1g [3.5g]
Gan Cao (Radix et Rhizoma Glycyrrhizae)	1.5g [2.5g]

The source text states to prepare the ingredients as a decoction by cooking the herbs with 5 slices of *Sheng Jiang* (Rhizoma Zingiberis Recens) in 2 bowls of water until it is reduced to 1 bowl. Take the warm, strained decoction after meals.

Di Tan Tang (Scour Phlegm Decoction) eliminates phlegm and opens the sensory orifices. Clinically, this formula is indicated for patients with *zhong feng* (wind stroke) caused by phlegm obstruction, marked by a stiff tongue and speech difficulty.

Zhī Suō Èr Chén Tāng
(Two-Cured Decoction with Aurantium and Cardamon)
枳縮二陳湯
枳缩二陈汤

Pinyin Name: *Zhi Suo Er Chen Tang*
Literal Name: Two-Cured Decoction with Aurantium and Cardamon
Alternate Name: Chih-shih and Cardamon Combination
Original Source: *Wan Bing Hui Chun* (Restoration of Health from the Myriad Diseases) by Gong Ting-Xian in 1587

Zhi Shi (Fructus Aurantii Immaturus),	
chao (dry-fried) with bran	6g
Sha Ren [*Suo Sha*] (Fructus Amomi)	6g
Ban Xia (Rhizoma Pinelliae),	
zhi (prepared) with ginger juice	6g
Chen Pi (Pericarpium Citri Reticulatae)	6g
Fu Ling (Poria)	6g
Xiang Fu (Rhizoma Cyperi)	6g
Mu Xiang (Radix Aucklandiae)	1.5g
Cao Dou Kou (Semen Alpiniae Katsumadai)	1.5g
Gan Jiang (Rhizoma Zingiberis), *chao* (dry-fried)	1.5g
Hou Po (Cortex Magnoliae Officinalis),	
chao (dry-fried) with ginger juice	2.4g
Xiao Hui Xiang (Fructus Foeniculi),	
chao (dry-fried) with liquor	2.4g
Yan Hu Suo (Rhizoma Corydalis)	2.4g
Gan Cao (Radix et Rhizoma Glycyrrhizae)	0.9g

The source text states to cook the herbs with 3 slices of *Sheng Jiang* (Rhizoma Zingiberis Recens), and take the warm, strained decoction with *Zhu Li* (Succus Bambusae).

Zhi Suo Er Chen Tang (Two-Cured Decoction with Aurantium and Cardamon) treats phlegm stagnation above the diaphragm and beneath the heart area, which can cause violent nausea and vomiting accompanied by severe pain. Phlegm stagnation also leads to qi and blood stagnation, causing migrating and shooting pain throughout the upper and lower back.

To treat this condition, this formula has *Er Chen Tang* as the base formula to eliminate phlegm accumulation, while *Xiao Hui Xiang* (Fructus Foeniculi), *Yan Hu Suo* (Rhizoma Corydalis), *Xiang Fu* (Rhizoma Cyperi), and *Gan Jiang* (Rhizoma Zingiberis) are added to activate qi and blood circulation to relieve pain. *Zhi Shi* (Fructus Aurantii Immaturus), *Sha Ren* (Fructus Amomi), *Hou Po* (Cortex Magnoliae Officinalis), *Mu Xiang* (Radix Aucklandiae), and *Cao Dou Kou* (Semen Alpiniae Katsumadai) resolve dampness and eliminate phlegm. *Sheng Jiang* (Rhizoma Zingiberis Recens) and *Gan Cao* (Radix et Rhizoma Glycyrrhizae) harmonize the herbs in the formula and protect the middle *jiao*.

Èr Chén Tāng (Two-Cured Decoction)

Clinically, this formula has been used to treat gastritis, acid reflux, gastro-esophageal reflux disease, gastric ulcer, duodenal ulcer, gastroptosis, chest pain, and angina pectoris.

AUTHORS' COMMENTS

Er Chen Tang is the fundamental formula for treating damp and phlegm accumulation. Depending on the other pathogenic factors involved, additional herbs should be added for maximum effect. Please refer to the Modifications section for details.

Er Chen Tang, literally 'Two-Cured Decoction,' is so named because its two main ingredients [*Ban Xia* (Rhizoma Pinelliae) and *Ju Hong* (Exocarpium Citri Reticulatae)] are more effective when cured and aged.

Er Chen Tang, Dao Tan Tang (Guide Out Phlegm Decoction), *Di Tan Tang* (Scour Phlegm Decoction), and *Zhi Suo Er Chen Tang* (Two-Cured Decoction with Aurantium and Cardamon) all dry dampness and dissolve phlegm.

- *Er Chen Tang* is the standard formula and first choice for treating damp and phlegm accumulation. It treats a wide variety of disorders characterized by dampness and phlegm.

- *Dao Tan Tang* is a much stronger formula for eliminating phlegm. Not only can it eliminate phlegm from the chest, but also resolve phlegm that is accompanied by Liver wind.

- *Di Tan Tang* eliminates phlegm and opens the sensory orifices. It is used mostly for post-stroke patients with a stiff tongue and speech difficulties.

- *Zhi Suo Er Chen Tang* eliminates phlegm, regulates qi circulation, and relieves pain. It treats severe radiating pain in the chest with violent nausea and vomiting.

References

1. *Zhong Yao Ming Fang Yao Li Yu Ying Yong* (Pharmacology and Applications of Famous Herbal Formulas) 1989;567-570.
2. *Zhong Yao Xian Dai Yan Jiu Yu Ying Yong* (Modern Study of Traditional Chinese Medicine) 1993;165, 199, 388, 490.
3. *Zhong Yao Xian Dai Yan Jiu Yu Ying Yong* (Modern Study of Traditional Chinese Medicine) 1993;165, 199, 388, 490.
4. *Jiang Xi Zhong Yi Yao* (Jiangxi Chinese Medicine and Herbology) 1988;1:16.
5. *Zhong Ji Yi Kan* (Medium Medical Journal) 1994;12:45.
6. *Bei Jing Zhong Yi* (Beijing Chinese Medicine) 1990;1:5.
7. *Zhe Jiang Zhong Yi Za Zhi* (Zhejiang Journal of Chinese Medicine) 1994;1:9.
8. *Shi Yong Zhong Yi Nei Ke Za Zhi* (Journal of Practical Chinese Internal Medicine) 1994;2:17.
9. *Zhe Jiang Zhong Yi Za Zhi* (Zhejiang Journal of Chinese Medicine) 1966;1:17.

Wēn Dǎn Tāng (Warm the Gallbladder Decoction)

溫膽湯
温胆汤

Pinyin Name: *Wen Dan Tang*
Literal Name: Warm the Gallbladder Decoction
Alternate Names: *Wen Tan Tang,* Gallbladder Warming Decoction, Gallbladder-Warming Decoction, Hoelen and Bamboo Combination
Original Source: *San Yin Ji Yi Bing Zheng Fang Lun* (Discussion of Illnesses, Patterns, and Formulas Related to the Unification of the Three Etiologies) by Chen Yan in 1174

COMPOSITION

Ban Xia (Rhizoma Pinelliae), *xi* (washed) with liquid 7 times	6g
Zhu Ru (Caulis Bambusae in Taenia)	6g
Zhi Shi (Fructus Aurantii Immaturus), *chao* (dry-fried) with bran	6g
Chen Pi (Pericarpium Citri Reticulatae)	9g
Fu Ling (Poria)	4.5g
Zhi Gan Cao (Radix et Rhizoma Glycyrrhizae Praeparata cum Melle)	3g

DOSAGE / PREPARATION / ADMINISTRATION

The source text states to grind the ingredients into powder.

Cook 12g of the powder with 5 slices of *Sheng Jiang* (Rhizoma Zingiberis Recens) and 1 piece of *Da Zao*

Wēn Dǎn Tāng (Warm the Gallbladder Decoction)

(Fructus Jujubae) in 1.5 large bowls of water until the liquid is reduced to 70%. Take the strained decoction before meals.

CHINESE THERAPEUTIC ACTIONS
1. Regulates qi and dissolves phlegm
2. Clears heat in the Gallbladder
3. Harmonizes the Gallbladder and Stomach

CLINICAL MANIFESTATIONS
Gallbladder and Stomach disharmony accompanied by heat-phlegm: irritability, insomnia, palpitations, seizures, epilepsy, nausea, vomiting, thirst, and a bitter taste in the mouth.

CLINICAL APPLICATIONS
Meniere's syndrome, vertigo, psychiatric disorders (schizophrenia, bipolar disorders, and reactive psychosis), melancholia, nephropathy, diabetes mellitus, diabetic microvascular complications (diabetic retinopathy, diabetic nephropathy, and diabetic foot), cardiovascular disorders, stroke, pneumonia, asthma, and organophosphorus poisoning.

EXPLANATION
Wen Dan Tang (Warm the Gallbladder Decoction) treats disharmony of the Gallbladder and Stomach, accompanied by heat-phlegm in the interior. The Gallbladder, which belongs to the wood element, has a dispersing and discharging characteristic. Stagnation inhibits the dispersing and discharging nature of the Gallbladder, which in turn may cause it to overact on the Stomach and produce disharmony between the two organs. This disharmony eventually creates heat-phlegm, which manifests in symptoms such as irritability, insomnia, and palpitations. Nausea and vomiting arise when heat-phlegm blocks the normal descension of Stomach qi, forcing it to move adversely upward. In severe cases, heat-phlegm may obstruct the sensory orifices and cause seizures and epilepsy. The bitter taste in the mouth signifies heat in the Liver or Gallbladder, and slight thirst may occur as a result of interior heat consuming body fluids.

This formula has *Ban Xia* (Rhizoma Pinelliae) to dry dampness, dissolve phlegm, harmonize the Stomach, and redirect reversed flow of Stomach qi downward. *Zhu Ru* (Caulis Bambusae in Taenia) clears heat, dissolves phlegm, and relieves irritability. *Zhi Shi* (Fructus Aurantii Immaturus) breaks up qi stagnation and dispels phlegm. *Chen Pi* (Pericarpium Citri Reticulatae) regulates qi flow and dries dampness. *Fu Ling* (Poria) strengthens the Spleen to eliminate dampness and phlegm. *Sheng Jiang* (Rhizoma Zingiberis Recens), *Da Zao* (Fructus Jujubae), and *Zhi Gan Cao* (Radix et Rhizoma Glycyrrhizae Praeparata cum Melle) strengthen the Spleen and harmonize the Stomach.

MODIFICATIONS
- With dry mouth and throat, add *Wu Wei Zi* (Fructus Schisandrae Chinensis), *Mai Dong* (Radix Ophiopogonis), and *Tian Hua Fen* (Radix Trichosanthis); and remove *Ban Xia* (Rhizoma Pinelliae).
- With dark, yellow urine and dysuria, add *Yin Chen* (Herba Artemisiae Scopariae) and *Tong Cao* (Medulla Tetrapanacis).

Wen Dan Tang (Warm the Gallbladder Decoction)

Diagnosis	Signs and Symptoms	Treatment	Herbs
Disharmony of the Gallbladder and Stomach accompanied by heat-phlegm	• Irritability, insomnia, and palpitations: heat-phlegm rising upward • Seizures and epilepsy: heat-phlegm obstructing the sensory orifices • Nausea and vomiting: reversed flow of Stomach qi • Thirst: interior heat consuming body fluids • Bitter taste in the mouth: heat in the Liver and/or Gallbladder	• Regulates qi and dissolves phlegm • Clears heat in the Gallbladder • Harmonizes the Gallbladder and Stomach	• *Ban Xia* (Rhizoma Pinelliae) dries dampness, dissolves phlegm, and harmonizes the Stomach. • *Zhu Ru* (Caulis Bambusae in Taenia) clears heat, dissolves phlegm, and relieves irritability. • *Zhi Shi* (Fructus Aurantii Immaturus) breaks up qi stagnation and dispels phlegm. • *Chen Pi* (Pericarpium Citri Reticulatae) regulates qi flow and dries dampness. • *Fu Ling* (Poria) strengthens the Spleen to eliminate dampness and phlegm. • *Sheng Jiang* (Rhizoma Zingiberis Recens), *Da Zao* (Fructus Jujubae), and *Zhi Gan Cao* (Radix et Rhizoma Glycyrrhizae Praeparata cum Melle) strengthen the Spleen and harmonize the Stomach.

1214

Wēn Dǎn Tāng (Warm the Gallbladder Decoction)

Chinese Herbal Formulas and Applications

- With vomiting, add *Zi Su Ye* (Folium Perillae) and *Huang Lian* (Rhizoma Coptidis).
- With nausea, vomiting, and chest oppression, add *Huo Xiang* (Herba Agastaches) and *Shi Chang Pu* (Rhizoma Acori Tatarinowii).
- With irritability due to interior heat, add *Zhi Zi* (Fructus Gardeniae).
- With irritability and a bitter taste in the mouth, add *Huang Lian* (Rhizoma Coptidis).
- With insomnia due to excess worries, add *Xiao Yao San* (Rambling Powder).
- With insomnia due to depression, add *Yue Ju Wan* (Escape Restraint Pill).
- With insomnia and palpitations due to fear and fright, add *Suan Zao Ren* (Semen Ziziphi Spinosae).
- With palpitations, add *Yuan Zhi* (Radix Polygalae) and *Shi Chang Pu* (Rhizoma Acori Tatarinowii).
- For epilepsy, add *Yu Jin* (Radix Curcumae) and *Shi Chang Pu* (Rhizoma Acori Tatarinowii).
- For epilepsy and convulsions, add *Dan Nan Xing* (Arisaema cum Bile), *Gou Teng* (Ramulus Uncariae cum Uncis), and *Quan Xie* (Scorpio).
- For hearing difficulty caused by damp-heat attacking the Gallbladder channel, add *Chai Hu* (Radix Bupleuri), *Huang Qin* (Radix Scutellariae), *Shi Chang Pu* (Rhizoma Acori Tatarinowii), and *Tong Cao* (Medulla Tetrapanacis).
- With dizziness and vertigo, add *Ju Hua* (Flos Chrysanthemi) and *Huang Qin* (Radix Scutellariae).

CAUTIONS / CONTRAINDICATIONS

Wen Dan Tang is contraindicated in the following cases: insomnia caused by Heart deficiency, palpitations caused by blood deficiency, dizziness and vertigo caused by yin deficiency, and vomiting or nausea caused by Stomach cold.

CLINICAL STUDIES AND RESEARCH

1. **Meniere's syndrome**: *Wen Dan Tang* has been shown in two studies to effectively treat Meniere's syndrome. According to one study, use of modified *Wen Dan Tang* was associated with complete recovery in 41 of 48 patients. Modifications to the original formula included addition of *Zhi Zi* (Fructus Gardeniae) and *Huang Qin* (Radix Scutellariae) for headache, irritability, and tinnitus; *Yuan Zhi* (Radix Polygalae) and *Da Zao* (Fructus Jujubae) for insomnia with excessive dreaming; *Chai Hu* (Radix Bupleuri) and *Yu Jin* (Radix Curcumae) for belching and acid reflux; *Shen Qu* (Massa Fermentata) and charred *Shan Zha* (Fructus Crataegi) for indigestion; *Huo Xiang* (Herba Agastaches) and *Jing Jie* (Herba Schizonepetae) for exterior conditions; *Tian Ma* (Rhizoma Gastrodiae) and *Zhe Shi* (Haematitum) for severe dizziness and

vertigo; *Tian Nan Xing* (Rhizoma Arisaematis) and *Shi Chang Pu* (Rhizoma Acori Tatarinowii) for abundant damp and phlegm; and substitution of *Sheng Jiang* (Rhizoma Zingiberis Recens) with *Gan Jiang* (Rhizoma Zingiberis) for Stomach cold.[1]

According to another study, use of modified *Wen Dan Tang* was associated with 92% effectiveness for treating Meniere's syndrome. The herbal treatment consisted of *Wen Dan Tang* plus *Tian Ma* (Rhizoma Gastrodiae) for dizziness; *Zhe Shi* (Haematitum) and *Zhu Ru* (Caulis Bambusae in Taenia) for nausea and vomiting; and *Cong Bai* (Bulbus Allii Fistulosi) for severe tinnitus. The herbs were cooked together with *Du Huo* (Radix Angelicae Pubescentis) and eggs, and administered in decoction. Of 42 patients, the study reported complete recovery in 17 cases, improvement in 22 cases, and no response in 3 cases.[2]

2. **Vertigo**: Administration of *Wen Dan Tang* was reported in one study to effectively treat vertigo. Of 53 patients, 35 had complete recovery, 13 had improvement, and 5 had no effect. Modifications to the original formula included the addition of *Xuan Fu Hua* (Flos Inulae) and *Zhe Shi* (Haematitum) for nausea and vomiting; *Shi Chang Pu* (Rhizoma Acori Tatarinowii) and *Ju Hua* (Flos Chrysanthemi) for tinnitus; *Chuan Xiong* (Rhizoma Chuanxiong) and *Man Jing Zi* (Fructus Viticis) for headache; *Long Dan* (Radix et Rhizoma Gentianae) and *Huang Qin* (Radix Scutellariae) for a bitter taste in the mouth; *Suan Zao Ren* (Semen Ziziphi Spinosae) and *He Huan Pi* (Cortex Albiziae) for insomnia; *Gui Ban* (Plastrum Testudinis) and *Du Zhong* (Cortex Eucommiae) for soreness and weakness of the lower back and knees; and *Gou Teng* (Ramulus Uncariae cum Uncis), *Shi Jue Ming* (Concha Haliotidis), and *Niu Xi* (Radix Achyranthis Bidentatae) for hypertension.[3]

3. **Psychiatric disorders**: *Wen Dan Tang* has been shown in several clinical studies to have a beneficial effect in treating various psychiatric disorders. According to one study, it has a 96% effectiveness in treating 149 patients with severe psychiatric disorders such as schizophrenia, bipolar disorders, reactive psychosis, and others. The duration of treatment ranged from 3 to 12 packs of herbs in most cases.[4]

4. **Melancholia:** Use of *Wen Dan Tang* was associated with 87.5% effectiveness in treating melancholia, a syndrome caused by emotional stress and Liver qi stagnation, affecting the Heart and Spleen, and leading to disharmony of qi of the *zang fu* organs. Of 40 patients, 19 cases were cured, 16 improved, and 5 showed no improvement.[5]

5. ***Dian kuang* (mania and withdrawal)**: Thirty patients with *dian kuang* (mania and withdrawal) were treated with 87% effectiveness using *Wen Dan Tang* plus *Mu Li*

PHLEGM-DISPELLING FORMULAS

18

1215

Wēn Dǎn Tāng (Warm the Gallbladder Decoction)

(Concha Ostreae), *Zhen Zhu Mu* (Concha Margaritiferae), and *Mai Dong* (Radix Ophiopogonis). Of 30 patients, the study reported recovery in 13 cases, significant improvement in 5 cases, moderate improvement in 8 cases, and no effect in 4 cases. The average duration of treatment was 78.7 days, with a range of 16-224 days.[6]

6. **Impotence**: Use of modified *Wen Dan Tang* was associated with 97% effectiveness in treating impotence in 35 men. The herbal treatment contained this formula plus *Tu Fu Ling* (Rhizoma Smilacis Glabrae), *Wu Gong* (Scolopendra), and *She Chuang Zi* (Fructus Cnidii). Patients were instructed to avoid sexual activity, smoking, alcohol, and spicy, greasy, oily and pungent foods during herbal treatment. Of 35 patients, the study reported complete recovery in 21 cases, improvement in 13 cases, and no effect in 1 case.[7]

7. **Epigastric pain**: One study reported good results using modified *Wen Dan Tang* to treat epigastric pain characterized by damp-heat. Modifications to this formula included the addition of *Cang Zhu* (Rhizoma Atractylodis) and *Pei Lan* (Herba Eupatorii) for more damp than heat; and *Lian Qiao* (Fructus Forsythiae), *Pu Gong Ying* (Herba Taraxaci), and *Zhe Bei Mu* (Bulbus Fritillariae Thunbergii) for more heat than damp; *Huang Lian* (Rhizoma Coptidis) and *Wu Zhu Yu* (Fructus Evodiae) for acid reflux; *Dan Shen* (Radix et Rhizoma Salviae Miltiorrhizae) and charred *Shan Zha* (Fructus Crataegi) for blood stagnation; and *Tai Zi Shen* (Radix Pseudostellariae) and *Sha Shen* (Radix Glehniae seu Adenophorae) for qi and yin deficiencies due to damp-heat. Of 42 patients, the study reported complete recovery in 33 cases, improvement in 7 cases, and no effect in 2 cases.[8]

8. **Stroke**: *Wen Dan Tang* has been used successfully to treat both acute episodes and sequelae of stroke. According to one study on treatment of acute stroke in 35 patients, use of herbs was associated with complete recovery in 15 cases, improvement in 17 cases, and no effect in 3 cases. The herbal formula contained *Chen Pi* (Pericarpium Citri Reticulatae), *Fu Ling* (Poria), *Ban Xia* (Rhizoma Pinelliae), *Zhi Shi* (Fructus Aurantii Immaturus), *Zhu Ru* (Caulis Bambusae in Taenia), *Shi Chang Pu* (Rhizoma Acori Tatarinowii), and *Gan Cao* (Radix et Rhizoma Glycyrrhizae). Additional modifications were made as needed.[9] According to another study, 34 patients with sequelae of stroke were treated with significant improvement in 10 cases, improvement in 22 cases, and no effect in 2 cases. The herbal formula contained *Wen Dan Tang* plus *San Qi* (Radix et Rhizoma Notoginseng), *Huang Qi* (Radix Astragali), and *Di Long* (Pheretima).[10]

9. **Diabetic microvascular complications**: Administration of modified *Wen Dan Tang* was effective in treating diabetic retinopathy, diabetic nephropathy, and "diabetic foot," which are three diabetic microvascular complications characterized by qi and phlegm stagnation.[11]

10. **Organophosphorus poisoning**: Use of modified *Wen Dan Tang* was associated with marked success in treating organophosphorus poisoning with symptoms such as headache, irritability, insomnia, excessive dreaming, chest oppression, fatigue, nausea, vomiting, depression, inability to concentrate, memory impairment, and others. Of 42 patients, the study reported complete recovery in 34 cases and improvement in 8 cases. The duration of treatment ranged from 3 to 32 days, with an average of 14.5 days.[12]

RELATED FORMULA

Shí Wèi Wēn Dǎn Tāng
(Ten-Ingredient Decoction to Warm the Gallbladder)

十味溫膽湯
十味温胆汤

Pinyin Name: *Shi Wei Wen Dan Tang*

Literal Name: Ten-Ingredient Decoction to Warm the Gallbladder

Original Source: *Zheng Zhi Zhun Sheng* (Standards of Patterns and Treatments) by Wang Ken-Tang in 1602

Ban Xia (Rhizoma Pinelliae), *xi* (washed) with liquid	6g
Zhi Shi (Fructus Aurantii Immaturus), *chao* (dry-fried) with bran	6g
Chen Pi (Pericarpium Citri Reticulatae)	6g
Fu Ling (Poria)	4.5g
Suan Zao Ren (Semen Ziziphi Spinosae), *chao* (dry-fried)	3g
Yuan Zhi (Radix Polygalae), *zhu* (boiled) with licorice juice and *chao* (dry-fried) with ginger juice	3g
Wu Wei Zi (Fructus Schisandrae Chinensis)	3g
Shu Di Huang (Radix Rehmanniae Praeparata), *xi* (washed) with liquor and *bei* (stone-baked)	3g
Ren Shen (Radix et Rhizoma Ginseng)	3g
Zhi Gan Cao (Radix et Rhizoma Glycyrrhizae Praeparata cum Melle)	1.5g

The source text states to prepare the ingredients as a decoction with 5 slices of *Sheng Jiang* (Rhizoma Zingiberis Recens) and 1 piece of *Da Zao* (Fructus Jujubae).

Shi Wei Wen Dan Tang (Ten-Ingredient Decoction to Warm the Gallbladder) dissolves phlegm and tranquilizes the Heart. Clinically, the patient may have Heart and Gallbladder deficiencies, with symptoms such as palpitations, restlessness, irritability, fidgeting, mild swelling of the extremities, and decreased appetite. Historically, this formula has been used to treat individuals who always exhibit fear when faced with challenging circumstances

1216

Wēn Dǎn Tāng (Warm the Gallbladder Decoction)

(Gallbladder deficiency). These individuals usually experience palpitations when they try to solve these issues, and they become easily discouraged by any difficulties (Heart deficiency).

Wen Dan Tang and *Shi Wei Wen Dan Tang* (Ten-Ingredient Decoction to Warm the Gallbladder) both dissolve phlegm.

- *Wen Dan Tang* treats Gallbladder and Stomach disharmony with obstruction of heat-phlegm.
- *Shi Wei Wen Dan Tang* treats Heart and Gallbladder deficiencies with phlegm disturbing the mind and *shen* (spirit).

References
1. *Hu Bei Zhong Yi Za Zhi* (Hubei Journal of Chinese Medicine) 1990;1:17.
2. *Zhe Jiang Zhong Yi Xue Yuan Xue Bao* (Journal of Zhejiang University of Chinese Medicine) 1998;3:25.
3. *Zhong Yi Ming Fang Lin Chuang Xin Yong* (Contemporary Clinical Applications of Classic Chinese Formulas) 2001;696.
4. *Zhe Jiang Zhong Yi Za Zhi* (Zhejiang Journal of Chinese Medicine) 1958;5:5.
5. Wu J, An H, Li Y, Duan L. TCM treatment with the modified wendan tang in 40 cases of melancholia. Journal of Traditional Chinese Medicine 1999 Dec;19(4):296-7.
6. *Zhong Yi Za Zhi* (Journal of Chinese Medicine) 1984;11:831.
7. *Shi Yong Zhong Yi Nei Ke Za Zhi* (Journal of Practical Chinese Internal Medicine) 1992;4:188.
8. *Nei Meng Gu Zhong Yi Yao* (Traditional Chinese Medicine and Medicinals of Inner Mongolia) 1998;3:19.
9. *Xin Zhong Yi* (New Chinese Medicine) 1994;26(8):45.
10. *Shan Xi Zhong Yi* (Shanxi Chinese Medicine) 1995;16(9):393.
11. Gao L. Qi-promoting and phlegm-resolving method for treatment of diabetic microvascular complications. Journal of Traditional Chinese Medicine 2000 Jun;20(2):104-9.
12. *Hu Nan Zhong Yi* (Hunan Journal of Traditional Chinese Medicine) 1976;3(3):46.

Zhú Rú Wēn Dǎn Tāng (Bamboo Decoction to Warm the Gallbladder)
竹茹溫膽湯
竹茹温胆汤

Pinyin Name: *Zhu Ru Wen Dan Tang*
Literal Name: Bamboo Decoction to Warm the Gallbladder
Alternate Name: Bamboo and Ginseng Combination
Original Source: *Wan Bing Hui Chun* (Restoration of Health from the Myriad Diseases) by Gong Ting-Xian in 1587

COMPOSITION

Chai Hu (Radix Bupleuri)	6g
Zhu Ru (Caulis Bambusae in Taenia)	6g
Jie Geng (Radix Platycodonis)	6g
Zhi Shi (Fructus Aurantii Immaturus), *chao* (dry-fried) with bran	6g
Huang Lian (Rhizoma Coptidis)	1.5g
Ren Shen (Radix et Rhizoma Ginseng)	15g
Chen Pi (Pericarpium Citri Reticulatae)	2.4g
Ban Xia (Rhizoma Pinelliae)	2.4g
Fu Ling (Poria)	2.4g
Xiang Fu (Rhizoma Cyperi)	2.4g
Gan Cao (Radix et Rhizoma Glycyrrhizae)	0.9g

DOSAGE / PREPARATION / ADMINISTRATION

The source text states to grind the ingredients into a coarse powder, and decoct it in water with 3 slices of *Sheng Jiang* (Rhizoma Zingiberis Recens) and 1 piece of *Da Zao* (Fructus Jujubae).

CHINESE THERAPEUTIC ACTIONS

1. Clears heat and dissolves phlegm
2. Regulates qi and calms the *shen* (spirit)

PHLEGM-DISPELLING FORMULAS

18

1217

Chapter 18 – Phlegm-Dispelling Formulas   *Section 1 – Damp-Drying and Phlegm-Dissolving Formulas*

Zhú Rú Wēn Dǎn Tāng (Bamboo Decoction to Warm the Gallbladder)

CLINICAL MANIFESTATIONS

Accumulation of heat and phlegm in the Heart and Gallbladder: tendency to get easily frightened and scared, palpitations, insomnia, mild and persistent fever, and copious phlegm in the chest.

CLINICAL APPLICATIONS

Insomnia, neurotic palpitations, alcohol poisoning, and neurasthenia.

EXPLANATION

Zhu Ru Wen Dan Tang (Bamboo Decoction to Warm the Gallbladder) is designed for patients with chronic febrile disorders, in which the heat consumes yin and fluids and gives rise to heat and phlegm accumulation. Patients often complain of mild and persistent fever, as well as copious phlegm and discomfort in the chest. Moreover, the heat and phlegm usually disturb the *shen* (spirit); thus, patients are easily frightened and scared, and experience palpitations and insomnia.

This formula contains herbs with many different functions, with the overall goals of clearing heat and phlegm from the Liver and Gallbladder, calming the *shen* (spirit), and regulating qi. *Chai Hu* (Radix Bupleuri) enters the *shaoyang* level, and is an excellent herb for treating patients with long-term illnesses such as chronic febrile

disorders. *Zhu Ru* (Caulis Bambusae in Taenia) dissolves phlegm and clears heat in the Gallbladder. *Jie Geng* (Radix Platycodonis) eliminates phlegm and relieves chest congestion. *Zhi Shi* (Fructus Aurantii Immaturus) breaks up qi stagnation and dispels phlegm. *Huang Lian* (Rhizoma Coptidis) clears damp-heat.

Because patients with chronic febrile disorders often have qi deficiency and excessive consumption of body fluids, *Ren Shen* (Radix et Rhizoma Ginseng) is added to tonify qi and generate body fluids. It also has the additional benefit of calming the *shen* (spirit). *Chen Pi* (Pericarpium Citri Reticulatae) regulates qi circulation and dries dampness. *Ban Xia* (Rhizoma Pinelliae) dissolves phlegm and guides reversed flow of Stomach qi downward. *Fu Ling* (Poria) strengthens the Spleen and eliminates dampness. *Xiang Fu* (Rhizoma Cyperi) regulates Liver qi. *Sheng Jiang* (Rhizoma Zingiberis Recens), *Da Zao* (Fructus Jujubae), and *Gan Cao* (Radix et Rhizoma Glycyrrhizae) strengthen the Spleen and harmonize the Stomach.

MODIFICATIONS

- With insomnia, add *Shou Wu Teng* (Caulis Polygoni Multiflori) and *Yuan Zhi* (Radix Polygalae).
- With delirium and confusion, add *Long Gu* (Os Draconis) and *Mu Li* (Concha Ostreae).

Zhu Ru Wen Dan Tang (Bamboo Decoction to Warm the Gallbladder)

Diagnosis	Signs and Symptoms	Treatment	Herbs
Accumulation of heat and phlegm in the Heart and Gallbladder	• Fear, fright, palpitations, and insomnia: heat and phlegm disturbing the *shen* (spirit) • Mild and persistent fever, copious phlegm, and chest discomfort: accumulation of heat and phlegm in the chest with damage to yin and fluids	• Clears heat and dissolves phlegm • Regulates qi and calms the *shen* (spirit)	• *Chai Hu* (Radix Bupleuri) and *Xiang Fu* (Rhizoma Cyperi) regulate Liver and Gallbladder. • *Zhu Ru* (Caulis Bambusae in Taenia) dissolves phlegm and clears heat from the Gallbladder. • *Jie Geng* (Radix Platycodonis) eliminates phlegm and relieves chest congestion. • *Zhi Shi* (Fructus Aurantii Immaturus) and *Chen Pi* (Pericarpium Citri Reticulatae) regulate qi circulation and break up qi stagnation. • *Huang Lian* (Rhizoma Coptidis) clears damp-heat. • *Ren Shen* (Radix et Rhizoma Ginseng) and *Fu Ling* (Poria) strengthen the Spleen and tonify qi. • *Ban Xia* (Rhizoma Pinelliae) dissolves phlegm and redirects reversed flow of Stomach qi. • *Sheng Jiang* (Rhizoma Zingiberis Recens), *Da Zao* (Fructus Jujubae), and *Gan Cao* (Radix et Rhizoma Glycyrrhizae) harmonize the Stomach.

1218

Chinese Herbal Formulas and Applications

Fú Líng Wán (Poria Pill)

茯苓丸
茯苓丸

Pinyin Name: *Fu Ling Wan*
Literal Name: Poria Pill
Original Source: *Fu Ren Da Quan Liang Fang* (Complete Fine Formulas for Women) by Chen Zi-Ming in 1237

COMPOSITION

Ban Xia (Rhizoma Pinelliae)	60g [9g]
Fu Ling (Poria)	30g [6g]
Zhi Qiao (Fructus Citri Aurantii), *chao* (dry-fried) with bran	15g [3g]
Po Xiao (Sal Glauberis)	0.3g [3g]

DOSAGE / PREPARATION / ADMINISTRATION

The source text states to grind the ingredients into powder, and form into small pills using the juice of *Sheng Jiang* (Rhizoma Zingiberis Recens). The pills should resemble the size of *Wu Tong Zi* (Semen Firmianae), a small seed approximately 5 mm in diameter. Take 20 pills (6g) after meals with a decoction made from *Sheng Jiang* (Rhizoma Zingiberis Recens). Today, this formula may be prepared as a decoction with the doses suggested in brackets.

CHINESE THERAPEUTIC ACTIONS

1. Dries dampness and activates qi
2. Softens nodules and dissolves phlegm

CLINICAL MANIFESTATIONS

Phlegm stagnation in the epigastrium: pain in both arms, edema of the extremities, a white, greasy tongue coating, and a wiry, slippery pulse.

CLINICAL APPLICATIONS

Muscle aches and pains, edema, and cough.

EXPLANATION

Fu Ling Wan (Poria Pill) treats damp and phlegm stagnation in the epigastrium, which arises from an underlying Spleen deficiency. Spleen deficiency leads to damp accumulation and, ultimately, to phlegm stagnation in the chest and epigastrium. Dampness and phlegm may travel via the channels and collaterals, causing pain in the arms or edema of the extremities. A white, greasy tongue coating and a wiry, slippery pulse indicate damp and phlegm accumulation.

This formula has *Ban Xia* (Rhizoma Pinelliae) to dry dampness and dispel phlegm. *Fu Ling* (Poria) strengthens

the Spleen and dispels dampness. *Zhi Qiao* (Fructus Aurantii) activates qi to dispel phlegm. *Po Xiao* (Sal Glauberis) softens nodules and facilitates the elimination of phlegm. The juice of *Sheng Jiang* (Rhizoma Zingiberis Recens) dissolves phlegm and detoxifies *Ban Xia* (Rhizoma Pinelliae).

MODIFICATIONS

- With swelling and pain of the limbs, add *Sang Zhi* (Ramulus Mori) and *Di Long* (Pheretima).
- For cough with thick sputum, add *Ge Qiao* (Concha Meretricis seu Cyclinae) and *Gua Lou* (Fructus Trichosanthis).

CAUTIONS / CONTRAINDICATIONS

- *Fu Ling Wan* should be used with caution in patients with generalized deficiencies.
- This formula is contraindicated for prolonged use. It should be discontinued as soon as the desired effect is achieved.

AUTHORS' COMMENTS

It is important to note that the arm pain in this syndrome is caused by damp and phlegm stagnation in the epigastrium. From the epigastrium, dampness and phlegm travel via the channels and collaterals to the extremities to cause pain and edema. Optimal treatment requires the use of herbs to dry dampness and dispel phlegm. Since wind-damp-cold factors are **not** the cause of this syndrome, herbs that dispel wind-damp-cold should not be used, as they will only consume qi and complicate the illness.

Fu Ling Wan also treats cough with profuse sputum, accompanied by a feeling of fullness and distention in the chest and epigastrium.

PHLEGM-DISPELLING FORMULAS

18

Chapter 18 – Phlegm-Dispelling Formulas   *Section 1 – Damp-Drying and Phlegm-Dissolving Formulas*

Fú Líng Wán (Poria Pill)

Fu Ling Wan (Poria Pill)

Diagnosis	Signs and Symptoms	Treatment	Herbs
Phlegm stagnation in the epigastrium	• Pain in both arms and edema of the extremities: phlegm stagnation in the channels and collaterals • White, greasy tongue coating and a wiry, slippery pulse: damp and phlegm accumulation	• Dries dampness and activates qi • Softens nodules and dissolves phlegm	• *Ban Xia* (Rhizoma Pinelliae) dries dampness and dispels phlegm. • *Fu Ling* (Poria) strengthens the Spleen and dispels dampness. • *Zhi Qiao* (Fructus Aurantii) activates qi to dispel phlegm. • *Po Xiao* (Sal Glauberis) softens nodules and facilitates the elimination of phlegm. • *Sheng Jiang* (Rhizoma Zingiberis Recens) dissolves phlegm and detoxifies *Ban Xia* (Rhizoma Pinelliae).

Xiǎo Bàn Xià Jiā Fú Líng Tāng (Minor Pinellia and Poria Decoction)
小半夏加茯苓湯
小半夏加茯苓汤

Pinyin Name: *Xiao Ban Xia Jia Fu Ling Tang*
Literal Name: Minor Pinellia and Poria Decoction
Alternate Names: *Hsiao Pan Hsia Chia Fu Ling Tang*, Minor Pinellia plus Hoelen Decoction, Minor Pinellia and Hoelen Combination
Original Source: *Jin Gui Yao Lue* (Essentials from the Golden Cabinet) by Zhang Zhong-Jing in the Eastern Han Dynasty

COMPOSITION

Ban Xia (Rhizoma Pinelliae)	1 cup [12g]
Sheng Jiang (Rhizoma Zingiberis Recens)	24g
Fu Ling (Poria)	9g

DOSAGE / PREPARATION / ADMINISTRATION

The source text states to cook the ingredients in 7 cups [1,400 mL] of water until the liquid is reduced to 1.5 cups [300 mL]. Take the warm, strained decoction in two equally-divided doses.

CHINESE THERAPEUTIC ACTIONS

1. Dispels phlegm
2. Regulates water circulation
3. Disperses qi stagnation

CLINICAL MANIFESTATIONS

Nausea and vomiting caused by phlegm stagnation and water accumulation: nausea, vomiting, a feeling of oppression in the epigastrium, dizziness, and dysuria.

CLINICAL APPLICATIONS

Nausea, vomiting, morning sickness during pregnancy, acute enteritis, gastric prolapse, and viral myocarditis.

EXPLANATION

Xiao Ban Xia Jia Fu Ling Tang (Minor Pinellia and Poria Decoction) treats nausea and vomiting caused by phlegm stagnation and water accumulation in the epigastrium. In this syndrome, the normal functions of the Spleen and Stomach are compromised due to phlegm stagnation and water accumulation, thus nausea and vomiting occur. In addition, phlegm and water stagnation creates a feeling of oppression in the epigastrium, affects urination, and causes dysuria. Other symptoms may include dizziness, absence of thirst, and palpitations.

1220

Chinese Herbal Formulas and Applications

Xiǎo Bàn Xià Jiā Fú Líng Tāng (Minor Pinellia and Poria Decoction)

Xiao Ban Xia Jia Fu Ling Tang (Minor Pinellia and Poria Decoction)

Diagnosis	Signs and Symptoms	Treatment	Herbs
Phlegm stagnation and water accumulation	• Nausea and vomiting: phlegm stagnation and water accumulation affecting the Spleen and Stomach • Feeling of oppression in the epigastrium: phlegm stagnation and water accumulation	• Dispels phlegm • Regulates water circulation • Disperses qi stagnation	• *Ban Xia* (Rhizoma Pinelliae) dries dampness, dispels phlegm, and alleviates nausea and vomiting. • *Sheng Jiang* (Rhizoma Zingiberis Recens) warms the middle *jiao* and reduces the toxicity of *Ban Xia* (Rhizoma Pinelliae). • *Fu Ling* (Poria) drains water accumulation and promotes normal urination.

Ban Xia (Rhizoma Pinelliae) acts as the chief herb to dry dampness, dispel phlegm, and redirect the reversed flow of Stomach qi downwards to alleviate nausea and vomiting. *Sheng Jiang* (Rhizoma Zingiberis Recens) serves two purposes in this formula. First, it warms the middle *jiao* and helps *Ban Xia* (Rhizoma Pinelliae) disperse stagnation. Second, it reduces the toxicity of *Ban Xia* (Rhizoma Pinelliae). The third herb, *Fu Ling* (Poria), drains water accumulation and promotes normal urination.

MODIFICATIONS

• For nausea and vomiting caused by Stomach deficiency, add *Dang Shen* (Radix Codonopsis) and *Chen Pi* (Pericarpium Citri Reticulatae).
• For nausea and vomiting caused by food stagnation, add *Zhi Qiao* (Fructus Aurantii), *Shen Qu* (Massa Fermentata), and *Mai Ya* (Fructus Hordei Germinatus).
• For nausea and vomiting caused by phlegm stagnation, add *Er Chen Tang* (Two-Cured Decoction).
• For nausea and vomiting caused by water accumulation, add *Wei Ling Tang* (Calm the Stomach and Poria Decoction).

• For morning sickness during pregnancy, add *Dang Gui* (Radix Angelicae Sinensis) and *Chuan Xiong* (Rhizoma Chuanxiong).

CLINICAL STUDIES AND RESEARCH

1. **Morning sickness**: Administration of *Xiao Ban Xia Jia Fu Ling Tang* was associated with relief of nausea and vomiting in pregnant women. Out of 66 patients, 42 had complete recovery within 5 to 8 doses, 12 had marked improvement after 5 doses, 7 had slight improvement after 9 doses, and 5 had no improvement. The overall effectiveness was 92.4%.[1]

2. **Viral myocarditis**: Use of modified *Xiao Ban Xia Jia Fu Ling Tang* showed marked effectiveness in treating 11 patients with viral myocarditis. The duration of treatment ranged from 15 to 150 doses of herbs. Out of 11 patients, symptomatic improvement was reported in all cases, and EKG readings improved in 10 cases.[2]

References
1. *Guang Xi Zhong Yi Yao* (Guangxi Chinese Medicine and Herbology) 1992;2:16.
2. *Shang Hai Zhong Yi Yao Za Zhi* (Shanghai Journal of Chinese Medicine and Herbology) 1983;9:267.

PHLEGM-DISPELLING FORMULAS

18

1221

Chapter 18 – Phlegm-Dispelling Formulas　　　*Section 2 – Heat-Clearing and Phlegm-Dissolving Formulas*

Section 2

清热化痰剂

— Heat-Clearing and Phlegm-Dissolving Formulas

Qīng Qi Huà Tán Wán (Clear the Qi and Transform Phlegm Pill)
清氣化痰丸
清气化痰丸

Pinyin Name: *Qing Qi Hua Tan Wan*
Literal Name: Clear the Qi and Transform Phlegm Pill
Alternate Name: Pinellia and Scute Formula
Original Source: *Yi Fang Kao (Investigation of Medical Formulas)* by Wu Kun in 1584

COMPOSITION

Dan Nan Xing (Arisaema cum Bile)	45g [9g]
Huang Qin (Radix Scutellariae), *chao* (dry-fried) with liquor	30g [6g]
Gua Lou Zi (Semen Trichosanthis), oil removed	30g [6g]
Zhi Shi (Fructus Aurantii Immaturus), *chao* (dry-fried) with bran	30g [6g]
Chen Pi (Pericarpium Citri Reticulatae)	30g [6g]
Fu Ling (Poria)	30g [6g]
Ku Xing Ren (Semen Armeniacae Amarum)	30g [6g]
Ban Xia (Rhizoma Pinelliae), *zhi* (prepared)	45g [9g]

DOSAGE / PREPARATION / ADMINISTRATION

The source text states to grind the ingredients into powder and form into pills with fresh juice from *Sheng Jiang* (Rhizoma Zingiberis Recens). Take 6g of pills per dose with warm, boiled water. Today, this formula may be prepared as a decoction with the doses suggested in brackets.

CHINESE THERAPEUTIC ACTIONS

1. Clears heat and dissolves phlegm
2. Regulates qi and stops coughing

CLINICAL MANIFESTATIONS

Phlegm-heat stagnation in the Lung: cough with thick, yellow sputum that cannot be completely expectorated; a feeling of fullness and distention in the chest and diaphragm; scanty, dark urine; a red tongue body with yellow, greasy tongue coating; and a slippery, rapid pulse.

CLINICAL APPLICATIONS

Hemoptysis, coughing, pneumonia, bronchitis, and respiratory tract infections.

EXPLANATION

Qing Qi Hua Tan Wan (Clear the Qi and Transform Phlegm Pill) treats phlegm-heat syndromes accompanied by thick, yellow sputum and a slippery, rapid pulse. The origin of these syndromes can be traced to the presence of internal fire, which dries and thickens the body fluids, turning them into phlegm. When phlegm accumulates in the Lung, it produces Lung qi stagnation and cough. The sputum is thick and yellowish as a result of internal fire. The feeling of fullness and distention in the chest is caused by qi stagnation in the chest area; and scanty, dark urine is the result of the internal fire affecting the lower *jiao*. A red tongue body with a yellow, greasy tongue coating and a slippery, rapid pulse suggest phlegm and heat accumulation in the interior.

This formula has *Dan Nan Xing* (Arisaema cum Bile) to clear heat and dissolve phlegm. *Huang Qin* (Radix Scutellariae) and *Gua Lou Zi* (Semen Trichosanthis) clear Lung heat and eliminate phlegm. Since phlegm obstructs the flow of qi, *Zhi Shi* (Fructus Aurantii Immaturus) and *Chen Pi* (Pericarpium Citri Reticulatae) remove qi

1222

Chinese Herbal Formulas and Applications

Qīng Qì Huà Tán Wán (Clear the Qi and Transform Phlegm Pill)

Qing Qi Hua Tan Wan (Clear the Qi and Transform Phlegm Pill)

Diagnosis	Signs and Symptoms	Treatment	Herbs
Phlegm-heat in the Lung	• Cough, thick, yellow sputum that cannot be completely expectorated, and a feeling of fullness and distention in the chest and diaphragm: phlegm-heat stagnation in the Lung • Scanty, dark urine: internal fire affecting the lower *jiao* • Red tongue body with yellow, greasy tongue coating, and slippery, rapid pulse: phlegm-heat accumulation in the interior	• Clears heat and dissolves phlegm • Regulates qi and stops cough	• *Dan Nan Xing* (Arisaema cum Bile) clears heat and dissolves phlegm. • *Huang Qin* (Radix Scutellariae) and *Gua Lou Zi* (Semen Trichosanthis) clear Lung heat and eliminate phlegm. • *Zhi Shi* (Fructus Aurantii Immaturus) and *Chen Pi* (Pericarpium Citri Reticulatae) remove qi stagnation and dissolve phlegm. • *Fu Ling* (Poria) strengthens the Spleen and drains dampness to prevent the formation of more phlegm. • *Ku Xing Ren* (Semen Armeniacae Amarum) causes the Lung qi to descend and relieves cough. • *Ban Xia* (Rhizoma Pinelliae) breaks up phlegm stagnation and dries dampness.

stagnation and dissolve phlegm. Because the Spleen is the organ that produces dampness and phlegm, *Fu Ling* (Poria) is used to strengthen the Spleen and drain dampness, preventing the formation of more phlegm. *Ku Xing Ren* (Semen Armeniacae Amarum) causes the Lung qi to descend and relieves cough, and *Ban Xia* (Rhizoma Pinelliae) breaks up phlegm stagnation and dries dampness.

MODIFICATIONS
• With cough and thirst due to severe Lung heat, add *Shi Gao* (Gypsum Fibrosum) and *Zhi Mu* (Rhizoma Anemarrhenae), or combine with *Ma Huang Xing Ren Gan Cao Shi Gao Tang* (Ephedra, Apricot Kernel, Licorice, and Gypsum Decoction).
• With profuse sputum and hurried respiration, add *Yu Xing Cao* (Herba Houttuyniae) and *Sang Bai Pi* (Cortex Mori).
• If there is constipation, add *Mang Xiao* (Natrii Sulfas).

CAUTIONS / CONTRAINDICATIONS
• *Qing Qi Hua Tan Wan* is contraindicated in patients with yin deficiency, dryness, or wind-cold conditions.
• Use of this formula is contraindicated during pregnancy.[1]

RELATED FORMULA
Huà Tán Wán (Transform Phlegm Pill)
化痰丸
化痰丸
Pinyin Name: *Hua Tan Wan*
Literal Name: Transform Phlegm Pill
Original Source: *Tian Jin Zhong Yi Xue Yuan* (Tianjin University of Chinese Medicine) in 1989

Gua Lou Zi (Semen Trichosanthis)
Yu Xing Cao (Herba Houttuyniae)
Chen Pi (Pericarpium Citri Reticulatae)
Yi Yi Ren (Semen Coicis)
Huang Qin (Radix Scutellariae)
Ku Xing Ren (Semen Armeniacae Amarum)
Zhi Shi (Fructus Aurantii Immaturus)
Fu Ling (Poria)
Tian Nan Xing (Rhizoma Arisaematis)
Ban Xia (Rhizoma Pinelliae)
Zhu Ru (Caulis Bambusae in Taenia)
Ting Li Zi (Semen Descurainiae seu Lepidii)
Da Zao (Fructus Jujubae)

Hua Tan Wan (Transform Phlegm Pill) clears heat, dissolves phlegm, and regulates qi circulation. Clinically, it treats accumulation of heat and phlegm in the chest, with symptoms such as cough, dyspnea, chest congestion, and abundant yellow, sticky phlegm.

AUTHORS' COMMENTS
Fresh juice from *Sheng Jiang* (Rhizoma Zingiberis Recens) has a strong dispersing property, which helps transform phlegm, therefore it is added to the herbs and made into pills.

Reference
1. *Zhong Yao Ming Fang Yao Li Yu Ying Yong* (Pharmacology and Applications of Famous Herbal Formulas) 1989;591-2.

PHLEGM-DISPELLING FORMULAS

18

1223

Chapter 18 – Phlegm-Dispelling Formulas　　　*Section 2 – Heat-Clearing and Phlegm-Dissolving Formulas*

Qīng Fèi Yǐn (Clear the Lung Drink)

清肺飲
清肺饮

Pinyin Name: *Qing Fei Yin*
Literal Name: Clear the Lung Drink
Alternate Names: *Ching Fai Yin, Qing Fai Yin*, Lung-Clearing Drink, Platycodon and Apricot Seed Formula
Original Source: *Yi Fang Ji Jie* (Analytical Collection of Medical Formulas) by Wang Ang in 1682

COMPOSITION

Ku Xing Ren (Semen Armeniacae Amarum)	3g
Bei Mu (Bulbus Fritillariae)	3g
Wu Wei Zi (Fructus Schisandrae Chinensis)	1.5g
Fu Ling (Poria)	3g
Ju Hong (Exocarpium Citri Reticulatae)	1.5g
Jie Geng (Radix Platycodonis)	1.5g
Gan Cao (Radix et Rhizoma Glycyrrhizae)	1.5g

DOSAGE / PREPARATION / ADMINISTRATION

The source text states to cook the herbs with *Sheng Jiang* (Rhizoma Zingiberis Recens). Take the warm, strained decoction between meals.

CHINESE THERAPEUTIC ACTIONS

Clears the Lung and dissolves phlegm

CLINICAL MANIFESTATIONS

Cough caused by phlegm and damp accumulation: cough with sputum, chest discomfort, and fatigue.

CLINICAL APPLICATIONS

Cough due to common cold and influenza, bronchial asthma, cough due to tuberculosis, and cough with sore throat.

EXPLANATION

Qing Fei Yin (Clear the Lung Drink) treats cough caused by phlegm and damp accumulation. As a result of the accumulation, the Lung qi cannot descend, causing qi reversal and cough. The presence of sputum indicates dampness and phlegm.

This formula contains herbs to clear the Lung, dissolve phlegm, and moisten the Lung. *Ku Xing Ren* (Semen Armeniacae Amarum) causes Lung qi to descend, and is commonly used to treat cough and dyspnea. *Bei Mu* (Bulbus Fritillariae) clears fire, dissolves phlegm, and moistens the Lung. *Wu Wei Zi* (Fructus Schisandrae Chinensis) stabilizes and binds to preserve the Lung

from further loss of qi. *Fu Ling* (Poria) strengthens the Spleen and dissolves dampness. *Ju Hong* (Exocarpium Citri Reticulatae) activates qi and relieves stagnation. *Jie Geng* (Radix Platycodonis) clears the Lung and eliminates phlegm. *Gan Cao* (Radix et Rhizoma Glycyrrhizae) and *Sheng Jiang* (Rhizoma Zingiberis Recens) harmonize the formula. In short, this formula treats mild to moderate cases of cough caused by damp and phlegm accumulation.

MODIFICATIONS

- If there is clear nasal discharge due to wind, add *Bo He* (Herba Menthae), *Fang Feng* (Radix Saposhnikoviae), and *Zi Su Ye* (Folium Perillae).
- With thirst and sore throat due to heat, add *Shi Gao* (Gypsum Fibrosum) and *Zhi Mu* (Rhizoma Anemarrhenae).
- For chronic cough caused by Lung deficiency, add *Ren Shen* (Radix et Rhizoma Ginseng) and *Huang Qi* (Radix Astragali).
- For cough and hoarseness, add *Di Gu Pi* (Cortex Lycii).
- For cough and dyspnea accompanied by profuse phlegm, add *Sang Bai Pi* (Cortex Mori) and *Di Gu Pi* (Cortex Lycii).
- With phlegm due to food stagnation, add *Shan Zha* (Fructus Crataegi), *Xiang Fu* (Rhizoma Cyperi), and *Zhi Shi* (Fructus Aurantii Immaturus).
- With phlegm and dryness, add *Zhi Mu* (Rhizoma Anemarrhenae), *Tian Dong* (Radix Asparagi), and *Gua Lou* (Fructus Trichosanthis).
- With Stomach fire, add *Shi Gao* (Gypsum Fibrosum) and *Huang Lian* (Rhizoma Coptidis).

1224

Qīng Fèi Yǐn (Clear the Lung Drink)

Qing Fei Yin (Clear the Lung Drink)

Diagnosis	Signs and Symptoms	Treatment	Herbs
Cough due to accumulation of phlegm and dampness	Cough with sputum, chest discomfort and fatigue: reversed qi flow due to accumulation of phlegm and dampness	Clears the Lung and dissolves phlegm	• *Ku Xing Ren* (Semen Armeniacae Amarum) causes qi to descend to treat cough and dyspnea. • *Bei Mu* (Bulbus Fritillariae) clears fire, dissolves phlegm, and moistens the Lung. • *Wu Wei Zi* (Fructus Schisandrae Chinensis) stabilizes and binds Lung qi. • *Fu Ling* (Poria) strengthens the Spleen and dissolves dampness. • *Ju Hong* (Exocarpium Citri Reticulatae) activates qi and relieves stagnation. • *Jie Geng* (Radix Platycodonis) clears the Lung and eliminates phlegm. • *Gan Cao* (Radix et Rhizoma Glycyrrhizae) and *Sheng Jiang* (Rhizoma Zingiberis Recens) harmonize the formula.

Qīng Fèi Tāng (Clear the Lung Decoction)

清肺湯
清肺汤

Pinyin Name: *Qing Fei Tang*
Literal Name: Clear the Lung Decoction
Alternate Names: *Ching Fei Tang*, Lung-Clearing Decoction, Platycodon and Fritillaria Decoction, Platycodon and Fritillaria Combination
Original Source: *Wan Bing Hui Chun* (Restoration of Health from the Myriad Diseases) by Gong Ting-Xian in 1587

COMPOSITION

Huang Qin (Radix Scutellariae)	4.5g
Zhi Zi (Fructus Gardeniae)	2.1g
Ku Xing Ren (Semen Armeniacae Amarum)	2.1g
Zhe Bei Mu (Bulbus Fritillariae Thunbergii)	3g
Zhu Ru (Caulis Bambusae in Taenia)	3g
Sang Bai Pi (Cortex Mori)	3g
Jie Geng (Radix Platycodonis)	3g
Mai Dong (Radix Ophiopogonis)	2.1g
Tian Dong (Radix Asparagi)	2.1g
Dang Gui (Radix Angelicae Sinensis)	2.1g
Gan Cao (Radix et Rhizoma Glycyrrhizae)	0.9g
Chen Pi (Pericarpium Citri Reticulatae)	3g
Fu Ling (Poria)	3g
Wu Wei Zi (Fructus Schisandrae Chinensis)	7 pieces

Chapter 18 – Phlegm-Dispelling Formulas   *Section 2 – Heat-Clearing and Phlegm-Dissolving Formulas*

Qīng Fèi Tāng (Clear the Lung Decoction)

DOSAGE / PREPARATION / ADMINISTRATION

The source text states to grate and cook the herbs with *Sheng Jiang* (Rhizoma Zingiberis Recens) and *Da Zao* (Fructus Jujubae). Take the warm, strained decoction after meals.

CHINESE THERAPEUTIC ACTIONS

1. Dispels heat and phlegm from the chest
2. Moistens the Lung and relieves cough

CLINICAL MANIFESTATIONS

Chronic cough caused by heat and phlegm in the Lung: severe cough, thick and sticky phlegm, sore and itchy throat, and hoarseness.

CLINICAL APPLICATIONS

Chronic bronchitis, pneumonia, aspiration pneumonia, bronchiectasis, laryngitis, tuberculosis, and cardiac asthma.

EXPLANATION

Qing Fei Tang (Clear the Lung Decoction) addresses chronic cases of heat and phlegm attacking the Lung, leading to phlegm accumulation with underlying deficiency.

When heat and phlegm obstruct the Lung, the flow of qi is reversed, resulting in severe cough. In addition, phlegm accumulation can cause thick, sticky sputum, with color varying from white to yellow to green. The chronic nature of this illness also contributes to yin and fluid deficiencies, leading to sore, itchy throat, and hoarseness.

This formula contains herbs to dispel heat and phlegm, moisten the Lung, and relieve cough. *Huang Qin* (Radix Scutellariae) and *Zhi Zi* (Fructus Gardeniae) clear damp-heat from the upper *jiao*, thereby addressing the heat and phlegm condition in the Lung. *Ku Xing Ren* (Semen Armeniacae Amarum), *Zhe Bei Mu* (Bulbus Fritillariae Thunbergii), *Zhu Ru* (Caulis Bambusae in Taenia), and *Sang Bai Pi* (Cortex Mori) clear the Lung and cause qi to descend. *Jie Geng* (Radix Platycodonis) eliminates the accumulation of sputum and phlegm. *Mai Dong* (Radix Ophiopogonis) and *Tian Dong* (Radix Asparagi) have a synergistic effect to moisten the Lung and nourish yin. *Dang Gui* (Radix Angelicae Sinensis) and *Gan Cao* (Radix et Rhizoma Glycyrrhizae) nourish the blood, and balance the bitter and cold nature of *Huang Qin* (Radix Scutellariae) and *Zhi Zi* (Fructus Gardeniae). *Chen Pi* (Pericarpium Citri Reticulatae) regulates the proper flow

Qing Fei Tang (Clear the Lung Decoction)

Diagnosis	Signs and Symptoms	Treatment	Herbs
Chronic cough due to heat and phlegm in the Lung	• Cough with thick, sticky sputum: reversed qi flow due to heat and phlegm obstructing the Lung • Sore, itchy throat and hoarseness: yin and fluid deficiencies	• Dispels heat and phlegm from the chest • Moistens the Lung and relieves cough	• *Huang Qin* (Radix Scutellariae) and *Zhi Zi* (Fructus Gardeniae) clear damp-heat from the Lung in the upper *jiao*. • *Ku Xing Ren* (Semen Armeniacae Amarum), *Zhe Bei Mu* (Bulbus Fritillariae Thunbergii), *Zhu Ru* (Caulis Bambusae in Taenia) and *Sang Bai Pi* (Cortex Mori) clear the Lung and cause Lung qi to descend. • *Jie Geng* (Radix Platycodonis) eliminates the accumulation of sputum and phlegm. • *Mai Dong* (Radix Ophiopogonis) and *Tian Dong* (Radix Asparagi) moisten the Lung and nourish yin. • *Dang Gui* (Radix Angelicae Sinensis) and *Gan Cao* (Radix et Rhizoma Glycyrrhizae) nourish the blood. • *Chen Pi* (Pericarpium Citri Reticulatae) regulates the proper flow of qi. • *Fu Ling* (Poria) strengthens the Spleen to dry dampness and reduce phlegm production. • *Wu Wei Zi* (Fructus Schisandrae Chinensis) stabilizes and binds the Lung to prevent further loss of Lung qi. • *Sheng Jiang* (Rhizoma Zingiberis Recens) and *Da Zao* (Fructus Jujubae) harmonize the formula.

Chinese Herbal Formulas and Applications

Qīng Fèi Tāng (Clear the Lung Decoction)

of qi. *Fu Ling* (Poria) strengthens the Spleen to dry dampness and reduce phlegm production. *Wu Wei Zi* (Fructus Schisandrae Chinensis) stabilizes and binds the Lung to prevent further loss of Lung qi. *Sheng Jiang* (Rhizoma Zingiberis Recens) and *Da Zao* (Fructus Jujubae) harmonize the formula.

MODIFICATIONS

- With sore, dry throat due to heat, add *Shi Gao* (Gypsum Fibrosum) and *Zhi Mu* (Rhizoma Anemarrhenae).
- With irritability, swelling, and pain, add *Jin Yin Hua* (Flos Lonicerae Japonicae) and *Lian Qiao* (Fructus Forsythiae).
- With stubborn phlegm that is difficult to expectorate, add *Gua Lou* (Fructus Trichosanthis), *Zhi Shi* (Fructus Aurantii Immaturus), and *Zhu Li* (Succus Bambusae). Remove *Wu Wei Zi* (Fructus Schisandrae Chinensis).
- With cough, asthma, and increased respiration, add *Zi Su Zi* (Fructus Perillae) and *Zhu Li* (Succus Bambusae). Remove *Jie Geng* (Radix Platycodonis).
- With chronic cough with spontaneous perspiration, add *Bai Zhu* (Rhizoma Atractylodis Macrocephalae), *Bai Shao* (Radix Paeoniae Alba), and *Di Huang* (Radix Rehmanniae). Remove *Jie Geng* (Radix Platycodonis), *Zhe Bei Mu* (Bulbus Fritillariae Thunbergii), and *Ku Xing Ren* (Semen Armeniacae Amarum).
- With high fever, flushed face, and blood in the sputum, add *Bai Shao* (Radix Paeoniae Alba), *Di Huang* (Radix Rehmanniae), *Zi Wan* (Radix et Rhizoma Asteris), *E Jiao* (Colla Corii Asini), and *Zhu Li* (Succus Bambusae). Remove *Wu Wei Zi* (Fructus Schisandrae Chinensis), *Ku Xing Ren* (Semen Armeniacae Amarum), *Zhe Bei Mu* (Bulbus Fritillariae Thunbergii), and *Jie Geng* (Radix Platycodonis).

PHARMACOLOGICAL EFFECTS

1. **Expectorant**: According to one study, administration of 500 mg/kg of *Qing Fei Tang* in powder extract via oral ingestion was associated with a marked expectorant effect, with the onset of action beginning after 3 hours. No expectorant effect was observed when the formula was given at lower doses, such as 50 and 100 mg/kg.[1,2]
2. **Antiallergic**: This formula has an inhibitory effect on leukotriene (LT) B4 synthesis of human alveolar macrophages. In one study, two-week cultured basophil levels identified by alcian blue-safranin staining and those histamine contents assayed fluorometrically were inhibited by this formula in a dose-dependent manner. Since *Qing Fei Tang* modulates basophil growth and differentiation *in vitro* and/or *in vivo*, the study suggested that the formula has an antiallergic effect and may be useful for controlling allergic diseases including bronchial asthma.[3]

3. **Respiratory**: Administration of *Qing Fei Tang* was associated with various effects on the respiratory system, including but not limited to inhibited release of slow reacting substance of anaphylaxis from the lung, suppressed chemiluminescence of oxygen radicals, increased output volume and fatty acid contents in respiratory tract fluid, and facilitated tracheal mucociliary transport.[4] According to one study in mice, use of *Qing Fei Tang* was associated with reduced mortality for aspiration pneumonia artificially-induced with *Streptococcus pneumoniae* and gastric juice. The mechanism of this effect was attributed to the decreased activity of xanthine oxidase and reduction of oxygen radical production in inflamed lungs.[5]
4. **Anti-inflammatory**: *Qing Fei Tang* can be used to treat inflammatory lung diseases through its anti-inflammatory action to inhibit the oxidative and arachidonate metabolism of local inflammatory lung cells.[6]

CLINICAL STUDIES AND RESEARCH

Aspiration pneumonia: According to a randomized, controlled clinical trial, 15 patients with relapsing aspiration pneumonia were divided into two groups. Eight patients were treated with conventional Western medicine, and 7 were treated with *Qing Fei Tang*. After a study period of 16 weeks, the study reported a significant reduction of relapse of aspiration pneumonia and reduction in antibiotic use in patients treated with *Qing Fei Tang*, in comparison with drug therapy group. Swallowing reflex, however, did not change in patients treated with *Qing Fei Tang*. No adverse reactions were reported in either group. The study concluded that *Qing Fei Tang* is an effective therapy for treatment of aspiration pneumonia. It improved the defense mechanism or excessive inflammation caused by pneumonia in the lower airway, but did not improve the swallowing reflex.[7]

RELATED FORMULA

Qīng Fèi Tāng (Clear the Lung Decoction)

清肺湯
清肺汤

Pinyin Name: *Qing Fei Tang*
Literal Name: Clear the Lung Decoction
Original Source: *Han Fang Yi Xue* (Kampo Medicine)

Huang Qin (Radix Scutellariae)
Jie Geng (Radix Platycodonis)
Fu Ling (Poria)
Chen Pi (Pericarpium Citri Reticulatae)
Bei Mu (Bulbus Fritillariae)
Sang Bai Pi (Cortex Mori)
Dang Gui (Radix Angelicae Sinensis)
Tian Dong (Radix Asparagi)

PHLEGM-DISPELLING FORMULAS

18

1227

Chapter 18 – Phlegm-Dispelling Formulas   *Section 2 – Heat-Clearing and Phlegm-Dissolving Formulas*

Qīng Fèi Tāng (Clear the Lung Decoction)

Zhi Zi (Fructus Gardeniae)
Ku Xing Ren (Semen Armeniacae Amarum)
Mai Dong (Radix Ophiopogonis)
Wu Wei Zi (Fructus Schisandrae Chinensis)
Gan Cao (Radix et Rhizoma Glycyrrhizae)
Zhu Ru (Caulis Bambusae in Taenia)

These two formulas have essentially the same ingredients and functions. *Qing Fei Tang* (Clear the Lung Decoction), which appeared in *Wan Bing Hui Chun* (Restoration of Health from the Myriad Diseases), is the original formulation. *Qing Fei Tang* (Clear the Lung Decoction), from *Han Fang Yi Xue* (Kampo Medicine), is the revised formulation, with the addition of *Zhu Ru* (Caulis Bambusae in Taenia), which clears heat and dissolves thick, yellow phlegm.

AUTHORS' COMMENTS

According to Dr. Chang Wei-Yen, *Qing Fei Tang* can be combined with *Sang Ju Yin* (Mulberry Leaf and Chrysanthemum Decoction), *Hu Yao Huang* (Herba Leucas Mollissimae), *Pao Zai Cao* (Herba Physalis Angulatae), and *Zhu Zi Cao* (Herba Euphorbiae Thymifoliae) to treat cough and dyspnea associated with wind-heat invasion.

Qing Fei Tang (Clear the Lung <u>Decoction</u>) and *Qing Fei Yin* (Clear the Lung <u>Drink</u>) are two formulas with similar names, but have different functions and indications.

- *Qing Fei Tang* is a potent formula that treats chronic cough with both excess (heat and phlegm) and deficiency (underlying yin and fluid deficiencies). It clears heat, dispels phlegm, moistens the Lung, and relieves cough.
- *Qing Fei Yin* is a mild to moderate formula that treats cough characterized by only excess (phlegm and dampness). It dissolves dampness, dispels phlegm, and relieves coughing.

References

1. *Guo Wai Yi Xue Zhong Yi Zhong Yao Fen Ce* (Monograph of Chinese Herbology from Foreign Medicine) 1986;4:18.
2. *Zhong Yi Fang Ji Xian Dai Yan Jiu* (Modern Study of Medical Formulae in Traditional Chinese Medicine) 1997;1496.
3. Tanno Y, Shindoh Y, Takishima T. Modulation of human basophil growth in vitro by xiao-qing-long-tang (syo-seiryu-to), chai-pu-tang (saiboku-to), qing-fei-tang (seihai-to), baicalein and ketotifen. American Journal of Chinese Medicine 1989;17(1-2):45-50.
4. Miyamoto K, Furusawa K, Kuroiwa A, Saito M, Miyata T, Furukawa T. Effects of qing-fei-tang on the airway inflammation and clearance. Am J Chin Med 1990;18(1-2):5-18.
5. Iwasaki K, Wang Q, Satoh N, Yoshida S, Akaike T, Sekizawa K, Maeda H, Sasaki H. Effects of qing fei tang (TJ-90) on aspiration pneumonia in mice. Phytomedicine 1999 May;6(2):95-101.
6. Tanno Y, Kakuta Y, Aikawa T, Shindoh Y, Ohno I, Takishima T. Effects of Qing-Fei-Tang (seihai-to) and baicalein, its main component flavonoid, on lucigenin-dependent chemiluminescence and leukotriene B4 synthesis of human alveolar macrophages. Am J Chin Med 1988;16(3-4):145-54.
7. Mantani N, Kasahara Y, Kamata T, Sekiya N, Shimada Y, Usuda K, Sakakibara I, Hattori N, Terasawa K. Effect of Seihai-to, a Kampo medicine, in relapsing aspiration pneumonia--an open-label pilot study. Phytomedicine 2002 Apr;9(3):195-201.

Chinese Herbal Formulas and Applications

Zǐ Wǎn Tāng (Aster Decoction)

紫苑湯
紫苑汤

Pinyin Name: *Zi Wan Tang*
Literal Name: Aster Decoction
Alternate Names: *Tzu Wan Tang*, Aster Combination
Original Source: *Yi Fang Ji Jie* (Analytical Collection of Medical Formulas) by Wang Ang in 1682

COMPOSITION

Zhi Mu (Rhizoma Anemarrhenae)

Zi Wan (Radix et Rhizoma Asteris)

Bei Mu (Bulbus Fritillariae)

Jie Geng (Radix Platycodonis)

Ren Shen (Radix et Rhizoma Ginseng)

Fu Ling (Poria)

Wu Wei Zi (Fructus Schisandrae Chinensis)

E Jiao (Colla Corii Asini)

Gan Cao (Radix et Rhizoma Glycyrrhizae)

DOSAGE / PREPARATION / ADMINISTRATION

The source text states to grind all of the ingredients into a coarse powder, and cook it with *Sheng Jiang* (Rhizoma Zingiberis Recens) in water to make a decoction, which then should be strained and taken while warm. Note: The source text did not specify the doses for the ingredients.

CHINESE THERAPEUTIC ACTIONS

1. Clears heat and dissolves phlegm
2. Relieves cough
3. Protects the Lung

CLINICAL MANIFESTATIONS

Chronic cough caused by Lung heat and yin deficiency: chronic cough, excess phlegm, fever due to overexertion, lung abscesses, and blood in the sputum.

CLINICAL APPLICATIONS

Pulmonary tuberculosis, asthma, emphysema, cough in chronic smokers, and cough due to chronic pulmonary disorders.

EXPLANATION

Zi Wan Tang (Aster Decoction) treats chronic Lung disorders characterized by heat and underlying yin deficiency. When chronic heat attacks the Lung, it causes cough, profuse phlegm and sputum, dyspnea, and fever. Furthermore, as heat consumes yin and body fluids, patients may experience chest tightness, discomfort, abscess, and blood in the sputum.

This formula has herbs that treat both the cause and the symptoms. *Zhi Mu* (Rhizoma Anemarrhenae) clears heat while preserving the integrity of yin and body fluids. *Zi Wan* (Radix et Rhizoma Asteris) regulates Lung qi and relieves cough. *Bei Mu* (Bulbus Fritillariae) and *Jie Geng* (Radix Platycodonis) dissolve phlegm, relieve cough, and drain pus. *Ren Shen* (Radix et Rhizoma Ginseng) tonifies Lung qi, while *Fu Ling* (Poria) tonifies Spleen qi. *Wu Wei Zi* (Fructus Schisandrae Chinensis) stabilizes and binds the Lung to prevent further loss of qi through coughing. *E Jiao* (Colla Corii Asini) tonifies the blood and stops bleeding. Lastly, *Gan Cao* (Radix et Rhizoma Glycyrrhizae) harmonizes the formula.

MODIFICATIONS

- With more pus and sputum, add *Ting Li Zi* (Semen Descurainiae seu Lepidii) and *Da Zao* (Fructus Jujubae).
- With more sputum and blood, add *Zhu Ru* (Caulis Bambusae in Taenia) and *Di Huang* (Radix Rehmanniae).
- For chronic non-productive cough, add *Mai Dong* (Radix Ophiopogonis) and *Zhi Shi* (Fructus Aurantii Immaturus).
- For cough and dyspnea caused by qi deficiency, add *Chen Pi* (Pericarpium Citri Reticulatae) and *Ku Xing Ren* (Semen Armeniacae Amarum).
- With hemoptysis due to lung abscess, add *San Huang Xie Xin Tang* (Three-Yellow Decoction to Sedate the Epigastrium).

PHLEGM-DISPELLING FORMULAS

18

1229

Chapter 18 – Phlegm-Dispelling Formulas　　　　　*Section 2 – Heat-Clearing and Phlegm-Dissolving Formulas*

Zǐ Wăn Tāng (Aster Decoction)

Zi Wan Tang (Aster Decoction)

Diagnosis	Signs and Symptoms	Treatment	Herbs
Chronic cough caused by Lung heat and yin deficiency	• Cough and dyspnea with profuse phlegm and sputum and fever: Lung heat • Chest tightness and discomfort with abscess and blood in the sputum: Lung heat consuming yin and body fluids	• Clears heat and dissolves phlegm • Relieves cough • Protects the Lung	• *Zhi Mu* (Rhizoma Anemarrhenae) clears heat while preserving yin and body fluids. • *Zi Wan* (Radix et Rhizoma Asteris) regulates Lung qi and relieves cough. • *Bei Mu* (Bulbus Fritillariae) and *Jie Geng* (Radix Platycodonis) dissolve phlegm, relieve cough, and drain pus. • *Ren Shen* (Radix et Rhizoma Ginseng) tonifies Lung qi and *Fu Ling* (Poria) tonifies Spleen qi. • *Wu Wei Zi* (Fructus Schisandrae Chinensis) stabilizes and binds the Lung. • *E Jiao* (Colla Corii Asini) tonifies blood and stops bleeding. • *Gan Cao* (Radix et Rhizoma Glycyrrhizae) harmonizes all of the herbs.

Jié Gěng Tāng (Platycodon Decoction)

桔梗湯
桔梗汤

Pinyin Name: *Jie Geng Tang*
Literal Name: Platycodon Decoction
Alternate Names: *Chieh Keng Tang*, Platycodon Combination
Original Source: *Shang Han Lun* (Discussion of Cold-Induced Disorders) by Zhang Zhong-Jing in the Eastern Han Dynasty

COMPOSITION

Jie Geng (Radix Platycodonis)	3g
Gan Cao (Radix et Rhizoma Glycyrrhizae)	6g

DOSAGE / PREPARATION / ADMINISTRATION

The source text states to cook the herbs in 3 cups of water until the liquid is reduced to 1 cup. Strain and take the decoction while warm.

CHINESE THERAPEUTIC ACTIONS

1. Eliminates phlegm and pus
2. Clears deficiency fire and toxins

CLINICAL MANIFESTATIONS

Phlegm stagnation: coughing, swelling and pain of the throat, and thick, sticky sputum with mucus and blood.

Patients may also experience chills and aversion to cold, fullness and congestion in the chest, a dry mouth without thirst, and thick, sticky sputum with a foul odor.

CLINICAL APPLICATIONS

Pulmonary gangrene, pulmonary abscess, bronchitis, and tonsillitis.

EXPLANATION

Jie Geng Tang (Platycodon Decoction) treats phlegm stagnation in the chest with deficiency fire rising. Phlegm stagnation will produce a sensation of fullness and

1230

Chinese Herbal Formulas and Applications

Jié Gěng Tāng (Platycodon Decoction)

Jie Geng Tang (Platycodon Decoction)

Diagnosis	Signs and Symptoms	Treatment	Herbs
Phlegm stagnation in the chest with deficiency fire rising	• Chest fullness and congestion: phlegm stagnation in the chest • Thick, sticky sputum with blood and mucus: deficiency fire consuming body fluids and damaging the internal organs • Cough and sore throat with swelling and pain: deficiency fire traveling upward	• Eliminates phlegm and pus • Clears deficiency fire and toxins	• *Jie Geng* (Radix Platycodonis) disperses phlegm stagnation and regulates Lung qi circulation. • *Gan Cao* (Radix et Rhizoma Glycyrrhizae) resolves phlegm stagnation and tonifies Lung qi.

congestion in the chest. When phlegm stagnation is complicated by fire that dries body fluids, the sputum becomes thick and sticky. In addition, if deficiency fire dries the fluids and damages the internal organs, there may be blood and mucus in the sputum. As deficiency fire travels upward, it may cause cough and sore throat with swelling and pain.

Jie Geng Tang is a simple formula with only two ingredients: *Jie Geng* (Radix Platycodonis), a bitter and acrid herb that opens and disperses phlegm stagnation; and *Gan Cao* (Radix et Rhizoma Glycyrrhizae), a sweet

and neutral herb that resolves phlegm stagnation. The combination of these two herbs has a synergistic effect to eliminate phlegm stagnation in the chest. Furthermore, *Jie Geng* (Radix Platycodonis) regulates qi and relieves cough, while *Gan Cao* (Radix et Rhizoma Glycyrrhizae) tonifies Lung qi and enhances overall recovery.

MODIFICATION

For severe conditions, heat-clearing and toxin-eliminating herbs should be added, since *Jie Geng Tang* simply treats phlegm stagnation.

Rén Shēn Xiè Fèi Tāng (Ginseng Decoction to Sedate the Lung)
人參瀉肺湯
人参泻肺汤

Pinyin Name: *Ren Shen Xie Fei Tang*
Literal Name: Ginseng Decoction to Sedate the Lung
Alternate Name: Ginseng and Scute Combination
Original Source: *Tai Ping Hui Min He Ji Ju Fang* (Imperial Grace Formulary of the Tai Ping Era) by the Imperial Medical Department in 1078-85

COMPOSITION

Huang Qin (Radix Scutellariae)

Zhi Zi (Fructus Gardeniae)

Bo He (Herba Menthae)

Zhi Qiao (Fructus Citri Aurantii)

Ku Xing Ren (Semen Armeniacae Amarum)

Lian Qiao (Fructus Forsythiae)

Sang Bai Pi (Cortex Mori)

Jie Geng (Radix Platycodonis)

Da Huang (Radix et Rhizoma Rhei)

Ren Shen (Radix et Rhizoma Ginseng)

Gan Cao (Radix et Rhizoma Glycyrrhizae)

PHLEGM-DISPELLING FORMULAS

18

1231

Chapter 18 – Phlegm-Dispelling Formulas *Section 2 – Heat-Clearing and Phlegm-Dissolving Formulas*

Rén Shēn Xiè Fèi Tāng (Ginseng Decoction to Sedate the Lung)

DOSAGE / PREPARATION / ADMINISTRATION
The source text states to grind equal amounts of all of the ingredients into a coarse powder. Cook 30g of the powder in 2 cups of water until the liquid is reduced to 1 cup. Take the warm, strained decoction after meals.

CHINESE THERAPEUTIC ACTIONS
1. Clears heat and sedates the Lung
2. Eliminates phlegm and regulates qi

CLINICAL MANIFESTATIONS
Lung heat with phlegm accumulation: wheezing, dyspnea, fullness and distention in the chest and epigastrium, cough with profuse sputum, and constipation.

CLINICAL APPLICATIONS
Upper respiratory tract infection, bronchitis, pneumonia, bronchial asthma, and pulmonary abscess.

EXPLANATION
Ren Shen Xie Fei Tang (Ginseng Decoction to Sedate the Lung) treats Lung heat accompanied by phlegm accumulation and qi flow obstruction. The presence of phlegm is evident in the yellow sputum discharge. Heat and phlegm create the feeling of fullness and distention in the chest; they also obstruct the normal qi flow to cause wheezing, dyspnea, and cough.

In this formula, *Huang Qin* (Radix Scutellariae), *Zhi Zi* (Fructus Gardeniae), and *Bo He* (Herba Menthae) clear heat in the Lung and address the excess condition. *Zhi*

Qiao (Fructus Aurantii) regulates qi, while *Ku Xing Ren* (Semen Armeniacae Amarum) guides Lung qi downward. Together, these two herbs restore the normal flow of Lung qi to relieve wheezing, dyspnea, and cough. *Lian Qiao* (Fructus Forsythiae), *Sang Bai Pi* (Cortex Mori), and *Jie Geng* (Radix Platycodonis) clear heat and phlegm to dispel sputum and relieve congestion and fullness. *Da Huang* (Radix et Rhizoma Rhei) purges downward, and enables the elimination of heat via defecation. *Ren Shen* (Radix et Rhizoma Ginseng) strengthens the Lung and Spleen and prevents the bitter and cold herbs in the formula from damaging these two organs. Lastly, *Gan Cao* (Radix et Rhizoma Glycyrrhizae) reduces inflammation in the Lung and harmonizes the herbs within the formula.

MODIFICATIONS
- For cough with profuse sputum, add *Fu Ling* (Poria) and *Chen Pi* (Pericarpium Citri Reticulatae).
- For cough due to wind-cold, add *Hua Gai San* (Canopy Powder).
- For cough due to tuberculosis, add *Qing Fei Tang* (Clear the Lung Decoction).
- For cough with phlegm and fluid retention, add *Er Chen Tang* (Two-Cured Decoction).
- With fullness and distention in the chest and epigastrium, add *Huang Lian* (Rhizoma Coptidis) and *Hou Po* (Cortex Magnoliae Officinalis).
- With feeling of both cold and heat in the chest, add *Chai Hu* (Radix Bupleuri) and *Di Gu Pi* (Cortex Lycii).
- For recurrent bronchitis, add *Shi Gao* (Gypsum Fibrosum) and *Zhi Mu* (Rhizoma Anemarrhenae).

Ren Shen Xie Fei Tang (Ginseng Decoction to Sedate the Lung)

Diagnosis	Signs and Symptoms	Treatment	Herbs
Lung heat with phlegm accumulation	• Wheezing, dyspnea and cough with a feeling of fullness and distention in the chest: heat and phlegm affecting Lung qi circulation • Yellow sputum: heat and phlegm condition	• Clears heat and sedates the Lung • Eliminates phlegm and regulates qi	• *Huang Qin* (Radix Scutellariae), *Zhi Zi* (Fructus Gardeniae), and *Bo He* (Herba Menthae) clear heat in the Lung and address the excess condition. • *Zhi Qiao* (Fructus Aurantii) and *Ku Xing Ren* (Semen Armeniacae Amarum) regulate and cause Lung qi to descend. • *Lian Qiao* (Fructus Forsythiae), *Sang Bai Pi* (Cortex Mori), and *Jie Geng* (Radix Platycodonis) clear heat and phlegm to dispel sputum and relieve congestion and fullness. • *Da Huang* (Radix et Rhizoma Rhei) purges heat downward. • *Ren Shen* (Radix et Rhizoma Ginseng) strengthens the Lung and Spleen and prevents the bitter and cold herbs in the formula from damaging these two organs. • *Gan Cao* (Radix et Rhizoma Glycyrrhizae) harmonizes the herbs.

1232

Guā Lóu Zhǐ Shí Tāng
(Trichosanthes Fruit and Immature Bitter Orange Decoction)

瓜蔞枳實湯
瓜蒌枳实汤

Pinyin Name: *Gua Lou Zhi Shi Tang*
Literal Name: Trichosanthes Fruit and Immature Bitter Orange Decoction
Alternate Names: *Kua Lou Chih Shih Tang*, Trichosanthes and Chih-shih Decoction, Trichosanthes and Aurantium Combination
Original Source: *Wan Bing Hui Chun* (Restoration of Health from the Myriad Diseases) by Gong Ting-Xian in 1587

COMPOSITION

Gua Lou (Fructus Trichosanthis)	3g
Bei Mu (Bulbus Fritillariae)	3g
Chen Pi (Pericarpium Citri Reticulatae)	3g
Zhi Shi (Fructus Aurantii Immaturus), *chao* (dry-fried) with bran	3g
Jie Geng (Radix Platycodonis)	3g
Mu Xiang (Radix Aucklandiae)	1.5g
Sha Ren (Fructus Amomi)	1.5g
Fu Ling (Poria)	3g
Zhi Zi (Fructus Gardeniae)	3g
Huang Qin (Radix Scutellariae)	3g
Dang Gui (Radix Angelicae Sinensis)	1.8g
Gan Cao (Radix et Rhizoma Glycyrrhizae)	0.9g

DOSAGE / PREPARATION / ADMINISTRATION

The source text states to cook the ingredients with 1 slice of *Sheng Jiang* (Rhizoma Zingiberis Recens) and the juices of *Zhu Li* (Succus Bambusae) and *Sheng Jiang* (Rhizoma Zingiberis Recens) in water. Take the strained decoction while warm.

CHINESE THERAPEUTIC ACTIONS

1. Breaks up stagnation and dissolves phlegm
2. Clears heat and moistens dryness
3. Relieves chest congestion

CLINICAL MANIFESTATIONS

Phlegm-heat stagnation in the chest: accumulation of phlegm in the chest that is difficult to expectorate, pain in the chest, difficulty rotating the trunk due to pain in the chest, a feeling of fullness and stifling sensation in the chest and hypochondriac region, fever, aversion to cold, labored breathing, and delirious speech.

CLINICAL APPLICATIONS

Acute and chronic bronchitis, pneumonia, asthma, pulmonary emphysema, pulmonary tuberculosis, cough, chest pain, profuse sputum in chronic smokers, and intercostal neuralgia.

EXPLANATION

Phlegm-heat stagnation is often described as stubborn or viscous in nature, such that the phlegm cannot be coughed or expectorated out. Phlegm stagnation in the chest immediately affects the local area, causing chest pain and a feeling of fullness and a stifling sensation in the chest and hypochondriac region. The chest pain is sometimes so severe that the patient usually exhibits labored breathing and difficulty in rotating the trunk. If phlegm attacks the Heart and blocks the *shen* (spirit), the patient will exhibit delirious speech.

The two main actions of *Gua Lou Zhi Shi Tang* (Trichosanthes Fruit and Immature Bitter Orange Decoction) are to clear heat and dissolve phlegm. *Gua Lou* (Fructus Trichosanthis), *Bei Mu* (Bulbus Fritillariae), and *Zhu Li* (Succus Bambusae) soften phlegm, relieve chest congestion, and benefit the diaphragm. *Chen Pi* (Pericarpium Citri Reticulatae), *Zhi Shi* (Fructus Aurantii Immaturus), *Jie Geng* (Radix Platycodonis), and *Mu Xiang* (Radix Aucklandiae) regulate qi, dissolve phlegm, and eliminate stagnation. *Sha Ren* (Fructus Amomi) and *Fu Ling* (Poria) strengthen the Spleen, dry dampness, and stop the production of phlegm. *Zhi Zi* (Fructus Gardeniae)

Chapter 18 – Phlegm-Dispelling Formulas　　　　*Section 2 – Heat-Clearing and Phlegm-Dissolving Formulas*

Guā Lóu Zhǐ Shí Tāng
(Trichosanthes Fruit and Immature Bitter Orange Decoction)

Gua Lou Zhi Shi Tang (Trichosanthes Fruit and Immature Bitter Orange Decoction)

Diagnosis	Signs and Symptoms	Treatment	Herbs
Phlegm-heat stagnation in the chest	• Chest pain, a feeling of fullness and a stifling sensation in the chest and hypochondriac region, and stagnant phlegm that cannot be coughed or expectorated out: phlegm-heat stagnation in the chest • Delirious speech: phlegm affecting the Heart and disturbing the *shen* (spirit)	• Breaks up stagnation and dissolves phlegm • Clears heat and moistens dryness • Relieves chest congestion	• *Gua Lou* (Fructus Trichosanthis), *Bei Mu* (Bulbus Fritillariae), and *Zhu Li* (Succus Bambusae) soften phlegm, relieve chest congestion, and benefit the diaphragm. • *Chen Pi* (Pericarpium Citri Reticulatae), *Zhi Shi* (Fructus Aurantii Immaturus), *Jie Geng* (Radix Platycodonis), and *Mu Xiang* (Radix Aucklandiae) regulate qi, dissolve phlegm, and eliminate stagnation. • *Sha Ren* (Fructus Amomi) and *Fu Ling* (Poria) strengthen the Spleen, dry dampness, and stop the production of phlegm. • *Zhi Zi* (Fructus Gardeniae) and *Huang Qin* (Radix Scutellariae) clear damp-heat. • *Dang Gui* (Radix Angelicae Sinensis) activates blood circulation and prevents blood stagnation. • *Gan Cao* (Radix et Rhizoma Glycyrrhizae) and *Sheng Jiang* (Rhizoma Zingiberis Recens) harmonize all of the herbs.

and *Huang Qin* (Radix Scutellariae), both bitter and cold herbs, clear damp-heat, which occurs frequently with phlegm stagnation. *Dang Gui* (Radix Angelicae Sinensis) activates blood circulation and prevents blood stagnation. *Gan Cao* (Radix et Rhizoma Glycyrrhizae) and *Sheng Jiang* (Rhizoma Zingiberis Recens) harmonize all of the herbs in this formula.

MODIFICATIONS

• With delirious speech due to phlegm affecting the Heart and blocking the *shen* (spirit), add *Shi Chang Pu* (Rhizoma Acori Tatarinowii) and remove *Mu Xiang* (Radix Aucklandiae).

• With wheezing and dyspnea, add *Sang Bai Pi* (Cortex Mori) and *Zi Su Zi* (Fructus Perillae).

1234

Chinese Herbal Formulas and Applications

Xiǎo Xiàn Xiōng Tāng (Minor Sinking into the Chest Decoction)

小陷胸湯
小陷胸汤

Pinyin Name: *Xiao Xian Xiong Tang*
Literal Name: Minor Sinking into the Chest Decoction
Alternate Names: *Hsiao Hsien Hsiung Tang*, Minor Chest-Congestion Decoction, Minor Trichosanthes Decoction, Minor Trichosanthes Combination
Original Source: *Shang Han Lun* (Discussion of Cold-Induced Disorders) by Zhang Zhong-Jing in the Eastern Han Dynasty

COMPOSITION

Gua Lou (Fructus Trichosanthis)	1 big fruit [20-30g]
Huang Lian (Rhizoma Coptidis)	3g [6g]
Ban Xia (Rhizoma Pinelliae), *xi* (washed)	0.5 cup [12g]

DOSAGE / PREPARATION / ADMINISTRATION

The source text states to first cook *Gua Lou* (Fructus Trichosanthis) with 6 cups [1,200 mL] of water until the liquid is reduced to 3 cups [600 mL]. Filter and discard the residue, add the other herbs, and cook until the strained decoction is further reduced to 2 cups [400 mL]. Take the warm, strained decoction in three equally-divided doses. Today, this formula may be prepared as a decoction with the doses suggested in brackets.

CHINESE THERAPEUTIC ACTIONS

1. Clears heat and dissolves phlegm
2. Opens the chest and disperses stagnation

CLINICAL MANIFESTATIONS

Phlegm-heat stagnation in the chest: distention and fullness in the chest and epigastric regions with pain upon palpation; cough with yellow, sticky sputum; a yellow, greasy tongue coating; and a slippery, rapid pulse.

CLINICAL APPLICATIONS

Gastritis, erosive gastritis, acid reflux, epigastric pain, reflux esophagitis, acute bronchitis, bronchitis, pneumonia, silicosis, pulmonary heart disease, tuberculous pleurisy, pleurisy with effusion, exudative pleurisy, chronic hepatitis, and cholelithiasis.

EXPLANATION

Xiao Xian Xiong Tang (Minor Sinking into the Chest Decoction), first cited in *Shang Han Lun* (Discussion of Cold-Induced Disorders), is designed to treat patients who have exterior syndrome and who have been incorrectly treated with downward draining herbs, which cause heat and phlegm to sink into the interior of the chest. As a result, heat and phlegm become stagnated in the chest and cause qi stagnation. Consequently, chest and epigastric distention, fullness, and pain occur. The Lung qi, after being stagnant for a period of time, may rise adversely and cause coughing. Since the heat and phlegm factors are predominant, the sputum appears yellow and sticky. Yellow, greasy tongue coating and slippery, rapid pulse are typical signs of interior heat and phlegm.

Gua Lou (Fructus Trichosanthis), the chief herb, clears heat, dissolves phlegm, and relieves pain in the chest and epigastrium. *Huang Lian* (Rhizoma Coptidis) sedates heat

Xiao Xian Xiong Tang (Minor Sinking into the Chest Decoction)

Diagnosis	Signs and Symptoms	Treatment	Herbs
Phlegm-heat stagnation in the chest	• Chest and epigastric distention and pain: phlegm-heat stagnation in the chest • Cough with yellow, sticky sputum: phlegm-heat stagnation in the chest blocking qi circulation • Yellow, greasy tongue coating, and a slippery, rapid pulse: interior heat and phlegm	• Clears heat and dissolves phlegm • Opens the chest and disperses stagnation	• *Gua Lou* (Fructus Trichosanthis) clears heat, dissolves phlegm, and relieves pain in the chest. • *Huang Lian* (Rhizoma Coptidis) sedates heat and relieves epigastric distention. • *Ban Xia* (Rhizoma Pinelliae) eliminates phlegm and breaks up qi stagnation to relieve chest distention.

PHLEGM-DISPELLING FORMULAS

18

1235

Chapter 18 – Phlegm-Dispelling Formulas　　　　*Section 2 – Heat-Clearing and Phlegm-Dissolving Formulas*

Xiǎo Xiàn Xiōng Tāng (Minor Sinking into the Chest Decoction)

and relieves epigastric distention. *Ban Xia* (Rhizoma Pinelliae) eliminates phlegm and breaks up qi stagnation to relieve chest distention.

MODIFICATIONS

- With intercostal or hypochondriac pain, add *Yu Jin* (Radix Curcumae) and *Chai Hu* (Radix Bupleuri).
- With thick sputum that is difficult to expectorate, add *Dan Nan Xing* (Arisaema cum Bile) and *Chuan Bei Mu* (Bulbus Fritillariae Cirrhosae).
- With vomiting and nausea, add *Zhu Ru* (Caulis Bambusae in Taenia) and *Sheng Jiang* (Rhizoma Zingiberis Recens).
- For disorders characterized by phlegm-fire, add *Gan Cao* (Radix et Rhizoma Glycyrrhizae) and *Sheng Jiang* (Rhizoma Zingiberis Recens).

CAUTIONS / CONTRAINDICATIONS

- Use of *Xiao Xian Xiong Tang* may be associated with loose stools and diarrhea, as the formula is cold and lubricating in nature.[1]
- This formula is not recommended for individuals with deficiency and cold of the Spleen and Stomach.[2]

PHARMACOLOGICAL EFFECTS

1. **Expectorant and antitussive**: Ingredients of *Xiao Xian Xiong Tang* have been shown to have marked expectorant and antitussive effects.[3]
2. **Gastrointestinal**: Administration of *Xiao Xian Xiong Tang* has a marked inhibitory effect on the production of gastric acid in mice.[4]

CLINICAL STUDIES AND RESEARCH

1. **Bronchitis**: In one study, 100 pediatric patients with acute bronchitis were divided into two groups and treated with herbs. Group one of 50 patients received both *Xiao Xian Xiong Tang* plus *Ma Huang Xing Ren Gan Cao Shi Gao Tang* (Ephedra, Apricot Kernel, Licorice, and Gypsum Decoction). The study reported complete recovery in 37 cases, improvement in 7 cases, and no effect in 6 cases. Group two of 50 patients received only *Ma Huang Xing Ren Gan Cao Shi Gao Tang* (Ephedra, Apricot Kernel, Licorice, and Gypsum Decoction). The study reported complete recovery in 26 cases, improvement in 5 cases, and no effect in 19 cases. The study concluded that the combination of these two formulas was more effective for treating acute bronchitis in pediatric patients.[5]
2. **Silicosis**: According to one study, concurrent use of *Xiao Xian Xiong Tang* and *Gua Lou Xie Bai Ban Xia Tang* (Trichosanthes Fruit, Chinese Chive, and Pinellia Decoction) was associated with a marked effect in treating coal miners with silicosis. The treatment protocol was to administer the herbs daily in decoction, for 20 days

per course of treatment, for 2-3 courses total. Out of 33 patients, the study reported marked effect in 28 cases, improvement in 3 cases, and no effect in 2 cases. The overall effectiveness was 93.93%.[6]

3. **Pulmonary heart disease**: According to one study, 112 patients with pulmonary heart disease were treated with modified *Xiao Xian Xiong Tang*. The study used this formula with *Zhi Shi* (Fructus Aurantii Immaturus), *Ze Xie* (Rhizoma Alismatis), and *Zhi Gan Cao* (Radix et Rhizoma Glycyrrhizae Praeparata cum Melle) as the base formula. In addition, *Da Huang* (Radix et Rhizoma Rhei) was added for constipation, and *Hua Shi* (Talcum) was added for burning urination with yellow urine. Out of 112 patients, the study reported complete recovery in 12 cases, marked improvement in 52 cases, improvement in 40 cases, and no effect in 8 cases. The overall effectiveness was 92.9%.[7]

4. **Tuberculous pleurisy**: According to one study, 24 patients with tuberculous pleurisy were treated with good results using *Xiao Xian Xiong Tang* plus *Xie Bai* (Bulbus Allii Macrostemonis) and others. Improvements included reduction of fever and resolution of other symptoms.[8]

5. **Exudative pleurisy**: Modified *Xiao Xian Xiong Tang* was used with good results for treatment of 22 patients with exudative pleurisy. The treatment was to administer the herbs daily in decoction, for 30 days per course of treatment. Drug treatment was incorporated when necessary. Out of 22 patients, the study reported significant improvement in 13 cases, moderate improvement in 17 cases, and no effect in 2 cases. The overall effectiveness was 90.9%.[9]

6. **Erosive gastritis**: According to one study, 101 patients with acute erosive gastritis were divided into two groups: group one received modified *Xiao Xian Xiong Tang* and group two received pharmaceutical drug treatment. Herbal treatment used *Xiao Xian Xiong Tang* with *Hai Piao Xiao* (Endoconcha Sepiae) and *Xian He Cao* (Herba Agrimoniae) as the base formula, plus *Di Yu* (Radix Sanguisorbae) for hematochezia; *Zhe Shi* (Haematitum) for hematemesis; calcined *Mu Li* (Concha Ostreae) for acid reflux; *Qing Mu Xiang* (Radix Aristolochiae), *Bai Shao* (Radix Paeoniae Alba) and *Yan Hu Suo* (Rhizoma Corydalis) for severe pain; and *Pu Gong Ying* (Herba Taraxaci) and *Yu Xing Cao* (Herba Houttuyniae) for superficial ulceration. Patients in group two were treated with drugs (the names of drugs were not available at the time of publication). The study reported 90.8% effectiveness for the herb group (65 cases: 48 with complete recovery, 11 with improvement, and 6 with no effect) and 86.1% effectiveness for the drug group (36 cases: 9 with complete recovery, 22 with improvement, and 5 with no effect).[10]

1236

Xiǎo Xiàn Xiōng Tāng (Minor Sinking into the Chest Decoction)

7. **Epigastric pain**: *Xiao Xian Xiong Tang* has been shown to effectively relieve epigastric pain in several studies. According to one report, use of this formula in 83 patients with epigastric pain was associated with complete recovery in 52 cases, improvement in 29 cases, and no effect in 2 cases. The causes of epigastric pain included gastritis, peptic ulcers, and others.[11]

8. **Reflux esophagitis**: According to one study, 54 patients with reflux esophagitis were treated with good results using *Xiao Xian Xiong Tang* and *Xiao Chai Hu Tang* (Minor Bupleurum Decoction) together. In addition to these two formulas, the treatment added *Zhi Qiao* (Fructus Aurantii), *Tan Xiang* (Lignum Santali Albi), and *Hou Po* (Cortex Magnoliae Officinalis) for chest and epigastric fullness and distention; *Hai Piao Xiao* (Endoconcha Sepiae) and calcined *Wa Leng Zi* (Concha Arcae) for acid reflux; dry-fried *Bai Shao* (Radix Paeoniae Alba) and *Sha Ren* (Fructus Amomi) for nausea and vomiting; *Jie Geng* (Radix Platycodonis) and *Zhe Shi* (Haematitum) for difficulties in swallowing; and *Mai Dong* (Radix Ophiopogonis), *Sha Shen* (Radix Glehniae seu Adenophorae), and *Shi Hu* (Caulis Dendrobii) for dry mouth, dry throat, and constipation. The treatment protocol was to administer the herbs daily in decoction, for 15 days per course of treatment. All other herbs/drugs/supplements were discontinued through the duration of the study. Out of 54 patients, the study reported complete recovery in 26 cases, marked improvement in 18 cases, moderate improvement in 8 cases, and no effect in 2 cases.[12]

9. **Chronic hepatitis**: In one study, modified *Xiao Xian Xiong Tang* was used to treat patients with chronic hepatitis progressing into liver cirrhosis. The treatment protocol was to administer one dose of the herbs daily in decoction, for 30 days per course of treatment. Out of 72 patients, 41 had resolution of symptoms and restoration of normal liver functions, 29 had varying degrees of improvement, and 2 required modification of treatment. Furthermore, 53 cases showed improvement within 1 course, and 17 cases within 2 courses of treatment.[13]

RELATED FORMULA

Chái Hú Xiàn Xiōng Tāng
(Bupleurum Decoction for Sinking into the Chest)
柴胡陷胸湯
柴胡陷胸汤
Pinyin Name: *Chai Hu Xian Xiong Tang*
Literal Name: Bupleurum Decoction for Sinking into the Chest
Original Source: *Chong Ding Tong Su Shang Han Lun* (Revised Popular Guide to the Discussion of Cold-Induced Disorders) by Yu Gen-Chu in the Qing Dynasty

Chai Hu (Radix Bupleuri)	3g
Ban Xia (Rhizoma Pinelliae), *zhu* (boiled) with ginger	9g
Huang Lian (Rhizoma Coptidis)	2.4g
Jie Geng (Radix Platycodonis)	3g
Huang Qin (Radix Scutellariae)	4.5g
Gua Lou Zi (Semen Trichosanthis)	15g
Zhi Shi (Fructus Aurantii Immaturus)	4.5g
Sheng Jiang (Rhizoma Zingiberis Recens), *chong fu* (take drenched)	4 drops of juice

The source text states to prepare the ingredients as a decoction. This formula clears heat, dissolves phlegm, opens the chest and diaphragm, and harmonizes the *shaoyang*. Clinically, this formula may be used for *shaoyang* syndrome with alternating chills and fever, distention and fullness in the chest and diaphragm regions with pain upon palpation, cough with sticky sputum, a bitter taste in the mouth, a yellow tongue coating, and a wiry, rapid pulse.

Chai Hu Xian Xiong Tang (Bupleurum Decoction for Sinking into the Chest) is formulated by combining *Xiao Chai Hu Tang* (Minor Bupleurum Decoction) and *Xiao Xian Xiong Tang* (Minor Sinking into the Chest Decoction), and removing tonic herbs such as *Ren Shen* (Radix et Rhizoma Ginseng), *Gan Cao* (Radix et Rhizoma Glycyrrhizae), and *Da Zao* (Fructus Jujubae). *Chai Hu Xian Xiong Tang* is designed to concurrently harmonize *shaoyang* syndrome and treat phlegm-heat stagnation in the chest.

AUTHORS' COMMENTS

Xiao Xian Xiong Tang is the representative formula for treating chest pain and discomfort due to stagnation of phlegm-heat in the chest. The three diagnostic criteria include phlegm, heat, and stagnation, with key signs and symptoms such as distention and fullness in the chest and epigastrium, pain that intensifies with pressure, a yellow, greasy tongue coating, and a slippery, rapid pulse.

Xiao Xian Xiong Tang and *Da Xian Xiong Tang* (Major Sinking into the Chest Decoction) both treat stagnation in the chest.

- *Xiao Xian Xiong Tang* treats less serious conditions characterized by stagnation of heat and phlegm in the chest. Clinical manifestations include a feeling of fullness in the chest and epigastrium, and pain upon palpation.

- *Da Xian Xiong Tang* treats more serious conditions characterized by stagnation of heat and water in the chest. Clinical manifestations include a hardened epigastrium with a sensation of fullness, and severe pain upon palpation.

Chapter 18 – Phlegm-Dispelling Formulas　　　　*Section 2 – Heat-Clearing and Phlegm-Dissolving Formulas*

Xiǎo Xiàn Xiōng Tāng (Minor Sinking into the Chest Decoction)

References

1. *Zhong Yao Ming Fang Yao Li Yu Ying Yong* (Pharmacology and Applications of Famous Herbal Formulas) 1989;573-4.
2. *Zhong Yao Ming Fang Yao Li Yu Ying Yong* (Pharmacology and Applications of Famous Herbal Formulas) 1989;573-4.
3. *Zhong Yi Fang Ji Xian Dai Yan Jiu* (Modern Study of Medical Formulae in Traditional Chinese Medicine) 1997.
4. *Zhong Cheng Yao Yan Jiu* (Research of Chinese Patent Medicine) 1985;8:23.
5. *Shang Hai Zhong Yi Yao Za Zhi* (Shanghai Journal of Chinese Medicine and Herbology) 1986;1:26.
6. *Bei Jing Zhong Yi Yao Da Xue Xue Bao* (Journal of Beijing University of Medicine and Medicinals) 1994;17(1):37.

7. *Nei Meng Gu Zhong Yi Yao* (Traditional Chinese Medicine and Medicinals of Inner Mongolia) 1998;3:18.
8. *Shang Hai Yi Yao Za Zhi* (Shanghai Journal of Medicine and Herbology) 1986;1:36.
9. *Shan Xi Zhong Yi* (Shanxi Chinese Medicine) 1994;15(8):368.
10. *Jiang Xi Zhong Yi Yao* (Jiangxi Chinese Medicine and Herbology) 1998;6:22.
11. *Hu Bei Zhong Yi Za Zhi* (Hubei Journal of Chinese Medicine) 1984;1:33.
12. *Hu Bei Zhong Yi Za Zhi* (Hubei Journal of Chinese Medicine) 1997;3:20.
13. *Ji Lin Zhong Yi Yao* (Jilin Chinese Medicine and Herbology) 1992;1:37.

Gǔn Tán Wán (Vaporize Phlegm Pill)

滚痰丸
滚痰丸

Pinyin Name: *Gun Tan Wan*
Literal Name: Vaporize Phlegm Pill
Alternate Name: *Meng Shi Gun Tan Wan* (Lapis Micae and Chloriti Pill to Vaporize Phlegm)
Original Source: *Dan Xi Xin Fa Fu Yu* (Additions to the Teachings for [Zhu] Dan-Xi) by Fang Guang-Lei in 1536

COMPOSITION

Meng Shi (Lapis Micae seu Chloriti), *duan* (calcined) at high temperature and *fen sui* (pulverized)		30g [3g]
Da Huang (Radix et Rhizoma Rhei), *zheng* (steamed) with liquor		240g [15g]
Huang Qin (Radix Scutellariae), *xi* (washed) with liquor		240g [15g]
Chen Xiang (Lignum Aquilariae Resinatum)		15g [2g]

DOSAGE / PREPARATION / ADMINISTRATION

The source text states to grind the ingredients into a fine powder and form into small pills with water. The pills should resemble the size of *Wu Tong Zi* (Semen Firmianae), a small seed approximately 5 mm in diameter. Take 40-50 pills with tea or warm, boiled water after meals and at bedtime. Adjust the dose depending on the severity of the condition.

Today, this formula may be taken as pills or decoction. For pills, grind the herbs into powder and form into small pills with water, and take 5-9g of pills with warm water one to two times daily. For decoction, use the suggested doses in brackets.

CHINESE THERAPEUTIC ACTIONS

Purges fire and eliminates phlegm

CLINICAL MANIFESTATIONS

Old (chronic and stubborn) phlegm with excess heat: *dian kuang* (mania and withdrawal), or manic-depressive psychosis; severe palpitations with unconsciousness; coughing and wheezing with thick sputum; chest and epigastric fullness and oppression; dizziness, vertigo, and tinnitus; nodules around the neck; peristalsis-like movements of the eyes and mouth; insomnia or disturbed sleep with bizarre dreams; severe stabbing pain in the joints; dysphagia with irritability and a feeling of oppression in the chest and epigastrium; constipation; yellow, thick tongue coating, and a slippery, rapid and forceful pulse.

CLINICAL APPLICATIONS

Stroke, epilepsy, schizophrenia, and migraines.

EXPLANATION

Gun Tan Wan (Vaporize Phlegm Pill) treats old (chronic and stubborn) phlegm with excess heat. Old phlegm and

1238

Chinese Herbal Formulas and Applications

Gŭn Tán Wán (Vaporize Phlegm Pill)

Gun Tan Wan (Vaporize Phlegm Pill)

Diagnosis	Signs and Symptoms	Treatment	Herbs
Old (chronic and stubborn) phlegm with excess heat	• *Dian kuang* (mania and withdrawal), manic-depressive psychosis, insomnia and disturbed sleep with bizarre dreams: old phlegm and excess heat surround the Heart and inhibit *shen* (spirit) • Coughing with thick phlegm, wheezing, or chest fullness: old phlegm and excess heat obstructing Lung qi flow • Dizziness and tinnitus: old phlegm and excess heat traveling upward to the head • Joint pain, nodules, and peristalsis-like movements of the eyes: old phlegm and excess heat affecting the muscles • Irritability and constipation: old phlegm and excess heat consuming body fluids • Thick, yellow tongue coating and a slippery, rapid and forceful pulse: phlegm and excess heat in the interior	Purges fire and eliminates phlegm	• *Meng Shi* (Lapis Micae seu Chloriti) removes chronic, stubborn phlegm. • *Da Huang* (Radix et Rhizoma Rhei) drains excess heat. • *Huang Qin* (Radix Scutellariae) sedates phlegm-heat in the upper *jiao*. • *Chen Xiang* (Lignum Aquilariae Resinatum) guides Lung qi downward to stop coughing and eliminate phlegm.

excess heat may cause a number of different clinical manifestations. They may surround the Heart and inhibit the *shen* (spirit), causing insomnia, disturbed sleep with bizarre dreams, *dian kuang* (mania and withdrawal), manic-depressive psychosis, or severe palpitations with unconsciousness. The phlegm and excess heat also can obstruct the flow of Lung qi, causing coughing with thick phlegm, wheezing, or chest fullness. If the phlegm and heat travel to the head, dizziness, tinnitus, or peristalsis-like movements of the eyes and mouth may occur. Phlegm and heat may also obstruct the qi flow in the joints, causing severe stabbing pain. It may become lodged in the muscles to form nodules around the neck. Irritability and constipation are due to consumption of body fluids by excess heat. Thick, yellow tongue coating and a slippery, rapid and forceful pulse are signs of phlegm and excess heat in the interior.

Meng Shi (Lapis Micae seu Chloriti), the chief herb of this formula, removes chronic, stubborn phlegm. *Da Huang* (Radix et Rhizoma Rhei), a bitter and cold herb, drains excess heat. *Huang Qin* (Radix Scutellariae) sedates phlegm-heat in the upper *jiao*. *Chen Xiang* (Lignum Aquilariae Resinatum) guides Lung qi downward to stop coughing and eliminate phlegm.

CAUTIONS / CONTRAINDICATIONS

• *Gun Tan Wan* is very strong, and should be reserved only for strong robust patients who have excess conditions.

• Because this formula is designed for old (chronic and stubborn) phlegm caused by excess heat, it is contraindicated during pregnancy and in patients with generalized deficiency.

PHARMACOLOGICAL EFFECTS

Antitussive and expectorant: Administration of *Gun Tan Wan* at 4.2 g/kg was associated with a marked effect to suppress cough and eliminate sputum.[1]

CLINICAL STUDIES AND RESEARCH

1. **Stroke**: One study reported an 87.5% effectiveness using modified *Gun Tan Wan* to treat 24 patients with stroke. Herbal treatment varied depending on the traditional Chinese medical diagnosis. In addition to *Gun Tan Wan*, *Da Cheng Qi Tang* (Major Order the Qi Decoction) was added for wind, yang, phlegm, and fire; *Tiao Wei Cheng Qi Tang* (Regulate the Stomach and Order the Qi Decoction) for wind, yang, and phlegm; and *Zeng Ye Cheng Qi Tang* (Increase the Fluids and Order the Qi Decoction) for rising wind and yang.[2]

2. **Seizures and epilepsy**: One study reported stabilization in 27 of 32 patients using modified *Gun Tan Wan* to treat seizures and epilepsy caused by inflammation, fever, physical trauma, and other causes.[3]

References

1. *Zhong Cheng Yao* (Study of Chinese Patent Medicine) 1988;9:27.
2. *Si Chuan Zhong Yi* (Sichuan Chinese Medicine) 1995;2:20.
3. *An Hui Zhong Yi Xue Yuan Xue Bao* (Journal of Anhui University School of Medicine) 1988;3:33.

PHLEGM-DISPELLING FORMULAS

18

1239

Chapter 18 – Phlegm-Dispelling Formulas   *Section 3 – Dryness-Moistening and Phlegm-Dissolving Formula*

Section 3

润燥化痰剂

— Dryness-Moistening and Phlegm-Dissolving Formula

Bèi Mǔ Guā Lóu Sǎn (Fritillaria and Trichosanthes Fruit Powder)

贝母瓜蒌散

贝母瓜蒌散

Pinyin Name: *Bei Mu Gua Lou San*
Literal Name: Fritillaria and Trichosanthes Fruit Powder
Alternate Name: Fritillaria and Trichosanthes Fruit Formula
Original Source: *Yi Xue Xin Wu* (Medical Revelations) by Cheng Guo-Peng in 1732

COMPOSITION

Bei Mu (Bulbus Fritillariae)	4.5g
Gua Lou (Fructus Trichosanthis)	3g
Tian Hua Fen (Radix Trichosanthis)	2.4g
Fu Ling (Poria)	2.4g
Ju Hong (Exocarpium Citri Reticulatae)	2.4g
Jie Geng (Radix Platycodonis)	2.4g

DOSAGE / PREPARATION / ADMINISTRATION

The source text states to prepare the ingredients as a decoction.

CHINESE THERAPEUTIC ACTIONS

1. Moistens the Lung and clears heat
2. Regulates qi and dissolves phlegm

CLINICAL MANIFESTATIONS

Lung dryness with phlegm accumulation: coughing, thick, sticky sputum that is difficult to expectorate, and dry throat.

CLINICAL APPLICATIONS

Bronchitis, sore throat, and dry cough.

EXPLANATION

Bei Mu Gua Lou San (Fritillaria and Trichosanthes Fruit Powder) treats Lung dryness with phlegm accumulation. Lung dryness may consume fluids and create phlegm. Because the pathogenic factor in this syndrome is dryness, the phlegm is thick, sticky, and not easily expectorated. Dryness of the throat is due to injury of the body fluids.

This formula has *Bei Mu* (Bulbus Fritillariae) to clear heat, moisten the Lung, dispel phlegm, and stop coughing. *Gua Lou* (Fructus Trichosanthis) clears heat, moistens dryness, regulates qi, and breaks up phlegm stagnation. *Tian Hua Fen* (Radix Trichosanthis) clears heat, dissolves phlegm, promotes the generation of body fluids, and moistens dryness. *Fu Ling* (Poria) strengthens the Spleen and removes dampness. *Ju Hong* (Exocarpium Citri Reticulatae) activates qi circulation and dissolves phlegm. *Jie Geng* (Radix Platycodonis) ventilates the Lung to stop cough and eliminate phlegm.

MODIFICATIONS

- With exterior wind invasion, add *Sang Ye* (Folium Mori), *Ku Xing Ren* (Semen Armeniacae Amarum), *Qian Hu* (Radix Peucedani), and *Niu Bang Zi* (Fructus Arctii).
- With voice hoarseness or blood-streaked sputum due to yin deficiency, add *Sha Shen* (Radix Glehniae seu Adenophorae), *Mai Dong* (Radix Ophiopogonis), *Lu Gen* (Rhizoma Phragmitis), *Xian He Cao* (Herba Agrimoniae), *Mu Hu Die* (Semen Oroxyli), and *Qian Cao* (Radix et Rhizoma Rubiae). Remove *Ju Hong* (Exocarpium Citri Reticulatae).

1240

Bèi Mǔ Guā Lóu Sǎn (Fritillaria and Trichosanthes Fruit Powder)

Bei Mu Gua Lou San (Fritillaria and Trichosanthes Fruit Powder)

Diagnosis	Signs and Symptoms	Treatment	Herbs
Lung dryness with phlegm accumulation	• Coughing with thick, sticky sputum that is difficult to expectorate: dryness consuming and turning fluids into phlegm • Dry throat: dryness injuring body fluids	• Moistens the Lung and clears heat • Regulates qi and dissolves phlegm	• *Bei Mu* (Bulbus Fritillariae) clears heat, moistens the Lung, dispels phlegm, and stops coughing. • *Gua Lou* (Fructus Trichosanthis) clears heat, moistens dryness, regulates qi, and breaks up phlegm stagnation. • *Tian Hua Fen* (Radix Trichosanthis) clears heat, dissolves phlegm, promotes the generation of body fluids, and moistens dryness. • *Fu Ling* (Poria) strengthens the Spleen and removes dampness. • *Ju Hong* (Exocarpium Citri Reticulatae) activates qi to dissolve phlegm. • *Jie Geng* (Radix Platycodonis) ventilates the Lung to stop cough and eliminate phlegm.

- For cough with thick, yellow sputum, add *Huang Lian* (Rhizoma Coptidis), *Zhi Zi* (Fructus Gardeniae), *Dan Nan Xing* (Arisaema cum Bile), and *Gan Cao* (Radix et Rhizoma Glycyrrhizae). Remove *Tian Hua Fen* (Radix Trichosanthis), *Fu Ling* (Poria), and *Jie Geng* (Radix Platycodonis).
- With tidal fever, *wu xin re* (five-center heat), and other signs of yin deficiency, add *Mai Men Dong Tang* (Ophiopogonis Decoction) or *Bai He Gu Jin Tang* (Lily Bulb Decoction to Preserve the Metal).

- With dry, itchy throat, add *Qian Hu* (Radix Peucedani) and *Niu Bang Zi* (Fructus Arctii).
- With dry mouth and sore throat, add *Xuan Shen* (Radix Scrophulariae), *Di Huang* (Radix Rehmanniae), *Mai Dong* (Radix Ophiopogonis), and *Lu Gen* (Rhizoma Phragmitis).

CAUTIONS / CONTRAINDICATIONS

Bei Mu Gua Lou San is contraindicated for cough due to Kidney yin deficiency, or deficiency-heat rising.

PHLEGM-DISPELLING FORMULAS

18

1241

Chapter 18 – Phlegm-Dispelling Formulas　　　　　*Section 4 – Warm Formulas that Dissolve Cold Phlegm*

Section 4

温化寒痰剂
— Warm Formulas that Dissolve Cold Phlegm

Líng Gān Wǔ Wèi Jiāng Xīn Tāng
(Poria, Licorice, Schisandra, Ginger, and Asarum Decoction)

苓甘五味姜辛湯
苓甘五味姜辛汤

Pinyin Name: *Ling Gan Wu Wei Jiang Xin Tang*
Literal Name: Poria, Licorice, Schisandra, Ginger, and Asarum Decoction
Original Source: *Jin Gui Yao Lue* (Essentials from the Golden Cabinet) by Zhang Zhong-Jing in the Eastern Han Dynasty

COMPOSITION

Gan Jiang (Rhizoma Zingiberis)	9g
Xi Xin (Radix et Rhizoma Asari)	9g [3g]
Fu Ling (Poria)	12g
Wu Wei Zi (Fructus Schisandrae Chinensis)	0.5 cup [3-6g]
Gan Cao (Radix et Rhizoma Glycyrrhizae)	9g

DOSAGE / PREPARATION / ADMINISTRATION

The source text states to cook the ingredients with 8 cups [1,600 mL] of water until the liquid is reduced to 3 cups [600 mL]. Take 0.5 cup [100 mL] of the warm, strained decoction three times daily. Today, this formula may be prepared as a decoction with the doses suggested in brackets.

CHINESE THERAPEUTIC ACTIONS

Warms the Lung and resolves *yin* (invisible phlegm)

CLINICAL MANIFESTATIONS

Retention of cold-type *yin* (invisible phlegm): coughing with profuse, white, watery sputum, discomfort in the chest and diaphragm regions, white, slippery tongue coating, and a wiry, slippery pulse.

CLINICAL APPLICATIONS

Bronchitis and cough.

EXPLANATION

Ling Gan Wu Wei Jiang Xin Tang (Poria, Licorice, Schisandra, Ginger, and Asarum Decoction) treats retention of cold-type *yin* (invisible phlegm) due to yang deficiency and yin excess, with accumulation of water and dampness. Spleen yang deficiency compromises the Spleen's normal functioning, and may lead to interior cold formation and damp accumulation, which precipitate retention of cold-type *yin* (invisible phlegm). This phlegm may be stored in the Lung and affect the Lung's qi flow. Consequently, coughing with profuse, white, watery sputum occurs. A white, slippery tongue coating and a wiry, slippery pulse are signs of interior cold and phlegm.

Gan Jiang (Rhizoma Zingiberis), the chief herb in this formula, warms the Lung, dispels cold, dissolves dampness, and resolves *yin* (invisible phlegm). *Xi Xin* (Radix et Rhizoma Asari), an acrid and warm herb, warms the Lung, disperses cold, and assists *Gan Jiang* (Rhizoma Zingiberis) in resolving *yin* (invisible phlegm). *Fu Ling* (Poria) strengthens the Spleen and resolves dampness. *Wu Wei Zi* (Fructus Schisandrae Chinensis) astringes Lung qi to stop coughing. Moreover, the astringent effect of *Wu Wei Zi* (Fructus Schisandrae Chinensis) moderates the dispersing function of *Xi Xin* (Radix et Rhizoma Asari) to effectively relieve cough. *Gan Cao* (Radix et Rhizoma Glycyrrhizae) harmonizes all of the herbs in the formula.

1242

Chinese Herbal Formulas and Applications

Líng Gān Wǔ Wèi Jiāng Xīn Tāng
(Poria, Licorice, Schisandra, Ginger, and Asarum Decoction)

Ling Gan Wu Wei Jiang Xin Tang (Poria, Licorice, Schisandra, Ginger, and Asarum Decoction)

Diagnosis	Signs and Symptoms	Treatment	Herbs
Retention of cold-type *yin* (invisible phlegm)	• Coughing with profuse, white, watery sputum: accumulation of phlegm obstructing Lung qi circulation • White, slippery tongue coating and a wiry, slippery pulse: interior cold and phlegm	Warms the Lung and resolves *yin* (invisible phlegm)	• *Gan Jiang* (Rhizoma Zingiberis) warms the Lung, dispels cold, dissolves dampness, and resolves *yin* (invisible phlegm). • *Xi Xin* (Radix et Rhizoma Asari) warms the Lung and disperses cold. • *Fu Ling* (Poria) strengthens the Spleen and resolves dampness. • *Wu Wei Zi* (Fructus Schisandrae Chinensis) astringes the Lung qi to stop coughing. • *Gan Cao* (Radix et Rhizoma Glycyrrhizae) harmonizes all of the herbs.

MODIFICATIONS

• With profuse phlegm and nausea or vomiting, add *Ban Xia* (Rhizoma Pinelliae).

• With severe coughing, add *Ku Xing Ren* (Semen Armeniacae Amarum).

• If there are signs of exterior wind condition, replace *Gan Jiang* (Rhizoma Zingiberis) with *Sheng Jiang* (Rhizoma Zingiberis Recens), and add *Zi Su Ye* (Folium Perillae).

• With Spleen deficiency and decreased food intake, add *Dang Shen* (Radix Codonopsis), *Bai Zhu* (Rhizoma Atractylodis Macrocephalae), and *Chen Pi* (Pericarpium Citri Reticulatae).

• With epigastric fullness and distention, add *Chen Pi* (Pericarpium Citri Reticulatae) and *Zhi Qiao* (Fructus Aurantii).

CAUTIONS / CONTRAINDICATIONS

Ling Gan Wu Wei Jiang Xin Tang contains many warm and drying herbs, and is contraindicated in cases of cough or dyspnea caused by Lung heat, dryness, yin deficiency, or phlegm-fire accumulation.

RELATED FORMULAS

Lěng Xiào Wán (Cold Wheezing Pill)

冷哮丸

Pinyin Name: Leng Xiao Wan
Literal Name: Cold Wheezing Pill
Original Source: *Zhang Shi Yi Tong* (Comprehensive Medicine According to Master Zhang) by Zhang Lu-Xuan in 1695

Ma Huang (Herba Ephedrae), *pao* (blast-fried)	30g
Zhi Chuan Wu (Radix Aconiti Praeparata)	30g
Xi Xin (Radix et Rhizoma Asari)	30g

Hua Jiao (Pericarpium Zanthoxyli)	30g
Bai Fan (Alumen)	30g
Zao Jiao (Fructus Gleditsiae), *zhi* (fried with liquid) until crisp	30g
Ban Xia Qu (Rhizoma Pinelliae Massa Fermentata)	30g
Dan Nan Xing (Arisaema cum Bile)	30g
Ku Xing Ren (Semen Armeniacae Amarum)	30g
Gan Cao (Radix et Rhizoma Glycyrrhizae)	30g
Zi Wan (Radix et Rhizoma Asteris)	60g
Kuan Dong Hua (Flos Farfarae)	60g

The source text states to grind the ingredients into a fine powder and form into pills with powdered *Shen Qu* (Massa Fermentata) and fresh juice of *Sheng Jiang* (Rhizoma Zingiberis Recens). At the onset of this syndrome, take 6g (3g for weak patients) of pills at bedtime with tea made from 6g of *Sheng Jiang* (Rhizoma Zingiberis Recens). Furthermore, apply *San Jian Gao* (Three Constructive Paste) topically to *Feishu* (BL 13).

Today, this formula is prepared by grinding the ingredients into powder and mixing it with fresh juice from *Sheng Jiang* (Rhizoma Zingiberis Recens) to form pills. Take 6g of pills twice daily with warm, boiled water or a decoction of *Sheng Jiang* (Rhizoma Zingiberis Recens). In addition, apply *San Jian Gao* (Three Constructive Paste) topically to *Feishu* (BL 13) for optimal results.

According to the source text, ingestion of *Leng Xiao Wan* (Cold Wheezing Pill) will help to expectorate stubborn phlegm and unblock the stagnation in the chest and diaphragm. After the resolution of the acute condition, herbs that tonify the Spleen and Stomach should be prescribed.

PHLEGM-DISPELLING FORMULAS

18

1243

Chapter 18 – Phlegm-Dispelling Formulas　　　　　*Section 4 – Warm Formulas that Dissolve Cold Phlegm*

Líng Gān Wǔ Wèi Jiāng Xīn Tāng
(Poria, Licorice, Schisandra, Ginger, and Asarum Decoction)

Leng Xiao Wan (Cold Wheezing Pill) dispels cold and expels phlegm, and can be used to treat individuals with cold invasion to the upper back, with symptoms such as coughing and wheezing after exposure to cold, feeling of distention and fullness in the chest and diaphragm, and inability to lie down flat because of dyspnea. For best results, apply *San Jian Gao* (Three Constructive Paste) topically to the following acupuncture points: *Feishu* (BL 13), *Huagai* (CV 20), and *Shanzhong* (CV 17).

Sān Jiàn Gāo (Three Constructive Paste)

三建膏

Pinyin Name: *San Jian Gao*

Literal Name: Three Constructive Paste

Original Source: *Zhang Shi Yi Tong* (Comprehensive Medicine According to Master Zhang) by Zhang Lu-Xuan in 1695

Zhi Cao Wu (Radix Aconiti Kusnezoffii Praeparata)	60g
Fu Zi (Radix Aconiti Lateralis Praeparata)	60g
Zhi Chuan Wu (Radix Aconiti Praeparata)	60g
Gui Xin (Cortex Rasus Cinnamomi)	60g
Rou Gui (Cortex Cinnamomi)	60g
Gui Zhi (Ramulus Cinnamomi)	60g
Xi Xin (Radix et Rhizoma Asari)	60g
Gan Jiang (Rhizoma Zingiberis)	60g
Hua Jiao (Pericarpium Zanthoxyli)	60g

This herbal paste is prepared by cooking the herbs with 1,000 grams of sesame oil. After the initial cooking

and extraction process, the herb residue is filtered and discarded. The dense herbal extract is cooked again at low temperature for a prolonged period of time until it turns into a thick herbal paste. Lastly, add a small amount of *She Xiang* (Moschus) before applying the herbal paste to acupuncture points or the affected areas.

Note: *She Xiang* (Moschus) is derived from an endangered animal, and is rarely used as a medicinal substance today. Its discussion here is included primarily for academic purposes, to reflect the historical use of this substance in its original formulation. Most herbal products today have removed it completely, or replaced it with substitutes with similar functions.

San Jian Gao (Three Constructive Paste) contains only warm and hot herbs to treat disorders characterized by cold. Clinical applications are as follows:

- For cough, wheezing, and dyspnea, apply this formula to *Feishu* (BL 13), *Huagai* (CV 20), and *Shanzhong* (CV 17).
- For yin-type deep-rooted sores and lesions, apply this formula to the affected area.
- For abdominal pain with poor appetite and diarrhea due to cold, apply topically to the umbilicus and *Zhongwan* (CV 12).
- For sexual and reproductive disorders due to yang deficiency, apply this formula to the umbilicus and *Dantian* (an area 3 *cun* below the umbilicus).
- For masses in the abdomen due to cold accumulation, apply this formula to the affected area.

1244

Chinese Herbal Formulas and Applications

Sān Zǐ Yǎng Qīn Tāng
(Three-Seed Decoction to Nourish One's Parents)

三子養親湯
三子养亲汤

Pinyin Name: *San Zi Yang Qin Tang*
Literal Name: Three-Seed Decoction to Nourish One's Parents
Alternate Name: Three-Seed Combination
Original Source: *Han Shi Yi Tong* (Comprehensive Medicine According to Master Han) by Han Mao in 1522

COMPOSITION

Bai Jie Zi (Semen Sinapis)	[6g]
Zi Su Zi (Fructus Perillae)	[9g]
Lai Fu Zi (Semen Raphani)	[9g]

DOSAGE / PREPARATION / ADMINISTRATION

The source text states to dry-fry the ingredients and crush open the seeds. Place a maximum of 9g of the herbs into a silk sack, and cook it with a large amount of water. Do not overcook.* Take the decoction in small sips frequently throughout the day. The source text recommends adding honey for patients with constipation, and to include 3 slices of *Sheng Jiang* (Rhizoma Zingiberis Recens) in the winter. Today, this formula is prepared by crushing the seeds (using the suggested doses in brackets), placing them all in a cheesecloth bag, and cooking them in water. Take the decoction frequently in small amounts throughout the day. [*Please see Authors' Comments for explanation.]

CHINESE THERAPEUTIC ACTIONS

1. Redirects Lung qi and soothes the diaphragm
2. Dissolves phlegm and promotes food digestion

CLINICAL MANIFESTATIONS

Phlegm retention with qi stagnation: coughing with profuse sputum, wheezing, dyspnea, a feeling of distention in the chest, indigestion even with decreased intake of food, white, greasy tongue coating, and a slippery pulse.

CLINICAL APPLICATIONS

Chronic bronchitis, pulmonary emphysema, asthma, bronchial asthma, cardiopulmonary disease, and cough.

EXPLANATION

San Zi Yang Qin Tang (Three-Seed Decoction to Nourish One's Parents) was originally designed to treat geriatric patients with phlegm retention and qi stagnation. Because geriatric patients often have qi deficiency, overeating or consumption of cold or raw food easily leads to stagnation of food and qi. If the qi becomes stagnated, the fluids will not be distributed properly, and dampness and phlegm may accumulate as a result. Phlegm retention may cause reversed flow of Lung qi, resulting in coughing, dyspnea, and chest oppression. Stagnation of food and Stomach qi may lead to lack of appetite and indigestion. The white, greasy tongue coating and slippery pulse suggest qi deficiency and phlegm retention.

This formula has *Bai Jie Zi* (Semen Sinapis) to warm the Lung, dissolve phlegm, and soothe the diaphragm. *Zi Su Zi* (Fructus Perillae) disperses phlegm and guides reversed flow of Lung qi downward to relieve coughing and wheezing. *Lai Fu Zi* (Semen Raphani) activates Stomach qi, resolves food stagnation, and eliminates phlegm.

San Zi Yang Qin Tang (Three-Seed Decoction to Nourish One's Parents)

Diagnosis	Signs and Symptoms	Treatment	Herbs
Phlegm retention with qi stagnation	• Coughing, dyspnea and chest oppression: phlegm retention in the Lung causing reversed qi flow and qi stagnation • Lack of appetite and indigestion: phlegm retention in the Stomach affecting digestive functions • White, greasy tongue coating and slippery pulse: qi deficiency and phlegm retention	• Descends Lung qi and soothes the diaphragm • Dissolves phlegm and promotes digestion of food	• *Bai Jie Zi* (Semen Sinapis) dissolves phlegm. • *Zi Su Zi* (Fructus Perillae) redirects qi downward to relieve coughing and wheezing. • *Lai Fu Zi* (Semen Raphani) resolves food stagnation and eliminates phlegm.

PHLEGM-DISPELLING FORMULAS

18

1245

Chapter 18 – Phlegm-Dispelling Formulas

Section 4 – Warm Formulas that Dissolve Cold Phlegm

Sān Zǐ Yǎng Qīn Tāng
(Three-Seed Decoction to Nourish One's Parents)

PHARMACOLOGICAL EFFECTS

1. **Antiasthmatic**: *San Zi Yang Qin Tang* has been shown in many studies to effectively reverse airway obstruction. The mechanism of this action is attributed to its ability to relax the smooth muscles and reverse bronchial constriction.[1]

2. **Antitussive**: According to one study, administration of *San Zi Yang Qin Tang* was associated with a marked antitussive effect in mice with artificially-induced cough. The antitussive effect began approximately 1 hour after oral ingestion.[2]

3. **Expectorant**: One study reported marked expectorant and antitussive effects using *San Zi Yang Qin Tang* at 20 g/kg given in decoction via oral ingestion.[3]

CLINICAL STUDIES AND RESEARCH

1. **Cough**: One study used *San Zi Yang Qin Tang* to treat 40 patients with chronic and stubborn cough. Out of 40 patients, 14 had cough for more than 10 years, and 15 were geriatric persons 60 years of age and older. The study reported successful treatment of cough in 25 cases within 3-5 days, and 15 cases within 14 days.[4]

2. **Pediatric cough**: Daily usage of modified *San Zi Yang Qin Tang* successfully treated 25 children with chronic cough. The herbal treatment included *Lai Fu Zi* (Semen Raphani), *Zi Su Zi* (Fructus Perillae), *Ting Li Zi* (Semen Descurainiae seu Lepidii), *Zi Wan* (Radix et Rhizoma Asteris), *Jing Jie* (Herba Schizonepetae), *Qian Hu* (Radix Peucedani), *Ku Xing Ren* (Semen Armeniacae Amarum), *Wu Wei Zi* (Fructus Schisandrae Chinensis), and *Gan Cao* (Radix et Rhizoma Glycyrrhizae) as the base formula. Modifications were made by adding *Dang Shen* (Radix Codonopsis), *Fu Ling* (Poria), and *Bai Zhu* (Rhizoma Atractylodis Macrocephalae) for Spleen and Lung qi deficiencies; *Sha Shen* (Radix Glehniae seu Adenophorae), *Mai Dong* (Radix Ophiopogonis), and *Chuan Bei Mu* (Bulbus Fritillariae Cirrhosae) for qi and yin deficiencies; *Mao Dong Qing* (Radix Ilicis Pubescentis), *Dan Shen* (Radix et Rhizoma Salviae Miltiorrhizae), *Chi Shao* (Radix Paeoniae Rubra), and *Jiang Can* (Bombyx Batryticatus) for phlegm and blood stagnation. The herbs were given in decoction daily. The study reported successful treatment in all 25 patients.[5]

3. **Bronchial asthma**: Administration of modified *San Zi Yang Qin Tang* via oral inhalation was successful in treating 53 patients with bronchial asthma. Improvements included relief of wheezing, dyspnea, lowered heartbeat, and resolution of 3 concave signs. Out of 53 patients, 39 had complete recovery within 1-2 days and 14 within 3-4 days. The average time required to achieve complete recovery was 2.08 days.[6]

4. **Bronchitis**: Eighty-eight children with acute bronchitis were treated successfully using *San Zi Yang Qin Tang* plus *San Ao Tang* (Three-Unbinding Decoction). Improvement was noted in most cases within 3 packs of herbs. The study reported a 65.9% rate of recovery, 86.4% rate of significant improvement, and 96.6% effectiveness. Those who did not respond to the treatment also had Spleen and Lung qi deficiencies with a suppressed immune system.[7]

5. ***Mei he qi* (plum-pit qi)**: Modified *San Zi Yang Qin Tang* was used to treat 32 patients with plum-pit *qi* with complete recovery in 15 cases, marked improvement in 13 cases, and no effect in 4 cases. The overall effectiveness was 87.5%.[8,9]

TOXICOLOGY

San Zi Yang Qin Tang has very little toxicity. According to one study, the LD_{50} for oral administration of this formula in mice cannot be measured. Oral administration of up to 120 g/kg (maximum capacity of the stomach) of this formula did not cause any fatality.[10]

AUTHORS' COMMENTS

San Zi Yang Qin Tang treats the symptoms (phlegm retention with qi stagnation), not the cause (qi deficiency) of the illness. Thus, once the acute clinical manifestations are relieved, some qi-tonic herbs should be added to strengthen the qi. Moreover, the doses of the three herbs in the formula are frequently adjusted depending on the symptoms presented by the patient. Because this formula is relatively strong and is aimed at treating the symptoms, it is cooked with a large amount of water for only a short period of time to ensure that the potency of the decoction is not too strong. Furthermore, the decoction is not to be taken all at once, but in small amounts throughout the day for sustained symptomatic relief.

References

1. *Zhong Yao Yao Li Yu Lin Chuang* (Pharmacology and Clinical Applications of Chinese Herbs) 1992;8(3):15.
2. *Zhong Yao Yao Li Yu Lin Chuang* (Pharmacology and Clinical Applications of Chinese Herbs) 1992;8(3):15.
3. *Si Chuan Zhong Yi* (Sichuan Chinese Medicine) 1989;7(11):10.
4. *Zhong Yao Tong Bao* (Journal of Chinese Herbology) 1986;8:56.
5. *Xin Zhong Yi* (New Chinese Medicine) 1995;9:50.
6. *Shan Xi Zhong Yi* (Shanxi Chinese Medicine) 1995;4:148.
7. *Shang Hai Yi Yao Za Zhi* (Shanghai Journal of Medicine and Herbology) 1991;10:22.
8. *Hei Long Jiang Zhong Yi Yao* (Heilongjiang Chinese Medicine and Herbology) 1992;6:31.
9. *Guang Xi Zhong Yi Yao* (Guangxi Chinese Medicine and Herbology) 1988;11(3):43.
10. *Zhong Yao Yao Li Yu Lin Chuang* (Pharmacology and Clinical Applications of Chinese Herbs) 1992;8(3):15.

Chinese Herbal Formulas and Applications

Section 5

治风化痰剂
— Wind-Expelling and Phlegm-Dissolving Formulas

Bàn Xià Bái Zhú Tiān Má Tāng
(Pinellia, Atractylodes Macrocephala, and Gastrodia Decoction)

半夏白朮天麻湯
半夏白术天麻汤

Pinyin Name: *Ban Xia Bai Zhu Tian Ma Tang*
Literal Name: Pinellia, Atractylodes Macrocephala, and Gastrodia Decoction
Alternate Names: *Pan Hsia Tien Ma Pai Shu Tang, Ban Xia Tian Ma Bai Shu Tang*, Pinellia, Gastrodia, and Atractylodes Decoction; Pinellia, Gastrodia and Bighead Atractylodes Decoction; Pinellia and Gastrodia Combination
Original Source: *Yi Xue Xin Wu* (Medical Revelations) by Cheng Guo-Peng in 1732

COMPOSITION

Ban Xia (Rhizoma Pinelliae)	4.5g [9g]
Tian Ma (Rhizoma Gastrodiae)	3g [6g]
Bai Zhu (Rhizoma Atractylodis Macrocephalae)	9g [15g]
Fu Ling (Poria)	3g [6g]
Ju Hong (Exocarpium Citri Reticulatae)	3g [6g]
Gan Cao (Radix et Rhizoma Glycyrrhizae)	1.5g [3g]

DOSAGE / PREPARATION / ADMINISTRATION

The source text states to prepare the ingredients as a decoction with 1 slice of *Sheng Jiang* (Rhizoma Zingiberis Recens) and 2 pieces of *Da Zao* (Fructus Jujubae). Today, this formula may be prepared as a decoction with the doses suggested in brackets.

CHINESE THERAPEUTIC ACTIONS

1. Dries dampness and dissolves phlegm
2. Soothes the Liver and subdues Liver wind

CLINICAL MANIFESTATIONS

Wind and phlegm rising upward: dizziness, vertigo, heaviness of the head, headache, a stifling sensation in the chest, nausea, vomiting, a white, greasy tongue coating, and a wiry, slippery pulse.

CLINICAL APPLICATIONS

Habitual headache, migraine headache, tension headache, Meniere's syndrome, cerebellitis, dizziness, vertigo, gastroatonia, gastroptosis, facial paralysis, and nasosinusitis.

EXPLANATION

Ban Xia Bai Zhu Tian Ma Tang (Pinellia, Atractylodes Macrocephala, and Gastrodia Decoction) treats rising of wind and phlegm with key symptoms such as dizziness and vertigo, heaviness of the head, nausea and vomiting, and a white, greasy tongue coating. Wind and phlegm syndrome occurs as a result of a combination of Spleen and Liver disorders. Spleen deficiency results in the formation of dampness and phlegm. The phlegm can be accompanied by Liver wind rising. Together, these factors rise and disturb many parts of the upper body. Dizziness, vertigo, and heaviness of the head are due to the turbid dampness, phlegm, and Liver wind traveling to the head. A stifling sensation in the chest is due to damp-phlegm obstruction in the chest. Nausea and vomiting are caused by damp-phlegm obstruction in the middle *jiao*.

The treatment plan is to dissolve phlegm, subdue Liver wind, strengthen the Spleen, and dispel dampness. *Ban Xia* (Rhizoma Pinelliae) dries dampness, dissolves phlegm, and redirects the reversed flow of Stomach qi

PHLEGM-DISPELLING FORMULAS

18

1247

Chapter 18 – Phlegm-Dispelling Formulas   *Section 5 – Wind-Expelling and Phlegm-Dissolving Formulas*

Bàn Xià Bái Zhú Tiān Má Tāng
(Pinellia, Atractylodes Macrocephala, and Gastrodia Decoction)

Ban Xia Bai Zhu Tian Ma Tang (Pinellia, Atractylodes Macrocephala, and Gastrodia Decoction)

Diagnosis	Signs and Symptoms	Treatment	Herbs
Wind and phlegm rising	• Dizziness, vertigo and heaviness of the head: phlegm and Liver wind rising to the head • A stifling sensation in the chest: damp-phlegm obstruction in the chest • Nausea and vomiting: damp-phlegm obstruction in the middle *jiao* • White, greasy tongue coating, and a wiry, slippery pulse: damp-phlegm in the interior	• Dries dampness and dissolves phlegm • Soothes the Liver and subdues Liver wind	• *Ban Xia* (Rhizoma Pinelliae) dries dampness and dissolves phlegm. • *Tian Ma* (Rhizoma Gastrodiae) subdues Liver wind. • *Bai Zhu* (Rhizoma Atractylodis Macrocephalae) and *Fu Ling* (Poria) strengthen the Spleen and dispel dampness. • *Ju Hong* (Exocarpium Citri Reticulatae) regulates qi and dissolves phlegm. • *Sheng Jiang* (Rhizoma Zingiberis Recens) and *Da Zao* (Fructus Jujubae) harmonize the Spleen and Stomach. • *Gan Cao* (Radix et Rhizoma Glycyrrhizae) harmonizes all of the herbs.

downward to stop nausea and vomiting. *Tian Ma* (Rhizoma Gastrodiae) subdues Liver wind and alleviates dizziness and vertigo. These two chief herbs are essential in treating dizziness, vertigo, headache, and other symptoms caused by wind and phlegm. *Bai Zhu* (Rhizoma Atractylodis Macrocephalae) strengthens the Spleen and dries dampness, while *Fu Ling* (Poria) strengthens the Spleen and dispels dampness. *Ju Hong* (Exocarpium Citri Reticulatae) regulates qi and dissolves phlegm. *Sheng Jiang* (Rhizoma Zingiberis Recens) and *Da Zao* (Fructus Jujubae) harmonize the Spleen and Stomach, while *Gan Cao* (Radix et Rhizoma Glycyrrhizae) harmonizes all of the herbs.

MODIFICATIONS

- With headache, add *Man Jing Zi* (Fructus Viticis) and *Ji Li* (Fructus Tribuli).
- With headache caused by wind-cold, add *Fang Feng* (Radix Saposhnikoviae) and *Qiang Huo* (Rhizoma et Radix Notopterygii).
- With headache caused by blood deficiency, add *Dang Gui* (Radix Angelicae Sinensis) and *Chuan Xiong* (Rhizoma Chuanxiong).
- With headache and dizziness caused by cold and phlegm, add *Zhen Wu Tang* (True Warrior Decoction).
- With migraine headache, add *Chuan Xiong* (Rhizoma Chuanxiong) and *Man Jing Zi* (Fructus Viticis).
- With dizziness and vertigo due to qi deficiency, add *Ren Shen* (Radix et Rhizoma Ginseng) and *Huang Qi* (Radix Astragali).
- If there is severe dizziness or vertigo due to Liver excess, add *Jiang Can* (Bombyx Batryticatus), *Gou Teng* (Ramulus

Uncariae cum Uncis), and *Dan Nan Xing* (Arisaema cum Bile).
- With profuse phlegm and damp accumulation, add *Ze Xie* (Rhizoma Alismatis) and *Gui Zhi* (Ramulus Cinnamomi).
- With sinusitis or rhinitis, add *Xin Yi Hua* (Flos Magnoliae).
- For arteriostenosis in the brain, add *Gou Teng* (Ramulus Uncariae cum Uncis).

CAUTIONS / CONTRAINDICATIONS

Ban Xia Bai Zhu Tian Ma Tang should not be used for dizziness caused by Liver and Kidney yin deficiencies, or dizziness or vertigo caused by Liver yang rising.

CLINICAL STUDIES AND RESEARCH

1. **Meniere's syndrome**: One study evaluated the efficacy of *Ban Xia Bai Zhu Tian Ma Tang* in treating Meniere's syndrome in 32 patients (18 males and 14 females) with 1 to 5 years history of illness. The base formula contained *Ban Xia Bai Zhu Tian Ma Tang* plus *Ze Xie* (Rhizoma Alismatis), *Zhu Ru* (Caulis Bambusae in Taenia), and *Jiang Can* (Bombyx Batryticatus). Modifications were made by adding *Zhe Shi* (Haematitum) and *Xuan Fu Hua* (Flos Inulae) for frequent nausea and vomiting; *Ci Shi* (Magnetitum), *Shi Chang Pu* (Rhizoma Acori Tatarinowii) and *Hu Tao Ren* (Semen Juglandis) for severe tinnitus; and *Long Gu* (Os Draconis) and *Mu Li* (Concha Ostreae) for severe dizziness. Of 32 patients, the study reported complete recovery in 6 cases, improvement in 21 cases, and no effect in 5 cases. The overall effectiveness was 84.4%.[1]

1248

Bàn Xià Bái Zhú Tiān Má Tāng
(Pinellia, Atractylodes Macrocephala, and Gastrodia Decoction)

Another study also reported marked results using a modification of this formula to treat 70 patients with Meniere's syndrome with severe dizziness, vertigo, nausea, vomiting, and tinnitus. The formula used contained *Ban Xia* (Rhizoma Pinelliae), *Bai Zhu* (Rhizoma Atractylodis Macrocephalae), *Tian Ma* (Rhizoma Gastrodiae), *Ze Xie* (Rhizoma Alismatis), *Fu Ling* (Poria), *Xuan Fu Hua* (Flos Inulae), *Shi Chang Pu* (Rhizoma Acori Tatarinowii), *Sha Ren* (Fructus Amomi), *Zhe Shi* (Haematitum), and *Dan Shen* (Radix et Rhizoma Salviae Miltiorrhizae) as the base formula. Modifications included the addition of *Dang Gui* (Radix Angelicae Sinensis) and *Huang Qi* (Radix Astragali) for blood deficiency; and *Long Chi* (Dens Draconis) and *Shou Wu Teng* (Caulis Polygoni Multiflori) for insomnia. The duration of treatment ranged from 3-35 packs of herbs.[2]

2. **Dizziness and vertigo**: *Ban Xia Bai Zhu Tian Ma Tang* has been shown in many studies to effectively treat dizziness and vertigo due to various causes. According to one study, use of the formula plus *Zi Su Ye* (Folium Perillae) and *Ze Xie* (Rhizoma Alismatis) in decoction daily was very effective in treating acute onset of dizziness and vertigo accompanied by nausea, vomiting, and tinnitus.[3]

   Another study reported 98% effectiveness using modified *Ban Xia Bai Zhu Tian Ma Tang* to treat dizziness and vertigo due to inner ear imbalance. Of 50 patients, 28 had complete recovery (resolution of all symptoms without recurrence within 1 year of follow-ups), significant improvement in 21 cases (resolution of all symptoms with recurrence associated with stress, fatigue, and other causes) and no effect in 1 case.[4]

   Lastly, one study combined *Ban Xia Bai Zhu Tian Ma Tang* and *Wen Dan Tang* (Warm the Gallbladder Decoction) to treat dizziness in 80 patients with complete recovery in 51 cases, improvement in 20 cases, and no effect in 9 cases. The composition of the herbal treatment included these two formulas without *Bai Zhu* (Rhizoma Atractylodis Macrocephalae) and *Gan Cao* (Radix et Rhizoma Glycyrrhizae), and with the addition of *Gou Teng* (Ramulus Uncariae cum Uncis), *Zhu Ru* (Caulis Bambusae in Taenia), *Ci Shi* (Magnetitum), and others as deemed necessary.[5]

3. **Tension headache**: Use of modified *Ban Xia Bai Zhu Tian Ma Tang* to treat tension headache in 68 patients was associated with complete recovery in 49 cases, improvement in 18 cases, and no effect in 1 case. Modifications to the base formula included *Shi Chang Pu* (Rhizoma Acori Tatarinowii) and *Gou Teng* (Ramulus Uncariae cum Uncis) for numbness in the head; *Gua Lou Pi* (Pericarpium Trichosanthis) and *Zhu Ru* (Caulis Bambusae in Taenia) for fullness and distention in the chest and epigastrium with sensations of nausea and vomiting; *Gou Teng* (Ramulus Uncariae cum Uncis), *Huang Qin* (Radix Scutellariae), and *Chai Hu* (Radix Bupleuri) for headache accompanied by dizziness, tinnitus, and vertigo; and removal of *Ban Xia* (Rhizoma Pinelliae) and the addition of *Dang Gui* (Radix Angelicae Sinensis), *Chuan Xiong* (Rhizoma Chuanxiong), *Shou Wu Teng* (Caulis Polygoni Multiflori), and *Ji Xue Teng* (Caulis Spatholobi) for headache with poor facial complexion, palpitations, and a fine, weak pulse.[6]

4. **Cerebellitis**: One study reported 94% effectiveness using modified *Ban Xia Bai Zhu Tian Ma Tang* to treat acute cerebellitis. Of 17 patients, the study reported significant improvement in 9 cases, moderate improvement in 7 cases, and no effect in 1 case. The herbal formula contained *Ban Xia Bai Zhu Tian Ma Tang* without *Gan Cao* (Radix et Rhizoma Glycyrrhizae) and *Da Zao* (Fructus Jujubae), and with the addition of *Gou Teng* (Ramulus Uncariae cum Uncis) and *Shi Chang Pu* (Rhizoma Acori Tatarinowii). Furthermore, *Di Long* (Pheretima) and *Quan Xie* (Scorpio) were added for difficulty in walking; and *Dan Nan Xing* (Arisaema cum Bile) and *Yuan Zhi* (Radix Polygalae) were added for profuse phlegm.[7]

5. **Facial paralysis**: According to one study, 17 patients with facial paralysis characterized by deviation of the eyes and mouth were treated with modified *Ban Xia Bai Zhu Tian Ma Tang* with complete recovery in 10 cases, significant results in 4 cases, moderate results in 2 cases, and no effect in 1 case. The overall effectiveness was 94%. The herbal treatment contained this formula plus *Qiang Huo* (Rhizoma et Radix Notopterygii), *Bai Jie Zi* (Semen Sinapis), *Hong Hua* (Flos Carthami), *Quan Xie* (Scorpio), and *Wu Gong* (Scolopendra). The treatment protocol was to grind all herbs into a fine powder, and administer with a small amount of warm grain-based alcohol.[8]

6. **Nasosinusitis**: Administration of modified *Ban Xia Bai Zhu Tian Ma Tang* was associated with marked success in treating 50 patients with nasosinusitis. The herbal formula contained *Ban Xia* (Rhizoma Pinelliae) 10g, *Tian Ma* (Rhizoma Gastrodiae) 10g, *Cang Er Zi* (Fructus Xanthii) 10g, *Bai Zhi* (Radix Angelicae Dahuricae) 10g, *Yan Hu Suo* (Rhizoma Corydalis) 10g, *Gan Cao* (Radix et Rhizoma Glycyrrhizae) 10g, *Bai Zhu* (Rhizoma Atractylodis Macrocephalae) 15-30g, *Huang Qi* (Radix Astragali) 15-30g, *Xi Xin* (Radix et Rhizoma Asari) 4g, *Huang Qin* (Radix Scutellariae) 12g, *Yu Xing Cao* (Herba Houttuyniae) 30g, *Chuan Xiong* (Rhizoma Chuanxiong) 15g, *Lian Qiao* (Fructus Forsythiae) 15g, *Dan Shen* (Radix et Rhizoma Salviae Miltiorrhizae) 15g, *Niu Xi* (Radix Achyranthis Bidentatae) 15g, *Bai Shao* (Radix Paeoniae Alba) 15g, and *Huo Xiang* (Herba Agastaches)

Chapter 18 – Phlegm-Dispelling Formulas   *Section 5 – Wind-Expelling and Phlegm-Dissolving Formulas*

Bàn Xià Bái Zhú Tiān Má Tāng
(Pinellia, Atractylodes Macrocephala, and Gastrodia Decoction)

6g. The herbal formula was given in decoction daily. Of 50 patients, the study reported complete recovery in 35 cases and improvement in 15 cases. The duration of treatment ranged from 10-30 days.[9]

RELATED FORMULA

Bàn Xià Bái Zhú Tiān Má Tāng (Pinellia, Atractylodes Macrocephala, and Gastrodia Decoction)

半夏白朮天麻湯
半夏白术天麻汤

Pinyin Name: *Ban Xia Bai Zhu Tian Ma Tang*

Literal Name: Pinellia, Atractylodes Macrocephala, and Gastrodia Decoction

Original Source: *Pi Wei Lun* (Discussion of the Spleen and Stomach) by Li Gao in 1249

Huang Bo (Cortex Phellodendri Chinensis)	0.6g [1g]
Gan Jiang (Rhizoma Zingiberis)	0.6g [1g]
Tian Ma (Rhizoma Gastrodiae)	1.5g [2.5g]
Cang Zhu (Rhizoma Atractylodis)	1.5g [2.5g]
Fu Ling (Poria)	1.5g [2.5g]
Huang Qi (Radix Astragali)	1.5g [2.5g]
Ze Xie (Rhizoma Alismatis)	1.5g [2.5g]
Ren Shen (Radix et Rhizoma Ginseng)	1.5g [2.5g]
Bai Zhu (Rhizoma Atractylodis Macrocephalae)	3g [5g]
Shen Qu (Massa Fermentata), *chao* (dry-fried)	3g [5g]
Ban Xia (Rhizoma Pinelliae),	
xi (washed) in liquid 7 times	4.5g [7.5g]
Mai Ya (Fructus Hordei Germinatus)	4.5g [7.5g]
Chen Pi (Pericarpium Citri Reticulatae)	4.5g [7.5g]

The source text states to cook the herbs in 2 bowls of water until it is reduced down to 1 bowl. Take the warm,

strained decoction after meals. Today, this formula may be prepared as a decoction with the doses suggested in brackets.

This formula has functions to dry dampness, dissolve phlegm, benefit qi, and harmonize the Stomach. It is designed to treat headache due to phlegm retention with signs and symptoms such as nausea, vomiting, thick and sticky saliva and sputum, dizziness and vertigo, irritability, a stifling sensation in the chest, shortness of breath, severe headache, heavy sensations in the body, cold extremities, and restless sleep.

AUTHORS' COMMENTS

Ban Xia Bai Zhu Tian Ma Tang is one of the most essential formulas for treating dizziness and vertigo caused by Liver wind and phlegm rising. The key signs and symptoms include dizziness, vertigo, headache, a white, greasy tongue coating, and a wiry, slippery pulse.

References

1. *Shi Yong Zhong Xi Yi Jie He Za Zhi* (Practical Journal of Integrated Chinese and Western Medicines) 1991;1:37.
2. *Shi Yong Zhong Yi Za Zhi* (Journal of Practical Chinese Medicine) 1998;7:22.
3. *Shi Yong Zhong Yi Nei Ke Za Zhi* (Journal of Practical Chinese Internal Medicine) 1993;4:190.
4. *Tian Jin Zhong Yi* (Tianjin Chinese Medicine) 1995;2:16.
5. *Bei Jing Zhong Yi* (Beijing Chinese Medicine) 1997;5:50.
6. *Zhong Yi Yao Xue Bao* (Report of Chinese Medicine and Herbology) 1999;3:27.
7. *Shan Dong Zhong Yi Za Zhi* (Shandong Journal of Chinese Medicine) 1999;5:232.
8. *Bei Jing Zhong Yi* (Beijing Chinese Medicine) 1991;6:31.
9. *Shan Xi Zhong Yi* (Shanxi Chinese Medicine) 1995;16(2):63.

1250

Chinese Herbal Formulas and Applications

Ding Xiān Wán (Arrest Seizures Pill)

定癇丸
定痫丸

Pinyin Name: *Ding Xian Wan*
Literal Name: Arrest Seizures Pill
Alternate Name: Succinum Combination
Original Source: *Yi Xue Xin Wu* (Medical Revelations) by Cheng Guo-Peng in 1732

COMPOSITION

Dan Nan Xing (Arisaema cum Bile), *zhi* (prepared) 9 times	15g [3g]
Ban Xia (Rhizoma Pinelliae), *chao* (dry-fried) with ginger juice	30g [6g]
Chen Pi (Pericarpium Citri Reticulatae), *xi* (washed)	21g [4.5g]
Chuan Bei Mu (Bulbus Fritillariae Cirrhosae)	30g [6g]
Fu Ling (Poria), *zheng* (steamed)	30g [6g]
Mai Dong (Radix Ophiopogonis)	60g [12g]
Dan Shen (Radix et Rhizoma Salviae Miltiorrhizae), *zheng* (steamed) with liquor	60g [12g]
Shi Chang Pu (Rhizoma Acori Tatarinowii), *chu* (pestled) to powder	15g [3g]
Quan Xie (Scorpio), remove the tails and *xi* (washed) with licorice water	15g [3g]
Jiang Can (Bombyx Batryticatus), *xi* (washed) with licorice water and *chao* (dry-fried)	15g [3g]
Tian Ma (Rhizoma Gastrodiae)	30g [6g]
Zhu Sha (Cinnabaris), *shui fei* (refined with water) and *yan* (ground) into thin particles	9g [2g]
Hu Po (Succinum), *zhu* (boiled) till soft and *yan* (ground) with *Deng Xin Cao* (Medulla Junci)	15g [3g]
Yuan Zhi (Radix Polygalae), *pao* (blast-fried) with licorice water	21g [4.5g]
Fu Shen (Poria Pararadicis), *zheng* (steamed)	30g [6g]

Note: *Zhu Sha* (Cinnabaris) is a potentially toxic heavy metal, and is rarely used as a medicinal substance today. Its discussion here is included primarily for academic purposes, to reflect the historical use of this substance in its original formulation. Most herbal products today have removed it completely, or replaced it with substitutes with similar functions. For additional information on the toxicity, please refer to *Chinese Medical Herbology and Pharmacology* by John Chen and Tina Chen.

DOSAGE / PREPARATION / ADMINISTRATION

The source text states to grind the ingredients into powder and form into pills using the resultant mixture of the following liquids: a small bowl [100 mL] of *Zhu Li* (Succus Bambusae), a small cup [50 mL] of fresh juice of *Sheng Jiang* (Rhizoma Zingiberis Recens), and a thick herbal paste made from condensing 120g of *Gan Cao* (Radix et Rhizoma Glycyrrhizae). The pills are coated with *Zhu Sha* (Cinnabaris), and should resemble a large bullet in size [approximately 6g]. Take one pill per dose with warm, boiled water in the morning and at night.

CHINESE THERAPEUTIC ACTIONS

Eliminates phlegm and subdues Liver wind

CLINICAL MANIFESTATIONS

Phlegm and heat rising: sudden onset of seizures and epilepsy in young children, loss of balance, semi-unconsciousness or complete loss of consciousness, falling down, tonic-clonic seizures, upward-rolling of the eyes, deviation of the mouth, involuntary salivation or dripping saliva, and sudden shrieking. It is also used for *dian kuang* (mania and withdrawal) conditions.

CLINICAL APPLICATIONS

Seizures, epilepsy, and convulsions.

EXPLANATION

Ding Xian Wan (Arrest Seizures Pill) treats seizures and epilepsy caused by Liver wind rising and hot phlegm obstructing the sensory orifices. According to traditional Chinese medicine, seizures and epilepsy can be caused by many factors, such as phlegm stagnation, emotional imbalance, irregular diet, and overexertion or overwork. Seen more commonly in children, seizures and epilepsy occur when Liver wind and hot phlegm rise together to the head. As phlegm rises, it blocks the sensory orifices, causing sudden loss of consciousness, loss of balance, upward-rolling of the eyes, deviation of the mouth, and involuntary salivation or dripping saliva. If Liver wind and phlegm block the channels and collaterals, patients will have tonic-clonic type of convulsions.

PHLEGM-DISPELLING FORMULAS

18

1251

Chapter 18 – Phlegm-Dispelling Formulas   *Section 5 – Wind-Expelling and Phlegm-Dissolving Formulas*

Dìng Xiān Wán (Arrest Seizures Pill)

Ding Xian Wan (Arrest Seizures Pill)

Diagnosis	Signs and Symptoms	Treatment	Herbs
Rising of phlegm and heat	• Seizures and epilepsy: Liver wind and hot phlegm rise together to the head • Sudden loss of consciousness and loss of balance: hot phlegm blocking the sensory orifices • Convulsions: hot phlegm obstructing the channels and collaterals	Eliminates phlegm and subdues Liver wind	• *Zhu Li* (Succus Bambusae) clears heat, dissolves phlegm, and opens the sensory orifices. • *Dan Nan Xing* (Arisaema cum Bile) clears heat and dissolves phlegm. • *Ban Xia* (Rhizoma Pinelliae), *Chen Pi* (Pericarpium Citri Reticulatae), *Chuan Bei Mu* (Bulbus Fritillariae Cirrhosae), *Fu Ling* (Poria) and *Mai Dong* (Radix Ophiopogonis) dispel phlegm, direct qi downwards, and prevent yin damage. • *Dan Shen* (Radix et Rhizoma Salviae Miltiorrhizae) eliminates blood stagnation. • *Shi Chang Pu* (Rhizoma Acori Tatarinowii) warms and opens the sensory orifices. • *Quan Xie* (Scorpio), *Jiang Can* (Bombyx Batryticatus) and *Tian Ma* (Rhizoma Gastrodiae) subdue Liver wind and stop muscle convulsions. • *Zhu Sha* (Cinnabaris), *Hu Po* (Succinum), *Yuan Zhi* (Radix Polygalae), *Deng Xin Cao* (Medulla Junci) and *Fu Shen* (Poria Paradicis) calm the *shen* (spirit) and enhance the treatment of seizures and epilepsy. • *Sheng Jiang* (Rhizoma Zingiberis Recens) and *Gan Cao* (Radix et Rhizoma Glycyrrhizae) harmonize all of the herbs.

Zhu Li (Succus Bambusae) clears heat, dissolves phlegm, and opens the sensory orifices. *Dan Nan Xing* (Arisaema cum Bile) clears heat and dissolves phlegm. Together, these two herbs treat all types of seizures, convulsions, and stroke disorders. *Ban Xia* (Rhizoma Pinelliae), *Chen Pi* (Pericarpium Citri Reticulatae), *Chuan Bei Mu* (Bulbus Fritillariae Cirrhosae), *Fu Ling* (Poria), and *Mai Dong* (Radix Ophiopogonis) dispel phlegm and direct qi downward. They also prevent the warm and drying herbs from damaging yin. *Dan Shen* (Radix et Rhizoma Salviae Miltiorrhizae) eliminates blood stagnation. *Shi Chang Pu* (Rhizoma Acori Tatarinowii) warms and opens the sensory orifices. *Quan Xie* (Scorpio) and *Jiang Can* (Bombyx Batryticatus) subdue Liver wind and stop muscle convulsions. *Tian Ma* (Rhizoma Gastrodiae) subdues Liver wind and dissolves phlegm. *Zhu Sha* (Cinnabaris), *Hu Po* (Succinum), *Deng Xin Cao* (Medulla Junci), *Yuan Zhi* (Radix Polygalae), and *Fu Shen* (Poria Paradicis) calm the *shen* (spirit) and enhance the overall function of treating seizures and epilepsy. Lastly, *Sheng Jiang*

(Rhizoma Zingiberis Recens) and *Gan Cao* (Radix et Rhizoma Glycyrrhizae) harmonize all of the herbs.

MODIFICATIONS
• With chronic and frequent seizure attacks due to deficiency of *zheng* (upright) *qi*, add *Ren Shen* (Radix et Rhizoma Ginseng).
• With constipation, add *Da Huang* (Radix et Rhizoma Rhei) and *Mang Xiao* (Natrii Sulfas).
• With continuous twitching and spasms, add *Gou Teng* (Ramulus Uncariae cum Uncis).

CAUTIONS / CONTRAINDICATIONS
• *Ding Xian Wan* treats seizures and epilepsy caused by Liver wind rising and hot phlegm. It should not be used indiscriminately to treat seizures and epilepsy caused by other factors, such as Liver fire, Liver and Kidney yin deficiencies, and Spleen and Stomach deficiencies.
• This formula treats acute cases of seizures and epilepsy. Once the condition is stabilized, this formula should be discontinued, and additional supportive therapy started.

1252

Dìng Xián Wán (Arrest Seizures Pill)

RELATED FORMULA

Hé Chē Wán Fāng

河車丸方
河车丸方

Pinyin Name: He Che Wan Fang
Literal Name: Placenta Pill Formula
Original Source: *Yi Xue Xin Wu* (Medical Revelations) by Cheng Guo-Peng in 1732

Zi He Che (Placenta Hominis)	1 piece
Fu Ling (Poria)	30g
Fu Shen (Poria Paradicis)	30g
Yuan Zhi (Radix Polygalae)	30g
Ren Shen (Radix et Rhizoma Ginseng)	15g
Dan Shen (Radix et Rhizoma Salviae Miltiorrhizae)	21g

The source text states to prepare the herbs with honey to make pills. Take 9g of pills with water every morning.

He Che Wan Fang (Placenta Pill Formula) is to be used after the seizures and epilepsy have been treated with *Ding Xian Wan*. According to the source text, *He Che Wan Fang* tonifies the Kidney, nourishes the Heart, and strengthens the Spleen to terminate the recurrence of seizures and epilepsy.

Note: Human placenta is generally not used, for many reasons. Instead, placentae from pigs and cattle are used as substitutes.

AUTHORS' COMMENTS

Ding Xian Wan is designed to treat acute onsets of seizures and epilepsy, characterized by rising of phlegm, heat, and Liver wind. Although effective, the use of this formula alone is insufficient for the overall management of seizures and epilepsy. Optimal treatment of seizures and epilepsy must focus on treating both the symptoms and the cause. During seizures and epilepsy attacks, the emphasis is on treating the symptoms, which entails eliminating phlegm and Liver wind. During remission, the emphasis is on treating the cause, which could mean strengthening the Spleen, nourishing the Heart, benefiting the Liver and/or Kidney, or regulating qi and blood circulation. Furthermore, long-term care of patients with seizures and epilepsy must also include dietary and lifestyle adjustments.

PHLEGM-DISPELLING FORMULAS

18

1253

Chapter 18 – Phlegm-Dispelling Formulas

Chapter 18 — Summary

— Phlegm-Dispelling Formulas

SECTION 1: DAMP-DRYING AND PHLEGM-DISSOLVING FORMULAS

Name	Similarities	Differences
Er Chen Tang (Two-Cured Decoction)		Regulates qi, harmonizes the middle *jiao*
Wen Dan Tang (Warm the Gallbladder Decoction)		Clears Gallbladder heat, harmonizes the Stomach
Zhu Ru Wen Dan Tang (Bamboo Decoction to Warm the Gallbladder)	Dry dampness, dissolve phlegm	Clears heat, calms the *shen* (spirit)
Fu Ling Wan (Poria Pill)		Activates qi, softens nodules
Xiao Ban Xia Jia Fu Ling Tang (Minor Pinellia and Poria Decoction)		Regulates water circulation, disperses qi stagnation

Er Chen Tang (Two-Cured Decoction) is the most basic formula to dry dampness and dissolve phlegm. Internal dampness and phlegm stagnation due to Spleen deficiency produce coughing with profuse sputum, chest congestion, nausea, and vomiting.

Wen Dan Tang (Warm the Gallbladder Decoction) treats Gallbladder and Stomach disharmony with phlegm heat. The main clinical manifestations include irritability, palpitations, insomnia, nausea and vomiting, dizziness and vertigo, and seizures and epilepsy.

Zhu Ru Wen Dan Tang (Bamboo Decoction to Warm the Gallbladder) clears heat, dissolves phlegm, regulates qi, and calms the *shen* (spirit). It is used for accumulation of heat and phlegm in the Heart and Gallbladder, with signs and symptoms such as tendency to get easily frightened, palpitations, insomnia, mild and persistent fever, and copious phlegm in the chest.

Fu Ling Wan (Poria Pill) dispels phlegm, regulates qi, and softens nodules. Due to phlegm stagnation in the middle *jiao* that travels via the channels and collaterals, manifestations of painful arms and edema of the extremities can be seen.

Xiao Ban Xia Jia Fu Ling Tang (Minor Pinellia and Poria Decoction) dispels phlegm, regulates water circulation, and disperses qi stagnation. It mostly treats nausea and vomiting caused by phlegm stagnation and water accumulation in the epigastrium. Clinical manifestations include nausea, vomiting, stifling sensations in the epigastrium, dizziness, and dysuria.

Chinese Herbal Formulas and Applications

Chapter 18 — Summary

SECTION 2: HEAT-CLEARING AND PHLEGM-DISSOLVING FORMULAS

Name	Similarities	Differences
Qing Qi Hua Tan Wan (Clear the Qi and Transform Phlegm Pill)	Clear heat, dissolve phlegm in the Lung	Regulates qi circulation, relieves cough
Qing Fei Yin (Clear the Lung Drink)		Resolves dampness and phlegm
Qing Fei Tang (Clear the Lung Decoction)	Clear heat, dissolve phlegm in the Lung, treat deficiencies	Nourishes yin and body fluids
Zi Wan Tang (Aster Decoction)		Nourishes yin and body fluids, stops bleeding
Jie Geng Tang (Platycodon Decoction)		Tonifies Lung qi
Ren Shen Xie Fei Tang (Ginseng Decoction to Sedate the Lung)		Tonifies qi, regulates qi circulation
Gua Lou Zhi Shi Tang (Trichosanthes Fruit and Immature Bitter Orange Decoction)	Clear heat, dissolve phlegm, relieve the feeling of fullness and the stifling sensation	Breaks up stagnation
Xiao Xian Xiong Tang (Minor Sinking into the Chest Decoction)		Opens the chest
Gun Tan Wan (Vaporize Phlegm Pill)	Purges fire, eliminates phlegm	Eliminates old (chronic and stubborn) phlegm with excess heat

Qing Qi Hua Tan Wan (Clear the Qi and Transform Phlegm Pill) and *Qing Fei Yin* (Clear the Lung Drink) both clear heat and dissolve phlegm in the Lung.
- *Qing Qi Hua Tan Wan* clears heat, eliminates phlegm, regulates qi and arrests cough. It treats phlegm-heat congestion in the chest, accompanied by coughing with copious, yellow sputum that cannot be easily expectorated.
- *Qing Fei Yin* dissolves dampness and phlegm, and clears the Lung. It treats cough caused by accumulation of phlegm and dampness, with symptoms such as coughing with sputum, chest discomfort, and fatigue.

Qing Fei Tang (Clear the Lung Decoction), *Zi Wan Tang* (Aster Decoction), *Jie Geng Tang* (Platycodon Decoction), and *Ren Shen Xie Fei Tang* (Ginseng Decoction to Sedate the Lung) have similar functions to clear heat, dissolve phlegm, and support underlying deficiencies. They are used frequently to address Lung phlegm-heat, accompanied by qi, yin and/or body fluid deficiencies.
- *Qing Fei Tang* dispels phlegm-heat from the chest, moistens the Lung, and relieves cough. It treats chronic cough due to phlegm-heat in the Lung with yin and body fluid deficiencies. Clinical manifestations include severe cough, thick and sticky phlegm, sore and itchy throat, and voice hoarseness.
- *Zi Wan Tang* clears heat, dissolves phlegm, and nourishes yin and body fluids. It treats chronic cough due to Lung heat and yin deficiency, with symptoms such as chronic cough, excess phlegm, fever due to over-exertion, and the presence of lung abscesses and blood in the sputum.
- *Jie Geng Tang* eliminates pus and phlegm, dispels toxins, and clears deficiency fire. It is commonly used to treat Lung phlegm stagnation, with symptoms such as cough, and swelling and pain of the throat. Because the phlegm consumes yin and body fluids, deficiency fire arises and leads to symptoms such as thick, sticky sputum with mucous and blood or with foul odor, and a dry mouth without thirst.
- *Ren Shen Xie Fei Tang* clears heat, sedates the Lung, eliminates phlegm, and regulates qi circulation. It treats Lung heat with wheezing, dyspnea, fullness and distention in the chest and epigastrium, cough with profuse sputum, and constipation. This formula contains *Ren Shen* (Radix et Rhizoma Ginseng) to tonify qi, strengthen the Lung and Spleen, and prevent the draining herbs from consuming body fluids.

PHLEGM-DISPELLING FORMULAS

18

1255

Chapter 18 – Phlegm-Dispelling Formulas

Chapter 18 — Summary

Gua Lou Zhi Shi Tang (Trichosanthes Fruit and Immature Bitter Orange Decoction) and **Xiao Xian Xiong Tang** (Minor Sinking into the Chest Decoction) both have strong effects to clear heat and dissolve phlegm. These formulas commonly treat excess cases of phlegm-heat in the Lung with a feeling of fullness and a stifling sensation in the chest.

- *Gua Lou Zhi Shi Tang* treats severe phlegm-heat stagnation in the chest with chest congestion, difficult breathing and expectoration, and occasional severe chest and epigastric pain.
- *Xiao Xian Xiong Tang* is used for phlegm-heat stagnation with chest pain upon application of pressure. It clears heat, eliminates phlegm, expands the chest, and disperses stagnation. In addition to chest pain, other important clinical manifestations include coughing with yellow and thick, sticky sputum.

Gun Tan Wan (Vaporize Phlegm Pill) purges fire and eliminates phlegm. This formula is used for more severe cases in which the stubborn, chronic phlegm-fire surrounds the Heart and causes *shen* (spirit) disturbance conditions, such as manic-depressive psychosis and severe palpitations with unconsciousness.

SECTION 3: DRYNESS-MOISTENING AND PHLEGM-DISSOLVING FORMULA

Name	Similarities	Differences
Bei Mu Gua Lou San (Fritillaria and Trichosanthes Fruit Powder)	Moistens the Lung, dissolves phlegm	Clears Lung heat, regulates Lung qi

Bei Mu Gua Lou San (Fritillaria and Trichosanthes Fruit Powder) moistens the Lung, dissolves phlegm, clears heat, and regulates qi circulation. It is indicated for dry, sore throat, hoarse voice, and coughing with thick, sticky sputum that cannot be expectorated easily.

SECTION 4: WARM FORMULAS THAT DISSOLVE COLD PHLEGM

Name	Similarities	Differences
Ling Gan Wu Wei Jiang Xin Tang (Poria, Licorice, Schisandra, Ginger, and Asarum Decoction)	Dissolve cold phlegm	Warms and tonifies the Lung and Spleen
San Zi Yang Qin Tang (Three-Seed Decoction to Nourish One's Parents)		Guides Lung qi downward, resolves food stagnation

Ling Gan Wu Wei Jiang Xin Tang (Poria, Licorice, Schisandra, Ginger, and Asarum Decoction) warms the Lung and dispels cold-phlegm accumulation. Key clinical manifestations include coughing with profuse, white, watery sputum, a white, greasy tongue coating, and a wiry, slippery pulse.

San Zi Yang Qin Tang (Three-Seed Decoction to Nourish One's Parents) dispels phlegm retention, unblocks qi stagnation, and resolves food stagnation. Clinical manifestations include coughing with profuse sputum, chest distention, lack of appetite with indigestion, a white, greasy tongue coating, and a slippery pulse.

Chinese Herbal Formulas and Applications

Chapter 18 — Summary

SECTION 5: WIND-EXPELLING AND PHLEGM-DISSOLVING FORMULAS

Name	Similarities	Differences
Ban Xia Bai Zhu Tian Ma Tang (Pinellia, Atractylodes Macrocephala, and Gastrodia Decoction)	Calm Liver wind, dissolve phlegm	Treats headache, dizziness, and vertigo
Ding Xian Wan (Arrest Seizures Pill)		Treats seizures and epilepsy

Ban Xia Bai Zhu Tian Ma Tang (Pinellia, Atractylodes Macrocephala, and Gastrodia Decoction) dries dampness, dissolves phlegm, smoothes the Liver, and subdues Liver wind. In addition to the usual phlegm manifestations, headache, dizziness, and vertigo caused by Liver wind rising can also be seen.

Ding Xian Wan (Arrest Seizures Pill) eliminates phlegm and subdues Liver wind. It primarily treats rising of Liver wind and phlegm-heat. Clinical manifestations include sudden onset of seizures and epilepsy, semi-unconsciousness or complete loss of consciousness, tonic-clonic seizures, upward-rolling of the eyes, deviation of the mouth, involuntary salivation or dripping saliva, and *dian kuang* (mania and withdrawal).

PHLEGM-DISPELLING FORMULAS

18

Chapter 19

— Reducing, Guiding, and Dissolving Formulas

消
导
化
积
剂

李杲 Lǐ Gǎo

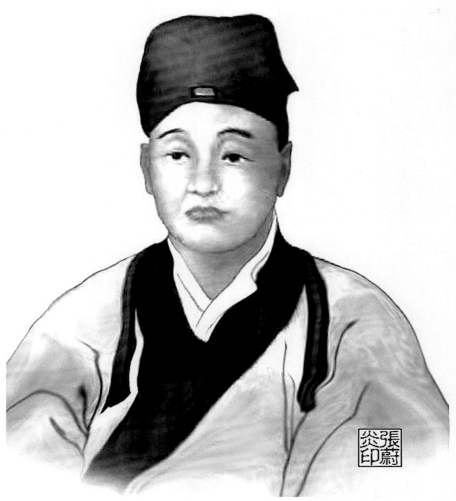

李杲 Lǐ Gǎo, also known as
李东垣 Lǐ Dóng-Héng, 1180 – 1251.

李杲 Lǐ Gǎo

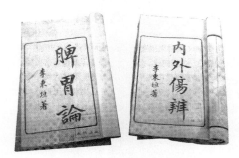

脾胃论 *Pi Wei Lun* (Discussion of the Spleen and Stomach) and
内外伤辨惑论 *Nei Wai Shang Bian Huo Lun* (Clarifying Doubts about Injury from Internal and External Causes).

Li Gao, also known as Li Dong-Heng, was born into a very wealthy family. Yet, unlike many of the very rich, he never hesitated to share his wealth to help those who were less fortunate during times of famine from drought or flood. However, no amount of money helped his mother when she was seriously ill. She was seen by numerous physicians, all of whom made conflicting diagnoses, and prescribed differing treatments. Li blamed himself for not knowing medicine, and watched helplessly as his mother's health continued to deteriorate and she eventually died. Li vowed to study and practice medicine, so no others would ever have to die from inadequate care.

Li Gao is best known for treating disorders of the Spleen and Stomach. He believed that the Spleen and Stomach are the source of *yuan* (source) *qi*, and adequate *yuan* (source) *qi* is the key to health. Conversely, when the Spleen and Stomach are deficient, *yuan* (source) *qi* is weakened and diseases begin to surface. He proposed that three main factors damage the Spleen and Stomach: 1) inappropriate diet, 2) excessive physical labor, and 3) unbalanced emotions. From this base of understanding, Li demonstrated that damage to the Spleen and Stomach contributed to the rise of hundreds of different disorders. Li specialized in using tonic herbs to selectively supplement the Spleen and Stomach, and developed the famous formula *Bu Zhong Yi Qi Tang* (Tonify the Middle and Augment the Qi Decoction).

Li Gao wrote many books throughout his life. The three most well-known are 脾胃论 *Pi Wei Lun* (Discussion of the Spleen and Stomach), 兰室秘藏 *Lan Shi Mi Cang* (Secrets from the Orchid Chamber) and 内外伤辨惑论 *Nei Wai Shang Bian Huo Lun* (Clarifying Doubts about Injury from Internal and External Causes). Many formulas from these references are still used today, such as:

- *Run Chang Wan* (Moisten the Intestines Pill)
- *Qing Wei San* (Clear the Stomach Powder)
- *Sheng Mai San* (Generate the Pulse Powder)
- *Bu Zhong Yi Qi Tang* (Tonify the Middle and Augment the Qi Decoction)
- *Dang Gui Bu Xue Tang* (Tangkuei Decoction to Tonify the Blood)
- *Hou Po Wen Zhong Tang* (Magnolia Bark Decoction for Warming the Middle)
- *Tian Tai Wu Yao San* (Top-Quality Lindera Powder)
- *Qiang Huo Sheng Shi Tang* (Notopterygium Decoction to Overcome Dampness)
- *Dang Gui Nian Tong Tang* (Tangkuei Decoction to Lift the Pain)
- *Zhi Shi Dao Zhi Wan* (Immature Bitter Orange Pill to Guide Out Stagnation)
- *Zhi Shi Xiao Pi Wan* (Immature Bitter Orange Pill to Reduce Focal Distention)
- *Zhi Zhu Wan* (Immature Bitter Orange and Atractylodes Macrocephala Pill)

Dynasties & Kingdoms	Year
Xia Dynasty 夏	2100-1600 BCE
Shang Dynasty 商	1600-1100 BCE
Zhou Dynasty 周	1100-221 BCE
Qin Dynasty 秦	221-207 BCE
Han Dynasty 汉	206 BCE-220
Three Kingdoms 三国	220-280
Western Jin Dynasty 西晋	265-316
Eastern Jin Dynasty 东晋	317-420
Northern and Southern Dynasties 北南朝	420-581
Sui Dynasty 隋	581-618
Tang Dynasty 唐	618-907
Five Dynasties 五代	907-960
Song Dynasty 宋	960-1279
Liao Dynasty 辽	916-1125
Jin Dynasty 金	**1115-1234**
Yuan Dynasty 元	1271-1368
Ming Dynasty 明	1368-1644
Qing Dynasty 清	1644-1911
Republic of China 中華民國	1912-Present Day
People's Republic of China 中華人民共和國	1949-Present Day

Chapter 19 – Reducing, Guiding, and Dissolving Formulas

Table of Contents

Chapter 19. Reducing, Guiding, and Dissolving Formulas ⋯⋯⋯⋯⋯⋯⋯⋯⋯⋯ **1259**

Biography of Li Gao ⋯⋯⋯⋯⋯⋯⋯⋯⋯⋯⋯⋯⋯⋯⋯⋯⋯⋯⋯⋯⋯⋯⋯⋯⋯⋯⋯⋯⋯⋯⋯⋯ 1260

Section 1. Reducing, Guiding, and Dissolving Formulas that Treat Food Stagnation ⋯⋯⋯ **1266**

Bao He Wan (Preserve Harmony Pill) ⋯⋯⋯⋯⋯⋯⋯⋯⋯⋯⋯⋯⋯⋯⋯⋯⋯⋯⋯⋯⋯⋯⋯⋯ 1266

 Da An Wan (Great Tranquility Pill) ⋯⋯⋯⋯⋯⋯⋯⋯⋯⋯⋯⋯⋯⋯⋯⋯⋯⋯⋯⋯⋯⋯⋯ 1268

 Shan Zha Tang (Crataegus Decoction) ⋯⋯⋯⋯⋯⋯⋯⋯⋯⋯⋯⋯⋯⋯⋯⋯⋯⋯⋯⋯⋯ 1268

 Shan Zha Hua Tan Tang (Crataegus Decoction to Transform Phlegm) ⋯⋯⋯⋯⋯⋯⋯ 1269

Zhi Shi Dao Zhi Wan (Immature Bitter Orange Pill to Guide Out Stagnation) ⋯⋯⋯⋯⋯ 1270

Mu Xiang Bing Lang Wan (Aucklandia and Betel Nut Pill) ⋯⋯⋯⋯⋯⋯⋯⋯⋯⋯⋯⋯⋯⋯ 1272

Zhi Zhu Wan (Immature Bitter Orange and Atractylodes Macrocephala Pill) ⋯⋯⋯⋯⋯⋯ 1274

 Zhi Zhu Tang (Immature Bitter Orange and Atractylodes Macrocephala Decoction) ⋯⋯⋯ 1275

 Qu Mai Zhi Zhu Wan (Medicated Leaven, Barley Sprout, Immature Bitter Orange, and Atractylodes Macrocephala Pill) ⋯⋯⋯ 1275

 Ju Ban Zhi Zhu Wan (Tangerine Peel, Pinellia, Immature Bitter Orange, and Atractylodes Macrocephala Pill) ⋯⋯⋯ 1276

 Xiang Sha Zhi Zhu Wan (Aucklandia, Amomum, Immature Bitter Orange, and Atractylodes Macrocephala Pill) ⋯⋯⋯⋯⋯ 1276

Jian Pi Wan (Strengthen the Spleen Pill) ⋯⋯⋯⋯⋯⋯⋯⋯⋯⋯⋯⋯⋯⋯⋯⋯⋯⋯⋯⋯⋯⋯ 1277

 Zi Sheng Wan (Nourish Life Pill) ⋯⋯⋯⋯⋯⋯⋯⋯⋯⋯⋯⋯⋯⋯⋯⋯⋯⋯⋯⋯⋯⋯⋯⋯ 1278

Section 2. Reducing, Guiding, and Dissolving Formula that Relieves Distention ⋯⋯⋯⋯⋯ **1280**

Zhi Shi Xiao Pi Wan (Immature Bitter Orange Pill to Reduce Focal Distention) ⋯⋯⋯⋯ 1280

Reducing, Guiding, and Dissolving Formulas (Summary) ⋯⋯⋯⋯⋯⋯⋯⋯⋯⋯⋯⋯⋯ **1283**

Chinese Herbal Formulas and Applications

Chapter 19 — Overview

— Reducing, Guiding, and Dissolving Formulas

Definition: Reducing, guiding, and dissolving formulas consist of herbs that reduce (digest) foods, guide out stagnation, and dissolve accumulations. These formulas generally treat food stagnation, abdominal rigidity, and various types of stagnation, accumulation, and masses. This method of treatment is known as *xiao fa* (reducing), one of the *ba fa* (eight treatment methods) described in the *Huang Di Nei Jing* (Yellow Emperor's Inner Classic) in the first or second century, A.D.

Reducing, guiding, and dissolving formulas treat two main types of disorders: food stagnation due to indigestion and distention due to accumulation.

- Food stagnation usually occurs as a result of inappropriate diet with overindulgence in foods that damage the Spleen and Stomach, or constitutional Spleen and Stomach deficiencies with inability to digest foods. Under either circumstance, two types of herbs are generally prescribed at the same time: herbs that promote digestion of foods and herbs that strengthen the Spleen and Stomach.
- Distention may occur due to prolonged accumulation and stagnation of qi, blood, cold, heat, food, or phlegm. Because the feeling of distention may be caused by many different types of accumulation and stagnation, it is often necessary to add herbs to activate the qi and blood circulation, dispel dampness and phlegm, soften masses, and relieve distention and fullness.

Note: Reducing, guiding, and dissolving formulas and downward draining formulas are both used to dispel abnormal accumulation in the interior. However, reducing, guiding, and dissolving formulas are mild in nature, and are suitable for treating chronic syndromes with mild symptoms. In addition, these formulas are most effective for hardness and nodules that cannot be quickly eliminated, but require long-term use of herbs to gradually soften and dissolve the mass. Downward draining formulas, on the other hand, are drastic in nature, and should be reserved only for acute syndromes with severe symptoms. These formulas are most useful in treating accumulations that can and must be purged immediately and quickly, such as acute constipation or intestinal obstruction.

SUBCATEGORIES OF ACTION

Reducing, guiding, and dissolving formulas are divided into two subcategories to accurately differentiate the nature of the disorders and the characteristics of the corresponding formulas.

1. Reducing, Guiding, and Dissolving Formula that Treats Food Stagnation

These formulas commonly treat food stagnation with clinical manifestations of chest and epigastric fullness and distention, belching, acid regurgitation with a foul smell, abdominal pain, nausea, vomiting, and diarrhea. Herbs commonly used to treat food stagnation include *Shan Zha* (Fructus Crataegi), *Shen Qu* (Massa Fermentata), and *Lai Fu Zi* (Semen Raphani). Exemplar formulas include *Bao He Wan* (Preserve Harmony Pill) and *Zhi Shi Dao Zhi Wan* (Immature Bitter Orange Pill to Guide Out Stagnation).

Spleen and Stomach deficiencies and food stagnation often occur together, because either pre-existing deficiencies of the Spleen and Stomach contribute to food stagnation, or prolonged food stagnation damages the Spleen and Stomach. In these cases, it is necessary to use

---

> Distention may occur due to prolonged accumulation and stagnation of qi, blood, cold, heat, food, or phlegm.

> Food stagnation, abdominal rigidity, accumulation and masses cannot be quickly purged outward or drained downwards. They must be slowly reduced and dissolved in size, and gently guided out.

REDUCING, GUIDING, AND DISSOLVING FORMULAS

19

1263

Chapter 19 – Reducing, Guiding, and Dissolving Formulas

Chapter 19 — Overview

qi-tonifying herbs to strengthen the Spleen and Stomach and reducing herbs to treat food stagnation at the same time. The emphasis on tonifying or reducing may be adjusted according to the constitution of the patient and the severity of the food stagnation. Commonly used herbs that strengthen the Spleen and Stomach include *Ren Shen* (Radix et Rhizoma Ginseng), *Bai Zhu* (Rhizoma Atractylodis Macrocephalae) and *Fu Ling* (Poria). Exemplar formulas include *Jian Pi Wan* (Strengthen the Spleen Pill) and *Zhi Zhu Wan* (Immature Bitter Orange and Atractylodes Macrocephala Pill).

> Use of decoction is not appropriate. Stagnation and accumulation in these cases can only be slowly moved, not quickly purged by immediate and potent decoctions.

2. Reducing, Guiding, and Dissolving Formula that Relieves Distention

This type of formula is used mainly for distention, accompanied by signs and symptoms of general accumulation and stagnation, such as epigastric and abdominal fullness, immobile masses in the abdomen and hypochondrium, poor appetite, decreased intake of food, and wasting of muscles. Optimal treatment for this condition includes use of herbs that activate qi circulation, invigorate blood circulation, resolve dampness, dissolve phlegm and soften hardness. A representative formula is *Zhi Shi Xiao Pi Wan* (Immature Bitter Orange Pill to Reduce Focal Distention).

CAUTIONS / CONTRAINDICATIONS

- Reducing, guiding, and dissolving formulas are generally given in pill form to gradually treat food stagnation and relieve distention. The use of decoction in these cases is not appropriate because the stagnation and accumulation can only be slowly reduced, guided out, or dissolved, not quickly purged out by the immediate, potent actions of a decoction.
- Reducing, guiding, and dissolving formulas are relatively mild, but they nonetheless consume qi and may cause weakness and deficiency with long-term use. Therefore, these formulas should be used with caution in individuals who have underlying weakness and deficiency.

PHARMACOLOGICAL EFFECTS & CLINICAL APPLICATIONS

> Reducing, guiding, and dissolving formulas are commonly used to treat gastrolithiasis, cholelithiasis and various gastrointestinal disorders.

While reducing, guiding, and dissolving formulas commonly treat gastrointestinal disorders, they also effectively treat gastrolithiasis and cholelithiasis.

- **Gastrointestinal disorders**: Pharmacological effects demonstrated by these herbs and formulas include increased production of gastric acid,[1] increased production of bile acid,[2] and increased intestinal peristalsis.[3] Clinically, these formulas have been used successfully to treat digestive disorders such as indigestion,[4,5] anorexia,[6] intestinal obstruction,[7] stenosis of the colon and rectum,[8] chronic gastritis,[9] atrophic gastritis,[10] constipation,[11] and acute abdomen.[12] Exemplar formulas that treat gastrointestinal disorders include *Bao He Wan* (Preserve Harmony Pill), *Zhi Shi Dao Zhi Wan* (Immature Bitter Orange Pill to Guide Out Stagnation), and *Zhi Zhu Wan* (Immature Bitter Orange and Atractylodes Macrocephala Pill).
- **Gastrolithiasis and cholelithiasis**: Reducing, guiding, and dissolving formulas can also be used to treat stomach and gallbladder stones.[13,14] The exact mechanisms of action are unclear, but can probably be attributed to the ability of these herbs and formulas to stimulate the production and release of gastric and bile acids, increase gastric emptying time, and increase intestinal peristalsis.[15,16] Exemplar formulas that treat stomach and gallbladder stones include *Bao He Wan* (Preserve Harmony Pill) and *Zhi Shi Xiao Pi Wan* (Immature Bitter Orange Pill to Reduce Focal Distention).

1264

Chapter 19 — Overview

References

1. *Ying Yang Xue Bao* (Report of Nutrition) 1984;6(2):109.
2. *Zhong Yao Yao Li Yu Lin Chuang* (Pharmacology and Clinical Applications of Chinese Herbs) 1991;7(4):1.
3. *Zhong Hua Yi Xue Za Zhi* (Chinese Journal of Medicine) 1956;42:946.
4. *Fu Jian Zhong Yi Yao* (Fujian Chinese Medicine and Herbology) 1985;3(8):18.
5. *Zhong Yi Za Zhi* (Journal of Chinese Medicine) 1959;9:630.
6. *Liao Ning Zhong Yi Za Zhi* (Liaoning Journal of Chinese Medicine) 1996;12:550.
7. *Zhong Yi Ming Fang Lin Chuang Xin Yong* (Contemporary Clinical Applications of Classic Chinese Formulas) 2001;502.
8. *Guang Xi Zhong Yi Yao* (Guangxi Chinese Medicine and Herbology) 1999;2:33.
9. *Zhong Yi Yao Xue Bao* (Report of Chinese Medicine and Herbology) 1991;3:39.
10. *Shan Xi Zhong Yi* (Shanxi Chinese Medicine) 1997;7:304.
11. *Zhe Jiang Zhong Yi Xue Yuan Xue Bao* (Journal of Zhejiang University of Chinese Medicine) 1996;2:28.
12. *Jiang Su Zhong Yi* (Jiangsu Chinese Medicine) 1982;6:3.
13. *Shan Dong Zhong Yi Za Zhi* (Shandong Journal of Chinese Medicine) 1993;4:21.
14. *Hu Bei Zhong Yi Za Zhi* (Hubei Journal of Chinese Medicine) 1998;5:38.
15. *Zhong Yao Yao Li Yu Lin Chuang* (Pharmacology and Clinical Applications of Chinese Herbs) 1991;7(1):8.
16. *Hu Bei Zhong Yi Za Zhi* (Hubei Journal of Chinese Medicine) 1998;5:38.

Chapter 19 – Reducing, Guiding, and Dissolving Formulas   *Section 1 – Reducing, Guiding, and Dissolving Formulas that Treat Food Stagnation*

Section 1

消食化积剂

— Reducing, Guiding, and Dissolving Formulas that Treat Food Stagnation

Băo Hé Wán (Preserve Harmony Pill)

保和丸

Pinyin Name: *Bao He Wan*
Literal Name: Preserve Harmony Pill
Alternate Names: Harmony-Preserving Pill, Citrus and Crataegus Formula
Original Source: *Dan Xi Xin Fa* (Teachings of [Zhu] Dan-Xi) by Zhu Zhen-Heng in 1481

COMPOSITION

Shan Zha (Fructus Crataegi)	180g [18g]
Shen Qu (Massa Fermentata)	60g [6g]
Lai Fu Zi (Semen Raphani)	30g [6g]
Ban Xia (Rhizoma Pinelliae)	90g [9g]
Chen Pi (Pericarpium Citri Reticulatae)	30g [6g]
Fu Ling (Poria)	90g [9g]
Lian Qiao (Fructus Forsythiae)	30g [6g]

DOSAGE / PREPARATION / ADMINISTRATION

The source text states to grind the ingredients into powder, and form into small pills. The pills should resemble the size of *Wu Tong Zi* (Semen Firmianae), a small seed approximately 5 mm in diameter. Take 70-80 pills between meals with warm, boiled water. Today, this formula may be taken in pills or decoction. For pills, grind the herbs into powder and form into pills with water. Take 6-9g of pills per dose with warm, boiled water. For decoction, use the suggested doses in brackets.

CHINESE THERAPEUTIC ACTIONS

Reduces food stagnation and harmonizes the Stomach

CLINICAL MANIFESTATIONS

Food stagnation and indigestion: epigastric and abdominal fullness, distention and pain; acid regurgitation, belching with a rotten smell, nausea, vomiting, possible diarrhea, aversion to food, thick, greasy tongue coating, and a slippery pulse.

CLINICAL APPLICATIONS

General gastrointestinal disorders, such as atrophic gastritis, gastrolithiasis, indigestion, acid regurgitation, nausea, vomiting, belching, diarrhea, abdominal pain, and poor appetite.

EXPLANATION

Bao He Wan (Preserve Harmony Pill) is one of the most commonly used formulas to treat all types of food stagnation. This condition is usually caused by inappropriate diet, overeating, or excessive drinking. Excessive intake of food that remains undigested will stagnate in the stomach and impair the digestive function. Food stagnation causes qi stagnation, which may result in fullness, distention, and pain in the epigastrium and abdomen. When Stomach qi stagnates and cannot descend, acid regurgitation, nausea, and vomiting occur. When Spleen qi stagnates and cannot ascend, diarrhea results.

Shan Zha (Fructus Crataegi) functions as the chief herb to digest any kind of food stagnation; it is especially effective in dissolving meat (protein) and fatty, greasy foods. *Shen Qu* (Massa Fermentata) dissolves food stagnation and strengthens the Spleen; it is effective for the digestion of alcohol and spoiled or rotten food that arise from chronic food stagnation. *Lai Fu Zi* (Semen Raphani) guides qi downward; it is best for digesting starch and

1266

Chinese Herbal Formulas and Applications

Bǎo Hé Wán (Preserve Harmony Pill)

Bao He Wan (Preserve Harmony Pill)

Diagnosis	Signs and Symptoms	Treatment	Herbs
Food stagnation	• Indigestion with epigastric and abdominal fullness, distention, and pain: food stagnation • Acid regurgitation, belching, aversion to food, nausea, vomiting: reversed flow of Stomach qi • Thick, greasy tongue coating and slippery pulse: food stagnation	• Reduces food stagnation • Harmonizes the Stomach	• *Shan Zha* (Fructus Crataegi) promotes digestion of foods (meat and fatty, greasy foods). • *Shen Qu* (Massa Fermentata) strengthens the Spleen and dissolves foods (alcohol and spoiled or rotten foods). • *Lai Fu Zi* (Semen Raphani) guides qi downward and dissolves foods (starch and carbohydrates). • *Ban Xia* (Rhizoma Pinelliae) and *Chen Pi* (Pericarpium Citri Reticulatae) activate qi circulation and harmonize the Stomach. • *Fu Ling* (Poria) strengthens the Spleen and dispels dampness. • *Lian Qiao* (Fructus Forsythiae) clears heat associated with food stagnation.

carbohydrates. Combined together, these three herbs can treat any type of food stagnation. *Ban Xia* (Rhizoma Pinelliae) and *Chen Pi* (Pericarpium Citri Reticulatae) activate qi circulation and harmonize the Stomach to relieve nausea and vomiting. *Fu Ling* (Poria) dispels dampness, strengthens the Spleen, and stops diarrhea. Food stagnation is often accompanied by heat, which is cleared by *Lian Qiao* (Fructus Forsythiae).

MODIFICATIONS

- For severe food stagnation and constipation, add *Bing Lang* (Semen Arecae), *Zhi Shi* (Fructus Aurantii Immaturus), *Da Fu Pi* (Pericarpium Arecae) and *Da Huang* (Radix et Rhizoma Rhei).
- For food stagnation turning into heat, evident by a red tongue body and a yellow tongue coating, and a rapid pulse, add *Huang Lian* (Rhizoma Coptidis) and *Huang Qin* (Radix Scutellariae).
- For indigestion accompanied by an exterior condition (e.g., a superficial, rapid pulse and a white, greasy tongue coating), add *Huo Xiang* (Herba Agastaches), *Zi Su Ye* (Folium Perillae), and *Jin Yin Hua* (Flos Lonicerae Japonicae).
- With severe nausea and vomiting, add *Sha Ren* (Fructus Amomi) and *Huo Xiang* (Herba Agastaches).
- With vomiting and diarrhea, add *Huo Xiang* (Herba Agastaches) and *Pei Lan* (Herba Eupatorii).
- To enhance the overall digestive function, add *Mai Ya* (Fructus Hordei Germinatus), *Gu Ya* (Fructus Setariae Germinatus), and *Ji Nei Jin* (Endothelium Corneum Gigeriae Galli).

CAUTIONS / CONTRAINDICATIONS

- *Bao He Wan* is not suitable for food stagnation due to Spleen deficiency.
- Avoid oily, greasy, or fatty foods while taking this formula.
- This formula should be used with caution during pregnancy.[1]

CLINICAL STUDIES AND RESEARCH

1. **Indigestion**: According to one study, *Bao He Wan* effectively treated indigestion in 69 children. Those with indigestion characterized by food stagnation were treated with only *Bao He Wan*. Additions to this base formula included *Bai Zhu* (Rhizoma Atractylodis Macrocephalae) for chronic diarrhea with deficiency; and *Ji Nei Jin* (Endothelium Corneum Gigeriae Galli) and *He Ye* (Folium Nelumbinis) for poor appetite associated with diarrhea and/or nausea. Of 69 patients, the study reported complete recovery in 61 cases, improvement in 5 cases, and no effect in 3 cases. The overall effectiveness was 95.65%.[2]

2. **Atrophic gastritis**: One study reported a marked effect using modified *Bao He Wan* to treat 34 patients with chronic atrophic gastritis. In addition to this formula, modifications were made by adding *Huang Qi* (Radix Astragali) and *Tai Zi Shen* (Radix Pseudostellariae) for qi deficiency; *Gui Zhi* (Ramulus Cinnamomi) and *Gao Liang Jiang* (Rhizoma Alpiniae Officinarum) for presence of cold; *Dan Shen* (Radix et Rhizoma Salviae Miltiorrhizae) and *Tan Xiang* (Lignum Santali Albi) for blood stagnation; and *Zhe Shi* (Haematitum) for belching. The herbs were cooked in water, and the decoction given in two equally-divided doses, for 3 months per course of treatment. The study reported significant improvement in 25 of 34 cases.[3]

REDUCING, GUIDING, AND DISSOLVING FORMULAS

19

1267

Chapter 19 – Reducing, Guiding, and Dissolving Formulas   Section 1 – Reducing, Guiding, and Dissolving Formulas that Treat Food Stagnation

Bǎo Hé Wán (Preserve Harmony Pill)

3. **Gastrolithiasis**: One study reported that the combination of *Bao He Wan* and *Xiao Cheng Qi Tang* (Minor Order the Qi Decoction) was effective in treating stomach stones in 29 of 33 patients (18 males and 15 females). The herbal formula contained charred *Shan Zha* (Fructus Crataegi), charred *Shen Qu* (Massa Fermentata), charred *Mai Ya* (Fructus Hordei Germinatus), *Ji Nei Jin* (Endothelium Corneum Gigeriae Galli), *Ban Xia* (Rhizoma Pinelliae), *Chen Pi* (Pericarpium Citri Reticulatae), *Hou Po* (Cortex Magnoliae Officinalis), *Zhi Shi* (Fructus Aurantii Immaturus), and *Da Huang* (Radix et Rhizoma Rhei). In addition, *San Leng* (Rhizoma Sparganii), *E Zhu* (Rhizoma Curcumae), and *Bing Lang* (Semen Arecae) were added for individuals who were otherwise healthy, as they are too strong for individuals with deficiencies. The duration of treatment ranged from 20-30 days. The largest stone identified was 12 x 20 cm.[4]

HERB-DRUG INTERACTION

Chemotherapy-induced gastrointestinal side-effects: Use of modified *Bao He Wan* relieved gastrointestinal side effects associated with chemotherapy in cancer patients in one study. In addition to *Bao He Wan*, modifications were made by adding *Huang Qi* (Radix Astragali) and *Bai Zhu* (Rhizoma Atractylodis Macrocephalae) for fatigue and poor appetite; *Da Huang* (Radix et Rhizoma Rhei) [processed with grain-based liquor] for yellow tongue coating with constipation; *Sha Shen* (Radix Glehniae seu Adenophorae), *Mai Dong* (Radix Ophiopogonis), and *Shi Hu* (Caulis Dendrobii) for thirst and red tongue body with dry tongue coating. The treatment protocol was to administer the herbs in decoction for 10 days. Of 110 patients, 105 had complete recovery and 5 had improvement.[5]

TOXICOLOGY

According to one study on acute toxicology, administration of *Bao He Wan* at 120 g/kg via oral ingestion twice daily for 7 days did not contribute to any abnormal reactions in mice. Similarly, administration of this formula in adults at 650 times the normal dose did not contribute to any abnormal reactions. Furthermore, in one study on chronic toxicology, daily administration of this formula at 8, 16 and 32 g/kg one time daily for 4 weeks caused no abnormalities in blood tests or internal organs such as liver, kidneys, heart, stomach, and intestines.[6]

RELATED FORMULAS

Dà Ān Wán (Great Tranquility Pill)
大安丸
Pinyin Name: *Da An Wan*
Literal Name: Great Tranquility Pill

Original Source: *Yi Fang Ji Jie* (Analytical Collection of Medical Formulas) by Wang Ang in 1682

Shan Zha (Fructus Crataegi)	180g [18g]
Shen Qu (Massa Fermentata)	60g [6g]
Ban Xia (Rhizoma Pinelliae)	90g [9g]
Fu Ling (Poria)	90g [9g]
Chen Pi (Pericarpium Citri Reticulatae)	30g [6g]
Lian Qiao (Fructus Forsythiae)	30g [6g]
Lai Fu Zi (Semen Raphani)	30g [6g]
Bai Zhu (Rhizoma Atractylodis Macrocephalae)	60g [6g]

The instructions for preparation and administration of this formula are the same as *Bao He Wan*. *Da An Wan* (Great Tranquility Pill) is composed of *Bao He Wan* plus *Bai Zhu* (Rhizoma Atractylodis Macrocephalae). The addition of *Bai Zhu* (Rhizoma Atractylodis Macrocephalae) enhances the overall function of the formula to tonify and strengthen the Spleen. Clinically, it may be used for patients with food stagnation and indigestion accompanied by qi deficiency. This formula is also appropriate for children with the same clinical manifestations.

Shān Zhā Tāng (Crataegus Decoction)
山楂湯
山楂汤
Pinyin Name: *Shan Zha Tang*
Literal Name: Crataegus Decoction
Original Source: *Guang An Men Yi Yuan* (Guang An Men Hospital) in 1990

Shan Zha (Fructus Crataegi)
Ze Xie (Rhizoma Alismatis)
Yi Yi Ren (Semen Coicis)
Jue Ming Zi (Semen Cassiae)
Cha Ye (Folium Camelliae)
Hu Zhang (Rhizoma et Radix Polygoni Cuspidati)
Dan Shen (Radix et Rhizoma Salviae Miltiorrhizae)
Ge Gen (Radix Puerariae Lobatae)
He Ye (Folium Nelumbinis)
Ju Hua (Flos Chrysanthemi)
He Shou Wu (Radix Polygoni Multiflori)
Zao Jiao Ci (Spina Gleditsiae)
Cang Zhu (Rhizoma Atractylodis)

Shan Zha Tang (Crataegus Decoction) treats chronic damp and phlegm accumulation in the body. This formula strengthens the Spleen and Stomach, reduces dampness, and eliminates phlegm. Clinically, this formula is most useful in treating such disorders as elevated cholesterol levels, hyperlipidemia, and atherosclerosis.

1268

Băo Hé Wán (Preserve Harmony Pill)

Shān Zhā Huà Tán Tāng

(Crataegus Decoction to Transform Phlegm)

山楂化痰湯
山楂化痰汤

Pinyin Name: Shan Zha Hua Tan Tang
Literal Name: Crataegus Decoction to Transform Phlegm
Original Source: Guang An Men Yi Yuan (Guang An Men Hospital) in 1990

Yin Chen (Herba Artemisiae Scopariae)

Ge Gen (Radix Puerariae Lobatae)

Dan Shen (Radix et Rhizoma Salviae Miltiorrhizae)

Huang Qin (Radix Scutellariae)

Jue Ming Zi (Semen Cassiae)

Shan Zha (Fructus Crataegi)

Ze Xie (Rhizoma Alismatis)

Yu Jin (Radix Curcumae)

Hai Zao (Sargassum)

Da Huang (Radix et Rhizoma Rhei)

Shan Zha Hua Tan Tang (Crataegus Decoction to Transform Phlegm) has been used to treat accumulation of dampness, turbidity, and phlegm in the body. It dissolves dampness, eliminates phlegm, and invigorates blood circulation. Clinical manifestations include fatigue, lack of energy, a feeling of heaviness in the body and extremities, and obesity. Today, it is commonly used to treat individuals with a generalized condition of obesity with high cholesterols and triglycerides.

AUTHORS' COMMENTS

Bao He Wan is designed for mild and moderate cases of food stagnation and indigestion with zheng (upright) qi not yet damaged. Key signs and symptoms include epigastric and abdominal fullness, distention and pain, acid regurgitation, belching with a rotten smell, nausea, vomiting, aversion to food, and a slippery pulse.

Classic texts use the term "dissolve" to describe herbs that treat indigestion and food stagnation. However, these herbs do not literally "dissolve" foods; rather, they stimulate the gastrointestinal tract and facilitate food digestion, thereby reducing accumulation and stagnation.

References

1. Zhong Yao Ming Fang Yao Li Yu Ying Yong (Pharmacology and Applications of Famous Herbal Formulas) 1989;619-20.
2. Fu Jian Zhong Yi Yao (Fujian Chinese Medicine and Herbology) 1985;3(8):18.
3. Hu Bei Zhong Yi Za Zhi (Hubei Journal of Chinese Medicine) 1992;6:10.
4. Shan Dong Zhong Yi Za Zhi (Shandong Journal of Chinese Medicine) 1993;4:21.
5. Zhong Yi Yao Xin Xi (Information on Chinese Medicine and Herbology) 1995;12(6):45.
6. Zhong Yi Yao Xin Xi (Information on Chinese Medicine and Herbology) 1995;11:25.

REDUCING, GUIDING, AND DISSOLVING FORMULAS

19

Chapter 19 – Reducing, Guiding, and Dissolving Formulas   *Section 1 – Reducing, Guiding, and Dissolving Formulas that Treat Food Stagnation*

Zhǐ Shí Dǎo Zhì Wán

(Immature Bitter Orange Pill to Guide Out Stagnation)

枳實導滯丸
枳实导滞丸

Pinyin Name: *Zhi Shi Dao Zhi Wan*
Literal Name: Immature Bitter Orange Pill to Guide Out Stagnation
Original Source: *Nei Wai Shang Bian Huo Lun* (Clarifying Doubts about Injury from Internal and External Causes) by Li Gao in 1247

COMPOSITION

Da Huang (Radix et Rhizoma Rhei)	30g [9g]
Zhi Shi (Fructus Aurantii Immaturus), *chao* (dry-fried) with bran	15g [9g]
Huang Lian (Rhizoma Coptidis)	9g [6g]
Huang Qin (Radix Scutellariae)	9g [6g]
Fu Ling (Poria)	9g [6g]
Ze Xie (Rhizoma Alismatis)	6g [6g]
Bai Zhu (Rhizoma Atractylodis Macrocephalae)	9g [6g]
Shen Qu (Massa Fermentata), *chao* (dry-fried)	15g [9g]

DOSAGE / PREPARATION / ADMINISTRATION

The source text states to grind the ingredients into a fine powder, and form into small pills with water. The pills should resemble the size of *Wu Tong Zi* (Semen Firmianae), a small seed approximately 5 mm in diameter. Take 50-70 pills per dose between meals with warm water. Adjust the dose depending on the severity of the condition. Today, this formula may be taken in pills or decoction. For pills, grind the herbs into powder and form into small pills with water. Take 6-9g of pills per dose with warm, boiled water twice daily. For decoction, use the suggested doses in brackets.

CHINESE THERAPEUTIC ACTIONS

1. Reduces, guides out, and dissolves stagnation
2. Clears heat and dispels dampness

CLINICAL MANIFESTATIONS

Food stagnation and damp-heat accumulation in the Stomach and Intestines: fullness and pain in the epigastric and abdominal regions, diarrhea or constipation, scanty, dark urine, a yellow, greasy tongue coating, and a deep, forceful pulse.

CLINICAL APPLICATIONS

Acute or chronic gastroenteritis, diarrhea, dysentery, hepatitis, liver cirrhosis, urinary tract infection, chronic constipation, and trigeminal pain.

EXPLANATION

Zhi Shi Dao Zhi Wan (Immature Bitter Orange Pill to Guide Out Stagnation) treats food stagnation and damp-heat accumulation in the Stomach and Intestines. Stagnation of food and damp-heat may lead to qi stagnation, which may result in fullness and pain in the epigastric and abdominal regions. Diarrhea may occur as a result of indigestion and formation of damp-heat in the Intestines, while constipation may occur as a result of interior heat drying body fluids. Scanty, dark urine may result from consumption of body fluids by interior heat. Yellow, greasy tongue coating and a deep, forceful pulse indicate stagnation of food and damp-heat.

This formula has *Da Huang* (Radix et Rhizoma Rhei) to purge stagnant food and damp-heat, and to remove any harmful retention through defecation. *Zhi Shi* (Fructus Aurantii Immaturus) breaks down qi and food stagnation to reduce epigastric and abdominal fullness and pain. *Huang Lian* (Rhizoma Coptidis) and *Huang Qin* (Radix Scutellariae) clear heat, dry dampness, and relieve diarrhea. *Fu Ling* (Poria) and *Ze Xie* (Rhizoma Alismatis) regulate water circulation and dispel dampness. *Bai Zhu* (Rhizoma Atractylodis Macrocephalae) strengthens the Spleen and dries dampness. In addition, *Bai Zhu* (Rhizoma Atractylodis Macrocephalae) prevents the bitter and cold herbs from damaging the body. *Shen Qu* (Massa Fermentata) helps to digest stagnant food and harmonizes the middle *jiao*.

MODIFICATIONS

• For more severe fullness, distention, and rectal tenesmus due to qi stagnation, add *Mu Xiang* (Radix Aucklandiae) and *Bing Lang* (Semen Arecae).

1270

Zhǐ Shí Dǎo Zhì Wán
(Immature Bitter Orange Pill to Guide Out Stagnation)

Zhi Shi Dao Zhi Wan (Immature Bitter Orange Pill to Guide Out Stagnation)

Diagnosis	Signs and Symptoms	Treatment	Herbs
Food stagnation and damp-heat accumulation in the Stomach and Intestines	• Fullness and pain in the epigastric and abdominal regions: food and qi stagnation • Diarrhea: damp-heat in the Intestines • Constipation: interior heat drying body fluids • Scanty, dark urine: interior heat consuming body fluids • Yellow, greasy tongue coating with a deep, forceful pulse: damp-heat in the interior	• Reduces, guides out, and dissolves stagnation • Clears heat and dispels dampness	• *Da Huang* (Radix et Rhizoma Rhei) purges the stagnant food and clears excess heat. • *Zhi Shi* (Fructus Aurantii Immaturus) breaks up qi and food stagnation. • *Huang Lian* (Rhizoma Coptidis) and *Huang Qin* (Radix Scutellariae) clear heat and dry dampness. • *Fu Ling* (Poria) and *Ze Xie* (Rhizoma Alismatis) regulate water circulation and dispel dampness. • *Bai Zhu* (Rhizoma Atractylodis Macrocephalae) strengthens the Spleen and dries dampness. • *Shen Qu* (Massa Fermentata) helps to digest stagnant food and harmonizes the middle *jiao*.

• With diarrhea and dysentery due to toxic heat, add *Jin Yin Hua* (Flos Lonicerae Japonicae) and *Bai Tou Weng* (Radix Pulsatillae).

• With nausea and vomiting, add *Zhu Ru* (Caulis Bambusae in Taenia).

CAUTIONS / CONTRAINDICATIONS

• *Zhi Shi Dao Zhi Wan* is contraindicated in patients with loose stools or diarrhea who do not have food stagnation. Such patients have deficient conditions without excess, and the use of formulas that contain *Da Huang* (Radix et Rhizoma Rhei) is not appropriate as it may cause damages to the body.

• This formula should be used with caution in patients with food stagnation and indigestion due to Spleen deficiency, as many herbs in this formula are bitter and cold to clear heat, and may further injure the Spleen.

• Use of this formula is contraindicated during pregnancy.

• Avoid consumption of raw and cold foods while taking this formula.[1]

CLINICAL STUDIES AND RESEARCH

1. **Chronic constipation**: One study evaluated the effectiveness of treating chronic constipation in 60 patients (mostly women, with history of chronic constipation for up to 20 years) via herbs and control group. The herb group had 31 patients, and the control group had 29 patients. The patients in the herb group were given *Zhi Shi Dao Zhi Wan* for 5 days. Of 31 patients in the herb group, 25 had significant improvement, 3 had moderate improvement, and 3 had no effect (90% effectiveness). Of 29 patients in the control group, 12 had significant improvement, 8 had moderate improvement, and 9 had no effect (70% effectiveness). The difference between the two groups was statistically significant ($p<0.05$).[2] The treatment protocol for the control group was unavailable at the time of publication.

2. **Trigeminal pain**: Administration of modified *Zhi Shi Dao Zhi Wan* was associated with good results in treating trigeminal pain in 11 patients (4 males and 7 females, between 5-60 years of age, 1 month to 21 years history of illness). In addition to the base formula, modifications included increasing the dose of *Da Huang* (Radix et Rhizoma Rhei) for constipation; adding *Di Huang* (Radix Rehmanniae) for yin deficiency; and *Tao Ren* (Semen Persicae) and *Hong Hua* (Flos Carthami) for chronic illness with blood stagnation. Of 11 patients, the study reported recovery (complete relief of pain) in 6 cases, improvement (partial relief of pain) in 4 cases, and no effect in 1 case.[3]

References

1. *Zhong Yao Ming Fang Yao Li Yu Ying Yong* (Pharmacology and Applications of Famous Herbal Formulas) 1989;623.

2. *Zhe Jiang Zhong Yi Xue Yuan Xue Bao* (Journal of Zhejiang University of Chinese Medicine) 1996;2:28.

3. *Nei Meng Gu Zhong Yi Yao* (Traditional Chinese Medicine and Medicinals of Inner Mongolia) 1993;3:44.

Chapter 19 – Reducing, Guiding, and Dissolving Formulas   *Section 1 – Reducing, Guiding, and Dissolving Formulas that Treat Food Stagnation*

Mù Xiāng Bīng Láng Wán (Aucklandia and Betel Nut Pill)

木香檳榔丸
木香槟榔丸

Pinyin Name: *Mu Xiang Bing Lang Wan*
Literal Name: Aucklandia and Betel Nut Pill
Alternate Name: Saussurea and Areca Seed Formula, Aucklandia and Areca Seed Formula
Original Source: *Ru Men Shi Qin* (Confucians' Duties to their Parents) by Zhang Cong-Zheng in 1228

COMPOSITION

Mu Xiang (Radix Aucklandiae)	30g [3g]
Bing Lang (Semen Arecae)	30g [3g]
Qian Niu Zi (Semen Pharbitidis)	120g [10g]
Da Huang (Radix et Rhizoma Rhei)	90g [5g]
Qing Pi (Pericarpium Citri Reticulatae Viride)	30g [3g]
Chen Pi (Pericarpium Citri Reticulatae)	30g [3g]
Xiang Fu (Rhizoma Cyperi), *chao* (dry-fried)	120g [10g]
E Zhu (Rhizoma Curcumae), *shao* (burned)	30g [3g]
Huang Lian (Rhizoma Coptidis), *chao* (dry-fried) with bran	30g [3g]
Huang Bo (Cortex Phellodendri Chinensis)	90g [5g]

DOSAGE / PREPARATION / ADMINISTRATION

The source text states to grind the ingredients into a fine powder, and form into small pills with water. The pills should resemble small beans in size. Take 30 pills [6g] after meals with a decoction made from *Sheng Jiang* (Rhizoma Zingiberis Recens). Today, this formula may be taken as pills or decoction. For pills, grind the herbs into powder and form into small pills with water, and take 3-6g of pills per dose with warm, boiled water twice daily. For decoction, use the suggested doses in brackets.

CHINESE THERAPEUTIC ACTIONS

1. Activates qi circulation and guides out stagnation
2. Attacks accumulation and purges heat

CLINICAL MANIFESTATIONS

Food stagnation and damp-heat accumulation: fullness, distention, and pain in the epigastric and abdominal regions, dysentery with red (blood) or white (mucus) stools, rectal tenesmus, constipation, a yellow, greasy tongue coating, and a deep, excess pulse.

CLINICAL APPLICATIONS

Dysentery, gastroenteritis, stenosis of colon and rectum, acute abdomen, liver cirrhosis with ascites, chronic nephritis, and tuberculous peritonitis.

EXPLANATION

Mu Xiang Bing Lang Wan (Aucklandia and Betel Nut Pill) treats qi stagnation and damp-heat accumulation due to food stagnation. Food stagnation can cause qi stagnation, which may lead to fullness, distention, and pain in the epigastric and abdominal regions, as well as constipation. Food stagnation may also lead to damp-heat accumulation, which often descends to the lower *jiao* to cause dysentery and tenesmus. A yellow, greasy tongue coating suggests damp-heat in the interior, and the deep, excess pulse is a sign of constipation and food stagnation.

In this formula, *Mu Xiang* (Radix Aucklandiae) and *Bing Lang* (Semen Arecae) activate qi circulation and break up stagnation to relieve epigastric and abdominal fullness, distention, and pain. *Qian Niu Zi* (Semen Pharbitidis) and *Da Huang* (Radix et Rhizoma Rhei) purge damp-heat and reduce stagnation and accumulation. *Qing Pi* (Pericarpium Citri Reticulatae Viride) and *Chen Pi* (Pericarpium Citri Reticulatae) activate qi circulation to relieve qi stagnation. *Xiang Fu* (Rhizoma Cyperi) and *E Zhu* (Rhizoma Curcumae) smooth the qi flow to relieve pain. *Huang Lian* (Rhizoma Coptidis) and *Huang Bo* (Cortex Phellodendri Chinensis) clear heat and dry dampness to stop dysentery.

MODIFICATIONS

• With qi stagnation in the chest and food retention in the abdomen, add *Zhi Qiao* (Fructus Aurantii).
• For severe constipation, add *Mang Xiao* (Natrii Sulfas) and *Zhi Qiao* (Fructus Aurantii).
• For damp-heat dysentery, remove *Chen Pi* (Pericarpium Citri Reticulatae), *E Zhu* (Rhizoma Curcumae), *Qian Niu Zi* (Semen Pharbitidis), and add *Qin Pi* (Cortex Fraxini) and *Bai Tou Weng* (Radix Pulsatillae).

1272

Mù Xiāng Bīng Láng Wán (Aucklandia and Betel Nut Pill)

Mu Xiang Bing Lang Wan (Aucklandia and Betel Nut Pill)

Diagnosis	Signs and Symptoms	Treatment	Herbs
Food stagnation and damp-heat accumulation	• Fullness, distention, and pain in the epigastric and abdominal regions: food and qi stagnation • Dysentery and tenesmus with red [blood] or white [mucus] stools: damp-heat accumulation in the lower *jiao* • Constipation: food stagnation • Yellow greasy tongue coating: damp-heat in the interior • Deep, excess pulse: excess heat condition in the interior	• Activates qi circulation and guides out stagnation • Attacks accumulation • Sedates heat	• *Mu Xiang* (Radix Aucklandiae) and *Bing Lang* (Semen Arecae) activate qi circulation and break up stagnation. • *Qian Niu Zi* (Semen Pharbitidis) and *Da Huang* (Radix et Rhizoma Rhei) purge damp-heat and reduce stagnation and accumulation. • *Qing Pi* (Pericarpium Citri Reticulatae Viride) and *Chen Pi* (Pericarpium Citri Reticulatae) activate qi circulation to relieve qi stagnation. • *Xiang Fu* (Rhizoma Cyperi) and *E Zhu* (Rhizoma Curcumae) smooth the qi flow to relieve pain. • *Huang Lian* (Rhizoma Coptidis) and *Huang Bo* (Cortex Phellodendri Chinensis) clear heat and dry dampness.

- With phlegm accumulation, add *Ban Xia* (Rhizoma Pinelliae) and *Fu Ling* (Poria).
- With damp-heat accumulation, add *Yin Chen* (Herba Artemisiae Scopariae) and *Zhi Zi* (Fructus Gardeniae).

CAUTIONS / CONTRAINDICATIONS

- *Mu Xiang Bing Lang Wan* contains potent herbs to activate qi circulation, clear heat, and eliminate stagnation and accumulation. It should be reserved for patients with excess conditions without underlying deficiencies. The use of this formula is contraindicated in deficient patients (especially those with Spleen and Stomach deficiencies), as this formula will injure *zheng* (upright) *qi* and complicate the illness.
- This formula is contraindicated during pregnancy. It should be used with caution in geriatric individuals with generalized weakness and deficiencies.[1]

CLINICAL STUDIES AND RESEARCH

1. **Stenosis of colon and rectum**: Administration of 10g of *Mu Xiang Bing Lang Wan* twice daily in 23 patients with stenosis of colon and rectum was associated with good results. Depending on the severity of the condition, the duration of treatment ranged from 3 months to 1 year. Of 23 patients, 13 had complete recovery, 7 had improvement, and 3 had no response. The overall effectiveness was 87%.[2]

2. **Acute abdomen**: Administration of *Mu Xiang Bing Lang Wan* was reported in 2 case studies to be effective for treatment of acute abdomen.[3]

AUTHORS' COMMENTS

Mu Xiang Bing Lang Wan is one of the stronger formulas for dispelling stagnation; it treats cases involving epigastric and abdominal distention and pain.

Zhi Shi Dao Zhi Wan (Immature Bitter Orange Pill to Guide Out Stagnation) and *Mu Xiang Bing Lang Wan* both treat food stagnation with damp-heat accumulation.

- *Zhi Shi Dao Zhi Wan* has a stronger action to dispel dampness. It is used for mild to moderate cases of stagnation and accumulation, with abdominal distention but not fullness.
- *Mu Xiang Bing Lang Wan* has a stronger action to activate qi and treat qi stagnation. It is used for more serious cases of stagnation and accumulation, with severe abdominal fullness, distention, and pain.

References

1. *Zhong Yao Ming Fang Yao Li Yu Ying Yong* (Pharmacology and Applications of Famous Herbal Formulas) 1989;624.
2. *Guang Xi Zhong Yi Yao* (Guangxi Chinese Medicine and Herbology) 1999;2:33.
3. *Jiang Su Zhong Yi* (Jiangsu Chinese Medicine) 1982;6:3.

REDUCING, GUIDING, AND DISSOLVING FORMULAS

19

Chapter 19 – Reducing, Guiding, and Dissolving Formulas   Section 1 – Reducing, Guiding, and Dissolving Formulas that Treat Food Stagnation

Zhǐ Zhú Wán

(Immature Bitter Orange and Atractylodes Macrocephala Pill)

枳术丸
枳术丸

Pinyin Name: *Zhi Zhu Wan*
Literal Name: Immature Bitter Orange and Atractylodes Macrocephala Pill
Original Source: *Nei Wai Shang Bian Huo Lun* (Clarifying Doubts about Injury from Internal and External Causes) by Li Gao in 1247

COMPOSITION

Bai Zhu (Rhizoma Atractylodis Macrocephalae)	60g [10g]
Zhi Shi (Fructus Aurantii Immaturus), *chao* (dry-fried) with bran	30g [5g]

DOSAGE / PREPARATION / ADMINISTRATION

The source text states to grind the ingredients into a fine powder, and form into small pills with cooked rice wrapped in *He Ye* (Folium Nelumbinis). The pills should resemble the size of *Wu Tong Zi* (Semen Firmianae), a small seed approximately 5 mm in diameter. Take 50 pills per dose with warm, boiled water any time during the day. Today, this formula may be taken in pills or decoction. For pills, grind the herbs into powder and form into small pills with water, and take 6-9g of pills per dose twice daily with warm, boiled water or with a decoction made from *He Ye* (Folium Nelumbinis). For decoction, use the suggested doses in brackets.

CHINESE THERAPEUTIC ACTIONS

1. Strengthens the Spleen
2. Reduces distention

CLINICAL MANIFESTATIONS

Spleen qi deficiency with qi stagnation and food retention: distention and fullness in the chest and epigastric regions, and decreased appetite.

CLINICAL APPLICATIONS

Gastric prolapse, rectal prolapse, chronic gastritis, anorexia, indigestion, and hepatitis.

EXPLANATION

Zhi Zhu Wan (Immature Bitter Orange and Atractylodes Macrocephala Pill) treats qi stagnation and food retention due to Spleen qi deficiency. If the Spleen qi is deficient, then food will not be digested properly, causing qi stagnation and food retention. The resulting symptoms would be distention and fullness of the chest and epigastrium and lack of appetite.

This formula contains *Bai Zhu* (Rhizoma Atractylodis Macrocephalae) to strengthen the Spleen and dry dampness, and *Zhi Shi* (Fructus Aurantii Immaturus) to break up qi stagnation and remove food stagnation. Because the main purpose of this formula is to strengthen the Spleen to prevent further indigestion, the dose of *Bai Zhu* (Rhizoma Atractylodis Macrocephalae) is twice that of *Zhi Shi* (Fructus Aurantii Immaturus). Finally, *He Ye* (Folium Nelumbinis) nourishes the Stomach and helps the Spleen ascend nutrients and clear yang.

MODIFICATIONS

- With Spleen deficiency or generalized weakness, add *Dang Shen* (Radix Codonopsis) and *Fu Ling* (Poria).
- With more food stagnation, add *Shan Zha* (Fructus Crataegi), *Shen Qu* (Massa Fermentata), and *Mai Ya* (Fructus Hordei Germinatus).

Zhi Zhu Wan (Immature Bitter Orange and Atractylodes Macrocephala Pill)

Diagnosis	Signs and Symptoms	Treatment	Herbs
Spleen qi deficiency with qi stagnation and food retention	• Distention and fullness in the chest and epigastric regions: qi and food stagnation • Decreased appetite: Spleen qi deficiency	• Strengthens the Spleen • Reduces distention	• *Bai Zhu* (Rhizoma Atractylodis Macrocephalae) strengthens the Spleen and dries dampness. • *Zhi Shi* (Fructus Aurantii Immaturus) breaks down qi stagnation and removes food stagnation. • *He Ye* (Folium Nelumbinis) nourishes the Stomach and ascends clear yang.

Zhǐ Zhú Wán

(Immature Bitter Orange and Atractylodes Macrocephala Pill)

CAUTIONS / CONTRAINDICATIONS

While taking *Zhi Zhu Wan*, patients should avoid food that is raw, cold, and stimulating (not bland) in nature.

PHARMACOLOGICAL EFFECTS

1. **Gastrointestinal**: According to one study, *Zhi Zhu Wan* administered in decoction to dogs stimulated the smooth muscles of the gastrointestinal tract and increased its peristalsis.[1]
2. **Cholagogic**: *Zhi Zhu Wan* has been shown to stimulate the production and release of bile acids in rats.[2]

CLINICAL STUDIES AND RESEARCH

1. **Anorexia**: Administration of *Zhi Zhu Wan* was associated with successful treatment of anorexia in 70 patients. The dose was 1g per dose for children between 1-3 years of age, 1.5g per dose for children between 4-5 years of age, and 2g per dose for children between 6-9 years of age. The herbs were given twice daily for 2 weeks per course of treatment.[3]
2. **Indigestion**: Administration of *Zhi Zhu Wan* was associated with good results for treating food retention and indigestion in children. The treatment protocol was to administer this formula in pills along with an herbal decoction made from *Chen Pi* (Pericarpium Citri Reticulatae), *Gu Ya* (Fructus Setariae Germinatus), and *Mai Ya* (Fructus Hordei Germinatus).[4]

RELATED FORMULAS

Zhǐ Zhú Tāng (Immature Bitter Orange and Atractylodes Macrocephala Decoction)

枳朮湯
枳术汤

Pinyin Name: *Zhi Zhu Tang*
Literal Name: Immature Bitter Orange and Atractylodes Macrocephala Decoction
Original Source: *Jin Gui Yao Lue* (Essentials from the Golden Cabinet) by Zhang Zhong-Jing in Eastern Han

Zhi Shi (Fructus Aurantii Immaturus),
   chao (dry-fried) with bran   7 pieces [12g]
Bai Zhu (Rhizoma Atractylodis Macrocephalae) 60g [6g]

The source text states to cook the herbs in 5 cups [1,000 mL] of water until it is reduced down to 3 cups [600 mL]. Take the warm, strained decoction in three equally-divided doses. *Zhi Zhu Tang* (Immature Bitter Orange and Atractylodes Macrocephala Decoction) has functions to activate qi circulation and reduce distention. Clinically, it is used for qi stagnation and water accumulation with a feeling of hardness and distention beneath the heart area.

Zhi Zhu Wan (Immature Bitter Orange and Atractylodes Macrocephala Pill) and *Zhi Zhu Tang* (Immature Bitter Orange and Atractylodes Macrocephala Decoction) are both designed to treat distention, and both formulas contain *Zhi Shi* (Fructus Aurantii Immaturus) and *Bai Zhu* (Rhizoma Atractylodis Macrocephalae).

- *Zhi Zhu Wan* has a larger dose of *Bai Zhu* (Rhizoma Atractylodis Macrocephalae) to strengthen the Spleen, and a smaller dose of *Zhi Shi* (Fructus Aurantii Immaturus) to reduce distention. Furthermore, it is given in pill form for sustained and moderate effect.
- *Zhi Zhu Tang* contains a higher dose of *Zhi Shi* (Fructus Aurantii Immaturus) to reduce distention, and a smaller dose of *Bai Zhu* (Rhizoma Atractylodis Macrocephalae) to strengthen the Spleen. In addition, it is given in decoction for more potent and immediate effect.

Qū Mài Zhǐ Zhú Wán
(Medicated Leaven, Barley Sprout, Immature Bitter Orange, and Atractylodes Macrocephala Pill)
曲糵枳朮丸
曲糵枳术丸
Pinyin Name: *Qu Mai Zhi Zhu Wan*
Literal Name: Medicated Leaven, Barley Sprout, Immature Bitter Orange, and Atractylodes Macrocephala Pill
Original Source: *Nei Wai Shang Bian Huo Lun* (Clarifying Doubts about Injury from Internal and External Causes) by Li Gao in 1247

Zhi Shi (Fructus Aurantii Immaturus),
   chao (dry-fried) with bran   30g [5g]
Bai Zhu (Rhizoma Atractylodis Macrocephalae) 60g [10g]
Shen Qu (Massa Fermentata), *chao* (dry-fried)   30g [5g]
Mai Ya (Fructus Hordei Germinatus),
   chao (dry-fried)   30g [5g]

The source text states to grind the ingredients into a fine powder, and form into small pills with cooked rice wrapped in *He Ye* (Folium Nelumbinis). The pills should resemble the size of *Wu Tong Zi* (Semen Firmianae), a small seed approximately 5 mm in diameter. Take 50 pills per dose with warm, boiled water on an empty stomach.

Qu Mai Zhi Zhu Wan (Medicated Leaven, Barley Sprout, Immature Bitter Orange, and Atractylodes Macrocephala Pill) is composed of *Zhi Zhu Wan* plus *Shen Qu* (Massa Fermentata) and *Mai Ya* (Fructus Hordei Germinatus). The main functions of this formula are to strengthen the Spleen and promote digestion. Clinically, it is often used for patients with inappropriate diet (overeating) that damages the Spleen and Stomach, which, in turn, causes

Zhǐ Zhú Wán
(Immature Bitter Orange and Atractylodes Macrocephala Pill)

food retention, phlegm stagnation, and epigastric and abdominal fullness and stifling sensations.

Jú Bàn Zhǐ Zhú Wán (Tangerine Peel, Pinellia, Immature Bitter Orange, and Atractylodes Macrocephala Pill)

橘半枳求丸
橘半枳术丸

Pinyin Name: *Ju Ban Zhi Zhu Wan*
Literal Name: Tangerine Peel, Pinellia, Immature Bitter Orange, and Atractylodes Macrocephala Pill
Original Source: *Yi Xue Ru Men* (Introduction to Medicine) by Li Ting in 1575

Zhi Shi (Fructus Aurantii Immaturus), *chao* (dry-fried) with bran	30g [5g]
Bai Zhu (Rhizoma Atractylodis Macrocephalae)	60g [10g]
Chen Pi (Pericarpium Citri Reticulatae)	30g [5g]
Ban Xia (Rhizoma Pinelliae)	30g [5g]

The source text states to grind the ingredients into a fine powder, and form into small pills with cooked rice wrapped in *He Ye* (Folium Nelumbinis). The pills should resemble the size of *Wu Tong Zi* (Semen Firmianae), a small seed approximately 5 mm in diameter. Take 50-60 pills per dose with warm, boiled water on an empty stomach.

Ju Ban Zhi Zhu Wan (Tangerine Peel, Pinellia, Immature Bitter Orange and Atractylodes Macrocephala Pill) is composed of *Zhi Zhu Wan* plus *Chen Pi* (Pericarpium Citri Reticulatae) and *Ban Xia* (Rhizoma Pinelliae). This formula strengthens the Spleen to dissolve phlegm and regulate qi to relieve distention in the chest and epigastrium. Clinically, it may be used for patients who have Spleen qi deficiency due to an inappropriate diet, with phlegm accumulation, and a feeling of distention and a stifling sensation in the heart and chest regions.

Xiāng Shā Zhǐ Zhú Wán (Aucklandia, Amomum, Immature Bitter Orange, and Atractylodes Macrocephala Pill)

香砂枳求丸
香砂枳术丸

Pinyin Name: *Xiang Sha Zhi Zhu Wan*
Literal Name: Aucklandia, Amomum, Immature Bitter Orange, and Atractylodes Macrocephala Pill
Original Source: *She Sheng Mi Pou* (Secrets Investigations into Obtaining Health) by Hong Ji in 1638

Bai Zhu (Rhizoma Atractylodis Macrocephalae), *chao* (dry-fried) with soil	480g
Zhi Shi (Fructus Aurantii Immaturus)	240g
Mu Xiang (Radix Aucklandiae)	30g
Sha Ren (Fructus Amomi)	30g

The source text states to grind the ingredients into a fine powder, and form into small pills with cooked rice wrapped in *He Ye* (Folium Nelumbinis). The pills should resemble *Jiao Mu* (Semen Zanthoxyli Bungeani) in size. Take 9g of pills per dose with warm, boiled water.

Xiang Sha Zhi Zhu Wan (Aucklandia, Amomum, Immature Bitter Orange, and Atractylodes Macrocephala Pill) is composed of *Zhi Zhu Wan* plus *Mu Xiang* (Radix Aucklandiae) and *Sha Ren* (Fructus Amomi). This formula strengthens the Spleen and activates qi. Clinically, it may be used for Spleen deficiency and qi stagnation characterized by symptoms such as decreased food intake, food stagnation, chronic indigestion, and a feeling of distention and oppression in the chest and epigastrium.

AUTHORS' COMMENTS

All five formulas listed above contain *Zhi Shi* (Fructus Aurantii Immaturus) and *Bai Zhu* (Rhizoma Atractylodis Macrocephalae) to strengthen the Spleen and reduce distention. Their differences are as follows:

- *Zhi Zhu Wan* (Immature Bitter Orange and Atractylodes Macrocephala Pill) has a stronger function to strengthen the Spleen, and weaker effect to reduce distention. It is given in pill form for sustained effect and moderate potency.

- *Zhi Zhu Tang* (Immature Bitter Orange and Atractylodes Macrocephala Decoction) has a stronger effect to reduce distention, and a weaker effect to strengthen the Spleen. It is given in decoction form for more potent effect and faster onset of action.

- *Qu Mai Zhi Zhu Wan* (Medicated Leaven, Barley Sprout, Immature Bitter Orange, and Atractylodes Macrocephala Pill) contains *Shen Qu* (Massa Fermentata) and *Mai Ya* (Fructus Hordei Germinatus) to promote digestion of foods.

- *Ju Ban Zhi Zhu Wan* (Tangerine Peel, Pinellia, Immature Bitter Orange and Atractylodes Macrocephala Pill) contains *Chen Pi* (Pericarpium Citri Reticulatae) and *Ban Xia* (Rhizoma Pinelliae), and has extra functions to move qi and dissolve phlegm.

- *Xiang Sha Zhi Zhu Wan* (Aucklandia, Amomum, Immature Bitter Orange, and Atractylodes Macrocephala Pill) contains *Mu Xiang* (Radix Aucklandiae) and *Sha Ren* (Fructus Amomi), and has additional effect to regulate qi circulation and dry dampness.

Chinese Herbal Formulas and Applications

Zhĭ Zhú Wán

(Immature Bitter Orange and Atractylodes Macrocephala Pill)

References

1. *Zhong Hua Yi Xue Za Zhi* (Chinese Journal of Medicine) 1956;42:946.
2. *Zhong Yao Yao Li Yu Lin Chuang* (Pharmacology and Clinical Applications of Chinese Herbs) 1991;7(1):8.
3. *Liao Ning Zhong Yi Za Zhi* (Liaoning Journal of Chinese Medicine) 1996;12:550.
4. *Zhong Yi Za Zhi* (Journal of Chinese Medicine) 1959;9:630.

Jiàn Pí Wán (Strengthen the Spleen Pill)

健脾丸

Pinyin Name: *Jian Pi Wan*
Literal Name: Strengthen the Spleen Pill
Alternate Names: *Chian Pi Wan*, Spleen-Strengthening Pill
Original Source: *Zheng Zhi Zhun Sheng* (Standards of Patterns and Treatments) by Wang Ken-Tang in 1602

COMPOSITION

Ren Shen (Radix et Rhizoma Ginseng)	45g [9g]
Bai Zhu (Rhizoma Atractylodis Macrocephalae), *chao* (dry-fried)	75g [15g]
Fu Ling (Poria)	60g [10g]
Gan Cao (Radix et Rhizoma Glycyrrhizae)	22.5g [6g]
Shan Yao (Rhizoma Dioscoreae)	30g [6g]
Rou Dou Kou (Semen Myristicae), oil removed	30g [6g]
Shan Zha (Fructus Crataegi)	30g [6g]
Shen Qu (Massa Fermentata), *chao* (dry-fried)	30g [6g]
Mai Ya (Fructus Hordei Germinatus), *chao* (dry-fried)	30g [6g]
Mu Xiang (Radix Aucklandiae), *yan* (ground) to small particles	22.5g [6g]
Sha Ren (Fructus Amomi)	30g [6g]
Chen Pi (Pericarpium Citri Reticulatae)	30g [6g]
Huang Lian (Rhizoma Coptidis), *chao* (dry-fried) with liquor	22.5g [6g]

DOSAGE / PREPARATION / ADMINISTRATION

The source text states to grind the ingredients into a fine powder. Steam the powder and form it into pills, which should resemble *Lu Dou* (Semen Phaseoli Radiati) in size. Take 50 pills per dose twice daily with rice soup on an empty stomach. Today this formula may be taken as pills or decoction. For pills, grind the herbs into powder and form into pills with water, and take 6-9g of pills per dose with warm, boiled water twice daily. For decoction, use the suggested doses in brackets.

CHINESE THERAPEUTIC ACTIONS

1. Strengthens the Spleen and harmonizes the Stomach
2. Reduces food stagnation and stops diarrhea

CLINICAL MANIFESTATIONS

Food stagnation and interior heat accumulation due to Spleen and Stomach deficiencies: decreased food intake, chronic indigestion and food stagnation, abdominal and epigastric distention and fullness, loose stools and diarrhea, a greasy and slightly yellow tongue coating, and a deficient, weak pulse.

CLINICAL APPLICATIONS

Indigestion and chronic enteritis.

EXPLANATION

When the Spleen and Stomach are deficient, food cannot be digested properly. The undigested food may accumulate and stagnate in the middle *jiao*. As a result of food stagnation, there will be poor appetite and abdominal and epigastric distention and fullness. Food stagnation creates damp accumulation, which may travel downward and cause loose stools and diarrhea with undigested food. Food stagnation may also create interior heat, which may cause the tongue coating to appear slightly yellow. A

REDUCING, GUIDING, AND DISSOLVING FORMULAS

19

1277

Chapter 19 – Reducing, Guiding, and Dissolving Formulas *Section 1 – Reducing, Guiding, and Dissolving Formulas that Treat Food Stagnation*

Jiàn Pí Wán (Strengthen the Spleen Pill)

Jian Pi Wan (Strengthen the Spleen Pill)

Diagnosis	Signs and Symptoms	Treatment	Herbs
Food stagnation and interior heat accumulation due to Spleen and Stomach deficiencies	• Abdominal and epigastric distention and fullness: food stagnation • Poor appetite, decreased food intake and undigested food in the stools: Spleen and Stomach deficiencies • Loose stools and diarrhea: dampness traveling downward • Greasy and slightly yellow tongue coating: presence of dampness and heat • Deficient, weak pulse: deficiency condition	• Strengthens the Spleen and harmonizes the Stomach • Reduces food stagnation and stops diarrhea	• *Ren Shen* (Radix et Rhizoma Ginseng), *Bai Zhu* (Rhizoma Atractylodis Macrocephalae), *Fu Ling* (Poria) and *Gan Cao* (Radix et Rhizoma Glycyrrhizae) tonify qi, strengthen the Spleen and Stomach, dispel dampness, and relieve diarrhea. • *Shan Yao* (Rhizoma Dioscoreae) and *Rou Dou Kou* (Semen Myristicae) strengthen the Spleen and stop diarrhea. • *Shan Zha* (Fructus Crataegi), *Shen Qu* (Massa Fermentata) and *Mai Ya* (Fructus Hordei Germinatus) promote digestion and reduce food stagnation. • *Mu Xiang* (Radix Aucklandiae), *Sha Ren* (Fructus Amomi) and *Chen Pi* (Pericarpium Citri Reticulatae) activate qi and harmonize the Stomach. • *Huang Lian* (Rhizoma Coptidis) clears interior heat and dries dampness.

greasy tongue coating suggests dampness and food accumulation, and a deficient, weak pulse reflects Spleen and Stomach deficiencies.

Jian Pi Wan (Strengthen the Spleen Pill) is formulated following the principles of *Si Jun Zi Tang* (Four-Gentlemen Decoction): *Ren Shen* (Radix et Rhizoma Ginseng), *Bai Zhu* (Rhizoma Atractylodis Macrocephalae), *Fu Ling* (Poria), and *Gan Cao* (Radix et Rhizoma Glycyrrhizae) tonify qi, strengthen the Spleen and Stomach, dispel dampness, and relieve diarrhea. *Shan Yao* (Rhizoma Dioscoreae) and *Rou Dou Kou* (Semen Myristicae) strengthen the Spleen and stop diarrhea. *Shan Zha* (Fructus Crataegi), *Shen Qu* (Massa Fermentata), and *Mai Ya* (Fructus Hordei Germinatus) promote digestion and reduce food stagnation. *Mu Xiang* (Radix Aucklandiae), *Sha Ren* (Fructus Amomi), and *Chen Pi* (Pericarpium Citri Reticulatae) activate qi circulation and harmonize the Stomach. *Huang Lian* (Rhizoma Coptidis) clears interior heat and dries dampness.

MODIFICATIONS
• With Spleen qi deficiency accompanied by coldness and food stagnation, remove *Huang Lian* (Rhizoma Coptidis) and add *Gan Jiang* (Rhizoma Zingiberis).
• With severe damp accumulation, add *Che Qian Zi* (Semen Plantaginis) and *Ze Xie* (Rhizoma Alismatis).

• With nausea and vomiting, add *Ban Xia* (Rhizoma Pinelliae) and *Ding Xiang* (Flos Caryophylli).

CAUTIONS / CONTRAINDICATIONS
Jian Pi Wan is designed to treat food stagnation due to Spleen and Stomach deficiencies. It should not be used to treat food stagnation due to overindulgence in foods, which is an excess condition.

RELATED FORMULA
Zī Shēng Wán (Nourish Life Pill)
資生丸
资生丸
Pinyin Name: Zi Sheng Wan
Literal Name: Nourish Life Pill
Original Source: *Xian Xing Zhai Yi Xue Guang Bi Ji* (Wide-Ranging Medical Notes from the First-Awakened Studio) by Miao Xi-Yong in 1613

Bai Zhu (Rhizoma Atractylodis Macrocephalae)	90g
Ren Shen (Radix et Rhizoma Ginseng)	90g
Yi Yi Ren (Semen Coicis)	45g
Fu Ling (Poria)	45g
Shan Zha (Fructus Crataegi)	60g
Ju Hong (Exocarpium Citri Reticulatae)	60g
Huang Lian (Rhizoma Coptidis)	9g
Dou Kou (Fructus Amomi Rotundus)	10g
Ze Xie (Rhizoma Alismatis)	10g

Chinese Herbal Formulas and Applications

Jiàn Pí Wán (Strengthen the Spleen Pill)

Jie Geng (Radix Platycodonis)	15g
Huo Xiang Ye (Folium Agastaches)	15g
Zhi Gan Cao (Radix et Rhizoma Glycyrrhizae Praeparata cum Melle)	15g
Bai Bian Dou (Semen Lablab Album)	45g
Lian Zi (Semen Nelumbinis)	45g
Shan Yao (Rhizoma Dioscoreae), *chao* (dry-fried)	45g
Qian Shi (Semen Euryales), *chao* (dry-fried)	45g
Mai Ya (Fructus Hordei Germinatus), *chao* (dry-fried)	30g

The source text states to grind the ingredients into a fine powder and form into pills with honey. Chew and swallow 1 pill [6g] with boiled water, rice soup, or decoction made from *Chen Pi* (Pericarpium Citri Reticulatae) or dry-fried *Sha Ren* (Fructus Amomi). The source text recommends avoiding peaches, plums, clams, and food that is raw or cold in nature while taking the formula.

Zi Sheng Wan (Nourish Life Pill) strengthens the Spleen, reduces food stagnation, increases appetite, and stops diarrhea. Clinically, it may be used for patients with Spleen deficiency characterized by symptoms such as lack of appetite, nausea, vomiting, and diarrhea. This formula may also be used for pregnant women in their first trimester with deficiency of the *yangming* channel and instability of the fetus. Lastly, it can be used in pediatric patients to treat lack of energy, fatigue, loose stools, lack of appetite and decreased food intake.

AUTHORS' COMMENTS

Jian Pi Wan literally means "Strengthen the Spleen Pill," because the primary function of this formula is to strengthen the Spleen, which in turn carries out the functions of transportation and transformation.

Zhi Zhu Wan (Immature Bitter Orange and Atractylodes Macrocephala Pill) and *Jian Pi Wan* both tonify the Spleen and treat food stagnation.

- *Zhi Zhu Wan* has moderate potency to tonify the Spleen and eliminate food stagnation.
- *Jian Pi Wan*, in addition to having a stronger effect of tonifying the Spleen and eliminating food stagnation, also dispels damp-heat and stops diarrhea.

Jian Pi Wan and *Si Jun Zi Tang* (Four-Gentlemen Decoction) both contain *Ren Shen* (Radix et Rhizoma Ginseng), *Bai Zhu* (Rhizoma Atractylodis Macrocephalae), *Fu Ling* (Poria) and *Gan Cao* (Radix et Rhizoma Glycyrrhizae) to tonify qi and strengthen the Spleen. The differences are as follows:

- *Jian Pi Wan* contains large doses of *Bai Zhu* (Rhizoma Atractylodis Macrocephalae) and *Fu Ling* (Poria) to strengthen the Spleen, resolve dampness, and stop diarrhea.
- *Si Jun Zi Tang* contains larger doses of *Ren Shen* (Radix et Rhizoma Ginseng) to greatly tonify *yuan* (source) *qi*, strengthen the Spleen, and nourish the Stomach.

REDUCING, GUIDING, AND DISSOLVING FORMULAS

19

1279

Section 2

消痞化积剂
— Reducing, Guiding, and Dissolving Formula that Relieves Distention

Zhǐ Shí Xiāo Pǐ Wán
(Immature Bitter Orange Pill to Reduce Focal Distention)

枳實消痞丸
枳实消痞丸

Pinyin Name: *Zhi Shi Xiao Pi Wan*
Literal Name: Immature Bitter Orange Pill to Reduce Focal Distention
Original Source: *Lan Shi Mi Cang* (Secrets from the Orchid Chamber) by Li Gao in 1336

COMPOSITION

Zhi Shi (Fructus Aurantii Immaturus)	15g
Hou Po (Cortex Magnoliae Officinalis), *zhi* (fried with liquid)	12g
Huang Lian (Rhizoma Coptidis)	15g
Ban Xia Qu (Rhizoma Pinelliae Massa Fermentata)	9g
Gan Jiang (Rhizoma Zingiberis)	3g
Ren Shen (Radix et Rhizoma Ginseng)	9g
Bai Zhu (Rhizoma Atractylodis Macrocephalae)	6g
Fu Ling (Poria)	6g
Mai Ya Qu (Fructus Hordei Germinatus Massa Fermentata)	6g
Zhi Gan Cao (Radix et Rhizoma Glycyrrhizae Praeparata cum Melle)	6g

DOSAGE / PREPARATION / ADMINISTRATION

The source text states to grind the ingredients into a fine powder and form into small pills with water. The pills should resemble the size of *Wu Tong Zi* (Semen Firmianae), a small seed approximately 5 mm in diameter. Take 50-70 pills with warm, boiled water between meals. Today, the ingredients are grind into powder and form into small pills with water. Take 6-9g of pills per dose with warm, boiled water twice daily.

CHINESE THERAPEUTIC ACTIONS

1. Activates qi circulation and reduces fullness and distention
2. Strengthens the Spleen and harmonizes the Stomach

CLINICAL MANIFESTATIONS

Spleen deficiency complicated by qi stagnation and interlocking of interior heat and cold: epigastric fullness and distention, lack of appetite, lethargy, and irregular bowel movements with mild constipation.

CLINICAL APPLICATIONS

Chronic gastritis, chronic atrophic gastritis, indigestion, intestinal obstruction, cholelithiasis, and cholecystitis.

EXPLANATION

Zhi Shi Xiao Pi Wan (Immature Bitter Orange Pill to Reduce Focal Distention) treats epigastric fullness and distention complicated with both deficiency and excess conditions. This condition begins with Spleen deficiency and compromised digestive functioning. As the food stagnates, it slowly causes phlegm accumulation, qi stagnation, and interlocking of heat and cold (more heat). Clinical manifestations include epigastric fullness and distention, lethargy, lack of appetite, and constipation.

The treatment plan for this syndrome is to activate qi, strengthen the Spleen, and regulate the cold and heat. This formula contains *Zhi Shi* (Fructus Aurantii Immaturus) to break up qi stagnation and reduce epigastric distention.

Chinese Herbal Formulas and Applications

Zhǐ Shí Xiāo Pǐ Wán
(Immature Bitter Orange Pill to Reduce Focal Distention)

Zhi Shi Xiao Pi Wan (Immature Bitter Orange Pill to Reduce Focal Distention)

Diagnosis	Signs and Symptoms	Treatment	Herbs
Spleen deficiency complicated by qi stagnation and interlocking of interior heat and cold	• Lack of appetite and lethargy: Spleen deficiency • Epigastric fullness and distention: qi stagnation and phlegm accumulation • Irregular bowel movements: interlocking of heat and cold • Mild constipation: interior heat drying fluids	• Strengthens the Spleen and harmonizes the Stomach • Reduces fullness and distention	• *Zhi Shi* (Fructus Aurantii Immaturus) and *Hou Po* (Cortex Magnoliae Officinalis) activate qi circulation and relieve epigastric fullness and distention. • *Huang Lian* (Rhizoma Coptidis) clears heat and dries dampness. • *Ban Xia Qu* (Rhizoma Pinelliae Massa Fermentata) disperses interior damp and cold, breaks up clumps, and harmonizes the Stomach. • *Gan Jiang* (Rhizoma Zingiberis) warms the Spleen and dispels cold. • *Ren Shen* (Radix et Rhizoma Ginseng), *Bai Zhu* (Rhizoma Atractylodis Macrocephalae) and *Fu Ling* (Poria) strengthen the Spleen and dry dampness. • *Mai Ya Qu* (Fructus Hordei Germinatus Massa Fermentata) improves digestion and harmonizes the Stomach. • *Zhi Gan Cao* (Radix et Rhizoma Glycyrrhizae Praeparata cum Melle) harmonizes the herbs.

Hou Po (Cortex Magnoliae Officinalis) activates qi circulation to relieve epigastric fullness. As a pair, *Zhi Shi* (Fructus Aurantii Immaturus) and *Hou Po* (Cortex Magnoliae Officinalis) have a synergistic effect to regulate qi and relieve both fullness and distention. *Huang Lian* (Rhizoma Coptidis) clears heat and dries dampness. *Ban Xia Qu* (Rhizoma Pinelliae Massa Fermentata) disperses interior damp and cold, breaks up clumps, and harmonizes the Stomach. A small amount of *Gan Jiang* (Rhizoma Zingiberis) warms the Spleen and dispels cold. *Ren Shen* (Radix et Rhizoma Ginseng), *Bai Zhu* (Rhizoma Atractylodis Macrocephalae), and *Fu Ling* (Poria) strengthen the Spleen and dry dampness. *Mai Ya Qu* (Fructus Hordei Germinatus Massa Fermentata) improves digestion and harmonizes the Stomach. *Zhi Gan Cao* (Radix et Rhizoma Glycyrrhizae Praeparata cum Melle) harmonizes all of the herbs in the formula.

MODIFICATIONS

• With epigastric and abdominal pain due to cold, reduce the dose of *Huang Lian* (Rhizoma Coptidis), increase the dose of *Gan Jiang* (Rhizoma Zingiberis), and add *Rou Gui* (Cortex Cinnamomi) and *Gao Liang Jiang* (Rhizoma Alpiniae Officinarum).

• With feelings of distention and a stifling sensation in the chest and diaphragm, add *Sha Ren* (Fructus Amomi),

Chen Pi (Pericarpium Citri Reticulatae), and *Jie Geng* (Radix Platycodonis).

• With intestinal parasitic infestation, add *Shi Jun Zi* (Fructus Quisqualis), *He Zi* (Fructus Chebulae), and *Bing Lang* (Semen Arecae).

CAUTIONS / CONTRAINDICATIONS

Although *Zhi Shi Xiao Pi Wan* has dual effects to purge excess (food stagnation) and tonify deficiency (Spleen deficiency), the main emphasis is to purge excess and clear heat. Therefore, it should be used with caution in patients with severe Spleen deficiency.

PHARMACOLOGICAL EFFECTS

Gastrointestinal: Use of *Zhi Shi Xiao Pi Wan* was associated with stimulating the gastrointestinal tract to increase peristalsis of the intestines and gastric emptying time.[1]

CLINICAL STUDIES AND RESEARCH

1. **Chronic gastritis:** One study reported good results using modified *Zhi Shi Xiao Pi Wan* to treat chronic gastritis in 30 patients (22 males and 8 females, between 25-70 years of age, with 1-30 years history of illness). Modifications to the base herbal formula were made as needed. For Liver qi overacting on the Stomach, *Chai Hu* (Radix Bupleuri), *Chen Pi* (Pericarpium Citri Reticulatae), and *Dan Shen*

REDUCING, GUIDING, AND DISSOLVING FORMULAS

19

1281

Zhǐ Shí Xiāo Pǐ Wán
(Immature Bitter Orange Pill to Reduce Focal Distention)

(Radix et Rhizoma Salviae Miltiorrhizae) were added, and *Gan Jiang* (Rhizoma Zingiberis) was removed. For deficiency and cold of the Spleen and Stomach, *Pao Jiang* (Rhizoma Zingiberis Praeparatum) and *Gui Zhi* (Ramulus Cinnamomi) were added, and *Huang Lian* (Rhizoma Coptidis) and *Dan Shen* (Radix et Rhizoma Salviae Miltiorrhizae) were removed. For damp-heat affecting the Spleen and Stomach, *Mu Dan Pi* (Cortex Moutan) and *Zhi Zi* (Fructus Gardeniae) were added. Of 30 patients, the study reported a marked effect in 26 cases, improvement in 3 cases, and no effect in 1 case.[2]

2. **Chronic atrophic gastritis**: One study reported good results using modified *Zhi Shi Xiao Pi Wan* to treat chronic atrophic gastritis in 45 patients. The herbal treatment contained this formula, with modifications based on the condition of the individual patients. For excess heat, the dose of *Huang Lian* (Rhizoma Coptidis) was increased and the dose of *Gan Jiang* (Rhizoma Zingiberis) was reduced. For excess cold, the dose of *Huang Lian* (Rhizoma Coptidis) was decreased and the dose of *Gan Jiang* (Rhizoma Zingiberis) was increased. For frequent belching, *Xuan Fu Hua* (Flos Inulae) was added. The herbs were given three times daily for 1 month per course of treatment, and the patients were monitored for 1 year. Of 45 patients, the study reported significant improvement in 23 cases, improvement in 20 cases, and no effect in 2 cases. The overall effectiveness was 95.6%.[3]

3. **Indigestion**: Use of *Zhi Shi Xiao Pi Wan* was associated with 94.74% effectiveness in treating non-ulcerative indigestion. In addition to the base formula, modifications were made as needed. For Stomach yin deficiency, *Yu Zhu* (Rhizoma Polygonati Odorati) and *Shi Hu* (Caulis Dendrobii) were added, and *Ban Xia* (Rhizoma Pinelliae) and *Sheng Jiang* (Rhizoma Zingiberis Recens) were removed. For constipation, *Da Huang* (Radix et Rhizoma Rhei) and *Gua Lou* (Fructus Trichosanthis) were added. For pain in the upper abdominal area, *Mu Xiang* (Radix Aucklandiae) and *Yan Hu Suo* (Rhizoma Corydalis) were added. For burning sensations in the stomach with acid reflux, *Zuo Jin Wan* (Left Metal Pill) was added. For thick, greasy, white tongue coating, *Dou Kou* (Fructus Amomi Rotundus) was added, and *Bai Zhu* (Rhizoma Atractylodis Macrocephalae) was replaced with *Cang Zhu* (Rhizoma Atractylodis). The herbs were given for 4 weeks per course of treatment. Of 76 patients, the study reported complete recovery in 20 cases, significant improvement in 24 cases, moderate improvement in 28 cases, and no effect in 4 cases.[4]

4. **Intestinal obstruction**: *Zhi Shi Xiao Pi Wan* was used to treat 12 hospitalized patients (between 18-65 years of age) with intestinal obstruction for 1-3 days, associated with inappropriate diet. Modifications to the original formula included substitution of *Ren Shen* (Radix et Rhizoma Ginseng) with *Xi Yang Shen* (Radix Panacis Quinquefolii). Furthermore, *Chuan Lian Zi* (Fructus Toosendan) and *Yan Hu Suo* (Rhizoma Corydalis) were added for severe abdominal pain; *Shen Qu* (Massa Fermentata) and *Shan Zha* (Fructus Crataegi) for severe food stagnation; and *Shi Hu* (Caulis Dendrobii) and *Tian Hua Fen* (Radix Trichosanthis) for severe damage to body fluids. The treatment protocol was to cook the herbs and administer the formula in decoction twice daily. Of 12 patients, 11 had complete recovery, and 1 who did not respond was treated with surgery.[5]

5. **Cholelithiasis and cholecystitis**: Administration of modified *Zhi Shi Xiao Pi Wan* was associated with complete recovery in all 19 patients with cholelithiasis and cholecystitis. Modifications to the base formula included the addition of a larger dose of *Da Huang* (Radix et Rhizoma Rhei) for excess heat; *Chai Hu* (Radix Bupleuri) and *Yu Jin* (Radix Curcumae) for stabbing pain in the hypochondrium; *Zhu Ru* (Caulis Bambusae in Taenia) for nausea and vomiting; *Da Huang* (Radix et Rhizoma Rhei) and *Gua Lou* (Fructus Trichosanthis) for constipation with dry stools; and *Yin Chen* (Herba Artemisiae Scopariae) and *Zhi Zi* (Fructus Gardeniae) for jaundice. Each course of treatment was 5 days.[6]

AUTHORS' COMMENTS

Zhi Zhu Wan (Immature Bitter Orange and Atractylodes Macrocephala Pill), *Jian Pi Wan* (Strengthen the Spleen Pill) and *Zhi Shi Xiao Pi Wan* all treat indigestion using both tonifying and reducing methods.

- *Zhi Zhu Wan* and *Jian Pi Wan* primarily tonify the Spleen and secondarily remove stagnation.

- *Zhi Shi Xiao Pi Wan* removes stagnation and relieves fullness and distention, more so than strengthens the Spleen and Stomach.

References

1. *An Hui Zhong Yi Xue Yuan Xue Bao* (Journal of Anhui University School of Medicine) 1991;19(3):47.
2. *Zhong Yi Yao Xue Bao* (Report of Chinese Medicine and Herbology) 1991;3:39.
3. *Shan Xi Zhong Yi* (Shanxi Chinese Medicine) 1997;7:304.
4. *Si Chuan Zhong Yi* (Sichuan Chinese Medicine) 1998;7:26.
5. *Zhong Yi Ming Fang Lin Chuang Xin Yong* (Contemporary Clinical Applications of Classic Chinese Formulas) 2001;502.
6. *Hu Bei Zhong Yi Za Zhi* (Hubei Journal of Chinese Medicine) 1998;5:38.

Chinese Herbal Formulas and Applications

Chapter 19 — Summary

— Reducing, Guiding, and Dissolving Formulas

SECTION 1: REDUCING, GUIDING, AND DISSOLVING FORMULAS THAT TREAT FOOD STAGNATION

Name	Similarities	Differences
Bao He Wan (Preserve Harmony Pill)	Promotes digestion, harmonizes the Stomach	Treats food stagnation, indigestion and other digestive disorders
Zhi Shi Dao Zhi Wan (Immature Bitter Orange Pill to Guide Out Stagnation)	Reduce and dissolve stagnation, clear damp-heat	Moderate potency, stronger to dispel dampness
Mu Xiang Bing Lang Wan (Aucklandia and Betel Nut Pill)		Strong potency, stronger to activate qi circulation
Zhi Zhu Wan (Immature Bitter Orange and Atractylodes Macrocephala Pill)	Strengthen the Spleen, reduce food stagnation	Moderate potency, activates qi circulation
Jian Pi Wan (Strengthen the Spleen Pill)		Strong potency, harmonizes the Stomach, stops diarrhea

Bao He Wan (Preserve Harmony Pill) is the principal formula used for any kind of food stagnation with symptoms of epigastric and abdominal fullness and distention, aversion to food, and belching with a foul smell. It activates digestion and harmonizes the Stomach.

Zhi Shi Dao Zhi Wan (Immature Bitter Orange Pill to Guide Out Stagnation) and **Mu Xiang Bing Lang Wan** (Aucklandia and Betel Nut Pill) have similar functions of activating qi circulation, and reducing and dissolving stagnation.

- *Zhi Shi Dao Zhi Wan* has a stronger damp-eliminating action. This formula is indicated for patients with stagnation of food and damp-heat in the Stomach and Intestines causing abdominal pain and diarrhea.
- *Mu Xiang Bing Lang Wan* has a stronger action in breaking up stagnation. It is reserved for a more severe form of stagnation with both abdominal fullness and pain.

Zhi Zhu Wan (Immature Bitter Orange and Atractylodes Macrocephala Pill) and **Jian Pi Wan** (Strengthen the Spleen Pill) have similar effects to treat indigestion via tonifying and reducing methods. Both formulas tonify the Spleen to improve its digestive functioning. They also utilize reducing and dissolving methods to treat stagnation and accumulation.

- *Zhi Zhu Wan* strengthens the Spleen and activates qi circulation. It is used for qi and food stagnation with underlying Spleen qi deficiency. Clinical manifestations include lack of appetite, and fullness and distention in the chest and epigastric regions.
- *Jian Pi Wan* strengthens the Spleen, harmonizes the Stomach, promotes digestion, and stops diarrhea. It resolves heat and food stagnation with underlying Spleen deficiency. Clinical manifestations include poor appetite, epigastric and abdominal fullness, diarrhea, and a greasy and slightly yellow tongue coating.

REDUCING, GUIDING, AND DISSOLVING FORMULAS

19

1283

Chapter 19 – Reducing, Guiding, and Dissolving Formulas

Chapter 19 — Summary

SECTION 2: REDUCING, GUIDING, AND DISSOLVING FORMULA THAT RELIEVES DISTENTION

Name	Similarities	Differences
Zhi Shi Xiao Pi Wan (Immature Bitter Orange Pill to Reduce Focal Distention)	Reduces, guides, and dissolves accumulation	Relieves epigastric and abdominal fullness and distention

Zhi Shi Xiao Pi Wan (Immature Bitter Orange Pill to Reduce Focal Distention) relieves epigastric and abdominal fullness and distention, strengthens the Spleen, and harmonizes the Stomach. This formula treats Spleen deficiency with interior heat, cold, damp, and phlegm stagnation. Clinical manifestations include epigastric and abdominal fullness and distention, lack of appetite, lethargy, and mild constipation.

1284

Chapter 20

— Antiparasitic Formulas

Chapter 20 – Antiparasitic Formulas

葛洪 Gē Hōng

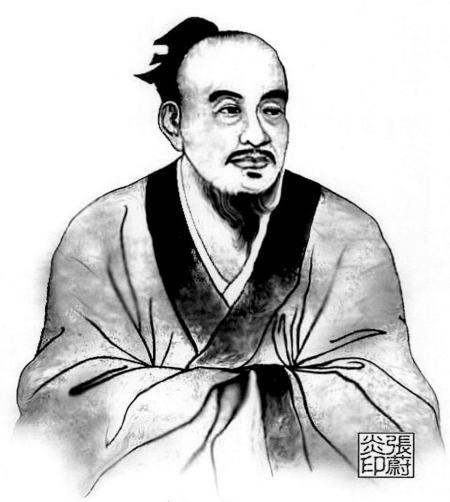

葛洪 Gē Hōng, 284 – 364.

葛洪 Gē Hōng

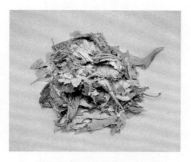

Ai Ye (Folium Artemisiae Argyi), the main ingredient used in moxa sticks.

Ge Hong was born into a poor family. When he was thirteen years old, his father died, and his family suffered extreme financial hardship. He began to work to support his family, and during his spare time, he borrowed books and studied diligently. He later became a famed physician and alchemist.

As a physician, he compiled his clinical experiences and published 肘后备急方 *Zhou Hou Bei Ji Fang* (Emergency Formulas to Keep Up One's Sleeve) in 341 CE. This is a valuable text that described in detail many diseases and their corresponding treatments using herbs that are simple, readily-available, inexpensive, and effective. For example, he is credited as the first person to treat jaundice with *Qing Hao* (Herba Artemisiae Annuae),[1] leg *qi* with milk from cows and sheep,[2] and bites from rabid dogs with the brain marrow from the attacking dog.[3]

As an alchemist, he experimented with various substances to prepare special pills, such as *Xiong Huang* (Realgar), *Liu Huang* (Sulfur), *Dan Fan* (Chalcanthitum), *Xiao Shi* (Niter), *Ci Shi* (Magnetitum), *Zhu Sha* (Cinnabaris), and others. Although many of these substances are no longer used today, he emphasized the use of pills and the concept that many dosage forms are available beyond decoction. Ge Hong demonstrated that there are many other viable preparation methods and effective forms of delivery of medicinal substances.

Ge Hong's wife, 鲍姑 Bao Gu, was also a skilled physician. Bao Gu is credited for the discovery of moxa and its medicinal properties. Moxa is made by rolling *Ai Ye* (Folium Artemisiae Argyi) into a stick. Since this herb grows all over China, her discovery follows the same principles put forth by her husband, that medicines should be simple, readily-available, inexpensive and effective.

1. Artemisinin from *Qing Hao* (Herba Artemisiae Annuae) is now a standard medication for treating malaria.
2. 脚气 Leg *qi* is a term that describes beriberi, which was treated with beans and milk which contain ample supply of vitamin B_1.
3. The brain marrow of rabid dogs contains antibodies, and has been confirmed to effectively prevent/treat rabies.

Dynasties & Kingdoms	Year
Xia Dynasty 夏	2100-1600 BCE
Shang Dynasty 商	1600-1100 BCE
Zhou Dynasty 周	1100-221 BCE
Qin Dynasty 秦	221-207 BCE
Han Dynasty 漢	206 BCE-220
Three Kingdoms 三國	220-280
Western Jin Dynasty 西晉	**265-316**
Eastern Jin Dynasty 東晉	317-420
Northern and Southern Dynasties 北南朝	420-581
Sui Dynasty 隋	581-618
Tang Dynasty 唐	618-907
Five Dynasties 五代	907-960
Song Dynasty 宋	960-1279
Liao Dynasty 潦	916-1125
Jin Dynasty 金	1115-1234
Yuan Dynasty 元	1271-1368
Ming Dynasty 明	1368-1644
Qing Dynasty 清	1644-1911
Republic of China 中華民國	1912-Present Day
People's Republic of China 中華人民共和國	1949-Present Day

Chapter 20 – Antiparasitic Formulas

Table of Contents

Chapter 20. Antiparasitic Formulas ·· **1285**
Biography of Ge Hong ··· 1286

Wu Mei Wan (Mume Pill) ·· 1292
   Li Zhong An Hui Tang (Regulate the Middle and Calm Roundworms Decoction) ·········· 1295
   Lian Mei An Hui Tang (Picrorhiza and Mume Decoction to Calm Roundworms) ··········· 1295
Fei Er Wan (Fat Child Pill) ·· 1296
   Jin Jian Fei Er Wan (Golden Pill to Construct a Fat Child) ···························· 1298
Bu Dai Wan (Cloth Sack Pill) ·· 1299
Hua Chong Wan (Dissolve Parasites Pill) ·· 1300
Fa Mu Wan (Quell Wood Pill) ··· 1302

Antiparasitic Formulas (Summary) ·· **1303**

Chinese Herbal Formulas and Applications

Chapter 20 — Overview

— Antiparasitic Formulas

Definition: Antiparasitic formulas consist mainly of herbs that calm, expel and/or kill various types of parasites affecting the human body. There are many different types of parasites, all with different clinical manifestations, and all require different treatment. This chapter emphasizes the treatment of intestinal parasites, such as ascariasis (roundworms), oxyuriasis (pinworms), cestodiasis (tapeworms), ancylostomiasis (hookworms), and others.

The common clinical manifestations of intestinal parasitic infestations include intermittent abdominal pain around the umbilical region, ability to eat despite pain, a sallow facial appearance, a greenish or pale face, development of white spots or red streaks on the face, nighttime teeth grinding, nausea, vomiting of clear fluids, a peeled tongue coating, and a big or small pulse. If the condition is untreated or treated inappropriately, there may be emaciation, loss of muscle mass, lack of appetite, lassitude, poor vision, dry and dull hair, enlarged and distended abdomen, protrusion of veins, and malnutrition.

SUBCATEGORIES OF ACTION

Antiparasitic formulas are usually not divided into subcategories. Clinical manifestations vary, however, with different types of parasitic infestations. Examples of parasitic infestation, associated signs and symptoms, and commonly used herbs, are as follows:

- Ascariasis (roundworms) is characterized by itching of the ears, nose and mouth accompanied by red and white spots on the mucous membranes of the mouth and lips, and white flakes and worm segments in the stools. Ascariasis may be treated with herbs such as *Shi Jun Zi* (Fructus Quisqualis), *Ku Lian Pi* (Cortex Meliae), *Bing Lang* (Semen Arecae), and *Lei Wan* (Omphalia).
- Oxyuriasis (pinworms) is characterized by an itching anus that is often worse at night. Oxyuriasis may be treated with *Shi Jun Zi* (Fructus Quisqualis), *Ku Lian Pi* (Cortex Meliae), *Bing Lang* (Semen Arecae), *Fei Zi* (Semen Torreyae), and *Mian Ma Guan Zhong* (Rhizoma Dryopteridis Crassirhizomatis).
- Cestodiasis (tapeworms) is characterized by stools containing white particles (parasite bodies). Cestodiasis may be treated with herbs such as *Bing Lang* (Semen Arecae), *Nan Gua Zi* (Semen Cucurbitae Moschatae), *Fei Zi* (Semen Torreyae), *He Shi* (Fructus Carpesii), and *Wu Yi* (Fructus Ulmi Praeparatus).
- Ancylostomiasis (hookworms) is characterized by a pale or sallow facial appearance, cravings for unusual foods, a marked change in appetite, uncharacteristic weakness, and swelling with edema. Ancylostomiasis may be treated with *Ku Lian Pi* (Cortex Meliae), *Fei Zi* (Semen Torreyae), *He Shi* (Fructus Carpesii), *Lei Wan* (Omphalia), and *Mian Ma Guan Zhong* (Rhizoma Dryopteridis Crassirhizomatis).

In addition, antiparasitic herbs and formulas have different characteristics, and are used for different general conditions.

- Parasitic infestations characterized by cold should be treated with warm herbs and formulas, such as *Gan Jiang* (Rhizoma Zingiberis), *Hua Jiao* (Pericarpium Zanthoxyli), and *Li Zhong An Hui Tang* (Regulate the Middle and Calm Roundworm Decoction).

~

Antiparasitic formulas calm, kill and/or expel various intestinal parasites, such as roundworm, pinworm, tapeworm, and hookworm.

~

It is best to verify [via stool examination] what parasites are present before administering a formula.

~

ANTIPARASITIC FORMULAS

20

1289

Chapter 20 – Antiparasitic Formulas

Chapter 20 — Overview

- Parasitic infestations characterized by heat should be treated with the addition of cold herbs and formulas, such as *Hu Huang Lian* (Rhizoma Picrorhizae), *Huang Bo* (Cortex Phellodendri Chinensis), and *Lian Mei An Hui Tang* (Picrorhiza and Mume Decoction to Calm Roundworms).
- Parasitic infestations characterized by both cold and heat signs and symptoms should be treated with two types of herbs: acrid and warm herbs to dispel cold (e.g., *Gan Jiang* (Rhizoma Zingiberis) and *Fu Zi* (Radix Aconiti Lateralis Praeparata)), and bitter and cold herbs to clear heat (e.g., *Huang Lian* (Rhizoma Coptidis) and *Huang Bo* (Cortex Phellodendri Chinensis)). One exemplar formula is *Wu Mei Wan* (Mume Pill).

~

Antiparasitic formulas must be dosed properly: large doses may cause toxic side effects, but small doses may yield no therapeutic benefit.

~

- Chronic parasitic infestation characterized by malnutrition and Spleen dysfunction should be treated with three types of herbs: herbs that strengthen and harmonize the middle *jiao*, such as *Shen Qu* (Massa Fermentata) and *Mai Ya* (Fructus Hordei Germinatus); herbs that regulate qi and awaken the Stomach, such as *Rou Dou Kou* (Semen Myristicae) and *Mu Xiang* (Radix Aucklandiae); and herbs that clear heat and kill parasites, such as *Huang Lian* (Rhizoma Coptidis), and *Zhu Dan* (Fel Porcus). A representative formula is *Fei Er Wan* (Fat Child Pill).
- Lastly, parasitic infestation characterized by Spleen deficiency should be treated with antiparasitic and tonic herbs, such as *Ren Shen* (Radix et Rhizoma Ginseng), *Fu Ling* (Poria), *Bai Zhu* (Rhizoma Atractylodis Macrocephalae), and *Gan Cao* (Radix et Rhizoma Glycyrrhizae). One exemplar formula is *Bu Dai Wan* (Cloth Sack Pill).

CAUTIONS / CONTRAINDICATIONS

- To ensure efficacy of the treatment, it is best to examine the stools and verify what parasites are present before administering a formula.
- Because these herbs have purgative actions, they should be used cautiously or not at all for weak, pregnant, or elderly patients.
- Because some antiparasitic herbs are toxic in nature, they must be dosed properly. Large doses may be associated with adverse effects, but small doses may yield little or no antiparasitic benefit.
- These formulas should be taken on an empty stomach. Greasy or oily foods should be avoided when taking these formulas, as digestion and absorption of the formulas could be affected.
- These formulas may cause Spleen and Stomach deficiencies, in which case tonic herbs may be indicated to address the underlying deficiency.

PHARMACOLOGICAL EFFECTS & CLINICAL APPLICATIONS

~

Certain antiparasitic formulas may also be used to treat other gastrointestinal disorders, such as diarrhea, ulcerative colitis, and irritable bowel syndrome.

~

Antiparasitic formulas are commonly used to treat various types of intestinal parasitic infestations.

- **Parasitic infestations**: The mechanisms of antiparasitic formulas are attributed to two actions: they directly kill parasites,[1] or they paralyze the muscles of the parasites, inhibit their mobility, and thereby facilitate their elimination from the intestines (parasites with paralyzed muscles cannot physically attach to the intestines of the host, and will be expelled).[2,3] Clinical applications of these formulas include ascariasis (roundworms),[4,5] oxyuriasis (pinworms),[8] cestodiasis (tapeworms),[6] ancylostomiasis (hookworms),[6] biliary ascariasis (roundworms),[7] schistosomiasis (trematode worms),[8] and blood flukes.[9] *Wu Mei Wan* (Mume Pill) is one of the most commonly used formulas in treatment of intestinal parasites.
- **Others**: In addition to treating parasites, certain antiparasitic formulas may also be used to treat other gastrointestinal disorders, such as diarrhea,[10] ulcerative colitis,[11] and irritable bowel syndrome.[12]

1290

Chapter 20 — Overview

References

1. *Zhe Jiang Yi Ke Da Xue Xue Bao* (Journal of Zhejiang Province School of Medicine) 1980;9(1):1.
2. *Fu Jian Zhong Yi Yao* (Fujian Chinese Medicine and Herbology) 1960;6:29.
3. *Zhong Cao Yao* (Chinese Herbal Medicine) 1987;4:28.
4. *Fu Jian Zhong Yi Yao* (Fujian Chinese Medicine and Herbology) 1960;4:20.
5. *Jiang Su Zhong Yi* (Jiangsu Chinese Medicine) 1959;9:64.
6. *Zhe Jiang Zhong Yi Za Zhi* (Zhejiang Journal of Chinese Medicine) 1960;2:65.
7. *Xin Zhong Yi* (New Chinese Medicine) 1995;1:49.
8. *Zhe Jiang Zhong Yi Za Zhi* (Zhejiang Journal of Chinese Medicine) 1984;1:15.
9. *Guang Dong Zhong Yi* (Guangdong Chinese Medicine) 1959;4(7):307.
10. *Jiang Xi Zhong Yi Yao* (Jiangxi Chinese Medicine and Herbology) 1990;6:45.
11. *Xin Zhong Yi* (New Chinese Medicine) 1981;6:26.
12. *Gan Su Zhong Yi* (Gansu Chinese Medicine) 1995;4:24.

Chapter 20 – Antiparasitic Formulas

Wū Méi Wán (Mume Pill)

烏梅丸
乌梅丸

Pinyin Name: *Wu Mei Wan*
Literal Name: Mume Pill
Alternate Name: Mume Formula
Original Source: *Shang Han Lun* (Discussion of Cold-Induced Disorders) by Zhang Zhong-Jing in the Eastern Han Dynasty

COMPOSITION

Wu Mei (Fructus Mume)	300 pieces or 480g [30g]
Hua Jiao (Pericarpium Zanthoxyli), *chao* (dry-fried) till aromatic	120g [6g]
Xi Xin (Radix et Rhizoma Asari)	180g [3g]
Huang Lian (Rhizoma Coptidis)	480g [6g]
Huang Bo (Cortex Phellodendri Chinensis)	180g [6g]
Gan Jiang (Rhizoma Zingiberis)	300g [9g]
Gui Zhi (Ramulus Cinnamomi)	180g [6g]
Fu Zi (Radix Aconiti Lateralis Praeparata), *pao* (blast-fried)	180g [6g]
Ren Shen (Radix et Rhizoma Ginseng)	180g [6g]
Dang Gui (Radix Angelicae Sinensis)	120g [6g]

DOSAGE / PREPARATION / ADMINISTRATION

The source text states to steep *Wu Mei* (Fructus Mume) in a 50% vinegar solution overnight, then remove the pit and mash the fruit. Dry the mashed fruit under the sun, then mix it with the rest of the ingredients and grind them into powder, and form into pills with honey. The pills should resemble the size of *Wu Tong Zi* (Semen Firmianae), a small seed approximately 5 mm in diameter. Take 10 pills [9g] three times daily on an empty stomach with warm, boiled water. Today, this formula may be prepared as a decoction with the doses suggested in brackets. The source text states to avoid cold, raw, or spoiled foods during medication.

CHINESE THERAPEUTIC ACTIONS

1. Warms the internal organs
2. Calms roundworms

CLINICAL MANIFESTATIONS

Ascariasis (roundworms) characterized by heat in the Stomach and cold in the Intestines: irritability, recurrent nausea and vomiting, ingestion of food followed by vomiting of roundworms, extremely cold hands and feet, and abdominal pain; also for chronic dysentery and diarrhea.

CLINICAL APPLICATIONS

Ascariasis (biliary ascariasis, intestinal ascariasis, and ascariasis in children), hookworms, schistosomiasis, chronic gastritis, bacterial dysentery, chronic dysentery, ulcerative colitis, irritable bowel syndrome, chronic diarrhea, cholecystitis, and cholelithiasis.

EXPLANATION

Wu Mei Wan (Mume Pill) treats roundworms characterized by heat in the Stomach and cold in the Intestines. According to traditional Chinese medicine, roundworms prefer warmth and have aversion to cold. So while they reside in the intestines, they constantly move toward the stomach in search of warmth and food. However, their presence and movement disrupt the normal qi flow in the Stomach and Intestines, causing symptoms such as abdominal pain, irritability, recurrent nausea and vomiting, and ingestion of food followed by vomiting of ascaris. In cases of severe pain, the flow of yin and yang qi will be disrupted, causing extremely cold hands and feet.

Treatment of intestinal parasites follows the principle that "sweet taste [of herbs] induces movement [of the parasites], sour taste induces tranquility, acrid taste induces suppression, and bitter taste induces downward movement." *Wu Mei* (Fructus Mume), a sour herb processed with vinegar, calms parasites. *Hua Jiao* (Pericarpium Zanthoxyli) and *Xi Xin* (Radix et Rhizoma Asari) are acrid and warm herbs that warm the interior, dispel cold, and suppress the movement of parasites. *Huang Lian* (Rhizoma Coptidis) and *Huang Bo* (Cortex Phellodendri Chinensis) are bitter and cold herbs that clear heat and drain parasites downward. *Gan Jiang* (Rhizoma Zingiberis), *Gui Zhi* (Ramulus Cinnamomi), and *Fu Zi* (Radix Aconiti Lateralis Praeparata) are acrid and hot herbs that warm the interior and dispel cold. In using herbs that are sour, acrid and bitter, this formula effectively calms the parasites, suppresses their movement,

Chinese Herbal Formulas and Applications

Wū Méi Wán (Mume Pill)

Wu Mei Wan (Mume Pill)

Diagnosis	Signs and Symptoms	Treatment	Herbs
Ascariasis infection characterized by heat and cold	• Irritability, recurrent nausea and vomiting, ingestion of food followed by vomiting: roundworms • Severe pain and cold limbs: disrupted yin and yang qi circulation • Chronic dysentery and diarrhea: underlying deficiency	• Warms the internal organs • Calms parasites	• *Wu Mei* (Fructus Mume) calms parasites. • *Hua Jiao* (Pericarpium Zanthoxyli) and *Xi Xin* (Radix et Rhizoma Asari) warm the interior, dispel cold, and suppress the movement of parasites. • *Gan Jiang* (Rhizoma Zingiberis), *Gui Zhi* (Ramulus Cinnamomi), and *Fu Zi* (Radix Aconiti Lateralis Praeparata) warm the interior and dispel cold. • *Huang Lian* (Rhizoma Coptidis) and *Huang Bo* (Cortex Phellodendri Chinensis) clear heat and drain parasites downward. • *Ren Shen* (Radix et Rhizoma Ginseng) and *Dang Gui* (Radix Angelicae Sinensis) tonify qi and blood.

and drains them out of the body via defecation. Moreover, it uses both cold herbs to clear heat in the Stomach and hot herbs to dispel cold in the Intestines. Since chronic parasitic infestation often causes generalized weakness and deficiency, this formula contains *Ren Shen* (Radix et Rhizoma Ginseng) and *Dang Gui* (Radix Angelicae Sinensis) to tonify qi and blood.

Interestingly, this formula can treat chronic dysentery and diarrhea with deficiency of *zheng* (upright) *qi*, because such cases are often complicated by the simultaneous presence of cold and heat.

MODIFICATIONS

• To enhance the antiparasitic effect, add *Shi Jun Zi* (Fructus Quisqualis), *Ku Lian Pi* (Cortex Meliae), *Fei Zi* (Semen Torreyae), and *Bing Lang* (Semen Arecae).
• With vomiting, add *Wu Zhu Yu* (Fructus Evodiae) and *Ban Xia* (Rhizoma Pinelliae).
• With severe abdominal pain, add *Mu Xiang* (Radix Aucklandiae) and *Chuan Lian Zi* (Fructus Toosendan).
• With constipation, add *Da Huang* (Radix et Rhizoma Rhei) and *Bing Lang* (Semen Arecae).
• For patients without deficiencies, remove *Ren Shen* (Radix et Rhizoma Ginseng) and *Dang Gui* (Radix Angelicae Sinensis).
• With more heat, remove *Fu Zi* (Radix Aconiti Lateralis Praeparata) and *Gan Jiang* (Rhizoma Zingiberis).
• With more cold, remove *Huang Lian* (Rhizoma Coptidis) and *Huang Bo* (Cortex Phellodendri Chinensis).

CAUTIONS / CONTRAINDICATIONS

• *Wu Mei Wan* may be used to treat chronic dysentery and diarrhea with deficiency of *zheng* (upright) *qi*, if it is

characterized by the presence of cold and heat at the same time. Do not use this formula, however, if the dysentery and diarrhea are due to damp-heat.
• This formula should be used with caution during pregnancy.[1]

PHARMACOLOGICAL EFFECTS

1. **Antiparasitic**: *Wu Mei Wan* has been shown to have marked antiparasitic effects against roundworms. The mechanism of this action is attributed to the paralyzing effect of the formula, as the herbs do not actually kill the parasites. It has been suggested that the herbs paralyze the muscles of the parasites, inhibit their mobility, and thereby facilitate the elimination from the intestines.[2,3]
2. **Cholagogic**: *Wu Mei Wan* has been shown to have a stimulating effect on the liver and gallbladder. It increases the production of bile acid by the liver, and stimulates the contraction of the gallbladder.[4,5]
3. **Antibiotic**: Many herbs in *Wu Mei Wan* have shown marked inhibitory effects against various micro-organisms.[6]

CLINICAL STUDIES AND RESEARCH

1. **Intestinal ascariasis (roundworms)**: In one study of 8 patients, intestinal obstruction caused by ascariasis was treated effectively using *Wu Mei Wan*. Most patients experienced relief of abdominal pain within 1-2 doses, and complete resolution of the condition in 3 days.[7] Another study of patients also reported marked success expelling roundworms using modified *Wu Mei Wan*, with the addition of *Shi Jun Zi* (Fructus Quisqualis) and *Chuan Lian Zi* (Fructus Toosendan). The treatment protocol was to administer modified *Wu Mei Wan* first to paralyze the roundworms, followed by purgative herbs to expel them with the stools from the intestines.[8]

ANTIPARASITIC FORMULAS

20

1293

Chapter 20 – Antiparasitic Formulas

Wū Méi Wán (Mume Pill)

2. **Biliary ascariasis (roundworms)**: One study of 48 patients reported marked success within 2-13 days using both acupuncture and *Wu Mei Wan* to treat biliary ascariasis.[9] Another study reported good results to relieve pain within 1-3 packs of herbs in 30 of 31 patients using *Wu Mei Wan* plus *Mu Xiang* (Radix Aucklandiae), *Bing Lang* (Semen Arecae) and others.[10] Furthermore, use of modified *Wu Mei Wan* in 40 patients with biliary ascariasis was associated with a 95% effectiveness. The duration of treatment varied between 2-6 doses.[11] Lastly, one study reported successful treatment of biliary ascariasis in 10 of 11 patients. The herbal treatment was based on *Wu Mei Wan*, with removal of *Huang Bo* (Cortex Phellodendri Chinensis), and the addition of *Wu Zhu Yu* (Fructus Evodiae), *Chuan Lian Zi* (Fructus Toosendan), *Zhi Gan Cao* (Radix et Rhizoma Glycyrrhizae Praeparata cum Melle), and others.[12]

3. **Ascariasis (roundworms) in children**: Complete recovery was reported in 24 patients with intestinal ascariasis when treated with modified *Wu Mei Wan*. Modifications were made based on the presentation of the individuals. For excess heat, *Huang Qin* (Radix Scutellariae) was added, the dose of *Huang Lian* (Rhizoma Coptidis) was increased, and the doses of *Gan Jiang* (Rhizoma Zingiberis) and *Hua Jiao* (Pericarpium Zanthoxyli) were reduced. For excess cold, the doses of *Gan Jiang* (Rhizoma Zingiberis) and *Hua Jiao* (Pericarpium Zanthoxyli) were increased, and the dose of *Huang Lian* (Rhizoma Coptidis) was reduced. For severe abdominal pain, the doses of *Hua Jiao* (Pericarpium Zanthoxyli) and *Gan Cao* (Radix et Rhizoma Glycyrrhizae) were increased, and *Yan Hu Suo* (Rhizoma Corydalis), *Wu Zhu Yu* (Fructus Evodiae), and *Bai Shao* (Radix Paeoniae Alba) were added. For severe nausea and vomiting, the doses of *Wu Mei* (Fructus Mume), *Ban Xia* (Rhizoma Pinelliae), and *Hua Jiao* (Pericarpium Zanthoxyli) were increased, and *Dou Kou* (Fructus Amomi Rotundus) and *Zhu Ru* (Caulis Bambusae in Taenia) were added.[13]

4. **Ancylostomiasis (hookworms)**: One study reported 53.2% effectiveness using *Wu Mei Wan* to treat 60 patients with hookworm infestation.[14]

5. **Schistosomiasis (trematode worms)**: Three hundred and nineteen patients with schistosomiasis were treated with 92.4% effectiveness and 75.9% rate of recovery using *Wu Mei Wan* plus *Da Chai Hu Tang* (Major Bupleurum Decoction) in decoction or pills. The decoction was given once every other day. The pills were made by grinding all the herbs into a fine powder and mixing with honey to make pills. Ten grams of pills were taken per dose, twice daily. The treatment protocol was to use decoctions for acute cases, and pills for chronic cases.[15]

6. **Chronic diarrhea**: Rectal instillation of *Wu Mei Wan* showed 97.8% effectiveness in treating 47 patients with chronic diarrhea of 2-20 years. The treatment protocol was to cook the herbs to yield 200 mL of herbal solution and instill 100 mL of the herbal solution rectally twice daily in the morning and at night.[16]

7. **Bacterial dysentery**: Use of modified *Wu Mei Wan* was associated with complete recovery in 53 of 60 patients with bacterial dysentery. The herbal treatment contained *Wu Mei Wan* plus *Hua Shi* (Talcum) as the base formula. Furthermore, *Gui Zhi* (Ramulus Cinnamomi) and *Xi Xin* (Radix et Rhizoma Asari) were added for aversion to cold; *Ban Xia* (Rhizoma Pinelliae) for nausea and vomiting; *Chi Shao* (Radix Paeoniae Rubra) and *Mu Xiang* (Radix Aucklandiae) for abdominal pain; and *Da Huang* (Radix et Rhizoma Rhei) for rectal tenesmus.[17]

8. **Ulcerative colitis**: According to one study, 25 patients with chronic ulcerative colitis were treated with modified *Wu Mei Wan* with complete recovery in 16 cases, improvement in 7 cases, and no effect in 2 cases.[18]

9. **Irritable bowel syndrome (IBS)**: Use of modified *Wu Mei Wan* was associated with 91% effectiveness in treating IBS in 34 patients (23 males and 11 females). Modifications to *Wu Mei Wan* included the addition of *Ying Su Ke* (Pericarpium Papaveris) and *Yan Hu Suo* (Rhizoma Corydalis) for abdominal pain; dry-fried *Yi Yi Ren* (Semen Coicis) and *Bu Gu Zhi* (Fructus Psoraleae) for diarrhea; *Bai Shao* (Radix Paeoniae Alba) and *Huo Ma Ren* (Fructus Cannabis) for constipation; ginger-processed *Ban Xia* (Rhizoma Pinelliae) and *Zhe Shi* (Haematitum) for nausea and belching. Of 34 patients, the study reported complete recovery in 18 cases, significant improvement in 6 cases, and no response in 3 cases.[19]

10. **Cholecystitis**: One study reported 97.5% effectiveness in treating cholecystitis using modified *Wu Mei Wan*. For acute cholecystitis, *Jin Qian Cao* (Herba Lysimachiae) was added and *Dang Shen* (Radix Codonopsis) was removed from the formula. For chronic illness, *Ji Nei Jin* (Endothelium Corneum Gigeriae Galli) was added. The treatment protocol was to cook the herbs and administer the decoction in two to three equally-divided doses, followed by 10-30 mL of rice vinegar. Of 40 patients, the study reported complete recovery in 12 cases, marked improvement in 15 cases, moderate improvement in 12 cases, and no effect in 1 case.[20]

11. **Cholelithiasis**: Use of modified *Wu Mei Wan* was associated with good result in treating 40 cases of cholelithiasis. In addition to the base formula, *Da Huang* (Radix et Rhizoma Rhei) and *Pu Gong Ying* (Herba Taraxaci) were added for excess heat; larger doses of *Fu*

1294

Wū Méi Wán (Mume Pill)

Zi (Radix Aconiti Lateralis Praeparata) and *Gan Jiang* (Rhizoma Zingiberis) were used for excess cold; *Jiang Huang* (Rhizoma Curcumae Longae) and *Chuan Lian Zi* (Fructus Toosendan) for severe hypochondriac pain; *Ban Xia* (Rhizoma Pinelliae) and *Ru Xiang* (Gummi Olibanum) for nausea and vomiting; and *Yin Chen* (Herba Artemisiae Scopariae) and *Yu Jin* (Radix Curcumae) for jaundice. The duration of treatment was 1-3 courses, with 30 days per course. Of 47 patients, the study reported complete resolution in 5 cases, marked improvement in 16 cases, moderate improvement in 20 cases, and no effect in 6 cases. The overall effectiveness was 87.23%.[21]

RELATED FORMULAS

Lǐ Zhōng Ān Huí Tāng
(Regulate the Middle and Calm Roundworms Decoction)

理中安蛔湯
理中安蛔汤

Pinyin Name: *Li Zhong An Hui Tang*
Literal Name: Regulate the Middle and Calm Roundworms Decoction
Original Source: *Wan Bing Hui Chun* (Restoration of Health from the Myriad Diseases) by Gong Ting-Xian in 1587

Ren Shen (Radix et Rhizoma Ginseng)	2.1g
Bai Zhu (Rhizoma Atractylodis Macrocephalae)	3g
Fu Ling (Poria)	3g
Hua Jiao (Pericarpium Zanthoxyli)	0.9g [3g]
Wu Mei (Fructus Mume)	0.9g [3g]
Gan Jiang (Rhizoma Zingiberis), *chao* (dry-fried) to black	1.5g [2g]

The source text states to prepare the ingredients as a decoction. Today this formula can be prepared in pill form by proportionally increasing the doses of the ingredients, grinding them into a fine powder, and mixing the powder with honey to form pills. Take 5g of the pills three times daily with boiled water on an empty stomach. This formula may be prepared as a decoction with the doses suggested in brackets.

Li Zhong An Hui Tang (Regulate the Middle and Calm Roundworms Decoction) warms the middle *jiao* and expels internal parasites (namely ascariasis infestation). Clinically, it is often used for patients with ascaris and yang deficiency and cold in the middle *jiao*, characterized by loose stools, clear urine, polyuria, abdominal pain, borborygmus, cold limbs, a thin, white tongue coating, and a deficient, moderate pulse. Sometimes ascaris may even be found in the vomitus or stool.

Lián Méi Ān Huí Tāng
(Picrorhiza and Mume Decoction to Calm Roundworms)

連梅安蛔湯
连梅安蛔汤

Pinyin Name: *Lian Mei An Hui Tang*
Literal Name: Picrorhiza and Mume Decoction to Calm Roundworms
Original Source: *Tong Su Shang Han Lun* (Plain Version of Discussion of Cold-Induced Disorders) by Yu Gen-Chu in the Qing Dynasty

Hu Huang Lian (Rhizoma Picrorhizae)	3g
Hua Jiao (Pericarpium Zanthoxyli), *chao* (dry-fried)	10 pieces [1.5g]
Lei Wan (Omphalia)	9g
Wu Mei (Fructus Mume)	2 pieces [6g]
Huang Bo (Cortex Phellodendri Chinensis)	2.4g
Bing Lang (Semen Arecae), *qie* (sliced)	2 pieces [9g]

The source text states to prepare the ingredients as a decoction. Cook the herbs in water and decoct three times, then mix all three batches of the decoction together. Take the herbs on an empty stomach three times daily (twice in the morning and one time in the afternoon).

Lian Mei An Hui Tang (Picrorhiza and Mume Decoction to Calm Roundworms) clears heat and expels internal parasites. Clinical manifestations include abdominal pain, lack of appetite, vomiting with ascaris upon eating, fidgeting, irritability, a red face, feverish sensations, dry mouth, a red tongue body, and a rapid pulse.

AUTHORS' COMMENTS

Wu Mei Wan is the representative formula for treating ascariasis. The key signs and symptoms include abdominal pain, recurrent nausea and vomiting, ingestion of food followed by vomiting of ascaris, and cold limbs.

Wu Mei Wan, *Li Zhong An Hui Tang* (Regulate the Middle and Calm Roundworms Decoction) and *Lian Mei An Hui Tang* (Picrorhiza and Mume Decoction to Calm Roundworms) are three formulas that treat ascariasis.

- *Wu Mei Wan* is the most potent formula that treats severe cases of ascariasis characterized by underlying deficiency and excess, with interlocking of heat (in the Stomach) and cold (in the Intestines).
- *Li Zhong An Hui Tang* warms yang and dispels cold to treat ascariasis characterized by deficiency and cold of the middle *jiao*.
- *Lian Mei An Hui Tang* clears heat to treat cases of ascariasis characterized by Liver fire and Stomach heat.

Chapter 20 – Antiparasitic Formulas

Wū Méi Wán (Mume Pill)

References

1. *Zhong Yao Ming Fang Yao Li Yu Ying Yong* (Pharmacology and Applications of Famous Herbal Formulas) 1989;636-7.
2. *Fu Jian Zhong Yi Yao* (Fujian Chinese Medicine and Herbology) 1960;6:29.
3. *Zhong Cao Yao* (Chinese Herbal Medicine) 1987;4:28.
4. *Fu Jian Zhong Yi Yao* (Fujian Chinese Medicine and Herbology) 1960;6:29.
5. *Zhong Cao Yao* (Chinese Herbal Medicine) 1987;4:28.
6. *Zhong Yi Fang Ji Xian Dai Yan Jiu* (Modern Study of Medical Formulae in Traditional Chinese Medicine) 1997;1555.
7. *Fu Jian Zhong Yi Yao* (Fujian Chinese Medicine and Herbology) 1960;4:20.
8. *Jiang Su Zhong Yi* (Jiangsu Chinese Medicine) 1959;9:64.
9. *Zhong Hua Wai Ke Za Zhi* (Chinese Journal of External Medicine) 1959;6:547.
10. *Guang Xi Zhong Yi Yao* (Guangxi Chinese Medicine and Herbology) 1981;3:47.
11. *Shan Xi Zhong Yi* (Shanxi Chinese Medicine) 1985;1:37.
12. *Xin Zhong Yi* (New Chinese Medicine) 1995;1:49.
13. *Cheng Du Zhong Yi Xue Yuan Xue Bao* (Journal of Chengdu University of Traditional Chinese Medicine) 1960;1:45.
14. *Zhe Jiang Zhong Yi Za Zhi* (Zhejiang Journal of Chinese Medicine) 1960;2:65.
15. *Zhe Jiang Zhong Yi Za Zhi* (Zhejiang Journal of Chinese Medicine) 1984;1:15.
16. *Jiang Xi Zhong Yi Yao* (Jiangxi Chinese Medicine and Herbology) 1990;6:45.
17. *Guang Xi Zhong Yi Yao* (Guangxi Chinese Medicine and Herbology) 1981;3:21.
18. *Xin Zhong Yi* (New Chinese Medicine) 1981;6:26.
19. *Gan Su Zhong Yi* (Gansu Chinese Medicine) 1995;4:24.
20. *Shan Xi Zhong Yi* (Shanxi Chinese Medicine) 1993;7:316.
21. *Zhong Yi Ming Fang Lin Chuang Xin Yong* (Contemporary Clinical Applications of Classic Chinese Formulas) 2001;153-4.

Féi Ér Wán (Fat Child Pill)
肥兒丸
肥儿丸

Pinyin Name: *Fei Er Wan*
Literal Name: Fat Child Pill
Original Source: *Tai Ping Hui Min He Ji Ju Fang* (Imperial Grace Formulary of the Tai Ping Era) by the Imperial Medical Department in 1078-85

COMPOSITION

Shen Qu (Massa Fermentata), *chao* (dry-fried)	300g
Mai Ya (Fructus Hordei Germinatus), *chao* (dry-fried)	150g
Huang Lian (Rhizoma Coptidis)	300g
Rou Dou Kou (Semen Myristicae), *wei* (roasted)	150g
Mu Xiang (Radix Aucklandiae)	60g
Bing Lang (Semen Arecae), *cuo* (grated) into thin particles and sun-dried 20 pieces [120g]	
Shi Jun Zi (Fructus Quisqualis)	150g

DOSAGE / PREPARATION / ADMINISTRATION

The source text states to grind the ingredients into a fine powder and form into small pills using bile from a pig's gallbladder. The pills should resemble *Su Mi* (Semen Setariae) in size. Take 30 pills daily on an empty stomach with warm, boiled water. Adjust the dose depending on the age of the patient.

Today, this formula is prepared by grinding the ingredients and sifting the resultant powders together. The mixed powder is then formed into small pills [3g each] using fresh bile from the gallbladder of a pig. Dissolve 1 pill in boiled water and take it on an empty stomach. Reduce the dose for infants under one year of age.

1296

Féi Ér Wán (Fat Child Pill)

CHINESE THERAPEUTIC ACTIONS

1. Kills parasites
2. Reduces accumulation
3. Strengthens the Spleen
4. Clears heat

CLINICAL MANIFESTATIONS

Intestinal parasites and *gan ji* (infantile malnutrition): abdominal pain, poor digestion, sallow and yellowish facial complexion, thin or emaciated appearance, lack of appetite, decreased food ingestion, loose stools, enlarged abdomen with swelling and fullness, weak constitution, low-grade fever, constant fatigue, possible nausea and vomiting, dry mouth and thirst, and foul breath.

CLINICAL APPLICATIONS

Parasitic infestation and infantile malnutrition.

EXPLANATION

Fei Er Wan (Fat Child Pill) treats patients with intestinal parasites with abdominal pain and poor digestion. Chronic parasitic infestation may cause *gan ji* (infantile malnutrition) characterized by Spleen deficiency and Stomach heat, with symptoms such as thin or emaciated appearance, enlarged abdomen, fever, foul breath, and loose stools.

This formula contains *Shen Qu* (Massa Fermentata) and *Mai Ya* (Fructus Hordei Germinatus) to strengthen the Spleen, harmonize the middle *jiao*, and reduce food stagnation. *Huang Lian* (Rhizoma Coptidis) clears Stomach heat. *Rou Dou Kou* (Semen Myristicae), an aromatic herb, strengthens the Spleen and relieves loose stools. *Mu Xiang* (Radix Aucklandiae) regulates qi to relieve abdominal pain. *Bing Lang* (Semen Arecae) and *Shi Jun Zi* (Fructus Quisqualis) kill and expel parasites. Lastly, bile from a pig's gallbladder helps *Huang Lian* (Rhizoma Coptidis) clear heat from the Liver and Stomach.

MODIFICATIONS

- With dry mouth, thirst, and irritability, add *Mai Dong* (Radix Ophiopogonis) and *Wu Wei Zi* (Fructus Schisandrae Chinensis).
- With nausea, vomiting, and diarrhea, add *Ban Xia* (Rhizoma Pinelliae) and *Chen Pi* (Pericarpium Citri Reticulatae).
- With weak body constitution accompanied by alternating spells of chills and fever, add *Chai Hu* (Radix Bupleuri) and *Bai Shao* (Radix Paeoniae Alba).
- Without interior heat, remove *Huang Lian* (Rhizoma Coptidis).
- With Spleen and Stomach deficiencies, add *Ren Shen* (Radix et Rhizoma Ginseng) and *Bai Zhu* (Rhizoma Atractylodis Macrocephalae).
- With constipation, add *Da Huang* (Radix et Rhizoma Rhei) and *Zhi Shi* (Fructus Aurantii Immaturus).

CAUTIONS / CONTRAINDICATIONS

- *Fei Er Wan* should **not** be used in cases of *gan ji* (infantile malnutrition) due to Spleen and Stomach deficiencies, as many herbs that expel parasites are rather harsh and may cause more deficiencies.
- Avoid foods that are raw, cold, oily, or greasy while taking this formula.[1]

Fei Er Wan (Fat Child Pill)

Diagnosis	Signs and Symptoms	Treatment	Herbs
Intestinal parasites and *gan ji* (infantile malnutrition)	Abdominal pain and poor digestion, sallow and yellowish facial complexion, thin or emaciated appearance, enlarged abdomen, fever, foul breath, and loose stools: malnutrition due to parasitic infestation	• Kills parasites • Reduces accumulation • Strengthens the Spleen • Clears heat	• *Shen Qu* (Massa Fermentata) and *Mai Ya* (Fructus Hordei Germinatus) strengthen the Spleen, harmonize the middle *jiao*, and reduce food stagnation. • *Bing Lang* (Semen Arecae) and *Shi Jun Zi* (Fructus Quisqualis) kill and expel parasites. • *Huang Lian* (Rhizoma Coptidis) sedates Stomach heat. • *Rou Dou Kou* (Semen Myristicae) strengthens the Spleen and relieves loose stools. • *Mu Xiang* (Radix Aucklandiae) regulates qi to relieve abdominal pain.

Chapter 20 – Antiparasitic Formulas

Féi Ér Wán (Fat Child Pill)

RELATED FORMULA

Jīn Jiàn Féi Ér Wán
(Golden Pill to Construct a Fat Child)

金鑑肥兒丸
金鉴肥儿丸

Pinyin Name: *Jin Jian Fei Er Wan*
Literal Name: Golden Pill to Construct a Fat Child
Alternate Name: Ginseng and Hoelen Formula
Original Source: *Yi Zong Jin Jian* (Golden Mirror of the Medical Tradition) by Wu Qian in 1742

Ren Shen (Radix et Rhizoma Ginseng)
Bai Zhu (Rhizoma Atractylodis Macrocephalae)
Fu Ling (Poria)
Huang Lian (Rhizoma Coptidis)
Hu Huang Lian (Rhizoma Picrorhizae)
Shi Jun Zi (Fructus Quisqualis)
Shen Qu (Massa Fermentata)
Mai Ya (Fructus Hordei Germinatus)
Shan Zha (Fructus Crataegi)
Gan Cao (Radix et Rhizoma Glycyrrhizae)
Lu Hui (Aloe)

Jin Jian Fei Er Wan (Golden Pill to Construct a Fat Child) treats malnutrition in children or infants due to parasitic infestation. Intestinal parasites, transmitted via oral-anal route, create internal heat and then affect the gastrointestinal tract. Immediate signs and symptoms of parasitic infestation include lack of appetite, decreased food ingestion, dry mouth, thirst, and possibly nausea and vomiting. With chronic parasitic infestation, proper digestion and absorption of food will be compromised, leading to malnutrition characterized by a sallow facial appearance, muscle wasting, weak constitution, low-grade fever, and constant fatigue. The abdomen is often enlarged due to parasites.

Jin Jian Fei Er Wan incorporates *Si Jun Zi Tang* (Four-Gentlemen Decoction) as the base to strengthen the Spleen and tonify qi. In this formula, *Ren Shen* (Radix et Rhizoma Ginseng) tonifies *yuan* (source) qi as well as Spleen and Stomach qi. *Bai Zhu* (Rhizoma Atractylodis Macrocephalae), in addition to tonifying Spleen qi, also dries dampness in the middle *jiao* to strengthen digestion. *Fu Ling* (Poria) tonifies and dispels dampness in the middle *jiao* through diuresis. *Gan Cao* (Radix et Rhizoma Glycyrrhizae) tonifies Spleen qi and harmonizes the herbs in this formula. *Shan Zha* (Fructus Crataegi), *Mai Ya* (Fructus Hordei Germinatus), and *Shen Qu* (Massa Fermentata) promote digestion and eliminate food stagnation. *Shan Zha* (Fructus Crataegi) is most effective in digesting meat (protein) and fatty food; *Mai Ya* (Fructus Hordei Germinatus) is most effective in digesting carbohydrates; and *Shen Qu* (Massa Fermentata) is most effective in digesting alcohol and spoiled or rotten food. *Huang Lian* (Rhizoma Coptidis) clears damp-heat, which is common with food stagnation. *Shi Jun Zi* (Fructus Quisqualis), *Hu Huang Lian* (Rhizoma Picrorhizae), and *Lu Hui* (Aloe) have antiparasitic effects. They kill and expel intestinal parasites, treating the underlying cause of malnutrition.

Fei Er Wan (Fat Child Pill) and *Jin Jian Fei Er Wan* (Golden Pill to Construct a Fat Child) have similar names and functions to treat *gan ji* (infantile malnutrition) associated with parasitic infestation.

- *Fei Er Wan* focuses more on killing parasites and reducing accumulation, and less on strengthening the Spleen.
- *Jin Jian Fei Er Wan* emphasizes primarily on strengthening the Spleen and promoting digestion. Killing and expelling parasites are secondary functions.

Reference
1. *Zhong Yao Ming Fang Yao Li Yu Ying Yong* (Pharmacology and Applications of Famous Herbal Formulas) 1989;638.

1298

Chinese Herbal Formulas and Applications

Bù Dài Wán (Cloth Sack Pill)

布袋丸

Pinyin Name: *Bu Dai Wan*
Literal Name: Cloth Sack Pill
Original Source: *Bu Yao Xiu Zhen Xiao Er Fang Lun* (Supplement to the Pocket-Sized Discussion of Formulas for Children)

COMPOSITION

Wu Yi (Fructus Ulmi Praeparatus), *chao* (dry-fried)	60g
Shi Jun Zi (Fructus Quisqualis), *chao* (dry-fried)	60g
Lu Hui (Aloe), *yan* (ground) into thin particles	15g
Ye Ming Sha (Faeces Vespertilionis Murini), *jing* (cleaned)	60g
Ren Shen (Radix et Rhizoma Ginseng)	15g
Bai Zhu (Rhizoma Atractylodis Macrocephalae)	15g
Fu Ling (Poria)	15g
Gan Cao (Radix et Rhizoma Glycyrrhizae)	15g

DOSAGE / PREPARATION / ADMINISTRATION

The source text states to grind the ingredients into a fine powder, and form into large pills with water. Each pill should resemble a large bullet, and weigh approximately 10g. For administration, place 1 pill in a cheesecloth and cook it with 60g of pork in water until the pork is thoroughly cooked. The pork and the soup are given to children as medication. The pill in the cheesecloth may be used again the next day.

Today, this formula is normally prepared as a powder by proportionally adjusting all of the ingredients and grinding them into powder. Take 3g of powder with pork soup on an empty stomach in the morning upon awakening.

CHINESE THERAPEUTIC ACTIONS

1. Dispels roundworms and treats *gan ji* (infantile malnutrition)
2. Tonifies and strengthens the Spleen and Stomach

CLINICAL MANIFESTATIONS

Parasitic infestation with *gan ji* (infantile malnutrition) in infants and children: feeling of warmth in the body, sallow facial appearance, enlarged and distended abdomen, skinny arms and legs, dry, lusterless hair, and dull eyes.

CLINICAL APPLICATIONS

Parasitic infestation and malnutrition.

EXPLANATION

Bu Dai Wan (Cloth Sack Pill) treats parasitic infestation in infants and children with Spleen deficiency. Chronic infestation of parasites may lead to Spleen and Stomach deficiencies, leading to skinny limbs. With chronic illness, deficiency heat rises to cause the feeling of warmth in the body. The abdominal distention is due to Spleen and Stomach qi deficiencies and stagnation. Because of decreased absorption of nutrients due to Spleen and Stomach deficiencies, less blood is produced, resulting

Bu Dai Wan (Cloth Sack Pill)

Diagnosis	Signs and Symptoms	Treatment	Herbs
Parasitic infestation and *gan ji* (infantile malnutrition)	Sallow facial appearance, enlarged and distended abdomen, skinny arms and legs, dry and lusterless hair, and dull eyes: malnutrition due to parasitic infestation	• Dispels roundworms and treats *gan ji* (infantile malnutrition) • Tonifies and strengthens the Spleen and Stomach	• *Wu Yi* (Fructus Ulmi Praeparatus) and *Shi Jun Zi* (Fructus Quisqualis) expel roundworms and treat *gan ji* (infantile malnutrition). • *Lu Hui* (Aloe) expels parasites by purging them out of the body through the bowels. • *Ye Ming Sha* (Faeces Vespertilionis Murini) clears Liver heat and brightens the vision. • *Ren Shen* (Radix et Rhizoma Ginseng), *Bai Zhu* (Rhizoma Atractylodis Macrocephalae), *Fu Ling* (Poria), and *Gan Cao* (Radix et Rhizoma Glycyrrhizae) tonify the Spleen and Stomach.

ANTIPARASITIC FORMULAS

20

1299

Chapter 20 – Antiparasitic Formulas

Bù Dài Wán (Cloth Sack Pill)

in a sallow facial appearance, dry, lusterless hair, and dull eyes.

Acrid, bitter, and warm *Wu Yi* (Fructus Ulmi Praeparatus) is combined with sweet and warm *Shi Jun Zi* (Fructus Quisqualis) in this formula to expel roundworms and treat *gan ji* (infantile malnutrition). Bitter and cold *Lu Hui* (Aloe) expels the parasites by purging them out of the body through the bowels. *Ye Ming Sha* (Faeces Vespertilionis Murini) clears Liver heat and brightens the vision. Since the root of this syndrome is Spleen and Stomach deficiencies, *Ren Shen* (Radix et Rhizoma Ginseng), *Bai Zhu* (Rhizoma Atractylodis Macrocephalae), *Fu Ling* (Poria), and *Gan Cao* (Radix et Rhizoma Glycyrrhizae) are used to tonify the Spleen and Stomach. Indeed, this formula functions on both tonic and sedative levels. It safely and effectively sedates heat and removes parasites without injuring the Spleen and Stomach.

MODIFICATIONS

- With more heat, add *Huang Lian* (Rhizoma Coptidis).
- With food stagnation, add *Shen Qu* (Massa Fermentata) and *Ji Nei Jin* (Endothelium Corneum Gigeriae Galli).

AUTHORS' COMMENTS

Bu Dai Wan is a formula that treats chronic parasitic infestation in infants and children with malnutrition. While the parasites are considered as an excess condition, the underlying malnutrition represents a deficiency condition. Because of the complexity of this condition, antiparasitic herbs that expel parasites must be used together with tonic herbs to address the underlying deficiencies. Lastly, this formula is prepared with pork for two reasons: 1) to mask the taste of the herbs and improve compliancy in infants and children who often dislike taking bitter herbs, and 2) its nourishing effect enhances the tonic herbs to treat *gan ji* (infantile malnutrition).

Huà Chóng Wán (Dissolve Parasites Pill)

化蟲丸
化虫丸

Pinyin Name: *Hua Chong Wan*
Literal Name: Dissolve Parasites Pill
Original Source: *Tai Ping Hui Min He Ji Ju Fang* (Imperial Grace Formulary of the Tai Ping Era) by the Imperial Medical Department in 1078-85

COMPOSITION

He Shi (Fructus Carpesii)	1,500g
Ku Lian Pi (Cortex Meliae)	1,500g
Bing Lang (Semen Arecae)	1,500g
Bai Fan (Alumen)	375g
Qian Dan (Minium), *chao* (dry-fried)	1,500g

Note: *Qian Dan* (Minium) is a potentially toxic heavy metal, and is rarely used as a medicinal substance today. Its discussion here is included primarily for academic purposes, to reflect the historical use of this substance in its original formulation. Most herbal products today have removed it completely, or replaced it with substitutes with similar functions. For additional information on the toxicity, please refer to *Chinese Medical Herbology and Pharmacology* by John Chen and Tina Chen.

DOSAGE / PREPARATION / ADMINISTRATION

The source text states to grind the ingredients into a fine powder and form into very small pills with flour. The pills should resemble *Huo Ma Ren* (Fructus Cannabis) in size. For infant around one year of age, take 5 pills anytime during the day. The pills may be taken with warm rice soup, or warm, boiled water plus 1-2 drops of sesame oil.

1300

Chinese Herbal Formulas and Applications

Huà Chóng Wán (Dissolve Parasites Pill)

CHINESE THERAPEUTIC ACTIONS
Expels and kills various intestinal parasites

CLINICAL MANIFESTATIONS
Intestinal parasites: intermittent severe pain migrating up and down the abdomen, nausea, and vomiting of clear fluids or parasites.

CLINICAL APPLICATIONS
Ascariasis (roundworms), oxyuriasis (pinworms), cestodiasis (tapeworms), cysticercosis (bladder worms), and fasciolopsiasis (intestinal flukes).

EXPLANATION
Hua Chong Wan (Dissolve Parasites Pill) is designed to treat retention of parasites in the intestines. The intermittent severe pain migrating up and down the abdomen is due to upward movement of the parasites. If the parasites affect the Stomach qi flow and cause rising Stomach qi, vomiting of clear fluids or parasites will occur.

This formula contains bitter, acrid, and slightly toxic *He Shi* (Fructus Carpesii) to kill and expel roundworms, pinworms and tapeworms. Bitter, cold, and toxic, *Ku Lian Pi* (Cortex Meliae) relieves abdominal pain and has a strong effect to kill roundworms, hookworms and pinworms. *Bing Lang* (Semen Arecae) activates qi to expel roundworms, tapeworms, hookworms and pinworms from the body. The astringent *Bai Fan* (Alumen) relieves toxicity and calms the parasites. Lastly, the toxic *Qian Dan* (Minium) kills all kinds of parasites.

Today, this formula is used to treat various types of parasitic infections. It can be used as a general formula to clear the intestinal pathways and expel various parasites. However, since the herbs in this formula are strong in nature, caution should be exercised in administering this formula.

To prevent possible injury to the qi, it is advisable to use Spleen and Stomach qi-tonifying herbs after administering this formula.

MODIFICATIONS
- With more abdominal pain, add *Zhi Qiao* (Fructus Aurantii) and *Mu Xiang* (Radix Aucklandiae).
- With more heat, add *Huang Lian* (Rhizoma Coptidis) or *Huang Bo* (Cortex Phellodendri Chinensis).
- With intestinal obstruction due to ascariasis (roundworms), add *Hou Po* (Cortex Magnoliae Officinalis), *Zhi Shi* (Fructus Aurantii Immaturus), *Mu Xiang* (Radix Aucklandiae), and *Da Xue Teng* (Caulis Sargentodoxae).

CAUTIONS / CONTRAINDICATIONS
- *Hua Chong Wan* is an extremely potent and slightly toxic formula for treatment of intestinal parasites. It must be used with caution in elderly patients and children. It should not be used in large doses, or for a prolonged period of time. Lastly, it should be discontinued once the desired effects are achieved. If the parasites are not completely expelled after the first dose, another dose may be given after one week of rest.
- Use of this formula is contraindicated during pregnancy, and in patients with loose stools or diarrhea.
- Because this is a potent formula that may injury the body, tonic herbs should be administered after the parasites are cleared to restore the patient's *zheng* (upright) *qi*.

AUTHORS' COMMENTS
Hua Chong Wan is a potent antiparasitic formula that may be used to treat various types of intestinal infestation of parasites, including but not limited to ascariasis (roundworms), oxyuriasis (pinworms), cestodiasis (tapeworms), cysticercosis (bladder worms), and fasciolopsiasis (intestinal flukes).

Hua Chong Wan (Dissolve Parasites Pill)

Diagnosis	Signs and Symptoms	Treatment	Herbs
Intestinal parasites	• Intermittent severe pain migrating up and down the abdomen: intestinal parasites • Nausea and vomiting: intestinal parasites affecting Stomach qi circulation	Expels and kills various intestinal parasites	• *He Shi* (Fructus Carpesii), *Ku Lian Pi* (Cortex Meliae) and *Bing Lang* (Semen Arecae) kill and expel various parasites. • *Bai Fan* (Alumen) relieves toxicity and calms the parasites. • *Qian Dan* (Minium) kills all kinds of parasites.

ANTIPARASITIC FORMULAS

20

1301

Chapter 20 – Antiparasitic Formulas

Fá Mù Wán (Quell Wood Pill)

伐木丸

Pinyin Name: *Fa Mu Wan*
Literal Name: Quell Wood Pill
Alternate Name: *Zhu Fan Wan* (Atractylodes and Melanterite Pill)
Original Source: *Zhang San Feng Xian Chuan Fang* (Divine Formulas from Zhang San-Feng)

COMPOSITION

Cang Zhu (Rhizoma Atractylodis), *jin* (soaked) in rice water and *qie* (sliced)	1,000g
Jiu Qu (Leaven), *chao* (dry-fried) to deep-red	120g
Zao Fan (Melanterite), *ban* (blended) with vinegar and *duan* (calcined) at high temperature	500g

DOSAGE / PREPARATION / ADMINISTRATION

The source text states to first prepare all three ingredients separately. Soak *Cang Zhu* (Rhizoma Atractylodis) in rice water for two nights, and then slice and dry the herb. Dry-fry *Jiu Qu* (Leaven) with the processed *Cang Zhu* (Rhizoma Atractylodis) until *Jiu Qu* (Leaven) becomes deep-red in color. Blend *Zao Fan* (Melanterite) with vinegar, allow it to dry, and calcine it at high temperature with fire. Grind all of the processed ingredients into a fine powder and form into small pills with vinegar. Take 30-40 pills two to three times daily with grain-based liquor or rice soup. Today this formula is prepared the same way, but the suggested administration has been changed to 8g of pills per dose once a day after meal with rice soup.

CHINESE THERAPEUTIC ACTIONS

1. Reduces accumulation
2. Dries dampness
3. Drains the Liver
4. Expels parasites

CLINICAL MANIFESTATIONS

Parasitic infestation (usually hookworms): a sallow facial appearance, edema, palpitations, hurried respiration, fatigue, and lack of energy.

CLINICAL APPLICATIONS

Parasitic infestation and malnutrition.

EXPLANATION

Fa Mu Wan (Quell Wood Pill) treats individuals with parasitic infestations accompanied by food accumulation and damp obstruction. Clinical presentations include a sallow facial appearance, edema, palpitations, hurried respiration, and fatigue.

This formula contains *Cang Zhu* (Rhizoma Atractylodis), a bitter and warm herb, to dry dampness. *Jiu Qu* (Leaven) promotes digestion and reduces food accumulation. *Zao Fan* (Melanterite) dissolves dampness, sedates the Liver, and expels parasites.

MODIFICATIONS

With indigestion or food stagnation, add *Ping Wei San* (Calm the Stomach Powder).

CAUTIONS / CONTRAINDICATIONS

Use of *Fa Mu Wan* has been associated with nausea and vomiting.[1]

AUTHORS' COMMENTS

This formula is called "Quell Wood Pill" because one of its main functions is to drain the Liver and soothe the wood element to prevent the Liver (wood) from overacting on the Spleen (earth).

Reference
1. *Zhong Yao Ming Fang Yao Li Yu Ying Yong* (Pharmacology and Applications of Famous Herbal Formulas) 1989;638-9.

Fa Mu Wan (Quell Wood Pill)

Diagnosis	Signs and Symptoms	Treatment	Herbs
Parasitic infestation (usually hookworms)	Sallow facial appearance, edema, palpitations, hurried respiration, and fatigue: parasites with food accumulation and damp obstruction	• Reduces accumulation • Dries dampness • Drains the Liver • Expels parasites	• *Cang Zhu* (Rhizoma Atractylodis) dries dampness. • *Jiu Qu* (Leaven) promotes digestion and reduces food accumulation. • *Zao Fan* (Melanterite) dispels dampness, sedates the Liver, and expels parasites.

1302

Chinese Herbal Formulas and Applications

Chapter 20 — Summary

— Antiparasitic Formulas

Name	Similarities	Differences
Wu Mei Wan (Mume Pill)		Tonifies deficiency
Fei Er Wan (Fat Child Pill)		Strengthens the Spleen, clears Stomach heat
Bu Dai Wan (Cloth Sack Pill)	Expel and/or kill parasites	Tonifies Spleen and Stomach deficiencies
Hua Chong Wan (Dissolve Parasites Pill)		Strongly expels and kills intestinal parasites
Fa Mu Wan (Quell Wood Pill)		Reduces food accumulation, dries dampness

Wu Mei Wan (Mume Pill) is generally used to treat ascariasis (roundworms) complicated by heat and cold, and excess and deficiency. It warms the interior, tonifies the middle *jiao*, dispels cold, and expels the parasites. It is most effective for ascariasis characterized by irritability, recurrent nausea and vomiting, ingestion of food followed by vomiting with ascaris, abdominal pain, and extremely cold limbs.

Fei Er Wan (Fat Child Pill) and *Bu Dai Wan* (Cloth Sack Pill) both treat *gan ji* (infantile malnutrition) associated with parasitic infestations.
• *Fei Er Wan* clears heat, kills parasites, and strengthens the Spleen to treat *gan ji* (infantile malnutrition). Clinically, it is used to treat *gan ji* (infantile malnutrition) characterized by Spleen deficiency and Stomach heat.
• *Bu Dai Wan* expels parasites, strengthens the Spleen, and relieves *gan ji* (infantile malnutrition). This formula contains more tonic herbs, and is more suitable for *gan ji* (infantile malnutrition) with Spleen and Stomach deficiencies.

Hua Chong Wan (Dissolve Parasites Pill) expels and kills intestinal parasites. It has potent antiparasitic effects, and may be used to treat a wide variety of parasites, including ascariasis (roundworms), oxyuriasis (pinworms), cestodiasis (tapeworms), cysticercosis (bladder worms), and fasciolopsiasis (intestinal flukes).

Fa Mu Wan (Quell Wood Pill) reduces food accumulation, dries dampness, and expels parasites. It may be used for parasitic infestation (usually hookworms) with food stagnation and damp accumulation in the middle *jiao*, with signs and symptoms such as a thin, sallow facial appearance, edema, palpitations, hurried respiration, and lack of energy.

ANTIPARASITIC FORMULAS

20

Chapter 21

— Emetic Formulas

张从正 Zhāng Cōng-Zhèng

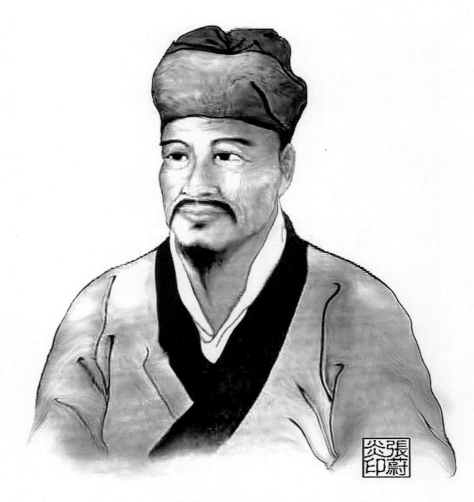

张从正 Zhāng Cōng-Zhèng, also known as
张子和 Zhāng Zǐ-Hé, 1151 – 1231.

张从正 Zhāng Cōng-Zhèng

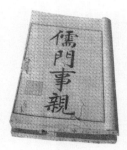

儒门事亲 *Ru Men Shi Qin* (Confucians' Duties to their Parents), published in 1228.

Zhang Cong-Zheng, also known as Zhang Zi-He, is one of the four famous physicians from the period of the Jin and Yuan dynasties. Heavily influenced by Liu Yuan-Su's theories of 火热论 *huo re lun* (discussion of fire and heat), Zhang developed 攻邪论 *gong xie lun* (discussion on attacking evil). Zhang proposed that all evils are derived from three sources: heaven (wind, cold, summer-heat, dampness, dryness and fire), earth (fog, dew, rain, ice, water and soil) and human (inappropriate diet of excessive sour, bitter, sweet, acrid, salty or bland foods). Correspondingly, all evils can be treated with three methods: *han fa* (sweating) to dispel evil at the exterior, *tu fa* (vomiting) to expel evil from upper body, and *xia fa* (draining downward) to purge evil from the lower body. In contrast to his aggressive treatment methods, Zhang also emphasized the importance of nutrition, and proposed the use of food and herbs to supplement diet and promote longevity. He was the first to establish clear guidelines for nutritional therapy.

Zhang was one of the first to establish the relationship among illnesses, the social environment and emotions. Zhang lived and practiced medicine during the end of the Jin dynasty and beginning of the Yuan dynasty, when there was extreme political instability and constant turmoil in the country. Because of this social unrest, people suffered from extreme emotional disturbances, including anger, joy, sadness, fear, worry, and other stressors.

Because of his skills and fame, Zhang was brought to the Imperial Palace as a supreme physician to treat the royal family and court officials. However, he resigned after five years, and opted to live a rambling and leisurely lifestyle that allowed him to read books, write poetry, and travel around the world. Zhang wrote many works in his lifetime, and is best known for *Ru Men Shi Qin* (Confucians' Duties to their Parents), published in 1228.

Mu Xiang Bing Lang Wan (Aucklandia and Betel Nut Pill) and *Gua Di San* (Melon Pedicle Powder) are two formulas created by Zhang Cong-Zheng that are still in use today.

Dynasties & Kingdoms	Year
Xia Dynasty 夏	2100-1600 BCE
Shang Dynasty 商	1600-1100 BCE
Zhou Dynasty 周	1100-221 BCE
Qin Dynasty 秦	221-207 BCE
Han Dynasty 漢	206 BCE-220
Three Kingdoms 三國	220-280
Western Jin Dynasty 西晉	265-316
Eastern Jin Dynasty 東晉	317-420
Northern and Southern Dynasties 北南朝	420-581
Sui Dynasty 隋	581-618
Tang Dynasty 唐	618-907
Five Dynasties 五代	907-960
Song Dynasty 宋	960-1279
Liao Dynasty 遼	916-1125
Jin Dynasty 金	**1115-1234**
Yuan Dynasty 元	1271-1368
Ming Dynasty 明	1368-1644
Qing Dynasty 清	1644-1911
Republic of China 中華民國	1912-Present Day
People's Republic of China 中華人民共和國	1949-Present Day

Chapter 21 – Emetic Formulas

Table of Contents

Chapter 21. Emetic Formulas · **1305**
Biography of Zhang Cong-Zheng · 1306

Gua Di San (Melon Pedicle Powder) · 1311
  San Sheng San (Three-Sage Powder) · 1312
Jiu Ji Xi Xian San (Urgent Powder to Dilute Saliva) · 1313
Yan Tang Tan Tu Fang (Salt Decoction to Induce Vomiting) · 1314

Emetic Formulas (Summary) · **1315**

Chinese Herbal Formulas and Applications

Chapter 21 — Overview

— Emetic Formulas

Definition: Emetic formulas induce vomiting to treat phlegm stagnation, food accumulation, and the ingestion of poisonous substances. This method of treatment is known as *tu fa* (vomiting), one of the *ba fa* (eight treatment methods) described in the *Huang Di Nei Jing* (Yellow Emperor's Inner Classic) in the first or second century, A.D.

These formulas are mainly used to dispel foreign substances from the throat, chest, diaphragm, or epigastrium. Their clinical applications include food stagnation, phlegm stagnation, ingestion of poisonous substances, convulsions, *zhong feng* (wind stroke), *bi zheng* (closed disorder) syndrome, *dian kuang* (mania and withdrawal), and *hou bi* (painful obstruction of the throat).

CAUTIONS / CONTRAINDICATIONS

- Emetic formulas are strong and harsh in nature. Therefore, they should be used with extreme caution during pregnancy, in pediatric or geriatric patients, and in cases of blood deficiency, palpitations with shortness of breath, dizziness and vertigo, wheezing and dyspnea, and generalized weakness and deficiency. Furthermore, these formulas must be discontinued once the desired effect is achieved.

- Some patients may not vomit immediately after ingestion of emetic formulas. To facilitate emesis, the patient should take the formula with warm water, and then physically induce vomiting by inserting a finger into the back of his or her throat. If the patient does not respond to emetic herbs, or if relief is not evident, he or she must immediately seek emergency medical treatment.

- The potent and harsh nature of emetic formulas can cause continuous vomiting and injure the Stomach qi. For patients who do not cease vomiting after taking the formula, general antidotes such as fresh juice of *Sheng Jiang* (Rhizoma Zingiberis Recens), cold congee, or cold water should be administered. If general antidotes do not work, specific antidotes are given. Specific antidotes vary, and are listed in each individual formula monograph.

- Proper care must be given after emesis to ensure recovery and avoid complications. In order to restore the normal functions of the Spleen and Stomach, patients should consume only congee and other easy-to-digest foods, and avoid greasy, spicy, processed foods, or other foods that are hard to digest. Also, patients should avoid exposure to wind during and after vomiting to prevent contracting an exterior condition.

- Accidental poisonings manifest in different symptoms and signs, depending on the substance ingested. The use of emetic formulas is justified within a short period of time following ingestion of a poisonous substance, when the injurious matter is still in the stomach and can be ejected by vomiting.

- Emetic formulas should **not** be used to induce vomiting if corrosive substances have been ingested; this would only cause additional damage to the upper gastrointestinal tract when the corrosive elements are ejected as vomitus. Select other methods to neutralize or remove the corrosive substances, and have the patient seek immediate emergency medical treatment.

> Emetic formulas induce vomiting and dispel foreign substances from the throat, chest, diaphragm, or epigastrium.

> Proper care must be given after emesis to ensure recovery and avoid complications.

EMETIC FORMULAS

21

1309

Chapter 21 – Emetic Formulas

Chapter 21 — Overview

PHARMACOLOGICAL EFFECTS & CLINICAL APPLICATIONS

Poisoning: The emetic effect of these formulas has been attributed in part to stimulation of the central nervous system and the gastrointestinal tract by herbs such as *Gua Di* (Pedicellus Cucumeris) and *Chang Shan* (Radix Dichroae). Emetic formulas are generally reserved for acute, urgent cases, such as the use of *Gua Di San* (Melon Pedicle Powder) for acute poisoning.[1]

Reference
1. *Zhong Yao Xue* (Chinese Herbology) 1998;908-909.

Chinese Herbal Formulas and Applications

Guā Dì Sǎn (Melon Pedicle Powder)

瓜蒂散

Pinyin Name: *Gua Di San*
Literal Name: Melon Pedicle Powder
Original Source: *Shang Han Lun* (Discussion of Cold-Induced Disorders) by Zhang Zhong-Jing in the Eastern Han Dynasty

COMPOSITION

Gua Di (Pedicellus Cucumeris), *ao* (simmered) until yellow	[1-2g]
Chi Xiao Dou (Semen Phaseoli)	[1-2g]

DOSAGE / PREPARATION / ADMINISTRATION

The source text states to grind equal amounts of the two herbs into a fine powder and sift together. Take 1 spoonful (1-3g) of the powder with a warm, strained decoction made from 6-9g of *Dan Dou Chi* (Semen Sojae Praeparatum). If vomiting is not induced, increase the dose slightly until vomiting is achieved. In addition to using the herbs, vomiting can also be induced physically via the gag reflex. Discontinue the formula when vomiting occurs.

CHINESE THERAPEUTIC ACTIONS

Induces vomiting of phlegm or stagnant food

CLINICAL MANIFESTATIONS

Phlegm or food stagnation in the chest and epigastrium: chest or epigastric distention and hardness, feelings of discomfort, a feeling of qi rising to the throat causing difficulty in breathing, restlessness, and a slightly superficial pulse at the *cun* position.

CLINICAL APPLICATIONS

Acute poisoning, mania, hepatitis, and jaundice.

EXPLANATION

Gua Di San (Melon Pedicle Powder) treats acute and severe phlegm accumulation in the chest, or food stagnation in the epigastrium. The phlegm accumulation and food stagnation may obstruct the proper flow of qi, causing distention and hardness in the chest or epigastrium.

Moreover, qi stagnation may lead to reversed flow of qi, which produces a feeling of qi rising to the throat and causing difficulty in breathing. Because the stagnation is most severe in the chest region, a slightly superficial pulse at the *cun* position may be felt.

This formula contains *Gua Di* (Pedicellus Cucumeris) to induce vomiting of phlegm and stagnant food. *Gua Di* (Pedicellus Cucumeris) also works with *Chi Xiao Dou* (Semen Phaseoli) to expel phlegm and relieve distention and hardness. *Dan Dou Chi* (Semen Sojae Praeparatum) ventilates the Lung, disperses qi stagnation in the chest, and relieves irritability. It also harmonizes the Stomach and regulates the middle *jiao* to prevent vomiting from damaging the Spleen and Stomach.

CAUTIONS / CONTRAINDICATIONS

• Since *Gua Di* (Pedicellus Cucumeris) is toxic and can easily injure the qi and Stomach, it is contraindicated in patients who have Spleen and Stomach deficiencies.

• *Gua Di San* is contraindicated if there is lack of stagnant phlegm in the chest. Do not use this formula to induce vomiting if the stagnant food has already passed from the stomach to the intestines.

• This formula should only be used in acute and excess conditions. It should be used with extreme caution in children, the elderly, postpartum patients with blood deficiency, and those with dizziness and palpitations caused by qi and blood deficiencies.

EMETIC FORMULAS

21

Gua Di San (Melon Pedicle Powder)

Diagnosis	Signs and Symptoms	Treatment	Herbs
Phlegm or food stagnation in the chest and epigastrium	• Distention and hardness in the chest or epigastrium: phlegm accumulation and food stagnation • Difficult breathing: obstructed qi circulation due to phlegm accumulation and food stagnation	Induces vomiting of phlegm or stagnant food	• *Gua Di* (Pedicellus Cucumeris) induces vomiting of phlegm and stagnant food. • *Chi Xiao Dou* (Semen Phaseoli) expels phlegm and relieves distention and hardness. • *Dan Dou Chi* (Semen Sojae Praeparatum) ventilates the Lung, disperses qi stagnation in the chest, and relieves irritability.

1311

Guā Dì Sǎn (Melon Pedicle Powder)

Chapter 21 – Emetic Formulas

- *Gua Di San* must be discontinued when the desired effect is achieved. Do not use it for a prolonged period of time.

Do not use this formula to induce vomiting of corrosive substances - this causes additional damage to the upper gastrointestinal tract when the corrosive elements are ejected as vomitus.

CLINICAL STUDIES AND RESEARCH

1. **Acute poisoning**: Acute poisoning treated with a modified *Gua Di San* preparation was associated with successful emptying of the stomach in 56 of 58 patients. The overall effectiveness was 96.55%. The average time to empty the stomach of the offending agent was 20.7 minutes. The herbal treatment contained *Gua Di* (Pedicellus Cucumeris), *Sheng Ma* (Rhizoma Cimicifugae), and *Gan Cao* (Radix et Rhizoma Glycyrrhizae). In comparison with other treatment modalities, 58 patients treated with gastric lavage needed an average of 46.4 minutes to empty the stomach, and 56 patients treated with warm water to induce vomiting had only 71.42% effectiveness.[1]

2. **Hepatitis**: Use of *Gua Di San* via intranasal administration has been shown in many studies to effectively treat acute or chronic viral hepatitis.[2] In one study, 153 of 188 patients with acute icteric viral hepatitis showed significant improvement with intranasal administration of 0.1g of *Gua Di San* bilaterally, one time daily, for 3 days per course of treatment.[3]

TOXICOLOGY

Administration of a small dose of *Gua Di San* has not been associated with significant changes to respiration, blood pressure, or heartbeat. However, administration of a large dose has been associated with irregular respiration, decreased blood pressure, reduced heart rate, and eventually, weakened and collapsed respiration.[4] Fatality was reported in one individual eight hours after ingestion of 30g of *Gua Di* (Pedicellus Cucumeris) and 15g of *Chi Xiao Dou* (Semen Phaseoli) on an empty stomach with warm water.[5] Another reported case of fatality involved an individual who ingested *Gua Di San* (actual dose unknown), which subsequently caused gastrointestinal bleeding and eventual fatality on the same day.[6]

TREATMENT OF OVERDOSE

Gua Di San should be used with extreme caution and only when needed. It must be discontinued when the desired effects are achieved. If vomiting persists after the herbs are discontinued, an antidote must be given immediately. Persistent vomiting associated with the use of *Gua Di San* can be relieved with 0.03-0.06 gram of *She Xiang* (Moschus) or 0.3-0.6 gram of *Ding Xiang* (Flos Caryophylli).

RELATED FORMULA

Sān Shèng Sǎn (Three-Sage Powder)

三聖散
三圣散

Pinyin Name: *San Sheng San*
Literal Name: Three-Sage Powder
Original Source: *Ru Men Shi Qin* (Confucians' Duties to their Parents) by Zhang Cong-Zheng in 1228

Fang Feng (Radix Saposhnikoviae)	90g [5g]
Gua Di (Pedicellus Cucumeris), *chao* (dry-fried) till yellow	90g [5g]
Li Lu (Radix et Rhizoma Veratri)	0.75-30 g [1-3g]

The source text states to grind the ingredients into a coarse powder and prepare as a decoction. Sip the decoction slowly, and stop when vomiting begins. Today, this formula may be prepared as a decoction with the doses suggested in brackets. It may also be administered via a nasogastric tube.

This formula induces vomiting and dispels wind-phlegm. Clinically, it may be used for patients with *zhong feng* (wind stroke) and *bi zheng* (closed disorder), showing symptoms such as loss of voice, facial paralysis with deviation of the eyes and mouth, unconsciousness, locked jaws, and a superficial, slippery and excess pulse. This formula is also good for treating poisoning when the offending agent is still in the stomach.

San Sheng San (Three-Sage Powder) should be used with extreme caution and only when needed. It must be discontinued when the desired effects are achieved. If vomiting persists after the herbs are discontinued, an antidote must be given immediately. Persistent vomiting associated with the use of *San Sheng San* can be alleviated with a decoction of *Cong Bai* (Bulbus Allii Fistulosi).

Gua Di San and *San Sheng San* (Three-Sage Powder) both induce vomiting.

- *Gua Di San* eliminates food and phlegm stagnation, and treats chest distention and hardness with qi rising to the throat, causing difficulty breathing.
- *San Sheng San* has more potent emetic action. It eliminates wind-phlegm to treat *zhong feng* (wind stroke), *bi zheng* (closed disorder), and *dian kuang* (mania and withdrawal).

1312

Guā Dì Sǎn (Melon Pedicle Powder)

AUTHORS' COMMENTS

Gua Di San is generally regarded as the standard formula for inducing vomiting. Historically, it has been used to treat severe phlegm accumulation in the chest or food stagnation in the epigastrium. Today, it is also used to treat food poisoning. This formula helps to eliminate offending agents from the stomach, and minimizes their further absorption in the digestive tract.

References

1. *Zhong Yi Ming Fang Lin Chuang Xin Yong* (Contemporary Clinical Applications of Classic Chinese Formulas) 2001;289.
2. *Zhong Yi Ming Fang Lin Chuang Xin Yong* (Contemporary Clinical Applications of Classic Chinese Formulas) 2001;289.
3. *Ji Lin Zhong Yi Yao* (Jilin Chinese Medicine and Herbology) 1986;3:12.
4. *Shan Xi Zhong Yi* (Shanxi Chinese Medicine) 1989;6:39.
5. *Liao Ning Zhong Yi Za Zhi* (Liaoning Journal of Chinese Medicine) 1978;3:50.
6. *Yao Xue Tong Bao* (Report of Herbology) 1986;1:42.

Jiù Jí Xī Xián Sǎn (Urgent Powder to Dilute Saliva)
救急稀涎散

Pinyin Name: *Jiu Ji Xi Xian San*
Literal Name: Urgent Powder to Dilute Saliva
Original Source: *Sheng Ji Zong Lu* (General Collection for Holy Relief) by a staff of court physicians in the Northern Song Dynasty around 1111-1117

COMPOSITION

Zao Jiao (Fructus Gleditsiae)	15g
Bai Fan (Alumen)	30g

DOSAGE / PREPARATION / ADMINISTRATION

The source text states to grind the ingredients into an extremely fine powder. Take 1.5g of the powder with warm water that has been boiled. The dose may be increased (up to 3g) for severe condition. However, do not overdose as it may cause weakness and deficiency.

CHINESE THERAPEUTIC ACTIONS

1. Opens the sensory orifices
2. Dispels phlegm
3. Induces vomiting

CLINICAL MANIFESTATIONS

Zhong feng (wind stroke) and *bi zheng* (closed disorder) syndrome: profuse amount of phlegm and saliva with a rattling sound in the throat, obstruction of qi circulation, a feeling of oppression, decreased muscle tone in the four limbs, altered consciousness or unconsciousness, deviation of the mouth, and a slippery, excess and forceful pulse. It is also used for *hou bi* (painful obstruction of the throat).

CLINICAL APPLICATIONS

Sudden unconsciousness.

EXPLANATION

Jiu Ji Xi Xian San (Urgent Powder to Dilute Saliva) treats individuals with *zhong feng* (wind stroke) and *bi zheng* (closed disorder) syndromes characterized by phlegm accumulation. The primary functions of this formula are to dissolve phlegm and open the sensory orifices, and the secondary function is to induce vomiting. As a result of

Jiu Ji Xi Xian San (Urgent Powder to Dilute Saliva)

Diagnosis	Signs and Symptoms	Treatment	Herbs
Zhong feng (wind stroke) and *bi zheng* (closed disorder) syndromes	• Profuse amount of phlegm and saliva with a rattling sound in the throat: phlegm obstructing the airways • Altered consciousness or unconsciousness: phlegm obstructing the sensory orifices • Decreased muscle tone in the four limbs and deviation of the mouth: phlegm obstructing the channels and collaterals • Slippery, excess and forceful pulse: phlegm accumulation	• Opens the sensory orifices • Induces vomiting	• *Zao Jiao* (Fructus Gleditsiae) opens the orifices by dispelling phlegm. • *Bai Fan* (Alumen) induces vomiting and dissolves phlegm.

EMETIC FORMULAS

21

1313

Chapter 21 – Emetic Formulas

Jiù Jí Xī Xián Sǎn (Urgent Powder to Dilute Saliva)

zhong feng (wind stroke), phlegm and saliva begin to accumulate in the interior, producing qi stagnation with a feeling of chest oppression, breathing difficulty, and, in severe cases, *bi zheng* (closed disorder) syndrome with altered consciousness or unconsciousness.

Zao Jiao (Fructus Gleditsiae) opens the orifices by dispelling phlegm, while *Bai Fan* (Alumen) induces vomiting and dissolves phlegm. Once the excessive phlegm and saliva are eliminated, the acute condition of their accumulation will be resolved, hence this formula's name: "Urgent Powder to Dilute Saliva."

CAUTIONS / CONTRAINDICATIONS

Jiu Ji Xi Xian San is designed to treat an urgent situation characterized by acute accumulation of phlegm and saliva. Once this condition is resolved, other herbs and formulas should be used to treat the underlying cause.

Yán Tāng Tàn Tù Fāng (Salt Decoction to Induce Vomiting)

鹽湯探吐方
盐汤探吐方

Pinyin Name: *Yan Tang Tan Tu Fang*
Literal Name: Salt Decoction to Induce Vomiting
Original Source: *Bei Ji Qian Jin Yao Fang* (Thousands of Golden Prescriptions for Emergencies) by Sun Si-Miao in Tang Dynasty

COMPOSITION

Shi Yan (Sodium Chloride)

DOSAGE / PREPARATION / ADMINISTRATION

The source text states to dissolve a large amount of *Shi Yan* (Sodium Chloride) in 3 bowls of hot water to make it extremely salty and concentrated. Take 1 bowl per dose while warm, and repeat with additional doses until all the stagnant food are removed via vomiting.

Today, this formula is prepared by dissolving *Shi Yan* (Sodium Chloride) in warm, boiled water until the solution becomes fully saturated. Take 2,000 mL of this preparation per dose to induce vomiting.

CHINESE THERAPEUTIC ACTIONS

Induces vomiting of stagnant food or poisonous substances

CLINICAL MANIFESTATIONS

Food stagnation, and sudden turmoil disorder with inability to vomit or defecate.

CLINICAL APPLICATIONS

Ingestion of poisonous substances.

EXPLANATION

Yan Tang Tan Tu Fang (Salt Decoction to Induce Vomiting) treats food stagnation characterized by the patient's inability to vomit. In this syndrome, the patient may have the desire to vomit, but is unable to do so.

This formula uses salt to induce vomiting and relieve stagnation in the body. It is a mild and convenient formula. If the patient does not respond immediately, try administering more salt water, or insert a finger in the back of the throat to induce vomiting.

This formula may also be used for sudden turmoil disorder with severe abdominal pain, in which the patient cannot vomit or defecate. Lastly, it may be used for unconsciousness syndromes that are caused by overeating or Liver qi stagnation.

Yan Tang Tan Tu Fang (Salt Decoction to Induce Vomiting)

Diagnosis	Signs and Symptoms	Treatment	Herbs
Food stagnation	Food stagnation with a desire to vomit	Induces vomiting	*Shi Yan* (Sodium Chloride) induces vomiting and relieves stagnation

1314

Chinese Herbal Formulas and Applications

Chapter 21 — Summary

— Emetic Formulas

Name	Similarities	Differences
Gua Di San (Melon Pedicle Powder)		Strongest emetic effect
Jiu Ji Xi Xian San (Urgent Powder to Dilute Saliva)	Induce vomiting	Mildest emetic effect
Yan Tang Tan Tu Fang (Salt Decoction to Induce Vomiting)		Moderate and gentle emetic effect

Gua Di San (Melon Pedicle Powder) has the strongest emetic action. It resolves food accumulation in the Stomach and phlegm stagnation in the chest or diaphragm. Clinical manifestations include chest or epigastric fullness and hardness, heartburn, irritability, a feeling of obstruction in the throat, and a slightly superficial pulse at the *cun* position.

Jiu Ji Xi Xian San (Urgent Powder to Dilute Saliva) has the mildest emetic action. This formula treats *zhong feng* (wind stroke) and *bi zheng* (closed disorder) syndromes with profuse amount of phlegm, obstruction of saliva, and stagnation of qi. Clinical manifestations include a feeling of oppression, decreased muscle tone in the four extremities, altered consciousness or unconsciousness, deviation of the mouth, and a slippery, excess and forceful pulse.

Yan Tang Tan Tu Fang (Salt Decoction to Induce Vomiting) has a gentle and moderate emetic function. It treats the presence of stagnant food or ingestion of poisonous substances. It is also used for sudden turmoil disorder characterized by the presence of abdominal pain with inability to vomit or defecate.

EMETIC FORMULAS

21

1315

Chapter 22

— Formulas that Treat Abscesses and Sores

痈
疡
剂

龚廷贤 Gǒng Tíng-Xiān

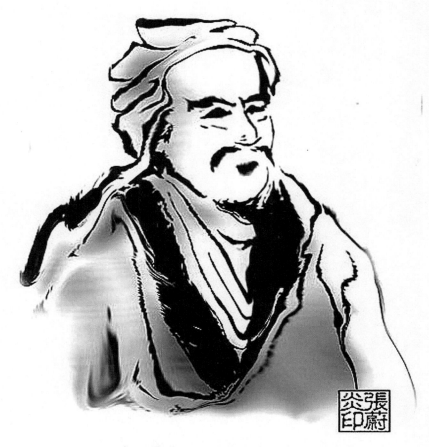

龚廷贤 Gǒng Tíng-Xiān, 1522 – 1619.

龚廷贤 Gŏng Tíng-Xiān

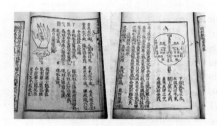

万病回春 Wan Bing Hui Chun (Restoration of Health from the Myriad Diseases) in 1587.

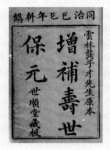

寿世保元 Shou Shi Bao Yuan (Achieving Longevity by Guarding the Source) in 1615.

Gong Ting-Xian was one of the most famous physicians of the Ming dynasty in the 16th century. Gong's father was a supreme physician in the Imperial Palace, and subsequently trained him to also become a supreme physician. Gong studied many aspects of medicine, and published many books in his lifetime.

His most famous works include *Wan Bing Hui Chun* (Restoration of Health from the Myriad Diseases) in 1587 and *Shou Shi Bao Yuan* (Achieving Longevity by Guarding the Source) in 1615. The former text totaled 8 volumes, and contained detailed information on differential diagnosis, pathology, treatment, and prevention of, as the name of the text suggests, a myriad of diseases. The latter text contained 10 volumes, and discussed the diagnosis and treatment of internal medicine, external medicine, gynecology, pediatrics and more.

These texts presented many formulas that are commonly prescribed today, such as
- *Jing Jie Lian Qiao Tang* (Schizonepeta and Forsythia Decoction)
- *Shu Gan Tang* (Spread the Liver Decoction)
- *Qing Shang Fang Feng Tang* (Clear the Upper and Guard the Wind Decoction)
- *Wen Qing Yin* (Warming and Clearing Decoction)
- *Fen Xiao Tang* (Separate and Reduce Decoction)
- *Shu Jing Huo Xue Tang* (Relax the Channels and Invigorate the Blood Decoction)
- *Qing Fei Tang* (Clear the Lung Decoction)
- *Qian Jin Nei Tuo San* (Drain-the-Interior Powder Worthy of a Thousand Gold)
- *Shi Liu Wei Liu Qi Yin* (Sixteen-Ingredient Decoction to Flow Qi)
- *San Zhong Kui Jian Tang* (Disperse the Swelling and Break the Hardness Decoction)

Dynasties & Kingdoms	Year
Xia Dynasty 夏	2100-1600 BCE
Shang Dynasty 商	1600-1100 BCE
Zhou Dynasty 周	1100-221 BCE
Qin Dynasty 秦	221-207 BCE
Han Dynasty 漢	206 BCE-220
Three Kingdoms 三國	220-280
Western Jin Dynasty 西晉	265-316
Eastern Jin Dynasty 東晉	317-420
Northern and Southern Dynasties 北南朝	420-581
Sui Dynasty 隋	581-618
Tang Dynasty 唐	618-907
Five Dynasties 五代	907-960
Song Dynasty 宋	960-1279
Liao Dynasty 遼	916-1125
Jin Dynasty 金	1115-1234
Yuan Dynasty 元	1271-1368
Ming Dynasty 明	**1368-1644**
Qing Dynasty 清	1644-1911
Republic of China 中華民國	1912-Present Day
People's Republic of China 中華人民共和國	1949-Present Day

Chapter 22 – Formulas that Treat Abscesses and Sores

Table of Contents

Chapter 22. Formulas that Treat Abscesses and Sores ⋯⋯⋯⋯ **1317**
Biography of Gong Ting-Xian ⋯⋯⋯⋯⋯⋯⋯⋯⋯⋯⋯⋯⋯⋯⋯⋯⋯ 1318

Section 1. External Abscesses and Sores ⋯⋯⋯⋯⋯⋯⋯⋯⋯⋯ **1325**
Xian Fang Huo Ming Yin (Sublime Formula for Sustaining Life) ⋯⋯⋯⋯⋯⋯⋯ 1325
  Zhen Ren Huo Ming Yin (True Man's Decoction to Revitalize Life) ⋯⋯⋯⋯⋯ 1330
  Huo Ming Yin (Revitalize Life Decoction) ⋯⋯⋯⋯⋯⋯⋯⋯⋯⋯⋯⋯ 1330
  Lian Qiao Bai Du San (Forsythia Powder to Overcome Pathogenic Influences) ⋯⋯ 1331
Niu Bang Jie Ji Tang (Arctium Decoction to Release the Muscle Layer) ⋯⋯⋯⋯ 1332
Jing Fang Bai Du San (Schizonepeta and Saposhnikovia Powder to Overcome Pathogenic Influences) ⋯ 1334
  Jing Fang Bai Du San (Schizonepeta and Saposhnikovia Powder to Overcome Pathogenic Influences) ⋯ 1335
  Jing Fang Bai Du San (Schizonepeta and Saposhnikovia Powder to Overcome Pathogenic Influences) ⋯ 1336
Wu Wei Xiao Du Yin (Five-Ingredient Decoction to Eliminate Toxins) ⋯⋯⋯⋯ 1337
  Yin Hua Jie Du Tang (Honeysuckle Decoction to Relieve Toxicity) ⋯⋯⋯⋯ 1340
Shi Wei Bai Du Tang (Ten-Ingredient Decoction to Overcome Pathogenic Influences) ⋯ 1341
  Bai Du Tang (Overcome Pathogenic Influences Decoction) ⋯⋯⋯⋯⋯⋯⋯ 1343
Si Miao Yong An Tang (Four-Valiant Decoction for Well-Being) ⋯⋯⋯⋯⋯⋯ 1344
  Wu Shen Tang (Five-Miracle Decoction) ⋯⋯⋯⋯⋯⋯⋯⋯⋯⋯⋯⋯ 1347
  Shen Xiao Tuo Li San (Miraculous Powder for Supporting the Interior) ⋯⋯⋯ 1347
Zi Cao Gen Mu Li Tang (Arnebia and Oyster Shell Decoction) ⋯⋯⋯⋯⋯⋯ 1348
Xi Huang Wan (Cattle Gallstone Pill) ⋯⋯⋯⋯⋯⋯⋯⋯⋯⋯⋯⋯⋯⋯ 1350
  Xing Xiao Wan (Awake and Disperse Pill) ⋯⋯⋯⋯⋯⋯⋯⋯⋯⋯⋯ 1351
  Chan Su Wan (Toad Venum Pill) ⋯⋯⋯⋯⋯⋯⋯⋯⋯⋯⋯⋯⋯⋯ 1351
Hai Zao Yu Hu Tang (Sargassum Decoction for the Jade Flask) ⋯⋯⋯⋯⋯⋯ 1352
Xiao Luo Wan (Reduce Scrofula Pill) ⋯⋯⋯⋯⋯⋯⋯⋯⋯⋯⋯⋯⋯⋯ 1355
San Zhong Kui Jian Tang (Disperse the Swelling and Break the Hardness Decoction) ⋯ 1357
  San Zhong Kui Jian Tang (Disperse the Swelling and Break the Hardness Decoction) ⋯ 1358
  Xiao San Tang Yi Hao (Dissolve and Disperse Decoction Formula One) ⋯⋯⋯ 1359
  Xiao San Tang Er Hao (Dissolve and Disperse Decoction Formula Two) ⋯⋯⋯ 1359
Shi Liu Wei Liu Qi Yin (Sixteen-Ingredient Decoction to Flow Qi) ⋯⋯⋯⋯⋯ 1360
  Shi Liu Wei Liu Qi Yin (Sixteen-Ingredient Decoction to Flow Qi) ⋯⋯⋯⋯ 1361
Tou Nong San (Discharge Pus Powder) ⋯⋯⋯⋯⋯⋯⋯⋯⋯⋯⋯⋯⋯⋯ 1362
  Tuo Li Tou Nong Tang (Drain the Interior and Discharge Pus Decoction) ⋯⋯⋯ 1363
Pai Nong San (Drain the Pus Powder) ⋯⋯⋯⋯⋯⋯⋯⋯⋯⋯⋯⋯⋯⋯ 1364
Qian Jin Nei Tuo San (Drain the Interior Powder Worthy of a Thousand Gold) ⋯⋯ 1365
Tuo Li Xiao Du Yin (Drain the Interior and Detoxify Decoction) ⋯⋯⋯⋯⋯⋯ 1367
  Tuo Li Xiao Du Yin (Drain the Interior and Detoxify Decoction) ⋯⋯⋯⋯⋯ 1368
Nei Bu Huang Qi Tang (Tonify the Interior Decoction with Astragalus) ⋯⋯⋯⋯ 1369
Yang He Tang (Yang-Heartening Decoction) ⋯⋯⋯⋯⋯⋯⋯⋯⋯⋯⋯⋯ 1370
  Zhong He Tang (Middle-Heartening Decoction) ⋯⋯⋯⋯⋯⋯⋯⋯⋯⋯ 1373
Xiao Jin Dan (Minor Gold Special Pill) ⋯⋯⋯⋯⋯⋯⋯⋯⋯⋯⋯⋯⋯⋯ 1374

Section 2. Internal Abscesses and Sores ⋯⋯⋯⋯⋯⋯⋯⋯⋯⋯ **1377**
Wei Jing Tang (Reed Decoction) ⋯⋯⋯⋯⋯⋯⋯⋯⋯⋯⋯⋯⋯⋯⋯⋯ 1377
Da Huang Mu Dan Tang (Rhubarb and Moutan Decoction) ⋯⋯⋯⋯⋯⋯⋯⋯ 1378
  Qing Chang Yin (Clear the Intestines Drink) ⋯⋯⋯⋯⋯⋯⋯⋯⋯⋯⋯ 1381
Yi Yi Fu Zi Bai Jiang San (Coicis, Prepared Aconite, and Patrinia Powder) ⋯⋯⋯ 1382
  Yi Yi Ren Tang (Coicis Decoction) ⋯⋯⋯⋯⋯⋯⋯⋯⋯⋯⋯⋯⋯⋯ 1383

Formulas that Treat Abscesses and Sores (Summary) ⋯⋯⋯⋯⋯ **1385**

Chinese Herbal Formulas and Applications

Chapter 22 — Overview

— Formulas that Treat Abscesses and Sores

Definition: Formulas that treat abscesses and sores generally clear heat, eliminate toxins, reduce swellings, drain the interior, discharge pus, promote the generation of new flesh, and astringe ulcerations. Clinically, their applications are not restricted to treating abscesses and sores. Rather, they may treat both external conditions (including abscesses, sores, cellulitis, boils, erysipelas, multiple abscesses, carbuncles, furuncles, scrofula, goiter, and tumor), and internal disorders (such as abscesses of the organs).

Abscesses and sores are either externally contracted or internally generated. External causes of abscesses and sores include *liu yin* (six exogenous factors), insect or animal bites, cuts and burns, and various sport injuries or traumas. Internal causes of abscesses and sores include damage caused by imbalance of the *qi qing* (seven emotions), or an improper diet consisting of too much acrid or hot food. These etiological factors lead to stagnation within the channels and collaterals and disharmony between qi and blood. If this stagnation is left untreated, heat formation results, and abscesses and sores eventually form. Other factors, such as cold, dampness, or phlegm, can also stagnate in the muscles, tendons, ligaments, and channels and collaterals, to cause either *yin* (deep-rooted) or *yang* (superficial) type of abscesses and sores.

Differential diagnosis of abscesses and sores begins with assessment of whether the condition is externally contracted or internally generated.

> Internal and external abscesses and sores may be treated via oral ingestion and/or topical application.

- Diagnostic criteria for externally-contracted abscesses and sores include the differentiation of yin and yang. For example, *yang* (superficial) abscesses and sores are characterized by prominent swelling and inflammation, limited size or surface area with defined borders, redness, and warm, burning sensations in the affected area. On the other hand, *yin* (deep-rooted) abscesses and sores are usually characterized by very slight swelling (almost flat) that may be hard or soft. The affected area is widespread, involves a large surface area, and shows no change in skin color.
- Diagnostic criteria for internally-generated abscesses and sores include differentiation of cold or heat, deficiency or excess, and the presence or absence of pus. Lung and intestinal abscesses are the most common internal abscess disorders affecting the *zang fu* organs.

External abscesses and sores are treated internally with three main treatment methods: *xiao fa* (reducing method) in the early stage, *tuo fa* (draining method) in the middle stage when pus has formed, and *bu fa* (tonifying method) in the late stage involving ulcerations.

- *Xiao fa* (reducing method) is used in early stage abscesses and sores, prior to the formation of pus, to disperse heat and toxins, reduce swelling, and terminate the illness. Specific types of *xiao fa* (reducing method) include the use of herbs that release the exterior, clear heat, warm and unblock, resolve phlegm, move qi, activate blood circulation, and eliminate stagnation.
- *Tuo fa* (draining method) is used in the early to middle stages of abscesses and sores, marked by pus formation in the presence of heat and toxins, or generalized weakness and deficiency with inability to discharge the pus. *Tuo fa* (draining method) brings the heat and toxins from the deep aspects of the body to the superficial, and facilitates the perforation and discharge of pus. However, because this stage is usually characterized by underlying weakness and deficiency, the use of *bu fa* (tonifying method) may also be necessary to facilitate the healing process.

FORMULAS THAT TREAT ABSCESSES AND SORES

22

1321

Chapter 22 — Overview

Some formulas emphasize treatment based on differentiation of yin or yang, hot or cold, and excess or deficiency; others focus on the physical location of sores.

- *Bu fa* (tonifying method) is employed in the late stage when the abscesses and sores have perforated and ulcerated, and pus is being discharged. However, the area of ulceration may not have reduced in size, and the pus may continue to discharge and not heal because of underlying deficiencies of qi and blood, the Spleen and Stomach, or the Liver and Kidney. In these circumstances, *bu fa* (tonifying method) is used to tonify deficiencies, astringe the ulcerations, dry the pus, promote the generation of tissue, and facilitate healing.

Internal abscesses and sores affecting the interior *zang fu* organs should be treated with multiple methods to clear heat, eliminate toxins, and dispel stagnation to reduce swelling. Depending on the individual condition, it may be necessary to add herbs to drain pus and tonify the underlying deficiencies.

SUBCATEGORIES OF ACTION

Formulas that treat abscesses and sores are divided into two subcategories to indicate their use in treating external and internal abscesses and sores.

1. **External Abscesses and Sores**
   External abscesses and sores can have various presentations, and require formulas of corresponding characteristics for treatment. Some formulas emphasize treatment based on differentiation of yin or yang, hot or cold, and excess or deficiency, others focus on the physical location of the abscesses and sores.
   - External abscesses and sores characterized by excess, heat, and yang should be treated with formulas that clear heat, eliminate toxins, break hardness, and reduce swelling, such as *Xian Fang Huo Ming Yin* (Sublime Formula for Sustaining Life).
   - External abscesses and sores characterized by deficiency, cold, and yin should be treated with formulas that tonify, warm and disperse cold, such as *Yang He Tang* (Yang-Heartening Decoction) and *Xiao Jin Dan* (Minor Gold Special Pill).

   Moreover, depending on the nature of the disease (excess or deficiency) and the underlying constitution of the patient, formulas with various functions may be used.
   - Exemplar formulas that drain the interior and discharge pus include *Xian Fang Huo Ming Yin* (Sublime Formula for Sustaining Life) and *Wu Wei Xiao Du Yin* (Five-Ingredient Decoction to Eliminate Toxins).
   - Exemplar formulas that tonify the underlying deficiencies and drain abscesses and sores include *Nei Bu Huang Qi Tang* (Tonify the Interior Decoction with Astragalus) and *Yang He Tang* (Yang-Heartening Decoction).

Internal abscesses and sores generally affect the lungs and the intestines.

   Lastly, external abscesses and sores may affect different parts of the body, and thus require formulas that treat these affected areas. Formulas in this subcategory include formulas from other chapters that also treat abscesses and sores.
   - Formulas that disperse and clear wind-heat are often used to treat abscesses and sores affecting the upper parts of the body (head, face, neck, and shoulders), such as *Niu Bang Jie Ji Tang* (Arctium Decoction to Release the Muscle Layer).
   - Formulas that regulate Liver qi circulation, purge fire and eliminate toxins are incorporated to treat abscesses and sores affecting the middle parts of the body (chest, back, and abdomen), such as *Jia Wei Xiao Yao San* (Augmented Rambling Powder) and *Huang Lian Jie Du Tang* (Coptis Decoction to Relieve Toxicity).
   - Formulas that clear heat, eliminate toxins, and activate qi and blood circulation in the peripheral channels and collaterals are frequently deployed to treat abscesses and sores affecting the limbs (arms and legs), such as *Si Miao Yong An Tang* (Four-Valiant Decoction for Well-Being).

Chinese Herbal Formulas and Applications

Chapter 22 — Overview

2. Internal Abscesses and Sores

Internal abscesses and sores generally affect the lungs and intestines. Lung abscesses characterized by phlegm, heat, and blood stagnation are treated with formulas such as *Wei Jing Tang* (Reed Decoction). Intestinal abscesses characterized by damp-heat accumulation and qi and blood stagnation are treated with formulas such as *Da Huang Mu Dan Tang* (Rhubarb and Moutan Decoction).

CAUTIONS / CONTRAINDICATIONS

Accurate differential diagnosis and proper selection of treatment methods are essential to obtaining successful results. Incorrect diagnosis or use of inappropriate treatment methods will delay healing, or possibly worsen the condition.

- *Xiao fa* (reducing method) is used for early stage abscesses and sores. Use of this strong method is inappropriate in late stage abscesses and sores with underlying deficiencies, as it will damage qi and blood, leading to prolonged duration of the illness due to the inability of the ulcerations to heal.

- *Tuo fa* (draining method) is used in the middle stage of abscesses and sores. This method is not recommended if the abscesses and sores are characterized by the presence of excess heat and toxins, which should be treated with herbs that clear heat and eliminate toxins.

- *Bu fa* (tonifying method) is employed in the late stage of abscesses and sores. This method should not be used during the early stage, or in cases of accumulation of heat and toxins in the interior, because this method will contribute to more excess and stagnation.

PHARMACOLOGICAL EFFECTS & CLINICAL APPLICATIONS

Although these formulas are known for treating abscesses and sores, they have a wide variety of pharmacological effects and clinical applications. These formulas can treat disorders characterized by infections and inflammations that come with abscesses, sores, nodules, and hardness.

- **Dermatological disorders**: These formulas may be used to treat various disorders affecting the skin, such as carbuncles and sores,[1,2] cellulitis,[3] acne vulgaris,[4] gangrene,[5] and erysipelas.[6] Exemplar formulas include *Xian Fang Huo Ming Yin* (Sublime Formula for Sustaining Life), *Si Miao Yong An Tang* (Four-Valiant Decoction for Well-Being), and *Shi Wei Bai Du Tang* (Ten-Ingredient Decoction to Overcome Pathogenic Influences).

- **Blood vessel disorders**: These formulas are effective in treating inflammatory conditions of the blood vessels, such as phlebitis,[7] thrombophlebitis,[8,9,10] thromboangiitis obliterans,[11,12,13] and thrombosis of the iliofemoral vein.[14] Representative formulas include *Xian Fang Huo Ming Yin* (Sublime Formula for Sustaining Life), *Si Miao Yong An Tang* (Four-Valiant Decoction for Well-Being), and *Yang He Tang* (Yang-Heartening Decoction).

- **Breast disorders**: These formulas demonstrate effectiveness in treating various types of breast disorders, such as mastitis,[15,16] breast abscesses,[17] hyperplasia of the mammary glands,[18,19] and cystic hyperplasia of the breast.[20] Representative formulas include *Xian Fang Huo Ming Yin* (Sublime Formula for Sustaining Life), *Xiao Luo Wan* (Reduce Scrofula Pill), *Yang He Tang* (Yang-Heartening Decoction), and *Hai Zao Yu Hu Tang* (Sargassum Decoction for the Jade Flask).

- **Throat disorders**: *Xian Fang Huo Ming Yin* (Sublime Formula for Sustaining Life) and *Wu Wei Xiao Du Yin* (Five-Ingredient Decoction to Eliminate Toxins) are formulas commonly used to treat parotitis, tonsillitis, and peritonsillar abscesses.[21,22,23,24]

- **Others**: Some of these formulas treat other inflammatory diseases, such as pelvic inflammatory disease,[25,26] appendicular abscess,[27] osteomyelitis,[28,29] and myelitis.[30]

Formulas that treat internal abscesses and sores treat various infections and inflammation of the internal organs with abscesses and sores.

- **Pulmonary disorders**: *Wei Jing Tang* (Reed Decoction) has been shown to effectively treat infection and inflammation of the lungs. The clinical applications of this formula include pulmonary abscesses,[31,32] pneumonia (lobar pneumonia, lobular pneumonia, bronchopneumonia,

> Formulas that treat abscesses and sores have antibiotic and anti-inflammatory effects on infections and inflammations affecting superficial tissues and internal organs.

FORMULAS THAT TREAT ABSCESSES AND SORES

22

1323

Chapter 22 — Overview

and mycoplasmal pneumonia),[33] and bronchitis (bronchitis in children, suppurative bronchitis, and chronic bronchitis).[34,35,36]

- **Appendicitis:** These formulas have been used successfully to treat acute appendicitis,[37] chronic appendicitis,[38] ruptured appendix with peritonitis,[39] and periappendicular abscess.[40] Two representative formulas are *Da Huang Mu Dan Tang* (Rhubarb and Moutan Decoction) and *Yi Yi Fu Zi Bai Jiang San* (Coicis, Prepared Aconite, and Patrinia Powder).

- **Others:** Formulas that treat internal abscesses and sores have also been shown to treat other diseases characterized by infection and/or inflammation of the internal organs, such as pelvic inflammatory disease,[41,42] acute cholecystitis,[43] ulcerative colitis,[44] chronic prostatitis,[45] and suppurative tonsillitis.[46]

References

1. *He Nan Zhong Yi* (Henan Chinese Medicine) 1988;5:31.
2. *Hu Bei Zhong Yi Za Zhi* (Hubei Journal of Chinese Medicine) 1988;6:23.
3. *Liao Ning Zhong Yi Za Zhi* (Liaoning Journal of Chinese Medicine) 1994;21(5):222.
4. Higaki S, Kitagawa T, Kagoura M, Morohashi M, Yamagishi T. Relationship between Propionibacterium acnes biotypes and Jumi-haidoku-to. Journal of Dermatology 2000 Oct;27(10):635-8.
5. *Xin Zhong Yi* (New Chinese Medicine) 1990;2:27.
6. *Hu Bei Zhong Yi Za Zhi* (Hubei Journal of Chinese Medicine) 1998;5:32.
7. *Shan Xi Zhong Yi* (Shanxi Chinese Medicine) 1998;2:74.
8. *Liao Ning Zhong Yi Za Zhi* (Liaoning Journal of Chinese Medicine) 1991;5:34.
9. *Xin Zhong Yi* (New Chinese Medicine) 1992;10:24.
10. *Si Chuan Zhong Yi* (Sichuan Chinese Medicine) 1992;9:37.
11. *Zhong Yi Za Zhi* (Journal of Chinese Medicine) 1980;1:42.
12. *Tian Jin Yi Yao Za Zhi* (Journal of Tianjin Medicine and Herbology) 1960;1:1.
13. *Zhe Jiang Zhong Yi Za Zhi* (Zhejiang Journal of Chinese Medicine) 1982;2:82.
14. *Hei Long Jiang Zhong Yi Yao* (Heilongjiang Chinese Medicine and Herbology) 1997;3:1.
15. *Nei Meng Gu Zhong Yi Yao* (Traditional Chinese Medicine and Medicinals of Inner Mongolia) 1994;2:7.
16. *Shi Yong Zhong Yi Yao Za Zhi* (Journal of Practical Chinese Medicine and Medicinals) 1997;6:13.
17. *Shan Xi Zhong Yi* (Shanxi Chinese Medicine) 1989;8:366.
18. *Shi Yong Zhong Yi Yao Za Zhi* (Journal of Practical Chinese Medicine and Medicinals) 1998;11:9.
19. *Shi Yong Zhong Yi Yao Za Zhi* (Journal of Practical Chinese Medicine and Medicinals) 1999;3:14.
20. *Xin Zhong Yi* (New Chinese Medicine) 1997;2:18.
21. *Zhong Xi Yi Jie He Za Zhi* (Journal of Integrated Chinese and Western Medicine) 1989;9(10):612.
22. *He Nan Zhong Yi* (Henan Chinese Medicine) 1995;5:35.
23. *Shan Dong Zhong Yi Za Zhi* (Shandong Journal of Chinese Medicine) 1992;11(5):15.
24. *Shang Hai Zhong Yi Yao Za Zhi* (Shanghai Journal of Chinese Medicine and Herbology) 1994;4:24.
25. *Jiang Su Zhong Yi* (Jiangsu Chinese Medicine) 1996;6:18.
26. *Fu Jian Yi Yao Za Zhi* (Fujian Journal of Medicine and Herbology) 1994;4:58.
27. *Zhong Hua Wai Ke Za Zhi* (Chinese Journal of External Medicine) 1960;2:171.
28. *He Bei Zhong Yi* (Hebei Chinese Medicine) 1989;3:108.
29. *Jiang Su Zhong Yi* (Jiangsu Chinese Medicine) 1963;4.
30. *Jiang Xi Zhong Yi Yao* (Jiangxi Chinese Medicine and Herbology) 1997;5:44.
31. *He Nan Zhong Yi* (Henan Chinese Medicine) 1991;11(5):24.
32. *Shi Yong Zhong Xi Yi Jie He Za Zhi* (Practical Journal of Integrated Chinese and Western Medicines) 1992;5(2):83.
33. *Shan Xi Zhong Yi* (Shanxi Chinese Medicine) 1994;15(8):342.
34. *Shang Hai Zhong Yi Yao Za Zhi* (Shanghai Journal of Chinese Medicine and Herbology) 1983;10:26.
35. *Shang Hai Zhong Yi Yao Za Zhi* (Shanghai Journal of Chinese Medicine and Herbology) 1959;2:15.
36. *Jiang Su Zhong Yi* (Jiangsu Chinese Medicine) 1982;5:14.
37. *Guang Xi Zhong Yi Yao* (Guangxi Chinese Medicine and Herbology) 1986;3:10.
38. *Tian Jin Yi Yao Za Zhi* (Journal of Tianjin Medicine and Herbology) 1959;11:411.
39. *Nei Meng Gu Zhong Yi Yao* (Traditional Chinese Medicine and Medicinals of Inner Mongolia) 1993;2:23.
40. *Yun Nan Zhong Yi Za Zhi* (Yunan Journal of Chinese Medicine) 1995;2:11.
41. *Guang Xi Zhong Yi Yao* (Guangxi Chinese Medicine and Herbology) 1992;5:6.
42. *Shan Xi Zhong Yi* (Shanxi Chinese Medicine) 1993;14(12):533.
43. *Shi Yong Zhong Yi Nei Ke Za Zhi* (Journal of Practical Chinese Internal Medicine) 1992;3:127.
44. *He Nan Zhong Yi* (Henan Chinese Medicine) 1998;1:22.
45. *Zhe Jiang Zhong Yi Za Zhi* (Zhejiang Journal of Chinese Medicine) 1993;8:368.
46. *Liao Ning Zhong Yi Za Zhi* (Liaoning Journal of Chinese Medicine) 1991;6:36.

Chinese Herbal Formulas and Applications

Section 1

外痈疡剂
— External Abscesses and Sores

Xiān Fāng Huó Mìng Yǐn (Sublime Formula for Sustaining Life)
仙方活命飲
仙方活命饮

Pinyin Name: *Xian Fang Huo Ming Yin*
Literal Name: Sublime Formula for Sustaining Life
Original Source: *Jiao Zhu Fu Ren Liang Fang* (Revised Fine Formulas for Women) by Bi Li-Zhai in the 16th century

COMPOSITION

Jin Yin Hua (Flos Lonicerae Japonicae)	9g
Fang Feng (Radix Saposhnikoviae)	3g
Bai Zhi (Radix Angelicae Dahuricae)	3g
Dang Gui Wei (Extremitas Radix Angelicae Sinensis)	3g
Chi Shao (Radix Paeoniae Rubra)	3g
Ru Xiang (Gummi Olibanum)	3g
Mo Yao (Myrrha)	3g
Bei Mu (Bulbus Fritillariae)	3g
Tian Hua Fen (Radix Trichosanthis)	3g
Chuan Shan Jia (Squama Manis), *zhi* (fried with liquid)	3g
Zao Jiao Ci (Spina Gleditsiae), *chao* (dry-fried)	3g
Chen Pi (Pericarpium Citri Reticulatae)	9g
Gan Cao (Radix et Rhizoma Glycyrrhizae)	3g

DOSAGE / PREPARATION / ADMINISTRATION

The source text states to cook the ingredients with 1 large bowl of grain-based liquor and bring it to a boil 5-7 times. Today, it is prepared as a decoction with water or with a 50:50 mixture of water and grain-based liquor.

CHINESE THERAPEUTIC ACTIONS

1. Clears heat and eliminates toxins
2. Reduces swelling and breaks the hardness
3. Activates blood circulation and stops pain

CLINICAL MANIFESTATIONS

Early onset of abscesses and sores characterized by accumulation of heat and toxins and stagnation of qi and blood: local redness; swelling and pain with or without fever and chills; a thin and white or yellow tongue coating; and a rapid, forceful pulse.

CLINICAL APPLICATIONS

Carbuncles, furuncles, sores, breast abscesses, appendicular abscesses, acute appendicitis, thrombophlebitis, mastitis, mammary abscess, pelvic inflammatory disease, cervicitis, vaginitis, tonsillitis, peritonsillar abscesses, anal sinusitis, stye, post-herpetic neuralgia, psoriasis, reflux esophagitis, peptic ulcer disease, ulcerative colitis, osteoradionecrosis, osteomyelitis, pneumonia, and tumors.

EXPLANATION

Xian Fang Huo Ming Yin (Sublime Formula for Sustaining Life) treats early onset of abscesses and sores characterized by accumulation of heat and toxins and stagnation of qi and blood. It is suitable for early onset of abscesses and sores, in which pus has not yet formed. In this syndrome, heat and toxins in the skin and muscles may cause local redness and swelling, while qi and blood stagnation may cause pain. Since the disease is still located at the exterior,

FORMULAS THAT TREAT ABSCESSES AND SORES

22

1325

Chapter 22 – Formulas that Treat Abscesses and Sores | *Section 1 – External Abscesses and Sores*

Xiān Fāng Huó Mìng Yǐn (Sublime Formula for Sustaining Life)

Xian Fang Huo Ming Yin (Sublime Formula for Sustaining Life)

Diagnosis	Signs and Symptoms	Treatment	Herbs
Early onset of abscesses and sores	• Abscesses, sores, local redness and swelling: heat and toxins in the skin and muscles • Local pain: qi and blood stagnation • Fever and chills: exterior condition • Thin and white or yellow tongue coating: early stage of heat • Rapid, forceful pulse: excess heat condition	• Clears heat and eliminates toxins • Reduces swelling and breaks the hardness • Activates blood circulation and stops pain	• *Jin Yin Hua* (Flos Lonicerae Japonicae) clears heat and eliminates toxins. • *Fang Feng* (Radix Saposhnikoviae) and *Bai Zhi* (Radix Angelicae Dahuricae) disperse and dispel heat toxins. • *Dang Gui Wei* (Extremitas Radix Angelicae Sinensis), *Chi Shao* (Radix Paeoniae Rubra), *Ru Xiang* (Gummi Olibanum), and *Mo Yao* (Myrrha) activate blood circulation and remove blood stagnation. • *Bei Mu* (Bulbus Fritillariae) and *Tian Hua Fen* (Radix Trichosanthis) resolve phlegm, clear heat, reduce swelling, dispel pus, and break the hardness. • *Chuan Shan Jia* (Squama Manis) and *Zao Jiao Ci* (Spina Gleditsiae) drain abscesses and soften nodules. • *Chen Pi* (Pericarpium Citri Reticulatae) regulates the qi flow. • *Gan Cao* (Radix et Rhizoma Glycyrrhizae) clears heat, eliminates toxins and harmonizes the Stomach.

fever and chills are present. A thin and white or yellow tongue coating indicates that the heat has not yet progressed to the interior organs, while a rapid, forceful pulse suggests excess heat in the body.

Jin Yin Hua (Flos Lonicerae Japonicae) clears heat and eliminates toxins. *Fang Feng* (Radix Saposhnikoviae) and *Bai Zhi* (Radix Angelicae Dahuricae) disperse and dispel heat and toxins from the superficial parts of the body. *Dang Gui Wei* (Extremitas Radix Angelicae Sinensis), *Chi Shao* (Radix Paeoniae Rubra), *Ru Xiang* (Gummi Olibanum), and *Mo Yao* (Myrrha) activate blood circulation and remove blood stagnation to reduce the redness, swelling, and pain. *Bei Mu* (Bulbus Fritillariae) and *Tian Hua Fen* (Radix Trichosanthis) resolve phlegm, clear heat, reduce swelling, dispel pus, and disperse nodules. *Chuan Shan Jia* (Squama Manis) and *Zao Jiao Ci* (Spina Gleditsiae) open the channels and collaterals to drain the abscesses and soften the nodules. *Chen Pi* (Pericarpium Citri Reticulatae) regulates the qi flow. *Gan Cao* (Radix et Rhizoma Glycyrrhizae) clears heat, eliminates toxins and harmonizes the Stomach. The use of grain-based liquor helps to activate blood circulation and open the channels and collaterals.

MODIFICATIONS

• For abscesses and sores in the head region, add *Chuan Xiong* (Rhizoma Chuanxiong).
• For abscesses and sores in the chest region, add *Gua Lou* (Fructus Trichosanthis).
• For abscesses and sores in the hypochondriac area, add *Chai Hu* (Radix Bupleuri).
• For abscesses and sores in the waist and back regions, add *Qin Jiao* (Radix Gentianae Macrophyllae).
• For abscesses and sores in the lower extremities, add *Niu Xi* (Radix Achyranthis Bidentatae).
• With swelling and pain, add *Zi Hua Di Ding* (Herba Violae) and *Pu Gong Ying* (Herba Taraxaci).
• With damaged body fluids caused by high fever, increase the dose of *Tian Hua Fen* (Radix Trichosanthis).
• With heat in the *xue* (blood) level, add *Di Huang* (Radix Rehmanniae), *Xuan Shen* (Radix Scrophulariae), and *Mu Dan Pi* (Cortex Moutan).
• With qi deficiency, add *Huang Qi* (Radix Astragali).
• With constipation, add *Mang Xiao* (Natrii Sulfas) and *Da Huang* (Radix et Rhizoma Rhei).

CAUTIONS / CONTRAINDICATIONS

• *Xian Fang Huo Ming Yin* should be used with caution in

1326

Xiān Fāng Huó Mìng Yǐn (Sublime Formula for Sustaining Life)

patients with Spleen and Stomach deficiencies, or qi and blood deficiencies.

- This formula is indicated for early stages of abscesses and sores. It is contraindicated for *yin* (deep-rooted) sores, or if the lesions have already ulcerated.

CLINICAL STUDIES AND RESEARCH

1. **Abscesses and sores**: One study reported 100% effectiveness using modified *Xian Fang Huo Ming Yin* to treat generalized sores and abscesses.[1] Another study reported 96.3% effectiveness in treating 54 patients with swelling and deep-rooted sores.[2]

2. **Breast abscesses**: Researchers reported complete recovery in 29 of 30 patients with breast abscesses using both oral and topical applications of herbs. Oral formulation was given as a decoction daily, for 7 days per course of treatment, for 1-2 courses total. The formula contained *Jin Yin Hua* (Flos Lonicerae Japonicae) 20g, *Bai Zhi* (Radix Angelicae Dahuricae) 10g, *Dang Gui* (Radix Angelicae Sinensis) 10g, *Chuan Bei Mu* (Bulbus Fritillariae Cirrhosae) 10g, *Fang Feng* (Radix Saposhnikoviae) 10g, *Gan Cao* (Radix et Rhizoma Glycyrrhizae) 10g, *Ru Xiang* (Gummi Olibanum) 6g, *Mo Yao* (Myrrha) 6g, *Zao Jiao Ci* (Spina Gleditsiae) 10g, *Tian Hua Fen* (Radix Trichosanthis) 10g, and *Chen Pi* (Pericarpium Citri Reticulatae) 10g. The treatment protocol was to administer the herbs in decoction with a small amount of grain-based liquor. The topical formulation contained 60g each of *Da Huang* (Radix et Rhizoma Rhei) and *Mang Xiao* (Natrii Sulfas). These two herbs were cooked in 8,000 mL of water for 40 minutes, and the decoction was given as a room-temperature herbal wash to the affected area.[3]

3. **Mastitis**: One hundred and eight patients with acute mastitis were treated with modified *Xian Fang Huo Ming Yin*, with complete recovery in 82 cases, marked improvement in 15 cases, slight improvement in 10 cases, and no effect in 1 case. The herbal formula contained *Jin Yin Hua* (Flos Lonicerae Japonicae) 20g, *Fang Feng* (Radix Saposhnikoviae) 10g, *Bai Zhi* (Radix Angelicae Dahuricae) 10g, *Zhe Bei Mu* (Bulbus Fritillariae Thunbergii) 20g, *Tian Hua Fen* (Radix Trichosanthis) 10g, dry-fried *Ru Xiang* (Gummi Olibanum) 10g, dry-fried *Mo Yao* (Myrrha) 10g, vinegar-fried *Chai Hu* (Radix Bupleuri) 20g, vinegar-fried *Xiang Fu* (Rhizoma Cyperi) 12g, *Huang Qin* (Radix Scutellariae) 10g, *Wang Bu Liu Xing* (Semen Vaccariae) 10g, and others as deemed necessary. The treatment protocol was to cook the herbs in water, drink the decoction, and apply the warm herb residue topically to the affected area.[4]

4. **Appendicular abscess**: Use of *Xian Fang Huo Ming Yin* was effective in treating 27 of 30 patients with appendicular abscess. The formula effectively reduced

inflammation, relieved pain, and lowered body temperature.[5]

5. **Thrombophlebitis**: Two studies reported good results using modified *Xian Fang Huo Ming Yin* to treat thrombophlebitis. According to the first study, 12 patients were treated with both oral and topical applications of herbs on a daily basis. The herbal formula contained *Jin Yin Hua* (Flos Lonicerae Japonicae) 50g, *Pu Gong Ying* (Herba Taraxaci) 30g, *Lian Qiao* (Fructus Forsythiae) 15g, *Tian Hua Fen* (Radix Trichosanthis) 15g, *Dang Gui* (Radix Angelicae Sinensis) 15g, *Ji Xue Teng* (Caulis Spatholobi) 15g, *Xiang Fu* (Rhizoma Cyperi) 15g, *Chen Pi* (Pericarpium Citri Reticulatae) 15g, *Si Gua Luo* (Retinervus Luffae Fructus) 15g, *Wei Ling Xian* (Radix et Rhizoma Clematidis) 10g, *Fang Feng* (Radix Saposhnikoviae) 10g, *Chuan Shan Jia* (Squama Manis) 10g, *Bai Zhi* (Radix Angelicae Dahuricae) 10g, *Chi Shao* (Radix Paeoniae Rubra) 10g, *Hong Hua* (Flos Carthami) 10g, *Ru Xiang* (Gummi Olibanum) 10g, *Mo Yao* (Myrrha) 10g, *Mu Xiang* (Radix Aucklandiae) 10g, *Cang Zhu* (Rhizoma Atractylodis) 10g, *Huang Bo* (Cortex Phellodendri Chinensis) 10g, *Gan Cao* (Radix et Rhizoma Glycyrrhizae) 10g, *Niu Xi* (Radix Achyranthis Bidentatae) 25g, and 50 mL of grain-based liquor. The treatment protocol was to cook the herbs in water, and drink the decoction. The herb residue was placed inside a cheese cloth which was applied topically to the affected area while warm. Of 12 patients, the study reported complete recovery in 9 cases and marked improvement in 3 cases.[6] In another study, 111 patients with thrombophlebitis were also treated with good results using modified *Xian Fang Huo Ming Yin*. Of 60 patients diagnosed with damp-heat, 49 had complete recovery and 11 had improvement. Of 51 patients diagnosed with blood stagnation, 28 had complete recovery and 20 had improvement.[7]

6. **Tonsillitis**: Use of modified *Xian Fang Huo Ming Yin* was associated with complete recovery in all 36 patients with acute tonsillitis (19 males and 17 females, between 4-65 years of age). The duration of treatment ranged from 3-8 days, with improvement noted in most patients within the first 1-2 days. The herbal formula contained *Jin Yin Hua* (Flos Lonicerae Japonicae) 9-30g, *Dang Gui Wei* (Extremitas Radix Angelicae Sinensis) 6-15g, *Chi Shao* (Radix Paeoniae Rubra) 6-15g, processed *Ru Xiang* (Gummi Olibanum) 3-15g, processed *Mo Yao* (Myrrha) 6-15g, *Zhe Bei Mu* (Bulbus Fritillariae Thunbergii) 3-15g, *Tian Hua Fen* (Radix Trichosanthis) 6-15g, processed *Chuan Shan Jia* (Squama Manis) 3-15g, dry-fried *Zao Jiao Ci* (Spina Gleditsiae) 3-15g, *Chen Pi* (Pericarpium Citri Reticulatae) 6-18g, *Gan Cao* (Radix et Rhizoma Glycyrrhizae) 3-9g, *Fang Feng* (Radix Saposhnikoviae) 3-15g, *Bai Zhi* (Radix Angelicae Dahuricae) 6-15g, and

Chapter 22 – Formulas that Treat Abscesses and Sores   *Section 1 – External Abscesses and Sores*

Xiān Fāng Huó Mìng Yǐn (Sublime Formula for Sustaining Life)

others as needed. The herbs were cooked in water, and the decoction administered in three equally-divided doses.[8]

7. **Peritonsillar abscesses**: One study reported complete recovery in 57 of 60 patients (54 males and 6 females, between 18-55 years of age) with peritonsillar abscesses using modified *Xian Fang Huo Ming Yin*. The duration of treatment ranged from 3-7 packs of herbs. The herbal formula contained 10 grams each of *Jin Yin Hua* (Flos Lonicerae Japonicae), *Bai Zhi* (Radix Angelicae Dahuricae), *Bei Mu* (Bulbus Fritillariae), *Fang Feng* (Radix Saposhnikoviae), *Chi Shao* (Radix Paeoniae Rubra), *Dang Gui* (Radix Angelicae Sinensis), *Zao Jiao Ci* (Spina Gleditsiae), *Chuan Shan Jia* (Squama Manis) and *Tian Hua Fen* (Radix Trichosanthis); and 6 grams each of *Ru Xiang* (Gummi Olibanum), *Mo Yao* (Myrrha), *Chen Pi* (Pericarpium Citri Reticulatae), and *Gan Cao* (Radix et Rhizoma Glycyrrhizae). Additional modifications were made if necessary.[9]

8. **Anal sinusitis**: One hundred and fifty-six patients with anal sinusitis showed marked improvement using oral and topical application of herbs. The formula for oral ingestion contained *Jin Yin Hua* (Flos Lonicerae Japonicae), *Chen Pi* (Pericarpium Citri Reticulatae), *Gan Cao* (Radix et Rhizoma Glycyrrhizae), *Tian Hua Fen* (Radix Trichosanthis), *Ru Xiang* (Gummi Olibanum), *Mo Yao* (Myrrha), *Dang Gui Wei* (Extremitas Radix Angelicae Sinensis), *Bai Zhi* (Radix Angelicae Dahuricae), *Fang Feng* (Radix Saposhnikoviae), *Chi Shao* (Radix Paeoniae Rubra), *Zao Jiao Ci* (Spina Gleditsiae), processed *Chuan Shan Jia* (Squama Manis), *Da Huang* (Radix et Rhizoma Rhei), and *Huang Bo* (Cortex Phellodendri Chinensis). The herbs used as a topical wash included *Ku Shen* (Radix Sophorae Flavescentis), *Da Huang* (Radix et Rhizoma Rhei), *Mang Xiao* (Natrii Sulfas) and *Huang Bo* (Cortex Phellodendri Chinensis). The duration of treatment was 10-20 days.[10]

9. **Stye**: One study evaluated the use of *Xian Fang Huo Ming Yin* in treating styes in 30 patients (21 males and 9 females, between 8-35 years of age; 24 were affected in one eye, 6 in both eyes). The herbs were administered in decoction daily, with complete recovery in 28 of 30 cases. The duration of treatment was 4-5 days in most patients, and up to 6-7 days in 3 cases. The herbal formula included *Jin Yin Hua* (Flos Lonicerae Japonicae) 25g, *Bai Zhi* (Radix Angelicae Dahuricae) 10g, *Fang Feng* (Radix Saposhnikoviae) 10g, *Dang Gui* (Radix Angelicae Sinensis) 10g, *Chen Pi* (Pericarpium Citri Reticulatae) 10g, *Zhe Bei Mu* (Bulbus Fritillariae Thunbergii) 9g, processed *Chuan Shan Jia* (Squama Manis) 10g, *Chi Shao* (Radix Paeoniae Rubra) 15g, *Tian Hua Fen* (Radix Trichosanthis) 15g, *Zi Hua Di Ding* (Herba Violae) 15g, *Ru Xiang* (Gummi Olibanum) 6g, *Mo Yao* (Myrrha)

6g, and *Gan Cao* (Radix et Rhizoma Glycyrrhizae) 3g. Furthermore, *Pu Gong Ying* (Herba Taraxaci) was added for toxic heat, and *Da Huang* (Radix et Rhizoma Rhei) for constipation. The treatment protocol was to give one pack of herbs in decoction daily.[11]

10. **Pelvic inflammatory disease**: One study reported good results using modified *Xian Fang Huo Ming Yin* to treat pelvic inflammatory disease. The duration of illness varied from 5-22 days among 34 patients (between 21-44 years of age). The herbal formula contained *Chuan Shan Jia* (Squama Manis) 12g, *Tian Hua Fen* (Radix Trichosanthis) 20g, *Gan Cao* (Radix et Rhizoma Glycyrrhizae) 6g, *Ru Xiang* (Gummi Olibanum) 6g, *Mo Yao* (Myrrha) 6g, *Bai Zhi* (Radix Angelicae Dahuricae) 6g, *Chi Shao* (Radix Paeoniae Rubra) 12g, *Zhe Bei Mu* (Bulbus Fritillariae Thunbergii) 12g, *Fang Feng* (Radix Saposhnikoviae) 10g, *Zao Jiao Ci* (Spina Gleditsiae) 12g, *Dang Gui Wei* (Extremitas Radix Angelicae Sinensis) 12g, *Chen Pi* (Pericarpium Citri Reticulatae) 10g, and *Jin Yin Hua* (Flos Lonicerae Japonicae) 30g. *Pu Gong Ying* (Herba Taraxaci), *Gua Lou* (Fructus Trichosanthis), *Huang Bo* (Cortex Phellodendri Chinensis), and *Chi Fu Ling* (Poria Rubra) were added for excess heat; and *Hong Hua* (Flos Carthami), *San Leng* (Rhizoma Sparganii), and *E Zhu* (Rhizoma Curcumae) were added for inflammation and abscesses. The treatment protocol was to cook the herbs in water and drink the decoction in four equally-divided doses daily. In addition, the herb residue was fried with vinegar, placed inside a cheese cloth, and applied topically to the abdominal area for 30 minutes. Of 34 patients, the study reported complete recovery in 15 cases, marked effect in 9 cases, improvement in 8 cases, and no effect in 2 cases. The overall effectiveness was 94.1%.[12]

11. **Cervicitis and vaginitis**: Modified *Xian Fang Huo Ming Yin* was reported to successfully treat 21 patients with cervicitis and 30 patients with vaginitis. In addition to *Xian Fang Huo Ming Yin* as the base formula, *Da Xue Teng* (Caulis Sargentodoxae) and *Bai Jiang Cao* (Herba cum Radice Patriniae) were added for lower abdominal pain; *Tao Ren* (Semen Persicae), *Hong Hua* (Flos Carthami), *San Leng* (Rhizoma Sparganii) and *E Zhu* (Rhizoma Curcumae) were added for lower abdominal hardness and pain that intensify with pressure; and *Gua Lou Zi* (Semen Trichosanthis) and *Dong Gua Zi* (Semen Benincasae) for itching and leukorrhea. Patients were instructed to soak the affected area in an herbal solution made from *Er Cha* (Catechu), *Wu Bei Zi* (Galla Chinensis), *Tong Lu* (Verdigris), *Xiong Huang* (Realgar), *Qing Dai* (Indigo Naturalis), *Bing Pian* (Borneolum Syntheticum), *Hua Jiao* (Pericarpium Zanthoxyli), *She Chuang Zi* (Fructus Cnidii), and *Di Fu Zi* (Fructus Kochiae).[21]

1328

Chinese Herbal Formulas and Applications

Xiān Fāng Huó Mìng Yǐn (Sublime Formula for Sustaining Life)

12. **Post-herpetic neuralgia**: One study reported complete recovery in all 44 patients (26 males and 18 females, between 45-85 years of age) with post-herpetic neuralgia using modified *Xian Fang Huo Ming Yin*. The herbal formula contained *Jin Yin Hua* (Flos Lonicerae Japonicae) 12g, *Ru Xiang* (Gummi Olibanum) 6g, *Mo Yao* (Myrrha) 6g, *Zao Jiao Ci* (Spina Gleditsiae) 6g, *Bai Zhi* (Radix Angelicae Dahuricae) 6g, *Chi Shao* (Radix Paeoniae Rubra) 10g, *Dang Gui Wei* (Extremitas Radix Angelicae Sinensis) 10g, *Tian Hua Fen* (Radix Trichosanthis) 10g, *Chen Pi* (Pericarpium Citri Reticulatae) 10g, *Tao Ren* (Semen Persicae) 10g, *Yan Hu Suo* (Rhizoma Corydalis) 10g, *Chuan Shan Jia* (Squama Manis) 3g, *Gan Cao* (Radix et Rhizoma Glycyrrhizae) 3g, *Dan Shen* (Radix et Rhizoma Salviae Miltiorrhizae) 30g, and *Hong Hua* (Flos Carthami) 5g. Moreover, *Chuan Lian Zi* (Fructus Toosendan) 10g, *Yu Jin* (Radix Curcumae) 12g, and *Chai Hu* (Radix Bupleuri) 6g were added for shingles affecting the trunk; *Jiang Huang* (Rhizoma Curcumae Longae) 12g was added for upper extremities; *Chuan Niu Xi* (Radix Cyathulae) for lower extremities; and *Quan Xie* (Scorpio) for prolonged duration of pain. The herbs were given in decoction daily, with duration varying from 9-26 packs of herbs.[13]

13. **Psoriasis**: Use of *Xian Fang Huo Ming Yin* to treat psoriasis in 25 patients was associated with a 72% rate of recovery and 92% effectiveness. The herbal formula contained *Jin Yin Hua* (Flos Lonicerae Japonicae), *Fang Feng* (Radix Saposhnikoviae), *Bai Zhi* (Radix Angelicae Dahuricae), *Zao Jiao Ci* (Spina Gleditsiae), *Chuan Shan Jia* (Squama Manis), *Tian Hua Fen* (Radix Trichosanthis), *Ru Xiang* (Gummi Olibanum), *Mo Yao* (Myrrha), *Chi Shao* (Radix Paeoniae Rubra), and *Chen Pi* (Pericarpium Citri Reticulatae). The patients were given 6g of pills made from herbal extract, three times daily, for 30 days per course of treatment, for 2 courses total.[14]

14. **Reflux esophagitis**: One study reported complete recovery in 78 of 104 patients with reflux esophagitis who were treated with modified *Xian Fang Huo Ming Yin*. The base formula contained *Jin Yin Hua* (Flos Lonicerae Japonicae) 30g, *Zao Jiao Ci* (Spina Gleditsiae) 30g, *Dang Gui* (Radix Angelicae Sinensis) 12g, *Chen Pi* (Pericarpium Citri Reticulatae) 10g, *Chi Shao* (Radix Paeoniae Rubra) 10g, *Tian Hua Fen* (Radix Trichosanthis) 10g, *Bei Mu* (Bulbus Fritillariae) 6g, processed *Chuan Shan Jia* (Squama Manis) 6g, *Ru Xiang* (Gummi Olibanum) 6g, *Mo Yao* (Myrrha) 6g, and *Gan Cao* (Radix et Rhizoma Glycyrrhizae) 6g. In addition, *Hai Piao Xiao* (Endoconcha Sepiae) 10g and *Wa Leng Zi* (Concha Arcae) 10g were added for acid reflux and belching; *Xian He Cao* (Herba Agrimoniae) 15g and *Ou Jie* (Nodus Nelumbinis Rhizomatis) 10g for bleeding; and *She Gan* (Rhizoma Belamcandae) 10g and

Xuan Shen (Radix Scrophulariae) 10g for soreness and pain of the throat. The duration of treatment ranged from 1-3 weeks.[15]

15. **Peptic ulcer disease**: One study reported 94.3% effectiveness using modified *Xian Fang Huo Ming Yin* to treat peptic ulcers in 53 patients (39 males and 14 females, between 20-60 years of age). The herbal formula contained 15g each of *Dang Gui Wei* (Extremitas Radix Angelicae Sinensis), *Chi Shao* (Radix Paeoniae Rubra), *Zhe Bei Mu* (Bulbus Fritillariae Thunbergii), *Tian Hua Fen* (Radix Trichosanthis), and *Jin Yin Hua* (Flos Lonicerae Japonicae); 10g each of *Fang Feng* (Radix Saposhnikoviae), *Bai Zhi* (Radix Angelicae Dahuricae), *Chen Pi* (Pericarpium Citri Reticulatae), and *Zao Jiao Ci* (Spina Gleditsiae); and 6g each of *Ru Xiang* (Gummi Olibanum), *Mo Yao* (Myrrha), *Chuan Shan Jia* (Squama Manis), and *Gan Cao* (Radix et Rhizoma Glycyrrhizae). The treatment protocol was to administer the herbs in decoction daily, for 30 days per course of treatment. Of 53 patients, the study reported complete recovery in 35 cases, improvement in 15 cases, and no effect in 3 cases.[16]

16. **Ulcerative colitis**: Modified *Xian Fang Huo Ming Yin* was effective in treating chronic ulcerative colitis in 42 patients (24 male, 18 female, between 16-67 years of age). The history of illness ranged from 6 months to 5 years. The base herbal formula contained *Jin Yin Hua* (Flos Lonicerae Japonicae) 30g, *Zao Jiao Ci* (Spina Gleditsiae) 30g, *Chuan Shan Jia* (Squama Manis) 30g, *Fang Feng* (Radix Saposhnikoviae) 9g, *Tian Hua Fen* (Radix Trichosanthis) 9g, *Mo Yao* (Myrrha) 9g, *Huai Hua* (Flos Sophorae) 9g, *Dang Gui* (Radix Angelicae Sinensis) 10g, *Gan Cao* (Radix et Rhizoma Glycyrrhizae) 10g, *Chuan Bei Mu* (Bulbus Fritillariae Cirrhosae) 6g, *Ru Xiang* (Gummi Olibanum) 6g, and *Bai Ji* (Rhizoma Bletillae) 6g. Furthermore, *He Zi* (Fructus Chebulae) 6g and *Ying Su Ke* (Pericarpium Papaveris) 6g were added for severe diarrhea; *Mu Xiang* (Radix Aucklandiae) 6g and *Zhi Qiao* (Fructus Aurantii) 6g for severe abdominal pain; *Huang Bo* (Cortex Phellodendri Chinensis) 9g and *Huang Lian* (Rhizoma Coptidis) 9g for rectal tenesmus; and *Mu Dan Pi* (Cortex Moutan) 9g and *Ce Bai Ye* (Cacumen Platycladi) 9g for hematochezia. The duration of treatment ranged from 10-20 days. Of 42 patients, the study reported complete recovery in 24 cases, improvement in 10 cases, and no effect in 8 cases.[17]

17. **Osteoradionecrosis**: Concurrent Western and herbal treatments showed good results in treating 42 patients with bone necrosis following irradiation. The base formula included *Dang Gui* (Radix Angelicae Sinensis) 12g, *Chuan Shan Jia* (Squama Manis) 12g, *Jin Yin Hua* (Flos Lonicerae Japonicae) 10g, *Tian Hua Fen*

FORMULAS THAT TREAT ABSCESSES AND SORES

22

1329

Chapter 22 – Formulas that Treat Abscesses and Sores

Section 1 – External Abscesses and Sores

Xiān Fāng Huó Mìng Yǐn (Sublime Formula for Sustaining Life)

(Radix Trichosanthis) 10g, *Bai Zhi* (Radix Angelicae Dahuricae) 10g, *Fang Feng* (Radix Saposhnikoviae) 10g, *Zao Jiao Ci* (Spina Gleditsiae) 10g, *Chen Pi* (Pericarpium Citri Reticulatae) 10g, *Zhe Bei Mu* (Bulbus Fritillariae Thunbergii) 10g, *Ru Xiang* (Gummi Olibanum) 9g, *Mo Yao* (Myrrha) 9g, *Chi Shao* (Radix Paeoniae Rubra) 8g, and *Gan Cao* (Radix et Rhizoma Glycyrrhizae) 8g. Additional modifications were made as deemed necessary. The treatment protocol was to cook the herbs in water, and administer the decoction twice daily in two equally-divided doses before breakfast and at bedtime, for 7 days per course of treatment, for 3-4 courses total. Of 42 patients, the study reported complete recovery in 23 cases, improvement in 14 cases, and no effect in 5 cases.[18] Note: Details of the Western treatment were unavailable at the time of publication.

18. **Osteomyelitis**: Individuals with osteomyelitis were treated with good results using *Xian Fang Huo Ming Yin* and *Yang He Tang* (Yang-Heartening Decoction), plus topical application of other medicine(s). Of 28 patients, the study reported complete recovery in 19 cases after 3-4 months, 4 cases after 5-6 months, and unsatisfactory effect in 5 cases.[19] Note: Details of the medicine(s) used topically were unavailable at the time of publication.

19. **Pneumonia**: Use of modified *Xian Fang Huo Ming Yin* was associated with 87% effectiveness in treating pneumonia in 46 patients (28 males and 18 females, between 18-67 years of age). The herbal formula contained *Jin Yin Hua* (Flos Lonicerae Japonicae) 30g, *Chuan Shan Jia* (Squama Manis) 20g, *Fang Feng* (Radix Saposhnikoviae) 10g, *Bai Zhi* (Radix Angelicae Dahuricae) 12g, *Dang Gui* (Radix Angelicae Sinensis) 10g, *Chen Pi* (Pericarpium Citri Reticulatae) 10g, *Bei Mu* (Bulbus Fritillariae) 10g, *Huang Qin* (Radix Scutellariae) 10g, *Zao Jiao Ci* (Spina Gleditsiae) 20g, *Tian Hua Fen* (Radix Trichosanthis) 15g, *Gan Cao* (Radix et Rhizoma Glycyrrhizae) 5g, *Sang Bai Pi* (Cortex Mori) 12g, and *Jie Geng* (Radix Platycodonis) 12g. *Yu Xing Cao* (Herba Houttuyniae) 30g was added for dark, thick phlegm; and *Gua Lou* (Fructus Trichosanthis) 15g for chest pain. The herbs were given in decoction daily, for 7 days per course of treatment. Of 46 patients, 29 had significant improvement, 11 had moderate improvement, and 6 had no effect.[20]

RELATED FORMULAS

Zhēn Rén Huó Mìng Yǐn

(True Man's Decoction to Revitalize Life)

真人活命飲
真人活命饮

Pinyin Name: *Zhen Ren Huo Ming Yin*
Literal Name: True Man's Decoction to Revitalize Life
Alternate Name: Angelica and Mastic Combination

Original Source: *Yi Fang Ji Jie* (Analytical Collection of Medical Formulas) by Wang Ang in 1682

Bai Zhi (Radix Angelicae Dahuricae)	3g
Bei Mu (Bulbus Fritillariae)	3g
Fang Feng (Radix Saposhnikoviae)	3g
Dang Gui Wei (Extremitas Radix Angelicae Sinensis)	3g
Gan Cao (Radix et Rhizoma Glycyrrhizae)	3g
Zao Jiao Ci (Spina Gleditsiae), *chao* (dry-fried)	3g
Chuan Shan Jia (Squama Manis), *zhi* (fried with liquid)	3g
Tian Hua Fen (Radix Trichosanthis)	3g
Mo Yao (Myrrha)	3g
Ru Xiang (Gummi Olibanum)	3g
Jin Yin Hua (Flos Lonicerae Japonicae)	9g
Chen Pi (Pericarpium Citri Reticulatae)	9g

Xian Fang Huo Ming Yin and *Zhen Ren Huo Ming Yin* (True Man's Decoction to Revitalize Life) are essentially the same formula, except that *Xian Fang Huo Ming Yin* contains *Chi Shao* (Radix Paeoniae Rubra), while *Zhen Ren Huo Ming Yin* (True Man's Decoction to Revitalize Life) does not.

According to Dr. Chang Wei-Yen, male infertility caused by spermophlebectasia (varicocele) or inflammation can be treated with *Zhen Ren Huo Ming Yin* (True Man's Decoction to Revitalize Life) combined with *Da Ding Huang* (Caulis Euonymi), *Zao Jiao Ci* (Spina Gleditsiae), *Ma Bian Cao* (Herba Verbenae), and *Cha Chi Huang* (Herba Stellariae Aquaticae). Also according to Chang, prostate enlargement can be effectively treated with the combination of *Zhen Ren Huo Ming Yin* (True Man's Decoction to Revitalize Life), *San Zhong Kui Jian Tang* (Disperse the Swelling and Break the Hardness Decoction), and *Shi Liu Wei Liu Qi Yin* (Sixteen-Ingredient Decoction to Flow Qi). This can be done by combining prepared formulas together, such as with extracts in granular or capsule forms.

Huó Mìng Yǐn (Revitalize Life Decoction)

活命飲
活命饮

Pinyin Name: *Huo Ming Yin*
Literal Name: Revitalize Life Decoction
Original Source: *Jian Tai Zhen Suo Fang* (Herbal Prescriptions from *Jiantai* Clinic) by Chang Wei-Yen in 1981

Bai Zhi (Radix Angelicae Dahuricae)
Zhe Bei Mu (Bulbus Fritillariae Thunbergii)
Fang Feng (Radix Saposhnikoviae)
Dang Gui (Radix Angelicae Sinensis)

1330

Xiān Fāng Huó Mìng Yǐn (Sublime Formula for Sustaining Life)

Chi Shao (Radix Paeoniae Rubra)

Gan Cao (Radix et Rhizoma Glycyrrhizae)

Zao Jiao Ci (Spina Gleditsiae), *chao* (dry-fried)

Tian Hua Fen (Radix Trichosanthis)

San Leng (Rhizoma Sparganii)

E Zhu (Rhizoma Curcumae)

Jin Yin Hua (Flos Lonicerae Japonicae)

Chen Pi (Pericarpium Citri Reticulatae)

Kun Bu (Thallus Eckloniae)

Tong Cao (Medulla Tetrapanacis)

Xia Ku Cao (Spica Prunellae)

Xian Fang Huo Ming Yin and *Huo Ming Yin* (Revitalize Life Decoction) are very similar formulas. *Huo Ming Yin* contains *Kun Bu* (Thallus Eckloniae), *Tong Cao* (Medulla Tetrapanacis), and *Xia Ku Cao* (Spica Prunellae) to enhance the formula's ability to eliminate stagnation and soften nodules and hardness. *Chuan Shan Jia* (Squama Manis) has been removed, since it is derived from an endangered animal.

Lián Qiào Bài Dú Sǎn

(Forsythia Powder to Overcome Pathogenic Influences)

連翹敗毒散
连翘败毒散

Pinyin Name: *Lian Qiao Bai Du San*

Literal Name: Forsythia Powder to Overcome Pathogenic Influences

Alternate Names: *Lien Jiao Pai Tu San*, Forsythia Detoxifying Formula

Original Source: *Shang Han Quan Sheng Ji* (All New Collection of Cold-Induced Disorders)

Lian Qiao (Fructus Forsythiae)	[9g]
Zhi Zi (Fructus Gardeniae)	[9g]
Qiang Huo (Rhizoma et Radix Notopterygii)	[8g]
Xuan Shen (Radix Scrophulariae)	[12g]
Bo He (Herba Menthae)	[5g]
Fang Feng (Radix Saposhnikoviae)	[5g]
Chai Hu (Radix Bupleuri)	[6g]
Jie Geng (Radix Platycodonis)	[5g]
Sheng Ma (Rhizoma Cimicifugae)	[5g]
Chuan Xiong (Rhizoma Chuanxiong)	[6g]
Dang Gui (Radix Angelicae Sinensis)	[8g]
Huang Qin (Radix Scutellariae)	[9g]
Bai Shao (Radix Paeoniae Alba)	[10g]
Niu Bang Zi (Fructus Arctii)	[6g]

The source text states to cook the ingredients with *Hong Hua* (Flos Carthami) to make a decoction. However, the doses of the ingredients are unavailable from the source text. Today, the decoction is prepared by using the doses suggested in brackets.

The main actions of *Lian Qiao Bai Du San* (Forsythia Powder to Overcome Pathogenic Influences) are to release wind-heat, clear heat, and eliminate heat and toxins. Clinically, this formula has been used to treat mumps. In addition to the base formula, modifications can be made as follows: *Tian Hua Fen* (Radix Trichosanthis) for thirst; *Bai Zhi* (Radix Angelicae Dahuricae) for swelling in the face; *Wei Ling Xian* (Radix et Rhizoma Clematidis) for swelling on the neck; *Da Huang* (Radix et Rhizoma Rhei) and *Chuan Shan Jia* (Squama Manis) for constipation due to excess; and *Ren Shen* (Radix et Rhizoma Ginseng) for deficiency.

AUTHORS' COMMENTS

Xian Fang Huo Ming Yin is one of the most commonly used formulas for treating all sorts of abscesses, sores, nodules or swellings that are red, hot, hard, and painful to the touch. The lesions may or may not contain pus. The effect of this formula can be maximized by both oral and topical use of herbs. After serving the decoction, the herb residue can be applied topically to ease pain and swelling.

Xian Fang Huo Ming Yin and *Pu Ji Xiao Du Yin* (Universal Benefit Decoction to Eliminate Toxin) both clear heat and eliminate toxins.

- *Xian Fang Huo Ming Yin*, besides clearing heat and eliminating toxins, also moves qi and blood to disperse the initial stages of nodules, swellings, carbuncles, and sores.
- *Pu Ji Xiao Du Yin* focuses on treating toxic heat affecting the upper *jiao*, manifesting in symptoms such as redness, swelling and pain of the face, difficulty in opening the eyes, sore throat, thirst, and fever. It disperses wind-heat as well as toxins lodged in the head.

References

1. *He Nan Zhong Yi* (Henan Chinese Medicine) 1988;5:31.
2. *Hu Bei Zhong Yi Za Zhi* (Hubei Journal of Chinese Medicine) 1988;6:23.
3. *Shan Xi Zhong Yi* (Shanxi Chinese Medicine) 1989;8:366.
4. *Nei Meng Gu Zhong Yi Yao* (Traditional Chinese Medicine and Medicinals of Inner Mongolia) 1994;2:7.
5. *Zhong Hua Wai Ke Za Zhi* (Chinese Journal of External Medicine) 1960;2:171.
6. *Liao Ning Zhong Yi Za Zhi* (Liaoning Journal of Chinese Medicine) 1991;5:34.
7. *Xin Zhong Yi* (New Chinese Medicine) 1992;10:24.
8. *He Nan Zhong Yi* (Henan Chinese Medicine) 1995;5:35.
9. *Shan Dong Zhong Yi Za Zhi* (Shandong Journal of Chinese Medicine) 1992;11(5):15.
10. *Hu Nan Zhong Yi Xue Yuan Xue Bao* (Journal of Hunan University of Traditional Chinese Medicine) 1994;2:24.
11. *Hu Bei Zhong Yi Za Zhi* (Hubei Journal of Chinese Medicine) 1989;4.
12. *Jiang Su Zhong Yi* (Jiangsu Chinese Medicine) 1996;6:18.
13. *Si Chuan Zhong Yi* (Sichuan Chinese Medicine) 1996;12:49.

Xiān Fāng Huó Mìng Yǐn (Sublime Formula for Sustaining Life)

14. *Hu Nan Zhong Yi Xue Yuan Xue Bao* (Journal of Hunan University of Traditional Chinese Medicine) 1998;3:50.
15. *Zhe Jiang Zhong Yi Za Zhi* (Zhejiang Journal of Chinese Medicine) 1990;4:155.
16. *Si Chuan Zhong Yi* (Sichuan Chinese Medicine) 1990;8(8):22.
17. *Zhe Jiang Zhong Yi Za Zhi* (Zhejiang Journal of Chinese Medicine) 1996;1:16.

18. *Xin Zhong Yi* (New Chinese Medicine) 1999;10:24.
19. *Xin Zhong Yi* (New Chinese Medicine) 1990;4:37.
20. *Fu Jian Zhong Yi Yao* (Fujian Chinese Medicine and Herbology) 1997;4:37.
21. *Xin Zhong Yi* (New Chinese Medicine) 1986;11:7.

Niú Bàng Jiě Jī Tāng
(Arctium Decoction to Release the Muscle Layer)

牛蒡解肌湯
牛蒡解肌汤

Pinyin Name: *Niu Bang Jie Ji Tang*
Literal Name: Arctium Decoction to Release the Muscle Layer
Original Source: *Yang Ke Xin De Ji* (Collection of Personal Expertise Concerning Skin Lesions) by Gao Bing-Jun in 1805

COMPOSITION

Niu Bang Zi (Fructus Arctii)	[10g]
Bo He (Herba Menthae)	[6g]
Jing Jie (Herba Schizonepetae)	[6g]
Lian Qiao (Fructus Forsythiae)	[10g]
Mu Dan Pi (Cortex Moutan)	[10g]
Xia Ku Cao (Spica Prunellae)	[12g]
Zhi Zi (Fructus Gardeniae)	[10g]
Xuan Shen (Radix Scrophulariae)	[10g]
Shi Hu (Caulis Dendrobii)	[12g]

DOSAGE / PREPARATION / ADMINISTRATION

The source text states to prepare the ingredients as a decoction. However, the doses of the ingredients are unavailable from the source text. Today, the decoction is prepared by using the doses suggested in brackets.

CHINESE THERAPEUTIC ACTIONS

1. Disperses exterior wind and clears heat
2. Cools the blood and reduces swelling

CLINICAL MANIFESTATIONS

Localized abscesses and swelling due to exterior wind-heat invasion: phlegm and toxins in the neck, toothache caused by wind-heat, abscesses with redness, swelling, and pain; chills and fever (more fever than chills), mild perspiration, thirst, yellow urine, a white or yellow tongue coating, and a superficial, rapid pulse.

CLINICAL APPLICATIONS

Cellulitis, mastitis, and various abscesses and sores.

EXPLANATION

Niu Bang Jie Ji Tang (Arctium Decoction to Release the Muscle Layer) treats localized abscesses and swellings (mostly on the face and neck) accompanied by exterior wind-heat. Local accumulation of heat and toxins may cause redness and pain. Chills and fever, with more fever than chills, suggest an exterior wind-heat syndrome. Mild perspiration, thirst, toothache, and yellowish urine indicate that the heat has damaged the body fluids. The yellow tongue coating and a superficial, rapid pulse signify a wind-heat syndrome.

Niu Bang Zi (Fructus Arctii) disperses wind-heat, eliminates toxins, and reduces swelling, especially from

1332

Chinese Herbal Formulas and Applications

Niú Bàng Jiě Jī Tāng
(Arctium Decoction to Release the Muscle Layer)

Niu Bang Jie Ji Tang (Arctium Decoction to Release the Muscle Layer)

Diagnosis	Signs and Symptoms	Treatment	Herbs
Localized abscesses and swelling due to exterior wind-heat	• Abscesses with redness, swelling and pain: accumulation of heat and toxins • Chills and fever: exterior wind-heat condition • Mild perspiration, thirst and yellow urine: heat damaging the body fluids • Yellow tongue coating and a superficial, rapid pulse: wind-heat condition	• Disperses exterior wind and clears heat • Cools the blood and reduces swelling	• *Niu Bang Zi* (Fructus Arctii) disperses wind-heat, eliminates toxins, and reduces swelling. • *Bo He* (Herba Menthae) and *Jing Jie* (Herba Schizonepetae) disperse the wind-heat factor and release exterior symptoms. • *Lian Qiao* (Fructus Forsythiae) clears heat, eliminates toxins, disperses nodules, and reduces abscesses. • *Mu Dan Pi* (Cortex Moutan), *Xia Ku Cao* (Spica Prunellae), and *Zhi Zi* (Fructus Gardeniae) sedate fire and cool the blood. • *Xuan Shen* (Radix Scrophulariae) sedates heat and eliminates toxins. • *Shi Hu* (Caulis Dendrobii) nourishes yin and body fluids.

the head and face. *Bo He* (Herba Menthae) and *Jing Jie* (Herba Schizonepetae) disperse the wind-heat and release exterior symptoms. *Lian Qiao* (Fructus Forsythiae) clears heat, eliminates toxins, disperses nodules, and reduces abscesses. *Mu Dan Pi* (Cortex Moutan), *Xia Ku Cao* (Spica Prunellae), and *Zhi Zi* (Fructus Gardeniae) sedate fire and cool the blood. *Xuan Shen* (Radix Scrophulariae) sedates heat and eliminates toxins; also, it is combined with *Shi Hu* (Caulis Dendrobii) to clear heat and nourish yin and body fluids.

CAUTIONS / CONTRAINDICATIONS

Niu Bang Jie Ji Tang should be used with caution in patients with underlying yin and body fluid deficiencies, or those without excess heat or fire.

AUTHORS' COMMENTS

Niu Bang Jie Ji Tang was used originally for localized abscesses and swellings on the face and neck. Today, its application has been expanded to include most regions of the body, as long as the condition is characterized by localized abscesses and swellings accompanied by exterior wind-heat invasion.

FORMULAS THAT TREAT ABSCESSES AND SORES

22

1333

Jīng Fáng Bài Dú Sǎn
(Schizonepeta and Saposhnikovia Powder to Overcome Pathogenic Influences)

荆防敗毒散
荆防败毒散

Pinyin Name: *Jing Fang Bai Du San*
Literal Name: Schizonepeta and Saposhnikovia Powder to Overcome Pathogenic Influences
Alternate Names: *Ching Fang Pai Tu San*, Schizonepeta and Siler Detoxifying Formula, Schizonepeta and Siler Formula
Original Source: *She Sheng Zhong Miao Fang* (Marvelous Formulas for the Health of Multitudes) by Zhang Shi-Che in 1550

COMPOSITION

Chai Hu (Radix Bupleuri)	4.5g
Qian Hu (Radix Peucedani)	4.5g
Jing Jie (Herba Schizonepetae)	4.5g
Fang Feng (Radix Saposhnikoviae)	4.5g
Qiang Huo (Rhizoma et Radix Notopterygii)	4.5g
Du Huo (Radix Angelicae Pubescentis)	4.5g
Jie Geng (Radix Platycodonis)	4.5g
Chuan Xiong (Rhizoma Chuanxiong)	4.5g
Fu Ling (Poria)	4.5g
Zhi Qiao (Fructus Citri Aurantii)	4.5g
Gan Cao (Radix et Rhizoma Glycyrrhizae)	1.5g [3g]

DOSAGE / PREPARATION / ADMINISTRATION

Prepare the ingredients as a decoction.

CHINESE THERAPEUTIC ACTIONS

1. Releases the exterior and induces diaphoresis
2. Treats skin and external diseases
3. Relieves pain

CLINICAL MANIFESTATIONS

Early stage of skin and external diseases: abscesses and sores with redness, swelling and pain, aversion to cold, fever, absence of perspiration, no thirst, a thin, white tongue coating, and a superficial, rapid pulse.

CLINICAL APPLICATIONS

Carbuncles, pustules, boils, urticaria, eczema, dermatitis, abscesses, sores, suppuration, mastitis, eye disorders, syphilis, and scabies.

EXPLANATION

Jing Fang Bai Du San (Schizonepeta and Saposhnikovia Powder to Overcome Pathogenic Influences) primarily treats skin and external disorders, such as abscesses and sores. Local signs and symptoms include redness, swelling and pain of the affected area, and systemic signs and symptoms include aversion to cold, fever, absence of perspiration, and lack of thirst.

Chai Hu (Radix Bupleuri) and *Qian Hu* (Radix Peucedani) are exterior-releasing herbs that dispel wind and heat. *Jing Jie* (Herba Schizonepetae), *Fang Feng* (Radix Saposhnikoviae), *Qiang Huo* (Rhizoma et Radix Notopterygii), and *Du Huo* (Radix Angelicae Pubescentis) release the exterior, eliminate toxins, and relieve pain. *Jie Geng* (Radix Platycodonis), *Chuan Xiong* (Rhizoma Chuanxiong), and *Fu Ling* (Poria) reduce swelling and inflammation, move the blood, and eliminate pus. *Zhi Qiao* (Fructus Aurantii) regulates qi circulation and removes stagnation. *Gan Cao* (Radix et Rhizoma Glycyrrhizae) harmonizes the herbs.

MODIFICATIONS

- If there is swelling and pain caused by more heat, add *Huang Qin* (Radix Scutellariae) and *Huang Lian* (Rhizoma Coptidis).
- If there is swelling and pain caused by more formation of pus, add *Bai Zhi* (Radix Angelicae Dahuricae) and *Zao Jiao* (Fructus Gleditsiae).
- For allergic dermatitis, add *Wen Qing Yin* (Warming and Clearing Decoction).
- For eczema or rashes, add *Xiao Feng San* (Eliminate Wind Powder).
- If there is exterior cold and interior heat with symptoms of sore throat, a red tongue tip, and a dry mouth, add *Jin Yin Hua* (Flos Lonicerae Japonicae), *Lian Qiao* (Fructus Forsythiae), *Niu Bang Zi* (Fructus Arctii), *Ban Lan Gen*

Chinese Herbal Formulas and Applications

Jīng Fáng Bài Dú Sǎn
(Schizonepeta and Saposhnikovia Powder to Overcome Pathogenic Influences)

Jing Fang Bai Du San (Schizonepeta and Saposhnikovia Powder to Overcome Pathogenic Influences)

Diagnosis	Signs and Symptoms	Treatment	Herbs
Early stages of skin and external diseases	• Abscesses and sores with redness, swelling and pain: wind, cold and dampness in the muscle layer • Aversion to cold, fever and absence of perspiration: presence of wind at the exterior • Thin, white tongue coating, and a superficial, rapid pulse: exterior condition	• Releases the exterior and induces diaphoresis • Treats skin and external diseases	• *Chai Hu* (Radix Bupleuri) and *Qian Hu* (Radix Peucedani) release wind and heat from the exterior parts of the body. • *Jing Jie* (Herba Schizonepetae), *Fang Feng* (Radix Saposhnikoviae), *Qiang Huo* (Rhizoma et Radix Notopterygii), and *Du Huo* (Radix Angelicae Pubescentis) release the exterior, eliminate toxins, and relieve pain. • *Jie Geng* (Radix Platycodonis), *Chuan Xiong* (Rhizoma Chuanxiong), and *Fu Ling* (Poria) reduce swelling and inflammation, move the blood, and eliminate pus. • *Zhi Qiao* (Fructus Aurantii) regulates qi circulation and removes stagnation. • *Gan Cao* (Radix et Rhizoma Glycyrrhizae) harmonizes the herbs.

(Radix Isatidis); and remove *Du Huo* (Radix Angelicae Pubescentis) and *Chuan Xiong* (Rhizoma Chuanxiong).

• For infectious parotitis with severe redness, swelling and burning pain of the tonsils, add *Niu Bang Zi* (Fructus Arctii), *Ma Bo* (Lasiosphaera seu Calvatia), and *She Gan* (Rhizoma Belamcandae).

CAUTIONS / CONTRAINDICATIONS

Avoid foods that are raw, cold, oily, or greasy while taking *Jing Fang Bai Du San*.[1]

CLINICAL STUDIES AND RESEARCH

High fever: One study reported success in the treatment of high fever in 36 of 45 patients using modified *Jing Fang Bai Du San*. The causes of high fever included postpartum illness, nephritis, respiratory tract infection, and others. The herbal treatment contained *Jing Jie* (Herba Schizonepetae) 30g, *Chai Hu* (Radix Bupleuri) 15g, *Fang Feng* (Radix Saposhnikoviae) 10g, and *Bo He* (Herba Menthae) 10g as the base formula. Modifications varied depending on the causes of fever. For postpartum fever, *Dang Shen* (Radix Codonopsis) and *Dang Gui* (Radix Angelicae Sinensis) were added. For nephritis and fever, *Jin Qian Cao* (Herba Lysimachiae) and *Qu Mai* (Herba Dianthi) were added. For exterior cold with fever, *Huo Xiang* (Herba Agastaches) and *Hou Po* (Cortex Magnoliae Officinalis) were added. The treatment protocol was to cook the herbs in water and administer the decoction in two equally-divided doses daily.[2]

RELATED FORMULAS

Jīng Fáng Bài Dú Sǎn (Schizonepeta and Saposhnikovia Powder to Overcome Pathogenic Influences)

荊防毒散
荆防败毒散

Pinyin Name: *Jing Fang Bai Du San*
Literal Name: Schizonepeta and Saposhnikovia Powder to Overcome Pathogenic Influences
Original Source: *Qi Xiao Liang Fang* (Fine Formulas with Miraculous Results)

Chai Hu (Radix Bupleuri)	3g
Chuan Xiong (Rhizoma Chuanxiong)	3g
Du Huo (Radix Angelicae Pubescentis)	3g
Fang Feng (Radix Saposhnikoviae)	3g
Fu Ling (Poria)	3g
Jie Geng (Radix Platycodonis)	3g
Jing Jie (Herba Schizonepetae)	3g
Qian Hu (Radix Peucedani)	3g
Qiang Huo (Rhizoma et Radix Notopterygii)	3g
Sheng Jiang (Rhizoma Zingiberis Recens)	3g
Zhi Qiao (Fructus Aurantii)	3g
Gan Cao (Radix et Rhizoma Glycyrrhizae)	1.5g
Bo He (Herba Menthae)	1g

This formula induces perspiration, releases the exterior, disperses wind, and dispels dampness. It is used to treat wind, cold and dampness at the exterior, leading to signs and symptoms such as fever, aversion to cold, headache, neck stiffness, and body aches and pain.

FORMULAS THAT TREAT ABSCESSES AND SORES

22

1335

Chapter 22 – Formulas that Treat Abscesses and Sores

Section 1 – External Abscesses and Sores

Jīng Fáng Bài Dú Sǎn
(Schizonepeta and Saposhnikovia Powder to Overcome Pathogenic Influences)

Jīng Fáng Bài Dú Sǎn (Schizonepeta and Saposhnikovia Powder to Overcome Pathogenic Influences)

荊防敗毒散
荆防败毒散

Pinyin Name: *Jing Fang Bai Du San*

Literal Name: Schizonepeta and Saposhnikovia Powder to Overcome Pathogenic Influences

Original Source: *Wan Bing Hui Chun* (Restoration of Health from the Myriad Diseases) by Gong Ting-Xian in 1587

Jing Jie (Herba Schizonepetae)

Fang Feng (Radix Saposhnikoviae)

Qiang Huo (Rhizoma et Radix Notopterygii)

Du Huo (Radix Angelicae Pubescentis)

Chai Hu (Radix Bupleuri)

Qian Hu (Radix Peucedani)

Jie Geng (Radix Platycodonis)

Zhi Qiao (Fructus Aurantii)

Chuan Xiong (Rhizoma Chuanxiong)

Bo He (Herba Menthae)

Jin Yin Hua (Flos Lonicerae Japonicae)

Lian Qiao (Fructus Forsythiae)

Chi Fu Ling (Poria Rubra)

Grind equal proportions of all the ingredients into powder and prepare as a decoction with *Sheng Jiang* (Rhizoma Zingiberis Recens) and *Bo He* (Herba Menthae).

This formula treats skin and external disorders with suppuration caused by wind-heat and toxins. Suppuration may occur at various parts of the body, including, but not limited to, the skin and glands. The presence of wind is characterized by such exterior signs and symptoms as aversion to wind and cold, and headache; and the presence of heat is characterized by fever and soreness and swelling of the throat. As the disease progresses, suppuration develops as swelling and inflammation at the affected area begin to form and discharge pus. At this time, treatment must focus on dispelling exterior wind and heat, reducing swelling and inflammation, and eliminating toxins and pus.

Clinical applications of this formula include carbuncles, pustules, boils, urticaria, eczema, dermatitis, abscesses, sores, suppuration, mastitis, protitis, eye disorders, syphilis, and scabies.

AUTHORS' COMMENTS

These three formulas have identical names, but are derived from different sources and have slightly different compositions and applications.

- *Jing Fang Bai Du San* from *She Sheng Zhong Miao Fang* (Marvelous Formulas for the Health of Multitudes) primarily treats early-stage skin and external disorders characterized by wind, cold, and dampness.

- *Jing Fang Bai Du San* from *Qi Xiao Liang Fang* (Fine Formulas with Miraculous Results) also treats early-stage skin and external disorders characterized by wind, cold, and dampness. This formula contains *Sheng Jiang* (Rhizoma Zingiberis Recens) and *Bo He* (Herba Menthae), and is slightly stronger than the previous formula.

- *Jing Fang Bai Du San* from *Wan Bing Hui Chun* (Restoration of Health from the Myriad Diseases) mainly treats skin and external disorders with suppuration, caused by wind, heat, and toxins.

Bai Du San (Overcome Pathogenic Influences Powder) and *Jing Fang Bai Du San* are two very commonly used formulas with similar actions and functions. Both formulas treat external abscesses and sores, but have the following differences:

- *Bai Du San* is more suitable for deficient patients because it contains *Ren Shen* (Radix et Rhizoma Ginseng), which strengthens *yuan* (source) *qi*. In addition, it has only a mild exterior-releasing action, which is all that a weak patient can withstand.

- *Jing Fang Bai Du San* is a potent formula that contains many exterior-releasing herbs, but no tonic herbs to moderate its exterior-releasing actions. *Jing Fang Bai Du San* is indicated for patients who have no deficiencies.

References

1. *Zhong Yao Ming Fang Yao Li Yu Ying Yong* (Pharmacology and Applications of Famous Herbal Formulas) 1989;69-70.

2. *Guang Xi Zhong Yi Yao* (Guangxi Chinese Medicine and Herbology) 1989;4:9.

Chinese Herbal Formulas and Applications

Wŭ Wèi Xiāo Dú Yĭn
(Five-Ingredient Decoction to Eliminate Toxins)

五味消毒飲
五味消毒饮

Pinyin Name: *Wu Wei Xiao Du Yin*
Literal Name: Five-Ingredient Decoction to Eliminate Toxins
Alternate Names: Dandelion and Wild Chrysanthemum Combination, Five-Ingredient Decoction to Eliminate Pathogenic Influences
Original Source: *Yi Zong Jin Jian* (Golden Mirror of the Medical Tradition) by Wu Qian in 1742

COMPOSITION

Jin Yin Hua (Flos Lonicerae Japonicae)	9g [20g]
Zi Hua Di Ding (Herba Violae)	3.6g [15g]
Pu Gong Ying (Herba Taraxaci)	3.6g [15g]
Ye Ju Hua (Flos Chrysanthemi Indici)	3.6g [15g]
Tian Kui Zi (Radix Semiaquilegiae)	3.6g [15g]

DOSAGE / PREPARATION / ADMINISTRATION

The source text states to cook the ingredients with 2 large bowl of water until the liquid is reduced to 80%. Add 0.5 bowl of grain-based liquor and bring it to a boil 2-3 times. Take the hot, strained decoction, and cover the body with blankets to promote sweating.

Today, it is prepared as a decoction, with the doses suggested in brackets, and taken with 1-2 spoonfuls of grain-based liquor. The herb residue is crushed into a paste and applied topically to the affected area.

CHINESE THERAPEUTIC ACTIONS

1. Clears heat and eliminates toxins
2. Disperses external carbuncles and furuncles

CLINICAL MANIFESTATIONS

Carbuncles, furuncles, and other types of epithelial inflammations due to accumulation of fire and toxins: local redness, swelling, heat and pain sensations, fever, aversion to cold, carbuncles and furuncles that are hard and deeply rooted, a red tongue body with a yellow tongue coating, and a rapid pulse.

CLINICAL APPLICATIONS

Cellulitis, febrile disorder, viral hepatitis, acute cholecystitis, acute pyelonephritis, chronic pyelonephritis, glomerulonephritis, pelvic inflammation, bartholinitis, urinary tract infection, tonsillitis, pericoronitis, burns, myelitis, shingles, eczema, boils, acne, carbuncles, and furuncles.

EXPLANATION

Wu Wei Xiao Du Yin (Five-Ingredient Decoction to Eliminate Toxins) treats carbuncles, furuncles, and other types of epithelial inflammations characterized by accumulation of fire and toxins. Accumulation of fire and toxins in the interior *zang fu* organs may result in nail-like carbuncles and furuncles that are hard and deeply rooted, and are characterized by local redness, swelling, heat, and pain. A red tongue body with a yellow tongue coating

Wu Wei Xiao Du Yin (Five-Ingredient Decoction to Eliminate Toxins)

Diagnosis	Signs and Symptoms	Treatment	Herbs
Carbuncles, furuncles, and other types of epithelial inflammations	• Nail-like nodules that are hard and deeply rooted: stagnation of fire and toxins • Local redness, swelling, heat, and pain: qi and blood stagnation • Red tongue body with a yellow tongue coating: heat and toxins • Rapid pulse: heat and toxins	• Clears heat, fire, and toxins • Disperses carbuncles and furuncles	• *Jin Yin Hua* (Flos Lonicerae Japonicae) clears heat and eliminates toxins from both the *qi* (energy) and *xue* (blood) levels. • *Zi Hua Di Ding* (Herba Violae), *Pu Gong Ying* (Herba Taraxaci), *Ye Ju Hua* (Flos Chrysanthemi Indici), and *Tian Kui Zi* (Radix Semiaquilegiae) clear heat, eliminate toxins, cool the blood, disperse nodules, and relieve pain.

FORMULAS THAT TREAT ABSCESSES AND SORES

22

1337

Wǔ Wèi Xiāo Dú Yǐn
(Five-Ingredient Decoction to Eliminate Toxins)

and a rapid pulse suggest that the heat toxins are located mainly in the interior.

This formula contains *Jin Yin Hua* (Flos Lonicerae Japonicae) to clear heat and eliminate toxins from both the *qi* (energy) and *xue* (blood) levels. *Zi Hua Di Ding* (Herba Violae), *Pu Gong Ying* (Herba Taraxaci), *Ye Ju Hua* (Flos Chrysanthemi Indici), and *Tian Kui Zi* (Radix Semiaquilegiae) clear heat, eliminate toxins, cool the blood, disperse nodules, and relieve pain. Grain-based liquor helps to activate blood circulation, and distribute the herbs to the affected area of the body.

MODIFICATIONS

- With more fire and toxins, add *Lian Qiao* (Fructus Forsythiae), *Ban Zhi Lian* (Herba Scutellariae Barbatae), and *Huang Lian* (Rhizoma Coptidis).
- With more swelling and inflammation, add *Fang Feng* (Radix Saposhnikoviae) and *Chan Tui* (Periostracum Cicadae).
- With heat in the *xue* (blood) level, add *Chi Shao* (Radix Paeoniae Rubra) and *Mu Dan Pi* (Cortex Moutan).
- For swelling with pus that does not perforate, or sores that have perforated and ulcerated but do not heal, add *Zao Jiao Ci* (Spina Gleditsiae).
- For acute tonsillitis, add *Jie Geng* (Radix Platycodonis), *She Gan* (Rhizoma Belamcandae), and *Gan Cao* (Radix et Rhizoma Glycyrrhizae).
- For breast abscess with swelling, redness, and pain, add *Gua Lou* (Fructus Trichosanthis), *Bei Mu* (Bulbus Fritillariae), and *Qing Pi* (Pericarpium Citri Reticulatae Viride).
- For infection or inflammation in constitutionally-deficient individuals, add *Ren Shen* (Radix et Rhizoma Ginseng) or *Dang Gui Bu Xue Tang* (Tangkuei Decoction to Tonify the Blood).
- For acute nephritis with edema, swelling, dysuria, red tongue body, and a rapid pulse, add *Ze Xie* (Rhizoma Alismatis), *Zhi Zi* (Fructus Gardeniae), and *Che Qian Zi* (Semen Plantaginis).

CAUTIONS / CONTRAINDICATIONS

- *Wu Wei Xiao Du Yin* should be used with caution in patients with Spleen and Stomach deficiencies, or qi and blood deficiencies.
- This formula is contraindicated for *yin* (deep-rooted) type of abscesses and sores with underlying deficiencies.

PHARMACOLOGICAL EFFECTS
Antibacterial: According to *in vitro* studies, *Wu Wei Xiao Du Yin* has an inhibitory effect against *Staphylococcus albus*, *Staphylococcus aureus*, *alpha-hemolytic streptococcus*, *beta-hemolytic streptococcus*, *Salmonella typhi* and *Bacillus proteus*. At high doses, it has an inhibitory effect against *Pseudomonas aeruginosa*. It is ineffective against *E. coli*.[1,2]

CLINICAL STUDIES AND RESEARCH

1. **Cellulitis**: Forty-five patients with cellulitis were treated successfully using modified *Wu Wei Xiao Du Yin*. The herbal formula contained *Jin Yin Hua* (Flos Lonicerae Japonicae) 25g, *Ye Ju Hua* (Flos Chrysanthemi Indici) 20g, *Pu Gong Ying* (Herba Taraxaci) 20g, *Zi Hua Di Ding* (Herba Violae) 20g, *Lian Qiao* (Fructus Forsythiae) 25g, *Shi Gao* (Gypsum Fibrosum) 30g, *Bo He* (Herba Menthae) 5g, *Niu Bang Zi* (Fructus Arctii) 15g, *Jiang Can* (Bombyx Batryticatus) 10g, *Mu Dan Pi* (Cortex Moutan) 10g, *Sheng Ma* (Rhizoma Cimicifugae) 10g, and *Zao Jiao Ci* (Spina Gleditsiae) 10g. Furthermore, modifications were made by adding *Da Huang* (Radix et Rhizoma Rhei) 5g and *Xuan Ming Fen* (Natrii Sulfas Exsiccatus) 5g for constipation; *Jing Jie* (Herba Schizonepetae) 15g for aversion to cold; *Gu Sui Bu* (Rhizoma Drynariae) 10g and *Xuan Shen* (Radix Scrophulariae) 10g for chronic illness; and *Ban Lan Gen* (Radix Isatidis) 20g and *Ku Shen* (Radix Sophorae Flavescentis) 15g for severe inflammation. The treatment protocol was to give the herbs in decoction for 6-18 packs of herbs. Of 45 patients, the study reported complete recovery in 30 cases, significant improvement in 10 cases, moderate improvement in 1 case, and no effect in 4 cases. The overall effectiveness was 91.11%.[3]

2. **Shingles**: Administration of 3-6 packs of herbs in decoction was effective in treating all 38 patients with shingles. The herbal treatment contained *Wu Wei Xiao Du Yin* and *Si Wu Tang* (Four-Substance Decoction) as the base formula, with the addition of *Lian Qiao* (Fructus Forsythiae) and *Ban Lan Gen* (Radix Isatidis) for toxic heat; *Long Dan* (Radix et Rhizoma Gentianae) for a bitter taste in the mouth and dysuria; *Da Huang* (Radix et Rhizoma Rhei) for constipation; and *Tu Fu Ling* (Rhizoma Smilacis Glabrae) and a large dose of *Di Huang* (Radix Rehmanniae) for itching and pain.[4]

3. **Febrile disorder**: Use of modified *Wu Wei Xiao Du Yin* was associated with 81.1% effectiveness in treating externally-contracted febrile disorders. In addition to the base formula, modifications were made based on the differential diagnosis of the condition. For exterior wind-heat, *Lian Qiao* (Fructus Forsythiae), *Bo He* (Herba Menthae), and *Lu Gen* (Rhizoma Phragmitis) were added. For exterior wind-cold, *Jing Jie* (Herba Schizonepetae), *Fang Feng* (Radix Saposhnikoviae), and *Qiang Huo* (Rhizoma et Radix Notopterygii) were added. For Lung heat,

1338

Wǔ Wèi Xiāo Dú Yǐn
(Five-Ingredient Decoction to Eliminate Toxins)

Ma Huang (Herba Ephedrae), *Ku Xing Ren* (Semen Armeniacae Amarum), and *Shi Gao* (Gypsum Fibrosum) were added. For Stomach heat, *Shi Gao* (Gypsum Fibrosum) and *Zhi Mu* (Rhizoma Anemarrhenae) were added. For Gallbladder heat, *Chai Hu* (Radix Bupleuri), *Huang Qin* (Radix Scutellariae), and *Bai Jiang Cao* (Herba cum Radice Patriniae) were added. For Large Intestine heat, *Ge Gen* (Radix Puerariae Lobatae), *Huang Qin* (Radix Scutellariae), and *Huang Lian* (Rhizoma Coptidis) were added. For Urinary Bladder damp-heat, *Mu Tong* (Caulis Akebiae), *Hua Shi* (Talcum), and *Shi Wei* (Folium Pyrrosiae) were added. For constipation, *Da Huang* (Radix et Rhizoma Rhei) was added. Of 122 patients, the study reported complete recovery in 81 cases, marked improvement in 18 cases, moderate improvement in 16 cases, and no effect in 7 cases.[5]

4. **Viral hepatitis**: Administration of modified *Wu Wei Xiao Du Yin* in decoction daily was effective in treating 248 hepatitis patients (183 hepatitis A cases and 65 hepatitis B). Most patients received 60-100 packs of herbs. However, those with severe conditions required up to 200-300 packs.[6]

5. **Acute cholecystitis**: According to one study, 20 patients with acute cholecystitis were treated with modified *Wu Wei Xiao Du Yin* with 75% effectiveness.[7] Another study reported satisfactory results in all 60 patients (21 males and 39 females) with acute cholecystitis treated with modified *Wu Wei Xiao Du Yin*. The formula was modified by adding *Ze Lan* (Herba Lycopi) and *Fu Ling* (Poria) for dampness; *Dang Gui* (Radix Angelicae Sinensis) and *Tao Ren* (Semen Persicae) for chronic illness; *Da Huang* (Radix et Rhizoma Rhei) and *Po Xiao* (Sal Glauberis) for constipation; *Yan Hu Suo* (Rhizoma Corydalis), *Ru Xiang* (Gummi Olibanum), and *Mo Yao* (Myrrha) for severe pain; *Chen Pi* (Pericarpium Citri Reticulatae) and *Ban Xia* (Rhizoma Pinelliae) for nausea and vomiting; *Yin Chen* (Herba Artemisiae Scopariae) and *Jin Qian Cao* (Herba Lysimachiae) for jaundice; and others as deemed necessary.[8]

6. **Acute pyelonephritis**: Administration of modified *Wu Wei Xiao Du Yin* in decoction daily was associated with 91.4% effectiveness in treating acute pyelonephritis. The duration of treatment ranged from 1-2 courses, with 7 days per course. Of 58 patients with acute pyelonephritis, the study reported complete recovery in 41 cases, improvement in 12 cases, and no effect in 5 cases.[9]

7. **Chronic pyelonephritis**: Administration of modified *Wu Wei Xiao Du Yin* in 13 patients with chronic pyelonephritis was associated with complete recovery in 8 cases, improvement in 3 cases, and no effect in 2 cases.[10]

8. **Glomerulonephritis**: Use of modified *Wu Wei Xiao Du Yin* was associated with marked success in treating glomerulonephritis in children. The herbal treatment contained *Wu Wei Xiao Du Yin* plus *Mu Tong* (Caulis Akebiae) and *Gan Cao* (Radix et Rhizoma Glycyrrhizae) as the base formula. Furthermore, modifications were made as follows: *Ma Huang* (Herba Ephedrae) and *Shi Gao* (Gypsum Fibrosum) for wind and water accumulation; *Wu Ling San* (Five-Ingredient Powder with Poria) for water and damp accumulation; and *Shi Gao* (Gypsum Fibrosum), *Bai Mao Gen* (Rhizoma Imperatae), *Dan Zhu Ye* (Herba Lophatheri), and *Xiao Ji* (Herba Cirsii) for damp-heat accumulation. Of 36 patients, the study reported complete recovery in 30 cases, improvement in 4 cases, and no effect in 2 cases. The overall effectiveness was 94.4%.[11]

9. **Pelvic inflammation**: Use of modified *Wu Wei Xiao Du Yin* in solution at 37°C / 98.6°F via rectal instillation one time per day for 10 days was associated with complete recovery in 52 of 55 patients. The overall rate of effectiveness was 94.5%.[12]

10. **Bartholinitis**: Acute inflammation of the Bartholin's glands was successfully treated using modified *Wu Wei Xiao Du Yin*. The herbal treatment contained *Wu Wei Xiao Du Yin* plus *Ru Xiang* (Gummi Olibanum), *Mo Yao* (Myrrha), *Chi Shao* (Radix Paeoniae Rubra), *Mu Dan Pi* (Cortex Moutan), and *Gan Cao* (Radix et Rhizoma Glycyrrhizae) as the base formula. *Chai Hu* (Radix Bupleuri) was added for aversion to cold with fever. *Huang Qi* (Radix Astragali) was added for formation of abscesses. *Dong Gua Zi* (Semen Benincasae) and *Yi Yi Ren* (Semen Coicis) were added for pus. *Da Huang* (Radix et Rhizoma Rhei) [post-decocted] and *Zhi Shi* (Fructus Aurantii Immaturus) were added for constipation. Lastly, an herbal wash was applied topically using *Ku Shen* (Radix Sophorae Flavescentis), *Da Huang* (Radix et Rhizoma Rhei), *Huang Bo* (Cortex Phellodendri Chinensis), and *Pu Gong Ying* (Herba Taraxaci). Of 48 patients, the study reported complete recovery in 35 cases, improvement in 11 cases, and no effect in 2 cases. The rate of effectiveness was 95.8%.[13]

11. **Tonsillitis**: One study reported complete recovery in all 38 patients with acute tonsillitis when treated with modified *Wu Wei Xiao Du Yin* in decoction twice daily for 2-5 days. In addition to the base formula, *Lian Qiao* (Fructus Forsythiae) and *Niu Bang Zi* (Fructus Arctii) were added for exterior wind-heat; *Jing Jie* (Herba Schizonepetae) and *Fang Feng* (Radix Saposhnikoviae) for exterior wind-cold; and *Huang Qin* (Radix Scutellariae) and *Huang Lian* (Rhizoma Coptidis) for high fever.[14]

Chinese Herbal Formulas and Applications

FORMULAS THAT TREAT ABSCESSES AND SORES

22

1339

Wǔ Wèi Xiāo Dú Yǐn
(Five-Ingredient Decoction to Eliminate Toxins)

12. **Pericoronitis**: Administration of modified *Wu Wei Xiao Du Yin* was associated with 94.7% effectiveness in treating 150 patients with acute inflammation around the crown of a partially-erupted tooth. The herbs were cooked in water to yield an herbal decoction. Patients were instructed to gargle with the decoction before swallowing twice daily. The herbal formula contained *Wu Wei Xiao Du Yin* plus *Huang Qin* (Radix Scutellariae) as the base formula, with the addition of *Shi Gao* (Gypsum Fibrosum) and *Lu Gen* (Rhizoma Phragmitis) for fever; and *Di Huang* (Radix Rehmanniae) and *Sha Ren* (Fructus Amomi) for severe pain.[15]

13. **Burns**: Fourteen of 15 patients with various degrees of burns were treated successfully with modified *Wu Wei Xiao Du Yin* for prevention and treatment of infection. Depending on the severity of burns and infection, the duration of treatment ranged from 7-21 days. The herbal formula contained *Wu Wei Xiao Du Yin* as the base formula, with the addition of *Dang Shen* (Radix Codonopsis), *Huang Qi* (Radix Astragali), and *Mai Dong* (Radix Ophiopogonis) for qi and yin deficiencies; *Huang Lian Jie Du Tang* (Coptis Decoction to Relieve Toxicity) or *Si Miao San* (Four-Marvel Powder) for fire and toxins; and *Dan Shen* (Radix et Rhizoma Salviae Miltiorrhizae) and *Chi Shao* (Radix Paeoniae Rubra) during the middle stage of recovery.[16]

14. **Myelitis**: Thirteen patients with inflammation of the spinal cord or the bone marrow were treated successfully using both antibiotic drugs and modified *Wu Wei Xiao Du Yin*. Concurrent drug and herb treatment was employed for 3-4 days to control acute infection and inflammation, followed by use of herbs to maintain and consolidate the condition. All 13 patients reported significant improvement or complete recovery within one month. The herbal formula was based on *Wu Wei Xiao Du Yin*, with the removal of *Tian Kui Zi* (Radix Semiaquilegiae), and the addition of processed *Chuan Shan Jia* (Squama Manis) and *Lian Qiao* (Fructus Forsythiae). *Huang Qi* (Radix Astragali) was added for qi deficiency when necessary.[17]

15. **Urinary tract infection**: One study reported 94.6% effectiveness using modified *Wu Wei Xiao Du Yin* to treat 37 children with acute urinary tract infection. In addition to *Wu Wei Xiao Du Yin*, *Chai Hu* (Radix Bupleuri) was added for more heat; *Bai Mao Gen* (Rhizoma Imperatae), *Da Ji* (Herba Cirsii Japonici), and *Xiao Ji* (Herba Cirsii) for hematuria; *Che Qian Zi* (Semen Plantaginis) and *Mu Tong* (Caulis Akebiae) for frequent urination with urgency; and *Huang Qi* (Radix Astragali) for qi deficiency. Of 37 patients, the study reported complete recovery in 26 cases, improvement in 9 cases, and no effect in 2 cases.[18]

16. ***Re lin* (heat dysuria)**: One hundred and fourteen patients out of 128 were successfully treated using modified *Wu Wei Xiao Du Yin*. In addition to the base formula, *Che Qian Zi* (Semen Plantaginis) and *Fu Ling* (Poria) were added for dysuria; *Da Huang* (Radix et Rhizoma Rhei) and *Zhi Shi* (Fructus Aurantii Immaturus) for constipation with a yellow, greasy tongue coating; *Di Huang* (Radix Rehmanniae) and *Bai Mao Gen* (Rhizoma Imperatae) for damp-heat damaging yin; and *Dang Shen* (Radix Codonopsis) and *Huang Qi* (Radix Astragali) for generalized deficiency.[19]

RELATED FORMULA
Yín Huā Jiě Dú Tāng
(Honeysuckle Decoction to Relieve Toxicity)

銀花解毒湯
银花解毒汤

Pinyin Name: Yin Hua Jie Du Tang
Literal Name: Honeysuckle Decoction to Relieve Toxicity
Original Source: *Yang Ke Xin De Ji* (Collection of Personal Expertises Concerning Skin Lesions) by Gao Bing-Jun in 1805

Jin Yin Hua (Flos Lonicerae Japonicae)
Zi Hua Di Ding (Herba Violae)
Xi Jiao (Cornu Rhinoceri)
Chi Fu Ling (Poria Rubra)
Lian Qiao (Fructus Forsythiae)
Mu Dan Pi (Cortex Moutan)
Huang Lian (Rhizoma Coptidis)
Xia Ku Cao (Spica Prunellae)

Note: *Xi Jiao* (Cornu Rhinoceri) is derived from an endangered animal, and is rarely used as a medicinal substance today. Its discussion here is included primarily for academic purposes, to reflect the historical use of this substance in its original formulation. Most herbal products today have removed it completely, or replaced it with substitutes with similar functions.

The doses of herbs were not given in the source text. The main actions of *Yin Hua Jie Du Tang* (Honeysuckle Decoction to Relieve Toxicity) are to clear heat, eliminate toxins, purge fire, and cool the blood. Clinically, this formula may be used to treat carbuncles, cellulitis, boils, and other types of epithelial inflammations caused by dampness, heat, wind, and fire. In patients with exterior signs and symptoms, this formula should be modified accordingly.

1340

Wŭ Wèi Xiāo Dú Yĭn
(Five-Ingredient Decoction to Eliminate Toxins)

Wu Wei Xiao Du Yin and *Yin Hua Jie Du Tang* (Honeysuckle Decoction to Relieve Toxicity) have very similar functions:

- *Wu Wei Xiao Du Yin* focuses on clearing heat and eliminating toxins.
- *Yin Hua Jie Du Tang* emphasizes clearing heat, eliminating toxins, purging fire, and cooling the blood.

References

1. *Zhe Jiang Zhong Yi Za Zhi* (Zhejiang Journal of Chinese Medicine) 1978;1:3.
2. *He Bei Zhong Yi* (Hebei Chinese Medicine) 1980;2:46.
3. *Liao Ning Zhong Yi Za Zhi* (Liaoning Journal of Chinese Medicine) 1994;21(5):222.
4. *Yun Nan Zhong Yi Za Zhi* (Yunan Journal of Chinese Medicine) 1994;3:10.
5. *Hu Bei Zhong Yi Za Zhi* (Hubei Journal of Chinese Medicine) 1989;4:13.
6. *Shi Zhen Guo Yao Yan Jiu* (Research of Shizhen Herbs) 1994;1:7.
7. *Hu Bei Zhong Yi Za Zhi* (Hubei Journal of Chinese Medicine) 1989;4:13.
8. *Shi Zhen Guo Yao Yan Jiu* (Research of Shizhen Herbs) 1993;2:7.
9. *Shi Yong Zhong Xi Yi Jie He Za Zhi* (Practical Journal of Integrated Chinese and Western Medicines) 1992;8:466.
10. *Jiang Xi Zhong Yi Yao* (Jiangxi Chinese Medicine and Herbology) 1993;2:31.
11. *Hu Nan Zhong Yi Za Zhi* (Hunan Journal of Chinese Medicine) 1999;3:59.
12. *Fu Jian Yi Yao Za Zhi* (Fujian Journal of Medicine and Herbology) 1994;4:58.
13. *Jiang Xi Zhong Yi Yao* (Jiangxi Chinese Medicine and Herbology) 1995;2:16.
14. *Shang Hai Zhong Yi Yao Za Zhi* (Shanghai Journal of Chinese Medicine and Herbology) 1994;4:24.
15. *Hu Nan Zhong Yi Xue Yuan Xue Bao* (Journal of Hunan University of Traditional Chinese Medicine) 1998;2:39.
16. *Guang Xi Zhong Yi Yao* (Guangxi Chinese Medicine and Herbology) 1996;3:24.
17. *Jiang Xi Zhong Yi Yao* (Jiangxi Chinese Medicine and Herbology) 1997;5:44.
18. *Si Chuan Zhong Yi* (Sichuan Chinese Medicine) 1995;8:47.
19. *Fu Jian Zhong Yi Yao* (Fujian Chinese Medicine and Herbology) 1996;2:17.

Shí Wèi Bài Dú Tāng
(Ten-Ingredient Decoction to Overcome Pathogenic Influences)

十味敗毒湯
十味败毒汤

Pinyin Name: *Shi Wei Bai Du Tang*
Literal Name: Ten-Ingredient Decoction to Overcome Pathogenic Influences
Alternate Name: Bupleurum and Schizonepeta Formula
Original Source: Seiju Hanaoka's experience formula

COMPOSITION

Chai Hu (Radix Bupleuri)	3g
Sheng Jiang (Rhizoma Zingiberis Recens)	1g
Du Huo (Radix Angelicae Pubescentis)	3g
Fang Feng (Radix Saposhnikoviae)	3g
Fu Ling (Poria)	4g
Jie Geng (Radix Platycodonis)	3g
Chuan Xiong (Rhizoma Chuanxiong)	3g
Jing Jie (Herba Schizonepetae)	1g
Ye Ying Pi (Pericarpium Prunus Pseudocerasus)	3g
Gan Cao (Radix et Rhizoma Glycyrrhizae)	1g

Chapter 22 – Formulas that Treat Abscesses and Sores　　　　　*Section 1 – External Abscesses and Sores*

Shí Wèi Bài Dú Tāng
(Ten-Ingredient Decoction to Overcome Pathogenic Influences)

DOSAGE / PREPARATION / ADMINISTRATION

The source text states to prepare the ingredients as a decoction. Today, the decoction may be prepared using a higher dose of ingredients (approximately 2-3 times higher).

CHINESE THERAPEUTIC ACTIONS

1. Dispels wind
2. Eliminates toxins

CLINICAL MANIFESTATIONS

Accumulation of heat and toxin at the exterior: various types of suppurative skin disorders, such as acne, eczema, urticaria, boils, carbuncles, furuncles, lymphadenitis, mastitis, sinusitis, and otitis media.

CLINICAL APPLICATIONS

Acne vulgaris, acne rash, eczema, urticaria, boils, carbuncles, furuncles, lymphadenitis, mastitis, sinusitis, otitis media, tinea pedis (athlete's foot), and allergic ophthalmia.

EXPLANATION

Accumulation of heat and toxin at the exterior is often characterized by redness, swelling and pain in the early stages. As the disease progresses, the heat and toxins turn into pus and abscess, leading to the discharge of fluids. This formula may be used to treat heat and toxins in the early to late stage in various parts of the body.

Shi Wei Bai Du Tang (Ten-Ingredient Decoction to Overcome Pathogenic Influences) contains herbs to clear heat and eliminate toxins from the exterior. *Chai Hu* (Radix Bupleuri) and *Sheng Jiang* (Rhizoma Zingiberis Recens)

work as a pair to harmonize the interior and release the exterior. *Du Huo* (Radix Angelicae Pubescentis), *Fang Feng* (Radix Saposhnikoviae), and *Fu Ling* (Poria) dispel wind and resolve dampness. *Jie Geng* (Radix Platycodonis) and *Chuan Xiong* (Rhizoma Chuanxiong) activate blood circulation and drain pus and phlegm. *Jing Jie* (Herba Schizonepetae) and *Ye Ying Pi* (Pericarpium Prunus Pseudocerasus) eliminate toxins. *Gan Cao* (Radix et Rhizoma Glycyrrhizae) harmonizes all of the herbs in the formula. In short, this formula treats various suppurative dermatological conditions characterized by heat and toxins.

MODIFICATIONS

- With more heat and toxins, add *Lian Qiao* (Fructus Forsythiae) and *Jin Yin Hua* (Flos Lonicerae Japonicae).
- With more pus, add *Yi Yi Ren* (Semen Coicis).
- With thirst, add *Shi Gao* (Gypsum Fibrosum).
- With more itching, add *Shui Ding Xiang* (Herba Ludwigiae Prostratae) and *Huang Shui Qie* (Herba Solani); or *Xiao Feng San* (Eliminate Wind Powder).
- With constipation, add *Da Huang* (Radix et Rhizoma Rhei) or *Da Cheng Qi Tang* (Major Order the Qi Decoction).
- For ulcerations accompanied by swelling and pus, add *Tuo Li Xiao Du Yin* (Drain the Interior and Detoxify Decoction) or *Wu Wei Xiao Du Yin* (Five-Ingredient Decoction to Eliminate Toxins).
- For hypertrophic rhinitis, add *Xin Yi Hua* (Flos Magnoliae) and *Ge Gen* (Radix Puerariae Lobatae); or *Xin Yi San* (Magnolia Flower Powder).
- For urticaria, add *Lian Qiao* (Fructus Forsythiae), *Yi Yi Ren* (Semen Coicis), *Yin Chen* (Herba Artemisiae Scopariae), and *Zhi Zi* (Fructus Gardeniae).

Shi Wei Bai Du Tang (Ten-Ingredient Decoction to Overcome Pathogenic Influences)

Diagnosis	Signs and Symptoms	Treatment	Herbs
Accumulation of heat and toxin at the exterior	Suppurative skin disorders with redness, swelling, and pain in the early stages, and the formation of pus and abscess in the later stages: heat and toxin accumulation at the exterior	• Dispels wind • Eliminates toxins	• *Chai Hu* (Radix Bupleuri) and *Sheng Jiang* (Rhizoma Zingiberis Recens) harmonize the interior and release the exterior. • *Du Huo* (Radix Angelicae Pubescentis), *Fang Feng* (Radix Saposhnikoviae), and *Fu Ling* (Poria) dispel wind and resolve dampness. • *Jie Geng* (Radix Platycodonis) and *Chuan Xiong* (Rhizoma Chuanxiong) activate blood circulation and drain pus and phlegm. • *Jing Jie* (Herba Schizonepetae) and *Ye Ying Pi* (Pericarpium Prunus Pseudocerasus) eliminate toxins. • *Gan Cao* (Radix et Rhizoma Glycyrrhizae) harmonizes all of the herbs.

1342

Shí Wèi Bài Dú Tāng
(Ten-Ingredient Decoction to Overcome Pathogenic Influences)

- For cellulitis that is warm and swollen, add *Huang Lian Jie Du Tang* (Coptis Decoction to Relieve Toxicity).
- For acne with redness and pus, add *Yi Yi Ren* (Semen Coicis), *Lian Qiao* (Fructus Forsythiae), and *Da Huang* (Radix et Rhizoma Rhei).
- For measles and eczema, add *Sheng Ma Ge Gen Tang* (Cimicifuga and Kudzu Decoction).

CLINICAL STUDIES AND RESEARCH

1. **Acne vulgaris (pimples)**: Administration of *Shi Wei Bai Du Tang* was associated with a suppressed production of propionic acid and butyric acid by all strains of *Propionibacterium acnes* tested. No significant difference in the rate of suppressed production was noted between different *P. acnes* biotype, nor between isolates from mild skin rash and more severe skin rash. Based on this information, the researchers concluded that the clinical effectiveness of *Shi Wei Bai Du Tang* did not seem to be influenced by the degree of acne rash or the *P. acnes* biotype.[1]

2. **Acne rashes**: One study showed *Shi Wei Bai Du Tang* to be an effective therapy for the treatment of acne rashes as well as incidental symptoms.[2]

RELATED FORMULA

Bài Dú Tāng
(Overcome Pathogenic Influences Decoction)

敗毒湯
败毒汤

Pinyin Name: *Bai Du Tang*
Literal Name: Overcome Pathogenic Influences Decoction

Original Source: *Guang An Men Yi Yuan* (Guang An Men Hospital) in 1990

Bai Xian Pi (Cortex Dictamni)
Niu Bang Zi (Fructus Arctii)
Da Qing Ye (Folium Isatidis)
Ban Lan Gen (Radix Isatidis)
Jin Yin Hua (Flos Lonicerae Japonicae)
Ban Zhi Lian (Herba Scutellariae Barbatae)
Zi Hua Di Ding (Herba Violae)
Yi Yi Ren (Semen Coicis)
Ku Shen (Radix Sophorae Flavescentis)
Pu Gong Ying (Herba Taraxaci)
Chi Shao (Radix Paeoniae Rubra)
He Shou Wu (Radix Polygoni Multiflori)
Mu Dan Pi (Cortex Moutan)
Gan Cao (Radix et Rhizoma Glycyrrhizae)

Bai Du Tang (Overcome Pathogenic Influences Decoction) treats heat and toxins affecting the exterior parts of the body. It contains herbs to release the exterior, clear heat, and eliminate toxins. Clinical applications include cellulitis, sores, carbuncles, furuncles, psoriasis, and other types of skin disorders characterized by heat and toxins.

References

1. Higaki S, Kitagawa T, Kagoura M, Morohashi M, Yamagishi T. Relationship between Propionibacterium acnes biotypes and Jumi-haidoku-to. Journal of Dermatology 2000 Oct;27(10):635-8.
2. Higaki S, Toyomoto T, Morohashi M. Seijo-bofu-to, Jumi-haidoku-to and Toki-shakuyaku-san suppress rashes and incidental symptoms in acne patients. Drugs Under Experimental & Clinical Research 2002;28(5):193-6.

FORMULAS THAT TREAT ABSCESSES AND SORES

22

1343

Chapter 22 – Formulas that Treat Abscesses and Sores　　　　　　*Section 1 – External Abscesses and Sores*

Si Miào Yǒng Ān Tāng (Four-Valiant Decoction for Well-Being)

四妙勇安湯
四妙勇安汤

Pinyin Name: *Si Miao Yong An Tang*
Literal Name: Four-Valiant Decoction for Well-Being
Original Source: *Yan Fang Xin Bian* (New Compilation of Time-Tested Formulas) by Bao Xiang-Ao in 1846

COMPOSITION

Jin Yin Hua (Flos Lonicerae Japonicae)	90g [30-90g]
Xuan Shen (Radix Scrophulariae)	90g [30-90g]
Dang Gui (Radix Angelicae Sinensis)	60g [15-30g]
Gan Cao (Radix et Rhizoma Glycyrrhizae)	30g [10-15g]

DOSAGE / PREPARATION / ADMINISTRATION

The source text states to prepare the ingredients as a decoction. The source text specifically emphasizes to use all four herbs in decoction for a total of 10 packs of herbs. Today, this formula may be prepared as a decoction with the doses suggested in brackets.

CHINESE THERAPEUTIC ACTIONS

1. Clears heat and eliminates toxins
2. Activates blood circulation and relieves pain

CLINICAL MANIFESTATIONS

Gangrene: gangrene of the extremities with purulent abscess, dark red discoloration, local inflammation and swelling, a burning sensation, sometimes severe pain, possible fever, thirst, a red tongue body, and a rapid pulse.

CLINICAL APPLICATIONS

Thromboangiitis obliterans, thrombophlebitis, phlebitis, iliofemoral vein thrombosis, arteriosclerotic gangrene, chronic hepatitis, chronic gastritis, sciatica, prostatic hypertrophy, carpal tunnel syndrome, gout, and erysipelas.

EXPLANATION

Si Miao Yong An Tang (Four-Valiant Decoction for Well-Being) treats gangrene in the extremities, especially the lower legs, characterized by severe accumulation of heat and toxins. Severe heat and toxin accumulation may injure the body tissues and damage the qi and blood, causing gangrene of the extremities with local inflammation, purulent abscess, dark red color, swelling, and a burning sensation. In acute conditions, there may be severe pain. Fever, thirst, red tongue body, and a rapid pulse suggest interior heat.

This formula contains a large dose of *Jin Yin Hua* (Flos Lonicerae Japonicae) to clear heat and eliminate toxins. *Xuan Shen* (Radix Scrophulariae) purges fire and eliminates toxins. *Dang Gui* (Radix Angelicae Sinensis) activates blood circulation and disperses stagnation. *Gan Cao* (Radix et Rhizoma Glycyrrhizae) assists *Jin Yin Hua* (Flos Lonicerae Japonicae) in clearing heat and eliminating toxins.

MODIFICATIONS

- With severe pain, add *Ru Xiang* (Gummi Olibanum) and *Mo Yao* (Myrrha).
- With more blood stagnation, add *Tao Ren* (Semen Persicae) and *Hong Hua* (Flos Carthami).
- With qi deficiency, add *Huang Qi* (Radix Astragali) and *Dang Shen* (Radix Codonopsis).
- With cold excess and yang deficiency, add *Fu Zi* (Radix Aconiti Lateralis Praeparata), *Gui Zhi* (Ramulus Cinnamomi), and *Lu Jiao Shuang* (Cornu Cervi Degelatinatum).
- With severe swelling and inflammation due to damp-heat, add *Fang Ji* (Radix Stephaniae Tetrandrae), *Huang Bo* (Cortex Phellodendri Chinensis), and *Cang Zhu* (Rhizoma Atractylodis).
- For gangrene in the lower extremities, add *Niu Xi* (Radix Achyranthis Bidentatae) and *Yi Yi Ren* (Semen Coicis).
- For gangrene in the upper extremities, add *Chuan Xiong* (Rhizoma Chuanxiong).
- For gangrene in the trunk of the body, add *Du Zhong* (Cortex Eucommiae).
- For thromboangiitis obliterans, add *Mao Dong Qing* (Radix Ilicis Pubescentis), *Pu Gong Ying* (Herba Taraxaci), *Dan Shen* (Radix et Rhizoma Salviae Miltiorrhizae), *Chi Xiao Dou* (Semen Phaseoli), *Chuan Shan Jia* (Squama Manis), and *Di Long* (Pheretima).

CAUTIONS / CONTRAINDICATIONS

- The source text states to avoid scratching the affected area while taking this formula.

1344

Sì Miào Yŏng Ān Tāng (Four-Valiant Decoction for Well-Being)

Si Miao Yong An Tang (Four-Valiant Decoction for Well-Being)

Diagnosis	Signs and Symptoms	Treatment	Herbs
Gangrene	• Gangrene in the extremities, local inflammation, purulent abscess, dark red color, swelling and a burning sensation: severe heat and toxins damaging the qi and blood • Thirst: heat consuming body fluids • Red tongue body and a rapid pulse: interior heat	• Clears heat and eliminates toxins • Activates blood circulation and relieves pain	• *Jin Yin Hua* (Flos Lonicerae Japonicae) clears heat and eliminates toxins. • *Xuan Shen* (Radix Scrophulariae) purges fire and eliminates toxins. • *Dang Gui* (Radix Angelicae Sinensis) activates the blood and disperses stagnation. • *Gan Cao* (Radix et Rhizoma Glycyrrhizae) clears heat, eliminates toxins, and harmonizes all of the herbs.

- *Si Miao Yong An Tang* is designed for gangrene characterized by heat and toxins. It is inappropriate for gangrene characterized by cold.
- In severe cases of gangrene in which there is confirmed necrosis of the tissues, use of this formula is not sufficient. Instead, surgery, or possibly even amputation, is necessary to remove the necrotic tissue.

PHARMACOLOGICAL EFFECTS

1. **Analgesic**: Administration of *Si Miao Yong An Tang* was associated with marked analgesic effects in mice, starting 40 minutes after oral ingestion.[1]
2. **Effect on coagulation**: Administration of *Si Miao Yong An Tang* did not affect coagulation or bleeding time in rabbits and mice.[2]

CLINICAL STUDIES AND RESEARCH

1. **Arteriosclerotic gangrene**: One study used modified *Si Miao Yong An Tang* to treat 28 patients with arteriosclerotic gangrene. In addition to the base formula, *Quan Xie* (Scorpio), *Wu Gong* (Scolopendra), and *Bai Shao* (Radix Paeoniae Alba) were added for severe pain; *Pu Gong Ying* (Herba Taraxaci), *Huang Bo* (Cortex Phellodendri Chinensis), and *An Gong Niu Huang Wan* (Calm the Palace Pill with Cattle Gallstone) for heat and toxins; *Dan Shen* (Radix et Rhizoma Salviae Miltiorrhizae), *Tao Ren* (Semen Persicae), and *Hong Hua* (Flos Carthami) for blood stagnation; *Huang Qi* (Radix Astragali), *Bai Zhu* (Rhizoma Atractylodis Macrocephalae), and *Fu Ling* (Poria) for qi deficiency; and *Jue Ming Zi* (Semen Cassiae) for constipation. Of 28 patients, the study reported complete recovery in 19 cases, marked improvement in 3 cases, and no effect in 2 cases.[3]
2. **Thromboangiitis obliterans**: Thirty-three patients (32 males and 1 females) with thromboangiitis obliterans were treated with complete recovery in 16 cases, improvement in 11 cases, and no effect in 6 cases. The herbal formula contained *Si Miao Yong An Tang* plus *Huang Qin* (Radix Scutellariae), *Ban Lan Gen* (Radix Isatidis), and *Chuan Niu Xi* (Radix Cyathulae).[4] Another study reported complete recovery in 28 of 30 patients with thromboangiitis obliterans using *Si Miao Yong An Tang*.[5]

3. **Thrombophlebitis**: Twenty-eight patients with thrombophlebitis were treated with complete recovery in 22 cases, significant effect in 5 cases, and no effect in 1 case. The herbal treatment used *Si Miao Yong An Tang* as the base formula. In addition, depending on the affected area, the following additions were made: *Chuan Xiong* (Rhizoma Chuanxiong) for upper extremities, *Niu Xi* (Radix Achyranthis Bidentatae) for lower extremities, *Du Zhong* (Cortex Eucommiae) for the trunk of the body, and *Chuan Shan Jia* (Squama Manis) for obvious swelling and inflammation.[6]

4. **Phlebitis**: One study reported marked effectiveness using modified *Si Miao Yong An Tang* to treat 32 patients with phlebitis in the lower extremities. Modifications to the base formula included: *Che Qian Zi* (Semen Plantaginis), *Bai Hua She She Cao* (Herba Hedyotis), and *Chuan Niu Xi* (Radix Cyathulae) for early-stage phlebitis; and *Shui Zhi* (Hirudo), *Huang Qi* (Radix Astragali), and *E Zhu* (Rhizoma Curcumae) for late-stage phlebitis. The herbs were cooked in water and the decoction was given orally to the patient. In addition, the herb residue was cooked again in water, and the solution was used as an herbal wash and applied to the affected area. Of 32 patients, the study reported complete recovery in 29 cases and marked improvement in 3 cases.[7]

5. **Thrombosis of iliofemoral vein**: Integrative treatment was found to be effective in 97.2% of patients with iliofemoral vein thrombosis. The herbal treatment contained *Si Miao Yong An Tang*, modified by removing *Gan Cao* (Radix et Rhizoma Glycyrrhizae) and adding *Chuan Xiong* (Rhizoma Chuanxiong), *Da Huang* (Radix et Rhizoma Rhei) and others as needed. In addition, patients also received an intravenous infusion of *Dan Shen* (Radix et Rhizoma Salviae Miltiorrhizae) and oral

Sì Miào Yǒng Ān Tāng (Four-Valiant Decoction for Well-Being)

ingestion of aspirin (300 mg/day for five days, followed by 100 mg/day daily). Antibiotic drugs were given if necessary. Of 36 patients, the study reported complete recovery in 28 cases, marked improvement in 7 cases, and no effect in 1 case.[8]

6. **Chronic hepatitis**: One study reported 94% effectiveness using modified *Si Miao Yong An Tang* to treat chronic hepatitis. Of 33 patients, 25 had significant improvement, 6 had moderate improvement, and 2 had no effect. The herbal formula contained *Si Miao Yong An Tang* plus *Bai Mao Gen* (Rhizoma Imperatae), *Huang Qi* (Radix Astragali), *Tu Fu Ling* (Rhizoma Smilacis Glabrae), and others as the base formula. Modifications included the addition of *Yin Chen* (Herba Artemisiae Scopariae) and *Ku Shen* (Radix Sophorae Flavescentis) for jaundice; *Ji Nei Jin* (Endothelium Corneum Gigeriae Galli) and processed *Chuan Shan Jia* (Squama Manis) for splenomegaly; *Gan Jiang* (Rhizoma Zingiberis), *Cang Zhu* (Rhizoma Atractylodis), and *Bai Zhu* (Rhizoma Atractylodis Macrocephalae) for damp-cold in the Spleen; *Dan Shen* (Radix et Rhizoma Salviae Miltiorrhizae) and *Chuan Xiong* (Rhizoma Chuanxiong) for blood stagnation; and *Xian He Cao* (Herba Agrimoniae) and *San Qi* (Radix et Rhizoma Notoginseng) for bleeding. The herbs were given in decoction daily for 30 days per course of treatment.[9]

7. **Chronic gastritis**: Use of modified *Si Miao Yong An Tang* to treat 64 patients with chronic gastritis was associated with significant improvement in 54 cases, moderate improvement in 5 cases, and no effect in 5 cases. The overall effectiveness was 92.18%. The treatment protocol was to use *Si Miao Yong An Tang* plus *Pu Gong Ying* (Herba Taraxaci), *Yan Hu Suo* (Rhizoma Corydalis), and *Sha Ren* (Fructus Amomi) as the base formula. Furthermore, modifications included the addition of *Cang Zhu* (Rhizoma Atractylodis), *Hou Po* (Cortex Magnoliae Officinalis), and dry-fried *Lai Fu Zi* (Semen Raphani) for nausea and abdominal distention; *Gao Liang Jiang* (Rhizoma Alpiniae Officinarum) and *Xiang Fu* (Rhizoma Cyperi) for qi stagnation with cold; *Chai Hu* (Radix Bupleuri), *Sheng Ma* (Rhizoma Cimicifugae), and *Huang Qi* (Radix Astragali) for Spleen deficiency and *zhong* (central) *qi* deficiency; and *Wa Leng Zi* (Concha Arcae) or *Zuo Jin Wan* (Left Metal Pill) for belching and acid reflux.[10]

8. **Sciatica**: Use of modified *Si Miao Yong An Tang* in 30 patients with sciatica was associated with complete recovery in 21 cases, marked improvement in 8 cases, and no effect in 1 case. The herbal treatment included *Si Miao Yong An Tang* plus *Wei Ling Xian* (Radix et Rhizoma Clematidis), *Qian Nian Jian* (Rhizoma Homalomenae) and *Chuan Niu Xi* (Radix Cyathulae) as the base formula. Furthermore,

modifications to the original formula included the addition of *Huang Bo* (Cortex Phellodendri Chinensis) and *Di Long* (Pheretima) for soreness, heaviness and pain due to damp-heat; *Fu Zi* (Radix Aconiti Lateralis Praeparata) and *Xi Xin* (Radix et Rhizoma Asari) for cold extremities and aversion to cold due to damp-cold; *Du Zhong* (Cortex Eucommiae) and *Sang Ji Sheng* (Herba Taxilli) for low back pain; and *Bai Shao* (Radix Paeoniae Alba), *Yu Zhu* (Rhizoma Polygonati Odorati), and *Shen Jin Cao* (Herba Lycopodii) for muscle spasms, cramps and/or atrophy.[11]

9. **Prostatic hypertrophy**: One study reported good results using modified *Si Miao Yong An Tang* to treat prostatic hypertrophy. The base formula included *Si Miao Yong An Tang* plus *Tao Ren* (Semen Persicae), *Niu Xi* (Radix Achyranthis Bidentatae), *Ze Xie* (Rhizoma Alismatis), *Ju He* (Semen Citri Reticulatae), *Rou Gui* (Cortex Cinnamomi), and *Chuan Shan Jia* (Squama Manis). Furthermore, *Yan Hu Suo* (Rhizoma Corydalis) and *Mu Xiang* (Radix Aucklandiae) were added for testicular swelling and pain; *Mang Xiao* (Natrii Sulfas) for constipation; *Yin Yang Huo* (Herba Epimedii) and *Du Zhong* (Cortex Eucommiae) for weakness and soreness of lower back and knees; *Mo Han Lian* (Herba Ecliptae) and *Bai Mao Gen* (Rhizoma Imperatae) for hematuria; and *Bie Jia* (Carapax Trionycis) and *Hong Hua* (Flos Carthami) for hardness and nodules in the prostate area. Of 28 patients, the study reported significant improvement in 13 cases, moderate improvement in 12 cases, and no effect in 3 cases.[12]

10. **Carpal tunnel syndrome**: Use of modified *Si Miao Yong An Tang* was associated with 94.74% effectiveness in treating 19 patients with carpal tunnel syndrome. The herbal treatment included *Si Miao Yong An Tang* plus *Wei Ling Xian* (Radix et Rhizoma Clematidis), processed *Ru Xiang* (Gummi Olibanum), and *Dan Shen* (Radix et Rhizoma Salviae Miltiorrhizae). After cooking the herbs in water, the patients were instructed to drink the decoction and apply the herb residue topically to the affected area for 20-30 minutes. The duration was 15 days per course of treatment. Of 19 patients, the study reported complete recovery in 15 cases (complete resolution of numbness, pain, and other symptoms), moderate improvement in 3 cases (over 50% relief of symptoms) and no effect in 1 case.[13]

11. **Gout**: Sixteen patients with gout were treated with herbs resulting in complete recovery in 9 cases, improvement in 6 cases, and no effect in 1 case. The overall effectiveness was 93.7%. The herbal formula included *Si Miao Yong An Tang*, *Si Miao San* (Four-Marvel Powder), *Jin Qian Cao* (Herba Lysimachiae), *Ru Xiang* (Gummi Olibanum), and *Mo Yao* (Myrrha). Modifications included the addition

Sì Miào Yǒng Ān Tāng (Four-Valiant Decoction for Well-Being)

of *Shi Gao* (Gypsum Fibrosum) for heat; *Bai Zhi* (Radix Angelicae Dahuricae) for headache; *Da Huang* (Radix et Rhizoma Rhei) [post-decocted] for constipation; *Tu Fu Ling* (Rhizoma Smilacis Glabrae) for swelling and pain of the joints; *Wu Gong* (Scolopendra), and *Chuan Shan Jia* (Squama Manis) to enhance the efficacy of the herbal formula; and *Jin Qian Cao* (Herba Lysimachiae) for urinary stones. In addition, an herbal solution was applied topically to the affected area to treat redness, swelling, and pain. The topical solution was made from *Shang Lu* (Radix Phytolaccae), *Gan Sui* (Radix Kansui), and *Ze Lan* (Herba Lycopi).[14]

12. **Erysipelas**: Use of modified *Si Miao Yong An Tang* as a decoction in 31 patients was associated with complete recovery in 19 cases after 2-3 days, 10 cases after 4-6 days, and 2 cases after 1 week.[15] Another study reported marked effect in all 28 patients with erysipelas of the lower extremities when treated with *Si Miao Yong An Tang* plus *Huang Bo* (Cortex Phellodendri Chinensis), *Chuan Niu Xi* (Radix Cyathulae), *Di Long* (Pheretima), and others.[16]

RELATED FORMULAS

Wǔ Shén Tāng (Five-Miracle Decoction)

五神湯
五神汤

Pinyin Name: *Wu Shen Tang*
Literal Name: Five-Miracle Decoction
Original Source: *Dong Tian Ao Zhi* (Profound Purpose from the Heavenly Abode) by Chen Shi-Duo in 1694

Fu Ling (Poria)	30g [20g]
Che Qian Zi (Semen Plantaginis)	30g [15g]
Jin Yin Hua (Flos Lonicerae Japonicae)	90g [45g]
Niu Xi (Radix Achyranthis Bidentatae)	15g [10g]
Zi Hua Di Ding (Herba Violae)	30g [20g]

The source text states to prepare the ingredients as a decoction. Today, the decoction may be prepared using the doses suggested in brackets.

Wu Shen Tang (Five-Miracle Decoction) clears heat, eliminates toxins, and drains damp-heat. It is used to treat abscesses of the bones and legs, erysipelas, and toxic rash around *Weizhong* (BL 40) [popliteal region].

Shén Xiào Tuō Lǐ Sǎn
(Miraculous Powder for Supporting the Interior)

神效托裡散

Pinyin Name: *Shen Xiao Tuo Li San*
Literal Name: Miraculous Powder for Supporting the Interior

Alternate Name: *Si Miao San* (Four-Marvel Powder)
Original Source: *Tai Ping Hui Min He Ji Ju Fang* (Imperial Grace Formulary of the Tai Ping Era) by the Imperial Medical Department in 1078-85

Ren Dong Teng (Caulis Lonicerae Japonicae)	150g
Huang Qi (Radix Astragali)	150g
Dang Gui (Radix Angelicae Sinensis)	36g
Zhi Gan Cao (Radix et Rhizoma Glycyrrhizae Praeparata cum Melle)	240g

The source text states to grind the ingredients into a fine powder. Cook 6g of the powder with 1.5 bowls of grain-based liquor until the liquid is reduced to 0.5 bowl. If the affected area is in the upper body, take the formula after meals. If the affected area is in the lower body, take the formula before meals. Apply the herb residue topically to the affected area.

Shen Xiao Tuo Li San (Miraculous Powder for Supporting the Interior) tonifies qi, nourishes the blood, promotes the generation of flesh, and eliminates toxins. Clinically, it is used to treat individuals with qi and blood deficiencies with intestinal abscesses, breast abscesses, and any other types of swelling, sores, and abscesses, accompanied by fever and chills.

AUTHORS' COMMENTS

Si Miao Yong An Tang is the representative formula for treating gangrene, with such key diagnostic symptoms as localized inflammation, purulent abscess, dark red color, swelling, and a burning sensation. The original text notes that successful treatment of gangrene requires the use of this formula in large doses for a prolonged duration (at least 10 packs of herbs). The use of this formula at a low dose or for a short period of time will not be effective.

Si Miao Yong An Tang, *Wu Shen Tang* (Five-Miracle Decoction), and *Shen Xiao Tuo Li San* (Miraculous Powder for Supporting the Interior) all clear heat and eliminate toxins. The differences are as follows:

• *Si Miao Yong An Tang* eliminates toxins, clears heat, activates the blood, and disperses blood stasis. It is most effective for gangrene due to heat and toxins with underlying yin and blood deficiencies.

• *Wu Shen Tang* eliminates toxins, clears heat, and drains damp-heat. It is best for abscesses and erysipelas due to heat, toxins and damp-heat.

• *Shen Xiao Tuo Li San* clears heat and eliminates toxins, as well as tonifies qi and blood. It treats chronic abscesses and sores with underlying qi and blood deficiencies.

Chapter 22 – Formulas that Treat Abscesses and Sores　　　　　　　*Section 1 – External Abscesses and Sores*

Sì Miào Yŏng Ān Tāng (Four-Valiant Decoction for Well-Being)

References

1. *Zhe Jiang Yi Xue* (Zhejiang Journal of Medicine) 1960;36.
2. *Zhe Jiang Yi Xue* (Zhejiang Journal of Medicine) 1960;36.
3. *Xin Zhong Yi* (New Chinese Medicine) 1990;2:27.
4. *Zhong Yi Za Zhi* (Journal of Chinese Medicine) 1980;1:42.
5. *Tian Jin Yi Yao Za Zhi* (Journal of Tianjin Medicine and Herbology) 1960;1:1.
6. *Si Chuan Zhong Yi* (Sichuan Chinese Medicine) 1992;9:37.
7. *Shan Xi Zhong Yi* (Shanxi Chinese Medicine) 1998;2:74.
8. *Hei Long Jiang Zhong Yi Yao* (Heilongjiang Chinese Medicine and Herbology) 1997;3:1.
9. *Jiang Su Zhong Yi Za Zhi* (Jiangsu Journal of Chinese Medicine) 1983;5:272.
10. *Liao Ning Zhong Yi Za Zhi* (Liaoning Journal of Chinese Medicine) 1999;1:24.
11. *Hu Bei Zhong Yi Za Zhi* (Hubei Journal of Chinese Medicine) 1993;2:19.
12. *Shan Xi Zhong Yi* (Shanxi Chinese Medicine) 1991;5:15.
13. *Shi Yong Zhong Yi Za Zhi* (Journal of Practical Chinese Medicine) 1999;6:7.
14. *Hu Bei Zhong Yi Xue Yuan Xue Bao* (Journal of Hubei University of Medicine) 1996;1:18.
15. *Hei Long Jiang Zhong Yi Yao* (Heilongjiang Chinese Medicine and Herbology) 1986;4:41.
16. *Hu Bei Zhong Yi Za Zhi* (Hubei Journal of Chinese Medicine) 1998;5:32.

Zǐ Cǎo Gēn Mǔ Lì Tāng (Arnebia and Oyster Shell Decoction)

紫草根牡蠣湯
紫草根牡蛎汤

Pinyin Name: *Zi Cao Gen Mu Li Tang*
Literal Name: Arnebia and Oyster Shell Combination
Alternate Name: *Zi Gen Mu Li Tang*, Lithospermum and Oyster Shell Decoction
Original Source: *Bai Rai Shin Shu* (A New Study of Dermatomycosis and Dermatitis) by Tsursure Katakura

COMPOSITION

Zi Cao (Radix Arnebiae)	3g
Jin Yin Hua (Flos Lonicerae Japonicae)	1.5g
Sheng Ma (Rhizoma Cimicifugae)	2g
Mu Li (Concha Ostreae)	4g
Huang Qi (Radix Astragali)	2g
Dang Gui (Radix Angelicae Sinensis)	5g
Bai Shao (Radix Paeoniae Alba)	3g
Chuan Xiong (Rhizoma Chuanxiong)	3g
Da Huang (Radix et Rhizoma Rhei)	1.5g
Gan Cao (Radix et Rhizoma Glycyrrhizae)	1g

Note: *Zi Cao* (Radix Arnebiae) may be derived from three sources: *Arnebiae euchroma*, *Arnebiae guttata*, and *Lithospermum erythrorhizon*. All three herbs have similar functions, and have been used interchangeably in the history of Chinese herbal medicine. However, *Zhong Hua Ren Min Gong He Guo Yao Dian* (Pharmacopoeia of People's Republic of China) in 2005 identifies the arnebia genus as the official source of *Zi Cao*. Therefore, we have adopted arnebia as the standard nomenclature for both single herbs and herbal formulas throughout this text.

DOSAGE / PREPARATION / ADMINISTRATION

The source texts states to cook the herbs in 5 cups of water until the liquid is reduced to 2.5 cups. Take the warm, strained decoction in three equally-divided doses daily. Today, the decoction may be prepared using a higher dose of the ingredients (approximately 2-3 times higher).

CHINESE THERAPEUTIC ACTIONS

1. Clears heat and eliminates toxins
2. Reduces swelling and disperses nodules and hardness

1348

Zǐ Cǎo Gēn Mǔ Lì Tāng (Arnebia and Oyster Shell Decoction)

CLINICAL MANIFESTATIONS

Malignant abscesses and sores: various types of abscesses, sores, nodules, hardness, and dermatological disorders of unknown origin.

CLINICAL APPLICATIONS

Breast cancer, mastitis, lymphadenitis, gangrene, herpes, and skin lesions from syphilis.

EXPLANATION

Zi Cao Gen Mu Li Tang (Arnebia and Oyster Shell Decoction) treats various types of dermatological disorders characterized by heat and toxins. It has a broad range of effects, and is effective against sores, abscesses, nodules, and hardness.

Zi Cao (Radix Arnebiae) and *Jin Yin Hua* (Flos Lonicerae Japonicae) clear heat and eliminate toxins from the blood. They are also effective in treating various types of chronic and stubborn abscesses and sores due to infection. *Sheng Ma* (Rhizoma Cimicifugae) raises and disperses yang qi while eliminating heat and toxins. *Mu Li* (Concha Ostreae) softens hardness and disperses nodules. *Huang Qi* (Radix Astragali) tonifies qi and promotes healing, and

is one of the most important herbs for treating patients with suppurative disorders. *Dang Gui* (Radix Angelicae Sinensis), *Bai Shao* (Radix Paeoniae Alba), and *Chuan Xiong* (Rhizoma Chuanxiong) tonify blood and strengthen the body. *Da Huang* (Radix et Rhizoma Rhei) drains damp-heat. *Gan Cao* (Radix et Rhizoma Glycyrrhizae) harmonizes all of the herbs in the formula.

MODIFICATIONS

- With painful bruises and swelling, add *Ru Xiang* (Gummi Olibanum) and *Mo Yao* (Myrrha).
- With swelling caused by wind and dampness, add *Bai Zhi* (Radix Angelicae Dahuricae) and *Bai Zhu* (Rhizoma Atractylodis Macrocephalae).
- For herpes, add *Jing Jie* (Herba Schizonepetae), *Fang Feng* (Radix Saposhnikoviae), and *Lian Qiao* (Fructus Forsythiae).
- For herpes with neuralgia, add *Gui Zhi* (Ramulus Cinnamomi), *Qian Niu Zi* (Semen Pharbitidis), and *Fu Zi* (Radix Aconiti Lateralis Praeparata).
- For herpes affecting the eyes, add *Ju Hua* (Flos Chrysanthemi), *Che Qian Zi* (Semen Plantaginis), *Jie Geng* (Radix Platycodonis), *Fang Feng* (Radix Saposhnikoviae), and *Lian Qiao* (Fructus Forsythiae).

Zi Cao Gen Mu Li Tang (Arnebia and Oyster Shell Decoction)

Diagnosis	Signs and Symptoms	Treatment	Herbs
Malignant abscesses and sores	Abscesses, sores, nodules and hardness: heat and toxins accumulation	• Clears heat and eliminates toxins • Reduces swelling and disperses nodules and hardness	• *Zi Cao* (Radix Arnebiae) and *Jin Yin Hua* (Flos Lonicerae Japonicae) clear heat and eliminate toxins from the blood. • *Sheng Ma* (Rhizoma Cimicifugae) raises and disperses yang qi while eliminating heat and toxins. • *Mu Li* (Concha Ostreae) softens hardness and disperses nodules. • *Huang Qi* (Radix Astragali) tonifies qi and promotes healing. • *Dang Gui* (Radix Angelicae Sinensis), *Bai Shao* (Radix Paeoniae Alba) and *Chuan Xiong* (Rhizoma Chuanxiong) tonify blood and strengthen the body. • *Da Huang* (Radix et Rhizoma Rhei) drains damp-heat. • *Gan Cao* (Radix et Rhizoma Glycyrrhizae) harmonizes all of the herbs.

Chapter 22 – Formulas that Treat Abscesses and Sores　　　　　*Section 1 – External Abscesses and Sores*

Xī Huáng Wán (Cattle Gallstone Pill)

犀黃丸
犀黃丸

Pinyin Name: *Xi Huang Wan*
Literal Name: Cattle Gallstone Pill
Original Source: *Wai Ke Zheng Zhi Quan Sheng Ji* (Complete Collection of Patterns and Treatments in External Medicine) by Wang Wei-De in 1740

COMPOSITION

Niu Huang (Calculus Bovis)	0.9g [15g]
She Xiang (Moschus)	4.5g [75g]
Ru Xiang (Gummi Olibanum), oil removed and *yan* (ground) into fine powder	30g [500g]
Mo Yao (Myrrha), oil removed and *yan* (ground) into fine powder	30g [500g]

Although this formula is called *Xi Huang Wan*, literally "Rhinoceros Gallstone Pill," it is *Niu Huang* (Calculus Bovis), **not** *Xi Huang* (Calculus Rhinoceri), that is used in this formula. Therefore, to more accurately state the composition of this formula, the literal name is translated as "Cattle Gallstone Pill," **not** "Rhinoceros Gallstone Pill."

Note: *She Xiang* (Moschus) is derived from an endangered animal, and is rarely used as a medicinal substance today. Its discussion here is included primarily for academic purposes, to reflect the historical use of this substance in its original formulation. Most herbal products today have removed it completely, or replaced it with substitutes with similar functions.

DOSAGE / PREPARATION / ADMINISTRATION

The source text states to grind the ingredients into fine powder and form into pills with mashed, cooked rice. Allow the pills to sun-dry naturally. Do not dry the pills by baking or exposing them to fire. Take 9g of pills per dose with aged, grain-based liquor. If the disease is in the upper body, take the formula before bedtime. If the disease is in the lower body, take it on an empty stomach.

Today, this formula is prepared using the doses suggested in brackets. Steam 350g of rice and all of the ingredients, except *Niu Huang* (Calculus Bovis) and *She Xiang* (Moschus), until the rice is well-cooked. Oven-dry the herbs and grind them into a fine powder. Separately grind *Niu Huang* (Calculus Bovis) and *She Xiang* (Moschus) into a fine powder. Mix and sift all the powders evenly. Form the powder into pills with water, and dry the pills in a cool place without direct exposure to sunlight.

CHINESE THERAPEUTIC ACTIONS

1. Eliminates toxins and reduces abscesses
2. Dissolves phlegm and disperses nodules
3. Activates blood circulation and dispels blood stasis

CLINICAL MANIFESTATIONS

Yang-type abscesses and sores: breast cancer, buboes, scrofula, subcutaneous nodules, multiple abscesses, lung abscesses, and intestinal abscesses.

EXPLANATION

Xi Huang Wan (Cattle Gallstone Pill) treats various yang-type abscesses and sores characterized by accumulation and stagnation of fire, phlegm, heat, and toxins. As a result of such accumulation and stagnation, yin

Xi Huang Wan (Cattle Gallstone Pill)

Diagnosis	Signs and Symptoms	Treatment	Herbs
Yang-type abscesses and sores	Breast cancer, buboes, scrofula, subcutaneous nodules, multiple abscesses, lung abscesses, and intestinal abscesses: accumulation of fire, phlegm, heat, and toxins	• Eliminates toxins and reduces abscesses • Dissolves phlegm and disperses nodules • Activates blood and dispels blood stasis	• *Niu Huang* (Calculus Bovis) clears heat, eliminates toxins, dissolves phlegm, and disperses nodules. • *She Xiang* (Moschus) disperses and unblocks stagnation and nodules. • *Ru Xiang* (Gummi Olibanum) and *Mo Yao* (Myrrha) activate the blood, dispel blood stasis, reduce swelling, and relieve pain.

1350

Xī Huáng Wán (Cattle Gallstone Pill)

Chinese Herbal Formulas and Applications

and yang become unbalanced, channels and collaterals become obstructed, and the *zang fu* organs cannot perform their functions. Over time, abscesses and sores form at various parts of the body.

In this formula, *Niu Huang* (Calculus Bovis) clears heat, eliminates toxins, dissolves phlegm, and disperses nodules. *She Xiang* (Moschus) disperses and unblocks stagnation and nodules. *Ru Xiang* (Gummi Olibanum) and *Mo Yao* (Myrrha) activate blood circulation, dispel blood stasis, reduce swelling, and relieve pain. Rice nourishes the Stomach and protects it from the harsh characteristics of the other herbs in this formula. Lastly, this formula is taken with aged grain-based liquor to enhance the blood-activating function.

CAUTIONS / CONTRAINDICATIONS

- *Xi Huang Wan* treats nodules and abscesses while they are still hard. It should not be used for individuals with qi, yin and blood deficiencies, or in conditions in which the nodules and abscesses have already broken into open lesions and ulcerations with discharge of fluids and pus. Use of *Xi Huang Wan* under these circumstances will only consume *zheng* (upright) *qi*.
- This formula should only be given as pills for two reasons. First, pills are more appropriate than decoction as pills provide consistent and continuous effect needed to slowly dissolve phlegm and disperse nodules. Second, many ingredients in this formula cannot be prepared in decoction because they are acrid and aromatic, and contain volatile oils which evaporate easily during cooking.
- This formula should not be taken for a prolonged period of time, as it contains many herbs that are acrid and drying in nature.
- This formula is contraindicated during pregnancy.

RELATED FORMULAS

Xǐng Xiāo Wán (Awake and Disperse Pill)
醒消丸
Pinyin Name: Xing Xiao Wan
Literal Name: Awake and Disperse Pill
Original Source: *Wai Ke Zheng Zhi Quan Sheng Ji* (Complete Collection of Patterns and Treatments in External Medicine) by Wang Wei-De in 1740

Ru Xiang (Gummi Olibanum), oil removed	30g
Mo Yao (Myrrha), oil removed	30g
She Xiang (Moschus), *yan* (ground) into fine powder	4.5g
Xiong Huang (Realgar), *yan* (ground) into fine powder	15g

Note: *Xiong Huang* (Realgar) is a potentially toxic heavy metal, and *She Xiang* (Moschus) is derived from an

endangered animal. They are rarely used as medicinal substances today. Their discussion here is included primarily for academic purposes, to reflect the historical use of these substances in their original formulations. Most herbal products today have removed them completely, or replaced them with substitutes with similar functions. For additional information on the toxicity of *Xiong Huang* (Realgar), please refer to *Chinese Medical Herbology and Pharmacology* by John Chen and Tina Chen.

The source text states to mash the ingredients and form into pills with 30g of cooked rice. The pills should resemble *Lai Fu Zi* (Semen Raphani) in size. Allow the pills to sun-dry naturally. Do not dry the pills by baking or exposing them to fire. Take 9g of pills per dose with aged, grain-based liquor. The patient should be covered with blankets to promote sweating.

Xing Xiao Wan (Awake and Disperse Pill) activates the blood, disperses nodules, and eliminates toxins. It can be used for all types of abscesses characterized by redness and swelling. This formula is potentially toxic, and should be used with extreme caution and only for a short period of time. This formula is contraindicated during pregnancy.

Chán Sū Wán (Toad Venum Pill)
蟾酥丸
Pinyin Name: Chan Su Wan
Literal Name: Toad Venum Pill
Original Source: *Wai Ke Zheng Zong* (True Lineage of External Medicine) by Chen Shi-Gong in 1617

Chan Su (Venenum Bufonis), *hua* (dissolved) with liquor	6g
Qing Fen (Calomelas)	1.5g
Bai Fan (Alumen)	3g
Han Shui Shi (Mirabilite), *duan* (calcined)	3g
Tong Lu (Verdigris)	3g
Ru Xiang (Gummi Olibanum)	3g
Mo Yao (Myrrha)	3g
Dan Fan (Chalcanthitum)	3g
She Xiang (Moschus)	3g
Xiong Huang (Realgar)	6g
Wo Niu (Eulota)	21 pieces
Zhu Sha (Cinnabaris)	9g

Note: *Zhu Sha* (Cinnabaris) and *Qing Fen* (Calomelas) are potentially toxic heavy metals, and *She Xiang* (Moschus) is derived from an endangered animal. They are rarely used as medicinal substances today. Their discussion here is included primarily for academic purposes, to reflect the historical use of these substances in their original

FORMULAS THAT TREAT ABSCESSES AND SORES

22

1351

Chapter 22 – Formulas that Treat Abscesses and Sores　　　　　*Section 1 – External Abscesses and Sores*

Xī Huáng Wán (Cattle Gallstone Pill)

formulations. Most herbal products today have removed them completely, or replaced them with substitutes with similar functions. For additional information on the toxicity, please refer to *Chinese Medical Herbology and Pharmacology* by John Chen and Tina Chen.

The source text states to mash *Wo Niu* (Eulota) with *Chan Su* (Venenum Bufonis) and grind them together. Separately grind the other ingredients into powder. Mix all the powders together thoroughly, and form into pills that resemble the size of *Lu Dou* (Semen Phaseoli Radiati). For administration, chew 5 *cun* (approximately 5 inches) of *Cong Bai* (Bulbus Allii Fistulosi) first, then take 3 pills with 1 bowl of hot, grain-based liquor, and cover the body with blankets to promote sweating.

Chan Su Wan (Toad Venum Pill) eliminates toxins, reduces swellings, activates blood circulation, and relieves pain. It treats furuncles, lumbodorsal cellulitis, carbuncles of the nape, breast abscesses, pyogenic infection of the bone, deep-rooted carbuncles of the hips and legs, and all other

types of abscesses and sores. This formula is potentially toxic. It should *not* be used at a large dose or for a prolonged period of time. It should be used with extreme caution for individuals with underlying qi and blood deficiencies. This formula is contraindicated during pregnancy.

AUTHORS' COMMENTS

Xi Huang Wan, *Xing Xiao Wan* (Awake and Disperse Pill), and *Chan Su Wan* (Toad Venum Pill) all activate blood circulation, reduce swelling, eliminate toxins, and disperse nodules and hardness.

- *Xi Huang Wan* potently clears heat and eliminates toxins, and is primarily used to treat yang-type abscesses and sores.
- *Xing Xiao Wan* moderately clears heat and eliminates toxins, and is primarily used to treat yang-type abscesses characterized by redness and swelling.
- *Chan Su Wan* clears heat and eliminates toxins via its warming and dispersing herbs. It may be used for both superficial or deep-rooted abscesses.

Hǎi Zǎo Yù Hú Tāng (Sargassum Decoction for the Jade Flask)
海藻玉壺湯
海藻玉壶汤

Pinyin Name: *Hai Zao Yu Hu Tang*
Literal Name: Sargassum Decoction for the Jade Flask
Alternate Name: Sargassum Combination for the Jade Flask
Original Source: *Yi Zong Jin Jian* (Golden Mirror of the Medical Tradition) by Wu Qian in 1742

COMPOSITION

Hai Zao (Sargassum), *xi* (washed)	3g
Kun Bu (Thallus Eckloniae)	3g
Hai Dai (Thallus Laminariae)	1.5g
Bei Mu (Bulbus Fritillariae)	3g
Ban Xia (Rhizoma Pinelliae), *zhi* (prepared)	3g
Qing Pi (Pericarpium Citri Reticulatae Viride)	3g
Chen Pi (Pericarpium Citri Reticulatae)	3g
Dang Gui (Radix Angelicae Sinensis)	3g
Chuan Xiong (Rhizoma Chuanxiong)	3g
Du Huo (Radix Angelicae Pubescentis)	3g
Lian Qiao (Fructus Forsythiae)	3g
Gan Cao (Radix et Rhizoma Glycyrrhizae)	3g

Hǎi Zǎo Yù Hú Tāng (Sargassum Decoction for the Jade Flask)

DOSAGE / PREPARATION / ADMINISTRATION

The source text states to prepare the ingredients as a decoction by cooking the herbs in 2 cups of water until it is reduced down to 80%. Take the decoction before meals if the affected area is in the upper body, and after meals for lower body.

CHINESE THERAPEUTIC ACTIONS

1. Dissolves phlegm and softens hardness
2. Reduces and disperses goiter and tumor

CLINICAL MANIFESTATIONS

Goiter due to Liver and Spleen disharmony and qi and phlegm stagnation: immobile goiter in the neck region that is hard as a rock, with no pain, no change in skin color, and no inflammation.

CLINICAL APPLICATIONS

Goiter, thyroid adenocarcinoma, hyperthyroidism, lymphadenitis, hyperplasia of mammary glands, and panniculitis.

EXPLANATION

Hai Zao Yu Hu Tang (Sargassum Decoction for the Jade Flask) treats goiter caused by qi and phlegm stagnation, which often arises from the disharmony between the Liver and Spleen. The local qi and phlegm stagnation can then produce blood stagnation. The nodule is usually located on the neck, and is immobile, with no color change, no pain, does not perforate, and is often described as "hard as rock."

This formula has *Hai Zao* (Sargassum), *Kun Bu* (Thallus Eckloniae), and *Hai Dai* (Thallus Laminariae) to dissolve phlegm and soften nodules. *Bei Mu* (Bulbus Fritillariae) and *Ban Xia* (Rhizoma Pinelliae) dry dampness and resolve phlegm. *Qing Pi* (Pericarpium Citri Reticulatae Viride) and *Chen Pi* (Pericarpium Citri Reticulatae) regulate the qi and spread the Liver. *Dang Gui* (Radix Angelicae Sinensis), *Chuan Xiong* (Rhizoma Chuanxiong), and *Du Huo* (Radix Angelicae Pubescentis) activate blood circulation and disperse the nodule. *Lian Qiao* (Fructus Forsythiae) disperses nodules and reduces swelling. *Gan Cao* (Radix et Rhizoma Glycyrrhizae) harmonizes all of the herbs in the formula.

MODIFICATIONS

- For rock-hard nodules, add *San Leng* (Rhizoma Sparganii) and *E Zhu* (Rhizoma Curcumae).
- For nodules associated with Liver qi stagnation, add *Chai Hu* (Radix Bupleuri) and *Xiang Fu* (Rhizoma Cyperi).
- With a stifling sensation in the chest due to phlegm accumulation and qi stagnation, add *Xiang Fu* (Rhizoma Cyperi), *Zi Su Geng* (Caulis Perillae), *Yu Jin* (Radix Curcumae), and *Ge Qiao* (Concha Meretricis seu Cyclinae).
- With palpitations and sweating caused by blood deficiency and heat, add *Di Huang* (Radix Rehmanniae), *Shu Di Huang* (Radix Rehmanniae Praeparata), *Fu Shen* (Poria Paradicis), and *Suan Zao Ren* (Semen Ziziphi Spinosae).
- With hand and tongue tremors due to Liver wind, add *Zhen Zhu Mu* (Concha Margaritiferae), *Gou Teng* (Ramulus Uncariae cum Uncis), *Bai Shao* (Radix Paeoniae

Hai Zao Yu Hu Tang (Sargassum Decoction for the Jade Flask)

Diagnosis	Signs and Symptoms	Treatment	Herbs
Goiter	Hard, immobile goiter in the neck region: Liver and Spleen disharmony accompanied by qi and phlegm stagnation	• Dissolves phlegm and softens hardness • Reduces and disperses goiter and tumor	• *Hai Zao* (Sargassum), *Kun Bu* (Thallus Eckloniae), and *Hai Dai* (Thallus Laminariae) dissolve phlegm and soften nodules. • *Bei Mu* (Bulbus Fritillariae) and *Ban Xia* (Rhizoma Pinelliae) dry dampness and resolve phlegm. • *Qing Pi* (Pericarpium Citri Reticulatae Viride) and *Chen Pi* (Pericarpium Citri Reticulatae) regulate qi and smooth the Liver. • *Dang Gui* (Radix Angelicae Sinensis), *Chuan Xiong* (Rhizoma Chuanxiong) and *Du Huo* (Radix Angelicae Pubescentis) activate blood circulation and disperse the nodule. • *Lian Qiao* (Fructus Forsythiae) disperses nodules and reduces swelling. • *Gan Cao* (Radix et Rhizoma Glycyrrhizae) harmonizes all of the herbs.

FORMULAS THAT TREAT ABSCESSES AND SORES

22

Chapter 22 – Formulas that Treat Abscesses and Sores　　　　　*Section 1 – External Abscesses and Sores*

Hǎi Zǎo Yù Hú Tāng (Sargassum Decoction for the Jade Flask)

Alba), *Mu Li* (Concha Ostreae), and *Xia Ku Cao* (Spica Prunellae).

- With loose stools due to Spleen deficiency, add *Bai Zhu* (Rhizoma Atractylodis Macrocephalae), *Shan Yao* (Rhizoma Dioscoreae), and *Bai Bian Dou* (Semen Lablab Album).
- With frequent thirst and hunger due to Stomach heat, add *Shi Gao* (Gypsum Fibrosum), *Zhi Mu* (Rhizoma Anemarrhenae), and *Tian Hua Fen* (Radix Trichosanthis).
- With irregular menstruation, add *Lu Jiao* (Cornu Cervi), *Rou Cong Rong* (Herba Cistanches), *Yi Mu Cao* (Herba Leonuri), and *Tu Si Zi* (Semen Cuscutae).

CAUTIONS / CONTRAINDICATIONS

While taking *Hai Zao Yu Hu Tang*, patients should avoid foods that are sweet, fatty, or heavy in nature.

CLINICAL STUDIES AND RESEARCH

1. **Hyperthyroidism**: Use of modified *Hai Zao Yu Hu Tang* in 23 patients with hyperthyroidism was associated with 87% effectiveness. The herbal treatment contained *Hai Zao* (Sargassum), *Kun Bu* (Thallus Eckloniae), *Zhe Bei Mu* (Bulbus Fritillariae Thunbergii), *Qing Pi* (Pericarpium Citri Reticulatae Viride), *Chen Pi* (Pericarpium Citri Reticulatae), *Di Huang* (Radix Rehmanniae), *Bai Shao* (Radix Paeoniae Alba), *Tian Dong* (Radix Asparagi), *Xuan Shen* (Radix Scrophulariae), *Xia Ku Cao* (Spica Prunellae), *Huang Qin* (Radix Scutellariae), and *Mu Li* (Concha Ostreae). Clinical results included both subjective and objective improvements, with resolution of signs and symptoms and normalization of T3 and T4. Of 23 patients, the study reported recovery in 11 cases, improvement in 9 cases, and no effect in 3 cases.[1]

2. **Hyperplasia of mammary glands**: One study reported 94.2% effectiveness using modified *Hai Zao Yu Hu Tang* to treat hyperplasia of mammary glands in 52 women (2 women younger than 18 years of age, 43 women between 19-45 years of age, and 7 women older than 46 years of age). The herbal treatment contained *Hai Zao* (Sargassum), *Kun Bu* (Thallus Eckloniae), *Xia Ku Cao* (Spica Prunellae), *Zhe Bei Mu* (Bulbus Fritillariae Thunbergii), *Xiang Fu* (Rhizoma Cyperi), *Ban Xia* (Rhizoma Pinelliae), *Shui Zhi* (Hirudo), *Tu Bie Chong* (Eupolyphaga seu Steleophaga), *San Leng* (Rhizoma Sparganii), *E Zhu* (Rhizoma Curcumae), *Lian Qiao* (Fructus Forsythiae), and *Bai Hua She She Cao* (Herba Hedyotis). Overall, the study reported a reduction in the number and size of breast nodules by more than 50%. Of 52 patients, 32 had complete recovery, 17 had marked improvement, and 3 had no effect.[2] Another study reported marked results (92.1% effectiveness) using modified *Hai*

Zao Yu Hu Tang to treat 26 women with hyperplasia of mammary glands. Guidelines for modifications were to add *Chai Hu* (Radix Bupleuri), *Xiang Fu* (Rhizoma Cyperi) and *Jie Geng* (Radix Platycodonis) for qi stagnation with distention and pain; *San Leng* (Rhizoma Sparganii) and *Chuan Shan Jia* (Squama Manis) for blood stagnation; *Gua Lou* (Fructus Trichosanthis) and *Bai Jie Zi* (Semen Sinapis) for a white, greasy tongue coating with a wiry, slippery pulse; *Huang Qi* (Radix Astragali), *Bai Zhu* (Rhizoma Atractylodis Macrocephalae), and *Fu Ling* (Poria) for lack of energy; *Lu Jiao Jiao* (Colla Cornus Cervi) and *Yin Yang Huo* (Herba Epimedii) for aversion to cold with low back soreness; and other modifications as needed. Of 26 patients, the study reported complete recovery in 16 patients, significant improvement in 5 cases, moderate improvement in 3 cases, and no effect in 2 cases.[3]

3. **Panniculitis**: One study reported satisfactory results using modified *Hai Zao Yu Hu Tang* to treat 12 patients with painful inflammatory and necrotic nodules in the subcutaneous tissues affecting the extremities, buttocks, and other areas of the body. The herbal formula contained *Hai Zao* (Sargassum) 10g, *Kun Bu* (Thallus Eckloniae) 10g, *Lian Qiao* (Fructus Forsythiae) 10g, *Bei Mu* (Bulbus Fritillariae) 10g, *Dang Gui* (Radix Angelicae Sinensis) 10g, *Hai Dai* (Thallus Laminariae) 10g, *Du Huo* (Radix Angelicae Pubescentis) 10g, *Tao Ren* (Semen Persicae) 10g, *Yi Yi Ren* (Semen Coicis) 10g, *Si Gua Luo* (Retinervus Luffae Fructus) 10g, *Qing Pi* (Pericarpium Citri Reticulatae Viride) 5g, *Chen Pi* (Pericarpium Citri Reticulatae) 5g, *Ban Xia* (Rhizoma Pinelliae) 5g, *Chuan Xiong* (Rhizoma Chuanxiong) 5g, and *Gan Cao* (Radix et Rhizoma Glycyrrhizae) 5g. Modifications were made by adding *Ren Dong Teng* (Caulis Lonicerae Japonicae) and *Chi Xiao Dou* (Semen Phaseoli) for early stage inflammation with redness, swelling and pain; and *Tu Bie Chong* (Eupolyphaga seu Steleophaga) and *Chi Shao* (Radix Paeoniae Rubra) for middle stage inflammation with hardness and stiffness of the affected tissues and dark discoloration. The treatment protocol was to administer the herbs for 15 days per course of treatment, for 1-2 courses total. Of 12 patients, the study reported complete recovery in 10 cases, improvement in 1 case, and no response in 1 case.[4]

4. **Vocal cord nodule**: One study reported good success using modified *Hai Zao Yu Hu Tang* to treat formation of vocal cord nodules in 37 patients (3 males and 34 females). The herbal formula contained *Hai Zao* (Sargassum), *Kun Bu* (Thallus Eckloniae), *Mu Li* (Concha Ostreae), *Dang Gui* (Radix Angelicae Sinensis), *Chi Shao* (Radix Paeoniae Rubra), *Chuan Xiong* (Rhizoma Chuanxiong), *Mai Dong* (Radix Ophiopogonis), *Pu Gong*

1354

Hǎi Zǎo Yù Hú Tāng (Sargassum Decoction for the Jade Flask)

Ying (Herba Taraxaci), *Jin Yin Hua* (Flos Lonicerae Japonicae), *Zhe Bei Mu* (Bulbus Fritillariae Thunbergii), and *Chen Pi* (Pericarpium Citri Reticulatae). The herbs were given in decoction daily. Clinical improvements included normalization of voice, reduced redness and swelling, and reduction or resolution of vocal nodules. Of 37 patients, the study reported complete recovery in 26 cases, significant recovery in 9 cases, and no effect in 2 cases.[5]

AUTHORS' COMMENTS

Hai Zao Yu Hu Tang is one of the most commonly used formulas today for various thyroid disorders with enlargement of the thyroid glands, such as goiter and thyroid tumor. The duration of treatment necessary for improvement ranges from 3-6 months. Should the nodule remain the same size or increase in size, surgery should be considered.

According to *Shi Ba Fan* (Eighteen Incompatibles), *Hai Zao* (Sargassum) and *Gan Cao* (Radix et Rhizoma Glycyrrhizae) are not compatible with each other and should not be used together. However, this formula has been prescribed since 1742, and there has been no reported toxicity or side effects associated with its use. Furthermore, when prescribed, this formula is usually given for approximately 3-6 months. Thus, it is presumed that the use of these two herbs together in this formula is considered safe.

References

1. *Nei Meng Gu Zhong Yi Yao* (Traditional Chinese Medicine and Medicinals of Inner Mongolia) 1993;4:9.
2. *Zhong Yi Za Zhi* (Journal of Chinese Medicine) 1993;8:610.
3. *Shi Yong Zhong Yi Yao Za Zhi* (Journal of Practical Chinese Medicine and Medicinals) 1999;3:14.
4. *Zhe Jiang Zhong Yi Za Zhi* (Zhejiang Journal of Chinese Medicine) 1993;28(6):254.
5. *Zhong Yi Za Zhi* (Journal of Chinese Medicine) 1984;7:504.

Xiāo Luǒ Wán (Reduce Scrofula Pill)

消瘰丸

Pinyin Name: *Xiao Luo Wan*
Literal Name: Reduce Scrofula Pill
Alternate Name: Scrophularia and Fritillaria Combination
Original Source: *Yi Xue Xin Wu* (Medical Revelations) by Cheng Guo-Peng in 1732

COMPOSITION

Xuan Shen (Radix Scrophulariae), *zheng* (steamed)	120g
Bei Mu (Bulbus Fritillariae), *zheng* (steamed)	120g
Mu Li (Concha Ostreae), *duan* (calcined) and *yan* (ground) with vinegar	120g

DOSAGE / PREPARATION / ADMINISTRATION

The source text states to first steam *Xuan Shen* (Radix Scrophulariae) and *Bei Mu* (Bulbus Fritillariae), and calcine and grind *Mu Li* (Concha Ostreae) with vinegar. Then, grind all of the ingredients into powder, mix with honey, and form into pills. Take 9g of pills with boiled water twice daily.

CHINESE THERAPEUTIC ACTIONS

1. Reduces scrofula
2. Nourishes yin
3. Dissolves phlegm and softens hardness

CLINICAL MANIFESTATIONS

Hardness and nodules: hard lumps or nodules anterior or posterior to the ear or on the neck; dry mouth and throat; and a bitter taste in the mouth.

CLINICAL APPLICATIONS

Goiter, scrofula, hyperthyroidism, thyroiditis, acute simple lymphadenitis, parotitis, and hyperplasia of mammary glands.

EXPLANATION

Xiao Luo Wan (Reduce Scrofula Pill) treats lumps and nodules around the ears and the neck. Such nodules or

FORMULAS THAT TREAT ABSCESSES AND SORES

22

1355

Chapter 22 – Formulas that Treat Abscesses and Sores   Section 1 – External Abscesses and Sores

Xiāo Luǒ Wán (Reduce Scrofula Pill)

Xiao Luo Wan (Reduce Scrofula Pill)

Diagnosis	Signs and Symptoms	Treatment	Herbs
Hardness and nodules	Lumps, hardness, and nodules around the ears and neck	• Reduces scrofula • Nourishes yin • Dissolves phlegm and softens hardness	• *Xuan Shen* (Radix Scrophulariae) nourishes yin and guides fire downward. • *Bei Mu* (Bulbus Fritillariae) dissolves phlegm and reduces swelling. • *Mu Li* (Concha Ostreae) softens hardness and disperses nodules.

hardness is often caused by inflammation of the lymph nodes or enlargement of the thyroid glands. Patients may or may not have any subjective symptoms or complaints.

Although this formula contains only three herbs, it is very effective. *Xuan Shen* (Radix Scrophulariae) nourishes yin and guides fire downward. *Bei Mu* (Bulbus Fritillariae) dissolves phlegm and reduces swelling. *Mu Li* (Concha Ostreae) softens hardness and disperses nodules. When combined together, these three herbs treat various hardness and nodules, from early to late stages.

MODIFICATIONS

- With excess phlegm and fire, increase the dose of *Bei Mu* (Bulbus Fritillariae), and add *Gua Lou* (Fructus Trichosanthis), *Qing Dai* (Indigo Naturalis), and *Ge Qiao* (Concha Meretricis seu Cyclinae).
- With anger, restlessness, and irritability, add *Zhi Zi* (Fructus Gardeniae), *Huang Lian* (Rhizoma Coptidis), and *Huang Qin* (Radix Scutellariae).
- With Liver qi stagnation, add *Chai Hu* (Radix Bupleuri), *Xiang Fu* (Rhizoma Cyperi), and *Qing Pi* (Pericarpium Citri Reticulatae Viride).
- With yin-deficient fire, add *Di Gu Pi* (Cortex Lycii), *Mu Dan Pi* (Cortex Moutan), and *Zhi Mu* (Rhizoma Anemarrhenae).
- For enlarged thyroid gland, add *Kun Bu* (Thallus Eckloniae), *Hai Zao* (Sargassum), and *Xia Ku Cao* (Spica Prunellae).
- For swellings that are large and hard, increase the dose of *Mu Li* (Concha Ostreae), and add *Kun Bu* (Thallus Eckloniae), *Hai Zao* (Sargassum,) and *Xia Ku Cao* (Spica Prunellae).

CAUTIONS / CONTRAINDICATIONS

Xiao Luo Wan should be used with caution in patients with Spleen deficiency and loose stools.

CLINICAL STUDIES AND RESEARCH

1. **Parotitis**: One study reported improvement in all 406 patients with acute infectious parotitis using oral and topical applications of herbs. *Xiao Luo Wan* was used orally, and *Qing Dai* (Indigo Naturalis) was applied topically to the affected area. Of 290 patients who had unilateral parotitis, the study reported complete recovery in 186 cases, significant recovery in 96 cases, and improvement in 8 cases. Of 116 patients with bilateral parotitis, the study reported complete recovery in 68 cases, significant recovery in 36 cases, and improvement in 12 cases.[1]

2. **Hyperplasia of mammary glands**: One study reported 99.42% effectiveness using *Xiao Luo Wan* plus *Xiao Yao San* (Rambling Powder) to treat 118 patients with unilateral or bilateral hyperplasia of mammary glands. Of 118 patients, the study reported complete recovery in 78 cases, improvement in 34 cases, and no effect in 6 cases.[2]

AUTHORS' COMMENTS

Xiao Luo Wan is the representative formula for treating various types of hardness and nodules. Although this formula is literally called "Reduce Scrofula Pill," it may be used for many other types of hardness and nodules. Clinical applications include scrofula, goiter, hyperthyroidism, thyroiditis, lymphadenitis, parotitis, and hyperplasia of mammary glands.

For the purpose of dissolving nodules, calcined *Mu Li* (Concha Ostreae) should be used instead of the unprocessed form.

References

1. *Zhong Xi Yi Jie He Za Zhi* (Journal of Integrated Chinese and Western Medicine) 1989;9(10):612.
2. *Shi Yong Zhong Yi Yao Za Zhi* (Journal of Practical Chinese Medicine and Medicinals) 1998;11:9.

Chinese Herbal Formulas and Applications

Sàn Zhǒng Kùi Jiān Tāng
(Disperse the Swelling and Break the Hardness Decoction)

散腫潰堅湯
散肿溃坚汤

Pinyin Name: *San Zhong Kui Jian Tang*
Literal Name: Disperse the Swelling and Break the Hardness Decoction
Alternate Names: *San Tsung Kuei Chien Tang*, Forsythia and Laminaria Decoction, Forsythia and Laminaria Combination
Original Source: *Wan Bing Hui Chun* (Restoration of Health from the Myriad Diseases) by Gong Ting-Xian in 1587

COMPOSITION

Hai Zao (Sargassum), *chao* (dry-fried)	15g
Kun Bu (Thallus Eckloniae), *xi* (washed) with cold water	15g
Jie Geng (Radix Platycodonis)	15g
San Leng (Rhizoma Sparganii), *jin* (soaked) in liquor	9g
E Zhu (Rhizoma Curcumae), *jin* (soaked) in liquor	9g
Bai Shao (Radix Paeoniae Alba), *chao* (dry-fried) with liquor	9g
Dang Gui Wei (Extremitas Radix Angelicae Sinensis)	1.5g
Huang Qin (Radix Scutellariae), *chao* (dry-fried) with liquor	9g
Huang Lian (Rhizoma Coptidis)	9g
Long Dan (Radix et Rhizoma Gentianae)	9g
Lian Qiao (Fructus Forsythiae)	9g
Zhi Mu (Rhizoma Anemarrhenae), *jin* (soaked) in liquor	15g
Huang Bo (Cortex Phellodendri Chinensis), *chao* (dry-fried) with liquor	15g
Tian Hua Fen (Radix Trichosanthis)	15g
Chai Hu (Radix Bupleuri)	1.5g
Sheng Ma (Rhizoma Cimicifugae)	1.5g
Ge Gen (Radix Puerariae Lobatae)	9g
Zhi Gan Cao (Radix et Rhizoma Glycyrrhizae Praeparata cum Melle)	15g

DOSAGE / PREPARATION / ADMINISTRATION

The source text states to first soak all of the ingredients in water for half a day, then cook until the liquid is reduced by 50%. Take the strained decoction while warm.

CHINESE THERAPEUTIC ACTIONS

1. Disperses stagnation and softens hardness
2. Reduces swelling and drains pus

CLINICAL MANIFESTATIONS

Suppurative sores, ulcerations, and swellings that remain hard after discharge of pus and abscess.

CLINICAL APPLICATIONS

Lymphadenitis, hyperthyroidism, goiter, carbuncles, and furuncles.

EXPLANATION

San Zhong Kui Jian Tang (Disperse the Swelling and Break the Hardness Decoction) treats nodules, swelling, and hardness on various parts of the body, especially below the ears, under the cheeks, around the shoulders, and beneath the armpits. It contains many herbs that drain swelling and pus, and disperse hardness and stagnation.

Hai Zao (Sargassum), *Kun Bu* (Thallus Eckloniae) and *Jie Geng* (Radix Platycodonis) eliminate phlegm to soften hardness and disperse nodules. *San Leng* (Rhizoma Sparganii) and *E Zhu* (Rhizoma Curcumae) move the blood and eliminate blood stasis to break the hardness. Because these two herbs are rather potent, *Bai Shao* (Radix Paeoniae Alba) and *Dang Gui Wei* (Extremitas Radix Angelicae Sinensis) are added to nourish blood and moderate their effect. *Huang Qin* (Radix Scutellariae), *Huang Lian* (Rhizoma Coptidis), and *Long Dan* (Radix et Rhizoma Gentianae) clear damp-heat from the upper, middle and lower *jiao*. *Lian Qiao* (Fructus Forsythiae) clears heat and eliminates toxins. Since these bitter and cold herbs are drying in nature, *Zhi Mu* (Rhizoma Anemarrhenae), *Huang Bo* (Cortex Phellodendri Chinensis) and *Tian Hua Fen* (Radix Trichosanthis) are used to clear deficiency heat and protect yin and fluids. *Chai Hu* (Radix Bupleuri), *Sheng Ma* (Rhizoma Cimicifugae) and *Ge Gen* (Radix Puerariae Lobatae) activate qi circulation, and

FORMULAS THAT TREAT ABSCESSES AND SORES

22

1357

Chapter 22 – Formulas that Treat Abscesses and Sores   Section 1 – External Abscesses and Sores

Sàn Zhŏng Kùi Jiān Tāng
(Disperse the Swelling and Break the Hardness Decoction)

San Zhong Kui Jian Tang (Disperse the Swelling and Break the Hardness Decoction)

Diagnosis	Signs and Symptoms	Treatment	Herbs
Suppurative sores, ulcerations, and swellings	Nodules, swelling, and hardness with pus and abscess	• Disperses stagnation and softens hardness • Reduces swelling and drains pus	• *Hai Zao* (Sargassum), *Kun Bu* (Thallus Eckloniae) and *Jie Geng* (Radix Platycodonis) eliminate phlegm, soften hardness, and disperse nodules. • *San Leng* (Rhizoma Sparganii) and *E Zhu* (Rhizoma Curcumae) move the blood and eliminate blood stasis to break the hardness. • *Bai Shao* (Radix Paeoniae Alba) and *Dang Gui Wei* (Extremitas Radix Angelicae Sinensis) nourish blood and promote blood circulation. • *Huang Qin* (Radix Scutellariae), *Huang Lian* (Rhizoma Coptidis), and *Long Dan* (Radix et Rhizoma Gentianae) clear damp-heat from the upper, middle and lower *jiao*. • *Lian Qiao* (Fructus Forsythiae) clears heat and eliminates toxins. • *Zhi Mu* (Rhizoma Anemarrhenae), *Huang Bo* (Cortex Phellodendri Chinensis) and *Tian Hua Fen* (Radix Trichosanthis) clear deficiency heat and protect yin and fluids. • *Chai Hu* (Radix Bupleuri), *Sheng Ma* (Rhizoma Cimicifugae) and *Ge Gen* (Radix Puerariae Lobatae) guide the formula to upper parts of the body. • *Zhi Gan Cao* (Radix et Rhizoma Glycyrrhizae Praeparata cum Melle) harmonizes all of the herbs.

guide the formula to the upper parts of the body. *Zhi Gan Cao* (Radix et Rhizoma Glycyrrhizae Praeparata cum Melle) harmonizes all of the herbs.

MODIFICATIONS
- For nodules and hardness prior to the formation of pus, add *Jin Yin Hua* (Flos Lonicerae Japonicae) and *Zhi Shi* (Fructus Aurantii Immaturus).
- For nodules and hardness after the formation of pus, add *Huang Qi* (Radix Astragali) and *Bai Zhi* (Radix Angelicae Dahuricae).
- For nodules and hardness with redness, swelling, and pain, add *Shi Gao* (Gypsum Fibrosum) and *Zhi Zi* (Fructus Gardeniae).

RELATED FORMULAS
Sàn Zhŏng Kùi Jiān Tāng (Disperse the Swelling and Break the Hardness Decoction)

散腫潰堅湯
散肿溃坚汤

Pinyin Name: *San Zhong Kui Jian Tang*
Literal Name: Disperse the Swelling and Break the Hardness Decoction
Original Source: *Lan Shi Mi Cang* (Secrets from the Orchid Chamber) by Li Gao in 1336

Huang Qin (Radix Scutellariae), *xi* (washed) with liquor and *chao* (dry-fried)	12g
Huang Qin (Radix Scutellariae)	12g
Long Dan (Radix et Rhizoma Gentianae), *xi* (washed) with liquor and *chao* (dry-fried)	15g
Tian Hua Fen (Radix Trichosanthis), *xi* (washed) with liquor	15g
Huang Bo (Cortex Phellodendri Chinensis), *zhi* (fried with liquid)	15g
Zhi Mu (Rhizoma Anemarrhenae), *zhi* (fried with liquid)	15g
Jie Geng (Radix Platycodonis)	15g
Kun Bu (Thallus Eckloniae)	15g
Chai Hu (Radix Bupleuri)	12g

1358

Sàn Zhǒng Kùi Jiān Tāng
(Disperse the Swelling and Break the Hardness Decoction)

Zhi Gan Cao (Radix et Rhizoma Glycyrrhizae Praeparata cum Melle)	9g
San Leng (Rhizoma Sparganii), *xi* (washed) with liquor	9g
E Zhu (Rhizoma Curcumae), *xi* (washed) with liquor and *chao* (dry-fried)	9g
Lian Qiao (Fructus Forsythiae)	9g
Ge Gen (Radix Puerariae Lobatae)	6g
Bai Shao (Radix Paeoniae Alba)	6g
Dang Gui Wei (Extremitas Radix Angelicae Sinensis)	6g
Huang Lian (Rhizoma Coptidis)	6g
Sheng Ma (Rhizoma Cimicifugae)	1.8g

This formula clears heat, eliminates toxins, softens hardness, and disperses stagnations. It treats nodules, swellings and hardness along the hand *shaoyang* or foot *yangming* channels, such as regions below the ears, around the shoulders, and beneath the armpits.

These two formulas have identical names, and very similar compositions and functions.

- *San Zhong Kui Jian Tang* (Disperse the Swelling and Break the Hardness Decoction) from *Wan Bing Hui Chun* (Restoration of Health from the Myriad Diseases) uses *Hai Zao* (Sargassum) and *Kun Bu* (Thallus Eckloniae) as chief herbs, and therefore, has stronger effect to soften hardness and disperse nodules.

- *San Zhong Kui Jian Tang* (Disperse the Swelling and Break the Hardness Decoction) from *Lan Shi Mi Cang* (Secrets from the Orchid Chamber) contains larger doses of *Huang Qin* (Radix Scutellariae) and *Long Dan* (Radix et Rhizoma Gentianae), and thus, has better function to clear heat and eliminate toxins.

Xiāo Sàn Tāng Yī Haò
(Dissolve and Disperse Decoction Formula One)

消散湯一號
消散汤一号

Pinyin Name: *Xiao San Tang Yi Hao*
Literal Name: Dissolve and Disperse Decoction Formula One
Original Source: *Guang An Men Yi Yuan* (Guang An Men Hospital) in 1990

Chai Hu (Radix Bupleuri)
Hou Po (Cortex Magnoliae Officinalis)
Qing Pi (Pericarpium Citri Reticulatae Viride)
Dan Shen (Radix et Rhizoma Salviae Miltiorrhizae)
Wang Bu Liu Xing (Semen Vaccariae)
Zhi Zi (Fructus Gardeniae)

Zi Hua Di Ding (Herba Violae)
Ban Zhi Lian (Herba Scutellariae Barbatae)
Gua Lou (Fructus Trichosanthis)
Niu Bang Zi (Fructus Arctii)
Pu Gong Ying (Herba Taraxaci)
Tu Fu Ling (Rhizoma Smilacis Glabrae)
Zhe Bei Mu (Bulbus Fritillariae Thunbergii)
Zao Jiao (Fructus Gleditsiae)

This formula dissolves and disperses nodules and hardness in the upper *jiao* by activating qi and blood circulation, clearing heat, and eliminating phlegm. Clinically, it is effective for fibrocystic disorders in the upper half of the body, palpable masses in the breast, breast distention, lymphadenopathy with swollen and enlarged lymph nodes, and mastitis with nodules or fibroids.

Xiāo Sàn Tāng Èr Haò
(Dissolve and Disperse Decoction Formula Two)

消散湯二號
消散汤二号

Pinyin Name: *Xiao San Tang Er Hao*
Literal Name: Dissolve and Disperse Decoction Formula Two
Original Source: *Guang An Men Yi Yuan* (Guang An Men Hospital) in 1990

Gui Zhi (Ramulus Cinnamomi)
Fu Ling (Poria)
Mu Dan Pi (Cortex Moutan)
Tao Ren (Semen Persicae)
Chi Shao (Radix Paeoniae Rubra)
Pu Huang (Pollen Typhae)
Hong Hua (Flos Carthami)
San Leng (Rhizoma Sparganii)
E Zhu (Rhizoma Curcumae)
Mu Li (Concha Ostreae)
Zao Jiao (Fructus Gleditsiae)
Zhe Bei Mu (Bulbus Fritillariae Thunbergii)
Chuan Xiong (Rhizoma Chuanxiong)
Dan Shen (Radix et Rhizoma Salviae Miltiorrhizae)
San Qi (Radix et Rhizoma Notoginseng)
Yan Hu Suo (Rhizoma Corydalis)

This formula dissolves and disperses nodules and hardness in the lower *jiao* by activating qi and blood circulation, clearing heat, and eliminating phlegm. Clinically, it is effective for fibrocystic disorders in the lower half of the body, fibroids and cysts in the uterus and ovaries, and complications of fibroids and cysts.

Chapter 22 – Formulas that Treat Abscesses and Sores   *Section 1 – External Abscesses and Sores*

Sàn Zhŏng Kùi Jiān Tāng
(Disperse the Swelling and Break the Hardness Decoction)

AUTHORS' COMMENTS

According to Dr. Chang Wei-Yen, prostate enlargement can be treated with *San Zhong Kui Jian Tang* combined with *Zhen Ren Huo Ming Yin* (True Man's Decoction to Revitalize Life) and *Shi Liu Wei Liu Qi Yin* (Sixteen-Ingredient Decoction to Flow Qi).

Shi Liù Wèi Liú Qi Yǐn (Sixteen-Ingredient Decoction to Flow Qi)
十六味流氣飲
十六味流气饮

Pinyin Name: *Shi Liu Wei Liu Qi Yin*
Literal Name: Sixteen-Ingredient Decoction to Flow Qi
Alternate Name: Tangkuei Sixteen Herbs Combination
Original Source: *Wan Bing Hui Chun* (Restoration of Health from the Myriad Diseases) by Gong Ting-Xian in 1587

COMPOSITION

Ren Shen (Radix et Rhizoma Ginseng)
Huang Qi (Radix Astragali)
Gan Cao (Radix et Rhizoma Glycyrrhizae)
Dang Gui (Radix Angelicae Sinensis)
Bai Shao (Radix Paeoniae Alba)
Chuan Xiong (Rhizoma Chuanxiong)
Mu Xiang (Radix Aucklandiae)
Bing Lang (Semen Arecae)
Zhi Qiao (Fructus Citri Aurantii)
Hou Po (Cortex Magnoliae Officinalis)
Zi Su Ye (Folium Perillae)
Fang Feng (Radix Saposhnikoviae)
Wu Yao (Radix Linderae)
Bai Zhi (Radix Angelicae Dahuricae)
Gui Zhi (Ramulus Cinnamomi)
Jie Geng (Radix Platycodonis)

DOSAGE / PREPARATION / ADMINISTRATION

The source text states to grate equal proportions of all of the ingredients and prepare as a decoction.

CHINESE THERAPEUTIC ACTIONS

1. Tonifies qi and blood
2. Activates qi and blood circulation
3. Disperses stagnation and drains pus

CLINICAL MANIFESTATIONS

Nodules and hardness due to qi, blood, and phlegm stagnation: nodules and hardness in various parts of the body, such as the neck, breast, and abdominal region.

CLINICAL APPLICATIONS

Breast cancer, fibrocystic disease, goiter, and inflammation of the lymph glands.

EXPLANATION

Shi Liu Wei Liu Qi Yin (Sixteen-Ingredient Decoction to Flow Qi) is one of the best formulas for dispersing nodules and softening hardness. These nodules and lumps may be caused by inflammation of the lymph glands, goiter, tumor, sores, or abscess of unknown origin.

This formula focuses on treating both the underlying deficiencies (qi and blood) and the stagnations (qi, blood, and phlegm). *Ren Shen* (Radix et Rhizoma Ginseng), *Huang*

1360

Chinese Herbal Formulas and Applications

Shí Liù Wèi Liú Qì Yǐn (Sixteen-Ingredient Decoction to Flow Qi)

Shi Liu Wei Liu Qi Yin (Sixteen-Ingredient Decoction to Flow Qi)

Diagnosis	Signs and Symptoms	Treatment	Herbs
Nodules and hardness	Nodules and hardness in various parts of the body: stagnation with underlying deficiency	• Tonifies qi and blood • Activates qi and blood circulation • Disperses stagnation and drains pus	• *Ren Shen* (Radix et Rhizoma Ginseng), *Huang Qi* (Radix Astragali) and *Gan Cao* (Radix et Rhizoma Glycyrrhizae) tonify qi. • *Dang Gui* (Radix Angelicae Sinensis), *Bai Shao* (Radix Paeoniae Alba) and *Chuan Xiong* (Rhizoma Chuanxiong) tonify blood and activate blood circulation. • *Mu Xiang* (Radix Aucklandiae), *Bing Lang* (Semen Arecae), *Zhi Qiao* (Fructus Aurantii), *Hou Po* (Cortex Magnoliae Officinalis), *Zi Su Ye* (Folium Perillae) and *Fang Feng* (Radix Saposhnikoviae) regulate the proper flow of qi. • *Wu Yao* (Radix Linderae), *Zhi Qiao* (Fructus Aurantii) and *Hou Po* (Cortex Magnoliae Officinalis) break up qi stagnation. • *Bai Zhi* (Radix Angelicae Dahuricae) and *Gui Zhi* (Ramulus Cinnamomi) warm and open the channels and collaterals. • *Jie Geng* (Radix Platycodonis) dispels phlegm and drains pus and abscess. • *Gan Cao* (Radix et Rhizoma Glycyrrhizae) harmonizes all of the herbs.

Qi (Radix Astragali), and *Gan Cao* (Radix et Rhizoma Glycyrrhizae) tonify qi. *Dang Gui* (Radix Angelicae Sinensis), *Bai Shao* (Radix Paeoniae Alba), and *Chuan Xiong* (Rhizoma Chuanxiong) tonify blood and activate blood circulation. *Mu Xiang* (Radix Aucklandiae), *Bing Lang* (Semen Arecae), *Zhi Qiao* (Fructus Aurantii), *Hou Po* (Cortex Magnoliae Officinalis), *Zi Su Ye* (Folium Perillae), and *Fang Feng* (Radix Saposhnikoviae) regulate the proper flow of qi. *Wu Yao* (Radix Linderae), *Zhi Qiao* (Fructus Aurantii), and *Hou Po* (Cortex Magnoliae Officinalis) break up stubborn qi stagnation. *Bai Zhi* (Radix Angelicae Dahuricae) and *Gui Zhi* (Ramulus Cinnamomi) warm and open the channels and collaterals. *Jie Geng* (Radix Platycodonis) dispels phlegm and drains pus and abscess. Lastly, *Gan Cao* (Radix et Rhizoma Glycyrrhizae) harmonizes all of the herbs in the formula.

MODIFICATIONS
• For various swellings, nodules, lumps, fibroids, and carbuncles, add *San Zhong Kui Jian Tang* (Disperse the Swelling and Break the Hardness Decoction).
• For fibrocystic growth related to estrogen intake, add *Zi Cao* (Radix Arnebiae) and *Tian Hua Fen* (Radix Trichosanthis).

RELATED FORMULAS
Shí Liù Wèi Liú Qì Yǐn

(Sixteen-Ingredient Decoction to Flow Qi)

十六味流氣飲
十六味流气饮

Pinyin Name: Shi Liu Wei Liu Qi Yin
Literal Name: Sixteen-Ingredient Decoction to Flow Qi
Alternate Name: Tangkuei Sixteen Herbs Combination
Original Source: *Yi Xue Ru Men* (Introduction to Medicine) by Li Ting in 1575

Ren Shen (Radix et Rhizoma Ginseng)
Huang Qi (Radix Astragali)
Gan Cao (Radix et Rhizoma Glycyrrhizae)
Dang Gui (Radix Angelicae Sinensis)
Bai Shao (Radix Paeoniae Alba)
Chuan Xiong (Rhizoma Chuanxiong)
Mu Xiang (Radix Aucklandiae)
Bing Lang (Semen Arecae)
Zhi Qiao (Fructus Citri Aurantii)
Hou Po (Cortex Magnoliae Officinalis)
Zi Su Ye (Folium Perillae)
Fang Feng (Radix Saposhnikoviae)
Wu Yao (Radix Linderae)

FORMULAS THAT TREAT ABSCESSES AND SORES

22

1361

Chapter 22 – Formulas that Treat Abscesses and Sores

Section 1 – External Abscesses and Sores

Shí Liù Wèi Liú Qì Yǐn (Sixteen-Ingredient Decoction to Flow Qi)

Bai Zhi (Radix Angelicae Dahuricae)
Rou Gui (Cortex Cinnamomi)
Jie Geng (Radix Platycodonis)

These two formulas have identical names, and essentially the same ingredients and functions.
- Shi Liu Wei Liu Qi Yin from Wan Bing Hui Chun (Restoration of Health from the Myriad Diseases) by Gong Ting-Xian in 1587 contains Gui Zhi (Ramulus Cinnamomi), and is a more commonly used formulation today.

- Shi Liu Wei Liu Qi Yin from Yi Xue Ru Men (Introduction to Medicine) by Li Ting in 1575 contains Rou Gui (Cortex Cinnamomi), and is the original formulation.

AUTHORS' COMMENTS

According to Dr. Chang Wei-Yen, prostate enlargement can be treated by combining Shi Liu Wei Liu Qi Yin with Zhen Ren Huo Ming Yin (True Man's Decoction to Revitalize Life) and San Zhong Kui Jian Tang (Disperse the Swelling and Break the Hardness Decoction).

Tòu Nóng Sǎn (Discharge Pus Powder)

透膿散
透脓散

Pinyin Name: Tou Nong San
Literal Name: Discharge Pus Powder
Original Source: Wai Ke Zheng Zong (True Lineage of External Medicine) by Chen Shi-Gong in 1617

COMPOSITION

Huang Qi (Radix Astragali)	12g
Dang Gui (Radix Angelicae Sinensis)	6g
Chuan Xiong (Rhizoma Chuanxiong)	9g
Chuan Shan Jia (Squama Manis), chao (dry-fried)	3g
Zao Jiao Ci (Spina Gleditsiae)	4.5g

DOSAGE / PREPARATION / ADMINISTRATION

The source text states to cook the ingredients in 2 large bowls of water until the liquid is reduced by 50%. Take the decoction with a cup of grain-based liquor.

CHINESE THERAPEUTIC ACTIONS

1. Drains toxins
2. Breaks and dispels pus

CLINICAL MANIFESTATIONS

Abscesses and sores accompanied by swelling and pain with underlying qi deficiency: diffused presentation of abscesses and sores with swelling, burning sensations, pain, and formation of pus without ulceration.

CLINICAL APPLICATIONS

Abscesses, sores, carbuncles, and boils.

EXPLANATION

Tou Nong San (Discharge Pus Powder) treats abscesses and sores accompanied by swelling and pain with underlying qi deficiency. In this condition, pus has already formed inside, and has begun to cause swelling, inflammation, and pain. However, because of qi deficiency, the body is unable to dispel the toxins or drain the pus. The abscesses and sores stay diffused and stagnant inside the tissues.

This formula contains Huang Qi (Radix Astragali) to tonify qi and drain toxins. Dang Gui (Radix Angelicae Sinensis) and Chuan Xiong (Rhizoma Chuanxiong) nourish the blood, activate blood circulation and relieve pain. Chuan Shan Jia (Squama Manis) and Zao Jiao Ci (Spina Gleditsiae) soften hardness and drain pus and abscesses. A small amount of grain-based liquor activates the blood and enhances the overall effect of the formula.

1362

Tòu Nóng Săn (Discharge Pus Powder)

Tou Nong San (Discharge Pus Powder)

Diagnosis	Signs and Symptoms	Treatment	Herbs
Abscesses and sores accompanied by swelling and pain	• Abscesses and sores with swelling, inflammation and pain: accumulation of toxins • Diffused abscesses and sores with pus that do not perforate: underlying qi deficiency	• Drains toxins • Breaks and dispels pus	• *Huang Qi* (Radix Astragali) tonifies qi and drains toxins. • *Dang Gui* (Radix Angelicae Sinensis) and *Chuan Xiong* (Rhizoma Chuanxiong) nourish the blood, activate blood circulation and relieve pain. • *Chuan Shan Jia* (Squama Manis) and *Zao Jiao Ci* (Spina Gleditsiae) soften hardness and drain pus and abscesses.

MODIFICATIONS

- With more qi deficiency, increase the dose of *Huang Qi* (Radix Astragali).
- For abscesses and sores with swelling and pain, add *Jin Yin Hua* (Flos Lonicerae Japonicae), *Lian Qiao* (Fructus Forsythiae), *Zi Hua Di Ding* (Herba Violae), and *Pu Gong Ying* (Herba Taraxaci).

RELATED FORMULA

Tuō Lĭ Tòu Nóng Tāng

(Drain the Interior and Discharge Pus Decoction)

托裏透膿湯
托里透脓汤

Pinyin Name: *Tuo Li Tou Nong Tang*
Literal Name: Drain the Interior and Discharge Pus Decoction
Original Source: *Yi Zong Jin Jian* (Golden Mirror of the Medical Tradition) by Wu Qian in 1742

Ren Shen (Radix et Rhizoma Ginseng)	3g
Bai Zhu (Rhizoma Atractylodis Macrocephalae), *chao* (dry-fried) with soil	3g
Chuan Shan Jia (Squama Manis), *chao* (dry-fried) and *yan* (ground) to small particles	3g
Bai Zhi (Radix Angelicae Dahuricae)	3g
Sheng Ma (Rhizoma Cimicifugae)	1.5g
Gan Cao (Radix et Rhizoma Glycyrrhizae)	1.5g
Dang Gui (Radix Angelicae Sinensis)	6g
Huang Qi (Radix Astragali)	9g
Zao Jiao Ci (Spina Gleditsiae)	4.5g
Qing Pi (Pericarpium Citri Reticulatae Viride), *chao* (dry-fried)	1.5g

The source text states to cook the ingredients with 3 large bowls of water until the liquid is reduced to 1 bowl. If the disease is in the upper part of the body, take 1 bowl of hot grain-based liquor before the decoction. If the disease is in the lower part of the body, take the decoction first, followed by 1 bowl of hot, grain-based liquor. If the disease is in the middle part of the body, take the decoction with half a bowl of hot, grain-based liquor.

Tuo Li Tou Nong Tang (Drain the Interior and Discharge Pus Decoction) supports the righteous qi, dispels pathogenic factors, drains the interior, and discharges pus. Clinically, it is used to treat all kinds of abscesses with qi and blood deficiencies, in which the lesions and ulcerations do not heal, and continue to expand in size and depth.

Tou Nong San and *Tuo Li Tou Nong Tang* (Drain the Interior and Discharge Pus Decoction) both treat abscesses and sores in individuals with underlying deficiency.

- *Tou Nong San* focuses primarily on draining toxins, dispelling pus, and eliminating abscesses, and secondarily on benefiting qi and nourishing the blood.
- *Tuo Li Tou Nong Tang* emphasizes tonifying and supporting righteous qi, with a secondary focus on draining the interior and discharging pus.

Chapter 22 – Formulas that Treat Abscesses and Sores　　　　　　　*Section 1 – External Abscesses and Sores*

Pái Nóng Săn (Drain the Pus Powder)

排膿散
排脓散

Pinyin Name: *Pai Nong San*
Literal Name: Drain the Pus Powder
Alternate Names: *Pai Nung San*, Pus-Expelling Powder, Platycodon and Chih-shih Formula
Original Source: *Jin Gui Yao Lue* (Essentials from the Golden Cabinet) by Zhang Zhong-Jing in the Eastern Han Dynasty

COMPOSITION

Zhi Shi (Fructus Aurantii Immaturus)	16 pieces
Jie Geng (Radix Platycodonis)	1.5g
Bai Shao (Radix Paeoniae Alba)	4.5g

DOSAGE / PREPARATION / ADMINISTRATION

The source text states to grind all of the ingredients into a fine powder. Mix one egg yolk with an equal portion of the herb powder, and take this mixture one time daily with warm water.

CHINESE THERAPEUTIC ACTIONS

1. Dispels pus and eliminates toxins
2. Reduces nodules and disperses stagnation

CLINICAL MANIFESTATIONS

Abscesses and sores: carbuncles, furuncles, cellulitis, boils, and other conditions characterized by formation of pus, abscess, and discharge.

CLINICAL APPLICATIONS

Carbuncles, furuncles, boils, sores, lymphadenitis, tonsillitis, otitis media, and mastitis.

EXPLANATION

Pai Nong San (Drain the Pus Powder) is designed to treat heat and toxins attacking various parts of the body. While the early stage of heat and toxins is in the form of nodules and hardness, the mid- to late-stages are often characterized by the formation of abscess and discharge of pus.

This formula contains herbs that dispel pus, eliminate toxins, reduce nodules, and disperse stagnation. *Zhi Shi* (Fructus Aurantii Immaturus), one of the strongest herbs for breaking up stagnant qi and activating qi circulation, reduces the size of the nodules. *Jie Geng* (Radix Platycodonis) is an excellent herb for draining and dispelling pus. Because heat and toxins may consume the blood, *Bai Shao* (Radix Paeoniae Alba) and egg yolk are added to nourish the body.

MODIFICATIONS

- For nodules without ulceration, add *Jin Yin Hua* (Flos Lonicerae Japonicae) and *Lian Qiao* (Fructus Forsythiae).
- For nodules with ulceration, add *Huang Qi* (Radix Astragali) and *Dang Gui* (Radix Angelicae Sinensis).
- With redness, warmth, swelling, and pain, add *Huang Lian* (Rhizoma Coptidis) and *Zhi Zi* (Fructus Gardeniae).
- For carbuncles and furuncles, add *Zhen Ren Huo Ming Yin* (True Man's Decoction to Revitalize Life).
- For sores and cellulitis, add *Tuo Li Xiao Du Yin* (Drain the Interior and Detoxify Decoction).

Pai Nong San (Drain the Pus Powder)

Diagnosis	Signs and Symptoms	Treatment	Herbs
Abscesses and sores	Nodules and hardness with formation of abscess and discharge of pus: heat and toxins attacking the body	• Dispels pus and eliminates toxins • Reduces nodules and disperses stagnation	• *Zhi Shi* (Fructus Aurantii Immaturus) activates qi circulation and breaks up stagnant qi. • *Jie Geng* (Radix Platycodonis) drains and dispels pus. • *Bai Shao* (Radix Paeoniae Alba) and egg yolk tonify the blood and nourish the body.

1364

Qiān Jīn Nèi Tuō Sǎn

(Drain the Interior Powder Worthy of a Thousand Gold)

千金內托散
千金內托散

Pinyin Name: *Qian Jin Nei Tuo San*
Literal Name: Drain the Interior Powder Worthy of a Thousand Gold
Alternate Name: Astragalus and Platycodon Formula
Original Source: *Wan Bing Hui Chun* (Restoration of Health from the Myriad Diseases) by Gong Ting-Xian in 1587

COMPOSITION

Ren Shen (Radix et Rhizoma Ginseng)	6g
Huang Qi (Radix Astragali), *mi zhi* (fried with honey)	6g
Dang Gui (Radix Angelicae Sinensis), *xi* (washed) with liquor	6g
Chuan Xiong (Rhizoma Chuanxiong)	3g
Bai Zhi (Radix Angelicae Dahuricae)	3g
Rou Gui (Cortex Cinnamomi)	3g
Fang Feng (Radix Saposhnikoviae)	3g
Jie Geng (Radix Platycodonis)	3g
Bo He (Herba Menthae)	3g
Hou Po (Cortex Magnoliae Officinalis), *chao* (dry-fried) with ginger juice	3g
Gan Cao (Radix et Rhizoma Glycyrrhizae)	3g

DOSAGE / PREPARATION / ADMINISTRATION

The source text states to grind all of the ingredients into powder, and take 6g of the powder with grain-based liquor or a decoction made from *Mu Xiang* (Radix Aucklandiae). This formula may also be prepared as a decoction by cooking the herbs with water or grain-based liquor.

CHINESE THERAPEUTIC ACTIONS

1. Activates qi and blood circulation
2. Harmonizes the Stomach and tonifies qi and blood
3. Clears heat and eliminates toxins

CLINICAL MANIFESTATIONS

Suppurative diseases with heat and toxins and underlying deficiencies: hardness and nodules with pus and discharge.

CLINICAL APPLICATIONS

Carbuncles, furuncles, sores, boils, hemorrhoids, suppurative mastitis, suppurative otitis media, and lymphadenitis.

EXPLANATION

Qian Jin Nei Tuo San (Drain the Interior Powder Worthy of a Thousand Gold) contains herbs that clear heat and eliminate toxins while tonifying the underlying qi and blood deficiencies. While early-stage heat-toxin accumulation is characterized by nodules and hardness, mid- to late-stage is characterized by the presence of pus and discharge. In the early stage, herbs that disperse the nodule and soften the hardness are used. In mid- to late-stage,

herbs that expedite the drainage of pus and facilitate the healing process are helpful.

Ren Shen (Radix et Rhizoma Ginseng) and *Huang Qi* (Radix Astragali) tonify qi and facilitate the generation of new tissues. *Dang Gui* (Radix Angelicae Sinensis) and *Chuan Xiong* (Rhizoma Chuanxiong) tonify and activate the blood. *Bai Zhi* (Radix Angelicae Dahuricae) and *Rou Gui* (Cortex Cinnamomi) have a dispersing property to promote pus drainage. *Fang Feng* (Radix Saposhnikoviae) disperses toxins, while *Jie Geng* (Radix Platycodonis) dispels phlegm. *Bo He* (Herba Menthae) clears heat and eliminates toxins. *Hou Po* (Cortex Magnoliae Officinalis) and *Gan Cao* (Radix et Rhizoma Glycyrrhizae) harmonize the middle *jiao* and minimize injury to the Stomach.

MODIFICATIONS

- With inability to eat due to swelling and pain, add *Sha Ren* (Fructus Amomi) and *Xiang Fu* (Rhizoma Cyperi).
- With severe pain, add *Ru Xiang* (Gummi Olibanum) and *Mo Yao* (Myrrha).
- With constipation, add *Da Huang* (Radix et Rhizoma Rhei) and *Zhi Qiao* (Fructus Aurantii).
- With dysuria, add *Mai Dong* (Radix Ophiopogonis), *Che Qian Zi* (Semen Plantaginis), *Mu Tong* (Caulis Akebiae), and *Deng Xin Cao* (Medulla Junci).
- With cough, add *Ban Xia* (Rhizoma Pinelliae), *Chen Pi* (Pericarpium Citri Reticulatae), and *Ku Xing Ren* (Semen Armeniacae Amarum).

Chapter 22 – Formulas that Treat Abscesses and Sores

Section 1 – External Abscesses and Sores

Qiān Jīn Nèi Tuō Săn

(Drain the Interior Powder Worthy of a Thousand Gold)

Qian Jin Nei Tuo San (Drain the Interior Powder Worthy of a Thousand Gold)

Diagnosis	Signs and Symptoms	Treatment	Herbs
Suppurative disorders	• Hardness and nodules: heat and toxins attacking the body • Pus and discharge: deficiency condition	• Activates qi and blood circulation • Harmonizes the Stomach and tonifies qi and blood • Reduces inflammation and eliminates heat and toxins	• *Ren Shen* (Radix et Rhizoma Ginseng) and *Huang Qi* (Radix Astragali) tonify qi and generate new tissues. • *Dang Gui* (Radix Angelicae Sinensis) and *Chuan Xiong* (Rhizoma Chuanxiong) tonify blood and activate blood circulation. • *Bai Zhi* (Radix Angelicae Dahuricae) and *Rou Gui* (Cortex Cinnamomi) have dispersing property to promote pus drainage. • *Fang Feng* (Radix Saposhnikoviae) disperses toxins. • *Jie Geng* (Radix Platycodonis) dispels phlegm. • *Bo He* (Herba Menthae) clears heat and eliminates toxins. • *Hou Po* (Cortex Magnoliae Officinalis) and *Gan Cao* (Radix et Rhizoma Glycyrrhizae) harmonize the middle *jiao* and minimize harm to the Stomach.

CAUTIONS / CONTRAINDICATIONS

• Avoid the consumption of alcohol while taking this formula.

AUTHORS' COMMENTS

According to the source text, this formula is "worthy of a thousand gold." It reduces abscesses and sores in their early stage, drains pus in their middle stage, and helps to resolve the necrosed tissues in their late stage.

1366

Tuō Lǐ Xiāo Dú Yǐn (Drain the Interior and Detoxify Decoction)

托裏消毒飲
托里消毒饮

Pinyin Name: *Tuo Li Xiao Du Yin*
Literal Name: Drain the Interior and Detoxify Decoction
Alternate Names: *Tuo Li Hsiao Tu Yin*, Interior-Drawing and Detoxifying Drink, Drain the Interior and Eliminate Pathogenic Influences Decoction, Gleditsia Combination
Original Source: *Yi Fang Ji Jie* (Analytical Collection of Medical Formulas) by Wang Ang in 1682

COMPOSITION

Ren Shen (Radix et Rhizoma Ginseng)	3g
Bai Zhu (Rhizoma Atractylodis Macrocephalae)	3g
Fu Ling (Poria)	3g
Gan Cao (Radix et Rhizoma Glycyrrhizae)	1.5g
Dang Gui (Radix Angelicae Sinensis)	3g
Bai Shao (Radix Paeoniae Alba)	3g
Chuan Xiong (Rhizoma Chuanxiong)	3g
Huang Qi (Radix Astragali)	3g
Jin Yin Hua (Flos Lonicerae Japonicae)	3g
Jie Geng (Radix Platycodonis)	1.5g
Bai Zhi (Radix Angelicae Dahuricae)	1.5g
Zao Jiao Ci (Spina Gleditsiae)	1.5g

DOSAGE / PREPARATION / ADMINISTRATION

The source text states to cook the ingredients in 2 cups of water until the liquid is reduced to 80%. Take the warm, strained decoction after meals.

CHINESE THERAPEUTIC ACTIONS

1. Tonifies qi and blood
2. Reduces swelling, drains pus, and promotes generation of new tissues

CLINICAL MANIFESTATIONS

Suppurative disorders in individuals with qi and blood deficiencies: nodules and hardness with or without discharge of pus and abscess, generalized deficiency, and weakness.

CLINICAL APPLICATIONS

Carbuncles, bed sores, pus, abscesses, lymphadenitis, otitis media, chronic osteomyelitis, and conjunctivitis.

EXPLANATION

Tuo Li Xiao Du Yin (Drain the Interior and Detoxify Decoction) treats various types of suppurative disorders with underlying qi and blood deficiencies. It contains herbs to reduce swelling and drain pus to treat abscesses and sores. It also contains herbs to tonify qi, nourish blood and promote generation of new tissues.

Ren Shen (Radix et Rhizoma Ginseng), *Bai Zhu* (Rhizoma Atractylodis Macrocephalae), *Fu Ling* (Poria), and *Gan Cao* (Radix et Rhizoma Glycyrrhizae) tonify qi, following the concept of *Si Jun Zi Tang* (Four-Gentlemen Decoction). *Dang Gui* (Radix Angelicae Sinensis), *Bai Shao* (Radix Paeoniae Alba), and *Chuan Xiong* (Rhizoma Chuanxiong) tonify the blood, following the original concept of *Si Wu Tang* (Four-Substance Decoction). *Huang Qi* (Radix Astragali), in addition to tonifying qi, can promote generation of new tissues, thereby facilitating recovery. *Jin Yin Hua* (Flos Lonicerae Japonicae) clears heat, eliminates toxins, and treats all types of suppurative disorders. *Jie Geng* (Radix Platycodonis), *Bai Zhi* (Radix Angelicae Dahuricae), and *Zao Jiao Ci* (Spina Gleditsiae) drain pus and eliminate toxins.

MODIFICATIONS

• For ulcerations with constant discharge of pus, add *Ge Gen* (Radix Puerariae Lobatae) and *Huang Lian* (Rhizoma Coptidis).
• With swelling and pain accompanied by fever, add *Huang Lian Jie Du Tang* (Coptis Decoction to Relieve Toxicity).
• With severe pain, add *Ru Xiang* (Gummi Olibanum) and *Mo Yao* (Myrrha).
• For cellulitis with swelling and pain, add *Pai Nong San* (Drain the Pus Powder).
• For itching, add *Chan Tui* (Periostracum Cicadae) and *Wu Shao She* (Zaocys).

FORMULAS THAT TREAT ABSCESSES AND SORES

22

Chapter 22 – Formulas that Treat Abscesses and Sores　　　　　　　*Section 1 – External Abscesses and Sores*

Tuō Lǐ Xiāo Dú Yǐn (Drain the Interior and Detoxify Decoction)

Tuo Li Xiao Du Yin (Drain the Interior and Detoxify Decoction)

Diagnosis	Signs and Symptoms	Treatment	Herbs
Suppurative disorders in individuals with qi and blood deficiencies	• Nodules and hardness: heat and toxins attacking the body • Discharge of pus and abscess, and generalized deficiency and weakness: qi and blood deficiencies	• Strengthens the qi and blood • Reduces swelling, drains pus, and promotes generation of new tissues	• *Ren Shen* (Radix et Rhizoma Ginseng), *Bai Zhu* (Rhizoma Atractylodis Macrocephalae), *Fu Ling* (Poria) and *Gan Cao* (Radix et Rhizoma Glycyrrhizae) tonify qi. • *Dang Gui* (Radix Angelicae Sinensis), *Bai Shao* (Radix Paeoniae Alba) and *Chuan Xiong* (Rhizoma Chuanxiong) tonify the blood. • *Huang Qi* (Radix Astragali) tonifies qi and promotes generation of new tissues. • *Jin Yin Hua* (Flos Lonicerae Japonicae) clears heat and eliminates toxins. • *Jie Geng* (Radix Platycodonis), *Bai Zhi* (Radix Angelicae Dahuricae) and *Zao Jiao Ci* (Spina Gleditsiae) drain pus and eliminate toxins.

RELATED FORMULA

Tuō Lǐ Xiāo Dú Yǐn

(Drain the Interior and Detoxify Decoction)

托裏消毒飲
托里消毒饮

Pinyin Name: Tuo Li Xiao Du Yin

Literal Name: Drain the Interior and Detoxify Decoction

Alternate Names: *Tuo Li Hsiao Tu Yin*, Interior-Drawing and Detoxifying Drink

Original Source: *Wan Bing Hui Chun* (Restoration of Health from the Myriad Diseases) by Gong Ting-Xian in 1587

Huang Qi (Radix Astragali)	6g
Tian Hua Fen (Radix Trichosanthis)	6g
Fang Feng (Radix Saposhnikoviae)	3g
Dang Gui (Radix Angelicae Sinensis)	3g
Chuan Xiong (Rhizoma Chuanxiong)	3g
Bai Zhi (Radix Angelicae Dahuricae)	3g
Jie Geng (Radix Platycodonis)	3g
Hou Po (Cortex Magnoliae Officinalis)	3g
Chuan Shan Jia (Squama Manis)	3g
Zao Jiao (Fructus Gleditsiae)	3g
Jin Yin Hua (Flos Lonicerae Japonicae)	9g
Chen Pi (Pericarpium Citri Reticulatae)	9g

The source text states to cook the ingredients with equal portions of water and grain-based liquor until the liquid is reduced to 70%. Take the warm, strained decoction after meals if the affected area is located on the upper parts of the body, and on an empty stomach before meals if the affected area is located on the lower parts of the body. After the first two decoctions, the remaining decoctions utilize water only to cook the herbs.

This formula tonifies qi and blood, reduces swelling and pus, and promotes generation of new tissues. Clinically, it treats various abscesses and sores that do not heal after 6-7 days.

The principal and related formulas have the same names but are derived from different sources. They have similar functions to treat suppurative disorders in individuals with qi and blood deficiencies.

• *Tuo Li Xiao Du Yin* from *Yi Fang Ji Jie* (Analytical Collection of Medical Formulas) by Wang Ang in 1682 has a stronger effect to tonify qi and blood, and thus can better address the underlying deficiencies.

• *Tuo Li Xiao Du Yin* from *Wan Bing Hui Chun* (Restoration of Health from the Myriad Diseases) by Gong Ting-Xian in 1587 has a better function to regulate qi circulation and resolve nodules and hardness.

1368

Nèi Bǔ Huáng Qí Tāng

(Tonify the Interior Decoction with Astragalus)

內補黃耆湯
内补黄芪汤

Pinyin Name: Nei Bu Huang Qi Tang
Literal Name: Tonify the Interior Decoction with Astragalus
Original Source: Wai Ke Fa Hui (External Medicine Elaboration) by Xue Yi in 1528

COMPOSITION

Ren Shen (Radix et Rhizoma Ginseng)	3g [10g]
Fu Ling (Poria)	3g [10g]
Zhi Gan Cao (Radix et Rhizoma Glycyrrhizae Praeparata cum Melle)	0.9g [3g]
Dang Gui (Radix Angelicae Sinensis), ban (blended) with liquor	1.5g [5g]
Bai Shao (Radix Paeoniae Alba), chao (dry-fried)	1.5g [5g]
Shu Di Huang (Radix Rehmanniae Praeparata), ban (blended) with liquor	3g [10g]
Chuan Xiong (Rhizoma Chuanxiong)	1.5g [5g]
Huang Qi (Radix Astragali), chao (dry-fried) with salted water	3g [10g]
Rou Gui (Cortex Cinnamomi)	1.5g [5g]
Mai Dong (Radix Ophiopogonis)	3g [10g]
Yuan Zhi (Radix Polygalae), chao (dry-fried)	1.5g [5g]

DOSAGE / PREPARATION / ADMINISTRATION

The source text states to cook the ingredients with 3 slices of Sheng Jiang (Rhizoma Zingiberis Recens) and 1 piece of Da Zao (Fructus Jujubae) in 2 large bowls of water until the liquid is reduced to 80%. Take the decoction between meals. Today, the decoction may be prepared using the doses suggested in brackets.

CHINESE THERAPEUTIC ACTIONS

1. Tonifies qi and blood
2. Nourishes yin
3. Promotes generation of flesh

CLINICAL MANIFESTATIONS

Late-stage abscesses and sores with qi and blood deficiencies: localized pain at the affected area, lethargy, lack of desire to speak, disturbed sleep, spontaneous perspiration, intermittent or persistent fever, dry mouth, pale tongue with a thin coating, and a fine, weak pulse.

CLINICAL APPLICATIONS

Chronic abscesses and sores.

EXPLANATION

Nei Bu Huang Qi Tang (Tonify the Interior Decoction with Astragalus) is designed to treat late-stage abscesses and sores that have perforated and ulcerated, but do not heal because of underlying qi and blood deficiencies. Abscesses and sores are accompanied by localized pain.

Spontaneous perspiration indicates qi deficiency, disturbed sleep suggests blood deficiency, and lethargy and lack of desire to speak reflect Spleen and Stomach deficiencies. Furthermore, intermittent or persistent fever and dry mouth indicate deficiency-heat rising with yin damage.

Ren Shen (Radix et Rhizoma Ginseng), Fu Ling (Poria), and Zhi Gan Cao (Radix et Rhizoma Glycyrrhizae Praeparata cum Melle) tonify qi. Dang Gui (Radix Angelicae Sinensis), Bai Shao (Radix Paeoniae Alba), Shu Di Huang (Radix Rehmanniae Praeparata), and Chuan Xiong (Rhizoma Chuanxiong) tonify the blood. Huang Qi (Radix Astragali) and Rou Gui (Cortex Cinnamomi) tonify qi, warm yang, and promote regeneration of flesh. Mai Dong (Radix Ophiopogonis) nourishes yin and body fluids. Yuan Zhi (Radix Polygalae) stabilizes the shen (spirit).

MODIFICATIONS

- For abscesses and sores with severe pain, add Yan Hu Suo (Rhizoma Corydalis), Ru Xiang (Gummi Olibanum), and Mo Yao (Myrrha).
- For hardened abscesses and sores, add Chuan Shan Jia (Squama Manis) and Zao Jiao Ci (Spina Gleditsiae).

CAUTIONS / CONTRAINDICATIONS

Nei Bu Huang Qi Tang treats late-stage abscesses and sores with qi and blood deficiencies. It is contraindicated for early-stage abscesses and sores characterized by heat toxins.

Chapter 22 – Formulas that Treat Abscesses and Sores   *Section 1 – External Abscesses and Sores*

Nèi Bǔ Huáng Qí Tāng
(Tonify the Interior Decoction with Astragalus)

Nei Bu Huang Qi Tang (Tonify the Interior Decoction with Astragalus)

Diagnosis	Signs and Symptoms	Treatment	Herbs
Late-stage abscesses and sores with qi and blood deficiencies	• Abscesses and sores that do not heal: presence of heat and toxins with underlying deficiencies • Lethargy, lack of desire to speak, disturbed sleep, spontaneous perspiration: qi and blood deficiencies • Intermittent or persistent fever and dry mouth: deficiency-heat rising with yin damage	• Tonifies qi and blood • Nourishes yin • Promotes generation of flesh	• *Ren Shen* (Radix et Rhizoma Ginseng), *Fu Ling* (Poria) and *Zhi Gan Cao* (Radix et Rhizoma Glycyrrhizae Praeparata cum Melle) tonify qi. • *Dang Gui* (Radix Angelicae Sinensis), *Bai Shao* (Radix Paeoniae Alba), *Shu Di Huang* (Radix Rehmanniae Praeparata), and *Chuan Xiong* (Rhizoma Chuanxiong) tonify the blood. • *Huang Qi* (Radix Astragali) and *Rou Gui* (Cortex Cinnamomi) tonify qi, warm yang, and promote regeneration of flesh. • *Mai Dong* (Radix Ophiopogonis) nourishes yin and body fluids. • *Yuan Zhi* (Radix Polygalae) stabilizes the *shen* (spirit).

Yáng Hé Tāng (Yang-Heartening Decoction)
陽和湯
阳和汤

Pinyin Name: *Yang He Tang*
Literal Name: Yang-Heartening Decoction
Original Source: *Wai Ke Zheng Zhi Quan Sheng Ji* (Complete Collection of Patterns and Treatments in External Medicine) by Wang Wei-De in 1740

COMPOSITION

Shu Di Huang (Radix Rehmanniae Praeparata)	30g
Lu Jiao Jiao (Colla Cornus Cervi)	9g
Pao Jiang (Rhizoma Zingiberis Praeparatum), *tan* (charred to ash)	1.5g
Rou Gui (Cortex Cinnamomi), *yan* (ground) into powder	3g
Ma Huang (Herba Ephedrae)	1.5g
Bai Jie Zi (Semen Sinapis)	6g
Gan Cao (Radix et Rhizoma Glycyrrhizae)	3g

DOSAGE / PREPARATION / ADMINISTRATION
The source text states to prepare the ingredients as a decoction.

CHINESE THERAPEUTIC ACTIONS
1. Warms yang and tonifies the blood
2. Disperses cold and eliminates stagnation

CLINICAL MANIFESTATIONS
Yin-type (deep-rooted) sores due to yang deficiency and interior cold stagnation: general swelling, soreness, and pain without local heat sensation on the body and extremities, no change of skin color, no thirst, pale white tongue coating, and a deep, fine pulse. This formula may be applied for cellulitis, gangrene of the fingers and toes, multiple abscesses, subcutaneous nodules, and arthroncus of the knee.

1370

Yáng Hé Tāng (Yang-Heartening Decoction)

CLINICAL APPLICATIONS

Cellulitis, gangrene, frostbite, multiple abscesses, mastitis, cystic hyperplasia of the breast, endometriosis, oophoritic cyst, Raynaud's disease, peripheral neuritis, thromboangiitis obliterans, tuberculosis of the lung and bone, chronic bronchitis, osteomyelitis, inflammation and pain, prolapse of lumbar intervertebral disk, sciatica, and rheumatoid arthritis.

EXPLANATION

Yang He Tang (Yang-Heartening Decoction) treats *yin*-type (deep-rooted) sores due to yang deficiency and interior cold stagnation. Deficiency of yang may lead to formation of interior cold, which binds to the bones, muscles, tendons, vessels, or joints. Because of yang deficiency and cold excess, there is an absence of warm or heat sensations. Since the abscesses and sores are deeper in the tissues, there is no change of skin color. Lastly, *yin*-type (deep-rooted) sores are usually harder to treat since they are anchored deep into the tissues.

This formula contains *Shu Di Huang* (Radix Rehmanniae Praeparata) to warm and nourish the blood. *Lu Jiao Jiao* (Colla Cornus Cervi) tonifies *jing* (essence) and strengthens bones and tendons. *Pao Jiang* (Rhizoma Zingiberis Praeparatum) and *Rou Gui* (Cortex Cinnamomi) warm the body, tonify the yang, and disperse cold accumulation. A small amount of *Ma Huang* (Herba Ephedrae) opens skin pores to help disperse the interior cold through the superficial level. *Bai Jie Zi* (Semen Sinapis) warms the interior and disperses phlegm and cold. It also prevents the warm tonic herbs from creating stagnation in the body. *Gan Cao* (Radix et Rhizoma Glycyrrhizae) eliminates toxins and harmonizes all of the herbs in the formula.

Indeed, this formula both tonifies the body and disperses the cold stagnation.

MODIFICATIONS

- With more cold, add *Fu Zi* (Radix Aconiti Lateralis Praeparata).
- With more qi deficiency, add *Dang Shen* (Radix Codonopsis) and *Huang Qi* (Radix Astragali).
- With damp and cold accumulation, add *Xi Xin* (Radix et Rhizoma Asari).

CAUTIONS / CONTRAINDICATIONS

- *Yang He Tang* is contraindicated in the following cases: *yang*-type sores that affect only the superficial parts of the body, and are characterized by redness, swelling, burning sensations, and pain; *yin*-type (deep-rooted) sores that have already perforated and ulcerated; and chronic ulceration with heat.
- Once the sores are perforated and ulcerated, *Ma Huang* (Herba Ephedrae) should be removed from this formula to prevent damage to qi and blood.

CLINICAL STUDIES AND RESEARCH

1. **Frostbite**: One study reported good results using modified *Yang He Tang* to treat 30 patients with frostbite. In addition to the base formula, modifications were made by adding *Ban Zhi Lian* (Herba Scutellariae Barbatae) for open wounds with discharge, and *Huang Qi* (Radix Astragali) for chronic illness. Most patients recovered within 3-6 packs of herbs, with some needing up to 15 packs.[1]

2. **Thromboangiitis obliterans**: Use of modified *Yang He Tang* in decoction daily was associated with complete

Yang He Tang (Yang-Heartening Decoction)

Diagnosis	Signs and Symptoms	Treatment	Herbs
Yin-type (deep-rooted) sores	• Sores with swelling, soreness, and pain without local heat sensation on the body and extremities, and no change in skin color: stagnation of cold and phlegm with underlying yang and blood deficiencies • Pale, white tongue coating and a deep, fine pulse: presence of deficiency and excess conditions	• Warms the yang and tonifies blood • Disperses cold and eliminates stagnation	• *Shu Di Huang* (Radix Rehmanniae Praeparata) warms and nourishes the blood. • *Lu Jiao Jiao* (Colla Cornus Cervi) tonifies *jing* (essence) and strengthens bones and tendons. • *Pao Jiang* (Rhizoma Zingiberis Praeparatum) and *Rou Gui* (Cortex Cinnamomi) warm the body, tonify yang, and disperse cold accumulation. • *Ma Huang* (Herba Ephedrae) opens the skin pores to help disperse the interior cold. • *Bai Jie Zi* (Semen Sinapis) warms the interior and disperses phlegm and cold. • *Gan Cao* (Radix et Rhizoma Glycyrrhizae) eliminates toxins and harmonizes all of the herbs in the formula.

Yáng Hé Tāng (Yang-Heartening Decoction)

Chapter 22 – Formulas that Treat Abscesses and Sores

Section 1 – External Abscesses and Sores

recovery in 12 cases and improvement in 8 cases of thromboangiitis obliterans. The herbal treatment contained *Yang He Tang* plus *Dang Gui* (Radix Angelicae Sinensis) and *Dan Shen* (Radix et Rhizoma Salviae Miltiorrhizae). *Jin Yin Hua* (Flos Lonicerae Japonicae) and *Xuan Shen* (Radix Scrophulariae) were added for heat; *Dang Shen* (Radix Codonopsis), *Huang Qi* (Radix Astragali), *Ba Ji Tian* (Radix Morindae Officinalis), and *Yin Yang Huo* (Herba Epimedii) were added for chronic cases.[2]

3. **Raynaud's disease**: One study reported good results for treating Raynaud's disease using *Yang He Tang* and *Si Ni San* (Frigid Extremities Powder). Additional modifications were made as necessary. Of 30 patients (28 female and 2 male), the study reported complete recovery in 21 cases, significant improvement in 8 cases, and no effect in 1 case.[3]

4. **Peripheral neuritis**: One study reported 90.4% effectiveness using modified *Yang He Tang* to treat 63 patients with peripheral neuritis. The herbal treatment contained *Yang He Tang* plus *Dang Gui* (Radix Angelicae Sinensis) and *Huang Qi* (Radix Astragali) as the base formula. Additional modifications included *Cang Zhu* (Rhizoma Atractylodis) for damp; *Ji Xue Teng* (Caulis Spatholobi) for blood stagnation; *Quan Xie* (Scorpio) and *Wu Gong* (Scolopendra) for wind and phlegm obstructing the channels and collaterals. Of 63 patients, the study reported complete recovery in 43 cases, improvement in 14 cases, and no effect in 6 cases.[4]

5. **Sciatica**: One hundred and sixty-eight patients with sciatica were treated with complete recovery in 130 cases, improvement in 28 cases, and no effect in 10 cases. The herbal treatment contained *Fu Zi* (Radix Aconiti Lateralis Praeparata), *Shu Di Huang* (Radix Rehmanniae Praeparata), *Lu Jiao Jiao* (Colla Cornus Cervi), *Fang Ji* (Radix Stephaniae Tetrandrae), *Xi Xin* (Radix et Rhizoma Asari), *Hong Hua* (Flos Carthami), *Wu Shao She* (Zaocys), and others. The treatment protocol was to cook the herbs in water, and drink the decoction in two equally-divided doses. In addition, the herb residue was placed inside a cloth bag and applied topically to the affected area at bedtime. The duration was 10 days per course of treatment.[5]

6. **Mastitis**: One study reported effective treatment for all 21 patients with yin-type mastitis using modified *Yang He Tang*. The base herbal formula contained *Yang He Tang* plus *Zao Jiao Ci* (Spina Gleditsiae), *Huang Qi* (Radix Astragali) and processed *Chuan Shan Jia* (Squama Manis). Modifications included the addition of *Fu Zi* (Radix Aconiti Lateralis Praeparata) for yang qi deficiency; *Gou Qi Zi* (Fructus Lycii) and *Dang Gui* (Radix Angelicae Sinensis) for Liver and Kidney deficiencies; and *Quan Xie* (Scorpio) and *Wu Gong* (Scolopendra)

for prolonged swelling and hardness without resolution. Of 21 patients, the study reported complete recovery in 15 cases and improvement in 6 cases. The duration of treatment ranged from 12-60 days, with an average of 32 days.[6]

7. **Cystic hyperplasia of the breast**: One study reported 88.7% effectiveness using modified *Yang He Tang* to treat cystic hyperplasia of the breast. Of 62 cases, 38 had complete recovery, 17 had significant improvement, and 7 had no effect. The herbal treatment contained *Yang He Tang* as the base formula, with the addition of *Chai Hu* (Radix Bupleuri) and *Qing Pi* (Pericarpium Citri Reticulatae Viride) for qi stagnation; *Mu Li* (Concha Ostreae) and *Zhe Bei Mu* (Bulbus Fritillariae Thunbergii) for phlegm stagnation; *San Leng* (Rhizoma Sparganii) and *E Zhu* (Rhizoma Curcumae) for blood stagnation; *Wang Bu Liu Xing* (Semen Vaccariae) and *Chuan Shan Jia* (Squama Manis) for obstructed flow of breast milk; *Dang Gui* (Radix Angelicae Sinensis) and *Tao Ren* (Semen Persicae) for infertility; and other herbs as necessary. For women who have cystic hyperplasia of the breast within one month after labor, *Yang He Tang* was modified by removing *Shu Di Huang* (Radix Rehmanniae Praeparata) and *Ma Huang* (Herba Ephedrae), doubling the dose of *Rou Gui* (Cortex Cinnamomi), and adding *Chuan Xiong* (Rhizoma Chuanxiong), *Xiang Fu* (Rhizoma Cyperi) and *Ze Lan* (Herba Lycopi).[7]

8. **Endometriosis**: Modified *Yang He Tang* was used to treat 27 patients with endometriosis characterized by blood stagnation, cold obstruction in the Liver channel, and deficiencies of Kidney yang, *jing* (essence), and blood. The herbal treatment contained *Yang He Tang* plus *Fu Zi* (Radix Aconiti Lateralis Praeparata), *Chuan Shan Jia* (Squama Manis), *Bai Zhu* (Rhizoma Atractylodis Macrocephalae), *Dang Gui* (Radix Angelicae Sinensis), *Wu Ling Zhi* (Faeces Trogopteri), *Xi Xin* (Radix et Rhizoma Asari), and *Wu Zhu Yu* (Fructus Evodiae). Of 27 patients, the study reported complete recovery in 19 cases, significant improvement in 4 cases, moderate improvement in 3 cases, and no response in 1 case.[8]

9. **Oophoritic cyst**: One study reported good results using modified *Yang He Tang* to treat 26 patients with unilateral oophoritic cyst up to 10 cm in diameter in size. The herbal formula used *Yang He Tang* as the base formula, with the elimination of *Gan Jiang* (Rhizoma Zingiberis) and *Gan Cao* (Radix et Rhizoma Glycyrrhizae), and the addition of *Tao Ren* (Semen Persicae), *Hai Zao* (Sargassum), and *E Zhu* (Rhizoma Curcumae). Other herbs were added as necessary. Of 26 patients, the study reported complete recovery in 23 cases, improvement in 2 cases, and no effect in 1 case. The duration of treatment ranged from 5-36 packs of herbs.[9]

Yáng Hé Tāng (Yang-Heartening Decoction)

10. **Inflammation and pain**: *Yang He Tang* has been shown in many studies to effectively treat inflammation and pain affecting many parts of the body. According to one study, neck pain in 64 patients was treated with 92.2% effectiveness using *Yang He Tang* plus *Gui Zhi* (Ramulus Cinnamomi), *Ge Gen* (Radix Puerariae Lobatae), *Sang Zhi* (Ramulus Mori) and others as needed.[10] According to another study, shoulder pain in 220 patients was treated at 95% effectiveness using *Yang He Tang* plus *Ru Xiang* (Gummi Olibanum), *Mo Yao* (Myrrha), *Bai Shao* (Radix Paeoniae Alba), *Jin Qian Bai Hua She* (Bungarus Parvus), and others.[11] Lastly, 60 patients with chronic lower back pain were treated with good results using modified *Yang He Tang*.[12]

11. **Prolapse of lumbar intervertebral disk**: Use of modified *Yang He Tang* was associated with marked success in treating prolapse of a lumbar intervertebral disk. Of 210 patients, the study reported complete recovery in 148 cases, significant improvement in 28 cases, moderate improvement in 16 cases, and no effect in 18 cases. The overall effectiveness was 91.4%. Most patients responded within 1 month. The herbal formula contained *Yang He Tang* plus *Tu Bie Chong* (Eupolyphaga seu Steleophaga), *Huang Lian* (Rhizoma Coptidis) and *Wu Gong* (Scolopendra) as the base formula. Furthermore, modifications were made by adding processed *Ru Xiang* (Gummi Olibanum), processed *Mo Yao* (Myrrha) and *Di Long* (Pheretima) for severe pain; *Wei Ling Xian* (Radix et Rhizoma Clematidis), *Niu Xi* (Radix Achyranthis Bidentatae), and *Xu Duan* (Radix Dipsaci) for severe lower back pain; *Mu Gua* (Fructus Chaenomelis) and *Du Huo* (Radix Angelicae Pubescentis) for severe leg pain; *Fu Zi* (Radix Aconiti Lateralis Praeparata) for cold; *Cang Zhu* (Rhizoma Atractylodis) and *Fu Ling* (Poria) for dampness; and *Du Zhong* (Cortex Eucommiae) and *Sang Ji Sheng* (Herba Taxilli) for Kidney deficiency.[13]

12. **Osteomyelitis**: Use of *Yang He Tang* has been shown in several studies to effectively treat osteomyelitis. According to one study, use of modified *Yang He Tang* was associated with 95% effectiveness in treating 560 patients with osteomyelitis characterized by yin deficiency and blood stagnation.[14] Another study reported 100% effectiveness using modified *Yang He Tang* to treat osteomyelitis characterized by yang deficiency with cold accumulation.[15] Lastly, suppurative and chronic osteomyelitis have also been treated with good results using this formula.[16,17]

13. **Pain from metastatic carcinoma of bone**: Use of modified *Yang He Tang* was effective in relieving pain associated with metastatic carcinoma of bone. The herbal formula contained *Shu Di Huang* (Radix Rehmanniae Praeparata) 30g, *Rou Gui* (Cortex Cinnamomi) 3g, *Pao Jiang* (Rhizoma Zingiberis Praeparatum) 3g, *Ma Huang* (Herba Ephedrae) 3g, *Lu Jiao Shuang* (Cornu Cervi Degelatinatum) 10g, *Bai Jie Zi* (Semen Sinapis) 6g, *Fu Zi* (Radix Aconiti Lateralis Praeparata) 6g, and *Gan Cao* (Radix et Rhizoma Glycyrrhizae) 5g. The herbs were given in decoction daily, for 1 week per course of treatment.[18]

RELATED FORMULA

Zhōng Hé Tāng (Middle-Heartening Decoction)

中和湯
中和汤

Pinyin Name: *Zhong He Tang*
Literal Name: Middle-Heartening Decoction
Original Source: *Zheng Zhi Zhun Sheng* (Standards of Patterns and Treatments) by Wang Ken-Tang in 1602

Ren Shen (Radix et Rhizoma Ginseng)	6g
Chen Pi (Pericarpium Citri Reticulatae)	6g
Huang Qi (Radix Astragali)	4.5g
Bai Zhu (Rhizoma Atractylodis Macrocephalae)	4.5g
Dang Gui (Radix Angelicae Sinensis)	4.5g
Bai Zhi (Radix Angelicae Dahuricae)	4.5g
Fu Ling (Poria)	3g
Chuan Xiong (Rhizoma Chuanxiong)	3g
Zao Jiao Ci (Spina Gleditsiae), *chao* (dry-fried)	3g
Ru Xiang (Gummi Olibanum)	3g
Mo Yao (Myrrha)	3g
Jin Yin Hua (Flos Lonicerae Japonicae)	3g
Gan Cao (Radix et Rhizoma Glycyrrhizae)	3g

The source text states to cook the herbs in a solution comprised of equal portions of water and grain-based liquor.

This formula tonifies qi, drains the interior, harmonizes the blood, and reduces abscesses and sores. It treats half-yin and half-yang type of abscesses and sores, that seem to perforate but actually do not. The affected area has diffused swelling with a pale red color, mild pain, absence of warmth at the affected area, and qi deficiency signs.

Yang He Tang and *Zhong He Tang* (Middle-Heartening Decoction) both tonify qi and blood to treat abscesses and sores.

• *Yang He Tang* warms yang, tonifies the blood, dissolves phlegm, and dispels cold. It is used to treat *yin*-type (deep-rooted) sores caused by yang deficiency and interior cold stagnation.

• *Zhong He Tang* tonifies qi, drains the interior, and reduces abscesses and sores. It is used to treat half-yin and half-yang abscesses and sores with underlying qi deficiency.

Chapter 22 – Formulas that Treat Abscesses and Sores

Section 1 – External Abscesses and Sores

Yáng Hé Tāng (Yang-Heartening Decoction)

AUTHORS' COMMENTS

Yang He Tang treats *yin*-type (deep-rooted) sores due to yang deficiency and interior cold stagnation. This formula has a large dose of *Shu Di Huang* (Radix Rehmanniae Praeparata) to tonify yin and nourish the blood. *Ma Huang* (Herba Ephedrae), however, must be used in a small dose (as specified in this formula) to facilitate the ulceration of *yin*-type (deep-rooted) sores. The combination of these two herbs also provides mutual checks and balances. The dispersing nature of *Ma Huang* (Herba Ephedrae) prevents the heavy nature of *Shu Di Huang* (Radix Rehmanniae Praeparata) from creating stagnation; and the heavy nature of *Shu Di Huang* (Radix Rehmanniae Praeparata) prevents the dispersing nature of *Ma Huang* (Herba Ephedrae) from damaging yin and body fluids.

References

1. *Xin Zhong Yi* (New Chinese Medicine) 1989;3:42.
2. *Zhe Jiang Zhong Yi Za Zhi* (Zhejiang Journal of Chinese Medicine) 1982;2:82.

3. *Si Chuan Zhong Yi* (Sichuan Chinese Medicine) 1997;8:31.
4. *Shan Xi Zhong Yi* (Shanxi Chinese Medicine) 1991;4:160.
5. *Liao Ning Zhong Yi Za Zhi* (Liaoning Journal of Chinese Medicine) 1982;11:36.
6. *Shi Yong Zhong Yi Yao Za Zhi* (Journal of Practical Chinese Medicine and Medicinals) 1997;6:13.
7. *Xin Zhong Yi* (New Chinese Medicine) 1997;2:18.
8. *Zhe Jiang Zhong Yi Za Zhi* (Zhejiang Journal of Chinese Medicine) 1997;5:208.
9. *Zhong Yi Za Zhi* (Journal of Chinese Medicine) 1989;11:40.
10. *Shan Xi Zhong Yi* (Shanxi Chinese Medicine) 1996;4:162.
11. *Shan Xi Zhong Yi* (Shanxi Chinese Medicine) 1997;10:444.
12. *Zhe Jiang Zhong Yi Za Zhi* (Zhejiang Journal of Chinese Medicine) 1998;4:164.
13. *An Hui Zhong Yi Xue Yuan Xue Bao* (Journal of Anhui University School of Medicine) 1994;13(1):31.
14. *Bei Jing Zhong Yi Xue Yuan Xue Bao* (Journal of Beijing University School of Medicine) 1991;14(2):25.
15. *Shan Xi Zhong Yi* (Shanxi Chinese Medicine) 1989;3:108.
16. *He Bei Zhong Yi* (Hebei Chinese Medicine) 1989;3:108.
17. *Jiang Su Zhong Yi* (Jiangsu Chinese Medicine) 1963;4.
18. *Xin Zhong Yi* (New Chinese Medicine) 1994;26(9):51.

Xiǎo Jīn Dān (Minor Gold Special Pill)

小金丹

Pinyin Name: *Xiao Jin Dan*
Literal Name: Minor Gold Special Pill
Original Source: *Wai Ke Zheng Zhi Quan Sheng Ji* (Complete Collection of Patterns and Treatments in External Medicine) by Wang Wei-De in 1740

COMPOSITION

Zhi Cao Wu (Radix Aconiti Kusnezoffii Praeparata)	[150g]
Wu Ling Zhi (Faeces Trogopteri)	[150g]
Ru Xiang (Gummi Olibanum), oil removed	[75g]
Mo Yao (Myrrha), oil removed	[75g]
Dang Gui Shen (Corpus Radix Angelicae Sinensis), *chao* (dry-fried) with liquor	[75g]
Di Long (Pheretima)	[150g]
She Xiang (Moschus)	[30g]
Feng Xiang Zhi (Resina Liquidambaris)	[150g]
Mu Bie Zi (Semen Momordicae), oil removed	[150g]
Mo Tan (Chinese ink cake)	[12g]

Note: *She Xiang* (Moschus) is derived from an endangered animal, and is rarely used as a medicinal substance today. Its discussion here is included primarily for academic purposes, to reflect the historical use of this substance in its original formulation. Most herbal products today have removed it completely, or replaced it with substitutes with similar functions.

1374

Xiǎo Jīn Dān (Minor Gold Special Pill)

DOSAGE / PREPARATION / ADMINISTRATION

The source text states to grind the ingredients into a fine powder, mix it evenly with *Nuo Mi* (Oryza Glutinosa) [36g], and form into 250 pills. The pills should resemble *Qian Shi* (Semen Euryales) in size. Take one pill with aged, grain-based liquor and cover the body with blankets to promote sweating.

Today, this formula is prepared by grinding *She Xiang* (Moschus) separately from the rest of the ingredients, then mixing the powders together. Combine 100g of the herbal powder and 25g of starch to form pills. Take 2-5 pills twice daily. Reduce the dose for children.

CHINESE THERAPEUTIC ACTIONS

1. Dissolves phlegm and dispels dampness
2. Dispels stagnation and opens the channels and collaterals

CLINICAL MANIFESTATIONS

Yin-type (deep-rooted) sores due to obstruction by cold, dampness, phlegm, and blood stasis: multiple abscesses, subcutaneous nodules, scrofula, mammary "rock," buboes, cellulitis, and others. The affected area in these conditions is characterized by swelling, hardening, and pain. There is usually no change in skin color in the early stages.

CLINICAL APPLICATIONS

Multiple abscesses, subcutaneous nodules, scrofula, mammary "rock," buboes, cellulitis, and other abscesses and sores.

EXPLANATION

Xiao Jin Dan (Minor Gold Special Pill) is formulated to treat *yin*-type (deep-rooted) sores due to obstruction by cold, dampness, phlegm, and blood stasis. The treatment strategies are to warm, unblock, dissolve, and disperse nodules and hardness.

Zhi Cao Wu (Radix Aconiti Kusnezoffii Praeparata) dispels wind and dampness, warms the channels and collaterals, and dispels cold. *Wu Ling Zhi* (Faeces Trogopteri), *Ru Xiang* (Gummi Olibanum), and *Mo Yao* (Myrrha) activate the blood, dispel blood stasis, reduce swelling, and relieve pain. *Dang Gui Shen* (Corpus Radix Angelicae Sinensis) tonifies the blood. *Di Long* (Pheretima) opens the channels and collaterals. *She Xiang* (Moschus) unblocks the channels and collaterals to disperse nodules. *Feng Xiang Zhi* (Resina Liquidambaris) regulates qi and blood to dissolve carbuncles and furuncles. *Mu Bie Zi* (Semen Momordicae) dispels phlegm and toxins to disperse swelling and nodules. *Mo Tan* (Chinese ink cake) reduces swelling and dissolves phlegm. *Nuo Mi* (Oryza Glutinosa)

Xiao Jin Dan (Minor Gold Special Pill)

Diagnosis	Signs and Symptoms	Treatment	Herbs
Yin-type (deep-rooted) sores	Deep-rooted nodules and hardness with swelling, hardening and pain: obstruction by cold, dampness, phlegm and blood	• Dissolves phlegm and dispels dampness • Dispels stagnation and opens the channels and collaterals	• *Zhi Cao Wu* (Radix Aconiti Kusnezoffii Praeparata) dispels wind and dampness, warms the channels and collaterals, and dispels cold. • *Wu Ling Zhi* (Faeces Trogopteri), *Ru Xiang* (Gummi Olibanum) and *Mo Yao* (Myrrha) activate the blood, dispel blood stasis, reduce swelling, and relieve pain. • *Dang Gui Shen* (Corpus Radix Angelicae Sinensis) tonifies the blood. • *Di Long* (Pheretima) opens the channels and collaterals. • *She Xiang* (Moschus) unblocks the channels and collaterals to disperse nodules. • *Feng Xiang Zhi* (Resina Liquidambaris) regulates qi and blood to dissolve carbuncles and furuncles. • *Mu Bie Zi* (Semen Momordicae) dispels phlegm and toxins to disperse swelling and nodules. • *Mo Tan* (Chinese ink cake) reduces swelling and dissolves phlegm.

Xiǎo Jīn Dān (Minor Gold Special Pill)

nourishes the Stomach. Grain-based liquor potentiates the formula by increasing its distribution to the affected area of the body.

CAUTIONS / CONTRAINDICATIONS

- *Xiao Jin Dan* should be used with caution in individuals with underlying deficiency, as it has strong effects.
- This formula is contraindicated during pregnancy.

AUTHORS' COMMENTS

Yang He Tang (Yang-Heartening Decoction) and *Xiao Jin Dan* both treat *yin*-type (deep-rooted) sores.

- *Yang He Tang* addresses sores characterized by both excess and deficiency. However, it is more specific for yang and blood deficiencies, giving rise to cold invasion.
- *Xiao Jin Dan* treats sores characterized by excess factors, such as cold, dampness, and phlegm.

Chinese Herbal Formulas and Applications

Section 2

内痈疡剂
— Internal Abscesses and Sores

Wĕi Jīng Tāng (Reed Decoction)
葦莖湯
苇茎汤

Pinyin Name: *Wei Jing Tang*
Literal Name: Reed Decoction
Original Source: *Bei Ji Qian Jin Yao Fang* (Thousands of Golden Prescriptions for Emergencies) by Sun Si-Miao in Tang Dynasty

COMPOSITION

Wei Jing (Herba Phragmitis), *qie* (sliced)	2 cups [30g]
Dong Gua Zi (Semen Benincasae)	0.5 cup [24g]
Yi Yi Ren (Semen Coicis)	0.5 cup [30g]
Tao Ren (Semen Persicae)	30 pieces [9g]

DOSAGE / PREPARATION / ADMINISTRATION

The source text states to first cook 2 cups [30g] of *Wei Jing* (Herba Phragmitis) in 20 cups of water until it is reduced to 5 cups. Add the other ingredients, and further reduce the decoction from 5 to 2 cups. Take 1 cup of decoction per dose to induce vomiting of pus and abscesses.

CHINESE THERAPEUTIC ACTIONS

1. Clears the Lung and dissolves phlegm
2. Dispels stagnation and drains pus

CLINICAL MANIFESTATIONS

Lung abscess: coughing, foul-smelling yellow sputum with pus and blood, dull pain in the chest, squamous, dry skin; red tongue body with a yellow, greasy tongue coating, and a slippery, rapid pulse.

CLINICAL APPLICATIONS

Pulmonary abscesses, pneumonia, and bronchitis.

EXPLANATION

Wei Jing Tang (Reed Decoction) treats lung abscess with stagnation of heat, toxins, and phlegm. Stagnation in the Lung affects Lung qi circulation, causing coughing and chest pain. Stagnation of heat, toxins, and phlegm also damages the Lung, resulting in foul-smelling yellow

sputum with pus and blood. Squamous, dry skin suggests malnourishment of the skin due to lung abscess and obstructed qi and blood circulation.

This formula has *Wei Jing* (Herba Phragmitis) to clear the Lung and dispel heat. *Dong Gua Zi* (Semen Benincasae) and *Yi Yi Ren* (Semen Coicis) clear heat, dissolve phlegm, dispel dampness, and drain pus. *Tao Ren* (Semen Persicae) activates the blood and breaks up blood stagnation.

MODIFICATIONS

- With cough, sputum, and chest congestion, add *Ting Li Zi* (Semen Descurainiae seu Lepidii).
- With lingering heat accompanied by cough and profuse sputum, add *Si Gua Luo* (Retinervus Luffae Fructus) and *Gua Lou Pi* (Pericarpium Trichosanthis).
- With cough and dyspnea due to pneumonia, combine with *Ma Huang Xing Ren Gan Cao Shi Gao Tang* (Ephedra, Apricot Kernel, Licorice, and Gypsum Decoction).
- For lung abscess that has not yet turned into pus, add *Jin Yin Hua* (Flos Lonicerae Japonicae) and *Yu Xing Cao* (Herba Houttuyniae).
- For lung abscess with a profuse amount of pus, add *Jie Geng* (Radix Platycodonis), *Gan Cao* (Radix et Rhizoma Glycyrrhizae), and *Bei Mu* (Bulbus Fritillariae).

FORMULAS THAT TREAT ABSCESSES AND SORES

22

Chapter 22 – Formulas that Treat Abscesses and Sores　　　　　*Section 2 – Internal Abscesses and Sores*

Wĕi Jīng Tāng (Reed Decoction)

Wei Jing Tang (Reed Decoction)

Diagnosis	Signs and Symptoms	Treatment	Herbs
Lung abscess	• Coughing and chest pain: stagnation in the Lung with reversed flow of Lung qi • Foul-smelling yellow sputum with pus and blood: heat, toxins and phlegm damaging the Lung • Red tongue with a yellow, greasy tongue coating, a slippery, rapid pulse: heat and phlegm in the interior	• Clears the Lung and dissolves phlegm • Dispels stagnation and drains pus	• *Wei Jing* (Herba Phragmitis) clears the Lung, dispels heat, eliminates phlegm, and drains abscesses. • *Dong Gua Zi* (Semen Benincasae) and *Yi Yi Ren* (Semen Coicis) clear heat, dissolve phlegm, dispel dampness, and drain pus. • *Tao Ren* (Semen Persicae) activates the blood and breaks up blood stagnation.

CLINICAL STUDIES AND RESEARCH

1. **Pulmonary abscesses**: An integrative treatment using drugs and *Wei Jing Tang* (Reed Decoction) was associated with a marked effect in treating pulmonary abscesses. Of 110 patients, the study reported complete recovery in 68 cases, improvement in 29 cases, and no effect in 13 cases.[1] According to another study, complete recovery was reported in 24 of 26 patients with pulmonary abscesses using *Wei Jing Tang*, *Huang Lian Jie Du Tang* (Coptis Decoction to Relieve Toxicity), and intravenous administration of penicillin.[2]

2. **Pneumonia**: *Wei Jing Tang* has been shown to effectively treat many different types of pneumonia, including but not limited to lobar pneumonia, lobular pneumonia, bronchopneumonia, and mycoplasmal pneumonia.[3]

3. **Bronchitis**: *Wei Jing Tang* has been shown to successfully treat bronchitis in children,[4] suppurative bronchitis,[5] and chronic bronchitis.[6]

AUTHORS' COMMENTS

It is safe to use *Wei Jing Tang* at various stages of lung abscess, either before or after the formation of pus.

References

1. *He Nan Zhong Yi* (Henan Chinese Medicine) 1991;11(5):24.
2. *Shi Yong Zhong Xi Yi Jie He Za Zhi* (Practical Journal of Integrated Chinese and Western Medicines) 1992;5(2):83.
3. *Shan Xi Zhong Yi* (Shanxi Chinese Medicine) 1994;15(8):342.
4. *Shang Hai Zhong Yi Yao Za Zhi* (Shanghai Journal of Chinese Medicine and Herbology) 1983;10:26.
5. *Shang Hai Zhong Yi Yao Za Zhi* (Shanghai Journal of Chinese Medicine and Herbology) 1959;2:15.
6. *Jiang Su Zhong Yi* (Jiangsu Chinese Medicine) 1982;5:14.

Dà Huáng Mŭ Dān Tāng (Rhubarb and Moutan Decoction)

大黃牡丹湯
大黄牡丹汤

Pinyin Name: *Da Huang Mu Dan Tang*
Literal Name: Rhubarb and Moutan Decoction
Alternate Names: *Ta Huang Mu Tan Pi Tang*, *Da Huang Mu Dan Pi Tang*, Rhubarb and Moutan Combination
Original Source: *Jin Gui Yao Lue* (Essentials from the Golden Cabinet) by Zhang Zhong-Jing in the Eastern Han Dynasty

COMPOSITION

Da Huang (Radix et Rhizoma Rhei)	12g [18g]
Mang Xiao (Natrii Sulfas)	0.3 cup [9g]
Tao Ren (Semen Persicae)	50 pieces [12g]
Mu Dan Pi (Cortex Moutan)	3g [9g]
Dong Gua Zi (Semen Benincasae)	0.5 cup [30g]

1378

Chinese Herbal Formulas and Applications

Dà Huáng Mǔ Dān Tāng (Rhubarb and Moutan Decoction)

DOSAGE / PREPARATION / ADMINISTRATION

The source text states to cook the ingredients, except *Mang Xiao* (Natrii Sulfas), with 6 cups [1,200 mL] of water until the liquid is reduced to 1 cup [200 mL]. Discard the herb residue, add *Mang Xiao* (Natrii Sulfas) to the strained decoction, bring to a quick boil, and take the decoction immediately. Today, the decoction may be prepared using the doses suggested in brackets.

CHINESE THERAPEUTIC ACTIONS

1. Drains heat and breaks up stagnation
2. Disperses nodules and reduces swellings

CLINICAL MANIFESTATIONS

Early onset of intestinal abscess: swelling and distention of the abdomen; abdominal pain that is worse with palpation (pain resembles that of *lin zheng* [dysuria syndrome], but urination is normal); abdominal pain that decreases when the right leg is flexed, but increases when the right leg and hip are extended; fever; perspiration; aversion to cold; and a thin, greasy, yellow tongue coating.

CLINICAL APPLICATIONS

Acute appendicitis, uncomplicated appendicitis, ruptured appendicitis with peritonitis, chronic appendicitis, peri-appendicular abscess, pelvic inflammatory disease, acute cholecystitis, ulcerative colitis, chronic prostatitis, suppurative tonsillitis, mesenteric lymphadenitis, colitis, ulcerative colitis, hemorrhoids, rectal prolapse, and incarcerated internal hemorrhoids.

EXPLANATION

Da Huang Mu Dan Tang (Rhubarb and Moutan Decoction) treats early-stage intestinal abscess caused by accumulation of damp-heat and stagnation of qi and blood in the Intestines. Because stagnation of qi and blood in the Intestines may cause disharmony between the *ying* (nutritive) and *wei* (defensive) levels, fever, perspiration,

and aversion to cold may occur. The thin, greasy, yellow tongue coating signifies damp-heat in the interior.

This formula consists of cold downward draining, damp-heat clearing, and blood-activating herbs. *Da Huang* (Radix et Rhizoma Rhei) quickly purges damp-heat and disperses stagnation. *Mang Xiao* (Natrii Sulfas) softens nodules and reduces swellings. *Tao Ren* (Semen Persicae) and *Mu Dan Pi* (Cortex Moutan) activate blood circulation and cool the blood. *Dong Gua Zi* (Semen Benincasae) clears damp-heat and drains pus from the Intestines.

MODIFICATIONS

- With severe abdominal pain, add *Chuan Lian Zi* (Fructus Toosendan), *Yan Hu Suo* (Rhizoma Corydalis), *Ru Xiang* (Gummi Olibanum) and *Mo Yao* (Myrrha).
- With abdominal fullness, add *Zhi Shi* (Fructus Aurantii Immaturus), *Hou Po* (Cortex Magnoliae Officinalis), and *Bing Lang* (Semen Arecae).
- With high fever, add *Huang Lian* (Rhizoma Coptidis) and *Shi Gao* (Gypsum Fibrosum).
- With palpable mass in the lower abdomen, add *Dang Gui* (Radix Angelicae Sinensis), *Chi Shao* (Radix Paeoniae Rubra), and *Zi Hua Di Ding* (Herba Violae).
- Prior to the formation of pus or ulceration, add *Jin Yin Hua* (Flos Lonicerae Japonicae), *Pu Gong Ying* (Herba Taraxaci), *Bai Jiang Cao* (Herba cum Radice Patriniae), *Lian Qiao* (Fructus Forsythiae), *Chi Shao* (Radix Paeoniae Rubra), and *Da Xue Teng* (Caulis Sargentodoxae).
- With a feeling of incomplete evacuation of the stools caused by yin deficiency, add *Xuan Shen* (Radix Scrophulariae) and *Di Huang* (Radix Rehmanniae).
- For intestinal abscess without pus, add *Zao Jiao Ci* (Spina Gleditsiae) and *Bai Zhi* (Radix Angelicae Dahuricae).
- For intestinal abscess with pus, add *Jin Yin Hua* (Flos Lonicerae Japonicae), *Pu Gong Ying* (Herba Taraxaci), and *Bai Hua She She Cao* (Herba Hedyotis).

Da Huang Mu Dan Tang (Rhubarb and Moutan Decoction)

Diagnosis	Signs and Symptoms	Treatment	Herbs
Early onset of intestinal abscess	• Swelling and distention of the abdomen, abdominal pain that worsens with palpation: damp-heat accumulation and qi and blood stagnation in the Intestines • Fever, perspiration, and aversion to cold: disharmony between the *ying* (nutritive) and *wei* (defensive) levels • Greasy, yellow tongue coating: damp-heat	• Drains heat and breaks up stagnation • Disperses nodules and reduces swellings	• *Da Huang* (Radix et Rhizoma Rhei) quickly purges damp-heat and disperses stagnation. • *Mang Xiao* (Natrii Sulfas) softens nodules and reduces swellings. • *Tao Ren* (Semen Persicae) and *Mu Dan Pi* (Cortex Moutan) activate blood circulation and cool the blood. • *Dong Gua Zi* (Semen Benincasae) clears Intestinal damp-heat and drains pus.

FORMULAS THAT TREAT ABSCESSES AND SORES

22

1379

Chapter 22 – Formulas that Treat Abscesses and Sores   *Section 2 – Internal Abscesses and Sores*

Dà Huáng Mǔ Dān Tāng (Rhubarb and Moutan Decoction)

• For appendicitis, add *Jin Yin Hua* (Flos Lonicerae Japonicae), *Lian Qiao* (Fructus Forsythiae), *Dang Gui* (Radix Angelicae Sinensis), and *Zhi Qiao* (Fructus Aurantii).

CAUTIONS / CONTRAINDICATIONS

• Intestinal abscesses are generally classified as either damp-heat or damp-cold. Patients with intestinal abscesses caused by damp-cold should *not* take this formula.

• *Da Huang Mu Dan Tang* is not suitable for pregnant women, elderly patients, or individuals with general weakness or deficiency.

• When preparing this formula in decoction, *Da Huang* (Radix et Rhizoma Rhei) does not need to be post-decocted as the emphasis is to clear damp-heat, not to drain or purge downwards. *Mang Xiao* (Natrii Sulfas) should be dissolved in the decoction immediately before serving.

PHARMACOLOGICAL EFFECTS

1. **Antibacterial**: According to *in vitro* studies, *Da Huang Mu Dan Tang* has a potent inhibitory effect against *Staphylococcus* species, and a moderate inhibitory effect against *E. coli*.[1]

2. **Anti-inflammatory**: Both the formula and its ingredients have been shown to reduce inflammation and swelling.[2]

3. **Gastrointestinal**: Administration of *Da Huang Mu Dan Tang* was associated with a stimulatory effect on the gastrointestinal tract; it was shown to increase the intestinal peristalsis and contraction of the appendix.[3,4]

4. **Antioxidant**: One study evaluated several Chinese herbal formulas and found *Da Huang Mu Dan Tang* to have the strongest scavenging activity against three types of free radicals: 1,1-diphenyl-2-picrylhydrazyl (DPPH), superoxide anion radical (O2-.) and hydroxyl radical (OH.). The study suggested that use of *Da Huang Mu Dan Tang* may play a role in treating cerebral ischemia and brain damage, because these disorders are associated with highly reactive oxygen-derived free radicals.[5]

CLINICAL STUDIES AND RESEARCH

1. **Acute appendicitis**: Modified *Da Huang Mu Dan Tang* was used with excellent results to treat 224 patients with acute appendicitis. The study included 121 male and 103 female patients, between 7-84 years of age. Out of 224 cases, the study reported complete recovery in 206 cases, and ineffectiveness in 18 cases. The herbal formula was modified as follows: *Chuan Lian Zi* (Fructus Toosendan) and *Chi Shao* (Radix Paeoniae Rubra) were added for stagnation and accumulation; *Jin Yin Hua* (Flos Lonicerae Japonicae) and *Yi Yi Ren* (Semen Coicis) were added for damp-heat; *Huang Lian* (Rhizoma Coptidis) and *Bai Jiang Cao* (Herba cum Radice Patriniae) were added for

heat and toxins; *Huang Lian* (Rhizoma Coptidis) and *Hu Zhang* (Rhizoma et Radix Polygoni Cuspidati) for toxic sores; and *Chuan Shan Jia* (Squama Manis) and *Chi Shao* (Radix Paeoniae Rubra) for damp-heat masses.[6]

2. **Chronic appendicitis**: One study reported 99% effectiveness using modified *Da Huang Mu Dan Tang* to treat 150 patients with appendicitis.[7] Another study reported 89.5% effectiveness using *Da Huang Mu Dan Tang* plus *Bai Jiang Cao* (Herba cum Radice Patriniae) to treat 200 patients with appendicitis.[8]

3. **Ruptured appendicitis with peritonitis**: Modified *Da Huang Mu Dan Tang* and antibiotic drugs were successfully used together to treat 123 patients with ruptured appendicitis and peritonitis. The herbal formula used *Da Huang Mu Dan Tang* plus *Jin Yin Hua* (Flos Lonicerae Japonicae), *Chuan Lian Zi* (Fructus Toosendan), and *Tao Ren* (Semen Persicae) as the base formula, with the addition of *Shi Gao* (Gypsum Fibrosum) and *Tian Hua Fen* (Radix Trichosanthis) for high fever; *Zhu Ru* (Caulis Bambusae in Taenia) and *Lu Gen* (Rhizoma Phragmitis) for nausea and vomiting; *Ru Xiang* (Gummi Olibanum), *Mo Yao* (Myrrha), and *Yan Hu Suo* (Rhizoma Corydalis) for severe pain; and *Bing Pian* (Borneolum Syntheticum) and *Mang Xiao* (Natrii Sulfas) for abscess and swelling in the appendix area. Out of 123 patients, the study reported complete recovery in 75 cases, marked improvement in 44 cases, and no effect in 4 cases.[9]

4. **Periappendicular abscess**: Administration of modified *Da Huang Mu Dan Tang* along with antibiotic drugs showed good success in treating periappendicular abscess. The herbal formula used *Da Huang Mu Dan Tang* as the base formula, and added *Yan Hu Suo* (Rhizoma Corydalis) and *Chi Shao* (Radix Paeoniae Rubra) for stagnation and accumulation; and *Jin Yin Hua* (Flos Lonicerae Japonicae), *Zhi Zi* (Fructus Gardeniae), and *Pu Gong Ying* (Herba Taraxaci) for excess heat. In addition, patients also received intravenous antibiotics and fluids. Out of 36 cases, the study reported complete recovery in 28 cases, improvement in 7 cases, and no effect in 1 case.[10]

5. **Pelvic inflammation**: Fifty-three patients with pelvic inflammation were treated with marked success using modified *Da Huang Mu Dan Tang* plus antibiotic drugs. The herbal formula contained *Da Huang* (Radix et Rhizoma Rhei), *Mu Dan Pi* (Cortex Moutan), *Tao Ren* (Semen Persicae), *Dong Gua Zi* (Semen Benincasae), *Jin Yin Hua* (Flos Lonicerae Japonicae), *Lian Qiao* (Fructus Forsythiae), *Huang Bo* (Cortex Phellodendri Chinensis), *Pu Gong Ying* (Herba Taraxaci), *Di Huang* (Radix Rehmanniae), *Bai Jiang Cao* (Herba cum Radice Patriniae) and *Gan Cao* (Radix et Rhizoma Glycyrrhizae). Out of 53 patients, the study reported complete recovery in 50 cases and improvement in 3 cases.[11]

1380

Dà Huáng Mǔ Dān Tāng (Rhubarb and Moutan Decoction)

6. **Acute cholecystitis**: Eighty-eight patients with acute cholecystitis (3 hours to 5 days) were treated with *Da Huang Mu Dan Tang* with good success. Most patients had resolution of symptoms and signs within 36 hours. Those who did not respond were referred out for emergency treatment. Out of 88 patients, the study reported complete recovery in 57 cases, marked improvement in 22 cases, and no effect in 9 cases.[12]

7. **Ulcerative colitis**: *Da Huang Mu Dan Tang* effectively treated ulcerative colitis in one study. The treatment protocol was to instill the decoction rectally twice daily for one month per course of treatment. Out of 30 patients, the study reported complete recovery in 9 cases, marked improvement in 16 cases, and no effect in 5 cases. The overall effectiveness was 80.3%.[13]

8. **Chronic prostatitis**: Rectal instillation of modified *Da Huang Mu Dan Tang* was effective in treating patients with chronic prostatitis. In addition to the formula, *Bian Xu* (Herba Polygoni Avicularis) and *Qu Mai* (Herba Dianthi) were added for frequent and painful urination; *Chuan Lian Zi* (Fructus Toosendan) and *Yan Hu Suo* (Rhizoma Corydalis) were added for testicular pain; *Du Zhong* (Cortex Eucommiae) and *Xu Duan* (Radix Dipsaci) were added for lower abdominal pain; *Chuan Shan Jia* (Squama Manis) and *E Zhu* (Rhizoma Curcumae) were added for hardness and nodules of the prostate; and *Pu Gong Ying* (Herba Taraxaci) and *Mo Han Lian* (Herba Ecliptae) were added for presence of white or red blood cells in the seminal fluids. The treatment protocol was to cook the herbs in water, and instill the solution in the rectum one time daily for seven days per course of treatment, for a total of 1-8 courses. Out of 60 patients, the study reported complete recovery in 47 cases, and marked improvement in 13 cases.[14]

9. **Suppurative tonsillitis**: Modified *Da Huang Mu Dan Tang* was used with good success in treating suppurative tonsillitis in 50 young children. The herbal treatment used *Da Huang Mu Dan Tang* plus *Lian Qiao* (Fructus Forsythiae), *Huang Lian* (Rhizoma Coptidis), *Jin Yin Hua* (Flos Lonicerae Japonicae), and *Gan Cao* (Radix et Rhizoma Glycyrrhizae) as the base formula. Furthermore, it added *Gou Teng* (Ramulus Uncariae cum Uncis) and *Quan Xie* (Scorpio) for seizures and epilepsy; *Mu Xiang* (Radix Aucklandiae) and *Yan Hu Suo* (Rhizoma Corydalis) for abdominal pain; and *Chuan Shan Jia* (Squama Manis) and *Xia Ku Cao* (Spica Prunellae) for submandibular lymphadenitis. The duration of treatment ranged from 4 to 12 packs of herbs. The study reported complete recovery in all 50 patients.[15]

10. **Incarcerated internal hemorrhoids**: One study reported good results using modified *Da Huang Mu Dan Tang* to treat incarcerated internal hemorrhoids. The herbal formula contained *Da Huang* (Radix et Rhizoma Rhei) 30g, *Mu Dan Pi* (Cortex Moutan) 15g, *Tao Ren* (Semen Persicae) 10g, *Dong Gua Zi* (Semen Benincasae) 30g, *Mang Xiao* (Natrii Sulfas) 9g, *Pu Gong Ying* (Herba Taraxaci) 30g, *Hong Hua* (Flos Carthami) 10g, *Di Yu* (Radix Sanguisorbae) 12g, and *Zhi Shi* (Fructus Aurantii Immaturus) 15g. The treatment protocol was to cook the herbs in water twice, and mix the two resultant decoctions together, and administer the liquid in two equally-divided doses, twice daily. In addition to oral therapy, patients were also advised to take sitz bath twice daily using an herbal solution made by cooking 30g of *Da Huang* (Radix et Rhizoma Rhei) and 15g of *Hua Jiao* (Pericarpium Zanthoxyli) in 2,000 mL of water for 5 minutes. Of 30 patients, the study reported recovery in 12 cases within 24 hours, 16 cases after 48 hours, and 2 cases after 72 hours. The average time to recovery was 1.67 days.[16]

RELATED FORMULA

Qīng Cháng Yǐn (Clear the Intestines Drink)

清腸飲
请肠饮

Pinyin Name: *Qing Chang Yin*

Literal Name: Clear the Intestines Drink

Original Source: *Bian Zheng Lun* (Records of Differential Diagnosis)

Jin Yin Hua (Flos Lonicerae Japonicae)	90g
Dang Gui (Radix Angelicae Sinensis)	60g
Di Yu (Radix Sanguisorbae)	30g
Mai Dong (Radix Ophiopogonis)	30g
Xuan Shen (Radix Scrophulariae)	30g
Gan Cao (Radix et Rhizoma Glycyrrhizae)	9g
Yi Yi Ren (Semen Coicis)	15g
Huang Qin (Radix Scutellariae)	6g

The source text states to prepare the ingredients as a decoction. *Qing Chang Yin* (Clear the Intestines Drink) activates the blood, eliminates toxins, nourishes yin, and purges fire. Its main indication is for treating abscesses in the large intestine.

AUTHORS' COMMENTS

Da Huang Mu Dan Tang has been used successfully to treat acute and/or uncomplicated appendicitis. However, the use of this formula alone is ***not*** appropriate for ruptured appendix with peritonitis or other complications. These cases are medical emergencies that are best treated in hospitals.

Chapter 22 – Formulas that Treat Abscesses and Sores　　　　　*Section 2 – Internal Abscesses and Sores*

Dà Huáng Mǔ Dān Tāng (Rhubarb and Moutan Decoction)

References

1. *Zhong Yi Za Zhi* (Journal of Chinese Medicine) 1955;10:36.
2. *Zhong Yi Fang Ji Xian Dai Yan Jiu* (Modern Study of Medical Formulae in Traditional Chinese Medicine) 1997;1600.
3. *Shan Dong Yi Xue Yuan Xue Bao* (Journal of Shandong University School of Medicine) 1959;4:25.
4. *Zhong Yi Fang Ji Xian Dai Yan Jiu* (Modern Study of Medical Formulae in Traditional Chinese Medicine) 1997;1600.
5. Department of Pharmacy, Tokushima University Hospital, Japan. Studies on attenuation of post-ischemic brain injury by kampo medicines-inhibitory effects of free radical production. Yakugaku Zasshi 1994 Jun;114(6):388-94.
6. *Guang Xi Zhong Yi Yao* (Guangxi Chinese Medicine and Herbology) 1986;3:10.
7. *Ha Er Bing Zhong Yi* (Haerbing Chinese Medicine) 1959;2(1):20.
8. *Tian Jin Yi Yao Za Zhi* (Journal of Tianjin Medicine and Herbology) 1959;11:411.
9. *Nei Meng Gu Zhong Yi Yao* (Traditional Chinese Medicine and Medicinals of Inner Mongolia) 1993;2:23.
10. *Yun Nan Zhong Yi Za Zhi* (Yunan Journal of Chinese Medicine) 1995;2:11.
11. *Guang Xi Zhong Yi Yao* (Guangxi Chinese Medicine and Herbology) 1992;5:6.
12. *Shi Yong Zhong Yi Nei Ke Za Zhi* (Journal of Practical Chinese Internal Medicine) 1992;3:127.
13. *He Nan Zhong Yi* (Henan Chinese Medicine) 1998;1:22.
14. *Zhe Jiang Zhong Yi Za Zhi* (Zhejiang Journal of Chinese Medicine) 1993;8:368.
15. *Liao Ning Zhong Yi Za Zhi* (Liaoning Journal of Chinese Medicine) 1991;6:36.
16. *Zhong Yao Xian Dai Yan Jiu Yu Ying Yong* (Modern Study of Traditional Chinese Medicine) 1997;1601.

Yi Yǐ Fù Zǐ Bài Jiàng Sǎn

(Coicis, Prepared Aconite, and Patrinia Powder)

薏苡附子敗醬散
薏苡附子败酱散

Pinyin Name: *Yi Yi Fu Zi Bai Jiang San*
Literal Name: Coicis, Prepared Aconite, and Patrinia Powder
Original Source: *Jin Gui Yao Lue* (Essentials from the Golden Cabinet) by Zhang Zhong-Jing in the Eastern Han Dynasty

COMPOSITION

Yi Yi Ren (Semen Coicis)	[30g]
Bai Jiang Cao (Herba cum Radice Patriniae)	[15g]
Fu Zi (Radix Aconiti Lateralis Praeparata)	[6g]

DOSAGE / PREPARATION / ADMINISTRATION

The source text states to grind the ingredients into powder. Cook 1 large spoonful [6-9g] of the powder with 2 cups [400 mL] of water until the liquid is reduced by half. Take the decoction immediately.

CHINESE THERAPEUTIC ACTIONS

Drains pus and reduces swelling

CLINICAL MANIFESTATIONS

Intestinal abscess with pus: absence of fever, squamous, dry skin; abdominal swelling that feels soft with the application of pressure, and a rapid pulse.

CLINICAL APPLICATIONS

Appendicitis and pelvic inflammatory disease.

EXPLANATION

Yi Yi Fu Zi Bai Jiang San (Coicis, Prepared Aconite, and Patrinia Powder) treats intestinal abscess with pus formation characterized by interlocking of interior cold, dampness, and blood stasis. A rapid pulse without fever suggests interior abscess and pus. The abdomen feels soft upon palpation since there is no constipation. Squamous, dry skin is the result of lack of nourishment.

This formula contains a large dose of *Yi Yi Ren* (Semen Coicis) to resolve dampness and reduce swelling. *Bai*

1382

Chinese Herbal Formulas and Applications

Yì Yǐ Fù Zǐ Bài Jiàng Sǎn
(Coicis, Prepared Aconite, and Patrinia Powder)

Yi Yi Fu Zi Bai Jiang San (Coicis, Prepared Aconite, and Patrinia Powder)

Diagnosis	Signs and Symptoms	Treatment	Herbs
Intestinal abscess with pus	Abdominal swelling that feels soft with the application of pressure, absence of fever and a rapid pulse: interlocking of interior cold, dampness, and blood stasis	Drains pus and reduces swelling	• *Yi Yi Ren* (Semen Coicis) drains pus and reduces swelling. • *Bai Jiang Cao* (Herba cum Radice Patriniae) clears heat, reduces abscesses, drains pus and disperses blood stasis. • *Fu Zi* (Radix Aconiti Lateralis Praeparata) activates yang and qi, and disperses cold and damp stagnation.

Jiang Cao (Herba cum Radice Patriniae) clears heat, reduces abscesses, drains pus and disperses blood stasis. A small dose of *Fu Zi* (Radix Aconiti Lateralis Praeparata) is used to disperse cold and damp stagnation and activate the yang and qi. The hot property of *Fu Zi* (Radix Aconiti Lateralis Praeparata) balances the cold property of *Bai Jiang Cao* (Herba cum Radice Patriniae) and prevents damages to the middle *jiao*.

MODIFICATIONS
• For late-stage intestinal abscess with heat and toxins and yang qi deficiency manifesting in abdominal mass, add *Tao Ren* (Semen Persicae) and *Mu Dan Pi* (Cortex Moutan).
• With Spleen qi deficiency, add *Dang Shen* (Radix Codonopsis) and *Fu Ling* (Poria).
• With regional burning pain, add *Huang Qin* (Radix Scutellariae) and increase the dose of *Bai Jiang Cao* (Herba cum Radice Patriniae).

CLINICAL STUDIES AND RESEARCH
1. **Appendicitis**: *Yi Yi Fu Zi Bai Jiang San* has been shown to effectively treat both acute and chronic appendicitis. According to one study of 25 patients with acute or chronic appendicitis, use of modified *Yi Yi Fu Zi Bai Jiang San* was associated with complete recovery in 21 cases, significant improvement in 2 cases, and no effect in 2 cases.[1] According to another study, use of modified *Yi Yi Fu Zi Bai Jiang San* in 93 patients with chronic appendicitis was associated with complete recovery in 78 cases, improvement in 11 cases, and no effect in 4 cases (who were subsequently treated with surgery).[2]
2. **Pelvic inflammatory disease**: One study reported 94.6% effectiveness using modified *Yi Yi Fu Zi Bai Jiang San* to treat 56 patients with pelvic inflammatory disease. The herbal formula contained *Yi Yi Ren* (Semen Coicis) 30g, *Bai Jiang Cao* (Herba cum Radice Patriniae) 30g, *Yi Mu Cao* (Herba Leonuri) 30g, processed *Xiang Fu* (Rhizoma

Cyperi) 15g, *Bai Shao* (Radix Paeoniae Alba) 15g, *Fu Zi* (Radix Aconiti Lateralis Praeparata) 10g, *Dang Gui* (Radix Angelicae Sinensis) 6g, *Hu Po* (Succinum) 1g, and *Chuan Shan Jia* (Squama Manis) 1g. *Hu Po* (Succinum) and *Chuan Shan Jia* (Squama Manis) were not cooked, but ingested in powder form with the herbal decoction. These two herbs were not used during menstruation. Additional modifications were made if necessary. The treatment protocol was to administer the herbs in decoction for 4 weeks per course of treatment, for 1-3 courses total. Of 56 patients, the study reported complete recovery in 31 cases, significant improvement in 12 cases, moderate improvement in 10 cases, and no effect in 3 cases.[3]

RELATED FORMULA
Yì Yǐ Rén Tāng (Coicis Decoction)

薏苡仁湯
薏苡仁汤

Pinyin Name: *Yi Yi Ren Tang*
Literal Name: Coicis Decoction
Original Source: *Zheng Zhi Zhun Sheng* (Standards of Patterns and Treatments) by Wang Ken-Tang in 1602

Yi Yi Ren (Semen Coicis)	9g
Gua Lou Zi (Semen Trichosanthis)	9g
Mu Dan Pi (Cortex Moutan)	6g
Tao Ren (Semen Persicae)	6g

The source text states to cook the ingredients with 3 large bowls of water until the liquid is reduced to 1 bowl. Take the decoction any time during the day.

Yi Yi Ren Tang (Coicis Decoction) resolves dampness, moistens the Intestines, activates the blood, and relieves pain. It is commonly used to treat early-stage intestinal abscesses characterized by damp accumulation and blood stagnation, with symptoms such as abdominal fullness and pain, poor appetite, and dysuria. It may also be used

FORMULAS THAT TREAT ABSCESSES AND SORES

22

Chapter 22 – Formulas that Treat Abscesses and Sores   Section 2 – Internal Abscesses and Sores

Yī Yǐ Fù Zǐ Bài Jiàng Sǎn
(Coicis, Prepared Aconite, and Patrinia Powder)

for abdominal pain associated with menstruation, or for postpartum women whose pain is characterized by damp and blood stagnation.

AUTHORS' COMMENTS

There are two formulas called *Yi Yi Ren Tang* (Coicis Decoction) discussed in this text. Though they have identical names, their compositions and clinical applications are different, and must not be confused with each others.

- *Yi Yi Ren Tang* (Coicis Decoction), from *Zhang Shi Yi Tong* (Comprehensive Medicine According to Master Zhang) by Zhang Lu-Xuan in 1695, dispels wind-dampness from the exterior to treat *bi zheng* (painful obstruction syndrome).

- *Yi Yi Ren Tang* (Coicis Decoction), from *Zheng Zhi Zhun Sheng* (Standards of Patterns and Treatments) by Wang Ken-Tang in 1602, dispels dampness from the Intestines to treat intestinal abscess.

Da Huang Mu Dan Tang (Rhubarb and Moutan Decoction) and *Yi Yi Fu Zi Bai Jiang San* are two formulas commonly used to treat early stage of intestinal abscesses without underlying deficiencies.

- *Da Huang Mu Dan Tang* is a bitter and cold formula that has functions to drain downwards, clear heat, disperse blood stagnation and reduce swelling. It is a stronger formula that is more suitable for intestinal abscesses characterized by damp-heat with qi and blood stagnation.

- *Yi Yi Fu Zi Bai Jiang San* resolves dampness and moistens the intestines. It has moderate potency and is more appropriate for intestinal abscesses characterized by dampness.

References

1. *Bei Jing Zhong Yi* (Beijing Chinese Medicine) 1987;5:32.
2. *Nei Meng Gu Zhong Yi Yao* (Traditional Chinese Medicine and Medicinals of Inner Mongolia) 1992;11(3):26.
3. *Shan Xi Zhong Yi* (Shanxi Chinese Medicine) 1993;14(12):533.

1384

Chapter 22 — Summary

— Formulas that Treat Abscesses and Sores

SECTION 1: EXTERNAL ABSCESSES AND SORES

Name	Similarities	Differences
Xian Fang Huo Ming Yin (Sublime Formula for Sustaining Life)		Reduces swelling, break the hardness, activates blood circulation, stops pain
Niu Bang Jie Ji Tang (Arctium Decoction to Release the Muscle Layer)	Clear heat, eliminate toxins, release the exterior	Cools the blood, nourishes yin, reduces swelling
Jing Fang Bai Du San (Schizonepeta and Saposhnikovia Powder to Overcome Pathogenic Influences)		Strongly releases the exterior, regulates qi and blood circulation
Wu Wei Xiao Du Yin (Five-Ingredient Decoction to Eliminate Toxins)		Disperses external carbuncles and furuncles
Shi Wei Bai Du Tang (Ten-Ingredient Decoction to Overcome Pathogenic Influences)	Clear heat, eliminate toxins	Treats suppurative skin disorders
Si Miao Yong An Tang (Four-Valiant Decoction for Well-Being)		Treats gangrene with heat, fire and toxins
Zi Cao Gen Mu Li Tang (Arnebia and Oyster Shell Decoction)		Treats malignant sores and abscesses
Xi Huang Wan (Cattle Gallstone Pill)		Treats various abscesses and sores, such as breast cancer, buboes, scrofula
Hai Zao Yu Hu Tang (Sargassum Decoction for the Jade Flask)		Treats goiter affecting the neck
Xiao Luo Wan (Reduce Scrofula Pill)	Dissolve phlegm, soften hardness, disperse nodules	Treats hardness and nodules around the ears and neck
San Zhong Kui Jian Tang (Disperse the Swelling and Break the Hardness Decoction)		Treats hardness and nodules, especially around the ears, cheeks, and shoulders
Shi Liu Wei Liu Qi Yin (Sixteen-Ingredient Decoction to Flow Qi)		Treats hardness and nodules, especially in the neck, breast and abdominal regions
Tou Nong San (Discharge Pus Powder)		Tonifies qi
Pai Nong San (Drain the Pus Powder)		Tonifies the blood
Qian Jin Nei Tuo San (Drain the Interior Powder Worthy of a Thousand Gold)	Tonify deficiencies, drain pus from abscesses and sores	Tonifies qi and blood
Tuo Li Xiao Du Yin (Drain the Interior and Detoxify Decoction)		Strongly tonifies qi and blood
Nei Bu Huang Qi Tang (Tonify the Interior Decoction with Astragalus)		Tonifies qi and blood, nourishes yin
Yang He Tang (Yang-Heartening Decoction)	Warm yang, dispel cold, treat *yin* (deep-rooted) abscesses and sores	Warms yang, tonifies the blood
Xiao Jin Dan (Minor Gold Special Pill)		Dispels dampness and phlegm, opens the channels and collaterals

FORMULAS THAT TREAT ABSCESSES AND SORES

22

1385

Chapter 22 – Formulas that Treat Abscesses and Sores

Chapter 22 — Summary

Xian Fang Huo Ming Yin (Sublime Formula for Sustaining Life), ***Niu Bang Jie Ji Tang*** (Arctium Decoction to Release the Muscle Layer) and ***Jing Fang Bai Du San*** (Schizonepeta and Saposhnikovia Powder to Overcome Pathogenic Influences) have similar functions to release the exterior, clear heat, and eliminate toxins.

- *Xian Fang Huo Ming Yin* treats early onset of abscesses and sores characterized by accumulation of heat and toxins at the exterior with stagnation of qi and blood.
- *Niu Bang Jie Ji Tang* treats abscesses and sores in the head and facial regions due to wind-heat. It releases wind, clears heat, cools the blood, and reduces swelling.
- *Jing Fang Bai Du San* strongly releases the exterior to treat sores and abscesses with exterior symptoms, such as fever, aversion to cold, and absence of sweating.

Wu Wei Xiao Du Yin (Five-Ingredient Decoction to Eliminate Toxins), ***Shi Wei Bai Du Tang*** (Ten-Ingredient Decoction to Overcome Pathogenic Influences), ***Si Miao Yong An Tang*** (Four-Valiant Decoction for Well-Being), and ***Zi Cao Gen Mu Li Tang*** (Arnebia and Oyster Shell Decoction) clear heat and eliminate toxins to treat various conditions with abscesses and sores.

- *Wu Wei Xiao Du Yin* treats carbuncles, furuncles, and other types of epithelial inflammation.
- *Shi Wei Bai Du Tang* treats various types of suppurative skin disorders at the exterior.
- *Si Miao Yong An Tang* treats gangrene of the extremities with local swelling and pus formation.
- *Zi Cao Gen Mu Li Tang* treats malignant abscesses, sores, and ulcers.

Xi Huang Wan (Cattle Gallstone Pill), ***Hai Zao Yu Hu Tang*** (Sargassum Decoction for the Jade Flask), ***Xiao Luo Wan*** (Reduce Scrofula Pill), ***San Zhong Kui Jian Tang*** (Disperse the Swelling and Break the Hardness Decoction), and ***Shi Liu Wei Liu Qi Yin*** (Sixteen-Ingredient Decoction to Flow Qi) have similar functions to dissolve phlegm, soften hardness, and disperse nodules.

- *Xi Huang Wan* treats various types of abscesses and nodules, such as lymph edema, lymphadenitis, breast cancer, buboes, scrofula, subcutaneous nodules, and multiple abscesses.
- *Hai Zao Yu Hu Tang* treats enlarged thyroid glands in goiter and hyperthyroidism.
- *Xiao Luo Wan* was originally designed to treat scrofula, but may also be used for goiter, thyroiditis, lymphadenitis, parotitis, and hyperplasia of the mammary glands.
- *San Zhong Kui Jian Tang* treats hardness and nodules throughout the body, but is especially effective for areas below the ears and around the shoulders. Clinical applications include lymphadenitis, hyperthyroidism, goiter, carbuncles, and furuncles.
- *Shi Liu Wei Liu Qi Yin* treats hardness and nodules throughout the body, but is especially effective for neck, breast and abdominal regions. Clinical applications include breast cancer, fibrocystic disease, goiter, and inflammation of the lymph glands.

Tou Nong San (Discharge Pus Powder), ***Pai Nong San*** (Drain the Pus Powder), ***Qian Jin Nei Tuo San*** (Drain the Interior Powder Worthy of a Thousand Gold), ***Tuo Li Xiao Du Yin*** (Drain the Interior and Detoxify Decoction), and ***Nei Bu Huang Qi Tang*** (Tonify the Interior Decoction with Astragalus), all treat mid-to-late stages of abscesses and sores, when affected individuals begin to show more underlying deficiencies.

- *Tou Nong San* tonifies qi and enhances pustulation. It is effective in the middle or late stage of abscesses and sores, in which there is a proliferation of pus in the interior with qi deficiency.
- *Pai Nong San* nourishes the blood, drains pus, and reduces nodules. It is used to treat middle or late stage of abscesses and sores with blood deficiency.
- *Qian Jin Nei Tuo San* tonifies qi and blood and promotes the generation of flesh. It is used to treat late stage of abscesses and sores with qi and blood deficiencies.
- *Tuo Li Xiao Du Yin* tonifies qi and blood, strengthens the Spleen and Stomach, and drains pus and swellings. It is used to treat late stage of abscesses and sores with severe qi and blood deficiencies.
- *Nei Bu Huang Qi Tang* tonifies qi and blood, nourishes yin, and promotes generation of flesh. It is especially applicable in the late stage of abscesses and sores with generalized weakness and deficiency.

1386

Chapter 22 — Summary

Yang He Tang (Yang-Heartening Decoction) and *Xiao Jin Dan* (Minor Gold Special Pill) have similar effects to warm yang, dispel cold, and drain pus from abscesses and sores. These two formulas are most effective for *yin*-type (deep-rooted) abscesses and sores with yang deficiency and cold accumulation.

- *Yang He Tang* focuses primarily on warming yang and tonifying the blood to treat *yin* (deep-rooted) abscesses and sores.
- *Xiao Jin Dan*, on the other hand, works by dispelling dampness and phlegm, dispersing cold, and warming the channels and collaterals to treat *yin* (deep-rooted) abscesses and sores.

SECTION 2: INTERNAL ABSCESSES AND SORES

Name	Similarities	Differences
Wei Jing Tang (Reed Decoction)	Resolve internal abscesses and sores	Treats lung abscesses
Da Huang Mu Dan Tang (Rhubarb and Moutan Decoction)		Treats intestinal abscesses
Yi Yi Fu Zi Bai Jiang San (Coicis, Prepared Aconite, and Patrinia Powder)		Treats intestinal abscesses with pus

Wei Jing Tang (Reed Decoction) clears heat, eliminates toxins, and drains pus. It treats lung abscesses with stagnation of blood, heat, toxins, and phlegm.

Da Huang Mu Dan Tang (Rhubarb and Moutan Decoction) purges stagnant heat and eliminates toxins. It is excellent for treating early onset of intestinal abscesses.

Yi Yi Fu Zi Bai Jiang San (Coicis, Prepared Aconite, and Patrinia Powder) strongly drains pus and reduces swellings. It treats intestinal abscesses with pus formation.

Part III

— Additional Resources

吴尚先 Wú Shàng-Xían

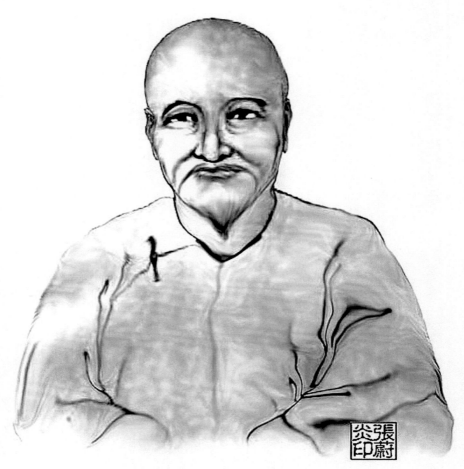

吴尚先 Wú Shàng-Xían, 1806 – 1886.

吴尚先 Wú Shàng-Xian

Chinese Herbal Formulas and Applications

Wu Shang-Xian specialized in treating both local and systemic disorders via topical applications of herbs. His exploration of topical approaches was motivated by his concern for patients who could not or would not take herbs by oral ingestion, and by his desire to minimize the side effects associated with oral use. In many years of research, Wu explored many different routes of administration, such as oral inhalation, nasal inhalation, topical application, and ophthalmic instillation. He also developed many different dosage forms for medicines, including creams, ointments, plasters, inhalation solutions, and more. Because of his unique treatment methods and uncommon success, he literally treated 4,000 to 5,000 patients per month, and 50,000 to 60,000 patients per year. Wu's style of medicine introduced new options for treatment, and influenced generations of physicians and herbalists, shaping the practice of medicine to this day.

Dynasties & Kingdoms	Year
Xia Dynasty 夏	2100-1600 BCE
Shang Dynasty 商	1600-1100 BCE
Zhou Dynasty 周	1100-221 BCE
Qin Dynasty 秦	221-207 BCE
Han Dynasty 漢	206 BCE-220
Three Kingdoms 三國	220-280
Western Jin Dynasty 西晉	265-316
Eastern Jin Dynasty 東晉	317-420
Northern and Southern Dynasties 北南朝	420-581
Sui Dynasty 隋	581-618
Tang Dynasty 唐	618-907
Five Dynasties 五代	907-960
Song Dynasty 宋	960-1279
Liao Dynasty 遼	916-1125
Jin Dynasty 金	1115-1234
Yuan Dynasty 元	1271-1368
Ming Dynasty 明	1368-1644
Qing Dynasty 清	**1644-1911**
Republic of China 中華民國	1912-Present Day
People's Republic of China 中華人民共和國	1949-Present Day

Table of Contents

PART III ADDITIONAL RESOURCES

Appendix 1 Cross-reference Based on Traditional Chinese Medicine Diagnosis ············· 1393
Appendix 2 Cross-reference Based on Western Medicine Diagnosis ······························· 1397
Appendix 3 Formulas Offering Beneficial Effects to Support Pregnancy ······················· 1433
Appendix 4 Formulas Offering Beneficial Effects for Postpartum Care ························· 1434
Appendix 5 Cautions / Contraindications for the Use of Formulas During Pregnancy ······ 1435
Appendix 6 Dosing Guidelines ·· 1437
Appendix 7 Weights and Measures: Chinese, British and Metric Systems ···················· 1439
Appendix 8 Convention on International Trade in Endangered Species (CITES) ············· 1441
Appendix 9 Cross-reference of Single Herb Names ··· 1442
Appendix 10 Cross-reference of Herbal Formula Names ··· 1464
Appendix 11 Tables of Famous Doctors ·· 1481
Bibliography of Historical Texts ··· 1485
Bibliography of Contemporary References ·· 1493
Glossary ·· 1505
Index ·· 1529
About the Authors ··· 1619

Chinese Herbal Formulas and Applications

Appendix 1

— Cross-reference Based on Traditional Chinese Medicine Diagnosis

1. 奔豚 *ben tun* (running piglet)
2. 崩漏 *beng lou* (flooding and spotting)
3. 痹证 *bi zheng* (painful obstruction syndrome)
4. 癫狂 *dian kuang* (mania and withdrawal)
5. 霍乱 *huo luan* (sudden turmoil)
6. 脚气 *jiao qi* (leg qi)
7. 积聚 *ji ju* (accumulation)
8. 淋证 *lin zheng* (dysuria syndrome)
9. 梅核气 *mei he qi* (plum-pit qi)

10. 痿证 *wei zheng* (atrophy syndrome)
11. 五心热 *wu xin re* (five-center heat)
12. 消渴 *xiao ke* (wasting and thirsting)
13. 胸痹 *xiong bi* (painful obstruction of the chest)
14. 虚劳 *xu lao* (deficiency and debilitation)
15. 血瘀 *xue yu* (blood stasis)
16. 脏燥 *zang zao* (restless organ)
17. 中风 *zhong feng* (wind stroke)

1. 奔豚 *BEN TUN* (RUNNING PIGLET)
- *Xuan Fu Dai Zhe Shi Tang* (Inula and Hematite Decoction), 851
- *Hei Xi Dan* (Lead Special Pill), 492

2. 崩漏 *BENG LOU* (FLOODING AND SPOTTING)
Kidney deficiency
- *Zuo Gui Wan* (Restore the Left [Kidney] Pill), 645

Spleen deficiency
- *Gu Chong Tang* (Stabilize Chong [Thoroughfare Channel] Decoction), 803
- *Sheng Mai San* (Generate the Pulse Powder), 554

3. 痹证 *BI ZHENG* (PAINFUL OBSTRUCTION SYNDROME)
Xing bi (mobile painful obstruction)
- *Gui Zhi Shao Yao Zhi Mu Tang* (Cinnamon Twig, Peony, and Anemarrhena Decoction), 1186

Zhuo bi (fixed painful obstruction)
- *Yi Yi Ren Tang* (Coicis Decoction), 1173

Re bi (heat painful obstruction)
- *Bai Hu Jia Gui Zhi Tang* (White Tiger plus Cinnamon Twig Decoction), 323

Xue bi (blood painful obstruction)
- *Shen Tong Zhu Yu Tang* (Drive Out Blood Stasis from a Painful Body Decoction), 893

Wan bi (stubborn painful obstruction)
- *Da Huo Luo Dan* (Major Invigorate the Collaterals Special Pill), 1179
- *Xiao Huo Luo Dan* (Minor Invigorate the Collaterals Special Pill), 1177

- *Shen Tong Zhu Yu Tang* (Drive Out Blood Stasis from a Painful Body Decoction), 893

Wei bi (atrophic painful obstruction)
- *San Bi Tang* (Three-Painful Obstruction Decoction), 1167
- *Huang Qi Gui Zhi Wu Wu Tang* (Astragalus and Cinnamon Twig Five-Substance Decoction), 500

Zhou bi (generalized painful obstruction)
- *Juan Bi Tang* (Remove Painful Obstruction Decoction), 1158
- *Shang Zhong Xia Tong Yong Tong Feng Wan* (Upper, Middle, and Lower General Use Pill for Wind-Pain), 1175

4. 癫狂 *DIAN KUANG* (MANIA AND WITHDRAWAL)
Qi and blood deficiencies
- *Yang Xin Tang* (Nourish the Heart Decoction), 735

Phlegm stagnation
- *Di Tan Tang* (Scour Phlegm Decoction), 1212
- *Gun Tan Wan* (Vaporize Phlegm Pill), 1238

Fire and phlegm disturbing the Heart
- *San Sheng San* (Three-Sage Powder), 1312
- *Sheng Tie Luo Yin* (Iron Filings Decoction), 711
- *Kong Xian Dan* (Control Mucus Special Pill), 182

With *shen* (spirit) disturbance
- *Ding Zhi Wan* (Settle the Emotions Pill), 723

5. 霍乱 *HUO LUAN* (SUDDEN TURMOIL DISORDER)
Cold
- *Huo Xiang Zheng Qi San* (Agastache Powder to Rectify the Qi), 1079

1393

Appendix 1 – Cross-reference Based on Traditional Chinese Medicine Diagnosis

Appendix 1 — Cross-reference Based on Traditional Chinese Medicine Diagnosis

- *Fu Zi Li Zhong Wan* (Prepared Aconite Pill to Regulate the Middle), 463

Heat

- *Can Shi Tang* (Silkworm Droppings Decoction), 1101
- *Xing Jun San* (Troop-Marching Powder), 756

6. 脚气 *JIAO QI* (LEG *QI*)

- *Ji Ming San* (Powder to Take at Cock's Crow), 1183

7. 积聚 *JI JU* (ACCUMULATION)

Liver qi stagnation

- *Zuo Jin Wan* (Left Metal Pill), 389
- *Gan Mai Da Zao Tang* (Licorice, Wheat, and Jujube Decoction), 731

Food and phlegm stagnation

- *Ban Xia Hou Po Tang* (Pinellia and Magnolia Bark Decoction), 827
- *Xiang Sha Liu Jun Zi Tang* (Six-Gentlemen Decoction with Aucklandia and Amomum), 531

Qi and blood stagnation

- *Wu Ji San* (Five-Accumulation Powder), 301
- *Shi Xiao San* (Sudden Smile Powder), 911
- *Ge Xia Zhu Yu Tang* (Drive Out Blood Stasis Below the Diaphragm Decoction), 885
- *Bie Jia Jian Wan* (Soft-Shelled Turtle Shell Pill), 935
- *Da Huang Zhe Chong Wan* (Rhubarb and Eupolyphaga Pill), 937

8. 淋证 *LIN ZHENG* (DYSURIA SYNDROME)

Re lin (heat dysuria)

- *Ba Zheng San* (Eight-Herb Powder for Rectification), 1103

Qi lin (qi dysuria)

- *Bu Zhong Yi Qi Tang* (Tonify the Middle and Augment the Qi Decoction), 542

Xue lin (bloody dysuria)

- *Xiao Ji Yin Zi* (Cirsium Decoction), 946
- *Zhi Bai Di Huang Wan* (Anemarrhena, Phellodendron, and Rehmannia Pill), 636

Gao lin (cloudy dysuria)

- *Bi Xie Fen Qing Yin* (Dioscorea Hypoglauca Decoction to Separate the Clear), 1140
- *Liu Wei Di Huang Wan* (Six-Ingredient Pill with Rehmannia), 627

Lao lin (fatigue dysuria)

- *Bu Zhong Yi Qi Tang* (Tonify the Middle and Augment the Qi Decoction), 542
- *Zhi Bai Di Huang Wan* (Anemarrhena, Phellodendron, and Rehmannia Pill), 636

9. 梅核气 *MEI HE QI* (PLUM-PIT *QI*)

- *Ban Xia Hou Po Tang* (Pinellia and Magnolia Bark Decoction), 827
- *Er Chen Tang* (Two-Cured Decoction), 1209

10. 痿证 *WEI ZHENG* (ATROPHY SYNDROME)

Damp-heat

- *Er Miao San* (Two-Marvel Powder), 1188

Blood stasis blocking channels and collaterals

- *Sheng Yu Tang* (Sage-Like Healing Decoction), 567

Lung heat with damaged body fluids

- *Qing Zao Jiu Fei Tang* (Eliminate Dryness and Rescue the Lung Decoction), 1029
- *Sha Shen Mai Dong Tang* (Glehnia and Ophiopogonis Decoction), 1047

Spleen and Stomach deficiency and cold

- *Shen Ling Bai Zhu San* (Ginseng, Poria, and Atractylodes Macrocephala Powder), 535
- *Bu Zhong Yi Qi Tang* (Tonify the Middle and Augment the Qi Decoction), 542
- *Qiong Yu Gao* (Beautiful Jade Paste), 1041

Liver and Kidney deficiencies

- *Hu Qian Wan* (Hidden Tiger Pill), 651

11. 五心热 *WU XIN RE* (FIVE-CENTER HEAT)

Yin deficiency

- *Qing Gu San* (Cool the Bones Powder), 418

Blood deficiency

- *Si Wu Tang* (Four-Substance Decoction), 562 and *Di Gu Pi* (Cortex Lycii)

Deficiency heat in the *ying* (nutritive) level

- *Qing Hao Bie Jia Tang* (Artemisia Annua and Soft-Shelled Turtle Shell Decoction), 412

Stagnant fire with blocked circulation of yang qi

- *Sheng Yang San Huo Tang* (Raise the Yang and Disperse the Fire Decoction), 858

12. 消渴 *XIAO KE* (WASTING AND THIRSTING)

Upper *jiao*

- *Bai Hu Jia Ren Shen Tang* (White Tiger plus Ginseng Decoction), 325
- *Yu Quan Wan* (Jade Spring Pill), 1052
- *Yu Ye Tang* (Jade Fluid Decoction), 1049

Middle *jiao*

- *Yu Nu Jian* (Jade Woman Decoction), 398
- *Bai Hu Jia Ren Shen Tang* (White Tiger plus Ginseng Decoction), 325

Lower *jiao*

- *Liu Wei Di Huang Wan* (Six-Ingredient Pill with Rehmannia), 627

Appendix 1 — Cross-reference Based on Traditional Chinese Medicine Diagnosis

- *Jin Gui Shen Qi Wan* (Kidney Qi Pill from the Golden Cabinet), 668

13. 胸痹 *XIONG BI* (PAINFUL OBSTRUCTION OF THE CHEST)

Cold stagnation in the Heart channel
- *Dang Gui Si Ni Tang* (Tangkuei Decoction for Frigid Extremities), 494
- *Su He Xiang Wan* (Liquid Styrax Pill), 758

Heat and fire
- *Xiao Xian Xiong Tang* (Minor Sinking into the Chest Decoction), 1235

Qi stagnation
- *Chai Hu Shu Gan San* (Bupleurum Powder to Spread the Liver), 238
- *Si Ni San* (Frigid Extremities Powder), 233
- *Xiao Yao San* (Rambling Powder), 247

Blood stagnation
- *Xue Fu Zhu Yu Tang* (Drive Out Stasis in the Mansion of Blood Decoction), 879
- *Dan Shen Yin* (Salvia Decoction), 917

Phlegm stagnation
- *Gua Lou Xie Bai Ban Xia Tang* (Trichosanthes Fruit, Chinese Chive, and Pinellia Decoction), 832
- *Wen Dan Tang* (Warm the Gallbladder Decoction), 1213
- *Su He Xiang Wan* (Liquid Styrax Pill), 758

Heart qi deficiency
- *Bao Yuan Tang* (Preserve the Basal Decoction), 525
- *Gan Mai Da Zao Tang* (Licorice, Wheat, and Jujube Decoction), 731

Heart yin deficiency
- *Tian Wang Bu Xin Dan* (Emperor of Heaven's Special Pill to Tonify the Heart), 725
- *Suan Zao Ren Tang* (Sour Jujube Decoction), 722
- *Zhi Gan Cao Tang* (Honey-Fried Licorice Decoction), 589

Heart yang deficiency
- *Shen Fu Tang* (Ginseng and Prepared Aconite Decoction), 489

14. 虚劳 *XU LAO* (DEFICIENCY AND DEBILITATION)

Qi deficiency
- *Si Jun Zi Tang* (Four-Gentlemen Decoction), 522
- *Liu Jun Zi Tang* (Six-Gentlemen Decoction), 527
- *Shen Ling Bai Zhu San* (Ginseng, Poria, and Atractylodes Macrocephala Powder), 535
- *Bu Fei Tang* (Tonify the Lung Decoction), 560

Blood deficiency
- *Si Wu Tang* (Four-Substance Decoction), 562

- *Dang Gui Bu Xue Tang* (Tangkuei Decoction to Tonify the Blood), 580
- *Gui Pi Tang* (Restore the Spleen Decoction), 583

Yin deficiency
- *Liu Wei Di Huang Wan* (Six-Ingredient Pill with Rehmannia), 627
- *Zuo Gui Wan* (Restore the Left [Kidney] Pill), 645
- *Yi Guan Jian* (Linking Decoction), 657

Yang deficiency
- *Jin Gui Shen Qi Wan* (Kidney Qi Pill from the Golden Cabinet), 668
- *You Gui Wan* (Restore the Right [Kidney] Pill), 678
- *Huan Shao Dan* (Return to Youth Pill), 681

15. 血瘀 *XUE YU* (BLOOD STASIS)

In the head region
- *Tong Qiao Huo Xue Tang* (Unblock the Orifices and Invigorate the Blood Decoction), 877

In the upper *jiao*
- *Xue Fu Zhu Yu Tang* (Drive Out Stasis in the Mansion of Blood Decoction), 879

In the middle *jiao*
- *Ge Xia Zhu Yu Tang* (Drive Out Blood Stasis Below the Diaphragm Decoction), 885

In the lower *jiao*
- *Shao Fu Zhu Yu Tang* (Drive Out Blood Stasis in the Lower Abdomen Decoction), 889

Blocking the channels and collaterals
- *Shen Tong Zhu Yu Tang* (Drive Out Blood Stasis from a Painful Body Decoction), 893
- *Huo Luo Xiao Ling Dan* (Fantastically Effective Pill to Invigorate the Collaterals), 914

Blocking the blood vessels
- *Tao Hong Si Wu Tang* (Four-Substance Decoction with Safflower and Peach Pit), 571 and *Yang He Tang* (Yang-Heartening Decoction), 1370

16. 脏躁 *ZANG ZAO* (RESTLESS ORGAN)
- *Gan Mai Da Zao Tang* (Licorice, Wheat, and Jujube Decoction), 731

17. 中风 *ZHONG FENG* (WIND STROKE)

Affecting the channels and collaterals
- *Da Qin Jiao Tang* (Major Gentiana Macrophylla Decoction), 988
- *Qian Zheng San* (Lead to Symmetry Powder), 977
- *Zhen Gan Xi Feng Tang* (Sedate the Liver and Extinguish Wind Decoction), 999

Affecting the *zang fu* organs: *bi zheng* (closed disorder)
- *Zhi Bao Dan* (Greatest Treasure Special Pill), 749

1395

Appendix 1 – Cross-reference Based on Traditional Chinese Medicine Diagnosis

Appendix 1 — Cross-reference Based on Traditional Chinese Medicine Diagnosis

- *Su He Xiang Wan* (Liquid Styrax Pill), 758
- *Di Tan Tang* (Scour Phlegm Decoction), 1212

Affecting the *zang fu* organs: *tuo zheng* (abandoned syndrome)

- *Shen Fu Tang* (Ginseng and Prepared Aconite Decoction), 489

- *Di Huang Yin Zi* (Rehmannia Decoction), 693

Sequelae

- *Bu Yang Huan Wu Tang* (Tonify the Yang to Restore Five Decoction), 905
- *Di Huang Yin Zi* (Rehmannia Decoction), 693
- *Qian Zheng San* (Lead to Symmetry Powder), 977

Appendix 2

— Cross-reference Based on Western Medicine Diagnosis

1. Abdominal pain
2. Acid reflux
3. Acne
4. Adrenocortical insufficiency (Addison's disease)
5. Aldosteronism, primary
6. Allergy
7. Alopecia
8. Amenorrhea
9. Anemia, aplastic
10. Anemia, hemolytic
11. Anemia, iron deficiency
12. Angina
13. Anorexia
14. Aphonia
15. Appendicitis
16. Arrhythmia
17. Arthritis
18. Ascites
19. Asthma
20. Atherosclerosis
21. Bedwetting
22. Behcet's disease
23. Bell's palsy
24. Bleeding
25. Breast abscess
26. Bronchiectasis
27. Bronchitis
28. Cancer (colon and rectum)
29. Cancer (esophagus)
30. Cancer (liver)
31. Cancer (lung)
32. Cancer (pancreas)
33. Cancer (stomach)
34. Carbuncles
35. Cardiomyopathy, dilated
36. Cerebral embolism
37. Cerebral hemorrhage
38. Cerebral infarction
39. Cerebrovascular disease
40. Chemotherapy, support for
41. Chest pain
42. Cholecystitis
43. Cholelithiasis
44. Colitis, ulcerative
45. Coma

46. Common cold
47. Congestive heart failure
48. Conjunctivitis
49. Constipation
50. Convulsions
51. Coronary artery disease
52. Cough
53. Crohn's disease
54. Cystitis
55. Deafness
56. Delirium
57. Dementia
58. Depression
59. Dermatitis
60. Diabetes insipidus
61. Diabetes mellitus
62. Diarrhea
63. Diphtheria
64. Disseminated intravascular coagulation (DIC)
65. Dizziness
66. Dysentery
67. Dysmenorrhea
68. Dysuria
69. Eczema
70. Edema
71. Emphysema
72. Endocarditis, infective
73. Endometriosis
74. Enteritis
75. Enuresis
76. Epigastric pain
77. Erysipelas
78. Fever
79. Forgetfulness
80. Freckles
81. Frostbite
82. Furuncles
83. Gastrectasis
84. Gastritis, chronic
85. Gastroenteritis
86. Gastroptosis
87. Gingivitis
88. Glaucoma
89. Glomerulonephritis, acute
90. Glomerulonephritis, chronic

Appendix 2 — Cross-reference Based on Western Medicine Diagnosis

91. Goiter
92. Gonorrhea
93. Gout
94. Halitosis
95. Headache
96. Heat stroke
97. Hemiplegia
98. Hemorrhoids
99. Hepatitis
100. Hepato-cirrhosis
101. Hernial pain
102. Herpes
103. Hiccups
104. Hypercortisolism
105. Hyperlipidemia
106. Hypersomnia
107. Hypertension, primary
108. Hyperthyroidism
109. Hypochondriac pain
110. Hypotension
111. Hypothyroidism
112. Hysteromyoma
113. Impetigo
114. Impotence
115. Indigestion
116. Infection (upper respiratory tract)
117. Infertility, female
118. Infertility, male
119. Influenza
120. Insomnia
121. Intestinal abscess
122. Intestinal obstruction
123. Irritable bowel syndrome
124. Jaundice
125. Kyphosis
126. Laryngitis
127. Leukemia
128. Leukemia, granulocytic
129. Leukemia, lymphocytic
130. Leukopenia
131. Leukorrhea
132. Loss of voice
133. Low back pain
134. Lung abscess
135. Lung atrophy
136. Lung distention
137. Lymphadenitis
138. Lymphoma
139. Maculae and papules
140. Malaria
141. Mania

142. Mastitis
143. Meniere's disease
144. Menopause
145. Menstruation, early
146. Menstruation, irregular
147. Menstruation, late
148. Menstruation, prolonged
149. Migraine
150. Motion sickness
151. Myasthenia gravis
152. Myocardial infarction
153. Nausea
154. Nephrotic syndrome
155. Neurasthenia
156. Neuropathy
157. Neuritis
158. Neurosis
159. Nocturia
160. Numbness
161. Obesity
162. Osteoarthritis
163. Osteoporosis
164. Otitis media
165. Palpitations
166. Pancreatitis
167. Parasitic infestation
168. Parkinson's disease
169. Parotitis
170. Pelvic inflammatory disease
171. Peptic ulcer
172. Pericarditis
173. Perspiration
174. Pheochromocytoma
175. Pleuritis
176. Pneumonia
177. Pneumothorax
178. Poisoning, alcohol
179. Pregnancy
180. Pregnancy, postpartum care
181. Premenstrual syndrome (PMS)
182. Prostatitis
183. Psoriasis
184. Purpura, allergic
185. Purpura, thrombocytopenic
186. Pyelonephritis
187. Radiation, support for
188. Rash
189. Raynaud's syndrome
190. Rectal prolapse
191. Reflux esophagitis
192. Renal failure

Chinese Herbal Formulas and Applications

Appendix 2 — Cross-reference Based on Western Medicine Diagnosis

193. Restless fetus
194. Retinitis
195. Rheumatoid arthritis
196. Rhinitis
197. Rosacea
198. Schizophrenia
199. Sciatica
200. Scleroderma
201. Seizures and epilepsy
202. Sinusitis
203. Spermatorrhea
204. Stomatitis
205. Systemic lupus erythematosus
206. Testitis
207. Tetanus
208. Thirst
209. Thyroiditis
210. Tidal fever
211. Tinnitus
212. Tonsillitis

213. Toothache
214. Tracheobronchitis
215. Tracheitis
216. Transient ischemic attack (TIA)
217. Trauma
218. Tremor
219. Trigeminal neuralgia
220. Tuberculosis (intestine)
221. Tuberculosis (lung)
222. Tuberculosis (peritoneum)
223. Urethritis
224. Urinary incontinence
225. Urinary tract infection
226. Uroschesis
227. Uterine prolapse
228. Vascular dementia
229. Vertigo
230. Vision, blurred
231. Vomiting
232. Wheezing and dyspnea

1. ABDOMINAL PAIN

Cold
- *Liang Fu Wan* (Galangal and Cyperus Pill), 841
- *Da Huang Fu Zi Tang* (Rhubarb and Prepared Aconite Decoction), 166

Heat
- *Da Cheng Qi Tang* (Major Order the Qi Decoction), 152
- *Xiao Cheng Qi Tang* (Minor Order the Qi Decoction), 158

Deficiency and cold
- *Xiao Jian Zhong Tang* (Minor Construct the Middle Decoction), 471
- *Da Jian Zhong Tang* (Major Construct the Middle Decoction), 480
- *Fu Zi Li Zhong Wan* (Prepared Aconite Pill to Regulate the Middle), 463

Qi stagnation
- *Chai Hu Shu Gan San* (Bupleurum Powder to Spread the Liver), 238
- *Si Ni San* (Frigid Extremities Powder), 233

Blood stagnation
- *Shao Fu Zhu Yu Tang* (Drive Out Blood Stasis in the Lower Abdomen Decoction), 889

Food stagnation
- *Bao He Wan* (Preserve Harmony Pill), 1266
- *Zhi Shi Dao Zhi Wan* (Immature Bitter Orange Pill to Guide Out Stagnation), 1270

Parasites
- *Wu Mei Wan* (Mume Pill), 1292

2. ACID REFLUX

Heat
- *Zuo Jin Wan* (Left Metal Pill), 389

Cold
- *Xiang Sha Liu Jun Zi Tang* (Six-Gentlemen Decoction with Aucklandia and Amomum), 531

3. ACNE
- *Qing Shang Fang Feng Tang* (Clear the Upper and Guard the Wind Decoction), 349
- *Huang Lian Shang Qing Wan* (Coptis Pill to Clear the Upper), 347
- *Jing Jie Lian Qiao Tang* (Schizonepeta and Forsythia Decoction), 120
- *Shi Wei Bai Du Tang* (Ten-Ingredient Decoction to Overcome Pathogenic Influences), 1341
- *Wu Wei Xiao Du Yin* (Five-Ingredient Decoction to Eliminate Toxins), 1337

4. ADRENOCORTICAL INSUFFICIENCY (ADDISON'S DISEASE)

Qi deficiency
- *Shi Quan Da Bu Tang* (All-Inclusive Great Tonifying Decoction), 609

CROSS-REFERENCE BASED ON WESTERN MEDICINE DIAGNOSIS

A2

1399

Appendix 2 – Cross-reference Based on Western Medicine Diagnosis

Appendix 2 — Cross-reference Based on Western Medicine Diagnosis

Blood deficiency
- *Si Wu Tang* (Four-Substance Decoction), 562

Spleen and Kidney yang deficiencies
- *You Gui Wan* (Restore the Right [Kidney] Pill), 678
- *Fu Zi Li Zhong Wan* (Prepared Aconite Pill to Regulate the Middle), 463

Liver and Kidney yin deficiencies
- *Liu Wei Di Huang Wan* (Six-Ingredient Pill with Rehmannia), 627
- *Da Bu Yin Wan* (Great Tonify the Yin Pill), 649

5. ALDOSTERONISM, PRIMARY
Damp-heat
- *Er Miao San* (Two-Marvel Powder), 1188

Spleen and Stomach deficiencies
- *Shen Ling Bai Zhu San* (Ginseng, Poria, and Atractylodes Macrocephala Powder), 535

Liver and Kidney deficiencies
- *Liu Wei Di Huang Wan* (Six-Ingredient Pill with Rehmannia), 627

6. ALLERGY
- *Xin Yi San* (Magnolia Flower Powder), 84
- *Cang Er Zi San* (Xanthium Powder), 82
- *Xiao Feng San* (Eliminate Wind Powder), 967

7. ALOPECIA
- *Qi Bao Mei Ran Dan* (Seven-Treasure Special Pill for Beautiful Whiskers), 690
- *Shou Wu Pian* (Polygonum Pill), 692

8. AMENORRHEA
Kidney deficiency
- *Zuo Gui Wan* (Restore the Left [Kidney] Pill), 645

Spleen deficiency
- *Shen Ling Bai Zhu San* (Ginseng, Poria, and Atractylodes Macrocephala Powder), 535

Qi and blood stagnation
- *Ge Xia Zhu Yu Tang* (Drive Out Blood Stasis Below the Diaphragm Decoction), 885
- *Shao Fu Zhu Yu Tang* (Drive Out Blood Stasis in the Lower Abdomen Decoction), 889

Blood stagnation with cold
- *Wen Jing Tang* (Warm the Channels Decoction), 919

9. ANEMIA, APLASTIC
Heat in *ying* (nutritive) and *xue* (blood) levels
- *Xi Jiao Di Huang Tang* (Rhinoceros Horn and Rehmannia Decoction), 333
- *Qing Ying Tang* (Clear the Nutritive Level Decoction), 330

Qi and blood deficiencies
- *Sheng Yu Tang* (Sage-Like Healing Decoction), 567

Spleen and Kidney yang deficiencies
- *You Gui Wan* (Restore the Right [Kidney] Pill), 678

Liver and Kidney yin deficiencies
- *Zuo Gui Wan* (Restore the Left [Kidney] Pill), 645 and *Er Zhi Wan* (Two-Ultimate Pill), 654

10. ANEMIA, HEMOLYTIC
Damp-heat in the interior
- *Yin Chen Hao Tang* (Artemisia Scoparia Decoction), 1086

Qi and blood deficiencies
- *Gui Pi Tang* (Restore the Spleen Decoction), 583

Spleen and Kidney deficiencies
- *Shi Quan Da Bu Tang* (All-Inclusive Great Tonifying Decoction), 609

Qi and blood stagnation
- *Xue Fu Zhu Yu Tang* (Drive Out Stasis in the Mansion of Blood Decoction), 879

11. ANEMIA, IRON DEFICIENCY
Liver blood deficiency
- *Si Wu Tang* (Four-Substance Decoction), 562 and *Dang Gui Bu Xue Tang* (Tangkuei Decoction to Tonify the Blood), 580

Heart and Spleen deficiencies
- *Si Wu Tang* (Four-Substance Decoction), 562 and *Gui Pi Tang* (Restore the Spleen Decoction), 583

Spleen and Stomach deficiencies
- *Xiang Sha Liu Jun Zi Tang* (Six-Gentlemen Decoction with Aucklandia and Amomum), 531

Spleen and Kidney deficiencies
- *You Gui Wan* (Restore the Right [Kidney] Pill), 678

Blood stagnation
- *Tao Hong Si Wu Tang* (Four-Substance Decoction with Safflower and Peach Pit), 571

12. ANGINA
Cold stagnation in the Heart channel
- *Dang Gui Si Ni Tang* (Tangkuei Decoction for Frigid Extremities), 494

Qi stagnation
- *Chai Hu Shu Gan San* (Bupleurum Powder to Spread the Liver), 238

Phlegm stagnation
- *Gua Lou Xie Bai Ban Xia Tang* (Trichosanthes Fruit, Chinese Chive, and Pinellia Decoction), 832

Blood stagnation
- *Xue Fu Zhu Yu Tang* (Drive Out Stasis in the Mansion of Blood Decoction), 879

Chinese Herbal Formulas and Applications

Appendix 2 — Cross-reference Based on Western Medicine Diagnosis

Heart qi deficiency
- *Bao Yuan Tang* (Preserve the Basal Decoction), 525
- *Gan Mai Da Zao Tang* (Licorice, Wheat, and Jujube Decoction), 731

Heart yin deficiency
- *Tian Wang Bu Xin Dan* (Emperor of Heaven's Special Pill to Tonify the Heart), 725

Heart yang deficiency
- *Shen Fu Tang* (Ginseng and Prepared Aconite Decoction), 489

13. ANOREXIA
- *Bao He Wan* (Preserve Harmony Pill), 1266
- *Xiang Sha Liu Jun Zi Tang* (Six-Gentlemen Decoction with Aucklandia and Amomum), 531
- *Fei Er Wan* (Fat Child Pill), 1296

14. APHONIA
- *Xiang Sheng Po Di San* (Loud Sound Powder for a Broken Flute), 388
- *Bei Mu Gua Lou San* (Fritillaria and Trichosanthes Fruit Powder), 1240

15. APPENDICITIS
- *Da Huang Mu Dan Tang* (Rhubarb and Moutan Decoction), 1378
- *Da Cheng Qi Tang* (Major Order the Qi Decoction), 152

16. ARRHYTHMIA

Heart qi deficiency
- *Sheng Mai San* (Generate the Pulse Powder), 554

Heart yin deficiency
- *Tian Wang Bu Xin Dan* (Emperor of Heaven's Special Pill to Tonify the Heart), 725

Heart and Spleen deficiencies
- *Gui Pi Tang* (Restore the Spleen Decoction), 583

Liver and Kidney yin deficiencies
- *Yi Guan Jian* (Linking Decoction), 657 and *Suan Zao Ren Tang* (Sour Jujube Decoction), 722

Spleen and Kidney yang deficiencies
- *Li Zhong Tang* (Regulate the Middle Decoction), 462 and *Zhen Wu Tang* (True Warrior Decoction), 1135

Heart and Gallbladder deficiencies
- *Ding Zhi Wan* (Settle the Emotions Pill), 723

Heart yang deficiency
- *Gui Zhi Jia Long Gu Mu Li Tang* (Cinnamon Twig Decoction plus Dragon Bone and Oyster Shell), 798

Water and *yin* (invisible phlegm) accumulation affecting the Heart
- *Ling Gui Zhu Gan Tang* (Poria, Cinnamon Twig, Atractylodes Macrocephala, and Licorice Decoction), 1131

Blood stagnation
- *Xue Fu Zhu Yu Tang* (Drive Out Stasis in the Mansion of Blood Decoction), 879

17. ARTHRITIS

General
- *Juan Bi Tang* (Remove Painful Obstruction Decoction), 1158
- *San Bi Tang* (Three-Painful Obstruction Decoction), 1167
- *Shang Zhong Xia Tong Yong Tong Feng Wan* (Upper, Middle, and Lower General Use Pill for Wind-Pain), 1175

Neck
- *Ge Gen Tang* (Kudzu Decoction), 59
- *Er Zhu Tang* (Two-Atractylodes Decoction), 1195

Shoulder
- *Ge Gen Tang* (Kudzu Decoction), 59
- *Wu Yao Shun Qi San* (Lindera Powder to Smooth the Flow of Qi), 990

Back
- *Du Huo Ji Sheng Tang* (Angelica Pubescens and Taxillus Decoction), 1161
- *Huan Shao Dan* (Return to Youth Pill), 681

Limbs
- *Shu Jing Huo Xue Tang* (Relax the Channels and Invigorate the Blood Decoction), 1169
- *Shu Jin Li An San* (Relax the Tendons and Instill Peace Powder), 1171

Joints
- *Dang Gui Nian Tong Tang* (Tangkuei Decoction to Lift the Pain), 1191
- *Ma Xing Yi Gan Tang* (Ephedra, Apricot Kernel, Coicis, and Licorice Decoction), 43
- *Yi Yi Ren Tang* (Coicis Decoction), 1173
- *Yue Bi Jia Zhu Tang* (Maidservant from Yue Decoction plus Atractylodes), 102
- *Gui Zhi Shao Yao Zhi Mu Tang* (Cinnamon Twig, Peony, and Anemarrhena Decoction), 1186

18. ASCITES
- *Shi Zao Tang* (Ten-Jujube Decoction), 181
- *Zhou Che Wan* (Vessel and Vehicle Pill), 184
- *Shu Zao Yin Zi* (Spread and Unblock Decoction), 185

CROSS-REFERENCE BASED ON WESTERN MEDICINE DIAGNOSIS

A2

1401

Appendix 2 – Cross-reference Based on Western Medicine Diagnosis

Appendix 2 — Cross-reference Based on Western Medicine Diagnosis

19. ASTHMA
Cold
- *She Gan Ma Huang Tang* (Belamcanda and Ephedra Decoction), 80
- *Xiao Qing Long Tang* (Minor Bluegreen Dragon Decoction), 74
- *Su Zi Jiang Qi Tang* (Perilla Fruit Decoction for Directing Qi Downward), 842

Heat
- *Ding Chuan Tang* (Arrest Wheezing Decoction), 845
- *Ma Huang Xing Ren Gan Cao Shi Gao Tang* (Ephedra, Apricot Kernel, Licorice, and Gypsum Decoction), 96
- *San Zi Yang Qin Tang* (Three-Seed Decoction to Nourish One's Parents), 1245

Lung deficiency
- *Yu Ping Feng San* (Jade Windscreen Powder), 773

Spleen deficiency
- *Liu Jun Zi Tang* (Six-Gentlemen Decoction), 527
- *Shen Ling Bai Zhu San* (Ginseng, Poria, and Atractylodes Macrocephala Powder), 535

Kidney deficiency
- *Jin Gui Shen Qi Wan* (Kidney Qi Pill from the Golden Cabinet), 668
- *Du Qi Wan* (Capital Qi Pill), 644
- *Ren Shen Ge Jie San* (Ginseng and Gecko Powder), 557

20. ATHEROSCLEROSIS
Phlegm obstruction
- *Dao Tan Tang* (Guide Out Phlegm Decoction), 1211
- *Gua Lou Xie Bai Ban Xia Tang* (Trichosanthes Fruit, Chinese Chive, and Pinellia Decoction), 832

Qi and blood stagnation
- *Xue Fu Zhu Yu Tang* (Drive Out Stasis in the Mansion of Blood Decoction), 879
- *Tao Hong Si Wu Tang* (Four-Substance Decoction with Safflower and Peach Pit), 571
- *Dan Shen Yin* (Salvia Decoction), 917

Liver and Kidney deficiencies
- *Liu Wei Di Huang Wan* (Six-Ingredient Pill with Rehmannia), 627
- *Jin Gui Shen Qi Wan* (Kidney Qi Pill from the Golden Cabinet), 668

21. BEDWETTING
Lung and Spleen qi deficiencies
- *Bu Zhong Yi Qi Tang* (Tonify the Middle and Augment the Qi Decoction), 542

Heart and Kidney disharmony
- *Sang Piao Xiao San* (Mantis Egg-Case Powder), 792

Damp-heat
- *Ba Zheng San* (Eight-Herb Powder for Rectification), 1103

Blood stagnation
- *Shao Fu Zhu Yu Tang* (Drive Out Blood Stasis in the Lower Abdomen Decoction), 889

22. BEHCET'S DISEASE
Damp-heat
- *Long Dan Xie Gan Tang* (Gentiana Decoction to Drain the Liver), 371

Yin-deficient heat
- *Zhi Bai Di Huang Wan* (Anemarrhena, Phellodendron, and Rehmannia Pill), 636

Spleen and Kidney yang deficiencies
- *Bu Zhong Yi Qi Tang* (Tonify the Middle and Augment the Qi Decoction), 542 and *Jin Gui Shen Qi Wan* (Kidney Qi Pill from the Golden Cabinet), 668

23. BELL'S PALSY
Wind-cold affecting the channels and collaterals
- *Xiao Xu Ming Tang* (Minor Prolong Life Decoction), 983

Wind-heat affecting the channels and collaterals
- *Da Qin Jiao Tang* (Major Gentiana Macrophylla Decoction), 988

Wind-damp obstructing the channels and collaterals
- *Qian Zheng San* (Lead to Symmetry Powder), 977

Qi deficiency and blood stagnation
- *Bu Yang Huan Wu Tang* (Tonify the Yang to Restore Five Decoction), 905

24. BLEEDING
Hemoptysis
- *Sang Xing Tang* (Mulberry Leaf and Apricot Kernel Decoction), 1027
- *Xie Bai San* (Drain the White Powder), 383
- *Bai He Gu Jin Tang* (Lily Bulb Decoction to Preserve the Metal), 1036

Epistaxis
- *Sang Ju Yin* (Mulberry Leaf and Chrysanthemum Decoction), 89
- *Yu Nu Jian* (Jade Woman Decoction), 398
- *Long Dan Xie Gan Tang* (Gentiana Decoction to Drain the Liver), 371

Gum bleeding
- *Qing Wei San* (Clear the Stomach Powder), 393 and *San Huang Xie Xin Tang* (Three-Yellow Decoction to Sedate the Epigastrium), 359
- *Yu Nu Jian* (Jade Woman Decoction), 398

1402

Chinese Herbal Formulas and Applications

Appendix 2 — Cross-reference Based on Western Medicine Diagnosis

Hematemesis
- *San Huang Xie Xin Tang* (Three-Yellow Decoction to Sedate the Epigastrium), 359 and *Shi Hui San* (Ten Partially-Charred Substances Powder), 939
- *Long Dan Xie Gan Tang* (Gentiana Decoction to Drain the Liver), 371

Hematochezia
- *Huang Tu Tang* (Yellow Earth Decoction), 948
- *Huai Hua San* (Sophora Japonica Flower Powder), 944

Hematuria
- *Xiao Ji Yin Zi* (Cirsium Decoction), 946
- *Dao Chi San* (Guide Out the Red Powder), 365

Subcutaneous bleeding
- *Shi Hui San* (Ten Partially-Charred Substances Powder), 939
- *Gui Pi Tang* (Restore the Spleen Decoction), 583

25. BREAST ABSCESS
- *Yi Yi Ren Tang* (Coicis Decoction), 1383
- *Pai Nong San* (Drain the Pus Powder), 1364
- *Shi Liu Wei Liu Qi Yin* (Sixteen-Ingredient Decoction to Flow Qi), 1360
- *Tuo Li Xiao Du Yin* (Drain the Interior and Detoxify Decoction), 1367
- *Xian Fang Huo Ming Yin* (Sublime Formula for Sustaining Life), 1325

26. BRONCHIECTASIS
Wind-heat affecting the Lung
- *Sang Ju Yin* (Mulberry Leaf and Chrysanthemum Decoction), 89

Liver fire affecting the Lung
- *Xie Bai San* (Drain the White Powder), 383

Phlegm and heat affecting the Lung
- *Wei Jing Tang* (Reed Decoction), 1377 and *Xiao Xian Xiong Tang* (Minor Sinking into the Chest Decoction), 1235

Yin deficiency and dryness affecting the Lung
- *Bai He Gu Jin Tang* (Lily Bulb Decoction to Preserve the Metal), 1036
- *Mai Men Dong Tang* (Ophiopogonis Decoction), 1043

27. BRONCHITIS
Damp and phlegm
- *Er Chen Tang* (Two-Cured Decoction), 1209 and *San Zi Yang Qin Tang* (Three-Seed Decoction to Nourish One's Parents), 1245

Cold phlegm in the Lung
- *Xiao Qing Long Tang* (Minor Bluegreen Dragon Decoction), 74

Wind and phlegm affecting the Lung
- *Zhi Sou San* (Stop Coughing Powder), 116

Hot phlegm in the Lung
- *Qing Qi Hua Tan Wan* (Clear the Qi and Transform Phlegm Pill), 1222

Lung qi deficiency
- *Bu Fei Tang* (Tonify the Lung Decoction), 560

Lung and Spleen qi deficiencies
- *Liu Jun Zi Tang* (Six-Gentlemen Decoction), 527

Spleen and Kidney yang deficiencies
- *Si Jun Zi Tang* (Four-Gentlemen Decoction), 522 and *Du Qi Wan* (Capital Qi Pill), 644

28. CANCER (COLON AND RECTUM)
Damp-heat
- *Qing Chang Yin* (Clear the Intestines Drink), 1381 and *Huai Hua San* (Sophora Japonica Flower Powder), 944

Spleen and Kidney yang deficiencies
- *Fu Zi Li Zhong Wan* (Prepared Aconite Pill to Regulate the Middle), 463 and *Si Shen Wan* (Four-Miracle Pill), 784

Qi and blood deficiencies
- *Ba Zhen Tang* (Eight-Treasure Decoction), 604 and *Dang Gui Bu Xue Tang* (Tangkuei Decoction to Tonify the Blood), 580

Liver and Kidney yin deficiencies
- *Zhi Bai Di Huang Wan* (Anemarrhena, Phellodendron, and Rehmannia Pill), 636

29. CANCER (ESOPHAGUS)
Qi and phlegm stagnation
- *Xuan Fu Dai Zhe Shi Tang* (Inula and Hematite Decoction), 851

Heat and toxins damaging yin
- *Sha Shen Mai Dong Tang* (Glehnia and Ophiopogonis Decoction), 1047
- *Mai Men Dong Tang* (Ophiopogonis Decoction), 1043

Qi and blood deficiencies
- *Ba Zhen Tang* (Eight-Treasure Decoction), 604

30. CANCER (LIVER)
Spleen qi deficiency
- *Liu Jun Zi Tang* (Six-Gentlemen Decoction), 527

Qi and blood stagnation
- *Xiao Yao San* (Rambling Powder), 247 and *Tao Hong Si Wu Tang* (Four-Substance Decoction with Safflower and Peach Pit), 571

CROSS-REFERENCE BASED ON WESTERN MEDICINE DIAGNOSIS

A2

1403

Appendix 2 – Cross-reference Based on Western Medicine Diagnosis

Appendix 2 — Cross-reference Based on Western Medicine Diagnosis

Blood stagnation with accumulation of dampness, heat and toxins

- *Yin Chen Hao Tang* (Artemisia Scoparia Decoction), 1086 and *Ge Xia Zhu Yu Tang* (Drive Out Blood Stasis Below the Diaphragm Decoction), 885

Heat and toxins damaging yin

- *Xi Jiao Di Huang Tang* (Rhinoceros Horn and Rehmannia Decoction), 333

Liver and Kidney yin deficiencies

- *Zhi Bai Di Huang Wan* (Anemarrhena, Phellodendron, and Rehmannia Pill), 636

31. CANCER (LUNG)

Qi and blood stagnation

- *Xue Fu Zhu Yu Tang* (Drive Out Stasis in the Mansion of Blood Decoction), 879

Accumulation of dampness, phlegm and toxins

- *Dao Tan Tang* (Guide Out Phlegm Decoction), 1211
- *Ting Li Da Zao Xie Fei Tang* (Descurainia and Jujube Decoction to Drain the Lung), 384

Lung and Spleen qi deficiencies

- *Liu Jun Zi Tang* (Six-Gentlemen Decoction), 527
- *Bu Zhong Yi Qi Tang* (Tonify the Middle and Augment the Qi Decoction), 542

Lung and Kidney yin deficiencies

- *Bai He Gu Jin Tang* (Lily Bulb Decoction to Preserve the Metal), 1036
- *Liu Wei Di Huang Wan* (Six-Ingredient Pill with Rehmannia), 627

Qi and yin deficiencies

- *Sheng Mai San* (Generate the Pulse Powder), 554

32. CANCER (PANCREAS)

Liver and Stomach disharmony

- *Chai Hu Shu Gan San* (Bupleurum Powder to Spread the Liver), 238 and *Xuan Fu Dai Zhe Shi Tang* (Inula and Hematite Decoction), 851

Qi and blood stagnation

- *Ge Xia Zhu Yu Tang* (Drive Out Blood Stasis Below the Diaphragm Decoction), 885

Qi and blood deficiencies

- *Shi Quan Da Bu Tang* (All-Inclusive Great Tonifying Decoction), 609

Yin-deficient heat

- *Yi Guan Jian* (Linking Decoction), 657 and *Gan Lu Yin* (Sweet Dew Decoction), 401

33. CANCER (STOMACH)

Liver and Stomach disharmony

- *Chai Hu Shu Gan San* (Bupleurum Powder to Spread the Liver), 238 and *Xuan Fu Dai Zhe Shi Tang* (Inula and Hematite Decoction), 851

Stomach heat

- *Qing Wei San* (Clear the Stomach Powder), 393

Food and phlegm stagnation

- *Hai Zao Yu Hu Tang* (Sargassum Decoction for the Jade Flask), 1352
- *Bao He Wan* (Preserve Harmony Pill), 1266

Blood and phlegm stagnation

- *Ge Xia Zhu Yu Tang* (Drive Out Blood Stasis Below the Diaphragm Decoction), 885

Spleen and Stomach deficiency and cold

- *Huang Qi Jian Zhong Tang* (Astragalus Decoction to Construct the Middle), 475

Qi and blood deficiencies

- *Ba Zhen Tang* (Eight-Treasure Decoction), 604

34. CARBUNCLES

- *Wu Wei Xiao Du Yin* (Five-Ingredient Decoction to Eliminate Toxins), 1337
- *Shi Wei Bai Du Tang* (Ten-Ingredient Decoction to Overcome Pathogenic Influences), 1341
- *Tou Nong San* (Discharge Pus Powder), 1362
- *Niu Bang Jie Ji Tang* (Arctium Decoction to Release the Muscle Layer), 1332
- *Xian Fang Huo Ming Yin* (Sublime Formula for Sustaining Life), 1325

35. CARDIOMYOPATHY, DILATED

Heart toxins

- *Yin Qiao San* (Honeysuckle and Forsythia Powder), 92

Blood stagnation with Heart qi deficiency

- *Sheng Yu Tang* (Sage-Like Healing Decoction), 567 and *Tao Hong Si Wu Tang* (Four-Substance Decoction with Safflower and Peach Pit), 571

Yang deficiency with water accumulation

- *Zhen Wu Tang* (True Warrior Decoction), 1135

36. CEREBRAL EMBOLISM

Wind, phlegm and fire rising

- *Tian Ma Gou Teng Yin* (Gastrodia and Uncaria Decoction), 1004

Qi deficiency with blood stagnation

- *Bu Yang Huan Wu Tang* (Tonify the Yang to Restore Five Decoction), 905

1404

Chinese Herbal Formulas and Applications

Appendix 2 — Cross-reference Based on Western Medicine Diagnosis

Liver wind rising with phlegm obstructing sensory orifices
* *Su He Xiang Wan* (Liquid Styrax Pill), 758

37. CEREBRAL HEMORRHAGE
Affecting the channels and collaterals
* *Da Qin Jiao Tang* (Major Gentiana Macrophylla Decoction), 988
* *Zhen Gan Xi Feng Tang* (Sedate the Liver and Extinguish Wind Decoction), 999

Affecting the *zang fu* organs – *bi zheng* (closed disorder)
* *Zhi Bao Dan* (Greatest Treasure Special Pill), 749
* *Su He Xiang Wan* (Liquid Styrax Pill), 758

Affecting the *zang fu* organs – *tuo zheng* (abandoned syndrome)
* *Shen Fu Tang* (Ginseng and Prepared Aconite Decoction), 489 and *Sheng Mai San* (Generate the Pulse Powder), 554

38. CEREBRAL INFARCTION
Wind, phlegm and fire rising
* *Tian Ma Gou Teng Yin* (Gastrodia and Uncaria Decoction), 1004

Qi deficiency with blood stagnation
* *Bu Yang Huan Wu Tang* (Tonify the Yang to Restore Five Decoction), 905

Liver wind rising with yin deficiency
* *Zhen Gan Xi Feng Tang* (Sedate the Liver and Extinguish Wind Decoction), 999

Wind attacking the channels and collaterals
* *Da Qin Jiao Tang* (Major Gentiana Macrophylla Decoction), 988

Liver wind rising with phlegm obstructing sensory orifices
* *Su He Xiang Wan* (Liquid Styrax Pill), 758 and *Di Tan Tang* (Scour Phlegm Decoction), 1212

39. CEREBROVASCULAR DISEASE
Liver wind rising with Liver and Kidney yin deficiencies
* *Tian Ma Gou Teng Yin* (Gastrodia and Uncaria Decoction), 1004

Wind and phlegm rising with Liver and Kidney yin deficiencies
* *Su He Xiang Wan* (Liquid Styrax Pill), 758
* *Di Tan Tang* (Scour Phlegm Decoction), 1212

Qi deficiency with blood stagnation blocking the channels and collaterals
* *Bu Yang Huan Wu Tang* (Tonify the Yang to Restore Five Decoction), 905

40. CHEMOTHERAPY, SUPPORT FOR
* *Shi Quan Da Bu Tang* (All-Inclusive Great Tonifying Decoction), 609
* *Bu Zhong Yi Qi Tang* (Tonify the Middle and Augment the Qi Decoction), 542
* *Ba Zhen Tang* (Eight-Treasure Decoction), 604

41. CHEST PAIN
Qi stagnation
* *Si Ni San* (Frigid Extremities Powder), 233

Blood stagnation
* *Xue Fu Zhu Yu Tang* (Drive Out Stasis in the Mansion of Blood Decoction), 879

Cold stagnation
* *Si Ni Tang* (Frigid Extremities Decoction), 486

Heat and phlegm obstruction
* *Xiao Xian Xiong Tang* (Minor Sinking into the Chest Decoction), 1235
* *Gua Lou Xie Bai Ban Xia Tang* (Trichosanthes Fruit, Chinese Chive, and Pinellia Decoction), 832

42. CHOLECYSTITIS
Liver and Gallbladder qi stagnation
* *Xiao Chai Hu Tang* (Minor Bupleurum Decoction), 206
* *Da Chai Hu Tang* (Major Bupleurum Decoction), 283

Liver and Gallbladder blood stagnation
* *Fu Yuan Huo Xue Tang* (Revive Health by Invigorating the Blood Decoction), 897
* *Ge Xia Zhu Yu Tang* (Drive Out Blood Stasis Below the Diaphragm Decoction), 885

Liver and Gallbladder damp-heat
* *Long Dan Xie Gan Tang* (Gentiana Decoction to Drain the Liver), 371

Heat and toxins in the Liver
* *Yin Chen Hao Tang* (Artemisia Scoparia Decoction), 1086 and *Huang Lian Jie Du Tang* (Coptis Decoction to Relieve Toxicity), 341

43. CHOLELITHIASIS
Liver and Gallbladder qi stagnation
* *Da Chai Hu Tang* (Major Bupleurum Decoction), 283

Liver and Gallbladder blood stagnation
* *Ge Xia Zhu Yu Tang* (Drive Out Blood Stasis Below the Diaphragm Decoction), 885

Liver and Gallbladder damp-heat
* *Long Dan Xie Gan Tang* (Gentiana Decoction to Drain the Liver), 371

CROSS-REFERENCE BASED ON WESTERN MEDICINE DIAGNOSIS

A2

1405

Appendix 2 – Cross-reference Based on Western Medicine Diagnosis

Appendix 2 — Cross-reference Based on Western Medicine Diagnosis

Heat and toxins in the Liver
- *Yin Chen Hao Tang* (Artemisia Scoparia Decoction), 1086 and *Huang Lian Jie Du Tang* (Coptis Decoction to Relieve Toxicity), 341

44. COLITIS, ULCERATIVE
Damp-heat accumulation
- *Bai Tou Weng Tang* (Pulsatilla Decoction), 408

Spleen deficiency with dampness
- *Shen Ling Bai Zhu San* (Ginseng, Poria, and Atractylodes Macrocephala Powder), 535
- *Bu Zhong Yi Qi Tang* (Tonify the Middle and Augment the Qi Decoction), 542

Spleen and Kidney yang deficiencies
- *Si Shen Wan* (Four-Miracle Pill), 784

Liver qi stagnation and Spleen deficiency
- *Tong Xie Yao Fang* (Important Formula for Painful Diarrhea), 257

Blood stagnation
- *Ge Xia Zhu Yu Tang* (Drive Out Blood Stasis Below the Diaphragm Decoction), 885

45. COMA
Bi zheng (closed disorder)
- *Zhi Bao Dan* (Greatest Treasure Special Pill), 749
- *Zi Xue* (Purple Snow), 752
- *An Gong Niu Huang Wan* (Calm the Palace Pill with Cattle Gallstone), 746
- *Ling Jiao Gou Teng Tang* (Antelope Horn and Uncaria Decoction), 993
- *Su He Xiang Wan* (Liquid Styrax Pill), 758

Tuo zheng (abandoned syndrome)
- *Sheng Mai San* (Generate the Pulse Powder), 554
- *Shen Fu Tang* (Ginseng and Prepared Aconite Decoction), 489
- *Di Huang Yin Zi* (Rehmannia Decoction), 693

46. COMMON COLD
Wind-cold
- *Cong Chi Tang* (Scallion and Prepared Soybean Decoction), 112
- *Jing Fang Bai Du San* (Schizonepeta and Saposhnikovia Powder to Overcome Pathogenic Influences), 1334
- *Qiang Huo Sheng Shi Tang* (Notopterygium Decoction to Overcome Dampness), 1156
- *Xing Su San* (Apricot Kernel and Perilla Leaf Powder), 1025

Wind-heat
- *Yin Qiao San* (Honeysuckle and Forsythia Powder), 92
- *Xiang Ru San* (Mosla Powder), 436

- *Sang Xing Tang* (Mulberry Leaf and Apricot Kernel Decoction), 1027

Summer-heat
- *Xin Jia Xiang Ru Yin* (Newly-Augmented Mosla Decoction), 439

Exterior wind with interior deficiency
- *Shen Su Yin* (Ginseng and Perilla Leaf Decoction), 128
- *Bai Du San* (Overcome Pathogenic Influences Powder), 124
- *Cong Bai Qi Wei Yin* (Scallion Decoction with Seven Ingredients), 135
- *Jia Jian Wei Rui Tang* (Modified Polygonatum Odoratum Decoction), 137

47. CONGESTIVE HEART FAILURE
Heart and Lung qi deficiencies with phlegm and blood stagnation
- *Sheng Yu Tang* (Sage-Like Healing Decoction), 567 and *Xiao Xian Xiong Tang* (Minor Sinking into the Chest Decoction), 1235

Heart and Kidney yang deficiencies with phlegm accumulation
- *Shen Fu Tang* (Ginseng and Prepared Aconite Decoction), 489 and *Ting Li Da Zao Xie Fei Tang* (Descurainia and Jujube Decoction to Drain the Lung), 384

Heart and Kidney yang deficiencies with water accumulation
- *Zhen Wu Tang* (True Warrior Decoction), 1135 and *Wu Ling San* (Five-Ingredient Powder with Poria), 1109

48. CONJUNCTIVITIS
- *Xi Gan Ming Mu San* (Wash the Liver and Brighten the Eyes Powder), 381
- *Yue Bi Jia Zhu Tang* (Maidservant from Yue Decoction plus Atractylodes), 102
- *San Huang Xie Xin Tang* (Three-Yellow Decoction to Sedate the Epigastrium), 359
- *Qing Shang Fang Feng Tang* (Clear the Upper and Guard the Wind Decoction), 349
- *Long Dan Xie Gan Tang* (Gentiana Decoction to Drain the Liver), 371

49. CONSTIPATION
Excess
- *Da Cheng Qi Tang* (Major Order the Qi Decoction), 152
- *Xiao Cheng Qi Tang* (Minor Order the Qi Decoction), 158
- *Tiao Wei Cheng Qi Tang* (Regulate the Stomach and Order the Qi Decoction), 160
- *Da Huang Fu Zi Tang* (Rhubarb and Prepared Aconite Decoction), 166

1406

Chinese Herbal Formulas and Applications

Appendix 2 — Cross-reference Based on Western Medicine Diagnosis

Deficiency
- *Ma Zi Ren Wan* (Hemp Seed Pill), 174
- *Run Chang Wan* (Moisten the Intestines Pill), 177
- *Ji Chuan Jian* (Benefit the River [Flow] Decoction), 179
- *Zeng Ye Tang* (Increase the Fluids Decoction), 1054

50. CONVULSIONS
Exterior wind
- *Qiang Huo Sheng Shi Tang* (Notopterygium Decoction to Overcome Dampness), 1156

Liver wind rising with heat
- *Ling Jiao Gou Teng Tang* (Antelope Horn and Uncaria Decoction), 993

Liver yang and wind rising
- *Zeng Ye Cheng Qi Tang* (Increase the Fluids and Order the Qi Decoction), 190

Yin deficiency with Liver wind rising
- *San Jia Fu Mai Tang* (Three-Shell Decoction to Restore the Pulse), 1011

Wind and phlegm affecting the channels and collaterals
- *Di Tan Tang* (Scour Phlegm Decoction), 1212

Heat in *ying* (nutritive) level
- *Qing Ying Tang* (Clear the Nutritive Level Decoction), 330

Blood stagnation
- *Tong Qiao Huo Xue Tang* (Unblock the Orifices and Invigorate the Blood Decoction), 877

Qi and blood deficiencies
- *Ba Zhen Tang* (Eight-Treasure Decoction), 604

Wind and toxins attacking the channels and collaterals
- *Yu Zhen San* (True Jade Powder), 981
- *Wu Hu Zhui Feng San* (Five-Tiger Powder to Pursue Wind), 982

51. CORONARY ARTERY DISEASE
Yang qi obstruction
- *Gua Lou Xie Bai Ban Xia Tang* (Trichosanthes Fruit, Chinese Chive, and Pinellia Decoction), 832

Blood stagnation
- *Tao Hong Si Wu Tang* (Four-Substance Decoction with Safflower and Peach Pit), 571
- *Xue Fu Zhu Yu Tang* (Drive Out Stasis in the Mansion of Blood Decoction), 879

Qi and yin deficiencies
- *Sheng Mai San* (Generate the Pulse Powder), 554

52. COUGH
Wind-cold
- *Xing Su San* (Apricot Kernel and Perilla Leaf Powder), 1025

- *San Ao Tang* (Three-Unbinding Decoction), 43
- *Jin Fei Cao San* (Inula Powder), 49

Wind-heat
- *Sang Ju Yin* (Mulberry Leaf and Chrysanthemum Decoction), 89
- *Ning Sou Wan* (Quiet the Cough Pill), 113

Dry-heat
- *Sang Xing Tang* (Mulberry Leaf and Apricot Kernel Decoction), 1027
- *Zhi Sou San* (Stop Coughing Powder), 116

Heat and fire
- *Liang Ge San* (Cool the Diaphragm Powder), 351

Phlegm in the Lung
- *Er Chen Tang* (Two-Cured Decoction), 1209
- *San Zi Yang Qin Tang* (Three-Seed Decoction to Nourish One's Parents), 1245

Lung deficiency
- *Sha Shen Mai Dong Tang* (Glehnia and Ophiopogonis Decoction), 1047
- *Ren Shen Ge Jie San* (Ginseng and Gecko Powder), 557

Lung heat
- *Dun Sou San* (Long-Bout Cough Powder), 115

53. CROHN'S DISEASE
Damp-cold affecting the Spleen
- *Wei Ling Tang* (Calm the Stomach and Poria Decoction), 1113

Damp-heat affecting the Spleen and Stomach
- *Ge Gen Huang Qin Huang Lian Tang* (Kudzu, Coptis, and Scutellaria Decoction), 295

Toxic heat affecting the Intestines
- *Wu Wei Xiao Du Yin* (Five-Ingredient Decoction to Eliminate Toxins), 1337 and *Xiao Cheng Qi Tang* (Minor Order the Qi Decoction), 158

Blood stagnation affecting the Intestines
- *Xue Fu Zhu Yu Tang* (Drive Out Stasis in the Mansion of Blood Decoction), 879

Spleen deficiency with qi sinking downwards
- *Bu Zhong Yi Qi Tang* (Tonify the Middle and Augment the Qi Decoction), 542

54. CYSTITIS
- *Ba Zheng San* (Eight-Herb Powder for Rectification), 1103
- *Long Dan Xie Gan Tang* (Gentiana Decoction to Drain the Liver), 371

55. DEAFNESS
- *Ci Zhu Wan* (Magnetite and Cinnabar Pill), 714
- *Er Long Zuo Ci Wan* (Pill for Deafness that Is Kind to the Left [Kidney]), 633

CROSS-REFERENCE BASED ON WESTERN MEDICINE DIAGNOSIS

A2

1407

Appendix 2 – Cross-reference Based on Western Medicine Diagnosis

Appendix 2 — Cross-reference Based on Western Medicine Diagnosis

- *Tong Qiao Huo Xue Tang* (Unblock the Orifices and Invigorate the Blood Decoction), 877
- *Qi Ju Di Huang Wan* (Lycium Fruit, Chrysanthemum, and Rehmannia Pill), 640

56. DELIRIUM

- *Chai Hu Jia Long Gu Mu Li Tang* (Bupleurum plus Dragon Bone and Oyster Shell Decoction), 715
- *An Gong Niu Huang Wan* (Calm the Palace Pill with Cattle Gallstone), 746
- *Zi Xue* (Purple Snow), 752
- *Xi Jiao Di Huang Tang* (Rhinoceros Horn and Rehmannia Decoction), 333

57. DEMENTIA

Spleen and Kidney deficiencies
- *Huan Shao Dan* (Return to Youth Pill), 681

Liver and Kidney yin deficiencies
- *Zhi Bai Di Huang Wan* (Anemarrhena, Phellodendron, and Rehmannia Pill), 636

Blood stagnation
- *Tong Qiao Huo Xue Tang* (Unblock the Orifices and Invigorate the Blood Decoction), 877

58. DEPRESSION

Liver qi stagnation
- *Chai Hu Shu Gan San* (Bupleurum Powder to Spread the Liver), 238
- *Yue Ju Wan* (Escape Restraint Pill), 822
- *Xiao Yao San* (Rambling Powder), 247

Liver heat and fire rising
- *Jia Wei Xiao Yao San* (Augmented Rambling Powder), 254
- *Zuo Jin Wan* (Left Metal Pill), 389

Qi and phlegm stagnation
- *Ban Xia Hou Po Tang* (Pinellia and Magnolia Bark Decoction), 827
- *Wen Dan Tang* (Warm the Gallbladder Decoction), 1213

Blood stagnation
- *Xue Fu Zhu Yu Tang* (Drive Out Stasis in the Mansion of Blood Decoction), 879

Deficiency
- *Gan Mai Da Zao Tang* (Licorice, Wheat, and Jujube Decoction), 731
- *Gui Pi Tang* (Restore the Spleen Decoction), 583
- *Tian Wang Bu Xin Dan* (Emperor of Heaven's Special Pill to Tonify the Heart), 725
- *Qi Ju Di Huang Wan* (Lycium Fruit, Chrysanthemum, and Rehmannia Pill), 640

59. DERMATITIS

Heat and toxins affecting the skin
- *Wu Wei Xiao Du Yin* (Five-Ingredient Decoction to Eliminate Toxins), 1337

Damp-cold blocking the channels and collaterals
- *Yang He Tang* (Yang-Heartening Decoction), 1370

Dampness and phlegm blocking the channels and collaterals
- *Er Miao San* (Two-Marvel Powder), 1188

Qi and blood deficiencies
- *Ba Zhen Tang* (Eight-Treasure Decoction), 604

Spleen and Kidney yang deficiencies
- *Jin Gui Shen Qi Wan* (Kidney Qi Pill from the Golden Cabinet), 668

Liver and Kidney yin deficiencies
- *Mai Wei Di Huang Wan* (Ophiopogonis, Schisandra and Rehmannia Pill), 642

60. DIABETES INSIPIDUS

Lung and Stomach yin deficiencies
- *Bai Hu Jia Ren Shen Tang* (White Tiger plus Ginseng Decoction), 325

Lung and Kidney yin deficiencies
- *Sha Shen Mai Dong Tang* (Glehnia and Ophiopogonis Decoction), 1047

Qi and body fluid deficiencies
- *Sheng Mai San* (Generate the Pulse Powder), 554

Kidney yin deficiency
- *Liu Wei Di Huang Wan* (Six-Ingredient Pill with Rehmannia), 627

Kidney yin and yang deficiencies
- *Jin Gui Shen Qi Wan* (Kidney Qi Pill from the Golden Cabinet), 668

61. DIABETES MELLITUS

Yin deficiency with dryness and heat
- *Xiao Ke Fang* (Wasting and Thirsting Formula), 1051

Qi and yin deficiencies
- *Sheng Mai San* (Generate the Pulse Powder), 554

Stomach heat
- *Yu Nu Jian* (Jade Woman Decoction), 398

Kidney yin deficiency
- *Liu Wei Di Huang Wan* (Six-Ingredient Pill with Rehmannia), 627

Kidney yin and yang deficiencies
- *Jin Gui Shen Qi Wan* (Kidney Qi Pill from the Golden Cabinet), 668

Qi and blood stagnation
- *Tao Hong Si Wu Tang* (Four-Substance Decoction with Safflower and Peach Pit), 571

1408

Chinese Herbal Formulas and Applications

Appendix 2 — Cross-reference Based on Western Medicine Diagnosis

• *Xue Fu Zhu Yu Tang* (Drive Out Stasis in the Mansion of Blood Decoction), 879

62. DIARRHEA
Damp-cold from the exterior
• *Huo Xiang Zheng Qi San* (Agastache Powder to Rectify the Qi), 1079
• *Ping Wei San* (Calm the Stomach Powder), 1068
Damp-heat from the exterior
• *Ge Gen Huang Qin Huang Lian Tang* (Kudzu, Coptis, and Scutellaria Decoction), 295
• *Xin Jia Xiang Ru Yin* (Newly-Augmented Mosla Decoction), 439
• *Liu Yi San* (Six-to-One Powder), 441
Food stagnation
• *Bao He Wan* (Preserve Harmony Pill), 1266
Liver overacting on the Spleen and Stomach
• *Tong Xie Yao Fang* (Important Formula for Painful Diarrhea), 257
Spleen and Stomach deficiencies
• *Shen Ling Bai Zhu San* (Ginseng, Poria, and Atractylodes Macrocephala Powder), 535
• *Fu Zi Li Zhong Wan* (Prepared Aconite Pill to Regulate the Middle), 463
• *Bu Zhong Yi Qi Tang* (Tonify the Middle and Augment the Qi Decoction), 542
Kidney yang deficiency
• *Si Shen Wan* (Four-Miracle Pill), 784

63. DIPHTHERIA
• *Liu Shen Wan* (Six-Miracle Pill), 363
• *Yang Yin Qing Fei Tang* (Nourish the Yin and Clear the Lung Decoction), 1033

64. DISSEMINATED INTRAVASCULAR COAGULATION (DIC)
Heat in *ying* (nutritive) and *xue* (blood) level
• *Xi Jiao Di Huang Tang* (Rhinoceros Horn and Rehmannia Decoction), 333
Blood stagnation in the channels and collaterals
• *Xue Fu Zhu Yu Tang* (Drive Out Stasis in the Mansion of Blood Decoction), 879
Blood stagnation with yin deficiency
• *Sheng Yu Tang* (Sage-Like Healing Decoction), 567
Blood stagnation with yang deficiency
• *Hui Yang Jiu Ji Tang* (Restore and Revive the Yang Decoction), 490

65. DIZZINESS
Liver wind rising
• *Tian Ma Gou Teng Yin* (Gastrodia and Uncaria Decoction), 1004
• *Da Ding Feng Zhu* (Major Arrest Wind Pearl), 1009
Liver fire rising
• *Long Dan Xie Gan Tang* (Gentiana Decoction to Drain the Liver), 371
• *Dang Gui Long Hui Wan* (Tangkuei, Gentiana, and Aloe Pill), 379
Phlegm accumulation
• *Ban Xia Bai Zhu Tian Ma Tang* (Pinellia, Atractylodes Macrocephala, and Gastrodia Decoction), 1247
• *Wen Dan Tang* (Warm the Gallbladder Decoction), 1213
Blood stagnation
• *Tong Qiao Huo Xue Tang* (Unblock the Orifices and Invigorate the Blood Decoction), 877
• *Xue Fu Zhu Yu Tang* (Drive Out Stasis in the Mansion of Blood Decoction), 879
Qi and blood deficiencies
• *Gui Pi Tang* (Restore the Spleen Decoction), 583
• *Ba Zhen Tang* (Eight-Treasure Decoction), 604
• *Shi Quan Da Bu Tang* (All-Inclusive Great Tonifying Decoction), 609
Kidney deficiency
• *Zuo Gui Wan* (Restore the Left [Kidney] Pill), 645
• *You Gui Wan* (Restore the Right [Kidney] Pill), 678

66. DYSENTERY
Damp-heat
• *Shao Yao Tang* (Peony Decoction), 402
• *Ge Gen Huang Qin Huang Lian Tang* (Kudzu, Coptis, and Scutellaria Decoction), 295
• *Bai Tou Weng Tang* (Pulsatilla Decoction), 408
Damp-cold
• *Wei Ling Tang* (Calm the Stomach and Poria Decoction), 1113
• *Bu Huan Jin Zheng Qi San* (Rectify the Qi Powder Worth More than Gold), 1075
Deficiency and cold
• *Li Zhong Tang* (Regulate the Middle Decoction), 462
• *Fu Zi Li Zhong Wan* (Prepared Aconite Pill to Regulate the Middle), 463
• *Tao Hua Tang* (Peach Blossom Decoction), 787
• *Zhen Ren Yang Zang Tang* (True Man's Decoction for Nourishing the Organs), 781

CROSS-REFERENCE BASED ON WESTERN MEDICINE DIAGNOSIS

A2

1409

Appendix 2 – Cross-reference Based on Western Medicine Diagnosis

Appendix 2 — Cross-reference Based on Western Medicine Diagnosis

67. DYSMENORRHEA

Qi and blood deficiencies
- *Huang Qi Jian Zhong Tang* (Astragalus Decoction to Construct the Middle), 475 with *Dang Gui* (Radix Angelicae Sinensis) and *Dang Shen* (Radix Codonopsis)

Qi and blood stagnation
- *Ge Xia Zhu Yu Tang* (Drive Out Blood Stasis Below the Diaphragm Decoction), 885
- *Shao Fu Zhu Yu Tang* (Drive Out Blood Stasis in the Lower Abdomen Decoction), 889

Blood stagnation with cold
- *Wen Jing Tang* (Warm the Channels Decoction), 919

68. DYSURIA

Re lin (heat dysuria)
- *Ba Zheng San* (Eight-Herb Powder for Rectification), 1103

Qi lin (qi dysuria)
- *Bu Zhong Yi Qi Tang* (Tonify the Middle and Augment the Qi Decoction), 542

Xue lin (bloody dysuria)
- *Xiao Ji Yin Zi* (Cirsium Decoction), 946
- *Zhi Bai Di Huang Wan* (Anemarrhena, Phellodendron, and Rehmannia Pill), 636

Gao lin (cloudy dysuria)
- *Bi Xie Fen Qing Yin* (Dioscorea Hypoglauca Decoction to Separate the Clear), 1140
- *Liu Wei Di Huang Wan* (Six-Ingredient Pill with Rehmannia), 627

Lao lin (fatigue dysuria)
- *Bu Zhong Yi Qi Tang* (Tonify the Middle and Augment the Qi Decoction), 542
- *Zhi Bai Di Huang Wan* (Anemarrhena, Phellodendron, and Rehmannia Pill), 636

69. ECZEMA
- *Xiao Feng San* (Eliminate Wind Powder), 967
- *Wen Qing Yin* (Warming and Clearing Decoction), 575
- *Dang Gui Yin Zi* (Tangkuei Decoction), 970
- *Qing Shang Fang Feng Tang* (Clear the Upper and Guard the Wind Decoction), 349

70. EDEMA

Wind affecting the Lung
- *Yue Bi Jia Zhu Tang* (Maidservant from Yue Decoction plus Atractylodes), 102

Heart yang deficiency
- *Zhen Wu Tang* (True Warrior Decoction), 1135

Water accumulation in the Urinary Bladder
- *Wu Ling San* (Five-Ingredient Powder with Poria), 1109
- *Wei Ling Tang* (Calm the Stomach and Poria Decoction), 1113

Kidney yang deficiency
- *Ji Sheng Shen Qi Wan* (Kidney Qi Pill from Formulas that Aid the Living), 675

Spleen yang deficiency
- *Shen Ling Bai Zhu San* (Ginseng, Poria, and Atractylodes Macrocephala Powder), 535
- *Shi Pi San* (Bolster the Spleen Powder), 1138

Spleen deficiency and damp accumulation
- *Wu Pi San* (Five-Peel Powder), 1121

71. EMPHYSEMA

Phlegm and heat in the Lung
- *Ma Huang Xing Ren Gan Cao Shi Gao Tang* (Ephedra, Apricot Kernel, Licorice, and Gypsum Decoction), 96 and *Qing Qi Hua Tan Wan* (Clear the Qi and Transform Phlegm Pill), 1222
- *She Gan Ma Huang Tang* (Belamcanda and Ephedra Decoction), 80

Exterior cold and interior *yin* (invisible phlegm)
- *Xiao Qing Long Tang* (Minor Bluegreen Dragon Decoction), 74

Phlegm and blood stasis in the interior
- *Ting Li Da Zao Xie Fei Tang* (Descurainia and Jujube Decoction to Drain the Lung), 384 and *Tao Hong Si Wu Tang* (Four-Substance Decoction with Safflower and Peach Pit), 571

Lung and Kidney deficiencies
- *Ren Shen Hu Tao Tang* (Ginseng and Walnut Decoction), 559
- *Ren Shen Ge Jie San* (Ginseng and Gecko Powder), 557 and *Bu Fei Tang* (Tonify the Lung Decoction), 560

Water accumulation and yang deficiency
- *Zhen Wu Tang* (True Warrior Decoction), 1135 and *Wu Ling San* (Five-Ingredient Powder with Poria), 1109

72. ENDOCARDITIS, INFECTIVE

Wind-heat
- *Yin Qiao San* (Honeysuckle and Forsythia Powder), 92

Heat in *qi* (energy) level
- *Bai Hu Tang* (White Tiger Decoction), 321

Heat in *ying* (nutritive) level
- *Qing Ying Tang* (Clear the Nutritive Level Decoction), 330

Zheng (upright) *qi* deficiency
- *Zhu Ye Shi Gao Tang* (Bamboo Leaves and Gypsum Decoction), 326

Chinese Herbal Formulas and Applications

Appendix 2 — Cross-reference Based on Western Medicine Diagnosis

73. ENDOMETRIOSIS

- *Shao Fu Zhu Yu Tang* (Drive Out Blood Stasis in the Lower Abdomen Decoction), 889
- *Gui Zhi Fu Ling Wan* (Cinnamon Twig and Poria Pill), 928
- *Shi Xiao San* (Sudden Smile Powder), 911

74. ENTERITIS

- *Ge Gen Huang Qin Huang Lian Tang* (Kudzu, Coptis, and Scutellaria Decoction), 295
- *Huo Xiang Zheng Qi San* (Agastache Powder to Rectify the Qi), 1079
- *Bai Tou Weng Tang* (Pulsatilla Decoction), 408
- *Shao Yao Tang* (Peony Decoction), 402
- *Tong Xie Yao Fang* (Important Formula for Painful Diarrhea), 257

75. ENURESIS

Lung and Spleen qi deficiencies
- *Bu Zhong Yi Qi Tang* (Tonify the Middle and Augment the Qi Decoction), 542

Heart and Kidney disharmony
- *Sang Piao Xiao San* (Mantis Egg-Case Powder), 792

Damp-heat
- *Ba Zheng San* (Eight-Herb Powder for Rectification), 1103

Blood stagnation
- *Shao Fu Zhu Yu Tang* (Drive Out Blood Stasis in the Lower Abdomen Decoction), 889

76. EPIGASTRIC PAIN

Stomach cold
- *Liang Fu Wan* (Galangal and Cyperus Pill), 841
- *Xiang Su San* (Cyperus and Perilla Leaf Powder), 67
- *Ban Xia Xie Xin Tang* (Pinellia Decoction to Drain the Epigastrium), 261

Food stagnation
- *Bao He Wan* (Preserve Harmony Pill), 1266

Liver overacting on the Spleen and Stomach
- *Chai Hu Shu Gan San* (Bupleurum Powder to Spread the Liver), 238

Stomach heat
- *Zuo Jin Wan* (Left Metal Pill), 389

Blood stagnation
- *Ge Xia Zhu Yu Tang* (Drive Out Blood Stasis Below the Diaphragm Decoction), 885
- *Shi Xiao San* (Sudden Smile Powder), 911 and *Dan Shen Yin* (Salvia Decoction), 917

Spleen and Stomach deficiency and cold
- *Huang Qi Jian Zhong Tang* (Astragalus Decoction to Construct the Middle), 475

- *Da Jian Zhong Tang* (Major Construct the Middle Decoction), 480

Spleen and Stomach yin deficiencies
- *Zhu Ye Shi Gao Tang* (Bamboo Leaves and Gypsum Decoction), 326 and *Mai Men Dong Tang* (Ophiopogonis Decoction), 1043

77. ERYSIPELAS

- *Long Dan Xie Gan Tang* (Gentiana Decoction to Drain the Liver), 371
- *Huang Lian Jie Du Tang* (Coptis Decoction to Relieve Toxicity), 341
- *Shi Wei Bai Du Tang* (Ten-Ingredient Decoction to Overcome Pathogenic Influences), 1341
- *Pu Ji Xiao Du Yin* (Universal Benefit Decoction to Eliminate Toxin), 355

78. FEVER

Exterior condition
- *Jing Fang Bai Du San* (Schizonepeta and Saposhnikovia Powder to Overcome Pathogenic Influences), 1334
- *Yin Qiao San* (Honeysuckle and Forsythia Powder), 92

Lung heat
- *Ma Huang Xing Ren Gan Cao Shi Gao Tang* (Ephedra, Apricot Kernel, Licorice, and Gypsum Decoction), 96

Stomach heat
- *Bai Hu Tang* (White Tiger Decoction), 321

Liver heat
- *Long Dan Xie Gan Tang* (Gentiana Decoction to Drain the Liver), 371

Gallbladder heat
- *Da Chai Hu Tang* (Major Bupleurum Decoction), 283

Yin-deficient heat
- *Qing Gu San* (Cool the Bones Powder), 418
- *Da Bu Yin Wan* (Great Tonify the Yin Pill), 649
- *Zhi Bai Di Huang Wan* (Anemarrhena, Phellodendron, and Rehmannia Pill), 636

Qi and blood deficiencies
- *Bu Zhong Yi Qi Tang* (Tonify the Middle and Augment the Qi Decoction), 542
- *Gui Pi Tang* (Restore the Spleen Decoction), 583
- *Dang Gui Bu Xue Tang* (Tangkuei Decoction to Tonify the Blood), 580

Stagnant heat in the Liver channel
- *Jia Wei Xiao Yao San* (Augmented Rambling Powder), 254
- *Long Dan Xie Gan Tang* (Gentiana Decoction to Drain the Liver), 371

Blood stagnation in the interior
- *Xue Fu Zhu Yu Tang* (Drive Out Stasis in the Mansion of Blood Decoction), 879

CROSS-REFERENCE BASED ON WESTERN MEDICINE DIAGNOSIS

A2

1411

Appendix 2 – Cross-reference Based on Western Medicine Diagnosis

Appendix 2 — Cross-reference Based on Western Medicine Diagnosis

79. FORGETFULNESS
Heart and Spleen deficiencies
- *Gui Pi Tang* (Restore the Spleen Decoction), 583

Kidney *jing* (essence) deficiency
- *Liu Wei Di Huang Wan* (Six-Ingredient Pill with Rehmannia), 627

Phlegm accumulation
- *Wen Dan Tang* (Warm the Gallbladder Decoction), 1213
- *Dao Tan Tang* (Guide Out Phlegm Decoction), 1211

Liver qi stagnation
- *Chai Hu Shu Gan San* (Bupleurum Powder to Spread the Liver), 238

80. FRECKLES
- *Dang Gui Shao Yao San* (Tangkuei and Peony Powder), 594 with *Yi Yi Ren* (Semen Coicis)
- *Gui Zhi Fu Ling Wan* (Cinnamon Twig and Poria Pill), 928 with *Yi Yi Ren* (Semen Coicis)

81. FROSTBITE
- *Gui Zhi Tang* (Cinnamon Twig Decoction), 51
- *Dang Gui Si Ni Tang* (Tangkuei Decoction for Frigid Extremities), 494

82. FURUNCLES
- *Wu Wei Xiao Du Yin* (Five-Ingredient Decoction to Eliminate Toxins), 1337
- *Shi Wei Bai Du Tang* (Ten-Ingredient Decoction to Overcome Pathogenic Influences), 1341
- *Niu Bang Jie Ji Tang* (Arctium Decoction to Release the Muscle Layer), 1332
- *Xian Fang Huo Ming Yin* (Sublime Formula for Sustaining Life), 1325

83. GASTRECTASIS
- *Li Zhong Wan* (Regulate the Middle Pill), 459
- *Fu Zi Li Zhong Wan* (Prepared Aconite Pill to Regulate the Middle), 463

84. GASTRITIS, CHRONIC
Liver and Stomach disharmony
- *Chai Hu Shu Gan San* (Bupleurum Powder to Spread the Liver), 238

Spleen and Stomach deficiencies
- *Xiang Sha Liu Jun Zi Tang* (Six-Gentlemen Decoction with Aucklandia and Amomum), 531

Stomach yin deficiency
- *Mai Men Dong Tang* (Ophiopogonis Decoction), 1043

Blood stagnation
- *Shi Xiao San* (Sudden Smile Powder), 911 and *Dan Shen Yin* (Salvia Decoction), 917

Liver and Stomach damp-heat
- *Wen Dan Tang* (Warm the Gallbladder Decoction), 1213 and *Zuo Jin Wan* (Left Metal Pill), 389

85. GASTROENTERITIS
Damp accumulation
- *Ping Wei San* (Calm the Stomach Powder), 1068

Stomach cold with heat in the chest
- *Huang Lian Tang* (Coptis Decoction), 271

Exterior wind-cold with interior dampness
- *Huo Xiang Zheng Qi San* (Agastache Powder to Rectify the Qi), 1079

86. GASTROPTOSIS
Spleen deficiency with qi sinking downward
- *Bu Zhong Yi Qi Tang* (Tonify the Middle and Augment the Qi Decoction), 542

Liver overacting on the Stomach
- *Chai Hu Shu Gan San* (Bupleurum Powder to Spread the Liver), 238

87. GINGIVITIS
- *Bai Hu Tang* (White Tiger Decoction), 321
- *Yu Nu Jian* (Jade Woman Decoction), 398
- *Gan Lu Yin* (Sweet Dew Decoction), 401
- *Qing Wei San* (Clear the Stomach Powder), 393

88. GLAUCOMA
- *Liu Wei Di Huang Wan* (Six-Ingredient Pill with Rehmannia), 627
- *Ba Wei Di Huang Wan* (Eight-Ingredient Pill with Rehmannia), 672
- *Ming Mu Di Huang Wan* (Improve Vision Pill with Rehmannia), 633
- *Zi Shen Ming Mu Tang* (Nourish the Kidney to Brighten the Eyes Decoction), 664

89. GLOMERULONEPHRITIS, ACUTE
Wind and water accumulation
- *Yue Bi Jia Zhu Tang* (Maidservant from Yue Decoction plus Atractylodes), 102

Water and dampness accumulation
- *Wei Ling Tang* (Calm the Stomach and Poria Decoction), 1113

Damp-heat in the interior
- *Shu Zao Yin Zi* (Spread and Unblock Decoction), 185

Damp-heat in the Urinary Bladder
- *Xiao Ji Yin Zi* (Cirsium Decoction), 946

1412

Chinese Herbal Formulas and Applications

Appendix 2 — Cross-reference Based on Western Medicine Diagnosis

90. GLOMERULONEPHRITIS, CHRONIC

Spleen deficiency with dampness
- *Fang Ji Huang Qi Tang* (Stephania and Astragalus Decoction), 1118

Kidney qi deficiency
- *Ji Sheng Shen Qi Wan* (Kidney Qi Pill from Formulas that Aid the Living), 675

Liver and Kidney yin deficiencies
- *Liu Wei Di Huang Wan* (Six-Ingredient Pill with Rehmannia), 627

Damp-heat accumulation
- *San Ren Tang* (Three-Nut Decoction), 1092

91. GOITER
- *Hai Zao Yu Hu Tang* (Sargassum Decoction for the Jade Flask), 1352
- *Dao Tan Tang* (Guide Out Phlegm Decoction), 1211
- *Xiao Luo Wan* (Reduce Scrofula Pill), 1355

92. GONORRHEA
- *Bi Xie Fen Qing Yin* (Dioscorea Hypoglauca Decoction to Separate the Clear), 1140
- *Er Miao San* (Two-Marvel Powder), 1188
- *Ba Zheng San* (Eight-Herb Powder for Rectification), 1103
- *Long Dan Xie Gan Tang* (Gentiana Decoction to Drain the Liver), 371

93. GOUT

Wind-cold-damp obstruction
- *Juan Bi Tang* (Remove Painful Obstruction Decoction), 1158
- *Shang Zhong Xia Tong Yong Tong Feng Wan* (Upper, Middle, and Lower General Use Pill for Wind-Pain), 1175

Wind-heat obstruction
- *Bai Hu Jia Gui Zhi Tang* (White Tiger plus Cinnamon Twig Decoction), 323
- *Gui Zhi Shao Yao Zhi Mu Tang* (Cinnamon Twig, Peony, and Anemarrhena Decoction), 1186

Liver and Kidney deficiencies
- *Du Huo Ji Sheng Tang* (Angelica Pubescens and Taxillus Decoction), 1161

94. HALITOSIS
- *Qing Wei San* (Clear the Stomach Powder), 393
- *Ban Xia Xie Xin Tang* (Pinellia Decoction to Drain the Epigastrium), 261
- *Gan Cao Xie Xin Tang* (Licorice Decoction to Drain the Epigastrium), 269

95. HEADACHE

Wind-cold
- *Chuan Xiong Cha Tiao San* (Ligusticum Chuanxiong Powder to be Taken with Green Tea), 973
- *Wu Zhu Yu Tang* (Evodia Decoction), 467

Wind-heat
- *Huang Lian Shang Qing Wan* (Coptis Pill to Clear the Upper), 347

Wind-damp
- *Qiang Huo Sheng Shi Tang* (Notopterygium Decoction to Overcome Dampness), 1156

Liver yang rising
- *Tian Ma Gou Teng Yin* (Gastrodia and Uncaria Decoction), 1004

Kidney deficiency
- *Qi Ju Di Huang Wan* (Lycium Fruit, Chrysanthemum, and Rehmannia Pill), 640

Qi and blood deficiencies
- *Ba Zhen Tang* (Eight-Treasure Decoction), 604

Phlegm obstruction
- *Ban Xia Bai Zhu Tian Ma Tang* (Pinellia, Atractylodes Macrocephala, and Gastrodia Decoction), 1247

Blood stasis
- *Tong Qiao Huo Xue Tang* (Unblock the Orifices and Invigorate the Blood Decoction), 877
- *Xue Fu Zhu Yu Tang* (Drive Out Stasis in the Mansion of Blood Decoction), 879

96. HEAT STROKE

***Bi zheng* (closed disorder)**
- *Bai Hu Tang* (White Tiger Decoction), 321

***Tuo zheng* (abandoned syndrome)**
- *Sheng Mai San* (Generate the Pulse Powder), 554

Unconsciousness
- *An Gong Niu Huang Wan* (Calm the Palace Pill with Cattle Gallstone), 746
- *Zhi Bao Dan* (Greatest Treasure Special Pill), 749
- *Zi Xue Dan* (Purple Snow Pill), 752

Liver wind rising
- *San Jia Fu Mai Tang* (Three-Shell Decoction to Restore the Pulse), 1011

97. HEMIPLEGIA
- *Bu Yang Huan Wu Tang* (Tonify the Yang to Restore Five Decoction), 905
- *Qian Zheng San* (Lead to Symmetry Powder), 977

98. HEMORRHOIDS
- *Yi Zi Tang* (Yi Word Decoction), 164
- *Qing Chang Tang* (Clear the Intestines Decoction), 165

CROSS-REFERENCE BASED ON WESTERN MEDICINE DIAGNOSIS

A2

1413

Appendix 2 – Cross-reference Based on Western Medicine Diagnosis

- *Huai Hua San* (Sophora Japonica Flower Powder), 944
- *Huai Jiao Wan* (Sophora Japonica Fruit Pill), 946

99. HEPATITIS

Damp-heat in the Liver
- *Xiao Chai Hu Tang* (Minor Bupleurum Decoction), 206
- *Da Chai Hu Tang* (Major Bupleurum Decoction), 283

Damp-heat in the Liver and Gallbladder
- *Yin Chen Hao Tang* (Artemisia Scoparia Decoction), 1086
- *Yin Chen Wu Ling San* (Artemisia Scoparia and Five-Ingredient Powder with Poria), 1090

Liver qi stagnation
- *Chai Hu Shu Gan San* (Bupleurum Powder to Spread the Liver), 238

Liver yin deficiency
- *Yi Guan Jian* (Linking Decoction), 657

100. HEPATO-CIRRHOSIS

Qi stagnation
- *Xiao Chai Hu Tang* (Minor Bupleurum Decoction), 206 and *Jia Wei Xiao Yao San* (Augmented Rambling Powder), 254

Qi stagnation and dampness accumulation
- *Chai Hu Shu Gan San* (Bupleurum Powder to Spread the Liver), 238 and *Ping Wei San* (Calm the Stomach Powder), 1068

Water and dampness accumulation
- *Wei Ling Tang* (Calm the Stomach and Poria Decoction), 1113
- *Shi Pi San* (Bolster the Spleen Powder), 1138

Liver and Spleen blood stagnation
- *Ge Xia Zhu Yu Tang* (Drive Out Blood Stasis Below the Diaphragm Decoction), 885
- *Bie Jia Jian Wan* (Soft-Shelled Turtle Shell Pill), 935

Spleen and Kidney yang deficiencies
- *Fu Zi Li Zhong Wan* (Prepared Aconite Pill to Regulate the Middle), 463 and *Wu Ling San* (Five-Ingredient Powder with Poria), 1109

Liver and Kidney yin deficiencies
- *Yi Guan Jian* (Linking Decoction), 657 and *Zhu Ling Tang* (Polyporus Decoction), 1115

101. HERNIAL PAIN

Deficiency and cold
- *Nuan Gan Jian* (Warm the Liver Decoction), 838

Damp-cold
- *Wu Ling San* (Five-Ingredient Powder with Poria), 1109

Damp and phlegm accumulation
- *Ju He Wan* (Tangerine Seed Pill), 833

Liver qi stagnation
- *Tian Tai Wu Yao San* (Top-Quality Lindera Powder), 835

Heat and phlegm accumulation
- *Long Dan Xie Gan Tang* (Gentiana Decoction to Drain the Liver), 371 and *Ju He Wan* (Tangerine Seed Pill), 833

102. HERPES

Wind-heat (oral)
- *Yin Qiao San* (Honeysuckle and Forsythia Powder), 92

Damp-heat (genital)
- *Long Dan Xie Gan Tang* (Gentiana Decoction to Drain the Liver), 371

Qi and blood stagnation (neuralgia)
- *Chai Hu Shu Gan San* (Bupleurum Powder to Spread the Liver), 238
- *Tao Hong Si Wu Tang* (Four-Substance Decoction with Safflower and Peach Pit), 571

103. HICCUPS

- *Ju Pi Zhu Ru Tang* (Tangerine Peel and Bamboo Shaving Decoction), 854
- *Ding Xiang Shi Di Tang* (Clove and Persimmon Calyx Decoction), 856

104. HYPERCORTISOLISM

Damp-heat in the Liver and Gallbladder
- *Long Dan Xie Gan Tang* (Gentiana Decoction to Drain the Liver), 371

Liver and Kidney yin deficiencies
- *Zhi Bai Di Huang Wan* (Anemarrhena, Phellodendron, and Rehmannia Pill), 636

Yin and yang deficiencies
- *Zuo Gui Wan* (Restore the Left [Kidney] Pill), 645 and *You Gui Wan* (Restore the Right [Kidney] Pill), 678

105. HYPERLIPIDEMIA

Phlegm accumulation
- *Dao Tan Tang* (Guide Out Phlegm Decoction), 1211

Stomach heat
- *Bao He Wan* (Preserve Harmony Pill), 1266 and *Xiao Cheng Qi Tang* (Minor Order the Qi Decoction), 158

Qi and blood stagnation
- *Xue Fu Zhu Yu Tang* (Drive Out Stasis in the Mansion of Blood Decoction), 879

Liver qi stagnation
- *Xiao Yao San* (Rambling Powder), 247

1414

Chinese Herbal Formulas and Applications

Appendix 2 — Cross-reference Based on Western Medicine Diagnosis

Liver and Kidney yin deficiencies
- *Qi Ju Di Huang Wan* (Lycium Fruit, Chrysanthemum, and Rehmannia Pill), 640

Spleen and Kidney yang deficiencies
- *Fu Zi Li Zhong Wan* (Prepared Aconite Pill to Regulate the Middle), 463

106. HYPERSOMNIA

Phlegm accumulation
- *Wen Dan Tang* (Warm the Gallbladder Decoction), 1213

Spleen qi deficiency
- *Xiang Sha Liu Jun Zi Tang* (Six-Gentlemen Decoction with Aucklandia and Amomum), 531

Yang qi deficiency
- *Fu Zi Li Zhong Wan* (Prepared Aconite Pill to Regulate the Middle), 463

Blood stagnation
- *Tong Qiao Huo Xue Tang* (Unblock the Orifices and Invigorate the Blood Decoction), 877

107. HYPERTENSION, PRIMARY

Liver yang rising
- *Tian Ma Gou Teng Yin* (Gastrodia and Uncaria Decoction), 1004

Liver heat and fire rising
- *Long Dan Xie Gan Tang* (Gentiana Decoction to Drain the Liver), 371

Wind and phlegm rising
- *Ban Xia Bai Zhu Tian Ma Tang* (Pinellia, Atractylodes Macrocephala, and Gastrodia Decoction), 1247

Liver and Kidney yin deficiencies
- *Yi Guan Jian* (Linking Decoction), 657
- *Qi Ju Di Huang Wan* (Lycium Fruit, Chrysanthemum, and Rehmannia Pill), 640

Yin and yang deficiencies
- *Er Xian Tang* (Two-Immortal Decoction), 684

Blood stagnation
- *Xue Fu Zhu Yu Tang* (Drive Out Stasis in the Mansion of Blood Decoction), 879

108. HYPERTHYROIDISM

Liver fire rising
- *Long Dan Xie Gan Tang* (Gentiana Decoction to Drain the Liver), 371
- *Zhen Gan Xi Feng Tang* (Sedate the Liver and Extinguish Wind Decoction), 999

Qi stagnation and phlegm accumulation
- *Xiao Yao San* (Rambling Powder), 247 and *Er Chen Tang* (Two-Cured Decoction), 1209

Heart and Liver yin deficiencies
- *Yi Guan Jian* (Linking Decoction), 657

Heart and Kidney yin deficiencies
- *Zhi Bai Di Huang Wan* (Anemarrhena, Phellodendron, and Rehmannia Pill), 636

Liver and Kidney yin deficiencies with yang rising
- *San Jia Fu Mai Tang* (Three-Shell Decoction to Restore the Pulse), 1011

Qi and yin deficiencies
- *Sheng Mai San* (Generate the Pulse Powder), 554

109. HYPOCHONDRIAC PAIN

Liver qi stagnation
- *Chai Hu Shu Gan San* (Bupleurum Powder to Spread the Liver), 238
- *Jin Ling Zi San* (Melia Toosendan Powder), 825
- *Zuo Jin Wan* (Left Metal Pill), 389

Blood stasis
- *Fu Yuan Huo Xue Tang* (Revive Health by Invigorating the Blood Decoction), 897
- *Xue Fu Zhu Yu Tang* (Drive Out Stasis in the Mansion of Blood Decoction), 879
- *Ge Xia Zhu Yu Tang* (Drive Out Blood Stasis Below the Diaphragm Decoction), 885

Damp-heat in the Liver and Gallbladder
- *Long Dan Xie Gan Tang* (Gentiana Decoction to Drain the Liver), 371

Liver yin deficiency
- *Yi Guan Jian* (Linking Decoction), 657

110. HYPOTENSION

Qi deficiency
- *Si Jun Zi Tang* (Four-Gentlemen Decoction), 522
- *Bu Zhong Yi Qi Tang* (Tonify the Middle and Augment the Qi Decoction), 542

Blood deficiency
- *Dang Gui Shao Yao San* (Tangkuei and Peony Powder), 594

Qi and blood deficiencies
- *Shi Quan Da Bu Tang* (All-Inclusive Great Tonifying Decoction), 609

Yang deficiency
- *Zhen Wu Tang* (True Warrior Decoction), 1135
- *Ba Wei Di Huang Wan* (Eight-Ingredient Pill with Rehmannia), 672

111. HYPOTHYROIDISM

Spleen qi deficiency
- *Si Jun Zi Tang* (Four-Gentlemen Decoction), 522

CROSS-REFERENCE BASED ON WESTERN MEDICINE DIAGNOSIS

A2

1415

Appendix 2 – Cross-reference Based on Western Medicine Diagnosis

Appendix 2 — Cross-reference Based on Western Medicine Diagnosis

Spleen and Kidney yang deficiencies
- *Si Jun Zi Tang* (Four-Gentlemen Decoction), 522 and *Ji Sheng Shen Qi Wan* (Kidney Qi Pill from Formulas that Aid the Living), 675

Heart and Kidney yang deficiencies
- *Ji Sheng Shen Qi Wan* (Kidney Qi Pill from Formulas that Aid the Living), 675 and *Bao Yuan Tang* (Preserve the Basal Decoction), 525

Yang qi deficiency
- *Si Ni Jia Ren Shen Tang* (Frigid Extremities Decoction plus Ginseng), 488
- *Jin Gui Shen Qi Wan* (Kidney Qi Pill from the Golden Cabinet), 668

112. HYSTEROMYOMA
- *Gui Zhi Fu Ling Wan* (Cinnamon Twig and Poria Pill), 928
- *Shao Fu Zhu Yu Tang* (Drive Out Blood Stasis in the Lower Abdomen Decoction), 889

113. IMPETIGO
- *Huang Lian Jie Du Tang* (Coptis Decoction to Relieve Toxicity), 341
- *Wu Wei Xiao Du Yin* (Five-Ingredient Decoction to Eliminate Toxins), 1337

114. IMPOTENCE
Ming men (life gate) fire deficiency
- *You Gui Wan* (Restore the Right [Kidney] Pill), 678

Heart and Spleen deficiencies
- *Gui Pi Tang* (Restore the Spleen Decoction), 583

Liver qi stagnation
- *Xiao Yao San* (Rambling Powder), 247

Damp-heat
- *Long Dan Xie Gan Tang* (Gentiana Decoction to Drain the Liver), 371

115. INDIGESTION
Food stagnation
- *Bao He Wan* (Preserve Harmony Pill), 1266
- *Ping Wei San* (Calm the Stomach Powder), 1068

Qi stagnation
- *Yue Ju Wan* (Escape Restraint Pill), 822

Spleen and Stomach deficiencies
- *Xiang Sha Liu Jun Zi Tang* (Six-Gentlemen Decoction with Aucklandia and Amomum), 531
- *Shen Ling Bai Zhu San* (Ginseng, Poria, and Atractylodes Macrocephala Powder), 535

Liver overacting on the Spleen and Stomach
- *Chai Hu Shu Gan San* (Bupleurum Powder to Spread the Liver), 238
- *Zuo Jin Wan* (Left Metal Pill), 389

116. INFECTION (UPPER RESPIRATORY TRACT)
Wind-cold
- *Jing Fang Bai Du San* (Schizonepeta and Saposhnikovia Powder to Overcome Pathogenic Influences), 1334
- *Qiang Huo Sheng Shi Tang* (Notopterygium Decoction to Overcome Dampness), 1156
- *Xing Su San* (Apricot Kernel and Perilla Leaf Powder), 1025

Wind-heat
- *Yin Qiao San* (Honeysuckle and Forsythia Powder), 92

Summer-heat
- *Xin Jia Xiang Ru Yin* (Newly-Augmented Mosla Decoction), 439

Exterior cold and interior heat
- *Shuang Jie Tong Sheng San* (Double Relieve Powder that Sagely Unblocks), 294

With interior deficiency
- *Shen Su Yin* (Ginseng and Perilla Leaf Decoction), 128
- *Jia Jian Wei Rui Tang* (Modified Polygonatum Odoratum Decoction), 137

117. INFERTILITY, FEMALE
Kidney deficiency
- *Zuo Gui Wan* (Restore the Left [Kidney] Pill), 645
- *You Gui Wan* (Restore the Right [Kidney] Pill), 678

Deficiency and cold
- *Ai Fu Nuan Gong Wan* (Mugwort and Cyperus Pill for Warming the Womb), 923

Qi and blood stagnation
- *Shao Fu Zhu Yu Tang* (Drive Out Blood Stasis in the Lower Abdomen Decoction), 889

118. INFERTILITY, MALE
Kidney deficiency
- *Zuo Gui Wan* (Restore the Left [Kidney] Pill), 645
- *You Gui Wan* (Restore the Right [Kidney] Pill), 678
- *Huan Shao Dan* (Return to Youth Pill), 681

Liver qi stagnation
- *Ju He Wan* (Tangerine Seed Pill), 833
- *Tian Tai Wu Yao San* (Top-Quality Lindera Powder), 835

119. INFLUENZA
Wind-cold
- *Cong Chi Tang* (Scallion and Prepared Soybean Decoction), 112
- *Jing Fang Bai Du San* (Schizonepeta and Saposhnikovia Powder to Overcome Pathogenic Influences), 1334
- *Qiang Huo Sheng Shi Tang* (Notopterygium Decoction to Overcome Dampness), 1156

Chinese Herbal Formulas and Applications

Appendix 2 — Cross-reference Based on Western Medicine Diagnosis

Wind-heat
- *Yin Qiao San* (Honeysuckle and Forsythia Powder), 92
- *Sang Xing Tang* (Mulberry Leaf and Apricot Kernel Decoction), 1027
- *Xin Jia Xiang Ru Yin* (Newly-Augmented Mosla Decoction), 439

Exterior wind with interior deficiency
- *Shen Su Yin* (Ginseng and Perilla Leaf Decoction), 128
- *Bai Du San* (Overcome Pathogenic Influences Powder), 124
- *Jia Jian Wei Rui Tang* (Modified Polygonatum Odoratum Decoction), 137

120. INSOMNIA

Heart fire
- *Zhu Sha An Shen Wan* (Cinnabar Pill to Tranquilize the Spirit), 710

Liver heat and fire rising
- *Jia Wei Xiao Yao San* (Augmented Rambling Powder), 254
- *Long Dan Xie Gan Tang* (Gentiana Decoction to Drain the Liver), 371

Heat and phlegm
- *Wen Dan Tang* (Warm the Gallbladder Decoction), 1213

Yin-deficient fire
- *Tian Wang Bu Xin Dan* (Emperor of Heaven's Special Pill to Tonify the Heart), 725
- *Zhi Bai Di Huang Wan* (Anemarrhena, Phellodendron, and Rehmannia Pill), 636

Heart and Spleen deficiencies
- *Gui Pi Tang* (Restore the Spleen Decoction), 583

Heart and Gallbladder qi deficiencies
- *Ding Zhi Wan* (Settle the Emotions Pill), 723
- *Suan Zao Ren Tang* (Sour Jujube Decoction), 722

121. INTESTINAL ABSCESS

Early stage of abscesses
- *Da Huang Mu Dan Tang* (Rhubarb and Moutan Decoction), 1378

Middle stage of abscesses
- *Xian Fang Huo Ming Yin* (Sublime Formula for Sustaining Life), 1325 and *Da Huang Mu Dan Tang* (Rhubarb and Moutan Decoction), 1378

Late stage of abscesses
- *Fu Fang Da Cheng Qi Tang* (Revised Major Order the Qi Decoction), 155

122. INTESTINAL OBSTRUCTION
- *Da Cheng Qi Tang* (Major Order the Qi Decoction), 152

- *Da Xian Xiong Tang* (Major Sinking into the Chest Decoction), 161
- *Da Chai Hu Tang* (Major Bupleurum Decoction), 283

123. IRRITABLE BOWEL SYNDROME

Liver qi stagnation with Spleen deficiency
- *Tong Xie Yao Fang* (Important Formula for Painful Diarrhea), 257

Yin and fluids deficiencies in the Intestines
- *Yi Guan Jian* (Linking Decoction), 657

Damp-heat obstruction
- *Ban Xia Xie Xin Tang* (Pinellia Decoction to Drain the Epigastrium), 261

Damp-cold obstruction
- *Hou Po Wen Zhong Tang* (Magnolia Bark Decoction for Warming the Middle), 840

Spleen qi deficiency
- *Shen Ling Bai Zhu San* (Ginseng, Poria, and Atractylodes Macrocephala Powder), 535

Spleen and Kidney yang deficiencies
- *Si Shen Wan* (Four-Miracle Pill), 784

124. JAUNDICE

Damp-heat
- *Yin Chen Hao Tang* (Artemisia Scoparia Decoction), 1086
- *Yin Chen Wu Ling San* (Artemisia Scoparia and Five-Ingredient Powder with Poria), 1090
- *Gan Lu Xiao Du Dan* (Sweet Dew Special Pill to Eliminate Toxins), 1096
- *Da Chai Hu Tang* (Major Bupleurum Decoction), 283

Damp-cold
- *Yin Chen Si Ni Tang* (Artemisia Scoparia Decoction for Frigid Extremities), 1089

Liver blood stagnation
- *Bie Jia Jian Wan* (Soft-Shelled Turtle Shell Pill), 935

Qi and blood deficiencies
- *Xiao Jian Zhong Tang* (Minor Construct the Middle Decoction), 471

125. KYPHOSIS
- *Yu Zhen San* (True Jade Powder), 981
- *Wu Hu Zhui Feng San* (Five-Tiger Powder to Pursue Wind), 982

126. LARYNGITIS
- *Yin Qiao San* (Honeysuckle and Forsythia Powder), 92
- *Xiang Sheng Po Di San* (Loud Sound Powder for a Broken Flute), 388
- *Ban Xia Hou Po Tang* (Pinellia and Magnolia Bark Decoction), 827

CROSS-REFERENCE BASED ON WESTERN MEDICINE DIAGNOSIS

A2

1417

127. LEUKEMIA

Heat and toxins
- *Huang Lian Jie Du Tang* (Coptis Decoction to Relieve Toxicity), 341 and *Qing Ying Tang* (Clear the Nutritive Level Decoction), 330

Yin-deficient fire
- *Zhi Bai Di Huang Wan* (Anemarrhena, Phellodendron, and Rehmannia Pill), 636 and *Er Zhi Wan* (Two-Ultimate Pill), 654

Damp-heat accumulation and blood stagnation
- *Wen Dan Tang* (Warm the Gallbladder Decoction), 1213 and *Tao Hong Si Wu Tang* (Four-Substance Decoction with Safflower and Peach Pit), 571

Damp-heat in the interior
- *Ge Gen Huang Qin Huang Lian Tang* (Kudzu, Coptis, and Scutellaria Decoction), 295

128. LEUKEMIA, GRANULOCYTIC

Heat and toxins
- *Qing Ying Tang* (Clear the Nutritive Level Decoction), 330 and *Xi Jiao Di Huang Tang* (Rhinoceros Horn and Rehmannia Decoction), 333

Blood stagnation
- *Ge Xia Zhu Yu Tang* (Drive Out Blood Stasis Below the Diaphragm Decoction), 885

Qi and blood deficiencies
- *Ba Zhen Tang* (Eight-Treasure Decoction), 604

129. LEUKEMIA, LYMPHOCYTIC

Blood stagnation
- *Tao Hong Si Wu Tang* (Four-Substance Decoction with Safflower and Peach Pit), 571

Qi and yin deficiencies
- *Si Jun Zi Tang* (Four-Gentlemen Decoction), 522 and *Sha Shen Mai Dong Tang* (Glehnia and Ophiopogonis Decoction), 1047

130. LEUKOPENIA

Qi and blood deficiencies
- *Gui Pi Tang* (Restore the Spleen Decoction), 583
- *Ba Zhen Tang* (Eight-Treasure Decoction), 604

Spleen and Kidney deficiencies
- *Huang Qi Jian Zhong Tang* (Astragalus Decoction to Construct the Middle), 475 and *You Gui Wan* (Restore the Right [Kidney] Pill), 678

Qi and yin deficiencies
- *Sheng Mai San* (Generate the Pulse Powder), 554

Liver and Kidney yin deficiencies
- *Liu Wei Di Huang Wan* (Six-Ingredient Pill with Rehmannia), 627

131. LEUKORRHEA

Damp-heat
- *Er Miao San* (Two-Marvel Powder), 1188
- *Ba Wei Dai Xia Fang* (Eight-Ingredient Formula for Leukorrhea), 810

Yin-deficient fire
- *Gu Jing Wan* (Stabilize the Menses Pill), 802

Liver qi stagnation
- *Xiao Yao San* (Rambling Powder), 247
- *Jia Wei Xiao Yao San* (Augmented Rambling Powder), 254

Spleen qi deficiency and Liver qi stagnation
- *Wan Dai Tang* (End Discharge Decoction), 806

132. LOSS OF VOICE

Exterior
- *San Ao Tang* (Three-Unbinding Decoction), 43
- *Xing Su San* (Apricot Kernel and Perilla Leaf Powder), 1025
- *Xiang Sheng Po Di San* (Loud Sound Powder for a Broken Flute), 388
- *Sang Xing Tang* (Mulberry Leaf and Apricot Kernel Decoction), 1027

Interior
- *Qing Zao Jiu Fei Tang* (Eliminate Dryness and Rescue the Lung Decoction), 1029
- *Mai Wei Di Huang Wan* (Ophiopogonis, Schisandra and Rehmannia Pill), 642

133. LOW BACK PAIN

Damp-cold
- *Du Huo Ji Sheng Tang* (Angelica Pubescens and Taxillus Decoction), 1161

Damp-heat
- *Er Miao San* (Two-Marvel Powder), 1188

Blood stagnation
- *Shen Tong Zhu Yu Tang* (Drive Out Blood Stasis from a Painful Body Decoction), 893

Kidney deficiency
- *You Gui Wan* (Restore the Right [Kidney] Pill), 678
- *Zuo Gui Wan* (Restore the Left [Kidney] Pill), 645
- *Huan Shao Dan* (Return to Youth Pill), 681

134. LUNG ABSCESS

Early stage of abscesses
- *Yin Qiao San* (Honeysuckle and Forsythia Powder), 92

Middle stage of abscesses
- *Wei Jing Tang* (Reed Decoction), 1377

Late stage of abscesses
- *Jie Geng Tang* (Platycodon Decoction), 1230 and *Wei Jing Tang* (Reed Decoction), 1377

Chinese Herbal Formulas and Applications

Appendix 2 — Cross-reference Based on Western Medicine Diagnosis

Recovery stage of abscesses
- *Qing Zao Jiu Fei Tang* (Eliminate Dryness and Rescue the Lung Decoction), 1029
- *Zhu Ye Shi Gao Tang* (Bamboo Leaves and Gypsum Decoction), 326

135. LUNG ATROPHY
- *Zhu Ye Shi Gao Tang* (Bamboo Leaves and Gypsum Decoction), 326
- *Mai Men Dong Tang* (Ophiopogonis Decoction), 1043
- *Bai He Gu Jin Tang* (Lily Bulb Decoction to Preserve the Metal), 1036

136. LUNG DISTENTION
Phlegm accumulation in the Lung
- *Su Zi Jiang Qi Tang* (Perilla Fruit Decoction for Directing Qi Downward), 842
- *San Zi Yang Qin Tang* (Three-Seed Decoction to Nourish One's Parents), 1245

Heat and phlegm in the Lung
- *Qing Qi Hua Tan Wan* (Clear the Qi and Transform Phlegm Pill), 1222
- *Di Tan Tang* (Scour Phlegm Decoction), 1212

Cold and phlegm in the Lung
- *Xiao Qing Long Tang* (Minor Bluegreen Dragon Decoction), 74

Phlegm blocking sensory orifices
- *Di Tan Tang* (Scour Phlegm Decoction), 1212
- *An Gong Niu Huang Wan* (Calm the Palace Pill with Cattle Gallstone), 746
- *Zhi Bao Dan* (Greatest Treasure Special Pill), 749

Lung and Kidney deficiencies
- *Ren Shen Ge Jie San* (Ginseng and Gecko Powder), 557
- *Bu Fei Tang* (Tonify the Lung Decoction), 560

137. LYMPHADENITIS
- *Pu Ji Xiao Du Yin* (Universal Benefit Decoction to Eliminate Toxin), 355
- *Xiao Luo Wan* (Reduce Scrofula Pill), 1355

138. LYMPHOMA
Toxic heat
- *Qing Wen Bai Du Yin* (Clear Epidemics and Overcome Pathogenic Influences Decoction), 337

Cold and phlegm obstruction
- *Yang He Tang* (Yang-Heartening Decoction), 1370

Heat and phlegm obstruction
- *Wen Dan Tang* (Warm the Gallbladder Decoction), 1213 and *Tao Hong Si Wu Tang* (Four-Substance Decoction with Safflower and Peach Pit), 571

Blood stagnation and phlegm obstruction
- *Er Chen Tang* (Two-Cured Decoction), 1209 and *Tao Hong Si Wu Tang* (Four-Substance Decoction with Safflower and Peach Pit), 571

Liver and Kidney yin deficiencies
- *Qi Ju Di Huang Wan* (Lycium Fruit, Chrysanthemum, and Rehmannia Pill), 640

Qi and blood deficiencies
- *Ba Zhen Tang* (Eight-Treasure Decoction), 604 and *Xiao Luo Wan* (Reduce Scrofula Pill), 1355

139. MACULAE AND PAPULES
- *Huang Lian Jie Du Tang* (Coptis Decoction to Relieve Toxicity), 341
- *Qing Wen Bai Du Yin* (Clear Epidemics and Overcome Pathogenic Influences Decoction), 337
- *Qing Ying Tang* (Clear the Nutritive Level Decoction), 330
- *Xi Jiao Di Huang Tang* (Rhinoceros Horn and Rehmannia Decoction), 333

140. MALARIA
- *Xiao Chai Hu Tang* (Minor Bupleurum Decoction), 206
- *Bai Hu Jia Gui Zhi Tang* (White Tiger plus Cinnamon Twig Decoction), 323
- *Chai Hu Gui Zhi Gan Jiang Tang* (Bupleurum, Cinnamon Twig, and Ginger Decoction), 304
- *Bie Jia Jian Wan* (Soft-Shelled Turtle Shell Pill), 935
- *Bu Huan Jin Zheng Qi San* (Rectify the Qi Powder Worth More than Gold), 1075

141. MANIA
Qi and blood deficiencies
- *Yang Xin Tang* (Nourish the Heart Decoction), 735

Phlegm stagnation
- *Di Tan Tang* (Scour Phlegm Decoction), 1212
- *Gun Tan Wan* (Vaporize Phlegm Pill), 1238

Fire and phlegm disturbing the Heart
- *San Sheng San* (Three-Sage Powder), 1312
- *Sheng Tie Luo Yin* (Iron Filings Decoction), 711
- *Kong Xian Dan* (Control Mucus Special Pill), 182

With shen (spirit) disturbance
- *Ding Zhi Wan* (Settle the Emotions Pill), 723

142. MASTITIS
- *Shi Liu Wei Liu Qi Yin* (Sixteen-Ingredient Decoction to Flow Qi), 1360
- *Tou Nong San* (Discharge Pus Powder), 1362 and *Wu Wei Xiao Du Yin* (Five-Ingredient Decoction to Eliminate Toxins), 1337

CROSS-REFERENCE BASED ON WESTERN MEDICINE DIAGNOSIS

A2

1419

Appendix 2 – Cross-reference Based on Western Medicine Diagnosis

Appendix 2 — Cross-reference Based on Western Medicine Diagnosis

143. MENIERE'S DISEASE
- *Tian Ma Gou Teng Yin* (Gastrodia and Uncaria Decoction), 1004
- *Ban Xia Bai Zhu Tian Ma Tang* (Pinellia, Atractylodes Macrocephala, and Gastrodia Decoction), 1247

144. MENOPAUSE
Kidney yin deficiency
- *Liu Wei Di Huang Wan* (Six-Ingredient Pill with Rehmannia), 627
- *Yi Guan Jian* (Linking Decoction), 657

Kidney yang deficiency
- *You Gui Wan* (Restore the Right [Kidney] Pill), 678
- *Er Xian Tang* (Two-Immortal Decoction), 684

Yin-deficient heat
- *Zhi Bai Di Huang Wan* (Anemarrhena, Phellodendron, and Rehmannia Pill), 636

Kidney *jing* (essence) deficiency
- *Gui Lu Er Xian Jiao* (Tortoise Shell and Deer Antler Syrup), 687

145. MENSTRUATION, EARLY
Qi deficiency
- *Bu Zhong Yi Qi Tang* (Tonify the Middle and Augment the Qi Decoction), 542
- *Ju Yuan Jian* (Lift the Source Decoction), 548
- *Gui Pi Tang* (Restore the Spleen Decoction), 583

Liver qi stagnation with heat
- *Jia Wei Xiao Yao San* (Augmented Rambling Powder), 254
- *Xiao Yao San* (Rambling Powder), 247

Blood stagnation
- *Tao Hong Si Wu Tang* (Four-Substance Decoction with Safflower and Peach Pit), 571

146. MENSTRUATION, IRREGULAR
Spleen deficiency
- *Gui Pi Tang* (Restore the Spleen Decoction), 583

Liver qi stagnation
- *Xiao Yao San* (Rambling Powder), 247

147. MENSTRUATION, LATE
Blood deficiency
- *Ren Shen Yang Ying Tang* (Ginseng Decoction to Nourish the Nutritive Qi), 615

Cold
- *Wen Jing Tang* (Warm the Channels Decoction), 919

Damp and phlegm accumulation
- *Er Chen Tang* (Two-Cured Decoction), 1209 with *Chuan Xiong* (Rhizoma Chuanxiong) and *Dang Gui* (Radix Angelicae Sinensis)

Blood stagnation
- *Tao Hong Si Wu Tang* (Four-Substance Decoction with Safflower and Peach Pit), 571

148. MENSTRUATION, PROLONGED
Qi deficiency
- *Gui Pi Tang* (Restore the Spleen Decoction), 583

Blood heat
- *Gu Jing Wan* (Stabilize the Menses Pill), 802

149. MIGRAINE
Wind-cold attacking the head
- *Chuan Xiong Cha Tiao San* (Ligusticum Chuanxiong Powder to be Taken with Green Tea), 973
- *Huang Lian Shang Qing Wan* (Coptis Pill to Clear the Upper), 347

Liver fire rising
- *Long Dan Xie Gan Tang* (Gentiana Decoction to Drain the Liver), 371

Dampness and phlegm attacking the head
- *Ban Xia Bai Zhu Tian Ma Tang* (Pinellia, Atractylodes Macrocephala, and Gastrodia Decoction), 1247

Blood stagnation blocking the channels and collaterals
- *Tong Qiao Huo Xue Tang* (Unblock the Orifices and Invigorate the Blood Decoction), 877

150. MOTION SICKNESS
Nausea and vomiting due to reversed flow of Stomach qi
- *Ju Pi Zhu Ru Tang* (Tangerine Peel and Bamboo Shaving Decoction), 854

Qi and blood deficiencies
- *Gui Pi Tang* (Restore the Spleen Decoction), 583

Dampness and phlegm obstructing the middle *jiao*
- *Ban Xia Bai Zhu Tian Ma Tang* (Pinellia, Atractylodes Macrocephala, and Gastrodia Decoction), 1247

151. MYASTHENIA GRAVIS
Spleen deficiency with qi sinking downwards
- *Bu Zhong Yi Qi Tang* (Tonify the Middle and Augment the Qi Decoction), 542

Spleen deficiency with *ying* (nutritive) *qi* insufficiency
- *Gui Pi Tang* (Restore the Spleen Decoction), 583

Spleen and Kidney yang deficiencies
- *Zuo Gui Wan* (Restore the Left [Kidney] Pill), 645

Qi deficiency and blood stagnation
- *Bu Yang Huan Wu Tang* (Tonify the Yang to Restore Five Decoction), 905

Damp-heat obstructing the channels and collaterals
- *Er Miao San* (Two-Marvel Powder), 1188

Chinese Herbal Formulas and Applications

Appendix 2 — Cross-reference Based on Western Medicine Diagnosis

152. MYOCARDIAL INFARCTION

Blood stagnation with qi and yin deficiencies
- *Xue Fu Zhu Yu Tang* (Drive Out Stasis in the Mansion of Blood Decoction), 879 and *Sheng Mai San* (Generate the Pulse Powder), 554

Cold stagnation with yang and qi deficiencies
- *Shen Fu Tang* (Ginseng and Prepared Aconite Decoction), 489 and *Zhi Shi Xie Bai Gui Zhi Tang* (Immature Bitter Orange, Chinese Chive, and Cinnamon Twig Decoction), 831

153. NAUSEA

Exterior condition
- *Huo Xiang Zheng Qi San* (Agastache Powder to Rectify the Qi), 1079
- *Xin Jia Xiang Ru Yin* (Newly-Augmented Mosla Decoction), 439

Stomach cold
- *Li Zhong Tang* (Regulate the Middle Decoction), 462
- *Li Zhong Wan* (Regulate the Middle Pill), 459

Stomach heat
- *Xiao Cheng Qi Tang* (Minor Order the Qi Decoction), 158
- *Zhu Ye Shi Gao Tang* (Bamboo Leaves and Gypsum Decoction), 326

Phlegm obstruction
- *Ling Gui Zhu Gan Tang* (Poria, Cinnamon Twig, Atractylodes Macrocephala, and Licorice Decoction), 1131
- *Xuan Fu Dai Zhe Shi Tang* (Inula and Hematite Decoction), 851
- *Dao Tan Tang* (Guide Out Phlegm Decoction), 1211

Food stagnation
- *Bao He Wan* (Preserve Harmony Pill), 1266

Blood stagnation
- *Ge Xia Zhu Yu Tang* (Drive Out Blood Stasis Below the Diaphragm Decoction), 885

Spleen and Stomach deficiency and cold
- *Li Zhong Wan* (Regulate the Middle Pill), 459
- *Xiang Sha Liu Jun Zi Tang* (Six-Gentlemen Decoction with Aucklandia and Amomum), 531

Stomach yin deficiency
- *Sha Shen Mai Dong Tang* (Glehnia and Ophiopogonis Decoction), 1047
- *Mai Men Dong Tang* (Ophiopogonis Decoction), 1043

Liver overacting on the Spleen and Stomach
- *Ban Xia Hou Po Tang* (Pinellia and Magnolia Bark Decoction), 827
- *Zuo Jin Wan* (Left Metal Pill), 389

154. NEPHROTIC SYNDROME

Wind and water accumulation
- *Yue Bi Tang* (Maidservant from Yue Decoction), 101 and *Wu Pi San* (Five-Peel Powder), 1121
- *Yue Bi Jia Zhu Tang* (Maidservant from Yue Decoction plus Atractylodes), 102

Damp-heat
- *Bi Xie Fen Qing Yin* (Dioscorea Hypoglauca Decoction to Separate the Clear), 1140

Liver and Kidney yin deficiencies
- *Zhi Bai Di Huang Wan* (Anemarrhena, Phellodendron, and Rehmannia Pill), 636

Spleen and Kidney yang deficiencies
- *Zhen Wu Tang* (True Warrior Decoction), 1135 and *Shi Pi San* (Bolster the Spleen Powder), 1138

Qi and yin deficiencies
- *Mai Wei Di Huang Wan* (Ophiopogonis, Schisandra and Rehmannia Pill), 642

Blood stagnation with water accumulation
- *Dang Gui Shao Yao San* (Tangkuei and Peony Powder), 594 and *Wu Pi San* (Five-Peel Powder), 1121
- *Gui Zhi Fu Ling Wan* (Cinnamon Twig and Poria Pill), 928 and *Wu Pi San* (Five-Peel Powder), 1121

155. NEURASTHENIA

Liver qi stagnation
- *Xiao Yao San* (Rambling Powder), 247

Liver qi stagnation with heat and fire
- *Jia Wei Xiao Yao San* (Augmented Rambling Powder), 254

Liver fire rising with *shen* (spirit) disturbance
- *Chai Hu Jia Long Gu Mu Li Tang* (Bupleurum plus Dragon Bone and Oyster Shell Decoction), 715

Shen (spirit) disturbance due to phlegm and heat
- *Wen Dan Tang* (Warm the Gallbladder Decoction), 1213

Yin-deficient fire
- *Zhu Sha An Shen Wan* (Cinnabar Pill to Tranquilize the Spirit), 710

Heart and Spleen deficiencies
- *Gui Pi Tang* (Restore the Spleen Decoction), 583

Heart and Kidney disharmony
- *Tian Wang Bu Xin Dan* (Emperor of Heaven's Special Pill to Tonify the Heart), 725

156. NEUROPATHY
- *Chuan Xiong Cha Tiao San* (Ligusticum Chuanxiong Powder to be Taken with Green Tea), 973
- *Shu Jing Huo Xue Tang* (Relax the Channels and Invigorate the Blood Decoction), 1169

CROSS-REFERENCE BASED ON WESTERN MEDICINE DIAGNOSIS

A2

1421

Appendix 2 – Cross-reference Based on Western Medicine Diagnosis

Appendix 2 — Cross-reference Based on Western Medicine Diagnosis

- *Shu Jin Li An San* (Relax the Tendons and Instill Peace Powder), 1171
- *Shen Tong Zhu Yu Tang* (Drive Out Blood Stasis from a Painful Body Decoction), 893
- *Tao He Cheng Qi Tang* (Peach Pit Decoction to Order the Qi), 873

157. NEURITIS
Wind-cold affecting the channels and collaterals
- *Xiao Xu Ming Tang* (Minor Prolong Life Decoction), 983
Wind-heat affecting the channels and collaterals
- *Da Qin Jiao Tang* (Major Gentiana Macrophylla Decoction), 988
Wind-damp obstructing the channels and collaterals
- *Qian Zheng San* (Lead to Symmetry Powder), 977
Qi deficiency and blood stagnation
- *Bu Yang Huan Wu Tang* (Tonify the Yang to Restore Five Decoction), 905

158. NEUROSIS
Liver qi stagnation
- *Xiao Yao San* (Rambling Powder), 247
- *Chai Hu Shu Gan San* (Bupleurum Powder to Spread the Liver), 238
- *Yi Gan San* (Restrain the Liver Powder), 245
Liver qi stagnation with heat
- *Jia Wei Xiao Yao San* (Augmented Rambling Powder), 254
Liver qi stagnation with *shen* (spirit) disturbance
- *Chai Hu Jia Long Gu Mu Li Tang* (Bupleurum plus Dragon Bone and Oyster Shell Decoction), 715

159. NOCTURIA
- *Jin Gui Shen Qi Wan* (Kidney Qi Pill from the Golden Cabinet), 668
- *Ba Wei Di Huang Wan* (Eight-Ingredient Pill with Rehmannia), 672
- *Suo Quan Wan* (Shut the Sluice Pill), 795

160. NUMBNESS
Qi deficiency
- *Bu Zhong Yi Qi Tang* (Tonify the Middle and Augment the Qi Decoction), 542
- *Bu Yang Huan Wu Tang* (Tonify the Yang to Restore Five Decoction), 905
Blood deficiency
- *Si Wu Tang* (Four-Substance Decoction), 562
- *Dang Gui Bu Xue Tang* (Tangkuei Decoction to Tonify the Blood), 580

Wind-damp blocking channels and collaterals
- *Juan Bi Tang* (Remove Painful Obstruction Decoction), 1158
- *San Miao Wan* (Three-Marvel Pill), 1190 and *Si Wu Tang* (Four-Substance Decoction), 562
Phlegm blocking channels and collaterals
- *Qian Zheng San* (Lead to Symmetry Powder), 977
- *Kong Xian Dan* (Control Mucus Special Pill), 182
- *Er Chen Tang* (Two-Cured Decoction), 1209

161. OBESITY
Stomach heat
- *Xiao Cheng Qi Tang* (Minor Order the Qi Decoction), 158 and *Bao He Wan* (Preserve Harmony Pill), 1266
- *Fang Feng Tong Sheng San* (Saposhnikovia Powder that Sagely Unblocks), 291
Spleen deficiency with dampness accumulation
- *Shen Ling Bai Zhu San* (Ginseng, Poria, and Atractylodes Macrocephala Powder), 535 and *Fang Ji Huang Qi Tang* (Stephania and Astragalus Decoction), 1118
Damp and phlegm accumulation
- *Dao Tan Tang* (Guide Out Phlegm Decoction), 1211
Spleen and Kidney yang deficiencies
- *Zhen Wu Tang* (True Warrior Decoction), 1135 and *Ling Gui Zhu Gan Tang* (Poria, Cinnamon Twig, Atractylodes Macrocephala, and Licorice Decoction), 1131
Qi and blood stagnation
- *Xue Fu Zhu Yu Tang* (Drive Out Stasis in the Mansion of Blood Decoction), 879 and *Shi Xiao San* (Sudden Smile Powder), 911

162. OSTEOARTHRITIS
Blood stagnation
- *Shen Tong Zhu Yu Tang* (Drive Out Blood Stasis from a Painful Body Decoction), 893
Kidney deficiency
- *San Bi Tang* (Three-Painful Obstruction Decoction), 1167
Damp-heat
- *Si Miao Wan* (Four-Marvel Pill), 1190

163. OSTEOPOROSIS
Kidney yin deficiency
- *Zuo Gui Wan* (Restore the Left [Kidney] Pill), 645
Kidney yang deficiency
- *You Gui Wan* (Restore the Right [Kidney] Pill), 678
Kidney *jing* (essence) deficiency
- *Gui Lu Er Xian Jiao* (Tortoise Shell and Deer Antler Syrup), 687

1422

Chinese Herbal Formulas and Applications

Appendix 2 — Cross-reference Based on Western Medicine Diagnosis

Spleen qi deficiency
- *Shen Ling Bai Zhu San* (Ginseng, Poria, and Atractylodes Macrocephala Powder), 535

164. OTITIS MEDIA
- *Shi Wei Bai Du Tang* (Ten-Ingredient Decoction to Overcome Pathogenic Influences), 1341
- *Qian Jin Nei Tuo San* (Drain the Interior Powder Worthy of a Thousand Gold), 1365
- *Pai Nong San* (Drain the Pus Powder), 1364
- *Tuo Li Xiao Du Yin* (Drain the Interior and Detoxify Decoction), 1367
- *Jing Jie Lian Qiao Tang* (Schizonepeta and Forsythia Decoction), 120

165. PALPITATIONS
Heart and Gallbladder deficiencies
- *Ding Zhi Wan* (Settle the Emotions Pill), 723
- *Zhi Gan Cao Tang* (Honey-Fried Licorice Decoction), 589

Heart and Spleen deficiencies
- *Gui Pi Tang* (Restore the Spleen Decoction), 583
- *Zhi Gan Cao Tang* (Honey-Fried Licorice Decoction), 589

Heart yin deficiency
- *Tian Wang Bu Xin Dan* (Emperor of Heaven's Special Pill to Tonify the Heart), 725

Heart yang deficiency
- *Gui Zhi Jia Long Gu Mu Li Tang* (Cinnamon Twig Decoction plus Dragon Bone and Oyster Shell), 798

Water accumulation
- *Ling Gui Zhu Gan Tang* (Poria, Cinnamon Twig, Atractylodes Macrocephala, and Licorice Decoction), 1131

Blood stagnation
- *Xue Fu Zhu Yu Tang* (Drive Out Stasis in the Mansion of Blood Decoction), 879

166. PANCREATITIS
Liver qi stagnation
- *Chai Hu Shu Gan San* (Bupleurum Powder to Spread the Liver), 238
- *Xiao Chai Hu Tang* (Minor Bupleurum Decoction), 206

Excess heat in the Spleen and Stomach
- *Da Cheng Qi Tang* (Major Order the Qi Decoction), 152

Liver and Gallbladder damp-heat
- *Long Dan Xie Gan Tang* (Gentiana Decoction to Drain the Liver), 371

Qi and yin deficiencies
- *Zeng Ye Cheng Qi Tang* (Increase the Fluids and Order the Qi Decoction), 190

Blood stagnation
- *Ge Xia Zhu Yu Tang* (Drive Out Blood Stasis Below the Diaphragm Decoction), 885

167. PARASITIC INFESTATION
- *Lian Mei An Hui Tang* (Picrorhiza and Mume Decoction to Calm Roundworms), 1295
- *Li Zhong An Hui Tang* (Regulate the Middle and Calm Roundworms Decoction), 1295
- *Hua Chong Wan* (Dissolve Parasites Pill), 1300
- *Wu Mei Wan* (Mume Pill), 1292
- *Fa Mu Wan* (Quell Wood Pill), 1302

168. PARKINSON'S DISEASE
Yin deficiency with Liver wind rising
- *Da Ding Feng Zhu* (Major Arrest Wind Pearl), 1009

Blood deficiency with Liver wind rising
- *Si Wu Tang* (Four-Substance Decoction), 562 and *Zhi Jing San* (Stop Spasms Powder), 979

Liver wind and yang rising
- *Tian Ma Gou Teng Yin* (Gastrodia and Uncaria Decoction), 1004

Liver wind rising with hot phlegm
- *Dao Tan Tang* (Guide Out Phlegm Decoction), 1211

Wind and phlegm blocking the channels and collaterals
- *Ban Xia Bai Zhu Tian Ma Tang* (Pinellia, Atractylodes Macrocephala, and Gastrodia Decoction), 1247 and *Qian Zheng San* (Lead to Symmetry Powder), 977

Blood stagnation in the head
- *Tong Qiao Huo Xue Tang* (Unblock the Orifices and Invigorate the Blood Decoction), 877

Kidney *jing* (essence) deficiency
- *Zuo Gui Wan* (Restore the Left [Kidney] Pill), 645

169. PAROTITIS
- *Yin Qiao San* (Honeysuckle and Forsythia Powder), 92
- *Jing Fang Bai Du San* (Schizonepeta and Saposhnikovia Powder to Overcome Pathogenic Influences), 1334
- *Pu Ji Xiao Du Yin* (Universal Benefit Decoction to Eliminate Toxin), 355
- *Qing Xin Li Ge Tang* (Clear the Epigastrium and Benefit the Diaphragm Decoction), 386

170. PELVIC INFLAMMATORY DISEASE
- *Da Huang Mu Dan Tang* (Rhubarb and Moutan Decoction), 1378

CROSS-REFERENCE BASED ON WESTERN MEDICINE DIAGNOSIS

A2

1423

- *Long Dan Xie Gan Tang* (Gentiana Decoction to Drain the Liver), 371
- *Gui Zhi Fu Ling Wan* (Cinnamon Twig and Poria Pill), 928

171. PEPTIC ULCER

Liver and Stomach disharmony
- *Chai Hu Shu Gan San* (Bupleurum Powder to Spread the Liver), 238

Liver and Stomach heat
- *Zuo Jin Wan* (Left Metal Pill), 389

Spleen and Stomach deficiency and cold
- *Huang Qi Jian Zhong Tang* (Astragalus Decoction to Construct the Middle), 475 and *Li Zhong Tang* (Regulate the Middle Decoction), 462

Stomach yin deficiency
- *Yi Guan Jian* (Linking Decoction), 657

Blood stagnation
- *Shi Xiao San* (Sudden Smile Powder), 911 and *Dan Shen Yin* (Salvia Decoction), 917

172. PERICARDITIS

Yin (invisible phlegm) accumulation
- *Xiao Xian Xiong Tang* (Minor Sinking into the Chest Decoction), 1235

Yin (invisible phlegm) accumulation with yin deficiency
- *Xie Bai San* (Drain the White Powder), 383 and *Bai He Gu Jin Tang* (Lily Bulb Decoction to Preserve the Metal), 1036

Yin (invisible phlegm) accumulation with yang deficiency
- *Ting Li Da Zao Xie Fei Tang* (Descurainia and Jujube Decoction to Drain the Lung), 384 and *Ling Gui Zhu Gan Tang* (Poria, Cinnamon Twig, Atractylodes Macrocephala, and Licorice Decoction), 1131

Blood stagnation and *zheng* (upright) *qi* deficiency
- *Ge Xia Zhu Yu Tang* (Drive Out Blood Stasis Below the Diaphragm Decoction), 885 and *Dang Gui Bu Xue Tang* (Tangkuei Decoction to Tonify the Blood), 580

173. PERSPIRATION

Spontaneous sweating
- *Gui Zhi Tang* (Cinnamon Twig Decoction), 51
- *Yu Ping Feng San* (Jade Windscreen Powder), 773
- *Mu Li San* (Oyster Shell Powder), 776

Night sweating
- *Gui Pi Tang* (Restore the Spleen Decoction), 583
- *Dang Gui Liu Huang Tang* (Tangkuei and Six-Yellow Decoction), 420
- *Mu Li San* (Oyster Shell Powder), 776

174. PHEOCHROMOCYTOMA

Liver yang rising
- *Tian Ma Gou Teng Yin* (Gastrodia and Uncaria Decoction), 1004

Liver and Kidney yin deficiencies
- *Yi Guan Jian* (Linking Decoction), 657

Phlegm accumulation
- *Ban Xia Bai Zhu Tian Ma Tang* (Pinellia, Atractylodes Macrocephala, and Gastrodia Decoction), 1247

Yin and yang deficiencies
- *Er Xian Tang* (Two-Immortal Decoction), 684

175. PLEURITIS

- *Chai Hu Xian Xiong Tang* (Bupleurum Decoction for Sinking into the Chest), 1237
- *Xiao Xian Xiong Tang* (Minor Sinking into the Chest Decoction), 1235
- *Da Qing Long Tang* (Major Bluegreen Dragon Decoction), 45
- *Ting Li Da Zao Xie Fei Tang* (Descurainia and Jujube Decoction to Drain the Lung), 384

176. PNEUMONIA

Wind-heat affecting the Lung
- *Sang Ju Yin* (Mulberry Leaf and Chrysanthemum Decoction), 89
- *San Ao Tang* (Three-Unbinding Decoction), 43

Lung heat
- *Ma Huang Xing Ren Gan Cao Shi Gao Tang* (Ephedra, Apricot Kernel, Licorice, and Gypsum Decoction), 96
- *Wei Jing Tang* (Reed Decoction), 1377

Heat and phlegm affecting the Lung
- *Chai Hu Xian Xiong Tang* (Bupleurum Decoction for Sinking into the Chest), 1237

Heat obstructing sensory orifices
- *Qing Ying Tang* (Clear the Nutritive Level Decoction), 330
- *An Gong Niu Huang Wan* (Calm the Palace Pill with Cattle Gallstone), 746
- *Zhi Bao Dan* (Greatest Treasure Special Pill), 749

177. PNEUMOTHORAX

Exterior wind-cold and Lung qi deficiency
- *Xiang Su San* (Cyperus and Perilla Leaf Powder), 67

Heat and phlegm
- *Chai Hu Xian Xiong Tang* (Bupleurum Decoction for Sinking into the Chest), 1237

Spleen deficiency with phlegm accumulation
- *Si Jun Zi Tang* (Four-Gentlemen Decoction), 522

Chinese Herbal Formulas and Applications

Appendix 2 — Cross-reference Based on Western Medicine Diagnosis

Qi, blood and phlegm stagnation
- *Si Mo Tang* (Four Milled-Herbs Decoction), 849 and *Xue Fu Zhu Yu Tang* (Drive Out Stasis in the Mansion of Blood Decoction), 879

Yang deficiency in the chest
- *Zhi Shi Xie Bai Gui Zhi Tang* (Immature Bitter Orange, Chinese Chive, and Cinnamon Twig Decoction), 831

Liver and Lung qi stagnation, with upper excess and lower deficiency
- *Chai Hu Shu Gan San* (Bupleurum Powder to Spread the Liver), 238 and *Su Zi Jiang Qi Tang* (Perilla Fruit Decoction for Directing Qi Downward), 842

178. POISONING, ALCOHOL
- *Ge Hua Jie Cheng San* (Pueraria Flower Powder for Detoxification and Awakening), 1084
- *Di Huang Yin Zi* (Rehmannia Decoction), 693
- *Xiao Yao San* (Rambling Powder), 247

179. PREGNANCY
Abdominal pain, with
- *Dang Gui Shao Yao San* (Tangkuei and Peony Powder), 594
- *Jiao Ai Tang* (Ass-Hide Gelatin and Mugwort Decoction), 950
- *Xiao Yao San* (Rambling Powder), 247 with *Zi Su Geng* (Caulis Perillae) and *Chen Pi* (Pericarpium Citri Reticulatae)

Breech presentation of the fetus
- *Ba Zhen Tang* (Eight-Treasure Decoction), 604 with *Huang Qi* (Radix Astragali), *Xu Duan* (Radix Dipsaci) and *Zhi Qiao* (Fructus Aurantii)

Cough, with
- *Bai He Gu Jin Tang* (Lily Bulb Decoction to Preserve the Metal), 1036
- *Liu Jun Zi Tang* (Six-Gentlemen Decoction), 527

Ectopic pregnancy, to terminate
- *Gong Wai Yun Fang* (Ectopic Pregnancy Formula), 917

Edema and generalized swelling, with
- *Wu Ling San* (Five-Ingredient Powder with Poria), 1109

Irritability, with
- *Qi Ju Di Huang Wan* (Lycium Fruit, Chrysanthemum, and Rehmannia Pill), 640
- *Ba Zhen Tang* (Eight-Treasure Decoction), 604
- *Ban Xia Bai Zhu Tian Ma Tang* (Pinellia, Atractylodes Macrocephala, and Gastrodia Decoction), 1247

Miscarriage, prevention of
- *Bao Chan Wu You Fang* (Preserve Pregnancy and Care-Free Decoction), 621

- *Tai Shan Pan Shi San* (Powder that Gives the Stability of Mount Tai), 618

Nausea and vomiting, with
- *Xiang Sha Liu Jun Zi Tang* (Six-Gentlemen Decoction with Aucklandia and Amomum), 531
- *Wen Dan Tang* (Warm the Gallbladder Decoction), 1213
- *Ju Pi Zhu Ru Tang* (Tangerine Peel and Bamboo Shaving Decoction), 854

Restless fetus, with
- *Bao Chan Wu You Fang* (Preserve Pregnancy and Care-Free Decoction), 621
- *Dang Gui Shao Yao San* (Tangkuei and Peony Powder), 594

Seizures and epilepsy, with
- *Ling Jiao Gou Teng Tang* (Antelope Horn and Uncaria Decoction), 993
- *Ban Xia Bai Zhu Tian Ma Tang* (Pinellia, Atractylodes Macrocephala, and Gastrodia Decoction), 1247 and *An Gong Niu Huang Wan* (Calm the Palace Pill with Cattle Gallstone), 746

Uterine bleeding, with
- *Gui Zhi Fu Ling Wan* (Cinnamon Twig and Poria Pill), 928
- *Bao Chan Wu You Fang* (Preserve Pregnancy and Care-Free Decoction), 621

180. PREGNANCY, POSTPARTUM CARE
Blood stagnation (retention of lochia)
- *Sheng Hua Tang* (Generation and Transformation Decoction), 925

Qi and blood deficiencies
- *Ba Zhen Tang* (Eight-Treasure Decoction), 604

Lactation, insufficient
- *Tong Ru Wan* (Unblock the Breast Pill), 927

Lactation, excessive
- *Bu Zhong Yi Qi Tang* (Tonify the Middle and Augment the Qi Decoction), 542 with *Qian Shi* (Semen Euryales) and *Wu Wei Zi* (Fructus Schisandrae Chinensis)
- *Jia Wei Xiao Yao San* (Augmented Rambling Powder), 254 with *Mu Li* (Concha Ostreae) and *Xia Ku Cao* (Spica Prunellae)

Lactation, termination of
- *Mai Ya* (Fructus Hordei Germinatus) 60g

181. PREMENSTRUAL SYNDROME (PMS)
Edema and swelling
- *Ling Gui Zhu Gan Tang* (Poria, Cinnamon Twig, Atractylodes Macrocephala, and Licorice Decoction), 1131

CROSS-REFERENCE BASED ON WESTERN MEDICINE DIAGNOSIS

A2

1425

Appendix 2 — Cross-reference Based on Western Medicine Diagnosis

Breast distention and pain
- *Chai Hu Shu Gan San* (Bupleurum Powder to Spread the Liver), 238
- *Si Wu Tang* (Four-Substance Decoction), 562 and *Er Chen Tang* (Two-Cured Decoction), 1209

Emotional instability
- *Gan Mai Da Zao Tang* (Licorice, Wheat, and Jujube Decoction), 731
- *Xiao Yao San* (Rambling Powder), 247
- *Jia Wei Xiao Yao San* (Augmented Rambling Powder), 254
- *Wen Dan Tang* (Warm the Gallbladder Decoction), 1213

Stomatitis
- *Zhi Bai Di Huang Wan* (Anemarrhena, Phellodendron, and Rehmannia Pill), 636
- *Liang Ge San* (Cool the Diaphragm Powder), 351

182. PROSTATITIS

Damp-heat
- *Ba Zheng San* (Eight-Herb Powder for Rectification), 1103
- *Long Dan Xie Gan Tang* (Gentiana Decoction to Drain the Liver), 371

Dampness
- *Bi Xie Fen Qing Yin* (Dioscorea Hypoglauca Decoction to Separate the Clear), 1140

Kidney yang deficiency
- *Ba Wei Di Huang Wan* (Eight-Ingredient Pill with Rehmannia), 672

183. PSORIASIS
- *Dang Gui Yin Zi* (Tangkuei Decoction), 970
- *Shi Wei Bai Du Tang* (Ten-Ingredient Decoction to Overcome Pathogenic Influences), 1341
- *Wu Wei Xiao Du Yin* (Five-Ingredient Decoction to Eliminate Toxins), 1337

184. PURPURA, ALLERGIC

Heat and toxins
- *Xi Jiao Di Huang Tang* (Rhinoceros Horn and Rehmannia Decoction), 333 and *Si Sheng Wan* (Four-Fresh Pill), 942

Yin-deficient fire
- *Yu Nu Jian* (Jade Woman Decoction), 398

Damp-heat in the interior
- *Xiao Ji Yin Zi* (Cirsium Decoction), 946

Qi deficiency with aimless movement of blood
- *Gui Pi Tang* (Restore the Spleen Decoction), 583 and *Bao Yuan Tang* (Preserve the Basal Decoction), 525

Blood stagnation
- *Xue Fu Zhu Yu Tang* (Drive Out Stasis in the Mansion of Blood Decoction), 879

185. PURPURA, THROMBOCYTOPENIC

Qi deficiency with aimless movement of blood
- *Gui Pi Tang* (Restore the Spleen Decoction), 583 and *Bao Yuan Tang* (Preserve the Basal Decoction), 525

Heat in the blood causing reckless movement of blood
- *Xi Jiao Di Huang Tang* (Rhinoceros Horn and Rehmannia Decoction), 333
- *Qing Ying Tang* (Clear the Nutritive Level Decoction), 330

Yin-deficient fire
- *Yu Nu Jian* (Jade Woman Decoction), 398

Blood stagnation
- *Tao Hong Si Wu Tang* (Four-Substance Decoction with Safflower and Peach Pit), 571

186. PYELONEPHRITIS

Damp-heat
- *Ba Zheng San* (Eight-Herb Powder for Rectification), 1103

Damp-heat in the Liver and Gallbladder
- *Long Dan Xie Gan Tang* (Gentiana Decoction to Drain the Liver), 371

Heat and toxins
- *Xiao Ji Yin Zi* (Cirsium Decoction), 946

Lung and Stomach heat
- *Bai Hu Tang* (White Tiger Decoction), 321 and *Qing Fei Yin* (Clear the Lung Drink), 1224

Yin-deficient fire
- *Zhi Bai Di Huang Wan* (Anemarrhena, Phellodendron, and Rehmannia Pill), 636

Qi and blood stagnation with damp-heat accumulation
- *Wu Lin San* (Five-Ingredient Powder for Painful Urinary Dysfunction), 1107

187. RADIATION, SUPPORT FOR
- *Shi Quan Da Bu Tang* (All-Inclusive Great Tonifying Decoction), 609
- *Bu Zhong Yi Qi Tang* (Tonify the Middle and Augment the Qi Decoction), 542
- *Ba Zhen Tang* (Eight-Treasure Decoction), 604

188. RASH
- *Xiao Feng San* (Eliminate Wind Powder), 967
- *Wen Qing Yin* (Warming and Clearing Decoction), 575
- *Dang Gui Yin Zi* (Tangkuei Decoction), 970
- *Qing Shang Fang Feng Tang* (Clear the Upper and Guard the Wind Decoction), 349

Chinese Herbal Formulas and Applications

Appendix 2 — Cross-reference Based on Western Medicine Diagnosis

189. RAYNAUD'S SYNDROME

Yin and cold stagnation

- *Dang Gui Si Ni Tang* (Tangkuei Decoction for Frigid Extremities), 494

Blood stagnation

- *Xue Fu Zhu Yu Tang* (Drive Out Stasis in the Mansion of Blood Decoction), 879
- *Shen Tong Zhu Yu Tang* (Drive Out Blood Stasis from a Painful Body Decoction), 893

Blood stagnation with heat

- *Si Miao Yong An Tang* (Four-Valiant Decoction for Well-Being), 1344

190. RECTAL PROLAPSE

- *Bu Zhong Yi Qi Tang* (Tonify the Middle and Augment the Qi Decoction), 542
- *Yi Zi Tang* (Yi Word Decoction), 164

191. REFLUX ESOPHAGITIS

Reversed flow of Stomach qi

- *Xuan Fu Dai Zhe Shi Tang* (Inula and Hematite Decoction), 851

Liver overacting on the Spleen and Stomach

- *Chai Hu Shu Gan San* (Bupleurum Powder to Spread the Liver), 238
- *Zuo Jin Wan* (Left Metal Pill), 389

Stomach yin deficiency

- *Mai Men Dong Tang* (Ophiopogonis Decoction), 1043

Spleen and Stomach deficiency and cold

- *Si Jun Zi Tang* (Four-Gentlemen Decoction), 522

192. RENAL FAILURE

Spleen yang deficiency

- *Fu Zi Li Zhong Wan* (Prepared Aconite Pill to Regulate the Middle), 463 and *Wu Ling San* (Five-Ingredient Powder with Poria), 1109

Kidney yang deficiency

- *Ji Sheng Shen Qi Wan* (Kidney Qi Pill from Formulas that Aid the Living), 675 and *Zhen Wu Tang* (True Warrior Decoction), 1135

Liver and Kidney yin deficiencies

- *Qi Ju Di Huang Wan* (Lycium Fruit, Chrysanthemum, and Rehmannia Pill), 640

Yin and yang deficiencies

- *Ji Sheng Shen Qi Wan* (Kidney Qi Pill from Formulas that Aid the Living), 675

193. RESTLESS FETUS

- *Bao Chan Wu You Fang* (Preserve Pregnancy and Care-Free Decoction), 621

- *Tai Shan Pan Shi San* (Powder that Gives the Stability of Mount Tai), 618
- *Dang Gui Shao Yao San* (Tangkuei and Peony Powder), 594

194. RETINITIS

- *Ci Zhu Wan* (Magnetite and Cinnabar Pill), 714
- *Liu Wei Di Huang Wan* (Six-Ingredient Pill with Rehmannia), 627
- *Qi Ju Di Huang Wan* (Lycium Fruit, Chrysanthemum, and Rehmannia Pill), 640
- *Ming Mu Di Huang Wan* (Improve Vision Pill with Rehmannia), 633
- *Zi Shen Ming Mu Tang* (Nourish the Kidney to Brighten the Eyes Decoction), 664

195. RHEUMATOID ARTHRITIS

Wind-cold-damp obstruction

- *Juan Bi Tang* (Remove Painful Obstruction Decoction), 1158

Heat obstruction

- *Bai Hu Jia Gui Zhi Tang* (White Tiger plus Cinnamon Twig Decoction), 323

Blood stagnation and phlegm obstruction

- *Xiao Huo Luo Dan* (Minor Invigorate the Collaterals Special Pill), 1177

Liver and Kidney deficiencies

- *Hu Qian Wan* (Hidden Tiger Pill), 651

Yin-deficient heat

- *Zhi Bai Di Huang Wan* (Anemarrhena, Phellodendron, and Rehmannia Pill), 636

Kidney yang deficiency

- *Jin Gui Shen Qi Wan* (Kidney Qi Pill from the Golden Cabinet), 668

196. RHINITIS

Wind-cold

- *Xin Yi San* (Magnolia Flower Powder), 84

Wind-heat

- *Cang Er Zi San* (Xanthium Powder), 82

Damp-heat

- *Qing Bi Tang* (Clear the Nose Decoction), 86

Lung heat

- *Xin Yi Qing Fei Yin* (Magnolia Decoction to Clear the Lung), 122

Spleen qi deficiency

- *Bu Zhong Yi Qi Tang* (Tonify the Middle and Augment the Qi Decoction), 542

CROSS-REFERENCE BASED ON WESTERN MEDICINE DIAGNOSIS

A2

1427

Appendix 2 — Cross-reference Based on Western Medicine Diagnosis

197. ROSACEA
- *Si Wu Tang* (Four-Substance Decoction), 562
- *Tao Hong Si Wu Tang* (Four-Substance Decoction with Safflower and Peach Pit), 571
- *Tong Qiao Huo Xue Tang* (Unblock the Orifices and Invigorate the Blood Decoction), 877

198. SCHIZOPHRENIA
Heart and Spleen deficiencies
- *Yang Xin Tang* (Nourish the Heart Decoction), 735
- *Gan Mai Da Zao Tang* (Licorice, Wheat, and Jujube Decoction), 731
Qi and phlegm stagnation
- *Dao Tan Tang* (Guide Out Phlegm Decoction), 1211
Liver fire rising
- *Dang Gui Long Hui Wan* (Tangkuei, Gentiana, and Aloe Pill), 379
Shen (spirit) disturbance
- *Chai Hu Jia Long Gu Mu Li Tang* (Bupleurum plus Dragon Bone and Oyster Shell Decoction), 715

199. SCIATICA
- *Du Huo Ji Sheng Tang* (Angelica Pubescens and Taxillus Decoction), 1161
- *Qiang Huo Sheng Shi Tang* (Notopterygium Decoction to Overcome Dampness), 1156

200. SCLERODERMA
Wind-damp obstruction
- *Du Huo Ji Sheng Tang* (Angelica Pubescens and Taxillus Decoction), 1161
- *Qiang Huo Sheng Shi Tang* (Notopterygium Decoction to Overcome Dampness), 1156
Spleen and Kidney yang deficiencies
- *Yang He Tang* (Yang-Heartening Decoction), 1370
- *Shen Fu Tang* (Ginseng and Prepared Aconite Decoction), 489
Qi deficiency with blood stagnation
- *Bu Yang Huan Wu Tang* (Tonify the Yang to Restore Five Decoction), 905

201. SEIZURES AND EPILEPSY
Liver wind rising with phlegm
- *Ding Xian Wan* (Arrest Seizures Pill), 1251
- *Tian Ma Gou Teng Yin* (Gastrodia and Uncaria Decoction), 1004
Liver fire rising with phlegm
- *Long Dan Xie Gan Tang* (Gentiana Decoction to Drain the Liver), 371
- *Di Tan Tang* (Scour Phlegm Decoction), 1212

Heat and phlegm rising
- *Wen Dan Tang* (Warm the Gallbladder Decoction), 1213
Deficiency
- *Zuo Gui Wan* (Restore the Left [Kidney] Pill), 645

202. SINUSITIS
Wind-cold
- *Xin Yi San* (Magnolia Flower Powder), 84
Wind-heat
- *Cang Er Zi San* (Xanthium Powder), 82
Damp-heat
- *Qing Bi Tang* (Clear the Nose Decoction), 86
Lung heat
- *Xin Yi Qing Fei Yin* (Magnolia Decoction to Clear the Lung), 122
Spleen qi deficiency
- *Bu Zhong Yi Qi Tang* (Tonify the Middle and Augment the Qi Decoction), 542

203. SPERMATORRHEA
Kidney yin deficiency
- *Zuo Gui Wan* (Restore the Left [Kidney] Pill), 645
- *Liu Wei Di Huang Wan* (Six-Ingredient Pill with Rehmannia), 627
Kidney yang deficiency
- *You Gui Wan* (Restore the Right [Kidney] Pill), 678
- *Ba Wei Di Huang Wan* (Eight-Ingredient Pill with Rehmannia), 672
Kidney jing (essence) deficiency
- *Jin Suo Gu Jing Wan* (Metal Lock Pill to Stabilize the Essence), 789
- *Shui Lu Er Xian Dan* (Water and Earth Two Immortals Special Pill), 790
Yin-deficient fire
- *Zhi Bai Di Huang Wan* (Anemarrhena, Phellodendron, and Rehmannia Pill), 636
- *Ding Zhi Wan* (Settle the Emotions Pill), 723
Liver fire
- *Long Dan Xie Gan Tang* (Gentiana Decoction to Drain the Liver), 371
Damp-heat in the interior
- *Bi Xie Fen Qing Yin* (Dioscorea Hypoglauca Decoction to Separate the Clear), 1140

204. STOMATITIS
Heart and Spleen heat
- *Xie Huang San* (Drain the Yellow Powder), 396 and *Dao Chi San* (Guide Out the Red Powder), 365

1428

Chinese Herbal Formulas and Applications

Appendix 2 — Cross-reference Based on Western Medicine Diagnosis

Lung and Stomach heat
- *Liang Ge San* (Cool the Diaphragm Powder), 351 and *Qing Wei San* (Clear the Stomach Powder), 393
- *Gan Lu Yin* (Sweet Dew Decoction), 401

Yin-deficient fire
- *Zhi Bai Di Huang Wan* (Anemarrhena, Phellodendron, and Rehmannia Pill), 636

205. SYSTEMIC LUPUS ERYTHEMATOSUS
Toxic heat
- *Qing Wen Bai Du Yin* (Clear Epidemics and Overcome Pathogenic Influences Decoction), 337

Heart and Spleen deficiencies
- *Gui Pi Tang* (Restore the Spleen Decoction), 583

Qi and yin deficiencies
- *Sheng Mai San* (Generate the Pulse Powder), 554

Spleen and Kidney deficiencies
- *Zhen Wu Tang* (True Warrior Decoction), 1135

Spleen deficiency with Liver excess
- *Xiao Yao San* (Rambling Powder), 247

206. TESTITIS
- *Ju He Wan* (Tangerine Seed Pill), 833
- *Tian Tai Wu Yao San* (Top-Quality Lindera Powder), 835

207. TETANUS
- *Yu Zhen San* (True Jade Powder), 981
- *Zhi Jing San* (Stop Spasms Powder), 979
- *Wu Hu Zhui Feng San* (Five-Tiger Powder to Pursue Wind), 982

208. THIRST
- *Mai Men Dong Tang* (Ophiopogonis Decoction), 1043
- *Sha Shen Mai Dong Tang* (Glehnia and Ophiopogonis Decoction), 1047
- *Zeng Ye Tang* (Increase the Fluids Decoction), 1054

209. THYROIDITIS
Liver and Gallbladder damp-heat
- *Long Dan Xie Gan Tang* (Gentiana Decoction to Drain the Liver), 371

Yin-deficient fire
- *Qing Gu San* (Cool the Bones Powder), 418

Phlegm accumulation
- *Hai Zao Yu Hu Tang* (Sargassum Decoction for the Jade Flask), 1352

Spleen yang deficiency
- *Shi Pi San* (Bolster the Spleen Powder), 1138

210. TIDAL FEVER
- *Da Bu Yin Wan* (Great Tonify the Yin Pill), 649
- *Qing Gu San* (Cool the Bones Powder), 418
- *Qing Hao Bie Jia Tang* (Artemisia Annua and Soft-Shelled Turtle Shell Decoction), 412

211. TINNITUS
Qi and yang deficiencies
- *Yi Qi Cong Ming Tang* (Augment the Qi and Increase Acuity Decoction), 551
- *Bu Zhong Yi Qi Tang* (Tonify the Middle and Augment the Qi Decoction), 542

Yin and blood deficiencies
- *Ba Zhen Tang* (Eight-Treasure Decoction), 604
- *Ren Shen Yang Ying Tang* (Ginseng Decoction to Nourish the Nutritive Qi), 615

Liver and Kidney deficiencies
- *Er Long Zuo Ci Wan* (Pill for Deafness that Is Kind to the Left [Kidney]), 633
- *Qi Ju Di Huang Wan* (Lycium Fruit, Chrysanthemum, and Rehmannia Pill), 640

Phlegm stagnation
- *Di Tan Tang* (Scour Phlegm Decoction), 1212
- *Gun Tan Wan* (Vaporize Phlegm Pill), 1238

Liver fire
- *Long Dan Xie Gan Tang* (Gentiana Decoction to Drain the Liver), 371

212. TONSILLITIS
- *Yin Qiao San* (Honeysuckle and Forsythia Powder), 92
- *Qing Xin Li Ge Tang* (Clear the Epigastrium and Benefit the Diaphragm Decoction), 386
- *Chai Hu Qing Gan Tang* (Bupleurum Decoction to Clear the Liver), 243
- *Ban Xia Hou Po Tang* (Pinellia and Magnolia Bark Decoction), 827

213. TOOTHACHE
- *Qing Wei San* (Clear the Stomach Powder), 393
- *Huang Lian Jie Du Tang* (Coptis Decoction to Relieve Toxicity), 341
- *Gan Lu Yin* (Sweet Dew Decoction), 401
- *Tiao Wei Cheng Qi Tang* (Regulate the Stomach and Order the Qi Decoction), 160

214. TRACHEOBRONCHITIS
Wind-cold affecting the Lung
- *Xing Su San* (Apricot Kernel and Perilla Leaf Powder), 1025
- *Jin Fei Cao San* (Inula Powder), 49

CROSS-REFERENCE BASED ON WESTERN MEDICINE DIAGNOSIS

A2

1429

Appendix 2 – Cross-reference Based on Western Medicine Diagnosis

Appendix 2 — Cross-reference Based on Western Medicine Diagnosis

Wind-heat affecting the Lung
- *Sang Ju Yin* (Mulberry Leaf and Chrysanthemum Decoction), 89
- *Liu Yi San* (Six-to-One Powder), 441

Dryness affecting the Lung
- *Sang Xing Tang* (Mulberry Leaf and Apricot Kernel Decoction), 1027

Wind and phlegm affecting the Lung
- *Zhi Sou San* (Stop Coughing Powder), 116

Phlegm and heat affecting the Lung
- *Qing Qi Hua Tan Wan* (Clear the Qi and Transform Phlegm Pill), 1222
- *Er Chen Tang* (Two-Cured Decoction), 1209 and *San Zi Yang Qin Tang* (Three-Seed Decoction to Nourish One's Parents), 1245

215. TRACHEITIS
- *Ma Huang Xing Ren Gan Cao Shi Gao Tang* (Ephedra, Apricot Kernel, Licorice, and Gypsum Decoction), 96
- *Qing Qi Hua Tan Wan* (Clear the Qi and Transform Phlegm Pill), 1222
- *Bei Mu Gua Lou San* (Fritillaria and Trichosanthes Fruit Powder), 1240

216. TRANSIENT ISCHEMIC ATTACK (TIA)
Liver yang rising with Liver and Kidney yin deficiencies
- *Zhen Gan Xi Feng Tang* (Sedate the Liver and Extinguish Wind Decoction), 999

Qi deficiency with blood stagnation
- *Bu Yang Huan Wu Tang* (Tonify the Yang to Restore Five Decoction), 905

Blood stagnation with phlegm obstruction
- *Wen Dan Tang* (Warm the Gallbladder Decoction), 1213 and *Tao Hong Si Wu Tang* (Four-Substance Decoction with Safflower and Peach Pit), 571

217. TRAUMA
- *Fu Yuan Huo Xue Tang* (Revive Health by Invigorating the Blood Decoction), 897
- *Zheng Gu Zi Jin Dan* (Purple and Gold Pill for Righteous Bones), 901
- *Shen Tong Zhu Yu Tang* (Drive Out Blood Stasis from a Painful Body Decoction), 893
- *Qi Li San* (Seven-Thousandths of a Tael Powder), 903
- *Tao He Cheng Qi Tang* (Peach Pit Decoction to Order the Qi), 873

218. TREMOR
Liver and Kidney deficiencies
- *Da Bu Yin Wan* (Great Tonify the Yin Pill), 649 and *Liu Wei Di Huang Wan* (Six-Ingredient Pill with Rehmannia), 627

Qi and blood deficiencies
- *Ba Zhen Tang* (Eight-Treasure Decoction), 604 and *Tian Ma Gou Teng Yin* (Gastrodia and Uncaria Decoction), 1004

Liver wind rising with phlegm and heat accumulation
- *Tian Ma Gou Teng Yin* (Gastrodia and Uncaria Decoction), 1004 and *Dao Tan Tang* (Guide Out Phlegm Decoction), 1211

219. TRIGEMINAL NEURALGIA
Wind-cold affecting the channels and collaterals
- *Chuan Xiong Cha Tiao San* (Ligusticum Chuanxiong Powder to be Taken with Green Tea), 973

Wind-heat affecting the channels and collaterals
- *Shi Gao Tang* (Gypsum Decoction), 299 with *Chuan Xiong* (Rhizoma Chuanxiong) and *Bai Zhi* (Radix Angelicae Dahuricae)

Wind and phlegm blocking the channels and collaterals
- *Dao Tan Tang* (Guide Out Phlegm Decoction), 1211 with *Chuan Xiong* (Rhizoma Chuanxiong) and *Xi Xin* (Radix et Rhizoma Asari)

Stomach fire rising
- *Qing Wei San* (Clear the Stomach Powder), 393

Liver and Gallbladder fire rising
- *Long Dan Xie Gan Tang* (Gentiana Decoction to Drain the Liver), 371

Yin deficiency with fire rising
- *Zhen Gan Xi Feng Tang* (Sedate the Liver and Extinguish Wind Decoction), 999

Blood stagnation
- *Tong Qiao Huo Xue Tang* (Unblock the Orifices and Invigorate the Blood Decoction), 877

220. TUBERCULOSIS (INTESTINE)
Yin-deficient heat
- *Qing Gu San* (Cool the Bones Powder), 418

Damp-heat
- *Ge Gen Huang Qin Huang Lian Tang* (Kudzu, Coptis, and Scutellaria Decoction), 295

Spleen and Stomach deficiencies
- *Shen Ling Bai Zhu San* (Ginseng, Poria, and Atractylodes Macrocephala Powder), 535

Kidney yang deficiencies
- *Si Shen Wan* (Four-Miracle Pill), 784

Qi and blood stagnation
- *Shao Fu Zhu Yu Tang* (Drive Out Blood Stasis in the Lower Abdomen Decoction), 889

221. TUBERCULOSIS (LUNG)
Lung yin deficiency
- *Yue Hua Wan* (Moonlight Pill), 1040

1430

Chinese Herbal Formulas and Applications

Appendix 2 — Cross-reference Based on Western Medicine Diagnosis

- *Mai Men Dong Tang* (Ophiopogonis Decoction), 1043
- *Sha Shen Mai Dong Tang* (Glehnia and Ophiopogonis Decoction), 1047

Yin-deficient fire
- *Bai He Gu Jin Tang* (Lily Bulb Decoction to Preserve the Metal), 1036
- *Qing Gu San* (Cool the Bones Powder), 418
- *Qin Jiao Bie Jia San* (Gentiana Macrophylla and Soft-Shelled Turtle Shell Powder), 416

Qi and yin deficiencies
- *Sheng Mai San* (Generate the Pulse Powder), 554

222. TUBERCULOSIS (PERITONEUM)

***Yangming* heat**
- *Da Cheng Qi Tang* (Major Order the Qi Decoction), 152

Qi and yin deficiencies
- *Si Jun Zi Tang* (Four-Gentlemen Decoction), 522 and *Qing Gu San* (Cool the Bones Powder), 418

Blood and phlegm stagnation
- *Xue Fu Zhu Yu Tang* (Drive Out Stasis in the Mansion of Blood Decoction), 879

223. URETHRITIS

- *Ba Zheng San* (Eight-Herb Powder for Rectification), 1103
- *Long Dan Xie Gan Tang* (Gentiana Decoction to Drain the Liver), 371

224. URINARY INCONTINENCE

Lung and Spleen qi deficiencies
- *Bu Zhong Yi Qi Tang* (Tonify the Middle and Augment the Qi Decoction), 542

Heart and Kidney disharmony
- *Sang Piao Xiao San* (Mantis Egg-Case Powder), 792

Damp-heat
- *Ba Zheng San* (Eight-Herb Powder for Rectification), 1103

Blood stagnation
- *Shao Fu Zhu Yu Tang* (Drive Out Blood Stasis in the Lower Abdomen Decoction), 889

225. URINARY TRACT INFECTION

Damp-heat in the lower *jiao*
- *Ba Zheng San* (Eight-Herb Powder for Rectification), 1103

Liver and Gallbladder heat
- *Long Dan Xie Gan Tang* (Gentiana Decoction to Drain the Liver), 371

226. UROSCHESIS

Damp-heat
- *Ba Zheng San* (Eight-Herb Powder for Rectification), 1103
- *Dao Chi San* (Guide Out the Red Powder), 365

Lung heat
- *Qing Fei Yin* (Clear the Lung Drink), 1224

Spleen deficiency
- *Bu Zhong Yi Qi Tang* (Tonify the Middle and Augment the Qi Decoction), 542

Kidney deficiency
- *Ji Sheng Shen Qi Wan* (Kidney Qi Pill from Formulas that Aid the Living), 675

227. UTERINE PROLAPSE

- *Bu Zhong Yi Qi Tang* (Tonify the Middle and Augment the Qi Decoction), 542

228. VASCULAR DEMENTIA

Phlegm misting the Heart and disturbing the *shen* (spirit)
- *Dao Tan Tang* (Guide Out Phlegm Decoction), 1211

Phlegm blocking the sensory orifices
- *Tong Qiao Huo Xue Tang* (Unblock the Orifices and Invigorate the Blood Decoction), 877

Heart qi deficiency
- *Ren Shen Yang Ying Tang* (Ginseng Decoction to Nourish the Nutritive Qi), 615

229. VERTIGO

Liver wind rising
- *Tian Ma Gou Teng Yin* (Gastrodia and Uncaria Decoction), 1004
- *Da Ding Feng Zhu* (Major Arrest Wind Pearl), 1009

Liver fire rising
- *Long Dan Xie Gan Tang* (Gentiana Decoction to Drain the Liver), 371
- *Dang Gui Long Hui Wan* (Tangkuei, Gentiana, and Aloe Pill), 379

Phlegm accumulation
- *Ban Xia Bai Zhu Tian Ma Tang* (Pinellia, Atractylodes Macrocephala, and Gastrodia Decoction), 1247
- *Wen Dan Tang* (Warm the Gallbladder Decoction), 1213

Blood stagnation
- *Tong Qiao Huo Xue Tang* (Unblock the Orifices and Invigorate the Blood Decoction), 877
- *Xue Fu Zhu Yu Tang* (Drive Out Stasis in the Mansion of Blood Decoction), 879

Qi and blood deficiencies
- *Gui Pi Tang* (Restore the Spleen Decoction), 583

CROSS-REFERENCE BASED ON WESTERN MEDICINE DIAGNOSIS

A2

1431

Appendix 2 – Cross-reference Based on Western Medicine Diagnosis

Appendix 2 — Cross-reference Based on Western Medicine Diagnosis

- *Ba Zhen Tang* (Eight-Treasure Decoction), 604
- *Shi Quan Da Bu Tang* (All-Inclusive Great Tonifying Decoction), 609

Kidney deficiency
- *Zuo Gui Wan* (Restore the Left [Kidney] Pill), 645
- *You Gui Wan* (Restore the Right [Kidney] Pill), 678

230. VISION, BLURRED

Deficiency
- *Ming Mu Di Huang Wan* (Improve Vision Pill with Rehmannia), 633
- *Qi Ju Di Huang Wan* (Lycium Fruit, Chrysanthemum, and Rehmannia Pill), 640
- *Zi Shen Ming Mu Tang* (Nourish the Kidney to Brighten the Eyes Decoction), 664

Excess
- *Xi Gan Ming Mu San* (Wash the Liver and Brighten the Eyes Powder), 381

231. VOMITING

Exterior condition
- *Huo Xiang Zheng Qi San* (Agastache Powder to Rectify the Qi), 1079
- *Xin Jia Xiang Ru Yin* (Newly-Augmented Mosla Decoction), 439

Stomach cold
- *Li Zhong Tang* (Regulate the Middle Decoction), 462
- *Li Zhong Wan* (Regulate the Middle Pill), 459

Stomach heat
- *Xiao Cheng Qi Tang* (Minor Order the Qi Decoction), 158
- *Zhu Ye Shi Gao Tang* (Bamboo Leaves and Gypsum Decoction), 326

Phlegm obstruction
- *Ling Gui Zhu Gan Tang* (Poria, Cinnamon Twig, Atractylodes Macrocephala, and Licorice Decoction), 1131
- *Xuan Fu Dai Zhe Shi Tang* (Inula and Hematite Decoction), 851
- *Dao Tan Tang* (Guide Out Phlegm Decoction), 1211

Food stagnation
- *Bao He Wan* (Preserve Harmony Pill), 1266

Blood stagnation
- *Ge Xia Zhu Yu Tang* (Drive Out Blood Stasis Below the Diaphragm Decoction), 885

Spleen and Stomach deficiency and cold
- *Li Zhong Wan* (Regulate the Middle Pill), 459
- *Xiang Sha Liu Jun Zi Tang* (Six-Gentlemen Decoction with Aucklandia and Amomum), 531

Stomach yin deficiency
- *Sha Shen Mai Dong Tang* (Glehnia and Ophiopogonis Decoction), 1047
- *Mai Men Dong Tang* (Ophiopogonis Decoction), 1043

Liver overacting on the Spleen and Stomach
- *Ban Xia Hou Po Tang* (Pinellia and Magnolia Bark Decoction), 827
- *Zuo Jin Wan* (Left Metal Pill), 389

232. WHEEZING AND DYSPNEA

Wind-cold invading the Lung
- *Ma Huang Tang* (Ephedra Decoction), 39

Wind-heat invading the Lung
- *Ma Huang Xing Ren Gan Cao Shi Gao Tang* (Ephedra, Apricot Kernel, Licorice, and Gypsum Decoction), 96

Phlegm in the Lung
- *Er Chen Tang* (Two-Cured Decoction), 1209
- *San Zi Yang Qin Tang* (Three-Seed Decoction to Nourish One's Parents), 1245

Lung heat
- *Ding Chuan Tang* (Arrest Wheezing Decoction), 845

Lung cold
- *She Gan Ma Huang Tang* (Belamcanda and Ephedra Decoction), 80
- *Xiao Qing Long Tang* (Minor Bluegreen Dragon Decoction), 74

Lung deficiency
- *Sheng Mai San* (Generate the Pulse Powder), 554
- *Yu Ping Feng San* (Jade Windscreen Powder), 773
- *Bu Fei Tang* (Tonify the Lung Decoction), 560

Spleen deficiency
- *Liu Jun Zi Tang* (Six-Gentlemen Decoction), 527

Kidney deficiency
- *Jin Gui Shen Qi Wan* (Kidney Qi Pill from the Golden Cabinet), 668
- *Du Qi Wan* (Capital Qi Pill), 644
- *Ren Shen Ge Jie San* (Ginseng and Gecko Powder), 557

1432

Appendix 3

— Formulas Offering Beneficial Effects to Support Pregnancy

The following formulas have been shown to offer beneficial effects during pregnancy. However, these formulas should be used only under supervision of a qualified healthcare professional, and only when the benefits of using the herbs outweigh the risks.

Symptoms	Formulas
Abdominal pain	• *Dang Gui Shao Yao San* (Tangkuei and Peony Powder), 594 • *Jiao Ai Tang* (Ass-Hide Gelatin and Mugwort Decoction), 950
Breech presentation of the fetus	• *Ba Zhen Tang* (Eight-Treasure Decoction), 604 with *Huang Qi* (Radix Astragali), *Xu Duan* (Radix Dipsaci) and *Zhi Qiao* (Fructus Aurantii)
Cough	• *Bai He Gu Jin Tang* (Lily Bulb Decoction to Preserve the Metal), 1036 • *Liu Jun Zi Tang* (Six-Gentlemen Decoction), 527
Edema and swelling	• *Wu Ling San* (Five-Ingredient Powder with Poria), 1109
Irritability	• *Qi Ju Di Huang Wan* (Lycium Fruit, Chrysanthemum, and Rehmannia Pill), 640 • *Ba Zhen Tang* (Eight-Treasure Decoction), 604 • *Ban Xia Bai Zhu Tian Ma Tang* (Pinellia, Atractylodes Macrocephala, and Gastrodia Decoction), 1247
Miscarriage, prevention of	• *Bao Chan Wu You Fang* (Preserve Pregnancy and Care-Free Decoction), 621 • *Tai Shan Pan Shi San* (Powder that Gives the Stability of Mount Tai), 618
Nausea and vomiting	• *Xiang Sha Liu Jun Zi Tang* (Six-Gentlemen Decoction with Aucklandia and Amomum), 531 • *Wen Dan Tang* (Warm the Gallbladder Decoction), 1213 • *Ju Pi Zhu Ru Tang* (Tangerine Peel and Bamboo Shaving Decoction), 854
Restless fetus	• *Bao Chan Wu You Fang* (Preserve Pregnancy and Care-Free Decoction), 621 • *Dang Gui Shao Yao San* (Tangkuei and Peony Powder), 594
Uterine bleeding	• *Gui Zhi Fu Ling Wan* (Cinnamon Twig and Poria Pill), 928 • *Bao Chan Wu You Fang* (Preserve Pregnancy and Care-Free Decoction), 621

Appendix 4 – Formulas Offering Beneficial Effects for Postpartum Care

Appendix 4

— Formulas Offering Beneficial Effects for Postpartum Care

The following formulas have been shown to offer beneficial effects for postpartum care. However, these formulas should be used only under supervision of a qualified healthcare professional, and only when the benefits of using the herbs outweigh the risks.

Symptoms	Formulas
Blood stagnation (retention of lochia)	• *Sheng Hua Tang* (Generation and Transformation Decoction), 925
Qi and blood deficiencies	• *Ba Zhen Tang* (Eight-Treasure Decoction), 604
Lactation, insufficient	• *Tong Ru Wan* (Unblock the Breast Pill), 927
Lactation, excessive	• *Bu Zhong Yi Qi Tang* (Tonify the Middle and Augment the Qi Decoction), 542 with *Qian Shi* (Semen Euryales) and *Wu Wei Zi* (Fructus Schisandrae Chinensis) • *Jia Wei Xiao Yao San* (Augmented Rambling Powder), 254 with *Mu Li* (Concha Ostreae) and *Xia Ku Cao* (Spica Prunellae)
Lactation, termination of	• *Mai Ya* (Fructus Hordei Germinatus) 60g

Appendix 5

— Cautions / Contraindications for the Use of Formulas During Pregnancy

The following formulas have a recognized potential to endanger or cause harm to a fetus during pregnancy, thus possibly causing birth defects or miscarriages. As a general rule, formulas with potent effects to regulate qi, move blood, or drain downward should be avoided during pregnancy. These formulas are **contraindicated,** or if absolutely necessary, used with **caution** in treatment of pregnant women. Please note that this is not a comprehensive list - additional information is listed in each formula monograph.

An Gong Niu Huang Wan (Calm the Palace Pill with Cattle Gallstone)	746
Ba Wei Di Huang Wan (Eight-Ingredient Pill with Rehmannia)	672
Ba Zheng San (Eight-Herb Powder for Rectification)	1103
Bao He Wan (Preserve Harmony Pill)	1266
Ci Zhu Wan (Magnetite and Cinnabar Pill)	714
Da Cheng Qi Tang (Major Order the Qi Decoction)	152
Da Huang Mu Dan Tang (Rhubarb and Moutan Decoction)	1378
Da Huang Zhe Chong Wan (Rhubarb and Eupolyphaga Pill)	937
Da Jian Zhong Tang (Major Construct the Middle Decoction)	480
Da Xian Xiong Tang (Major Sinking into the Chest Decoction)	161
Dang Gui Long Hui Wan (Tangkuei, Gentiana, and Aloe Pill)	379
Du Huo Ji Sheng Tang (Angelica Pubescens and Taxillus Decoction)	1161
Fang Feng Tong Sheng San (Saposhnikovia Powder that Sagely Unblocks)	291
Fu Yuan Huo Xue Tang (Revive Health by Invigorating the Blood Decoction)	897
Fu Zi Li Zhong Wan (Prepared Aconite Pill to Regulate the Middle)	463
Ge Xia Zhu Yu Tang (Drive Out Blood Stasis Below the Diaphragm Decoction)	885
Gong Wai Yun Fang (Ectopic Pregnancy Formula)	917
Gun Tan Wan (Vaporize Phlegm Pill)	1238
Guo Qi Yin (Delayed Menstruation Decoction)	578
Hei Xi Dan (Lead Special Pill)	492
Hua Chong Wan (Dissolve Parasites Pill)	1300
Huo Luo Xiao Ling Dan (Fantastically Effective Pill to Invigorate the Collaterals)	914
Ji Ming San (Powder to Take at Cock's Crow)	1183
Jia Wei Xiao Yao San (Augmented Rambling Powder)	254
Jin Gui Shen Qi Wan (Kidney Qi Pill from the Golden Cabinet)	668
Jin Ling Zi San (Melia Toosendan Powder)	825
Li Zhong Wan (Regulate the Middle Pill)	459
Liang Ge San (Cool the Diaphragm Powder)	351

Appendix 5 — Cautions / Contraindications for the Use of Formulas During Pregnancy

Liu Shen Wan (Six-Miracle Pill)	363
Liu Yi San (Six-to-One Powder)	441
Ma Huang Fu Zi Xi Xin Tang (Ephedra, Asarum, and Prepared Aconite Decoction)	132
Ma Zi Ren Wan (Hemp Seed Pill)	174
Mu Xiang Bing Lang Wan (Aucklandia and Betel Nut Pill)	1272
Ping Wei San (Calm the Stomach Powder)	1068
Qi Li San (Seven-Thousandths of a Tael Powder)	903
Qian Zheng San (Lead to Symmetry Powder)	977
Qing Qi Hua Tan Wan (Clear the Qi and Transform Phlegm Pill)	1222
Run Chang Wan (Moisten the Intestines Pill)	177
San Huang Xie Xin Tang (Three-Yellow Decoction to Sedate the Epigastrium)	359
San Wu Bei Ji Wan (Three-Substance Pill for Emergencies)	171
Shao Fu Zhu Yu Tang (Drive Out Blood Stasis in the Lower Abdomen Decoction)	889
Shen Ling Bai Zhu San (Ginseng, Poria, and Atractylodes Macrocephala Powder)	535
Shen Tong Zhu Yu Tang (Drive Out Blood Stasis from a Painful Body Decoction)	893
Sheng Hua Tang (Generation and Transformation Decoction)	925
Shi Xiao San (Sudden Smile Powder)	911
Shi Zao Tang (Ten-Jujube Decoction)	181
Su He Xiang Wan (Liquid Styrax Pill)	758
Tao He Cheng Qi Tang (Peach Pit Decoction to Order the Qi)	873
Tao Hong Si Wu Tang (Four-Substance Decoction with Safflower and Peach Pit)	571
Wu Mei Wan (Mume Pill)	1292
Wu Yao Shun Qi San (Lindera Powder to Smooth the Flow of Qi)	990
Xi Huang Wan (Cattle Gallstone Pill)	1350
Xiao Huo Luo Dan (Minor Invigorate the Collaterals Special Pill)	1177
Xiao Jin Dan (Minor Gold Special Pill)	1374
Xiao Yao San (Rambling Powder)	247
Xing Jun San (Troop-Marching Powder)	756
Xue Fu Zhu Yu Tang (Drive Out Stasis in the Mansion of Blood Decoction)	879
Yin Chen Hao Tang (Artemisia Scoparia Decoction)	1086
Yu Zhen San (True Jade Powder)	981
Zhi Bao Dan (Greatest Treasure Special Pill)	749
Zhi Shi Dao Zhi Wan (Immature Bitter Orange Pill to Guide Out Stagnation)	1270
Zhou Che Wan (Vessel and Vehicle Pill)	184
Zhu Sha An Shen Wan (Cinnabar Pill to Tranquilize the Spirit)	710
Zi Jin Ding (Purple Gold Special Pill)	760
Zi Xue (Purple Snow)	752
Zuo Jin Wan (Left Metal Pill)	389

Appendix 6

— Dosing Guidelines

DOSING

The dosages listed in this text refer to the daily dose for an adult of average height and weight, when using dehydrated herbs. However, the actual prescribed dosage will vary significantly, based not only on the characteristics of the illness and overall condition of the patient, but also on his or her size and age. Generally speaking, single herbs used individually require higher dosages, while herbs used as part of an herbal formula are chosen in smaller amounts. Treatment of an acute condition necessitates higher dosages, and treatment of a mild condition, smaller dosages. One must also consider the constitution of the patient. Those who are basically healthy and strong may tolerate larger doses, while weak and/or deficient patients will need a smaller dose.

Recommended ingestion levels must be adjusted to reflect variations in age and body weight. The principle behind the *Age-to-Dose Dosing Guidelines* is based on assessment of the maturity of the internal organs and their capacity to metabolize, utilize and eliminate herbs. This highly-detailed chart is especially useful for infants and younger children. The recommendations are taken from *Zhong Cao Yao* (Chinese Herbal Medicine), published by the Nanjing College of Traditional Chinese Medicine.

The principle behind the *Weight-to-Dose Dosing Guidelines* is based on the effective concentration of the herbal medicine once it is distributed throughout different areas of the body. This dosing strategy is especially useful for patients whose body weight falls outside of the normal range. All calculations are based on Clark's Rule in *Pharmaceutical Calculations*, written by Mitchell Stoklosa and Howard Ansel.

These charts provide herbal practitioners a handy reference for dosing those patients who fall outside the definition of an "average adult." It is important to remember, however, that the charts serve only as guidelines--not as absolute rules. One must always remember to treat each patient as a unique individual, not as a statistic on a chart!

Appendix 6 – Dosing Guidelines

Appendix 6 — Dosing Guidelines

AGE-TO-DOSE DOSING GUIDELINE

Age	Recommended Daily Dosage
0 – 1 month	1/18 - 1/14 of adult dose
1 – 6 month	1/14 - 1/7 of adult dose
6 – 12 month	1/7 - 1/5 of adult dose
1 – 2 years	1/5 - 1/4 of adult dose
2 – 4 years	1/4 - 1/3 of adult dose
4 – 6 years	1/3 - 2/5 of adult dose
6 – 9 years	2/5 - 1/2 of adult dose
9 – 14 years	1/2 - 2/3 of adult dose
14 – 18 years	2/3 - full adult dose
18 – 60 years	**adult dose**
60 years and over	3/4 or less of adult dose

WEIGHT-TO-DOSE DOSING GUIDELINE

Weight	Recommended Daily Dosage
30 – 40 lbs	20% - 27% of adult dose
40 – 50 lbs	27% - 33% of adult dose
50 – 60 lbs	33% - 40% of adult dose
60 – 70 lbs	40% - 47% of adult dose
70 – 80 lbs	47% - 53% of adult dose
80 – 100 lbs	53% - 67% of adult dose
100 – 120 lbs	67% - 80% of adult dose
120 – 150 lbs	80% - 100% of adult dose
150 lbs	**adult dose**
150 – 200 lbs	100% - 133% of adult dose
200 – 250 lbs	133% - 167% of adult dose
250 – 300 lbs	167% - 200% of adult dose

Chinese Herbal Formulas and Applications

Appendix 7

— Weights and Measures: Chinese, British and Metric Systems

CHINESE SYSTEM

1. Measure of Weight

1 *jin* (斤) = 16 *liang* (两)
1 *liang* (两) = 10 *qian* (钱)
1 *qian* (钱) = 10 *fen* (分)
1 *fen* (分) = 10 *li* (厘)

2. Measure of Volume

1 *shi* (石) = 10 *dou* (斗)
1 *dou* (斗) = 10 *sheng* (升)
1 *sheng* (升) = 10 *he* (合)
1 *he* (合) = 10 *shao* (勺)

BRITISH SYSTEM

1. Measure of Weight (Apothecary)

20 grains = 1 scruple
3 scruples (60 grains) = 1 drachm or dram
8 drachms (480 grains) = 1 ounce
12 ounces (5760 grains) = 1 pound

2. Measure of Weight (Avoirdupois)

437½ or 437.5 grains = 1 ounce
16 ounces (7,000 grains) = 1 pound

3. Measure of Volume (Apothecary)

60 minims = 1 fluidrachm or fluidram
8 fluidrachms (480 minims) = 1 fluidounce
16 fluidounces = 1 pint
2 pints (32 fluidounces) = 1 quart
4 quarts (8 pints) = 1 gallon

METRIC SYSTEM

1. Measure of Weight

1 kilogram (kg) = 1,000.000 grams
1 hectogram (hg) = 100.000 grams
1 dekagram (dag) = 10.000 grams
1 gram (g or gm) = 1.000 gram
1 decigram (dg) = 0.100 gram
1 centigram (cg) = 0.010 gram
1 milligram (mg) = 0.001 gram
1 microgram (μg or mcg) = 0.000,001 gram

1 gram (g or gm) = 0.001 kilogram
= 0.010 hectogram
= 0.100 dekagram
= 10 decigrams
= 100 centigrams
= 1,000 milligrams
= 1,000,000 micrograms

2. Measure of Volume

1 kiloliter (kL) = 1,000.000 liters
1 hectoliter (hL) = 100.000 liters
1 dekaliter (daL) = 10.000 liters
1 liter (L) = 1.000 liter
1 deciliter (dL) = 0.100 liter
1 centiliter (cL) = 0.010 liter
1 milliliter (mL) = 0.001 liter
1 microliter (μL) = 0.000,001 liter

1 liter = 0.001 kiloliter
= 0.010 hectoliter
= 0.100 dekaliter
= 10 deciliters
= 100 centiliters
= 1,000 milliliters
= 1,000,000 microliters

Appendix 7 – Weights and Measures: Chinese, British and Metric Systems

Appendix 7 — Weights and Measures: Chinese, British and Metric Systems

METRIC SYSTEM

Multiples and Submultiples		Prefix	Symbols
1,000,000,000,000	(10^{12})	*tera-*	T
1,000,000,000	(10^{9})	*giga-*	G
1,000,000	(10^{6})	*mega-*	M
1,000	(10^{3})	*kilo-*	k
100	(10^{2})	*hecto-*	h
10	(10)	*deka-*	da
0.1	(10^{-1})	*deci-*	d
0.01	(10^{-2})	*centi-*	c
0.001	(10^{-3})	*milli-*	m
0.000,001	(10^{-6})	*micro-*	μ or mc
0.000,000,001	(10^{-9})	*nano-*	n
0.000,000,000,001	(10^{-12})	*pico-*	p
0.000,000,000,000,001	(10^{-15})	*femto-*	f
0.000,000,000,000,000,001	(10^{-18})	*atto-*	a

CONVERSIONS

Weight Conversion
(Chinese Units : Metric : Avoirdupois)

Chinese Units	Grams	Ounces
1 *jin*	500	17.87
1 *liang*	31.25	1.116875
1 *qian*	3.125	0.111688
1 *fen*	0.3125	0.011169
1 *li*	0.03125	0.001117

Volume Conversion
(Chinese Units : Metric : Apothecary)

Chinese Units	Liter	Fluid Ounces
1 *sheng*	1	33.815

Note: Chinese units of weights and measures vary from dynasty to dynasty. Therefore, the conversion of Chinese units to another system is not always simple or straight forward. For additional information, please see pages 22 to 23.

1440

Appendix 8

Chinese Herbal Formulas and Applications

— Convention on International Trade in Endangered Species (CITES)

Trade in herbs and animals listed in Appendix I of Convention on International Trade in Endangered Species (CITES) is strictly prohibited. The discussion of these substances in this text is included only to offer 1) the accurate history of their critically important usage in traditional herbal medicine, and 2) models for appropriate usage of effective substitute substances and alternatives. The information should not be interpreted as condoning illegal use of these endangered species. Additional and updated information may be obtain from www.cites.org.

Endangered Species	Status	Alternatives
Chuan Shan Jia (Squama Manis)	Appendix II	*Wang Bu Liu Xing* (Semen Vaccariae)
Hu Gu (Os Tigris)	Appendix I	*Zhu Gu* (Os Porcus)
She Xiang (Moschus)	Appendix I/II	*Bing Pian* (Borneolum Syntheticum) or *Su He Xiang* (Styrax)
Xi Jiao (Cornu Rhinoceri)	Appendix I	*Shui Niu Jiao* (Cornu Bubali)
Xiong Dan (Fel Ursi)	Appendix I	*Niu Dan* (Fel Bovis)

CONVENTION ON INTERNATIONAL TRADE IN ENDANGERED SPECIES (CITES)

A8

1441

Appendix 9 – Cross-reference of Single Herb Names

Appendix 9

— Cross-reference of Single Herb Names

Pinyin Names	Pharmaceutical Names	Chinese Names
A Wei	Resina Ferulae	阿魏
Ai Di Cha	Herba Ardisiae Japonicae	矮地茶
Ai Ye	Folium Artemisiae Argyi	艾叶
Ai Ye Tan	Folium Artemisiae Argyi Carbonisatum	艾叶炭
An Xi Xiang	Benzoinum	安息香
Ba Dou	Semen Crotonis	巴豆
Ba Dou Shuang	Semen Crotonis Pulveratum	巴豆霜
Ba Ji Tian	Radix Morindae Officinalis	巴戟天
Ba Jiao Feng	Radix Alangii	八角枫
Ba Jiao Hui Xiang	Fructus Anisi Stellati	八角茴香
Ba Li Ma	Fructus Rhododendri	八里麻
Ba Qia	Rhizoma Smilacis Chinae	菝葜
Bai Bian Dou	Semen Lablab Album	白扁豆
Bai Bu	Radix Stemonae	百部
Bai Fan	Alumen	白矾
Bai Fu Ling	Poria Alba	白茯苓
Bai Fu Zi	Rhizoma Typhonii	白附子
Bai Guo	Semen Ginkgo	白果
Bai He	Bulbus Lilii	百合
Bai Hua She She Cao	Herba Hedyotis	白花蛇舌草
Bai Ji	Rhizoma Bletillae	白及
Bai Jiang Cao	Herba cum Radice Patriniae	败酱草
Bai Lian	Radix Ampelopsis	白蔹
Bai Long Chuan Hua Tou	Radix Clerodendron Paniculatum	白龙船花头
Bai Mao Gen	Rhizoma Imperatae	白茅根
Bai Mao Hua	Flos Imperatae	白茅花
Bai Mu Er	Fructificatio Tremellae Fuciformis	白木耳
Bai Mu Tong	Caulis Akebiae Trifoliatae	白木通
Bai Qian	Rhizoma et Radix Cynanchi Stauntonii	白前
Bai Qu Cai	Herba Chelidonii	白屈菜
Bai Shao	Radix Paeoniae Alba	白芍
Bai Tou Weng	Radix Pulsatillae	白头翁
Bai Tou Weng Jing	Caulis Pulsatillae	白头翁茎
Bai Tou Weng Ye	Folium Pulsatillae	白头翁叶
Bai Wei	Radix et Rhizoma Cynanchi Atrati	白薇
Bai Xian Pi	Cortex Dictamni	白鲜皮

1442

Chinese Herbal Formulas and Applications

Appendix 9 — Cross-reference of Single Herb Names

Pinyin Names	Pharmaceutical Names	Chinese Names
Bai Zhi	Radix Angelicae Dahuricae	白芷
Bai Zhu	Rhizoma Atractylodis Macrocephalae	白术
Bai Zi Ren	Semen Platycladi	柏子仁
Ban Bian Lian	Herba Lobeliae Chinensis	半边莲
Ban Lan Gen	Radix Isatidis	板蓝根
Ban Mao	Mylabris	斑蝥
Ban Xia	Rhizoma Pinelliae	半夏
Ban Xia Qu	Rhizoma Pinelliae Massa Fermentata	半夏曲
Ban Zhi Lian	Herba Scutellariae Barbatae	半枝莲
Bao Ma Zi Pi	Cortex Syringae Amurensis	暴马子皮
Bei Chai Hu	Radix Bupleurum Chinensis	北柴胡
Bei Dou Gen	Rhizoma Menispermi	北豆根
Bei Mu	Bulbus Fritillariae	贝母
Bei Sha Shen	Radix Glehniae	北沙参
Bei Ting Li Zi	Semen Lepidii	北葶苈子
Bi Bo	Fructus Piperis Longi	荜茇
Bi Cheng Qie	Fructus Litseae	荜澄茄
Bi Ma Zi	Semen Ricini	蓖麻子
Bi Zi Cao	Herba Pogonantheri Criniti	笔仔草
Bian Dou Hua	Flos Lablab Album	扁豆花
Bian Dou Yi	Pericarpium Lablab Album	扁豆衣
Bian Xu	Herba Polygoni Avicularis	萹蓄
Bie Jia	Carapax Trionycis	鳖甲
Bie Jia Jiao	Gelatinum Carapax Trionycis	鳖甲胶
Bing Lang	Semen Arecae	槟榔
Bing Pian	Borneolum Syntheticum	冰片
Bo He	Herba Menthae	薄荷
Bo He Nao	Mentholum	薄荷脑
Bo Luo Hui	Herba Macleayae	博落回
Bu Gu Zhi	Fructus Psoraleae	补骨脂
Can Sha	Faeces Bombycis	蚕砂
Cang Er Cao	Herba Xanthii	苍耳草
Cang Er Gen	Radix Xanthii	苍耳根
Cang Er Zi	Fructus Xanthii	苍耳子
Cang Zhu	Rhizoma Atractylodis	苍术
Cao Dou Kou	Semen Alpiniae Katsumadai	草豆蔻
Cao Guo	Fructus Tsaoko	草果
Cao Wu	Radix Aconiti Kusnezoffii	草乌
Cao Wu Ye	Folium Aconiti Kusnezoffii	草乌叶
Ce Bai Ye	Cacumen Platycladi	侧柏叶
Ce Bai Ye Tan	Cacumen Platycladi Carbonisatum	侧柏叶炭

CROSS-REFERENCE OF SINGLE HERB NAMES

A9

1443

Appendix 9 – Cross-reference of Single Herb Names

Appendix 9 — Cross-reference of Single Herb Names

Pinyin Names	Pharmaceutical Names	Chinese Names
Cha Chi Huang	Herba Stellariae Aquaticae	茶匙癀
Cha Ye	Folium Camelliae	茶叶
Chai Hu	Radix Bupleuri	柴胡
Chan Su	Venenum Bufonis	蟾酥
Chan Tui	Periostracum Cicadae	蝉蜕
Chang Shan	Radix Dichroae	常山
Chang Zui Lao Guan Cao	Herba Erodii	长嘴老鹳草
Chao Gua Lou Zi	Semen Trichosanthis Tostum	炒瓜蒌子
Che Qian Cao	Herba Plantaginis	车前草
Che Qian Zi	Semen Plantaginis	车前子
Chen Pi	Pericarpium Citri Reticulatae	陈皮
Chen Xiang	Lignum Aquilariae Resinatum	沉香
Chi Fu Ling	Poria Rubra	赤茯苓
Chi Shao	Radix Paeoniae Rubra	赤芍
Chi Shi Zhi	Halloysitum Rubrum	赤石脂
Chi Xiao Dou	Semen Phaseoli	赤小豆
Chong Bai La	Cera Chinensis	虫白蜡
Chong Lou	Rhizoma Paridis	重楼
Chong Wei Zi	Fructus Leonuri	茺蔚子
Chou Wu Tong	Folium Clerodendri Trichotomi	臭梧桐
Chu Chong Ju	Flos Pyrethri	除虫菊
Chu Shi Zi	Fructus Broussonetiae	楮实子
Chuan Bei Mu	Bulbus Fritillariae Cirrhosae	川贝母
Chuan Lian Zi	Fructus Toosendan	川楝子
Chuan Mu Tong	Caulis Clematidis Armandii	川木通
Chuan Mu Xiang	Radix Vladimiriae	川木香
Chuan Niu Xi	Radix Cyathulae	川牛膝
Chuan Shan Jia	Squama Manis	穿山甲
Chuan Shan Long	Rhizoma Dioscoreae Nipponicae	穿山龙
Chuan She Gan	Rhizoma Iridis Tectori	川射干
Chuan Wu	Radix Aconiti	川乌
Chuan Xin Lian	Herba Andrographis	穿心莲
Chuan Xiong	Rhizoma Chuanxiong	川芎
Chui Pen Cao	Herba Sedi	垂盆草
Chun Gen	Radix Ailanthi	椿根
Chun Pi	Cortex Ailanthi	椿皮
Ci Shi	Magnetitum	磁石
Ci Wu Jia	Radix et Rhizoma seu Caulis Acanthopanacis Senticosi	刺五加
Cong	Herba Allii Fistulosi	葱
Cong Bai	Bulbus Allii Fistulosi	葱白
Da Ding Huang	Caulis Euonymi	大丁癀

Appendix 9 — Cross-reference of Single Herb Names

Pinyin Names	Pharmaceutical Names	Chinese Names
Da Dou Huang Juan	Semen Glycines Germinatum	大豆黄卷
Da Feng Zi	Semen Hydnocarpi	大风子
Da Fu Pi	Pericarpium Arecae	大腹皮
Da Huang	Radix et Rhizoma Rhei	大黄
Da Huang Tan	Radix et Rhizoma Rhei Carbonisatus	大黄炭
Da Ji	Radix Euphorbiae seu Knoxiae	大戟
Da Ji	Herba Cirsii Japonici	大蓟
Da Ji Gen	Radix Cirsii Japonici	大蓟根
Da Ji Tan	Herba Cirsii Japonici Carbonisatum	大蓟炭
Da Ji Ye	Folium Cirsii Japonici	大蓟叶
Da Ma Yao	Radix Dolichi	大麻药
Da Qing Ye	Folium Isatidis	大青叶
Da Suan	Bulbus Alli Sativi	大蒜
Da Xiao Ji	Herba Cirsii	大小蓟
Da Xue Teng	Caulis Sargentodoxae	大血藤
Da Ye Ma Dou Ling	Caulis Aristolochiae Kaempferi	大叶马兜铃
Da Zao	Fructus Jujubae	大枣
Dai Mao	Carapax Eretmochelydis Imbricatae	玳瑁
Dan Dou Chi	Semen Sojae Praeparatum	淡豆豉
Dan Fan	Chalcanthite	胆矾
Dan Nan Xing	Arisaema cum Bile	胆南星
Dan Shen	Radix et Rhizoma Salviae Miltiorrhizae	丹参
Dan Zhu Ye	Herba Lophatheri	淡竹叶
Dang Gui	Radix Angelicae Sinensis	当归
Dang Gui Shen	Corpus Radix Angelicae Sinensis	当归身
Dang Gui Tou	Caput Radix Angelicae Sinensis	当归头
Dang Gui Wei	Extremitas Radix Angelicae Sinensis	当归尾
Dang Shen	Radix Codonopsis	党参
Dao Di Wu Gong	Rhizoma Heliminthostachytis	倒地蜈蚣
Dao Diao Jin Zhong	Melothria Maderospatana	倒吊金钟
Dao Dou	Semen Canavaliae	刀豆
Dao Ya	Fructus Oryzae Germinatus	稻芽
Deng Xin Cao	Medulla Junci	灯心草
Deng Zhan Hua	Herba Erigerontis	灯盏花
Di Feng Pi	Cortex Illicii	地枫皮
Di Fu Zi	Fructus Kochiae	地肤子
Di Gu Pi	Cortex Lycii	地骨皮
Di Huang	Radix Rehmanniae	地黄
Di Jin Cao	Herba Euphorbiae Humifusae	地锦草
Di Long	Pheretima	地龙
Di Yu	Radix Sanguisorbae	地榆

1445

Appendix 9 – Cross-reference of Single Herb Names

Appendix 9 — Cross-reference of Single Herb Names

Pinyin Names	Pharmaceutical Names	Chinese Names
Di Yu Tan	Radix Sanguisorbae Carbonisatum	地榆炭
Dian Qie Cao	Herba Belladonnae	颠茄草
Ding Gong Teng	Caulis Erycibes	丁公藤
Ding Jing Cao	Herba Linderniae	定经草
Ding Shu Xiu	Herba Elephantopus Scaber	丁竖朽
Ding Xiang	Flos Caryophylli	丁香
Ding Xiang Pi	Cortex Caryophylli	丁香皮
Dong Chong Xia Cao	Cordyceps	冬虫夏草
Dong Gua Pi	Exocarpium Benincasae	冬瓜皮
Dong Gua Zi	Semen Benincasae	冬瓜子
Dong Kui Guo	Fructus Malvae	冬葵子
Dong Ling Cao	Herba Rabdosiae	冬凌草
Dong Qing Ye	Folium Ilexis	冬青叶
Dong Yang Shen	Radix et Rhizoma Ginseng Japonica	东洋参
Dou Kou	Fructus Amomi Rotundus	豆蔻
Dou Kou Ke	Pericarpium Amomi Rotundus	豆蔻壳
Du Huo	Radix Angelicae Pubescentis	独活
Du Yi Wei	Herba Lamiophlomis	独一味
Du Zhong	Cortex Eucommiae	杜仲
Du Zhong Ye	Folium Eucommiae	杜仲叶
Duan Ge Qiao	Concha Meretricis seu Cyclinae Calcinata	煅蛤壳
Duan Mu Li	Concha Ostreae Calcinata	煅牡蛎
Duan Shi Gao	Gypsum Fibrosum Praeparatum	煅石膏
Duan Shi Jue Ming	Concha Haliotidis Calcinata	煅石决明
Duan Wa Leng Zi	Concha Arcae Calcinata	煅瓦楞子
Duan Xue Liu	Herba Clinopodii	断血流
Duan Zhen Zhu Mu	Concha Margaritiferae Calcinata	煅珍珠母
Duan Zui Lao Guan Cao	Herba Geranii	短嘴老鹳草
E Bu Shi Cao	Herba Centipedae	鹅不食草
E Jiao	Colla Corii Asini	阿胶
E Zhu	Rhizoma Curcumae	莪术
Er Cha	Catechu	儿茶
Fa Ban Xia	Rhizoma Pinelliae Praeparatum	法半夏
Fan Xie Ye	Folium Sennae	番泻叶
Fang Feng	Radix Saposhnikoviae	防风
Fang Ji	Radix Stephaniae Tetrandrae	防己
Fang Jie Shi	Calcitum	方解石
Fei Zi	Semen Torreyae	榧子
Fen Bi Xie	Rhizoma Dioscoreae Hypoglaucae	粉萆薢
Fen Gen	Radix Puerariae Thomsonii	粉葛
Feng Fang	Nidus Vespae	蜂房

1446

Chinese Herbal Formulas and Applications

Appendix 9 — Cross-reference of Single Herb Names

Pinyin Names	Pharmaceutical Names	Chinese Names
Feng Jiao	Propolis	峰胶
Feng La	Cera Flava	峰蜡
Feng Mi	Mel	蜂蜜
Feng Wei Cao	Herba Pteris	凤尾草
Feng Xiang Zhi	Resina Liquidambaris	风香脂
Fo Shou	Fructus Citri Sarcodactylis	佛手
Fo Shou Hua	Flos Citri Sarcodactylis	佛手花
Fu Fang Teng	Herba Euonymi	扶芳藤
Fu Hai Shi	Pumice	浮海石
Fu Ling	Poria	茯苓
Fu Ling Pi	Cortex Poria	茯苓皮
Fu Long Gan	Terra Flava Usta	伏龙肝
Fu Pen Zi	Fructus Rubi	覆盆子
Fu Ping	Herba Spirodelae	浮萍
Fu Rong	Radix Hibisci	芙蓉
Fu Rong Ye	Folium Hibisci	芙蓉叶
Fu Shen	Poria Paradicis	茯神
Fu Shou Cao	Herba Adonis	福寿草
Fu Xiao Mai	Fructus Tritici Levis	浮小麦
Fu Zi	Radix Aconiti Lateralis Praeparata	附子
Gan Cao	Radix et Rhizoma Glycyrrhizae	甘草
Gan Jiang	Rhizoma Zingiberis	干姜
Gan Qi	Resina Toxicodendri	干漆
Gan Qing Qing Lan	Herba Dracoephali Tangutici	甘青青兰
Gan Song	Radix et Rhizoma Nardostachydis	甘松
Gan Sui	Radix Kansui	甘遂
Gang Ban Gui	Herba Polygoni Perfoliati	杠板归
Gao Ben	Rhizoma et Radix Ligustici	藁本
Gao Liang Jiang	Rhizoma Alpiniae Officinarum	高良姜
Ge Gen	Radix Puerariae Lobatae	葛根
Ge Hua	Flos Puerariae	葛花
Ge Jie	Gecko	蛤蚧
Ge Qiao	Concha Meretricis seu Cyclinae	蛤壳
Geng Mi	Semen Oryzae	粳米
Geng Tong Cao	Ramulus Aeschynomene Indica	梗通草
Gong Lao Mu	Caulis Mahoniae	功劳木
Gong Lau Ye	Folium Mahoniae	功劳叶
Gou Gu	Os Canitis	狗骨
Gou Gu Ye	Folium Ilicis Cornutae	枸骨叶
Gou Ji	Rhizoma Cibotii	狗脊
Gou Qi Gen	Radix Lycii	枸杞根

CROSS-REFERENCE OF SINGLE HERB NAMES

A9

1447

Appendix 9 – Cross-reference of Single Herb Names

Appendix 9 — Cross-reference of Single Herb Names

Pinyin Names	Pharmaceutical Names	Chinese Names
Gou Qi Ye	Folium Lycii	枸杞叶
Gou Qi Zi	Fructus Lycii	枸杞子
Gou Teng	Ramulus Uncariae cum Uncis	钩藤
Gou Wen	Herba Gelsemii Elegantis	钩吻
Gu Jing Cao	Flos Eriocauli	谷精草
Gu Sui Bu	Rhizoma Drynariae	骨碎补
Gu Ya	Fructus Setariae Germinatus	谷芽
Gua Di	Pedicellus Cucumeris	瓜蒂
Gua Lou	Fructus Trichosanthis	瓜蒌
Gua Lou Pi	Pericarpium Trichosanthis	瓜蒌皮
Gua Lou Zi	Semen Trichosanthis	瓜蒌子
Guan Bai Fu	Radix Aconiti Coreani	关白附
Guan Huang Bo	Cortex Phellodendri Amurensis	关黄柏
Guan Mu Tong	Caulis Aristolochiae Manshuriensis	关木通
Guan Ye Jin Si Tao	Herba Hyperici Perforati	贯叶金丝桃
Guang Fang Ji	Radix Aristolochiae Fangchi	广防己
Guang Huo Xiang	Herba Pogostemonis	广藿香
Guang Jin Qian Cao	Herba Desmodii Styracifolii	广金钱草
Guang Zao	Fructus Choerospondiatis	广枣
Gui Ban	Plastrum Testudinis	龟板
Gui Ban Jiao	Gelatinum Plastrum Testudinis	龟板胶
Gui Jia	Carapax et Plastrum Testudinis	龟甲
Gui Jia Jiao	Colla Carapax et Plastrum Testudinis	龟甲胶
Gui Xin	Cortex Rasus Cinnamomi	桂心
Gui Zhen Cao	Herba Bidentis Bipinnatae	鬼针草
Gui Zhi	Ramulus Cinnamomi	桂枝
Hai Dai	Thallus Laminariae	海带
Hai Feng Teng	Caulis Piperis Kadsurae	海风藤
Hai Fu Rong	Herba Limonium Wrightii	海芙蓉
Hai Gou Shen	Testes et Penis Otariae	海狗肾
Hai Jin Sha	Spora Lygodii	海金砂
Hai Long	Syngnathus	海龙
Hai Ma	Hippocampus	海马
Hai Piao Xiao	Endoconcha Sepiae	海螵蛸
Hai Shen	Strichopus Japonicus	海参
Hai Tong Pi	Cortex Erythrinae	海桐皮
Hai Zao	Sargassum	海藻
Han Shui Shi	Mirabilite	寒水石
He Cao Ya	Gemma Agrimoniae	鹤草芽
He Di	Calyx Nelumbinis	荷蒂
He Geng	Caulis Nelumbinis	荷梗

Appendix 9 — Cross-reference of Single Herb Names

Pinyin Names	Pharmaceutical Names	Chinese Names
He Huan Hua	Flos Albiziae	合欢花
He Huan Pi	Cortex Albiziae	合欢皮
He Shi	Fructus Carpesii	鹤虱
He Shou Wu	Radix Polygoni Multiflori	何首乌
He Tao Qiu Pi	Cortex Juglandis	核桃楸皮
He Tao Ren	Semen Juglandis	核桃仁
He Ye	Folium Nelumbinis	荷叶
He Zi	Fructus Chebulae	诃子
Hei Da Zao	Fructus Jujubae Nigrum	黑大枣
Hei Dou	Semen Sojae	黑豆
Hei Xi	Lead	黑锡
Hei Zhi Ma	Semen Sesami Nigrum	黑芝麻
Hei Zhong Cao Zi	Semen Nigellae	黑种草子
Hong Da Ji	Radix Knoxiae	红大戟
Hong Dou Kou	Fructus Galangae	红豆蔻
Hong Fen	Hydrargyri Oxydum Rubrum	红粉
Hong Gu She	Radix Kadsura Japonicae	红骨蛇
Hong Han Lian	Herba Hypericum Ascyron	红旱莲
Hong Hua	Flos Carthami	红花
Hong Jing Tian	Radix et Rhizoma Rhodiolae Crenulatae	红景天
Hong Qi	Radix Hedysari	红芪
Hong Qu	Monascus	红曲
Hong Shen	Radix et Rhizoma Ginseng Rubra	红参
Hong Shi Gao	Gypsum Rubrae	红石膏
Hou Po	Cortex Magnoliae Officinalis	厚朴
Hou Po Hua	Flos Magnoliae Officinalis	厚朴花
Hu Bei Bei Mu	Bulbus Fritillariae Hupehensis	湖北贝母
Hu Gu	Os Tigris	虎骨
Hu Huang Lian	Rhizoma Picrorhizae	胡黄连
Hu Ji Sheng	Herba Visci	槲寄生
Hu Jiao	Fructus Piperis	胡椒
Hu Lu Ba	Semen Trigonellae	胡芦巴
Hu Po	Succinum	琥珀
Hu Yao Huang	Herba Leucas Mollissimae	虎咬癀
Hu Zhang	Rhizoma et Radix Polygoni Cuspidati	虎杖
Hua Jiao	Pericarpium Zanthoxyli	花椒
Hua Ju Hong	Exocarpium Citri Grandis	化橘红
Hua Rui Shi	Ophicalcitum	花蕊石
Hua Shan Shen	Radix Physochlainae	华山参
Hua Shi	Talcum	滑石
Hua Shi Cao	Herba Orthosiphon Aristatus	化石草

Appendix 9 – Cross-reference of Single Herb Names

Appendix 9 — Cross-reference of Single Herb Names

Pinyin Names	Pharmaceutical Names	Chinese Names
Hua Shi Fen	Pulvis Talci	滑石粉
Huai Hua	Flos Sophorae	槐花
Huai Hua Tan	Flos Sophorae Carbonisatum	槐花炭
Huai Jiao	Fructus Sophorae	槐角
Huai Mi	Flos Sophorae Immaturus	槐米
Huai Tong Ma Dou Ling	Caulis Aristolochiae Moupinensis	淮通马兜铃
Huang Bo	Cortex Phellodendri Chinensis	黄柏
Huang Hua Jia Zhu Tao	Semen Thevetiae	黄花夹竹桃
Huang Jie Zi	Semen Brassicae	黄芥子
Huang Jin	Gold	黄金
Huang Jin Gui	Caulis Vanieriae	黄金桂
Huang Jing	Rhizoma Polygonati	黄精
Huang Jing Zi	Fructus Viticis Negundis	黄荆子
Huang Lian	Rhizoma Coptidis	黄连
Huang Niu Jiao	Cornus Bovis	黄牛角
Huang Qi	Radix Astragali	黄芪
Huang Qin	Radix Scutellariae	黄芩
Huang Shui Qie	Herba Solani	黄水茄
Huang Teng	Caulis Fibraureae	黄藤
Huang Yang Jiao	Cornu Procapra Gutturosa	黄羊角
Huang Yao Zi	Herba Dioscoreae Bulbiferae	黄药子
Huo Ma Ren	Fructus Cannabis	火麻仁
Huo Xiang	Herba Agastaches	藿香
Huo Xiang Ye	Folium Agastaches	藿香叶
Ji Gu Cao	Herba Abri	鸡骨草
Ji Guan Hua	Flos Celosiae Cristatae	鸡冠花
Ji Li	Fructus Tribuli	蒺藜
Ji Nei Jin	Endothelium Corneum Gigeriae Galli	鸡内金
Ji Xiang Teng	Caulis Paederiae	鸡香藤
Ji Xing Zi	Semen Impatientis	急性子
Ji Xue Cao	Herba Centellae	积雪草
Ji Xue Teng	Caulis Spatholobi	鸡血藤
Ji Zi Huang	Galli Vitellus	鸡子黄
Jia Zhu Tao	Folium Cortex et Radix Nerii	夹竹桃
Jian Shen Qu	Massa Fermentata Praeparata	建神曲
Jiang Can	Bombyx Batryticatus	僵蚕
Jiang Huang	Rhizoma Curcumae Longae	姜黄
Jiang Xiang	Lignum Dalbergiae Odoriferae	降香
Jiao Bing Lang	Semen Arecae Praeparata	焦槟榔
Jiao Gu Lan	Rhizoma seu Herba Gynostemmatis	绞股蓝
Jiao Mu	Semen Zanthoxyli Bungeani	椒目

Chinese Herbal Formulas and Applications

Appendix 9 — Cross-reference of Single Herb Names

Pinyin Names	Pharmaceutical Names	Chinese Names
Jiao Zhi Zi	Fructus Gardeniae Praeparatus	焦栀子
Jie Geng	Radix Platycodonis	桔梗
Jie Lie Xiao Hui Xiang	Herba Hypecoe Leptocarpe	节裂小茴香
Jie Zi	Semen Sinapis	芥子
Jin Bo	Gold foil	金箔
Jin Deng Long	Calyx seu Fructus Physalis	锦灯笼
Jin Fei Cao	Herba Inulae	金沸草
Jin Guo Lan	Radix Tinosporae	金果榄
Jin Meng Shi	Lapis Micae Aureus	金礞石
Jin Qian Bai Hua She	Bungarus Parvus	金钱白花蛇
Jin Qian Cao	Herba Lysimachiae	金钱草
Jin Qiao Mai	Rhizoma Fagopyri Dibotryis	金荞麦
Jin Yin Hua	Flos Lonicerae Japonicae	金银花
Jin Ying Gen	Radix Rosae Laevigatae	金樱根
Jin Ying Zi	Fructus Rosae Laevigatae	金樱子
Jing Da Ji	Radix Euphorbiae Pekinensis	京大戟
Jing Jie	Herba Schizonepetae	荆芥
Jing Jie Sui	Spica Schizonepetae	荆芥穗
Jing Jie Sui Tan	Spica Schizonepetae Carbonisatum	荆芥穗炭
Jing Jie Tan	Herba Schizonepetae Carbonisatum	荆芥炭
Jing Tian San Qi	Herba seu Radix Sedum Aizoom	景天三七
Jiu Cai Zi	Semen Allii Tuberosi	韭菜子
Jiu Ceng Ta	Herba Ocimi Basilici	九层塔
Jiu Jie Chang Pu	Rhizoma Anemones Altaicae	九节菖蒲
Jiu Li Xiang	Folium et Cacumen Murrayae	九里香
Jiu Xiang Chong	Aspongopus	九香虫
Ju He	Semen Citri Reticulatae	橘核
Ju Hong	Exocarpium Citri Rubrum	橘红
Ju Hua	Flos Chrysanthemi	菊花
Ju Ju	Herba et Radix Cichorii	菊苣
Ju Luo	Vascular Citri Reticulatae	橘络
Ju Ye	Folium Citri Reticulatae	橘叶
Ju Ye San Qi	Herba seu Radix Gynura Segetum	菊叶三七
Juan Bai	Herba Selaginellae	卷柏
Jue Ming Zi	Semen Cassiae	决明子
Ku Di Ding	Herba Corydalis Bungeanae	苦地丁
Ku Dou Cao	Herba Sophora Alopecuroidies	苦豆草
Ku Fan	Alumen Exsiccatum	苦矾
Ku Lian Pi	Cortex Meliae	苦楝皮
Ku Lian Zi	Fructus Meliae	苦楝子
Ku Mu	Ramulus et Folium Picrasmae	苦木

CROSS-REFERENCE OF SINGLE HERB NAMES

A9

1451

Appendix 9 – Cross-reference of Single Herb Names

Appendix 9 — Cross-reference of Single Herb Names

Pinyin Names	Pharmaceutical Names	Chinese Names
Ku Shen	Radix Sophorae Flavescentis	苦参
Ku Shen Zi	Fructus Sophorae Flavescentis	苦参子
Ku Xing Ren	Semen Armeniacae Amarum	苦杏仁
Ku Xuan Shen	Herba Picriae	苦玄参
Kuan Dong Hua	Flos Farfarae	款冬花
Kun Bu	Thallus Eckloniae	昆布
Lai Fu Zi	Semen Raphani	莱菔子
Lang Du	Radix Euphorbiae Fischerianae	狼毒
Lao Guan Cao	Herba Erodii seu Geranii	老鹳草
Lei Gong Teng	Radix Tripterygii Wilfordii	雷公藤
Lei Wan	Omphalia	雷丸
Li Lu	Radix et Rhizoma Veratri	黎芦
Li Pi	Pericarpium Pyri	梨皮
Li Zhi He	Semen Litchi	荔枝核
Lian Fang	Receptaculum Nelumbinis	莲房
Lian Qian Cao	Herba Glechomae	连钱草
Lian Qiao	Fructus Forsythiae	连翘
Lian Xu	Stamen Nelumbinis	莲须
Lian Zi	Semen Nelumbinis	莲子
Lian Zi Xin	Plumula Nelumbinis	莲子心
Liang Mian Zhen	Radix Zanthoxyli	两面针
Liang Tou Jian	Rhizoma Anemones Raddeanae	两头尖
Liao Da Qing Ye	Folium Polygoni Tinctorii	蓼大青叶
Ling Xiao Hua	Flos Campsis	凌霄花
Ling Yang Jiao	Cornu Saigae Tataricae	羚羊角
Ling Yin Chen	Herba Siphonostegia Chinensis	铃茵陈
Ling Zhi	Ganoderma	灵芝
Liu Huang	Sulfur	硫黄
Liu Ji Nu	Herba Artemisiae Anomalae	刘寄奴
Liu Ye	Folium Salicis Babylonicae	柳叶
Liu Zhi Huang	Herba Solidaginis	柳枝癀
Long Chi	Dens Draconis	龙齿
Long Dan	Radix et Rhizoma Gentianae	龙胆
Long Gu	Os Draconis	龙骨
Long Kui	Herba Solanum Nigrum	龙葵
Long Yan He	Semen Longan	龙眼核
Long Yan Hua	Flos Longan	龙眼花
Long Yan Rou	Arillus Longan	龙眼肉
Lou Lu	Radix Rhapontici	漏芦
Lu Dou	Semen Phaseoli Radiati	绿豆
Lu Dou Yi	Pericarpium Phaseoli Radiati	绿豆衣

Appendix 9 — Cross-reference of Single Herb Names

Pinyin Names	Pharmaceutical Names	Chinese Names
Lu Gan Shi	Galamina	炉甘石
Lu Gen	Rhizoma Phragmitis	芦根
Lu Hui	Aloe	芦荟
Lu Jiao	Cornu Cervi	鹿角
Lu Jiao Jiao	Colla Cornus Cervi	鹿角胶
Lu Jiao Shuang	Cornu Cervi Degelatinatum	鹿角霜
Lu Lu Tong	Fructus Liquidambaris	路路通
Lu Rong	Cornu Cervi Pantotrichum	鹿茸
Lu Song Jiu Mao	Pilus Fructi Malloti	吕宋揪毛
Lu Xian Cao	Herba Pyrolae	鹿衔草
Luo Bu Ma	Herba Apocyni Veneti	罗布麻
Luo Bu Ma Ye	Folium Apocyni Veneti	罗布麻叶
Luo Han Guo	Fructus Momordicae	罗汉果
Luo Han Guo Ye	Folium Momordicae	罗汉果叶
Luo Shi Teng	Caulis Trachelospermi	络石藤
Luo Tuo Peng Zi	Semen Pegani Harmalae	骆驼蓬子
Ma An Teng	Herba Ipomoea Pes-caprae	马鞍藤
Ma Bian Cao	Herba Verbenae	马鞭草
Ma Bo	Lasiosphaera seu Calvatia	马勃
Ma Chi Xian	Herba Portulacae	马齿苋
Ma Dou Ling	Fructus Aristolochiae	马兜铃
Ma Huang	Herba Ephedrae	麻黄
Ma Huang Gen	Radix et Rhizoma Ephedrae	麻黄根
Ma Li Jin	Herba Asclepii	马利筋
Ma Qian Zi	Semen Strychni	马钱子
Ma Qian Zi Fen	Semen Strychni Pulveratum	马钱子粉
Ma Sang	Radix et Folium Coriariae	马桑
Ma Sang Gen	Radix Coriariae	马桑根
Ma Sang Ye	Folium Coriariae	马桑叶
Ma Ti Jin	Herba Dichondrae Repentis	马蹄金
Mai Dong	Radix Ophiopogonis	麦冬
Mai Jiao	Ergota	麦角
Mai Ya	Fructus Hordei Germinatus	麦芽
Mai Ya Qu	Fructus Hordei Germinatus Massa Fermentata	麦芽曲
Man Jing Zi	Fructus Viticis	蔓荆子
Man Shan Hong	Folium Rhododendri Daurici	满山红
Mang Cao	Fructus Illicium Lanceolatum	莽草
Mang Xiao	Natrii Sulfas	芒硝
Mao Dong Qing	Radix Ilicis Pubescentis	毛冬青
Mao Gen	Herba Ranunculi Japonici	毛茛
Mao He Zi	Fructus Terminaliae Billericae	毛诃子

Appendix 9 – Cross-reference of Single Herb Names

Appendix 9 — Cross-reference of Single Herb Names

Pinyin Names	Pharmaceutical Names	Chinese Names
Mao Zhao Cao	Radix Ranunculi Ternati	猫爪草
Mao Zi Dun Tou	Herba Abutilon Indicum	帽仔盾头
Mei Gui Hua	Flos Rosae Rugosae	玫瑰花
Mei Hua	Flos Mume	梅花
Meng Chong	Tabanus	蛇虫
Meng Shi	Lapis Micae seu Chloriti	礞石
Mi Jiao	Cornu Elaphurus	麋角
Mi Meng Hua	Flos Buddlejae	密蒙花
Mi Rong	Cornu Elaphurus Parvum	麋茸
Mi Tuo Seng	Lithargyum	密陀僧
Mian Bi Xie	Rhizoma Dioscoreae Septemlobae	绵萆薢
Mian Hua Zi	Semen Gossypi	棉花子
Mian Ma Guan Zhong	Rhizoma Dryopteridis Crassirhizomatis	绵马贯众
Mian Ma Guan Zhong Tan	Rhizoma Dryopteridis Crassirhizomatis Carbonisatum	绵马贯众炭
Ming Dang Shen	Radix Changii	明党参
Mo Gu Xiao	Caulis Hyptis Capitatae	有骨消
Mo Han Lian	Herba Ecliptae	墨旱莲
Mo Yao	Myrrha	没药
Mu Bie Zi	Semen Momordicae	木鳖子
Mu Dan Pi	Cortex Moutan	牡丹皮
Mu Dan Ye	Folium Moutan	牡丹叶
Mu Ding Xiang	Fructus Caryophylli	母丁香
Mu Fang Ji	Radix Cocculi Trilobi	木防己
Mu Gua	Fructus Chaenomelis	木瓜
Mu Hu Die	Semen Oroxyli	木蝴蝶
Mu Jing Ye	Folium Viticis Negundo	牡荆叶
Mu Li	Concha Ostreae	牡蛎
Mu Ma Dou	Herba Thermopsis Lanceolatae	牧马豆
Mu Tong	Caulis Akebiae	木通
Mu Xiang	Radix Aucklandiae	木香
Mu Zei	Herba Equiseti Hiemalis	木贼
Nan Ban Lan Gen	Rhizoma et Radix Baphicacanthis Cusiae	南板蓝根
Nan Chai Hu	Radix Bupleurum Scorzonerifolfium	南柴胡
Nan Gua Zi	Semen Cucurbitae Moschatae	南瓜子
Nan He Shi	Fructus Carotae	南鹤虱
Nan Sha Shen	Radix Adenophorae	南沙参
Nan Ting Li Zi	Semen Descurainiae	南葶苈子
Nan Wu Wei Zi	Fructus Schisandrae Sphenantherae	南五味子
Nao Yang Hua	Flos Rhododendri Mollis	闹羊花
Niao Bu Su	Ramus Kalopanax Pictus	鸟不宿
Niu Bang Gen	Radix Arctii	牛蒡根

1454

Chinese Herbal Formulas and Applications

Appendix 9 — Cross-reference of Single Herb Names

Pinyin Names	Pharmaceutical Names	Chinese Names
Niu Bang Zi	Fructus Arctii	牛蒡子
Niu Dan	Fel Bovis	牛胆
Niu Huang	Calculus Bovis	牛黄
Niu Xi	Radix Achyranthis Bidentatae	牛膝
Nu Zhen Zi	Fructus Ligustri Lucidi	女贞子
Nuo Mi	Oryza Glutinosa	糯米
Ou Jie	Nodus Nelumbinis Rhizomatis	藕节
Pang Da Hai	Semen Sterculiae Lychnophorae	胖大海
Pao Jiang	Rhizoma Zingiberis Praeparatum	炮姜
Pao Zai Cao	Herba Physalis Angulatae	炮仔草
Pei Lan	Herba Eupatorii	佩兰
Peng Sha	Borax	硼砂
Pi Pa Ye	Folium Eriobotryae	枇杷叶
Pi Shi	Arsenolite	砒石
Pian Jiang Huang	Rhizoma Wenyujin Concisum	片姜黄
Ping Bei Mu	Bulbus Fritillariae Ussuriensis	平贝母
Po Bu Zi Ye	Folium Cordia Dichotoma	破布子叶
Po Xiao	Sal Glauberis	朴硝
Pu Gong Ying	Herba Taraxaci	蒲公英
Pu Huang	Pollen Typhae	蒲黄
Pu Huang Tan	Pollen Typhae Carbonisatum	蒲黄炭
Pu Tao Zi	Semen Vitis Viniferae	葡萄子
Pu Yin	Radix Wikstroemia Indica	埔银
Qi Dai	Corda Umbilicalis Hominis	脐带
Qi She	Agkistrodon	蕲蛇
Qi Ye Lian	Radix Schefflerae	七叶莲
Qian Cao	Radix et Rhizoma Rubiae	茜草
Qian Cao Tan	Radix et Rhizoma Rubiae Carbonisatus	茜草炭
Qian Ceng Ta	Herba Lycopodii Serrati	千层塔
Qian Dan	Minium	铅丹
Qian Hu	Radix Peucedani	前胡
Qian Jin Zi	Semen Euphorbiae	千金子
Qian Jin Zi Shuang	Semen Euphorbiae Pulveratum	千金子霜
Qian Li Guang	Herba Senecionis Scandens	千里光
Qian Nian Jian	Rhizoma Homalomenae	千年健
Qian Niu Zi	Semen Pharbitidis	牵牛子
Qian Shi	Semen Euryales	芡实
Qiang Huo	Rhizoma et Radix Notopterygii	羌活
Qiao Mai	Semen Fagopyri Esculenti	荞麦
Qin Jiao	Radix Gentianae Macrophyllae	秦艽
Qin Pi	Cortex Fraxini	秦皮

CROSS-REFERENCE OF SINGLE HERB NAMES

A9

1455

Appendix 9 – Cross-reference of Single Herb Names

Appendix 9 — Cross-reference of Single Herb Names

Pinyin Names	Pharmaceutical Names	Chinese Names
Qing Dai	Indigo Naturalis	青黛
Qing Fen	Calomelas	轻粉
Qing Feng Teng	Caulis Sinomenii	青风藤
Qing Ge Qiao	Concha Cyclinae	青蛤壳
Qing Guo	Fructus Canarii	青果
Qing Guo Gen	Radix Canarii	青果根
Qing Hao	Herba Artemisiae Annuae	青蒿
Qing Ma Zi	Semen Abutili	苘麻子
Qing Meng Shi	Lapis Chloriti	青礞石
Qing Mu Xiang	Radix Aristolochiae	青木香
Qing Niu Jiao Fen	Cornus Bovis	青牛角粉
Qing Pi	Pericarpium Citri Reticulatae Viride	青皮
Qing Xiang Zi	Semen Celosiae	青葙子
Qing Ye Dan	Herba Swertiae Mileensis	青叶胆
Qu Mai	Herba Dianthi	瞿麦
Quan Shen	Rhizoma Bistortae	拳参
Quan Xie	Scorpio	全蝎
Ren Dong Cao	Herba Lonicerae Japonicae	忍冬草
Ren Dong Teng	Caulis Lonicerae Japonicae	忍冬藤
Ren Gong Niu Huang	Calculus Bovis Artifactus	人工牛黄
Ren Shen	Radix et Rhizoma Ginseng	人参
Ren Shen Ye	Folium Ginseng	人参叶
Ren Zhong Bai	Urinae Hominis Sedimen	人中白
Rou Cong Rong	Herba Cistanches	肉苁蓉
Rou Dou Gen	Radix Myristicae	肉豆根
Rou Dou Kou	Semen Myristicae	肉豆蔻
Rou Gui	Cortex Cinnamomi	肉桂
Ru Xiang	Gummi Olibanum	乳香
Rui Ren	Nux Prinsepiae	蕤仁
San Bai Cao	Herba Saururi	三白草
San Leng	Rhizoma Sparganii	三棱
San Qi	Radix et Rhizoma Notoginseng	三七
San Qi Ye	Folium Notoginseng	三七叶
Sang Bai Pi	Cortex Mori	桑白皮
Sang Ji Sheng	Herba Taxilli	桑寄生
Sang Piao Xiao	Ootheca Mantidis	桑螵蛸
Sang Shen	Fructus Mori	桑椹
Sang Ye	Folium Mori	桑叶
Sang Zhi	Ramulus Mori	桑枝
Sha Ji	Fructus Hippophae	沙棘
Sha Ren	Fructus Amomi	砂仁

Chinese Herbal Formulas and Applications

Appendix 9 — Cross-reference of Single Herb Names

Pinyin Names	Pharmaceutical Names	Chinese Names
Sha Ren Ke	Pericarpium Amomi	砂仁壳
Sha Shen	Radix Glehniae seu Adenophorae	沙参
Sha Yuan Zi	Semen Astragali Complanati	沙苑子
Shan Ci Gu	Pseudobulbus Cremastrae seu Pleiones	山慈姑
Shan Dou Gen	Radix et Rhizoma Sophorae Tonkinensis	山豆根
Shan Geng Cai	Herba Lobeliae Sessilifoliae	山梗菜
Shan Ma Ti	Radix Rauvolfiae Hainanensis	山马蹄
Shan Mai Dong	Radix Liriopes	山麦冬
Shan Nai	Rhizoma Kaempferiae	山奈
Shan Pu Tao	Radix Vitis Amurensis	山葡萄
Shan Yang Jiao	Cornu Naemorhedis	山羊角
Shan Yao	Rhizoma Dioscoreae	山药
Shan Yin Hua	Flos Lonicerae	山银花
Shan Zha	Fructus Crataegi	山楂
Shan Zha Tan	Fructus Crataegi Carbonisatum	山楂炭
Shan Zha Ye	Folium Crataegi	山楂叶
Shan Zhu Yu	Fructus Corni	山茱萸
Shang Lu	Radix Phytolaccae	商陆
She Chuang Zi	Fructus Cnidii	蛇床子
She Dan	Fel Serpentis	蛇胆
She Gan	Rhizoma Belamcandae	射干
She Tui	Periostracum Serpentis	蛇蜕
She Xiang	Moschus	麝香
Shen Jin Cao	Herba Lycopodii	伸筋草
Shen Qu	Massa Fermentata	神曲
Sheng Fu Zi	Radix Aconiti Lateralis	生附子
Sheng Jiang	Rhizoma Zingiberis Recens	生姜
Sheng Jiang Pi	Pericarpium Zingiberis Recens	生姜皮
Sheng Ma	Rhizoma Cimicifugae	升麻
Sheng Tie Luo	Frusta Ferri	生铁落
Shi Chang Pu	Rhizoma Acori Tatarinowii	石菖蒲
Shi Di	Calyx Kaki	柿蒂
Shi Gao	Gypsum Fibrosum	石膏
Shi Hu	Caulis Dendrobii	石斛
Shi Jue Ming	Concha Haliotidis	石决明
Shi Jun Zi	Fructus Quisqualis	使君子
Shi Lian Zi	Herba Sinocrassulae Indicae	石莲子
Shi Liu Gen Pi	Cortex Radix Granati	石榴根皮
Shi Liu Guo	Fructus Granati	石榴果
Shi Liu Pi	Pericarpium Granati	石榴皮
Shi Liu Pi Tan	Pericarpium Granati Carbonisatum	石榴皮炭

CROSS-REFERENCE OF SINGLE HERB NAMES

A9

1457

Appendix 9 — Cross-reference of Single Herb Names

Pinyin Names	Pharmaceutical Names	Chinese Names
Shi Luo	Fructus Anethum Graveolens	莳萝
Shi Nan Teng	Ramulus Piper	石南藤
Shi Nan Ye	Folium Photiniae	石南叶
Shi Suan	Bulbus Lycoris	石蒜
Shi Wei	Folium Pyrrosiae	石韦
Shi Xian Tao	Pseudobulbus Pholidotae Chinensis	石仙桃
Shou Wu Teng	Caulis Polygoni Multiflori	首乌藤
Shu Di Huang	Radix Rehmanniae Praeparata	熟地黄
Shu Hua Sha Shen	Radix Adenophorae Remotiflora	疏花沙参
Shu Qi	Folium Dichroae	蜀漆
Shu Wei Huang	Herba Rostellulariae	鼠尾癀
Shuang Liu Huang	Herba Vernoniae Patulae	双柳黄
Shui Ban Xia	Rhizoma Typhonii Flagelliformis	水半夏
Shui Ding Xiang	Herba Ludwigiae Prostratae	水丁香
Shui Fei Ji	Fructus Silybi	水飞蓟
Shui Hong Hua Zi	Fructus Polygoni Orientalis	水红花子
Shui Niu Jiao	Cornu Bubali	水牛角
Shui Yin	Hydrargyrum	水银
Shui Zhi	Hirudo	水蛭
Si Chuan Da Jin Qian Cao	Herba Lysimachia Christinae	四川大金钱草
Si Gua Luo	Retinervus Luffae Fructus	丝瓜络
Song Guo	Fructus Pini	松果
Song Hua Fen	Pollen Pini	松花粉
Song Jie	Lignum Pini Nodi	松节
Song Luo	Herba Usneae	松萝
Song Ye	Folium Pini	松叶
Su He Xiang	Styrax	苏合香
Su Mu	Lignum Sappan	苏木
Suan Zao Ren	Semen Ziziphi Spinosae	酸枣仁
Suo Luo Zi	Semen Aesculi	娑罗子
Suo Yang	Herba Cynomorii	锁阳
Tai Zi Shen	Radix Pseudostellariae	太子参
Tan Xiang	Lignum Santali Albi	檀香
Tao Ren	Semen Persicae	桃仁
Teng Huang	Resina Garciniae	藤黄
Tian Dong	Radix Asparagi	天冬
Tian Hua Fen	Radix Trichosanthis	天花粉
Tian Kui Zi	Radix Semiaquilegiae	天葵子
Tian Ma	Rhizoma Gastrodiae	天麻
Tian Nan Xing	Rhizoma Arisaematis	天南星
Tian Ran Bing Pian	Borneolum	天然冰片

Chinese Herbal Formulas and Applications

Appendix 9 — Cross-reference of Single Herb Names

Pinyin Names	Pharmaceutical Names	Chinese Names
Tian Shan Xue Lian	Herba Saussureae Involucratae	天山雪莲
Tian Xian Teng	Herba Aristolochiae	天仙藤
Tian Xian Zi	Semen Hyoscyami	天仙子
Tian Zhu Huang	Concretio Silicea Bambusae	天竺黄
Tian Zhu Zi	Fructus Nandinae Domesticae	天竹子
Ting Li Zi	Semen Descurainiae seu Lepidii	葶苈子
Tong Bian	Infantis Urina	童便
Tong Cao	Medulla Tetrapanacis	通草
Tou Gu Cao	Caulis Impatientis	透骨草
Tu Bei Mu	Rhizoma Bolbostematis	土贝母
Tu Bie Chong	Eupolyphaga seu Steleophaga	土鳖虫
Tu Fu Ling	Rhizoma Smilacis Glabrae	土茯苓
Tu Jing Jie	Herba Chenopodii	土荆芥
Tu Jing Pi	Cortex Pseudolaricis	土荆皮
Tu Mu Xiang	Radix Inulae	土木香
Tu Niu Xi	Radix Achyranthis Longifoliae	土牛膝
Tu Rou Gui	Cortex Cinnamomum Burmannium	土肉桂
Tu Si Zi	Semen Cuscutae	菟丝子
Tu Xi Xin	Herba Asari Forbesii	土细辛
Wa Leng Zi	Concha Arcae	瓦楞子
Wa Song	Herba Orostachyis Fimbriati	瓦松
Wan Dian Jin	Radix Ilicis Asprellae	万点金
Wan Nian Qing	Rhizoma et Herba Rohdea	万年青
Wang Bu Liu Xing	Semen Vaccariae	王不留行
Wei Ling Cai	Herba Potentillae Chinensis	委陵菜
Wei Ling Xian	Radix et Rhizoma Clematidis	威灵仙
Wen Ge Qiao	Concha Meretricis	文蛤壳
Wu Bei Zi	Galla Chinensis	五倍子
Wu Gong	Scolopendra	蜈蚣
Wu Jia Pi	Cortex Acanthopanacis	五加皮
Wu Jiu	Cortex Radix Sapii	乌桕
Wu Ling Zhi	Faeces Trogopteri seu Pteromi	五灵脂
Wu Long Cha	Folium Camellia Fermentata	乌龙茶
Wu Mei	Fructus Mume	乌梅
Wu Ming Yi	Pyrolusitum	无名异
Wu Shao She	Zaocys	乌蛸蛇
Wu Teng	Ramulus Linderae	乌藤
Wu Tian	Radix et Folium Viticis Quinatae	乌甜
Wu Tong Zi	Semen Firmianae	梧桐子
Wu Wei Zi	Fructus Schisandrae Chinensis	五味子
Wu Yao	Radix Linderae	乌药

1459

Appendix 9 – Cross-reference of Single Herb Names

Appendix 9 — Cross-reference of Single Herb Names

Pinyin Names	Pharmaceutical Names	Chinese Names
Wu Ye Mu Tong	Caulis Quinata	五叶木通
Wu Yi	Fructus Ulmi Praeparatus	芜荑
Wu Zhu Yu	Fructus Evodiae	吴茱萸
Xi Gua	Fructus Citrulli	西瓜
Xi Gua Cui Pi	Exocarpium Citrulli	西瓜翠皮
Xi Gua Pi	Pericarpium Citrulli	西瓜皮
Xi Gua Shuang	Mirabilitum Praeparatum	西瓜霜
Xi He Liu	Cacumen Tamaricis	西合柳
Xi Hong Hua	Stigma Croci	西红花
Xi Huang	Calculus Bovis	犀黄
Xi Jiao	Cornu Rhinoceri	犀角
Xi Qing Guo	Fructus Chebulae Immaturus	西青果
Xi Shu	Camptotheca	喜树
Xi Xian Cao	Herba Siegesbeckiae	豨莶草
Xi Xin	Radix et Rhizoma Asari	细辛
Xi Yang Shen	Radix Panacis Quinquefolii	西洋参
Xia Ku Cao	Spica Prunellae	夏枯草
Xia Ku Hua	Flos Prunellae	夏枯花
Xia Tian Wu	Rhizoma Corydalis Decumbentis	夏天无
Xian Di Huang	Radix Rehmanniae Recens	鲜地黄
Xian Feng Cao	Herba Bidentis	咸丰草
Xian He Cao	Herba Agrimoniae	仙鹤草
Xian Mao	Rhizoma Curculiginis	仙茅
Xiang Fu	Rhizoma Cyperi	香附
Xiang Jia Pi	Cortex Periplocae	香加皮
Xiang Ru	Herba Moslae	香薷
Xiang Si Cao	Herba Eupatorii Formosani	相思草
Xiang Si Zi	Semen Abrus Precatoris	相思子
Xiang Yuan	Fructus Citri	香橼
Xiao Hui Xiang	Fructus Foeniculi	小茴香
Xiao Ji	Herba Cirsii	小蓟
Xiao Jin Ying	Fructus Rosae Cymosae	小金樱
Xiao Mai	Fructus Tritici	小麦
Xiao Tong Cao	Medulla Stachyuri seu Helwingiae	小通草
Xiao Ye Lian	Fructus Podophylli	小叶莲
Xie Bai	Bulbus Allii Macrostemonis	薤白
Xie Cao	Radix et Rhizoma Valerianae	缬草
Xin Yi	Flos Magnoliae	辛夷
Xing Ren Shu Pi	Cortex Pruni Armeniacae	杏仁树皮
Xiong Dan	Fel Ursi	熊胆
Xiong Huang	Realgar	雄黄

Chinese Herbal Formulas and Applications

Appendix 9 — Cross-reference of Single Herb Names

Pinyin Names	Pharmaceutical Names	Chinese Names
Xu Chang Qing	Radix et Rhizoma Cynanchi Paniculati	徐长卿
Xu Duan	Radix Dipsaci	续断
Xuan Diao Zi Jing	Ramulus Rubi	悬钩子茎
Xuan Fu Hua	Flos Inulae	旋覆花
Xuan Ming Fen	Natrii Sulfas Exsiccatus	玄明粉
Xuan Shen	Radix Scrophulariae	玄参
Xue Jie	Sanguis Draconis	血竭
Xue Shang Yi Zhi Hao	Radix Aconiti Brachypodi	雪上一枝蒿
Xue Yu Tan	Crinis Carbonisatus	血余炭
Xun Gu Feng	Herba Aristolochiae Mollissimae	寻骨风
Ya Dan Zi	Fructus Bruceae	鸦胆子
Ya Hu Nu	Herba Cissampelotis	亚乎奴
Ya Ma Zi	Semen Lini	亚麻子
Ya She Huang	Herba Lippiae	鸭舌癀
Ya Zhi Cao	Herba Commelinae	鸭跖草
Yan Hu Suo	Rhizoma Corydalis	延胡索
Yang Dan	Fel Capra seu Ovis	羊胆
Yang Jiao Ao	Fructus Strophanthi	羊角拗
Yang Jin Hua	Flos Daturae	洋金花
Yang Qi Shi	Actinolitum	阳起石
Yang Ti	Radix Rumicis Japonici	羊蹄
Ye Ju Hua	Flos Chrysanthemi Indici	野菊花
Ye Ming Sha	Faeces Vespertilionis Murini	夜明砂
Ye Ying Pi	Pericarpium Prunus Pseudocerasus	野樱皮
Yi Bei Mu	Bulbus Fritillariae Pallidiflorae	伊贝母
Yi Mu Cao	Herba Leonuri	益母草
Yi Tang	Maltosum	饴糖
Yi Tiao Gen	Radix Moghaniae	一条根
Yi Wu Gen	Radix Elaeagni	宜梧根
Yi Ye Qiu	Radix Securinegae Suffruticosae	一叶萩
Yi Yi Gen	Radix Coicis	薏苡根
Yi Yi Ren	Semen Coicis	薏苡仁
Yi Zhi	Fructus Alpiniae Oxyphyllae	益智
Yi Zhi Xiang	Herba Vernoniae Cinereae	一枝香
Yin Bo	Silver foil	银箔
Yin Chai Hu	Radix Stellariae	银柴胡
Yin Chen	Herba Artemisiae Scopariae	茵陈
Yin Xing Ye	Folium Ginkgo	银杏叶
Yin Yang Huo	Herba Epimedii	淫羊藿
Yin Yu	Caulis et Folium Skimmiae	茵芋
Ying Su Ke	Pericarpium Papaveris	罂粟壳

CROSS-REFERENCE OF SINGLE HERB NAMES

A9

1461

Appendix 9 – Cross-reference of Single Herb Names

Appendix 9 — Cross-reference of Single Herb Names

Pinyin Names	Pharmaceutical Names	Chinese Names
You Chong Zhu	Blattela	油虫珠
Yu Gan Zi	Fructus Phyllanthi	余甘子
Yu Jin	Radix Curcumae	郁金
Yu Li Ren	Semen Pruni	郁李仁
Yu Mi Xu	Stigma Maydis	玉米须
Yu Teng	Radix seu Herba Derridis Trifoliatae	鱼藤
Yu Xing Cao	Herba Houttuyniae	鱼腥草
Yu Yu Liang	Limonitum	禹余粮
Yu Zhi Zi	Fructus Akebiae	预知子
Yu Zhou Lou Lu	Radix Echinopsis	禹州漏芦
Yu Zhu	Rhizoma Polygonati Odorati	玉竹
Yuan Hua	Flos Genkwa	芫花
Yuan Zhi	Radix Polygalae	远志
Yue Ji Hua	Flos Rosae Chinensis	月季花
Yun Zhi	Coriolus	云芝
Zang Chang Pu	Rhizoma Acori Calami	藏菖蒲
Zao Jiao	Fructus Gleditsiae	皂角
Zao Jiao Ci	Spina Gleditsiae	皂角刺
Ze Lan	Herba Lycopi	泽兰
Ze Qi	Herba Euphorbiae Helioscopiae	泽漆
Ze Xie	Rhizoma Alismatis	泽泻
Zhang Mu Xiang	Radix Inulae Racemosae	藏木香
Zhang Nao	Camphora	樟脑
Zhang Ya Cai	Herba Swertae	獐牙菜
Zhao Shan Bai	Folium Rhododendri Micranthi	照山白
Zhe Bei Mu	Bulbus Fritillariae Thunbergii	浙贝母
Zhe Shi	Haematitum	赭石
Zhen Zhu	Margarita	珍珠
Zhen Zhu Mu	Concha Margaritiferae	珍珠母
Zhi Cao Wu	Radix Aconiti Kusnezoffii Praeparata	制草乌
Zhi Chuan Wu	Radix Aconiti Praeparata	制川乌
Zhi Gan Cao	Radix et Rhizoma Glycyrrhizae Praeparata cum Melle	炙甘草
Zhi He Shou Wu	Radix Polygoni Multiflori Praeparata cum Succo Glycines Sojae	炙何首乌
Zhi Hong Qi	Radix Hedysari Praeparata cum Melle	炙红芪
Zhi Huang Qi	Radix Astragali Praeparata cum Melle	炙黄芪
Zhi Ju Zi	Fructus Hoveniae	枳椇子
Zhi Ma Huang	Herba Ephedrae Praeparata	炙麻黄
Zhi Mu	Rhizoma Anemarrhenae	知母
Zhi Qiao	Fructus Aurantii	枳壳
Zhi Qiao Tan	Fructus Aurantii Carbonisatum	枳壳炭

1462

Appendix 9 — Cross-reference of Single Herb Names

Chinese Herbal Formulas and Applications

Pinyin Names	Pharmaceutical Names	Chinese Names
Zhi Shi	Fructus Aurantii Immaturus	枳实
Zhi Xie Mu Zi	Semen Holarrhena Antidysentericae	止泻木子
Zhi Zi	Fructus Gardeniae	栀子
Zhi Zi Pi	Pericarpium Gardeniae	栀子皮
Zhi Zi Ren	Semen Gardeniae	栀子仁
Zhong Jie Feng	Herba Sarcandrae	肿节风
Zhong Ru Shi	Stalactitum	钟乳石
Zhu Dan	Fel Porcus	猪胆
Zhu Dan Fen	Pulvis Fellis Suis	猪胆粉
Zhu Fan Hua Tou	Rhizoma Mirabilidis	煮饭花头
Zhu Gu	Os Porcus	猪骨
Zhu Jie Shen	Rhizoma Panacis Japonici	竹节参
Zhu Li	Succus Bambusae	竹沥
Zhu Ling	Polyporus	猪苓
Zhu Ru	Caulis Bambusae in Taenia	竹茹
Zhu Sha	Cinnabaris	朱砂
Zhu Sha Gen	Radix Ardisiae Crenatae	朱砂根
Zhu Ya Zao	Fructus Gleditsiae Abnormalis	猪牙皂
Zhu Ye	Herba Phyllostachys	竹叶
Zhu Zi Cao	Herba Euphorbiae Thymifoliae	珠仔草
Zhu Zi Shen	Rhizoma Panacis Majoris	珠子参
Zi Bei Tian Kui	Herba Semiaquilegiae	紫背天葵
Zi Cao	Radix Arnebiae	紫草
Zi He Che	Placenta Hominis	紫河车
Zi Hua Di Ding	Herba Violae	紫花地丁
Zi Jin Pi	Radix Tripterygii Hypoglauci	紫金皮
Zi Ran Tong	Pyritum	自然铜
Zi Shi Ying	Fluoritum	紫石英
Zi Su Geng	Caulis Perillae	紫苏梗
Zi Su Ye	Folium Perillae	紫苏叶
Zi Su Zi	Fructus Perillae	紫苏子
Zi Wan	Radix et Rhizoma Asteris	紫菀
Zi Zhu	Folium Callicarpae	紫珠
Zong Lu	Petiolus Trachycarpi	棕榈
Zong Lu Zi	Fructus Trachycarpi	棕榈子
Zou Ma Tai	Rhizoma Ardisiae	走马胎
Zu Shi Ma	Cortex Daphnes	祖师麻

CROSS-REFERENCE OF SINGLE HERB NAMES

A9

1463

Appendix 10

— Cross-reference of Herbal Formula Names

Pinyin Names (Literal Names)	Chinese Names
Ai Fu Nuan Gong Wan (Mugwort and Cyperus Pill for Warming the Womb)	艾附暖宫丸
An Gong Niu Huang Wan (Calm the Palace Pill with Cattle Gallstone)	安宫牛黄丸
An Shen Tang (Tranquilize the Spirit Decoction)	安神汤
An Zhong San (Calm the Middle Powder)	安中散
Ba Wei Dai Xia Fang (Eight-Ingredient Formula for Leukorrhea)	八味带下方
Ba Wei Di Huang Wan (Eight-Ingredient Pill with Rehmannia)	八味地黄丸
Ba Zhen Tang (Eight-Treasure Decoction)	八珍汤
Ba Zheng San (Eight-Herb Powder for Rectification)	八正散
Bai Du San (Overcome Pathogenic Influences Powder)	败毒散
Bai Du Tang (Overcome Pathogenic Influences Decoction)	败毒汤
Bai He Gu Jin Tang (Lily Bulb Decoction to Preserve the Metal)	百合固金汤
Bai Hu Jia Cang Zhu Tang (White Tiger plus Atractylodes Decoction)	白虎加苍术汤
Bai Hu Jia Gui Zhi Tang (White Tiger plus Cinnamon Twig Decoction)	白虎加桂枝汤
Bai Hu Jia Ren Shen Tang (White Tiger plus Ginseng Decoction)	白虎加人参汤
Bai Hu Tang (White Tiger Decoction)	白虎汤
Bai Mao Gen Tang (Imperata Decoction)	白茅根汤
Bai Tong Tang (White Penetrating Decoction)	白通汤
Bai Tou Weng Jia Gan Cao E Jiao Tang (Pulsatilla Decoction plus Licorice and Ass-Hide Gelatin)	白头翁加甘草阿胶汤
Bai Tou Weng Tang (Pulsatilla Decoction)	白头翁汤
Bai Zi Yang Xin Wan (Biota Seed Pill to Nourish the Heart)	柏子养心丸
Ban Xia Bai Zhu Tian Ma Tang (Pinellia, Atractylodes Macrocephala, and Gastrodia Decoction)	半夏白术天麻汤
Ban Xia Hou Po Tang (Pinellia and Magnolia Bark Decoction)	半夏厚朴汤
Ban Xia Xie Xin Tang (Pinellia Decoction to Drain the Epigastrium)	半夏泻心汤
Bao Chan Wu You Fang (Preserve Pregnancy and Care-Free Decoction)	保产无忧方
Bao He Wan (Preserve Harmony Pill)	保和丸
Bao Yuan Tang (Preserve the Basal Decoction)	保元汤
Bei Mu Gua Lou San (Fritillaria and Trichosanthes Fruit Powder)	贝母瓜蒌散
Bi Xie Fen Qing Yin (Dioscorea Hypoglauca Decoction to Separate the Clear)	萆薢分清饮
Bi Yu San (Jasper Powder)	碧玉散
Bie Jia Jian Wan (Soft-Shelled Turtle Shell Pill)	鳖甲煎丸
Bu Dai Wan (Cloth Sack Pill)	布袋丸
Bu Fei E Jiao Tang (Tonify the Lung Decoction with Ass-Hide Gelatin)	补肺阿胶汤
Bu Fei Tang (Tonify the Lung Decoction)	补肺汤
Bu Gu Wan (Tonify the Bone Pill)	补骨丸

Chinese Herbal Formulas and Applications

Appendix 10 — Cross-reference of Herbal Formula Names

Pinyin Names (Literal Names)	Chinese Names
Bu Huan Jin Zheng Qi San (Rectify the Qi Powder Worth More than Gold)	不换金正气散
Bu Shen Tang (Tonify the Kidney Decoction)	补肾汤
Bu Shen Wan (Tonify the Kidney Pill)	补肾丸
Bu Yang Huan Wu Tang (Tonify the Yang to Restore Five Decoction)	补阳还五汤
Bu Zhong Yi Qi Tang (Tonify the Middle and Augment the Qi Decoction)	补中益气汤
Can Shi Tang (Silkworm Droppings Decoction)	蚕矢汤
Cang Er Zi San (Xanthium Powder)	苍耳子散
Cang Lin San (Old Rice Granary Powder)	仓廪散
Chai Ge Jie Ji Tang (Bupleurum and Kudzu Decoction to Release the Muscle Layer)	柴葛解肌汤
Chai Hu An Shen Tang (Bupleurum Decoction to Tranquilize the Spirit)	柴胡安神汤
Chai Hu Da Yuan Yin (Bupleurum Decoction to Reach the Membrane Source)	柴胡达原饮
Chai Hu Gui Zhi Gan Jiang Tang (Bupleurum, Cinnamon Twig, and Ginger Decoction)	柴胡桂枝乾姜汤
Chai Hu Gui Zhi Tang (Bupleurum and Cinnamon Twig Decoction)	柴胡桂枝汤
Chai Hu Jia Long Gu Mu Li Tang (Bupleurum plus Dragon Bone and Oyster Shell Decoction)	柴胡加龙骨牡蛎汤
Chai Hu Jie Du Tang (Bupleurum Decoction to Relieve Toxicity)	柴胡解毒汤
Chai Hu Qing Gan Tang (Bupleurum Decoction to Clear the Liver)	柴胡清肝汤
Chai Hu Shu Gan San (Bupleurum Powder to Spread the Liver)	柴胡疏肝散
Chai Hu Tang (Bupleurum Decoction)	柴胡汤
Chai Hu Xian Xiong Tang (Bupleurum Decoction for Sinking into the Chest)	柴胡陷胸汤
Chai Hu Zhi Jie Tang (Bupleurum, Bitter Orange, and Platycodon Decoction)	柴胡枳桔汤
Chai Ling Tang (Bupleurum and Poria Decoction)	柴苓汤
Chai Ping Tang (Bupleurum and Calm the Stomach Decoction)	柴平汤
Chai Xian Tang (Bupleurum Decoction to Raise the Sunken)	柴陷汤
Chan Su Wan (Toad Venum Pill)	蟾酥丸
Cheng Qi Yang Ying Tang (Order the Qi and Nourish the Nutritive Qi Decoction)	承气养营汤
Chi Shi Zhi Yu Yu Liang Tang (Halloysitum and Limonite Decoction)	赤石脂禹余粮汤
Chuan Xiong Cha Tiao San (Ligusticum Chuanxiong Powder to be Taken with Green Tea)	川芎茶调散
Ci Zhu Wan (Magnetite and Cinnabar Pill)	磁朱丸
Cong Bai Qi Wei Yin (Scallion Decoction with Seven Ingredients)	葱白七味饮
Cong Chi Jie Geng Tang (Scallion, Prepared Soybean, and Platycodon Decoction)	葱豉桔梗汤
Cong Chi Tang (Scallion and Prepared Soybean Decoction)	葱豉汤
Cui Sheng Tang (Birth-Hastening Decoction)	催生汤
Da An Wan (Great Tranquility Pill)	大安丸
Da Bu Tang (Great Tonifying Decoction)	大补汤
Da Bu Yin Wan (Great Tonify the Yin Pill)	大补阴丸
Da Chai Hu Tang (Major Bupleurum Decoction)	大柴胡汤
Da Cheng Qi Tang (Major Order the Qi Decoction)	大承气汤
Da Ding Feng Zhu (Major Arrest Wind Pearl)	大定风珠

CROSS-REFERENCE OF HERBAL FORMULA NAMES

A10

1465

Appendix 10 — Cross-reference of Herbal Formula Names

Pinyin Names (Literal Names)	Chinese Names
Da Fang Feng Tang (Major Saposhnikovia Decoction)	大防风汤
Da Huang Fu Zi Tang (Rhubarb and Prepared Aconite Decoction)	大黄附子汤
Da Huang Mu Dan Tang (Rhubarb and Moutan Decoction)	大黄牡丹汤
Da Huang Zhe Chong Wan (Rhubarb and Eupolyphaga Pill)	大黄䗪虫丸
Da Huo Luo Dan (Major Invigorate the Collaterals Special Pill)	大活络丹
Da Jian Zhong Tang (Major Construct the Middle Decoction)	大建中汤
Da Qiang Huo Tang (Major Notopterygium Decoction)	大羌活汤
Da Qin Jiao Tang (Major Gentiana Macrophylla Decoction)	大秦艽汤
Da Qing Long Tang (Major Bluegreen Dragon Decoction)	大青龙汤
Da Xian Xiong Tang (Major Sinking into the Chest Decoction)	大陷胸汤
Da Xian Xiong Wan (Major Sinking into the Chest Pill)	大陷胸丸
Da Yuan Yin (Reach the Membrane Source Decoction)	达原饮
Dan Shen Yin (Salvia Decoction)	丹参饮
Dang Gui Bu Xue Tang (Tangkuei Decoction to Tonify the Blood)	当归补血汤
Dang Gui Jian Zhong Tang (Tangkuei Decoction to Construct the Middle)	当归建中汤
Dang Gui Liu Huang Tang (Tangkuei and Six-Yellow Decoction)	当归六黄汤
Dang Gui Long Hui Wan (Tangkuei, Gentiana, and Aloe Pill)	当归龙荟丸
Dang Gui Nian Tong Tang (Tangkuei Decoction to Lift the Pain)	当归拈痛汤
Dang Gui San (Tangkuei Powder)	当归散
Dang Gui Shao Yao San (Tangkuei and Peony Powder)	当归芍药散
Dang Gui Si Ni Jia Wu Zhu Yu Sheng Jiang Tang (Tangkuei Decoction for Frigid Extremities plus Evodia and Fresh Ginger)	当归四逆加吴茱萸生姜汤
Dang Gui Si Ni Tang (Tangkuei Decoction for Frigid Extremities)	当归四逆汤
Dang Gui Yin Zi (Tangkuei Decoction)	当归饮子
Dao Chi San (Guide Out the Red Powder)	导赤散
Dao Qi Tang (Conduct the Qi Decoction)	导气汤
Dao Shui Fu Ling Tang (Poria Decoction to Drain Water)	导水茯苓汤
Dao Tan Tang (Guide Out Phlegm Decoction)	导痰汤
Di Huang Yin Zi (Rehmannia Decoction)	地黄饮子
Di Tan Tang (Scour Phlegm Decoction)	涤痰汤
Ding Chuan Tang (Arrest Wheezing Decoction)	定喘汤
Ding Xian Wan (Arrest Seizures Pill)	定痫丸
Ding Xiang Shi Di Tang (Clove and Persimmon Calyx Decoction)	丁香柿蒂汤
Ding Zhi Wan (Settle the Emotions Pill)	定志丸
Du Huo Ji Sheng Tang (Angelica Pubescens and Taxillus Decoction)	独活寄生汤
Du Qi Wan (Capital Qi Pill)	都气丸
Dun Sou San (Long-Bout Cough Powder)	顿嗽散
Duo Ming Wan (Life-Taking Pill)	夺命丸
E Jiao Ji Zi Huang Tang (Ass-Hide Gelatin and Egg Yolk Decoction)	阿胶鸡子黄汤
Er Chen Tang (Two-Cured Decoction)	二陈汤
Er Long Zuo Ci Wan (Pill for Deafness that Is Kind to the Left [Kidney])	耳聋左慈丸

Chinese Herbal Formulas and Applications

Appendix 10 — Cross-reference of Herbal Formula Names

Pinyin Names (Literal Names)	Chinese Names
Er Miao San (Two-Marvel Powder)	二妙散
Er Xian Bu Shen Tang (Two-Immortal Decoction to Tonify the Kidney)	二仙补肾汤
Er Xian Tang (Two-Immortal Decoction)	二仙汤
Er Zhi Wan (Two-Ultimate Pill)	二至丸
Er Zhu Tang (Two-Atractylodes Decoction)	二术汤
Fa Mu Wan (Quell Wood Pill)	伐木丸
Fang Feng Tong Sheng San (Saposhnikovia Powder that Sagely Unblocks)	防风通圣散
Fang Ji Fu Ling Tang (Stephania and Poria Decoction)	防己茯苓汤
Fang Ji Huang Qi Tang (Stephania and Astragalus Decoction)	防己黄芪汤
Fei Er Wan (Fat Child Pill)	肥儿丸
Fen Xiao Tang (Separate and Reduce Decoction)	分消汤
Fu Fang Ba Zheng San (Revised Eight-Herb Powder)	复方八正散
Fu Fang Da Cheng Qi Tang (Revised Major Order the Qi Decoction)	复方大承气汤
Fu Ling Tang (Poria Decoction)	茯苓汤
Fu Ling Wan (Poria Pill)	茯苓丸
Fu Ling Yin (Poria Decoction)	茯苓饮
Fu Tu Dan (Poria and Cuscuta Special Pill)	茯菟丹
Fu Yuan Huo Xue Tang (Revive Health by Invigorating the Blood Decoction)	复元活血汤
Fu Zheng Yi Yan Tang (Support the Upright and Suppress Cancer Decoction)	扶正抑癌汤
Fu Zi Li Zhong Wan (Prepared Aconite Pill to Regulate the Middle)	附子理中丸
Fu Zi Tang (Prepared Aconite Decoction)	附子汤
Gan Cao Gan Jiang Fu Ling Bai Zhu Tang (Licorice, Ginger, Poria and Atractylodes Macrocephala Decoction)	甘草乾姜茯苓白术汤
Gan Cao Xie Xin Tang (Licorice Decoction to Drain the Epigastrium)	甘草泻心汤
Gan Jiang Ren Shen Ban Xia Wan (Ginger, Ginseng, and Pinellia Pill)	乾姜人参半夏丸
Gan Lu Xiao Du Dan (Sweet Dew Special Pill to Eliminate Toxins)	甘露消毒丹
Gan Lu Yin (Sweet Dew Decoction)	甘露饮
Gan Mai Da Zao Tang (Licorice, Wheat, and Jujube Decoction)	甘麦大枣汤
Ge Gen Huang Qin Huang Lian Tang (Kudzu, Coptis, and Scutellaria Decoction)	葛根黄芩黄连汤
Ge Gen Huo Xiang Shao Yao Tang (Kudzu, Pogostemon, and Peony Decoction)	葛根藿香芍药汤
Ge Gen Tang (Kudzu Decoction)	葛根汤
Ge Hua Jie Cheng San (Pueraria Flower Powder for Detoxification and Awakening)	葛花解醒散
Ge Xia Zhu Yu Tang (Drive Out Blood Stasis Below the Diaphragm Decoction)	膈下逐瘀汤
Gong Wai Yun Fang (Ectopic Pregnancy Formula)	宫外孕方
Gou Teng San (Uncaria Powder)	钩藤散
Gou Teng Yin (Uncaria Decoction)	钩藤饮
Gu Chong Tang (Stabilize *Chong* [Thoroughfare Channel] Decoction)	固冲汤
Gu Jing Wan (Stabilize the Menses Pill)	固经丸
Gua Di San (Melon Pedicle Powder)	瓜蒂散
Gua Lou Xie Bai Bai Jiu Tang (Trichosanthes Fruit, Chinese Chive, and Wine Decoction)	瓜蒌薤白白酒汤

1467

Appendix 10 — Cross-reference of Herbal Formula Names

Pinyin Names (Literal Names)	Chinese Names
Gua Lou Xie Bai Ban Xia Tang (Trichosanthes Fruit, Chinese Chive, and Pinellia Decoction)	瓜蒌薤白半夏汤
Gua Lou Zhi Shi Tang (Trichosanthes Fruit and Immature Bitter Orange Decoction)	瓜蒌枳实汤
Guan Xin Su He Wan (Coronary Styrax Pill)	冠心苏合丸
Gui Ling Gan Lu Yin (Cinnamon and Poria Sweet Dew Decoction)	桂苓甘露饮
Gui Lu Er Xian Jiao (Tortoise Shell and Deer Antler Syrup)	龟鹿二仙胶
Gui Pi An Shen Tang (Restore the Spleen and Tranquilize the Spirit Decoction)	归脾安神汤
Gui Pi Tang (Restore the Spleen Decoction)	归脾汤
Gui Qi Jian Zhong Tang (Tangkuei and Astragalus Decoction to Construct the Middle)	归芪建中汤
Gui Zhi Fu Ling Wan (Cinnamon Twig and Poria Pill)	桂枝茯苓丸
Gui Zhi Jia Ge Gen Tang (Cinnamon Twig Decoction plus Kudzu)	桂枝加葛根汤
Gui Zhi Jia Hou Po Xing Zi Tang (Cinnamon Twig Decoction plus Magnolia Bark and Apricot Kernel)	桂枝加厚朴杏子汤
Gui Zhi Jia Long Gu Mu Li Tang (Cinnamon Twig Decoction plus Dragon Bone and Oyster Shell)	桂枝加龙骨牡蛎汤
Gui Zhi Jia Shao Yao Tang (Cinnamon Twig Decoction plus Peony)	桂枝加芍药汤
Gui Zhi Ma Huang Ge Ban Tang (Combined Cinnamon Twig and Ephedra Decoction)	桂枝麻黄各半汤
Gui Zhi Ren Shen Tang (Cinnamon Twig and Ginseng Decoction)	桂枝人参汤
Gui Zhi Shao Yao Zhi Mu Tang (Cinnamon Twig, Peony, and Anemarrhena Decoction)	桂枝芍药知母汤
Gui Zhi Tang (Cinnamon Twig Decoction)	桂枝汤
Gun Tan Wan (Vaporize Phlegm Pill)	滚痰丸
Guo Qi Yin (Delayed Menstruation Decoction)	过期饮
Hai Zao Yu Hu Tang (Sargassum Decoction for the Jade Flask)	海藻玉壶汤
Hao Qin Qing Dan Tang (Artemisia Annua and Scutellaria Decoction to Clear the Gallbladder)	蒿芩清胆汤
He Che Wan Fang (Placenta Pill Formula)	河车丸方
Hei Xi Dan (Lead Special Pill)	黑锡丹
Hei Xiao Yao San (Black Rambling Powder)	黑逍遥散
Hou Po Qi Wu Tang (Seven-Substance Decoction with Magnolia Bark)	厚朴七物汤
Hou Po Wen Zhong Tang (Magnolia Bark Decoction for Warming the Middle)	厚朴温中汤
Hu Qian Wan (Hidden Tiger Pill)	虎潜丸
Hua Ban Tang (Transform Blotches Decoction)	化斑汤
Hua Chong Wan (Dissolve Parasites Pill)	化虫丸
Hua Gai San (Canopy Powder)	华盖散
Hua Tan Wan (Transform Phlegm Pill)	化痰丸
Huai Hua San (Sophora Japonica Flower Powder)	槐花散
Huai Jiao Wan (Sophora Japonica Fruit Pill)	槐角丸
Huan Shao Dan (Return to Youth Pill)	还少丹
Huan Shao Di Huang Wan (Rehmannia Pill to Return to Youth)	还少地黄丸

Chinese Herbal Formulas and Applications

Appendix 10 — Cross-reference of Herbal Formula Names

Pinyin Names (Literal Names)	Chinese Names
Huang Lian Jie Du Tang (Coptis Decoction to Relieve Toxicity)	黄连解毒汤
Huang Lian Shang Qing Wan (Coptis Pill to Clear the Upper)	黄连上清丸
Huang Lian Tang (Coptis Decoction)	黄连汤
Huang Long Tang (Yellow Dragon Decoction)	黄龙汤
Huang Qi Fang Feng Tang (Astragalus Decoction to Guard the Wind)	黄芪防风汤
Huang Qi Gui Zhi Wu Wu Tang (Astragalus and Cinnamon Twig Five-Substance Decoction)	黄芪桂枝五物汤
Huang Qi Jian Zhong Tang (Astragalus Decoction to Construct the Middle)	黄芪建中汤
Huang Qin Hua Shi Tang (Scutellaria and Talcum Decoction)	黄芩滑石汤
Huang Qin Tang (Scutellaria Decoction)	黄芩汤
Huang Tu Tang (Yellow Earth Decoction)	黄土汤
Hui Yang Jiu Ji Tang (Restore and Revive the Yang Decoction)	回阳救急汤
Huo Luo Xiao Ling Dan (Fantastically Effective Pill to Invigorate the Collaterals)	活络效灵丹
Huo Ming Yin (Revitalize Life Decoction)	活命饮
Huo Po Xia Ling Tang (Agastache, Magnolia Bark, Pinellia, and Poria Decoction)	藿朴夏苓汤
Huo Ren Cong Chi Tang (Scallion and Prepared Soybean Decoction from the Book to Safeguard Life)	活人葱豉汤
Huo Xiang Zheng Qi San (Agastache Powder to Rectify the Qi)	藿香正气散
Huo Xue Shun Qi Tang (Invigorate the Blood and Smooth the Qi Decoction)	活血顺气汤
Huo Xue Tong Lin Tang (Invigorate the Blood to Unblock Dysuria Decoction)	活血通淋汤
Huo Xue Zhi Tong Tang (Invigorate the Blood and Stop Pain Decoction)	活血止痛汤
Ji Chuan Jian (Benefit the River [Flow] Decoction)	济川煎
Ji Ming San (Powder to Take at Cock's Crow)	鸡鸣散
Ji Sheng Shen Qi Wan (Kidney Qi Pill from Formulas that Aid the Living)	济生肾气丸
Ji Su San (Peppermint Powder)	鸡苏散
Ji Tong Tang (Spine Pain Decoction)	脊痛汤
Jia Jian Cheng Qi Tang (Modified Order the Qi Decoction)	加减承气汤
Jia Jian Fu Mai Tang (Modified Restore the Pulse Decoction)	加减复脉汤
Jia Jian Wei Rui Tang (Modified Polygonatum Odoratum Decoction)	加减葳蕤汤
Jia Jian Xiao Qing Long Tang (Modified Minor Bluegreen Dragon Decoction)	加减小青龙汤
Jia Wei Ba Zheng San (Augmented Eight Herb Powder for Rectification)	加味八正散
Jia Wei Gua Lou Xie Bai Tang (Augmented Trichosanthes Fruit and Chinese Chive Decoction)	加味瓜蒌薤白汤
Jia Wei Huo Luo Dan (Augmented Invigorate the Collaterals Special Pill)	加味活络丹
Jia Wei Ma Xing Gan Shi Tang (Augmented Ephedra, Apricot Kernel, Licorice, and Gypsum Decoction)	加味麻杏甘石汤
Jia Wei Ping Wei San (Modified Calm the Stomach Powder)	加味平胃散
Jia Wei Qian Zheng San (Augmented Lead to Symmetry Powder)	加味牵正散
Jia Wei Shao Yao Gan Cao Tang (Augmented Peony and Licorice Decoction)	加味芍药甘草汤
Jia Wei Si Wu Tang (Augmented Four-Substance Decoction)	加味四物汤
Jia Wei Xiang Su San (Augmented Cyperus and Perilla Leaf Powder)	加味香苏散
Jia Wei Xiao Yao San (Augmented Rambling Powder)	加味逍遥散

CROSS-REFERENCE OF HERBAL FORMULA NAMES

A10

1469

Appendix 10 — Cross-reference of Herbal Formula Names

Pinyin Names (Literal Names)	Chinese Names
Jia Wei Xin Yi San (Augmented Magnolia Flower Powder)	加味辛夷散
Jia Wei You Gui Wan (Augmented Restore the Right [Kidney] Pill)	加味右归丸
Jia Wei Zuo Gui Wan (Augmented Restore the Left [Kidney] Pill)	加味左归丸
Jian Bi Tang (Remove Painful Obstruction in the Shoulders Decoction)	肩痹汤
Jian Ling Tang (Construct Roof Tiles Decoction)	建瓴汤
Jian Pi Wan (Strengthen the Spleen Pill)	健脾丸
Jiao Ai Tang (Ass-Hide Gelatin and Mugwort Decoction)	胶艾汤
Jie Geng Tang (Platycodon Decoction)	桔梗汤
Jin Fei Cao San (Inula Powder)	金沸草散
Jin Gui Shen Qi Wan (Kidney Qi Pill from the Golden Cabinet)	金匮肾气丸
Jin Jian Fei Er Wan (Golden Pill to Construct a Fat Child)	金鉴肥儿丸
Jin Ling Zi San (Melia Toosendan Powder)	金铃子散
Jin Suo Gu Jing Wan (Metal Lock Pill to Stabilize the Essence)	金锁固精丸
Jing Fang Bai Du San (Schizonepeta and Saposhnikovia Powder to Overcome Pathogenic Influences)	荆防败毒散
Jing Fang Er Hao (Neck Formula Two)	颈方二号
Jing Fang Yi Hao (Neck Formula One)	颈方一号
Jing Jie Lian Qiao Tang (Schizonepeta and Forsythia Decoction)	荆芥连翘汤
Jiu Ji Xi Xian San (Urgent Powder to Dilute Saliva)	救急稀涎散
Jiu Wei Bing Lang Jia Wu Fu Tang (Areca Nine Decoction plus Evodia and Poria)	九味槟榔加吴茯汤
Jiu Wei Qiang Huo Tang (Nine-Herb Decoction with Notopterygium)	九味羌活汤
Jiu Xian San (Nine-Immortal Powder)	九仙散
Ju Ban Zhi Zhu Wan (Tangerine Peel, Pinellia, Immature Bitter Orange, and Atractylodes Macrocephala Pill)	橘半枳术丸
Ju Fang Zhi Bao San (Greatest Treasure Powder from the Imperial Grace Formulary)	局方至宝散
Ju He Wan (Tangerine Seed Pill)	橘核丸
Ju Hua Cha Tiao San (Chrysanthemum Powder to be Taken with Green Tea)	菊花茶调散
Ju Pi Zhu Ru Tang (Tangerine Peel and Bamboo Shaving Decoction)	橘皮竹茹汤
Ju Yuan Jian (Lift the Source Decoction)	举元煎
Juan Bi Tang (Remove Painful Obstruction Decoction)	蠲痹汤
Ke Xue Fang (Coughing of Blood Formula)	咳血方
Kong Xian Dan (Control Mucus Special Pill)	控涎丹
Leng Xiao Wan (Cold Wheezing Pill)	冷哮丸
Li Zhong An Hui Tang (Regulate the Middle and Calm Roundworms Decoction)	理中安蛔汤
Li Zhong Hua Tan Wan (Regulate the Middle and Transform Phlegm Pill)	理中化痰丸
Li Zhong Wan (Regulate the Middle Pill)	理中丸
Lian Mei An Hui Tang (Picrorhiza and Mume Decoction to Calm Roundworms)	连梅安蛔汤
Lian Po Yin (Coptis and Magnolia Bark Decoction)	连朴饮
Lian Qiao Bai Du San (Forsythia Powder to Overcome Pathogenic Influences)	连翘败毒散
Lian Qiao Jie Du Tang (Forsythia Decoction to Relieve Toxicity)	连翘解毒汤

Chinese Herbal Formulas and Applications

Appendix 10 — Cross-reference of Herbal Formula Names

Pinyin Names (Literal Names)	Chinese Names
Liang Fu Wan (Galangal and Cyperus Pill)	良附丸
Liang Ge San (Cool the Diaphragm Powder)	凉膈散
Ling Gan Wu Wei Jiang Xin Tang (Poria, Licorice, Schisandra, Ginger, and Asarum Decoction)	苓甘五味姜辛汤
Ling Gui Zhu Gan Tang (Poria, Cinnamon Twig, Atractylodes Macrocephala, and Licorice Decoction)	苓桂术甘汤
Ling Jiao Gou Teng Tang (Antelope Horn and Uncaria Decoction)	羚角钩藤汤
Liu He Tang (Harmonize the Six Decoction)	六和汤
Liu Jun Zi Tang (Six-Gentlemen Decoction)	六君子汤
Liu Shen Wan (Six-Miracle Pill)	六神丸
Liu Wei Di Huang Wan (Six-Ingredient Pill with Rehmannia)	六味地黄丸
Liu Wei Gu Jing Wan (Rehmannia Six and Lotus Stamen Pill)	六味固精丸
Liu Yi San (Six-to-One Powder)	六一散
Long Dan Jiang Ya Pian (Gentiana Pill to Lower [Blood] Pressure)	龙胆降压片
Long Dan Jie Du Tang (Gentiana Decoction to Relieve Toxicity)	龙胆解毒汤
Long Dan Xie Gan Tang (Gentiana Decoction to Drain the Liver)	龙胆泻肝汤
Ma Huang Fu Zi Gan Cao Tang (Ephedra, Prepared Aconite, and Licorice Decoction)	麻黄附子甘草汤
Ma Huang Fu Zi Xi Xin Tang (Ephedra, Asarum, and Prepared Aconite Decoction)	麻黄附子细辛汤
Ma Huang Jia Zhu Tang (Ephedra Decoction plus Atractylodes)	麻黄加术汤
Ma Huang Tang (Ephedra Decoction)	麻黄汤
Ma Huang Xing Ren Gan Cao Shi Gao Tang (Ephedra, Apricot Kernel, Licorice, and Gypsum Decoction)	麻黄杏仁甘草石膏汤
Ma Xing Yi Gan Tang (Ephedra, Apricot Kernel, Coicis, and Licorice Decoction)	麻杏苡甘汤
Ma Zi Ren Wan (Hemp Seed Pill)	麻子仁丸
Ma Zi Run Chang Wan (Hemp Seed Pill to Moisten the Intestines)	麻子润肠丸
Mai Men Dong Tang (Ophiopogonis Decoction)	麦门冬汤
Mai Men Yang Yin Tang (Ophiopogonis Decoction to Nourish the Yin)	麦门养阴汤
Mai Wei Di Huang Wan (Ophiopogonis, Schisandra, and Rehmannia Pill)	麦味地黄丸
Ming Mu Di Huang Wan (Improve Vision Pill with Rehmannia)	明目地黄丸
Mu Fang Ji Tang (Cocculus Decoction)	木防己汤
Mu Li San (Oyster Shell Powder)	牡蛎散
Mu Xiang Bing Lang Wan (Aucklandia and Betel Nut Pill)	木香槟榔丸
Nao Wei Kang Wan (Benefit Brain Atrophy Pill)	脑姜康丸
Nei Bu Huang Qi Tang (Tonify the Interior Decoction with Astragalus)	内补黄芪汤
Nian Tong Tang (Lift the Pain Decoction)	拈痛汤
Ning Sou Wan (Quiet the Cough Pill)	宁嗽丸
Niu Bang Jie Ji Tang (Arctium Decoction to Release the Muscle Layer)	牛蒡解肌汤
Niu Huang Qing Xin Wan (Cattle Gallstone Pill to Clear the Heart)	牛黄清心丸
Nu Ke Bai Zi Ren Wan (Platycladus Seed Pill for Females)	女科柏子仁丸
Nuan Gan Jian (Warm the Liver Decoction)	暖肝煎

CROSS-REFERENCE OF HERBAL FORMULA NAMES

A10

1471

Appendix 10 – Cross-reference of Herbal Formula Names

Appendix 10 — Cross-reference of Herbal Formula Names

Pinyin Names (Literal Names)	Chinese Names
Pai Nong San (Drain the Pus Powder)	排脓散
Ping Wei San (Calm the Stomach Powder)	平胃散
Po Bu Zi Ye Tang (Cordia Decoction)	破布子叶汤
Pu Ji Xiao Du Yin (Universal Benefit Decoction to Eliminate Toxin)	普济消毒饮
Qi Bao Mei Ran Dan (Seven-Treasure Special Pill for Beautiful Whiskers)	七宝美髯丹
Qi Ju Di Huang Wan (Lycium Fruit, Chrysanthemum, and Rehmannia Pill)	杞菊地黄丸
Qi Li San (Seven-Thousandths of a Tael Powder)	七厘散
Qi Pi Wan (Guide the Spleen Pill)	启脾丸
Qi Wei Bai Zhu San (Seven-Ingredient Powder with Atractylodes Macrocephala)	七味白术散
Qian Jin Nei Tuo San (Drain the Interior Powder Worthy of a Thousand Gold)	千金内托散
Qian Zheng San (Lead to Symmetry Powder)	牵正散
Qiang Huo Sheng Shi Tang (Notopterygium Decoction to Overcome Dampness)	羌活胜湿汤
Qiao He Tang (Forsythia and Mint Decoction)	翘荷汤
Qin Jiao Bie Jia San (Gentiana Macrophylla and Soft-Shelled Turtle Shell Powder)	秦艽鳖甲散
Qing Bi Tang (Clear the Nose Decoction)	清鼻汤
Qing Chang Tang (Clear the Intestines Decoction)	清肠汤
Qing Chang Yin (Clear the Intestines Drink)	清肠饮
Qing Dai Tang (Clear the Discharge Decoction)	清带汤
Qing Fei Tang (Clear the Lung Decoction)	清肺汤
Qing Fei Yin (Clear the Lung Drink)	清肺饮
Qing Gu San (Cool the Bones Powder)	清骨散
Qing Hao Bie Jia Tang (Artemisia Annua and Soft-Shelled Turtle Shell Decoction)	青蒿鳖甲汤
Qing Liang Yin (Clearing and Cooling Decoction)	清凉饮
Qing Luo Yin (Clear the Collaterals Decoction)	清络饮
Qing Pi Yin (Clear the Spleen Decoction)	清脾饮
Qing Qi Hua Tan Wan (Clear the Qi and Transform Phlegm Pill)	清气化痰丸
Qing Re Jie Du Tang (Clear Heat Relieve Toxicity Decoction)	清热解毒汤
Qing Re Liang Xue Tang (Clear Heat and Cool the Blood Decoction)	清热凉血汤
Qing Re Tong Lin Tang (Clear Heat to Unblock Dysuria Decoction)	清热通淋汤
Qing Shang Fang Feng Tang (Clear the Upper and Guard the Wind Decoction)	清上防风汤
Qing Shu Yi Qi Tang (Clear Summer-Heat and Augment the Qi Decoction)	清暑益气汤
Qing Wei San (Clear the Stomach Powder)	清胃散
Qing Wei Tang (Clear the Stomach Decoction)	清胃汤
Qing Wen Bai Du Yin (Clear Epidemics and Overcome Pathogenic Influences Decoction)	清瘟败毒饮
Qing Xin Li Ge Tang (Clear the Epigastrium and Benefit the Diaphragm Decoction)	清心利膈汤
Qing Xin Lian Zi Yin (Lotus Seed Decoction to Clear the Heart)	清心莲子饮
Qing Ying Tang (Clear the Nutritive Level Decoction)	清营汤
Qing Zao Jiu Fei Tang (Eliminate Dryness and Rescue the Lung Decoction)	清燥救肺汤
Qiong Yu Gao (Beautiful Jade Paste)	琼玉膏

1472

Chinese Herbal Formulas and Applications

Appendix 10 — Cross-reference of Herbal Formula Names

Pinyin Names (Literal Names)	Chinese Names
Qu Feng San (Dispel Wind Powder)	祛风散
Qu Mai Zhi Zhu Wan (Medicated Leaven, Barley Sprout, Immature Bitter Orange, and Atractylodes Macrocephala Pill)	曲蘗枳术丸
Ren Shen Bai Du San (Ginseng Powder to Overcome Pathogenic Influences)	人参败毒散
Ren Shen Chong Cao Tang (Ginseng and Cordyceps Decoction)	人参虫草汤
Ren Shen Da Bu Tang (Ginseng Great Tonifying Decoction)	人参大补汤
Ren Shen Dang Shao San (Ginseng, Tangkuei, and Peony Powder)	人参当芍散
Ren Shen Ge Jie San (Ginseng and Gecko Powder)	人参蛤蚧散
Ren Shen Hu Tao Tang (Ginseng and Walnut Decoction)	人参胡桃汤
Ren Shen Tang (Ginseng Decoction)	人参汤
Ren Shen Xie Fei Tang (Ginseng Decoction to Sedate the Lung)	人参泻肺汤
Ren Shen Yang Ying Tang (Ginseng Decoction to Nourish the Nutritive Qi)	人参养荣汤
Run Chang Wan (Moisten the Intestines Pill)	润肠丸
San Ao Tang (Three-Unbinding Decoction)	三拗汤
San Bi Tang (Three-Painful Obstruction Decoction)	三痹汤
San Ceng Hui Xiang Wan (Fennel Seed Pill with Three Levels)	三层茴香丸
San Huang Shi Gao Tang (Three-Yellow and Gypsum Decoction)	三黄石膏汤
San Huang Xie Xin Tang (Three-Yellow Decoction to Sedate the Epigastrium)	三黄泻心汤
San Jia An Shen Wan (Three-Shell Pill to Tranquilize the Spirit)	三甲安神丸
San Jia Fu Mai Tang (Three-Shell Decoction to Restore the Pulse)	三甲复脉汤
San Jian Gao (Three Constructive Paste)	三建膏
San Jiao Zhu Yu Tang (Drive Out Blood Stasis in Three *Jiaos* Decoction)	三焦逐瘀汤
San Jin Pai Shi Tang (Three Gold Decoction to Expel Stone)	三金排石汤
San Miao Wan (Three-Marvel Pill)	三妙丸
San Ren Tang (Three-Nut Decoction)	三仁汤
San Sheng San (Three-Sage Powder)	三圣散
San Wu Bai San (Three-Substance White Powder)	三物白散
San Wu Bei Ji Wan (Three-Substance Pill for Emergencies)	三物备急丸
San Wu Xiang Ru Yin (Mosla Three Decoction)	三物香薷饮
San Zhong Kui Jian Tang (Disperse the Swelling and Break the Hardness Decoction)	散肿溃坚汤
San Zi Jiang Qi Tang (Three-Seed Decoction for Directing Qi Downward)	三子降气汤
San Zi Yang Qin Tang (Three-Seed Decoction to Nourish One's Parents)	三子养亲汤
Sang Ju Yin (Mulberry Leaf and Chrysanthemum Decoction)	桑菊饮
Sang Ma Wan (Mulberry Leaf and Sesame Seed Pill)	桑麻丸
Sang Piao Xiao San (Mantis Egg-Case Powder)	桑螵蛸散
Sang Xing Tang (Mulberry Leaf and Apricot Kernel Decoction)	桑杏汤
Sang Zhi Shi Gao Zhi Mu Tang (Mulberry Twig, Gypsum, and Anemarrhena Decoction)	桑枝石膏知母汤
Sha Shen Mai Dong Tang (Glehnia and Ophiopogonis Decoction)	沙参麦冬汤
Shan Zha Hua Tan Tang (Crataegus Decoction to Transform Phlegm)	山楂化痰汤

CROSS-REFERENCE OF HERBAL FORMULA NAMES

A10

1473

Appendix 10 – Cross-reference of Herbal Formula Names

Appendix 10 — Cross-reference of Herbal Formula Names

Pinyin Names (Literal Names)	Chinese Names
Shan Zha Tang (Crataegus Decoction)	山楂汤
Shang Zhong Xia Tong Yong Tong Feng Wan (Upper, Middle, and Lower General Use Pill for Wind-Pain)	上中下通用痛风丸
Shao Fu Zhu Yu Tang (Drive Out Blood Stasis in the Lower Abdomen Decoction)	少腹逐瘀汤
Shao Yao Gan Cao Tang (Peony and Licorice Decoction)	芍药甘草汤
Shao Yao Hou Po Tang (Peony and Magnolia Bark Decoction)	芍药厚朴汤
Shao Yao Tang (Peony Decoction)	芍药汤
Shao Yao Yi Yi Ren Tang (Peony and Coicis Decoction)	芍药薏苡仁汤
She Gan Ma Huang Tang (Belamcanda and Ephedra Decoction)	射干麻黄汤
Shen Fu Tang (Ginseng and Prepared Aconite Decoction)	参附汤
Shen Ling Bai Zhu San (Ginseng, Poria, and Atractylodes Macrocephala Powder)	参苓白术散
Shen Ling San (Ginseng and Poria Powder)	参苓散
Shen Mi Tang (Mysterious Decoction)	神秘汤
Shen Su Yin (Ginseng and Perilla Leaf Decoction)	参苏饮
Shen Tong Zhu Yu Tang (Drive Out Blood Stasis from a Painful Body Decoction)	身痛逐瘀汤
Shen Xi Dan (Magical Rhinoceros Special Pill)	神犀丹
Shen Xiao Tuo Li San (Miraculous Powder for Supporting the Interior)	神效托里散
Sheng Hua Tang (Generation and Transformation Decoction)	生化汤
Sheng Jiang Xie Xin Tang (Fresh Ginger Decoction to Drain the Epigastrium)	生姜泻心汤
Sheng Ma Ge Gen Tang (Cimicifuga and Kudzu Decoction)	升麻葛根汤
Sheng Mai San (Generate the Pulse Powder)	生脉散
Sheng Tie Luo Yin (Iron Filings Decoction)	生铁落饮
Sheng Xian Tang (Raise the Sinking Decoction)	升陷汤
Sheng Yang San Huo Tang (Raise the Yang and Disperse the Fire Decoction)	升阳散火汤
Sheng Yu Tang (Sage-Like Healing Decoction)	圣愈汤
Shi Bu Wan (Ten-Tonic Pill)	十补丸
Shi Di Tang (Persimmon Calyx Decoction)	柿蒂汤
Shi Gao Tang (Gypsum Decoction)	石膏汤
Shi Hu Ye Guang Wan (Dendrobium Pill for Night Vision)	石斛夜光丸
Shi Hui San (Ten Partially-Charred Substances Powder)	十灰散
Shi Liu Wei Liu Qi Yin (Sixteen-Ingredient Decoction to Flow Qi)	十六味流气饮
Shi Pi San (Bolster the Spleen Powder)	实脾散
Shi Quan Da Bu Tang (All-Inclusive Great Tonifying Decoction)	十全大补汤
Shi Shen Tang (Ten-Immortal Decoction)	十神汤
Shi Wei Bai Du Tang (Ten-Ingredient Decoction to Overcome Pathogenic Influences)	十味败毒汤
Shi Wei Di Huang Wan (Ten-Ingredient Pill with Rehmannia)	十味地黄丸
Shi Wei Wen Dan Tang (Ten-Ingredient Decoction to Warm the Gallbladder)	十味温胆汤
Shi Wei Xiang Ru Yin (Ten-Ingredient Decoction with Mosla)	十味香薷饮
Shi Wei Xiao Yao San (Ten-Ingredient Rambling Powder)	十味逍遥散
Shi Xiao San (Sudden Smile Powder)	失笑散

1474

Chinese Herbal Formulas and Applications

Appendix 10 — Cross-reference of Herbal Formula Names

Pinyin Names (Literal Names)	Chinese Names
Shi Zao Tang (Ten-Jujube Decoction)	十枣汤
Shou Nian San (Pinch Powder)	手拈散
Shou Wu Pian (Polygonum Pill)	首乌片
Shu Gan Tang (Spread the Liver Decoction)	疏肝汤
Shu Jin Li An San (Relax the Tendons and Instill Peace Powder)	疏筋立安散
Shu Jing Huo Xue Tang (Relax the Channels and Invigorate the Blood Decoction)	疏经活血汤
Shu Zao Yin Zi (Spread and Unblock Decoction)	疏凿饮子
Shuang Jie Tong Sheng San (Double Relieve Powder that Sagely Unblocks)	双解通圣散
Shui Lu Er Xian Dan (Water and Earth Two Immortals Special Pill)	水陆二仙丹
Si Jun Zi Tang (Four-Gentlemen Decoction)	四君子汤
Si Ling San (Four-Ingredient Powder with Poria)	四苓散
Si Miao Wan (Four-Marvel Pill)	四妙丸
Si Miao Yong An Tang (Four-Valiant Decoction for Well-Being)	四妙勇安汤
Si Mo Tang (Four Milled-Herbs Decoction)	四磨汤
Si Ni Jia Ren Shen Tang (Frigid Extremities Decoction plus Ginseng)	四逆加人参汤
Si Ni San (Frigid Extremities Powder)	四逆散
Si Ni Tang (Frigid Extremities Decoction)	四逆汤
Si Shen Wan (Four-Miracle Pill)	四神丸
Si Sheng Wan (Four-Fresh Pill)	四生丸
Si Wu Tang (Four-Substance Decoction)	四物汤
Su He Xiang Wan (Liquid Styrax Pill)	苏合香丸
Su Zi Jiang Qi Tang (Perilla Fruit Decoction for Directing Qi Downward)	苏子降气汤
Suan Zao Ren Tang (Sour Jujube Decoction)	酸枣仁汤
Suo Quan Wan (Shut the Sluice Pill)	缩泉丸
Tai Shan Pan Shi San (Powder that Gives the Stability of Mount Tai)	泰山磐石散
Tao He Cheng Qi Tang (Peach Pit Decoction to Order the Qi)	桃核承气汤
Tao Hong Si Wu Tang (Four-Substance Decoction with Safflower and Peach Pit)	桃红四物汤
Tao Hua Tang (Peach Blossom Decoction)	桃花汤
Tian Ma Gou Teng Yin (Gastrodia and Uncaria Decoction)	天麻钩藤饮
Tian Ma Jiang Ya Pian (Gastrodia Pill to Lower [Blood] Pressure)	天麻降压片
Tian Tai Wu Yao San (Top-Quality Lindera Powder)	天台乌药散
Tian Wang Bu Xin Dan (Emperor of Heaven's Special Pill to Tonify the Heart)	天王补心丹
Tiao Jing Er Hao (Regulate Menses Formula Two)	调经二号
Tiao Jing San Hao (Regulate Menses Formula Three)	调经三号
Tiao Jing Si Hao (Regulate Menses Formula Four)	调经四号
Tiao Jing Yi Hao (Regulate Menses Formula One)	调经一号
Tiao Wei Cheng Qi Tang (Regulate the Stomach and Order the Qi Decoction)	调胃承气汤
Ting Li Da Zao Xie Fei Tang (Descurainia and Jujube Decoction to Drain the Lung)	葶苈大枣泻肺汤
Tong Feng Wan (Wind-Pain Pill)	痛风丸
Tong Mai Si Ni Tang (Unblock the Pulse Decoction for Frigid Extremities)	通脉四逆汤

CROSS-REFERENCE OF HERBAL FORMULA NAMES

A10

1475

Appendix 10 – Cross-reference of Herbal Formula Names

Appendix 10 — Cross-reference of Herbal Formula Names

Pinyin Names (Literal Names)	Chinese Names
Tong Qiao Huo Xue Tang (Unblock the Orifices and Invigorate the Blood Decoction)	通窍活血汤
Tong Ru Wan (Unblock the Breast Pill)	通乳丸
Tong Xie Yao Fang (Important Formula for Painful Diarrhea)	痛泻要方
Tou Nong San (Discharge Pus Powder)	透脓散
Tuo Li Tou Nong Tang (Drain the Interior and Discharge Pus Decoction)	托里透脓汤
Tuo Li Xiao Du Yin (Drain the Interior and Detoxify Decoction)	托里消毒饮
Wan Dai Tang (End Discharge Decoction)	完带汤
Wei Jing Tang (Reed Decoction)	苇茎汤
Wei Ling Tang (Calm the Stomach and Poria Decoction)	胃苓汤
Wei Rui Tang (Polygonatum Odoratum Decoction)	葳蕤汤
Wen Dan Tang (Warm the Gallbladder Decoction)	温胆汤
Wen Jing Tang (Warm the Channels Decoction)	温经汤
Wen Jing Zhi Tong Tang (Warm the Channel and Stop Pain Decoction)	温经止痛汤
Wen Pi Tang (Warm the Spleen Decoction)	温脾汤
Wen Qing Yin (Warming and Clearing Decoction)	温清饮
Wu Hu Zhui Feng San (Five-Tiger Powder to Pursue Wind)	五虎追风散
Wu Ji San (Five-Accumulation Powder)	五积散
Wu Ji Wan (Wu Ji Pill)	戊己丸
Wu Lin San (Five-Ingredient Powder for Painful Urinary Dysfunction)	五淋散
Wu Ling San (Five-Ingredient Powder with Poria)	五苓散
Wu Mei Wan (Mume Pill)	乌梅丸
Wu Mo Yin Zi (Five Milled-Herbs Decoction)	五磨饮子
Wu Pi San (Five-Peel Powder)	五皮散
Wu Ren Wan (Five-Seed Pill)	五仁丸
Wu Shen Tang (Five-Miracle Decoction)	五神汤
Wu Wei Xiao Du Yin (Five-Ingredient Decoction to Eliminate Toxins)	五味消毒饮
Wu Yao Shun Qi San (Lindera Powder to Smooth the Flow of Qi)	乌药顺气散
Wu Zhu Yu Tang (Evodia Decoction)	吴茱萸汤
Xi Gan Ming Mu San (Wash the Liver and Brighten the Eyes Powder)	洗肝明目散
Xi Huang Wan (Cattle Gallstone Pill)	犀黄丸
Xi Jiao Di Huang Tang (Rhinoceros Horn and Rehmannia Decoction)	犀角地黄汤
Xi Tong Fang Er Hao (Knee Pain Formula Two)	膝痛方二号
Xi Tong Fang Yi Hao (Knee Pain Formula One)	膝痛方一号
Xia Yu Xue Tang (Drain Blood Stasis Decoction)	下血瘀汤
Xian Fang Huo Ming Yin (Sublime Formula for Sustaining Life)	仙方活命饮
Xiang Fu Wan (Cyperus Pill)	香砂丸
Xiang Lian Wan (Aucklandia and Coptis Pill)	香连丸
Xiang Ru San (Mosla Powder)	香薷散
Xiang Sha Liu Jun Zi Tang (Six-Gentlemen Decoction with Cyperus and Amomum)	香砂六君子汤

1476

Chinese Herbal Formulas and Applications

Appendix 10 — Cross-reference of Herbal Formula Names

Pinyin Names (Literal Names)	Chinese Names
Xiang Sha Liu Jun Zi Tang (Six-Gentlemen Decoction with Aucklandia and Amomum)	香砂六君子汤
Xiang Sha Ping Wei San (Cyperus and Amomum Powder to Calm the Stomach)	香砂平胃散
Xiang Sha Yang Wei Tang (Nourish the Stomach Decoction with Aucklandia and Amomum)	香砂养胃汤
Xiang Sha Zhi Zhu Wan (Aucklandia, Amomum, Immature Bitter Orange, and Atractylodes Macrocephala Pill)	香砂枳术丸
Xiang Sheng Po Di San (Loud Sound Powder for a Broken Flute)	响声破笛散
Xiang Su Cong Chi Tang (Cyperus, Perilla Leaf, Scallion, and Prepared Soybean Decoction)	香苏葱豉汤
Xiang Su San (Cyperus and Perilla Leaf Powder)	香苏散
Xiao Ban Xia Jia Fu Ling Tang (Minor Pinellia and Poria Decoction)	小半夏加茯苓汤
Xiao Chai Hu Tang (Minor Bupleurum Decoction)	小柴胡汤
Xiao Cheng Qi Tang (Minor Order the Qi Decoction)	小承气汤
Xiao Ding Feng Zhu (Minor Arrest Wind Pearl)	小定风珠
Xiao Er Hui Chun Dan (Return of Spring Special Pill [Pediatric])	小儿回春丹
Xiao Feng San (Eliminate Wind Powder)	消风散
Xiao Huo Luo Dan (Minor Invigorate the Collaterals Special Pill)	小活络丹
Xiao Ji Yin Zi (Cirsium Decoction)	小蓟饮子
Xiao Jian Zhong Tang (Minor Construct the Middle Decoction)	小建中汤
Xiao Jin Dan (Minor Gold Special Pill)	小金丹
Xiao Ke Fang (Wasting and Thirsting Formula)	消渴方
Xiao Luo Wan (Reduce Scrofula Pill)	消瘰丸
Xiao Qing Long Jia Shi Gao Tang (Minor Bluegreen Dragon Decoction plus Gypsum)	小青龙加石膏汤
Xiao Qing Long Tang (Minor Bluegreen Dragon Decoction)	小青龙汤
Xiao San Tang Er Hao (Dissolve and Disperse Decoction Formula Two)	消散汤二号
Xiao San Tang Yi Hao (Dissolve and Disperse Decoction Formula One)	消散汤一号
Xiao Xian Xiong Tang (Minor Sinking into the Chest Decoction)	小陷胸汤
Xiao Xu Ming Tang (Minor Prolong Life Decoction)	小续命汤
Xiao Yao San (Rambling Powder)	逍遥散
Xie Bai San (Drain the White Powder)	泻白散
Xie Huang San (Drain the Yellow Powder)	泻黄散
Xie Qing Wan (Drain the Green Pill)	泻青丸
Xin Jia Huang Long Tang (Newly-Augmented Yellow Dragon Decoction)	新加黄龙汤
Xin Jia Xiang Ru Yin (Newly-Augmented Mosla Decoction)	新加香薷饮
Xin Yi Qing Fei Yin (Magnolia Decoction to Clear the Lung)	辛夷清肺饮
Xin Yi San (Magnolia Flower Powder)	辛夷散
Xin Zhi Ju Pi Zhu Ru Tang (Newly-Formulated Tangerine Peel and Bamboo Shaving Decoction)	新制橘皮竹茹汤
Xing Jun San (Troop-Marching Powder)	行军散

CROSS-REFERENCE OF HERBAL FORMULA NAMES

A10

1477

Appendix 10 – Cross-reference of Herbal Formula Names

Pinyin Names (Literal Names)	Chinese Names
Xing Su San (Apricot Kernel and Perilla Leaf Powder)	杏苏散
Xing Su Yin (Apricot Kernel and Perilla Leaf Decoction)	杏苏饮
Xing Xiao Wan (Awake and Disperse Pill)	醒消丸
Xiong Gui Tiao Xue Yin (Cnidium and Tangkuei Decoction to Regulate Blood)	芎归调血饮
Xu Ming Tang (Prolong Life Decoction)	续命汤
Xuan Du Fa Biao Tang (Dissipate Toxins and Release the Exterior Decoction)	宣毒发表汤
Xuan Fu Dai Zhe Shi Tang (Inula and Hematite Decoction)	旋覆代赭石汤
Xue Fu Zhu Yu Tang (Drive Out Stasis in the Mansion of Blood Decoction)	血府逐瘀汤
Yan Hu Er Hao (Corydalis Formula Two)	延胡二号
Yan Hu Suo San (Corydalis Powder)	延胡素散
Yan Hu Yi Hao (Corydalis Formula One)	延胡一号
Yan Tang Tan Tu Fang (Salt Decoction to Induce Vomiting)	盐汤探吐方
Yang He Tang (Yang-Heartening Decoction)	阳和汤
Yang Xin Dan (Nourish the Heart Pill)	养心丹
Yang Xin Tang (Nourish the Heart Decoction)	养心汤
Yang Yin Qing Fei Tang (Nourish the Yin and Clear the Lung Decoction)	养阴清肺汤
Yao Tong Fang Er Hao (Low Back Formula Two)	腰痛方二号
Yao Tong Fang Yi Hao (Low Back Formula One)	腰痛方一号
Yi Gan San (Restrain the Liver Powder)	抑肝散
Yi Gong San (Extraordinary Merit Powder)	异功散
Yi Guan Jian (Linking Decoction)	一贯煎
Yi Huang Tang (Change the Yellow [Discharge] Decoction)	易黄汤
Yi Qi Cong Ming Tang (Augment the Qi and Increase Acuity Decoction)	益气聪明汤
Yi Yi Fu Zi Bai Jiang San (Coicis, Prepared Aconite, and Patrinia Powder)	薏苡附子败酱散
Yi Yi Ren Tang (Coicis Decoction)	薏苡仁汤
Yi Yuan San (Benefit the Basal Powder)	益元散
Yi Zi Tang (Yi Word Decoction)	乙字汤
Yin Chen Hao Tang (Artemisia Scoparia Decoction)	茵陈蒿汤
Yin Chen Pai Shi Tang (Artemisia Scoparia Decoction to Expel Stone)	茵陈排石汤
Yin Chen Si Ni Tang (Artemisia Scoparia Decoction for Frigid Extremities)	茵陈四逆汤
Yin Chen Wu Ling San (Artemisia Scoparia and Five-Ingredient Powder with Poria)	茵陈五苓散
Yin Hua Jie Du Tang (Honeysuckle Decoction to Relieve Toxicity)	银花解毒汤
Yin Qiao Jie Du San (Honeysuckle and Forsythia Powder to Relieve Toxicity)	银翘解毒散
Yin Qiao San (Honeysuckle and Forsythia Powder)	银翘散
Yin Qiao Tang (Honeysuckle and Forsythia Decoction)	银翘汤
You Bi Tang (Benefit the Nose Decoction)	优鼻汤
You Gui Wan (Restore the Right [Kidney] Pill)	右归丸
You Gui Yin (Restore the Right [Kidney] Decoction)	右归饮
Yu Nu Jian (Jade Woman Decoction)	玉女煎
Yu Ping Feng San (Jade Windscreen Powder)	玉屏风散

1478

Chinese Herbal Formulas and Applications

Appendix 10 — Cross-reference of Herbal Formula Names

Pinyin Names (Literal Names)	Chinese Names
Yu Quan Wan (Jade Spring Pill)	玉泉丸
Yu Ye Tang (Jade Fluid Decoction)	玉液汤
Yu Zhen San (True Jade Powder)	玉真散
Yue Bi Jia Zhu Tang (Maidservant from Yue Decoction plus Atractylodes)	越婢加术汤
Yue Bi Tang (Maidservant from Yue Decoction)	越婢汤
Yue Hua Wan (Moonlight Pill)	月华丸
Yue Ju Wan (Escape Restraint Pill)	越鞠丸
Zai Zao San (Renewal Powder)	再造散
Zeng Ye Cheng Qi Tang (Increase the Fluids and Order the Qi Decoction)	增液承气汤
Zeng Ye Tang (Increase the Fluids Decoction)	增液汤
Zhe Chong Yin (Break the Conflict Decoction)	折冲饮
Zhen Gan Xi Feng Tang (Sedate the Liver and Extinguish Wind Decoction)	镇肝熄风汤
Zhen Ling Dan (Rouse the Spirits Special Pill)	震灵丹
Zhen Ren Huo Ming Yin (True Man's Decoction to Revitalize Life)	真人活命饮
Zhen Ren Yang Zang Tang (True Man's Decoction for Nourishing the Organs)	真人养脏汤
Zhen Wu Tang (True Warrior Decoction)	真武汤
Zhen Zhong Dan (Pillow Special Pill)	枕中丹
Zhen Zhu Mu Wan (Mother of Pearl Pill)	珍珠母丸
Zheng Gu Zi Jin Dan (Purple and Gold Pill for Righteous Bones)	正骨紫金丹
Zhi Bai Di Huang Wan (Anemarrhena, Phellodendron, and Rehmannia Pill)	知柏地黄丸
Zhi Bao Dan (Greatest Treasure Special Pill)	至宝丹
Zhi Gan Cao Tang (Honey-Fried Licorice Decoction)	炙甘草汤
Zhi Jing San (Stop Spasms Powder)	止痉散
Zhi Ke Tang (Stop Coughing Decoction)	止咳汤
Zhi Shi Dao Zhi Wan (Immature Bitter Orange Pill to Guide Out Stagnation)	枳实导滞丸
Zhi Shi Shao Yao San (Immature Bitter Orange and Peony Powder)	枳实芍药散
Zhi Shi Xiao Pi Wan (Immature Bitter Orange Pill to Reduce Focal Distention)	枳实消痞丸
Zhi Shi Xie Bai Gui Zhi Tang (Immature Bitter Orange, Chinese Chive, and Cinnamon Twig Decoction)	枳实薤白桂枝汤
Zhi Sou San (Stop Coughing Powder)	止嗽散
Zhi Suo Er Chen Tang (Two-Cured Decoction with Aurantium and Cardamon)	枳缩二陈汤
Zhi Xue Tang (Stop Bleeding Decoction)	止血汤
Zhi Zhu Tang (Immature Bitter Orange and Atractylodes Macrocephala Decoction)	枳术汤
Zhi Zhu Wan (Immature Bitter Orange and Atractylodes Macrocephala Pill)	枳术丸
Zhi Zhuo Gu Ben Wan (Treat the Turbidity and Guard the Root Pill)	治浊固本丸
Zhi Zi Bo Pi Tang (Gardenia and Phellodendron Decoction)	栀子柏皮汤
Zhi Zi Chi Tang (Gardenia and Soja Decoction)	栀子豉汤
Zhi Zi Jiang Huo Tang (Gardenia Decoction to Descend Fire)	栀子降火汤
Zhi Zi Qing Gan Tang (Gardenia Decoction to Clear the Liver)	栀子清肝汤
Zhong He Tang (Middle-Heartening Decoction)	中和汤

CROSS-REFERENCE OF HERBAL FORMULA NAMES

A10

Appendix 10 — Cross-reference of Herbal Formula Names

Pinyin Names (Literal Names)	Chinese Names
Zhou Che Wan (Vessel and Vehicle Pill)	舟车丸
Zhu Ling Tang (Polyporus Decoction)	猪苓汤
Zhu Ru Wen Dan Tang (Bamboo Decoction to Warm the Gallbladder)	竹茹温胆汤
Zhu Sha An Shen Wan (Cinnabar Pill to Tranquilize the Spirit)	朱砂安神丸
Zhu Ye Liu Bang Tang (Lophatherum, Tamarisk and Arctium Decoction)	竹叶柳蒡汤
Zhu Ye Shi Gao Tang (Bamboo Leaves and Gypsum Decoction)	竹叶石膏汤
Zhu Yu Tang (Drive Out Blood Stasis Decoction)	逐瘀汤
Zhuang Jin Tang (Strengthen the Tendon Decoction)	壮筋汤
Zi Cao Gen Mu Li Tang (Arnebia and Oyster Shell Decoction)	紫草根牡蛎汤
Zi Jin Ding (Purple Gold Special Pill)	紫金锭
Zi Shen Ming Mu Tang (Nourish the Kidney to Brighten the Eyes Decoction)	滋肾明目汤
Zi Shen Tong Er Tang (Nourish the Kidney to Unblock the Ears Decoction)	滋肾通耳汤
Zi Sheng Wan (Nourish Life Pill)	资生丸
Zi Wan Tang (Aster Decoction)	紫菀汤
Zi Xue (Purple Snow)	紫雪
Zi Yin Di Huang Wan (Rehmannia Pill to Nourish Yin)	滋阴地黄丸
Zi Yin Jiang Huo Tang (Nourish Yin and Descend the Fire Decoction)	滋阴降火汤
Zi Yin Qing Re Tang (Nourish Yin and Clear Heat Decoction)	滋阴清热汤
Zuo Gui Wan (Restore the Left [Kidney] Pill)	左归丸
Zuo Gui Yin (Restore the Left [Kidney] Decoction)	左归饮
Zuo Jin Wan (Left Metal Pill)	左金丸

Chinese Herbal Formulas and Applications

Appendix 11

— Tables of Famous Doctors

Table 1. Famous Doctors – in Chapter Order

Chapters	Names
Part I. Overview	黄帝 Huang Di (Yellow Emperor), dates unknown.
Part II. Formula Monographs	神农 Shen Nong (Divine Husbandman), dates unknown.
1. Exterior-Releasing Formulas	张仲景 Zhang Zhong-Jing, also known as 张机 Zhang Ji, 150-219 CE.
2. Downward Draining Formulas	张景岳 Zhang Jing-Yue, also known as 张介宾 Zhang Jie-Bin, 1563-1640.
3. Harmonizing Formulas	吴有性 Wu You-Xing, also known as 吴又可 Wu You-Ke, 1580's-1660's.
4. Exterior- and Interior-Releasing Formulas	刘完素 Liu Yuan-Su, 1120-1200.
5. Heat-Clearing Formulas	叶桂 Ye Gui, also known as 叶天士 Ye Tian-Shi, 1666-1745.
6. Summer-Heat Dispelling Formulas	吴塘 Wu Tang, also known as 吴鞠通 Wu Ju-Tong, 1758-1836.
7. Interior-Warming Formulas	王叔和 Wang Shu-He, third century.
8. Tonic Formulas	钱乙 Qian Yi, 1032-1113.
9. *Shen*-Calming Formulas	扁鹊 Bian Que, also known as 秦越人 Qin Yue-Ren, 407-310 BCE.
10. Orifice-Opening Formulas	华佗 Hua Tuo, 110-207 CE.
11. Astringent Formulas	傅山 Fu Shan, also known as 傅青主 Fu Qing-Zhu, 1607-1684.
12. Qi-Regulating Formulas	李时珍 Li Shi-Zhen, 1518-1593.
13. Blood-Regulating Formulas	王清任 Wang Qing-Ren, 1768-1831.
14. Wind-Expelling Formulas	王焘 Wang Tao, 670-755.
15. Dryness-Relieving Formulas	陶弘景 Tao Hong-Jing, 456-536.
16. Damp-Dispelling Formulas	王肯堂 Wang Ken-Tang, 1549-1613.
17. Wind-Damp Dispelling Formulas	孙思邈 Sun Si-Miao, 581-682.
18. Phlegm-Dispelling Formulas	朱震亨 Zhu Zhen-Heng, also known as 朱丹溪 Zhu Dan-Xi, 1281-1358.
19. Reducing Guiding and Dissolving Formulas	李杲 Li Gao, also known as 李东垣 Li Dong-Heng, 1180-1251.
20. Antiparasitic Formulas	葛洪 Ge Hong, 284-364.
21. Emetic Formulas	张从正 Zhang Cong-Zheng, also known as 张子和 Zhang Zi-He, 1151-1231.
22. Formulas that Treat Abscesses and Sores	龚廷贤 Gong Ting-Xian, 1522-1619.
Part III. Additional Resources	吴尚先 Wu Shang-Xian, 1806-1886.

TABLES OF FAMOUS DOCTORS

A11

1481

Appendix 11 – Tables of Famous Doctors

Appendix 11 — Tables of Famous Doctors

Table 2. Famous Doctors – According to Chronology of Chinese Dynasties

Dynasties & Kingdoms		Year	Names
Xia Period 夏		2100-1600 BCE	黄帝 Huang Di (Yellow Emperor), dates unknown. 神农 Shen Nong (Divine Husbandman), dates unknown.
Shang Period 商		1600-1100 BCE	
Zhou Period 周	Western Zhou Period 西周	1100-771 BCE	扁鹊 Bian Que, also known as 秦越人 Qin Yue-Ren, 407-310 BCE.
	Eastern Period 东周	770-256 BCE	
	Spring and Autumn Period 春秋	770-476 BCE	
	Warring States 战国	475-221 BCE	
Qin Dynasty 秦		221-207 BCE	
Han Dynasty 汉	Western Han 西汉	206 BCE- 24	华佗 Hua Tuo, 110-207 CE. 张仲景 Zhang Zhong-Jing, also known as 张机 Zhang Ji, 150-219 CE.
	Eastern Han 东汉	25-220	
Three Kingdoms 三国	Wei 魏	220-265	王叔和 Wang Shu-He, third century.
	Shu 蜀	221-263	
	Wu 吴	222-280	
Western Jin Dynasty 西晋		265-316	葛洪 Ge Hong, 284-364.
Eastern Jin Dynasty 东晋		317-420	
Northern and Southern Dynasties 北南朝	Southern 南朝	420-589	陶弘景 Tao Hong-Jing, 456-536.
	Northern 北朝	386-581	
Sui Dynasty 隋		581-618	孙思邈 Sun Si-Miao, 581-682.
Tang Dynasty 唐		618-907	王焘 Wang Tao, 670-755.
Five Dynasties 五代	Later Liang 后梁	907-923	
	Later Tang 后唐	923-936	
	Later Jin 后晋	936-947	
	Later Han 后汉	947-950	
	Later Zhou 后周	951-960	
Song Dynasty 宋	Northern Song 北宋	960-1127	
	Southern Song 南宋	1127-1279	

Chinese Herbal Formulas and Applications

Appendix 11 — Tables of Famous Doctors

Dynasties & Kingdoms	Year	Names
Liao Dynasty 遼	916-1125	钱乙 Qian Yi, 1032-1113.
Jin Dynasty 金	1115-1234	刘完素 Liu Yuan-Su, 1120-1200. 张从正 Zhang Cong-Zheng, also known as 张子和 Zhang Zi-He, 1151-1231. 李杲 Li Gao, also known as 李东垣 Li Dong-Heng, 1180-1251.
Yuan Dynasty 元	1271-1368	朱震亨 Zhu Zhen-Heng, also known as 朱丹溪 Zhu Dan-Xi, 1281-1358.
Ming Dynasty 明	1368-1644	李时珍 Li Shi-Zhen, 1518-1593. 龚廷贤 Gong Ting-Xian, 1522-1619. 王肯堂 Wang Ken-Tang, 1549-1613. 张景岳 Zhang Jing-Yue, also known as 张介宾 Zhang Jie-Bin, 1563-1640. 吴有性 Wu You-Xing, also known as 吴又可 Wu You-Ke, 1580's-1660's. 傅山 Fu Shan, also known as 傅青主 Fu Qing-Zhu, 1607-1684.
Qing Dynasty 清	1644-1911	叶桂 Ye Gui, also known as 叶天士 Ye Tian-Shi, 1666-1745. 吴塘 Wu Tang, also known as 吴鞠通 Wu Ju-Tong, 1758-1836. 王清任 Wang Qing-Ren, 1768-1831. 吴尚先 Wu Shang-Xian, 1806-1886.
Republic of China 中华民国	1911-Present Day	
People's Republic of China 中华人民共和国	1949-Present Day	

TABLES OF FAMOUS DOCTORS

A11

1483

Appendix 11 – Tables of Famous Doctors

Appendix 11 — Tables of Famous Doctors

Table 3. Famous Doctors – in Alphabetic Order

Names	Chapters
扁鹊 Bian Que, also known as 秦越人 Qin Yue-Ren, 407-310 BCE.	9. *Shen*-Calming Formulas
傅山 Fu Shan, also known as 傅青主 Fu Qing-Zhu, 1607-1684.	11. Astringent Formulas
葛洪 Ge Hong, 284-364.	20. Antiparasitic Formulas
龚廷贤 Gong Ting-Xian, 1522-1619.	22. Formulas that Treat Abscesses and Sores
华佗 Hua Tuo, 110-207 CE.	10. Orifice-Opening Formulas
黄帝 Huang Di (Yellow Emperor), dates unknown.	Part I. Overview
李杲 Li Gao, also known as 李东垣 Li Dong-Heng, 1180-1251.	19. Reducing Guiding and Dissolving Formulas
李时珍 Li Shi-Zhen, 1518-1593.	12. Qi-Regulating Formulas
刘完素 Liu Yuan-Su, 1120-1200.	4. Exterior- and Interior-Releasing Formulas
钱乙 Qian Yi, 1032-1113.	8. Tonic Formulas
神农 Shen Nong (Divine Husbandman), dates unknown.	Part II. Formula Monographs
孙思邈 Sun Si-Miao, 581-682.	17. Wind-Damp Dispelling Formulas
陶弘景 Tao Hong-Jing, 456-536.	15. Dryness-Relieving Formulas
王肯堂 Wang Ken-Tang, 1549-1613.	16. Damp-Dispelling Formulas
王清任 Wang Qing-Ren, 1768-1831.	13. Blood-Regulating Formulas
王叔和 Wang Shu-He, third century.	7. Interior-Warming Formulas
王焘 Wang Tao, 670-755.	14. Wind-Expelling Formulas
吴尚先 Wu Shang-Xian, 1806-1886.	Part III. Additional Resources
吴塘 Wu Tang, also known as 吴鞠通 Wu Ju-Tong, 1758-1836.	6. Summer-Heat Dispelling Formulas
吴有性 Wu You-Xing, also known as 吴又可 Wu You-Ke, 1580's-1660's.	3. Harmonizing Formulas
叶桂 Ye Gui, also known as 叶天士 Ye Tian-Shi, 1666-1745.	5. Heat-Clearing Formulas
张从正 Zhang Cong-Zheng, also known as 张子和 Zhang Zi-He, 1151-1231.	21. Emetic Formulas
张景岳 Zhang Jing-Yue, also known as 张介宾 Zhang Jie-Bin, 1563-1640.	2. Downward Draining Formulas
张仲景 Zhang Zhong-Jing, also known as 张机 Zhang Ji, 150-219 CE.	1. Exterior-Releasing Formulas
朱震亨 Zhu Zhen-Heng, also known as 朱丹溪 Zhu Dan-Xi, 1281-1358.	18. Phlegm-Dispelling Formulas

1484

Chinese Herbal Formulas and Applications

Bibliography of Historical Texts

Pinyin Names (Translated Names)	Chinese Names
Bai Rai Shin Shu (A New Study of Dermatomycosis and Dermatitis) by Tsursure Katakura	
Bai Yi Xuan Fang (Selected Formulas)	百一选方
Bao Ying Cuo Yao (Synopsis of Caring for Infants) by Xue Kai in 1555	保婴撮要
Bei Ji Qian Jin Yao Fang (Thousands of Golden Prescriptions for Emergencies) by Sun Si-Miao in Tang Dynasty	备急千金要方
Ben Cao Bei Yao (Essentials of the Materia Medica) by Wang Ang in 1751	本草备要
Ben Cao Cong Xin (Thoroughly Revised Materia Medica) by Wu Yi-Luo in 1751	本草从新
Ben Cao Fa Hui (Elaboration of the Materia Medica) by Xu Yan-Chun in Ming Dynasty	本草发挥
Ben Cao Gang Mu (Materia Medica) by Li Shi-Zhen in 1578	本草纲目
Ben Cao Gang Mu Shi Yi (Omissions from the Grand Materia Medica) by Zhao Xue-Min in 1765	本草纲目拾遗
Ben Cao Hui Yan (Treasury of Words on the Materia Medica) by Ni Zhu-Mo in 1624	本草汇言
Ben Cao Jing Ji Zhu (Collection of Commentaries on the Classic of the Materia Medica) by Tao Hong-Jing in 480-498 B.C.	本草经集注
Ben Cao Meng Quan (Hidden Aspects of the Materia Medica) by Chen Jia-Mo in 1565	本草蒙荃
Ben Cao Pin Hui Jing Yao (Essentials of Materia Medica) by Liu Wen-Tai in 1505	本草品汇精要
Ben Cao Qiu Zheng (Verification of Materia Medica) by Huang Gong-Xiu in 1769	本草求正
Ben Cao Shi Yi (Omissions from the [Classic of the] Materia Medica) by Chen Cang-Qi in 741 A.D.	本草拾遗
Ben Cao Yan Yi (Extension of the Materia Medica) by Kou Zong-Shi in 1116	本草衍义
Ben Cao Yan Yi Bu Yi (Supplement to the Extension of the Materia Medica) by Zhu Zhen-Heng in 1347	本草衍义补遗
Ben Cao Yuan Shi (Origins of the Materia Medica) by Li Zhong-Li in Ming Dynasty	本草原始
Ben Cao Zai Xin (Renewed Materia Medica)	本草再新
Ben Cao Zheng (Rectification of the Materia Medica)	本草正
Ben Cao Zheng Yi (Truth and False Information of Materia Medica) by Zhang Shan-Lei in 1920	本草正义
Ben Jing (Divine Husbandman's Classic of the Materia Medica) in the second century	本经
Ben Jing Feng Yuan (Journey to the Origin of the Classic of Materia Medica) by Zhang Lu in 1670	本经逢原
Bian Zheng Lun (Records of Differential Diagnosis)	辨证论
Bo Ai Xin Jian (Manual of Universal Lover from the Heart) by Wei Zhi in 1525	博爱心鉴
Bu Yao Xiu Zhen Xiao Er Fang Lun (Supplement to the Pocket-Sized Discussion of Formulas for Children)	补要袖诊小儿方论
Chang Yong Zhong Cao Yao Shou Ce (Handbook of Commonly Used Traditional Chinese Herbs) by Guangzhou People's Liberation Army Medical Brigade	常用中草药手册
Cheng Fang Bian Du (Convenient Reader of Established Formulas) by Zhang Bing-Cheng in 1904	成方便读
Cheng Fang Qie Yong (Practical Formulas) by Wu Yi-Luo in 1761	成方切用
Chong Ding Ji Sheng Fang (Revised Formulas to Aid the Living)	重订济生方
Chong Ding Tong Su Shang Han Lun (Revised Popular Guide to the Discussion of Cold-Induced Disorders) by Yu Gen-Chu in Qing Dynasty	重订通俗伤寒论
Chong Ding Yan Shi Ji Sheng Fang (Revised Formulas to Aid the Living from Yan's Family)	重订严氏济生方
Chong Lou Yu Yao (Jade Key to Many Towers) by Zheng Mei-Run in 1838	重楼玉钥

BIBLIOGRAPHY OF HISTORICAL TEXTS

B

1485

Bibliography of Historical Texts

Pinyin Names (Translated Names)	Chinese Names
Ci Shi Nan Zhi (Hard-Won Knowledge) by Wang Hao-Gu in 1308	此事难知
Dan Xi Xin Fa (Teachings of [Zhu] Dan-Xi) by Zhu Zhen-Heng in 1481	丹溪心法
Dan Xi Xin Fa Fu Yu (Additions to the Teachings for [Zhu] Dan-Xi) by Fang Guang-Lei in 1536	丹溪心法附余
De Pei Ben Cao (Materia Medica of Combinations)	得配本草
Dong Heng Shi Xiao Fang (Tested and Effective Formulas by Dong Heng) by Dong Heng in 1266	东恒试效方
Dong Tian Ao Zhi (Profound Purpose from the Heavenly Abode) by Chen Shi-Duo in 1694	洞天奥旨
Dong Yi Bao Jian (Precious Mirror of Oriental Medicine) by Xu Sun in 1611	东医宝鉴
Dou Zhen Shi Yi Xin Fa (Teachings of Generations of Physicians about Pox) by Wan Quan in 1568	痘疹世医心法
Fang Ji Xue (Traditional Chinese Medical Formulas) by Shanghai College of Traditional Chinese Medicine in 1975	方剂学
Fu Ke Chan Lun Fang (Discussion of Formulas for Obstetrics and Gynecology)	妇科常论方
Fu Qing Zhu Nu Ke (Women's Diseases According to Fu Qing-Zhu) by Fu Shan in 1827	傅青主女科
Fu Ren Da Quan Liang Fang (Complete Fine Formulas for Women) by Chen Zi-Ming in 1237	妇人大全良方
Fu Ren Liang Fang (Fine Formulas for Women) by Chen Zi-Ming in 1237	妇人良方
Fu Shou Jing Fang (Exquisite Formulas for Fostering Longevity) by Wu Min in 1530	扶寿精防
Gan Zheng Ji Yao (Essential Compilation of Infectious Syndromes) by Yan Hong-Zhi in 1920	感证辑要
Gu Jin Ming Fang (Famous Classic and Contemporary Formulas) by Luo Mei in 1675	古今名方
Gu Jin Yi Jian (Medical Mirror of the Past and Present) by Gong Xin-Zuan in Ming Dynasty	古今医鉴
Gu Jin Yi Tong Da Quan (Comprehensive Collection of Medicine Past and Present) by Xu Chun-Fu in 1556	古今医通大全
Guang Wen Yi Lun (Discussion of Widespread Warm Epidemics) by Dai Tian-Zhang in 1722	广温疫论
Guangxi Zhong Yao Zhi (Guangxi Journal of Chinese Herbal Medicines)	广西中药志
Guizhou Min Jian Yao Wu (Folk Medicina from Guizhou)	贵州民间药物
Hai Jing Ben Cao (Materia Medica from the Ocean)	海经本草
Hai Yao Ben Cao (Materia Medica of Herbs from [Across the] Seas) by Li Xun in 907-960 A.D.	海药本草
Han Shi Yi Tong (Comprehensive Medicine According to Master Han) by Han Mao in 1522	韩氏医通
Hong Shi Ji Yan Fang (Time-Tested Formulas of Hong Family)	洪氏集验方
Huang Di Nei Jing (Yellow Emperor's Inner Classic) in the second century A.D.	黄帝内经
Huang Di Su Wen Xuan Ming Lun Fang (Formulas from the Discussion Illuminating the Yellow Emperor's Basic Questions) by Liu Yuan-Su in 1172	黄帝素问宣明论方
Huo Luan Lun (Discussion of Sudden Turmoil Disorders) by Wan Shi-Xiong in 1862	霍乱论
Ji Sheng Fang (Formulas to Aid the Living) by Yan Yong-He in 1253	济生方
Ji Yin Gang Mu (Materia Medica to Aid Yin) by Wu Zhi-Wang in 1620	济阴纲目
Jia You Ben Cao (Materia Medica of the Jia You Era) by Zhang Yu-Xi and Su Song in 1057-1060	嘉佑本草
Jiang Su Zhi Wu Zhi (Jiangsu Journal of Botany)	江苏植物志
Jiao Zhu Fu Ren Liang Fang (Revised Fine Formulas for Women) by Bi Li-Zhai in 16th century	校注妇人良方
Jin Gui Yao Lue (Essentials from the Golden Cabinet) by Zhang Zhong-Jing in Eastern Han	金匮要略
Jing Shi Zheng Lei Bei Ji Ben Cao (Differentiation and Application of Materia Medica) by Tang Shen-Wei in 1082	经史证类备急本草

Chinese Herbal Formulas and Applications

Bibliography of Historical Texts

Pinyin Names (Translated Names)	Chinese Names
Jing Xiu Tang Yao Shuo (Herbal Teachings from the Respectfully Decorated Hall) by Qian Shu-Tian	敬修堂药说
Jing Yue Quan Shu (Collected Treatises of [Zhang] Jing Yue) by Zhang Jie-Bin (Zhang Jing-Yue) in 1624	景岳全书
Jiu Huang Ben Cao (Materia Medica to Rescue Emergencies)	救荒本草
Ju Fang (Imperial Formulary) by the Imperial Medical Department in 1078-85	局方
Kai Bao Ben Cao (Materia Medica of the Kai Bao Era) by Ma Zhi in 973-974 A.D.	开宝本草
Lan Shi Mi Cang (Secrets from the Orchid Chamber) by Li Gao in 1336	兰室秘藏
Lan Tai Gui Fan (Guidelines from Lan-Tai) by Xu Da-Chun in 1764	兰台轨范
Lei Bian Zhu Shi Ji Yan Yi Fang (Effective Medical Formulas Arranged by Category by Doctor Zhu) by Zhu Zuo in 1266	类编朱氏集验医方
Lei Gong Pao Zhi Lun (Grandfather Lei's Discussions of Herb Preparation) by Lei Xiao in 470 A.D.	雷公炮制抡
Lei Zheng Huo Ren Shu (Book to Safeguard Life Arranged According to Pattern) by Zhu Gong in 1108	类证活人书
Liang Fang Yi Ye (Small Collection of Fine Formulas) by Xie Yuan-Qing in 1842	良方集腋
Lin Zheng Zhi Nan Yi An (Case Histories from the Compass of Clinical Patterns) by Ye Tian-Shi in 1746	临证指南医案
Ling Nan Cai Yao Lu (Records of Picking Herbs in Guangdong)	岭南采药录
Ling Shu (Magic Pivot) in the second century A.D.	灵枢
Liu Zhou Yi Hua (Medical Dialogues from Liuzhou) by Wei Zhi-Xiu in mid-16th century	柳州医话
Lu Chan Yan Ben Cao (Materia Medica from Steep Mountain-sides)	履巉岩本草
Meika Hosen (A Selection of Famous Physicians' Prescriptions) by Yoshine Hirai	名家方选
Ming Yi Bie Lu (Miscellaneous Records of Famous Physicians) by Tao Hong-Jing in 500 A.D.	名医别录
Ming Yi Za Zhu (Miscellaneous Books of Ming Medicine) by Wang Lun in 1549 A.D.	明医杂著
Ming Yi Zhi Zhang (Displays of Enlightened Physicians) by Huang Fu-Zhong in 16th century	名医指掌
Nanning Shi Yao Wu Zhi (Nanning City Medicines)	南宁市药物志
Nei Jing (Inner Classic) in the second century A.D.	内经
Nei Jing Shi Yi Fang Lun (Enumeration of Formulas Omitted from the Inner Classic) by Luo Long-Ji in Song Dynasty	内经拾遗方论
Nei Ke Zhai Yao (Summary of Internal Medicine) by Wen Sheng in mid-19th century	内科摘要
Nei Wai Shang Bian Huo Lun (Clarifying Doubts about Injury from Internal and External Causes) by Li Gao in 1247	内外伤辨惑论
Pi Wei Lun (Discussion of the Spleen and Stomach) by Li Gao in 1249	脾胃论
Pian Yu Xin Shu (Text from Heart of Jade) by Wu Quan in the mid-16th century	片玉心书
Pin Hui Jing Yao (Essentials of (Herbal) Distinctions)	品汇精要
Pu Ji Ben Shi Fang (Formulas of Universal Benefit from My Practice) by Xu Shu-Wei in 1132	普济本事方
Pu Ji Fang (Formulas of Universal Benefit) by Teng Hong in Ming Dynasty	普济方
Qi Xiao Hai Shang Xian Fang Mi Ben (Secret Text of Extraordinary Effective Beneficial Formulas from Across the Seas)	奇效海上仙方秘本
Qi Xiao Liang Fang (Fine Formulas with Miraculous Results)	奇效良方
Qian Jin Yao Fang (Thousand Ducat Prescriptions) by Sun Si-Miao in 581-685 A.D.	千金要方
Qian Jin Yi Fang (Supplement to the Thousand Ducat Formulas) by Sun Si-Miao in 682 A.D.	千金翼方

BIBLIOGRAPHY OF HISTORICAL TEXTS

B

1487

Bibliography of Historical Texts

Pinyin Names (Translated Names)	Chinese Names
Qian Tian Jia Fang (Family Formulas of Qian Tian-Jia)	浅田家方
Qing Cao Shi Jie (The World of Herbs) by Zhong Ding-Chuan in 1992	青草世界
Qing Cao Yao Han Shou Jiao Cai (Textbook of Botanical Medicine) by Zhong Ding-Chuan in 1992	青草药函授教材
Quan Guo Zhong Cheng Yao Chu Fang Ji (National Collection of Chinese Herbal Prepared Medicines) in 1949	全国中成药处方剂
Ren Zhai Zhi Zhi (Straight Directions of Benevolent Aid) by Yang Tu-Ying in 1264	仁斋直指
Ri Hua Zi Ben Cao (Materia Medica of Ri Hua-Zi) by Ri Hua-Zi in 713 A.D.	日华子本草
Ri Yong Ben Cao (Household Materia Medica) by Wu Rui in 1330	日用本草
Ru Men Shi Qin (Confucians' Duties to their Parents) by Zhang Cong-Zheng in 1228	儒门事亲
San Yin Ji Yi Bing Zheng Fang Lun (Discussion of Illnesses, Patterns, and Formulas Related to the Unification of the Three Etiologies) by Chen Yan in 1174	三因即一病证方论
Shang Hai Shi Zhong Cheng Yao Zhi Ji Gui Fan (Shanghai Municipal Standards for the Manufacturing of Chinese Prepared Medicines) in 1970	上海市中成药制剂规范
Shang Han Biao Ben Xin Fa Lei Cui (Collection of Methods Related to the Manifestation and Root of Cold-Induced Disorders)	伤寒标本心法类萃
Shang Han Liu Shu (Six Texts on Cold-Induced Disorders) by Tao Hua in 1445	伤寒六书
Shang Han Lun (Discussion of Cold-Induced Disorders) by Zhang Zhong-Jing in Eastern Han	伤寒论
Shang Han Lun Ming Li Lun (Clarification of the Theory of Cold Induced Disorders) by Cheng Wu-Ji in 1156	伤寒论明理论
Shang Han Ming Li Yao Fang Lun (Clarification of the Formulas and Herbs of Cold Induced Disorders) by Cheng Wu-Ji	伤寒明理药方论
Shang Han Quan Sheng Ji (All-New Collection of Cold Induced Disorders)	伤寒全生集
Shang Han Za Bing Lun (Discussion of Cold-Induced Disorders and Miscellaneous Diseases) by Zhang Zhong-Jing in Eastern Han	伤寒杂病论
Shang Han Zhi Ge Fang Lun (Direct Investigations of Formulas for Cold-Induced Disorders) by Liu Yuan-Su in Jin Dynasty	伤寒直格方论
She Sheng Mi Pou (Secrets Investigations into Obtaining Health) by Hong Ji in 1638	摄生秘剖
She Sheng Zhong Miao Fang (Marvelous Formulas for the Health of Multitudes) by Zhang Shi-Che in 1550	摄生众妙方
Shen Nong Ben Cao Jing (Divine Husbandman's Classic of the Materia Medica) in the second century	神农本草经
Shen Nong Ben Cao Jing Shu (Revised Divine Husbandman's Classic of the Materia Medica) by Miao Xi-Yong in 1625	神农本草经书
Shen Shi Yao Han (Scrutiny of the Priceless Jade Case) by Fu Ren-Yu in 1644	审视瑶函
Shen Shi Zun Sheng Shu (Master Shen's Book for Revering Life) by Shen Jin-Ao in 1773	沈氏尊生书
Sheng Ji Jing (Holy Relief Reference) by Zhao Ji in Jin Dynasty	圣济经
Sheng Ji Zong Lu (General Collection for Holy Relief) by a staff of court physicians of Northern Song Dynasty around 1111-1117	圣剂总录
Shi Bing Lun (Discussion of Seasonal Diseases) by Lei Feng in 1882	时病论
Shi Chuan En Jia Chuan Fang (Family Formulas from Shi Chuan-En)	史传恩家传方
Shi Fang Ge Kuo (Collected Songs about Contemporary Formulas) by Chen Nian-Zi in 1801	时方歌括
Shi Liao Ben Cao (Materia Medica of Diet Therapy) by Meng Shan in the seventh century	食疗本草
Shi Wu Ben Cao (Food as Materia Medica) by Lu He-Ming in 701-704 A.D.	食物本草

Bibliography of Historical Texts

Pinyin Names (Translated Names)	Chinese Names
Shi Yao Shen Shu (Miraculous Book of Ten Remedies) by Ge Qian-Sun in 1348	十药神书
Shi Yi De Xiao Fang (Effective Formulas from Generations of Physicians) by Wei Yi-Lin in 1345	世医得效方
Shi Yong Tian Ran Yao Wu (Practical Natural Medicine) by Zheng Bing-Chuan in 1997	实用天然药物
Shou Shi Bao Yuan (Achieving Longevity by Guarding the Source) by Gong Ting-Xian in early 17th century	寿世保元
Shu Ben Cao (Materia Medica of Sichuan) by Han Bao-Sheng in 935-960 A.D.	蜀本草
Si He Ting Ji Fang (Collection of Formulas of Si He-Ting)	饲鹤亭集方
Sichuan Zhong Yao Zhi (Sichuan Journal of Chinese Herbal Medicines)	四川中药志
Su Shen Liang Fang (Fine Formulas by Su and Shen) in Song Dynasty	苏沈良方
Su Wen (Basic Questions) in the second century A.D.	素问
Su Wen Bing Ji Qi Yi Bao Ming Ji (Collection of Writings on the Mechanism of Illness, Suitability of Qi, and the Safeguarding of Life as Discussed in the Basic Questions) by Zhang Yuan-Su in 1186	素问病机气宜保命集
Tai Ping Hui Min He Ji Ju Fang (Imperial Grace Formulary of the Tai Ping Era) by the Imperial Medical Department in 1078-85	太平惠民和济局方
Tai Ping Sheng Hui Fang (Holy Grace Formulary of the Tai Ping Era) by Wang Huai-Yin in Song Dynasty	太平圣惠方
Tai Wan Min Jian Yao (Folk Medicine of Taiwan) by Gao Mu-Chun in 1985	台湾民间药
Tai Wan Zhi Wu Yao Cai Zhi (Medicinal Plants of Taiwan)	台湾植物药材志
Tang Ben Cao (Tang Materia Medica) by Su Jing in 659 A.D.	唐本草
Tang Ye Ben Cao (Materia Medica for Decoctions) by Wang Hao-Gu in 1306	汤液本草
Ti Ren Hui Bian (Compilation of Materials of Benevolence for the Body) by Peng Yong-Guang in 1549	体仁汇编
Tong Su Shang Han Lun (Plain Version of Discussion of Cold-Induced Disorders)	通俗伤寒论
Tu Jing Ben Cao (Illustrated Classic of the Materia Medica) by Su Song in 1061	图经本草
Wai Dan Ben Cao (Materia Medica for External Elixirs)	外丹本草
Wai Ke Fa Hui (External Medicine Elaboration) by Xue Yi in 1528	外科发挥
Wai Ke Zheng Zhi Quan Sheng Ji (Complete Collection of Patterns and Treatments in External Medicine) by Wang Wei-De in 1740	外科症治全生集
Wai Ke Zheng Zhi Zhun Sheng (Standards of Patterns and Treatments in External Medicine) by Wang Ken-Tang in Ming Dynasty	外科症治准绳
Wai Ke Zheng Zong (True Lineage of External Medicine) by Chen Shi-Gong in 1617	外科正宗
Wai Tai Mi Yao (Arcane Essentials from the Imperial Library) by Wang Tao in 752 A.D.	外台秘要
Wan Bing Hui Chun (Restoration of Health from the Myriad Diseases) by Gong Ting-Xian in 1587	万病回春
Wei Sheng Bao Jian (Precious Mirror of Health) by Luo Tian-Yi in Yuan Dynasty	卫生宝鉴
Wei Yao Tiao Bian (Cataloged Differentiation of Erroneous Medicines)	伪药条辩
Wen Bing Tiao Bian (Systematic Differentiation of Warm Disease) by Wu Ju-Tong in 1798	温病条辨
Wen Re Jing Wei (Warp and Woof of Warm-Febrile Diseases) by Wang Meng-Ying in 1852	温热经纬
Wen Yi Lun (Discussion of Epidemic Warm Disease) by Wu You-Xing in 1642	温疫论
Wu Pu Ben Cao (Wu Pu's Materia Medica)	吴普本草
Wu Shi Er Bing Fang (Prescriptions for Fifty-Two Kinds of Diseases) in approximately third century B.C.	五十二病方

Bibliography of Historical Texts

Pinyin Names (Translated Names)	Chinese Names
Xi Yuan Ji Lu Jiao Yi (Correction and Explanation of the Wrongly Accused)	洗冤集录校译
Xian Dai Shi Yong Zhong Yao (Modern Practical Chinese Medicines)	现代实用中药
Xian Shou Li Shang Xu Duan Mi Fang (Secret Recipes of Treating Wounds and Bone-Setting Taught by Celestials) by Taoist Lin in 846 A.D.	仙授理伤续断秘方
Xian Xing Zhai Yi Xue Guang Bi Ji (Wide-Ranging Medical Notes from the First-Awakened Studio) by Miao Xi-Yong in 1613	先醒斋医学广笔记
Xiao Er Yao Zheng Zhi Jue (Craft of Medicinal Treatment for Childhood Disease Patterns) by Qian Yi in 1119	小儿药症直决
Xin Xiu Ben Cao (Newly Revised Materia Medica) by Su Jing in 657-659 A.D.	新修本草
Xu Ming Yi Lei An (Continuation of Famous Physicians' Cases Organized by Categories) by Wei Zhi-Xiu in 1770	续名医类案
Xuan Ming Lun Fang (Discussion of Dispersing and Brightening Formulas) by Liu Yuan-Su in Jin and Yuan Dynasties	宣明论方
Yan Fang Xin Bian (New Compilation of Time-Tested Formulas) by Bao Xiang-Ao in 1846	验方新编
Yang Ke Xin De Ji (Collection of Personal Expertises Concerning Skin Lesions) by Gao Bing-Jun in 1805	疡科心得集
Yang Shi Jia Zang Fang (Collected Formulas of the Yang Family) by Yang Tan in 1178	杨氏家藏方
Yang Shi Mi Fang (Secret Formulas of Yang Family)	杨氏秘方
Yao Cai Xue (Study of Medicinal Substances)	药材学
Yao Pu (Medicinal Recipes) by Hou Ning-Ji	药谱
Yao Xing Ben Cao (Materia Medica of Medicinal Properties) by Zhen Quan in 600 A.D.	药性本草
Ye Shi Nu Ke (Ye's Women's Diseases)	叶氏女科
Yi Bian (Ordinary Medicine) by Wang San-Cai in 1587	医便
Yi Fang Ji Jie (Analytical Collection of Medical Formulas) by Wang Ang in 1682	医方集解
Yi Fang Kao (Investigation of Medical Formulas) by Wu Kun in 1584	医方考
Yi Fang Xin Jie (New Explanations of Medical Formulas) by Ma You-Du in 1980	医方新解
Yi Guan (Thorough Knowledge of Medicine) by Zhao Xian-Ke in 1617	医贯
Yi Guan Tang (Linking Clinic)	一贯堂
Yi Ji (Levels of Medicine)	医级
Yi Ji Bao Jian (Precious Mirror for Advancement of Medicine) by Dong Xi-Yuan in 1777	医籍宝鉴
Yi Lin Gai Cuo (Corrections of Errors Among Physicians) by Wang Qing-Ren in 1830	医林改错
Yi Lue Liu Shu (Six Texts on the Essentials of Medicine)	医略六书
Yi Men Fa Lu (Precepts for Physicians) by Yu Chang in 1658	医门法律
Yi Xue Fa Ming (Medical Innovations) by Li Gao in Jin Dynasty	医学发明
Yi Xue Qi Yuan (Origins of the Medicine) by Zhang Yuan-Su in Yuan Dynasty	医学启原
Yi Xue Quan Shu (Complete Book of Medicine) by Xu Si-He	医学全书
Yi Xue Ru Men (Introduction to Medicine) by Li Ting in 1575	医学入门
Yi Xue Xin Wu (Medical Revelations) by Cheng Guo-Peng in 1732	医学心悟
Yi Xue Zheng Zhuan (True Lineage of Medicine) by Yu Tian-Min in 1515	医学正传
Yi Xue Zhong Zhong Can Xi Lu (Records of Heart-Felt Experiences in Medicine With Reference to the West) by Zhang Xi-Chun in 1918-34	医学衷中参西录
Yi Yuan (Bases of Medicine) by Shi Shou-Tang in 1861	医原

Chinese Herbal Formulas and Applications

Bibliography of Historical Texts

Pinyin Names (Translated Names)	Chinese Names
Yi Zhen Yi De (Achievements Regarding Epidemic Rashes) by Yu Shi-Yu in 1794	疫疹一得
Yi Zong Jin Jian (Golden Mirror of the Medical Tradition) by Wu Qian in 1742	医宗金鉴
Yin Pian Xin Can (New References of Prepared Medicines)	饮片新参
Yin Shan Zheng Yao (Correct Guide to Eating and Drinking)	饮膳正要
Yong Lei Qian Fang (Everlasting Categorization of Seal Formulas)	永类钤方
Yuan Ji Qi Wei (Explanation of the Subtitles of the Original Mechanism) by Ni Wei-De in 1370	原机启微
Yuan Nan Yang (Asada's Prescriptions) by Sohaku Asada	
Za Bing Yuan Liu Xi Zhu (Wondrous Lantern for Peering into Origin and Development of Miscellaneous Diseases) by Shen Jin-Ao in 1773	杂病源流犀烛
Za Bing Zheng Zhi Xin Yi (New Significance of Patterns and Treatment in Miscellaneous Diseases)	杂病证治新义
Zeng Bu Nei Jing Shi Yi (Supplement to the Formulas Omitted from the Inner Classic)	增补内经拾遗
Zhang San Feng Xian Chuan Fang (Divine Formulas from Zhang Sanfeng)	张三丰仙传方
Zhang Shi Yi Tong (Comprehensive Medicine According to Master Zhang) by Zhang Lu-Xuan in 1695	张氏医通
Zhen Nan Ben Cao (Materia Medica of South Yunnan) by Lan Mao in Qing Dynasty	滇南本草
Zhen Zhu Nang (Pouch of Pearls) by Zhang Yuan-Su in 1186	珍珠囊
Zheng He Sheng Ji Zong Lu (Comprehensive Recording of Sage-Like Benefit from the Zheng He Era) by Sheng Fu in 1122	政和圣济总录
Zheng Lei Ben Cao (Materia Medica Arranged According to Pattern) by Tang Shen-Wei in 1082	证类本草
Zheng Shi Jia Chuan Nu Ke Wan Jin Fang (Zheng's Family Formulas for Women's Disorders)	郑氏家传女科万金方
Zheng Ti Lei Yao (Catalogued Essentials for Correcting the Body) by Bi Li-Zhai (Ji) in 1529	正体类要
Zheng Yin Mai Zhi (Pattern, Cause, Pulse, and Treatment) by Qin Jing-Ming in 1702	证因脉治
Zheng Zhi Zhun Sheng (Standards of Patterns and Treatments) by Wang Ken-Tang in 1602	症治准绳
Zhi Wu Ming Shi Tu Kao (Illustrated Guide for Nomenclature and Identification of Botanical Products)	植物名实图考
Zhong Guo Guo Yao Gu You Cheng Fang Xuan Ji (A Selection of Traditional Prescriptions of Chinese Medicine) by Chinese Herbal Medicine Committee of the Ministry of the Interior in 1967	中国国药故有成方选集
Zhong Guo Yao Dian (Dictionary of Chinese Medicine) in 1977	中国药典
Zhong Guo Yao Yong Zhi Wu Zi (Chinese Journal of Medicinal Botanicals)	中国药用植物志
Zhong Guo Zhi Wu Zi (Chinese Journal of Botany)	中国植物志
Zhong Xi Yi Jie He Zhi Liao Ji Fu Zheng (Combined Chinese and Western Medical Treatment of the Acute Abdomen) by Nankai Hospital of Tianjin in 1973	中西医结合治疗急腹症
Zhong Yao Yao Ming Ci Dian (Dictionary on Nomenclature of Chinese Herbs)	中药药名词典
Zhong Yao Zhi (Journal of Traditional Chinese Herbal Medicines)	中药志
Zhong Yao Zhi Ji Shou Ce (Handbook of Traditional Chinese Medicinal Preparations)	中药制剂手册
Zhong Yi Fu Ke Zhi Liao Xue (Traditional Chinese Medical Treatment of Women's Disorders) by Chengdu College of Traditional Chinese Medicine in 1970	中医妇科治疗学
Zhong Yi Nei Ke Xue (Traditional Chinese Internal Medicine) by Shanghai College of Traditional Chinese Medicine in 1970	中医内科学

BIBLIOGRAPHY OF HISTORICAL TEXTS

B

1491

Bibliography of Historical Texts

Bibliography of Historical Texts

Pinyin Names (Translated Names)	Chinese Names
Zhong Yi Shang Ke Xue (Traditional Chinese Traumatology) in 1949	中医伤科学
Zhong Yi Yan Ke Xue (Traditional Chinese Opthalmology) by Chengdu College of Traditional Chinese Medicine in 1970	中医眼科学
Zhong Zang Jing (Treasury Classic) by Hua-Tuo in the Han Dynasty	中藏经
Zhou Hou Bei Ji Fang (Emergency Formulas to Keep Up One's Sleeve) by Ge Hong in 341 A.D.	肘后备急方
Zhou Hou Fang (Formulas to Keep Up One's Sleeve)	肘后方

Chinese Herbal Formulas and Applications

Bibliography of Contemporary References

Pinyin Names (Translated Names)	Chinese Names
Ai Zheng (Cancer)	癌症
An Hui Yi Xue (Anhui Medicine)	安徽医学
An Hui Zhong Yi Lin Chuang Za Zi (Anhui Journal of Clinical Chinese Medicine)	安徽中医临床杂志
An Hui Zhong Yi Xue Yuan Xue Bao (Journal of Anhui University School of Medicine)	安徽中医学院学报
An Yi Xue Bao (Anyi Medical Journal)	安医学报
Bai Qiu En Yi Ke Da Xue Xue Bao (Journal of Baiqiuen University of Medicine)	白求恩医科大学学报
Bei Jing Yi Ke Da Xue Xue Bao (Journal of Beijing University of Medicine)	北京医科大学学报
Bei Jing Yi Xue (Beijing Medicine)	北京医学
Bei Jing Yi Xue Yuan Xue Bao (Journal of Beijing School of Medicine)	北京医学院学报
Bei Jing Zhong Yi (Beijing Chinese Medicine)	北京中医
Bei Jing Zhong Yi Xue Yuan Xue Bao (Journal of Beijing University School of Medicine)	北京中医学院学报
Bei Jing Zhong Yi Yao Da Xue Xue Bao (Journal of Beijing University of Medicine and Medicinals)	北京中医药大学学报
Bei Jing Zhong Yi Za Zhi (Beijing Journal of Chinese Medicine)	北京中医杂志
Ben Cao Cong Xin (Revised Herbal Materia Medica)	本草从新
Chang Chun Zhong Yi Xue Yuan Xue Bao (Journal of Changchun University of Chinese Medicine)	长春中医学院学报
Chang Yong Zhong Cao Yao Zhong Du Yu Ji Jiu (Poisoning and Treatment of Commonly-Used Chinese Herbs)	常用中草药中毒与急救
Chang Yong Zhong Yao Cheng Fen Yu Yao Li Shou Ce (A Handbook of the Composition and Pharmacology of Common Chinese Drugs)	常用中药成分与药理手册
Chang Yong Zhong Yao De Ying Yong (Application of Commonly-Used Chinese Herbs)	常用中药的应用
Chang Yong Zhong Yao Xian Dai Yan Jiu Yu Lin Chuang (Recent Study & Clinical Application of Common Traditional Chinese Medicine)	常用中药现代研究与临床
Chen Tzu Yen Chiu (Acupuncture Research)	针灸研究
Cheng Du Zhong Yi Xue Yuan Xue Bao (Journal of Chengdu University of Traditional Chinese Medicine)	成都中医学院学报
Chi Jiao Yi Sheng Za Zhi (Journal of Barefoot Doctors)	赤脚医生杂志
Chong Qing Yi Yao (Chongching Medicine and Herbology)	重庆医药
Chong Qing Zhong Yi Yao Za Zi (Chongching Journal of Chinese Medicine and Medicinals)	重庆中医药杂志
Chuan Dong Zhong Yi Za Zhi (Chuandong Journal of Chinese Medicine)	川东中医杂志
Da Zhong Yi Xue (Public Medicine)	大众医学
Dang Dai Ming Yi Lin Zhen Jing Hua Zhong Liu Juan Ji (Essential Clinical Experience of Famous Modern Doctors - Cancer Volume)	当代明医临证精华-肿瘤卷辑
Di Er Jun Yi Da Xue Xue Bao (Journal of Second Military University of Medicine)	第二军医大学学报
Di Yi Jun Yi Da Xue Xue Bao (Journal of First Military University of Medicine)	第一军医大学学报
Dong Bei Zhi Wu Zhi (Northeast Journal of Herbal Medicine)	东北植物志
Dong Jing Yi Shi Xin Zhi (Tokyo Journal of Medicine)	东京医师新知
Dong Wu Xue Za Zhi (Journal of Zoology)	动物学杂志
Fang Ji Xue (Chinese Herbal Formulas)	方剂学
Fang She Yi Xue (Journal of Radiology)	放射医学
Fu Chan Ke Bing Shi Yong Fang (Practical Formulas for Obstetrics and Gynecology Disorders)	妇产科病实用方

BIBLIOGRAPHY OF CONTEMPORARY REFERENCES

B

1493

Bibliography of Contemporary References

Pinyin Names (Translated Names)	Chinese Names
Fu Chan Ke Qing Bao Zi Liao (Journal of Gynecology)	妇产科情报资料
Fu Jian Jun Qu Wei Sheng Bu (Health Department of Fujian Military)	福建军区卫生部
Fu Jian Min Jian Cao Yao (Local Herbs of the Fujian)	福建民间草药
Fu Jian Sheng Yi Yao Yan Jiu Suo (Fujian Province Institute of Medicine and Herbal Research)	福建生医药研究所
Fu Jian Yi Xue Yuan Xue Bao (Journal of Fujian University of Medicine)	福建医学院学报
Fu Jian Yi Yao Za Zhi (Fujian Journal of Medicine and Herbology)	福建医药杂志
Fu Jian Yi Za Zhi (Fujian Journal of Chinese Medicine)	福建医杂志
Fu Jian Zhong Yi Yao (Fujian Chinese Medicine and Herbology)	福建中医药
Fu Ke Jing Sui (Essence of Obstetrics and Gynecology)	妇科精髓
Fu Ke Lin Chuang Jing Hua (Clinical Pearl of Obstetrics and Gynecology)	妇科临床精华
Fu Zhou Yi Yao (Fuzhou Medicine and Medicinals)	福州医药
Gan Su Zhong Yi (Gansu Chinese Medicine)	甘肃中医
Gan Su Zhong Yi Xue Yuan Xue Bao (Journal of Gansu University of Chinese Medicine)	甘肃中医学院学报
Guang Dong Yi Xue (Guangdong Medicine)	广东医学
Guang Dong Yi Yao Za Zhi (Guangdong Journal of Medicine and Herbology)	广东医药杂志
Guang Dong Zhong Yi (Guangdong Chinese Medicine)	广东中医
Guang Ming Zhong Yi (Guangming Chinese Medicine)	光明中医
Guang Xi Ben Cao (Guangxi Materia Medica)	广西本草
Guang Xi Chi Jiao Yi Sheng (Guangxi Barefoot Doctor)	广西赤脚医生
Guang Xi Wei Sheng (Guangxi Province Public Health)	广西卫生
Guang Xi Yi Xue (Guangxi Medicine)	广西医学
Guang Xi Yi Xue Yuan Xue Bao (Journal of Guangxi University of Medicine)	广西医学院学报
Guang Xi Zhi Wu (Guangxi Plants)	广西植物
Guang Xi Zhi Wu Tu Zhi (Illustrated Guide of Guangxi Plants)	广西植物图志
Guang Xi Zhong Yi Yao (Guangxi Chinese Medicine and Herbology)	广西中医药
Guang Zhou Yi Yao (Guangzhou Medicine and Medicinals)	广州医药
Guang Zhou Zhong Yi Xue Yuan Xue Bao (Journal of Guangzhou University of Chinese Medicine)	广州中医学院学报
Gui Yang Yi Xue Yuan Xue Bao (Journal of Guiyang Medical University)	贵阳医学院学报
Gui Yang Zhong Yi Xue Yuan Xue Bao (Journal of Guiyang Chinese Medical University)	贵阳中医学院学报
Gui Zhou Cao Yao (Guizhou Herbology)	贵州草药
Gui Zhou Yao Xun (Guizhou Journal of Herbology)	贵州药讯
Gui Zhou Yi Yao (Medicine and Medicinals from Guizhou)	贵州医药
Guo Wai Yao Xue Zhi Wu Yao Fen Ce (Foreign Study of Medicine: Herbology)	国外药学植物药分册
Guo Wai Yi Xue (Foreign Medicine)	国外医学
Guo Wai Yi Xue Can Kao Za Zhi (Foreign Journal of Medicine)	国外医学参考杂志
Guo Wai Yi Xue Can Kao Zi Liao (Foreign Reference of Medicine)	国外医学参考资料
Guo Wai Yi Xue Zhong Yi Zhong Yao Fen Ce (Monograph of Chinese Herbology from Foreign Medicine)	国外医学中医中药分册
Guo Wai Yi Yao Zhi Wu Yao Fen Ce (Monograph of Foreign Botanical Medicine)	国外医药植物药分册
Guo Yao De Yao Li Xue (Pharmacology of Chinese Herbs)	国药的药理学

Bibliography of Contemporary References

Pinyin Names (Translated Names)	Chinese Names
Ha Er Bing Yi Ke Da Xue (Haerbing University of Medicine)	哈尔滨医科大学
Ha Er Bing Yi Ke Da Xue Xue Bao (Journal of Haerbing University of Medicine)	哈尔滨医科大学学报
Ha Er Bing Zhong Yi (Haerbing Chinese Medicine)	哈尔滨中医
Ha Yi Da Xue Bao (Journal of Ha Medical University)	哈医大学报
Hai Jun Yi Xue (Navy Medicine)	海军医学
Hai Yang Yao Wu Za Zhi (Journal of Herbs from the Sea)	海洋药物杂志
Hai Yao Ben Cao (Sea of Herbal Pharmacopia)	海药本草
Han Fang Yi Xue (Kampo Medicine)	汉方医学
He Bei Xin Yi Yao (Hebei New Medicine and Herbology)	河北新医药
He Bei Yi Yao (Hebei Medicine and Herbology)	河北医药
He Bei Zhong Yi (Hebei Chinese Medicine)	河北中医
He Bei Zhong Yi Za Zhi (Hebei Journal of Chinese Medicine)	河北中医杂志
He Han Yi Yao Xue Hui Zhi (Hehan Journal of Medicine and Herbology)	和汉医药学会志
He Nan Yi Ke Da Xue Xue Bao (Journal of Henan University School of Medicine)	河南医科大学学报
He Nan Yi Xue Yuan Xue Bao (Journal of Henan University of Medicine)	河南医学院学报
He Nan Yi Yao (Henan Medicine and Herbology)	河南医药
He Nan Zhong Yi (Henan Chinese Medicine)	河南中医
He Nan Zhong Yi Xue Yuan Xue Bao (Journal of University of Henan School of Medicine)	河南中医学院学报
Hei Long Jiang Zhong Yi Yao (Heilongjiang Chinese Medicine and Herbology)	黑龙江中医药
Hu Bei Wei Sheng (Hubei Health)	湖北卫生
Hu Bei Yi Sheng (Hubei Doctor)	湖北医生
Hu Bei Yi Xue Yuan Xue Bao (Journal of Hubei College of Medicine)	湖北医学院学报
Hu Bei Zhong Yi Xue Yuan Xue Bao (Journal of Hubei University of Medicine)	湖北中医学院学报
Hu Bei Zhong Yi Za Zhi (Hubei Journal of Chinese Medicine)	湖北中医杂志
Hu Nan Sheng Jie He Bing Yan Jiu Yuan (Hunan Treatment and Research Center of Tuberculosis)	湖南省结核病研究院
Hu Nan Wei Sheng Fang Yi Tong Xun (Hunan Journal of Preventative Health)	湖南卫生防疫通讯
Hu Nan Yi Cao Gong Ye Yan Jiu (Hunan Research and Industry of Medicine and Medicinals)	湖南医草工业研究
Hu Nan Yi Ke Da Xue Xue Bao (Journal of Hunan University School of Medicine)	湖南医科大学学报
Hu Nan Yi Xue (Hunan Medicine)	湖南医学
Hu Nan Yi Xue Yuan Xue Bao (Medical Journal of Hunan University of Medicine)	湖南医学院学报
Hu Nan Yi Yao Za Zhi (Hunan Journal of Medicine and Herbology)	湖南医药杂志
Hu Nan Zhong Yi (Hunan Journal of Traditional Chinese Medicine)	湖南中医
Hu Nan Zhong Yi Xue Yuan Xue Bao (Journal of Hunan University of Traditional Chinese Medicine)	湖南中医学院学报
Hu Nan Zhong Yi Za Zhi (Hunan Journal of Chinese Medicine)	湖南中医杂志
Hua Xi Kou Qiang Yi Xue Za Zhi (Huaxi Journal of Stomatology)	华西口腔医学杂志
Hua Xi Yao Xue Za Zhi (Huaxi Herbal Journal)	华西药学杂志
Hua Xi Yi Xue Za Zhi (Huaxi Medical Journal)	华西医学杂志
Hua Xue Xue Bao (Journal of Chemistry)	化学学报
Huo Xue Hua Yu Yan Jiu (Research on Blood-Activating and Stasis-Eliminating Herbs)	活血化瘀研究
Ji Lin Wei Sheng (Jilin Public Health)	吉林卫生

Bibliography of Contemporary References

Pinyin Names (Translated Names)	Chinese Names
Ji Lin Yi Sheng (Jilin Doctor)	吉林医生
Ji Lin Yi Xue (Jilin Medicine)	吉林医学
Ji Lin Yi Xue Yuan Xue Bao (Journal of Jilin University of Medicine)	吉林医学院学报
Ji Lin Zhong Yi (Jilin Chinese Medicine)	吉林中医
Ji Lin Zhong Yi Yao (Jilin Chinese Medicine and Herbology)	吉林中医药
Jiang Su Xin Yi Xue Yuan (New Jiangsu University of Medicine)	江苏新医学院
Jiang Su Yi Ke Da Xue Xue Bao (Journal of Jiangsu University of Medicine)	江苏医科大学学报
Jiang Su Yi Xue (Jiangsu Medical Journal)	江苏医学
Jiang Su Yi Yao (Jiangsu Journal of Medicine and Herbology)	江苏医药
Jiang Su Zhong Yi (Jiangsu Chinese Medicine)	江苏中医
Jiang Su Zhong Yi Yao (Jiangsu Medicine and Herbology)	江苏中医药
Jiang Su Zhong Yi Za Zhi (Jiangsu Journal of Chinese Medicine)	江苏中医杂志
Jiang Xi Xin Yi Yao (Jiangxi New Medicine and Herbology)	江西新医药
Jiang Xi Yi Xue Yuan Xue Bao (Medical Journal of Jiangxi University of Medicine)	江西医学院学报
Jiang Xi Yi Yao (Jiangxi Medicine and Herbology)	江西医药
Jiang Xi Yi Yao Za Zhi (Jiangxi Journal of Medicine and Herbology)	江西医药杂志
Jiang Xi Zhong Yi Yao (Jiangxi Chinese Medicine and Herbology)	江西中医药
Jing Xian Dai 25 Wei Zhong Yi Ming Jia Fu Ke Jing Yan (Experiences of 25 Modern Obstetrics and Gynecology Experts)	近现代二十五位中医名家妇科经验
Jin Yi Ke Ji (Jinyi Science and Technology)	锦医科技
Jin Zhou Yi Xue Yuan Xue Bao (Journal of Jinzhou University of Medicine)	锦州医学院学报
Jing Fang Yan Jiu (Research of Experienced Formulas)	经方研究
Jun Shi Yi Xue Jian Xun (Military Medicine Notes)	军事医学简讯
Kang Sheng Su (Antibiotic)	抗生素
Ke Ji Tong Bao (Newspaper of Science and Technology)	科技通报
Ke Ji Tong Xun (Journal of Science and Technology)	科技通讯
Ke Ji Zi Liao (Scientific Techniques and Knowledge)	科技资料
Ke Xue Chu Ban She (Scientific Press)	科学出版社
Ke Xue Tong Bao (Journal of Science)	科学通报
Ke Yan Tong Xun (Journal of Science and Research)	科研通讯
Lan Zhou Yi Xue Yuan Xue Bao (Journal of Lanzhou University of Medicine)	兰州医学院学报
Lao Nian Xue Za Zhi (Journal of Geriatrics)	老年学杂志
Liao Ning Yi Xue (Liaoning Medicine)	辽宁医学
Liao Ning Yi Xue Za Zhi (Liaoning Journal of Medicine)	辽宁医学杂志
Liao Ning Yi Yao (Liaoning Medicine and Herbology)	辽宁医药
Liao Ning Zhong Ji Yi Kan (Liaoning Journal of Medium Medicine)	辽宁中级医刊
Liao Ning Zhong Yi (Liaoning Chinese Medicine)	辽宁中医
Liao Ning Zhong Yi Za Zhi (Liaoning Journal of Chinese Medicine)	辽宁中医杂志
Lin Chuang Gan Dan Bing Za Zhi (Clinical Journal of Hepatic and Gallbladder Diseases)	临床肝胆病杂志
Lin Chuang Pi Fu Ke Za Zhi (Journal of Clinical Dermatology)	临床皮肤科杂志
Lin Chuang Shou Ce You Du Zhong Yao Shi Yong (Clinical Handbook on Applications of Toxic Chinese Herbs)	临床手册有毒中药实用

Bibliography of Contemporary References

Pinyin Names (Translated Names)	Chinese Names
Lin Chuang Yi Shi Zhen Liao Ji Qiao (Clinical Treatment & Techniques)	临床医师诊疗技巧
Lin Chuang Zhong Yao Xue (Clinical Chinese Pharmacology)	临床中药学
Liu Feng Wu Fu Ke Jing Yen (Experience of Obstetrics and Gynecology from Master Liu Feng Wu)	刘奉五妇科经验
Lu Zhou Yi Xue Yuan Xue Bao (Journal of Luzhou Institution of Medicine)	泸州医学院学报
Mei Rong Mei Fa Zhong Yi Gu Fang (Ancient Chinese Formulas for Beautiful Face and Hair)	美容美发中医古方
Mei Rong Yu Wu Guan Bing Wai Zhi Du Te Xin Liao Fa (New Treatments for Cosmetology and the Five Senses)	美容与五官病外之独特新疗法
Meika Hosen (A Selection of Famous Physicians' Prescriptions)	名家方选
Min Guo Yi Xue Za Zhi (Medical Journal of People's Republic of China)	民国医学杂志
Ming Yi Bie Lun (Theories of Famous Doctors)	名医别论
Nan Jing Yi Xue Yuan Xue Bao (Journal of Nanjing University of Medicine)	南京医学院学报
Nan Jing Zhong Yi Xue Yuan Xue Bao (Journal of Nanjing University of Traditional Chinese Medicine)	南京中医学院学报
Nan Jing Zhong Yi Yao Da Xue Xue Bao (Journal of Nanjing University of Traditional Chinese Medicine and Medicinals)	南京中医药大学学报
Nei Ke (Internal Medicine)	内科
Nei Meng Gu Zhong Yi Yao (Traditional Chinese Medicine and Medicinals of Inner Mongolia)	内蒙古中医药
Nei Meng Gu Zhong Yi Za Zi (Inner Mongolia Journal of Traditional Chinese Medicine)	内蒙古中医杂志
Pi Fu Bing Fang Zhi Yan Jiu Tong Xun (Research Journal on Prevention and Treatment of Dermatological Disorders)	皮肤病防治研究通讯
Qing Dao Yi Xue Yuan Bao Dao (Medical Journal of Qingdao Institution)	青岛医学院报导
Qing Dao Yi Xue Yuan Xue Bao (Journal of Qingdao Institution of Medicine)	青岛医学院学报
Qing Hai Yi Yao Za Zhi (Qinghai Journal of Medicine and Herbology)	青海医药杂志
Quan Guo Zhong Yi Er Ke Xue (National Chinese Pediatrics)	全国中医儿科学
Ren Min Jun Yi (Military Reserve Medicine)	人民军医
Ren Min Wei Sheng Chu Ban She (Journal of People's Public Health)	人民卫生出版社
Ri Ben Yao Li Xue Za Zhi (Japanese Journal of Herbology)	日本药理学杂志
Ri Ben Yao Wu Xue Za Zhi (Japanese Journal of Pharmacology)	日本药物学杂志
Shan Dong Ke Xue Ji Shu Chu Ban She (Shandong Science Publication)	山东科学技术出版社
Shan Dong Yi Kan (Shandong Medical Journal)	山东医刊
Shan Dong Yi Ke Da Xue Xue Bao (Journal of Shandong University of Medicine)	山东医科大学学报
Shan Dong Yi Xue Yuan Xue Bao (Journal of Shandong University School of Medicine)	山东医学院学报
Shan Dong Yi Yao (Shandong Medicine and Herbology)	山东医药
Shan Dong Yi Yao Gong Ye (Shandong Pharmaceutical Industry)	山东医药工业
Shan Dong Zhong Cao Yao Shou Ce (Handbook of Shandong Herbs)	山东中草药手册
Shan Dong Zhong Yi Xue Yuan Xue Bao (Journal of Shandong University School of Chinese Medicine)	山东中医学院学报
Shan Dong Zhong Yi Za Zhi (Shandong Journal of Chinese Medicine)	山东中医杂志
Shan Xi Xin Yi Yao (New Medicine and Herbology of Shanxi)	陕西新医药
Shan Xi Xin Zhong Yi (New Shanxi Chinese Medicine)	陕西新中医
Shan Xi Yi Kan (Shanxi Journal of Medicine)	陕西医刊

Bibliography of Contemporary References

Pinyin Names (Translated Names)	Chinese Names
Shan Xi Yi Xue Za Zhi (Shanxi Journal of Medicine)	陕西医学杂志
Shan Xi Yi Yao (Shanxi Medicine and Herbology)	陕西医药
Shan Xi Yi Yao Za Zhi (Shanxi Journal of Medicine and Herbology)	陕西医药杂志
Shan Xi Zhong Yi (Shanxi Chinese Medicine)	陕西中医
Shan Xi Zhong Yi Xue Yuan Xue Bao (Journal of Shanxi University School of Chinese Medicine)	陕西中医学院学报
Shan Xi Zhong Yi Za Zhi (Shanxi Journal Chinese Medicine)	陕西中医杂志
Shang Hai Chi Jiao Yi Sheng Za Zhi (Shanghai Journal of Barefoot Doctors)	上海赤脚医生杂志
Shang Hai Di Er Yi Ke Da Xue Xue Bao (Journal of Second Shanghai University College of Medicine)	上海第二医科大学学报
Shang Hai Di Yi Xue Yuan Xue Bao (Journal of First Shanghai Medical College)	上海第一学院学报
Shang Hai Ke Xue Ji Shu Chu Ban She (Shanghai Science and Technology Publishing Company)	上海科学技术出版社
Shang Hai Ren Min Chu Ban She (People's Press of Shanghai)	上海人民出版社
Shang Hai Yao Wu Shi Yan (Shanghai Research of Medicine)	上海药物实验
Shang Hai Yi Ke Da Xue Xue Bao (Journal of Shanghai University of Medicine)	上海医科大学学报
Shang Hai Yi Xue (Shanghai Medicine)	上海医学
Shang Hai Yi Yao Za Zhi (Shanghai Journal of Medicine and Herbology)	上海医药杂志
Shang Hai Zhong Yi Xue Yuan Xue Bao (Journal of Shanghai University of Chinese Medicine)	上海中医学院学报
Shang Hai Zhong Yi Yao Za Zhi (Shanghai Journal of Chinese Medicine and Herbology)	上海中医药杂志
Shang Hai Zhong Yi Za Zhi (Shanghai Journal of Chinese Medicine)	上海中医杂志
Shen De Yan Jiu (Research of Kidney)	肾的研究
Shen Jing Jing Shen Ji Bing Za Zhi (Journal of Psychiatric Disorders)	神经精神疾病杂志
Shen Nong Ben Cao Jing (Shen Nong Materia Medica)	神农本草经
Shen Yang Yao Xue Yuan Xue Bao (Journal of Shenyang College of Pharmacy)	沈阳药学院学报
Shen Yang Yi Xue Yuan Xue Bao (Journal of Shenyang University of Medicine)	沈阳医学院学报
Sheng Cao Yao Xing Bei Yao (Essentials of Raw Herbal Medicine)	生草药性备要
Sheng Li Xue Bao (Physiology News)	生理学报
Sheng Wu Hua Xue Yu Sheng Wu Wu Li Xue Bao (Journal of Biochemistry and Biophysiology)	生物化学与生物物理学报
Sheng Yao Xue Za Zhi (Journal of Raw Herbology)	生药学杂志
Shi Yong Kou Qiang Yi Xue Za Zhi (Journal of Medical Stomatology)	实用口腔医学杂志
Shi Yong Nei Ke Za Zhi (Practical Journal of Internal Medicine)	实用内科杂志
Shi Yong Yi Xue Za Zhi (Practical Journal of Medicine)	实用医学杂志
Shi Yong Zhong Liu Xue Za Zhi (Practical Journal of Cancer)	实用肿瘤学杂志
Shi Yong Zhong Xi Yi Jie He Fu Ke Xue (Practical Integrated Medicine: Obstetrics and Gynecology)	实用中西医结合妇科学
Shi Yong Zhong Xi Yi Jie He Za Zhi (Practical Journal of Integrated Chinese and Western Medicines)	实用中西医结合杂志
Shi Yong Zhong Xi Yi Jie He Zhen Duan Zhi Liao Xue (Practical Diagnostic and Therapeutics of Integrated Traditional Chinese and Western Medicine)	实用中西医结合诊断治疗学
Shi Yong Zhong Yi Mei Rong Jian Shen 3,000 Fang (3,000 Practical TCM Cosmetology Formulas)	实用中医美容健身3000方

Chinese Herbal Formulas and Applications

Bibliography of Contemporary References

Pinyin Names (Translated Names)	Chinese Names
Shi Yong Zhong Yi Nei Ke Za Zhi (Journal of Practical Chinese Internal Medicine)	实用中医内科杂志
Shi Yong Zhong Yi Yao Za Zhi (Journal of Practical Chinese Medicine and Medicinals)	实用中医药杂志
Shi Yong Zhong Yi Za Zhi (Journal of Practical Chinese Medicine)	实用中医杂志
Shi Zhen Guo Yao Yan Jiu (Research of Shizhen Herbs)	时珍国药研究
Shi Zhen Guo Yi Guo Yao (Shizhen National Herbs and Medicine)	时珍国医国药
Shou Pi Guo Jia Ji Ming Lao Zhong Yi Xiao Yan Mi Fang Jing Xuan (Experienced Secret Formulas from Nationally Famous TCM Doctors)	首批国家级名老中医效验秘方精选
Si Chuan Sheng Zhong Liu Fang Zhi Zi Liao Xuan Bian (Sichuan Journal of Cancer Prevention and Treatment)	四川省肿瘤防治资料选编
Si Chuan Yi Xue (Sichuan Medicine)	四川医学
Si Chuan Yi Xue Yuan Xue Bao (Journal of Sichuan School of Medicine)	四川医学院学报
Si Chuan Zhong Cao Yao Tong Xun (Sichuan Journal of Chinese Herbology)	四川中草药通讯
Si Chuan Zhong Yi (Sichuan Chinese Medicine)	四川中医
Su Zhou Yi Xue Yuan Xue Bao (Journal of Suzhou University of Medicine)	苏州医学院学报
Tai Wan Yi Xue Hui Za Zhi (Journal of Taiwan Medical Association)	台湾医学会杂志
Tai Wan Zhi Wu Yao Cao (Manual of Vegetable Drugs in Taiwan)	台湾植物药草
Te Chan Ke Xue Shi Yan (Research of Special Scientific Projects)	特产科学实验
Tian Jin Yi Xue Za Zhi (Journal of Tianjin Medicine and Herbology)	天津医学杂志
Tian Jin Yi Yao (Tianjin Medicine and Herbology)	天津医药
Tian Jin Yi Yao Tong Xun (Publication of Tianjin Medicine and Herbology)	天津医药通讯
Tian Jin Yi Yao Za Zhi (Journal of Tianjin Medicine and Herbology)	天津中医药杂志
Tian Jin Zhong Yi (Tianjin Chinese Medicine)	天津中医
Tie Dao Yi Xue (Tiedao Medicine)	铁道医学
Tong Ji Yi Ke Da Xue Xue Bao (Journal of Tongji University of Medicine)	同济医科大学学报
Wu Han Xin Yi Yao (Wuhan New Medicine and Herbology)	武汉新医药
Wu Han Xin Zhong Yi (Wuhan New Chinese Medicine)	武汉新中医
Wu Han Yi Xue Yuan Xue Bao (Journal of Wuhan University School of Medicine)	武汉医学院学报
Wu Han Yi Xue Za Zhi (Wuhan Journal of Medicine)	武汉医学杂志
Wu Shi Er Bing Fang (Fifty-two Disease Patterns & Formulas)	五十二病方
Xi An Yi Ke Da Xue Xue Bao (Journal of Xian University School of Medicine)	西安医科大学学报
Xi An Yi Xue Yuan Xue Bao (Journal of Xian University School of Medicine)	西安医学院学报
Xi Bei Yi Yao Za Zhi (Northwest Journal of Herbal Medicine)	西北医药杂志
Xi Xue Xue Bao (Academic Journal of Medicine)	西学学报
Xi Yao Yan Jiu Tong Xun (Research Journal of Medicine and Herbology)	西药研究通讯
Xian Dai Ben Cao Gang Mu (Contemporary Materia Medica)	现代本草纲目
Xian Dai Shi Yong Yao Xue (Practical Applications of Modern Herbal Medicine)	现代实用药学
Xian Dai Zhong Yao Yao Li Xue (Contemporary Pharmacology of Chinese Herbs)	现代中药药理学
Xiang Cun Yi Xue (Suburban Medicine)	乡村医学
Xiang Gang Zhong Yi Yao Nian Jian (Chinese Medicine and Medicinals of Hong Kong)	香港中医药年鉴
Xin Hua Ben Cao Gang Mu (New Chinese Materia Medica)	新华本草纲目
Xin Jiang Zhong Cao Yao Shou Ce (Xinjiang Handbook of Chinese Herbs)	新疆中草药手册
Xin Jiang Zhong Yi Yao (Xinjiang Chinese Medicine and Herbology)	新疆中医药

1499

Bibliography of Contemporary References

Pinyin Names (Translated Names)	Chinese Names
Xin Yao Yu Lin Chuang (New Medicine and the Clinical Application)	新药与临床
Xin Yi Xue (New Medicine)	新医学
Xin Yi Yao Tong Xun (Journal of New Medicine and Herbology)	新医药通讯
Xin Yi Yao Xue Za Zhi (New Journal of Medicine and Herbology)	新医药学杂志
Xin Zhang Xue Guan Ji Bing (Cardiovascular Diseases)	心脏血管疾病
Xin Zhong Yao Xue (New Chinese Herbal Medicine)	新中药学
Xin Zhong Yi (New Chinese Medicine)	新中医
Xin Zhong Yi Yao (New Chinese Medicine and Medicinals)	新中医药
Yan Ke Tong Xun (Journal of Ophthalmology)	眼科通讯
Yao Jian Gong Zuo Tong Xun (Journal of Herbal Preparations)	药检工作通讯
Yao Li Shi Yan Fang Fa Xue (Research Methodology of Herbal Medicine)	药理实验方法学
Yao Li Xue (Pharmacology)	药理学
Yao Wu Fen Xi Za Zhi (Journal of Herbal Analysis)	药物分析杂志
Yao Xue Qing Bao Tong Xun (Journal of Herbal Information)	药学情报通讯
Yao Xue Tong Bao (Report of Herbology)	药学通报
Yao Xue Xue Bao (Journal of Herbology)	药学学报
Yao Xue Za Zhi (Journal of Medicinals)	药学杂志
Yao Yong Zhi Wu Da Ci Dian (Dictionary of Medicinal Herbs)	药用植物大辞典
Yi Fang Xin Jie (New Explanation for Medical Formulas)	医方新解
Yi Xue Ji Shu Zi Liao (Resource of Medical Techniques)	医学技术资料
Yi Xue Qing Kuang Jiao Liu (Medical Information Exchange)	医学情况交流
Yi Xue Wei Sheng Tong Xun (Journal of Medicine and Sanitation)	医学卫生通讯
Yi Xue Xue Bao (Report of Medicine)	医学学报
Yi Xue Yan Jiu Tong Xun (Report of Medical Studies)	医学研究通讯
Yi Xue Zhong Yang Za Zhi (Central Journal of Medicine)	医学中央杂志
Yi Yao Gong Ye (Pharmaceutical Industry)	医药工业
Yi Yao Ke Ji Za Zhi (Journal of Medical Technology)	医药科技杂志
Yi Yao Wei Sheng (Medicine, Medicinals, and Sanitation)	医药卫生
Yi Yao Xue (Study of Medicine and Medicinals)	医药学
Yi Yao Yan Jiu Tong Xun (Research Journal of Medicine and Medicinals)	医药研究通讯
Yi Yao Za Zhi (Journal of Medicine and Herbology)	医药杂志
Ying Yang Xue Bao (Report of Nutrition)	营养学报
You Du Zhong Yao Jian Bie Pao Zhi Yu Bao Guan (Identification, Preparation and Storage of Toxic Chinese Herbs)	有毒中药鉴别泡制与保管
Yu Bei Yi Xue Zhuan Ke Xue Xiao (Yubei University of Medicine)	预备医学专科学校
Yun Nan Yi Xue Za Zhi (Yunan Journal of Medicine)	云南医学杂志
Yun Nan Yi Yao (Yunan Medicine and Herbology)	云南医药
Yun Nan Zhong Yao Zhi (Yunan Journal of Chinese Herbal Medicine)	云南中药志
Yun Nan Zhong Yi (Yunnan Journal of Traditional Chinese Medicine)	云南中医
Yun Nan Zhong Yi Xue Yuan Xue Bao (Journal of Yunnan University School of Medicine)	云南中医学院学报
Yun Nan Zhong Yi Za Zhi (Yunan Journal of Chinese Medicine)	云南中医杂志
Yun Nan Zhong Yi Zhong Yao Za Zhi (Yunan Journal of Chinese Medicine and Medicinals)	云南中医中药杂志

Chinese Herbal Formulas and Applications

Bibliography of Contemporary References

Pinyin Names (Translated Names)	Chinese Names
Zhe Jiang Min Jian Chang Yong Cao Yao (Commonly Used Herbs in Zhejiang)	浙江民间常用草药
Zhe Jiang Wei Sheng Shi Yan Yuan (Zhejiang Department of Health Research)	浙江卫生实验院
Zhe Jiang Yao Xue (Zhejiang Journal of Chinese Herbology)	浙江药学
Zhe Jiang Yi Ke Da Xue Xue Bao (Journal of Zhejiang Province School of Medicine)	浙江医科大学学报
Zhe Jiang Yi Xue (Zhejiang Journal of Medicine)	浙江医学
Zhe Jiang Zhong Yi Xue Yuan Xue Bao (Journal of Zhejiang University of Chinese Medicine)	浙江中医学院学报
Zhe Jiang Zhong Yi Yao (Zhejiang Chinese Medicine and Herbology)	浙江中医药
Zhe Jiang Zhong Yi Za Zhi (Zhejiang Journal of Chinese Medicine)	浙江中医杂志
Zhi Wu Yao You Xiao Cheng Fen Shou Ce (Manual of Plant Medicinals and Their Active Constituents)	植物药有效成份手册
Zhi Wu Zi Yuan Yu Huan Jing (Source and Environment of Plants)	植物资源与环境
Zhong Cao Tong Xun (Journal of Chinese Herbs)	中草通讯
Zhong Cao Yao (Chinese Herbal Medicine)	中草药
Zhong Cao Yao Cheng Fen Hua Xue (Composition and Chemistry of Chinese Herbs)	中草药成分化学
Zhong Cao Yao Fang Ji De Ying Yong (Applications of Chinese Herbal Formulas)	中草药方剂的应用
Zhong Cao Yao Tong Xun (Journal of Chinese Herbal Medicine)	中草药通讯
Zhong Cao Yao Xue (Study of Chinese Herbal Medicine)	中草药学
Zhong Cao Yao Yao Li Xue (Herbology of Chinese Medicinals)	中草药药理学
Zhong Cheng Yao (Study of Chinese Patent Medicine)	中成药
Zhong Cheng Yao Yan Jiu (Research of Chinese Patent Medicine)	中成药研究
Zhong Guo Bing Li Sheng Li Za Zhi (Chinese Journal of Pathology and Biology)	中国病理生理杂志
Zhong Guo Fang Lao (Chinese Prevention of Tuberculosis)	中国防痨
Zhong Guo Fang Lao Za Zhi (Chinese Journal on Prevention of Tuberculosis)	中国防痨杂志
Zhong Guo Gang Chang Bing Za Zhi (Chinese Journal of Proctology)	中国肛肠病杂志
Zhong Guo Gang Chang Za Zhi (Chinese Journal of Anus and Intestines)	中国肛肠杂志
Zhong Guo Kang Fu Yi Xue Za Zhi (Chinese Journal of Rehabilitation)	中国康复医学杂志
Zhong Guo Mian Yi Xue Za Zhi (Chinese Journal of Immunology)	中国免疫学杂志
Zhong Guo Nong Cun Yi Xue (Chinese Agricultural Medicine)	中国农村医学
Zhong Guo Shen Jing Jing Shen Ke Za Zhi (Chinese Journal of Psychiatric Disorders)	中国神经精神科杂志
Zhong Guo Sheng Li Ke Xue Hui, Di Er Ci Hui (Chinese Convention on Biophysiology, 2nd Annual Convention)	中国生理科学会第二次会
Zhong Guo Shi Yong Nei Ke Za Zhi (Chinese Journal of Practical Internal Medicine)	中国实用内科杂志
Zhong Guo Shou Yi Za Zhi (Chinese Journal of Husbandry)	中国兽医杂志
Zhong Guo Xiang Cun Xin Xi (Suburb Doctors of China)	中国乡村信息
Zhong Guo Yao Chai Xue (Chinese Herbal Botany)	中国药材学
Zhong Guo Yao Ci Dian (Dictionary of Chinese Medicinal Plants)	中国药辞典
Zhong Guo Yao Ke Da Xue Xue Bao (Journal of University of Chinese Herbology)	中国药科大学学报
Zhong Guo Yao Li Tong Xun (Journal of Chinese Herbal Studies)	中国药理通讯
Zhong Guo Yao Li Xue Bao (Chinese Herbal Pharmacology Journal)	中国药理学报
Zhong Guo Yao Li Xue Tong Bao (Journal of Chinese Herbal Pharmacology)	中国药理学通报
Zhong Guo Yao Li Xue Yu Du Li Xue Za Zhi (Journal of Herbology and Toxicology)	中国药理学与毒理学杂志
Zhong Guo Yao Xue Da Ci Dian (Grand Dictionary of Chinese Herbal Medicine)	中国药学大辞典

BIBLIOGRAPHY OF CONTEMPORARY REFERENCES

B

1501

Bibliography of Contemporary References

Pinyin Names (Translated Names)	Chinese Names
Zhong Guo Yi Ke Da Xue Xue Bao (Journal of University of Chinese Medicine)	中国医科大学学报
Zhong Guo Yi Xue Da Ci Dian (Grand Dictionary of Chinese Medicine)	中国医学大辞典
Zhong Guo Yi Xue Ke Xue Xue Bao (Journal of Chinese Medical Science University)	中国医学科学学报
Zhong Guo Yi Yao Bao (Chinese Journal of Medicine and Medicinals)	中国医药报
Zhong Guo Yi Yao Ke Xue Yuan Lun Wen Zhai Yao (Abstract from Chinese University of Medicine and Science)	中国医药科学院论文摘要
Zhong Guo Yi Yao Xue Bao (Chinese Journal of Medicine and Herbology)	中国医药学报
Zhong Guo Yi Yuan Yao Xue Za Zhi (Chinese Hospital Journal of Herbology)	中国医院药学杂志
Zhong Guo Zhong Xi Yi Jie He Za Zhi (Chinese Journal of Integrative Chinese and Western Medicine)	中国中西医结合杂志
Zhong Guo Zhong Yao Za Zhi (People's Republic of China Journal of Chinese Herbology)	中国中药杂志
Zhong Guo Zhong Yi Yao Xue Bao (Chinese Journal of Chinese Medicine and Herbology)	中国中医药学报
Zhong Hua Bing Li Xue Za Zhi (Chinese Journal of Pathology)	中华病理学杂志
Zhong Hua Er Bi Hou Ke Za Zhi (Chinese Journal of Otolaryngology)	中华耳鼻喉科杂志
Zhong Hua Er Ke Za Zhi (Chinese Journal of Pediatrics)	中华儿科杂志
Zhong Hua Fu Chan Ke Za Zhi (Chinese Journal of Obstetrics and Gynecology)	中华妇产科杂志
Zhong Hua Ji Sheng Chong Chuan Ran Bing Za Zhi (Chinese Journal of Infectious Parasitic Diseases)	中华寄生虫传染病杂志
Zhong Hua Jie He Bing Ke Za Zhi (Chinese Journal of Tuberculosis)	中华结核病科杂志
Zhong Hua Kou Qiang Ke Za Zhi (Chinese Journal of Stomatology)	中华口腔科杂志
Zhong Hua Mi Niao Wai Ke (Chinese Journal of Urology and External Medicine)	中华泌尿外科
Zhong Hua Nei Ke Xue Za Zhi (Journal of Chinese Internal Medicine)	中华内科学杂志
Zhong Hua Nei Ke Za Zhi (Chinese Journal of Internal Medicine)	中华内科杂志
Zhong Hua Pi Fu Ke Xue Za Zhi (Chinese Journal of Dermatology)	中华皮肤科学杂志
Zhong Hua Ren Min Gong He Guo Yao Dian (Chinese Herbal Pharmacopoeia by People's Republic of China)	中华人民共和国药典
Zhong Hua Shen Jing Jing Shen Ke Za Zhi (Chinese Journal of Neurology and Psychiatry)	中华神经精神科杂志
Zhong Hua Wai Ke Za Zhi (Chinese Journal of External Medicine)	中华外科杂志
Zhong Hua Xin Xue Guan Bing Za Zhi (Chinese Journal of Cardiology)	中华心血管病杂志
Zhong Hua Xin Yi Xue Bao (Chinese Journal of New Medicine)	中华新医学报
Zhong Hua Xue Yi Xue Za Zhi (Chinese Journal on Study of Hematology)	中华血液学杂志
Zhong Hua Xue Yi Za Zhi (Chinese Journal of Hematology)	中华血液杂志
Zhong Hua Yan Ke Za Zhi (Chinese Journal of Ophthalmology)	中华眼科杂志
Zhong Hua Yi Liao Za Zhi (Journal of Chinese Therapies)	中华医疗杂志
Zhong Hua Yi Xue Za Zhi (Chinese Journal of Medicine)	中华医学杂志
Zhong Hua Yi Yao Xue Bao (Chinese Journal of Medicinal and Herbology)	中华医药学报
Zhong Hua Yu Fang Yi Xue Za Zhi (Chinese Journal of Preventative Medicine)	中华预防医学杂志
Zhong Hua Zhong Liu Za Zhi (Chinese Journal of Cancer)	中华肿瘤杂志
Zhong Ji Yi Kan (Medium Medical Journal)	中级医刊
Zhong Liu Bian Bing Zhuan Fang Zhi Liao (Differential Diagnosis and Treatment for Cancer)	肿瘤辨病专方治疗
Zhong Liu Yu Fang Yan Jiu (Tumor Prevention and Research)	肿瘤预防研究
Zhong Liu Yu Zhi Tong Xun (Journal of Prevention and Treatment of Cancer)	肿瘤预治通讯

Chinese Herbal Formulas and Applications

Bibliography of Contemporary References

Pinyin Names (Translated Names)	Chinese Names
Zhong Xi Yi Jie He Fang Zhi Yan Jiu Xue Guan Zhi Liao (Research on Prevention and Treatment of Cardiovascular Disorders Using Integrated Chinese and Western Medicines)	中西医结合防治研究血管治疗
Zhong Xi Yi Jie He Yan Jiu Zi Liao (Research Information on Integration of Chinese and Western Medicine)	中西医结合研究资料
Zhong Xi Yi Jie He Za Zhi (Journal of Integrated Chinese and Western Medicine)	中西医结合杂志
Zhong Xi Yi Yao Za Zhi (Journal of Chinese and Western Medicine)	中西医药杂志
Zhong Yao Bu Liang Fan Ying Yu Zhi Liao (Adverse Reactions and Treatment of Chinese Herbal Medicine)	中药不良反应与治疗
Zhong Yao Cai (Study of Chinese Herbal Material)	中药材
Zhong Yao Cai Ke Ji (Science and Technology of Chinese Herbal Material)	中药材科技
Zhong Yao Ci Hai (Encyclopedia of Chinese Herbs)	中药辞海
Zhong Yao Da Ci Dian (Dictionary of Chinese Herbs)	中药大辞典
Zhong Yao Du Li Xue (Toxicology of Chinese Herbs)	中药毒理学
Zhong Yao Lin Zheng Ying Yong (Clinical Applications of Chinese Herbs)	中药淋症应用
Zhong Yao Tong Bao (Journal of Chinese Herbology)	中药通报
Zhong Yao Xian Dai Yan Jiu Yu Ying Yong (Modern Study of Traditional Chinese Medicine)	中药现代研究与应用
Zhong Yao Xue (Chinese Herbology)	中药学
Zhong Yao Yan Jiu (Research of Chinese Herbology)	中药研究
Zhong Yao Yao Li Du Li Yu Lin Chuang (Pharmacology, Toxicology and Clinical Applications of Chinese Herbs)	中药药理毒理与临床
Zhong Yao Yao Li Xue (Study of Chinese Herbology)	中药药理学
Zhong Yao Yao Li Yu Du Li Za Zhi (Journal of Pharmacology and Toxicology of Chinese Herbs)	中药药理与毒理杂志
Zhong Yao Yao Li Yu Lin Chuang (Pharmacology and Clinical Applications of Chinese Herbs)	中药药理与临床
Zhong Yao Yao Li Yu Ying Yong (Pharmacology and Applications of Chinese Herbs)	中药药理与应用
Zhong Yao Yu Jian Mei (Chinese Herbs and Cosmotology)	中药与健美
Zhong Yao Zhi (Chinese Herbology Journal)	中药志
Zhong Yao Zhong Du Yu Ji Jiu (Poisoning and Treatment of Chinese Herbs)	中药中毒与急救
Zhong Yi Er Ke Za Zhi (Chinese Medical Journal of Pediatrics)	中医儿科杂志
Zhong Yi Fang Ji Da Ci Dian (Grand Dictionary of Chinese Herbal Formulas)	中医方剂大辞典
Zhong Yi Fang Ji De Yao Li Yu Ying Yong (Pharmacology and Applications of Chinese Herbal Formulas)	中医方剂的药理与应用
Zhong Yi Fang Ji Lin Chuan Shou Ce (Clinical Handbook of Chinese Herbal Formulae)	中医方剂临床手册
Zhong Yi Fang Ji Xian Dai Yan Jiu (Modern Study of Medical Formulae in Traditional Chinese Medicine)	中医方剂现代研究
Zhong Yi Fu Ke Xue (Traditional Chinese Medicine of Obstetrics and Gynecology)	中医妇科学
Zhong Yi Han Shou Tong Xun (Reports of Chinese Medicine)	中医函授通讯
Zhong Yi Lin Chuan Fang Ji Xue (Clinical Study of Chinese Herbal Formulas)	中医临床方剂学
Zhong Yi Ming Fang Lin Chuang Xin Yong (Contemporary Clinical Applications of Classic Chinese Formulas)	中医名方临床新用
Zhong Yi Xue (Chinese Herbal Medicine)	中医学
Zhong Yi Yan Jiu Yuan (Research Hospital of Chinese Medicine)	中医研究院

Bibliography of Contemporary References

Bibliography of Contemporary References

Pinyin Names (Translated Names)	Chinese Names
Zhong Yi Yao Li (Pharmacology of Chinese Herbs)	中医药理
Zhong Yi Yao Xin Xi (Information on Chinese Medicine and Herbology)	中医药信息
Zhong Yi Yao Xue Bao (Report of Chinese Medicine and Herbology)	中医药学报
Zhong Yi Yao Yan Jiu (Research of Chinese Medicine and Herbology)	中医药研究
Zhong Yi Yao Yan Jiu Can Kao (Research and Discussion of Chinese Medicine and Herbology)	中医药研究参考
Zhong Yi Yao Yan Jiu Zi Liao (Research and Resource of Chinese Medicine and Herbology)	中医药研究资料
Zhong Yi Za Zhi (Journal of Chinese Medicine)	中医杂志
Zhong Yuan Yi Kan (Resource Journal of Chinese Medicine)	中原医刊

Glossary

Chinese Herbal Formulas and Applications

The first column consists of the terms used in the body of the text. Subsequent columns provide correlation to the Chinese characters, pinyin transliteration, previous translation by Wiseman and Feng, and finally, a definition of the term. When a Chinese term is important to the understanding of a theoretical or clinical concept, or when it is a term familiar to many students and practitioners of Chinese Herbal Medicine, that term is given in pinyin in the text, with an accompanying translation, if needed. However, for lesser-known terms, English translations have been used in the body of the text, with the glossary provided to assist interested individuals in making connections with the Chinese. The authors have carefully considered the translation of each term and have offered the clearest and most practical translation they could discover, based on the consideration of both the Chinese terminology and nuances of standard American English usage. In some cases, this differs slightly from translations offered by Wiseman and Feng, which we have included here for purposes of assisting readers already familiar with their work. These small differences in no way diminish our respect for and appreciation of the diligence with which our esteemed colleagues have worked to provide thorough, extensive and effective bridges in understanding via their work.

Terminology	Chinese	Pinyin	Wiseman & Feng	Definition
5 a.m. diarrhea	五更泄	*wu geng xie*	fifth-watch diarrhea	Characterized by early morning (approximately 5 a.m.) diarrhea, this is often caused by Kidney deficiency.
Accumulation	积聚	*ji ju*	accumulation and gathering	An inclusive term describing the accumulation of *ji* (yin substances) and *ju* (yang substances), that may occur in any organ. Clinical presentation differs, depending on the area(s) and organ(s) affected.
Ah shi point	阿是穴	*ah shi xue*	a-shi point	A type of acupuncture point having no fixed location or name, but corresponding to an underlying disorder. Stimulating an *ah shi* point elicits tenderness and pain.
Ao (simmer)	熬	*ao*		A method that slowly cooks the herbs using low heat, extracts active constituents, and removes excess water.
Ba gang bian zheng (eight principle differentiation)	八纲辨证	*ba gang bian zheng*	eight-principle pattern identification	A system of differential diagnosis based on patterns of imbalance or disharmony of the eight factors: exterior and interior location, cold and hot attributes, deficiency and excess states, and yin and yang qualities.
Ba hui (eight meeting) points	八会穴	*ba hui xue*	eight meeting points	A set of eight points corresponding to *zang* (solid organs), *fu* (hollow organs), qi, blood, tendons, vessels, bones and marrows.
Ban (blend)	拌	*ban*		To mix medicinal substances.
Bang (scrape)	镑	*bang*	flaking	A method used to process horn substances to obtain thin flakes. This method increases the surface area and enhances extraction of active ingredients.
Bei (stone-bake)	焙	*bei*	stone-baking	A method to indirectly dry the herbs without changing their color by placing the herbs on a heated stone.
Ben tun (running piglet)	奔豚	*ben tun*	running piglet	A sensation of qi rushing upwards from the lower abdomen to the chest, epigastrium and throat. There will generally be concurrent pain, discomfort, alternation of heat and cold, and palpitations.
Beng lou (flooding and spotting)	崩漏	*beng lou*	flooding and spotting	A condition that includes massive uterine bleeding at irregular intervals and incessant dripping of blood from the uterus.

GLOSSARY

G

1505

Glossary

Terminology	Chinese	Pinyin	Wiseman & Feng	Definition
Bi zheng (closed disorder)	闭证	*bi zheng*	block pattern	Characterized by clenched jaws, tight fists, unconsciousness, a warm body and cold extremities; this generally occurs in wind stroke or febrile disorders, with heat attacking the *ying* (nutritive) and *xue* (blood) levels.
Bi zheng (painful obstruction syndrome)	痹证	*bi zheng*	impediment pattern	A pain condition characterized by stagnation and obstruction that may affect any tissue and/or organ.
Big pulse	大脉	*da mai*	big pulse	A broad pulse.
Blood	血	*xue*	blood	The red, viscous fluid in the body that comprises nutrients, body fluids and Kidney *jing* (essence).
Blood deficiency	血虚	*xue xu*	blood vacuity	Pale, lusterless face, pale lips, dizziness, vertigo, palpitations, insomnia, coldness and numbness of the extremities, and a fine, weak pulse illustrate this condition, caused by loss of blood, excessive thinking and worrying, the presence of parasites, or injury to the internal organs.
Blood desiccation	血枯	*xue ku*	blood desiccation	Following profuse loss of blood, a condition characterized by dizziness, a feeling of weightlessness of the extremities, and amenorrhea.
Blood stagnation/stasis	血瘀	*xue yu*	blood stasis	A condition characterized by obstructed blood flow, leading to dark purplish skin color, dried or scaly skin, pain at a fixed location, pain that intensifies with pressure, fullness and distention of the lower abdomen, amenorrhea, black, tarry stools, and a dark purple tongue with black spots. Blood stagnation/stasis may be caused by external injuries, menstrual irregularities, qi stagnation and cold stagnation. Blood stagnation refers to mild to moderate obstruction of blood circulation. Blood stasis refers to moderate to severe obstruction of blood circulation, possibly with clotting.
Bo (open)	擘	*bo*		To open the medicinal substances to allow maximum extraction of active ingredients.
Body fluids	津液	*jin ye*	fluids	An all-inclusive term that describes all the fluids in the body, including tears, saliva, sweat, blood and fluids that lubricate the joints.
Bound pulse	结脉	*jie mai*	bound pulse	A slow pulse with pulses at irregular intervals.
Bowl	盅	*zhong*		A traditional unit of measurement for volume. The exact unit varies depending on the place and time in history.
Breast abscess	乳痈	*ru yong*	mammary welling-abscess	A hard breast abscess accompanied by distention and pain, chills and fever, and obstructed flow of breast milk; this is generally caused by Liver qi stagnation, Stomach fire, or stasis of breast milk.
Bu fa (tonifying)	补法	*bu fa*	supplementation	A method of treatment that nourishes, enriches, supplements, and benefits qi, blood, yin, and yang in the *zang fu* organs.
Chang feng (intestinal wind)	肠风	*chang feng*	intestinal wind	A condition caused by wind attacking the intestines, leading to the presence of bright red blood in the stools.

Chinese Herbal Formulas and Applications

Glossary

Terminology	Chinese	Pinyin	Wiseman & Feng	Definition
Chao (dry-fry)	炒	*chao*	stir-frying	Parching or tossing medicinal substances in a heated wok. This method increases the warmth of the herb, harmonizes and moderates therapeutic effects, and facilitates extraction of active constituents.
Chao huang (dry-fry to yellow)	炒黄	*chao huang*		Parching or tossing medicinal substances in a heated wok until they become yellow in color.
Chao jiao (dry-fry to burnt)	炒焦	*chao jiao*	scorch-frying	Parching or tossing at high temperature until the medicinal substances are burnt on the outside.
Chao tan (dry-fry to ash)	炒炭	*chao tan*	char-frying	Parching or tossing at high temperature until the medicinal substances turn into ash.
Chen yao (deputy herb)	臣药	*chen yao*	minister	The second of four guiding principles in herbal formulation: *Jun Chen Zuo Shi* (Chief, Deputy, Assistant, Envoy). This herb serves two main functions: 1) to reinforce the effect of *jun yao* (chief herb) to treat the key disease or symptom; and 2) to treat the associated or coexisting diseases or symptoms.
Chi position	尺	*chi*	cubit	The third (most proximal) position on the wrist for pulse diagnosis; it represents Kidney yang (right hand) and Kidney yin (left hand).
Chong (thoroughfare) channel	冲脉	*chong mai*	thoroughfare vessel	One of the eight extraordinary vessels which controls the twelve channels. Also known as the "sea of blood," as it has functions related to blood and gynecology.
Chong fu (take drenched)	冲服	*chong fu*	take drenched	Infusing the medicinal substances into water, decoction or other liquid before ingestion.
Chu (pestle)	杵	*chu*		Using a club-shaped implement to pound or grind medicinal substances in a mortar. This method increases the surface area and enhances extraction of active ingredients.
Clumping	结	*jie*	bind	This describes the formation of a solid mass or masses from one or more substances, such as phlegm, heat or cold.
Cold	寒	*han*	cold	Cold is a yin pathogenic factor that attacks both the outside and inside of the body and is characterized by contraction and stagnation. Clinical presentation of cold includes chills, shivering, aversion to cold, cold extremities, pale face and lips, the presence of undigested food in the stools, and clear urine.
Collapse	厥	*jue*	reversal	A condition of sudden collapse and loss of consciousness that generally can be reversed. The causes of collapse include cold, heat, phlegm and dietary injury, among others.
Controlling sequence	相克	*xiang ke*	restraining	A concept of *wu xing* (five element) theory that describes the orderly sequence in which one element controls the growth of another.
Cui (quench)	淬	*cui*	calcining and quenching	Heating medicinal substances at high temperature until they turn red, followed by dipping them in cold water or vinegar. This method makes the substances brittle to facilitate pulverization.

GLOSSARY

G

1507

Glossary

Terminology	Chinese	Pinyin	Wiseman & Feng	Definition
Cun position	寸	*cun*	cun	The first (most distal) position on the wrist for pulse diagnosis; it represents the Lung (right hand) and the Heart (left hand).
Cuo (grate)	锉	*cuo*	grating	To reduce hard medicinal substances into small particles. This method increases the surface area and enhances extraction of active ingredients.
Cup	升	*sheng*		A traditional unit of measurement for both volume (approximately 200 mL) and weight (approximately 18-30g). Today, *sheng* has been standardized to 1,000 mL.
Da tou wen (swollen head epidemic)	大头瘟	*da tou wen*	massive head scourge	An epidemic disease characterized by redness and swelling of the face and sore throat, caused by wind, heat and toxins attacking the face and head.
Dai (girdle) channel	带脉	*dai mai*	girdling vessel	Another of the eight extraordinary vessels, this one serves to bind all of the channels together, and influences lower extremity function.
Damp	湿	*shi*	damp	Damp is a pathogenic factor that occurs mainly in the late summer or in places with high humidity. Dampness is characterized by heaviness and turbidity, which may lead to such symptoms as feeling heaviness in the head and extremities, general fatigue, and fullness in the chest and epigastrium. Dampness is also characterized by increased viscosity of substances and stagnation, such as in cases of abscesses, oozing ulcers, leukorrhea with foul discharge, and arthritis.
Damp rash	湿疹	*shi zhen*		Red eruption of the skin characterized by wind, dampness and heat.
Dao (pound)	捣	*dao*	crushing	To reduce medicinal substances into particles by crushing or grinding. This method increases the surface area and enhances extraction of active ingredients.
De qi (arrival of qi)	的气	*de qi*	obtaining qi	Qi sensation (numbness, pressure, swelling, warmth or other) that follows insertion and manipulation of acupuncture needles.
Debilitation	劳	*lao*	taxation	Generalized weakness resulting from persistent mental and physical wear and tear on the body.
Deep pulse	沉脉	*chen mai*	sunken pulse	A pulse that is distinct at the deep level.
Deficiency	虚	*xu*	vacuity	Deficiency refers to a state of insufficiency (such as deficiency of qi, blood, yin or yang), or decreased ability of the organ to carry out its normal physiological functioning (Spleen deficiency, Kidney deficiency, and so on). Deficiency occurs due to congenital deficiency, lack of nourishment, or long-term illness.
Deficient pulse	虚脉	*xu mai*	vacuous pulse	A soggy pulse that is also fine and forceless.
Dian kuang (mania and withdrawal)	癫狂	*dian kuang*	mania and withdrawal	An inclusive term for various types of mental illness. *Dian* (withdrawal) represents yin disorders: the individual is quiet and socially inactive. *Kuang* (mania) represents yang disorders: the individual is irritable, restless, and physically active.

Chinese Herbal Formulas and Applications

Glossary

Terminology	Chinese	Pinyin	Wiseman & Feng	Definition
Do not expose to heat	不见火	*bu jian huo*		To avoid direct or indirect contact with fire or high temperature.
Drooling phlegm	痰涎	*tan xian*	phlegm-drool	Characterized by profuse dripping of saliva in children; this is generally caused by wind-heat attacking the Spleen, resulting in its inability to properly process water.
Drum skin pulse	革脉	*ge mai*	drum skin pulse	A pulse that is string-like and empty in the middle.
Drum-like abdominal distention	鼓胀	*gu zhang*	drum distention	Characterized by severe fullness and distention, resulting in the abdomen resembling a drum; this may be caused by emotional constraint, inappropriate diet, excessive use of alcohol, or intestinal parasites.
Dryness	乾	*gan*	dry	Dryness is a pathogenic factor that invades the body in late autumn when there is a lack of moisture in the environment. Dryness consumes yin and body fluids, and may lead to clinical presentations such as dry and chapped skin, dryness of the mouth and throat, thirst, dry cough with little sputum, and so on.
Du (governing) channel	督脉	*du mai*	governing vessel	Confluence of all yang vessels, one of the eight extraordinary vessels, also known as the "sea of yang qi." It influences brain and spinal column functioning.
Duan (calcine)	煅	*duan*	calcination	A preparation method to make medicinal substances crisp and brittle by burning them directly or indirectly in a container. This method is often reserved for minerals or shell-like substances to facilitate pulverization.
Dun (stew)	炖	*dun*	double-boiling	To boil slowly or with simmering heat.
Dysentery	痢疾	*li ji*	dysentery	A disorder characterized by abdominal pain, increased frequency but decreased volume of bowel movements, tenesmus, and the presence of undigested food, mucus, and blood in the stool.
Earth	土	*tu*	earth	Another of the five elements, earth corresponds to ripeness and late summer, to sweet flavors, transformation, and centeredness. The corresponding organ is the Spleen.
Epidemic toxin	疫毒	*yi du*	epidemic toxin	An epidemic pathogenic factor that attacks and affects the entire community, regardless of individual health and constitution.
Epilepsy	痫证	*xian zheng*	epilepsy pattern	Characterized by altered consciousness and muscle convulsions, this disorder occurs frequently in children because they have not yet gained fully-developed defenses against external pathogens. Factors commonly causing seizure include wind, heat, phlegm and inappropriate diet.
Excess	实	*shi*	repletion	Excess refers to the state of surplus or overload that creates a pathologic condition in the body, such as when there is excess heat, formation or accumulation of phlegm, or blood stagnation, among others. Excess conditions occur in the case of invasion of exogenous pathogenic factors or in disharmony of the internal organs.
Excess pulse	实脉	*shi mai*	replete pulse	A broad, large and forceful pulse upon arrival and departure.

GLOSSARY

G

1509

Glossary

Terminology	Chinese	Pinyin	Wiseman & Feng	Definition
Exterior	表	biao	exterior	The outside of the body, such as the skin, mouth, nose and nostrils. Pathogenic factors are often said to attack the exterior prior to invading the interior. The clinical presentation of an exterior syndrome includes headache, muscle aches and pain, nasal congestion, coughing and so on.
Exterior and interior	表里	biao li	exterior and interior	A term used to indicate differentiation between the exterior and interior parts of the body.
Faint pulse	微脉	wei mai	faint pulse	A pulse that is extremely fine, forceless, and indistinct.
Febrile diseases	热病	re bing	heat disease	A term that describes all externally-contracted diseases characterized by heat.
Fen sui (pulverize)	粉碎	fen sui		To reduce medicinal substances by crushing, beating, or grinding into powder. This method increases the surface area and enhances extraction of active ingredients.
Feng lao bing (wind consumption disease)	风劳病	feng lao bing	wind taxation disease	A yin-deficient heat syndrome characterized by tidal fever and steaming bones sensation, caused by maltreatment of an exterior condition leading to formation of heat in the interior damaging yin and blood.
Feng shi (wind-damp)	风湿	feng shi	wind-damp	A condition caused by invasion of wind-dampness, leading to pain and limited movements of the joints, muscles and bones.
Feng shui (wind water)	风水	feng shui	wind water	A condition caused by invasion of wind to the exterior parts of the body, leading to swelling and water accumulation.
Filth and fetidness	秽	hui	foulness	Terms used to describe things that are dirty, foul, or turbid, such as foods or pathogenic factors.
Fine pulse	细脉	xi mai	fine pulse	A small and well-defined pulse.
Fire	火	huo	fire	Fire is one of the five elements, associated with upward movement of energy, the sparkling flaring of fire, and summer. The corresponding organ is the Heart. In disease terminology, fire is a yang pathogenic factor representing a severe form of heat.
Firm pulse	牢脉	lao mai	firm pulse	A pulse that is deep and forceful.
Five elements	五行	wu xing	five phases	A theory which evaluates all things according to elements of water, wood, fire, earth and metal. The theory is also used to explain anatomy, physiology, and pathology of the human body, as well as treatment strategies.
Floating edema	浮肿	fu zhong	puffy swelling	A symptom characterized by fluid accumulation in superficial parts of the body. This is generally caused by Lung, Spleen or Kidney deficiency, and the consequent inability to properly regulate water metabolism pathways.
Focal distention	痞满	pi man	glomus fullness	Fullness, distention and oppression in the chest and abdomen, caused by food retention, phlegm stagnation, and/or damp-heat accumulation.
Fright and palpitations	惊悸	jing ji	fright palpitations	A condition of emotional instability and increased sensitivity to stimulus caused by Heart qi deficiency.

Chinese Herbal Formulas and Applications

Glossary

Terminology	Chinese	Pinyin	Wiseman & Feng	Definition
Frightened wind	惊风	*jing feng*	fright wind	Literally "frightened wind," this describes seizures and convulsions in children. It is most common in children under the age of five, with incidence gradually decreasing with increased age. Clinical presentations include high fever, red eyes, convulsion, opisthotonos, clenched jaws, tight fists, eyes rolled upward, and urinary and bowel incontinence.
Fu (hollow organ)	腑	*fu*	bowel	The hollow organs of the body are the Small Intestine, Large Intestine, Gallbladder, Stomach and Urinary Bladder.
Gallbladder	胆	*dan*	gallbladder	Paired with the Liver, the Gallbladder stores bile and excretes it to the intestines to facilitate digestion.
Gan ji (infantile malnutrition)	疳疾	*gan ji*	gan disease	A disorder characterized by the inability of the Spleen and Stomach to properly transform and transport food. Generally occurring in children under five years of age, *gan ji* is characterized by a sallow facial appearance, weight loss, thin hair, poor appetite, abdominal distention, and irregular bowel movements.
Gao lin (cloudy dysuria)	膏淋	*gao lin*	unctuous strangury	A urinary tract disorder in which the urine has a milky or cloudy appearance, and may be slightly pink (an indication of bleeding). This is caused by damp-heat attacking the Urinary Bladder, leading to the bladder's inability to clear turbid substances.
Generating sequence	相生	*xiang sheng*	engendering	A concept of *wu xing* (five element) theory that describes the orderly sequence in which one element promotes the generation of another.
Gu (food) *qi*	谷气	*gu qi*		Qi that is derived from the ingestion and absorption of food.
Guan position	关	*guan*	bar	The second (middle) position on the wrist for pulse diagnosis represents the Spleen (right hand) and the Liver (left hand).
Half-body perspiration	半身汗	*ban shen han*		Half-body perspiration refers to sweating only on half of the body, such as the left or right side, or upper or lower half. This condition occurs because of obstruction of the channels and collaterals caused by wind-phlegm or wind-dampness. It may also be caused by disharmony of qi and blood, or of *ying* (nutritive) and *wei* (defensive) levels.
Han fa (sweating)	汗法	*han fa*	diaphoresis	A method of treatment that induces a mild sweat by ventilating and dispersing Lung qi, and regulating and harmonizing the *ying* (nutritive) and *wei* (defensive) levels. Sweating is primarily used to expel pathogenic factors at the exterior (skin) level to treat common cold, influenza, the early stage of measles, acute edema (especially above the waist), abscesses and sores with fever and chills, dysentery with exterior signs and symptoms, and many others.
He (uniting) point	合穴	*he xue*	uniting point	Known as "uniting" or "sea" point, this point represents the flow of qi where it is vast and deep, near the elbows or knees.

GLOSSARY

G

1511

Glossary

Terminology	Chinese	Pinyin	Wiseman & Feng	Definition
He fa (harmonizing)	和法	he fa	harmonization	A method of treatment that regulates and accords complicated patterns of disease that affect multiple parts of the body. Harmonizing is generally used to treat such disorders as *shaoyang* syndrome, *mo yuan* (membrane source) disorders, disharmony of the Liver and Spleen, concurrent presentation of heat in the Stomach and cold in the Intestines, irregularities of qi and blood, and disharmony of the nutritive and defensive levels.
He xi feng (crane's knee wind)	鹤膝风	he xi feng	crane's-knee wind	A condition in which the knees are swollen and enlarged, but the muscles above and below the knees are atrophied.
Heart	心	xin	heart	The Heart functions to control the blood channels and house the *shen* (spirit). It connects to the Small Intestine and opens to the tongue, and is associated with the fire element.
Heat	热	re	heat	Heat is a yang pathogenic factor that attacks both external and internal aspects of the body; it is characterized by the tendency to disperse outwards and to consume yin and fluids. Clinical presentations of heat include a wide variety of signs and symptoms, such as fever, inflammation, infection, bleeding, and others.
Heat in the blood	血热	xue re	blood heat	A condition characterized by nosebleeds, coughing of blood, and late-afternoon fever, because of heat affecting the *xue* (blood) level.
Hernial disorder	疝气	shan qi	mounting qi	Historically, this term covers a wide variety of disorders related to both internal and external genitalia, in men and women. More recently, it refers specifically to disorders of the male external genitalia (testicles and scrotum).
Hidden pulse	伏脉	fu mai	hidden pulse	A pulse that is distinct at the deep level, deeper than the deep pulse.
Hong (bake)	烘	hong		A method to directly dry the herbs at low temperature without charring it.
Hou bi (painful obstruction of the throat)	喉痹	hou bi	throat impediment	Redness, swelling and pain of the throat caused mainly by wind-cold at the exterior, or Liver or Lung fire in the interior.
Hua (dissolve)	化	hua	transform	To cause to pass into solution.
Hui (influential) point	会穴	hui xue	meeting point	Referred to as "meeting" or "influential" points, these eight points individually represent one of the following: *zang*, *fu*, qi, blood, tendons, channels, bones or marrow.
Hun (ethereal soul)	魂	hun	ethereal soul	Similar to the Western interpretation of "soul" or "spirit," the *hun* functions to maintain mental and psychological health and well-being. It has been said that the Liver stores blood, and blood contains *hun*. Therefore, disorders of the *hun* are often secondary to the inability of the Liver to store blood; or, secondary to deficiency of Liver blood.

Glossary

Chinese Herbal Formulas and Applications

Terminology	Chinese	Pinyin	Wiseman & Feng	Definition
Insulting sequence	相侮	*xiang wu*	rebellion	A concept of *wu xing* (five element) theory that describes the situation in which an element normally controlled by another reverses the sequence and suppresses or reduces what is normally the controlling element.
Interior	里	*li*	interior	Internal aspects of the body, such as organs, bone marrow, and the *qi* (energy) and *xue* (blood) levels. Pathogenic factors may affect the interior of the body directly or indirectly (via the exterior). Clinical presentation of interior conditions varies significantly, depending on the area and/or organs affected.
Intermittent pulse	代脉	*dai mai*	intermittent pulse	A pulse interspersed with more relatively regular pauses.
Intestinal abscess	肠痈	*chang yong*	intestinal welling-abscess	Intestinal abscesses generally arise from inappropriate diet or emotional disturbances (excessive anger or worry), and are characterized by abdominal pain.
Irritability	烦	*fan*	vexation	A state of impatience, anger, annoyance, and increased sensitivity to stimulus.
Jian (decoct)	煎	*jian*	decoct, brew	To boil medicinal substances in water to extract their active ingredients.
Jie xiong (stagnant chest)	结胸	*jie xiong*	chest bind	A condition caused by stagnation in the chest of pathogenic heat or cold with retention of fluid, phlegm or blood.
Jin (soak)	浸	*jin*	soaking, steeping	To infuse or steep medicinal substances in water or other fluids over a period of time.
Jin (thin body fluid)	津	*jin*	liquid	An inclusive term that describes body fluids of lesser density, such as tears, saliva and sweat.
Jing (clean)	净	*jing*		To remove unwanted or non-medicinal parts from medicinal substances.
Jing (essence)	精	*jing*	essence	The basic substance that makes up the human body and sustains the vital functions of the internal organs. Derived prenatally from one's parents, and postnatally from food, essence is stored in the Kidney.
Jing (river) point	经穴	*jing xue*	river point	Commonly referred to as either "traversing" or "river" points, these points suggest that the flow of qi at the forearms or lower legs has attained a large volume.
Jing (well) point	井穴	*jing xue*	well point	"Well" points represent the beginning of qi circulation within channels, at the most distal parts of the body, where qi flow is still small and shallow.
Jueyin	厥阴	*jue yin*	reverting yin	The last of six stages in the paradigm of yin and yang. This describes the degree of pathology of disease according to the *Shang Han Lun* (Discussion of Cold-Induced Disorders) text. It also identifies the level attributed to the Liver and Pericardium channels that travel throughout the body.
Jun yao (chief herb)	君药	*jun yao*	sovereign	The first of four guiding principles in herbal formulation: *Jun Chen Zuo Shi* (Chief, Deputy, Assistant, Envoy). It is the essential ingredient used at a large dosage to maximize the effect and treat the key disease or symptom.

1513

Glossary

Terminology	Chinese	Pinyin	Wiseman & Feng	Definition
Kidney	肾	*shen*	kidney	The Kidney controls growth, maturation, reproduction and aging. It produces marrow that forms the brain and spinal cord, and it promotes production of bones and blood. Furthermore, it dominates body fluids and receives qi from air via the Lung. Associated with the water element, the Kidney connects with the Urinary Bladder, opens to the ears, and houses the faculty of *zhi* (will power).
Lao lin (fatigue dysuria)	劳淋	*lao lin*	taxation strangury	A urinary tract disorder involving increased frequency of urination, especially with physical stress and exertion. Accompanying symptoms include fatigue, lower back and knee soreness and pain, with dribbling urine, but no pain during urination. This is caused when prolonged exertion leads to Spleen and Kidney exhaustion and inability to control the normal flow of water and urination.
Large Intestine	大肠	*da chang*	large intestine	Connected to the Small Intestine, the Large Intestine absorbs nutrients and water from food.
Large spoon	方寸匕	*fang cun bi*		A large spoon that contains approximately 6-9 grams of powdered herbs.
Leg *qi*	脚气	*jiao qi*	leg qi	A disorder of the leg(s) characterized by numbness, soreness, pain, weakness, possible swelling and cramps, and possible atrophy of leg muscles. Accompanying symptoms may include nausea, vomiting, dyspnea, incoherent speech, and palpitations. Generally caused by wind, damp, and toxins attacking the legs, it overlaps in symptomology with beriberi.
Li feng (dysenteric wind)	痢风	*li feng*		A condition of constitutional weakness and deficiency caused by chronic dysentery, in which wind attacks the legs leading to weakness, pain, paralysis, and inability to walk.
Lin zheng (dysuria syndrome)	淋证	*lin zheng*	strangury pattern	Dysuria syndrome refers to a condition of frequent and painful urination, abdominal pain, and/or pain radiating to the lower back.
Liu jing bian zheng (six stages differentiation)	六经辨证	*liu jing bian zheng*	six-channel pattern identification	A system of differential diagnosis based on identifying patterns of disharmony by relationship to the energetic stages *taiyang, yangming, shaoyang, taiyin, shaoyin,* and *jueyin*.
Liu yin (six exogenous factors)	六淫	*liu yin*	six excesses	The six exogenous climatic conditions that may cause illness when in excess, including wind, cold, summer-heat, dampness, dryness, and fire.
Liver	肝	*gan*	liver	The Liver stores blood, maintains proper flow of qi, and controls tendons. It connects to the Gallbladder, opens to the eyes, and is associated with the wood element.
Long pulse	长脉	*chang mai*	long pulse	A pulse that can be felt beyond the *cun* and *chi* positions.
Loss of qi with hemorrhage	气随血脱	*qi sui xue tuo*	qi deserting with the blood	A dangerous dynamic in which qi is lost because it flows out with the blood in severe bleeding.
Lower *jiao*	下焦	*xia jiao*	lower burner	The lower *jiao* represents the hypogastrium, and includes the functions of the Kidney and the Urinary Bladder.
Lung	肺	*fei*	lung	The Lung controls breathing and the flow of air, regulates water passages, and dominates the skin and hair. It connects with the Large Intestine, opens to the nose, and is associated with the metal element.

1514

Glossary

Chinese Herbal Formulas and Applications

Terminology	Chinese	Pinyin	Wiseman & Feng	Definition
Lung abscess	肺痈	*fei yong*	pulmonary welling-abscess	A disorder characterized by cough, chest fullness, fever and chills, rapid pulse, dry throat without thirst, foul-smelling sputum, and profuse discharge of sputum. It is generally caused by wind-heat attacking the Lung.
Luo (connecting) point	络穴	*luo xue*	network point	Known as "connecting" or "vessel" points, these points assist communication between the yang external and yin internal channels. Fifteen points in all represent each of the twelve channels and one on each of the front, back and side of the trunk.
Malaria	疟疾	*nue ji*	malaria	An infectious disorder characterized by alternation of chills, fever and perspiration. This disorder occurs most frequently in summer and fall, and is diagnosed as wind, cold, summer-damp, and damp attacking the *ying* (nutritive) and *wei* (defensive) levels.
Mammary aggregation	乳癖	*ru pi*	mammary aggregation	A breast nodule of variable size, slightly mobile, not painful, not of cold or hot origin, does not cause a change in local skin color, nor erupt or cause ulceration. These form primarily because of Liver qi stagnation.
Mammary 'rock'	乳岩	*ru yan*	mammary rock	Single or multiple breast nodules similar in size to jujubes, that do not cause pain, itching, redness or heat sensations, and may continue to grow in size. Most common in women past middle age, this is caused by emotional constraint and obstructed flow of Liver and Spleen qi.
Man (fullness)	满	*man*	fullness	*Man* (fullness) is the feeling of bloating and fullness in the epigastric and abdominal regions.
Metal	金	*jin*	metal	One of the five elements, metal has inward or contracting movement, represents autumn and harvest, and is associated with the Lung.
Middle *jiao*	中焦	*zhong jiao*	middle burner	The middle *jiao* represents the epigastrium, and includes the functions of the Spleen and Stomach.
Ming men (life gate)	命门	*ming men*	life gate	This is key to the overall vitality of the individual. A strong *ming men* (life gate) often indicates that an individual is in great health and will age slowly. A weak *ming men* is often evident in persons who look older than their actual age, and suffer from numerous age-related illnesses.
Moderate pulse	缓脉	*huan mai*	moderate pulse	A slow pulse with approximately three or more beats per respiration.
Mo yuan (membrane source)	膜原	*mo yuan*	membrane source	A term used in *wen bing* (warm disease) to describe a space situated midway between the exterior and the interior of the body where warm disease factors tend to settle.
Mu (collecting) point	募穴	*mu xue*	alarm point	Commonly referred to as "alarm" or "collecting" points, these twelve points individually represent where the qi of a specific internal organ passes on the chest and abdomen.

GLOSSARY

G

1515

Glossary

Terminology	Chinese	Pinyin	Wiseman & Feng	Definition
Mumps	痄腮	zha sai	mumps	An acute infectious disorder commonly seen in children. Clinical presentations include swelling and pain of the parotid glands, chills and fever, difficulty chewing, and discomfort of the entire body. Most common in winter and spring, it may occur in any season, and is caused by wind-heat (entering the body through the mouth and nose) that becomes blocked in the *shaoyang* channels.
Night perspiration	盗汗	dao han	night sweating	Night perspiration refers to sweating that occurs during sleep, and stops when one awakens. It is an indication of yin deficiency.
Over-acting sequence	相乘	xiang cheng	overwhelming	A concept of *wu xing* (five element) theory that describes a situation in which a controlling element suppresses or reduces the controlled element instead of controlling its growth or activity.
Pao (blast-fry)	炮	pao	blast-drying	To stir fry medicinal substances in an iron wok over intense fire until their surface becomes dark-brown, burnt, or cracked open.
Pericardium	心包	xin bao	pericardium	The Pericardium is the external covering of the Heart. It functions as the protective barrier of the Heart against pathological factors, and connects with the *San Jiao*.
Persistent, indeterminate hunger	嘈杂	cao za	clamoring stomach	An uncomfortable sensation that mimics pain yet is not painful, that mimics hunger yet the person is not hungry. This condition is usually caused by fire, phlegm accumulation, qi stagnation, or food retention.
Perspiration of the palms and soles	手足心汗	shou zhu xin han	sweating in the (heart of the) palms and soles	Profuse perspiration of the hands and feet is an indication of yin deficiency with heat. It is often caused by excessive thinking and worrying that leads to injuries of the Heart and Spleen.
Phlegm	痰	tan	phlegm	Phlegm is a by-product formed from water and damp stagnation. The presence of phlegm may obstruct healthy flow and cause illness throughout the body, damaging the Lung, Heart, Stomach, peripheral channels and collaterals, throat and skin.
Pi (distention)	痞	pi	glomus	*Pi* (distention) is the feeling of oppression, obstruction, and increased pressure in the chest and epigastric regions.
Pi shui (skin water)	皮水	pi shui	skin water	Severe and generalized edema due to Spleen deficiency and damp accumulation, with symptoms such as pitting edema and heaviness and pain of the body and limbs.
Piao (rinse)	漂	piao	long rinsing	To steep or soak medicinal substances with frequent change of water to remove dirt, odor or toxicity.
Plum-pit *qi*	梅核气	mei he qi	plum-pit qi	The feeling of having a foreign substance, such as a plum pit, obstructing the throat which cannot be expectorated or swallowed.
Po (break open)	破	po		To force open.

Glossary

Chinese Herbal Formulas and Applications

Terminology	Chinese	Pinyin	Wiseman & Feng	Definition
Po (corporeal soul)	魄	*po*	corporeal soul	A term that refers to basic human instinct and reaction, such as the ability to smell, taste, see, distinguish between cold and hot, and the ability of the newborn to nurse and feed. The main function of *po*, which resides in the Lung, is to maintain physical awareness in order to react and adapt to the external environment.
Post-decoct	后下	*hou xia*	add at end	A specific instruction when preparing a decoction, to add specific herbs near the end of the cooking process and then continue cooking the herbs for approximately 5 to 10 additional minutes.
Pre-decoct	先煎	*xian jian*	predecoct	Instruction to cook a certain herb or herbs first (usually for 30 minutes, but this varies) before adding the rest of the herbs to cook a decoction.
Profuse sweating	大汗	*da han*	great sweating	Profuse perspiration often leads to depletion of body fluids. It may occur because of excessive heat or yang collapse.
Qi	气	*qi*	qi	Qi represents the vital energy needed for proper functioning and existence of the organs and the body.
Qi (energy) level	气分	*qi fen*	qi aspect	Qi (energy) level refers to the second of four levels of febrile infections. Heat attacking the *qi* level may affect such organs as the Stomach, Lung, Intestines, Gallbladder and Spleen. Clinical presentations will vary depending on the organ(s) affected.
Qi and blood deficiency	气血两虚	*qi xue liang xu*	dual vacuity of qi and blood	Insufficiency of both qi and blood, which influences basic organ functions more strongly than insufficiency of either one alone.
Qi and blood stagnation	气滞血瘀	*qi zhi xue yu*	qi stagnation and blood stasis	Obstructed flow of both qi and blood.
Qi collapse	气陷	*qi xian*	qi fall	Severe insufficiency of qi results in collapse of vital functions.
Qi deficiency	气虚	*qi xu*	qi vacuity	A condition in which insufficient quantity of qi affects body or organ functions.
Qi deficiency bleeding	气虚失血	*qi xu shi xue*	qi vacuity bleeding	Bleeding caused by insufficiency of qi, and its consequent inability to properly guide the flow of blood.
Qi lin (qi dysuria)	气淋	*qi lin*	qi strangury	A urinary tract disorder characterized by obstructed urinary flow, lower abdominal distention and pain, and green-blue tongue color. It is caused by Liver stagnation leading to obstructed flow of qi and urine.
Qi qing (seven emotions)	七情	*qi qing*	seven affects	The seven emotional factors that may cause illness when out of balance, including joy, anger, melancholy, thought (over-thinking), grief, fear and fright.
Qi stagnation	气滞	*qi zhi*	qi stagnation	Obstructed qi flow in internal organs or peripheral channels and collaterals, caused by a variety of factors, including inappropriate diet, emotional disturbance, environmental factors, or external injuries.
Qi xue jin ye bian zheng (qi, blood, and body fluid differentiation)	气血津液辨证	*qi xue jin ye bian zheng*	qi, blood and fluids pattern identification	A system of differential diagnosis based on patterns of disharmony of qi, blood, and body fluids.

1517

Glossary

Terminology	Chinese	Pinyin	Wiseman & Feng	Definition
Qie (slice)	切	qie	cutting	To cut open. This method increases the surface area, creates standard portion weights and sizes, facilitates drying, and prolongs shelf life.
Qing fa (clearing)	清法	qing fa	clearing	A method of treatment that clears heat, purges fire and cools the blood to treat diseases characterized by warmth, heat, fire, and toxins.
Racing pulse	疾脉	ji mai	racing pulse	A fast pulse with seven or more beats per respiration.
Rapid pulse	数脉	shu mai	rapid pulse	A fast pulse with six or more beats per respiration.
Re bi (heat painful obstruction)	热痹	re bi	heat impediment	One type of *bi zheng* (painful obstruction syndrome) characterized by local redness, swelling, burning sensations and pain. The development of heat is often caused by prolonged obstruction of the channels and collaterals by wind, cold or damp.
Re jue (heat reversal)	热厥	re jue	heat reversal	A morbid condition in which excessive pathogenic heat leads to consumption of body fluids which impairs the normal circulation of yang qi and results in cold extremities.
Re lin (heat dysuria)	热淋	re lin	heat strangury	A urinary tract disorder characterized by frequent urination, painful and burning sensations upon urination, yellow urine, muscle cramps and pain in the lower abdomen, and a bitter taste in the mouth. This condition is caused by damp-heat attacking the lower *jiao*.
Rebellious qi	气逆	qi ni	qi counterflow	Rebellious qi is the flow of qi opposite of its normal or appropriate direction, such as the flow of Lung qi upwards, that leads to coughing.
Ren (conception) channel	任脉	ren mai	conception vessel	The confluence of all yin vessels, one of the eight extraordinary vessels. Also known as the "sea of yin qi," it relates to urogenital, gynecological and obstetrical functions.
Restless fetus	胎动不安	tai dong bu an	stirring fetus	Constant downward movement of the fetus, abdominal pain, sore back, and perhaps bleeding, are generally caused by qi deficiency, blood deficiency, Kidney deficiency, heat in the blood, or external injuries.
Rock-like breast abscess	乳石痈	ru shi yong	rock-like mammary welling-abscess	A rock-hard breast abscess.
Rough pulse	涩脉	se mai	rough pulse	A pulse that does not flow smoothly.
Run (moisten)	润	run		To soak the herbs in water to soften the substances prior to slicing, or to ensure complete extraction prior to cooking in decoctions.
San Jiao	三焦	san jiao	triple burner	The *San Jiao* is not an anatomical organ, but a generalization of different sections of the body compartment. The *San Jiao* is divided into upper, middle and lower sectors.
San Jiao bian zheng (triple burner differentiation)	三焦辨证	san jiao bian zheng	triple burner pattern identification	A system of differential diagnosis based on locating patterns of disharmony in the upper *jiao*, middle *jiao*, or lower *jiao*.
Scallion-stalk pulse	芤脉	kou mai	scallion-stalk pulse	A large superficial pulse that feels empty in the middle upon pressure.
Scattered pulse	散脉	san mai	scattered pulse	A large superficial pulse without root.

Glossary

Chinese Herbal Formulas and Applications

Terminology	Chinese	Pinyin	Wiseman & Feng	Definition
Scoop	合子	*he zi*		A device used to measure herbs, such as *Dan Dou Chi* (Semen Sojae Praeparatum).
Seven emotions	七情	*qi qing*	seven affects	Joy, anger, melancholy, thought (over-thinking), grief, fear and fright. An excess of any of the seven emotions may create illness.
Sha zhang (acute filthy disease)	痧胀	*sha zhang*	sand distention	A disease contracted primarily via ingestion of filthy (raw, dirty or unclean) foods, leading to fever, chest oppression, abdominal distention, nausea, vomiting and diarrhea.
Shang han (cold damage)	伤寒	*shang han*	cold damage	A collective term for disorders caused by cold externally-contracted pathogens, diagnosed and treated via *Liu Jing Bian Zheng* (Six Stages Differentiation).
Shang Han Lun (Discussion of Cold-Induced Disorders)	伤寒论	*shang han lun*	on cold damage	A text written by Zhang Zhong-Jing in the Eastern Han dynasty that focuses on diagnosis and treatment of cold-induced disorders. The basic principles of diagnosis and treatment are based on *Liu Jing Bian Zheng* (Six Stages Differentiation).
Shao (burn)	烧	*shao*	burn	To treat the medicinal substances with heat or fire.
Shaoyang	少阳	*shao yang*	lesser yang	Third of six stages in the paradigm of yin and yang. This term identifies the degree of pathology of disease according to the *Shang Han Lun* (Discussion of Cold-Induced Disorders) text. It also describes the level attributed to the Gallbladder and *San Jiao* channels that travel throughout the body.
Shaoyin	少阴	*shao yin*	lesser yin	The fifth of six stages in the paradigm of yin and yang. This term describes the degree of pathology of disease according to the *Shang Han Lun* (Discussion of Cold-Induced Disorders) text. It also identifies the level attributed to the Heart and Kidney channels that travel throughout the body.
Shen (spirit)	神	*shen*	spirit	A term that refers to the entire presentation of the human being, including energy levels, the state of consciousness, and the ability to think and reason. Because it is housed in the Heart, disorders affecting the Heart may also lead to disturbance of the *shen* (spirit).
Shi (hardness)	实	*shi*	repletion	*Shi* (hardness) is the excess condition in which the dry hard stools are interlocked with heat, causing constipation and abdominal pain that intensifies with palpation.
Shi lin (stone dysuria)	石淋	*shi lin*	stone strangury	A urinary tract disorder characterized by lower abdominal tightness and pain, the presence of sandy particles (and possibly blood) in the urine, difficult and painful urination, or sudden termination of the stream of urine. This is caused by damp-heat attacking the lower *jiao*, drying fluids, and leading to the formation of stones.
Shi yao (envoy herb)	使药	*shi yao*	courier	The fourth of four guiding principles in herbal formulation: *Jun Chen Zuo Shi* (Chief, Deputy, Assistant, Envoy). This herb has two main functions: 1) it acts as a channel-guiding herb to direct the formula to the affected channels/areas of the body; and 2) it harmonizes all of the herbs within the formula. *Shi yao* (envoy herb) is usually used only in small doses.

GLOSSARY

G

1519

Glossary

Terminology	Chinese	Pinyin	Wiseman & Feng	Definition
Shi-re lin (damp-heat dysuria)	湿热淋	*shi re lin*	damp-heat strangury	A urinary tract disorder characterized by frequent urination, painful and burning sensations upon urination, yellow urine, muscle cramps and pain in the lower abdomen, and a bitter taste in the mouth, all caused by damp-heat attacking the lower *jiao*. Other symptoms of damp-heat may include nausea, vomiting, constipation, a yellow, greasy tongue coating, and a slippery, rapid pulse.
Shivering perspiration	战汗	*zhan han*	shivering	Shivering perspiration is a phenomenon that occurs when the body fights against pathogenic factors. The prognosis is good if the patient has a normal temperature after perspiring. The prognosis is poor if the patient becomes fidgety and irritable after perspiring.
Short pulse	短脉	*duan mai*	short pulse	A pulse that can be felt only at *guan* position.
Shu (stream) point	输穴	*shu xue*	stream point	Commonly referred to as "stream" points, these are usually located near the wrists or ankles and suggest that the flow of qi is now of sufficient quantity to carry out these functions.
Shu (transport) point	俞穴	*shu xue*	transport point	Known as "associated points of the back," or "transporting" points, these are twelve points on the upper and lower back where the qi of the internal organs passes. Each represents an organ.
Shui fei (refine with water)	水飞	*shui fei*	water-grinding	A technique to reduce medicinal substances into fine particles by repeatedly grinding them in water.
Skipping pulse	促脉	*cu mai*	skipping pulse	A relatively fast pulse that is broken up by regular pauses.
Slippery pulse	滑脉	*hua mai*	slippery pulse	A pulse that feels smooth and flowing.
Slow pulse	迟脉	*chi mai*	slow pulse	A pulse with three or less beats per respiration.
Small Intestine	小肠	*xiao chang*	small intestine	Connecting to the Stomach and Large Intestine, the Small Intestine absorbs nutrients from food.
Small pulse	小脉	*xiao mai*	small pulse	A fine and well-defined pulse. Same as fine pulse.
Small spoon	钱匕	*qian bi*		A small spoon that contains approximately 1.5-1.8 grams of powdered herbs.
Soggy pulse	濡脉	*ru mai*	soggy pulse	A pulse that is fine and floating.
Sores	疮疡	*chuang yang*	sore	An inclusive term for skin lesions, boils, ulcers, carbuncles and furuncles.
Spleen	脾	*pi*	spleen	The Spleen governs the transportation and transformation of food, controls blood, and dominates muscle. It connects with the Stomach, opens to the mouth, and represents the earth element.
Spontaneous sweating	自汗	*zi han*	spontaneous sweating	Spontaneous perspiration, especially after only mild physical activities, is an indication of *wei* (defensive) *qi* deficiency.
Steaming bones sensation	骨蒸	*gu zheng*	steaming bone	A Kidney disorder characterized by heat and steaming sensations originating from the bone marrow. Accompanying symptoms include bodily coldness in the mornings and warm sensations in the evenings, irritability, restlessness, disturbed sleep, red urine, low back pain, cold hands and feet, and warm palms and soles.

Glossary

Chinese Herbal Formulas and Applications

Terminology	Chinese	Pinyin	Wiseman & Feng	Definition
Stifling sensation	闷	*men*	oppression	An oppressive and congested feeling in the chest that leads to difficulties in breathing deeply.
Stirred pulse	动脉	*dong mai*	stirred pulse	A forceful rapid slippery pulse.
Stomach	胃	*wei*	stomach	Connecting to the mouth through the esophagus, the Stomach receives and decomposes food to facilitate digestion and absorption.
Sudden turmoil	霍乱	*huo luan*	sudden turmoil	An acute disorder characterized by sudden onset of nausea, vomiting, and chest and abdominal pain. Generally occurring in summer and fall, it is usually caused by inappropriate diet, leading to dysfunction of the stomach and intestines.
Summer heat	暑	*shu*	summerheat	Summer heat is a yang pathogenic factor that occurs only in the summer, and is comprised of both heat and damp characteristics, including upward direction and dispersion. Clinical presentations of summer heat include excessive perspiration, thirst, shortness of breath, fatigue, elevated body temperature, heavy sensations in the extremities, poor appetite, and a feeling of congestion in the chest.
Superficial pulse	浮脉	*fu mai*	floating pulse	A pulse that is more pronounced at the superficial level.
Supreme physician	太医	*tai yi*	supreme physician	Physicians that practice in the Imperial Palace to treat the royalties and their court members.
Surging pulse	洪脉	*hong mai*	surging pulse	A pulse that is broad, large and forceful at all three levels.
Sweaty head	头汗	*tou han*	sweating head	Head perspiration generally arises from heat affecting the upper and middle *jiao*s, possibly accompanied by irritability, thirst, a yellow tongue coating, and a rapid pulse.
Taiyang	太阳	*tai yang*	greater yang	First of six stages in the paradigm of yin and yang, identifying the degree of pathology of disease according to the *Shang Han Lun* (Discussion of Cold-Induced Disorders) text. It also names the level attributed to the Small Intestine and Urinary Bladder channels that travel throughout the body.
Taiyin	太阴	*tai yin*	greater yin	The fourth of six stages in the paradigm of yin and yang. This term describes the degree of pathology of disease according to the *Shang Han Lun* (Discussion of Cold-Induced Disorders) text. It also identifies the level attributed to the Spleen and Lung channels that travel throughout the body.
Tan (char to ash)	炭	*tan*		Charring at high temperature until the medicinal substances turn into ash. This method harmonizes and moderates therapeutic effects, reduces side effects, and potentiates the 'stop bleeding' properties of specific substances.
Tan yin (phlegm retention)	痰饮	*tan yin*	phlegm-rheum	Phlegm retention caused by accumulation of water and dampness, this may occur at various organs and tissues in the body, leading to different illnesses and clinical presentations.
Tight pulse	紧脉	*jin mai*	tight pulse	A pulse that is forceful and string-like.

GLOSSARY

G

1521

Glossary

Terminology	Chinese	Pinyin	Wiseman & Feng	Definition
Tong bi (extremely painful obstruction)	痛痹	tong bi	painful impediment	One type of *bi zheng* (painful obstruction syndrome) characterized by cold. Similar to cold that is stationary and constricting, *tong bi* is distinguished by severe pain at a fixed location. This type of pain intensifies with exposure to cold, and is relieved by exposure to warmth.
Toxin	毒	du	toxin	A toxin is any substance that is potentially harmful to the body. 'Toxin' also describes a pathogenic factor that may cause illness either on the exterior or in the interior of the body. Clinical manifestations of toxicity include pus, abscesses, sores, ulcerations, swelling and inflammation.
Tu fa (vomiting)	吐法	tu fa	ejection	A method of treatment that induces emesis to eliminate phlegm, stagnant food, or toxic matters from the throat, chest and diaphragm, or epigastrium. Vomiting induces qi to move upwards and outwards to treat ingestion of poisonous substances, severe cases of food stagnation, sudden turmoil disorder with vomiting and diarrhea, mania and withdrawal caused by phlegm accumulation, and *zhong feng* (wind stroke) with phlegm accumulation.
Tuo zheng (abandoned syndrome)	脱证	tuo zheng	desertion pattern	Characterized by profuse sweating, cold extremities, open mouth and closed eyes, and urinary incontinence, this condition occurs when there is severe exhaustion of yin, yang, qi and blood.
Upper *jiao*	上焦	shang jiao	upper burner	The upper *jiao* represents the chest, and includes functions of the Heart and the Lung.
Urinary Bladder	膀胱	pang guang	bladder	The Urinary Bladder stores and excretes urine.
Uroschesis	癃闭	long bi	dribbling urinary block	A disorder in which there is little or no urination, brought about by any of the following: heat in the Urinary Bladder, Kidney yang deficiency, qi deficiency, qi stagnation, or body fluid deficiencies.
Wan bi (stubborn painful obstruction)	顽痹	wan bi	insensitive impediment	One type of *bi zheng* (painful obstruction syndrome) that generally occurs after chronic or repetitive injuries to the same areas, causing stiffness, numbness, and lack of mobility.
Warm epidemics	温疫	wen yi	warm epidemic	Contagious diseases characterized by heat, with clinical manifestations such as fever, headache, irritability, thirst, vomiting, and with or without sweating.
Water	水	shui	water	Water is one of the five elements, associated with winter, with the Kidney, downward movement, and the ability to store or accumulate.
Water and fluid stagnation	水液停滞	shui ye ting zhi		Obstructed flow of water and thick fluids in the body.
Weak pulse	弱脉	ruo mai	weak pulse	A deep and forceless pulse.
Wei (defensive) level	卫分	wei fen	defense aspect	The first of four levels affected by febrile infections. Heat attacking the *wei* (defensive) level is characterized by disorders of the Lung, with such symptoms as fever, headache, dry mouth, thirst, cough, and sore throat, and a red tongue, and superficial, rapid pulse.

Glossary

Chinese Herbal Formulas and Applications

Terminology	Chinese	Pinyin	Wiseman & Feng	Definition
Wei (defensive) *qi*	卫气	*wei qi*	defense qi	A type of yang qi responsible for warming the exterior, nourishing the skin and muscles, circulating under the skin to prevent invasion by external pathogenic factors, and controlling the skin pores and perspiration. It is generated by the Spleen and Stomach from the essence of food, controlled by the Lung, and resides in the upper *jiao*.
Wei (roast)	煨	*wei*		To cook and parch by wrapping the herbs in wet cloth, paper, or mud, and heating this bundle in hot cinders until the coating has turned black or burned away. This method reduces toxicity or moderates the drastic actions of some herbs.
Wei bi (atrophic painful obstruction)	痿痹	*wei bi*	wilting impediment	One type of *bi zheng* (painful obstruction syndrome) caused by deficiency of the Liver and Kidney, with such presentations as atrophy, weakness and pain of the muscles and bones.
Wei qi ying xue bian zheng (defensive, qi, nutritive, blood differentiation)	卫气营血辨证	*wei qi ying xue bian zheng*	four aspect pattern identification	A system of differential diagnosis based on patterns of disharmony found in the *wei* (defensive) level, *qi* (energy) level, *ying* (nutritive) level or *xue* (blood) level.
Wei zheng (atrophy) syndrome)	痿证	*wei zheng*	wilting pattern	A condition involving decreasing muscle mass and physical strength of the extremities, especially the legs; generally caused by the concurrent presence of excess and deficiency factors.
Wen bing (warm disease)	温病	*wen bing*	warm disease	Acute illnesses caused by externally contracted heat factors: diagnosed and treated based on *Wei Qi Ying Xue Bian Zheng* (Defensive, Qi, Nutritive, Blood Differentiation) and *San Jiao Bian Zheng* (Triple Burner Differentiation).
Wen fa (warming)	温法	*wen fa*	warming	A method of treatment that warms the interior, dispels cold, restores yang, and unblocks channels and collaterals. Warming is usually used to treat the presence of cold affecting the normal functions of *zang fu* organs, or stagnation of cold blocking the channels and collaterals.
Wheezing and dyspnea	哮喘	*xiao chuan*	wheezing and panting	A disorder characterized by wheezing, dyspnea and hurried respiration.
Wind	风	*feng*	wind	Wind is a pathogenic factor that attacks the body through the pores. Wind is a yang pathogenic factor characterized by upward, outward dispersion. Clinical presentation of exterior wind includes headache, nasal obstruction, sore throat, aversion to wind and sweating.
Wind rash	风疹	*feng zhen*	wind papules	An infectious skin disorder commonly seen during winter and spring in children under five years of age. Generally caused by wind-heat attack, it is characterized by itching, rashes and wheals of various sizes.
Wiry pulse	弦脉	*xian mai*	wiry pulse	A pulse that feels like a string of a musical instrument.

GLOSSARY

G

1523

Glossary

Terminology	Chinese	Pinyin	Wiseman & Feng	Definition
Wood	木	*mu*	wood	One of the five elements, wood represents the expansive energy of Spring, moving outward in all directions, and is associated with the Liver.
Wu shu (five transport) points	五輸穴	*wu shu xue*	five transport points	Located below the knees and elbows, these points represent the growth of qi from small to large volume. Their name suggests images of the flow of water. It starts with only a small quantity in a *jing* (well), gushes out into a *ying* (spring), flows from shallow to deep as a *shu* (stream), traverses like a *jing* (river) through the continent, and finally unites with the *he* (sea).
Wu xin re (five-center heat)	五心热	*wu xin re*	vexing heat in the five hearts	A condition characterized by yin-deficient heat in which there is a warm sensation in the middle of the chest, palms and soles.
Xi (cleft) point	郄穴	*xi xue*	cleft point	"Accumulating" or "cleft" points represent the holes or crevices where circulating qi accumulates. There are a total of sixteen such points, one for each of the twelve regular channels, as well as the *yangqiao*, *yinqiao*, *yangwei* and *yinwei* channels.
Xi (wash)	洗	*xi*		To remove unwanted substances or odor with water.
Xia fa (draining downwards)	下法	*xia fa*	precipitation	A method of treatment that cleanses the Stomach and Intestines, induces defecation, and eliminates pathogenic accumulation from the body. This method is generally used to treat stagnant food, dry stools, cold accumulation, hot accumulation, blood stasis, phlegm stagnation, water stagnation, and parasitic infestation.
Xiao fa (reducing)	消法	*xiao fa*	dispersion	A method of treatment that dissolves and disperses hardness and nodules to treat accumulation and stagnation of various substances, such as food, qi, blood, phlegm, water, and parasites. Reducing may be used to treat a wide variety of illness due to various causes.
Xiao ke (wasting and thirsting)	消渴	*xiao ke*	dispersion-thirst	A pathological condition characterized by increased intake of water and food, increased frequency of urination, and decreased body weight.
Xing bi (mobile painful obstruction)	行痹	*xing bi*	moving impediment	One type of *bi zheng* (painful obstruction syndrome) caused by wind attacking the body. Similar to wind that is light and mobile, *xing bi* is characterized by pain in the upper body, specifically pain that travels from one area to another.
Xiong bi (painful obstruction of the chest)	胸痹	*xiong bi*	chest impediment	Characterized by feelings of chest congestion, pain and discomfort, this condition is usually caused by factors such as cold excess, yang deficiency, or phlegm stagnation.
Xuan yin (pleural effusion)	悬饮	*xuan yin*	suspended rheum	Accumulation of *yin* (invisible phlegm) in the chest and hypochondrium causing pain with coughing, breathing, and rotation of the trunk.
Xue (blood) level	血分	*xue fen*	blood aspect	*Xue* (blood) level refers to the fourth level of febrile infections. Heat attacking the *xue* level is characterized by disorders of the Heart and Liver, with such symptoms as high fever, anger, mania, various types of bleeding, delirium, convulsions and clenched jaws.

Chinese Herbal Formulas and Applications

Glossary

Terminology	Chinese	Pinyin	Wiseman & Feng	Definition
Xue bi (blood painful obstruction)	血痹	*xue bi*	blood impediment	One type of *bi zheng* (painful obstruction syndrome) that is related to blood. Dull pain may be caused by blood deficiency and the inability to nourish the tendons and bones. Sharp pain is often related to blood stagnation blocking the channels and collaterals.
Xue lin (bloody dysuria)	血淋	*xue lin*	blood strangury	A urinary tract disorder characterized by the presence of blood or blood clots in the urine, and burning sensations and pain during urination. Accompanying symptoms may include fatigue, back pain, a pale red tongue, and a fine, rapid pulse. This condition is caused by damp-heat attacking the lower *jiao*, leading to bleeding and obstructed flow of qi and urine.
Ya (press)	軋	*ya*		To push or squeeze into small particles. This methods increases the surface area and enhances extraction of active ingredients.
Yan (drown)	淹	*yan*		To soak or steep in water or other liquids.
Yan (grind)	研	*yan*	grinding	To reduce into small particles with a mortar and pestle. This methods increases the surface area and enhances extraction of active ingredients.
Yang	阳	*yang*	yang	Yang is the complement to and opposite of yin. Anatomically, it represents the upper, posterior and exterior parts of the body. Physiologically, it represents body functioning, such as the energy level, rate of metabolism, and state of awareness. Pathologically, it represents disharmony or imbalance of body organs.
Yang (melt)	烊	*yang*		To dissolve or disintegrate in water or other liquids.
Yangming	阳明	*yang ming*	yang brightness	Second of the six stages in the paradigm of yin and yang, this term describes the degree of pathology of disease according to the *Shang Han Lun* (Discussion of Cold-Induced Disorders) text. It also identifies the level given the Stomach and Large Intestine channels that travel throughout the body.
Yangqiao (movement) channel	阳跷脉	*yang qiao mai*	yang springing vessel	Of the eight extraordinary vessels, this one pairs with *yinqiao* to maintain proper sleep cycles and control movement and balance.
Yangwei (linking) channel	阳维脉	*yang wei mai*	yang linking vessel	Of the eight extraordinary vessels, this one dominates the exterior in cooperation with *yinwei*, to balance yin and yang in the four extremities.
Ye (thick body fluid)	液	*ye*	humor	An inclusive term that describes body fluids of higher density, such as the fluid that lubricates the joints and moistens the bone marrow.
Yi (intellect)	意	*yi*	intellect	The ability to think, study, memorize, focus, understand, and all other cognitive activities. It resides in the Spleen. Therefore, excessive use of *yi* may consume the Spleen, and deficiency of the Spleen may interfere with the optimal performance of *yi* (intellect).

GLOSSARY

G

1525

Glossary

Terminology	Chinese	Pinyin	Wiseman & Feng	Definition
Yin	阴	*yin*	yin	Yin is the complement to and opposite of yang. Anatomically, it represents the lower, anterior and interior parts of the body. Physiologically, it represents the substances of the body, such as blood, sweat, saliva and body fluids. Pathologically, it represents the disharmony or imbalance of body organs.
Yin (invisible phlegm)	饮	*yin*	rheum	*Yin* (invisible phlegm) is the by-product formed from stagnation of water and dampness. *Yin* is the less viscous form of *tan* (phlegm).
Yin shui (yin edema)	阴水	*yin shui*	yin water	A type of edema caused by yang qi deficiency, with generalized deficiency and cold manifestations such as cold hands and feet and loose stools.
Ying (nutritive) level	营分	*ying fen*	construction aspect	The *ying* (nutritive) level refers to the third of four levels of febrile infections. Heat attacking the *ying* level is characterized by disorders of the Heart, with such symptoms as fever, thirst, irritability, delirium, red tongue and fine, rapid pulse.
Ying (nutritive) qi	营气	*ying qi*	construction qi	The qi produced by Spleen and Stomach and circulates within blood vessels to nourish the entire body.
Ying (spring) point	荥穴	*ying xue*	spring point	"Gushing" or "spring" points are located in distal parts of the body; their name suggests that qi has begun to flow in larger quantity.
Yinqiao (movement) channel	阴跷脉	*yin qiao mai*	yin springing vessel	Of the eight extraordinary vessels, this one pairs with *yangqiao* to maintain proper sleep cycles and control movement and balance.
Yinwei (linking) channel	阴维脉	*yin wei mai*	yin linking vessel	Another of the eight extraordinary vessels: in cooperation with *yangwei*, this one dominates the interior; to balance yin and yang in the four extremities.
Yuan (source) point	原穴	*yuan xue*	source point	Known as "source" points, these are locations to which the qi of the organs flows and is retained. There are twelve such points, each representing a channel and an organ.
Yuan (source) qi	原气	*yuan qi*	source qi	The most basic and most important qi in the body, *yuan* (source) *qi* is derived prenatally from the *jing* (essence) of one's parents, and postnatally from the essence of food. It is distributed throughout the body to maintain health and well-being.
Zang (solid organ)	脏	*zang*	viscus	Solid organs of the body, including the Heart, Lung, Spleen, Liver and Kidney.
Zang du (solid organ toxin)	脏毒	*zang du*	visceral toxin	A condition caused by presence of toxin attacking the solid organ leading to dysentery with presence of dark black blood in the stools.
Zang fu	脏腑	*zang fu*	bowels and viscera	The general term for the five *zang* (solid) and six *fu* (hollow) organs.
Zang fu bian zheng (organ pattern differentiation)	脏腑辨证	*zang fu bian zheng*	organ pattern identification	A system of differential diagnosis based on patterns of disharmony of *zang* (solid) organs and *fu* (hollow) organs.

Glossary

Chinese Herbal Formulas and Applications

Terminology	Chinese	Pinyin	Wiseman & Feng	Definition
Zang zao (restless organ)	脏躁	zang zao	visceral agitation	In middle-aged to geriatric women, this disorder is characterized by symptomology such as emotional instability, mental confusion, crying, episodes of extreme sadness or happiness, and increased sensitivity to stimulus.
Zao (dryness)	燥	zao	dryness	*Zao* (dryness) refers to the dry compacted stool, which feels hard upon abdominal palpation.
Zha (crush)	砸	zha		To reduce medicinal substances into particles by pounding. This method increases the surface area and enhances extraction of active ingredients.
Zheng (steam)	蒸	zheng	steam	A preparation method to heat the medicinal substances with steam. This method indirectly introduces heat and water to the herbs to alter the therapeutic effect or reducing toxicity.
Zheng (upright) *qi*	正气	zheng qi	right qi	A term that summarizes the positive strength generated by healthy functioning of the organs. In comparison to the pathogenic factors, *zheng* (upright) *qi* also represents one's immunity.
Zhi (fry with liquid)	炙	zhi	mix-frying	Stir-frying with liquid to improve effectiveness, enhance smell, or reduce side effects. Liquids used for frying include honey, grain-based liquor, vinegar, ginger juice, and salt water.
Zhi (prepared)	制	zhi	prepare	To process medicinal substances with different methods.
Zhi (will-power)	志	zhi	mind	A term that encompasses will-power and memory. Stored by the Kidney, *zhi* controls drive, determination, motivation, memory and will-power.
Zhong (central) *qi*	中气	zhong qi	center qi	The qi of the middle *jiao* represents the healthy functioning of the Spleen and Stomach to transport and transform food and nutrients.
Zhong feng (wind stroke)	中风	zhong feng	wind stroke	An acute disorder of semi- or un-consciousness, deviation of the eyes or mouth, hemiparalysis, and difficulty with speech. The cause of the illness is predominantly wind, but this may be accompanied by blood deficiency, phlegm, fire, or other pathogens.
Zhong qi (qi stroke)	中气	zhong qi	qi stroke	A condition characterized by stagnated or reversed flow of qi, caused by internal injuries, accumulation of dampness and phlegm, or imbalance of the seven emotions.
Zhou bi (generalized painful obstruction)	周痹	zhou bi	generalized impediment	One type of *bi zheng* (painful obstruction syndrome) characterized by generalized pain that also affects the bones and joints.
Zhu (boiling)	煮	zhu	boil	Cooking certain medicinal substances in boiling water or another medium to enhance the therapeutic effect or reduce toxicity.
Zhuo bi (fixed painful obstruction)	著痹	zhuo bi	fixed impediment	One type of *bi zheng* (painful obstruction syndrome) that often occurs when dampness affects specific, fixed areas. Similar to dampness that is heavy and sinking, *zhuo bi* is characterized by pain and swelling in the lower extremities.

Glossary

Terminology	Chinese	Pinyin	Wiseman & Feng	Definition
Zong (essential) *qi*	宗气	*zong qi*	ancestral qi	*Zong* (essential) *qi* is derived from air taken in by the Lung, and nutrients absorbed by the Spleen and Stomach. It functions to maintain proper ventilation of the Lung and circulation of the Heart.
Zuo yao (assistant herb)	佐药	*zuo yao*	assistant	The third of four guiding principles in herbal formulation: *Jun Chen Zuo Shi* (Chief, Deputy, Assistant, Envoy). This herb has three main functions: 1) it reinforces the effect of *jun yao* (chief herb) or *chen yao* (deputy herb) to treat the disease, or directly treats the secondary symptoms; 2) it counteracts the toxicity or minimizes the drastic effects of the *jun yao* (chief herb) or *chen yao* (deputy herb); and 3) it has an opposite effect as, but works in synergy with, the *jun yao* (chief herb) to treat the most serious and complex disorders.

Index

Words in bold indicate primary formula and chapter names.
Page numbers in **bold** indicate main entries.
Page numbers in ***bold italics*** indicate entries in Appendix or Glossary.

3 TC. *See* Lamivudine
5 FU. *See* 5-fluorouracil
5-fluorouracil, 214, 612, 617
A New Study of Dermatomycosis and Dermatitis, 1348
A Selection of Famous Physicians' Prescriptions, 810
A Selection of Traditional Prescriptions of Chinese Medicine, 113
Abandoned syndrome, 743, ***1522***. *See also Tuo zheng* (abandoned syndrome)
Abdomen
  acute, **167, 1273**
  enlarged, 1297
  enlarged and distended, 1299
Abdominal
  coldness, **482**
  coldness and pain, 282, 479
  distention and pain, 149, 159, 578
  distention, drum-like, 1127, ***1509***
  fullness
    damp-heat, 1086
    damp-warmth, 1096
    overview, 149, 281, 1264
    taiyang and *yangming* syndromes, 289
  fullness and distention
    dampness, 1068, 1076
    food stagnation with heat, 1277
    interior excess heat, 152, 158
    overview, 149, 819, 1064
    severe, 1127
  fullness and pain, 463, 531, 571
    excess cold accumulation, 171
    food stagnation, 1270
    overview, 202, 455
    qi stagnation, 822
  fullness, distention and oppression, 1127
  fullness, distention and pain
    damp-cold in the Spleen and Stomach, 840
    food stagnation, 1266
    food stagnation and damp-heat accumulation, 1272
  hardness and pain, 187
  mass, 885, 889
  pain, ***1399***
    acute, 911
    blood accumulation in the lower *jiao*, 873
    blood and yin deficiencies, 593
    blood deficiency and heat, 575
    blood stagnation, 885, 933
    in children, **264**
    cold *bi zheng* (closed disorder), 759
    damp accumulation, 1072
    damp-heat, 403, 406, 1101
    deficiency and cold, 459, 471, 476, 784, 787
    excess cold accumulation, 166
    fixed area, 885
    gastric pain, **601**
    heat in the chest and cold in the Stomach, 271
    in infants and children, **473**
    intermittent, severe, 1301
    due to intestinal parasites, 481, 1297, 1301
    Kidney yang deficiency, 668, 673
    Liver qi stagnation, 238

    lower abdomen, 889
    overview, 149, 316, 456, 1263, 1289
    palpation, worse with, 1379
    postpartum, 911
    post-surgical, 482
    during pregnancy, 594, **596**
    pressure and warmth, relieved by, 471, 476, 781
    qi and blood stagnation, 915
    qi deficiency with dampness and phlegm, **528**
    qi stagnation with heat, 825
    due to roundworms, 1292
    shaoyin syndrome, 233, 486
    sharp, 911
    Spleen and Stomach deficiencies, 541
    Spleen and Stomach disharmony, 1074
    Spleen deficiency and Liver excess, 257
    Spleen qi deficiency, **524**
    Spleen yang deficiency with cold, 169
    toxic heat, 408
    water accumulation, 1125
    yang deficiency with excess cold, 491
    yang deficiency with water accumulation, 1135
    yin and yang deficiencies, 798
    yin, blood and body fluid deficiencies, 600
  pulsations on the skin, 481
  rigidity, 152
  swelling and distention, 1379
Abortion. *See* Miscarriage; Pregnancy
Abscesses. *See also* Sores
  appendicular, 1325, **1327**
  bones, 1347
  breast, **1327**, 1347, ***1403, 1506***
  breast, rock-like, ***1518***
  chronic, 479, 1369
  cold, dampness, phlegm and blood stasis, 1375
  damp-heat in all three *jiaos*, 359
  early onset/stage, 1325, 1334
  face and neck, 1332
  generalized, **1327**
  heat and toxins, 291, 1325
  heat, fire and toxins in all three *jiaos*, 341
  hepatic, **898**
  intestinal, 1347, 1350, 1379, 1382, 1383, ***1417, 1513***
  late-stage, 1369
  legs, 1347
  localized, 1332
  lower extremities, **344**
  lung/pulmonary, 1229, 1230, 1232, 1350, 1377, **1378, *1418, 1515***
  malignant, 1349
  mid- to late-stages, 1364
  multiple, 1350, 1370, 1375
  overview, 1321
  periappendicular, **1380**
  peritonsillar, **1328**
  with pus, 1362
  with pus and discharge, 479, 1364
  qi and blood deficiencies, 479, 1367, 1369
  qi deficiency, 1362
  red, hot, hard and painful, 1331

1529

Index

with redness, localized, 1325
with redness, swelling and pain, 1332, 1334
with swelling, burning sensations and pain, 1362
wind-heat, 1332
yang (superficial), 1321, 1350
yin (deep-rooted), 1321, 1375
Abscesses and sores
external, 1321
internal, 1322
intestines, 1323
lungs, 1323
overview, 1321
Absent-mindedness, 731, 735
Accumulation, *1394*, *1505*
blood, 302
cold, 302
cold, dampness, qi, blood and phlegm, 302
dampness, 302
five types of, 301
overview, 1263
phlegm, 302
qi, 302
ACE inhibitors. *See* Angiotensin-converting enzyme inhibitors
Acetaminophen, 62
Acetylcholine, 344, 846
Aches. *See also* Pain
general, 1167
throughout the body, 1175
Achievements Regarding Epidemic Rashes, 7, 337
Achieving Longevity by Guarding the Source, 1319
Acid reflux/regurgitation, *1399*
accumulations in the interior, 302
damp accumulation, 1068, 1076
deficiency and cold of the Stomach, 467
deficiency and cold with qi stagnation, 484
food stagnation, 1266
heat in the chest and cold in the Stomach, 271
Liver fire overacting on the Stomach, 389
overview, 455, 819, 820, 1064, 1263
phlegm and dampness, 1077
phlegm-heat, 1235
qi deficiency with phlegm stagnation, 851
qi stagnation, 822
taiyang and *shaoyang* syndromes, 219
yin deficiency with qi stagnation and blood dryness, 657
Acne, *1399*. *See also* Pimples
excess fire in the Liver and Gallbladder channels, **380**
fire and toxins, 1337
heat and toxins, 291, 1342
heat, fire and toxins in all three *jiaos*, **344**
rashes, 597, **1343**
wind, heat and toxins in the upper body, 349
wind-heat, 120
Acne vulgaris, 576, **1343**
Aconite, Ginger and Licorice Combination, 486
Aconite, Ginseng and Ginger Combination, 463
Aconite, Ginseng and Ginger Decoction (Pill), 463
Aconite Middle-Regulating Decoction (Pill), 463
Aconitine, 235, 296, 590, 629
ACTH. *See* Adrenocorticotropic hormone
Acute filthy disease, 757, *1519*. *See also Sha zhang* (acute filthy disease)
Adaptogenic effect, 544, 629, 658, 679, 688
ADD. *See* Attention deficit disorder; Concentration
Addiction, **586**
drug, **470**

withdrawal reactions from, **470**
Addison's disease, *1399*
Additions to the Teachings for [Zhu] Dan-Xi, 1238
Adenocarcinoma, thyroid, 1353
Adenoids, 243
Adenoma, thyroid, **630**
Adenomyosis, 929, 931
Adnexitis, **236**, **597**, **930**
Adrenal cortex, effect on the, 76
Adrenal glands, 461. *See* Adrenocorticotropic hormone; Adrenergic effect
Adrenalin. *See* Epinephrine
Adrenaline, 296, 590, 629
Adrenergic effect, 1044
Adrenoceptors, 76, 98
Adrenocortical
effect, 461
insufficiency, *1399*
Adrenocorticotropic hormone (ACTH), 76, 223, 266, 530, 830
Adriamycin, 612
Adverse reactions. *See* individual formula monographs
Affective disorders, 255
Affective psychosis, 249
Agastache Formula, 1079
Agastache Genuine-Qi Powder (Pill), 1079
Agastache Powder to Rectify the Qi, 1079
Agastache Qi-Regulating Formula (Pill), 1079
Agastache, Magnolia Bark, Pinellia, and Poria Decoction, 1095
Aging, premature, 682, 690. *See also* Antiaging effect
Agoraphobia, 830
Ah shi point, 1151, *1505*
Ai Fu Nuan Gong Wan (Mugwort and Cyperus Pill for Warming the Womb), 923
vs. Wen Jing Tang (Warm the Channels Decoction), 924
Ai Ye (Folium Artemisiae Argyi), 1287
Alanine aminotransferase (ALT), 60. *See also* Serum glutamic pyruvic transaminase (SGPT)
Alcohol
intoxication, 1085
liver damage, 223
poisoning, 1218, *1425*
Aldosteronism, *1400*
All New Collection of Cold-Induced Disorders, 1331
Allergic
colitis, 403
dermatitis, drug-induced, 334
ophthalmia, 1342
purpura, *1426*
blood stagnation, 895
exterior-deficient, wind-cold, 54
Heart and Spleen deficiencies, 584
heat in the *xue* (blood) level, 333
rhinitis
acute or chronic, 83
blood deficiency, **567**
blood deficiency and blood stagnation, **573**
blood deficiency with wind-cold, **497**
damp-heat, **375**
deficiency and cold of the middle *jiao*, **477**
exterior-deficient, wind-cold, 51
exterior-excess, wind-cold, 39
perennial, **85**
qi and blood deficiencies, **479**
shaoyang syndrome, **212**
Spleen and Stomach qi deficiencies, **547**
wei (defensive) *qi* deficiency, **775**

1530

Index

wind-cold, 59
wind-cold with interior heat, **47**
wind-cold with water accumulation, **77**
sinusitis, **1137**
Allergy, 84, 441, 444, *1400*. *See also* Antiallergic effect
All-Inclusive Great Tonifying Decoction, 609
Alopecia, **691**, **972**, **1031**, *1400*. *See also* Hair
Alpha-naphthylisothiocyanate, 244
ALT (alanine aminotransferase), 60. *See also* Serum glutamic
pyruvic transaminase (SGPT)
Altitude stress, **1094**
Alumen, xxv
Alzheimer's disease, **556**, **998**. *See also* Dementia; Antiamnestic
effect; Antidementia effect
Amenorrhea, *1400*
due to abnormal development of the uterus, **581**
blood accumulation in the lower *jiao*, 873
blood and yin deficiencies, 593
blood stagnation, **883**, 885, 889, **930**, 933
blood stasis, 911, 932
deficiency and cold, 919, **921**
deficiency and injury, 562
interior cold with yang qi and blood deficiencies, **497**
Kidney yang deficiency, **1136**
Kidney yin and *jing* (essence) deficiencies, **647**
Kidney yin and yang deficiencies with fire, 684
Liver qi stagnation, 238
overview, 867
qi and blood deficiencies, 619
Amoebic dysentery, **297**, 787
Ampicillin, 969
An Chung San, 484
An Gong Niu Huang Wan **(Calm the Palace Pill with Cattle**
Gallstone), 746
vs. Zhi Bao Dan (Greatest Treasure Special Pill), 749
vs. Zi Xue Dan (Purple Snow Pill), 749
An Shen Tang **(Tranquilize the Spirit Decoction)**, 733
An Shen Wan (Tranquilize the Spirit Pill), 710
An Zhong San **(Calm the Middle Powder)**, 484
An Zhung San, 484
Anal
fissures, **191**, 945
sinusitis, **1328**
Analgesic effect, 53, 65, 94, 220, 263, 343, 464, 487, 576, 600, 894,
904, 975, 1163, 1170, 1178, 1345
Analytical Collection of Medical Formulas, 13, 85, 104, 371, 479,
533, 653, 654, 656, 663, 672, 690, 789, 800, 976, 985, 1036,
1084, 1141, 1224, 1229, 1268, 1330, 1367
Anaphylaxis, 133
Ancylostomiasis (hookworms), 1289, **1294**, 1302
Androgen, 673
Anemarrhena, Phellodendron and Rehmannia Formula, 636
Anemarrhena, Phellodendron, and Rehmannia Pill, 636
Anemia
aplastic, **655**, **686**, **692**, *1400*
blood deficiency, 562
deficiency and cold of the middle *jiao*, 471
deficiency and damage, 951
Heart blood deficiency, 735
hemolytic, *1400*
hypochromic, 594, **597**
iron deficiency, **586**, *1400*
pernicious, 476, 542
postpartum, 562, 625
qi and blood deficiencies, 580, **605**, **617**
qi, blood and yang deficiencies, **611**

Anemone Combination, 408
Angelica and Mastic Combination, 1330
Angelica Pubescens and Taxillus Decoction, 1161
Anger, 707. *See also* Irritability
Angina, *1400*
blood stagnation, 879
cold *bi zheng* (closed disorder), 759
and coronary artery disease, **913**
and coronary heart disease, 591
decreased blood perfusion, **597**
Heart and Kidney deficiencies, **727**
heat and toxins, 363
qi and blood stagnation, 915
qi and phlegm stagnation, 760
qi and yin deficiencies, **555**
shaoyang syndrome, **212**
taiyang, yangming and *shaoyang* disorders, 716
Angioneurotic headache, **975**
Angiotensin-converting enzyme inhibitors, 1042
Anhidrosis, 39, **47**
Ankylosing spondylitis, **1163**, **1189**
Ano-rectal anomaly, 482
Anorexia, *1401*. *See also* Appetite
in children, **252**, **477**, **533**, **1070**, **1275**
qi, blood, yang and *jing* (essence) deficiencies, 682
shaoyang syndrome with water accumulation, 222
Anovulation, **224**, **921**
Antelope Horn and Uncaria Decoction, 993
Antiaging effect, 544, 611, 669
Antiallergic effect, 76, 133, 209, 372, 544, 829, 968, 1227
Antiamnestic effect, 997
Antiandrogenic effect, 673
Antiarrhythmic effect, 235, 293, 296, 590, 629
Antiasthmatic effect, 76, 81, 98, 844, 846, 1211, 1246
Antibacterial effect, 46, 60, 296, 357, 372, 1081, 1104, 1338, 1380
Antibiotic effect, 41, 53, 93, 154, 158, 258, 285, 332, 357, 372,
394, 404, 409, 544, 1034, 1293. *See also* Antibacterial effect;
Antiviral effect; Antifungal effect; specific pathogens
Anticancer effect, 544, 611
Anticoagulant effect, 655, 869, 874, 881, 907, 926
Anticonvulsant effect, 997
Antidementia effect, 997
Antidepressant effect, 246, 544, 717
Antidiabetic effect, 325
Antidiarrheal effect, 343, 785
Antidiuretic effect, 795
Antidote. *See* Poisoning
Antiemetic effect, 468, 1081
Antiepileptic effect, 978
Antifibrotic effect, 1087
Antihyperglycemic effect, 285
Antihyperlipidemic effect, 285, 343, 572, 617, 688, 874, 881, 907,
1088
Antihypertensive effect, 343, 673, 685, 718, 1000, 1005, 1111
Anti-inflammatory effect, 53, 60, 65, 90, 93, 133, 209, 220, 285,
343, 372, 394, 404, 487, 555, 564, 572, 576, 748, 808, 844, 875,
890, 894, 904, 920, 929, 975, 1055, 1157, 1159, 1163, 1170,
1193, 1227, 1380
Antimetastatic effect, 209, 610
Antineoplastic effect, 523, 528, 610
Antinociceptive effect, 246, 544, 717
Antioxidant effect, 343, 564, 595, 685, 929, 997, 1380
Antiparasitic effect, 1289, 1293
Antiparasitic formulas, 1289
Antiplatelet effect, 564, 581, 655, 679, 869, 874, 881, 907, 912, 918,
929, 997, 1163

Index

Antipruritic effect, 326, 564, 576
Antipsychotic drugs, 175, 256, 482
Antipyretic effect, 60, 65, 129, 296, 322, 332, 334, 342, 748, 975, 1055, 1097, 1157
Antirheumatic effect, 1183
Antispasmodic effect, 285, 1081
Antitumor effect, 209, 272, 564, 610, 611
Antitussive effect, 41, 81, 98, 129, 844, 846, 1044, 1211, 1236, 1239, 1246
Antiulcer effect, 209, 220, 263, 285, 343, 460, 472, 532, 576, 585, 658
Antiviral effect, 41, 60, 76, 357, 544, 771, 774
Anuria
    damp-heat, 1103
    Kidney yang deficiency, 668, 673
    postpartum, 191, 542
    water and damp accumulation, 186
Anus
    burning sensations, 403, 408
    eczema, 344
Anxiety. See also Anxiolytic effect
    blood and yin deficiencies, 593
    Heart fire, 710
    Liver qi stagnation, 247
    Liver qi stagnation with heat, 254
    phlegm retention with yang deficiency, 1131
    taiyang, yangming and shaoyang disorders, 716
Anxiolytic effect, 255, 829
Ao (simmer), 1505
Aphasia, 694, 1002
Aphonia, 1401
Aphtha, 577
Aplastic anemia, 655, 686, 692, 1400
Apnea, sleep, 360, 829
Apoplexy, 999
Apothecary, 1439
Appendicitis, 1401
    acute, 154, 158, 160, 171, 233, 1325, 1380
    acute and chronic, 1383
    chronic, 219, 839, 1380
    exterior-deficient, wind-cold, 51
    heat and toxins, 363
    overview, 1324
    ruptured, 1380
Appendicular abscesses, 1325, 1327
Appetite
    decreased/low/poor
        damp-cold in the Spleen and Stomach, 840
        dampness, 1068, 1076
        dampness and phlegm, 1077
        food stagnation, 1266
        Heart and Spleen deficiencies, 583
        Liver qi stagnation, 849
        overview, 513, 819, 1064, 1264
        qi and blood deficiencies, 604
        qi deficiency, 522
        qi deficiency with dampness, 536
        qi stagnation and food retention, 1274
        qi, blood and yang deficiencies, 609
        Spleen and Stomach deficiencies, 541
        Spleen deficiency, 534
    lack of/loss of
        damp-heat, 1085
        deficiency and cold, 459
        deficiency and cold of the Spleen and Kidney, 784
        heat and cold, interlocked, 1280
        due to intestinal parasites, 1297

overview, 201, 202, 455, 513, 1021
    qi deficiency, 522
    qi deficiency with cold and dampness, 531
    qi deficiency with dampness and phlegm, 527
    Spleen and Stomach disharmony, 1074
    summer-heat damaging qi and body fluids, 446
    weakness and deficiency, 370
Apprehension. See Stress; Anxiety
Apraxia, 1002
Apricot and Perilla Powder, 1025
Apricot Kernel and Perilla Leaf Decoction, 70
Apricot Kernel and Perilla Leaf Powder, 1025
Apricot Seed and Linum Formula, 174
Apricot Seed and Perilla Formula, 1025
Apricot Seed and Perilla Pediatric Formula, 70
Aqueous flare, 343, 382
    post-surgical, 62, 345
Arcane Essentials from the Imperial Library, 6, 135, 299, 341, 752, 847, 961, 986
Arctium Combination, 386
Arctium Decoction to Release the Muscle Layer, 1332
Areca Nine Decoction plus Evodia and Poria, 1123
Areca Seed and Chaenomeles Formula, 1183
Areca Seed Combination, 1123
Arms
    aches and pain, 1175
    pain, 915, 1159, 1195, 1219
    pain, severe, 1171
Arnebia and Oyster Shell Decoction, 1348
Arrest Seizures Pill, 1251
Arrest Wheezing Decoction, 845
Arrhythmia, 1401. See also Antiarrhythmic effect
    aconitine-induced, 293, 296
    adrenaline-induced, 296
    and coronary heart disease, 590
    Heart fire, 710
    qi and blood deficiencies, 589
    qi and yin deficiencies, 555
    various types, 221
    yang deficiency with water accumulation, 1135
Arrival of qi, 1508. See also De qi (arrival of qi)
Artemisia and Hoelen Five Formula, 1090
Artemisia Annua and Scutellaria Decoction to Clear the Gallbladder, 227
Artemisia Annua and Soft-Shelled Turtle Shell Decoction, 412
Artemisia Annua Decoction, 412
Artemisia Combination, 1086
Artemisia Scoparia and Five-Ingredient Powder with Poria, 1090
Artemisia Scoparia Decoction, 1086
Artemisia Scoparia Decoction for Frigid Extremities, 1089
Artemisia Scoparia Decoction to Expel Stone, 1089
Arteries
    hardening of, 996
    restenosis of coronary artery, 719
Arteriosclerosis. See also Atherosclerosis
    cerebral, 551
    damp-heat in all three jiaos, 359
    Liver excess, 996
    prevention of, 343
    wind-heat with interior heat, 291
Arteriosclerosis obliterans, 908
Arteriosclerotic gangrene, 1345
Arteriostenosis, 668, 673
Arthralgia
    accumulations in the interior, 302
    damp-heat, 1192

Chinese Herbal Formulas and Applications

Index

exterior excess with interior deficiency, 1169
paclitaxel-induced, 602
throughout the body, 1175
wind, 991
wind, cold, dampness and heat, 1172
wind, heat and dampness, 1188
wind-dampness, 1173
Arthritis, *1401. See also* Analgesic effect; Anti-inflammatory
effect; *Bi zheng* (painful obstruction syndrome); specific
conditions
accumulations in the interior, 302
blood stagnation, **894**
chronic, 652
cold and dampness, 1134
damp-heat, **1189**, 1190, 1192
damp-warmth, 1092
exterior excess with interior deficiency, 1169
fire in the Liver and Gallbladder channels, 379
gout, **639**, 1159, 1186, **1189**, *1413*
osteoarthritis, *1422*
overview, 1155
qi and blood deficiencies, **582**
rheumatoid, 64, 101, **133**, **224**, **323**, 494, 877, **895**, 1101, **1120**,
1135, 1156, 1159, **1163**, 1173, 1182, 1186, *1427*
throughout the body, 1175
wind and heat with qi and blood deficiencies, 986
wind attacking the channels and collaterals, 988
wind with interior qi deficiency, **1120**
wind with qi deficiency, 984
wind, cold and dampness, 1167, **1179**, 1182
wind, cold, dampness and heat, 64, 1172
wind, heat and dampness, 1186, 1188
wind-cold with interior heat, 45
wind-dampness, 1173
Arthroncus, knee, 1370
Asada's Prescriptions, 164
Ascariasis (roundworms), 1292
biliary, **170**, **235**, **285**, 380, 482, 826, **1294**
in children, **1294**
heat in the Stomach and cold in the Intestines, 1292
intestinal, 1301
intestinal obstruction, **1293**
overview, 1289
Ascites, *1401*
cold damaging the Stomach and Spleen, 1113
excess water retention in the interior, 181
exterior wind with interior qi deficiency, 1118
heat formation and qi stagnation, 184
due to liver cirrhosis, **1111**, 1127
overview, 150
qi stagnation and damp-heat accumulation, 1272
water accumulation, 1129
water and damp accumulation, 186
water stagnation, 1127
yang deficiency, 1138
Aspartate aminotransferase (AST). *See* Serum glutamic
oxaloacetic transaminase (SGOT)
Aspirin, 287, 345, 360, 390, 391
Ass-Hide Gelatin and Egg Yolk Decoction, 1007
Ass-Hide Gelatin and Mugwort Decoction, 950
Ass-Hide Gelatin Powder, 1039
Assistant herb, 14, *1528. See also Zuo yao* (assistant herb)
AST (aspartate aminotransferase). *See* Serum glutamic
oxaloacetic transaminase (SGOT)
Aster Combination, 1229
Aster Decoction, 1229

Asthenopia, 665
Asthma, *1402. See also* Wheezing; Dyspnea; Antiasthmatic effect
bronchial
chronic, **211**, **847**
deficiency heat, 558
heat, lingering or residual, 327
in infants, 53
Kidney deficiency, **630**
Kidney yang deficiency, **1137**
Kidney yin deficiency, 644
Lung heat, 96
Lung heat with phlegm accumulation, 1232
Lung yin deficiency with heat, 1039
phlegm and damp accumulation, 1224
phlegm retention and qi stagnation, **1246**
prevention of, **680**
qi and phlegm stagnation, 848
shaoyang syndrome with phlegm stagnation, 226
shaoyin with *taiyang* syndrome, 132
upper excess and lower deficiency, 842
water accumulation, 1125
due to bronchitis, 80, **846**
cardiac, 1125, 1226
chronic, 558
exterior-excess, wind-cold, 39
heat-phlegm, 1214
Kidney and Lung yin deficiencies, 643
Kidney yang deficiency, **670**, 673
Kidney yin deficiency, 644
Liver qi stagnation, **849**
Lung and Kidney yin deficiencies, 1036
Lung heat, **98**, 383
Lung heat and yin deficiency, 1229
Lung qi deficiency, 560
Lung yin deficiency with heat, 1039
overview, 36
phlegm retention, **82**
phlegm retention and qi stagnation, 1245
phlegm-heat, 1233
qi and blood stagnation, **899**
qi and phlegm stagnation, 848
severe, **846**
summer-heat damaging qi and body fluids, 446
warm-dryness, 1030
water accumulation, 1125
wind-cold, 55
wind-cold attacking the Lung, 48, 49
wind-cold with interior heat, **46**
wind-cold with water accumulation, 74
Asthma-Relieving Decoction, 845
Asthma-Stopping Decoction, 845
Astragalus and Atractylodes Combination, 446
Astragalus and Cinnamon Five Herb Combination, 500
Astragalus and Cinnamon Twig Five-Substance Decoction, 500
Astragalus and Peony Combination, 905
Astragalus and Platycodon Formula, 1365
Astragalus and Siler Formula, 773
Astragalus and Zizyphus Combination, 735
Astragalus Centre-Fortifying Decoction, 475
Astragalus Combination, 475
Astragalus Decoction to Construct the Middle, 475
Astragalus Decoction to Guard the Wind, 775
Astragalus Five Decoction, 500
Astragalus Five-Component Decoction, 500
Astragalus Five-Herbs Decoction, 500
Astragalus Middle-Strengthening Decoction, 475

INDEX

I

1533

Index

Astringent formulas, 769
Atherosclerosis, *1402*. *See also* Arteriosclerosis
  cerebral, **882**, **908**
  in coronary stenosis, **719**
  Liver excess, 996
  prevention of, 154, 285, 718
  taiyang, *yangming* and *shaoyang* disorders, 716
Athlete's foot, 1342
Athletic performance, **478**
Atractylodes and Arisaema Combination, 1195
Atractylodes and Dioscorea Combination, 806
Atractylodes and Melanterite Pill, 1302
Atractylodes and Phellodendron Formula, 1190
Atractylodes Combination, 102
Atractylodes Macrocephala and Peony Powder, 257, 259
Atractylodes Macrocephala Powder, 539
Atrioventricular block, **53**
Atrophic gastritis
  chronic, **601**, **606**, **611**, **630**, **918**, **1045**, **1047**, **1211**, **1267**, **1282**
  cold and dampness, 1134
  Liver and Kidney yin deficiencies, **658**
  Liver qi stagnation, **240**
  Spleen and Stomach deficiencies and dampness, **263**
Atrophic painful obstruction, 1064, 1153, 1180, *1523*. *See also Wei bi* (atrophic painful obstruction); *Bi zheng* (painful obstruction syndrome)
Atrophy
  bones and tendons, 651
  legs, 1182, 1188
  limbs, lower, 654
  lung, 558, 589, *1419*
  muscles, **652**, 988, 1186, 1190
  muscles, sinews, and bones, 651
  nervous system, 651
  optic nerve, **252**, **573**, 640
  post-stroke, 906
  reproductive system, 651
  sebaceous glands, 970
  skin, 970
  sweat glands, 970
Atrophy syndrome, *1394*, *1522*. *See also Wei zheng* (atrophy) syndrome
Atropine, 209
Attention deficit disorder, 726
Aucklandia and Amomum Gentlemen Decoction, 531
Aucklandia and Areca Seed Formula, 1272
Aucklandia and Betel Nut Pill, 1272
Aucklandia and Coptis Pill, 391
Aucklandia, Amomum, Immature Bitter Orange, and Atractylodes Macrocephala Pill, 1276
Auditory
  compromised functions, 551
  impaired, 666
Augment the Qi and Increase Acuity Decoction, 551
Augmented Cyperus and Perilla Leaf Powder, 69
Augmented Eight Herb Powder for Rectification, 1105
Augmented Ephedra, Apricot Kernel, Licorice, and Gypsum Decoction, 99
Augmented Four-Substance Decoction, 568
Augmented Invigorate the Collaterals Special Pill, 1180
Augmented Kidney Qi Pill, 675, 677
Augmented Lead to Symmetry Powder, 980
Augmented Magnolia Flower Powder, 85
Augmented Peony and Licorice Decoction, 603
Augmented Rambling Powder, 254
Augmented Restore the Left [Kidney] Pill, 647

Augmented Restore the Right [Kidney] Pill, 680
Augmented Trichosanthes Fruit and Chinese Chive Decoction, 832
Avoirdupois, *1439*
Awake and Disperse Pill, 1351
Azidothymidine. *See* Zidovudine
AZT (azidothymidine). *See* Zidovudine
B-lymphocytes, 610
Ba Dou (Semen Crotonis), xxiii
Ba fa (eight treatment methods), 9
Ba Gang Bian Zheng (Eight Principle Differentiation), *1505*
Ba hui (eight meeting) points, *1505*
Ba Jiao Hui Xiang (Fructus Anisi Stellati), xxiii
Ba Wei Dai Xia Fang (**Eight-Ingredient Formula for Leukorrhea**), 810
Ba Wei Di Huang Wan (**Eight-Ingredient Pill with Rehmannia**), 672, 674
  vs. Jin Gui Shen Qi Wan (Kidney Qi Pill from the Golden Cabinet), 674
  vs. Liu Wei Di Huang Wan (Six-Ingredient Pill with Rehmannia), 635
  vs. You Gui Wan (Restore the Right [Kidney] Pill), 648, 681
Ba Wei Xiao Yao San, 254
Ba Xian Chang Shou Wan (Eight-Immortal Pill for Longevity), 642
Ba Zhen (Eight Arrays of Formulas), 12, 147
Ba Zhen Tang (**Eight-Treasure Decoction**), 604
  vs. Ren Shen Yang Ying Tang (Ginseng Decoction to Nourish the Nutritive Qi), 607
  vs. Shi Quan Da Bu Tang (All-Inclusive Great Tonifying Decoction), 607
  vs. Tai Shan Pan Shi San (Powder that Gives the Stability of Mount Tai), 620
Ba Zhen Tang (*Wan*), 604
Ba Zheng San (**Eight-Herb Powder for Rectification**), 1103
  vs. Wu Lin San (Five-Ingredient Powder for Painful Urinary Dysfunction), 1108
Bacillus, 409
Bacillus Calmette-Guerin, 235
Bacillus dysenteriae, 154, 258, 296, 404, 1081, 1104
Bacillus paratyphosus, 154, 332, 1104
Bacillus proteus, 93, 332, 404, 1081, 1104, 1338
Bacillus subtilis, 93
Back
  heavy sensation, 1192
  pain and stiffness, 1156
  pain, acute, **601**
  soreness, 644
  stiffness, 59
Back, lower
  coldness and pain, 1134
  heavy sensation, 1134
  pain, 1418
    cold and dampness, 1134
    Kidney yang deficiency, 668, 673
  soreness, 637, 784
  soreness and pain, 593, 1161
  soreness and weakness, 651
    Kidney yin and *jing* (essence) deficiencies, 645
    Liver and Kidney deficiencies, 690
    Liver and Kidney yin deficiencies, 627, 640, 654
    yin, yang, blood and *jing* (essence) deficiencies, 687
  weakness, 678
Back, upper, stiffness, 48
Back to the Spleen Decoction, 583
Bacteria. *See* individual bacteria; Antibacterial effect; Antibiotic effect

Index

Bacterial dysentery, 1294
acute, **297**
damp-heat, 1099
with diarrhea, **787**
heat in the Stomach and cold in the Intestines, 1292
Bai Bian Dou (Semen Lablab Album), xxiii
Bai Du San **(Overcome Pathogenic Influences Powder)**, 124
vs. *Jing Fang Bai Du San* (Schizonepeta and Saposhnikovia Powder to Overcome Pathogenic Influences), 127, 1336
vs. *Shen Su Yin* (Ginseng and Perilla Leaf Decoction), 130
Bai Du Tang **(Overcome Pathogenic Influences Decoction)**, 1343
Bai Fan (Alumen), xxv
Bai He Gu Jin Tang **(Lily Bulb Decoction to Preserve the Metal)**, 1036
vs. *Bu Fei E Jiao Tang* (Tonify the Lung Decoction with Ass-Hide Gelatin), 1038
vs. *Mai Men Dong Tang* (Ophiopogonis Decoction), 1038
vs. *Qing Zao Jiu Fei Tang* (Eliminate Dryness and Rescue the Lung Decoction), 1032
vs. *Qiong Yu Gao* (Beautiful Jade Paste), 1038
vs. *Yang Yin Qing Fei Tang* (Nourish the Yin and Clear the Lung Decoction), 1035
Bai Hu Jia Cang Zhu Tang **(White Tiger plus Atractylodes Decoction)**, 323
Bai Hu Jia Gui Zhi Tang **(White Tiger plus Cinnamon Twig Decoction)**, 323
Bai Hu Jia Ren Shen Tang **(White Tiger plus Ginseng Decoction)**, 325
vs. *Zhu Ye Shi Gao Tang* (Bamboo Leaves and Gypsum Decoction), 328
Bai Hu Tang **(White Tiger Decoction)**, 321
vs. *Zhu Ye Shi Gao Tang* (Bamboo Leaves and Gypsum Decoction), 328
Bai Hua She She Cao (Herba Hedyotis), xxiii
Bai Mao Gen Tang **(Imperata Decoction)**, 1112
Bai Qian (Rhizoma et Radix Cynanchi Stauntonii), xxiii
Bai Rai Shin Shu (A New Study of Dermatomycosis and Dermatitis), 1348
Bai San (White Powder), 172
Bai Tong Tang **(White Penetrating Decoction)**, 489
Bai Tou Weng Jia Gan Cao E Jiao Tang **(Pulsatilla Decoction plus Licorice and Ass-Hide Gelatin)**, 410
Bai Tou Weng Tang **(Pulsatilla Decoction)**, 408
vs. *Ge Gen Huang Qin Huang Lian Tang* (Kudzu, Coptis, and Scutellaria Decoction), 298, 783
vs. *Shao Yao Tang* (Peony Decoction), 298, 405, 410, 783
vs. *Zhen Ren Yang Zang Tang* (True Man's Decoction for Nourishing the Organs), 783
Bai Wei (Radix et Rhizoma Cynanchi Atrati), xxiii
Bai Yi Xuan Fang (Selected Formulas), 1158
Bai Zhu San (Atractylodes Macrocephala Powder), 539
Bai Zhu Shao Yao San (Atractylodes Macrocephala and Peony Powder), 257, 259
Bai Zi Ren Wan (Platycladus Seed Pill), 592
Bai Zi Yang Xin Wan **(Biota Seed Pill to Nourish the Heart)**, 729
Bake, *1512*. *See also* Hong (bake)
Baked Licorice Decoction, 589
Balance, loss of, 1251
Balanoposthitis, **969**
Baldness. *See* Hair loss
Bamboo and Ginseng Combination, 1217
Bamboo Decoction to Warm the Gallbladder, 1217
Bamboo Leaves and Gypsum Combination, 326
Bamboo Leaves and Gypsum Decoction, 326

Ban (blend), *1505*
Ban Xia Bai Zhu Tian Ma Tang **(Pinellia, Atractylodes Macrocephala, and Gastrodia Decoction)**, 1247, 1250
Ban Xia Hou Po Tang **(Pinellia and Magnolia Bark Decoction)**, 827
Ban Xia Hou Pu Tang, 827
Ban Xia Tian Ma Bai Shu Tang, 1247
Ban Xia Xie Xin Tang **(Pinellia Decoction to Drain the Epigastrium)**, 261
vs. *Gan Cao Xie Xin Tang* (Licorice Decoction to Drain the Epigastrium), 266
vs. *Huang Lian Tang* (Coptis Decoction), 273
vs. *Sheng Jiang Xie Xin Tang* (Fresh Ginger Decoction to Drain the Epigastrium), 266
Ban Xia Xieh Xin Tang, 261
Bang (scrape), *1505*
Bao Chan Wu You Fang **(Preserve Pregnancy and Care-Free Decoction)**, 621
vs. *Tai Shan Pan Shi San* (Powder that Gives the Stability of Mount Tai), 623
Bao Gu, 1287
Bao He Wan **(Preserve Harmony Pill)**, 1266
Bao jian (decocted in gauze), 20
Bao Xiang-Ao, 1344
Bao Ying Cuo Yao (Synopsis of Caring for Infants), 245
Bao Yuan Tang **(Preserve the Basal Decoction)**, 525
Bartholinitis, **374**, **1339**
Basic Questions, 3, 5
Beautiful Jade Paste, 1041
Bedwetting, *1402*. *See also* Enuresis
Behavioral disorders
abnormal, 731
marked changes in, 996
overview, 708
Behcet's disease, **339**, **375**, **576**, *1402*
Bei (stone-bake), *1505*
Bei Ho Gu Jin Tang (Wan), 1036
Bei Ji Qian Jin Yao Fang (Thousands of Golden Prescriptions for Emergencies), 6, 138, 169, 333, 714, 729, **1151**, 1161, 1314, 1377
Bei Mu (Bulbus Fritillariae), xxiii
Bei Mu Gua Lou San **(Fritillaria and Trichosanthes Fruit Powder)**, 1240
Bei Xie Fen Qing Yin, 1140
Belamcanda and Ephedra Decoction, 80
Belamcanda and Mahuang Combination, 80
Belching
damp accumulation, 1068, 1076
dampness and phlegm, 1077
deficiency and cold of the Stomach, 467
food stagnation, 1266
heat and water, interlocked, 268
Liver fire overacting on the Stomach, 389
overview, 819, 1064, 1263
qi deficiency with cold and dampness, 531
qi deficiency with phlegm stagnation, 851
qi stagnation, 822
with a rotten smell, 1266
Spleen and Stomach disharmony, 1074
Bell's palsy, **61**, 991, *1402*. *See also* Facial paralysis; Eyes, deviated; Mouth, deviated
Ben Cao Gang Mu (Materia Medica), **817**
Ben Cao Jing Ji Zhu (Collection of Commentaries on the Classic of the Materia Medica), **1019**
Ben Cao Yan Yi (Extension of the Materia Medica), 792
Ben tun (running piglet), 493, *1393*, *1505*

1535

Index

Benefit Brain Atrophy Pill, 909
Benefit the Basal Powder, 443
Benefit the Nose Decoction, 87
Benefit the River [Flow] Decoction, 179
Beng lou (flooding and spotting), *1393*, *1505*
    blood deficiency, **565**
    blood stagnation, 889
    deficiency, 609
    deficiency and cold, 805, 949
    deficiency and damage, 950
    deficiency heat, 802
    Heart and Spleen deficiencies, **586**
    overview, 770
    qi deficiency, 542
    yin deficiency and heat in the blood, **803**
Benign prostatic hypertrophy. *See* Prostatic hypertrophy, benign
Benzene, poisoning, **586**
Benzodiazepines, 221
Beriberi
    blood deficiency, 594
    damp-heat, 1190
    dampness and cold, 1184
    water accumulation, 1124, 1129
    wind with water accumulation, 101
    wind-dampness, 1173
    xue bi (blood painful obstruction), 500
Bi Bo (Fructus Piperis Longi), xxiii
Bi Li-Zhai, 489, 604, 725, 1325
Bi Xie Fen Ching Yin, 1140
***Bi Xie Fen Qing Yin* (Dioscorea Hypoglauca Decoction to Separate the Clear)**, 1140, 1141, 1142
***Bi Yu San* (Jasper Powder)**, 443
Bi zheng (closed disorder), *1506*
    cold, 759
    overview, 743, 1309
    phlegm accumulation, 1313
    phlegm and heat obstruction, 750
    wind-phlegm, 1312
Bi zheng (painful obstruction syndrome), *1393*, *1506*
    classification, 1153
    damp-heat in the lower body, 1188
    deficiency, 1161
    exterior excess with interior deficiency, 1169
    generalized, 1175
    overview, 1064, 1153
    qi and blood stagnation, **894**, **915**
    throughout the body, **1193**
    wind, cold, and dampness with deficiencies, **1164**, 1167
    wind, cold, dampness and heat, 1171
    wind, dampness, and heat, 323
    wind-dampness, 1173
    wind-dampness with deficiency, 1158
    wind-dampness with heat, 1186
    yang deficiency and cold invasion, **501**
Bian Que, 705, 1481, 1482, 1484. *See also* Qin Yue-Ren
Bian Que Nei Jing (Internal Medicine according to Bian Que), **705**
Bian Que Wai Jing (External Medicine according to Bian Que), **705**
Bian Zheng Lun (Records of Differential Diagnosis), 1381
***Bie Jia Jian Wan* (Soft-Shelled Turtle Shell Pill)**, 935
Bie Xie Fen Qing Yin, 1140
Big pulse, *1506*
Bile acid. *See also* Gallbladder; Cholagogic effect; Choleretic effect
    to increase, 209, 239, 482, 485, 1087, 1275, 1293
    regurgitation of, 263, 390, 545, 857
Bile duct, 154, 240. *See also* Gallbladder; Cholagogic effect; Choleretic effect

Biliary ascariasis (roundworms), **170**, **235**, **285**, **380**, **482**, **826**, **1294**
Biliary atresia, **1088**
Biota and Cyathula Formula, 592
Biota Seed Pill to Nourish the Heart, 729
Bipolar disorders, 1214. *See also* Mania; Depression
Birth-Hastening Decoction, 931
Black Rambling Powder, 252
Bladder. *See* Gallbladder; Urinary Bladder
Bladder worms, 1301
Blast-fry, *1516. See also* Pao (blast-fry)
Bleeding, *1402. See also* specific types and locations of bleeding; Hemorrhage; Hemostatic effect
    damp-heat in all three *jiaos*, 359
    defecation, before or after, 945
    deficiency and cold, 948
    duodenal, **949**, **952**
    epistaxis, **91**, 160, **191**, 333, **334**, 337, 351, **353**, 359, **384**, 396, **399**, 459, **639**, 942, 948, **1031**, **1034**
    gastrointestinal, **334**, 359, **360**, 802, 911
        lower, **360**
        upper, **264**, **360**, **373**, **399**, **941**, **949**
    gums, 393, 398
    heat in the *xue* (blood) level, 333, 939, 942
    heat, fire and toxins in all three *jiaos*, 341
    hematemesis, 160, 333, 337, 351, **940**, 942, 948
    hematochezia, 333, 459, 584, 654, 945, 948
    hemoptysis, 359, 654, 939, 942, 943, 951, **1031**, 1036, 1039, 1042, 1222
    hemorrhoids, 359, 945, **949**, 951
    interior heat and toxins, 361
    intestinal, 359
    Liver and Kidney yin deficiencies, 654
    menstrual, **524**, **547**, 571, 575, 654, 802, **803**, 805, 948, 950
    occult, 576
    overview, 315, 317, 770, 868, 870, 1023
    postpartum, 951
    qi deficiency, *1517*
    rectal, 951
    Spleen deficiency, 584
    subcutaneous, 359
    uterine, 359, 368, 459, 542, 576, 580, 584, **586**, 594, **596**, 604, 616, 625, **647**, **803**, 805, **891**, 911, **912**, **921**, **926**, 949, **951**
    yang deficiency, 459
Blend, *1505. See also* Ban (blend)
Bloating, 1077. *See also* Fullness; Distention
Blockage-Relieving Decoction, 1158
Blood (TCM), *1506*
    accumulation, 302
    accumulation in the lower *jiao*, 873
    circulation, 867
    deficiency, 512, 562, *1506*
    deficiency and heat, 575
    deficiency with blood stagnation, 571
    deficiency with deficiency heat, 722
    dessication, *1506*
    heat in the, *1512*
    overview, 867
    qi and blood deficiencies, 580, 589, 604, *1517*
    qi and blood stagnation, 578, 893, 915, *1517*
    qi, blood and yang deficiencies, 609
    stagnation, 867, *1395*
        chest, 879
        diaphragm, 885
        head, 877
        lower abdomen, 889, 933
        with blood deficiency, 571

Index

stasis, 867, *1395*
  stasis in the body, 911
  stasis in the uterus, 928
Blood disorders (WM). *See* specific disorders; Hematological
  disorders
Blood glucose. *See* Glucose; Diabetes mellitus; Hypoglycemic
  effect; Metabolic effect
Blood level, *1524*. *See also* Xue (blood) level
Blood painful obstruction, 500, 1153, *1525*. *See also* Xue bi (blood
  painful obstruction); *Bi zheng* (painful obstruction syndrome)
Blood pressure. *See* Hypertension; Hypotension
Blood stagnation syndrome, *1506*
Blood stasis syndrome, *1506*
Blood sugar. *See* Glucose; Diabetes mellitus; Hypoglycemic effect;
  Metabolic effect
Blood urea nitrogen (BUN), 461, 1066, 1111
Blood vessel disorders, 1323. *See also* Arteries; Veins; Vasodilative
  effect; specific disorders
Blood-House Blood Stasis-Dispelling Decoction, 879
Blood-Producing and Clotting-Cleaning Decoction, 925
Blood-Regenerating and Stasis-Resolving Decoction, 925
Blood-regulating formulas, 867
Bloody dysuria, 947, 1103, 1107, 1115, *1525*. *See also* Xue lin
  (bloody dysuria); *Lin zheng* (dysuria syndrome)
Bo (open), *1506*
Bo Ai Xin Jian (Manual of Universal Lover from the Heart), 525
Bo Gao, 3
Body
  aches and pain, 124, 1175
  blood stasis, 911
  cold, 463, 466
Body fluids, *1506*
  deficiency, 512
  thick, *1525*
  thin, *1513*
Boiling, *1527*. *See also* Zhu (boiling)
Boils
  dampness, heat, wind and fire, 1340
  early stage, 1334
  fire and toxins, 1337
  heat and toxins, 103, 1342
  heat and toxins with underlying deficiencies, 1365
  heat, fire and toxins in all three *jiaos*, 341
  overview, 315, 1321
  with pus and discharge, 1364
  qi deficiency, 1362
  wind, heat and toxins, 356
  wind, heat and toxins in the upper body, 349
Bolster the Spleen Powder, 1138
Bone marrow toxicities, cis-diamminedichloroplatinum-induced,
  612
Bones
  abscesses, 1347
  aches and pains, 1188
  degeneration, 1166
  fractures, **573, 899**, 901, **904, 1120**
  loss of density, 544, 611
  metastatic carcinoma, *1373*
  necrosis, 1329
  osteoporosis, 673, 921
  tuberculosis, 1371
  weakness and atrophy, 651
Book to Safeguard Life Arranged According to Pattern, 113, 324
Borborygmus
  deficiency and cold, 463
  heat and water, interlocked, 268

heat in the chest and cold in the Stomach, 271
  overview, 202
  post-surgical, 482
  qi deficiency with dampness, 535
  Spleen deficiency and Liver excess, 257
  Stomach deficiency and interlocking of heat and cold, 270
  Stomach qi disharmony, 261
Bound pulse, *1506*
Bowel movement. *See also* Constipation; Diarrhea
  irregular, 1280
  uncontrollable, 781, 788
Bowel-Nourishing Decoction, 178
Bowl, *1506*
BPH (benign prostatic hypertrophy). *See* Prostatic hypertrophy,
  benign
Bradyarrhythmia, **881**
Bradykinin, 133
Brain
  ischemia, 343, **719**, **931**
  trauma, **908**
Break open, *1516*. *See also* Po (break open)
Break the Conflict Decoction, 933
Breast disorders, 1323. *See also* specific disorders
  abscesses, *1327*, *1347*, *1403*, *1506*
  abscesses, rock-like, *1518*
  benign tumor, 250
  cancer, 1349, 1350, 1360
  cystic hyperplasia, *1372*
  distention, 247
  distention and pain, **240**
  fibrocystic, 254
  proliferation disease, **250**
  swollen, painful, 238
Breath, foul
  fire in the Spleen and Stomach, 396
  heat, 268
  heat in the upper and middle *jiaos*, 354
  overview, 316
  Stomach heat, 393
Breath, shortness of. *See also* Wheezing; Dyspnea; Asthma
  damp accumulation, 1121
  Kidney and Lung yin deficiencies, 643
  Lung yin and Spleen qi deficiencies, 1042
  overview, 512, 513, 769, 820
  phlegm, 1109
  phlegm retention with yang deficiency, 1131
  qi and blood deficiencies, 589, 604, 616
  qi and yin deficiencies with dryness, 1050
  Spleen and Stomach qi deficiencies, 542
  summer-heat damaging qi and body fluids, 446
  summer-heat with damaged qi and body fluids, 554
  upper excess and lower deficiency, 842
  warm-dryness, 1030
  water accumulation, 1125
  wind-cold with interior phlegm, 128
  yang deficiency, 459
  yin and qi deficiencies, 776
Breathing
  labored, 1233
  more exhalation than inhalation, 842
  rapid, 845, 1121
Breech presentation, **565, 596, 606**
Bromocriptine, 674
Bronchial asthma. *See also* Asthma
  chronic, **211**, **847**
  deficiency heat, 558

1537

Index

heat, lingering or residual, 327
in infants, **53**
Kidney deficiency, **630**
Kidney yin deficiency, 644
Lung heat, 96
Lung heat with phlegm accumulation, 1232
Lung yin deficiency with heat, 1039
phlegm and damp accumulation, 1224
phlegm retention and qi stagnation, **1246**
prevention of, **680**
qi and phlegm stagnation, 848
shaoyang syndrome with phlegm stagnation, 226
shaoyin with *taiyang* syndrome, 132
upper excess and lower deficiency, 842
water accumulation, 1125
Bronchiectasis, *1403*
exterior cool-dryness, 1025
heat in the *xue* (blood) level, 942
heat-phlegm, 1226
with hemoptysis, **353**, **1037**
Liver fire invading the Lung, 943
qi deficiency with cold and dampness, 531
warm-dryness, 1030
wind-cold with water accumulation, 74
Bronchiolitis, 845, **1211**
Bronchitis, *1403*
acute, 89, **98**, **118**, 1235, **1236**, **1246**
acute and chronic, 1233
asthmatic, 80, **846**
in children, 77, 81, **1378**
chronic, **98**, **118**, 416, 423, **529**, 542, 554, 558, 668, 673, 779, 842, 1036, **1045**, 1131, 1226, 1378
cold phlegm, 1242
cool-dryness, 1025
with cough, 114
dryness with damaged yin, 1047
dryness with phlegm, 1240
exterior-excess, wind-cold, 39
heat, lingering or residual, 327
Lung heat, 383
Lung heat with phlegm accumulation, 1232
Lung yin deficiency with heat, 1039
overview, 36
phlegm retention, **81**
phlegm stagnation, 1230
phlegm-heat, 1222
qi deficiency with cold and dampness, 531
shaoyang syndrome, 206, 304
shaoyang syndrome with phlegm stagnation, 226
shaoyin with *taiyang* syndrome, 132
suppurative, 1378
uncomplicated, **1211**
warm-dryness, 1030
wind-cold and interior phlegm-heat, 845
wind-cold attacking the Lung, 48, 49
wind-cold with interior heat, 45
wind-cold with interior phlegm, 128
wind-cold with water accumulation, **76**
yin-deficient heat and fire, 420
Bronchopneumonia, **847**
Bronchorelaxation, 76
Bruises, 901, 915. *See also* Trauma; Injuries
Bu Dai Wan (Cloth Sack Pill), 1299
Bu fa (tonifying), **11**, 512, 1322, *1506*
Bu Fei E Jiao San (Tonify the Lung Powder with Ass-Hide Gelatin), 1039

Bu Fei E Jiao Tang (**Tonify the Lung Decoction with Ass-Hide Gelatin**), 1039
  vs. *Bai He Gu Jin Tang* (Lily Bulb Decoction to Preserve the Metal), 1038
  vs. *Da Bu Yin Wan* (Great Tonify the Yin Pill), 1041
  vs. *Ren Shen Ge Jie San* (Ginseng and Gecko Powder), 1041
  vs. *Sheng Mai San* (Generate the Pulse Powder), 1041
Bu Fei San (Tonify the Lung Powder), 1039
Bu Fei Tang (**Tonify the Lung Decoction**), 560
Bu Gu Wan (**Tonify the Bone Pill**), 689
Bu Huan Jin Zheng Qi San (**Rectify the Qi Powder Worth More than Gold**), 1075
Bu Shen Tang (**Tonify the Kidney Decoction**), 683
Bu Shen Wan (**Tonify the Kidney Pill**), 689
Bu Yang Huan Wu Tang (**Tonify the Yang to Restore Five Decoction**), 905
Bu Yao Xiu Zhen Xiao Er Fang Lun (Supplement to the Pocket-Sized Discussion of Formulas for Children), 1299
Bu Zhong Yi Chi Tang (*Wan*), 542
Bu Zhong Yi Qi Tang (**Tonify the Middle and Augment the Qi Decoction**), 542
  vs. *Gui Pi Tang* (Restore the Spleen Decoction), 588
Buboes, 1350, 1375
Bulbus Fritillariae, xxiii
BUN. *See* Blood urea nitrogen
Bungarus Parvus, xxiii
Bupleurum and Calm the Stomach Decoction, 1071
Bupleurum and Chih-shih Formula, 233
Bupleurum and Cinnamon Combination, 219
Bupleurum and Cinnamon Twig Decoction, 219
Bupleurum and Cyperus Combination, 238
Bupleurum and Dragon Bone Combination, 715
Bupleurum and Evodia Combination, 241
Bupleurum and Ginseng Combination, 858
Bupleurum and Hoelen Combination, 222
Bupleurum and Kudzu Decoction to Release the Muscle Layer, 107, 110
Bupleurum and Peony Formula, 254
Bupleurum and Poria Decoction, 222
Bupleurum and Pueraria Combination, 107
Bupleurum and Pueraria Decoction for Relieving Muscles, 107
Bupleurum and Rehmannia Combination, 243
Bupleurum and Schizonepeta Formula, 1341
Bupleurum and Scute Combination, 226
Bupleurum and Tangkuei Formula, 247
Bupleurum Chest Bind Decoction, 226
Bupleurum Cinnamon and Ginger Combination, 304
Bupleurum Decoction, 287
Bupleurum Decoction for Sinking into the Chest, 1237
Bupleurum Decoction to Clear the Liver, 243, 244
Bupleurum Decoction to Raise the Sunken, 226
Bupleurum Decoction to Reach the Membrane Source, 230
Bupleurum Decoction to Relieve Toxicity, 215
Bupleurum Decoction to Spread the Liver, 238
Bupleurum Decoction to Tranquilize the Spirit, 720
Bupleurum Formula, 245
Bupleurum Liver-Clearing Decoction, 243
Bupleurum plus Dragon Bone and Oyster Shell Decoction, 715
Bupleurum Powder to Spread the Liver, 238
Bupleurum, Bitter Orange, and Platycodon Decoction, 215
Bupleurum, Cinnamon Twig, and Ginger Decoction, 304
Burn (cooking method), *1519*. *See also Shao* (burn)
Burns (injury), **1340**
Bursitis, 59, 1159, 1195
CAD. *See* Coronary artery disease
Cai Hu Gui Zhi Tang, 219

Chinese Herbal Formulas and Applications

Index

Cai Xian Tang, 226
Calamus and Carthamus Formula, 760
Calcine, *1509. See also Duan* (calcine)
Calcium, plasma level, 652
Calculi. *See* Stones
Calculus Bovis Artifactus, xxv
Calluses, 494
Calm the Middle Powder, 484
Calm the Palace Pill with Cattle Gallstone, 746
Calm the Stomach and Poria Decoction, 1113
Calm the Stomach Powder, 1068
Camptosar. *See* Irinotecan
Can Sha (Faeces Bombycis), xxiii
Can Shi Tang (Silkworm Droppings Decoction), 1101
  vs. Lian Po Yin (Coptis and Magnolia Bark Decoction), 1102
Cancer. *See also* names and sites of specific tumors; Anticancer
    effect; Antineoplastic effect; Antimetastatic effect
  breast, 1349, 1350, 1360
  colon and rectum, *1403*
  esophagus, *1403*
  with fever, 210, 413
  genitourinary tract, **617**
  liver, **659**, 935, 937, *1403*
  lung, **1038**, **1048**, *1404*
  pain, **496**, **529**
  pancreas, *1404*
  stomach, 527, *1404*
  supportive treatments of, 515, **611**
  throat, 363
Candida albicans, 93, 808
Candidiasis, 351
Cang Er San, 82
Cang Er Zi San (Xanthium Powder), 82
  vs. Qing Bi Tang (Clear the Nose Decoction), 88
  vs. Xin Yi San (Magnolia Flower Powder), 88
Cang Lin San (Old Rice Granary Powder), 127
Canker sores, 92, 354
Canopy Powder, 48
Cao Cao, 741
Cape Jasmine and Prepared Soybean Decoction, 370
Capillaries and Hoelen Five Formula, 1090
Capital Qi Pill, 644
Capsaicin, 1045
Capsule, 18
Caput Radix Angelicae Sinensis, xxiv
Carafate. *See* Sucralfate
Carbamazepine, 77, 214, 720
Carbon monoxide poisoning, **878**
Carbon tetrachloride, 214, 235, 244, 249, 581, 629, 655, 658
Carboplatin, 612
Carbuncles, *1404*
  damp-heat in all three *jiaos*, 359
  dampness, heat, wind and fire, 1340
  early stage, 1334
  fire and toxins, 1337
  hard and deeply rooted, 1337
  heat and toxins, 291, 1325, 1342
  heat and toxins, with underlying deficiencies, 1365
  localized with redness, swelling, heat and pain, 1337
  overview, 1321
  with pus and discharge, 1364
  qi and blood deficiencies, 1367
  qi deficiency, 1362
  with swelling and hardness, 1357
  wind with blood deficiency, 970
  wind, heat and toxins, 356

Carcinoma. *See also* names and sites of specific cancers;
    Anticancer effect; Antineoplastic effect; Antimetastatic effect
  bone, **1373**
  liver, **210**, **547**
  lung, **617**
Cardamon Combination, 1082
Cardiac. *See also* Heart; Cardiovascular disorders
  asthma, 1125, 1226
  edema, 1121
  failure, 486, 491, 554, **1132**, **1136**
  infarction, 457, **487**, 491
  ischemia, **881**
Cardiomyopathy, 1133, *1404*
Cardioprotective effect, 555
Cardiopulmonary diseases
  chronic, **1094**
  phlegm retention and qi stagnation, 1245
  yang deficiency with water accumulation, 1135
Cardiotonic effect, 235, 555
Cardiovascular disorders, 869, 1065, 1066, 1214. *See also* specific
    disorders; Cardiovascular effect
Cardiovascular effect, 41, 53, 60, 235, 239, 285, 293, 373, 487, 555,
    564, 572, 590, 691, 727, 881, 907, 912, 918, 978, 997, 1132. *See
    also* Cardiotonic effect; Chronotropic effect; Inotropic effect;
    Circulatory effect; Vasodilative effect
Carditis, viral, 710
Carpal tunnel syndrome, **1346**
Carphology, 187
Case Histories from the Compass of Clinical Patterns, **311**
Cassia Twig Decoction, 51
Catalogued Essentials for Correcting the Body, 489, 604
Cataract
  blood deficiency and blood stagnation, **573**
  deficiency, 551
  in geriatrics, **547**, **671**
  Heart and Kidney disharmony, 714
  post-surgical complications, **62**, **345**
  qi, blood and yin deficiencies, 665
  to delay the appearance, **674**
  yin deficiency with internal fire and wind, 661
Cattle Gallstone Pill, 746, 1350
Cattle Gallstone Pill to Clear the Heart, 748
Caulis Dendrobii, xxv
Caulis Fibraureae, xxiv
Caulis Lonicerae Japonicae, xxv
Caulis Perillae, xxv
Caulis Polygoni Multiflori, xxvi
Caulis Sargentodoxae, xxiv
Cells. *See* specific types of cells
Cellulitis
  cold, dampness, phlegm and blood stasis, 1375
  dampness, heat, wind and fire, 1340
  fire and toxins, **1338**
  heat in the Liver, Gallbladder, and *San Jiao* channels, 243
  heat, fire and toxins in all three *jiaos*, 341
  overview, 1321
  with pus and discharge, 1364
  wind-heat, 1332
  yang deficiency and interior cold stagnation, 1370
Central nervous system, effect on, 249, 555, 717, 723, 727, 732,
    748, 907
Central *qi*, *1527. See also Zhong* (central) *qi*
Cephalanoplos Decoction, 946
Cerebellitis, **1249**
Cerebral
  arteriosclerosis, 551

INDEX

1539

Index

atherosclerosis, **882**, **908**
embolism, *1404*
  acute, **989**
  Liver wind rising, 1008
  Liver yang and wind excess, 1004
hemorrhage, *1405*
  Liver wind rising, 993
  Liver yang and wind excess, 1004
  Liver yang and wind rising, **1001**
  due to stroke, **990**, 991
  taiyang, *yangming* and *shaoyang* disorders, 716
infarction, *1405*
  asymptomatic, **998**
  blood deficiency with blood stagnation, **573**
  damaged qi and body fluids, **555**
  Liver yang and wind excess, 1004
  due to stenosis of the artery, **907**
ischemia, 343
thrombosis, **1001**
Cerebrospinal meningitis, **343**
Cerebrovascular accident. *See also* Stroke
  blood stagnation, 877
  cold *bi zheng* (closed disorder), 759
  damp-heat in all three *jiaos*, 359
  excess heat, fire and toxins, **343**
  hot *bi zheng* (closed disorder), 747
  overview, 744
  post-stroke sequelae, 991
  prevention, 1003
  qi and blood stagnation, 915
Cerebrovascular diseases, *1405*
  ischemic, **907**
  qi deficiency and blood stagnation, **907**
  supportive treatments of, **695**
Cervical disorders, **1157**
Cervical spondylosis, **916**
Cervicitis
  chronic, **375**, **808**
  with vaginitis, **1328**
Cestodiasis (tapeworms), 1289, 1301
Cha ji (tea), 18
Cha Ye (Folium Camelliae), xxv
Chai Chao San, 130
Chai Ge Jie Ji Tang (**Bupleurum and Kudzu Decoction to Release the Muscle Layer**), 107, 110
  vs. Gui Zhi Tang (Cinnamon Twig Decoction), 110
Chai Hu An Shen Tang (**Bupleurum Decoction to Tranquilize the Spirit**), 720
Chai Hu Da Yuan Yin (**Bupleurum Decoction to Reach the Membrane Source**), 230
  vs. Hao Qin Qing Dan Tang (Artemisia Annua and Scutellaria Decoction to Clear the Gallbladder), 232
Chai Hu Gui Zhi Gan Jiang Tang (**Bupleurum, Cinnamon Twig, and Ginger Decoction**), 304
Chai Hu Gui Zhi Tang (**Bupleurum and Cinnamon Twig Decoction**), 219
Chai Hu Jia Long Gu Mu Li Tang (**Bupleurum plus Dragon Bone and Oyster Shell Decoction**), 715
Chai Hu Jia Long Mu Tang, 715
Chai Hu Jie Du Tang (**Bupleurum Decoction to Relieve Toxicity**), 215
Chai Hu Qing Gan Tang (**Bupleurum Decoction to Clear the Liver**), 243, 244
Chai Hu Shu Gan San (**Bupleurum Powder to Spread the Liver**), 238
  vs. Shu Gan Tang (Spread the Liver Decoction), 242

vs. Si Ni San (Frigid Extremities Powder), 241
vs. Xiao Yao San (Rambling Powder), 253
Chai Hu Shu Gan Tang (Bupleurum Decoction to Spread the Liver), 238
Chai Hu Tang (**Bupleurum Decoction**), 287
Chai Hu Xian Xiong Tang (**Bupleurum Decoction for Sinking into the Chest**), 1237
Chai Hu Zhi Jie Tang (**Bupleurum, Bitter Orange, and Platycodon Decoction**), 215
Chai Ling Tang (**Bupleurum and Poria Decoction**), 222
Chai Ping Tang (**Bupleurum and Calm the Stomach Decoction**), 1071
Chai Xian Tang (**Bupleurum Decoction to Raise the Sunken**), 226
Chan Su Wan (**Toad Venum Pill**), 1351
Chancre, 371
Chang feng (intestinal wind), 291, *1506*
Change the Yellow [Discharge] Decoction, 809
Channels and collaterals, 3
Channel-Warming Decoction, 919
Chao (dry-fry), *1507*
Chao huang (dry-fry to yellow), *1507*
Chao jiao (dry-fry to burnt), *1507*
Chao tan (dry-fry to ash), *1507*
Charring to ash, *1521*. *See also Tan* (char to ash)
Cheeks
  painful and swollen, 393
  red, 416, 418
  swelling of, 1096
Cheilitis, **1055**
Chemoprotective effect, 515
Chemotherapy, 530, 539, 582, 612, 633, 855, 1268, *1405*. *See also* Chemoprotective effect
Chen Nian-Zi, 917
Chen Shi-Duo, 1347
Chen Shi-Gong, 122, 244, 967, 981, 1351, 1362
Chen Wu Tang, 1135
Chen Yan, 182, 1213
Chen yao (deputy herb), 14, *1507*
Chen Zi-Ming, 7, 527, 592, 795, 931, 942, 1167, 1219
Cheng Fang Bian Du (Convenient Reader of Established Formulas), 1190
Cheng Guo-Peng, 69, 110, 116, 711, 1040, 1142, 1240, 1247, 1251, 1253, 1355
Cheng Ku Tzu Chin Tan, 901
Cheng Qi Yang Ying Tang (**Order the Qi and Nourish the Nutritive Qi Decoction**), 192
Cheng Wu-Ji, 7
Cheng's Bupleurum and Kudzu Decoction to Release the Muscle Layer, 110
Cheng's Chai Ge Jie Ji Tang (Cheng's Bupleurum and Kudzu Decoction to Release the Muscle Layer), 110
Chest
  blood stagnation, 879
  congestion, 72
  discomfort, 1224, 1242
  distention, 819, 1063, 1245
  distention and hardness, 1311
  distention and oppression, 822, 1099
  distention and stifling sensations, 1209
  fullness
    phlegm retention with yang deficiency, 1131
    shaoyang and *yangming* syndromes, 283
    shaoyang syndrome, 716
    warm-dryness, 1030
  fullness and clumping, 304
  fullness and discomfort, 48, 201, 206, 226

Chinese Herbal Formulas and Applications

Index

fullness and distention
  damp accumulation, 1082
  damp and phlegm obstruction, 230
  deficiency and cold of the Stomach, 467
  deficiency and cold with qi stagnation, 484
  interior excess heat, 158
  Lung heat with phlegm accumulation, 1232
  phlegm-heat, 1222, 1235
  qi stagnation and food retention, 1274
  qi and phlegm stagnation, 848
  Spleen and Stomach disharmony, 1074
  taiyang, yangming and *shaoyang* disorders, 716
  water accumulation, 1125
  wind-cold with interior phlegm, 128
  wind-cold with qi stagnation, 67
fullness and oppression, 842, 1079
fullness and pain, 831
fullness and stifling sensation, 49, 80, 536, 1233
fullness, distention and oppression, 1127
heat and water accumulation, 162, 163
heat in the chest with cold in the Stomach, 271
jie xiong (stagnant chest), 161, 172
oppression
  damp accumulation, 1072
  damp-heat in all three *jiaos*, 359
  damp-warmth, 1096
  Liver qi stagnation, 849
oppression and discomfort, 1092
oppression and distention, 527
pain, **1405**. *See also* Angina; Angina pectoris; *Xiong bi* (painful
  obstruction of the chest)
  dull pain, 1377
  extreme, 759
  fixed location, 879
  overview, 867, 1206
  phlegm-heat, 1233
  qi stagnation with heat, 825
  radiating to the back, 831
  severe coldness and pain, 481
  sharp, 911
  stabbing, 171, 879
  yin deficiency with qi stagnation and blood dryness, 657
phlegm stagnation and water retention, 183
phlegm-heat, 1233, 1235
stifling sensation, 202
  Gallbladder damp-heat, 228
  heat in the chest and cold in the Stomach, 271
  wind and phlegm rising, 1247
  wind-cold with water accumulation, 74
stifling sensation and distention, 327, 1206
swelling and pain, 897
yang deficiency, phlegm accumulation and qi stagnation, 831
Chi Chu Ti Huang Wan, 640
Chi Fu Ling (Poria Rubra), xxiii
Chi Ju Di Huang Wan, 640
Chi Ming San, 1183
Chi Pao Mei Jan Tan, 690
Chi position, **1507**
Chi Shao (Radix Paeoniae Rubra), xxiii
Chi Sheng Shen Qi Wan, 675
Chi Shi Zhi Yu Liang Shi Tang, 788
Chi Shi Zhi Yu Yu Liang Tang (Halloysitum and Limonite
  Decoction), 788
Chia Wei Hsiao Yao San, 254
Chian Pi Wan, 1277
Chiang Huo Sheng Shih Tang, 1156

Chiang-huo Dampness-Overcoming Decoction, 1156
Chickenpox, 105
Chief herb, 14, **1513**. *See also Jun yao* (chief herb)
Chief, Deputy, Assistant, Envoy, 14
Chieh Keng Tang, 1230
Chih Cho Ku Pen Wan, 800
Chih Kan Tsao Tang, 589
Chih Po Ti Huang Wan, 636
Chih Sou San, 116
Chih Tzu Ku Tang, 370
Chih Yin Ti Huang Wan, 663
Chih-shih and Cardamon Combination, 1212
Chills. *See also* Cold, aversion to
  heat in the Liver, Gallbladder, and *San Jiao* channels, 243
  morning, 316
  taiyang and *shaoyang* syndromes, 219
Chills and fever
  alternating
    diagnosis, 216
    Gallbladder damp-heat, 227
    Liver qi stagnation, 238, 247
    Liver qi stagnation with heat, 254
    overview, 201
    shaoyang and *yangming* syndromes, 283
    shaoyang syndrome, 206
    shaoyang syndrome with phlegm stagnation, 226
    shaoyang syndrome with water accumulation, 222
  intermittent, 230
Chin Chiu Pieh Chia San, 416
Chin Fei Tsao San, 49
Chin Jiao Bie Jia San, 416
Chin Suo Ku Ching Wan, 789
Chin-chiu and Tu-huo Decoction, 1167
Chin-chiu and Turtle Shell Formula, 416
Chin-chiu Formula, 416
Chinese Angelica and Six Yellow Herbs Decoction, 420
Chinese Angelica Blood-Tonifying Decoction, 580
Chinese Angelica Cold Limbs Decoction, 494
Chinese Angelica, Gentiana and Aloe Pill, 379
Ching Chieh Lien Chiao Tang, 120
Ching Fai Yin, 1224
Ching Fang Pai Tu San, 1334
Ching Fei Tang, 1225
Ching Hsin Li Ke Tang, 386
Ching Hsin Lien Tzu Yin, 368
Ching Shu I Chi Tang, 446
Ching Shu Yi Chi Tang, 446
Ching Tsao Chiu Fei Tang, 1029
Ching Wei San, 393
Ching Xin Lian Zi Yin, 368
Ching Zao Jiu Fei Tang, 1029
Chiu Wei Qiang Huo Tang, 64
Chiung Kuei Jiao Ai Tang, 950
Chloasma, **252**, **574**, **597**, **1001**
Chloroform, 629
Chlorpromazine, 482
Cholagogic effect, 209, 239, 485, 1087, 1275, 1293
Cholecystitis, **1405**. *See also* Cholagogic effect; Choleretic effect
  acute, **154**, 158, 160, 370, 371, **373**, **1294**, **1339**, **1381**
  acute or chronic, **210**, **252**, **875**
  blood stagnation, 885
  with cholelithiasis, **210**, **1282**
  chronic, **235**, **239**, **257**, **265**
  damp-heat, 1086
  damp-warmth, **1094**, 1096
  excess cold accumulation, 166

1541

Index

fire in the Liver and Gallbladder channels, 379
heat and fire in the upper and middle *jiaos*, 351
qi stagnation, 822
shaoyang syndrome, 304
shaoyang syndrome with phlegm stagnation, 226
shaoyang syndrome with water accumulation, 222
taiyang and *shaoyang* syndromes, 219
yang deficiency and interior cold, 481
yang deficiency, phlegm accumulation and qi stagnation, 831
yin, blood and body fluid deficiencies, **602**
yin-deficient heat and fire, 420
Cholelithiasis, *1405*. *See also* Cholagogic effect; Choleretic effect
with bile duct infection, **240**
with cholecystitis, **210**, **1282**
chronic, **265**
damp-heat, 1086
fire in the Liver and Gallbladder channels, 379
Gallbladder damp-heat, **229**
gallbladder removal, **285**
heat and fire in the upper and middle *jiaos*, 351
heat in the Stomach and cold in the Intestines, **1294**
overview, 1264
phlegm-heat, 1235
qi stagnation, 822
shaoyang syndrome with phlegm stagnation, 226
shaoyin syndrome, **235**
taiyang and *shaoyang* syndromes, 219
yang deficiency and interior cold, 481
Choleretic effect, 244, 1087
Cholestasis, 244
Cholesterols. *See also* Antihyperlipidemic effect; Metabolic effect
elevated, 209, 252, 285, 293, 343, 572, 629, 655, 669, 718, 881, 883, 907, 1088
high-density lipoproteins (HDL), 285, 629, 1088
low-density lipoprotein (LDL), 1088
triglycerides, 209, 252, 285, 293, 572, 617, 629, 655, 669, 718, 874, 883, 1088
very low-density lipoprotein (VLDL), 285
Chondritis, costal, **899**
Chong (thoroughfare) channel, *1507*
deficiency, 593
deficiency and cold, 805, 919, 923
deficiency and damage, 950
deficiency and injury, 562
heat, 206, 802
unstable, 804
Chong Ding Ji Sheng Fang (Revised Formulas to Aid the Living), 1138
Chong Ding Tong Su Shang Han Lun (Revised Popular Guide to the Discussion of Cold-Induced Disorders), 215, 227, 230, 1237
Chong Ding Yan Shi Ji Sheng Fang (Revised Formulas to Aid the Living from the Yan Family), 970
Chong fu (take drenched), 21, *1507*
Chong fu ji (granule or powder), 18
Chong Lou Yu Yao (Jade Key to Many Towers), 1033
Chong Wei Zi (Fructus Leonuri), xxiii
Chorea, 733, **982**
Chorea minor, **1010**
Choroidopathy, **586**
Chronic fatigue syndrome
overview, 515
qi and blood deficiencies, **617**
qi deficiency, 522
shaoyang syndrome, **213**
Spleen and Stomach qi deficiencies, **544**
Spleen qi deficiency with dampness, **447**

Chronotropic effect, 60, 235, 1119
Chrysanthemum Combination, 664
Chrysanthemum Powder to be Taken with Green Tea, 976
Chu (pestle), *1507*
Chu He Pi (*Wan*), 833
Chu Ling Tang, 1115
Chu Pi Tsu Ju Tang, 854
Chu Yeh Shih Kao Tang, 326
Chuan Chiung and Tea-Regulating Formula, 973
Chuan Chiung Cha Tiao San, 973
Chuan Pi Tang, 1158
Chuan Xiong (Rhizoma Chuanxiong), xxiii
***Chuan Xiong Cha Tiao San* (Ligusticum Chuanxiong Powder to be Taken with Green Tea)**, 973
Chun Pi (Cortex Ailanthi), xxiii
Ci Shi Nan Zhi (Hard-Won Knowledge), 64, 66
Ci Wu Jia (Radix et Rhizoma seu Caulis Acanthopanacis Senticosi), xxiii
***Ci Zhu Wan* (Magnetite and Cinnabar Pill)**, 714
vs. Zhu Sha An Shen Wan (Cinnabar Pill to Tranquilize the Spirit), 715
Cimetidine, 209, 287, 345
Cimicifuga and Kudzu Decoction, 103, 104
Cimicifuga and Pueraria Combination, 103
Cimicifuga and Pueraria Decoction, 103
Cimicifuga Combination, 164
Cinnabar Pill to Tranquilize the Spirit, 710
Cinnamon and Anemarrhena Combination, 1186
Cinnamon and Angelica Formula, 1175
Cinnamon and Angelica Pill, 1175
Cinnamon and Dragon Bone Combination, 798
Cinnamon and Ginseng Combination, 466
Cinnamon and Hoelen Formula, 928
Cinnamon and Mahuang Combination, 56
Cinnamon and Persica Combination, 933
Cinnamon and Poria Sweet Dew Decoction, 444
Cinnamon Combination, 51
Cinnamon Decoction, 51
Cinnamon Twig and Ginseng Decoction, 466
Cinnamon Twig and Hoelen Pill, 928
Cinnamon Twig and Poria Pill, 928
Cinnamon Twig Decoction, 51
Cinnamon Twig Decoction plus Dragon Bone and Oyster Shell, 798
Cinnamon Twig Decoction plus Kudzu, 55
Cinnamon Twig Decoction plus Magnolia Bark and Apricot Kernel, 55
Cinnamon Twig Decoction plus Peony, 55
Cinnamon Twig, Peony, and Anemarrhena Decoction, 1186
Circulatory effect, 495, 1136, 1163
Cirrhosis, liver, *1414*
alcohol-induced, 223
with ascites, **1111**, **1127**
blood stagnation, 885
damp-heat accumulation, 1270
deficiency with dampness, 536
due to five consumptive lifestyles, 937
with gynecomastia, **61**
heat formation and qi stagnation, 184
Liver qi stagnation, **251**
Liver qi stagnation with heat, 254
qi and blood stagnation with damp and phlegm accumulation, 935
qi deficiency with cold and dampness, 531
qi stagnation and damp-heat accumulation, 1272
shaoyin syndrome, **235**
Stomach deficiency and interlocking of heat and cold, 270
Stomach qi disharmony, 261

Index

taiyang and *shaoyang* syndromes, 219
water and damp accumulation, 186
yang deficiency, 1138
Cirrhosis, renal, 1090
Cirsium Decoction, 946
Cis-diamminedichloroplatinum, 612
Cisplatin, 266, 612
CITES (Convention on International Trade in Endangered Species), *1441*
Citrus and Apricot Seed Formula, 116
Citrus and Bamboo Combination, 854
Citrus and Bamboo Shaving Decoction, 854
Citrus and Crataegus Formula, 1266
Citrus and Pinellia Combination, 1209
Citrus Seed Formula, 833
Civilian fire, 19
Clarification of the Theory of Cold-Induced Disorders, 7
Clarifying Doubts about Injury from Internal and External Causes, 554, 580, 840, 858, 1156, **1261**, 1270, 1274, 1275
Clean, *1513. See also Jing* (clean)
Clear Epidemics and Overcome Pathogenic Influences Decoction, 337
Clear Heat and Cool the Blood Decoction, 335
Clear Heat and Relieve Toxicity Decoction, 350
Clear Heat to Unblock Dysuria Decoction, 1108
Clear Summer-Heat and Augment the Qi Decoction, 446, 448
Clear the Collaterals Decoction, 435
Clear the Discharge Decoction, 809
Clear the Epigastrium and Benefit the Diaphragm Decoction, 386, 387
Clear the Intestines Decoction, 164, 165, 1381
Clear the Intestines Drink, 1381
Clear the Lung Decoction, 1225, 1227
Clear the Lung Drink, 1224
Clear the Nose Decoction, 86
Clear the Nutritive Level Decoction, 330
Clear the Qi and Transform Phlegm Pill, 1222
Clear the Spleen Decoction, 231
Clear the Stomach Decoction, 392
Clear the Stomach Powder, 393
Clear the Upper and Guard the Wind Decoction, 349
Clearing, *1518. See also Qing fa* (clearing)
Clearing and Cooling Decoction, 354
Clearing method, **10**, 281, 314, 743
Cleft point, *1524. See also Xi* (cleft) point
Clematis and Carthamus Combination, 1171
Clematis and Stephania Blood-Activating Decoction, 1169
Clematis and Stephania Combination, 1169
Clinical Handbook of Chinese Herbal Formulae, 684
Clomid. *See* Clomiphene
Clomiphene, 224, 922
Clonic convulsions, 1009
Closed disorder, *1506. See also Bi zheng* (closed disorder)
cold, 759
overview, 743, 1309
phlegm accumulation, 1313
wind-phlegm, 1312
Cloth Sack Pill, 1299
Clotting disorders, 869. *See also* Thrombosis; Embolism; Anticoagulant effect; Antiplatelet effect; Thrombolytic effect
Cloudy dysuria, 1142, *1511. See also Gao lin* (cloudy dysuria); *Lin zheng* (dysuria syndrome)
Clove and Persimmon Calyx Decoction, 856
Clumping, *1507*
Cnidium and Notopterygium Combination, 893
Cnidium and Rehmannia Combination, 624

Cnidium and Tangkuei Decoction to Regulate Blood, 624
Cnidium and Tangkuei Decoction to Tonify Blood, 624
Cnidium and Tea Formula, 973
Cnidium, Tangkuei, Gelatin and Artemisia Decoction, 950
Cnidium, Tangkuei, Gelatin and Mugwort Leaf Decoction, 950
Cocculus and Ginseng Combination, 1125
Cocculus Decoction, 1125
Cock's Crow Powder, 1183
Cognition, deteriorated, **552**
Cognitive deficits, scopolamine-induced, 567
Cognitive effect, 564, 585, 679
Cognitive impairment, **538**
Coicis Decoction, 1173, 1383
Coicis, Prepared Aconite, and Patrinia Powder, 1382
Coix Combination, 1173
Col-Benemid. *See* Colchicine
Colchicine, 598
Cold, *1507*
accumulation, 302
in the channels and collaterals, 456, 494
interior, 455
interior cold with yang qi and blood deficiencies, 494
interior excess, 166, 171
intolerance of, 560
overview, 455
in *taiyin, shaoyin,* and *jueyin,* 491
with yang deficiency, 456
Cold damage, 31, 199, 311, *1519. See also Shang han* (cold damage)
Cold Limbs Decoction, 486
Cold Limbs Powder, 233
Cold sores. *See* Herpes
Cold Wheezing Pill, 1243
Cold, aversion to
exterior cool-dryness, 1025
exterior-excess, wind-cold, 39
Kidney yang deficiency, 678
overview, 34, 35, 281, 455, 456, 514, 1021, 1063
severe, 132, 291, 491
shaoyin syndrome, 486
shaoyin with *taiyang* syndrome, 132
summer-heat with cold and dampness, 436, 439
wei (defensive) *qi* deficiency, 773
wind, 973
wind, cold and dampness with interior heat, 64
wind, cold and dampness with qi deficiency, 124
wind-cold, 59, 67, 70, 72
wind-cold and interior dampness, 1079
wind-cold turning into heat, 108
wind-cold with interior deficiency and cold, 466
wind-cold with interior heat, 45
wind-cold with interior phlegm, 128
wind-cold with water accumulation, 74
wind-cold with yang qi deficiency, 131
wind-cold with yin and blood deficiencies, 136
wind-heat, 92
wind-heat with yin deficiency, 137
wind-warmth, 111
Colic, intestinal, 494
Colitis
acute, 403, 1079
acute or chronic, **404**
allergic, 403
chronic, **167**, **259**, **537**, **601**, **783**, 787, **808**, 840, **887**
chronic nonspecific, 448

Index

damp-heat, 406
damp-heat with qi and blood stagnation, 1379
deficiency and cold, 459
with diarrhea, **786**
toxic heat, **409**
ulcerative, *1406*
    blood stagnation, **892**
    chronic, **236, 265, 297, 469, 524, 581, 1294, 1329**
    damp accumulation in the Spleen and Stomach, **1070**
    damp-heat, **404**
    damp-heat with qi and blood stagnation, 1379, **1381**
    deficiency and cold, **464**
    deficiency and cold of the Stomach, **469**
    heat in the Stomach and cold in the Intestines, 1292
    qi deficiency, **524**
    shaoyang syndrome with water accumulation, **224**
    Spleen deficiency, **553**
    Spleen deficiency and Liver excess, **259**
    toxic heat, 408
    wind, heat and toxins, 945
Colla Cornus Cervi, xxv
Collapse, *1507*
    qi, *1517*
Collected Formulas of the Yang Family, 977
Collected Songs about Contemporary Formulas, 917
Collected Treatises of [Zhang] Jing Yue, 12, **147,** 179, 184, 238,
    257, 398, 548, 618, 645, 647, 678, 680, 836, 838, 1071
Collecting point, *1515. See also Mu* (collecting) point
Collection of Commentaries on the Classic of the Materia
    Medica, **1019**
Collection of Formulas of Si He-Ting, 347
Collection of Personal Expertise Concerning Skin Lesions, 1332,
    1340
Collection of Writings on the Mechanisms of Illness, Suitability
    of Qi, and the Safeguarding of Life as Discussed in the Basic
    Questions, 825, 988
Colon
    cancer, *1403*
    stenosis, *1273*
Colony-stimulating factor (CSF), 203, 209, 564, 617
Col-Probenecid. *See* Colchicine
Coma, *1406*
    hot *bi zheng* (closed disorder), 747
    Liver wind rising, 993
    overview, 964
    phlegm and heat obstruction, 750
Combined Cinnamon Twig and Ephedra Decoction, 56
Common cold, *1406*
    in children, 69
    with constitutional deficiencies, **546**
    with cough and phlegm, 114
    exterior-excess, wind-cold, 39
    in geriatrics, 69, **130,** 132
    heat and fire in the upper and middle *jiaos,* **352**
    heat, lingering or residual, 327
    interior heat, 321
    overview, 37
    phlegm and damp accumulation, 1224
    shaoyang syndrome, 206, 304
    shaoyang syndrome with phlegm stagnation, 226
    shaoyang syndrome with water accumulation, 222
    in the summer, **53,** 435, **440,** 446, 1079
    summer-heat, 438
    summer-heat with exterior cold and interior dampness, 436
    taiyang and *shaoyang* syndromes, **220**
    wind, 973

wind, cold and dampness with interior heat, 64
wind, cold and dampness with qi deficiency, 124
wind, heat and toxins, 356
wind-cold, 59, 67, 70, 72
wind-cold attacking the Lung, 48, 49
wind-cold turning into heat, 108
wind-cold with interior deficiency and cold, 466
wind-cold with interior heat, 45, 295
wind-cold with water accumulation, 74
wind-cold with yang qi deficiency, 131
wind-cold with yin and blood deficiencies, 136
wind-dampness, 1156
wind-heat, **94**
wind-heat with interior heat, 291
wind-heat with yin deficiency, 137
wind-warmth, 89, 111
yin deficiency, **414**
Compilation of Materials of Benevolence for the Body, 729
Complete Book of Medicine, 12
Complete Collection of Patterns and Treatments in External
    Medicine, 1350, 1351, 1370, 1374
Complete Fine Formulas for Women, 7, 1219
Complete Nourishment Decoction (Pill), 609
Composition, 14
Comprehensive Medicine According to Master Han, 1245
Comprehensive Medicine According to Master Zhang, 1173,
    1243, 1244
Concentration, poor, 735. *See also* Forgetfulness; Memory;
    Cognitive effect
Conception channel, *1518. See also Ren* (conception) channel
Concha Margaritiferae, xxvi
Concha Meretricis seu Cyclinae, xxiv
Concussion, **878, 882, 899, 1001**
Conduct the Qi Decoction, 837
Confucians' Duties to their Parents, 7, 1272, **1307,** 1312
Confusion, post-stroke, 986
Cong Bai Qi Wei Yin **(Scallion Decoction with Seven**
    Ingredients), 135
Cong Chi Jie Geng Tang **(Scallion, Prepared Soybean, and**
    Platycodon Decoction), 111
    vs. Sang Ju Yin (Mulberry Leaf and Chrysanthemum
        Decoction), 113
Cong Chi Tang **(Scallion and Prepared Soybean Decoction),** 112
Congestion, sinus, 84
Congestive heart disease, 584
Congestive heart failure, 74, 554, *1406*
Conjunctivitis, *1406*
    acute, **293, 351, 357, 371, 410**
    damp-heat in all three *jiaos,* 359
    damp-heat in the Spleen and Stomach, 401
    heat accumulation in all three *jiaos,* 347
    qi and blood deficiencies, 1367
    wind, heat and toxins in the upper body, 349
    wind-cold with interior heat, 295
    wind-heat, 381
Connecting point, *1515. See also Luo* (connecting) point
Connective tissue disorders, **617,** 1186. *See also* specific locations
    and disorders
Consciousness, altered, 187, 753. *See also* Unconsciousness
Constipation, *1406. See also* Laxative effect; Purgative effect
    in anemic persons, 177
    blood deficiency, 177
    body fluid deficiency, 176
    chronic, 179, **1271**
    chronic, habitual, **473**
    deficiency, **477**

Index

deficiency and cold, 784, **786**
drug-induced
  antipsychotics, 175, 482
  morphine, **483**
  opioids, 159
  phenothiazine, 191
with dry, immobile stools, 190
dryness and heat, 160, 174, **175**
excess cold accumulation, 166, 171
excess heat with qi and blood deficiencies, 187
fire in the Liver and Gallbladder channels, 379, **380**
in geriatric/elderly persons, 177, 179, **212**, **794**
habitual, 152, 174, 177, 179, 289, 291, 359, **601**
heat and toxins in the lower *jiao*, 164
heat in the Stomach and Intestines, 160
interior excess heat, 152, 158
interior heat and toxins, 361
Kidney yang deficiency, 179
overview, 149, 151, 281, 315, 819, 1021, 1022
post-operative/post-surgical, 152, **159**, **175**
postpartum, 174
qi and blood deficiencies, **545**
severe, 152
shaoyang and *yangming* syndromes, 283
Spleen yang deficiency with cold, 169
taiyang and *yangming* syndromes, 289
with watery fluids, 152, 187
yin and body fluids, damaged, 190, 1054, **1056**
yin-deficient heat and fire, 420
Construct Roof Tiles Decoction, 1002
Continuation of Famous Physicians' Cases Organized by
  Categories, 1096
Continuation of Famous Physicians' Patients Organized by
  Categories, 657
Control Mucus Special Pill, 182
Controlling sequence, *1507*
Convenient Reader of Established Formulas, 1190
Convention on International Trade in Endangered Species
  (CITES), *1441*
Convulsions, *1407*. *See also* Seizures; Epilepsy; Anticonvulsant
  effect
  clonic, 1009
  excess heat and toxins, 337
  external wind, 980
  hot *bi zheng* (closed disorder), 747
  infantile, 363, 747, 755
    chronic, 459
  Liver wind rising, 993
  Liver wind rising with yin deficiency, 1009
  overview, 744, 1309
  Pericardium heat and Liver wind, 753
  phlegm and heat rising, 1251
  post-stroke, 984
  re jue (heat reversal), 152
  tetanus, 983
  theophylline-induced, 720
  yin, blood and body fluid deficiencies, 600
Cooked and Dried Rehmannia Pill, 663
Cool the Bones Powder, 418
Cool the Diaphragm Powder, 351
Coptis and Magnolia Bark Combination, 1099
Coptis and Magnolia Bark Decoction, 1099
Coptis and Rehmannia Formula, 393
Coptis and Rhubarb Combination, 359
Coptis and Scute Combination, 341
Coptis and Scute Detoxifying Decoction, 341

Coptis Combination, 271
Coptis Decoction, 271
Coptis Decoction to Relieve Toxicity, 341
Coptis Phellodendron and Mint Formula, 347
Coptis Pill to Clear the Upper, 347
Coptis Up-Clearing Pill, 347
Cor pulmonale, 1036
Cordia Decoction, 900
Corneal ulcer, **606**
Corns, 494
Cornu Cervi Degelatinatum, xxv
Cornu Elaphuri, xxv
Cornu Elaphuri Pantotrichum, xxv
Coronary artery disease, *1407*
  cold *bi zheng* (closed disorder), 759
  in geriatrics, **670**
  Kidney yang deficiency, 673
  qi and blood deficiencies, **606**
  qi and blood stagnation, 915
  qi and yin deficiencies, **555**
  with angina, **913**, **1132**
Coronary heart disease
  blood stagnation, 879
  Heart and Kidney deficiencies, **727**
  Kidney deficiency, **630**
  qi and blood deficiencies, 589
  qi and yin deficiencies, **555**
  qi deficiency and blood stagnation, **908**
Coronary Styrax Pill, 760
Corporeal soul, *1517*. *See also* Po (corporeal soul)
Corpus luteum, 673
Corpus Radix Angelicae Sinensis, xxiv
Corrections of Errors Among Physicians, **865**, **877**, 879, 885, 889,
  893, 905
Cortex Ailanthi, xxiii
Cortex Periplocae, xxiii
Cortex Phellodendri Chinensis, xxiv
Corticosteroids, 680
Corticosterone, 717
Corticotropin-releasing factor, 223
Cortisol, 76, 266, 530, 830
Corydalis Formula One, 826
Corydalis Formula Two, 826
Corydalis Powder, 826
Corynebacterium diphtheriae, 1034
Cough, **117**, *1407*. *See also* Antitussive effect
  with blood, 649, 943, 1042
  with blood in the sputum, 1036
  bronchitis, 114, 115
  with chest pain, 226
  chronic, **384**, 554, 558, 560, 1226, 1229
    persistent, 779
    stubborn, 1246
  in children, **384**, **1048**, **1246**
  cold and phlegm, 1244
  cold phlegm, 1242
  common cold, 114, 115
  damaged qi and body fluids, 554
  drug-induced, 1042
    angiotensin-converting enzyme inhibitors, 1042
    capsaicin, 1045
    enalapril, 1045
  dry, 589, **1048**, 1240
    exterior warm-dryness, 1028
    Lung yin and Spleen qi deficiencies, 1042
    overview, 513

INDEX

I

1545

Index

warm-dryness, 1030
with damaged yin, 1047
dryness and heat, **1037**
dryness with phlegm, 1240
with dyspnea, **98**, 1027
excessive, 80
exterior cool-dryness, 1025, **1026**
heat, 115
heat-phlegm, 1226
influenza, 115
interstitial pneumonia, **1045**
Kidney and Lung yin deficiencies, 643
Kidney yin deficiency, 644
lung abscess, 1377
Lung and Kidney yin deficiencies, 1036
Lung heat, 96, 383, **1031**
Lung heat and yin deficiency, 1229
Lung heat with phlegm accumulation, 1232
Lung qi deficiency, 560
Lung yin and qi deficiencies, 779
Lung yin deficiency, **1040**, 1043, **1045**
Lung yin deficiency with heat, 1039
overview, 35, 36, 316, 769, 771, 820, 1021, 1205, 1206
in pediatrics, **91**
persistent or violent, 115
phlegm, 1230
phlegm and damp accumulation, 1224
phlegm retention, 80
phlegm retention and qi stagnation, 1245
phlegm retention with yang deficiency, 1131
phlegm-heat, 1222, 1233, 1235
postinfectious, **1045**
qi deficiency with dampness and phlegm, 527
severe, 779, 1226
shaoyang syndrome, **211**
in smokers, 1229
with sputum, difficult-to-expectorate, 1043
with sputum, yellow and foul-smelling, 1377
with sputum, thin, 1025
stubborn, **41**
due to tuberculosis, 1224
upper excess and lower deficiency, 842
with wheezing, 844
whooping, 74, 80, **98**, 115, **117**, 351, **384**, **442**, 1028
wind, **117**
wind invading the Lung, 116
wind, cold and dampness with qi deficiency, 124
wind-cold, 70, 72, **77**
wind-cold and interior phlegm-heat, 845
wind-cold attacking the Lung, 48, 49
wind-cold with interior phlegm, 128
wind-cold with water accumulation, 74
wind-heat, 114
wind-heat with yin deficiency, 137
wind-warmth, 89, 111
yang deficiency with water accumulation, 1135
yin-deficient fire, 422
Coughing of Blood Formula, 943
Cough-Stopping Pill, 113
Cough-Stopping Powder, 116
Counterflow Cold Combination, 486
Counterflow Cold Formula, 233
Coxarthritis, pyogenic, **339**
Cr. *See* Creatinine
Craft of Medicinal Treatment for Childhood Disease Patterns, 7, 103, 124, 365, 376, 383, 396, **509**, 525, 539, 627, 1039

Cramps. *See also* Spasms; Antispasmodic effect
calf, 601
during hemodialysis, **601**
Liver wind rising, 1008
Liver wind rising with yin deficiency, 1009
overview, 963, 964
stomach, 731, **1044**
uterine, 731
wind, 980
wind, cold and dampness, 1177
yin, blood and body fluid deficiencies, 600
Crane's knee wind, 1182, 1186, *1512*. *See also He xi feng* (crane's knee wind)
Crataegus Decoction, 1268
Crataegus Decoction to Transform Phlegm, 1269
Creatinine (Cr), 774, 1066, 1111
Crohn's disease, *1407*
Crush, *1527*. *See also Zha* (crush)
Crying
in children, 246
constant, 471
in infants, 731
night, 731
urges, 731
CSF. *See* Colony-stimulating factor
Cui (quench), *1507*
***Cui Sheng Tang* (Birth-Hastening Decoction)**, 931
Cun position, *1508*
Cuo (grate), *1508*
Cup, *1508*
Curculigo and Epimedium Combination, 684
CVA. *See* Cerebrovascular accident; Stroke
Cyathula and Plantago Formula, 675
Cyathula and Rehmannia Formula, 645
Cyclophosphamide, 548, 612, 617
Cyperus and Amomum Powder to Calm the Stomach, 1073, 1075
Cyperus and Atractylodes Combination, 822
Cyperus and Atractylodes Pill, 822
Cyperus and Carthamus Combination, 578
Cyperus and Cluster Combination, 534
Cyperus and Perilla Formula, 67
Cyperus and Perilla Leaf Powder, 67
Cyperus and Perilla Powder, 67
Cyperus Cardamon and Atractylodes Formula, 1073
Cyperus Pill, 824
Cyperus, Perilla Leaf, Scallion, and Prepared Soybean Decoction, 69
Cyst
oophoritic, **250**, **891**, 928, **930**, **1372**
ovarian, 889, 928
Cysteamine, 220
Cysticercosis (bladder worms), 1301
Cystitis, *1407*
acute, **1117**
blood deficiency and heat, 576
chronic, 800
damp-heat, 1103
deficiency and cold, 1140
fire in the Heart channel, 365
fire in the Liver and Gallbladder, 371
fire in the Liver and Gallbladder channels, 379
Heart and Kidney deficiencies, 793
Heart fire with damp-heat in the lower *jiao*, 368
heat, 1107
Liver qi stagnation with heat, 254
Cytochrome P450 enzymes, 214, 224, 548
Cytotoxic drugs, 345

Chinese Herbal Formulas and Applications

Index

Cytoxan. *See* Cyclophosphamide
Da An Wan (Great Tranquility Pill), 1268
Da Bu Tang (Great Tonifying Decoction), 613
Da Bu Wan (Great Tonify Pill), 649
Da Bu Yin Wan (Great Tonify the Yin Pill), 649
   vs. Bu Fei E Jiao Tang (Tonify the Lung Decoction with
      Ass-Hide Gelatin), 1041
   vs. Hu Qian Wan (Hidden Tiger Pill), 653
   vs. Liu Wei Di Huang Wan (Six-Ingredient Pill with
      Rehmannia), 634, 650
   vs. Sheng Mai San (Generate the Pulse Powder), 1041
Da Chai Hu Tang (Major Bupleurum Decoction), 283
   vs. Da Cheng Qi Tang (Major Order the Qi Decoction), 287
   vs. Hou Po Qi Wu Tang (Seven-Substance Decoction with
      Magnolia Bark), 290
   vs. Xiao Chai Hu Tang (Minor Bupleurum Decoction), 216, 288
Da Cheng Chi Tang, 152
Da Cheng Qi Tang (Major Order the Qi Decoction), 152
   vs. Da Chai Hu Tang (Major Bupleurum Decoction), 287
   vs. Da Xian Xiong Tang (Major Sinking into the Chest
      Decoction), 157, 163
   vs. Tiao Wei Cheng Qi Tang (Regulate the Stomach and Order
      the Qi Decoction), 156
   vs. Xiao Cheng Qi Tang (Minor Order the Qi Decoction), 156
Da Ding Feng Zhu (Major Arrest Wind Pearl), 1009
   vs. E Jiao Ji Zi Huang Tang (Ass-Hide Gelatin and Egg Yolk
      Decoction), 1012
Da Fang Feng Tang (Major Saposhnikovia Decoction), 1181
**Da Huang Fu Zi Tang (Rhubarb and Prepared Aconite
Decoction)**, 166
   vs. San Wu Bei Ji Wan (Three-Substance Pill for Emergencies),
      168
   vs. Wen Pi Tang (Warm the Spleen Decoction), 168, 170
Da Huang Mu Dan Pi Tang, 1378
Da Huang Mu Dan Tang (Rhubarb and Moutan Decoction), 1378
   vs. Yi Yi Fu Zi Bai Jiang San (Coicis, Prepared Aconite, and
      Patrinia Powder), 1384
Da Huang Zhe Chong Wan (Rhubarb and Eupolyphaga Pill), 937
**Da Huo Luo Dan (Major Invigorate the Collaterals Special
Pill)**, 1179
Da Ji (Herba Cirsii Japonici), xxiii
Da Jian Zhong Tang (Major Construct the Middle Decoction), 480
   vs. Dang Gui Jian Zhong Tang (Tangkuei Decoction to
      Construct the Middle), 474
   vs. Huang Qi Jian Zhong Tang (Astragalus Decoction to
      Construct the Middle), 474
   vs. Xiao Jian Zhong Tang (Minor Construct the Middle
      Decoction), 474, 483
Da Jian Zhung Tang, 480
Da Qiang Huo Tang (Major Notopterygium Decoction), 66
Da Qin Jiao Tang (Major Gentiana Macrophylla Decoction), 988
Da Qing Long Tang (Major Bluegreen Dragon Decoction), 45
   vs. Ma Huang Xing Ren Gan Cao Shi Gao Tang (Ephedra,
      Apricot Kernel, Licorice, and Gypsum Decoction), 100
   vs. Xiao Qing Long Tang (Minor Bluegreen Dragon
      Decoction), 79
Da Qing Tang (Isatis Decoction), 358
Da tou wen (swollen head epidemic), 355, *1508*
Da Xian Xiong Tang (Major Sinking into the Chest Decoction), 161
   vs. Da Cheng Qi Tang (Major Order the Qi Decoction), 157, 163
   vs. Xiao Xian Xiong Tang (Minor Sinking into the Chest
      Decoction), 163, 1237
Da Xian Xiong Wan (Major Sinking into the Chest Pill), 163
Da Xue Teng (Caulis Sargentodoxae), xxiv
Da Yuan Yin (Reach the Membrane Source Decoction), 231
Dai (girdle) channel, *1508*

Dai Tian-Zhang, 633
Damp, *1508*
   accumulation, 302
   damp-cold, 1064
      hernia, 834
      jaundice, 1089
      Spleen and Stomach, 840
   damp-heat, 1064
      with food stagnation, 1272
      Gallbladder, 227, 1086
      in all three *jiaos*, 359
      in the lower *jiao*, 368, 371, 810, 1103
      Spleen and Stomach, 401, 1085
      Stomach and Intestines, 1270
      Urinary Bladder, 800
   damp-phlegm, 1209
   damp-warmth, 1092, 1096
   external, 1063
   internal, 1063
   middle *jiao*, 1076
   overview, 1063
   Spleen and Stomach, 1064, 1068, 1072, 1082
   Spleen deficiency, 1121, 1127
   water and dampness accumulation, 1064, 1109
   with wind-cold, 1079
Damp rash, *1508*
Damp-dispelling formulas, 1063
Damp-heat dysuria, *1520*. *See also Shi-re lin* (damp-heat dysuria);
   Lin zheng (dysuria syndrome)
Dan ji (pellet), 17
Dan Shen (Radix et Rhizoma Salviae Miltiorrhizae), xxiv
Dan Shen Yin (Salvia Decoction), 917
Dan Xi Xin Fa (Teachings of [Zhu] Dan-Xi), 7, 379, 389, 649, 651,
   773, 822, 943, 946, 1113, 1140, 1175, 1188, **1203**, 1266
Dan Xi Xin Fa Fu Yu (Additions to the Teachings for [Zhu]
   Dan-Xi), 1238
Dan Zhi Xiao Yao San (Moutan and Gardenia Rambling Powder),
   254
Danazol, 214
Dandelion and Wild Chrysanthemum Combination, 1337
Dang Gui (Radix Angelicae Sinensis), xxiv
**Dang Gui Bu Xue Tang (Tangkuei Decoction to Tonify the
Blood)**, 580
**Dang Gui Jian Zhong Tang (Tangkuei Decoction to Construct
the Middle)**, 474
   vs. Da Jian Zhong Tang (Major Construct the Middle
      Decoction), 474
   vs. Huang Qi Jian Zhong Tang (Astragalus Decoction to
      Construct the Middle), 474
   vs. Xiao Jian Zhong Tang (Minor Construct the Middle
      Decoction), 474
**Dang Gui Liu Huang Tang (Tangkuei and Six-Yellow
Decoction)**, 420
   vs. Mu Li San (Oyster Shell Powder), 421, 778
Dang Gui Long Hui Wan (Tangkuei, Gentiana, and Aloe Pill), 379
   vs. Long Dan Xie Gan Tang (Gentiana Decoction to Drain the
      Liver), 377
   vs. Xie Qing Wan (Drain the Green Pill), 377
**Dang Gui Nian Tong Tang (Tangkuei Decoction to Lift the
Pain)**, 1191
Dang Gui San (Tangkuei Powder), 623
Dang Gui Shao Yao San (Tangkuei and Peony Powder), 594
Dang Gui Shen (Corpus Radix Angelicae Sinensis), xxiv
**Dang Gui Si Ni Jia Wu Zhu Yu Sheng Jiang Tang (Tangkuei
Decoction for Frigid Extremities plus Evodia and Fresh
Ginger)**, 498

INDEX

1547

Index

Dang Gui Si Ni Tang (**Tangkuei Decoction for Frigid Extremities**), 494
  vs. *Si Ni San* (Frigid Extremities Powder), 499
  vs. *Si Ni Tang* (Frigid Extremities Decoction), 499
Dang Gui Tou (Caput Radix Angelicae Sinensis), xxiv
Dang Gui Wei (Extremitas Radix Angelicae Sinensis), xxiv
Dang Gui Yin Zi (**Tangkuei Decoction**), 970
  vs. *Xiao Feng San* (Eliminate Wind Powder), 972
Danocrine. *See* Danazol
Dao (pound), *1508*
Dao Chi San (**Guide Out the Red Powder**), 365
Dao Qi Tang (**Conduct the Qi Decoction**), 837
Dao Shui Fu Ling Tang (**Poria Decoction to Drain Water**), 1129
Dao Tan Tang (**Guide Out Phlegm Decoction**), 1211
De qi (arrival of qi), *1508*
Deafness, *1407*
  deficiency, 551, 666
  fire in the Liver and Gallbladder, 371
  Heart and Kidney disharmony, 714
  Kidney deficiency, 633
  Liver and Kidney yin deficiencies, 627
  yin deficiency with internal fire and wind, 661
Debilitation, *1508*
Debility
  deficiency and cold of the middle *jiao*, 471
  generalized, 1042
  qi deficiency with dampness, 536
  severe illness, 542
Decoct, *1513. See also Jian* (decoct)
  in gauze, 20
  post, *1517*
  pre, *1517*
Decoction, 16
  administration, 21
  equipment, 19
  method, 19
  preparation, 19
  temperature, 19
  water, 19
Deep pulse, *1508*
Deep vein thrombosis, **908**
Defensive level, *1522. See also Wei* (defensive) level
Defensive *qi*, *1523. See also Wei* (defensive) *qi*
Defensive, Qi, Nutritive, Blood Differentiation, 311, 431, *1523*.
  See also Wei qi ying xue bian zheng (defensive, qi, nutritive, blood differentiation)
Deficiency, *1508*
  blood, 513, 562, *1506*
  blood and yin, 593
  blood deficiency and heat, 575
  blood deficiency with blood stagnation, 571
  body fluids, 512
  chong (thoroughfare) and *ren* (conception) channels, 562
  du (governing) and *ren* (conception) channels, 687
  exhaustion of the body, 615
  extreme, 937
  generalized, 609, 725, 1042
  Heart and Kidney, 792
  Heart and Kidney with yin and blood, 725
  Heart and Spleen, 583
  Heart blood, 735
  jing (essence), 512
  Kidney and Liver yin, 654
  Kidney yang, 493, 668, 673
  Kidney yang with diminished *ming men* (life gate) fire, 678
  Kidney yang with water accumulation, 675

  Kidney yin, 644
  Kidney yin and yang deficiencies with fire, 684
  Kidney yin, marrow and *jing* (essence), 645
  Kidney yin, yang, blood and *jing* (essence), 687
  Liver and Kidney yin, 627, 640, 643
  Liver and Kidney yin deficiencies with deficiency fire, 649
  Liver blood and Kidney *jing* (essence), 690
  Lung qi, 560
  Lung yin, 1043
  Lung yin and qi, 779
  overview, 512, 769
  during pregnancy, 619, 621, 623
  qi, 512, *1517*
  qi and blood, 513, 580, 589, 604, *1517*
  qi and body fluids, 554
  qi, blood and yang, 609
  qi, blood, yang and *jing* (essence), 682
  Spleen and Kidney, 682
  Spleen and Stomach deficiencies with dampness, 535
  Spleen and Stomach qi, 522, 542
  Spleen and Stomach qi with cold and dampness, 531
  Spleen and Stomach qi with dampness and phlegm, 527
  Stomach yin, 1043
  wei (defensive) qi, 773
  yang, 513
  yang qi and blood, 494
  yin, 513
  yin and qi, 776
  yin and yang, 514, 798
  yin, blood and body fluids, 600
Deficiency and cold
  chong (thoroughfare) and *ren* (conception) channels, 919
  lower *jiao*, 795, 1140
  middle *jiao*, 455, 459, 471, 476, 484, 787
  postpartum, 925
  Spleen and Kidney, 781, 784
  Spleen and Stomach, 455, 463, 484
  Stomach, 467, 857
  uterus, 923
  with wind-cold, 466
Deficiency and debilitation, *1395*
Deficient pulse, *1508*
Degeneration, 1166. *See also* Atrophy
Delayed Menstruation Decoction, 578
Delirium, *1408*
  blood accumulation in the lower *jiao*, 873
  excess heat accompanied by qi and blood deficiencies, 187
  excess heat and toxins, 337
  heat in the *ying* (nutritive) level, 333
  heat, fire and toxins in all three *jiaos*, 341
  hot *bi zheng* (closed disorder), 747
  interior excess heat, 152, 158
  interior heat and toxins, 361
  interior heat in all three *jiaos*, 299
  overview, 315, 744
  Pericardium heat and Liver wind, 753
  phlegm and heat obstruction, 750
  shaoyang syndrome, 716
  taiyang, yangming and *shaoyang* disorders, 716
Dementia, **695**, *1408. See also* Alzheimer's disease; Antidementia effect; Antiamnestic effect
  vascular, 997, **998**, *1431*
Dendrobium Pill for Night Vision, 661
Depression, *1408. See also* Antidepressant effect
  Heart fire, 368, 710
  Liver qi stagnation, **249**

1548

Index

qi deficiency, **547**
qi stagnation, 823
severe, **473**
shaoyang syndrome, **213**
with stress, **265**, **529**, **830**
taiyang, yangming and *shaoyang* disorders, **718**
Deputy herb, 14, *1507*. *See also Chen yao* (deputy herb)
Dermatitis, *1408*
atopic, 326
blood deficiency, 562
blood deficiency and heat, 576
cosmetics-induced, 574
damp-heat, 1192
drug-induced, 92, 334, 567
early stage, 1334
heat and toxins, 291
heat in the *ying* (nutritive) level, 331
Lung yin and Spleen qi deficiencies, 1042
seborrheic, 576, **1088**
wind, 967
Dermatological disorders, 338, 359, 516, **577**, 1323, 1349. *See also* specific disorders; Dermatological effect
Dermatological effect, 576
Descurainia and Jujube Decoction to Drain the Lung, 384
Detoxification. *See* Poisoning
D-galactosamine, 214
Di Huang (Radix Rehmanniae), xxv
Di Huang Wan, 627
Di Huang Yin Zi (Rehmannia Decoction), 693
Di Tan Tang (Scour Phlegm Decoction), 1212
Diabetes insipidus, 668, 673, 1052, *1408*
Diabetes mellitus, *1408*. *See also* Antidiabetic effect; Hypoglycemic effect
adult-onset, **400**, 630
complications, **1216**
foot, 1214
nephropathy, 224, 929, 1214
neuropathy, **502**, **573**, **676**
obesity, **373**
retinopathy, 1214
damp-heat, **1211**
dryness with yin deficiency, **1048**
excess interior heat, 323
Heart and Kidney deficiencies, 793
Heart and Kidney disharmony, 797
heat, lingering or residual, 327
heat-phlegm, 1214
Kidney and Lung yin deficiencies, **643**
Kidney yang deficiency, 673, 678
Kidney yang deficiency with water accumulation, 675
Liver and Kidney yin deficiencies, **629**, 641
Lung and Kidney yin deficiencies, **1038**
Lung yin and Spleen qi deficiencies, 1042
non-insulin dependant, 629
overview, 317, 517, 1023
qi and yin deficiencies, **695**, **1050**
qi, yin and body fluid deficiencies, **556**
Stomach heat, **326**
type II, **369**, **638**, **670**, **875**, **1053**, **1056**
yin, blood and body fluid deficiencies, **602**
yin-deficient fire, 423
Dian kuang (mania and withdrawal), *1393*, *1508*
heat-phlegm, **1215**
old phlegm and excess heat, 1238
overview, 1205, 1309
phlegm and fire, 712

qi stagnation and phlegm obstruction, **830**
Dianthus Formula, 1103
Dianthus Plus Formula, 1105
Diaphragm
blood stagnation, 885
discomfort, 1242
distention and oppression, 822
fullness and discomfort, 48
fullness and distention
damp accumulation, 1082
damp and phlegm obstruction, 230
deficiency and cold of the Stomach, 467
phlegm-heat, 1222
wind-cold with interior phlegm, 128
fullness and oppression, 842, 1079
fullness and stifling sensation, 49, 80
heat and water accumulation, 162
oppression, 849
phlegm stagnation and water retention, 183
Diarrhea, *1409*. *See also* Antidiarrheal effect
5 a.m., *1505*
acute, **265**, **1114**
anus, burning sensations of the, 295
with blood and mucus, 169
with blood and pus, 408, 781
in children, **407**, **487**
chronic, 169, 536, 541, 542, 781, 784, 787, 788, **790**, 805, **1294**
cold and dampness, 1134
cold damaging the Stomach and Spleen, 1113
constant, 466
damp accumulation, 1072, 1076, 1082
damp-heat, 406, **445**, **1101**
damp-warmth, 1096
deficiency and cold, 459, 463, **788**
deficiency and cold of the middle *jiao*, 787
deficiency and cold of the Spleen and Kidney, 781, 784, **785**
drug-induced
cisplatin, 266
irinotecan, 266
early morning, 784
enteritis, 296
excessive, 1099
food poisoning, 296
food stagnation, 1270, 1277
food, undigested, 270
foul-smelling, 295
in geriatrics, **546**
hands and feet, extremely cold, 467
heat and fire in the upper and middle *jiaos*, 351
heat and water, interlocked, 268
heat in the chest and cold in the Stomach, 271
infantile, **442**, 444, **465**, 536, **905**, **1081**
infection, 296
overview, 202, 281, 455, 456, 513, 770, 771, 1063, 1064, 1263
postpartum, 296
post-surgical, **533**
during pregnancy, **297**
qi deficiency with dampness, 535, **537**
qi deficiency with dampness and phlegm, 527
recurrent, **783**
shaoyin syndrome, 467, 486
Spleen and Stomach deficiencies, 541
Spleen and Stomach disharmony, 1074
Spleen deficiency and Liver excess, 257, **258**
Spleen qi deficiency and Liver qi stagnation, 807
Stomach qi disharmony, 261

1549

Index

summer-heat, 438
summer-heat and dampness, 441, 444
summer-heat with exterior cold and interior dampness, 436
traveler's, 406, 757
wind-cold, 59
wind-cold and interior dampness, 1079
wind-cold with interior heat, *296*
yang deficiency with excess cold, 491
yang deficiency with water accumulation, 1135
DIC (disseminated intravascular coagulation), *1409*
Digestion, poor, 1297. *See also* Indigestion; Digestive effect
Digestive effect, 154
Din Chuan Tang, 845
***Ding Chuan Tang* (Arrest Wheezing Decoction)**, 845
Ding ji (lozenge), 18
***Ding Xian Wan* (Arrest Seizures Pill)**, 1251
***Ding Xiang Shi Di Tang* (Clove and Persimmon Calyx Decoction)**, 856
    vs. *Ju Pi Zhu Ru Tang* (Tangerine Peel and Bamboo Shaving Decoction), 853
    vs. *Xuan Fu Dai Zhe Shi Tang* (Inula and Hematite Decoction), 853
***Ding Zhi Wan* (Settle the Emotions Pill)**, 723
Dioscorea and Achyranthes Combination, 1002
Dioscorea Hypoglauca Decoction to Separate the Clear, 1140, 1141, 1142
Diphtheria, 96, 363, 1033, *1409*
Diplococcus pneumoniae, 296
Direct Investigations of Formulas for Cold-Induced Disorders, **279**, 441, 443
Discharge. *See* Nasal discharge; Vaginal discharge
Discharge Pus Powder, 1362
Discomfort, generalized, 484. *See* specific locations
Discouraged, easily, 1217
Discussion of Cold-Induced Disorders, 6, **31**, 39, 45, 51, 55, 56, 59, 74, 96, 132, 134, 152, 158, 160, 161, 163, 172, 174, 181, 206, 219, 233, 261, 268, 269, 271, 295, 304, 321, 325, 326, 370, 406, 408, 453, 459, 466, 467, 471, 486, 488, 489, 494, 498, 589, 599, 715, 787, 788, 851, 873, 1086, 1089, 1109, 1115, 1135, 1137, 1230, 1235, 1292, 1311, *1519*. *See also Shang Han Lun* (Discussion of Cold-Induced Disorders)
Discussion of Cold-Induced Disorders and Miscellaneous Diseases, 5, **31**, **453**
Discussion of Dispersing and Brightening Formulas, 7, **279**, 442
Discussion of Epidemic Warm Disease, 192, **199**, 231
Discussion of fire and heat, 279, 1307
Discussion of Formulas for Obstetrics and Gynecology, 933
Discussion of Illnesses, Patterns, and Formulas Related to the Unification of the Three Etiologies, 182, 1213
Discussion of Sudden Turmoil Disorders, 756, 1099, 1101
Discussion of the Spleen and Stomach, 7, 177, 448, 492, 542, 1250, **1261**
Discussion of Warm and Hot Disorders, 311
Discussion of Widespread Warm Epidemics, 633
Discussion on attacking evil, 1307
Disease. *See* specific diseases
Disharmony
    Gallbladder and Stomach, 1214
    half-interior, half-exterior, 201
    Heart and Kidney, 714, 797
    Liver and Spleen, 202, 233
    overview, 201
    shaoyang, 201
    Spleen and Stomach, 1074
    Stomach and Intestines, 202
    Stomach qi, 261
    ying (nutritive) and *wei* (defensive) levels, 51, 798

Disk, prolapse, **1164**, **1373**
Disorder. *See* specific disorders
Disorientation, 731
Dispel Wind Powder, 969
Disperse the Swelling and Break the Hardness Decoction, 1357, 1358
Displays of Enlightened Physicians, 1112
Disseminated intravascular coagulation (DIC), *1409*
Dissipate Toxins and Release the Exterior Decoction, 104
Dissolution, 20
Dissolve, *1512*. *See also Hua* (dissolve)
Dissolve and Disperse Decoction Formula One, 1359
Dissolve and Disperse Decoction Formula Two, 1359
Dissolve Parasites Pill, 1300
Distention, *1516*. *See also* specific locations; *Pi* (distention)
    abdominal, 149, 159
        drum-like, *1509*
    definition, 156
    epigastric, **269**
    focal, *1510*
    lung, *1419*
    overview, 1263, 1264
Distillation, 18
Diuretic effect, 162, 223, 442, 1091, 1111, 1116
Divine Formulas from Zhang San-Feng, 1302
Divine Husbandman, 27, 1481, 1482, 1484
Divine Husbandman's Classic of the Materia Medica, 5, 27, **1019**
Dizziness, *1409*
    acute, **212**
    blood and yin deficiencies, 593
    blood deficiency, 562
    blood stagnation, 877
    damp-heat, 1085
    fire in the Liver and Gallbladder channels, 379
    with headache, **585**
    Heart and Kidney disharmony, 714
    Heart and Spleen deficiencies, **585**
    due to inner ear imbalance, **1006**
    Kidney yin and *jing* (essence) deficiencies, 645
    Kidney yin deficiency, 644
    Liver and Kidney yin deficiencies, 627, 640, 654
    Liver blood deficiency, 722
    Liver excess, 996
    Liver wind rising, 1008
    Liver yang and wind excess, 1004
    Liver yang and wind rising, 999
    Liver yang hyperactivity, 713
    Liver yang rising, 1002
    overview, 513, 514, 963, 964, 1205, 1206
    phlegm retention with yang deficiency, 1131
    qi and blood deficiencies, 604, 616
    qi, blood and yang deficiencies, 609
    with vertigo, **597**, **1133**, **1249**
    wind and phlegm rising, 1247
    wind-heat with interior heat, 291
    yang deficiency with water accumulation, 1135
    yin deficiency with internal fire and wind, 661
    yin, yang, blood and *jing* (essence) deficiencies, 687
Do not expose to heat, *1509*
Dong Heng Shi Xiao Fang (Tested and Effective Formulas by Dong Heng), 355, 551
Dong Tian Ao Zhi (Profound Purpose from the Heavenly Abode), 1347
Dopamine, 717
Dosage forms, 15, 16
Dosages, 15, *1437*
Dosing, *1437*

Index

Chinese Herbal Formulas and Applications

age, according to, *1438*
weight, according to, *1438*
Dou (measure of volume), 22
Dou Kou (Fructus Amomi Rotundus), xxiii
Dou Kou Ke (Pericarpium Amomi Rotundus), xxiii
Dou Zhen Shi Yi Xin Fa (Teachings of Generations of Physicians about Pox), 748
Double Relieve Powder that Sagely Unblocks, 294
Downbearing. *See* Prolapse
Downward draining formulas, 149
Doxorubicin. *See* Adriamycin
Drain Blood Stasis Decoction, 876
Drain the Epigastrium Decoction, 359
Drain the Green Pill, 376
Drain the Interior and Detoxify Decoction, 1367, 1368
Drain the Interior and Discharge Pus Decoction, 1363
Drain the Interior and Eliminate Pathogenic Influences Decoction, 1367
Drain the Interior Powder Worthy of a Thousand Gold, 1365
Drain the Lung Powder, 383
Drain the Pus Powder, 1364
Drain the Spleen Powder, 396
Drain the White Powder, 383
Drain the Yellow Powder, 396
Draining, 1321. *See also Tuo fa* (draining method)
Draining downward method, **10**, 149, 281, 1307, *1524*. *See also Xia fa* (draining downwards)
Dreams
 bizarre, 1238
 excessive, 654, 1002
 frequent, 710
 of sex, 798
Drive Out Blood Stasis Below the Diaphragm Decoction, 885
Drive Out Blood Stasis Decoction, 895
Drive Out Blood Stasis from a Painful Body Decoction, 893
Drive Out Blood Stasis in the Lower Abdomen Decoction, 889
Drive Out Blood Stasis in Three *Jiaos* Decoction, 883
Drive Out Stasis in the Mansion of Blood Decoction, 879
Drooling phlegm, *1509*
Drown, *1525*. *See also Yan* (drown)
Drowsiness, 486
Drug-herb interactions, **24**. *See also* drug and formula names
Drum skin pulse, *1509*
Drum-like abdominal distention, *1509*
Dry-fry, *1507*. *See also Chao* (dry-fry)
 to ash, *1507*. *See also Chao tan* (dry-fry to ash)
 to burnt, *1507*. *See also Chao jiao* (dry-fry to burnt)
 to yellow, *1507*. *See also Chao huang* (dry-fry to yellow)
Dryness, *1509, 1527*. *See also Zao* (dryness)
 cool-dryness, 1021
 definition, 156
 exterior
  cool-dryness, 1025
  warm-dryness, 1028
 external, 1021
 in geriatric, **639**
 internal, 1021
 Lung, 1030
 Lung and Stomach yin, damaged, 1047
 in the organs, 1022
 overview, 1021
 with qi and yin deficiencies, 1050
 Stomach and Intestines, 174
 warm-dryness, 1021
 with yin and body fluid deficiencies, 1054
 with yin deficiency and heat, 1052

Dryness-Clearing and Lung-Rescuing Decoction, 1029
Dryness-relieving formulas, 1021
Du (governing) channel, 687, *1509*
Du Huo Ji Sheng Tang (Angelica Pubescens and Taxillus Decoction), 1161
 vs. San Bi Tang (Three-Painful Obstruction Decoction), 1168
Du Qi Wan (Capital Qi Pill), 644
 vs. Liu Wei Di Huang Wan (Six-Ingredient Pill with Rehmannia), 635
Duan (calcine), *1509*
Duan Chang Cao, 27
Duan Shi Gao (Gypsum Fibrosum Praeparatum), xxiv
Dun (stew), *1509*
Dun Sou San (Long-Bout Cough Powder), 115
 vs. Ning Sou Wan (Quiet the Cough Pill), 119
 vs. Zhi Sou San (Stop Coughing Powder), 119
Duo Ming Wan (Life-Taking Pill), 931
Duodenal ulcer. *See also* Antiulcer effect
 bleeding, **949**, **952**
 cold and dampness, 1134
 damp accumulation, 1068
 damp-heat, 1099
 deficiency and cold, 459
 deficiency and cold with qi stagnation, 484
 Heart and Spleen deficiencies, 584
 heat in the chest and cold in the Stomach, 271
 Liver qi stagnation, 248
 qi deficiency with cold and dampness, 531
 qi deficiency with dampness, 536
 qi deficiency with dampness and phlegm, **529**
 shaoyang and *yangming* syndromes, **286**
 Spleen deficiency, 534
 taiyang and *shaoyang* syndromes, 219
 wind-cold with interior deficiency and cold, 466
 yang deficiency and interior cold, 481
 yin deficiency with qi stagnation and blood dryness, **658**
Dysenteric wind, 1182, *1514*. *See also Li feng* (dysenteric wind)
Dysentery, *1409, 1509*
 amoebic, 297, 403, **409**, 787
 with anorexia, 127
 bacterial, **297**, 341, **344**, **404**, **409**, 436, **787**, 1099, 1292, **1294**
 chronic, **461**, 542, 781, **783**, 787, 1292
 damp-heat, 391, 392, 403, **404**, 406, 1101
 damp-heat accumulation, 1270
 damp-heat in all three *jiaos*, 359
 deficiency and cold of the middle *jiao*, 787
 deficiency and cold of the Spleen and Kidney, 781
 excess cold accumulation, 166
 fasting, 127
 food stagnation and damp-heat accumulation, 1272
 Liver stagnation and Spleen deficiency, **785**
 overview, 770, 771
 with rectal tenesmus, 158
 with red (blood) or white (mucus) stools, 392, 781, 1272
 shaoyang and *yangming* syndromes, 283
 summer-heat, 438
 summer-heat and dampness, 444
 toxic heat, 408, 410
Dysmenorrhea, *1410*
 blood accumulation in the lower *jiao*, 873
 blood stagnation, 885, 933
 blood stasis, 928, 932
 cold and blood stagnation, **891**
 deficiency and cold, 919
 deficiency and cold with qi stagnation, 484
 heat, 243

1551

INDEX

I

Index

Liver qi stagnation, 238
overview, 819, 867
painful, **912**
primary, **213**, **596**
qi and blood stagnation, 579
recurrent, **596**, **602**
stagnation, **572**
Dyspepsia
drug-induced, 1112
qi deficiency with dampness, 536
Dysphagia, 977, 1238
Dysphasia, 963, 991
Dyspnea. *See also* Wheezing; Asthma
with cough, **98**, **1027**
deficiency heat, 558
exterior-excess, wind-cold, 39
Lung and Kidney deficiencies, 559
Lung heat, 96, 383
Lung heat with phlegm accumulation, 1232
Lung qi deficiency, 560
lying down, 1125
overview, 36, 281, 316, 820
phlegm retention, 80
phlegm retention and qi stagnation, 1245
qi and blood deficiencies, 616
qi and phlegm stagnation, 848
qi flow, reversed, 55
in summer, **447**
in tracheitis, **46**
upper excess and lower deficiency, 842
warm-dryness, 1030
water accumulation, 1129
with wheezing, **77**, **1432**
wind-cold, 72
wind-cold and interior phlegm-heat, 845
wind-cold attacking the Lung, 48, 49
wind-heat, 114
yin-deficient fire, 422
Dyspnea and wheezing, *1523*
Dystonia, autonomic, 731
Dysuria, *1394*, *1410*, *1514*. *See also* Diuretic effect; *Lin zheng*
(dysuria syndrome)
damp-heat, 371, 1086, 1090, 1103, 1192
deficiency and cold, 787, 1140, **1141**
fire in the Heart and Small Intestine channels, **366**
fire in the Liver and Gallbladder channels, 379
heat, fire and toxins in all three *jiaos*, **344**
infection, **1104**
interior heat and toxins, 361
Kidney yang deficiency, 668, 673
Kidney yang deficiency with water accumulation, 675
overview, 433, 1063
postpartum, **546**
shaoyang syndrome, 716
summer-heat and dampness, 441, 444
taiyang, *yangming* and *shaoyang* disorders, 716
water accumulation, 102, 1129
water and heat, interlocked, 1115
E Jiao Ji Zi Huang Tang (**Ass-Hide Gelatin and Egg Yolk Decoction**), 1007
vs. *Da Ding Feng Zhu* (Major Arrest Wind Pearl), 1012
vs. *Ling Jiao Gou Teng Tang* (Antelope Horn and Uncaria Decoction), 1008
E Jiao San (Ass-Hide Gelatin Powder), 1039
E. coli, 41, 46, 60, 158, 258, 285, 404, 1104, 1380
Ear disorders, 318. *See also* specific disorders

diminished acuity, 551
impaired hearing, 666
suppuration, 120
swelling, 1002
swelling and pain, 371
swelling, inflammation and infection, 120
Earth, *1509*
Ectopic Pregnancy Formula, 917
Eczema, *1410*. *See also* Rashes; Itching; Urticaria
acute, **155**
anus, **344**
blood deficiency and heat, 576
blood deficiency with blood stagnation, **574**
damp-heat, **1190**
early stage, 1334
exterior-deficient, wind-cold, 51
fire and toxins, 1337
heat and toxins, 1342
overview, 963
scrotum, **375**
wind, **967**, **969**
wind with blood deficiency, 970
wind with water accumulation, 101
wind, cold and dampness with qi deficiency, 124
wind, heat and toxins in the upper body, 349
ED (erectile disorder). *See* Impotence
Edema, *1410*. *See also* Diuretic effect
cardiac, 1113
cardiac and nephritic, 1121
cold damaging the Stomach and Spleen, 1113
damp accumulation, 1121
dampness and cold, **1184**
extremities, 1219
floating, *1510*
generalized, 101, 181, 186, 1121, 1129
heat formation and qi stagnation, 184
due to hypothyroidism, 1137
idiopathic, **1119**
leg, 1118
lower half of the body, 1138
due to nephritis, 45, 101, 1113, 1125, 1129
overview, 150, 1063, 1064, 1065
phlegm retention with yang deficiency, 1131
pitting, 1124, 1125, 1127
pregnancy, during, 594, 807, **1105**
pulmonary, 1173
qi deficiency with dampness, **538**
severe, 675, 1138
shaoyang syndrome with water accumulation, 222
Spleen deficiency and damp accumulation, **1122**
water accumulation, 102, 1129
water and dampness accumulation, 186, 1109
water and heat, interlocked, **1116**
water stagnation, 1127
wind with interior qi deficiency, 1118
wind with water accumulation, 101
wind-cold with water accumulation, 74
wind-dampness, **1157**
yang deficiency, 1138
yang deficiency with water accumulation, 1135
Effective Formulas from Generations of Physicians, 176, 728
Effective Medical Formulas Arranged by Category by Doctor Zhu, 1183
Eight Arrays of Formulas, 12, 147
Eight Corrections Powder, 1103
Eight Jewel Decoction (Pill), 604

1552

Index

Chinese Herbal Formulas and Applications

Eight meeting points, **1505**. *See also Ba hui* (eight meeting) points
Eight Principle Differentiation, **1505**. *See also Ba gang bian zheng* (eight principle differentiation)
Eight Treasures Decoction (Pill), 604
Eight treatment methods, 9
Eight-Flavour Rehmannia Pill, 672
Eight-Herb Powder for Rectification, 1103
Eight-Immortal Pill for Longevity, 642
Eight-Ingredient Formula for Leukorrhea, 810
Eight-Ingredient Pill with Anemarrhena and Phellodendron, 636
Eight-Ingredient Pill with Rehmannia, 672, 674
Eight-Ingredient Rambling Powder, 254
Eight-Taste Discharging Formula, 810
Eight-Treasure Decoction, 604
Ejaculation
   premature
      Heart and Kidney disharmony, 797
      Kidney yang deficiency, 668, 673, 678
      overview, 514
      yin and yang deficiencies, 798
   unable to, 374
Elbow
   pain, 893, 1195
   tennis, 1159
Eliminate Dryness and Rescue the Lung Decoction, 1029
Eliminate Wind Powder, 967
Elsholtzia Drink, 436
Emaciation. *See also* Face
   blood deficiency and heat, 575
   qi and blood deficiencies, 616
   yin-deficient heat, 418
Embolism, 879. *See also* Thrombosis; Anticoagulant effect; Antiplatelet effect; Thrombolytic effect
   cerebral, 989, 1004, 1008, **1404**
Emergency Formulas to Keep Up One's Sleeve, 6, 112, 438, **1287**
Emetic formulas, 1309
Emissions
   nocturnal, 708, **723**
      Heart and Kidney deficiencies, 725
      Kidney deficiency, 789
      Liver and Kidney deficiencies, 690
      Liver and Kidney yin deficiencies, 654
      overview, 770
      yin and yang deficiencies, 798
      yin, yang, blood and *jing* (essence) deficiencies, 687
      yin-deficient fire, 423, 649
   seminal
      damp-heat in the lower *jiao*, 368
      Heart and Kidney deficiencies, 792
      Kidney deficiency, 789, 791
      Kidney yang deficiency, 678
      Kidney yin and *jing* (essence) deficiencies, 645
      Liver and Kidney deficiencies, 690
      Liver and Kidney yin deficiencies, 627
      due to mental and physical exhaustion, 791
      due to neurasthenia, 791
      overview, 513, 514
      due to prostatitis, 791
      qi, blood and yang deficiencies, 609
      qi, blood, yang and *jing* (essence) deficiencies, 682
      Spleen and Kidney yang deficiencies, **786**
      yin, yang, blood and *jing* (essence) deficiencies, 687
      yin-deficient fire, 637, 649
   spontaneous, 423
Emotional disorders. *See also* specific disorders; *Shen* (spirit) disturbance

changes, marked, 996
distress, 247, 254
instability, 253, 254, 713, 849
overview, 708, 820
unable to control, 731
Emotions, seven, **1519**
Emperor of Heaven's Special Pill to Tonify the Heart, 725, 728
Emphysema, **1410**
   damp-phlegm, 1209
   deficiency heat, 558
   exterior cool-dryness, 1025
   Kidney yang deficiency, 668, 673
   Kidney yin deficiency, 644
   Lung heat and yin deficiency, 1229
   phlegm retention, 80
   phlegm retention and qi stagnation, 1245
   phlegm-heat, 1233
   upper excess and lower deficiency, 842
   wind-cold with water accumulation, 74
Enalapril, 1045
Encephalitis
   complications of, 1008, **1011**
   damp-warmth, **1098**
   epidemic, 92
   excess heat and toxins, 338
   excess heat, fire and toxins, **343**
   excess interior heat, 323, 325
   heat and fire in the upper and middle *jiaos*, 351
   heat in the *xue* (blood) level, 333
   hot *bi zheng* (closed disorder), 747
   Liver wind rising, 993
   phlegm and heat obstruction, 750
   wind-cold, 59
End Discharge Decoction, 806
Endangered species, **1441**
Endocarditis, 589, **1410**
Endocrine, 717
Endocrine disorders. *See* specific diseases, glands or hormones; Endocrine effect
Endocrine effect, 223, 249, 595, 669, 673, 685, 921, 929
Endometriosis, **1411**
   blood deficiency, **565**
   blood stagnation, **883**, 885, **912**, **930**, 933
   cold obstruction and blood stagnation, **891**
   deficiency and damage, 951
   fire in the Liver and Gallbladder, 371
   interior cold with yang qi and blood deficiencies, **497**
   yang deficiency and interior cold, **1372**
Endometrorrhagia, 584
Energy level, **1517**. *See also Qi* (energy) level
Energy, low, 560, 678. *See also* Fatigue
ENT. *See* Ear; Nose; Throat; specific conditions
Enteritis, **1411**
   acute
      cold damaging the Stomach and Spleen, 1113
      damp-heat, 403, 406
      with diarrhea, 1109
      with diarrhea and severe pain, **259**
      heat, fire and toxins in all three *jiaos*, 341
      phlegm stagnation and water accumulation, 1220
      qi stagnation, **830**
      during the summer and fall, **1081**
      wind-cold with interior heat, 295
   acute or chronic, 302, **461**
   chronic
      damp-cold in the Spleen and Stomach, 840

1553

INDEX
I

Index

deficiency and cold of the Spleen and Kidney, 781
food stagnation with heat, 1277
Spleen deficiency and Liver excess, **259**
yang deficiency with water accumulation, 1135
deficiency and cold, 459, 787
excess cold accumulation, 166
in infants, **297**
postpartum, 408
shaoyang syndrome with water accumulation, 222
summer-heat, 438
toxic heat, 409
Enteroparalysis, **154, 875**
Enuresis, *1411*
in children, **42, 54, 786, 794, 796**
cold and dampness, 1134
deficiency and cold, **733, 795**
deficiency and cold of the middle *jiao*, 471
Heart and Kidney deficiencies, 792
Kidney deficiency, 789
overview, 770
yin and yang deficiencies, 798
Envoy herb, 14, *1519*. See also *Shi yao* (envoy herb)
Enzymes. *See* specific enzymes
Eosinophils, 36, 76, 846
Ephedra Decoction, 39
Ephedra Decoction plus Atractylodes, 42
Ephedra, Apricot Kernel, Coicis and Licorice Decoction, 43
Ephedra, Apricot Kernel, Gypsum and Licorice Decoction, 96
Ephedra, Apricot Kernel, Licorice and Gypsum Decoction, 96
Ephedra, Apricot, Coix and Licorice Decoction, 43
Ephedra, Apricot, Licorice and Gypsum Decoction, 96
Ephedra, Asarum, and Prepared Aconite Decoction, 132
Ephedra, Prepared Aconite, and Licorice Decoction, 134
Ephedrine, 133
Epidemic toxin, *1509*
Epidemics, warm, *1522*
Epididymitis, **650,** 834
Epigastric
coldness and pain, 282, 481
cramps and pain, 484
discomfort or distention, 534
distention, **269,** 270, 389, 1063
distention and fullness, 202, 1274
distention and hardness, 268, 851, 1311
distention and oppression, 1099
distention and pain, 158
distention and stifling sensations, 1206, 1209
fullness and distention
damp accumulation, 1068, 1121
food stagnation with heat, 1277
heat and cold, interlocked, 1280
interior excess heat, 152
Liver qi stagnation, 849
Lung heat with phlegm accumulation, 1232
overview, 149, 819, 1064, 1263
phlegm-heat, 1235
Stomach qi disharmony, 261
water accumulation, 1125
wind-cold with qi stagnation, 67
fullness and pain, 171, 202, 455, 463, 531, 822, 1270
fullness and stifling sensations, 536
fullness, distention and hardness, 270
fullness, distention and pain, 283, 840, 1266, 1272
hardness and pain, 187
hardness, fullness and pain, 161
oppression, 1220

overview
coldness and pain
distention
distention and stifling sensations
distention, fullness and pain
fullness, 1264
fullness and distention
fullness and pain
pain, *1411*
damp-heat, **1216**
deficiency and cold, **461**
deficiency and cold of the middle *jiao*, **473**
deficiency and cold of the Stomach, 467
due to gastritis, 1070
heat in the chest and cold in the Stomach, **272**
Liver fire overacting on the Stomach, **391**
overview, 867
phlegm-heat, **1237**
qi and blood stagnation, 917, **918**
shaoyin syndrome, 233, **236**
Spleen qi deficiency, **524**
Stomach yin deficiency, **1051**
with vomiting, 841
yang deficiency, phlegm accumulation and qi stagnation, 831
yin deficiency, **1047**
yin deficiency with qi stagnation and blood dryness, 657
phlegm stagnation, 1219
rigidity, 169
stifling sensation and distention, 327
Epilepsy, *1428, 1509*. See also Seizures; Convulsions; Antiepileptic effect
blood deficiency with heat, 245
in children, **1005,** 1251
Heart and Kidney disharmony, 714
heat-phlegm, 1214
in infants, 755
Liver yang and wind rising, 999
overview, 707, 1205, 1206, 1207
Pericardium heat and Liver wind, 753
phlegm and heat obstruction, 750
phlegm and heat rising, 1251
with seizures, **547, 719, 1239**
sudden onset, 1251
taiyang and *shaoyang* syndromes, 219
Epinephrine, 235
Epistaxis, *1402*
chronic, **334**
damp-heat in all three *jiaos*, 359
deficiency and cold, 948
excess heat and toxins, 337
heat and fire in the upper and middle *jiaos*, 351, **353**
heat in the Stomach and Intestines, 160
heat in the *xue* (blood) level, 333, 942
heat with damaged yin and body fluids, **191**
latent fire of the Spleen and Stomach, 396
Lung heat, **384**
overview, 315, 868
Stomach heat, **399**
stubborn, 639
warm-dryness, **1031**
wind-warmth, **91**
yang deficiency, 459
yin deficiency with heat, **1034**
Epithelial inflammations, 1337
Epivir. *See* Lamivudine

Index

Chinese Herbal Formulas and Applications

Er Chen Tang (Two-Cured Decoction), 1209
Er Chen Wan, 1209
Er Ke Xing Su Yin (Pediatric Apricot Kernel and Perilla Leaf Decoction), 70
Er Ke Zheng Zhi Zhun Sheng (Standards of Patterns and Treatments in Pediatrics), **1061**
Er Long Zuo Ci Wan (Pill for Deafness that Is Kind to the Left [Kidney]), 633
Er Miao San (Two-Marvel Powder), 1188
Er Shi Er Ji (Twenty-Two Types of Formulas), 13
Er Shi Si Ji (Twenty-Four Types of Formulas), 12
Er Xian Bu Shen Tang (Two-Immortal Decoction to Tonify the Kidney), 686
Er Xian Tang (Two-Immortal Decoction), 684
Er Zhi Wan (Two-Ultimate Pill), 654
  vs. Liu Wei Di Huang Wan (Six-Ingredient Pill with Rehmannia), 634
Er Zhu Tang (Two-Atractylodes Decoction), 1195
Erectile disorders. *See* Impotence
Erh Chen Tang (Wan), 1209
Eriobotrya and Ophiopogon Combination, 1029
Erysipelas, *1411*
  heat and toxins, 291, **1347**
  overview, 1321
  wind, heat, and toxins, **358**
  wind-cold with interior heat, 45, 295
Erythematosis, **373**
Erythrocytes, 524
Erythromelalgia, **1190**
Escape Restraint Pill, 822
Esophageal
  cancer, *1403*
  hemorrhage, 333
  spasms, 828
  varices, 937
Esophagitis
  chronic, **630**
  erosive, **855**
  heat, 370
  reflux, **211**, 261, **264**, **1237**, **1329**, *1427*
Essence, *1513*. *See also Jing* (essence)
Essential Compilation of Infectious Syndromes, 1095
Essential *qi*, *1528*. *See also Zong* (essential) *qi*
Essentials from the Golden Cabinet, 6, **31**, 42, 78, 80, 101, 102, 166, 171, 237, 283, 289, 323, 359, 384, 410, 453, 462, 475, 480, 500, 594, 623, 668, 722, 731, 798, 827, 831, 832, 853, 854, 876, 919, 928, 935, 937, 948, 950, 1043, 1077, 1090, 1118, 1120, 1125, 1131, 1133, 1186, 1220, 1242, 1275, 1364, 1378, 1382
Estradiol, 54, 256, 595, 598, 602, 630, 673, 685, 876, 921, 931
Estrogen, 596
Ethereal soul, 707, *1512*. *See also Hun* (ethereal soul)
Ethylamine hydrochloride, 390
Etoposide, 612
Eucommia and Rehmannia Formula, 678
Eupolyphaga seu Steleophaga, xxiv
Everlasting Categorization of Seal Formulas, 560
Everyone's Detoxifying Decoction, 355
Evodia and Coptis Pill, 389
Evodia Combination, 467
Evodia Decoction, 467
Evodia Fruit Decoction, 467
Excess, 158, *1509*
  heat, 321
  heat and toxins, 337
  heat with qi and body fluid deficiencies, 325
  interior cold, 166, 171

interior heat, 152, 187
water accumulation, 181
water accumulation with heat and qi stagnation, 184
water and damp accumulation, 186
Excess pulse, *1509*
Expectorant effect, 81, 129, 846, 1211, 1227, 1236, 1239, 1246
Explanation of the Subtitles of the Original Mechanism, 661
Extension of the Materia Medica, 792
Exterior, *1510*
  cool-dryness, 1021, 1025
  dampness, 1063
  dryness, 1021
  exterior and interior, 281, *1510*
  exterior-deficient, wind-cold, 51
  exterior-excess, wind-cold, 39
  heat, 314
  heat and toxins, 1342
  with interior deficiency, 35
  with interior heat in all three *jiaos*, 299
  overview, 34
  taiyang syndrome with wind-cold, 59
  warm-dryness, 1021, 1028
  wen bing (warm disease), 92
  wind, 963
  wind with water accumulation, 101
  wind, cold and dampness with interior heat, 64
  wind, cold and dampness with qi deficiency, 124
  wind-cold, 34, 72
  wind-cold in children, 70
  wind-cold turning into heat, 108
  wind-cold with five accumulations, 301
  wind-cold with interior dampness, 1079
  wind-cold with interior deficiency and cold, 466
  wind-cold with interior heat, 45, 295
  wind-cold with interior phlegm-heat, 845
  wind-cold with phlegm, 128
  wind-cold with qi stagnation, 67
  wind-cold with water accumulation, 74
  wind-cold with yang qi deficiency, 131
  wind-cold with yin and blood deficiencies, 136
  wind-dampness, 1156
  wind-heat, 35, 114
  wind-heat attacking the upper *jiao*, 120
  wind-heat with interior heat, 291
  wind-heat with yin deficiency, 137
  wind-warmth, 89, 111
Exterior- and interior-releasing formulas, 281
Exterior-releasing formulas, 34
External Medicine according to Bian Que, **705**
External Medicine Elaboration, 1369
Extraordinary Merit Powder, 525
Extremely painful obstruction, 1153, *1522*. *See also Tong bi* (extremely painful obstruction); *Bi zheng* (painful obstruction syndrome)
Extremitas Radix Angelicae Sinensis, xxiv
Extremities
  cold
    excess cold accumulation, 166
    Kidney yang deficiency, 678
    overview, 149, 455
    shaoyin syndrome, 486
    wind-cold with interior deficiency and cold, 466
    yang deficiency with excess cold, 491
  edema, 1219
  gangrene, 1344
  heaviness and warmth, 859

INDEX

1555

Index

numbness, 500
numbness and pain, 1173
pain, 1177
paralysis, 1182
swelling and edema, 578
weakness
    damp-phlegm, 1209
    qi deficiency, 522
    qi deficiency with dampness, 536
    Spleen and Stomach qi deficiencies, 542
Exudative pleurisy, **1236**
Eye disorders, 1334. *See also* specific disorders; Ocular effect
acuity, diminished, 551
deviated
    external wind, 977, 988
    overview, 963
    post-stroke, 906, 984
dry, 640
infection, 381
itching and tearing, excessive, 665
lacrimal gland, inflammation of, 295
light, increased sensitivity to, 663
optic nerve atrophy, **252**
overview, 318
painful, 108
pupils, dilated, 663
red
    damp-heat in all three *jiaos*, 359
    fire in the Liver and Gallbladder, 371
    heat accumulation in all three *jiaos*, 347
    Liver excess, 996
    Liver fire rising with deficiencies, 663
    wind, heat and toxins in the upper body, 349
red and painful, 291
red and swollen, 355
red, swollen and painful, 381, 641
swollen, 999
swollen and painful, 359
tearing, excessive, 634, 640
upward-rolling, 1251
vision, blurred, 633, 634, 640, 661, 663, 665
wind-heat, 381
yellow sclera, 1086
Fa Mu Wan (Quell Wood Pill), 1302
Face. *See also* specific disorders
abscesses and swellings, 1332
cyanotic, 171
dark, 1125
emaciated, 1297
flushed, 321, 325, 349
pale, 512, 513, 522, 542, 560, 562, 604, 609, 773
red, 349, 365, 420, 580, 999
red, swollen and painful, 355
sallow, 484, 522, 536, 562, 575, 583, 604, 609, 615, 1289
sallow and dull, 471, 476
spasms, 977, **1006**
Facial paralysis
overview, 965
post-stroke, **908**
shaoyin with *taiyang* syndrome, **133**
wei (defensive) *qi* deficiency, **775**
wind and phlegm rising, **1249**
wind invading the channels and collaterals, **981**
wind-cold, **61**, **990**
xue bi (blood painful obstruction), 500
zhong feng (wind stroke), **978**

Faeces Bombycis, xxiii
Faeces Trogopteri, xxvi
Faeces Vespertilionis Murini, xxvi
Faint pulse, *1510*
Fainting. *See* Unconsciousness
Fairy Decoction, 398
Fallopian tubes
blocked, 236, 572, **835**
infected, 371
Family Formulas from Shi Chuan-En, 982
Family Formulas of Qian Tian-Jia, 1123
Famous Classic and Contemporary Formulas, 363, 531
***Fang Feng Tong Sheng San* (Saposhnikovia Powder that Sagely Unblocks)**, 291
Fang Feng Tung Sheng San, 291
Fang Guang-Lei, 1238
Fang Ji (Radix Stephaniae Tetrandrae), xxiv
***Fang Ji Fu Ling Tang* (Stephania and Poria Decoction)**, 1120
***Fang Ji Huang Qi Tang* (Stephania and Astragalus Decoction)**, 1118
Fantastically Effective Pill to Invigorate the Collaterals, 914
Fasciolopsiasis (intestinal flukes), 1301
Fat Child Pill, 1296
Fatigue. *See also* Energy
chronic fatigue syndrome, **213**, **447**, 522, **544**, **617**
damp accumulation, 1068
Kidney yin and yang deficiencies with fire, 684
Lung yin and Spleen qi deficiencies, 1042
overview, 433, 455, 456, 513, 515, 1064
qi, blood, yang and *jing* (essence) deficiencies, 682
Spleen and Stomach qi deficiencies, 542
water accumulation, 1124
Fatigue dysuria, *1514*. *See also* Lao lin (fatigue dysuria); *Lin zheng* (dysuria syndrome)
Fear, 707, 708, 710, 1216
Febrile disorders, *1510*. *See also* Fever; Antipyretic effect
acute, 289, 361
excess interior heat, 325
externally-contracted, **1338**
heat and fire, 347
heat, fire and toxins in all three *jiaos*, 341
in summer, **440**
summer-heat damaging qi and body fluids, 446
yin-deficient heat and fire, 420
Feet
cold
    interior cold with yang qi deficiency, 494
    overview, 456
    roundworms, 1292
    shaoyin syndrome, 233
pain, 494
pain, severe, 481
***Fei Er Wan* (Fat Child Pill)**, 1296
Female disorders, 318
Fen (measure of weight), 22, 1439
Fen Bi Xie (Rhizoma Dioscoreae Hypoglaucae), xxiii
Fen sui (pulverize), *1510*
***Fen Xiao Tang* (Separate and Reduce Decoction)**, 1127
Feng Fang (Nidus Vespae), xxv
Feng lao bing (wind consumption disease), 416, *1510*
Feng shi (wind damp), 1118, *1510*
Feng shui (wind water), 1118, *1510*
Fennel and Galanga Formula, 484
Fennel Seed and Corydalis Combination, 889
Fennel Seed Pill with Three Levels, 836
Fertility. *See* Infertility

1556

Index

Chinese Herbal Formulas and Applications

Fetidness and filth, *1510*
Fetus. *See also* Pregnancy
  dead, 931
  restless, 619, 623, *1427*, *1518*
  unstable, 928
Fever, *1411*. *See also* Febrile disorders; Antipyretic effect
  afternoon, 919
  blood deficiency and heat, 575
  in cancer, 210, 412, **413**, **659**, **748**
  in children, 41, **61**, 216, **297**, **397**
  in children and infants, **109**
  chronic illness, **328**
  damp-warmth, 1092, 1096
  dryness with damaged yin, 1047
  enteric, 1096
  epidemic hemorrhagic, **323**, **339**, **357**
  exterior-deficient, wind-cold, 51
  exterior-excess, wind-cold, 39
  infection, **53**, **99**, **126**, **221**, **229**, **1098**
  heat and fire in the upper and middle *jiaos*, 351
  heat in the Liver, Gallbladder, and *San Jiao* channels, 243
  heat, lingering or residual, 327
  hemorrhagic, 333
  high
    in cancer, **748**
    excess heat, 321, 325
    excess interior heat, **323**
    exterior wind, **1335**
    exterior wind-heat with interior heat, 291
    heat, 337
    heat and toxins, 363
    heat, fire and toxins in all three *jiaos*, 341
    hot *bi zheng* (closed disorder), 747
    infection, **94**
    interior heat in all three *jiaos*, 299
    Liver wind rising, 993
    Pericardium heat and Liver wind, 753
    persistent, 993
    shaoyang syndrome, **210**
    wind-cold turning into heat, **109**
  low-grade
    due to bone fracture, **419**
    deficiency and cold of the middle *jiao*, 471
    qi, blood, yang and *jing* (essence) deficiencies, 682
    unremitting, 418
  Lung heat, 96
  mild, 406, 735
  mild and persistent, 1218
  night, 330
  overview, 34, 35, 36, 149, 281, 314, 315, 316, 317, 318, 433,
    434, 744, 964, 1021, 1063
  perspiration, without, **46**
  pharyngo-conjunctival, 92
  postpartum, **213**
  qi and blood deficiencies, **546**
  scarlet, 103
  Stomach heat, 393
  in summer, **437**, **440**
  summer-heat, 435
  summer-heat and dampness, 441, 444
  summer-heat damaging qi and body fluids, 446
  summer-heat with exterior cold and interior dampness, 436, 439
  surgery, after, 412, **414**
  taiyang and *shaoyang* syndromes, 219
  taiyang and *yangming* syndromes, 289
  tidal, *1429*

  blood and yin deficiencies, 593
  in pulmonary tuberculosis, **643**
  Kidney and Lung yin deficiencies, 643
  overview, 513, 514
  yin-deficient fire, 637, 649
  yin-deficient heat, 416, 418, 627
  warm-dryness, 1028, 1030
  water and heat, interlocked, 1115
  wind, 973
  wind, cold and dampness with interior heat, 64
  wind, cold and dampness with qi deficiency, 124
  wind-cold, 45, 67, 70, 72
  wind-cold and interior dampness, 1079
  wind-cold turning into heat, 108
  wind-cold with interior deficiency and cold, 466
  wind-cold with interior heat, 295
  wind-cold with interior phlegm, 128
  wind-cold with water accumulation, 74
  wind-cold with yang qi deficiency, 131
  wind-cold with yin and blood deficiencies, 136
  wind, heat and toxins, 355
  wind-heat, 92
  wind-heat with yin deficiency, 137
  wind-warmth, 89, 111
  yin-deficient fire, 422
  yin-deficient heat and fire, 420
Fever and chills, alternating
  diagnosis, 216
  Gallbladder damp-heat, 227
  Liver qi stagnation, 238, 247
  Liver qi stagnation with heat, 254
  overview, 201
  shaoyang and *yangming* syndromes, 283
  shaoyang syndrome, 206
  shaoyang syndrome with phlegm stagnation, 226
  shaoyang syndrome with water accumulation, 222
Fever and chills, intermittent, 230
Fibrocystic
  breasts, 254
  disease, 1360
Fibroids, uterine, 928
Fibromyalgia
  wind attacking the channels and collaterals, 988
  wind, heat and dampness, 1188
  yang qi and blood deficiencies, 494
Fibrosis
  liver, 937, **1010**
  pancreatic, 220
Fidgeting
  deficiency and cold of the middle *jiao*, 471
  fire in the Heart channel, 365
  heat, fire and toxins in all three *jiaos*, 341
  hot *bi zheng* (closed disorder), 747
  interior heat in all three *jiaos*, 299
  Liver qi stagnation, 238
  overview, 316, 433, 707
  yin-deficient fire, 649
Filariasis, 1184
Filth and fetidness, *1510*
Fine Formulas for Women, 527, 592, 795, 931, 942, 1167
Fine Formulas with Miraculous Results, 913, 1335
Fine pulse, *1510*
Fingers, gangrene, 1370
Fire, *1510*
  attacking the head, 347
  Heart, 710

INDEX

1557

Index

Heart channel, 365
  in all three *jiaos*, 341
  in the upper and middle *jiaos*, 351
  Liver and Gallbladder, 371
  Liver and Gallbladder channels, 379
  overview, 314
  Spleen and Stomach, 396
  yin-deficient, 422
  yin-deficient fire, 637
Fire-Inducing Powder, 365
Firm pulse, *1510*
Fissures, anal, *191*, 945
Five Accumulations Powder, 301, 303
Five Animal Frolics, 741
Five elements, 3, *1510*
Five Kinds of Peels Drink, 1121
Five Milled-Herbs Decoction, 850
Five transport points, *1524. See also Wu shu* (five transport) points
Five-Accumulation Powder, 301, 303
Five-center heat, 316, 513, *1394*, *1524. See also Wu xin re* (five-center heat)
Five-Ingredient Decoction to Eliminate Pathogenic Influences, 1337
Five-Ingredient Decoction to Eliminate Toxins, 1337
Five-Ingredient Powder for Painful Urinary Dysfunction, 1107
Five-Ingredient Powder with Poria, 1109
Five-Ling Formula, 1109
Five-Miracle Decoction, 1347
Five-Peel Powder, 1121, 1123
Five-Pi Drink, 1121
Five-Seed Pill, 176
Five-Strangury Formula, 1107
Five-Tiger Powder to Pursue Wind, 982
Fixed painful obstruction, 1153, *1527. See also Zhuo bi* (fixed painful obstruction); *Bi zheng* (painful obstruction syndrome)
Flashes, hot, 329, 415, 630, 684, 701
Flatulence. *See* Fullness; Distention
Floating edema, *1510*
Flonase. *See* Fluticasone
Flooding and spotting, 542, **565**, **586**, 609, 770, 802, 805, 889, 950, *1393*, *1505. See also Beng lou* (flooding and spotting)
Flos Lonicerae Japonicae, xxiv
Flovent. *See* Fluticasone
Floxin. *See* Ofloxacin
Flu. *See* Influenza
Fluid and water stagnation, *1522*
Fluids, body, 1055, *1506*
Flukes, intestinal, 1301
Fluticasone, 77
Focal distention, *1510*
Focus. *See* Attention; Concentration
Folium Agastaches, xxiv
Folium Camelliae, xxv
Folium Camelliae Fermentata, xxvi
Folium Camelliae Nigrum, xxiv
Folium Citri Reticulatae, xxv
Folium Ginkgo, xxvi
Folium Perillae, xxv
Follicle-stimulating hormone (FSH), 224, 630, 921, 929
Fontanel, delayed closing, 627
Food *qi*, *1511. See also Gu* (food) *qi*
Food stagnation, 1266. *See also* Indigestion; Digestive effect
  chest and epigastrium, 1311
  damp-heat accumulation, 1270
  overview, 1263, 1309
  qi deficiency with qi stagnation, 1274

qi stagnation and damp-heat accumulation, 1272
Spleen and Stomach deficiencies, 541
Spleen and Stomach deficiencies with heat, 1277
unable to vomit, 1314
Foot, athlete's, 1342
Forearm, pain, 1195
Forgetfulness, *1412. See also* Memory; Concentration; Cognitive effect
  Heart and Kidney deficiencies, 725
  Heart and Kidney disharmony, 714
  Heart and Spleen deficiencies, 583
  Heart blood deficiency, 735
  Heart fire, 710
  Liver yang rising, 1002
  overview, 708
  qi, blood, yang and *jing* (essence) deficiencies, 682
  yin and yang deficiencies, 798
Formulas from the Discussion Illuminating the Yellow Emperor's Basic Questions, 279, 291, 444, 693
Formulas of Universal Benefit, 7, 127
Formulas of Universal Benefit from My Practice, 712, 944, 996
Formulas that treat abscesses and sores, 1321
Formulas to Aid the Living, 82, 84, 185, 231, 559, 583, 671, 675, 826, 833, 849, 855, 858, 1211
Formulation, 14
Forsythia and Acorus Formula, 1096
Forsythia and Laminaria Combination, 1357
Forsythia and Laminaria Decoction, 1357
Forsythia and Mint Decoction, 1028
Forsythia and Rhubarb Formula, 351
Forsythia Decoction to Relieve Toxicity, 345
Forsythia Detoxifying Formula, 1331
Forsythia Powder to Overcome Pathogenic Influences, 1331
Four Component Decoction, 562
Four Herbs Decoction, 562
Four Major Herb Decoction, 522
Four Milled-Herbs Decoction, 849
Four-Fresh Pill, 942
Four-Gentlemen Decoction, 522
Four-Ingredient Powder with Poria, 1112
Four-Marvel Pill, 1190
Four-Marvel Powder, 1190, 1347
Four-Miracle Pill, 784
Four-Substance Decoction, 562
Four-Substance Decoction with Safflower and Peach Pit, 571
Four-Valiant Decoction for Well-Being, 1344
Freckles, *1412*
Free radicals, 343, 555, 595, 685, 719, 882, 931, 997, 1380. *See also* Antioxidant effect
Fresh Ginger Decoction to Drain the Epigastrium, 268
Fright and palpitations, *1510*
Frightened
  abnormal, 710
  easily, 245, 735, 1218
  Liver yang hyperactivity, 713
  overview, 707
Frightened wind, *1511*
Frigid Extremities Decoction, 486
Frigid Extremities Decoction plus Ginseng, 488
Frigid Extremities Powder, 233
Fritillaria and Platycodon Formula, 113
Fritillaria and Trichosanthes Fruit Formula, 1240
Fritillaria and Trichosanthes Fruit Powder, 1240
Frostbite, **54**, **496**, **502**, **1371**, *1412*
Frozen shoulder, **497**. *See also* Shoulders
Fructus Akebiae, xxiii

1558

Index

Fructus Alpiniae Oxyphyllae, xxvi
Fructus Amomi Rotundus, xxiii
Fructus Anisi Stellati, xxiii
Fructus Aurantii, xxvi
Fructus Galangae, xxiv
Fructus Leonuri, xxiii
Fructus Mori, xxv
Fructus Perillae, xxv
Fructus Piperis, xxiv
Fructus Piperis Longi, xxiii
Fructus Tribuli, xxiii
Fructus Trichosanthis, xxiv
Fructus Tritici Levis, xxiv
Fry with liquid, *1527*. *See also* Zhi (fry with liquid)
FSH. *See* Follicle-stimulating hormone
Fu (hollow organ), *1511*. *See also* specific organs
Fu Fang Ba Zheng San (**Revised Eight-Herb Powder**), 1105
Fu Fang Da Cheng Qi Tang (**Revised Major Order the Qi Decoction**), 155
Fu Ke Chan Lun Fang (Discussion of Formulas for Obstetrics and Gynecology), 933
Fu Ke Zheng Zhi Zhun Sheng (Standards of Patterns and Treatments in Gynecology), **1061**
Fu Ling Gui Zhi Bai Zhu Gan Cao Tang, 1131
Fu Ling Tang (**Poria Decoction**), 1112
Fu Ling Wan (**Poria Pill**), 1219
Fu Ling Yin (**Poria Decoction**), 1077
Fu Mai Tang (Restore the Pulse Decoction), 589, 591
Fu Qing Zhu Nan Ke (Men's Diseases According to Fu Qing-Zhu), **767**
Fu Qing Zhu Nu Ke (Women's Diseases According to Fu Qing-Zhu), 621, **767**, 806, 809, 925
Fu Qing-Zhu, **767**, 1481, 1483, 1484. *See also* Fu Shan
Fu Ren Da Quan Liang Fang (Complete Fine Formulas for Women), 7, 1219
Fu Ren Liang Fang (Fine Formulas for Women), 527, 592, 795, 931, 942, 1167
Fu Ren-Yu, 633
Fu Shan, 621, **767**, 806, 809, 925, 1481, 1483, 1484. *See also* Fu Qing-Zhu
Fu Tu Dan (**Poria and Cuscuta Special Pill**), 797
Fu Tzu Li Chung Tang (*Wan*), 463
Fu Xiao Mai (Fructus Tritici Levis), xxiv
Fu Yuan Huo Hsieh Tang, 897
Fu Yuan Huo Xieh Tang, 897
Fu Yuan Huo Xue Tang (**Revive Health by Invigorating the Blood Decoction**), 897
Fu Zheng Yi Yan Tang (**Support the Upright and Suppress Cancer Decoction**), 336
Fu Zi Li Zhong Tang (*Wan*), 463
Fu Zi Li Zhong Wan (**Prepared Aconite Pill to Regulate the Middle**), 463
  vs. Li Zhong Wan (Regulate the Middle Pill), 465
Fu Zi Tang (**Prepared Aconite Decoction**), 1137
Fullness, 156, 1263, *1515*. *See also* specific locations; *Man* (fullness)
Fullness and distention, 1274, 1277, 1280
Fungal infection, **1081**, **1190**. *See also* Antifungal effect
Furuncles, *1412*
  damp-heat in all three *jiaos*, 359
  external wind with blood deficiency, 970
  fire and toxins, 1337
  hard and deeply rooted, 1337
  heat and toxins, 1325, 1342
  heat and toxins with underlying deficiencies, 1365
  with localized redness, swelling, heat and pain, 1337

overview, 1321
  with pus and discharge, 1364
  with swelling and hardness, 1357
GABA receptor, 221, 255
Galacturia, **632**, **1117**, **1141**
Galangal and Cyperus Pill, 841
Gallbladder (TCM), *1511*
  damp-heat, 227, 1086
  excess fire, 371, 379
  heat, 243
  heat-phlegm, 1214, 1218
Gallbladder disorders (WM), **285**. *See also* Chole- and specific disorders
  effect on, 482
  infection, **154**
  overview, 203, 282, 318, 870, 1065
Gallbladder Warming Decoction, 1213
Gallstones. *See* Cholelithiasis
Gambir Combination, 1004
Gambir Formula, 996
Gan Cao (Radix et Rhizoma Glycyrrhizae), xxiv
Gan Cao Gan Jiang Fu Ling Bai Zhu Tang (**Licorice, Ginger, Poria and Atractylodes Macrocephala Decoction**), 1133
  vs. Ling Gui Zhu Gan Tang (Poria, Cinnamon Twig, Atractylodes Macrocephala, and Licorice Decoction), 1134
Gan Cao Xiao Mai Da Zao Tang, 731
Gan Cao Xie Xin Tang (**Licorice Decoction to Drain the Epigastrium**), 269
  vs. Ban Xia Xie Xin Tang (Pinellia Decoction to Drain the Epigastrium), 266
  vs. Sheng Jiang Xie Xin Tang (Fresh Ginger Decoction to Drain the Epigastrium), 266
Gan ji (infantile malnutrition), 1297, 1299, *1511*
Gan Jiang Ren Shen Ban Xia Wan (**Ginger, Ginseng, and Pinellia Pill**), 853
Gan Lu Xiao Du Dan (**Sweet Dew Special Pill to Eliminate Toxins**), 1096
  vs. San Ren Tang (Three-Nut Decoction), 1098
Gan Lu Yin (**Sweet Dew Decoction**), 401
Gan Mai Da Zao Tang (**Licorice, Wheat, and Jujube Decoction**), 731
  vs. Suan Zao Ren Tang (Sour Jujube Decoction), 724
  vs. Tian Wang Bu Xin Dan (Emperor of Heaven's Special Pill to Tonify the Heart), 724
Gan Song (Radix et Rhizoma Nardostachydis), xxiv
Gan Sui (Radix Kansui), xxiv
Gan Zao Xiao Mai Da Zao Tang, 731
Gan Zheng Ji Yao (Essential Compilation of Infectious Syndromes), 1095
Gangrene
  arteriosclerotic, **1345**
  deficiency and cold of the middle *jiao*, 476
  extremities, 1344
  fingers and toes, 1370
  heat and toxins, 1349
  pulmonary, 1230
  purulent abscess, 1344
  yang deficiency and interior cold stagnation, 1370
Gao Ben (Rhizoma et Radix Ligustici), xxiv
Gao Bing-Jun, 1332, 1340
Gao ji (soft extract), 17
Gao lin (cloudy dysuria), 1142, *1511*
Gardenia and Fermented Soybean Decoction, 370
Gardenia and Hoelen Formula, 1107
Gardenia and Phellodendron Decoction, 1089
Gardenia and Soja Combination, 370

Index

Gardenia and Soja Decoction, 370
Gardenia and Vitex Combination, 381
Gardenia Decoction to Clear the Liver, 245
Gardenia Decoction to Descend Fire, 377
Gas, 1077
Gasping Formula, 388
Gastrectasis, 851, 1068, *1412*
Gastric
  acid
    hypersecretion of, 261, 270
    to decrease, 209, 220, 234, 258, 285, 343, 360, 469, 472, 476,
      485, 532, 576, 585, 1211, 1236
    to increase, 154, 249, 543
  cramps, 731
  distention, post-surgical, 482
  lesions, aspirin- and ethanol-induced, 287, 345
  neuralgia, 233
  neurosis
    cold damaging the Stomach and Spleen, 1113
    damp accumulation, 1068, 1072, 1076
    Liver qi stagnation and blood dryness, 657
    qi stagnation, 822
  pain, 211, 600, **601**
  prolapse. *See also* Gastroptosis
    damp accumulation, 1072
    deficiency and cold, 463
    deficiency and cold with qi stagnation, 484
    phlegm and dampness, 1077
    phlegm stagnation and water accumulation, 1220
    qi and blood deficiencies, **611**
    qi deficiency with qi stagnation, 1274
    shaoyang and *yangming* syndromes, **286**
    shaoyang syndrome, **211**
    shaoyin syndrome, **488**
    Spleen and Stomach deficiencies, **544**
    wind-cold with interior deficiency and cold, 466
  ulcer
    bile reflux, 390
    blood deficiency and heat, 576
    damp accumulation, 1068
    deficiency and cold, 459
    deficiency and cold with qi stagnation, 484
    Heart and Spleen deficiencies, 584
    heat in the chest and cold in the Stomach, 271
    Liver qi stagnation, 248
    qi deficiency with cold and dampness, 531
    qi deficiency with dampness and phlegm, 527
    shaoyang and *yangming* syndromes, 283
    Spleen deficiency, 534
    taiyang and *shaoyang* syndromes, 219
    wind-cold with interior deficiency and cold, 466
    yang deficiency and interior cold, 481
    yin deficiency with qi stagnation and blood dryness, **658**
Gastrin, 262, 528
Gastritis
  acute, 370
  acute or chronic, 467, **529**
  antral, **211**, **477**
  atrophic
    chronic, 272, 532, 601, 606, 611, 630, 918, 1045, 1047,
      1211, 1267, 1282
    cold and dampness, 1134
    deficiency and cold of the middle *jiao*, **477**
    Liver and Kidney yin deficiencies, **658**
    Liver qi stagnation, **240**
    Spleen and Stomach deficiencies and dampness, **263**

due to bile acid regurgitation, **211, 229, 236, 263, 390, 545, 857**
chronic, *1412*
  antral, **477**
  cold damaging the Stomach and Spleen, 1113
  damp-cold in the Spleen and Stomach, 840
  deficiency and cold of the middle *jiao*, **473**
  deficiency and cold with qi stagnation, 484
  heat and cold, interlocked, **1281**
  heat and toxins, **1346**
  heat in the Stomach and cold in the Intestines, 1292
  interior excess heat, **159**
  Liver qi stagnation, 248
  phlegm retention with yang deficiency, 1131
  qi and blood stagnation, **918**
  qi deficiency with dampness and phlegm, 527
  qi stagnation and food retention, 1274
  Spleen deficiency, 534
  Stomach deficiency and interlocking of heat and cold, 270
  Stomach qi disharmony, **263**
  superficial, **297, 524**
  wind-cold with qi stagnation, **68**
  yin deficiency, **1044, 1051**
  yin deficiency with qi stagnation and blood dryness, 657
cold and dampness, 1134
damp accumulation in the Spleen and Stomach, **1069**
damp-heat, 373, **1097**, 1099
deficiency and cold, 461, 463
deficiency and cold of the middle *jiao*, 476
with epigastric pain, **1070**
erosive, 391, **1236**
fire in the Liver and Gallbladder channels, 379
phlegm and dampness, 1077
phlegm-heat, 1235
qi flow, reversed, 854
shaoyang and *yangming* syndromes, 283
shaoyang syndrome with water accumulation, 222
superficial, **235, 263, 537**, 1099, 1134
yang deficiency and interior cold, 481
Gastroatonia
  damp accumulation, 1068
  deficiency and cold, 463
  qi stagnation, 828
  wind and phlegm rising, 1247
Ge Gen (Radix Puerariae Lobatae), xxiv
Gastrodia and Uncaria Decoction, 1004
Gastrodia Pill to Lower [Blood] Pressure, 1006
Gastroenteritis, *1412*
  accumulations in the interior, 302
  acute
    damp accumulation, 1076
    damp-heat, 1099, 1101
    damp-warmth, **1094**, 1096
    heat and water, interlocked, 268
    heat in the Stomach and Intestines, 160
    interior excess heat, **159**
    Stomach qi disharmony, **264**
    wind-cold and interior dampness, **1081**
    wind-cold with interior heat, 295
    wind-cold with qi stagnation, 67
  acute or chronic, 466, 1270
  chronic, 536, 541, 1076
  damp-heat in all three *jiaos*, 359
  deficiency and cold, 459, 463
  fire in the Liver and Gallbladder channels, 379
  food stagnation, 1270
  heat in the chest and cold in the Stomach, 271

1560

Index

qi deficiency with cold and dampness, 531
qi stagnation and damp-heat accumulation, 1272
shaoyang and *yangming* syndromes, 283
shaoyang syndrome with water accumulation, 222
shaoyin syndrome, 486
Spleen deficiency, 534
Stomach deficiency and interlocking of heat and cold, 270
summer-heat, 438
summer-heat with exterior cold and interior dampness, 436
taiyang and *yangming* syndromes, 289
toxic heat, **409**
Gastroesophageal reflux disease. *See* Acid reflux/regurgitation
Gastrointestinal
   bleeding
      acute, profuse, **360**
      blood stasis, 911
      damp-heat in all three *jiaos*, **360**
      deficiency and cold, **949**
      deficiency heat, 802
      fire in the Liver and Gallbladder, **373**
      due to gastric or duodenal ulcers, **941**
      Stomach heat, **334**
      Stomach qi disharmony, **264**
      yin deficiency, **399**
   infection, 757
   neurosis, 851, 1209
Gastrointestinal disorders, 151, **159**, 257, 282, 359, **472**, **529**,
      1099, 1266. *See also* specific disorders; Gastrointestinal effect;
      Gastroprotective effect
   overview, 203, 204, 434, 457, 514, 517, 820, 821, 1023, 1065,
      1207, 1264
Gastrointestinal effect, 154, 158, 162, 167, 170, 175, 209, 234, 249,
      258, 262, 285, 296, 342, 390, 404, 468, 472, 476, 482, 485, 523,
      528, 532, 537, 543, 1047, 1211, 1236, 1275, 1281, 1380
Gastrolithiasis, 1264, **1268**
Gastroprotective effect, 287, 345, 360, 528
Gastroptosis, *1412*. *See also* Gastric prolapse
   deficiency, **264**
   deficiency and cold, 459
   deficiency and cold of the Stomach, 467
   phlegm and dampness, 1077
   qi deficiency, 522
   qi deficiency with cold and dampness, 531
   qi deficiency with dampness, 536
   qi deficiency with dampness and phlegm, 527
   qi stagnation, 828
   Spleen deficiency, 534
   Stomach deficiency and interlocking of heat and cold, 270
   wind and phlegm rising, 1247
***Ge Gen Huang Qin Huang Lian Tang* (Kudzu, Coptis, and
   Scutellaria Decoction)**, 295
   vs. Bai Tou Weng Tang (Pulsatilla Decoction), 298, 783
   vs. Shao Yao Tang (Peony Decoction), 298, 783
   vs. Zhen Ren Yang Zang Tang (True Man's Decoction for
      Nourishing the Organs), 783
***Ge Gen Huo Xiang Shao Yao Tang* (Kudzu, Pogostemon, and
   Peony Decoction)**, 298
Ge Gen Qin Lian Tang, 295
***Ge Gen Tang* (Kudzu Decoction)**, 59
Ge Hong, 6, 112, 438, **1287**, 1481, 1482, 1484
***Ge Hua Jie Cheng San* (Pueraria Flower Powder for
   Detoxification and Awakening)**, 1084
Ge Qian-Sun, 939
Ge Qiao (Concha Meretricis seu Cyclinae), xxiv
***Ge Xia Zhu Yu Tang* (Drive Out Blood Stasis Below the
   Diaphragm Decoction)**, 885

vs. Shao Fu Zhu Yu Tang (Drive Out Blood Stasis in the Lower
   Abdomen Decoction), 884
vs. Shen Tong Zhu Yu Tang (Drive Out Blood Stasis from a
   Painful Body Decoction), 884
vs. Xue Fu Zhu Yu Tang (Drive Out Stasis in the Mansion of
   Blood Decoction), 884
General Collection for Holy Relief, 6, 1313
Generalized painful obstruction, 1153, *1527*. *See also Zhou
   bi* (generalized painful obstruction); *Bi zheng* (painful
   obstruction syndrome)
Generate the Pulse Decoction, 554
Generate the Pulse Powder, 554
Generating sequence, *1511*
Generation and Transformation Decoction, 925
Genital
   herpes, 318
   itching, 810, 1192
   swelling and itching, 371
Genitourinary disorders. *See* specific disorders
Gentiana Combination, 371
Gentiana Decoction to Drain the Liver, 371
Gentiana Decoction to Relieve Toxicity, 376
Gentiana Liver-Draining Decoction (Pill), 371
Gentiana Liver-Purging Decoction (Pill), 371
Gentiana Macrophylla and Soft-Shelled Turtle Shell Powder, 416
Gentiana Pill to Lower [Blood] Pressure, 376
GERD (gastroesophageal reflux disease). *See* Acid reflux/
   regurgitation
Gestational disorders, 562, 598. *See also* Pregnancy
Ginger, Aconite Hoelen and Peony Combination, 1135
Ginger, Ginseng, and Pinellia Pill, 853
Gingivitis, *1412*
   damp-heat in the Spleen and Stomach, 401
   excess interior heat, 321, 325
   heat and fire in the upper and middle *jiaos*, 351
   heat in the *xue* (blood) level, 942
   heat, lingering or residual, 327
   Stomach heat, **394**, 398
   ulcerative, 393
   wind, heat and toxins in the upper body, 349
Ginseng and Aster Combination, 560
Ginseng and Astragalus Combination, 542
Ginseng and Atractylodes Combination, 535
Ginseng and Cordyceps Decoction, 559
Ginseng and Gecko Combination, 557
Ginseng and Gecko Powder, 557
Ginseng and Ginger Combination, 459
Ginseng and Gypsum Combination, 325
Ginseng and Hoelen Formula, 1298
Ginseng and Longan Combination, 583
Ginseng and Longan Decoction, 583
Ginseng and Mentha Formula, 124
Ginseng and Ophiopogon Formula, 554
Ginseng and Perilla Combination, 128
Ginseng and Perilla Decoction, 128
Ginseng and Perilla Drink, 128
Ginseng and Perilla Leaf Decoction, 128
Ginseng and Poria Powder, 539
Ginseng and Prepared Aconite Decoction, 489
Ginseng and Rehmannia Combination, 615
Ginseng and Scute Combination, 1231
Ginseng and Tangkuei Formula, 598
Ginseng and Tangkuei Ten Combination, 609
Ginseng and Walnut Decoction, 559
Ginseng and Zizyphus Formula, 725
Ginseng Antiphlogistic Powder, 124

Index

Ginseng Decoction, 462
Ginseng Decoction to Nourish the Nutritive Qi, 615
Ginseng Decoction to Sedate the Lung, 1231
Ginseng Detoxifying Formula, 124
Ginseng Great Tonifying Decoction, 613
Ginseng Nutrition Decoction (Pill), 615
Ginseng Nutritive Decoction (Pill), 615
Ginseng plus White Tiger Decoction, 325
Ginseng Powder to Overcome Pathogenic Influences, 124, 126
Ginseng, Astragalus and Pueraria Decoction, 551
Ginseng, Poria and Bighead Atractylodes Powder, 535
Ginseng, Poria, and Atractylodes Macrocephala Powder, 535
Ginseng, Tangkuei, and Peony Powder, 598
Girdle channel, *1508*. See also *Dai* (girdle) channel
Glaucoma, *1412*
　chronic, 641
　damp-heat, 1106
　Heart and Kidney disharmony, 714
　Liver stagnation, *573*
　wind-heat, 381
　yin deficiency with internal fire and wind, 661
Gleditsia Combination, 1367
Glehnia and Ophiopogon Combination, 1047
Glehnia and Ophiopogonis Decoction, 1047
Globus hystericus, 820, 821, 828. See also *Mei he qi* (plum-pit *qi*)
Globus pharyngeus, **68**
Glomerulonephritis
　acute, 369, 947, 1118, *1412*
　chronic, 170, **671**, 684, *1413*
　damp-heat, 1103, 1106
　damp-warmth, **1094**
　deficiency and cold, 461
　fire and toxins, **1339**
　fire in the Heart channel, 365
　Spleen qi deficiency and Liver qi stagnation, 807
Glomerulosclerosis, 673
Glucocorticoids, 555
Glucose, plasma, 285, 325, 328, 343, 369, 629, 641, 643, 655, 676, 875, 1023, 1044, 1050, 1053, 1056. See also Diabetes mellitus; Hypoglycemic effect; Metabolic effect
Goiter, *1413*. See also Thyroid; Hyperthyroidism; Hypothyroidism
　damp-phlegm, **1211**
　immobile, 1353
　overview, 1321
　phlegm, 1355
　qi and phlegm stagnation, 1353
　qi, blood, and phlegm stagnation, 1360
　with swelling and hardness, 1357
Gold foil, xxiv
Golden Lock Essence-Securing Pill, 789
Golden Lock Pill for Consolidating the Essence, 789
Golden Mirror of the Medical Tradition, 70, 105, 294, 567, 571, 636, 901, 995, 1075, 1298, 1337, 1352, 1363
Golden Pill to Construct a Fat Child, 1298
Gonadotropin, 54, 224, 256, 596, 598, 602, 876, 921, 922, 931
Gonadotropin-releasing hormone, 595
Gong Ting-Xian, 120, 178, 241, 349, 381, 388, 422, 534, 540, 575, 624, 664, 666, 1073, 1127, 1169, 1171, 1195, 1212, 1217, 1225, 1233, 1295, **1319**, 1336, 1357, 1360, 1365, 1368, 1481, 1483, 1484
Gong Wai Yun Fang (Ectopic Pregnancy Formula), 917
Gong xie lun (discussion on attacking evil), 1307
Gonorrhea, *1413*
　damp-heat, 1192
　fire in the Liver and Gallbladder, 371
　heat, 1107

　with leukorrhea, 810
Gou Teng San (Uncaria Powder), 996
　vs. *Gou Teng Yin* (Uncaria Decoction), 998
Gou Teng Yin (Uncaria Decoction), 995
　vs. *Gou Teng San* (Uncaria Powder), 998
Gou Wen (Herba Gelsemii Elegantis), 27
Gout, *1413*
　accumulations in the interior, 302
　acute, **1189**
　cold, heat, dampness, phlegm, and stagnation, 1175
　damp-heat, **1105**, 1106, **1193**
　exterior excess with interior deficiency, 1169
　heat and toxins, **1346**
　wind, heat and dampness, 1186, 1188
　wind-dampness with deficiency, 1159
　yin-deficient fire, **639**
Governing channel, *1509*. See also *Du* (governing) channel
Grand Dictionary of Chinese Medicine, 387
Granule, 18
Granulocyte colony-stimulating factor (G-CSF), 547
Grate, *1508*. See also *Cuo* (grate)
Great Tonify Pill, 649
Great Tonify the Yin Pill, 649
Great Tonifying Decoction, 613
Great Tranquility Pill, 1268
Greatest Treasure Powder from the Imperial Grace Formulary, 751
Greatest Treasure Special Pill, 749
Grind, *1525*. See also *Yan* (grind)
Groin, sweating, 371
Growth, retarded, 627
Gu (food) *qi*, 455, *1511*
Gu Chong Tang (Stabilize *Chong* [Thoroughfare Channel] Decoction), 803
Gu Jin Ming Fang (Famous Classic and Contemporary Formulas), 363, 531
Gu Jing Wan (Stabilize the Menses Pill), 802
　vs. *Gui Pi Tang* (Restore the Spleen Decoction), 588, 804
Gua Di San (Melon Pedicle Powder), 1311
Gua Lou (Fructus Trichosanthis), xxiv
Gua Lou Xie Bai Bai Jiu Tang (Trichosanthes Fruit, Chinese Chive, and Wine Decoction), 832
　vs. *Gua Lou Xie Bai Ban Xia Tang* (Trichosanthes Fruit, Chinese Chive, and Pinellia Decoction), 833
　vs. *Zhi Shi Xie Bai Gui Zhi Tang* (Immature Bitter Orange, Chinese Chive, and Cinnamon Twig Decoction), 833
Gua Lou Xie Bai Ban Xia Tang (Trichosanthes Fruit, Chinese Chive, and Pinellia Decoction), 832
　vs. *Gua Lou Xie Bai Bai Jiu Tang* (Trichosanthes Fruit, Chinese Chive, and Wine Decoction), 833
　vs. *Zhi Shi Xie Bai Gui Zhi Tang* (Immature Bitter Orange, Chinese Chive, and Cinnamon Twig Decoction), 833
Gua Lou Zhi Shi Tang (Trichosanthes Fruit and Immature Bitter Orange Decoction), 1233
Gua Lou Zi (Semen Trichosanthis), xxiv
Guan Bai Fu (Radix Aconiti Coreani), xxiv
Guan position, *1511*
Guan Xin Su He Wan (Coronary Styrax Pill), 760
Guan Ye Jin Si Tao (Herba Hyperici Perforati), xxiv
Guan Yu, 741
Guang Wen Yi Lun (Discussion of Widespread Warm Epidemics), 633
Gui Ling Gan Lu Yin (Cinnamon and Poria Sweet Dew Decoction), 444
　vs. *Liu Yi San* (Six-to-One Powder), 445
Gui Lu Er Xian Gao (Tortoise Shell and Deer Antler Paste), 687
Gui Lu Er Xian Jiao (Tortoise Shell and Deer Antler Syrup), 687

Index

Chinese Herbal Formulas and Applications

vs. Qi Bao Mei Ran Dan (Seven-Treasure Special Pill for Beautiful Whiskers), 693

Gui Pi An Shen Tang (Restore the Spleen and Tranquilize the Spirit Decoction), 587

Gui Pi Tang (Restore the Spleen Decoction), 583

  vs. Bu Zhong Yi Qi Tang (Tonify the Middle and Augment the Qi Decoction), 588

  vs. Gu Jing Wan (Stabilize the Menses Pill), 588, 804

  vs. Si Wu Tang (Four-Substance Decoction), 587

  vs. Suan Zao Ren Tang (Sour Jujube Decoction), 587

  vs. Tian Wang Bu Xin Dan (Emperor of Heaven's Special Pill to Tonify the Heart), 587, 730

Gui Qi Jian Zhong Tang (Tangkuei and Astragalus Decoction to Construct the Middle), 479

  vs. Xiao Jian Zhong Tang (Minor Construct the Middle Decoction), 480

Gui Zhi Fu Ling Wan (Cinnamon Twig and Poria Pill), 928

Gui Zhi Jia Ge Gen Tang (Cinnamon Twig Decoction plus Kudzu), 55

Gui Zhi Jia Hou Po Xing Zi Tang (Cinnamon Twig Decoction plus Magnolia Bark and Apricot Kernel), 55

Gui Zhi Jia Long Gu Mu Li Tang (Cinnamon Twig Decoction plus Dragon Bone and Oyster Shell), 798

Gui Zhi Jia Long Mu Tang, 798

Gui Zhi Jia Shao Yao Tang (Cinnamon Twig Decoction plus Peony), 55

Gui Zhi Ma Huang Ge Ban Tang (Combined Cinnamon Twig and Ephedra Decoction), 56

Gui Zhi Ren Shen Tang (Cinnamon Twig and Ginseng Decoction), 466

Gui Zhi Shao Yao Zhi Mu Tang (Cinnamon Twig, Peony, and Anemarrhena Decoction), 1186

Gui Zhi Tang (Cinnamon Twig Decoction), 51

  vs. Chai Ge Jie Ji Tang (Bupleurum and Kudzu Decoction to Release the Muscle Layer), 110

  vs. Ma Huang Tang (Ephedra Decoction), 44

  vs. Xiao Jian Zhong Tang (Minor Construct the Middle Decoction), 58, 474

  vs. Yu Ping Feng San (Jade Windscreen Powder), 57, 775

Guide Out Phlegm Decoction, 1211

Guide Out the Red Powder, 365

Guide the Spleen Pill, 540

Guidelines from Lan-Tai, 1179

Gums

  bleeding, 393, 398, *1402*

  inflammation and bleeding, 254

  overview, 316

  swelling, 682

  swelling and pain, 393, 399

  swelling, inflammation and suppuration, 401

  ulcerations, 393

Gun Tan Wan (Vaporize Phlegm Pill), 1238

Guo Qi Yin (Delayed Menstruation Decoction), 578

Gynecological disorders, 206, 253, 515, 516, *577*, 771, 869. *See also* specific disorders

Gynecomastia

  Kidney yang deficiency, 673

  in liver cirrhosis, **61**

  Liver qi stagnation, **251**, **849**

  unilateral or bilateral, **670**

Gypsum Combination, 321

Gypsum Coptis and Scute Combination, 361

Gypsum Decoction, 299, 321

Gypsum Fibrosum Praeparatum, xxiv

H. pylori, 53, **391**, 544

Haematitum, xxiv

Hai Jin Sha (Spora Lygodii), xxiv

Hai Zao Yu Hu Tang (Sargassum Decoction for the Jade Flask), 1352

Hair, 63

  loss, 798, 877

  premature gray, 654, 690

Half-body perspiration, *1511*

Halitosis, **395**, 396, 398, *1413*. *See also* Breath, foul

Halotan. *See* Halothane

Halothane, 214

Han fa (sweating), **9**, 34, 281, 1307, *1511*

Han Fang Yi Xue (Kampo Medicine), 1227

Han Mao, 1245

Han Shi Yi Tong (Comprehensive Medicine According to Master Han), 1245

Hands, cold

  interior cold with yang qi deficiency, 494

  overview, 456

  roundworms, 1292

  shaoyin syndrome, 233, 467

  Spleen yang deficiency with cold, 169

Hangover. *See also* Alcohol poisoning

  damp accumulation, 1082

  damp-heat, 1085

  damp-phlegm, 1209

  heat in the chest and cold in the Stomach, 271

  wind-cold with interior heat, 295

Hao Qin Qing Dan Tang (Artemisia Annua and Scutellaria Decoction to Clear the Gallbladder), 227

  vs. Chai Hu Da Yuan Yin (Bupleurum Decoction to Reach the Membrane Source), 232

  vs. Xiao Chai Hu Tang (Minor Bupleurum Decoction), 217, 229

Harada's syndrome, **332**

Hardness, *1519*. *See also* Lumps; Nodules; Masses; *Shi* (hardness)

  abdomen, 1360

  breast, 1360

  definition, 156

  heat and toxins, 1349

  neck, 1360

  overview, 1205

  posterior to the ear or on the neck, 1355

  with pus and discharge, 1365, 1367

  qi, blood and phlegm stagnation, 1360

Hard-Won Knowledge, 64, 66

Harmonize the Six Decoction, 1082, 1083

Harmonizing, *1512*. *See also* *He fa* (harmonizing)

Harmonizing formulas, 201

Harmonizing method, **10**, 201

Harmony-Preserving Pill, 1266

HDL (high-density lipoproteins). *See* Cholesterols

He (measure of volume), 22

He (uniting) point, *1511*

He Che Wan Fang (Placenta Pill Formula), 1253

He fa (harmonizing), **10**, 201, *1512*

He Han Yi Yao Xue Hui Zhi (Hehan Journal of Medicine and Herbology), 577

He xi feng (crane's knee wind), 1182, 1186, *1512*

Head. *See also* specific disorders

  blood stagnation, 877

  heaviness, 1247

  old phlegm and excess heat, 1239

  red, swollen and painful, 355

  sweaty, *1521*

  wind, heat, and toxins, 349, 355

Headache, *1413*

1563

Index

accumulations in the interior, 302
alcohol intoxication, 1085
angioneurotic, **975**
blood deficiency, 562
blood stagnation, 877, **881**
damp-heat, 1085
damp-warmth, 1092
deficiency and cold of the Stomach, 469
with dizziness, **585**
exterior cool-dryness, 1025
exterior wind, 973, **975**
exterior wind, cold and dampness with qi deficiency, 124
exterior-deficient, wind-cold, 51
exterior-excess, wind-cold, 39
fire in the Liver and Gallbladder, 371
fixed location, 879
frontal, 83, 973
habitual, 467, 1247
hypertension, 293
jueyin syndrome, 467
Liver excess, 996
Liver qi stagnation, 247
Liver yang and wind excess, 1004
Liver yang and wind rising, 999
Liver yang rising, 1002, **1005**
migraine, 64, **212**, 293, **373**, 467, **824**, **975**, **979**, 1247, *1420*
nasal obstruction, 83, 84, 86
neurogenic, **566**, 661, 973
neurotic, 467
occipital, 973
overview, 34, 35, 516, 963, 1154, 1206
phlegm, 1250
qi and blood deficiencies, **606**
severe, 481
shaoyin with *taiyang* syndrome, 132
sinus, 84, 977
sinus infection, 293
splitting, 337
stabbing, 879
Stomach heat, 398
stubborn, **293**, **496**
summer-heat and dampness, 444
summer-heat with exterior cold and interior dampness, 436, 439
temporal, 83, 393, 973
tension, **61**, 293, 973, **1249**
trauma, **566**, **875**
vascular, **566**, **573**, 877, **881**, **908**, 977, **1001**
vertex, 468, 973
warm-dryness, 1030
wind and phlegm rising, 1247
wind, cold and dampness with interior heat, 64
wind-cold, 67, 70, 72
wind-cold and interior dampness, 1079
wind-cold turning into heat, 108
wind-cold with interior phlegm, 128
wind-cold with yang qi deficiency, 131
wind-cold with yin and blood deficiencies, 136
wind-dampness, **65**, 1156
wind-heat, 92
wind-heat with yin deficiency, 137
wind-warmth, 111
Hearing, poor/impaired/loss of
blood stagnation, 877
fire in the Liver and Gallbladder channels, 379
heat in the Liver, Gallbladder, and *San Jiao* channels, 243
Kidney and blood deficiencies, 666

Kidney deficiency, 633
Heart (TCM), *1512*
blood and Kidney yin deficiencies, 726
blood deficiency, 735
blood deficiency and Liver qi stagnation, 731
deficiency, due to over-thinking, 583
disharmony with Kidney, 714, 797
fire, 365
fire with qi and yin deficiencies, 368
fire with yin and blood deficiencies, 710
Heart and Kidney deficiencies, 792
heat, 333
heat-phlegm, 1218
old phlegm and excess heat, 1239
Heart disorders (WM). *See also* Cardiovascular and specific disorders
congestive heart disease, 584
congestive heart failure, 554, 1124, **1126**, 1129, *1406*
coronary restenosis, **719**
failure, 74, 1124, **1126**, 1129
pain, 915
Heartburn. *See* Acid reflux/regurgitation
Heart-Clearing Diaphragm-Relieving Decoction, 386
Heart-Nourishing Decoction, 735
Heat, *1512*
in all three *jiaos*, 299, 341, 347
attacking the Pericardium, 747, 753
aversion to, 314, 321
in the blood, *1512*
deficiency heat, 316
do not expose to, *1509*
exterior heat and toxins, 363
Heart, 333
heat and phlegm rising, 1251
heat, fire and toxins, 315
interior excess, 187
interior heat and toxins, 361, 363
in the Liver, Gallbladder, and *San Jiao* channels, 243
Lung, 96, 383
in the Lung and throat, 386
overview, 314
in the organs, 315
in the *qi* (energy) and *xue* (blood) levels, 315, 337
in the *qi* (energy) level, 314
Stomach, 393, 398
Stomach and Intestines, 160, 174
summer-heat, 433
in the upper and middle *jiaos*, 351, 354
Urinary bladder, 1107
in the *xue* (blood) level, 333
in the *ying* (nutritive) and *xue* (blood) levels, 314
in the *ying* (nutritive) level, 330, 333
yangming, 321
yangming with qi and body fluid deficiencies, 325
yin-deficient heat, 316, 627
Heat dysuria, 1064, 1103, 1340, *1518*. *See also Re lin* (heat dysuria); *Lin zheng* (dysuria syndrome)
Heat painful obstruction, 1153, 1194, *1518*. *See also Re bi* (heat painful obstruction); *Bi zheng* (painful obstruction syndrome)
Heat reversal, 152, *1518*. *See also Re jue* (heat reversal)
Heat stroke, *1413*
damp accumulation, 1082
excess interior heat, 321, 325
phlegm and heat obstruction, 750
shaoyang syndrome with water accumulation, 222
summer-heat, 435

1564

Chinese Herbal Formulas and Applications

Index

summer-heat damaging qi and body fluids, 446
summer-heat with exterior cold and interior dampness, 436
wind-cold and interior dampness, 1079
Heat-clearing formulas, 314
Heaves, dry
  Gallbladder damp-heat, 228
  qi flow, reversed, 854
  Stomach deficiency and interlocking of heat and cold, 270
  Stomach qi disharmony, 261
Heaviness
  damp accumulation, 1068, 1121
  damp-heat, 1192
  damp-warmth, 1092
  overview, 433, 1063, 1154
  sensations, 436
  wind and phlegm rising, 1247
  wind with interior qi deficiency, 1118
  wind-dampness, 1156
  yang deficiency with water accumulation, 1135
Heel pain, **581**, **601**, **632**, **915**
Hehan Journal of Medicine and Herbology, 577
Hei Cha (Folium Camelliae Nigrum), xxiv
Hei Dou (Semen Sojae), xxiv
***Hei Xi Dan* (Lead Special Pill)**, 492
***Hei Xiao Yao San* (Black Rambling Powder)**, 252
Helicobacter pylori, 53, 391, 544
Hemangioma, hepatic, **887**
Hematemesis, *1403*
  in bronchiectasis, **940**
  deficiency and cold, 948
  excess heat and toxins, 337
  heat and fire in the upper and middle *jiaos*, 351
  heat in the Stomach and Intestines, 160
  heat in the *xue* (blood) level, 333, 942
  overview, 315, 868
  in pulmonary tuberculosis, **940**
Hematite and Scrophularia Combination, 999
Hematochezia, *1403*
  deficiency and cold, 948
  heat in the *xue* (blood) level, 333
  Liver and Kidney yin deficiencies, 654
  overview, 868
  Spleen deficiency, 584
  wind, heat and toxins, 945
  yang deficiency, 459
Hematocrit, 524
Hematological disorders, 515. *See also* specific disorders
Hematopoietic effect, 524, 564, 581, 605, 610
Hematoporphyria, **887**
Hematuria, *1403*
  damp-heat, 1192
  damp-heat in all three *jiaos*, 359
  deficiency and damage, 951
  fire in the Heart and Small Intestine channels, 365
  heat in the lower *jiao*, 947
  heat in the Urinary Bladder, 1107
  heat in the *xue* (blood) level, 333
  Liver and Kidney yin deficiencies, 654
  due to urinary infection, **948**
  water and heat, interlocked, **1116**
Hemiplegia, *1413*
  exterior excess with interior deficiency, 1169
  external wind, 977
  Liver yang and wind excess, 1004
  overview, 867, 964
  post-stroke, 906, 984, 986, 988, 991, 1180

taiyang, *yangming* and *shaoyang* disorders, 716
wind, cold and dampness, 1178, 1182
wind, cold, dampness and heat, 1172
xue bi (blood painful obstruction), 500
Hemodialysis, with muscle cramps, **601**
Hemodynamic effect, 595
Hemoglobin, 610
Hemoptysis, *1402*
  due to bronchiectasis, 1037
  damp-heat in all three *jiaos*, 359
  deficiency and damage, 951
  heat in the *xue* (blood) level, 939, 942
  Liver and Kidney yin deficiencies, 654
  Liver fire invading the Lung, 943
  Lung and Kidney yin deficiencies, 1036
  Lung yin and Spleen qi deficiencies, 1042
  Lung yin deficiency with heat, 1039
  overview, 868
  phlegm-heat, 1222
  warm-dryness, **1031**
Hemorrhage. *See also* Bleeding; Hemostatic effect; specific types and locations of bleeding
  cerebral, 716, **990**, 991, 993, **1001**, 1004, *1405*
  esophageal, 333
  ocular, **899**
  postpartum, 606
Hemorrhagic fever, **323**, **333**, **339**, **357**
Hemorrhoids, *1413*
  bleeding, 165, 945, **949**, 951
  damp-heat in all three *jiaos*, 359
  damp-heat with qi and blood stagnation, 1379
  heat and toxins, 291
  heat and toxins in the lower *jiao*, 164
  heat and toxins with underlying deficiencies, 1365
  internal or external, 165
  internal, incarcerated, **1381**
  Lung heat, 96
  wind, heat and toxins, 945
  yin and body fluid damage, 1054
Hemospermia, **638**
Hemostatic effect, 870, 940
Hemp Seed Pill, 174
Hemp Seed Pill to Moisten the Intestines, 178
Hepatic disorders. *See also* Liver; Hepatoprotective effect; specific disorders
  hepatocellular carcinoma, **547**
  hepato-cirrhosis, *1414*
  hepatoma, **547**
  hepatomegaly, 254, 935
Hepatitis, *1414*
  acute
    icteric, **286**, **371**, **747**, **1088**, **1094**, 1312
    infectious, **1088**, **1097**
    viral, **126**, **1312**
  alcohol-induced, 223
  chemical-induced, 1087
  chronic, 221, 223, 270, 363, **524**, **547**, **631**, **727**, **807**, **881**, 937, **1237**, **1346**
    active, **209**, **265**, **875**, **887**
    infectious, **692**
    viral, **1312**
  damp-heat accumulation, 1270
  damp-heat in all three *jiaos*, 359
  damp-warmth, 1096
  drug-induced, 1087
  fire in the Liver and Gallbladder channels, 379

1565

Index

hepatitis A, 1339
hepatitis B, 210, **240**, **251**, **473**, **655**, 1339
hepatitis C, 210, **617**
hot *bi zheng* (closed disorder), 747
with hypochondriac pain, 235
icteric, **286**, 371, **373**, 747, **1088**, **1094**, 1312
infectious, 243, **692**, 822, **1088**, **1097**
with jaundice, **334**, **1091**
Liver fire overacting on the Stomach, 389
Liver qi stagnation with heat, 254
non-icteric, **373**
qi and blood stagnation with damp and phlegm accumulation, 935
qi deficiency with dampness, 536
qi stagnation and food retention, 1274
shaoyang syndrome, 304
shaoyang syndrome with phlegm stagnation, 226
shaoyin syndrome, **235**
with thrombopenia, **585**
viral, **126**, **159**, 210, 243, **913**, **1312**, **1339**
yin-deficient heat and fire, 420
Hepatoprotective effect, 60, 208, 220, 235, 244, 249, 285, 343, 581, 611, 629, 655, 658, 679, 1087, 1091, 1097, 1111
Herb-drug interactions, **24**. *See also* specific drug and formula names
Herba Agastaches, xxiv
Herba Artemisiae Scopariae, xxvi
Herba Cirsii, xxvi
Herba Cirsii Japonici, xxiii
Herba Ecliptae, xxiv
Herba Gelsemii Elegantis, 27
Herba Hedyotis, xxiii
Herba Hyperici Perforati, xxiv
Herba Lonicerae Japonicae, xxv
Herba Moslae, xxvi
Herba Pyrolae, xxv
Herba Selaginellae, xxv
Herbal Teachings from the Respectfully Decorated Hall, 754
Hernia
accumulations in the interior, 302
cold, 837
cold accumulation and qi stagnation, 836
cold in the Liver and Kidney channels, 838, **839**
cold-type, 493
damp-cold, 834
exterior-deficient, wind-cold, 51
overview, 819, 820
pain, 836, *1414*
shaoyin syndrome, 233
small intestine, 836
yin deficiency with qi stagnation and blood dryness, 657
Hernial disorder, *1512*
Herpes, *1414*
genital, 318
heat and toxins, 1349
labiales, 351
neuralgia, post-herpetic, 571, **1329**
oral, 354, **366**
overview, 318
pharyngitis, herpetic, **353**
simplex, 105
wind, heat and toxins, 356
zoster, **104**, **364**, 367, 371, **905**
Herpetiformis, impetigo, 1193
Hiccups, *1414*
constant, 857

deficiency and cold of the Stomach, 467, 857
Gallbladder damp-heat, 228
overview, 819, 820
phlegm and dampness, 1077
qi deficiency with phlegm stagnation, 851
qi flow, reversed, 854, 855, 856
Stomach cold, 858
unremitting, 858
Hidden pulse, *1512*
Hidden Tiger Pill, 651, 653
Hips, pain, 494
Hircismus, **1120**
Hirschsprung's disease, 482
Histamine, 76, 98, 133, 209, 544, 846, 968
Hives. *See* Rashes; Eczema; Itching; Urticaria
HMG-CoA reductase inhibition, 343
Hoelen and Alisma Combination, 1127
Hoelen and Areca Combination, 1121
Hoelen and Atractylodes Combination, 1131
Hoelen and Bamboo Combination, 1213
Hoelen and Cuscuta Formula, 797
Hoelen and Polyporus Formula, 800
Hoelen Combination, 1077
Hoelen Five Herb Formula, 1109
Hoelen, Atractylodes, and Areca Decoction, 1129
Hoelen, Cinnamon Twig, Atractylodes and Licorice Decoction, 1131
Hollow organ, *1511*. *See also Fu* (hollow organ)
Holy Grace Formulary of the Tai Ping Era, 6
Honey-Fried Licorice Decoction, 589
Honeysuckle and Forsythia Decoction, 94
Honeysuckle and Forsythia Powder, 92
Honeysuckle and Forsythia Powder to Relieve Toxicity, 95
Honeysuckle Decoction to Relieve Toxicity, 1340
Hong (bake), *1512*
Hong Dou Kou (Fructus Galangae), xxiv
Hong Ji, 728, 1276
Hong Shi Ji Yan Fang (Time-Tested Formulas of the Hong Family), 790, 1041
Hookworms, 1289, **1294**, 1302
Hormone replacement therapy, 255
Hormones. *See* individual hormones
Hot flashes. *See* Menopause
Hou bi (painful obstruction of the throat), 1309, 1313, *1512*
***Hou Po Qi Wu Tang* (Seven-Substance Decoction with Magnolia Bark)**, 289
vs. Da Chai Hu Tang (Major Bupleurum Decoction), 290
***Hou Po Wen Zhong Tang* (Magnolia Bark Decoction for Warming the Middle)**, 840
Hou xia (post-decoction), 20
Hsiang Ju Yin, 436
Hsiang Sha Liu Chun Tzu Tang, 531
Hsiang Sheng Po Ti Wan, 388
Hsiang Su San, 67
Hsiao Cheng Chi Tang, 158
Hsiao Chien Chung Tang, 471
Hsiao Ching Lung Tang, 74
Hsiao Feng San, 967
Hsiao Hsien Hsiung Tang, 1235
Hsiao Hsu Ming Tang, 983, 985
Hsiao Pan Hsia Chia Fu Ling Tang, 1220
Hsiao Tsai Hu Tang, 206
Hsiao Yao San, 247
Hsieh Fu Chu Yu Tang, 879
Hsin I Ching Fei Tang, 122
Hsin I San, 84
Hsing Su San, 1025

1566

Index

Chinese Herbal Formulas and Applications

Hsuan Fu Tai Che Shih Tang, 851
Hu Jiao (Fructus Piperis), xxiv
Hu Qian Wan (Hidden Tiger Pill), 651, 653
   vs. Da Bu Yin Wan (Great Tonify the Yin Pill), 653
   vs. Liu Wei Di Huang Wan (Six-Ingredient Pill with
     Rehmannia), 634
Hu Zhang (Rhizoma et Radix Polygoni Cuspidati), xxiv
Hua (dissolve), **1512**
Hua Ban Tang (Transform Blotches Decoction), 339
Hua Chong Wan (Dissolve Parasites Pill), 1300
Hua Gai San (Canopy Powder), 48
   vs. Jin Fei Cao San (Inula Powder), 50
Hua Kai San, 48
Hua Tan Wan (Transform Phlegm Pill), 1223
Hua Tuo, **741**, 1481, 1482, 1484
Huai Hua San (Sophora Japonica Flower Powder), 944
Huai Jiao Wan (Sophora Japonica Fruit Pill), 946
Huan Shao Dan (Return to Youth Pill), 681
**Huan Shao Di Huang Wan (Rehmannia Pill to Return to
   Youth)**, 683
Huan Shao Tan, 681
Huang Bo (Cortex Phellodendri Chinensis), xxiv
Huang Chi Chien Chung Tang, 475
Huang Chi Wu Wu Tang, 500
Huang Di, **3**, 1481, 1482, 1484
Huang Di Nei Jing (Yellow Emperor's Inner Classic), 3, 5
Huang Di Su Wen Xuan Ming Lun Fang (Formulas from
   the Discussion Illuminating the Yellow Emperor's Basic
   Questions), **279**, 291, 444, 693
Huang Fu-Zhong, 1112
Huang Lian Jie Du Tang (Coptis Decoction to Relieve Toxicity), 341
   vs. San Huang Xie Xin Tang (Three-Yellow Decoction to Sedate
     the Epigastrium), 361
Huang Lian Shang Qing Wan (Coptis Pill to Clear the Upper), 347
Huang Lian Tang (Coptis Decoction), 271
   vs. Ban Xia Xie Xin Tang (Pinellia Decoction to Drain the
     Epigastrium), 273
Huang Lian Chieh Tu Tang, 341
Huang Lian Shang Ching Wan, 347
Huang Lian Tang, 271
Huang Long Tang (Yellow Dragon Decoction), 187
**Huang Qi Fang Feng Tang (Astragalus Decoction to Guard the
   Wind)**, 775
**Huang Qi Gui Zhi Wu Wu Tang (Astragalus and Cinnamon
   Twig Five-Substance Decoction)**, 500
**Huang Qi Jian Zhong Tang (Astragalus Decoction to Construct
   the Middle)**, 475
   vs. Da Jian Zhong Tang (Major Construct the Middle
     Decoction), 474
   vs. Dang Gui Jian Zhong Tang (Tangkuei Decoction to
     Construct the Middle), 474
   vs. Xiao Jian Zhong Tang (Minor Construct the Middle
     Decoction), 474
Huang Qi Jian Zhung Tang, 475
Huang Qi Wu Wu Tang, 500
Huang Qin Hua Shi Tang (Scutellaria and Talcum Decoction),
   1095
   vs. Huo Po Xia Ling Tang (Agastache, Magnolia Bark, Pinellia
     and Poria Decoction), 1095
   vs. San Ren Tang (Three-Nut Decoction), 1095
Huang Qin Tang (Scutellaria Decoction), 406
Huang Teng (Caulis Fibraureae), xxiv
Huang Tu Tang (Yellow Earth Decoction), 948
Hua-Tuo, 1121
Hui (influential) point, **1512**
Hui Chun Dan (Return of Spring Special Pill), 754

Hui Yang Jiu Ji Tang (Restore and Revive the Yang Decoction), 490
Hun (ethereal soul), 707, **1512**
Hunger
   excess, 398
   frequent, 396
   increased, 1052
   overview, 1022
   persistent, indeterminate, **1516**
Huo Hsiang Cheng Qi San (*Wan*), 1079
Huo luan (sudden turmoil disorder), 459, **1393**, **1521**. *See also*
   Sudden turmoil disorder
Huo Luan Lun (Discussion of Sudden Turmoil Disorders), 756,
   1099, 1101
Huo Luo Dan (Invigorate the Collaterals Special Pill), 1177
**Huo Luo Xiao Ling Dan (Fantastically Effective Pill to
   Invigorate the Collaterals)**, 914
Huo Ming Yin (Revitalize Life Decoction), 1330
**Huo Po Xia Ling Tang (Agastache, Magnolia Bark, Pinellia, and
   Poria Decoction)**, 1095
   vs. Huang Qin Hua Shi Tang (Scutellaria and Talcum
     Decoction), 1095
   vs. San Ren Tang (Three-Nut Decoction), 1095
Huo re lun (discussion of fire and heat), 279, 1307
**Huo Ren Cong Chi Tang (Scallion and Prepared Soybean
   Decoction from the Book to Safeguard Life)**, 112
Huo Xiang (Herba Agastaches), xxiv
Huo Xiang Ye (Folium Agastaches), xxiv
Huo Xiang Zheng Qi San (Agastache Powder to Rectify the Qi),
   1079
   vs. Liu He Tang (Harmonize the Six Decoction), 1081
Huo Xiang Zheng Qi San (*Wan*), 1079
**Huo Xue Shun Qi Tang (Invigorate the Blood and Smooth the
   Qi Decoction)**, 900
**Huo Xue Tong Lin Tang (Invigorate the Blood to Unblock
   Dysuria Decoction)**, 1107
**Huo Xue Zhi Tong Tang (Invigorate the Blood and Stop Pain
   Decoction)**, 902
Hydramnios, **1139**
Hydrocele
   damp-cold, 834
   exterior wind with interior qi deficiency, 1118
   exterior wind with water accumulation, 101
Hydrocephalus, **1111**
Hydrocortisone, 487, 572, 605, 655, 890
Hydronephrosis, **1117**, **1120**, **1133**
Hydrothorax, 150
Hydroxyl radical, 1380
Hyperacidity, **182**. *See also* Acid reflux/regurgitation
Hyperactivity, **54**, 589. *See also* Attention; Concentration
Hyperaldosteronism, 668, 673
Hypercholesterolemia, 209, 285, 718. *See also* Lipoproteins;
   Cholesterols; Antihyperlipidemic effect
Hypercortisolism, **1414**
Hyperemia, 641
Hyperglycemia. *See* Diabetes mellitus; Glucose; Hypoglycemic effect
Hyperlipidemia, **1414**. *See also* Lipoproteins; Cholesterols;
   Antihyperlipidemic effect
   aging-induced, 285
   blood deficiency and blood stagnation, 571
   blood stagnation, **883**
   damp-heat, **1088**
   effect on, 209
   Liver qi stagnation, **252**
   overview, 869
   shaoyang and *yangming* syndromes, **286**
   wind-heat with interior heat, **293**

1567

Index

Hyperlipoproteinemia, **718**, 1090, **1091**. *See also* Lipoproteins; Cholesterols; Antihyperlipidemic effect

Hypermenorrhea
  deficiency and injury, 562
  deficiency heat, 802
  Liver and Kidney yin deficiencies, 654
  qi and blood deficiencies, 580
  Spleen deficiency, 584

Hyperosteogeny. *See also* Bones
  knees, **1163**
  lumbar spine, 895
  yin, blood and body fluid deficiencies, **602**

Hyperprolactinemia, 602, 674

Hypersomnia, 877, 1112, *1415*

Hypertension, *1415*. *See also* Antihypertensive effect; Hypotensive effect; Vasodilative effect
  with arteriosclerosis and high cholesterol, 1125
  blood deficiency and blood stagnation, 571
  blood stagnation, 879
  deficiency and cold of the Stomach, **469**
  with edema, 1125
  gestational, **596**, **659**, **1111**
  Heart and Kidney deficiencies, 726
  Heart and Kidney disharmony, 714
  heat, fire and toxins in all three *jiaos*, 341
  interior excess heat, 158
  Kidney yang deficiency, 673
  Kidney yin and yang deficiencies with fire, 684
  Liver excess, **997**
  Liver fire rising, **373**
  Liver yang hyperactivity, 713
  Liver yang rising, **1003**
  overview, 517, 965
  primary, **630**, **642**, **670**, **1001**, **1005**, *1415*
  qi deficiency, **546**
  taiyang, *yangming* and *shaoyang* disorders, 716
  water accumulation, 1124
  wind-heat with interior heat, 291
  yang deficiency, **1136**
  yin deficiency with internal fire and wind, 661
  yin-deficient fire, **638**

Hyperthermia. *See* Fever; Antipyretic effect

Hyperthyroidism, *1415*
  Heart and Kidney deficiencies, 726
  Liver and Kidney yin deficiencies, **630**
  Liver yang and wind rising, 999
  phlegm, 1355
  qi and blood deficiencies, 589
  qi and phlegm stagnation, **1354**
  with swelling and hardness, 1357
  T3 and T4, elevated, **373**
  taiyang, *yangming* and *shaoyang* disorders, 716
  yin deficiency with qi stagnation and blood dryness, **659**
  yin-deficient heat and fire, 420

Hypertrophic myelitis, **497**

Hyphema, **941**

Hypnotic effect, 708, 718, 1132

Hypocalcemia, **652**

Hypochondriac
  distention, 72
  fullness, **283**, 1131
  fullness and clumping, 304
  fullness and discomfort, 206, 226
  fullness and distention, 233, 484, 848
  fullness and pain, 238, 242, 389
  fullness and stifling sensation, 1233

neuralgia, 657
oppression and distention, 527
overview, 201, 819
pain, *1415*
  bilateral, 247, 254
  chronic, stabbing, 879
  excess cold accumulation, 166
  fire in the Liver and Gallbladder, 371
  due to hepatitis, **235**
  Liver and blood stagnation, **899**
  overview, 202, 316
  qi stagnation with heat, 825
  warm-dryness, 1030
  yang deficiency, phlegm accumulation and qi stagnation, 831
  yin deficiency with qi stagnation and blood dryness, 657
pain and swelling, 897

Hypoglycemia, 476

Hypoglycemic effect, 325, 328, 369, 399, 629, 641, 643, 655, 676, 874, 1044, 1050, 1053

Hypokalemia, **437**

Hypomenorrhea, 562

Hypoperistalsis, chlorpromazine-induced, **482**

Hypopituitarism, 606

Hypopnea, sleep, **829**

Hypotension, *1415*
  Kidney yang deficiency, 668, 673
  qi and blood deficiencies, **591**
  qi and yin deficiencies, **556**
  radiation-induced, 548
  yin, yang, blood and *jing* (essence) deficiencies, **689**

Hypotensive effect, 629, 748

Hypothalamo-pituitary-adrenal system, 717

Hypothyroidism, *1415*
  Kidney yang deficiency, 668, 673
  yang deficiency with water accumulation, 1135
  yin, yang, blood and *jing* (essence) deficiencies, 687

Hysteria
  blood deficiency with heat, 246
  Heart blood deficiency and Liver qi stagnation, **733**
  phlegm retention with yang deficiency, 1131
  phlegm stagnation, **830**
  taiyang, *yangming* and *shaoyang* disorders, 716

Hysteromyoma, *1416*
  blood deficiency with cold, **926**
  blood stasis, **929**
  cold obstruction and blood stagnation, **891**
  qi and blood stagnation, **916**

I Chi Chung Ming Tang, 551

I Chi Tang, 164

I Kan San, 245

IBS. *See* Irritable bowel syndrome

I-Character Decoction, 164

Ichthyosis, **972**

Ig. *See* Immunoglobulins

IL. *See* Interleukin

Ileus, post-operative, **482**

Immature Bitter Orange and Atractylodes Macrocephala Decoction, 1275

Immature Bitter Orange and Atractylodes Macrocephala Pill, 1274

Immature Bitter Orange and Peony Powder, 236

Immature Bitter Orange Pill to Guide Out Stagnation, 1270

Immature Bitter Orange Pill to Reduce Focal Distention, 1280

Immature Bitter Orange, Chinese Chive, and Cinnamon Twig Decoction, 831

Immune, compromised, **538**, **546**, **1042**

Chinese Herbal Formulas and Applications

Index

Immunoglobulins
  IgA, 76, 532, 774, 1136
  IgE, 98, 544
  IgG, 774, 1136
  IgM, 532, 930, 1136
Immunomodulatory effect, 76
Immunostimulant effect, 60, 209, 220, 285, 322, 372, 394, 476,
  487, 523, 532, 544, 555, 581, 595, 605, 610, 616, 629, 641, 655,
  669, 679, 771, 774, 1034
Immunosuppressant effect, 576, 673, **968**
Immunosuppression
  corticosteroid-induced, 680
  cyclophosphamide-induced, **612**, 617
  mitomycin-induced, 548
  prednisolone-induced, 617
Impediment-Alleviating Decoction, 1158
Imperata Decoction, 1112
Imperial Grace Formulary of the Tai Ping Era, 6, 43, 48, 49, 67,
  72, 126, 128, 247, 303, 351, 368, 391, 401, 436, 463, 484, 522,
  535, 562, 609, 615, 751, 758, 776, 781, 797, 805, 842, 911, 946,
  973, 990, 1068, 1075, 1079, 1082, 1103, 1105, 1107, 1123, 1177,
  1181, **1203**, 1209, 1231, 1296, 1300, 1347
Impetigo, 344, **1193**, *1416*
Important Formula for Painful Diarrhea, 257
Important Formula for Painful Purging, 257
Impotence, *1416*
  cold and dampness, 1134
  damp accumulation in the Spleen and Stomach, **1070**
  damp-heat, **1216**
  Heart and Kidney deficiencies, **727**
  Kidney yang deficiency, **670**, 673, 678
  Kidney yin and *jing* (essence) deficiencies, 645
  Liver and Kidney deficiencies, 690
  Liver and Kidney yin deficiencies, **632**
  Liver qi stagnation, **251**
  overview, 514
  due to prostatitis, **1141**
  qi, blood, yang and *jing* (essence) deficiencies, **682**
  shaoyin syndrome, **236**
  yin and yang deficiencies, 798
  yin, yang, blood and *jing* (essence) deficiencies, 687, **688**
Improve Vision Pill with Rehmannia, 633
Incontinence
  overview, 770
  postpartum, **547**
  post-surgical, **547**
  rectal, 770
  urinary, *1431*
    Kidney deficiency, 789
    Kidney yang deficiency, **671**, 673, 678
    post-stroke, **796**, 906
Increase the Fluids and Order the Qi Decoction, 190
Increase the Fluids Decoction, 1054
Indigestion, *1416*. *See also* Digestive effect
  in children, **1275**
  chronic, 1277
  damp accumulation, 1068, 1072, 1076
  deficiency and cold, 463
  food stagnation, 1266, **1267**
  food stagnation with heat, 1277
  in infants, **264**
  non-ulcerative, **1282**
  qi blood, dampness, phlegm, and food stagnation, 824
  qi deficiency with dampness and phlegm, **529**
  qi stagnation, 822
  Spleen and Stomach deficiencies, 541

Spleen and Stomach disharmony, 1074
  summer-heat, 438
Indocin. *See* Indomethacin
Indomethacin, 360
Infantile
  convulsions, 755
  epilepsy, 755
  malnutrition, 1074, 1297, 1299, *1511*. *See also Gan ji* (infantile
    malnutrition)
  seizures, 750, 755
Infarction
  acute, **487**
  cardiac, 491
  cerebral, **555**, **573**, **907**, **998**, 1004, *1405*
  myocardial, **555**, *1421*
  overview, 457
Infection. *See also* specific infections; Antibiotic effect;
  Antibacterial effect; Antiviral effect; Antifungal effect
  bacterial, 321, 325
  bile duct, **154**, **240**
  epidemic, **109**
  eye, 381
  fallopian tube, 371
  with fever, **126**
  frequent, **129**
  fungal, **1081**, **1190**
  gallbladder, **154**
  gastrointestinal, 757
  H. pylori, **391**
  heat and fire in the upper and middle *jiaos*, 351
  Helicobacter pylori, **391**
  ofloxacin-resistant, 133
  oral cavity, 365
  overview, 37, 317, 318, 1023, 1065
  postpartum, **213**
  post-surgical, **344**
  prevention, 771, **774**
  pyogenic, **339**
  respiratory tract, *1416*
    acute, **94**
    in children, **417**
    damp-phlegm, 1209
    deficiency heat, 558
    exterior-deficient, wind-cold, 51
    with fever, **357**
    heat and fire in the upper and middle *jiaos*, 351
    phlegm accumulation, 1232
    phlegm-heat, 1222
    upper, **41**, **61**, **70**, **91**, **94**, **98**, **109**, **126**, **129**, *1416*
    viral, **126**
    warm-dryness, 1030
    wind, **118**
    wind-cold, 70
    wind-cold with yin and blood deficiencies, 136
    wind-heat, **94**
  salmonella, **297**
  suppurative, 124
  urinary tract, *1431*
    acute, 947, **1340**
    acute or chronic, **373**
    blood deficiency and heat, 576
    damp-heat, 800, **1104**
    damp-heat accumulation, 1270
    fire in the Heart and Small Intestine channels, **366**
    Heart fire with damp-heat in the lower *jiao*, 368
    heat accumulation in all three *jiaos*, 347

INDEX

I

1569

Index

heat, fire and toxins in all three *jiaos*, 341
Kidney yin and yang deficiencies with fire, 684
Liver qi stagnation with heat, 254
toxic heat, **410**
water and dampness accumulation, 1109
water and heat, interlocked, 1115
yin-deficient fire, **650**
yin-deficient heat and fire, 420
viral, **109**, 321, 325, **417**, **1056**
Infertility. *See also* Reproductive effect
female, *1416*
anovulation, **556**, 922
blood deficiency, **565**, 596
blood deficiency and heat, 576
blood stagnation, **890**
blood stasis, 911
deficiency and cold, 919, **921**, 923
fallopian tubes, blocked, **236**, **572**, **835**
hyperprolactinemic, **674**
Kidney yang deficiency with diminished *ming men* (life gate) fire, 679
menstruation, irregular, **685**
Liver and Kidney yin deficiencies, 631
Liver qi stagnation, **251**
Liver qi stagnation with heat, 254
ovarian failure, **646**
prolactin, elevated, **670**
male, *1416*
cold obstruction and blood stagnation, **891**
Kidney yang deficiency with diminished *ming men* (life gate) fire, **679**
Liver and Kidney deficiencies, **691**
Liver and Kidney yin deficiencies, **631**
prostatitis, 367
seminal vesiculitis, 367
sperm disorders, **461**, **547**, **617**, **670**, **677**, **891**
varicocele, **930**
yin-deficient fire, **637**
overview, 516
Inflammation. *See also* specific disorders; Anti-inflammatory effect
damp-heat, 1192
joints, 1173, 1192
overview, 1023
with pain, **1373**
qi and blood stagnation, 901
due to trauma, **1122**
Inflammatory bowel syndrome, 476, 840
Inflammatory disorders. *See* specific disorders; Anti-inflammatory effect
Influential point, *1512*. *See also Hui* (influential) point
Influenza, *1416*
cool-dryness, 1025
exterior-deficient, wind-cold, 51
exterior-excess, wind-cold, 39
heat and fire in the upper and middle *jiaos*, **352**
heat, lingering or residual, 327
interior heat, 321, 325
Lung heat, 96
overview, 37
phlegm and damp accumulation, 1224
shaoyang syndrome, 206, 304
shaoyang syndrome with phlegm stagnation, 226
shaoyang syndrome with water accumulation, 222
shaoyin with *taiyang* syndrome, 132
stomach flu, 67
in summer, 435, **440**, 1079

summer-heat, 438
taiyang and *shaoyang* syndromes, **220**
warm-dryness, 1030
wind, 973
wind, cold and dampness with interior heat, 64
wind, cold and dampness with qi deficiency, 124
wind, heat and toxins, 356
wind-cold, 59, 70, 72
wind-cold and interior deficiency and cold, 466
wind-cold attacking the Lung, 48, 49
wind-cold turning into heat, 108
wind-cold with interior heat, 45, 295
wind-cold with water accumulation, 74
wind-cold with yang qi deficiency, 131
wind-cold with yin and blood deficiencies, 136
wind-dampness, 1156
wind-heat, **94**
wind-heat with interior heat, 291
wind-heat with yin deficiency, 137
wind-warmth, **91**, 111
Influenza virus, 76, 544
A virus, 76, 774
B virus, 76
Ingredients, 15
Injection, 18
Injuries. *See also* Trauma
overview, 867
qi and blood stagnation, 900
soft tissues, **61**, **1178**
with swelling and pain, 903
Inner Classic, 3. *See also Huang Di Nei Jing* (Yellow Emperor's Inner Classic)
Inotropic effect, 60, 235, 1119
Insomnia, *1417*. *See also* Sleep; Hypnotic effect; Sedative effect
blood deficiency, 562, **566**
blood deficiency with deficiency heat, **723**
blood deficiency with heat, 245
Heart and Kidney deficiencies, 725, **727**
Heart and Kidney disharmony, 714
Heart and Spleen deficiencies, 583
Heart blood deficiency, 735
Heart blood deficiency and Liver qi stagnation, **733**
Heart fire, 710
heat in the *ying* (nutritive) level, 330
heat, fire and toxins in all three *jiaos*, 341
heat, lingering or residual, 327
heat-phlegm, 1214, 1218
Kidney yin and yang deficiencies with fire, 684
Liver and Kidney yin deficiencies, 654
Liver blood deficiency, 722
Liver excess, 996
Liver yang and wind excess, 1004
Liver yang hyperactivity, 713
Liver yang rising, 1002
overview, 314, 513, 707, 708
post-stroke, **1010**
qi and blood deficiencies, 616
qi, blood and yang deficiencies, 609
severe, **585**
shaoyang syndrome, **719**
stubborn, **240**, **882**
taiyang, *yangming* and *shaoyang* disorders, 716
water and heat, interlocked, 1115
with weakness and irritability, 370
yang deficiency with water accumulation, 1135
yin and yang deficiencies, 798

1570

Index

Insulting sequence, *1513*
Intellect, *1525*. See also Yi (intellect)
Interactions (drugs), 24. See also specific drug and formula names
   5-fluorouracil, 214, 612, 617
   acetaminophen, 62
   adriamycin, 612
   ampicillin, 969
   angiotensin-converting enzyme inhibitors, 1042
   antipsychotic drugs, 175, 256, 482
   aspirin, 287, 345, 391
   benzodiazepines, 221
   capsaicin, 1045
   carbamazepine, 77, 214, 720
   carbon tetrachloride, 214
   carboplatin, 612
   chemotherapy, 530, 539, 582, 612, 633, 855, 1268
   chlorpromazine, 482
   cis-diamminedichloroplatinum, 612
   cisplatin, 266, 612
   clomiphene, 922
   colchicine, 598
   corticosteroids, 680
   cyclophosphamide, 548, 612, 617
   cytotoxic drugs, 345
   danazol, 214
   D-galactosamine, 214
   enalapril, 1045
   etoposide, 612
   fluticasone, 77
   gonadotropin, 54, 256, 598, 602, 876, 931
   halothane, 214
   interferon, 42, 47, 214, 612
   interleukin, 214
   irinotecan, 266
   lamivudine, 214
   levofloxacin, 530, 613
   mitomycin, 548, 612
   morphine, 483
   neuroleptics, 602
   ofloxacin, 133, 214, 225, 530
   opioids, 159
   paclitaxel, 602
   penicillin, 567
   pentobarbital, 214, 221
   phenothiazine, 191
   prednisolone, 612, 617
   prednisone, 671
   radiation, 539, 548, 582, 612
   rifampin, 613
   scopolamine, 567, 617
   selective serotonin reuptake inhibitors, 1112
   streptomycin, 639
   theophylline, 720
   tolbutamide, 214
   zidovudine, 214
Interactions (formulas), 24. See also specific drug and formula names
   Ban Xia Xie Xin Tang (Pinellia Decoction to Drain the Epigastrium), 266
   Bao He Wan (Preserve Harmony Pill), 1268
   Bu Zhong Yi Qi Tang (Tonify the Middle and Augment the Qi Decoction), 548
   Chai Hu Gui Zhi Tang (Bupleurum and Cinnamon Twig Decoction), 221
   Chai Hu Jia Long Gu Mu Li Tang (Bupleurum plus Dragon Bone and Oyster Shell Decoction), 720

   Chai Ling Tang (Bupleurum and Poria Decoction), 225
   Da Chai Hu Tang (Major Bupleurum Decoction), 287
   Da Jian Zhong Tang (Major Construct the Middle Decoction), 482
   Da Qing Long Tang (Major Bluegreen Dragon Decoction), 47
   Dang Gui Bu Xue Tang (Tangkuei Decoction to Tonify the Blood), 582
   Dang Gui Shao Yao San (Tangkuei and Peony Powder), 598
   Ge Gen Tang (Kudzu Decoction), 62
   Gui Zhi Fu Ling Wan (Cinnamon Twig and Poria Pill), 931
   Gui Zhi Tang (Cinnamon Twig Decoction), 54
   Huang Lian Jie Du Tang (Coptis Decoction to Relieve Toxicity), 345
   Jia Wei Xiao Yao San (Augmented Rambling Powder), 256
   Jin Gui Shen Qi Wan (Kidney Qi Pill from the Golden Cabinet), 671
   Ju Pi Zhu Ru Tang (Tangerine Peel and Bamboo Shaving Decoction), 855
   Liu Jun Zi Tang (Six-Gentlemen Decoction), 530
   Liu Wei Di Huang Wan (Six-Ingredient Pill with Rehmannia), 633
   Ma Huang Fu Zi Xi Xin Tang (Ephedra, Asarum, and Prepared Aconite Decoction), 133
   Ma Huang Tang (Ephedra Decoction), 42
   Ma Zi Ren Wan (Hemp Seed Pill), 175
   Mai Men Dong Tang (Ophiopogonis Decoction), 1045
   Qiong Yu Gao (Beautiful Jade Paste), 1042
   Ren Shen Yang Ying Tang (Ginseng Decoction to Nourish the Nutritive Qi), 617
   Shao Yao Gan Cao Tang (Peony and Licorice Decoction), 602
   Shen Ling Bai Zhu San (Ginseng, Poria, and Atractylodes Macrocephala Powder), 539
   Shi Quan Da Bu Tang (All-Inclusive Great Tonifying Decoction), 612
   Si Wu Tang (Four-Substance Decoction), 567
   Tao He Cheng Qi Tang (Peach Pit Decoction to Order the Qi), 876
   Wen Jing Tang (Warm the Channels Decoction), 922
   Wu Ling San (Five-Ingredient Powder with Poria), 1112
   Xiao Chai Hu Tang (Minor Bupleurum Decoction), 214
   Xiao Cheng Qi Tang (Minor Order the Qi Decoction), 159
   Xiao Feng San (Eliminate Wind Powder), 969
   Xiao Qing Long Tang (Minor Bluegreen Dragon Decoction), 77
   You Gui Wan (Restore the Right [Kidney] Pill), 680
   Zeng Ye Cheng Qi Tang (Increase the Fluids and Order the Qi Decoction), 191
   Zhi Bai Di Huang Wan (Anemarrhena, Phellodendron, and Rehmannia Pill), 639
   Zuo Jin Wan (Left Metal Pill), 391
Intercostal
   neuralgia, 242, 1233
   pain, 242
Interferon, 42, 47, 214, 544, 546, 612
Interior, *1513*
   accumulation, 149
   cold, 149, 455
   dampness, 1063
   dryness, 1021
   excess, 149
   excess and deficiency, 150
   excess cold, 166, 171
   excess heat, 152
   excess heat with qi and blood deficiencies, 187
   exterior and interior, 281, *1510*
   heat, 149, 314
   heat and dryness, 150
   heat and toxins, 361

1571

Index

heat with exterior wind-cold, 295
heat with exterior wind-heat, 291
overview, 149
phlegm-heat with exterior wind-cold, 845
water accumulation and heat, 150
wind, 964
Interior Comforting Formula, 484
Interior-Drawing and Detoxifying Drink, 1367, 1368
Interior-Nourishing and Qi-Increasing Decoction (Pill), 542
Interior-warming formulas, 455
Interleukin
herb-drug interactions, 214
IL-1alpha, 564, 611
IL-2, 544
IL-4, 133, 210
IL-5, 210
IL-10, 210
IL-12, 60
Intermittent pulse, *1513*
Internal Medicine according to Bian Que, **705**
Interstitial pneumonia, 118, **1045**
Intestinal disorders
abscesses, 1321, 1347, 1350, 1379, 1383, *1417*, *1513*
abscesses with pus, 1382
adhesion, **498, 899**
ascariasis, **1293**
bleeding, 945
colic, 494
cramps, 600
flukes, 1301
motility, decreased, 481
obstruction, *1417*
acute, 160, **162**
antipsychotics-induced, 482
excess heat, 155
excess heat with qi and blood deficiencies, 187
in hospitalized patients, **1282**
interior excess heat, **154, 158, 172**
overview, 151
shaoyin syndrome, 233
yang deficiency and interior cold, **482**
overview, 318
parasites, 1292, 1297, 1299, 1301
peristalsis
absence of, 159, 1072
to decrease, 258, 263, 296, 342, 472, 771, 785
to increase, 154, 158, 162, 167, 175, 209, 1275, 1281, 1380
to regulate, 523, 528, 532, 537, 543
spasms, 481
tuberculosis, 541, 784
Intestinal wind, 291, *1506. See also Chang feng* (intestinal wind)
Intestines. *See also* Small Intestine; Large Intestine
damp-heat, 1270
dryness and heat, 160, 174
heat with damaged yin and body fluids, 190
tuberculosis, **892**, *1430*
Intoxication, 486
Introduction to Medicine, 802, 1276, 1361
Intropine. *See* Dopamine
Inula and Hematite Combination, 851
Inula and Hematite Decoction, 851
Inula and Red Ochre Decoction, 851
Inula Powder, 49
Investigation of Medical Formulas, 1083, 1222
Invigorate the Blood and Smooth the Qi Decoction, 900
Invigorate the Blood and Stop Pain Decoction, 902

Invigorate the Blood to Unblock Dysuria Decoction, 1107
Invigorate the Collaterals Special Pill, 1177
Invigorating Recuperation Decoction, 905
Invisible phlegm, *1526. See also Yin* (invisible phlegm)
Irinotecan, 266
Iritis, 381
Iron Filings Decoction, 711
Iron Flute Pill, 388
Irritability, *1513. See also* Stress; Anxiety; related conditions
blood accumulation in the lower *jiao*, 873
blood deficiency with heat, 245, 575
damp-heat, 1101
damp-heat in all three *jiaos*, 359
deficiency and cold of the middle *jiao*, 471
fire in the Heart channel, 365
fire in the Spleen and Stomach, 396
Heart and Kidney deficiencies, 725
Heart fire, 368, 710
heat and fire, 347
heat and fire in the upper and middle *jiaos*, 351
heat in the chest and cold in the Stomach, 271
heat, fire and toxins in all three *jiaos*, 341
heat, lingering or residual, 327
heat-phlegm, 1214
hot *bi zheng* (closed disorder), 747
interior heat, 321, 325
interior heat and toxins, 361
interior heat in all three *jiaos*, 299
Kidney yin and yang deficiencies with fire, 684
Liver blood deficiency, 722
Liver excess, 996
Liver qi stagnation, 238, 849
Liver qi stagnation with deficiencies, 254
Liver wind rising, 993
Liver yang rising, 1002
overview, 201, 281, 314, 315, 316, 433, 707, 708
Pericardium heat and Liver wind, 753
phlegm and heat obstruction, 750
qi and blood deficiencies, 580
shaoyang syndrome, 206, 716
Stomach heat, 398
summer-heat and dampness, 441, 444
summer-heat damaging qi and body fluids, 446
summer-heat with damaged qi and body fluids, 554
taiyang, yangming and *shaoyang* disorders, 716
warm-dryness, 1030
water and heat, interlocked, 1115
wind-cold with interior heat, 45
with weakness, 370
yin and qi deficiencies, 776
yin-deficient fire, 637, 649
yin-deficient heat, 418
yin-deficient heat and fire, 420
Irritable bowel syndrome (IBS), *1417*
deficiency and cold, 459
deficiency and cold of the middle *jiao*, **477**
deficiency and cold of the Spleen and Kidney, **786**
heat in the Stomach and cold in the Intestines, **1294**
Liver qi stagnation, **252**
qi deficiency, **524**
qi deficiency with cold and dampness, **532**
qi deficiency with dampness, **537**
Spleen deficiency and Liver excess, **259**
Spleen qi deficiency and Liver qi stagnation, **808**
Stomach qi disharmony, **264**
Isatis Decoction, 358

Index

Ischemia
 brain injury, due to, **719**, **931**
 cardiac, **881**
 cerebral, transient, **343**
 cerebrovascular, **907**
 stroke, **916**, **1006**
Itching. *See also* Rashes; Eczema; Urticaria
 blood deficiency, **566**
 blood deficiency with blood stagnation, **574**
 constant, **606**, **972**
 genital, 810, 1192
 in geriatrics, **54**, **293**, **1031**
 Liver and Kidney deficiencies, **695**
 vaginal, 164
 wind, 967
 wind-heat, **293**
 wind with blood deficiency, 970
Jade Fluid Decoction, 1049
Jade Key to Many Towers, 1033
Jade Screen Powder, 773
Jade Source Combination, 1052
Jade Spring Pill, 1052
Jade Wind-Barrier Formula, 773
Jade Windscreen Powder, 773
Jade Woman Decoction, 398
Jade-Spring Pill, 1052
Jasper Powder, 443
Jaundice, **1088**, *1417*
 acute, 338, 341, 370
 blood stagnation, 885
 damp-cold, 1089
 damp-heat, 1086, 1090
 damp-heat in all three *jiaos*, 359
 damp-heat in the Spleen and Stomach, 401
 damp-warmth, 1096
 overview, 1063, 1064
 phlegm accumulation, 1311
 shaoyang syndrome, 206
 taiyang and *shaoyang* syndromes, 219
Jaws, clenched, 744. *See also* Lockjaw
Jen Shen Pai Tu San, 124
Jen Shen Yang Yung Tang (*Wan*), 615
***Ji Chuan Jian* (Benefit the River [Flow] Decoction)**, 179
Ji ju (accumulation), *1394*
Ji Li (Fructus Tribuli), xxiii
***Ji Ming San* (Powder to Take at Cock's Crow)**, 1183
Ji Sheng Fang (Formulas to Aid the Living), 82, 84, 185, 231, 559, 583, 671, 675, 826, 833, 849, 855, 858, 1211
***Ji Sheng Shen Qi Wan* (Kidney Qi Pill from Formulas that Aid the Living)**, 675
 vs. Jin Gui Shen Qi Wan (Kidney Qi Pill from the Golden Cabinet), 677
***Ji Su San* (Peppermint Powder)**, 443
***Ji Tong Tang* (Spine Pain Decoction)**, 1165
Ji Yin Gang Mu (Materia Medica to Aid Yin), 931
***Jia Jian Cheng Qi Tang* (Modified Order the Qi Decoction)**, 156
***Jia Jian Fu Mai Tang* (Modified Restore the Pulse Decoction)**, 591
***Jia Jian Wei Rui Tang* (Modified Polygonatum Odoratum Decoction)**, 137
***Jia Jian Xiao Qing Long Tang* (Modified Minor Bluegreen Dragon Decoction)**, 78
***Jia Wei Ba Zheng San* (Augmented Eight Herb Powder for Rectification)**, 1105
***Jia Wei Gua Lou Xie Bai Tang* (Augmented Trichosanthes Fruit and Chinese Chive Decoction)**, 832

***Jia Wei Huo Luo Dan* (Augmented Invigorate the Collaterals Special Pill)**, 1180
***Jia Wei Ma Xing Gan Shi Tang* (Augmented Ephedra, Apricot Kernel, Licorice, and Gypsum Decoction)**, 99
***Jia Wei Ping Wei San* (Modified Calm the Stomach Powder)**, 1072
***Jia Wei Qian Zheng San* (Augmented Lead to Symmetry Powder)**, 980
***Jia Wei Shao Yao Gan Cao Tang* (Augmented Peony and Licorice Decoction)**, 603
Jia Wei Shen Qi Wan (Augmented Kidney Qi Pill), 675, 677
***Jia Wei Si Wu Tang* (Augmented Four-Substance Decoction)**, 568
***Jia Wei Xiang Su San* (Augmented Cyperus and Perilla Leaf Powder)**, 69
***Jia Wei Xiao Yao San* (Augmented Rambling Powder)**, 254
***Jia Wei Xin Yi San* (Augmented Magnolia Flower Powder)**, 85
***Jia Wei You Gui Wan* (Augmented Restore the Right [Kidney] Pill)**, 680
***Jia Wei Zuo Gui Wan* (Augmented Restore the Left [Kidney] Pill)**, 647
Jian (decoct), *1513*
***Jian Bi Tang* (Remove Painful Obstruction in the Shoulders Decoction)**, 1160
***Jian Ling Tang* (Construct Roof Tiles Decoction)**, 1002
 vs. Zhen Gan Xi Feng Tang (Sedate the Liver and Extinguish Wind Decoction), 1003
***Jian Pi Wan* (Strengthen the Spleen Pill)**, 1277
 vs. Si Jun Zi Tang (Four-Gentlemen Decoction), 1279
 vs. Zhi Shi Xiao Pi Wan (Immature Bitter Orange Pill to Reduce Focal Distention), 1282
 vs. Zhi Zhu Wan (Immature Bitter Orange and Atractylodes Macrocephala Pill), 1279, 1282
Jiao. See also specific conditions
 lower, *1514*
  accumulation of dampness, heat and toxins, 164
  blood accumulation, 873
  blood stagnation, 933
  damp-heat, 371, 810, 1103
  deficiency and cold, 795, 1140
 middle, *1515*
  dampness, 1076
  deficiency and cold, 455, 459, 471, 476, 484, 787
  heat, 354
  heat and fire, 351
  yang deficiency, 481, 1131
 San Jiao, *1518*
  damp-heat, 359
  excess heat, fire and toxins, 341
  heat, 243
  heat accumulation, 347
 upper, *1522*
  heat, 354
  water accumulation, 1125
  wind, heat, and toxins, 355
***Jiao Ai Tang* (Ass-Hide Gelatin and Mugwort Decoction)**, 950
Jiao nang ji (capsule), 18
Jiao qi (leg qi), *1394*
Jiao Zhu Fu Ren Liang Fang (Revised Fine Formulas for Women), 725, 1325
***Jie Geng Tang* (Platycodon Decoction)**, 1230
Jie xiong (stagnant chest), 161, 163, 172, *1513*
Jin (measure of weight), 22, 1439
Jin (soak), *1513*
Jin (thin body fluid), *1513*
Jin Bo (gold foil), xxiv
***Jin Fei Cao San* (Inula Powder)**, 49

INDEX

1573

Index

vs. Hua Gai San (Canopy Powder), 50

vs. Zhi Sou San (Stop Coughing Powder), 119

Jin Gui Shen Qi Wan (Kidney Qi Pill from the Golden Cabinet), 668

vs. Ba Wei Di Huang Wan (Eight-Ingredient Pill with Rehmannia), 674

vs. Ji Sheng Shen Qi Wan (Kidney Qi Pill from Formulas that Aid the Living), 677

vs. Liu Wei Di Huang Wan (Six-Ingredient Pill with Rehmannia), 635

Jin Gui Yao Lue (Essentials from the Golden Cabinet), 6, **31**, 42, 78, 80, 101, 102, 166, 171, 237, 283, 289, 323, 359, 384, 410, 453, 462, 475, 480, 500, 594, 623, 668, 722, 731, 798, 827, 831, 832, 853, 854, 876, 919, 928, 935, 937, 948, 950, 1043, 1077, 1090, 1118, 1120, 1125, 1131, 1133, 1186, 1220, 1242, 1275, 1364, 1378, 1382

Jin Jian Fei Er Wan (Golden Pill to Construct a Fat Child), 1298

Jin Ling Zi San (Melia Toosendan Powder), 825

Jin Qian Bai Hua She (Bungarus Parvus), xxiii

Jin Suo Gu Jing Wan (Metal Lock Pill to Stabilize the Essence), 789

vs. Sang Piao Xiao San (Mantis Egg-Case Powder), 794

Jin Yin Hua (Flos Lonicerae Japonicae), xxiv

Jing (clean), *1513*

Jing (essence), 512, 645, *1513*

Jing (river) point, *1513*

Jing (well) point, *1513*

Jing Fang Bai Du San (Schizonepeta and Saposhnikovia Powder to Overcome Pathogenic Influences), 1334, 1335, 1336

vs. Bai Du San (Overcome Pathogenic Influences Powder), 127, 1336

Jing Fang Er Hao (Neck Formula Two), 62

Jing Fang Yi Hao (Neck Formula One), 62

Jing Jie Lian Chiao Tang, 120

Jing Jie Lian Qiao Tang (Schizonepeta and Forsythia Decoction), 120

Jing Jie Sui (Spica Schizonepetae), xxiv

Jing Xiu Tang Yao Shuo (Herbal Teachings from the Respectfully Decorated Hall), 754

Jing Yue Quan Shu (Collected Treatises of [Zhang] Jing Yue), 12, **147**, 179, 184, 238, 257, 398, 548, 618, 645, 647, 678, 680, 836, 838, 1071

Jiu ji (medicinal wine), 17

Jiu ji (moxa), 18

Jiu Ji Xi Xian San (Urgent Powder to Dilute Saliva), 1313

Jiu Wei Bing Lang Jia Wu Fu Tang (Areca Nine Decoction plus Evodia and Poria), 1123

Jiu Wei Chiang Huo Tang, 64

Jiu Wei Qiang Huo Tang (Nine-Herb Decoction with Notopterygium), 64

vs. Qiang Huo Sheng Shi Tang (Notopterygium Decoction to Overcome Dampness), 67, 1158

Jiu Xian San (Nine-Immortal Powder), 779

Joints. *See also* Arthritis; *Bi zheng* (painful obstruction syndrome); specific conditions

dislocation, 901

mobility, reduced/limited, 456, 1177

pain, 124, 1167, 1169, 1171

pain and swelling, 1186, 1190

range of motion, decreased/limited, 1161, 1167

swelling, burning pain, 323

swelling, inflammation and decreased mobility, 1173

swelling, inflammation and pain, 1192

Ju Ban Zhi Zhu Wan (Tangerine Peel, Pinellia, Immature Bitter Orange, and Atractylodes Macrocephala Pill), 1276

Ju Fang Zhi Bao San (Greatest Treasure Powder from the Imperial Grace Formulary), 751

Ju He (Semen Citri Reticulatae), xxiv

Ju He Pi (*Wan*), 833

Ju He Wan (Tangerine Seed Pill), 833

vs. Nuan Gan Jian (Warm the Liver Decoction), 835

vs. Tian Tai Wu Yao San (Top-Quality Lindera Powder), 835, 837

Ju Hua Cha Tiao San (Chrysanthemum Powder to be Taken with Green Tea), 976

Ju Luo (Vascular Citri Reticulatae), xxiv

Ju Pi Zhu Ru Tang (Tangerine Peel and Bamboo Shaving Decoction), 854, 855

vs. Ding Xiang Shi Di Tang (Clove and Persimmon Calyx Decoction), 853

vs. Xuan Fu Dai Zhe Shi Tang (Inula and Hematite Decoction), 853

Ju Pi Zu Ru Tang, 854

Ju Ye (Folium Citri Reticulatae), xxv

Ju Yuan Jian (Lift the Source Decoction), 548

Juan Bai (Herba Selaginellae), xxv

Juan Bi Tang (Remove Painful Obstruction Decoction), 1158

Jueyin, *1513*

headache, 467

toxic heat, 408

yang deficiency with cold, 491

Jun Chang Tang, 178

Jun Chen Zuo Shi (Chief, Deputy, Assistant, Envoy), 14

Jun yao (chief herb), 14, *1513*

Kampo Medicine, 1227

Kan Lu Hsiao Tu Tan, 1096

Kan Lu Yin, 401

Kan Mai Ta Tsao Tang, 731

Kan Tsao Hsiao Mai Ta Tsao Tang, 731

Ke Ken Huang Chin Huang Lien Tang, 295

Ke Xue Fang (Coughing of Blood Formula), 943

Keratitis, 101, 381

Keratosis, 43

Keratosis plantaris, 43

Keshan disease, **1133**

Kidney (TCM), *1514*. *See also* specific disorders

deficiency and cold, 781, 784

deficiency with phlegm in the Lung, 842

disharmony with Heart, 714, 797

Heart and Kidney deficiencies, 792

jing (essence) and Liver blood deficiencies, 691

Liver and Kidney yin deficiencies, 627, 654, 643, 657

yang deficiency, 493, 668, 673

yang deficiency with diminished *ming men* (life gate) fire, 678

yang deficiency with water accumulation, 1135, 1138

yin and Heart blood deficiencies, 726

yin and yang deficiencies with fire, 684

yin deficiency, 644, 1036

yin, marrow and *jing* (essence) deficiencies, 645

yin, yang, blood and *jing* (essence) deficiencies, 687

yin-deficient fire, 637, 649

Kidney disorders (WM). *See also* Renal-; Nephro-; specific disorders

compromised function, 461

function, effect on, 461

overview, 203, 318, 517, 518, 870, 1065, 1066

polycystic, 461, 684

tuberculosis, 412, 461

Kidney Fixity Decoction, 1133, 1134

Kidney Qi Formula from the Golden Cabinet, 668

Kidney Qi Pill, 668, 672

Kidney Qi Pill from Formulas that Aid the Living, 675

Kidney Qi Pill from the Golden Cabinet, 668

Knee Pain Formula One, 1165

Knee Pain Formula Two, 1165

Chinese Herbal Formulas and Applications

Index

Knees
  arthroncus, 1370
  atrophy and weakness, 649
  atrophy of the bones and tendons, 651
  overview, 513, 514
  red, swollen and painful, 1188
  soreness, 637
  soreness and pain, 1161
  soreness and weakness
    Kidney yin and *jing* (essence) deficiencies, 645
    Liver and Kidney deficiencies, 690
    Liver and Kidney yin deficiencies, 627, 640, 654
    yin, yang, blood and *jing* (essence) deficiencies, 687
  synovitis, **501**
  weak
    Kidney yang deficiency, 678
    Kidney yin deficiency, 644
    qi and blood deficiencies, 1182
Ko Ken Tang, 59
Kong Xian Dan (Control Mucus Special Pill), 182
Kou Teng San, 996
Kou Zong-Shi, 12, 792
Ku Shen (Radix Sophorae Flavescentis), xxv
Ku Xing Ren (Semen Armeniacae Amarum), xxvi
Kua Lou Chih Shih Tang, 1233
Kudzu Decoction, 59
Kudzu, Coptis, and Scutellaria Decoction, 295
Kudzu, Pogostemon, and Peony Decoction, 298
Kuei Chih Fu Ling Wan, 928
Kuei Chih Shao Yao Chih Mu Tang, 1186
Kuei Chih Tang, 51
Kuei Pi Tang, 583
Kun Bu (Thallus Eckloniae), xxv
Kyphosis, 963, 981, 983, *1417*
Labor, difficult, 621, 623
Lacrimal gland, inflammation, 295
Lactation
  difficulties, **250**
  insufficient, **581**, 625
Lamivudine, 214
Lan Shi Mi Cang (Secrets from the Orchid Chamber), 393, 420, 567, 1191, **1261**, 1280, 1358
Lan Tai Gui Fan (Guidelines from Lan-Tai), 1179
Lao lin (fatigue dysuria), *1514*
Lapis Micae and Chloriti Pill to Vaporize Phlegm, 1238
Largactil. *See* Chlorpromazine
Large Intestine (TCM), *1514*
Large Intestine disorders (WM). *See* Intestinal disorders; specific disorders
Large spoon, *1514*
Large-Leaf Gentian and Turtle Shell Powder, 416
Laryngitis, *1417*
  chronic, 828, **1034**
  heat and fire in the upper and middle *jiaos*, 351
  heat-phlegm, 1226
  Lung heat, 388
  voice, loss of, **1031**
Laryngopharyngitis, **1097**
Laryngopharynx, swelling of, 393
Lassitude
  damp accumulation, 1068
  damp-phlegm, 1209
  Heart and Kidney deficiencies, 725
  Heart and Spleen deficiencies, 583
  Kidney yin and yang deficiencies with fire, 684
  overview, 434, 512, 1206

qi and blood deficiencies, 615
qi deficiency, 522
qi, blood and yang deficiencies, 609
shaoyin syndrome, 486
summer-heat damaging qi and body fluids, 446
yang deficiency, 459
Laxative effect, 175
LDL (low-density lipoprotein). *See* Cholesterols
Lead poisoning, **155**
Lead Special Pill, 492
Lead to Symmetry Formula, 977
Lead to Symmetry Powder, 977
Learning impairment, colchicine-induced, 598
Left Metal Pill, 389
Leg *qi*, *1394*, *1514*
  dampness and cold, 1183
  Kidney yang deficiency, 668, 673
  overview, 1064
  with weakness and difficulty walking, 991
Legs
  abscesses, 1347
  aches and pain, 1175
  atrophy and weakness, 649
  edema, 1118
  numbness, 1190
  numbness and pain, 1172, 1182
  pain, 494, 893, 915
    severe, 1171
  paralysis, 694
  restless, **502**, **601**, **659**, 1092, **1137**, **1184**
  swelling, heaviness, weakness, numbness, coldness and pain, 1184
  weakness, 668, 673
  weakness and atrophy, 1188
  weakness and paralysis, 1182
  weakness and soreness, 651
Lei Bian Zhu Shi Ji Yan Yi Fang (Effective Medical Formulas Arranged by Category by Doctor Zhu), 1183
Lei Gong, 3
Lei Zheng Huo Ren Shu (Book to Safeguard Life Arranged According to Pattern), 113, 324
Leiomyoma, 931
  uterine, **602**, **930**, 937
Leng Xiao Wan (Cold Wheezing Pill), 1243
Leptospirosis, **339**, 1096
Lethargy
  damp-cold in the Spleen and Stomach, 840
  damp-warmth, 1096
  Kidney yang deficiency, 678
  overview, 455
  summer-heat with damaged qi and body fluids, 446, 554
  summer-heat with exterior cold and interior dampness, 436
  yin and qi deficiencies, 776
Leucopenia. *See* Leukopenia
Leukemia, *1418*
  acute, **373**
  granulocytic, *1418*
  heat and toxins, 363
  leukocytic, 333
  lymphocytic, *1418*
  myelogenous, 379
  yin-deficient heat, **419**
Leukocytes, 524
Leukopenia, *1418*
  5-fluorouracil-induced, 617
  chemotherapy-induced, 582

1575

Index

cyclophosphamide-induced, 548, 617
deficiency and cold of the middle *jiao*, **478**
qi and blood deficiencies, **581**
qi, yin and body fluid deficiencies, **556**
radiation-induced, 582
Spleen and Stomach qi deficiencies, **546**
Leukorrhea, *1418*
  acute or chronic, 810
  blood deficiency, 594
  blood deficiency and heat, 576
  cold accumulation and qi stagnation, 836
  damp-cold in the Spleen and Stomach, 840
  damp-heat, 1188
  damp-heat in the lower *jiao*, 368, 810
  deficiency and cold, 795, 805, 923
  gonorrheal, 810
  odorless, clear, and thin, 807
  overview, 770
  Spleen and Stomach qi deficiencies, 542
  Spleen deficiency, 809
  Spleen qi deficiency and Liver qi stagnation, **808**
  toxic heat, 408
  trichomonal, 810
  with white or light yellow discharge, 807
  with white, yellow, or red discharge, 810
  yang deficiency with water accumulation, 1135
Levaquin. *See* Levofloxacin
Levels of Medicine, 640, 642
Levofloxacin, 530, 613
LH. *See* Luteinizing hormone
Li (measure of weight), 22, 1439
Li Dong-Heng, 355, 551, **1261**, 1481, 1483, 1484. *See also* Li Gao
Li feng (dysenteric wind), 1182, *1514*
Li Gao, 7, 177, 355, 393, 420, 448, 492, 542, 551, 554, 567, 580,
  710, 835, 840, 858, 897, 1156, 1191, 1250, **1261**, 1270, 1274,
  1275, 1280, 1358, 1481, 1483, 1484. *See also* Li Dong-Heng
Li qi (perverse qi), 199
Li Shi-Zhen, **817**, 1481, 1483, 1484
Li Ting, 802, 1276, 1361
Li Zhong An Hui Tang (Regulate the Middle and Calm
  Roundworms Decoction), 1295
Li Zhong Hua Tan Wan (Regulate the Middle and Transform
  Phlegm Pill), 462
Li Zhong Tang (Regulate the Middle Decoction), 462
Li Zhong Wan (Regulate the Middle Pill), 459
  vs. Fu Zi Li Zhong Wan (Prepared Aconite Pill to Regulate the
    Middle), 465
  vs. Si Jun Zi Tang (Four-Gentlemen Decoction), 462, 526
  vs. Wu Zhu Yu Tang (Evodia Decoction), 470
  vs. Xiao Jian Zhong Tang (Minor Construct the Middle
    Decoction), 474
Lian Ke San, 351
Lian Mei An Hui Tang (Picrorhiza and Mume Decoction to
  Calm Roundworms), 1295
Lian Po Yin (Coptis and Magnolia Bark Decoction), 1099
  vs. Can Shi Tang (Silkworm Droppings Decoction), 1102
Lian Qiao Bai Du San (Forsythia Powder to Overcome
  Pathogenic Influences), 1331
Lian Qiao Jie Du Tang (Forsythia Decoction to Relieve
  Toxicity), 345
Liang (measure of weight), 22, 1439
Liang Fang Yi Ye (Small Collection of Fine Formulas), 841, 903
Liang Fu Wan (Galangal and Cyperus Pill), 841
Liang Ge San (Cool the Diaphragm Powder), 351
Libido, decreased, 682. *See also* Sexual disorders
Lichen planus, oral, **375**

Licorice and Jujube Combination, 731
Licorice Combination, 589
Licorice Decoction to Drain the Epigastrium, 269
Licorice, Ginger, Poria and Atractylodes Macrocephala
  Decoction, 1133
Licorice, Wheat, and Date Decoction, 731
Licorice, Wheat, and Jujube Decoction, 731
Lien Jiao Pai Tu San, 1331
Life gate, *1515. See also* Ming men (life gate)
Life-Preserving Kidney-Qi Pill, 675
Life-Saving Renal Chi Pill, 675
Life-Taking Pill, 931
Lift the Pain Decoction, 1193
Lift the Source Decoction, 548
Ligaments, degeneration, 1166
Lightheadedness. *See* Dizziness; Vertigo
Ligusticum Chuanxiong and Atractylodes Pill, 822
Ligusticum Chuanxiong Powder to be Taken with Green Tea, 973
Ligustrum and Eclipta Combination, 654
Lily Bulb Decoction to Preserve the Metal, 1036
Lily Combination, 1036
Lily Gold-Firming Decoction (Pill), 1036
Lily Metal-Consolidation Decoction (Pill), 1036
Limbs
  cold, 784
  heaviness and pain, 1135
  weak, 604
Lin zheng (dysuria syndrome), *1394*, *1514. See also* specific
  disorders
  deficiency and cold, **1141**
  fire in the Heart and Small Intestine channels, **366**
  gao lin (cloudy dysuria), *1511*
  heat, fire and toxins in all three *jiaos*, **344**
  due to infection, **1104**
  lao lin (fatigue dysuria), *1514*
  overview, 1063
  qi lin (qi dysuria), *1517*
  re lin (heat dysuria), *1518*
  shi lin (stone dysuria), *1519*
  shi-re lin (damp-heat dysuria), *1520*
  xue lin (bloody dysuria), *1525*
Lin Zheng Zhi Nan Yi An (Case Histories from the Compass of
  Clinical Patterns), *311*
Lindera Chi-Regulating Formula, 990
Lindera Chi-Regulating Powder, 990
Lindera Formula, 990
Lindera Powder to Smooth the Flow of Qi, 990
Ling dun (separately simmered), 20
Ling Gan Wu Wei Jiang Xin Tang (Poria, Licorice, Schisandra,
  Ginger, and Asarum Decoction), 1242
Ling Gui Shu Gan Tang, 1131
Ling Gui Zhu Gan Tang (Poria, Cinnamon Twig, Atractylodes
  Macrocephala, and Licorice Decoction), 1131
  vs. Gan Cao Gan Jiang Fu Ling Bai Zhu Tang (Licorice, Ginger,
    Poria and Atractylodes Macrocephala Decoction), 1134
Ling jian (separately decocted), 20
Ling Jiao Gou Teng Tang (Antelope Horn and Uncaria
  Decoction), 993
  vs. E Jiao Ji Zi Huang Tang (Ass-Hide Gelatin and Egg Yolk
    Decoction), 1008
Ling Kuei Shu Kan Tang, 1131
Ling Shu (Magic Pivot), 3, 5
Linking channel, *1525*, *1526. See also* Yinwei (linking) channel;
  Yangwei (linking) channel
Linking Clinic, 243
Linking Decoction, 657

Index

Chinese Herbal Formulas and Applications

Linum and Rhubarb Formula, 178
Lipid biosynthesis, effect on, 285
Lipid peroxidation, 343
Lipids. *See* Cholesterols
Lipolysis, 293
Lipoproteins, elevated, 874. *See* Cholesterols
Lips
    dry, 396, 420
    painful and swollen, 393
    pale, 562
Liquid Styrax Pill, 758
Lithiasis. *See* Stones
Lithospermum and Oyster Shell Decoction, 1348
Liu Chun Tzu Tang (Wan), 527
Liu He Tang (Harmonize the Six Decoction), 1082, 1083
    vs. Huo Xiang Zheng Qi San (Agastache Powder to Rectify the
        Qi), 1081
Liu Jing Bian Zheng (Six Stages Differentiation), 311, *1514*
Liu Jun Zi Tang (Six-Gentlemen Decoction), 527
Liu Shen Wan (Six-Miracle Pill), 363
Liu Wei Di Huang Wan (Six-Ingredient Pill with Rehmannia),
    509, 627
    vs. Ba Wei Di Huang Wan (Eight-Ingredient Pill with
        Rehmannia), 635
    vs. Da Bu Yin Wan (Great Tonify the Yin Pill), 634, 650
    vs. Du Qi Wan (Capital Qi Pill), 635
    vs. Er Zhi Wan (Two-Ultimate Pill), 634
    vs. Hu Qian Wan (Hidden Tiger Pill), 634
    vs. Jin Gui Shen Qi Wan (Kidney Qi Pill from the Golden
        Cabinet), 635
    vs. Mai Wei Di Huang Wan (Ophiopogonis, Schisandra, and
        Rehmannia Pill), 634
    vs. Qi Ju Di Huang Wan (Lycium Fruit, Chrysanthemum, and
        Rehmannia Pill), 634
    vs. Shi Hu Ye Guang Wan (Dendrobium Pill for Night Vision), 634
    vs. Yi Guan Jian (Linking Decoction), 634
    vs. Yu Ye Tang (Jade Fluid Decoction), 1051
    vs. Zhi Bai Di Huang Wan (Anemarrhena, Phellodendron, and
        Rehmannia Pill), 634
    vs. Zuo Gui Wan (Restore the Left [Kidney] Pill), 634, 648
Liu Wei Gu Jing Wan (Rehmannia Six and Lotus Stamen Pill),
    791
Liu Wei Ti Huang Wan, 627
Liu Yi San (Six-to-One Powder), 441, 442
    vs. Gui Ling Gan Lu Yin (Cinnamon and Poria Sweet Dew
        Decoction), 445
Liu yin (six exogenous factors), 34, 1321, *1514*
Liu Yuan-Su, 7, **279**, 291, 441, 442, 443, 444, 693, 1481, 1483, 1484
Liu Zhou Yi Hua (Medical Dialogues from Liuzhou), 657
Liver (TCM), *1514*
    blood and Kidney *jing* (essence) deficiencies, 691
    blood deficiency with deficiency heat, 722
    blood deficiency with heat, 245
    disharmony with Spleen, 233
    excess fire in the Liver and Gallbladder, 371, 379
    fire overacting on the Stomach, 389
    heat, 243
    heat with blood deficiency, 245
    Liver and Kidney yin deficiencies, 627, 643, 654, 657
    Liver excess, 996
    Liver heat and wind rising, 993
    Liver wind rising due to yin and blood deficiencies, 1008
    Liver wind rising due to yin deficiency, 1009
    Liver yang and wind rising, 1004
    Liver yang and wind rising due to yin deficiencies, 999
    Liver yang rising, 1002

qi stagnation, 238, 247, 849
qi stagnation with blood and Spleen deficiencies, 247, 254
qi stagnation with blood deficiency, 731
qi stagnation with blood stasis, 242
qi stagnation with heat, 254, 825
qi stagnation with heat and underlying blood and Spleen
    deficiencies, 254
yang hyperactivity with yin and blood deficiencies, 713
yin-deficient fire, 637, 649
Liver disorders (WM). *See also* Hepato- and specific disorders
    abscesses, **898**
    cancer, **659**, 935, 937, *1403*
    carcinoma, **210**, **547**
    cirrhosis
        alcohol-induced, 223
        in ascites, **1111**, 1127
        blood stagnation, 885
        damp-heat accumulation, 1270
        deficiency with dampness, 536
        due to five consumptive lifestyles, 937
        in gynecomastia, **61**
        heat formation and qi stagnation, 184
        Liver qi stagnation, **251**
        Liver qi stagnation with heat, 254
        qi and blood stagnation with damp and phlegm
            accumulation, 935
        qi deficiency with cold and dampness, 531
        qi stagnation and damp-heat accumulation, 1272
        shaoyin syndrome, **235**
        Stomach deficiency and interlocking of heat and cold, 270
        Stomach qi disharmony, 261
        taiyang and *shaoyang* syndromes, 219
        water and damp accumulation, 186
        yang deficiency, 1138
    damage, drug-induced, 214
    enzymes, elevated, 285
    fatty, 223, **286**
    fibrosis, **210**, 937, **1010**
    hemangioma, **887**
    overview, 203, 282, 318, 517, 870, 1065
    tumor, 885
Liver-Repressing Formula, 245
Lochia, retention of
    blood accumulation, 873
    blood deficiency with cold, **926**
    blood stasis, 911
    overview, 867
    postpartum, 625
Lochioschesis, 928
Lockjaw
    cold *bi zheng* (closed disorder), 759
    excess cold accumulation, 171
    overview, 963
    tetanus, 983
    wind invading the channels and collaterals, 981
Long Dan (Radix et Rhizoma Gentianae), xxv
**Long Dan Jiang Ya Pian (Gentiana Pill to Lower [Blood]
    Pressure)**, 376
**Long Dan Jie Du Tang (Gentiana Decoction to Relieve
    Toxicity)**, 376
**Long Dan Xie Gan Tang (Gentiana Decoction to Drain the
    Liver)**, 371
    vs. Dang Gui Long Hui Wan (Tangkuei, Gentiana, and Aloe
        Pill), 377
    vs. Wan Dai Tang (End Discharge Decoction), 809
    vs. Xie Qing Wan (Drain the Green Pill), 377

1577

Index

Long pulse, *1514*
Long-Bout Cough Powder, 115
Lonicera and Forsythia Formula, 92
Lophatherum, Tamarisk and Arctium Decoction, 106
Loss of qi with hemorrhage, *1514*
Loss of voice, *1418*
Lotus and Citrus Formula, 540
Lotus Seed Combination, 368
Lotus Seed Decoction to Clear the Heart, 368
Lotus Seed Drink, 368
Lotus Stamen Formula, 789
Loud Sound Powder for a Broken Flute, 388
Loud Sound Resembling Broken Bamboo Powder, 388
Low back. *See* Back; Lumbago
Low Back Pain Formula One, 1164
Low Back Pain Formula Two, 1164
Lower *jiao*, *1514*. *See also Jiao*, lower
Lozenge, 18
Lu Jiao Jiao (Colla Cornus Cervi), xxv
Lu Jiao Shuang (Cornu Cervi Degelatinatum), xxv
Lu Xian Cao (Herba Pyrolae), xxv
Lumbago. *See also* Back, lower
  acute, **895**
  cold and dampness, 1134
  deficiency, **566**
  deficiency and cold, 795
  exterior excess with interior deficiency, 1169
  Kidney yang deficiency, **670**, 673, 678
  Kidney yang deficiency with water accumulation, 675
  Liver and Kidney deficiencies, 690
  Liver and Kidney yin deficiencies, 627
  qi and blood deficiencies, 604
  weakness and atrophy, 652
  wind-dampness with deficiency, 1159
  yin, yang, blood and *jing* (essence) deficiencies, 687
Lumps. *See also* Nodules; Masses
  posterior to the ear or on the neck, 1355
  qi, blood and phlegm stagnation, 1360
Lung (TCM), *1514*. *See also* specific disorders
  damp-phlegm, 1209
  deficiency heat, 558
  dryness with phlegm, 1240
  heat, 96, 383, 386
  heat with phlegm accumulation, 1232
  heat with yin deficiency, 1229
  heat-phlegm, 1226
  old phlegm and excess heat, 1239
  phlegm accumulation with Kidney deficiency, 842
  phlegm-heat, 1222
  qi and phlegm stagnation, 848
  qi deficiency, 560
  summer-heat, 435
  warm-dryness, 1028, 1030
  yin and qi deficiencies, 779
  yin and Spleen qi deficiencies, 1042
  yin deficiency, 1036, 1043
  yin deficiency with heat, 1039
Lung disorders (WM). *See also* Pulmonary disorders; Respiratory disorders; specific disorders
  abscesses, 1229, 1350, 1377, *1418*, *1515*
  atrophy, 558, 589, *1419*
  cancer, **1038**, **1048**, *1404*
  carcinoma, **617**
  chronic consumptive disease, 558
  cough and dyspnea, 96
  distention, *1419*

overview, 317, 1321
  tuberculosis, 1371, *1430*
Lung Tan Hsieh Kan Tang, 371
Lung-Clearing Decoction, 1225
Lung-Clearing Drink, 1224
Luo (connecting) point, *1515*
Luo Mei, 363, 531
Luo Tian-Yi, 416, 557, 1089
Luo Zhi-Ti, 1203
Lupus. *See* Systemic lupus erythematosus (SLE)
Luteal insufficiency, **596**
Luteal phase defects, **921**
Luteinizing hormone (LH), 224, 595, 596, 921, 929
Luteinizing hormone-releasing hormone (LHRH), 685
Lycium Formula, 681
Lycium Fruit, Chrysanthemum, and Rehmannia Pill, 640
Lycium, Chrysanthemum and Rehmannia Formula, 640
Lycium, Chrysanthemum and Rehmannia Pill, 640
Lymph
  glands, inflammation, 1360
  nodes, swollen, 243
Lymphadenitis, *1419*
  acute, simple, 1355
  damp-warmth, 1092
  heat, 243
  heat and toxins, 1342, 1349, 1364
  heat and toxins with underlying deficiencies, 1365
  mesenteric, 1379
  qi and blood deficiencies, 1367
  qi and phlegm stagnation, 1353
  with swelling and hardness, 1357
  wind, heat and toxins, 356
Lymphangitis, 363
Lymphatic effect, 605
Lymphocytes, 220, 595, 605, 669
  B-lymphocytes, 610
  T-lymphocytes, 523, 544, 555, 610, 655
Lymphoma, *1419*
Ma Fei San (Numbing and Boiling Powder), 741
Ma Hsing I Kan Tang, 43
Ma Hsing Kan Shih Tang, 96
Ma Huang Fu Tzu Hsi Hsin Tang, 132
Ma Huang Fu Zi Gan Cao Tang (Ephedra, Prepared Aconite, and Licorice Decoction), 134
Ma Huang Fu Zi Xi Xin Tang (Ephedra, Asarum, and Prepared Aconite Decoction), 132
  vs. *Zai Zao San* (Renewal Powder), 134
Ma Huang Gen (Radix et Rhizoma Ephedrae), xxv
Ma Huang Jia Zhu Tang (Ephedra Decoction plus Atractylodes), 42
  vs. *Ma Xing Yi Gan Tang* (Ephedra, Apricot Kernel, Coicis, and Licorice Decoction), 44
Ma Huang Tang (Ephedra Decoction), 39
  vs. *Gui Zhi Tang* (Cinnamon Twig Decoction), 44
  vs. *Xiao Qing Long Tang* (Minor Bluegreen Dragon Decoction), 79
Ma Huang Xing Ren Gan Cao Shi Gao Tang (Ephedra, Apricot Kernel, Licorice, and Gypsum Decoction), 96
  vs. *Da Qing Long Tang* (Major Bluegreen Dragon Decoction), 100
  vs. *Sang Ju Yin* (Mulberry Leaf and Chrysanthemum Decoction), 100
  vs. *Xie Bai San* (Drain the White Powder), 100, 385
  vs. *Yue Bi Tang* (Maidservant from Yue Decoction), 102
Ma Huang Xing Ren Yi Yi Gan Cao Tang, 43
Ma Xing Gan Shi Tang (Ephedra, Apricot Kernel, Licorice, and

1578

Chinese Herbal Formulas and Applications

Index

Gypsum Decoction), 96
Ma Xing Shi Gan Tang (Ephedra, Apricot Kernel, Gypsum, and Licorice Decoction), 96
Ma Xing Yi Gan Tang (Ephedra, Apricot Kernel, Coicis, and Licorice Decoction), 43
    vs. Ma Huang Jia Zhu Tang (Ephedra Decoction plus Atractylodes), 44
Ma Zi Ren Wan (Hemp Seed Pill), 174
    vs. Run Chang Wan (Moisten the Intestines Pill), 178
    vs. Xiao Cheng Qi Tang (Minor Order the Qi Decoction), 176
Ma Zi Run Chang Wan (Hemp Seed Pill to Moisten the Intestines), 178
Macrophages, 133, 394, 523, 528, 544, 581, 605, 610, 679
Maculae, *1419*
    excess heat and toxins, 337
    heat in the *qi* (energy) and *xue* (blood) levels, 339
    heat in the Stomach and Intestines, 160
    overview, 315
Magic Pivot, 3, 5
Magical Rhinoceros Special Pill, 335
Magnetite and Cinnabar Pill, 714
Magnolia and Ginger Formula, 1068
Magnolia and Ginger Formula Modified, 1072
Magnolia and Gypsum Combination, 122
Magnolia and Hoelen Combination, 1113
Magnolia Bark Decoction for Warming the Middle, 840
Magnolia Combination, 840
Magnolia Decoction to Clear the Lung, 122
Magnolia Flower and Gypsum Decoction, 122
Magnolia Flower Formula, 84
Magnolia Flower Powder, 84, 85
Magnolia Seven Combination, 289
Mahuang and Apricot Seed Combination, 96
Mahuang and Apricot Seed Decoction, 96
Mahuang and Asarum Decoction, 132
Mahuang and Cimicifuga Combination, 72
Mahuang and Coix Combination, 43
Mahuang and Coix Decoction, 43
Mahuang and Ginkgo Combination, 845
Mahuang and Ginseng Combination, 983
Mahuang and Magnolia Combination, 847
Mahuang and Morus Formula, 48
Mahuang and Peony Combination, 983
Mahuang and Peony Decoction, 983, 985
Mahuang Combination, 39
Mahuang Decoction, 39
Mahuang, Aconite and Asarum Combination, 132
Mahuang, Aconite and Asarum Decoction, 132
Mai Dong (Radix Ophiopogonis), xxv
Mai Jing (Pulse Classics), 453
Mai Men Dong Tang (Ophiopogonis Decoction), 1043
    vs. Bai He Gu Jin Tang (Lily Bulb Decoction to Preserve the Metal), 1038
    vs. Qing Zao Jiu Fei Tang (Eliminate Dryness and Rescue the Lung Decoction), 1046
    vs. Qiong Yu Gao (Beautiful Jade Paste), 1038
Mai Men Yang Yin Tang (Ophiopogonis Decoction to Nourish the Yin), 1045
Mai Wei Di Huang Wan (Ophiopogonis, Schisandra, and Rehmannia Pill), 642
    vs. Liu Wei Di Huang Wan (Six-Ingredient Pill with Rehmannia), 634
Mai Wei Ti Huang Wan (Ophiopogon-Flavoured Rehmannia Pill), 642
Maidservant from Yue Decoction, 101
Maidservant from Yue Decoction plus Atractylodes, 102

Major Arrest Wind Pearl, 1009
Major Blue Dragon Combination, 45
Major Bluegreen Dragon Decoction, 45
Major Bupleurum Combination, 283
Major Bupleurum Decoction, 283
Major Centre-Fortifying Decoction, 480
Major Chi-Infusing Decoction, 152
Major Chin-chiu Combination, 988
Major Construct the Middle Decoction, 480
Major Four Herb Combination, 522
Major Gentiana Macrophylla Decoction, 988
Major Invigorate the Collaterals Special Pill, 1179
Major Middle-Strengthening Decoction, 480
Major Notopterygium Decoction, 66
Major Order the Qi Decoction, 152
Major Purgative Decoction, 152
Major Rhubarb Combination, 152
Major Saposhnikovia Decoction, 1181
Major Siler Combination, 1181
Major Sinking into the Chest Decoction, 161
Major Sinking into the Chest Pill, 163
Major Six Herb Combination, 527
Major Yin-Nourishing Pill, 649
Major Zanthoxylum Combintion, 480
Malaria, *1419*, *1515*. See also Antimalarial effect
    damp accumulation, 1077
    damp and phlegm obstruction, 230
    dampness and phlegm, 232
    dampness and turbidity obstruction, 231
    shaoyang syndrome, 206, 304
    with splenomegaly, 935
Malignancy. See names and sites of specific cancers; Anticancer effect; Antineoplastic effect; Antimetastatic effect
Malnutrition
    in children, 1298, 1299
    deficiency and cold of the middle *jiao*, 471
    hookworms, 1302
    infantile, 541, 1074. See also *Gan ji* (infantile malnutrition)
    parasites, 1289, 1297, 1298, 1299
Maltosum, xxvi
Mammary
    aggregation, *1515*
    hardness, rock-like, 1375
    hyperplasia, **250**, **882**, **899**, **1354**, **1356**
    rock, *1515*
Man (fullness), 156, *1515*
Mania, *1419*
    blood accumulation in the lower *jiao*, 873
    excess heat and toxins, 337
    heat in the *ying* (nutritive) level, 333
    overview, 315
    phlegm accumulation, 1311
    re jue (heat reversal), 152
Mania and withdrawal, **830**, 1205, **1215**, 1238, 1309, *1393*, *1508*. See also *Dian kuang* (mania and withdrawal)
Manic-depressive psychosis, 1238
Mantis Egg-Case Formula, 792
Mantis Egg-Case Powder, 792
Mantis Formula, 792
Manual of Universal Lover from the Heart, 525
Marvelous Formulas for the Health of Multitudes, 845, 1334
Masses. See also Nodules; Lumps
    abdominal, 885, 889
    hypochondriac, 935
    overview, 1263, 1264
    yin deficiency with qi stagnation and blood dryness, 657

1579

Index

Mast cells, 76, 98, 133, 968
Mastadenoma, 247, **250**
Master Shen's Book for Revering Life, 222, 226, 577, 837
Mastitis, *1419*
    acute, **42**, **293**, **1327**
    early stage, 1334
    heat and toxins, 363, 1342, 1349, 1364
    with redness, swelling and pain, **375**
    suppurative, 1365
    wind-heat, 1332
    yin-type (deep-rooted), **1372**
Materia Medica, **817**
Materia Medica to Aid Yin, 931
MCTD (mixed connective tissue disease), 617
Measles, **104**, 106
    early stage, 103, 104, 105
    heat, 243
    heat, lingering or residual, 327
    interior heat and toxins, 361
    Lung heat, 96
    shaoyang syndrome, 206
    wind-cold with interior heat, 45, 295
Measures, *1439*
Medical Dialogues from Liuzhou, 657
Medical Innovations, 710, 835, 897
Medical Revelations, 69, 110, 116, 711, 1040, 1142, 1240, 1247,
    1251, 1253, 1355
Medicated Leaven Pill, 714
Medicated Leaven, Barley Sprout, Immature Bitter Orange, and
    Atractylodes Macrocephala Pill, 1275
Medicinal wine, 17
Mei qi he (plum-pit *qi*), 827, **829**, *1394*
    phlegm retention and qi stagnation, **1246**
    qi stagnation, **823**
    upper excess and lower deficiency, **844**
Meika Hosen (A Selection of Famous Physicians' Prescriptions), 810
Melancholia, **1215**
Melanoma, 209
Melasma, **1001**
Melia Toosendan Powder, 825
Melon Pedicle Powder, 1311
Melt, *1525*. *See also Yang* (melt)
Membrane source, 230, *1515*. *See also Mo yuan* (membrane
    source)
Memory. *See also* Forgetfulness; Concentration; Cognitive effect
    deteriorated, **552**
    improved, 679
Meng Shi Gun Tan Wan (Lapis Micae and Chloriti Pill to Vaporize
    Phlegm), 1238
Meniere's disease, *1420*
    cold damaging the Stomach and Spleen, **1114**
    damp-phlegm, 1209
    deficiency and cold of the Stomach, **469**
    heat-phlegm, **1215**
    Liver excess, 996
    overview, 1207
    phlegm and damp accumulation, **1111**
    phlegm retention with yang deficiency, **1132**
    qi deficiency with phlegm stagnation, 851
    qi, blood and yang deficiencies, **611**
    shaoyang syndrome, **212**
    taiyang, *yangming* and *shaoyang* disorders, 716
    wind and phlegm rising, **1248**
    yang deficiency with water accumulation, **1137**
Meningitis
    cerebrospinal, **343**

    excess heat and toxins, 338
    excess interior heat, 321, 325
    heat and fire in the upper and middle *jiaos*, 351
    heat in the *xue* (blood) level, 333
    hot *bi zheng* (closed disorder), 747
    infectious, **61**, 343
    overview, 744
    purulent, 333
    wind-cold with interior heat, 45
Menopause, *1420*. *See also* specific symptoms
    blood deficiency, **596**
    blood deficiency and heat, 576
    blood stagnation, 885
    drug-induced, 54, 256, 598, 602, 876, 931
    Heart and Spleen deficiencies, **586**
    Heart blood deficiency and Liver qi stagnation, **732**
    heat with yin and body fluid deficiencies, 412
    hot flashes, 329, 415, 630, 684, 701
    Kidney yin and yang deficiencies with fire, **685**
    Liver and Kidney deficiencies, 690
    Liver and Kidney yin deficiencies, **630**, 642
    Liver blood deficiency, 722
    Liver qi stagnation, **250**
    Liver qi stagnation with heat, **255**
    Liver yang and wind rising, **1001**
    overview, 318
    taiyang, *yangming* and *shaoyang* disorders, 716
    yin deficiency with internal fire and wind, 661
    yin-deficient fire, 637
    yin-deficient heat and fire, **421**
Menorrhagia, 950
Men's Diseases According to Fu Qing-Zhu, **767**
Menstrual disorders, 593, 598
    bleeding
        black and purplish with blood clots, 578, 889
        continuous, 802, 805
        dark red blood, 802
        deficiency and cold, 948
        excessive, 571, 654
        excessive and continuous, 950
        multiple cycles of, 889
        overview, 770, 868
        profuse, **524**, **547**, 575
        purplish-black blood clots, 802
        red or purplish black blood, 805
        scanty, 578
    overview, 515, 771
    pain
        acute, **602**
        blood deficiency, **564**
        blood stagnation, 889
        Liver qi stagnation, **249**
        qi and blood deficiencies, 619
        qi and blood stagnation, 826
    pain and cramps, 254, 484
Menstruation
    delayed, *1420*
        deficiency and injury, 562
        qi and blood stagnation, 578
    early, *1420*
        blood deficiency and blood stagnation, 571
        Spleen deficiency, 584
    irregular, *1420*
        with abdominal pain, 253
        accumulations in the interior, 302
        blood accumulation in the lower *jiao*, 873

Index

blood and yin deficiencies, 593
blood deficiency, 562, **565**, 594
blood deficiency and blood stagnation, 571
blood stagnation/stasis, 889, 911, 928, 932, 933
deficiency and cold, 919, 923
deficiency and damage, 950
Kidney yin deficiency with deficiency heat, **803**
Liver qi stagnation, 238, **250**
with profuse bleeding, 575
qi and blood deficiencies, 604, 616
qi and blood stagnation, 578
overview, 513, 819
prolonged, *1420*
Mental disorders, 203, 708. *See also* specific diseases
Mental instability, 726
Meridians-Warming Decoction, 919
Merry Life Powder, 247
Metabolic disorders. *See* specific diseases; Metabolic effect
Metabolic effect, 293, 343, 629, 655, 718
Metal, *1515*
Metal Lock Pill to Stabilize the Essence, 789
Methicillin-resistant *Staphylococcus aureus* (MRSA), **546**
Methylprednisolone, 209
Metrorrhagia, 770
Metrypertrophia, **926**
Mi Lu Jiao (Cornu Elaphuri), xxv
Mi Lu Rong (Cornu Elaphuri Pantotrichum), xxv
Mian Ma Guan Zhong (Rhizoma Dryopteridis Crassirhizomatis), xxiv
Miao Xi-Yong, 106, 1278
Miasma, 1077
Microadenoma, pituitary, 674
Micturition syncope, **617**
Middle *jiao*, *1515*. *See also* Jiao, middle
Middle-Heartening Decoction, 1373
Middle-Reinforcing and Qi-Benefiting Decoction, 542
Migraine, *1420*
blood deficiency and blood stagnation, 571
deficiency, **975**
deficiency and cold of the Stomach, 467
exterior wind with qi deficiency, 984
fire in the Liver and Gallbladder, **373**
Liver excess, 996
old phlegm and excess heat, 1238
qi stagnation, **824**
shaoyang syndrome, **212**
stubborn, **979**
wind and phlegm rising, 1247
wind, cold and dampness with interior heat, 64
wind-heat with interior heat, **293**
Military fire, 19
Ming men (life gate), 676, 678, *1515*
**Ming Mu Di Huang Wan (Improve Vision Pill with
Rehmannia)**, 633
vs. Xi Gan Ming Mu San (Wash the Liver and Brighten the
Eyes Powder), 382
Ming Yi Za Zhu (Miscellaneous Books of Ming Medicine), 462
Ming Yi Zhi Zhang (Displays of Enlightened Physicians), 1112
Minor Arrest Wind Pearl, 1011
Minor Blue Dragon Combination, 74
Minor Blue Dragon Decoction, 74
Minor Bluegreen Dragon Decoction, 74
Minor Bluegreen Dragon Decoction plus Gypsum, 78
Minor Bupleurum Combination, 206
Minor Bupleurum Decoction, 206
Minor Centre-Fortifying Decoction, 471
Minor Chest-Congestion Decoction, 1235

Minor Cinnamon and Peony Combination, 471
Minor Construct the Middle Decoction, 471
Minor Gold Special Pill, 1374
Minor Invigorate the Collaterals Special Pill, 1177
Minor Middle-Strengthening Decoction, 471
Minor Order the Qi Decoction, 158
Minor Pinellia and Hoelen Combination, 1220
Minor Pinellia and Poria Decoction, 1220
Minor Pinellia plus Hoelen Decoction, 1220
Minor Prolong Life Decoction, 983, 985
Minor Purgative Decoction, 158
Minor Qi-Infusing Decoction, 158
Minor Rhubarb Combination, 158
Minor Sinking into the Chest Decoction, 1235
Minor Trichosanthes Combination, 1235
Minor Trichosanthes Decoction, 1235
Miraculous Book of Ten Remedies, 939
Miraculous Powder for Supporting the Interior, 1347
Miscarriage. *See also* Pregnancy
autoimmunity-related, **224**
habitual, **596**, 623
history of, **631**
prevention of, **606**, **620**, 621, **656**, 951
qi and blood deficiencies, 619
recurrent, **224**, 542
Miscellaneous Books of Ming Medicine, 462
Mitomycin, 548, 612
Mixed connective tissue disease (MCTD), 617
Mo Han Lian (Herba Ecliptae), xxiv
Mo yuan (membrane source), 230, *1515*
Mobile painful obstruction, 1153, *1524*. *See also Xing bi* (mobile
painful obstruction); *Bi zheng* (painful obstruction syndrome)
Moderate pulse, *1515*
Modified Calm the Stomach Powder, 1072
Modified Merry Life Powder, 254
Modified Minor Bluegreen Dragon Decoction, 78
Modified Order the Qi Decoction, 156
Modified Polygonatum Odoratum Decoction, 137
Modified Restore the Pulse Decoction, 591
Moisten the Intestines Pill, 177, 178
Moistening, *1518*. *See also Run* (moisten)
Mood swings, 684. *See also* Emotional disorders
Moonlight Pill, 1040
Morning sickness. *See also* Pregnancy
deficiency and cold of the Stomach, 467
overview, 515
phlegm stagnation and water accumulation, **1221**
qi deficiency with cold and dampness, **533**
qi deficiency with dampness and phlegm, **529**
qi deficiency with phlegm stagnation, **852**
qi flow, reversed, 854
shaoyang syndrome, **213**
Stomach qi disharmony, **264**
upper excess and lower deficiency, **844**
yin and body fluid damage, **1056**
yin deficiency, **1044**
Morphine, 483
Morpholinosydnonimine, 170
Morus and Chrysanthemum Combination, 89
Morus and Lycium Formula, 383
Morus and Platycodon Formula, 115
Morus Leaves and Chrysanthemum Drink, 89
Mosla Powder, 436
Mosla Three Decoction, 438
Mother of Pearl Pill, 712
Motilin, 262

INDEX

1581

Index

Motion sickness, 270, *1420*. *See also* Nausea; Vomiting; Antiemetic effect
Motor dysfunction, 1131
Moutan and Gardenia Rambling Powder, 254
Mouth disorders, 318. *See also* specific disorders
 deviated
  external wind, 977, 988
  Liver yang and wind rising, 999
  overview, 963, 964
  phlegm and heat rising, 1251
  post-stroke, 906, 984
 dry
  fire in the Spleen and Stomach, 396
  heat and toxins, 291
  heat, fire and toxins in all three *jiaos*, 341
  heat, lingering or residual, 327
  Liver blood deficiency, 722
  Lung yin deficiency, 1043
  overview, 513, 1021, 1022
  Stomach heat, **326**, 398
  warm-dryness, 1030
  yin deficiency, **1044**
  yin deficiency with qi stagnation and blood dryness, 657
  yin-deficient fire, 422
  yin-deficient heat, 627, 1052
  yin-deficient heat and fire, 420
 swelling and soreness, 160
 taste, bitter
  chronic gastritis, **529**
  damp-heat, 406
  fire in the Liver and Gallbladder, 371
  Gallbladder and Stomach disharmony, 1214
  Gallbladder damp-heat, 228
  heat and toxins, 291
  Liver fire overacting on the Stomach, 389
  Liver qi stagnation, 825
  overview, 201, 316
  shaoyang syndrome, 206
  shaoyang syndrome with phlegm stagnation, 226
  shaoyang syndrome with water accumulation, 222
 taste, bland, 455
 taste, decreased sense of, 1068
 ulcerations
  damp-heat in all three *jiaos*, 359
  fire in the Heart channel, 365
  fire in the Spleen and Stomach, 396
  heat and fire, 347
  heat and fire in the upper and middle *jiaos*, 351
Movement channel, *1525, 1526*. *See also Yinqiao* (movement) channel; *Yangqiao* (movement) channel
Moxa, 18, 1287
MRSA (methicillin-resistant *Staphylococcus aureus*), **546**
Mu (collecting) point, *1515*
Mu Fang Chi Tang, 1125
Mu Fang Ji (Radix Cocculi Trilobi), xxv
***Mu Fang Ji Tang* (Cocculus Decoction)**, 1125
Mu Hu Die (Semen Oroxyli), xxiv
***Mu Li San* (Oyster Shell Powder)**, 776
 vs. Dang Gui Liu Huang Tang (Tangkuei and Six-Yellow Decoction), 421, 778
 vs. Yu Ping Feng San (Jade Windscreen Powder), 777
***Mu Xiang Bing Lang Wan* (Aucklandia and Betel Nut Pill)**, 1272
 vs. Zhi Shi Dao Zhi Wan (Immature Bitter Orange Pill to Guide Out Stagnation), 1273
Mucositis, drug-induced, 345
Mugwort and Cyperus Combination, 923

Mugwort and Cyperus Pill for Warming the Womb, 923
Mulberry and Chrysanthemum Decoction, 89
Mulberry Leaf and Apricot Kernel Decoction, 1027
Mulberry Leaf and Chrysanthemum Decoction, 89
Mulberry Leaf and Sesame Seed Pill, 656
Mulberry Twig, Gypsum, and Anemarrhena Decoction, 1187
Multiple neuritis, **647**, 1124
Mume Formula, 1292
Mume Pill, 1292
Mumps, 367, *1516*
Muscles. *See also* specific disorders
 aches and pain, 64, 1219
 atrophy
  damp-heat, 1190
  post-stroke, 988
  severe, 651
  wind, dampness and heat, 1186
  yin and yang deficiencies, **652**
 numbness, 1167
 pain, 323, 1169, 1171
 paralysis, 500
 spasms and contraction, 245
 spasms and cramps, 600, 1177
 stiffness, 59
 tension, 55
 wasting, 1042, 1264
Musculoskeletal disorders, 1155, 1195. *See also* specific locations and disorders
Musculoskeletal effect, 732
Musculoskeletal injuries, 897
Mutamycin. *See* Mitomycin
Myalgia, paclitaxel-induced, 602
Myasthenia gravis, 547, 584, **790**, *1420*
Mycobacterium tuberculosis, 53
Myelanalosis, **695**
Myelitis, **1340**
 acute, 906
 hypertrophic, 494, **497**, **680**
Myelosuppression
 carboplatin-induced, 612
 cisplatin-induced, 612
Myocardial infarction, 555, *1421*
Myocarditis
 qi and yin deficiencies, **556**
 viral, **94**, 556, 591, 727, **1221**
  acute, **357**
 water accumulation, 1124
 yin-deficient heat and fire, 420
Myomas, uterine, 597, **930**
Myrrh and Aconite Formula, 1177
Mysterious Decoction, 847
Nails
 dry and dull, 513
 pale, 562
 spoon-shaped, 597
***Nao Wei Kang Wan* (Benefit Brain Atrophy Pill)**, 909
Nasal disorders, 36
 congestion
  exterior cool-dryness, 1025
  exterior-deficient, wind-cold, 51
  wind, cold and dampness with qi deficiency, 124
 discharge
  clear, white, 84
  sticky, yellow, 86
  thick, sticky, yellow, 122
  thick, yellow, 83

1582

Index

obstruction
damp-heat, 86
Lung heat, 122
wind, 83, 973
wind, cold and dampness with qi deficiency, 124
wind-cold, 72, 84
wind-cold attacking the Lung, 48
wind-cold with interior phlegm, 128
polyps, **976**
Nasosinusitis, **99**, **1249**. *See also* Rhinitis; Sinusitis
Natrii Sulfas Exsiccatus, xxvi
Natural killer cells, 60, 203, 209, 523, 528, 544, 546, 610, 616, 774
Nausea, *1421*. *See also* Vomiting; Antiemetic effect
alcohol intoxication, 1085
cancer of the gastrointestinal tract, **469**
chemotherapy-induced, 855
damp accumulation, 1068, 1072, 1082
damp-heat, 1085
dampness and phlegm, 1077, 1209
damp-phlegm, 1209
deficiency and cold, 463
deficiency and cold with qi stagnation, 484
deficiency with accumulation of cold, **469**
drug-induced, 1112
food stagnation, 1266
gastrointestinal infection, 761
heat in the chest and cold in the Stomach, 271
heat, lingering or residual, 327
heat-phlegm, 1214
Liver fire overacting on the Stomach, 389
motion sickness, 270
neurogenic, 854
opioid-induced, 159
overview, 202, 455, 819, 820, 1063, 1064, 1205, 1206, 1263
with pain, 1212
phlegm stagnation and water accumulation, 1220
postpartum, 625
post-surgical, 854
during pregnancy, 213, 264, 529, 533, 621, 844, 852, 853, 1044, 1056, 1221, *1433*
qi deficiency with dampness and phlegm, 527
qi flow, reversed, 854
qi stagnation, 822
roundworms, 1292
Spleen and Stomach deficiencies, 541
Spleen and Stomach disharmony, 1074
Stomach yin deficiency, 1043
stubborn, **1044**
summer-heat with exterior cold and interior dampness, 436
with vomiting, **545**, **852**, **857**
wind and phlegm rising, 1247
Neck
abscesses and swellings, 1332
pain, **61**, 1159, **1160**, **1163**
and shoulder pain, **61**, **501**
and shoulder stiffness, 59
stiffness, 55
exterior-excess, wind-cold, 39
wind, cold and dampness with interior heat, 64
wind, cold and dampness with qi deficiency, 124
wind-cold, 48, 59
Neck Formula One, 62
Neck Formula Two, 62
Nei Bu Huang Qi Tang (**Tonify the Interior Decoction with Astragalus**), 1369

Nei Jing (Inner Classic), 3. *See also Huang Di Nei Jing* (Yellow Emperor's Inner Classic)
Nei Ke Zhai Yao (Summary of Internal Medicine), 254, 256
Nei Wai Shang Bian Huo Lun (Clarifying Doubts about Injury from Internal and External Causes), 554, 580, 840, 858, 1156, **1261**, 1270, 1274, 1275
Neoplasm. *See* names and sites of specific cancers; Anticancer effect; Antineoplastic effect; Antimetastatic effect
Nephritic edema, 1121
Nephritis
acute
in children, **1114**
damp-heat, **1105**
exterior-excess, wind-cold, 39
heat and fire in the upper and middle *jiaos*, 351
phlegm and damp accumulation, **1111**
wind with water accumulation, 101
wind-cold with interior heat, **47**
wind-cold with water accumulation, 74
acute or chronic, 181, **211**
chronic
blood deficiency, 594
damp accumulation, 1121
exterior wind with interior qi deficiency, 1118
Heart and Kidney deficiencies, 793
with hypertension and proteinuria, **630**
Kidney yang deficiency, 678
Kidney yang deficiency with water accumulation, 675
Liver and Kidney yin deficiencies with heat, **655**
Liver excess, 996
phlegm retention with yang deficiency, 1131
with proteinuria and hematuria, **566**
qi deficiency and blood stagnation, **909**
qi stagnation and damp-heat accumulation, 1272
water accumulation, 1129
yang deficiency, 1138
yin-deficient fire, 423
damp-heat, 1090, 1106
edema, 101, 1125, 1129, **1136**
fire in the Liver and Gallbladder, 371
Heart fire with damp-heat in the lower *jiao*, 368
heat and toxins, 338, 363
heat, fire and toxins in all three *jiaos*, 341
with hypertension and proteinuria, 630
Kidney yang deficiency, 668, 673
Kidney yin and yang deficiencies with fire, 684
overview, 771
qi and blood deficiencies, **617**
qi deficiency with dampness, **538**
proteinuria and hematuria, **566**
taiyang and *shaoyang* syndromes, 219
water and heat, interlocked, 1115
water stagnation, 1127
wei (defensive) *qi* deficiency, **775**
wind-dampness, 1173
yin-deficient heat and fire, 420
Nephrolithiasis, 368, **442**. *See also* Stones
Nephropathy
in children, **685**
deficiency and cold, 459
diabetic, **224**, 461, 929, 1214
heat-phlegm, 1214
shaoyang syndrome with water accumulation, 222, **223**
Nephroprotective effect, 170, 223, 629, 673, 774, 929, 1111, 1116, 1136
Nephroptosis, **545**

1583

Index

Nephrosclerosis, 668, 673, 1129
Nephrotic syndrome, *1421*
    deficiency and cold, 1140
    edema and proteinuria, **631**
    Kidney yang deficiency with water accumulation, **676**
    Kidney yin deficiency, **369**
    severe, **1133**
    steroid-dependent, **224**
    steroids, unresponsive to, **679**
    yin-deficient fire, **638**
Nephrotoxicity, cis-diamminedichloroplatinum-induced, 612
Nerve
    atrophy and degeneration, 651
    numbness and paralysis, **976**
Nervousness. *See also* Anxiety; Stress
    blood deficiency with heat, 245
    Kidney yin and yang deficiencies with fire, 684
    qi stagnation, 828
    taiyang, *yangming* and *shaoyang* disorders, 716
Neuralgia
    accumulations in the interior, 302
    damp and phlegm, 1195
    damp-heat, 1192
    exterior excess with interior deficiency, 1169
    gastric, 233
    hypochondriac, 657
    intercostal, 233, 242, 822, 897, 1233
    post-herpetic, 571, **1329**
    trigeminal, *1430*
        accumulations in the interior, 302
        damp-heat in all three *jiaos*, 359
        deficiency and cold of the Stomach, 468
        external wind, **979**, 991
        Liver yang and wind excess, 1004
        Liver yang rising, 1002
        shaoyin with *taiyang* syndrome, 132
        Stomach heat, 393, **400**
        taiyang and *shaoyang* syndromes, **221**
        wind-cold turning into heat, 108
        yin, blood and body fluid deficiencies, **600**
    wind and heat with qi and blood deficiencies, 986
    wind, cold and dampness, 1182
    wind, cold, dampness and heat, 1172
    yin, blood and body fluid deficiencies, **601**
Neurasthenia, *1421*
    blood deficiency with heat, 246
    damp-heat in all three *jiaos*, 359
    deficiency and cold of the middle *jiao*, 471, 476
    Heart and Kidney deficiencies, **727**, 793
    Heart and Kidney disharmony, 714
    Heart and Spleen deficiencies, **585**
    Heart blood deficiency, 735
    Heart fire, 710
    headache and insomnia, **733**
    heat, 370
    heat-phlegm, 1218
    Liver and Kidney yin deficiencies, 654
    Liver blood deficiency, 722
    Liver qi stagnation, 247
    Liver qi stagnation with heat, 254
    Liver yang hyperactivity, 713
    Liver yang rising, **1006**
    qi and blood deficiencies, 580
    qi deficiency with dampness and phlegm, 527
    qi stagnation, 828
    taiyang and *shaoyang* syndromes, **221**

taiyang, *yangming* and *shaoyang* disorders, 716
Neuritis, *1422*
    chronic, 637
    damp-heat, 1192
    multiple, **647**, 1124
    optic, **332**, **573**, **607**, 627
    peripheral, **496**, **502**, **607**, **1372**
    retrobulbar, 640
Neurodermatitis
    blood deficiency and heat, 576
    damp-heat, **1190**, **1193**
    external wind with blood deficiency, **972**
    overview, 1155
Neurogenic
    headache, 661, 973
    nausea and vomiting, 854
Neuroleptics, 602
Neurologic disorders. *See* specific disorders
Neuropathy, *1421*
    diabetic, **502**, **573**, **676**
    peripheral, **41**, 500, 573
Neuroprotective effect, 997
Neurosis, *1422*
    blood deficiency with heat, 246
    damp-heat in all three *jiaos*, 359
    functional, 879
    gastric, 657, 822, 1068, 1072, 1076, 1113
    gastrointestinal, 851, 1209
    Heart blood deficiency and Liver qi stagnation, 731
    Liver excess, 996
    Liver qi stagnation, **249**
    pharyngeal, 853
    phlegm retention with yang deficiency, 1131
    qi stagnation, 823
    taiyang, *yangming* and *shaoyang* disorders, **718**
    water accumulation, 1124
    yin and yang deficiencies, 798
Neurosyphilis, 695
Neurotic palpitations, 716, 1218
Neutropenia
    chemotherapy-induced, 612
    qi, blood and yang deficiencies, 609
    radiation-induced, 612
    rifampin-induced, 613
Neutrophils, 98, 214, 576, 921
New Compilation of Time-Tested Formulas, 1344
New Significance of Patterns and Treatment in Miscellaneous
    Diseases, 1004
Newly-Augmented Mosla Decoction, 439
Newly-Augmented Yellow Dragon Decoction, 189
Newly-Formulated Tangerine Peel and Bamboo Shaving
    Decoction, 856
Ni Wei-De, 661
Nian Tong Tang (**Lift the Pain Decoction**), 1193
Nidus Vespae, xxv
Night sweat. *See* Sweating; Perspiration
Night Vision Formula, 661
Nine-Flavour Chiang-hou Decoction, 64
Nine-Herb Decoction with Notopterygium, 64
Nine-Immortal Powder, 779
Ning Sou Wan (**Quiet the Cough Pill**), 113
    vs. Dun Sou San (Long-Bout Cough Powder), 119
    vs. Zhi Sou San (Stop Coughing Powder), 119
Nitric oxide, 203, 223, 235, 528, 576, 965, 997, 998
Niu Bang Jie Ji Tang (**Arctium Decoction to Release the Muscle
    Layer**), 1332

1584

Index

Niu Huang Qing Xin Wan (**Cattle Gallstone Pill to Clear the Heart**), 748

Niu Huang Wan (**Cattle Gallstone Pill**), 746

Niu Xi (Radix Achyranthis Bidentatae), xxiv, xxv

NK cells. *See* Natural killer cells

N-nitrosomorpholine, 220

Nocturia, 668, 673, 789, *1422*

Nodules. *See also* Lumps; Masses
  abdominal, 1360
  breast, 1360
  heat and toxins, 1349
  neck, 1238, 1360
  overview, 1205
  posterior to the ear or on the neck, 1355
  with pus and discharge, 1365, 1367
  qi, blood and phlegm stagnation, 1360
  red, hot, hard and painful, 1331
  subcutaneous, 1350, 1370
  vocal cord, 1354

Norepinephrine, 60, 1119

Nose disorders, 318. *See also* specific disorders
  dry, 299, 1030
  stuffy, 83, 84, 86, 122, 1025
  suppuration, 120
  swelling, inflammation and infection, 120

Nosebleeds. *See* Bleeding; Epistaxis

Notopterigium Nine Herb Combination, 64

Notopterygium and Tuhuo Combination, 1156

Notopterygium and Turmeric Combination, 1158

Notopterygium Damp-Expelling Decoction, 1156

Notopterygium Decoction to Overcome Dampness, 1156

Notopterygium Decoction with Nine Herbs, 64

Nourish Life Pill, 1278

Nourish the Heart Decoction, 735

Nourish the Heart Pill, 729

Nourish the Kidney to Brighten the Eyes Decoction, 664

Nourish the Kidney to Unblock the Ears Decoction, 666

Nourish the Nutritive Qi Decoction, 615

Nourish the Stomach Decoction with Aucklandia and Amomum, 534

Nourish the Yin and Clear the Lung Decoction, 1033

Nourish Yin and Clear Heat Decoction, 414

Nourish Yin and Descend the Fire Decoction, 422

Nu Ke Bai Zi Ren Wan (**Platycladus Seed Pill for Females**), 592

Nuan Gan Jian (**Warm the Liver Decoction**), 838
  vs. Ju He Wan (Tangerine Seed Pill), 835
  vs. Tian Tai Wu Yao San (Top-Quality Lindera Powder), 835, 839

Numbing and Boiling Powder, 741

Numbness, *1422*
  exterior excess with interior deficiency, 1169
  extremities, 500, 1173
  legs, 1172, 1182, 1190
  muscles, 1167
  overview, 456, 963
  peripheral nerves, **976**
  qi deficiency and blood stagnation, **909**
  water accumulation, 1124
  wind, dampness and heat, 1186
  wind-dampness, 1161
  wind-dampness with deficiency, 1159

Nursing. *See* Pregnancy; Postpartum

Nutritive level, *1526. See also Ying* (nutritive) level

Nutritive qi, *1526. See also Ying* (nutritive) *qi*

Nux Prinsepiae, xxv

Obesity, *1422*

damp-warmth, 1092
  interior excess heat, 158
  shaoyang and *yangming* syndromes, 283
  wind-heat with interior heat, **293**

Obliterans, thromboangiitis, 494, **1345**, **1371**

Obstetric disorders, 516, 869. *See also* specific disorders

Obstructive bowel disease, **482**

Occult bleeding, 576

Ocular effect, 343, 382

Ocular hemorrhage, **899**

Ofloxacin, 133, 214, 225, 530

Old Rice Granary Powder, 127

Oliguria, 675, 1129

Omnipen. *See* Ampicillin

Oophoritic cyst, **250**, **891**, 928, 930, **1372**

Opacity, vitreous, **641**

Open, *1506. See also Bo* (open)

Operation, recovery from, **188**. *See also* Surgery

Ophiopogon Combination, 1043

Ophiopogon-Flavoured Rehmannia Pill, 642

Ophiopogonis Decoction, 1043

Ophiopogonis Decoction to Nourish the Yin, 1045

Ophiopogonis, Schisandra, and Rehmannia Pill, 642

Ophthalmia, allergic, 1342

Ophthalmic disorders. *See* specific disorders

Opioids, 159

Oppression. *See* specific locations

Optic
  nerve atrophy, **252**, **573**, 640
  neuritis, **573**, 627
    acute, **332**
    orbital, **607**

Orchitis
  acute, **374**
  chronic, **251**
  damp-cold, 834
  Liver qi stagnation, **240**

Order the Qi and Nourish the Nutritive Qi Decoction, 192

Ordinary Medicine, 687, 850

Organ
  hollow, *1511*
  solid, *1526*

Organ Pattern Differentiation, *1526. See also Zang fu bian zheng* (organ pattern differentiation)

Organophosphorus
  peripheral neuritis, **607**
  poisoning, 155, **1216**

Orifice-opening formulas, 743

Origins of the Medicine, 1193

Orinase. *See* Tolbutamide

Osteoarthritis, 1159, **1163**, *1422*

Osteomyelitis, **1330**, 1367, **1373**

Osteoporosis, **677**, **688**, **692**, *1422*

Osteoradionecrosis, **1329**

Otitis media, *1423*
  catarrhal, **1093**
  chronic, **478**, 479
  excess heat, fire and toxins, **344**
  fire in the Liver and Gallbladder channels, 379
  heat and toxins, 363, 1342, 1364
  pyogenic, chronic, **375**
  qi and blood deficiencies, 1367
  suppurative, **224**, 478, 553, 1365
  wind, heat and toxins in the upper body, 349
  wind-heat, 120

Ouabain, 629

INDEX

1585

Index

Ovarian
cyst, 889, 928
dysfunction, **658**
failure, **646**
Ovaries, inflammation of, 933
Ovaritis, 371
Over-acting sequence, *1516*
Overcome Pathogenic Influences Decoction, 1343
Overcome Pathogenic Influences Powder, 124
Overdose. *See also* individual formulas; Poisoning
drug, 161
Overweight, 824. *See also* Obesity
Ovulation, 595
Ovulatory effect, 595
Oxyuriasis (pinworms), 1289, 1301
Oyster Shell Powder, 776
Pa Chen Tang (Wan), 604
Pa Cheng San, 1103
Pa Wei Tai Hsia Fang, 810
Pa Wei Ti Huang Wan, 672
Paclitaxel, 602
Pai Ho Ku Chin Tang (Wan), 1036
Pai Hu Chia Jen Shen Tang, 325
Pai Hu Tang, 321
Pai Nong San (Drain the Pus Powder), 1364
Pai Nung San, 1364
Pain. *See also* Analgesic effect; Antinociceptive effect; specific
locations and diseases for differential diagnosis
abdominal, *1399*
body, **495**, 893, 1175
bones and tendons, 1188
cancer, **496**, **529**, **1373**
chest, *1405*
chest, abdominal and hypochondriac, 825
chest, epigastric and hypochondriac, 657
cold and blood stagnation, 913
epigastric, 917, *1411*
extremities, 1173, 1177
gastric, **211**
gastric and abdominal, **601**
heel, **581**, **601**, **632**, **915**
hypochondriac, *1415*
with inflammation, *1373*
intercostal, 242
joints, 1167, 1169, 1186
legs, 1182
lower back, *1418*
lower back and knees, 1161
lower back and legs, **895**
migratory, 1177
muscles, 64, 1169
muscles and joints, 1167, 1171
neck, **1160**, **1163**
neck and shoulder, **61**, **501**
overview, 149, 456, 457, 867, 869, 963, 965, 1063, 1153, 1154,
1155, 1263
qi and blood stagnation, 893, 897, 901
severe, 897, 1171
shoulder and back, 1156
spinal cord, 695
stomach, **264**
testicular, 53
trunk, 1169
waist, hips, legs, and feet, 494
wind, cold and dampness with interior heat, 64
wind-dampness with deficiency, 1159

wrist, forearm, elbow, and shoulder, 1195
Painful obstruction of the chest, **133**, 831, 832, **899**, *1395*, *1524*.
See also Xiong bi (painful obstruction of the chest)
Painful obstruction of the throat, 1309, 1313, *1512*. *See also Hou
bi* (painful obstruction of the throat)
Painful obstruction syndrome, 501, 894, 915, 1153, **1164**, **1193**,
1393, *1506*. *See also Bi zheng* (painful obstruction syndrome)
Palmaris, 43
Palmoplantar pustulosis, 576
Palms, warm/heat sensations, 627, 1036
Palpitations, *1423*
blood deficiency, 562, 594
deficiency and cold of the middle *jiao*, 471
Heart and Kidney deficiencies, 725
Heart and Kidney disharmony, 714
Heart and Spleen deficiencies, 583
Heart blood deficiency, 735
heat-phlegm, 1214, 1218
Kidney yin and yang deficiencies with fire, 684
Liver and Kidney yin deficiencies, 654
Liver blood deficiency, 722
Liver excess, 996
Liver yang hyperactivity, 713
Liver yang rising, 1002
neurotic, 716, 1218
overview, 513, 707, 708
phlegm retention with yang deficiency, 1131
qi and blood deficiencies, 589, 604, 616
qi, blood and yang deficiencies, 609
severe, 710, 1238
taiyang, yangming and *shaoyang* disorders, 716
water accumulation, 1124
yin and qi deficiencies, 776
Palpitations and fright, *1510*
Pan Hsia Hou Pu Tang, 827
Pan Hsia Hsieh Hsin Tang, 261
Pan Hsia Tien Ma Pai Shu Tang, 1247
Pancreatic disorders
cancer, *1404*
enzymes, 154
fibrosis, 220
overview, 203, 870
Pancreatitis, *1423*
acute, 154, 162, 210, 286, 747
blood stagnation, **881**
chronic, **221**, 840
Liver qi stagnation with blood stasis, 242
overview, 282
yang deficiency and interior cold, 481
Panic disorder, **256**, **830**
Panniculitis, **1354**
Pao (blast-fry), *1516*
Pao Chan Wu You Fang, 621
Pao Jiang (Rhizoma Zingiberis Praeparatum), xxv
Papules, *1419*
Paraesthesia, pharyngeal, **829**
Paralysis
extremities, 1182
facial
post-stroke, **908**
shaoyin with *taiyang* syndrome, **133**
wei (defensive) *qi* deficiency, 775
wind and phlegm rising, 1249
wind invading the channels and collaterals, **981**
wind-cold, **61**, **990**
xue bi (blood painful obstruction), 500

Index

zhong feng (wind stroke), **978**
  intestinal, 159
  leg, 694
  muscle, 500, 991
  overview, 965
  periodic, **631**
  peripheral nerves, **976**
  post-stroke, 908, 984, 986, 988, **1010**, 1180
  wind, cold and dampness, 1178
Paraplatin. *See* Carboplatin
Parasites, *1423*. *See also* Antiparasitic effect; individual parasites
  ancylostomiasis (hookworms), 1289
  ascariasis (roundworms), 1289
  cestodiasis (tapeworms), 1289
  in children, 1297
  intestinal, 481, 1292, 1297, 1299, 1301
  overview, 1289, 1290
  oxyuriasis (pinworms), 1289
Parkinson's disease, 829, *1423*
Parkinsonism, antipsychotic-induced, 256
Parlodel. *See* Bromocriptine
Parotitis, *1423*
  acute, 212
  acute, infectious, 1356
  chronic, suppurative, **126**
  infectious, 59, 212, 351, 357, 367, **1356**
  Lung heat, 386
  wind-heat, 92
Pattern. *See* specific conditions
Pattern, Cause, Pulse, and Treatment, 856
PCOS. *See* Polycystic ovary syndrome
Peach Blossom Decoction, 787
Peach Kernel and Safflower plus Four Herbs, 571
Peach Kernel Purgative Decoction, 873
Peach Pit Decoction to Order the Qi, 873
Pediatric Apricot Kernel and Perilla Leaf Decoction, 70
Pediatrics, Sage of, 509
Pellet, 17
Pelvic inflammatory disease, *1423*
  acute, **375**, **410**, 873
  blood deficiency, **565**
  blood stagnation, **892**, **929**, 933
  chronic, 597, 719, 882, 887, 1140
  damp-heat with qi and blood stagnation, **1380**
  excess heat, fire and toxins, **344**
  fire and toxins, **1339**
  heat and toxins, **1328**
  interior cold with yang qi and blood deficiencies, **497**
  interior cold, dampness, and blood stasis, **1383**
  Liver qi stagnation, 247
  Liver qi stagnation with heat, 254
Peng Yong-Guang, 729
Penicillin, 567
Penis, cold sensations of the, 798
Pentobarbital, 214, 221
Pen-Vee-K. *See* Penicillin
Peony and Coicis Decoction, 405
Peony and Licorice Combination, 599
Peony and Licorice Decoction, 599
Peony and Magnolia Bark Decoction, 405
Peony Combination, 402
Peony Decoction, 402
Peppermint Powder, 443
Peptic ulcer disease, *1424*. *See also* Gastric ulcer, Duodenal ulcer; Antiulcer effect
  accumulations in the interior, 302

blood stagnation, **888**
  damp accumulation in the Spleen and Stomach, **1070**
  damp-cold in the Spleen and Stomach, 840
  damp-phlegm, 1209
  deficiency and cold, **464**
  deficiency and cold of the middle *jiao*, **473**, **476**
  heat and toxins, **1329**
  heat and water, interlocked, 268
  Liver qi stagnation, **240**
  Liver yang rising with phlegm accumulation, **852**
  qi deficiency, **524**
  qi stagnation, **823**
  qi stagnation with heat, **826**
  shaoyin syndrome, **236**
  Spleen yang deficiency with cold, **170**
  Stomach qi disharmony, **263**
  yin deficiency, **1045**
  yin, blood and body fluid deficiencies, **601**
Performance, athletic, **478**
Periappendicular abscess, **1380**
Periarthritis, shoulders
  blood deficiency, **566**
  blood deficiency with wind-cold, **496**
  wind, cold and dampness, 1178
  wind, dampness and heat, 1186
  wind-cold, **61**
  wind-dampness with deficiency, **1159**
  wind with interior qi deficiency, **1120**
  xue bi (blood painful obstruction), **501**
Pericarditis, *1424*
Pericardium, 747, 753, *1516*
Pericarpium Amomi Rotundus, xxiii
Pericoronitis, **1340**
Peridonitis, 942
Perilla Fruit Decoction for Directing Qi Downward, 842
Perilla Seed Combination, 842
Perilla Seed Decoction, 842
Perimenopause, with uterine leiomyomas, **602**, **930**
Period. *See* Menstruation; Amenorrhea; Dysmenorrhea; specific conditions
Periodontal disease, 395, 398, **399**
Periodontitis
  acute, **394**
  excess interior heat, 321, 325
  heat and toxins, 363
Peripheral neuritis, **502**, **607**, **1372**
Peritoneum, tuberculosis, *1431*
Peritonitis
  acute, **163**
  appendicitis, ruptured, **1380**
  taiyang and *shaoyang* syndromes, 219
  taiyang and *yangming* syndromes, 289
  tubercular, 937
  tuberculous, 1272
  water stagnation, 1127
Peritonsillar abscesses, **1328**
Peroxynitrite, 170
Persica and Carthamus Combination, 879
Persica and Rhubarb Combination, 873
Persica Qi-Infusing Decoction, 873
Persica, Carthamus and Tangkuei Decoction, 571
Persimmon Calyx Decoction, 858
Persistent, indeterminate hunger, *1516*
Perspiration, *1424*. *See also* Sweating
  abnormal, **421**
  absence of

INDEX

I

1587

Index

exterior-excess, wind-cold, 39
    wind, cold and dampness with interior heat, 64
    wind-cold, 59, 67, 72
    wind-cold with interior heat, 45
exterior-deficient, wind-cold, 51
half-body, *1511*
mild, 463
night, *1516*
    Kidney and Lung yin deficiencies, 643
    in pulmonary tuberculosis, 643
    qi and blood deficiencies, 479
overview, 34, 35, 433, 456, 769
palms and soles, *1516*
profuse, 327, 446, **775**, **1119**
shivering, *1520*
spontaneous, *1520*
    damaged qi and yin, 554
    Lung qi deficiency, 560
    qi and blood deficiencies, 479
spontaneous and night, **777**
wind with water accumulation, 101
wind-cold with interior deficiency and cold, 466
wind-cold with water accumulation, 74
wind-heat, 92
yin-deficient fire, **639**
Pertussis. *See* Whooping cough
Perverse qi, 199
Pesticide poisoning, **442**
Pestle, *1507*. *See also Chu* (pestle)
Petiolus Trachycarpi, xxvi
Peyer's patch lymphocyte, 76
Pharmacopoeia of People's Republic of China, 634, 760
Pharyngeal
    neurosis, 853
    paraesthesia, **829**
Pharyngeus, globus, **68**
Pharyngitis
    acute, **99**, **875**
    blood accumulation in the lower *jiao*, 873
    chronic, **400**, **1055**
    fire in the Liver and Gallbladder channels, 379
    heat and toxins, 363
    herpetic, **353**
    Lung and Kidney yin deficiencies, 1036
    yin-deficiency with wind-heat, 138
Pharyngo-conjunctival fever, 92
Pharyngoneurosis, **853**
Phellodendron Combination, 422
Phellodendron Decoction, 422
Phellodendron Formula, 651
Phenothiazine, 191
Pheochromocytoma, *1424*
Phlebitis, **882**, **1345**
Phlegm, *1516*
    accumulation, 302
    chest, 1233, 1235
    chest and epigastrium, 1311
    cold-phlegm, 1206
    copious, 1218
    damp accumulation, 1224
    damp-phlegm, 1206
    deficiency fire, 1230
    drooling, *1509*
    dry phlegm, 1206
    epigastrium, 1219
    heat and phlegm rising, 1251

heat-phlegm, 1206, 1218
    invisible, *1526*
    Lung, 1222, 1226
    Lung dryness, 1240
    Lung heat, 1232
    obstructing the orifices, 747
    old phlegm and excess heat, 1238
    overview, 1205, 1309
    phlegm-heat with exterior wind-cold, 845
    qi stagnation, 1245
    Stomach qi deficiency, 851
    syncope, 761
    tan (visible phlegm), 1205
    thick, sticky, 1226
    wind and phlegm rising, 1247
    wind-phlegm, 1206
    water accumulation, 1220
    yang deficiency and yin excess, 1242
    yin (invisible phlegm), 1205
Phlegm retention, 80, 1064, 1109, 1131, *1521*. *See also Tan yin*
    (phlegm retention)
Phlegm-dispelling formulas, 1205
Phosphodiesterase, 293
Photophobia, 634, 640, 661
Photosensitivity, 640
Physical injuries, 901
Physician, supreme, *1521*
Pi (distention), 156, *1516*
Pi (distention), *man* (fullness), *zao* (dryness) and *shi* (hardness),
    156
Pi Hsieh Fen Ching Yin, 1140
Pi shui (skin water), 1121, *1516*
Pi Wei Lun (Discussion of the Spleen and Stomach), 7, 177, 448,
    492, 542, 1250, **1261**
Pian ji (tablet), 18
Pian Yu Xin Shu (Text from Heart of Jade), 760
Piao (rinse), *1516*
Picrorhiza and Mume Decoction to Calm Roundworms, 1295
Picrotoxine, 997
Picryl chloride, 235
PID. *See* Pelvic inflammatory disease
Pill, 16
    extract pills, 17
    glue pills, 17
    honey pills, 17
    water pills, 17
Pill for Deafness that Is Kind to the Left [Kidney], 633
Pillow Special Pill, 729
Pimples. *See also* Acne
    heat and fire, 347
    heat and toxins, **1343**
    wind, heat and toxins in the upper body, 349
Pinch Powder, 913
Pinellia and Gastrodia Combination, 1247
Pinellia and Ginger Combination, 268
Pinellia and Licorice Combination, 269
Pinellia and Magnolia Bark Decoction, 827
Pinellia and Magnolia Combination, 827
Pinellia and Magnolia Decoction, 827
Pinellia and Scute Formula, 1222
Pinellia Atractylodes and Agastache Formula, 1075
Pinellia Combination, 261
Pinellia Decoction to Drain the Epigastrium, 261
Pinellia Heart-Draining Decoction, 261
Pinellia, Atractylodes Macrocephala, and Gastrodia Decoction,
    1247, 1250

Index

Pinellia, Gastrodia and Bighead Atractylodes Decoction, 1247
Pinellia, Gastrodia, and Atractylodes Decoction, 1247
Ping Wei San (Calm the Stomach Powder), 1068
Ping Wei San (Wan), 1068
Pinworms, 1289, 1301
Pituitary gland
    microadenoma, 674
    necrosis, 606
Placenta Pill Formula, 1253
Plain Version of Discussion of Cold-Induced Disorders, 69, 111, 137, 993, 1007, 1295
Plaque. *See* Atherosclerosis; Arteriosclerosis
Platelets. *See* specific disorders; Antiplatelet effect
Platinol. *See* Cisplatin
Platycladus Seed Pill, 592
Platycladus Seed Pill for Females, 592
Platycodon and Apricot Seed Formula, 1224
Platycodon and Chih-shih Formula, 1364
Platycodon and Fritillaria Combination, 1225
Platycodon and Fritillaria Decoction, 1225
Platycodon and Schizonepeta Formula, 116
Platycodon Combination, 1230
Platycodon Decoction, 1230
Pleural
    adhesion, **887**
    effusion, 181, *1524*. *See also Xuan yin* (pleural effusion)
Pleurisy
    effusion, 1235
    exudative, **1236**
    shaoyang syndrome with phlegm stagnation, 226
    tuberculous, **1236**
    wind-dampness, 1173
Pleuritis, **182**, 831, *1424*
Plum-pit *qi*, 823, 827, **829**, 844, 1246, *1394*, *1516*. *See also Mei he qi* (plum-pit *qi*)
PMS. *See* Premenstrual syndrome
Pneumonia, *1424*
    aspiration, 829, **1227**
    in children, **94**, **98**, **384**, **1048**
    chronic, 416
    damp-warmth, **1093**
    exterior-excess, wind-cold, 39
    heat accumulation in all three *jiaos*, 347
    heat and toxins, **1330**
    heat, lingering or residual, 327
    heat-phlegm, 1214, 1226
    interstitial, **118**, **1045**
    lobar, **323**, 325, **352**
    Lung heat with phlegm accumulation, 1232
    Lung yin deficiency with heat, 1039
    overview, 36, 744
    phlegm-heat, 1222, 1233, 1235
    shaoyang syndrome, 206, 304
    shaoyang syndrome with phlegm stagnation, 226
    summer-heat damaging qi and body fluids, **447**
    toxic heat, **409**
    viral, 338, **344**
    warm-dryness, **1031**
    wind-cold with interior heat, 45
    wind-cold with interior phlegm, 128
    wind-cold with water accumulation, **77**
    with abscesses, **1378**
    yin-deficient fire, 423
Pneumothorax, **881**, **1038**, *1424*
Po (break open), *1516*
Po (corporeal soul), *1517*

Po Bu Zi Ye Tang (Cordia Decoction), 900
Pogostemon Formula, 1079
Pogostemon Powder to Rectify the Qi, 1079
Poisoning
    acute, 271, **1312**
    alcohol, 1218, *1425*
    benzene, **498**, **586**
    carbon monoxide, **878**
    drug overdose, 161
    food, 152, 158, 160, 291, 438, 467, 1076, **1081**
    lead, **155**, **478**
    organophosphorus, **155**, **1216**
    overview, 744, 1309, 1310
    pesticide, **442**
    to induce vomiting, 1311, 1312, 1314
Polio, sequelae, 651
Poliomyelitis, 295, **908**
Polycillin. *See* Ampicillin
Polycystic kidneys, 461, 684
Polycystic ovary syndrome, **224**, 371, **375**
Polydipsia, 1050. *See also* Diabetes mellitus; *Xiao ke* (wasting and thirsting)
Polygonatum Odoratum Decoction, 138
Polygonum Pill, 692
Polyhydramnios, **1133**
Polyneuritis, **647**, **908**, 1192
Polyneuropathy, 500
Polyphagia. *See* Diabetes mellitus; *Xiao ke* (wasting and thirsting)
Polyporus Combination, 1115
Polyporus Decoction, 1115
Polyps, nasal, **976**
Polyuria. *See also* Diabetes mellitus; *Xiao ke* (wasting and thirsting)
    damp-heat, 800
    Kidney yang deficiency, 668, 673
    in *xiao ke* (wasting and thirsting) syndrome, 1050
Poria and Cuscuta Special Pill, 797
Poria Decoction, 1077, 1112
Poria Decoction to Drain Water, 1129
Poria Pill, 1219
Poria Powder with Five Herbs, 1109
Poria Rubra, xxiii
Poria, Cinnamon Twig, Atractylodes Macrocephala, and Licorice Decoction, 1131
Poria, Cinnamon, Bighead Atractylodes and Licorice Decoction, 1131
Poria, Licorice, Schisandra, Ginger, and Asarum Decoction, 1242
Post-decoction, 20, *1517*
Postnasal drip. *See* Nasal discharge
Postpartum
    abdominal pain, 911
    aches and pains, **1164**
    anemia, 562
    anuria, **191**, 542
    bleeding, 562, 580, 625, 911, 925, 951
    care/recovery, **926**, *1425*
    complications, 625
    constipation, 174
    deficiency and weakness, 474, 479
    disorders, 928
    dysuria, **546**
    emotional instability, 625
    enteritis, 408
    fever, **213**
    hemorrhage, 606
    hypochondriac fullness and distention, 625

1589

Index

illnesses, 542
infection, **213**
lactation, *1434*
lochia, retention of, *1434*
menstruation, irregular, 625
pain, 925, 1169
perspiration, 625
qi and blood deficiencies, *1434*
qi and blood stagnation, 237
recovery, **626**
sweating, 776
tinnitus, 625
weakness and anemia, 623
Potassium
excretion, 162
low, 437
Pound, *1508. See also Dao* (pound)
Powder, 16, 18
Powder that Gives the Stability of Mount Tai, 618
Powder to Take at Cock's Crow, 1183
Precepts for Physicians, 1029
Precious Mirror of Health, 416, 557, 1089
Pre-decoction, 20, *1517*
Prednisolone, 612, 617, 629
Prednisone, 671
Pregnancy, *1425. See also* Postpartum
abdominal pain, 621, 928, *1433*
abdominal pain and cramps, 594
anemia, 594
bleeding, 928, 951, *1433*
blood deficiency, 623
blood stasis in the uterus, 928
breech presentation, **565, 596, 606,** *1433*
cautions and contraindications, *1435*
cough, *1433*
diarrhea, 297
dizziness, 594
ectopic, 562, **887, 891,** 911, **916, 917, 926,** 928
edema, 594, 807, **1105,** 1121, *1433*
general weakness, 621
hypertension, **596, 659, 1111**
irritability, *1433*
lower back pain, 621
miscarriage, prevention of, *1433*
nausea and vomiting, 213, 264, 529, 533, 621, 844, 852, 853, 1044, 1056, 1221, *1433*
palpitations, 594
qi and blood deficiencies, 619, 621
restless fetus, 928, 1279, *1433*
tinnitus, 594
unstable, 594, 619, 623
urination, frequent, **546**
vertigo, 594
vomiting, pernicious, **620**
weakness, general, 621
Pregnancy Carefree Formula, 621
Pregnanediol, 596
Premature aging. *See* Aging, premature; Antiaging effect
Premature ejaculation. *See* Ejaculation, premature
Premelle, 255
Premenstrual syndrome (PMS), *1425*
blood stagnation, **930**
Liver qi stagnation, 238, 247, **249**
Liver qi stagnation with heat, 254
Liver yang and wind rising, 999
shaoyang syndrome, **213**

Spleen qi deficiency, **524**
Prepared, *1527. See also Zhi* (prepared)
Prepared Aconite Decoction, 1137
Prepared Aconite Pill to Regulate the Middle, 463
Prescriptions for Fifty-Two Kinds of Diseases, 5
Preserve Harmony Pill, 1266
Preserve Pregnancy and Care-Free Decoction, 621
Preserve the Basal Decoction, 525
Press, *1525. See also Ya* (press)
Priapism, **1094**
Priceless Chi-Regulating Formula, 1075
Principen. *See* Ampicillin
Proctitis, chronic, **538**
Profound Purpose from the Heavenly Abode, 1347
Progesterone, 595, 673, 921
Prolactin, 596, 670
Prolapse
gastric
damp accumulation, 1072
deficiency and cold, 463
deficiency and cold with qi stagnation, 484
phlegm and dampness, 1077
phlegm stagnation and water accumulation, 1220
qi and blood deficiencies, **611**
qi deficiency with qi stagnation, 1274
shaoyang and *yangming* syndromes, **286**
shaoyang syndrome, **211**
shaoyin syndrome, **488**
Spleen and Stomach deficiencies, **544**
wind-cold with interior deficiency and cold, 466
lumbar intervertebral disk, **1164, 1373**
rectal, *1427*
damp-heat with qi and blood stagnation, 1379
deficiency and cold of the Spleen and Kidney, 781
due to dysentery, chronic, **783**
qi deficiency, 542
qi stagnation and food retention, 1274
Spleen and Stomach deficiencies, **545**
renal, **545**
uterine, 375, 542, **545,** *1431*
Prolong Life Decoction, 986
Propionibacterium acnes, 344
Prostaglandins, 343, 673, 921
Prostate disorders, 518, 673
Prostatic hypertrophy
benign, **673**
blood stagnation, **887, 930**
damp-heat, 800
in geriatrics, **909, 1105**
Heart fire with damp-heat in the lower *jiao,* 368
heat and toxins, **1346**
interior cold with yang qi and blood deficiencies, **497**
Kidney yang deficiency, **670,** 673
Urination, frequent and difficult, **677**
Prostatitis, *1426*
chronic, **118,** 251, **909, 1381**
chronic non-bacterial, **632**
damp-heat, **374,** 1103
deficiency and cold, **1141**
water and heat, interlocked, 1115
Prostration, 486, 491
Proteinuria
heat in the lower *jiao,* **948**
Kidney yang deficiency, 668, 673
in nephritis, 566
in nephropathy, 224

Index

in nephrotic syndrome, 224
Prothrombin time, 929
Pruritus, 576
Pseudobulbus Cremastrae seu Pleiones, xxv
Pseudomonas aeruginosa, 93, 394, 404, 1338
  drug-resistant, 134
Psoriasis, *1426*
  blood deficiency, **567**
  blood deficiency with blood stagnation, **574**
  blood deficiency with wind-cold, **497**
  external wind, **969**
  external wind with blood deficiency, 970
  heat and toxins, **1329**
  heat in the *ying* (nutritive) level, **332**
  vulgaris, 576
Psychiatric disorders, 247, 714, **823**, **1215**. *See also* specific disorders
Psychological disorders, 708. *See also* specific disorders
Psychosis
  affective, **249**
  heat-phlegm, 1214
  manic-depressive, 1238
Psycho-somatic disorders, 253
Pu Chi Hsiao Tu Yin, 355
Pu Chung I Chi Tang (Wan), 542
Pu Huan Chin Cheng Chi San, 1075
Pu Ji Ben Shi Fang (Formulas of Universal Benefit from My Practice), 712, 944, 996
Pu Ji Fang (Formulas of Universal Benefit), 7, 127
Pu Ji Xiao Du Dan, 1096
***Pu Ji Xiao Du Yin* (Universal Benefit Decoction to Eliminate Toxin)**, 355
  vs. Xian Fang Huo Ming Yin (Sublime Formula for Sustaining Life), 358, 1331
Pu Yang Huan Wu Tang, 905
Pubescent Angelica and Loranthus Decoction, 1161
Pueraria Combination, 59
Pueraria Coptis and Scute Combination, 295
Pueraria Decoction, 59
Pueraria Flower Formula, 1084
Pueraria Flower Powder for Detoxification and Awakening, 1084
Pueraria Nasal Combination, 86
Pueraria, Scute, and Coptis Decoction, 295
Pueraria, Scutellaria and Coptis Decoction, 295
Pulmonary disorders, **76**. *See also* specific disorders; Respiratory effect
  abscesses, 1230, 1232, **1378**
  edema, 1173
  gangrene, 1230
  heart disease, **503**, **1236**
  overview, 1323
  tuberculosis
    coughing of blood, **650**
    Kidney yin deficiency, 644
    Liver fire invading the Lung, 943
    Lung heat and yin deficiency, 1229
    Lung qi deficiency, 560
    Lung yin and qi deficiencies, 779
    Lung yin deficiency with heat, 1039
    phlegm-heat, 1233
    qi and yin, damaged, 554
    qi and yin deficiencies, **1038**
    shaoyang syndrome, 206
    tidal fever, **417**
    warm-dryness, 1030
    wind-cold with water accumulation, 74

yin-deficient fire, 423
yin-deficient heat and fire, 420
Pulpitis, 363
Pulsatilla Decoction, 408
Pulsatilla Decoction plus Licorice and Ass-Hide Gelatin, 410
Pulse
  big, *1506*
  bound, 591, *1506*
  bound or intermittent, 589
  deep, *1508*
  deficient, *1508*
  drum skin, *1509*
  excess, *1509*
  faint, *1510*
  fine, *1510*
  firm, *1510*
  hidden, *1512*
  intermittent, *1513*
  knotted, 591
  long, *1514*
  moderate, *1515*
  racing, *1518*
  rapid, *1518*
  rough, *1518*
  scallion-stalk, *1518*
  scattered, *1518*
  short, *1520*
  skipping, *1520*
  slippery, *1520*
  slow, *1520*
  small, *1520*
  soggy, *1520*
  stirred, *1521*
  superficial, *1521*
  surging, *1521*
  tight, *1521*
  weak, *1522*
  wiry, *1523*
Pulse Classics, 453
Pulverizing, *1510*. *See also Fen sui* (pulverize)
Pupils, dilated, 661
Purgative effect, 874
Purple and Gold Pill for Righteous Bones, 901
Purple Gold Special Pill, 760
Purple Snow, 752
Purple Snow Pill, 752
Purpura
  allergic, *1426*
    blood stagnation, **895**
    exterior-deficient, wind-cold, **54**
    Heart and Spleen deficiencies, 584
  exterior excess with interior deficiency, 1169
  heat in the *xue* (blood) level, 333
  heat in the *ying* (nutritive) level, 331
  thrombocytopenic, *1426*
    deficiency and damage, **951**
    Heart and Spleen deficiencies, 586
    primary, **334**, **586**
    qi and blood deficiencies, **581**, **606**
    yin-deficient heat and fire, 420
Pus-Expelling Powder, 1364
Pustules, early stage, 1334
Pyelitis, 368
Pyelonephritis, *1426*
  acute, **1339**
  chronic, 412, 684, **875**, 1140, **1339**

1591

Index

damp-warmth, 1092, 1096
deficiencies with damp-heat, **369**
in women, **1105**
Pyloric
  obstruction, 851, 854
  stenosis, 484
Pyonephritis, 1103
Qi, *1517*
  accumulation, 302
  deficiency, 512, 522, *1517*
  deficiency with cold and dampness, 531
  deficiency with dampness and phlegm, 527
  gu (food) *qi*, 455, *1511*
  li qi (perverse qi), 199
  Liver qi stagnation, 238, 849
  Liver qi stagnation with blood stasis, 242
  Liver qi stagnation with heat, 825
  loss of qi with hemorrhage, *1514*
  Lung qi, reversed flow of, 74, 80, 96, 383, 558, 845, 848
  overview, 819
  qi and blood deficiencies, 580, 589, 604, *1517*
  qi and blood stagnation, 578, 893, 915, *1517*
  qi deficiency with bleeding, *1517*
  qi flow, reversed, 819
  qi stagnation, 819, 822, *1517*
  qi stagnation with phlegm retention, 1245
  qi, blood and yang deficiencies, 609
  rebellious, *1518*
  Spleen and Stomach qi deficiencies, 542
  Stomach qi, reversed flow of, 389, 852, 854, 857
  wei (defensive) *qi*, 773, *1523*
  yuan (source) *qi*, *1526*
  zheng (upright) *qi*, 984, *1527*
  zhong (central) *qi*, *1527*
  zong (essential) *qi*, *1528*
Qi (energy) level, *1517*
  damp-warmth, 1092, 1096
  summer-heat, 435
Qi Bao Mei Ran Dan (Seven-Treasure Special Pill for Beautiful Whiskers), 690
  vs. Gui Lu Er Xian Jiao (Tortoise Shell and Deer Antler Syrup), 693
Qi Bao Mei Ran Wan, 690
Qi Bo, 3
Qi collapse, *1517*
Qi dysuria, *1517*. *See also Qi lin* (qi dysuria); *Lin zheng* (dysuria syndrome)
Qi Fang (Seven Types of Formulas), 11
Qi Ju Di Huang Wan (Lycium Fruit, Chrysanthemum, and Rehmannia Pill), 640
  vs. Liu Wei Di Huang Wan (Six-Ingredient Pill with Rehmannia), 634
Qi Li San (**Seven-Thousandths of a Tael Powder**), 903
Qi lin (qi dysuria), *1517*
Qi Pi Wan (Guide the Spleen Pill), 540
Qi qing (seven emotions), 1321, *1517*
Qi stroke, *1527*. *See also Zhong qi* (qi stroke)
Qi Wei Bai Zhu San (Seven-Ingredient Powder with Atractylodes Macrocephala), 539
Qi Xiao Liang Fang (Fine Formulas with Miraculous Results), 913, 1335
Qi Xue Jin Ye Bian Zheng (Qi, Blood, and Body Fluid Differentiation), *1517*
Qi, Blood, and Body Fluid Differentiation, *1517*
Qian (measure of weight), 22, 1439
Qian Cao (Radix et Rhizoma Rubiae), xxv

Qian Jin Nei Tuo San (Drain the Interior Powder Worthy of a Thousand Gold), 1365
Qian Jin Yao Fang (Thousand Ducat Prescriptions), 983, **1151**
Qian Jin Yi Fang (Supplement to the Thousand Ducat Formulas), 6, 474, **1151**
Qian Jin Zi (Semen Euphorbiae), xxv
Qian Shu-Tian, 754
Qian Tian Jia Fang (Family Formulas of Qian Tian-Jia), 1123
Qian Yi, 7, 103, 124, 365, 376, 383, 396, **509**, 525, 539, 627, 1039, 1481, 1483, 1484
Qian Zheng San (Lead to Symmetry Powder), 977
  vs. Yu Zhen San (True Jade Powder), 983
Qiang Huo Sheng Shi Tang (Notopterygium Decoction to Overcome Dampness), 1156
  vs. Jiu Wei Qiang Huo Tang (Nine-Herb Decoction with Notopterygium), 67, 1158
Qiao He Tang (Forsythia and Mint Decoction), 1028
Qie (slice), *1518*
Qin Jiao Bie Jia San (Gentiana Macrophylla and Soft-Shelled Turtle Shell Powder), 416
  vs. Qing Gu San (Cool the Bones Powder), 415
  vs. Qing Hao Bie Jia Tang (Artemisia Annua and Soft-Shelled Turtle Shell Decoction), 415
Qin Jing-Ming, 856
Qin Yue-Ren, 704, 1482. *See also* Bian Que.
Qing Bi Tang (Clear the Nose Decoction), 86
  vs. Cang Er Zi San (Xanthium Powder), 88
  vs. Xin Yi San (Magnolia Flower Powder), 88
Qing Chang Tang (Clear the Intestines Decoction), 164, 165
Qing Chang Yin (Clear the Intestines Drink), 1381
Qing Dai Tang (Clear the Discharge Decoction), 809
  vs. Wan Dai Tang (End Discharge Decoction), 809
  vs. Yi Huang Tang (Change the Yellow [Discharge] Decoction), 809
Qing fa (clearing), **10**, 281, 314, 743, *1518*
Qing Fai Yin, 1224
Qing Fei Tang (Clear the Lung Decoction), 1225, 1227
  vs. Qing Fei Yin (Clear the Lung Drink), 1228
Qing Fei Yin (Clear the Lung Drink), 1224
  vs. Qing Fei Tang (Clear the Lung Decoction), 1228
Qing Gu San (Cool the Bones Powder), 418
  vs. Qin Jiao Bie Jia San (Gentiana Macrophylla and Soft-Shelled Turtle Shell Powder), 415
  vs. Qing Hao Bie Jia Tang (Artemisia Annua and Soft-Shelled Turtle Shell Decoction), 415
Qing Hao Bie Jia Tang (Artemisia Annua and Soft-Shelled Turtle Shell Decoction), 412
  vs. Qin Jiao Bie Jia San (Gentiana Macrophylla and Soft-Shelled Turtle Shell Powder), 415
  vs. Qing Gu San (Cool the Bones Powder), 415
  vs. Zhu Ye Shi Gao Tang (Bamboo Leaves and Gypsum Decoction), 415
Qing Liang Yin (Clearing and Cooling Decoction), 354
Qing Luo Yin (Clear the Collaterals Decoction), 435
Qing Pi Tang, 231
Qing Pi Yin (Clear the Spleen Decoction), 231
Qing Qi Hua Tan Wan (Clear the Qi and Transform Phlegm Pill), 1222
Qing Re Jie Du Tang (Clear Heat and Relieve Toxicity Decoction), 350
Qing Re Liang Xue Tang (Clear Heat and Cool the Blood Decoction), 335
Qing Re Tong Lin Tang (Clear Heat to Unblock Dysuria Decoction), 1108
Qing Shang Fang Feng Tang (Clear the Upper and Guard the Wind Decoction), 349

1592

Index

Qing Shu Yi Qi Tang (Clear Summer-Heat and Augment the Qi Decoction), 446, 448
Qing Wei San (Clear the Stomach Powder), 393
  vs. Xie Huang San (Drain the Yellow Powder), 395
  vs. Yu Nu Jian (Jade Woman Decoction), 395, 400
Qing Wei Tang (Clear the Stomach Decoction), 392
Qing Wen Bai Du Yin (Clear Epidemics and Overcome Pathogenic Influences Decoction), 337
Qing Xin Li Ge Tang (Clear the Epigastrium and Benefit the Diaphragm Decoction), 386, 387
Qing Xin Lian Zi Yin (Lotus Seed Decoction to Clear the Heart), 368
Qing Ying Tang (Clear the Nutritive Level Decoction), 330
  vs. Xi Jiao Di Huang Tang (Rhinoceros Horn and Rehmannia Decoction), 336
Qing Zao Jiu Fei Tang (Eliminate Dryness and Rescue the Lung Decoction), 1029
  vs. Bai He Gu Jin Tang (Lily Bulb Decoction to Preserve the Metal), 1032
  vs. Mai Men Dong Tang (Ophiopogonis Decoction), 1046
  vs. Sang Xing Tang (Mulberry Leaf and Apricot Kernel Decoction), 1027, 1032
  vs. Sha Shen Mai Dong Tang (Glehnia and Ophiopogonis Decoction), 1049
  vs. Xing Su San (Apricot Kernel and Perilla Leaf Powder), 1027
Qiong Gui Jiao Ai Tang, 950
Qiong Yu Gao (Beautiful Jade Paste), 1041
  vs. Bai He Gu Jin Tang (Lily Bulb Decoction to Preserve the Metal), 1038
  vs. Mai Men Dong Tang (Ophiopogonis Decoction), 1038
Qi-regulating formulas, 819
Qu Feng San (Dispel Wind Powder), 969
Qu Mai Zhi Zhu Wan (**Medicated Leaven, Barley Sprout, Immature Bitter Orange, and Atractylodes Macrocephala Pill**), 1275
Quell Wood Pill, 1302
Quenching, *1507*. See also *Cui* (quench)
Qui Zhi Fu Ling Wang, 928
Quiet the Cough Pill, 113
Racing pulse, *1518*
Radiation, 539, 548, 582, 612, *1426*. See also Radioprotective effect
Radioprotective effect, 41, 209, 515, 524, 544, 564, 577, 595, 985
Radix Achyranthis Bidentatae, xxiv, xxv
Radix Achyranthis Longifoliae, xxv
Radix Aconiti Coreani, xxiv
Radix Angelicae Sinensis, xxiv
Radix Arnebiae, xxvi
Radix Asparagi, xxv
Radix Cocculi Trilobi, xxv
Radix et Rhizoma Asari, xxvi
Radix et Rhizoma Asteris, xxvi
Radix et Rhizoma Clematidis, xxv
Radix et Rhizoma Cynanchi Atrati, xxiii
Radix et Rhizoma Cynanchi Paniculati, xxvi
Radix et Rhizoma Ephedrae, xxv
Radix et Rhizoma Gentianae, xxv
Radix et Rhizoma Ginseng, xxv
Radix et Rhizoma Glycyrrhizae, xxiv
Radix et Rhizoma Glycyrrhizae Praeparata cum Melle, xxvi
Radix et Rhizoma Nardostachydis, xxiv
Radix et Rhizoma Notoginseng, xxv
Radix et Rhizoma Rubiae, xxv
Radix et Rhizoma Salviae Miltiorrhizae, xxiv
Radix et Rhizoma seu Caulis Acanthopanacis Senticosi, xxiii
Radix et Rhizoma Sophorae Tonkinensis, xxv

Radix Kansui, xxiv
Radix Ophiopogonis, xxv
Radix Paeoniae Rubra, xxiii
Radix Puerariae Lobatae, xxiv
Radix Rehmanniae, xxv
Radix Rehmanniae Praeparata, xxv
Radix Sophorae Flavescentis, xxv
Radix Stephaniae Tetrandrae, xxiv
Raise the Sinking Decoction, 549
Raise the Yang and Disperse the Fire Decoction, 858
Rambling Powder, 247
Rapid pulse, *1518*
Rash, *1426*. See also Eczema; Itching; Urticaria
  acne, **1343**
  ampicillin-induced, 969
  damp, *1508*
  damp-heat, 1190, **1193**
  diaper, **1081**
  external wind, 967
  external wind with blood deficiency, 970
Raynaud's disease, *1427*
  qi and blood deficiencies, **617**
  qi deficiency and blood stagnation, **908**
  yang deficiency and interior cold stagnation, **1372**
  yang qi and blood deficiencies, 494
Re bi (heat painful obstruction), 1153, 1194, *1518*
Re jue (heat reversal), 152, *1518*
Re lin (heat dysuria), 1064, 1103, **1340**, *1518*
Reach the Membrane Source Decoction, 231
Rebellious qi, *1518*
Records of Differential Diagnosis, 1381
Records of Heart-Felt Experiences in Medicine with Reference to the West, 549, 803, 809, 914, 999, 1002, 1049
Recovery
  from illness, 459
  post-surgical, **606, 611**
Recovery and Blood Activating Decoction, 897
Recovery Blood Activating Decoction, 897
Rectal
  bleeding, 945, 951
  cancer, **1403**
  prolapse, *1427*
    accumulation of dampness, heat and toxins, 164
    damp-heat with qi and blood stagnation, 1379
    deficiency and cold of the Spleen and Kidney, 781
    due to dysentery, **783**
    qi deficiency, 542
    qi stagnation and food retention, 1274
    Spleen and Stomach deficiencies, **545**
  stenosis, **1273**
  tenesmus, 403, 408, 781, 1272
Rectify the Qi Powder Worth More than Gold, 1075
Red blood cells, 524, 581, 605, 610, **931**
Reduce Scrofula Pill, 1355
Reducing, *1524*. See also *Xiao fa* (reducing)
Reducing method, **10**, 1263, 1321
Reducing, guiding, and dissolving formulas, 1263
Reed Decoction, 1377
Refine with water, *1520*. See also *Shui fei* (refine with water)
Reflux esophagitis, **211, 1237, 1329, *1427***
Reflux, acid, *1399*. See also Acid reflux/regurgitation
Regulate Menses Formula Four, 569
Regulate Menses Formula One, 568
Regulate Menses Formula Three, 569
Regulate Menses Formula Two, 568
Regulate the Middle and Calm Roundworms Decoction, 1295

Index

Regulate the Middle and Transform Phlegm Pill, 462
Regulate the Middle Decoction, 462
Regulate the Middle Pill, 459
Regulate the Stomach and Order the Qi Decoction, 160
Regurgitation, acid, *1399*. *See also* Acid reflux/regurgitation
Rehmannia and Akebia Formula, 365
Rehmannia and Gypsum Combination, 398
Rehmannia and Gypsum Decoction, 398
Rehmannia Bolus with Eight Herbs, 672
Rehmannia Bolus with Six Herbs, 627
Rehmannia Combination, 649
Rehmannia Decoction, 693
Rehmannia Eight Formula, 672
Rehmannia Four Formula, 942
Rehmannia Pill to Nourish Yin, 663
Rehmannia Pill to Return to Youth, 683
Rehmannia Six and Lotus Stamen Pill, 791
Rehmannia Six and Stamen Formula, 791
Rehmannia Six Formula, 627
Rehmannia Six Pill, 627
Rehmannia Vision Formula, 633
Rehmannia, Bupleurum and Scute Formula, 663
Relax the Channels and Invigorate the Blood Decoction, 1169
Relax the Tendons and Instill Peace Powder, 1171
Remove Painful Obstruction Decoction, 1158
Remove Painful Obstruction in the Shoulders Decoction, 1160
Ren (conception) channel, *1518*
    deficiency, 593, 687
    deficiency and cold, 805, 919, 923
    deficiency and damage, 950
    deficiency and injury, 562
    heat, 802
Ren Dong Cao (Herba Lonicerae Japonicae), xxv
Ren Dong Teng (Caulis Lonicerae Japonicae), xxv
Ren Gong Niu Huang (Calculus Bovis Artifactus), xxv
Ren Shen (Radix et Rhizoma Ginseng), xxv
Ren Shen Bai Du San, 124
Ren Shen Bai Du Sar: (Ginseng Powder to Overcome Pathogenic Influences), 126
Ren Shen Chong Cao Tang (Ginseng and Cordyceps Decoction), 559
Ren Shen Da Bu Tang (Ginseng Great Tonifying Decoction), 613
Ren Shen Dang Shao San (Ginseng, Tangkuei, and Peony Powder), 598
Ren Shen Ge Jie San (Ginseng and Gecko Powder), 557
    vs. Bu Fei E Jiao Tang (Tonify the Lung Decoction with Ass-Hide Gelatin), 1041
Ren Shen Hu Tao Tang (Ginseng and Walnut Decoction), 559
Ren Shen Tang (Ginseng Decoction), 462
Ren Shen Xie Fei Tang (Ginseng Decoction to Sedate the Lung), 1231
Ren Shen Yang Rong Tang (Wan), 615
Ren Shen Yang Ying Tang (Ginseng Decoction to Nourish the Nutritive Qi), 615
    vs. Ba Zhen Tang (Eight-Treasure Decoction), 607
    vs. Sheng Mai San (Generate the Pulse Powder), 775
    vs. Shi Quan Da Bu Tang (All-Inclusive Great Tonifying Decoction), 607
    vs. Yu Ping Feng San (Jade Windscreen Powder), 775
Ren Zhai Zhi Zhi (Straight Directions of Benevolent Aid), 735, 923
Renal. *See also* Kidney; Nephro-; specific disorders
    cirrhosis, 1090
    colic, **875**
    failure, **1111**, *1427*

    chronic, **167, 170, 265, 631, 1136**
    insufficiency, **191, 461, 875**
        chronic, **211**
    prolapse, **545**
    stones, 875
    tuberculosis, 423, 668, 673
Renewal Formula, 130
Renewal Powder, 130
Reproductive disorders, 204, 516, 517. *See also* specific disorders
Reproductive effect, 629, 646, 670
Reproductive system, atrophy, 652
Respiratory disorders, 36, **559**. *See also* Lung; Pulmonary; specific disorders; Respiratory effect
    overview, 434, 517, 821, 1022, 1207
    respiration, hurried
        Liver qi stagnation, 849
        Lung heat, 383
        overview, 316, 512, 1205
Respiratory effect, 844, 1044, 1211, 1227
Respiratory tract infection
    acute, **94**
    in children, **417**
    damp-phlegm, 1209
    deficiency heat, 558
    exterior-deficient, wind-cold, 51
    fever, high, **357**
    heat and fire in the upper and middle *jiaos*, 351
    Lung heat with phlegm accumulation, 1232
    phlegm-heat, 1222
    prevention, **774**
    upper, **41, 61, 91, 98, 109, 129, *1416***
    viral, **126**
    warm-dryness, 1030
    wind, **118**
    wind-cold, 70
    wind-cold with yin and blood deficiencies, 136
Restless fetus, *1427*, *1518*. *See also* Pregnancy
Restless leg syndrome, **502, 601, 659, 1184**
Restless organ, 731, *1395*, *1527*. *See also Zang zao* (restless organ)
Restlessness. *See also* Stress; Anxiety; related conditions
    blood deficiency with heat, 245
    damp-heat, 1101
    damp-heat in all three *jiaos*, 359
    fire in the Liver and Gallbladder channels, 379
    Heart blood deficiency, 735
    Heart fire, 368
    heat in the upper and middle *jiaos*, 354
    Liver qi stagnation with heat, 254
    Liver wind rising, 993
    Liver yang rising, 1002
    overview, 281, 707, 708
    Pericardium heat and Liver wind, 753
    phlegm and heat obstruction, 750
    wind-cold with interior heat, 45
Restoration of Health from the Myriad Diseases, 120, 178, 241, 349, 381, 388, 422, 534, 540, 575, 624, 664, 666, 1073, 1127, 1169, 1171, 1195, 1212, 1217, 1225, 1233, 1295, **1319**, 1336, 1357, 1360, 1365, 1368
Restore and Revive the Yang Decoction, 490
Restore the Left [Kidney] Decoction, 647
Restore the Left [Kidney] Pill, 645
Restore the Pulse Decoction, 589, 591
Restore the Right [Kidney] Decoction, 680
Restore the Right [Kidney] Pill, 678
Restore the Spleen and Tranquilize the Spirit Decoction, 587
Restore the Spleen Decoction, 583

1594

Index

Restrain the Liver Powder, 245
Retching, 854
Retinitis, *1427*
    yin deficiency, 627, **641**
    yin deficiency with fire, 661
Retinopathy, diabetic, 1214
Retrobulbar neuritis, 640
Retrovir. *See* Zidovudine
Return of Spring Special Pill, 754
Return of Spring Special Pill [Pediatric], 754
Return to Youth Pill, 681
Revised Eight-Herb Powder, 1105
Revised Fine Formulas for Women, 725, 1325
Revised Formulas to Aid the Living, 1138
Revised Formulas to Aid the Living from the Yan Family, 970
Revised Major Order the Qi Decoction, 155
Revised Popular Guide to the Discussion of Cold-Induced
    Disorders, 215, 227, 230, 1237
Revitalize Life Decoction, 1330
Revive Health by Invigorating the Blood Decoction, 897
Revive Health by Invigorating the Blood Decoction from the
    Trauma Department, 897
Rheumatic heart disease, 589, 879
Rheumatism
    damp-heat, 1190
    throughout the body, 1175
    wind with interior qi deficiency, 1118
    wind, cold and dampness with qi deficiency, 124
    wind, cold and dampness, 1167
Rheumatoid arthritis, *1427*
    blood stagnation, 877, **895**
    damp-heat, 1101
    excess interior heat, **323**
    exterior wind with interior qi deficiency, **1120**
    exterior wind with water accumulation, 101
    shaoyang syndrome with water accumulation, 224
    shaoyin with *taiyang* syndrome, **133**
    wind, cold and dampness, 1182
    wind, cold and dampness with interior heat, 64
    wind, dampness and heat, 1186
    wind-dampness, 1156, **1163**, 1173
    wind-dampness with deficiency, 1159
    yang deficiency with water accumulation, 1135
    yang qi and blood deficiencies, 494
Rhinalgia, 96
Rhinitis, *1427*. *See also* Sinusitis
    acute and chronic, 86
    allergic
        acute or chronic, 83
        blood deficiency, **567**
        blood deficiency and blood stagnation, **573**
        blood deficiency with wind-cold, **497**
        damp-heat, **375**
        deficiency and cold of the middle *jiao*, **477**
        exterior-deficient, wind-cold, 51
        exterior-excess, wind-cold, 39
        perennial, **85**
        qi and blood deficiencies, 479
        shaoyang syndrome, **212**
        Spleen and Stomach qi deficiencies, **547**
        wei (defensive) *qi* deficiency, **775**
        wind-cold, 59
        wind-cold with interior heat, **47**
        wind-cold with water accumulation, **77**
    atrophic, **1055**
    chronic, 59, **538**

exterior wind, 973
Lung heat, 122
wind-cold, 84, 85
wind-cold with water accumulation, **77**
wind-dampness, 1156
wind-heat, 120
Rhinoceros Horn and Rehmannia Decoction, 333
Rhizoma Acori Calami, xxv
Rhizoma Acori Tatarinowii, xxv
Rhizoma Anemarrhenae, xxvi
Rhizoma Bolbostematis, xxv
Rhizoma Chuanxiong, xxiii
Rhizoma Dioscoreae Hypoglaucae, xxiii
Rhizoma Dryopteridis Crassirhizomatis, xxiv
Rhizoma et Radix Cynanchi Stauntonii, xxiii
Rhizoma et Radix Ligustici, xxiv
Rhizoma et Radix Polygoni Cuspidati, xxiv
Rhizoma Zingiberis Praeparatum, xxv
Rhubarb and Carthamus Formula, 901
Rhubarb and Eupolyphaga Pill, 937
Rhubarb and Mirabilitum Combination, 160
Rhubarb and Moutan Combination, 1378
Rhubarb and Moutan Decoction, 1378
Rhubarb and Prepared Aconite Decoction, 166
Rifadin. *See* Rifampin
Rifampin, 613
Ringing in the ears. *See* Ears; Tinnitus
Rinse, 1516. *See also Piao* (rinse)
River point, *1513*. *See also Jing* (river) point
Roast, *1523*. *See also Wei* (roast)
Roasted Licorice Decoction, 589
Rock-like breast abscess, *1518*
Rong hua (dissolution), 20
Rosacea, 877, *1428*
Rough pulse, *1518*
Roundworms, 1292
    biliary, **1294**
    in children, **1294**
    heat in the Stomach and cold in the Intestines, 1292
    intestinal, **1293**
    overview, 1289
    pain, intermittent, severe, 1301
Rouse the Spirits Special Pill, 805
Ru Men Shi Qin (Confucians' Duties to their Parents), 7, 1272,
    1307, 1312
Rubella, 963, 967
Rui Ren (Nux Prinsepiae), xxv
Run (moisten), *1518*
Run Chang Wan (Moisten the Intestines Pill), 177, 178
    vs. Ma Zi Ren Wan (Hemp Seed Pill), 178
Running piglet, 493, *1393*, *1505*. *See also Ben tun* (running piglet)
Runny nose. *See* Nose; Nasal discharge
Sadness, 731. *See also* Depression; Melancholia
Sage-Like Healing Decoction, 567
Salivation
    dripping, 1251
    drooling, 459
    excessive, **461**
    foamy, 459, 491
    involuntary, 906, 1251
Salmonella infection, **297**
Salmonella typhi, 53, 154, 332, 1081, 1338
Salt Decoction to Induce Vomiting, 1314
Salvia Decoction, 917
San Ao Tang (Three-Unbinding Decoction), 43
San Bi Tang (Three-Painful Obstruction Decoction), 1167

1595

Index

vs. Du Huo Ji Sheng Tang (Angelica Pubescens and Taxillus Decoction), 1168

San Ceng Hui Xiang Wan (Fennel Seed Pill with Three Levels), 836

San Huang Hsieh Hsin Tang, 359

San Huang Shi Gao Tang (Three-Yellow and Gypsum Decoction), 361, 362

vs. Shi Gao Tang (Gypsum Decoction), 300

San Huang Xie Xin Tang (Three-Yellow Decoction to Sedate the Epigastrium), 359

vs. Huang Lian Jie Du Tang (Coptis Decoction to Relieve Toxicity), 361

San ji (powder), 16

San Jia An Shen Wan (Three-Shell Pill to Tranquilize the Spirit), 1011

San Jia Fu Mai Tang (Three-Shell Decoction to Restore the Pulse), 1011

San Jian Gao (Three Constructive Paste), 1244

San Jiao, **1518**. *See also Jiao*

San Jiao Bian Zheng (Triple Burner Differentiation), 431, **1518**

San Jiao Zhu Yu Tang (Drive Out Blood Stasis in Three Jiaos Decoction), 883

San Jin Pai Shi Tang (Three Gold Decoction to Expel Stone), 1106

San Miao San (Three-Marvel Powder), 1190

San Miao Wan (Three-Marvel Pill), 1190

San Pi Tang, 1167

San Qi (Radix et Rhizoma Notoginseng), xxv

San Ren Tang (Three-Nut Decoction), 1092

vs. Gan Lu Xiao Du Dan (Sweet Dew Special Pill to Eliminate Toxins), 1098

vs. Huang Qin Hua Shi Tang (Scutellaria and Talcum Decoction), 1095

vs. Huo Po Xia Ling Tang (Agastache, Magnolia Bark, Pinellia and Poria Decoction), 1095

San Sheng San (Three-Sage Powder), 1312

San Tsung Kuei Chien Tang, 1357

San Wu Bai San (Three-Substance White Powder), 172

San Wu Bei Ji Wan (Three-Substance Pill for Emergencies), 171

vs. Da Huang Fu Zi Tang (Rhubarb and Prepared Aconite Decoction), 168

vs. Wen Pi Tang (Warm the Spleen Decoction), 168

San Wu Xiang Ru Yin (Mosla Three Decoction), 438

San Yin Ji Yi Bing Zheng Fang Lun (Discussion of Illnesses, Patterns, and Formulas Related to the Unification of the Three Etiologies), 182, 1213

San Zhong Kui Jian Tang (Disperse the Swelling and Break the Hardness Decoction), 1357, 1358

San Zi Jiang Qi Tang (Three-Seed Decoction for Directing Qi Downward), 844

San Zi Yang Qin Tang (Three-Seed Decoction to Nourish One's Parents), 1245

Sang Chu Yin, 89

Sang Ju Yin (Mulberry Leaf and Chrysanthemum Decoction), 89

vs. Cong Chi Jie Geng Tang (Scallion, Prepared Soybean, and Platycodon Decoction), 113

vs. Ma Huang Xing Ren Gan Cao Shi Gao Tang (Ephedra, Apricot Kernel, Licorice, and Gypsum Decoction), 100

vs. Sang Xing Tang (Mulberry Leaf and Apricot Kernel Decoction), 91, 1029

vs. Yin Qiao San (Honeysuckle and Forsythia Powder), 91, 95

Sang Ma Wan (Mulberry Leaf and Sesame Seed Pill), 656

Sang Piao Hsiao San, 792

Sang Piao Xiao San (Mantis Egg-Case Powder), 792

vs. Jin Suo Gu Jing Wan (Metal Lock Pill to Stabilize the Essence), 794

vs. Suo Quan Wan (Shut the Sluice Pill), 796

Sang Shen (Fructus Mori), xxv

Sang Xing Tang (Mulberry Leaf and Apricot Kernel Decoction), 1027

vs. Qing Zao Jiu Fei Tang (Eliminate Dryness and Rescue the Lung Decoction), 1027, 1032

vs. Sang Ju Yin (Mulberry Leaf and Chrysanthemum Decoction), 91, 1029

vs. Sha Shen Mai Dong Tang (Glehnia and Ophiopogonis Decoction), 1049

vs. Xing Su San (Apricot Kernel and Perilla Leaf Powder), 1027, 1029

Sang Zhi Shi Gao Zhi Mu Tang (Mulberry Twig, Gypsum, and Anemarrhena Decoction), 1187

Saposhnikovia Powder that Sagely Unblocks, 291

Sargassum Combination for the Jade Flask, 1352

Sargassum Decoction for the Jade Flask, 1352

Saussurea and Areca Seed Formula, 1272

Saussurea and Cardamon Combination, 531

Saussurea and Six-Major-Herb Decoction, 531

Scabies, early stage, 1334

Scallion and Prepared Soybean Decoction, 112

Scallion and Prepared Soybean Decoction from the Book to Safeguard Life, 113

Scallion Decoction with Seven Ingredients, 135

Scallion, Prepared Soybean, and Platycodon Decoction, 111

Scallion-stalk pulse, **1518**

Scapulocostal syndrome, **899**

Scared, easily, 245, 1218

Scarlet fever, 103

Scattered pulse, **1518**

Schistosomiasis (trematode worms), **1294**

Schizonepeta and Forsythia Combination, 120

Schizonepeta and Forsythia Decoction, 120

Schizonepeta and Pinellia Formula, 49

Schizonepeta and Saposhnikovia Powder to Overcome Pathogenic Influences, 1334, 1335, 1336

Schizonepeta and Siler Detoxifying Formula, 1334

Schizonepeta and Siler Formula, 1334

Schizophrenia, **1428**

blood stagnation, **876, 883**

damp-heat in all three *jiaos*, 359

Heart blood deficiency and Liver qi stagnation, **733**

heat-phlegm, 1214

Liver qi stagnation, **249**

old phlegm and excess, 1238

qi stagnation, 823

shaoyang syndrome, **718**

Sciatica, **1428**

accumulations in the interior, 302

blood deficiency, **566**

blood stagnation, **895**

cold and dampness, 1134

damp-heat, **374**, 1192

deficiency and cold, 54

exterior excess with interior deficiency, 1169

heat and toxins, **1346**

Kidney yang deficiency, **680**

overview, 1155

qi and blood stagnation, **915**

qi deficiency and blood stagnation, **909**

shaoyin with *taiyang* syndrome, **133**

wind, cold and dampness, **1178**

wind, dampness and heat, 1186

wind-dampness, **65, 1163**

yang deficiency and interior cold, **1372**

yang qi and blood deficiencies, **496**

Scleroderma, **61**, 617, **931**, **1428**

1596

Index

Chinese Herbal Formulas and Applications

Sclerosis, spine, 652
Scoop, *1519*
Scopolamine, 567, 617
Scour Phlegm Decoction, 1212
Scrape, *1505*. *See also* Bang (scrape)
Scrofula
    cold, dampness, phlegm and blood stasis, 1375
    overview, 1321
    phlegm, 1355
    subcutaneous, 1375
    yang (superficial), 1350
Scrophularia and Fritillaria Combination, 1355
Scrotum
    eczema, acute, **375**
    enlarged, 837
Scrutiny of the Priceless Jade Patient, 633
Scute and Cimicifuga Combination, 355
Scute and Licorice Combination, 406
Scute and Mentha Combination, 354
Scute Combination, 666
Scutellaria and Talcum Decoction, 1095
Scutellaria Decoction, 406
Sebaceous glands, atrophy, 970
Secret Formulas of the Yang Family, 681
Secret Recipes for Treating Wounds and Bone-Setting Taught by
    Celestials, 301
Secrets from the Orchid Chamber, 393, 420, 567, 1191, **1261**,
    1280, 1358
Secrets Investigations into Obtaining Health, 728, 1276
Sedate the Liver and Extinguish Wind Decoction, 999
Sedative effect, 53, 708, 718, 829, 978, 1132, 1178
Seiju Hanaoka, 1341
Seizures, *1428*. *See also* Epilepsy; Convulsions; Antiseizure effect
    in children, 1251
    damp-phlegm, **1211**
    with epilepsy, **547**, **719**, **1239**
    Heart and Kidney disharmony, 714
    heat-phlegm, 1214
    hot *bi zheng* (closed disorder), 747
    infantile, 750, 753, 755
    Liver yang and wind excess, 1004
    overview, 1205, 1206, 1207
    phlegm and heat, 750, 1251
    sudden onset, 1251
    taiyang and *shaoyang* syndromes, 219
    tonic-clonic, 1251
Selected Formulas, 1158
Selective serotonin reuptake inhibitors, 1112
Selenium, deficiency, 1133
Semen. *See* Sperm
Semen Armeniacae Amarum, xxvi
Semen Citri Reticulatae, xxiv
Semen Crotonis, xxiii
Semen Euphorbiae, xxv
Semen Lablab Album, xxiii
Semen Oroxyli, xxiv
Semen Sojae, xxiv
Semen Trichosanthis, xxiv
Semen Ziziphi Spinosae, xxv
Seminal emissions
    damp-heat in the lower *jiao*, 368
    exhaustion, mental and physical, 791
    Heart and Kidney deficiencies, 792
    Kidney deficiency, 789, 791
    Kidney yang deficiency, 678
    Kidney yin and *jing* (essence) deficiencies, 645

Liver and Kidney deficiencies, 690
Liver and Kidney yin deficiencies, 627
    overview, 513, 514
    qi, blood and yang deficiencies, 609
    qi, blood, yang and *jing* (essence) deficiencies, 682
    Spleen and Kidney yang deficiencies, **786**
    yin, yang, blood and *jing* (essence) deficiencies, 687
    yin-deficient fire, 637, 649
Separate and Reduce Decoction, 1127
Separately decocted, 20
Separately simmered, 20
Septicemia
    heat and toxins, 363
    heat in the *xue* (blood) level, 333
    heat in the *ying* (nutritive) level, **332**
    heat, fire and toxins in all three *jiaos*, 341
    overview, 744
Serophene. *See* Clomiphene
Serotonin, 482, 717, 997
Serum glutamic oxaloacetic transaminase (SGOT), 209, 223, 244, 285
Serum glutamic pyruvic transaminase (SGPT), 209, 223, 244, 285
Settle the Emotions Pill, 723
Seven emotions, 1321, *1517*, *1519*. *See also* Qi qing (seven
    emotions)
Seven Treasures Formula, 690
Seven Types of Formulas, 11
Seven-Ingredient Powder with Atractylodes Macrocephala, 539
Seven-Substance Decoction with Magnolia Bark, 289
Seven-Thousandths of a Tael Powder, 903
Seven-Treasure Pill for Beautiful Whiskers, 690
Seven-Treasure Special Pill for Beautiful Whiskers, 690
Seven-Treasury Beard-Blackening Formula, 690
Sexual disorders, 204, 517, 798. *See also* specific disorders
Sexual dysfunction
    general, 797
    inability to ejaculate, **240**, **251**, **374**
    Kidney deficiency, **646**, 789
SGOT. *See* Serum glutamic oxaloacetic transaminase
SGPT. *See* Serum glutamic pyruvic transaminase
Sha Shen Mai Dong Tang (Glehnia and Ophiopogonis
    Decoction), 1047
    vs. Qing Zao Jiu Fei Tang (Eliminate Dryness and Rescue the
      Lung Decoction), 1049
    vs. Sang Xing Tang (Mulberry Leaf and Apricot Kernel
      Decoction), 1049
Sha zhang (acute filthy disease), 757, *1519*
Shaking. *See* Tremor
Shan Ci Gu (Pseudobulbus Cremastrae seu Pleiones), xxv
Shan Dou Gen (Radix et Rhizoma Sophorae Tonkinensis), xxv
Shan Xi Yi Xue Yuan Yan Fang, 917
Shan Xi Zhong Yi (Shanxi Chinese Medicine), 1011
Shan Zha Hua Tan Tang (Crataegus Decoction to Transform
    Phlegm), 1269
Shan Zha Tang **(Crataegus Decoction), 1268**
Shang Chung Hsia Tung Yung Tung Feng Wan, 1175
Shang Hai Zhong Yi Xue Yuan (Shanghai University of Chinese
    Medicine), 979
Shang han (cold damage), 31, 199, 311, *1519*
Shang Han Liu Shu (Six Texts on Cold-Induced Disorders), 107,
    130, 187, 362, 490
Shang Han Lun (Discussion of Cold-Induced Disorders), 6, **31**,
    39, 45, 51, 55, 56, 59, 74, 96, 132, 134, 152, 158, 160, 161, 163,
    172, 174, 181, 206, 219, 233, 261, 268, 269, 271, 295, 304, 321,
    325, 326, 370, 406, 408, 453, 459, 466, 467, 471, 486, 488, 489,
    494, 498, 589, 599, 715, 787, 788, 851, 873, 1086, 1089, 1109,
    1115, 1135, 1137, 1230, 1235, 1292, 1311, *1519*

INDEX

1597

Index

Shang Han Lun Ming Li Lun (Clarification of the Theory of Cold-Induced Disorders), 7

Shang Han Quan Sheng Ji (All New Collection of Cold-Induced Disorders), 1331

Shang Han Za Bing Lun (Discussion of Cold-Induced Disorders and Miscellaneous Diseases), 5, **31**, **453**

Shang Han Zhi Ge Fang Lun (Direct Investigations of Formulas for Cold-Induced Disorders), **279**, 441, 443

Shang Ke Fu Yuan Huo Xue Tang (Revive Health by Invigorating the Blood Decoction from the Trauma Department), 897

Shang Zhong Xia Tong Yong Tong Feng Wan (Upper, Middle, and Lower General Use Pill for Wind-Pain), 1175

Shanghai University of Chinese Medicine, 979

Shanxi Chinese Medicine, 1011

Shao (burn), **1519**

Shao Fu Zhu Yu Tang (Drive Out Blood Stasis in the Lower Abdomen Decoction), 889

    vs. Ge Xia Zhu Yu Tang (Drive Out Blood Stasis Below the Diaphragm Decoction), 884

    vs. Shen Tong Zhu Yu Tang (Drive Out Blood Stasis from a Painful Body Decoction), 884

    vs. Xue Fu Zhu Yu Tang (Drive Out Stasis in the Mansion of Blood Decoction), 884

Shao Yao Gan Cao Tang (Peony and Licorice Decoction), 599

Shao Yao Hou Po Tang (Peony and Magnolia Bark Decoction), 405

Shao Yao Kan Tsao Tang, 599

Shao Yao Tang (Peony Decoction), 402

    vs. Bai Tou Weng Tang (Pulsatilla Decoction), 298, 405, 410, 783

    vs. Ge Gen Huang Qin Huang Lian Tang (Kudzu, Coptis, and Scutellaria Decoction), 298, 783

    vs. Zhen Ren Yang Zang Tang (True Man's Decoction for Nourishing the Organs), 783

Shao Yao Yi Yi Ren Tang (Peony and Coicis Decoction), 405

Shao Yu, 3

Shaoyang, 206, 716, **1519**

    alternating fever and chills, 206

    overview, 201

    phlegm stagnation, 226

    taiyang syndrome, 219

    water accumulation, 222, 304

    yangming syndrome, 283

Shaoyin, 486, **1519**

    frigid extremities, 233

    taiyang syndrome, 132, 134

    yang deficiency, 489

    yang deficiency with cold, 491

She Gan Ma Huang Tang (Belamcanda and Ephedra Decoction), 80

    vs. Xiao Qing Long Tang (Minor Bluegreen Dragon Decoction), 82

She Sheng Mi Pou (Secrets Investigations into Obtaining Health), 728, 1276

She Sheng Zhong Miao Fang (Marvelous Formulas for the Health of Multitudes), 845, 1334

Sheehan's syndrome, **606**, **612**

Shen (spirit), 707, **1519**

Shen (spirit) disturbance, 316, 707

    deficient-type, 708

    excess-type, 707

    qi blood, dampness, phlegm, and food stagnation, 824

Shen Chu Tang, 1133

Shen Fu Tang (Ginseng and Prepared Aconite Decoction), 489

Shen Jin-Ao, 222, 226, 577, 723, 837, 1052

Shen Ling Bai Zhu San (Ginseng, Poria, and Atractylodes Macrocephala Powder), 535

    vs. Si Jun Zi Tang (Four-Gentlemen Decoction), 539

    vs. Si Shen Wan (Four-Miracle Pill), 260, 540, 786

    vs. Tong Xie Yao Fang (Important Formula for Painful Diarrhea), 260, 540, 786

Shen Ling Pai Chu San, 535

Shen Ling San (Ginseng and Poria Powder), 539

Shen Mi Tang (Mysterious Decoction), 847

Shen Nong, **27**, 1481, 1482, 1484

Shen Nong Ben Cao Jing (Divine Husbandman's Classic of the Materia Medica), 5, 27, **1019**

Shen Qi Wan (Kidney Qi Pill), 668, 672

Shen Qu Wan (Medicated Leaven Pill), 714

Shen Shi Yao Han (Scrutiny of the Priceless Jade Patient), 633

Shen Shi Zun Sheng Shu (Master Shen's Book for Revering Life), 222, 226, 577, 837

Shen Su Yin (Ginseng and Perilla Leaf Decoction), 128

    vs. Bai Du San (Overcome Pathogenic Influences Powder), 130

Shen Tong Zhu Yu Tang (Drive Out Blood Stasis from a Painful Body Decoction), 893

Shen Xi Dan (Magical Rhinoceros Special Pill), 335

Shen Xiao Tuo Li San (Miraculous Powder for Supporting the Interior), 1347

Shen Zhu Tang, 1133

Shen Zhuo Tang (Kidney Fixity Decoction), 1133, 1134

Shen-calming formulas, 707

Sheng (measure of volume), 22, 1439

Sheng Hua Tang (Generation and Transformation Decoction), 925

Sheng Ji Zong Lu (General Collection for Holy Relief), 6, 1313

Sheng Jiang Xie Xin Tang (Fresh Ginger Decoction to Drain the Epigastrium), 268

    vs. Ban Xia Xie Xin Tang (Pinellia Decoction to Drain the Epigastrium), 266

    vs. Gan Cao Xie Xin Tang (Licorice Decoction to Drain the Epigastrium), 266

Sheng Ma Ge Gen Tang (Cimicifuga and Kudzu Decoction), 103, 104

Sheng Ma Ke Ken Tang, 103

Sheng Mai San (Generate the Pulse Powder), 554

    vs. Bu Fei E Jiao Tang (Tonify the Lung Decoction with Ass-Hide Gelatin), 1041

    vs. Da Bu Yin Wan (Great Tonify the Yin Pill), 1041

    vs. Ren Shen Yang Ying Tang (Ginseng Decoction to Nourish the Nutritive Qi), 775

    vs. Yu Ping Feng San (Jade Windscreen Powder), 775

    vs. Zhi Gan Cao Tang (Honey-Fried Licorice Decoction), 591

Sheng Mai Yin (Generate the Pulse Decoction), 554

Sheng Tie Luo Yin (Iron Filings Decoction), 711

Sheng Xian Tang (Raise the Sinking Decoction), 549

Sheng Yang San Huo Tang (Raise the Yang and Disperse the Fire Decoction), 858

Sheng Yu Tang (Sage-Like Healing Decoction), 567

Shi (hardness), 156, **1519**

Shi (measure of volume), 22

Shi Bu Wan (Ten-Tonic Pill), 671

Shi Chang Pu (Rhizoma Acori Tatarinowii), xxv

Shi Chuan En Jia Chuan Fang (Family Formulas from Shi Chuan-En), 982

Shi Di Tang (Persimmon Calyx Decoction), 858

Shi Er Ji (Twelve Types of Formulas), 12

Shi Fang Ge Kuo (Collected Songs about Contemporary Formulas), 917

Shi Gao Tang (Gypsum Decoction), 299

    vs. San Huang Shi Gao Tang (Three-Yellow and Gypsum Decoction), 300

Index

Chinese Herbal Formulas and Applications

Shi Hu (Caulis Dendrobii), xxv
Shi Hu Ye Guang Wan (Dendrobium Pill for Night Vision), 661
   vs. Liu Wei Di Huang Wan (Six-Ingredient Pill with Rehmannia), 634
Shi Hui San (Ten Partially-Charred Substances Powder), 939
Shi Ji (Ten Types of Formulas), 12
Shi lin (stone dysuria), *1519*
Shi Liu Wei Liu Qi Yin (Sixteen-Ingredient Decoction to Flow Qi), 1360, 1361
Shi Pi San (Bolster the Spleen Powder), 1138
   vs. Zhen Wu Tang (True Warrior Decoction), 1139
Shi Quan Da Bu Tang (All-Inclusive Great Tonifying Decoction), 609
   vs. Ba Zhen Tang (Eight-Treasure Decoction), 607
   vs. Ren Shen Yang Ying Tang (Ginseng Decoction to Nourish the Nutritive Qi), 607
   vs. Tai Shan Pan Shi San (Powder that Gives the Stability of Mount Tai), 620
Shi Quan Da Bu Tang (*Wan*), 609
Shi Shen Tang (Ten-Immortal Decoction), 72
Shi Wei Bai Du Tang (Ten-Ingredient Decoction to Overcome Pathogenic Influences), 1341
Shi Wei Di Huang Wan (Ten-Ingredient Pill with Rehmannia), 639
Shi Wei Wen Dan Tang (Ten-Ingredient Decoction to Warm the Gallbladder), 1216
Shi Wei Xiang Ru Yin (Ten-Ingredient Decoction with Mosla), 438
Shi Wei Xiao Yao San (Ten-Ingredient Rambling Powder), 256
Shi Xiao San (Sudden Smile Powder), 911
Shi yao (envoy herb), 14, *1519*
Shi Yao Shen Shu (Miraculous Book of Ten Remedies), 939
Shi Yi De Xiao Fang (Effective Formulas from Generations of Physicians), 176, 728
Shi Zao Tang (Ten-Jujube Decoction), 181
Shi Zao Wan (Ten-Jujube Pill), 181
Shih Chuan Ta Pu Tang (*Wan*), 609
Shih Shen Tang, 72
Shingles, **374**, **994**, **1338**. *See also* Herpes
Shi-re lin (damp-heat dysuria), *1520*
Shivering, 491
Shivering perspiration, *1520*
Shixuan points, 1151
Shock
   due to infection, **556**
   shaoyin syndrome, 486
   yang deficiency with excess cold, 491
Short pulse, *1520*
Shortness of breath. *See* Breath, shortness of; Wheezing; Dyspnea; Asthma
Shou Gan Di Huang Wan, 663
Shou Nian San (Pinch Powder), 913
Shou Shi Bao Yuan (Achieving Longevity by Guarding the Source), **1319**
Shou Wu Pian (Polygonum Pill), 692
Shou Wu Teng (Caulis Polygoni Multiflori), xxvi
Shoulders
   bursitis, 59
   frozen, **221**, **497**, 1159, 1195
   heavy sensation, 1192
   pain
      damp and phlegm, 1195
      qi and blood stagnation, 893
      wind-cold, **61**
      wind-dampness with deficiency, 1159
      yang deficiency and invasion cold, **501**
   pain and stiffness, 1156

periarthritis
   blood deficiency, **566**
   blood deficiency with wind-cold, **496**
   wind with interior qi deficiency, **1120**
   wind, cold and dampness, 1178
   wind, dampness and heat, 1186
   wind-cold, **61**
   wind-dampness with deficiency, **1159**
   xue bi (blood painful obstruction), **501**
   tendonitis, 59
Shrieking, sudden, 1251
Shu (stream) point, *1520*
Shu (transport) point, *1520*
Shu Ching Huo Hsieh Tang, 1169
Shu Di Huang (Radix Rehmanniae Praeparata), xxv
Shu Gan Tang (Spread the Liver Decoction), 241
   vs. Chai Hu Shu Gan San (Bupleurum Powder to Spread the Liver), 242
Shu Jin Li An San (Relax the Tendons and Instill Peace Powder), 1171
Shu Jing Huo Xue Tang (Relax the Channels and Invigorate the Blood Decoction), 1169
Shu Zao Yin Zi (Spread and Unblock Decoction), 185
Shuang Jie Tong Sheng San (Double Relieve Powder that Sagely Unblocks), 294
Shui fei (refine with water), *1520*
Shui Lu Er Xian Dan (Water and Earth Two Immortals Special Pill), 790
Shut the Sluice Formula, 795
Shut the Sluice Pill, 795
Shwachman syndrome, **612**
Si He Ting Ji Fang (Collection of Formulas of Si He-Ting), 347
Si Jun Zi Tang (Four-Gentlemen Decoction), 522
   vs. Jian Pi Wan (Strengthen the Spleen Pill), 1279
   vs. Li Zhong Wan (Regulate the Middle Pill), 462, 526
   vs. Shen Ling Bai Zhu San (Ginseng, Poria, and Atractylodes Macrocephala Powder), 539
Si Jung Zi Tang, 522
Si Ling San (Four-Ingredient Powder with Poria), 1112
   vs. Wei Ling Tang (Calm the Stomach and Poria Decoction), 1112
   vs. Wu Ling San (Five-Ingredient Powder with Poria), 1112
   vs. Yin Chen Wu Ling San (Artemisia Scoparia and Five-Ingredient Powder with Poria), 1112
Si Miao San (Four-Marvel Powder), 1190, 1347
Si Miao Wan (Four-Marvel Pill), 1190
Si Miao Yong An Tang (Four-Valiant Decoction for Well-Being), 1344
Si Mo Tang (Four Milled-Herbs Decoction), 849
Si Ni Jia Ren Shen Tang (Frigid Extremities Decoction plus Ginseng), 488
Si Ni San (Frigid Extremities Powder), 233
   vs. Chai Hu Shu Gan San (Bupleurum Powder to Spread the Liver), 241
   vs. Dang Gui Si Ni Tang (Tangkuei Decoction for Frigid Extremities), 499
   vs. Si Ni Tang (Frigid Extremities Decoction), 237, 489, 499
   vs. Xiao Yao San (Rambling Powder), 253
   vs. Yi Guan Jian (Linking Decoction), 237, 660
Si Ni Tang (Frigid Extremities Decoction), 486
   vs. Dang Gui Si Ni Tang (Tangkuei Decoction for Frigid Extremities), 499
   vs. Si Ni San (Frigid Extremities Powder), 237, 489, 499
Si Shen Wan (Four-Miracle Pill), 784
   vs. Shen Ling Bai Zhu San (Ginseng, Poria, and Atractylodes Macrocephala Powder), 260, 540, 786

1599

Index

vs. Tong Xie Yao Fang (Important Formula for Painful Diarrhea), 260, 540, 786

vs. Zhen Ren Yang Zang Tang (True Man's Decoction for Nourishing the Organs), 786

Si Sheng Wan (Four-Fresh Pill), 942

Si Wu Tang (Four-Substance Decoction), 562

vs. Gui Pi Tang (Restore the Spleen Decoction), 587

Side effects. *See* individual formula monographs

Siler and Licorice Formula, 396

Siler and Platycodon Formula, 291

Siler and Platycodon Formula (Minus Rhubarb), 294

Siler Combination, 349

Siler Sage-Inspired Formula, 291

Silicosis, 420, **1236**

Silkworm Droppings Decoction, 1101

Simmer, *1505*. *See also Ao* (simmer)

Sinus

congestion, 84

headache, 84

Sinusitis, *1428*. *See also* Nasosinusitis; Rhinitis

acute and/or chronic, 83, 86

allergic, **1137**

anal, **1328**

heat and toxins, 1342

Lung heat, 122

qi and blood deficiencies, 479

wind, **976**

wind-cold, 84, 85

wind-cold with water accumulation, 74

wind-heat, 120

Six exogenous factors, 34, 1321, *1514*. *See also Liu yin* (six exogenous factors)

Six Gentlemen Decoction (Pill), 527

Six Major Herb Decoction (Pill), 527

Six Stages Differentiation, 311, *1514*. *See also Liu jing bian zheng* (six stages differentiation)

Six Texts on Cold-Induced Disorders, 107, 130, 187, 362, 490

Six Texts on the Essentials of Medicine, 252

Six-Flavour Rehmannia Pill, 627

Six-Gentlemen Decoction, 527

Six-Gentlemen Decoction with Aucklandia and Amomum, 531

Six-Gentlemen Decoction with Cyperus and Amomum, 533

Six-Ingredient Pill with Rehmannia, 509, 627

Six-Miracle Pill, 363

Sixteen-Ingredient Decoction to Flow Qi, 1360, 1361

Six-to-One Powder, 441, 442

Sjogren's syndrome, **1045**

Skin disorders. *See also* specific disorders; Dermatological effect

atrophy, 970

dry and coarse, 970

itching, 575, **972**

maculae, 299

maculae or red blotches, 339

overview, 965

scaling, 972

suppurative, 1342

yellow, 1086

wind, 967

wind with blood deficiency, 970

Skin water, 1121, *1516*. *See also Pi shui* (skin water)

Skipping pulse, *1520*

SLE. *See* Systemic lupus erythematosus

Sleep. *See also* Insomnia

apnea, **360**

apnea and hypopnea, **829**

dreams, bizarre, 1238

dreams, frequent, 649

restless, 731

Sleep-walking, 710, 731

Slicing, *1518*. *See also Qie* (slice)

Slippery pulse, *1520*

Slow pulse, *1520*

SMA (superior mesenteric artery) syndrome, 482

Small Collection of Fine Formulas, 841, 903

Small Intestine (TCM), *1520*

Small Intestine (WM). *See* Intestinal disorders; specific disorders

Small pulse, *1520*

Small spoon, *1520*

Smallpox, 105

Smell, decreased sense of, 86, 122

Sneezing

damp-heat, 86

wind, 973

wind-cold, 70

wind-heat, 114

Soak, *1513*. *See also Jin* (soak)

Sodium excretion, 162

Sodium hydroxide, 390

Soft extract, 17

Soft tissues injuries, **61**, 897, 901, **1178**

Soft-Shelled Turtle Shell Pill, 935

Soggy pulse, *1520*

Sohaku Asada, 164

Soles, hot/warm sensations, 627, 1036

Solid organ, *1526*. *See also Zang* (solid organ)

Solid organ toxin, *1526*. *See also Zang du* (solid organ toxin)

Somatostatin, 262, 528

Somnolence, 722

Sophora Flower Formula, 944

Sophora Flower Powder, 944

Sophora Japonica Flower Powder, 944

Sophora Japonica Fruit Pill, 946

Soreness. *See* specific locations

Sores, *1520*. *See also* Abscesses

bed, 1367

canker, 92, 354

chronic, 1369

cold, dampness, phlegm and blood stasis, 1375

damp-heat in all three *jiaos*, 359

early onset/stage, 1325, 1334

generalized, **1327**

heat and toxins, 291, 1325

heat and toxins with underlying deficiencies, 1365

heat, fire and toxins in all three *jiaos*, 341

late-stage, 1369

lower extremities, **344**

malignant, 1349

mid- to late-stages, 1364

overview, 315, 456, 1321

with pus, 1362

with pus and discharge, 1364

qi and blood deficiencies, 1369

qi deficiency, 1362

red, hot, hard and painful, 1331

redness, swelling and pain, 1325, 1334

suppurative, 1357

swelling, burning sensations, pain, 1362

temple area of the head, 244

wind-heat, 1332

yang deficiency and interior cold stagnation, 1370

yang (superficial), 1321, 1350

yin (deep-rooted), 1321, 1370, 1375

1600

Chinese Herbal Formulas and Applications

Index

Sour Jujube Decoction, 722
Source point, *1526*. *See also Yuan* (source) point
Source *qi*, *1526*. *See also Yuan* (source) *qi*
Spasms. *See also* Cramps; Antispasmodic effect
  facial, 977, **1006**
  intestinal, 481
  Liver excess, 996
  Liver wind rising, 993, 1008
  Liver wind rising with yin deficiency, 1009
  overview, 963, 964
  wind, 980
  wind invading the channels and collaterals, 981
  wind, cold and dampness, 1177
  yin, blood and body fluid deficiencies, 600
Speech
  abnormal, 731
  delirious, 330
  difficulties in, 988
  incoherent, 299, 361
  slurred, post-stroke, 906, 984, 986
Sperm disorders, **891**
  with blood, 638
  decreased motility, 690
  hemospermia, **638**
  increased count and motility, 670
  low count, 678, 690
Spermatorrhea, *1428*
  damp-heat, 800
  deficiency and cold, 795
  deficiency and cold of the Spleen and Kidney, 784
  exhaustion, mental and physical, 791
  Heart and Kidney disharmony, 797
  Kidney deficiency, 789, 791
  Kidney yin and *jing* (essence) deficiencies, 645
  overview, 770, 771
  qi, blood, yang and *jing* (essence) deficiencies, 682
  severe, **790**
  yin and yang deficiencies, 798
Spica Schizonepetae, xxiv
Spine
  pain, 695
  prolapse of lumbar intervertebral disk, **1164**
  sclerosis, 652
Spine Pain Decoction, 1165
Spirit, *1519*. *See also Shen* (spirit)
Spleen (TCM), *1520*
  damp-cold, 840
  damp-heat, 401
  damp-phlegm, 1209
  deficiency and cold, 781, 784
  deficiency and damp accumulation, 1121
  deficiency due to over-thinking, 583
  deficiency with damp accumulation, 1127
  deficiency with dampness, 535
  deficiency with poor appetite, 534
  disharmony with Liver, 233
  fire, latent, 396
  qi deficiency, 522, 542
  qi deficiency with cold and dampness, 531
  qi deficiency with dampness and phlegm, 527
  qi stagnation and food retention, 1274
  yang deficiency with cold, 169
  yang deficiency with water accumulation, 1135, 1138
Spleen and Stomach (TCM)
  damp-heat, 401, 1085
  dampness, 1068, 1072, 1082

deficiency and cold, 455, 463
deficiency and cold with qi and blood stagnation, 484
deficiency with dampness, 535
deficiency with indigestion and food stagnation, 541
deficiency with interlocking of heat and water, 268
disharmony, 1074
fire, latent, 396
qi deficiencies with cold and damp, 531
qi deficiencies with dampness and phlegm, 527
qi deficiency, 522, 542
Spleen disorders (WM). *See* specific disorders
Spleen-Effusing plus Atractylodes Decoction, 102
Spleen-Strengthening Pill, 1277
Splenomegaly, 885, 935
Spondylitis, ankylosing, **1163**, **1189**
Spondylosis, cervical, **916**
Spontaneous sweating, *1520*. *See also* Perspiration; Sweating
Spoon
  large, *1514*
  small, *1520*
Spora Lygodii, xxiv
Sports injuries, 897, 900, 901
Spread and Unblock Decoction, 185
Spread the Liver Decoction, 241
Spring point, *1526*. *See also Ying* (spring) point
Sputum. *See also* Phlegm; Expectorant effect
  with blood, 589, 1229
  with blood and mucus, 1230
  difficult to expectorate, 1233
  dry, sticky, 1047
  overview, 1206
  profuse, 1245
  profuse, white, 1209
  profuse, white, watery, 1242
  scanty, sticky, 1028
  thick, sticky, 1230, 1240
  thick, sticky, yellow and difficult to expectorate, 845
  thick, yellow, 1222
  yellow, sticky, 1235
SSRI. *See* Selective serotonin reuptake inhibitors
Stabilize *Chong* [Thoroughfare Channel] Decoction, 803
Stabilize the Menses Pill, 802
Stagnant chest, 161, 163, 172, *1513*. *See also Jie xiong* (stagnant chest)
Stagnation
  blood, *1506*
  food, 1266, 1270, 1272, 1274, 1277
  overview, 1263
  qi, 822, *1517*
  qi and blood, 578, 893, 897, 901, 903, 915, *1517*
  qi, blood, phlegm, heat, dampness and food, 822
  water and fluid, *1522*
Stagnation-Relieving Pill, 822
Standards of Patterns and Treatments, 354, 386, 402, 418, 438, 578, 784, **1061**, 1129, 1212, 1216, 1277, 1373, 1383
Standards of Patterns and Treatments in External Medicine, 361, **1061**
Standards of Patterns and Treatments in Gynecology, **1061**
Standards of Patterns and Treatments in Pediatrics, **1061**
Standards of Patterns and Treatments in Sores and Abscesses, **1061**
Staphylococcus albus, 332, 1338
Staphylococcus aureus, 41, 46, 53, 60, 93, 154, 158, 258, 285, 296, 332, 394, 404, 1081, 1104, 1338
  methicillin-resistant (MRSA), **546**
Staphylococcus species, 409, 1380
Stasis, blood, *1506*
Steaming, *1527*. *See also Zheng* (steam)

INDEX

1601

Index

Steaming bones sensations, *1520*
  Lung and Kidney yin deficiencies, 1036
  overview, 316, 513
  yin-deficient fire, 637, 649
  yin-deficient heat, 416, 418, 627
Stenosis
  colon and rectum, **1273**
  pyloric, 484
Stephania and Astragalus Combination, 1118
Stephania and Astragalus Decoction, 1118
Stephania and Poria Decoction, 1120
Steroidogenesis, 595
Steroids, 596. *See also* Adrenocorticotropic hormone; Adrenergic
  effect
Stew, *1509. See also Dun* (stew)
Stiffness. *See also* specific locations and disease
  muscle and tendon, 991
  neck, 39, 55, 64, 124
  neck and back, 48, 59
  neck and shoulder, 59
  shoulder and back, 1156
  wind invading the channels and collaterals, 981
Stifling sensations, *1521. See also* specific locations
Stigma Croci, xxvi
Stillbirth, 928
Stirred pulse, *1521*
Stomach (TCM), *1521*
  cold with heat in the chest, 271
  damp-cold, 840
  damp-heat, 401, 1270
  deficiency and cold, 467, 857
  deficiency with dampness, 535
  deficiency with interlocking of heat and cold, 270
  dryness and heat, 160, 174
  fire, latent, 396
  heat, 393
  heat with damaged yin and body fluids, 190
  heat with yin deficiency, 398
  heat-phlegm, 1214
  qi deficiency, 522, 542
  qi deficiency with cold and dampness, 531
  qi deficiency with dampness and phlegm, 527
  qi deficiency with phlegm, 851
  qi disharmony, 261
  qi flow, reversed, 854
  yin deficiency, 1043
Stomach disorders (WM), 318. *See also* Gastro-; Gastric-; specific
  disorders
  cancer, 527, *1404*
  cramps, 600, **1044**
  hyperacidity, **182**
  influenza, 67
  pain, **264**, 917
Stomach-Calming Powder, 1068
Stomach-Clearing Powder, 393
Stomach-Comforting Formula (Pill), 1068
Stomach-Comforting with Five-Ling Decoction, 1113
Stomach-Regulating and Purgative Decoction, 160
Stomach-Regulating and Qi-Infusing Decoction, 160
Stomatitis, *1428*
  in children, **397**
  damp-heat in all three *jiaos*, 359
  damp-heat in the Spleen and Stomach, 401
  in early or late stage, 60
  fire in the Heart channel, 365
  heat and fire in the upper and middle *jiaos*, 351

heat and toxins, 363
heat in the chest and cold in the Stomach, 271
heat in the upper and middle *jiaos*, 354
heat, lingering or residual, 327
Liver qi stagnation with heat, 254
qi deficiency with dampness and phlegm, **529**
due to radiation, **1055**
recurrent, **394**, **461**, **532**, **1097**
shaoyang syndrome, **212**
Stomach deficiency and interlocking of heat and cold, 270
Stomach heat, 398
Stomach qi disharmony, 261
ulcerative, 401
wind-cold with interior heat, 295
Stone dysuria, *1519. See also Shi lin* (stone dysuria); *Lin zheng*
  (dysuria syndrome)
Stone-bake, *1505. See also Bei* (stone-bake)
Stones
  cholelithiasis, *1405*
    bile duct infection, **240**
    cholecystitis, **210**, **1282**
    chronic, **265**
    damp-heat, 1086
    fire in the Liver and Gallbladder channels, 379
    Gallbladder damp-heat, **229**
    gallbladder removal, **285**
    heat and fire in the upper and middle *jiaos*, 351
    heat in the Stomach and cold in the Intestines, **1294**
    overview, 1264
    phlegm-heat, 1235
    qi stagnation, 822
    shaoyang syndrome with phlegm stagnation, 226
    shaoyin syndrome, **235**
    taiyang and *shaoyang* syndromes, 219
    yang deficiency and interior cold, 481
  gastrolithiasis, 1264, **1268**
  nephrolithiasis, 368, **442**
  urolithiasis
    damp-heat, 1103
    Heart fire with damp-heat in the lower *jiao*, 368
    heat, 1107
    interior excess heat, **155**
    Kidney yang deficiency, 668
    phlegm and damp accumulation, **1111**
    summer-heat and dampness, **442**
    water and heat, interlocked, **1116**
    yang deficiency and interior cold, 481
  vesical calculus, 668, 673
Stools
  dry, 176, 179, 725
  dry and hard, 177
  impacted, 152
  loose
    food stagnation with heat, 1277
    due to intestinal parasites, 1297
    Kidney yang deficiency, 678
    overview, 513
    qi deficiency with cold and dampness, 531
    qi deficiency with dampness, 535
    qi deficiency with dampness and phlegm, 527
    Spleen and Stomach qi deficiencies, 542
    water and dampness accumulation, 1109
  with undigested food, 1113
Stop Bleeding Decoction, 941
Stop Coughing Decoction, 118
Stop Coughing Powder, 116

Index

Stop Spasms Powder, 979
Straight Directions of Benevolent Aid, 735, 923
Stream point, *1520. See also Shu* (stream) point
Strengthen the Spleen Pill, 1277
Strengthen the Tendon Decoction, 568
Streptococcus
    alpha-hemolytic, 332, 1338
    beta-hemolytic, 332, 372, 1338
Streptomycin, 639
Stress. *See also* Adaptogenic effect; Sedative effect
    altitude, **1094**
    with depression, **265, 529, 830**
    Liver qi stagnation, 247
    Liver qi stagnation with heat, 254
Stroke. *See also* Cerebrovascular accident
    acute, **1216**
    cold stroke, 744
    exterior wind with qi deficiency, 984
    heat stroke, 222, 321, 325, 435, 436, 446, 750, 1082, *1413*
    ischemic, *343, 882*, **916, 1006**
    Liver wind rising, 993
    Liver yang and wind excess, 1004
    Liver yang and wind rising, **1000**
    old phlegm and excess heat, **1239**
    overview, 744, 965, 1207
    phlegm and heat obstruction, 750
    post-stroke sequelae, 571, **631**, 651, **695**, 906, **907**, 984, 986,
        988, 993, 999, **1010**, 1178, **1216**
    qi deficiency and blood stagnation, **907**
    qi stroke, *1527*
    summer-heat, 327
    wind stroke, 750, 977, 988, 991, 1177, 1312, 1313, *1395, 1527*
        overview, 744, 1309
Strychnine, 997
Stubborn painful obstruction, 1153, *1522. See also Wan bi*
    (stubborn painful obstruction); *Bi zheng* (painful obstruction
    syndrome)
Stye, *1328*
***Su He Xiang Wan* (Liquid Styrax Pill)**, 758
Su Ni San, 233
Su Ni Tang, 486
Su Tzu Chiang Chi Tang, 842
Su Wen (Basic Questions), 3, 5
Su Wen Bing Ji Qi Yi Bao Ming Ji (Collection of Writings on the
    Mechanism of Illness, Suitability of Qi, and the Safeguarding
    of Life as Discussed in the Basic Questions), 825, 988
Su Zi Jiang Chi Tang, 842
***Su Zi Jiang Qi Tang* (Perilla Fruit Decoction for Directing Qi
    Downward)**, 842
Suan Zao Ren (Semen Ziziphi Spinosae), xxv
***Suan Zao Ren Tang* (Sour Jujube Decoction)**, 722
    vs. *Gan Mai Da Zao Tang* (Licorice, Wheat, and Jujube
        Decoction), 724
    vs. *Tian Wang Bu Xin Dan* (Emperor of Heaven's Special Pill to
        Tonify the Heart), 724
Suan Zao Tang, 722
Subcutaneous bleeding, *1403*
Sublime Formula for Sustaining Life, 1325
Substance P, 576
Succinum Combination, 1251
Sucralfate, 209, 287, 345
Sudden Smile Formula, 911
Sudden Smile Powder, 911
Sudden turmoil disorder, 444, 459, 463, 757, 1076, 1099, 1109,
    1314, *1393, 1521. See also Huo luan* (sudden turmoil disorder)
Summary of Internal Medicine, 254, 256

Summer-heat, *1521*
    with damaged qi and body fluids, 434, 446, 554
    with dampness, 441, 444
    with exterior cold and interior dampness, 436, 439
    with internal dampness, 433
    Lung, 435
    overview, 433
    qi (energy) level, 435
    with wind-cold, 433
Summer-heat-clearing and Chi-tonifying Decoction, 446
Summer-heat-dispelling formulas, 433
Sun Si-Miao, 6, 138, 169, 474, 714, 729, 983, **1151**, 1161, 1314,
    1377, 1481, 1482, 1484
***Suo Quan Wan* (Shut the Sluice Pill)**, 795
    vs. *Sang Piao Xiao San* (Mantis Egg-Case Powder), 796
Superficial pulse, *1521*
Superior mesenteric artery (SMA) syndrome, 482
Superoxide anion radical, 1380
Supplement to the Pocket-Sized Discussion of Formulas for
    Children, 1299
Supplement to the Thousand Ducat Formulas, 6, 474, **1151**
Support the Upright and Suppress Cancer Decoction, 336
Suppuration
    ear and nose, 120
    early stage, **1334**
    glands, 1336
    skin, 1336
Suppurative disorders, 1365, 1367
Suppurative infection, 124
Supreme physician, *1521*
Surgery (post-operative or post-surgical)
    constipation, **175**
    diarrhea, **533**
    fever, **414**
    ileus, **482**
    infection, **344**
    intestinal adhesion, **498**
    intestinal obstruction, 482
    nausea and vomiting, 854
    recovery, **188, 606, 611, 1056**
    sweating, 776
    treatment, **482**
Surging pulse, *1521*
Swallowing disorder, **829**
Swallowing, difficult, 363, 827
Sweat glands, atrophy, 970
Sweating. *See also* Perspiration
    night
        Heart and Spleen deficiencies, 583
        Heart blood deficiency, 735
        Heart fire, 710
        Kidney and Lung yin deficiencies, 643
        Kidney yin and yang deficiencies with fire, 684
        Liver and Kidney yin deficiencies, 627
        Liver blood deficiency, 722
        Lung and Kidney yin deficiencies, 1036
        qi, blood, yang and *jing* (essence) deficiencies, 682
        yin and qi deficiencies, 776
        yin-deficient fire, 422, 637, 649
        yin-deficient heat, 416, 418
        yin-deficient heat and fire, 420
    overview, 314, 456, 513, 514, 708, 769, 771
    postpartum, 776
    post-surgical, 776
    profuse, 321, 325, *1517*
    profuse and continuous, 776

Index

spontaneous
  Kidney yin and *jing* (essence) deficiencies, 645
  Spleen and Stomach qi deficiencies, 542
  wei (defensive) *qi* deficiency, 773
  yin and qi deficiencies, 776
Sweating method, **9**, 34, 281, 1307, **1511**. *See also Han fa*
  (sweating)
Sweating regulation, effect on, 53
Sweaty head, *1521*
Sweet Combination, 401
Sweet Combination Drink, 401
Sweet Dew Decoction, 401
Sweet Dew Detoxication Pellet, 1096
Sweet Dew Special Pill to Eliminate Toxins, 1096
Swelling
  damp-heat, 1192
  joints, 1173, 1186, 1192
  localized, 1332
  qi and blood stagnation, 901
  suppurative, 1357
  trauma, 915, **1122**
  water accumulation, 102
  wind-heat, 1332
Swollen head epidemic, 355, *1508*. *See also Da tou wen* (swollen
  head epidemic)
Sympathomimetic effect, 76
Syncope
  micturition, **617**
  phlegm, 761, 1180
  post-stroke, 991
  shaoyin syndrome, 233
Syncytial virus, 41
Syndrome. *See* specific conditions
Synopsis of Caring for Infants, 245
Synovitis, **501**
Syphilis
  early stage, 1334
  fire in the Liver and Gallbladder, 371
  heat and toxins, 1349
Syrup, 18
Systematic Differentiation of Warm Disease, 7, 89, 92, 94, 189,
  190, 330, 339, 412, **431**, 435, 439, 591, 746, 856, 1009, 1011,
  1025, 1027, 1029, 1047, 1054, 1092, 1095
Systemic lupus erythematosus (SLE), 170, **224**, 243, 617, *1429*
Systremma, **601**
Szu Chun Tzu Tang, 522
Szu Wu Tang, 562
T cells, 76, 532
T-lymphocytes, 523, 544, 555, 610, 655
T3, 373, 1354
T4, 373, 1354
Ta Cheng Chi Tang, 152
Ta Chien Chung Tang, 480
Ta Huang Mu Tan Pi Tang, 1378
Ta Pu Yin Wan, 649
Ta Tsai Hu Tang, 283
Tablet, 18
Tachycardia
  supraventricular, 584
  theophylline-induced, 720
Tai Ping Hui Min He Ji Ju Fang (Imperial Grace Formulary of the
  Tai Ping Era), 6, 43, 48, 49, 67, 72, 126, 128, 247, 303, 351, 368,
  391, 401, 436, 463, 484, 522, 535, 562, 609, 615, 751, 758, 776,
  781, 797, 805, 842, 911, 946, 973, 990, 1068, 1075, 1079, 1082,
  1103, 1105, 1107, 1123, 1177, 1181, **1203**, 1209, 1231, 1296,
  1300, 1347

Tai Ping Sheng Hui Fang (Holy Grace Formulary of the Tai Ping
  Era), 6
***Tai Shan Pan Shi San* (Powder that Gives the Stability of Mount
  Tai)**, 618
  vs. Ba Zhen Tang (Eight-Treasure Decoction), 620
  vs. Bao Chan Wu You Fang (Preserve Pregnancy and Care-Free
    Decoction), 623
  vs. Shi Quan Da Bu Tang (All-Inclusive Great Tonifying
    Decoction), 620
Taiyang, *1521*
  with *shaoyang* syndrome, 219
  with *shaoyin* syndrome, 132, 134
  taiyang cold syndrome, 39
  taiyang cold syndrome with interior heat, 45
  taiyang cold syndrome, severe, 45
  taiyang wind syndrome, 51
  with wind-cold, 59
  with *yangming* syndrome, 289
Taiyin, *1521*
  with *taiyang* syndrome, 55
  yang deficiency with cold, 491
Take drenched, 21, *1507*. *See also Chong fu* (take drenched)
Talc and Scute Formula, 1096
Tan (char to ash), *1521*
Tan (visible phlegm), 1205
Tan yin (phlegm retention), 80, 668, 673, 1064, 1109, 1131, *1521*
Tang Gui Si Ni Tang, 494
Tang ji (decoction), 16
Tang jiang ji (syrup), 18
Tang Kuei Liu Huang Tang, 420
Tang Kuei Lung Hui Wan, 379
Tang Kuei Nien Tung Tang, 1191
Tang Kuei Pu Hsieh Tang, 580
Tang Kuei Shao Yao San, 594
Tang Kuei Su Ni Tang, 494
Tang Kuei Yin Tzu, 970
Tangerine Peel and Bamboo Shaving Decoction, 854, 855
Tangerine Peel, Pinellia, Immature Bitter Orange, and
  Atractylodes Macrocephala Pill, 1276
Tangerine Pip Pill, 833
Tangerine Seed Pill, 833
Tangkuei and Anemarrhena Combination, 1191
Tangkuei and Arctium Formula, 967
Tangkuei and Astragalus Combination, 580
Tangkuei and Astragalus Decoction to Construct the Middle, 479
Tangkuei and Bupleurum Formula, 247
Tangkuei and Corydalis Combination, 885
Tangkuei and Counterflow Cold Decoction, 494
Tangkuei and Evodia Combination, 919
Tangkuei and Gardenia Combination, 575
Tangkuei and Ginger Combination, 925
Tangkuei and Ginseng Eight Combination, 604
Tangkuei and Jujube Combination, 494
Tangkuei and Magnolia Five Formula, 301
Tangkuei and Pain-Assuaging Decoction, 1191
Tangkuei and Parsley Combination, 621
Tangkuei and Peony Formula, 594
Tangkuei and Peony Powder, 594
Tangkuei and Persica Combination, 897
Tangkuei and Six Huang Decoction, 420
Tangkuei and Six Yellow Combination, 420
Tangkuei and Six-Yellow Decoction, 420
Tangkuei and Tribulus Combination, 970
Tangkuei Blood-Nourishing Decoction, 580
Tangkuei Decoction, 970
Tangkuei Decoction for Frigid Extremities, 494

1604

Index

Tangkuei Decoction for Frigid Extremities plus Evodia and Fresh Ginger, 498
Tangkuei Decoction to Construct the Middle, 474
Tangkuei Decoction to Lift the Pain, 1191
Tangkuei Decoction to Tonify the Blood, 580
Tangkuei Drink, 970
Tangkuei Eight Herb Formula, 810
Tangkuei Formula, 623
Tangkuei Four and Persica Carthamus Combination, 571
Tangkuei Four Combination, 562
Tangkuei Four Plus Combination, 567
Tangkuei Gentiana and Aloe Formula, 379
Tangkuei Powder, 623
Tangkuei Sixteen Herbs Combination, 1360, 1361
Tangkuei, Astragalus and Peony Combination, 479
Tangkuei, Gentiana, and Aloe Pill, 379
Tangkuei, Lung-tan, and Aloe Pill, 379
Tao Chih San, 365
Tao He Cheng Chi Tang, 873
***Tao He Cheng Qi Tang* (Peach Pit Decoction to Order the Qi)**, 873
***Tao Hong Si Wu Tang* (Four-Substance Decoction with Safflower and Peach Pit)**, 571
Tao Hong-Jing, **1019**, 1481, 1482, 1484
Tao Hua, 107, 130, 187, 362, 490
***Tao Hua Tang* (Peach Blossom Decoction)**, 787
Tao Hung Szu Wu Tang, 571
Tao Jen Cheng Chi Tang, 873
Tao Ren Cheng Qi Tang, 873
Tao Shui Fu Ling Tang, 1129
Tao's Bupleurum and Kudzu Decoction to Release the Muscle Layer, 107
Tao's Chai Ge Jie Ji Tang, 107
Tapeworms, 1289, 1301
Taxol. *See* Paclitaxel
Tea, 18
Tea-Blended Ligusticum Powder, 973
Teachings of [Zhu] Dan-Xi, 7, 379, 389, 649, 651, 773, 822, 943, 946, 1113, 1140, 1175, 1188, **1203**, 1266
Teachings of Generations of Physicians about Pox, 748
Tearing, excessive, 641, 661
Teeth
    clenching, 245
    grinding at night, 1289
    loose, 690
Tegretol. *See* Carbamazepine
Temper, short, 254, 649
Temperature. *See* Fever
Temperature regulation, effect on, 41, 46, 53, 90, 93, 98, 209, 437
Ten Partially-Charred Substances Powder, 939
Ten Spirits Decoction, 72
Ten Strong Tonic Herbs Decoction (Pill), 609
Ten Types of Formulas, 12
Tendonitis, 59, 1195
Tendons
    aches and pains, 1188
    degeneration, 1166
    weakness and atrophy, 651
Tenesmus, rectal
    damp-heat, 403, 406, 1272
    in dysentery, 158
    in dysentery or diarrhea, 781
    overview, 202, 316
    toxic heat, 408
Teng Hong, 7, 127
Ten-Immortal Decoction, 72

Ten-Ingredient Decoction to Overcome Pathogenic Influences, 1341
Ten-Ingredient Decoction to Warm the Gallbladder, 1216
Ten-Ingredient Decoction with Mosla, 438
Ten-Ingredient Pill with Rehmannia, 639
Ten-Ingredient Rambling Powder, 256
Ten-Jujube Decoction, 181
Ten-Jujube Pill, 181
Tension. *See* Stress; Anxiety
Tension headache, **1249**
Ten-Tonic Pill, 671
Tested and Effective Formulas by Dong Heng, 355, 551
Testicles
    enlargement and hardening, 837
    hardening and pain, 834
    hardening of, 838
    increased weight of, 646
    pain, **53**
    pain and swelling, 836
    stimulation of, 673
    swelling and enlargement, 834
Testitis, 356, 834, **1429**
Testosterone, 646, 673, 685
Tetanus, **1429**
    mild to moderate, **155**
    overview, 963
    wind, 981, 983
Text from Heart of Jade, 760
Thallus Eckloniae, xxv
Theophylline, 720
Thermogenesis, 293
Thermogenic effect, 293
Thick body fluid, **1525**. *See also* Ye (thick body fluid)
Thin body fluid, **1513**. *See also* Jin (thin body fluid)
Thioacetamide, 629
Thirst, **1429**
    absence of, 34, 459
    blood deficiency and heat, 575
    damp-heat, 1086, 1101
    damp-warmth, 1096
    with desire to drink, 321, 325, 408
    dryness with damaged yin, 1047
    extreme, 337
    fire in the Heart channel, 365
    fire in the Spleen and Stomach, 396
    heat and fire in the upper and middle *jiaos*, 351
    heat in the upper and middle *jiaos*, 354
    heat, lingering or residual, 327
    heat-phlegm, 1214
    interior heat and toxins, 361
    Kidney yin and *jing* (essence) deficiencies, 645
    Lung heat, 96
    overview, 35, 314, 433, 1022
    qi and blood deficiencies, 580
    qi and yin deficiencies with dryness, 1050
    Spleen and Stomach qi deficiencies, 542
    Stomach heat, 398
    Stomach yin deficiency, 1043
    summer-heat, 435
    summer-heat and dampness, 441, 444
    summer-heat damaging qi and body fluids, 446
    summer-heat with damaged qi and body fluids, 554
    summer-heat with exterior cold and interior dampness, 439
    warm-dryness, 1028, 1030
    water and heat, interlocked, 1115
    wind, heat and toxins, 355

Index

yin and body fluid damage, 1054
yin deficiency with heat, 1052
yin-deficient heat, 418, 627
Thorazine. *See* Chlorpromazine
Thorough Knowledge of Medicine, 644
Thoroughfare channel, *1507*. *See also Chong* (thoroughfare)
channel
Thousand Ducat Prescriptions, 983, **1151**
Thousands of Golden Prescriptions for Emergencies, 6, 138, 169,
333, 714, 729, **1151**, 1161, 1314, 1377
Threatened miscarriage. *See* Pregnancy
Three Blockage Syndrome Decoction, 1167
Three Constructive Paste, 1244
Three Gold Decoction to Expel Stone, 1106
Three-Huang Heart-Draining Decoction, 359
Three-Marvel Pill, 1190
Three-Marvel Powder, 1190
Three-Nut Decoction, 1092
Three-Painful Obstruction Decoction, 1167
Three-Sage Powder, 1312
Three-Seed Combination, 1245
Three-Seed Decoction for Directing Qi Downward, 844
Three-Seed Decoction to Nourish One's Parents, 1245
Three-Shell Decoction to Restore the Pulse, 1011
Three-Shell Pill to Tranquilize the Spirit, 1011
Three-Substance Pill for Emergencies, 171
Three-Substance White Powder, 172
Three-Unbinding Decoction, 43
Three-Yellow and Gypsum Decoction, 361, 362
Three-Yellow Decoction to Sedate the Epigastrium, 359
Throat disorders, 829. *See also* specific disorders
cancer, 363
dry
exterior cool-dryness, 1025
exterior warm-dryness, 1028, 1030
heat in the upper and middle *jiaos*, 354
heat, fire and toxins in all three *jiaos*, 341
Liver and Kidney yin deficiencies, 654
Liver blood deficiency, 722
Lung yin and Spleen qi deficiencies, 1042
Lung yin deficiency, 1043
Lung yin deficiency with heat, 1039
overview, 513, 1022, 1206
with phlegm, 1240
Stomach yin deficiency, 1043
summer-heat with damaged qi and body fluids, 554
wind-cold turning into heat, 108
yin, damaged, 1047
yin and body fluid, damaged, 1054
yin-deficient heat, 418, 627
dry and scratchy, 388
dry and sore, 1036
dry mouth and throat, **326, 1044**
heat, 386
inflammation and pain, 401
overview, 318, 1323
with rattling sound, 80, 848
sore
damp-heat in the Spleen and Stomach, 401
damp-warmth, 1096
dryness with phlegm, 1240
fire in the Liver and Gallbladder channels, 379
heat accumulation in all three *jiaos*, 347
heat and fire in the upper and middle *jiaos*, 351
overview, 1021, 1206
Stomach heat, 393

warm-dryness, **1031**
wind, heat and toxins, 355
wind-heat, 92
wind-heat with interior heat, 291
wind-warmth, 111
yin deficiency with qi stagnation and blood dryness, 657
sore and itchy, 1226
sore and swollen, 363
strep, 386
swallowing, difficulty in, 827
swelling and pain, 160, 363, 386, 1033, 1230
swelling, inflammation and suppuration, 401
with white curd-like spots, 1033
Thromboangiitis obliterans, 494, 906, **916, 1345, 1371**
Thrombocytes, 524
Thrombocytopenic purpura, *1426*
deficiency and damage, **951**
primary, **334, 586**
qi and blood deficiencies, **581, 606**
yin-deficient heat and fire, 420
Thrombolytic effect, 869, 907
Thrombopenic purpura. *See* Thrombocytopenic purpura
Thrombophlebitis, **1327, 1345**
Thrombosis. *See also* Embolism; Anticoagulant effect; Antiplatelet
effect; Thrombolytic effect
blood stagnation, 879
cerebral, **1001**
deep vein, **908**
exterior excess with interior deficiency, 1169
iliofemoral vein, **1345**
Throwing up. *See* Nausea; Vomiting; Antiemetic effect
Thyroid disorders, 517. *See also* specific disorders
adenocarcinoma, 1353
adenoma, **630**
enlargement, 1211
thyroiditis, 1355, *1429*
tumor, 885
Ti Ren Hui Bian (Compilation of Materials of Benevolence for the
Body), 729
TIA. *See* Transient ischemic attack
Tian Dong (Radix Asparagi), xxv
Tian Jin Bai Lou Yi Yuan (Tianjin Bailou Hospital), 909
Tian Ma Gou Teng Yin **(Gastrodia and Uncaria Decoction),**
1004
Tian Ma Jiang Ya Pian **(Gastrodia Pill to Lower [Blood]**
Pressure), 1006
Tian Tai Wu Yao San **(Top-Quality Lindera Powder),** 835
vs. Ju He Wan (Tangerine Seed Pill), 835, 837
vs. Nuan Gan Jian (Warm the Liver Decoction), 835, 839
Tian Wang Bu Xin Dan **(Emperor of Heaven's Special Pill to**
Tonify the Heart), 725, 728
vs. Gan Mai Da Zao Tang (Licorice, Wheat, and Jujube
Decoction), 724
vs. Gui Pi Tang (Restore the Spleen Decoction), 587, 730
vs. Suan Zao Ren Tang (Sour Jujube Decoction), 587, 724
vs. Zhi Gan Cao Tang (Honey-Fried Licorice Decoction), 592, 730
Tianjin Bailou Hospital, 909
Tiao Jing Er Hao **(Regulate Menses Formula Two),** 568
Tiao Jing San Hao **(Regulate Menses Formula Three),** 569
Tiao Jing Si Hao **(Regulate Menses Formula Four),** 569
Tiao Jing Yi Hao **(Regulate Menses Formula One),** 568
Tiao Wei Cheng Chi Tang, 160
Tiao Wei Cheng Qi Tang **(Regulate the Stomach and Order the**
Qi Decoction), 160
vs. Da Cheng Qi Tang (Major Order the Qi Decoction), 156
vs. Xiao Cheng Qi Tang (Minor Order the Qi Decoction), 156

1606

Index

Chinese Herbal Formulas and Applications

Tidal fever, **1429**. *See also* Fever, tidal
Tie Di Wan (Iron Flute Pill), 388
Tight pulse, **1521**
Time-Tested Formulas from Shanxi Medical School, 917
Time-Tested Formulas of the Hong Family, 790, 1041
Tinea
    blood deficiency and heat, 576
    capitis, 967
    inguinal, 101
    pedis, 1342
Ting Chuen Tang, 845
***Ting Li Da Zao Xie Fei Tang* (Descurainia and Jujube Decoction to Drain the Lung)**, 384
Tinnitus, **1429**
    chronic, 877, **998**
    deficiency, 666
    fire in the Liver and Gallbladder channels, 379
    Heart and Kidney disharmony, 714
    Kidney deficiency, 633
    Kidney yin and *jing* (essence) deficiencies, 645
    Kidney yin deficiency, 644
    Liver and Kidney yin deficiencies, 627, 640
    Liver excess, 996
    Liver yang and wind rising, 999
    Liver yang rising, 1002
    Spleen and Stomach qi deficiencies, **547**
    Spleen deficiency, **552**
    yin deficiency with internal fire and wind, 661
    yin-deficient fire, 637
Tiredness. *See* Fatigue; Energy
TNF. *See* Tumor necrosis factor
Toad Venum Pill, 1351
Toes, gangrene, 1370
Tokoro Combination, 1140
Tokoro Turbidity-Clearing Drink, 1140
Tolbutamide, 214
Tong bi (extremely painful obstruction), 1153, **1522**
***Tong Feng Wan* (Wind-Pain Pill)**, 1176
Tong Jun, 3
***Tong Mai Si Ni Tang* (Unblock the Pulse Decoction for Frigid Extremities)**, 488
***Tong Qiao Huo Xue Tang* (Unblock the Orifices and Invigorate the Blood Decoction)**, 877
***Tong Ru Wan* (Unblock the Breast Pill)**, 927
Tong Su Shang Han Lun (Plain Version of Discussion of Cold-Induced Disorders), 69, 111, 137, 993, 1007, 1295
***Tong Xie Yao Fang* (Important Formula for Painful Diarrhea)**, 257
    vs. Shen Ling Bai Zhu San (Ginseng, Poria, and Atractylodes Macrocephala Powder), 260, 540, 786
    vs. Si Shen Wan (Four-Miracle Pill), 260, 540, 786
Tongue
    dry, 152, 161, 354, 554, 1030, 1052
    mirror-like, 645
    pale, 580
    pale, flabby, 668, 673
    purple, 578, 833
    red, 92, 111, 137, 228, 327, 337, 341, 351, 355, 383, 389, 393, 396, 398, 406, 408, 412, 418, 420, 435, 536, 649, 651, 710, 716, 731, 750, 802, 825, 879, 942, 947, 993, 1009, 1036, 1039, 1222, 1337, 1344, 1377,
    stiff, 694, 988
    swelling, inflammation and suppuration, 401
    ulcerations, 347, 351, 359, 365, 401, 710, 725
    yellow and dry, 398
Tonic formulas, 512

Tonic-clonic seizures, 1251
Tonify the Bone Pill, 689
Tonify the Interior Decoction with Astragalus, 1369
Tonify the Kidney Decoction, 683
Tonify the Kidney Pill, 689
Tonify the Lung Decoction, 560
Tonify the Lung Decoction with Ass-Hide Gelatin, 1039
Tonify the Lung Powder, 1039
Tonify the Lung Powder with Ass-Hide Gelatin, 1039
Tonify the Middle and Augment the Qi Decoction, 542
Tonify the Yang to Restore Five Decoction, 905
Tonifying method, 11, 512, 1322, **1506**. *See also Bu fa* (tonifying)
Tonsillitis, **1429**
    acute
        fire and toxins, **1339**
        heat and fire in the upper and middle *jiaos*, 352
        heat and toxins, **1327**
        shaoyang and *yangming* syndromes, **287**
        shaoyang syndrome, **212**
        suppurative, 109, **357**
        wind-heat, **94**
        wind-warmth, 89
        yin deficiency with heat, **1034**
    chronic, **524**
    in early or late stage, 60
    heat, 243
    heat and toxins, 103, **364**, 1364
    Lung heat, 386
    Lung yin deficiency with heat, 1039
    phlegm stagnation, 1230
    pustular, 363
    suppurative, **1381**
    unilateral or bilateral, 363
    wind-heat, 120
    yin-deficiency with wind-heat, 138
Toothache, **1429**
    blood accumulation, **875**
    damp-heat in the Spleen and Stomach, 401
    heat in the Stomach and Intestines, 160
    heat, lingering or residual, **328**
    overview, 316
    qi, blood, yang and *jing* (essence) deficiencies, 682
    Stomach heat, 393, 398
    wind-cold turning into heat, 108
    wind-cold with interior heat, 295
    wind-heat, 1332
    yin-deficient heat, 627
Top-Quality Lindera Powder, 835
Tortoise Shell and Deer Antler Paste, 687
Tortoise Shell and Deer Antler Syrup, 687
***Tou Nong San* (Discharge Pus Powder)**, 1362
Toxic uremia, 744
Toxins, **1522**
    in all three jiaos, 341
    epidemic, **1509**
    exterior heat and toxins, 363
    in the *qi* (energy) and *xue* (blood) levels, 337
    interior heat and toxins, 361, 363
Tracheitis, **1430**
    acute, 96
    chronic, 46
    damp-phlegm, 1209
    exterior cool-dryness, 1025
    qi stagnation, 828
    wind-cold and interior phlegm-heat, 845
    wind-heat, 114

INDEX

1607

Index

Tracheobronchitis, *1429*
Trachoma, 295
Tranquilize the Spirit Decoction, 733
Tranquilize the Spirit Pill, 710
Transform Blotches Decoction, 339
Transform Phlegm Pill, 1223
Transient ischemic attack, *1430*
Transport point, *1520. See also Shu* (transport) point
Trauma, *1430*
  brain, **908**
  joints, **904**
  overview, 867, 869
  qi and blood stagnation, 897, 901, 903
Traveler's diarrhea, 406, 757
Treasury Classic, 1121
Treat the Turbidity and Guard the Root Pill, 800
Treating Morbid Leukorrhea Decoction, 806
Trematode, *1294*
Tremor, *1430*
Trichomonal leukorrhea, 810
Trichosanthes and Aurantium Combination, 1233
Trichosanthes and Chih-shih Decoction, 1233
Trichosanthes Fruit and Immature Bitter Orange Decoction, 1233
Trichosanthes Fruit, Chinese Chive, and Pinellia Combination, 832
Trichosanthes Fruit, Chinese Chive, and Pinellia Decoction, 832
Trichosanthes Fruit, Chinese Chive, and Wine Decoction, 832
Trigeminal
  neuralgia, *1430*
    accumulations in the interior, 302
    damp-heat, 1192
    deficiency and cold of the Stomach, 467
    external wind, **979**, 991
    Liver yang and wind excess, 1004
    Liver yang rising, 1002
    Stomach heat, **400**
    taiyang and *shaoyang* syndromes, **221**
    wind-cold turning into heat, 108
    yin, blood and body fluid deficiencies, **600**
  pain, **976**, **1271**
Triglycerides, elevated, 209, 252, 285, 293, 572, 617, 629, 655, 669, 718, 874, 883, 1088. *See also* Cholesterols; Metabolic effect
Triple Burner Differentiation, 431, *1518. See also San Jiao bian zheng* (triple burner differentiation)
Triple Nut Combination, 1092
Troop-Marching Powder, 756
True Jade Powder, 981
True Lineage of External Medicine, 122, 244, 967, 981, 1351, 1362
True Lineage of Medicine, 779, 1190
True Man's Decoction for Nourishing the Organs, 781
True Man's Decoction to Revitalize Life, 1330
True Pearl Pill, 712
True Warrior Decoction, 1135
Tsai Hsien Tang, 226
Tsai Hu Chia Lung Ku Mu Li Tang, 715
Tsai Hu Ching Kan Tang, 243
Tsai Hu Kuei Chih Tang, 219
Tsai Ko Chieh Chi Tang, 107
Tsang Erh San, 82
Tsursure Katakura, 1348
Tu Bei Mu (Rhizoma Bolbostematis), xxv
Tu Bie Chong (Eupolyphaga seu Steleophaga), xxiv
Tu fa (vomiting), **9**, 1307, 1309, *1522*
Tu Huo Chi Sheng Tang, 1161
Tu Niu Xi (Radix Achyranthis Longifoliae), xxv

Tuberculosis
  bones, 649, 1371
  cough, 1224
  deficiency heat, 558
  heat in the *xue* (blood) level, 942
  heat-phlegm, 1226
  intestinal, 541, 784, **892**, *1430*
  peritoneal, *1431*
  peritonitis, 1272
  pleurisy, *1236*
  pulmonary, 74, 206, **417**, 420, 423, 554, 560, 644, **650**, 779, 943, 1030, **1038**, 1039, 1229, 1233, 1371, *1430*
  renal, 412, 423, 461, 649, 668, 673
  supportive treatment, **419**
  yin deficiency with heat, 1033
  yin-deficiency with wind-heat, 138
Tuhuo and Astragalus Combination, 1167
Tuhuo and Loranthus Decoction, 1161
Tuhuo and Taxillus Combination, 1161
Tumor. *See also* names and sites of specific cancers; Anticancer effect; Antineoplastic effect; Antimetastatic effect
  heat and toxins, 1325
  liver, 885
  overview, 1321
  thyroid gland, 885
  uterus, 885
Tumor necrosis factor (TNF), 76, 104, 209, 547, 564, 611
Tuo fa (draining method), 1321
Tuo Li Hsiao Tu Yin, 1367, 1368
***Tuo Li Tou Nong Tang* (Drain the Interior and Discharge Pus Decoction)**, 1363
***Tuo Li Xiao Du Yin* (Drain the Interior and Detoxify Decoction)**, 1367, 1368
Tuo zheng (abandoned syndrome), 743, *1522*
Turbidity-Curing Body-Securing Pill, 800
Twelve Types of Formulas, 12
Twenty-Four Types of Formulas, 12
Twenty-Two Types of Formulas, 13
Twitching. *See* Spasms; Cramps
Two Vintage Herbs Decoction, 1209
Two-Atractylodes Decoction, 1195
Two-Chen Decoction (Pill), 1209
Two-Cured Decoction, 1209
Two-Cured Decoction with Aurantium and Cardamon, 1212
Two-Immortal Decoction, 684
Two-Immortal Decoction to Tonify the Kidney, 686
Two-Marvel Powder, 1188
Two-Ultimate Pill, 654
Tylenol. *See* Acetaminophen
Tzu Wan Tang, 1229
Tzu Yin Chiang Huo Tang, 422
UC. *See* Ulcerative colitis
Ulcer. *See also* Duodenal ulcer; Gastric ulcer; Peptic ulcer
  duodenal ulcer, 219, 248, 271, **286**, 459, 466, 481, 484, **529**, 531, 534, 536, 584, **658**, **952**, 1068, 1099, 1134
  gastric ulcer, 219, 248, 271, 283, 390, 459, 466, 481, 484, 527, 531, 534, 576, 584, **658**, 1068
  peptic ulcer, **170**, **236**, **240**, **263**, 268, 302, **464**, **473**, **476**, **524**, **601**, **823**, **826**, 840, **852**, **888**, **1045**, **1070**, 1209, **1329**, *1424*
  perforating, **286**
Ulcerations
  chronic, 476, 479
  corneal, **606**
  external, **982**
  gum, 393
  mouth, 396

Index

mouth and tongue, 347, 351, 359, 365
oral cavity, **399**
overview, 315
qi and blood deficiencies, 479
with pus and discharge, 479
suppurative, 1357
temple area of the head, 244
tongue, 401, 710, 725
various, **918**
Ulcerative colitis, *1406*
blood stagnation, **892**
chronic, 236, 265, 297, 469, 524, 581, 1294, **1329**
damp accumulation in the Spleen and Stomach, **1070**
damp-heat, **404**
damp-heat with qi and blood stagnation, 1379, **1381**
deficiency and cold, **464**
deficiency and cold of the Stomach, **469**
heat in the Stomach and cold in the Intestines, 1292
qi deficiency, **524**
shaoyang syndrome with water accumulation, **224**
Spleen deficiency, **553**
Spleen deficiency and Liver excess, **259**
toxic heat, 408
wind, heat and toxins, 945
Ulcerative gingivitis, 393
Unblock the Breast Pill, 927
Unblock the Orifices and Invigorate the Blood Decoction, 877
Unblock the Pulse Decoction for Frigid Extremities, 488
Uncaria Decoction, 995
Uncaria Powder, 996
Unconsciousness
closed sensory orifices, 743
old phlegm and excess heat, 1238
overview, 744, 964, 1206
phlegm and heat, 750, 1251
due to stroke, 747
post-stroke, 984
sudden, 759, 1313
Uniting point, *1511*. *See also He* (uniting) point
Universal Benefit Decoction to Eliminate Toxin, 355
Universal Benefit Special Pill to Eliminate Toxin, 1096
Universal Salvation Detoxifying Drink, 355
Upper *jiao*, *1522*. *See also Jiao*, upper
Upper, Middle, and Lower General Use Pill for Wind-Pain, 1175
Upright *qi*, *1527*. *See also Zheng* (upright) *qi*
Uremia, **167**, 744, 747
Urethritis, *1431*
chronic, 800
damp-heat, **1104**
fire in the Heart channel, 365
fire in the Liver and Gallbladder, 371
fire in the Liver and Gallbladder channels, 379
heat, 1107
non-bacterial, **1141**
summer-heat and dampness, **442**, 444
water and heat, interlocked, 1115
Urgent Powder to Dilute Saliva, 1313
Urinary bladder (TCM), *1522*
damp-heat, 800
heat, 1107
Urinary disorders (WM), 518, 771, 1065, 1066, **1117**. *See also* specific disorders
Urinary tract infection, *1431*
acute, 947, **1340**
acute or chronic, **373**
blood deficiency and heat, 576

damp-heat, 800, **1104**
damp-heat accumulation, 1270
damp-heat in the lower *jiao* with Heart fire, 368
fire in the Heart and Small Intestine channels, **366**
heat accumulation in all three *jiaos*, 347
heat, fire and toxins in all three *jiaos*, 341
Kidney yin and yang deficiencies with fire, 684
Liver qi stagnation with heat, 254
overview, 318
toxic heat, **410**
water and dampness accumulation, 1109
water and heat, interlocked, 1115
yin-deficient fire, **650**
yin-deficient heat and fire, 420
Urination
difficult, 1115
damp accumulation, 1121
overview, 1064
water and dampness accumulation, 1109
wind with interior qi deficiency, 1118
yang deficiency with water accumulation, 1135
dripping, 795
frequent
with burning sensations and pain, 947
in children, 632, **794**, **795**
deficiency and cold, 795, 1140
deficiency and cold of the middle *jiao*, 471
in geriatrics, **679**
Heart and Kidney deficiencies, 792
Kidney deficiency, 789, 1050
Kidney yin and yang deficiencies with fire, 684
Liver and Kidney deficiencies, 690
post-stroke, 906
pregnancy, during, **546**
yin deficiency with heat, 1052
incontinent, *1431*
Kidney deficiency, 789
Kidney yang deficiency, **671**, 678
post-stroke, **796**
painful, 347, 1103, 1107, 1115
retention of, 1113
stones, 838, **892**, **1105**, 1116. *See also* Urolithiasis
Urine
with blood, 1107
clear, 795
cloudy, 792, 1107
dark-colored, 446
with protein, 461
red, 1103
turbid, 368, 371, 1050
white, thick, turbid, and cloudy, 1140
white, turbid, 797, 800
Urolithiasis
damp-heat, 1103
damp-heat in the lower *jiao* with Heart fire, 368
heat, 1107
interior excess heat, **155**
Kidney yang deficiency, 668
phlegm and damp accumulation, **1111**
summer-heat and dampness, **442**
water and heat, interlocked, **1116**
yang deficiency and interior cold, 481
yin, blood and body fluid deficiencies, **602**
Uroschesis, *1431*, *1522*
damp-heat, 1103
in geriatrics, **1116**

1609

Index

overview, 1064

Urticaria. *See also* Rashes; Eczema; Itching
  acute, 66
  acute or chronic, **567**
  blood deficiency and heat, 576
  chronic, 494, **573**, **972**
  damp-heat in all three *jiaos*, 359
  early stage, 1334
  exterior-deficient, wind-cold, 51
  heat and toxins, 1342
  wind, **968**
  wind, cold and dampness with qi deficiency, 124
  wind-cold, 59
  wind-cold with interior heat, 45
  wind-heat with interior heat, 291

Uterine
  adenomyosis, 929
  bleeding
    due to abortion or miscarriage, **912**, **926**
    blood deficiency, 594
    blood deficiency and heat, 576
    blood stasis, 911
    deficiency and cold, 805, **921**, 949
    excessive, **912**
    in functional disorder, **891**, **951**
    Kidney deficiency, **647**
    postpartum, 562, 625
    profuse, **586**
    qi and blood deficiencies, 580, 604, 616
    qi deficiency, 542
    Spleen deficiency, 584
    various causes, **596**
  cramps, 731
  fibroids, 928
  leiomyomas, **602**, **930**, 937
  myomas, **597**, **930**
  prolapse, 375, 542, 545, *1431*

Uterine effect, 482

Uteritis
  blood deficiency and heat, 576
  chronic, 243
  damp-heat in the lower *jiao*, 810

Uterus
  blood stasis, 805, 928
  deficiency and cold, 923
  effect on, 595, 912
  inflammation, 933
  tumor, 885

Uveitis, 331

Vaginal
  discharge
    abnormal, 536, 807
    thick, white, 584
    sticky with a foul odor, 809
    yellow, 809
  itching, 164

Vaginitis
  acute or chronic, **808**
  cervicitis, **1328**
  deficiency and cold, **922**
  fire in the Liver and Gallbladder channels, 379
  fungal, **344**
  heat and toxins, 363
  trichomonal, **344**

Valvular disease, 716

Vaporize Phlegm Pill, 1238

Varices, esophageal, 937

Varicocele, **930**

Varicose veins, **908**, **1056**

Vascular
  dementia, 997, *1431*
  headache, 881, **908**, **1001**

Vascular Citri Reticulatae, xxiv

Vasodilative effect, 1111

Vasodilatory effect, 41

Vasotec. *See* Enalapril

Veetids. *See* Penicillin

Veins, varicose, **908**, **1056**

Vepesid. *See* Etoposide

Veramyst. *See* Fluticasone

Vertigo, *1431*
  with dizziness, **597**, **1133**, **1249**
  fire in the Liver and Gallbladder channels, 379
  in geriatrics, 552
  heat-phlegm, **1215**
  Kidney yin and *jing* (essence) deficiencies, 645
  Liver and Kidney yin deficiencies, 627, 640
  Liver blood deficiency, 722
  Liver excess, 996
  Liver qi stagnation, 247
  Liver wind rising, 1008
  Liver yang and wind excess, 1004
  Liver yang and wind rising, 999
  Liver yang hyperactivity, 713
  Liver yang rising, 1002, **1006**
  Liver yang rising with phlegm accumulation, **852**
  overview, 201, 513, 514, 964, 1205, 1206
  phlegm, 1109
  phlegm retention with yang deficiency, **1131**
  severe, 996
  shaoyang syndrome, 206
  wind, 973
  wind and phlegm rising, **855**, 1247
  wind-heat with interior heat, 291
  yin deficiency, **414**
  yin deficiency with internal fire and wind, 661

Vesical calculus, 668, 673

Vesiculitis, seminal, 367

Vessel and Vehicle Pill, 184

Viral. *See also* specific disease; Antiviral effect
  hepatitis, **1339**
  infection, **1056**
  myocarditis, **556**, **591**, **1221**

Virus. *See* specific virus; Antiviral effect

Vision
  blurred, *1432*
    blood deficiency, 562
    deficiency, 551
    Heart and Kidney disharmony, 714
    Liver and Kidney deficiencies, 633
    Liver and Kidney yin deficiencies, 627, 640, 641, 654
    Liver fire rising with underlying qi, blood and yin deficiencies, 663
    overview, 513
    qi, blood and yin deficiencies, 665
    yin deficiency, 634
    yin deficiency with internal fire and wind, 661
    yin, yang, blood and *jing* (essence) deficiencies, 687
  compromised functions, 551

Vitiligo, 877

Vitreous opacity, **641**

Vladimiria and Cardamon Combination, 531

Index

Chinese Herbal Formulas and Applications

VLDL (very low-density lipoprotein). *See* Cholesterols
Vocal cord nodule, **1354**
Voice
    hoarse, 124, 388, 750
    loss of, 388, *1418*
    low, 522
    low and weak, 560
Volume, *1439*
Vomiting, *1432*. *See also* Nausea; Morning sickness; Antiemetic effect
    alcohol intoxication, 1085
    cancer of the gastrointestinal tract, **469**
    chemotherapy-induced, 855
    continuous, 283
    damp accumulation, 1068, 1072, 1076, 1082
    damp-heat, 1085, 1101
    damp-phlegm, 1209
    damp-warmth, 1096
    deficiency and cold, 459, 463
    deficiency and cold of the Stomach, 467
    deficiency and cold with qi stagnation, 484
    excessive, 1099
    food stagnation, 1266
    gastrointestinal infection, 761
    hands and feet, extremely cold, 467
    heat-phlegm, 1214
    Liver fire overacting on the Stomach, 389
    motion sickness, 270
    with nausea, **545, 852, 857**
    neurogenic, 854
    overview, 201, 202, 455, 456, 819, 820, 1021, 1063, 1064, 1205, 1206, 1263
    with pain, 1212
    phlegm stagnation and water accumulation, 1220
    postpartum, 625
    post-surgical, 854
    during pregnancy, 213, 264, 529, 533, 621, 844, 852, 853, 1044, 1056, 1221, *1433*
    qi deficiency with cold and dampness, 531
    qi deficiency with dampness, 535
    qi deficiency with dampness and phlegm, 527
    qi flow, reversed, 854, 855, 856
    qi stagnation, 822
    roundworms, 1292
    saliva, 467, 1109
    shaoyang and *yangming* syndromes, 283
    shaoyin syndrome, 467, 486
    Spleen and Stomach deficiencies, 541
    Spleen and Stomach disharmony, 1074
    Stomach deficiency and interlocking of heat and cold, 270
    Stomach qi disharmony, 261
    Stomach yin deficiency, 1043
    stubborn, **1044**
    summer-heat and dampness, 444
    summer-heat with exterior cold and interior dampness, 436
    wind and phlegm rising, 1247
    wind-cold and interior dampness, 1079
    yang deficiency and interior cold, 481
    yang deficiency with excess cold, 491
Vomiting method, 9, 1307, 1309, *1522*. *See also Tu fa* (vomiting)
Wai Ke Fa Hui (External Medicine Elaboration), 1369
Wai Ke Zheng Zhi Quan Sheng Ji (Complete Collection of Patterns and Treatments in External Medicine), 1350, 1351, 1370, 1374
Wai Ke Zheng Zhi Zhun Sheng (Standards of Patterns and Treatments in External Medicine), 361, **1061**
Wai Ke Zheng Zong (True Lineage of External Medicine), 122, 244, 967, 981, 1351, 1362

Wai Tai Mi Yao (Arcane Essentials from the Imperial Library), 6, 135, 299, 341, 752, 847, **961**, 986
Waist pain, 494, 893
Wan bi (stubborn painful obstruction), 1153, *1522*
Wan Bing Hui Chun (Restoration of Health from the Myriad Diseases), 120, 178, 241, 349, 381, 388, 422, 534, 540, 575, 624, 664, 666, 1073, 1127, 1169, 1171, 1195, 1212, 1217, 1225, 1233, 1295, **1319**, 1336, 1357, 1360, 1365, 1368
Wan Dai Tang (End Discharge Decoction), 806
    vs. *Long Dan Xie Gan Tang* (Gentiana Decoction to Drain the Liver), 809
    vs. *Qing Dai Tang* (Clear the Discharge Decoction), 809
    vs. *Yi Huang Tang* (Change the Yellow [Discharge] Decoction), 809
Wan ji (pill), 16
Wan Quan, 748
Wan Shi-Xiong, 756, 1099, 1101
Wan Tai Tang, 806
Wang Ang, 13, 85, 104, 371, 479, 533, 653, 654, 656, 663, 672, 690, 789, 800, 976, 985, 1036, 1084, 1141, 1224, 1229, 1268, 1330, 1367
Wang Hao-Gu, 64, 66
Wang Huai-Yin, 6
Wang Ken-Tang, 354, 361, 386, 402, 418, 438, 578, 784, **1061**, 1129, 1212, 1216, 1277, 1373, 1383, 1481, 1483, 1484
Wang Lun, 462
Wang Meng-Ying, 7, 335, 446
Wang Qing-Ren, **865**, 877, 879, 885, 889, 893, 905, 1481, 1483, 1484
Wang San-Cai, 687, 850
Wang Shu-He, **453**, 1481, 1482, 1484
Wang Tao, 6, 135, 299, 341, 752, 847, **961**, 986, 1481, 1482, 1484
Wang Wei-De, 1350, 1351, 1370, 1374
Warm disease, 92, 311, 431, *1523*. *See also Wen bing* (warm disease)
Warm epidemics, 199, 337, 340, *1522*
Warm the Channels and Stop Pain Decoction, 913
Warm the Channels Decoction, 919
Warm the Gallbladder Decoction, 1213
Warm the Liver Decoction, 838
Warm the Menses Decoction, 919
Warm the Spleen Decoction, 169
Warming, *1523*. *See also Wen fa* (warming)
Warming and Clearing Decoction, 575, 577
Warming and Clearing Drink, 575
Warming and Clearing Powder, 575
Warming method, **10**, 281, 455, 743
Warmth, 314. *See also* Heat; Fire
Warp and Woof of Warm-Febrile Diseases, 7, 335, 446
Warts, 43
Wash, *1524*. *See also Xi* (wash)
Wash the Liver and Brighten the Eyes Powder, 381
Wasting and thirsting, 398, 538, 627, 1021, 1022, 1050, 1052, *1394*, *1524*. *See also Xiao ke* (wasting and thirsting)
Wasting and Thirsting Formula, 1051
Water, *1522*. *See also* Edema; Ascites; specific conditions
    accumulation
        excess, 181
        heat formation and qi stagnation, 184
        in the upper *jiao*, 1125
        severe, 1129
        shaoyang syndrome, 304
        Spleen and Kidney yang deficiencies, 1135
    water and damp accumulation, 186, 1109
Water and Earth Two Immortals Special Pill, 790
Water and fluid stagnation, *1522*
Weak pulse, *1522*

Index

Weakness
    atrophy of the bones and tendons, 651
    generalized, 682, 725
    legs, 1188
    lower back and knees, 678
    overview, 512
    qi and blood deficiencies, 615
    water accumulation, 1124
Wei (atrophy) syndrome, *1522*
Wei (defensive) level, 51, 92, 798, *1522*
Wei (defensive) *qi*, 773, *1523*
Wei (roast), *1523*
Wei bi (atrophic painful obstruction), 1064, 1153, 1180, *1523*
Wei Jing Tang (Reed Decoction), 1377
Wei Ling Tang (Calm the Stomach and Poria Decoction), 1113
    vs. Si Ling San (Four-Ingredient Powder with Poria), 1112
    vs. Wu Ling San (Five-Ingredient Powder with Poria), 1112
    vs. Yin Chen Wu Ling San (Artemisia Scoparia and Five-Ingredient Powder with Poria), 1112
Wei Ling Xian (Radix et Rhizoma Clematidis), xxv
Wei Qi Ying Xue Bian Zheng (Defensive, Qi, Nutritive, Blood Differentiation), 311, 431, *1523*
Wei Rui Tang (Polygonatum Odoratum Decoction), 138
Wei Sheng Bao Jian (Precious Mirror of Health), 416, 557, 1089
Wei Yi-Lin, 176, 728
Wei zheng (atrophy syndrome), *1394*
Wei Zhi, 525
Wei Zhi-Xiu, 657, 1096
Weight loss, 687
Weights, *1439*
Weights and measurements, 22
Weiling Decoction, 1113
Well point, *1513*. *See also Jing* (well) point
Wen bing (warm disease), 92, 311, 431, 750, *1523*
Wen Bing Tiao Bian (Systematic Differentiation of Warm Disease), 7, 89, 92, 94, 189, 190, 330, 339, 412, **431**, 435, 439, 591, 746, 856, 1009, 1011, 1025, 1027, 1029, 1047, 1054, 1092, 1095
Wen Ching Tang, 919
Wen Ching Yin (Warming and Clearing Drink), 575
Wen Dan Tang (Warm the Gallbladder Decoction), 1213
Wen fa (warming), **10**, 281, 455, 743, *1523*
Wen huo (civilian fire), 19
Wen Jing Tang (Warm the Channels Decoction), 919
    vs. Ai Fu Nuan Gong Wan (Mugwort and Cyperus Pill for Warming the Womb), 924
Wen Jing Zhi Tong Tang (Warm the Channels and Stop Pain Decoction), 913
Wen Pi Tang (Warm the Spleen Decoction), 169
    vs. Da Huang Fu Zi Tang (Rhubarb and Prepared Aconite Decoction), 168, 170
    vs. San Wu Bei Ji Wan (Three-Substance Pill for Emergencies), 168
Wen Qing San (Warming and Clearing Powder), 575
Wen Qing Yin (Warming and Clearing Decoction), 575, 577
Wen Re Jing Wei (Warp and Woof of Warm-Febrile Diseases), 7, 335, 446
Wen Re Lun (Discussion of Warm and Hot Disorders), 311
Wen Sheng, 254, 256
Wen Tan Tang, 1213
Wen yi (warm epidemics), 199, 337, 340
Wen Yi Lun (Discussion of Epidemic Warm Disease), 192, **199**, 231
Wheezing. *See also* Dyspnea; Asthma
    in children, **1048**
    cold and phlegm, 1244
    with cough, **844**
    deficiency heat, 558

exterior-excess, wind-cold, 39
Kidney yin deficiency, 644
Liver qi stagnation, 849
Lung and Kidney deficiencies, 559
Lung heat with phlegm accumulation, 1232
Lung qi deficiency, 560
Lung yin deficiency with heat, 1039
overview, 36, 820, 1022, 1205
phlegm retention and qi stagnation, 1245
qi and phlegm stagnation, 848
in summer, **447**
in tracheitis, **46**
upper excess and lower deficiency, 842
water and damp accumulation, 186
wind-cold and interior phlegm-heat, 845
wind-cold attacking the Lung, 48, 49
wind-cold with water accumulation, 74
wind-heat, 114
Wheezing and dyspnea, **77**, *1432*, *1523*
Whiplash. *See* Neck
White blood cells, 478, 524, 555, 629, 655
White Penetrating Decoction, 489
White Powder, 172
White Tiger Decoction, 321
White Tiger plus Atractylodes Decoction, 324
White Tiger plus Cinnamon Twig Decoction, 323
White Tiger plus Ginseng Decoction, 325
White-Draining Formula, 383
Whooping cough
    heat, 115
    heat and fire in the upper and middle *jiaos*, 351
    Lung heat, **98**, **384**
    phlegm retention, 80
    summer-heat and dampness, **442**
    warm-dryness, 1028
    wind, **117**
    wind-cold with water accumulation, 74
Wide-Ranging Medical Notes from the First-Awakened Studio, 106, 1278
Will-power, 707, *1527*. *See also Zhi* (will-power)
Wind, *1523*
    external, 963
    internal, 964
    overview, 963
    wind-cold
        attacking the Lung, 48
        in children, 70
        exterior excess, 39
        exterior, 72
        exterior-deficient, 51
        five accumulations in the interior, 301
        interior deficiency and cold, 466
        interior heat, 45, 295
        Lung dysfunction, 49
        overview, **34**
        qi stagnation, 67
        taiyang syndrome, 59
        tan yin (phlegm retention), 128
        turning into heat, 108
        water accumulation, 74
        yang qi deficiency, 131
        yin and blood deficiencies, 136
    wind-damp, *1510*. *See also Feng shi* (wind-damp)
        cold, and dampness and pain, 1154
        damp-cold, 1154
        damp-heat, 1154

1612

Index

Chinese Herbal Formulas and Applications

damp-phlegm, 1154
  with deficiency, 1158
  exterior, 1156
  overview, 1153
  wind, cold and dampness, 1154
wind-heat
  attacking the eyes, 381
  attacking the upper *jiao*, 120
  exterior, 114
  with interior heat, 291
  overview, 35
  with yin deficiency, 137
wind-warmth, 89, 111
Wind, aversion to
  exterior wind with water accumulation, 101
  exterior-deficient, wind-cold, 51
  overview, 35
  wei (defensive) *qi* deficiency, 773
  wind-cold, 59
  wind-heat, 92
  wind-heat with yin deficiency, 137
  wind-warmth, 111
Wind consumption disease, 416, *1510*. *See also Feng lao bing*
  (wind consumption disease)
Wind rash, *1523*
Wind stroke, 977, 988, 991, 1177, 1309, 1312, 1313, *1395*, *1527*.
  See also Zhong feng (wind stroke)
Wind water syndrome, 1118, *1510*. *See also Feng shui* (wind water)
Wind-damp dispelling formulas, 1153
Wind-Dispelling Formula, 967
Wind-Dispelling Powder, 967
Wind-expelling formulas, 963
Wind-Pain Pill, 1176
Wiry pulse, *1523*
Wolfberry, Chrysanthemum and Rehmannia Pill, 640
Women's Diseases According to Fu Qing-Zhu, 621, **767**, 806,
  809, 925
Wondrous Lantern for Peering into Origin and Development of
  Miscellaneous Diseases, 723, 1052
Wood, *1524*
Worrying, excessive, 583, 722
Wounds, delayed healing, 476, 580
Wrist pain, 1195
Wu Chi San, 301, 303
Wu Chu Yu Tang, 467
Wu Hu Zhui Feng San (Five-Tiger Powder to Pursue Wind), 982
Wu huo (military fire), 19
Wu Ji Pill, 391
Wu Ji San (Five-Accumulation Powder), 301, 303
Wu Ji Wan (Wu Ji Pill), 391
Wu Ju-Tong, 7, 89, 92, 94, 189, 190, 330, 339, 412, **430**, 435, 439,
  591, 746, 856, 1009, 1011, 1025, 1027, 1029, 1047, 1054, 1092,
  1095, 1481, 1483, 1484. *See also* Wu Tang
Wu Kun, 1083, 1222
Wu Lin San (Five-Ingredient Powder for Painful Urinary
  Dysfunction), 1107
  vs. Ba Zheng San (Eight-Herb Powder for Rectification), 1108
  vs. Wu Ling San (Five-Ingredient Powder with Poria), 1108
Wu Ling San (Five-Ingredient Powder with Poria), 1109
  vs. Si Ling San (Four-Ingredient Powder with Poria), 1112
  vs. Wei Ling Tang (Calm the Stomach and Poria Decoction), 1112
  vs. Wu Lin San (Five-Ingredient Powder for Painful Urinary
    Dysfunction), 1108
  vs. Yin Chen Wu Ling San (Artemisia Scoparia and Five-Ingredient
    Powder with Poria), 1112
  vs. Zhu Ling Tang (Polyporus Decoction), 1117

Wu Ling Zhi (Faeces Trogopteri), xxvi
Wu Long Cha (Folium Camelliae Fermentata), xxvi
Wu Mei Wan (Mume Pill), 1292
Wu Mo Yin Zi (Five Milled-Herbs Decoction), 850
Wu Pi San (Five-Peel Powder), 1121, 1123
Wu Pi Yin, 1121
Wu Qian, 70, 105, 294, 567, 571, 636, 901, 995, 1075, 1298, 1337,
  1352, 1363
Wu Qin Xi (Five Animal Frolics), 741
Wu Quan, 760
Wu Ren Wan (Five-Seed Pill), 176
Wu Shang-Xian, 1391, 1481, 1483, 1484
Wu Shen Tang (Five-Miracle Decoction), 1347
Wu Shi Er Bing Fang (Prescriptions for Fifty-Two Kinds of
  Diseases), 5
Wu shu (five transport) points, *1524*
Wu Tang, **431**, 1481, 1483, 1484. *See also* Wu Ju-Tong
Wu Wei Xiao Du Yin (Five-Ingredient Decoction to Eliminate
  Toxins), 1337
Wu xin re (five-center heat), 316, 513, *1394*, *1524*
Wu Yao Chun Chi San, 990
Wu Yao Shun Chi San, 990
Wu Yao Shun Qi San (Lindera Powder to Smooth the Flow of
  Qi), 990
Wu You-Ke, **198**, 1481, 1483, 1484. *See also* Wu You-Xing
Wu You-Xing, 192, **199**, 231, 1481, 1483, 1484. *See also* Wu You-Ke
Wu Zhi-Wang, 931
Wu Zhu Yu Tang (Evodia Decoction), 467
  vs. Li Zhong Wan (Regulate the Middle Pill), 470
Xanthium Formula, 82
Xanthium Powder, 82
Xi (cleft) point, *1524*
Xi (wash), *1524*
Xi Gan Ming Mu San (Wash the Liver and Brighten the Eyes
  Powder), 381
  vs. Ming Mu Di Huang Wan (Improve Vision Pill with
    Rehmannia), 382
Xi Hong Hua (Stigma Croci), xxvi
Xi Huang Wan (Cattle Gallstone Pill), 1350
Xi Jiao Di Huang Tang (Rhinoceros Horn and Rehmannia
  Decoction), 333
  vs. Qing Ying Tang (Clear the Nutritive Level Decoction), 336
Xi Tong Fang Er Hao (Knee Pain Formula Two), 1165
Xi Tong Fang Yi Hao (Knee Pain Formula One), 1165
Xi Xin (Radix et Rhizoma Asari), xxvi
Xia fa (draining downward), **10**, 149, 281, 1307, *1524*
Xia Yu Xue Tang (Drain Blood Stasis Decoction), 876
Xian Fang Huo Ming Yin (Sublime Formula for Sustaining
  Life), 1325
  vs. Pu Ji Xiao Du Yin (Universal Benefit Decoction to
    Eliminate Toxin), 358, 1331
Xian jian (pre-decoction), 20
Xian Shou Li Shang Xu Duan Mi Fang (Secret Recipes for Treating
  Wounds and Bone-Setting Taught by Celestials), 301
Xian Xing Zhai Yi Xue Guang Bi Ji (Wide-Ranging Medical Notes
  from the First-Awakened Studio), 106, 1278
Xiang Fu Wan (Cyperus Pill), 824
Xiang Jia Pi (Cortex Periplocae), xxiii
Xiang Lian Wan (Aucklandia and Coptis Pill), 391
Xiang Ru (Herba Moslae), xxvi
Xiang Ru San (Mosla Powder), 436
  vs. Xin Jia Xiang Ru Yin (Newly-Augmented Mosla
    Decoction), 440
Xiang Ru Yin, 436
Xiang Sha Liu Jun Zi Tang (Six-Gentlemen Decoction with
  Cyperus and Amomum), 533

1613

Index

Xiang Sha Liu Jun Zi Tang (Six-Gentlemen Decoction with Aucklandia and Amomum), 531

Xiang Sha Ping Wei San (Cyperus and Amomum Powder to Calm the Stomach), 1073, 1075

Xiang Sha Yang Wei Tang (Nourish the Stomach Decoction with Aucklandia and Amomum), 534

Xiang Sha Zhi Zhu Wan (Aucklandia, Amomum, Immature Bitter Orange, and Atractylodes Macrocephala Pill), 1276

Xiang Sheng Po Di San (Loud Sound Powder for a Broken Flute), 388

Xiang Sheng Po Di Wan, 388

Xiang Su Cong Chi Tang (Cyperus, Perilla Leaf, Scallion, and Prepared Soybean Decoction), 69

Xiang Su San (Cyperus and Perilla Leaf Powder), 67

Xiao Ban Xia Jia Fu Ling Tang (Minor Pinellia and Poria Decoction), 1220

Xiao Chai Hu Tang (Minor Bupleurum Decoction), 206
   vs. Da Chai Hu Tang (Major Bupleurum Decoction), 216, 288
   vs. Hao Qin Qing Dan Tang (Artemisia Annua and Scutellaria Decoction to Clear the Gallbladder), 217, 229
   vs. Xiao Yao San (Rambling Powder), 216

Xiao Cheng Qi Tang (Minor Order the Qi Decoction), 158
   vs. Da Cheng Qi Tang (Major Order the Qi Decoction), 156
   vs. Ma Zi Ren Wan (Hemp Seed Pill), 176
   vs. Tiao Wei Cheng Qi Tang (Regulate the Stomach and Order the Qi Decoction), 156

Xiao Ching Long Tang, 74

Xiao Ding Feng Zhu (Minor Arrest Wind Pearl), 1011

Xiao Er Hui Chun Dan (Return of Spring Special Pill [Pediatric]), 754

Xiao Er Yao Zheng Zhi Jue (Craft of Medicinal Treatment for Childhood Disease Patterns), 7, 103, 124, 365, 376, 383, 396, **509**, 525, 539, 627, 1039

Xiao fa (reducing method), **10**, 1263, 1321, *1524*

Xiao Feng San (Eliminate Wind Powder), 967
   vs. Dang Gui Yin Zi (Tangkuei Decoction), 972

Xiao Huo Luo Dan (Minor Invigorate the Collaterals Special Pill), 1177

Xiao Ji (Herba Cirsii), xxvi

Xiao Ji Yin Zi (Cirsium Decoction), 946

Xiao Jian Zhong Tang (Minor Construct the Middle Decoction), 471
   vs. Da Jian Zhong Tang (Major Construct the Middle Decoction), 474, 483
   vs. Dang Gui Jian Zhong Tang (Tangkuei Decoction to Construct the Middle), 474
   vs. Gui Qi Jian Zhong Tang (Tangkuei and Astragalus Decoction to Construct the Middle), 480
   vs. Gui Zhi Tang (Cinnamon Twig Decoction), 58, 474
   vs. Huang Qi Jian Zhong Tang (Astragalus Decoction to Construct the Middle), 474
   vs. Li Zhong Wan (Regulate the Middle Pill), 474

Xiao Jian Zhung Tang, 471

Xiao Jin Dan (Minor Gold Special Pill), 1374
   vs. Yang He Tang (Yang-Heartening Decoction), 1376

Xiao ke (wasting and thirsting), *1394*, *1524*. See also Diabetes mellitus
   Kidney yang deficiency, 668, 673
   overview, 1021, 1022
   qi and yin deficiencies with dryness, 1050
   Spleen and Stomach deficiencies with damp accumulation, **538**
   with excess hunger, 398
   yin deficiency with heat, 627, 1052

Xiao Ke Fang (Wasting and Thirsting Formula), 1051

Xiao Luo Wan (Reduce Scrofula Pill), 1355

Xiao Qing Long Jia Shi Gao Tang (Minor Bluegreen Dragon Decoction plus Gypsum), 78

Xiao Qing Long Tang (Minor Bluegreen Dragon Decoction), 74
   vs. Da Qing Long Tang (Major Bluegreen Dragon Decoction), 79
   vs. Ma Huang Tang (Ephedra Decoction), 79
   vs. She Gan Ma Huang Tang (Belamcanda and Ephedra Decoction), 82

Xiao San Tang Er Hao (Dissolve and Disperse Decoction Formula Two), 1359

Xiao San Tang Yi Hao (Dissolve and Disperse Decoction Formula One), 1359

Xiao Xian Xiong Tang (Minor Sinking into the Chest Decoction), 1235
   vs. Da Xian Xiong Tang (Major Sinking into the Chest Decoction), 163, 1237

Xiao Xu Ming Tang (Minor Prolong Life Decoction), 983, 985
   vs. Xu Ming Tang (Prolong Life Decoction), 987

Xiao Yao San (Rambling Powder), 247
   vs. Chai Hu Shu Gan San (Bupleurum Powder to Spread the Liver), 253
   vs. Si Ni San (Frigid Extremities Powder), 253
   vs. Xiao Chai Hu Tang (Minor Bupleurum Decoction), 216
   vs. Yi Guan Jian (Linking Decoction), 253, 660

Xie Bai San (Drain the White Powder), 383
   vs. Ma Huang Xing Ren Gan Cao Shi Gao Tang (Ephedra, Apricot Kernel, Licorice, and Gypsum Decoction), 100, 385

Xie Fei San, 383

Xie Huang San (Drain the Yellow Powder), 396
   vs. Qing Wei San (Clear the Stomach Powder), 395
   vs. Yu Nu Jian (Jade Woman Decoction), 395

Xie Pi San (Drain the Spleen Powder), 396

Xie Qing Wan (Drain the Green Pill), 376
   vs. Dang Gui Long Hui Wan (Tangkuei, Gentiana, and Aloe Pill), 377
   vs. Long Dan Xie Gan Tang (Gentiana Decoction to Drain the Liver), 377

Xie Xin Tang (Drain the Epigastrium Decoction), 359

Xie Yuan-Qing, 841, 903

Xin Jia Huang Long Tang (Newly-Augmented Yellow Dragon Decoction), 189

Xin Jia Xiang Ru Yin (Newly-Augmented Mosla Decoction), 439
   vs. Xiang Ru San (Mosla Powder), 440

Xin Yi Ching Fei Tang, 122

Xin Yi Qing Fei Yin (Magnolia Decoction to Clear the Lung), 122

Xin Yi San (Magnolia Flower Powder), 84, 85
   vs. Cang Er Zi San (Xanthium Powder), 88
   vs. Qing Bi Tang (Clear the Nose Decoction), 88

Xin Zhi Ju Pi Zhu Ru Tang (Newly-Formulated Tangerine Peel and Bamboo Shaving Decoction), 856

Xing bi (mobile painful obstruction), 1153, *1524*

Xing Jun San (Troop-Marching Powder), 756

Xing Su San (Apricot Kernel and Perilla Leaf Powder), 1025
   vs. Qing Zao Jiu Fei Tang (Eliminate Dryness and Rescue the Lung Decoction), 1027
   vs. Sang Xing Tang (Mulberry Leaf and Apricot Kernel Decoction), 1027, 1029

Xing Su Yin (Apricot Kernel and Perilla Leaf Decoction), 70

Xing Xiao Wan (Awake and Disperse Pill), 1351

Xiong bi (painful obstruction of the chest), **133**, 831, 832, **899**, *1395*, *1524*. See also Angina

Xiong Gui Bu Xue Tang (Cnidium and Tangkuei Decoction to Tonify Blood), 624

Xiong Gui Jiao Ai Tang, 950

Xiong Gui Tiao Xue Yin (Cnidium and Tangkuei Decoction to Regulate Blood), 624

Xiong Zhu Wan (Cyperus and Atractylodes Pill), 822

Xu Chang Qing (Radix et Rhizoma Cynanchi Paniculati), xxvi

Index

Xu Da-Chun, 1179
Xu lao (deficiency and debilitation), **1395**
Xu Ming Tang (Prolong Life Decoction), 986
   vs. Xiao Xu Ming Tang (Minor Prolong Life Decoction), 987
Xu Ming Yi Lei An (Continuation of Famous Physicians' Cases
   Organized by Categories), 1096
Xu Shu-Wei, 712, 944, 996
Xu Si-He, 12
Xu Zhi-Cai, 12
Xuan Du Fa Biao Tang (Dissipate Toxins and Release the
   Exterior Decoction), 104
Xuan Fu Dai Zhe Shi Tang (Inula and Hematite Decoction), 851
   vs. Ding Xiang Shi Di Tang (Clove and Persimmon Calyx
     Decoction), 853
   vs. Ju Pi Zhu Ru Tang (Tangerine Peel and Bamboo Shaving
     Decoction), 853
Xuan Ming Fen (Natrii Sulfas Exsiccatus), xxvi
Xuan Ming Lun Fang (Discussion of Dispersing and Brightening
   Formulas), 7, **279**, 442
Xuan yin (pleural effusion), 181, **1524**
Xue (blood) level, 333, 939, 942, **1524**
Xue bi (blood painful obstruction), 500, 1153, **1525**
Xue Fu Zhu Yu Tang (Drive Out Stasis in the Mansion of Blood
   Decoction), 879
   vs. Ge Xia Zhu Yu Tang (Drive Out Blood Stasis Below the
     Diaphragm Decoction), 884
   vs. Shao Fu Zhu Yu Tang (Drive Out Blood Stasis in the Lower
     Abdomen Decoction), 884
   vs. Shen Tong Zhu Yu Tang (Drive Out Blood Stasis from a
     Painful Body Decoction), 884
Xue Kai, 245
Xue lin (bloody dysuria), 947, 1103, 1107, 1115, **1525**
Xue Yi, 1369
Xue yu (blood stasis), **1395**
Ya (press), **1525**
Yan (drown), **1525**
Yan (grind), **1525**
Yan Fang Xin Bian (New Compilation of Time-Tested Formulas),
   1344
Yan Hong-Zhi, 1095
Yan Hu Er Hao (Corydalis Formula Two), 826
Yan Hu Suo San (Corydalis Powder), 826
Yan Hu Yi Hao (Corydalis Formula One), 826
Yan Tang Tan Tu Fang (Salt Decoction to Induce Vomiting),
   1314
Yan Yong-He, 82, 84, 185, 231, 559, 583, 671, 675, 826, 833, 849,
   855, 858, 1211
Yang, **1525**
   deficiency, 512
   deficiency in the middle *jiao*, 481
   deficiency, extreme, 491
   depletion, 486
   qi, blood and yang deficiencies, 609
Yang (melt), **1525**
Yang He Tang (Yang-Heartening Decoction), 1370
   vs. Xiao Jin Dan (Minor Gold Special Pill), 1376
Yang Hsin Tang, 735
Yang Ke Xin De Ji (Collection of Personal Expertise Concerning
   Skin Lesions), 1332, 1340
Yang Nourishing Five Returning Decoction, 905
Yang Shi Jia Zang Fang (Collected Formulas of the Yang Family),
   977
Yang Shi Mi Fang (Secret Formulas of the Yang Family), 681
Yang Tan, 977
Yang Tu-Ying, 735, 923
Yang Xin Dan (Nourish the Heart Pill), 729

Yang Xin Tang (Nourish the Heart Decoction), 735
Yang Yin Qing Fei Tang (Nourish the Yin and Clear the Lung
   Decoction), 1033
   vs. Bai He Gu Jin Tang (Lily Bulb Decoction to Preserve the
     Metal), 1035
Yang Ying Tang, 615
Yang-Heartening Decoction, 1370
Yangming, **1525**
   fu (hollow organ) syndrome, 152, 158, 160, 187, 189, 190, 1054
   jing (channel) syndrome, 321, 325
   mild, 94
   qi (energy) level, 321
   qi (energy) level with qi and body fluid deficiencies, 325
   with *shaoyang* syndrome, 283
   with *taiyang* syndromes, 289
Yangqiao (movement) channel, **1525**
Yangwei (linking) channel, **1525**
Yao lu (distillation), 18
Yao Tong Fang Er Hao (Low Back Pain Formula Two), 1164
Yao Tong Fang Yi Hao (Low Back Pain Formula One), 1164
Ye (thick body fluid), **1525**
Ye Gui, 311, 1481, 1483, 1484. *See also* Ye Tian-Shi
Ye Ming Sha (Faeces Vespertilionis Murini), xxvi
Ye Tian-Shi, **311**, 1481, 1483, 1484. *See also* Ye Gui
Yellow Dragon Decoction, 187
Yellow Earth Decoction, 948
Yellow Emperor, 3, 1481, 1482, 1484
Yellow Emperor's Inner Classic, 3, 5
Yi (intellect), **1525**
Yi Bian (Ordinary Medicine), 687, 850
Yi Chi Cong Ming Tang, 551
Yi Fang Ji Jie (Analytical Collection of Medical Formulas), 13, 85,
   104, 371, 479, 533, 653, 654, 656, 663, 672, 690, 789, 800, 976,
   985, 1036, 1084, 1141, 1224, 1229, 1268, 1330, 1367
Yi Fang Kao (Investigation of Medical Formulas), 1083, 1222
Yi Gan San (Restrain the Liver Powder), 245
Yi Gong San (Extraordinary Merit Powder), 525
Yi Guan (Thorough Knowledge of Medicine), 644
Yi Guan Jian (Linking Decoction), 657
   vs. Liu Wei Di Huang Wan (Six-Ingredient Pill with
     Rehmannia), 634
   vs. Si Ni San (Frigid Extremities Powder), 237, 660
   vs. Xiao Yao San (Rambling Powder), 253, 660
Yi Guan Tang (Linking Clinic), 243
Yi Huang Tang (Change the Yellow [Discharge] Decoction), 809
   vs. Qing Dai Tang (Clear the Discharge Decoction), 809
   vs. Wan Dai Tang (End Discharge Decoction), 809
Yi Ji (Levels of Medicine), 640, 642
Yi Lin Gai Cuo (Corrections of Errors Among Physicians), **865**,
   877, 879, 885, 889, 893, 905
Yi Lue Liu Shu (Six Texts on the Essentials of Medicine), 252
Yi Men Fa Lu (Precepts for Physicians), 1029
Yi Qi Cong Ming Tang (Augment the Qi and Increase Acuity
   Decoction), 551
Yi Tang (Maltosum), xxvi
Yi Word Decoction, 164
Yi Xue Fa Ming (Medical Innovations), 710, 835, 897
Yi Xue Qi Yuan (Origins of the Medicine), 1193
Yi Xue Quan Shu (Complete Book of Medicine), 12
Yi Xue Ru Men (Introduction to Medicine), 802, 1276, 1361
Yi Xue Xin Wu (Medical Revelations), 69, 110, 116, 711, 1040,
   1142, 1240, 1247, 1251, 1253, 1355
Yi Xue Zheng Zhuan (True Lineage of Medicine), 779, 1190
Yi Xue Zhong Zhong Can Xi Lu (Records of Heart-Felt
   Experiences in Medicine with Reference to the West), 549,
   803, 809, 914, 999, 1002, 1049

Index

Yi Yi Fu Zi Bai Jiang San (Coicis, Prepared Aconite, and Patrinia Powder), 1382
  vs. Da Huang Mu Dan Tang (Rhubarb and Moutan Decoction), 1384
Yi Yi Ren Tang (Coicis Decoction), 1173, 1383
Yi Yuan San (Benefit the Basal Powder), 443
Yi Zhen Yi De (Achievements Regarding Epidemic Rashes), 7, 337
Yi Zhi (Fructus Alpiniae Oxyphyllae), xxvi
Yi Zi Tang (Yi Word Decoction), 164
Yi Zong Jin Jian (Golden Mirror of the Medical Tradition), 70, 105, 294, 567, 571, 636, 901, 995, 1075, 1298, 1337, 1352, 1363
Yin, *1526*
  deficiency, 512
  deficiency with fire, 422
  Liver and Kidney yin deficiencies, 627, 640, 643
  Lung and Kidney yin deficiencies, 1036
  yin-deficient fire, 637
  yin-deficient heat, 627
Yin (invisible phlegm), 1205, *1526*
Yin Chen (Herba Artemisiae Scopariae), xxvi
Yin Chen Hao Tang (Artemisia Scoparia Decoction), 1086
  vs. Yin Chen Wu Ling San (Artemisia Scoparia and Five-Ingredient Powder with Poria), 1091
  vs. Zhi Zi Bai Pi Tang (Gardenia and Phellodendron Decoction), 1091
Yin Chen Pai Shi Tang (Artemisia Scoparia Decoction to Expel Stone), 1089
Yin Chen Si Ni Tang (Artemisia Scoparia Decoction for Frigid Extremities), 1089
Yin Chen Wu Ling San (Artemisia Scoparia and Five-Ingredient Powder with Poria), 1090
  vs. Si Ling San (Four-Ingredient Powder with Poria), 1112
  vs. Wei Ling Tang (Calm the Stomach and Poria Decoction), 1112
  vs. Wu Ling San (Five-Ingredient Powder with Poria), 1112
  vs. Yin Chen Hao Tang (Artemisia Scoparia Decoction), 1091
  vs. Zhi Zi Bai Pi Tang (Gardenia and Phellodendron Decoction), 1091
Yin edema, 1138, *1526*. See also *Yin shui* (yin edema)
Yin Hua Jie Du Tang (Honeysuckle Decoction to Relieve Toxicity), 1340
Yin Jiao San, 92
Yin Qiao Jie Du San (Honeysuckle and Forsythia Powder to Relieve Toxicity), 95
Yin Qiao San (Honeysuckle and Forsythia Powder), 92
  vs. Sang Ju Yin (Mulberry Leaf and Chrysanthemum Decoction), 91, 95
Yin Qiao Tang (Honeysuckle and Forsythia Decoction), 94
Yin shui (yin edema), 1138, *1526*
Yin Xing Ye (Folium Ginkgo), xxvi
Yin yang, 3
Ying (nutritive) level, *1526*
  disharmony with *wei* (defensive) level, 51, 798
  heat, 330, 333
Ying (nutritive) *qi*, *1526*
Ying (spring) point, *1526*
Yin-Nourishing Rehmannia Pill, 663
Yin-Nourishing Style, 1203
Yinqiao (movement) channel, *1526*
Yinwei (linking) channel, *1526*
Yong Ke Zheng Zhi Zhun Sheng (Standards of Patterns and Treatments in Sores and Abscesses), **1061**
Yong Lei Qian Fang (Everlasting Categorization of Seal Formulas), 560
Yoshine Hirai, 810
You Bi Tang (Benefit the Nose Decoction), 87

You Gui Wan (Restore the Right [Kidney] Pill), 678
  vs. Ba Wei Di Huang Wan (Eight-Ingredient Pill with Rehmannia), 648, 681
  vs. Zuo Gui Wan (Restore the Left [Kidney] Pill), 648, 681
You Gui Yin (Restore the Right [Kidney] Decoction), 680
Youth-Returning Formula, 681
Yu Chang, 1029
Yu Chuan Wan, 1052
Yu Gen-Chu, 69, 111, 137, 215, 227, 230, 993, 1007, 1237, 1295
Yu Lian Wan (Evodia and Coptis Pill), 389
Yu Nu Chien, 398
Yu Nu Jian (Jade Woman Decoction), 398
  vs. Qing Wei San (Clear the Stomach Powder), 395, 400
  vs. Xie Huang San (Drain the Yellow Powder), 395
Yu Ping Feng San (Jade Windscreen Powder), 773
  vs. Gui Zhi Tang (Cinnamon Twig Decoction), 57, 775
  vs. Mu Li San (Oyster Shell Powder), 777
  vs. Ren Shen Yang Ying Tang (Ginseng Decoction to Nourish the Nutritive Qi), 775
  vs. Sheng Mai San (Generate the Pulse Powder), 775
Yu Quan Wan (Jade Spring Pill), 1052
  vs. Yu Ye Tang (Jade Fluid Decoction), 1053
Yu Shi-Yu, 7, 337
Yu Tian-Min, 779, 1190
Yu Ye Tang (Jade Fluid Decoction), 1049
  vs. Liu Wei Di Huang Wan (Six-Ingredient Pill with Rehmannia), 1051
  vs. Yu Quan Wan (Jade Spring Pill), 1053
Yu Zhen San (True Jade Powder), 981
  vs. Qian Zheng San (Lead to Symmetry Powder), 983
Yu Zhi Zi (Fructus Akebiae), xxiii
Yuan (source) point, *1526*
Yuan (source) *qi*, 127, 548, 1261, *1526*
Yuan Ji Qi Wei (Explanation of the Subtitles of the Original Mechanism), 661
Yue Bi Jia Zhu Tang, 102
Yue Bi Jia Zhu Tang (Maidservant from Yue Decoction plus Atractylodes), 102
Yue Bi Tang (Maidservant from Yue Decoction), 101
  vs. Ma Huang Xing Ren Gan Cao Shi Gao Tang (Ephedra, Apricot Kernel, Licorice, and Gypsum Decoction), 102
Yue Chu Wan (Stagnation-Relieving Pill), 822
Yue Hua Wan (Moonlight Pill), 1040
Yue Ju Wan (Escape Restraint Pill), 822
Yueh Pi Chia Shu Tang, 102
Za Bing Yuan Liu Xi Zhu (Wondrous Lantern for Peering into Origin and Development of Miscellaneous Diseases), 723, 1052
Za Bing Zheng Zhi Xin Yi (New Significance of Patterns and Treatment in Miscellaneous Diseases), 1004
Zai Zao San (Renewal Powder), 130
  vs. Ma Huang Fu Zi Xi Xin Tang (Ephedra, Asarum, and Prepared Aconite Decoction), 134
Zang (solid organ), *1526*. See also specific organs
Zang Chang Pu (Rhizoma Acori Calami), xxv
Zang du (solid organ toxin), *1526*
Zang fu, 3, *1526*. See also specific organs and disorders
Zang Fu Bian Zheng (Organ Pattern Differentiation), *1526*
Zang zao (restless organ), 731, **732**, *1395*, **1527**
Zao (dryness), 156, *1527*
Zeng Ye Cheng Qi Tang (Increase the Fluids and Order the Qi Decoction), 190
Zeng Ye Tang (Increase the Fluids Decoction), 1054
Zha (crush), *1527*
Zhang Bing-Cheng, 1190
Zhang Cong-Zheng, 7, 1272, **1307**, 1312, 1481, 1483, 1484. *See also* Zhang Zi-He

Index

Chinese Herbal Formulas and Applications

Zhang Ji, 31, 1481, 1482, 1484. *See also* Zhang Zhong-Jing

Zhang Jie-Bin, **146**, 179, 184, 238, 257, 398, 548, 618, 645, 647, 678, 680, 836, 838, 1071, 1481, 1483, 1484. *See also* Zhang Jing-Yue

Zhang Jing-Yue, 12, **147**, 179, 184, 238, 257, 398, 548, 618, 645, 647, 678, 680, 836, 838, 1071, 1481, 1483, 1484. *See also* Zhang Jie-Bin

Zhang Lu-Xuan, 1173, 1243, 1244

Zhang San Feng Xian Chuan Fang (Divine Formulas from Zhang San-Feng), 1302

Zhang Shi Yi Tong (Comprehensive Medicine According to Master Zhang), 1173, 1243, 1244

Zhang Shi-Che, 845, 1334

Zhang Xi-Chun, 549, 803, 809, 914, 999, 1002, 1049

Zhang Yuan-Su, 825, 988, 1193

Zhang Zhong-Jing, 5, **31**, 39, 42, 45, 51, 55, 56, 59, 74, 78, 80, 96, 101, 102, 132, 134, 152, 158, 160, 161, 163, 166, 171, 172, 174, 181, 206, 219, 233, 237, 261, 268, 269, 271, 283, 289, 295, 304, 321, 323, 325, 326, 359, 370, 384, 406, 408, 410, 459, 462, 466, 467, 471, 475, 480, 486, 488, 489, 494, 498, 500, 589, 594, 599, 623, 668, 715, 722, 731, 787, 788, 798, 827, 831, 832, 851, 853, 854, 873, 876, 919, 928, 935, 937, 948, 950, 1043, 1077, 1086, 1089, 1090, 1109, 1115, 1118, 1120, 1125, 1131, 1133, 1135, 1137, 1186, 1220, 1230, 1235, 1242, 1275, 1292, 1311, 1364, 1378, 1382, 1481, 1482, 1484. *See also* Zhang Ji

Zhang Zi-He, **1307**, 1481, 1483, 1484. *See also* Zhang Cong-Zheng

Zhao Xian-Ke, 644

***Zhe Chong Yin* (Break the Conflict Decoction)**, 933

Zhe Shi (Haematitum), xxiv

***Zhen Gan Xi Feng Tang* (Sedate the Liver and Extinguish Wind Decoction)**, 999

  vs. Jian Ling Tang (Construct Roof Tiles Decoction), 1003

Zhen ji (injection), 18

***Zhen Ling Dan* (Rouse the Spirits Special Pill)**, 805

***Zhen Ren Huo Ming Yin* (True Man's Decoction to Revitalize Life)**, 1330

***Zhen Ren Yang Zang Tang* (True Man's Decoction for Nourishing the Organs)**, 781

  vs. Bai Tou Weng Tang (Pulsatilla Decoction), 783

  vs. Ge Gen Huang Qin Huang Lian Tang (Kudzu, Coptis, and Scutellaria Decoction), 783

  vs. Shao Yao Tang (Peony Decoction), 783

  vs. Si Shen Wan (Four-Miracle Pill), 786

***Zhen Wu Tang* (True Warrior Decoction)**, 1135

  vs. Shi Pi San (Bolster the Spleen Powder), 1139

***Zhen Zhong Dan* (Pillow Special Pill)**, 729

Zhen Zhu Mu (Concha Margaritiferae), xxvi

***Zhen Zhu Mu Wan* (Mother of Pearl Pill)**, 712

Zhen Zhu Wan (True Pearl Pill), 712

Zheng (steam), *1527*

Zheng (upright) *qi, 1527*

***Zheng Gu Zi Jin Dan* (Purple and Gold Pill for Righteous Bones)**, 901

Zheng Mei-Run, 1033

Zheng Ti Lei Yao (Catalogued Essentials for Correcting the Body), 489, 604

Zheng Yin Mai Zhi (Pattern, Cause, Pulse, and Treatment), 856

Zheng Zhi Zhun Sheng (Standards of Patterns and Treatments), 354, 386, 402, 418, 438, 578, 784, **1061**, 1129, 1212, 1216, 1277, 1373, 1383

Zhi (fry with liquid), *1527*

Zhi (prepared), *1527*

Zhi (will-power), 707, *1527*

Zhi Bai Ba Wei Wan, 636

***Zhi Bai Di Huang Wan* (Anemarrhena, Phellodendron, and Rehmannia Pill)**, 636

  vs. Liu Wei Di Huang Wan (Six-Ingredient Pill with Rehmannia), 634

***Zhi Bao Dan* (Greatest Treasure Special Pill)**, 749

  vs. An Gong Niu Huang Wan (Calm the Palace Pill with Cattle Gallstone), 749

  vs. Zi Xue Dan (Purple Snow Pill), 749

Zhi Bo Di Huang Wan, 636

Zhi Gan Cao (Radix et Rhizoma Glycyrrhizae Praeparata cum Melle), xxvi

***Zhi Gan Cao Tang* (Honey-Fried Licorice Decoction)**, 589

  vs. Sheng Mai San (Generate the Pulse Powder), 591

  vs. Tian Wang Bu Xin Dan (Emperor of Heaven's Special Pill to Tonify the Heart), 592, 730

***Zhi Jing San* (Stop Spasms Powder)**, 979

***Zhi Ke Tang* (Stop Coughing Decoction)**, 118

Zhi Mu (Rhizoma Anemarrhenae), xxvi

Zhi Qiao (Fructus Aurantii), xxvi

***Zhi Shi Dao Zhi Wan* (Immature Bitter Orange Pill to Guide Out Stagnation)**, 1270

  vs. Mu Xiang Bing Lang Wan (Aucklandia and Betel Nut Pill), 1273

***Zhi Shi Shao Yao San* (Immature Bitter Orange and Peony Powder)**, 236

***Zhi Shi Xiao Pi Wan* (Immature Bitter Orange Pill to Reduce Focal Distention)**, 1280

  vs. Jian Pi Wan (Strengthen the Spleen Pill), 1282

  vs. Zhi Zhu Wan (Immature Bitter Orange and Atractylodes Macrocephala Pill), 1282

***Zhi Shi Xie Bai Gui Zhi Tang* (Immature Bitter Orange, Chinese Chive, and Cinnamon Twig Decoction)**, 831

  vs. Gua Lou Xie Bai Bai Jiu Tang (Trichosanthes Fruit, Chinese Chive, and Wine Decoction), 833

  vs. Gua Lou Xie Bai Ban Xia Tang (Trichosanthes Fruit, Chinese Chive, and Pinellia Decoction), 833

***Zhi Sou San* (Stop Coughing Powder)**, 116

  vs. Dun Sou San (Long-Bout Cough Powder), 119

  vs. Jin Fei Cao San (Inula Powder), 119

  vs. Ning Sou Wan (Quiet the Cough Pill), 119

***Zhi Suo Er Chen Tang* (Two-Cured Decoction with Aurantium and Cardamon)**, 1212

***Zhi Xue Tang* (Stop Bleeding Decoction)**, 941

***Zhi Zhu Tang* (Immature Bitter Orange and Atractylodes Macrocephala Decoction)**, 1275

***Zhi Zhu Wan* (Immature Bitter Orange and Atractylodes Macrocephala Pill)**, 1274

  vs. Jian Pi Wan (Strengthen the Spleen Pill), 1279, 1282

  vs. Zhi Shi Xiao Pi Wan (Immature Bitter Orange Pill to Reduce Focal Distention), 1282

***Zhi Zhuo Gu Ben Wan* (Treat the Turbidity and Guard the Root Pill)**, 800

***Zhi Zi Bai Pi Tang* (Gardenia and Phellodendron Decoction)**, 1089

  vs. Yin Chen Hao Tang (Artemisia Scoparia Decoction), 1091

  vs. Yin Chen Wu Ling San (Artemisia Scoparia and Five-Ingredient Powder with Poria), 1091

Zhi Zi Bo Pi Tang, 1089

***Zhi Zi Chi Tang* (Gardenia and Soja Decoction)**, 370

Zhi Zi Gu Tang, 370

***Zhi Zi Jiang Huo Tang* (Gardenia Decoction to Descend Fire)**, 377

***Zhi Zi Qing Gan Tang* (Gardenia Decoction to Clear the Liver)**, 245

Zhong (central) *qi, 1527*

Zhong feng (wind stroke), 744, 750, 977, 988, 991, 1177, 1309, 1312, 1313, **1395**, *1527*

Zhong Guo Guo Yao Gu You Cheng Fang Xuan Ji (A Selection of Traditional Prescriptions of Chinese Medicine), 113

1617

INDEX

Index

Zhong Guo Yi Xue Da Ci Dian (Grand Dictionary of Chinese Medicine), 387

Zhong He Tang (Middle-Heartening Decoction), 1373

Zhong Hua Ren Min Gong He Guo Yao Dian (Pharmacopoeia of People's Republic of China), 634, 760

Zhong qi (qi stroke), **1527**

Zhong Yi Fang Ji Lin Chuan Shou Ce (Clinical Handbook of Chinese Herbal Formulae), 684

Zhong Zang Jing (Treasury Classic), 1121

Zhou bi (generalized painful obstruction), 1153, **1527**

Zhou Che Wan (Vessel and Vehicle Pill), 184

Zhou Hou Bei Ji Fang (Emergency Formulas to Keep Up One's Sleeve), 6, 112, 438, **1287**

Zhu (boiling), **1527**

Zhu Dan-Xi, **1202**, 1481, 1483, 1484. *See also* Zhu Zhen-Heng

Zhu Fan Wan (Atractylodes and Melanterite Pill), 1302

Zhu Gong, 113, 324

Zhu Ling Tang (Polyporus Decoction), 1115
   vs. Wu Ling San (Five-Ingredient Powder with Poria), 1117

Zhu Ru Wen Dan Tang (Bamboo Decoction to Warm the Gallbladder), 1217

Zhu Sha An Shen Wan (Cinnabar Pill to Tranquilize the Spirit), 710
   vs. Ci Zhu Wan (Magnetite and Cinnabar Pill), 715

Zhu Ye Liu Bang Tang (Lophatherum, Tamarisk and Arctium Decoction), 106

Zhu Ye Shi Gao Tang (Bamboo Leaves and Gypsum Decoction), 326
   vs. Bai Hu Jia Ren Shen Tang (White Tiger plus Ginseng Decoction), 328
   vs. Bai Hu Tang (White Tiger Decoction), 328
   vs. Qing Hao Bie Jia Tang (Artemisia Annua and Soft-Shelled Turtle Shell Decoction), 415

Zhu Yu Tang (Drive Out Blood Stasis Decoction), 895

Zhu Zhen-Heng, 7, 379, 389, 649, 651, 773, 822, 943, 946, 1113, 1140, 1175, 1188, **1203**, 1266, 1481, 1483, 1484. *See also* Zhu Dan-Xi

Zhu Zuo, 1183

Zhuang Jin Tang (Strengthen the Tendon Decoction), 568

Zhuo bi (fixed painful obstruction), 1153, **1527**

Zi Bo Di Huang Wan, 636

Zi Cao (Radix Arnebiae), xxvi

Zi Cao Gen Mu Li Tang (Arnebia and Oyster Shell Decoction), 1348

Zi Gen Mu Li Tang, 1348

Zi Jin Ding (Purple Gold Special Pill), 760

Zi Shen Ming Mu Tang (Nourish the Kidney to Brighten the Eyes Decoction), 664

Zi Shen Tong Er Tang (Nourish the Kidney to Unblock the Ears Decoction), 666

Zi Sheng Wan (Nourish Life Pill), 1278

Zi Su Geng (Caulis Perillae), xxv

Zi Su Ye (Folium Perillae), xxv

Zi Su Zi (Fructus Perillae), xxv

Zi Wan (Radix et Rhizoma Asteris), xxvi

Zi Wan Tang (Aster Decoction), 1229

Zi Xue (Purple Snow), 752
   vs. An Gong Niu Huang Wan (Calm the Palace Pill with Cattle Gallstone), 749
   vs. Zhi Bao Dan (Greatest Treasure Special Pill), 749

Zi Xue Dan (Purple Snow Pill), 752

Zi Yin Di Huang Wan (Rehmannia Pill to Nourish Yin), 663

Zi Yin Jiang Huo Tang (Nourish Yin and Descend the Fire Decoction), 422

Zi Yin Qing Re Tang (Nourish Yin and Clear Heat Decoction), 414

Zidovudine, 214

Zizyphus Combination, 722

Zong (essential) *qi*, **1528**

Zong Lu (Petiolus Trachycarpi), xxvi

Zuo Gui Wan (Restore the Left [Kidney] Pill), 645
   vs. Liu Wei Di Huang Wan (Six-Ingredient Pill with Rehmannia), 634, 648
   vs. You Gui Wan (Restore the Right [Kidney] Pill), 648, 681

Zuo Gui Yin (Restore the Left [Kidney] Decoction), 647

Zuo Jin Wan (Left Metal Pill), 389

Zuo yao (assistant herb), 14, **1528**

1618

About the Authors

John K. Chen, Ph.D., Pharm.D., O.M.D., L.Ac.

Dr. John Chen actively participates in education, research and the frontiers of contemporary application of herbal medicine. In addition to developing professional continuing education seminars and serving as a senior lecturer through the widely-respected Lotus Institute of Integrative Medicine, Dr. Chen speaks at seminars and conferences for universities and local, state, national and international educational and professional organizations. A professor at the University of Southern California School of Pharmacy and numerous colleges/universities of traditional Chinese medicine, Dr. Chen is also a member of the Herbal Medicine Committee for the American Association of Acupuncture and Oriental Medicine (AAAOM) and an herbal consultant for the California State Oriental Medicine Association (CSOMA). A recognized authority on Chinese herbal medicine and western (allopathic) pharmacology, Dr. Chen has written extensively on Oriental medicine and alternative complementary/integrative medicine for professional publications, journals and texts, drawing on his wealth of specialty post-graduate training and experience in mainland China in herbology as applied in internal medicine, and on his doctoral degrees from the University of Southern California (USC) School of Pharmacy and South Baylo University of Oriental Medicine. An editorial board member for the peer-reviewed journal of the American Academy of Medical Acupuncture (AAMA), *Medical Acupuncture*, John Chen was also a board member of the 1999 *Los Angeles Times* Festival Honorary Committee and speaker on Herbal Medicine for the City of Los Angeles First Annual Festival of Health. Appearing in the Discovery Channel 1999 six-hour documentary on alternative and complementary medicine, Dr. Chen served as the expert resource on Traditional Chinese Medicine. He also was a guest speaker on herb-drug interactions in 1998 for the annual USC Bergen Brunswig convention, during which he addressed over 400 pharmacists and medical doctors. Dr. Chen maintains his consulting practice in Southern California.

Tina T. Chen, M.S., L.Ac.

Tina Chen is an active and respected educator in Oriental medicine and Chinese herbal medicine. In addition to lecturing on TCM Gynecology and Cosmetology across North America through the widely-respected Lotus Institute of Integrative Medicine, Ms. Chen is active on the faculty of South Baylo University of Oriental Medicine and has been an active contributor to professional journals and publications. She has served as Southern California Chair of the Education Committee for the California State Oriental Medical Association (CSOMA), and as an examiner for the California State License Exam for acupuncturists, and from 1996-2001 maintained private practice of acupuncture and herbal medicine through Chen's Clinic in La Puente, California. Her teaching and consulting is grounded in extensive post-graduate training in herbal medicine, and TCM gynecology and cosmetology in numerous hospitals in mainland China. This included concentrated training sponsored by the World Health Organization (WHO) in Guang-An-Men Hospital of Traditional Chinese Medicine, Beijing, in the People's Republic of China, specializing in internal medicine, acupuncture and gynecology; also intensive clinical training in internal medicine and gynecology at First Tien-Jin Hospital, People's Republic of China; and at An-Hui Hospital, People's Republic of China, advanced training in internal medicine. Tina Chen's expertise in translation includes serving as translation specialist for the International Association of Integrating East-West Medicine from 1996-2000, the 1996 Third Annual International Acupuncture and Massage Conference sponsored by the Acupuncture and Massage Institute of America, and the California State Association of Oriental Medicine (CSOMA) in 1990. Licensed by the Acupuncture Board in California, Tina Chen also holds certification from the World Health Organization in internal medicine and gynecology. A graduate of South Baylo University of Oriental Medicine, she also earned a B.A. from the University of California at Irvine School of Humanities, in East Asian Language and Literature. She maintains a consulting practice in Southern California.

Notes

Notes

Notes